TEXTBOOK OF THERAPEUTICS:
DRUG AND DISEASE MANAGEMENT

SIXTH EDITION

TEXTBOOK OF THERAPEUTICS: DRUG AND DISEASE MANAGEMENT

SIXTH EDITION

EDITORS

ERIC T. HERFINDAL, Pharm.D., M.P.H.

SENIOR VICE PRESIDENT
AXION HEALTHCARE INC.
SAN BRUNO, CALIFORNIA

PROFESSOR EMERITUS
SCHOOL OF PHARMACY
UNIVERSITY OF CALIFORNIA
SAN FRANCISCO, CALIFORNIA

DICK R. GOURLEY, Pharm.D.

PROFESSOR AND DEAN
DEPARTMENT OF PHARMACY AND PHARMACOECONOMICS
UNIVERSITY OF TENNESSEE COLLEGE OF PHARMACY
MEMPHIS, TENNESSEE

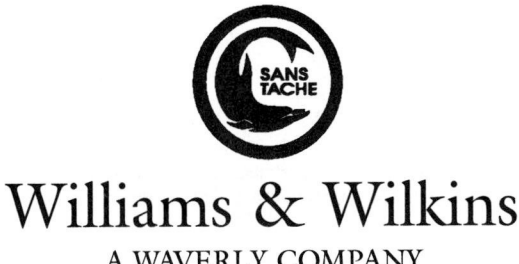

Williams & Wilkins

A WAVERLY COMPANY

BALTIMORE • PHILADELPHIA • LONDON • PARIS • BANGKOK
HONG KONG • MUNICH • SYDNEY • TOKYO • WROCLAW

1996

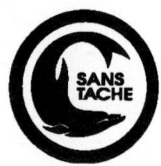

Editor: Donna M. Balado
Managing Editor: Victoria Rybicki Vaughn
Production Coordinator: Danielle Santucci
Project Editor: Jennifer Weir
Cover Designer: Tom Scheuerman
Typesetter: Graphic World, Inc.
Printer: RR Donnelley and Sons
Binder: RR Donnelley and Sons

Copyright © 1996
Williams & Wilkins
351 West Camden Street
Baltimore, Maryland 21201-2436 USA

Rose Tree Corporate Center
1400 North Providence Road
Building II, Suite 5025
Media, Pennsylvania 19063-2043 USA

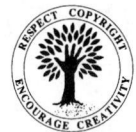

Accurate indications, adverse reactions, and dosage schedules for
drugs are provided in this book, but it is possible that they may
change. The reader is urged to review the package information data of
the manufacturers of the medications mentioned.

Printed in the United States of America

Textbook of therapeutics : drug and disease management/ editors: Eric
 T. Herfindal, Dick R. Gourley. -- 6th ed.   p.   cm.
   Rev. ed. of: Clinincal pharmacy and therapeutics / editors. Eric T.
 Herfindal, Dick R. Gourley. Linda Lloyd Hart. 5th ed. c1992
   Includes bibliographical references and index.
   ISBN 0-683-03969-5
   1.Chemotherapy. 2. Therapeutics. I. Herfindal, Eric T. II. Gourley,
 D.R.H., 1922-   . III.Clinical pharmacy and therapeutics.
   (DNLM: 1. Drug Therapy. WB 330 T3555 1996)
 RM262.C5 1996
 615.5'8--dc20
 DNLM/DLC   96-5665
 for Library of Congress   CIP

To purchase additional copies of this book, call our customer service department at (800) 638-0672 or fax
orders to (800) 447-8438. For other book services, including chapter reprints and large quantity sales, ask
for the Special Sales Department.

Canadian customers should call (800) 268-4178 or fax (905) 470-6780. For all other calls originating outside
the United States, please call (410) 528-4223 or fax us at (410) 528-8550.

Visit Williams & Wilkins on the Internet http://www.wwilkins.com or contact our customer service department
at http://custserv@wwilkins.com. Williams & Wilkins customer service representatives are available from 8:30am
to 6:00pm EST, Monday through Friday, for either telephone or Internet access.

CONSULTING EDITORS

PREFACE

The publication of the sixth edition of this textbook coincides with a period of revolutionary changes in the health care system and the treatment of disease. This revolution has many causes: significant technological advances in the diagnosis and treatment of disease: the high cost of new technology; the struggle for market share and control by payers, providers, and suppliers of health care; and the blurring of roles among health care practitioners. With health care consuming approximately 14% of the gross domestic product, and the recognition that health care as a benefit is one of their greatest expenses, employers are asking difficult questions about the quality and cost of this very expensive benefit.

The traditional approach to managing disease has been to focus mainly on the episodes of care. Payers have attempted to minimize expenses through individual cost components such as hospitalization, professional services, home care, laboratories, etc. This approach has been unsuccessful due to cost shifting by providers. For example, in attempting to reduce hospitalization, care has been shifted to the outpatient arena, and without adequate control, costs will continue to escalate. According to the Boston Consulting Group, "Disease management is an approach to managed care that coordinates resources across the entire care delivery system and throughout the life cycle of a disease." By taking a systemic approach and focusing on the patient as the relevant unit of management, with an equal emphasis on quality and costs, we believe that disease management will lead to greatly improved outcomes as measured by improved clinical results, reduced costs, and greater patient satisfaction. Achieving success in disease management requires a broad array of capabilities that can only be achieved in a multidisciplinary environment. This textbook focuses on the management of disease through appropriate therapeutics guided by the health care practitioner.

Reflecting this focus on drug and disease management, this edition of the textbook is organized by disease groups and gives the student and health care practitioner the tools to manage the disease, establish rational treatment plans, establish realistic outcome goals, and provide the parameters to monitor the progress of the disease. Also, particular attention is paid to the involvement of patients in their own therapy. As in the last three editions, the accompanying workbook is designed to simulate typical cases and is organized to be consistent with the textbook.

We are pleased to welcome to this edition six Consulting Editors who have worked with us in redesigning the structure of the textbook and provided valuable editorial assistance throughout the editorial process. The Consulting Editors are Drs. Richard Helms, Shal Lynch, David Quan, Nathan Rawls, Donna Schroeder, and Timothy Self.

In addition, we are grateful to our staff who helped us keep track of the progress of the authors and the flow of correspondence and revisions necessary to successfully complete this complex undertaking. We would particularly like to recognize Sylvia Pass and Amy Baker who were primarily responsible for overall coordination of the editoral process. Our gratitude also to the proofreaders for a job well done: Dorothy Nicholson, Syliva Pass, Sue Hatton, and Karin Ingram. We also would like to express our appreciation to our colleagues at Williams & Wilkins for being flexible and responsive to our needs as editors.

E.T.H. and D.R.G.

CONTRIBUTORS

SHAWN R. AKKERMAN, Pharm.D., BCPS
Assistant Director, Clinical Pharmaceutical Research Program
Clinical Specialist, Research and Infectious Diseases
Emory University
Atlanta, Georgia

BRIAN K. ALLDREDGE, Pharm.D.
Associate Professor of Clinical Pharmacy and Neurology
Departments of Clinical Pharmacy and Neurology
University of California, San Francisco
San Francisco, California

ANN B. AMERSON, Pharm.D.
Professor
Division of Pharmacy Practice and Science
College of Pharmacy
University of Kentucky
Lexington, Kentucky

ROBERT J. ANDERSON, Pharm.D.
Professor
Department of Pharmacy Practice
Mercer University
Atlanta, Georgia

ARASB ATESHKADI, Pharm.D.
Assistant Professor
Pharmacy Practice
University of Utah
Salt Lake City, Utah

LISA M. AVERY, Pharm.D.
Assistant Professor
Pharmacy Practice and Administration
Rutgers University College of Pharmacy
Piscataway, New Jersey

FRANCESCA T. AWEEKA, Pharm.D.
Associate Clinical Professor
Department of Pharmacy Practice
School of Pharmacy
University of California, San Francisco
San Francisco, California

NEETA BAHAL O'MARA, Pharm.D., BCPS
Assistant Professor
Department of Pharmacy Practice
Butler University
College of Pharmacy and Health Sciences
Family Practice–Clinical Pharmacist
Methodist Hospital of Indiana
Indianapolis, Indiana

JEFFREY N. BALDWIN, Pharm.D.
Associate Professor
Pharmacy Practice and Pediatrics
University of Nebraska Medical Center
Omaha, Nebraska

CAROL BALMER, Pharm.D.
Associate Professor
Department of Pharmacy Practice
University of Colorado School of Pharmacy
Denver, Colorado

JOSEPH A. BARONE, Pharm.D., FCCP
Associate Professor and Chair
Department of Pharmacy Practice and Administration
Rutgers University College of Pharmacy
Piscataway, New Jersey

STEVEN L. BARRIERE, Pharm.D.
Associate Director, Anti-Infectives
Clinical Research and Development
Rhône Poulenc Rorer
Collegeville, Pennsylvania

RITA G. BATES, Pharm.D.
Assistant Professor
Adult Therapeutics
Baptist Memorial Hospital
Memphis, Tennessee

ELIZABETH A. BELTZ, Pharm.D.
Clinical Pharmacy Specialist–M.I.C.U./Pulmonary
Pharmacy Department
The University of Iowa Hospitals and Clinics
Adjunct Assistant Professor
College of Pharmacy
University of Iowa
Iowa City, Iowa

ROSEMARY R. BERARDI, Pharm.D., FASHP
Professor of Pharmacy
College of Pharmacy
University of Michigan
Ann Arbor, Michigan

CONSTANTINE G. BERBATIS, MSc, FPS
Deputy Administrator
Queen Victoria Medical Center
Melbourne, Australia

STEPHEN C. BERGQUIST, MS
Clinical Pharmacy Specialist–Infectious Diseases
Pharmacy Department
The University of Iowa Hospitals and Clinics
Adjunct Assistant Professor
College of Pharmacy
University of Iowa
Iowa City, Iowa

KIMBERLY A. BERGSTROM, Pharm.D.
Director
Disease Management
Axion HealthCare Inc.
San Bruno, California

KATHY BIRD, Pharm.D.
Pharmacy Practice Resident
Clinical Pharmacy
Veterans Affairs Medical Center
Memphis, Tennessee

KATHRYN BLAKE, Pharm.D.
Department of Research
Nemours Children's Clinic
Jacksonville, Florida

LAURA BOEHNKE-MICHAUD, Pharm.D.
Oncology Clinical Pharmacy Specialist
Division of Pharmacy
University of Texas Cancer Center
Houston, Texas

BRADLEY A. BOUCHER, Pharm.D.
Professor of Clinical Pharmacy
College of Pharmacy
University of Tennessee
Memphis, Tennessee

ERIC G. BOYCE, Pharm.D.
Associate Professor of Clinical Pharmacy
Department of Pharmacy Practice and Pharmacy Administration
Philadelphia College of Pharmacy and Science
Philadelphia, Pennsylvania

J. CHRIS BRADBERRY, Pharm.D.
Professor and Chair
Department of Pharmacy Practice
University of Oklahoma
Oklahoma City, Oklahoma

RONALD L. BRADEN, Pharm.D.
Clinical Pharmacy Specialist, Critical Care
Department of Pharmacy
Veterans Affairs Medical Center
Associate Professor
Department of Clinical Pharmacy
University of Tennessee
Memphis, Tennessee

RICHARD BROWN, Pharm.D., BCPS, FASHP
Clinical Pharmacy Specialist
Medical Service Department
Veterans Affairs Medical Center
Associate Professor
College of Pharmacy
University of Tennessee
Memphis, Tennessee

REX O. BROWN, Pharm.D., BCNSP
Professor of Clinical Pharmacy
College of Pharmacy
University of Tennessee
Memphis, Tennessee

BETH BRUMBAUGH BREADY, Pharm.D.
Division of Pharmacy
University of Texas M.D. Anderson Cancer Center
Houston, Texas

HOWARD A. BURRIS III, MD
Director of Drug Development
Hematology/Oncology Service
Brooke Army Medical Center
San Antonio, Texas

R. KEITH CAMPBELL, RPh, B. Pharm., MBA
Associate Dean/Professor of Pharmacy
College of Pharmacy
Washington State University
Pullman, Washington

JANNET M. CARMICHAEL, Pharm.D., BCPS, FCCP
Clinical Pharmacy Coordinator
Department of Pharmacy
VA Medical Center
Associate Professor of Medicine
Department of Internal Medicine
University of Nevada
Reno, Nevada

DONNA CARR, Pharm.D.
Assistant Professor of Clinical Pharmacy
College of Pharmacy
Clinical Pharmacist
Veterans Affairs Medical Center
University of Tennessee
Memphis, Tennessee

MARSHALL CATES, Pharm.D.
Assistant Professor of Pharmacy Practice
Samford University School of Pharmacy
Birmingham, Alabama

JUDY L. CHASE, Pharm.D.
Clinical Pharmacy Specialist
Division of Pharmacy
UT University of Texas Cancer Center
Houston, Texas

BRUCE D. CLAYTON, Pharm.D., R.Ph.
Associate Dean and Professor of Pharmacy Practice
Department of Pharmacy Practice
Butler University College of Pharmacy and Health Sciences
Indianapolis, Indiana

G. DENNIS CLIFTON, Pharm.D.
Associate Professor
Division of Pharmacy Practice and Science
University of Kentucky
Lexington, Kentucky

STEPHEN C. COOKE, Pharm.D.
Assistant Professor
Department of Pharmacy Practice and Pharmacoeconomics
University of Tennessee College of Pharmacy
Director of Pharmacy
Memphis Mental Health Institute
Memphis, Tennessee

CATHY E. CORBETT, MD
Assistant Professor of Medicine
College of Medicine
University of Tennessee
Department of the Veterans Affairs Medical Center
Memphis, Tennessee

WILLIAM R. CROM, Pharm.D., FCCP, BCPS
Associate Member
Pharmaceutical Department
St. Jude Children's Research Hospital
Memphis, Tennessee

MONICA CYR, Pharm.D.
Assistant Professor of Clinical Pharmacy
University of Tennessee
College of Pharmacy
Memphis, Tennessee

BETTY J. DONG, Pharm.D.
Professor of Clinical Pharmacy and Family and Community Medicine
Division of Clinical Pharmacy and Department of Family and
  Community Medicine
University of California, San Francisco
School of Pharmacy
San Francisco, California

ANTON C. DREYER, DSc
Professor
Department of Pharmacy Practice
Potchefstroom University for Christian Higher Education
Potchefstroom, South Africa

JAMES C. EOFF III, Pharm.D.
Executive Associate Dean
Professor of Clinical Pharmacy
College of Pharmacy
University of Tennessee
Memphis, Tennessee

WILLIAM E. EVANS, Pharm.D.
First Tennessee Professor and Chair
Pharmaceutical Sciences, Clinical Pharmacy and Pediatrics
St. Jude Children's Research Hospital and University of Tennessee
Memphis, Tennessee

SUZANNE M. FIELDS JONES, Pharm.D.
Outpatient Infusion Center
Tyler Hematology-Oncology
Tyler, Texas

REBECCA S. FINLEY, Pharm.D., MS
Associate Professor
Pharmacy Practice and Science
University of Maryland School of Pharmacy
Baltimore, Maryland

CLARENCE L. FORTNER, MS
Executive Scientific and Medical Affairs
Adria Laboratories
Joppa, Maryland

CARLA B. FRYE, Pharm.D., BCPS, R.Ph.
Assistant Professor and Director, Pharmacy Practice
College of Pharmacy and Health Science
Butler University
Indianapolis, Indiana

DARLENE FUJIMOTO, Pharm.D.
Assistant Clinical Professor
Pharmaceutical Services
University of California, Irvine
Orange, California

STEPHEN H. FULLER, Pharm.D., BCPS
Associate Professor
Department of Pharmacy Practice
Campbell University
Fayetteville, North Carolina

MARIE E. GARDNER, Pharm.D.
Associate Professor, Pharmacy Practice
Department of Pharmacy Practice
The University of Arizona College of Pharmacy
Tucson, Arizona

MARTHA L. GARDNER, Pharm.D.
Pharmacy Clinical Practice Specialist
Pediatric Oncology
Pharmacy
University of Texas M.D. Anderson Cancer Center
Houston, Texas

MARK W. GARRISON, Pharm.D.
Assistant Professor of Pharmacy
College of Pharmacy
Washington State University at Spokane
Spokane, Washington

ASHKAN GHORBANI, MD
Resident
Department of Dermatology
University of Tennessee, Memphis
Memphis, Tennessee

MARK A. GILL, Pharm.D., FASHP, FCCP
Professor of Clinical Pharmacy
Department of Clinical Pharmacy
University of Southern California
Los Angeles, California

TRACEY L. GOLDSMITH, Pharm.D.
Clinical Manager
Department of Pharmacy Services
Hermann Hospital
Houston, Texas

EDGAR R. GONZALEZ, Pharm.D., FASCP
Associate Professor of Medicine and Pharmacy
Department of Pharmacy and Pharmaceutics
Virginia Commonwealth University
MCV Campus
Richmond, Virginia

DICK R. GOURLEY, Pharm.D.
Professor and Dean
Department of Pharmacy and Pharmacoeconomics
University of Tennessee College of Pharmacy
Memphis, Tennessee

GRETA K. GOURLEY, M.S.N., Ph.D., Pharm.D.
Assistant Professor
Department of Pharmacy Practice and Pharmacoeconomics
University of Tennessee College of Pharmacy
Memphis, Tennessee

ANDRIES G. GOUS, Pharm.D.
Clinical Pharmacist
Baragwanath Hospital
Johannesburg, South Africa

HERMIEN GOUS, Pharm.D.
Clinical Pharmacist
Baragwanath Hospital
Johannesburg, South Africa

WILLIAM L. GREENE, Pharm.D., BCPS, FASHP
Assistant Director for Clinical Services
Department of Pharmacy
Methodist Hospitals of Memphis
Associate Professor
Department of Clinical Pharmacy
University of Tennessee College of Pharmacy
Memphis, Tennessee

EMILY B. HAK, Pharm.D.
Associate Professor of Clinical Pharmacy
College of Pharmacy
The University of Tennessee, Memphis
Memphis, Tennessee

LAWRENCE J. HAK, Pharm.D., FCCP
Professor and Chairman
Department of Clinical Pharmacy
University of Tennessee
Memphis, Tennessee

THOMAS C. HARDIN, Pharm.D.
Clinical Coordinator
Pharmacy Service
Audie L. Murphy Memorial Veterans Hospital
San Antonio, Texas

JEANNE HAWKINS VAN TYLE, MS, Pharm.D.
Associate Professor
Department of Pharmacy Practice
Butler University
College of Pharmacy and Health Sciences
Indianapolis, Indiana

RICHARD A. HELMS, Pharm.D., BCNSP
Professor, Clinical Pharmacy and Vice Chair
Department of Clinical Pharmacy
College of Pharmacy
LeBonheur Children's Medical Center
The University of Tennessee, Memphis
Memphis, Tennessee

ROBERT P. HENDERSON, Pharm.D., FASHP, BCPS
Professor of Pharmacy Practice
School of Pharmacy
Samford University
Clinical Pharmacy Specialist
Pharmacy Department
Birmingham Baptist Medical Center Princeton
Birmingham, Alabama

ERIC T. HERFINDAL, Pharm.D., M.P.H.
Senior Vice President
Axion HealthCare Inc.
San Bruno, California
Professor Emeritus
School of Pharmacy
University of California
San Francisco, California

KATHERINE C. HERNDON, Pharm.D.
Assistant Professor of Pharmacy Practice
Department of Pharmacy Practice
Samford University School of Pharmacy
Birmingham, Alabama

RICHARD N. HERRIER, Pharm.D.
Assistant Professor
Department of Pharmacy Practice
University of Arizona
College of Pharmacy
Tucson, Arizona

VALERIE W. HOGUE, Pharm.D., CDE
Associate Professor
Department of Clinical and Administrative Pharmacy Sciences
College of Pharmacy and Pharmaceutical Sciences
Howard University
Washington, D.C.

JOHN M. HOLBROOK, Ph.D.
Professor, Pharmaceutical Sciences
Mercer University
Southern School of Pharmacy
Atlanta, Georgia

MARTIN J. JINKS, Pharm.D.
Professor of Pharmacy
College of Pharmacy
Washington State University
Pullman, Washington

MARTIN L. JOB, Pharm.D., MA, BCPS, FASHP, FCCP
Professor and Vice Chair
Department of Pharmacy Practice
Mercer University School of Pharmacy
Atlanta, Georgia

JANNIFER J. JOHNSON, Pharm.D.
Medical Services Associate
Medical and Professional Services
Solvay Pharmaceuticals
Marietta, Georgia

JULIE A. JOHNSON, Pharm.D.
Associate Professor of Clinical Pharmacy
Department of Clinical Pharmacy
College of Pharmacy
University of Tennessee, Memphis
Memphis, Tennessee

ARCELIA M. JOHNSON-FANNIN, Pharm.D.
Associate Professor
Clinical Pharmacy Division
College of Pharmacy
Florida A&M University
Tallahassee, Florida

STANLEY G. KAILIS, Ph.D., FPS
Associate Professor of Pharmaceutical Biology and Clinical Pharmacy
Curtin University of Technology
Perth, Western Australia

ALAN K. KAMADA, Pharm.D.
Assistant Professor
Department of Pediatrics
Clinical Pharmacy Division
National Jewish Center for Immunology and Respiratory Disease
Denver, Colorado

JOAN E. KAPUSNIK-UNER, Pharm.D.
Associate Clinical Professor
Division of Clinical Pharmacy
University of California
San Francisco, California

STEVEN R. KAYSER, Pharm.D.
Clinical Professor of Pharmacy
Director, Anticoagulation Clinic
Department of Clinical Pharmacy
University of California, San Francisco
San Francisco, California

WENDY KLEIN-SCHWARTZ, Pharm.D.
Associate Professor
Department of Pharmacy Practice
School of Pharmacy
University of Maryland
Baltimore, Maryland

PETER J. S. KOO, Pharm.D.
Associate Clinical Professor
School of Pharmacy
University of California, San Francisco
San Francisco, California

S. CASEY LAIZURE, Pharm.D., BCPS
Associate Professor of Clinical Pharmacy
Department of Clinical Pharmacy
College of Pharmacy
University of Tennessee, Memphis
Memphis, Tennessee

VICTOR LAMPASONA, Pharm.D.
Associate Director
Department of Pharmaceutical Services
Emory University Hospital
Atlanta, Georgia

ROGER D. LANDER, Pharm.D., BCPS, FASHP, FCCP
Professor and Vice Chair
Department of Pharmacy Practice
Samford University School of Pharmacy
Clinical Pharmacy Specialist
Birmingham Veterans Administration Medical Center
Birmingham, Alabama

RICHARD D. LEFF, Pharm.D., FCCP
Professor of Pharmacy Practice
School of Pharmacy
University of Kansas
Lawrence, Kansas

LAWRENCE J. LEVANTHAL, MD, FACP, FACR
Clinical Assistant Professor of Medicine
University of Pennsylvania
Associate Chief of Rheumatology
Graduate Hospital
Philadelphia, Pennsylvania

ROBERT H. LEVIN, Pharm.D., FASHP, FCSHP
Professor of Clinical Pharmacy and Pediatrics
Division of Clinical Pharmacy
University of California School of Pharmacy
San Francisco, California.

JANET A. LYLE, Pharm.D.
Clinical Oncology Pharmacist
Department of Pharmacy
Alta Bates Medical Center
Berkeley, California

SHALINI LYNCH, Pharm.D.
Drug Experience Associate
Medical and Safety Services
Alza Corporation
Palo Alto, California

JANELLE M. MAHONEY, Pharm.D.
Medical Services Manager
Medical Services
Bristol-Myers Squibb
Leawood, Kansas

PIERRE A. MALOLEY, Pharm.D.
Assistant Professor
Pharmacy Practice, Internal Medicine
University of Nebraska Medical Center
Omaha, Nebraska

MARGARET MALONE, Ph.D., MRPharms, BCNSP
Professor
Department of Pharmacy Practice
Albany College of Pharmacy
Albany, New York

EDITH C. MARTINGANO, Pharm.D., R.Ph.
Clinical Coordinator, Hematology/Oncology Pharmacy
Texas Children's Hospital
Houston, Texas

HEWITT W. MATTHEWS, Ph.D.
Dean and Hood-Meyer Professor
Department of Pharmaceutical Sciences
Mercer University Southern Shcool of Pharmacy
Atlanta, Georgia

WILLIAM J. McINTYRE, Pharm.D.
Assistant Professor
Department of Pharmacy Practice
University of Arkansas for Medical Sciences
Little Rock, Arkansas

CONSTANCE McKENZIE, Pharm.D.
Assistant Professor and Director
Drug Information
Campbell University
Buies Creek, North Carolina

KELLIE D. McQUEEN, Pharm.D.
Adjunct, Assistant Professor
Department of Pharmacy Practice
University of Colorado School of Pharmacy
Executive Director
Pediatric Pharmacy Advocacy Group
Denver, Colorado

GAIL W. McSWEENEY, Pharm.D.
Clinical Pharmacy Consultant
San Francisco, California

HELEN MELDRUM, Ph.D.
Associate Professor of Psychology and Communications
Massachusetts College of Pharmacy and Allied Health Sciences
Boston, Massachusetts

MADHAVI MENON, MD
Chief Resident
Department of Dermatology
University of Tennessee
Memphis, Tennessee

SUSAN W. MILLER, Pharm.D., FASCP
Professor
Department of Pharmacy Practice
Mercer University School of Pharmacy
Atlanta, Georgia

JAY F. MOUSER, Pharm.D.
Research Fellow
Department of Clinical Pharmacy
The University of Tennessee, Memphis
College of Pharmacy
Memphis, Tennessee

ALAN H. MUTNICK, Pharm.D.
Senior Assistant Director Clinical Practice
Pharmacy Department
The University of Iowa Hospital and Clinics
Adjunct Associate Professor
College of Pharmacy
University of Iowa
Iowa City, Iowa

JEAN K. NOGUCHI, Pharm.D.
Assistant Professor of Clinical Pharmacy
University of Southern California
School of Pharmacy
Los Angeles, California

PAUL E. NOLAN, Jr., Pharm.D., FCCP, FASHP
Associate Professor
Department of Pharmacy Practice
The University of Arizona College of Pharmacy
Associate Clinical Scientist
University Heart Center
The University of Arizona
Tucson, Arizona

DIANE NYKAMP McCARTER, Pharm.D.
Professor of Pharmacy
Director of Clinical Clerkships
Mercer University
Southern School of Pharmacy
Atlanta, Georgia

GARY M. ODERDA, Pharm.D., M.P.H.
Professor and Chair
Department of Pharmacy Practice
University of Utah College of Pharmacy
Salt Lake City, Utah

MICHAEL A. OSZKO, Pharm.D., BCPS
Associate Professor
Department of Pharmacy Practice
The University of Kansas School of Pharmacy
Kansas City, Kansas

MICHAEL D. PARR, Pharm.D.
Director of Pharmacy
Department of Inpatient Pharmacy
University of Arkansas for Medical Sciences
Little Rock, Arkansas

DANIEL PATERSON
Director, Clinical Affairs
Axion HealthCare Inc.
South San Francisco, California

ANGELA PENTECOST, Pharm.D.
Arden, North Carolina

CONSTANCE M. PFEIFFER, Pharm.D.
Assistant Professor
Pharmacy Practice and Administration
Rutgers University College of Pharmacy
Piscataway, New Jersey

STEPHANIE J. PHELPS, Pharm.D.
Associate Professor of Clinical Pharmacy
College of Pharmacy
Pediatric Therapeutics
LeBonhuer Children's Medical Center
The University of Tennessee, Memphis
Memphis, Tennessee

FRANK M. POMPILIO, Pharm.D.
Assistant Professor
Department of Pharmacy Practice
School of Pharmacy
University of Southern California
Los Angeles, California

DAVID J. QUAN, Pharm.D.
Critical Care Pharmacist
Department of Pharmacy
Mount Zion Medical Center of UC San Francisco
San Francisco, California

NATHAN RAWLS, Pharm.D.
Associate Professor
College of Pharmacy
University of Tennessee
Clinical Specialist
VA Medical Center
Memphis, Tennessee

CYNTHIA L. RAEHL, Pharm.D.
Professor and Chair
Department of Pharmacy Practice
School of Pharmacy
Texas Tech University Health Sciences Center
Amarillo, Texas

LORI A. REISNER-KELLER, Pharm.D.
Clinical Pharmacist/Assistant Professor
Department of Clinical Pharmacy
University of California
San Francisco, California

BETH H. RESMAN-TARGOFF, Pharm.D.
Clinical Assistant Professor
Department of Pharmacy Practice
University of Oklahoma
Oklahoma City, Oklahoma

TED L. RICE, MS
Clinical Assistant Professor and Clinical Pharmacist
Department of Pharmacy Services
University of Michigan Medical Center
Ann Arbor, Michigan

KEVIN M. RODONDI, Pharm.D.
Director, Corporate Operations
OnCare, Inc.
San Bruno, California
Associate Clinical Professor of Pharmacy
University of California
Division of Clinical Pharmacy
San Francisco, California

REBECCA ROGERS PREVOST, Pharm.D., BCPS
Clinical Specialist for Ob/Gyn and Neonatology and
    Associate Professor, University of Tennessee College of Pharmacy
Regional Medical Center
Memphis, Tennessee

DIANE R. ROMAC, Pharm.D., FCSHP
Clinical Pharmacist
Department of Pharmacy
University of California, Davis
Sacramento, California
Assistant Clinical Professor
School of Pharmacy
University of California, San Francisco
San Francisco, California

RONALD J. RUGGIERO, Pharm.D.
Clinical Professor
Division of Clinical Pharmacy and Department of Obstetrics,
    Gynecology and Reproductive Sciences
University of California
San Francisco, California

GORDON S. SACKS, Pharm.D.
Nutrition Support Specialist
Clinical Pharmacy
Huntsville Hospital
Huntsville, Alabama

MICHELLE H. SANDERS, Pharm.D., BCNSP
Clinical Specialist
Pharmaceutical Department
St. Jude Children's Research Hospital
Memphis, Tennessee

PETER SANTALUCIA, MD
Resident
Department of Dermatology
University of Tennessee, Memphis
Memphis, Tennessee

MICHAEL L. SCHMITZ, MD
Resident, Orthopedic Surgery
Department of Orthopedics
Boston University School of Medicine
Boston, Massachusetts

DONNA J. SCHROEDER, Pharm.D.
Manager, Clinical Services
Axion HealthCare Inc.
Assistant Clinical Professor
University of California, San Francisco
San Francisco, California

CHARLES F. SEIFERT, Pharm.D., FCCP, BCPS
Director of Clinical Pharmacy Services
Rapid City Regional Hospital
Adjunct Professor of Clinical Pharmacy
College of Pharmacy
South Dakota State University
Rapid City, South Dakota

TIMOTHY SELF, Pharm.D.
Professor of Clinical Pharmacy
College of Pharmacy
University of Tennessee, Memphis
Memphis, Tennessee

MARK S. SHAEFER, Pharm.D.
Clinical Research Scientist
Clinical Support
Burroughs Wellcome Co.
Research Triangle Park, North Carolina

SAM K. SHIMOMURA, Pharm.D.
Professor of Clinical Pharmacy
Division of Clinical Pharmacy
School of Pharmacy
University of California, San Francisco
San Francisco, California

STEPHEN D. SILBERSTEIN, MD, F.A.C.P.
Adjunct Professor
Rutgers, The State University of New Jersey
College of Pharmacy
Busch Campus
Piscataway, New Jersey

RENU F. SINGH, Pharm.D.
Clinical Assistant Professor
Division of Clinical Pharmacy
University of California, San Francisco
San Francisco, California

LUKE SLOAN, MD
Resident
Department of Dermatology
University of Tennessee, Memphis
Memphis, Tennessee

KEVIN M. SOWINSKI, Pharm.D.
Assistant Professor
Department of Clinical Pharmacy
University of Tennessee, Memphis
Memphis, Tennessee

ROBERT J. STAGG, Pharm.D.
Director, Clinical Research
Department of Clinical Affairs
Gilead Sciences
Foster City, California

MARK STEPHENS, Pharm.D., BCPS
Ambulatory Care Specialist
Regional Medical Center at Memphis
Assistant Professor
University of Tennessee College of Pharmacy
Memphis, Tennessee

GLEN L. STIMMEL, Pharm.D.
Professor of Clinical Pharmacy and Psychiatry
University of Southern California
Schools of Pharmacy and Medicine
Los Angeles, California

CINDY D. STOWE, Pharm.D.
Assistant Professor
Department of Pharmacy Practice
University of Arkansas for Medical Sciences
Little Rock, Arkansas

ELIZABETH STUBITS SHLOM, Pharm.D.
Director of Clinical Pharmacy Programs
GNYHA Services, Inc.
New York, New York

JANICE L. STUMPF, Pharm.D.
Clinical Pharmacist and Clinical Assistant Professor
Department of Pharmacy Services
University of Michigan Medical Center and College of Pharmacy
Ann Arbor, Michigan

ALAN H. TANENBAUM, MD
Resident
Department of Dermatology
University of Tennessee, Memphis
Memphis, Tennessee

DAVID S. TATRO, Pharm.D.
Drug Information Consultant
San Carlos, California

MARY E. TERESI, Pharm.D.
Post Doctoral Associate
Department of Pediatrics
The University of Iowa–College of Medicine
Iowa City, Iowa

G. WILLIAM THATCHER, MD
Staff Psychiatrist
Inpatient Psychiatry Unit
Veterans Affairs Medical Center
Salt Lake City, Utah

PAULA A. THOMPSON, MS, Pharm.D., BCPS
Assistant Professor
Department of Pharmacy Practice
Samford University School of Pharmacy
Birmingham, Alabama

THEODORE G. TONG, Pharm.D.
Professor of Pharmacy Practice, Pharmacology and Toxicology
Associate Dean for Academic Affairs
College of Pharmacy
University of Arizona
Tucson, Arizona

KEVIN A. TOWNSEND, Pharm.D.
Clinical Pharmacist–Internal Medicine and Clinical Assistant
   Professor of Pharmacy
University of Michigan
Ann Arbor, Michigan

SHIRLEY M. TSUNODA, Pharm.D.
Assistant Professor Clinical Pharmacy
Department of Pharmacy Practice
Bouve College of Pharmacy and Health Sciences
Northeastern University
Boston, Massachusetts

J. EDWIN UNDERWOOD, Jr., Pharm.D.
Assistant Professor, Clinical Pharmacist
Department of Pharmacy Practice
Samford University and Lloyd Noland Hospital
Birmingham, Alabama

MARY L. WAGNER, MS, Pharm.D.
Assistant Professor
Pharmacy Practice and Administration
Rutgers, The State University of New Jersey
College of Pharmacy
Piscataway, New Jersey

JEFFREY J. WEBER, Pharm.D., BCPS
Clinical Specialist
Department of Pharmacy Services
Hermann Hospital
Houston, Texas

ROBERT T. WEIBERT, Pharm.D.
Clinical Professor
Division of Clinical Pharmacy
University of California, San Diego
UCSD Medical Center
San Diego, California

BARBARA G. WELLS, Pharm.D.
Professor and Dean
College of Pharmacy
Idaho State University
Pocatello, Idaho

JOHN R. WHITE, Jr., Pharm.D.
Assistant Professor
Washington State University/SHMC Drug Studies
Spokane, Washington

KARI A. WIELAND, Pharm.D.
Clinical Ambulatory Specialist
Pharmacy Service
Veterans Affairs Medical Center
Clinical Assistant Professor
Department of Medicine
Reno, Nevada

MICHAEL Z. WINCOR, Pharm.D.
Assistant Professor of Clinical Pharmacy, Psychiatry and
   the Behavioral Sciences
Schools of Pharmacy and Medicine
University of Southern California
Los Angeles, California

THOMAS H. WISER, Pharm.D.
Professor and Dean
College of Pharmacy and Allied Health Professions
St. John's University
Jamaica, New York

DAWN G. ZAREMBSKI, Pharm.D.
Assistant Professor
Department of Pharmacy Practice
Chicago College of Pharmacy
Midwestern University
Downers Grove, Illinois

CAROLINE S. ZEIND, Pharm.D.
Assistant Professor of Clinical Pharmacy
Massachusetts College of Pharmacy and Allied Health Sciences
Boston, Massachusetts

CONTENTS

SECTION 15 : INFECTIOUS DISEASES

SECTION 16 : NEOPLASTIC DISORDERS

SECTION 17 : PEDIATRIC AND NEONATAL THERAPY

SECTION 18 : OB–GYN DISORDERS

SECTION 19 : GERONTOLOGY

SECTION 20 : CRITICAL CARE

CHAPTER 1

CLINICAL PHARMACOKINETICS

S. CASEY LAIZURE and WILLIAM E. EVANS

Clinical pharmacokinetics is the application of pharmacokinetic principles in a patient care setting. Probably the most difficult aspect of clinical pharmacokinetics is understanding both the full potential and the practical limitations of using specific models of drug disposition to attain target concentrations based on only one or two measured serum drug concentrations (SDCs). While a good understanding of common pharmacokinetic models (e.g., first-order elimination and Michaelis-Menten kinetics) is crucial, the competent clinician will have knowledge of not only the mathematics of these models, but the principles, assumptions, and potential errors underlying their clinical application. Furthermore, a broad therapeutic knowledge is also necessary, as measured SDCs must be interpreted with respect to the clinical condition of the patient and the pharmacodynamics of the therapeutic agent. This chapter presents a pragmatic approach to clinical pharmacokinetics, focusing on the utilization of measured SDCs for the adjustment of patient drug therapy.

BASIC PHARMACOKINETIC PARAMETERS

The three basic pharmacokinetic parameters of the one-compartment open model are volume of distribution (V), clearance (Cl), and half-life ($t_{1/2}$). These parameters are derived from the mathematical model describing a monoexponential first-order elimination and do not have a direct correlation with anatomic structures or physiologic functions responsible for drug elimination.

Volume of Distribution

The volume of distribution (V) is a proportionality constant that equates the SDC to the total amount of drug in the body (1). This concept is depicted in Figure 1.1 by using drug distribution in a conical flask containing 70 mL of water and 30 mL of oil. In this example the concentration of drug is measured only in the water phase, analogous to the measurement of drug in the blood (serum or plasma) of patients. The following examples are thus analogous to the common practice of measuring drug in serum and calculating the V based on the one-compartment open model, with the assumption of homogeneous distribution of drug throughout the body, equivalent to the measured serum concentration.

When drug is added to the flask, it partitions between the oil and water, depending on its lipophilicity. Hydrophilic compounds will tend to remain in the water phase, while lipophilic compounds will distribute more extensively into the oil phase. The *apparent* volume of distribution of drug in the flask is determined by measuring the concentration of drug in the water phase (drug in the oil phase does not contribute to the measured concentration in the water phase) and determining the volume that would be required to account for all the drug put in the flask. One hundred milligrams of a hydrophilic drug is put in one flask, and 90 mg distributes into the water and 10 mg into the oil. The measured concentration of hydrophilic drug in water is the total amount of drug in the water phase divided by the volume of water (i.e., 90 mg ÷ 70 mL = 1.29 mg/mL). Thus, accounting for all the drug in the flask, if it exists at the concentration measured in the water phase, the apparent volume is 100 mg ÷ 1.29 mg/mL = 78 mL (apparent volume of distribution). The apparent volume is close to the volume of water in the flask, because the hydrophilic drug distributes primarily into the water phase. In contrast, when 100 mg of a lipophilic drug is put into the other flask, 90 mg distributes into the oil phase and only 10 mg remains in the water phase. The measured concentration of lipophilic drug in the water is the total amount of drug in the water phase divided by the volume of water (i.e., 10 mg ÷ 70 mL = 0.14 mg/mL). Thus, accounting for all the drug in the flask, assuming it exists at the concentration measured in the water phase, the apparent volume is 100 mg ÷ 0.14 mg/mL = 714 mL (apparent volume of distribution). The apparent volume is much greater than the actual volume of the container, because most of the drug has distributed outside the water phase. Hence, the apparent volume is a function of the amount of drug put in the flask (or body) and the measured concentration of drug in the water phase (or serum), and is unrelated to any physical volume.

As can be appreciated from the above discussion, the V has no physiologic basis, and is not related to the volume of serum, blood, total body water, and so on. Theoretically, if V is determined experimentally from multiple SDCs after a single dose of a drug and the calculated V equals the volume of serum in the patient's body, then all the drug

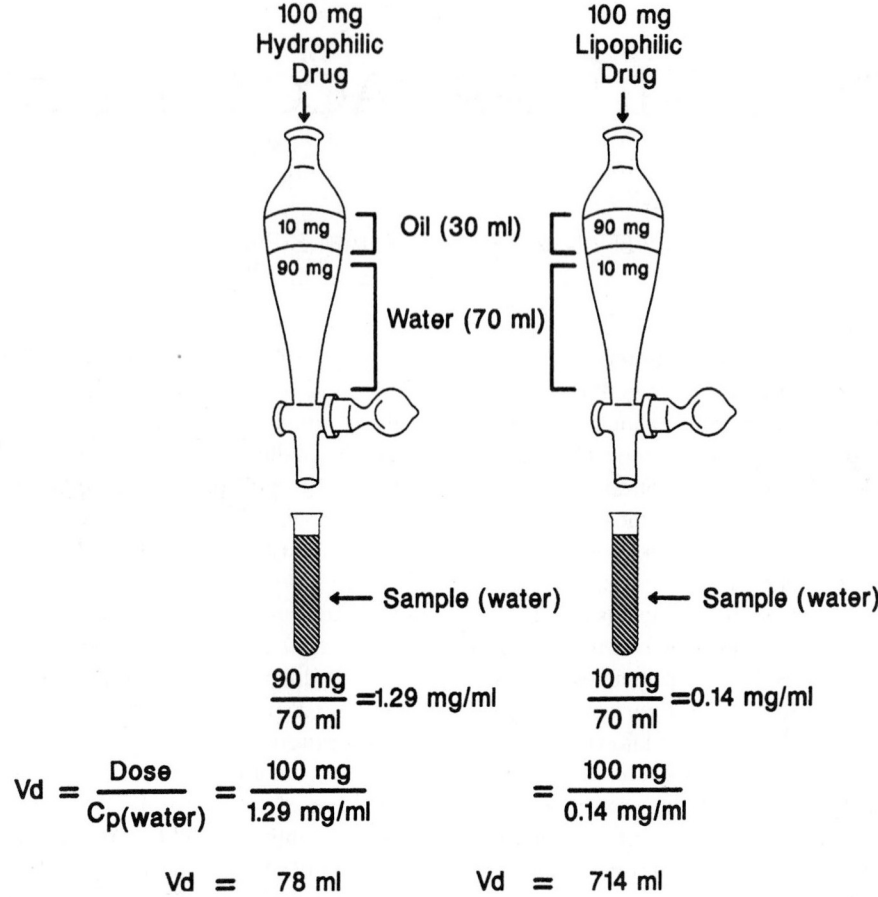

Figure 1.1   Volume of distribution does not correlate to any anatomical space. It is a proportionality constant that relates a measured serum concentration to the total amount of drug in the body (see text).

must be in the patient's serum (assuming a uniform concentration). When the V is greater than the serum volume, this means simply that to equate the SDC with the total amount of drug in the body, a value greater than the serum volume is required. A V greater than the serum volume indicates that some portion of the drug is located outside the serum. Though it is common to speculate on where a drug distributes, based on its V, technically such speculation is not possible. If a drug has a V of 0.7 L/kg, it is tempting to assume that the drug distributes in total body water, since total body water is approximately 70% of total body weight. However, the V could just as easily be increased because of distribution or binding to some other body tissue. The fact that the V is 0.7 L/kg only indicates that the drug distributes outside the serum. Determining where the drug has distributed requires data other than V.

After a single dose (X_O) of drug with first-order elimination (rate constant k), the total amount (X_t) of the drug remaining in the body after some time interval t can be converted to the serum concentration by dividing both sides of Equation (1.1) by V.

$$X_t = X_0 e^{-kt} \tag{1.1}$$

$$\frac{X_t}{V} = \frac{X_0 e^{-kt}}{V} \tag{1.2}$$

$$C_t = C_0 e^{-kt} \tag{1.3}$$

For a specific drug, if the V of the drug and an SDC are known, then the total amount of drug in the patient's body can be estimated. For example, if the measured SDC of theophylline is 12 mg/L and the V is 35 liters, then the total amount of drug in the body can be estimated as follows:

$$\text{Amount} = (SDC)(V)$$
$$= (12 \text{ mg/L})(35 \text{ L}) = 420 \text{ mg} \tag{1.4}$$

This same equation can also be used to calculate the loading dose necessary to achieve a specific peak SDC after a single dose. "Amount" in this case refers to the amount of the loading dose. Thus, to calculate the loading dose necessary to achieve an initial theophylline SDC of 15 mg/L in a patient with a V equal to 35 liters, we have

$$\text{Loading Dose} = (\text{SDC}_{\text{target}})(V)$$

$$= (15 \text{ mg/L})(35 \text{ L})$$

$$= 525 \text{ mg} \qquad (1.5)$$

This equation assumes that the SDC of theophylline before the loading dose was zero. Patients with drug already in their body (e.g., a patient in status epilepticus with a phenytoin SDC of 5 mg/L) may only need a partial loading dose. If the desired target SDC is 20 mg/L, then a loading dose that will raise the SDC from 5 to 20 mg/L is needed. The following equation takes into account drug present in the patient when the loading dose is determined:

$$\text{Loading Dose} = \frac{(\text{SDC}_{\text{target}} - \text{SDC}_{\text{observed}})(V)}{(S)(F)}$$

$$= \frac{(20 \text{ mg/L} - 5 \text{ mg/L})(70 \text{ L})}{(0.92)(1.0)} \ 1141 \text{ mg} \qquad (1.6)$$

where $\text{SDC}_{\text{observed}}$ is the SDC before the partial loading dose is given, S is the fraction of active drug by weight in the salt formulation (parenteral phenytoin is a sodium salt that is 92% phenytoin), and F is the bioavailability ($F = 1$ for the IV route). This latter equation is appropriate for calculating a partial or full loading dose for most drugs given by either the parenteral or oral route.

Clearance

Clearance is a proportionality constant that relates the rate of drug elimination to the SDC (1). Clearance should not be equated with the drug elimination rate, since Cl is a flow rate measured in units of volume per time (e.g., mL/min). However, if the Cl of a drug is known, then the rate of drug elimination can be calculated by multiplying the Cl by the SDC (assuming first-order drug elimination).

$$\text{Rate of drug elimination} = (\text{SDC})(\text{Cl}) \qquad (1.7)$$

The rate of drug elimination applies only to the SDC used in the calculation. If a different SDC value is used, a different rate of drug elimination will be calculated. Thus, the rate of drug elimination is constantly changing and directly proportional to the change in the SDC for a first-order process (i.e., as the SDC increases, the rate of drug elimination increases proportionately).

If a patient receives a drug by constant IV infusion, intermittent IV infusion, or oral dosing at regular intervals, the steady-state SDC is determined by the dose and the Cl. The steady-state SDC occurs when the rate of drug in (i.e., dose rate) is equivalent to the rate of drug out (i.e., rate of drug elimination). The SDC at which the rate in equals the rate out is determined solely by the Cl parameter and dose.

CASE #1

L.L. presents to the emergency room diaphoretic and complaining of sharp substernal chest pain radiating to the left shoulder. The EKG shows bigeminy. The patient is admitted to rule out a myocardial infarction. L.L.'s physician begins a constant IV infusion of an antiarrhythmic drug at a rate of 4 mg/min. The following kinetic parameters are estimated from measured SDCs in this patient. Estimate the steady-state concentration that will occur with this dose.

$t_{1/2}$ 1.5 hours
V 130 liters
Cl 1 L/min

The steady-state SDC is reached when the administration rate of the drug equals the rate of drug elimination (Equation 1.7). Multiplying the SDC by the Cl gives the rate of drug elimination. The volume unit (L) cancels out, leaving the units as mg/min, the same units as those for the administration rate. When the SDC reaches 4 mg/L, the rate of drug elimination equals the rate of drug administration (4 mg/min), and steady state is achieved (input equals output).

SDC (mg/L)		Cl (L/min)		Rate of Drug Elimination (mg/min)
1	×	1	=	1
2	×	1	=	2
3	×	1	=	3
4	×	1	=	4 (steady state)

Since the rate of drug elimination equals the rate of drug administration at steady state, the steady-state concentration can be calculated by substituting rate of drug administration for rate of drug elimination in Equation (1.7) and rearranging to equation to solve for SDC. This gives the following equation:

$$C_{ss} = \frac{ko}{\text{Cl}} \qquad (1.8)$$

where C_{ss} is the steady-state SDC, ko equals the rate of drug administration (amount/time), and Cl is the clearance. For a drug given by intermittent IV infusion or oral dosing, the mean steady-state SDC that will be achieved can be calculated using

$$\overline{C_{ss}} = \frac{(F)(D)}{(\text{Cl})(\tau)} \qquad (1.9)$$

where $\overline{C_{ss}}$ is the mean steady-state SDC, F is the bioavailability, D is the dose (maintenance dose), Cl is the clearance, and τ is the dosing interval. Note that the mean steady-state concentration is defined as

$$\overline{C_{ss}} = \frac{\text{AUC}\tau}{\tau} \qquad (1.10)$$

where $\text{AUC}\tau$ is the area under the concentration time curve for a single steady-state dosing interval and τ is the time duration of the dosing interval. The C_{ss} calculated from this equation is *not* equivalent to taking the average of the peak and trough from a dosing interval.

Half-Life

The half-life is the time required for the serum concentration to decrease by one half (1). Half-life is a transformation of the elimination rate constant to a form more easily interpreted. Do not confuse k or $t_{1/2}$ with the drug elimination rate (Equation 1.7). The parameter k is a mathematical variable that defines a constant exponential rate of change. The k can be estimated from two measured SDCs (e.g., a measured peak and trough) drawn within the same dosing interval. Assuming a one-compartment model with first-order elimination, k is estimated by plotting the natural log (ln) of the concentration versus time and determining the slope of the line passing through the peak and trough. The calculated slope will be equal to $-k$. The k may be calculated by taking the natural log of the quotient of the peak divided by the trough and dividing by the time interval between the peak and trough. This solution for k can be derived from the standard calculation for the slope of a line from two points:

$$
\begin{aligned}
k &= -m \\
&= -\left[\frac{(\ln \text{SDC}_{\text{trough}} - \ln \text{SDC}_{\text{peak}})}{(T_{\text{trough}} - T_{\text{peak}})}\right] \\
&= -\left[\frac{\ln\left(\dfrac{\text{SDC}_{\text{trough}}}{\text{SDC}_{\text{peak}}}\right)}{T_{\text{trough}} - T_{\text{peak}}}\right] \\
&= \frac{\ln\left(\dfrac{\text{SDC}_{\text{peak}}}{\text{SDC}_{\text{trough}}}\right)}{T_{\text{trough}} - T_{\text{peak}}}
\end{aligned}
\tag{1.11}
$$

where m is the slope of the line of a semilog plot of the natural log of the SDCs versus time. The SDC_{peak} and $\text{SDC}_{\text{trough}}$ are Y values, and the T_{trough} and T_{peak} are the corresponding times the trough and peak were collected, or the X values. Clinically, the last expression in Equation (1.11) is used to calculate k. The penultimate expression differs from the last expression only in that the SDC_{peak} and $\text{SDC}_{\text{trough}}$ have been flipped, which only changes the sign of the answer from negative to positive. Obviously, there are limitations in estimating the slope of a line from only two measured SDCs, as any error in the measured SDCs or the time of collection will create error in the estimate of k. To avoid excessive error in the estimate of k, the SDC_{peak} should be at least two times greater than the $\text{SDC}_{\text{trough}}$.

CASE #2

G.W. is a 55-year-old female patient receiving gentamicin, 80 mg every 8 hours. A peak SDC of 5.2 µg/mL is drawn 30 min after the end of a 30-min infusion, and a trough SDC of 1.7 µg/mL is drawn 7 hours after the end of the infusion. Calculate the half-life of gentamicin in this patient.

First, determine k:

$$
k = \frac{\ln\left(\dfrac{5.2 \text{ µg/mL}}{1.7 \text{ µg/mL}}\right)}{(7.5 \text{ hr} - 1.0 \text{ hr})} = 0.172 \text{ hr}^{-1}
\tag{1.12}
$$

To compute the half-life from k, divide the ln 2 (i.e., 0.693) by k.

$$
t_{1/2} = \frac{\ln 2}{k} = \frac{0.693}{0.172 \text{ hr}^{-1}} = 4.0 \text{ hours}
\tag{1.13}
$$

Measured peak and trough concentrations allow an estimation of $t_{1/2}$. The half-life provides information about specific aspects of drug disposition, such as how long it will take to reach steady state once maintenance dosing is started and how long it will take for "all" the drug to be eliminated from the body once dosing is stopped (usually considered to be five half-lives). Also, once the k and SDC are known, there are three calculations that will aid in the individualization of a patient's dosing regimen: (a) extrapolation, (b) back-extrapolation, and (c) determination of the time required for the concentration to decrease to some specified SDC. These functions are defined by solving for the appropriate variable in the following equation:

$$
C_t = C_0 e^{-kt}
\tag{1.14}
$$

where C_t is the concentration after time t has elapsed, C_0 is a measured SDC, k is the elimination rate constant, and t is some specified time interval. In the previous gentamicin example ($\text{SDC}_{\text{peak}} = 5.2$ µg/mL, $\text{SDC}_{\text{trough}} = 1.7$ µg/mL, $k = 0.172$ hr^{-1}, $t = 8$ hr), Equation (1.14) can be used to calculate (a) the C_{min}, defined as the theoretical SDC at the end of the dosing interval (extrapolation), (b) the C_{max}, defined as the theoretical SDC at the instant the infusion is complete (back-extrapolation), and (c) the time interval required for the concentration to fall from the C_{max} to some lower SDC (e.g., 0.5 µg/mL).

a. The concentration at the end of the dosing interval is calculated by extrapolating from the SDC_{peak} to the end of the dosing interval ($t = 7$ hr) using equation (1.14).

$$
\begin{aligned}
C_t &= C_0 e^{-kt} \\
&= (5.2 \text{ µg/mL}) e^{(-0.172 \text{ hr}^{-1})(7.0 \text{ hr})} \\
&= 1.5 \text{ µg/mL}
\end{aligned}
\tag{1.15}
$$

b. Equation (1.14) can be rearranged to back-extrapolate, that is, determine the concentration that occurred at some earlier time. The theoretical peak concentration, C_{max}, which occurs at the instant the infusion is complete, is determined by back-extrapolating from the SDC_{peak} to the time the infusion ended (30 min).

$$
C_t = \frac{C_0}{e^{-kt}} = \frac{5.2 \text{ µg/mL}}{e^{(-0.172 \text{ hr}^{-1})(0.5 \text{ hr})}} = 5.7 \text{ µg/mL}
\tag{1.16}
$$

c. The time interval for the concentration to drop from 5.7 µg/mL (C_{max}) to 0.5 µg/mL is determined by solving for t in Equation (1.14).

Table 1.1.
Clinical Utility of the Three Basic Pharmacokinetic Parameters of the One-Compartment Open Model

Parameter	Use	Equation
Volume of distribution, V (units: volume, e.g., liter)	Determine a loading dose	(1.6)
	Determine amount of drug in body	(1.4)
	Make qualitative assessment of distribution of drug in the body	
Clearance, Cl (units: volume/time, e.g., liter/hour)	Determine the steady-state concentration that will be achieved from a specific maintenance dose	(1.8) and (1.9)
Elimination rate constant, k (units: reciprocal time, e.g., hr^{-1})	Determine how long it will take to reach steady-state once maintenance dosing started	$5 \times t_{1/2}$
Half-life, $t_{1/2}$ (units: time, e.g., hours)	Determine how long it will take for the concentration to drop from some specified concentration to some lower concentration	(1.17)

The three basic pharmacokinetic parameters of first-order elimination are clearance, volume, and half-life. These parameters have specific, well-defined clinical utility.

$$t = \frac{\ln\left(\dfrac{C_0}{C_t}\right)}{k} = \frac{\ln\left(\dfrac{5.7\ \mu g/mL}{0.5\ \mu g/mL}\right)}{0.172\ hr^{-1}} = 14.1\ \text{hours} \qquad (1.17)$$

The three pharmacokinetic parameters, Cl, V, and $t_{1/2}$ do not correlate to anatomic structures or physiologic functions in the body; however, they define specific characteristics of drug disposition that are well defined. Table 1.1 summarizes the clinical utility of each pharmacokinetic parameter.

RELATIONSHIP BETWEEN $T_{1/2}$, CLEARANCE, VOLUME, AND STEADY-STATE CONCENTRATION

Clearance and V are independent pharmacokinetic parameters. This means Cl may change without affecting V, and V may change without affecting Cl. Half-life is a dependent function whose value depends on both Cl and V. If $t_{1/2}$ changes, then Cl, V, or both must have changed.

An often inappropriately applied equation is

$$Cl = (k)(V) \qquad (1.18)$$

which is frequently interpreted to mean that Cl depends on V. A mathematical equation can be algebraically rearranged in many ways, but it should not be deduced that one parameter depends on another simply because of the way the equation is written. For example, if an experiment demonstrated that an increase in blood pressure (BP) correlates with increasing age, and a linear regression of BP

(dependent variable) as a function of age (independent variable) is performed; an equation for the estimation of BP from age is derived:

$$BP = (Age)(m) + b \qquad (1.19)$$

where m is the slope of the regression line and b is the intercept. Equation (1.19) could be algebraically rearranged to give the following equation:

$$Age = \frac{BP - b}{m} \qquad (1.20)$$

It is obviously absurd to conclude from this equation that decreasing a patient's BP will decrease the patient's age. Thus, an equation does not necessarily define the interrelationships among the variables within the equation. This same situation exists for Cl $= kV$. The form of the equation that correctly reflects the interrelationship among the parameters is

$$k = \frac{Cl}{V} \qquad (1.21)$$

Clearance and V are the primary pharmacokinetic parameters that determine drug disposition. Clearance can be thought of as representing the sum of all drug elimination processes in the body, while V represents the distribution of drug. The steady-state concentration of a drug achieved after constant IV infusion or the mean steady-state concentration achieved after multiple oral or multiple intermittent IV infusions depends on Cl only (Equations 1.8 and 1.9, respectively). Changes in the V have no effect on the steady-state or mean steady-state concentration. Intuitively, it may seem that a decrease in the V will mean that the same amount of drug is distributed in a smaller volume, and the concentration will increase. However, the basic principle, which states that Cl and V are independent, would be violated, as the only way the steady-state concentration can increase is for the Cl to decrease (Equations 1.8 and 1.9). The question then arises as to exactly what effect changes in the V have on drug disposition. The patient on the antiarrhythmic (Case #1) can be used to illustrate the consequence of a decrease in V.

CASE #1 (Revisited)

The patient is admitted to the hospital with chest pain. Subsequent clinical examination and laboratory data confirm a myocardial infarction (MI) complicated by congestive heart failure. The patient's condition improves over the next two days, the IV antiarrhythmic is discontinued, and an oral antiarrhythmic is prescribed. Two days later the patient again develops runs of premature ventricular depolarizations (PVDs) despite adequate oral antiarrhythmic therapy. The patient is put back on a continuous IV infusion of the same antiarrhythmic as before. However, the patient's congestive heart failure (CHF) has responded to therapy, which has lead to a diuresis of edematous fluid. The antiarrhythmic is distributed into total body water, with the result that the V of the antiarrhythmic has decreased by one third. Clearance has remained unchanged. Describe how the drug disposition from the start of the 4 mg/min IV infusion to steady state will be altered.

The Cl and V before and after diuresis are as follows:

	Before Treatment	After Treatment
Cl	1 L/min	1 L/min
V	130 L	87 L

The rate of drug elimination can be calculated by taking the SDC and multiplying by the Cl (Equation 1.7). Though the V has decreased, the fact remains that at an SDC of 4 mg/L and a Cl of 1 L/min, the rate of drug elimination will be 4 mg/min (4 mg/min = 4 mg/L × 1 L/min). No matter how V changes, the rate of drug elimination at an SDC of 4 mg/L will always be 4 mg/min as long as the Cl remains unchanged. On the other hand, k is a dependent function that will change with changes in Cl and V. How the k changes and what effect it has on drug disposition is more easily interpreted if k is expressed as $t_{1/2}$. Since $k = Cl/V$ (Equation 1.21) and $k = 0.693/t_{1/2}$ (rearrangement of Equation 1.13), then

$$\frac{0.693}{t_{1/2}} = \frac{Cl}{V} \qquad (1.22)$$

Solving for $t_{1/2}$ gives the following:

$$t_{1/2} = \frac{0.693\, V}{Cl} \qquad (1.23)$$

This equation can be used to calculate the change in $t_{1/2}$ when the V decreases from 130 to 87 liters:

$$t_{1/2_{130L}} = \frac{(0.693)(130\text{ L})}{1\text{ L/min}} = 90\text{ min} \qquad (1.24)$$

$$t_{1/2_{87L}} = \frac{(0.693)(87\text{ L})}{1\text{ L/min}} = 60\text{ min} \qquad (1.25)$$

The decrease in V results in a decrease in the $t_{1/2}$, with no change in the steady-state concentration. The time to reach steady state will decrease from 7.5 hours (1.5 hr × 5) to 5.0 hours (1.0 hr × 5), but the steady-state concentration achieved will be unchanged. Table 1.2 gives the relative changes in $t_{1/2}$ and Css that occur when Cl and V change.

In the case of multiple intermittent IV infusions or oral dosing, the C_{ss} in Table 1.2 refers to the $\overline{C_{ss}}$ as defined in Equation (1.10). Though it is true that changes in V do not alter the C_{ss}, changes in V do affect the peak and trough concentrations within the dosing interval. Figure 1.2 compares and contrasts changes in Cl and V for a constant IV infusion and an intermittent IV infusion. As Figure 1.2B illustrates, a decrease in V for intermittent IV infusions leads to greater fluctuations between the peak and trough. It is possible that the

Table 1.2.
The Effect of Changes in Clearance and Volume on Half-Life and Steady-State Concentration

Independent Parameters		Dependent Parameters	
Clearance	Volume	Half-Life	C_{ss}
↑	↔	↓	↓
↓	↔	↑	↑
↔	↑	↑	↔
↔	↓	↓	↔
↑	↑	?	↓
↑	↓	↓	↓
↓	↑	↑	↑
↓	↓	?	↑

Clearance and volume are independent parameters whose values determine the apparent elimination rate (or half-life) of drug from the serum and the steady-state concentration achieved after maintenance dosing. The half-life is affected by both the clearance (inversely proportional) and volume (directly proportional), as depicted in Equation (1.23). The steady-state concentration is only affected by the clearance, as shown in Equations (1.8) and (1.9). The "?" in the table indicates that the effect on half-life cannot be determined without knowing the specific changes in Cl and V.

increased fluctuation between the peak and trough could result in transient toxicities associated with high peaks or periods of subtherapeutic concentrations associated with low troughs. The actual effect of alterations in V will depend on the degree of change in V and the pharmacodynamic characteristics of the particular drug in question.

USING SERUM DRUG CONCENTRATIONS FOR OPTIMIZATION OF DRUG THERAPY
Rationale for Therapeutic Drug Monitoring
Routine clinical monitoring utilizing SDCs is reserved for therapeutic agents that have a "defined" therapeutic range and a low therapeutic index. A "defined" therapeutic range is characterized by both upper and lower limits, where exceeding the upper limit is associated with a high probability of unacceptable toxicity and falling below of the lower limit is associated with a low probability of achieving a clinical therapeutic benefit. A low therapeutic index indicates that the serum concentrations necessary to achieve the therapeutic effect are close to serum concentrations that result in significant clinical toxicity. The implication is that dosing patients using population-average pharmacokinetic parameters will result in an unacceptable frequency of therapeutic failures or clinical toxicity directly attributable to low or high serum concentrations, respectively. The therapeutic ranges given in Table 1.3 are by no means supported by unequivocal evidence. Also, controversy surrounds the use of therapeutic ranges for drugs that have only a few well-controlled pharmacodynamic studies to establish

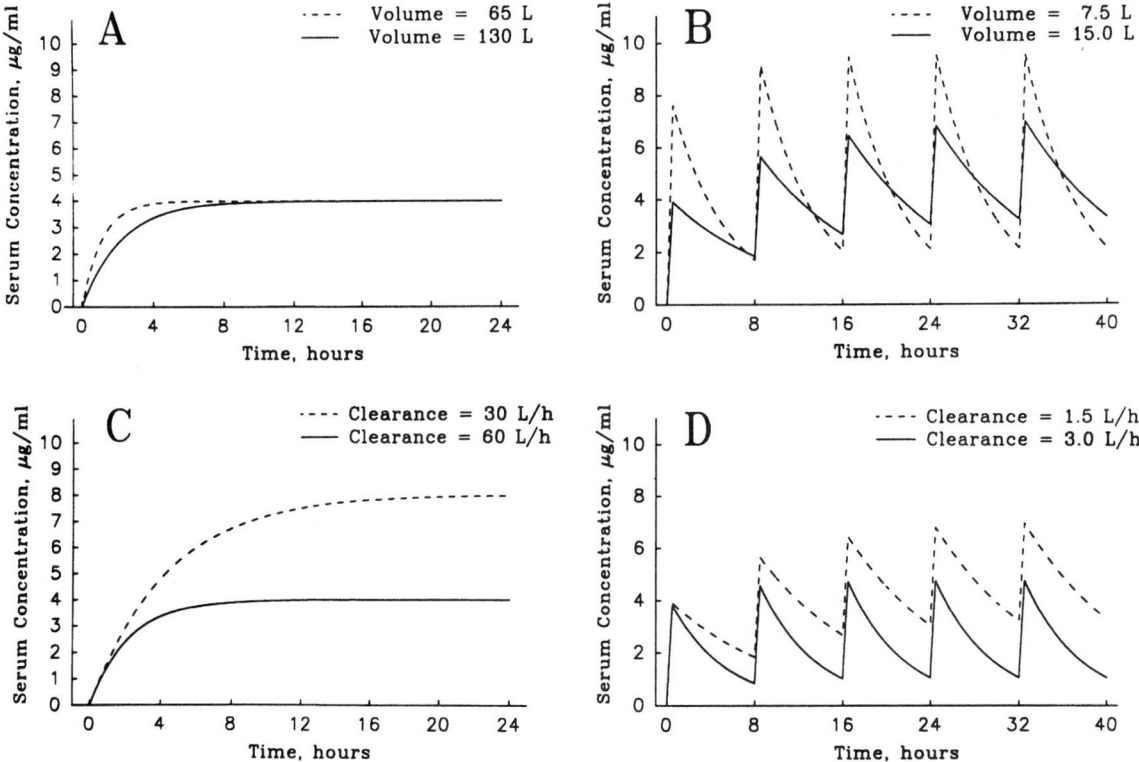

Figure 1.2 The effect of clearance and volume changes on the concentration–time profile of a continuous and intermittent IV drug infusion. **A** and **B** depict an IV constant infusion and an IV intermittent infusion, respectively. The dashed line represents the change in the concentration–time plot if the volume is decreased by one-half with no change in clearance. For both **A** and **B**, the time to reach steady-state is decreased. For graph **A**, the steady state concentration is unchanged. For graph **B**, the mean steady-state concentration is unchanged, but the peak will be higher and the trough lower. **C** and **D** depict an IV constant infusion and an IV intermittent infusion, respectively. The dashed line represents the change in the concentration–time plot if the clearance decreases by one-half with no change in the volume. The time to reach steady-state is increased, and the steady-state concentration is doubled.

Table 1.3.
Drugs Commonly Monitored in the Clinical Setting[a]

Drug	Therapeutic Range	Half-Life (hours)	Volume (liter/kg)	Clearance	SDC Type	Disposition	References
Digoxin	0.8–2.0 ng/mL	41	7.0	180 mL/min/1.73 m^2	$C_{ss\text{-}trough}$	Two-compt	9, 10
Theophylline	5–20 µg/mL	8	0.5	0.65 mL/min/kg	$C_{ss\text{-}trough}$	Two-compt	11
Lidocaine	1.5–5.0 µg/mL	2	1.2	15.6 mL/min/kg	C_{ss}	Two-compt	12, 13, 14
Procainamide	4–12 µg/mL	3.3	2.0	8.6 mL/min/kg	$C_{ss\text{-}trough}$	Two-compt	15
Lithium[b]	0.6–1.4 mEq/L	21	0.8	10–40 mL/min	$C_{ss\text{-}12\ hour}$	Two-compt	16, 17
Quinidine	2–5 µg/mL	7	2.5	4.5 mL/min/kg	$C_{ss\text{-}trough}$	Two-compt	18, 19
Gentamicin[c]	5–10 µg/mL peak	2	0.21	—	Zaske Eqn	One-compt	20, 21
Tobramycin[c]	<2 µg/mL trough	2.1	0.27	—	Zaske Eqn	One-compt	20
Amikacin[c]	20–30 µg/mL peak	2.2	0.25	—	Zaske Eqn	One-compt	21
	<5 µg/mL trough						
Carbamazepine[d]	4–12 µg/mL	12.3	1.0	0.91 mL/min/kg	$C_{ss\text{-}trough}$	—	22, 23
Phenobarbital	15–40 µg/mL	100	0.58	2.5 mL/min/m^2	$C_{ss\text{-}trough}$	Two-compt	23, 24
Phenytoin	10–20 µg/mL	N/A[e]	0.7	N/A	$C_{ss\text{-}trough}$	Nonlinear	25
Valproic acid	50–100 µg/mL	13	0.24	4–6 mL/min/m^2	$C_{ss\text{-}trough}$	Two-compt	23, 26
Vancomycin	25–40 µg/mL peak	7	0.72	1.2 mL/min/kg	Zaske Eqn	Two-compt	27, 28
	5–15 µg/mL trough						

[a]This table is not all-inclusive, covering only the most commonly monitored drugs. The stated therapeutic ranges and the pharmacokinetic parameters are for patients with normal hepatic and renal function and have significant variability, as reported in the literature.
[b]Lithium clearance averages 20% of creatinine clearance.
[c]Aminoglycoside clearance is dependent on renal function. Half-life given assumes young patient with normal renal function.
[d]Carbamazepine parameter values after autoinduction.
[e]N/A = not applicable.

such ranges. However, these ranges are generally accepted as an initial starting point for therapy and represent the current standards of practice.

A therapeutic range must not be used as the primary determinant of a patient's drug regimen. It would be inappropriate to consider achievement of a specific serum concentration as the clinical end point of therapy. The end point of therapy is always defined by a clinical response. If the clinical response is achieved when the SDC is outside the commonly stated therapeutic range, the patient's clinical condition rather than the SDC should be considered. For example, if a patient taking digoxin for chronic atrial fibrillation did not respond when the steady-state trough SDC ($SDC_{ss\text{-}trough}$) was below 2.0 ng/mL but is now responding with a $SDC_{ss\text{-}trough}$ of 2.3 ng/mL (therapeutic range 0.8–2.0 ng/mL), as evidenced by an acceptable ventricular response and no drug toxicity, then this should be considered a clinically acceptable digoxin concentration with no need to change the dosage regimen. Only a limited number of therapeutic agents are routinely monitored and doses adjusted by utilization of SDCs (Table 1.3). The methods by which dosing adjustments based on SDCs are made include the following:

1. Collection of steady-state peak and trough SDCs after multiple intermittent IV infusions and application of one-compartment equations
2. Collection of a single SDC at steady state during a constant IV infusion
3. Collection of a single trough SDC concentration at steady state during multiple oral dosing
4. Collection of two SDCs at two different steady-state concentrations achieved while on two different doses of a drug exhibiting Michaelis-Menten kinetics

One-Compartment Model

The most widely accepted clinical use of the one-compartment model was first proposed by Sawchuk and Zaske and originally used to adjust aminoglycoside doses in burn patients (2). However, this dosing adjustment method can be used for any drug that fulfills the following criteria:

1. Drug disposition can be adequately described by a one-compartment model.
2. The serum drug concentrations are determined after steady state has been achieved.
3. Drug is given by an intermittent intravenous infusion.
4. Sufficient SDCs are available (minimum one peak and one trough).

The first criterion should not be misconstrued to imply that the pharmacokinetic disposition must be monoexponential. The aminoglycosides are known to exhibit multicompartmental disposition, as does vancomycin, which may also be adjusted by this method. Multicompartment disposition does not preclude using the one-compartment

model. However, if the disposition of the drug is complicated by a significant distribution phase or other multicompartment nature, then the clinical relevance of this simplification must be understood. The caveat to using one-compartment equations for dosage adjustment of drugs exhibiting multicompartment disposition is recognizing the possible errors involved. When applying this method, the distribution phase of a two-compartment drug such as vancomycin is ignored. This means that the predicted peak concentration will be lower than the actual peak concentration and indirectly implies that the actual peak during the distribution phase is not clinically important. Also, if a one-compartment model is assumed for a drug like vancomycin, then the peak concentration must not be collected in the distribution phase, as this will result in unacceptable error in the calculation of V and k (see Fig. 1.3).

Applying one-compartment equations for the adjustment of IV intermittent infusions is often viewed as excessively complicated. However, a better description would be that this method is lengthy because the actual step-by-step process is straightforward.

1. Determine the amount and times of doses given to the patient and the values and times of the measured SDCs.

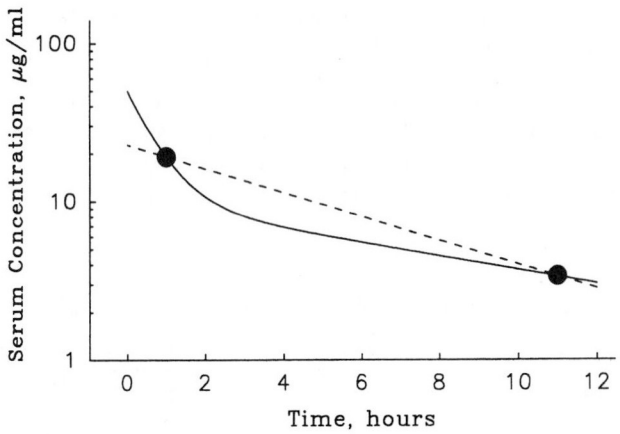

Figure 1.3 Consequence of sampling in the distribution phase and applying the Sawchuk/Zaske method of dosage adjustment. The dashed line illustrates the error incurred if the Sawchuk/Zaske equations are used to adjust dosage for a drug that exhibits two-compartment disposition and the peak SDC sample is collected in the distribution phase. The steeper slope calculated when the peak sample is collected in the distribution phase. The steeper slope calculated when the peak sample is collected in the α phase results in an overestimation of the terminal elimination rate constant, k (the estimated $t_{1/2}$ will be shorter than the actual $t_{1/2}$). The high peak and overestimated k will both contribute to underestimation of the volume. The error in clearance will be unpredictable, as the underestimated volume and overestimated k will counteract each other. The larger the elevation of the peak, the greater the underestimation of the dose and τ, leading to low peaks and high troughs.

2. Calculate the elimination rate constant (half-life) from peak and trough.
3. Determine C_{max} (concentration at instant the infusion is completed).
4. Determine C_{min} (concentration at the end of the dosing interval).
5. Calculate the volume of distribution.
6. Decide the target peak and trough desired for patient's therapy.
7. Calculate τ.
8. Calculate dose.
9. Calculate the theoretical peak and trough that will be achieved from the dose and τ recommended.

CASE #3

Patient J.L. is a 55-year-old female with a suspected nosocomial acquired pneumonia. Gentamicin, 100 mg given as a 30-min infusion every 8 hours is started. Peak and trough serum drug concentrations are determined around the third dose. The actual times of the doses and measured SDCs are as follows:

Time	Dose
0810	Dose #1: 100 mg IV infusion over 30 min
1550	Dose #2: 100 mg IV infusion over 30 min
2245	SDC #1: 1.8 µg/mL
2355	Dose #3: 100 mg IV infusion over 30 min
0115	SDC #2: 5.1 µg/mL

For a nosocomial pneumonia a peak concentration of 8.0 µg/mL and a trough around 1.0 µg/mL is desired. Calculate the dose and τ that will achieve the desired peak and trough concentrations in this patient.

STEP 1

Time Line

0810	1550	2245	2355	0115
Dose #1	Dose #2	SDC #1	Dose #3	SDC #2

It is common practice to determine the trough and peak concentrations around the third aminoglycoside dose, as depicted on the time line. The trough SDC sample is collected near the end of the second dosing interval, then the third dose is given, and a peak SDC sample is collected 30 minutes after the end of a 30-min infusion.

	Value	Time from Start of Last Infusion to the SDC
SDC #1 (trough)	1.8 µg/mL	1550 → 2245 = 6:55 (6.92 hr)
SDC #2 (peak)	5.1 µg/mL	2355 → 0115 = 1:20 (1.33 hr)

Since the trough and peak samples are collected during different dosing intervals, the time intervals between the peak and trough SDCs and the start of their respective dosing infusions are determined. Obtaining the trough and peak in this fashion is common practice. However, this method is not optimal, and good arguments can be made for collecting samples for peak and trough determinations within the same dosing interval. The former method is more efficient and generally considered adequate for dosing adjustments of aminoglycosides.

STEP 2

Because the SDCs are collected under steady-state conditions, they are treated as if they were collected within the same dosing interval. The time interval calculated above is based on the principle that at steady state, dosing regimens are superimposable, so 6.92 hours after the start of each dosing infusion the SDC will be 1.8 µg/mL and 1.33 hours after the start of the dosing infusion the SDC will be 5.1 µg/mL. Therefore, the time required for the concentration to decrease from 5.1 µg/mL to 1.8 µg/mL will be the time different between the two intervals, or 5.59 hours (6.92 hr – 1.33 hr). If a semilog plot of the natural log of the SDCs and the time intervals is constructed, the elimination rate constant (k) is defined as the negative slope of the line, or the k and $t_{1/2}$ may be calculated mathematically as previously discussed (Equations 1.12 and 1.13):

$$k = \frac{\ln\left(\dfrac{SDC_{peak}}{SDC_{trough}}\right)}{(T_{trough} - T_{peak})}$$

$$= \frac{\ln\left(\dfrac{5.1\ \mu g/mL}{1.8\ \mu g/mL}\right)}{(6.92\ hr - 1.33\ hr)} = 0.186\ hr^{-1} \qquad (1.26)$$

$$t_{1/2} = \frac{\ln 2}{k} = \frac{0.693}{0.186\ hr^{-1}} = 3.7\ hours \qquad (1.27)$$

where SDC_{trough} and SDC_{peak} are the measured trough and peak concentrations, and T_{trough} and T_{peak} are the time intervals calculated in step 1. Do not confuse the time interval with the clock time at which samples for the peak and trough determinations were collected.

STEP 3

The C_{max}, which is the theoretical peak concentration within the dosing interval occurring at the instant the infusion is complete, is calculated by back-extrapolation from the SDC_{peak} to the end of the infusion.

$$C_{max} = \frac{SDC_{peak}}{e^{(-k)(T_{peak} - T_{infusion})}}$$

$$= \frac{5.1\ \mu g/mL}{e^{(-0.186\ hr^{-1})(1.33\ hr - 0.5\ hr)}} = 6\ \mu g/mL \qquad (1.28)$$

where T_{peak} is the time interval from the start of the dosing infusion to the time the peak sample was collected and $T_{infusion}$ is the length of the infusion.

STEP 4

The C_{min}, which is the theoretical trough concentration within the dosing interval occurring at the end of the dosing interval, is calculated by extrapolating from the C_{max} to the end of the dosing interval. The t used in this equation is the scheduled dosing interval, which is not necessarily the actual dosing interval as documented in the patient's medication administration records.

$$C_{min} = C_{max}e^{(-k)(\tau - T_{infusion})}$$

$$= (6 \ \mu g.mL) \ e^{(-0.186 \ hr^{-1})(8 \ hr - 0.5 \ hr)} \quad (1.29)$$

$$= 1.5 \ \mu g/mL$$

STEP 5

The calculation of V uses the C_{max} and C_{min} calculated previously.

$$V = \frac{Dose(1 - e^{-kT_{infusion}})}{(T_{infusion})(k)[C_{max} - (C_{min}e^{-kT_{infusion}})]}$$

$$= \frac{100mg(1 - e^{-(0.186hr^{-1})(0.5hr)})}{(0.5 \ hr)(0.186 \ hr^{-1})(5.95 \ mg/L - 1.47 \ mg/L \ e^{(-0.186hr^{-1})(0.5hr)})} \quad (1.30)$$

$$= 20.7 \ liters$$

STEP 6

The target peak and trough are 8.0 µg/mL and 1.0 µg/mL, respectively.

STEP 7

A new dosing interval is calculated based on the desired steady-state peak and trough concentrations and the k calculated in step 2.

$$\tau = \frac{\ln\left(\frac{C_{max-target}}{C_{min-target}}\right)}{k} + T_{infusion}$$

$$= \frac{\ln\left(\frac{8.0 \ \mu g/mL}{1.0 \ \mu g/mL}\right)}{0.186 \ hr^{-1}} + 0.5 \ hr = 11.7 \ hr \quad (1.31)$$

STEP 8

The new τ calculated in step 7 is rounded to a convenient dosing interval (12 hr) and used with the calculated k from step 2 and calculated V from step 5 to determine a new dose to achieve the desired peak and trough concentrations (step 6).

Dose

$$= (T_{infusion})(k)(V)(C_{max-target})\left(\frac{(1 - e^{-k\tau})}{(1 - e^{-kT_{infusion}})}\right) \quad (1.32)$$

Dose

$$= (0.5 \ hr)(0.186 \ hr-1)(20.7 \ L)(8.0 \ mg/mL)$$

$$\times \left(\frac{(1 - e^{(-0.186hr^{-1})(12hr)})}{1 - e^{(-0.186hr^{-1})(0.5hr)}}\right) \quad (1.33)$$

$$= 155 \ mg$$

Because our calculations represent an *estimation*, the dose should be rounded down to the nearest 10-mg increment (e.g., 150 mg).

STEP 9

Both the τ and the dose have been rounded to convenient values (recommendation is 150 mg q12h); therefore, the theoretical peak and trough SDCs at steady state will be slightly different from the target values (from step 6).

$$C_{max-ss} = \frac{ko(1 - e^{-kT_{infusion}})}{(k)(V)(1 - e^{-k\tau})}$$

$$= \frac{\left(\frac{150 \ mg}{0.5 \ hr}\right)(1 - e^{(-0.186hr^{-1})(0.5hr)})}{(0.186 \ hr^{-1})(20.7 \ L)(1 - e^{(-0.186hr^{-1})(12hr)})} \quad (1.34)$$

$$= 7.8 \ \mu g/mL$$

$$C_{min-ss} = C_{max-ss}e^{(-k)(\tau - T_{infusion})}$$

$$= (7.75 \ \mu g/mL)(e^{(-0.186hr^{-1})(12hr - 0.5hr)}) \quad (1.35)$$

$$= 0.9 \ \mu g/mL$$

Note that C_{max-ss} and C_{min-ss} are the concentrations occurring at the instant the infusion is complete and the end of the scheduled dosing interval, respectively. If the predicted clinical peak (30 min postinfusion) and trough (30 min preinfusion) are desired, they may be calculated by extrapolating 0.5 hours from the C_{max} and back-extrapolating 0.5 hours from the C_{min}, respectively.

Constant IV Infusions

From Table 1.3 there are two drugs commonly given by a continuous intravenous infusion, lidocaine and theophylline. The most appropriate time to draw a sample for SDC determination for estimation of the patient's clearance is after steady-state conditions have been achieved ($5 \times t_{1/2}$). A steady-state C_{ss} allows the calculation of Cl, which in turn allows the determination of the dose that must be given to achieve a specific target steady-state concentration (refer to Table 1.1 and Equation 1.8).

CASE #4

Patient K.N. has received several boluses of lidocaine, and a continuous IV infusion at a rate of 2 mg/min has been started. Ten hours after the start of the infusion a SDC is collected. K.N. has responded well to the lidocaine infusion, but is still having occasional brief runs of PVDs (premature ventricular depolarizations). The SDC reported by the laboratory is 2.7 μg/mL. Calculate a new administration rate to achieve the desired steady-state concentration of 4.0 μg/mL.

Equation (1.8) could be used to solve for clearance, and then using the calculated Cl and target C_{ss} a new ko could be calculated. However, this type of problem can also be solved without determining the Cl directly. First recognize that the ratio of the administration rate ko to the C_{ss} must be constant if the Cl is unchanged.

$$Cl = \frac{ko}{C_{ss}} \tag{1.36}$$

Thus, for any infusion rate the ko divided by the C_{ss} must equal the Cl. Given a known infusion rate and a measured steady-state SDC, a new infusion rate can be computed that will achieve a new target steady-state concentration

$$\frac{ko_1}{SDCss} - \frac{ko_2}{C_{ss-target}} \tag{1.37}$$

$$ko_2 = \frac{(ko_1)(C_{ss-target})}{SDC_{ss}} \tag{1.38}$$

where ko_1 is the administration rate of the IV continuous infusion that achieved the measured steady-state concentration (SDC_{ss}), ko_2 is the new administration rate, and $C_{ss\text{-target}}$ is the new estimated SDC achieved when ko_2 reaches steady-state conditions. Thus, for K.N. the new administration rate is calculated as follows:

$$\frac{2.0 \text{ mg/min}}{2.7 \text{ mg/L}} = \frac{ko_2}{4.0 \text{ mg/L}} \tag{1.39}$$

$$ko_2 = \frac{(2.0 \text{ mg/min})(4.0 \text{ mg/L})}{2.7 \text{ mg/L}} \tag{1.40}$$

$$= 3.0 \text{ mg/min}$$

This allows an easy and quick method for the adjustment of a continuous IV infusion, based on a steady-state SDC determination. However, the assumptions underlying this process, namely, that the measured SDC is a steady-state concentration, that the drug is eliminated by a first-order process, and that Cl has not changed, must always be remembered.

If an SDC is determined before steady-state conditions have been achieved, then its usefulness for dosage adjustment is limited, as the Cl cannot be calculated from an SDC that is not a steady-state concentration. It is possible to glean some information from a non-steady-state SDC, though the necessity of using a population-based rather than an individualized pharmacokinetic parameter makes specific dosage estimations much less reliable. The non-steady-state SDC can only be interpreted by assuming a value for the $t_{1/2}$. The $t_{1/2}$ is needed to estimate how close to steady-state conditions the SDC was drawn.

CASE #5

Patient D.E. is a 33-year-old nonsmoking female who has been on a theophylline constant IV infusion at a rate of 35 mg/hr for 12 hours. A theophylline SDC determined at this time (12 hr after the start of the infusion) is 16.2 μg/mL. Decide if the administration rate should be changed.

The real question being asked is, what will the serum concentration of theophylline be at steady-state? To answer this question the population value for $t_{1/2}$ will be assumed (Table 1.3, $t_{1/2} = 8$ hr). Remember that the $t_{1/2}$ determines how long it takes to reach steady-state (see Table 1.1). Usually this is considered to be $5 \times t_{1/2}$; thus, steady-state would be achieved at 40 hours into the constant IV infusion. At 12 hours into the infusion, the SDC is between 50% ($t_{1/2} = 8$ hr) and 75% ($2 \times t_{1/2} = 16$ hr) of the steady-state concentration. The estimated fraction of the steady-state concentration the SDC at 12 hours represents is determined as follows:

$$\begin{aligned} \text{Fraction of } C_{ss} &= 1 - e^{-kt} \\ &= 1 - e^{(-0.087\text{hr}^{-1})(12\text{hr})} \\ &= 0.648 \end{aligned} \tag{1.41}$$

So, at 12 hours into the infusion, the SDC has accumulated to a concentration about 65% of what it will be when it reaches steady-state. To calculate the predicted concentration that will be achieved if the infusion is continued at the same rate to steady-state conditions the SDC is divided by the fraction of C_{ss},

$$C_{ss} = \frac{SDC_t}{1 - e^{-kt}} = \frac{16.2 \text{ μg/mL}}{1 - e^{(-0.087\text{hr}^{-1})(12\text{hr})}} \tag{1.42}$$

$$= 25.0 \text{ μg/mL}$$

where SDC_t is the measured SDC at time t, and t is the time interval from the start of the IV infusion to collection of the sample. Thus, it would be prudent to reduce the administration rate to avoid accumulation of drug to concentrations associated with theophylline toxicity. The rate could be adjusted using Equation (1.38), assuming the C_{ss} achieved at an administration rate of 35 mg/hr will be 25 μg/mL.

When applying the one-compartment model equations to measured peak and trough SDCs or adjusting a constant IV infusion based on a single measured steady-state SDC, patient-specific pharmacokinetic parameters are estimated from the SDCs. In case #5 it is impossible to determine any patient-specific pharmacokinetic parameters, and thus, a population-based pharmacokinetic parameter must be used. This reduces the probability that the predicted steady-state concentration will be accurate; however, it is the best estimate that can be made from the available data.

Multiple Oral Dosing

The majority of therapeutic agents monitored by SDCs are drugs given by mouth. Unlike a drug administered by IV infusion, the Cl cannot be estimated based on a single measured SDC, nor can the one-compartment model equations be applied to measured peak and trough concentrations. The fraction or percentage of the amount of drug absorbed after oral administration (F) and the time of the C_{max} (T_{max}) are highly variable, which makes estimation of patient-specific pharmacokinetic parameters such as Cl and V infeasible. In this situation a measured steady-state trough concentration ($SDC_{ss\text{-}trough}$) is used for dosage adjustment. For a drug that exhibits first-order elimination, dosage adjustment is based on an equation analogous to equation (1.37):

$$\frac{Dose_1}{SDC_{ss-trough}} = \frac{Dose_2}{C_{ss-trough}} \qquad (1.43)$$

where ($SDC_{ss\text{-}trough}$) is the measured SDC corresponding to $Dose_1$ and $Dose_2$ is some new dose, with the corresponding ($SDC_{ss\text{-}trough}$) being the steady-state trough concentration that will be achieved given $Dose_2$. As in Equation (1.37) the measured SDC is assumed to be a steady-state concentration, the drug is assumed to be eliminated by a first-order process, and the Cl is assumed to remain constant. Equation (1.43) also assumes that bioavailability *(F)* and the absorption rate *(ka)* remain constant, and that τ has not been changed.

CASE #6

Patient E.T. is a 55-year-old male who has been on digoxin p.o. q.d. 0.125 mg for the past month. You would like the digoxin SDC to reach 1.6 ng/mL. An SDC sample drawn this morning was reported by the clinical chemistry laboratory as 0.8 ng/mL. The physician requests your assistance in adjusting E.T.'s regimen to achieve the desired target concentration of 1.6 ng/mL.

Using Equation (1.43) a recommendation can be quickly determined.

$$\frac{0.125 \text{ mg}}{0.8 \text{ ng/mL}} = \frac{Dose_2}{1.6 \text{ ng/mL}} \qquad (1.44)$$

$$Dose_2 = \frac{(0.125 \text{ mg})(1.6 \text{ ng/mL})}{0.8 \text{ ng/mL}} = 0.25 \text{ mg} \quad (1.45)$$

Thus, if the dose is increased to 0.25 mg every day, then the serum concentration should increase to 1.6 ng/mL. Caution should be exercised in applying this equation because of the number of assumptions necessary for the estimation to remain valid. Additionally, nothing is known about the peak concentration achieved within the dosing interval. If peak concentrations are unrelated to clinical efficacy and toxicity (digoxin), or if the half-life of the drug is extremely long, such that there is very little fluctuation between the peak and trough concentrations within a dosing interval (digoxin, phenobarbital, phenytoin, lithium), then this assumption is reasonable. However, if the peak concentration is clinically important and $t_{1/2}$ is short relative to the dosing interval (e.g., theophylline, procainamide, carbamazepine, valproic acid), then careful consideration must be given to the possibility of high peak concentrations when increasing the dose based on measured trough SDCs.

CASE #7

Patient F.N. is an outpatient taking a generic brand of carbamazepine, 400 mg q8h. A measured steady state trough concentration determined early this afternoon (7 hr after the last dose) was 6.3 µg/mL. The patient is complaining of transient headache, dizziness, and diplopia with an onset about 30 minutes after taking each dose and persisting for about 30 minutes to 1 hours. F.N. has been on this dosing schedule for the past month, and previous to this was taking 300 mg q8h. However, on this lower dosage the patient was having approximately two grand mal seizure episodes per month. The patient has not experienced any seizures on the higher dosing regimen.

In F.N., the peak concentration achieved is unknown, though the side effects experienced shortly after each dose would suggest that the peak concentration after each dose is causing transiently toxic concentrations. This would indicate a need to reduce the dose, but a lower dose may not control F.N.'s seizures. In fact, reducing the patient's dosage may not be appropriate in this circumstance, given the past history of seizure activity while on 300 mg q8h. Instead, the same daily dose of carbamazepine (1200 mg) could be given, but the dosage interval reduced from 8 to 6 hours (i.e., 300 mg q6h). This will reduce the peak concentration and increase the trough concentration, thereby reducing the fluctuation between the highest and lowest concentration within the dosing interval. The mean steady-state concentration should remain unchanged, as the total daily dose has not changed. The peak concentration will be reduced enough to ameliorate the transient concentration-dependent toxicities F.N. is experiencing.

Michaelis-Menten Kinetics (Phenytoin)

The pharmacokinetic parameters, Cl and $t_{1/2}$, and the methods of dosage adjustment discussed up to this point apply only to drugs that are eliminated by a first-order process. The individualization of phenytoin dosing in patients cannot be done with any of the three methods previously described because phenytoin obeys Michaelis-Menten kinetics (MMK) (3). The most significant clinical implication of MMK is that disproportionate changes in steady-state SDC occur with changes in dosage. Although the ratio between the dose and C_{ss} is constant for first-order elimination processes for MMK, the ratio of dose to C_{ss} decreases with increasing doses.

Note that the V was not included in our list of pharmacokinetic parameters that are not applicable to MMK. This is because MMK pertains particularly to the elimination of drug from the body, and not the distribution of drug in the body. The volume of distribution is not related (independent of Cl) to the elimination mechanisms of drug from the body; however, the relationship of V to the total amount of drug in the body remains valid for drugs that obey MMK.

The best way to understand the concepts and clinical implications of MMK is to compare and contrast it with first-order elimination. For MMK the elimination rate of drug from the body is described by the following equation:

$$\text{Rate of Drug Elimination} = \frac{(V_{max})(C)}{k_m + C} \qquad (1.46)$$

where C is the serum concentration (mg/L), V_{max} is the maximum rate of drug elimination (mg/day), and k_m is the serum concentration at which the elimination rate is equal

Table 1.4.
Michaelis-Menten Kinetics: Dependence of Nonlinear Elimination on k_m

SDC (mg/L)	Rate of Drug Elimination (mg/day)	Clearance (L/day)
Drug A ($k_m = 7$ mg/L; $V_{max} = 600$ mg/day		
1	75	75
5	250	50
10	353	35
15	409	27
20	444	22
Drug B ($k_m = 300$ mg/L; $V_{max} = 600$ mg/day)		
1	2	2.0
5	10	2.0
10	19	1.9
15	28	1.9
20	38	1.9

Drug A is representative of k_m and V_{max} values within the normal range expected for phenytoin. Drug B represents a hypothetical drug whose V_{max} is identical to that of drug A, but for which the k_m is much greater. The rate of elimination is calculated using Equation (1.46). The clearance is calculated by dividing the rate of drug elimination (mg/day) by the SDC (mg/L), which is an algebraic rearrangement of Equation (1.7). Drug B behaves in a first-order manner (clearance remains approximately constant), demonstrating that the most important parameter determining the extend to MMK seen in the therapeutic serum concentration range is the k_m. If for drug A and drug B the V_{max} were doubled to 1200 mg/day, then the rate of drug elimination would be doubled and the clearance would be doubled, but drug A would still obey MMK and drug B first-order kinetics.

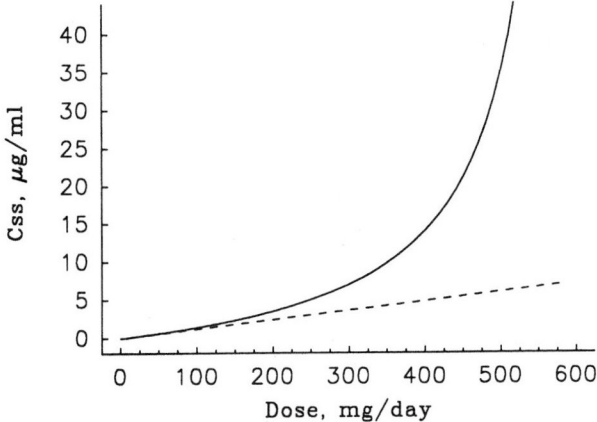

Figure 1.4 Relationship between dose and steady-state concentration for a drug exhibiting Michaelis-Menten kinetics. The relationship between steady-state concentration and dose for a drug that demonstrates Michaelis-Menten kinetics in the normal therapeutic serum concentration range ($k_m = 7$ µg/mL; $V_{max} = 600$ mg/day). At low concentrations ($C_p \ll k_m$) the drug obeys first-order elimination, as the concentration approaches and exceeds the k_m, there is a disproportionate increase in the steady-state concentration when the dose is increased. When the serum concentration is much greater than the k_m, the elimination approaches zero-order elimination. Zero-order is characterized by an infinitely increasing serum concentration; as such, steady-state concentration will never occur.

to half the maximum rate. Compare this equation with Equation (1.7), the calculation for rate of drug elimination for a drug that obeys first-order elimination. The most important parameter determining the clinical significance of MMK is k_m. If the normal therapeutic concentrations are much lower than the k_m, then Equation (1.46) simplifies to a first-order process. As the k_m approaches therapeutic serum concentration, MMK becomes clinically important and must be considered. All drugs eliminated by liver metabolism must have some k_m and V_{max}, but fortunately the majority of drugs have k_m values that are much greater than the normal therapeutic concentrations. Table 1.4 compares the average value of k_m and V_{max} for phenytoin with a hypothetical drug for which k_m is much greater than the normal serum concentrations (approximating first-order elimination).

Table 1.4 shows the decreasing Cl of phenytoin as the serum concentration increases. A decreasing Cl does not imply a decreasing rate of drug elimination; the rate of drug elimination increases with increasing serum concentration for drugs that obey MMK, but the increase in drug elimination is not proportional to the increase in the dose (capacity limited metabolism). This concept of a decreasing clearance with increasing serum concentration has two very important implications for dosage adjustment. An elimination rate constant k cannot be

defined. Since Cl decreases as serum concentration increases, k decreases as the serum concentration increases (Equation 1.21). Thus, it is not possible to extrapolate or back-extrapolate if two SDCs are known, as the semilog plot of drug elimination is not linear. The ratio between a dose and its C_{ss} decreases as the dose increases. Again, this can be deduced by noting that the Cl decreases with increasing serum concentration and examining the effect of decreasing the Cl on Equations (1.8) and (1.9) (Fig. 1.4).

Several methods have been proposed for adjusting phenytoin dosage based on steady-state SDCs. These methods require two SDCs determined from samples collected while the patient is on two different maintenance doses. The algebraic method derived by solving two simultaneous equations (4) is preferable because it allows the new dosage to be estimated without graphing. Thus,

$$k_m = \frac{\text{Dose}_2 - \text{Dose}_1}{\dfrac{\text{Dose}_1}{C_{ss_1}} - \dfrac{\text{Dose}_2}{C_{ss_2}}} \tag{1.47}$$

$$V_{max} = \text{Dose}_1 + \left(k_m \times \frac{\text{Dose}_1}{C_{ss_1}} \right) \tag{1.48}$$

where Dose$_1$ and Dose$_2$ are two different maintenance doses of phenytoin in mg per day and C_{ss_1} and C_{ss_2} are their respective steady-state concentrations. The k_m is calculated first and then used in the calculation of the V_{max}.

CASE #8

Patient C.W. has a long-standing seizure disorder controlled with phenytoin, 600 mg/day. However, at this dosage the patient experiences an unacceptable level of side effects, the most debilitating of which is ataxia. The steady-state concentration on this regimen is 26 mg/L. He had been on 300 mg/day before the increase to 600 mg/day; however, on the lower dosage, which produced a steady-state concentration of 6 mg/L, the patient experienced approximately one grand mal seizure episode per month. The patient's physician had hoped that the increase to 600 mg/day would produce a steady-state concentration around 16 mg/L and result in good seizure control without unacceptable side effects. Recommend a dose to achieve a steady-state concentration of 16 mg/L.

To estimate the dose required to achieve the target steady-state concentration of 16 mg/L, first estimate k_m and V_{max} using Equations (1.47) and (1.48), respectively.

$$k_m = \frac{600\,\text{mg/day} - 300\,\text{mg/day}}{\dfrac{600\,\text{mg/day}}{26\,\text{mg/L}} - \dfrac{300\,\text{mg/day}}{6\,\text{mg/L}}} \qquad (1.49)$$

$$= 11\,\text{mg/L}$$

$$V_{max} = 3200\,\text{mg/day} + \left(11\,\text{mg/L} \times \frac{300\,\text{mg/day}}{6\,\text{mg/L}}\right) \qquad (1.50)$$

$$= 850\,\text{mg/day}$$

The estimates of k_m and V_{max} are used to calculate a new maintenance dose to achieve a C_{ss} of 16 mg/L using the following equation:

$$\text{Dose} = \frac{V_{max}}{\left(1 + \dfrac{k_m}{C_{ss}}\right)}$$

$$= \frac{850\,\text{mg/day}}{\left(1 + \dfrac{11\,\text{mg/L}}{16\,\text{mg/L}}\right)} = 503.7 \approx 500\,\text{mg/day} \qquad (1.51)$$

Three assumptions underlying this method are:

1. Both SDCs were determined from samples collected under steady-state conditions.
2. The same dosage form (must be same brand name product) was administered.
3. Protein binding remains constant.

These assumptions must be followed strictly to avoid excessive error in the new dosage estimation. The clinical utility of this method is limited by the requirement for two SDCs determined on samples collected while the patient is on two different steady-state dosing regimens. In an inpatient setting, it is unlikely that two SDCs on two different steady-state dosing regimens will be available. This method is most likely to be used in a clinic for the adjustment of phenytoin in an ambulatory population. This introduces a fourth assumption, 100% patient compliance.

PHYSIOLOGIC VARIABLES AFFECTING DRUG CLEARANCE

Hepatic Drug Elimination

The disposition of drugs eliminated primarily by hepatic metabolism can be affected by alterations in protein binding, liver enzymes, and liver blood flow. It is important to understand the mechanism by which changes in protein binding, liver enzymes, or liver blood flow can affect drug disposition in order to predict when such changes may be of clinical importance in a specific patient. Compartmental mathematical models are inadequate for this purpose because they describe changes in total drug concentration, using hybrid parameters that do not correlate with the physiologic processes responsible for drug elimination. To evaluate changes in these determinants of hepatic drug clearance, a model that includes them as parameters and defines their mathematical relationship to clearance can be used. One such model is the venous equilibrium model (VEM). The VEM is an attempt to construct a pharmacokinetic model for drug clearance, using model parameters that correspond to specific physiologic determinants of drug elimination.

For drugs cleared predominantly by hepatic metabolic processes (phenytoin, phenobarbital, theophylline, valproic acid, carbamazepine), the Cl of the drug from the body is approximately equivalent to the hepatic drug clearance. In these cases, drug elimination is the difference between the amount of drug entering the liver and the amount of drug exiting the liver, as illustrated in Figure 1.5. C_{in} is the concentration of drug in the blood entering the liver, C_{out} is the concentration of drug in

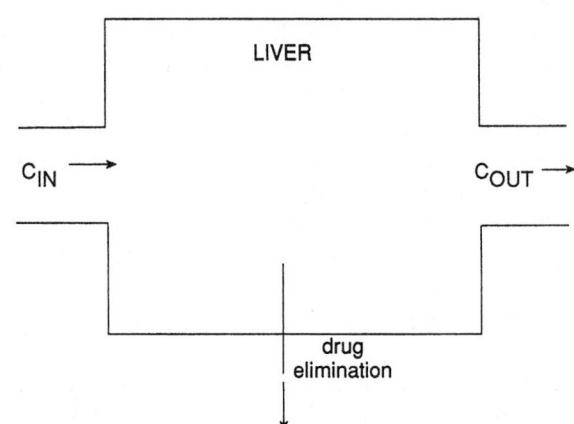

Figure 1.5 Venous equilibrium model of hepatic drug elimination. A hepatically eliminated drug enters the liver where it is metabolized. The difference between C_{IN} and C_{OUT} represents the amount of drug eliminated from the blood as it passes through the liver. From this simple scheme the concept of organ clearance is illustrated and used to explain the derivation of Equations (1.47) and (1.48).

the blood exiting the liver. Thus, the rate of drug elimination would be described by

$$\text{Rate of Drug Elimination} = (Q)(C_{\text{in}}) - (Q)(C_{out}) \qquad (1.52)$$

where Q equals the liver blood flow (approximately 1.5 L/min in humans), and C_{in} and C_{out} are as previously defined. Since blood flow into the liver must be equivalent to blood flow out of the liver (it is within a closed system), Equation (1.52) simplifies to $(Q)(C_{\text{in}} - C_{\text{out}})$. This is the mg/min rate of drug eliminated by the liver. Dividing this by the mg/min rate of drug entering the liver gives a unitless parameter known as the extraction ratio (ER).

$$\text{ER} = \frac{(Q)(C_{\text{in}} - C_{\text{out}})}{(Q)(C_{\text{in}})} = \frac{C_{\text{in}} - C_{\text{out}}}{C_{\text{in}}} \qquad (1.53)$$

The ER is an indicator of the efficiency of the processes responsible (e.g. metabolism) for eliminating drug from the blood as it passes through the liver. The ER can range from 0 to 1. An ER of 1 means 100% of the drug entering the liver is eliminated, while an ER of 0 means none of the drug entering the liver is eliminated. The hepatic clearance (Cl_H) of a drug is the liver blood flow multiplied by the ER, $Cl_H = (Q)(\text{ER})$. The ER as defined in Equation (1.53) assumes that the drug is not bound to any proteins in the blood. When protein binding is considered, the ER is best described by the following equation (5, 6):

$$\text{ER} = \frac{(f_u)(Cl_{\text{int}})}{Q + (f_u)(Cl_{\text{int}})} \qquad (1.54)$$

where f_u is the fraction of the total drug in the blood that is unbound, Q is the liver blood flow, and Cl_{int} is the intrinsic clearance of the drug. Cl_{int} is the theoretical value for clearance of the drug by the liver if it is not protein bound, and is an indication of the liver's enzymatic capacity to eliminate a drug if access is not impeded by protein binding or blood flow.

High-Clearance Drugs (Hepatic Elimination)

A high-clearance drug is one that has an extraction ratio greater than or equal to 0.7. For the purpose of qualitative prediction of the effect of changes in f_u, Cl_{int}, and Q on $C_{ss\text{-total}}$ and $C_{ss\text{-free}}$, the extraction ratio is assumed to be 1.0. Thus, the Cl of the drug simplifies to $Cl_H = Q$. which means that the clearance depends on the rate of presentation of drug to the liver (i.e., the liver blood flow). For a high-extraction drug given by the IV route, alterations in protein binding and enzyme induction or inhibition have no effect on the clearance of drug. The elimination of drug by the liver is so efficient that protein-bound drug is stripped from its protein-binding sites and metabolized. Concomitant administration of drugs that inhibit or induce hepatic enzymes also has little effect on drug elimination, because the metabolic capacity of the liver is so great that

the small changes secondary to enzyme induction or inhibition are clinically irrelevant. Though protein-binding changes do not alter clearance of a high-extraction drug, they may alter the relationship between total drug concentration and therapeutic and toxic effects.

The free drug in the blood is the pharmacologically active portion of drug. Drug molecules bound to proteins are usually considered pharmacologically inactive because the steric interference of the protein molecule inhibits binding of the drug molecule to the active receptor site and protein-bound drug cannot easily diffuse from the blood compartment to the site of action. Thus, the therapeutic effect is more closely related to the free drug concentration than to the total drug concentration. The use of total concentration is strictly for purposes of feasibility, and in fact the underlying assumption is that the inter- and intraindividual variability in protein binding (or f_u) is relatively small. In the case of a high-extraction drug, a change in protein binding secondary to displacement from protein-binding sites (increase in f_u) or an increase in protein-binding receptor sites (decrease in f_u) will cause the free concentration of drug to increase or decrease, respectively, with no change in the total drug concentration, thus altering the relationship between total concentration and therapeutic or toxic effects. Such alterations in f_u can lead to changes in the "therapeutic range," which is based on total SDC.

Low-Clearance Drugs

A low-clearance drug is one for which the hepatic elimination is restricted by the enzymatic capacity of the liver rather than by the liver blood flow. In this case, clearance depends on both the intrinsic free clearance of drug by the liver, Cl_{int}, and the free fraction of drug in the blood f_u such that $Cl_H = f_u Cl_{\text{int}}$. Alterations in liver blood flow Q have no effect on clearance of a low-extraction drug, as the rate of presentation of drug to the liver exceeds the ability of the liver to eliminate the drug. Decreased protein binding will result in an increase in hepatic clearance, and an increase in protein binding will cause a decrease in hepatic clearance, whereas enzyme induction increases hepatic clearance and enzyme inhibition decreases hepatic clearance. Changes in f_u are particularly important because of the alteration in the total concentration-response relationship.

CASE #9

Patient E.W. is a 55-year-old male with a long-standing seizure disorder treated successfully with phenytoin, 200 mg b.i.d. Random levels in clinic have run between 12 and 19 mg/L over the last 2 years. Six months ago E.W. was diagnosed with prostate cancer. The patient's prognosis remains good despite a weight loss of 35 pounds over the last 6 months. Today E.W. comes in to clinic with nystagmus upon lateral gaze and mild ataxia. A stat phenytoin drug level is reported as 18.7 mg/L. The only other clinically significant laboratory value is a low albumin, 2.9 g/dL. E.W.'s physician says levels from past visits have been as high and even higher without any signs or symptoms of toxicity, and requests your expertise in speculating on the reason for this patient's apparent phenytoin toxicity.

Phenytoin is a highly protein-bound (90%), hepatically eliminated, low-extraction drug. The major plasma protein to which phenytoin binds is albumin. The effect of a low albumin level is fewer protein-binding sites in the plasma, which results in an increase in the f_u. Normally, phenytoin is 90% protein bound ($f_u = 0.10$), which is equivalent to a free phenytoin therapeutic range of 1.0 to 2.0 µg/mL. In the case of E.W., this would be equivalent to a free phenytoin concentration of 1.87 mg/L. However, since the f_u is increased via a reduced number of albumin protein-binding sites in the plasma, the proportion of the measured total concentration that is free drug is increased such that the free concentration will be more than 10% of the measured total concentration.

A formula has been proposed for estimating the free concentration, based on the degree of hypoalbuminemia (7):

$$C_{free} = \frac{(SDC_{total})(0.1)}{(0.2)(Alb) + 0.1} \qquad (1.55)$$

where C_{free} is the estimated free concentration of phenytoin in the blood, SDC_{total} is the measured SDC, and Alb is the serum albumin level in mg/dL. For E.W. the estimated free concentration would be

$$C_{free} = \frac{(18.7\mu g/mL)(0.1)}{(0.2)(2.9) + 0.1} = 2.8 \text{ mg/L} \qquad (1.56)$$

This estimate of the free phenytoin concentration would be equivalent to a total serum concentration of 28 mg/L if the patient had a normal serum albumin. The f_u has increased from the presumed normal of 0.1 to 0.15:

$$f_u = \frac{C_{free}}{C_{total}} = \frac{2.8 \text{ mg/L}}{18.7 \text{ mg/L}} = 0.15 \qquad (1.57)$$

demonstrating that small increases in the f_u can have a significant effect on the relationship between the total measured phenytoin serum concentration and the free serum concentration. In the case of E.W., the phenytoin dose should be reduced and free phenytoin concentrations measured instead of total concentrations, if available. Monitoring free phenytoin concentrations circumvents the need to apply Equation (1.50), which should not be used for dosage adjustment because of the unreliability of this free concentration estimate.

The perturbations in drug disposition for high- and low-extraction drugs that are hepatically eliminated are summarized in Table 1.5. Protein-binding changes affect the f_u, alterations in intrinsic metabolic capacity through enzyme induction or inhibition affect the Cl_{int}, and changes in blood flow secondary to hemodynamic changes are represented by changes in Q. This table only describes VEM predictions for high-extraction drugs given IV (lidocaine) and low-extraction drugs given by the IV or oral

Table 1.5.

Venous Equilibrium Model: Effect of Changes in Q, f_u, and Cl_{int} on Steady-State Free and Total Drug Concentration

Independent Parameters			Dependent Parameters	
Q	f_u	Cl_{int}	$C_{ss\text{-}total}$	$C_{ss\text{-}free}$
High-clearance drug (IV route only)				
↑	↔	↔	↓	↓
↓	↔	↔	↑	↑
↔	↑	↔	↔	↑
↔	↓	↔	↔	↓
↔	↔	↑	↔	↔
↔	↔	↓	↔	↔
Low-clearance drug (IV or p.o. route)				
↑	↔	↔	↔	↔
↓	↔	↔	↔	↔
↔	↑	↔	↓	↔
↔	↓	↔	↑	↔
↔	↔	↑	↓	↓
↔	↔	↓	↑	↑

The parameters of the venous equilibrium model are liver blood flow (Q), fraction of drug unbound in the blood (f_u), and the free intrinsic clearance (Cl_{int}). These three parameters determine the total steady-state concentration ($C_{ss\text{-}total}$) and the free or unbound steady-state concentration ($C_{ss\text{-}free}$) of drug in the blood. For a high-extraction drug (IV route), $C_{ss\text{-}total}$ and $C_{ss\text{-}free}$ are equally affected by changes in liver blood flow with f_u remaining constant; while changes in f_u are directly related to $C_{ss\text{-}free}$, but do not affect $C_{ss\text{-}total}$. Changes in Cl_{int} secondary to enzyme induction or inhibition do not affect $C_{ss\text{-}total}$ or $C_{ss\text{-}free}$. For a low-clearance drug, changes in liver blood flow do not affect $C_{ss\text{-}total}$ or $C_{ss\text{-}free}$; while changes in f_u are inversely related to changes in $C_{ss\text{-}total}$, but do not affect $C_{ss\text{-}free}$. Alterations in Cl_{int} effect an inversely related change in $C_{ss\text{-}total}$ and $C_{ss\text{-}free}$ equally (f_u is unchanged). For both a high-extraction drug given IV and a low-extraction drug given IV or p.o., changes in f_u will alter the relationship between total serum drug concentration and free serum drug concentration at steady-state. This subsequently can result in a significant alteration in the relationship between total serum drug concentration at steady-state and the therapeutic and toxic effects, i.e., a change in the therapeutic range (e.g., case #9).

route (phenytoin, phenobarbital, valproic acid, carbamazepine, theophylline). For drugs with intermediate extraction ratios (between 0.3 and 0.7), simplification of these equations results in poor approximations, and since the parameters of the VEM are impractical to determine clinically, this physiologic model is not useful.

Renal Drug Elimination

The renal route of drug elimination is important for digoxin, procainamide, lithium, gentamicin, amikacin, tobramycin, and vancomycin. Unlike hepatic drug elimination, which cannot be quantitatively assessed, renal function can be estimated from a measured 24-hr urinary creatinine level or from a measured serum creatinine level using the Cockcroft-Gault equation (8):

$$CrCl = \frac{(140 - Age)(Weight)}{(72)(SCr)} \qquad (1.58)$$

where CrCl is the estimated creatinine clearance in milliliters per minute, age is in years, weight is in kilograms (and refers to the lean body weight), and SCr is the serum

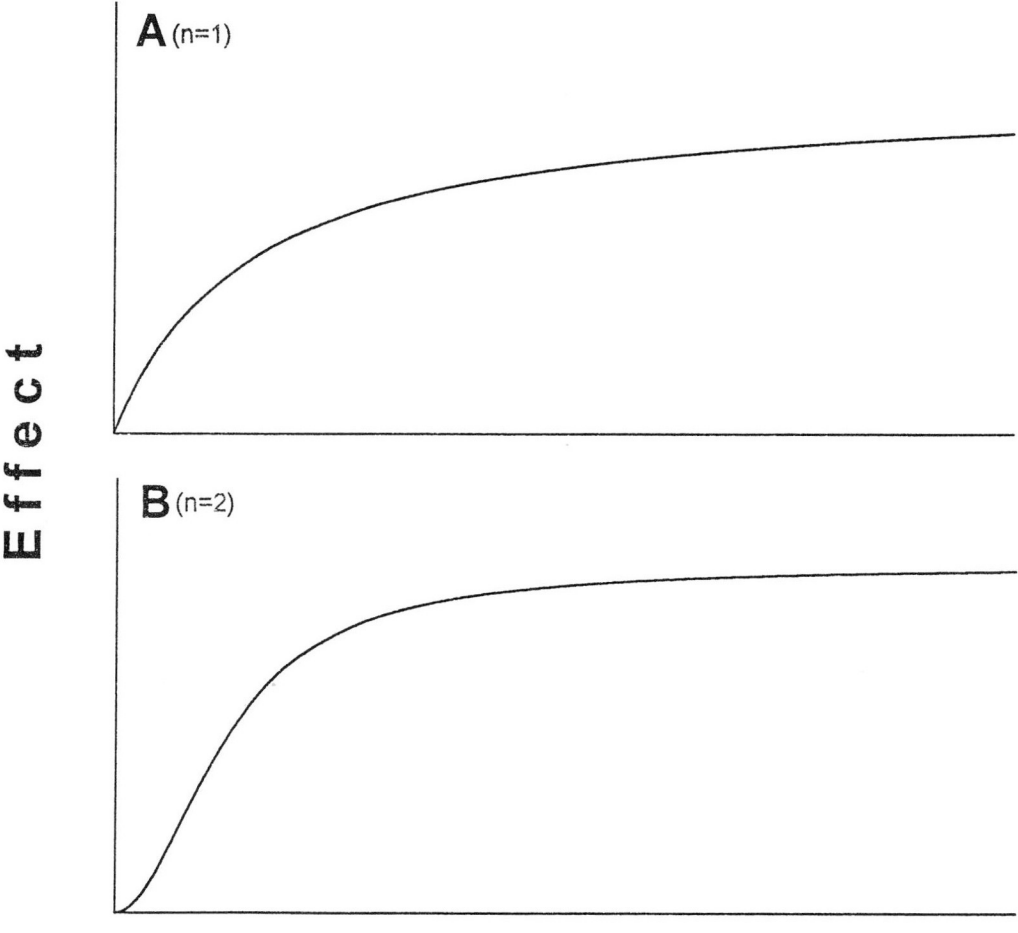

Figure 1.6 These graphs show plots of *E*, a measured effect, versus drug concentration measured in plasma. Graph A shows a hyperbolic concentration-effect relationship (n = 1), where the effect increases in a smooth arc as plasma drug concentration increases until E_{max} is achieved, after which further increasing the drug plasma concentration does not cause any increase in effect (*E*). Graph B shows the case where *E* increases very gradually at first and then increases rapidly (n = 2) and levels off rapidly once the E_{max} is achieved. This S-shaped function is the reason for referring to the model as sigmoidal.

creatinine level in mg/dL. Equation (1.58) is an estimation of creatinine clearance in males based on serum creatinine level. If the patient is female, the same calculation is performed, but the answer is then multiplied by 0.85. The estimated creatinine clearance is an indication of the patient's kidney function and correlates with the renal elimination of drugs. Assessment of a patient's renal function is particularly important for the initial maintenance dosing with drugs that are eliminated by the kidney. Once measured SDCs are available, the patient's drug therapy can be individualized based on these SDCs. Various dosing nomograms have been developed for the adjustment of maintenance doses in patients with renal impairment (29-32). Using nomograms that estimate doses based on renal function is subject to significant error, and follow-up SDCs should be done.

Pharmacodynamics

The clinical utility of pharmacokinetic modeling is limited by the fact that it only provides predictions about the SDC achieved when a patient is given a certain dose of drug (i.e., it is a model of the dose-concentration relationship). However, even in patients in which identical SDCs occur there is usually a significant difference in response. The purpose of pharmacodynamic modeling is to describe and predict this variability of response (i.e., it is a model of the concentration-effect relationship). When pharmacokinetic and pharmacodynamic modeling are combined, they provide a powerful tool for quantifying the clinical effects of drugs. For example, it is known that the elderly are more sensitive to the opiate agonistic effects of morphine. This increased sensitivity could be due either to differences in the SDC achieved

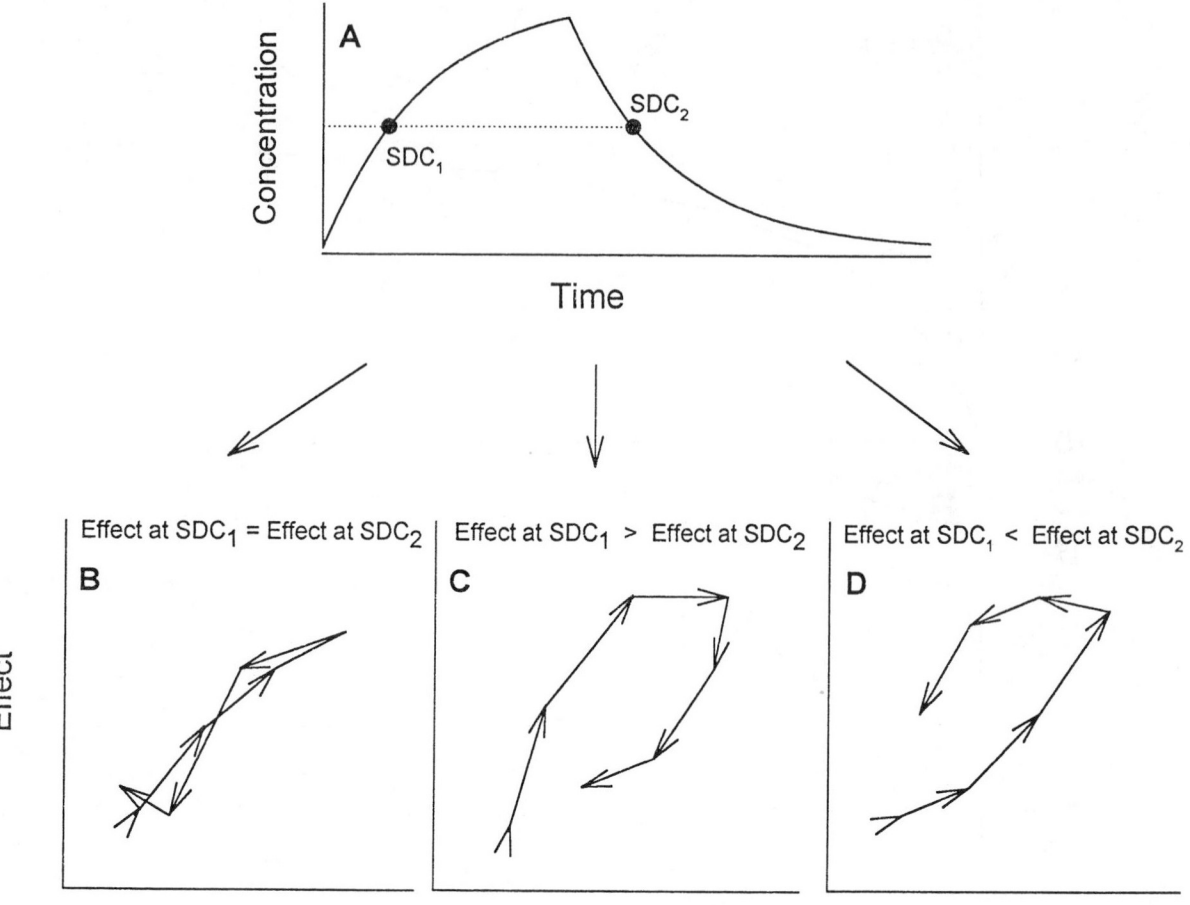

Figure 1.7 Graph A shows the concentration-time profile after a single dose of drug with SDC_1 and SDC_2. If a response is measured at two time points, then the concentration-effect relationship can be compared between the two points (typically this is done for many points). If the response at SDC_1 equals the response at SDC_2, neither tolerance nor sensitization occurs (Graph B: no hysteresis). If the response at SDC_1 is greater than the response at SDC_2, tolerance occurs (Graph C: clockwise hysteresis). If the response at SDC_1 is less than SDC_2, sensitization occurs (Graph D: counterclockwise hysteresis).

in young and elderly patients given the same mg/kg dose, or due to differences in the clinical effects achieved in the elderly and young patients with identical SDCs. The former is evaluated by comparing their pharmacokinetic parameters (Cl, V, and $t_{1/2}$), while the latter is evaluated by comparing their pharmacodynamic parameters (Emax and EC50).

The most common pharmacodynamic model fit to concentration-effect data is the sigmoid Emax model (33):

$$E = \frac{(E_{max})(C^n)}{EC_{50} + C^n} \qquad (1.59)$$

where E is some measured clinical effect, E_{max} is the maximum response possible, C is the SDC that caused E, EC_{50} is the SDC at which the measured effect is at one-half of E_{max}, and n determines the sigmoidal shape of the

concentration-effect relationship (see Fig. 1.6). Conducting a pharmacodynamic analysis involves measuring a clinical effect such as blood pressure and determining the plasma concentration at the time the blood pressure measurement is made. Then blood pressure is plotted against the SDC. The E_{max}, EC_{50}, and n are estimated by a computer program that determines the values of these parameters that give the best fit between the predicted effect, determined by solving Equation (1.59), and the actual observed effect.

Tolerance and Increased Sensitivity

The relationship between concentration and effect for a specific drug action often changes over time, causing either a reduction (tolerance) or increase (sensitization) in the drug's effects. How a drug's effects change over time can

Table 1.6.
Information Necessary for Clinical Interpretation of Measured SDCs

Drug monitored	Dose
	Route of administration
	History: Length of time on this drug and length of time on present dosing regimen
Measured SDC	Exact time measured SDC sample collected
	Postdose time: Time interval between administration of last dose and collection of SDC.
	Reason for SDC determination
Patient information	Demographics: Age, sex, weight, height
	History of present illness
	Past medical history
	Laboratory data: SCr, liver function tests, any other abnormal lab values
	Pertinent clinical parameters: most common include heart rate, blood pressure, temperature, chest x-ray, nutritional status, mental status
Other drug therapy	Drug-drug interactions
	Drug-disease interactions
	Drug-food interactions

The information needed to properly assess a patient's drug therapy will be highly variable and depend on the drug and clinical circumstances. This table is not all-inclusive, but represents a basic starting point.

significantly alter patient response. A classic example would be the dosing of nitroglycerin sustained-release preparations for angina. Around-the-clock dosing results in tolerance to the beneficial effects of nitroglycerin for anginal pain. This tolerance can be avoided by having the patient take the medication only while awake. The nitrate-free interval that occurs during sleep reduces the development of tolerance. Such changes in the concentration-effect relationship are evaluated by plotting the SDC for a drug against an effect measured at the time of the SDC determination. The occurrence of tolerance and sensitization is determined from the hysteresis of the curve (Fig. 1.7).

CONCLUSION

The practice of clinical pharmacokinetics requires a broad therapeutic knowledge and a careful clinical assessment of the patient, in addition to a solid foundation in the pharmacokinetic principles. Too often, it is assumed that a measured SDC stands alone as an indicator of the adequacy or inadequacy of a patient's drug therapy. However, a SDC cannot be interpreted without a clinical assessment of the patient, including the disease state being treated, the clinical condition of the patient, a complete drug dosing history, the exact time at which the SDC was collected, pertinent laboratory data, and assessment of concomitant drug therapy (Table 1.6). Collection of this information is often difficult, and the clinical pharmacist must be prepared to perform a hands-on assessment, talk to the patient, and consult with physicians, nurses, and other health care providers associated with the patient's care.

REFERENCES

1. Gibaldi M, Pemer D. Pharmacokinetics, 2nd ed. New York: Marcel Dekker, 1982, ch 1–5.

2. Sawchuk RJ, Zaske DE. Pharmacokinetics of dosing regimens which utilize multiple intravenous infusions: gentamicin in burn patients. J Pharmacokinet Biopharm 4:183–195, 1976.

3. Martin E, Tozer TN, Sheiner LB, Riegelman S. The clinical pharmacokinetics of phenytoin. J Pharmacokinet Biopharm 5:579, 1977.

4. Shargel L, Yu ABC. Nonlinear pharmacokinetics. In: Applied biopharmaceutics and pharmacokinetics, 3rd ed. Norwalk, CT: Appleton and Lange, 1993:375–398.

5. Wilkinson GR, Shand DC. A physiologic approach to hepatic drug clearance. Clin Pharmacol Ther 18:377, 1975.

6. Shand DG, Cotham RH, Wilkinson GR. Perfusion-limited effects of plasma drug binding on hepatic drug extraction. Life Sci 19:125, 1976.

7. Sheiner LB, Tozer TN. Clinical pharmacokinetics: the use of plasma concentrations of drugs. In: Melmon KL, Morrelli HF, eds. Clinical pharmacology: basic principles in therapeutics. New York: Macmillan, 1978:71–109.

8. Cockcroft D, Gault M. Prediction of creatinine clearance from serum creatinine. Nephron 16:31–34, 1976.

9. Keys PW. Digoxin. In: Evans WE, Schentag JJ, Jusko WJ, eds. Applied pharmacokinetics. Spokane, WA: Applied Therapeutics, 1980:319.

10. Reuning RH, Garaets DR. Digoxin. In: Evans WE, Sehentag JJ, Jusko WJ, eds. Applied pharmacokinetics, 2nd ed. Spokane, WA: Applied Therapeutics, 1986:570.

11. Hendeles L, Massanan M, Weinberger M. Theophylline. In: Evans WE, Schentag JJ, Jusko WJ, eds. Applied pharmacokinetics, 2nd ed. Spokane, WA: Applied Therapeutics, 1986:1105.

12. Benowitz NL, Meister W. Clinical pharmacokinetics of lignocaine. Clin Pharmacokinet 3:177–201, 1978.

13. Rowland M, Thomson PD, Guichard A, Melmon KL. Disposition of lignocaine in normal subjects. Ann N Y Acad Sci 179:383–398, 1971.

14. Pieper JA, Rodman JH. Lidocaine. In: Evans WE, Schentag JJ, Jusko WJ, eds. Applied pharmacokinetics, 2nd ed. Spokane, WA: Applied Therapeutics, 1986:639.

15. Coyle JD, Lima JJ. Procainamide. In: Evans WE, Schentag JJ, Jusko WJ, eds. Applied pharmacokinetics, 2nd ed. Spokane, WA: Applied Therapeutics, 1986:698.

16. Nielsen-Kudsk F, Amdisen A. Analysis of the pharmacokinetics of lithium in man. Eur J Clin Pharmacol 16:271–277, 1979.

17. Amdisen A, Carson SW. Lithium. In: Evans WE, Schentag JJ, Jusko WJ, eds. Applied pharmacokinetics, 2nd ed. Spokane, WA: Applied Therapeutics, 1986:978.

18. Ochs HR, Grub EE, Greenblatt DJ, Woo E, Bodem G. Intravenous quinidine: pharmacokinetic properties and effects on left ventricular performance in humans. Am Heart J 99:468–475, 1980.

19. Ueda CT. Quinidine. In: Evans WE, Schentag JJ, Jusko WJ, eds. Applied pharmacokinetics, 2nd ed. Spokane, WA: Applied Therapeutics, 1986:712.

20. Sehentag JJ. Aminoglycoside. In: Evans WE, Schentag JJ, Jusko WJ, eds. Applied pharmacokinetics. Spokane, WA: Applied Therapeutics, 1980:174.

21. Zaske D. Aminoglycosides. In: Evans WE, Schentag JJ, Jusko WJ, eds. Applied pharmacokinetics, 2nd ed. Spokane, WA: Applied Therapeutics, 1986:331.

22. Bertilsson L, Tomson T. Clinical pharmacokinetics and pharmacological effects of carbamazepine and carbamazepine-10,11-epoxide. Clin Pharmacokinet 11:177–198, 1986.

23. Levy RH, Wilensky AJ, Fnel PN. Other antiepileptic drugs. In: Evans WE, Schentag JJ, Jusko WJ, eds. Applied pharmacokinetics, 2nd ed. Spokane, WA: Applied Therapeutics, 1986:540.

24. Wilenskv AJ, Friel PN, Levy RH, Comfort CP, Kaluzny SP. Kinetics of phenobarbital in normal subjects and epileptic patients. Eur J Clin Pharmacol 23:87–92, 1982.

25. Winter ME, Tozer TN. Phenytoin. In: Evans WE, Schentag JJ, Jusko WJ, eds. Applied pharmacokinetics, 2nd ed. Spokane, WA: Applied Therapeutics, 1986:493.

26. Klotz U, Antonin KH. Pharmacokinetics and bioavailability of sodium valproate. Clin Pharmacol Ther 21:736–743, 1977.

27. Matzke GR, McGory RW, Halstenson CE, Keane WF. Pharmacokinetics of vancomycin inpatients with various degrees of renal function. Antimicrob Agents Chemother 25:433–437, 1984.

28. Matzke GR. Vancomycin. In: Evans WE, Schentag JJ, Jusko WJ, eds. Applied pharmacokinetics, 2nd ed. Spokane, WA: Applied Therapeutics, 1986:399.

29. Dobbs SM, Mawer GE, Rodgers EM, Woodcock BG, Lucas SB. Can digoxin dose requirements be predicted? Br J Clin Pharmacol 3:231237, 1976.

30. Hull JH, Sarubbi FA. Gentamicin serum concentrations: pharmacokinetic predictions. Ann Intern Med 85:183–189, 1976.

31. Sarubbi FA, Hull JH. Amikacin serum concentrations: prediction of levels and dosage guidelines. Ann Intern Med 89:612–618, 1978.

32. Como JA, Farringer JA. Vancomycin dosing recommendations. Drug Information Bull 22:5, 1988.

33. LaLonde RL. Pharmacodynamics. In: Evans WE, Jusko WJ, Schentag JJ, eds. Applied pharmacokinetics, 3rd ed. Spokane, WA: Applied Therapeutics, 1992:4-1–4-33.

CHAPTER 2

ADVERSE DRUG REACTIONS AND DRUG-INDUCED DISEASES

DONNA J. SCHROEDER and JOSEPH A. BARONE

BACKGROUND

Adverse drug reactions contribute to overall health care costs by increasing morbidity, and even mortality in severe cases. An estimated $3 billion is spent annually in the United States on ADR screening and treatment functions (1). The Joint Commission on Accreditation of Healthcare Organizations (JCAHO) and the Food and Drug Administration (FDA) place a high priority on the recognition and reporting of ADRs by health care professionals in order to improve the quality of life of patients receiving drug therapy.

To demonstrate the impact of ADRs on the cost of health care, one can use the number of hospital admissions that are drug related. Approximately 5% (range 2–20%) of reported hospitalizations are a result of an ADR (2). Many ADR admissions are acute in nature and require expensive emergency room care. Drug classes frequently involved in ADR-related admissions include drugs of abuse, anticonvulsants, antibiotics, respiratory drugs, and pain medications (3). ADRs can also occur in hospitalized patients and require an increase in length of stay and treatment with medical and pharmacologic interventions.

DRUG REACTIONS DEFINED

Confusion exists regarding the terms *adverse drug reaction, side effect,* and *drug allergy.* The World Health Organization (WHO) endorses an ADR definition that many health care practitioners have also adopted; it reads as follows: "any response to a drug which is noxious and unintended, and which occurs at doses used in man for prophylaxis, diagnosis, or treatment" (4). An ADR may therefore include any of the following: (a) an exaggerated drug response, (b) an unwanted effect on an organ system different from that being treated, (c) an allergic or hypersensitivity reaction, (d) an idiosyncratic reaction, or (e) a drug interaction that causes either an increased or diminished response (5). A side effect and a drug allergy are both types of ADRs. A side effect is an example of a dose-related, predictable reaction to a drug (6). It is typically accepted that a side effect of a drug is known to occur in a given percentage of the population and has been observed with regular frequency. A side effect is also expected based on the pharmacologic activity of the agent in question. A drug allergy is an example of a non-dose-related, unpredictable adverse effect to a drug. Some side effects that are not drug allergies are inappropriately classified as such. For example, nausea secondary to narcotic use is not immunologically mediated and should not be considered an allergy; however, an anaphylactic reaction to penicillin is an adverse reaction that should be categorized as a true allergic reaction (7). Unfortunately, reactions reported to health care professionals by patients or caregivers during the course of history taking are frequently mislabeled as an "allergy." This mislabeled diagnosis is often perpetuated throughout the patient's medical record. If not corrected, this may result in inadequate medical care in future circumstances.

In addition to applying an appropriate definition, ADRs need to be further classified in terms of severity, causality, and preventability. Most institutions and community providers follow published algorithms that assist in this task (8–10). Preventable ADRs should be a focus of any ADR reporting system in both the ambulatory care and hospital settings. By identifying trends, risk factors and circumstances that contribute to a preventable ADR, programs can be implemented to decrease the occurrence (11, 12). Refer to Table 2.1 for severity definitions and Table 2.2 for preventable definitions.

NATIONAL ADR REPORTING SYSTEMS

The FDA requirements on ADR reporting vary depending on the source of the report. Health care professionals may participate in the reporting structure on a voluntary basis. Pharmaceutical manufacturers are legally required to report all ADRs to the FDA. However, this reporting requirement is not fulfilled by the manufacturers through information submission alone, the manufacturers must also use the reported data to verify the reaction and analyze additional reports for trends (13–15).

The question of what constitutes a reportable adverse drug reaction can be answered by examining the FDA's definition of an ADR and the types of reactions the FDA is most interested in reviewing (Table 2.3). With the increasing speed of some drug approvals, the FDA has become increasingly dependent on postmarketing surveillance to monitor reactions involving new chemical entities.

Table 2.1.
Severity Definitions

Severity	Definition
Minor	• No antidote, therapy or prolongation of hospitalization required
Moderate	• A change in drug therapy, specific treatment or an increase in hospitalization by at least one day
Severe	• Potentially life-threatening, caused permanent damage or required intensive medical care
Lethal	• Directly or indirectly contributed to the death of the patient

Adapted from Anon. ASHP Guidelines on adverse drug reaction monitoring and reporting. Am J Hosp Pharm. 49:336–337, 1989.

Table 2.2.
Preventable Reactions

Elements of a Preventable Adverse Drug Reaction
• Inappropriate drug utilization based on the patient's clinical condition
• Inappropriate dose, route or frequency of administration based on patient specific variables (e.g., age, weight, underlying disease)
• Omission of appropriate laboratory monitoring
• Previous allergy or drug reaction history
• Known drug-drug interactions
• Known administration technique error (i.e., rapid vancomycin administration leading to red man syndrome)

Adapted from Schumock GT, Thornton JP. Focusing on preventability of adverse drug reactions. Clin Pharmacol Ther 30:239–245, 1992.

Table 2.3.
Reportable Adverse Drug Reactions[a]

• New and unexpected reactions,[b] particularly from new chemical entities[c,d]
• All serious reactions,[e] particularly from new chemical entities[c,d]
• Unusual increases in the frequency or severity of reactions
• Reports of therapeutic failure which may suggest bioavailability problems

[a] Modified from Baum C, Anello C: The spontaneous reporting system in the United States. In: Strom BL. Pharmaco-epidemiology. New York: Churchill Livingstone, 1989 107–118; and Johnson JM. Contributing to drug safety (editorial). Am J Hosp Pharm 47:1280, 1990.
[b] Unexpected reactions are those not found in the current product labeling.
[c] New chemical entities are products not previously marketed in the US either as single agents or in combination products.
[d] Emphasis should be placed on *newly approved* new chemical entities, i.e., those marketed for 3 years or less.
[e] Any reaction that causes hospitalization or significant or permanent disability, is life-threatening or fatal, or results in cancer, congenital anomaly, or overdose is considered serious.

Thus, any reaction to a new drug (e.g., a drug on the market 3 years or less), whether or not it is included in the product labeling and regardless of its severity, should be reported. The FDA places particular emphasis on unexpected and serious reactions. Reactions of these types should be reported for any medications, not only those which are newly approved (16, 17). The FDA also oversees ADR

reporting for biologic agents (e.g., vaccines) as well as devices, and any reactions for these agents or products should be reported as well.

MedWatch

Due to the complex nature of adverse event reporting for drugs, biologics, and devices, the FDA launched the Medwatch program (see Figure 2.1). One goal of the MedWatch program is to simplify and standardize drug product and device reporting. To this end, MedWatch uses one telephone number so that health care practitioners can report events efficiently and do not have to identify a particular department to call (e.g., devices, drugs, biologics, or vaccines). Because of the increased efficiency of the system, the FDA can now focus on serious outcomes associated with the reported ADRs more rapidly. By making it easier for practitioners to report, the number of ADRs received should increase. The four methods for submitting information to the FDA via MedWatch are as follows: (a) by using a prepaid U.S. mail reporting form (FDA 3500), (b) by dialing a WATTS 24-hour toll-free telephone number (1-800-FDA-1088), (c) by facsimile transmission to 1-800-FDA-0178 and (d) by modem transmission at 1-800-FDA-7737.

In addition to an increase in report volume, the quality of the report should also be improved. The new form has specific patient information areas that will assist the reporter in gathering pertinent information before ADR submission. Key fields have also been included on the form that will allow for more useful information to be provided by the system. Both the American Medical Association and the American Society of Health Systems Pharmacists endorse the new format.

The FDA has compiled recommendations to assist health care providers in determining what types of adverse reports to submit. Their guidelines suggest an event is serious and should be reported when it

1. resulted in death.
2. was life-threatening.
3. required prolonged hospitalization.
4. directly resulted in disability.
5. resulted in congenital anomaly.

HOSPITAL-BASED REPORTING SYSTEMS

The Joint Committee on Accreditation of Healthcare Organizations (JCAHO), an independent hospital accrediting body, has placed a great deal of emphasis on ADR reporting and analysis in recent years. In addition, the FDA has recognized that hospitals can play an important role in postmarketing surveillance (18, 19). Although adverse reaction monitoring is the joint responsibility of the medical and pharmacy staffs, it often becomes the obligation of the pharmacy department to develop, initiate, and manage the ADR reporting (20).

MEDWATCH
THE FDA MEDICAL PRODUCTS REPORTING PROGRAM

For VOLUNTARY reporting
by health professionals of adverse
events and product problems

Page ___ of ___

Form approved: OMB No. 0910-0291 Expires: 12/31/94
See OMB statement on reverse

FDA Use Only

Triage unit sequence #

A. Patient information

1. Patient identifier	2. Age at time of event: ___ or Date of birth:	3. Sex ☐ female ☐ male	4. Weight ___ lbs or ___ kgs

In confidence

B. Adverse event or product problem

1. ☐ Adverse event and/or ☐ Product problem (e.g., defects/malfunctions)

2. Outcomes attributed to adverse event
(check all that apply)
☐ death ___ (mo/day/yr)
☐ life-threatening
☐ hospitalization – initial or prolonged
☐ disability
☐ congenital anomaly
☐ required intervention to prevent permanent impairment/damage
☐ other: ___

3. Date of event (mo/day/yr)	4. Date of this report (mo/day/yr)

5. Describe event or problem

6. Relevant tests/laboratory data, including dates

7. Other relevant history, including preexisting medical conditions
(e.g., allergies, race, pregnancy, smoking and alcohol use, hepatic/renal dysfunction, etc.)

C. Suspect medication(s)

1. **Name** (give labeled strength & mfr/labeler, if known)
#1
#2

2. **Dose, frequency & route used** #1 #2	3. **Therapy dates** (if unknown, give duration) from/to (or best estimate) #1 #2

4. **Diagnosis for use** (indication)
#1
#2

6. **Lot #** (if known) #1 #2	7. **Exp. date** (if known) #1 #2

9. **NDC #** (for product problems only)
- -

5. **Event abated after use stopped or dose reduced**
#1 ☐ yes ☐ no ☐ doesn't apply
#2 ☐ yes ☐ no ☐ doesn't apply

8. **Event reappeared after reintroduction**
#1 ☐ yes ☐ no ☐ doesn't apply
#2 ☐ yes ☐ no ☐ doesn't apply

10. **Concomitant medical products** and therapy dates (exclude treatment of event)

D. Suspect medical device

1. **Brand name**

2. **Type of device**

3. **Manufacturer name & address**	4. **Operator of device** ☐ health professional ☐ lay user/patient ☐ other: ___

6. model # ___ catalog # ___ serial # ___ lot # ___ other #

5. **Expiration date** (mo/day/yr)

7. **If implanted, give date** (mo/day/yr)

8. **If explanted, give date** (mo/day/yr)

9. **Device available for evaluation?** (Do not send to FDA)
☐ yes ☐ no ☐ returned to manufacturer on ___ (mo/day/yr)

10. **Concomitant medical products** and therapy dates (exclude treatment of event)

E. Reporter (see confidentiality section on back)

1. **Name, address & phone #**

2. **Health professional?** ☐ yes ☐ no	3. **Occupation**	4. **Also reported to** ☐ manufacturer
5. **If you do NOT want your identity disclosed to the manufacturer, place an "X" in this box.** ☐		☐ user facility ☐ distributor

FDA
Mail to: **MEDWATCH**
5600 Fishers Lane
Rockville, MD 20852-9787

or **FAX** to:
1-800-FDA-0178

FDA Form 3500 (6/93) **Submission of a report does not constitute an admission that medical personnel or the product caused or contributed to the event.**

Figure 2.1

Most effective ADR programs contain four fundamental components: (a) a definition of an ADR that clearly describes reportable adverse drug reactions; (b) a concurrent method of monitoring and reporting adverse drug events; (c) a system for evaluating ADRs for severity and causality (probability); and (d) a system for using the results of the ADR program to improve patient care. Each of these components should be reviewed by the Pharmacy and Therapeutics Committee. Approval of the ADR program should be obtained prior to initiating the program, since JCAHO requires hospitals to follow written procedures in reporting ADRs.

OUTPATIENT-BASED REPORTING SYSTEMS

With the emphasis in health care switching to the ambulatory care setting, detecting ADRs in this arena will gain importance. The current postmarketing surveillance programs will continue to detect clusters of ADRs and to develop accurate ADR profiles of newly released drugs. In addition, a move toward changing the status of medications from prescription to over the counter (OTC) will require all health care professionals to increase their questioning of total medication use when obtaining patient histories. In Europe, the number of ADRs reported secondary to H_2-antagonist use declined as the drugs were switched to OTC status. However, this does not necessarily mean the true number of events actually decreased. It has been speculated that the number decreased secondary to decreased health care professional monitoring and lack of consumer reporting strategies. Prescription to OTC switches are being considered for NSAIDs, birth control pills, and acyclovir, to name a few examples. Obviously, these are not innocuous agents and the burden should be placed on the ambulatory care professional to monitor patients for ADRs associated with nonprescription medications.

ADRS IN CLINICAL TRIALS AND PHARMACOVIGILENCE

Safety profiles are an important aspect of a drug submission that must be reviewed prior to FDA approval of a new molecular entity. However, generating sufficient numbers to detect rare and serious ADRs is difficult. Even phase III trials may not enroll enough patients or be carried out over a long enough period of time to detect a rare ADR that may occur in less than 1 in 1000 patients (22–24). A good example of this dilemma is illustrated by the agent felbamate, an anticonvulsant that was FDA approved for use in 1993 in patients with partial and generalized tonic-clonic seizures. Felbamate represented one of only two new anticonvulsant therapies approved in the past 20 years. Less than 6 months after it was marketed, 27 cases of aplastic anemia were reported at incidences much higher than those reported in the clinical trials. The FDA immediately issued a warning to all health care providers urging them to reconsider felbamate therapy in their patients unless it was absolutely necessary.

In addition to the relatively small numbers of subjects in clinical trials as compared to the general population that will use the drug, clinical trials often do not include patient populations that may be at a higher risk of developing an ADR. Such populations include the elderly, women, and children. Also at risk of developing ADRs are patients with underlying metabolic dysfunction (e.g., renal or hepatic disorders). Efforts are being undertaken to increase the inclusion of these subgroups of the population in clinical trials; however, postmarketing surveillance still provides the majority of information regarding ADRs and drug safety in these patients.

VARIABLES AFFECTING ADR INCIDENCE AND SEVERITY

Certain variables predispose individuals to developing ADRs. These variables can be patient or drug focused. In terms of patient variables, age, underlying disease, and genetic factors may influence the likelihood of developing an ADR. Drug variables that also may affect the incidence of adverse reactions are the route of administration, product formulation, and the duration of therapy.

Patient Variables

ELDERLY

Since both hepatic and renal function decline with age, the elderly are subject to changes in metabolism that affect the clearance of drugs and active metabolites (25). Decreased hepatic blood flow can lead to an increased bioavailability of active metabolites and ultimately increased serum concentrations of certain drugs with high first-pass clearance characteristics. Drugs that do not undergo high hepatic clearance may be affected by decreased microsomal enzyme activity, especially of the phase I metabolism type. The result is a decreased metabolism in general, which again leads to increased serum drug levels (26, 27). The amount of albumin available for protein binding also decreases with age, which places the elderly population at a higher risk for developing ADRs when prescribed highly protein bound drugs. This can be avoided by obtaining an albumin level and reducing the dose or choosing another agent (28).

As opposed to hepatic function, the decline in renal function is more readily apparent in the elderly. A decline in glomerular filtration rates (GFR) of approximately 35% is not uncommon (29). The GFR may be decreased despite a normal serum creatinine, which can be misleading. Drugs that are excreted unchanged in the urine should be have doses adjusted and be carefully monitored to avoid excessive serum drug concentrations.

NEONATES

As reported by Knight (30), neonates experience ADRs for several reasons, which include the following: (a) placental transfer of drugs, which results in exposure in utero, (b) a lack of information on drug use in neonates, and (c) altered drug disposition, metabolism, and excretion profiles. As a further complication, many neonates are born in critical condition with multiple organ compromise. Neonates are also susceptible to developing adverse reactions to environmental agents that are not meant for therapeutic use (e.g., antiseptics containing phenol and disinfectants).

Drug metabolism and excretion are crucial components of successful drug therapy in neonates. The neonate is not born with full capacity to process exogenous substrates. For example, the hepatic microsomal enzyme system can take up to 3 days postpartum to become functional. Gray baby syndrome can develop if agents dependent on the glucuronyl transferase pathway are administered sooner than 1 to 2 weeks postpartum. A full-term newborn has approximately 33% of the glomerular filtration rate of an adult. Kidney function continues to improve rapidly, and by the time a child is 9 to 12 months of age, the kidney function is equivalent to that of an adult. Until the organ systems have a chance to develop, neonates and infants are at a higher risk of developing ADRs due to the immaturity of their organs. (See Chapter 88 "Pediatric and Neonatal Therapy.")

PATIENTS WITH HUMAN IMMUNODEFICIENCY VIRUS DISEASE (HIV)

The incidence of ADRs in patients infected with HIV appears to be higher than the incidence occurring in the general population (31–33). Severe immunosuppression,

Table 2.4.
Combined Rates of Hypersensitivity Reactions in Patients with HIV Infection

Drug	Rates of Occurrence with HIV (percent range)
Amoxicillin	17–40
Amphotericin B	4–15
Antituberculosis medications	3–20
Ciprofloxacin	5.7
Clindamycin and Pyrimethamine	21–33
Trimethoprim-Sulfamethoxazole	37–69
Fluconazole	6–13
Pentamidine	5–15
Sulfadiazine-Pyrimethamine	13–34

Adapted from Harb GE, Jacobson MA. Human Immunodeficiency Virus (HIV) infection: Does it increase susceptibility to adverse drug reactions? Drug Safety. 9:1–8, 1993.

development of drug-specific antibodies, and impaired capacity to clear drugs and unchanged metabolites results in an increased sensitivity to drug toxicity. In most cases, the drug reactions are not life-threatening, but they often lead to suboptimal changes in therapy, which may limit the number of effective treatment plans. A classic example of increased hypersensitivity in patients infected with HIV is illustrated by the use of trimethoprim/sulfamethoxazole (TMP/SMX). In a study conducted at San Francisco General Hospital, 83% (29 of 35 patients) experienced some level of toxicity to TMP/SMX as they were being treated for pneumocystis carinii pneumonia (PCP) (34). This figure is much higher than was reported in a group of hospitalized patients with no known HIV history (2–8%) (see Table 2.4) (35).

GENETICS

The rates of metabolism and elimination of various substances may be influenced by genetic factors (e.g., G-6PD deficiency resulting in drug-induced hemolytic anemia; acetylator status and drug-induced SLE) (36). It has been reported that some degree of genetic polymorphism is present in up to 50% of the enzyme systems involved in drug metabolism. Unfortunately, screening tests for genetically susceptible patients are often not easily performed and clinical decisions must be based on the available epidemiologic data.

Drug Variables
ROUTE OF ADMINISTRATION

The route of administration and drug formulation have been shown to be variables associated with the increased or decreased likelihood of developing an ADR (37). Intravenous administration may be associated with side effects local to the site of injection, such as phlebitis and extravasation, as well as with systemic adverse effects secondary to rapid increases in drug blood levels and accelerated clinical response. Oral administration, which is generally associated with relatively decreased bioavailability, may be associated with somewhat milder adverse events (38). Variability in absorption of oral agents subsequent to drug-drug or drug-food interactions can also change side effect profiles. Local adverse effects, such as irritation to gastrointestinal mucosa, may also occur following oral administration.

PRODUCT FORMULATION

Product formulations that alter the extent and the rate of absorption may also affect the incidence of ADRs. For example, sustained release products may avoid the potential for adverse effects due to excessive peaks and inadequate troughs associated with immediate release products. Sustained release nifedipine, for example, provides a steady serum concentration of drug compared with the immediate release formulation. The sustained release product results in less variation in serum drug concentrations and, therefore, a decrease in the incidence of trough periods, which provide inadequate blood pressure control, and peak periods associated with lightheadedness and other side effects. Flushing secondary to niacin has been a major contributor to noncompliance and, therefore, therapeutic failures with this agent. The sustained release product, which avoids the peak serum concentrations of the immediate release preparations, is associated with a decreased incidence of flushing and increased patient tolerance.

DURATION OF THERAPY

The duration of therapy has also been implicated in the determination of the rate of ADR occurrence. For example, in patients greater than 60 years of age, an increased duration of therapy with nonsteroidal antiinflammatory drugs (NSAIDs) was associated with an increased risk of upper gastrointestinal toxicity (39). Meperidine is known to possess an active metabolite, normeperidine, which accumulates in patients with renal dysfunction. Normeperidine accumulation may ultimately result in seizure activity. This, is most likely to occur with chronic administration, however, rather than with single dose or intermittent therapy.

DRUG INDUCED DISEASES

Disease management, collective management of all aspects of a patient's disease, rather than isolated drug treatment of a disease is rapidly becoming the accepted practice in health care. Adverse drug monitoring and management should be thought of in a similar fashion. It is impossible to consider the desired outcomes of drug therapy without taking into consideration all adverse, as well as beneficial, consequences of treatment. The remaining sections of this chapter will focus on major organ systems most commonly associated with adverse pharmacologic reactions. Throughout the remainder of this chapter, the reader may be referred to other chapters in this book that describe in detail the mechanism of specific drug-induced diseases.

Hypersensitivity Reactions

Many drug reactions are often erroneously referred to as hypersensitivity or allergic reactions (40, 41). True hypersensitivity reactions are immunologically mediated through a series of reproducible steps. The four classic hypersensitivity reactions as described by Gell and Coombs (42) are outlined in Table 2.5.

Type I hypersensitivity reactions are most frequently associated with β-lactam antibiotics, which include penicillins and cephalosporins (43). While allergic reactions to penicillin have been reported to occur in 0.7 to 8% of the general population, anaphylaxis only occurs in 0.01% of identified treatment courses. The true immunochemistry of the penicillin reaction has been characterized, and cross-sensitivity to cephalosporins has been postulated based on chemical structure similarities, typically a 4-membered β-lactam ring. Hypersensitivity reactions that are IgE mediated show clinical cross-reactivity between penicillins and cephalosporins in approximately 5% of patients (44). Imipenem (a carbapenem antibiotic) has a bicyclic nucleus and has been shown to be associated with a cross-reactivity in approximately 50% of penicillin allergic patients (45). Aztreonam, a monocyclic β-lactam antibiotic, is poorly immunogenic. β-lactam allergic patients have been given aztreonam and have not demonstrated any clinical signs of cross reactivity. Structural differences may

Table 2.5.
Classic Hypersensitivity Reactions

Type	Antibody	Mechanism	Example and Causative Agent
I	IgE	• Anaphylactic • Antigen-antibody reaction on mast cells leading to histamine, leukotriene, platelet-activating factor release	• True systemic anaphylactic reaction. • Penicillins and cephalosporins • Represents classic example of the hapten hypothesis
II	IgG IgM	• Cytotoxic • Antigen-specific antibodies directed against antigens on cell surface	• Hemolytic anemia. • Penicillin and quinine are examples of causative agents
III	IgG IgM	• Complex mediated • Immune complexes interact with antibodies	• Serum sickness • Penicillins, cephalosporins, isoniazid, phenytoin, etc
IV	T cells	• Delayed hypersensitivity • Generally takes more than 12 hours to develop • Antigen interacts directly with sensitized T cells	• Typically seen with topical therapies rather than systemic • Characterized clinically by rash which worsens on subsequent or repetitive administration

Adapted from Coombs RRA, Gell PGH. Classification of allergic reactions responsible for clinical hypersensitivity and disease. In: Coombs RRA, Gell PGH, eds. Clinical Aspects of Immunology, 2nd ed. New York: FA Davis, 1968:575–596.

Table 2.6.
Six β-Lactam Containing Groups and Representative Agents

Penicillins	Cephalosporins
• Penicillin G	• Cephalothin
• Penicillin V	• Cefazolin
• Methicillin	• Cephalexin
• Oxacillin	• Cephradine
• Cloxacillin	• Cefamandole
• Nafcillin	• Cefuroxime
• Ampicillin	• Cefixime
• Amoxicillin	• Cefonicid
• Carbenicillin	• Cefotetan
• Ticarcillin	• Cefotaxime
• Azlocillin	• Ceftixozime
• Mezlocillin	• Ceftriaxone
• Piperacillin	• Cefoperazone
	• Ceftazidime
Monobactams	*Clavams*
• Aztreonam	• Clavulanic acid
Carbapenems	
• Imipenem	

Reproduced with permission from Blanca et al. New aspects of allergic reactions to betalactams: crossreactions and unique specificities. Clin Exp Allergy 24:407–415, 1994.

therefore be a significant determinant in the incidence of hypersensitivity reactions (see Table 2.6).

Hypersensitivity reactions may manifest as acute urticaria, rhinitis, bronchial asthma, and angioedema. Depending on the severity of the reaction, there may also be peripheral circulatory collapse; therefore, immediate medical care should be sought. The offending agent should be removed. Epinephrine should be administered 0.1–0.2 mg IV over 2 to 3 minutes. This dose may be repeated every 15 to 20 minutes as needed up to 3 doses. Oxygen should be administered if available. Since the patient may be experiencing vascular collapse, fluid therapy should be initiated as needed to maintain blood pressure. If the patient is unresponsive to fluid replacement, a dopamine infusion may be necessary at a rate of 2 to 15 μg/kg/min. β-Agonists, diphenhydramine, and hydrocortisone should also be administered after the emergent situation is controlled.

Hepatotoxicity

Drug-induced hepatotoxicity has been associated with over 600 drugs. Hepatotoxicity can be difficult to diagnose because the literature consists primarily of case reports and because injury can present acutely or after prolonged drug administration (46). Table 2.7 illustrates some of the risk factors associated with developing hepatotoxic reactions.

Acute liver injury can be cytotoxic or cholestatic. Cytotoxic injury involves direct injury to the hepatocytes with necrosis that can be localized or diffuse throughout

Table 2.7.
Risk Factors Associated with Developing Hepatotoxic Reactions

Factor	Example
Age	
• Adult > Children	Isoniazid, halothane
• Elderly > others	NSAIDs
• Children > Adults	Valproic acid, aspirin
Sex	
• Female > Male	Methyldopa, Drug-induced chronic active hepatitis
Drugs	
• Alcohol	Can induce cytochrome P 450 system and enhance the toxicity of agents converted to active metabolites
• Phenobarbitol	See above
Pathological State	
• AIDS	Incresed susceptibility to hepatotoxic effects of sulfamethoxazole-trimethoprim
• Diabetes	Enhances toxicity of carbon tetrachloride
• Hyperthyroidism	Enhances toxicity of carbon tetrachloride
• Arthritis	Active rheumatoid arthritis, rheumatic fever, and SLE enhance the hepatic effects of aspirin.

Adapted from Zimmerman HJ. Hepatoxicity. Disease-a-Month 39:675–787, 1993.

Table 2.8.
Drugs Implicated in Causing Chronic Active Hepatitis

Acetaminophen	Isoniazid	Papaverine
Dantrolene	Nitrofurantoin	Propylthiouracil
Diclofenac	Methyldopa	Sulfonamides

Adapted from Zimmerman HJ. Hepatoxicity. Disease-a-Month 39:675–787, 1993.

the liver. Aminotransferase levels can be elevated to up to 500 times the normal levels. Prominent signs and symptoms include fatigue, anorexia, nausea, and jaundice. Drug-induced cytotoxic injury can progress to fulminant hepatic failure. Isoniazid, methyldopa, and phenytoin have been associated with direct cytotoxic reactions that have led to mortality rates of 10% or higher (47).

Cholestatic injury results in a characteristic decrease in bile flow. Hepatic injury of this type leads to jaundice and pruritus, and aminotransferase levels are only moderately elevated. Cholestatic hepatic injury has a much better prognosis as compared to cytotoxic injury with a mortality rate of less than 1%.

Chronic liver damage consists of a group of disorders including chronic hepatitis, steatosis, pseudo-alcoholic liver disease, granulomatous disease, and cirrhosis. Chronic lesions can result from continued or repeated exposure to hepatotoxic agents. Table 2.8 lists a number of drugs that have been implicated in causing chronic active hepatitis.

Most cases of drug-induced hepatotoxicity involve the transformation of the parent drug to an active intermediate that may be inherently toxic or evoke an immune response. Some drugs implicated in hepatic injury include

Table 2.9.
Drug-Induced Pancreatitis

Criteria for Drug-Induced Pancreatitis
- Pancreatitis developed during treatment with the drug
- Pancreatitis disappeared upon withdrawal of the drug
- Pancreatitis recurred upon rechallenge

Elements of Classification (based on above criteria)

Definite: Literature report met all three criteria
Probable: Literature reports did not meet all three criteria but an association with thought to exist
Doubtful: Published evidence was either inadequate or contradictory

Adapted from Underwood TW, Frye CB. Drug-induced pancreatitis. Clin Pharm 12:400–448, 1993.

Table 2.10.
Examples of Drugs Suspected in Drug-Induced Pancreatitis

Drug	Comments
Asparginase	• Frequently reported to cause pancreatitis • Possible direct cytotoxic effect
Azathioprine	• Mechanism of injury unknown but thought to be related to the immunosuppressive effect of azathioprine
Didanosine	• Pancreatitis detected as high as 9% in the Phase I trials • Dosages higher than 10 mg/kg/day are more likely to cause pancreatitis
Estrogens	• Estrogen use is known to cause hyperlipidemia, a risk factor for pancreatitis development
Furosemide	• Suggested direct toxic effect • A similar outcome was observed upon bumetanide administration
Mercaptopurine	• Mechanism may be Type II or Type IV hypersensitivity reaction
Pentamidine	• Mechanism may be direct toxic effect • Also often administered after exposure to sulfonamides (see below)
Sulfonamides	• Pancreatitis accompanied by fever, chills, pruritus and rash • Possible allergic reaction
Sulindac	• Most reports received through the voluntary ADR reporting system
Tetracyclines	• Occurred primarily in patients with preexisting liver disease
Thiazides	• Among the first class of drugs to be associated with pancreatitis • Possible direct toxic effect
Valproic Acid	• Can occur within normal dosages of the drug • Has occurred in children • Possible direct toxic effect

Adapted from Underwood TW, Frye CB. Drug-induced pancreatitis. Clin Pharm 12:440–448, 1993. Mallary A, Kern F. Drug-induced pancreatitis: a critical review. Gastroenterology 78:813–820, 1980.

anesthetic agents (e.g., halothane), chlorpromazine, anticonvulsants (e.g., phenytoin and valproic acid), NSAIDs, and allopurinol. Herbal products and teas have also been implicated in several cases of severe hepatotoxicity (48). The specific hepatotoxicity profiles associated with each of these agents are beyond the scope of this chapter. Health care practitioners should be aware that a plethora of agents can cause hepatotoxicity and that careful history taking is crucial in a patient who presents with nonspecific symptoms.

Pancreatitis

Pancreatitis can also be characterized as being either acute or chronic. A recent literature review by Underwood and Frye (49) revealed that a large number of medications can cause acute pancreatitis, while relatively few cause chronic pancreatitis. Clinical symptoms of pancreatitis include acute abdominal pain and increased blood and urine pancreatic enzyme concentrations. Morphologic changes in the pancreas itself are minor or absent. Based on a system originally developed by Mallory and Kern (50), implicated drugs can be classified into one of three categories (see Table 2.9. Table 2.10 illustrates the results of the literature review with a focus on the agents that have a definite association with pancreatitis.

Nephrotoxicity

Drug-induced nephrotoxicity depends on the concentration of drug presented to the kidney and the biochemical or physiologic effect of the drug on the affected tissue (51). Factors that influence the concentration of given drugs in the kidney include mechanisms for the transport of drugs across the tubular epithelium, the rate of water versus drug reabsorption, plasma protein binding, and rate of urine flow. Some of the most common drugs associated with nephrotoxicity include the aminoglycosides, amphotericin B, cisplatin, cephalosporins, cyclosporin A, and NSAIDs (52–55).

Four types of lesions are used to describe drug-induced kidney damage: (a) acute tubular necrosis (ATN), (b) acute tubulointerstitial disease (ATID), (c) chronic tubulointerstitial disease (CTID), and (d) glomerulonephritis (GN). A list of drugs and chemicals associated with each of these lesions is provided in Table 2.11. A complete discussion of drug-induced nephrotoxicity can be found in Chapters 2 and 21.

From an ADR reporting system standpoint, drug-induced nephrotoxicity should be closely monitored, since the majority of these types of ADRs are preventable. For example, underlying renal dysfunction necessitates a dose adjustment of many drugs. Compromise to the nephron can be avoided by carefully monitoring drug levels and altering drug doses accordingly.

Table 2.11.
Drugs Associated with Nephrotoxicity

Acute tubular necrosis	Phenylbutazone
Antibiotics	Tolmetin
Aminoglycosides	Metals
Amphotericin B	Bismuth
Bacitracin	Gold
Cephalosporins	Miscellaneous
Polymixins	Allopurinol
Sulfonamides	Azathioprine
Metals	Captopril
Antimony	Cimetidine
Bismuth	Clofibrate
Mercurials	Furosemide
Platinum	Phenytoin
Chelates	Thiazides
Dimercaprol	Glomerulonephritis
EDTA	Allopurinol
Contrast media	Ampicillin
Miscellaneous agents	Captopril
Acetaminophen	Cocaine
Aminocaproic acid	Cyclophosphamide
Carbamazepine	Daunorubicin
Cisplastin	Fenoprofen
Cyclosporine	Gold
Methotrexate	Heroin
Methoxyflurane	Hydralazine
Phenazopyridine	Methicillin
Streptozocin	Penicillamine
Acute tubulointerstital disease	Penicillin
Penicillins	Rifampin
Amoxicillin	Sodium diatrizoate
Ampicillin	Sulfonamides
Carbenicillin	Thiazides
Methicillin	Trimethadione
Nafcillin	Chronic tubulointerstitial disease
Oxacillin	Acetaminophen
Penicillin	Aspirin
Other antibiotics	Lithium
Cephalosporins	Methyl-CCNU
Cotrimoxazole	Phenacetin
Erythromycin	Miscellaneous mechanisms
p-aminosalicylate	Prerenal azotemia
Polymixins	NSAIDs
Rifampin	Renal tubular acidosis and concentration defects
Sulfonamides	Lithium
NSAIDs	Amphotericin B
Fenoprofen	Postrenal obstruction
Ibuprofen	Methysergide
Indomethacin	
Mefanamic acid	

Hematologic Disorders

Drug-induced hematologic disorders encompass a wide variety of disorders, only some of which are mechanistically understood. The reader is referred to the chapters in this book describing anemias, where aplastic anemia, agranulocytosis, hemolytic anemia, megoblastic anemia, and thrombocytopenia are discussed. All of these hematologic disorders have been associated with drug-induced etiologies.

Cardiovascular Effects

The scope of this topic is much larger than can be covered in a chapter focusing on ADRs. The reader is referred to the chapters in this textbook that discuss cardiovascular disorders and critical care issues. Some aspects of adverse reactions associated with cardiovascular drug therapy, however, require specific attention.

Adverse drug reactions involving the cardiovascular system are not specifically limited to those agents used to treat cardiovascular disease. For example, bronchodilator therapy and sympathomimetic effects of various cough and cold remedies often negatively affect cardiac rate and rhythm regulation. Many antiarrhythmic agents may also be proarrhythmic (56, 57). Tricyclic antidepressants in an overdose situation cause ECG changes that can be life-threatening (58). In addition to certain cardiac medications, bradycardia can also be induced by agents such as carbamazepine, methyldopa, and H_2 antagonists (59–61). Some agents used in chemotherapy regimens, such as the anthracyclines, have a dose limiting side effect of causing congestive cardiomyopathy (62). Additionally, some diuretics and β-blockers may adversely affect lipid risk profiles, the clinical outcome of which remains to be elucidated (63). Careful monitoring of patients for cardiovascular ADRs is crucial, since the potential for negative sequelae is enormous.

Pulmonary Effects

Pulmonary injury secondary to pharmacologic treatment has been shown to occur with the administration of over 150 medications (64–66). Table 2.12 lists agents known to cause pulmonary disease. Four mechanisms for drug induced pulmonary disease have been described: (a) direct cytotoxic effect on alveolar endothelial cells, (b) deposition of phospholipid with the alveolar macrophages, (c) oxidized injury by drugs, and (d) immune-mediated injury (e.g., drug-induced systemic lupus erythematosus) (67).

Bronchospasm can occur commonly as a drug-induced effect. Angiotensin converting enzyme (ACE) inhibitors cause cough in approximately 15% of the population with a 2:1 ratio of women to men. This ADR has been identified with all of the β-blockers and is reversible within 1 to 7 days of discontinuation. Symptoms include a dry, unproductive cough. Aspirin administration can also lead to bronchospasm in approximately 4 to 20% of all patients with asthma (68). The pathogenesis is thought to be related to cyclooxygenase inhibition and subsequent destabilization of mast cells and bronchial smooth muscle constriction (69). All NSAIDs, which inhibit cyclooxygenase, can produce reactions, and the degree of cross-reactivity is related to the degree of cyclooxygenase inhibition. β-Blockade can precipitate asthmatic attacks, even when a cardioselective agent such as atenolol or metoprolol

Table 2.12.
Agents Known to Cause Pulmonary Disease

Cardiovascular	Antiinflammatory	Chemotherapeutic Agents
• Amiodarone	• Aspirin	• Azathioprine
• ACE inhibitors	• Gold	• Bleomycin
• Anticoagulants	• Methotrexate	• Busulfan
• β-Blockers	• NSAIDs	• Chlorambucil
• Dipyridamole	Penicillamine	• Cyclophosphamide
• Tocainide	Miscellaneous	• Etoposide
Antibiotics	• Bromocriptine	• Melphalan
• Amphotericin B	• Dantrolene	• Mitomycin
• Nitrofuantoin	• Oral Contraceptives	• Nitrosoureas
• Sulfasalazine	• Hydrochlorthiazide	• Procarbazine
• Sulfonamides	• Tricyclic Antidepressants	• Vinvlastine
• Pentamidine		• Ifosfamide

Adapted from Rosenow ECIII. Drug-induced pulmonary disease. Disease-a-Month. 5:258–310, 1994.

is used (70). Aggravation of chronic obstructive pulmonary disease with subsequent death has been reported secondary to topical timolol, since the drug can be systemically absorbed (71).

Noncardiogenic pulmonary edema can develop secondary to narcotic use, as cases have been reported with heroin, methadone, and propoxyphene administration (72). The mechanism of this reaction is unclear but could be related to a hypoxemic state. Other possible mechanisms include a direct toxic effect on the alveolar-capillary membrane, CNS effects resulting in a neurogenic pulmonary edema, and immunologic activation. The pulmonary edema generally improves within 24 to 48 hours and radiologic clearing results after approximately 2 to 4 days.

Sexual Dysfunction

Normal sexual function is mediated by various physiologic mechanisms including neurogenic, psychogenic, vascular, and hormonal factors (73). These functions are coordinated by the hypothalamus, limbic system, and cerebral cortex. It is expected, then, that medications that interfere with any of these systems may also interfere with sexual function.

Sexual dysfunction is often associated with antihypertensive and antipsychotic medications. Antihypertensive agents are reported to be associated with sexual dysfunction more than any other type of drug. However, the majority of associations between antihypertensive therapy and sexual dysfunction are from case reports (74). Thiazide diuretics, peripheral and central sympatholytics, and β-blockers have all been associated with a decline in sexual function. The adverse events range from loss of libido to impotence, ejaculatory failure, and anorgas-

mia, with impotence being the most frequently reported. Calcium channel blockers and ACE inhibitors appear to have a relatively decreased potential for causing sexual dysfunction (75). Combination therapy appears to be associated with a higher incidence of sexual dysfunction than monotherapy.

Antipsychotic or antidepressant medications are also associated with a variety of effects on sexual function (e.g., impotence, priapism, anorgasmia, and diminished libido); however, ejaculatory failure is the most frequently reported (76). These agents may impair sexual function due to anticholinergic and sympatholytic activity, through effects on neurotransmitters or hormonal secretion (e.g., increased serum prolactin concentrations secondary to amoxapine), or by causing sedation.

It is important to realize that the disease states for which these medications are prescribed may independently be associated with an alteration in normal sexual function. For example, sexual dysfunction has been shown to occur frequently (up to 17%) in untreated hypertensive men (77). Hypertensive diabetics have an even higher incidence of impotence (25–60%) (78). In regard to the psychiatric population, impotence in untreated patients can be as high as 70% and varies with the particular diagnosis. The high incidence of sexual dysfunction associated with these disease states is an important consideration when evaluating the relationship of drug administration to an alteration in sexual function, and baseline data on sexual function prior to the institution of therapy may be helpful in differentiating disease versus drug effects.

Additional medications that have been associated with sexual dysfunction, although less frequently than the aforementioned agents, are the H_2 antagonists (e.g., cimetidine and ranitidine), metoclopramide, anticonvulsants (e.g., carbamazepine, phenytoin, phenobarbital, and primidone), and opioids when used chronically.

CONCLUSION

Adverse drug reactions are an important cause of morbidity and mortality. Drug-induced disease is common in certain patient populations such as the elderly, the newborn, HIV infected patients, and patients with impaired organ of elimination function. Many adverse drug reactions are both reversible and preventable. Because they are reversible, early identification and treatment are of extreme importance. The preventable nature of adverse reactions is the motivation for current reporting programs. It is through reporting that high-risk patient populations are identified so that certain medications can be avoided. The monitoring program currently in place relies on voluntary reporting from health care professionals and mandatory reporting from pharmaceutical manufacturers. System innovations such as the MedWatch program should increase the efficiency of adverse event reporting and improve outcomes of drug therapy.

REFERENCES

1. Rieder MJ. Immunopharmacology and adverse drug reactions. J Clin Pharmacol 33:316–323, 1993.
2. Einarson TR. Drug-related hospital admissions. Ann Pharmacother 27:832–840, 1993.
3. Prince BS, Goetz CM, Rihn TL, Olsky M. Drug-related emergency department visits and hospital admissions. Am J Hosp Pharm 49:1696–1700, 1992.
4. Karch FE, Lasagna L. Adverse drug reactions: a critical review. JAMA 234:1236–1241, 1975.
5. Fincham JE. An overview of adverse drug reactions. Am Pharm NS31:47–52, 1991.
6. Berkow R, Fletcher AJ, et al, eds. The Merck Manual of Diagnosis and Therapy, 16th ed. Rahway, NJ: Merck Research Laboratories, 1992:2642–2644.
7. Anderson JA. Allergic reactions to drugs and biological agents. JAMA 268:2845–2857, 1992.
8. Anon. ASHP guidelines on adverse drug reaction monitoring and reporting. Am J Hosp Pharm 46:336–337, 1989.
9. Naranjo CA, Busto U, Sellers EM, et al. A method for estimating the probability of adverse drug reactions. Clin Pharmacol Ther 30:239–245, 1981.
10. Pearson TF, Pittman DG, Longley JM, Grapes ZT, Vigliotti DJ, Mullis SR. Factors associated with preventable adverse drug reactions. Am J Hosp Pharm 51:2268–2272, 1994.
11. Burnum JF. Preventability of adverse drug reactions [Letter]. Ann Intern Med 85:80, 1976.
12. Melmon KL. Preventable drug reactions-causes and cures. N Engl J Med 284:1361–1368, 1971.
13. Faich GA. National adverse drug reaction reporting: 1984–1989. Arch Intern Med 151:1645–1647, 1991.
14. Rossi AC, Knapp DE. Discovery of new adverse drug reactions: a review of the Food and Drug Administration's spontaneous reporting system. JAMA 252:1030–1033, 1986.
15. McQueen K. ADR monitoring: rationale, impact and cost issues. Calif J Hosp Pharm 2:5–7, 1990.
16. Edlavitch SA. Adverse drug event reporting. Improving the low US reporting rates [Editorial]. Arch Intern Med 148:1499–1503, 1988.
17. Baum C, Anello C. The spontaneous reporting system in the United States. In: Strom BL, ed. Pharmacoepidemiology. New York: Churchill Livingstone, 1989:107–118.
18. Johnson JM. Contributing to drug safety [Editorial]. Am J Hosp Pharm 47:1280, 1990.
19. Hoffman RP. Adverse drug reactions revisited-JCAHO. Hosp Pharm 23:685–686, 1988.
20. Middleton RK. Adverse drug reactions and drug-induced diseases. In: Herfindal ET, Gourley DR, Hart LL, eds. Clinical pharmacy and therapeutics, 5th ed. Baltimore: Williams & Wilkins, 1992.
21. Wallander MA. The way towards adverse event monitoring in clinical trials. Drug Safety 8:251–262, 1993.
22. Stang PE, Fox JL. Adverse drug events and the Freedom of Information act: an apple in Eden. Ann Pharmacother 26:238–243, 1992.
23. Edwards IR, Biriell C. Harmonisation in pharmacovigilance. Drug Safety 10:93–102, 1994.
24. Auriche M, Loupi E. Does proof of causality ever exist in pharmacovigilance? Drug Safety 9:230–235, 1993.
25. French EH. ADRs and metabolic changes in the elderly. U S Pharmacist 5:H1–H28, 1994.
26. Koch-Weser J, Greemblatt DJ, Sellers EM, Shader RI. Drug disposition in old age. N Engl J Med 306:1081–1088, 1982.
27. Brawn LA, Castelden CM. Adverse drug reactions: an overview of special considerations in the management of the elderly patient. Drug Safety 5:421–435, 1990.
28. Antal EJ, Kramer PA, Merick SA, Chapron DJ, Lawson IR. Theophylline pharmacokinetics in advanced age. Br J Clin Pharmacol 12:637–645, 1981.
29. Rowe JW, Andres R, Tobin JP, Norris AH, Shock NW. The effects of age on creatinine clearance in man: a cross sectional and longitudinal study. J Gerontol 31:155–163, 1976.
30. Knight M. Adverse drug reactions in neonates. J Clin Pharmacol 34:128–135, 1994.
31. Bayard PJ, Berger TG, Jacobson MA. Drug hypersensitivity reactions and human immunodeficiency virus disease. J Acquir Immune Defic Syndr 5:1237–57, 1992.
32. Peters BS, Carlin E, Weston RJ, Loveless SJ, Sweeney J, Weber J, et al. Adverse effects of drugs used in the management of opportunistic infections associated with HIV infection. Drug Safety 10:439–454, 1994.
33. Harb GE, Jacobson M. Human inmmunodeficiency virus (HIV) infection: does it increase susceptibility to adverse drug reactions? Drug Safety 9:1–8, 1993.
34. Gordin FM, Simon GL, Wofsy CB, Mills J. Adverse reactions to trimethoprim-sulfamethoxazole in patients with the acquired immunodeficiency syndrome. Ann Intern Med 100, 495–499, 1984.
35. Jick J. Adverse reactions to trimethoprim-sulfamethoxazole in hospitalized patients. Rev Infect Dis 4:426–428, 1982.
36. Goedde HW. Ethnic differences in reactions to drugs and other xenobiotics: outlooks of a geneticist. In: Kalow W, Goedde HW, Agerwal DP, eds. Ethnic differences in reactions to drugs and xenobiotics. New York: Alan R. Liss, 1986.
37. Florence AT, Jani PU. Novel oral drug formulations. Their potential in modulation adverse effects. Drug Safety 10:233–266, 1994.
38. Benet LZ, Mitchell JR, Sheiner LB. Pharmacokinetics: the dynamics of drug absorption, distribution, and elimination. In: Gilman AG, Rall TW, Nies AS, Taylor P, eds. Goodman and Gilman's the pharmacologic basis of therapeutics. Elmsford: Pergamon Press, 1990.
39. Carson JL, Willett LR. Toxicity of nonsteroidal anti-inflammatory drugs: an overview of the epidemiological evidence. Drugs 46(suppl 1):243–248, 1993.
40. Preston SL, Briceland LL, Lesar TS. Accuracy of penicillin allergy reporting. Am J Hosp Pharm 51:79–84, 1994.
41. Lin RY. A perspecitve on penicillin allergy. Arch Intern Med 152:930–937, 1992.
42. Coombs RRA, Gell PGH. Classification of allergic reactions responsible for clinical hypersensitivity and disease. In: Coombs RRA, Gell PGH, eds. Clinical aspects of immunology, 2nd ed. New York: FA Davis, 1968:575–596.
43. Kishiyama JL, Adelman DC. The cross-reactivity and immunology of β-lactam antibiotics. Drug Safety 10:318–327, 1994.
44. Thompson JW, Jacobs RF. Adverse effects of newer cephalosporins. Drug Safety 9:132–142, 1993.
45. Saxon A, Adelman DA, Patel A, Hadju R, Calandra GB, et al. Imipenem cross-reactivity with penicillin in humans. J Allergy Clin Immunol 82:213–217, 1988.
46. Dossing M, Sonne J. Drug-induced hepatic disorders. Drug Safety 9:441–449, 1993.
47. Zimmerman HJ. Hepatotoxicity. Disease-a-Month 39:675–787, 1993.
48. Larrey D, Vial T, Pauwells A, Castot A, Biour M, et al. Hepatitis after germander (teucrium chamaedrys) administration: another instance of herbal medicine hepatotoxicity. Ann Intern Med 117:129–132, 1992.
49. Underwood TW, Frye CB. Drug-induced pancreatitis. Clin Pharm 12:440–448, 1993.

50. Mallory A, Kern F. Drug-induced pancreatitis: a critical review. Gastroenterology 78:813–820, 1980.

51. Walker RJ, Duggin GG. Drug nephrotoxicity. Annu Rev Pharmacol Toxicol 28:331–345, 1988.

52. Schlondorff D. Renal complications of nonsteroidal antiinflammatory drugs. Kidney Int 44:643–653, 1993.

53. Clive DM, Stoff JS. Renal syndromes associated with nonsteroidal antiinflammatory drugs. N Engl J Med 310:563–572, 1984.

54. Whelton A, Hamilton CW. Nonsteroidal anti-inflammatory drugs: effects on kidney function. J Clin Pharmacol 31:588–598, 1991.

55. Humes HD. Aminoglycoside nephrotoxicity. Kidney Int 33:900–911, 1988.

56. CAST (Cardiac Arrhythmia Suppression Trial Investigators). Increased morbidity due to encainide or flecaninide in a randomized trial of arrhythmia suppression after myocardial infarction. N Engl J Med 321:406, 1989.

57. Roden DM. Risks and benefits of antiarrhythmic therapy. N Engl J Med 331:785–791, 1994.

58. Pellinen TJ, Farkkilae M, Keikrila J, Luumanmaki K. Electorcardiographic and clinical factors of tricyclic antidepressant intoxication. Ann Clin Res 19:12, 1987.

59. Bernassi E, Bo G, Cocito L, Maffini M, Loeb C. Carbamazepine and cardiac conduction disturbances. Ann Neurol 22:280, 1987.

60. Rosen B, Ovsyshcher IA, Zimlichman R. Complete atrioventriucular block induced by methyldopa. PACE 11:1555, 1988.

61. Hart A. Cardiac arrest associated with ranitidine. Br Med J 299:519, 1989.

62. Rhoden W, Hasleton P, Brooks N. Anthracyclines and the heart. Br Heart J 1993;70:499–502.

63. Henkin Y, Como J, Oberman A. Secondary dyslipidemia. Inadvertent effects of drugs in clinical practice. JAMA 267:961–968, 1992.

64. Rosenow EC III, Myers JL, Swensen SJ. Drug-induced pulmonary disease: an update. Chest 102:239–250, 1992.

65. Gregory SA, Grippi MA. The clinical diagnosis of drug-induced pulmonary disorders. J Thorac Imaging 6:8–18,1991.

66. Goodwin DS, Glenny RW. Nonsteroidal anti-inflammatory drug-associated pulmonary infiltrates with eosinophilia. Arch Intern Med 152:1521–1524, 1992.

67. Rosenow EC III. Drug-induced pulmonary disease. Disease-a-Month 5:258–310, 1994.

68. Settipane GA. Aspirin and allergic diseases: a review. Am J Med 74(suppl 6a):102–109, 1983.

69. Szczeklik A, Gryglewski RJ. Asthma and antiinflammatory drugs: mechanisms and clincial patterns. Drugs 25:533–543, 1983.

70. Kelly HW. Drug-induced pulmonary diseases. In: DiPiro JT, Talbert RL, Hayes PE, Yee GC, Matzke GR, Posey LM, eds. Pharmacotherapy: a pathophysiologic approach. Norwalk, CT: Appleton & Lange, 1993.

71. Dunn TL, Gerber MJ, Shen AS, Fernandez E, Iseman MD, Cherniack RM. The effect of topical ophthalmic instillation of timolol and betaxolol on lung function in asthmatic subjects. Am Rev Resp Dis 133:264–268, 1986.

72. Cooper JAD, White DA, Matthay RA. Drug-induced pulmonary disease. Part 2: noncytotoxic drugs. Am Rev Respir Dis 133:488–505, 1986.

73. Smith PJ, Talbert RL. Sexual dysfunction with antihypertensive and antipsychotic agents. Clin Pharm 5:373–384, 1986.

74. Prisant LM, Carr AA, Bottini PB, Solursh DS, Solursh LP. Sexual dysfunction with antihypertensive drugs. Arch Intern Med 154:730–736, 1994.

75. Abramowicz M, ed. Drugs that cause sexual dysfunction: an update. In: The Medical Letter on Drugs and Therapeutics 34:73–77, 1992.

76. Deamer RL, Thompson JF. The role of medications in geriatric sexual function. Clin Geriatr Med 7:95–110, 1991.

77. Bulpitt CJ, Dollery CT, Carne S. Change in symptoms of hypertensive patients after referral to hospital clinic. Br Heart J 38:121–128, 1976.

78. Buvat J, Lamaire A, Buvat-Herbaut M, et al. Comparative investigations in 26 impotent and 26 non-impotent diabetic patients. J Urol 133:34–38, 1985.

CHAPTER 3

DRUG INTERACTIONS

DAVID S. TATRO

A drug interaction can be defined as the modification of the effects of one drug (i.e., the object drug) by the prior or concomitant administration of another (i.e., the precipitant drug) (1). Adverse drug interactions can cause a loss in therapeutic effect, toxicity, or unexpected increases in pharmacologic activity. The basic definition of a drug interaction should focus on patient outcomes that are of potential clinical importance and not on additive or beneficial effects occurring with simultaneous drug administration. Thus, one should be seeking a response that is greater than the sum of the independent actions of the drugs (e.g., potentiation) or an action that is less than expected (e.g., antagonism).

This chapter does not consider physical or chemical interactions (e.g., intravenous incompatibilities) or beneficial interactions (e.g., clinically useful or intended interactions such as coadministration of probenecid and penicillin).

In a study involving 9,900 patients with 83,200 drug exposures, 234 (6.5%) of 3,600 adverse drug reactions were attributed to drug interactions (2). The incidence of potential drug interactions has been observed to be 17% in surgical patients, 22% in patients on medical wards, 19% in nursing home patients, and 23% in outpatient clinics (3–6). In a prospective study involving 2,422 patients, 113 patients were taking potentially interacting drugs; however, only 7 patients developed clinical evidence of a drug interaction (0.3% of the total number of patients) (7). This does not preclude the more frequent occurrence of certain clinically significant drug interactions (8).

Knowledge of drug interactions may allow early recognition and prevention of adverse consequences. The most comprehensive understanding of clinically important drug interactions can be achieved by combining knowledge of the mechanism(s) with the recognition of high-risk patients and the identification of drugs with a narrow therapeutic index (9).

MECHANISMS OF DRUG INTERACTIONS

Understanding the pharmacology of a drug and the mechanism by which a drug may interact can assist in predicting or allowing early recognition of a drug interaction. In a drug interaction, the drug for which the effect is altered (either increased or decreased) is referred to as the object drug, while the drug that induces the interaction is the precipitant drug.

Drug interactions are frequently characterized as being either pharmacokinetic or pharmacodynamic. Pharmacokinetic interactions influence the disposition of a drug in the body and involve the effects of one drug on the absorption, distribution, metabolism, and excretion of another. Due to large inter- and intrapatient variability in drug disposition, pharmacokinetic interactions seldom produce serious clinical consequences. Pharmacokinetic interactions are frequently associated with changes in plasma drug concentrations, and when feasible, observing the clinical status of the patient as well as monitoring serum drug levels may provide useful information about potential interactions. Pharmacodynamic interactions are related to the pharmacologic activity of the interacting drugs. This category is the most frequent mechanism by which drugs interact. Mechanisms of pharmacodynamic interactions include synergism, antagonism, altered cellular transport, and effects on receptor sites.

Pharmacokinetic Interactions

Pharmacokinetic interactions are characterized by changes in the kinetics of the object drug, including absorption, distribution, metabolism, and excretion.

ALTERED GASTROINTESTINAL (GI) ABSORPTION

Changes in drug absorption from the GI tract can result from various mechanisms, including altered pH, altered bacterial flora, formation of drug chelates or complexes, drug-induced mucosal damage, and altered gastrointestinal motility. These changes may produce either a decrease or increase in drug absorption. The former is more common. Frequently interactions affecting absorption require the simultaneous presence of both drugs in the stomach; therefore, separating the administration times of the two agents by at least 2 hours will often prevent these interactions. Drug interactions affecting the absorption rate of a drug are most clinically significant when the drug has a short half-life or if a rapid peak plasma level is needed to achieve a therapeutic effect (9). In the latter instance, a decrease in the rate of absorption of the object drug may produce subtherapeutic concentrations. Unless the bioavailability of a drug is significantly altered, interactions changing the absorption rate of a drug with a long half-life will usually be of little clinical consequence. Cancer patients receiving chemotherapy may experience drug-induced mucosal damage, decreasing the bioavailability of poorly absorbed medications (9).

Altered pH. The nonionized form of a drug is more lipid soluble and more readily absorbed from the gastrointestinal tract into the systemic circulation than the ionized form. Most drugs are weak acids or bases. Therefore, acidic drugs that have dissolved tend to be absorbed in the upper portion of the GI tract, where they are in an acidic medium. The opposite is true of weak bases. Drugs, such as antacids, that increase the gastric pH may delay the absorption of certain drugs (e.g., ciprofloxacin).

Clinical Consideration. Clinically significant interactions occurring by this mechanism are rare. This interaction may be avoided by adjusting the administration times of the two agents. Separating the administration times of each agent by at least 2 hours will often prevent these interactions.

Clinically Important Examples. The administration of an aluminum-magnesium hydroxide antacid with ciprofloxacin may decrease the absorption of the antibiotic, resulting in a decrease in the pharmacologic effect (10–12). If antacids are administered during ciprofloxacin therapy, the antacid should be given at least 6 hours before or 2 hours after the antibiotic dose (12). In addition to antacids, H_2-antagonists may significantly alter gastric pH.

Altered Intestinal Bacterial Flora. Antibiotic administration may decrease the number of bacteria in the GI tract. The greatest numbers of bacteria are found in the large intestine. Some drugs have been shown to be affected by changes in the intestinal flora (13).

Clinical Considerations. This mechanism of interaction appears to be rare. Drug interactions resulting from changes in the intestinal bacterial flora tend to involve drugs that are either incompletely absorbed from the upper GI tract or undergo enterohepatic recirculation (13). The onset and reversal of this interaction are delayed, requiring up to several weeks. Thus, adjusting the administration times of the two drugs would not alter interactions occurring by this mechanism.

Clinically Important Example. In approximately 10% of the patients receiving digoxin, 40% or more of an orally administered dose of the drug is metabolized by gastrointestinal flora to inactive digoxin reduction products (10, 14, 15). Erythromycin appears to reverse this process by altering GI bacteria, allowing more digoxin to be absorbed. Digoxin toxicity may occur (15). The effects of this interaction may persist for weeks to months after erythromycin is discontinued.

Complexation or Chelation. Certain drugs (e.g., tetracycline) can combine with other drugs (e.g., iron preparations) or food (e.g., milk) in the GI tract to form poorly absorbed complexes.

Clinical Considerations. Although different mechanisms may cause changes in the absorption of the object drug from the GI tract, clinically significant interactions are uncommon. Administration of the object drug in the absence of the precipitant will minimize the occurrence of this interaction. Therefore, it may be necessary to lengthen the interval between administration of the two drugs by as much as possible, preferably by 2 to 4 hours.

Clinically Important Examples. Magnesium and aluminum cations in the buffers in didanosine tablets decrease GI absorption of ciprofloxacin by forming a chelate with the antibiotic (16). Tetracycline forms an insoluble chelate with iron salts, decreasing absorption and serum levels of both drugs (10). The antiinfective response may be decreased. A similar mechanism has been proposed for the decreased absorption of ciprofloxacin and norfloxacin occurring during coadministration of sucralfate (17–19). The binding resin cholestyramine decreases the absorption of exogenously administered thyroid by binding thyroid hormone in the GI tract (19). Other agents that can interfere with drug absorption by binding to the object drug or by forming complexes or chelates with the object drug include activated charcoal, antacids, colestipol, and various polyvalent cations (e.g., iron salts).

Drug-Induced Mucosal Damage. Drugs that damage the GI mucosa may reduce the absorption of certain drugs (9, 20).

Clinical Considerations. Antineoplastic agents are most frequently implicated. This mechanism remains to be confirmed.

Clinically Important Example. Reduced GI absorption of certain digoxin preparations has been attributed to alterations in the intestinal mucosa induced by chemotherapy regimens (e.g., cyclophosphamide, vincristine, procarbazine, and prednisone) (21, 22). The effects of this interaction appear to be minimized by administration of digoxin capsules or digitoxin (22, 23).

Altered Motility. Increased absorption can occur when the drug is retained at the site of optimal absorption for a prolonged period of time. Due to the large absorptive area of the small intestine, it is the primary site of drug absorption from the gastrointestinal tract. Changes in GI motility may increase or decrease absorption. Increasing GI motility may decrease absorption by reducing the amount of time that an orally administered drug is in contact with the absorbing surface (20). A decrease in bioavailability may be seen as a result of slowing dissolution or delaying gastric emptying.

Clinical Considerations. Clinically significant interactions due to this mechanism are rare. Interactions occurring as a result of altered GI motility result from systemic administration of the precipitant drug. Therefore, separating the administration times of the interacting drugs would not circumvent this interaction.

Clinically Important Examples. The increase in cyclosporine absorption occurring with concurrent administration of metoclopramide has been attributed to an increase in stomach emptying time. This may result in an increase in the immunologic and toxic effects of cyclosporine (24). Conversely, by increasing GI motility, metoclopramide may decrease the absorption of orally administered digoxin (25). This interaction may not occur with digoxin formulations that have high bioavailability (e.g., digoxin capsules or elixir) (26). Anticholinergic drugs are an example of a class of drugs that slow gastrointestinal transit time.

DISPLACED PROTEIN BINDING

Many drugs are reversibly bound to plasma proteins. Concurrent administration of more than one drug bound to the same protein fraction may displace either agent from its binding site, increasing the free concentration of the displaced drug. The drug with the higher affinity (i.e., association constant) for the binding site will displace the drug with the lower association constant (13). Following displacement from the protein binding site, there is immediate redistribution to the tissues. Subsequently, there is a compensatory increase in metabolism or excretion, resulting in a steady-state free plasma level similar to the level that existed prior to the displacement (20, 27). Drugs bound to plasma protein are pharmacologically inactive, since they are not available to extravascular receptor sites. In addition, the bound form is not available for metabolism or excretion. Thus, once the object drug is displaced from the protein binding site, not only is more drug free to exert its pharmacologic action, but additional drug becomes available for metabolism, excretion and redistribution to other tissues. The absolute concentration of unbound drug is referred to as the free concentration while the fraction of the total concentration of unbound drug is the free fraction (13).

The total plasma concentration of drug is the sum of the bound form and the free (unbound) drug. When drug is released from plasma protein, the increase in free drug concentration that occurs is transient. As the free fraction increases, it becomes available for metabolism and the total drug concentration will decrease. Because drugs that are highly bound to plasma protein tend to remain in the vascular space, the volume of distribution of these drugs is frequently small (13). An equilibrium is maintained between the free drug in the circulation and the protein-bound drug, and, as the drug is metabolized and excreted, the agent is released from its protein binding site. The fact that one drug displaces another is not sufficient to predict the pharmacologic outcome of a potential interaction. The overall pharmacologic effect of protein displacement is usually minimal. Clinically significant interactions may result from protein displacement if displacement is accompanied by enzyme inhibition or if the displaced drug has a small apparent volume of distribution, a narrow therapeutic index and a rapid onset of action (9).

Table 3.1.
Drug Protein Binding Sites

Binding Site	Drug
Plasma Protein	
Albumin	Warfarin
α-1-acid glycoprotein	Amitriptyline
	Disopyramide
	Lidocaine
	Propranolol
Lipoprotein	Cyclosporine
Transcortin	Corticosteroids
Tissue	
Sodium-potassium ATPase	Digoxin

Plasma proteins serve as a storage site or reservoir, limiting extravascular distribution. Examples of protein binding sites are listed in Table 3.1 (13).

The systemic clearance of certain drugs (e.g., lidocaine, propranolol) is independent of protein binding. Since both the bound and unbound forms of these drugs are removed from the plasma, their clearance is determined by hepatic blood flow. Thus, changes in protein binding will not affect the clearance of these drugs.

Clinical Considerations. Clinically important drug interactions involving displacement from protein binding are uncommon because once the object drug is displaced from plasma protein it is rapidly cleared from the body (8). Significant interactions occur when displacement is accompanied by enzyme inhibition, as occurs during coadministration of warfarin and phenylbutazone. In addition, a protein displacement interaction may be clinically significant if the displaced drug has a small apparent volume of distribution, a narrow therapeutic index, and a rapid onset of action (9).

Clinical Examples. Examples of drugs that are highly protein bound include phenytoin (90%), tolbutamide (96%), and warfarin (99%) (8). Common precipitant drugs include sulfonamides (e.g., sulfisoxazole), aspirin, and phenylbutazone (8, 27). The metabolite of chloral hydrate, trichloroacetic acid, displaces warfarin from its protein binding site, increasing the hypoprothrombinemic effect of warfarin (28, 29). However, the effect is slight and transient. With continued coadministration of the drugs, the free warfarin levels return to the concentrations that existed prior to the interaction. Although phenylbutazone displaces warfarin from plasma protein, it also inhibits the metabolism of the more potent S(−) warfarin enantiomorph, increasing the anticoagulant response to warfarin (30, 31).

ALTERED METABOLISM

The effects of one drug on the metabolism of a second are well documented. The concurrent administration of one drug with another may lead to an increase or decrease in the metabolic rate. These modifications may affect both the intensity and duration of activity. The major site of drug metabolism is the liver; however, other tissues, including white blood cells, skin, lung, and GI tract, are involved in drug metabolism. Drug metabolizing enzymes primarily convert lipophilic drugs into water-soluble metabolites, which may be more readily excreted. Drug metabolism may be divided into two types: Phase I, which includes hydroxylation, oxidation and reduction, and Phase II, which includes glucuronide, glycine, and sulfate conjugation. Phase II metabolism is frequently preceded by Phase I, preparing the drug for conjugation (32). The major hepatic enzyme system consists of the microsomal P-450 mixed-function oxygenases; however, there are numerous forms of cytochrome P-450 (CYP) (9).

It is estimated that there are between 20 and 200 different CYP human genes (32). According to the current classification, the entire group represents a superfamily (cytochrome-P450, also CYP) consisting of families (designated by a roman numeral) and subfamilies (designated by a capital letter) based on the similarity of the amino acid sequences of the encoded P450 isozyme protein (32, 33). The individual gene is designated by an arabic numeral (32, 33). Of the CYP genes that have been identified, families CYPI, CYPII, CYPIII, and CYPIV are involved with drug metabolism (32). Numerous drugs have been identified as substrates for the metabolism by subfamilies of these cytochrome P-450 enzymes (see Table 3.2) (32–37). However, it is not known which CYP isozyme is responsible for oxidation of most drugs. Over the past 15 years, the CYPIID6 isozyme has been the most extensively studied. This enzyme is not present in 5 to 10% of Caucasians, who have been designated as poor metabolizers. More than one isozyme may be involved in the metabolism of a drug (e.g.,

Table 3.2.
Drugs Identified as Being Metabolized by CYP Isozymes (32–37)

Drug	CYPIA2	CYPIIC8	CYPIIC9	CYPIIC10	CYPIID6	CYPIIIA3	CYPIIIA4	CYPIIIA5
Amitriptyline					x			
Clomipramine					x			
Codeine					x			
Cyclosporine							x	
Desipramine					x			
Dextromethorphan					x			
Diazepam		x						
Diltiazem							x	
Encainide					x			
Erythromycin						x	x	
Flecainide					x			
Fluoxetine					x			
Hexobarbital			x	x				
Hydrocortisone							x	
Imipramine					x			
Lidocaine							x	
Mephenytoin			x					
Metoprolol					x			
Midazolam							x	
Nifedipine							x	x
Nortriptyline					x			
Paroxetine					x			
Perphenazine					x			
Phenformin					x			
Phenacetin	x							
Progesterone							x	
Propafenone					x			
Propranolol					x			
Quinidine							x	
Testosterone							x	
Theophylline	x							
Thioridazine					x			
Timolol					x			
Tolbutamide		x	x	x				
Triazolam							x	
Warfarin			x					

Table 3.3.
Drugs that Induce Hepatic Enzymes

Barbiturates
  Phenobarbital
Carbamazepine
Griseofulvin
Ethanol (chronic ingestion)
Phenytoin
Primidone
Rifampin (CYPIIIA and CYPIID6)[8]
Environmental agents
  Cigarette smoking
  Diet

tolbutamide). Furthermore, a drug may act as a competitive inhibitor of one isozyme while being metabolized by another (32). For example, quinidine inhibits the CYPIID6 isozyme but is metabolized (i.e., oxidized) by CYPIIIA4. Drug interactions involving this enzyme system occur only if both drugs bind to the active site of the same form of the enzyme. Due to inter- and intrapatient variability, it is difficult to anticipate the clinical significance of potential interactions that occur by alterations in metabolism.

Increased Metabolism (Enzyme Induction). This interaction mechanism results from increased production of drug metabolizing enzymes (i.e., enzyme binding sites) and primarily involves Phase I metabolism (13). Since protein synthesis is involved, this interaction typically has a slow onset and may require up to 3 weeks before the maximum effect is observed. Although the precipitant drug usually induces the enzymes that enhance the metabolism of the object drug, some drugs (e.g., carbamazepine) increase their own metabolism. When the drug responsible for enzyme induction (i.e., the precipitant drug) is discontinued, the process will reverse. However, reversal of enzyme induction is frequently a slower process than the onset. As the number of enzymes decrease, the serum concentration of the object drug will gradually increase if the dose is not decreased. Thus, for example, in patients receiving warfarin and phenytoin concurrently, bleeding could occur if the enzyme inducer, phenytoin, is discontinued without adjusting the anticoagulant dose.

Clinical Considerations. This mechanism of interaction has a slow onset because protein synthesis is involved and may take up to several weeks before the maximum effect is seen. If an interaction occurs, the serum levels of the object drug may be reduced, producing a decrease in therapeutic activity. To compensate for this interaction, when practical, monitor serum drug concentrations and observe the patient for loss of therapeutic effects. Frequently, it is necessary to increase the dose of the object drug or select a noninteracting alternative. When a patient is stabilized on both drugs, if the precipitant drug is discontinued or the dose is decreased, serum levels of the object drug may increase and toxicity could occur. Dissipation of the effects of the interaction after discontinuation of the precipitant drug is also slow. Once again, patients should be monitored for changes in clinical response.

Clinically Important Examples. Phenytoin increases the hepatic metabolism of mexiletine, producing a decrease in steady-state plasma mexiletine levels and a reduction in efficacy (38). Similarly, theophylline and phenytoin appear to increase the metabolism of each other. When both drugs are administered concomitantly, serum drug concentrations may decrease and loss of seizure control or an exacerbation of pulmonary symptoms may result (10). Examples of other drugs that induce hepatic enzymes are listed in Table 3.3.

Decreased Metabolism (Enzyme Inhibition). As occurs with enzyme induction, enzyme inhibition usually involves the liver and results from competition between the precipitant and object drugs for binding sites on the enzyme. However, since this mechanism involves direct competition, the onset of interactions is more rapid than with enzyme induction, frequently occurring within hours. Unless the precipitant drug has a long half-life, enzyme inhibition will reach a maximum effect within 24 hours (39). Less commonly, a noncompetitive mechanism, which suspends the metabolic activity of an enzyme, may be involved (13). Drug interactions involving enzyme inhibition will often result in clinical effects that are protracted or intensified as the object drug reaches a steady-state plasma level. The enzymes most frequently involved are mono-oxygenase enzymes (9).

Table 3.4.
Drugs that Inhibit Hepatic Enzymes (33–36, 43)

Allopurinol
Amiodarone (CYPIID6)
Chloramphenicol
Cimetidine
Ciprofloxacin
Disulfiram
Diltiazem
Erythromycin
Isoniazid
Ketoconazole
Metronidazole
Monoamine oxidase inhibitors
Omeprazole
Paroxetine (CYPIID6)
Propoxyphene (CYPIID6)
Phenylbutazone
Quinidine (CYPIID6)
Sertraline (CYPIID6)
Sulfonamides
Troleandomycin
Verapamil

When metabolism of the object drug is inhibited, new steady-state serum levels are achieved in approximately five half-lives. However, the inhibitory effect of the precipitant drug on the metabolism of the object drug is usually maximal within three half-lives. Upon discontinuation of the enzyme inhibiting drug (i.e., precipitant drug), plasma concentrations of the object drug will decrease, resulting in loss of efficacy unless appropriate action is taken. The time frame for reversal of the interaction depends on the half-life of the object drug but will usually occur within 24 hours. As with most pharmacokinetic interactions, enzyme inhibition appears to be dose related, with higher doses producing greater inhibition.

Clinical Considerations. Enzyme induction is one of the most common mechanisms of drug interactions. The onset and reversal of this interaction often occur within 24 hours. This interaction usually produces an increase in serum drug concentration, resulting in a possible augmentation of both the pharmacologic and toxic effects of the object drug. Clinically significant interactions will be most frequent with those drugs that have a narrow therapeutic index and when the serum level is near the upper end of the therapeutic range. When a hepatic microsomal enzyme inducing drug (e.g., carbamazepine) is coadministered with an enzyme inhibitor (e.g., verapamil), the effect of the inhibitor appears to predominate and the effect of the inducer is attenuated. Stereospecific drug interactions involving warfarin metabolism are most clinically significant when the greatest effect occurs with the more potent $S(-)$ enantiomer (8).

Clinically Important Examples. Erythromycin and other macrolide antibiotics can inhibit the metabolism of astemizole and terfenadine, increasing the serum concentrations of the antihistamines as well as the risk of life-threatening cardiotoxicity (10). Omeprazole appears to inhibit the oxidative metabolism of diazepam, resulting in increased serum levels of the benzodiazepine and producing an increase the pharmacologic effect (40). Similarly, isoniazid inhibits the hepatic metabolism of phenytoin, producing an increase in serum phenytoin levels and a corresponding increase in the pharmacologic and toxic effects of the drug (41, 42). Phenytoin toxicity appears to be most significant in patients who are slow acetylators of isoniazid (42). Other drugs that significantly inhibit metabolic enzymes are listed in Table 3.4 (33–36, 43).

First-Pass Metabolism. Some drugs are metabolized extensively during the first pass through the wall of the gastrointestinal tract and liver (9, 20). In this instance, relatively small amounts of a drug will reach the systemic circulation (e.g., 10% of an orally administered dose of propranolol). Thus, drugs that increase or decrease liver blood flow may have profound effects on the bioavailability of the object drug. In addition, drugs with a high first-pass metabolism tend to compete for metabolic enzyme sites,

enhancing each others bioavailability (20). In other instances oral bioavailability may be decreased due to increased first-pass metabolism in the presence of enzyme induction.

Clinical Considerations. The object drug must be given orally. A clinically significant interaction will be seen when the precipitant drug is either an enzyme inducer or inhibitor.

Clinically Important Examples. Propafenone increases plasma levels of both metoprolol and propranolol by decreasing first-pass metabolism and reducing systemic clearance. Propafenone and the β-blockers are metabolized by the hepatic cytochrome P-450 oxidase system (i.e., CYPIID6), and propafenone appears to inhibit metoprolol and propranolol metabolism (44, 45). The pharmacologic and toxic effects of these β-blockers may be increased. Rifampin lowers serum verapamil levels by increasing first-pass hepatic metabolism of verapamil (46, 47). In addition, rifampin appears to induce the hepatic microsomal enzymes responsible for the metabolism of verapamil.

RENAL EXCRETION

The renal excretion of one drug may be increased or decreased by the coadministration of another drug. Most lipid-soluble drugs are metabolized by the liver to inactive, water-soluble metabolites prior to renal excretion. Various mechanisms may be involved with interactions affecting renal elimination, including competition for active tubular secretion and pH-dependent renal tubular transport.

Active Tubular Secretion. Active tubular secretion of drug molecules occurs in the proximal portion of the renal tubule. In order for the drug to pass from the systemic circulation to the tubular lumen, the drug is transported, by combining with a protein, through the basolateral and brush border membranes. Although each protein has a unique affinity for an anion or cation, drugs that use a similar system for transport appear to interact by competitive inhibition of transport proteins (13). Saturation of the transport system by the precipitant drug may decrease the tubular secretion of the object drug.

Table 3.5.
Drugs with a Narrow Therapeutic Index (8, 9)

Aminoglycoside antibiotics
Cyclosporine
Digoxin
Hypoglycemic agents
Lithium
Phenytoin
Theophylline
Tricyclic antidepressants
Warfarin

Clinical Considerations. Interactions resulting from this mechanism tend to occur rapidly. Plasma levels of the object drug may be increased, producing an increase in therapeutic and toxic effects.

Clinically Important Examples. Cyclosporine may decrease etoposide renal clearance by inhibiting drug transport in the brush border of the proximal renal tubule, increasing serum etoposide concentrations and the risk of toxicity (48). Probenecid appears to impair the tubular secretion of methotrexate. Methotrexate serum levels have been reported to be increased three- to fourfold during concurrent administration of probenecid (49). Quinidine reduces the renal and biliary clearance of digoxin by 30 to 40%, increasing serum digoxin levels in approximately 90% of the patients receiving both drugs (10, 50).

Passive Tubular Reabsorption. The excretion and reabsorption of many drugs from the renal tubules occur by passive diffusion, which is regulated by the concentration and lipid solubility of the drug on both sides of the cell membrane (13). Nonionized drug molecules are preferentially reabsorbed over ionized drugs with the ratio being determined by the pH and pK_a of the drug (13). Although strongly acidic and basic drugs tend to be ionized in the usual range of urinary pH (i.e., 5 to 8), the degree of ionization of weak acids and bases will vary with the pH of the urine. Therefore, an increased amount of weakly acidic drug will be reabsorbed from an acidic urine, while basic drugs will be excreted. The opposite is true in an alkaline urine (1).

Clinical Considerations. Interference with renal elimination may be clinically important if the fraction of unmetabolized drug is large, and if the drug has a narrow therapeutic index (e.g., thiazide diuretics decrease renal lithium clearance, producing toxicity).

Clinically Important Examples. Administration of sodium bicarbonate, 245 mEq administered over 5 hours, has been reported to increase renal lithium clearance, possibly decreasing the clinical effectiveness of lithium (51). Chronic antacid therapy with a magnesium and aluminum hydroxide combination has been associated with increased salicylate clearance and a 30 to 70% decrease in serum salicylate levels (10).

Pharmacodynamic Interactions

In contrast to pharmacokinetic interactions, pharmacodynamic interactions have not been amply studied or reported. Pharmacodynamic interactions involve changes in the response of the patient to a drug combination without alterations in the serum concentration or pharmacokinetics of the object drug. Inasmuch as pharmacologic responses to a drug may be difficult to assess, pharmacodynamic studies are difficult to perform (13). Investigations are further complicated because pharmacokinetic and pharmacodynamic drug interactions may occur simultaneously. Since pharmacodynamic interactions often involve drugs with similar or opposing pharmacologic activity, many of these interactions can be anticipated by an understanding of the pharmacology of each of the drugs (1). Frequently, observing patients for changes in their clinical condition and making the appropriate dosage adjustment will correct the situation.

Synergistic and Antagonistic Effects. When a drug interaction involves synergistic or antagonistic effects, the therapeutic or toxic effects of two concurrently administered agents are greater or less, respectively, than the sum or the difference of their individual activity. These interactions frequently involve drugs acting on the same organ system (e.g., central nervous system) or site.

Clinical Considerations. Synergism is probably the most common mechanism by which drug interactions occur.

Clinically Important Examples. Synergism: Propranolol and verapamil have synergistic or additive cardiovascular effects (10). Both drugs have direct negative inotropic and chronotropic effects. Propranolol does not affect verapamil kinetics, and verapamil has only minimal effects on propranolol concentration. The pharmacologic as well as the toxic effects of propranolol and verapamil may be enhanced. Aminoglycosides have been reported to stabilize the postjunctional membrane and impair prejunctional calcium influx and acetylcholine output, thereby potentiating the neuromuscular effects of succinylcholine (10). *Antagonism:* The pharmacologic effects of fluoxetine may be reversed by concurrent administration of cyproheptadine. Fluoxetine has serotonergic activity while cyproheptadine is a serotonin antagonist (52). The capacity of warfarin to interfere with the activation of the vitamin

Table 3.6.
Patients at Increased Risk of Drug Interactions (9, 13, 53)

Increased Risk Due to Severity of the Disease State Being Treated
   Cardiac arrhythmia
   Epilepsy
   Diabetes
   Asthma
   Hypothyroidism
   Aplastic anemia
   Hepatic precoma
Increased Risk Due to Drug Interaction Potential of Therapy
   Cardiovascular disease
   Connective tissue disorders
   Gastrointestinal disease
   Infection
   Metabolic disorders
   Psychiatric illness
   Respiratory ailments
   Seizure disorders

K-dependent clotting factors is reversed by vitamin K administration, allowing possible thrombus formation.

Altered Transport System and Effects at Receptor Sites. These drug interactions involve interference with physiologic transport systems, limiting the access of certain drugs into cells.

Clinical Considerations. The serum level of the drugs will be unchanged unless a pharmacokinetic interaction occurs simultaneously.

Clinically Important Examples. Both phenothiazines (eg, chlorpromazine) and tricyclic antidepressants (e.g., amitriptyline) inhibit the neuronal uptake of guanethidine, preventing the antihypertensive activity of guanethidine.(10)

HIGH-RISK DRUGS

Drugs having the highest risk of being involved in a clinically significant drug interaction frequently have a narrow therapeutic index, a steep dose-response curve and potent pharmacologic effects (1, 7, 9). When a drug has a narrow therapeutic index, the toxic dose may be only slightly more than the therapeutic dose. Similarly, when a drug has a steep dose-response curve, a small change in dose may result in a large increase in clinical effect. Therefore, a small increase in the serum concentration of drugs with these characteristics may produce an exaggerated pharmacologic response or toxicity. Patients receiving drugs with a narrow therapeutic index should be routinely monitored for possible drug interactions. Examples of drugs with a narrow therapeutic index are listed in Table 3.5. Conversely, a slight decrease in the plasma level of drugs with a steep dose-response curve may result in significant loss of therapeutic effects, examples include corticosteroids, carbamazepine, quinidine, oral contraceptives, and rifampin (9). Drugs with a wider therapeutic index are less likely to be involved in clinically significant interactions.

HIGH-RISK PATIENTS

Drug interactions that would be of minor clinical significance in most patients with less severe forms of a disease could cause significant exacerbation of the clinical condition in patients with more severe forms of the disease (see Table 3.6). Loss of therapeutic activity can be particularly important in situations that could result in an unwanted outcome (e.g., pregnancy), or where a serious pathologic condition is being suppressed (e.g., connective tissue disorder or a malignancy) (9). Since the risk of experiencing a drug interaction increases with the number of drugs a patient receives, severely ill or the elderly who are taking multiple drugs may also be at an increased risk for drug interactions (9). Additionally, patients being treated for certain diseases appear to be at an increased risk of experiencing a drug interaction because of the drug therapy prescribed for their disorder (see Table 3.6) (13, 53).

ONSET

There is considerable variation in the time of onset of drug interactions, ranging from seconds to weeks (13). Knowledge of the onset can assist in minimizing the adverse effects associated with interactions by enabling the clinician to select the most appropriate monitoring parameters. Interactions that occur with the administration of the first dose or within 24 hours of administration of the precipitant drug may require immediate attention. Since protein synthesis is involved in enzyme induction, it may be 2 weeks or more before the full potential for a clinically significant interaction is evident. Thus, an interaction would not be expected to occur by this mechanism in a patient receiving 1 or 2 days of treatment with an enzyme inducing drug (13). Conversely, enzyme inhibition results from competition between two drugs for the same enzyme site and may occur rapidly after administration of the precipitant drug. Patients should be monitored for changes in their clinical status soon after initiation of an interacting combination.

The time of onset of an interaction may be affected by the half-lives of the respective drugs. When the precipitant drug has a long half-life, it may take several days for plasma levels to reach steady state, delaying the onset of the interaction. The half-life of the object drug may also influence the onset of the interaction. Drug interactions occurring by similar mechanisms may have a more rapid onset when the object drug has a shorter half-life, since new steady-state plasma levels will be achieved sooner. For example, cimetidine inhibits the metabolism of warfarin and theophylline. The latter drug has a considerably shorter half-life than the former. Therefore, a clinically significant interaction may occur within a few days of adding cimetidine to the drug regimen of a patient stabilized on theophylline but may require a week or longer for a patient receiving warfarin.

The mechanism by which a drug interaction occurs can influence the onset of clinical effects. When relevant, the effect of the mechanism on the onset of an interaction was described in the clinical considerations section for the specific mechanism of interaction (see "Mechanisms of Drug Interaction").

CIRCUMVENTING AN INTERACTION

Many drug interactions can be avoided if adequate precautions are taken. Monitoring therapy and making appropriate adjustments in the drug regimen may circumvent a potentially serious drug interaction. Patients receiving drugs with a narrow therapeutic index should be routinely monitored for possible drug interactions. Drug interactions in this category may be life-threatening or have serious clinical consequences. Hospitalized patients are frequently given warfarin with an interacting agent without the occurrence of clinical consequences. In the hospital setting, a patient's prothrombin times are monitored daily and appropriate adjustments are made in the warfarin dosage whether or not a potential drug interaction is suspected. No symptoms of an interaction are observed. However, in order to avoid possible bleeding or the risk of exacerbating the condition being treated, adjustments in the warfarin dosage are necessary if the interacting drug is discontinued after the patient is discharged from the hospital.

DRUG INTERACTION RESOURCES

It is not surprising that the administration of one drug may modify the action of another drug given simultaneously. Whenever a patient receives multiple drug therapy, the possibility of a drug-drug interaction exists. In addition, as the number of drugs a patient receives increases, so does the potential for a drug interaction. Fortunately, those interactions with the greatest clinical significance are infrequent.

It would be impractical for pharmacists or physicians to be aware of all possible drug interactions. However, over the past two decades, drug interactions have received considerable attention. The medical literature is replete with anecdotal case reports, controlled clinical trials, and review articles concerning this subject. In addition, new interactions are constantly being reported. Comprehensive textbooks have been written on drug interactions, detailing the clinical effects, mechanisms and management of potential drug interactions (10, 13). Computer systems for storage and retrieval of drug interaction information as well as for patient monitoring have been developed (54, 55). Other available sources of drug interaction information include meetings, continuing education programs, and professional seminars. Even the manufacturer's package brochure contains a section regarding known and suspected drug interactions.

However, it is frequently difficult to interpret the relevance of much of the drug interaction data, since they are derived from animal or in vitro studies, investigations involving healthy volunteers given a single dose of a drug, and anecdotal case reports (9). In addition, studies may illustrate and emphasize pharmacokinetic findings without demonstrating clinically significant changes in patient outcome.

Problems Associated with Using the Medical Literature to Determine Clinical Significance
(10, 13, 56)

ANIMAL STUDIES

It may not be possible to extrapolate interactions based on animal studies to humans. Animals frequently receive much higher doses on a mg/kg basis than would be administered to humans.

ANECDOTAL CASE REPORTS

Drug interactions based on a single case report require additional controlled studies to determine their clinical significance. One must rule out other alternative explanations for the observed event (e.g., natural progression of the disease being treated).

HEALTHY VOLUNTEERS

Results of studies involving healthy volunteers or a small number of patients may not allow adequate evaluation of a potential interaction. Some pharmacokinetic interactions may be determined in normal, healthy volunteers but may not be clinically important when observed in patients. In other instances, healthy volunteers may not exhibit an interaction that is observed in patients. For example, the ability of erythromycin to reduce warfarin clearance is significantly more pronounced in patients than in healthy subjects.

MAGNITUDE OF EFFECT

A study may fail to identify or accurately describe a potential drug interaction based upon the magnitude of the effect of that interaction. Factors that may interfere with assessing the degree of effect are discussed below.

1. *Order of Administration.* Treatment with the object drug is started after the patient is stabilized on the precipitant drug. No interaction may be observed in this instance until the precipitant drug is discontinued. Thus, in a patient receiving chronic cimetidine treatment prior to the initiation of warfarin therapy, no interaction would be observed. However, if cimetidine was discontinued after the warfarin dosage was stabilized, a higher dose of anticoagulant may be required. Clinically significant interactions are more likely to occur when the precipitant drug is added to the regimen of a patient stabilized on the object drug.
2. *Duration of Treatment.* An interaction with a delayed onset may not be observed if the study is not conducted for an adequate period of time. Neurotoxicity occurring with concurrent administration of lithium and carbamazepine may only be observed after the drug combination is given for several days.
3. *Adequate Dose.* Most drug interactions are dose related. Larger doses of the precipitant drug tend to produce greater effects in the object drug. If an adequate dose of the drug is not administered, one may fail to observe an interaction. Thus, while high-dose salicylates (e.g., aspirin >3 g/day) antagonize the uricosuric action of probenecid, occasional low doses do not.
4. *Dosage Form.* It is necessary, for example, to consider the effects of food on theophylline absorption on an individual product basis. Although food can be ingested with many theophylline preparations without the occurrence of an interaction, Theo-24 taken less than 1 hour before a high-fat

meal may cause a significant increase in both theophylline absorption and peak serum concentrations.

5. *Presence of Multiple Drugs.* In a preliminary investigation, the presence of propylene glycol in IV nitroglycerin preparations was reported to interfere with the anticoagulant effect of heparin. Subsequent studies have demonstrated the effect on heparin to be due to the nitroglycerin.

EXTRAPOLATION TO CHEMICALLY OR PHARMACOLOGICALLY RELATED DRUGS

Based upon pharmacokinetic (e.g., elimination) or pharmacodynamic differences, not all members of a drug class may interact in the same manner. Cimetidine inhibits the hepatic microsomal enzymes involved in the metabolism of diazepam; however, famotidine does not appear to affect diazepam metabolism. In addition, cimetidine does not alter oxazepam metabolism.

MEAN VALUES

For drug interactions that occur in a small number of patients, no statistically significant difference in response may be observed between the control group and the study group. However, if one analyzes the results for individual subjects, there may be a clinically significant change in a small number of patients. For example, some patients exhibit a fivefold increase in serum digoxin concentrations during concurrent administration of quinidine, while in others, the effect is minimal.

VARIABILITY IN PATIENT RESPONSE

In well-controlled drug interaction studies, it is not unusual to find a wide variation in the response of patients to the same drug regimen. Thus, while one patient may experience a life-threatening reaction, a second patient may not experience any adverse effects. Frequently it is not possible to explain these differences; however, the factors listed below account for some of the variability.

1. *Age.* The very young and the elderly may be at increased risk of experiencing drug interactions. Studies have indicated that elderly patients receive approximately 25% of all prescription drugs dispensed. In addition, this age group extensively uses over-the-counter medications. Furthermore, elderly patients may have other chronic diseases or decreased renal or hepatic function necessitating careful monitoring of drug therapy. However, irrespective of age, drug therapy should be closely monitored in any patient with decreased organ function. Drug interactions involving enzyme induction may occur less frequently in elderly patients (57).

2. *Genetic Factors.* Certain drug interactions may be more significant in some patients due to genetic factors. For example, the toxicity resulting from the inhibitory effect of isoniazid on phenytoin metabolism appears to be more significant in slow acetylators of isoniazid than in those patients who metabolize the drug more rapidly.

3. *Disease States.* Various diseases such as impaired renal function, hepatic dysfunction, hypoalbuminemia may adversely influence the response to various drugs used concurrently. In addition, patients with certain disease states, including cardiovascular, connective tissue, GI, lipid, infectious, psychiatric, respiratory, or seizure disorders may be at an increased risk of experiencing moderate-to-severe drug interactions (13). This may be related either to changes in the disposition of the drug as a result of the disease or, more commonly, to the types of drugs used in the treatment of the disease.

4. *Alcohol Consumption.* Acute alcohol intolerance (disulfiram reaction) may occur in patients consuming alcohol while taking other drugs, including cefamandole, cefoperazone, cefotetan, and moxalactam.

5. *Smoking.* Smoking has been shown to increase the activity of drug-metabolizing enzymes in the liver (58). Smoking stimulates the metabolism of theophylline and mexiletine. Compared to nonsmokers, smokers may require larger doses of these drugs in order to maintain therapeutic serum levels. In addition, the administration of an enzyme inducing drug may not have as significant an effect on the object drug as might occur in a nonsmoking patient receiving the same drug combination. There is evidence indicating that the effects of administering multiple enzyme inducing drugs to the same patient are less than additive (59).

When evaluating the medical literature for a drug interaction, it is important to be aware of the type of documentation supporting the proposed interaction (i.e., case report, animal study, controlled study). If the citing is a controlled study, one must evaluate the study design, including sample size, route of drug administration, duration of therapy, and type of subjects (e.g., normal volunteers vs. clinical patients).

SUMMARY

It is important to understand the clinical significance of potentially interacting drug combinations. Although one does not want the choice of therapy to be detrimental to the patient, it is equally important not to deprive a patient of worthwhile treatment by overreacting to a potential interaction that lacks clinical significance or that can be easily circumvented. Most interacting drug combinations can be administered concurrently if the patient is monitored appropriately and corresponding adjustments are made in the drug dose, dosing interval, or route of administration. Understanding the mechanisms by which drugs interact as well as having a knowledge of those drugs and patients at increased risk of experiencing potentially significant drug interactions will allow the physician to anticipate and prevent clinically significant problems. Careful attention should be given to those interactions involving drugs that have a narrow therapeutic index (e.g., cyclosporine, digoxin, phenytoin, theophylline, warfarin). When a patient's clinical condition changes unexpectedly, all drug treatment should be reviewed. When possible, a suspected interaction should be placed in clinical perspective and one should be prepared to offer recommendations for minimizing possible consequences.

Factors that will help minimize the occurrence of drug interactions include (a) awareness of over-the-counter drugs that the patient may take, (b) avoidance of unnecessary therapy, (c) observing the patient for unexpected changes in clinical response, and (d) monitoring serum drug levels, particularly for drugs with a narrow therapeutic index.

The importance of educating patients about potential drug interactions that may be associated with their treatment regimens should not be overlooked. Patient knowledge of unexpected reactions that could occur with coadministration of their current medications with other prescription and over-the-counter drugs could lead to the early detection or prevention of possibly significant drug interactions.

REFERENCES

1. Berkow R, ed. The merck manual of diagnosis and therapy, 16th ed. Rahway, NJ: Merck Sharp & Dohme Research Laboratories, 1992:2634–2640.
2. Boston Collaborative Drug Surveillance Program. Adverse drug interactions. JAMA 220:1238–1239, 1972.
3. Durrence CW, DiPiro JT, May JR, et al. Potential drug interactions in surgical patients. Am J Hosp Pharm 42:1553–1555, 1985.
4. Borda IT, Slone D, Jick H. Assessment of adverse reactions within a drug surveillance program. JAMA 205:645–647, 1968.
5. Blaschke TF, Cohen SN, Tatro DS. Drug-drug interactions and aging. In: Jarvik LF, Greenblatt DJ, Harman D, eds. Clinical pharmacology in the aged patient. New York: Raven Press, 16:11–26, 1981.
6. Stanaszek WF, Franklin CE. Survey of potential drug interaction incidence in an outpatient clinic population. Hosp Pharm 13:255–263, 1978.
7. Puckett WH, Visconti JA. An epidemiological study of the clinical significance of drug-drug interactions in a private community hospital. Am J Hosp Pharm 28:247–53, 1971.
8. Aronson JK, Grahame-Smith DG. Adverse drug interactions. Br Med J 282:288–291, 1981.
9. McInnes GT, Brodie MJ. Drug interactions that matter: a critical reappraisal. Drugs 36:83–110, 1988.
10. Tatro DS, ed. Drug interaction facts. St. Louis, MO: Wolters Kluwer Co, 1995. 110, 110b, 164, 281, 290, 353, 365, 615, 627, 691, 735.
11. Hoffken G, Borner K, Glatzel PD, et al. Reduced enteral absorption of ciprofloxacin in the presence of antacids. Eur J Clin Microbiol 4:345, 1985.
12. Nix DE, Watson WA, Lener ME, et al. Effects of aluminum and magnesium antacids and ranitidine on the absorption of ciprofloxacin. Clin Pharmacol Ther 46:700–705, 1989.
13. Hansten PD. Drug interactions & updates. Vancouver, WA: Applied Therapeutics, 1994.
14. Lindenbaum J, Rund DG, Butler VP, et al. Inactivation of digoxin by the gut flora: reversal by antibiotic therapy. N Engl J Med 305:789–794, 1981.
15. Morton MR, Cooper JW. Erythromycin-induced digoxin toxicity. DICP Ann Pharmacother 23:668–670, 1989.
16. Sahai J, Gallicano K, Oliveras L, et al. Cations in the didanosine tablet reduce ciprofloxacin bioavailability. Clin Pharmacol Ther 53:292–297, 1993.
17. Parpia SH, Nix DE, Hejmanowski LG, et al. Sucralfate reduces the gastrointestinal absorption of norfloxacin. Antimicrob Agents Chemother 33:99–102, 1989.
18. Nix DE, Watson WA, Handy L, et al. The effect of sucralfate pretreatment on the pharmacokinetics of ciprofloxacin. Pharmacotherapy 9:377–380, 1989.
19. Garrelts JC, Godley PJ, Peterie JD, et al. Sucralfate significantly reduces ciprofloxacin concentrations in serum. Antimicrob Agents Chemother 34;931–933, 1990.
20. Brodie MJ, Feely J. Adverse drug interactions. Br Med J 296:845–9, 1988.
21. Kuhlman J, Zilly W, Wilke J. Effects of cytotoxic drugs on plasma level and renal excretion of beta-acetyldigoxin. Clin Pharmacol Ther 30:518–527, 1981.
22. Kuhlman J, Wilke J, Rietbrock N. Cytostatic drugs are without significant effect on digitoxin plasma level and renal excretion. Clin Pharmacol Ther 32:646–651, 1982.
23. Bjornsson TD, Huang AT, Roth P, et al. Effects of high-dose cancer chemotherapy on the absorption of digoxin in two different formulations. Clin Pharmacol Ther 39:25–28, 1986.
24. Wadhwa NK, Schroeder TJ, O'Flaherty E, et al. The effect of oral metoclopramide on the absorption of cyclosporine. Transplant Proc 19:1730–1733, 1987.
25. Manninen V, Melin J, Apajalahti A, et al. Altered absorption of digoxin in patients given propantheline and metoclopramide. Lancet 1:398–399, 1973.
26. Johnson BF, Bustrack JA, Urbach DR, et al. Effect of metoclopramide on digoxin absorption from tablets and capsules. Clin Pharmacol Ther 36:724–730, 1984.
27. Rolan PE. Plasma protein binding displacement interaction-why are they still regarded as clinically important? Br J Clin Pharmacol 37:125–128, 1994.
28. Boston Collaborative Drug Surveillance Program. Interaction between chloral hydrate and warfarin. N Engl J Med 286:53–55, 1972.
29. Udall JA. Warfarin-chloral hydrate interaction: pharmacological activity and clinical significance. Ann Intern Med 81:341–344, 1974.
30. Banfield C, O'Reilly R, Chan E, et al. Phenylbutazone-warfarin interaction in man: further stereochemical and metabolic considerations. Br J Clin Pharmacol 16:669–675, 1983.
31. O'Reilly RA, Trager WF, Motley CH, et al. Stereoselective interaction of phenylbutazone with [^{12}C/^{13}C]warfarin pseudoracemates in man. J Clin Invest 65:746–753, 1980.
32. Brosen K. Recent developments in hepatic drug oxidation: implications for clinical pharmacokinetics. Clin Pharmacokinet 18:220–239, 1990.
33. Gonzalez FJ, Idle JR. Pharmacogenetic phenotyping and genotyping: present status and future potential. Clin Pharmacokinet 26:59–70, 1994.
34. Murray M. P450 enzymes: inhibition mechanisms, genetic regulation and effects of liver disease. Clin Pharmacokinet 23:132–146, 1992.
35. Tucker GT. The rational selection of drug interaction studies: implications of recent advances in drug metabolism. Int J Clin Pharmacol Ther Toxicol 30:550–553, 1992.
36. van Harten J. Clinical pharmacokinetics of selective serotonin reuptake inhibitors. Clin Pharmacokinet 24:203–220, 1993.
37. Andersson T. Omeprazole drug interaction studies. Clin Pharmacokinet 21:195–212, 1991.
38. Begg EJ, Chinwah PM, Webb C, et al. Enhanced metabolism of mexiletine after phenytoin administration. Br J Clin Pharmacol 14:219–223, 1982.

39. Dossing M, et al. Time course of phenobarbital and cimetidine mediated changes in hepatic drug metabolism. Eur J Clin Pharmacol 25:215–222, 1983.

40. Gugler R, Jensen JC. Omeprazole inhibits oxidative drug metabolism. Gastroenterology 89:1235–1241, 1985.

41. Murray FJ. Outbreak of unexpected reactions among epileptics taking isoniazid. Am Rev Respir Dis 86:729–732, 1962.

42. Brennan RW, Dehejia H, Kutt H, et al. Diphenylhydantoin intoxication attendant to slow inactivation of isoniazid. Neurology 20:687–693, 1970.

43. Humphries TJ. Clinical implications of drug interactions with the cytochrome P-450 enzyme system associated with omeprazole. Dig Dis Sci 36:1665–1669, 1991.

44. Wagner F, Kalusche D, Trenk D, et al. Drug interaction between propafenone and metoprolol. Br J Clin Pharmac 24:213–220, 1987.

45. Kowey PR, Kirsten EB, Fu CHJ, et al. Interaction between propranolol and propafenone in healthy volunteers. J Clin Pharmacol 29:512–517, 1989.

46. Mooy JJ, Bohm R, van Kemenade J, et al. The influence of antituberculosis drugs on plasma level of verapamil. Eur J Clin Pharmacol 32:107–109, 1987.

47. Barbarash RA, Bauman JL, Fischer JH, et al. Near-total reduction in verapamil bioavailability by rifampin: electrocardiographic correlates. Chest 94:954–959, 1988.

48. Lum BL, Kaubisch S, Yahanda AM, et al. Alteration of etoposide pharmacokinetics and pharmacodynamics by cyclosporine in a Phase I trial of modulate multidrug resistance. J Clin Oncol 10:1635–1642, 1992.

49. Aherne GW, Piall E, Marks V, et al. Prolongation and enhancement of serum methotrexate concentrations by probenecid. Br Med J 1:1097–1099, 1978.

50. Hedman A, Angelin B, Arvidsson A, et al. Interactions in the renal and biliary elimination of digoxin: stereoselective differences between quinine and quinidine. Clin Pharmacol Ther 47:20–26, 1990.

51. Thomsen K, Schou M, et al. Renal lithium excretion in man. Am J Physiol 215:823–827, 1968.

52. Feder R. Reversal of antidepressant activity of fluoxetine by cyproheptadine in three patients. J Clin Psychiatry 52:163–164, 1991.

53. Tatro DS. Drugs interfering with control of the diabetic patient: hypoglycemic drug-drug interactions. Rev Drug Interaction 1:3–34, 1974.

54. Tatro DS, Briggs RL, Chavez-Pardo R, et al. Detection and prevention of drug interactions utilizing an online computer system. Drug Info J 9:10–17, 1975.

55. Tatro DS, Briggs RL, Chavez-Pardo R, et al. Online drug interaction surveillance. Am J Hosp Pharm 32:417–420, 1975.

56. Tatro DS. Understanding drug interactions. Facts and Comparisons Drug Newsletter 7:57–59, 1988.

57. Salem SAM, et al. Reduced induction of drug metabolism in the elderly. Age Ageing 7:68, 1978.

58. Tatro DS. Effects of smoking on drug therapy. Facts and Comparisons Drug Newsletter 13:49–51, 1994.

59. Perucca E, Hedges A, Makki A, et al. A comparative study of the relative enzyme-inducing properties of anticonvulsant drugs in epileptic patients. Br J Clin Pharmacol 18:401–410, 1984.

CHAPTER 4

CLINICAL TOXICOLOGY

GARY M. ODERDA and WENDY KLEIN-SCHWARTZ

Clinical toxicology deals with the assessment and medical management of persons exposed acutely or chronically to potentially harmful agents. Because of the diverse nature of the substances involved in poisonings as well as the wide range of clinical manifestations and their treatment, optimal management of the poisoned patient is achieved through an interdisciplinary approach to patient care. Expertise provided by physicians, nurses, pharmacists, social workers, and paraprofessionals contributes greatly to the care of these patients.

GENERAL INFORMATION

Poisoning is a serious problem in the United States today. The American Association of Poison Control Centers (AAPCC) Toxic Exposure Surveillance System (TESS) reported 1,751,476 human poison exposures in 1993 (1). This figure does not reflect the actual number reported to poison centers nationally, since reporting is voluntary. Although it is difficult to be certain of the true magnitude of the problem, it is estimated that each year, 2.1 to 4.6 million poison exposures occur nationally, with accidental poisoning accounting for 5803 deaths in 1990 (1, 2).

Poisoning is a common pediatric medical emergency. Fifty-six percent of poisonings occur in children less than 6 years of age (1). Most childhood poisonings are unintentional and occur via the oral route. Children's natural curiosity can at times have disastrous consequences. The most common substances involved in poison exposures in children under 6 years of age are drugs, household products, personal care products, and plants. The drugs most commonly involved are analgesics and antipyretics, antihistamines, cough and cold products, vitamins, and topical preparations.

Thirty years ago, aspirin was the leading cause of unintentional poisonings and poisoning deaths in children under 5 years of age. There has been a progressive decline in both ingestions and deaths since the mid-1960s (3). The percentage of ingestions of aspirin in those under 5 years of age decreased steadily from approximately 25% in 1966 to 3.9% in 1979 (4). In 1993, AAPCC data showed that ingestions of aspirin alone in children 5 years of age and under accounted for 0.13% of exposures (1). Many factors are responsible for this decrease, including an increased awareness on the part of the general public of the dangers of aspirin. The child resistant container (CRC) requirement for all products containing aspirin and all liquid preparations containing methylsalicylate played a major role in the decline. Hopefully, CRCs will further decrease the number of intoxications from other products on which these closures are now required. The limit of 36 tablets (each 81 mg) per bottle of children's aspirin has helped reduce the severity of the ingestions that still occur.

Approximately 24% of poisonings occur in adults 19 years of age or older and are often the result of an intentional exposure (suicide or drug abuse), but may also be unintentional (e.g., occupational exposure) (1). Although poison prevention activities may decrease the number of pediatric exposures and minimize the severity of childhood intoxications, these efforts generally have little impact on intentional poisonings in adults. One possible exception is poisoning in the elderly. Many of these ingestions are unintentional and are amenable to poison prevention efforts (5). Poisonings in adults are generally responsible for more significant morbidity and mortality than those in children.

ROLE AND STATUS OF POISON CENTERS

The first poison center was established in Chicago in 1953. Today, poison centers exist in most major U.S. metropolitan areas. During the 1970s, the concept of regionalization of poison centers developed in an attempt to more efficiently and effectively meet the needs of the poisoned patients. Many large centers serve as regional centers and provide information to a large population or geographic area. This may involve a major metropolitan area, a portion of a large state, an entire state, or several states. It is not unusual for these regional centers to handle 15,000 to 30,000 or more calls per year. Fifty to one hundred regional poison centers could adequately serve the entire United States. In this way, duplication of information sources and staff would be avoided. In addition, regional poison center staff would handle large numbers of cases to develop extensive expertise. Poison centers receive calls relating to drugs, chemicals, household products, personal care products, plants, animal toxins, fish toxins, food poisoning, and others. Approximately 40% of calls involve exposures to drugs. The majority of calls to the poison center come from the general public and can be managed in a non-health care facility setting.

The American Association of Poison Control Centers has developed standards for poison centers and certifies regional centers. According to a survey conducted in 1989, there were 104 poison centers in the United States, of which 35 are certified as regional poison centers by the American Association of Poison Control Centers (6). At the beginning of 1995 there were 40 certified regional poison centers in the United States serving just more than half of the population of the United States.

A regional poison center provides telephone information 24 hours a day utilizing comprehensive information sources and management protocols, and has access to regional treatment facilities for patient referral and transport. Additional components include a regional system for providing poisoning care, public and health professional education programs, and a regional data collection and reporting system.

Clinical pharmacists or nurses are often administratively responsible for the day-to-day operation of the center as well as providing professional input into the management of the poisoned patient. Specialists in poison information, usually pharmacists or nurses, are responsible for providing primary telephone consultations.

During the early 1990s, problems with poison center funding caused a crisis, with several regional poison centers closing or being threatened with closure. A Congressional hearing was held in March 1994 to address the problem. However, a long-range solution to the funding problem has not been identified, even though every $1 spent on poison center services saves almost $8 in unnecessary emergency care (7).

Poison information and drug information centers differ in several respects. Poison centers usually provide services both to professionals and to the general public, whereas drug information centers usually provide information only to health professionals. The volume of calls to poison centers is usually higher than to drug information centers. Rapid retrieval of information is necessary in poison centers because of the potential emergency nature of calls. Therefore, the information sources used for handling the majority of cases are mainly secondary resources. The assessment and recommendations are provided during the initial call to the center. As a result, the depth of research performed in a poison center is less than in a drug information center.

POISON PREVENTION

A major component of poison center activity is in the area of poison prevention education. All prescription drugs should be dispensed in CRCs unless specifically excluded by law. Recent regulations require CRCs on mouthwashes containing higher than 5% ethanol. A proposal to require CRCs on iron products with 30 mg and higher concentration of elemental iron per tablet is under consideration by the FDA. In those few instances in which a patient requires a non-CRC, both the dispensing pharmacist and

prescriber should warn the patient to store the container properly to avoid an unintentional poisoning. Elderly patients who request non-CRCs may not have young children of their own, but many have grandchildren who come to visit.

Health care providers should promote the distribution of syrup of ipecac by providing information and urging families to purchase one ounce of ipecac syrup for each young child. Parents should be cautioned to contact their poison center or health care provider before giving the ipecac so that the situation can be evaluated to determine the appropriateness of administering an emetic. If syrup of ipecac is indicated, the health professional can review dosing with the caller, follow up to determine if the person has vomited, and provide additional instructions regarding the side effects of ipecac or symptoms to watch for that might indicate the need for additional evaluation and treatment. If ipecac is not indicated, the health professional can discourage its use and recommend other treatment if necessary.

ANALYSIS OF A POISONING SITUATION-TYPES OF QUESTIONS ASKED

In many poisoning calls, the caller does not volunteer enough information initially for the health care provider to assess the situation. The fact that an overdose has occurred is not always obvious. Occasionally a poisoning situation can be uncovered only by persistent questioning. Inquiries relating to tablet identification or other general information may involve a poisoning, and this information can be elicited by determining why the caller needs the information. In addition, poisoning should be considered in the differential diagnosis whenever there is an abrupt onset of illness with multiple organ system involvement, especially if the patient is a child under 5 years of age or has a history of a previous ingestion (8).

When a poisoning is suspected, the following information must be obtained to "analyze" a poisoning situation:

1. **Substance.** This information should include ingredients and their percentages. Examples of situations where the substance involved may be unknown include patients who are unable to give a history (e.g., patient is comatose), who ingest tablets or capsules from an unmarked container, or who ingest an unidentified plant.
2. **Amount.** If an accurate determination of the amount ingested is impossible and the product is potentially toxic, one must assume that a potentially toxic amount was ingested or that the total amount originally in the container was ingested. In intentional exposures the history of the amount ingested should be considered suspect.
3. **Time Since Exposure.** By knowing about the onset and duration of action of the substance, one can determine whether the symptoms are consistent with the history of the amount ingested and the time since exposure. In addition, treatment recommendations, such as whether or not to empty

the stomach, may be influenced by the length of time since ingestion.

4. **Symptoms.** Determine whether symptoms are consistent with the substance involved; if they are not, determine what other substances or medical conditions may be responsible for these symptoms. Severe signs and symptoms, such as respiratory and cardiovascular collapse, necessitate immediate treatment. Some treatment modalities are contraindicated when certain signs or symptoms are present (e.g., emetics in the comatose patient).

5. **Age and Weight of Patient.** These are important considerations in determining the toxicity of the substance as well as for dosing antidotes.

6. **Past Medical History and Prior Therapy.** The patient's medical history may influence the severity of the intoxication or treatment. Some home remedies may complicate therapy, whereas other prior treatment may influence subsequent recommendations.

INFORMATION SOURCES

After obtaining the poisoning history and the patient's current clinical status, consult appropriate information sources. The major toxicologic information sources are secondary sources designed to allow rapid retrieval of toxicity and management information. The current primary literature should be consulted in some cases.

The following references are strictly toxicology oriented and do not include other important references, such as pharmacology or drug interaction texts that are available in pharmacies, poison centers, and drug information centers.

Poisindex

Poisindex (B. Rumack, editor; published by Micromedex, Englewood, Colorado; new edition published four times yearly) is a computer-generated system with information on most commercial products and other agents including biologics such as plants and venomous animals. It is usually used as a computer accessible database, either as a compact disk (CD-ROM) system (standalone or on a network) or a multiuser mainframe computer system. It also is available on microfiche, although using the microfiche version is more cumbersome and is not recommended. The editorial board is comprised of individuals actively involved with poisoning and poison centers throughout the United States. For each product, the manufacturer's name, the type of product, ingredients, percentages (if available), and tablet imprint (if applicable) are listed. Specific toxicity information may also be included.

For all agents the user is referred to the appropriate managements. Managements are preceded by "overviews" that contain summaries of emergency treatment and toxicity information, eliminating the need to scan many screens of information initially. The overview is followed by the complete management, which includes information on

available forms, pharmacology, clinical effects, kinetics, range of toxicity, laboratory (blood levels, etc.), treatment, and major references. The major advantages of this system are (a) ease of use; (b) storage of a large amount of data in a small space; (c) information kept up to date; (d) detailed management protocols; (e) information on drugs, chemicals, household products, food poisoning, mushrooms, snakes, and drug imprint codes; and (f) cross-referenced product information. It is an essential resource for poison centers and is also useful for other health care providers.

Textbooks

Toxicology of the Eye (3rd ed. W.G. Grant. Springfield, Illinois: Charles C Thomas, 1986) is an excellent resource on the effects of various agents on contact with the eye. In addition, those agents for which systemic intoxication produces ocular effects (e.g., methanol) are included. Specific human information is discussed where available. A separate treatment section is included.

Patty's Industrial Hygiene and Toxicology (3rd ed. G.D. Clayton and F.E. Clayton, eds. New York: John Wiley & Sons, 1981) is a series published in three volumes. Volume 1 discusses general principles, Volumes 2A, 2B, and 2C provide specific toxicology information; and Volume 3 describes industrial hygiene practice. Poison centers find Volumes 2A, 2B, and 2C the most useful. Both chronic and acute exposures to industrial chemicals are described. For each chemical, information such as the following is provided: (a) source, use, and industrial exposure; (b) physical and chemical properties; (c) determination in the atmosphere; (d) physiologic response; (e) hygiene standard of permissible exposure; (f) flammability; and (g) odor and warning properties.

Medical Toxicology. Diagnosis and Treatment of Human Poisoning (M.J. Ellenhorn and D.G. Barceloux. New York: Elsevier, 1988), *Clinical Management of Poisoning and Drug Overdose* (2nd ed. L.M. Haddad and J.F. Winchester eds. Philadelphia: WB Saunders, 1990), and *Goldfrank's Toxicology Emergencies* (5th ed. L.R. Goldfrank, N.E. Flomenbaum, N.A. Lewin, et al., eds. Norwalk, CT: Appleton-Lange, 1994) are textbooks of clinical toxicology that provide brief reviews of poisoning by drugs, chemicals, and biologics and their management.

Hazardous Materials Toxicology: Clinical Principles of Environmental Health (J.B. Sullivan and G.R. Krieger. Baltimore: Williams & Wilkins, 1992) begins by discussing general principles of hazardous materials toxicology. It then moves into regulatory, health, and safety aspects of hazardous materials and emergency medical response and hazardous materials. Specific information on toxic materials is provided in two ways. Section IV describes toxic hazards by industrial site. For example, chemical hazards in the tire and rubber manufacturing industry are covered. The remaining section covers specific toxins. This text is an excellent reference to help manage occupational and environmental exposures.

Proctor and Hughes' Chemical Hazards of the Workplace (3rd ed. G.J. Hathaway, N.H. Proctor, J.P. Hughes, et al. New York: Van Nostrand Reinhold, 1991). Deals with general toxicologic concepts in the introductory chapters. The majority of the book consists of short monographs on 542 chemicals most likely to be encountered in the workplace. It is well referenced and an excellent start to obtain information on common and obscure chemicals found in the workplace.

Clinical Toxicology of Commercial Products (5th ed. R.E. Gosselin, R.P. Smith, and H.C. Hodge, eds. Baltimore: Williams & Wilkins, 1984) is divided into seven sections: First Aid and General Emergency Treatment, Ingredients Index, Therapeutics Index, Supportive Treatment, Trade Name Index, General Formulations, and Manufacturers' Names and Addresses. Most commonly, one looks up the name of a product in the trade name index, which lists the ingredients and their percentages. One then looks up each ingredient in the ingredients index for specific toxicity information. The therapeutics index has detailed toxicity and treatment information on general categories such as antihistamines. The general formulations index is very useful in those situations where a brand name is unavailable. If, for example, one is dealing with a child who drank an unknown brand of furniture polish, one could find the ingredients usually found in furniture polishes.

SUPPORTIVE CARE

Supportive care is the most important component of managing the seriously intoxicated patient. Close attention to airway, breathing, level of consciousness, and blood pressure is critical. While some clinical toxicologists may argue about the value of some gastrointestinal decontamination procedures or disagree over the specific indications for extracorporeal removal of toxins, there is no disagreement about the value of supportive care. In many serious intoxications, supportive care sustains the patient while the toxin is being detoxified by liver metabolism or renal elimination.

All patients with CNS depression should be given intravenous dextrose (50 mL D50W) and naloxone (0.4-2.0 mg) in case altered mental status is the result of either hypoglycemia or opioid intoxication. Dextrose and naloxone will rapidly reverse CNS depression from these causes and will help "rule in" certain substances responsible for the intoxication but will have no serious consequences if given to patients without hypoglycemia or opioid intoxication. If respirations are compromised the patient should be placed on a ventilator. Hypotension is treated initially with intravenous fluids and positioning. If blood pressure remains low, vasopressors such as dopamine or norepinephrine should be administered. Overdoses with poten-

tially cardiotoxic agents or unknown agents should be on a cardiac monitor. Fluid and electrolyte status should be monitored and intravenous fluids adjusted accordingly.

The need for supportive care and the level of supportive care required will depend on the toxin and the patient. Similarly, the time period during which supportive care is required will vary from one individual to the next. Decisions regarding extubation and discontinuing vasopressors will be based on continuing assessment of the patient's level of consciousness and blood pressure.

DECREASING ABSORPTION

The toxic potential of an ingestion can be decreased by minimizing the absorption of the ingested agent from the gastrointestinal tract. Emptying the stomach, administering an adsorbent, and inducing catharsis are potential treatments that should be considered when a sufficient amount of a potentially toxic substance has been ingested within a reasonable time period. For most substances, this time period is within the past 4 hours. Drugs for which gastrointestinal (GI) decontamination may be warranted up to 10 to 12 hours after ingestion include salicylates, which delay gastric emptying; anticholinergics, which decrease GI motility; and phenytoin, which is slowly and erratically absorbed from the GI tract.

Activated charcoal has become the primary treatment modality to prevent absorption from the GI tract in emergency department treated patients. The use of ipecac syrup or gastric lavage may be appropriate in some of these patients. For example, patients who have taken agents not adsorbed by activated charcoal may benefit from ipecac or lavage. The major role of ipecac syrup is for use in the home to remove toxic agents from the GI tract and prevent absorption. The use of ipecac syrup has decreased from 13.4% of all exposures reported to TESS in 1983 to 3.7% of all exposures in 1993, while use of activated charcoal increased from 4.0% of all exposures in 1983 to 7.3% of all exposures in 1993 (1). Some of the decrease in ipecac syrup use may be attributable to a decrease in the percentage of children included in the TESS system. In 1983, 64% of all reported exposures were in children under 6 years of age as compared with 56% in 1993 (1).

The efficacy of ipecac syrup-induced emesis was evaluated in 20 children between 12 and 20 months of age who had ingested salicylates (9). Lavage was performed and emesis induced in each patient, and the amount of salicylates returned by each method was measured. Approximately half of the patients were lavaged first; the other half were given syrup of ipecac first. Overall, ipecac removed significantly more salicylate than lavage, even when emesis was induced after lavage was completed. The study concluded that "ipecac-induced emesis is superior to gastric lavage for emptying the stomach per os of unwanted contents . . . ipecac-induced emesis leaves little or no salicylate which could potentially be removed by lavage."

Goldstein (10) reported two acute overdoses in adults seen 10 to 15 minutes after ingestion. Each patient was lavaged with 3 liters of normal saline through a 20 French (Fr) tube. Both patients were then given ipecac and vomited successfully. In one case 25 tablets were found in the vomitus and in the other 10 to 15 tablets.

In many of the studies comparing emesis and lavage, either the size of the lavage tube is not mentioned or it is smaller than is currently recommended. The size of the lavage tube is one of the most important factors determining the effectiveness with which the stomach will be emptied. Optimally a 36 French (12 mm or about ½ inch in diameter) or larger Ewald or Lavacuator tube should be used by the oral route in adults. Nasogastric tubes usually are smaller and therefore less effective. Smaller tubes (16–18 French) must be used in children, markedly limiting the effectiveness of the procedure. A prospective study of 88 patients seen in an emergency department for drug overdose found gastric lavage superior to ipecac-induced emesis when thiamine was used as a marker of recovery of gastric samples (11). A controlled study in 18 fasting normal adult volunteers who ingested 25 100-µg cyanocobalamin tablets on two separate occasions reported a mean return of 28% with ipecac-induced emesis compared with 45% after gastric lavage with a modified 32 French orogastric tube (12). Potential methodologic biases leave this issue unresolved (13).

Following lavage with a 33 French tube, 88% of poisoned patients still had residual intragastric solids (14). In a subsequent study, Suetta gave 20 poisoned patients 20 polyethylene pellets impregnated with barium sulfate. Approximately half of the pellets were retained following 3.5 to 6 liters of fluid, with one third of those in the small intestine half an hour after ingestion of the pellets (15).

Another important clinical consideration is that the percentage return with both emesis and lavage is low. In 14 humans given magnesium hydroxide as a marker and then ipecac, a mean return of $28 \pm 7.0\%$ was found, with a range of 0 to 78% (16). Arnold et al. (17) found that under optimal conditions dogs given sodium salicylate returned 38% (range 2–69%) after lavage and 45%, (range 7–75%) after ipecac-induced emesis. When the administration of ipecac was delayed until 30 minutes after ingestion and lavage was not performed until 1 hour after ingestion, only 13% (range 0–40%) was removed by lavage and 39% (range 5–74%) by emesis (17). A small 16 French tube was used for lavage. A similar study in dogs using barium sulfate found that $29 \pm 10\%$ (range 10–62%) was returned with gastric lavage, $19 \pm 9\%$ (range 2–31%) with ipecac, and $74 \pm 5\%$ (range 54–87%) with apomorphine (18).

In situations where gastric emptying is warranted (e.g., home management, ingestion of an agent not adsorbed by activated charcoal), emesis with syrup of ipecac should be the procedure of first choice in children. In those cases where emetics are contraindicated (e.g., the CNS depressed patient), lavage is preferred. Lavage should be performed in adults who are treated early after the ingestion of substances with high inherent toxicity (e.g. cyclic antidepressants). Lavage should also be performed if induction of emesis with ipecac fails. Ipecac syrup should not be administered to patients who will be receiving activated charcoal, since many of these patients will vomit the charcoal.

Although induction of emesis or gastric lavage has been considered standard procedure for gastric emptying, the role of these procedures in gastrointestinal decontamination has been questioned. Several studies comparing ipecac and/or lavage with activated charcoal have found activated charcoal superior (19–21). A crossover study in 12 adult volunteers given twenty-four 81-mg aspirin tablets and randomly assigned to a control group (no further treatment), ipecac group, activated charcoal/cathartic group, or ipecac/activated charcoal/cathartic group found that aspirin absorption was decreased in both the ipecac group and the activated charcoal/cathartic group (19). Analysis of the effectiveness of ipecac/activated charcoal/cathartic was not possible, since 8 of 10 volunteers vomited the charcoal and cathartic. However, activated charcoal/cathartic was significantly more effective than ipecac, and it was concluded that activated charcoal/cathartic used alone is superior to other treatment. Similarly, a randomized crossover study in six healthy adult volunteers comparing ipecac with activated charcoal following therapeutic doses of acetaminophen, tetracycline, and aminophylline found activated charcoal significantly more effective than ipecac in reducing drug absorption (20). In both of these studies therapeutic or subtoxic doses were given, so extrapolation of these results to the overdosed patient may not be appropriate.

Tenenbein et al. (21) compared prevention of ampicillin absorption in human volunteers. Each volunteer was given 5 grams of ampicillin and then gastric lavage, ipecac, or activated charcoal and a cathartic in a crossover design with a washout period between each phase. The amount absorbed was compared to a control phase, which used no procedures to limit absorption. Charcoal and cathartic were most effective, preventing absorption of 57%, followed by ipecac, 38%, and gastric lavage, 32%.

A prospective, randomized, unblinded trial comparing charcoal alone versus ipecac and charcoal was performed in 70 children over a 2-year period. A statistically significant increase was seen in the hours in the emergency department (ED) prior to charcoal administration, the proportion of patients who vomited charcoal, and the amount of time discharged patients spend in the ED in the ipecac and charcoal groups as compared with charcoal alone (22).

There was not a statistically significant difference in either the proportion of patients admitted or the proportion that improved in the ED between groups. The number of patients evaluated was small, and it is likely that there was insufficient power to determine whether there was, in fact, a difference.

Several studies have attempted to evaluate outcomes of overdosed patients given different GI decontamination procedures. Kulig et al. performed a prospective randomized study of ipecac or lavage plus activated charcoal and a cathartic versus activated charcoal and a cathartic in 592 acute oral drug overdose patients (23). There were no differences between the two groups in the number of hospital days, number of days in the intensive care unit, clinical deterioration, and morbidity and mortality. This study has been criticized, since the seven sickest patients were assigned to the lavage group in an unrandom manner and patients were excluded if they took agents not adsorbed by charcoal (24). Both maneuvers biased the study against showing a benefit for gastric emptying.

Merigian et al. prospectively studied presumed overdose patients (25). Symptomatic patients were randomly assigned to receive either gastric emptying or activated charcoal. Asymptomatic patients were either just observed or given activated charcoal. The authors concluded that activated charcoal provided no benefit in asymptomatic patients and that gastric emptying did not improve outcome and increased the likelihood of aspiration pneumonitis. As Perrone points out, however, there was a bias toward nonemptying, since the population had limited toxicity and patients who took agents not well adsorbed by charcoal, or with delayed toxicity, were excluded (24).

Albertson compared ipecac syrup and activated charcoal to activated charcoal alone in 200 overdose patients (26). The only statistically significant difference was in the mean time the patients spent in the emergency room, with a mean of 6.8 hours in the ipecac and charcoal group and 6.0 hours in the activated charcoal alone group. There was no difference in the percentage hospitalized, the percentage admitted to an ICU or the number of hospital or ICU days. A difference was seen in the percentage of patients developing complications with 5.4% in the ipecac and charcoal group (primarily aspiration pneumonitis) as compared with 0.9% in the charcoal alone group.

Overall, these data suggest a limited role for gastric emptying. The majority of patients treated in a health care facility can be managed with activated charcoal alone. Gastric lavage should be considered in adults who present early and have taken potentially life-threatening substances. GI decontamination with activated charcoal and a cathartic appears to be as effective as, or superior to, gastric emptying with ipecac or lavage. Some poison centers have adopted protocols that recommend activated charcoal and a cathartic only for GI decontamination in

hospital treated patients. Ipecac syrup continues to have a significant role in patients who do not require treatment in a health care facility.

Emetics

Emetics are agents that induce vomiting. Although emetics can act locally on the GI tract or centrally through stimulation of the chemoreceptor trigger zone and the vomiting center, vomiting occurs only if the medullary centers are still responsive. Emetics are absolutely contraindicated in the following situations:

1. Patients with significant CNS depression manifested by severe lethargy, loss of the gag reflex, or unconsciousness, since the risk of aspiration of the vomitus into the lungs, a potentially severe complication, is significant.
2. Patients who are seizing or in whom seizures are imminent, since aspiration is a significant risk.
3. Patients who have ingested a caustic agent, since strong acids and bases may produce severe burns of the mucous membranes of the mouth and esophagus. Inducing emesis will reexpose these tissues to the caustic agent and further damage may occur. In addition, the force of vomiting may cause perforation of the damaged esophagus.

There has been some concern that emetics may be ineffective in patients who have overdosed on drugs with antiemetic properties. Two studies concluded that antiemetics do not significantly interfere with the effectiveness of emetics (27, 28). However, both studies failed to address such issues as the amount of antiemetic ingested and the time between ingestion and emesis, or document through laboratory analysis whether a sufficient quantity of the ingested agent was present to produce an antiemetic effect. Three cases of serious toxicity related to ipecac administration involved patients who ingested a phenothiazine, failed to vomit with ipecac, and developed cardiac toxicity (29, 30). Therefore, caution may be warranted in phenothiazine ingestions, and ipecac should be reserved for asymptomatic patients who have ingested the antiemetic within the past hour.

Another controversial issue involves the use of emetics in hydrocarbon (e.g., kerosene, gasoline) exposures. Because of their low viscosity, low surface tension, and high volatility, hydrocarbons are likely to be aspirated and produce significant pulmonary toxicity. When aliphatic hydrocarbons are ingested, emptying the stomach is unnecessary, since absorption from the GI tract does not appear to be responsible for toxicity. Ingestions of aromatic hydrocarbons, halogenated hydrocarbons, or potentially dangerous chemicals (such as pesticides in a hydrocarbon solvent) may require gastric emptying. Two retrospective studies have concluded that ipecac-induced emesis does not increase the risk of aspiration of hydrocarbons (31, 32). Based on these studies and recent clinical experience, syrup of ipecac can be safely administered under medical supervision following the ingestion of a systemically toxic hydrocarbon; however, in many of these instances it is unnecessary and activated charcoal is preferred.

Syrup of ipecac is considered the emetic of choice both in the home and in hospital settings. It is a local and centrally acting emetic, and is available without prescription in 15- and 30-mL containers. Analysis of reports from various sources suggests that syrup of ipecac is almost 100% effective in producing emesis when 15 mL or more are given (33, 34). Although the use of ipecac syrup at home in children under 1 year of age has been questioned, several studies have demonstrated that ipecac syrup is effective at inducing vomiting and safe in this age group (35–37). It is, however, not recommended in infants less than 6 months of age.

Vomiting usually occurs about 18 minutes after administration of a 15- to 30-mL dose (33). The dose of syrup of ipecac is 10 mL in children under 1 year of age, 15 mL in older children, and 30 mL in adolescents and adults. Fluid administration is generally recommended. Although milk has been shown to delay vomiting from syrup of ipecac in adult volunteers (38), another study failed to demonstrate a delay in clinical situations involving children (39). At least 4 to 6 ounces of fluid are recommended in children and 12 to 16 ounces in adults. If vomiting does not occur in 15 to 20 minutes, the initial dose may be repeated one time. If vomiting still does not occur, the decision to lavage or administer activated charcoal in a health care facility would be based primarily on the condition of the patient and the potential danger of the ingested agent, and not on the fact that the ipecac remains in the stomach.

The most common side effects of therapeutic doses of ipecac are diarrhea and mild drowsiness. The adverse effects in children between 6 and 11 months of age and 12 and 35 months of age who were given ipecac syrup for a potentially toxic ingestion are summarized in Table 4.1 (35). Protracted vomiting (persistent vomiting for more than 3 hours after the initial episode) was seen in 4.2% of all patients. This is of concern because persistent vomiting may delay the administration of activated charcoal. Therefore, ipecac should not be given to patients who will be receiving activated charcoal.

Toxic reactions to large doses of syrup of ipecac or due to the inadvertent use of the fluid extract of ipecac, which is 14 times stronger than ipecac syrup, have been reported. The most frequent complications are GI and cardiovascular. In large doses, ipecac is a cardiotoxin and has been shown to cause reversible depression of T waves, bradycardia, atrial fibrillation, and hypotension. Death has been reported following ingestion of as little as 10 mL of the fluid extract in a 4-year-old child (40). A 14-month-old child died following a therapeutic dose of ipecac syrup, but death was attributed to an anatomic defect (41). A fatal intracerebral hemorrhage has been reported in an 84-year-old female

Table 4.1.

Development of Side Effects Possibly Related to Ipecac Administration

Side Effect	Patients with Side Effect (%)	
	6–11 Months	12–35 Months
Diarrhea	25.7	25.8
Drowsiness	19.0	19.5
Irritability/Hyperactivity	5.7	2.6
Coughing/Choking	2.9	3.6
Diaphoresis/Flushing	1.0	0.0
Fever	4.8	0.7

Modified from Reference 35.

given ipecac syrup and activated charcoal following a non-toxic amount of boric acid (42). Fatalities have also been reported in adults with bulimia or anorexia nervosa who take large amounts of ipecac chronically to lose weight (43).

Other potential emetics that could be considered to empty the stomach in a poisoning include apomorphine, copper and zinc sulfate, salt water and mustard water. These agents are not recommended because of lack of effectiveness or toxicity.

It has been noted that children frequently vomit following the ingestion of liquid dishwashing detergents. An evaluation of liquid dishwashing detergents as emetics found them to be effective in producing vomiting (44). However, poor palatability resulted in a high rate of refusal to drink the solution; 6 of 15 patients refused it or only drank half of it, and only one of these people vomited. The use of liquid dishwashing detergent as an emetic should be limited to home managed situations where syrup of ipecac can not be obtained within 30 minutes.

Gastric Lavage

Gastric lavage is a procedure in which a tube is inserted into the stomach through the nose or the mouth. The patient should be in the left lateral decubitus position with the head forward and down. The contents of the stomach are first aspirated through this tube. Fluid is then instilled into the tube, allowed to mix with gastric contents, and then removed via the same tube. The process is repeated until the gastric washings are clear. The procedure usually takes 20 to 30 minutes to complete.

Lavage may be performed in comatose patients. The patient's airway should be protected by prior insertion of a cuffed endotracheal tube to prevent aspiration. Patients with convulsions may be lavaged once their seizures have been controlled. Although lavage is generally not recommended in caustic ingestions because of the risk of perforation, there is some debate that the benefit of lavage with a small nasogastric tube by mouth may outweigh the risks following large ingestions of some caustics (e.g. acids).

Initial management of a caustic ingestion is limited to dilution with milk or water followed by an evaluation of the extent and degree of burns.

The lavage solution is usually tap water or a normal saline solution. In children, however, it is safer to use normal or one-half normal saline instead of water because of the child's limited tolerance for electrolyte-free solutions. Water intoxication, tonic and clonic seizures, and coma can result from a 5% increase in body water from absorption of electrolyte free solutions. Each wash is approximately 200 to 300 mL in adults or 10 mL/kg (usually 50–100 mL) in children. The procedure usually requires several liters of fluid in adults.

Activated Charcoal

As the only modality to decrease GI absorption, or following lavage, activated charcoal adsorbs any of the ingested agent remaining in the GI tract. Activated charcoal is an odorless, tasteless, fine black powder that is an effective nonspecific adsorbent of a wide variety of drugs and chemicals. Two characteristics are necessary for activated charcoal to be effective: (a) small particle size and large surface area, and (b) low mineral content (vegetable origin). For these reasons neither burnt toast nor charcoal tablets are effective. Activated charcoal products with higher surface areas have been developed (45). Activated charcoal has been shown to be relatively ineffective for cyanide, iron, ethanol, methanol, caustic alkalis, and mineral acids (46).

The dose of charcoal is approximately 10 times the amount of the ingested agent. Since this does not take into account that tablet excipients or food may bind to the charcoal, which decreases its adsorptive capacity, it is a good idea to give an excess of charcoal. The usual doses of activated charcoal are 60 to 100 grams in adults or 15 to 30 grams in children. One level measuring tablespoonful of activated charcoal contains between 5 and 6 grams. If commercially packaged charcoal products are not used, the pharmacy should prepackage weighed charcoal, since the density of charcoal products may vary. Activated charcoal should be stored in tightly sealed glass or metal containers. Prolonged exposure to vapors of the atmosphere will decrease adsorptive capability. Activated charcoal is mixed with water to the consistency of a slurry and is administered either orally or by lavage tube. Charcoal does not mix well with water and must be shaken vigorously. This is not as great a problem with commercially packaged products, which contain sorbitol or a suspending agent.

Although generally only one dose of a cathartic is recommended, in some cases the activated charcoal is repeated. It is critically important to know whether a cathartic is present in a commercial activated charcoal product. A 55-year-old salicylate poisoned patient inadvertently received 30 grams of magnesium sulfate every 6 hours for four doses, 120 mL of 70% sorbitol for two doses, and an activated charcoal preparation containing 70% sorbitol for four doses (47). She developed an acute abdomen and died. Postmortem examination revealed a profoundly dilated bowel containing fluid and activated charcoal with a perforation at the hepatic flexure. This case illustrates that when multiple doses of activated charcoal are given, it is essential that an activated charcoal preparation that does not contain a cathartic be available.

Cathartics

Cathartics are used in conjunction with activated charcoal to further decrease the absorption of the ingested agent from the GI tract. By enhancing transit of gastric contents, the likelihood of absorption is decreased. A study in rats demonstrated that sodium sulfate enhanced the effect of activated charcoal in preventing the absorption of the drugs tested (48). There are no clinical studies in overdose patients to document the efficacy of cathartics, and studies in human volunteers have shown conflicting findings. Two studies in human volunteers found that cathartics had no effect on aspirin absorption when used with activated charcoal (49, 50). A study utilizing sorbitol as the cathartic demonstrated that activated charcoal and sorbitol significantly reduced aspirin absorption compared with activated charcoal alone (51). An additional effect of cathartics has been demonstrated when the ingested agent is a sustained release product (52).

Saline cathartics, such as magnesium sulfate and magnesium citrate, or hyperosmotic cathartics, such as sorbitol, are the agents of choice. Irritant cathartics, such as aloes or cascara, and oil-based cathartics, such as castor oil, are not recommended.

Magnesium sulfate is administered orally in approximately a 10% concentration at 250 mg/kg or 15 to 20 grams in an adult. Magnesium sulfate is available as epsom salts or as a sterile 10 or 50% solution. Magnesium citrate is used in a dose of 200 mL in adolescents and adults or 5 mL/kg in children. The adult dose of sorbitol is usually 1 to 3 g/kg as a 35-70% solution and the children's dose is 1 to 1.5 g/kg as a 35% solution. Cathartics are administered orally or via lavage tube. If charcoal has been administered, the appearance of a charcoal stool indicates that the charcoal (and hopefully the toxic agent) has passed through the GI tract. A study in human volunteers demonstrated that sorbitol enhanced gastrointestinal transit of charcoal to a greater extent than magnesium citrate or magnesium sulfate (53). The onset time of sorbitol is most rapid, followed by magnesium citrate and then magnesium sulfate. These cathartics are generally considered safe. However, the patient's hydration and electrolyte balance should be monitored, especially if repeated doses of the cathartic are administered. Cathartics containing magnesium should not be used in patients with decreased renal function, since absorbed magnesium may accumulate and produce toxicity. Hypermagnesemia has been reported following a single 17.5-g dose of magnesium citrate in a 77-year-old theophylline intoxicated woman with poor renal function (54).

HASTENING EXCRETION

If a poison has been absorbed in potentially dangerous quantities, multiple-dose activated charcoal, forced diuresis, alteration of urine pH, dialysis, and hemoperfusion can be considered. These procedures are not warranted in the majority of poisoned patients and do not replace supportive care.

Multiple-Dose Activated Charcoal

Elimination via the GI tract can be augmented for drugs that are secreted into the stomach or undergo biliary secretion. The use of multiple doses of activated charcoal has also been termed "gastrointestinal dialysis." Multiple doses of activated charcoal are routinely recommended for theophylline and phenobarbital overdose. The excretion half-life for theophylline has been reported to decrease by from 50 to 75% following multiple doses of activated charcoal (55, 56). A randomized trial in patients with phenobarbital overdose demonstrated a reduction in phenobarbital half-life in the multiple-dose versus single-dose charcoal groups, but found no differences in the time until extubation or patient outcome (57). With the cyclic antidepressants, which undergo enterohepatic recycling, the effectiveness of multiple-dose charcoal has not been convincingly demonstrated (58–61). Conflicting evidence has been presented for salicylates. Most recently Mayer et al. have shown that multiple-dose charcoal did not enhance excretion of salicylate in human volunteers (62).

Based primarily on human volunteer and animal studies multiple-dose activated charcoal may be considered to increase the clearance of

Amitriptyline	Digoxin	Phenylbutazone
Carbamazepine	Doxepin	Phenytoin
Cyclosporine	Glutethimide	Piroxicam
Dapsone	Meprobamate	Porphyrins
Desmethyldiazepam	Methotrexate	Proscillaridin
Dextropropoxyphene	Nadolol	Quinine
Diazepam	Nortriptyline	Sotalol
Digitoxin	Phenobarbital	Theophylline

Inclusion in the above list does not necessarily imply that multiple-dose activated charcoal is necessary to treat poisonings from these agents or has been adequately studied. A review of studies on multiple-dose charcoal found that increased clearance from multiple-dose charcoal has been demonstrated for only a few drugs and improved outcome has not been demonstrated for any

drugs (63). Aspiration of charcoal and charcoal-induced bowel obstruction are potential complications. A 39-year-old female on methadone maintenance therapy was given multiple doses of activated charcoal for an amitriptyline overdose (64). Peritoneal signs developed, and a laparoscopy revealed a 4-cm perforation in the sigmoid colon and a 120-g obstructing charcoal mass. Multiple-dose charcoal appears to provide the opportunity to increase clearance for some agents. Further studies are needed to demonstrate benefit before routinely recommending multiple-dose charcoal.

In multiple-dose activated charcoal regimens, activated charcoal is administered every 4 to 6 hours. A cathartic is administered with the first dose but is generally not administered with subsequent doses. When multiple doses of cathartics have been administered, fluid and electrolyte problems including hypernatremia and hypermagnesemia have been reported (60, 65–68).

Alteration of Urine pH

Therapeutic maneuvers to enhance the renal elimination of drugs can be considered when managing the poisoned patient. Despite the theoretical advantages of removing the drug from the body more quickly, there are no controlled trials documenting changes in patient outcome.

Only the un-ionized forms of weak acids and bases are capable of crossing membranes and being reabsorbed. For some drugs, adjusting the pH of the tubular filtrate will increase the amount of drug in the ionized form, thereby decreasing tubular reabsorption. The effectiveness of urine pH alteration will depend on the pK_a of the drug and the extent of renal elimination of active drug.

Urine alkalinization will increase the renal elimination of phenobarbital (not short-acting barbiturates, such as pentobarbital and secobarbital) and salicylate. Sodium bicarbonate is administered. Usually in adults, 88 mEq is added to the first liter of intravenous fluid; in children 2 mEq/kg is added to initial intravenous fluids and infused over 1 hour; subsequent doses of 1 to 2 mEq/kg as needed, with a goal of a urine pH of 7.0 to 8.0. An alkaline urine may be difficult to achieve in severely salicylate poisoned children and is not recommended by some clinicians in this subset of patients (69). Tromethamine and acetazolamide are no longer recommended as alkalinizing agents, since their potential toxicities may worsen the course of the intoxication.

Urine acidification will increase the renal elimination of amphetamines, phencyclidine, and strychnine; however, it is no longer recommended. Overdoses with these drugs, especially phencyclidine, can produce muscle injury resulting in rhabdomyolysis and myoglobinuria; in the presence of an acid urine, myoglobin can precipitate in the tubules, leading to acute renal failure.

Dialysis and Hemoperfusion

In the severely intoxicated patient hemodialysis or hemoperfusion may be considered to rapidly remove certain toxins from the blood. Hemodialysis removes drugs from the blood by diffusion across a synthetic semipermeable membrane. The dialysate is replaced, continuously or intermittently, with fresh solution of carefully defined composition. This is a specialized technique that is not available at all hospitals.

The use of dialysis in poisoning cases is limited to situations in which the ingested agent is dialyzable, distributed in or rapidly equilibrated with plasma water, and removed at a rate significantly higher than by normal metabolism and renal excretion. Because a drug is dialyzable does not mean that dialysis is indicated.

Dialysis may be considered in those patients who are severely intoxicated with a dialyzable drug and are not responding to conservative therapy. Dialysis may be indicated for severe intoxications with ethanol, isopropanol, lithium, phenobarbital, theophylline, and salicylates. Occasionally dialysis is considered when the agent ingested is not dialyzable, but the procedure will correct hyperosmolarity or severe acid-base or electrolyte abnormalities not responding to fluid therapy.

Two examples where dialysis may be indicated before significant toxicity develops are methanol and ethylene glycol ingestion. In both cases, these alcohols are metabolized to compounds more toxic than the parent compound. Methanol is metabolized to formaldehyde and formic acid; ethylene glycol is metabolized to glycolaldehyde, glycolate, glyoxylate, and oxalic acid. If the methanol and ethylene glycol can be removed by dialysis before metabolism, toxicity will be minimized.

Hemoperfusion involves pumping blood from the patient through a cartridge containing coated activated charcoal or uncoated activated charcoal in a fixed-bed system. For the treatment to be effective, not only must the toxin be adsorbed by the material in the column, but the amount removed by hemoperfusion must significantly reduce the total body burden of the ingested agent. For some drugs that are effectively adsorbed, such as the cyclic antidepressants, a large volume of distribution results in a relatively small proportion of the total body burden being eliminated, even if the blood is completely cleared of the drug after passing through the column. Theophylline is an example of a drug for which hemoperfusion has been found to be extremely effective, producing a marked drop in blood levels and a rapid improvement in the clinical picture (70). Potential complications include bleeding, destruction of blood cells (including a significant drop in the platelet count immediately following the procedure), removal of plasma proteins, and hypothermia (71).

As with dialysis, hemoperfusion should be limited to those severely intoxicated patients who have ingested a hemoperfusable drug and are not responding to conservative therapy. In most situations, aggressive supportive care should be adequate to maintain the patient until his or her own body is able to detoxify and eliminate the toxin.

SYSTEMIC ANTIDOTES

Systemic antidotes are available for only a few commonly ingested agents. Antidotes act by a variety of mechanisms to antagonize the effects of a systemically absorbed toxin. Antidotes do not replace supportive care and other previously described treatment modalities. If an antidote is available for a particular intoxicant, specific indications should be considered before its use. Included in Table 4.2 is a list of major systemic antidotes. Naloxone, deferoxamine, digoxin immune Fab, and N-acetylcysteine are also discussed below.

Naloxone

Naloxone is a pure opiate antagonist without opiate agonist properties. The use of nalorphine and levallorphan has been abandoned because they have both opiate agonist and antagonist properties. Naloxone is one of the most commonly used antidotes.

Naloxone directly competes with the opiate for the receptor site, reversing CNS and respiratory depression. The antagonistic effects can be as short as 30 minutes but may last as long as 1 to 4 hours. It is important to note that the antagonistic action of naloxone may be shorter than the duration of action of the ingested opiate, especially methadone and diphenoxylate. It is very important that these patients be monitored closely so that naloxone boluses can be readministered or a naloxone infusion be started if needed.

Naloxone antagonizes naturally occurring and synthetic opiates, including heroin, morphine, codeine, meperidine, propoxyphene, pentazocine, diphenoxylate, and dextromethorphan. For some opiates, particularly propoxyphene, larger than usual doses of naloxone may be required. Naloxone is indicated in opiate intoxications with CNS and respiratory depression. It is also frequently used diagnostically, along with glucose and thiamine, in all comatose patients presenting to an emergency treatment facility. If given at a high enough dose, naloxone will rapidly reverse any opiate-induced symptoms. Since naloxone has no opiate agonist activity, administration to patients in whom the coma is not opiate induced will produce no adverse effects.

The usual adult dose is 0.4 to 2 mg intravenously. Doses of 0.1 mg/kg or 0.4 to 2 mg have been recommended in children. If no response is seen, the dose should be repeated. At least 10 mg total of naloxone should be administered before ruling out opiates as the cause of toxicity. A continuous infusion of naloxone can be considered after the initial bolus dose of naloxone reverses the

Table 4.2.
Major Systemic Antidotes

Antidote	Poison	Usual Dosage and Route	Comments
Atropine	Carbamate insecticides. Organophosphate insecticides. Other anticholinesterases	Test dose of 2 mg IV in an adult and 0.05 mg/kg in a child up to 2 mg; anticholinergic symptoms will be seen only if poisoning is not present. Doses are repeated as needed (up to 2000 mg/day in severe cases), with the end point being cessation of secretions	In severe organophosphate ingestion usually given in combination with pralidoxime.
BAL	Arsenic, gold, mercury, lead	Given by deep IM. Dosage variable depending on the agent being chelated and severity of intoxication. Usually 3–5 mg/kg/dose.	Contraindicated in iron, cadmium, or selenium since complex is toxic. For lead, used in combination with other agents.
Cyanide antidote kit (amyl nitrite, sodium nitrite, sodium thiosulfate)	Cyanide	Amyl nitrite—breathe 30 sec of each 60 sec until sodium nitrite is ready. Use a new ampule every 3 min. For adults 300 mg sodium nitrite (10 mL) is usually given IV, over at least 5 min, followed by 12.5 g of sodium thiosulfate IV. If symptoms persist, one half the above dosage of sodium nitrite is repeated. The dose of sodium nitrite for children depends on the hemoglobin level and is included in the package literature. Children are given 1.65 mg/kg of sodium thiosulfate.	Overzealous administration of sodium nitrite especially in children can produce severe methemoglobinemia.
Deferoxamine	Iron	15 mg/kg/hr IV (see text). A maximum of 6.0 g in either children or adults/24 hr should not generally be exceeded.	Indications: serum iron ≥ 90 umol/liter (500 µg/dL) and/or symptomatic patients. Pink-red urine indicates the presence of the deferoxamine-iron chelate; urine color change is not always present.
Digoxin immune Fab (Digibind)	Digoxin Digitoxin	Administered IV. Dose = body load (mg)/0.6 (mg/vial) See package insert for dosing. Tables based on amount ingested or levels.	Only indicated in severe cases unresponsive to standard antiarrhythmics (see text). Total serum digoxin level will increase dramatically after administration but the digoxin is bound to the Fab fragment and is not toxic.
Diphenhydramine	Phenothiazine induced extrapyramidal symptoms	Adults: 50 mg IV. Children: 1–2 mg/kg up to a total of 50 mg IV.	
d-Penicillamine	Copper, gold, mercury, lead, arsenic	Children 20–100 mg/kg/day PO (depends on the metal being chelated). Adults: 1–1.5 g/day.	Avoid in patients with penicillin allergy. Inhibits enzymes that are pyridoxal dependent, thus pyridoxine usually given concurrently (10–25 mg/day).
Ca-EDTA	Lead, zinc, cadmium, manganese, copper	75 mg/kg/day IV or IM given in 3–6 divided doses for up to 5 days. May repeat course after at least 2 days.	May produce renal tubular necrosis. If decreased renal function present dialysis may be necessary to remove chelate.
Ethanol	Ethylene glycol, methanol	Ethanol is given to maintain a 22 mmol/L (100 mg/dL) blood level. Loading dose (oral) is 0.8 mL/kg of 95% ethanol given over 30 min followed by an average maintenance dose of 0.15 mL/kg/hr PO. Loading dose (IV) of 10% ethanol is 7.6 mL/kg IV over 30–60 min followed by an average maintenance dose of 1.4 mL/kg/hr IV. Monitor blood levels of ethanol and adjust accordingly.	Chronic drinkers may require higher doses and nondrinkers may require lower doses. Dose must be increased if dialysis is used. Glucose usually simultaneously administered.

(continued)

Table 4.2. *(Continued)*

Antidote	Poison	Usual Dosage and Route	Comments
Flumazenil	Benzodiazepines	Initial dose 0.2 mg IV. If adequate consciousness not obtained in 30 seconds inject another 0.3 mg IV over 30 seconds. Further doses of 0.5 mg may be administered IV at 1-min intervals up to a maximum total dose of 3 mg. Most patients respond to 1–3 mg.	Contraindicated in patients who have taken tricyclic antidepressants or other cardiosensitizing drugs or who have been given benzodiazepines to treat seizures. Seizures may occur if patients are benzodiazepine dependent.
Methylene blue	Nitrates and nitrites	0.2 ml/kg IV of a 1% solution over 5 min.	
N-acetylcysteine	Acetaminophen	140 mg/kg orally diluted 1:3 with Coke, Fresca, grapefruit juice, or water as a loading dose. Then 70 mg/kg every 4 hours for a total of 17 maintenance doses.	Intravenous use is investigational (see text).
Naloxone	Opiates	0.1 mg/kg/dose IV in children; 2–4 mg in adults (see text)	Should be given several times if no effect before ruling out opiates as the cause of symptoms. Short duration of action.
Physostigmine	Anticholinergics	Children: 0.5 mg slow IV. If no response and no cholinergic symptoms, give 0.5 mg every 5 min until a response is seen or 2 mg is reached. Repeat lowest effective trial dose if severe symptoms recur. Adults: 1–2 mg slow IV. May repeat up to 4 mg total if no response and no cholinergic symptoms. 1–4 mg may be needed for severe symptoms.	Short duration of action. Atropine should be available to reverse cholinergic effects should they occur. Must be given slowly. Of limited usefulness. Avoid in patients where cyclic antidepressants may be involved or in patients with cardiac conduction defects.
Pralidoxime	Organophosphates, severe carbamate ingestions, but not carbaryl	Adults: 1 g IV over 2 min. Children: 25–50 mg/kg slow IV. Either dose may be repeated every 8–12 hours as needed.	Given in combination with atropine. Little benefit if administered more than 36 hours after poisoning.
Succimer (DMSA)	Lead	Children: 10 mg/kg PO every 8 hr for 5 days.	Monitor liver function at least weekly.

narcotic effects if (a) long-acting agents such as methadone or diphenoxylate are involved, (b) poorly antagonized agents such as propoxyphene have been taken, (c) large doses of naloxone were required to reverse the initial opiate effects, or (d) the naloxone needs to be repeated frequently to reverse recurring opiate effects. The infusion is initiated at two thirds of the naloxone bolus dose per hour. At 15 minutes after initiation of the infusion, half of the bolus dose should be readministered. The infusion rate is titrated against the patient's response. If the patient becomes symptomatic at a given infusion rate, symptoms should be reversed with a naloxone bolus and the infusion rate should be increased. In adults, the naloxone concentration in D_5W is usually adjusted to deliver the required dose in 100 mL of solution per hour.

Deferoxamine

Deferoxamine is a chelating agent that binds with ferric iron. The iron-deferoxamine complex (ferrioxamine) is less toxic and more easily excreted than iron alone. Ferrioxamine produces a pink-red colored urine in some patients. The presence of a color change indicates that free iron was present and chelated. However, the absence of a urine color change does not rule out iron poisoning.

Deferoxamine should be given in iron intoxications when free iron is present in the serum. This usually occurs at serum iron levels of 63–90 μmol/L (350–500 μg/dL) or greater. In iron-intoxicated patients whose clinical status suggests a severe iron intoxication (severe vomiting, coma, hypotension, acidosis) the use of deferoxamine should be considered before serum iron levels are available.

Deferoxamine is given intravenously at a dose of 90 mg/kg every 8 hours at a rate of 15 mg/kg/hr. Hypotension may occur at higher infusion rates. Higher infusion rates have been used in severe iron poisonings (72). In those cases where hypotension occurred, it responded to decreasing the infusion rate. The maximum recommended dose is 6 g/day, although there is no evidence to support this limitation.

The most common adverse reactions to deferoxamine include generalized erythema, urticaria, and hypotension. Four patients treated with 15 mg/kg/hr of deferoxamine for 65 to 92 hours developed adult respiratory distress syndrome (ARDS) (73). A further review of treated patients revealed that pulmonary toxicity was only of concern in patients treated with deferoxamine for longer than 24 hours (72).

Digoxin Immune Fab

Digoxin immune Fab (Digibind) can be lifesaving in digitalis glycoside poisoning (73). Digoxin immune Fab has a high binding affinity for digoxin, and the complex is renally excreted. Although digoxin immune Fab will bind digitoxin, its affinity for digitoxin is approximately one tenth of its affinity for digoxin.

Digoxin immune Fab should be considered in life-threatening digoxin or digitoxin poisoning from either acute or chronic exposure. Although serum concentrations of digoxin may be helpful in evaluating digoxin poisoned patients, determination of whether digoxin immune Fab should be used is based on the patient's clinical status. Digoxin immune Fab is indicated in patients with life-threatening arrhythmias (e.g., ventricular arrhythmias), conduction defects or progressive bradyarrhythmias (e.g., severe sinus bradycardia), or third-degree heart block, or in severe hyperkalemia resistant to treatment. Life-threatening digitalis toxicity was reversed in 21 of 26 patients in one series and 52 of 56 patients in another series with digoxin immune Fab administration (74, 75). The failures were the result of inadequate supply of digoxin immune Fab ($n = 2$), refractory low cardiac output ($n = 5$), anoxic CNS damage ($n = 1$), or multiple drug overdose with uncertain diagnosis of digitalis toxicity ($n = 1$). A potential complication of digoxin immune Fab is heart failure in patients with intrinsically poor cardiac function who depend on digoxin's inotropic effect.

Each vial of digoxin immune Fab contains 40 mg, which will bind 0.6 mg of digoxin or digitoxin. The dose can be determined either from the amount of digoxin or digitoxin ingested in acute poisonings or by the serum level in chronic intoxications. In general, the number of vials required equals the body load (in milligrams) divided by 0.6 (mg per vial). Tables to determine the dose in children and adults based either on the amount ingested or the serum concentration are included in the package insert. The total serum digoxin level will increase markedly after administration of digoxin immune Fab but the digoxin is bound to the Fab fragment and is not toxic. The serum potassium level will drop. Digoxin immune FAB was used in 174 (7.6%) of the 2,285 cardiac glycoside ingestions reported to the TESS database in 1993 (1).

N-acetylcysteine

N-acetylcysteine is indicated for the treatment of acetaminophen poisoning and was used in 7,493 (7.9% of all acetaminophen exposures) patients captured by TESS in 1993 (1). The major toxic effect of acetaminophen overdose is hepatic necrosis, which results from saturation of the enzymes in the nontoxic sulfate and glucuronide conjugation pathways and increased formation of the toxic metabolite by the cytochrome P_{450} mixed function oxidase system. Glutathione, which detoxifies the toxic metabolite in therapeutic doses, is depleted in overdoses. The protective effect of N-acetylcysteine relates to its activity as a glutathione substitute or precursor or to enhancement of the activity of the sulfate conjugation pathway.

N-acetylcysteine therapy should be initiated in adults with a history of ingesting 7.5 grams or more of acetaminophen, in children ingesting 200 mg/kg or more of acetaminophen, or in any patient in whom the amount ingested is unknown. N-acetylcysteine therapy can be initiated up to 24 hours postingestion but is most effective if started early. A study of 2540 patients with acetaminophen overdoses treated with oral N-acetylcysteine found that N-acetylcysteine therapy is most efficacious if initiated within 8 hours of the ingestion but that an effect on liver enzyme elevations could be demonstrated up to 24 hours postingestion (76). Improved survival rate and fewer complications have been demonstrated following late administration of N-acetylcysteine in patients with acetaminophen induced hepatic failure (77). A plasma acetaminophen concentration at 4 hours or more postingestion should be obtained and interpreted utilizing the modified Matthew-Rumack nomogram to determine whether to continue N-acetylcysteine (Figure 4.1). The nomogram, a semilogarithmic plot of plasma acetaminophen level vs. time, has two lines which define the plasma acetaminophen level as "no hepatic toxicity" (below the lower line), "possible hepatic toxicity" (between the two lines), and "probable hepatic toxicity" (above the upper solid line). A 4-hr plasma acetaminophen concentration of 992 µmol/L (150 µg/mL) is considered possibly hepatotoxic. A plasma acetaminophen concentration which falls at or above the lower line is an indication for the full course of N-acetylcysteine even if the level subsequently falls below the lower line. If the initial plasma acetaminophen concentration is below the lower line, N-acetylcysteine is not necessary.

N-acetylcysteine is approved for use in the United States in an oral dosing regimen consisting of a loading dose of 140 mg/kg followed by 17 maintenance doses of 70 mg/kg. Available in a 10% or 20% concentration, the solution should be diluted to a 5% solution before the patient drinks it or it is administered via a nasogastric tube. The main side effects of N-acetylcysteine are nausea and vomiting. Patients may have difficulty retaining N-acetylcysteine, which should be readministered if the patient vomits within 1 hour of the dose. Another consideration is the potential interaction between oral N-acetylcysteine and activated charcoal. The 39% decrease in the plasma N-acetylcysteine area under the curve when 140 mg/kg of

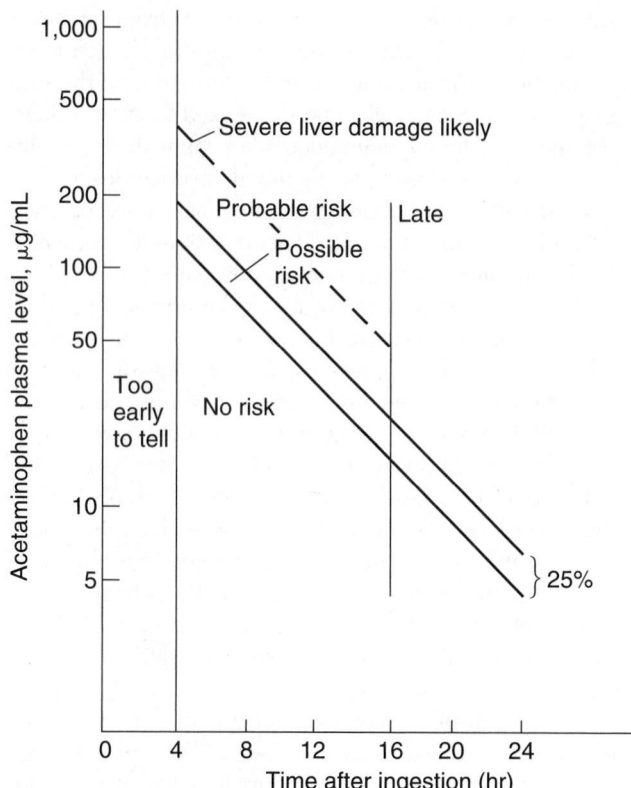

Figure 4.1. Rumack-Matthew nomogram for acetaminophen poisoning. Note: Plasma levels drawn before 4 hours may not represent peak levels. The nomogram should be used for single acute ingestions only. Adapted from Arch Intern Med 141:380-385, 1981. Copyright 1981.

N-acetylcysteine was administered 30 minutes after 100 grams of activated charcoal in one study (78) could be reversed by increasing the N-acetylcysteine dose by 40% (79). However, any adsorption of N-acetylcysteine by activated charcoal is generally considered to be clinically insignificant, since the dose of N-acetylcysteine is so large. Therefore, adjustment of the N-acetylcysteine dose is considered unnecessary, even when charcoal is administered concomitantly.

In Europe and Canada, intravenous administration of N-acetylcysteine is standard, with a dosage regimen consisting of 300 mg/kg over a 20-hr period. A 48-hr intravenous regimen was found to be superior to the 20-hr course but less effective than the 72-hr oral regimen in high-risk patients (80).

SUMMARY

Clinical toxicology provides challenging opportunities. To effectively function as an information resource, it is essential to remain up to date on new developments in this growing field. Management of the poisoned patient may involve providing supportive care, terminating the exposure, hastening excretion of the toxin, and administering

antidotes. A thorough evaluation of the patient and application of these general treatment principles to the specific poisoning situation are essential for definitive treatment.

REFERENCES

1. Litovitz TL, Clark LR, Soloway RA. 1993 annual report of the American Association of Poison Control Centers toxic exposure surveillance system. Am J Emerg Med 12:546–584, 1994.
2. National Center for Health Statistics. Vital Statistics of the United States. Washington, D.C.: U.S. Department of Health and Human Services. 2 (Part A):298, 1990.
3. Done AK. Aspirin overdosage: incidence, diagnosis and management. Pediatrics 62(suppl):890, 1978.
4. Anon. Tabulation of 1979 reports. U.S. Department of Health, Education and Welfare. Washington, D.C. Natl Clgh Poison Control Cent Bull 25:1, 1981.
5. Klein-Schwartz W, Oderda GM, Booze L. Poisoning in the elderly. J Am Geriatr Soc 31:195, 1983.
6. Manoguerra A. The status of poison control centers in the United States-1989: a report from the AAPCC. Vet Hum Toxicol 33(2):131–150, 1991.
7. Miller, T. Statement of Ted Miller, Ph.D., National Public Services Research Institute. Poison control centers: is there an antidote for budget cuts? Hearing Before the Human Resources and Intergovernmental Relations Subcommittee of the Committee on Government Operations, House of Representatives, One Hundred Third Congress, March 15, 1994, U.S. Government Printing Office ISBN 0-16-045845-5.
8. Mofenson HC, Greensher J. The unknown poison. Pediatrics 54:336, 1974.
9. Boxer L, Anderson FP, Rowe DS. Comparison of ipecac-induced emesis with gastric lavage in the treatment of acute salicylate ingestion. J Pediatr 74:800, 1969.
10. Goldstein L. Emesis vs. lavage for drug ingestion. JAMA 208:2162, 1969.
11. Auerbach PS, Osterloh J, Braun O, et al. Efficacy of gastric emptying: gastric lavage versus emesis induced with ipecac. Ann Emerg Med 15:692, 1986.
12. Tandberg D, Diven BG, McLeod JW. Ipecac-induced emesis versus gastric lavage: a controlled study in normal adults. Am J Emerg Med 4:205, 1986.
13. Litovitz TL. Emesis versus lavage for poisoning victims. Am J Emerg Med 4:294, 1986.
14. Suetta JP, Aminton DN. Residual gastric content after gastric lavage and ipecacuanha-induced emesis in self-poisoned patients. J R Soc Med 84:35–38, 1991.
15. Suetta JP, Marsh S, Gaunt ME, et al. Gastric emptying procedures in the self-poisoned patients, are we forcing gastric contents beyond the pylorus? J R Soc Med 84:274–276, 1991.
16. Corby D, Decker W, Moran M, et al. Clinical comparison of pharmacologic emetics in children. Pediatrics 42:361, 1968.
17. Arnold FJ Jr, Hodges JF Jr, Barta RA Jr. Evaluation of the efficacy of lavage and induced emesis in treatment of salicylate poisoning. Pediatrics 23:286, 1959.
18. Corby D, Lisciandro R, Lehman R, et al. The efficacy of methods used to evacuate the stomach after acute ingestions. Pediatrics 40:871, 1967.
19. Curtis RA, Barone J, Giacona N. Efficacy of ipecac and activated charcoal/cathartic. Prevention of salicylate absorption in a simulated overdose. Arch Intern Med 144:48, 1984.
20. Neuvonen PJ, Vartiainen M, Tokola O. Comparison of activated charcoal and ipecac syrup in prevention of drug absorption. Eur J Clin Pharmacol 24:557, 1983.

21. Tenenbein M, Cohen S, Sitar OS. Efficacy of ipecac, induced emesis, orogastric lavage and activated charcoal for drug overdose. Ann Emerg Med 16:838–41, 1987.

22. Kornberg AE, Dolgin J. Pediatric ingestions: charcoal alone versus ipecac and charcoal. Ann Emerg Med 20:648–651, 1991.

23. Kulig K, Bar-Or D, Cnatrill SV, et al. Management of acutely poisoned patients without gastric emptying. Ann Emerg Med 14:562, 1985.

24. Perrone J, Hoffman RS, Goldfrank LR. Special considerations in gastrointestinal decontamination. Concepts and controversies in toxicology. Emerg Med Clin North Am 12:285–299, 1994.

25. Merigian KS, Woodward M, Hedges JR, et al. Prospective evaluation of gastric emptying in the self-poisoned patient. Am J Emerg Med 8:479–483, 1990.

26. Albertson TE, Derlet RW, Foulke GE, et al. Superiority of activated charcoal alone compared with ipecac and activated charcoal in the treatment of acute toxic ingestions. Ann Emerg Med 18:56–59, 1989.

27. Thomas M, Verhulst H. Ipecac syrup in antiemetic ingestions. JAMA 195:147, 1966.

28. Manoguerra AS, Krenzelok EP. Rapid emesis from high-dose ipecac syrup in adults and children intoxicated with antiemetics and other drugs. Am J Hosp Pharm 35:1360, 1978.

29. Bourianoff G. No time for ipecac. Emerg Med 3:5, 1971.

30. MacLeod J. Ipecac intoxication-use of a cardiac pacemaker in management. N Engl J Med 268:146, 1963.

31. Molinas S. A note on the use of syrup of ipecac by poison control centers. Washington, D.C. U.S. Department of Health, Education and Welfare. Natl Clgh Poison Control Cent Bull (March-April):4–6, 1966.

32. Ng R, Darwish H, Stewart D. Emergency treatment of petroleum distillate and turpentine ingestion. Can Med Assoc J 111:537, 1974.

33. Robertson W. Syrup of ipecac—a slow or fast emetic? Am J Dis Child 103:136, 1962.

34. MacLean W. A comparison of ipecac syrup and apomorphine in the immediate treatment of ingestion of poison. J Pediatr 82:121, 1973.

35. Litovitz TL, Klein-Schwartz W, Oderda GM, et al. Safety and efficacy of ipecac administration in children younger than one year of age. Pediatrics 76:761, 1985.

36. McCray EA, Bonfiglio JF, Sigell LT. Home administration of syrup of ipecac to infants. Drug Intel Clin Pharm 18:792, 1984.

37. Gaudreault P, McCormick MA, Lacouture PG, et al. Poisoning exposures and use of ipecac in children less than 1 year old. Ann Emerg Med 15:808, 1986.

38. Varipapa RJ, Oderda GM. Effect of milk on ipecac induced emesis. N Engl J Med 296:112, 1977.

39. Grbcich PA, Lacouture PG, Lewander WJ, et al. Does milk delay the onset of ipecac induced emesis? [Abstract]. Vet Hum Toxicol 28:499, 1986.

40. Bates B, Grunwaldt E. Ipecac poisoning. Am J Dis Child 103:1, 1962.

41. Robertson WO. Syrup of ipecac associated fatality: a case report. Vet Hum Toxicol 21:87, 1979.

42. Klein-Schwartz W, Gorman RL, Oderda GM, et al. Ipecac use in the elderly: the unanswered question. Ann Emerg Med 13:1152, 1984.

43. Adler AG, Walinsky P, Krall RA, et al. Death resulting from ipecac syrup. JAMA 243:1927, 1980.

44. Geiseker DR, Troutman WG. Emergency induction of emesis using liquid detergent product: a report of 15 cases. Clin Toxicol 18:283, 1981.

45. Cooney DO. A "superactive" charcoal for antidotal use in poisonings. Clin Toxicol 11:387, 1977.

46. Picchioni AL. Charcoal and saline laxatives for treatment of poison ingestion. Vet Hum Toxicol 21:132, 1979.

47. Brent J, Kulig K, Rumack BH. Iatrogenic death from sorbitol and magnesium sulfate during treatment for salicylism [Abstract]. Vet Hum Toxicol 31:334, 1989.

48. Chin L, Picchioni AL. Charcoal and saline laxatives for treatment of poison ingestion. Vet Hum Toxicol 21:132, 1979.

49. Sketris IS, Mowry JB, Czajka PA, et al. Saline catharsis: effect on aspirin bioavailability in combination with activated charcoal. J Clin Pharmacol 22:59, 1982.

50. Easom JM, Caraccio TR, Lovejoy FH. Evaluation of activated charcoal and magnesium citrate in the prevention of aspirin absorption in humans. Clin Pharm 1:154, 1982.

51. Keller RE, Schwab RA, Krenzelok EP. Contribution of sorbitol combined with activated charcoal in prevention of salicylate absorption. Ann Emerg Med 19:654–6, 1990.

52. Goldberg MJ, Spector R, Park GD, et al. The effect of sorbitol and activated charcoal on serum theophylline concentrations after slow-release theophylline. Clin Pharmacol Ther 41:108, 1987.

53. Krenzelok EP, Keller R, Stewart RD. Gastrointestinal transit times of cathartics combined with charcoal. Ann Emerg Med 14:1152, 1985.

54. Weber WA, Santiago R. Hypermagnesemia: a potential complication during treatment of theophylline intoxication with oral activated charcoal and magnesium-containing cathartics. Chest 95:56, 1989.

55. Berlinger WG, Spector R, Goldberg MJ, et al. Enhancement of theophylline clearance by oral activated charcoal. Clin Pharmacol Ther 33:351, 1983.

56. Ohning BL, Reed MD, Blumer JL. Continuous nasogastric administration of activated charcoal for the treatment of theophylline intoxication. Pediatric Pharmacol 5:241, 1986.

57. Pond SM, Olson KR, Osterloh JD, et al. Randomized study of the treatment of phenobarbital overdose with repeated doses of activated charcoal. JAMA 251:3104, 1984.

58. Goldberg, et al. Lack of effect of oral activated charcoal on imipramine clearance. Clin Pharmacol Ther 38:350–353, 1985.

59. Karkkainen S, Neuvonen PJ. Pharmacokinetics of amitriptyline influenced by oral charcoal and urine pH. Int J Clin Pharmacol Ther Toxicol 24:326–332, 1986.

60. Scheinin M, Virtanen R, Iisalo E. Effect of single and repeated doses of activated charcoal on the pharmacokinetics of doxepin. Int J Clin Pharmacol Ther Toxicol 23:38–42, 1985.

61. Swartz CM, Sherman A. The treatment of tricyclic antidepressant overdose with repeated charcoal. J Clin Pyschopharmacol 4:336–340, 1984.

62. Mayer AL, Sitar DS, Tennenbein M. Multiple-dose charcoal and whole bowel irrigation do not increase clearance of absorbed salicylate. Arch Intern Med 152:393–396, 1992.

63. Tennenbein M. Multiple doses of activated charcoal: time for reappraisal? Ann Emerg Med 20:529–531, 1991.

64. Gomez HF, Brent JA, Munoz DC, et al. Charcoal stercolith with intestinal perforation in a patient treated for amitryptyline ingestion. J Emerg Med 12:57–60, 1994.

65. Caldwell JW, Nowa AJ, Dehaass DD. Hypernatremia associated with cathartics in overdose management. West J Med 147:593–596, 1987.

66. Garrelts JC, Watson WA, Sweet DE, et al. Magnesium toxicity secondary to catharsis during management of theophylline poisoning. Am J Emerg Med 7:34–37, 1989.

67. Gren J, Woolf A. Hypermagnesemia associated with catharsis in a salicylate-intoxicated patient with anorexia nervosa. Ann Emerg Med 8:200–203, 1989.

68. McCord MM. Toxicity of sorbitol-charcoal suspension. J Ped 307–308, 1987.

69. Elenbaas RM. Critical review of forced alkaline diuresis in acute salicylism. Crit Care Q 4:89, 1982.

70. Russo M. Management of theophylline intoxication with charcoal-column hemoperfusion. N Engl J Med 300:24, 1979.

71. Pond S, Rosenberg J, Benowitz NL, et al. Pharmacokinetics of hemoperfusion for drug overdose. Clin Pharmacokinet 4:329, 1979.

72. Boehnert M, Lacouture PG, Guttmacher A, et al. Massive iron overdose treated with high-dose deferoxamine infusion [Abstract]. Vet Hum Toxicol 27:291, 1985.

73. Tenenbein M, Kowalski S, Sienko A, Bowden DH, Adamson IY. Pulmonary toxic effects of continuous desferrioxamine administration in acute iron poisoning. Lancet 339(8795):699–701, 1992.

74. Smith TW, Butler VP, Habert E, et al. Treatment of life-threatening digitalis intoxication with digoxin-specific Fab antibody fragments. Experience in 26 cases. N Engl J Med 307:1357, 1982.

75. Wenger TL, Butler VP, Haber E, Smith TW. Treatment of 63 severely digitalis-toxic patients with digoxin-specific antibody fragments. J Am Coll Cardiol 5:118A–123A, 1984.

76. Smilkstein MJ, Knapp GL, Kulig KW, Rumack BH. Efficacy of oral N-acetylcysteine in the treatment of acetaminophen overdose. Analysis of the national multicenter study (1976 to 1985). N Engl J Med 319:1557, 1988.

77. Keays R, Harrison PM, Wendon JA, Forbes A, Gove C, Alexander GJ, et al. Intravenous acetylcysteine paracetamol induced fulminant hepatic necrosis: a prospective controlled trial. Br Med J 303(6809): 1026–9, 1991.

78. Ekin BR, Ford DC, Thompson MIB, Bridges RR, Rollins DE, Jenkins RD. The effect of activated charcoal on N-acetylcysteine absorption in normal subjects. Am J Emerg Med 5:483, 1987.

79. Chamberlain JM, Gorman RL, Oderda GM, Klein-Schwartz W, Klein BL. The use of activated charcoal in a simulated poisoning with acetaminophen: A new loading dose for N-acetylcysteine. Ann Emerg Med 22:1398–1402, 1993.

80. Smilkstein MJ, Bronstein AC, Linden C, Augenstein WL, Kulig KW, Rumack BH. Acetaminophen overdose: a 48 hour intravenous N-acetylcysteine treatment protocol. Ann Emerg Med 20(10):1058–63, 1991.

CHAPTER 5

CLINICAL LABORATORY TESTS AND INTERPRETATION

CHARLES F. SEIFERT, J. CHRIS BRADBERRY, and BETH H. RESMAN-TARGOFF

Patient evaluation based on information obtained through laboratory data should support a good history and physical examination. If the laboratory data does not match the history and physical examination, the results should be suspect and the tests repeated. Several steps are involved in the collection, evaluation, and reporting of laboratory data. These multiple steps allow for an increased chance of error. Therapeutic and management decisions may be made daily based solely on a misleading laboratory value. Examples of errors of this type include estimations of creatinine clearances based on non-steady-state serum creatinine values, normal hematocrits in dehydrated patients, and the evaluation of total phenytoin concentrations in hypoalbuminemic patients. This chapter reviews routinely encountered laboratory tests not thoroughly covered in other parts of this text, including their regulation, critical ranges, clinical application, and drug interference. Sodium, potassium, chloride, carbon dioxide content, calcium, magnesium, phosphate, and urinalysis are more than adequately covered in the chapters on fluid and electrolytes, acid-base disorders, and renal diseases.

GENERAL PRINCIPLES

Specimen Collection

Blood and urine are by far the body fluids most frequently used for analytic purposes. Phlebotomists should be familiar with the test being performed and know the appropriate container for collection and how the collection procedure affects the results. Verification that computer-printed labels match requisitions at the nurses' station and the patient's wrist band is essential. Specimens should never be drawn without first identifying the patient. Proper techniques help avoid hemolysis and bacterial contamination. Particular attention should be paid to tests where timing is important (e.g., in relation to ingestion of food or drugs). Special precautions are necessary for blood cultures and specimens obtained from indwelling catheters, especially central venous access catheters. Urine collection must also follow a very strict procedure to ensure valid results. A freshly obtained urine specimen is crucial when testing for bilirubin, red cells, and white cells, as these undergo decomposition when

standing at room temperature. Unpreserved urine specimens are also predisposed to microbial overgrowth at room temperature. A good rule for all specimens is to deliver them to the laboratory within 1 hour of collection or refrigerate them. Proper techniques for performing each method of collection can be found in *Clinical Diagnosis and Management by Laboratory Methods* (1) or other textbooks on laboratory methods.

Methods of Analysis

Several methods are available in the clinical laboratory to assay desired substances in body fluids. Two commonly employed techniques are chromatography and immunoassays. The type of compound to be measured determines which assay is used. Certain methods are used for qualitative measurements and others for quantitative measurements. Qualitative measurements detect only whether the substance is present and not the quantity of substance. A urine toxicology screen is an example of a qualitative test in which knowing if a substance is present is usually more important than knowing its amount. Sensitivity and specificity are important determinants of a clinical laboratory test. Sensitivity is commonly defined as the lowest detectable value of a substance, and specificity as the ability to accurately quantitate the substance of interest in the presence of other interfering substances. Sensitivity and specificity are calculated by the formulas below.

$$\text{Sensitivity} = \frac{\text{True positives}}{\text{True positives} + \text{False negatives}} \times 100$$

$$\text{Specificity} = \frac{\text{True negatives}}{\text{True negatives} + \text{False positives}} \times 100$$

Ideally, sensitivity and specificity should each be at least 95%. Most clinical laboratories have strict performance criteria set for their assay techniques. These criteria vary widely between institutions and can greatly affect the accuracy of individual patient results. Most clinical laboratories use the most accurate method with the best automation at a reasonable cost. For each individual clinical laboratory, particular attention to accuracy, precision, and quality control is essential for reliable reproducible results.

Reference Values

Normal ranges are provided as a guideline, but individual laboratory results may vary considerably. Values outside of the quoted normal range may be considered abnormal but not important, whereas certain values in the normal range with a particular disease state are actually abnormal (e.g., normal hemoglobin in a patient with chronic obstructive airway disease). Laboratories may evaluate substances with different assays that are more or less precise. Certain tests are time dependent, and the time at which the sample is drawn is crucial in determining if the patient sample is truly within the reference range. This is especially true for most serum drug concentrations. Most of the normal reference ranges quoted in this chapter are reproduced with permission from D.S. Young (2).

Drug Interference

Medications affect laboratory test results in two major ways. Due to a drug's intrinsic pharmacokinetic, pharmacologic, or toxicologic properties, it may alter the formation, regulation, release, or elimination of the substance being tested (e.g., hydrochlorothiazide blocking the tubular secretion of uric acid, exogenous insulin effect on serum glucose, or toxic acetaminophen concentration effect on serum transaminases). Medications may also directly interfere with the assay used to detect the substance (e.g., ascorbic acid causes false-negative results with urine glucose by the glucose oxidase method). Each laboratory test discussed in this chapter will include a brief section on common medications that affect the test results.

Système Internationale d'Unités (SI units)

The impetus to convert all measurements of body fluid substances to a molar concentration unit is based on the fact that substances in the body interact on a molar basis. It also standardizes units internationally. Several societies including the American Medical Association and the American College of Physicians and their official journals (*JAMA* and *Annals of Internal Medicine*) have adopted SI units as their sole reference standard. Other journals still accept both sets of units. Reference laboratories in most hospitals and most clinicians in the United States have not accepted this change willingly and still use the old conventional reference standards. For each laboratory test in this chapter, both SI units and conventional units with conversion factors will be given. To convert from conventional units to SI units, multiply the results in conventional units by the conversion factor.

Laboratory Tests

SERUM CREATININE, SCR

(SI units: males = 50–110 μmol/L, females = 10 μmol/L lower [males = 0.6–1.2 mg/dL, females 0.1 mg/dL lower]; Conversion Factor [CF] = 88.40.)

Creatinine is an amino acid formed as a waste product of creatine, an important energy storage substance in

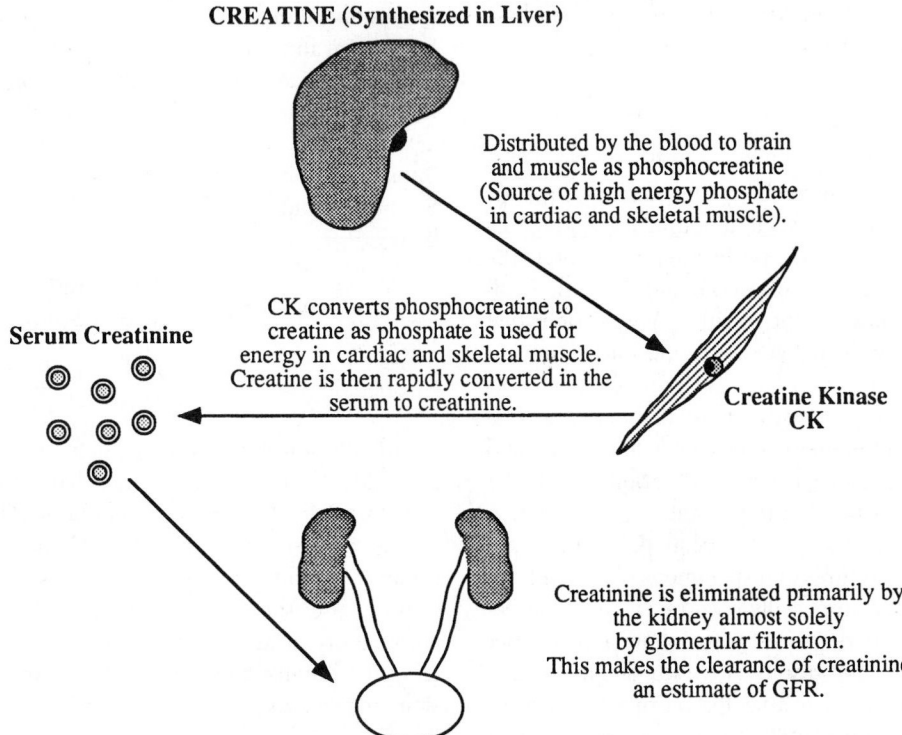

Figure 5.1. Creatinine production.

muscle metabolism. Creatinine is an anhydride of creatine and is not used in the body (3). Formation of creatinine is relatively constant, with about 1 to 2% of creatine transformed to creatinine each 24 hours (Fig. 5.1). This is in turn depends on the total muscle content of creatine and creatine phosphate. The serum concentration of creatinine is also relatively constant, and urinary excretion is the result of glomerular filtration, with only a small amount excreted by active tubular secretion.

Factors that affect creatine levels, such as diet, fever, and muscle damage, do not readily influence serum creatinine level. Since serum creatinine production is relatively constant and excretion is primarily by glomerular filtration, the serum creatinine level is a good index of renal function and is a more reliable indicator of renal function than the blood urea nitrogen (BUN).

Serum creatinine concentration increases in the presence of impaired renal function. Since up to 50% of renal function is lost before the serum creatinine level becomes abnormally elevated, it is not a good indicator of early renal dysfunction. Creatinine clearance based on 24-hr urinary excretion of creatinine is the most reliable clinically available test to evaluate glomerular filtration. Several methods exist for the rapid estimation of creatinine clearance based on the patient's age, ideal body weight, and serum creatinine level. The methods are discussed in more detail in Chapters 21, "Acute and Chronic Renal Diseases" and 1, "Clinical Pharmacokinetics." A steady-state serum creatinine level is necessary for an accurate estimation. Certain methods are more inaccurate in the elderly and in patients with decreased muscle mass (4). Other causes of increased serum creatinine include ingestion of creatinine in the diet, muscle disease, acromegaly, and pre- and postrenal azotemia. Decreases in serum creatinine are usually not clinically significant, but they can occur as an artifact when the serum bilirubin is markedly elevated.

Drugs that may cause an increased serum creatinine level due to interference with tubular secretion of creatinine are acetohexamide, cephalosporins, cimetidine, salicylates, and trimethoprim. Drugs such as ascorbic acid, levodopa, p-aminohippurate, and phenolsulfonphthalein may cause increases by interference with the analytic methodology of the serum creatinine determination (5).

BLOOD UREA NITROGEN, BUN

(SI units = 3.0–6.5 mmol/L [8–18 mg/dL]; CF = 0.357.)

Urea is the predominant end product of protein and amino acid catabolism and is made in the liver through the urea cycle. It is the main nonprotein nitrogen (NPN) constituent in the blood. Other NPN substances include amino acids, uric acid, creatinine, and ammonia. Total NPN determinations are no longer used clinically. Urea is distributed to all intra- and extracellular fluids and is freely diffusible across most cell membranes (3). Urea is excreted

mostly by the kidneys, with only small amounts excreted in sweat and in the intestines.

When there is a large increase of nonprotein compounds such as urea in the blood, the condition of azotemia is present. Azotemia can be categorized as prerenal, renal, and postrenal. Prerenal azotemia is the result of inadequate perfusion of kidneys with otherwise normal renal function. Causes of prerenal azotemia include dehydration, decreased blood volume, shock, and heart failure. Renal azotemia refers to decreased glomerular filtration as a result of acute or chronic renal disease. Postrenal azotemia is most commonly the result of urinary tract obstruction. There are two analytic procedures for the determination of urea nitrogen, a direct calorimetric method and an indirect enzymatic procedure. The enzymatic method is used today on most automated analyzers (3).

BUN can be used as a rough guide to renal function. As with creatinine levels, a clinically important elevation will not be observed until glomerular filtration is decreased by at least 50%. A decreased BUN is usually not clinically significant; however, a few conditions may cause a significant decrease. These include poor nutrition, high fluid intake, and severe liver disease in which urea synthesis is decreased. Drugs that may increase BUN by methodologic interference are chloral hydrate, chloramphenicol, ammonium salts, aminophenol, asparagine, acetohexamide, and sulfonylureas, and those that decrease it are chloramphenicol and streptomycin (5).

BUN and serum creatinine concentrations may be evaluated simultaneously. To give more information than either alone, the BUN is divided by the SCr. This is termed the BUN:creatinine ratio; the normal ratio ranges from 40 to 60:1. Table 5.1 indicates clinical causes of elevated BUN and serum creatinine with increased or normal BUN.

PLASMA GLUCOSE

(Fasting SI units = 3.9–6.1 mmol/L [70–110 mg/dL], but normal ranges depend on the method; CF = 0.05551.)

Laboratory determinations of glucose level are usually performed on venous plasma specimens. Whole blood determinations are only used for capillary blood used in

Table 5.1.

BUN:Creatinine Ratio in Clinical Conditions with Elevated BUN and Serum Creatinine

≥60:1	Prerenal azotemia (e.g., heart failure, dehydration)
	Postrenal azotemia (e.g., obstructive uropathy)
	Impaired renal function plus excess protein intake or tissue breakdown
	Drugs such as tetracycline and glucocorticosteroids
<60:1	Prerenal azotemia in hepatic cirrhosis
	Renal dialysis
	Renal failure in muscular patients
	Decreased urea production (e.g. low protein intake, severe diarrhea, or vomiting)

finger stick devices. Serum and plasma glucose concentrations are identical and are 10 to 15% higher than whole blood measurements. Along with fructose and galactose, glucose is one of the clinically important carbohydrates. Disorders of carbohydrate metabolism such as diabetes are evaluated in part by measurement of plasma glucose in either the fasting state or after suppression or stimulation. The concentration of glucose in the blood is regulated within narrow limits by hormones produced by the pancreas as well as through other mechanisms mediated by the adrenergic and cholinergic nervous systems (6). Glucose is a major source of energy for brain, muscle, and fat. The brain is the only tissue not requiring insulin for glucose utilization. If glucose is not available exogenously (fasting state), the body, through hormonal mechanisms (counter-regulatory hormones: glucagon, epinephrine, cortisol, and somatostatin), will form its own glucose by tissue and hepatic gluconeogenesis as well as hepatic glycogenolysis. Glucose is therefore carefully regulated by glucagon and

Table 5.2.
Classification of Hyperglycemia

Primary
  Insulin-dependent diabetes mellitus
  Non-insulin-dependent diabetes mellitus
Secondary
  Hyperglycemia resulting from disease of the pancreas
    Inflammation
      Acute pancreatitis (rare)
      Chronic pancreatitis
      Pancreatitis due to mumps
      ?Cell damage due to coxsackievirus B_4 infection
      ?Autoimmune disease
    Pancreatectomy
    Pancreatic infiltration
      Hemochromatosis
      Tumors
    Trauma to pancreas (rare)
  Hyperglycemia related to other major endocrine diseases
    Acromegaly
    Cushing's syndrome
    Thyrotoxicosis
    Pheochromocytoma
    Hyperaldosteronism
    Glucagonoma
    Somatostatinoma
  Hyperglycemia caused by drugs
    Steroids
    Thiazide diuretics, β-blockers, phenytoin, and diazoxide
    Oral contraceptives
    Alloxan and streptozotocin
  Hyperglycemia related to other major disease states
    Chronic renal failure
    Chronic liver disease
    Infection
  Miscellaneous hyperglycemia
    Pregnancy
    Related to insulin receptor antibodies (acanthosis nigricans)

Table 5.3.
Classification of Common Causes of Hypoglycemia

No anatomic lesion present
  Fasting plasma glucose normal
    Reactive hypoglycemia
      Functional hypoglycemia
      Alimentary hypoglycemia
      Diabetic and impaired glucose tolerance
  Fasting plasma glucose low
    Drug-induced hypoglycemia
      Sulfonylureas
      Phenformin
      Insulin
      Ethanol
      Salicylates
      Combinations of the above
  Factitious-fasting glucose normal or low
Anatomic lesion present
  Insulinoma
  Extrapancreatic neoplasms
  Adrenocortical insufficiency
  Hypopituitarism
  Massive liver disease

insulin secretion which compensate for food ingestion and fasting. (Please refer to Chapter 19, "Diabetes Mellitus" for a detailed discussion of carbohydrate metabolism in normal and diabetic patients.)

Methods for clinical determination of glucose are either chemical or enzymatic. Chemical analysis is based on the reducing properties of glucose and uses a color change reaction that is measured spectrophotometrically. The enzymatic method is based on the reaction of glucose and glucose oxidase. This is a very specific method and is generally inexpensive. Ascorbic acid can interfere with this method and produce decreased values.

Elevated plasma glucose concentrations, or hyperglycemia, can be caused by a number of syndromes and diseases. The classification of hyperglycemia is shown in Table 5.2 (6). A fasting plasma glucose of 7.7 mmol/L (140 mg/dL) or greater is considered abnormal.

Hypoglycemia is a syndrome of low plasma glucose with related symptoms. In the adult an overnight fasting plasma glucose below 2.5 mmol/L (45 mg/dL) is considered abnormal and above 3.0 mmol/L (55 mg/dL) is considered normal. In neonates less than 1.9 mmol/L (35 mg/dL) is abnormal and in infants and children less than 2.5 mmol/L (45 mg/L) is abnormal. Table 5.3 shows the classification of common causes of hypoglycemia (6).

URIC ACID
(SI units = 120–420 µmol/L [2.0–7.0 mg/dL]; CF = 59.48; see chapter on gout and hyperuricemia.)

Uric acid is the end product of purine metabolism. The major rate-limiting step in the synthesis of uric acid is the intracellular concentration of 5-phosphoribosyl-1-

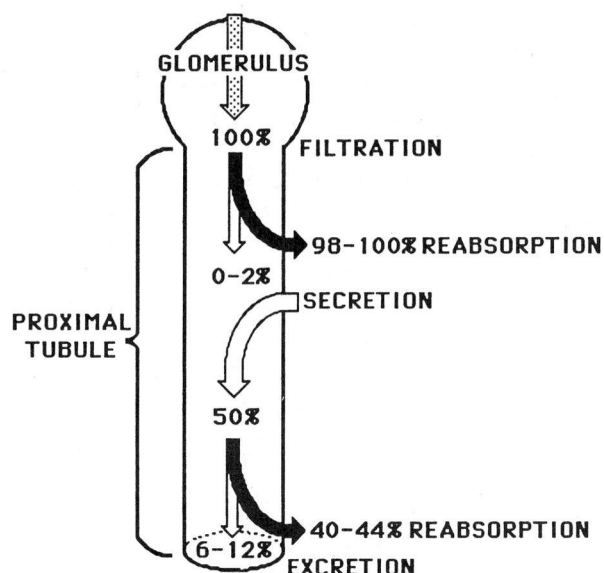

Figure 5.2. Uric acid excretion.

pyrophosphate (PRPP). Uric acid serves no biologic function. Approximately two thirds of uric acid is excreted renally and one third through the gastrointestinal tract. Assuming that the uric acid filtered through the glomerulus equates to 100%, 98 to 100% of this glomerular filtrate is reabsorbed in the proximal portion of the proximal convoluted tubule (Fig. 5.2) (7). Fifty percent of the original amount is secreted into the distal portion of the proximal convoluted tubule, but 40 to 44% subsequently reabsorbed, and 6 to 12% of the original glomerular filtrate eventually excreted.

Hyperuricemia is due either to an overproduction of uric acid (increased destruction of nucleoproteins, high-protein diets, or inborn enzymatic defects) or an underexcretion (renal defect). Since the serum is saturated with urate at a concentration of 420 µmol/L (7 mg/dL), as serum urate concentrations exceed this saturation point, monosodium urate crystals deposit in and around the joints and cartilage and in the kidneys, sometimes eliciting the disease known as gout. As urinary pH is increased, the solubility of uric acid is increased; decreasing urinary pH may precipitate urate nephrolithiasis in patients with high urine uric acid concentrations. Asymptomatic hyperuricemia is classified as an elevated serum uric acid without symptoms of acute gouty arthritis (7). With increasing uric acid levels, there is an increased risk of developing acute gout. There is a 2.0 to 4.1% 5-year cumulative incidence of gouty arthritis in adult males with prior serum urate levels ranging from 416 to 529 µmol/L (7.0–8.9 mg/dL) as compared to a 5-year cumulative incidence of 0.5 to 0.6% with prior serum urate levels of 410 µmol/L or lower (≤6.9 mg/dL). The incidence of gouty arthritis increases tremendously as urate levels rise above 535 µmol/L (9.0 mg/dL).

The 5-year cumulative incidence for adult males with prior serum urate levels of 535 to 589 µmol/L (9.0–9.9 mg/dL) and 595 µmol/L or greater (≥10.0 mg/dL) were 19.8 and 30.5% respectively (8). After one attack of gout, a patient may never have another or may have a recurrence from 3 to 42 years later (mean = 11.4 years) (8).

Agents that have a cytotoxic effect causing an increased turnover of nucleic acids may increase uric acid concentrations (e.g., antimetabolite and chemotherapeutic agents used to treat neoplastic diseases, such as methotrexate, busulfan, vincristine, prednisone, and azathioprine) (5). Agents that decrease the renal clearance or block tubular secretion may cause a substantial elevation in serum urate concentrations (e.g., thiazide and loop diuretics, pyrazinamide, and ethambutol) (5, 9). Diuretic-induced hyperuricemia accounts for 95% of acute attacks of gout in women over 60 years of age and 56% of men (10). Some agents, such as salicylates, probenecid, sulfinpyrazone, and phenylbutazone, inhibit the tubular secretion of urate at low doses, but at high doses also inhibit tubular reabsorption, inducing a marked uricosuric effect (3). Allopurinol therapeutically lowers serum uric acid by inhibiting xanthine oxidase (the enzyme that converts xanthine to uric acid in purine metabolism), while uricosuric agents such as probenecid are also used therapeutically to lower serum uric acid by blocking proximal tubular reabsorption. Ascorbic acid, glucose, levodopa, methyldopa, and theophylline may interfere with the analytic technique and cause false high results (3, 5).

Enzymes

Enzymes are located in all body tissues and are responsible for the organic catalytic conversion of chemicals throughout the body. When enzymatically active cells are lysed or destroyed, certain enzymes are released into the serum. These enzymes are measured to assess which tissue is damaged. Only active cells release high quantities of enzymes in the serum. The more acute and extensive tissue injury is, the greater the rise in enzymes released from that tissue. Chronic smoldering damage causes moderate release of similar enzymes, with patterns usually different from those in acute injury.

Isoenzymes are proteins with different amino acid sequences, arising primarily from different tissues, that have the same enzymatic action. Clinically these isoenzyme fractions are used to determine which tissue is damaged, and through their particular patterns clinical diagnoses are made. Isoenzymes are usually separated by gel electrophoresis. For example, creatine kinase has two enzymatic subunits, MM and BB. BB is found predominantly in brain and travels very rapidly to the anode, whereas MM, which is predominantly found in skeletal muscle, moves very slowly toward the anode (11). Even though the two isoenzymes have the same enzymatic activity, they are of different sizes and electronegativity and predominate in different tissues.

Enzymatic units are determined on a micromolar catalytic basis. One international unit (IU) is the amount of enzyme that catalyzes the conversion of one micromole of substrate per minute. The SI unit for enzymatic activity is known as the katal (kat). One katal is equal to one mole catalyzed per second (11). One μkat is equal to one micromole of substrate catalyzed per second; therefore, one μkat = 60 IU.

CREATINE KINASE, CK

(SI units = 0–2.16 μkat/L [0–130 IU/L]; however, normal ranges vary considerably with method, CF = 0.01667.)

Creatine kinase (CK), formerly known as creatine phosphokinase, catalyzes the conversion of phosphocreatine to creatine, releasing high-energy phosphate to skeletal and cardiac muscle (Fig. 5.1). Creatine is an unstable molecule and is converted very rapidly to creatinine. Creatine kinase is a dimer consisting of two subunits, M and B. Brain tissue yields approximately 90% BB (CK1) and 10% MM (CK3), cardiac tissue yields approximately 40% MB (CK2) and 60% MM, whereas normal serum contains virtually 100% MM, as does skeletal muscle. Clinical conditions causing elevated serum CK primarily involve skeletal muscle or cardiac tissue. The brain fraction is almost never observed in serum, even after a cerebrovascular accident, since the enzyme does not readily cross the blood-brain barrier (11).

Almost any damage to skeletal muscle will cause an elevation in serum CK. Severe acute rhabdomyolysis secondary to trauma, prolonged coma, or overdoses of various drugs may cause dramatic rises of CK, ranging from 167 to 1670 μkat/L (10,000 to 100,000 IU/L) (12). Other conditions damaging skeletal muscle such as progressive muscular dystrophy, polymyositis/dermatomyositis, delirium tremens, seizures, or hypothyroidism may cause significant elevations in CK.

CK is the first enzyme to increase in an acute myocardial infarction (MI). Serum concentrations begin to rise approximately 4 to 8 hours after the acute event, peak at 12 to 24 hours, and may persist throughout the initial 72-hr period (13). An MB fraction greater than 6% of the total is indicative of myocardial injury (14). Several studies have shown that patients with a history of angina compatible with acute MI in whom total peak CK serum concentrations were normal but MB isoenzyme fractions were greater than 6% of the total had true acute microinfarctions (15–20).

Intramuscular injections of medications may cause a variable increase in CK of 2 to 6 times the normal concentration. These elevations return to normal within 48 hours after cessation of the injections. CK rises in over 50% of patients receiving countershock or defibrillation but

usually returns to normal in 48 to 72 hours (5). Several medications have been reported to cause rhabdomyolysis in therapeutic and overdose situations, including opiates, cocaine, phencyclidine, amphetamines, theophylline, antihistamines, fibric acid derivatives, barbiturates, aminocaproic acid, certain antibiotics, chloroquine, colchicine, corticosteroids, and vincristine (12). Patients receiving therapeutic doses of neuroleptics may rarely experience the neuroleptic malignant syndrome, which may cause severe elevations in CK (21). Lovastatin has also been reported to cause severe rhabdomyolysis alone (0.5%) or in combination with gemfibrozil (5%), niacin, cyclosporine (as high as 30%), and erythromycin (22).

LACTATE DEHYDROGENASE, LDH

(SI units = 0.82–2.66 μkat/L [100–190 IU/L]; CF = 0.01667.)

Lactate dehydrogenase (LDH) catalyzes the conversion of pyruvate to lactate anaerobically to generate ATP (23). LDH occurs in high concentrations in cardiac and skeletal muscle, liver, kidney, lung parenchyma, and erythrocytes. It is essential to have prompt analysis of the sample, which has to be hemolysis free for an accurate LDH measurement. LDH can be separated into five distinct components. The five LDH isoenzymes are all approximately the same molecular weight but have different charges. LDH_5 has the greatest mobility and LDH_1 the least. Table 5.4 lists the LDH isoenzymes and their relative activity in each tissue (11).

Serum LDH is almost always increased after an acute MI. The serum LDH begins to rise 10 to 12 hours after the acute event, reaching a peak in 48 to 72 hours with prolonged elevation for up to 10 to 14 days (5). Increased serum LDH level, with LDH_1 greater than LDH_2 (flipped enzymes), occurs in acute myocardial infarction in approximately 80% of patients, but also occurs in acute renal infarction, pernicious anemia, and hemolysis (5). In a large myocardial infarction with biventricular failure, LDH_5 levels may also be elevated due to liver congestion.

LDH_5 may be markedly increased in hepatitis and may also be increased in other hepatic disorders. LDH elevations may occur 50% of the time in malignant tumors, usually with a nonspecific isoenzyme pattern. LDH is elevated in approximately 60% of patients with lymphomas and 90% of patients with leukemias. Marked increases in LDH_5 levels are seen in patients with skeletal muscle damage, including extensive burns and trauma. Pulmonary embolus and infarction may cause elevations in LDH_2 and LDH_3; if cor pulmonale is present, LDH_5 will also rise. In nephrotic syndrome, LDH_4 and LDH_5 will rise, but in nephritis and renal infarction LDH_1 and LDH_2 rise. All forms of hemolysis, including sickle cell crisis and drug-induced hemolysis, will cause elevations in LDH_1 and LDH_2 (24, 25).

Table 5.4.
Lactate Dehydrogenase Isoenzymes Nomenclature[a]

Nomenclature of Isoenzyme Starting with Most Anodic	Composition: Proportion of Monomers[b] in Each Isoenzyme	Relative Content[c] of Isoenzyme						
		Lung	Myocardium	Liver	Skeletal Muscle	Brain	Kidney	RBC
1	HHHH	+	++++	±	±	++	+	+++
2	HHHM	+++	++++	±	±	++	+	+++
3	HHMM	++++	+	+	+	++	++	+
4	HMMM	±	±	++	++	++	++	±
5	MMMM	±	±	++++	++++	±	++	±

[a]From Pincus MR, Zimmerman HJ, Henry JB. Clinical enzymology. In: Henry JB, ed. Clinical Diagnosis and Management by Laboratory Methods, 18th ed. Philadelphia: WB Saunders, 1991:250–284.
[b]Monomer H (myocardial). Monomer M (skeletal muscle).
[c]Content graded from ±, which represents almost no activity, to ++++, which represents high activity.

All drugs causing damage to the above-mentioned tissues will cause elevations in LDH. Hepatotoxic agents and agents inducing hemolysis will increase serum LDH concentrations (25, 26).

ASPARTATE AMINOTRANSFERASE, AST
(SI units = 0–0.58 µkat/L [0–35 IU/L]; CF = 0.01667.)

Aspartate aminotransferase (AST), formerly known as serum glutamic oxaloacetic transaminase (SGOT), is one of several transaminases responsible for transfer of amino groups in gluconeogenesis. AST is responsible for transferring an amino group from aspartate to α, β-glutaric acid forming glutamate and oxaloacetate (23). The highest concentrations of AST are located in cardiac and hepatic tissues.

AST is the second enzyme to increase after an acute MI, usually appearing within 6 to 8 hours after onset, peaking in 24 hours, and returning to baseline in 4 to 6 days (5). AST rises in virtually all types of hepatic diseases. Its peak concentration and ratio to other enzymes reflect the type of hepatic damage. These differences will be discussed later under hyperbilirubinemia.

Several medications may cause elevations in AST levels because of either direct hepatocellular damage or cholestasis (26–28). Anticholinergics and opioids cause elevation of transaminases due to spasm of the sphincter of Oddi (29). Several agents (commonly isoniazid and rifampin) may cause transient elevations in transaminase levels (26, 30, 31). Initially, dye binding techniques were used to assay for transaminases, which accounted for several drug interferences including isoniazid, but with newer ultraviolet techniques very little interacts with the assay (29).

ALANINE AMINOTRANSFERASE, ALT
(SI units = 0–0.58 µkat/L [0–35 IU/L]; CF = 0.01667.)

Alanine aminotransferase (ALT), formerly known as serum glutamate pyruvate transaminase (SGPT), transfers an amino group from alanine to α-ketoglutarate, forming glutamate and pyruvate (23). ALT is very specific for hepatic tissue and is almost always absent in acute myocardial infarction. It is much more sensitive to hepatic damage, and levels rise faster and higher than those of AST in most types of hepatocellular damage.

γ-GLUTAMYL TRANSFERASE, GGT
(SI units = 0–0.50 µkat/L [0–30 IU/L]; CF = 0.01667.)

γ-Glutamyl transferase (GGT) catalyzes the transfer of a γ-glutamyl group from one peptide to another (23). The kidneys, liver, and pancreas contain large quantities of GGT. Several isoenzymes of GGT have been isolated, but to date, no clinical utility for them has been found (11).

The elevation of GGT parallels that of alkaline phosphatase and rises higher in cholestatic and obstructive diseases than in acute hepatocellular diseases. It is always elevated in acute pancreatitis, and its rise is faster and greater than that of alkaline phosphatase in obstructive jaundice. GGT is the most sensitive biochemical indicator of alcohol exposure, since elevation exceeds that of other commonly monitored liver enzymes. In alcoholic hepatitis, GGT is usually the enzyme that rises fastest and has the highest peaks. Agents such as phenytoin and phenobarbital that induce the cytochrome P-450 enzyme system may cause elevations in GGT (5).

PHOSPHATASES

Phosphatases are primarily responsible for catalyzing cleavage of monophosphate esters and may be acid or alkaline (23). Acid phosphatases have optimal enzymatic activity at a pH of 5, and alkaline phosphatases have an optimal enzymatic activity at a pH of 9 (11). Acid phosphatase (SI units = 0–90 nkat/L [0–5.5 IU/L]; CF = 16.67) is primarily found in prostate, erythrocytes, and platelets. Approximately 60 to 75% of men with prostate cancer have elevated acid phosphatase concentrations (5).

Alkaline phosphatase (ALP), (SI units = 0.5–2.0 µkat/L [30–120 IU/L]; CF = 0.01667) is found in most tissues but is derived predominantly from hepatic, osseous, and intestinal cells (5). The placenta produces high concentrations of ALP in the third trimester as a result of high fetal osteoblastic activity. Children in the active growth phase produce ALP at two to five times adult rates. Serum isoenzymes may be separated through electrophoresis with acrylamide gel; however, this technique is not widely available clinically and separation of osseous and hepatic isoenzymes is still difficult with this technique (11). Heating of serum to 56° C will inactivate 90% of the osseous isoenzyme, and separation of the hepatic and osseous isoenzymes is readily achieved clinically with this method.

ALP is elevated in most disorders of bone involving osteoblastic activity. Metastatic disease to bone may cause substantial elevations in ALP levels. ALP is also elevated in acute fractures, hyperparathyroidism, osteogenic sarcoma, and Paget's disease (11).

ALP is secreted into bile, and an elevation may be the first clue to intra- and extrahepatic cholestasis (14, 32). Separation of intra- and extrahepatic disease cannot be separated by the peak height of the serum ALP concentration (32). When biliary obstruction is complete, ALP serum concentrations are almost always 3 to 8 times normal, whereas, in incomplete obstruction, concentrations are only 2 to 3 times normal (33).

AMYLASE

(SI units = 0–2.17 µkat/L [0–70 Somogyi units/dL; 0–130 IU/L]; CF: Somogyi to IU = 1.85, Somogyi to SI units = 0.031, IU to SI units = 0.01667.)

Amylase enzymatically cleaves large polysaccharides into oligo- and monosaccharides in the gastrointestinal tract through salivary and pancreatic stimulation. Amylase is present as α-, β-, and γ-amylase, but only α-amylase is of clinical interest. Amylase is present in a variety of human tissues including the pancreas, salivary glands, muscle, adipose tissue, kidney, brain, lung, fallopian tubes, intestine, spleen, and heart (34). Normal serum amylase is composed of approximately 40% pancreatic isoenzyme (P-type isoamylase) and 60% salivary isoenzyme (S-type isoamylase) (35). This percentage changes with age such that after the age of 70, P-type isoamylase comprises only 20% of total serum amylase (34).

Serum amylase concentrations rise within 6 to 48 hours after the onset of acute pancreatitis in over 80% of patients (35). Values over 4 times the upper limit of normal are highly suggestive of the diagnosis (34). This is a sensitive measure of acute pancreatitis, but it is not highly specific, since several other conditions may present with acute abdominal pain and elevated serum amylase levels, including biliary colic, perforated peptic ulcer, and mesenteric infarction (35). In acute pancreatitis the urinary clearance of amylase is increased, possibly because of altered renal tubular function. A urinary amylase to creatinine ratio of greater than 0.04 suggests acute pancreatitis; however, this method is unreliable because elevated ratios may also be

seen with other conditions, such as burns, renal insufficiency, and ketoacidosis (34, 35). The usefulness of isoenzyme separation is limited, since other intestinal sources also account for P-type isoamylase. Patients with acute alcoholic pancreatitis have normal serum amylase levels approximately 30% of the time (35).

Parotitis and mumps cause elevations of S-type isoamylase. Chronic alcohol consumption may also increase S-type isoamylase. This is an important consideration because alcohol is the most common cause of acute pancreatitis. Macroamylase is a circulating complex of normal amylase bound to either IgG or IgA (34). Analysis of macroamylase reveals variable amounts of both P-type and S-type isoamylase. Macroamylasemia is an acquired benign condition that must be separated from other causes of hyperamylasemia.

Medications that cause spasm of the sphincter of Oddi, such as narcotics and cholinergic agents, may cause elevations in serum amylase (5). Agents that precipitate acute pancreatitis include azathioprine, estrogens, thiazide diuretics, furosemide, sulfonamides, and tetracycline. With all of these agents, acute pancreatitis occurred within approximately 2 weeks to 4 months after initiating therapy (36). Certain pancreatic enzyme preparations contain amylase and lipase, which may elevate serum amylase and lipase values (5).

LIPASE

(SI units = 0–2.66 µkat/L [0–0.6 Cherry-Crandal units/mL; 0–160 IU/L]; CF: Cherry-Crandal to IU = 278, Cherry-Crandal to SI units = 4.63.)

Lipase hydrolyzes glycerol esters of long-chain fatty acids at the 1 and 3 positions, producing β-monoglyceride and 2 mol free fatty acid. Serum lipase should not be confused with lipoprotein lipase; since these are entirely different enzymes. Lipase is located in stomach, intestine, leukocytes, fat cells, and milk, but predominates in the pancreas (34). Serum lipase concentrations are usually elevated in patients with acute pancreatitis and are more predictive than amylase, but technical difficulty in measurement because of the long incubation period limits widespread clinical use (34, 35). Serum lipase increases at approximately the same time as amylase in acute pancreatitis, but elevations may persist for much longer than serum amylase. Serum lipase concentrations may also be elevated in other acute abdominal illnesses (35). Medications that may elevate serum lipase concentrations are very similar to those that elevate serum amylase.

BILIRUBIN

(SI units = Total 2–18 µmol/L, Direct 0–4 µmol/L [Total 0.1–1.0 mg/dL, Direct 0–0.2 mg/dL]; CF = 17.10.)

Bilirubin is a metabolic byproduct of the lysis of erythrocytes by the reticuloendothelial system (Fig. 5.3). The reticuloendothelial system catabolizes hemoglobin

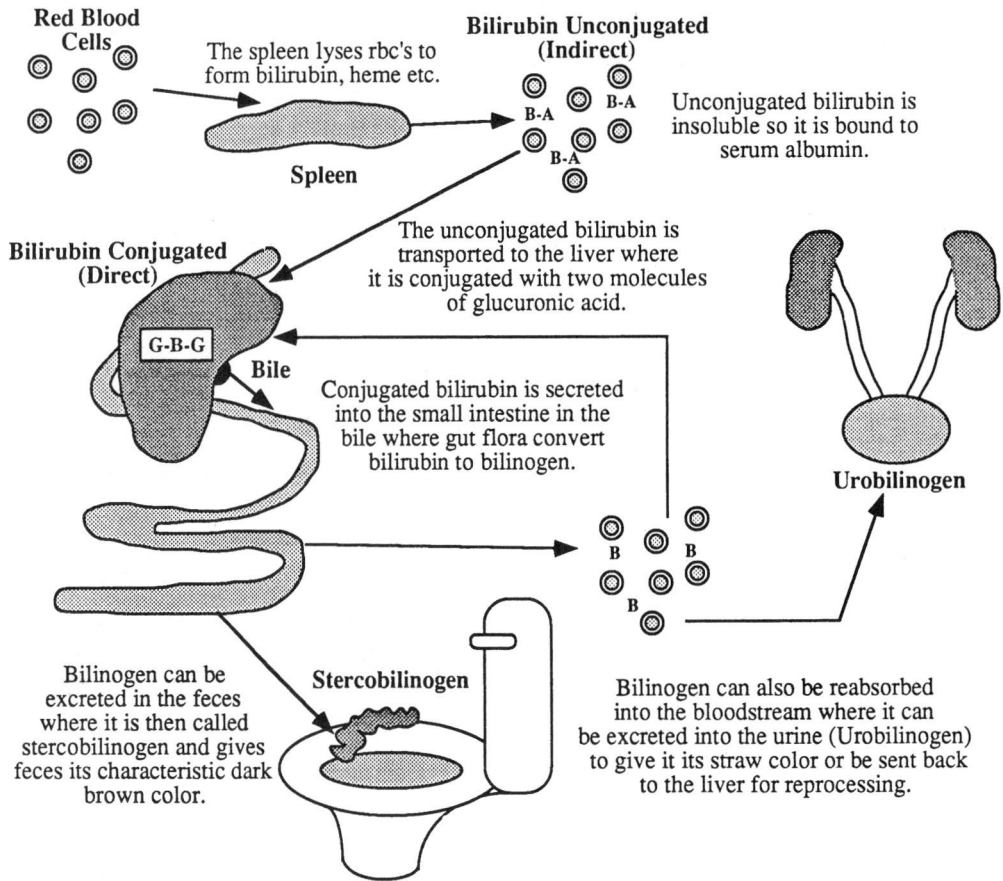

Figure 5.3. Bilirubin formation, metabolism, and excretion.

into free iron, globin, and biliverdin, which is rapidly converted to bilirubin. Unconjugated bilirubin is poorly soluble in serum, so it is transported to the liver bound to albumin. This unconjugated form is also known as indirect or prehepatic bilirubin. In the liver, glucuronyl transferase conjugates bilirubin with two molecules of glucuronic acid, forming bilirubin diglucuronide (33). This form of bilirubin is highly soluble in serum and is known as direct or hepatic bilirubin. Direct bilirubin is transported through the biliary tree with bile acids and stored in the gall bladder as bile. When bile is released during the digestive process, intestinal bacteria convert bilirubin into several compounds, collectively referred to as bilinogen. An estimated 10% of bilinogen is reabsorbed from the intestine into the bloodstream and resecreted by the liver. Small amounts of bilinogen are then excreted in the urine (urobilinogen), accounting for the urine's straw color. Most bilinogen, however, is directly eliminated in the feces (stercobilinogen), accounting for their characteristic dark brown color. Small portions of bilinogen are converted to bilins by intestinal flora which are also eliminated in the feces. The presence of bilirubin in the urine implies direct bilirubin, since indirect bilirubin is bound to serum albumin, which should normally not be filtered by the glomerulus (32). δ-Bilirubin is a protein-bound pigment that may falsely

raise total bilirubin measurements during hepatobiliary disease.

Causes of hyperbilirubinemia can be classified into three broad categories: (a) prehepatic (hemolysis), (b) hepatic (defective removal of bilirubin from the blood or defective conjugation), and (c) posthepatic (obstruction of the extrahepatic biliary tree), also referred to as cholestatic or obstructive (33). As serum bilirubin concentrations rise above approximately 34 μmol/L, classic scleral icterus and jaundice develop. Table 5.5 summarizes the enzymatic patterns of the common etiologies of hyperbilirubinemia.

Hemolytic jaundice results from the rapid destruction of erythrocytes, overwhelming the ability of the liver to process excess bilirubin concentration. Tissue hematomas or collection of blood in body cavities may increase the serum bilirubin. Severe sepsis or malignancy-induced disseminated intravascular coagulation, sickle cell crisis, or certain medications may induce hemolytic anemia. Drug-induced hemolytic anemia may be immune mediated (25) (methyldopa, penicillins, cephalosporins, quinidine, ibuprofen, and triamterene); hemoglobin oxidation mediated (37) (dapsone, antimalarials, sulfonamides, aspirin, nitrates, methylene blue, and ascorbic acid); megaloblastic mediated (38) (antineoplastics, anticonvulsants, and alco-

Table 5.5.
Usual Enzymatic Patterns in Hyperbilirubinemia

	Fecal Bilinogen	Urine Bilirubin	Direct Bili (% total)	AST	ALT	ALP	GGTP	LDH
Hemolysis	↑	–	<20%	nl	nl	nl	nl	↑↑↑ LDH$_1$>LDH$_2$
Hepatocellular Damage (Viral or Toxin)	↓	+	>40%	↑↑↑↑	↑↑↑↑↑	↑↑	↑↑	↑↑ LDH$_5$
Alcoholic Hepatitis	↓	+	<30%	↑↑	↑	↑	↑↑↑	nl
Obstructive or Cholestatic Jaundice	↓	+	>50%	↑	↑	↑↑↑	↑↑↑	↑ LDH$_5$
Alcoholic Cirrhosis	nl	±	<30%	↑↑ nl (25%)	↑ nl (50%)	↑	↑	nl

hol); or sideroblastic mediated with bone marrow suppression (39) (chloramphenicol, alcohol, lead, and antituberculous agents).

Hepatocellular injury from viral hepatitis, alcoholic hepatitis, toxin mediated hepatitis, or cirrhosis may elevate serum bilirubin concentrations. Viral hepatitis usually causes elevations in direct bilirubin levels. Viral hepatitis may cause extreme elevations in transaminases (167 to 334 μkat/L, 10,000 to 20,000 IU/L), with ALT levels usually greater than those of AST. Medications commonly reported to cause direct hepatocellular damage include acetaminophen, halothane, tetracycline, valproic acid, isoniazid, rifampin, methyldopa, labetalol, and tacrine (26–28). Drug-induced hepatocellular damage may be indistinguishable from acute viral hepatitis. Alcoholic hepatitis presents in patients with either acute or chronic alcohol ingestion. Transaminase elevations are only a fraction of those seen in viral or toxin-induced hepatitis. AST concentration is usually greater than ALT, but GGT levels may be markedly elevated due to the effects of alcohol on GGT release.

Patients with obstructive jaundice usually present with light clay-colored stools and dark cola-colored urine due to reabsorption of conjugated bilirubin from the biliary ducts, with redistribution to the urine and lack of bilinogen in the stool. The lack of bile acids in the gastrointestinal tract because of obstruction may cause steatorrhea. Transaminase levels are usually only mildly elevated unless severe obstruction occurs, causing hepatocellular damage. ALP and GGT concentrations are usually quite high. The most common cause of biliary obstruction is choledocholithiasis (gallstones) obstructing the common bile duct. Obese, middle aged women are highly predisposed to choledocholithiasis; however, it may occur in both sexes at any age. Other causes of obstructive jaundice include carcinoma of the head of the pancreas, pancreatitis, or other neoplastic invasion of the papilla of Vater. Cholestatic changes may be

due to an intrahepatic defect of the transport of bilirubin into hepatic canaliculi (33). Cholestatic jaundice closely resembles posthepatic biliary obstruction, except the stools are only somewhat lighter than normal due to less exclusion of bilirubin from the duodenum. Common medications that induce obstructive or cholestatic jaundice include C-17 alkyl steroids, estrogens, chlorpromazine, and erythromycin estolate. Other medications may cause a mixed picture of hepatic injury through an atypical (phenytoin) or granulomatous pattern (quinidine, allopurinol) (26).

Common pitfalls in the application of liver function tests in the etiology of hyperbilirubinemia include (a) dependence on single tests rather than patterns of abnormality; (b) normal results, implying no disease (cirrhosis has normal AST in 25% and ALT in 50%); (c) abnormal liver function tests, suggesting only liver disease; (d) failure to recognize hepatocellular disease with low transaminase and high ALP levels, or failure to recognize cholestasis or obstruction with high transaminase and low ALP levels; or (e) failure to repeat tests that did not correlate with clinical results (33).

Serum Proteins

TOTAL PROTEIN

(SI units = 60–80 g/L [6.0–8.0 g/dL]; CF = 10.)

Serum proteins are separated by serum protein electrophoresis into prealbumin, albumin, and globulin fractions.

Prealbumin. Prealbumin makes up a very small percentage of total protein (<1%) and is not widely used for clinical management. Prealbumin contains retinol binding protein, which plays a role in the transport and metabolism of vitamin A (40).

Albumin. (SI units = 40–60 g/L [4.0–6.0 g/dL]; CF = 10) Albumin is by far the most abundant serum protein. Albumin is synthesized in the liver and accounts for up to 65% of total protein. Albumin has three major functions: (a) controlling oncotic pressure in the plasma, (b) transporting amino acids synthesized in the liver to other tissues, and (c) transporting poorly soluble organic and inorganic ligands (40).

Albumin accounts for 80% of the oncotic pressure of the plasma. Capillary hemodynamics are controlled by four major forces: intravascular oncotic pressure, interstitial oncotic pressure, capillary hydrostatic pressure, and interstitial hydrostatic pressure (Fig. 5.4). Intravascular oncotic pressure and interstitial hydrostatic pressure are the forces holding fluid in the intravascular space, while capillary hydrostatic pressure and interstitial oncotic pressure force fluid into tissue spaces. Normally intravascular oncotic pressure overrides capillary hydrostatic pressure, having a net hemodynamic flow into the vasculature. These forces may be disrupted, causing local edema, ascites, or anasarca. Malnutrition, malignancy, severe trauma, or burns cause a net catabolic state, decreasing serum albumin and oncotic pressure. In hepatic cirrhosis there is decreased synthesis of albumin and increased portal capillary pressure, resulting in ascites. In severe sepsis, toxin mediated increases in capillary permeability allow intravascular albumin to escape into the interstitial tissues, accounting for increases in interstitial oncotic pressure. Nephrotic syndrome and protein-losing enteropathies cause increased losses of serum albumin resulting in anasarca. Congestive heart failure alters pulmonary capillary hydrostatic pressure, resulting in pulmonary edema. Table 5.6 summarizes changes in capillary hemodynamics resulting from various disease states. Dehydration and hemodilution may increase or decrease serum albumin concentrations.

Albumin acts as a carrier protein for both organic and inorganic molecules, which may bind ionically or covalently (40, 41). Several common medications that are highly insoluble in serum bind over 90% to albumin, including phenytoin, salicylates, phenylbutazone, first-generation sulfonylureas, valproic acid, warfarin, and certain sulfonamides (41). Since free drug is thought to be the active portion, changes in serum albumin concentrations may have a large influence on drug distribution and pharmacologic effect (42).

GLOBULIN

(SI units = 20–40 g/L [2.0–4.0 g/dL]; CF = 10.)

The globulin fraction comprises one third of total protein and is composed of four major components including α_1, α_2, β and γ (40). Important proteins located in the α_1 zone are α_1 antitrypsin, which is a scavenger enzyme for lysosomal proteases, and $\alpha 1$ acid glycoprotein (AAG). Young patients with homozygous α_1 antitrypsin deficiency develop severe pulmonary emphysema due to protein lysis by elastase. AAG is an acute-phase reactant that acts as a carrier protein for certain poorly soluble medications. AAG is increased transiently in a variety of clinical conditions, including burns, chronic pain, enzyme induction, rheumatoid arthritis, morbid obesity, myocardial infarction, malignancy, surgery, or trauma. Several common medications bind to AAG, including amitriptyline, chlorpromazine, dipyridamole, disopyramide, erythromycin, imipramine, lidocaine, meperidine, methadone, nortriptyline, phencyclidine, propranolol, and quinidine (41). The transient elevations in AAG levels during the previously mentioned conditions may cause important changes in the binding and pharmacologic effect of these medications.

The α_2 portion consists primarily of α_2-macroglobulin, haptoglobin, and ceruloplasmin. α_2-Macroglobulin is another major protease inhibitor; haptoglobin is a carrier protein for hemoglobin; and ceruloplasmin is a copper-binding protein. The β portion is composed of low density lipoprotein (LDL), transferrin, C3, and fibrinogen (40). LDL is the major transport protein for cholesterol to tissues; transferrin transports ferric iron stores to bone marrow for erythropoiesis; C3 is a major component of the

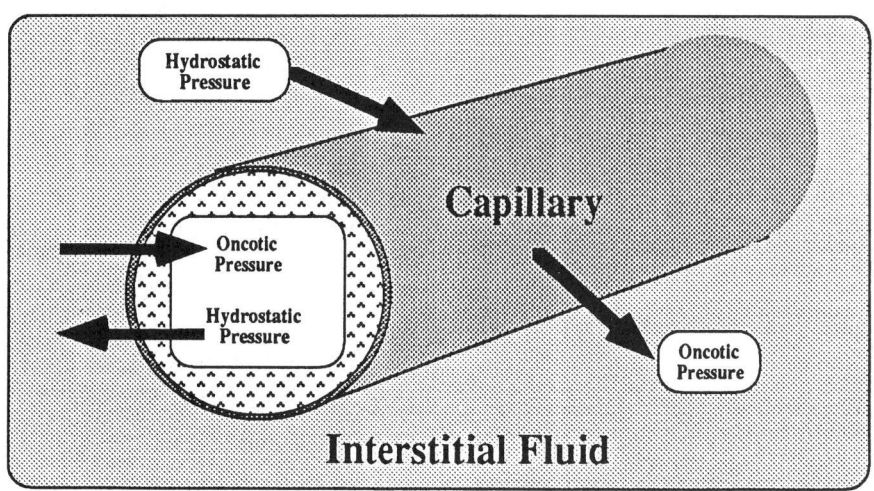

Figure 5.4. Capillary hemodynamic forces.

Table 5.6.
Common Disease States Resulting in Altered Capillary Hemodynamics

Disease	Mechanism	Serum Albumin	Capillary Hydrostatic Pressure	Interstitial Oncotic Pressure
Malnutrition	Decreased protein synthesis; increased protein catabolism	↓↓↓	nl	nl
Malignancy	Increased protein catabolism	↓↓	nl, ↑ Tumor Compression	nl
Burns	Increased protein catabolism; altered skin capillary permeability	↓↓↓	nl	↑↑, Skin
Hepatic Cirrhosis	Decreased albumin synthesis; increased portal capillary hydrostatic pressure	↓↓↓	↑↑↑, Portal	nl, ↑
Sepsis	Toxin altered capillary permeability	↓↓↓	nl	↑↑↑
Congestive Heart Failure	Increased pulmonary and systemic capillary hydrostatic pressure due to biventricular failure	nl, ↓ Malnutrition Due to Cardiac Cachexia	↑↑↑, Pulmonary and/or Systemic	nl
Nephrotic Syndrome	Loss of albumin into the urine due to glomerular damage and leakage	↓↓↓	nl	nl

Symbols: nl, normal; ↓↓↓, dramatically decreased; ↑↑↑, dramatically increased.

complement system; and fibrinogen is a coagulation precursor for fibrin. The gamma globulin portion is composed of antibody immunoglobulins IgA, IgE, IgG, and IgM. IgA is responsible for surface immunity; IgE binds to mast cells and is responsible for hypersensitivity reactions; IgM is responsible for initial humoral immunity and IgG for sustained humoral immunity (40). The primary disorder associated with hypergammaglobulinemia is multiple myeloma.

Complete Blood Count with Differential, CBC with Diff

The complete blood count (CBC) provides information about the erythrocytes, leukocytes, and platelets. The number of parameters provided with a CBC depends on the type of machine used for the analysis. Any other desired tests may be ordered separately.

In the normal adult, blood cells are predominantly made in the bone marrow of the sternum, ribs, vertebral bodies, pelvic bones, and proximal portions of the long bones (humerus and femur). The pathways of hematopoiesis from the pluripotential stem cell and the relationship between the different cell lines are shown in Figure 5.5 (43, 44).

ERYTHROCYTES, ERCS

(Males = $4.3–5.9 \times 10^{12}$/L [$4.3–5.9 \times 10^6$/mm³]; females = $3.5–5.0 \times 10^{12}$/L [$3.5–5.0 \times 10^6$/mm³]; CF = 1.)

The main function of erythrocytes, or red blood cells, is to carry oxygen from the lungs to the tissues. Anemia occurs when the hemoglobin, hematocrit, and/or erythrocytes are below the normal range. This can be a result of impaired erythrocyte production, increased erythrocyte destruction, or blood loss. The extent of anemia is generally described by the hemoglobin or hematocrit values. The red blood cell indices may be used to further characterize the anemia by cell morphology or color. Normal-sized Ercs are called normocytes, small ones are microcytes, and large Ercs are macrocytes. If there is abnormal variation in size, the patient is said to have anisocytosis, which is a feature of most anemias. Those with normal amounts of hemoglobin are said to be normochromic; those with decreased, hypochromic; and those with increased hemoglobin, hyperchromic. Abnormally shaped cells are poikilocytes (45). Polycythemia means "many blood cells" but usually refers to an increased red blood cell mass (43).

Red cell production is regulated by tissue oxygenation. Tissues receive inadequate oxygen if there is an insufficient supply in inspired air, impaired oxygen transport from the alveoli into the blood stream, inadequate hemoglobin to carry oxygen, abnormal blood flow, or a failure of hemoglobin to release bound oxygen at tissue sites (43). This can occur in diseases such as anemia, in cardiac or pulmonary disease, or with decreased oxygen tension in the air, such as occurs at high altitudes (44). Smokers tend to have a mild stimulation of erythrocyte production. Hypoxia or decreased oxygenation stimulates the production of erythropoietin, with about 90% being produced by the kidneys. A small amount of erythropoietin is produced by the liver. Erythropoietin stimulates and accelerates all aspects of Erc

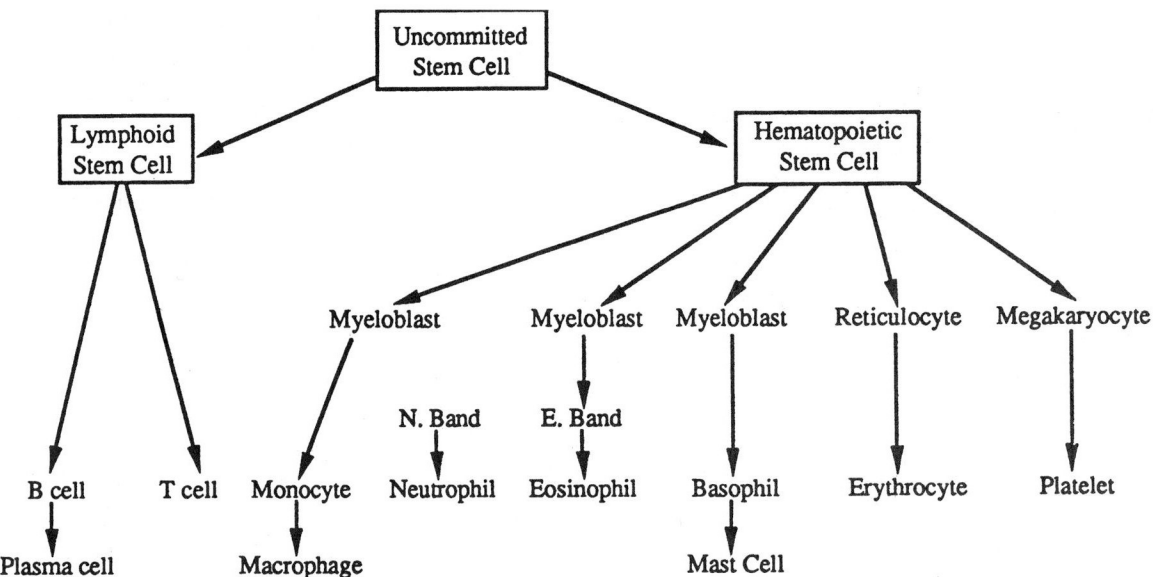

Figure 5.5. Hematopoiesis.

production and release (46). Erythropoietin increases in most anemias, but not adequately in those associated with chronic diseases (47). If tissue oxygen concentrations are perceived as inadequate, erythrocyte production continues, regardless of the erythrocyte count or hemoglobin concentration, and secondary or reactive polycythemia can occur (43).

The life span of erythrocytes in circulation is 120 days. They are removed by the reticuloendothelial system. With an abnormally large spleen, there is increased destruction of normal cells. The spleen may be enlarged in conditions such as liver disease, congestive heart failure, leukemias, lymphomas, or protozoal infections. There can be accelerated destruction of erythrocytes by a normal spleen when they contain abnormal hemoglobin or have abnormal membranes or enzymes. Increased destruction can also occur with abnormal physical, chemical, microbiologic, or immunologic conditions (43).

Hemolysis refers to the disruption of the mature erythrocyte membrane and release of hemoglobin before the end of the usual life span. It can take place in the spleen or vasculature. This accelerated destruction of cells can occur in response to physical trauma or massive exertion, severe burns, infections such as malaria, or toxic insults such as *Clostridium* infections or brown recluse spider bites. Hemolysis can also occur with drugs and chemicals such as arsine gas or copper salts. With oxidizing drugs such as nitrites or nitrates, methemoglobin can be formed and lead to severe cases of erythrocyte destruction (43).

Destruction of erythrocytes may be mediated by antibodies. Various types of antibody mediated hemolysis are associated with drugs (e.g., methyldopa, penicillin). The erythrocytes may also be destroyed as "innocent

bystanders." Drug-antibody complexes can settle on the surface of erythrocytes and attract complement, which hemolyzes the cells (43). This has been reported with quinine derivatives, *p*-aminosalicylic acid, phenacetin, sulfonamides, and insecticides (48).

Patients with chronic diseases such as infections, renal or liver disease, various endocrine disorders, rheumatoid arthritis, or neoplasms often have anemia. Aplastic anemia involves a pancytopenia or a depression of erythrocytes, neutrophils, and platelets. About 12% of cases can be attributed to drug or chemical exposure (48). It can occur secondary to infections, neoplasms, radiation, or drugs such as chloramphenicol, gold, phenylbutazone, sulfonamides, anticonvulsants, or antineoplastic drugs (43, 48). Reports of aplastic anemia with felbamate led the FDA to recommend that patients be withdrawn from that drug (49). Up to 70% of cases are primary or idiopathic, where there is no known predisposing cause. This may lead to leukemia (48). Polycythemia vera is a myeloproliferative syndrome in which there is a spontaneous increase in erythrocytes. The predominant picture is one of erythrocyte proliferation, but other elements of the blood are also hyperactive. It usually occurs in older adults and is slightly more common in men than in women. Thrombosis and hemorrhage are common complications (43).

HEMOGLOBIN, HB

(Males = 8.45–10.65 mmol/L or 136–172 g/L [13.6–17.2 g/dL]; females = 7.45–9.30 mmol/L or 120–150 g/L [12.0–15.0 g/dL]; CF = 0.6206 for mmol/L and 10 for g/L.)

Hemoglobin, the primary component of erythrocytes, transports oxygen and carbon dioxide (45). Hemoglobinopathies occur when genes code for abnormal amino acid sequences. The most common abnormal hemoglobin is sickle hemoglobin. Thalassemias are characterized by decreased synthesis of globin chains (43).

The preferred assay for hemoglobin is the cyanmethemoglobin method. Errors in venipuncture technique can lead to hemoconcentration, which results in falsely elevated values for hemoglobin and cell counts. The difference in the normal range between men and women is thought to result mainly from androgen stimulation of erythropoiesis and its effect on the marrow. Estrogen probably has a slight suppressive effect on erythrocyte production (45). Menstrual blood loss is also a contributing factor (43). In older men, the hemoglobin tends to fall. This occurs to a lesser extent in women, who may even have a slight increase in the value. As a result, there is a less than 0.62 mmol/L (1 g/dL) sex difference in hemoglobin in older individuals. There is a diurnal variation of approximately 8 to 9% in hemoglobin concentrations, with the highest value in the morning and the lowest in the evening (45). Hemoglobin values are approximately 0.62 mmol/L (1 g/dL) lower in blacks than in whites. Some attribute this to a higher incidence of iron deficiency anemia in blacks (50).

HEMATOCRIT, HCT

(Males = 0.39–0.49 [39–49%]; females = 0.33–0.43 [33–43%]; CF = 0.01.)

The hematocrit is the ratio of the volume of erythrocytes to that of whole blood or the packed erythrocyte volume (45). It increases when more fluid is lost than erythrocytes and dehydration occurs, as is seen in patients with vomiting, diarrhea, or prolonged fever. An inappropriate polycythemia occurs with renal cancer, hepatomas, pheochromocytomas, or adrenal adenomas where there is increased erythropoietin and increased hematocrit (46). The hematocrit is unreliable for patient assessment immediately after blood loss or transfusion (45).

RETICULOCYTES

(0.001–0.024 [0.1–2.4% erythrocytes]; CF = 0.01.)

Reticulocytes are immature erythrocytes. Generally, the absolute reticulocyte count is more useful than the percentage of erythrocytes. Reticulocytes provide an estimate of erythrocyte production; however, as the hematocrit drops, increasingly immature reticulocytes are released into the blood. These cells take longer to mature in circulation as indicated below:

Hct (%)	Reticulocyte Maturation Time (days)
0.45 (45)	1.0
0.35 (35)	1.5
0.25 (25)	2.0
0.15 (15)	2.5

To accurately estimate erythrocyte production in response to anemia, a correction factor must be used to account for this longer maturation time and avoid overestimating the erythropoietic response. The corrected reticulocyte count can be calculated by

$$\text{Corrected count} = \frac{\text{Reticulocyte count}}{\text{Normal reticulocyte count}} \times \frac{\text{Patient's Hct}}{\text{Normal Hct}} \div \text{Maturation time}$$

This value can then be compared to the average normal reticulocyte count to estimate how much Erc production has actually increased (44). The reticulocytes are most markedly increased in patients with hemolysis or acute blood loss and also increase when iron or vitamin B12 is administered to a deficient patient. If the reticulocyte count is normal but the hemoglobin low, there is an inadequate response to anemia, such as may be seen in iron deficiency. If the reticulocytes are increased but the hemoglobin is normal, there is probably some destruction or loss of erythrocytes occurring, and the body is appropriately compensating for the loss (43).

ERYTHROCYTE INDICES

The size and hemoglobin content of erythrocytes can be quantitated by the erythrocyte indices.

The *mean corpuscular volume* (MCV) is the average volume of erythrocytes. It can be measured by machines or calculated by the formula MCV = Hct/Ercs. The normal range is 76–100 femtoliters (fL) in SI units (a femtoliter is 10^{-15} liter or 76–100 μm^3). The MCV is decreased in microcytic anemia and increased in macrocytic anemia. Young erythrocytes and reticulocytes are larger than mature cells, so when there is rapid cell production, the MCV will be increased. This type of macrocytosis can be observed in compensated hemolytic conditions or when a patient is recovering from acute blood loss. Megaloblastic changes can occur when DNA production is impaired but RNA production is normal. This causes nuclear maturation to lag behind cytoplasmic maturation. This change occurs in all cells, but is most dramatic and can be most easily diagnosed in erythrocyte precursors. The most common causes of megaloblastosis are deficiencies of vitamin B12 or folic acid, which are required for DNA synthesis. Drugs that interfere with DNA synthesis such as folate antagonists (e.g., methotrexate, trimethoprim, or triamterene), those interfering with vitamin B12 absorption (e.g., colchicine or cholestyramine), or inhibitors of purine or pyrimidine synthesis (e.g., azathioprine or 5-fluorouracil) may also cause megaloblastosis (51). It may also result from drugs that decrease folate absorption such as oral contraceptives, phenytoin, and cycloserine. Alcohol can impair folic acid absorption and interfere with folate-dependent enzymatic reactions. Megaloblastic anemia can also be associated with hypothyroidism, multiple myeloma, myeloproliferative disease, and enzyme defects such as in Lesch-Nyhan syndrome. A microcytic anemia is associated with iron deficiency anemia, thalassemias, anemia of chronic disease, and sideroblastic anemia (43).

The *mean corpuscular hemoglobin* (MCH) is the weight of the hemoglobin in the average red blood cell. It is calculated by MCH = Hb/Ercs (45). The normal range is 1.70–2.05 femtomoles (fmol) in SI units or 27–33 picograms (pg) (CF = 0.06206). In microcytic anemia it is decreased, and in macrocytic anemia, increased (45). Hypochromic cells are associated with iron deficiency anemia, thalassemias, anemia of chronic disease, and sideroblastic anemia (43).

The *mean corpuscular hemoglobin concentration* (MCHC) is the average concentration of hemoglobin in a given volume of packed erythrocytes and is described by MCHC = Hb/Hct (45). The normal range is 20–23 mmol/L or, in SI units, 330–370 g/L or 33–37 g/dL (CF = 0.6206 for mmol/L and 10 for g/L). In microcytic anemia it is decreased. In macrocytic anemia it may be normal or decreased. In hypochromic anemias, both the MCH and MCHC are decreased (43).

The red cell distribution width (RDW) quantitates the extent of variation in the size of erythrocytes. The reference value is 11.5 to 14.5 (5). It may be calculated by RDW = (standard deviation of Erc size)/MCV.

ERYTHROCYTE SEDIMENTATION RATE, ESR

(Males = 0–20 mm/h; females = 0–30 mm/h, Westergren technique.)

The erythrocyte sedimentation rate is the length of fall of the top of a column of erythrocytes in anticoagulated blood in a given period of time. It is directly proportional to the weight of the cell aggregates and inversely proportional to the surface area. Microcytes settle slower than macrocytes. The ESR generally increases in anemia and following an injury, and decreases if there are abnormal or irregularly shaped erythrocytes. The ESR gradually increases with age and modestly increases during pregnancy. The ESR is used mainly as an indicator of active inflammatory diseases (e.g., rheumatoid arthritis), chronic infection (e.g., tuberculosis), collagen disease, or neoplastic disease (e.g., multiple myeloma), and may be used to monitor the disease course. It is particularly useful in the diagnosis and monitoring of temporal arteritis and polymyalgia rheumatica. The Westergren technique is widely used as the standard for determining ESR. Alternatives are the Wintrobe method and the Zeta Sedimentation Ratio (43, 45).

LEUKOCYTES, LKCS

(3.2–9.8×10^9/L [3200–9800 mm^{-3}]; CF = 0.001.)

Laboratories commonly report six types of leukocytes or white blood cells found in the peripheral blood:

neutrophils, bands, lymphocytes, monocytes, eosinophils, and basophils. Less mature or abnormal forms may be observed in certain disease states. The differential white count indicates the fraction of the total leukocyte count that is accounted for by each type (addition of the differential should total 1.00). The leukocyte and differential counts can change within minutes to hours of stimulation (43). Cigarette smokers have a higher average leukocyte count. It is about 30% higher in heavy smokers who inhale, with an increase in neutrophils, lymphocytes, and monocytes. In leukocytosis, the total Lkc count is increased above the normal range. Exercise can lead to a leukocytosis with an increase in neutrophils due to shifting of cells and lymphocyte drainage into blood (45). The leukocyte count tends to be lower in blacks than in whites (50).

The leukocyte count and/or the differential count may be abnormal in patients with sepsis, but this is not always the case and normal values would not rule out an infection. False results may occur with hemorrhage, hemolysis, trauma, diabetic ketoacidosis, and sickle cell crisis. The differential is often abnormal after surgery (50).

Leukemias are malignant diseases characterized by abnormal leukocytes, which may be greatly increased in number (although they may also be decreased). A massive increase in leukocytes as a systemic response to various conditions (e.g., tuberculosis, diabetic ketoacidosis, heavy metal poisoning) is called a "leukemoid reaction" because the hematologic picture strongly resembles that seen in chronic leukemia. Different cell lines may predominate depending on the cause (43).

GRANULOCYTES

Granulocytes are leukocytes with granules in their cytoplasm. They develop from the same precursor cell as monocytes in the bone marrow (Fig. 5.5). Their synthesis is stimulated by the hormone colony-stimulating factor for granulocytes (G-CSF) and granulocytes-monocytes (GM-CSF) (43). Unlike erythrocytes, granulocytes retain their nuclei. Mature cells remain in the marrow for about 10 days and serve as a "storage pool." The cells can be released within minutes of a stimulus. Granulocytes usually spend less than a day in circulating blood (44). Their primary site of activity is in tissues. There are three main types of granulocytes: neutrophils (including bands), eosinophils, and basophils (43).

NEUTROPHILS

(1.8–7.8×10^9/L [1800–7800 mm^{-3}]; CF = 0.001.)

In normal adults, about 0.51 ± 0.15 of leukocytes are neutrophils (5), also called polymorphonuclear (meaning many forms of nuclei) leukocytes, PMNs, polys, segmented neutrophilic granulocytes, or segs. The lower limit of the normal range is 1.8×10^9/L (1800 mm^{-3}) for white adults and 1.1×10^9/L (1100 mm^{-3}) for blacks. There is some diurnal variation in neutrophils, with higher values in the afternoon and lower in the morning.

The nuclei of neutrophils have two to five lobes connected by thin filaments (45). Their cytoplasm is packed with enzyme-containing granules that react with both acidic and basic stains. Bands or stabs are the immature form of neutrophils. They have thicker strands connecting their nuclear lobes or U-shaped nuclei that look like curved bands (45). Band neutrophils normally average 0.08 ± 0.03 of leukocytes (5). A "shift to the left" means there is an increase in bands and immature neutrophils in the blood. The term is derived from a time when the differential was reported on a grid that listed the immature forms on the left and the mature neutrophils on the right (43). When tissue is damaged or foreign material enters the body, substances are released that stimulate neutrophils to move to that area. This is called chemotaxis. Chemotaxis can be abnormal in some diseases such as Hodgkin's disease, cirrhosis, rheumatoid arthritis, and diabetes mellitus. The neutrophils then phagocytize and destroy microorganisms and other materials at the site enzymatically.

The neutrophils must attach to the particles before they can engulf them. This attachment is enhanced by the presence of antibodies or complement coating the surface of the particles. It is decreased by exposure to alcohol, aspirin, prednisone, or nonsteroidal antiinflammatory drugs (43). This action of neutrophils is important in host defense against infection, but when enzymes are released outside the cell, it may also play a part in causing tissue damage to the host in other diseases (44). Neutrophils are stored in the bone marrow and in the marginal granulocyte pool along the vessel walls or in capillary beds. In response to stress, they can be released from these sites into the circulating pool, resulting in a neutrophilia. In an acute infection, the neutrophils leave the circulation and migrate into the tissues. Production of neutrophils will also increase, in which case, more immature forms will be seen. If supply cannot keep up with demand, a neutropenia may occur. A toxic suppression of the bone marrow may also be involved in this process (52).

An increase in neutrophils is associated with some infections (especially bacterial), various inflammatory diseases (e.g., rheumatoid arthritis, vasculitis), tissue necrosis (e.g., as in myocardial infarction or burns), metabolic disorders (e.g., uremia, diabetic ketoacidosis, thyroid storm), and tumors. Endogenous or exogenous adrenal corticosteroids cause lymphocytes and eosinophils to disappear from circulation within 4 to 8 hours, with circulating granulocytes increasing later (43). Prolonged use of corticosteroids can lead to chronic neutrophilia by decreasing the rate at which neutrophils leave circulation (52). Epinephrine can cause granulocytosis within minutes and probably is the mediator of neutrophilic leukocytosis associated with physiologic stimuli such as exercise, emotional stress, or exposure to extreme temperatures. Other drugs that can stimulate neutrophilia include lithium, histamine, heparin, digitalis, and many toxins, venoms, and heavy metals (e.g., lead, mercury) (43, 52).

Neutropenia is a result of impaired production, increased destruction, or altered distribution of neutrophils. It occurs when the absolute neutrophil count is below the normal range and is associated with certain bacterial (e.g., typhoid, tularemia, brucellosis), viral, and protozoal (especially malaria) infections, or an overwhelming infection of any kind. It can be caused by drugs interfering with DNA synthesis (e.g., phenothiazines, phenytoin, antibiotics, sulfonamides), idiosyncratic drug reactions (e.g., chloramphenicol, gold salts, propylthiouracil, phenylbutazone, quinidine), or treatment with cytotoxic drugs or radiation (43, 52). There can be increased destruction of neutrophils through immunologic mechanisms in patients receiving drugs such as aminopyrine, phenylbutazone, or sulfapyridine (52). Neutropenia is also seen with hypersplenism due to liver or storage diseases, some collagen-vascular diseases (e.g., lupus erythematosus), and folic acid or vitamin B12 deficiency.

A more severe form of neutropenia is agranulocytosis, in which the granulocytes suddenly disappear. Often other blood elements are also affected.(43) Agranulocytosis can occur as a complication of drug therapy (e.g., clozapine) (53). The absolute neutrophil count (ANC) is calculated by multiplying the total leukocyte count by the sum of the percentage of mature neutrophils (segs) plus the percentage of immature neutrophils (bands): ANC = Total Lkcs $\times$ (% segs + % bands). When the ANC is below 1.0×10^9/L (1000 mm^{-3}), there is an increased risk of infection, and when it is less than 0.5×10^9/L (500 mm^{-3}), this risk is very high (52).

EOSINOPHILS
$(0–0.45 \times 10^9$/L [0–450 mm^{-3}]; CF = 0.001.)

Eosinophils are structurally similar to neutrophils, but their cytoplasm contains larger round or oval granules that contain enzymes and have a strong affinity for acid (red) stains. Their nuclei usually contain two connected segments (43, 45). Eosinophils normally average 0.027 of leukocytes (5). The count is higher in allergic individuals (45). Eosinophils are capable of phagocytosis but are not bactericidal. They modulate activities associated with immunologically mediated inflammation and can damage the larvae of some helminth parasites. Eosinophils are increased in allergic diseases (e.g., asthma, hay fever), parasitic infections (e.g., trichinosis), certain skin disorders (e.g., atopic dermatitis, eczema, pemphigus), neoplastic diseases, collagen vascular diseases, adrenal cortical hypofunction, ulcerative colitis, and "hypereosinophilic" syndromes (43, 52). Eosinophils are decreased during acute stress or other conditions with increased epinephrine secretion or elevated levels of adrenal corticosteroids, and in acute inflammatory states (52).

BASOPHILS

($0–0.2 \times 10^9$/L [0–200 mm^{-3}]; CF = 0.001.)

Basophils look similar to neutrophils, except that their nuclei are less segmented and their cytoplasmic granules are larger and have a strong affinity for basic (blue) stains (45). They average about 0.005 of total leukocytes (5). They show diurnal variation, with levels highest during the night and lowest in the morning (52). Tissue basophils are called mast cells and have immunoglobulin E receptors on their cell membranes. They react with allergens and cause release of histamine and other substances from the basophil granules, producing allergic reactions. Basophils may be increased in chronic hypersensitivity states in the absence of the specific allergen, in myeloproliferative disorders, and in hypothyroidism (43, 52). They may be decreased with chronic corticosteroid therapy, acute infection or stress, or in patients with hyperthyroidism (52).

LYMPHOCYTES

($1.0–4.8 \times 10^9$/L [1000–4800 mm^{-3}]; CF = 0.001.)

Lymphocytes are mononuclear cells without cytoplasmic granules (45). They average 0.34 ± 0.10 of leukocytes in adults (5). They may form plasma cells, which are not normally present in blood (45). Plasma cells may be found in patients with neoplasms (e.g., multiple myeloma), chronic infections, and allergic states (52). Lymphocytes and plasma cells are important for the immune defenses of the body. Normally, about 75 to 80% of circulating lymphocytes are T cells, which are responsible for cell mediated immunity including delayed hypersensitivity, graft rejection, graft-versus-host reactions, defense against intracellular organisms, and probably defense against neoplasms (43, 44). They have a life span of months to years. They are named for the thymus gland, where they differentiate (44).

B lymphocytes account for 10 to 15% of circulating lymphocytes and are responsible for humoral immunity (43). They are named for the bursa of Fabricius, where they develop· in birds. In humans, the bursal equivalent is thought to be in fetal liver and bone marrow, with further differentiation occurring in secondary lymphoid organs. These organs, important for postnatal lymphocyte production, include the spleen, lymph nodes, and intestine-associated lymphoid tissue. B cells have a life span of days and can differentiate into antibody-producing plasma cells (44).

There are also "null" lymphocytes that cannot be classified. Although lymphocytes can be found in circulation, they mainly concentrate in the lymph nodes, spleen, mucosa of alimentary and respiratory tracts, bone marrow,

liver, skin, and chronically inflamed tissue (43).

Changes in the proportion of lymphocytes in the total leukocyte count usually reflect changes in numbers of granulocytes. An absolute or relative increase in lymphocytes occurs with some viral or other infections (e.g., tuberculosis, infectious mononucleosis, cytomegalovirus, pertussis, toxoplasmosis), inflammatory or immunologic diseases, and hypersensitivity reactions to drugs (e.g., phenytoin, paraaminosalicylic acid) (43, 52). When the number of lymphocytes is decreased abnormally (lymphocytopenia) or function is impaired, the patient suffers from immunodeficiency. This can be an inherited disorder or may be associated with immunodeficiency syndromes (e.g., acquired immune deficiency syndrome or AIDS), diseases such as congestive heart failure, renal failure, malnutrition, or advanced tuberculosis, or with defects of lymphatic circulation (43). Lymphocytopenia can also occur after administration of antineoplastic drugs or high-dose corticosteroids, or after irradiation (52).

MONOCYTES

($0–0.8 \times 10^9$/L [0–800 mm^{-3}]; CF = 0.001.)

Monocytes are the largest cells in normal blood, with a diameter two to three times that of erythrocytes. They have a single nucleus that is partly lobulated and may appear round or oval. Their cytoplasm contains fine granules (45). Monocytes average 0.04 of leukocytes (5). After circulating briefly, they enter the tissues, transform into the larger macrophages, and remain there for several months. Macrophages are capable of motility, phagocytosis, enzyme secretion, particle recognition, and interactions with the immune system. They have important functions in host defense and control of hematopoiesis. They remove old or defective blood cells in the marrow and inhaled particles in the lungs (44). They are increased in some infectious diseases (e.g., mycotic, rickettsial, protozoal, and viral infections; tuberculosis; subacute bacterial endocarditis; and hepatitis), and granulomatous, collagen-vascular, and neoplastic diseases (43, 44). The circulating monocytes and tissue macrophages together compose the mononuclear phagocyte or reticuloendothelial system (44).

PLATELETS

($130–400 \times 10^9$/L [$130–400 \times 10^3$/mm^3]; CF = 1.)

Platelets maintain the integrity of blood vessels and play a key role in hemostasis. The precursors of platelets are megakaryocytes (Fig. 5.5) (43). Their proliferation and maturation are controlled by megakaryocyte colony-stimulating factor (Meg-CSF) and thrombopoietin. Normally, about two thirds of platelets are in circulation and one third in the spleen. When the spleen is enlarged, however, up to 80 to 90% may be sequestered there. In patients without a spleen, all are in circulation. Platelets circulate for about 8 to 11 days (44).

The major sites for destruction of platelets are the spleen and liver (54). Antibodies may also destroy platelets. They may be directed against the platelets, or the platelets may be "innocent bystanders" that are destroyed when an immune complex attaches to them. This may occur with exposure to drugs such as quinine, quinidine, or heparin (43).

Thrombocytopenia, a reduced number of circulating platelets, can occur as a congenital or acquired disorder. It may result from decreased production, abnormal distribution or dilution, or increased destruction of platelets. These may be associated with factors such as neoplasms; immune processes; infections; exposure to drugs, chemicals, or toxins; or an enlarged spleen; and may be combined with abnormalities of other blood elements such as in aplastic anemia. Thrombocytosis, an increased number of circulating platelets, can be part of a reactive process or a myeloproliferative disorder (55). Half of patients with an otherwise unexplained increase in platelets are found to have a malignancy (5).

Platelets are activated at times of vascular injury by exposure to substances such as collagen and thrombin. They adhere to exposed surfaces and aggregate in the presence of calcium (55). They release adenosine diphosphate (ADP), which promotes further aggregation, and platelet plugs are formed (43). Aggregation is also stimulated by thromboxane A_2 from platelets and inhibited by prostacyclin (prostaglandin I_2) from vascular endothelium. Both are products of platelet arachidonic acid metabolism mediated by cyclooxygenase (Fig. 5.6). Platelets also release various substances that activate or allow progression of the clotting cascade. These actions lead to the formation of thrombi. Overall platelet function may be assessed by the bleeding time, and various in vitro techniques employing activator substances may also be used to assess platelet aggregation. Platelet contraction within thrombi is responsible for clot retraction (55).

If the count is 20 to 50×10^9/L [20 to 50×10^3/mm^3], the patient is at a high risk for minor bruising and bleeding after surgery, and if it is less than 20×10^9/L [20×10^3/ mm^3], spontaneous bruising and bleeding become more common (56). Platelet function is impaired in various diseases such as severe uremia or liver disease, or when there are high levels of abnormal serum proteins. Numerous drugs can also interfere with platelet function (43). Most affect the arachidonic pathway shown in Figure 5.6. Aspirin irreversibly acetylates platelet cyclooxygenase, thus inhibiting aggregation for the life of the platelet by decreasing formation of thromboxane A_2. This effect is observed for up to ten days following ingestion of aspirin. Most other nonsteroidal antiinflammatory drugs will also affect platelet cyclooxygenase, but it is a reversible effect observed only while the drug is present. Other drugs inhibit platelet effects by activating adenylate cyclase (e.g., prostaglandins) or inhibiting phosphodiesterase (e.g., dipyridamole), both of which result in increased cyclic-AMP (55). Ticlopidine is a drug that inhibits the ADP pathway (57). Examples of additional drugs that may inhibit aggregation include dextran, antimicrobial agents, membrane stabilizing agents, and β-adrenergic blocking agents (55). Synthesis of platelets is inhibited by many antineoplastic agents. Ethyl alcohol can inhibit both synthesis and function of platelets (43).

Coagulation Tests
CLOTTING CASCADE

The clotting cascade involves the progressive activation of clotting factors, with the end result of a fibrin clot. Platelets and other substances help or accelerate this progression. A

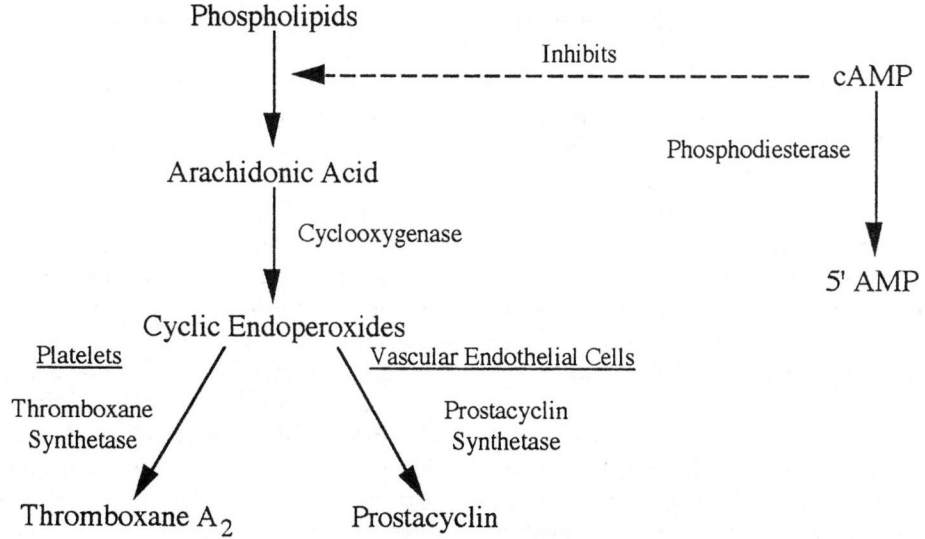

Figure 5.6. Arachidonic acid pathway.

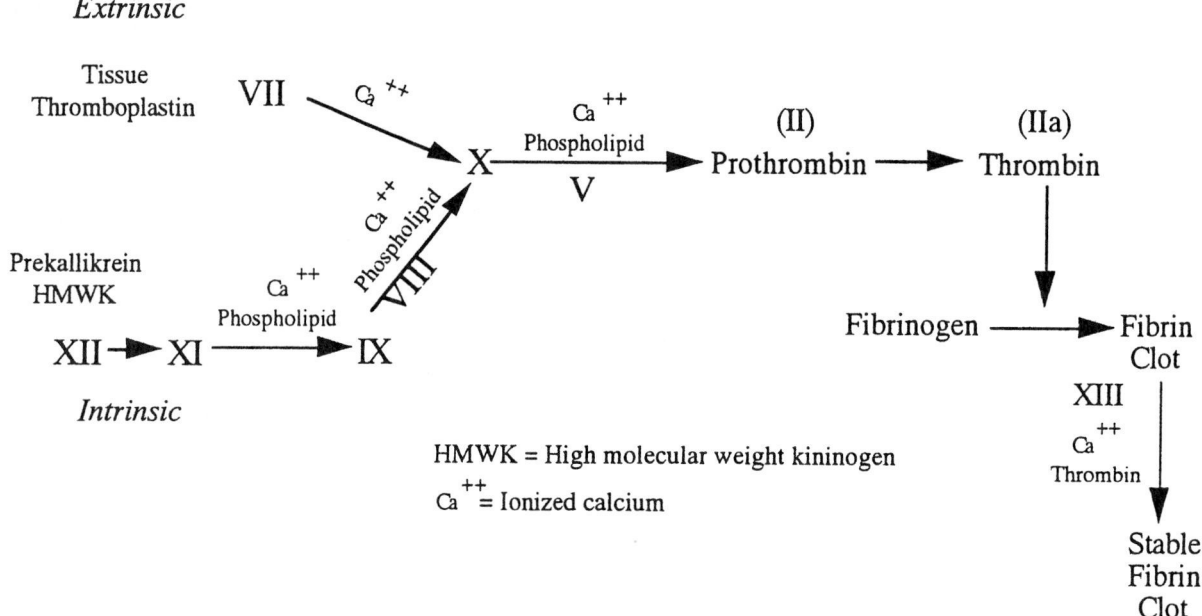

Figure 5.7. Clotting cascade.

simplified diagram of the traditional clotting cascade is shown in Figure 5.7. The process is actually much more complex, with additional points of factor interaction. The clotting factors are identified by Roman numerals, although they also have other names (58). Each factor must be activated before it can in turn activate other factors in the sequence. The active forms of most factors are serine proteases, except V and VIII, which act as cofactors. Factors II, VII, IX, and X require vitamin K for their synthesis. The main source of phospholipid is platelets. Ionized calcium is required for some of the steps to proceed. The intrinsic pathway is initiated by contact activation, for example, by exposure to damaged vascular endothelium. The extrinsic pathway is stimulated by factors released from damaged tissue. The two pathways come together at factor X to form the common pathway (43).

Different tests are used to assess the body's ability to form a clot, by evaluating the function of different parts of the pathways, and they are also used to monitor drug therapy. For most coagulation tests, the blood is centrifuged to remove platelets and citrate is added to bind calcium and thus prevent the cascade from progressing. Patients with defective or deficient clotting factors can experience bleeding. This may be a congenital disorder such as hemophilia, where there is a deficiency of factor VIII or IX, an acquired disorder such as the impaired factor synthesis seen in liver disease, or an effect of drugs (58).

ACTIVATED PARTIAL THROMBOPLASTIN TIME, aPTT (25–38 SEC)

The aPTT is used to assess the integrity of the intrinsic and common coagulation pathways. It is performed by adding

a contact activating agent (e.g., kaolin, ellagic acid, or celite), phospholipid, and calcium to citrated plasma, then measuring the time required for a clot to form. It will be prolonged if there is a deficiency of factor XII, XI, IX, VIII, X, V, or II; or of fibrinogen, prekallikrein, or high molecular weight kininogen; or if an inhibitor of one of those is present. It is not affected by abnormal factor VII (58). It is usually prolonged when the concentration of the clotting factors is less than 30% of normal (43). It is also abnormal in patients with a lupuslike anticoagulant and sometimes in those with liver failure, since many clotting factors are manufactured in the liver. It may be shortened in an active coagulopathy. It is the main test used to monitor heparin therapy and will be prolonged in the presence of thrombolytic drugs or coumarin derivatives (58).

PROTHROMBIN TIME, PT (11–16 SEC)

The PT is used to evaluate the extrinsic and common pathways. Tissue thromboplastin (e.g., brain or lung extract or human recombinant tissue factor with phospholipid) and calcium are added to citrated plasma, and the time to clot formation is measured (59). In the United States, rabbit brain thromboplastin is commonly used, which is much less sensitive to changes in clotting factor concentrations than the thromboplastin used in other countries (60). The PT is prolonged by a deficiency of factor VII, X, V, or II, or fibrinogen, or the presence of an inhibitor to one of those factors. It is not affected by abnormal factor VIII or IX (58). The PT is sometimes expressed as the International Normalized Ratio (INR). This is calculated by the formula $INR = R^c$, where R is the ratio of patient's PT : mean control PT, and c is the International Sensitivity Index

(ISI), which relates an individual batch of thromboplastin to the World Health Organization international reference preparation (59). For example, a quoted therapeutic range for warfarin in the treatment of deep venous thrombosis in this country (rabbit brain thromboplastin with an ISI of 2.8) would be 1.3 to 1.5 times the control value; the corresponding INR would be 2.0–3.0. The PT is prolonged in liver disease, in patients with a vitamin K deficiency, and in widespread intravascular coagulation or fibrinolysis. It is used to monitor coumarin (e.g., warfarin) treatment but may be prolonged by the presence of heparin or a thrombolytic drug (43). An extensive discussion of drugs that affect the clotting tests is found in Chapter 40, "Thromboembolic Diseases."

THROMBIN TIME, TT (17–25 SEC)

The TT is used to appraise the body's ability to convert fibrinogen to fibrin. Thrombin is added to citrated plasma, and the time for clotting is measured. The time is prolonged if there is a deficiency or abnormality of fibrinogen, if an inhibitor is present, or if heparin or fibrin-fibrinogen degradation products are present (58). It may be used in monitoring thrombolytic therapy (e.g., streptokinase, urokinase, alteplase, or anistreplase).

BLEEDING TIME (120–480 SEC)

The bleeding time is the best screening test to assess platelet function, although it is imprecise. It is performed by making a uniform incision on the arm. Blood that beads up is removed by filter paper, with care taken not to touch the wound and disturb platelet plugs. The blood is removed to prevent fibrin from forming and stopping the bleeding. The end point of the test is when there is no longer a spot on the filter paper after blotting. The test is prolonged when there is platelet dysfunction, when the number of platelets is less than 100×10^9/L (100×10^3/mm^3), or when a platelet-inhibiting drug is present. If the bleeding time is shorter than expected, many young, active platelets may be present (43).

CONCLUSION

This chapter has reviewed commonly encountered clinical laboratory tests including serum creatinine, blood urea nitrogen, plasma glucose, uric acid, enzymes, bilirubin, serum proteins, clotting tests, and complete blood count with differential. Reliable measurements are an integral component in the management of any patient. Laboratory test values that do not correlate with a patient's clinical picture should be suspect and repeated. Reference values should be used from the given clinical laboratory in which the test was performed. Critical or treatment values for a given test in a clinical situation should be considered rather than just normal or abnormal values. Drugs may alter a particular laboratory test, and medication histories and administration profiles should be thoroughly reviewed for potential drug causes of these alterations. Clinical laboratory tests are a major component of the diagnosis and treatment of patients. Understanding their regulation, critical ranges, clinical applications, and limitations is vital.

REFERENCES

1. Woo J, Henry JB. Clinical pathology/laboratory medicine purposes and practice. In: Henry JB, ed. Clinical diagnosis and management by laboratory methods, 18th ed. Philadelphia: WB Saunders, 1991:3–26.
2. Young DS. Implementation of SI units for clinical laboratory data. Style specifications and conversion tables. Ann Intern Med 106:114–129, 1987.
3. Woo J, Cannon DC. Metabolic intermediates and inorganic ions. In: Henry JB, ed. Clinical diagnosis and management by laboratory methods, 18th ed. Philadelphia: WB Saunders, 1991:140–171.
4. Smith CL, Hampton EM. Using estimated creatinine clearance for individualizing drug therapy: a reassessment. DICP Ann Pharmacother 24:1185–1190, 1990.
5. Wallach J. Interpretation of diagnostic tests: a synopsis of laboratory medicine, 5th ed. Boston: Little, Brown, 1992:ch 1–20.
6. Howanitz PJ, Howanitz JH, Henry JB. Carbohydrates. In: Henry JB, ed. Clinical diagnosis and management by laboratory methods, 18th ed. Philadelphia: WB Saunders, 1991:172–187.
7. Stanaszek WF, Seifert CF. Arthritis in the elderly: presentation, treatment and monitoring aspects. J Geriatr Drug Ther 3:5–89, 1989.
8. Campion EW, Clynn RJ, DeLabry LO. Asymptomatic hyperuricemia. Risks and consequences in the normative aging study. Am J Med 82:421–426, 1987.
9. Steele MA, Des Prez RM. The role of pyrazinamide in tuberculosis chemotherapy. Chest 94:845–850, 1988.
10. Borg EJT, Rasker JJ. Gout in the elderly. A separate entity? Ann Rheum Dis 46:72–76, 1987.
11. Pincus MR, Zimmerman HJ, Henry JB. Clinical enzymology. In: Henry JB, ed. Clinical diagnosis and management by laboratory methods, 18th ed. Philadelphia: WB Saunders, 1991:250–284.
12. Koppel C. Clinical features, pathogenesis and management of drug-induced rhabdomyolysis. Med Toxicol Adv Drug Exp 4:108–126, 1989.
13. Zeller FP, Bauman JL. Current concepts in clinical therapeutics: acute myocardial infarction. Clin Pharm 5:553–572, 1986.
14. Young LY, Smith GH. Interpretation of clinical laboratory tests. In: Koda-Kimble MA, Young LY, eds. Applied therapeutics: the clinical use of drugs, 5th ed. Vancouver, WA: Applied Therapeutics, 1992:3-1–3-17.
15. Heller GV, Blaustein AS, Wei JY, et al. Implications of increased myocardial isoenzyme level in the presence of normal serum creatine kinase activity. Am J Cardiol 51:24–27, 1983.
16. Ingwall JS, Kramer MF, Fifer MA, et al. The creatine kinase system in normal and diseased human myocardium. N Engl J Med 313:1050–1054, 1985.
17. White RD, Grande P, Califf L, et al. Diagnostic and prognostic significance of minimally elevated creatine kinase-MB in suspected acute myocardial infarction. Am J Cardiol 55:1478–1484, 1985.
18. Hong RA, Licht JD, Wei JY, et al. Elevated CK-MB with normal total creatine kinase in suspected myocardial infarction: associated clinical findings and early prognosis. Am Heart J 111:1041–1047, 1986.
19. Lee TH, Weisberg MC, Cook F, et al. Evaluation of creatine kinase and creatine kinase-MB for diagnosing myocardial infarction. Clinical impact in the emergency room. Arch Intern Med 147:115–121, 1987.
20. Yusuf S, Collins R, Lin L, et al. Significance of elevated MB isoenzyme with normal creatine kinase in acute myocardial infarction. Am J Cardiol 59:245–250, 1987.

21. Pearlman CA. Neuroleptic malignant syndrome: a review of the literature. J Clin Psychopharmacol 6:257–273, 1986.

22. Henwood JM, Heel RC. Lovastatin. A preliminary review of its pharmacodynamic properties and therapeutic use in hyperlipidaemia. Drugs 36:429–454, 1988.

23. Montgomery R, Dryer RL, Conway TW, et al. Biochemistry. A case-oriented approach, 2nd ed. Saint Louis: CV Mosby, 1977.

24. Diggs LW. Sickle cell crises. Am J Clin Pathol 44:1–19, 1965.

25. Petz LD. Drug-induced immune haemolytic anaemia. Clin Haematol 9:455–483, 1980.

26. Kaplowitz N, Aw TY, Simon FR, et al. Drug-induced hepatotoxicity. Ann Intern Med 104:826–839, 1986.

27. Clark JA, Zimmerman HJ, Tanner LA. Labetalol hepatotoxicity. Ann Intern Med 113:210–213, 1990.

28. Davis KL, Thal LJ, Gamzu ER, et al. A double-blind, placebo-controlled multicenter study of tacrine for Alzheimer's disease. N Engl J Med 327:1253–1259, 1992.

29. Sher PP. Drug interferences with clinical laboratory tests. Drugs 24:24–63, 1982.

30. Girling DJ. The hepatic toxicity of antituberculosis regimens containing isoniazid, rifampicin, and pyrazinamide. Tubercle 59:13–32, 1978.

31. Mitchell JR, Zimmerman HJ, Ishak KG, et al. Isoniazid liver injury: clinical spectrum, pathology, and probable pathogenesis. Ann Intern Med 84:181–192, 1976.

32. Chopra S, Griffin PH. Laboratory tests and diagnostic procedures in evaluation of liver disease. Am J Med 79:221–230, 1985.

33. Schaffner JA, Schaffner F. Assessment of the status of the liver. In: Henry JB, ed. Clinical diagnosis and management by laboratory methods, 18th ed. Philadelphia: WB Saunders, 1991:229–249.

34. Kao YS, Liu FJ. Laboratory diagnosis of gastrointestinal tract and exocrine pancreatic disorders. In: Henry JB, ed. Clinical diagnosis and management by laboratory methods, 18th ed. Philadelphia: WB Saunders, 1991:519–549.

35. Geokas MC, Baltaxe HA, Banks PA, et al. Acute pancreatitis. Ann Intern Med 103:86–100, 1985.

36. Mallory A, Kern F. Drug-induced pancreatitis: a critical review. Gastroenterology 78:813–820, 1980.

37. Gordon-Smith EC. Drug-induced oxidative haemolysis. Clin Haematol 9:557–586, 1980.

38. Scott JM, Weir DG. Drug-induced megaloblastic change. Clin Haematol 9:587–619, 1980.

39. Yunis AA, Salem Z. Drug-induced mitochondrial damage and sideroblastic change. Clin Haematol 9:607–619, 1980.

40. McPherson RA. Specific proteins. In: Henry JB, ed. Clinical diagnosis and management by laboratory methods, 18th ed. Philadelphia: WB Saunders, 1991:215–228.

41. MacKichan JJ. Influence of protein binding and use of unbound (free) drug concentrations. In: Evans WE, Schentag JJ, Jusko WJ, eds. Applied pharmacokinetics principles of therapeutic drug monitoring, 3rd ed. Vancouver, WA: Applied Therapeutics, 1992: 5-1–5-48.

42. Zini R, Riant P, Barre J, et al. Disease-induced variations in plasma protein levels. Implications for drug dosage regimens (part I). Clin Pharmacokinet 19:147–159, 1990.

43. Sacher RA, McPherson RA. Widmann's clinical interpretation of laboratory tests, 10th ed. Philadelphia: FA Davis, 1991: ch 1–6.

44. Nelson DA, Davey FR. Hematopoiesis. In: Henry JB, ed. Clinical diagnosis and management by laboratory methods, 18th ed. Philadelphia: WB Saunders, 1991:604–626.

45. Nelson DA, Morris MW. Basic examination of blood. In: Henry JB, ed. Clinical diagnosis and management by laboratory methods, 18th ed. Philadelphia: WB Saunders, 1991:553–603.

46. McGuire MJ, Spivak JL. Erythrocytosis and polycythemia. In: Spivak JL, Eichner ER. The fundamentals of clinical hematology, 3rd ed. Baltimore: Johns Hopkins University Press, 1993:117–128.

47. Mladenovic J, Roodman GD. Normocytic anemia. In: Spivak JL, Eichner ER, eds. The fundamentals of clinical hematology, 3rd ed. Baltimore: Johns Hopkins University Press, 1993:91–100.

48. Nelson DA, Davey FR. Erythrocytic disorders. In: Henry JB, ed. Clinical diagnosis and management by laboratory methods, 18th ed. Philadelphia: WB Saunders, 1991:627–676.

49. Anon. Recommendation for the immediate withdrawal of patients from treatment with Felbatol (felbamate). FDA Med Bull 24(2):5, 1994.

50. Shapiro MF, Greenfield S. The complete blood count and leukocyte differential count. An approach to their rational application. Ann Intern Med 106:65–74, 1987.

51. Eichner ER. Macrocytic anemia. In: Spivak JL, Eichner ER, eds. The fundamentals of clinical hematology, 3rd ed. Baltimore: Johns Hopkins University Press, 1993:27–46.

52. Davey FR, Nelson DA. Leukocytic disorders. In: Henry JB, ed. Clinical diagnosis and management by laboratory methods, 18th ed. Philadelphia: WB Saunders, 1991:677–716.

53. Alvir JMJ, Lieberman JA, Safferman AZ, et al. Clozapine-induced agranulocytosis: incidence and risk factors in the United States. N Engl J Med 329:162–167, 1993.

54. Tsan MF, Pasquale D, McIntyre PA. Nuclear hematology. In: Spivak JL, Eichner ER, eds. The fundamentals of clinical hematology, 3rd ed. Baltimore: Johns Hopkins University Press, 1993:449–468.

55. Miller JL. Blood platelets. In: Henry JB, ed. Clinical diagnosis and management by laboratory methods, 18th ed. Philadelphia: WB Saunders, 1991:717–733.

56. Murphy S. Platelets. In: Spivak JL, Eichner ER, eds. The fundamentals of clinical hematology, 3rd ed. Baltimore: Johns Hopkins University Press, 1993:343–365.

57. Flores-Runk P, Raasch RH. Ticlopidine and antiplatelet therapy. Ann Pharmacother 27:1090–1098, 1993.

58. Miller JL. Blood coagulation and fibrinolysis. In: Henry JB, ed. Clinical diagnosis and management by laboratory methods, 18th ed. Philadelphia: WB Saunders, 1991:734–757.

59. Hirsh J, Poller L. The international normalized ratio: a guide to understanding and correcting its problems. Arch Intern Med 154:282–288, 1994.

60. Hirsh J, Dalen JE, Deykin D, et al. Oral anticoagulants: mechanism of action, clinical effectiveness, and optimal therapeutic range. Chest 102(suppl):312s–326s, 1992.

CHAPTER 6

RACIAL AND ETHNIC DIFFERENCES IN RESPONSE TO DRUGS

HEWITT W. MATTHEWS and JANNIFER J. JOHNSON

The premise that a drug will act identically in two different people or in two different racial, ethnic, or gender groups has been proven to be incorrect. For a growing number of drugs, the percentage of patients who react differently or adversely is determined by their racial and ethnic background as well as sexual differences. The adage that "one size does not fit all" well illustrates the increasingly recognized fact that racial and ethnic differences must be taken into account in prescribing drug therapy. Factors that affect drug response based on racial and ethnic differences basically fall into three major categories: environmental, social (psychosocial), and genetic. Age and gender are other factors that may also affect drug response. The major drugs/classes that show varying effects among racial and ethnic groups are the antipsychotics, benzodiazepines, antidepressants, cardiovascular/antihypertensives, atropine, analgesics, antidiabetic agents, and alcohol. Even though therapeutic response, metabolism, and side effects may differ with various medicines due to racial and ethnic differences, clinical significance is often not established. This chapter will focus primarily on the effects that racial and ethnic differences have on drug responses.

FACTORS AFFECTING DRUG RESPONSE

Environmental

Environmental factors may have significant influences on drug response, metabolism, disposition, and excretion. Some of these factors are shown in Table 6.1. It is well known that ethnic variations in diet may play a major role in the absorption, and therefore plasma levels, of a drug. Studies comparing the metabolism of antipyrine between Asian Indians and Indian immigrants in England revealed that as immigrants adopted the life-style and dietary habits of the British, their drug metabolism became more rapid (1). Similar findings were observed among Sudanese and Western Africans (2, 3). Cigarette smoking, as well as heavy drinking, are known to activate liver enzymes, thus fostering drug metabolism (4). Pregnancy, stress, diurnal rhythms, and fever may operate independently or simultaneously in the same individual, thus affecting in different ways and to different degrees, the processes of drug absorption, distribution, biotransformation, and excretion.

Cultural (Psychosocial)

Drug efficacy and compliance are affected by cultural or psychosocial factors such as beliefs, attitudes, and therapy expectations, as well as communication skills and family influences. Noncompliance in medication utilization is a major problem in the treatment of chronic medical conditions. Contrasting cultural beliefs across ethnic groups can affect medication compliance and hence drug effectiveness. For example, Kinzie et al. reported that 61% of depressed medicated refugee patients from Southeast Asia showed no evidence of tricyclic antidepressants (TCAs) in the blood, although they were all adequately treated with TCA dosages (5). The majority of these patients reported not taking the prescribed TCAs and pretended to comply with medication regimens for a number of reasons. In a South African study involving a long-term regimen of oral phenothiazines among black, white, and "colored" patients, rates of compliance varied: 33% for black, 50% for colored, and 75% for white patients (6).

Cultural beliefs among racial and ethnic groups may affect their attitudes toward the perceived benefits of medicines. This concept may best be illustrated by the fact that there is a therapeutic effect observed in the use of placebos in clinical trials. It is not known why a placebo has a therapeutic effect; however, a positive attitude about the potential benefit of the medication taken, albeit a placebo, may be a factor in drug response.

Expectations of medications also play an important role in patient compliance. Clinicians working with refugees and other Asian populations report that these patients typically expect medicines from the Western culture to work quickly, to have a high potential for severe side effects, and to be effective only for the control of the "superficial" manifestations, not underlying conditions of the diseases (7). The investigators concluded that Asian refugees, unless carefully counseled, often have difficulty appreciating the need for maintenance therapy in most psychiatric conditions (7).

Gender

The gender of an individual is a factor that can often lead to interindividual differences in the metabolism of

Table 6.1.
Factors Affecting Drug Responses in Different Racial and Ethnic Groups

I. Environmental
- Chronic alcohol ingestion
- Multiple Disease States
- Diet
- Fever
- Cigarette smoking
- Pregnancy
- Stress
- Diurnal rhythms

II. Cultural (Psychosocial)
- Attitudes
- Beliefs
- Family influence
- Therapy expectations

III. Genetic
- Pharmacogenetics
- Genetic polymorphism

Table 6.2.
Some Drugs That Show Genetic Polymorphism in Drug Metabolism

Debrisoquine Polymorphism	Acetylation Polymorphism	Mephenytoin Polymorphism
Amitriptyline	Clonazepam	Diazepam
Imipramine	Nitrazepam	Imipramine
Clomipramine	Hydralazine	Mephobarbital
Nortriptyline	Procainamide	Hexobarbital
Chlorpromazine	Isoniazid	Omeprazol
Haloperidol	Caffeine	
Labetolol	Phenelzine	
Metoprolol		
Timolol		
Propranolol		

Adapted from Relling MV, Evans WE. Genetic polymorphisms of drug metabolism. In Evans WE, Schentag JJ, Josko WJ, Relling MV, eds. Applied pharmacokinetics: principles of therapeutic drug monitoring, 3rd ed. Chap 7. Vancouver, WA. Applied Therapeutics, 1992; and Meyer UA. Drugs in special patient groups: clinical importance of genetics in drug effects. In: Melman KL, Morrelli HF, Hoffman BB, Nierenberg DW, eds. Melman and morrelli clinical pharmacology: basic principles in therapeutics, 3rd ed. Chap 32 New York: McGraw-Hill, 1992:875–894.

drugs (8). Studies done to assess sex differences in drug metabolism are inconclusive, because confounding factors, such as menstrual cycle and the use of oral contraceptives, frequently were not taken into consideration (9). However, in those studies where gender differences in metabolism/pharmacokinetics exist, women tend to have higher plasma concentrations than men. When the pharmacokinetics of lidocaine and chlordiazepoxide were examined with respect to gender differences, it was found that the elimination half-life in females was larger compared to males due to either increased volume of distribution or decreased clearance (10).

In general, drugs that are metabolized by hepatic oxidation have impaired metabolic clearance and prolonged elimination half-lives in females who are on oral contraceptives compared to those who are not (9). The clinical significance of gender-related differences in the pharmacokinetic properties of some drugs has not been clearly established. Giudicelli and Tillement concluded that it is unnecessary to change dose or frequency of administration of a drug based on gender-related differences in metabolism (8).

Physiologic differences between the sexes in hormone and enzyme levels and basal metabolism influence the metabolism of various drugs (11). For example, gender differences in muscle mass, disposition of muscle tissue, and vascular resistance could cause variation in response to intramuscular injections. Gender differences in gastric motility and secretion and metabolic rate may influence plasma levels of orally administered drugs. However, it must be pointed out that the clinical significance of these influencing factors remains to be established.

Gender differences in drug therapy probably have been studied the most with the psychotropic agents. This could be due in part to the observation that females have higher admission rates than males for mental disorders and a greater degree of severity of symptoms (12, 13). In one

study, male schizophrenic patients required less medication than females (14). Another study showed that male schizophrenic patients generally require less medication, lower doses, and have a more favorable outcome to psychotropic therapy than female patients (15). However, findings from a more recent study by Yonkers et al. indicate that women have greater efficacy with antipsychotic agents and a greater likelihood of adverse reactions (16). It is clear that the gender differences require more extensive controlled studies.

Pharmacogenetics

Pharmacogenetics is the study of genetically determined variations in drug response (17). In healthy individuals, genetically controlled differences in the way individuals metabolize (i.e., oxidize and acetylate) drugs are major determinants of racial and ethnic differences in response to medicines. Genetic polymorphisms (multiple forms of enzymes governing drug metabolism) account for interindividual differences in their ability to metabolize drugs that are controlled by a single gene. The focus of this discussion will be on pharmacogenetic metabolism related to the cytochrome P40 enzymes catalyzing the biotransformation of debrisoquine (debrisoquin hydroxylase, known as CYP2D6) and mephenytoin (mephenytoin hydroxylase, known as CYP2C19), and the acetylation polymorphisms (Table 6.2) (17, 18). These are the most important clinical polymorphisms, because many drugs are metabolized by their pathways.

Debrisoquine Polymorphism. Debrisoquine is an antihypertensive agent that was found to exhibit a genetic polymorphism in its oxidated metabolism (19). Two distinct phenotypes were observed in the population with a urinary ratio of debrisoquine to its main 4-hydroxy metabolite. Those individuals who were deficient in their ability to oxidize the substrate are called poor metabolizers (PMs), whereas extensive metabolizers (EMs) biotransform a substantial amount of the drug to its metabolite.

The importance of debrisoquine polymorphic oxidation lies in the fact that more than 30 commonly prescribed medications are metabolized by this pathway (20). Drugs metabolized by this pathway include antidepressants, anticonvulsants, antipsychotics, opioids, antiarrhythmics, and β-blockers (Table 6.2). Poor metabolizers (PMs) and extensive metabolizers (EMs) may experience problems when being treated with these agents. PMs do not metabolize the drugs in question well and will often develop elevated plasma concentrations, leading to adverse effects. EMs, however, do not respond to recommended doses because drug concentrations are too low (17). The prevalence of the PM phenotype in all ethnic groups studied ranges on an average between 2 and 10%, with Asians being identified with no or very few poor metabolizers (Table 6.3) (21).

Mephenytoin Polymorphism. The polymorphism of mephenytoin hydroxylation varies according to racial and ethnic differences. Drug categories affected by mephenytoin polymorphism include antidepressants as well as antianxiety agents (Table 2). The incidence of poor metabolizers (PMs) is 2 to 5% among Caucasians and 15 to 20% in Japanese, and no PMs were found among Panamanian Cuna Amerindians (Table 6.3) (22, 23). A study in an elderly unmedicated population showed an increased incidence of slow metabolizers among African-Americans (18.5%) as compared to Caucasians (4.1%) (24). It was not determined if these differences were due to genetic or environmental factors.

Acetylation Polymorphism. Polymorphic N-acetylation was first studied when serum concentrations of isoniazid showed substantial interindividual variability (25). Patients were classified as slow acetylators (SA) and rapid acetylators (RA) according to their ability to metabolize isoniazid. American and European Caucasians and American blacks have approximately equal numbers of SAs and RAs, whereas in Japanese and Canadian Eskimo subjects, the percentage of RAs is high and that of SAs is low (Table 6.4) (26). Commonly prescribed medications that are metabolized by this pathway include procainamide, hydralazine, phenelzine, and clonazepam (Table 6.2).

DRUG RESPONSE TO RACIAL AND ETHNIC DIFFERENCES

The drug categories that have been studied the most and shown to be most clinically significant in their actions with regard to racial and ethnic differences are cardiovascular (antihypertensives, atropine) and central nervous system agents (psychotropics, analgesics, alcohol).

Variations in Effects of Cardiovascular Drugs
ANTIHYPERTENSIVE AGENTS

Essential hypertension is considered to be a multifactorial disorder. Recent studies have identified characteristics that may help predict the efficacy of monotherapy in controlling this disease. These characteristics include physiologic factors, such as sodium sensitivity, plasma renin activity, sympathetic nervous system activity, and demographic environmental factors (27). These characteristics of individual patients are important considerations in antihypertensive drug selection because of the increasing numbers and classes of antihypertensive agents and the difference in response among varied ethnic and racial groups.

Table 6.3.
Incidence of Poor/Slow Metabolizers in Different Racial Groups

Metabolic Polymorphism	Drug Examples	Poor/Slow Metabolizers (%)	
		Caucasian	Asian
Debrisoquine	desipramine amitriptyline haloperidol metaprolol phenacetin	5–10	<1
Acetylation	caffeine hydralazine procainamide isoniazid	50	7–22
Mephenytoin	diazepam imipramine	2–5	15–20

Adapted from Levy RA. Ethnic and racial differences in response to medicines. Preserving individualized therapy in managed pharmaceutical programs. Reston, VA: National Pharmaceutical Council, 1993:1–42; and Nakamura K, Goto F, Ray WA, et al. Interethnic differences in genetic polymorphism of debrisoquine and mephenytoin hydroxylation between Japanese and Caucasian populations. Clin Pharmacol Ther 38:402–408, 1985.

Table 6.4.
Incidence of Slow Acetylators in Some Racial and Ethnic Groups

Group	Slow Acetylators (%)
Caucasians	50
American Blacks	50
Japanese	10
Canadian Eskimo	5
Egyptians	80–90
Moroccans	80–90
Chinese	15

Adapted from Nakamura K, Goto F, Ray WA, et al. Interethnic differences in genetic polymorphism of debrisoquine and mephenytoin hydroxylation between Japanese and Caucasian populations. Clin Pharmacol Ther 38:402–408, 1985.

Table 6.5.
Racial and Ethnic Differences in Response to Antihypertensive Agents

Comparison Groups	Drug Class/Agent	Clinical Response	Reference
African American/Caucasian	Calcium Channel Blockers	African-Americans respond to monotherapy as well as whites.	27
African American/Caucasian	Beta-Blockers	Blacks respond less than whites. No difference if diuretic is added.	27, 29
African American/Caucasian	Propranolol	African-Americans have a higher oral clearance of propranolol.	36
Chinese/Caucasian	Propranolol	Chinese are twice as sensitive to the effects on blood pressure.	29
African American/Caucasian	Diuretics	African-Americans respond better to diuretics.	21
African American/Caucasian	Labetolol (combined α- and β-blocker)	African-Americans respond the same as Caucasians.	37
African American/Caucasian	ACE Inhibitors	Monotherapy more effective in Caucasians. No difference if diuretic is added.	29

Although all antihypertensive agents can be effective in the general population, with regard to specific racial and ethnic racial groups, some are more predictable than others and some require different doses for an equivalent effect (Table 6.5).

DIURETICS

The pathophysiology of hypertension in a large segment of the black population is characterized, among other things, by enhanced sodium retention and expanded plasma volume. Diuretics are useful as monotherapy and in combination with other agents in the treatment of hypertension in black patients. Diuretics are effective in this racial group because they reduce plasma volume and intracellular sodium concentrations. The reduction in blood pressure with diuretics is due to a decrease in total peripheral resistance that is related to a decreased sensitivity of the vascular wall to pressor substances and possibly to stimulation of the prostacyclin and kallikrein-kinin vasodilator systems (28).

Monotherapy with diuretics tends to cause a greater reduction in blood pressure in black than in white hypertensives. Studies by the Veterans Administration documented an average decrease in blood pressure in black males of approximately 20/13 mm Hg as opposed to an average decrease of 15/11 mm Hg in white men, despite a lower dose of diuretic in the black male hypertensives (29).

β-Blockers. The Veterans Administration Cooperative Study Group on Antihypertensive Agents showed that fewer black than white subjects reached their blood pressure goal while taking β-blockers (30). It has also been shown that differences in plasma renin activity are believed to underlie many of the cross-racial and ethnic differences in response to β-blockers. A greater proportion of white people than black people have elevated plasma renin activity, hence requiring lower therapeutic doses of a β-blocker. The reasons for these differences may be due to differences in renal physiology, which may be genetically determined. For example, the renin-angiotensin system is more frequently suppressed relative to sodium intake and excretion in blacks than in whites (31). It has been shown that 36 to 62% of black hypertensives have relatively suppressed plasma renin activities as compared to 19 to 55% of white hypertensives (32). Even in normotensive patients, plasma renin activity is lower in blacks than in whites (33, 34). Therefore, β-blockers, which are believed to work in part by lowering plasma renin, would be less effective in blacks who already have lowered renin levels. Even though blacks tend to fall into the low-renin category, with a volume-dependent, salt-sensitive type of hypertension, there are subgroups within the black population that do respond to β-blockers.

Pharmacokinetic and pharmacodynamic factors may also explain the difference in response to β-blockers. Racial differences in affinity for the lymphocyte β receptor may explain documented differences in response. For example, a study by Johnson showed that the affinity for the β receptor for propranolol was greater in white than in black patients (35). Another study concluded that black patients may be less responsive to the effects of β-blockers than whites because of observed higher renal clearance of propranolol (36).

Evidence exists that Blacks may even respond differently to different β-blockers. For example, labetalol (a combined α-β-blocker), unlike propranolol, is equally effective in controlling blood pressure in black and white patients (37). It was also shown that bisoprolol produced significant decreases in both systolic and diastolic blood pressure in black patients, and there also was a trend for atenolol to decrease blood pressure (38). Also, Blacks respond to β-blockers in combination with diuretics equally as well as whites (27, 29, 39). Therefore, pharmacotherapy with β-blockers must be specifically directed toward the individual patient.

It seems as though Chinese patients also exhibit altered sensitivity to β-blockers, but conversely to black Americans. A study involving the pharmacokinetic and pharmacodynamic of propranolol compared men of Chinese descent and white American men (40). The Chinese exhibited a twofold greater sensitivity to the effect of propranolol on blood pressure and heart rate as compared to Caucasians. The investigators concluded that the increased sensitivity to β-blockers results, possibly through the β-receptor-mediated suppression of plasma renin activity, and this increased sensitivity to plasma renin activity suppression in Chinese subjects may partially explain their increased sensitivity to the hypotensive effects of propranolol.

ACE Inhibitors. Angiotensin-converting enzyme (ACE) inhibitors act through a renin-dependent mechanism. Therefore, the major determinant in response to ACE inhibitors in hypertensive patients is their renin status. Individuals with high plasma renin have a much greater response to the antihypertensive effects of ACE inhibitors than do low renin patients. Therefore, one would generally expect the ACE inhibitors to be less effective in black than white patients. This difference was observed with captopril and enalapril; however, when the diuretic hydrochlorothiazide was added, the racial difference in response was abolished (41).

Calcium Channel Blockers. The hypotensive effect of calcium channel blockers as monotherapy in Blacks is comparable to that observed in white patients and significantly greater than that observed in Blacks treated with β-blockers or ACE inhibitors (28). Blacks, elderly, and low-renin hypertensive patients tend to have an enhanced calcium influx-dependent vasoconstriction (42). This may explain, in part, the excellent antihypertensive effectiveness of monotherapy with calcium channel blockers in black patients.

In summary, regarding the antihypertensive agents, the low-renin profile, salt retention, expanded plasma volume, and increased intracellular concentrations of sodium and calcium found in many black hypertensives may provide the pathophysiologic basis for the significant differences observed in response to antihypertensive agents. When used as monotherapy to treat black hypertensives, diuretics and calcium channel blockers tend to produce a greater reduction in blood pressure when compared to β-blockers and ACE inhibitors.

Atropine. Paskind reported over 70 years ago that initial bradycardia, attributed to central vagal stimulation prior to peripheral cholinergic blockade, after parenteral administration of atropine does not occur in African-

Americans at doses that cause bradycardia in Caucasians (43). Similar results were reported in a study from South Africa (44). However, the black patients were more susceptible to the late bradycardia effect, which occurs about an hour after the dose. They also observed that the tachycardia effect was significantly more pronounced in African blacks when compared to whites (44).

Zhou and Wood reported that healthy Chinese subjects showed a greater increase in heart rate than Caucasians after receiving intravenous atropine. There was no difference in the bradycardia effect that occurred in both groups (45).

Variation in Effects of CNS Drugs
PSYCHOTROPIC AGENTS

Racial and/or ethnic differences need to be considered in decisions regarding the use of psychotropic drugs (Table 6.6). Growing evidence seems to indicate that the pharmacodynamic and pharmacokinetic influences of these agents may undoubtedly differ between races, and these differences can affect clinical outcome.

Antipsychotics. Comparisons of antipsychotic activity among different racial groups reveal both similarities and potentially important differences (Table 6.6). Blacks, Caucasians, and Hispanics do not differ in their pharmacokinetics or dosage requirements of antipsychotic drugs; however, Asians seem to have a lower threshold than whites for both the therapeutic and adverse effects of these agents (46). Increased absorption, reduced hepatic hydroxylation, and pharmacodynamic factors all play a role in dosage differences (47). Midha et al. and Jann et al. showed that Chinese patients showed higher haloperidol plasma concentrations than in Caucasians, Hispanics, and Blacks (48, 49). Lam et al., 1995, showed intra- and interethnic variability among Blacks, Caucasians, Chinese, and Mexican-Americans in reduced haloperidol to haloperidol ratios compared with the other three ethnic groups. The Chinese patients had the lowest ratio (50). Additionally, the haloperidol dosage required for the black and white groups were significantly greater than the Chinese group to achieve comparable plasma levels. This observation that Asian patients require lower dosages than do other groups is strengthened by pharmacokinetic studies that report higher plasma or serum drug concentrations in Asian patients, even when weight and body surface area are controlled (49). Additionally, other investigators have reported that lower antipsychotic dosages are required in Asian populations when compared to Caucasians (51–53). Cultural, environmental, and genetic factors may all be involved in this difference in dosage requirement (1). Therefore, it seems prudent to use lower than usual initial dosages of antipsychotic drugs in the treatment of Asian patients.

Table 6.6.
Racial and Ethnic Differences in Response to Psychotropic Agents

Comparison Groups	Drug Class/Agent	Clinical Response	Reference
Chinese/African-American/ Hispanic/Caucasian	Haloperidol	Chinese showed higher plasma concentrations.	49
Asian/Caucasian	Antipsychotics	Lower dosages are required in Asian population.	51, 52, 53
African-American/Caucasian	Chlorpromazine	African-Americans showed more rapid improvement.	56
African-American/Caucasian	Nortriptyline	African-Americans had steady-state plasma concentrations that were 50% higher.	58
African-American/Caucasian	Imipramine	African-Americans showed more rapid improvement.	56
Hispanics/Caucasian	Antidepressants	Hispanics appeared to experience more overall side effects.	60
Asian/Caucasian	Antidepressants	Asians achieved significantly higher plasma concentrations and had lower clearance rates.	63
Chinese/Caucasians/Hispanics	Antidepressants	Chinese and Hispanics require lower doses; side effects greater in Hispanics than Caucasians.	22
Asian/Caucasian	Alprazolam	Asians exhibit higher serum concentrations, decreased clearance, and longer half-lives.	53
Chinese/Caucasian	Diazepam	Chinese showed smaller volumes of distribution and higher mean serum concentrations.	64
Asian/Caucasian	Diazepam	Caucasians showed higher clearance rates.	1

It should be noted that the use of antipsychotics in Blacks is more frequent than in other racial groups (54). This may be explained, in part, by the fact that black patients generally receive more severe diagnoses, such as schizophrenia as opposed to an anxiety or mood disorder (55). Perhaps for similar reasons, Blacks tend to receive substantially higher doses of antipsychotics. This may also be due to the stereotype that Blacks are more difficult to manage and less compliant (54).

Raskin and Cook studied the effects of chlorpromazine and imipramine in black and white inpatients (56). In general, black patients showed greater clinical improvement than whites on measured psychiatric illnesses, irrespective of treatment. However, these differences were more apparent early in treatment (i.e., at 1 week) than at 2 or 3 weeks. Significant differences were found in drug effects when comparing black men and women. Chlorpromazine was more efficacious for treating black women, and black men were therapeutically more responsive to imipramine. Methodologic concerns include an overrepresentation of patients with the diagnosis of schizophrenia among African-Americans (especially black males) and the fact that black patients were much younger and significantly more educationally and economically disadvantaged than their white counterparts.

Lieberman et al observed a genetically determined increased risk of agranulocytosis during clozapine therapy in about 20% of Ashkenazi Jewish patients (57). This adverse reaction developed only in about 1% of chronic schizophrenic patients. The investigators used human leukocyte antigen (HLA) typing to identify the haplotype (a cluster of genes that are involved in immune recognition and autoimmunity) that is associated with the development of clozapine-induced agranulocytosis.

Antidepressant Agents. There is not much published information regarding differences in antidepressant pharmacology among black, Caucasian, Hispanic, and Asian patients. Additional controlled pharmacokinetic and pharmacodynamic studies with these classes of drugs need to be carried out before clinical applications of tricyclic antidepressants in different racial groups can be made.

General findings seem to indicate that, for a given dose of tricyclic antidepressants, African-American patients show higher blood levels and faster therapeutic response than Caucasians. Also, black patients tend to manifest a greater degree of toxic effects than white patients (54). An often cited study by Ziegler and Biggs reported that steady-state plasma levels of nortriptyline in patients treated with equal oral dosages were 50%

higher in black patients than in white patients (58). It should be noted, however, that the study has been criticized for improper correction of plasma concentrations on the basis of weight (59). Also, the investigators did not employ a fixed dose protocol or clearly outline diagnostic criteria or description of gender distribution (54).

While many studies indicated that Hispanic and Asian patients required lower doses of tricyclic antidepressants, the results were inconsistent. Hispanic patients also appeared to experience more overall side effects with antidepressants than Caucasians; however, a single-dose study comparing plasma nortriptyline levels and clearance rates in healthy Hispanic and Caucasian volunteers failed to demonstrate any major differences between the two groups (60, 61).

Regarding Asian patients, survey data collected from multiple Asian countries indicate that both imipramine and amitriptyline are used in much lower dosage ranges than is typical in the United States (62). Additionally, single-dose pharmacokinetic studies indicated that Asians achieve significantly higher plasma concentrations of TCAs and have lower clearance rates than do Caucasians (63). However, it should be noted that some of the research did not adjust for patient weight (63). Therefore, the role of racial and ethnic differences in response to antidepressants remains unclear because of limited, and sometimes conflicting, data.

Antianxiety Agents. A single-dose pharmacokinetic study using alprazolam showed that Asians manifested significantly higher plasma concentrations, decreased clearance, and longer half-lives than did Caucasians (53). Lin et al. showed in 1986 that the clearance rate of diazepam was higher in Caucasians, suggesting that diazepam is metabolized at a significantly higher rate in Caucasians than Asians (1). Another study showed that healthy male Chinese subjects showed smaller volumes of distribution and higher mean serum concentrations than their white counterparts (64). Pharmacokinetic differences in the metabolism of these benzodiazepines may be because Asians (e.g., Japanese) have a higher incidence of poor metabolizers (PMs) than Caucasians (1).

Based on the data observed, it is suggested that Asian psychiatric patients will require smaller initial and continuing doses of benzodiazepines (e.g., alprazolam and diazepam) for similar clinical effects than Caucasian patients (65).

Bipolar Agents. There is little evidence for claims of racial and ethnic differences in response to lithium. However, one study reported that African-Americans have a significantly longer plasma half-life of lithium compared to Caucasians and Chinese (66). It has also been reported that Japanese patients require lower dosages of lithium and respond to lower plasma lithium levels than their U.S. counterparts for the treatment of bipolar illness (67). Honda and Suzuki reported in 1979 that Caucasians in the United States have higher lithium clearances and larger volumes of distribution than do Japanese (68).

In summary, regarding psychotropic agents, Asians in general need lower doses and exhibit adverse effects at lower doses than whites when given psychotropic drugs. Hispanics tend to require less antidepressant medications and report more adverse effects at lower doses than Caucasians. Blacks, in general, respond better than whites to antidepressants, have higher plasma levels, and show a greater degree of adverse effects.

Analgesics. Racial and ethnic differences have been demonstrated for the metabolism of codeine. Wood and Zhou showed that Chinese patients were less able to metabolize codeine than Caucasian patients (21). Another study comparing Swedish Caucasians and Chinese healthy subjects revealed that the excretion of unchanged codeine was significantly higher in Chinese compared with Caucasians (69). The clinical consequences of these differences in the pharmacokinetics of codeine must be considered in establishing dosing levels in patients for the treatment of pain.

Mucklow et al. observed racial and ethnic differences in the metabolism of paracetamol (acetaminophen) (70). Asian immigrants had lower acetaminophen clearance and longer half-life when compared to Caucasians. It has also been observed that the mean combined recovery of paracetamol metabolites in Caucasians was twice that observed in Ghanians and Kenyan blacks (39). This finding was attributed to a reduced level of microsomal oxidation in Africans and Asians.

Alcohol. North American Indians, Chinese, and Japanese show a faster rate of alcohol metabolism (i.e., conversion to the aldehyde) and less tolerance than do Caucasians (71). Asians of Mongoloid heritage, American Indians, Japanese, and Chinese show more symptoms of intoxication after alcohol use than Caucasians and are much more sensitive to its adverse effects, including facial flushing, palpitations, and tachycardia. Facial flushing occurs in 45 to 85% of Asians versus 3 to 29% of Caucasians (72). The flushing is caused by the accumulation of acetaldehyde due to an unusual less-active liver aldehyde dehydrogenase (39, 72). An "atypical" alcohol dehydrogenase that has higher alcohol metabolism is present in 85 to 90% of Asians and may also contribute to increased blood levels of acetaldehyde (72).

Jewish men and women have one of the lowest percentages of severe alcohol-related problems of any group. One reason proposed is that Jewish men and women may have an increased sensitivity to relatively low doses of alcohol. This might serve as an internal checkpoint in order to avoid high intake of alcoholic beverages (73).

CONCLUSIONS

The premise that a drug will act identically in two different people or in two different races, ethnic groups, or cultures has been challenged and found to be flawed. Therefore, racial and ethnic representation in clinical trials must be broadened. For a growing number of drugs, the percentage of patients who react differently or adversely is determined by their racial and ethnic background. The study of racial and ethnic differences in response to medicines has been primarily limited to a few classes of drugs. However, future studies will likely reveal significant data regarding these differences in the action of many additional drugs.

Cost is often the driving force in a managed care environment with a restricted formulary. The formulary must not be so restrictive that it ignores the fact that patients in specific groups metabolize drugs differently, have different clinical responses, and experience different side effects. Therefore, racial, ethnic, and gender differences require us to balance control of drug cost with the need for individualized therapy.

REFERENCES

1. Lin K-M, Poland RE, Lesser IM. Ethnicity and psychopharmacology. Cult Med Psychiatry 10:151–165, 1986.
2. Branch RA, Salih SY, Momeida M. Racial differences in drug metabolizing ability: a study with antipyrine in the Sudan. Clin Pharmacol Ther 24:283–286, 1978.
3. Fraser HS, Mucklow JC, Bulpitt CJ, et al. Environmental effects on antipyrine half-life in man. Clin Pharmacol Ther 22:799–808, 1977.
4. Robinson R. Individualization of drug therapy: considering ethnic differences. Consult Pharm 5(6):328–334, 1990.
5. Kinzie JD, Leung P, Boehnlein J, et al. Tricyclic antidepressant plasma levels in Indochinese refugees clinical implications. J Nerv Ment Dis 175:480–485, 1987.
6. Gillis LS, Trollip D, Jakoet A, et al. Noncompliance with psychotropic medication. S Afr Med J 72:602–606, 1987.
7. Lin K-H, Shen WW. Pharmacotherapy for Southeast Asian psychiatric patients. J Nerv Ment Dis 197:346–350, 1991.
8. Giudicelli JF, Tillement JP. Influences of sex on drug kinetics in man. Clin Pharmacokinet 2:157–166, 1977.
9. Bonate DL. Gender-related differences in xenobiotic metabolism. J Clin Pharmacol 31:684–690, 1991.
10. Wings IMH, Miner JO, Birkett J, et al. Lidocaine disposition-sex differences and effects of cimetidine. Clin Pharmacol Ther 35:695–701, 1984.
11. Proksch RA, Lamy PP. Sex variation and drug therapy. Drug Intell Clin Pharm 2:398–406, 1977.
12. Kramer M. Cross-national study of diagnosis of the mental disorders: origins of the problem. Am J Psychiatry 125(suppl 10):1–11, 1969.
13. Weich MJ. Behavioral differences between groups of acutely psychotic males and females. Psychiatr Q 42(1):107–122, 1968.
14. Taylor MA, Levine R. Influence of sex of hospitalized schizophrenia on therapeutic dosage levels of neuroleptics. Dis Nerv Syst 32(2):131–134, 1971.
15. Demer HC, Bird EG. Chlorpromazine in the treatment of mental illness. IV Final results with analysis of data on 1,523 patients. Am J Psychiatry 113:972–978, 1957.
16. Yonkers KA, Kando JC, Cole JO, et al. Gender differences in pharmacokinetics and pharmacodynamics of psychotropic medication. Am J Psychiatr 149(5):587–595, 1992.
17. Meyer UA. Drugs in special patient groups: clinical importance of genetics in drug effects. In: Melman KL, Morrelli HF, Hoffman BB, Nierenberg DW, eds. Melman and Morrelli Clinical Pharmacology: Basic Principles in Therapeutics, 3rd ed. New York: McGraw-Hill, 1992:875–94.
18. Relling MV, Evans WE. Genetic polymorphisms of drug metabolism. In: Evans WE, Schentag JJ, Josko WJ, Relling MV, eds. Applied Pharmacokinetics: Principles of Therapeutic Drug Monitoring, 3rd ed. Vancouver, WA: Applied Therapeutics, 1992:1–32.
19. Mahgoub A, Idle JR, Dring LG, et al. Polymorphic hydroxylation of debrisoquine in man. Lancet 2:584–586, 1977.
20. Evans WE, Relling MV, Rahman A, et al. Genetic basis for a lower prevalence of deficient CYP2D6 oxidative drug metabolism phenotypes in Black Americans. J Clin Invest 91:2150–2154, 1993.
21. Wood AJ, Zhou HH. Ethnic differences in drug disposition and responsiveness. Clin Pharmacokinet 20:350–373, 1991.
22. Levy RA. Ethnic and racial differences in response to medicines. Preserving individualized therapy in managed pharmaceutical programs. Reston, VA: National Pharmaceutical Council, 1993:1–42.
23. Nakamura K, Goto F, Ray WA, et al. Interethnic differences in genetic polymorphism of debrisoquine and mephenytoin hydroxylation between Japanese and Caucasian populations. Clin Pharmacol Ther 38:402–408, 1985.
24. Pollock BG, Perel JM, Kirshner M, et al. S-mephenytoin 4-hydroxylation in older Americans. Eur J Clin Pharmcol 40:609–611, 1991.
25. Mitchell RS, Bell JC. Clinical implications of isoniazid blood levels in pulmonary tuberculosis. N Engl J Med 257:1066–1071, 1957.
26. Weber WW, Hein DW. N-acetylation pharmacogenetics. Pharmacol Rev 35:25–79, 1985.
27. Weinberger MH. Racial differences in antihypertensive therapy: evidence and implications. Cardiovasc Drugs Ther 4:379–382, 1990.
28. Hall WD. Pathophysiology of hypertension in blacks. Am J Hypertens 3:12:366S–371S, 1990.
29. Veterans Administration Cooperative Study Group on Antihypertensive Agents. Comparison of propranolol and hydrochlorothiazide for the initial treatment of hypertension: I. Results of short-term titration with emphasis on racial differences in response. JAMA 248:1996–2003, 1982.
30. Veterans Administration Cooperative Study Group on Antihypertensive Agents. Racial differences in response to low-dose captopril are abolished by the addition of hydrochlorothiazide. Br J Clin Pharmacol 14:97S–101S, 1982.
31. Gillum RF. Pathophysiology of hypertension in Blacks and whites. Hypertension 1(5):468–475, 1979.
32. Wisenbaugh PE, Garst JB, Hull C, et al. Renin, aldosterone, sodium and hypertension. Am J Med 52(2):175–186, 1972.
33. Levy SB, Lilley JJ, Frigon RP, et al. Urinary kallikrein and plasma renin activity as determinants of renal blood flow. The influence of race and dietary sodium intake. J Clin Invest 60(1):129–138, 1977.
34. Luft FC, Grim CE, Higgins JT, et al. Differences in response to sodium administration in normotensive white and Black subjects. J Lab Clin Med 90(3):555–562, 1977.
35. Johnson JA. Racial differences in lymphocyte beta-receptor sensitivity to propranolol. Life Sci 53(4):297–304, 1993.
36. Johnson JA, Burlew BS. Racial differences in propranolol pharmacokinetics. Clin Pharmacol Ther 51:495–500, 1992.
37. Oster G, Huse DM, Deles TE, et al. Cost effectiveness of labetolol and propranolol in the treatment of hypertensive Black patients. Natl Med Assoc 79:1049–1055, 1987.
38. Neutel JM, Smith DHG, Ram VS, et al. Comparison of bisoprolol with atenolol for systematic hypertension in four population groups using ambulatory blood pressure monitoring. Am J Cardiol 72:41–46, 1993.

39. Kitler ME. Clinical trials and transethnic pharmacology. Drug Saf (5):378–391, 1994.

40. Zhou H, Koshakji RP, Silberstein DJ, et al. Racial differences in response: altered sensitivity to and clearance of propranolol in men of Chinese descent as compared with American Whites. N Engl J Med 320:565–570, 1989.

41. 1988 report of the joint national committee on detection, evaluation, and treatment of high blood pressure. Arch Intern Med 148:1023–1038, 1988.

42. Buhler FR. Antihypertensive treatment according to age, plasma renin and race. Drugs 35:495–503, 1988.

43. Paskind HA. Some differences in response to atropine in White and colored races. J Lab Clin Med 7:104–108, 1921.

44. Meyer EC, Sommers DK, Schoeman HS. The effect of atropine on heart-rate: a comparison between two ethnic groups. Br J Clin Pharmacol 25:776–777, 1988.

45. Zhou HA, Wood AJ. Atropine produces a greater increase in heart rate in Chinese than Caucasians [Abstract]. Clin Res 38:7A, 1990.

46. Bond WS. Ethnicity and psychotropic drugs. Clin Pharm 10:467–470, 1990.

47. Jann MW, Grimsley SR. Pharmacogenetics of agents on the central nervous system. J Pharm Pract 6(1):2–16, 1993.

48. Midha KK, Chahraborty BS, Ganes DA, et al. Intersubject variation in the pharmacokinetics of haloperidol and reduced haloperidol. J Clin Psychopharmacol 9:98–104, 1988.

49. Jann MW, Chang WH, Lam YM, et al. Comparison of haloperidol and reduced haloperidol plasma levels in four different ethnic populations. Prog Neuropsychopharmacol Biol Psychiatry 16:193–202, 1992.

50. Lam YW, Jann MW, Chang WH, et al. Intra- and interethnic variability in reduced haloperidol to haloperidol ratios. J Clin Pharmacol 35:128–136, 1995.

51. Lin KM, Finder EJ. Neuroleptic dosage in Asians. Am J Psychiatry 140:490–491, 1983.

52. Potkin SG, Shen Y, Pardes H, et al. Haloperidol concentrations elevated in Chinese patients. Psychiatry Res 12:167–172, 1984.

53. Lin K-M, Lau JK, Smith R, et al. Comparison of alprazolam plasma levels in normal Asian and Caucasian male volunteers. Psychopharmacology 96:365–369, 1988.

54. Strickland TL, Raiganath V, Lin K-M, et al. Psychopharmacologic considerations in the treatment of Black American populations. Psychopharmacol Bull 27(4):441–448, 1991.

55. Bell CC, Mehta H. Misdiagnosis of Black patients with manic depressive illness: second in the series. J Natl Med Assoc 73:101–107, 1980.

56. Raskin A, Cook TH. Antidepressants in Black and White inpatients. Arch Gen Psychiatry 32:643–649, 1975.

57. Lieberman JA, Yunis J, Egea E, et al. HLA-B38, DR4, DQw3 and clozapine-induced agranulocytosis in Jewish patients with schizophrenia. Arch Gen Psychiatr 47:945–948, 1990.

58. Ziegler VE, Biggs JT. Tricyclic plasma levels: effects of age, race, sex, and smoking. JAMA 238(20):2167–2169, 1977.

59. Rifkin A, Kline DF, Quitkin F. Possible effects of race on tricyclic plasma level [Letter]. JAMA 239:1845–1846, 1978.

60. Mendoza R, Smith MW, Poland RE, et al. Ethnic psychopharmacology: the Hispanic and Native American perspective. Psychopharmacol Bull 27(4):449–461, 1991.

61. Gaviria M, Gil AA, Javard JI. Nortriptyline kinetics in Hispanic and Anglo subjects. J Clin Psychopharmacol 6:227–231, 1986.

62. Yamashita I, Yutaka A. Tricyclic antidepressants: therapeutic plasma level. Psychopharmacol Bull 15:40–41, 1979.

63. Rudorfer MB, Lane EA, Chang W-H, et al. Desipramine pharmacokinetics in Chinese and Caucasian volunteers. Br J Clin Pharmacol 17:433–440 1984.

64. Kumana CR, Lauder IJ, Chan M, et al. Differences in diazepam pharmacokinetics in Chinese and White Caucasians-relation to body lipid stores. J Clin Pharmacol 32:211–215, 1987.

65. Lin K-M, Poland RE, Smith MW, et al. Pharmacokinetic and other related factors affecting psychotropic responses in Asians. Psychopharmacol Bull 27(4):427–439, 1991.

66. Chang SS, Pandey GN, Zhang MY, et al. Racial differences in plasma and RBC lithium levels. Paper presented at the American Psychiatric Association. Los Angeles, CA. Continuing Medical Education Syllabus and Scientific Proceedings, 1984:239–240.

67. Takashshi R. Lithium treatment in affective disorders: therapeutic plasma level. Psychopharmacol Bull 15(4):32–35, 1979.

68. Honda Y, Suzuki T. Transcultural pharmacokinetic study on Li concentration in plasma and saliva. Psychopharmacol Bull 156(4):37–39, 1979.

69. Yue QY, Svensson JO, Alm C, et al. Interindividual and interethnic differences in the demethylation and glucuronidation of codeine. Br J Clin Pharmacol 28:629–637, 1989.

70. Mucklow JC, Fraser HS, Bulpitt CJ, et al. Environmental factors affecting paracetamol metabolism in London factory and office workers. Br J Clin Pharmacol 10:67–74, 1980.

71. Kalow W. Ethnic differences in drug metabolism. Clin Pharmacokinet 7:373–400, 1992.

72. Chan AW. Racial differences in alcohol sensitivity. Alcohol 21(1):93–104, 1986.

73. Monteiro MG, Klein JL, Schuckit MA. High levels of sensitivity to alcohol in young adult Jewish men: a pilot study. J Stud Alcohol 52:464–469, 1991.

CHAPTER 7

BIOTECHNOLOGY

KIMBERLY BERGSTROM and DANIEL PATERSON

Recombinant DNA technology has enabled us to produce commercially viable quantities of biologically active substances that are normally found in the body, many of which have specific therapeutic benefits. This has helped to spawn an entire industry that uses this and other tools of biotechnology to study the molecular biology of living systems and produce therapeutic products. Two of the most commercially successful products of the biotechnology industry are recombinant tissue plasminogen activator and recombinant human insulin. These products are reviewed extensively in Chapters 19 and 41. This chapter will focus on the impact that biotechnology is having on our understanding of the immune system and the products that are resulting from that understanding.

Although much has been learned in the last decade concerning the workings of the immune system, much remains to be explained. Undoubtedly, the acquired immune deficiency syndrome (AIDS) epidemic has been responsible for the increased focus on the immune system. This attention has yielded virtually daily breakthroughs that are exposing new pieces of a very complex and important puzzle. It is clear that many diseases, including cancer, infections, and genetic diseases, are influenced by the immune system.

The primary function of the immune system is to defend the host from foreign substances. The immune system must first recognize the foreign substance as "nonself" and then proceed to destroy or neutralize it (1). The immune system has two functional divisions of defense against foreign substances: specific and nonspecific.

NONSPECIFIC IMMUNE RESPONSE

The nonspecific (innate) immune response is stimulated the first time a foreign substance (antigen) enters the host (1). Components of the nonspecific response perform functions that provide both physical and biochemical defenses (2). Physical defenses are provided by the skin, the mucous membranes, and the cilia of the respiratory tract. The biochemical defenses include the process of inflammation, release of lysozyme, and the initiation of the complement cascade (2). *Inflammation* is a complex series of events that occur when tissue is injured. Vasoactive substances such as histamine are released, stimulating neutrophil and macrophage migration to the area of tissue injury to ingest (phagocytose) the antigen that is responsible (2).

Complement is set in motion by the recognition of either an antigen-antibody complex or bacteria or viruses. The cascading effect of activated complement stimulates biologic activities, including chemotaxis of monocytes, neutrophils, basophils, and eosinophils; the release of hydrolytic enzymes; and ultimately the destruction or inactivation of the invading antigen (2). Lysozyme (a bactericidal substance) is also released from nasal mucosa, saliva, and tears in high concentrations in response to bacterial invasion.

Nonspecific cellular components of the innate system include granulocytes (neutrophils, 60 to 70% of white blood cell counts [WBCs]; basophils, <1% of WBCs; eosinophils, 1 to 3% of WBCs) and mononuclear phagocytes (monocytes and macrophages). Eosinophils ingest immune complexes (antigen-antibody complexes) and clear parasitic organisms (2). Basophils help to mediate immune responses by releasing substances such as histamine in response to antigen-antibody complexes. Macrophages and neutrophils are primarily responsible for the ingestion of particles, a process termed phagocytosis.

Phagocytosis is an important component of the nonspecific immune response. Macrophages (phagocytes) envelop the antigen and expose it to internal enzymes that degrade and inactivate the antigen. The antigen then either is completely digested by degradative enzymes or appears on the surface of the macrophage, where T lymphocytes (from the specific immune system) can recognize the antigen and react to it (3).

SPECIFIC IMMUNE RESPONSE

The specific immune system recognizes and eliminates antigens with specialized and sophisticated cells, primarily macrophages and T and B lymphocytes. T lymphocytes are primarily responsible for cell-mediated immunity, delayed hypersensitivity, organ transplant rejection, and tumor surveillance (Fig. 7.1). B lymphocytes are responsible for humoral, or antibody-mediated, immunity.

There are four types of T lymphocytes: helper T cells, suppressor T cells, cytotoxic T cells, and memory T cells. *Helper T cells* regulate the cell-mediated response to antigens. When macrophages of the nonspecific immune system present antigen to the helper T cells, a series of events are set into motion: The helper T cells release interleukin-2 (IL-2) and γ-interferon, which in turn

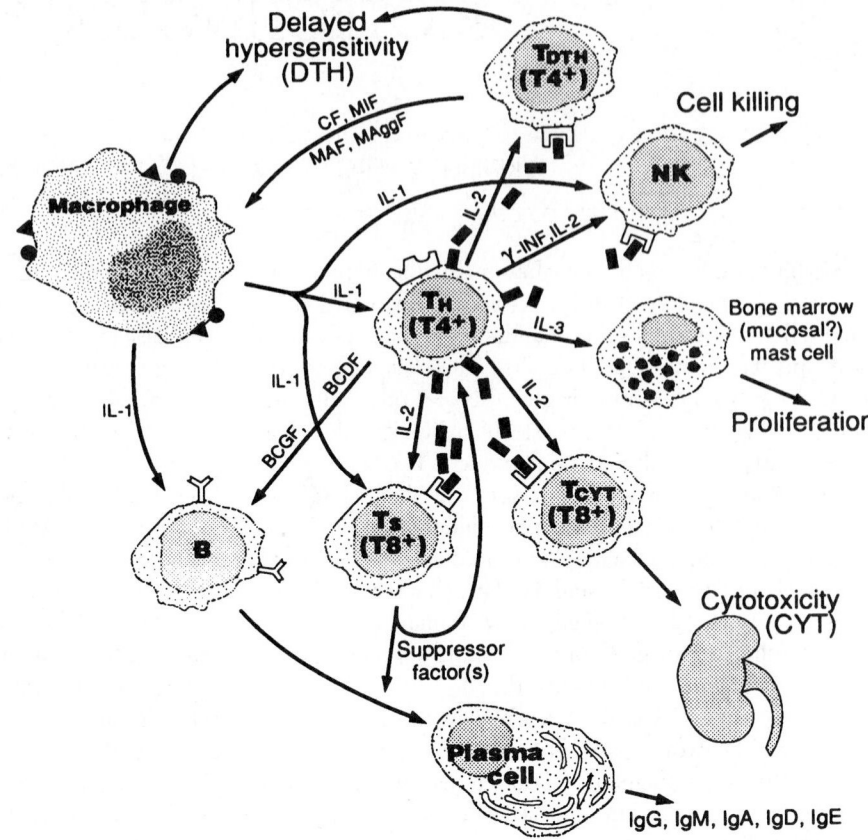

Figure 7.1. Cellular events of cell-mediated immunity and response. (Source: From Bellanti JA, Rocklin RE. Cell-mediated immune reactions. In: Immunology III. Philadelphia: WB Saunders: 181, 1985, with permission.)

stimulate other helper T cells and natural killer T cells, respectively. IL-2 also stimulates *cytotoxic T cells*, which attack the antigen-presenting cells, causing cellular lysis and death by boring holes through the cell membrane and releasing lysing enzymes (2).

Suppressor T cells have the opposite effect on cells. They act on cytotoxic cells and plasma cells to inhibit their proliferation and the production of antibodies. Suppressor T cells play a critical role in the development of tolerance, which is particularly important in cases of autoimmune disease and some types of drug therapy.

Memory T cells are integrally involved in delayed hypersensitivity reactions. They secrete macrophage-chemotactic factor, which stimulates chemotaxis of monocytes and macrophages to the antigen contact site, and macrophage inhibitory factor, which helps to keep macrophages in the area. The delayed hypersensitivity reaction occurs 24 to 48 hr after initial contact, because of the time required to accumulate these cells.

B lymphocytes are responsible for antibody-mediated or humoral immunity. Each mature B lymphocyte carries on its surface an antibody that is specific for one particular antigen (1). If a mature B lymphocyte comes into contact with its specific antigen, it will be stimulated to differentiate into an antibody-producing cell called a plasma cell. Plasma cells that encounter helper T cells may differentiate

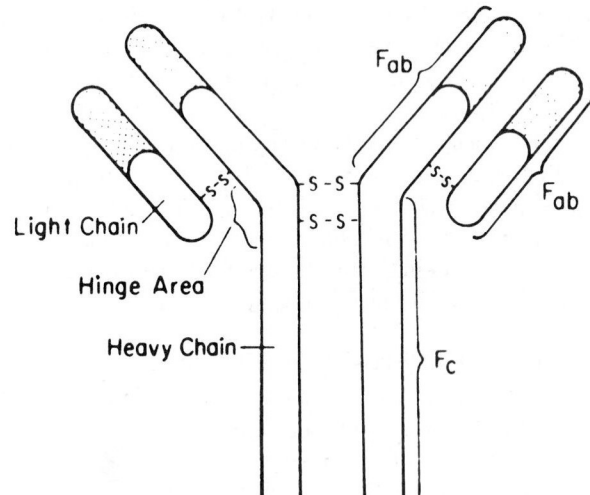

Figure 7.2. Basic structure of an antibody. (Source: From Campion J. A basic review of the immune system. US Pharmacist 15(8):19–26, 1990, with permission.)

further into memory cells, which have a long lifespan. On future encounters with that specific antigen, memory cells can more quickly mount a heightened immune response (1). Antibody production is the primary responsibility of the B lymphocyte.

Table 7.1.
Characteristics of the Five Classes of Human Immunoglobulins

Variable	Immunoglobulin Class				
	IgG	IgM	IgA	IgE	IgD
Heavy chain	γ	μ	α	ε	δ
Subclasses	γ 1, 2, 3, 4	μ 1, 2	α 1, 2	None	None
Extra chains	None	Joining	Joining and secretory	None	None
Serum Concentration (mg/100 mL)	1000	100	250	0.01	3
Plasma half-life (days)	21	5	6	2	3
Molecular weight	150,000	900,000 (polymer)	350,000 (polymer)	190,000	180,000
Major function	Primary or secondary response	Primary response	Secretory response	Allergic response	Membrane receptor (?)

Source: Reprinted with permission from Tami JA, Parr M, Thompson JS. The immune system. Am J Hosp Pharm 43:2485, 1986.

Antibodies are made up of four polypeptide chains: two light chains and two heavy chains. The basic structure of an antibody is similar to a "Y" (Fig. 7.2). The top portion binds to a specific antigen and is known as the Fab (fragment of antigen binding) portion. The base of the antibody, called the Fc (crystallizable fragment) portion, is the part that determines the biologic function of the antibody, such as complement activation and opsonization (2). Opsonization is the ability of antibodies to increase their adherence to foreign antigens to facilitate phagocytosis. Antibodies are generally divided into five distinct classes: IgG, IgM, IgA, IgE, and IgD. Each class of antibody has its own specific function and response to antigen (Table 7.1).

A third type of lymphoid cells that are important to the specific immune system are killer cells and natural killer cells. Killer cells recognize and destroy antigen bound to antibodies (antibody-dependent cell-mediated cytotoxicity). Natural killer cells also have the ability to recognize and destroy tumors and other foreign antigens. This cytotoxicity is independent of antibody-antigen binding.

Antibody-dependent cell-mediated cytotoxicity requires the orchestration of many substances, including lymphokines, monokines, colony-stimulating factors, interleukins, and others to communicate between cells and to elicit the checks and balances of the immune system. In the absence of a normally functioning immune system, the host is susceptible to infection, tumors, and eventually death.

RECOMBINANT DNA TECHNOLOGY

Many of the cellular mediators of the immune system can now be produced in clinically useful quantities by recombinant DNA technology. With this technology the natural genetic processes that take place in mammalian, bacterial, and yeast cells can be manipulated to produce human proteins, such as erythropoietin, in large enough quantities to be useful in the treatment of human disease.

Recombinant DNA technology entails isolating the gene (i.e., a specific segment of DNA) that contains the

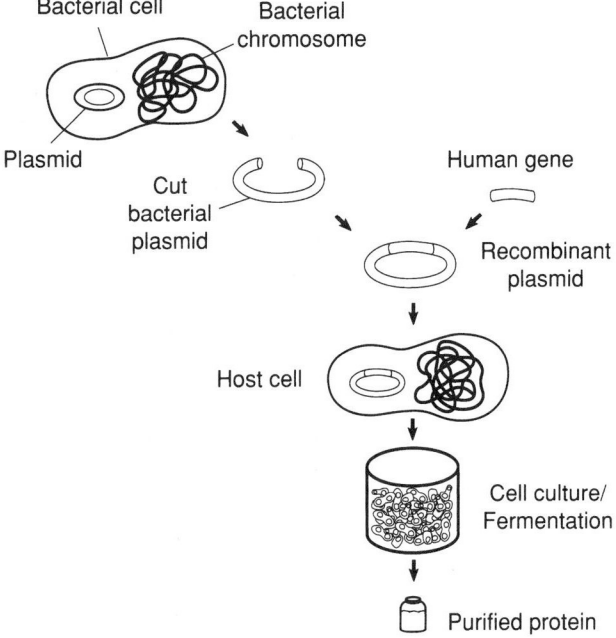

Figure 7.3. Summary of the steps typically involved in the formation of a recombinant DNA molecule. (Source: Reprinted from Anon. An introduction to pharmaceutical biotechnology. Regents of the University of Wisconsin System, 1990, with permission.)

genetic code for a desired protein and inserting it into a cell that can reproduce that protein rapidly. The result is large quantities of the desired protein.

Yeast cells, *Escherichia coli* bacteria, and mammalian cells (Chinese hamster ovary cells, human myeloma cells) are most commonly used to reproduce human proteins. These cell types are used because they can be genetically manipulated easily and quickly, they multiply and divide rapidly, and they yield large quantities of protein (4).

E. coli cells are genetically simple and well-understood cell types, so they are ideal host cells for recombinant DNA molecules. However, they cannot perform some of the

Table 7.2.
Recombinant DNA Pharmaceutical Products in the Pipeline

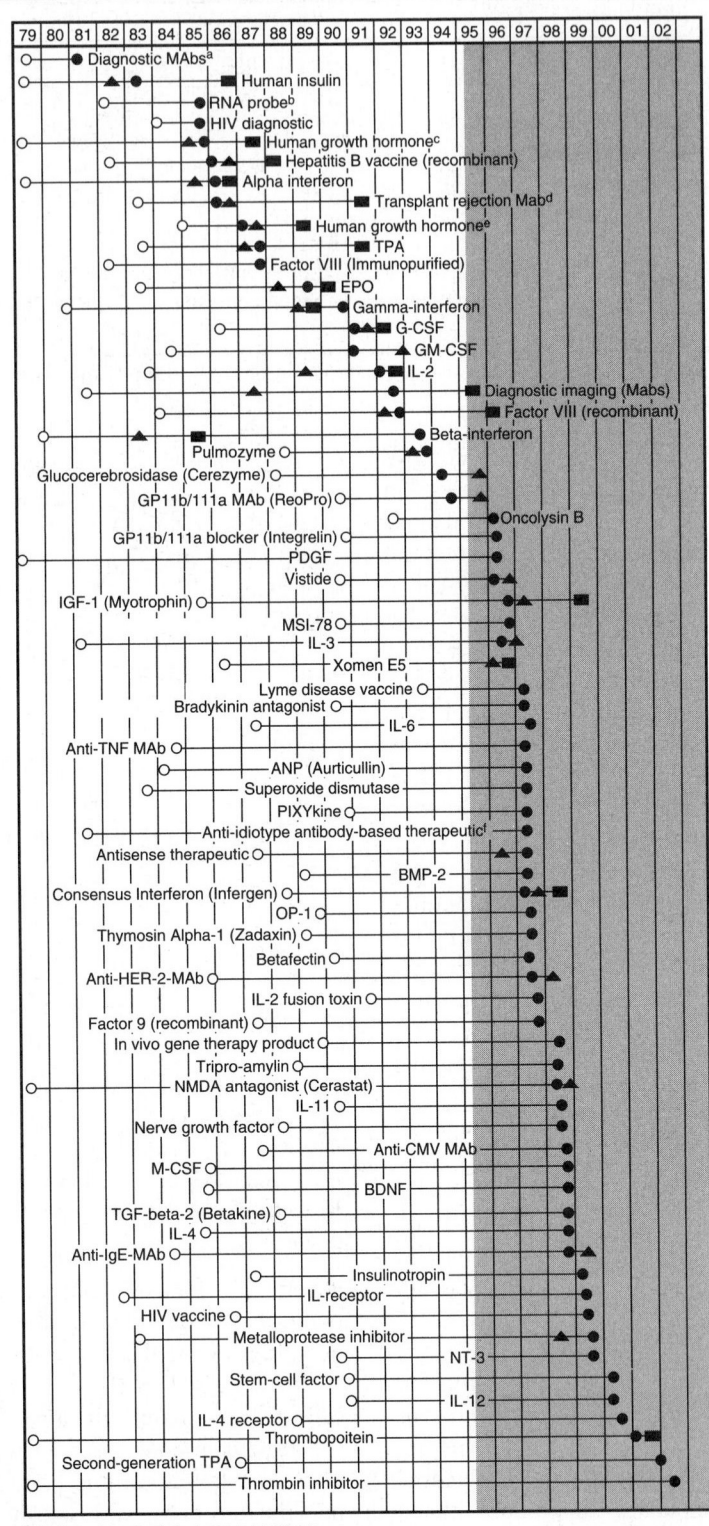

a. MAb-based test to detect serum IgE levels.
b. Nucleic-acid-probe-based test to detect *Legionella* infection.
c. Genentech's methionine human growth hormone (Protropin).
d. Johnson & Johnson's therapeutic MAb. Orthoclone OKT3.
e. Eli Lilly's nonmethionine human growth hormone (Humatrope).
f. IDEC Pharmaceutical's pan-B antibody.

Source: From Vivian Lee and Decision Resources, Inc.
           1995 Update: Timelines to Commercialization for Biomedical Products.
           Spectrum Pharmaceutical Industry Dynamics Portfolio, May 1995.

more complicated processes of fine-tuning proteins, such as glycosylation, that the more advanced cells can perform. If glycosylation is not necessary, as with interferons, *E. coli* is a less expensive and simpler choice for a host cell (4).

To produce a specific protein, the corresponding gene from the DNA strand must be isolated. A gene can be isolated easily if the amino acid sequence of the desired protein is known. If not, a DNA probe may be used to isolate the specific gene. The desired gene is then cut precisely from the DNA molecule by restriction enzymes.

The isolated gene is then inserted into the host cell, with a plasmid, to produce the desired protein (Fig. 7.3). A plasmid is a circular strand of DNA that can replicate freely inside a host cell. Plasmids are found in *E. coli*, where they are isolated and cut open (4). The human gene is then spliced to the plasmid by DNA ligase to form the recombinant DNA molecule. The DNA molecule is inserted into the host cell through a process called transformation (the uptake of foreign DNA into a cell) (4). As host cell division and replication take place, the plasmid-containing human gene is also replicated. The host cell replicates into millions of genetically identical cells that are capable of producing the desired protein. The protein is secreted, harvested, purified, and formulated into the final commercial product (4).

Among the commercially available pharmaceuticals that have been developed through recombinant DNA technology are human insulin, human growth hormone, interferons (α, β, and γ), tissue plasminogen activator, hepatitis B vaccine, and hematopoietic growth factors (granulocyte colony-stimulating factor, granulocyte-macrophage colony-stimulating factor, erythropoietin). Many more are in clinical trials (Table 7.2).

IMMUNOTHERAPEUTICS

Immunization

When an antigen enters an organism, the specific immune system stimulates antibody production against that specific antigen. It retains memory of that antigen exposure, so on reexposure to the antigen, it can mount a rapid and complete immune response. *Active immunization* uses this basic principle to help develop a complete and long-lasting immunity to certain diseases by exposing the body to a harmless portion of the antigen. (See Chapter 61, "Immunizations," for a more complete discussion of active and passive immunization.)

Recombinant Vaccines

With recombinant DNA technology a vaccine that is devoid of both pathogenic potential and extraneous material can be produced. Recombinant DNA technology has also made it possible to develop vaccines from organisms that are difficult to grow, such as cancer cells and the AIDS virus.

One example of a biotechnologically produced recombinant vaccine is the hepatitis B vaccine. The gene encoding the hepatitis B surface antigen polypeptide has been incorporated into a plasmid and cloned in yeast, *E. coli*, and mammalian cells. The ability of the recombinant hepatitis B vaccine to confer immunity is similar to that of the plasma-derived vaccine. Other recombinant vaccines that have been produced and are being studied include malaria, cholera, typhoid fever, influenza, and rabies (2).

Biologic Response Modifiers

Cytokines are responsible for the growth and differentiation of the cells of the immune system (Fig. 7.4). Cytokines that are products of monocytes and macrophages are termed monokines; those derived from lymphocytes are termed lymphokines. Cytokines have a broad range of overlapping immunologic, inflammatory, and physiologic properties. The cytokines that have been produced through recombinant DNA technology are broadly termed *biologic response modifiers*. They include interleukins, colony-stimulating factors, and interferons. These immunomodulators may be specific (e.g., target identifiable tumor antigens) or nonspecific (alter the response and function of the immune system against a stimulus without reference to a specific antigen).

INTERLEUKINS

The interleukins have been called the hormones of the immune system. They are the molecular mediators of immune system cells and induce replication and differentiation of those cells and activate the expression of certain functions. At least 15 different interleukins have been identified, each with its own cell targets and functions. Some of the interleukins have been cloned through recombinant DNA technology and are undergoing clinical trials to determine their clinical usefulness. One interleukin, IL-2, has been approved by the U.S. Food and Drug Adminstration (FDA) for use in treating patients with metastatic renal cell carcinoma.

IL-1. Interleukin-1 is a potent hematopoeitic agent that also has effects on other organ systems. It is actually two distinct molecules: interleukin-1-alpha (IL-1α) and interleukin-1-beta (IL-1β). Although IL-1α and IL-1β are structurally different molecules with only 45% homology at the nucleotide level and 26% homology at the peptide level, they have virtually identical biologic effects (5). Il-1 is produced by a number of cells, including mononuclear phagocytes, fibroblasts, natural killer cells, and T lymphocytes (6, 7). The in vitro hematologic effects of IL-1 include the activation of T cells, granulocyte-macrophage colony-stimulating factor, granulocyte colony-stimulating factor, macrophage colony-stimulating factor, interleukins-2, -3, -4, -5, and -6, and interferon-γ. In vivo, IL-1 has been shown to enhance the generation of myeloid, megakaryocytic, and early erythroid progenitors in mice (5, 8). In mice, IL-1 has been shown to act as a radioprotector, increasing the survival after lethal irradiation. In primates, IL-1 has shown enhanced myeloid recovery following treatment with 5-fluorouracil, doxorubicin, or cyclophosphamide (5). IL-1 has been well tolerated in clinical studies, hypotension being the dose-limiting toxicity. Hematologic effects consist of an early transient decrease in leukocyte count, followed by a dose-dependent leukocytosis. Patients also experience a transient minor decrease in platelet count followed by a sustained thrombocytosis (8).

IL-2. Interleukin-2 was the first of the interleukins to receive FDA approval, with an initial indication as a treatment for metastatic renal cell carcinoma. Also known as T cell growth factor, IL-2 has been shown to increase the proliferation of a subset of T lymphocytes called lymphocyte-activated killer cells (LAK cells), which lyse a broad range of tumor targets. In patients with metastatic renal cell carcinoma, IL-2 alone has an objective response rate of approximately 20%, with 5% of patients achieving a complete response. Response duration varies but can be quite prolonged (>12 months), with some patients remaining in complete remission for more than 60 months (9). Recommended dosing is 6×10^{15} IU/kg given intravenously as a 15-min bolus every 8 hr for up to a total of 14 doses (9). IL-2 given in combination with LAK cells has shown similar clinical results. The combination of IL-2 and LAK cells is termed adoptive immunotherapy, which means the transfer of active immunologic reagents (LAK cells stimulated by IL-2) to a tumor-bearing host. The goal of adoptive immunotherapy is to have the tumor-targeted immunologic agents destroy the tumor specifically. In metastatic malignant melanoma, IL-2 monotherapy has shown an average objective response rate of 13%, but when given in combination with other agents, it has shown an objective response rate of 30% (range: 4 to 59%) (9). IL-2 has also been studied in the treatment of colorectal cancer, ovarian cancer, bladder cancer, non-Hodgkin's lymphoma, and acute myeloid leukemia. The major drawback to IL-2 therapy is its toxicity. Patients who were treated with the original IL-2 regimens required intensive care, and treatment was associated with mortality rates of 1 to 6% in clinical trials. IL-2 produces a severe capillary leak syndrome that leads to fluid retention, prerenal azotemia, respiratory distress, and interstitial edema. A great deal of effort has been expended in managing and limiting the side effects of IL-2 treatment. More recently developed regimens with moderate and low dosages and subcutaneous rather than intravenous administration have resulted in better tolerability (9).

IL-3. Interleukin-3 has been called multi-colony-stimulating factor because of its ability to stimulate the proliferation and activity of every member of the hemato-

poeitic cell line (6). In vitro IL-3 acts directly on progenitor stem cells to amplify their response to more lineage-specific factors (granulocyte colony-stimulating factor, macrophage colony-stimulating factor, erythropoietin), resulting in erythroid, granulocytic, monocytic, and megakaryocytic proliferation. In clinical studies, IL-3 has shown stimulatory effects on leukocytes, neutrophils, eosinophils, monocytes, reticulocytes, and platelets. It has been shown to be effective in reducing the length of neutropenia and thrombocytopenia after chemotherapy with frequent but tolerable side effects (10). Current studies are evaluating the effects of IL-3 in combination with later-acting colony-stimulating factors such as granulocyte-macrophage colony-stimulating factor and exploring effects of timing and duration of administration.

IL-4. Interleukin-4 is a pleiotropic cytokine that was first identified in 1982 as a B-cell growth factor (11). IL-4 affects a wide variety of cell types, including B and T lymphocytes, natural killer (NK) cells, lymphokine-activated killer (LAK) cells, monocytes/macrophages, mast cells, eosinophils, basophils and fibroblasts, and endothelial cells. IL-4 is produced primarily by activated T helper cells and mast cells. In vitro IL-4 has been shown to inhibit the growth of malignant melanoma, breast carcinoma, ovarian carcinoma, mesothelioma, neurofibrosarcoma, and renal cell carcinoma. In initial clinical studies, IL-4 has caused mild fever, headache, sinus congestion, nausea, and elevated hepatic enzymes at low doses and causes a dose-limiting vascular leak syndrome (11).

IL-5. Interleukin-5 is derived from a T-cell subset and is known as T-cell-replacing factor, B-cell growth factor II, and eosinophil-differentiating factor (6). IL-5 acts primarily on B cells to stimulate the production of IgA. Since IgA is responsible for inducing a secretory response to gastrointestinal or respiratory pathogens, IL-5 may play an important role in mucosal immunity, one of the first defense mechanisms of the nonspecific immune system (6). IL-5 has also been shown to induce eosinophilic differentiation of acute myelogenous leukemia (AML) blasts, suggesting the presence of specific IL-5 receptors on AML cells (12).

IL-6. Interleukin-6 is a pleiotropic cytokine that may be a pivotal mediator in the progression of shock and sepsis, in modulating megakaryocytopoiesis, and in the inhibition of tumor growth (13). IL-6 is synthesized by blood monocytes, granulocytes, blood vessel endothelial cells, smooth muscle cells, connective tissue fibroblasts, chondrocytes of the cartilage, osteoblasts, keratinocytes of the skin, mesangial cells of the kidney, brain astrocytes, microglial cells, pituitary cells, and stromal endometrium cells (13). The physiologic effects of IL-6 include induction of fever, induction of immunoglobulin synthesis in activated B cells, activation of T cells and natural killer cells, stimulation of megakaryopoiesis, induction of acute-phase protein syn-

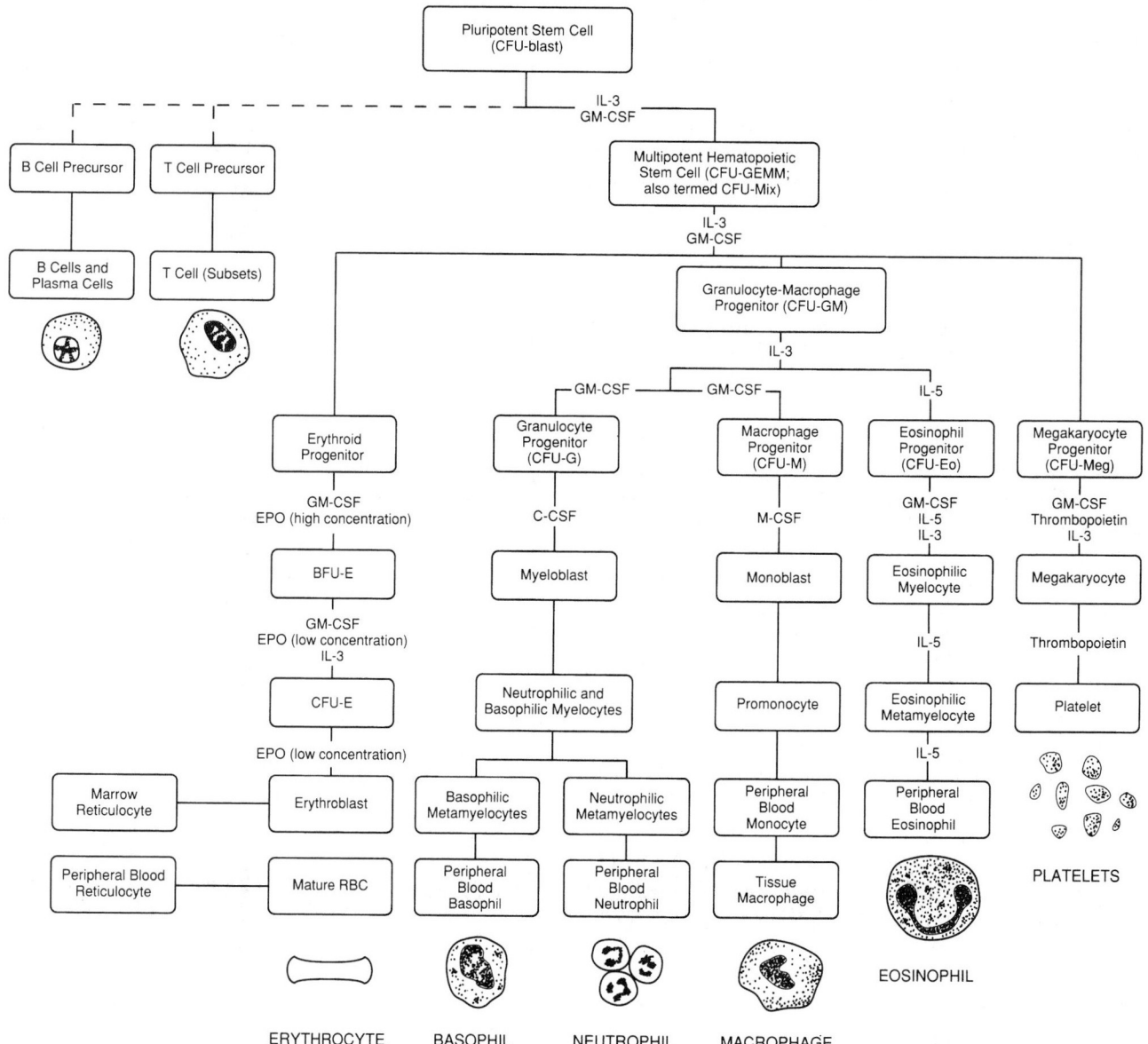

Figure 7.4. Differentiation of the hematopoietic stem cell from the pluripotent form to the highly differentiated macrophages, lymphocytes, erythrocytes, and granulocytes, and the growth factors that are responsible for their differentiation.

(Source: From Shriner DA. Colony-stimulating factors: clinical trials in humans. Highlights on Antineoplastic Drugs 8:6–14, 1990, with permission.)

thesis by the liver, and corticotropin release by the pituitary gland. IL-6 production is induced by a number of acute inflammatory responses and may also be associated with some chronic disease processses such as rheumatoid arthritis (13).

IL-7. Interleukin-7 is produced by bone marrow stromal cells and has growth-promoting and possibly differentiative effects on pre-B cells and immature thymocytes. In vitro, IL-7 has been shown to have a proliferative effect on T cells and LAK cells, as well as stimulating tumoricidal activity in monocytes and macrophages. In vivo studies in mice have

shown an increase in B-cell precursors, numbers of immature and mature B cells, and numbers of CD8+ and CD4+ cells in the spleen. However, the effects on myeloid progenitors have not been consistent (14).

IL-8. Interleukin-8 is a cytokine with potent and specific neutrophil activation and chemoattractant properties. It has been detected in the circulation during septic shock and endotoxemia and after the administration of IL-1α. IL-8 is released from neutrophils after phagocytosis; this suggests a role in the amplification of neutrophil recruitment to sites of tissue inflammation (15).

IL-11. Interleukin-11 is a multifunctional cytokine with a hypothesized role in regulating the growth and development of cells in the hematopoeitic and lymphoid systems. It is produced by bone marrow stromal cells. IL-11 has been shown in vitro to synergize with other cytokines to enhance colony formation by progenitors committed to the megakaryocyte lineage and promote megakaryocyte maturation. This may indicate that IL-11 regulates megakaryocytopoiesis at multiple points. It has also been shown to stimulate erythropoiesis (16).

IL-12. Interleukin-12 is a heterodimeric cytokine, which makes it unique among the known interleukins. The IL-12 protein consists of two disulfide bonded subunits that are encoded by two distinct genes. IL-12, which was originally called natural killer cell stimulatory factor, has been shown in vitro to exert a number of immunoenhancing effects on the activities of NK/LAK cells and T lymphocytes, as well as inducing interferon-gamma (IFN-γ) production from peripheral blood lymphocytes (PBLs) and augmenting the lytic activity of PBL against a variety of targets. The biologic activities of IL-12 suggest that it may have a role as an antitumor agent (17, 18).

IL-13. Interleukin-13 is a recently described protein that is secreted by activated human T cells and is closely related to IL-4 (19).

COLONY-STIMULATING FACTORS (CSFS)

The colony-stimulating factors (granulocyte-macrophage colony-stimulating factor [GM-CSF], granulocyte colony-stimulating factor [G-CSF], macrophage colony-stimulating factor [M-CSF], and erythropoietin [EPO]) are the most promising of the cytokines because of their broad range of clinical applications (20). These glycoproteins have been cloned through DNA technology, and the FDA has approved three (GM-CSF, G-CSF, and EPO) for clinical use. Colony-stimulating factors help to regulate the growth and differentiation of hematopoietic cells. There are two main classes of colony-stimulating factors. Class 1 CSFs such as IL-3 or GM-CSF act at the partially committed stem cell level to cause differentiation and proliferation of multiple cell lines (monocytes, granulocytes, eosinophils, etc.). Class 2 CSFs such as G-CSF, M-CSF, and EPO act on already differentiated cell lines to stimulate proliferation of more specific cell types (21).

Granulocyte-Macrophage Colony-Stimulating Factor (GM-CSF). GM-CSF supports the expansion of both monocytic and granulocytic cell lines and also cell lines containing myeloid, erythroid, and megakaryocytic cells when combined with erythropoietin. GM-CSF received FDA approval for use in bone marrow transplantation on the basis of a pivotal trial of 128 patients that was randomized, placebo-controlled, and multicenter. Patients receiving high-dose chemotherapy and autologous bone marrow transplants for lymphoid malignancies were ran-

domized to receive placebo or 250 $\mu g/m^2$/day of GM-CSF administered as a 2-hr infusion for 21 days after transplant. The patients receiving GM-CSF experienced a neutrophil recovery 7 days earlier than the placebo-treated group (19 versus 26 days). It was also noted that days of hospitalization, days of antibiotic use, and the incidence of documented infection were all reduced in the GM-CSF treated group. In addition to its indication for accelerating myeloid recovery in patients with lymphoid cancers undergoing autologous bone marrow transplantation, it has also received FDA approval for use in treating patients who have bone marrow transplant failure or engraftment delay in both the allogeneic and autologous setting.

GM-CSF has also been used to accelerate myeloid recovery in patients undergoing chemotherapy for AML (22–24). In one uncontrolled trial, GM-CSF reduced the median recovery time of neutrophils by 4 days in patients receiving 6-thioguanine, standard dose cytarabine, and daunorubicin and by 9 days in patients receiving high-dose cytarabine and mitoxantrone (23). In a larger, randomized, placebo-controlled trial, 124 patients undergoing induction and consolidation therapy for AML were randomized to receive GM-CSF or placebo on day 11 if a day 10 bone marrow sample was aplastic. The median time to recover an absolute neutrophil count of ≥500/μL was 11 days in the GM-CSF group and 14 days in the placebo group (P = 0.01). The median survival time was 325 days in the GM-CSF group and 135 days in the placebo group (P = 0.035). GM-CSF is also being studied in the treatment of AIDS patients and patients with myelodysplastic and aplastic anemia and for the purpose of increasing the concentration of peripheral-blood progenitor cells before bone marrow transplantation.

The most commonly reported adverse effects of GM-CSF in early trials included fever, nausea, vomiting, diarrhea, malaise, myalgia, rash, peripheral edema, and weight gain (21). The higher doses that were used in these early trials contributed to these side effects. With currently recommended doses, these side effects are not often seen. Other less commonly seen but more severe adverse effects include renal and hepatic dysfunction in patients with preexisting dysfunction and respiratory distress. At higher doses of 16 to 32 μg/kg/day, a large vessel thrombosis has occurred in one patient (25), and a capillary leak syndrome has been seen in conjunction with adult respiratory distress syndrome. Other side effects that have been noted with higher doses include renal failure and hypotension.

Granulocyte Colony-Stimulating Factor (G-CSF). G-CSF is a cell-lineage-specific colony-stimulating factor that stimulates granulocyte progenitor cells to differentiate into granulocytes. G-CSF received FDA approval following a Phase III trial in which 211 patients were randomized to receive 200 μg/m^2 of G-CSF or placebo after chemotherapy with cyclophosphamide, doxorubicin, and etoposide. G-CSF reduced the duration of neutropenia from 6 days to 3 days in the first cycle as well as the incidence of febrile neutropenia (57% versus 28% in cycle 1), the length of first cycle hospital stay, and the days of intravenous antibiotic use, compared to placebo (24). Additional studies have consistently shown a significantly shorter duration of leukopenia than in placebo controls (25–27). Small studies of G-CSF have shown reductions in infection, mucositis, and fever and greater adherence to scheduled chemotherapy regimens (26, 28). G-CSF has also received approval for use in bone marrow transplantation to reduce the duration of neutropenia and neutropenia-related clinical sequelae in patients with nonmyeloid malignancies who are undergoing myeloablative chemotherapy followed by marrow transplantation and to reduce the incidence and duration of sequelae of neutropenia (e.g., fever, infection, oropharyngeal ulcers) in symptomatic patients with congenital neutropenia, cyclic neutropenia, or idiopathic neutropenia. G-CSF continues to be studied for other indications, including peripheral-blood progenitor mobilization, the treatment of febrile neutropenia following chemotherapy, and use in treating AIDS patients.

The American Society of Clinical Oncology recently published CSF guidelines with a principal goal of creating a useful, practical document that would help clinicians improve patient outcomes and medical practice. The guidelines state that in consideration of both efficacy and cost-modeling analyses, the primary administration of CSFs should be as a prophylactic measure only when the chemotherapy that is being administered is expected to have an incidence of febrile neutropenia associated with it greater than 40% of the time. However, some high-risk patients, including those with bone marrow compromise, preexisting neutropenia, substantial irradiation of the pelvic area, history of recurrent febrile neutropenia during previous chemotherapy exposure, or open wounds, would benefit from treatment with CSFs even when a relatively nonmyelosuppressive chemotherapy regimen is used. The guidelines recommend that CSFs not be used to treat patients who are neutropenic but afebrile, patients who are undergoing cerebrospinal fluid priming, or patients with myelodysplastic syndromes or to treat febrile neutropenic patients unless they are high-risk patients such as those with pneumonia, hypotension, multiorgan dysfunction, or fungal infections (29).

Macrophage Colony-Stimulating Factor (M-CSF). M-CSF, also called CSF-1, selectively stimulates the proliferation and differentiation of the macrophage cell line. It has been studied in the treatment of cancer patients with invasive fungal infections following bone marrow transplant. Forty-six patients received M-CSF at doses ranging from 100 to 2000 $\mu g/m^2/day$. The M-CSF did not affect monocyte, neutrophil, or lymphocyte counts. When compared to historical controls, there was a significant difference in survival in patients who received M-CSF compared with historical control patients who received antifungal agents (27% versus 5%). However, the difference was entirely due to better patient survival in patients with a Karnofsky score greater than 20% with invasive candidiasis. Thrombocytopenia was the dose-limiting toxicity seen in 11 of the 46 patients. M-CSF continues to be studied in phase II trials.

Erythropoietin (EPO). EPO is the primary regulator of red blood cell production and thus is an important cytokine for the erythroid cell line. Recombinant human erythropoietin alpha (rHEPO) is produced through recombinant DNA technology and is approved for use in the treatment of anemia associated with chronic renal failure in patients on dialysis as well as in treating predialysis patients, severe anemia associated with zidovudine (AZT) therapy in AIDS, and treatment of anemia in patients receiving cancer chemotherapy.

EPO was the first of the recombinant stimulating factors to be approved for use in humans. Many trials have confirmed its benefit for transfusion-dependent patients. While the use of erythropoietin in treating anemia in renal failure patients and AIDS patients is discussed in Chapter 14, "Other Anemias," and Chapter 72, "Human Immunodeficiency Virus (HIV) infection and the Acquired Immunodeficiency Syndrome (AIDS)," it is important to be aware of the studies regarding its use in treating the anemia of patients who are undergoing cancer chemotherapy. In double-blind trials involving 124 patients with cancer-induced anemia, 132 patients receiving a cisplatin-containing regimen, and 157 patients receiving other chemotherapy not containing cisplatin, the mean weekly hematocrit level in EPO-treated patients in all three treatment groups increased from 28.6% to 32.1%. The mean weekly hematocrit level for the placebo-treated group remained essentially unchanged over the same time period (28.4% to 28.8%). The transfusion requirements during the second and third months of therapy for EPO-treated patients were less than those of placebo-treated patients, although the difference did not reach statistical significance (24).

The common adverse effects that are associated with EPO therapy are generally mild and include hypertension, rash, headache, arthralgias, and nausea and vomiting. A rapid rise in red blood cell count due to EPO administration can also result in severe hypertension, thrombosis, and seizures.

PIXY321 (GM-CSF/IL-3 Fusion Protein). PIXY321 is a genetically engineered molecule that combines yeast-derived GM-CSF with IL-3 via an amino acid linker protein. The products were combined to take advantage of their complementary hematopoietic effects in vivo. While GM-CSF produces a rapid increase in neutrophil count, IL-3 induces a slower, more sustained response with broader hematopoietic activity. PIXY321 has been studied in pediatric patients receiving ifosfamide, cisplatin, etoposide (ICE) therapy for solid tumors. In this phase II trial, PIXY321 was compared to historic control patients who received ICE therapy with no cytokine. The median number of days of platelet counts less than 20,000/μL was 13.5 days for the historic control patients and only 4 days for patients receiving PIXY321 therapy (24).

PIXY321 has also been studied in phase II trials of high-dose chemotherapy followed by autologous bone marrow transplant. While it demonstrated equivalent neutrophil engraftment compared to historical control patients treated with GM-CSF (days to absolute neutrophil count [ANC] ≥500/μL, 19 days each), it showed a decrease in the time to platelet independence (GM-CSF, 26 days; PIXY321, 17 days) (24). Phase III trials are now underway to confirm these early results in the areas of chemotherapy-induced cytopenias and high-dose chemotherapy followed by autologous bone marrow transplantation.

TUMOR NECROSIS FACTOR

There are two types of tumor necrosis factor (TNF): α and β. TNF-α, or cachectin, is produced primarily by activated macrophages but also by lymphocytes, natural killer cells, astrocytes, and microglial cells of the brain. It is available for investigational use as a recombinant product produced by *E. coli* (6). TNF-α is the principal host mediator of septic shock and the cachexia of chronic disease. TNF-β, or lymphotoxin, is a cytotoxic protein that was discovered as a substance produced by T-lymphocytes and some transformed B lymphoblastoid and monocytic cell lines and is associated with the 24-hr inflammatory response known as delayed-type hypersensitivity. TNF-β is 28% homologous at the nucleotide level and approximately 52% homologous with TNF-α in amino acid sequence (30). TNF-β is also available for clinical trials work as a recombinant *E. coli* product that is nonglycosylated but fully active. The TNFs are not species-specific in their biologic activity, although the level of activity may vary from species to species (31).

Septic Shock. TNF-α is the main host mediator of the metabolic and vascular changes that occur in septic shock. It is produced very early in the process and coincides with the onset of fever, rigors, myalgia, headache, and nausea. Anti-TNF-α monoclonal antibodies are being developed and tested in clinical trials to thwart the effects of TNF-α in septic shock.

Cachexia. TNF-α has been strongly implicated in the cachexia associated with cancers, AIDS, and some infectious processes. Cachectin, also called TNF-α, depresses the activity of lipoprotein lipase activity in fatty tissue. Monoclonal antibodies against TNF-α are also being developed to prevent the cachexia that develops in chronic inflammatory and neoplastic diseases (31).

Malignancy. TNF-α and -β are both capable of causing rapid necrosis of tumors. Preliminary studies have begun in humans because animal studies have shown marked tumor regression in high-tumor-burden mouse sarcomas. Phase II trials are now underway after phase I trials involving 27 patients with advanced solid tumors, primarily colorectal and soft tissue sarcoma, showed tumor regression (31). The toxicities that were seen in these early trials are significant and included fever, rigors (occasionally with hypertension), nausea, vomiting, fatigue, headache, and hypotension. TNF-α is also being studied in phase I trials, in which it has been successfully combined with IFN-γ to establish maximum tolerated doses in cancer patients.

INTERFERONS

The interferons are a group of naturally occurring glycoproteins that are produced by a variety of cell types in response to viral, antigenic, or mitogenic stimuli. They were originally discovered in 1957 when Isaacs and Lindenmann observed that virus-infected cells produced a protein that rendered them resistant to other viruses (32). In addition to their antiviral action, interferons affect a number of vital cellular and body functions, including hormone stimulation, immunity, metabolism, and tumor development.

Interferons have been categorized into two classes: type 1 (interferon-α, -β, and -ω) and type 2 (interferon-γ). The type 1 interferons are produced by many cell types in response to many different factors, including infectious agents. The type 2 interferons are produced only by T lymphocytes and natural killer cells stimulated by antigens/mitogens and interleukin-2 (33). While naturally occurring interferons are glycosylated, recombinant interferons produced in *E. coli* are not. However, activity does not seem to be diminished by their unglycosylated state. While interferon-α and interferon-β are similar in structure, cell receptor site interactions, and biologic effects, interferon-γ interacts at a different receptor site, has a different structure, and appears to have greater antitumor, immunosuppressive, and cytolytic effects (34).

To date, interferon-α has been approved for use in the treatment of chronic viral hepatitis B, chronic hepatitis non-A and non-B/C, condyloma acuminata, hairy cell leukemia, and AIDS-related Kaposi's sarcoma. Interferon-β has been approved for use in treating ambulatory patients with relapsing-remitting multiple sclerosis to reduce the frequency of clinical exacerbations of the disease. Interferon-γ is approved by the FDA to reduce the frequency and severity of serious infections associated with chronic granulomatous disease.

α-Interferon. Interferon-α was the first of the interferons to be approved for clinical use. In addition to its FDA-approved indications, it has been widely used as first-line or adjuvant treatment for several other solid tumors and hematologic malignancies. Hairy cell leukemia was the first malignancy against which interferon-α was found to have significant activity. Although up to 90% of patients will respond to interferon-α treatment, up to 50% will relapse within a short period of time. Studies have shown that continuous treatment with interferon-α will lead to a long-term survival up to 6 years in 82% of patients when doses of 2×10^6 U/M^2 are used (35).

In the early 1980s, interferon-α was recognized as an effective agent in the treatment of chronic myelogenous leukemia (CML). It is now a first-line agent in doses of 3 to 6×10^6 units/m^2 and can result in remission rates of up to 79% (36). The interferons have also been used to treat other hematologic malignancies, including multiple myeloma, chronic lymphocytic leukemia, macroglobulinemia, and essential thrombocythemia.

In solid tumors, interferon-α's efficacy has been clinically documented in treatment of malignant melanoma, metastatic renal cell carcinoma, bladder cancer, and AIDS-related Kaposi's sarcoma, for which it was also approved. Since 1978 there have been more than 12 phase II trials documenting the antitumor activity of interferon-α against malignant melanoma. Response rates of up to 16% have been reported. Higher response rates are seen in patients with minimal disease involving lymph nodes or cutaneous sites. Doses of interferon-α2 of 10×10^6 units/m^2 daily and 50×10^6 units/m^2 every other day have been used. The combination of interferon-α and IL-2 has shown very favorable results. Response rates of up to 43% have been reported (33).

Interferon-α has been studied in the treatment of renal cell cancer; response rates of 10 to 15% have been reported (2% complete response rates). When interferon-α is combined with IL-2, response rates of 38% have been noted (33). The role of sequential interferon-α followed by interferon-γ is also being studied. Interferon-α has also been studied in treating breast cancer, ovarian cancer, colorectal cancer, and superficial bladder cancer. While response rates of only 5 to 10% have been seen in treatment of breast cancer and ovarian cancer, three trials involving colorectal cancer combining 5FU and interferon-α have produced response rates between 26 and 63%, and trials in superficial bladder cancer have produced response rates of 43% (36). These encouraging results have led to other trials of gastrointestinal malignancies with this combination of products. In a review of interferon-α, Spiegel (37) reported the incidence of adverse effects in 1403 patients (Table 7.3).

Interferon-β. Interferon-β was approved in 1994 for the treatment of patients with exacerbating-remitting ambulatory multiple sclerosis on the basis of the results of a multicenter, randomized, double-blind, placebo-controlled trial. In that trial, interferon-β resulted in fewer exacerbations, fewer severe exacerbations, and less progression of T2 signal abnormalities seen on yearly MRI scans (38).

In both solid and hematologic malignancies, interferon-β has shown modest results overall. Its activity against renal cell, malanoma, and colorectal cancers, as well

Table 7.3.

Incidence (%) of Adverse Experiences with Interferon-α

Adverse Effects	All Patients ($n = 1403$)	
	Any Severity	Grades III, IV
Flulike symptoms	96	37
Nausea/vomiting	42	5
Other gastrointestinal symptoms	24	2
Central nervous system	33	7
Cardiovascular	12	2
Skin	13	1
Respiratory	6	1
Alopecia	6	<1
Weight loss	5	1
Hepatic	<1	0

Source: From Spiegel RJ. The alpha interferons: clinical overview. Semin Oncol 14:1–12, 1987, with permission.

as its activity against hairy cell leukemia, chronic myelogenous leukemia, and non-Hodgkin's lymphoma, does not seem to offer any advantage over interferon-α (34). The best clinical responses to interferon-β have been seen in treatment of Kaposi's sarcoma (39), with a 40 to 50% response rate, and glioma brain tumors, in which a 10 to 20% response rate has been reported (34).

Interferon-γ. Interferon-γ has been FDA-approved to reduce infectious complications in patients with chronic granulomatous disease, an inherited immunodeficiency syndrome. A study of 128 patients who received either interferon-γ or placebo (subcutaneously three times a week for 1 year) had two study endpoints. The first was the time to serious infection (defined as a clinical event leading to hospitalization and parenteral antibiotic administration). The second was the number of serious infections, length of hospitalization, and effect on existing infection. After 1 year, 77% of patients treated with interferon-γ were infection-free compared to 30% of the placebo-treated group. There was also a twofold reduction in the number of serious infections in the interferon-γ group compared to placebo.

The toxicities of interferon-γ appear to be similar to those of interferon-α and interferon-β, although headaches appear to be more severe and may be dose-limiting. Interferon-γ has also been shown to increase serum triglyceride levels by inhibiting lipoprotein lipase.

MONOCLONAL ANTIBODIES

Although they are derived from relatively new technology, monoclonal antibodies have far-reaching therapeutic applications in the treatment of cancers, AIDS, organ transplant rejection, drug toxicities, infectious diseases, insulin-dependent diabetes mellitus, rheumatoid arthritis, Reye's syndrome, and other diseases. The clinical applications of monoclonal antibodies for diagnostic imaging are also extensive, particularly for cancer, infectious diseases, and cardiovascular disease. This has recently led to FDA approval of a monoclonal imaging agent used to detect the presence, location, and extent of myocardial necrosis in acute ischemic heart disease. While the theoretical applications seem endless, the practical applications have been somewhat slow in developing, partly because of the difficulties inherent in monoclonal antibody production.

Monoclonal antibody production begins with the identification of the B lymphocyte that is responsible for the production of a specific antibody to a specific antigen (40). Antigen to which the desired antibody will respond is first injected into a mouse (Fig. 7.5). The antigen stimulates B lymphocytes (the precursor of the antibody-secreting plasma cell) to produce a specific antibody against that antigen. B lymphocytes are then recovered from the spleen of the mouse. Only a few of the B lymphocytes recovered from the mouse spleen actually secrete the desired antibody. Those B lymphocytes are then mixed with myeloma cells (an immortal cell line that can live forever in culture) in polyethylene glycol, resulting in the membranes of the two cell types being fused together.

The technique of fusing myeloma cells and B lymphocytes together, developed by Kohler and Milstein in the mid-1970s, results in a hybridoma. The hybridomas are grown for several weeks. Either enzyme-linked immunosorbent assay (ELISA) or radio immunoassay (RIA) methods are then used to select the appropriate antibody-secreting hybridoma. The target antigen is chemically bound to the bottom of the testing tray in wells, and the hybridoma cells are added to each of the wells. Antibodies produced inside the wells that are specific for the target antigen will bind to the antigen at the bottom of the wells. Radioactive or enzyme-labeled secondary antibodies that are specific for the primary antibodies are then added to the wells, and the mixture is incubated and rewashed. The wells that show radioactivity or a color reaction due to the enzyme are those that contain the desired antibody. Once identified, the hybridomas containing the desired antibody can be cloned.

Monoclonal antibodies exert their killing effect on cells primarily in three ways. The first is through antibody-dependent cell-mediated cytotoxicity. As with the rest of the immune system, when an antibody attaches to an antigen, effector cells such as monocytes, macrophages, granulocytes, and some lymphocytes will bind to the constant region (Fc) of the antibody and cause enzymatic puncture of the antigenic cell membrane, ultimately resulting in cell death.

A second mechanism of monoclonal antibody action is to target molecules on the cell surface that are critical to that cell's growth or differentiation. For example, monoclonal antibodies have been prepared against epidermal growth factor to inhibit growth of epidermal carcinomas. Antibodies against bombesin, an autocrine growth factor for small-cell lung cancer, have helped to inhibit tumor

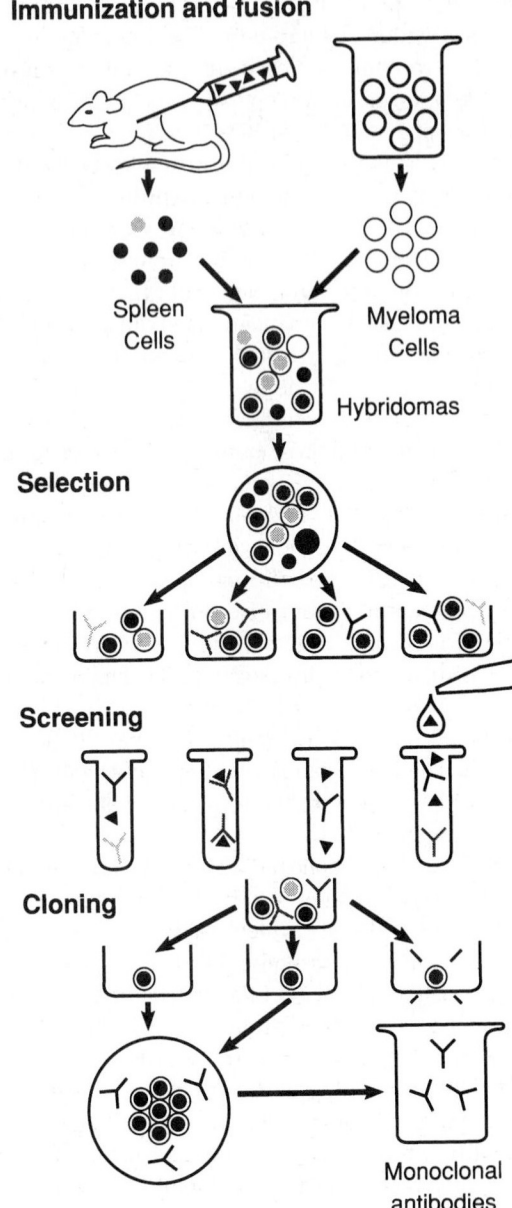

Figure 7.5. Summary of the steps involved in the production of monoclonal antibodies. (Source: Reprinted from Chisolm R. On the trail of the magic bullet. High Technology Business 3:57–63, 1983, with permission.)

growth of this cancer. A third method of killing is through complement-mediated cytotoxicity. Monoclonal antibodies, primarily IgM, invoke the release of complement, which sets off the complement cascade to mediate cell destruction.

Researchers have also been able to augment the effectiveness of monoclonal antibodies by conjugating them with radioisotopes, toxins, chemotherapeutic agents, and drug-filled liposomes (Fig. 7.6). Radioconjugates used in the treatment of malignancies have been successful

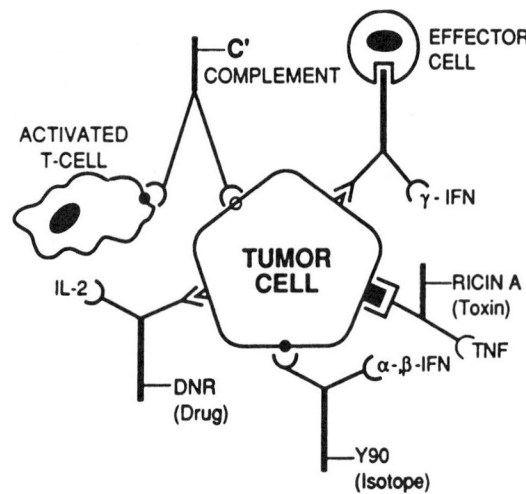

Figure 7.6. Various uses of monoclonal antibodies. (Source: From Dillman R. Monoclonal antibodies for treating cancer. Ann Intern Med 111:592–603, 1989, with permission.)

because they do not have to enter the cells to induce a killing effect. Instead, they can exert their energy over several cells (the field effect). Nearby healthy tissue, especially in areas in which the conjugate may be detained, such as the liver and spleen, may be injured (41). Radioconjugate monoclonal antibodies have been used in clinical trials to treat leukemias, lymphomas, and melanoma.

Monoclonal antibodies that are fused with all or part of plant or bacterial toxins are called immunoconjugates. Monoclonal antibodies that are conjugated with ricin-A, a plant toxin, have been used to treat melanoma, lymphoma, rheumatoid arthritis, and leukemia.

Antineoplastic-monoclonal antibody conjugates are also being used to deliver antineoplastics to specific areas of the body. This helps to improve the therapeutic-to-toxic ratio of systemic chemotherapy. Antineoplastic conjugates have been tried in treating colorectal, breast, and ovarian cancers and in malignant melanoma and glioma. Researchers have developed a doxorubicin-conjugated monoclonal antibody, yielding a drug that is ten times more cytotoxic than doxorubicin alone. Liposome-carrying drugs conjugated to monoclonal antibodies have also shown promise. The liposomes concentrate the drug in cells of the reticuloendothelial system, liver, and spleen and thus reduce drug uptake to other critical organs, such as the heart, kidney, and gastrointestinal tract. Liposome-containing doxorubicin has been developed to reduce the cardiotoxic potential of this drug.

Another advance in the mechanistic development of monoclonal antibodies is the engineering of bispecific monoclonal antibodies-antibodies that can be bidirected to both a tumor cell and an effector cell such as a monocyte or lymphocyte (42). Bispecific monoclonal antibodies can bind two different antigenic determinants simultaneously

to bring effector cells into close contact with tumor cells for improved cellular cytotoxicity. These monoclonal antibodies have been developed by cross-linking hybridomas. Antibodies directed against the CD3T-cell receptor subunit of cytotoxic T cells help to trigger the effector function once it is brought into contact with the tumor cell. These bispecific antibodies have so far been tested in phase II clinical trials against ovarian cancer cells and have clearly been successful.

Genetically engineered monoclonal antibody fragments directed to site-specific antigens have also been developed. The rationale for developing these fragments is based on their greater ability to gain access to tumors because of their smaller size and more rapid clearance from the circulation (42). Digoxin-specific Fab antibody fragments are commercially available for the treatment of digitalis toxicity. The digoxin antibody fragments bind specifically to unbound (free) digoxin in the intravascular space, preventing and reversing the glycoside's toxic effect. The Fab fragment has advantages over the intact antibody in that it causes less immunogenicity because it lacks the antigenic Fc fragment and is cleared from the circulation more rapidly.

Transplantation. Muromonab-CD3 (Orthoclone OKT3, Ortho) is the only monoclonal antibody that is commercially available for the treatment of acute renal allograft rejection. It has also been used prophylactically to prevent acute rejection. Muromonab-CD3 is a murine (mouse) IgG monoclonal antibody that directs its action against the CD3 molecule present on the surface of thymocytes and mature T lymphocytes. CD3 forms a complex with the T-cell antigen receptor to induce T-cell function (activation and proliferation) and activation of cytotoxic cells that contribute to graft-versus-host disease. It has been shown in vivo that administration of this antibody results in the coating of circulatory T cells and their subsequent disappearance from the circulation. By interfering with the CD3, muromonab-CD3 does not allow the complex to form, rendering the T cells inactive.

In the first controlled trial involving 123 patients with acute rejection of cadaveric transplants, the rejection reversal rate was 94% with muromonab-CD3, compared to 75% with high-dose steroids. The 1-year graft survival rate was also improved with muromonab CD3 (62%) versus high-dose steroids (45%) (42).

Side effects of muromonab-CD3 include pyrexia, dyspnea, headache, nausea and vomiting, and diarrhea. These effects generally begin within 1 hr of administration of the first dose of the drug and diminish over the next several hours. On days 2 through 5 of treatment, pruritis, rash, aseptic meningitis, and altered mental status have been reported to occur. The side effects are probably due to muromonab-CD3-induced increases in tumor necrosis factor and IL-2.

Patients can also develop human antimouse antibodies (HAMA) to the monoclonal antibody, which can lead to an abrogated therapeutic response. In general, most patients can undergo two to three courses of muromonab-CD3 without developing a decreased response.

Another monoclonal antibody that is close to FDA approval for use in transplant rejection is Zolimomab aritex (MA-2) (OrthoZyme-CD5 Plus, Ortho). This monoclonal is an anti-pan T-lymphocyte murine monoclonal antibody ricin A-chain immunoconjugate that is used for the treatment of steroid-resistant acute graft-versus-host disease in patients undergoing bone marrow transplant. It is also being investigated for first-line treatment of acute graft-versus-host disease and for treating rheumatoid arthritis. The immunoconjugate specifically binds to the CD5 receptor on mature T lymphocytes and destroys them, thus preventing or reducing the effects of graft-versus-host disease.

In one study of Zolimomab aritex, 37 patients with steroid-resistant acute graft-versus-host disease in one to four organ systems were treated in a dose escalation, open label study (43). Fifty percent of patients had either a complete or partial response; the other 50% had either stable disease, progression, or a mixed response. In another study, which compared Zolimomab-treated patients with historical control patients, Zolimomab-treated patients achieved a 52% response rate compared to a 31% response rate for the control group (44).

Cancer Treatment. The initial studies involving monoclonal antibodies in the treatment of cancers primarily involved hematologic malignancies. More than 25 trials involving 135 patients resulted in complete remission rates in approximately 5% of patients, partial response rates in 16%, and minor response rates in an additional 17% of patients (42).

Most of the patients who were treated in these studies had refractory disease and compromised immune systems, making it difficult for them to respond to immunotherapy. Additionally, these earlier studies were done with mouse monoclonal antibodies, leading to a significant HAMA response that limited the duration of treatment. Other problems that were identified in these earlier trials included (a) heterogeneous antigens expressed on the surface of tumor cells, (b) immune complex formation between free, circulating antigens and monoclonal antibodies, (c) the disappearance or modulation of antigens on the tumor cell surface, and (d) the relatively short half-life of the mouse monoclonal in the human circulation.

With these problems identified, researchers set out to minimize these problems and (a) achieve site-specific delivery of monoclonal antibodies to the tumor cells with minimal disruption to normal tissue and (b) produce a more stable monoclonal conjugate, resulting in a longer half-life of the monoclonal antibody (42).

More recent studies of monoclonal antibodies used to treat malignancies have focused on the use of immunoconjugates, radioconjugates, and chemotherapy conjugates. In one trial, using radioconjugates to treat non-Hodgkin's lymphoma, nine out of ten patients obtained complete responses that lasted from 4 to 30 months. Immunoconjugates such as ricin A-chain armed monoclonal antibodies have been used to treat patients with cutaneous T-cell lymphomas; partial responses were seen in 29% of patients. The major toxicity seen was a capillary leak syndrome (45). Current studies using immunotoxins or radioisotopes as conjugates have demonstrated fairly good response rates, but they have not been long-standing. The best role for these agents may be their use in combination with other antitumor treatments, such as chemotherapy, to obtain a sustained response without overlapping toxicity (45). Table 7.4 summarizes the majority of monoclonal antibodies being studied in various cancers and their developmental status (46).

Infectious Diseases. The use of monoclonal antibodies in the treatment of Gram-negative septic shock has yielded disappointing results. Two monoclonals, nebacumab (HA1A, Centocor) and E5 monoclonal antibody (XOMA), were studied in Phase III trials that were double-blind and placebo-controlled. The results of the HA1A trial found only one subset of patients for whom the monoclonal was significantly effective (47). XOMA studied its product in two independent trials that ended in conflicting results: One study showed a trend toward benefit in Gram-negative bacteremic patients who were not yet in shock, and one study showed no difference in mortality in the bacteremic nonshock subset. Because of the unimpressive results of these studies, neither product has yet received FDA approval. With the multiplicity of events ultimately leading to septic shock, investigators are going to have to delineate more clearly the process before a monoclonal antibody can be produced that will augment the host's normal response to the presence of Gram-negative organisms in the blood.

Cardiovascular Therapeutics. The FDA recently approved abciximab (ReoPro, Centocor B.V., and Eli Lilly) for the prevention of acute ischemic complications in patients with percutaneous transluminal coronary angioplasty (PTCA) who were at high risk for abrupt closure of the treated vessel. Abciximab is the Fab fragment of the chimeric human-murine monoclonal antibody 7E3 with antiplatelet activity designed to reduce arterial thrombus formation after PTCA. It acts by binding to an adhesion receptor involved in platelet aggregation and preventing the binding of fibrinogen, von Willebrand factor, and other adhesive molecules to receptor sites on activated platelets (48).

Abciximab was studied in a multicenter, double-blind, placebo-controlled trial involving 2099 patients who were at high risk for abrupt closure of the treated coronary vessel. The primary endpoint was the occurrence of any of

Table 7.4.
Monoclonal Antibody Therapeutics in Development for Cancer

Cancer	Company	Status
Bladder cancer	Cytogen	R&D
Breast cancer (ERB-2)	Genentech	Phase 1
Breast cancer (ERB-2)	Chiron	Phase 1
Breast cancer (ERB-2)	Protein Design Labs	Preclinical
Colorectal cancer (ADCC)	Centocor	Phase 2
Colorectal cancer	XOMA	Phase 1, 2
Colorectal cancer	Immunomedics	Phase 1, 2
Colorectal cancer	NeoRx	Phase 1
Colorectal cancer	Hybritech	Phase 1
Colorectal cancer (ADCC + cytokine)	NeoRx	Phase 1
Colorectal cancer	ImmunoGen	Preclinical
Colorectal cancer (rhenium)	Immunomedics	Preclinical
Liver cancer	Hybritech (Lilly)	Phase 2
Liver cancer	Immunomedics	Preclinical
Lung cancer	NeoRx	Phase 1
Lung cancer	Hybritech	Phase 1
Small cell lung cancer	ImmunoGen	Phase 1, 2
Lymphoma	Techniclone	Phase 2
Lymphoma	Immunomedics	Phase 1, 2
Lymphoma/leukemia	Protein Design Labs	Phase 1
B-cell lymphoma	IDEC	Phase 3
Non-Hodgkin's lymphoma/lymphocytic leukemia	ImmunoGen	Phase 2
Myelogenous leukemia	ImmunoGen	Phase 1, 2
Myelogenous leukemia	Protein Design Labs	Preclinical
Melanoma	XOMA	Phase 2
Melanoma	ImmunoGen	Preclinical
Melanoma	Hybritech (Lilly)	Preclinical
Ovarian cancer	Cytogen	Phase 1, 2
Ovarian cancer—radiation	NeoRx	Phase 1, 2
Ovarian cancer	Chiron	Phase 1
Ovarian cancer	XOMA	Preclinical
Ovarian cancer (ERB-2)	Genentech	Phase 1
Ovarian cancer	ImmunoGen	Preclinical
Neuroblastoma	Genetics Institute	Preclinical
Prostate cancer	Cytogen	IND filed
Prostate cancer	Techniclone	Phase 1
Solid tumor (lung/breast/colon/ovarian)	Bristol-Myers Squibb	Phase 1, 2
Solid tumor (lung/breast/colon)	Protein Design Labs	Preclinical

Source: Adapted from Merrill Lynch. A biotechnology score-card. Leading products and companies as of January 1992.

the following events within 30 days of PTCA: death, myocardial infarction, or the need for urgent intervention for recurrent ischemia. There was a 4.5% lower incidence of the primary endpoint in the monoclonal antibody treated group versus placebo. This difference was statistically significant (48).

Abciximab is associated with an increased frequency of major bleeding complications, which limits its use by patients who are at high risk for bleeding. It has also been shown to cause allergic reactions (anaphylaxis), thrombocytopenia, hypotension (mostly due to bleeding complications), anemia, pleural effusions, pain at the injection site, and peripheral edema (48).

GENE THERAPY

The underlying cause of many human diseases can be traced back to genetic abnormalities. Whether the abnor-

mality is the lack of a receptor, a defective feedback loop, or the overproduction or underproduction of some pharmacologically active substance, many times the cause is a defect in the genetic code. Traditional therapeutic approaches focus on providing the missing substance or blocking the action of a substance that is overproduced or to which the body is overly sensitive. The aim of genetic therapy is to correct the underlying defect.

Genetic therapy involves the introduction of foreign genetic material into selected cells in the body to treat disease. It has been made possible by advances in our understanding of how tumor viruses achieve oncogenic transformation by integration of viral genomes into the DNA of target cells, development of effective ways to transfer DNA into mammalian cells, and advances in recombinant DNA technologies that gave us the ability to isolate and generate large amounts of pure genetic material

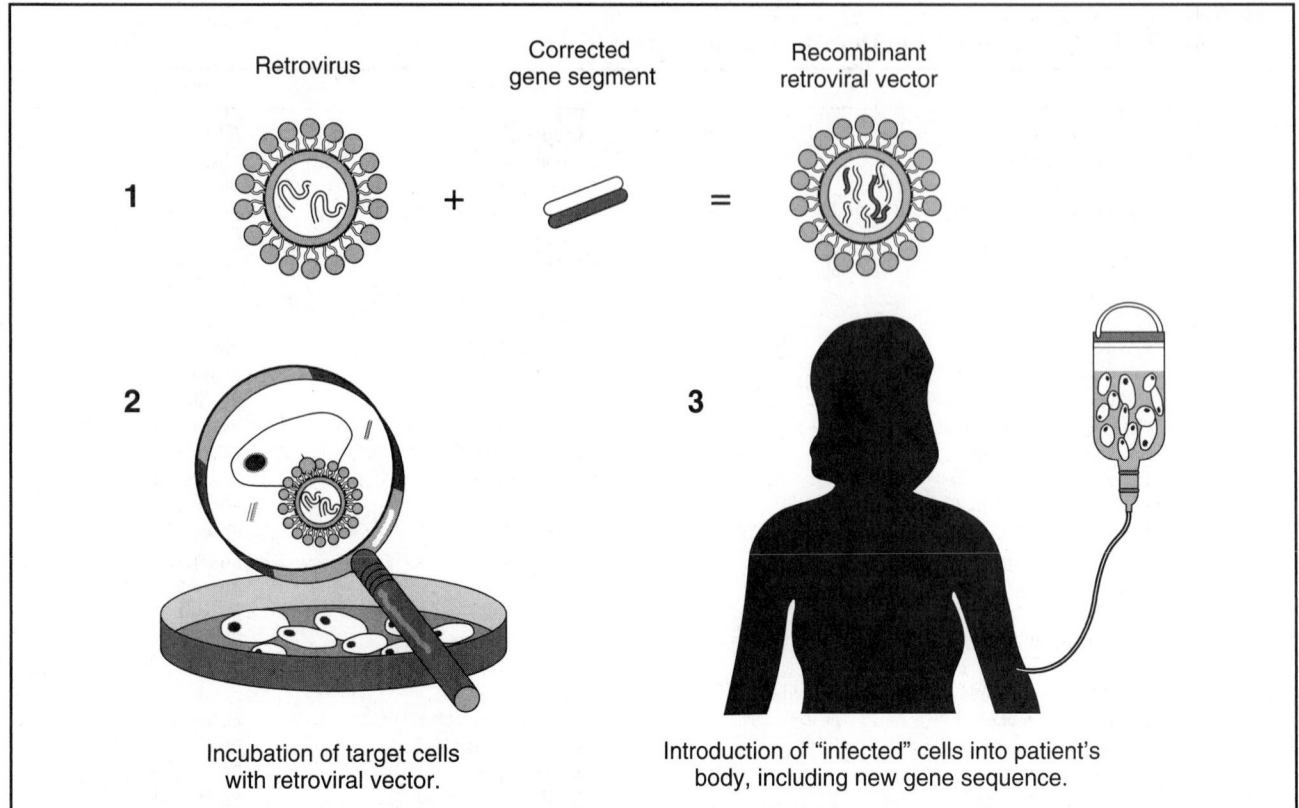

Retrovirus   Corrected   Recombinant
                    gene segment   retroviral vector

Incubation of target cells   Introduction of "infected" cells into patient's
with retroviral vector.   body, including new gene sequence.

1. The retrovirus is altered through recombinant DNA technology to add the gene sequence that is to be delivered to the patient.
2. The retroviral vector is incubated with the target cells and the desired gene is inserted into the target cells.
3. The target cells with the desired gene are infused into the patient.

Figure 7.7. Ex vivo gene transfer process. 1. The retrovirus is altered through recombinant DNA technology to add the gene sequence that is to be delivered to the patient. 2. The retroviral vector is incubated with the target cells, and the desired gene is inserted into the target cells. 3. The target cells with the desired gene are infused into the patient.

(49). Current approaches involve only somatic cells, not germ cells. Therefore the therapeutic effects are not passed on to future generations.

Genetic material can be introduced into mammalian cells by a variety of methods that fall into two major categories. One category involves the use of the physical properties of accompanying salts, lipids, or inorganic particles. These methods rely on chemical properties to stimulate the uptake of the introduced genetic material into the target cells. The more widely used methods of gene transfer involve biologic vectors, adenoviruses and retroviruses being the predominant vectors. The major difference between these two methods is that retroviruses permanently introduce genes into the chromosomes of infected cells, and adenoviruses do not. Most clinical gene therapy trials to date have used retroviral vectors (50). Retroviruses are ribonucleic acid (RNA) viruses that replicate through reverse transcription to produce a deoxyribonucleic acid (DNA) intermediate called a provirus. The DNA provirus is then incorporated into the host DNA, thus transferring the genetic material from the retrovirus to the host cell (51). In genetic therapy the

genes that encode for viral functions are replaced by genes that encode for the desired therapeutic function. In addition to introducing the desired genetic material, the retroviruses that are altered in this way are incapable of viral replication, thus providing a safe means of genetic transfer. The most common method of human gene therapy is to remove the target cells from the body, expose them to the altered retrovirus in vitro, and then reinfuse the "infected" target cells (Fig. 7.7). This approach has been favored for early trials because it is technically less complicated, and there is the ability to monitor and control the modified cells before administration to a patient. Genetic material can also be delivered directly to the target area for in vivo exposure, although this is a less well developed method. The in vivo approach involves a host of additional technical and safety issues, including the consideration of complex multicompartmental pharmacokinetics.

Therapeutic trials have been undertaken involving cancer, genetic diseases, and infectious diseases. Genetic diseases that have been targeted include severe combined immune deficiency, Gaucher's disease, Franconi's anemia, cystic fibrosis, and hypercholesterolemia (50). To date, the only infectious disease that has been targeted by gene therapy has been AIDS.

Genetic Diseases. In September 1990 a therapeutic trial was begun that was designed to treat adenosine deaminase (ADA) deficiency in children with severe combined immune deficiency (49). The protocol called for the isolation of peripheral lymphocytes from a patient with ADA deficiency. In vitro the human ADA gene was introduced into the lymphocytes with a retroviral vector. The modified lymphocytes were multiplied and then reintroduced into the patient. Patients were retreated at 6- to 8-week intervals. Researchers were able to show the presence of substantial numbers of gene-corrected T cells and improved immune function (49).

Familial hypercholesterolemia, a disease characterized by extraordinary high levels of cholesterol, has also been treated with gene therapy. The disease is caused by defective or absent receptors for low-density lipoprotein (LDL). The gene therapy protocol calls for a portion of the patient's liver to be removed. The hepatocytes that are obtained from the liver then undergo retroviral-mediated gene transfer of the LDL receptor genes. The altered liver cells are then returned directly to the patient's liver via a catheter (49, 52). Initial results have been encouraging, with the first patient tolerating the procedure well, showing evidence of engraftment and an improvement in LDL/HDL ratio from 10 to 13 pretreatment to 5 to 8 posttreatement (53).

Cancer. The first human trial of genetic therapy conducted in the United States began in May 1989 and was designed not as a direct therapeutic trial but as a method of marking cells that are critical to the treatment of cancer. The trial used a retroviral vector to genetically mark a class of lymphocytes in cancer patients called tumor-infiltrating lymphocytes (TIL) (49). In TIL therapy, which is used for treating metastatic melanoma and renal cell carcinoma, part of the tumor is removed, and the lymphoid cells that had successfully infiltrated the tumor are harvested. These TIL cells are then cultured with interleukin-2 to stimulate growth. The large numbers of TIL are then reinfused into the patient. The TIL were marked by inserting the genetic code for the bacterial antibiotic resistance gene, neomycin phosphotransferase, thus making it possible to track them (54).

Oncogenes, or tumor-promoting genes, have been implicated in a number of cancers. A number of researchers have pursued methods to replace or deactivate overexpressed tumor-promoting genes. The most common method is to introduce antisense RNA into the cell to stop expression of the oncogene. More recent efforts have included both antisense RNA to stop the activity of the tumor-promoting oncogene and a mutant antisense-resistant oncogene with the desired activity. This method is theorized to inhibit the expression of the endogenous oncogene, while the "corrected" oncogene restores regulated DNA synthesis (54).

Tumor suppressor genes, for example p53, are responsible for maintaining normal cell replication. A malfunctioning or missing tumor suppressor gene results in the uncontrolled proliferation of malignancy. By introducing a suppressor gene, it may be possible to reverse the malignant potential of the tumor cells (54).

Since retroviral DNA will be incorporated into rapidly dividing cancer cells more rapidly than into normal cells, it is possible to preferentially introduce genetic material into cancer cells. By introducing genes that make the tumor susceptible to substances that will not normally harm cells or will metabolize harmless substances into toxic substances, tumor cells can be preferentially killed. An example of a common suicide gene is the herpes simplex thymidine kinase gene. Nucleoside analogs such as acyclovir and ganciclovir will bind to this gene product and kill the cell but will not bind to endogenous thymidine kinase. Another example is the *E. coli* cytosine deaminase (cd) gene. This gene, which is not present in normal mammalian cells, causes the cell to metabolize 5-fluorocytosine, a relatively nontoxic substance, into 5-fluorouracil, which is toxic to cells. When this gene is inserted into cancer cells, they become suceptible to a substance that will not harm normal cells (53, 54).

The host immune response can be enhanced by introducing tumor-killing cytokines into tumor cells. This can be accomplished in vivo, where the genes for cytokine production are introduced into the tumor, or in vitro, where the cytokine gene is introduced into the tumor cells in culture and the tumor cells are reinfused into the patient. Tumor necrosis factor (TNF) has been shown to induce tumor regression, but its general use has been limited by systemic toxicity. Another gene therapy approach is to enhance the tumor-killing ability of TIL by inserting the gene for TNF into harvested TIL and reinfusing them. This localizes the therapeutic effect of TNF and limits systemic exposure (55).

CONCLUSIONS

A thorough knowledge of the immune system is a prerequisite to the understanding of many human diseases. With the availability of new knowledge about the regulation of the immune system coupled with the powerful tools offered by biotechnology, a new era in the diagnosis and treatment of many diseases that have eluded effective intervention is beginning. Although only a handful of products are currently commercially available, many more are in development, and they will undoubtedly significantly alter the way in which we treat many diseases.

REFERENCES

1. Tami JA, Parr M, Thompson J. The immune system. Am J Hosp Pharm 43:2483–93, 1986.

2. Koeller J, Tami J. Concepts in immunology and immunotherapeutics. Bethesda, MD: ASHP Publication, 1990. Campion J. A basic review of the immune system. US Pharmacist 15(8):19–26, 1990.

3. Campion J. A basic review of the immune system. US Pharmacist 15(8):19–26, 1990.

4. Anon. An introduction to pharmaceutical biotechnology. Madison, WI: Regents of the University of Wisconsin System, 1990.

5. Johnson CS, Interleukin-1: therapeutic potential for solid tumors. Cancer Invest 11:600–08, 1993.

6. Staren E, Essner R, Economou JS. Overview of biological response modifiers. Semin Surg Oncol 5:379–84, 1989.

7. Kirkpatrick C. Biological response modifiers: interferons, interleukins, and transfer factor. Ann Allergy 62:170–76, 1989.

8. Crown J, Jakubowski A, Gabrilove J. Interleukin-1: biological effects in human hematopoiesis. Leuk Lymphoma 9:433–40, 1993.

9. Whittington R, Faulds D. Interleukin-2: a review of its pharmacological properties and therapeutic use in patients with cancer. Drugs 46:446–514, 1993.

10. de Vries EG, van Gameren MM, Willemse PH. Recombinant human interleukin-3 in clinical oncology. Stem Cells 11:72–80, 1993.

11. Puri RK, Siegel JP. Interleukin-4 and cancer therapy. Cancer Invest 11:473–86, 1993.

12. Baumann MA, Paul CC, Grace MJ. Effects of interleukin-5 on acute myeloid leukemias. Am J Hematol 39:269–74, 1992.

13. Bauer J, Herrman F. Interleukin-6 in clinical medicine. Ann Hematol 62:203–10, 1991.

14. Appasamy PM. Interleukin-7: biology and potential clinical applications. Cancer Invest 11:487–499, 1993.

15. Van Zee KJ, Fischer E, Hawes AS, Hebert A, Terrell TG, Baker JB, Lowry SF, Moldawer LL. Effects of intravenous IL-8 administration in nonhuman primates. J Immunol 148:1746–52, 1992.

16. Neben S, Turner K. The biology of interleukin 11. Stem Cells 11(suppl 2):156–62, 1993.

17. Gately MK. Interleukin-12: a recently discovered cytokine with potential for enhancing cell-mediated immune responses to tumors. Cancer Invest 11:500–06, 1993.

18. Tahara H, Lotze MT. Antitumor effects of interleukin-12: applications for the immunotherapy and gene therapy of cancer. Gene Therapy 2:96–106, 1995.

19. Nilsson G, Nilsson K. Effects of interleukin-13 on immediate-early response gene expression, phenotype and differentiation of human mast cells: comparison with IL-4. Eur J Immunol 25:870–73, 1995.

20. Gabrilove J. Introduction and overview of hematopoietic growth factors. Semin Hematol 26:1–4, 1989.

21. Yee GC. Focus on GM-CSF and G-CSF: promising biotherapeutics for use in hematology and oncology. Hosp Formul 25:943–48, 1990.

22. Bettelheim P, Muhm M, Valent P, et al. GM-CSF in combination with cytotoxic chemotherapy in AML patients. Bone Marrow Transplant 1:127–30, 1990.

23. Buechner T, Hiddemann W, Koenigsmann M, et al. Recombinant human GM-CSF following chemotherapy in high-risk AML. Bone Marrow Transplant 1:131–33, 1990.

24. Vose JM, Armitage JO. Clinical applications of hematopoietic growth factors. J Clin Oncol 13(4):1023–35, 1995.

25. Moore M. Hematopoietic growth factors in cancer. Cancer 65:836–44, 1990.

26. Appelbaum FR. The clinical use of hematopoietic growth factors. Semin Hematol 26:7–14, 1989.

27. Morstyn G, Lieschke G, Sheridan W, et al. Clinical experience with recombinant human granulocyute colony-stimulating factor and granulocyte macrophage colony-stimulating factor. Semin Hematol 26:9–13, 1989.

28. Glaspy J, Golde D. Clinical applications of the myeloid growth factors. Semin Hematol 26:14–17, 1989.

29. American Society of Clinical Oncology. Recommendations for the use of hematopoietic colony-stimulating factors: evidence-based, clinical practice guidelines. J Clin Oncol 12:2471–2508, 1994.

30. Porter AG. The prospects for therapy with tumour necrosis factors and their antagonists. Trends Biotchnol 9(5):158–62, 1991.

31. Goh CR. Tumour necrosis factors in clinical practice. Ann Acad Med 19:235–39, 1990.

32. Tyring SK. Interferons: biochemistry and mechanisms of action. Am J Obstet Gynecol 172:1350–53, 1995.

33. Agarwala S, Kirkwood J. Interferons in the therapy of solid tumors. Oncology 51:129–36, 1994.

34. McManus BC. Clinical use of biologic response modifiers in cancer treatment. Ann Pharmacother 24:761–67, 1990.

35. Takaku F. Clinical application of cytokines for cancer treatment. Oncology 51:123–28, 1994.

36. Urabe A. Interferons for the treatment of hematological malignancies. Oncology 51:137–41, 1994.

37. Spiegel RJ. The alpha interferons: clinical overview. Semin Oncol 14:1–12, 1987.

38. Weinstock-Guttman B, Ransohoff RM, Kinkel RP, Rudick RA. The interferons: biological effects, mechanisms of action and use in multiple sclerosis. Ann Neurol 37:7–13, 1995.

39. Triozzi P, Rinehart J. The role of IFN-beta in cancer therapy. Cancer Surv 8:799–807, 1989.

40. Vaickus L. Antitumor antibodies as therapeutic reagents. P&T 15(12):143–61, 1990.

41. Dillman RO. Monoclonal antibodies for treating cancer. Ann Intern Med 111:592–603, 1989.

42. Reisfeld RA. Monoclonal antibodies in cancer immunotherapy. Clin Lab Med 12(2):201–16, 1992.

43. Byers VS, Henslee J, Kernan NA, et al. Use of an anti-pan T-lymphocyte ricin A chain immunotoxin in steroid-resistant acute graft-versus-host disease. Blood 75:1426–32, 1990.

44. Lomen PL, Stewart KK, Saks SR, et al. Safety and efficacy of H65–RTA in the treatment of steroid-resistant acute graft-versus-host disease after allogeneic Bone Marrow Transplant [Abstract 911]. Blood 78(1):230a, 1991.

45. Matthews OC, Smith FO, Bernstein ID. Monoclonal antibodies in the study and therapy of hematopoietic cancers. Curr Opin Immunol 4(5):641–6, 1992.

46. Merrill Lynch. A biotechnology scorecard. Leading Products and Companies as of January 1992.

47. Ziegler ET, Fisher CJ, Sprung CL, et al. Treatment of gram-negative bacteremia and septic shock with HA-1A human monoclonal antibody against endotoxin. N Engl J Med 324:429–36, 1991.

48. Anon. ReoPro package insert. Centocor. Philadelphia: Eli Lilly and Company, 1995.

49. Tolstoshev P. Gene therapy, concepts, current trials and future direction. Annu Rev Pharmacol 32:573–96, 1993.

50. Kerr WG, Mule JJ. Gene therapy: current status and future prospects. J Leukemia Bio 56:210–14, 1994.

51. Blattner WA. Retroviruses that cause human disease. In: Wyngaarden JB, Smith LH, Bennett JC, eds. Cecil textbook of medicine, 19th ed. Philadelphia: WB Saunders, 1992:1845.

52. Ledley FD. Hepatic gene therapy: present and future. Hepatology 18:1263–73, 1993.

53. Grossman M, Raper SE, Kozarsky K, Stein EA, et al. Successful ex vivo gene therapy directed to liver in a patient with familial hypercholesteroleaemia. Nat Genet 6(4):335–41, 1994.

54. Tolaza EM, Economou JS. Gene therapy of cancer. In: Haskell CM, ed. Cancer treatment, 4th ed. Philadelphia: WB Saunders, 1995:305.

55. Rosenberg SA. Immunotherapy and gene therapy of cancer. Cancer Research 51(suppl):5074s–5079s, 1991.

CHAPTER 8

PATIENT COMMUNICATION IN CLINICAL PHARMACY PRACTICE

MARIE E. GARDNER, RICHARD N. HERRIER, and HELEN MELDRUM

The health care professions are founded on both strong technical and people skills. Although all health professionals are well versed in the technical aspects of their profession, most are not as skilled with regard to interpersonal communication. In contemporary clinical practice, good communication skills are critical to achieving optimal patient outcomes. The goal of this chapter is to briefly summarize some of the skills required to provide quality patient consultation and education. It is obvious that these techniques are very important in improving outcomes for the patient and for increasing practitioners' satisfaction with their professional roles. Although there is much to expand on in regard to this topic, the focus of this chapter will be limited to a review of essential communication skills, clinical interviewing and medication history guidelines, symptomatology assessments, basic medication consultation skills, and strategies for interviewing to improve compliance and monitor clinical progress.

In this era of technologic wonders, clear, direct and sensitive communication between people seems to be in short supply. And yet, from extensive research on customer service and patient education, we know that when providers communicate well, patients are more likely to comply with treatment plans and less likely to complain or entertain thoughts of legal retribution because of perceived mistreatment. Additionally, Bolton has stated that 80 percent of professionals who "fail" at their jobs do so because of poor human relations skills (1). Humanistic psychologist Carl Rogers concludes that people seek counseling because of poor communication with others in their lives. Effective interpersonal communication may be the most important skill we can develop. Practitioners must not only maintain an open attitude of ongoing learning about human relations, but to function as professionals, they must also master the basic skills of questioning, empathic response, responsible language use, assertiveness, and conflict management, and integrate these into applied communications.

BASIC COMMUNICATION SKILLS
Skills in Asking Questions

Most people are not very conscious about the types of questions they ask. If practitioners are lacking in question-

ing skills, much damage to the patient can result from a poorly conducted patient interview or medication history. Questions can be organized on a continuum from highly open to restricted to leading. Closed questions narrow the patients' options and evoke minimal "recall levels" of information instead of thoughtful elaborated responses. Some examples are:

Very Open:	What have you noticed about how you have been feeling since you started this medication?
Open:	What exactly has changed since you have been on this medication?
Moderately Open:	How do you feel about trying a generic version of your regular medication?
Moderately Closed:	Of the drugs we have tried for relief of your pain, which did you think worked the best for you?
Highly Closed:	Is this dosage OK for you?
Closed and Leading:	You're not having any side effects, are you?

When seeking information from *most* patients, it is best to begin questioning with open-ended questions. These start with *who, what, where, when, how,* and *why,* as they did in the examples above. Questions phrased like this allow the patient to answer in any number of ways. For example, a question like "How have you been feeling since starting this new medication?" can elicit a response from the patient that indicates either that the patient is improved (and happy with the medication) or that side effects are present (and presumably the patient is unhappy with the medication). This type of question is obviously preferred over "Are you feeling better?" and "The medicine hasn't made you sick, has it?" When conducting the medication history interview and prescription consultation activities, the use of open-ended questions is of paramount importance, as will be seen later in this chapter.

It is important to remember that not all open questions are created equal. "Why didn't you finish your antibiotic?" implies strong criticism and will provoke a defensive reaction from the patient. In most cases, when you are trying to elicit the patient's reasoning it is better to *start with a universal statement and transition to an open question.* For example, "Most people don't realize how important it is to finish an antibiotic because an infection can appear to be gone but actually be lingering. What has been your experience in trying to take antibiotics?" Although many pharmacists fear this approach will consume too much time, when we ask "quick" questions in ways that produce defensiveness, patients learn to hide the real and truthful answers because they do not trust their providers.

Empathic Responding and Why It Is Essential

Many health practitioners have had no coursework in basic counseling and communication skills. Providers are often held captive by a fear that they won't know what to do if the patient has a deeply emotional reaction. "I'm sorry" sounds pretty empty and inadequate in the face of such feeling. Yet empathic communication is a key skill that helps patients open up and share their concerns. Empathic responding, also called *reflective responding,* is a type of active listening that reflects the thought and/or feeling content of the speaker's communication. Practitioners may fear opening up "Pandora's box" by encouraging patients to elaborate on issues that they might not otherwise discuss in a direct fashion. If practitioners do not use this essential skill, patients may conclude that the provider is not interested or that the discussion is bothersome or too time-consuming. However, these skills are part of the necessary tools pharmacists need to provide quality pharmaceutical care. Extensive research links empathic communication to patient satisfaction, improved diagnostic assessment, less litigation and better outcomes (2–4).

Sometimes, the professional demeanor of pharmacists appears to be unconsciously cultivated to protect the provider from his or her own discomfort. Unfortunately, it serves at the same time to prevent genuine expression with the patient. Every provider has heard "Don't let it get to you," or the equivalent from mentors and colleagues. On some level, this advice could be translated as "Don't have feelings about the patient." Without use of empathy skills, providers often report feeling like "sitting ducks in a shooting gallery," being blown away by their patients' or co-workers' emotional reactions with no clue about what to do or say except "stay calm and professional."

Effective empathic skills help patients feel a sense of safety in discussing their concerns with providers. When trust is established, the patient is more likely to reveal clinically relevant data. Much of the theory on empathic facilitation is based on the work of Carl Rogers (5, 6). Rogers and colleagues came to believe that there were three conditions necessary for the maintenance of mental health:

1. Congruence: Patients would not feel the need to develop a protective facade.
2. Unconditional positive regard: Patients would feel warmth, interest, respect, and liking from their providers.
3. Nonjudgmental understanding: Patients get the most benefit when they feel they can share their perceptions, which will be

accepted as valid without feedback that communicates approval or disapproval.

Because most of us experience a shortage of these conditions in our lives, we have become socialized into expressing our feelings indirectly. Indirect messages are hard to decode, and the listener's interpretation of the speaker's message generally goes unspoken. Indirect communication is one reason why needs and expectations are often unmet.

This indirect expression of concerns is replicated in patients' patterns of questions about medications. For instance, they may present secondary concerns ("What if I forget to take this with food?") that mask the presence of a deeper concern ("What if this makes me more sick?"). The presentation of peripheral concerns may be a "test" of the provider. If the provider heedlessly launches into a lecture about how to remember to take the medicine at mealtime, then he or she is missing the deeper meaning. Given this response, the patient may be afraid to ask if the medicine will cause illness because such a question could be interpreted as an insult to the pharmacist who is providing the medicine. Empathic mirroring reduces the emotional charge present during medication counseling. With the emotional tone decreased, the patient is able to process the information in a more conscious manner (7). Patients who are quite upset may need three or more cycles of empathy to de-escalate their affect to the point that information can be exchanged. Often, it is easier to learn about this type of reflective listening by examining what is *not* an empathic response. For instance, if the patient says to the pharmacist "Why won't anybody tell me what's wrong with me?" a variety of responses are possible. Table 8.1 shows examples of response types that are not recommended. Judgmental responses imply judgment

Table 8.1.
Reflecting and Other Response Types

Patient's Statement:
  How come nobody will give me a straight answer about what is wrong with me?
Possible Responses:
  Judgmental Response
    Example: Dr. Morsello is a good doctor. I'm sure she has things under control.
  Diverting Response
    Example: Gee, I don't know, but I have your medication here. Let's go over how you should take it.
  Advising Response
    Example: What you should do is, next time you see your doctor, write down some specific questions you want to ask.
  Questioning Response
    Example: Did you actually ask the doctor what you have?
  Reflecting Response
    Example: Sounds like you would like to know more about your illness.

---

against what the patient is saying; diverting responses change the subject; advice giving moves to problem solving before the real concern is even known; questioning seeks to probe the issue but neglects the emotional tone. Actually, these four responses avoid an open, nonjudgmental discussion of what is really bothering the patient. A fifth type of response, the reflecting or empathic response, attempts to open the discussion of the problem as perceived by the patient.

Making a reflecting response initially is difficult for some pharmacists, again because most of us have not been raised using these skills. Reflecting responding attempts to "reflect" in words what the patient is saying or feeling. The reflection may be based on the *content* or thought expressed by the patient, and/or the *feelings* associated with it, which are often not outwardly expressed. Reflecting responses are called for, especially when the patient is demonstrating emotions. Angry looks, pounding fists, averted eye contact, and head drooping all convey certain emotional states. Hesitating gestures or remarks like "Well . . . I *guess* I could try it" all suggest concerns that need to be gently brought to light. The *first* step in effective reflective responding when emotions are at issue, is to identify and label the emotional state. The four basic emotional states are *mad, sad, glad,* and *scared.* As you observe the patient during consultation, certain nonverbal signs, or verbal ones (e.g., hesitating words), may suggest one of the four feeling states. The *second* step is to put the word describing the feeling state into a sentence to use as a response to the patient. Some basic structures for sentences include "Sounds like you're getting pretty *frustrated*" and "I can see that you're *frustrated.*" Using remarks such as these indicates to patients that you are listening and truly attempting to understand their concerns. Thus, patients and their concerns remain the focus of the encounter. It is important to remember that skills in empathy do not come naturally. Rubin, Judd, and Connie showed that untrained allied health students could not recognize what constitutes an empathic response (8). If health care providers do not master the skill of providing accurate empathy, communication will remain controlled by and centered on the practitioner. Empowerment of patients and retention of a sense of personal control is more likely if patients can express their feeling in an atmosphere of acceptance (9). This is accomplished with nonjudgmental, empathic responding.

Responsible Language Use

In everyday discussion, it is all too easy to blame other people for our own negative feelings or, conversely, to pretend our emotions and thoughts are not important. The goal of communicators is to continuously "own up" to our messages and to analyze them for tones of blaming or denial. For example, pharmacists have increased visibility as part of the interdisciplinary medical team, and each member of the team is responsible for analyzing breakdowns in communication and assessing their own part in causing and fixing the breakdown. Particularly when offering advice, when making a complaint, or when there is conflict of views, careless choice of language can create a destructive communication climate. For example, when working with an asthma patient who is noncompliant, the pharmacist could say "You are trying to overuse your medication now to make up for not using it correctly when you should have known better" (*blaming*) or "Oh, well, I guess as long as your attacks aren't too serious" (*denial*). *Responsible language* is the appropriate alternative. An example to the above patient would be "I'm concerned about your having three more asthma attacks this month than last. Let's look at how you have been using the medication." Responsible language incorporates *first* a statement of your concern citing specifics of the case, and *second* a statement or question about what to do next. Notice that the pharmacist's comment neither places blame nor denies that a potentially serious situation exists. It focuses on the problem (more frequent attacks) as perceived by the pharmacist, and proposes to problem-solve in a joint effort with the patient. The skills of responsible ownership language and specificity come together when we attempt to send assertive messages.

Assertiveness

With patients and co-workers alike, pharmacists must sometimes set limits on behavior that is too demanding, inappropriate, or uncompromising. For example, a consultant pharmacist recently had a case in which a 26-year-old drug-dependent male was admitted to a nursing home for total parenteral nutrition after a case of alcoholic pancreatitis. The pharmacist was present at the nursing station and had to deal with his constant demands for intravenous narcotics, which were not clinically indicated. The pharmacist decided to use the C.L.E.A.R. system. This mnemonic device is a way to remember steps in formulating an assertive message (10).

Clear description: "This is the fifth time this hour you have asked for morphine."
Listen: "I'm ready to listen if something new has come up."
Emotional reaction: "I'm finding it difficult to get my work done with the disruptions."
Assert: "I need you to not keep asking."
Results expected: "If you can do this for us, we will be able to work with you more during the time that you are here" or "we will be able to respond more quickly when you really need us."

The assertive message above incorporates the elements of a specific description of the problem behavior, a sharing of feelings that the behavior provokes, and a description of the consequences if the behavior does not stop. Sending clear, responsible messages is usually enough to help patients understand what kind of dilemma these difficult communications create for the pharmacist.

Conflict Management

When faced with an emotionally charged situation, most professionals either try to avoid the other person, become too passive and accommodating, give in to the urge to fight in a competitive fashion, or compromise their needs prematurely. It is difficult to lower the emotional temperature of an interpersonal conflict to the point where the two parties can collaborate effectively. The assertiveness and empathy skills discussed previously are helpful when used with appropriate timing and with sensitivity to the setting. Additionally, pharmacists have the option of deflection, a kind of partial agreement. For example, it is more effective to say to a nurse, "You've got a good point. It would be great if we had more techs, then we could get special orders up to you much faster" than to feel the need to defend yourself and the pharmacy in the face of accusations about slow response.

Also, some of the criticism that comes in the direction of the pharmacy is very vague. "You guys have got to get your act together" is one of those typically annoying criticisms to which it is too easy to respond in kind. Instead, a strategy of inquiry is needed. "What is it exactly that makes it hard for you to do your job?" could go a long way toward pulling out useful information. When your colleagues provide the information, empathic responding can address their concerns. As a last resort, if tempers are running too high, you should wisely defer further talk until after a cool down period.

With improved skills of empathic/reflective responding, assertiveness, deflection, and inquiry, a strategy of deferral will rarely be needed. Competently using an appropriate combination of these conflict management skills will keep difficult situations from escalating. Additional case studies on conflict resolution in pharmacy practice can be found in other sources (10).

CLINICAL INTERVIEWING SKILLS

Many of the basic communication skills discussed in the section above are applicable to the clinical interviewing and medication consultation processes. This section discusses clinical interviewing skills as they relate to pharmacy practice.

The term *interviewing* means getting "into view" the patient's problems and associated issues. The skills associated with interviewing can be applied to a highly structured, complete assessment of medication use, as well as to a brief conversation with the patient about an adverse drug reaction, and each of these will be discussed below in more detail.

Medication History

A thorough, detailed, up-to-date medication history provides the necessary background for consultation with the patient. Pharmacists are in the ideal position of having the most knowledge about the medication use patterns and outcomes of their patients. This allows pharmacists to effectively interact between patients and medical providers on matters of drug therapy. Obtaining a detailed history of medication use means more than giving patients a form to complete about medication usage. Knowledge of what history content to obtain, as well as what process skills to use when interviewing, is fundamental to providing good pharmaceutical care in this area. Research shows that skills in medication history interviewing are improved with training on specific techniques (11, 12). The following is a step-by-step guide to conducting a comprehensive medication history.

1. *Open the interview.* The first of the core skills is opening the interview. Depending on the setting you are in, you may have been requested to conduct the interview, or perhaps this is a service you offer to all your patients. Greet the patient warmly. Identify yourself to the patient. Verify the patient's identity and others (e.g., care givers) who are present. Keep in mind that care givers may be needed to assist in clarifying information. On the other hand, if the patient is alert and oriented, and can give valid information, address your remarks to that individual. State the purpose of the interview and relate it to expected outcomes for that patient. For example, "Mrs. Smith, Dr. Welsh asked me to speak with you about your medications so we can get a complete picture of what medications you are taking and how they are working."

2. *Set the stage for good communication.* Let the patient know about how long the interview will take to determine if the interview can be completed at that time. If so, arrange furniture to allow face to face communication at eye level. Sit two to four feet from the patient, if at all possible. One study showed patients perceived pharmacists who used these nonverbal skills as more "available" to them, thus facilitating good rapport and better information exchange (13). Maintain good nonverbal communication throughout the interview, have a slightly forward lean and open body posture, and maintain good eye contact.

3. *Control the flow of information.* The pharmacist must maintain control of the interview without appearing brusque or asking questions in an authoritarian style. Using appropriate questioning skills and having a structured framework are imperative to obtain complete information in a manner that facilitates dialogue while allowing the pharmacist to maintain control. Begin by asking the patient, "Tell me about the medications you are currently taking." Use open-ended, broad questions to start data gathering, and proceed to closed-ended and forced-choice questions for discriminating details. Recall that open-ended questions start with *who, what, where, when, why,* and *how* as opposed to closed-ended questions, which can be answered with a yes or no. Indeed, if the patient answers inappropriately to these, the pharmacist should

suspect some barrier to communication, whether it be language, hearing, or mental abilities. After obtaining information about the current medications, proceed to ask about past medication usage, allergies and adverse reactions, and last, life-style questions. Use as many open-ended questions as possible, minimizing the use of closed-ended questions. For example, ask "What medications for diabetes have you taken in the past?" rather than "Have you ever taken tolazamide? Or glipizide?" It may be necessary to ask them specifically, but questions like these should not be used to open discussion of past medications, since they really limit the patient's responses and do not allow for other information to be revealed. Such questions are helpful, however, if the patient admits to taking medication but can't recall the name. Using a closed-ended statement like "Have you ever taken tolazamide?" at that time is appropriate. It can be very helpful to ask such questions at the very end of an interview in which you may be asked to help select therapy. You may be planning to suggest a specific medication to be used for the patient. In that case, it is helpful to ask specifically whether the patient has ever taken it. Patients with chronic conditions often have taken numerous medications with both good and disastrous results. It is not uncommon to have the patient say "Oh, I've had that and it doesn't work," or some other revealing response.

After obtaining a block of related information, give a brief summary or paraphrase of pertinent points. For example, "Mrs. Smith, you've told me you currently take hydrochlorothiazide and digoxin for your heart, and you used to take potassium, but you're not on it now and you're concerned that you need it. Is that correct?" Between subsections of the history, use *transitional* statements to let the patient know you are asking about a different type of information. After making the above statement, the pharmacist might say "Now I'd like to ask about any allergies or reactions to medications you've had." Again, open the discussion with an open-ended statement like "Tell me about your allergies." Keep using open-ended statements like "What other reactions have you had?" to obtain further information. When clarification is needed, it is often necessary to used closed-ended questions. For example, the pharmacist might say "You mentioned being allergic to 'mycin' but can't recall the name of the medication. Could it be erythromycin?"

The pharmacist needs to keep control of the interview to maximize effort while being efficient. When a long interview is expected, invariably the dialogue strays from the topic at hand. The patient may ramble or ask a lot of questions or wish to discuss matters not related to drug therapy. The pharmacist must keep the framework of questioning in mind, know what needs to be asked, and politely defer topics that are not germane to the drug history. Look for openings to bring the subject into focus. For example, "Mr. Jones, you've been telling me how unpleasant it is to be in the hospital and I'd like to focus on how this medicine can help you stay out of the hospital."

When it is necessary at times to interrupt, address the patient by name and simply state your need to ask a certain question. Remember that the goal is not to have a social conversation with the patient, but to obtain the medication history.

4. *Obtain complete information.* Table 8.2 shows a framework for the content of a complete medication history. Begin by asking for information about the current prescribed medications. As noted above, a broad opening allows the patient to note any or all of the medications currently prescribed. For each of the medications, ask specifically for the purpose, dosage, duration of use, some assessment of how the drug is working, and any problems the patient perceives due to the medication. For medications taken as needed, question the patient to determine the amount used per day and per dose. Also, it may be important to know for what symptoms or in what context the patient uses the as-needed medications. Be attentive to vague responses given by the patient. For example, a patient may state that she uses the β-agonist inhaler "only when I really need it." Question specifically how many times a day and how much each dose is used. Similarly, when the patient's responses include words such as *sometimes, not often,* and *occasionally,* probe for more specifics and document amounts of medications used.

After asking about prescribed routine and as-needed medications, next ask about nonprescription medications

Table 8.2.
Content Items for a Comprehensive Medication History

1. Current Prescribed Medications
   Drug name
   Purpose
   Dose
   Duration
   Beneficial effects
   Adverse effects
2. Current Nonprescription Medications
   Drug name
   Purpose/symptoms treated
   Dose and frequency of use
   Duration
   Assessment of effects
3. Past Medication Usage
   Drug name
   Purpose
   Time period of use
   Reason for discontinuation
4. Drug Allergies and Adverse Reactions
   Drug name
   Date of reaction
   Type and severity of reaction
5. Life-style Factors
   Nicotine usage
   Alcohol usage
   Illicit drug usage
   Dietary habits
   Occupation
   Stressors

used on a regular basis. Since patients may not perceive vitamins or cold products as medications, it may be necessary to specifically ask "What medications do you take for a cold? For your stomach problems? For a headache? What other medications or health products of any kind might you be taking?" Another approach is to query the patient using an approach similar to the review of systems used by physicians. Begin by asking about medications used for disorders of the head, eyes, ears, nose, and throat. Next, ask about products for respiratory, gastrointestinal, genitourinary, and skin conditions. When the patient notes using any medication, ask specifically about the amounts used, duration of use, and outcome of treatment. After this lengthy discussion, the pharmacist will have a complete history of the medications currently being used by the patient.

Past medication use constitutes the next large block of data to be obtained. Ask about the medications previously used to treat conditions the patient has at the present time. This is important, since the pharmacist would not want to recommend medications that were ineffective or caused adverse reactions. It is useful to ask "Why was that medication stopped?" and "Who stopped that medication?" It is important for the pharmacist to know whether the physician advised stopping the medication or whether the patient made the decision alone. Before proceeding to the next history section, summarize significant points in past drug history to allow the patient to clarify information or add history data.

Obtain complete information on drug sensitivities. Remember that many patients think of any adverse reaction as an "allergy," so it is important to clearly define the nature of the drug reaction. Begin with an open-ended statement like "Tell me about any drug allergies and other problems you've had from medications." Follow with asking for details of the reaction—when did it occur, what exactly happened—to provide a clear picture.

Last, ask about life-style issues that may affect drug therapy. These include dietary habits, tobacco and alcohol consumption, and illicit drug use. Since nicotine and alcohol are a factor in response to many drug therapies, it is important to quantify their intake, even though it may be uncomfortable for the pharmacist to do so. A useful suggestion is to open the discussion with a statement describing the importance of that information to you. For example, "Mr. Smith, I'd like to ask about your intake of alcohol and tobacco, since these can affect the way your medicines work. How much alcohol do you drink?" Quantify the amount as well as the type of alcohol used. Note whether the patient smokes, and how much. If the patient has stopped, it may be useful to know when. Other factors may be important to probe. For example, it is helpful to know the stressors for patients with heart or ulcer disease, or the job environment of the asthma patient.

5. *Close the interview.* When you feel you have obtained all necessary and important information, it is time to close the interview. Begin the closure with a brief summary of only the most important points, noting any concerns that you or the patient has regarding the medications and recommendations for resolution of problems. Ask the patient to verify agreement on the issues and tell the patient what to expect next. Ask the patient if there is anything he or she wants to add, or if he or she has any other questions. If not, the interview is ended. Here is an example of a good closure: "Mr. Smith, we've talked about your heart and diabetes medications, and you mentioned some 'weak spells,' which I think may be caused by one of your medications. You're concerned about them. I am going to discuss them with your doctor. Is there anything else you would like to add or discuss?"

Symptom-Based Interview

During a lengthy interview, at a bedside visit, over the telephone, or at the prescription counter, the patient may mention symptoms that could be related to drug therapy. Knowing how to explore the patient's symptoms and evaluate their relationship to either the disease or its treatment is a key component of the pharmacist's assessment skills. The first step is to get the patient to more fully reveal information regarding the symptom. An introductory statement ("Tell me more about it.") will get the patient to provide more specific details. The *Key Symptom Questions* can also be used to explore symptoms mentioned by the patient. These seven, focused, open-ended questions, based on medical interviewing techniques, seek specifics that will help define whether the symptom is related to drug therapy (14, 15). Depending on the patient's response to "Tell me more about it," it may not be necessary or appropriate to ask all seven questions every time a symptom is noted. Listed below are seven specific points to be addressed and an open-ended question that could be used to probe for that information.

Onset/Timing: When did you notice this? When did it start?
Duration: How long have you had this problem?
Content: Under what circumstances does this symptom appear?
Quality: What does it feel like?
Quantity: How much, how often do you notice it?
Treatment: What makes it better? What have you done about it?
Associated Symptoms: What other symptoms are you having?

Without proper attention to detail, many practitioners make assumptions that the symptom expressed is due to a disease state and do not adequately address it. Or, they may jump to conclusions about the cause of the symptom and recommend a treatment without knowing the real cause. For example, a patient taking a nonsteroidal antiinflammatory drug who complains of fatigue might be recommended a vitamin if the pharmacist thinks the patient is tired from inadequate nutrition, whereas probing the symptom of fatigue with the questions listed above may reveal that the fatigue started after the medication was begun and is accompanied by gastric distress, suggesting anemia from gastrointestinal blood loss as a possible cause for the fatigue.

The *Key Symptom Questions* are also important when there is a tendency to attribute *every* symptom to a medication, as sometimes patients are inclined to do. For instance, a pharmacy student reviewed the chart of a patient with bipolar illness, seizures, and Parkinsonism. The patient was on several medications including carbamazepine and carbidopa/levodopa. The patient complained of blurred vision and insomnia, which the student felt were due to the medications. When the patient was interviewed using the questioning technique described above, she indicated that she had blurred vision only out of the left eye, and that she had had insomnia "since the day I was born." Answers to further questions suggested that her symptoms were not likely related to her drug therapy.

Knowledge of each drug's side effect profile as well as the disease state symptomatology is essential to be able to differentiate whether the symptom is a drug-related adverse effect or not. In some cases, it could be either, in which case onset of the symptom will be very important to ascertain. If the symptom began or worsened after starting a new medication, then there is a higher likelihood of the problem being drug-related.

Students and new practitioners are often confused about what to do once the symptom has been explored. Determining the seriousness of the problem is sometimes difficult. It is helpful to ask yourself "What is the worst thing that can happen in this case? If this is an adverse reaction to the medication, what will happen if the medication is continued? What will happen to the patient (and disease process) if the medication is stopped?" Easily discernible side effects, such as dizziness from an antihypertensive, are managed by practical suggestions to the patient without discontinuation of drug therapy. Even so, the patient may elect to stop taking the medication, and the pharmacist must think ahead to those consequences and advise the patient accordingly. More serious toxicities require either calling the patient's physician or advising the patient to discuss the problem with his or her physician as soon as possible, rather than suggesting stopping the medication.

The most important aspect of addressing symptoms is to obtain enough information to make an informed clinical judgment. This is accomplished by using the *Key Symptom Questions* outlined above.

BASIC MEDICATION CONSULTATION

Consultation on medication use is one of the most fundamental and important activities of the pharmacist, whether you practice in a community pharmacy, clinic, or institutional site. Consultation on new medications is mandated by the Omnibus Budget Reconciliation Act of 1990, and most states require counseling for all patients on either new or both new and refill prescriptions (16, 17).

The traditional method of consulting involved providing information—the pharmacist "told" and the patient "listened." There was little true dialogue, since often the pharmacist asked closed-ended questions such as "Do you understand?" and "Do you have any questions?" As was noted previously, such closed-ended questions tend to restrict the flow of information. When the pharmacist merely provides information and the conversation is basically one-way, there is no opportunity to ascertain what the patient may know or think about the medication.

The pharmacist-patient consultation techniques developed by the Indian Health Service three decades ago, and further refined in collaboration with colleagues around the country, teach an interactive method of consultation, one that seeks to verify what the patient knows about using the medication, and "fill in the gaps" with only the most basic information when needed (18). Research shows that people forget 90% of what is heard within 60 minutes of hearing it (1). Any counseling technique that is based on the pharmacist speaking most of the time will be ineffective, since patients will almost immediately forget what they heard. By making the patient an active participant in the process, increased learning will occur. Engaging patient participation in the exchange requires the use of specific, open-ended questions that seek to obtain what the patient already knows about the medication, then following up by providing new information to the patient and summarizing at the end of the consultation. These specific techniques are further discussed below.

Basic Medication Consultation Skills: The Prime Question Technique

The interactive technique for consulting on medications consists of two sets of open-ended questions. One set is for a new prescription (*Prime Questions*), and the other is for refill prescription consultation (*Show and Tell Questions*), as shown in Table 8.3. Using these questions when counseling provides an interactive process that engages the patient, thereby making him or her an active participant in the learning process. The questions provide an organized approach to ascertain what the patient already knows about the medication. Utilizing a systematic approach has been associated with improved recall of prescription instructions (19). The pharmacist can praise the patient for correct information recalled, clarify points misunderstood, and add new information when needed. It spares the pharmacist from repeating information already known by the patient, which is an inefficient use of time. The steps in the consultation process are described in detail below.

1. *Open the consultation.* When the prescription is ready and the patient is called for counseling, establish rapport by introducing yourself by name and stating the purpose of the

Table 8.3.
Medication Consultation Skills

Prime Questions
* What did your doctor tell you the medication is for?
  or
  What were you told the medication is for?
    What problem or symptom is it supposed to help?
    What is it supposed to do?
* How did your doctor tell you to take the medication?
  or
  How were you told to take the medication?
    How often did your doctor say to take it?
    How much are you supposed to take?
    What did your doctor say to do when you miss a dose?
    What does three times a day mean to you?
* What did your doctor tell you to expect?
  or
  What were you told to expect?
    What good effects are you supposed to expect?
    What bad effects did your doctor tell you to watch for?
    What should you do if a bad reaction occurs?
Show and Tell Questions
* What do you take the medication for?
* How do you take it?
* What kind of problems are you having?

consultation. Verify the patient's identity, either by asking for identification, or at least by asking "And you are . . . ?" after you identify yourself. If the patient is non-English speaking, hard of hearing, or otherwise unable to answer his or her name, you have identified a barrier in the consultation that must be overcome before discussing the medication.

If time and help permit and a private space is available, suggest that the consultation be conducted there and move to that area. This will be important for patients who have hearing problems and those needing extra privacy, such as the patient receiving a vaginal cream or the patient with AIDS. Sit facing the patient, and maintain the appropriate interpersonal distance (1½ to 2 feet) during the consultation.

2. *Conduct the counseling session.* Begin by asking the Prime Questions if the prescription is a new one, or the Show and Tell for a refill prescription. If the patient is able to tell you what the medication is for, you may choose to probe further or move to the next question. Probing further may be helpful when the patient answers in broad or vague terms. An example would be the patient receiving a β-blocker who tells you the medication is for "my heart." You may wish to ask in an open-ended fashion, "What is it supposed to do for your heart?" Avoid asking "Is it for chest pains?" or similar closed-ended questions, since you may alarm the patient by your suggestions and you might waste time if multiple questions are asked. If the patient does not know what the medication is for or says "Don't you know?" you should then ask why they visited the physician. They may describe symptoms of a condition known to be treatable with the medication in question. If so, indicate what symptoms the medication will help. If the patient is totally unaware, a referral

back to the physician is indicated, lest the pharmacist judge in error the indication for the medication.

After verifying that the patient knows what the medication is for, ask the second prime question. Often, patients are unaware of the dosage instructions or indicate "It's on the label, isn't it?" Be aware of the optimal dosing instructions, since the patient may respond correctly "twice a day," but you may still need to advise on exact timing or whether to take the drug with meals. Other questions to include under the second prime question are how long to take the medication, exactly how much or how often to take when the medication is prescribed as needed, what to do when a dose is missed, and how to store the medication. When possible, rather than providing facts, ask the patient "What did the doctor say about how long to take this medication?" or "What will you do if you miss a dose?" Asking a question of the patient prompts his or her attention, whereas "telling" the information is more passive for the patient, and the patient may not listen as well. Think of the counseling session as an opportunity to find out what the patient knows, rather than a place to showcase your knowledge. Keep the information you provide brief and to the point.

After reviewing information about how to take the medication, proceed to the third prime question. Most often, patients have been told nothing about side effects or beneficial effects. On the other hand, a patient may describe either beneficial or adverse results anticipated by taking the medication. If beneficial effects are mentioned, follow up with "What side effects were you warned about?" to determine the patient's knowledge of potential side effects. Other questions subsumed under this third prime question relate to how the patient will know if the medication is working, what precautions to take while taking the medication, and what to do if the medication doesn't work.

With regard to adverse effects from drug therapy, if the patient is unaware, mention the main or most serious adverse effects, and what to do if they occur. Research shows that patients want information about their medications, especially adverse effects, and that providing such information does not lead to the development of those reactions in most cases (20–23). Recent work on communicating about risk, in this case risk in terms of drug reactions, suggests a four-quadrant model in which each quadrant requires specific communications skills (24). The quadrants are shown having a combination of either high or low probability of occurrence with high or low magnitude. An example of high probability and high magnitude would be cancer chemotherapy, which entails frequent and severe toxicities. Empathic communication should be the lead skill in discussing risk of therapy in this case. The second case, high probability and low magnitude, might be exemplified by gastric complaints from erythromycin. Pharmacists often encounter patients with common, bothersome side effects. Useful communication skills include providing information about how the medication will work and why it is a good therapy for them, as well as how to manage expected side effects.

In the third quadrant, where there is low probability but high magnitude (e.g., stroke with an oral contraceptive), careful attention to and assessment of the patient's perceptions about the possible side effects are needed. Be aware of how the patient's perceptions may differ from your own. Since the patient may only hear "This is unlikely to happen but . . . " and tune out the specifics about the toxicity, it is helpful to ask the patient for feedback on the discussion of toxicity. In the fourth case, the low probability and low magnitude of risk may be associated with a perception that the medication may have little value to the patient. Again, heavy-handed tactics to convince, scare, or otherwise threaten the patient will not be effective. Questioning patients to determine their view of what benefits might accrue from taking the medication is necessary. Follow with comments to "match" their assessment. For example, when a patient says "Well, I could get an allergic reaction to this," the issue of the adverse effect is first and foremost in her mind, whereas the pharmacist may think "I've never seen anyone allergic to this." Rather than try to convince the patient that no one becomes allergic to it, one might say "Yes, that's possible. Which do you think is worse—putting up with the pain or taking a chance on the medication?" This brings into the open, the discussion of both the risks and benefits of treatment. If the pharmacist can "bring the patient along" the thought continuum with a discussion of potential benefits, the patient may decide to "give it a try." At times, the authors have found it useful to "contract" with the patient. For example, "Sam, we've discussed both the good and bad about taking this medicine, and I know you still have concerns about side effects. I really think this medicine is best for you. Would you be willing to try it for a week? I will check in with you after a few days to see how things are going." More often than not, the anticipated adverse effects do not appear.

Using skills described in the sections above for confronting adverse reactions or the fear of them will set the stage for better patient compliance. However, just the act of having to take a medication when one is not used to doing so poses a problem for compliance. When a patient has a new medication, and after using the Prime Questions to counsel him or her, it may be helpful to raise compliance concerns. A *universal statement* is a useful opener. It describes the situation for a group, then narrows down to focus on the individual. For example, "Mrs. Green, a lot of patients have trouble fitting taking medication into their daily schedule. What problems do you foresee in taking this?" It may be necessary to probe the patient's daily habits and help him or her find a way to tie medication taking into a particular activity. For instance, if the patient always makes coffee in the morning, having the medication nearby may be sufficient reminder to promote compliance. Be sure to use a partnership approach. Additional compliance-enhancing skills are discussed later in this chapter.

3. *Close the consultation.* Most consultations are a combination of the patient knowing some information and the pharmacist providing additional information as the Prime Questions are reviewed. Because of this, it is important to close the consultation with the *final verification.* Think of the final verification as asking the patient to "play back" everything he or she has learned in order to check that the information is complete and accurate. Say to the patient "Just to make sure I didn't leave anything out (explain things clearly), please go over with me how you are going to use the medication." Although the language seems bulky, if the question were phrased "Just to make sure you've got this . . . " the patient may feel embarrassed if he or she does not recall important facts. At this point, the patient should describe correct use of the medication. Any errors can be corrected and any omissions clarified. Then, ask the patient if there is anything else he or she needs and offer help as needed.

A similar process is used for refill prescriptions. The Show and Tell questions verify patient understanding of proper use of chronic medications, or medications that the patient has used in the past. The pharmacist begins the process by "showing" the medication to the patient (i.e., by opening the bottle and displaying the contents). Then, the patient "tells" the pharmacist how he or she uses the medication by answering the questions as shown in Table 8.3. Note that the doctor is omitted as a reference, since the patient should have been counseled properly before this and should have all information needed for proper medication usage. The Show and Tell technique allows the pharmacist to detect problems with compliance or unwanted drug effects. If the patient answers incorrectly to the second question, the patient may be noncompliant, or the physician may have changed the dosage. The pharmacist will need to further define the reason for the discrepancy. The second Show and Tell question also allows the pharmacist to ask the patient to demonstrate use of an inhaler or an injectable, or how to measure liquid doses to assure proper use.

Some pharmacists have difficulty asking the third question, fearing that they may arouse suspicion in the patient. However, research discounts this notion, as was previously mentioned. If potential adverse effects were discussed when the patient was initially counseled, it seems natural, and certainly relevant and important to query the patient about adverse effects at the refill visit. If new symptomatology is present, explore this further using the *Key Symptom Questions.* Clinical judgment will dictate whether the problem is medication related and how it should be managed.

Barriers in the Consultation

The clinical skills described above will be easily applied in situations where there are few or no barriers in communication between patient and pharmacist. In reality, there are often obstacles to overcome in the environment or within the pharmacist or the patient. Examples of problems within the pharmacy environment that deter patient consultation include lack of privacy, interruptions, high work load, and lack of sufficient staff. Barriers present within the pharmacist include lack of desire or lack of skills to adequately counsel patients, stereotyping patients and problems, and difficulty in maintaining control of concentration while counseling, especially when stress is a factor. A detailed analysis of these barriers is beyond the scope of this discussion but can be found in Reference 25. Barriers that the patient brings to the encounter will be discussed here insofar as overcoming them relates to the clinical communication skills discussed above.

The structured approach for obtaining a medication history and for medication counseling can be likened to knowing the road on which you are traveling. However, unforeseen events happen on every path. Within the context of the clinical encounter, unforeseen issues may arise at any time. Just as one must remove or negotiate around the obstacle on the highway, the pharmacist must recognize and manage barriers brought by the patient during the encounter for the consultation to reach the desired end. These are of two types—functional and emotional. Functional barriers include problems with hearing and vision that make it difficult for the patient to absorb information during the consultation. Also, language barriers and illiteracy are formidable obstacles to proper consultation. Recognizing these barriers is usually not difficult, as the signs of poor vision are easy to observe. So, too, language problems will become apparent early on in the counseling process. Strategies specific to each barrier are needed when these problems are identified. For instance, moving to a quiet area, repeating information and asking feedback of the patient are important when hearing is a problem. Giving clear verbal instructions and using large-type print materials are helpful when the patient has vision difficulties. Using translators and picture diagrams, and involving English-speaking care givers are important when language problems exist. In these cases, the barriers are usually permanent; however, with emotional barriers, they may be transitory or more longstanding.

Emotional barriers are common in everyday interactions, including pharmacist-patient communication, and when not handled properly, they give rise to further aggravation, break down communication, and thus inhibit effective consultation. Patients may express, directly or indirectly, anger, hostility, sadness, depression, fear, anxiety, or embarrassment during consultation with the pharmacist. They may also give the attitude of a "know-it-all," be suspicious of medications, and seem unmotivated or uninterested. Some of these barriers might be momentary, such as the frustration experienced when the prescription can't be filled because the medication is unavailable at that time. On the other hand, the patient with a chronic pain syndrome may at various times be less attentive due to being uncomfortable or in pain. The attitude of the patient who "knows" all about his or her medications likely will not change in time.

Unlike seeing the patient with a "white cane" and knowing a vision problem exists, emotional barriers can be more difficult to discern. Since most patients will not say "I'm angry and frustrated about feeling so ill" or "I'm upset that my doctor didn't spend that much time with me," their feelings surface in statements like "I don't know why it takes all day to put a few pills in the bottle!" and "I don't know why I have to take this stupid medicine. Nothing seems to help anyway." Unfortunately, we usually respond to the content of the message (e.g., "Well, I'll have this ready for you as soon as I can") and in doing so, overlook the opportunity to respond to the issues behind the statement, issues that may impact on the encounter and, more important, on the patient's decision to comply with therapy. In the beginning of this chapter, several nonverbal and verbal clues were mentioned that suggest different emotional tones (e.g., pounding fists associated with anger). It takes patience and practice to listen *beyond* the words. The first step is to notice these nonverbal and verbal clues, identify the feeling state they represent, and respond with a reflecting or empathic statement as has been described. To the patient in the second example, the pharmacist might say "Sounds like you've been frustrated with other things you've tried" rather than "This is a good medicine, Joe, and I really think it will help." Recall that a statement such as this can occur at any time throughout the consultation, and that this barrier of frustration should be dealt with before closing the consultation. Embarrassment is a factor when vaginal preparations, condom use, and similar topics are the subject of the consultation. Again, observe for signs of embarrassment, such as averted gaze or fidgeting, and respond with "This can be hard to talk about, but it's really important that we discuss . . . " Also, be matter-of-fact, move to a private space and speak in a normal tone of voice to alleviate the embarrassment.

Use of proper skills to remove the barriers during the consultation will allow for the consultation to proceed with both parties devoting attention to the primary issues of drug therapy and usage, rather than to the interpersonal difficulties that can arise. It is important to note that the consultation and medication interview processes explained in detail above do not exist in isolation. Indeed, they are part of the larger review of medication usage required by law and which comprises high-quality pharmaceutical care. Obtaining a comprehensive profile of the patient and his/her medications, and providing ongoing consultation on prescriptions are two key components of patient-focused care. The third is compliance and disease monitoring, which occur during subsequent visits. This is discussed in the following subsection.

COMPLIANCE AND DISEASE MONITORING

Nowhere else is the pharmacist's role in monitoring and managing medication use more vital than in the case of those patients requiring chronic drug therapy, especially with diseases that are asymptomatic. Many factors contribute to the pharmacist's success in assuring beneficial outcomes. Among them are practice site, pharmacist competence, support of administration, and breadth of responsibilities, including in some cases, prescriptive authority. Hatoum and Akhras have documented extensively the value of pharmacist's contributions to ambulatory care sites ranging from a community group practice to home health patients and others (26). The Indian Health Service has provided a full range of pharmaceutical care services to its patients for over three decades. Besides the traditional dispensing role, IHS pharmacists offer private consultations to all patients and have prescriptive authority for refilling chronic medications based on their assessment of the patient's needs (27, 28). Some pharmacists have been educated to provide primary medical care as pharmacist practitioners, and this movement has subsequently spread to other practice sites. Currently, several states have passed regulations that allow pharmacists to diagnose and prescribe (15). Whether your practice is a sophisticated one such as those just described or a more typical one in community, hospital, or long-term care, providing pharmaceutical care to patients requiring chronic drug therapy can have significant positive outcomes. To effectively provide long-term pharmaceutical care, several important factors need to be considered.

Who's Disease Is It Anyway?

One of the common misperceptions held by health professionals regarding a patient with a chronic disease is that the professional manages the patient's disease. Nothing could be further from the truth, and this medical myth is probably one of the major contributors to compliance problems among patients with chronic diseases. In the traditional model, health professionals perceive their roles to be in the diagnosis, treatment, and management of disease. As drug therapy managers, clinical pharmacists focus on blood levels, kinetic dosage calculations and drug interactions. Guided by this focus on technical aspects of patient care, health professionals often get frustrated and angry when patients don't follow instructions or, despite

the provider's best efforts, achieve only partially satisfactory results. In reality, the only time the health professional manages the treatment is during the very limited time when patients encounter the health care delivery system during an office visit or institutionalization in hospital or long-term-care facility. Most of the time, the patient controls the treatment of his or her disease, especially those that require continuous medication. Failure to recognize this basic truth has created (a) considerable tension in patient-provider relationships, (b) provider frustration and anger, (c) poor communication, (d) negative provider attitudes toward individual patients, (e) poor patient outcomes, (f) patient distrust of providers, and (g) legal consequences that have been a major contributor to rising health care costs (29–32).

One author strongly suggests that noncompliance in diabetes mellitus is due in large part to the failure of providers to recognize that their goal is not treating the disease, but *helping the patient treat their disease* (33). That contention is supported by current medical literature on compliance that links good communication and a partnership style of provider-patient relationship to increased satisfaction, increased compliance, and better patient outcomes (4, 31, 32).

To be successful in assisting patients achieve good outcomes, the provider and pharmacist must eschew the traditional medical myth regarding who manages the disease and adopt a partnership approach, acting as facilitators to help patients manage their disease (i.e., it's the *patient's* disease—the provider's job is to *help the patient manage it*).

Go Slow/Use Interactive Techniques

Patients can only absorb a limited amount of new information at each encounter. Too many times, in an attempt to do a thorough job, health professionals inadvertently overwhelm the patient with information at or near the time of diagnosis or treatment initiation. A patient's active listening abilities last less than a minute during a monologue presentation; therefore, they retain only a few pieces of information from a prolonged discussion and possibly miss key facts. In addition, a large volume of technical information may confuse or frighten patients, leading to the poor outcome that we hope to prevent with our educational efforts (34).

Successful patient educators do two things: (a) give patients information in small manageable increments, and (b) actively involve the patient in the educational process by creating an interactive dialogue and using other "hands-on" approaches that are consistent with adult learning principles (34). For the pharmacist, at the time of the initial prescription, this means focusing on verifying that the patient understands how to take the medicine and its most common side effects. For example, with hydrochlorothiazide 25 mg daily for hypertension, the pharmacist should verify that the patient knows what it's for, to take it once daily in the morning to prevent nighttime voiding, that it takes a while before any changes in blood pressure occur, and that the patient will notice increased urination the first week but it should lessen after that. Discussions about diet, exercise, and related issues can wait until later visits. Giving the patient a handout on hypertension and diuretics would be appropriate and can lead to questions and subsequent education at later visits or during a follow-up phone call.

Set the Stage for Future Encounters

Many providers initially explain to patients how they are going to monitor them for disease control and progression so that subsequent questions, lab tests, and examinations are viewed by the patients as a normal part of their care. However, few providers follow a similar process regarding compliance. Therefore, without previous explanation, provider questions about compliance are likely to be associated with parent-type sanctions from the provider. To avoid this "punishment," patients may avoid disclosing compliance problems when asked. This all-too-common problem can be prevented by remembering who ultimately manages the disease and by specific strategies during the initial patient contact. Explain that compliance is very important to successful outcomes, but that you know how hard it is to remember to take medication every day. Tell the patient that you expect that he or she will be like all patients and experience some difficulties remembering to take their medication. Ask patients to keep track of those instances if possible, and further explain that you will be asking them at each visit about what kind of problems they have had with the medication so that you can assist them to better remember to take the medication. This can easily be done in association with explanations about how the progress of the disease will be monitored.

Monitoring and Education of the Patient at Return Visits

Organizing an effective approach to evaluating and educating patients with chronic diseases at return visits may be problematic in a busy practice setting. One simple way to look at all patients returning for follow-up of a chronic disease is to use the three Cs: *Control, Complications,* and *Compliance.* The first C refers to control of the chronic disease. To evaluate the control, objective findings such as the blood pressure and range of motion can be coupled with subjective findings from the consultation, such as reports of dizziness, nocturnal voiding, and degree of morning stiffness. The second C refers to complications due to both disease progression and drug effects. As with the control parameters, a combination of subjective

findings from the interview with the patient and objective findings from the health record or patient profile, from physical findings during examination, and from pertinent lab and other tests can be used to quickly evaluate the presence of potential complications. For example, a patient with hypertension, diabetes mellitus, and osteoarthritis who takes captopril, chlorpropamide, and ibuprofen can be queried about the presence of cough, difficulty sleeping, and exercise tolerance. These are primarily directed at detecting congestive heart failure or renal failure due to hypertension and/or diabetes, but also will help detect drug-related problems such as cough due to the angiotensin-converting enzyme (ACE) inhibitor and renal effects from the ibuprofen. Checking recent lab values for creatinine, electrolytes, and blood glucose will help detect diabetes, hypertension or NSAID-induced renal impairment, excessive chlorpropamide dosage, and ACE inhibitor hyperkalemia.

The third C relates to compliance problems. Pharmacist actions can be broken up into three steps: *recognize* potential compliance problems, *identify* probable causes, and once the cause of the noncompliance is determined, *manage* the problem with specific steps. This RIM model is an easy process that can be used by pharmacists to enhance patient compliance (35). In this model (Table 8.4), subjective and objective findings are used to detect potential compliance problems. The health record or drug profile is reviewed for objective evidence of potential compliance before talking with the patient. During profile review, three items should alert the pharmacist to potential compliance problems. The first, and most common, is a discrepancy between the number of doses that should have been taken and the number of doses dispensed. Second, patients with incomplete refill requests (e.g., only one or two out of more chronic medications due at the same time) raise suspicion for noncompliance. Third is the prescribing of a new medication that may be taken to offset adverse effects from another medication, if the adverse effect is unrecognized as such. Many times, patients present to the medical provider with a new complaint. If the provider doesn't make the connection between the new symptom and the side effect, it may eventually result in compliance or therapeutic problems. Patients on ACE inhibitors with new or repeat prescriptions for cough suppressants or antibiotics for bronchitis should alert the pharmacist to potential ACE-inhibitor-induced cough. In extreme cases, patients may stop the needed drug and continue with the drug used to treat the side effects, which is unnecessary and could pose risks in itself.

Care must be taken in interpreting these signs. Positive findings during profile or chart review call for further exploration before a definite compliance problem can be ascertained. In some cases there are rational explanations

Table 8.4.
Steps in the RIM Model for Compliance Counseling

Recognize Potential Noncompliance
- For "objective evidence," use supportive compliance probes.
    - Examples: I noticed that this refill was due.
    - I'm concerned that you won't get the full benefits from your medication if it's not taken as prescribed.
- For "subjective evidence" use reflecting responses.
    - Examples: It sounds like you are worried about side effects.
    - So you feel that your medication is not working.

Identify/Categorize the Noncompliance
- "Knowledge deficits" are evidenced through a patient's statements, indicating a misunderstanding or lack of information.
- "Practical impediments" are revealed by a patient's description of lack of funds, inability to access the medication, forgetfulness, difficulty with a complicated dosing schedule or adverse reaction.
- "Attitudinal barriers" are disclosed by a patient's statements highlighting their lack of faith in medication.
    - Example: I hate to take pills.

Manage the Noncompliance
- "Knowledge deficits" are resolved by providing both verbal and written information, verifying the patient's understanding.
- "Practical impediments" are dealt with by providing corrective actions individualized for the problem, e.g., providing a dosing calendar developed with the patient, working with the physician to find easier dosing regimens, or using pill boxes. Adverse reactions require the use of the Key Symptoms Questions.
    - Example: When did your headaches start?
- "Attitudinal barriers" are rectified by maintaining an understanding of the patient's view and using empathy, open-ended questions, and universal statements.

for the objective findings. Gaps in refills may be due to patients getting refills at another location, or the doctor may have told the patient to change the dosage schedule or to stop the drug altogether.

When the profile indicates potential noncompliance, the best approach is to begin consultation using the Show and Tell technique for refill prescriptions. Possibly, the patient will provide you with one or more clues to confirm your suspicions. If not, the pharmacist must initiate a more direct approach using a *supportive compliance probe.* This is a specific type of statement that uses "I" language by the pharmacist, describes specifically what the pharmacist sees, and asks a question to probe the discrepancy. For example, "I noticed when I reviewed your profile that you hadn't had your prednisone refilled in about two weeks. I was concerned that there might have been some changes that I'm not aware of." This combination of "I noticed . . . and I'm concerned . . . " can be very effective in getting a dialogue started in a nonthreatening manner. Another useful approach is the *universal* statement (e.g., "Most of my patients have problems remembering to take every dose of their medication. What kinds of problems are you having?") Open the discussion of compliance problems

with nonthreatening language and there is a greater likelihood that the patient will disclose problems.

During the consultation, the patient may provide the pharmacist with clues to compliance problems not revealed by patient record review. Indeed, patients may refill their medications on time, but actually take only some of the doses. Patients who, during the Show and Tell questioning, tell the pharmacist that they are taking their medication differently than prescribed provide a strong indication of a potential compliance problem. Some may be quite obvious, such as when the patient asks "Why do I have to keep taking this medicine?" This might be called a red flag, since it seems fairly obvious that the patient wishes not to take the prescription. However, many statements are more subtle. Examples of these vague clues, called pink flags, include "My doctor says I *should* take it," "my doctor *wants* me to," or "I'm *supposed* to be taking . . . " These are usually picked up when the pharmacist asks the first two Show and Tell questions. Other pink flags are more closely associated with the third question, such as when a long pause occurs during the patient's reply, which may indicate potential problems. For example, "What kinds of problems are you having with the medication?" may prompt the following pink flag responses: "Well, . . . none, really" or a hesitation before saying "no, none." Reflecting responses previously discussed in this chapter are appropriate. Such would include "Seems like you're not too sure about taking that" or "Sounds like you think there may be a problem." These open the dialogue in a nonthreatening manner and focus on the patient's perceptions or suggestion that a problem exists.

Patients may ask "Does this medicine have any side effects? What kind of side effects does this have? or Is this anything like (specific drug)?" More often than not, pharmacists simply answer the question without really listening to the underlying concern. This point was mentioned in the section on basic communication skills. An appropriate response would be "Why do you ask?" especially if the patient looks hesitant or the intonation of the question suggests doubt about taking the medication. Often, when the authors have used this question, patients will disclose that a relative had it or something like it, or the media reports problems with it. These indirect experiences create enough doubt that the patient wavers about taking the medication. Obviously, if the pharmacist uses the Show and Tell solely, and does not *recognize* these pink flags, the consultation will be in vain, for the patient will leave without having the underlying doubt resolved. Therefore, it is crucial to develop keen active listening skills to denote the presence of the pink flags and use reflecting responses to probe the problem. During the Show and Tell questioning, patients may disclose symptoms that may indicate an adverse effect. This is sometimes a reason for premature discontinuation of treatment or for skipping doses. When such appears to be the case, use of the Key Symptom Questions if needed will help identify the exact nature of the problem. Resolution of the problem will be dictated by the clinical urgency of the problem.

Once the presence of the compliance problem has been confirmed, further use of reflecting and other responses can identify the nature of the problem. Compliance problems can be categorized within three groups. The first is a *knowledge* deficit. In these cases, patients have insufficient information, lack skills, or have misinformation that prevents compliance. Examples are a patient who put contraceptive jelly on toast and the patient who was never shown or has forgotten how to use an inhaler. The second group involves *practical impediments* or barriers, such as complex drug regimens involving multiple drugs and/or different dosage schedules, difficulty in developing routines that facilitate medication compliance, difficulty in opening containers, or insufficient mental aptitude to comply. The final category is *attitudinal barriers*. Among the most difficult to identify and manage, these include patient beliefs about health, disease, and/or treatment that are inconsistent with the prescribed regimen. These may reflect differences in cultural beliefs (36–38). As outlined by the health belief model, perceived severity of risk compared to the perceived benefit of treatment plays a large role in determining patient compliance (38). Other factors such as patient desire to be in control and belief that he or she can successfully implement the recommended treatment also strongly influence compliance (34). Finally, the most prevalent and potentially the most difficult belief differences to overcome are patient's *lay theories* (38). Common lay theories held by patients include "You need to give your body a rest from medicine or it will become immune to it. You only need to take medicine when you feel sick, not when you feel OK."or "If one dose is good, then two must be better."

Once the specific cause is identified, then a specific strategy to manage that problem can be attempted. Most knowledge and skill deficiencies can be successfully corrected with education and/or training. Practical impediments respond well to specific measures such as simplifying regimens, use of easy-open containers, and enlisting the aid of spouse or care giver. Attitudinal issues tend to be the most complex and difficult to solve. Even lay theories, which would seem easily fixed by correcting misinformation, are extremely difficult to overcome because the nature of lay theories makes them highly resistant to change. Again, it takes practice, careful listening, repeated conversations with the patients, and a supportive climate for the patient to acknowledge one of these barriers. They will only do so when they feel the pharmacist will not denigrate them or argue against their beliefs. Partnership language and gentle confrontation on the facts are indicated. Repeated efforts to enlighten may, over time, change the view of the patient.

CONCLUSION

Contemporary pharmacy practice is changing at a very rapid pace. Pharmaceutical care, that which focuses on the patient's outcomes of drug therapy, is the founding principle for practitioners. New systems for pharmaceutical care delivery are appearing almost daily. From the pioneering work done by the Indian Health Service, which uses pharmacists across the spectrum of care, model clinical pharmacy practices that incorporate IHS patient care principles into the community pharmacies are evolving (39–41). For today's pharmacist, whether he or she practices in a community, hospital, or other setting, the delivery of quality pharmaceutical care involves the skills and techniques discussed in this chapter, as well as others that support the pharmacist-patient interaction and medication use process. As direct patient contact and responsibility for drug therapy outcomes becomes the main task for the pharmacist, the skills of interpersonal communication, medication history interview and consultation, and compliance monitoring and enhancement become the "tools of the trade." The consistent application of a high level of interpersonal and applied clinical skills by the pharmacist will lead to optimal outcomes for the patient.

REFERENCES

1. Bolton R. People skills. New York: Simon & Schuster, 1979.
2. McWhinney I. The need for a transformed clinical method. In: Steward M, Roter D, eds. Communicating with medical patients. Thousand Oaks, CA: Sage Publications, 1989:25–40.
3. Henbest R, Stewart M. Patient-centeredness in the consultation, 2: does it really make a difference? In: Family practice. New York: Oxford Press, 1980.
4. Roter D, Hall J. Doctors talking with patients, patients talking with doctors. New York: Auburn House, 1992.
5. Rogers C. On becoming a person. Boston: Houghton Mifflin, 1961.
6. Lickhart W. Rogers' necessary and sufficient conditions revisited. Br J Guid Counsel 12:113–123, 1984.
7. Barrett-Lennard GT. The empathy cycle: refinement of a nuclear concept. J Counsel Psychol 28(2):91–100, 1981.
8. Rubin FL, Judd MM, Connie TA. Empathy: can it be learned and retained? Phys Ther 57:644–647, 1977.
9. Kalisch B. What is empathy? Am J Nurs 73:1541–1552, 1973.
10. Meldrum H. Interpersonal communication in pharmaceutical care. New York: Pharmaceutical Products Press, 1994.
11. Gardner ME, Burpeau-DiGregorio MY. Objective assessment of pharmacy students' interviewing skills. Am J Pharm Educ 49:137–144, 1985.
12. Gardner ME, McGhan WF. Objective assessment of interviewing skills: a comparison of two history types. Am J Pharm Educ 50:165–169, 1986.
13. Ranelli PL. The utility of nonverbal communication in the profession of pharmacy. Soc Sci Med 13A:733–736, 1979.
14. Billings JA, Stoeckle JD. The clinical encounter. Chicago: Year Book Medical Publishers, 1989.
15. Boyce RW, Herrier RN. Obtaining and using patient data. Am Pharm NS31:65–71, 1991.

16. Meade V. OBRA '90: how has pharmacy reacted? Am Pharm NS35:12–16, 1995.

17. Pugh CB. PreOBRA '90 Medicaid survey: how community pharmacy practice is changing. Am Pharm NS35:17–23, 1995.

18. Boyce RW, Herrier RN, Gardner ME. Pharmacist-Patient consultation program, unit 1: an interactive approach to verify patient understanding. New York: Pfizer Inc., 1991.

19. Gardner ME, Hurd PD, Slack MK. Effect of information organization on recall of medication instructions. J Clin Pharm Ther 14:1–7, 1989.

20. Morris LA, Grossman R, Barkdoll GL, Gordon E, Soviero C. A survey of patient sources of prescription drug information. AJPH 74 (10):1161–1162, 1984.

21. Lamb GC. Can physicians warn patients of potential side effects without fear of causing those side effects? Arch Intern Med 154:2753–2756, 1994.

22. Howland JS, Baker MG, Poe T. Does patient education cause side effects? J Fam Pract 31(1):62–64, 1990.

23. Gardner ME, Rulien N, McGhan WF, Mead RA. A study of perceived importance of medication information provided in a health maintenance organization setting. Drug Intell Clin Pharm 22:596–598, 1988.

24. Meldrum H, Hardy M. Challenges in communicating about risk. Proceedings of the Conference, United States Pharmacopeial Convention, Rockville, Maryland, 1995:36–49.

25. Pharmacist-Patient Consultation Program: Counseling Patients in Challenging Situations. New York: Pfizer Inc., 1993.

26. Hatoum HT, Akhras K. 1993 Bibliography: a 32-year literature review on the value and acceptance of ambulatory care provided by pharmacists. Ann Pharmacother 27:1106–19, 1993.

27. Church RM. Pharmacy practice in the Indian Health Service. Am J Hosp Pharm 44:771–5, 1987.

28. Herrier RN, Boyce RW, Apgar DA. Pharmacist-managed patient care services and prescriptive authority in the U.S. Public Health Service. Hosp Form 25:67–80, 1990.

29. Beckman HS, et al. The doctor patient relationship and malpractice: lessons from patient dispositions. Arch Intern Med 154:1365–70, 1994.

30. Anderson LA, Zimmerman MA. Patient and physician perceptions of their relationship and patient satisfaction: a study in chronic disease management. Patient Educ Counsel 20:27–36, 1993.

31. DiMatteo MR. The physician-patient relationship: effects on quality of health care. Clin Obstet Gynecol 37:149–61, 1994.

32. Viinamaki H. The patient-doctor relationship and metabolic control in patients with type 1 (insulin dependent) diabetes mellitus. Int J Psychiatry Med 23:265–74, 1993.

33. Anderson RM. Is the problem of noncompliance all in our heads? Diabetes Educ 11:31–34, 1985.

34. Herrier RN, Boyce RW. Compliance with prescribed drug regimens. In: Bressler R, Katz M, eds. Geriatric pharmacology. New York: McGraw-Hill, 1993, 63–77.

35. Pharmacist-Patient Consultation Program, Unit 3: Counseling to Enhance Compliance. New York: Pfizer Inc., 1995.

36. Eraker SA, Kirscht JP, Becker MH. Understanding and improving patient compliance. Ann Intern Med 100:258–68, 1984.

37. Becker MH. Patient adherence to prescribed therapies. Med Care 23:539–55, 1985.

38. Leventhal H. The role of theory in the study of adherence to treatment and doctor patient interactions. Med Care 23:556–63, 1985.

39. Meade V. Adapting to providing pharmaceutical care. Am Pharm NS34:37–42, 1994.

40. Meade V. Pharmacist in Richmond launches pharmaceutical care program. Am Pharm NS34:43–45, 1994.

41. Meade V. Helping pharmacists provide disease-based pharmaceutical care. Am Pharm NS35:45–48, 1995.

CHAPTER 9

FLUID AND ELECTROLYTE THERAPY AND ACID-BASE BALANCE

GAIL W. McSWEENEY

The body maintains its internal environment by balancing fluids, electrolytes, acids, and bases. Body weight is approximately 60% water; within this are dissolved or suspended the necessary elements and formed substances that are required to metabolize nutrients and drugs, generate energy, maintain and manufacture body components, and eliminate waste. These processes can be efficiently done only within very narrow limits of size, composition, and pH of the internal fluid. Disorders of body water, salts, and pH are not diseases; they are alterations in homeostasis during which the body cannot continue to function normally or protect and repair itself (1).

PHYSIOLOGY OF BODY WATER BALANCE

Body water is divided into three compartments: intracellular, interstitial, and vascular. The interstitial and vascular compartments taken together are referred to as the extracellular fluid (ECF). In the nonobese, well-conditioned 70-kg man, water inside the cells (intracellular fluid, ICF) comprises 40–45% (30 L) of body weight. Interstitial water, that between cells, accounts for 11–15% (10 L); vascular water, that inside the walls of the blood vessels, accounts for approximately 5% (3.5 L) (2). The actual amount of body water that is present varies according to age, sex, and body muscle/fat content; these factors must be taken into consideration in estimating body water in an individual person. At birth, the newborn is approximately 75% water; the slight weight loss that is seen shortly after birth is actually water loss as the infant adjusts to an air environment. By the end of the first year of life, the total body water (TBW) is about 60%. Men usually have a higher water content than do women of the same age, height, and weight because of men's greater amount of muscle mass. This difference is estimated to be about 5%. Obese people are less than 60% water, since fat has negligible intracellular water, the absolute decrease being a function of the degree of obesity. For practical purposes, estimations of TBW in obese patients are made by using ideal rather than actual body weight. Many elderly individuals are also less than 60% water, since because of decreases in endogenous anabolic sex hormones

and exercise, they are less muscular than younger people of the same body size (3).

Body water is constantly being circulated in the vascular system, the connections between the three compartments occurring at the level of the capillaries. Under usual conditions the volume of each compartment remains constant, but there is a continuous interchange of individual molecules across the water-permeable cell membranes. This is regulated by hydrostatic and protein (oncotic) pressures. Cardiac output and arterial tone determine the intravascular or "blood" pressure. At the level of the arterial capillary this hydrostatic pressure is approximately 17 mm Hg and pushes solute-free water out into the interstitial or "third" space. Proteins, primarily albumin, and negative hydrostatic pressure present in the third space simultaneously pull water from the vascular system. On the venule side of the capillary bed, intravascular oncotic pressure pulls 95% of the extruded water back into the vascular compartment. The remaining 5% is returned by the action of the lymphatic collecting system (see Figure 9.1).

The volume of the three compartments will remain normal only as long as these hydrostatic and oncotic forces

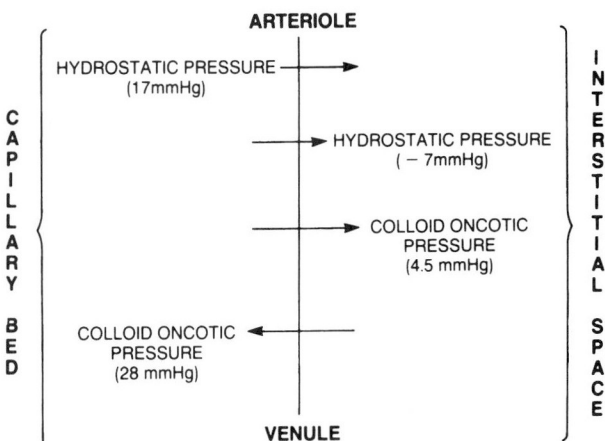

Figure 9.1. Forces regulating water movement in the extracellular fluid.

remain normal relative to each other. In assessing the appropriateness of body water content, it is crucial to evaluate not only the total volume but also its distribution among the three body spaces. Dehydration refers to the state in which the fluid volume, but not usually the amount of solute, is low in all three compartments. Hypovolemia is the state in which the intravascular volume is low; the word does not define in any way the volumes of the interstitial and intracellular spaces. "Total body water overload" means only that TBW is greater than 60% and also does not describe specifically the volume of any individual compartment. The term is often used imprecisely and incorrectly. When the phrase "TBW overload" is used, the real distribution of water must be determined before the appropriate action to be taken can be determined. Fluid will accumulate in the interstitial space if blood (hydrostatic) pressure is normal but oncotic pressure is low, as is the case with low levels of albumin; this condition is referred to as edema. The volume of the third space gradually expands at the expense of the vascular space. In the most severe cases, death results from too low a circulating blood volume (hypovolemia) in the presence of interstitial space overload (edema) and a TBW of greater than 60%. In this example the action to maintain life is to give more fluid to support the circulating vascular volume even if the edema worsens and the total body water continues to rise.

PHYSIOLOGY OF BODY SOLUTE BALANCE (2, 4)

Osmotic pressure keeps the volume of the three body fluid compartments constant; only solute-free water moves freely across cell membranes. It is the concentration of dissolved ions (electrolytes) in each compartment that creates the osmotic pressure that holds water in each space. These ions and their distribution are listed in Table 9.1. The normal serum osmolality (osmotic concentration) is 280 to 300 mmol/kg (280 to 300 mOsm/L). Sodium and chloride are the main ions in the ECF, and potassium and phosphate are the main ions in the ICF. Other ions are present, but their concentrations are too low to contribute significantly to the osmotic gradient. Other osmotically active substances that are present are glucose, urea, phospholipids, cholesterol, and neutral fats. Osmolality is determined by all the particles mentioned, but the nonelectrolytes contribute little; the effective osmolality is very close to twice the serum sodium in the ECF and twice the potassium in the ICF (see Table 9.1) (2, 4).

The equation that is used to determine osmolality is

$$\text{Osmolality (mmol/kg)} = 2 \times \text{Na (mmol/L)} + \text{glucose (mmol/L)}/18 + \text{urea (mmol/L)}/3$$

A molecule of glucose has one-eighteenth and urea has one-third the osmotic activity of an atom of an electrolyte. Body processes function best within a serum osmolality of 280 to 300 mmol/kg, so the kidneys will attempt to maintain

Table 9.1.
Approximate Composition of Body Fluid (mmol/L)

	Plasma (total = 300)	Interstitium (total = 304)	Cell (total = 300)
Na	141	144	16
K	4	4	150
Ca	2.5	2.5	—
Mg	2	2	34
Cl	100	114	—
HCO₃	25	30	10
PO₄	1	1.5	50
Protein or acid	25	6	40

this value and increase the excretion of glucose and urea when concentrations rise; if this is not possible or sufficient, they will also increase the excretion of sodium. In the physiologic sense, the need (biologic priority) to maintain a normal osmolality is greater than the need to maintain a normal body sodium (2, 4).

When the concentration of ions in any compartment changes, water will migrate across cell membranes to reestablish osmotic equilibrium. If the serum sodium rises, the osmolality of the vascular space will be momentarily higher than that of the interstitial and intracellular spaces. Water will move from these two areas to dilute the vascular space until the correct relative osmolalities of all three compartments are reestablished. The result is a decrease in the size of the interstitial and intracellular spaces and an increase in the volume of the vascular space. If the serum sodium falls, the opposite will happen, and the sizes of the interstitial and intracellular compartments will increase (2, 4).

MAINTENANCE FLUID AND ELECTROLYTE REQUIREMENTS

Salt and water balance in the body is maintained by the equilibrium between oral intake of fluid and electrolytes, by evaporation of solute-free water across the skin and lungs, and by controlled renal excretion of water and electrolytes. The amount of water that evaporates (insensible loss) is a function of body surface area and respiratory rate. In a 70-kg man the amount is approximately 1 L/day and remains constant. The kidneys increase or decrease their output by the action of antidiuretic hormone (ADH) and aldosterone; this compensates for daily variations in oral fluid and electrolyte intake. ADH regulates the amount of water that is reabsorbed in the distal tubule of the kidney by assessing the osmolality of the ECF. If the osmolality of the ECF is higher than normal, ADH will be released and water will be reabsorbed in the renal tubules; if the osmolality is low, the converse will be true. Another name for ADH is vasopressin. It will increase vascular tone and cause constriction of blood vessels, especially those leading to the kidneys. Aldosterone acts to increase sodium reabsorption;

release of this hormone is stimulated by a low circulating blood volume and a low total body sodium. These two hormones, along with stimulation of thirst centers in the brain, enable total body water and sodium to be maintained within 1% of normal over wide variations in daily intake. In the case of an extremely low circulating plasma volume, ADH and aldosterone acting together can cause the kidneys to reabsorb essentially all salt and water. This is the mechanism for acute tubular necrosis and renal failure, seen in hypovolemic shock. Renal failure from this cause can be reversed if the vascular volume is restored before permanent injury to the kidneys occurs. The amount of water and electrolytes that is needed to replace insensible loss, maintain adequate perfusion of the body cell mass, and result in a urine output sufficient to excrete metabolic waste varies nonlinearly according to body size. This is because the change in body surface area to body mass as an individual's size increases is not linear. The first 10 kg of body weight require 100 mL/kg, the next 10 kg of body weight require 100 mL/kg, the next 10 mL/kg require 50 mL/kg, and each kilogram beyond 20 requires 20 mL/kg. A 50-kg adult has a water requirement of 2100 mL/day; this is derived from 1000 mL for the first 10 kg of weight, 500 mL for the next 10 kg, and 600 mL for the remaining 30 kg. Calculation of requirements for children follows the same rule; a 15-kg child has a water requirement of 1250 mL/day. Remember to use "ideal" weight for obese individuals. Insensible loss of free water increases in febrile patients; a patient requires an extra 10% of the calculated need for water for each 1°C elevation in body temperature.

The amounts of electrolytes needed to maintain normal total body concentrations vary because the kidneys constantly adjust excretion. This adjustment is centered on increasing or decreasing sodium excretion to maintain a normal circulating vascular volume and composition (4). When necessary, the kidney can reduce sodium loss to zero by increasing potassium and hydrogen excretion (see Figure 9.2). For practical purposes the amounts of electrolytes that need to be ingested to maintain homeostasis without stimulating inordinate amounts of ADH and aldosterone are linearly related to the water requirement. The values that are used to determine daily maintenance fluid and electrolyte needs are listed in Table 9.2. Oral or intravenous replacement of maintenance needs should always include sodium and potassium. Deficiencies of the other electrolytes develop more slowly, and they are not always given during short-term therapy. For a 50-kg woman with normal TBW and electrolytes, an appropriate maintenance intravenous solution is D5 ¼ NS with KCl 20 mmol/L infused at 85 mL/hr. This provides 2040 mL of fluid, 79 mmol of sodium, and 41 mmol of potassium; these amounts are almost exactly those calculated by using Table 9.2. This

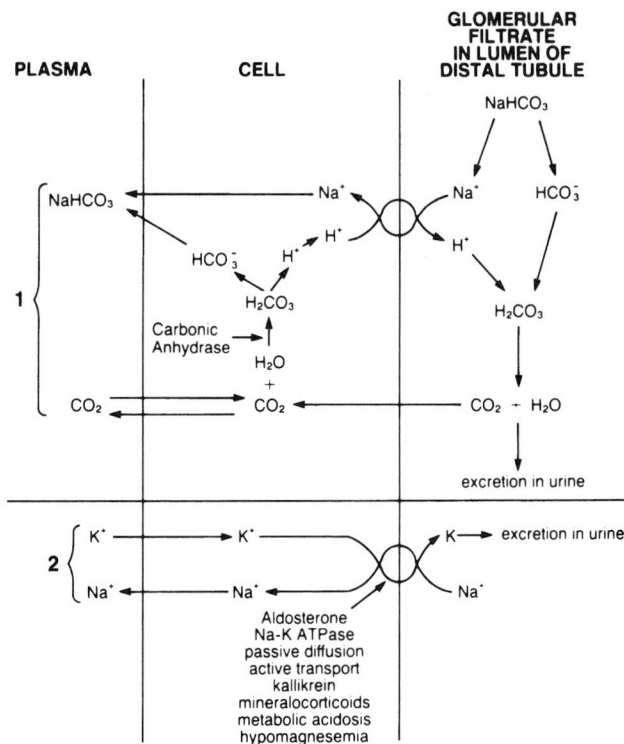

Figure 9.2. Mechanisms of Na-K exchange in the distal renal tubule.

Table 9.2.
Maintenance Requirements per 24 Hours[a]

	Water	
	0–10 kg	100 mL/kg
	10–20 kg	50 mL/kg
	>20 kg	20 mL/kg
	Electrolytes	
Na	3 mmol (3 mEq)/100 mL H_2O	
K	2 mmol (2 mEq)/100 mL H_2O	
Cl	2 mmol (2 mEq)/100 mL H_2O	
Ca	0.05–0.1 mmol (0.1–0.2 mEq)/kg	
Mg	0.05 mmol (0.1 mEq)/kg	
PO_4	0.1 mmol (2.8 mg)/kg	

[a]Use ideal body weight in obese patients.

patient will also receive Cl 120 mmol; cations must be given with an equal number of anions to maintain electrical neutrality, but hyperchloremia rarely occurs in patients with adequate renal function. Acetate salts of sodium and potassium are available and can be used if chloride anions must be avoided. Acetate is converted to bicarbonate in the body. Bicarbonate salts are not routinely added to intravenous solutions because they raise pH and may cause precipitation of electrolytes or drugs.

DISORDERS OF BODY WATER AND SOLUTE
Sodium

Serum sodium is the major determinant of the intravascular volume, since it is the osmotically active substance in greatest concentration in the compartment. Abnormalities in salt and water intake or excretion alter sodium concentration. This will affect the volume of the interstitial space because its major osmotic substance is also sodium and the two compartments are in equilibrium with each other.

The usual concentration of sodium in the serum is 135 to 147 mmol/L (135 to 147 mEq/L). Levels above and below this are referred to as hypernatremia and hyponatremia, respectively. The terms refer only to concentration and do not describe or define whether the abnormality is the result of increases or decreases in the total amounts of sodium, water, or both in the body. Hypernatremia is almost always the result of a free water deficit. An elevated total body sodium can result from an excessive intake of salt but is almost impossible to achieve if renal function is adequate. Clinically important symptoms of hypernatremia do not generally appear until the serum level is greater than 160 mmol/L and are the result of central nervous system (CNS) dehydration (see Table 9.3). Any treatment to correct an altered serum or total body sodium value should not

be so rapid and aggressive as to create new CNS problems. Equilibration across the blood-brain barrier is slower than that across other semipermeable membranes in the body, and rapid changes can cause seizures. The treatment for hypernatremia depends on whether the cause is too little water or too much sodium. Hypernatremia from water loss indicates a decrease in total body water, not just in intravascular volume. As the concentration of osmotically active substances across the three compartments is always in equilibrium, the interstitial sodium concentration and the intracellular potassium concentration will be as elevated as the intravascular sodium. Calculation of the amount of free water that is needed to correct all three electrolyte values and return the volumes of all three compartments to normal involves the use of the following equation:

Water deficit (L)
$$= [1 - 140/\text{measured serum Na (mmol/L)}] \\ \times \text{body weight (kg)} \times 0.6$$

Replacement of the deficit is done with electrolyte-free oral or intravenous solutions, such as D5W, given over 18 to 24 hr in addition to calculated maintenance fluid and electrolyte needs.

If hypernatremia is the result of an actual increase in the amount of sodium in the body, treatment is directed at removal of sodium from the body and involves the use of diuretics and D5W to increase renal elimination while maintaining a normal total body water (5–7).

Hyponatremia describes a serum sodium concentration less than 135 mmol/L, but clinically important symptoms do not usually appear until the level is below 120 mmol/L and are the result of CNS water intoxication (see Table 9.3). As with hypernatremia, the cause must be determined before treatment is begun. Hyponatremia can result from dilution or depletion or can be factitious. Dilutional hyponatremia is a condition in which the total body sodium is increased but TBW is increased to a greater degree; the result is a low serum sodium concentration. It occurs in conditions such as cirrhosis and congestive heart failure when effective cardiac output reaching the kidneys is diminished. This, along with the low sodium concentration, is a stimulus for ADH (8) and aldosterone secretion. The result is further salt and water retention, and the affected individuals are usually edematous because of the attendant increase in the size of the interstitial fluid compartment. Diuretics are not a primary treatment and may be contraindicated because they will exacerbate the hyponatremia by causing sodium excretion that exceeds water elimination. Salt and water restriction, bed rest (to increase venous return to the heart), and correction of the primary disorder are the initial treatments. However, these measures must not be so aggressive as to compromise intravascular volume or further decrease renal blood flow (9, 10).

Table 9.3.
Sodium

Serum level > 147 mmol/L (147 mEq/L)	Serum level < 135 mmol/L (135 mEq/L)
Cause	
Decreased water intake	Low-sodium diet with diuretics
Fever	Diuretics
Excessive salt intake	Congestive heart failure
Diabetes insipidus	Cirrhosis
Hyperventilation	Replacement of body secretion loss with electrolyte-free solutions
	Adrenal insufficiency
	Osmotic diuresis
Signs and Symptoms	
Thirst	Apathy/agitation
Dry mucous membranes	Fatigue
Decreased skin turgor	Anorexia/nausea
Acute weight loss	Headache
Confusion	Muscle cramps
Hallucinations	Tachycardia
Intracranial hemorrhage	Oliguria/anuria
Coma	Confusion
	Seizures
	Coma
	Shock
Treatment of Hypernatremia	
Water deficit (L) = [1 − (140/measured Na)] × Wt (kg) × 0.6	
Treatment of Hyponatremia	
Dilution: Sodium and water restriction	
Depletion: Na deficit (mmol) = (140 − measured Na) × Wt (kg) × 0.6	

Hyponatremia from depletion is a true decrease in the total body sodium, with or without a water deficit. It most commonly results from gastrointestinal losses from vomiting, excessive diuretic therapy, adrenal insufficiency, and replacement of losses from perspiration with electrolyte-free fluid. Patients will show signs of dehydration (dry mucous membranes, skin tenting, lethargy) and, in extreme cases, hypovolemia (11–13). Calculation of the amount of sodium needed to replace the total body deficit is made by use of the following equation:

Sodium deficit (mmol)
$$= [140 - \text{measured serum Na (mmol/L)}] \times \text{body weight (kg)} \times 0.6$$

Appropriate solutions to replace the sodium deficit are 0.9% saline (155 mmol of Na and Cl/L) or 3% saline (500 mmol of Na and Cl/L) given in addition to daily maintenance fluids and electrolytes. Because hyponatremia does not usually occur acutely, replacement of the deficit may be made over a period of several days if necessary to avoid intravascular volume overload, pulmonary edema, or congestive heart failure.

Factitious hyponatremia is the result of accumulation of osmotically active substances, such as glucose and lipids, in the intravascular space. Sodium is diluted as water moves from the interstitial to the vascular space to normalize the osmotic pressure. The degree of hyponatremia that is seen is usually mild. Serum sodium will fall only 1.6 mmol/L for every 5.3 mmol/L (100 mg/dL) increase in blood glucose, and treatment consists of correcting the underlying disorder.

Alterations in Fluid Compartment Integrity

Trauma, tissue ischemia, endotoxemia, hypoalbuminemia, and decreased cardiac output result in hypovolemia by damaging capillary membranes or by disrupting the hydrostatic and oncotic forces governing fluid movement across them. The symptoms of hypovolemia are tachycardia, low central venous pressure (CVP), low pulmonary wedge pressure, and decreased urine output. Blood pressure is not a good measure of this condition, since increases in sympathetic tone can maintain the blood pressure near normal in the presence of a decreased circulating volume.

In cases of trauma, ischemia, and endotoxemia, capillary pore size increases (capillary leak syndrome), and water, solute, and plasma proteins, primarily albumin, flow into the interstitial (third) space. This leak can be localized to an area of injury or ischemia (surgery, trauma) or generalized throughout the body (endotoxemic shock from Gram-negative sepsis). The amount of fluid that is lost from the intravascular space varies with the degree of injury but can result in hypovolemia that is severe enough to cause cardiovascular collapse and death if the circulating volume is not maintained. Treatment consists of correcting the underlying disorder to normalize capillary permeability and replacing the lost intravascular fluid with a solution of the same composition. Blood has no role in this therapy, since the formed elements of the intravascular fluid are not being lost to the third space. The two categories of replacement solutions are crystalloid and colloid. Crystalloid is a general term for any solution that contains electrolytes. Normal (0.9%) saline and lactated Ringer's solution are most commonly used for treatment of hypovolemia, since they are isotonic with the ECF and are most effective in maintaining the circulating volume. Colloid is a general term for a solution that contains plasma proteins or other colloidal molecules; three types are available. Plasma protein fraction (PPF) is approximately 85% albumin and 15% globulin; it is available as a 5% solution. Albumin is available as a 5% or 25% solution, and hetastarch is available as a 6% solution. Hetastarch is a mixture of ethoxylated amylopectin molecules having an average molecular weight of 450,000; they exert the same hemodynamic effect as albumin. It is not extracted from pooled human plasma and is much less expensive than PPF or albumin. All three products also contain 130 to 160 mmol of sodium and chloride per liter. The use of colloid infusions remains controversial. While some albumin does move into the third space when capillary pore size increases, it is proportionately much less than the amount of salt and water that leaks out; serum protein levels do not fall quickly or appreciably. Colloid will temporarily decrease the rate at which fluid migrates into the third space but may exacerbate hypovolemia 24 to 36 hr later as it moves into the interstitial space itself. Unless the actual serum albumin is below the level needed to maintain the capillary venule oncotic pressure gradient (20 to 25 g/L) or aggressive crystalloid therapy is not restoring intravascular volume, the routine use of colloid solutions is not recommended (14–16).

During the treatment of hypovolemia, the rate of fluid administration into the vascular space must meet or exceed the rate of loss to maintain tissue perfusion and can exceed 1 L/hr in extreme cases. Urine output should be kept at a minimum of 0.5 cc/kg/hr, the level at which a circulating volume sufficient to perfuse body tissues is present. Normalization of heart rate and CVP are also indicators of normal intravascular volume and can be monitored along with urine output. During the resuscitation process, the rate of fluid administration is adjusted hourly to maintain an adequate intravascular volume. It is important to remember that while edema can appear in some patients during this process, it is not the resuscitation process itself that is causing the edema. When healing begins, this extra fluid and solute will be returned to the vascular compartment and excreted. Diuretics have no role in the correction of edema caused by capillary leak syndromes, and their use can further deplete the intravascular volume.

Hypoalbuminemia without a concurrent capillary leak can result in hypovolemia with edema. Capillary venule oncotic pressure is low, and fluid that moved into the interstitial space on the arterial side of the capillary bed is not returned to the vascular system. Treatment for this condition consists of intravenous albumin or hetastarch in sufficient amounts to normalize the arteriovenous capillary oncotic pressure. Edema will resolve only if this can be done.

Hypovolemia due to a decreased cardiac output (congestive heart failure, cardiomyopathy, myocardial infarction) cannot be corrected by giving fluids. In these conditions, hypovolemia exists on the arterial side of the heart due to "pump failure"; the venous side of the circulatory system may be overloaded, and the patient may be edematous. Treatment options are confined to drugs that will improve cardiac output, such as inotropes.

If hypovolemia is the result of blood loss, then whole blood or packed red blood cells with normal saline or lactated Ringer's solution is indicated to reestablish the hematocrit above 0.25 (25%) and with a normal circulating volume.

Losses of Body Water and Solute

In prolonged vomiting, diarrhea, or losses through perforations in organs or the gastrointestinal tract leading to the skin (fistulas), water and solute are lost from the body. The composition of these fluids depends on the area affected and are listed in Table 9.4. When the exact site of origin of the fluid is not known, laboratory analysis of the fluid will help in the selection of an appropriate replacement solution. This analysis is often necessary in the case of entercutaneous (communication between the gastrointestinal tract and the skin) fistulas. They can make a circuitous tract through the body before reaching the skin, so the organ nearest to the exit site to the skin is not necessarily the one from which the fluid is draining. Diarrhea is most often of distal small bowel or colonic origin, but in cases of

secretory diarrhea, such as in giardiasis or acquired immunodeficiency syndrome (AIDS), the fluid may arise from the duodenum or the jejunum. In all cases of abnormal loss, the composition of the fluid should be determined. Appropriate replacement solutions, in addition to maintenance needs, are given at a rate to restore and maintain normal body water and solute.

ACID-BASE BALANCE (17–23)

For physiologic processes to occur at a normal rate, body pH must remain within a narrow range. It varies slightly among body compartments (the ICF has a pH of approximately 6.9, and some subcellular components, such as the mitochondria, have usual levels that are even lower), but normal total body acid-base balance is assumed to be present when the arterial pH is between 7.35 and 7.45.

Cellular metabolism, energy generation, and protein metabolism add large amounts of acid to the body daily. It is predominantly in the form of carbon dioxide (CO_2), but some hydrogen ions and weak organic and inorganic nonvolatile acids are also generated. Almost no alkaline substances result from metabolic processes, so body acid-base homeostatic mechanisms are designed only to buffer or eliminate acids. Hemoglobin, proteins, and phosphate buffer only nonvolatile acids. The amount of acid they can buffer cannot be altered because the amounts of them in the body are fixed; no adjustment can be made if the amount of acid in the body increases. These three systems contribute little to the overall buffering capacity of the body and so will not be discussed in detail here.

The bicarbonate–carbonic acid system buffers CO_2 and can adjust quickly to changes in the daily acid load. It keeps body pH in the normal range by maintaining the correct ratio between the concentrations of bicarbonate (HCO_3) and carbonic acid (H_2CO_3) in the blood. This relationship is described by the Henderson-Hasselbach equation:

$$pH = pKcarbonic\ acid + log\ [HCO_3/H_2CO_3]$$

When the HCO_3/H_2CO_3 (24 mmol/1.2 mmol) concentrations are at a ratio of 20:1, the pH will be 7.4, as the pKcarbonic acid is fixed at 6.1 and the log of 24/1.2 is 1.3. Carbonic acid concentrations are not obtained in the patient setting; the value reported by clinical laboratories is the partial pressure of CO_2 (pCO_2). A 40 mm Hg pCO_2 corresponds to a H_2CO_3 concentration of 1.2 mmol. The pCO_2 is maintained within the normal range because CO_2 generated by cellular metabolism is continuously diffused and eliminated across the lungs. The capacity of the lungs to excrete CO_2 is so great that it is saturated only in cases of severe pulmonary disease.

The kidneys are responsible for maintaining the serum HCO_3 within the normal range by reabsorbing bicarbonate ions from the glomerular filtrate and by generating new

Table 9.4.
Approximate Concentrations of Body Secretions[a] (mmol/L *and* mEq/L)

	Na	K	Cl	HCO₃
Saliva	10	25	10	15
Stomach	60	10	85	—
Bile	150	5	100	40
Pancreas	140	5	80	120
Small bowel	110	5	105	30
Terminal ileum	117	5	105	—
Sweat	45	5	60	—
Cerebrospinal fluid	140	3	130	—

[a]For specific values and/or ranges, refer to clinical laboratory standards for your institution.

HCO_3 ions in renal tubular cells. This generation is accomplished by the action of the enzyme carbonic anhydrase on carbon dioxide and water to form carbonic acid. Carbonic acid quickly dissociates into H and HCO_3; the H ion is secreted into the urine, and the HCO_3 is transported from the renal tubular cells into the vascular system. The capacity of this reaction to generate new HCO_3 cannot be saturated if renal function is normal. See Figure 9.2.

Acid-base disturbances begin as CO_2 or HCO_3 serum concentration changes. If the problem originates with CO_2, the resultant change in pH is referred to as being of respiratory origin; if it begins with HCO_3, the change is said to be of metabolic origin. A plasma pH below 7.35 is called acidosis and can be of respiratory or metabolic origin; a plasma pH above 7.45 is called alkalosis and can also be of respiratory or metabolic origin. When plasma pH goes outside the normal range, the lungs and the kidneys begin processes designed to compensate and normalize the pH value. When the respiratory center in the medulla oblongata perceives a change in pH, it causes the lungs to adjust the pCO_2 by increasing or decreasing the respiratory rate. While it occurs quickly, this process can correct the pH only when the change in HCO_3 concentration is minor; it is limited by how quickly or slowly an individual can breathe in and out and by the capacity of the intracellular hemoglobin and phosphate-buffering systems. The kidneys, by increasing or decreasing the plasma HCO_3, may take several days to fully compensate and normalize a pH that has been altered by a change in CO_2 concentration, but they have a much greater total buffering capacity (17).

It cannot be overemphasized that it is the ratio between CO_2 and HCO_3, not the absolute numbers, that determines pH. The body has a greater physiologic need (biologic priority) to have a plasma pH between 7.35 and 7.45 than it does to have "normal" levels of pCO_2 and HCO_3 (18, 19). A high plasma HCO_3 is not synonymous with metabolic alkalosis; it will also be seen in compensated respiratory acidosis. The alteration in one value is the appropriate physiologic response to a change in the other as long as the result is a normal pH. It is appropriate at these points to give bicarbonate to normalize the pH of the body without regard to the cause of the disturbance, since death may be imminent.

PRIMARY ACID-BASE DISTURBANCES
Metabolic Acidosis

Metabolic acidosis is the condition in which the plasma pH is below 7.35 as a result of a low bicarbonate concentration in the blood. As the bicarbonate concentration falls, the lungs attempt to lower the pCO_2 and maintain a normal pH by increasing the depth and rate of respiration (Kussmaul breathing). The symptoms of metabolic acidosis are cardio-

Table 9.5.
Metabolic Acidosis
(pH < 7.35, HCO_3 < 22 mmol (22 mEq)/L)

Cause	Signs and Symptoms
Ketoacidosis	Kussmaul breathing
Renal failure	Hyperkalemia
Hypoxia/anoxia	Ventricular arrhythmias
Diarrhea	Lethargy
Salicylates	Stupor
Methanol	Coma
Chloride loading	

Treatment (pH at or below 7.1)
HCO_3 deficit (mmol and mEq) = (22 − measured HCO_3) × Wt (kg) × 0.5

pulmonary or CNS symptoms but are not usually clinically important at a pH above 7.1 (see Table 9.5). A low serum bicarbonate results from increased HCO_3 losses from the body, decreased renal regeneration of HCO_3, or increased amounts of acid added to the body by ingestion or metabolic processes.

The number of positively charged ions in the body must always exactly equal the number of negatively charged ions. In the plasma this electrical neutrality is achieved with dissolved electrolytes and proteins in the following relationship:

$$Na^+ = Cl^- + HCO_3^- + \text{unmeasured anions}$$

Unmeasured anions consist of plasma proteins and small amounts of other negatively charged substances, such as SO_4 and PO_4, that are not "measured" by the tests usually done by clinical laboratories. The usual amounts of these anions in the blood have a combined ionic strength of 8 to 16 mmol/L (8 to 16 mEq/L); this value, referred to as the "anion gap," rarely changes. Assuming that Na remains constant, a change in the number of any one of the anions will necessitate a change in one or both of the others to maintain electrical neutrality. As the number of unmeasured anions is fixed, only the Cl or HCO_3 can change. With the addition of acid (Cl), the fall in the HCO_3 is actually an appropriate compensatory response to maintain the electrical neutrality of the blood (a condition with an even higher biologic priority than maintenance of a normal pH). Metabolic acidosis occurs when and because the HCO_3 goes down and the HCO_3/CO_2 ratio becomes abnormal.

Metabolic acidosis is divided into non-anion-gap and positive-anion-gap varieties. In non-anion-gap acidosis the number of unmeasured anions is the same as usual, so the decreased serum bicarbonate level is secondary to chloride loading, an actual loss of bicarbonate, or decreased bicarbonate generation. In positive-anion-gap acidosis the number of unmeasured anions has increased, and the

HCO_3 has dropped to maintain electrical neutrality. The cause of positive-anion-gap-acidosis is the contribution of nonvolatile acids to the blood. This can be from abnormal metabolic processes, such as diabetic ketoacidosis and hypoxia, or from poisonings by substances that dissociate at physiologic plasma pH. Salicylate and methanol overdoses commonly cause this particular kind of metabolic acidosis. It is important to make the distinction between these two types of metabolic acidosis before determining or beginning any treatment regimen.

TREATMENT OF NON-ANION-GAP METABOLIC ACIDOSIS

Loss of bicarbonate (prolonged diarrhea, upper gastrointestinal fistulas), inability to generate bicarbonate (renal failure), and chloride loading (normal saline infusions, NaCl overdoses) are the three causes of this type of metabolic acidosis. Treatment consists of correcting the underlying cause and replacing the bicarbonate deficit. Except in cases of renal failure or profound and continuing gastrointestinal (GI) losses, the kidneys will generate sufficient bicarbonate and normalize the pH when the cause of the acidosis has been corrected. Acute replacement of HCO_3 is done only when the plasma pH is 7.1 or the patient is exhibiting life-threatening symptoms of acidosis. The amount of the bicarbonate deficit can be determined by use of the following equation:

$$HCO_3 \text{ deficit (mmol)} = [24 - \text{measured } HCO_3 \text{ (mmol/L)} \times \text{body weight (kg)} \times 0.5$$

The volume of distribution of HCO_3 is estimated to be 10% less than the total body water, so the factor used is 0.5 rather than 0.6. One-half of the calculated dose is given. (This amount will usually change the pH by 0.2.) The goal of emergency bicarbonate replacement therapy is to correct existing cardiac or CNS disturbances and achieve a plasma pH of 7.2. Since the onset of acidosis has usually been gradual, the CNS has slowly equilibrated to a low pH. Rapidly changing the plasma pH relative to the CNS pH can cause seizures and death because the normalization of CNS pH lags behind. As the plasma pH normalizes over hours or days by renal bicarbonate generation, the CNS pH will equilibrate at a rate that is tolerable to the patient, and complications will be avoided. The additional risks of inducing alkalosis or hypernatremia from the administration of $NaHCO_3$ also often outweigh any benefit of quickly normalizing the pH.

Non-anion-gap acidosis in renal failure is the result of the reduced ability of damaged kidneys to generate bicarbonate. It is usually chronic and mild, and most patients are asymptomatic. Renal failure that is severe enough to cause acidosis almost always necessitates hemodialysis due to low or no urine output. Modifications in the composition of the dialysate are routinely made to improve serum HCO_3 concentrations and pH. Sodium bicarbonate is not routinely given (except as emergency therapy) because these patients are also chronically sodium- and water-overloaded. If the pH is at or below 7.1, bicarbonate will need to be given.

In cases of diarrheal or fistula outputs that have exceeded the ability of the kidneys to generate HCO_3, it will be necessary to give bicarbonate. This is usually done with sodium or potassium acetate rather than bicarbonate salts for reasons stated previously, but sodium bicarbonate can be used. The composition of the fluid being lost should be determined by laboratory analysis. The amount of base should be enough to correct the initial deficit and then should be continued in a quantity to match daily loss.

POSITIVE-ANION-GAP METABOLIC ACIDOSIS

Positive-anion-gap acidosis is the result of a rise in the number of unmeasured anions (nonvolatile acids) in the plasma with a resultant drop in HCO_3 concentration. These acids can be the by-products of metabolic processes seen in diabetes and prolonged starvation (ketosis), anaerobic carbohydrate metabolism, or accumulation of ingested acids (salicylate and methanol poisoning) or of acids that are normally produced in the body that cannot be eliminated, as is the case in renal failure.

During intracellular hypoglycemia, fat becomes the primary substrate for energy generation in the body. This quickly results in the production of ketone bodies. In diabetes the cause of the low intracellular glucose is a lack of insulin, since glucose transport from the blood to cells has been prevented. In starvation an absence of glucose from the body has occurred, which forces a change to fat metabolism. Ketone bodies dissociate and contribute hydrogen ions and the anion β-hydroxybutyrate. In cases of tissue hypoxia, insufficient oxygen to support the action of the Krebs' cycle results in the activation of an alternative pathway for energy generation: the Cori cycle. Its metabolic by-product is lactic acid; H ions and lactate accumulate after dissociation and acidosis results.

The treatment for anion-gap acidosis is always correction of the underlying problem. Intravenous insulin is given in the case of diabetes. In lactic acidosis, restoration of an appropriate circulating volume or plasma oxygen–carrying capacity is indicated. In poisoning, hemodialysis or gastric lavage may be necessary to remove toxic substances from the body. To reiterate, HCO_3 is given only if the pH is at or below 7.1 or if there are clinically important symptoms of acidosis.

Metabolic Alkalosis

Metabolic alkalosis is defined as a plasma pH above 7.45 due to a high bicarbonate concentration in the blood. The anion gap is never affected by this condition. As the HCO_3 rises, the lungs compensate by lowering the depth and rate

Table 9.6.
Metabolic Alkalosis
(pH > 7.45, HCO_3 > 28 mmol (28 mEq)/L)

Cause	Signs and Symptoms
Liver failure	Cheyne-Stokes breathing
Diuretics	Hypokalemia
Nasogastric suction	Muscle cramping
Hyponatremia	Seizures
Hyperaldosteronism	
Corticosteroids	

Treatment (pH at or above 7.6)
   HCl deficit (mmol and mEq) = (103 − measured Cl) × Wt (kg) × 0.2

Table 9.7.
Respiratory Acidosis
(pH < 7.35, pCO_2 > 4 mm Hg)

Cause	Signs and Symptoms
Emphysema	Anxiety
Airway obstruction	Disorientation
Bronchoconstriction	Vasodilation
Pneumonia	Increased cardiac output
Respiratory depression	Coma

Treatment
   Bronchodilators, antibiotics, respiratory support

of respiration (Cheyne-Stokes breathing) in an effort to increase the pCO_2 and thereby normalize the plasma pH. Important symptoms associated with alkalosis do not generally appear at a pH below 7.6 (see Table 9.6).

The most common causes of metabolic alkalosis are loss of chloride ion (nasogastric suction, loop diuretics, mineralocorticoid excess) or ECF depletion. Diuretics and mineralocorticoids stimulate exchange of hydrogen and potassium ions for sodium in the renal tubules; this induces both hypokalemia and alkalosis (see Figure 9.2). Diuretics cause volume depletion and hyponatremia, which further stimulate H and K loss. Volume depletion itself leads to alkalosis as the concentration of HCO_3 molecules occupying a smaller plasma space increases. This condition is referred to as contraction alkalosis. Because the body generates almost no basic substances during metabolism and base ingestion is uncommon, alkalosis from other causes is rare.

TREATMENT OF METABOLIC ALKALOSIS

Metabolic alkalosis that results from sodium and chloride loss along with volume contraction is referred to as "saline-responsive." Replacement of sodium will stop aldosterone-stimulated exchange of H for Na in the renal tubules. Replacement of chloride ions will stop the generation of HCO_3 to maintain electrical neutrality, and volume expansion will reduce HCO_3 concentration in the vascular space. Normal saline is the treatment of choice in this condition, as it is slightly higher in sodium (155 mmol/L) and much higher in chloride (155 mmol/L) than is the ECF. An amount of this solution that will restore the TBW deficit should normalize body sodium and chloride. Some patients with metabolic alkalosis present with TBW overload and may not be able to tolerate a sodium load. The alkalosis can be treated with an infusion of hydrochloric acid or arginine hydrochloride. HCl is preferred, as these patients commonly have severe hepatic dysfunction, and administration of arginine can precipitate hepatic coma. The dose of HCl to replace the hydrogen and chloride deficits can be determined by using the following equation:

$$HCl \ (mmol) = [103 - measured \ Cl \ (mmol/L)]$$
$$\times \ body \ weight \ (kg) \times 0.2$$

The volume of distribution of chloride is 33% of total body water, so the multiplication factor is 0.2. Giving one-half the HCl deficit over 12 to 24 hr should lower the plasma pH by 0.2 and not cause a significant CNS pH gradient. Hydrochloric acid solutions for intravenous use are not commercially available; extemporaneous compounding of a 0.1 to 0.2 N solution (10 to 20 mmol HCl/L) in D5W will be necessary. Infusion into a central venous catheter rather than a peripheral intravenous line is recommended to reduce the risk of phlebitis.

Metabolic alkalosis can be the result of hypokalemia secondary to ICF/ECF exchange of hydrogen for potassium ions and from mineralocorticoid excess. These types of alkalosis are "saline-resistant," and treatment consists of potassium replacement. Alkalosis caused by decreased aldosterone degradation (secondary hyperaldosteronism), which is seen in severe hepatic disease, may respond to the aldosterone antagonist spironolactone. Patients with mineralocorticoid-producing tumors of the adrenal or pituitary glands will require therapy with aminoglutethimide or surgery (22, 23).

Respiratory Acidosis

Respiratory acidosis is a plasma pH lower than 7.35 as the result of a pCO_2 higher than 40 mm Hg. The hemoglobin-buffering system is activated in acute respiratory acidosis and sequesters hydrogen ions inside red blood cells. It is a weak system, however, and can raise the HCO_3 by only 1 mmol/L for every 10 mm Hg rise in pCO_2. To correct the plasma pH, a 5-mmol/L rise in HCO_3 is needed for every 10 mm Hg rise in pCO_2. It is the slow generation of HCO_3 in the kidney that will eventually raise the plasma HCO_3 enough to compensate for the respiratory acidosis and normalize the pH.

Since the CO_2 excretion capacity of normal lungs is always greater than metabolic production, respiratory acidosis occurs only as a result of severe pulmonary disease (see Table 9.7).

Table 9.8.
Respiratory Alkalosis
(pH > 7.45, pCO$_2$ < 4 mm Hg)

Cause	Signs and Symptoms
Hyperventilation	Confusion
Respiratory stimulants	Tetany
Hypoxemia	Syncope
Treatment	
Rebreathing CO$_2$	

TREATMENT OF RESPIRATORY ACIDOSIS

Treatment always consists of correcting the underlying pulmonary disorder and may include antibiotics, bronchodilators, and steroids. Intubation and mechanical ventilation may be required if respiratory depression accompanies the acidosis. Rapid correction of the pH should be avoided, and administration of bicarbonate is indicated only if plasma pH is at or below 7.1. Chronic respiratory acidosis with emphysema and chronic obstructive pulmonary disease develops slowly and is rarely severe enough to require treatment. The stimulus for respiration in these patients may still be an elevated CO$_2$, but many have adapted to hypoxia as the respiratory drive; lowering the pCO$_2$ and raising the pO$_2$ acutely are not recommended, as apnea can result.

Respiratory Alkalosis

Respiratory alkalosis is a pCO$_2$ lower than 40 mm Hg causing a plasma pH higher than 7.45. The defense against this type of alkalosis is the movement of hydrogen ions (H$_2$PO$_4$ goes to HPO$_4$) from the intracellular to the vascular space. The phosphate-buffering system, like hemoglobin, is small in capacity and will not normalize the pH in severe respiratory alkalosis; it can lower the HCO$_3$ by only 3.5 mmol/L for every 10 mm Hg drop in pCO$_2$ (see Table 9.8).

TREATMENT OF RESPIRATORY ALKALOSIS

Voluntary hyperventilation, mechanical ventilation, and rapid breathing due to hypoxemia lower the pCO$_2$; correction of the disorder involves normalizing the pCO$_2$ by raising the CO$_2$ concentration of inspired air. This can be done by increasing the concentration of inspired CO$_2$ delivered by a ventilator or respirator or by having the patient breathe into a bag.

Compensatory Responses to Acid-Base Disturbances

All primary acid-base disturbances will engender a compensatory response; for example, metabolic acidosis will result in a drop in pCO$_2$ (compensating respiratory alkalosis). It can be difficult to determine the primary disturbance if the plasma pH has been returned to normal. It is also possible for two primary acid-base problems to

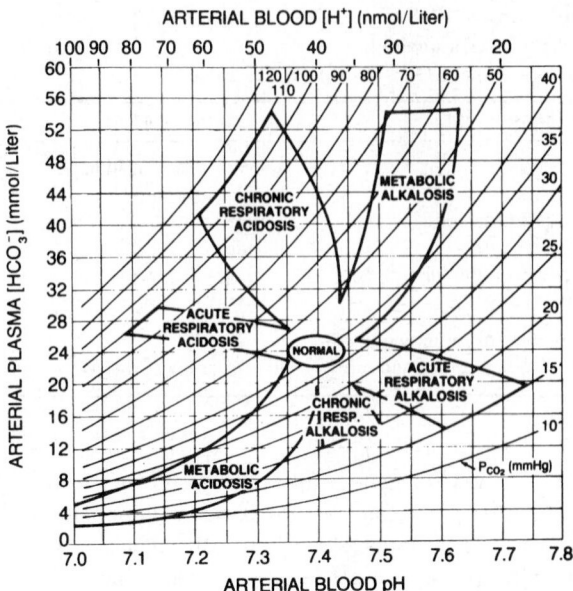

Figure 9.3. Acid-base nomogram. (Source: From Cogan MG, Rector FC. Acid-base disorders. In: Brenner BM, Rector FC, eds The Kidney, 3rd ed. Philadelphia: WB Saunders, 1986:457–518.)

occur together; the only exception is that respiratory acidosis and respiratory alkalosis cannot occur simultaneously. Correct diagnosis of the patient's diseases and a medication history are essential to establish the etiologies of an acid-base disorder and initiate treatment. No simple calculation using the arterial blood gases and serum electrolyte levels will suffice, given the complexity of the body buffering and compensatory mechanisms. Excellent nomograms by Arbus (18) and Cogan and Rector (19) (see Figure 9.3) exist that, within 95% confidence limits, aid the clinician in determining the constituents of an acid-base disturbance. This determination combined with the history guides treatment decisions (20, 21).

ELECTROLYTES

The major electrolytes in the body are sodium, chloride, bicarbonate, potassium, calcium, magnesium, and phosphate. Normal serum levels are listed in Table 9.1. Sodium is connected to total body water; maintenance of normal levels and correction of abnormalities were discussed above. The role of chloride in the body is as an osmotic substance and the major anion in the ECF; it has no inherent physiologic function. Bicarbonate is linked to the acid-base homeostatic system and was also discussed above. The physiologic functions of the remaining electrolytes are to maintain membrane potentials for nerve conduction and muscle contraction (K, Ca, Mg), to generate the energy needed to maintain these potentials, and to do the work of body functions and movement (PO$_4$). The main reservoirs of these ions are the intracellular space and bone. Serum levels fall slowly when intake goes down, as numerous hormonal and homeostatic mechanisms exist to keep serum levels within the normal range. The serum concentrations of these electrolytes are low in relation to sodium and to their own intracellular concentrations, but it is their intravascular concentrations that govern physiologic activities. Serum levels must be kept within a narrow range, or serious difficulties, such as arrhythmias, seizures, and tetany, will result.

Potassium (24–31)

The amount of potassium in the vascular space accounts for only 0.4% of the total amount in the body. With the normal serum concentration ranging from 3.5 to 5.0 mmol/L (3.5 to 5 mEq/L), potassium has major functions in impulse transmission, cardiac contractility, and aldosterone secretion. The major route of excretion of this cation is the kidney. Elimination can be increased when intake is high, but the kidneys have no mechanism to conserve potassium; a deficiency state will develop rapidly if intake drops. Hyponatremia will also cause potassium loss via renal processes discussed above in the subsection "Sodium" (see Figure 9.2). Serum levels of potassium do not totally depend on the relationship between intake/output and sodium homeostasis. The large intracellular pool of potassium is a source of ions for the intravascular compartment; a low serum level usually represents not just a low circulating amount of K but also an acquired intracellular deficit that can approach several hundred millimoles. Changes in acid-base status will alter the location of potassium ions in the body. In acidosis, potassium is exchanged across cell membranes with hydrogen ions in the body's attempt to hide and buffer protons (acid) in the intracellular space; this will help to maintain a normal pH. The converse is true in alkalosis. The serum potassium will rise (acidosis) or fall (alkalosis) by 0.6 mmol/L for every 0.1 change in pH from the value of 7.4 (22, 29).

HYPERKALEMIA

High serum potassium can be a true medical emergency and almost always manifests itself clinically as the sudden appearance of cardiac arrhythmias (25). This most often occurs at serum levels above 6 mmol/L. The symptoms and causes of hyperkalemia are listed in Table 9.9. Actual total body potassium can be high, normal, or (occasionally) low; it is the intravascular concentration that affects physiologic functions and causes the cardiac disorders seen (26). The life-threatening potential of the cardiac abnormality determines the type, complexity, and sequence of treatment given. Any exogenous sources of potassium such as intravenous fluids or drugs containing potassium should be discontinued immediately (27).

Measures that are employed to correct hyperkalemia act by either normalizing neuromuscular membrane potential, shifting ions back into the intracellular space, or removing potassium from the body. Membrane potential and therefore the strength of muscular contraction are

Table 9.9.
Potassium

Serum level > 5 mmol/L (5 mEq/L)	Serum level < 3.5 mmol/L (35 mEq/L)
Cause	
Renal failure	Amphotericin B
Acidosis	Diuretics
Crush injury	Diarrhea
Red cell hemolysis	Decreased intake
Potassium-sparing diuretics	Corticosteroids
Excess ingestion of potassium (salt substitutes)	Renal tubular acidosis
	Alkalosis
Adrenal insufficiency	Vomiting
Hypoaldosteronism	Fanconi's syndrome
	Hyperaldosteronism
	Licorice
Signs and Symptoms	
ECG findings:	ECG findings:
Peaked T waves	Flat or inverted T waves
Depressed S-T segment	Depressed S-T segment
Disappearance of P wave	Muscle weakness
Widened QRS complex	Diminished reflexes
Muscle weakness	Paralysis
Paresthesias	Weak pulse
GI hypermotility	Ileus
Flaccid paralysis	Depression
	Confusion
	Hypotension

Treatment of Hyperkalemia
  Calcium (as chloride or gluconate salt) 2–5 mmol over 5–10 min
  Na bicarbonate 50 mmol over 2–3 min
  Regular insulin 10 units in 50 g of dextrose over 5–10 min
  Kayexalate 30–60 g in 20% sorbitol by mouth or enema
Treatment of Hypokalemia
  KCl 10 mmol/hr × 4 doses, check serum K, repeat as necessary

determined by the relative concentrations of potassium, calcium, and magnesium at the cell membrane. If the potassium-induced arrhythmia is life-threatening, 2.5 to 5 mmol (5 to 10 mEq) of calcium is given over several minutes to temporarily correct the K-Ca ratio and eliminate the cardiac problem. If necessary to maintain good cardiac function until measures that permanently normalize the serum potassium take effect, a constant infusion of intravenous calcium at a rate determined by simultaneous electrocardiograph (ECG) monitoring is indicated. Calcium gluconate (2.3 mmol/g) and calcium chloride (6.8 mmol/g) are the products that are used, but therapy cannot continue for long periods because hypercalcemia will become a problem.

A different treatment approach is to shift potassium ions from the vascular to the intracellular space. Sodium bicarbonate administration will produce a temporary alkalosis and will lower serum potassium by 0.6 mmol/L for every 0.1 elevation in pH. This therapy, like calcium infusion, cannot be continued for long periods, as sodium overload and metabolic alkalosis will result. Fifty-milliliter vials and preloaded syringes of 8.4% (1 mmol/mL) and 500 mL containers of 5% (0.6 mmol/mL) sodium bicarbonate are commercially available.

Glucose/insulin infusions are another possible treatment. Potassium ions move with glucose across cell membranes in the presence of insulin. A ratio of 2 to 3 g glucose per unit of insulin is needed to maintain a normal blood glucose level during this process; 25 to 30 units of regular insulin per liter of 10% dextrose solution or 10 units in 50 mL of 50% dextrose are the commonly administered solutions. This is a temporizing measure, like Ca and $NaCO_3$ administration, because potassium ions are not removed from the body. It does, however, have the advantage that treatment can be continued without significant complication for long periods of time.

Two therapies remove potassium from the body but act slowly. While they should be initiated as soon as possible, they will not correct cardiac arrhythmias in a timely fashion and cannot be considered acute treatments for hyperkalemia. The cationic-anionic exchange resin Kayexalate (sodium polystyrene sulfonate) given orally or rectally binds potassium to itself by exchange with sodium in the gastrointestinal tract. One gram of Kayexalate will remove 1 mmol of potassium and add 2 to 3 mmol of sodium. The resin is very constipating, so it is given with sorbitol, an osmotic cathartic, and water to prevent fecal impaction. The oral route is preferred over rectal administration because the contact time with the GI mucosa is longer. The initial dose is 30 to 60 g of resin in 120–240 mL of 20% sorbitol and can be repeated every 1 to 2 hr if the serum potassium level remains high. Sodium overload can occur, so monitoring for congestive heart failure, edema, and pulmonary edema is required for patients who are at risk of developing these problems. Patients will complain about this therapy, as the resin has the consistency of sand and a very unpleasant taste. As a last resort in the treatment of hyperkalemia, peritoneal or hemodialysis can be used to remove potassium from the body. This procedure is very invasive and should not be used unless the patient's condition is life-threatening and other treatment methods have failed or will fail (31).

HYPOKALEMIA

Hypokalemia can also be a cardiac medical emergency, with rhythm disturbances appearing at serum levels below 3 mmol/L. Fortunately, the patient may exhibit muscle weakness and malaise before ECG changes appear. The symptoms and causes of hypokalemia are listed in Table 9.9. Correction of underlying diseases or discontinuation of drug therapy contributing to hypokalemia is a basic part of the initial treatment (30).

Hypokalemia secondary to hyponatremia is almost always accompanied by hypochloremic alkalosis, as the renal conservation of sodium causes secretion of potassium and hydrogen ions (see Figure 9.2). For every 3 mmol Na

that is reabsorbed, 2 mmol of K and 1 mmol of H will be lost in the urine. The hydrogen ion that is needed for the exchange with Na is generated from the action of carbonic anhydrase on H_2O and CO_2. Carbonic acid (H_2CO_3) in renal tubular cells dissociates into H and HCO_3, hydrogen ion is secreted into the urine, and bicarbonate is resorbed into the blood. When enough HCO_3 ions accumulate in serum, alkalosis results. Correction of any concomitant hyponatremia and alkalosis must accompany treatment of hypokalemia for the treatment to be successful. Administration of the chloride salt of potassium is the treatment of choice because correction of alkalosis is necessary. As chloride loading proceeds, bicarbonate excretion by the kidneys will increase, generation will decrease, and alkalosis will resolve. If a nonchloride salt of potassium is given, renal excretion and intracellular shifting of potassium will continue and will prevent correction of the hypokalemia (see Figure 9.2).

An intracellular deficit of potassium almost always precedes and accompanies an intravascular deficit; large amounts of potassium may need to be given before the total body and serum levels will normalize. Orally or intravenously administered potassium shifts slowly into the ICF to correct the deficit there, so the rate of KCl infusion must not be so rapid as to cause interim hyperkalemia. Under most conditions, intravenous KCl at 10 mmol/hr will not cause hyperkalemia in a patient with a serum level below 3.5 mmol/L. Infusion into a peripheral vein at a rate greater than 10 mmol/hr can also cause intolerable pain and phlebitis at the intravenous site. A 30 to 40 mmol dose given over 3 to 4 hr in D5W is the most common rate of potassium replacement. The serum potassium is checked 1 to 2 hr later, and the treatment is repeated until the level is 3.8 to 4.0 mmol/L. For patients with profound hypokalemia and continuing potassium wasting, such as those with renal tubular acidosis from amphotericin B therapy, replacement of the potassium deficit often requires very large doses. In these instances, 20 to 50 mmol/hr may need to be given; a central line is always necessary to avoid causing phlebitis.

Oral administration of KCl can correct hypokalemia, but many patients will experience considerable GI irritation and vomiting when given more than 20 mmol/dose or 60 mmol/day. They will also often refuse therapy because of the bad taste of KCl solutions. Wax-matrix tablets have greater patient acceptance than does oral potassium, but the problem of gastric irritation remains. Attempts to replace large potassium deficits by mouth are often unsuccessful; concomitant intravenous replacement may be needed (28).

Chloride

Chloride is the major anion in the ECF, but it has no inherent physiologic function (4). It will usually go up or down synchronously with total body sodium, but a change in chloride concentration will cause an acid-base disturbance. Because electrical neutrality must be maintained and the concentration of unmeasured ions is fixed, there will be an immediate change in the serum HCO_3 concentration. The effect will be metabolic acidosis or alkalosis, depending on the resultant increase or decrease in the HCO_3 to pCO_2 ratio.

The disorders of body chloride result from its loss from the body (vomiting, diuretics), hypernatremia, chloride loading (saline infusion), or changes in acid-base balance. In acidosis and alkalosis the change in the serum chloride concentration is almost always a compensatory response to an initial change in the bicarbonate value. In this instance the serum chloride will not normalize, nor should an effort be made to normalize it by giving or withholding chloride, until the cause of the acid-base abnormality is identified and corrected. When this occurs, the chloride concentration will be normalized naturally via renal homeostatic mechanisms (4).

HYPERCHLOREMIA

A serum level greater than 105 mmol/L is considered abnormal. Because it is the result of metabolic acidosis, hypernatremia, or chloride loading, treatment is aimed at correcting the underlying disorder. The composition of oral or intravenous fluids should be determined, and adjustments should be made if they appear to be the cause of the problem. Changing a normal saline infusion to lactated Ringer's solution or one-half normal saline or replacing NaCl with Na acetate may solve the problem. If the cause of the hyperchloremia is metabolic acidosis or respiratory alkalosis, correction of these disturbances is the only treatment. When hypernatremia due to overingestion of NaCl is the cause, treatment is free water replacement and diuresis; for hypernatremia due to water loss, the treatment is electrolyte-free water replacement (see the discussion above of sodium).

HYPOCHLOREMIA

A serum chloride level below 95 mmol/L is considered to be hypochloremia. As the ECF chloride changes with ECF sodium, hyponatremia will cause hypochloremia. This is an appropriate compensatory mechanism to maintain electrical neutrality, and the chloride will normalize with correction of the ECF sodium concentration.

The most common causes of hypochloremia are nasogastric suction, vomiting, and diuretic therapy. Large amounts of chloride and acid are lost with stomach fluid, so therapy consists of replacement of the volume of the nasogastric aspirate or vomiting with high-chloride-containing solutions such as normal saline or lactated Ringer's solution. Diuretics cause hypochloremia by mechanisms that are discussed in the section on hyponatremia. Therapy consists of liberalizing NaCl intake, reducing the diuretic dose, and correcting symptomatic hyponatremia and hypokalemia with saline and KCl solutions.

Calcium

The major repository of calcium in the body is bone; only 1% of the total amount in the body is in the fluid spaces. The normal serum concentration in the adult is 2.2 to 2.6 mmol/L (8.8 to 10.3 mg/dL), but only 50% is available to exert its physiologic effect; the other 50% is bound to albumin and other proteins. Serum calcium concentration does not fluctuate with daily intake and excretion. The synchronous activity of parathyroid hormone, vitamin D, and calcitonin regulates GI absorption, renal excretion, and skeletal deposition or resorption of calcium. These hormones establish and maintain the serum calcium (32). There is also an inverse relationship between serum calcium and phosphate; if one goes up or down, the other will change in the opposite direction.

Calcium has a variety of specific physiologic functions in the body. It is essential to neuromuscular conduction by stabilizing cell membrane permeability and excitability, it inhibits some enzymes in the Krebs' cycle, stimulates gastrin, reduces renal blood flow, and is active in the blood coagulation cascade as Factor IV. The normal range is narrow, and most laboratories measure total serum calcium, not just the active ionized 50%. This presents a problem in determining the physiologically active amount of the ion in the serum. Since 50% is protein bound, primarily to albumin, a low serum albumin will result in a low laboratory value; this does not necessarily mean that there is simultaneously a low ionized level. For each 10 gm/L change in the serum albumin concentration, total serum calcium will change 0.2 mmol/L in the same direction. For example, a patient with an albumin of 20 gm/L has a reported total calcium of 1.95 mmol/L; although the value is below normal, it does not represent a low ionized (free) level. Mathematically correcting the albumin to a normal of 40 gm/L raises the total calcium to 2.3 mmol/L. It can be assumed from this correction that the free calcium is normal and physiologic hypocalcemia is not present. If only the ionized calcium is reported, this correction need not be made.

Acid-base disturbances affect the ionized/bound calcium ratio but not total serum calcium. Some hydrogen ions circulate in the blood bound to albumin. In acidosis, more H ions are bound to albumin as the body attempts to buffer acid and normalize the plasma pH; this displaces calcium ions from their binding sites, and the amount of free calcium in the blood rises. The converse is true in alkalosis. For each 0.1 change in pH, the ionized calcium changes 0.42 mmol/L in the opposite direction (33).

HYPERCALCEMIA

Hypercalcemia is defined in adults as a corrected total serum calcium above 2.6 mmol/L (10.3 mg/dL) or an ionized value above 1.15 mmol/L. The symptoms and causes are listed in Table 9.10. Any sources of exogenous calcium should be immediately discontinued. It is important to note that the mental abberations seen with hypercalcemia can be profound and are not necessarily related in a linear fashion to the degree of hypercalcemia. Any evaluation of an apparently mentally ill or comatose patient should include a serum calcium level.

The therapies for hypercalcemia involve shifting ions back into the bone or removing calcium from the body (34). The removal therapies are given first because they work faster and are generally more effective in an acute situation. Loop diuretics, such as furosemide, increase renal excretion of calcium as well as sodium and chloride. The initial dose of furosemide is 1 mg/kg; it is given with an amount

Table 9.10.
Calcium

Serum level > 2.6 mmol/L (total, corrected) (10.3 mg/dL) 1.2 mmol/L (ionized) (2.3 mEq/L)	Serum level < 2.2 mmol/L (total corrected) (8.8 mg/dL) 1.0 mmol/L (ionized) (2.0 mEq/L)
Cause	
Bone neoplasms	Renal failure
Hyperparathyroidism	Hypoparathyroidism
Hypervitaminosis D	Vitamin D deficiency
Prolonged immobilization	Diuretics
Sarcoidosis	Mithramycin
Paget's disease	Transfusion with citrated blood
Lithium	Pancreatitis
Adrenal insufficiency	Hyperphosphatemia
Acidosis	Alkalosis
Idiopathic hypercalcemia of	Colchicine
infancy	Hypomagnesemia
Hypervitaminosis A	Fluoride poisoning
Aluminum osteodystrophy	
Signs and Symptoms	
Muscle weakness	Numbness/tingling of fingertips
Anorexia	and around mouth
Fatigue	Hyperactive reflexes
Nausea	Chvostek's sign
Lethargy	Trousseau's sign
Depression	Tetany
Psychosis	Lethargy
Stupor	Depression
Coma	Psychosis
	Stupor
	Coma

Treatment of Hypercalcemia
Normal saline and furosemide, calcitonin, gallium nitrate, etidronate, mithramycin, phosphate, steroids
Treatment of Hypocalcemia
Calcium (chloride or gluconate) IV 2–5 mmol (5–10 mEq) over 5–10 min and/or calcium carbonate PO 2–10 g/day

of normal saline that will maintain a normal body water and sodium when a urine output of 200 to 500 mL/hr is achieved.

Potassium must also be added in this therapy to avoid hypokalemia from the action of the loop diuretic. This "washout" therapy may need to be continued for extended periods if the cause of the hypercalcemia is severe and/or abnormally large amounts of calcium continue to appear in the vascular compartment (35). Treatments that shift calcium back into bone are hormone-based and slow and often become ineffective because of tachyphylaxis. Calcitonin is used because it increases bone uptake of calcium (36); salmon and human preparations are commercially available. While the hypocalcemic effect of calcitonin is rapid, it is of short duration and tachyphylaxis usually develops within days. The starting dose for treatment of hypercalcemia is 4 IU/kg of salmon calcitonin given every 12 hr by subcutaneous or intramuscular injection; after 2 days, this can be increased to a maximum dose of 8 IU/kg given every 6 hr, but additional hypocalcemic effect will not usually result. Human calcitonin is approved for use only in Paget's disease; dosing information for the treatment of hypercalcemia is not available. Intranasal salmon calcitonin has been evaluated in the treatment of osteoporosis and in pain associated with osteoporotic vertebral fractures but not in the treatment of hypercalcemia, and no intranasal product is available in the United States (37). Intravenous gallium nitrate is very occasionally used to treat hypercalcemia. In comparisons with salmon calcitonin in patients with hypercalcemia of malignancy, it more effectively reduced serum calcium levels and had a longer duration of action but can be very nephrotoxic. Adequate patient hydration is essential, and other potentially nephrotoxic agents should be avoided during the treatment period. The mechanism of action is not well understood, but gallium appears to inhibit bone turnover. It is given by continuous infusion in doses of 100 to 200 mg/m^2 for 5 days (38).

Etidronate disodium (Didronel) is a diphosphonate that inhibits osteoclastic bone resorption by binding hydroxyapatite (39). Initial treatment is with 7.5 mg/kg/day given intravenously once daily for 3 days. It is important that the infusion time be at least 2 hr. Therapy has been continued for as long as 7 days, but there is a risk of causing hypocalcemia. Once the serum calcium has been controlled, oral therapy with 20 mg/kg/day can be given if the hypercalcemia is expected to recur, for example, in the case of bone metastases in cancer patients. Pamidronate disodium (Aredia), a newer diphosphonate that is similar to etidronate, may offer the advantages of quicker onset and longer duration of action than etidronate without the disadvantage of inhibiting bone mineralization at high doses. It is dosed at 60 to 90 mg given intravenously over 24 hr; the treatment can be repeated at 7-day intervals if necessary. Steroids, such as prednisone, are useful in the management of chronic mild hypercalcemia. The initial dose of prednisone varies between 15 and 100 mg/day with an onset of action of 3 to 10 days. Steroids work by antagonizing activation of Vitamin D in the liver and by reducing bone resorption; for these reasons they are not effective in treating hypercalcemia secondary to hyperparathyroidism. Oral phosphate is a treatment option only in treating hypercalcemia that is the result of hypophosphatemia (a rare occurrence). As the ordinary reciprocal relationship between serum calcium and phosphate levels has not been maintained in hypercalcemia from all other causes, the amount that the serum calcium will fall when phosphate concentration rises is usually small. The risk of soft tissue calcification by $Ca-PO_4$ complexes often exceeds the benefit of this therapy. If raising the serum phosphate results in a calcium-phosphate product that exceeds 5 (multiply serum calcium and phosphate to get this value) precipitation can occur. In the rare instances when hypophosphatemia is the cause of hypercalcemia, administration of 30 to 100 mmol/day (1 to 3 g) of phosphorus should solve the problem. Replacement products that are available are Phospho-Soda (solution, 25 mmol (800 mg) P/5 mL) and Neutra-Phos (capsules, 8 mmol (250 mg) P and solution 32 mmol (1 g) P/300 mL). These products also contain considerable amounts of sodium and potassium as the obligate cations, so caution must be exercised with their use for this reason.

An effective but potentially toxic therapy for hypercalcemia is mithramycin; it is indicated only when other therapies fail. Mithramycin is a cancer chemotherapeutic agent that acts by inhibiting DNA-dependent bone osteoclast RNA synthesis. This will slow or stop bone resorption. The initial dose is 25 μg/kg/day up to a weekly maximum of 150 μg/kg. The onset of action is 12 to 48 hr, and the duration is 3 to 7 days. While these doses are considerably smaller than those used in cancer treatment, the risk of hematologic and GI toxicity remains.

HYPOCALCEMIA

Hypocalcemia in adults is defined as a corrected serum level below 2.20 mmol/L (8.8 mg/dL) or an ionized level below 1 mmol/L. The symptoms and etiologies are listed in Table 9.10. Acute treatment involves intravenous administration of calcium. The chloride salt contains 6.8 mmol/g (13.5 mEq Ca/g), and the gluconate and gluceptate salts contain 2.3 mmol/g (4.6 mEq Ca/g). The initial dose is 2.5 to 5 mmol of Ca followed by an infusion of 0.075 to 0.1 mmol Ca/kg/hr. Calcium level, blood pressure, and ECG should be monitored during this process to evaluate cardiac function and avoid hypercalcemia. Patients whose symptoms of hypocalcemia do not resolve with calcium replacement should be evaluated for hypomagnesemia, as the abnormalities can mimic each other and often appear together.

Treatment of chronic hypocalcemia is directed at correcting the underlying etiology. Most commonly, the etiology of chronic hypocalcemia is a low level of biologically active vitamin D. This appears in advanced hepatic or renal disease due to decreased transformation of cholecalciferol (D_3) by these organs to the active form, 1,25-dihydroxycholecalciferol. The serum level of calcium will not normalize until the level of 1,25-DHC is normal. Therapy usually involves calcium and vitamin D supplementation. Ergocalciferol (D_2) in a dose of 1.25 to 5 mg (50,000 to 200,000 IU/day) or dihydrotachysterol (DHT, Hytakerol) in a dose of 0.25 to 1 mg/day (equivalent to 30,000 to 120,000 IU of D_2) are most commonly used. The onset of action can be several weeks, and the effect can be prolonged because of the long half-life of vitamin D. Activated forms of vitamin D must be given if renal and/or hepatic transformation are absent or unreliable. 25-Hydroxycholecalciferol (calcifediol, Calderol) in doses of 25 to 200 μg/day or 1,25-dihydroxycholecalciferol (calcitriol, Rocaltrol, Calcijex) in doses of 0.25 to 1 μg/day are available. The active forms of vitamin D have an onset of action of 3 to 7 days and are preferred in treatment because their shorter half-lives make the risk of prolonged hypercalcemia less. Calcium supplementation with 25 to 100 mmol/day (1 to 4 g) elemental Ca is begun simultaneously. Several salts of calcium are available for oral therapy, but calcium carbonate contains the highest amount of elemental calcium, 10.2 mmol (400 mg) per 1000 mg $CaCO_3$. Calcium lactate is 1.5 mmol (60 mg) per 300 mg, calcium gluceptate contains 2.2 mmol (80 mg) per 1000 mg, and calcium gluconate contains 2.3 mmol (90 mg) per 1000 mg. Calcium carbonate is the preferred preparation as the number of tablets the patient must take is lower than with the other salts. Liquid $CaCO_3$ and Ca gluceptate are available for use by patients with achlorhydria or those receiving H_2 antagonist therapy because tablet dissolution in the GI tract may be incomplete without gastric acid. When hypocalcemia is due to hypoparathyroidism, parathyroid hormone replacement is indicated and is the only therapy that will raise the serum calcium (40–42).

Magnesium

The average adult body contains approximately 1000 mmol (2000 mEq) of magnesium; 99% of which is in bone and the intracellular compartment. Of the 1% remaining in the vascular space, 25% is bound to proteins; it is the ionized 75% that exerts the physiologic effect. Serum magnesium in adults is maintained in the normal range of 0.8 to 1.2 mmol/L (1.6 to 2.4 mEq/L) by efficient renal conservation/excretion mechanisms and by drawing on the intracellular space for "new" ions when intake falls. In conjunction with calcium and potassium, magnesium regulates neuromuscular excitability and conduction on the cell membrane; it also has a role in the release of parathyroid hormone.

Deviations from a normal serum magnesium rarely appear as an isolated problem. Most often, calcium, potassium, and phosphate levels are also abnormal, indicating a generalized abnormality in the solute concentration of the intracellular compartment. This pattern of electrolyte disturbances is most commonly seen in prolonged starvation (43).

HYPERMAGNESEMIA

Hypermagnesemia is defined as a serum level above 1.2 mmol/L (2.4 mEq/L), but serious symptoms do not usually occur until the level is above 3.0 mEq/L. The symptoms and causes of hypermagnesemia are listed in Table 9.11. Since large loads of magnesium can easily be excreted by the kidneys, hypermagnesemia is rarely seen without attendant severe renal dysfunction. Magnesium-containing antacids are often a contributing factor in this situation. All sources of exogenous magnesium should be discontinued. The treatments for an elevated magnesium involve eliminating it from the body or shifting it back into the intracellular space. Glucose and insulin can be used for brief periods of time, as in the treatment of hyperkalemia, but the only effective means of removing it from the body are peritoneal dialysis and hemodialysis.

HYPOMAGNESEMIA

Hypomagnesemia is defined as a serum level below 0.8 mmol/L (1.6 mEq/L); symptoms can appear at levels below 0.6. The symptoms and causes of hypomagnesemia are found in Table 9.11. Hypomagnesemia usually appears

Table 9.11.
Magnesium

Serum level > 1.2 mmol/L (2.4 mEq/L)	Serum level < 0.8 mmol/L (1.6 mEq/L)
Cause	
Renal failure	Amphotericin B
Hyperparathyroidism	Cis-platinum
Hypoaldosteronism	Diuretics
Adrenal insufficiency	Diarrhea
Lithium	Hypervitaminosis D
	Vitamin D deficiency
	Vomiting
	Hyperaldosteronism
	Aminoglycosides
Signs and Symptoms	
Weakness	Tremor
Nausea/vomiting	Hyperactive reflexes
Hypotension	Confusion
Respiratory depression	Seizures
Coma	
Treatment of Hypermagnesemia	
Dextrose and insulin, hemodialysis	
Treatment of Hypomagnesemia	
Magnesium SO$_4$ IV 0.15–0.25 mmol/kg/day	
Magnesium oxide 300–600 mg PO (6.25 mmol Mg) bid–tid	

with hypokalemia, hypocalcemia, and hypophosphatemia. Levels of these electrolytes should be measured when low levels of magnesium are found. As with the other intracellular electrolytes, there is almost always a generalized deficit present. The total body deficit of magnesium may be as much as 25 mmol before the serum level begins to fall. Therapy is with the sulfate or oxide salts of magnesium. The available product for intravenous administration is magnesium sulfate; each gram of the 50% solution contains 4 mmol (8 mEq) of magnesium. The initial dose is 0.25 mmol/kg/day if the serum level is less than 0.6 mmol/L and 0.15 mmol/kg/day if it is between 0.7 and 1.2 mmol/L. This amount should be given over 1 to 4 hr, and the serum level should be checked 1 to 2 hr later. The delay before measuring the serum concentration gives time for intracellular shifting; as is the case with potassium, an exact replacement dose cannot be determined from the serum level alone. Ideally, replacement should be completed slowly unless signs and symptoms are present. The oral replacement of large deficits can be difficult. Magnesium is a saline cathartic, and the large doses that are needed for replacement may produce diarrhea. When this route of administration is chosen, up to 20 mmol/day given in divided doses will usually be tolerated. Magnesium oxide capsules are most commonly given (6.2 mmol/250 mg MgO) because of convenience for the patient, but solutions of MgSO$_4$ are also available for oral administration (44).

Phosphorus

Of the total body phosphate, 99.99% is contained in bone and the intracellular space. The normal serum level in adults is 0.8 to 1.6 mmol/L (2.5 to 5 mg/dL). The equilibrium between serum calcium (reciprocal with PO$_4$), intracellular stores, parathyroid hormone, Vitamin D, renal conservation/excretion mechanisms, and oral intake maintains a normal serum level. The specific physiologic function of phosphate in the body is to form high-energy phosphate bonds of adenosine diphosphate and triphosphate in glycolysis (anaerobic metabolism) and the Krebs' cycle. Another important function of phosphate, as 2,3-diphosphoglycerate, is to facilitate the release of oxygen from hemoglobin.

HYPERPHOSPHATEMIA

Hyperphosphatemia is defined as a serum level above 1.6 mmol/L and almost always results from decreased excretion in the presence of severe renal dysfunction. Symptoms and causes of hyperphosphatemia are listed in Table 9.12. The major risk of hyperphosphatemia, and the reason it is most commonly corrected, is the hypocalcemia it reciprocally causes; a high phosphate level in and of itself does not cause significant negative physiologic consequences. Any patient with an elevated phosphate level needs a serum calcium check, as the physiologic disturbances from an abnormal calcium level can be serious. The only available treatments for hyperphosphatemia are decreasing PO_4 absorption from the GI tract by precipitating it with aluminum-containing antacids and with glucose-insulin infusions. Peritoneal dialysis or hemodialysis is used to lower serum phosphate levels when hypocalcemia is a problem, but they are not very efficient (45).

HYPOPHOSPHATEMIA

Hypophosphatemia is defined as a serum level below 0.8 mmol/L, but symptoms rarely appear if the level is above 0.3; the abnormality is usually simultaneous with starvation-induced deficits in other intracellular ions. Symptoms and causes are listed in Table 9.12. Therapy consists of replacement with the sodium or potassium salts of phosphate. Repletion must be slow, since calcium-phosphate precipitation in soft tissue, renal failure, and hyperphosphatemia can result from therapy that is too aggressive. The initial dose is 0.3 to 0.6 mmol/kg/day if the serum level is below 0.3 and 0.2 to 0.3 mmol/kg/day if it is between 0.4 and 0.8. Therapy should be given over at least 6 hr to allow for equilibration into the intracellular space; the serum level should be checked 3 to 4 hr after the end of the infusion. Oral replacement can be given with Phospho-Soda or Neutra-Phos in divided doses (46, 47).

Table 9.12.
Phosphorus

Serum level > 1.6 mmol/L (5.0 mg/dL)	Serum level < 0.8 mmol/L (2.5 mg/dL)
Cause	
Renal failure	Aluminum antacids
Hypoparathyroidism	Prolonged starvation
	Nutritional depletion
	Diuretics
	Vitamin D deficiency
	Hyperaldosteronism
	Corticosteroids
	Alkalosis
	Renal tubular defects
	SIADH
Signs and Symptoms	
Renal osteodystrophy	Muscle weakness
Ca-PO$_4$ complex deposition in soft tissue	Bone pain
	Paresthesias
	Irritability
	Respiratory insufficiency
	Hemolytic anemia
	Rhabdomyolysis
	Proximal muscle atrophy
	Cardiomyopathy
	Seizures
	Coma
Treatment of Hyperphosphotemia	
Dextrose and insulin, hemodialysis	
Treatment of Hypophosphatemia	
Na or K phosphate IV or PO 0.05–0.6 mmol PO$_4$/kg/day	

(Refer to the section on hypercalcemia for the phosphate content of these products.)

CONCLUSION

Identification and correction of disorders of fluids, electrolytes, and acid-base balance can be difficult. The body's internal environment is constantly changing and continuously adjusting to and correcting for internal and external forces that disturb homeostasis. Normal serum levels of electrolytes do not always reflect normal body water or pH status; abnormal values may be appropriate compensatory responses to maintain homeostasis, and the treatment of the patient consists of finding and correcting the primary disturbance. Normal body functions continue only within narrow ranges of ionic composition, pH, and intravascular volume and pressure. In evaluating any patient, establishing and maintaining a hemodynamic status sufficient to perfuse and oxygenate cells are the first priority and must be done quickly if the patient is to survive. With the exception of exsanguination (acute, massive blood loss), changes in fluids, electrolytes, and pH have usually occurred slowly, and some compensatory mechanisms are operating. Correcting an isolated abnormal laboratory value without regard to its cause and its contribution to overall patient status may further complicate the patient's condition without any benefit. Any therapy that is chosen must be given in a way and at a rate that will reestablish and support homeostasis without treatment-induced complications.

REFERENCES

1. Robertson GL, Berl T. Pathophysiology of water metabolism. In: Brenner BM, Rector FC, eds. The Kidney, 3rd ed. Philadelphia: WB Saunders, 1986:385–423.
2. Moore FD, McMurray JD. Total body water and electrolytes: intravascular and extravascular phase volumes. Metabolism 5:447, 1956.
3. Cohn SH, Vaswani A. Changes in body chemical composition with age measured by total-body neutron activation. Metabolism 25:85, 1976.
4. Earley LE, Daugharty TM. Sodium metabolism. N Engl J Med 281:72–86, 1969.
5. Feig PU, McCurdy DK. The hypertonic state. N Engl J Med 297:1444–1454, 1957.
6. Weitzman RE, Kleeman CR. The water depletion syndrome (hyperosmolar) and water excess (hyposmolar) syndromes. West J Med 132:16–38, 1980.
7. Hierholzer K, Wiederholt M. Some aspects of distal tubular solute and water transport. Kidney Int 9:198–218, 1976.
8. Bartter FE, Schwartz WB. The syndrome of inappropriate secretion of anti-diuretic hormone. Am J Med 42:790, 1967.
9. Narins RG, Jones ER. Diagnostic strategies in disorders of fluid, electrolyte and acid-base homeostasis. Am J Med 72:496, 1982.
10. Giebisch G, Stanton B. Potassium transport in the nephron. Ann Rev Physiol 41:241–256, 1979.
11. Field M, Rao M. Intestinal electrolyte transport and diarrheal disease, part 1. N Engl J Med 321:800–806, 1989.
12. Field M, Rao M. Intestinal electrolyte transport and diarrheal disease, part 2. N Engl J Med 321:879–883, 1989.

13. Good DW, Velazquez H. Luminal effects on potassium excretion: low sodium concentration. Am J Physiol 246:F46–F55, 1982.

14. Ross AD, Angaran DM. Colloids and crystalloids: a continuing controversy. Drug Intell Clin Pharm 18:202–212, 1984.

15. Lewis RT. Albumin: role and discriminative use in surgery. Can J Surg 23:322–333, 1980.

16. Hulse JD, Yacobi A. Hetastarch: an overview of the colloid and its metabolism. Drug Intell Clin Pharm 17:334–341, 1983.

17. Hyneck ML. Simple acid-base disorders. Am J Hosp Pharm 42:1992–2006, 1985.

18. Arbus GS. An in-vivo acid-base nomogram for clinical use. Can Med Assoc J 109:291, 1973.

19. Cogan MG, Rector FC. Acid-base disorders. In: Brenner BM, Rector FC, eds. The Kidney, 3rd ed. Philadelphia: WB Saunders, 1986:457–518.

20. McLaughlin M, Kassirer J. Rational treatment of acid-base disorders. Drugs 39(6):841–855, 1990.

21. Narins RG, Emmett M. Simple and mixed acid-base disorders: a practical approach. Medicine 59:161, 1980.

22. Adroque HJ, Madias NE. Changes in plasma potassium concentration during acute acid-base disturbances. Am J Med 71:456, 1981.

23. Weber JN. Treatment of metabolic alkalosis with intravenous administration of hydrochloric acid. CSHP Voice 13:1–3, 1986.

24. Brater DC. Serum electrolyte abnormalities caused by drugs. Prog Drug Res 30:9, 1986.

25. Surawicz B. Relationship between the ECG and electrolytes. Am Heart J 73:814, 1967.

26. Knochel JP. Neuromuscular manifestations of electrolyte disorders. Am J Med 72:521, 1982.

27. Pearson E, Fish H. Potassium content of selected medicines, foods and salt substitutes. Hosp Pharm 6(9):6–9, 1971.

28. Stanszek WF. Current approaches to management of potassium deficiency. Drug Intell Clin Pharm 19:176, 1985.

29. Cox M. Potassium homeostasis. Med Clin North Am 65:67–73, 1981.

30. Hollifield JW, Slaton PE. Thiazide diuretics, hypokalemia and cardiac arrhythmias. Acta Med Scand 647(Suppl):67–73, 1981.

31. DeFronzo RA, Bias M. Clinical disorders of hyperkalemia. Ann Rev Med 33:521, 1982.

32. Pederson KO. The effect of bicarbonate, CO_2 and pH on serum calcium fractions. Scand J Clin Lab Invest 27:147, 1979.

33. Suki WN, Rouse D. Hormonal regulation of calcium transport in the thick ascending limb renal tubules. Am J Physiol 241:F171, 1981.

34. Bell NH. Hypercalcemic and hypocalcemic disorders: diagnosis and treatment. Nephron 23:147, 1979.

35. Massry SG, Coburn JW. Role of serum Ca, parathyroid hormone, and NaCl infusion on renal Ca and Na clearance. Am J Physiol 214:1403, 1968.

36. Austin LA, Heath H. Calcitonin. N Engl J Med 304:269–280, 1981.

37. Pun KK, Chan LWL. Analgesic effect of intranasal salmon calcitonin in the treatment of osteoporotic vertebral fractures. Clin Ther 2:205–208, 1989.

38. Warrell JP, Israel R. Gallium nitrate for acute treatment of cancer-related hypercalcemia: a randomized, double-blind comparison to calcitonin. Ann Intern Med 108:669–674, 1988.

39. Ryzen E, Martodam RR. Intravenous etidronate in the management of malignant hypercalcemia. Arch Intern Med 145:449–452, 1985.

40. Bordier P. The effect of $1(OH)D_3$ and $1,25\ (OH)_2D_3$ on the bone of patients with renal osteodystrophy. Am J Med 64:101–107, 1978.

41. Kanis J. Vitamin D metabolism and its clinical application. J Bone Joint Surg 64B:542–557, 1982.

42. Bilezikian JP. Calcium and bone metabolism, part IV. In: Becker KL, ed. Principles and Practice of Endocrinology and Metabolism. Philadelphia: JP Lippincott, 1990.

43. Massry SG, Seelig MS. Hypomagnesemia and hypermagnesemia. Clin Nephrol 7:147, 1977.

44. Dickerson RN. Treating hypomagnesemia. Hosp Pharm 20:761–763, 1985.

45. Chernow B, Rainey TG. Iatrogenic hyperphosphatemia: a metabolic consideration in critical care medicine. Crit Care Med 9:772, 1981.

46. Vannatta JB, Whang R. Efficacy of intravenous phosphate therapy in the severely hypophosphatemic patient. Arch Intern Med 141:885, 1981.

47. Dickerson RN. Treating hypophosphatemia. Hosp Pharm 20:920–925, 1985.

CHAPTER 10

GENERAL NUTRITION

MARGARET MALONE

Clinicians practicing in either an institutional or community-based setting should be familiar with general nutritional guidelines, as their easy accessibility and availability provides an ideal opportunity to provide nutritional and health-promotion advice to the public. In this chapter general and certain population-specific nutritional recommendations will be addressed. The reader is referred to the chapters pertaining to particular disease states for additional information.

GENERAL NUTRITION GUIDELINES

The following section describes the current recommendations for healthy eating and dietary guidelines. These guidelines differ from the reference values for intakes of essential nutrients to maintain health, known as the *recommended dietary intakes* (RDIs), which vary for different ages, genders, and individual groups. RDIs are defined as "amounts of essential nutrients considered sufficient to meet the physiologic needs of practically all healthy persons in a specified group and the average amount of food sources of energy needed by members of the group" (1). In contrast, dietary guidelines and health policy recommendations are designed to promote the selection of foods to achieve a nutritionally adequate diet and include recommendations on nonnutrients such as fiber and advice regarding fat and cholesterol intake.

A healthy diet should follow three simple rules: moderation, variety, and balance. Advice on dietary selection from the basic food groups has been incorporated into a food guide pyramid by the U.S. Departments of Agriculture and of Health and Human Services (Fig. 10.1) (2). Individual diets are modified to take into account genetic variability. The general dietary guidelines that health care practitioners should advocate are presented in Table 10.1 (3).

Food Labeling Requirements

The 1994 FDA food labeling guidelines are designed to provide the consumer with straightforward information regarding the ingredients of food products. These guidelines have also required manufacturers to adhere to stricter definitions when applying terms such as *healthy*, *natural* or *low fat* in the labeling and advertising of products. All of these efforts are directed toward improving the nation's

health by modification of dietary intake (4) and promotion of the 5-A-Day for Better Health Program, which encourages people to eat five or more servings of fruit or vegetables per day (5).

Intake of Nutritional Supplements

Every year millions of consumers spend billions of dollars on multivitamin, mineral, and dietary supplements from health food stores and pharmacies. The majority of vitamin and mineral supplements contain the recommended daily intake and do not pose a direct hazard to health, though they are rarely indicated for adequately nourished individuals. Of more concern are the amino acid supplements, herbal and homeopathic preparations, and megadose vitamins that are promoted for specific disease treatment or prevention without any documented efficacy or indication. Currently the FDA is attempting to regulate dietary supplements and the procedure for substantiating health claims for these products. However, there is strong political opposition to these measures at a congressional level lobbied by both consumers and the dietary supplement industries (6).

POPULATION-SPECIFIC CONSIDERATIONS

As outlined in the following section, some populations and indications require particular attention due to their special needs and new data regarding nutritional recommendations. These include pregnancy, pediatrics, diabetes mellitus, and the elderly.

Pregnancy

FOLIC ACID REQUIREMENTS

Several studies have provided supportive evidence for the role of folic acid in the prevention of neural tube defects. Folate supplements during pregnancy have long been recommended as prophylaxis against megaloblastic anemia in the third trimester. When used for the reduction of neural tube defects, folate levels must be adequate in the first 4 weeks following conception prior to neural tube closure (7). Since many women do not realize they are pregnant until later than this time, difficulties arise in establishing the most appropriate method of supplementation. The U.S. Public Health Service has advised women of childbearing age to ensure that they have a daily folate intake of not less than 400 μg per day and that women with

145

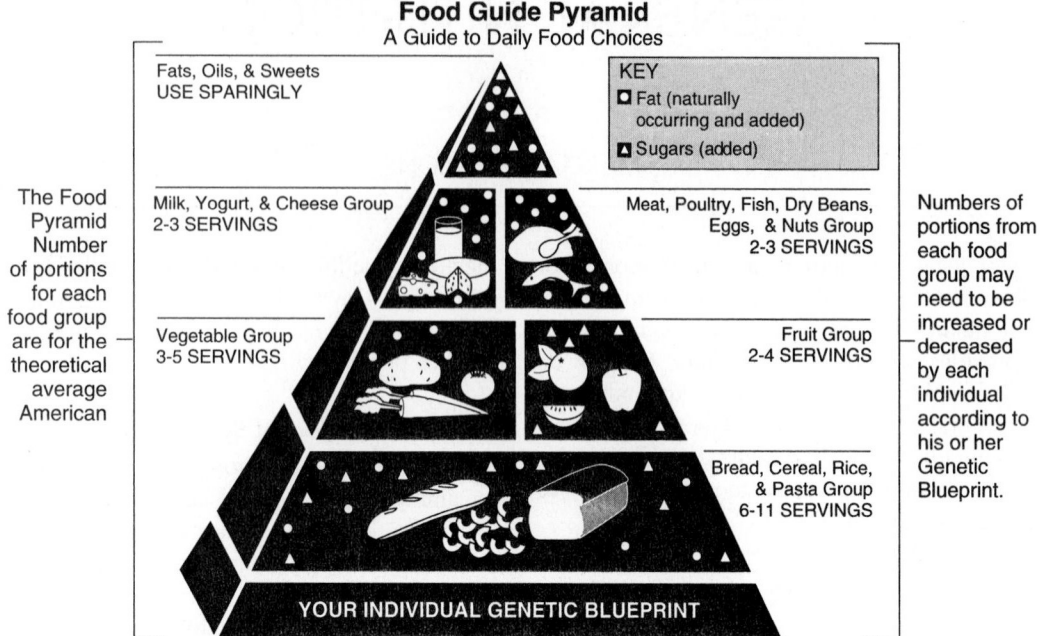

Figure 10.1   The U.S. food guide pyramid, modified to take genetic variability into account. (Courtesy of Victor Herbert.)

Table 10.1.
United States Dietary Guidelines for Adults

Eat a variety of foods.
Maintain a healthy weight.
Choose a diet low in fat (<30% total daily calories), saturated fat
   (<10% of daily fat calories), and cholesterol (<300 mg/day).
Eat plenty of fruits, vegetables, and whole grain products.
Use sugars in moderation.
Use salt and sodium in moderation.
If you drink alcoholic beverages, do so in moderation.

a previous neural tube defect baby take at least 4 μg/day as a supplement. Three possible approaches to increasing folic acid intake are increasing public awareness by health promotion campaigns, fortification of foods, in particular cereals, and recommending the use of supplements in women of childbearing age.

Food fortification has raised controversy due to the possible masking of pernicious anemia, especially in the elderly, antagonism of anticonvulsant therapy if ingested in large doses, hypersensitivity reactions to folate, and interference with zinc nutriture (8, 9). Food fortification is already used as a means of reaching the general population as demonstrated by the fortification of milk with vitamin D, which has been in practice since the 1930s to prevent rickets (10), although improved monitoring of the fortification process may be required (11). Also, the promotion of folate supplements has been criticized, as they need to be taken in the periconceptual period and made available to those who would perhaps receive the most benefit, namely economically disadvantaged women with limited access to health care.

IRON REQUIREMENTS

The use of iron supplements for all pregnant women has also been questioned. While many women develop anemia during pregnancy, for the majority it is clinically insignificant and iron stores return to baseline values postpartum without intervention. Iron therapy commonly causes gastrointestinal disturbance including nausea, vomiting, diarrhea, and constipation, exacerbating problems that are often associated with pregnancy. In practice, iron therapy should only be prescribed or recommended in the presence of clinically significant iron deficiency anemia.

Pediatrics

VITAMIN K SUPPLEMENTATION OF NEWBORNS

Controversy exists over the use of intramuscular vitamin K in neonates, which is given to prevent hemorrhagic disease, particularly intracranial bleeding. Golding et al. reported a twofold increase in childhood cancers associated with the use of intramuscular vitamin K at birth (12). Other studies have failed to confirm this finding and have cautioned against abandoning the practice of routine vitamin K supplementation for newborns, as the benefits associated with prophylaxis in reducing hemorrhagic disease have been well described (13, 14). At the present time insufficient evidence is available to resolve this important issue, though studies are in progress (15).

EFFECT OF SUGAR AND ARTIFICIAL SWEETENER INTAKE ON BEHAVIOR OF CHILDREN

Another controversial area relating to children is the possible role of refined sugar, especially sucrose, and aspartame in causing hyperactivity and behavioral problems. Proposed mechanisms include a raised blood sugar shortly after ingestion, hypoglycemia late after ingestion, or an allergic response to sucrose. It has been suggested that metabolism of aspartame to phenylalanine may alter amino acid transport into the brain. However, in a recent double-blind controlled trial 25 normal preschool children and 23 school-aged children were fed a different diet for three separate 3-week periods. These diets had a high sucrose content but no artificial sweeteners, a low sucrose content but containing aspartame, or a diet low in sucrose but sweetened with saccharin. No difference in activity or behavior between the groups was observed (16).

Diabetes Mellitus

RECOMMENDATIONS FOR DIETARY INTAKE AND FAT CONSUMPTION

The current American Diabetes Association nutrition guidelines for diabetic patients are similar to the current health promotion recommendations for the general population discussed earlier (17). The recommendations have departed from those previously put forward in the "diabetic diet." Logically this makes sense, since just as no one drug treatment regimen is applicable to all diabetic patients, neither is there one dietary recommendation that fits all. Obese patients are encouraged to lose weight and limit their intake of fat, especially saturated fat, and carbohydrate. Polyunsaturated fats or ideally monounsaturated fats are to be used in place of saturated fats. A recent small study reported that the composition of atherosclerotic plaques closely mirrors dietary fat intake, as has been previously demonstrated for adipose tissue (18). As polyunsaturated fatty acids are easily oxidized, this may lead to an increase rather than a decrease in cardiovascular disease. Monounsaturated fatty acids may be preferred, as they resist such oxidation. They appear to have no adverse effects on serum LDL cholesterol as has been observed with high-carbohydrate diets, which adversely affect triglycerides, very low density lipoproteins, and high density lipoproteins (19).

RECOMMENDATIONS FOR CARBOHYDRATE INTAKE

The concern that absorption of simple sugars is more rapid and thereby detrimental for the diabetic patient than the absorption from complex carbohydrates may be unfounded. A more fundamental approach appears to be evaluation of the total carbohydrate intake rather than the source. The new guidelines report no evidence that alternative sweeteners such as honey, corn syrup, fruit juice, sugar alcohols, or molasses have any advantage over sucrose in terms of limiting calorie intake or improvement in diabetic control.

RECOMMENDATIONS FOR PROTEIN INTAKE

The guidelines have moved away from defining the diet in terms of percentages of nutrients, except for protein, which is recommended to be between 10 and 20% of the daily intake. The issue relating to protein restriction in the diabetic population remains controversial. Diabetic nephropathy, which is present in 35% of insulin-dependent diabetic patients and 5 to 10% of patients with non-insulin-dependent diabetes mellitus may be reduced by protein restriction in the early phase of the incipient nephropathic process (20). However, in a large study with a mean follow-up period of 2.2 years, 840 patients with various chronic renal diseases were randomized to different dietary protein intakes. Five hundred and fifty-five patients with moderate renal impairment (GFR of 25 to 55 mL per minute) showed only limited benefit. This was manifested as a slower decline of renal function, 4 months after receiving a low-protein diet (0.58 g protein/kg/day), when compared to patients receiving a usual protein intake of 1.3 g/kg/day. In 255 patients with more severe renal impairment (GFR 13-24 mL/min) randomized to receive either a low-protein diet or a very low-protein diet (0.28 g/kg/day), no significant slowing in the progression of renal disease was observed (21). Others have proposed that protein restriction in diabetic patients may be detrimental, leading to protein malnutrition. It has been suggested that they may have increased catabolism, leading to increased rather than decreased requirements when compared to the normal population.

Geriatrics

Early in the next century 20% of Americans will be over the age of 65 years. Malnutrition in the elderly is a recognized problem caused by a variety of factors (Table 10.2). Polypharmacy is common in this population, as many elderly take both prescribed and OTC medications for chronic illness. For this reason, clinicians should be aware of the potential for drug-nutrient interactions, which may lead to deficiency of a particular nutrient or generalized weight loss due to inadequate food intake associated with medication use (22).

NUTRITION SCREENING INITIATIVE

Recognition of the problem of malnutrition in the elderly led to a national collaborative approach that developed a life-style screening tool, the Nutrition Screening Initiative Checklist (Fig. 10.2), to be used to identify elderly persons

Table 10.2.
Possible Causes of Malnutrition in the Elderly

A. Decreased intake:
  Problems with chewing and swallowing
  Poor dentition
  Dementia
  Depression, causing decreased interest in food
  Social isolation
  Lack of mobility, causing difficulty with shopping
  Poverty
B. Decreased absorption:
  Bowel surgery
  Malabsorption syndromes (e.g., lactose intolerance, atrophic gastritis)
C. Increased Requirements:
  Infection
  Inflammation
  Trauma
D. Drug Therapy:
  Drug-nutrient interactions
  Gastrointestinal side effects of medications (e.g., nausea, vomiting, diarrhea, constipation)
  Alterations in taste perception
  Difficulty swallowing due to dry mouth
  Central nervous system effects (e.g., sedation, confusion)

at risk for low nutrient intake (23). The best predictors of perceived poor health were taking three or more drugs per day and having changed one's diet because of illness. Lack of money, eating fewer than two meals per day, and not eating many fruits or vegetables were the strongest predictors of inadequate nutrient intake.

*ALTERATIONS IN NUTRIENT REQUIREMENTS
ASSOCIATED WITH AGING*

Digestion and absorption of most nutrients is qualitatively unaffected by aging. Although these functions are somewhat reduced, the capacity of the gastrointestinal tract is sufficient for this not to be significant (24). A more controversial area is the proposed alteration in micronutrient requirements for persons over 50 years. There is evidence that absorption of B12 may be impaired in the elderly due to atrophic gastritis and that achlorhydria may be present in 30 to 40% of this population. Elevated homocysteine levels associated with subclinical B12, B6, and folate deficiency may be implicated in the etiology of vascular disease and neuropsychiatric disorders including presenile dementia (25–27).

The elderly are also known to have lower levels of the active form of vitamin D, 1,25-dihydroxy vitamin D3. This may be due to a combination of factors, including low-level exposure to sunlight, reduced intake of dairy products, and decreased synthesis of active vitamin D by the kidney following parathyroid hormone stimulation. It has been proposed that the current RDI for vitamin D is too low to maintain bone health and that in elderly people not

exposed to sunlight, administration of a low-dose supplement is warranted. It has also been suggested that the current recommendations for vitamin A intake in the elderly are too high, possibly due to increased absorption from the gastrointestinal tract or decreased clearance in the liver of retinyl esters from chylomicron remnants (28).

Elderly individuals having a dietary intake of <125 mg/day of vitamin C were reported to have a fourfold increase in the incidence of cataracts when compared to those receiving 500 mg/day (29, 30). However, a dietary intake of vitamin C around 100 to 200 mg/day appears to be sufficient to saturate body stores. Vitamin E supplementation in short-term studies (3 months) has been shown to improve immune function in the elderly, though any long-term benefit from chronic supplementation has yet to be demonstrated (31).

Studies have suggested that in the oldest old (>85 years) exercise is important in maintaining or improving muscle strength, whereas the use of a multinutrient supplement in individuals with a nutritionally adequate diet provided no additional benefit (32).

RECOMMENDATIONS FOR SPECIFIC NUTRIENTS

The purpose of this section is to address some of the issues and controversies relating to particular nutrients and the proposed therapeutic benefits associated with their intake.

Dietary Fiber

The average daily intake of dietary fiber in most adults is around 11 grams per day. However current recommendations for normal healthy individuals suggest the intake should be between 10 and 17 grams per 1000 kilocalories or 20 to 35 grams per day. The majority of people find this level of fiber intake to be unpalatable. Some of the common problems, such as abdominal distension and gas, can be reduced by increasing intake over a period of 4 to 6 weeks. Evidence that fiber interferes with drug absorption is limited, but there may be reduced absorption of calcium, magnesium, zinc, and iron (33, 34). Dietary fiber may be defined as water insoluble, for example, the cellulosic polysaccharides lignin and cellulose, or water soluble, noncellulosic polysaccharides including pectins, gums, and mucilages. Each type of fiber has differing effects on gastrointestinal motility and function. Soluble fibers are fermented by colonic microflora, mainly in the cecum, to short-chain fatty acids, namely acetic, propionic, and butyric acids. These are important fuels for the colonic enterocyte and promote water and electrolyte absorption. Soluble fibers have been shown to delay gastric emptying and slow small intestinal transit time. This can be useful in reducing postprandial blood glucose concentrations, for example, in patients with dumping syndrome. The ability of the viscous gel matrix formed from soluble fibers such as guar gum, oat bran, and psyllium to bind bile acids and

The Warning Signs of poor nutritional health are often overlooked. Use this checklist to find out if you or someone you know is at nutritional risk.

Read the statements below. Circle the number in the yes column for those that apply to you or someone you know. For each yes answer, score the number in the box. Total your nutritional score.

DETERMINE YOUR NUTRITIONAL HEALTH

	YES
I have an illness or condition that made me change the kind and/or amount of food I eat.	2
I eat fewer than 2 meals per day.	3
I eat few fruits or vegetables, or milk products.	2
I have 3 or more drinks of beer, liquor or wine almost every day.	2
I have tooth or mouth problems that make it hard for me to eat.	2
I don't always have enough money to buy the food I need.	4
I eat alone most of the time.	1
I take 3 or more different prescribed or over-the-counter drugs a day.	1
Without wanting to, I have lost or gained 10 pounds in the last 6 months.	2
I am not always physically able to shop, cook and/or feed myself.	2
TOTAL	

Total Your Nutritional Score. If it's—

0–2   **Good!** Recheck your nutritional score in 6 months.

3-5   **You are at moderate nutritional risk.** See what can be done to improve your eating habits and lifestyle. Your office on aging, senior nutrition program, senior citizens center or health department can help. Recheck your nutritional score in 3 months.

8 or more   **You are at high nutritional risk.** Bring this checklist the next time you see your doctor, dietitian or other qualified health or social service professional. Talk with them about any problems you may have. Ask for help to improve your nutritional health.

These materials developed and distributed by the Nutrition Screening Initiative, a project of:

AMERICAN ACADEMY OF FAMILY PHYSICIANS

THE AMERICAN DIETETIC ASSOCIATION

NATIONAL COUNCIL ON THE AGING, INC.

Remember that warning signs suggest risk, but do not represent diagnosis of any condition. Turn the page to learn more about the Warning Signs of poor nutritional health.

Source. Reprinted with permission from the Nutrition Screening Initiative, Washington, DC (a project of the American Academy of Family Physicians, the American Dietetic Association, and the National Council on Aging, and funded in part by Ross Laboratories).

Figure 10.2. Revised Nutrition Screening Initiative Checklist. (Reprinted with permission from the Nutrition Screening Initiative, Washington, DC, a project of the American Academy of Family Physicians, The American Dietetic Association, and the National Council on Aging, and funded in part by Ross Laboratories.)

cholesterol may explain their cholesterol lowering properties. Insoluble fibers are less susceptible to degradation and due to their water retaining properties act to increase fecal bulk, leading to decreased colonic transit time and stimulation of the defecation reflex.

Cholesterol

A summary of the nutritional recommendations and identification of adults considered at high cardiovascular risk who may benefit from blood cholesterol management (35) is presented in Table 10.3. Positive risk factors for cardiovascular disease which have been identified include males over 45 years, females over 55 years or with untreated premature menopause, a family history of coronary heart disease, smoking, untreated hypertension, HDL levels below 35 mg/dL, and diabetes mellitus. Negative risk factors, which can be used to discount against any positive factors, include a HDL levels above 60 mg/dL, males under 35 years, premenopausal females, and postmenopausal females on estrogen therapy. In line with national guidelines discussed earlier, promotion of a diet low in saturated fat and cholesterol is warranted. Some

Table 10.3.
Recommendations for Management of High Blood Cholesterol in Adults

1. Low density lipoproteins (LDLs) identified as the primary target of cholesterol lowering therapy. Dietary intervention is recommended for patients without CHD and with < 2 risk factors° at LDL > 160 mg/dL, for patients without CHD but > 2 risk factors at LDL > 130 mg/dL, and for patients with CHD at LDL > 100 mg/dL.
2. Patients with prior history of atherosclerotic disease identified as highest risk. A lower target level of LDL cholesterol (100 mg/dL) has been established in this group.
3. Delay drug therapy in young adult men (< 35 years) and premenopausal women with moderately high LDL cholesterol (160–220 mg/dL) but no other risk factors.
4. Age: Men > 45 years and women > 55 years identified as a cardiovascular risk factor.
5. High-risk postmenopausal women and high-risk elderly in otherwise good health are candidates for cholesterol lowering therapy.
6. High HDL cholesterol (> 60 mg/dL) designated as a negative risk factor to be discounted against positive risk factors.
7. Emphasis on exercise and weight loss as part of dietary therapy.

°Risk factors defined in text.

consumers may seek advice regarding alternative approaches to cholesterol management, for example, the use of garlic as a cholesterol lowering agent. Data from a meta-analysis of controlled trials to reduce hypercholesterolemia showed that one half to one clove of garlic per day reduced total serum cholesterol levels by about 9% (36).

Calcium Supplements and Osteoporosis

Osteoporosis is characterized by a reduction in bone mineral density. The majority of white women are at risk of sustaining osteoporosis-related fractures, especially of the wrist, hip and spine. There is wide intraindividual variation in bone mineral density, as it is influenced by many dietary and life-style factors. To minimize fracture risk, young women should have regular menses, consume a nutritionally adequate diet, perform regular physical activity, only consume a moderate amount of alcohol, if any, and not smoke. The RDI for calcium for females between 11 and 24 years is 1200 to 1500 mg/day (37). As estrogen has a recognized protective effect, postmenopausal women should seriously consider estrogen replacement therapy (38). In the absence of estrogen replacement, calcium intake should be 1.5 grams per day (39). Aloia et al. (40) reported a prospective controlled randomized study in which early postmenopausal women received 400 IU of vitamin D daily and placebo, 1700 mg of calcium per day in divided doses, or 1700 mg of calcium and hormonal replacement therapy. They concluded that although less effective than calcium with hormonal replacement therapy, calcium alone significantly retarded bone loss and improved calcium balance. Calcium supplementation has also

been reported to be of value in reducing the risk of hip fractures and other nonvertebral fractures in healthy, elderly (mean age 84 years), ambulatory women. In this latter study, participants were randomized to receive placebo or 1200 mg of elemental calcium (as tricalcium phosphate) and 800 units (20 µg) per day of vitamin D3 (cholecalciferol) for an 18-month period (41).

Optimum calcium intake is best obtained from dietary sources; however, in practice an intake of 1200 to 1500 mg/day is difficult to achieve without supplements. Particular attention should be paid to vegetarians, as 70% of dietary calcium in the United States population comes from dairy products. Lactovegetarians have not been found to differ from omnivores in their risk for osteoporosis. However, vegans should be encouraged to take supplements, calcium fortified juices, or soy milk to meet the required daily intake (42). The solubility of different calcium salts is not a major determinant of absorbability, but absorption is increased if the supplements are taken with protein, lactose, vitamin D, and acidic foods, and in divided doses (43). Absorption is decreased by oxalate containing foods such as cocoa, spinach, kale, unpolished rice, wheat bran, and alkaline foods. Numerous calcium supplements are available as OTC products. Prior to advising individuals to take regular calcium supplements, clinicians must ensure there are no contraindications or drug interactions. Constipation is a common complaint of patients taking chronic calcium therapy of around 2400 mg/day. Calcium supplementation may cause problems with renal stone formation, arrhythmias or milk-alkali syndrome if renal function is compromised and doses are excessive (i.e., greater than 5-6 g/day).

Some authors have suggested that osteoporosis may be in part due to a long-term acid load imposed by the diet that is partially buffered by bases derived from bone. If this is borne out in larger, longer-term studies, supplementation of the diet with potassium bicarbonate may be beneficial in reducing osteoporosis (44).

Vitamins

Approximately 25% of all United States adults use vitamin supplements on a daily basis, and up to 50% use them to some extent. Pharmacists have been criticized for promoting supplements or at least passively advising consumers about the appropriate use of vitamin, mineral and nutritional supplements. Supplements are unnecessary for the majority of individuals taking a nutritionally adequate diet. However, certain groups, for example, the elderly, pregnant or lactating women, strict vegetarians, and those on very low-calorie diets, may benefit (45).

Megadose vitamin therapy is defined as treatment with one or more vitamins in amounts ten or more times the RDI. Vitamins are essential nutrients for which the human body has a minimum requirement; exceeding that require-

Table 10.4.
Toxicities Associated with Chronic Megadoses of Vitamins

Vitamin	Estmated Minimum Toxic Oral Dose	Possible Toxic Effect
Vitamin C	1000–5000 mg	Oxalate stones due to acidification of the urine (also, oxalate is a urinary metabolite of ascorbate teratogenesis + carcinogenesis), diarrhea
Vitamin B3	1000 mg	Peptic ulcer, alopecia, hepatotoxicity, pruritus, arrhythmias, hypotension
Vitamin B6	2000 mg	Neuropathies, ataxia, fatigue, depression
Vitamin B1	300 mg	Headache, irritability, insomnia, rapid pulse, weakness
Folic acid	400 mg	Diarrhea, sleep disturbance, hyperactivity, irritability
Vitamin A	25,000–50,000 IU	Hepatotoxicity, elevated intracranial pressure, alopecia, bone tenderness, birth defects. Skin changes: dryness, maculopapular rash, fissures, depigmentation, pruritus
Vitamin D	50,000 IU	Hypertension, anorexia, hypercalcemia
Vitamin E	1200 IU	Thrombophlebitis, pulmonary embolism, hypertension, hypertriglyceridemia, gynecomastia
Vitamin K	—	Hemolytic anemia, neonatal jaundice

ment is unlikely to provide additional benefit and may do harm. Megadoses of water soluble vitamins, even though they are readily excreted, may lead to toxicity. Some of the toxic effects associated with chronic megadoses of vitamins are presented in Table 10.4 (46).

Though there is no supportive evidence, megadoses of vitamins have been promoted to persons with HIV infection (47). These individuals may be susceptible, due to the weight loss and debilitation that are commonly associated with later stages of the disease, to claims made by fad diets suggesting improved immune resistance. Some commonly promoted diets of this type include "Weiner's Maximum Immunity Diet"; "Dr Berger's Immune Power Diet"; "Yeast Free Diets"; and "Macrobiotic diets" (48).

ERGOGENIC AIDS AND NUTRITIONAL SUPPLEMENTS IN SPORTS MEDICINE

Ergogenic aids in the form of nutritional supplements in sports and exercise are promoted as methods of enhancing athletic performance. The nutritional supplement market directed at amateur and professional athletes has been estimated to be on the order of billions of dollars. Some are suggested to promote weight loss or alter body composition by increasing lean body mass, for example, γ-oryzanol/ferulate and chromium (49). Multivitamin and mineral supplements are for the most part promoted to enhance metabolic efficiency. While a balanced diet should be adequate to provide most athletes' needs, nutritional supplements are often used in an attempt to gain a competitive advantage (50). However, lack of nutritional knowledge among athletes and coaches may lead to misconceptions regarding performance enhancement by diet and nutritional supplements (51). This is further promulgated by prominent advertisement campaigns for these supplements in body building magazines and their

widespread availability through mail order and retail stores. Some examples of the nutritional supplements that are commonly available are presented in Table 10.5.

A survey of advertisements in 12 health and body building magazines found 89 brands, 311 products, and 235 unique ingredients, the most frequent of which were unspecified amino acids primarily promoted for improving muscle growth (52). In a second study, which included 624 products from 33 companies, over 800 performance claims were identified that were unsupported by published research. Claims were found to be based on extrapolation of data from animal models, in vitro data, or epidemiologic studies (53). The majority of the studies that involve evaluation of ergogenic aids are flawed. Design problems include inadequate sample size, lack of appropriate control groups or control of nutrient intake, poorly designed training programs, and lack of proper analytic measures and control for possible placebo effects. Such deficiencies make the drawing of definitive conclusions difficult or impossible.

Protein Supplements

Under normal circumstances dietary protein provides the amino acids needed for energy production and muscle protein synthesis. There is a constant turnover of protein in the body, resulting in a daily loss of nitrogen in the form of urea and amino acids. When protein intake is excessive, there is increased formation of urea, which is excreted in urine and sweat, and enhanced gluconeogenesis, or conversion of the carbon skeleton, to fat and glycogen stores. The increase in the use of protein for energy during exercise is small. Only during strenuous endurance training has it been shown that athletes require more protein, accounting for 5 to 10% of energy production. The amount of excess protein in the average American diet is usually

Table 10.5.
Ergogenic Aids and Nutritional Supplements Promoted to Enhance Athletic Performance

Categories	Claims
Protein supplements	Improved lean body mass
Medium chain triglycerides	Increased energy and lean body mass due to easier absorption and oxidation than long chain triglycerides
Arginine	Increased growth hormone release leading to increased muscle mass
Inosine	Improved endurance by reduction of glycogen breakdown, vasodilation, and improved oxygen delivery to muscle
Carnitine	Improved endurance and fuel utilization by improving fatty acid transport into mitachondria for oxidation
Choline	Improved endurance and reduced body fat by improving incorporation of lipids into cell membranes and lipoproteins
Vitamins	Improved metabolic efficiency through activity as coenzymes, beneficial antioxidant effects to improve aerobic capacity
Minerals	
Chromium	Improved glucose utilization
Phosphate	Improved endurance due to its incorporation into high energy phosphate components
Boron	Increased weight and muscle gain due to increased testosterone

more than enough to cover this increase. Studies in long distance runners have documented that protein requirements are elevated 50 to 100% above the RDI during the first month of increased workload. Therefore, approximately 1.2 to 1.4 g/kg/day should result in a positive nitrogen balance, but it is unclear whether high protein intakes will actually improve endurance (54). The effect of protein loading on muscle mass and strength is less defined, and additional research is necessary before conclusions can be made. While protein intake can be increased by increasing overall food intake, particularly of foods containing high amounts of protein, this may lead to an unwanted increase in caloric intake for the individual. For this reason protein supplements in the form of protein hydrolysates and food-grade L-amino acids have become popular in the body building community. Nevertheless there remains no documented improvement in performance or muscle size or strength associated with the use of these supplements in normally nourished persons.

Arginine

Arginine is an amino acid that is known to have an effect on several physiologic functions important to exercise metabolism. Most notable is the increase in growth hormone concentrations observed after oral administration of l-ornithine, a precursor of arginine, at doses of 40, 100 or 170 mg/kg in body builders. An acute rise in growth hormone was noted 90 minutes after ingestion of the supplement. However, extrapolation of these findings to the effects on lean body mass and fat stores is difficult (18). The rate of creatine production, an energy source for muscle tissue, has been shown to increase with arginine supplementation, but the relatively small increase in creatine level may not be enough to affect exercise performance. Thus far, arginine supplementation at 2 to 10 g/day as an ergogenic agent appears promising, but

definitive conclusions are speculative until additional research is performed.

Carnitine

L-Carnitine is a nonessential amino acid synthesized in vivo from methionine and lysine. Its principal metabolic function is involved with the transport of long-chain fatty acids into the mitochondria, where they are oxidized (55). L-Carnitine is particularly important in skeletal muscle and the myocardium, which obtain their primary energy source from fatty acid oxidation. Several studies have been conducted in athletes to evaluate the effect of carnitine on performance and metabolic function but have been inconsistent in their results. Similar difficulties exist as described earlier regarding poor study design (56). At the present time L-carnitine supplementation does not appear to be warranted in this setting.

Vitamins/Minerals

Exercise has been shown to increase the need for certain vitamins and minerals, especially water soluble vitamins. However, studies in endurance athletes, who typically consume 1.5 to 3 times the average person's nutrient intake, from a variety of foods, suggest that their intake of vitamins whose requirement is related to energy intake should be adequate (57). At least two well-designed studies demonstrate the lack of effect on physical performance by multivitamin and mineral supplements (58, 59).

Vitamins are commonly taken singly in an attempt to affect more specific functions. One study in college age men showed that Vitamin B6 is not easily depleted in skeletal muscle and that supplementation does not significantly increase levels (60). Harmful effects have also been shown with vitamin B6 supplementation. Over a 2- to 40-month period, severe sensory nervous system dysfunction was seen in subjects self-dosing with between 2 and 6 grams (61). The dysfunction was not always reversed when the supplementation ceased.

Chromium

Chromium has been generally recognized for its ability to facilitate the insulin-tissue interaction, thereby decreasing the amount of insulin needed for glucose uptake by the tissues. In addition, chromium picolinate supplementation has been found to decrease serum cholesterol concentrations. Chromium is therefore often promoted as an ergogenic aid that will enhance metabolism, increase muscle, and decrease body fat. The amount of chromium in a typical U.S. diet is less than the estimated safe and adequate intake of 50 to 200 µg/dL. Following exercise, it has been shown that the serum chromium concentration is elevated and urinary chromium excretion increases significantly (62). This indicates that athletes may have a greater need for chromium in their diet. However, the benefits of chromium supplementation on athletic performance have yet to be documented.

Inosine

Inosine is used to synthesize adenosine nucleotides and is a precursor for the synthesis of adenosine triphosphate (ATP). ATP is the immediate energy source for muscle contraction. As a supplement, inosine is promoted as an energy enhancer and an aid to endurance, recuperation, and strength by promoting vasodilation, and oxygen availability to muscles by increasing 2,3-diphospho-glycerate (2,3-DPG) in red blood cells. One investigation has reported the lack of these effects finding no increases in 2,3-DPG in red blood cells, and no changes on time to exhaustion or treadmill performance (63). Excess inosine is not converted to adenosine nucleotidase but is metabolized by the enzyme xanthine oxidase to uric acid, contributing to gout in susceptible individuals. Xanthine oxidase is present in muscle tissue and generates free radicals, which are associated with fatigue during exercise. For these reasons inosine supplementation may be more detrimental than helpful for the enhancement of athletic performance (49).

In summary, there is little to support the use of nutritional ergogenic supplements to enhance athletic performance. While short-term use of these supplements is unlikely to be harmful, when the opportunity arises health practitioners should educate athletes and their coaches of basic nutritional concepts and the role of diet over unproven supplements.

ANTIOXIDANT NUTRIENTS

Antioxidant nutrients, β-carotene, vitamin E, vitamin C, and selenium, have been proposed to have a role in the prevention of cancer and cardiovascular disease. Support for this hypothesis comes primarily from animal studies and epidemiologic data. In cardiovascular disease, the role of antioxidants may be to limit the oxidation of LDL cholesterol, which is then taken up by macrophages to form foam cells, which are characteristic of early atherogenic disease. In the cancer model, it has been suggested that antioxidants act via a scavenging mechanism to prevent DNA damage by free radicals.

Cardiovascular Disease

Two large-scale studies, the Nurses Health Study (64) and the Health Professionals Follow Up Study (65), reported an inverse association between higher vitamin E (α-tocopherol) consumption and cardiovascular risk. The reduction in risk was only apparent after 2 to 4 years of taking supplements. However, in both groups the risk reduction was confined to a subgroup taking supplements. The maximum reduction in men was seen in those taking 100 to 249 IU per day. The authors suggested the lack of benefit seen with dietary vitamin E intake alone is consistent with experimental evidence, which suggests that resistance of LDL cholesterol to oxidation is only achieved at levels of vitamin E which are 10 to 100 times the RDI. In the same study no reduction in cardiovascular risk was associated with high intakes of vitamin C. β-Carotene intake was associated with a decreased risk of cardiovascular disease in former and current smokers but not in those who had never smoked. Despite the large numbers of individuals followed in these studies, it is difficult to interpret these types of epidemiologic data due to the multivariate nature of the population. In the absence of large, long-term controlled clinical trials of antioxidant supplementation to reduce cardiovascular risk that address both efficacy and toxicity, regular vitamin supplementation in healthy individuals cannot be supported at the present time (66).

Cancer Prevention

Data regarding the protective role of antioxidants in carcinogenesis and treatment of a variety of tumor types is also conflicting. Many studies that suggest potential benefit are also based on animal models or epidemiologic data showing lower levels of β-carotene, vitamins E and C, or selenium in patients with cancer compared to healthy controls (67). Extrapolation of these data and interpretations of single studies, regardless of their individual merit, to a policy that advocates routine supplementation is difficult. A good example comes from the controversial data reported from the Finnish Alpha Tocopherol, Beta Carotene (ATBC) Cancer Prevention Study, which evaluated the effect of vitamin E and β-carotene on the incidence primarily of lung cancer in male smokers (68). The study involved 29,000 middle aged male smokers randomly assigned to receive dietary supplementation with β-carotene (20 mg/day), α-tocopherol (50 mg/day), both, or placebo. Patients who received β-carotene had a higher incidence of lung cancer than those who did not. Patients who received α-tocopherol had no significant difference in the incidence of lung cancer. There were fewer cases of prostate cancer but an increased number of hemorrhagic strokes. Possible explanations are that these findings may have been due to chance, that the dose of vitamin E was too low to affect tumor development, or that, since the median duration of the study was 6 years, this was too short a time to provide protection against a carcinogenic process that may have been initiated decades earlier.

Further evidence for a conservative approach was reported by the Polyp Prevention Study Group. In a prospective randomized double-blind trial conducted over a 4-year period, 864 patients who had removal of a colonic adenoma received either β-carotene (25 mg/day), vitamin C (1 g/day), vitamin E (400 mg/day), or all three vitamins. In the 751 patients who completed the study there was no evidence that any of the vitamins alone or in combination reduced the incidence of new adenomas (69).

Vitamin C has an antioxidant role at levels normally obtained from the diet; however, larger doses (>500 mg/day) achieved with supplements may be harmful, acting as a pro-oxidant, particularly in the presence of iron (70). A number of studies have suggested that vitamin C plays a role in wound healing, the immune response, and protection from cancer, cataract prevention, and cholesterol metabolism. However, large intervention studies are also needed before supplements can be recommended (71). While it is tempting to recommend antioxidant supplements on the basis of possible beneficial effects and relative lack of toxicity, especially in those individuals with risk factors for cardiovascular disease and cancer, the data are unsupportive at this time (72).

CONCLUSION

Clinicians in all settings should take the opportunity to participate in preventive health care by promoting healthy dietary intake, exercise, and lifestyle to individual patients. Knowledge of the literature regarding specific patient groups should enable the pharmacist to make appropriate recommendations and provide improved pharmaceutical care.

REFERENCES

1. Harper AE. Recommended dietary intakes: current approaches and future directions. In Shils ME, Olson JA, Shike M, eds. Modern nutrition in health and disease, 8th ed. Philadelphia: Lea & Febiger, 1994:1475.
2. USDA's Food Guide Pyramid. Home and garden bulletin no. 249. Washington DC: U.S. Department of Agriculture, 1992.
3. Dietary Guidelines for Americans. USDA home and garden bulletin no. 232R, 3rd ed. Washington DC: Government Printing Office 1990:272–930).
4. Healthy People 2000: National health promotion and disease prevention objectives. DHHS publication no. (PHS) 91–50212. Washington, DC: U.S. Department of Health and Human Services, 1990.
5. Havas S, Heimendinger J, Reynolds K, et al. 5-A-Day for better health: a new research initiative. J Am Diet Assoc 94:32–36, 1994.
6. Mueller C, Nestle M. Regulation of medical foods: toward a rational policy. Nutr Clin Pract 10:8–15, 1995.
7. Czeizel AE, Dudas I. Prevention of the first occurence of neural tube defects by peri conceptional vitamin supplementation. N Engl J Med 327:1832–1835, 1992.
8. Wald NJ, Bower C. Folic acid, pernicious anaemia and prevention of neural tube defects. Lancet 343:307, 1994.
9. Zimmerman MB, Shane B. Supplemental folic acid. Am J Clin Nutr 58:127–128, 1993.
10. Jacobus CH, Holick MF, Shao Q, Chen TC, Holm IA, Kolodny JM, El Hajj Fuleihan G, Seely E. Hypervitaminosis D associated with drinking milk. N Engl J Med 326:1173–1177, 1992.
11. Holick MF, Qing Shao, Liu WW, Chen TC. The vitamin D content of fortified milk and infant formula. N Engl J Med 326:1178–1181, 1992.
12. Golding J, Greenwood R, Birmingham K, Mott M. Childhood cancer, intramuscular vitamin K and pethidine given during labour. Br Med J 305:341–346, 1992.
13. Klebanoff MA, Read JS, Mills JL, Shiono PH. The risk of childhood cancer after neonatal exposure to vitamin K. N Engl J Med 329:905–908, 1993.
14. Olsen JH, Hertz H, Blinkenberg K, Verder H. Vitamin K regimens and the incidence of childhood cancer in Denmark. Br Med J 308:895–896, 1994.
15. Draper G, McNinch A. Vitamin K for neonates: the controversy. Br Med J 308:867–868, 1994.
16. Wolraich ML, Lindgren SD, Stumbo PJ, Stegink LD, Appelbaum MI, Kiritsy MC. Effects of diets high in sucrose or aspartame on the behavior and cognitive performance of children. N Engl J Med 330:301–307, 1994.
17. American Dietetic Association. Nutrition recommendations and principles for people with diabetes mellitus. Diabetes Care 18(1): 16–19, 1995.
18. Felton CV, Crook D, Davies MJ, Oliver MF. Dietary polyunsaturated fatty acids and composition of human aortic plaques. Lancet 344:1195–1196, 1994.
19. Franz MJ. How enthusiastically should the use of monounsaturated fats be encouraged? Diabetes Educ 15(6):494–497, 1989.
20. Carella MJ, Gossain VV, Rovner DR. Early diabetic nephropathy. Emerging treatment options. Arch Intern Med 154(6):625–630, 1994.
21. Klahr S, Levey AS, Beck GJ, et al. The effect of dietary protein restriction and blood pressure control on the progression of renal disease. Modification of diet in renal disease study group. N Engl J Med 330(13):877–884, 1994.
22. Varma RN. Risk for drug induced malnutrition is unchecked in elderly patients in nursing homes. J Am Diet Assoc 94:192–194, 1994.
23. Posner BM, Jeete AM, Smith KW, Miller DR. Nutrition and health risks in the elderly: the nutrition screening initiative. Am J Public Health 83:972–978, 1993.
24. Hosoda S, Bamba T, Nakago S, Fujiyma Y, Senda S, Hirata M. Age related changes in the gastrointestinal tract. Nutr Rev 50:374–377, 1992.
25. Selhub J, Jacques PF, Wilson PWF, Rush D, Rosenberg IH. Vitamin status and intake as primary determinants of homocysteinemia in an elderly population. JAMA 270:2693–2698, 1993.
26. Pancharuniti N, Lewis CA, Sauberlich HE, et al. Plasma homocyst(e)ine, folate and vitamin B12 concentrations and risks for early onset coronary artery disease. Am J Clin Nutr 59:940–948, 1994.

27. Lindenbaum J, Healton EB, Savage DG, et al. Neuropsychiatric disorders caused by cobalamin deficiency in the absence of anemia or macrocytosis. N Engl J Med 318:1720–1728, 1988.

28. Russell RM, Suter PM. Vitamin requirements of elderly people: an update. Am J Clin Nutr 58:4–14, 1993.

29. Jacques PF, Chylack LT. Epidemiologic evidence of a role for the antioxidant vitamins and carotenoids in cataract prevention. Am J Clin Nutr 53:352s–355s, 1991.

30. Kneckt P, Heliovaara M, Rissanen A, Aromaa A, Aaran RK. Serum antioxidant vitamins and risk of cataract. Br Med J 305:1392–1394, 1992.

31. Russell RM. Micronutrient requirements of the elderly. Nutrition Rev 50:463–466, 1992.

32. Fiatarone MA, O Neill EF, Doyle Ryan N, Clements K, Solares GR, Nelson ME, Roberts SB, Kehayias JJ, Lipsitz LA, Evans WJ. Exercise training and nutritional supplementation for physical frailty in very elderly people. N Engl J Med 330:1769–1775, 1994.

33. Hunt R, Fedorak R, Frohlich J, McLennan C, Pavilanis A. Therapeutic role of dietary fibre. Can Fam Physician 39:897–910, 1993.

34. Koruda MJ. Dietary fiber and gastrointestinal disease. Surg Gynecol Obstet 177:209–214, 1993.

35. Expert Panel on Detection, Evaluation and Treatment of High Blood Cholesterol in Adults. Summary of the second report of the National Cholesterol Education Program (NCEP) Adult Treatment Panel LL. JAMA 269:3015–3023, 1993.

36. Warshafsky S, Kamer RS, Sivak SL. Effect of garlic on total serum cholesterol. Ann Intern Med 119:599–605, 1993.

37. NIH Consensus Development Panel on Optimal Calcium Intake. JAMA 272:1942–1948; 1994.

38. Wardlow GM. Putting osteoporosis into perspective. J Am Diet Assoc 93:1000–1006, 1993.

39. Recker RR. Current therapy for osteoporosis. J Clin Endocrin Metab 76:14–16, 1993.

40. Aloia JF, Vaswani A, Yeh JK, Ross PL, Flaster E, Dilmanian FA. Calcium supplementation with and without hormone replacement therapy to prevent postmenopausal bone loss. Ann Intern Med 120:97–103, 1994.

41. Chapuy MC, Arlot ME, Duboeuf F, Brun J, Crouzet B, Arnaud S, Delmas PD, Meunier PJ. Vitamin D3 calcium to prevent hip fractures in elderly women. N Engl J Med 327:1637–1642, 1992.

42. Weaver CM, Plawecki KL. Dietary calcium: adequacy of a vegetarian diet. Am J Clin Nutr 59:1238s–1241s, 1994.

43. Recker RR. Prevention of osteoporosis: calcium nutrition. Osteoporos Int 3(suppl 1):163–165, 1993.

44. Sebastian A, Harris ST, Ottaway JH, Todd KM, Morris RC. Improved mineral balance and skeletal metabolism in postmenopausal women treated with potassium bicarbonate. N Engl J Med 330:1776–1781, 1994.

45. O'Donnell JT. Nutrition fraud: vitamins and obesity-pharmacists' responsibilities. J Pharm Pract 1:131–149, 1988.

46. Bauernfeind JC. Nutrification of foods. In Shils ME, Olson JA, Shike M, eds. Modern nutrition in health and disease, 8th ed. Philadelphia: Lea & Febiger, 1994.

47. Gorbach SL, Knox TA, Roubenoff R. Interactions between nutrition and infection with the human immunodeficiency virus. Nutrition Rev 51:226–234, 1993.

48. Raiten DJ. Nutrition and HIV infection: a review and evaluation of the extent of the knowledge of the relationship between nutrition and HIV infection. Nutr Clin Pract 6:1s–94s, 1991.

49. Rosenbloom C, Millard–Stafford M, Lathrop J. Contemporary ergogenic aids used by strength/power athletes. J Am Diet Assoc 92:1264–1266, 1992.

50. Williams MH. Nutritional ergogenics: help or hype? J Am Diet Assoc 92:1213–1214, 1992.

51. Short SH, Marquart LF. Sports nutrition fraud. N Y State J Med 93:112–115, 1993.

52. Philen RM, Ortiz DI, Auerback SB, Falk H, et al. Survey of advertising for nutritional supplements in health and bodybuilding magazines. JAMA 268:1008–11, 1992.

53. Grunewald KK, Bailey RS. Commericaly marketed supplements for bodybuilding athletes. Sports Med 15:90–103, 1993.

54. Bucci LR. Nutrients as ergogenic aids for sports and exercise. Boca Raton, FL: CRC Press, 52:14–18, 1990.

55. Boehm KA, Helms RA, Christensen ML, Storm MC. Carnitine: a review for the pharmacy clinician. Hosp Pharm 2(8):843, 847–850, 1993.

56. Tonda ME, Hart LL. N, N Dimethylglycine and L-Carnitine as performance enhancers in athletes. Ann Pharmacother 26:935–937, 1992.

57. Singh A, Pelletier PA, Deuster PA. Dietary requirements for ultra endurance exercise. Sports Med 18(5):301–308, 1994.

58. Weight LM, Noakes TD, Labadarios D. Vitamin and mineral status of trained athletes including the effects of supplementation. Am J Clin Nutr 47:186–91, 1988.

59. Barnett DW, Conlee RK. The effects of a commercial dietary supplement on human performance. Am J Clin Nutr 40:586–90, 1984.

60. Guilland J, Penaranda T, Gallet C, et al. Vitamin status of young athletes including the effects of supplementation. Med Sci Sports Exerc 21:441–9, 1989.

61. Schaumburg H, Kaplan J, Windebank A, et al. Sensory neuropathy from pyridoxine abuse. N Engl J Med 309:445–8, 1983.

62. Clarkson PM. Nutritional ergogenic aids: chromium, exercise, and muscle mass. Int J Sport Nutr 1:289, 1991.

63. Williams MH, Kreider RB, Hunter DW, Somma CT, Shall LM, Woodhouse ML, Rokitski L. Effect of inosine supplementation on 3-mile treadmill run performance on VO2 peak. Med Sci Sports Exerc 22:517–522, 1990.

64. Stampfer MJ, Hennekens CH, Manson JE, Colditz GA, Rosner B, Willett WC. Vitamin E consumption and the risk of coronary disease in women. N Engl J Med 328:1444–1449, 1993.

65. Rimm EB, Stampfer MJ, Ascerio A, Giovannucci E, Colditz GA, Willett WC. Vitamin E consumption and the risk of coronary heart disease in men. N Engl J Med 328:1450–1456, 1993.

66. Steinberg D. Antioxidant vitamins and coronary heart disease. N Engl J Med 328:1487–1489, 1993.

67. Ozols RF. Chemoprevention of cancer. Curr Probl Cancer 18:1–69, 1994.

68. The ATBC Cancer Prevention Study Group. The effect of vitamin E and beta carotene on the incidence of lung cancer and other cancers in male smokers. N Engl J Med 330:1029–1035, 1994.

69. Greenberg ER, Baron JA, Tosteson TD, Freeman DH, Beck GJ, Bond JH, Colacchio TA, Coller JA, Frankl HD, Haile RW, Mandel JS, Nierenberg DW, Rothstein R, Snover DC, Stevens MM, Summers RW, van Stolk RU. A clinical trial of antioxidant vitamins to prevent colorectal adenoma. N Engl J Med 331:141–147, 1994.

70. Herbert V. The antioxidant supplement myth. Am J Clin Nutr 60:157–158, 1994.

71. Gershoff SN. Vitamin C: new roles, new requirements? Nutr Rev 51:313–326, 1993.

72. Voelker R. Recommendations for antioxidants: how much evidence is enough? JAMA 271(15):1148–1149, 1994.

CHAPTER 11

VITAMINS AND MINERALS

DIANE NYKAMP McCARTER and JOHN M. HOLBROOK

For several decades, the relationships between dietary insufficiencies and the occurrence of diseases such as scurvy, pellagra, and beriberi have been well known. More recently, researchers have discovered that a relationship exists between the maintenance of an optimal state of health and good nutritional practices. Proper nourishment improves the ability to learn, concentrate, participate in physical activities, and resist or overcome injury and disease. It is also critical to the prevention and management of heart disease, diabetes, hypertension, obesity, and other disorders.

The literature (both technical and lay) abounds with information about the use of nutrients to prevent or treat disorders. The public has become more concerned with nutrition, especially how good nutrition relates to self-care and wellness. People are also concerned with the amount of food they consume and the use of nutritional supplements. Controversy remains as to whether the U.S. Food and Drug Administration (FDA) has regulatory authority over vitamin supplement manufacturers who make unsubstantiated claims concerning the effectiveness of their products in the treatment or prevention of disease. This chapter focuses on the basic nutrients that the body requires for life.

VITAMINS

Vitamins are non-energy-producing organic substances that are essential in small amounts for the maintenance of normal metabolic functions. They are categorized into two groups: the fat-soluble vitamins—A, D, E, and K—and the water-soluble vitamins, B complex and C. All of the vitamins, with the exception of D, K, and biotin, must be supplied completely from dietary sources (1). The majority of vitamins are obtained from plant and animal sources with the exceptions of vitamin K and biotin, which are produced by microorganisms in the intestinal tract, and vitamin D, which is synthesized from cholesterol in the skin. The amount of vitamin K synthesized is sufficient to meet the body's needs, but some dietary supplementation of biotin is usually required. The amount of vitamin D produced in the skin may or may not be sufficient to meet the body's needs because its synthesis depends on exposure to ultraviolet light.

Vitamin Requirements

The recommended dietary allowance (RDA) is the nutritional standard that specifies the amounts and kinds of nutrients necessary to maintain a positive state of health. It is determined by the Food and Nutrition Board of the National Academy of Science National Research Council (NAS/NRC). The RDA has replaced the minimum daily requirement (MDR), since individual requirements vary due to sex, age, and physical condition (2). The RDA is believed to be adequate for known nutritional needs of healthy individuals. RDAs are not intended to cover therapeutic nutritional requirements in disease or other abnormal states. For example, extra allowances are needed for women during pregnancy and lactation, and allowances vary for age and sex as well.

The "official" listings of U. S. Recommended Daily Allowances (US-RDAs) differ from the RDA. US-RDAs serve as legal standards for nutritional labeling of products controlled by the U. S. Food and Drug Administration. Generally, they represent the higher value of the male or female RDA and are grouped into only four age categories instead of the usual six found with the RDAs. Table 11.1 lists vitamin and mineral RDA values for all age groups.

Vitamin Stability

In general, fat-soluble vitamins are not destroyed during cooking. However, water-soluble vitamins are easily dissolved in cooking water and may be destroyed through heating. Ascorbic acid (vitamin C) suffers the greatest loss in nutritive value through cooking. Riboflavin is only sparingly water soluble and is not removed as quickly (when cooked in water) as the other water-soluble vitamins. When meats are broiled or roasted, thiamin losses are 25% or less. Constant low-temperature cooking improves palatability of meat but decreases the nutritive value. Wilting of vegetables or dehydration of most foods results in considerable nutrient loss. Improper storage or dicing and cutting of fruits and vegetables prior to cooking in water also can result in vitamin loss. Fruits and vegetables should be consumed raw or cooked in a minimum amount of liquid to help retain their maximum vitamin content. Other vitamin-conserving cooking methods include steaming, microwaving, and stir frying (3). Steaming or microwaving

Table 11.1.
Recommended Dietary Allowances

RECOMMENDED DIETARY ALLOWANCES[1]

Age (years) or Condition	Weight[2] (kg)	Weight[2] (lb)	Height[2] (cm)	Height[2] (in)	Protein (g)	Vitamin A (μg RE[3])	Vitamin D (IU[4])	Vitamin E (IU[12])	Vitamin K (μg)	Ascorbic Acid (C) (mg)	Thiamine (B1) (mg)	Riboflavin (B2) (mg)	Niacin (B3) (mg)	Pyridoxine (B6) (mg)	Folate (μg)	Cyanocobalamin (B12) (μg)	Calcium (mg)	Phosphorus (mg)	Magnesium (mg)	Iron (mg)	Zinc (mg)	Iodine (μg)	Selenium (μg)
Infants																							
0.0–0.5	6	13	60	24	13	375	300	4	5	30	0.3	0.4	5	0.3	25	0.3	400	300	40	6	5	40	10
0.5	9	20	71	28	14	375	400	6	10	35	0.4	0.5	6	0.6	35	0.5	600	500	60	10	5	50	15
Children																							
1–8	13	29	90	35	16	400	400	9	15	40	0.7	0.8	9	1	50	0.7	800	800	80	10	10	70	20
4–6	20	44	112	44	24	500	400	10	20	45	0.9	1.1	12	1.1	75	1	800	800	120	10	10	90	20
7–10	28	62	132	52	28	700	400	10	30	45	1	1.2	13	1.4	100	1.4	800	800	170	10	10	120	30
Males																							
11–14	45	99	157	62	45	1000	400	15	45	50	1.3	1.5	17	1.7	150	2	1200	1200	270	12	15	150	40
15–18	66	145	176	69	59	1000	400	15	65	60	1.5	1.8	20	2	200	2	1200	1200	400	12	15	150	50
19–24	72	160	177	70	58	1000	400	15	70	60	1.5	1.7	19	2	200	2	1200	1200	350	10	15	150	70
25–50	79	174	176	70	63	1000	200	15	80	60	1.5	1.7	19	2	200	2	800	800	350	10	15	150	70
51+	77	170	173	68	63	1000	200	15	80	60	1.2	1.4	15	2	200	2	800	800	350	10	15	150	70
Females																							
11–14	46	101	157	62	46	800	400	12	45	50	1.1	1.3	15	1.4	150	2	1200	1200	280	15	12	150	45
15–18	55	120	163	64	44	800	400	12	55	60	1.1	1.3	15	1.5	180	2	1200	1200	300	15	12	150	50
19–24	58	128	164	65	46	800	400	12	60	60	1.1	1.3	15	1.6	180	2	1200	1200	280	15	12	150	55
25–50	63	138	163	64	50	800	200	12	60	60	1.1	1.3	15	1.6	180	2	800	800	280	15	12	150	55
51+	65	143	160	63	50	800	200	12	65	60	1	1.2	13	1.6	180	2	800	800	280	10	12	150	55
Pregnant					60	800	400	15	65	70	1.5	1.6	17	2.2	400	2.2	1200	1200	320	30	15	175	65
Lactating—1st 6 mo.					65	1300	400	18	65	95	1.6	1.8	20	2.1	280	2.6	1200	1200	355	15	19	200	75
2nd 6 mo.					62	1200	400	16	65	90	1.6	1.7	20	2.1	260	2.6	1200	1200	340	15	16	200	75

Reproduction from Recommended Dietary Allowances, 10th ed, 1989, National Academy of Sciences. National Academy Press, Washington, DC.

[1] The allowances, expressed as average daily intakes over time, are intended to provide for individual variations among most normal persons as they live in the US under usual environmental stresses. Diets should be based on a variety of common foods in order to provide other nutrients for which human requirements have been less well defined.

[2] Weights and heights of Reference Adults are actual medians for the U.S. population of the designated age, as reported by NHANES II. The median weights and heights of those under 19 years of age were taken from Hamill PV, et al. Am J Clin Nutr 32:607, 1979. The use of these figures does not imply that the height-to-weight ratios are ideal.

[3] Retinol equivalents. 1 retinol equivalent = 1 μg retinol or 6 μg β-carotene.

[4] As cholecalciferol. 10 μg cholecalciferol = 400 IU of vitamin D.

[5] α-Tocopherol equivalents. 1 mg d-α-tocopherol = α-TE = 1.49 IU.

is especially beneficial for vegetables containing thiamin, riboflavin, pyridoxine, folic acid, and ascorbic acid. Microwave cooking requires a shorter cooking time and less water, and generally results in greater retention of heat-labile nutrients (4).

Fat-Soluble Vitamins

Vitamins A, D, E, and K are classified as fat-soluble vitamins. Their absorption is facilitated by bile salts or dietary fat, and they are stored in moderate amounts in the body. Vitamins A and D function like hormones, interacting with specific intracellular receptors in their target tissues. Toxicity associated with the fat-soluble vitamins can occur, since fat-soluble vitamins can be stored with other lipids in fatty tissues and can accumulate. The characteristics of fat-soluble vitamins are found in Table 11.2.

VITAMIN A

Functions

Vitamin A is essential for vision, for dental development, and for growth and reproduction. Vitamin A is also necessary for the synthesis of hydrocortisone and for the regulation and differentiation of epithelial tissue. The integrity of the mucous membranes of the eyes, skin, mouth, gastrointestinal tract, and genitourinary tract is maintained by this vitamin, which is required for the production of mucus (5).

Properties

Vitamin A includes three natural compounds found in animal sources (retinol, retinal, and retinoic acid) and three provitamins found in plants (α-, β-, and γ-carotene). Retinol is apparently responsible for the actions of the vitamin in the reproductive process, and retinal is the functional compound of the visual cycle. Retinoic acid, the active form of vitamin A, is associated with growth and cell differentiation. Retinoic acid cannot replace retinal in the visual cycle and is not able to support reproduction (6). β-Carotene, the most abundant plant source, does not possess inherent vitamin A activity but yields retinol after absorption and metabolism. One international unit (IU) of vitamin A is equal to 0.3 μg retinol or 0.6 μg β-carotene. Large amounts of β-carotene can be ingested over a long period of time without development of toxic effects (other than skin pigmentation) because only one-half of absorbed carotene is converted to retinol (7, 8). When the dietary intake of retinol is in the range of the recommended dietary allowance, the majority will be absorbed; however, excess amounts ingested in the diet will be excreted.

Deficiency

A deficiency of vitamin A is usually due to fat malabsorption syndromes or malnutrition. Deficiency produces a variety of symptoms that include nyctalopia (night blindness), diminished production of corticosteroids, xerophthalmia (drying of the cornea), keratinization of the skin, growth failure, and fetal malformations. A deficiency of vitamin A can impair resistance to infections because of breakdown of mucous membranes (9).

Toxicity

Acute and chronic vitamin A toxicity is a well-recognized condition in adults. Acute poisoning may occur after a single dose in excess of 1,000,000 units. Chronic toxicity is mainly determined by the dose and duration of therapy. Usually a dose of more than 100,000 units daily for several months causes hypervitaminosis A (10). Prolonged daily use of vitamin A in doses of 25,000 units or more may result in a hypervitaminosis syndrome resembling a cirrhoticlike liver syndrome. Symptoms from chronic use of vitamin A include fatigue, vomiting, cheilosis, dizziness, nausea, and irritability, followed by generalized skin desquamation. Pruritus, dry scaly skin, bone pain, changes in texture of hair and nails, increased cerebrospinal fluid pressure, and hypercalcemia may also occur. Concern about an excess intake of vitamin A during pregnancy has increased in recent years because of its structural and metabolic relationship to other vitamin A analogs (retinoids), especially 13-cis-retinoic acid (isotretinoin), which is teratogenic. A daily dose lower than 10,000 IU is not thought to be teratogenic (11).

Therapeutic Uses

Vitamin A analogs (retinoids) have been developed to improve the therapeutic index of vitamin A. Isotretinoin and etretinate (12) were developed as less toxic and more effective agents. They have, however, caused embryopathy (13). Retinoids have had a major impact on the practice of dermatology and are under investigation in oncology (14, 15). Retinoids may play a role in cancer prophylaxis (16, 17) and in the treatment of skin lesions (18). Retinol supplements may reduce the risk of development of lung cancer in smokers and may also protect against cervical cancer (19). Also, a consistent relationship has been found with an above average intake of β-carotene and a lowered incidence of cancer, especially when β-carotene is used in combination with vitamins E and C (17, 20).

Until further research is conducted, advice to vitamin A users is understandably conservative. Doses higher than 10,000 units should not be recommended, and consumers should preferably rely on dietary intake of foods containing β-carotene. Excess use of retinol supplements may cause serious adverse reactions; however, increasing the dietary intake of retinol by eating more green and yellow vegetables may be beneficial and avoid toxicity. β-carotene is a vitamin A precursor that is less toxic because only 20 to 30% of a dose is absorbed from the gastrointestinal tract,

Table 11.2.
Summary of Fat-Soluble Vitamins

Vitamin	Function	Deficiency	Large Doses	Therapeutic Uses	Sources
Vitamin A Retinol Retinal Retinoic Acid β-Carotene	Growth Vision Dental development Reproduction Syntheses of hydrocortisone Epithelial tissue differentiation Maintenance of mucous membranes	Nyctalopia Xerophthalmia Faulty bone and tooth development Keratinization Fetal malformation Decreased production of cortical steroids Impaired resistance to infection	Acute Fatigue Cheilitis Dizziness Nausea and vomiting Irritability Desquamation Chronic Hypercalcemia Dry scaly skin Bone pain Changes in texture of hair and nails Increased cerebrospinal pressure Pruritis	Dermatology Oncology	Liver Milk Butter and margarine Dark-green leafy vegetables Carrots Sweet Potatoes
Vitamin D Ergocalciferol-D$_2$ Cholecalciferol-D$_3$	Bone mineralization Maintenance of normal neuromuscular activity Maintenance of serum calcium and phosphorus levels	Associated with inadequate calcium and phosphorus Rickets (Children) Osteomalacia (Adults) Secondary Hyperparathyroidism	Hypercalcemia (weakness, anorexia, vomiting, diarrhea, polydipsia, polyuria, & mental changes) Constipation Proteinuria Vague Aches Metallic or bad taste Renal failure Hypertension	Renal osteodystrophy Hypoparathyroidism	Sunlight Butter Egg yolk Fatty fish Liver Fortified milk and bread
Vitamin E dll-α-tocopherol (α-TE) (1 mg = 1.49 IU)	Antioxidant—maintains integrity of cell membrane Enhance vitamin A utilization Inhibition of prostaglandin production Cofactor in steroid metabolism Related to action of selenium	Neurologic Syndrome (ataxia, muscle weakness, nystagmus, loss of touch/pain) Anemia in premature infants Hemolysis of red blood	Increases the effects of oral anticoagulants	Intermittent claudication Retrolental fibroplasia	Wheat germ oil Nuts Green leafy vegetables
Vitamin K Phylloquinone-K$_1$ Menaquinone-K$_2$ Analog Menadione-K$_3$	Coagulation Formation of prothrombin and other clotting proteins	Prolonged clotting time Symptoms of deficiency can be produced by coumarin anticoagulants and by antibiotic therapy	Vomiting Toxicity can be induced by water-soluble analogs Neonatal jaundice Dietary supplements can block the effect of oral anticoagulant	Coagulation disorders Anticoagulant-induced prothrombin deficiency	Green leaves (spinach, cabbage) Liver Synthesis in intestine by bacteria Cheese, egg yolk

Adapted from Williams SR, ed. Nutrition and Diet Therapy. St. Louis: St. Louis Times Mirror/Mosby College Publishing, 1985; Luke B, ed. Principles of Nutrition and Diet Therapy. Boston: Little, Brown & Co., 1984; Robinson CH, Lawler MR, Chenoweth WL, Garwick AE, eds. Normal Therapeutic Nutrition, ed. 17. New York: Macmillan, 1986; Cataldo CB, DeBruyne LK, Chitney EN, eds. Nutrition & Diet Therapy; ed. 3. St. Paul, MN: West Publishing Company, 1992; and Sizer FS, Whitney EN, eds. Hamilton & Whitney's Nutrition—Concepts & Controversies, ed. 6. St. Paul, MN: West Publishing Company, 1994.

and it is metabolized at a rate of approximately 50 to 60% of normal dietary intake.

No definitive statement can be made at this time concerning the use of vitamin A in wound healing. Recent studies have reported a beneficial effect of vitamin A in promoting wound healing. No definitive statement can be made at this time concerning its use in this clinical applications until additional research has been completed.

VITAMIN D

Functions

Vitamin D is considered a hormone rather than a vitamin, although it is not a natural hormone. Vitamin D, in conjunction with parathyroid hormone (PTH) and calcitonin, is needed for calcium and phosphate metabolism. This in turn supports normal mineralization of bone and neuromuscular activity.

Properties

Vitamin D refers to both D_2 (calciferol, ergocalciferol) and D_3 (cholecalciferol). Vitamins D_2 and D_3 occur naturally and are equipotent. Either may supply the body's daily requirements. These forms have an onset of action time of 10 to 24 hours and may be stored in the body for prolonged periods.

Ninety percent of dietary vitamin D is absorbed from the small intestine. Vitamin D3 may be absorbed more rapidly and completely than vitamin D2.

The supply of vitamin D depends on ultraviolet light radiation for conversion of plant ergosterol to vitamin D_2 or for conversion of skin 7-dehydrocholesterol to vitamin D_3. Vitamins D_2 and D_3 require activation (hydroxylation) by both the liver and the kidney. Vitamin D_3 is absorbed into the circulation and converted by hepatic microsomal enzymes to 25-hydroxycholecalciferol, which in turn is hydroxylated in the kidney to its active metabolite, 1,25-dihydroxycholecalciferol (calcitrol). Calcitrol has pharmacologic activity that lasts from 3 to 5 days. The production rate of calcitrol is closely regulated by plasma calcium and parathyroid hormone. The active form of D_3 is responsible for promoting intestinal calcium absorption and mobilization of calcium from bone. Paradoxically, vitamin D mobilizes calcium from the bone to maintain proper plasma levels (21, 22).

Dihydrotachysterol (DHT) is a synthetic vitamin D analog activated in the liver that does not require renal hydroxylation. DHT has a rapid onset of action (2 hr), a shorter half-life, and a greater effect on mobilization of bone salts than does vitamin D.

Deficiency

Vitamin D deficiency may be induced by renal and hepatic disease, malabsorption syndromes, short bowel syndrome, hypoparathyroidism, and long-term anticonvulsant ther-apy. Vitamin D deficiency results in inadequate absorption of calcium and phosphorus from the intestinal tract. A deficiency of these minerals leads to faulty mineralization of bone and teeth, resulting in rickets in children and osteomalacia in adults. Also, increased parathyroid hormone secretion is seen due to a decreased serum calcium level, resulting in secondary hyperparathyroidism.

Toxicity

Large doses of vitamin D in the excess of 50,000 to 100,000 IU per day may result in toxicity, although tolerance to vitamin D varies widely. Initial manifestations of toxicity result from hypercalcemia and include weakness, anorexia, vomiting, diarrhea, polydipsia, polyuria, mental changes, and proteinuria. Prolonged hypercalcemia may result in calcification of soft tissue including the heart, blood vessels, renal tubules, and lungs. Death can result from cardiovascular or renal failure.

Therapeutic Uses

A vitamin D–resistant state exists in chronic renal failure. Renal osteodystrophy is characterized by a decreased ability of the kidney to convert 25-hydroxycholecalciferol to 1,25-dihydroxycholecalciferol. Active vitamin D (calcitrol) or dihydrotachysterol must be supplemented to lower the concentrations of PTH and raise the plasma calcium concentration of calcium (23). Vitamin D supplementation is also needed in hypoparathyroidism, which is characterized by hypocalcemia and hyperphosphatemia. Generally, if a patient has an inadequate diet and little exposure to sunlight, a vitamin D supplement may be appropriate.

An anticonvulsant-induced hypocalcemia is thought to be due to induction of the hepatic microsomal P-450 enzyme system and is treated with vitamin D, 25-hydroxycholecalciferol, and possibly calcium. Combination therapy is required because vitamin D obtained from the diet, supplements, or sun exposure is converted to inactive metabolites with prolonged anticonvulsant use. A favorable response is seen with a combination of both vitamin D and 25-hydroxycholecalciferol.

VITAMIN E

Functions

Many of the actions of vitamin E are related to its antioxidant properties. Vitamin E stabilizes the lipid portion of the cell membrane by preventing oxidation of polyunsaturated phospholipids, thereby maintaining the integrity of the cell membrane. Other functions of vitamin E include enhancement of vitamin A utilization, inhibition of prostaglandin production, and stimulation of an essential cofactor in steroid metabolism. Selenium acts synergistically with vitamin E to protect cell membranes from oxidative damage.

Properties

α-Tocopherol is the most active and abundant form of vitamin E, occurring naturally in substances such as wheat germ oil. Vitamin E is 20 to 40% absorbed from the gastrointestinal tract and is distributed to all tissues via the lymphatic system.

Deficiency

Vitamin E deficiency occurs primarily in premature infants and in patients with severe malabsorptive disease, such as cystic fibrosis. The neurologic syndrome of ataxia, muscle weakness, nystagmus, and loss of the senses of touch and pain has been attributed to vitamin E deficiency (24–26). Vitamin E deficiency may also lower the age of onset or increase the rate of progression in patients predisposed to Alzheimer's disease (27).

Toxicity

Current literature includes little evidence that vitamin E produces any harmful effects. A daily intake of 200 to 600 mg (1 IU = 0.6 mg d-α-tocopherol) appears to be innocuous in most people. The most commonly recurring complaint with large doses (300 to 3200 IU/day) is gastrointestinal upset (nausea, flatulence, or diarrhea), weakness or fatigue (28). Large doses of vitamin E may increase the incidence of sepsis and necrotizing enterocolitis when serum vitamin E levels are maintained at 5 mg/dL (normal range 1.0 to 3.0 mg/dL) in low-birth-weight infants and have been associated with a high mortality rate when given intravenously (29, 30). Vitamin E can also increase the effects of oral anticoagulants (31, 32).

Therapeutic Uses

Some therapeutic uses for vitamin E that have been proposed include treatment of cancer, aging, coronary heart disease, arthritis, cataracts, and tardive dyskinesia. However, its benefits in the healthy population are not known. Prolonged vitamin E therapy of 400 mg/day for at least 3 months has been reported to be beneficial to some patients with intermittent claudication (28, 33). Administration of 100 mg/kg/day appears to be effective in preventing retrolental fibroplasia in premature infants receiving oxygen therapy (34). Vitamin E supplements no longer appear to be necessary in premature infants for the treatment of hemolytic anemia because commercial infant formulas contain iron and the appropriate ratio of vitamin E to fatty acids to prevent the development of hemolytic anemia (35).

Vitamin E is reported to be beneficial in the treatment and/or prevention of a wide range of conditions. Scientists now believe that vitamin E serves with selenium as a cellular antioxidant, protecting cell membranes from peroxidase damage. However, there is no scientific basis for vitamin E supplementation in a host of conditions including infertility, cancer, angina, muscular dystrophy, diabetes, premenstrual syndrome, and nocturnal leg cramps, and in the enhancement of athletic performance.

VITAMIN K

Functions

The only rational use of vitamin K is for the correction of bleeding tendencies caused by its deficiency. Such a deficiency is unlikely to occur because of intestinal bacterial synthesis of the vitamin. For this reason, there are no dietary recommended allowances.

Properties

Vitamin K is essential for the hepatic synthesis of prothrombin and other clotting proteins. Vitamin K compounds are chemically referred to as *quiones* and include phylloquinone (K_1) and menaquione (K_2), which are synthesized by intestinal flora, and menadione (K_3), the water-soluble analog.

Deficiency

Vitamin K deficiency, clinically resulting in hemorrhage, may occur following destruction of intestinal flora associated with antibiotic use, and especially with prolonged poor dietary intake, as may be seen during hospitalization (36). The role of antibiotics, especially select third-generation cephalosporins, in producing hypoprothrombinemia is thought to be due to a common structural side chain that inhibits a vitamin K–dependent step in the synthesis of prothrombin in the liver. When antibiotics are used, prothrombin time should be monitored, and in many instances a prophylactic dose of vitamin K is given (37, 38). Also, large amounts of vitamins A and E interfere with absorption of vitamin K (39). Advanced liver damage, when caused by cancer and cirrhosis, results in a deficiency of clotting factors that can not be alleviated by the administration of vitamin K. However, increased prothrombin time as a result of vitamin K deficiency will respond to supplementation.

Infants are unable to synthesize vitamin K because they have a sterile intestinal tract at birth. A single prophylactic dose of vitamin K (0.5 to 1 mg intramuscularly or subcutaneously) should be given to infants to protect them until synthesis begins and to supplement dietary intake. Phylloquinone (phytonadione) is the agent of choice to prevent bleeding tendencies (40), but caution must be used with intravenous use.

Toxicity

Vitamin K is relatively nontoxic, even in massive doses. Too rapid an intravenous injection of phylloquinone may result in flushing and cause a sense of constriction in the chest. Menadione in doses of more than 10 mg parenterally may produce hemolysis, hyperbilirubinemia, and kernicterus in premature newborns. Large daily intakes of vitamin K (i.e., 250 mg of dietary vitamin K found in approximately 8 ounces of cauliflower, lettuce, spinach, or broccoli) may antagonize the hypoprothrombionic effect of oral anticoagulants.

WATER-SOLUBLE VITAMINS

The B complex vitamins and vitamin C are the water-soluble vitamins. The B complex includes thiamin, riboflavin, nicotinic acid, pyridoxine, pantothenic acid, biotin, folic acid, and cyanocobalamin.

Water-soluble vitamins serve as cofactors for specific enzyme systems in the body. Many water-soluble vitamins are not active until phosphorylation occurs after ingestion (thiamin, riboflavin, niacin, and pyridoxine) or until coupled to specific nucleotides (riboflavin, niacin).

Water-soluble vitamins are stored to a limited extent only, so a day-to-day supply is desirable. When excessive amounts are ingested, the unneeded portion is generally excreted, resulting in a minimal toxicity. However, even water-soluble vitamins can be toxic, especially when large amounts are ingested for prolonged periods.

Certain conditions or situations may cause depletion of water-soluble vitamins and result in the appearance of deficiency symptoms. These include fever, which may accelerate vitamin metabolism, the stress of injury or surgery, and hyperthyroidism. Deficiencies of water-soluble vitamins may begin as a depletion of body stores without evidence of clinical symptoms such as abnormal laboratory indices. Initial clinical symptoms include loss of appetite, weight loss, headache, apathy, insomnia or excitability. In severe deficiency states, specific clinical syndromes such as beriberi or pellagra occur. Characteristics of the water-soluble vitamins can be found in Table 11.3.

THIAMIN

The principle role of thiamin (B_1) is as a coenzyme in the form of thiamin pyrophosphate. This coenzyme plays a vital role in the intermediate metabolism of carbohydrates in decarboxylation (removal of carbon dioxide) and in transketolation (transfer of carbon units), such as the conversion of pyruvic acid into acetyl-CoA and in the synthesis of acetylcholine. Individual requirements for thiamin are related to metabolic rate and are greatest when carbohydrates are the primary source of calories. Thiamin is also necessary for the transmission of nerve impulses.

Thiamin deficiency results in beriberi characterized by peripheral neuritis. The symptoms of peripheral neuritis include sensory disturbances in the extremities, loss of muscle strength, muscle wasting (dry beriberi), edema (wet beriberi), tachycardia, and an enlarged heart.

In the United States, the most common cause of thiamin deficiency is excessive alcohol intake, which is frequently associated with poor dietary habits, decreased absorption of nutrients, and decreased activation of thiamin pyrophosphate. The Wernicke-Korsakoff syndrome, characterized by paralysis of eye muscles, nystagmus, and associated with excess alcohol intake, is primarily due to a thiamin deficiency (41).

RIBOFLAVIN

Riboflavin (vitamin B_2) is converted to two coenzymes, flavin mononucleotide (FMN) and flavin adenine dinucleotide (FAD), which are required for normal tissue respiration. Riboflavin is also required for activation of pyridoxine. Under normal conditions, Riboflavin like all B vitamins is readily absorbed from the gastrointestinal tract, specifically, the duodenum. Large doses may cause yellow discoloration of urine.

A deficiency of riboflavin such as with inadequate dietary intake, malabsorption syndromes, or alcohol will lead to singular stomatitis, cheilosis, corneal vascularization, or dermatoses.

Dietary sources of riboflavin include milk and daily products, meats, and green leafy vegetables.

NIACIN

Niacin, vitamin B_3, is a component of the coenzymes nicotinamide adenine dinucleotide (NAD) and nicotinamide adenine dinucleotide phosphate (NADP). These two coenzymes are important in the oxidation-reduction reactions essential for tissue respiration. Niacin (nicotinic acid) is essential for converting food to energy, fat synthesis, growth, and healthy skin. Niacin may be converted in the body to niacinamide (nicotinamide), but either form can be used by the body.

Both excessive intake of alcohol and protein-calorie malnutrition may lead to the niacin deficiency state known as *pellagra*, with initial symptoms of an erythematous eruption resembling sunburn. Later the "three Ds" of dermatitis, diarrhea, and dementia occur, followed by death if the deficiency is not corrected.

Therapeutic Uses

Niacin (but not niacinamide) is a peripheral vasodilator. It causes the release of histamine, resulting in a transient flushing of the skin as well as a tingling sensation, dizziness, nausea, gastrointestinal upset, and activation of peptic ulcer disease (42). The flushing sensation generally begins 20 minutes after ingestion and lasts 30 to 60 minutes. After 3 to 6 weeks of therapy, the flushing side effect usually decreases markedly (43). The adverse effects of niacin may be diminished by increasing the dose up slowly (100 mg, three times a day each week), administering with food or milk, or administering 60 minutes after a 325 mg dose of aspirin.

Nicotinic acid is also effective in lowering total cholesterol as well as low-density lipoprotein (LDL) levels, while concurrently increasing high-density lipoprotein (HDL) levels. Nicotinic acid is used in the treatment of lipid disorders, with doses from 3 to 6 grams each day.

Table 11.3.
Water-Soluble Vitamins

Vitamin	Function	Deficiency	Large Doses	Sources
Thiamin Vitamin B_1	Metabolism of carbohydrates Normal growth Functioning of nervous system Synthesis of acetylcholine	Beriberi Peripheral neuritis Loss of memory Depression Muscle wasting Edema Tachycardia Enlarged heart	Nontoxic even in very large doses of 100–500 mg parenterally	Milk Pork Liver Nuts Whole grains Enriched flour and cereals
Riboflavin Vitamin B_2 Flavin mono- nucleotide Flavin adenine dinucleotide	Building and maintaining body tissues	Cheilosis Glossitis Seborrheic dermatitis Burning and itching eyes Achlorhydria	No toxicity	Milk Eggs Meat Liver Green leafy vegetables
Niacin Nicotinic Acid Nicotinamide	Enzymes that convert food to energy Tissue respiration Fat synthesis Growth Healthy skin	Pellagra Erythematous eruptions Dermatitis Diarrhea Dementia	Transient flushing of skin and tingling sensation (vasodilation) Dizziness Nausea Gastrointestinal upset Peptic ulcer disease Liver toxicity Hyperuricemia Glucose intolerance	Lean meats Fish Whole grains Green vegetables
Pyridoxine Vitamin B_6 Pyridines: Pyridoxine Pyridoxamine Pyridoxal	Transformation of amino acids Metabolism of tryptophan to serotonin Modify action of steroid hormones	Seborrhea like skin Glossitis Stomatitis Peripheral neuropathy Anemia Drugs: hydralazine, penicilliamine, iso- niazid, cycloserine, and estrogen	Lower serum lipids with 3–6 g cholesterol and triglycerides Peripheral sensory neuropathy Ataxia	Wheat Corn Meat Potatoes

	Functions	Deficiency	Toxicity	Sources
Ascorbic Acid Vitamin C	Synthesis of collagen—important for wound healing and stress due to injury and infection; Synthesis of epinephrine from adrenal glands; Conversion of folic acid to folinic acid; Absorption of iron	Defect in collagen formation—poor wound healing, aching joints, increased susceptibility to infection, weakened cartilage and capillary walls; Scurvy	Possible kidney stones; Diarrhea with 4–15 g/day; Gout; Lower serum cholesterol; Rebound scurvy; Increased absorption of iron; Interference with oral anticoagulants; Treatment of pressure sores; Impaired bacterial activity	Citrus fruits; Tomatoes; Leafy vegetables; Melons
Pantothenic Acid	Metabolism of carbohydrates; Gluconeogenesis; Synthesis and degradation of fatty acids; Synthesis of steroids; Synthesis of steroid hormones; Synthesis of porphyrins	Usually only seen with severe multiple B-complex deficits	Essentially nontoxic in humans	Meat; Poultry; Fish; Cereals; Fruits and vegetables; Milk
Biotin	Carbohydrate metabolism; Fat metabolism	Seborrheic dermatitis; Algesia	Essentially nontoxic in humans	Liver; Egg yolk; Synthesized by intestinal bacteria
Folic Acid	Maturation of red blood cells; Interrelated with B_{12}	Megaloblastic anemia; Pregnancy	Essentially nontoxic in humans	Liver; Green leafy vegetables
Cobalamin B_{12}	Synthesis of DNA; Formation of red blood cells	Pernicious anemia; Peripheral neuropathy; Macrocytic anemia	Essentially nontoxic in humans	Liver, meat, milk, egg, cheese

Adapted from: Marcus R, Coulston AM. Water-soluble vitamins. In Gilman AG, Goodman LS, Rall TW, Murad F, eds. The Pharmacologic Basis of Therapeutics, ed. 7. New York: Macmillan, 1985; Tuckerman MM, Truco SJ, eds. Human Nutrition and Diet Therapy. Boston: Little, Brown & Co., 1984; Cataldo CB, DeBruyne LK, Whitney EN, eds. Nutrition & Diet Therapy, ed. 3. St. Paul, MN: 1992; Siaer FS, Whitney EN, eds. Hamilton & Whitney's Nutrition—Concepts & Controversies, ed. 6. St. Paul, MN: 1994.

Nicotinic acid is available at a relatively low cost, but it is not free of serious side effects. (See Chapter 20, "Hyperlipidemia.") Niacin may cause reversible hepatitis, glucose intolerance, and hyperuricemia. Fasting blood glucose levels, liver function values, and uric acid levels should be monitored during chronic therapy (44, 45).

Sustained-release nicotinic acid formulations have been used in the treatment of hyperlipidemia, because it was thought the gradual absorption of niacin would minimize adverse reactions and increase compliance. However, sustained-release formulations have not been proven to be successful. Flushing is not decreased, only delayed. Sustained formulations have also been shown to increase the incidence of gastrointestinal adverse effects (nausea, vomiting, and diarrhea). Niacin-induced elevated liver enzymes may be associated especially with extended-release forms (46, 47).

PYRIDOXINE

Vitamin B_6 consists of a group of related compounds known as the pyridines, which include pyridoxine, pyridoxamine, and pyridoxal. The pyridines are converted to the active form of vitamin B_6, pyridoxal phosphate, in the gastrointestinal tract.

Pyridoxal phosphate is a coenzyme involved in the metabolism of protein, carbohydrates, and fat. In protein metabolism, vitamin B_6 participates in the decarboxylation of amino acids and in the conversion of tryptophan to niacin or serotonin. Pyridoxine may also modify the actions of steroid hormones by interacting with steroid receptor complexes (48).

Vitamin B_6 deficiency due to dietary restrictions is seldom seen in adults, although deficiency in the alcoholic population may be as high as 30%. Symptoms of pyridoxine deficiency include seborrhealike skin lesions on the face, glossitis, stomatitis, peripheral neuropathy, and anemia. Drug-induced deficiencies have been observed with vitamin B_6 antagonists such as hydralazine, penicillamine, isoniazid, cycloserine, and estrogen. Pyridoxine has been reported to decrease phenobarbital and phenytoin serum levels when daily doses of 200 mg are administered for 4 weeks. Pyridoxine antagonizes the therapeutic action of levodopa by facilitating the conversion of levodopa to dopamine outside the CNS. Patients treated with levodopa should avoid supplemental B_6. Concurrent B_6 use does not adversely affect the levodopa/carbidopa combination, as carbidopa is a peripheral dopa decarboxylase inhibitor.

Large daily doses of 0.2 to 6 g/day for 2 months to 3 years may result in toxic symptoms of peripheral sensory neuropathies, with associated ataxia and numbness and clumsiness of the hands and feet (49, 50).

Pyridoxine supplementation has been reported to be beneficial in several clinical situations. Women who report symptoms of depression while taking oral contraceptives may be deficient in pyridoxine. Some studies suggest that these women may respond favorably to a daily supplement of 50 mg (51–53). Vitamin B_6 may be prescribed for those women who have decreased pyridoxine plasma levels.

In doses of 100 mg to 200 mg per day for a duration of at least 12 weeks, pyridoxine may relieve paresthesia and pain in hands of patients with carpal tunnel syndrome.

Pyridoxine may also be used to alleviate symptoms of premenstrual syndrome (PMS), such as depression, irritability, tension, breast tenderness, edema, headache, and acne, which may be related to abnormal tryptophan metabolism produced by pyridoxal phosphate deficiency. Side effects associated with pyridoxine, 25 to 100 mg, twice daily are minimal (54). Pyridoxine appears to be safe and effective in the majority of females studied for treatment of premenstrual syndrome (PMS) (55–58).

VITAMIN C (ASCORBIC ACID)

Ascorbic acid is involved in a variety of metabolic functions, including direct stimulation of peptide synthesis and hydroxylation of proline and lysine in the formation of collagen, synthesis of epinephrine, and conversion of folic acid to folinic acid. Vitamin C also facilitates the gastrointestinal absorption of iron. The adrenal cortex, leukocytes, and platelets contain high concentrations of vitamin C. The amount found in the leukocytes is less susceptible to depletion than that present in plasma (59). A deficiency of ascorbic acid results in defective collagen synthesis, joint pain, anemia, poor wound healing, and increased susceptibility to infection. The severe form of vitamin C deficiency is termed *scurvy*. The clinical findings in patients with scurvy include ecchymoses, petechial hemorrhages, easy bruising, loosening of the teeth secondary to gum inflammation, muscle weakness, and joint pains. Plasma levels of vitamin C may be lowered in cigarette smokers and women taking oral contraceptives (60, 61).

Large daily doses of 1 to 3 grams of ascorbic acid may result in formation of kidney stones because of excessive excretion of oxalate produced from the metabolism of ascorbic acid (62). Severe diarrhea and precipitation of gout as the result of excretion of uric acid in predisposed people may also occur (63).

Rebound scurvy may be seen in both infants and adults following cessation of the use of megadoses of vitamin C (64). An infant born to a mother taking large amounts of vitamin C can metabolize the vitamin at a more rapid rate than normal. Adults who abruptly stop high-dose therapy experience loosened teeth and bleeding gums. In both instances, an increased rate of vitamin C elimination results in a relative deficiency when large quantities are no longer available. Therefore, patients should be advised to taper the dose of vitamin C instead of suddenly discontinuing therapy.

Other adverse effects that have been reported with intake of megadoses of vitamin C include absorption of excessive amounts of iron (65), uricosuria with resultant stone formation (66), gastrointestinal disturbances, interference with anticoagulants, destruction of red blood cells (67), and impaired bactericidal activity of leukocytes (68, 69).

Ingestion of 1 to 3 g of vitamin C was advocated by Linus Pauling as a protective factor against the common cold. Some studies show a decrease in frequency and severity of symptoms of the common cold (70, 71), or enhance resistance to upper-respiratory infections (72). Others have found this not to be true (73–75). The claims of vitamin C for prevention of the common cold remain unsubstantiated by randomized, well-designed, double-blind clinical studies.

In addition, well-designed studies have proven that megadose vitamin C therapy is of no benefit in the survival of patients with terminal cancer.

PANTOTHENIC ACID

Pantothenic acid, a constituent of coenzyme A, is needed for enzyme-catalyzed reactions such as the metabolism of carbohydrates; gluconeogenesis; synthesis and metabolism of fatty acids; and synthesis of sterols, steroid hormones, and porphyrins. Since pantothenic acid is widely distributed in the diet, a deficiency is rare and would be expected to occur only in a malnourished individual.

BIOTIN

Biotin is important in carbohydrate and fat metabolism. Biotin is available from a wide variety of foods and is also synthesized by bacteria in the intestinal tract. A deficiency is rare but may occur due to inadequate synthesis. Exfoliative dermatitis is the primary deficiency symptom. Infants who are deficient in biotin because of malabsorption syndromes exhibit the symptoms of Leiner's disease. These infants should be treated with an intravenous form of biotin that is currently available as a compassionate investigational new drug.

VITAMIN B_{12}

Vitamin B_{12} participates as a coenzyme in DNA synthesis, cell reproduction, red blood cell formation, and nerve maintenance. It may also be required for the incorporation of folic acid into cells. Vitamin B_{12} also occurs in several forms designated as *cobalamins*. Commercially available cyanocobalamin is the most stable form.

Intrinsic factor is secreted by parietal cells in the stomach and regulates the amount of vitamin B_{12} absorbed in the terminal ileum. Because vitamin B_{12} is so well conserved by the body through enterohepatic recycling, signs of deficiency may not be seen for 3 to 5 years after absorption has ceased (76). Because cyanocobalamin is

important in cell production, the signs and symptoms of deficiency are manifested in organ systems with rapidly replicating cells. A deficiency results in megaloblastic anemia characterized by mature cells that lack oxygen-carrying capacity. Megaloblastic anemia may also occur following surgical removal of the stomach portion that produces intrinsic factor or part of the ileum where absorption of the vitamin occurs. Pernicious anemia, a genetic disorder, occurs when intrinsic factor is not produced and, consequently, vitamin B_{12} is not absorbed. In pernicious anemia, mature red blood cells are not produced due to a lack of DNA synthesis. The characteristic symptoms of the disorder include pallor, anorexia, dyspnea, prolonged bleeding time, weight loss, glossitis, and neurologic disturbances including depression and unsteady gait (see Chapters 13 and 14).

A vitamin B_{12} deficiency may exist in the geriatric patient, without the classic laboratory, hematologic, or clinical manifestations. This vitamin B_{12} deficiency appears to be due to an inability to absorb protein-bound vitamin B_{12}, despite a lack of gastric abnormalities. This vitamin B_{12} deficiency manifests itself by neurologic and psychiatric abnormalities without the classic hematologic abnormalities. Geriatric patients with a serum B_{12} level below 200 pg/mL should be treated initially with 1 μg per day of B_{12} until serum B_{12} is raised to above>300 pg/mL or B_{12} intramuscularly (100 μg i.m./day for 2 weeks, then 1000 μq i.m./month for life) if serum B_{12} does not come up to over 300 pg/mL (77). Vitamin B_{12} is available as a tablet, a solution for intramuscular injection, and an intranasal gel. The gel is reported by the manufacturer to have greater bioavailability then oral tablets and is easier to administer than an intramuscular injection.

Cyanocobalamin has no therapeutic value beyond that of correcting deficiencies. The use of vitamin B_{12} to boost energy is of no value.

FOLIC ACID

Folic acid is functionally related to cyanocobalamin because they are both essential for DNA synthesis. Folic acid is also important in cell reproduction, including red blood cell formation and protein synthesis.

Folacin is the generic term for folic acid (pteroylglutamic acid). Approximately 25% of the folacin found in food is in the active (tetrahydrofolic acid) form and is readily absorbed and stored in the liver. Ascorbic acid prevents its oxidation.

The usual causes of folic acid deficiency are similar to those previously discussed with other B vitamins. In addition, a deficiency may occur during pregnancy, causing birth defects such as neural tube defects—spina bifida and anencephaly (78). Women of childbearing age should have an intake of at least 0.4 mg of folic acid daily in order to reduce the risk of fetal neural tube defects. Currently the

FDA is proposing to require folic acid fortification in certain foods to prevent deficiency in pregnant women and the resulting birth defects (79). Deficiencies can also occur with oral contraceptive use, in the elderly as the result of a poor diet, and in infants whose formulas lack folic acid or vitamin C. A folic acid deficiency can also occur with anticonvulsants such as phenytoin or primidone. These agents lower serum folate by inhibiting deconjugase enzymes in the gastrointestinal tract. The anemia that results from folic acid deficiency is characterized by a reduction in the number of red blood cells, the release of large nucleated cells (macrocytic, megoblastic), low hemoglobin levels with a high color content in RBCs, and lowered leukocyte and platelet counts.

Folic acid therapy corrects the anemia associated with vitamin B_{12} deficiency, but it does not prevent or correct neurologic disturbances associated with vitamin B_{12} deficiency (see Chapter 13).

ANTIOXIDANTS

In 1993, retail vitamin sales in the United States reached a record high of 1.12 billion dollars, of which $658 million were from vitamin supplements sold in pharmacies. The sales of antioxidant vitamins (C, E, and β-carotene) are a growing segment of total vitamin sales because of the belief that supplementation with antioxidants may reduce the risk of certain types of cancer as well as cardiovascular disease. However, controversy exists regarding the efficacy of antioxidant supplements in disease prevention (80, 81). Antioxidants have been thought to reduce cancer risk and to protect the body against damage to biologic membranes because of their ability to reduce free radical formation. Antioxidants have also been proposed to prevent an increase in the amount of low-density lipoproteins which is linked to the etiology of stroke and heart disease. One study (80) tracked 29,000 men who were long-term smokers and reported that vitamin E and/or β-carotene failed to protect against lung cancer or heart disease in lifelong smokers and that significantly more new cases of lung cancer occurred in men who took supplements of β-carotene each day compared to men taking only vitamin E or placebo. A second study, which followed 751 patients for 4 years (81), failed to show efficacy of antioxidants in the prevention of colorectal adenoma.

The results of other large, controlled studies will be available soon and may provide more insight into the efficacy of antioxidant supplements in disease prevention. Until a sufficient amount of reliable information is available, a sufficient amount of antioxidants can be obtained through a nutritious diet that contains at least five daily servings of vegetables and fruits.

HEALTH FOOD FADS

Common compounds include garlic, bee pollen, tryptophan, and fish oil. Information regarding these types of vitamins can be found in Table 11.4.

Table 11.4.
Health Food Fads

Compound	Reported Function	Comment
Garlic	Control hypertension Treatment of high cholesterol Prevention of certain cancers Antiplatelet effect	May be more effective after fatty meal
Ginseng	Help handle stress Decrease allergic effects Antidiuretic effect Aphrodisiac	Adverse reactions of stimulation, nervousness, morning diarrhea, skin eruptions, sleeplessness, hypertension
Bee pollen	Improvement of athletic and sexual performance Prevent infection, allergies, and cancer Prolong life Promote weight loss or weight gain	Adverse reactions may occur if person is allergic to pollen. Adverse reactions reported to occur include asthma, urticaria, rhinitis, and anaphylactic shock after ingestion if allergic to pollens such as ragweed
Tryptophan	Effective antidepressant Effective in treating bipolar ailments and sleeping disorders	Nausea, anorexia, drowsiness
Fish oils	Treatment of coronary artery disease Control hypertension Treatment of rheumatoid arthritis Treatment of hypercholesteremia	May cause diarrhea, antiplatelet complications; fat-soluble vitamin toxicity, decreased insulin secretion

Table 11.5.
Minerals

Macronutrients	Micronutrients (trace elements)
Calcium	Iron
Phosphorus	Zinc
Magnesium	Iodine
Sodium	Copper
Potassium	Fluorine
Chloride	Manganese
Sulfur	Selenium
	Chromium
	Cobalt

MINERALS

Minerals are inorganic substances that are classed as either macro- or micronutrients. Macronutrients are required in daily amounts of 100 mg or more, whereas micronutrients are required in amounts of less than 100 mg daily. A list of essential minerals is included in Table 11.5. Other minerals are found widely in nature and in the human body, but their functions are uncertain, and many are considered to be contaminants. With all minerals, a narrow therapeutic index exists between general requirements and toxic levels.

Sources of minerals vary according to the composition of the soil in which they are found. In regions where the soil has been depleted of minerals, the population may experience deficiencies. Deficiencies may occur in individuals because of chronic ingestion of highly refined foods (flour and cereals) unless they have been fortified with the minerals lost during processing. Whole-grain foods are preferred to refined foods because of their higher content of zinc, copper, and iron as well as pyridoxine, pantothenic acid, biotin, folic acid and vitamin E.

In this section, emphasis is placed on a discussion of calcium, iron, and zinc because of their well-understood functions. Information regarding other minerals is summarized in Table 11.6. Table 11.7 lists the interactions that involve minerals.

CALCIUM

Calcium is essential for the functional integrity of the nervous and muscular systems, for normal cardiac function, for conversion of prothrombin into thrombin, and as the major mineral component of bone.

Ninety-nine percent of total body calcium is found in bone, and 1% is present in serum. Of the calcium found in serum, 45% is bound to plasma proteins and inactive. The calcium in bone serves as a reservoir to maintain normal plasma calcium levels (82). The interaction of PTH, vitamin D, and calcitonin is responsible for maintaining a normal calcium level of 2.12 to 2.62 mmol/L (8.5 to 10.5 mg/dL). Calcium absorption occurs in the small intestine at a relatively steady rate of 30% of intake, increasing to approximately 50% during growth periods, pregnancy, and lactation.

Hypocalcemia usually occurs when the plasma calcium level falls below 8 mg/dL. An exception to this is when there is a decreased concentration of plasma proteins. In this case, the calcium level will be reported lower than normal if there is a low concentration of plasma proteins. A corrected serum calcium concentration can be calculated, or ionized calcium can be measured (83). Chronic calcium deficiency, usually caused by inadequate dietary intake, results in osteoporosis or osteomalacia in adults and rickets in children. Chronic, excessive intake of calcium causes adverse effects that range from minor to life threatening and are clearly dose related. One to two grams of calcium per day are unlikely to cause problems in a healthy individual. However, possible adverse effects include nausea, bloating, constipation (which may be prevented by increased fiber and water consumption), and flatulence (especially with oral intake of calcium carbonate) (84). Symptoms of hypercalcemia generally occur with ingestion of greater than 4 to 5 g/day (85). Signs and symptoms of hypercalcemia include nausea, vomiting, anorexia, headache, muscle weakness, depression, apathy, fatigue, hypertension, nervousness, insomnia, and urolithiasis (86, 87).

Calcium supplements are suggested for prevention or control of osteoporosis (88–90), hypertension (91, 92), and colon cancer (93), but the only confirmed use is for correction of dietary deficiency. Of commercially available supplements, calcium carbonate (oyster shell) provides the greatest amount of elemental calcium (40%). In patients with achlorhydria (especially geriatric patients), calcium carbonate is not absorbed to a great extent on an empty stomach, but it is well absorbed with meals. Calcium citrate (21% elemental calcium) has been shown to have better solubility and absorption, particularly in patients with impaired acid secretion than calcium carbonate.

Two natural sources of calcium, bone meal and dolomite, should be avoided because of the risk of lead contamination. The risk of poisoning is especially great for pregnant/lactating women, infants, children, and possibly the elderly.

IRON

Iron is essential in the functioning of all biologic systems because it is the oxygen carrier in hemoglobin and myoglobin and also functions in the respiratory chain.

Iron in the body is either functional or stored. Functional iron is found in hemoglobin and myoglobin, whereas stored iron is found in association with transferrin, ferritin, and hemosiderin. The storage sites of ferritin and hemosiderin are the liver, spleen, and bone marrow.

Table 11.6.
Summary of Minerals

Minerals	Physiological Functions	Deficiency	Clinical Applications
Chlorine (chloride), major anion of the extracellular fluid	Required for fluid-electrolyte balance, acid-base balance, gastric acidity	Deficiency of chloride alone is rare	Losses occur in GI disorders, vomiting, diarrhea, and tube drainage
Chromium	Favors normal glucose tolerance	Impaired glucose clearance; peripheral neuropathy; ataxia	Required for normal glucose utilization; role in management of diabetes remains controversial; required for carbohydrate and lipid metabolism; lowers serum cholesterol and LDL; increases HDL
Cobalt	Integral part of B_{12}	Pernicious anemia	Excess leads to polycythemia
Copper 30% absorbed from diet; inversely related to zinc; essential for proper iron utilization	Synthesis of melanin, collagen, hemoglobin, and connective tissue	Decreased red blood cell production and poor wound healing	Menke's kinky hair syndrome; absorption disorder; toxicity; Wilson's disease
Fluoride	Contributes to structure of teeth and soft tissues	Dental carries	May be useful in osteoporosis, toxicity: fluorosis, mottled enamel
Iodine	Synthesis thyroxine and tridothyronine	Creatinism; goiter; myxedema	Regulation of basal metabolic rate growth, reproduction, cellular metabolism
Magnesium 25–65% absorbed primarily in small intestine. Efficiently absorbed and highly conserved: a person on a high magnesium diet will absorb only about ¼ of the intake, but on a low magnesium diet more than ¾ of the intake will be absorbed	Nerve cell function, enzyme activator, synthesis of skeleton	Occurs in alcoholics and diabetics, and with malabsorption syndrome; symptoms: tremor, spasm, irritability, lack of coordination, convulsions; excretion enhanced by mineralcorticoids, hypercalcemia, phosphate, depletion, alcohol ingestions	Uses in therapy include magnesium sulfate IV as anticonvulsant, electrolyte replenisher, uterine relaxant, magnesium gluconate for oral supplementation; magnesium citrate or sulfate as laxative; magnesium carbonate, oxide, hydroxide, trisilicate as antacid; hypermagnesemia is rare except in renal failure; excess may cause diarrhea
Manganese Substitute for magnesium in some reactions	Cofactor for enzyme systems involved in bone formation; required for formation of mucopolysaccharides	Has not been observed in humans	
Molybdenum	Cofactor for xanthine oxidase	Has not been observed in humans	
Phosphorus 70% absorbed from jenunum, maintained by renal resorption; normal plasma concentration: 3.0 mg/dL to 4.5 mg/dL	Skeletal synthesis, component of vitamins and essential for coenzyme formation; contributes to structure of teeth and soft tissue	Occurs if prolonged excessive use of alcohol or nonabsorbable antacids, prolonged vomiting, liver disease, hyperparathyroidism	Dibasic calcium phosphate is used orally; hyperphosphatemia is associated with chronic renal disease, hypoparathyroidism, tetany
Potassium Major cation of intracellular fluid; normal range: 3.5–5.0 mEq/liter 3–4.5 mg/dL	Required fluid-electrolyte balance, acid-base balance, muscle activity, carbohydrate metabolism, protein synthesis	Produces, sore, weak, or painful muscles	Losses occur in GI disorders and diarrhea; used in treatment of diabetic acidosis; required for fluid balance
Selenium 90% absorbed	Acts synergistically with vitamin E to protect cell membranes from oxidative damage	Thigh tenderness, deficiency due to TPN, malnutrition	Incidence of cancer may be due to low intake of selenium; marginal deficiency when soil content is low
Sodium Major cation of extracellular fluid; normal range: 136–145 mEq/L; under hormonal control of aldosterone	Required for fluid balance, acid-base balance, cell permeability, normal muscle irritability	Losses occur in GI disorders and diarrhea; weakness, mental confusion, nausea, lethargy, and muscle cramping may result	Fluid balance, blood pressure membrane permeability, neuromuscular function may be altered due to depletion or retention
Sulfur Obtained from protein	Structure of skin and cartilage; component of vitamins; important coenzyme formation		

Adapted from: Tuckerman MM, Turco SJ, eds. Human Nutrition. Philadelphia: Lea & Febiger, 1983; and Williams SR, ed. Nutrition and Diet Therapy. St Louis: Times Mirror/Mosby College Publishing, 1985.

Table 11.7.
Mineral Interactions

Mineral	Drug/Agent	Interaction/Effect
Calcium	Corticosteroids	Decreased calcium absorption
	Fiber	Decreased calcium absorption
	Iron	Decreased iron absorption
	Oxalic acid (found in rhubarb & spinach)	Decreased calcium absorption
	Phenytoin	Decreased absorption of phenytoin
	Phosphorus (found in dairy products)	Decreased calcium absorption
	Phytic acid (found in bran & cereals)	Decreased calcium absorption
	Quinidine	Decreased quinidine renal excretion and increased pharmacologic effects
	Salicylates	Increased salicylic acid renal excretion and decreased pharmacologic effects
	Tetracycline	Decreased serum levels of tetracycline
	Thiazide diuretics	Increased absorption of calcium
	Vitamin D	Increased absorption of calcium
Copper	Penicillamine	Copper deficiency
Iodine	Lithium	Additive or synergistic effect in inhibiting thyroid function
Iron	Antacids	Decreased iron absorption
	Ascorbic acid	200 mg ascorbic acid per 30 mg iron increases absorption of iron.
	Caffeine	Decreased absorption of iron
	Dairy products	Decreased absorption of iron
	Oxalic acid (found in rhubarb & spinach)	Decreased absorption of iron
	Phosphorus (found in dairy products)	Decreased absorption of iron
	Phytic acid (found in bran & cereals)	Decreased absorption of iron
Magnesium	Alcohol	Decreased absorption of magnesium
	Calcium	Decreased absorption of magnesium
	Diuretics	Increased absorption of magnesium
	Phosphorus	Decreased absorption of magnesium
Phosphorus	Antacids (Al or Mg)	Decreased absorption of phosphorus
	Calcium	Decreased absorption of phosphorus
	Iron	Decreased absorption of phosphorus
Zinc	Alcohol	Decreased serum zinc levels
	Bran or dairy products	Decreased zinc absorption
	Copper	An excess of either may cause a decreased absorption of the other.
	Diuretics	Increased zinc excretion
	Penicillamine	Zinc deficiency
	Phytic acid	Decreased zinc absorption
	Phosphorus	Decreased zinc absorption
	Tetracycline	Decreased tetracycline absorption

Dietary iron absorption is highly variable, ranging from 2 to 40% depending on the type and source. Heme iron and nonheme iron are the two forms of dietary iron. Heme iron is obtained from animal protein sources and is 15 to 35% absorbed (94). Meat may facilitate the absorption of heme iron by stimulating production of gastric acid (95). Nonheme iron constitutes most dietary iron found in grain products, vegetables, and dairy products and has an absorption rate of 2 to 20%. A healthy individual will absorb approximately 10% of dietary iron. Iron absorption may increase to 20% if iron stores are decreased or iron requirements are increased such as in menstruation, pregnancy, or growth stages. In the presence of iron deficiency anemia, absorption can increase to 30 to 40% (96). Absorption of nonheme iron is influenced by the levels of iron stores and by concomitantly consumed dietary components. A factor such as availability of ascorbic acid may increase the bioavailability of nonheme iron.

Iron deficiency is the most commonly recognized nutritional deficiency in the United States and is by far the major cause of anemia (97). Iron deficiency usually occurs in high-risk groups that include infants, children, adolescents, women of child-bearing age, frequent blood donors, and chronic aspirin users. Iron deficiency in these groups is usually treated or prevented with supplements.

ZINC

Zinc is important in the growth and maintenance of healthy skin and in the development and continued functioning of the male sex organs. It is also necessary for the synthesis of

DNA, RNA (98), and connective tissue and bone. It is necessary for the uptake of insulin by adipose tissue (99), normal sense of taste, increased oxygen-carrying capacity in normal and sickle red blood cells (100), spermatogenesis, ova formation, and the mobilization and transport of vitamin A from the liver. Zinc has an interaction with the immune system (101).

Ten to forty percent of dietary zinc is absorbed from the small intestine. The absorption of zinc, like that of iron, appears to be associated with the nutritional status of the individual (102). Decreased absorption of zinc has been associated with the formation of insoluble complexes with phytate (cereals), calcium, vitamin D, protein, and fiber. An increased copper intake can also suppress zinc absorption by competition for albumin binding sites (103). Zinc salts, acetate or sulfate, appear to have the highest degree of bioavailability (104). Zinc sulfate can be irritating to the gastrointestinal tract.

Zinc deficiency related to increased urinary excretion may be associated with surgery, diabetes, fever, alcohol consumption, and therapy with corticosteroids, estrogens, and thiazide diuretics. A zinc deficiency has also been associated with hypogonadal dwarfism (105). Clinical manifestations of zinc deficiency include loss of taste (hypogeusia) or smell (106), dermatitis, macular degeneration, and poor wound healing (107). Acrodermatitis enteropathica is the human genetic deficiency.

Zinc therapy may be of value in facilitating wound healing and in treating hypogeusia in zinc-deficient patients in dosages of 220 mg, 2 to 3 times daily.

Reported signs of zinc toxicity in humans include anorexia, nausea, lethargy, dizziness, and diarrhea. Vomiting may occur after ingestion of more than a 2-gram dose (108). Moderate doses of zinc (150 mg administered twice daily for 6 weeks) have been reported to increase the LDL/HDL ratio (109) and to impair cell-mediated immunity (110).

CHROMIUM

Chromium is required for appropriate glucose utilization, lipid metabolism, and insulin activity (111). Although the therapeutic role of chromium in the treatment of diabetes remains unknown, chromium is essential for the efficient use of insulin because it facilitates the binding of insulin to the cell membrane and is also required for normal glucose metabolism. Patients receiving total nutrition who develop glucose intolerance, insulin resistance, and central and peripheral nervous system disorders have regained normal function after chromium (not insulin) administration. Limited findings suggest a reduction in total serum cholesterol with chromium supplements. Chromium may also lower LDL cholesterol and increase HDL cholesterol. A deficiency in chromium is exhibited by hyperglycemia, glucosuria, peripheral neuropathy, and ataxia.

SELENIUM

Selenium, an antioxidant, is a component of the enzyme glutathione peroxidase, which is thought to deactivate lipid peroxidases, which are strong oxidizing agents that cause cell injury. The relationship between dietary selenium intake and incidence of cancer is being investigated. Limited epidemiologic evidence suggests that the risk of certain types of cancer, especially breast cancer, is inversely related to selenium intake. Because of the potential for toxicity, unsupervised use of selenium for cancer prevention should be discouraged. Selenium is being used (although claims remain unfounded) in heart disease, arthritis, heavy metal poisoning, sexual dysfunction, and aging. Selenium toxicity includes loss of hair, brittle fingernails, fatigue, irritability, and garlic odor or breath. A deficiency of selenium rarely occurs in humans, and supplementation is not recommended.

CONCLUSION

Vitamins are organic compounds that are essential for the body's biochemical processes. Vitamins, or their precursors, must be obtained through the diet, since they generally are not manufactured by the body and, under certain circumstances, are insufficiently produced. A positive relationship exists between the maintenance of optimal health and an optimal diet. Vitamin supplementation should not be a substitute for a well-balanced diet. For the normal population, the recommended number of daily servings from the five basic food groups (meats, vegetables, fruits, dairy products, and grains) provide the needed recommended dietary allowances. However, certain groups in the general population, with increased metabolic requirements, malabsorption syndromes, inadequate dietary intake, or stress require additional nutrients.

The fat-soluble vitamins—A, D, E, and K—are stored in the body for months. Therefore, toxicity due to fat-soluble vitamins is related to accumulation of vitamins in fatty tissues. The water-soluble vitamins, vitamin B complex and C, have very small reserves maintained in the body, and a day-to-day supply is desired. Water-soluble vitamins are usually nontoxic but can cause adverse effects when they are ingested for prolonged periods in larger than needed quantities.

Consumers often have questions about compounds that are not considered to be "true" or "real" vitamins. To protect the health as well as finances of the consumer, the pharmacist must be knowledgeable and provide the necessary information about vitaminlike substances.

Minerals are inorganic substances. Several of these elements, particularly calcium, iron, and zinc, have been found to be important catalysts in various enzymatic activities or play a role in hormonal metabolism. The importance of these elements must not be overlooked while investigators attempt to understand the nutritional importance of other minerals.

REFERENCES

1. Anon. Federal Register 44:16139, 1979.
2. Anon. Food and Drug Administration Drug Bulletin 13:27, 1983.
3. Sizer FS, Whitney EN, eds. Hamilton & Whitney's Nutrition-Concepts and Controversies, ed. 6. St. Paul, MN: West Publishing, 1994, 550–553.
4. Hoffman CJ, Zabik ME. Effects of microwave cooking/reheating on nutrients and food systems: a review of recent studies. J Am Diet Assoc 85:922–926, 1985.
5. Cataldo CB, DeBruyne LK, Whitney EN, eds. Nutrition & Diet Therapy, ed. 3. St. Paul, MN: West Publishing, 1992, 118.
6. Hathack JN, Hattan DG, Jenkins MY, et al. Evaluation of vitamin A toxicity. Am J Clin Nutr 52:183–202, 1990.
7. Luke B, ed. Principles of Nutrition and Diet Therapy. Boston: Little, Brown & Co., 1984, 137.
8. Stirling HF, Laing SC, Barr DG. Hypercarotenemia and vitamin A overdosage from proprietary baby food. Lancet 1:1089, 1986.
9. Sommer A, Djunaedi E, Loeden AA, Tarwotjo R. Impact of vitamin A supplementation on childhood mortality. Lancet 1:1169–1173, 1986.
10. Anon. Toxic effects of vitamin overdosage. Med Lett 26:73–74, 1984.
11. Kizer KW, Fan AM, Bankowska J, et al. Vitamin A-a pregnancy hazard alert. West J Med 152:78–81, 1990.
12. Ballag W. Vitamin A and retinoids: from nutrition to pharmacotherapy in dermatology and oncology. Lancet 1:860–863, 1983.
13. Lammer EJ, Chen DT, Hoar RM, Agnish ND, et al. Retinoic acid embryopathy. N Engl J Med 313:837–841, 1985.
14. Goodman DS. Vitamin A and the retinoids in health and disease. N Engl J Med 310:1023–1031, 1984.
15. Willett WC, Polk BF, Underwood BA, Stampfer MJ, et al. Relation of serum vitamins A and E and carotenoids to the risk of cancer. N Engl J Med 310:430–434, 1984.
16. Wald N, Idle M, Boreham J, Bailey A. Low serum vitamin-A and subsequent risk of cancer: preliminary results of a prospective study. Lancet 2:813–815, 1980.
17. Anon. Vitamin A and cancer. Lancet 2:325–326, 1984.
18. Kessler JF, Levine N, Meyskens FL Jr, Lynch PJ, et al. Treatment of cutaneous T-cell lymphoma (mycosis fungoides) with 13-cis-retinoic acid. Lancet 1:1345–1347, 1983.
19. Walker AR. Cancer of the cervix. Some aspects of epidemiology, screening, risk factors and survival. S Afr Med J 68(5):316–320, 1985.
20. Shekelle RB, Lepper M, Lius S, et al. Dietary vitamin A and risk of cancer in the Western Electric study. Lancet 2:1185–1190, 1981.
21. Haussler MR, McCain TA. Basic and clinical concepts related to vitamin D metabolism and action. N Engl J Med 18:974–983, 1977.
22. Deluca HF. Recent advances in metabolism of vitamin D. Annu Rev Physiol 43:199–209, 1981.
23. Johnson C. Acute and chronic renal failure. In Young LY, Koda-Kimble MA, eds. Applied Therapeutics, ed 6. Vancouver, BC: Applied Therapeutics, 1995, 14.
24. Muller DPR, Lloyd JK, Wolff OH. Vitamin E and neurological function. Lancet 1:227, 1983.
25. Sokol RJ, Guggenheim MA, Iannaccone ST, et al. Improved neurologic function after longterm correction of vitamin E deficiency in children with chronic cholestasis. N Engl J Med 313:1580–1586, 1985.
26. Satel SL, Riely CA. Vitamin E deficiency and neurologic dysfunction in children. N Engl J Med 314F:1389–1390, 1985.
27. Burns A, Holland T. Vitamin E deficiency. Lancet 1:805–806, 1986.
28. Bendich A, Machlin LJ. Safety of oral intake of vitamin E. Am J Clin Nutr 48:612–619, 1988.
29. Johnson B, Bowen FW Jr, Abbasi S, et al. Relationship of prolonged pharmacologic serum levels of vitamin E to incidence of sepsis and necrotizing enterocolitis in infants with birth weight 1,500 grams or less. Pediatrics 75:619–638, 1985.
30. Lorch V, Murphy D, Hoerstern LR, Harris E, Fitzgerald J, Sinha SN. Unusual syndrome among premature infants association with a new intravenous vitamin E product. Pediatrics 75:598–602, 1985.
31. Corrigan JJ, Marcus PI. Coagulopathy associated with vitamin E ingestion. JAMA 230:1300, 1974.
32. Evans CDH, Lacy JH. Toxicity of vitamins: complications of a health movement. Br Med J 292:510, 1986.
33. Haeger K. Long-time treatment of intermittent claudication with vitamin E. Am J Clin Nutr 27:1179–1181, 1974.
34. Hittner HM, Gadio LB, Rudolph AJ, et al. Retrolental fibroplasia: efficacy of vitamin E in a double-blind clinical study of preterm infants. N Engl J Med 305:1365, 1981.
35. Ehrenkranz RA. Vitamin E and the neonate. Am J Dis Child 134:1157–1166, 1980.
36. Lampe KF, McVeigh S, Rodgers BJ, eds. Drug Evaluations, ed. 6. Chicago: American Medical Association, 1986, 850.
37. Ne UHC. Adverse effects of new cephalosporins [Letter]. Ann Intern Med 98:415–416, 1983.
38. Lipsky JJ. N-methyl-thio-tetrazole inhibition of the gamma carboxylation of glutamic acid: possible mechanism for antibiotic associated hypoprothrombinemia. Lancet 2:192–193, 1983.
39. Robinson CH, Lawler MR, Chenoweth WL, Garwick AE, eds. Normal and Therapeutic Nutrition, ed. 7. New York: Macmillan, 1986, 170.
40. Mandel HG, Cohn VH. Fat-soluble vitamins. In Gilman AG, Goodman LS, eds. The Pharmacological Basis of Therapeutic Nutrition, ed. 7. New York: Macmillan, 1985, 1586.
41. Hoyumpa AM. Mechanisms of thiamine deficiency in chronic alcoholism. Am J Clin Nutr 33:2750, 1980.
42. Marcus R, Coulston AM. Water-soluble vitamins. The vitamin B complex ascorbic and ascorbic acid. In Gilman AG, Rall TW, Nies AS, Taylor P, eds. The Pharmacological Basis of Therapeutics, ed. 8. New York: Macmillan, 1990, 1536–1537.
43. Hoeg JM, Gregg RE, Brewer HB. An approach to the management of hyperlipoproteinemia. JAMA 255:512–521, 1986.
44. Grimm RH, Hunninghake OM. Lipids and hypertension. Implications of new guidelines for cholesterol management in the treatment of hypertension. Am J Med 80:56–62, 1986.
45. Figge HL, Figge J, Souney PF. Nicotinic acid: a review of its clinical use in the treatment of lipid disorders. Pharmcaotherapy 8(5):287–294, 1988.
46. McKenney JM, Proctor JD, Harris S. A comparison of the efficiency and toxic effects of sustained vs. immediate release Niacin in hypercholesterolemic patient. JAMA 271 (9):672, 1994.
47. Felicetta JV, Hayden CT. Why aren't we using more niacin? Arch Fam Med 3:324–326, 1994.
48. Marcus R, Coultston AM. Water-soluble vitamins. The vitamin B complex and ascorbic acid. In Gilman AG, Rall TW, Nies AS, Taylor P, eds. The Pharmacological Basis of Therapeutics, ed. 8. New York: Macmillan, 1990, 1539–1540.
49. Schaumburg H, Kaplan J, Windebank A, Vick N, et al. Sensory neuropathy with low dose pyridoxine abuse. A new megavitamin syndrome. N Engl J Med 310:445–448, 1983.
50. Parry G, Bredesen DE. Sensory neuropathy with low-dose pyridoxine. Neurology 35:1466, 1985.
51. Adams PW, Wynn V, Rose DP, Seed M, Folkard J, et al. Effect of pyridoxine hydrochloride (vitamin B6) upon depression with oral contraception. Lancet 1:897–904, 1973.

52. Adams PW, Wynn V, Seed M, et al. Vitamin B6, depression, and oral contraception. Lancet 2:516–517, 1974.

53. Miller LT. Do oral contraceptive agents affect nutrient requirements-Vitamin B6? J Nutr 116(7):1344–1345, 1986.

54. Williams MT, Harris RI, Dean BC. Management of premenstrual syndrome. J Int Med Res 13:174–179, 1985.

55. Abraham GE, Hargrove JT. Effect of vitamin B6 on premenstrual symptomatology in women with premenstrual tension syndromes: a double-blind crossover study. Infertility 3:155–165, 1980.

56. Brush MG, Perry M. Pyridoxine and the premenstrual syndrome [Letter]. Lancet 1:1399, 1985.

57. London RS, Bradley L, Chiamori NY. Effect of a nutritional supplement on premenstrual symptomatology in women with premenstrual syndrome: a double-blind longitudinal study. J Am Coll Nutr 10 (5):494–499, 1991.

58. Brush MG, Bennett T, Hansen K. Pyridoxine in the treatment of premenstrual syndrome. Br J Clin Pract 42 (11):448–52, 1988.

59. Matthews HW, Wells K. Vitamins, part IV: water soluble. J Natl Pharmaceut Assoc 27:8–13, 1982.

60. Kallner AB, Hartmann D, Hornig DH. On the requirements of ascorbic acid in man: steady-state turnover and body pool in smokers. Am J Clin Nutr 34:1347–1355, 1981.

61. Rivers JM. Oral contraceptives and ascorbic acid. Am J Clin Nutr 28:550–554, 1975.

62. Schmidt KH, Hagmaier V, Horning DH, Vuilleumier J, Ratishauser G. Urinary oxalate excretion after large intakes of ascorbic acid in man. Am J Clin Nutr 34:305–311, 1981.

63. Stein HB, Hasan A, Fox IH. Ascorbic acid-induced uricosuria: a consequence of megavitamin therapy. Ann Intern Med 84:385–388, 1976.

64. Tuckerman MM, Turco SJ, eds. Human Nutrition. Philadelphia: Lea & Febiger, 1983, 99.

65. Cook J, Monser ER. Vitamin C and the common cold and iron absorption. Am J Clin Nutr 30:235–241, 1977.

66. Stein HB, Fox IH. Ascorbic acid-induced uricosuria-a consequence of megavitamin therapy. Ann Intern Med 84:385–388, 1976.

67. Alhadeff L, et al. Toxicity and water-soluble vitamins. Nutr Rev 42:33–40, 1984.

68. Shilotri PG, Bhat KS. Effect of megadoses of vitamin C on bactericidal activity of leukocytes. Am J Clin Nutr 30:1077–1081, 1977.

69. Luke B, ed. Principles of Nutrition and Diet Therapy. Boston: Little, Brown & Co. 1984, 156.

70. Baird IM, Hughes RE, Wilson HK, Davies JEW, Howard AN. The effects of ascorbic acid and flavonoids on the occurrence of symptoms normally associated with a common cold. Am J Clin Nutr 32:1686–1690, 1979.

71. Schwartz J, Weiss ST. Dietary factors and chronic respiratory symptoms. Am J Epidemiol 132:67–76, 1990.

72. Peters EM, Goetzsche JM, Grobbelaar B, et al. Vitamin C supplementation reduces the incidence of postrace symptoms of upper-respiratory-tract infection in ultramarathon runners. Am J Clin Nutr 57:170–174, 1993.

73. Pitt HA, Costrini AM. Vitamin C prophylaxis in Marine recruits. JAMA 241:908–911, 1979.

74. Sperber SJ, Hayden FG. Chemotherapy of rhinovirus colds. Antimicrob Agents Chemother 32(4):409–419, 1988.

75. Coulehan JL. Ascorbic acid and the common cold: an evaluation of the evidence. Postgrad Med 66:153–160, 1979.

76. Cataldo CB, DeBruyne LK, Whitney EN, eds. Nutrition and Diet Therapy, ed. 3. St. Paul, MN: West Publishing, 1992, 133.

77. McRae TD, Freedman ML. Why vitamin B_{12} deficiency should be treated aggressively. Geriatrics 44(11):70–79, 1989.

78. Willett WC. Folic acid and neural tube defect: Can't we come to a closure? Am J Public Health 82:666–668, 1992.

79. FDA Medical Bulletin 24(1):9, 1994.

80. The Alpha-Tocopherol, Beta Carotene Cancer Prevention Study Group. The effect of vitamin E and beta carotene on the incidence of lung cancer and other cancers in male smokers. N Engl J Med 330:1029–35, 1994.

81. Greenberg ER, Baron JA, Tosteson TD, et al. A clinical trial of antioxidant vitamins to prevent colorectal adenoma. New Engl J Med 331(3):141–147, 1994.

82. Kesler D, Peterson CD. Oral calcium supplements. Postgrad Med 78(5):123–125, 1985.

83. Haynes RD Jr, Murad F. Agents affecting calcification: calcium, parathyroid hormone, calcitonin, vitamin D, and other compounds. In Gilman AG, Rall TW, Nies AS, Taylor P, eds. The Pharmacological Basis of Therapeutics, ed. 8. New York: Macmillan, 1990, 1497.

84. Precup AV, ed. United States Pharmacopeia Drug Information Advice for the Patient, vol. 2, ed. 9. 1994, 104.

85. Orwoll ES. The milk-alkali syndrome: current concepts. Ann Intern Med 97:242–248, 1982.

86. Randall RE, et al. The milk-alkali syndrome. Arch Intern Med 107:63, 1961.

87. Hunter H III, Callaway CW. Calcium tablets for hypertension [Editorial]. Ann Intern Med 103:946–947, 1985.

88. Nordin BEC, Heaney RP. Calcium supplementation on the diet: justified by present evidence. Br Med J 300:1056–1560, 1990.

89. Trachtenbarg DE. Treatment of osteoporosis. Postgrad Med 87(4):263–270, 1990.

90. Kanis JA. Calcium supplementation of the diet. II. Br Med J 298:205–208, 1989.

91. Grobbee DE, Waal-Manning HJ. The role of calcium supplementation in the treatment of hypertension. Drugs 39(1):7–18, 1990.

92. Henry HJ, McCarron DA, Morris CD, Parrott-Garcia M. Increasing calcium intake lowers blood pressure: the literature reviewed. J Am Diet Assoc 85:182–185, 1985.

93. Lipkin M, Newmark H. Effect of added dietary calcium on ionic epithelia-cell proliferation in subjects at high risk for familiar colonic cancer. N Engl J Med 313:1381–1384, 1985.

94. Monsen ER. Iron nutrition and absorption: dietary factors which impact iron bioavailability. J Am Diet Assoc 88(7):786–90, 1990.

95. Monsen ER, Hallberg L, Laurisse M, Hegsted M, Cook JD, et al. Estimation of available dietary iron. Am J Clin Nutr 31:131–141, 1978.

96. Bridges KR, Bunn HF. Anemias with disturbed iron metabolism. In Wilson JD, Braunwald E, Isselbacher KJ, et al, eds. Harrison's Principles of Internal Medicine, ed. 12. New York: McGraw-Hill, 1991, 1518–21.

97. Dallman PR. Iron deficiency: diagnosis and treatment. West J Med 134:496–504, 1981.

98. Taylor KB, Anthony LE. Clinical Nutrition. New York: McGraw-Hill, 1983, 518.

99. Kutsky RJ. Handbook of Vitamins, Minerals and Hormones, vol. I. New York: Van Nostrand Reinhold, 1981, 66.

100. Prasad AS, Cossack ZT. Zinc supplementation and growth in sickle cell disease. Ann Intern Med 100:367–371, 1984.

101. Cunningham-Rundles S, Bockman RS, Lin A, et al. Physiological and pharmacological effects of zinc on immune response. Ann N Y Acad Sci 587:113–22, 1990.

102. Taylor KB, Anthony LE. Clinical Nutrition. New York: McGraw-Hill, 1983, 517.

103. Sandstead HH. Copper bioavailability and requirements. Am J Clin Nutr 35:809–813, 1982.

104. Prasad AS. Zinc deficiency in man. In Hambidge KM, Nichols BL Jr, eds. Zinc and Copper in Clinical Medicine. New York: SP Medical and Scientific Books, 1978, 11.

105. Halsted JA, Smith JC Jr, Irwin MI. A conspectus of research on zinc requirements of man. J Nutr 104:345, 1974.

106. Prasad AS. Clinical, biochemical and nutritional spectrum of zinc deficiency in human subjects: an update. Nutr Rev 41:197–208, 1983.

107. Pories WJ, Henzel JH, Rob CG, Stain WH. Acceleration of wound healing in man with zinc sulfate given by mouth. Lancet 1:121–124, 1967.

108. Prasad AS. Zinc deficiency and toxicity. In Prasad AS, Oberleas D, eds. Trace Elements in Human Health and Disease. New York: Academic Press, 1976, 15–16.

109. Fosmire GJ. Zinc toxicity. Am J Clin Nutr 51:225–227, 1990.

110. Chandra RK. Excessive intake of zinc impairs immune response. JAMA 252:1443–1446, 1984.

111. Affenbacher EG, PL-Sunyer FX. Chromium in human nutrition. Am Rev Nutr 8:543–563, 1988.

CHAPTER 12

PARENTERAL AND ENTERAL NUTRITION IN ADULT PATIENTS

REX O. BROWN and GORDON S. SACKS

Specialized nutrition support includes parenteral and enteral nutrition. The practice of providing specialized nutrition support to patients is a relatively young discipline compared with other medical specialties. In 1968, Dudrick et al. reported that growth and development could be sustained with long-term parenteral nutrition in an infant who could not be fed via the gastrointestinal tract (1). Most practitioners consider this the beginning of modern clinical nutrition. During the last 30 years, many advances have been made to allow safe and efficacious delivery of parenteral and enteral nutrients.

Since the original report of Dudrick et al., the prevalence and complications of malnutrition have become more appreciated. Clearly, 30 to 50% of hospitalized patients in the United States have some malnutrition. Patients with malnutrition have poor wound healing, depressed immunocompetence, and an increased prevalence of septic and other postoperative complications.

Parenteral and enteral nutrition are powerful and relatively expensive interventions; however, they are not without complications. This has led to the development of nutrition support teams that assist in making specialized nutrition support safe and efficacious. Traditionally, the nutrition support team has consisted of multidisciplinary health care practitioners including a physician, pharmacist nurse, and dietitian. The pharmacist's role has ranged from ensuring provision of a properly compounded parenteral nutrition solution to being the director of the team. Most commonly, the pharmacist provides assistance in prescribing the parenteral or enteral nutrient formula, monitors the patient for metabolic complications, educates other practitioners about compatibilities and drug-nutrient interactions, and assists the institution/organization in developing a cost-effective formulary of nutrition products. In some institutions, the pharmacist is the director or coordinator of the nutrition support team with complete or nearly complete responsibility for parenteral and enteral nutrition prescribing, compounding, and delivery.

NUTRITIONAL ASSESSMENT

Nutritional assessment evaluates a patient's nutritional status (2), and can be used to detect and quantitate malnutrition in a variety of diseases. The ideal nutritional assessment would include a measurement of lean body mass or body cell mass. Body cell mass includes fat-free tissue such as skeletal muscle, smooth muscle, and solid organs. The lean body mass includes body cell mass and both extracellular water and solids. Unfortunately, it is difficult to measure these components using standard nutritional assessment methods. Delayed wound healing, impaired collagen formation, and decreased resistance to infection have all been associated with undernutrition (i.e., a depressed body cell mass). Patients with undernutrition can have this wasting process halted or reversed by specialized nutrition support.

Nutritional assessment has traditionally been divided into four parts: history and physical examination, anthropometric measurement, biochemical assessment of serum proteins, and evaluation of immune status.

History and Physical Examination

The history and physical examination should be used as a screening mechanism to identify patients who require a more thorough assessment. A history of unintentional weight loss, either chronic or acute, is usually a sign of suboptimal nutritional intake or altered metabolism. Chronic disease, gastrointestinal disease, certain social factors, or an abnormal metabolic state all may be risk factors for developing malnutrition (Table 12.1). Physical signs suggestive of malnutrition include edema, decubitus ulcers, muscle wasting, poor wound healing, and glossitis. Patients with documented unintentional weight loss, chronic disease, or physical signs as described above should have a thorough nutritional assessment.

Anthropometric Measurements

The anthropometric measurements are used to assess fat and somatic protein stores. The somatic protein stores include skeletal muscle and the visceral organs. Subcutaneous fat is often assessed by a series of skinfold measurements with an instrument called a Lange caliper. The most popular sites for skinfold measurement in the institutionalized patient are the triceps and subscapular area. These areas are usually available in a cooperative patient. Normal values exist for each measurement individually or as a sum in adult patients from ages 18 to 55 years. A value below the 40th percentile suggests some fat depletion. This method is attractive because it is relatively

Table 12.1.
Risk Factors for Undernutrition That Can Be Detected in a Patient History and Physical Examination

Chronic disease
   Renal failure
   Liver failure
   Chronic obstructive pulmonary disease
   Congestive heart failure
   Diabetes
Gastrointestinal disease
   Peptic ulcer disease
   Inflammatory bowel disease
   Pancreatitis
   Short bowel syndrome
Social factors
   Alcohol abuse
   Drug abuse
Abnormal metabolic state
   Cancer
   Sepsis
   Trauma or thermal injury

noninvasive and inexpensive. The assessment of skinfold measurements can be erroneous, however, if a patient has edema, if the equipment is not standardized, or if several observers are used. Also, some individuals may have very little subcutaneous fat and yet be in excellent physical condition (e.g., trained athletes such as runners or body builders).

The somatic protein compartment may be assessed indirectly by using body weight, midarm muscle circumference (MAMC), or arm muscle area (AMA). Chronic assessment of body weight is a relatively good marker of nutritional status in most patients. As mentioned earlier, acute or chronic weight loss is a harbinger of poor nutritional intake or altered metabolism. Fluid overload or edema results in a body weight greater than the patient's actual weight, which could mask impending undernutrition, especially in the critical care setting. Overhydrated patients often lose substantial weight during specialized nutrition support administration. This is actually desirable when excess fluid is mobilized. Conversely, other patients may retain excessive fluid and salt during specialized nutrition support intervention and gain weight very rapidly. Obviously weight fluctuations must be interpreted very carefully in all patients. Another way to assess body weight is to compare the patient's weight with the ideal body weight (Table 12.2). Somatic protein stores can also be assessed by calculation of the MAMC or AMA. The MAMC is calculated from the triceps skinfold (TSF) and midarm circumference (MAC) as follows:

$$MAMC \text{ (in cm)} = MAC \text{ (in cm)} - \pi TSF \text{ (in mm)}/10 \quad (12.1)$$

The AMA is calculated from the MAMC as follows:

$$AMA \text{ (in cm}^2) = (MAMC \text{ in cm})^2/4 \pi \quad (12.2)$$

Both of these methods are relatively easy, inexpensive, and noninvasive. The problems with skinfold measurements (edema, variation among observers) also exist with these assessments of somatic protein stores.

Biochemical Assessment of Serum Proteins

Serum concentrations of several constitutive proteins have been used initially and serially during specialized nutrition support intervention. Unfortunately, other factors such as metabolic stress, hydration status, and hepatic function may influence these serum concentration measurements. Although these serum markers lack sensitivity and specificity, some of them serve as very good prognostic indicators of patient outcome and therefore continue to be the subject of intense study. Albumin, transferrin, and prealbumin are the constitutive proteins used most frequently. Other serum proteins are being studied, but their role in nutritional assessment has not yet been determined.

Albumin is a protein with a half-life of 21 days and a large body pool compared with other secretory proteins. The normal serum concentration of albumin is 35 to 50 g/L (3.5 to 5.0 g/dL) in adults. A decrease in the serum concentration of albumin suggests inadequate protein intake, especially when the serum concentration is chronically depressed. An albumin concentration of 30 to 34 g/L (3.0 to 3.4 g/dL) suggests mild protein depletion; 25 to 29 (2.5 to 2.9), moderate depletion; and under 25 (2.5), severe depletion. Bed rest, overhydration, and transcapillary escape secondary to metabolic stress such as sepsis can all depress the serum concentration of albumin. Regardless of the cause, a depressed serum albumin concentration is associated with increased hospital morbidity and mortality. Therefore, many practitioners consider the serum albumin concentration to be very important. Because albumin has a long half-life and large body pool, it responds very slowly to specialized nutrition support intervention. In fact, some patients demonstrate a decrease in the serum albumin concentration during specialized nutrition support, presumably due to an increase in extracellular water and salt (3). Often, these patients have an ongoing septic process that increases aldosterone and antidiuretic hormone activity. Because factors other than nutrition can lower the serum concentration of albumin, its use as a nutritional marker must be interpreted cautiously. Its use as a prognostic indicator, however, cannot be ignored.

Transferrin is a secretory protein with a half-life of 8 days that serves as a carrier for iron. It has a much smaller

Table 12.2.
Formulas for Ideal Body Weight

Male	50 kg + 2.3 kg for each inch above 60 inches
Female	45.5 kg + 2.3 kg for each inch above 60 inches

body pool than albumin, and its normal serum concentration is 2 to 3.5 g/L (200 to 350 mg/dL). A serum concentration of transferrin of 1.5 to 2 g/L (150 to 200 mg/dL) suggests mild protein depletion; 1 to 1.5 g/L (100 to 150 mg/dL), moderate depletion; and under 1 g/L (<100 mg/dL), severe depletion. Because transferrin has a smaller body pool and shorter half-life than albumin, it is much more sensitive to protein-calorie deprivation or nutritional repletion. Therefore, it is used frequently in serial monitoring of patients receiving specialized nutrition support. Serum transferrin concentrations are attractive because they respond to nutritional repletion rather quickly (e.g., with weekly monitoring), are easy to measure, and are becoming available in many institutions. Iron deficiency anemia increases the transferrin serum concentration, while injury and sepsis depress it.

Prealbumin, also called *thyroxine-binding prealbumin* and *transthyretin*, has a normal serum concentration of 0.15 to 0.4 g/L (15 to 40 mg/dL). It is the major carrier protein for thyroxine and retinol-binding protein and has a half-life of 2 days. Because of the short half-life and relatively small body pool, prealbumin is quite sensitive to nutritional deprivation and repletion. Many institutions have added this laboratory test because it is inexpensive and relatively easy to perform. The serum concentration of prealbumin rises during nutrition support, even when the nitrogen balance remains negative. The correlation between improvement in nitrogen balance and increase in serum prealbumin concentration is highly significant; however, other events beside nutritional intake influence the prealbumin concentration. Acutely stressful events such as trauma or sepsis are known to depress, and chronic renal failure elevates serum prealbumin concentration.

Retinol-binding protein, fibronectin, and insulinlike growth factor I have all been studied for their role in documenting nutritional repletion. Retinol binding protein serum concentration is influenced by vitamin A status and the glomerular filtration rate. Its very short half-life of 12 hr may make it too sensitive to nutritional deprivation or intake. It may reflect the composition of the last meal instead of nutritional intake over a few days or weeks. Fibronectin is a glycoprotein nonspecific opsonin. It has a half-life of about 24 hr and is synthesized by the liver. Although fibronectin appears to respond positively during nutrition support, many other factors can alter its serum concentration (e.g., sepsis, trauma, shock). Insulinlike growth factor I is a growth hormone-dependent protein that possesses broad anabolic activity. The concentration correlates very well with nitrogen balance and increases during nutritional repletion (4). Human growth hormone and insulinlike growth factor I as adjunct therapy to nutrition support show promise.

Several acute-phase proteins (e.g., C-reactive protein) increase markedly during stressful events and decrease during recovery. The role of these proteins in nutrition support intervention is unclear; however, some of them are included in the Prognostic Inflammatory and Nutritional Index (5). This index includes the acute-phase proteins, α-1 acid glycoprotein and C-reactive protein, and the constitutive proteins, albumin and prealbumin. Other investigators have attempted to predict postoperative morbidity and mortality from preoperative nutritional status. One example of this is the Prognostic Nutritional Index, which includes serum albumin and transferrin concentrations, triceps skinfold, and cell-mediated immunity (6).

Evaluation of Immune Status

The relationship between malnutrition, depressed immune status, and infection has been appreciated for years. Many of these observations have been done in third-world countries where the prevalence of undernutrition is relatively high in the general population. Traditionally, assessments of immune stores (total lymphocyte count) and immune function (cell-mediated immunity) have been done in hospitalized patients who require specialized nutrition. Immune stores are usually assessed by determination of the total lymphocyte count (TLC), which includes predominantly thymus-derived lymphocytes (T cells). The TLC is calculated from the product of peripheral white blood cell count (WBC) and the percentage of lymphocytes.

$$\text{TCL (cells/L) (cells/mm}^3) \tag{12.3}$$

$$= \text{WBC (cells/L) (cells/mm}^3) \times \% \text{ lymphocytes/100}$$

A TLC above 2×10^9/L (>2000/mm^3) suggests adequate immune stores. A TLC of 1.2 to 2.0×10^9/L (1200 to 2000/mm^3) suggests mild depletion; 0.8 to 1.2 x 10^9/L (800 to 1200/mm^3), moderate depletion; and <0.8 x 10^9/L (<800/mm^3), severe depletion of immune reserves.

Immune function can be assessed by measuring the response to common antigens through skin testing. Antigens that have been used in this procedure include *Candida albicans*, mumps, streptokinase/streptodornase, tetanus, and *Trichophyton*. One product that is produced commercially includes seven antigens and a placebo that can be placed simultaneously (CMI Multitest, Merrieux). Most patients that have intact immune function will respond to both *Candida* and mumps skin tests; therefore, these are most commonly used. A positive test result is at least a 5-mm area of induration at the site of application within 24 to 48 hr. Geriatric patients may react slowly and not demonstrate a positive response until 72 hr after application. Many other factors, such as drug therapy (e.g., steroids, histamine antagonists, anesthetic agents), and certain disease states (e.g., cancer) can interfere with the body's cell-mediated immunity. The field of clinical immunology has experienced a resurgence in recent years, and this renewed interest has been carried over to specialized nutrition support. Several of the laboratory techniques used to assess immunologic function in immunodeficiency diseases are now being employed to characterize the impact of nutrition support on immune function. For instance, the concept of T lymphocyte subset analysis became widely recognized with the AIDS epidemic. Identification of CD4 (helper/inducer) and CD8 (suppressor/cytotoxic) T cell subsets and the CD4:CD8 ratio were used for staging and diagnosis of this disease. This technology is now being used in clinical trials to study the effects of parenteral and enteral nutrition on cell-mediated immunity of critically ill patients.

Lymphocyte proliferation is another assay used to measure cellular immunocompetence. This *in vitro* correlate of skin testing uses various mitogens, such as phytohemagglutinin or concanavalin A, to stimulate the proliferation of lymphocyte subsets. Under sterile conditions, peripheral mononuclear blood cells are incubated in the presence of mitogens for 5 to 7 days. The cells are then harvested and exposed to radioactive thymidine for 6 to 18 hours. A β-scintillation counter is used to measure the incorporation of thymidine into dividing cells, providing a quantitative measure of cellular proliferation. Low proliferative responses identify patients with deficiencies in cellular immune responses, possibly related to malnutrition. Measuring T lymphocyte responsiveness to mitogens may become an important tool for monitoring the nutritional status of patients receiving nutrition support.

Recent advancements in immunologic laboratory techniques have revealed further insight into the relationship between nutritional status and humoral immunity (B lymphocytes). With the development of enzyme-linked immunosorbent assays and fluorometric immunoassays, serum immunoglobulin concentrations and various complement components can be determined. Chemiluminescent assays, which measure the light energy generated after cell phagocytosis, are also being used to quantitate the bactericidal capacity of neutrophils. The recent growth and development in laboratory aspects of clinical immunology demonstrate the potential impact that specialized nutrition support can have on the immune system.

An alternative to a complete nutritional assessment is to use clinical judgment during the patient history and physical. Detsky et al. have suggested asking a short series of questions that include information about weight loss over the previous 6 months, recent dietary intake in relation to usual patterns, presence of significant gastrointestinal symptoms, and the patient's functional capacity (7). This technique has been called *subjective global assessment* and is easier and less expensive than a comprehensive nutritional assessment (8).

Another method of nutritional assessment that has gained considerable attention recently is bioelectric impedance. In this method a low-voltage electric current is introduced through distal electrodes on the hand and foot. After measurement of resistance and reactance, total body water and body cell mass can be determined. Using bioelectric impedance, one group has demonstrated maintenance of body cell mass in critically ill patients who received parenteral nutrition (9).

Types of Malnutrition

Marasmus is a form of undernutrition that results from chronic deprivation of protein and calories. Patients with this disorder are relatively easy to identify, as they have considerable wasting of somatic protein and fat. Their serum protein concentrations and immune status are often intact. This disorder is seen in patients who suffer from chronic disease and ingest a suboptimal amount of nutrition over a relatively long period of time (i.e., semistarvation). Table 12.3 contrasts the various types of malnutrition.

Kwashiorkor is traditionally classified as protein deficiency. Patients with kwashiorkor typically have adequate or excess caloric stores, as evidenced by sufficient body fat (Table 12.3). These patients often have a weight-for-height value that exceeds normal. Kwashiorkor patients have depressed serum concentrations of constitutive proteins and often have depressed immune function. The most common cause of this disorder is severe metabolic stress (e.g., trauma, sepsis, thermal injury). Less common are patients who ingest adequate calories and a low-protein diet over a long period of time. Kwashiorkor is often difficult to diagnose at the bedside because these patients appear to be well- or overnourished.

Kwashiorkor-marasmus mix results when a patient with marasmus is subjected to metabolic stress. These patients

Table 12.3.
Types of Malnutrition

Characteristic	Marasmus	Kwashiorkor	Kwashiorkor-Marasmus Mix	Obesity
Weight for height	↓	normal or ↑	↓	↑
Fat stores	↓	↑	↓	↑
Somatic protein stores	↓	normal or ↑	↓	↑
Serum protein concentrations	normal	↓	↓	normal
Immune function	normal	↓	↓	normal

have deficits in all categories of the nutritional assessment and have the highest risk for hospital morbidity and mortality (Table 12.3).

Patients with excess body weight secondary to fat are classified as obese if they are more than 20% above their ideal body weight. Obesity is a type of malnutrition that usually results from a prolonged increase in calories over what is needed or used. If subjected to metabolic stress, these patients can quickly develop kwashiorkor.

Because no one nutritional-assessment marker effectively identifies all patients at nutritional risk and because many nonnutritional factors alter the currently used tests, investigators continue to evaluate new methods of nutritional assessment. Some of the methods currently under investigation include underwater weighing, muscle-strength testing, magnetic resonance imaging, neutron-activation analysis, and radioisotope analysis. Some of these methods will be too expensive or invasive for general clinical use; however, bioelectric impedance analysis and muscle-strength testing show particular promise.

ENERGY AND PROTEIN REQUIREMENTS

After completion of the nutritional assessment in a patient who is going to receive specialized nutrition support, the nonprotein energy and protein goals must be determined. These goals will be different for each patient, based on the nutritional-assessment results, the purpose for initiating the specialized nutrition support, and the size of the patient.

Energy

The energy requirements for an individual patient may be predicted by several different methods. The degree of metabolic stress and any chronic disease afflicting the patient also help determine energy requirements. The most widely used method is the calculation of the basal energy expenditure (BEE) using the Harris-Benedict equations developed in 1919 (10). The BEE was developed by measuring oxygen consumption using direct calorimetry in 239 healthy male and female subjects. The two equations use the patient's gender, weight, height, and age.

Males: BEE = 66.4230 + 13.7516 Wt   (12.4)
+ 5.0033 Ht − 6.7550 Age

Females: BEE = 655.0955 + 9.5630 Wt   (12.5)
+ 1.8496 Ht − 4.6756 Age

BEE is in kilocalories per day, Wt is in kilograms, Ht is in centimeters, and Age is in years. BEE reflects the number of kilocalories expended during a 24-hr period in a subject at bed rest in a fasted state in a semidark room. This value can be multiplied by a factor that accounts for physical activity or stress to determine an energy goal (11). Examples of these factors appear in Table 12.4.

Table 12.4.
BEE Factors for Activity and Injury in Adult Patients

Condition	% by which to increase BEE
Confined to bed	↑20%
Elective surgery	↑20%
Ambulatory	↑30%
Traumatic injury	↑35%
Major septic episode	↑60%
Severe thermal injury	↑110%

From Long CL, Blakemore WS. Energy and protein requirements in the hospitalized patient. J Parenter Enteral Nutr 3:69–71, 1979.

In certain circumstances, all of the information required to calculate the BEE may not be available, so an alternative method may be used to determine the energy requirements. If the patient's weight is known, an estimated nonprotein energy goal may be calculated. A range of 25 to 35 kcal/kg/day is generally accepted for most patients (12). An energy goal of 25 kcal/kg/day would be used for an elective surgical patient who is otherwise healthy, whereas a septic or trauma patient would require at least 35 kcal/kg/day. A severely burned patient may require as much as 40 kcal/kg/day initially.

Patients who are older or have an abnormal body size create a particular dilemma when dosing energy on weight. For example, infusing energy to an obese patient at 35 kcal/kg/day will result in overfeeding and potential exacerbation of the obesity. Most practitioners would use an adjusted weight, for example, ideal body weight + 0.25 (actual body weight – ideal body weight), for energy and protein dosing. Undernourished patients should always be dosed on actual body weight, never ideal body weight. Dosing of energy in pediatrics and neonates is discussed in Chapter 85. Because of gradual loss of body cell mass over time, geriatric patients require a lower dose of energy based on body weight (e.g. 25 kcal/kg/day). It may be most prudent to determine energy doses in the elderly using the BEE formulas because age is a factor in the equations.

By using the Harris-Benedict equations with factors, patients receive energy based on their primary disease state or injuries. However, multiple stress factors may alter the energy requirement for a particular patient. Factors such as pulmonary toilet (pounding on the back to break up lung secretions) and pain can raise energy requirements, while sedation, immobilization, and pharmacologic paralyzation may lower them. Thus, the ideal way to determine an individual patient's energy requirement is to measure the resting energy expenditure (REE) of that patient. Indirect calorimetry may be used. This involves using a metabolic cart and measuring the concentration of oxygen consumed (VO_2) and carbon dioxide produced (VCO_2) over time (13). After measuring VO_2 and VCO_2, the complete Weir formula can be used to calculate the patient's REE (14).

$$REE = (3.941 \, VO_2 \qquad\qquad (12.6)$$
$$+ 1.106 \, VCO_2) \, 1.44 - 2.14 \, UUN$$

REE is in kcal/day, VO_2 is in mL/min, VCO_2 is in mL/min, and UUN is urinary urea nitrogen in g/24 hr. If a 24-hr urine sample is obtained the same day indirect calorimetry is performed, the nitrogen data are used in the calculation. The difference between the REE obtained from the complete Weir formula and the abbreviated Weir equation (without the UUN term) is less than 2% (14). Thus a 24-hr urine specimen is not required for each REE determination by indirect calorimetry. Many practitioners add 10 to 30% to the measured REE to allow for movement and patient interventions during the day (13). Information may also be gained about net substrate oxidation by using the respiratory quotient (RQ). RQ is the ratio of VCO_2 to VO_2. Carbohydrate is oxidized at an RQ of 1.0 (i.e., for every mole of oxygen consumed, one mole of carbon dioxide is produced), while fat is oxidized at an RQ of 0.7 (less carbon dioxide is produced for the oxygen consumed). In between these two quotients is the "theoretical" desired RQ of 0.85, where "mixed substrate" oxidation exists, or the mutual oxidation of carbohydrate and fat. Although protein can be oxidized for fuel (RQ = 0.8), the body proteins are not intended as energy sources because they are structural elements of functioning organs.

Protein

Protein requirements for an individual depend on many factors. In health, the recommended dietary allowance (RDA) for protein for an adult person is 0.8 g/kg/day. In a hospital environment patients are generally stressed and thus may require higher doses of protein. Depending on the clinical status of the patient, the protein requirement may range from 0.6 to 2.0 g/kg/day. As metabolic stress increases, the protein required to maintain adequate protein stores increases. An elective operative procedure such as cholecystectomy results in mild stress and a modest increase in protein requirements (Table 12.5). Patients with infections have a moderate degree of stress, while those who experience a traumatic injury or sepsis may be severely stressed (15). Severe thermal injury may require protein doses above 2.0 g/kg/day in selected situations.

Although the doses presented in Table 12.5 are reasonable, each patient should be monitored closely to

Table 12.5.
Protein Requirements for Adult Patients

Condition	Protein Dose (g/kg/day)
Maintenance	1.0
Mild stress	1.2
Moderate stress or repletion	1.5
Severe stress	2.0

Table 12.6.
Calculation of Nitrogen Balance

Nitrogen balance = $N_{IN} - N_{OUT}$

$$N_{IN} = \frac{\text{Protein intake (g)}}{6.25}$$

N_{OUT} = [UUN (g/liter) × 24-hr urine volume (liters)] + 4 g

determine whether the desired response is achieved (e.g., nutritional repletion, wound healing). During periods of metabolic stress, protein turnover is markedly increased, and urinary excretion of urea nitrogen is elevated, which can lead to rapid erosion of the body cell mass if adequate protein is not administered. Urinary 3-methylhistidine (3-MH), has been used as a noninvasive measurement of protein degradation. Although skeletal muscle proteins actin and myosin are a primary source of 3-MH, nonskeletal muscle sources of 3-MH (e.g., gastrointestinal tract) may contribute to the overall urinary amount excreted. Because of its questionable clinical applicability and expensive methodology, this technology is primarily used by research institutions. The "gold standard" to measure protein nutriture is nitrogen balance, with the obvious goal of achieving nitrogen equilibrium or a positive balance. This measurement is obtained by subtracting nitrogen output from nitrogen input during a 24-hr period (Table 12.6). Nitrogen input is calculated by dividing protein intake for 24 hr by 6.25 (protein is approximately 16% nitrogen). Nitrogen output is calculated by adding 4 g to the grams of urea nitrogen excreted by the kidneys during a 24-hr period. The 4 g represents nonmeasurable nitrogen losses such as stool losses, skin losses, and nonurea nitrogen losses in the urine. A nitrogen balance of 2 to 6 g/day suggests adequate intake of nonprotein energy and protein. A nitrogen balance between –2 and 2 g/day suggests that nitrogen equilibrium has been attained. A nitrogen balance below –2 g/day suggests more protein, more calories, or both are needed. Once the energy and protein requirements have been calculated and the nutrient formula has been prescribed, many practitioners calculate the nonprotein calorie (energy) to nitrogen ratio (NPC:N). Unstressed patients generally require a NPC:N of 150:1, while stressed patients require a ratio of 100:1. This reflects the increased protein needs of patients who are infected or injured.

PARENTERAL NUTRITION

Clinicians and investigators have long recognized the need for intravenous nutrition support in various patient populations. This is especially important in patients without a functional gastrointestinal tract. Over 100 years ago, six major dietary components were recognized: water, salt, vitamins, carbohydrates, fat, and protein. The landmark noted by Dr. Stanley Dudrick and colleagues in beagle puppies and later in humans in the late 1960s changed the medical world's perspective on parenteral nutrition support. They demonstrated successful administration of parenteral nutrition over a period of several weeks by documenting growth and improved nutritional status (1). Today, industry and clinical investigators continue to discover new parenteral nutrition products that improve on existing ones targeted to benefit specific patient populations.

Generally, parenteral nutrition should be reserved for patients who require specialized nutrition support and who do not have a functional or accessible gastrointestinal tract. With the multitude of available parenteral nutrient products, the practitioner needs sound guidelines so that patients may receive this therapy in a safe and efficacious way. Practice guidelines have been developed by the American Society for Parenteral and Enteral Nutrition (16) and they are summarized in Table 12.7. This group has also prepared guidelines for the use of parenteral and enteral nutrition in adult patients with cancer, acquired immune deficiency syndrome, liver failure, renal failure, pancreatitis, respiratory failure, inflammatory bowel disease, short-bowel syndrome, intestinal pseudo-obstruction, critical care, pregnancy, neurologic impairment, and geriatrics (17).

Types of Parenteral Nutrition

Parenteral nutrition may be given via a central or peripheral vein. Although central parenteral nutrition is more commonly used, peripheral parenteral nutrition is used by some institutions in certain patients.

Table 12.7.
Parenteral Nutrition Practice Guidelines

1. Patients who cannot receive enteral nutrition who already are or have the potential for becoming undernourished are candidates for parenteral nutrition.
2. Peripheral parenteral nutrition may be used in selected patients for up to 2 weeks, especially where central vein parenteral nutrition is not feasible.
3. Central vein parenteral nutrition should be used when parenteral nutrition will be needed for greater than 2 weeks, peripheral venous access is compromised, nutritional requirements are large, or fluid restriction is mandated.
4. Patients receiving this therapy should be monitored by health care professionals trained to detect the infectious, mechanical, metabolic, and nutritional complications of intravenous feeding at an early stage. Abnormalities detected during monitoring should be treated promptly.
5. The indications for home parenteral nutrition should be the same as for hospital parenteral nutrition, except that the patients no longer require an acute care setting.
6. The patients receiving home parenteral nutrition should be reevaluated periodically for the potential benefits of this therapy.

From Guidelines for Use of Parenteral and Enteral Nutrition in Adult and Pediatric Patients. J Parenter Enteral Nutr 17:9SA–11SA, 1993.

Peripheral parenteral nutrition can be used in patients who are being weaned from central parenteral nutrition to a normal diet, or as an adjunct to an oral or enteral diet. Generally, 900 mOsm/L is the maximum osmolality tolerated by peripheral veins (18). Actually, a solution of 600 mOsm/L is better tolerated and may lower the risk of phlebitis. It should be noted that the electrolytes added to parenteral nutrition contribute substantially to the osmolality of the parenteral nutrition solution (e.g., NaCl 50 mEq/L contributes 100 mOsm to each liter of solution). Concurrent infusion of fat emulsion with peripheral parenteral nutrition or subtherapeutic doses of heparin or hydrocortisone have been used in attempts to decrease the risk of phlebitis. Peripheral parenteral nutrition is intended to be used for short periods of time (e.g., 5 to 7 days) as adjunctive therapy. Dilute nutrient solutions must be used to maintain the osmolality of the solution within limits that the peripheral vein can tolerate. A solution with a final protein concentration of 3 to 5% and a dextrose concentration of 5 to 10% is commonly used for this type of therapy. It is extremely difficult, if not impossible, to meet a patient's nutritional requirements, because of the large volumes of fluid required. Also, the administration of peripheral parenteral nutrition has not demonstrated a significant benefit over 5% dextrose alone, which makes this therapy questionable (19).

Most patients receive parenteral nutrition via a large central vein. The superior vena cava is used most often after percutaneous catheterization of the subclavian, internal, or external jugular veins. The catheter may be placed in the operating room or at the patient's bedside using sterile technique and radiographic verification. A double or triple lumen catheter is used most often because patients who require parenteral nutrition often receive other intravenous medications or blood products. This provides access for the additional intravenous infusions without interrupting the administration of the parenteral nutrition. By having the catheter tip placed into the superior vena cava, very concentrated substrates may be infused because of the high rate of blood flow in this vein. Thus, required nutrients may be delivered in relatively small volumes without causing thrombophlebitis. This method is particularly effective in patients who have large energy and protein requirements or who require fluid restriction. If the catheter is properly cared for, it can be used indefinitely. The disadvantages of central parenteral nutrition include the increased prevalence of mechanical and metabolic complications.

PROTEIN

Parenteral Nutrition Formula Components

The initial protein products used in parenteral nutrition solutions were hydrolysates of naturally occurring proteins (fibrin, casein). Today, commercially available forms of parenteral protein are provided as crystalline amino acids.

Generally, the protein in a parenteral nutrition solution is not included in the energy intake, because ideally it should be used for protein synthesis. However, if protein is oxidized for energy, it will yield 4 kcal/g. Patients undergoing severe metabolic stress may require large doses of protein and actually use it as a preferential calorie source.

Currently marketed amino acid products in the United States are provided as standard or modified amino acids. Standard amino acid products are used for patients with normal organ function and relatively normal nutritional needs. The modified amino acid formulations are marketed for patients with hepatic failure, renal failure, fluid restriction, or high metabolic stress. Currently available amino acid products for parenteral nutrition are listed in Table 12.8.

The standard amino acid formulas are composed of physiologic mixtures of essential and nonessential amino acids. Although these products are commercially available in several concentrations, many institutions are now stocking only the 10 or 15% concentrations because lower concentrations can be made by adding sterile water with an automated compounder. These products are marketed with or without maintenance electrolytes.

Patients with severe liver failure develop many metabolic abnormalities, including disturbances in electrolyte and amino acid homeostasis (20). Some of these patients develop hepatic encephalopathy associated with decreased concentrations of branched-chain amino acids (BCAA) and elevated concentrations of aromatic amino acids (AAA) and methionine. The BCAAs include leucine, isoleucine, and valine, and the AAAs are phenylalanine, tyrosine, and tryptophan. In the absence of encephalopathy, liver failure patients who require parenteral nutrition may be maintained on standard amino acids. However, when hepatic encephalopathy is severe, the modified amino acid formula for hepatic failure may be used. Generally, patients should meet one of the following criteria to receive the modified amino acid: hepatic encephalopathy above grade 2, abnormal aminogram with a plasma molar ratio of BCAA:AAA of 2 or less, or hepatic encephalopathy associated with parenteral nutrition solutions containing standard amino acid solutions in doses

needed for nutritional support. The modified amino acid formula contains high concentration of BCAAs and low concentrations of AAAs and methionine. Although normalization of the amino acid profile has been shown with this product, an improvement in overall patient outcome has not been uniformly demonstrated in clinical trials. One randomized clinical trial (21) found a decrease in hepatic encephalopathy scores and a lower prevalence of mortality in patients receiving this formulation, while another study (22) failed to show any difference in encephalopathy scores and mortality with this product.

Patients with severe renal failure also have several metabolic changes, including electrolyte alterations and protein intolerance. Those who are not being dialyzed should have their daily protein dose restricted to 0.6 to 0.8 g/kg/day. Acute renal failure patients undergoing hemodialysis may be given 1.0 to 1.2 g protein/kg/day, while peritoneal dialysis patients may receive 1.2 to 1.5 g protein/kg/day. Patients receiving continuous arterial venous hemodialysis may receive protein doses in the range of 1.2 to 1.5 g/kg/day. Modified amino acids for renal failure, which contain primarily essential amino acids, are more expensive than standard amino acids. Prospective, randomized controlled studies have demonstrated that standard amino acids are as effective as modified amino acids in renal failure patients who require parenteral nutrition (23, 24). Thus, patients with severe renal failure should be given standard amino acids as part of parenteral nutrition in most clinical situations.

Some critically ill patients who require parenteral nutrition are markedly fluid-overloaded. In these patients, it is usually beneficial to use the smallest possible volume. Commercially available 15% amino acid products can be used to concentrate the parenteral nutrition formula in patients with overhydration or edema. These products are very expensive, so they should be reserved for patients who need severe fluid restriction.

Patients who are highly stressed have altered energy and protein metabolism. These patients take up BCAAs into skeletal muscle for energy. This has led to development of modified amino acid products with enhanced concentrations of the BCAAs. These products have been proposed to stimulate protein synthesis, decrease protein catabolism, and serve as a preferential fuel source. The many clinical trials using amino acids with an enhanced BCAA content have produced equivocal results. Some suggest that patients receiving these modified amino acids have decreased skeletal muscle catabolism and enhanced protein synthesis (25). In contrast, other studies have found a lack of clinical benefit when BCAA-enriched solutions were compared with standard amino acids (26). Given the expense of the products and the equivocal results of clinical trials, careful evaluation is needed when using these products.

Table 12.8.
Parenteral Amino Acid Categories with Examples

Patient Category	Example of Amino Acid Product
Normal (normal organ function)	Aminosyn, Aminosyn II, FreAmine III, Travasol
Fluid-restricted	Novamine 15%, Aminosyn-II 15%
Liver failure	HepatAmine
Renal failure	Aminosyn RF, NephrAmine, RenAmin, Aminess
Metabolic stress	FreAmine HBC, Branchamin, Aminosyn-HBC

CARBOHYDRATE

The nonprotein energy source in parenteral nutrition solutions may be carbohydrate only or a combination of carbohydrate and fat. The carbohydrate component of the nutrient solutions is usually dextrose. Other carbohydrates such as xylitol, fructose, or sorbitol have been studied, but have not gained wide acceptance in the United States. Each gram of hydrated dextrose provides 3.4 kcal. Dextrose stock solutions of 5 to 70% are available for use in parenteral nutrition solutions. Many institutions are stocking primarily the 70% dextrose solution because dilutions can be made using an automated compounder and sterile water. Final concentrations equal to or less than 10% dextrose in parenteral nutrition solutions may be infused peripherally. Solutions with higher concentrations should be administered through a large central vein.

Generally, dextrose infusion should not exceed 5 mg/kg/min (25 kcal/kg/day) during parenteral nutrition (27). This appears to be the maximum rate of dextrose utilization by the human body. Rates above 5 mg/kg/min are associated with lipogenesis, resulting in increased carbon dioxide production and hepatic steatosis.

Hospitalized patients receiving parenteral nutrition who have normal organ function often receive dextrose at a final concentration of 20 to 25% (Table 12.9). Therefore, a 70-kg patient would only receive 2 liters of parenteral nutrition if the dextrose infusion was held at 5 mg/kg/day as suggested above. Patients who are metabolically stressed may not tolerate this dose of carbohydrate, yet they have large requirements for protein. They often need to receive less dextrose, such as 15% final concentration of dextrose in the parenteral nutrition solution. Fluid-restricted patients (e.g., patients with congestive heart failure or liver failure) may receive smaller volumes of parenteral nutrition solutions when concentration dextrose is used. Patients with oliguric acute renal failure who are not undergoing dialysis often require fluid and protein restriction. High-calorie, low-protein parenteral nutrition formulas in small volumes are desired for these type of patients (Table 12.9).

FAT

The first intravenous fat emulsion product introduced into the United States contained cottonseed oil, but it was removed from the U.S. market in 1965 because of severe adverse reactions. Today, commercially available fat emulsions contain soybean oil or combinations of soybean and safflower oils. Unless contraindicated, fat emulsions should be given as part of a patient's parenteral nutrition regimen to prevent essential fatty acid deficiency or to serve as a calorie source (28). Essential fatty acid deficiency has both biochemical and clinical signs. Biochemical evidence usually becomes apparent within 1 to 3 weeks after fat-free parenteral nutrition is started. Biochemical evidence includes increased serum concentrations of saturated fatty acids, decreased concentrations of essential fatty acids, and a triene:tetraene ratio greater than 0.4. This ratio is the concentration of 5,8,11-eicosatrienoic acid (a fatty acid that appears in essential fatty acid deficiency) divided by the concentration of arachidonic acid. Clinical evidence of essential fatty acid deficiency does not usually appear until several weeks of glucose-based parenteral nutrition has been given. Manifestations of essential fatty acid deficiency include thrombocytopenia, delayed wound healing, fatty liver, alopecia, and dry, thick, desquamating skin.

Intravenous fat emulsions provide a concentrated source of calories (9 kcal/g of fat) and correct or prevent essential fatty acid deficiency. Absolute contraindications to the administration of fat emulsions include pathologic hyperlipemia, lipoid nephrosis, severe egg allergy, and acute pancreatitis associated with hyperlipidemia. Patients with acute pancreatitis who do not have hyperlipidemia may receive fat emulsions. Fat emulsions should be used cautiously in patients with severe liver disease, acute respiratory distress syndrome, high metabolic stress, or blood coagulation disorders. Most clinicians recommend administration of up to 30% of the nonprotein calories as fat, with the remainder being given as carbohydrate. The usual adult daily dose of fat is 0.5 to 1 g/kg/day, with the maximum dose being 2.5 g/kg/day. Table 12.10 lists commercially available fat emulsions, which are composed of either soybean or soybean/safflower oil mixtures and are generally referred to as *long-chain triglycerides*. Fat emulsion products are marketed in concentrations of 10% (1.1 kcal/mL), 20% (2.0 kcal/mL), and 30% (3.0 kcal/mL). The 30% product is not approved for direct infusion into patients, but only for preparation of total nutrient admixtures (TNAs). The 10% and 20% products can be infused at maximum rates of 125 mL/hr and 60 mL/hr respectively; however, this is rarely done. Currently, most clinicians infuse the daily dose of fat over a 24-hour period as a continuous infusion or as a component of a TNA. The lipid emulsions contain varying amounts of the essential fatty acids, linoleic and linolenic acid, and also contain egg yolk phospholipid as an emulsifying agent and glycerin, which makes the product isotonic.

If administered in the recommended doses, intravenous fat emulsions are very safe. Most side effects are caused by the administration of excessive doses of fat emulsions or excessive rates of infusion. Adverse reactions include nausea and vomiting, headache, fever, chills, chest or back pain, and irritation at the infusion site. Reactions that may be associated with long-term use include hepatomegaly, jaundice, splenomegaly, and thrombocytopenia. Fat-overload syndrome, reported with doses exceeding 4 g/kg/day, includes focal seizures, fever, leukocytosis, and shock.

Considerable controversy exists surrounding the ability of intravenous fat emulsions to modify immune function.

Table 12.9.
Examples of Some Total Nutrient Admixture Bases[a]

Components	Standard			Stress/Injury			Fluid Restricted			Liver Failure			Acute Renal Failure			Respiratory Failure		
	D70W	10% AA	20% IVFE	D70W	10% AA	30% IVFE	D70W	10% AA	30% IVFE	D70W	10% AA	20% IVFE	D70W	10% AA	20% IVFE	D70W	10% AA	20% IVFE
	360 mL	500 mL	100 mL	285 mL	600 mL	100 mL	425 mL	400 mL	100 mL	425 mL	500 mL[b]	100 mL	500 mL	250 mL[c]	100 mL	285 mL	500 mL	200 mL
Final Concentrations (%)																		
Dextrose	25			20			30			30			40			20		
Amino acids	5			6			6			5			3			5		
Lipids	2			3			3			2			2.5			4		
Nonprotein Energy (kcal/unit)[d]	1050			980			1320			1220			1390			1080		
Protein (g/unit)	50			60			60			50			25			50		

[a]Each patient's parenteral nutrition solution must be individualized, based on the metabolic state, fluid and electrolyte status, and patient size.
[b]The modified amino acid for liver failure (8% Hepatamine) is sometimes used if the patient has severe hepatic encephalopathy.
[c]When dialysis is instituted, the protein dose can usually be liberalized.
[d]A unit would be approximately 1 liter in all the above except the formula for acute renal failure (850 mL).

Table 12.10.
Intravenous Fat Emulsion Products

Product	Lipid Source	Linoleic Acid (%)	Linolenic Acid (%)
Intralipid	100% soybean	50	9
Soyacal	100% soybean	49–60	6–9
Liposyn II	50% soybean/ 50% safflower	65.8	4.2
Liposyn III	100% soybean	54.5	8.3

Table 12.11.
An Example of Adult Electrolyte Concentrations Used in Parenteral Nutrition Solutions of Patients with Normal Electrolyte Concentrations and Normal Organ Function

Sodium	50 mEq/liter
Potassium	40 mEq/liter
Chloride	40 mEq/liter
Acetate	30 mEq/liter
Phosphorous	15 mM/liter
Calcium	5 mEq/liter
Magnesium	12 mEq/liter

Because of the complexity associated with induction and control of the immune system, fat emulsions may alter different components of the immune response. Early experimental studies suggested that intravenous fat products impaired the bactericidal and migratory functions of polymorphonuclear cells and decreased bacterial clearance by the mononuclear phagocyte system. Most of these studies were associated with large bolus infusions of intravenous fat given over 1 to 6 hours. To date, controlled clinical trials have failed to demonstrate clinically significant alterations in neutrophil or monocyte/macrophage function in patients receiving continuous intravenous fat products. Inconsistent results have been demonstrated in studies assessing the influence of fat emulsions on cellular immunity, and further clinical trials are needed to determine the significance of these findings. No clinical trials to date have shown significant alterations in components of humoral immunity, such as serum immunoglobulin or complement factor concentrations, as a result of fat emulsion products.

Recent evidence suggests that fatty acid components of these products may also interfere with immune responses. Biochemical mediators derived from the Ω-6 family of fatty acids may induce inflammation and immunosuppression, while metabolic end products from the Ω-3 fatty acids may produce opposite effects. Other types of fats can also have unique and potent effects on the immune system. Medium-chain triglycerides may have less immunosuppressive property and serve as more rapidly available and high-energy lipid fuel sources than traditional intravenous fat emulsions. Currently, fat emulsion products are being developed that contain different fatty acid profiles, designed for better utilization of fat. Fat emulsions containing medium-chain triglycerides, short-chain triglycerides, or carnitine may become available after clinical trials are completed. Most likely, these new products will be marketed as a physical mixture of the different triglycerides (e.g., long-chain triglyceride, 25%, and medium-chain triglyceride, 75%) or as a structured triglyceride.

ELECTROLYTES

Electrolytes in maintenance or therapeutic doses must be added to the parenteral nutrition daily to maintain electrolyte homeostasis (Table 12.11). Requirements for individual electrolytes vary, depending on many factors in a patient's clinical course. Electrolyte imbalance may arise from insufficient intake, extraordinary losses, or a combination of both. Patients may have large renal or extrarenal losses of electrolytes and fluid. Occasionally these may need to be quantified by collecting the appropriate fluids and analyzing their electrolyte content. Extrarenal electrolyte losses may include losses from diarrhea, vomiting, fistulae, or nasogastric suctioning. In addition, various pharmacotherapeutic interventions may decrease or increase individual electrolyte requirements. For example, sodium ticarcillin administration delivers a substantial amount of sodium to the patient and causes renal potassium wasting. Amphotericin B therapy increases magnesium and potassium renal losses. Relative electrolyte deficiencies may develop as a result of intracellular shifts of electrolytes from the extracellular fluid compartments. For instance, intracellular shifts of potassium occur during metabolic alkalosis because intracellular hydrogen ions are exchanged for extracellular potassium ions. Also, refeeding chronically starved patients results in an intracellular shift of potassium, phosphorus, and magnesium (29).

Electrolytes are available as single- or multiple-entity products. Once the phosphorus dose has been determined and added, the remaining cations are given as chloride or acetate salts. Patients with metabolic acidosis should have the majority of electrolytes added as acetate salts, while patients with metabolic alkalosis should have most salts added as chlorides.

VITAMINS/TRACE ELEMENTS

Vitamins are an essential component of a patient's daily parenteral nutrition regimen, as they are necessary for normal metabolism and cellular function. Four fat-soluble and nine water-soluble vitamins are recognized as essential. The American Medical Association Nutrition Advisory Group established guidelines for daily parenteral administration of vitamins during parenteral nutrition (30). These amounts are shown for 12 of the vitamins in Table 12.12. These 12 vitamins are available in the suggested amounts from several commercial manufacturers as a multiple-

Table 12.12.
Recommended Adult Intravenous Doses of Vitamins

Vitamin	Daily Intravenous Doses
Fat-soluble vitamins	
A	3,300 I.U.[a]
D	200 I.U.
E	10 I.U.
Water-soluble vitamins	
B$_1$ (thiamine)	3 mg
B$_2$ (riboflavin)	3.6 mg
B$_3$ (pantothenic acid)	15 mg
B$_5$ (niacin)	40 mg
B$_6$ (pyridoxine)	4 mg
B$_{12}$ (cyanocobalamin)	5 µg
C (ascorbic acid)	100 mg
Folic acid	400 µg
Biotin	60 µg

[a]I.U., International Units.

entity product that is added to the parenteral nutrition solutions daily. Vitamin K is usually not included in adult, commercially available multiple-vitamin formulations to avoid complications in patients receiving warfarin. Patients not receiving anticoagulants may receive vitamin K as phytonadione 1 mg/day or 5 to 10 mg/week, during parenteral nutrition. Many of the vitamins are available as single-entity products that can be used for patients with documented vitamin deficiencies.

Trace elements are also a necessary part of a daily parenteral nutrition solution. Trace elements are metabolic cofactors essential to the proper functioning of several enzyme systems in the body. The American Medical Association Nutrition Advisory Group has also published guidelines for four trace elements known to be important in human nutrition (31): zinc, copper, manganese, and chromium. The suggested amounts are shown in Table 12.13. Since the original recommendations, substantial evidence for the essentiality of selenium has accumulated, and many clinicians now add this trace element to the parenteral nutrition on a daily basis. Zinc requirements are increased in metabolic stress or with large gastrointestinal losses. Zinc, chromium, and selenium are excreted by the kidneys, while manganese and copper are excreted through the biliary tract. Therefore, patients with cholestatic liver disease should have copper and manganese restricted or withheld from the parenteral nutrition solution. Selenium stores are depleted in patients with thermal injury, AIDS, and liver failure. Therefore, patients with these diseases should have selenium added initially to the parenteral nutrition solution. The trace elements are available as single- or multiple-entity products for admixture into parenteral nutrition solutions. Parenteral guidelines for molybdenum and iodine have not been established; however, these trace elements are available commercially.

Total Nutrient Admixtures (TNAs)

Traditionally, parenteral nutrition solutions have consisted of an admixture of dextrose and protein (two-in-one); however, intravenous fat is being added to these solutions at some institutions. The intravenous admixture of dextrose, amino acids, and fat emulsion is known as a TNA (32). Intravenous fat is a water-in-oil emulsion stabilized by the anionic emulsifier, egg yolk phospholipid. When properly prepared, the TNA is stable for at least 48 hr.

The use of TNA is increasing because it has several advantages. It may decrease the risk of infection because fewer central-line manipulations are involved. It also decreases the time spent by the nursing staff in parenteral nutrition administration. In addition, lipids mixed with dextrose and amino acids do not support bacterial growth as well as the fat emulsion alone. By giving the fat emulsion slowly and continuously over a 24-hr period, there is improved oxidation of the lipids and less potential for immunosuppression caused by the long-chain triglycerides.

Despite these advantages, there are some concerns about the total nutrient admixture system. It is not possible to detect particulate matter in a TNA. Also, because the fat particles are fairly large, the TNA cannot be filtered with a 0.22-micron filter. Furthermore, only a few medications are known to be compatible with and can be added to the TNAs. Those drugs that are known to be compatible include cimetidine, ranitidine, famotidine, heparin, and insulin. There is also potential for increased wastage using this method of parenteral nutrition administration because most pharmacies prepare one bag for each 24-hr period.

The order in which the three macronutrient substrates are admixed is important to ensure stability. The dextrose and amino acids should be mixed first, and then the fat emulsion should be added. Electrolytes, vitamins, and trace elements may be added before or after the fat emulsion is added, as long as they are not added directly to the fat emulsion. Creaming and coalescence of the fat emulsion results when electrolytes are added directly to it. The anionic emulsifier in the fat emulsion may be adversely affected by divalent cations and acidifying agents. Therefore, limitations exist on the doses of divalent cations that may be added to the TNA. Adding these electrolytes

Table 12.13.
Recommended Adult Intravenous Doses of Trace Elements

Element	Daily Intravenous Dose
Zinc[a]	2.5–4 mg
Copper	0.5–1.5 mg
Chromium[b]	10–15 µg
Manganese	0.15–0.8 mg
Selenium	40–120 µg

[a]Acute catabolic state, additional 2.0 mg.
[b]Intestinal losses, increase daily dose to 20 µg.

beyond the recommended amounts will neutralize the negative potential at the surface of the emulsion and cause the admixture to coalesce.

Complications of Parenteral Nutrition Support

The complications of parenteral nutrition support may be divided into three broad categories: infectious, technical, and metabolic. Catheter-related sepsis, the most common infectious complication, may occur as a result of contamination during line placement or poor catheter care. Catheter sepsis can be minimized by a strict protocol for line placement and catheter care. Many institutions have nutrition support nurses who assist in line placement and perform the central catheter dressing changes.

Technical complications, such as pneumothorax, hydrothorax, and arterial puncture, may occur during placement of the catheter. Proper training and careful technique minimize the chance of a technical complication.

Several metabolic complications may occur. Fluid overload may occur because patients receiving parenteral nutrition often require several other intravenous fluids. The macronutrient substrates are available in several concentrations; thus, the parenteral nutrition solution may be concentrated to decrease the volume of fluid administered when fluid problems exist or are anticipated. Metabolic acidosis or metabolic alkalosis occur with relative frequency in patients who receive parenteral nutrition. Metabolic acidosis may be treated by minimizing the chloride salts and maximizing the acetate salts in the parenteral nutrition solution. Metabolic alkalosis may be treated by administering KCl, maximizing the chloride salts, and restricting the acetate salts. Metabolic complications related to the carbohydrate component of parenteral nutrition include hyperglycemia, hyperosmolar coma, and adverse effects of overfeeding. Hyperglycemia is usually identified by frequent monitoring of serum glucose concentrations. This complication may be managed by the addition of insulin, by decreasing the dextrose concentration in the parenteral nutrition solution, or by decreasing the infusion rate. Carbohydrate overfeeding may cause excess carbon dioxide production leading to respiratory acidosis, elevations of liver function test results, and hepatic steatosis. These problems can usually be avoided by a dextrose infusion rate equal to or less than 5 mg/kg/min (25 kcal/kg/day). Disorders may occur with virtually all of the electrolytes. Malnourished patients who begin parenteral nutrition often experience hypokalemia and hypophosphatemia secondary to the intracellular shift of those ions, induced by dextrose. Vitamin and trace element disorders may also occur (e.g., vitamin A toxicity during parenteral nutrition in patients with renal failure and decreased serum zinc concentrations in severe metabolic stress). The doses of these micronutrients may be increased or decreased as necessary to alleviate metabolic complications.

Table 12.14.
Guidelines for Monitoring the Patient Receiving Parenteral Nutrition Support

1. Finger sticks for glucose q6h. If > 250 mg/dL, draw stat samples for serum glucose and potassium
2. Measures total fluid intake and output daily
3. Weigh patient one time per week
4. Sliding scale with regular human insulin
5. Draw samples for prealbumin or transferrin tests q. week
6. Draw samples for SMA-24 at least q. week, SMA-7 daily in ICU patient[a]
7. Draw samples for magnesium, phosphorus determinations two times per week
8. Collect 24-hour urine for nitrogen balance determination q. week

[a]The frequency of laboratory measurements will be dictated by the severity of the patient's illness.

Monitoring of Parenteral Nutrition Support Patients

Because many metabolic complications may occur in patients receiving parenteral nutrition support, the patients should be monitored daily. Table 12.14 lists some guidelines for monitoring patients receiving parenteral nutrition.

Drug Compatibility Considerations in Parenteral Nutrition Support

By using the parenteral nutrition solution as a drug vehicle, the overall amount of fluid administered and the number of line manipulations are decreased. Patients who are fluid restricted, receive home parenteral nutrition, or have limited venous access may benefit from receiving their medications in the parenteral nutrition solution.

Drugs that are added to the parenteral nutrition solution must be physically and chemically stable in it. It is not wise to add a drug to these solutions when frequent dosage changes are anticipated. When no dosage changes are anticipated and the drug is physically compatible, it could be added. Amino acid concentration, pH of the solution, and ambient room temperature all may affect the stability of the drug added to the parenteral nutrition solution. Also, drugs added to the parenteral nutrition solution may have an adverse effect on selected nutrients.

Numerous studies have been conducted on calcium and phosphorus compatibility in parenteral nutrition solutions. A number of factors may contribute to calcium-phosphate precipitation, such as the amount of calcium and phosphorus additives; the pH of the parenteral nutrient solution; the concentration of the amino acid solutions; and the mixing process used for preparation of parenteral nutrient admixtures. A recent safety alert published by the Food and Drug Administration (FDA) cautions that improper preparation of TNAs with automated compounding systems may result in calcium-phosphate precipitates. Life-threatening hazards such as microvascular pulmonary emboli and subacute interstitial pneumonitis have been

Table 12.15.
Summary of FDA Recommendations for Proper Compounding of Parenteral Nutrition Admixtures to Decrease Calcium and Phosphorus Precipitation

1. The solubility of the added calcium to the admixture should be calculated from the volume *at the time it is added*. It should not be based upon the final volume.
2. When adding calcium and phosphate to an admixture, the phosphate should be added first. The line should be flushed between the addition of any potentially incompatible components.
3. If a lipid emulsion is needed, (a) use a two-in-one admixture with the lipid infused separately, or (b) if a three-in-one admixture is used, add calcium before the lipid emulsion is added.
4. When using an automated compounding device, the above steps should be considered when programming the device.
5. During the mixing process, the pharmacist should periodically agitate the admixture and check for precipitates. Medical or home care personnel who start and monitor these infusions should carefully inspect for the presence of precipitates both before and during the infusion.
6. A filter should be used when infusing either central or peripheral parenteral nutrition admixtures. Standards of practice vary, but the following is suggested: 1.2-micron air-eliminating filter for lipid-containing admixtures and a 0.22-micro air-eliminating filter for non-lipid-containing admixtures.
7. Parenteral nutrition admixtures should be administered within the following time frames: if stored at room temperature, the infusion should be started within 24 hours after mixing; if stored at refrigerated temperatures, the infusion should be started within 24 hours of rewarming.
8. If symptoms of acute respiratory distress, pulmonary embolus, or interstitial pneumonitis develop, the infusion should be stopped immediately and thoroughly checked for precipitates. Appropriate medical interventions should be instituted.

linked to calcium-phosphate precipitates from parenteral nutrient solutions. Recommendations for proper compounding of TNAs have been suggested by the FDA (Table 12.15). Generally, solutions with amino acid concentrations above 2.5% and a pH of less than 6.0 favor solubility of calcium and phosphorus. Some studies have reported incompatibilities between therapeutic doses of iron and fat. Human albumin is reported to be compatible in most two-in-one solutions and TNAs by some manufacturers (e.g., Abbott). There is a lack of data on albumin compatibility with TNAs by other manufacturers. Whenever a question of compatibility arises, it is best to obtain information from a text on intravenous admixtures. If no data exist on a particular combination, the safest approach is to not add the medication to the parenteral nutrition solution.

ENTERAL NUTRITION

The use of enteral nutrition dates back to the ancient Egyptians, who used nutritional enemas to preserve health. Enteral nutrition by tube has been mentioned and used over the subsequent centuries; however, only during the last 20 years has it been used extensively in the hospital and home. Most practitioners feel that if the gastrointestinal tract is functional and accessible, it should be used for the delivery of specialized nutrition support. The development of new feeding tubes, modern equipment for administration, surgically placed enterostomies, and sophisticated enteral formulas have greatly improved this method of administering nutrients. A recent focus on the "gut" during critical illness has changed the role of enteral feeding. Stressful events such as major trauma, thermal injury, or sepsis appear to allow gastrointestinal bacteria to translocate across the gut lumen (33). In animal models these bacteria are taken up by the mesenteric lymph nodes, spleen, and liver. This translocation of gut organisms is thought to lead to sepsis and multiple organ dysfunction syndrome. Enteral feeding by tube is thought to preserve the gastrointestinal mass and prevent this translocation, resulting in fewer infections (34). Consequently, practitioners in specialized nutrition support are making extraordinary efforts to deliver enteral nutrients to the critically ill patient. Traditionally, pharmacists have not been involved extensively in this method of specialized nutrition support. This is changing because of the issues mentioned above, an appreciation of the many drug-nutrient interactions that occur in patients receiving enteral nutrition support, and the many hospital pharmacies that are becoming involved in the preparation and delivery of the enteral nutrient formulas.

The American Society for Parenteral and Enteral Nutrition has published practice guidelines for the rational use of enteral nutrition support (35). A summary of these recommendations appears in Table 12.16. Enteral nutrition should not be used when the gastrointestinal tract is not functional (e.g., postoperative ileus) or when enteral nutrients are undesirable (e.g., severe acute pancreatitis).

Types of Enteral Feeding Delivery

There are many ways to deliver enteral nutrients into the gastrointestinal tract, and enteral nutrition support can be delivered safely and efficaciously in most patients, as either short- or long-term therapy.

Table 12.16.
Summary of A.S.P.E.N. Guidelines for Enteral Nutrition

1. Enteral nutrition by tube feeding should be used in patients who are or will become undernourished and in whom oral feedings are inadequate.
2. Access to the gastrointestinal tract should be obtained in the most natural and least invasive manner.
3. During the administration of enteral nutrition, patients should be monitored by trained health care professionals knowledgeable in the potential pulmonary, mechanical, gastrointestinal, and metabolic complications of enteral tube feeding.
4. Candidates for home enteral nutrition should be evaluated by a multidisciplinary team of health care professionals.

Adapted from Anon. Enteral nutrition. J Parenter Enteral Nutr 17:8SA–9SA, 1993.

Table 12.17.
Types of Administration Devices for Enteral Feeding

Nasogastric and nasoduodenal tubes
    Flexiflo (Ross)
    Kangaroo (Cheeseborough-Ponds)
    Dobbhoff (Biosearch)
    Corpak (Corpak)
    Entriflex (Biosearch)
    ENtube (ENtech)
Gastrostomy
    Stamm gastrostomy
    Percutaneous endoscopic gastrostomy (PEG)
Jejunostomy
    Tube jejunostomy
    Needle catheter jejunostomy (NCJ)

[a]Examples of commonly used products

Nasogastric or nasoduodenal feeding tubes are used for patients who need enteral access for a short-term period (e.g., a few weeks). These soft, small-bore tubes have virtually replaced the large nasogastric tube, which is now only used for nasogastric suction. These tubes, made of polyurethane or silicone, have several advantages over the large nasogastric tubes. Many of them have a tungsten tip, which facilitates transpyloric passage of the tube into the small bowel. Irritation to the nose, pharynx, and esophagus is decreased when these smaller tubes are used over larger nasogastric tubes. Also, patients may eat food and swallow without difficulty when these softer tubes are used. These tubes are usually packaged with a stylet, which aids in proper placement during intubation. Several examples of these tubes are listed in Table 12.17.

A surgical gastrostomy provides the enteral route for a long-term period (months to years). The nutrients are infused directly into the stomach via the gastrostomy tube, bypassing the mouth, pharynx, and esophagus. The Stamm gastrostomy and percutaneous endoscopic gastrostomy (PEG) are the two most common types of gastrostomies for long-term use. The Stamm gastrostomy is usually done by a general surgeon in the operating room, using general anesthesia. PEGs are done by general surgeons or gastro-enterologists in a surgical suite or at the bedside, using local anesthesia.

Jejunostomies for enteral feeding administration are done for both short-term and long-term access (36). A tube jejunostomy is placed during a laparotomy and can be used for long-term enteral access. This type of jejunostomy is particularly effective in a patient who has severe, chronic gastroparesis (e.g., some diabetics). The chance of aspiration of nutrients is decreased, because both the pyloric and the lower esophageal sphincter protect the airway when feedings are delivered into the jejunum. The needle catheter jejunostomy (NCJ) is also placed surgically at the time of laparotomy, but this is used for short-term enteral access. Patients with an NCJ can be fed immediately after

placement. When supplemental enteral feedings are no longer needed and the patient is taking adequate nutrients by mouth, the NCJ can be removed at the bedside without surgical intervention.

Enteral Nutrition Products

Currently, more than 200 enteral products are marketed in the United States. Most organized health care settings (hospitals, nursing homes) that are involved in the administration of these products develop formularies by creating several categories and stocking one product in each one. (Table 12.18 lists 14 categories of enteral formulas and some examples in each category.) Patients with normal fluid requirements, normal nutritional needs, and normal electrolyte status can usually be treated with isotonic, nutritionally complete formulas. Several institutions use products with added dietary fiber as their standard enteral formula in the conditions above, presumably for improved gastrointestinal tolerance. Patients who are eating part of their diet orally can often be supplemented by ingestion of 16 to 32 ounces of an oral enteral supplement. This obviates placement of an enteral feeding tube. Fluid-restricted enteral formulas are reserved for patients who have a problem with overhydration and edema (e.g., congestive heart failure). These products are extremely low in free water and are potentially dangerous in a patient who does not need severe

Table 12.18.
Enteral Formula Categories with Examples of Commonly Used Products

Isotonic tube feeding	(Isocal, Osmolite)
Oral supplement	(Ensure, Ensure Plus, Sustacal)
Fluid-restricted tube feeding	(MagnaCal, Two Cal-HN, Isocal-HCN)
Chemically defined tube feeding	(Vital-HN, Criticare-HN, Vivonex-TEN)
Fiber-containing standard tube feeding	(Ultracal, Jevity)
Low-protein, low-electrolyte, or electrolyte-free tube feeding[a]	(AminAid, Travasorb-Renal, Supena, Nepro)
Modified protein, electrolyte-free or restricted tube feeding[b]	(HepaticAid, Nutrihep)
Low-carbohydrate, high-fat tube feeding[c]	(Pulmocare, Glucerna, Respi-lor)
High-protein tube feeding[d]	(Stresstein, Traumacal, Replete)
High-protein, fiber-containing tube feeding[d]	(Promote wth fiber, Replete with fiber, Isosource VHN)
Immune stimulating feeding	(Impact, Perative, ImmunAid)
Protein module	(Promod, Promix-RD)
Fat module	(Microlipid)
Carbohydrate module	(Polycose, Sumacal)

[a]Used occasionally in acute renal failure, chronic renal dysfunction, chronic renal failure.
[b]Used in liver failure with hepatic encephalopathy.
[c]Used occasionally in respiratory failure or diabetes.
[d]Used occasionally in trauma or sepsis.

fluid restriction. When gastrointestinal digestive capabilities are compromised, a chemically defined enteral formula is often used because most of the nutrients are in elemental or predigested form. Several products are marketed for patients with renal failure, liver failure, respiratory failure, diabetes, compromised immune function, and severe metabolic stress. These products all tend to be more expensive than standard enteral formulas. When a patient's specific needs cannot be met with commercially available enteral formulas, specific macronutrients (carbohydrate, fat, protein) can be added to these formulas to meet special needs. Several of these are listed in Table 12.18.

Administration of Enteral Feedings

There are essentially three ways to administer enteral feeding to institutionalized or home-bound patients: continuous, intermittent, and bolus. Continuous feeding, used preferentially in the institutionalized patient, involves an enteral pump so that the formula can be infused at a constant rate. The advantages of this method are less risk of aspiration, less nursing time, decreased gastrointestinal distension, and decreased diarrhea. Continuous feeding is more sophisticated and more expensive than the other methods. Intermittent feeding is used in the home setting and in some extended-care facilities. The desired volume of formula (usually 240 to 480 mL) is infused over a short period of time (e.g., 1 hr), several times each day. Bolus feeding consists of rapid administration of the desired volume of formula into the patient's ostomy tube. This method is most often used in the home-bound or nursing home patient who has a gastrostomy tube in place. When bolus feedings are administered into the stomach, the risk of aspiration, gastric distension, and diarrhea is higher. The bolus method is, however, the simplest method of administering enteral nutrients, making it attractive in the home setting when an enteral pump is not provided. In general, bolus feedings should not be given via jejunostomy.

Enteral nutrition support is usually started at a slow rate and increased gradually over time to the desired goal. Most patients can tolerate an initial rate of 25 to 50 mL/hr. The isotonic formulas can often be started at 50 mL/hr, while the more concentrated formulas (2 kcal/mL) are started at 25 mL/hr. Patients who are slowly regaining bowel function should be started at a more conservative rate (e.g., 25 mL/hr or less). Many institutions advance the infusion rate of the enteral nutrition formula by 25 mL/hr/day when gastrointestinal tolerance and fluid/electrolyte status are acceptable. This gets most patients to the desired rate within 3 to 4 days. It has been suggested that hyperosmolar enteral formulas be diluted when enteral tube feeding is initiated, to improve gastrointestinal tolerance, but this is not supported by published studies. In fact, in one study, patients who received an undiluted hyperosmolar enteral

formula received more calories and protein without any increase in gastrointestinal side effects than groups receiving diluted hyperosmolar formulas or isotonic formulas (37). Therefore, the use of diluted enteral formulas (e.g., half-strength) should be abandoned.

Complications of Enteral Nutrition Support

The complications of enteral nutrition support can be divided conveniently into four categories: pulmonary, gastrointestinal, mechanical, and metabolic. Aspiration of enteral nutrition formula into the lungs is a serious complication of this type of therapy. It occurs in the patient who has developed vomiting or impaired gastric emptying. This serious complication often results in pneumonia, requiring mechanical ventilation in an intensive care unit. Frequent examination of the abdomen and meticulous checking of gastric residuals aspirated through the feeding tube may help to identify patients who are at risk for aspiration. Prokinetic drugs such as metoclopramide, cisapride, and erythromycin have been used with some success in patients who have poor gastric emptying of enteral nutrition formulas. Diabetics and patients who have a septic process are particularly prone to delayed gastric emptying.

Gastrointestinal complications include vomiting and diarrhea. Vomiting can usually be prevented by advancing the enteral feeding rate slowly, as described earlier, and checking the patient's abdomen often. Most institutions elevate the head of the patient's bed at least 30° in gastric-fed patients. Diarrhea is a frequent problem in patients who receive enteral nutrition support; however, its cause is often elusive. Patients who have their enteral nutrient rate decreased by one-half often demonstrate decreased diarrhea. The rate may then be gradually increased to the desired goal, as tolerated. Suggested causes of diarrhea in association with enteral tube feeding include antibiotic administration, hypoalbuminemia, hyperosmolar formulas, lactase deficiency, and lack of a nutrition support team. The authors of an excellent report carefully examined diarrhea in tube-fed patients and found hyperosmolar drug solutions containing sorbitol (e.g., theophylline) to be the most likely cause (38). Therefore, all drugs administered via the gastrointestinal tract should be inspected in patients who have diarrhea associated with enteral tube feeding. Some patients demonstrate decreased stool volume and frequency when they are switched from a standard enteral formula to a chemically defined formula. Pharmacologic agents such as kaolin pectin may be helpful as first-line pharmacotherapy. Loperamide and diphenoxylate should be used as a last resort in treating diarrhea. A severe gastrointestinal complication of enteral nutrition via jejunostomy is pneumatosis intestinalis with bowel infarction/necrosis. This has been reported to occur in up to 5% of patients receiving enteral nutrition by this route. It appears that this is a complication of critically ill patients who are hemodynamically unstable (e.g., patients with hypotension, tachycardia, receiving intravenous pressor agents) and fed via jejunostomy (39). Regular abdominal examinations of patients receiving feedings by this route and stopping enteral nutrition during periods of instability are prudent approaches to help prevent this morbid complication.

Mechanical complications include a feeding tube that has become kinked or occluded. A kinked tube can be made functional by slowly withdrawing the tube until it straightens out. This should be done without the enteral formula infusing. Slow irrigation of the tube lumen with warm water administered by a 30-mL syringe will open some occluded feeding tubes. Cranberry juice, cola syrup, and pancreatic enzymes in water have also been used with some success. Occasionally, an occluded tube can be saved by passing the stylet back into the lumen of the tube. This may remove or "break up" any concretion formed within the lumen. This should be done by a physician and only in tubes that do not let the stylet exit through a side port.

Virtually all of the metabolic complications that happen with parenteral nutrition can occur with enteral nutrition. Hyperglycemia is usually not as severe with enteral nutrition support because the nutrients are being infused into the gastrointestinal tract rather than into a large vein. Some institutions where the pharmacy department prepares and dispenses the enteral formulas have programs that allow the addition of electrolytes (e.g., KCl, Fleet Phosphosoda) to help treat or prevent metabolic complications.

Monitoring of the Enteral Nutrition Support Patient

Patients who receive enteral nutrition support should be monitored frequently to ensure safety and efficacy. Many of the complications described above can be averted with meticulous patient monitoring. Some enteral tube feeding guidelines for monitoring are listed in Table 12.19.

Table 12.19.
Monitoring the Patient Receiving Enteral Nutrition Support

---

1. Raise head of bed at least 30° at all times
2. Check gastric residuals q6h. If > 150 mL, replace residual and hold feedings for 4 hours and recheck: if < 150 mL, restart, or if still > 150 mL, hold feedings
3. Finger stick for glucose q6h and regular human insulin to scale. If > 250 mg/dL, draw stat serum glucose and potassium samples
4. Draw samples for SMA-24, magnesium determination as needed[a]
5. Draw sample for prealbumin or transferrin determination q. week
6. Collect 24-hour urine for nitrogen balance q. week

---

[a]The frequency of laboratory measurements is dictated by the severity of the patient's illness.

Drug Compatibility Considerations in Enteral Nutrition Support

In many patients receiving enteral nutrition support, the feeding tube may be the only way to administer drugs. Therefore, any incompatibilities between drug and enteral formula or tube are of paramount importance. Phenytoin and warfarin have been reported to be altered during enteral nutrition administration. Patients who received both phenytoin (300 mg per day as the suspension) and enteral tube feeding were reported to have subtherapeutic serum concentrations, compared with patients who received the drug without enteral feedings (40). Interestingly, there does not appear to be a problem with this drug administered as a capsule to normal subjects who take oral enteral supplements concurrently (41). It is unclear what effect the difference in subjects (patients vs. normal subjects) or the effect of administering the drug through a tube has on this interaction. Difficulty has been reported in attaining a therapeutic prothrombin time with warfarin administration during concurrent enteral feeding. Initially this was thought to be caused by the large vitamin K content of some commercially available enteral formulas. The manufacturers have decreased the vitamin K content of most enteral formulas over the last 10 years; however, the problem with warfarin bioavailability and enteral formulas still exists. One study demonstrated reduced recovery of warfarin mixed with an enteral formula compared with it mixed with distilled water (42).

HOME CARE
Home Nutrition Therapy

Although most hospitalized patients on parenteral or enteral nutrition can be changed to an oral diet before discharge, some require continued specialized nutrition support at home. The hospital nutrition support team members work with one of the several home health care companies or a hospital-based home health service. The team devises a specialized nutrition support prescription that will meet the patient's nutritional requirements and an administration schedule that will be compatible with the patient's life-style. Parenteral or enteral nutrition formulations are often given as a nocturnal continuous drip over a 10- to 18-hr period. This allows patients to hold employment or participate in other activities during the day. Some patients on enteral nutrition, however, prefer periodic bolus feedings during the day. The home health service will compound the enteral or parenteral formula and provide the patient with the necessary equipment for its administration. Approximately 5 days prior to hospital discharge, clinicians from the home health service or nutrition support team will begin training the patient and family to administer the nutrition regimen. The patient and family are also trained to detect adverse effects that may occur during administration. In addition, the home health service works with the patient's physician to ensure that the patient is monitored between office visits. The home health service will visit the patient at home whenever necessary to solve any mechanical problems that might arise.

The patient and family must be willing and able to assume the added responsibility involved with home nutrition support for the therapy to be successful. This type of therapy is often cost-prohibitive for many patients; however, partial or complete reimbursement by third parties is frequently available. Provision of specialized nutrition support in the home setting remains costly, yet it is much more economic than keeping the patient hospitalized for extended periods of time. Specific guidelines have been developed to help identify those who may benefit from specialized nutrition support in the home (43). Examples include patients with extensive small bowel resection (short bowel syndrome), chronic enteritis from radiation therapy, or severe Crohn's disease. These patients receive parenteral nutrition via a permanent, centrally placed catheter (e.g., Hickman catheter, PortaCath). Patients who receive home enteral nutrition can absorb nutrients via the gastrointestinal tract, but are unable to consume adequate nutrients by mouth. Examples of patients who receive home enteral nutrition include patients with severe ulcerative colitis, colon cancer, cerebral trauma, or head and neck cancer. The administration route chosen for enteral feeding will depend on the patient's diagnosis and the estimated duration of enteral nutrition support. Surgical gastrostomy or jejunostomy is often used in these patients. Home nutrition programs have increased the quality of life for many patients who require these therapies and have allowed many to return to nearly normal life-styles.

PHARMACOKINETIC/PHARMACODYNAMIC CONSIDERATIONS

Altered disposition of drugs has been demonstrated with both malnutrition and changes in macronutrient intake (44). Much of this research has been performed in animal models; however, more clinical studies in patients are being conducted. In general, the systemic clearance of many drugs is decreased significantly in patients in an undernourished state, compared with that in well-nourished patients. One study demonstrated that elderly patients (usually with a reduced body weight) are given doses of drugs that are 30 to 45% higher than younger patients, when the doses are normalized for weight (45). This is of particular concern, since many elderly patients have a decreased creatinine clearance that makes them particularly susceptible to drug toxicity. Other drugs have increased clearance when they are given concurrently with aggressive doses of macronutrients (e.g., protein). Clearances of theophylline in children (46) and gentamicin in normal adult subjects (47) increased significantly when

they were given with relatively high protein diets. This may be clinically important, as there is a trend to give higher doses of protein to patients who require specialized nutrition support, especially in the critical care setting.

CONCLUSION

The pharmacist is an integral member of the nutrition support team and should be involved in the care of patients who receive specialized nutrition support. The Board of Pharmaceutical Specialties has approved a petition recognizing Nutritional Support Pharmacy Practice as a specialty, and over 300 pharmacists have become board certified through 1994.

Parenteral nutrition solutions are prepared in the pharmacy, using sterile technique. Because of this requirement, pharmacists will always be involved with the administration of parenteral nutrition and, more than likely, in the clinical monitoring of the patient receiving this therapy. The pharmacist must become more involved in enteral nutrition. There is an association between the use of enteral nutrition in critical illness and the development of morbidity. Clearly these patients receiving enteral nutrition have significantly less incidence of pneumonia and abdominal abscesses when compared to patients receiving parenteral nutrition. Most of this work has been done in trauma patients. It will be unfortunate if the pharmacist is not involved with this therapy as more data become available. Most likely an increased number of patients will receive enteral nutrition support and fewer parenteral nutrition over the next few years.

Specialized nutrition support in the acute care and home care setting continues to be a ripe area of specialized practice for the pharmacist. A sound base in sterile technique, nutrient metabolism, fluid and electrolytes, acid-base, and drug-nutrient interactions is needed to be effective in this area.

REFERENCES

1. Dudrick SJ, Wilmore DW, Vars HM, Rhoads JE. Long-term parenteral nutrition with growth, development, and positive nitrogen balance. Surgery 64:134–142, 1968.
2. Blackburn CL, Bistrian BR, Maini BS, Schlamm HT, Smith MF. Nutritional and metabolic assessment of the hospitalized patient. J Parenter Enteral Nutr 1:11–22, 1977.
3. Starker PM, Cump FE, Askanazi J, Elwyn DH, Kinney JM. Serum albumin levels as an index of nutritional support. Surgery 91:194–199, 1982.
4. Donahue SP, Phillips LS. Response of IGF-1 to nutritional support in malnourished hospital patients: a possible indicator of short-term changes in nutritional status. Am J Clin Nutr 50:962–969, 1989.
5. Ingenbleek Y, Carpentier YA. A prognostic inflammatory and nutritional index scoring critically ill patients. Int J Vitam Nutr Res 55:91–101, 1985.
6. Buzby CP, Mullen JL, Matthews DC, Hobbs CL, Rosato EF. Prognostic nutritional index in gastrointestinal surgery. Am J Surg 139:160–166, 1980.

7. Detsky AS, Smalley PS, Chang J. Is this patient malnourished? JAMA 217:54–58, 1994.

8. Baker JP, Detsky AS, Wesson DE, Wolman SL, Stewart S, Whitewell J, Langer B, Jeejeebhoy KN. Nutritional assessment: a comparison of clinical judgment and objective measurements. N Engl J Med 306:969–972, 1982.

9. Robert S, Zarowitz BJ, Hyzy R, et al. Bioelectrical impedance assessment of nutritional status in critically ill patients. Am J Clin Nutr 57:840–844, 1993.

10. Harris JA, Benedict FC. A biometric study of basal metabolism, publ. 279. Washington, DC: Carnegie Institute of Washington, 1919.

11. Long CL, Schaffel N, Geiger JW, et al.. Metabolic response and injury and illness: estimation of energy and protein needs from indirect calorimetry and nitrogen balance. J Parenter Enteral Nutr 3:452–456, 1979.

12. Long CL, Blakemore WS. Energy and protein requirements in the hospitalized patient. J Parenter Enteral Nutr 3:69–71, 1979.

13. Feurer I, Mullen JL. Bedside measurement of resting energy expenditure and respiratory quotient via indirect calorimetry. Nutr Clin Pract 2:43–49, 1986.

14. Weir JB de V. New methods for calculating metabolic rate with special reference to protein metabolism. J Physiol (Lond) 109:1–9, 1949.

15. Shaw JHF, Wildbore M, Wolfe RR. Whole body protein kinetics in severely septic patients: the response to glucose infusion and total parenteral nutrition. Ann Surg 205:288–294, 1987.

16. Anon. Parenteral nutrition. J Parenter Enteral Nutr 17(suppl):9SA-11SA, 1993.

17. Anon. Nutrition support for adults with specific diseases and conditions. J Parenter Enteral Nutr 17(suppl):12SA-26SA, 1993.

18. Daly JM, Masser E, Hansen L, et al. Peripheral vein infusion of dextrose-amino acid solutions ± 2% fat emulsion. J Parenter Enteral Nutr 9:296–299, 1985.

19. Figueras-Felip J, Rafecas-Renau A, Sitges-Serra A, et al. Does peripheral hypocaloric parenteral nutrition benefit the postoperative patient? Results of a multicenter randomized trial. Clin Nutr 5:117–121, 1986.

20. Blackburn CL, O'Keefe SJD. Nutrition in liver failure. Gastroenterology 97:1049–1051, 1989.

21. Cerra FB, Cheung NK, Fischer JF, et al. Disease-specific amino acid infusion (F080) in hepatic encephalopathy: a prospective, mixed double-blind, controlled trial. J Parenter Enteral Nutr 9:288–295, 1985.

22. Michel H, Bories P, Aubin JP, et al. Treatment of acute hepatic encephalopathy in cirrhotics with a branched-chain amino acids versus a conventional amino acids mixture. Liver 5:282–289, 1985.

23. Feinstein EL, Blumenkrantz MJ, Healy M, et al. Clinical and metabolic responses to parenteral nutrition in acute renal failure. Medicine 60:124–137, 1981.

24. Mirtallo JM, Schneider PS, Marko K, et al. A comparison of essential and general amino acid infusions in the nutritional support of patients with compromised renal function. J Parenter Enteral Nutr 6:109–113, 1982.

25. Oki JC, Cuddy PC. Branched-chain amino acid support of stressed patients. DICP Ann Pharmacother 23:399–410, 1989.

26. von Meyenfeldt MF, Soeters PB, Vente JP, et al. Effect of branched chain amino acid enrichment of total parenteral nutrition on nitrogen sparing and clinical outcome of sepsis and trauma. A prospective randomized double-blind trial. Br J Surg 77:924–929, 1990.

27. Burke JF, Wolfe RR, MuDancy CJ, et al. Glucose requirements following burn injury: parameters of optimal glucose infusion and possible hepatic and respiratory abnormalities following excessive glucose intake. Ann Surg 190:275–285, 1979.

28. Roesner M, Crant JP. Intravenous fat emulsions. Nutr Clin Pract 2:96–107, 1987.

29. Solomon SM, Kirby DF. The refeeding syndrome: a review. J Parenter Enteral Nutr 14:90–97, 1990.

30. Anon. Multivitamin preparations for parenteral use—a statement by the Nutrition Advisory Group. J Parenter Enteral Nutr 3:253–262, 1979.

31. Anon. Guidelines for essential trace element preparations for parenteral use—a statement by the Nutrition Advisory Group. J Parenter Enteral Nutr 3:263–267, 1979.

32. Driscoll DF. Clinical issues regarding the use of total nutrient admixtures. DICP Ann Pharmacother 24:296–303, 1990.

33. Wilmore DW, Smith RJ, O'Dwyer ST, Jacobs DO, Ziegler TR, Wang XD. The gut: a central organ after surgical stress. Surgery 104:917923, 1988.

34. Moore FA, Moore EE, Jones TN, McCroskey BL, Peterson VM. TEN versus TPN following major abdominal trauma—reduced septic morbidity. J Trauma 29:916–922, 1989.

35. Anon. Enteral nutrition. J Parenter Enteral Nutr 17(suppl):8SA-9SA, 1993.

36. Sarr MG, Mayo S. Needle catheter jejunostomy: an unappreciated and misunderstood advance in the care of patients after major abdominal operations. Mayo Clin Proc 63:565–572, 1988.

37. Keohane PP, Attrill H, Love M, Frost P, Silk DB. Relation between osmolality of diet and gastrointestinal side effects in enteral nutrition. Br Med J 288:678–680, 1984.

38. Edes TE, Walk BE, Austin JL. Diarrhea in tube-fed patients: feeding formula not necessarily the cause. Am J Med 88:91–93, 1990.

39. Delany HM, Lindine P. The pros and cons of needle catheter jejunostomy. Nutrition 4:119–124, 1988.

40. Bauer LA. Interference of oral phenytoin absorption by continuous nasogastric feedings. Neurology 32:570–572, 1982.

41. Nishimura LY, Armstrong EP, Plezia PM, Oacono RP. Influence of enteral feedings on phenytoin sodium absorption from capsules. Drug Intell Clin Pharm 22:130–133, 1988.

42. Kuhn TA, Garnett WR, Wells BK, Kames HT. Recovery of warfarin from an enteral nutrient formula. Am J Hosp Pharm 46:1395–1399, 1989.

43. Anon. Guidelines for use of home total parenteral nutrition. J Parenter Enteral Nutr 11:342–344, 1987.

44. Anderson KE. Influences of diet and nutrition on clinical pharmacokinetics. Clin Pharmacokinet 14:325–346, 1988.

45. Campion EW, Avorn J, Reder VA, Olins NJ. Overmedication of the low-weight elderly. Arch Intern Med 147:945–947, 1987.

46. Feldman CH, Hutchinson VE, Sher TH, Feldman BR, Davis WJ. Interaction between nutrition and theophylline metabolism in children. Ther Drug Monit 4:69–76, 1982.

47. Dickson CJ, Schwartzman MS, Bertino JS. Factors affecting aminoglycoside disposition: effects of circadian rhythm and dietary protein intake on gentamicin pharmacokinetics. Clin Pharmacol Ther 39:325–328, 1986.

CHAPTER 13

IRON DEFICIENCY AND MEGALOBLASTIC ANEMIAS

MARY E. TERESI, STANLEY G. KAILIS, and CONSTANTINE G. BERBATIS

Anemia is a hematologic condition in which there is quantitative deficiency of circulating hemoglobin, often accompanied by a reduced number of red blood cells (erythrocytes). Causes of anemia are blood loss, impaired erythropoiesis, and abnormal erythrocyte destruction.

Erythropoiesis is a controlled physiologic process. In response to changes in tissue oxygen availability the kidney regulates production and release of erythropoietin, which stimulates the bone marrow to produce and release red blood cells. Erythrocytes originate from pluripotent stem cells in the bone marrow and undergo multiple steps of differentiation and maturation. Early stages of red cell production consist of large cells with immature nuclei (pronormoblasts and basophilic normoblasts). As cells mature, hemoglobin is incorporated, the nucleus is extruded, and cell size decreases. Various nutrients are required for normal erythropoiesis. Lack of B_{12} or folate can interfere with the maturation of the cells, resulting in the release of megaloblasts (erythroid precursors with immature nuclei). Iron deficiency interferes with hemoglobin production and incorporation into the maturing cells, which continue to divide resulting in the release of smaller cells (microcytic).

In most cases the nutritional anemias are either preventable or treatable by providing the appropriate nutrient. For the effective treatment of these anemias the deficiency state must be documented, it must be confirmed that the anemia is due to the deficiency, the pathologic state responsible for the deficiency must be identified and where possible rectified, and the patient must comply with the treatment.

The number of erythrocytes in normal individuals varies with age, gender, and atmospheric pressure. People who live at high altitudes have more erythrocytes to compensate for the reduced oxygen in the air. At sea level the average normal adult male has 5.5×10^{12} erythrocytes/L ($5.5 \times 10^6/mm^3$). The erythrocytes occupy 47% of the blood, and this value is termed the packed cell volume (PCV) or hematocrit (Table 13.1). Blood from healthy adult males contains approximately 160 g/L (16 g/dL) of hemoglobin. All these parameters are lower for healthy adult women. Values for neonates, which show no gender differences, are higher at birth, but after several weeks they decrease to below those of adult women. Thereafter, the values rise gradually, and at puberty, male/female differences appear.

Anemia is not a single disease entity but a sign of disease, which has many causes. Regardless of the cause, anemia is associated with a reduction in circulating hemoglobin because of reduced numbers of erythrocytes, less hemoglobin per erythrocyte, or a combination of both.

The physiologic importance of low circulating hemoglobin is the reduced capacity for blood to carry oxygen. Consequently, less oxygen is available to tissues, including those of the heart, brain, and muscles, leading to the clinical manifestations of anemia. Anemia is generally associated with hemoglobin levels below 110 g/L for children 6 months to 6 years of age, 120 g/L (12 g/dL) for children 6 years to 14 years of age, 130 g/L (13 g/dL) for adult men, 120 g/L (12 g/dL) for adult women, and 110 g/L (11 g/dL) in pregnancy. However, lower hemoglobin levels are often tolerated with minimal symptoms if the anemia develops slowly and the body is able to adequately compensate for the reduction in oxygen.

GENERAL MANIFESTATION OF ANEMIAS

The term "anemia" denotes a complex of signs and symptoms that indicate an underlying disorder. Regardless of the cause of anemia, the clinical features depend on the rate of development and the ability of the cardiovascular-pulmonary system to compensate for the tissue hypoxia. Overt signs of anemia are pallor of the skin, mucous membranes (particularly the conjunctiva), and nail beds. Symptoms include faintness, malaise, dizziness, ease of fatigue, lack of concentration, irritability, headache, intermittent claudication, palpitations, ankle edema, and angina. Cardiomegaly and high-output heart failure are also possible in severe cases.

Even though the symptoms of anemia are distinctive, they can also be manifestations of other disorders. A comprehensive history and physical examination are important in the assessment of the anemic patient. More

Table 13.1.
Selected Hematologic and Biochemical Parameters

Component	Specimen[a]		Reference Range	
			Conventional	SI
Hematocrit (Hct)	B	M	45–52%	0.42–0.52
		F	37–48%	0.37–0.48
Hemoglobin (Hgb)	B	M	13–18 g/dL	8.1–11.2 mmol/L
		F	12–16 g/dL	7.4–9.9 mmol/L
Erythrocyte count (RBC)	B		$4.2–5.9 \times 10^6$/mm	$4.2–5.9 \times 10^6$/mm
Reticulocyte count	B		0.5–1.5% RBC	
Mean corpuscular volume (MCV)	Ery		80–94 fmol	80–94 fmol
Mean corpuscular hemoglobin (MCH)	Ery		27–32 pg	1.7–2.0 fmol
Mean corpuscular hemoglobin concentration (MCHC)	Ery		32–36 g/dL	19–22.8 mmol/L
Red cell distribution width (RDW)	Ery		11.5–14.5%	
Iron	S	M	80–180 µg/dL	14–32 µmol/L
		F	60–190 µg/dL	11–29 µmol/L
Transferrin	S		170–370 mg/dL	1.7–3.7 g/L
Total iron-binding capacity (TIBC)	S		250–410 g/mL	45–72 µmol/L
Transferrin saturation	S		20–55%	
Ferritin	S	M > F	2–20 µg/dL	20–200 µg/L
Folate (as pteroglutamic acid)				
Normal	S		2–10 ng/mL	4–22 nmol/L
Borderline	S		1–1.9 ng/mL	2.5–4 nmol/L
	Ery		150–800 ng/mL	
Vitamin B_{12}	S		200–1000 pg/mL	150–750 pmol/L

[a]B = whole blood, Ery = erythrocyte, S = serum, M = male, F = female.

specifically, dietary habits, drug histories, and occupation should be documented. Close questioning about blood loss, menses, gastrointestinal symptoms, and history of pregnancy provides useful information.

DIAGNOSIS OF ANEMIAS (1–3)

Hematologic and biochemical tests, including a full blood screen, are essential for identifying the type of anemia and in many cases directing the treatment. In most cases the full blood screen will reveal low hemoglobin and hematocrit, as well as information on cell size and color. Routine blood screens may reveal unsuspected hematologic abnormalities. As the nutritional anemias progress in stages (normal, negative nutrient balance, nutrient depletion, nutrient deficiency, anemia), monitoring early indicators of depletion may prevent the progression to overt anemia.

Many aspects of the cellular elements of blood can be quantified by automated blood analyzers, including blood hemoglobin concentration, cell counts, and the mean corpuscular volume (MCV). From these primary measurements the hematocrit, mean corpuscular hemoglobin (MCH), and mean corpuscular hemoglobin concentration (MCHC) are automatically calculated. The MCV, MCH, and MCHC are collectively known as the erythrocyte indices. The MCV correlates with cell size (smaller cells take up less volume) and is particularly valuable in differentiating microcytic anemias, which have

a reduced MCV (<80 fL), from macrocytic anemias, which have a greater than normal MCV (<95 fL). However, the MCV may appear normal in combination anemias, in which the microcytic cells of iron deficiency are counterbalanced by the macrocytic cells of a B_{12} or folate deficiency. In this instance a peripheral blood smear can aid in identifying the existence of a mixed anemia. The MCH and MCHC provide information on the color of the cells (lower hemoglobin, less color). Hypochromic anemias such as iron deficiency anemia have a low MCHC, indicating lower than normal hemoglobin concentrations. Another parameter, the red blood cell distribution width (RDW), which is expressed as the coefficient of variation of the volume of distribution width, gives an indication of the variation in erythrocyte size in a blood sample. A characteristic of iron deficiency anemia is an increased RDW, reflecting the anisocytosis seen in blood smears. Selected laboratory characteristics of iron deficiency anemia and megaloblastic anemias are summarized in Table 13.2.

Other hematologic investigations involve reticulocyte counts, differential white cell count, platelet count, and microscopic examination of peripheral blood smears and bone marrow aspirates. The normal life span of an erythrocyte is 120 days. As old erythrocytes are removed from the circulation by reticuloendothelial cells, they are replaced by young erythrocytes from the bone marrow.

Table 13.2.
Selected Laboratory Characteristics of Iron Deficiency Anemia and Megaloblastic Anemia

Type	MCV[a]	RDW	Peripheral Smear	Additional Investigations
Iron deficiency	L[b]	H	Hypochromic, microcytic	↓Fe, ↓ferritin, ↑transferrin, bone marrow iron stain
Vitamin B_{12} deficiency[c]	H	H	Macrocytic	↓S-vitamin B_{12}, achlorhydria, ↑antiparietal antibodies
Folate deficiency	H	H	Macrocytic	↓S-folate[d], ↓erythrocyte folate[e]
Chronic disease	L	H	Hypochromic, normocytic	↓Fe, ↓transferrin
	N	N	Normochromic, normocytic	
Blood loss	N	N	Normochromic, normocytic	Clinical evidence, occult blood loss

[a]N = normal, L = low, H = high.
[b]Normal in early iron deficiency.
[c]Includes pernicious anemia.
[d]Varies with diet.
[e]Provides a measure of tissue stores.

These immature cells, called reticulocytes, make up 1 to 1.5% of the total erythrocyte population in a normal individual. Reticulocyte identification and counting involve staining techniques that visualize endoplasmic reticular material, which is absent in mature erythrocytes. Because reticulocytes represent a young population of red blood cells, they are an important marker of bone marrow activity. Reticulocytosis, an increase in reticulocyte numbers, indicates increased bone marrow activity. Transient reticulocytosis often occurs in response to iron, B_{12}, or folic acid therapy for the respective deficiency states.

Biochemical tests for assessing anemias include measurement of serum iron, ferritin (stored iron), transferrin (iron transport protein), and transferrin saturation. Serum transferrin receptors (STR) may also be measured by using a monoclonal antibody assay. These receptors are normal during the early phase of iron depletion but increase in the later phase of iron and appear to correlate with the severity of iron deficiency. This is a relatively new test, and the exact role of STR in the diagnosis and management of iron deficiency anemia remains to be seen. Other specific tests can be directed toward the identification of a particular deficiency state or anemia. Serum B_{12} or folate as well as erythrocyte folate levels can be measured. However reduced levels of these nutrients must be addressed in conjunction with hematologic tests and the patient's clinical status.

GENERAL MANAGEMENT OF DEFICIENCY ANEMIAS

Treatment of nutritional anemia involves identification and correction of the cause if possible, replenishment of deficient nutrient(s), and reduction of symptoms. This may involve restoring missing nutrients, restoring blood volume by transfusions, or treating the cause by medical or surgical methods. Careful assessment of the patient's drug history may help to identify possible pharmacotherapeutic agents that could be involved in the cause. Because deficiency states of iron, vitamin B_{12}, or folic acid may require long-term or lifelong therapy, patients must be counseled appropriately.

IRON DEFICIENCY ANEMIA

Iron deficiency occurs when the body iron is insufficient for the normal formation of hemoglobin, iron-containing enzymes, and other functional iron compounds such as myoglobin and those of the cytochrome system. Iron deficiency can be classified according to its severity: normal stores, negative iron balance, iron store depletion (low serum ferritin), decreased serum iron (low serum iron, increased total iron-binding capacity (TIBC), and anemia (reduced hemoglobin with microcytic, hypochromic erythrocytes) (1). Erythrocytes of individuals with mild, early stage iron deficiency often appear to be normal in color and size (i.e., normochromic, normocytic).

Other conditions with reduced MCV and MCHC, such as thalassemia, sideroblastic anemia, and the anemia of chronic disease, can generally be differentiated from iron deficiency anemia by assessing iron stores. Ferritin is reduced in iron deficiency but normal to elevated in the other three conditions.

Occurrence of Iron Deficiency

Iron deficiency, estimated to occur in over 500 million people throughout the world, is the most common cause of anemia (4, 5). Data from the second Nutritional Health and Nutrition Examination Survey in the United States indicated that the prevalence of iron deficiency was 0.2% for men, 2.6% for premenopausal women, and 1.9% for postmenopausal women (5). Iron deficiency occurs more frequently in infants and menstruating or pregnant women.

Physiologic Importance of Iron

Iron is an essential element for many physiologic processes, including erythropoiesis, tissue respiration, and several enzyme-catalyzed reactions. Iron deficiency, in addition to its hematologic effects, may also be associated with diverse problems such as impaired work performance (6); low birth weight, prematurity, and increased perinatal mortality (7); impaired psychomotor behavior and cognitive function in infants and young children (8); and abnormalities of epidermal structures, heat production, catecholamine turnover, mentation, and resistance to infection (9). Oxidative metabolism by tissues is more effective when iron stores are normal (10). Behavioral effects associated with iron deficiency, best described in children, include decreased academic achievement, which can be reversed by giving iron (11).

The average adult body contains 3 to 5 g of elemental iron. Functional iron exists predominantly as hemoglobin (2.5 g) in circulating erythrocytes, with lesser amounts in myoglobin (130 mg) and tissue enzymes (8 mg). Circulating transferrin, the iron-binding protein that supplies iron to all tissues, contains 4 mg of iron in the ferric form.

Hemoglobin is the oxygen-binding protein in erythrocytes of vertebrates that transports oxygen absorbed from the lungs to the tissues. Each hemoglobin molecule consists of four heme groups surrounding a globin group forming a tetrahedral structure. Heme accounts for 4% by weight of the molecule and contains all the iron. Hemoglobin forms an unstable, reversible bond with oxygen, allowing for oxygen release at lower oxygen tension, as is encountered in the tissues. Globin consists of linked pairs of polypeptide chains. Fetal hemoglobin has two α and two γ globin chains. In normal erythrocyte development the γ chains are replaced by β chains, and a normal human adult has two α and two β chains. The composition of these chains differs in individuals with genetically determined disorders such as thalassemia and sickle cell anemia. (See Chapter 14, "Other Anemias.") In iron deficiency anemia, as well as other chronic anemias, hemoglobin has a reduced affinity for oxygen. This allows oxygen to transfer more readily from the erythrocytes than in normal states, resulting in more tolerable tissue oxygenation.

Myoglobin, a hemoprotein in muscle, accepts oxygen from hemoglobin in the periphery and acts as an oxygen store in muscle. If oxygen supply is limited, myoglobin releases its oxygen to cytochrome oxidase, the terminal enzyme in the mitochondrial respiratory chain, which has a higher affinity for oxygen than does myoglobin and so allows oxidative phosphorylation to occur.

Transferrin, a β-globulin that is synthesized by the liver, is a specific iron-binding protein in blood which transports iron through the plasma and extravascular spaces. Each molecule of transferrin can bind two molecules of iron in the ferric state. In normal circumstances it is only 30 to 50% saturated. The ability of transferrin to bind iron is called the iron-binding capacity. The total iron-binding capacity (TIBC), which reflects serum transferrin concentrations, is a well-recognized value in the investigation of anemias. It represents the amount of iron that can bind to transferrin to give 100% saturation of the binding sites. The TIBC is increased in iron deficiency and reduced in iron overload. Most cells obtain their iron from transferrin. In the case of reticulocytes and developing erythrocytes in the bone marrow, most of the iron that is taken up is used for hemoglobin synthesis.

Storage iron (1 g), in the form of ferritin and hemosiderin, which is located mainly in the parenchymal cells of the liver and the reticuloendothelial cells of the bone marrow, spleen, and liver, replenishes functional iron. Iron stores account for one-third of body iron in healthy adult males. Iron stores are more variable and are generally lower or absent in children and menstruating females. Low iron stores do not indicate iron deficiency and are not associated with abnormalities.

Iron Requirements

Body iron is usually kept constant by a delicate balance between the amounts lost and absorbed. There is no physiologic mechanism for excreting iron in humans; the quantity of iron that is lost daily is similar to the quantity that is absorbed. Consequently, there is only a limited ability to compensate for excessive loss or absorption of iron. Iron balance is a conservative system, and in the normal adult, even if iron intake is negligible, it takes at least 2 to 3 years to develop iron deficiency.

Iron requirements are determined by total losses from the body. Daily iron requirements vary according to age and gender. Total daily iron loss amounts to 1 mg/day (~14 µg/kg/day) in males. Iron losses in normal women are higher than those in men because of menstruation and pregnancy. Losses by postmenopausal or nonmenstruating women are similar to those of men. Iron losses occur from the gastrointestinal tract by sloughing of iron-containing mucosal cells and extravasation of erythrocytes, by exfoliation of skin, and by shedding of urinary tract epithelial cells. Loss of iron through sweat is minimal, so manual laborers working in humid conditions are not at risk. Normal men and postmenopausal women require only 1 mg of iron to be absorbed each day (Table 13.3).

Table 13.3.
Daily Iron Requirements[a]

Infant	
0–4 months	0.5 mg
5–12 months	1.0 mg
Children	1.0 mg
Adolescent male	1.8 mg
Adolescent female	2.4 mg
Menstruating female	2.8 mg
Adult male	1.0 mg
Postmenopausal female	1.0 mg
During pregnancy	3–4 mg

[a]Values represent actual iron absorbed.

Table 13.4.
Recommended Daily Allowances (RDAs) for Iron, Folic Acid, and Vitamin B_{12}[a]

Category	Iron		Folic Acid		Vitamin B_{12}	
	Age (yr)	Amount (mg)	Age (yr)	Amount (μg)	Age (yr)	Amount (μg)
Infants	0–0.5	6	0–0.5	25	0–0.5	0.3
	0.5–1	10	0.5–1	35	0.5–1	0.5
Children	1–10	10	1–3	50	1–3	0.7
			4–6	75	4–6	1
			7–10	100	7–10	1.4
Males	11–18[b]	12	11–14[b]	150	11+	2
	19+	10	15+	200		
Females	11–50	15	11–14[b]	200	11+	2
	51+	10	15+	180		
Pregnant		30		400		2.2
Lactating		15		260–280		2.6

[a]Values determined by the Food and Nutrition Board of the National Research Council. RDA provides adequate nutrition in most healthy persons under usual environmental stresses and are not minimum requirements. (See reference **26.**)
[b]Adolescents.

Blood loss in menstruating women varies, and if it is in excess of 80 mL, it can lead to iron deficiency. Average iron losses due to menstruation are about 0.6 mg/day; however, over 30% of menstruating women lose between 0.9 and 1.4 mg/day of iron. Daily iron loss for most menstruating women, which includes obligatory losses, is 1.5 to 2 mg/day. Menstrual iron losses are reduced by 50% in women taking oral contraceptives but are increased by up to 100% in women who are using an intrauterine device (12, 13).

Iron requirements increase to 3 to 4 mg/day during pregnancy because both maternal and fetal iron requirements must be met by the mother. Even though menstruation ceases, iron losses by the mother are still greater than in the nonpregnant state. Iron is needed for obligatory losses, for the expanded maternal erythrocyte mass that occurs in pregnancy, and for the placenta and fetus. Elemental iron requirements for a well-nourished 55-kg woman during pregnancy are at least 1000 mg (20 mg/kg). At term, 270 to 450 mg of this iron is in the fetus. Iron requirements are greatest in the second and third trimesters (5 to 6 mg/day), when the highest fetal erythrocyte requirements occur. Some of the iron that is incorporated in the expanded maternal erythrocyte mass returns to the iron pool after pregnancy, but peripartum blood loss partly nullifies this contribution. Because menstruation does not start until several weeks after delivery, iron losses are reduced. However, breast-feeding offsets some of the gain.

Maternal iron loss, estimated to be about 0.3 mg/day by the third month after delivery, should not pose a major problem to mothers, except for those in developing countries who continue to breast-feed well after menstruation has recommenced.

The need for iron is high in the first year of life and subsequent childhood years because of rapid growth and erythropoiesis during this period. Normal full-term infants need to absorb a minimum of 0.3 mg of iron daily in the first year of life. Premature infants can need up to 1 mg/day. With increasing age, the requirements for children increase progressively to 0.5 to 0.8 mg/day. The growth spurt of adolescence results in a daily iron requirement of about 1.6 mg/day. The recommended daily allowances for iron, to meet these levels of uptake, are summarized in Table 13.4. Normal infants need 1 mg/kg/day of dietary iron, and low-birth-weight infants require 2 mg/kg/day. Human breast milk is low in iron, and the usual infant diet does not provide sufficient quantities of iron. Therefore, iron supplementation of 10 mg/day is often necessary during the first year of life. For adolescent males and females during their growth spurt, 12 mg/day and 15 mg/day, respectively, are recommended. It is advised that women continue this supplementation throughout the reproductive years (14). Because the iron requirements of pregnancy, particularly during the second and third trimesters, cannot be met from dietary sources, 30 mg/day of elemental iron should be taken. The daily iron requirement of 10 mg/day for adult men and postmenopausal women can usually be met from dietary sources.

Iron Absorption (1, 15, 16)

Iron is present in a wide variety of foods, particularly red meats, poultry, brewer's yeast, wheat germ, some dried beans, and some vegetables. The iron content of food and its bioavailability determine whether the diet can meet physiologic requirements. Milk is a relatively poor source of iron, as is a diet that is high in cereal content and low in animal protein. An average Western diet contains 10 to 20 mg of iron per day, which can deliver 1 to 2 mg of iron to the body. The diet of poorer populations includes little animal meat and so contains very low amounts of iron.

The main sites of iron absorption are the duodenum and proximal jejunum, the upper parts of the small intestine. Only part of dietary iron is actually absorbed (15). This depends on a number of factors, including the amount of iron in the diet, the physiologic status of the small bowel where iron is absorbed, the composition of the diet, and the erythropoiesis rate. Adults with normal iron stores absorb 5 to 10% of dietary iron (1 to 2 mg/day). Iron absorption increases with decreasing levels of iron stores and, in those with severely depleted stores, may rise to 50% of the total intake.

Food iron is generally organically bound and must be freed from the bond for absorption. Dietary iron is present as two major pools: nonheme iron and heme iron. Ingested organic nonheme iron complexes and heme compounds are broken down in the acid environment of the stomach to ferric ions and heme molecules, respectively. The stomach's acidity promotes reduction of iron from the ferric state to the ferrous state, which is better absorbed. Patients with achlorhydria secondary to age or gastrectomy tend to absorb nonheme iron poorly. Iron is absorbed primarily in the upper duodenum. The iron-absorptive capacity is limited by the rate at which iron is transferred from the intestinal lumen to the plasma. The reduced iron (ferrous) binds to specific sites on the lumen and is actively carried across the intestinal membrane. Iron absorbed by these cells is incorporated into an iron-carrier pool, most of which is deposited as ferritin or used by the mitochondria for enzyme synthesis. It is then lost by sloughing during the usual intestinal cell turnover. A smaller proportion of the iron from the carrier pool is transferred to the plasma, where the ferric form binds tightly to transferrin.

A number of factors can inhibit or promote the absorption of nonheme iron (Table 13.5). Foods that can reduce iron absorption by forming less-soluble complexes include coffee, tea, milk and milk products, eggs, whole-grain breads and cereals, and any food that contains bicarbonates, carbonates, oxalates, or phosphates.

Enhancers of nonheme iron absorption include meat and food acids such as citric, lactic, or ascorbic acids. Ascorbic acid, the most powerful promoter, has a dose-related effect on nonheme iron absorption. In its presence, ferric iron is converted to the ferrous state, maintaining the solubility of the iron in the alkaline environment of the duodenum and upper jejunum. Ascorbic acid also forms an alkaline-stable chelate with ferric chloride in the stomach. Meat, itself a rich source of iron, promotes absorption of nonheme iron. Quantitatively, 1 g of meat enhances nonheme iron absorption to about the same extent as 1 mg of ascorbic acid. Citric acid, a common food additive and a less powerful promoter of iron absorption, has an additive effect to ascorbic acid.

Table 13.5.
Factors Associated with Iron Absorption

Factor	Associations
Favoring absorption	
Inorganic iron	Ionic iron, particularly in the ferrous form, is better absorbed than ferric iron and organically bound iron.
Ascorbic acid	Probably by assisting the conversion of ferric iron to ferrous iron.
Acid	Gastric HCl promotes the release and conversion of dietary iron to the ferrous form.
Chelates	Iron chelated to low-molecular-weight substances such as sugars (fructose and sucrose), amino acids, and succinate facilitates binding of iron to the intestinal mucosa.
Clinical states	Iron deficiency, increased erythropoiesis, pregnancy, anoxia, pyridoxine deficiency.
Reducing absorption	
Alkaline	Alkaline pancreatic secretions containing phosphate probably convert iron to insoluble ferric hydroxide, antacids.
Dietary	Dietary phosphates and phytates in cereals, tannins in tea (probably complex iron).
Clinical states	Chronic diarrhea, steatorrhea, adequate iron stores, decreased erythropoiesis, acute or chronic inflammation.

Heme iron is highly bioavailable (20 to 40%) in the iron-depleted patient because it is absorbed within the porphyrin ring and so is not exposed to inhibitory ligands in the diet. It is absorbed via specific, high-affinity, brush border binding sites. When the heme is absorbed, iron is released to the mucosal cell, where it enters the general iron pool. However, heme iron represents only a small fraction of dietary iron, particularly in poorer populations. Absorption of iron from heme increases when it is associated with hemoglobin, meat, protein, or soy proteins. Baking and prolonged frying significantly reduce heme iron absorption. Iron absorption from ferritin, hemosiderin, and ferric oxides is less than that from the nonheme dietary pool.

Iron absorption is regulated by iron need and stores of the body. When iron stores are low or depleted, a higher proportion of available iron is absorbed. Absorption is reduced when the stores are replete. The serum ferritin concentration, which reflects body iron stores, is inversely related to iron absorption. However, this feedback process can be overwhelmed when large amounts of iron are presented for absorption (e.g., in iron overdosing or toxicity cases). Malabsorption of iron, associated with mucosal abnormalities, has been reported for people living on and around the Indian subcontinent and Haiti. In some clinical states such as primary hemochromatosis, thalassemia, and sideroblastic anemia, iron absorption remains normal and even raised, despite increased iron stores. Giving additional iron to patients with these conditions is therefore inappropriate and potentially dangerous.

Etiology of Iron Deficiency (1, 2, 6, 17–21)

The primary causes of iron deficiency in adults are blood loss and pregnancy (Table 13.6). Blood loss from any body site is the major cause of iron deficiency in adult males and nonmenstruating females. Bleeding may be occult or overt. A common site of blood loss is the gastrointestinal tract. Iron deficiency anemia should be treated as a warning signal of gastrointestinal cancer and should not be passed off as a nutritional deficiency without adequate investigation. When bleeding is not obvious, a test for occult blood in the stool may give the first indication of blood loss. Common sources of blood loss in the gastrointestinal tract are peptic ulcers and esophageal varices. Nonsteroidal antiinflammatory agents such as aspirin and indomethacin are frequently responsible for gastrointestinal bleeding, especially if they are taken with warfarin. In the absence of upper gastrointestinal symptoms, investigations should be directed to the lower gastrointestinal tract. Bleeding hemorrhoids rarely result in anemia, but neoplasms are a common cause of bleeding, particularly in the elderly. Colonic cancer, which can cause bleeding, increases 40-fold between the ages of 40 and 80. Other causes of gastrointestinal blood loss include hookworm infestation, Meckel's diverticulum, and ulcerative colitis. Hookworm is a major cause of iron deficiency anemia in tropical areas.

Adolescent females are susceptible to iron deficiency because of the growth spurt associated with adolescence and menarche (6). Menorrhagia, heavy menstrual bleeding, is the chief cause of iron deficiency in fertile women.

Iron deficiency has also been noted in athletes, particularly adolescent women, marathon runners, and other endurance athletes. Up to 50% of adolescent female athletes demonstrate some degree of iron depletion; however, anemia is relatively uncommon. Blood loss is believed to result from ischemia of the gastrointestinal tract, as blood is shunted to muscles during prolonged exercise. Marathon runners can lose at least 3 mg of iron daily for several days after a marathon race. Another short-term anemia that is related to sport is the dilutional anemia that can result from plasma volume expansion in the early weeks of conditioning (21, 22).

Poor nutrition, defective intake, or decreased assimilation of iron rarely causes iron deficiency in people living in Western countries. Iron deficiency due to inadequate dietary iron intake is predominantly a problem of infants and children, for whom the daily requirements are increased. In some populations, however, whose diet is mainly of vegetable origin with little meat, women are likely to suffer from nutritional iron deficiency. Malabsorption of iron may occasionally cause iron deficiency, though it is rarely an important cause unless iron stores are low or there are other contributing factors such as blood loss, pregnancy, or poor nutrition. The two most common conditions in which iron absorption is a problem are gluten enteropathy (celiac disease) and gastrectomy. Other conditions that are associated with iron deficiency anemia include pernicious anemia, pica syndrome, and chronic inflammatory disease such as rheumatoid arthritis.

Clinical Findings and Manifestations

Iron deficiency precedes the manifestations of anemia. Most individuals with iron deficiency have minimal anemia and are asymptomatic. Progression of iron deficiency anemia is often insidious, although mildly lowered hemoglobin concentrations generally result in a decreased work capacity. The development of symptoms depends on the rate of iron loss and the body's ability to compensate. Symptoms generally becoming evident when the blood hemoglobin concentration falls below 100 g/L, though some patients remain asymptomatic even with hemoglobin concentrations of 70 g/L.

Table 13.6.
Factors Associated with Iron Deficiency

Factor	Association
Dietary	Starvation, poverty, vegetarianism, religious practice, food faddism
Blood loss	
Females	Menstruation, postmenopausal bleeding, pregnancy
General	Esophageal varices, peptic ulcer, drug-induced gastritis, carcinomas of stomach and colon, ulcerative colitis, hemorrhoids, renal or bladder lesions (hematuria), hookworm infestation, other organ bleeding (hemoptysis), frequent blood donors, athletes, widespread bleeding disorders
Malabsorption	Celiac disease (gluten-induced enteropathy), partial and total gastrectomy, chronic inflammation
Increased requirements	Rapid growth such as in childhood and adolescence, pregnancy

Table 13.7.
Features of Patients with Iron Deficiency

Clinical manifestations	
Appearance	Tired, listless, lifeless appearance
Skin and hair	Pale skin, inelastic and often dry; dry and often scanty hair
Mouth	Papillary atrophy and erythema of the tongue, angular stomatitis
Eye	Pearly white sclera
Nails	Flattened, longitudinally rigid, concave (koilonychia)
Cardiovascular system	Slight cardiomegaly, tachycardia, functional systolic murmur, ankle edema
Neurologic	Generally normal
Blood picture	
Hemoglobin	5–10 g/100 mL (moderate to severe)
MCV	Decreased
MCHC	Decreased
Marrow iron stores	Depleted
Serum iron	Reduced
Serum ferritin	Reduced
Serum transferrin	Increased

The usual signs and symptoms of iron deficiency anemia are often present (Table 13.7). Other problems due to the gross epithelial changes associated with chronic iron deficiency include brittle or spoon-shaped nails, angular stomatitis, atrophic tongue, and pharyngeal and esophageal webs causing dysphagia and atrophic gastric mucosa.

A common symptom of iron deficiency anemia is pica, a condition in which the individual craves unusual substances that are generally of little nutritional value. Pagophagia, or habitual ice eating, is a common form of pica in some communities. Other individuals consume earth and particles of clay cooking pots. Such ingestions have led to metabolic problems, including heavy metal poisoning (23).

Hematologic Changes in Iron Deficiency (1, 2)

In iron deficiency anemia, hematologic changes are evident only after all body iron stores have been depleted and there is insufficient iron to maintain normal erythrocyte morphology and mass (Table 13.8). Blood hemoglobin concentrations and erythrocyte numbers are normal in mild cases. Serum ferritin is the first parameter to change with iron deficiency. As the deficiency worsens, the MCV and erythrocyte count decrease markedly, the RDW increases, and eventually the hemoglobin decreases. When hemoglo-

bin concentrations are ≤70 g/L (7 g/dL) for females or ≤90 g/L (9 g/dL) for males, microscopic examination of peripheral blood smears shows hypochromia and poikilocytosis.

Examination of bone marrow aspirates shows moderate erythroid hypoplasia, and many of the erythroid precursors, such as normoblasts, have little cytoplasm. Peripherally, the proportion of reticulocytes is usually normal, but transient increases may follow acute hemorrhage or treatment with iron. The white cell count and platelet count are generally normal.

Diagnosis of Iron Deficiency Anemia (1, 2, 16, 18)

Identification of most cases of iron deficiency anemia is made on the basis of a full blood count and peripheral smears. The ultimate proof of iron deficiency is the absence of stainable iron in bone marrow aspirates. Since bone marrow aspiration is painful and expensive, it is not used routinely. Severe iron deficiency anemia (Fig. 13.1) is characterized by microcytosis (low MCV), reduced erythrocyte numbers, and cells of uneven size and shape (high RDW). Serum iron and ferritin concentrations are usually low, and serum TIBC and transferrin saturation are high and low, respectively (Table 13.8).

Table 13.8.
Laboratory Values in Various Stages of Iron Deficiency[a]

Stage	Serum Ferritin (µg/L)	Serum Iron	TIBC	Transferrin Saturation (%)	Hemoglobin
Normal	<15	nl	nl	>16	nl
Negative balance	<15	nl	nl	>16	nl
Depletion of stores	<15	↓	nl	>16	nl
Iron deficiency	<15	↓	nl	<16	nl
Iron deficiency anemia	<15	↓	↑	<16	↓
Anemia of chronic disease	nl or ↑	nl	nl or ↓	nl or ↓	↓

[a]nl = normal limits.

Figure 13.1. Photomicrographs of low-power views of peripheral blood showing (A) normal erythrocytes, (B) microcytosis and hypochromia typical of iron deficiency anemia, and (C) macrocytosis typical of megaloblastic anemia due to either vitamin B$_{12}$ or folic acid deficiency. In B, all cells depicted are erythrocytes, and anisocytosis is obvious. In C, oval (O) and bizarre (Z) shaped erythrocytes (poikilocytosis) can be seen. Hypersegmented or multilobed neutrophilic granulocytes (P), cells characteristic of megaloblastic anemia, can also be seen.

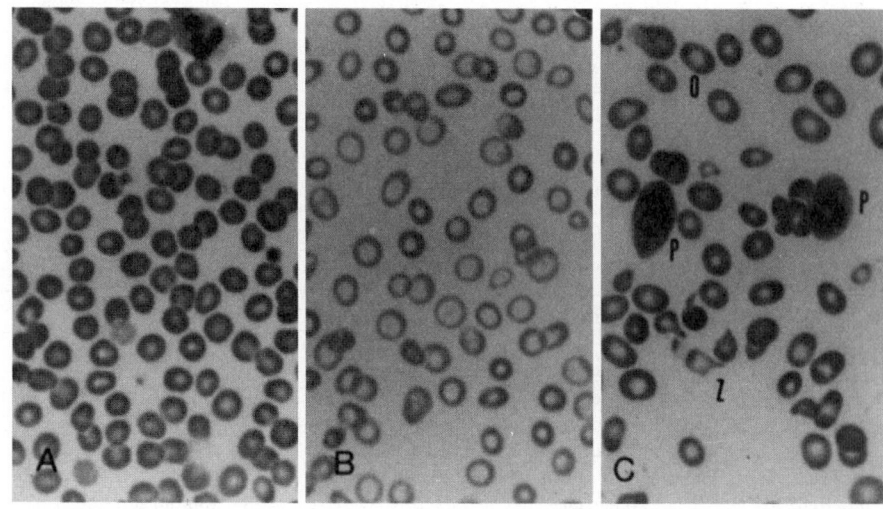

Once a microcytic anemia is detected, a number of potential causes must be explored. An elevated erythrocyte count and a normal RDW (as seen in thalassemia and hemoglobin E) exclude iron deficiency. Similarly, a peripheral blood smear showing hypochromia, erythrocyte targeting, and basophilic stippling is characteristic of thalassemia minor. Some cases of anemia of chronic disease are mildly microcytic, but these generally have a normal RWD. Sideroblastic anemia has both normal and hypochromic erythrocytes as well as an elevated RWD. Anemia due to acute blood loss is characterized by erythrocytes with a normal MCV and RDW.

Serum ferritin levels are an indirect but accurate index of body iron stores and are very useful in establishing the type of anemia. Ferritin concentrations fall in iron deficiency states and increase abnormally in iron storage conditions. Ferritin is an intracellular iron-storage protein, traces of which enter the plasma compartment. Serum ferritin concentrations of less than 15 µg/L (normal, 20 to 200 µg/L) are diagnostic for iron deficiency in adults. Iron deficiency can be differentiated from anemia of chronic diseases by evaluating the serum ferritin level and/or the absence of stainable iron in the bone marrow (Table 13.8). Interpretation of ferritin levels requires consideration of other patient factors, such as coexisting inflammatory processes, liver disease, or malignancy. A serum ferritin level below 12 µg/L indicates the absence of iron stores. Ferritin is an acute-phase reactant to inflammatory diseases such as rheumatoid arthritis. In these diseases, serum ferritin concentrations increase, the lower level of normal increasing to 50 µg/L. Subjects with levels between 12 µg/L and 50 µg/L should be investigated further for iron deficiency anemia. An abnormal release of ferritin from hepatocytes can also occur with acute hepatic necrosis or inflammation. To rule out iron deficiency anemia in individuals with liver disease, especially hepatitis, serum ferritin levels should be on the order of 200 µg/L (24, 25).

Determination of serum iron levels and the TIBC are other traditional methods of evaluating iron deficiency. However, these are less sensitive than ferritin determinations and are often normal in the early stages of iron deficiency. A low serum iron level and high TIBC level are generally characteristic of iron deficiency. Low serum iron levels with a high TIBC are associated with anemias of chronic disease. In thalassemia, hemoglobinopathies, and sideroblastic anemia, serum iron levels are normal or high. Transferrin saturation, another indicator of body iron stores, is below 16% in most cases of iron deficiency anemia. Transferrin saturation levels below 5% are found only in iron deficiency. However, there is considerable overlap with anemias of chronic disease.

Following depletion of iron stores, serum transferrin receptor (STR) levels increase, correlating with the degree of iron deficiency. Whereas ferritin is an early indicator of iron deficiency, STR measurement provides information on the later stages of iron deficiency (1).

Medical disorders can modify the clinical features of iron deficiency anemia. Individuals with polycythemia rubra vera or chronic obstructive airways disease and those who smoke tobacco heavily are predisposed to elevated blood hemoglobin concentrations. If they are also iron deficient, they have the typical features of iron deficiency anemia, except that their erythrocyte count is often above 6×10^{12}/L, and blood hemoglobin concentrations are within the normal range. In polycythemia, iron is lost through gastrointestinal bleeding and as a consequence of phlebotomy, a recognized treatment for this condition.

In the absence of a specialized hematology facility, a tentative diagnosis of iron deficiency can be made by giving a trial of iron therapy and monitoring hemoglobin concentrations and reticulocyte counts. Significant reticulocytosis occurs 7 to 10 days after the start of treatment, and the hemoglobin concentrations increase at a rate of 2 g/L/day over a period of 3 to 4 weeks. Inflammatory disease may retard reticulocytosis.

Prevention and Management of Iron Deficiency (1, 16, 18, 19)

Management is directed toward identifying and treating the cause of the iron deficiency. Treatment plans may involve giving pharmacologic agents such as cimetidine or ranitidine for bleeding stomach ulcers, performing surgery for neoplasms, or removing precipitants such as gluten in celiac disease. Prophylactic or therapeutic doses of iron are used as appropriate. As iron stores are replenished slowly, therapy is continued for at least a year. Some cases require blood transfusion.

Prophylaxis

In addition to ensuring a diet that is adequate in fish, meat, and vegetables, women with heavy menstrual periods or repeated pregnancies usually require iron supplementation. Fruit and vegetables that enhance iron bioavailability include lemons, oranges, tomatoes, beets, broccoli, cauliflower, pumpkin, and turnips.

In pregnancy a routine measurement of blood hemoglobin concentration at the first prenatal visit can guide the need for iron prophylaxis or therapy. Active prophylaxis with oral iron should be used during the second trimester, because even an iron-rich diet usually cannot provide sufficient iron. This will avert a negative iron balance during pregnancy. Ferrous sulfate is the least expensive form of iron therapy and the best salt for iron delivery. Daily prophylactic doses containing 50 to 100 mg of elemental iron, equivalent to 250 to 500 mg of ferrous sulfate, are given. If iron deficiency anemia occurs during pregnancy, it should be treated in the usual way.

To reduce the likelihood of iron deficiency in breast-fed babies, suitable iron-rich foods can be given from the age of 4 to 6 months. Low-birth-weight infants may be given liquid iron supplements from 3 months on. The usual prophylactic dose of ferrous sulfate oral solution is 5 mg/kg body weight.

In societies in which the diet lacks iron-rich food, iron supplementation as a public health measure, although controversial, is the only practical approach to the prevention and treatment of iron deficiency anemia (3, 4). This may be accomplished by either iron fortification of essential foods such as flour, sugar, salt, milk, and eggs; fortification of juices with ascorbic acid; or the daily ingestion of iron in solid or liquid dosage forms.

Treatment of Iron Deficiency (1, 16, 17, 19, 26–29)

Although improvements in diet may reduce the occurrence of iron deficiency, the poor absorption of iron from foods limits the usefulness of dietary therapy for correction of an existing deficiency. Therefore iron deficiency is generally corrected by the administration of either oral or parenteral iron. Since indiscriminate administration of iron may delay the diagnosis of underlying causes, a work-up should be done before initiating therapy. Most iron therapy is given by the oral route; few situations justify the use of parenteral iron. With appropriate therapy the hemoglobin levels improve within a few weeks, and the patient feels better. Adequate iron must be supplied in the early stages of treatment to optimize the response.

Oral Iron Therapy (1, 16, 26)

Solid and liquid oral dosage forms contain one of a variety of iron compounds, which vary in iron equivalence, cost, and effectiveness. Iron absorption from ferrous salts is considered better than that from ferric salts. Sustained-release, slow-release, or enteric-coated (16, 30, 31) preparations of iron, although useful for prophylaxis, are relatively ineffective in treating iron deficiency and should be avoided. Preparations of iron salts in combination with other minerals or vitamins is a wasteful way to treat iron deficiency. The dose of the iron product is based on the elemental iron content. Generally, 30 to 40 mg of elemental iron is used to treat iron deficiency states. These numbers are derived from calculating the maximum rate of hemoglobin regeneration:

$$\frac{0.25 \text{ g Hgb}}{100 \text{ mL}} \times \frac{5,000 \text{ mL}}{\text{blood}} \times \frac{3.4 \text{ mg Fe}}{1 \text{ g Hgb}} = 40 \text{ mg Fe/day}$$

Since only 10 to 20% of iron is absorbed, 200 to 400 mg of iron would need to be given for absorption of 40 mg of elemental iron. Oral iron preparations are salt forms. Ferrous sulfate tablets contain only 40% elemental iron (60 mg Fe/300 mg tablet). Therefore between 500 and 1000 mg of ferrous sulfate would need to be administered to provide 30 to 40 mg of absorbed elemental iron (200 mg/40% or 400 mg/40%). This accounts for the standard dosing of ferrous sulfate 300 mg three times a day (60 mg of elemental iron TID). In switching from one form of iron to another, care must be taken in calculating the doses of different salts to provide equivalent elemental iron quantities (Table 13.9).

Maximum absorption of iron occurs if it is given before or between meals. Large doses are more likely to cause gastric irritation (cramping, nausea, diarrhea, or constipation), which is thought to be due to free iron released in the stomach. This problem can be alleviated by either reducing the dose or taking the iron with food (at the expense of lower absorption). Some patients may also notice black stools during iron therapy, which should not be confused

Table 13.9.
Common Oral Iron Preparations

Proprietary Name	Active Ingredient	Elemental Iron	Iron (%)
Tablets			
Ferrous sulfate USP (generic)	Ferrous sulfate	60 mg/300 mg	20
		65 mg/325 mg	
Feosol	Ferrous sulfate dried	65 mg/200 mg	~32
Ferrous gluconate USP (generic)	Ferrous gluconate	35 mg/300 mg	11.6
Fergon	Ferrous gluconate	37 mg/320 mg	
Ferrous fumarate	Ferrous fumarate	66 mg/200 mg	33
Liquids			
Feosol elixir	Ferrous sulfate	8.8 mg/mL	
Fer-In-Sol syrup	Ferrous sulfate	3.6 mg/mL	
Fer-In-Sol drops	Ferrous sulfate	25 mg/mL	
Fer-Iron drops	Ferrous sulfate	25 mg/mL	
Fergon elixir	Ferrous gluconate	7 mg/mL	
Feostat suspension	Ferrous fumerate	6.6 mg/mL	
Feostat drops	Ferrous fumerate	25 mg/mL	

with darkened tarry stools, or melena, which occur with gastrointestinal bleeding. The therapeutic dose of oral ferrous sulfate solution is approximately 10 mg/kg body weight per day (rounded to the nearest dosage form available).

Drug Interactions and Related Problems with Oral Iron (16, 26)

Tetracyclines, pancrelipase, and antacids, particularly those containing carbonates or magnesium trisilicate, lower the bioavailability of iron. If these agents must be taken concurrently, dosing times should be separated by 1 to 2 hr.

Ascorbic acid in doses of 200 mg can increase iron absorption from 10 to 30%. Its routine use in such a high dose is usually unwarranted, as it is often possible to increase the dose of iron. This is also less expensive. Adding ascorbic acid may be beneficial in malabsorption states. High alcohol and ferric iron consumption for prolonged periods increases both iron absorption and hepatic storage of iron, resulting in iron toxicity. As foods can reduce iron absorption, oral iron supplements should be given 1 hr before or 2 hr after ingestion of food.

Parenteral Iron Therapy (16, 26, 32, 33)

Although the efficacy of parenteral iron therapy is similar to that of oral therapy, the potential for serious side effects limits its use. Indications for parenteral iron therapy include severe iron malabsorption, noncompliance with oral iron, severe intolerance that cannot be controlled by altering the dose or form of oral iron, excessive iron loss (e.g., bleeding hereditary hemorrhagic telangiectasia), and inflammatory bowel disease. Currently, iron dextran (INFeD), 50 mg/mL in 2-mL vials, is the only parenteral iron preparation available in the United States.

Iron dextran is a high-molecular-weight complex of ferric hydroxide (5%) and dextran (20%). In addition to the above indications, it has been used (a) to treat iron deficiency refractory to oral iron treatment and some cases of anemia associated with rheumatoid arthritis; (b) when normal serum iron and iron stores must be rapidly achieved, such as in emergency surgery in iron-deficient patients; (c) when iron deficiency is diagnosed in pregnancy; (d) to treat iron-deficient premature infants; and (e) to treat renal dialysis patients.

The amount of parenteral iron that is required to replenish iron stores and to restore hemoglobin levels in patients with iron deficiency anemia can be approximated by using the following formula:

$$\text{mg iron} = 0.3 \times \text{body weight (lb)} \times \frac{(100 - \text{Hgb (g/dL)} \times 100)}{14.8}$$

The formula can be modified to use kilograms instead of pounds:

$$\text{mg iron} = 0.66 \times \text{body weight (kg)} \times \frac{100 - \text{Hgb (g/dL)} \times 100}{14.8}$$

The mg iron calculated can be divided by 50 (50 mg iron/mL) to provide the volume of iron dextran injection needed. Therefore a 160-pound (73-kg) male with a hemoglobin level of 10 g/dL would require approximately 1560 mg of iron, or 31 mL of iron dextran. These formulas do not take into account active blood loss. To determine the iron replacement dose for these patients, one assumes that 1 mL of normochromic, normocytic erythrocytes contain 1 mg of elemental iron:

$$\text{Iron dextran (mg)} = 1 \text{ mg} \times \text{blood loss (mL)} \times \text{Hct}$$

An alternative method is giving periodic injections until the hemoglobin level has returned to a desired level. One milliliter of iron dextran (50 mg) is needed for each 1% decrease in hemoglobin for a 70-kg adult. Maximum daily doses for children are 0.5 mL for those weighing under 4 kg, 1 mL for those 4 to 10 kg, and 2 mL for those over 10 kg.

Parenteral iron is administered either by deep intramuscular injection into the ventrolateral aspect of the upper and outer quadrant of the buttock or intravenously, as either a bolus or a total dose infusion. The correct technique for intramuscular injections is the Z-track method. Before insertion of the needle, the subcutaneous tissue over the injection site is pulled aside. After administration of the iron, the tissue is released, covering the needle track, thus minimizing leakage through the needle track and staining of the skin. This technique is painful, and necrotic skin ulcerations have occurred after multiple intramuscular injections of iron dextran (32). Another limitation of intramuscular therapy is that only 2 mL (100 mg iron) can be delivered per injection. Therefore the male patient mentioned above would require 15 to 16 injections.

It is claimed that absorption of iron dextran from the injection site is virtually complete and that maximum serum levels are reached within 1 or 2 days, but variable amounts do bind locally for several months. Iron dextran is transported from the muscle by the lymphatic circulation to the blood and then to the liver, where it is taken up by the reticuloendothelial cells. These cells release iron, which is taken up by transferrin. The iron is used by the body or stored as ferritin or hemosiderin for later use. Some of the iron dextran remains trapped inside the reticuloendothelial cells, but it is gradually released. During the first week or so after injection the iron that is present in the plasma is largely iron dextran and unrelated to transferrin-bound iron.

Intravenous iron dextran use avoids deposition in skeletal muscle and local reactions. It is useful for patients who have gastrointestinal problems that prevent adequate iron absorption. Giving it by this route carries about a 10% prevalence of serious adverse effects, including anaphylactic and other allergic reactions. The dose can be delivered via multiple small bolus dose injections (maximum of 2 mL per injection) or by a continuous total dose infusion (TDI). The TDI method offers the advantages of providing the full therapeutic dose, minimizing patient discomfort, and increasing convenience and compliance. However, TDI does not have FDA approval. For TDI, iron dextran is diluted in 0.9% sodium chloride solution or in 5% dextrose solution and is administered over 6 to 8 hr. Local phlebitis is less likely to occur if 0.9% sodium chloride is used as the diluent rather than dextrose. Iron dextran has also been delivered in total parenteral nutrition solutions. Routine inclusion in nutritional replacement fluids is not recommended, as accumulation could occur. No physiochemical evidence of incompatibility or instability has been noted at concentrations of 100 mg iron dextran per liter of total parenteral nutrition (TPN) for 18 hrs. Longer periods or other concentrations have not been evaluated.

Regardless of the parenteral form used (intramuscular, intravenous, or TDI), a test dose of 25 mg (0.5 mL) should be administered to determine potential reactions. Iron dextran injections should not be given to patients with severe liver disease or acute kidney infections because of the risk of iron toxicity. Patients with a history of allergy should receive a trial of small doses followed by a gradual increase in the dose. Single large doses should not be administered to individuals with rheumatoid arthritis because this may exacerbate the disease.

Contraindications to Iron Therapy

Iron preparations should not be used in treating conditions such as hemochromatosis and hemosiderosis, which already signify iron overload. In thalassemias as well as anemic conditions with chronic inflammatory disease such as rheumatoid arthritis, iron is contraindicated, since these conditions have normal to excess iron stores because of impaired utilization of iron. Care must be exercised in giving iron to alcoholic subjects because increased iron store, with or without hemochromatosis, can occur in this group. Patients with alcoholic liver disease such as cirrhosis generally do not suffer from hemochromatosis, but those with marked increases in iron deposition and body stores are likely to have genetically determined hemochromatosis. Iron should be used carefully in treating enteritis, diverticulitis, colitis, and ulcerative colitis because of local effects. Individuals who receive repeated blood transfusions generally become iron overloaded because of the high erythrocytic iron content.

Iron Toxicity

Iron toxicity can be either acute, as in overdosage and accidental poisoning, or chronic, as in overload that occurs in hemochromatosis, hemosiderosis, and thalassemia. An iron-overloaded person usually has more than 4 g of body iron. Iron, which is ordinarily stored in reticuloendothelial cells, is deposited as ferritin and hemosiderin into hepatocytes of the liver and eventually other tissues and organs. Hemochromatosis is associated with severe iron overload. Recently, noninvasive methods such as computed tomography and magnetic resonance imaging have been used to determine hepatic iron content.

The pathogenesis of iron overload is associated with either increased mucosal iron absorption, the parenteral administration of iron as blood transfusions, or injections of therapeutic iron preparations. Diet is unlikely to cause iron overload unless other factors or problems are present. Normal individuals absorb the usual amounts of iron, even when the dietary iron load is increased 5 to 10 times. Amounts of 300 to 500 mg/day can be tolerated, although there are some exceptions. Worldwide, the consumption of alcoholic beverages is considered to be a common cause of iron overload. Another potential cause of iron overload is the controversial practice in some developed countries of fortifying food with iron. Although this addition may be useful for women, it may lead to a grossly excessive intake of iron by men. The prevalence of hemochromatosis is 0.5%, which is higher than that of iron deficiency in men. Indiscriminate use of iron supplements can be harmful. Intrinsic metabolic abnormalities may account for increased iron absorption from the small intestine. Such abnormalities occur in primary idiopathic hemochromatosis (hereditary hemochromatosis) and in some anemias.

Iron overload secondary to anemias can be divided into two classes: that in patients with hypoplastic bone marrow, in which the main source of iron is blood transfusion (e.g., aplastic anemia or sickle cell anemia) and that in patients with hyperplastic bone marrow, in whom the iron excess results from increased iron absorption secondary to ineffective erythropoiesis (e.g., thalassemia major, sideroblastic anemia, and some hemolytic anemias). Treatment of transfusional iron overload generally consists of chelation therapy, such as deferoxamine (34).

Monitoring Iron Therapy

Laboratory tests are especially useful in monitoring the response to iron therapy, including blood hemoglobin concentrations, reticulocyte counts, serum ferritin concentration, and, if necessary, serum iron level and the TIBC. In many centers, parameters of the hemograms are used as therapeutic indicators.

The initial aim of treatment of iron deficiency is to reverse the anemia. With treatment this should be achieved in the first 2 to 3 months. Once the hemoglobin reaches 100 g/L, the urgency for correcting the anemia decreases. Serial blood hemoglobin measurements should indicate a rise of 0.3 to 1.4 g/L/day. A speedy recovery generally indicates that the cause of iron loss is no longer present. Weekly reticulocyte counts give some indication of bone marrow activity, because in the early stages of treatment, reticulocytosis should occur. The rate of rise in blood hemoglobin concentration also depends on the severity of the anemia and on the usual range for an individual. The rate of rise for a male with a usual blood hemoglobin of 160 g/L will be faster than that for a pregnant subject, who would normally have a blood hemoglobin of about 105 g/L. Early in the treatment and depending on the severity of the deficiency, larger doses of iron should be used. Following a good hemoglobin response, doses can be reduced.

A second objective in instituting iron therapy is to replenish iron stores. Generally, this is a nonurgent phase of treatment, and iron replacement can be undertaken over 3 to 6 months. Serum ferritin concentration and iron saturation can be used as guides for this stage of therapy. Some patients will require long-term iron therapy because of blood loss or malabsorption problems. Doses of iron for these patients should be adjusted to the losses. Periodic serum ferritin determinations should be used as a guide to the patient's iron status.

Failure to respond to iron therapy can be due to a number of factors, including noncompliance, chronic disease, incorrect diagnosis, or an inadequate iron formulation.

MEGALOBLASTIC ANEMIAS (3, 19–21)

Megaloblastic anemia is characterized by a lowered blood hemoglobin mass because of reduced erythropoiesis secondary to defective DNA synthesis in the developing erythroid cells of the bone marrow. Other rapidly dividing tissue can also be affected, particularly the mucosal epithelium of the gastrointestinal tract. Because RNA synthesis continues in the developing erythroid cells, there is an increase in cytoplasmic mass. The resulting megaloblasts are characterized by an abnormal nucleus because of greater cytoplasmic (rather than nuclear) maturity. Cells that are released into the circulation are larger than normal (macrocytic). These erythrocytes have a reduced life span, so megaloblastic anemias have some of the features of hemolytic anemias, such as hyperbilirubinemia. In addition to the erythroid changes, similar effects on other hemopoietic cell lines in the bone marrow can lead to leukopenia, thrombocytopenia, or pancytopenia. Morphologic changes that are observed in the peripheral smear include macroovalocyte erythrocytes and multilobed neutrophilic granulocytes. Mitotic figures in developing erythroid cells in the bone marrow are another feature of megaloblastic anemias (Fig. 13.2).

Either B_{12} or folic acid is required for the synthesis of purine and pyrimidine nucleotides, precursors of DNA synthesis. Reduced availability or absence of one-carbon-unit coenzymes, such as methylcobalamin (active B_{12}) or formyltetrahydrofolic acid (active folic acid), results in impaired DNA synthesis in developing erythroid cells. These cells do not divide normally, and fewer, large, but well-hemoglobinized cells (megaloblasts) form in the bone marrow. When these cells lose their nuclei (the usual process going from nucleated erythroid precursors to the nonnucleated erythrocyte), they are released into the circulation as macrocytes (MCV >120 fL). The result is a macrocytic, normochromic anemia.

Causes of megaloblastic anemia include dietary deficiency, poor absorption, or impaired utilization of B_{12} or folic acid (Table 13.10). Worldwide, folic acid dietary deficiency is believed to be the most common cause of vitamin deficiency. Drug ingestion is the second common cause of megaloblastic anemia. The drugs can either affect the nutrient status of the patient or have a direct effect on DNA synthesis. For example, 5-fluorouracil inhibits thymidylate synthesis, hydroxyurea reduces dATP and dGTP by inhibiting ribonucleotide reductase, and cytosine arabinose competes with dTMP for binding sites on DNA polymerase.

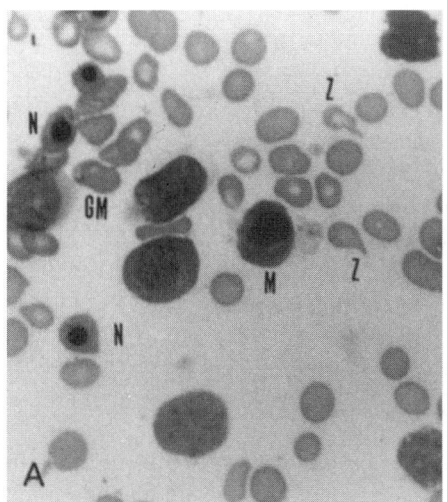
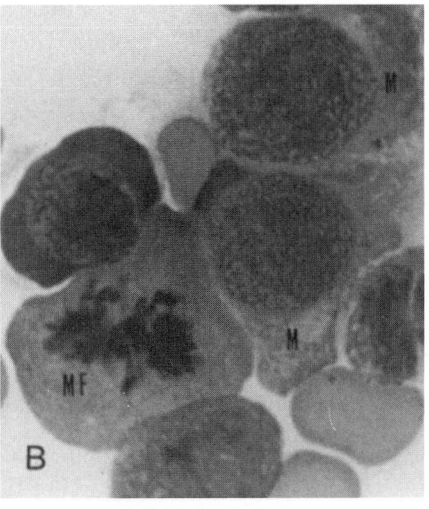

Figure 13.2. Photomicrographs of (A) medium and (B) high-power views of megaloblastic bone marrow. The nonnucleated erythrocytes are of abnormal shapes (Z), including some with a teardrop appearance. Megaloblasts (M) and a developing erythroid cell with mitotic figures (MF) characteristic of megaloblastic anemias are prominent. Other cells that are present include nucleated erythrocytes (N) and a giant metamyelocyte (GM).

Table 13.10.
Causes of Vitamin B$_{12}$ and Folic Acid Deficiencies

Vitamin B$_{12}$ deficiency	
Dietary	Inadequate intake
Malabsorption	Inadequate production of intrinsic factor, competition for vitamin B$_{12}$, disorders of terminal ileum, drug-related
Impaired transport	Transcobalamin II deficiency
Folic acid deficiency	
Dietary	Inadequate intake, unbalanced diet, excessive cooking
Malabsorption	Intestinal mucosal changes
Increased requirements	Pregnancy, infancy, malignancy, increased hematopoiesis
Impaired metabolism	Drug-related, enzyme deficiencies

General Management of Megaloblastic
Anemias (18, 19, 35)

Megaloblastic anemias exhibit the usual features of anemia. Before institution of therapy, the cause and pathophysiologic mechanism must be identified. The common megaloblastic anemias are corrected by replacement therapy (discussed in detail below). The leukopenia that is associated with megaloblastic anemia is rarely severe enough to predispose the patient to infection. Marked thrombocytopenia may occasionally result in life-threatening hemorrhage, which should be treated with platelet transfusions. Other manifestations include glossitis, dysphagia, anorexia, diminished levels of circulating immunoglobulins, and reduced lymphocyte reactivity.

Vitamin B$_{12}$ Absorption and Metabolism (35–37)

Vitamin B$_{12}$, also known as cobalamin, occurs in both synthetic and biologically active forms. It is a cobalt-containing vitamin that cannot be synthesized by mammalian tissue but only by microorganisms. Therefore it must be present in the diet. Some bacterial synthesis of B$_{12}$ occurs in the large bowel and the cecum, but there is no absorption at these sites. Unlike many vitamins, vitamin B$_{12}$ is not formed by higher plants. Methylcobalamin, deoxyadenosylcobalamin, and hydroxocobalamin are the major forms in foods. Cyanocobalamin, commonly used for therapeutic purposes, does not occur in the natural state but is an artifact of the isolation procedure.

For humans, dietary B$_{12}$ is present in most foods of animal origin, complexed to protein. Sources include fresh liver (the richest source) as well as eggs, meat, kidney, milk, other dairy products, fish, and shellfish. Fruits, vegetables, and grains lack the vitamin. Nonanimal sources, which contain relatively small amounts of the vitamin, include fermented soy products and yeasts. Because B$_{12}$ is water soluble and relatively heat stable, it is bioavailable from cooked food.

The daily requirement for humans is only 0.5 to 1.0 µg, and the total body stores amount to only 2 to 5 mg. The average diet in the United States supplies 15 µg/day, but there is a wide variation, from 1 to 100 µg/day. Some unusual diets, such as vegan-vegetarian, macrobiotic, or reducing diets that drastically restrict food selection, may not supply the minimum daily requirements. Supplementation is required for patients receiving total parenteral nutrition and those with malnutrition or malabsorption.

Vitamin B$_{12}$ uptake and transport are an orderly sequence of events involving three different binding proteins: intrinsic factor (IF), R proteins, and transcobalamin II. IF, a specific B$_{12}$-binding glycoprotein, is synthesized and secreted by the parietal cells of the stomach. Secretion of IF parallels the secretion of hydrochloric acid. The R proteins are a group of high-affinity, B$_{12}$-binding glycoproteins, produced by leukocytes (and probably other tissues), that are present in a variety of biologic secretions, including gastric fluid, plasma, saliva, tears, milk, and bile. Their function is not fully understood, but they appear to act as storage sites for the vitamin as well as providing a means of disposal for excess and unwanted vitamin B$_{12}$ analogs. Transcobalamin II is the plasma acceptor protein for recently absorbed B$_{12}$.

Vitamin B$_{12}$, particularly at the usual low levels in foods, is well absorbed from the gastrointestinal tract by a process involving interaction between the B$_{12}$ bound to IF and the mucosal cells of the distal ileum. The vitamin, which is protein-bound in foods, is released during gastric digestion. Although cobalamins can bind to R proteins or to IF, at the low gastric pH, binding to gastric R protein is favored. The relative binding of the vitamin may also depend on the dose, as well as on the amounts of R protein and IF secreted. The cobalamins remain bound to R protein in the upper small intestine until pancreatic proteases such as trypsin partially degrade the complex, releasing B$_{12}$, which then binds to IF. Individuals with pancreatic insufficiency could become B$_{12}$ deficient; however, few cases of megaloblastic anemia due to such a deficiency have been reported. The IF-B$_{12}$ complex, which is highly resistant to proteolysis, passes down the small intestine to the distal ileum, where it attaches to specific receptors on the luminal side of the mucosal cells (enterocytes). The attachment is non-energy-dependent; however, extracellular calcium and a pH greater than 5.4 are required. How cobalamins are transported across the enterocyte and the fate of IF are poorly understood. One possibility is that IF is released at the cell surface and the vitamin is taken up by the enterocyte. Recent animal studies support receptor-mediated endocytosis. Vitamin B$_{12}$ passes from the mucosa into the capillary circulation, but no IF passes into the blood.

Another mechanism for B$_{12}$ absorption involves diffusion and not IF. This mechanism is biologically important

Table 13.11.
Stages of Vitamin B_{12} Deficiency

Stage	B_{12} Level	MCV	Hgb	Signs and Symptoms
Normal	Normal	Normal	Normal	None
Negative balance	Normal	Normal	Normal	None
Depletion of stores	Slight decrease	Normal	Normal	Possible
B_{12} deficient erythropoiesis	Moderate decrease	Increased	Normal	Possible
B_{12} deficiency anemia	Severe decrease	Increased	Decreased	Probable

Source: Modified from Goodman KI, Salt WV. Vitamin B_{12} deficiency: important new concepts in recognition. Postgrad Med 88:147–158, 1990.

only when large amounts are ingested and generally provides only small quantities of the vitamin. However, this mechanism is being explored as a potential method of providing oral B_{12} therapy to people with low levels of IF (pernicious anemia) (38, 39).

Once in the circulation, cobalamins bind to transcobalamin II. There is increasing evidence that transcobalamin II plays an active role in transporting the vitamin from the enterocyte either by entering the cell or by attaching to its plasma membrane. Even though transcobalamin II accepts the newly absorbed vitamin, most circulating cobalamins are bound to transcobalamin I. An explanation for this is that B_{12} bound to transcobalamin II is quickly cleared from the blood ($t_{1/2}$ = 1 hr), whereas it takes several days to clear it from transcobalamin I.

The daily cellular requirements for B_{12} are low, and much of that ingested is stored in the liver. The amount in the liver is 2 to 5 mg, which represents 40 to 50% of the total body content. Vitamin B_{12} is conserved in the body by enterohepatic recycling. Biliary excretion of B_{12} is much higher than excretion in urine or feces. Vitamin B_{12} and its analogs in bile are excreted bound to biliary R protein. When the complex comes into contact with pancreatic enzymes in the upper small intestine, B_{12} and its analogs are released because of biliary R protein degradation. Only B_{12} binds to fresh intrinsic factor; the analogs are excreted in the feces. Bile, as well as being the major route of B_{12} analog excretion, possibly plays a role in enhancing B_{12} absorption. When the diet contains little or no B_{12}, as may be the case for strict vegans, biliary cobalamin is conserved to the extent that clinical deficiency may take up to 20 years to develop. When malabsorption occurs, as in pernicious anemia, endogenous as well as dietary B_{12} is lost, and deficiency develops within 3 to 6 years. This accounts for the slow and insidious course of pernicious anemia.

Vitamin B_{12} Deficiency

Deficiency occurs when the serum concentration of B_{12} is less than 150 pmol/L (200 pg/mL). Reduced erythropoiesis due to B_{12} deficiency also results in impaired utilization of iron and folic acid, leading to elevations in serum iron concentration, transferrin saturation, and ferritin and folate levels. Thus normal to elevated levels of serum folate and iron saturation in the presence of B_{12} deficiency strongly indicate accompanying deficiencies. The stages of B_{12} deficiency are outlined in Table 13.11.

Etiology of Vitamin B_{12} Deficiency (18, 20, 33, 34)

Causes of B_{12} deficiency include inadequate intake, malabsorption, B_{12} degradation, and increased requirement. Most cases of deficiency are secondary to malabsorption associated with pernicious anemia, gastric lesions, gastrectomy, and a number of small bowel disorders. Pernicious anemia is the most common specific type of B_{12} malabsorption in North America. Alcoholics are particularly vulnerable to B_{12} deficiency because of chronic gastritis, poor diet, folate deficiency, and pancreatic insufficiency.

Nutritional Deficiency of Vitamin B_{12}

Dietary causes of B_{12} deficiency are rare and are possibly important only in vegans (strict vegetarians who do not consume foods of animal origin, including milk, cheese, and eggs), breast-fed babies of vegan mothers, and people living in countries where poor nutrition is widespread. Vegetarians have serum B_{12} levels of 200 to 250 pmol/L (260 to 330 pg/mL), which on average are lower than those of omnivores. A number of years on a restricted unbalanced diet can result in deficiency. Deficiency is less likely in vegans who ingest sufficient calories from a wide selection of food. Here microbial contamination of foods can provide trace amounts of B_{12}. The elderly are also susceptible, particularly if they are living on tea and cereal, toast, or biscuits for financial reasons or because of unavailability of food or lack of interest in preparing meals. In addition, the incidence of pernicious anemia increases with age.

Gastric Disorders

Gastric disorders, most commonly gastrectomy, are the second most common cause of vitamin B_{12} malabsorption. Even when the diet is adequate, some abnormalities of the stomach prevent the release of the vitamin from foods. These include atrophic gastritis, achlorhydria, vagotomy, partial gastrectomy, and the use of H_2-receptor antagonists. Complete gastrectomy results in an absolute deficiency of

IF, and megaloblastic anemia develops 3 to 6 years after surgery unless supplementation is given. Partial gastrectomy is a variable cause of B_{12} deficiency. Deficiency is also possible if sufficient gastric mucosa has been destroyed by ingestion of corrosive chemicals, by tumors, or by chronic gastritis. A point worth noting is that the remaining amount of IF can often promote absorption of synthetic crystalline cyanocobalamin.

Intestinal Problems

Small intestine disorders are the third most common cause of B_{12} deficiency. Abnormal situations leading to malabsorption range from impaired transfer of the vitamin from R protein to competition for luminal B_{12} to a low pH in the ileum.

Absorption of B_{12}, as measured by the Schilling test (see later), is impaired in 50 to 70% of patients with pancreatic insufficiency. Defective absorption can be partly corrected by giving oral pancreatic preparations and/or sodium bicarbonate. B_{12} malabsorption also occurs in the Zollinger-Ellison syndrome if the associated hypersecretion of gastric acid is left uncontrolled. The resultant reduction of the pH in the duodenum inactivates pancreatic proteolytic enzymes.

Surgical resection or bypass of the ileum also increases the likelihood of malabsorption. Most people who have lost more than 5 cm of distal ileum have abnormal Schilling test results. Even in the presence of IF, B_{12} malabsorption occurs in conditions such as tropical sprue, Crohn's disease, celiac disease, lymphomas, and Whipple's disease, where alteration or destruction of the ileal absorptive surface occurs. In the recessive disorder, Imerslund-Grasbeck's disease, selective malabsorption of B_{12} by a poorly understood mechanism, occurs in association with proteinuria.

Bacterial overgrowth, particularly by *Bacteroides* and coliforms, in blind loops or diverticula result in B_{12} malabsorption. Absorption returns to normal when patients are given tetracycline, lincomycin, or metronidazole. The mechanism of B_{12} uptake by bacteria is unclear. Most intestinal bacteria avidly absorb the unbound vitamin, but only small amounts are taken up when it is bound to IF. Infestation by the tapeworm *Diphyllobothrium latum* (from eating undercooked freshwater fish), resulting in competition for the vitamin, is a potential problem in the Scandinavian countries, Japan, and Russia. Possibly, the parasite releases B_{12} from its IF complex.

Drug-Induced Vitamin B_{12} Deficiency

B_{12} deficiency has been associated with a number of pharmacotherapeutic agents, including colchicine, *p*-aminosalicylic acid, and the biguanide hypoglycemic agents. The latter are thought to affect transcellular transport of B_{12}. Agents that reduce B_{12} absorption in the ileum include ethanol and cholestyramine.

Exposure to nitrous oxide gas for prolonged periods of time also may result in megaloblastic marrow changes that can be corrected by B_{12} administration. Nitrous oxide may block the homocysteine-methionine reaction in cells of the bone marrow, nervous system, and other tissues. Peripheral neuropathy has also been reported in dentists who are chronically exposed to nitrous oxide.

Pernicious Anemia (35, 36)

Pernicious anemia (PA) is due to B_{12} malabsorption because of a lack of IF and hydrochloric acid secretion. The term "pernicious" is used because the anemia develops insidiously and progressively. Two types of PA have been described. The adult type, by far the more common of the two, occurs with a prevalence of 0.2 to 0.6%. It rarely occurs before 30 years of age and, between 45 and 60 years of age, affects women more frequently than men. There is a distinctive racial and geographic distribution of PA, which is far more common in temperate regions such as North America and northern Europe than in tropical countries. Juvenile PA is less common, and patients often develop clinical features of B_{12} deficiency during the second decade of life. Inherited conditions leading to PA in infancy or early childhood may be due to a lack of IF or the production of abnormal IF by an otherwise normal stomach.

Current evidence suggests that PA is caused by an autoimmune reaction against gastric parietal cells. PA has been linked with other immunologic problems. PA occurs more commonly in people with diseases that afflict the immune system, such as Graves' disease, myxedema, thyroiditis, idiopathic adrenocortical insufficiency, vitiligo, and hypoparathyroidism. Relatives of patients with PA also show a higher incidence of the disease. Most sufferers have increased levels of circulating antibodies, particularly those directed against antiparietal cells and IF. The latter antibodies are generally characteristic of PA.

Clinical Manifestations (20, 35, 40–42)

Many clinical manifestations are common to all forms of B_{12} deficiency, all of which are likely to occur in severe deficiency (Table 13.12). Clinical manifestations reflect abnormalities of the blood, gastrointestinal tract, and nervous system. In severe cases the peripheral blood smear exhibits severe macrocytic anemia, leukopenia with hypersegmentation of the polymorphonuclear cells, and thrombocytopenia. The diagnostic triad of symptoms is weakness, painful tongue, and numbness and tingling of extremities. In many instances at least two of these symptoms are encountered.

The onset of PA is insidious, and most patients present with signs and symptoms of anemia. Patients are generally well nourished, although they may have lost weight. The mucous membranes are usually pale, and in Caucasians the

Table 13.12.
Clinical Features of Pernicious Anemia[a]

Symptoms and physical appearance

Pallor, slight jaundice, and faint icterus of the sclera

Anorexia accompanied by a mild degree of weight loss; a flabby rather than a wasted appearance; diarrhea

Dyspnea, palpitations, sensation of extra heartbeats, weakness, vertigo, tinnitus, precordial pain, and heart murmurs

Paresthesia, difficulty in walking, loss of vibratory sense, incoordination of movements

Disturbed mentation, such as irritability, memory, disturbances, and mild depression. Serious mental symptoms may develop.

Mild pyrexia

Difficulty in urination

Organ involvement

Atrophic glossitis

Mild hepatosplenomegaly

Enlarged heart

Nervous system: spinal cord and periphreal nerve degeneration

Achylia gastrica

Gastric cancer

[a]Similar features occur in all types of vitamin B_{12} deficiency.

Table 13.13.
Laboratory Findings in Pernicious Anemia

Parameter	Comments
Hematocrit	Normal to decreased.
Peripheral smear	Macrocytic, occasional nucleated cells and a reticulocyte index well below 1.
Erythrocytes	Oval-shaped variations in size, some bizarre-shaped poikilocytes; MCV greater than normal, MCH is increased; MCHC is normal; increased hemolysis.
Leukocytes	Hypersegmentation of polymorphonuclear cell nuclei is a consistent finding; if more than 3 cells have 5 lobes or a single cell has 6 lobes, this is presumptive diagnosis of a megaloblastic anemia; there can be mild to moderate neutropenia.
Platelets	Reduced in number and bizarre in appearance on occasion.
Serum B_{12}	Decreased.
Serum folate	Normal; sometimes elevated because of folate metabolic trap.
Gastric secretion	Achlorhydria (histamine-fast achlorhydria found in most patients); total volume of the gastric secretion and its enzyme content are markedly reduced; increased serum gastrin.
Antibodies	Antiparietal and antiintrinsic factor antibodies present.
Others	Methylmalonic acid excretion is enhanced; plasma unconjugated bilirubin and lactic acid dehydrogenase (type 1) increased because of enhanced intramedullary destruction of erythrocytes; iron kinetic data is abnormal.

skin is pale and yellow-tinted because of the anemia and the mild jaundice of ineffective erythropoiesis.

Nonspecific symptoms related to coexisting anemia and neurologic involvement include apathy, weakness, fatigue, palpitations, and breathlessness. Gastrointestinal manifestations such as atrophic glossitis (sore and abnormally smooth tongue), anorexia, indigestion, and diarrhea occur because the normally rapidly proliferating epithelium is deprived of adequate amounts of B_{12}. In elderly patients the deficiency may manifest initially as postural hypotension or congestive heart failure. Other symptoms may complicate the picture, suggesting primary involvement of the gastrointestinal, cardiovascular, or genitourinary systems. Neurologic manifestations involving the spinal cord can develop before the anemia. Sometimes these are so advanced that primary neurologic disease is suspected. Because PA usually occurs in the elderly, it can be difficult to determine the extent to which age-related changes contribute to the clinical findings. The laboratory findings in PA are outlined in Table 13.13.

A long-standing lack of B_{12} results in distinct changes in the nervous system, beginning with demyelination of nerves and leading to neurologic abnormalities. Peripheral nerve damage results in symmetrical paresthesias (numbness and tingling of the extremities) and reduction of pain and temperature sensation. The most serious problem, subacute degeneration of the spinal cord, is associated with loss of position and vibration sense, resulting in ataxia and weakness. Lateral column disruption leads to weakness and spasticity, exemplified by myoclonus, hyperreflexia, and a positive Babinski's sign. If the condition remains untreated, instability of gait and virtual paralysis result.

Psychiatric manifestations include impaired mentation, delirium, paranoia, psychosis, irritability, depression, and personality changes. Psychiatric symptoms may occur in the absence of hematologic abnormalities or signs of neuropathy. The mechanism is unknown but could be secondary to folic acid deficiency.

Megaloblastosis and Neurologic Manifestations

In humans, B_{12} deficiency causes megaloblastic anemia that is indistinguishable from that found in folate deficiency, as well as subacute combined degeneration of the spinal cord. Although controversial, the most widely accepted view on the underlying biochemical mechanisms for these pathologies is an intracellular methylfolate trap due to reduced cellular methionine (Fig. 13.3). Methylcobalamin is an essential cofactor in the conversion of homocysteine to methionine. Impairment of this reaction results in deranged folate metabolism, thought to underlie defective DNA synthesis and the megaloblastosis in individuals who are deficient in B_{12}. It is proposed that in B_{12} deficiency states, unconjugated N-5-methyltetrahydrofolate taken up by cells from the plasma is a

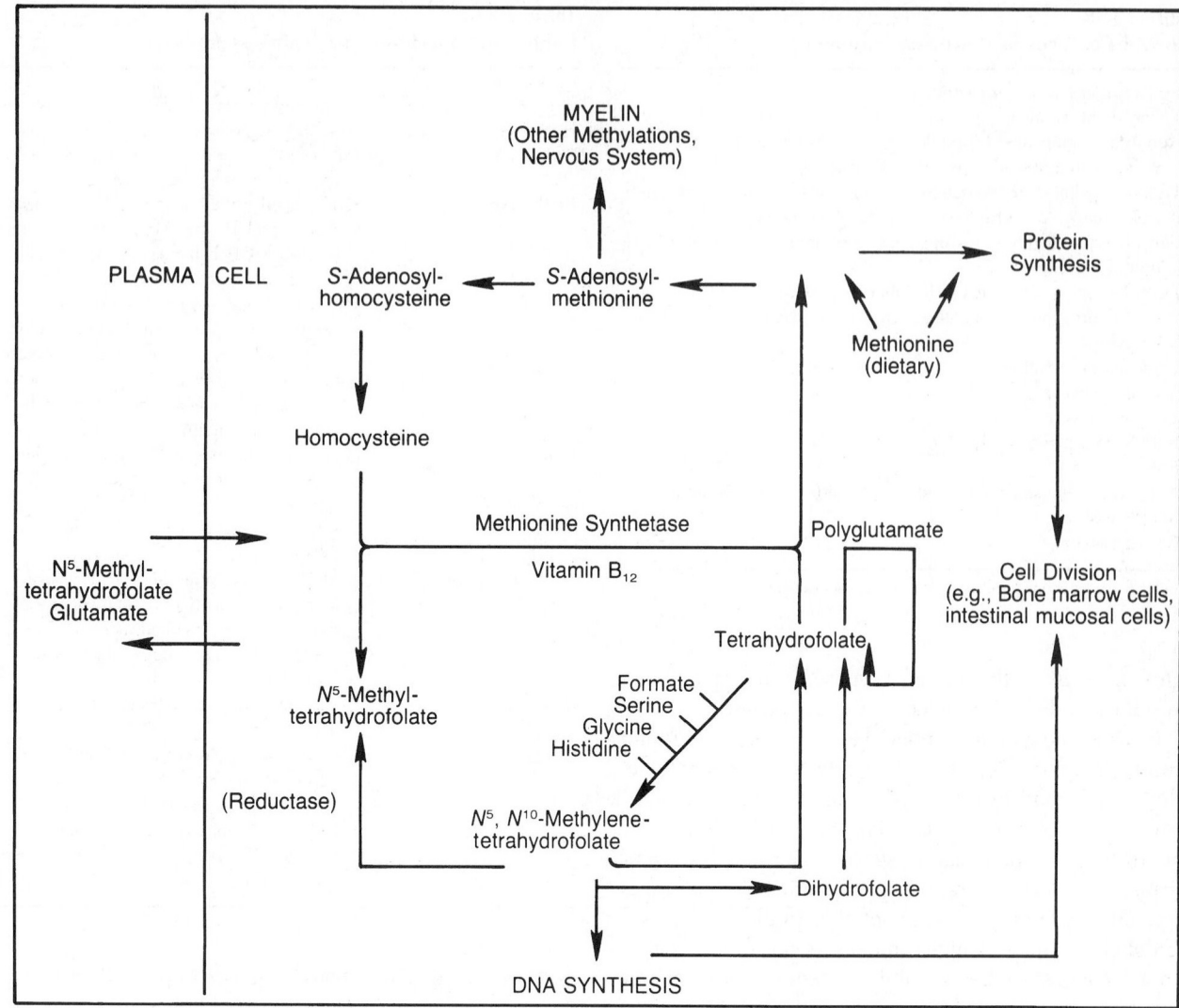

Figure 13.3.   Normal vitamin B_{12} and folate metabolism in mammalian cells.

poor substrate for conversion to other forms, such as N-5, 10-methylenetetrahydrofolate. Useful metabolites are used by cells for the most essential methylation reactions at the expense of DNA and protein synthesis and cell division. This in part explains why partial remission of the hematologic manifestations occurs if patients consume large quantities of folic acid. Although flooding the DNA synthetic pathways allows the bone marrow to return to normal, neurologic lesions do not respond readily in the short or long term. Without adequate treatment with B_{12} the methylating capacity of cells is ultimately reduced, resulting in subacute degeneration of the spinal cord.

Impaired conversion of homocysteine to methionine may in part cause the neurologic lesions of B_{12} deficiency. Methionine is required for the synthesis of choline and choline-containing phospholipids and for methylation of myelin proteins. Additionally, a lack of adenosylcobalamin, which is required for the conversion of methylmalonyl-

CoA to succinyl-CoA, leads to accumulation of methylmalonyl-CoA and propionyl-CoA. This leads to the synthesis of nonphysiologic odd-numbered fatty acids, which are subsequently incorporated into neuronal lipids.

During folate deficiency, cellular methionine synthesis is also diminished, which diverts folate from DNA synthesis, and megaloblastosis develops. Because folate is used selectively to conserve methionine and nerve tissue concentrates folate, subacute degeneration is absent in folate deficiency.

Diagnosis of Vitamin B_{12} Deficiency (20, 35, 37, 43, 44) The triad of anti-IF antibodies, low serum B_{12} level, and megaloblastic anemia is diagnostic for pernicious anemia. Macrocytic anemia, peripheral neuropathy, and dementia also suggest B_{12} deficiency. Clinical diagnosis can be confirmed by a complete blood count, serum B_{12} and folate measurements, and a reticulocyte count. The cause can be determined by the Schilling test. Serum B_{12} levels can be used for routine screening.

Hematologic tests revealing macrocytosis must be followed up with other tests to determine the cause. Macrocytosis may be an incidental finding when patients are being investigated for other problems, such as alcoholism or respiratory problems. Macrocytosis is also possible in association with liver disease, myxedema, acute myelogenous leukemia, acquired sideroblastic anemia, aplastic anemia, hemolytic anemia, posthemorrhagic states, and splenectomy and is seen in the aged.

Macrocytosis is not always present in B_{12} deficiency. It may be blocked by concurrent iron deficiency, underlying hematologic disorder (e.g., α-thalassemia), or anemia of chronic disease. Laboratory tests used for the differential diagnosis include serum B_{12} and folate determinations, erythrocyte folate determination, the Schilling test, and a test for IF antibodies. In pernicious anemia, serum concentrations of B_{12} are low, but the serum folate is within the normal range.

A number of independent factors can influence B_{12} test results. Falsely low values can occur in folic acid deficiency. Excluding laboratory errors and dietary factors, low results are obtained with the radioimmunoassay if radiopharmaceuticals have also been administered to the patient for investigations such as bone scanning, erythrocyte mass testing, thyroid function evaluation, or cardiac testing. Antibiotic therapy can falsely lower measurements obtained by the microbiologic method. In vitro decomposition of B_{12} is also possible if subjects have consumed high doses of ascorbic acid.

Lower B_{12} levels have also been observed in the elderly. However, this may not represent a true deficiency state, since most had a positive Schilling test. Elderly subjects with low serum B_{12} levels should be further evaluated. Low serum levels are also common in pregnancy. Reduced synthesis of transcobalamin I in many patients with multiple myeloma also leads to low levels. A Schilling test (with or without IF) should be performed in all cases of suspected B_{12} malabsorption to determine whether there is a lack of IF or an ileal defect. Several types of Schilling tests are available (37, 43). The standard test is divided into three stages. In stage I an oral dose of 1 μg of ^{57}Co-labeled B_{12} is given, followed by a 1-mg intramuscular flushing dose of unlabeled B_{12}, and the 24-hr urine excretion of the label is measured (Table 13.14). The large intramuscular dose of B_{12} saturates its binding proteins in the blood. Consequently, there are fewer binding sites for ^{57}Co-labeled B_{12}, and a substantial proportion is excreted in the urine. B_{12} absorption is considered to be impaired if less than 10% of the label is excreted in the urine. If less than 5% is excreted, the diagnosis is consistent with pernicious anemia. Note that this test depends on renal function and a complete 24-hr urine collection.

Table 13.14.
Summary of Schilling Test Results in Vitamin B_{12} Deficiency

Condition	Stage I	Stage II	Stage III
Normal	Normal		
Inadequate diet	Normal		
Pernicious anemia	Low	Normal	
Bacterial overgrowth	Low	Low	Normal
Ilial defect	Low	Low	Low

Stage II of the test distinguishes between the possible causes of the malabsorption (e.g., pernicious anemia, lack of ileal absorptive sites, or bacterial overgrowth proximal to the terminal ileum). This is performed by giving 10 mg of hog IF with the radiolabeled B_{12} and measuring excretion of the radiolabel. Previous exposure to hog IF (e.g., consumption of IF in some over-the-counter vitamin preparations) may give low results. In these cases, malabsorption can be detected by using normal human gastric juice rather than hog IF. If the results are inconclusive, stage III of the test is performed, which involves giving the patient antibiotics, usually tetracycline 250 mg orally four times a day, for 10 to 14 days, and then repeating the stage I test.

Vitamin B_{12} replacement therapy should be given for several weeks before repeating the Schilling test, to allow any intestinal megaloblastosis that accompanies deficiency states to resolve. Although this reversal may take several weeks, it is probably corrected in most patients over one cycle of intestinal epithelial cells. Megaloblastosis of the mucosal epithelium cells may cause secondary malabsorption and possibly a false-positive Schilling test. If malabsorption is not reversed with added IF, other causes should be explored.

Care must be taken in interpreting the Schilling test results for patients who are also taking H_2-antagonists such as cimetidine, ranitidine, or famotidine. Such agents may cause falsely abnormal results by preventing the degradation of R protein and decreasing the secretion of endogenous intrinsic factor. Reduced hydrochloric acid production caused by H_2-antagonists as well as other situations in which acid and intrinsic factor secretion is reduced, such as achlorhydria, vagotomy, or partial gastrectomy, can give falsely normal Schilling test results (45, 46). The problem here is that the aqueous, crystalline B_{12} that is used in the test differs in bioavailability from the usually food-bound vitamin that must be released to participate in the uptake process. A modified Schilling test, PBAT, using protein-bound B_{12}, more closely resembles the physiologic state.

Serum anti-IF antibodies should also be measured. This test has positive results in 50% of patients with pernicious anemia and, combined with a low serum B_{12}, is useful in the differential diagnosis. A disadvantage is that positive results can be associated with other autoimmune disorders. Less commonly used tests include thymidine uptake (dUST test) by bone marrow cells and serum methylmalonic acid or homocysteine measurements (45, 46).

Management of Vitamin B_{12} Deficiency (37, 40, 47)

Depending on the cause, either oral or parenteral B_{12} replacement therapy is used. A diagnosis of B_{12} deficiency should be confirmed by laboratory investigations before beginning therapy, although in seriously ill patients it may be necessary to administer both B_{12} and folic acid while awaiting confirmation.

The aims of treatment are hematologic remission, reversal or retardation of the nervous system complications, and replenishment of B_{12} stores. "Shotgun" treatments with hematinic combinations and the use of parenteral B_{12} injections as placebo injections should be discouraged, because there is no rational basis for their use. Dietary deficiencies can be treated with oral cyanocobalamin, but for malabsorption in pernicious anemia, intramuscular or deep subcutaneous injections of cyanocobalamin or hydroxocobalamin are used. Small amounts of cyanocobalamin are sometimes included in TPN solutions.

In severe cases of pernicious anemia the patient should be confined to bed until the hemoglobin has increased to about 70 g/L. The diet should be light, be easily digested, and contain protein, iron, and ascorbic acid. Blood transfusions are rarely indicated, but they have been used cautiously for patients who are dyspneic at rest, those who have not responded to B_{12}, and those who have a 20 to 30 g/L (2 to 3 g/dL) hemoglobin level. Packed cells (rather than whole blood) are used to prevent fluid overload and cardiovascular crisis.

Individuals with serum B_{12} levels of less than 150 pmol/L (200 pg/mL) should be treated, even in the absence of macrocytosis or a normal Schilling test result. A potential problem exists; therapeutic doses that are given before a diagnosis is made can mask some of the clinical manifestations of subacute degeneration of the spinal cord. Those with a normal Schilling test result and a serum B_{12} level of less than 150 pmol/L (200 pg/mL) should be given oral B_{12} (1 mg/day) until serum levels are raised to more than 250 pmol/L (330 pg/mL). If this response is not achieved or the results of a Schilling test are abnormal, the patient should be treated for pernicious anemia.

A number of different parenteral B_{12} regimens are in use. Because of the relative safety of these agents, large doses of 1000 μg of either cyanocobalamin or hydroxocobalamin can be given weekly, followed by monthly injections for a year to replenish stores. After this, injections (up to 3 months apart, based on the patient's response) are given for life to maintain remission. When patients with untreated pernicious anemia are given 1000 μg of cyanocobalamin, the serum concentration of the vitamin remains in the normal range for at least 1 week. The megaloblastosis can be transformed in a few hours, and the soreness of the tongue and affective disturbances recede in 1 day. Reversal of neurologic manifestations and dementia takes longer and may be incomplete. Although similar doses are used to treat both hematologic and neurologic problems, higher doses have been suggested for the latter.

Alternative lower dosing regimens can also be used. Single 80-μg doses completely reverse a megaloblastic bone marrow. However, doses under 15 μg are generally insufficient to completely correct the abnormality. If a low-dose regimen is used, more frequent administration is required. A suitable low-dose regimen for cyanocobalamin in the initial treatment of deficiency states is 100 μg/day for 6 to 7 days, followed by 100 μg/day every other day for 7 doses if clinical improvement and reticulocyte response occur. Then 100 μg/day is given every 3 to 4 days for another 2 to 3 weeks. Maintenance therapy is usually 100 to 200 μg/month. The regimen for hydroxocobalamin is similar. In pernicious anemia or after total gastrectomy or extensive ileal resection, parenteral therapy is required for life. The initial dose is low for children, but the maintenance dose is the same as that for adults. For children with intracellular defects of B_{12} metabolism, hydroxocobalamin is more effective for treatment than is cyanocobalamin and usually requires high doses, of the order of 500 to 1000 μg/day. For children with transcobalamin II deficiency, oral cyanocobalamin is the preferred treatment.

Hypokalemia is a potential problem of B_{12} therapy that is related to the rapid conversion of bone marrow from megaloblastic to normoblastic, particularly in patients with marked anemia, thrombocytopenia, and neutropenia. Sudden death is possible owing to the increased potassium requirements for erythropoiesis.

It was emphasized in the past that oral cyanocobalamin may be an effective way to treat B_{12} deficiency, including pernicious anemia (38, 39). When there is dietary deficiency or in vegans in whom absorption is normal, this is the preferred route. The oral dose of dietary cyanocobalamin for dietary supplementation is 1 μg/day and may be up to 25 μg/day for individuals with increased requirements. Because approximately 1% of an oral dose of B_{12} can be absorbed by a nonspecific process, even in the absence of IF, pernicious anemia can be treated by giving 1000 μg/day orally for 1 month, followed by 1000 μg/week orally to maintain remission. Such therapy may be erratic, so it should be assessed frequently.

Oral cyanocobalamin may be justified for patients with bleeding disorders or those who are allergic to parenterally administered B_{12} (rare). Oral administration means less frequent visits for injections, but careful compliance counseling about the importance of lifelong therapy is important. Before the availability of the crystalline forms of B_{12}, pernicious anemia was managed adequately with daily doses of liver containing 240 µg of B_{12}. Oral B_{12} is not useful in treating small bowel disease or malabsorption syndromes or following gastric or ileal resection.

Monitoring Therapy

The patient's progress should be monitored clinically and by appropriate laboratory testing (e.g., a full hemogram and reticulocyte count). Reticulocytosis with a maximum reticulocyte count occurs by about the fourth to seventh day after treatment has commenced. The neutrophil count also increases by this time, although the hypersegmented polymorphonuclear neutrophils will persist for 10 to 14 days. Macrocytosis may persist for several months after treatment is started because of the long half-life of erythrocytes. The serum iron concentration, which may be within the reference range or elevated before treatment, decreases to deficient levels within 24 hr of starting treatment. Some patients show a pause in the response to B_{12} 2 to 3 weeks after beginning therapy, and the hemoglobin fails to rise over 100 to 110 g/L (10 to 11 g/dL). This is probably due to a depletion of iron stores, resulting from the accelerated erythropoiesis, and it responds to oral ferrous sulfate, 200 mg three times a day.

The potential for life-threatening hypokalemia associated with rapid erythropoiesis necessitates close monitoring of serum potassium concentrations during the first 48 hr of treatment, particularly if potassium-depleting diuretics are also being used.

Synthetic Vitamin B_{12} (47)

The two synthetic forms of B_{12} that are incorporated into pharmaceuticals are cyanocobalamin and hydroxocobalamin. Indications for both of these agents are similar, although hydroxocobalamin may be preferred for treating B_{12} deficiencies because optic neuropathies may degenerate with the administration of cyanocobalamin. A disadvantage of hydroxocobalamin is that in rare cases, some people may develop antibodies to the transcobalamin-hydroxocobalamin complex, and therefore it must be discontinued.

Oral cyanocobalamin is well absorbed, peak serum levels being reached 8 to 12 hr after oral ingestion. In contrast, peak serum levels following intramuscular injection are reached in 1 hr. Following absorption, regardless of the route of administration, both forms of the vitamin are highly protein bound to the transcobalamins. Both are metabolized in the liver, followed by biliary and urinary excretion. Doses beyond the daily needs are excreted, largely unchanged, via the urine. Cyanocobalamin injected intramuscularly is excreted more rapidly than is hydroxocobalamin, which is more highly protein bound than the former. The half-life of synthetic B_{12} is about 6 days; its half-life in the liver is 400 days. With impaired liver or kidney function, more frequent dosing is necessary.

Synthetic B_{12} is usually well tolerated, and allergic reactions are rare. Medical attention should be sought if a rash or wheezing develops. Although anaphylactic reactions can occur after parenteral administration, they are rare. An intradermal test dose is recommended for patients with a history of suspected allergic reactions to B_{12}. Subjects who are intolerant to naturally occurring B_{12} in foods may be intolerant to the synthetic forms also. Other symptoms, such as mild diarrhea and transient itching, require medical attention only if they continue and worry the patient. A potential problem is that B_{12} therapy can mask the signs of polycythemia vera.

No adverse effects have been documented when the normal daily requirements for these agents have been administered during pregnancy. B_{12} crosses the placenta, and at birth the neonatal level can be two to five times that of the mother. Cyanocobalamin injection containing benzyl alcohol should not be used for neonates or immature infants because of possible toxicity of this preservative. B_{12} is excreted in breast milk, and no problems have been reported for humans taking the normal daily requirements. No geriatric problems have been reported.

Many pharmacologic agents can reduce the absorption of B_{12} from the gastrointestinal tract and thus increase the requirements. These include excessive consumption of ethanol for longer than 2 weeks, prolonged use of cholestyramine, colchicine, and in particular aminoglycoside antibiotics. Concurrent use of chloramphenicol may antagonize the hemopoietic response, so hematologic monitoring is necessary, and (if possible) an alternative antibiotic should be used. As large doses of ascorbic acid may destroy B_{12}, patients should avoid such ingestion within 1 hr of taking oral B_{12}. Large doses of folic acid may also reduce B_{12} concentrations in the blood.

Finally, megadoses of B_{12}, ten times or more the recommended daily allowances, have no proven value and should be discouraged. Cyanocobalamin has no proven value in the treatment of acute viral hepatitis, allergies, amblyopia, delayed growth, malnutrition or tardy appetite, fatigue, mental disorders, multiple sclerosis, sterility, trigeminal neuralgia, or other neurologic conditions or in retarding the aging process.

Prognosis (40, 42)

If correctly diagnosed and treated, cases of B_{12} deficiency and especially PA have an excellent prognosis. Anemia can be reversed, and early vigorous treatment is required to slow and reverse neurologic complications and neuropsychiatric manifestations.

FOLIC ACID DEFICIENCY (3, 20, 21)

Folate deficiency, like B_{12} deficiency, results in megaloblastic anemia and other hematologic abnormalities. However, malnourishment is more of a problem with folate deficiency. Folic acid is an important factor in cell division, and without it, division stops at metaphase. Adequate folic acid is required for normal erythropoiesis, including the maturation of megaloblasts into normoblasts in the bone marrow.

Absorption and Metabolism of Folic Acid (48)

Folic acid is present in many plant and animal foods, either as free folic acid or as polyglutamates, with the folic acid conjugated to glutamic acid. The best sources of folic acid include green leafy vegetables, fruits, and organ meats such as liver and kidney. Because heat destroys 50 to 90% of folic acid in foods, canned or overcooked food may be devoid of the vitamin.

The human requirement for folic acid, which depends on metabolic and cell turnover rates, varies from 25 to 35 µg/day in infancy to up to 100 µg/day in adults. Healthy individuals have total body folic acid stores of 5 to 10 mg, half of which is stored in the liver as N-5-methyltetrahydrofolate. More than 2% is degraded daily, so a continuous dietary supply is essential.

Active absorption of folic acid occurs mainly in the proximal part of the small intestine. Conjugated folic acid (such as in foods) is absorbed to a lesser degree than free folic acid; however, a conjugase in the epithelial cells converts the polyglutamates into absorbable monoglutamates. During absorption the folic acid is reduced and methylated to N-5-methyltetrahydrofolate. However, in malabsorption syndromes, absorption of folic acid from food is impaired. In contrast, folic acid from pharmaceutical products is almost completely absorbed in the upper duodenum, even in the presence of malabsorption. The principal circulating form of folic acid, N-5-methyltetrahydrofolate, is extensively bound to plasma proteins. There is no specific transport protein. Plasma levels vary from 3 to 21 ng/mL and closely reflect the dietary intake. Erythrocyte folate levels, 160 to 640 ng/mL of whole blood standardized to a hematocrit of 45%, are a better indicator of folate status than are the serum levels. Some enterohepatic cycling of folic acid occurs, although significant amounts are not reabsorbed from the bile.

Folic acid is excreted almost entirely as metabolites by the kidney. Amounts beyond the daily requirement are excreted, largely unchanged, in the urine. Because folic acid is removed by hemodialysis, dialysis patients should be given increased amounts (100 to 300% of the RDA).

Etiology of Folate Deficiency (19–21)

Folate deficiency is one of the common causes of nutritional anemias. Inadequate diet, alcoholism, pregnancy, and malabsorption syndromes are the most frequent causes of folate deficiency. Other causes include increased requirements, enhanced metabolism, and interference in the metabolism or clearance by other pharmacotherapeutic agents. The patient's diet, ethanol intake, or signs and symptoms associated with malabsorption may indicate the cause of folate deficiency.

Folic acid intake may be reduced if insufficient attention is paid to the diet and folic acid–rich foods are excluded or if food is poorly prepared or overheated. People who are at risk include alcoholics whose main caloric intake is in the form of ethanol; narcotic addicts who have a poor diet; the elderly, who often do not feel like eating or who eat commercially prepared foods; institutionalized people who have no control over their diet; adolescents and teenagers, who may skip meals and eat junk foods; and some infants. Megaloblastic anemia due to simple dietary deficiency of folic acid is common and sometimes severe among people living in the tropics or in underdeveloped countries. It is less common in more prosperous countries.

Several reasons have been suggested for folate deficiency in alcoholics. These include reduced dietary intake, inactivation of folate conjugase, impaired enterohepatic cycling, and depletion of liver folate stores. Malabsorption of folate in foods is frequently a problem in individuals with tropical sprue, a condition in which there is chronic inflammation of the bowel. Tropical sprue responds to either folic acid or oral antibiotic therapy. Regional ileitis, celiac disease, and resection of the small intestine may also lead to folic acid malabsorption.

Drugs are the most common cause of megaloblastic anemia after folate or B_{12} deficiency. Interference, either directly or indirectly, with DNA synthesis in developing erythroid cells is the most common effect of these drugs. Signs of folate deficiency often appear in epileptics, but these are due to dietary habits as much as to therapy. These agents, especially phenytoin and primidone, which possibly reduce intestinal absorption of folate, rarely induce megaloblastic anemia. Because the central nervous system effect of phenytoin may decrease with concurrent use of folic acid, an increase in the phenytoin dose may be necessary. The importance of the interaction can be determined by monitoring serum phenytoin levels.

Oral contraceptives and estrogen preparations may impair folate absorption in some women. Folate requirements are increased in long-term users of corticosteroids or analgesics. Antibiotics can interfere with the microbiologic assay of folate, giving falsely low results. Also, folic acid supplements should be taken 1 hr before or 4 to 6 hr after cholestyramine ingestion to avoid reduced absorption of the vitamin.

Chemotherapeutic agents such as 6-thioguanine, azathioprine, and 6-mercaptopurine, which are the purine analogs, act as direct inhibitors of DNA synthesis, resulting in drug-induced megaloblastic anemia. Similar effects occur with the pyrimidine analogs 5-fluorouracil and cytosine arabinoside and with hydroxyurea and procarbazine. Methotrexate and to a lesser extent pentamidine, pyrimethamine, and trimethoprim, when used for prolonged periods or at high doses, impair DNA synthesis by inhibiting dihydrofolate reductase. Giving leucovorin calcium (a folinic acid compound), particularly when methotrexate is being used, reduces the risk of megaloblastic anemia. Although oral sulfonamide agents can reduce the intestinal absorption of folic acid, supplementation is not generally given with the usual antibiotic courses. Patients who take sulfasalazine chronically may require supplementation.

An increased requirement for folic acid occurs during pregnancy, infancy, malignancy, and increased erythropoiesis and when there is a rapid cell turnover. During pregnancy a large increase in nucleic acid synthesis is associated with growth of the fetus, placenta, and uterus and the increased maternal erythrocyte mass. Folate requirements may increase threefold during pregnancy; and if supplements are not taken, particularly in the last trimester, the mother may develop megaloblastic anemia. Other problems that can affect folate status in the mother during pregnancy are urinary tract infections and nausea and vomiting, which may restrict food intake.

Folate deficiency is extremely common in myeloproliferative disorders such as chronic myeloid leukemia and myelofibrosis, often leading to thrombocytopenia or anemia. The increased folate requirements in chronic hemolytic anemia, exfoliative dermatitis, generalized psoriasis, or extensive burns can also lead to folate deficiency. In these cases, adequate supplementation is required. Anemia is more likely to occur if several contributing factors are present.

Clinical Features

Signs and symptoms of folate deficiency are similar to those of other megaloblastic anemias. Specifically, these include megaloblastosis, glossitis, diarrhea, weight loss, and neurologic manifestations. The disease progresses slowly, and the hemoglobin level may fall to an ominously low 20 to 30 g/L.

Diagnosis (3, 20)

In all patients with macrocytosis and in whom megaloblastosis is suspected, peripheral blood smears, both serum folate and B_{12} concentrations, and erythrocyte folate levels should be measured. Megaloblastosis possibly due to folic acid deficiency must be interpreted in the light of B_{12} status because of similar findings in B_{12} deficiency. Another problem is that some patients with pernicious anemia (PA) have low serum folate levels secondary to megaloblastosis of the intestinal epithelial cells. The diagnosis of megaloblastic anemia due to folate deficiency requires showing reduced folate tissue levels, as reflected by erythrocyte folate concentrations. Anemia occurs only when tissue levels are depleted. A normal serum folate concentration

does not exclude deficiency. Serum folate levels have the disadvantage of being sensitive to dynamic changes in folate metabolism, such as reflecting folate absorbed from a recent meal.

Bone marrow studies should be undertaken when a myeloproliferative disease or hemolytic anemia is suspected, to confirm the megaloblastosis. Also, because serum iron, iron saturation, and ferritin studies are unreliable in patients with folate or B_{12} deficiency, bone marrow studies are required to determine iron stores, particularly in cases of malabsorption.

Management of Folic Acid Deficiency (18, 19, 49)

Folic acid is indicated for the prevention and treatment of folic acid deficiencies. Dietary improvement is preferred over supplementation with pharmaceutical preparations. When possible, folic acid should not be given until B_{12} deficiency and PA have been excluded. The danger here is that large doses of folic acid (e.g., >1 mg/day) can reverse the hematologic aspects of PA but not the spinal cord degeneration, which can worsen. If it is essential to give some folic acid, doses of 100 µg/day are enough to meet the patient's minimal requirements but not enough to convert the megaloblastic marrow in PA.

Although folate levels are readily restored by 5 mg of folic acid daily, in practice much lower doses can be used. When absorption is normal, as little as 50 to 100 µg/day may suffice. In long-standing folate deficiency, secondary malabsorption due to megaloblastosis of intestinal epithelial cells increases requirements, and here 250 to 500 µg/day is usually sufficient. Severely ill patients with hemoglobin levels of less than 50 g/L need blood transfusions until folic acid therapy has increased erythropoiesis. To replenish depleted folate stores, a daily dose of 1 to 2 mg/day for 2 to 3 weeks should suffice.

The duration of therapy depends on the underlying cause. It can take 3 to 4 months to clear folate-deficient erythrocytes from the blood. Replacement therapy should be continued until the underlying problem has been corrected. If this is impossible, lifelong therapy is required. B_{12} studies should also be undertaken in this latter group, and prophylactic doses of B_{12} should be given if required. Long-term therapy may be required in chronic hemolytic states, myelofibrosis, and refractory malabsorption. Postgastrectomy states, prolonged stress or infection, chronic fever, and persistent diarrhea may also increase requirements. Supplementation is required for patients who are receiving TPN or undergoing rapid weight loss or those with malnutrition. Low doses of folic acid, 500 µg/day, can be given to patients with megaloblastic anemia due to antiepileptic agents, without stopping the antiepileptic therapy. Higher doses of folic acid rarely increase the risk of seizures. Use of folic acid in preventing mental disorders is of unproved benefit.

Prophylactic folate therapy during pregnancy, particularly in women with poor diets, multiple pregnancies, or thalassemia minor, is useful in preventing megaloblastic anemia. Folate deficiency is rare in well-nourished women with normal pregnancy. Because the greatest risk is in the latter part of the pregnancy, prophylaxis is achieved by giving 300 μg/day in the last trimester. This is generally given as a combination iron/folate preparation. Some authorities frown on giving this combination during the whole pregnancy. Subclinical maternal folate deficiency during pregnancy can result in underweight, premature infants and less than optimal health for the mother. Supplementation may be necessary for infants receiving unfortified formulas (e.g., evaporated milk), those being breast-fed by mothers with folic acid deficiency, or those with a low birth weight.

Monitoring Therapy

Response to treatment can be monitored by following the reticulocyte count, which peaks 5 to 8 days after commencing treatment. A rise in the erythrocyte count and blood hemoglobin level and a concurrent fall in the MCV are important monitoring signs. Measuring erythrocyte folate levels several times during the treatment can confirm replenishment of tissue stores. For patients with severe megaloblastic anemia, potassium levels should be monitored during the early stages of treatment.

Folic Acid (48)

The common pharmaceutical form of folic acid is dihydrofolate, which is available as either the acid or the sodium salt. Both oral and parenteral forms are available. Parenteral administration is indicated when oral administration is unacceptable (preoperatively, postoperatively, or if nausea or vomiting is a problem) or not possible (malabsorption syndromes or following gastric resection).

No major side effects have been reported with folic acid administration, even when ten times the RDA was taken for 1 month (49). Megadoses of folic acid taken for long periods should be discouraged unless some benefit is observed because zinc deficiency may occur. Rare side effects associated with allergic reactions include fever and rashes.

CONCLUSION

Anemia due to a deficiency of iron, B$_{12}$, or folic acid can usually be treated simply and effectively. Determining the primary cause and its subsequent management may be more difficult. When possible, dietary manipulation should be used as a maintenance strategy. In some cases, particularly with pernicious anemia, lifelong therapy is necessary. Compliance can be a major problem after the hemoglobin levels rise and the patient begins to feel better.

REFERENCES

1. Massey AC. Microcytic anemia: differential diagnosis and management of iron deficiency anemia. Med Clin North Am 76:549–66, 1992.
2. Brown RG. Determining the cause of anemia: general approach, with emphasis on microcytic hyprochromic anemias. Postgrad Med 89:161–70, 1991.
3. Brown RG. Normocytic and macrocytic anemias. Postgrad Med 89:125–36, 1991.
4. Mayer E, Adieles-Tegman M. The prevalence of anemia in the world. World Health Stat Q 38:302–16, 1985.
5. Cook JD, Skikne BS, Lynch SR, et al. Estimates of iron sufficiency in the US population. Blood 68:726–31, 1986.
6. Bertolone SJ. Anemia and coagulation defects in adolescents. Sem Reprod Endocrinol 6:35–43, 1988.
7. Murphy JF, O'Riordan J, Newcombe RG, Coles EC. Relation of hemoglobin levels in first and second trimesters to outcome of pregnancy. Lancet 1:992–94, 1986.
8. Walter T, De Andraca I, Chadud P, Perales CG. Iron deficiency anemia: adverse effects on infant psychomotor development. Pediatrics 84:7–17, 1989.
9. Dalman PR. Iron deficiency and the immune response. Am J Clin Nutr 46:329–34, 1987.
10. Dalman PR. Biochemical basis for manifestations of iron deficiency. Ann Rev Nutr 6:13–40, 1988.
11. Soemantri AG, Pollitt E, Kim I. Iron deficiency anaemia and educational achievement. Am J Clin Nutr 42:1221–28, 1986.
12. Cole SK, Billeweca WZ, Thomson AM. Sources of blood loss in menstrual blood loss. J Obstet Gynaecol Br Comm 78:933–39, 1971.
13. Nilsson L, Solvel L. Clinical studies on oral contraceptives: randomised double blind crossover study of four different populations. Acta Obstet Gynaecol Scand 46 (suppl 8):1–31, 1967.
14. Herbert V. Recommended dietary intakes (RDI) of iron in humans. Am J Clin Nutr 45:679–86, 1987.
15. Bothwell TH, Baynes RD, Macfarlane BJ, MacPhail APM. Nutritional iron requirements and food iron absorption. J Intern Med 226:357–65, 1989.
16. Harju E. Clinical pharmacokinetics of iron preparations. Clin Pharmacokinet 17:69–89, 1989.
17. Farley PC, Foland J. Iron deficiency anemia: how to diagnose and correct. Postgrad Med 87:89–101, 1990.
18. Finch C. Minisymposium. Introduction: knights of the oval table. J Intern Med 226:345–48, 1989.
19. McGrath K. Treatment of anaemia caused by iron, vitamin B$_{12}$ or folate deficiency. Med J Aust 151:695–97, 1989.
20. Mansouri A, Lipschitz DA. Anemia in the elderly patient. Med Clin North Am 76:619–30, 1992.
21. Beddall A. Anemias. Practitioner 234:714–15, 1990.
22. Rowland TW. Iron deficiency in the young athlete. Pediatr Clin North Am 37:1153–63, 1990.
23. Sayetta RB. Pica: an overview. Am Fam Physician 33(5):181–85, 1986.
24. Cook JD. Clinical evaluation of iron deficiency. Semin Hematol 19(1):6–18, 1982.
25. Jandl JH. The hypochromic anemias and other disorders of iron metabolism. In: Jandl JH, ed. Blood: text book of hematology. Boston: Little, Brown 1987:181–235.
26. Anon. Iron supplements (systemic) in USP DI. In: Drug information for the health care professional, 15th ed. Rockville, MD: United States Pharmacopeial Convention Inc, 1995:IB:1614–23.
27. Paparella P, Papadia LS, Brizio AM, Mancuso S. Effects of routine iron supplementation in pregnancy. Curr Ther Res 48:348–55, 1990.
28. Heese HD, Smith S, Watermeyer S, et al. Prevention of iron deficiency in preterm neonates during infancy. S Afr Med J 77:339–45, 1990.

29. Hibbard BM. Iron and folate supplements during pregnancy: supplementation is only valuable in some patients. Br Med J 197:1324–25, 1988.

30. Rudinskas L, Paton WP, Walker SE, et al. Case report: poor clinical response to enteric-coated iron preparations. Can Med Assoc J 141:565–66, 1989.

31. Walker SE, Paton TW, Cowan DH, Manuel MA, Dranitsaris G. Bioavailability of iron in oral ferrous sulfate preparations in healthy volunteers. Can Med Assoc J 141:543–47, 1989.

32. Kumpf VJ, Holland EG. Parenteral iron dextran therapy. DICP Ann Pharmacother 24:162–66, 1990.

33. Hanson DB, Hendeles L. Guide to total dose intravenous iron dextran therapy. Am J Hosp Pharm 31:592–95, 1974.

34. Cohen A. Treatment of transfusional iron overload. Am J Pediatr Hematol/Oncol 12:4–8, 1990.

35. Goodman KI, Salt WB. Vitamin B_{12} deficiency: important new concepts in recognition. Postgrad Med 88:147–58, 1990.

36. Schjonsby H. Vitamin B_{12} absorption and malabsorption. Gut 30:1686–91, 1989.

37. Carethers M. Diagnosing vitamin B_{12} deficiency, a common geriatric disorder. Geriatrics 43(3):89–112, 1989.

38. Hathcock JN, Troendle GJ. Oral cobalamin for treatment of pernicious anemia. JAMA 265:96–97, 1991.

39. Lederle FA. Oral cobalamin for pernicious anemia: medicine's best kept secret? JAMA 265:94–95, 1991.

40. McRae TD, Freedman ML. Why vitamin B_{12} deficiency should be managed aggressively. Geriatrics 44:70–79, 1989.

41. Martin DC. B_{12} and folate deficiency dementia. Clin Geriatr Med 4(4):841–53, 1988.

42. Healton EB, Savage DG, Brust JCM, Garrett TJ, Lindenbaum J. Neurologic aspects of cobalamin deficiency. Medicine 70:229–45, 1991.

43. Nickoloff E. Schilling test: physiologic basis and use as a diagnostic test. CRC Crit Rev Clin Lab Sci 26:263–76, 1988.

44. Bunting RW, Bitzer AM, Kenney RM, Ellman L. Prevalence of antibodies and vitamin B_{12} malabsorption in older patients admitted to a rehabilitation hospital. J Am Geriatr Soc 38:743–47, 1990.

45. Doscherholmen A, Swain WR. Impaired assimilation of egg Co57 vitamin B_{12} in patients with hypochlorhydria and achlorhydria after gastric resection. Gastroenterology 64:913–19, 1973.

46. Salom IL, Silvis SE, Doscherholmen A. Effect of cimetidine on the absorption of vitamin B_{12}. Scand J Gastroenterol 17:129–31, 1982.

47. Anon. Vitamin B_{12} (systemic) in USP DI. In: Drug information for the health care professional, 15th ed. Rockville, MD: United States Pharmacopeial Convention Inc., 1995:IB:2787–90.

48. Anon. Folic acid (systemic) in USP DI. In: Drug information for the health care professional, 15th ed. Rockville, MD: United States Pharmacopeial Convention Inc., 1995:IA:1365–68.

49. Butterworth CE, Tamura T. Folic acid safety and toxicity: a brief review. Am J Clin Nutr 50:353–58, 1989.

CHAPTER 14

OTHER ANEMIAS

JANICE L. STUMPF and KEVIN A. TOWNSEND

Although the clinical features of anemias resulting from many causes are often similar, treatment modalities and prognosis are quite distinct. In this chapter, a variety of anemias will be discussed, including the anemias of chronic disease and renal failure, aplastic anemia, sickle cell anemia, thalassemia, and hemolytic anemia.

ANEMIA OF CHRONIC DISEASE

The anemia of chronic disease is a mild, often asymptomatic condition that occurs in conjunction with a variety of infectious, inflammatory, and neoplastic disorders. The anemia develops 1 to 2 months following the onset of diseases (such as chronic osteomyelitis, tuberculosis, rheumatoid arthritis, systemic lupus erythematosus, and vasculitides) and carcinomas (including Hodgkin's disease and solid tumors). Although renal insufficiency is also a chronic disease, the associated anemia manifests differently and will therefore be discussed separately.

The common pathology of anemia of chronic disease appears to be a defect in iron transport from the reticuloendothelial system, hepatocytes, and intestinal epithelial cells to the plasma and erythroid precursor cells (1). In addition, a moderate shortening of red blood cell life-span may be noted that is unaccompanied by increased erythrocyte production. In fact, erythropoietin concentrations may be low relative to the measured hematocrit.

Although the reasons for these abnormalities are not presently known, it has been suggested that the cytokine interleukin-1 may be the primary mediator of the pathology that presents as anemia of chronic disease (1, 2). Interleukin-1 stimulates the elaboration of high concentrations of lactoferrin from leukocytes at sites of inflammation. This protein preferentially binds iron and prevents its mobilization to the plasma. Macrophages then take up the iron-lactoferrin complex, resulting in accumulation of iron in the cells of the reticuloendothelial system. Alternatively, interleukin-1 may induce the synthesis of ferritin, allowing increased iron storage and restricting the amount of iron available to the bone marrow. Other cytokines, including tumor necrosis factor and interferon, may also have a role in the suppression of erythropoiesis (2).

Because it is associated with many diseases and a unifying pathogenesis has not yet been elucidated, anemia of chronic disease remains a diagnosis of exclusion. The erythrocytes are typically normochromic and normocytic, but may be microcytic. The hematocrit concentration rarely falls below 0.30; if it does, other causes of anemia should be thoroughly investigated. The reticulocyte count is low or within normal limits, and serum iron levels and iron binding protein saturation are reduced. However, in contrast to the picture of iron deficiency anemia, ferritin levels are increased in the anemia of chronic disease. Anemia due to iron deficiency as a sole diagnosis or in conjunction with the anemia of chronic disease is unlikely if the serum ferritin concentration exceeds 50 to 60 g/L (1). These and other manifestations, including elevations in haptoglobin and fibrinogen levels and erythrocyte sedimentation rate, are known collectively as the "acute phase" reaction, a response to inflammation that may persist with chronic conditions.

Because the anemia of chronic disease is generally mild, no specific therapy is necessary in most cases. The degree of anemia correlates well with the severity of the associated disease state, and reversal of the underlying disorder will correct the anemia. If the patient becomes symptomatic, however, blood transfusions may be beneficial. Iron replacement regimens have been attempted, but have been uniformly ineffective and may place the patient at risk of iron toxicity. The anemia of chronic disease has responded to therapy with recombinant human erythropoietin; however, the role of this agent in the clinical setting remains to be established (1, 2).

ANEMIA OF RENAL FAILURE

The anemia that complicates end-stage renal disease is generally more severe than that associated with other chronic diseases. The severity of the anemia appears to correlate with the extent of the uremia, but not with the etiology of the underlying renal disease. Most patients with serum creatinine concentrations over 310 mol/L (3.5 mg/dL) and 97% of those on maintenance dialysis are affected. The cells are normochromic and normocytic, but are frequently irregular in shape. Although hematocrit levels may fall to 0.20 to 0.30 or less, not all patients become symptomatic. This tolerance of such low hematocrit concentrations may be explained by the compensatory reduction in oxygen-hemoglobin affinity, allowing improved delivery of oxygen to the tissues. Despite this adaptation, an estimated 25% of patients receiving dialysis required treatment with blood transfusions before the widespread use of recombinant erythropoietin (3). In addition to the commonly known symptoms of anemia such as fatigue, increasing angina, and shortness of breath, vague complaints of generalized coldness, anorexia, insomnia, and depression, which were not associated with anemia until recently, may be improved with adequate therapy.

Pathogenesis

The anemia of renal failure is a multifactorial process, but is primarily the result of reduced secretion of erythropoietin by the diseased kidneys. This hormone stimulates the proliferation and maturation of erythrocytes and is released when the availability of oxygen to the organs is diminished. Although to some extent synthesized extrarenally in the liver, serum erythropoietin concentrations in uremic patients are markedly lower than those measured in patients with similar degrees of anemia and normal renal function.

Other factors that contribute to the anemia are the accumulation of inhibitors of erythropoiesis, reduced red blood cell life-span, and chronic blood loss. In support of the presence of suppressive substances, erythropoietin-induced stimulation of erythroid progenitors is blunted in vitro by uremic serum. In addition, while erythropoietin levels remain stable, the anemia improves following dialysis, perhaps indicating removal of these substances. Parathyroid hormone and the polyamine spermine have both been implicated in reducing marrow responsiveness to erythropoietin, but data are conflicting and the identity of the inhibitory substances remains unknown.

Erythrocyte survival is also decreased to an average of one half of normal in uremia due to a mild, chronic hemolysis. The cause of the red cell destruction is unclear, but hypersplenism or increases in erythrocyte fragility induced by parathyroid hormone may contribute. This abnormality may not be corrected by dialysis, yet also does not appear to be a defect in the red cells. A similar reduction in erythrocyte life-span is noted after transfusion of blood products from nonuremic donors to renal failure patients.

Chronic blood loss both from a gastrointestinal source and during hemodialysis may also contribute to the anemia. Due to defects in platelet function, uremic patients have an elevated risk of bleeding; occult blood loss is reported in over 20% of dialysis patients (4). An estimated 2 grams of iron is lost annually during hemodialysis, increasing the likelihood of a concurrent iron deficiency anemia. In addition, the intestinal absorption of iron may be compromised by the chronic use of iron-chelating antacids. Other factors that may aggravate the anemia of end-stage renal disease include folic acid deficiency due to losses to the dialysate, the accumulation of the fat-soluble vitamin A, aluminum toxicity due to long-term hemodialysis, and the use of aluminum-containing phosphate binders and osteitis fibrosa, a complication of hyperparathyroidism in which myelofibrosis reduces viable erythroid cellular mass.

Treatment

Prior to the initiation of therapy aimed at the primary abnormality, other potential causes of anemia should be identified and addressed. Iron and folate supplementation should be provided as necessary, and blood loss and the use of aluminum-containing antacids minimized whenever possible. The treatment for acute symptoms of hypoxia consists of the transfusion of red blood cells. However, although transfusions may readily correct the anemia, they carry the risk of hypersensitivity reactions and the transmission of viral hepatitis. In addition, bone marrow suppression and iron overload requiring deferoxamine therapy may occur after multiple, chronic transfusions.

ANDROGENS

Traditionally, the administration of androgens has been recommended for treatment of anemia in selected patients with end-stage renal disease. These agents stimulate the synthesis of erythropoietin and/or the production of red blood cells in the bone marrow. However, they are not universally effective and rarely fully correct the anemia. Elevations in hematocrit concentrations of 0.05 or more compared to baseline were documented in 50% of patients able to tolerate the drugs in a 6-month controlled, crossover trial (4). Therapy with the injectable formulations nandrolone decanoate and testosterone enanthate resulted in significantly greater improvements in hematocrit levels than the two oral androgens studied, fluoxymesterone and oxymetholone. Transfusion requirements were not reduced during androgen therapy. Patients with lower pretreatment hematocrit concentrations, bilateral nephrectomies, or intact parathyroid glands had poorer response rates. Based on these results and the propensity for virilization effects such as hirsutism, changes in external genitalia, amenorrhea, acne, and voice deepening, the usefulness of androgens for this indication is limited. Injectable androgens are recommended over oral agents, and nandrolone decanoate is preferred in females because of its greater ratio of anabolic to androgenic activities. Nandrolone decanoate and testosterone enanthate are administered as weekly intramuscular injections of 1.5 to 2.5 mg/kg and 4 to 7 mg/kg, respectively. If an adequate response is not achieved after a 6-month trial, the agent should be discontinued. Therapy with oral androgens (fluoxymesterone 10 to 30 mg daily) may then be attempted. However, in addition to the adverse effects associated with the injectable agents, the oral androgens may also induce liver dysfunction and hepatic cancer.

RECOMBINANT HUMAN ERYTHROPOIETIN

Advances in recombinant technology have made possible the production of human erythropoietin (epoetin alfa, epoetin), a peptide whose 166-amino acid structure is identical to that of the native hormone. The availability of epoetin has revolutionized the therapy of anemia associated with end-stage renal disease and all but eliminated the use of androgen therapy.

In a multicenter study of the efficacy of epoetin, intravenous doses of 150 or 300 U/kg were administered to 333 anemic patients 3 times weekly after hemodialysis (5). Target hematocrit concentrations of 0.35 or 0.06 increases from baseline were achieved in over 97% of patients within 12 weeks. In addition, the need for routine red cell transfusions was eliminated within 2 months. Quality of life was enhanced as evidenced by increased energy and activity levels, cold tolerance, and appetite. A median dosage of 75 U/kg maintained these effects. Lack of response in the remaining patients was attributed to other causes of anemia, such as myelofibrosis and blood loss.

Patients with end-stage renal disease with hematocrit levels under 0.30 or requiring blood transfusions may be considered candidates for epoetin treatment. Although once commonly given as intravenous bolus doses of 50 to 100 U/kg 3 times weekly following hemodialysis, subcutaneous administration of epoetin is currently preferred and has been used successfully in predialysis and continuous ambulatory peritoneal dialysis (CAPD) populations as well. The bioavailability of epoetin after subcutaneous administration is approximately 48% (range, 14.5% to 96.5%); however, lower, more sustained plasma concentrations are achieved due to slow release from the subcutaneous depot (6). The elimination half-life after subcutaneous injection is approximately 28 hours, whereas that following intravenous administration ranges from 4 to 11 hours. Similarly, efficacy is provided by the subcutaneous route with epoetin doses 30 to 50% lower than those of the intravenous route. An initial subcutaneous regimen of 100 to 150 U/kg/week in 2 or 3 divided doses is recommended (6, 7). Alternatively, weekly subcutaneous injections of epoetin are also effective, yet allow no reduction in total dose as compared to intravenous therapy. The intraperitoneal route of administration is generally impractical because of the high doses required to produce plasma concentrations comparable to those following subcutaneous or intravenous administration (6).

Dose-dependent rises in hematocrit and reticulocyte counts are seen after 2 to 6 weeks of therapy (Fig. 14.1) (8). Hematocrit concentrations should be determined weekly; if the hematocrit has not increased to target range or by 5 or 6 percentage points after 8 weeks of therapy, the dose should be adjusted upward. Once a hematocrit of 0.30 is attained, the dose should be reduced by 50% and titrated every 2 to 4 weeks to maintain hematocrit concentrations of 0.33 to 0.38 (7). It should be noted that this goal hematocrit level remains controversial in that it provides for only partial correction of the anemia (7, 9). Preliminary data suggest that normalization of hematocrit concentra-

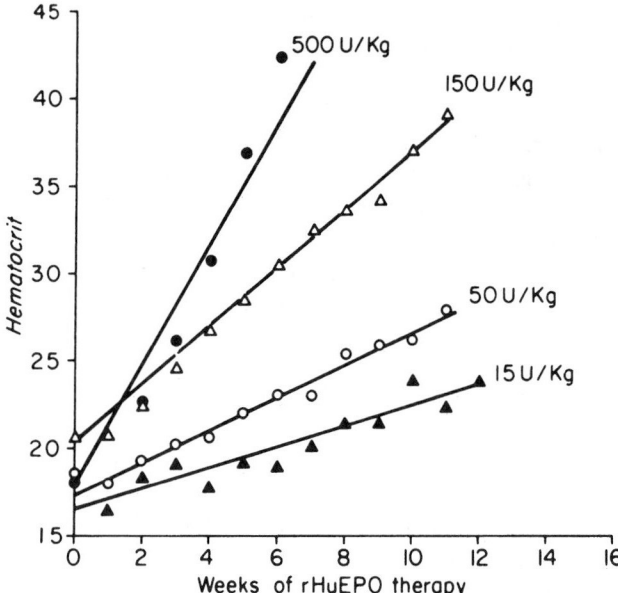

Figure 14.1 The rates at which hematocrit increases with various doses of epoetin. (From Eschbach JW, Egrie JC, Downing MR, et al. Correction of the anemia of end-stage renal disease with recombinant human erythropoietin. N Engl J Med 316:73–78, 1987, with permission.)

tions from 0.33 to 0.42 may result in significant improvements in physiologic and quality of life measures without compromising patient safety (9).

Adverse effects associated with epoetin therapy include myalgias, headache, flank pain, hypertension, and seizures. In addition, local reactions, such as burning, pain, and irritation, have been reported following subcutaneous injection. Increases in blood pressure appear to be a hemodynamic consequence of the rising hematocrit. As the anemia is corrected, compensatory vasodilation decreases and peripheral vascular resistance (and blood pressure) increases. Diastolic blood pressure elevations exceed 10 mm Hg or require the institution or upward adjustment of antihypertensive medications in 35% of patients within 3 months of epoetin initiation (5). Seizures may accompany uncontrolled hypertension. Therefore, close monitoring and control of blood pressure levels are essential.

Increases in predialysis concentrations of serum creatinine, potassium, and phosphate have also been documented. The reduced effectiveness of dialysis noted with higher hematocrit levels and increased dietary intake may account for these changes. In addition, clotting of arteriovenous access sites has occurred in up to 14% of epoetin-treated patients. In contrast, in another report, the incidence of graft thrombosis was no greater than that of a historical control hemodialysis population not receiving epoetin (6).

During the acute erythroid response, iron may be used more rapidly than it is released to transferrin from the reticuloendothelial system. A functional as well as an absolute iron deficiency may therefore develop, which may compromise further response to epoetin. Patients with pretreatment iron overload have experienced beneficial 39% reductions in serum ferritin levels within 6 months. Ferritin levels and transferrin saturation should be determined at baseline and monthly until the goal hematocrit is achieved; iron stores should be measured at 2- to 3-month intervals thereafter. If the ferritin concentration or transferrin saturation falls below 100 g/L or 20%, respectively, intravenous or oral iron supplementation should be initiated (6, 7).

The availability of epoetin offers clinicians the means to correct the anemia of renal disease on a long-term basis in both dialysis and predialysis patients. The high response rate indicates that the predominant cause of the anemia is erythropoietin deficiency. Other pathogenetic mechanisms, such as the presence of inhibitors of erythropoiesis, may also be operative, yet may be overwhelmed clinically by an excess of exogenous erythropoietin. The high cost of epoetin should be considered in the context of savings resulting from reductions in other interventions. Routine blood transfusions, androgen therapy, and hospitalizations due to complications of these modalities may be completely eliminated. In addition, improvements in quality of life parameters may represent a greater rehabilitation potential and a return to productive lives for more patients with end-stage renal disease.

APLASTIC ANEMIA

Aplastic anemia is distinguished by hypocellularity of the bone marrow and subsequent pancytopenia that is unrelated to malignancy or myeloproliferative disease. The characteristic anemia, neutropenia, and thrombocytopenia result from failure of the pluripotential stem cell due to congenital or acquired processes. Although the causative mechanisms remain unknown, advances in therapy have greatly improved the overall prognosis.

Pathogenesis

In normal hematopoiesis, three cell lines originate from the pluripotential stem cell, producing erythrocytes, agranulocytes, granulocytes, and platelets; however, these three are affected in bone marrow failure. Both cellular and humoral factors regulate the stem cells to maintain a balance between self-replication and differentiation into particular cell types. Aplastic anemia develops when hematopoiesis is interrupted because of deficient or defective stem cells. In addition to reduced numbers of progenitor cells, suggested pathophysiologic mechanisms include immune-mediated suppression of stem cell function, disturbances in the bone marrow microenvironment, and alterations in the cellular or humoral interactions that normally sustain hematopoiesis (10, 11). Current research

and the success of a variety of treatment modalities support the concept of aplastic anemia as a condition consisting of several pathogenetic abnormalities.

Etiology

Although numerous causes have been identified, up to 70% of cases of aplastic anemia are classified as idiopathic. Myelosuppression is a component of several congenital diseases, but is more commonly acquired after exposure to drugs, chemicals, ionizing radiation or viruses (Table 14.1).

Bone marrow suppression resulting from drugs or chemicals is often dose- and duration-dependent and may result from direct or immune-mediated stem cell toxicity. Chloramphenicol is the best-documented cause of drug-induced aplastic anemia. Reversible erythroid suppression is noted in approximately 50% of those receiving over 1 week of high-dose systemic therapy, but has been reported following even ophthalmic administration of the antibiotic. In contrast, rare idiosyncratic marrow suppression manifesting weeks to months after exposure is also associated with chloramphenicol. Before the availability of bone marrow transplantation and alternative treatments, this

Table 14.1.
Etiologies of Aplastic Anemia

Acquired
  Drugs and chemicals
    Acetazolamide
    Anticonvulsants
      Carbamazepine
      Phenytoin
      Primidone
    Arsenic
    Benzene
    Chloramphenicol
    Chlorpromazine
    Ethanol
    Gold salts
    Insecticides
    Phenylbutazone
    Quinacrine hydrochloride
    Sulfa drugs
  Viral
    Cytomegalovirus
    Epstein-Barr virus
    Hepatitis
    Herpes varicella-zoster
    Influenza
    Rubella
  Other
    Ionizing radiation
    Paroxysmal nocturnal hemoglobinuria
    Pregnancy
    Thymoma
Congenital
  Dyskeratosis congenita
  Fanconi's anemia
  Schwarchman-Diamond syndrome

Table 14.2.
Criteria for the Diagnosis of Severe Aplastic Anemia

Peripheral Blood Counts	*Two or three of the following:*
	Neutrophils $< 0.5 \times 10^9$/L
	Platelets $< 20 \times 10^9$/L
	Reticulocytes < 0.01
Bone Marrow Biopsy	*One of the following:*
	Severe hypocellularity (<25% normal)
	Moderate hypocellularity (25 to 50% normal) with < 30% of residual cells being hematopoietic

Adapted from references 10 and 11.

reaction was fatal in 90% of cases, often within 1 year of clinical presentation.

Aplastic anemia may also arise concurrently with or following viral infection. Hepatitis, most often non-A, non-B (including hepatitis C), precedes up to 5% of cases of aplastic anemia; however, the severity of the infection does not predict the subsequent development of bone marrow suppression. Myelosuppression is usually noted within 6 months of the onset of hepatitis.

Clinical Presentation

Stem cell dysfunction may be incomplete and result in unequal effects on each cell type. Therefore, the earliest clinical signs are determined by the cell line affected to the greatest degree. Often, features of a mild anemia, such as pallor and fatigue, will be reported initially and may be more pronounced if accompanied by bleeding due to thrombocytopenia. Ecchymoses and petechiae are also indicative of a low platelet count. Less commonly, infection due to the underlying neutropenia is the presenting manifestation of aplastic anemia. Signs of infection such as fever should be monitored closely as the neutropenia progresses, since inflammation may not be apparent.

Decreased numbers of morphologically normal cells are observed in the peripheral blood. The erythrocytes are normochromic and normocytic or slightly macrocytic. The corrected reticulocyte count is markedly reduced, as is the absolute granulocyte count. Bone marrow biopsy reveals extensive areas of hypocellularity interspersed with small patches of hematopoietic cells.

Epidemiology and Prognosis

The annual incidence of aplastic anemia in United States is estimated to be 2 to 5 cases per million population (10). The prevalence of disease is higher in Korea and Japan, perhaps reflecting increased exposure to viral hepatitis and environmental toxins. Two peaks are evident in the distribution of ages of onset; approximately 25% of those affected are younger than 15 years whereas 50 to 70% are over 40 years of age.

With supportive care alone, 80% of patients with severe aplastic anemia (Table 14.2) die within 1 to 2 years, with median survival of 6 months (10, 11). Advances in bone marrow transplantation and immunosuppressive therapy have dramatically improved this outcome. In some reports, long-term disease-free survival after transplantation is 70 to 80% (12). Six-year survival rates following immunosuppressive therapy range from 38 to 82% depending on age and absolute neutrophil count (ANC) at diagnosis, with best outcomes in patients under 20 years with ANC values over 200/mL (13).

Treatment

The management of patients with aplastic anemia includes removal of potential causative agents, supportive care, and the restoration of normal hematopoiesis with pharmacologic therapy or bone marrow transplantation (11). In mild cases, supportive care should be provided in anticipation of spontaneous recovery. Blood transfusions, preferably leukocyte-depleted products, should be reserved for patients with symptomatic anemia, to delay sensitization to alloantigens. Blood products from family members should not be used in candidates for marrow transplantation because of the development of antibodies to histocompatibility antigens of the donor, increasing the risk of graft rejection. Overall, nontransfused patients fare better after bone marrow transplantation than their transfused counterparts.

Antiplatelet antibodies that reduce platelet function and life-span also develop after 1 to 2 months of repeated transfusions. Patients often become refractory to subsequent transfusions, although a dose-response relationship has not been established. Platelets should be administered to maintain the platelet count over 20×10^9/L (20,000/mL) and to treat active bleeding.

Because of the risk of hematoma, intramuscular injections should be avoided whenever possible in patients with thrombocytopenia, as should aspirin, nonsteroidal antiinflammatory drugs, and other agents with antiplatelet properties. Menses should be hormonally suppressed to prevent menorrhagia in females with aplastic anemia.

Prompt recognition and treatment of infection is vital in the patient with aplastic anemia and severe neutropenia. Broad-spectrum antibiotics should be initiated in any patient with fever of unknown origin. If a pathogen is not identified and the patient continues to be febrile after 48 to 72 hours of treatment, empiric antifungal therapy with amphotericin B should be considered.

BONE MARROW TRANSPLANTATION

Bone marrow transplantation has become the treatment of choice for severe aplastic anemia, with greatest success achieved in younger patients undergoing the procedure soon after diagnosis (10–12). Initially, an HLA-compatible donor must be identified. There is a 25% chance that a sibling will be HLA-identical. Graft rejection may develop because of minor antigenic differences between donor and recipient marrow and previous sensitization by blood transfusions. Therefore, a course of immunosuppressive therapy is administered prior to transplantation. Most commonly, this "conditioning" regimen consists of intravenous cyclophosphamide (50 mg/kg daily for 4 days) combined with total body or total lymphoid irradiation or, alternatively, cyclophosphamide and cyclosporine with or without antithymocyte globulin (11, 12). These protocols have reduced graft rejection to 5% in some series (11, 12). Two to six weeks after intravenous infusion of marrow cells, the donor cells have engrafted and blood cells begin to be produced.

The interval between transplantation and the return of hematopoiesis and normal immune function poses the greatest threat to the patient. Supportive care should include isolation in a sterile environment, transfusions of blood products as required, and close monitoring for signs of infection. Prophylactic antifungal therapy and bowel sterilization with nonabsorbable oral antibiotics may be undertaken in attempts to reduce the incidence of systemic infections. Interstitial pneumonitis may complicate transplantation within the first 3 months and occurs in approximately 18% of patients with aplastic anemia. In over 39% of cases, cytomegalovirus was implicated and was associated with a mortality rate of over 70% (14). Infection with *Aspergillus, Candida, Pneumocystis carinii,* herpes simplex virus, and herpes varicella-zoster virus has also been reported. Trimethoprim-sulfamethoxazole and acyclovir prophylaxis are now frequently administered to inhibit activation of *Pneumocystis* and herpes viruses, respectively. In addition, the use of immune globulin to prevent cytomegalovirus activation is advocated at some centers.

Acute graft-versus-host-disease (GVHD), in which donor lymphocytes attack the host tissue, occurs in 30 to 60% of patients within 2 months after transplantation despite prophylactic immunosuppression (11). Regimens of methotrexate or cyclosporine alone or in combination are used to prevent GVHD; the addition of prednisone may further improve outcome (11, 12). Initial presenting signs of acute GVHD include skin rash and diarrhea. Elevations in liver function tests and severe immunodeficiency may also develop. Once established, GVHD may be managed with antithymocyte globulin, prednisone, or cyclosporine, with response rates of 30 to 50% (11).

Chronic GVHD manifests over 3 months posttransplantation in approximately 25% of surviving patients (12). The reaction is similar to a systemic autoimmune disease (e.g., systemic lupus erythematosus), with skin, gastrointestinal, hepatic, lymphoid, lung, and ophthalmic involvement. Eighty percent of afflicted patients recover following treatment regimens of prednisone and cyclosporine or azathioprine (11). The risk of acquiring and the severity of GVHD are directly correlated to the age of the patient. Therefore, most bone marrow transplants are performed in patients under the age of 40 years.

IMMUNOSUPPRESSION

Immunosuppressive therapy is generally reserved for older patients with aplastic anemia or those without an HLA-matched marrow donor. A variety of agents, both alone and in combination, have been used to treat the disease, including antithymocyte globulin (ATG), antilymphocyte globulin (ALG), corticosteroids, and cyclosporine (10, 11, 15).

ATG and ALG are prepared in animals and react against human thymocytes and lymphocytes, respectively. The mechanism by which these agents positively affect aplastic anemia is unknown, but they presumably inactivate cytotoxic lymphocytes responsible for suppression of hematopoiesis. In addition, proliferation and differentiation of hematopoietic progenitors may be stimulated. The overall efficacy of ATG/ALG is difficult to assess from current research because of variations in preparations, treatment protocols, and severity of illness in the study populations. However, improvements in blood indices are elicited in 40 to 70% of treated patients (15).

In a typical treatment protocol, a test dose is administered and, in the absence of anaphylaxis, is followed by an 8- to 10-day course of 10 to 20 mg/kg/day ATG or ALG infused intravenously over 4 to 12 hours. Response is usually observed within 1 to 3 months after therapy. A second course may be effective in those who fail initial therapy and in the 25 to 30% of patients who relapse.

Adverse effects of ATG/ALG include fever, chills, rash, headache, and hypotension. Serum sickness, manifesting with fever, rash, and arthralgias, may be evident 1 to 2 weeks after therapy; however, symptoms may be alleviated by concurrent corticosteroid therapy. Transient reductions in white blood cell and platelet counts are also reported. Hematologic complications, such as myelodysplasia, leukemia, and paroxysmal nocturnal hemoglobinuria, develop in 30 to 50% of patients, with the prevalence increasing with time.

Data regarding the usefulness of high-dose methylprednisolone in conjunction with ATG/ALG are conflicting, with response rates ranging from 20 to 83% (15). Steroids are frequently added to the regimen to control antiserum-induced toxicities. The efficacy of high-dose corticosteroids alone for the treatment of aplastic anemia has not been conclusively demonstrated.

In a recent controlled study, the addition of cyclosporine to the combination of ALG and methylprednisolone increased the rate of complete or partial remission from 39 to 65% at 3 months (10). Furthermore, therapy with cyclosporine alone has yielded response rates similar to those of ATG (10, 11). Effects are usually observed after 2 to 10 weeks of treatment. Long-term maintenance therapy with cyclosporine is often required, increasing the risk of renal toxicity and other adverse effects. Although at present cyclosporine appears to be a potential alternative to ATG or ALG treatment, further controlled studies are necessary to establish its place in therapy.

ANDROGENS

Androgens were once widely used for the treatment of aplastic anemia because of their stimulatory effects on hematopoiesis (predominantly red cell production). However, in patients with severe disease, oral oxymetholone and intramuscular nandrolone decanoate produced responses similar to those following supportive care alone. In addition, androgens do not potentiate the effects of ATG or ALG therapy. Although androgens have no apparent role in the management of severe forms of the disease, those with mild aplastic anemia or Fanconi's anemia not amenable to marrow transplantation may benefit from treatment. Initial responses are detected after 3 to 6 months of therapy; however, adverse effects such as virilization and hepatotoxicity may limit the prolonged courses required to achieve effects in all cell lines.

FUTURE DIRECTIONS: RECOMBINANT GROWTH FACTORS

Recombinant human granulocyte colony stimulating factor (G-CSF) and granulocyte-macrophage colony stimulating factor (GM-CSF) are growth factors that stimulate the proliferation of progenitor cells and thus may have applications to many hypoplastic disorders (16). Both intravenous and subcutaneous administration of growth factors to patients with aplastic anemia have produced marked elevations in leukocyte counts, primarily due to increases in neutrophils. Improvements in red cell and platelet counts were rare; the addition of recombinant human erythropoietin to the regimen may increase red blood cell counts. In general, response was dose dependent and inversely related to the severity of disease, and the effects did not persist after G-CSF or GM-CSF discontinuation. Because growth factors do not correct the underlying stem cell disorder, these agents should be used only in conjunction with definitive therapies for aplastic anemia (i.e., immunosuppression or bone marrow transplantation). The addition of G-CSF as supportive therapy has improved survival by reducing mortality due to infection (16).

Transient, but inconsistent, increases in reticulocyte, platelet, and leukocyte counts have also been demonstrated following daily subcutaneous injections of recombinant human interleukin-3 (17). Large-scale prospective clinical studies in aplastic anemia populations are necessary to determine optimal protocols for therapy with recombinant hematopoietic growth factors in combination with other treatment modalities.

SICKLE CELL ANEMIA

The term *sickle cell disease* encompasses a variety of hemoglobinopathies, including sickle cell anemia, sickle hemoglobin C (SC) disease, and sickle cell thalassemia. Although the clinical presentation of these disorders is often similar, the manifestations of sickle cell anemia are more severe and are therefore the focus of the following discussion.

Pathophysiology

The hemoglobin molecule is a tetramer comprised of four polypeptides linked to iron-carrying heme groups. Over 600 different types of hemoglobin have been distinguished, including hemoglobins A_1, A_2, C, F, and S. Only three variants are considered to be normal, hemoglobin A_1 (Hb A_1), hemoglobin A_2 (Hb A_2), and fetal hemoglobin (Hb F). Fetal hemoglobin accounts for 70 to 80% of the hemoglobin in the red cells of newborns. A gradual conversion occurs until the eighth postnatal month, when the normal adult pattern of 97% Hb A_1, 2.5% Hb A_2, and 1% Hb F is represented (18).

The Hb A_1 tetramer consists of two pairs of globin chains, α and β, which have distinct primary structures. Sickle cell anemia is a homozygous condition that results from the substitution of valine for glutamic acid in both of the β chains. Because each parent contributes a single β-chain gene, the heterozygous genotype AS is also possible and is expressed as the sickle cell trait phenotype.

Deoxygenation in the capillaries induces rapid polymerization of the sickling hemoglobin, Hb S, and results in the formation of helical strands of parallel fibers. The elongated, crescent-shaped cells characteristic of sickle cell anemia are thereby produced. The affected erythrocytes are rigid and are unable to pass through the microvasculature, leading to vaso-occlusion with subsequent painful ischemia and chronic organ damage. In general, the sickling is reversible on reexposure to oxygen; however, repeated sickling episodes will eventually damage the cell membrane. The sickled conformation will be sustained and the cells subject to hemolysis and removal by the liver or spleen.

The rate of Hb S polymerization depends on its concentration in the erythrocyte. The copolymerization of Hb S with Hb F inhibits further polymer growth; intracellular Hb F concentrations are inversely correlated with disease severity.

Epidemiology

The Hb S gene confers protection against *Plasmodium falciparum* infection in infancy. Therefore, populations residing in or originating from areas wherein malaria is endemic have the highest frequency of the AS and SS genotypes. The distribution of sickle disease is no longer restricted to Africa, Saudi Arabia, and India; however, areas of concentration remain. Up to 50% of individuals in west central Africa possess the Hb S gene. Among blacks in the United States, 0.17% have sickle cell anemia, whereas 8.6% have the sickle trait (18).

Diagnosis

The diagnosis of sickle cell diseases depends on hemoglobin electrophoresis, which reveals the types and proportion of hemoglobins present (18). This rapid, inexpensive screening test establishes the genotype of the individual, enabling appropriate genetic counseling and education. If both parents have the AS genotype, there is a 1 in 4 chance that their child will have homozygous SS disease. Prenatal diagnosis is also possible. Genotyping may be performed in the first trimester of pregnancy, using fetal cells obtained from amniotic fluid or a chorionic villus.

Clinical Presentation

Sickle cell anemia presents with constitutional, hematologic and vaso-occlusive manifestations (Table 14.3) late in the first postnatal year, after levels of the protective fetal hemoglobin have diminished. Skeletal growth and sexual maturation are impaired, although catch-up growth is apparent by adulthood.

Because of recurrent microinfarcts, the spleen is initially enlarged and then completely fibrosed by 6 years of age. This functional "autosplenectomy" and defects in other host defenses greatly increase the likelihood of infection, especially with *Streptococcus pneumoniae* and *Hemophilus influenzae*.

Hemolysis accompanied by inadequate erythropoiesis results in a normochromic, normocytic anemia, with hematocrit levels ranging from 0.18 to 0.30. The chronic anemia leads to a hyperdynamic circulatory system and subsequent cardiac hypertrophy and systolic ejection murmurs. The anemia is aggravated during aplastic crises, when erythropoiesis is further suppressed by acute infection or folate deficiency.

Painful vaso-occlusive crises produced by sludging of sickled cells in the microcirculation are the most common reason for hospitalization. The frequency and severity of painful crises vary greatly between individuals. Approximately 5% of those with sickle cell anemia require inpatient pain management over 40 times each year, whereas another 30% are rarely or never affected by severe pain (18). The episodes are sudden in onset and last for an average of 5 to 7 days. Pain is most often reported in the long bones, spine, pelvis, chest, and abdomen, and must be differentiated from infection and other acute processes. Factors that may precipitate vaso-occlusive crises include acidosis, heat or exercise (dehydration), cold (vasoconstriction), infection, stress, menses, and high altitudes.

Table 14.3.
Complications of Sickle Cell Anemia

Constitutional
  Impaired growth and development
  Increased risk of infection
    Meningitis
    Osteomyelitis
    Pneumonia
    Pyelonephritis
    Septicemia
Hematologic
  Hemolytic anemia
  Aplastic crises
  Splenic sequestration crises
Vaso-Occlusive
  Cardiovascular
    Cardiac enlargement
    Systolic murmur
  Gastrointestinal
    Autosplenectomy
    Gallstones/cholecystitis
    Hepatic crises/RUQ syndrome
    Hepatic insufficiency
    Intrahepatic cholelithiasis
  Genitourinary
    Hematuria
    Impotence
    Priapism
    Renal Insufficiency
  Neurologic
    Cerebral thrombosis
    Intracerebral hemorrhage
    Seizures
    Subarachnoid hemorrhage
  Ocular
    Retinopathy
    Secondary glaucoma
  Painful Crises
  Pulmonary
    Chronic obstructive disease
    Infarction
  Skin/Skeletal
    Arthropathy
    Aseptic necrosis
    Dactylitis
    Leg ulcers

Recurrent sickling and subsequent infarction produce chronic damage to many organ systems. Hematuria and an inability to concentrate urine progress in some patients to renal failure. Neurologic complications such as cerebrovascular accidents and seizures develop in up to 25% of patients. Chronic obstructive pulmonary disease and intrahepatic fibrosis are also reported. Impotence occurs in 25% of males with the disease, usually after multiple episodes of priapism.

In addition to indices of anemia, laboratory abnormalities include elevations in platelet count and leukocytosis due to demargination of granulocytes from vessel walls into the circulation. Irreversibly sickled cells are seen in the blood smear.

Individuals with sickle cell trait are generally asymptomatic, although sickling manifestations may occur at extreme levels of hypoxia or acidosis. Transient hematuria, renal papillary necrosis, pulmonary embolism, and splenic infarction have been rarely associated with the AS phenotype. Life expectancy is normal in sickle trait patients, in contrast to those with sickle cell anemia. However, patients with sickle cell anemia may now survive well into adulthood due to rapid recognition and management of complications.

Management of Major Complications

ANEMIA

Physiologic adaptations such as low Hb S-oxygen affinity allow patients with sickle cell anemia to tolerate relatively low hematocrit levels. Therefore, therapy is supportive, with blood transfusions reserved for acute, symptomatic exacerbations in the anemia. High folate utilization arising from continuously elevated red cell production may lead to folate deficiency and induce an aplastic crisis. Folate supplementation (1 mg p.o. daily) is recommended to maintain adequate stores. Aplastic crises may also develop from viral or bacterial infections, necessitating prompt diagnosis and treatment. Recovery of erythropoiesis generally occurs within 5 to 10 days, as the underlying infection resolves.

INFECTION

Bacterial infection is the leading cause of death in patients with sickle cell anemia. Therefore, a thorough search for an infectious source should be undertaken in any patient presenting with a painful crisis and fever.

Pneumonia may be treated empirically with parenteral cefuroxime, as its spectrum of activity includes the most likely pathogens, *S. pneumoniae* and *H. influenzae*. If a clinical response is not apparent after 24 to 48 hours, infection with *Mycoplasma pneumoniae* should be suspected and erythromycin added to the antibiotic regimen. Meningitis occurs 200 to 300 times more frequently in children with sickle cell anemia, with pneumococci being isolated in approximately 80% of cases (19).

Children over the age of 2 years should be immunized with polyvalent pneumococcal vaccine and a booster dose given after 3 to 5 years to children younger than 10 years at the time of revaccination. Although a 50% reduction in the incidence of pneumococcal infection has been demonstrated after immunization, the vaccine protects against a limited number of pneumococcal serotypes. Therefore, long-term prophylactic administration of oral penicillin is advisable. *H. influenzae* vaccination is also recommended.

Salmonella species are isolated in up to 80% of sickle cell disease patients with osteomyelitis. A 4- to 6-week course of treatment with ampicillin or a cephalosporin is required. Leg ulcers should receive local care and be monitored closely for potential progression to osteomyelitis.

PAINFUL CRISES

The goals of therapy for painful vaso-occlusive crises are to provide supportive care and effective analgesia, while eliminating potential precipitating factors (18, 19). Vigorous enteral or parenteral hydration should be initiated and oxygen administered if hypoxia from pulmonary involvement is evident. Both nonnarcotic and narcotic analgesics are used, depending on the severity of pain.

Those with mild to moderately painful crises should be managed as outpatients. Oral hydration with 3 to 5 L (100 mL/kg for children) of fluid daily should be encouraged and pain treated with acetaminophen, aspirin, or nonsteroidal antiinflammatory drugs. Pain unresponsive to these agents may be controlled by codeine or oxycodone, as single agents or in combination with acetaminophen. In addition, the efficacy of the parenteral nonsteroidal antiinflammatory drug ketorolac for the treatment of painful crises has been reported (20).

Inpatient management with parenteral hydration and narcotic analgesics is necessary for severe painful crises. Scheduled, around-the-clock narcotic administration is preferred over "prn" regimens. The pain-anxiety cycle is thereby diminished, and relief is often achieved with lower total doses. Oral narcotic protocols have been used, yet are not universally accepted by patients, especially if nausea and vomiting are present. Frequent intramuscular or subcutaneous injections cause local pain and promote the formation of abscesses and subsequent infection. In addition, drug absorption may be erratic. Peak effects associated with intravenous bolus administration may lead to excessive central nervous system depression. Continuous intravenous infusions are ideal for initial therapy, as a dosage range may be specified, allowing safe titration to pain control. Success with patient-controlled analgesia has also been reported (21).

Because narcotics have similar effects at equianalgesic doses, various regimens will alleviate symptoms. Agents with mixed agonist-antagonist properties (e.g., pentazocine, buprenorphine) are not recommended for patients with histories of outpatient narcotic use, since withdrawal may be precipitated. Although widely used, meperidine should be avoided, as its metabolite, normeperidine, accumulates after repeated high doses and may induce seizures, especially in the presence of renal insufficiency or underlying neurologic disease. The relatively short duration of action of meperidine of 2 to 4 hours also makes administration less practical. Morphine sulfate is the narcotic of choice. In patients unable to tolerate morphine because of nausea, vomiting, or pruritus, hydromorphone may be substituted. Adjuvant therapy with promethazine or hydroxyzine may promote analgesia and reduce narcotic requirements. However, adverse effects may also be potentiated. Recently, the efficacy of intravenous methylprednisolone in significantly reducing the duration of narcotic treatment was demonstrated in a study of 36 children and adolescents (22).

Analgesic dosages must be individualized and based on the degree of outpatient narcotic use and previous inpatient needs. The development of tolerance to narcotic analgesic effects after chronic administration may dramatically increase parenteral requirements. Although patients may appear manipulative and exhibit drug-seeking behavior, adequate analgesia should be provided; placebos should not be given.

A continuous intravenous infusion of morphine (100 mg/100 mL 5% dextrose) at a rate of 0.05 to 0.10 mg/kg/hr may be used for the first 24 to 48 hours (23). Alternatively, 0.10 to 0.15 mg/kg morphine doses may be administered as intravenous boluses every 2 to 3 hours. Adverse effects such as respiratory depression, oversedation, and blood pressure reductions should be monitored and the dosage decreased if indicated. As the pain subsides, the continuous infusion should be discontinued and the total daily morphine requirement divided into 4 to 6 intravenous bolus doses. The dosage should be tapered by 20 to 30% daily while the interval is maintained. Once the daily intravenous dose is 50% of that initially required, conversion to an equianalgesic dose of an oral narcotic can be made.

Because of the addictive potential, chronic oral narcotic use should be discouraged, although some feel that severe painful crises may be aborted by early treatment (23). Unfortunately, many become both psychologically and physically dependent on these agents. Continuity of care and communication between health care providers is therefore essential to eliminate the possibility of multiple sources of narcotic prescriptions. Psychosocial support and nonpharmacologic coping techniques, such as relaxation therapy, behavior modification, and self-hypnosis, should be thoroughly explored.

Management of the Sickle Cell Disease

Partial exchange transfusions, in which over 50% of the patient's erythrocytes are replaced by donor red cells, prevent vaso-occlusive crises. Hypertransfusion until the hematocrit level has doubled temporarily halts erythroid Hb S production and also inhibits sickling. Due to the inherent risks of hepatitis transmission and iron overload, however, transfusions are generally reserved for the management of acute complications such as strokes and priapism, and for prophylaxis preoperatively and in late pregnancy.

Table 14.4.
Agents Studied for the Treatment of Sickle Cell Anemia

5-Azacytidine	Medroxyprogesterone
Butyrate	Nifedipine
Cetiedil	Papaverine
Cytarabine	Pentoxifylline
Desmopressin	Piracetam
Dextran	Sodium cyanate
Epoetin alfa	Ticlopidine
Hydergine	Urea
Hydroxyurea	Zinc sulfate
Isoxsuprine	

Many pharmacologic modalities have been directed against the sickling abnormality (Table 14.4); until recently, these therapies have yielded minimal clinical benefit, in part due to limiting adverse effects (18). Inhibitors of Hb S polymerization, such as sodium cyanate and urea, are not dependably effective; in addition, sodium cyanate is associated with neurologic toxicity. Studies of cetiedil, a peripheral vasodilator that alters fluid and electrolyte transport across the red cell membrane, are underway. Cetiedil-induced increases in red cell volume functionally decrease intracellular Hb S concentrations and thereby reduce the polymerization rate. Pentoxifylline may prevent vaso-occlusive crises by increasing red cell deformability and decreasing blood viscosity. These effects improve blood flow through the microvasculature in peripheral vascular occlusive diseases. However, further studies are required to establish this agent's role in sickle cell anemia. The antineoplastics 5-azacytidine and cytarabine enhance production of the protective fetal hemoglobin. However, bone marrow suppression produced by these agents is problematic and long-term efficacy uncertain.

More promising are the results of clinical studies of hydroxyurea (24, 25). After treatment with hydroxyurea, the proportion of Hb F and the number of cells containing Hb F were increased, resulting in prolonged red cell survival. Clinical efficacy, including a 50% reduction in the frequency of painful crises and hospitalizations for sickling complications, has recently been demonstrated in 299 patients enrolled in the Multicenter Study of Hydroxyurea (25). These findings were so compelling that the placebo-controlled, double-blind study was halted prior to completion. Initial daily hydroxyurea doses of 15 mg/kg were increased by 5 mg/kg every 12 weeks until bone marrow toxicity was evident, to a maximum daily dose of 35 mg/kg. Reversible myelosuppression was the sole adverse effect reported. Data regarding the potential benefit of recombinant human erythropoietin in conjunction with hydroxyurea are conflicting (26, 27).

Bone marrow transplantation can cure patients of sickle cell anemia, and initial data indicate survival rates of up to 90% (28). At present, it remains unclear which patients would benefit most from this procedure. The risks of transplantation must be carefully considered in the light of reduced morbidity noted with improved management of complications and advances in antisickling drug therapy. In the future, however, genetic engineering may "cure" the disease by transferring normal hemoglobin genes into patients with sickle cell anemia.

THALASSEMIAS

The thalassemias are a group of hereditary disorders of hemoglobin synthesis characterized by impaired production of one or more of the normal polypeptide chains of globin. Any of the four polypeptides that occur in normal hemoglobin may be involved (α, β, γ, δ). However, the most prevalent thalassemia syndromes are those that involve diminished or absent synthesis of either the α (α-thalassemia) or β (β-thalassemia) globin chains of Hb A_1 (29, 30).

Pathogenesis

The imbalance in polypeptide chain production secondary to impaired synthesis of either the α chain or the β chain of globin is the underlying factor that accounts for the pathogenesis of all the clinically severe thalassemia syndromes. Reduced production of the normal $\alpha_2\beta_2$ tetramer of Hb A_1 results in the production of smaller erythrocytes with a low hemoglobin content. The synthesis and accumulation of normal globin chains within the red cell leads to the formation of unstable aggregates that may precipitate and cause cell membrane damage. These deformed cells undergo premature destruction either in the bone marrow (intramedullary hemolysis) or the peripheral circulation (31). Chronic hemolysis is a primary complication of the clinically significant α- and β-thalassemia syndromes (e.g., Hb H disease and β-thalassemia major). The "ineffective erythropoiesis" and microcytic, hypochromic anemia described above is associated with a compensatory increase in the absorption of dietary iron. This may contribute to the iron overload that can result in patients receiving therapy with blood transfusions. There is also an increase in erythropoietic activity in the bone marrow and in extramedullary sites (i.e., liver, spleen, and lymph nodes). In severe forms of thalassemia (e.g., β-thalassemia major) excessive erythropoiesis causes significant bone marrow hypertrophy, lymphadenopathy, and hepatosplenomegaly (31). Bone marrow expansion in untreated patients leads to skeletal deformities and fragility.

Epidemiology

The thalassemia syndromes are collectively one of the most common genetic disorders in humans. An estimated 190 million people throughout the world carry a hemoglobinopathy gene (i.e., 4% of the world's population), and greater than half of these are thalassemia genes (32).

Populations that are most affected include Asians, Africans, Eastern Indians, and Mediterraneans (29, 33). Since the geographic distribution of this disorder is similar to that of malaria, it is thought that certain types of thalassemia may offer protection from *Plasmodium falciparum* infection (30). The incidence of α-thalassemia is more common in Southeast Asia, China, and certain areas of Africa while β-thalassemia syndromes are concentrated in Mediterranean countries such as Greece and Italy. In North America, β-thalassemia is found primarily in people of Greek, Italian, and African ancestry. Genetic analysis studies indicate that approximately 30% of black Americans are "silent carriers" of α-thalassemia (29).

Because of their similar geographic distributions, coinheritance of sickle cell anemia with thalassemia is not uncommon. Detailed discussion of various sickle cell-thalassemia syndromes can be found elsewhere (29).

α-Thalassemia

There are four genes involved in the production of α-globin chains, with one pair occurring on each DNA strand ($\alpha\alpha/\alpha\alpha$). The most common forms of α-thalassemia result from deletion of one or more of these genes. Four such syndromes have been identified (Table 14.5).

The deletion of a single $\alpha\alpha$ gene is classified as a "silent carrier state" and is the most common single gene abnormality in the world. Up to 2% Hb Bart's, an abnormal hemoglobin containing a γ_4 polypeptide tetramer, can be isolated in cord blood of these individuals at birth. Hb Bart's disappears within the first year of life. Fortunately, there are virtually no clinical manifestations of the silent carrier state, and laboratory values such as hemoglobin concentration and mean corpuscular volume (MCV) are usually within normal limits (34). These individuals do not require treatment.

The deletion of two α genes is classified as "α-thalassemia trait" or "α-thalassemia minor." The most common genotype for this disorder is a homozygous α gene deletion ($-\alpha/-\alpha$). Individuals with α-thalassemia trait experience a mild microcytic, hypochromic anemia without hemolysis (34). In Southeast Asians, however, both α gene

Table 14.5.
Comparison of α-Thalassemia Syndromes

Syndrome	Genotypes	RBC Morphology	Clinical Manifestations
Silent Carrer	$-\alpha/\alpha\alpha$	Normal	None
α-Thalassemia Trait	$-\alpha/-\alpha$ or $--/\alpha\alpha$	Microcytic	Mild anemia
Hb H Disease	$--/-\alpha$	Microcytic; deformed	Chronic hemolysis; splenomegaly
Hydrops Fetalis	$--/--$	Nucleated RBC	Intrauterine or neonatal death

deletions frequently occur on the same chromosome ($-/\alpha\alpha$). This genotype is associated with a more pronounced microcytosis [MCV 70-80 fL (70–80 μm^3)] and mild hemolysis. In α-thalassemia trait, Hb Bart's (γ_4) constitutes 2 to 10% of hemoglobin in cord blood and disappears within the first year of life (29). Hemoglobin concentrations of adults with α-thalassemia trait are usually normal or only slightly decreased (34). Not surprisingly, this disorder is often identified in patients by chance during routine laboratory blood tests. Diagnosis is typically done through a DNA electrophoretic analysis technique known as Southern mapping (34). Because most patients are asymptomatic, treatment is seldom warranted.

Another α-thalassemia syndrome, more common in Asian populations, is Hb H disease. This disorder is associated with the deletion of three of the four α genes ($-/-\alpha$). Hemoglobin H is an unstable tetramer of β-globin chains (β_4) that is formed when there is a marked reduction of a globin production yielding a substantial surplus of β-globin chains. This hemoglobin variant constitutes 5 to 30% of total circulating hemoglobin in affected adults. In patients with Hb H disease, Hb Bart's represents 10 to 40% of the hemoglobin pool at birth and is found in trace amounts during adulthood (29). The unstable β_4 containing Hb H gradually undergoes oxidation and precipitates within the cell. These deformed cells are removed and hemolyzed primarily by the spleen.

Clinical manifestations associated with Hb H disease include microcytosis, mild to moderate chronic hemolytic anemia, mild jaundice, and splenomegaly (34). Enlargement of the spleen results from both the trapping of deformed red cells and extramedullary erythropoiesis in that organ. In most patients, Hb H disease is not severe enough to impair routine activities, interfere with reproductive function, or reduce longevity (34). However, circumstances such as infection, pregnancy, or exposure to oxidant drugs can precipitate severe exacerbations of the hemolytic anemia. In certain patients with Hb H disease, especially those with severe splenomegaly, splenectomy is often beneficial in reducing symptoms and slowing the rate of hemolysis. In rare instances, patients with severe forms of Hb H disease are blood transfusion dependent (34).

Deletion of all four α genes is classified as "Hb Bart's hydrops fetalis" and is incompatible with life (34). An affected fetus will be prematurely stillborn in the second or third trimester or will expire within hours after birth. Hemoglobin in an affected fetus will be greater than 80% Hb Bart's. Physical findings include massive edema (hydrops), ascites, and hepatomegaly, while peripheral blood examination reveals immature nucleated erythrocytes (erythroblasts), target cells, reticulocytosis, and hypochromia.

Since most α-thalassemia syndromes are associated with a relatively benign clinical course, prenatal diagnosis is usually not critical. An exception to this would be situations where couples are at risk of a hydrops pregnancy (e.g., Southeast Asians, Chinese, or prior α-thalassemic hydrops pregnancy). Prenatal diagnosis of the fetus involves gene mapping of DNA acquired by chorionic villus sampling (first trimester) or by amniocentesis (second trimester) (34). A positive diagnosis of Hb Bart's hydrops fetalis allows the option of early termination of the pregnancy which may protect the health of the mother by avoiding such problems as toxemia and peripartum hemorrhage.

β-Thalassemia

In contrast to α-thalassemia, in which gene deletion is the mechanism, β-thalassemia syndromes usually result from faulty mRNA transcription of the β gene (29). Since α- and δ-chain production is usually unaffected, increased levels of Hb A_2 ($\alpha_2 \delta_2$) are common to most of the β-thalassemias. There are a multitude of genetic mutations associated with β-thalassemia; however, patients can be classified as either heterozygous or homozygous for the β gene. Further distinction is then made based on clinical manifestations and severity (i.e., phenotype) of the syndrome (Table 14.6).

Heterozygous β-thalassemia is much less severe than homozygous forms of the disease. Patients either have a clinically undetectable disorder ("β-thalassemia minima") or one that results in only mild anemia ("β-thalassemia minor" or "β-thalassemia trait"). In general, patients with β-thalassemia minima are asymptomatic, have laboratory blood values (i.e., hemoglobin concentration and MCV) within normal limits, and require no treatment. Definitive diagnosis can be made by measuring the relative synthetic rates of β and α chains (29).

Table 14.6.
Comparison of β-Thalassemia Syndromes

Syndrome	Hb[a]	Clinical Manifestations	Conventional Treatment
Heterozygous			
Minima	Normal	None	None
Minor	>100	Mild anemia	Genetic/medical counseling
Homozygous			
Intermedia	70–100	Moderate to severe anemia; impaired growth and splenomegaly in severe cases	Intermittent blood transfusion and chelation therapy
Major	20–70	Severe anemia; abnormal skeletal growth; splenomegaly; iron overload complications	Chronic blood transfusion and chelation therapy

[a]Typical hemoglobin concentrations (g/L) in untreated patients.

Patients with β-thalassemia minor usually have a mild hypochromic, microcytic anemia. Hemoglobin concentration in these individuals is generally not less than 100 g/L (10 g/dL). Microcytosis is more pronounced, with MCV values of approximately 60 fL (60 μm^3). Clinical manifestations such as splenomegaly and hyperplastic marrow are usually absent. Nutritional deficiencies, infection, and pregnancy may exacerbate anemia in patients with β-thalassemia minor. However, since these individuals are predisposed to iron overload due to enhanced absorption of dietary iron, long-term iron supplementation and routine blood transfusions during pregnancy should be avoided if possible. Medical care for these individuals should also involve genetic counseling (29). Screening patients for β-thalassemia minor is often done through quantification of Hb A$_2$. Ranges of Hb A$_2$ levels in normal patients and those with β-thalassemia minor are 2 to 3% and 3.5 to 8%, respectively (29).

Homozygous forms of β-thalassemia can be classified as either "β-thalassemia intermedia" or "β-thalassemia major." The intermedia form is associated with moderate anemia and may require intermittent treatment with blood transfusions. Hemoglobin concentrations in patients with β-thalassemia intermedia usually range from 70 to 100 g/L (7 to 10 g/dL). In contrast, β-thalassemia major (Cooley's anemia) is associated with severe anemia and requires intensive chronic treatment. Hemoglobin concentration and MCV in these patients usually range from 20 to 70 g/L (2 to 7 g/dL) and 50 to 60 fL (50 to 60 μm^3), respectively (29, 35).

CLINICAL PRESENTATION OF β-THALASSEMIA MAJOR

Excessive erythropoiesis (secondary to severe anemia) in the bone marrow and extramedullary sites is a primary complication of untreated patients with β-thalassemia major. Bone marrow hypertrophy with subsequent abnormal skeletal growth usually develops in children from the second year of life through 10 years of age. Abnormal skeletal changes are most apparent in the craniofacial bones due to maxillary overgrowth, protrusion of teeth, and separation of orbits. Cortical thinning of weight bearing bones may lead to recurrent fractures in these patients. Fortunately, skeletal abnormalities are almost completely prevented if adequate blood transfusion therapy is initiated early in life. Excessive extramedullary erythropoiesis leads to significant lymphadenopathy and hepatosplenomegaly (31).

Red cell damage and subsequent chronic hemolysis that occurs in β-thalassemia major is due to precipitated intracellular aggregates of excess α chains. Removal of these deformed red cells by the spleen contributes to splenomegaly, which, if uncorrected by splenectomy, can significantly increase blood transfusion requirements of patients. Chronic hemolysis is also associated with gallstone formation, which is present in 70% of thalassemic children over 15 years of age (31, 35).

TREATMENT

Conventional treatment for most patients with β-thalassemia major continues to be supportive therapy with chronic blood transfusion and iron chelation regimens. The main goal of this approach is to avoid or reduce major complications of the disease. Experience with bone marrow transplantation in thalassemic patients has progressed substantially, and this approach offers a curative treatment for a small portion of patients. Research in gene therapy is ongoing and may eventually provide a more widely available cure of clinically significant thalassemias.

Transfusion and Chelation. The primary approach to treatment for patients with β-thalassemia major is chronic blood transfusions in conjunction with intensive iron chelation therapy. The goals of transfusion therapy are to suppress excessive erythropoiesis and prevent anemia. This can be accomplished by initiating aggressive (high) transfusion programs prior to 4 years of age. It is generally accepted that high transfusion programs (i.e., maintaining hemoglobin above 100 g/L) are clinically superior to low transfusion programs (i.e., maintaining hemoglobin above 70 g/L). Important advantages of the high transfusion approach include fewer skeletal abnormalities, normal or near normal growth prior to adolescence, less severe hepatosplenomegaly, and decreased incidence of cardiomegaly due to anemia. Furthermore, there is no evidence that iron accumulation and toxicity develop earlier in patients who receive high transfusion therapy as compared to those who receive low transfusion therapy (31).

Variations in transfusion protocols exist between institutions and different types of patients will have different requirements. However, a typical high transfusion program involves transfusing 12 to 15 mL/kg of packed red blood cells (PRBCs) over 4 to 5 hours every 3 to 4 weeks on an outpatient basis. This will usually cycle a patient's hemoglobin between 100 to 120 g/L (10 to 12 g/dL) and 150 to 170 g/L (15 to 17 g/dL). Longer intervals between transfusions (i.e., every 5 to 6 weeks) have been shown to increase iron accumulation, and therefore should be avoided. The adequacy of a given transfusion regimen is best evaluated by monitoring a patient's growth rate and serum hemoglobin concentrations (31, 35–37).

Important complications associated with chronic blood transfusions include sensitization reactions, transmission of viral infection, and iron overload. Febrile and urticarial reactions to PRBCs caused by sensitization to leukocyte surface antigens may occur. However, the incidence of these reactions has been greatly reduced through improved typing and matching techniques. Many institutions administer leukocyte-depleted RBC products to thalassemic patients in order to avoid this complication (31, 35, 37). A more hazardous problem of chronic blood transfusions is the transmission of viral infections. Careful screening of donors and donated blood products has reduced the risk of human immunodeficiency virus (HIV) transmission to less than 1 per 150,000 units transfused. Hepatitis B may be prevented through proper vaccination of uninfected thalassemic patients who are initiating or being maintained on chronic transfusion programs. Hepatitis C transmission remains a relatively common threat to transfused patients with an incidence of about 5%. The screening for donors infected with hepatitis C has reduced the risk of transmission of this disease (31, 35).

The primary cause of morbidity and mortality in patients with β-thalassemia major who receive adequate transfusion therapy is iron overload associated with the intensive administration of blood products. Each unit of PRBCs (450 mL) contains 200 to 250 mg of elemental iron. By 12 years of age, a properly transfused thalassemic has likely received 55 to 60 grams of iron. The normal iron content of the body is 2 grams, and there is no natural mechanism by which excess amounts may be excreted. Iron overload and subsequent toxicity occurs when the capacity of the storage proteins (ferritin and hemosiderin) and the transport protein (transferrin) is exceeded. The molecular mechanism of toxicity is thought to be due to the accumulation of unbound iron both intracellularly and in the circulation acting as a catalyst in Haber-Weiss and Fenton reactions which produce reactive oxygen species that oxidize membrane lipids and damage cells (31, 35, 37).

The clinical effects of iron overload are most pronounced on the liver, pancreas, and heart. Normal growth may also be impaired by an excess iron burden. In transfused thalassemic children, hepatic fibrosis often develops during the first decade of life, and older patients will often have histologic evidence of cirrhosis. Other than mild prolongations of clotting time, clinical problems associated with hepatic dysfunction in these individuals are uncommon. Diabetes mellitus secondary to the effects of hemochromatosis on the pancreas may occur and can be managed by standard insulin replacement therapy. The manifestations of iron overload on the heart include pericarditis, atrial and ventricular arrhythmias, and congestive heart failure. Cardiomegaly secondary to hypoxia is usually not significant in adequately transfused patients. In underchelated patients, cardiac dysfunction is the primary cause of death (31, 35). Growth and development failure associated with thalassemia is likely due to a combination of both the chronic disease process itself and the accumulation of iron associated with blood transfusion programs (31). For these reasons chronic iron chelation therapy must accompany standard blood transfusion regimens.

The only agent currently available for chelating and removing excess iron is deferoxamine, a polyhydroxamic acid introduced in 1961. Following parenteral administration, deferoxamine penetrates cell membranes and combines with free intracellular iron to form the complex ferrioxamine. Liver parenchymal cells serve as a large source of chelatable iron. Ferrioxamine is then transported extracellularly and is readily excreted in the urine and the bile. The general goal of treatment with deferoxamine is to create a "negative iron balance" in which measured urinary iron excretion exceeds the amount of iron administered during transfusions (31, 35, 37).

Chelation therapy is usually initiated in transfusion-dependent patients by 3 to 4 years of age. Due to poor oral absorption, deferoxamine must be given parenterally. The subcutaneous and intravenous routes are superior at promoting urinary iron excretion as compared to the intramuscular route. Furthermore, the half-life of deferoxamine in the blood following intravenous injection is very short (5 to 10 minutes). Therefore, continuous infusion is used to maximize exposure time between the drug and excess iron. Typical deferoxamine dosing regimens are 40 to 50 mg/kg/day infused subcutaneously over 8 to 12 hours, 5 to 7 days a week. Recently, intravenous deferoxamine dosing regimens of 50 to 80 mg/kg/day have been shown to be safe and efficacious (38). Larger doses of deferoxamine may also be administered on days of transfusion therapy. Treatment is usually administered with a portable infusion pump, infusing the drug at night while the patient is sleeping. Monitoring total body iron burden and chelation therapy efficacy should include the measurement of serum ferritin concentrations (normal: 18–300 µg/L [18–300 ng/mL]) and urinary iron excretion. However, urinary iron excretion may significantly underestimate the amount of iron being removed from the body when biliary excretion is high (31, 37, 39).

For patients who are poorly compliant, are extremely iron overloaded (i.e., serum ferritin > 5000 µg/L [>5000 ng/mL]), or have iron-induced cardiac disease prior to chelation therapy, high dose intravenous deferoxamine therapy has been used. Experience with doses of 6 to 12 grams daily for up to 41 months has been reported. Because rapid intravenous infusion may cause hypotension, the rate of administration should not exceed 15 mg/kg/hr. Because of the large amounts of deferoxamine being administered in this type of protocol, annual drug costs may range from $30,000 to $60,000 (37, 40).

The clinical benefits of regular transfusion and chelation therapy initiated at an early age include a reduced risk of complications from iron-induced organ damage (e.g. cardiac disease and impaired glucose tolerance) and a reduced risk of early death (36, 41). Patients who are treated in this manner and whose serum ferritin concentrations remain below 2500 µg/L (2500 ng/mL) have an excellent prognosis for prolonged survival without cardiac disease (41).

In most patients, deferoxamine used in typical chelation regimen doses is a relatively safe drug. Common side effects during subcutaneous infusion programs are mild and include local irritation and urticaria at the injection site, and abdominal discomfort. Some reports, however, have associated deferoxamine with a variety of adverse visual and auditory effects. The mechanism of this toxicity is not well understood, yet patients on deferoxamine should receive regular vision and hearing evaluations. Patients with lower iron burdens and patients receiving high doses of deferoxamine are likely to be at greater risk for toxicity (35, 40).

Because of the inconvenience, high cost, and frequent noncompliance with parenteral deferoxamine therapy, research efforts have focused on the development of a safe, effective, and inexpensive oral medication for iron chelation. The most promising compounds to date are those of the hydroxypyridone family. One agent of this class, deferiprone (L1), has shown similar efficacy to that of subcutaneous deferoxamine (42). However, more controlled clinical evaluation of these agents must be completed before their safety and efficacy are clearly established.

Patients with β-thalassemia intermedia are often not blood transfusion dependent. However, in severe forms of this syndrome, ineffective erythropoiesis and anemia are sometimes significant enough to inhibit growth and development and lead to skeletal fragility and injury. In these cases, patients with β-thalassemia intermedia should be treated with intermittent courses of transfusion and chelation therapy, as described above (35).

Splenectomy. Due to increased erythropoietic activity and trapping of red cells by the spleen, patients with β-thalassemia major develop splenomegaly. Proper transfusion therapy may slow the process, but gradual enlargement of the spleen usually occurs. In patients who receive chronic transfusion therapy, enlargement of the spleen is associated with increased transfusion requirements to maintain an adequate hemoglobin concentration. The administration of greater volumes of blood products increases the amount of iron a patient receives and makes successful chelation therapy more difficult. Therefore, when blood transfusion requirements reach approximately 200 to 250 mL/kg/year, splenectomy is indicated. Following spleen removal, requirements decrease substantially. Since splenectomized patients, especially young children, are predisposed to bacterial sepsis, removal of the spleen should be avoided until the age of 4 or 5 years, if possible. Prophylactic oral penicillin therapy (e.g., 250 mg twice daily) in splenectomized young children is appropriate. Furthermore, all splenectomized patients should be vaccinated against pneumococcus, *H. influenzae,* and meningococcus at the earliest appropriate age (31, 35, 37).

Bone Marrow Transplantation. Since the initial successful case in 1982, considerable experience has been gained with bone marrow transplantation (BMT) in patients with β-thalassemia major. Survival and disease-free survival rates reported from a group of 139 patients receiving BMT for thalassemia were 73% and 58%, respectively (43). A more recent report of a series of 89 patients ages 1 to 15 years demonstrated survival and rejection-free survival rates of 92% and 85%, respectively (44). Therefore, assuming an HLA-compatible donor exists, BMT offers thalassemic patients a reasonable chance for cure. The risk of graft failure and mortality associated with BMT varies among different institutions and different patients, and must be weighed against the high rate of survival and the good quality of life that is associated with conventional transfusion and chelation therapy for at least the first two decades. Thalassemic patients with the highest chances for rejection-free survival after BMT are those who are young, well-chelated, and in good clinical condition (43, 44).

Alternative Therapeutic Options. Gene therapy is another treatment approach that holds great potential for providing a definitive cure of patients with severe forms of thalassemia (45). Current limitations in the use of this therapy for the treatment of thalassemia include inefficient gene expression and regulation.

Another technique that has shown some success in treating patients with β-thalassemia major is to reduce transfusion requirements by increasing Hb F synthesis (46, 47). Agents currently available that have been investigated as clinical stimulators of Hb F synthesis include hydroxyurea, butyrate, and azacytidine. The adverse effects (i.e., bone marrow suppression and mutagenicity) and unknown long-term efficacy of these agents have limited their use in the treatment of thalassemia.

Prevention. Prevention is another effective approach in dealing with β-thalassemia major. Multifaceted programs involving education, genetic counseling, and prenatal diagnosis have led to a significant reduction in the incidence of this disease in certain areas. In Sardinia, for example, implementation of such a program was associated with a 95% reduction in the incidence of thalassemia major over a 16-year period (48). Inexpensive and simple DNA analysis techniques can provide a safe and accurate diagnosis at 8 to 14 weeks gestation (35).

PROGNOSIS

Prior to the implementation of adequate transfusion and chelation programs, children with β-thalassemia major suffered from skeletal deformities, growth and development retardation, progressive enlargement of the liver and spleen, congestive heart failure, and recurrent infections. More than 80% of these patients died within the first 5 years of life. The introduction and widespread use of regular transfusion programs along with effective chelation therapy has led to a significant improvement in the quality and duration of life for thalassemic patients who have such therapy accessible to them. Bone marrow transplantation is a currently available definitive cure of the disease in a small portion of affected patients. In the future, gene therapy may offer a widely available cure.

HEMOLYTIC ANEMIAS

Hemolytic anemias are due to an increased rate of red blood cell (RBC) destruction. The anemia is of greatest clinical concern when the rate of red cell destruction exceeds that of erythropoiesis. The hemolytic process may occur chronically or manifest as an acute episode depending on the causative mechanism. Acute hemolysis is generally a more clinically threatening event. Many anemias have a hemolytic component due to the production of defective or damaged red blood cells (e.g., megaloblastic anemias, thalassemias, sickle cell anemia) (49). As there are a multitude of causes of hemolytic anemia, this section will focus on those amenable to specific medical treatment and those that are drug-induced.

Etiology and Classification

Hemolytic anemias can be categorized as either inherited or acquired disorders. Inherited hemolytic anemias include defective globin synthesis, erythrocyte membrane defects, and erythrocyte enzyme deficiencies. Acquired hemolytic disorders are those caused by some extrinsic event and do not involve a genetic component. Typically, the acquired hemolytic anemias are either immune mediated, due to physical stress on the red cell, or are induced by certain infections (Table 14.7).

Epidemiology

The prevalence and distribution of sickle cell anemia and thalassemia have been discussed previously. With respect to other inherited hemolytic disorders, the incidence of hereditary spherocytosis and hereditary elliptocytosis in the United States is approximately 220 and 400 per million, respectively. Glucose-6-phosphate dehydrogenase (G6PD) deficiency is the most common inherited erythrocyte enzyme disorder worldwide, affecting close to 200 million people, but not all patients with G6PD deficiency are significantly predisposed to oxidative hemolysis (29, 50).

The majority of acquired hemolytic anemias are idiopathic. Many are due to immune reactions, collagen vascular disease, or malignancy. Drugs are the causative agents in under 10% of cases.

Pathophysiology

The average RBC life-span is 120 days. During severe hemolytic episodes this can be reduced to as low as 5 to 20 days. Red cells are hemolyzed within the circulation

Table 14.7.
Classification of Common Hemolytic Anemias

I. Inherited
   Globin synthesis defect
      Sickle cell anemia
      Thalassemia
      Unstable hemoglobin disease
   Erythrocyte membrane defect
      Hereditary spherocytosis
      Hereditary elliptocytosis
      Hereditary stomatocytosis
   Erythrocyte enzyme defect
      Hexose-monophosphate shunt defect (e.g., glucose-6-phosphate dehydrogenase)
      Glycolytic (Embden-Meyerhof) enzyme defect (e.g., pyruvate kinase)
      Other enzyme defect (e.g., adenylate kinase)
II. Acquired
   Immune mediated
      Warm reacting antibody (IgG)
         Secondary (e.g., collagen vascular disease, lymphoproliferative disorders)
         Drug induced
         Idiopathic
      Cold agglutinin disease (IgM)
         Acute (e.g., mycoplasma pneumonia, infectious mononucleosis)
         Chronic (e.g., lymphoid neoplasms, idiopathic)
      Transfusion reactions
      Hemolytic disease of newborns
   Microangiopathic and traumatic
      Disseminated intravascular coagulation
      Hemolytic-uremic syndrome
      Thrombotic thrombocytopenic purpura
      Prosthetic or diseased heart valves
   Infection
   Exogenous substances
   Other
      Paroxysmal nocturnal hemoglobinuria
      Liver disease
      Hypophosphatemia

(intravascular hemolysis) or taken up by the reticuloendothelial system (RES) and destroyed (extravascular hemolysis). Intravascular hemolysis may be caused by trauma to the RBC, complement fixation to the RBC (immune mediated), or by exposure to exogenous substances. Under normal circumstances, however, most RBC catabolism occurs extravascularly by the RES in the liver and spleen. Specific drug-induced mechanisms of RBC hemolysis are discussed later in the context of G6PD deficiency and immune-mediated hemolysis.

Following lysis of the RBC, hemoglobin is released into the blood, where it is bound by the plasma protein haptoglobin. Free heme molecules are bound by the plasma protein hemopexin. The hemoglobin-haptoglobin complex is rapidly cleared from the circulation by the RES, and the heme component is metabolized to unconjugated (indirect) bilirubin. In the liver, this is linked with glucuronic acid, forming conjugated (direct) bilirubin which passes from the bile duct into the intestine. Fecal bacteria then metabolize conjugated bilirubin to urobilinogen, which is primarily excreted in the feces. Iron from heme catabolism is stored as ferritin or hemosiderin.

During hemolysis, if the haptoglobin binding capacity is exceeded, unbound hemoglobin levels increase, resulting in hemoglobinemia. In this case, free hemoglobin is filtered through the glomerulus and is usually reabsorbed by the proximal tubules. In severe intravascular hemolysis, the reabsorptive capacity is exceeded, causing hemoglobinuria. Also during severe intravascular hemolysis, some heme molecules in the circulation are transferred from hemopexin to albumin forming methemalbumin. When the liver's conjugating capacity is exceeded during moderate or severe hemolysis, unconjugated (indirect) bilirubin serum levels increase (49).

Diagnosis

The primary diagnostic features of hemolytic anemia are a marked reticulocytosis along with jaundice (including scleral icterus) due to hyperbilirubinemia. A corrected reticulocyte count greater than 0.025 (2.5%) is a typical response to hemolysis. The severity of the anemia may also be judged by the extent to which the hematocrit is decreased. The enzyme lactate dehydrogenase (LDH) is released from the RBC during hemolysis, and plasma levels may be elevated. Red cells frequently undergo morphologic changes during hemolytic episodes, with spherocytosis being the most common abnormality. Splenomegaly is usually present in cases of chronic hemolysis. A summary

Table 14.8.
Common Diagnostic Features of Hemolytic Anemia

	Moderate Hemolysis	Severe Hemolysis
I. Physical Findings		
Jaundice	+	+
Hemoglobinuria	0	+
II. Laboratory Indices— Plasma Serum		
Reticulocytosis	+	++
Plasma Hemoglobin	+	++
RBC Hemoglobin	Decreased	Decreased
Hematocrit	Decreased	Decreased
Bilirubin (Unconjugated)	+	++
Haptoglobin	Decreased	Decreased or absent
Hemopexin	Normal or decreased	Decreased or absent
Methemalbumin	0	+
Lactate dehydrogenase	+ (Variable)	++ (Variable)
III. Laboratory Indices—Urine		
Hemoglobin	0	+
Hemosiderin	0	+

of important findings in hemolytic anemia is presented in Table 14.8.

With respect to immune-mediated hemolysis, diagnostic evaluation includes the direct antiglobulin test (DAT or Coomb's test) which detects the presence of IgG or C3 (complement) on the surface of a patient's RBCs. The indirect Coomb's test detects the presence of antibodies against RBCs in the serum rather than on the surface of the RBC itself. During oxidative hemolytic anemias, denatured hemoglobin precipitates within the RBC, forming Heinz bodies, which are visible during microscopic examination. Heinz bodies are rapidly removed by the spleen, creating "bite" cells, which are erythrocytes that appear to have a bite of cytoplasm removed.

Inherited Hemolytic Anemias

Hereditary spherocytosis, elliptocytosis, and stomatocytosis are all genetic disorders inherited in an autosomal dominant fashion and are associated with altered RBC morphology. Hemolysis and clinical sequelae tend to be more pronounced with hereditary spherocytosis than with the other two. Splenectomy usually corrects anemia in these individuals. Supplemental folic acid therapy (1 mg daily) is also recommended (49).

G6PD DEFICIENCY

The most prevalent inherited RBC enzyme defect is G6PD deficiency, a sex-linked (X-chromosome) disorder. Affected females are predominantly heterozygous and have both normal and G6PD-deficient RBCs. They are fairly resistant to RBC hemolysis. Men and homozygous women, however, have predominantly G6PD-deficient RBCs and are predisposed to more severe hemolytic episodes. Cultural distribution of this disorder is similar to that of thalassemia, as it occurs frequently in blacks and people of Mediterranean cultures. The A− variant of G6PD is found primarily in blacks. Enzyme activity in these individuals is 8 to 20% of normal. In the United States, approximately 13% of black males and 3% of black females are affected. The Mediterranean-type variant of G6PD has 0 to 4% of normal enzyme activity. Consequently, these individuals are generally at greater risk of developing hemolytic anemia and the associated clinical manifestations are more pronounced.

Hemolytic Mechanism. The G6PD enzyme, in conjunction with glutathione and nicotinamide adenine dinucleotide phosphate (NADPH), serves as a protective antioxidant for RBCs against external oxidative stresses (Fig. 14.2). In the presence of G6PD deficiency, oxidative stresses on the RBC such as drugs, infection, or acidosis can lead to denaturation of the globin chains. Denatured globin precipitates intracellularly onto the cell membrane as Heinz bodies, and premature hemolysis occurs (50, 51). This type of disorder is frequently referred to as oxidative hemolysis.

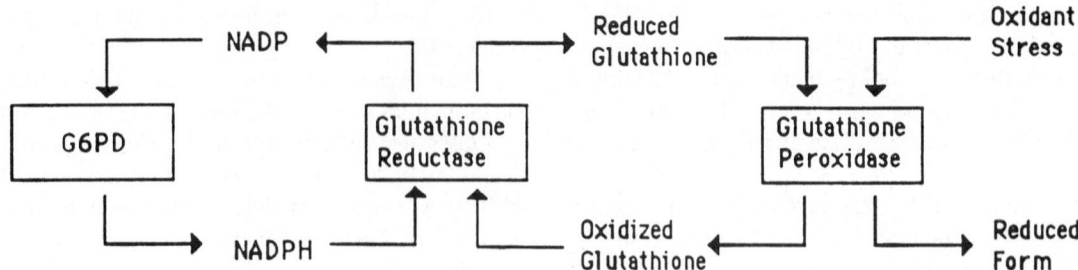

Figure 14.2 Antioxidant mechanism of G6PD. NADP, nicotinamide adenine dinucleotide phosphate.

Table 14.9.
Drugs and Substances Associated with Hemolytic Anemia in G6PD Deficiency

Primaquine	Sulfapyridine
Nalidixic acid	Phenazopyridine
Ciprofloxacin	Dapsone
Nitrofurantoin	Methylene blue
Sulfacetamide	Naphthalene (mothballs)
Sulfamethoxasole	Fava beans

Many drugs and substances have been associated with hemolytic anemia in G6PD-deficient individuals. However, the list of agents for which there is strong evidence of an association is relatively small and is presented in Table 14.9 (50, 51). A patient's susceptibility to oxidative stress of a particular drug varies according to several factors. The type of G6PD genetic variant present (i.e., type A– or Mediterranean-type) is a major determinant. Other factors include patient age, other sources of oxidant stress, dose of an offending drug, patient metabolism of an offending drug, and patient elimination of an offending drug. During hemolytic episodes in susceptible patients, signs and symptoms usually develop within 2 to 3 days of drug initiation. The hemolysis is primarily intravascular and generally results in pronounced hemoglobinuria.

Treatment. Withdrawal or avoidance of any potentially oxidant drugs or other substances is the most important component of treatment. In patients with A–variant G6PD deficiency, hemolysis is usually mild and self-limited, and therapy is seldom required. In patients with Mediterranean-type deficiency experiencing severe hemolysis, blood transfusions may occasionally be warranted. Folic acid supplementation should be given for 2 to 3 weeks following an acute hemolytic episode and may be necessary for extended periods in patients with chronic hemolysis. In patients who develop severe hemolytic anemia with hemoglobinuria, intravenous hydration to maintain adequate urine output may be necessary to prevent acute renal failure (50, 51).

The primary approach when caring for patients who have documented G6PD deficiency or those who may be

at risk (e.g., family history, ethnic background) is prevention. Several factors should be considered prior to initiating such patients on a potentially hemolyzing drug including patient age, renal function, type of G6PD variant that may be present, availability of alternative drugs, and severity of primary illness. A specific quantitative assay of G6PD is available for screening patients who may be deficient (51).

Acquired Hemolytic Anemias

Acquired hemolytic anemias are made up of a diverse group of disorders (Table 14.7). Microangiopathic hemolytic anemias including disseminated intravascular coagulation, hemolytic-uremic syndrome, and thrombotic thrombocytopenic purpura are generally caused by alterations such as fibrin deposition or narrowing of the microvasculature. Therapy for these disorders involves treatment of the underlying disease. Acquired hemolytic anemias secondary to RBC trauma occur in up to 10% of patients with prosthetic or diseased heart valves due to pressure gradient stresses placed on the RBC membrane. Beneficial treatment in these patients includes correcting iron deficiency and limiting exertional activity. Valve replacement may be necessary when less invasive measures fail.

AUTOIMMUNE HEMOLYSIS

Autoimmune hemolytic anemia results from the binding of complement or anti-RBC antibodies to the red cell membrane in affected individuals. These disorders are classified according to the temperature at which the antibodies have the greatest affinity for and interaction with red cells.

Cold Agglutinin Disease. Cold agglutinin disorders involve the binding of IgM antibodies to RBCs at low temperatures (4°C). This agglutination process is quickly reversed during warming. Most cold agglutinins do not appreciably shorten red cell survival. Acute cold agglutinin disease is frequently associated with mycoplasma pneumonia or infectious mononucleosis. Hemolysis typically begins 5 to 10 days after recovery from the infection and is mild and self-limited. Chronic cold agglutinin disease often occurs spontaneously in elderly patients, especially those with lymphoproliferative disorders, and results in poor peripheral circulation. Treatment of cold agglutinin disease involves preventing exposure to cold environments, folic acid supplementation, blood transfusions (if necessary), and treatment of any underlying diseases. Occasionally patients may respond to plasmapheresis or cytotoxic agents such as cyclophosphamide or chlorambucil. Splenectomy and corticosteroids are of questionable value (49).

Warm-Antibody Type. Warm reacting antibodies have the greatest affinity for red cells at room temperature (37°C) and are usually of the IgG or, occasionally, IgA type. This type of immunohemolytic anemia may be idiopathic, secondary to an underlying disease that affects the immune system (e.g., chronic lymphocytic leukemia, non-Hodgkin's lymphoma, or systemic lupus erythematosus), or secondary to certain drugs. Many of these patients have a chronic mild anemia and splenomegaly, but the clinical presentation of these patients varies widely. This disorder is more common in adults and in women. The direct Coomb's test is positive for IgG but usually not for C3. The indirect Coomb's test is usually negative (49).

Treatment of Warm-Antibody Immunohemolytic Anemia. Prior to treating patients with immunohemolytic anemia, drugs that have been associated with this condition (discussed below) should be excluded as the cause. Therapy should be guided based on the severity of the anemia. Patients with mild hemolysis usually do not require therapy. When hemolysis is clinically significant, corticosteroid therapy is usually effective and blood transfusions may be required. The mechanism of steroid action in immunohemolytic anemia is thought to involve a reduction in the clearance of IgG-coated red cells from the circulation and an inhibition of antibody synthesis. Typically, prednisone is administered in a dose of 1 mg/kg/day and continued until hemoglobin levels have normalized. Hemoglobin concentration usually begins to increase within 3 to 4 days after prednisone is initiated. Once hemoglobin has returned to baseline, prednisone therapy is tapered slowly over a period of several months. Approximately 60 to 70% of patients treated in this manner will have a sustained suppression of hemolysis. However, half of these patients will relapse as steroids are tapered or once they are withdrawn. Thirty to forty percent of patients will fail steroid therapy or will require excessive doses. Splenectomy is indicated in this group and will benefit 50 to 60% of these individuals. In patients who are refractory to steroids and splenectomy (about 10% of cases), alternative therapies for consideration include immunosuppressive agents (e.g., cyclophosphamide or azathioprine), danazol, intravenous immune globulin, and cyclosporine. Cross-matching patients with immunohemolytic anemia for blood transfusions is difficult because the antibody that is present will often react with all normal donor cells (49).

Table 14.10.
Examples of Drugs Associated with Immunohemolytic Anemia

Autoimmune (Methyldopa Type)	Drug Adsorption (Hapten Type)	Immune Complex Adsorption (Innocent Bystander Type)
Methyldopa	Penicillins	Quinidine
Levodopa	Cephalosporins	Quinine
Mefenamic acid	Tetracycline	Phenacetin
Cimetidine		Acetaminophen
Procainamide		

Drug-Induced Immunohemolytic Anemias. Examples of drugs that have been associated with immunohemolytic anemias are listed in Table 14.10. There are three proposed mechanisms by which drugs may initiate this condition.

Autoimmune (Methyldopa Type). Up to 10% of patients receiving methyldopa in daily doses of 2 grams develop a positive direct Coomb's test. Only a small percentage of these patients (<1%) will develop an extravascular hemolysis. The patient's red blood cells are coated with IgG. The mechanism of this condition is not well understood but may involve the inhibition of suppressor T cells. Hemolysis gradually subsides over a period of weeks after drug discontinuation, but the patient's Coomb's test may remain positive for more than a year.

Drug Adsorption (Hapten Type). In patients receiving large doses of penicillins (e.g., 15 to 20 million units per day) or cephalosporins, drug adsorbs to the RBC membrane, forming a hapten complex. Antibodies are then formed against this complex, resulting in extravascular hemolysis within 7 to 14 days following initiation of the drug. Red cells are Coomb's positive for IgG during therapy. Hemolysis subsides immediately after the drug is withdrawn.

Immune Complex Adsorption (Innocent Bystander Type). In this rare type of drug-induced immunohemolytic anemia, the offending agent induces the production of either IgG or IgM antibodies. A drug-antibody complex forms that then adheres nonspecifically to the red cell membrane. Complement (C3) is activated and fixes to the membrane surface. The drug-antibody complex dissociates from the RBC, and only C3 is detected by a Coomb's test. The hemolytic process may occur either extravascularly or intravascularly, and may be associated with hemoglobinemia, hemoglobinuria, and acute renal failure (49).

A fourth type of process may occur secondary to the administration of high-dose cephalosporins. In this case, the drug binds to the red cell membrane, causing it to be modified which results in the nonspecific adsorption of serum proteins. This process is not immune mediated, nor does hemolysis occur.

CONCLUSION

Anemia is a reduction in the concentration of viable erythrocytes or hemoglobin in the circulation, resulting in a reduced oxygen-carrying capacity of blood. There are several basic mechanisms discussed in this chapter by which anemia may occur, including impaired or absent erythropoiesis (e.g., anemia of chronic disease, aplastic anemia, anemia of renal failure), impaired hemoglobin synthesis (e.g., sickle cell anemia, thalassemia), and premature red cell destruction (e.g., hemolytic anemia). These mechanisms often coexist. Diseases or conditions that are frequently the primary cause of anemia include chronic infection or inflammation, neoplastic diseases, renal disease, exposure to certain pathogens or chemicals, exposure to certain drugs, inherited abnormalities, and autoimmune processes.

Anemia has many potential causes and is actually a symptom of an underlying condition. The treatment of patients should focus not only on correcting the anemia and its associated symptoms but also on identifying and correcting underlying causes when possible.

REFERENCES

1. Sears DA. Anemia of chronic disease. Med Clin North Am 76:567–579, 1992.
2. Means RT, Krantz SB. Progress in understanding the pathogenesis of the anemia of chronic disease. Blood 80:1639–1647, 1992.
3. Eschbach JW. The anemia of chronic renal failure: pathophysiology and the effects of recombinant erythropoietin. Kidney Int 35:134–148, 1989.
4. Neff MS, Goldberg J, Slifkin RF, et al. A comparison of androgens for anemia in patients on hemodialysis. N Engl J Med 304:871–875, 1981.
5. Eschbach JW, Abdulhadi MH, Browne JK, et al. Recombinant human erythropoietin in anemic patients with end-stage renal disease. Ann Intern Med 111:992–1000, 1989.
6. Zachee P. Controversies in selection of epoetin dosages. Drugs 49:536–547, 1995.
7. Humphries JE. Anemia of renal failure. Med Clin North Am 76:711–725, 1992.
8. Eschbach JW, Egrie JC, Downing MR, et al. Correction of the anemia of end-stage renal disease with recombinant human erythropoietin. N Engl J Med 316:73–78, 1987.
9. Eschbach JW. Erythropoietin: the promise and the facts. Kidney Int 45(suppl 44):570–576, 1994.
10. Bjorkholm M. Aplastic anaemia: pathogenetic mechanisms and treatment with special reference to immunomodulation. J Intern Med 231:575–582, 1992.
11. Stewart FM. Hypoplastic/aplastic anemia. Role of bone marrow transplantation. Med Clin North Am 76:683–697, 1992.
12. Storb R, Champlin RE. Bone marrow transplantation for severe aplastic anemia. Bone Marrow Transplant 8:69–72, 1991.
13. Bacigalupo A, Hows J, Gluckman E, et al. Bone marrow transplantation versus immunosuppression for the treatment of severe anaemia: a report of the EBMT SAA working party. Br J Haematol 70:177–182, 1988.
14. Weiner RS, Dicke KA. Risk factors for interstitial pneumonitis following allogeneic bone marrow transplantation for severe aplastic anemia: a preliminary report. Transplant Proc 19:2639–2642, 1987.
15. Camitta BM, Doney K. Immunosuppressive therapy for aplastic anemia: indications, agents, mechanisms and results. Am J Pediatr Hematol Oncol 12:411–424, 1990.
16. Bacigalupo A, Broccia G, Corda G. Antilymphocyte globulin, cyclosporine, and granulocyte colony stimulating factor in patients with acquired severe aplastic anemia (SAA): a pilot of the EBMT SAA working party. Blood 85:1348–1353, 1995.
17. Nimer SD, Paquette RL, Ireland P, et al. A phase I/II study of interleukin-3 in patients with aplastic anemia and myelodysplasia. Exp Hematol 22:875–880, 1994.
18. Hoffman R, Benz EJ, Shattil SJ, et al. Hematology: basic principles and practice. New York: Churchill Livingstone, 1991.
19. Steingart R. Management of patients with sickle cell disease. Med Clin North Am 76:669–682, 1992.
20. Pollack CV, Sanders DY, Severance HW. Emergency department analgesia without narcotics for adults with acute sickle cell pain crisis: case reports and review of crisis management. J Emerg Med 9:445–452, 1991.
21. Gonzalez ER, Bahal N, Hansen LA, et al. Intermittent injection vs patient-controlled analgesia for sickle cell crisis pain. Arch Intern Med 151:1373–1378, 1991.
22. Griffin TC, McIntire D, Buchanan GR. High-dose intravenous methylprednisolone therapy for pain in children and adolescents with sickle cell disease. N Engl J Med 330:733–737, 1994.
23. Shapiro BS. The management of pain in sickle cell disease. Pediatr Clin North Am 36:1029–1045, 1989.
24. Rodgers GP, Dover GJ, Noguchi CT, et al. Hematologic responses of patients with sickle cell disease to treatment with hydroxyurea. N Engl J Med 322:1037–1045, 1990.
25. Charache S, Terrin ML, Moore RD, et al. Effect of hydroxyurea on the frequency of painful crises in sickle cell anemia. N Engl J Med 332:1317–1322, 1995.
26. Goldberg MA, Brugnara C, Dover GJ, et al. Treatment of sickle cell anemia with hydroxyurea and erythropoietin. N Engl J Med 323:366–372, 1990.
27. Rodgers GP, Dover GJ, Uyesaka N, et al. Augmentation by erythropoietin of the fetal-hemoglobin response to hydroxyurea in sickle cell disease. N Engl J Med 328:73–80, 1993.
28. Vermylen C, Cornu G. Bone marrow transplantation for sickle cell disease. Am J Pediatr Hematol Oncol 16:18–21, 1994.
29. Jandl JH. Blood: textbook of hematology. Boston: Little, Brown, 1987.
30. Steinberg MH. Thalassemia: molecular pathology and management. Am J Med Sci 296:308–321, 1988.
31. Festa RS. Modern management of thalassemia. Pediatr Ann 14:597–606, 1985.
32. Wonke B. Prospects of β-thalassemia major. Indian Pediatr 24:969–975, 1987.
33. Huisman TH. Frequencies of common β-thalassemia alleles among different populations: variability in clinical severity. Br J Haematol 75:454–457, 1990.
34. Liebhaber SA. α-Thalassemia. Hemoglobin 13:685–721, 1989.
35. Fosburg MT, Nathan DG. Treatment of Cooley's anemia. Blood 76:435–444, 1990.
36. Brittenham GM, Griffith PM, Nienhuis AW, et al. Efficacy of deferoxamine in preventing complications of iron overload in patients with thalassemia major. N Engl J Med 331:567–573, 1994.
37. Lerner N. Medical management of β-thalassemia. Prog Clin Biol Res 309:14–22, 1989.
38. Olivieri NF, Berriman AM, Tyler BJ, et al. Reduction in tissue iron stores with a new regimen of continuous ambulatory intravenous deferoxamine. Am J Hematol 41:61–63, 1992.
39. Pippard MJ. Iron overload and iron chelation therapy in thalassemia and sickle cell haemoglobinopathies. Acta Haematol 78:206–211, 1987.

40. Cohen A. Current status of iron chelation therapy with deferoxamine. Semin Hematol 27:86–90, 1990.

41. Olivieri NF, Nathan DG, MacMillan JH, et al. Survival in medically treated patients with homozygous β-thalassemia. N Engl J Med 331:574–578, 1994.

42. Olivieri NF, Koren G, Matsui D, et al. Reduction of tissue iron stores and normalization of serum ferritin during treatment with the oral iron chelator L1 in thalassemia intermedia. Blood 79:2741–2748, 1992.

43. Barrett AJ, Lucarelli G, Gale RP, et al. Bone marrow transplantation for thalassemia—a preliminary report from the international bone marrow transplant registry. Prog Clin Biol Res 309:173–185, 1989.

44. Lucarelli G, Galimberti M, Polchi P, et al. Marrow transplantation in patients with thalassemia responsive to iron chelation therapy. N Engl J Med 329:840–844, 1993.

45. Steinberg MH. Prospects of gene therapy for hemoglobinopathies. Am J Med Sci 302:298–303, 1991.

46. Stamatoyannopoulos JA, Nienhuis AW. Therapeutic approaches to hemoglobin switching in treatment of hemoglobinopathies. Annu Rev Med 43:497–521, 1992.

47. Lowrey CH, Nienhuis AW. Treatment with azacitidine of patients with end-stage β-thalassemia. N Engl J Med 329:845–848, 1993.

48. Higgs DR. The thalassemia syndromes. Q J Med 86:559–564, 1993.

49. Tabbara IA. Hemolytic anemias: diagnosis and management. Med Clin North Am 76:649–668, 1992.

50. Beutler E. G6PD deficiency. Blood 84:3613–3636, 1994

51. Mehta AB. Glucose-6-phosphate dehydrogenase deficiency. Postgrad Med J 70:871–877, 1994.

CHAPTER 15

COAGULATION DISORDERS

JEAN K. NOGUCHI and MARK STEPHENS

HEMOSTASIS

Definitions and Components

The function of the hemostatic system is twofold: (a) to maintain blood in the fluid state while it is within the vasculature and (b) to minimize blood loss by promoting clotting when the blood is outside of the vasculature. This requires coordination of complex, highly integrated mechanisms with numerous components. Blood vessels, platelets, coagulation factors, natural inhibitors, and the fibrinolytic proteins exist in an overlapping system of checks and balances (1). Normal hemostasis requires three responses: the vascular response, formation of a platelet plug, and formation of a fibrin clot. At the same time, naturally occurring anticoagulant proteins inhibit the action of clotting factors in an attempt to control thrombosis, fibrinolysis, and inflammation. The fibrinolytic system also dissolves and removes excess fibrin deposits to preserve vascular patency.

The Vasculature

Normal intact vascular endothelium repels platelets and red blood cells (RBCs) and secretes substances to inhibit clotting. The initial vascular response to trauma is vasoconstriction, which shunts blood away from the damaged area. This response can assist in the hemostatic process, particularly in small vessels. Traumatic disruption of the vessel endothelial lining triggers formation, binding, and/or activation of various substances. Trauma also exposes substrates that facilitate attachment and formation of the platelet plug, which is the primary hemostatic mechanism. The secondary hemostatic mechanism controls the formation of a fibrin clot via the ordered interaction of a series of tissue and blood components or factors. Primary and secondary hemostasis operate simultaneously. During this time, inhibitor systems also operate to prevent propagation of the clot, and fibrinolysis is activated for eventual removal of the clot.

Platelet Physiology and Function

Platelets play a dominant role in the spontaneous prevention of blood loss from damaged blood vessels. Immediately after tissue injury, platelets clump together to form a primary hemostatic plug, stopping blood flow and maintaining vascular integrity. They play a major part in the ultimate formation of a permanent insoluble fibrin clot, which is essential for long-term hemostasis.

Platelets, or thrombocytes, are anucleate granular structures approximately 2 to 3 microns in diameter. Platelets are fragments of megakaryocytes, which are large stem cells formed in the bone marrow. These giant stem cells disintegrate into platelets, which are released into the peripheral blood. The normal platelet concentration is 150,000 to 400,000/mm^3 of blood, and production appears to be directly proportional to demand. This allows for the repair of minor ruptures that occur routinely in everyday life. After formation and release from the bone marrow, approximately 25 to 35% of platelets are found in the spleen and the remainder in the circulation. The average lifespan of platelets is 7 to 10 days, and younger platelets are more active physiologically than older cells (2).

The initial response to vascular injury, transient vasoconstriction, is caused by contraction of the vessel wall smooth muscle and instantaneously diminishes blood loss from the rupture. At the same time the vascular trauma disrupts the endothelium, causing platelets to come into contact with exposed subendothelial connective tissue and collagen fibers, elastin, adenosine diphosphate (ADP), epinephrine, and other substances of the vessel wall. Platelets do not adhere to intact endothelium.

Within seconds after tissue insult, the primary hemostatic plug is formed in a series of overlapping phases.

1. Adhesion. When platelets come into contact with exposed vessel subendothelium, they attach to this site of vascular injury via platelet adhesion receptors. Factor VIII and von Willebrand factor, proteins that circulate in plasma as a large complex, are required for normal platelet adhesion in areas of high shear (e.g., arterioles and the microcirculation). A deficiency in this protein complex leads to serious defects in platelet adhesiveness.
2. Aggregation. The initial adhesion of platelets to extruded substances of the injured vessel and the release of ADP stimulate platelet aggregation. The platelets become sticky, adhere, and recruit other passing platelets. This platelet mass forms the primary hemostatic plug. Aggregation requires platelet stimulation by physiologic agonists, which include thrombin and collagen; ADP, epinephrine, prostaglandin endoperoxides, thromboxane A$_2$, serotonin, and vasopressin are weak agonists. Adhesion and aggregation are dynamic processes that are controlled by the balance of agonist to antagonist effect at the cellular level (2).
3. Secretion of granules. Adhered platelets release the contents of their granules, including ADP, ATP, serotonin, platelet factor 4, calcium, lysosomal enzymes, prostaglandins, throm-

boxane A_2 (a platelet-derived growth factor), and platelet-specific proteins. This release attracts more platelets to the injured area.

4. Elaboration of procoagulant activity. Platelets also provide a staging surface for the assembly of coagulation protein complexes and the ultimate formation of activated thrombin via the coagulation cascade (3). In this function they serve as a nidus for the ultimate formation of the fibrin clot. Platelets also secrete factor V, a component of the coagulation cascade.

Arachidonic acid, which is stored in platelet phospholipids, plays an important role in the development of the normal hemostatic plug. Adhesion to collagen causes the cleavage of arachidonic acid from phospholipids by cyclooxygenase. This platelet enzyme converts free arachidonic acid into prostaglandin endoperoxides, which are converted into thromboxane A_2. Thromboxane A_2, a more potent stimulator of platelet release and aggregation than ADP, may prolong the vasospasm needed for normal hemostasis because of its arterial vasoconstrictor activity. Another prostaglandin metabolite of arachidonic acid,

prostacyclin, is synthesized by cyclooxygenase from the walls of arteries and veins. In contrast to thromboxane A_2, prostacyclin is a potent inhibitor of platelet aggregation and causes vasodilation. Its action may aid in localizing the hemostatic plug to the immediate area of tissue damage.

Formation of the platelet plug can rapidly stop bleeding, but reinforcement by fibrin is needed to produce a stable insoluble thrombus. Only through stimulation of the coagulation cascade can the loose aggregation of platelets be transformed into a permanent hemostatic plug. This occurs via formation of fibrin strands within 30 to 60 seconds after vessel damage, followed over several hours by fibrin accumulation and platelet disintegration, so that ultimately the platelet plug is replaced by fibrin (3).

Coagulation and Fibrinolysis

The nomenclature and characteristics of the factors that are involved in the coagulation cascade are summarized in Table 15.1. The Roman numeral designations for clotting factors generally correspond to their order of discovery.

Table 15.1.
Characteristics of Coagulation Factors[a]

Factor	Synonym(s)	Plasma Half-Life (hr)	Plasma Concentration (mg/dL)	Coagulation Pathway (E, I, C)	Biochemical Group
Procoagulants					
I	Fibrinogen	100–150	200–400	C	
II	Prothrombin, prethrombin	50–80	10	C	Vitamin K-dependent
III	Tissue factor, tissue thromboplastin	—	0	E	
IV	Calcium ion	—	9–10	E, I, C	
V	Proaccelerin, labile factor	24	1	C	
VII	Proconvertin, SPCA, stable factor	6	0.05	E	Vitamin K-dependent
VIII	Antihemophilic factor (AHF) Antihemophilic globulin Antihemophilic factor A Platelet cofactor I	12	0.01	I	
vWf	von Willebrand factor	24	1		
IX	Christmas factor Antihemophilic factor B Plasma thromboplastin component Platelet cofactor II	24	0.3	I	Vitamin K-dependent
X	Stuart-Prower factor	25–60	1	C	Vitamin K-dependent
XI	Plasma thromboplastin antecedent Antihemophilic factor C	40–80	0.5	I	Contact factor
XII	Hageman factor	50–70	3	I	Contact factor
XIII	Fibrin stabilizing factor	150	1–2	C	
Prekallikrein	Fletcher factor	35	5	I	Contact factor
HMW kininogen	Contact activation factor	150	6	I	Contact factor
Inhibitors/fibrinolysis					
Antithrombin III		24–36	18–30	I	Vitamin K-dependent
Protein C		16	0.4	I, C	Vitamin K-dependent
Protein S		42	2.3	I, C	Vitamin K-dependent
Plasminogen		48	20–40	C	

[a] Adapted from Saito H. Normal hemostatic mechanisms, and Bauer KA, Rosenberg RD. The hypercoagulable state. In: Ratnoff OD, Forbes CD, eds. Disorders of Hemostasis. Philadelphia: WB Saunders, 1991: 18–49, 267–291; and Comp PC. Production of plasma coagulation factors. In: Williams WJ, Beutler E, Erslev AJ, et al, eds. Hematology, 4th ed. New York: McGraw-Hill, 1983: 293.

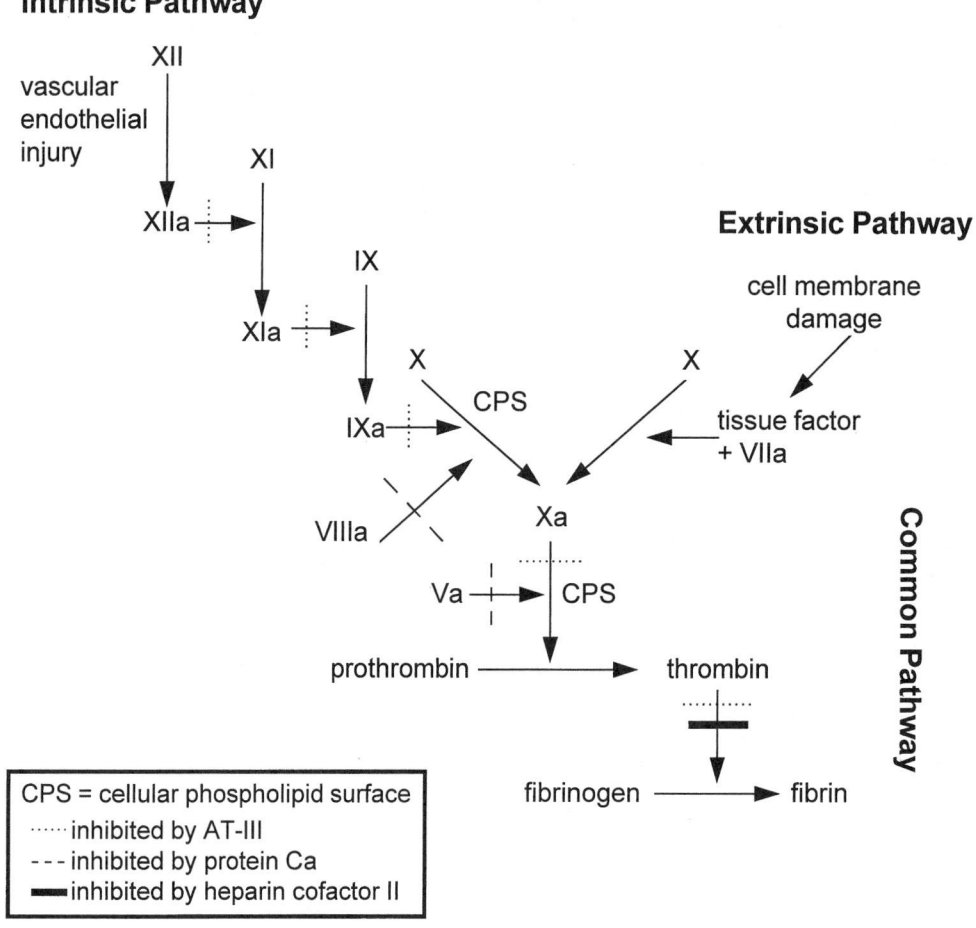

Figure 15.1.   Components and inhibitors of the intrinsic, extrinsic, and common coagulation pathways.

Many clotting factors fall into one of two major groups, based on their biochemical properties. Factors XI, XII, prekallikrein, and high-molecular-weight (HMW) kininogen are known as contact activation factors because they initiate the contact phase of coagulation pathway. Factors II, VII, IX, and X are vitamin K-dependent coagulation factors synthesized by the liver. Vitamin K is an essential cofactor for hepatic carboxylation of glutamic acid residues. The τ-carboxylglutamic acid residues allow the calcium binding that is essential for normal clotting activity. Vitamin K-deficient individuals continue to produce factors II, VII, IX, and X, but in inactive forms. Factor III (tissue factor) is found in many tissues; factor IV (calcium) comes from diet and bone. Hepatic biosynthesis provides the other factors listed in Table 15.1 (4).

The coagulation cascade is comprised of reaction complexes, each including an enzyme, a substrate, and a reaction accelerator. These complexes are linked in a series of catalytic reactions (Fig. 15.1). Components are assembled on specific lipid surfaces and are held together by calcium ions. Most coagulation factors are present as zymogens (inert precursor forms) and must be converted

to their active enzymatic forms during coagulation. Only very small amounts of factors are required to trigger the catalytic cascade. The numerous steps amplify the activation process, which ensures a rapid response at sites of injury. The product of these reactions is the potent enzyme thrombin, which is formed by the catalytic action of factor Xa (activated factor X) on prothrombin (Fig. 15.1). There are two classic pathways that lead to the generation of factor Xa, called the extrinsic and intrinsic pathways.

The extrinsic coagulation pathway is so designated because it is activated by tissue factor, which is not a normal component of the blood. Damage to the vessel causes release of tissue factor (Factor III, a lipoprotein). Tissue factor forms a calcium-dependent complex with factor VII that converts circulating factors IX and X to their active forms (1), as depicted in the right-hand column in Figure 15.1. The rate-limiting step in thrombin formation via the extrinsic pathway is the amount of tissue factor released at the site of injury.

The intrinsic pathway comprises a system in which all components are normal blood constituents (hence the name "intrinsic"). In this pathway, components from each reaction form the enzyme for the next. It is initiated when contact of blood with an abnormal surface (e.g., collagen fibers exposed in the subendothelial layer of traumatized blood vessels) activates factor XII (left-hand column, Fig. 15.1); this is called the contact phase of the intrinsic pathway. Interaction of factor XIIa, factor XI, prekallikrein, kallikrein, and HMW kininogen then forms factor XIa. Generation of factor XIa initiates the remainder of the intrinsic pathway, culminating in the formation of factor Xa.

The intrinsic and extrinsic pathways differ in how factor X is activated. Once factor Xa is formed, the common pathway is activated (Fig. 15.1, lower center column). Factor Xa cleaves prothrombin, forming thrombin, which has several crucial actions. At the site of endothelial injury, thrombin catalyzes the reaction that converts soluble fibrinogen into fibrin monomer. Fibrin monomer is then polymerized into fibrin, a highly cross-linked insoluble fibrous network. Thrombin also activates platelets. The platelets and attached fibrin clot act as a plug to minimize further blood loss.

Several control mechanisms limit the coagulation process to the site of vascular injury and maintain and/or restore blood flow. Blood flow itself washes away and dilutes active coagulation factors that are generated locally at the site of injury. The liver and/or reticuloendothelial system remove activated coagulants, fibrin, and plasminogen activators from the circulation. Feedback mechanisms in all coagulation pathways limit and control their activity, so at each step in the coagulation cascade, the factor may be activated or inhibited/lysed. For example, thrombin is able to promote its own production by activating factors V and VIII, while at the same time it inhibits its own formation by binding to thrombomodulin and activating protein C (5).

Naturally occurring inhibitors such as antithrombin III and protein C make up a second control mechanism. These hepatically synthesized proteins inhibit the activated clotting factors. Antithrombin III neutralizes thrombin and inhibits plasminogen, kallikrein, trypsin, and factors IXa, Xa, XIa, and XIIa. Activated protein C inhibits factors Va, VIIIa, and plasmin. Protein S is a cofactor in the action of protein C.

After the fibrin clot is formed, fibrinolysis is initiated to remove the clot and restore blood flow. Fibrinolysis is mediated by the enzyme plasmin. Plasmin circulates in the inactive form of plasminogen. Tissue plasminogen activators (t-PA) that are present in endothelial cells and other tissues activate plasminogen to form plasmin, which in turn cleaves fibrin into fibrin degradation products (FDP) (Fig. 15.2). Plasmin can also cleave other proteins, including fibrinogen, factors V, VIII, IX and XI. These control mechanisms help maintain fluid circulation during clotting, which prevents the massive thrombosis that would result if the clotting process were left unopposed. Plasmin is also a

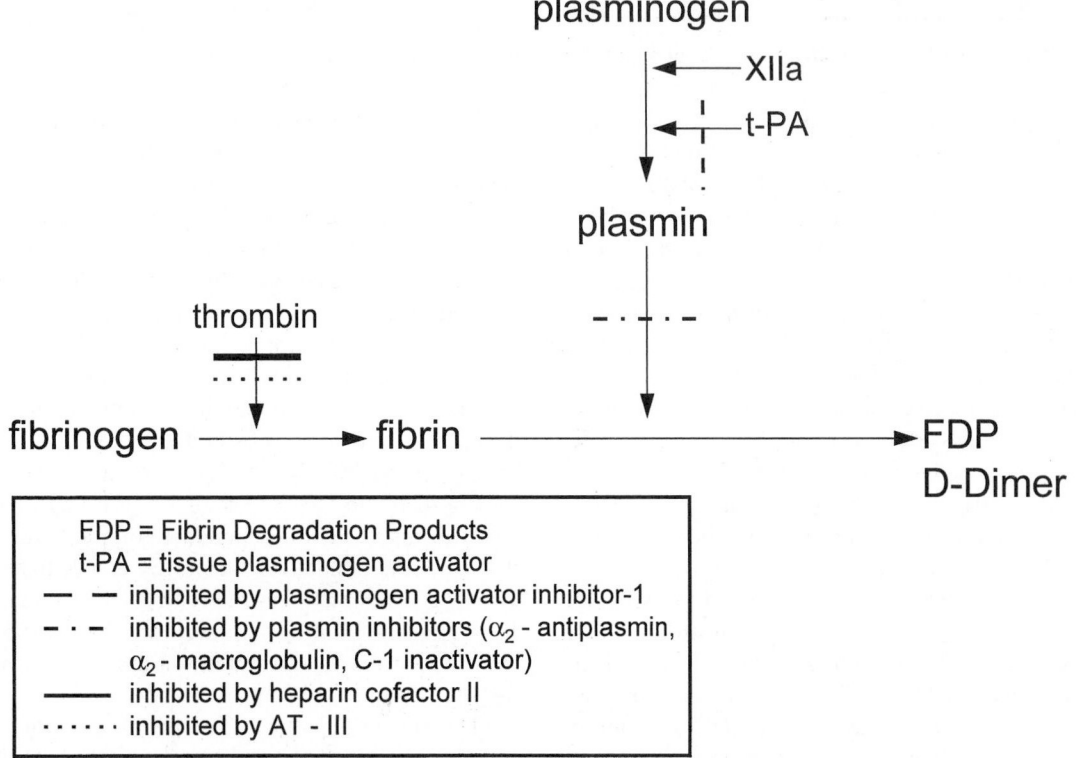

Figure 15.2. Components of fibrin formation and degradation.

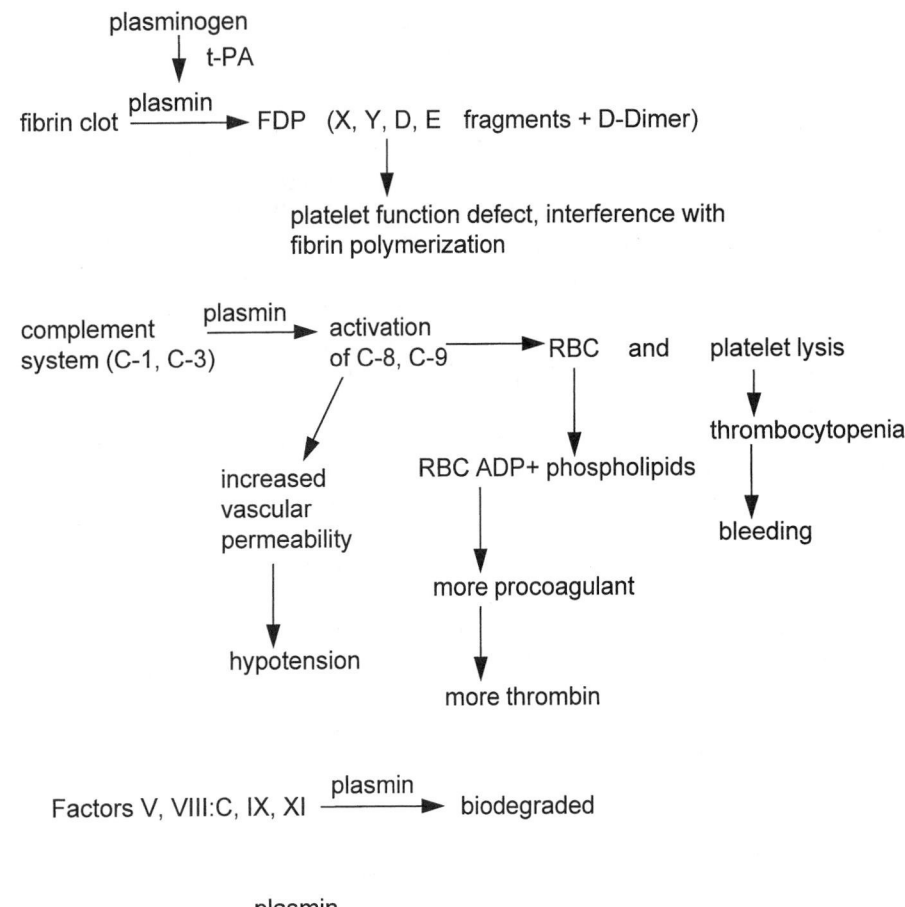

Figure 15.3 Additional actions of plasmin.

component of the complement and endocrine systems (Fig. 15.3).

Normal blood fluidity is therefore continuously maintained by the intact vessel endothelium and natural anticoagulants. Disruption of endothelial integrity or release of tissue factor after injury activates both the platelet and coagulation systems, resulting in an insoluble fibrin clot that limits further bleeding. The fibrinolytic system maintains vascular patency by breaking down the fibrin clot. Abnormalities in these systems may occur at virtually any step and may result in bleeding or coagulation disorders.

PLATELET DISORDERS

Thrombocytopenia

Thrombocytopenia is defined as a decrease in the number of blood platelets and is one of the most common causes of abnormal bleeding. A platelet count less than 100,000/mm^3 is considered mild thrombocytopenia and causes few symptoms. Counts less than 50,000/mm^3 constitute moderate thrombocytopenia and are associated with some bleeding potential. In severe thrombocytopenia (counts less than 10,000 to 20,000/mm^3), spontaneous life-threatening bleeding can occur. At platelet counts less than 100,000/mm^3 the bleeding time becomes progressively longer. However, it is important to note that the actual risk for bleeding depends on platelet function as well as number.

The symptoms of thrombocytopenia include symmetric petechiae and purpura on the extremities and trunk, mild to moderate bleeding of mucosal surfaces (oropharynx, nose, and the gastrointestinal, pulmonary, and genitourinary systems), and easy or spontaneous bleeding.

Thrombocytopenia has many causes, which should be distinguished to optimize the therapeutic approach. A decrease in the platelet count may occur from (a) a decrease in production, (b) altered distribution (sequestration), or (c) increased destruction of platelets.

A decrease in platelet production may occur from conditions that either alter normal thrombopoiesis or decrease the number of marrow megakaryocytes. Examples include marrow injury (e.g., myelosuppressive drugs, chemicals, radiation, or viral infections such as rubella, cytomegalovirus, Epstein-Barr virus, and human immunodeficiency virus), marrow failure (e.g., aplastic anemia, hereditary disorders), or marrow replacement (e.g., leukemia, tumor metastases, fibrosis). Ineffective thrombopoiesis caused by severe vitamin B_{12} or folate deficiency is characterized by a normal or increased number of megakaryocytes in the bone marrow but inadequate availability of platelets in the circulation. All of these disorders may be successfully treated with platelet transfusions.

Altered distribution of platelets can result from any disorder that causes splenomegaly (e.g., alcoholic liver disease, congestive heart failure, lymphomas, sickle cell disease, and myeloproliferative diseases). In this situation the actual number of total body platelets is normal, but their distribution in the body is altered. Normally, the spleen stores approximately one-third of the circulating platelets and also functions as a scavenger to remove nonfunctional platelets. When enlarged, the spleen can contain up to 80% of the circulating thrombocytes. Splenic sequestration alone does not usually cause platelet counts less than 50,000/mm³, and clinical bleeding is unusual. Treatment is therefore not generally indicated (6).

Increased destruction of platelets can result from increased platelet utilization and from immunologic and nonimmunologic mechanisms. Disseminated intravascular coagulation (DIC) is an example of a condition that causes increased platelet consumption. DIC occurs from widespread continuous activation of the clotting mechanisms, resulting in depletion of platelets and other clotting factors. Immunologic causes of thrombocytopenia include drug-induced immune thrombocytopenia (e.g., quinidine, quinine, gold, heparin); autoantibody production (e.g., systemic lupus erythematosus, autoimmune thrombocytopenic purpura); and alloantibody-produced thrombocytopenia (e.g., placental transfer, history of multiple transfusions).

Massive blood loss may result in dilutional thrombocytopenia when treated with large amounts of fluids having little or no platelets. Other miscellaneous causes of thrombocytopenia are thrombotic thrombocytopenic purpura (TTP), prosthetic heart valves, extracorporeal perfusion, hemodialysis, and snake envenomation.

Autoimmune Thrombocytopenic Purpura

Autoimmune thrombocytopenic purpura (AITP) is characterized by decreased numbers of circulating platelets, normal or increased numbers of megakaryocytes in the bone marrow, and clinical signs and symptoms related to the low platelet count. This syndrome is sometimes referred to as idiopathic thrombocytopenic purpura; however, the word "idiopathic" is actually a misnomer, since most research has indicated an autoimmune mechanism in the pathogenesis of AITP. Most cases of AITP involve shortened platelet survival due to immune-mediated platelet destruction by antiplatelet autoantibodies of the IgG or IgM subtypes.

EPIDEMIOLOGY

Clinically, AITP is divided into two forms: acute and chronic. The acute form most commonly occurs in young, previously healthy children 2 to 8 years of age and affects both sexes equally. Eighty percent of cases are preceded by an acute viral infection several weeks before the onset, most often an upper respiratory infection but also varicella, rubeola, or rubella. Immunizations have also been noted to precede the syndrome. The peak seasons of winter and spring correlate with the epidemiology of upper respiratory infections. Approximately 80% of patients will have a complete remission within several weeks to months, regardless of therapy. The annual incidence of the acute form is approximately 4:100,000 children, although many cases remain undiagnosed because of its transient and self-limiting nature. The chronic form occurs more often in females between 20 and 40 years of age, with a female:male ratio of 3:1 (6–8). It has an insidious onset and a lower rate of acute bleeding; in some cases the chronic form is detected as an incidental finding. It is sometimes associated with another underlying disease (e.g., systemic lupus erythematosus, other autoimmune disorders, chronic lymphocytic leukemia, lymphoma) (6, 8) and is not usually preceded by a viral infection. Chronic AITP undergoes remissions and exacerbations, persisting for more than 6 months and often for years. Only about 20% of patients will have a spontaneous remission, regardless of therapy. Although the exact incidence is unknown, chronic AITP is a relatively common hematologic disorder.

Human immunodeficiency virus (HIV)-associated thrombocytopenia is one of the most common hematologic complications of the infection, although it is not considered an acquired immunodeficiency syndrome (AIDS)-defining illness. Thrombocytopenia in patients with HIV infection resembles AITP in clinical and laboratory presentation. Patients have normal to increased numbers of megakaryocytes without evidence of splenomegaly.

PATHOGENESIS

Most researchers believe that antiplatelet IgG (with or without IgM) antibodies bound to the platelet surface are the underlying cause of the syndrome; other immune complexes may also be involved (6, 9). These immunoglobulins react with host platelets, which in turn bind firmly to receptors in the reticuloendothelial organs, especially the spleen and liver. This results in premature removal of the platelets from the circulation via phagocytosis. This theory is based on two findings: (a) Levels of platelet-associated IgG and/or IgM antibodies increase in more than 90% of patients with AITP, and (b) normal individuals develop thrombocytopenia when injected with plasma from patients with AITP (6).

SIGNS AND SYMPTOMS

Acute AITP is characterized by an abrupt onset, whereas the chronic form is insidious. In most cases the physical examination is remarkable only for the hemorrhagic abnormalities associated with the low platelet count. Small punctate red macules (petechiae) and a dark red-purple discoloration of the skin reflecting larger areas of hemorrhage (purpura) are the classic signs of AITP. These can occur anywhere on the external surface of the skin as well as internally, the gastrointestinal tract being the most common internal site. Bleeding of the nasal, oropharyngeal, and vaginal mucosa; easy bruising with ecchymoses; conjunctival hemorrhage; epistaxis; and menorrhagia are common. Hematuria, retinal hemorrhage, and joint bleeding are less common. Splenomegaly is absent. Central nervous system (CNS) bleeding is seen in approximately 1% of cases. Intracranial hemorrhage occurs early in the acute form of AITP, is most common in patients with platelet counts under 20,000/mm^3, and is considered the most serious risk in AITP, owing to its associated high morbidity and mortality. Manifestations include altered mental status and headache.

Patients with chronic AITP usually present with a higher platelet count compared to the acute form. Minor skin and mucous membrane bleeding may be the sole manifestations, and some patients are asymptomatic.

DIAGNOSIS AND CLINICAL FINDINGS

The diagnosis is usually a process of eliminating other disorders that also cause thrombocytopenia. This is especially true for children with signs and symptoms of acute AITP. The differential diagnosis of AITP includes a wide array of hematologic diseases including leukemia, marrow hypoplasia, disseminated intravascular coagulation, aplastic anemia, thrombotic thrombocytopenic purpura, and lymphoma. Nonhematologic causes of thrombocytopenia include systemic infection, thyroid disease, tuberculosis, and autoimmune diseases such as systemic lupus erythematosus (SLE). HIV infection should be considered as a possible diagnosis for patients who fit into high-risk categories. Drug-induced thrombocytopenia should also be excluded, and any drug that is capable of causing thrombocytopenia should be discontinued (Table 15.2). Splenomegaly, adenopathy, fever, and malaise are uncommon in acute AITP and may suggest other disorders when present.

Laboratory testing reveals isolated thrombocytopenia, unless bleeding has been sufficient to cause anemia. A complete blood examination shows a decreased number of platelets with an elevated mean platelet volume and platelet distribution width. On peripheral smear, the platelets

Table 15.2.
Drugs That Cause Thrombocytopenia

Amrinone (8)[a]	Ethanol (7)[a]
Antiinflammatory agents (1, 2, 3)[a]	Estrogens (7)[a]
Aspirin	Furosemide (1, 5)[a]
Fenoprofen	Gold salts (2)[a]
Indomethacin	Heparin (2)[a]
Phenylbutazone	Histamine H$_2$ antagonists (8)[a]
Piroxicam	Cimetidine
Tolmetin	Ranitidine
β-Blockers (3, 4, 8)[a]	Methyldopa (2)[a]
Alprenolol	Penicillins (3, 5, 8)[a]
Oxprenolol	Ampicillin
Propranolol	Carbenicillin
Carbamazepine (2, 8)[a]	Methicillin
Clofibrate (3)[a]	Penicillin G
Cytotoxic agents (7)[a]	Ticarcillin
Busulfan	Penicillamine (2, 8)[a]
Cytarabine	Phenytoin (2)[a]
Daunorubicin	Quinidine (2)[a]
Flucytosine	Quinine (2)[a]
Fluorouricin	Rifampin (8)[a]
Mechlorethamine	Sulfinpyrazone (1, 4)[a]
Mercaptopurine	Thiazide diuretics (8)[a]
Methotrexate	Chlorothiazide
Mithramycin	Hydrochlorothiazide
Mitomycin	Tocainide (8)[a]
Dextran(4, 8)[a]	
Digitoxin (2)[a]	Trimethoprim (8)[a]
Dipyridamole (3, 5, 6)[a]	Valproic acid (2)[a]

[a] Numbers in parentheses indicate confirmed and suspected mechanisms of thrombocytopenia: 1, Inhibits cyclo-oxygenase; 2, Drug-induced immune; 3, Inhibits aggregation; 4, Inhibits adhesion; 5, Inhibits release reaction; 6, Inhibits phosphodiesterase; 7, Myelosuppression; 8, Mechanism not documented.

are larger in size and appear to be less mature than normal. Thrombocytopenia in acute AITP may be severe (platelet count <10,000 to 20,000/mm^3), while patients with chronic AITP generally have higher counts (30,000 to 75,000/mm^3). Bleeding time is prolonged in proportion to the degree of thrombocytopenia. Of interest, the bleeding time for a given platelet count is shorter than that for thrombocytopenia caused by decreased platelet production, because the circulating platelets are young and "superactive." This accounts for the lack of bleeding symptoms in some patients despite severe thrombocytopenia. The prothrombin time, activated partial thromboplastin time, and erythrocyte sedimentation rate usually remain normal. Almost all patients have normal hemoglobin, hematocrit, and RBC indices, although chronic gastrointestinal hemorrhage or menorrhagia may occasionally cause iron-deficiency anemia. Bone marrow examination shows normal or increased numbers of immature megakaryocytes.

TREATMENT

The major goals in the treatment of AITP are to decrease the risk of hemorrhage and to obtain complete remission of the disease. Traditionally, these goals are met either by suppressing the production of antiplatelet antibodies or by inhibiting platelet phagocytosis. Supportive measures to reduce the risk of bleeding include restriction of physical activity and avoidance of drugs that alter platelet activity and should be implemented for all patients. For patients with chronic AITP secondary to another disorder, treatment of the underlying disease will benefit the AITP.

Acute AITP. More than 80% of patients with acute AITP will have a complete spontaneous recovery within a few weeks to months of the disease onset, irrespective of which (if any) treatment is given (2, 7). Considerable controversy exists regarding the decision to treat the disease or simply let it run its course. Intracranial hemorrhage is the primary concern of clinicians who prefer early treatment. Others choose not to treat because of adverse effects, cost, the low frequency of CNS bleeding, and the self-limiting nature of the disease. Some clinicians base the decision to treat on the platelet count, electing to treat when the count is less than 20,000/mm^3. Other factors in the treatment decision include days of hospitalization, the potential for outpatient treatment, and parental concern regarding intracranial hemorrhage and administration of blood products. Recent studies documenting a more rapid platelet response in treated compared to untreated patients (10), coupled with the known early occurrence of CNS bleeding, provide evidence favoring early treatment.

The goal of treatment is to rapidly increase the platelet count to hemostatically safe values (11). For many years, prednisone was considered the drug of choice in treating acute AITP. Hypothesized mechanisms of action include a prolongation of platelet lifespan by suppressing reticulo-endothelial system phagocytosis, inhibition of platelet-associated immunoglobulin production, and enhancement of bone marrow platelet production (12). At the traditional dose of 1 to 2 mg/kg/day, the onset of action is about 72 hr, with a return to normal platelet counts within 1 to 2 weeks in approximately 60 to 70% of patients (13). Some patients may take up to 4 weeks to demonstrate a maximal response. After a response is documented over 4 to 8 weeks, the dose is tapered; then the drug discontinued. A problem with the traditional doses is the discordance between the timing of drug effect and the maximal risk for CNS bleeding. Studies of higher doses (4 mg/kg/day) have resulted in a more rapid response (10, 11, 14); however, the optimal corticosteroid dose and route of administration have not been established. Adverse effects are minimal at low doses; higher doses have been associated with weight gain, epigastric discomfort, glycosuria, and behavioral changes (9, 11).

Intravenous high-dose immune globulins (IVIG) were discovered by serendipity to have efficacy in acute AITP (9). They are believed to inhibit Fc receptor-mediated platelet binding in the reticuloendothelial system (9, 12). This action prevents or slows phagocytosis of antibody-coated platelets and occurs immediately. IVIG also alters T- and B-cell numbers and function, a reduction in platelet-associated immunoglobulins being seen within 3 days. Another possible effect is an alteration in secretion and binding of interleukins. It is likely that IVIG has many simultaneous effects. The dose of IVIG is a total of 2 g/kg, given as either 0.4 g/kg/day for 5 days or 1 g/kg/day for 2 days. This usually results in a response in 1 to 3 days, with about 80% of patients having a platelet count greater than 50,000/mm^3 at 72 hours after treatment. If the effect is not sustained, repeat doses may be given. Adverse effects of IVIG include nausea, vomiting, headache, and fever, which appear to occur more often (50 to 60%) in patients who receive the total dose over 2 days (10, 11); these symptoms abate after about 1 day and are readily managed with acetaminophen. The long-term response to IVIG, assessed as maintenance of a platelet count greater than 20,000/mm^3 with no subsequent bleeding, is about 62% (9).

Short course high-dose IVIG therapy may also be of value when a temporary but rapid rise in platelet count is necessary (e.g., for surgery or during exposure to stressors such as infection). In children with severe bleeding and/or a high risk of intracranial hemorrhage, corticosteroids and IVIG may be given concomitantly. This combination has been shown to increase the platelet count more rapidly than either drug alone (8, 9, 12).

Small- and medium-scale comparative studies of IVIG and prednisone, sometimes with a "no-treatment" cohort, have yielded several interesting findings:

1. Both IVIG and prednisone (4 mg/kg/day, tapered over 21 days) caused fewer days of thrombocytopenia (<20,000/mm^3) compared to no treatment, and IVIG was significantly faster in attaining a platelet count greater than 50,000/mm^3 (10).
2. A trial comparing IVIG doses of 1 g/kg for 2 days and 0.8 g/kg once yielded similar responses as measured by days of thrombocytopenia and days to reach a "safer" platelet count (>50,000/mm^3) (11).
3. An early pilot study suggested that rapid responders had a better long-term prognosis compared to slow responders, and a trend favoring IVIG (15).

The decision whether to use prednisone or IVIG as initial therapy requires consideration of multiple factors. IVIG may be preferable because it has a more rapid onset of action compared to traditional dose prednisone; however, higher prednisone doses may yield comparable onset. Some investigators prefer IVIG, with the belief that it may have a disease-modifying role (12). Some practitioners consider prednisone to be the "gold standard" and favor its use because of familiarity with the drug. Much lower cost and parental concern regarding administration of blood products also favor prednisone, although some of the cost may be offset by a shortened hospital stay with IVIG. Additional studies are clearly necessary to clarify this clinical decision.

Splenectomy is avoided in treating children because of the risk of postsplenectomy sepsis. This is particularly true for children under 6 years of age and immunosuppressed patients, who carry the highest risk of overwhelming postsplenectomy infection. If splenectomy is contemplated, pneumococcal and *Haemophilus influenzae* immunizations should be given before the surgery.

Chronic AITP. Chronic AITP is primarily a disease of adults, but approximately 10 to 20% of children with acute AITP will respond poorly to treatment, and their AITP will evolve into the chronic form. Therapy for chronic AITP is usually begun with 1 mg/kg/day of prednisone, although 2 mg/kg/day has been used in severe cases. A positive response should be seen in 3 to 7 days, although 2 to 4 weeks may be needed for maximal response (12). Once the platelet count is greater than 100,000/mm^3, the dose of prednisone should be tapered slowly and reduced to the lowest effective dose, preferably on an alternate-day schedule. If no response is observed after 3 to 4 weeks, alternative treatment should be instituted. If a therapeutic response is obtained and the patient can tolerate the drug, prednisone is given on a long-term basis, because the disease is recurrent and spontaneous remission is uncommon. The initial response rate to steroid therapy may be as high as 50 to 80%, but fewer than 20% of patients will be maintained on long-term corticosteroids, owing to relapse or adverse reactions (12, 16).

In patients who are refractory to steroid treatment or unable to tolerate long-term treatment, or in cases of life-threatening hemorrhage, splenectomy is usually considered next. Postulated mechanisms for efficacy include a reduction in the phagocytosis of antibody-coated platelets and a reduction of platelet-associated antibody production. It is important that the operative procedure include a search for and removal of all accessory splenic tissues. Corticosteroids or IVIG are often given before surgery to boost the platelet count and reduce the risk of perioperative bleeding. Polyvalent pneumococcal vaccine should be administered preoperatively. Some clinicians also advocate daily oral penicillin therapy for several years after surgery (2). A complete remission of AITP has been reported in up to 80% of patients following splenectomy (2, 16, 17). Platelet kinetic studies may be performed to assess the degree of splenic sequestration; this may assist in the decision to perform splenectomy. In one study, a platelet count greater than 120,000/mm^3 at the time of discharge, age less than 30 years, preoperative corticosteroid dependence, and splenic sequestration (measured preoperatively) were associated with a more favorable response to splenectomy (16).

The role of IVIG in treating chronic AITP is limited by its short duration of action. Although 90% of patients have a brisk increase in platelet count, this effect usually lasts less than 3 weeks, only about 10% of patients achieving a long-term remission. Repeated infusions usually give equivalent response rates. However, maintenance therapy with IVIG is not cost-effective. IVIG is therefore generally reserved for patients who have symptomatic bleeding or to prepare the patient for surgery or other invasive procedures.

The treatment of patients who are refractory to corticosteroids and splenectomy is problematic. Immunosuppressive therapy is usually considered next. Azathioprine, cyclophosphamide, and the vinca alkaloids (vincristine and vinblastine) are the most commonly used agents. Azathioprine is believed to interfere with the response of T-cells to antigenic challenge, with an additional more generalized reduction in T-helper activity. It is given in a dose of 1 to 3 mg/kg/day (or 100 to 200 mg/day); the dose is reduced if the patient becomes leukopenic (13). It is usually given in conjunction with steroids and may have a steroid-sparing effect for some patients (12). Approximately one-half of patients show an adequate platelet response over several months. The long-term response is approximately 40% at one year and 32% at two or more years (12). Side effects are usually less serious than with cyclophosphamide, bone marrow suppression being the most important. Azathioprine is considered the safest agent for long-term therapy.

Cyclophosphamide is given in an oral dose of 2 to 3 mg/kg/m^2 daily or 600 to 1000 mg/m^2 intravenously every 3 to 4 weeks (12). Improvement is usually seen in 2 to 6 weeks, with a maximum response in platelet count seen in 8 weeks. Treatment is continued for 4 to 6 weeks after an adequate platelet count is achieved. Studies demonstrating complete remission in 30 to 40% of patients are an advantage with cyclophosphamide. Unfortunately, side effects, including bone marrow suppression, hemorrhagic cystitis, and bladder fibrosis, may limit its use.

Vinca alkaloids have been reported to be beneficial in more than 50% of patients who are refractory to steroids and splenectomy. Vincristine (0.25 mg/kg to a maximum dose of 2 mg) and vinblastine (0.125 mg/kg to a maximum dose of 10 mg) are given intravenously every 2 to 6 weeks (12). Response occurs more rapidly than with azathioprine or cyclophosphamide, but relapses usually occur in 3 to 4 weeks. These agents are believed to decrease the rate of destruction of platelets by inhibiting phagocytosis and decreasing antibody levels (6). Vincristine may also bind selectively to platelet tubulin, such that when the antibody-coated platelet is phagocytosed, the macrophages are poisoned. Vincristine and vinblastine have been loaded onto platelets in an attempt to deliver them selectively to macrophages that are responsible for platelet destruction, but this is not commonly done because of its impracticality and lack of advantage over conventional administration. The incidence of side effects is relatively high with the vinca alkaloids. Vincristine may cause transient malaise, fever after injection, temporary jaw pain, alopecia, and a variety of neuropathies. Leukopenia, abdominal pain, and headache are associated with vinblastine.

Danazol, an anabolic steroid, is thought to decrease phagocytosis of platelets by decreasing the number of phagocytic cell IgG Fc-receptors (6). Doses are usually between 400 to 800 mg/day initially, then tapered to 50 to 200 mg daily. Clinical response is normally seen within 8 weeks. Side effect frequency is low and includes virilization, fibrinolysis, and hepatic dysfunction. Danazol is contraindicated during pregnancy.

Intravenous anti-Rh(D) immunoglobulin has been used with moderate success in the treatment of autoimmune thrombocytopenic purpura and in a few cases of refractory HIV-associated thrombocytopenia. The mechanism of action appears to be inhibition of reticuloendothelial system function; however, it does not appear to be effective in Rhesus-negative or splenectomized patients (12, 13).

Other therapies that have been studied in limited numbers of patients include colchicine, high-dose ascorbic acid, cyclosporine, interferon-α, and anti-Fc receptor monoclonal antibodies. Plasma transfusion and plasma exchange (plasmapheresis) may have some merit, especially in life-threatening emergencies, but for chronic AITP they are of little value.

HIV-Associated Thrombocytopenia. Patients with this syndrome are generally treated only when the thrombocytopenia is symptomatic. One approach is to control the underlying disease via the use of zidovudine or other antiretroviral agents. This treatment is founded on the hypothesis that HIV-associated thrombocytopenia is caused by a direct effect of the virus on the bone marrow and/or immune system. Zidovudine doses of 200 mg every 6 hr have yielded an increase in the platelet count over 2 to 6 weeks (6).

Most studies of corticosteroids in HIV-associated thrombocytopenia have reported a moderate to excellent initial response but a return to pretreatment values when the dose is reduced. The high rate of steroid-induced adverse effects, the low rate of sustained response, and the possibility of opportunistic infections must all be considered before corticosteroid therapy is used in treating patients with HIV-associated thrombocytopenia.

The use of IVIG in the treatment of HIV-associated thrombocytopenia shows a high initial response rate, ranging from 70 to 100% (18, 19). Because it does not increase susceptibility to opportunistic infections, IVIG therapy may be the treatment of choice for HIV-associated thrombocytopenia. However, the effect is usually only transient.

The efficacy of splenectomy in patients with HIV-associated thrombocytopenia is not well established. The literature reports effects ranging from increased platelet counts in 80% of patients receiving corticosteroids plus splenectomy (2, 8) to patients who show no response (6). Splenectomy, like corticosteroid therapy, may increase the susceptibility to opportunistic infections in patients with HIV-induced thrombocytopenia and may also increase the risk of progression to AIDS.

PROGNOSIS

The prognosis for the acute childhood form of AITP is excellent, more than 80% of patients showing spontaneous remission within 3 to 6 months of diagnosis. The major concern for the clinician is whether or not to treat a disease that is generally benign and self-limiting. The principal cause of mortality is intracranial bleeding, which carries an incidence that is inversely proportional to the platelet count and occurs during the first 2 weeks of onset in 1% of cases.

Although spontaneous complete remission of chronic AITP is unusual, the long-term prognosis is usually favorable. Most patients will maintain stable, mild to moderate thrombocytopenia. The objective of therapy in chronic AITP is to maintain the patient hemostatically safe (i.e., platelet counts higher than 30,000 to 50,000/mm^3), not necessarily to obtain a complete remission. A review of the literature on patients with refractory disease showed a median death rate of 5.1%, caused either by uncontrolled bleeding or by complications of the therapy. High-risk groups included patients with a history of bleeding, those with the concomitant presence of other bleeding disorders, and those older than 60 years of age (16).

The prognosis for HIV-associated thrombocytopenia is poor because of the underlying illness.

Thrombotic Thrombocytopenic Purpura

Thrombotic thrombocytopenic purpura (TTP) is an uncommon but devastating disorder of multiorgan involvement. The original triad of clinical characteristics consisting of thrombocytopenia, microangiopathic hemolytic anemia (hemolysis secondary to RBC fragmentation), and neurologic abnormalities has been expanded to a pentad with the addition of fever and renal dysfunction. Extensive widespread occlusion by platelets and hyaline material in the capillaries and arterioles (but not the venules) of nearly all organs is the hallmark of the disease and is responsible for the high mortality.

ETIOLOGY

Despite many theories about the exact cause of TTP, the primary cause remains puzzling. Immunologic abnormalities have been suspected because of the hemolytic anemia and thrombocytopenic purpura associated with the disease and because TTP has occurred in other diseases of an immune nature, such as systemic lupus erythematosus

(SLE), scleroderma, Sjögren's syndrome, and rheumatoid arthritis.

Precipitating factors may be found in as many as 70% of cases (20). Bacterial or viral infection is the most common (including HIV infection at any stage), occurring in up to 40% of patients. Pregnancy is the comorbid condition in 10 to 25%, with the disease occurring either antepartum or postpartum. Other precipitating conditions include postoperative status, myocardial infarction, lymphoma, carcinoma, bee stings, and dog bites. Drugs such as penicillins, sulfonamides, cyclosporine-A, penicillamine, oral contraceptives, iodine, ticlopidine, mitomycin, cisplatinum, and bleomycin have also been implicated.

EPIDEMIOLOGY

Although TTP has been reported in all age groups, ranging from infants to the very old, it occurs most commonly between the ages of 30 and 40. It is found in both genders, most studies showing females having a slightly higher occurrence (female:male = 3:2) (20). Most patients have previously enjoyed good health. The overall incidence in the population is not known but is believed to be small.

PATHOGENESIS

The pathogenesis of TTP is unknown. Many believe that the diffuse microvascular thrombi are caused by abnormal platelet aggregation, adhesion, and release on the microarterial endothelial surfaces, without activation of the coagulation cascade. Occlusive hyaline microthrombi in arterioles and capillaries are composed of fibrin and platelets and occur most commonly in the brain, heart, adrenals, kidney, pancreas, and lymph nodes (2, 20).

The numerous defects in patients with TTP suggest that more than one factor plays a role in its pathogenesis. Evidence suggests that mechanisms may include the following (20, 21):

1. Absent fibrinolytic activity in the area of microvascular thrombi but normal activity in the circulating blood.
2. Prostacyclin deficiency or diminished release. Prostacyclin causes vasodilation and is a natural inhibitor of platelet aggregation and adhesion. The lack of this factor would therefore favor vasoconstriction and platelet aggregation. Increased destruction and altered binding of prostacyclin have also been postulated.
3. An unknown substance that precipitates platelet aggregation may be present in the blood.
4. An unknown substance that prevents platelet aggregation may be lacking.
5. A defect in the production of plasma von Willebrand factor may cause the formation of abnormal large multimer fragments.

SIGNS AND SYMPTOMS

Presenting signs and symptoms of TTP are variable and nonspecific, including complaints of malaise, weakness, fatigue, abdominal pain, nausea and vomiting, arthralgia, fever, and hemorrhage. Neurologic symptoms such as headache, syncope, vertigo, ataxia, aphasia, behavioral or mental status changes, and seizures are the most frequent complaints. Signs of hemorrhage, including petechiae and purpura, are the next most common. Target organ dysfunction may also be seen in the eyes, heart, and lungs. Not all patients present with symptoms in each element of the previously described pentad.

DIAGNOSIS AND CLINICAL FINDINGS

TTP should be suspected in patients who have the symptoms mentioned above. The diagnosis can usually be confirmed by biopsy findings of subendothelial and intraluminal occlusive accumulation in arterioles and capillaries of fragmented platelets and fibrin deposits. Hematologic, neurologic, renal, cardiovascular, gastrointestinal, and pulmonary abnormalities all appear to be secondary to occlusion in the microcirculation. Severe microangiopathic hemolytic anemia associated with a negative Coomb's test is seen in the majority of patients. Bilirubin and lactate dehydrogenase levels are markedly elevated due to RBC hemolysis. The hemoglobin concentration averages 8 to 9 g/dL. Peripheral blood smears reveal odd-shaped fragmented and nucleated red blood cells, with an abundance of reticulocytes. Severe thrombocytopenia is invariably present, with platelet counts usually below 30,000 to 50,000/mm^3 and bone marrow biopsies showing large numbers of megakaryocytes. The coagulation screen is normal except for mild elevations in fibrin degradation products in up to 70% (20); this is a useful parameter for distinguishing TTP from disseminated intravascular coagulation. Renal involvement is present in 40% of patients (6), with laboratory tests showing proteinuria, microscopic hematuria, and elevated blood urea nitrogen and serum creatinine levels.

TREATMENT

In the past, TTP was almost uniformly fatal; but in the last 20 years, researchers have had remarkable success in devising treatment strategies. Therapies include plasma infusion or exchange, corticosteroids, splenectomy, antiplatelet agents, immunosuppressive, and cytotoxic agents. Success is unpredictable, each approach showing some benefit in certain individuals but little benefit in others. The individual effectiveness of each modality is not known, since several or all are commonly administered simultaneously.

Plasmapheresis (exchange transfusion with fresh frozen plasma) is the treatment of choice for TTP, producing a response rate near 80% (2). When this procedure is not available, infusions of fresh frozen plasma are instituted, although this yields a lower overall response rate. The therapeutic rationale for plasmapheresis is to remove toxic substances and immune complexes and/or to replace deficient factor(s) that are responsible for the inhibition of platelet aggregation or stimulation of prostacyclin. The fact that some patients improve with plasma infusion alone suggests a deficiency of an unknown factor. Plasmapheresis has been associated with a higher response rate and lower mortality than plasma infusion, although it is technically more difficult and expensive. It should be initiated as soon as possible, with a single plasma volume exchange daily until clinical manifestations improve and the platelet count exceeds 150,000/mm^3 for 2 to 3 days (6, 20). Plasma exchange is then gradually replaced by plasma infusion. Adverse effects of plasma therapy include hypersensitivity reactions, acute infection, hepatitis, and volume overload (seen primarily with plasma infusion). Patients who respond poorly to plasmapheresis with fresh frozen plasma may benefit from the substitution of cryosupernatant as the replacement solution (20, 21).

Corticosteroids are of unknown benefit but are almost universally used, in part because the differential diagnosis often includes vasculitis or other steroid-responsive diseases. Prednisone is begun at 1 to 1.5 mg/kg/day (or its equivalent), in conjunction with other therapeutic modalities (6, 20, 21). The dose is then slowly tapered. Corticosteroids alone are not generally effective in treating the acute disease but may be useful in combination with other therapies. They are also used (alone or in combination) to reduce the remission rate and treat relapses.

Antiplatelet agents such as aspirin and dipyridamole are commonly administered in the acute phase. However, in some cases they may worsen bleeding without providing a beneficial effect (2, 6). After remission is achieved, maintenance doses of aspirin and dipyridamole may be given for prevention of relapse. The antiplatelet agent ticlopidine should not be used, since it has been implicated as a causative factor in some cases of TTP. Infusions of prostacyclin have been administered, since deficiencies of this vasodilator and platelet aggregation inhibitor have been observed in patients with TTP. The effectiveness of this modality has been questionable, and its use is restricted to patients who are unresponsive to other treatments. Sulfinpyrazone and dextran are also reserved for refractory patients.

Splenectomy is reserved for patients who fail to respond to other therapies and those who cannot be weaned off plasma therapy. It has also been shown to reduce the relapse rate. Vincristine may be given in severe cases at a dosage of 2 mg weekly (20, 21). IVIG has shown variable effect and is used only in refractory patients.

Platelet transfusions have been shown to worsen the microvascular occlusion and are therefore not given (2, 20, 21). Because TTP is a disease of the platelets, heparin has no beneficial effect and can even be harmful by increasing the risk of bleeding.

Supportive care for the associated symptoms should be provided. Hemodialysis may be necessary for patients with severe renal failure.

Relapses of TTP are generally milder in severity than the initial presentation. They are treated with plasma infusion (plasmapheresis is reserved for severe cases) or aspirin and dipyridamole combined with corticosteroids. To prevent relapse, aspirin, dipyridamole, and steroids may also be given as prophylaxis for patients with severe infections, postoperatively, and in subsequent pregnancies. Splenectomy is another useful measure for preventing relapses. Patient education is important to facilitate prompt evaluation and treatment of relapses.

PROGNOSIS

Before 1965, TTP was considered an infrequent, complicated, progressive, and nearly always fatal disease. Without treatment, TTP remains a fatal disorder in 80 to 90% of cases. Fortunately, with advances in the understanding and treatment of the disease, up to 70 to 80% of patients can now be expected to survive with appropriate treatment, most with few or no sequelae (20, 21). Early intervention minimizes the risk of long-term neurologic or renal sequelae.

The improved survival rate has resulted in larger numbers of patients with relapsed or chronic disease. Approximately 15 to 50% of TTP survivors will relapse (2, 20). Relapses are usually milder than the initial disease. They occur at intervals of months or years, and the patient is relatively healthy in the interim periods.

Platelet Function Disorders

Disorders of platelet function may cause bleeding or thrombosis independent of the platelet count. Congenital disorders of platelet function are rare and encompass defects in any of the four previously described actions. Acquired platelet function disorders are common, often associated with clinically significant bleeding, and may be caused by medical conditions as well as a variety of drugs.

Uremia is a commonly encountered medical condition that is associated with a variety of platelet function defects. Almost all uremic patients have prolonged bleeding times and abnormal in vitro platelet function (3), with a correlation between the bleeding time prolongation and the degree of renal insufficiency. The abnormalities are thought to be caused by unknown substances that are present in uremic plasma, since most defects abate with dialysis or improved renal function. Most patients experience bleeding, but this is rarely a cause of serious morbidity.

Cardiac bypass induces a platelet function disorder that is caused by factors related to the bypass procedure itself. Most defects correct spontaneously after completion of the bypass. Other conditions that are associated with abnormalities in platelet function include liver disease, dysproteinemias (e.g., multiple myeloma or macroglobulinemia), and myeloproliferative disorders.

The management of patients with platelet function disorders consists of both supportive care and administration of specific agents to improve platelet function. Supportive measures include avoidance of situations that are associated with a high risk of bleeding and medications that alter platelet function or numbers (Table 15.2). The underlying disorder should be corrected or treated when possible. Platelet transfusions are useful for postbypass patients but are otherwise avoided unless bleeding is life-threatening. For uremic patients with bleeding, desmopressin or conjugated estrogens will correct the bleeding time and slow clinical bleeding (3). Oral contraceptives may be given to reduce menorrhagia.

Drug-Induced Platelet Disorders

The pharmacist must recognize drugs that adversely affect platelets. Avoidance of their use entirely or close monitoring of platelet counts and function may be necessary for certain patients. Familiarity with these agents also facilitates assessment of drugs as potential causative factors in patients with platelet abnormalities. Although many drugs adversely affect platelet activity, the literature must be evaluated carefully before an "anti-platelet" label is placed on a therapeutic agent that only rarely produces clinically significant manifestations.

Drug-induced platelet disorders include those that alter platelet function and those that cause thrombocytopenia. Drug-induced disorders of platelet function are further subdivided (in descending order of prevalence) into drug interference with (1) platelet membranes or membrane receptor sites, (2) prostaglandin biosynthetic pathways, (3) phosphodiesterase activity, and (4) unknown mechanisms (22). Drug-induced thrombocytopenia may be caused by either decreased production or increased destruction of platelets. Table 15.2 lists commonly implicated drugs and their proposed mechanisms of action.

Aspirin is by far the most common and well-documented cause of drug-induced platelet dysfunction. This is mediated by aspirin-induced abnormalities on both platelets and endothelial cells. At the platelet level, aspirin irreversibly acetylates cyclooxygenase. This reduces platelet synthesis of cyclic endoperoxides and thromboxane A_2, resulting in loss of thromboxane A_2-mediated platelet stimulation and vasoconstriction. Endothelial cell cyclooxygenase activity is also inhibited, with a corresponding reduction in prostacyclin production and loss of platelet inhibition and vasodilation. Platelets cannot regenerate cyclooxygenase; therefore the effect of aspirin on thromboxane A_2 is irreversible. In contrast, endothelial cells can synthesize new cyclooxygenase; therefore prostacyclin synthesis resumes after the aspirin is metabolized. The

net effect of aspirin reflects its action on the platelets and endothelial cells. The irreversible loss of platelet cyclooxygenase often dominates, with a reduction in platelet stimulation. The peak effect of a single dose occurs in 2 to 4 hr, but because aspirin's effect on platelets is irreversible, its pharmacodynamic activity may last up to 10 days or the lifespan of the platelet. When aspirin is administered to a normal person, bleeding time is prolonged by a factor of 1.5 to 2 (3), but significant bleeding is uncommon. Aspirin may be associated with clinically significant hemorrhage when the hemostatic system is stressed (e.g., surgery or other invasive procedure), in the elderly, in hemophiliacs, in patients with coexisting thrombocytopenia or other bleeding risk (e.g., peptic ulcer disease), in patients taking other drugs with antiplatelet effect, or in patients undergoing neurologic or ophthalmic surgery. It should also be avoided late in pregnancy.

Other nonsteroidal antiinflammatory agents such as indomethacin, ibuprofen, naproxen, piroxicam, and ketorolac also prevent thromboxane A_2 generation by inhibiting platelet cyclooxygenase (3, 22). In these cases the platelet effect is reversible, occurring only while the drug is present in the circulation. The bleeding time is only slightly prolonged, and the effects abate as the drug is cleared from the plasma.

Dipyridamole is sometimes used therapeutically for its antithrombotic activity, usually in combination with aspirin. The mode of action is believed to be prevention of cyclic AMP breakdown by inhibition of phosphodiesterase activity. Increased platelet cyclic AMP levels inhibit platelet aggregation and release. Unlike aspirin, dipyridamole does not alter bleeding time or platelet survival.

Ticlopidine-induced antiplatelet effects occur via a mechanism that is not well established. Ticlopidine induces a thrombastheniclike state without altering the expression of platelet membrane receptors. This may occur via inhibition of common signal transduction pathways in platelets. The drug prolongs bleeding time; however, severe hemorrhage is not a prominent side effect (3).

Penicillin and related compounds prolong bleeding time and occasionally have clinically important effects on platelet function. These effects are mediated by an interaction with platelet membrane receptors that reduces responsiveness to stimulation by ADP and epinephrine and decreases platelet aggregation (3). Platelet dysfunction begins several days after initiation and abates several days after discontinuation of the drug. High-dose carbenicillin is the prototype example of this effect. Penicillin G, ampicillin, ticarcillin, piperacillin, methicillin, and nafcillin have all been implicated as having similar effects. Cephalosporins may also alter platelet function, although this effect is not as well documented. The clinical relevance of this effect is not well established. Significant bleeding is uncommon unless the patient has other risk factors such as renal failure or ulcer disease.

Dextran, a partially hydrolyzed polymer of glucose, is used as a plasma volume expander in certain types of shock, impaired renal function, and other conditions in which improved circulation is desirable. It also prolongs bleeding time, impairs fibrin polymerization, decreases blood viscosity, and alters platelet function. For these reasons, dextran is sometimes used in the prophylaxis of venous thrombosis and pulmonary thromboembolism. The mechanism of the antiplatelet activity is uncertain but may involve inhibition of platelet aggregation and reduced platelet agonist activity. Dextran should be used with caution in treating patients with coexisting thrombocytopenia.

Alcohol impairs platelet function and primary hemostasis. Large quantities of ethanol can inhibit prostaglandin endoperoxide synthesis and decrease thromboxane A_2 production, thereby causing a decrease in platelet aggregation and release. Alcohol ingestion may also directly suppress bone marrow thrombocyte production. Alcoholism can decrease ADP storage pools and platelet agonist (ADP, epinephrine) activity. Moreover, alcoholism is associated with other factors that may cause platelet dysfunction. Alcohol-mediated platelet dysfunction can occur in the absence of liver disease and is reversible; the platelet count returns to baseline 7 to 21 days after discontinuation (6).

Drug-induced immune thrombocytopenia is a relatively uncommon platelet disorder that is caused by a number of drugs. Two mechanisms have been postulated:

1. Formation of an immunoglobulin-drug immune complex that attaches to and destroys the platelet, via either accelerated reticuloendothelial system phagocytosis or complement-associated intravascular lysis. In this scenario the platelet is considered an "innocent bystander."
2. Binding of the drug to the platelet membrane, creating a hapten that induces a structural change, ultimately resulting in the formation of antiplatelet antibodies.

Drug-induced immune thrombocytopenia is more common in adults, is not dose-related, and is associated with antibody persistence for many years. The clinical presentation of petechiae, purpura, and mucous membrane bleeding is similar to the chronic form of autoimmune thrombocytopenia. However, its rapid onset (6 to 12 hr after reexposure), the severity of both symptoms and thrombocytopenia (commonly less than 10,000/mm^3), and the rapid sustained recovery after the drug is terminated are distinguishing features of the drug-induced form (2, 23). The primary management is discontinuation of the drug. Platelet destruction generally abates in 3 to 7 days but may persist for weeks to months after discontinuation in some patients. High-dose IVIG or a short course of

corticosteroids may be given to shorten the recovery period (23). Plasmapheresis may be used for critically ill patients. Drug-induced immune thrombocytopenia has been best documented with heparin, gold, quinidine, and quinine (which may be used therapeutically or found in soft drinks and street drugs). Other common drugs that cause this syndrome are listed in Table 15.2.

Heparin is the most common cause of drug-induced thrombocytopenia, with an overall incidence of 3 to 5% with intravenous therapy (23, 24) and fewer than 3% developing platelet counts less than 100,000/mm^3. The incidence is much lower with subcutaneous administration, yet this syndrome has been seen after the use of the small doses used in heparin flushes or even in patients with heparin-coated intravenous catheters. Thrombocytopenia is more common with bovine-derived heparin (versus porcine). Heparin causes two types of platelet disorders. In Type I a mild gradual thrombocytopenia develops over the first few days of treatment. Platelet counts rarely fall below 100,000/mm^3. The thrombocytopenia usually resolves spontaneously, even with continued heparin therapy. It is not dose-dependent and is thought to be caused by an induced platelet proaggregant effect that results in enhanced sequestration and destruction (25). Most patients are asymptomatic, and treatment is not indicated. Type II is much less common, appearing after 5 to 14 days of therapy (unless the patient has been previously exposed). Characteristics include platelet counts of 60,000 to 100,000/mm^3 that remain low until the drug is discontinued. After heparin is stopped, platelet counts return to normal values in 5 to 7 days. A common hypothesis proposes the formation of a platelet-associated IgG that reacts with heparin, forming a heparin-antibody immune complex. This complex binds to platelet Fc receptors, which causes in vivo platelet activation and aggregation (25). The resultant "paradoxical" thrombosis may be arterial (more common) or venous, may occur at multiple sites, and in some cases is devastating. Concomitant with the onset of thrombocytopenia, extensive arterial or venous thrombosis with limb ischemia or gangrene, myocardial infarction, stroke, recurrent pulmonary embolism, and skin necrosis have been observed. Treatment of Type I consists of monitoring the platelet count every 2 to 3 days. In Type II, heparin should be immediately discontinued, and alternative anticoagulants such as dextran, aspirin, thrombolytics, and/or warfarin should be initiated. Platelet counts should return to normal a few days after discontinuation (23). Unfortunately, thrombectomy or limb amputation may be necessary in some Type II cases, and mortality may be as high as 30% (25). A high in vitro cross-reaction rate has been reported with various low-molecular-weight heparins (25). These should therefore also be avoided unless a lack of cross-reactivity has been demonstrated.

Cytotoxic agents can cause thrombocytopenia because of their myelosuppressive action on the hematopoietic system. In contrast to other forms of drug-induced thrombocytopenia, which affect mature platelets in the circulation, antineoplastic agents cause a dose-dependent reduction in bone marrow platelet precursors. Precursors of all three cell lines (white blood cell (WBC), RBC, thrombocyte) are suppressed, the onset and severity being related to the lifespan of existing cells. In this regard, thrombocytopenia is intermediate, occurring gradually over 7 to 10 days (26). Host factors such as age, nutritional status, and preexisting bone marrow compromise affect the severity and symptoms. Drugs that may cause significant bone marrow suppression include cytarabine, the nitrosoureas, busulfan, methotrexate, cyclophosphamide, and mercaptopurine (6, 23). Busulfan may cause a severe prolonged thrombocytopenia due to an irreversible reduction in the number of marrow stem cells. Vincristine is an exception and may even stimulate thrombopoiesis (5, 23). The primary management consists of prophylactic platelet transfusions when the counts fall below 10,000 to 20,000/ mm^3, single-donor platelets being preferable because of a lower incidence of alloimmunization (26). When possible, chemotherapeutic regimens should be tailored to avoid the simultaneous administration of drugs that are known to cause this effect. A new therapeutic approach is the administration of interleukins; several have megakaryocyte stimulating properties.

Cocaine may also display a toxic effect on megakaryocytes, causing oropharyngeal and mucous membrane bleeding with platelet counts less than 10,000/mm^3 (6). This effect is unrelated to the route of administration. Bone marrow aspiration demonstrates a reduced number of megakaryocytes, without involvement of the WBC and RBC cell lines. The platelet count generally increases over 2 to 3 weeks after discontinuation of the drug.

Disseminated Intravascular Coagulation

PATHOGENESIS

Disseminated intravascular coagulation (DIC) is an intermediary syndrome caused by a second coexisting disease. The activating conditions encompass a broad spectrum of unrelated events (Table 15.3). Infection is the most common associated disorder, meningococcemia being the prototype. The precipitating conditions share as a common feature a breakdown of the intricate balance between coagulation and fibrinolysis, the systems that maintain blood in a fluid state within the vasculature. In DIC, simultaneous in vivo activation of the coagulation and fibrinolytic systems results in both thrombosis and hemorrhage. The clinical manifestations of DIC are highly variable and depend on the underlying disease process and the relative balance between coagulation and fibrinolysis in the individual patient.

Although the activating disease states are variable, once initiated, DIC results in the same pathophysiologic sequence: (1) In vivo activation of the coagulation system resulting in intravascular thrombin generation, (2) intravascular fibrin clot formation with end-organ ischemia, (3) activation of the fibrinolytic systems, and (4) depletion of blood coagulation proteins and platelets. The stronger the triggering process and the longer the process continues, the more severe the associated DIC.

In Vivo Activation of the Coagulation System. The triggering event for DIC is the release of procoagulant material into the circulation due to either vascular endothelial or tissue injury. The smooth layer lining the vascular endothelium normally repels clotting factors and platelets. Exposure to toxins or inflammatory mediators (e.g., endotoxins produced by Gram-negative bacteria) may disrupt the endothelium, resulting in platelet aggregation, activation of factor XII, and initiation of the intrinsic pathway. Activation of the extrinsic system may also occur when burns, trauma, obstetric accidents, or malignancies (especially leukemia) cause tissue injury or production of procoagulant material, resulting in the release of tissue thromboplastin (27). Activation of the intrinsic or extrinsic pathway results in intravascular thrombin generation.

Intravascular Fibrin Clot Formation with End-Organ Damage. In the presence of thrombin, fibrinogen is cleaved into fibrinopeptides A and B and fibrin monomer (Fig. 15.4, left column). Fibrin monomer is then polymerized to form a fibrin clot. Polymerized fibrin is deposited in the microvascular circulation and entraps platelets, forming microthrombi. Platelet-rich microthrombi are subsequently replaced by fibrin-rich hyaline microthrombi (28). Continued thrombin generation results in macrovascular thrombosis, ischemia, and eventual end-organ damage, which can be formidable.

Activation of the Fibrinolytic Systems. Fibrin clot activates the fibrinolytic system, beginning with plasminogen conversion to plasmin by tissue plasminogen activator (t-PA) (Fig. 15.3). Plasmin digests the fibrin clot by converting it to fibrin degradation products (FDP), which include X, Y, D, and E fragments, D-dimer, and other peptides. The D and E fragments induce a profound platelet function defect, which exacerbates bleeding. FDP also independently act as anticoagulants by interfering with fibrin polymerization and forming soluble fibrin monomer; this also worsens bleeding.

Plasmin is a broadly active serine protease that is also able to inactivate other substances. Activation of the complement system (Fig. 15.3) results in increased vascular permeability, hypotension, and RBC and platelet lysis (causing the production of more procoagulant and further worsening the thrombocytopenia). Plasmin is also capable of inactivating coagulation factors V, VIII:C, IX, and XI,

Table 15.3.
Conditions Associated with DIC

Acute (Fulminant)	Chronic (Low Grade)
Infection	Malignancy
Bacterial	Leukemia
Gram-negative (endotoxin)	Most metastatic solid malignancies
Gram-positive (mucopolysaccharides)	Cardiovascular disease
Viral	Aortic aneurysm
Cytomegalovirus	Giant hemangioma
Hepatitis	Collagen vascular disorders
Varicella	Systemic lupus erythematosus
Human immunodeficiency virus (HIV)	Rheumatoid arthritis
Rickettsial	Sjögren's syndrome
Rocky mountain spotted fever	Dermatomyositis
Others (mycoplasmal, chlamydial, fungal, mycobacterial, protozoal)	Renal vascular disorders
Obstetric accidents	Hematologic disorders
Amniotic fluid embolism	Polycythemia rubra vera
Placental abruption	Inflammatory disorders
Retained fetus syndrome	Crohn's disease
Eclampsia	Ulcerative colitis
Abortion	Sarcoidosis
Tissue injury	Eclampsia
Burns	
Crush injuries and tissue necrosis	
Multiple trauma	
Head trauma	
Extensive surgery	
Malignancy	
Leukemia	
Acute promyelocytic (M-3)	
Acute myelomonocytic (M-4)	
Most metastatic solid malignancies	
Others (pheochromocytoma, myeloma, neuroblastoma, sarcoma, histiocytosis X, polycythemia vera)	
Chemotherapy for leukemia (massive blast cell lysis)	
Intravascular hemolysis	
Hemolytic transfusion reaction	
Minor hemolysis	
Massive transfusion	
Acute liver disease	
Obstructive jaundice	
Acute hepatic failure	
Prosthetic devices	
LeVeen or Denver shunt	
Aortic balloon assist device	
Cardiovascular	
Postcardiac arrest	
Aortic aneurysm	
Giant hemangiomas	
Acute myocardial infarction	
Peripheral vascular disorders	
Pulmonary	
Adult respiratory distress syndrome (ARDS)	
Pulmonary embolism or infarction	
Hyaline membrane disease	
Miscellaneous	
Snake bite envenomation	
Hyperthermia or hypothermia	
Heat stroke	
Aspirin or organic solvent poisoning	

Adapted from (27, 28).

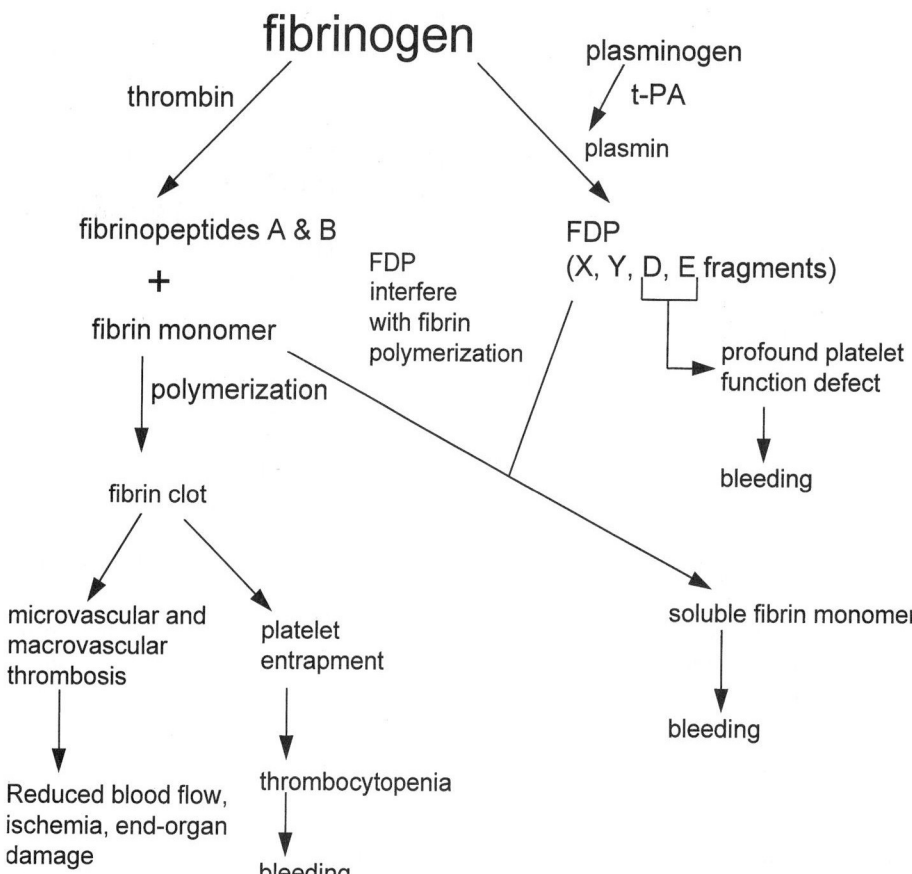

Figure 15.4. Pathogenesis of disseminated intravascular coagulation (DIC).

growth hormone, ACTH, and insulin (28). Plasmin also degrades both fibrinogen and fibrin with equal affinity. Breakdown of fibrinogen (Fig. 15.4, right column) results in even higher plasma concentrations of fibrinogen degradation products (also called FDP and including X, Y, D, and E fragments, but not D-dimer) with bleeding consequences as above.

Depletion of Blood Coagulation Proteins and Platelets. The ongoing processes of fibrin formation and breakdown result in consumptive depletion of coagulation factors, natural anticoagulants, and platelets. The intensity and duration of the DIC determine the degree of depletion.

The simultaneous presence of thrombin and plasmin in the systemic circulation generates a paradox of concurrent clotting and bleeding. Polymerized fibrin clot and microthrombi result in thrombosis and ischemia. At the same time, fibrinolysis, depletion of coagulation factors, natural anticoagulant proteins, and platelets, coupled with the platelet function disorder, cause hemorrhage. Hence DIC is sometimes called a "thrombo-hemorrhagic" disease, or "consumptive coagulopathy." Depending on the balance between coagulation and fibrinolysis, both processes may

be clinically evident in DIC, although sometimes one dominates over the other. In infection, thrombosis usually predominates. In acute leukemia, bleeding is the primary manifestation (27).

CLINICAL PRESENTATION AND DIAGNOSIS

The diagnosis of DIC is established when all four processes above occur in a patient who also has a condition that is known to be a precipitating cause. Prompt diagnosis requires a high index of suspicion and aggressive laboratory testing. Signs and symptoms are variable and confusing because of the wide spectrum of manifestations contributed by the coagulopathy and the underlying disease. In some patients the diagnosis is obvious (e.g., gangrene of the extremities, bleeding, and multiorgan failure in a patient with meningococcemia). In others there may be mild or no bleeding at all, clinically silent microvascular thrombosis, and only subtle laboratory abnormalities. A single patient may manifest one or more of these findings alone, simultaneously, or serially at different times in the disease process (29). The clinical presentation is further complicated by the signs and symptoms of the underlying disorder. The total picture for an individual patient therefore reflects both the DIC and the underlying disorder and depends on the tissues and organs that are involved and the severity of the DIC and disease processes. Vigilant correlation of physical examination and laboratory results is essential in the diagnosis, management, and evaluation of DIC.

In general, there are two modes of presentation of DIC: acute and chronic.

Acute ("fulminant") DIC is more common than the chronic form. In acute DIC the clinical and laboratory features develop rapidly (over a few hours to days), often with catastrophic consequences. The patient is critically ill from the underlying disease as well as the DIC. Acute DIC usually presents with both bleeding and thrombosis, bleeding being more clinically evident in most patients. Hemorrhage can range from low-grade oozing to massive bleeding. Bleeding from multiple sites is usually seen, since even small wounds lack normal hemostasis (Table 15.4). Areas of trauma, surgery, or other invasive procedures or pathology are common sources of bleeding. In the skin, microvascular thrombosis of end-arterioles with concurrent bleeding results in symptoms ranging from petechiae to gangrene. End-organ dysfunction secondary to microvascular and macrovascular thrombosis is also common, although it should be recognized that organ failure may also be due to the underlying disease. End-organ malfunction is often less evident clinically but

requires early identification and treatment to avoid irreversible damage. The most frequently affected organ systems (respiratory, renal, central nervous, cardiovascular, and hepatic) will exhibit progressive organ failure (Table 15.4). Fluid and electrolyte disorders and fever are also commonly seen. Pallor and jaundice secondary to microangiopathic hemolytic anemia are less common. The intermingling of these findings with those of the underlying disease make the diagnosis of DIC impossible without coagulation studies.

The coagulation laboratory findings associated with acute DIC encompass a wide spectrum. Unfortunately, there is no single test for DIC with acceptable specificity, sensitivity, and widespread availability. Specific criteria for the laboratory diagnosis of DIC have been published (28), but they rely on assays of biochemical markers that are often available only in research institutions (e.g., prothrombin fragment 1 + 2, fibrinopeptides A and B, thrombin-antithrombin complex, plasmin-antiplasmin complex, α_2-antiplasmin). The most useful readily available tests include the FDP (or D-dimer) level, platelet count, fibrinogen level, protamine sulfate test, and prothrombin time (PT) (Table 15.5) (28, 29). FDP levels are elevated to greater than 40 µg/mL in almost all patients. FDP levels are considered a sensitive but not specific test for DIC, since they do not distinguish between fibrin versus fibrinogen degradation. D-dimer is a specific biochemical

Table 15.4.
Signs and Symptoms of Acute DIC

Hemorrhage	Thrombosis
Surgical or trauma sites	Skin and soft tissue
Wound bleeding	Cyanosis of hands, feet, nose, cheeks
Internal bleeding	Acral cyanosis
Skin and soft tissue	Cold, mottled fingers, toes, hands, feet
Oozing at venipuncture, IV catheter insertion,	Purpura
and arterial-line sites	Infarction, necrosis or gangrene of digits, hands, feet, nose, earlobes
Petechiae, purpura	Venous thromboembolism
Ecchymoses	End-organ dysfunction
Spreading hematomas	Lung (hypoxia, acidosis, respiratory failure, adult respiratory distress syndrome [ARDS])
Hemorrhagic bullae	Kidney (elevated BUN, creatinine, oliguria, proteinuria, hematuria, acute renal failure)
Ear, nose, throat	Central nervous system (altered mental status, seizures, coma)
Gingival or oral mucosal bleeding	Cardiovascular (hypotension, shock, hemodynamic instability or failure)
Epistaxis	Liver (elevated ALT, AST)
Respiratory	Gastrointestinal (vomiting, diarrhea, abdominal distress, ileus)
Blood-tinged respiratory secretions	
Gastrointestinal	
Hematemesis	
Blood in nasogastric secretions (occult or gross)	
Fecal blood (occult or gross)	
Urinary	
Hematuria	

BUN = Blood urea nitrogen.
ALT = alanine aminotransferase.
AST = aspartate aminotransferase.
Adapted from (27, 29).

Table 15.5.
Laboratory Findings in Acute DIC

	Reference range	Findings in DIC
Fibrin degradation products	<10 µg/mL	Increased
D-dimer	<500 ng/mL	Increased
Platelet count	150,000–400,000/mm³	Decreased
Fibrinogen	200–400 mg/dL	Decreased
Protamine sulfate	Negative	Positive
Prothrombin time	0.88–1.12 INR	Increased

INR = international normalized ratio.
Adapted from (27, 29).

marker for fibrin breakdown; assays are therefore more useful, although they are not always available (27, 28). Thrombocytopenia is a cardinal finding. The platelet count is less than 50,000 to 60,000/mm³ in about 50% of cases (range: 2,000 to 100,000/mm³). Results of platelet function tests such as template bleeding time or platelet aggregation studies are abnormal in almost all patients as well (27, 28). The plasma fibrinogen level is less than 150 mg/dL in 70 to 80% of patients; levels less than 50 mg/dL are often associated with severe bleeding. A normal fibrinogen level may be observed in DIC associated with pregnancy, sepsis, or malignancy, since the baseline fibrinogen level may be elevated in these conditions (29–31). Conversely, liver disease is associated with low baseline fibrinogen levels. The protamine sulfate test measures the presence of circulating soluble fibrin monomer. It is usually positive in DIC, although it is not specific for this disease process. The prothrombin time (PT) is prolonged in 50 to 75% of patients with DIC, owing to factor consumption (27). Unfortunately, the PT may be normal or even shorter than the control in as many as 50% of patients; this test is therefore less useful in diagnosing DIC.

Other laboratory tests are commonly performed in the screening and evaluation of patients with suspected acute DIC but have limited value. These include the activated partial thromboplastin time (aPTT), thrombin clotting time (TCT or TT), euglobulin clot lysis time, coagulation factor assays, and peripheral blood smear examination. The aPTT is prolonged in 50 to 60% of patients with acute DIC, but it may also be normal or short (27, 28) and is therefore unreliable for patient assessment. Likewise, the TT may be prolonged, the euglobulin clot lysis time may be shortened, and blood coagulation factor levels are often low, but these findings are not reliable and do not add meaningful information. Examination of the peripheral blood smear provides evidence of RBC fragmentation, mild reticulocytosis, mild leukocytosis with a mild to moderate shift to immature neutrophil forms ("left shift"), and thrombocytopenia with large young platelets. Unfortunately, these findings also lack specificity and sensitivity.

Chronic ("low-grade" or "compensated") DIC is characterized by abnormal low-grade coagulation and fibrinolysis accompanying an array of less acute conditions (Table 15.4). It is often stated that chronic DIC is less common than the acute form. However, the subtle manifestations of this form may contribute to underdiagnosis. Many believe that acute and chronic DIC are simply different phases in the continuum of a single disease. Chronic DIC is not generally considered an emergency. Clinical findings are less florid, and laboratory abnormalities are more subtle. Enhanced turnover with increased production of platelets, fibrinogen, and coagulation proteins may yield normal or near-normal levels. If the rate of fibrinolysis is sufficient to balance the rate of fibrin formation, there may be no obvious clinical symptoms. Patients with chronic DIC uniformly have elevated D-dimer levels. Measurement of D-dimer (or FDP) levels are therefore very useful in establishing the diagnosis.

Over time these patients may develop overt problems, especially thrombotic complications such as thrombophlebitis, pulmonary embolism, or stroke (29, 31). Patients with metastatic malignancies often manifest DIC as a "hypercoagulable syndrome" with recurrent local or diffuse thrombotic events. Trousseau's syndrome, a recurrent migratory venous thrombosis, is a variant of this condition (31). Subacute or "bothersome" bleeding may also be seen. It is important to recognize that patients with chronic DIC may develop the acute form under hemostatic stress, such as surgery or invasive procedures.

In summary, no single physical finding or laboratory test is diagnostic for acute or chronic DIC. Careful physical examination and laboratory assessment, combined with vigilance and good judgment, are essential in establishing the diagnosis. Normal D-dimer (or FDP) levels make DIC unlikely. A combination of elevated D-dimer (or FDP) level, thrombocytopenia, low or falling fibrinogen (in the absence of liver disease), a positive protamine sulfate test, and a prolonged PT in a patient with a disease that is known to cause DIC will establish the diagnosis in most patients, the degree of abnormality roughly correlating with disease acuity. These tests are also the most useful in monitoring the response to therapy.

MANAGEMENT

The cornerstone of DIC management is treatment of the underlying disease and supportive therapy of the signs and symptoms. This along with careful observation and follow-up may be the only required measures for some patients.

Acute DIC with life-threatening hemorrhage and thrombosis requires complex management and intensive monitoring. Prompt and aggressive treatment to control or correct the underlying disorder is imperative. Without this, the stimulus for DIC will continue, and additional corrective measures might not be successful. Patients also require vigorous supportive therapy. Acid-base, fluid and electrolyte, hemodynamic, respiratory, and renal disturbances must be effectively managed. Intramuscular medications and venipunctures should be minimized to avoid additional sites of bleeding and hematoma formation. Frequent clinical and laboratory monitoring is essential. If treatment of the underlying disease and supportive therapy are timely and successful and the laboratory parameters are improving, the need for additional treatment should be transient; in some cases, no further therapy will be required. Aggressive antibiotic therapy for sepsis or evacuation of the uterus for an obstetric accident are examples in which successful treatment of the underlying disorder alone may resolve the DIC. In other situations, efforts to treat the precipitating disease are unsuccessful or inadequate, and/or the manifestations fail to improve. Patients with acute leukemia may even suffer an initial worsening of the DIC after administration of chemotherapy, due to massive blast cell lysis with subsequent generation of large amounts of procoagulant.

Specific treatment modalities for acute DIC beyond supportive care and treatment of the underlying diseases are highly controversial, are poorly documented, and lack consensus. A general lack of prospective randomized clinical trials exists, largely because of the complex spectrum of underlying diseases and clinical manifestations. Published trials are difficult to compare because of differences in diagnostic and outcome criteria. Moreover, patient outcomes are often contingent more on the underlying disease than on the DIC. Individualization of therapy is essential. Treatment may involve measures to (a) interrupt the coagulation process, (b) replace depleted coagulation factors and platelets, and/or (c) interrupt fibrinolysis.

Measures to interrupt the coagulation process include administration of anticoagulants and replacement of natural anticoagulant proteins. Although bleeding is often more obvious and alarming, thrombosis is more dangerous and has more impact on morbidity and mortality because of its potential to cause irreversible ischemic end-organ damage (28). Unfortunately, prospective, randomized studies of heparin use in DIC are lacking and impractical to perform because of variability in the clinical manifestations and precipitating disorders. Anecdotal evidence suggests that some patients benefit in terms of hemorrhage control and survival (29, 30). Heparin is clearly indicated for patients with thrombosis and has been associated with a reduction in mortality (31). All patients should be carefully monitored for evidence of microvascular and macrovascular thrombosis, including progressive organ failure (Table 15.4). Immediate heparin therapy is required if necrosis, gangrene, and irreversible end-organ damage are to be prevented.

The use of heparin in the treatment of patients with DIC and hemorrhage but no clear-cut evidence of fibrin deposition is controversial. Since bleeding in acute DIC is due to massive coagulation cascade activation with subsequent depletion of clotting factors and platelets, it seems reasonable to interrupt this process with heparin. Heparin will also inhibit the growth of existing thrombi, thereby stabilizing the coagulation system while the underlying disease is treated (28, 29, 31). However, heparin is also a potent anticoagulant and carries its own risks, including further bleeding. Patients with acute DIC and bleeding therefore usually receive heparin in conjunction with blood component replacement.

The timing of heparin administration relative to blood component replacement in patients with hemorrhage but no clinical evidence of thrombosis is debatable. Many clinicians recommend anticoagulants *before* blood component replacement therapy. This is based on the theory that administration of more coagulation factors and platelets will only fuel the fire unless the thrombosis has been interrupted; moreover, the exogenous blood components will be rapidly depleted and therefore ineffective in stopping the hemorrhage (28, 29). Others disagree, on the premise that early heparin may worsen bleeding. These clinicians base the initial treatment on the dominant abnormality (i.e., anticoagulants for thrombosis, replacement therapy for hemorrhage) (27).

Heparin dosing in acute DIC is also controversial (31). Many practitioners recommend full therapeutic dose heparin with a loading dose of 5,000 to 10,000 units followed by continuous infusion of 15 to 20 units/kg/hr (20,000 to 30,000 units/day). These doses are based on the theories that (a) the coagulation cascade has already been activated, (b) heparin-neutralizing components (e.g., platelet factor-4 and β-thromboglobulin) may be released from activated platelets, and (c) depletion of the natural anticoagulant antithrombin-III (AT-III) may limit heparin effect (29). Others recommend continuous administration of lower doses (5 to 10 units/kg/hr) without a loading dose. Another strategy is to give "low-dose" subcutaneous heparin (5000 units every 12 hr), with the belief that these doses are at least as effective as higher intravenous doses, they have been associated with a reduction in mortality, and the risk of excessive bleeding is reduced (28).

Specific aspects of the mechanism of action, pharmacokinetics and adverse drug reaction profile of heparin are reviewed in Chapter 42, "Thromboembolic Disease."

The potential for exacerbation of bleeding can be a significant deterrent to heparin use in treating acute DIC. Traditional heparin preparations are unfractionated mixtures containing several components. Purified low-molecular-weight heparins (LMWH) have been shown to have a lower incidence of bleeding and may therefore be advantageous in treating DIC patients. The anticoagulant effect of unfractionated heparin occurs via complexation with AT-III, which inhibits activated coagulation factors, principally thrombin and factor Xa. LMWH possess selective anti-Xa properties and do not inhibit thrombin. They do not markedly prolong the aPTT and have less effect on platelet activation and aggregation than unfractionated heparin does; these attributes have translated into a lower incidence of bleeding with LMWH. This offers attractive possibilities in treating patients with DIC, since LMWH may therefore abort thrombus formation without exacerbating bleeding. Several LMWH compounds have been identified, including enoxaparin (Lovenox or PK 10169), dalteparin (Fragmin, FR-860 or Kabi 2165), and fraxiparin (CY 216); enoxaparin and dalteparin are available in the United States. A double-blind randomized study of intravenous dalteparin versus unfractionated heparin in 126 patients suggested a more favorable profile for dalteparin with respect to improvement of clinical symptoms and safety, although there was no difference in overall efficacy (32). A dose-finding trial of dalteparin (33) and case studies using enoxaparin (34) have been reported with promising results. Large-scaled randomized comparative trials should be performed to establish the role of LMWH in acute DIC.

Contraindications to heparin in any form include CNS bleeding (e.g., intracranial or subarachnoid hemorrhage, subdural hematoma), bleeding into other closed spaces where vital functions might be compromised (e.g., intraspinal, pericardial, or peritracheal hemorrhage), and DIC associated with fulminant liver failure (28, 31). Caution should also be exercised in treating patients with a high risk of heparin-induced bleeding (e.g., intracranial metastases, severe hypertension, recent history of peptic ulcer disease).

Depletion of natural anticoagulant proteins (AT-III, proteins C and S) is another important contributor to clotting in acute DIC. AT-III depletion may be particularly significant, because it is both an anticoagulant (Fig. 15.1) and required for the in vivo activity of heparin. Restoration and maintenance of adequate AT-III levels may therefore ameliorate the coagulopathy via both direct and indirect mechanisms. AT-III administration may be especially useful in treating acute DIC patients with bleeding, since it does not exacerbate hemorrhage. Patients with apparent heparin resistance or those with severe bleeding may benefit from AT-III replacement via transfusion with fresh frozen plasma (FFP) or AT-III concentrate. FFP has the advantages of containing multiple coagulation proteins and derivation from a single donor, but the large volumes that are required may be a limitation. AT-III concentrate (Thrombate-III, ATnativ) is a purified heat-treated concentrate made from human plasma and is available in the United States as an orphan drug. It has been studied alone and in combination with heparin in treating acute DIC. Randomized trials of AT-III concentrate versus placebo

(35) or versus heparin alone or with AT-III (36) have demonstrated significantly shorter duration of DIC signs and symptoms in the AT-III groups. A significant effect on mortality was not observed (35). An important finding in one study (36) was a significantly higher RBC transfusion requirement in the group receiving both AT-III and heparin, yielding the conclusion that AT-III alone was effective and had a more favorable safety profile. Clinical improvement has also been demonstrated in a cohort of children (37) and in a patient with recurrent multisite arterial thrombosis refractory to heparin (38). Limited data also supports efficacy in DIC associated with pregnancy or acute fatty liver of pregnancy. Adverse effects have been minimal. On the basis of these data, some clinicians therefore advocate early initiation of AT-III replacement in fulminant DIC (28). Recognition of DIC as an FDA-approved use of AT-III concentrate is currently under study.

Specific dosing and adverse effect information regarding AT-III concentrate is reviewed in the section of this chapter entitled "Hypercoagulable States." Two important considerations specific to its use in treating acute DIC are a shorter half-life, which necessitates twice-daily initial administration (36), and the interaction between AT-III and heparin. Some clinicians administer heparin only after AT-III functional levels greater than 70% have been established (33, 36), because the efficacy of heparin depends on the presence of AT-III. Patients who are already receiving heparin before AT-III may demonstrate markedly enhanced heparin effect after AT-III is added. Careful monitoring of heparin dosing is therefore important in this scenario.

Protein C is another natural anticoagulant (Fig. 15.1) that is commonly depleted in acute DIC. Trials of protein C concentrate in limited numbers of patients with thrombosis have been quite favorable with respect to both efficacy and safety (39, 40); however, these represent only preliminary results. Protein C concentrate is available in the United States on an investigational basis; details regarding its use are found in the section of this chapter entitled "Hypercoagulable States."

Replacement of Depleted Coagulation Factors and Platelets. Blood component replacement therapy is indicated when the patient continues to bleed actively after initial supportive measures or when an invasive procedure or surgery is required. If coagulation factor and platelet depletion is believed to be a major cause of bleeding, replenishment may slow hemorrhage. It is unnecessary in most cases of chronic DIC (factors not usually depleted) and may even be harmful for patients with gross thrombosis (may cause thrombus extension).

Replacement therapy includes platelets, FFP, and cryoprecipitate. If bleeding is severe, administration of packed RBCs will also be necessary. Factor VIII concentrates are not appropriate, because DIC depletes multiple coagulation factors. Prothrombin complex ("factor IX") concentrates may actually worsen or induce DIC. Platelet transfusions are indicated for marked thrombocytopenia (platelet count less than 20,000/mm^3) or for ongoing hemorrhage. At least 5 to 10 units of platelet concentrate (or 0.1 unit/kg) should be given (27). One or two units of fresh frozen plasma (or 10 to 15 mL/kg) or 15 units of cryoprecipitate (or 0.2 bag/kg) usually improve factor deficiencies (27). FFP requires administration of larger volumes but is advantageous because it contains clotting factors plus AT-III and proteins C and S. Cryoprecipitate contains 10 times more fibrinogen per unit than FFP. It is indicated for patients with very low fibrinogen levels (<50 mg/dL) or those with fibrinogen levels less than 100 mg/dL who are bleeding.

As was previously discussed, the timing of blood component administration in the management strategy of acute DIC is controversial. If given while clotting is still ongoing, exogenous coagulation factors will simply be integrated into the coagulation process; this will not elevate factor levels and may even worsen the thrombosis. While this fuel-the-fire argument is theoretically possible and may rarely occur, it has not been well substantiated in clinical practice (30, 31). Nonetheless, many believe that factor replacement should be withheld until intravascular clotting has been suspended with heparin, especially in using components containing fibrinogen (28, 29). After intravascular clotting has been interrupted, any depleted component can be given and should raise factor levels and reduce bleeding. In situations in which heparin is contraindicated, products with high fibrinogen content (e.g., FFP and cryoprecipitate) should be avoided.

Vitamin K deficiency may occur in acute DIC patients, depending on the degree and duration of DIC, whether factor replacement is given, the type of nutrition support given to the patient, and other issues such as administration of broad-spectrum antibiotics. In deficient patients, supplementation will facilitate production of vitamin K-dependent clotting factors.

Interruption of Fibrinolysis. Fibrinolytic (or fibrinogenolytic) inhibitors such as ε-aminocaproic acid (Amicar) or tranexamic acid (Cyklokapron) are theoretically useful, since they will slow fibrinolysis of the microthrombi, thereby slowing bleeding. Successful use of intravenous tranexamic acid in acute DIC that is unresponsive to heparin, AT-III, and FFP has been reported (41). However, antifibrinolytics also carry a very significant danger. If intravascular clotting has not been suspended before use, they may cause catastrophic widespread fibrin deposition in the microcirculation, leading to irreversible ischemic multiorgan damage, which is sometimes fatal (31). These agents should be used with extreme caution and always with concurrent heparin therapy. They should be restricted

to last recourse situations with life-threatening bleeding or evidence of extensive secondary fibrinolysis and after failure of other therapies (27, 31). An exception to this is the patient with acute promyelocytic leukemia, who may have primary activation of both the coagulation and fibrinolytic systems caused by the malignancy. When antifibrolytics are used in conjunction with other modalities, the benefits may outweigh the risks for these patients.

Other Therapies. Exchange transfusions are sometimes used in the treatment of DIC. Plasma exchange, plasmapheresis, leucopheresis, and whole blood exchange have been used. Their efficacy is thought to be related to removal of FDP, activated clotting factors, and toxins from the patient's plasma, all of which aggravate bleeding (30). Replacement of AT-III, proteins C and S, and other proteins in the exchanged plasma may also contribute to a successful outcome by reestablishing the normal balance of circulating coagulation factors and natural anticoagulants. Exchange transfusion is not considered part of the routine management of DIC because of its associated risks and the need for specialized equipment and trained personnel.

A number of drugs are in clinical investigation in the management of acute DIC. These include gabexate mesilate (FOY), a synthetic inhibitor of serine proteases in the coagulation, fibrinolysis, and other systems (complement, kinins, prostaglandins, superoxide). Gabexate has antithrombin and antiplasmin effects that are independent of AT-III and account for its efficacy in acute DIC (42, 43). Dermatan sulfate (MF-701) enhances the antithrombin effect of heparin cofactor II via a mechanism that is analogous to the effect of AT-III on thrombin (44). Compounds that are undergoing preclinical trials include recombinant human soluble thrombomodulin (rhs-TM), recombinant hirudin (PEG hirudin), and an inhibitor of factor Xa (DX-9065).

Monitoring Parameters for Acute DIC. All patients with acute DIC should have regular monitoring of fibrinogen levels, D-dimer (or FDP) levels, the protamine sulfate test, and platelet counts. AT-III levels and other biochemical markers (prothrombin fragment 1+2, fibrinopeptides A and B) are also useful if available. Attainment and maintenance of adequate fibrinogen levels and platelet counts, with falling D-dimer (or FDP) levels, a negative protamine sulfate test, and stable hematocrit are indicators of successful interruption of the coagulopathy. Initial monitoring every 6 to 12 hr is appropriate, with once-daily assessment after the patient is stable. Changes in the balance between fibrinogen synthesis and consumption can be seen within hours, while platelet and D-dimer (or FDP) levels may take 1 to 2 days to show meaningful trends (30). In some cases, such as acute leukemia, D-dimer levels will increase initially, then fall. Clinical response begins shortly after laboratory improvement (28), with stabilization of bleeding, thrombosis, and end-organ dysfunction. Blood pressure, cardiac output, systemic vascular resistance, the Glasgow coma score, and urine output may be measured, as well as arterial blood gases, serum BUN, creatinine, ALT, and AST. Reduction in the need for continued use of pressor agents, ventilators, dialysis, and transfusion of coagulation factors, platelets, and packed RBCs also indicates improvement. It is essential to recognize that the patient's clinical status will also be influenced by improvement or deterioration in the underlying disease.

Patients who are receiving heparin require additional monitoring. aPTT, TT, PT, and hematocrit are measured 4 to 6 hr after initiation of heparin and every 12 to 24 hr thereafter. While the aPTT is a primary tool for monitoring and adjusting heparin therapy in other situations, most patients with acute DIC have an abnormal baseline aPTT. The aPTT therefore provides limited guidance, as do plasma heparin levels. Inability to ameliorate the general measures of acute DIC as described above (D-dimer, fibrinogen, etc.) can indicate a need to increase the heparin dose. In general, heparin should be continued until fibrinogen levels are above 100 mg/dL and platelet counts are above 100,000/mm^3. The hematocrit should also be monitored frequently to assess both beneficial and adverse effects of heparin.

Patients who are receiving AT-III via FFP or AT-III concentrate should have plasma AT-III levels drawn every 12 hr until they are stable, then daily. Clinical improvement should occur in 1 to 3 days.

Objective measures of successful management in patients who are receiving coagulation factor or platelet transfusions include an increase in platelet count and plasma fibrinogen concentration, as well as the criteria reviewed above in the general monitoring of acute DIC. Platelet and fibrinogen levels should be determined 30 to 60 min after a transfusion and every 6 to 12 hr thereafter until they are stable. With effective therapy the fibrinogen concentration and platelet count should stabilize and then increase. Similarly, clinical improvement, measured as a slowing then cessation of bleeding, occurs over several days. Subsequent need for transfusion will depend on clinical response, treatment of the underlying disorder, and the half-life of the platelets and clotting factors. Once consumption is interrupted, the bone marrow and liver usually take several days to replenish endogenous platelet and fibrinogen levels.

Chronic DIC should first be managed by treatment of the precipitating disorder and supportive therapy of clinical manifestations. For some patients, especially those who are asymptomatic and have a correctable underlying disease, this alone is adequate. Careful observation and follow-up are essential, since these patients can deteriorate into acute florid DIC when they are subjected to stressors such as

surgery, invasive procedures, infection, or disease progression (30, 31).

Patients who present with deep vein thrombosis should be managed with intravenous heparin at standard therapeutic doses (20,000 to 30,000 units/day via constant intravenous infusion). Special care should be exercised in treating patients with intracranial metastases or other risk factors for bleeding. It is important to recognize that patients with thrombotic complications of chronic DIC are only rarely successfully managed with oral anticoagulants. DIC associated with neoplastic disease is caused by direct activation of the extrinsic pathway via release of procoagulant material from the malignant cells. Warfarin and other coumarin derivatives are not effective in this situation because they simply reduce the amounts of activated vitamin K-dependent clotting factors but will not otherwise affect coagulation and fibrinolysis. Patients who require long-term secondary prophylaxis of thrombotic events in these situations should receive chronic subcutaneous heparin (29). Patients with untreatable malignancies and other persistent symptoms of DIC should also be managed with subcutaneous heparin. The use of antiplatelet agents (e.g., aspirin and/or dipyridamole) and pentoxifylline is controversial. Some advocates believe that they may correct coagulation parameters and reduce bleeding or thrombosis (28); others find no documented clinical benefit (31). Replacement therapy with blood components or antifibrinolytic drugs are rarely necessary in treating patients with chronic DIC.

Monitoring parameters for chronic DIC include routine assessment of signs and symptoms. If treatment is given, D-dimer (or FDP) and fibrinogen levels, the protamine sulfate test, and platelet counts should be monitored. Patients receiving long-term heparin should be monitored and counseled as described in Chapter 42, "Thromboembolic Disease."

PROGNOSIS

Much remains to be investigated to further clarify the pathophysiology and management of DIC. Randomized controlled large-scale trials have been difficult to perform because of the broad spectra of underlying diseases, diagnostic criteria, and outcome measurements. Most clinicians therefore base their treatment decisions on clinical judgment and prior experience.

Acute DIC may be an incidental preterminal event occurring in a variety of acute catastrophic illnesses. It may be brief and end promptly with effective treatment of the underlying disorder. Alternatively, patients may die from hemorrhage and progression of the underlying disorder. Mortality rates for patients with acute DIC are reported to be 50 to 85%. However, this may be more reflective of the mortality rates of the precipitating disorders rather than treatment of the DIC. Morbidity and mortality are reduced with early recognition and aggressive treatment of the DIC; however, the prognosis may not improve until better methods of prevention and treatment of the underlying disorders become available.

Some patients with chronic DIC may be asymptomatic with only laboratory evidence of the disorder. Others may have recurrent episodes of thromboembolism requiring long-term subcutaneous heparin for prophylaxis. In most cases the prognosis of patients with chronic DIC is related to that of the precipitating disease rather than the treatment strategy.

Hypercoagulable States

Hypercoagulable states comprise a number of conditions that share the common endpoint of inappropriate thrombus formation. Patients with these disorders are at higher risk for both venous and arterial thromboembolic disease. Disruption of coagulation may occur on an inherited (primary) or acquired (secondary) basis. *Inherited* hypercoagulable disorders are hereditary abnormalities in the synthesis or function of various proteins in the coagulation and fibrinolytic systems. Exaggerated formation or impaired breakdown of fibrin results in clotting, which may occur in the microvasculature or in large vessels such as the iliac veins. *Acquired* disorders include a wide spectrum of conditions associated with an enhanced risk of thromboembolism. Acquired risk factors for venous thromboembolism (Table 15.6) are various, including production of abnormal proteins, diseases, drugs, or clinical situations. This discussion will focus on the venous manifestations of hypercoagulable states; for a more detailed review of arterial diseases (myocardial infarction, cerebrovascular accident, peripheral vascular disease, etc.) the reader is referred to other chapters.

INHERITED HYPERCOAGULABLE STATES

Hemostasis is regulated by two major physiologic systems called the coagulation and fibrinolytic systems. Under normal conditions, both are intricately balanced to maintain the blood in a fluid state within the vessels while at the same time minimizing blood loss from the vasculature at sites of injury. Disruption of this intrinsic balance may result in either bleeding or thrombosis. Thrombosis occurs when large amounts of thrombin are produced via the coagulation cascade. Thrombin catalyzes the conversion of fibrinogen to fibrin, which then polymerizes to form an insoluble clot (Fig. 15.1). The fibrin clot is degraded by another endogenous cascade called the fibrinolytic system (Fig. 15.2). Physiologic inhibitors of coagulation act to either inhibit thrombin formation or enhance fibrinolysis. In this manner, almost every protein in the coagulation and fibrinolytic systems has a natural inhibitor or lytic mechanism.

Table 15.6.
Acquired Risk Factors for Venous Thromboembolism

Abnormal function of the coagulation cascade or fibrinolytic system
  Surgery (especially orthopedic surgery of the lower limb)
  Trauma
  Pregnancy
  Oral contraceptives
  Infection (associated with DIC)
  Nephrotic syndrome
  Antiphospholipid syndrome
  Hepatic insufficiency
Abnormal platelet number or function
  Myeloproliferative disorder (such as essential thrombocytosis)
  Paroxysmal nocturnal hemoglobinuria
Abnormal vessel endothelial cell function or blood rheology
  Stasis (prolonged sitting or bed rest, acute hemiplegia or paraplegia, congestive heart failure, varicose veins)
  Trauma
  Abnormal blood rheology (previous venous thrombosis, extrinsic compression)
  Hyperviscosity syndromes (including myeloproliferative syndromes such as polycythemia vera)
  Artificial surfaces (heart valves, vascular patches)
  Vasculitis
Miscellaneous
  Malignancy
  Obesity
  Drugs (heparin-associated thrombocytopenia, warfarin skin necrosis, antineoplastics)

DIC = disseminated intravascular coagulation.
Adapted from (5, 55, 56).

A number of endogenous proteins act as major deterrents to thrombin formation and are sometimes referred to as "natural" or "physiologic" anticoagulants. The best-understood include antithrombin-III (AT-III), protein C, and protein S. Each has a critical role in preventing the formation of pathologic amounts of thrombin, depicted in Figure 15.1. Patterns of inheritance, prevalence, and site(s) of endogenous production are summarized in Table 15.7. Other natural anticoagulants include heparin cofactor II and tissue factor pathway inhibitor; these proteins are relatively new discoveries, and their role in the pathogenesis of thrombus formation is less clear.

The fibrinolytic system is an enzymatic cascade that begins with the formation of plasmin. Plasmin digests fibrin, which lyses the thrombus (Fig. 15.2). Like the coagulation cascade, the fibrinolytic system is intricately regulated by a series of naturally produced proteins. Disorders of fibrinolysis include qualitative or quantitative abnormalities of fibrinogen, plasminogen, plasminogen activator, plasminogen activator inhibitor, or plasmin inhibitors (α_2-plasmin inhibitor, α_2-macroglobulin, and C1 inactivator) (Fig. 15.2). Integrity and regulation of the fibrinolytic system appear to have a less critical role in maintaining blood fluidity compared to the coagulation cascade; far fewer cases of thrombosis associated with these disorders have been reported.

Significant variation in the clinical expression of the genetic abnormalities results in a wide array of symptoms. Clues to a possible inherited disorder include thrombosis (a) in a familial pattern, (b) at a young age (under 40 years), (c) occurring spontaneously, (d) recurrence, and (e) at unusual sites (e.g., the kidney, eye, or cerebrum). Patients with these characteristics merit further investigation for a hereditary hypercoagulable condition. Most of the abnormalities are inherited in an autosomal dominant pattern, and most affected individuals are heterozygotes. Age is a particularly important variable; as many as 20 to 30% of patients with an initial thromboembolic episode before age 45 have deficiency or dysfunction of a physiologic anticoagulant or fibrinolytic protein (45, 46). It should be noted that standard tests used in blood coagulation screening, including the prothrombin time (PT), activated partial thromboplastin time (aPTT), fibrinogen, D-dimer, fibrin degradation products (FDP), platelet count, template bleeding time, and platelet aggregation are often normal in people with these conditions. Specific immunologic (antigenic) and functional assays of the individual proteins are required for detection.

Antithrombin-III Deficiency. Antithrombin-III (AT-III) is a serine protease inhibitor with a broad spectrum of activity in the coagulation cascade. AT-III irreversibly complexes with factors IXa, Xa, XIa, XIIa, thrombin, and plasmin (Fig. 15.1). Inactivation of factor Xa and thrombin is an especially important function. The entire process is markedly accelerated in the presence of heparin. AT-III is considered a crucial component in limiting ongoing activation of the coagulation cascade; it is sometimes called *primary physiologic inhibitor of in vivo coagulation.* Assays for both the quantity (antigen) and function of AT-III are reported as a percentage compared to normal pooled plasma; normal values for both assays range from 70 to 120% of control. AT-III levels in 20-week fetuses and term babies are about 25% and 50% of control, respectively; adult levels are achieved at about 6 months of age. In utero or neonatal clotting is uncommon because of a concurrent physiologic reduction in procoagulant factor levels. AT-III plasma levels may be measured in patients taking warfarin but should be avoided during heparin therapy and during acute thromboembolic events.

AT-III deficiency is inherited in an autosomal dominant pattern. Homozygotes die in utero or during infancy. The heterozygous AT-III-deficient population comprises two subtypes. Type I deficiency is more common and is characterized by decreased synthesis of a functionally normal AT-III molecule (i.e., a quantitative defect). In these individuals, functional and antigenic assays yield similar values; most individuals have approximately 40 to 70% of control levels (5, 47–49). Formation of a biologically dysfunctional form of AT-III (qualitative, or type II deficiency) is less common. These individuals have normal antigenic levels but abnormal AT-III activity as measured in functional assays. AT-III deficiency may be caused by more than one type of genetic abnormality; some investigators have suggested a relationship between specific aberrations and the prevalence and/or severity of thrombosis (45).

Diagnosis and Clinical Findings. The wide array of clinical manifestations reflect an inheritance pattern with variable expression. Only moderate reductions (50 to 70% of normal) of AT-III levels may induce thrombophilia. Some patients remain asymptomatic, although many clinically asymptomatic patients have laboratory evidence of a procoagulant state (49). In evaluations of AT-III-deficient families the prevalence of venous thromboembolism in heterozygotes is about 50% (50). The cumulative incidence of thrombosis increases with age; most patients have their

Table 15.7.
Natural Inhibitors of Coagulation

			Prevalence		
	Half-Life	Inheritance	General Population	8 Reports of Unselected Patients with Thrombosis[a]	Site of Synthesis
Antithrombin III	2.5 days	Autosomal dominant	1/2000 to 1/5000	0.5–8%, mean 4%	Hepatocyte; vitamin K-independent
Protein C	6–8 hours	Autosomal dominant	1/15,000	1.5–11.5%, mean 5.4%	Hepatocyte; vitamin K-dependent
		Autosomal recessive	1/200 to 1/300		
Protein S	Unknown	Autosomal dominant	Unknown	1.5–13.2%, mean 5.9%	Hepatocyte; vitamin K-dependent α-platelet granules Endothelial cells Megakaryocytes

Adapted from (5, 46, 47, 67).
[a] Bick RL: Hypercoagulability and thrombosis. Med Clin North Am 78(3):635–665, 1994.

first event in adolescence or young adulthood (10 to 35 years), by age 40 about 50% have had a thrombotic event, and by age 50 to 60 as many as 85 to 95% will have at least one episode (45, 50, 51). Recurrence is common (about 50 to 60%). Typically, the initial event is deep vein thrombosis of a lower extremity and/or pulmonary embolism. Thrombosis may also occur at unusual sites such as the upper extremity (axillary or brachial vein), viscera (mesenteric, renal, or retinal vein), cerebrum (the cerebral sinuses), or vena cava. Superficial thrombophlebitis and arterial thrombosis are relatively uncommon with AT-III deficiency. The initial event in AT-III deficiency usually occurs in the presence of a known thrombogenic risk factor (most commonly pregnancy or surgery/trauma but also during prolonged bed rest or exposure to other factors or drugs, as listed in Table 15.6). Apparent heparin resistance may rarely occur with AT-III deficiency and is an occasional clue to its presence. For a discussion of the clinical manifestations and diagnosis of venous thromboembolism refer to Chapter 42, "Thromboembolic Disease."

AT-III deficiency is also associated with a high risk of maternal and fetal complications during pregnancy; 42 to 68% of untreated pregnant AT-III deficient females will develop venous thrombosis during pregnancy or in the immediate postpartum period (48). Moreover, a significantly higher incidence of fetal morbidity and mortality is manifested as spontaneous abortions, intrauterine growth retardation, and preterm delivery. Widespread microvascular thrombosis with subsequent fibrosis of the placenta has been observed and is presumed to cause placental insufficiency (45, 52). It may occur at any stage of the pregnancy, and there is currently no way to prospectively identify that patients will develop these complications.

Treatment. The management of acute thromboembolism in AT-III-deficient individuals is the same as that for the general population. Heparin should be administered, the dose being titrated according to the activated partial thromboplastin time (aPTT). Heparin resistance is uncommon at the AT-III levels that are typically seen in deficient patients; the dose of heparin that is required to attain a therapeutic aPTT is not related to the degree of AT-III deficiency. Warfarin is initiated concomitant with the heparin, with a target prothrombin time INR (international normalized ratio) of 2.0 to 3.0. For further description of the management of acute deep vein thrombosis and pulmonary embolism, refer to Chapter 42, "Thromboembolic Disease."

AT-III concentrate (Thrombate-III, Miles Cutter Biological; ATnativ, KabiVitrum) is prepared as a purified (via heparin chromatography affinity) plasma concentrate that is then pasteurized to inactivate hepatitis B and HIV-1 viruses. One unit of AT-III concentrate is equal to the amount of AT-III present in 1 mL of normal plasma. AT-III concentrate is available in the United States as an orphan

drug. Its considerable expense and short half-life do not support long-term prophylaxis for AT-III deficient patients. Approved indications are therefore limited to short-term prophylaxis and treatment of thromboembolism in patients with inherited AT-III deficiency, with or without concomitant heparin therapy. Preventive indications include high-thrombosis-risk situations such as surgery, pregnancy and delivery, major trauma, and prolonged bed rest. After parturition and surgery, plasma AT-III levels are reduced for several days, concurrent with the high thrombotic risk (49, 53). The plasma level reduction is accentuated in congenital deficiency, and AT-III concentrate is therefore given just before (when able) and for a period of 5 to 7 days after exposure, depending on the situation. The lack of bleeding risk associated with AT-III administration makes it a particularly attractive alternative to traditional anticoagulants in preventing venous thrombosis. Randomized controlled trials of efficacy are limited by the rarity of congenital deficiency and ethical considerations. Several small-scale trials have yielded very promising results in preventing thrombosis, using AT-III concentrate either alone or with concurrent heparin (48–52). AT-III deficient patients with acute thrombosis may also benefit from the addition of AT-III concentrate to heparin therapy, especially those with thrombus extension while on heparin or apparent heparin resistance (45, 51). The use of AT-III concentration in *acquired* AT-III deficiency states far exceeds that in inherited conditions, and there are many more reported trials, although these are technically not approved uses (see the discussion below of acquired AT-III deficiency).

After intravenous administration, peak plasma AT-III levels are achieved in 15 to 30 min (49). *In vivo* recovery is variable, ranging from 60 to 100% after administration to patients with stable congenital AT-III deficiency (47, 48). Plasma AT-III activity levels can be expected to increase 1 to 2% for each unit per kilogram administered. Another dosing strategy is to set a desired plasma AT-III level of 80% to 125% as the goal, a plasma volume of 40 mL/kg, then calculate the dose as follows:

dose (units) =

$$\frac{(\text{desired } [\text{AT-III}]\%) - \text{pretreatment } [\text{AT-III}]\%}{\times 40 \text{ mL/kg} \times \text{weight (kg)}}{\text{fraction recovered} \times 100}$$

If the fraction recovered ranges from [0.6] to [1.0] and the desired AT-III level is 125%, then

dose (units) = (125% − pretreatment [AT-III]%)
                              × weight (kg) × [0.4]–[0.67]

If the pretreatment AT-III level is 50%, this corresponds to a loading dose of 30 to 50 units/kg (48, 49). Important dosing considerations include a lower goal concentration when used in treating neonates and highly variable fraction-recovered values, both between and within patients, which are related to the disease being treated and its acuity. It is therefore important to measure AT-III levels in dosage calculation, rather than using fixed dosing methods. In asymptomatic patients with inherited AT-III deficiency, elimination of initial doses is biphasic, when measured both immunologically and functionally the decline in AT-III activity and antigen. An initial half-life of AT-III activity of 22 hr has been reported (49), with terminal half-lives ranging from 60 to 90 hr (AT-III activity) and 53 to 59 hr (AT-III antigen) (49, 51). Prolonged administration yields single-phase second-order elimination. Once-daily administration is therefore usually sufficient, except in acute DIC, in which a 12-hr dosing interval is preferred because of a reduction in the half-life (4.5 hr) and fraction recovered (50%) (36, 49).

Adverse drug reactions reported with AT-III concentrate have been minimal. Rarely, chest tightness, dizziness, and fever have occurred (49, 51). An interesting finding in DIC patients who received AT-III plus heparin was a greater need for RBC transfusion compared to either drug alone (36). A higher incidence of wound hematoma and bleeding was also noted in postoperative joint replacement, compared to dextran-40 (53). Conversion of hepatitis B antigen and antibody has been reported; however, these patients were known to have received multiple other blood products (51). Hepatitis C and HIV-1 transmission has not been reported.

In administering AT-III concentrate and heparin concurrently, it is important to consider their interaction. Replenishment of AT-III to a deficient patient may result in a significantly lower dosage requirement for heparin. Empiric dosage reduction and/or frequent laboratory monitoring are appropriate when AT-III concentrate is added to heparin therapy.

Monitoring parameters for AT-III concentrate include plasma AT-III levels, hemoglobin, and hematocrit every 12 hr until stable, then every 24 hr. Care should be exercised during monitoring to ensure that AT-III functional rather than antigenic or immunologic levels are determined. Patients receiving heparin and warfarin should also have regular monitoring of the aPTT, PT, and TT. Other laboratory indicators of ongoing thrombin formation such as fibrinopeptide A, prothrombin fragment (F1+2), and thrombin-antithrombin complex levels should be assessed if available. The patient should be examined regularly for the signs and symptoms of thromboembolism such as lower extremity pain, swelling and warmth, shortness of breath, pleuritic chest pain, and hypoxemia. Occult blood monitoring of nasogastric aspirate, stools, and urine is appropriate.

Long-Term Management. Once a thrombotic event has occurred, the AT-III-deficient patient will have a significant lifelong risk of recurrence, which can occur spontaneously or in the presence of thrombosis risk factors. In a retrospective analysis of 238 patients from 73 families with inherited deficiency of either AT-III, protein C, or protein S, the incidence of an *initial* episode of venous thromboembolism was 1.3 per 100 patient-years; in contrast, the incidence of *recurrent* events was 4.8 per 100 patient-years (50). This finding emphasizes the importance of long-term secondary prophylaxis. Lifelong replacement therapy with AT-III concentrate is neither indicated nor practical. Most investigators therefore advise lifelong oral anticoagulants after a single thrombotic event, adjusted to a target prothrombin time INR of 2.0 to 3.0 (5, 46, 48). Some take a more conservative approach, advising lifelong therapy only for patients with recurrent deep vein thrombosis, or a single episode if life-threatening, or a single episode if spontaneous (50). The decision about long-term anticoagulants should be made individually. Patients with dementia, a history of frequent falls or trauma, poor or unreliable compliance, alcohol abuse, peptic ulcer disease, or chronic bleeding may not be suitable candidates for lifelong treatment.

The management of pregnant females (or those desiring pregnancy) merits special discussion. AT-III deficiency, whether inherited or acquired, is associated with both maternal and fetal complications. The incidence of maternal thrombosis during pregnancy is higher with AT-III deficiency than with protein C or S deficiency. Most investigators therefore recommend prophylaxis in all AT-III deficient patients, regardless of the thrombotic history (5, 50). Patients who are on warfarin should discontinue use in advance, if possible, because of its known teratogenic effects (54). Subcutaneous heparin should be initiated and maintained until the time of delivery. Patients with difficulty managing subcutaneous injections should receive heparin at least during the first trimester and the last 1 to 2 months of pregnancy, with oral anticoagulants during the remainder of the pregnancy (50, 54). Twice-weekly AT-III concentrate infusion plus subcutaneous heparin has been successfully used in treating two females with congenital AT-III deficiency and heparin resistance (49). For most patients, however, AT-III concentrate is withheld until the peripartum period, when it is given at the time of delivery and for several days thereafter (50, 51). Additionally, warfarin (usually with a few days of concurrent heparin) should be promptly reinitiated postpartum. Warfarin is considered safe for an infant whose mother is breast-feeding (54); however, it should be noted that this assessment of safety does not extend to other coumarin derivatives.

All AT-III deficient individuals who undergo surgery, incur trauma, or are exposed to other high-risk situations should receive prophylaxis with heparin, warfarin, and/or AT-III concentrate, whether or not they are taking long-term oral anticoagulants. Short-term prophylaxis should be given before, during, and for a few days after exposure to thrombosis risk factors (50).

The use of long-term oral anticoagulant prophylaxis in individuals with AT-III deficiency who have not experienced a thrombotic event (e.g., a person detected in family screening) is controversial. Short-term prophylaxis as described above during exposure to risk situations (including pregnancy) is appropriate. However, there are no studies demonstrating a definite benefit of long-term anticoagulant therapy for these patients (46, 55). The decision to initiate such treatment should therefore be individualized on the basis the family history and after patient consultation regarding the risks and benefits of treatment. If the patient and clinician elect to treat with warfarin, it may be initiated as an outpatient without concomitant heparin.

The value of a management strategy that incorporated short-term prophylaxis for all patients and long-term anticoagulants for symptomatic patients with inherited deficiencies of AT-III, protein C, or protein S was evaluated in a retrospective study of 238 patients from 73 families (50). At the time of diagnosis the incidence of recurrent venous thrombosis was 4.8 per 100 patient-years. This was reduced to 1.4/100 patient-years with the described treatment strategy; if poor compliers were excluded, the incidence was further reduced to 0.3/100 patient-years. Specific analysis of AT-III deficient patients yielded a reduction in the overall incidence (single event or recurrent, long-term prophylaxis or not) of major thrombotic events from 2.5 to 1.3 per 100 patient-years after implementation of the strategy (0.5 if poor compliers were excluded). Four AT-III-deficient females (two with and two without a prior history of thrombosis) became pregnant and were managed with heparin, with or without oral anticoagulants and AT-III concentrate; none had a thrombotic event. Six AT-III-deficient patients were given perioperative prophylaxis with heparin and/or AT-III concentrate, with no thrombotic events. During follow-up of 42 asymptomatic AT-III-deficient patients over a mean of 5.3 years, two developed major thrombotic manifestations. This last finding may argue for long-term prophylaxis for asymptomatic patients, although confirmation with larger patient populations is desirable.

Patient Education. Counseling for all patients with inherited AT-III deficiency should include a review of thrombosis risk settings and the importance of avoiding such situations. All patients should be informed of the symptoms of deep vein thrombosis and pulmonary embolism and the need for prompt medical evaluation should they occur. All patients should consider prophylaxis with short-term heparin, warfarin, and/or AT-III concentrate when risk factors are present. Patients who are on long-term warfarin therapy should be apprised of the rationale for treatment,

symptoms of bleeding, necessity to avoid contact sports or activities, importance of consistent dietary intake of vitamin K, necessity to avoid of aspirin in any form, abundance of drug interactions, and the need for regular coagulation studies and dosage adjustment (also refer to Chapter 42, "Thromboembolic Disease"). Females of childbearing age who are receiving long-term anticoagulants *must* be counseled regarding the teratogenic effects of coumarin derivatives and the need for effective contraception. Females who are not receiving long-term anticoagulants should be informed of the maternal and fetal risks during pregnancy and the advisability of prophylaxis during pregnancy and shortly thereafter.

Acquired Antithrombin-III Deficiency. In addition to congenital aberrations of the physiologic anticoagulant and fibrinolytic proteins, certain diseases may alter their levels or function, resulting in acquired deficiencies. This may occur in patients with increased AT-III consumption (DIC, preeclampsia, major surgery, extensive acute deep vein thrombosis or pulmonary embolism), decreased production (liver failure, fatty liver of pregnancy, malnutrition, preterm infants), or increased plasma loss (nephrotic syndrome, inflammatory bowel disease) (45, 56). Patients with malignancy may acquire AT-III deficiency via an uncertain mechanism. Most patients with acquired AT-III deficiency do not develop thrombosis. Although nephrotic syndrome is associated with a high thromboembolic risk, a causative relationship with AT-III deficiency remains unclear (56). Prophylaxis in acquired AT-III deficiency is therefore not generally necessary. In acute thromboembolism with known low plasma AT-III levels, DIC, fatty liver of pregnancy with DIC, or fulminant hepatic failure, the usefulness of AT-III concentrate has been demonstrated (36, 48, 52). Patient counseling regarding avoidance of high-risk situations is appropriate.

Two randomized double-blind trials of AT-III concentrate, either alone or in combination with heparin, have been reported involving patients with DIC. When compared to heparin (36) or placebo (35), a significantly shorter duration of DIC in groups receiving AT-III was observed. One trial found a trend toward a reduction in mortality in patients receiving AT-III concentrate that was not statistically significant (35). The need for RBC transfusion in patients receiving AT-III concentrate was higher in one study (36) and lower in the other (35). Uncontrolled trials or case reports have been published in patients with fatty liver of pregnancy and DIC (52), DIC in children (37), and DIC with arterial thrombosis that is unresponsive to heparin alone (38). While AT-III concentrate has been demonstrated to improve the clinical and laboratory markers for patients with DIC, the ultimate outcome as measured by mortality is primarily related to the underlying disease.

A third randomized trial of AT-III concentrate was performed in normal postoperative total hip or knee replacement patients (53). Patients in the AT-III plus heparin group (treated for 5 days) had a significantly lower incidence of venous thrombosis compared to those who received dextran-40. An interesting finding was the occurrence of venous thrombosis in 100% of patients with AT-III plasma levels less than 65%, suggesting that this value may represent an important threshold.

Drug-induced AT-III deficiency has been reported with L-asparaginase, oral contraceptives, and heparin. L-asparaginase is thought to cause thrombosis via reduced endogenous synthesis of the coagulation and fibrinolytic proteins and/or drug-induced endothelial damage. Thrombosis during or immediately after L-asparaginase administration is well documented, occurring in 3 to 5% of patients (57). AT-III concentrate has been evaluated in a small cohort of patients undergoing induction therapy for acute lymphoblastic leukemia, yielding a reduction in laboratory abnormalities and clinical thrombosis (57).

Oral contraceptives are the triggering event for the initial episode of venous thrombosis in 5 to 10% of AT-III-deficient patients and are generally avoided in this population (45, 50). To assess the additional risk of oral contraceptives in 48 patients with hereditary thrombophilia, a retrospective study of AT-III-deficient females compared those who had taken oral contraceptives at least once with age-matched AT-III-deficient controls (58). AT-III-deficient patients who had taken oral contraceptives incurred a significantly higher probability for thrombosis (48% and 77% after 12 and 60 months, respectively), with a yearly incidence of 27.5% compared to 3.4% of AT-III-deficient controls. It was concluded that oral contraceptives were contraindicated for patients with AT-III deficiency and that relatives of known AT-III-deficient individuals should be screened before initiation of contraception. A limitation of this study was a very small sample size of 15 AT-III-deficient patients.

Protein C Deficiency. Protein C is a vitamin K-dependent proenzyme that circulates as an inactive zymogen. Activation occurs when thrombomodulin, a vascular endothelial cell receptor, binds to thrombin, thereby altering thrombin's substrate affinity in two important ways: (a) Thrombomodulin-bound thrombin does not catalyze the conversion of fibrinogen to fibrin, and (b) the thrombomodulin-thrombin complex is a powerful activator of protein C, forming protein Ca. Protein Ca inhibits thrombin formation by proteolytic inactivation of Factors Va and VIIIa (Fig. 15.1), an effect that is markedly enhanced in the presence of a cofactor called protein S. Protein Ca also enhances fibrinolysis by inactivating tissue plasminogen activator inhibitor (PAI-1). In this capacity, protein Ca is a major physiologic modulator of blood fluidity and hemostasis.

Assays are available for determining both functional and immunologic (antigenic) protein C levels. The reference range of 65 to 130% that is used for both methods is expressed as a percentage of normal pooled plasma. Protein C levels are not affected by heparin. Assays in individuals taking oral anticoagulants are difficult to interpret because protein C production is vitamin K-dependent and therefore altered by the warfarin. If discontinuation of the oral anticoagulant is deemed harmful, the magnitude of protein C reduction may be compared to that of another vitamin K-dependent protein such as factor X, but this has less precision in identifying deficient individuals.

The inheritance pattern of protein C deficiency is intriguing. The commonly reported prevalence of 1:200 to 1:300 is not consistent with the pattern of clinical manifestations. This disparity may be due either to inheritance of a single congenital disorder with variable degrees of penetrance or to the existence of two separate phenotypes with different clinical manifestations. Recent research supports the latter hypothesis (59–61). In the autosomal-recessive form, heterozygotes have protein C antigen levels of 30 to 60%, but most remain asymptomatic for life (60, 61). Homozygotes with this form have nonmeasurable plasma levels associated with neonatal purpura fulminans or severe thrombosis in infancy. This form has a prevalence in the general population of 1:200 to 1:300 (Table 15.7). Heterozygotes with the autosomal-dominant form have similar protein C levels of 30 to 60% (59, 60, 62) but have a high incidence of recurrent thrombosis beginning in early adulthood. Homozygotes have very low levels (5 to 20%) but often remain completely asymptomatic until adolescence or young adulthood, when they develop recurrent thrombosis in a pattern similar to that of heterozygotes with the same autosomal-dominant form; some may even remain asymptomatic for life (62). The autosomal dominant form is found in about 60% of protein C-deficient individuals, with a prevalence in the general population estimated at 1:15,000 (60). This hypothesis therefore yields "healthy" (autosomal-recessive) and "thrombosis-prone" (autosomal-dominant) families (59) and at least partially explains the discordance between the prevalence of deficiency and the incidence of thrombotic manifestations. Heterozygotes in either group may have either reduced levels of functionally normal protein C (type I, quantitative; more common) or "normal" levels of dysfunctional protein C (type II, qualitative; less common).

A new type of congenital protein C abnormality has recently been described (59). In this form, antigenic and functional protein C levels are normal, but factor Va is resistant to the proteolytic action of protein Ca. The procoagulant activity of factor Va is retained, which therefore favors thrombosis in affected individuals. This disorder, called "activated protein C resistance" (APCR), is caused by a single point mutation of the gene for factor V and is inherited in an autosomal-dominant pattern. The prevalence of heterozygotes in the general population is very high (3 to 5%). Most are asymptomatic, which suggests that APCR alone is not a major thrombosis risk factor. However, a high thrombotic risk exists when APCR occurs concomitantly with a second abnormality such as AT-III, protein C or S deficiency, the lupus anticoagulant, or homozygous APCR. APCR may be found in as many as 50% of individuals with hereditary thrombophilia, compared to 3 to 7% of healthy controls (59). APCR is therefore the most common hereditary abnormality identified to date. An attractive hypothesis suggests that APCR, protein C deficiency, or protein S deficiency, if present alone, results in a moderate increase in thrombotic risk, whereas when two deficiencies coexist, the risk is markedly enhanced (59).

Diagnosis and Clinical Findings. Neonatal purpura fulminans: Homozygotes with the autosomal recessive form usually develop symptoms within hours after birth. Microvascular thrombosis with DIC is seen clinically as ecchymoses, purpura, and hemorrhagic bullae, followed by necrosis and gangrene, usually on the extremities, trunk, scalp, and pressure points (also occasionally in other organs) (60). Laboratory findings resemble those of DIC, except for nondetectable protein C antigenic and functional levels. Skin biopsies reveal extensive thrombosis of the arterioles and venules. CNS and vitreous or retinal thrombosis with hemorrhage may occur in utero, resulting in mental retardation, developmental delay, and blindness, although fortunately these complications are attenuated by reduced hepatic synthesis of vitamin K-dependent coagulation factors. Neonatal extension of this protected state may suppress purpura fulminans, with affected babies instead developing massive thrombosis later in infancy (60). Most reported infants with neonatal purpura fulminans have been the offspring of consanguineous parents.

Thromboembolic disease: Both heterozygotes and homozygotes with the autosomal dominant (thrombosis-prone) form may develop a wide spectrum of thrombotic diseases. Deep vein thrombosis and/or pulmonary embolism is the most frequent manifestation. Arterial events such as myocardial infarction, transient ischemic attacks, and ischemic stroke are uncommon overall, but the prevalence is higher in proteins C and S deficiency (8.4%) than in AT-III (1%) deficiency (50). Superficial thrombophlebitis is also relatively more common with protein C deficiency. Events begin in adolescence or young adulthood, 80% of cases occurring before the age of 40 years (50, 56, 62). About 50% of events occur during periods of thrombotic risk such as pregnancy or surgery. The risk is intensified in patients who are less than 40 years old; the incidence of thromboembolism before age 40 is 120-fold and 14-fold higher in protein C-deficient males and females, respectively, than in the general population (50). Thrombosis in unusual sites such as the upper extremities, viscera (renal, mesenteric veins) or brain (cerebral sinuses) occurs with a prevalence similar to that of other inherited deficiencies. Some individuals may have only a single thrombotic episode, but about 50% have recurrent events.

Warfarin-induced skin necrosis: This syndrome is characterized by the sudden onset of painful edematous erythema followed by hemorrhagic bullae, gangrene, and necrosis of the skin and subcutaneous tissues of the extremities, trunk, breasts, buttocks, or penis (63, 64). These symptoms typically occur 2 to 3 days after initiation and are more common with the older practice of large warfarin loading doses. Laboratory findings in severe cases resemble those of DIC. Histologic examination reveals microvascular thrombosis, a finding that was previously considered paradoxical, since the reaction was caused by an anticoagulant. It is now believed that warfarin-induced skin necrosis is caused by a transient hypercoagulable state that occurs because of the short half-life of protein C (6 to 8 hr) compared to the other vitamin K-dependent clotting factors, especially factors II, IX, and X (24 to 80 hr). When warfarin is begun, rapid depletion of protein C may be seen at a time when levels of factors II, IX, and X are almost normal (56, 63, 64). This exaggerated imbalance causes the thrombosis and may also explain the association with large loading doses. At steady state, the reduction in protein C levels is comparable to that of the other factors, and the thrombotic risk is therefore eliminated. Patients with inherited or acquired protein C deficiency are particularly susceptible to warfarin-induced skin necrosis because they have baseline low levels.

Treatment. Neonatal purpura fulminans: Prompt recognition and treatment are essential for survival. Protein C may be replaced by infusion of fresh frozen plasma (FFP) in doses of 8 to 12 mL/kg every 12 hr. This has been reported to halt the formation of new lesions and to induce regression of evolving lesions (60). Alternative sources of protein C include prothrombin complex concentrate (factor IX concentrate) and protein C concentrate if available. Heparin, factor VIII concentrate, AT-III concentrate, vitamin K, and antiplatelet agents are not useful (60). Supportive care for the dermatologic, neurologic, and ophthalmic manifestations should be provided. Replacement therapy should be continued until all lesions are healed. If the patient survives, healing occurs over 4 to 8 weeks, often with residual scarring and sometimes requiring plastic surgery or amputation.

Human protein C concentrate (manufacturer Immuno-AG; Austria) is available in the United States on an investigational basis. It is prepared as a monoclonal antibody-purified concentrate made from viral-inactivated prothrombin complex concentrate (factor IX concentrate). The product is then vapor heated for further virus inactivation. Protein C concentrate is undergoing trials in a number of conditions. In purpura fulminans, normalization of laboratory findings occurs over several days; actual resorption of retinal hemorrhage and healing of a necrotic leg lesion have also been reported (65). One International Unit of concentrate is equal to the protein C activity in 1 mL of normal pooled plasma. After intravenous administration the close correlation between antigenic and functional plasma levels suggests that the infused protein C retains its activity. Pharmacokinetic studies have demonstrated variability in the fraction recovered, depending on disease acuity. Biphasic elimination with initial and terminal half-lives of 6 and 11 hr, respectively, were observed in a neonate not receiving oral anticoagulants (65). When concentrate was given at the time of oral anticoagulant initiation, the half-life of protein C activity was about 12 hr after the first dose and 18 hr with subsequent dosing (62). Short- (4 days), medium- (32 days), and long-term (8 months) maintenance therapy has been administered without adverse effects (62, 65, 66).

Acute thromboembolism: Acute deep vein thrombosis and pulmonary embolism in protein C-deficient patients is managed with heparin and warfarin in doses to produce the same target laboratory values as the general population (refer to Chapter 42, "Thromboembolic Disease"). An important precaution in protein C-deficient patients is to ensure that therapeutic doses of heparin are being administered at the time of initial warfarin therapy and until a therapeutic prothrombin time INR is achieved. This reduces the risk of warfarin-induced skin necrosis. Resistance to heparin may rarely occur in protein C-deficient patients. This was managed in a homozygous male with acute deep vein thrombosis by infusion of protein C concentrate during the warfarin titration period (62).

Warfarin skin necrosis: Prompt diagnosis and management are required to avoid ischemic necrosis of the subcutaneous tissues. It is managed with heparin (to stop the clotting process), FFP or cryoprecipitate (to replace protein C), and vitamin K (to facilitate endogenous protein C production). Protein C concentrate with intravenous heparin administration has also been reported to induce a rapid improvement in laboratory abnormalities and clinical manifestations over 24 hr, with complete healing over 15 days (66). Appropriate supportive therapy to minimize complications such as infection is essential. Reconstructive surgery may be necessary in severe cases.

Long-Term Management. Until recently, neonatal purpura fulminans was considered a uniformly and rapidly fatal disorder. Advances in its diagnosis and management have improved short-term survival and allowed development of long-term treatment strategies. Protein C concentrate is not suitable for long-term maintenance use because of its short half-life and high cost. After complete resolution of the purpura fulminans, either FFP given daily or pro-

thrombin complex concentrate (factor IX complex) given every other day may be used to sustain protein C levels that are adequate to halt ongoing coagulation (60). Successful management for as long as 2 years has been reported (67). Unfortunately, both products have significant disadvantages including possible virus transmission and the need for venous access; hyperproteinemia, hypertension, or fluid overload and the need for daily infusions associated with FFP; and variable and unpredictable protein C content with the possibility of drug-induced thromboembolism with prothrombin complex concentrate. An alternative approach to long-term management is to reduce the levels of vitamin K-dependent coagulation factors (II, VII, IX, X) to a degree sufficient to suppress clot formation. Oral warfarin carefully titrated to a prothrombin INR that is adequate to maintain an asymptomatic state is the most common long-term treatment (60). Special considerations in the use of warfarin in protein C-deficient patients include delaying treatment until all lesions of purpura fulminans have healed and the need for 5 to 7 days of overlapping heparin or FFP when initiating therapy. The latter precaution is recommended to reduce the likelihood of warfarin skin necrosis. If the symptoms of purpura fulminans recur, prompt replacement of protein C with FFP or protein C concentrate is indicated (prothrombin complex concentrate may be harmful in this situation). Liver transplantation cured protein C deficiency in a single case report.

Patients with protein C deficiency or APCR associated with recurrent thrombosis should be managed with lifelong warfarin therapy to a prothrombin INR goal of 2.0 to 3.0 (or sometimes higher). Symptomatic patients with APCR and a second inherited deficiency (AT-III, protein C or S) should be similarly treated. LMW heparin (fraxiparin) has also been successfully used as long-term secondary prophylaxis in treating patients who have a history of warfarin skin necrosis (61). Patients who refuse or are not suitable candidates for long-term anticoagulant therapy should be counseled regarding avoidance of thrombosis risk situations and the advisability of short-term prophylaxis.

Management of asymptomatic individuals and those with a single thrombotic event is controversial because of variable and unpredictable clinical expression of the deficiency. The decision to maintain lifelong treatment is made only after individualized consultation regarding its potential risks and benefits. Many practitioners advise long-term prophylaxis after only one event if it is life-threatening or spontaneous. The value of this strategy was assessed in 141 protein C- or S-deficient patients who were followed for 598 patient-years (50). The overall incidence (initial or recurrent events, with or without long-term prophylaxis) was reduced from 1.4 (protein C) to 2.0 (protein S) per 100 patient-years before the strategy was initiated to 0.8 (combined) per 100 patient-years after implementation. If oral anticoagulants were given and poor compliers were excluded, this was further reduced to 0.5 per 100 patient-years. The reduction in recurrent thromboembolism was even more striking, from 4.8 per 100 patient-years (baseline incidence) to 1.4 after the strategy was initiated and 0.3 if poor compliers were excluded. A disturbing finding in this report was the occurrence of major thrombosis in 2 of 51 protein C-deficient patients and 2 of 16 protein S-deficient patients who were asymptomatic at presentation and therefore did not receive long-term prophylaxis. While this finding may support prophylaxis in all patients, it should be emphasized that the risk of treatment must also be considered in treating each patient. Patients who are unreliable, those who are subject to trauma, and those with bleeding risk such as ulcer disease should be carefully evaluated before long-term anticoagulants are given. An important therapeutic distinction in protein C-deficient patients is the need for either intravenous or subcutaneous heparin in doses to achieve a therapeutic aPTT before the first dose of warfarin and until a therapeutic prothrombin INR is achieved. Alternatively, FFP or protein C concentrate may be given during warfarin titration (62).

Approximately 50% of major thrombotic events occur in association with a risk situation. Short-term prophylaxis should be given to all patients during exposure to high-risk situations such as surgery, trauma, or prolonged immobilization, regardless of the thrombotic history. Heparin, warfarin, FFP, and/or protein C concentrate may be used. Limited evidence favors the use of replacement therapy, either alone or with heparin (50). Prophylaxis should be given before, during, and immediately after risk exposure and is especially important in patients under 40 years of age (50).

The risk of maternal and fetal complications during pregnancy in protein C-deficient females is not as high as that seen with AT-III deficiency but is nonetheless higher than that of the general population. All patients should therefore receive prophylaxis, regardless of thrombotic history. Pregnancy is managed as previously described in the discussin of AT-III deficiency, with the elimination of AT-III concentrate. FFP or protein C concentrate may be considered in the peripartum period. Warfarin should be initiated promptly after delivery, with overlapping heparin therapy.

Monitoring Parameters. Frequent clinical assessment of the affected areas should be performed. Relevant laboratory studies in patients with purpura fulminans include markers of DIC (Table 15.5). If available, levels of fibrinopeptide A, prothrombin fragment F(1+2), thrombin-antithrombin complex, and protein C are also useful in assessing response. Patients who receive FFP should be regularly assessed for fluid overload and hypertension, with periodic evaluation of cardiac, renal, and hepatic function. Indwelling intravenous catheters should be evaluated for function, patency, and infection. Patients who are on long-term warfarin should have regular monitoring of prothrombin INR, hematocrit, and bleeding signs. All patients should receive longitudinal assessment for recurrence of the thrombotic manifestations. Childhood growth and development should also be followed.

Patient Education. Patient counseling for individuals with protein C deficiency is similar to that described in the discussion of AT-III deficiency. Patients should be apprised of both the potential for reduction in subsequent events with treatment and the lack of effect with poor compliance. Family screening should be performed to identify additional deficient individuals. Females who desire oral contraceptives should be advised of the potential for drug-induced thromboembolism. Although the incremental risk in protein C-deficient females who have taken oral contraceptives appears to be less than that for AT-III deficiency (58), in one study oral contraceptives were the precipitating factor for five initial thrombotic events in 57 protein C-deficient patients (50). Other forms of contraception should therefore be advised.

Acquired Protein C Deficiency. Protein C levels may be reduced in severe liver disease, DIC, acute respiratory distress syndrome, malignancy, pregnancy, and postoperatively, but a causative relationship with thrombotic risk is unclear. Patients with previously normal protein C levels may have reduced levels during extensive deep vein thrombosis or pulmonary embolism due to consumption. Drugs that may alter levels include oral anticoagulants and L-asparaginase. Open trials of protein C concentrate in cohorts of children (39) and adults (40) with DIC have identified improvement in both clinical and laboratory parameters. The lack of bleeding risk with protein C is appealing and was found to be very useful in treating one patient with severe gastrointestinal bleeding.

Protein S Deficiency. Protein S is a vitamin K-dependent entity synthesized in the liver. It differs from protein C in that it does not require activation and is not itself an anticoagulant but rather a cofactor for the actions of other proteins. Binding of protein Ca to protein S markedly augments the proteolytic activity of protein Ca on factors Va and VIIIa. Protein S may also be a cofactor for the profibrinolytic actions of protein C. Approximately 30 to 50% of body stores circulate in the free (active) form (59). The remainder exists in an inactive membrane-bound complex with C4b binding protein, a regulator of the complement system. Protein S levels are altered by warfarin but not by heparin.

The prevalence of protein S deficiency in the general population is not known, nor is the exact genetic defect causing the syndrome (46, 55, 59). The prevalence in patients with venous thromboembolism is at least as high as that of AT-III and protein C deficiency (59). Three types of deficiency have been described:

1. Type I (quantitative) is the most common and is characterized by reduction in both total and free protein S antigen. The protein S produced is of normal or moderately reduced activity. C4b binding protein levels are also reduced.
2. Type II is a qualitative deficiency wherein normal amounts of protein S antigen are produced but it is functionally defective. This type is rare.
3. In type III, total protein S antigen and C4b binding protein levels are normal, but the levels of free protein S are reduced (59, 68). In general, the functional protein S levels in type III patients are higher than in type I patients (68).

Diagnosis and Clinical Findings. Like the other deficiency syndromes, protein S deficiency has variable clinical and biologic expression. Homozygous protein S deficiency manifests as death in utero or a syndrome similar to neonatal purpura fulminans as seen in protein C deficiency. Some heterozygotes are completely asymptomatic (even during exposure to risk factors). Deep vein thrombosis and/or pulmonary thrombosis account for 64% of initial events (68), which typically begin in young adulthood. Superficial thrombophlebitis (30% of events) occurs at a rate greater than that of AT-III deficiency and comparable to that of protein C deficiency. Venous thrombosis in unusual sites (axillary, cerebral sinuses, mesenteric, portal, jugular, etc.) is seen with a prevalence comparable to that of other deficiencies. Arterial thrombosis (primarily in the cerebrum or coronary arteries) occur in 5 to 8% (50, 68–70). Approximately one-half of initial events are spontaneous. Pregnancy is a common predisposing condition, especially for patients with combined protein S deficiency and APCR (69, 71). Recurrence is common, some reported patients having as many as 15 thrombotic episodes. Warfarin-induced skin necrosis has also been reported in protein S deficiency.

Thrombotic events appear to be more common in isolated protein S deficiency than in protein C deficiency (50), although some have suggested the high incidence may be due to selection of severely affected families (69) or misdiagnosis of patients who actually have APCR (59). At least 50 to 70% have their first episode before the age of 40 (50, 68, 69). Some investigators have suggested that with prolonged follow-up, all individuals with heterozygous protein S deficiency will eventually develop thrombosis (46, 69). There is no relationship between the type of deficiency, the levels of antigenic or functional protein S, and the incidence of thrombosis (68, 69), a finding that suggests that factors other than the antigenic or functional concentration regulate the degree of clinical expression. Evidence suggests that patients with both protein S deficiency and APCR have a significantly greater incidence of thrombosis than do patients with either alone (69, 71).

Treatment. The acute and long-term management of patients with protein S deficiency is similar to that for protein C deficiency. Because of the higher incidence of thrombotic events, however, there is a greater tendency to give lifelong oral anticoagulants in protein S deficiency after even one event. Conservative practitioners maintain a conservative approach, treating with long-term warfarin only patients with recurrent thrombosis (56). When given in doses titrated to the standard desired prothrombin INR, warfarin has been found to be effective in preventing subsequent events (68, 69); detailed documentation of value is discussed in the section above on protein C deficiency (50). Moreover, temporary discontinuation of warfarin resulted in recurrent thrombosis (69). Asymptomatic patients are generally not treated with long-term warfarin. The occurrence of initial thrombotic events in 2 of 16 previously asymptomatic patients who were followed for a mean of 5.3 years, coupled with the severity of these events (stroke in a 23-year-old and myocardial infarction in a 42-year-old) (50), suggests that further studies should be performed to assess the value of long-term warfarin in asymptomatic protein S-deficient patients. Replacement therapy with either FFP or prothrombin complex concentrate (factor IX concentrate) has been used both therapeutically and prophylactically (46). The use of FFP requires larger volumes; however, it may otherwise be advantageous, since it exposes the patient to fewer infectious complications and does not have the potential to enhance thrombosis risk by providing other coagulant factors.

On the basis of available data, all protein S-deficient individuals should receive short-term prophylaxis before, during, and immediately after exposure to risk situations such as surgery or trauma, regardless of thrombotic history. Pregnant females with isolated protein S deficiency are at lower thrombotic risk than are those with AT-III or protein C deficiency (58). Most clinicians nonetheless prefer to give prophylaxis to pregnant patients in the same fashion as for patients with protein C deficiency (50).

Acquired protein S deficiency: Liver disease, DIC, nephrotic syndrome, and pregnancy have all been associated with low protein S levels. Drug-induced reductions in protein S levels may occur during treatment with oral anticoagulants, oral contraceptives (70, 71), estrogens, and L-asparaginase. The C4b binding protein that complexes with protein S is an acute phase reactant; therefore levels will increase in acute inflammatory processes (e.g., postoperative states, infection). This may reduce levels of free (active) protein S, thereby partially explaining the high thrombotic risk associated with these conditions (5, 46). **Other Inherited Hypercoagulable States.** The miscellaneous causes of hypercoagulable states may be broadly grouped into impaired fibrinolysis, abnormal fibrinogen, or heparin cofactor II deficiency. Fibrinolysis is a complex process that is regulated by numerous proteins (Fig. 15.2).

Abnormalities in the fibrinolytic system are common in patients with acute thrombosis but in this context are probably due to the disease and are unlikely to be the cause of the thrombosis. Inherited deficiency, dysfunction, and impaired release of plasminogen, plasminogen activator (t-PA), plasminogen activator inhibitor (PAI-1), or factor XII have been reported (5, 46, 56) and occur in an autosomal-dominant pattern. Fibrinolysis may also be altered by acute ethanol ingestion, drugs (e.g., oral contraceptives), or diseases (e.g., acute myocardial infarction, postoperatively, malignancy, infection). The clinical presentation of thrombosis is similar to that of AT-III or protein C or S deficiency (5, 56). However, abnormalities in fibrinolysis appear to be much less important, since associated thrombosis is rare. An important therapeutic consideration in these patients is that abnormal plasminogen function or activation may preclude the use of thrombolytic agents.

Abnormal inherited fibrinogen defects may result in inadequate quantity or function, the latter condition being more common. Congenital fibrinogen disorders are clinically asymptomatic in most patients and more commonly cause bleeding rather than thrombosis when symptoms are seen (46, 56). Thrombosis is rare; when present, it is caused by the production of abnormal fibrinogen that is resistant to lysis by plasmin. Acquired quantitative abnormalities are more common than the inherited form. Low fibrinogen levels are one of the hallmark signs of DIC and contribute to its associated bleeding. Accelerated fibrinogen consumption by thrombolytic drugs and decreased production in liver disease are other causes of fibrinogenemia.

Heparin cofactor II has a specific antithrombin effect (Fig. 15.1) that is accelerated by heparin, dermatan sulfate, and dextran. Inherited deficiency may manifest clinically as arterial or venous thrombosis; however, the vast majority of heparin cofactor II-deficient individuals are asymptomatic. Low levels are also seen in DIC but not in nephrotic syndrome or acute venous thrombosis.

HEMOPHILIA

The hereditary deficiencies of factor VIII (antihemophilic factor, or AHF) or factor IX (plasma thromboplastin component, PTC, Christmas factor) procoagulant activity are known as the hemophilias. They occur in an estimated 10 to 25 males per 100,000 and are the most common congenital plasma coagulation defects. Hemophilia results in spontaneous or posttraumatic bleeding into muscles, joints, and body cavities.

Hemophilia A and B are caused by a defect or absence of the procoagulant portion of factor VIII or factor IX, respectively. Both are X-linked recessive disorders that are clinically indistinguishable. Lack of either functional factor decreases the conversion of factor X to factor Xa, diminishing the coagulation response to vascular injury.

The abnormality causes an increase in the activated partial thromboplastin time (aPTT) with no changes in prothrombin time (PT), bleeding time, or platelet count. Hemophilia A accounts for 80% of hemophilias.

Factor deficiency is not absolute in hemophilia. Factor VIII and factor IX procoagulant levels remain relatively constant in a patient and correspond to hemorrhagic frequency and severity. Factor VIII or factor IX levels of 100% correspond to factor VIII or factor IX activity of 1.0 U/ml. Factor VIII and factor IX levels in a normal person range from 50% to 200% (0.5 to 2.0 U/mL).

Although hemostasis occurs at 25 to 30% of normal factor VIII activity, most symptomatic patients with hemophilia A have factor VIII levels below 5%. Individuals with factor VIII levels less than 1% (0.01 U/mL) are classified as severe hemophiliacs. They average two to four hemorhagic episodes monthly, often occurring without discernible trauma. Patients with factor VIII levels greater than 5% are considered mild hemophiliacs. These patients usually hemorrhage only after trauma or surgery. Spontaneous bleeding may occur occasionally, especially in joints that have been damaged by previously undertreated posttraumatic hemorrhage. Patients with factor VIII levels between 1% and 5% are considered to be moderate hemophiliacs, with manifestations between the two extremes. Most patients with hemophilia A have factor VIII levels below 5%.

Clinical Manifestations

The clinical hallmarks of hemophilia A and B are (a) lack of excessive hemorrhage from minor cuts or abrasions, due to the normalcy of platelet function; (b) joint and muscle hemorrhages leading to the most difficult and disabling long-term sequelae; (c) easy bruising; (d) prolonged and potentially fatal postoperative hemorrhage; and (e) a panoply of social, psychological, vocational, and economic problems (72).

Hemarthrosis is the most common and often the most disabling manifestation of hemophilia. The joints that are most frequently involved include the knees, elbows, ankles, shoulders, hips, and wrists. The spine and hands are rarely involved.

An aura consisting of joint warmth and tingling often signals the onset of hemorrhage. Mild discomfort gives way to pain, swelling, erythema, and decreased range-of-motion over the next several hours. Young children often display guarding, irritability, and decreased movement in an affected joint. Classic symptoms in a reliable patient are a sufficient basis for immediate treatment.

Joint hemorrhage should be treated at the earliest symptoms to limit acute and prevent long-term sequelae. Within 8 to 12 hr of treatment, symptoms of hemarthrosis begin to improve. Initial treatment with factor VIII or factor IX concentrate requires that levels be increased to 30 to 50% (73). Maintenance at a level of 15 to 25% may be required for several days. Once bleeding has stopped, blood is resorbed, and the joint returns to normal over several days to weeks. Use of nonsteroidal antiinflammatory agents for joint pain should be avoided because of their disruptive effects on platelet function.

Many hemophiliac patients develop "target joints" that bleed more frequently. Frequent and undertreated hemarthrosis leads to synovitis, hemophilic arthropathy, joint capsule fibrosis, and chronic loss of joint mobility.

Microscopic and macroscopic hematuria is a common problem among hemophiliacs. Treatment usually includes bed rest, increased fluids, and corticosteroids (74). Treatment with factor concentrate to elevate levels to 40% for 2 to 4 days must be necessary if conservative treatment is unsuccessful. The use of ε-aminocaproic acid should be avoided, since decreasing clot lysis may prevent removal of a clot occluding the ureter (75).

Spontaneous and posttraumatic hematomas are frequent complications of hemophilia. Although most are small and resolve spontaneously, large soft-tissue bleeds may cause anemia and compartment syndromes with ischemic and neurologic complications (73).

Treatment of large hematomas requires factor concentrates to increase levels to 50 to 60% or more. Maintenance therapy for several days may be required to reduce rebleeding. Aggressive therapy can reduce the incidence of long-term complications, including pseudocysts, calcifications, and fibrosis (73).

Spontaneous or posttraumatic intracranial bleeding accounts for 25% of deaths of hemophiliac patients. Surviving patients are often left with mental retardation, seizure disorders, or motor impairment (76). Treatment of intracranial bleeding should be immediate and aggressive. Any patient with a history of head trauma and signs of head injury, including abrasions, lacerations, or scalp hematoma, should be treated. Factor VIII or factor IX concentrates should be used to increase and maintain the level to 100% (71, 72).

Minor lacerations are usually managed with conservative treatment. Factor replacement to raise the factor level to 30 to 50% is usually limited to minor lacerations that are unresponsive to conservative therapy or serious lacerations.

Falls, with mucosal lacerations to the mouth, are common among toddlers. Application of ice and pressure may be helpful but difficult. Factor replacement to a level of 40 to 50% is often indicated. Supplementation with ε-aminocaproic acid or tranexamic acid may be advantageous. Temporary restriction of oral intake and repeated treatment may be required if clot dislodgement is a problem (73).

Gastrointestinal bleeding, gingival bleeding, epistaxis, and other forms of bleeding occur less commonly.

Treatment

Currently available modes of hemophilia treatment center on increasing the concentration of deficient clotting factors or inhibiting fibrinolysis. Products that are used to increase clotting factor concentration include fresh-frozen plasma (FFP), cryoprecipitate, factor concentrates, and DDAVP. Antifibrinolytic agents include ε-aminocaproic acid and tranexamic acid.

FRESH-FROZEN PLASMA

FFP is the fluid portion of one unit of whole blood, taken from a single donor. It contains about 1 U of factor VIII and 1 U of factor IX per milliliter of plasma. One unit of FFP contains 200 to 300 U of both factors, a sufficient quantity to increase factor concentrations by 5 to 10% in a 60-kg man (73). Because of the large amount of fluid that would be required, FFP is not the optimal means of factor replacement. However, it is a readily available source of clotting factors that can be used until a more advantageous source is available.

CRYOPRECIPITATE

Cryoprecipitate is prepared by thawing FFP and removing the cell-free fluid remaining after centrifugation. The residual precipitate contains 40 to 50% of the original factor VIII concentration. Cryoprecipitate contains no factor IX. Although less volume would be required to restore hemostasis than with FFP, cryoprecipitate is not a primary means of hemophilia A treatment.

FACTOR VIII REPLACEMENT

Purified factor VIII is isolated from pooled plasma generated from thousands of donors. To decrease the risk of viral transmission, early lyophilized products were usually heat-treated to 60°C for 10 to 30 hr. This method was abandoned because of the continued reports of hepatitis and HIV. Current virucidal techniques include treating the concentrate with solvent/detergent to disrupt viral lipid coats, treatment to higher temperatures for longer time periods, pasteurization, and vapor heating.

Immunosuppression due to alloantigens or viruses in factor concentrates has been combated with the advent of highly purified factor concentrates. Purity refers to the amount of nonfactor VIII proteins in the final product. Those isolated by affinity chromatography with monoclonal antibody techniques produce high-purity concentrates. Although extraneous proteins are removed, increasing purity does not decrease the risk of viral transmission.

More recently, human factor VIII cDNA has been introduced into mammalian cell lines to produce recombinant factor VIII products that appear to be equivalent to plasma-derived concentrates. The obvious advantage of recombinant factor concentrate is the increased risk of viral

Table 15.8.
Factor VIII Concentrates

Product	Viral Inactivation	Manufacturer
Humate-P	Heat-treated, wet method; pasteurized	Armour
Melate	Solvent-detergent inactivation	Melville Biologics
Profilate OSD	Solvent-detergent inactivated	Alpha Therapeutics
Profilate SD	Heat-treated, wet method; solvent-detergent inactivated	Alpha Therapeutics
High-Purity		
Monoclate-P	Heat-treated, wet method; pasteurized, monoclonal antibody purified	Armour
Hemofil M, Method M	Solvent-detergent inactivated, monoclonal antibody purified	Hyland
Koate-HP	Solvent-detergent inactivated, gel-filtration purified	Miles
Antihemophilic factor (human)	Solvent-detergent inactivated, monoclonal antibody purified	American Red Cross
Recombinant		
Recombinate		
Kogenate		

From *American Hospital Formulary Service Drug Information,* American Society of Hospital Pharmacists, Inc., 1994.

transmission associated with plasma-derived factors. Currently, no recombinant factor IX is available. It is recommended that all patients with hemophilia, regardless of previous exposure to HIV or hepatitis, should receive treatment with high-purity concentrates or recombinant concentrates with the lowest possible risk of viral transmission (see Table 15.8). Cost, however, remains a factor since high purity and recombinant concentrates are more expensive.

The goal of factor replacement therapy is to achieve hemostasis by maintaining adequate levels of deficient factor. The level of clotting factor to achieve this goal depends on the indication for treatment.

Factor volume of distribution, baseline concentration, half-life, and the presence of inhibitors are four pharmacokinetic factors that influence the dose of factor replacement required.

Factor VIII distributes to plasma volume and initially to extravascular space. The volume of distribution is approximately 50 mL/kg. A simple dose calculation based on volume of distribution is that each unit of Factor VIII (equal to the amount found in 1 mL of plasma) infused per kilogram of body weight yields a 2% increase in plasma level (0.02 U/mL).

Dose in U/kg =

$$\frac{(\text{Desired concentration} - \text{baseline patient concentration})}{2}$$

The half-life of Factor VIII is biphasic. The early redistribution phase half-life is approximately 4 hr, and the biologic half-life is approximately 12 hr. Therefore 12 hr after an infusion, the plasma concentration of Factor VIII will decrease to one-half of its postinfusion concentration. Infusions of one-half the original dose given every 12 hr should restore the factor concentration to the desired level.

FACTOR IX REPLACEMENT

Since cryoprecipitate does not contain factor IX and DDAVP does not increase endogenous concentrations of factor IX, elevations in factor IX concentration are accomplished through infusions of either FFP or purified factor IX concentrates.

Prothrombin complex concentrates have been the mainstay of treatment for patients with hemophilia B. These concentrates contain not only factor IX, but also significant quantities of the other vitamin K–dependent clotting factors II, VII, and X. Although these agents are effective, they increase the risk of thrombosis, especially when used at high doses (77).

Highly purified factor IX concentrates are now available, containing only trace quantities of factors II, VII, and X. These concentrates should decrease the risk of thrombosis and myocardial infarction. Although more costly, they are the preferred source of factor IX in the treatment of hemophilia B (see Table 15.9).

Because the molecular size of factor IX is one-fifth that of factor VIII, the volume of distribution of factor IX is twice that of factor VIII. A simple dose calculation based on volume of distribution is that each unit of factor IX (equal to the amount found in 1 mL of plasma) infused per kilogram of body weight yields a 1% increase in plasma level (0.01 U/mL). The minimum hemostatic level is 10 to 25%, a range that is significantly lower than the estimated 30% minimum for factor VIII.

Factor IX dose in U/kg =

$$\frac{(\text{Desired concentration} - \text{baseline patient concentration})}{2}$$

The biologic half-life of factor IX is approximately 24 hr. Because of the long half-life, compared to factor VIII, subsequent doses of factor IX can be administered at a 24-hr dosing interval. Factor IX levels should be monitored every few days to ensure adequate concentrations.

Complications

Approximately 10 to 15% of patients with severe hemophilia A develop factor VIII inhibitors after repeated doses of factor concentrate. These inhibitors are immunoglobulin G (IgG) antibodies that bind to and inactivate factor VIII. Anti–factor VIII development (titers expressed as Bethesda units, BU) follow two patterns. Low responders (3 to 5 BU) have low inhibitor titers that do not rise after further exposure to factor VIII. High responders (65 to 75% of patients with inhibitors) have low inhibitor titers that rise markedly with further exposure to factor VIII (anamnestic response) (78). Inhibitor titers usually rise 2 to 3 days after exposure, reach a maximum in 7 to 21 days, then decline slowly. Inhibitors may persist for 1 to 2 years after exposure to factor VIII.

Options for treatment of patients producing inhibitors are to (1) administer sufficient quantities of human or porcine factor concentrate to overwhelm antibodies that are present with an excess to produce hemostasis, (2) restore hemostasis with factors other than factor VIII, and (3) remove antibodies by plasmaphoresis or extracorporeal adsorption.

Human factor VIII can be used to treat hemorrhages in either low or high responders with inhibitor levels less than 5 BU and in patients with inhibitor levels between 5 and 30 BU after inhibitor removal. To neutralize inhibitors and achieve therapeutic hemostatic concentrations of 30 to 50%, an adult patient can be given an initial factor VIII bolus of 70 to 140 U/kg followed by an infusion of 4 to 14 U/kg/hr (79). Alternatively, factor VIII can be given every 1 to 4 hr (40 U/kg + 20 U/kg/BU) (80). Factor VIII levels should be monitored regularly to ensure that therapeutic concentrations are maintained.

Cross-reactivity to porcine factor VIII is approximately 25%. After treatment with porcine VIII, antiporcine and antihuman factor VIII antibody concentrations rise, but less than is seen after the infusion of human factor VIII. Many patients who are unresponsive to human factor VIII respond to porcine factor VIII (81).

When factor VIII inhibitor levels are too high (>30 BU), an attempt to bypass factor VIII can be initiated with factor IX concentrate. Two types of factor IX concentrates are available: unactivated factor IX, as is used for the treatment of hemophilia B, and activated concentrate, with higher concentrations of "factor VIII–bypassing material." The activated concentrates, Autoplex and FEIBA, are designed specifically for treatment hemorrhages in patients with high factor VIII inhibitor concentrations. The efficacy of both types of factor IX is unpredictable. Infusion-induced hypercoagulability with resultant thromboembolic events are a possible complication (80).

Inhibitors to factor IX occur in approximately 12% patients with severe hemophilia B. Like factor VIII inhibitors, factor IX inhibitors are IgG antibodies. Treatment of patients with factor IX inhibitors is usually accomplished with factor IX concentrates. The role of immunosuppressive therapy is under investigation.

Infectious complications from viruses that are transmitted by transfusion were first noted in hemophiliacs in the late 1970s. Nearly all patients who are treated with concentrates before current viral inactivation methods were employed have developed antibodies to hepatitis C and/or hepatitis B. Patients who develop chronic carrier states are at increased risk for chronic liver disease and hepatocellular carcinoma. Despite current virucidal methods, sporadic cases of hepatitis are reported. Therefore all newly diagnosed patients with hemophilia should receive the HBV vaccination. Newly diagnosed infants should receive the series of three injections beginning soon after birth.

HIV was introduced into the U.S. blood supply in the 1970s. By 1982, 50% of hemophiliacs were infected with the virus (82). Since that time the virucidal treatment of concentrates has virtually eliminated the risk of HIV due to factor transfusion.

Table 15.9.
Factor IX Concentrates

Product	Viral Inactivation	Manufacturer
Factor IX Complex		
Bebulin VH Immuno	Heat-treated, wet method	Immuno-US
Konyne 80	Heat-treated, dry method	Miles
Profilnine Heat-Treated	Heat-treated, wet method; organic solvent	Alpha Therapeutics
Proplex T	Heat-treated, dry method	Baxter
Human		
AlphaNine SD	Solvent-detergent inactivated	Alpha Therapeutics
Mononine	Monoclonal antibody purified	Armour

From *American Hospital Formulary Service Drug Information*, American Society of Hospital Pharmacists, Inc., 1994.

Allergic reactions to factor concentrate is mild and uncommon. Patients who have had allergic reactions to cryoprecipitate usually do not react to concentrates. Large doses of factor VIII may cause hemolytic anemia in recipients with type A or B erythrocytes, owing to the presence of anti-A or anti-B antibodies in the concentrate. If red blood cell transfusion is necessary, type O cells should be given.

DESMOPRESSIN

Desmopressin (DDAVP) is a synthetic analog of the hormone vasopressin. Although the mechanism is unknown, DDAVP produces a twofold to fourfold increase in factor VIII concentrations in most mild hemophiliacs (83). DDAVP does not increase production of factor VIII but stimulates the release of stored factor VIII. DDAVP does not increase the concentration of factor IX. Therefore patients with severe hemophilia A or with hemophilia B do not benefit from this therapy.

To determine whether patients are responsive to DDAVP, a plasma factor concentration is obtained after an infusion. Testing for responsiveness is often conducted while a patient is asymptomatic. This prevents the decision to use more aggressive forms of therapy from being delayed while DDAVP response is being assessed. Most patients with mild hemophilia A and factor VIII levels greater than 10% respond to DDAVP.

For patients who are known to respond and who do not have life-threatening bleeding, DDAVP is the treatment of choice (73). The recommended intravenous dose is 0.3 to 0.4 µg/kg, diluted in 50 mL of normal saline (10 mL for children less than or equal to 10 kg) and infused 15 to 30 min. DDAVP may be administered daily for 2 to 3 days, after which tachyphylaxis may develop (84). DDAVP can be infused 30 min before a planned minor surgical procedure for prophylaxis. Blood pressure, fluids, electrolytes, and heart rate should be monitored in patients, since DDAVP may cause a slight pressor response and fluid retention. Seizures secondary to hyponatremia have also been reported (85).

ANTIFIBRINOLYTIC AGENTS

Epsilon aminocaproic acid (EACA) and tranexamic acid are antifibrinolytic agents that are used to help stabilize clots. Their primary role is as a single-dose prophylactic agent after dental procedures. EACA is administered orally as a loading dose of 200 mg/kg (maximum 10 g) followed by maintenance doses of 100 mg/kg every 6 hr (maximum 30 g over 24 hr) for 5 to 7 days. Tranexamic acid is administered orally at 25 mg/kg every 6 to 8 hr for 5 to 7 days. The two agents are generally well tolerated, gastrointestinal complaints being the most reported complication.

PROPHYLAXIS

Prophylactic factor VIII or factor IX infusions can eliminate or minimize most bleeding complications if therapy is initiated before joint disease (86). Once joint disease is present, prophylactic therapy in preventing progression is unproven (73). The expense and inconvenience of prophylactic regimens are also limiting factors.

FUTURE THERAPIES

The only documented cure for hemophilia to date is liver transplantation. One report describes liver transplants in four hemophiliac patients with end-stage liver disease. Of the three surviving patients, all had return of normal factor VIII production and resolution of hemophilia (87). The cloning of genes for factor VIII and factor IX ("gene therapy") may be the most practical cure currently under investigation. Transplanting human fibroblasts transfected with a human factor IX gene into mice has been successful in producing circulating human factor IX (88). Additional experiments are in progress.

REFERENCES

1. Saito H. Normal hemostatic mechanisms. In: Ratnoff OD, Forbes CD, eds. Disorders of hemostasis. Philadelphia: WB Saunders, 1991:18–47.
2. Goebel RA. Thrombocytopenia. Emerg Med Clin North Am 11(2):445–464, 1993.
3. Bennett JS, Kolodziej MA. Disorders of platelet function. Dis Mon 38:579–631, 1992.
4. Comp PC. Production of plasma coagulation factors. In: Williams WJ, Beutler E, Erslev AJ, et al, eds. Hematology, 4th ed. New York: McGraw-Hill, 1990:1285–1294.
5. Nachman RL, Silverstein R. Hypercoagulable states. Ann Intern Med 119(8):819–827, 1993.
6. Rutherford CJ, Frenkel EP. Thrombocytopenia: issues in diagnosis and therapy. Med Clin North Am 78(3):555–575, 1994.
7. Blanchette VS, Kirby MA, Turner C. Role of intravenous immunoglobulin G in autoimmune hematologic disorders. Semin Hematol 29(3 suppl 2):72–82, 1992.
8. Waters AH. Autoimmune thrombocytopenia: clinical aspects. Semin Hematol 29(1):18–25, 1992.
9. Imbach P. Immune thrombocytopenic purpura and intravenous immunoglobulin. Cancer 68(6 suppl):1422–1425, 1991.
10. Blanchette VS, Luke B, Andrew M, et al. A prospective, randomized trial of high-dose intravenous immune globulin G therapy, oral prednisone therapy, and no therapy in childhood acute immune thrombocytopenic purpura. J Pediatr 123(6):989–995, 1993.
11. Blanchette V, Imbach P, Andrew M, et al. Randomised trial of intravenous immunoglobulin G, intravenous anti-D, and oral prednisone in childhood acute immune thrombocytopenic purpura. Lancet 344(8924):703–707, 1994.
12. Collins PW, Newland AC. Treatment modalities of autoimmune blood disorders. Semin Hematol 29(1):64–74, 1992.
13. Warkentin TE, Kelton JG. Current concepts in the treatment of immune thrombocytopenia. Drugs 40:531–542, 1990.
14. Albayrak D, Islek I, Kalayci G, Gürses N. Acute immune thrombocytopenic purpura: A comparative study of very high oral doses of methylprednisolone and intravenously administered immune globulin. J Pediatr 125(6 Pt 1):1004–1007, 1994.

15. Imbach P, Berchtold W, Hirt A, et al. Intravenous immunoglobulin versus oral corticosteroids in acute immune thrombocytopenic purpura in childhood. Lancet 2(8453):464–468, 1985.

16. Naouri A, Feghali B, Chabal J, et al. Results of splenectomy for idiopathic thrombocytopenic purpura. Acta Haematol 89:200–203, 1993.

17. Schattner E, Bussel J. Mortality in immune thrombocytopenic purpura: report of seven cases and consideration of prognostic indicators. Am J Hematol 46:120–126, 1994.

18. Oksenhandler E, Bierling P, Farcet JP, et al. Response to therapy in 37 patients with HIV-related thrombocytopenic purpura. Br J Haematol 66:491–495, 1987.

19. Tertian G, Risler W, Lebras P, et al. Intravenous gammaglobulin treatment for thrombocytopenic purpura in patients with HIV infection. Eur J Hematol 39:180–181, 1987.

20. Rose M, Rowe JM, Eldor A. The changing course of thrombotic thrombocytopenic purpura and modern therapy. Blood Rev 7:94–103, 1993.

21. Dabrow MB, Wilkins JC. Hematologic emergencies. Postgrad Med 93(5):193–194, 197–199, 202, 1993.

22. Bick RL. Platelet function defects associated with hemorrhage or thrombosis. Med Clin North Am 78(3):577–607, 1994.

23. Salama A, Mueller-Eckhardt C. Immune-mediated blood cell dyscrasias related to drugs. Semin Hematol 29(1):54–63, 1992.

24. Schmitt BP, Adelman B. Heparin-associated thrombocytopenia: a critical review and pooled analysis. Am J Med Sci 305(4):208–215, 1993.

25. Chong BH. Heparin-induced thrombocytopenia. Aust NZ J Med 22:145–152, 1992.

26. Bodensteiner DC, Doolittle GC. Adverse haematological complications of anticancer drugs. Drug Safety 8(3):213–224, 1993.

27. Gilbert JA, Scalzi RP. Disseminated intravascular coagulation. Emer Med Clin North Am 11(2):465–480, 1993.

28. Bick RL. Disseminated intravascular coagulation: objective criteria for diagnosis and management. Med Clin North Am 78(3):511–543, 1994.

29. Rubin RN, Coleman RW. Disseminated intravascular coagulation: approach to treatment. Drugs 44(6):963–971, 1992.

30. Colman RW, Rubin RN. Disseminated intravascular coagulation due to malignancy. Semin Oncol 17:172–86, 1990.

31. Feinstein DI. Treatment of disseminated intravascular coagulation. Semin Thromb Hemostas 14:351–362, 1988.

32. Sakuragawa N, Hasegawa H, Maki M, et al. Clinical evaluation of low-molecular-weight heparin (FR-860) on disseminated intravascular coagulation (DIC): a multicenter co-operative double-blind trial in comparison with heparin. Thromb Res 72(6):475–500, 1993.

33. Oguma Y, Sakuragawa N, Maki M, et al. Treatment of disseminated intravascular coagulation with low molecular weight heparin. Semin Thromb Hemostas 16(suppl):34–40, 1990.

34. Gillis S, Dann EJ, Eldor A. Low molecular weight heparin in the prophylaxis and treatment of disseminated intravascular coagulation in acute promyelocytic leukemia. Eur J Haematol 54:59–60, 1995.

35. Fourrier F, Chopin C, Huart JJ, et al. Double-blind, placebo-controlled trial of antithrombin III concentrates in septic shock with disseminated intravascular coagulation. Chest 104(3):882–888, 1993.

36. Vinazzer H. Therapeutic use of antithrombin III in shock and disseminated intravascular coagulation. Semin Thromb Hemostas 15(3):347–352, 1989.

37. Hanada T, Abe T, Takita H. Antithrombin III concentrates for treatment of disseminated intravascular coagulation in children. Am J Pediatr Hematol Oncol 7(1):3–8, 1985.

38. Wisecarver JL, Haire WD. Disseminated intravascular coagulation with multiple arterial thromboses responding to antithrombin-III concentrate infusion. Thromb Res 54(6):709–717, 1989.

39. Rivard GE, David M, Farrell C, Schwarz HP. Treatment of purpura fulminans in meningococcemia with protein C concentrate. J Pediatr 126(4):646–652, 1995.

40. Okajima K, Imamura H, Koga S, et al. Treatment of patients with disseminated intravascular coagulation by protein C. Am J Hematol 33(4):277–278, 1990.

41. Takada A, Takada Y, Mori T, Sakaguchi S. Prevention of severe bleeding by tranexamic in a patient with disseminated intravascular coagulation. Thromb Res 58(2):101–108, 1990.

42. Tamaki S, Hiyoyama K, Minamikawa K, et al. Treatment of disseminated intravascular coagulation with gabexate mesilate. Clin Therapeut 15(6):1076–1084, 1993.

43. Okamura T, Niho Y, Itoga T, et al. Treatment of disseminated intravascular coagulation and its prodromal stage with gabaxate mesilate (FOY): a multi-center trial. Acta Haematol 90(3):120–124, 1993.

44. Cofrancesco E, Boschetti C, Leonardi P, et al. Dermatan sulphate for the treatment of disseminated intravascular coagulation (DIC) in acute leukaemia: a randomised, heparin-controlled pilot study. Thromb Res 74(1):65–75, 1994.

45. Hathaway WE. Clinical aspects of antithrombin III deficiency. Semin Hematol 28(1):19–23, 1991.

46. Bick RL. Hypercoagulability and thrombosis. Med Clin North Am 78(3):635–665, 1994.

47. Hassouna HI. Laboratory evaluation of hemostatic disorders. Hematol Oncol Clin North Am 7(6):1161–1249, 1993.

48. Menache D. Antithrombin III concentrates. Hematol Oncol Clin North Am 6(5):1115–1120, 1992.

49. Schwartz RS, Bauer KA, Rosenberg RD, et al. Clinical experience with antithrombin III concentrate in treatment of congenital and acquired deficiency of antithrombin. Am J Med 87(suppl 3B):53S–60S, 1989.

50. De Stefano V, Leone G, Mastrangelo S, et al. Clinical manifestations and management of inherited thrombophilia: retrospective analysis and follow-up after diagnosis of 238 patients with congenital deficiency of antithrombin III, protein C, protein S. Thromb Haemost 72(3):352–358, 1994.

51. Menache BD, O'Malley JP, Schorr JB, et al. Evaluation of the safety, recovery, half-life, and clinical efficacy of antithrombin III (human) in patients with hereditary antithrombin III deficiency. Blood 75(1):33–39, 1990; 76(2):649–550, 1990.

52. Owen J. Antithrombin III replacement therapy in pregnancy. Semin Hematol 28(1):46–52, 1991.

53. Francis CW, Pellegrini VD Jr, Harris CM, et al. Prophylaxis of venous thrombosis following total hip and total knee replacement using antithrombin III and heparin. Semin Hematol 28(1):39–45, 1991.

54. Briggs GG, Freeman RK, Yaffe SJ. Drugs in pregnancy and lactation. Baltimore MD: Williams & Wilkins, 1994:223c–229c.

55. Alving BM. The hypercoagulable states. Hosp Practice 28(2):109–114, 119–121, 1993.

56. Eby CS. A review of the hypercoagulable state. Hematol Oncol Clin North Am 7(6):1121–1142, 1993.

57. Pogliani EM, Parma M, Baragetti I, et al. L-asparaginase in acute lymphoblastic leukemia treatment: the role of human antithrombin III concentrates in regulating the prothrombotic state induced by therapy. Acta Haematol 93(1):5–8, 1995.

58. Pabinger I, Schneider B, and the GTH Study Group on Natural Inhibitors. Thrombotic risk of women with hereditary antithrombin III-, protein C- and protein S-deficiency taking oral contraceptive medication. Thromb Haemost 71(5):548–552, 1994.

59. Dahlbäck B. Molecular genetics of venous thromboembolism. Ann Med 27(2):187–192, 1995.

60. Marlar RA, Montgomery RR, Broekmans AW, and the Working Party. Diagnosis and treatment of homozygous protein C deficiency. J Pediatr 114(4 pt 1):528–534, 1989.

61. Pescatore P, Horellou HM, Conard J, et al. Problems of oral anticoagulation in an adult with homozygous protein C deficiency and late onset of thrombosis. Thromb Haemost 69(4):311–315, 1993.

62. De Stefano V, Mastrangelo S, Schwarz HP, et al. Replacement therapy with a purified protein C concentrate during initiation of oral anticoagulation in severe protein C congenital deficiency. Thromb Haemost 70(2):247–249, 1993.

63. Broekmans AW, Bertina RM, Loeliger EA, et al. Protein C and the development of skin necrosis during anticoagulant therapy [letter]. Thromb Haemost 49:251, 1983.

64. McGehee WG, Klotz TA, Epstein DJ, Rappaport SI. Coumarin necrosis associated with hereditary protein C deficiency. Ann Intern Med 101:59–60, 1984.

65. Dreyfus M, Magny JF, Bridey F, et al. Treatment of homozygous protein C deficiency and neonatal purpura fulminans with a purified protein C concentrate. N Engl J Med 325(22):1565–1568, 1991.

66. Schramm W, Spannagl M, Bauer KA, et al. Treatment of coumarin-induced skin necrosis with a monoclonal antibody purified protein C concentrate. Arch Dermatol 129(6):753–756, 1993.

67. Marlar RA, Sills RH, Groncy PK, et al. Protein C survival during replacement therapy in homozygous protein C deficiency. Am J Hematol 41(1):24–31, 1992.

68. Gouault-Heilmann M, Leroy-Matheron C, Levent M. Inherited protein S deficiency: clinical manifestations and laboratory findings in 63 patients. Thromb Res 76(3):269–279, 1994.

69. Zöller B, Berntsdotter A, Garcia de Frutos P, Dahlbäck B. Resistance to activated protein C as an additional genetic risk factor in hereditary deficiency of protein S. Blood 85(12):3518–3523, 1995.

70. Heistinger M, Rumpl E, Illiasch H, et al. Cerebral sinus thrombosis in a patient with hereditary protein S deficiency: case report and review of the literature. Ann Hematol 64(2):105–109.

71. Hellgren M, Svensson PJ, Dahlbäck B. Resistance to activated protein C as a basis for venous thromboembolism associated with pregnancy and oral contraceptives. Am J Obstet Gynecol 173(1):210–213, 1995.

72. Brettler DB, Levine PH. Clinical manifestations and therapy of inherited coagulation factor deficiencies. In: Coleman RW, Hirsch J, Marder VJ, et al, eds. Hemostasis and thrombosis, 3rd ed. Philadelphia: JB Lippincott, 1994:169.

73. Furie B, Limentani SA, Rosenfield CG. A practical guide to the evaluation and treatment of hemophilia. Blood 84:3, 1994.

74. Rizza CR, Kenoff PB, Matthews JM, et al. A comparison of coagulation factor replacement with and without prednisolone in the treatment of haematuria in haemophilia and Christmas disease. Thromb Haemost 37:86, 1977.

75. Hilgartner MW. Intrarenal obstruction in hemophilia. Lancet 2:486, 1966.

76. Eyster ME, Gill FM, Blatt PM, et al. Central nervous system bleeding in hemophiliacs. Blood 51:1179, 1978.

77. Abildgaard CF. Hazards of prothrombin complex concentrates in the treatment of hemophilia. N Engl J Med 304:671, 1981.

78. Feinstein DI. Acquired disorders of hemostasis. In: Coleman RW, Hirsch J, Marder VJ, et al, eds. Hemostasis and thrombosis, 3rd ed. Philadelphia: JB Lippincott, 1994:881.

79. Blatt PM, White GC, McMillan CW, et al. Treatment of antifactor VIII antibodies. Thromb Haemost 38:514, 1977.

80. Kasper CK. The therapy of factor VIII inhibitors. Prog Hemost Thromb 9:57, 1989.

81. Brettler DB, Forsberg AD, Levine PH, et al. The use of porcine factor VIII concentrate (hyate:C) in the treatment of patients with inhibitor antibodies to factor VIII. Arch Intern Med 149:1381, 1989.

82. Eyster EM, Goedert JJ, Sarngadhanan MG, et al. Development and natural history of HTLV-III antibodies in persons with hemophilia. JAMA 253:2219, 1985.

83. Mannucci PM, Ruggeri ZM, Pareti FI, et al. 1-Deamino-8-arginine vasopressin: a new pharmacologic approach to the management of hemophilia and von Willebrand's disease. Lancet 8:869, 1977.

84. Mannucci PM, Bettega D, Cattaneo M. Patterns of development of tachyphylaxis in patients with haemophilia and von Willebrand's disease after repeated doses of desmopressin (DDAVP). Blood 82:87, 1992.

85. Weinstein RE, Bona RD, Altman AJ, et al. Severe hyponatremia after repeated intravenous administration of desmopressin. Am J Hematol 32:258, 1989.

86. Nilsson IM. Experience with prophylaxis in Sweden. Semin Hematol 30(suppl 2):16, 1993.

87. Bontempo FA, Lewis JH, Gorenc TJ, et al. Liver transplantation in hemophilia. Blood 69:1721, 1987.

88. Palmer TD, Thompson AR, Miller AD. Production of human factor IX in animals by genetically modified skin fibroblasts. Blood 73:438, 1989.

CHAPTER 16

ADRENOCORTICAL DYSFUNCTION AND CLINICAL USE OF STEROIDS

ELIZABETH STUBITS SHLOM

Cortisol (hydrocortisone) is the prototype of the group of steroids that are referred to as glucocorticoids. Glucocorticoids maintain the body's homeostasis by regulating physiologic functions that are involved in stress as well as normal daily living. Cortisol and other steroid hormones such as androgens, aldosterone, and estrogens are manufactured and secreted from the cortex of the adrenal glands. These glands function on their own to provide the body with basal levels of steroid hormones and also respond to adrenocorticotropic hormone (ACTH) and the hypothalamic-pituitary-adrenocortical (HPA) feedback system. During nonstressful times, cortisol aids the body in the management of glucose and metabolic functioning. Cortisol also helps to maintain an adequate fluid and electrolyte balance. When the body is exposed to stresses such as pain, trauma, or infection, glucocorticoids are necessary to modulate inflammatory processes, immune reactions, and neurochemical imbalances.

Cortisol disorders involve either too much or too little cortisol in the body. When the adrenal cortex manufactures and secretes excess cortisol, the condition and symptom complex are called Cushing's syndrome. This usually occurs in response to pituitary microadenomas causing excess ACTH production (Cushing's disease) but could also be independent of ACTH, as when there are cortisol-producing tumors of the adrenal cortex. Addison's disease, or hypocortisolism, is often idiopathic and results from either insufficient ACTH or destruction of the adrenal gland itself. If not identified and treated early, both of these disorders are associated with a high mortality rate. Causes and clinical implications of these diseases will be discussed in this chapter, as will the use of exogenous glucocorticoids.

PHYSIOLOGY

The adrenal glands are triangle-shaped organs that weigh approximately 4 g each and are located directly above the poles of the kidneys. The adrenal gland is composed of two physiologically distinct organs: the adrenal medulla and the adrenal cortex. Both of these endocrine organs are responsible for producing substances that aid the body in

coping with stress. The adrenal medulla, which makes up the innermost portion of the adrenal gland, manufactures and secretes epinephrine and norepinephrine. These hormones are referred to as catecholamines. The secretion of catecholamines is under the control of the sympathetic nervous system.

The adrenal cortex is located on the outer portion and comprises 90% of the adrenal gland. The adrenal cortex is further subdivided into three zones: the outer zona glomerulosa, the medial zona fasciculata, and the inner zona reticularis. The zona fasciculata makes up 75% of the cortex, and the zona glomerulosa and zona reticularis comprise 15% and 10%, respectively. The zona fasciculata and zona reticularis are responsible for glucocorticoid and androgen synthesis; the zona glomerulosa manufactures aldosterone. Estrogen synthesis also occurs to a small degree in the zona fasciculata and zona reticularis. All of the adrenocortical hormones are derived from esterified cholesterol.

The activities of glucocorticoids provide energy in times of stress and regulate glucose metabolism. They increase the availability of glucose through hepatic gluconeogenesis, the release of glucose substrates through protein breakdown and inhibition of protein synthesis, and the release of glucose substrates (glycerol and lactate) from fat cells and muscle. Glucocorticoids inhibit the uptake of glucose by most body organs except the liver, heart, and brain. All of these actions contribute to hyperglycemia and hyperlipidemia when there are excess glucocorticoids. In a starved individual, however, glucocorticoids thus help to preserve vital body functions.

Glucocorticoids influence the body's inflammation and immunologic responses. When cortisol levels are elevated, the body's response to an infectious agent or physical trauma is blunted. Although the exact mechanisms are unclear, glucocorticoids are thought to inhibit cellular mediators of an inflammatory response, inhibit antigen processing, and decrease serum lymphocyte levels.

Glucocorticoids also affect the body in other ways. Cortisol enters the central nervous system by crossing the blood-brain barrier and results in mood changes. Cortisol decreases serum calcium levels when hypercalcemia is present. Glucocorticoids enhance gastric acid secretion when predisposing factors exist. Finally, excess glucocorticoids inhibit growth. All of these glucocorticoid actions help to explain the symptoms and clinical manifestations that are seen with cortisol excess and deficiency, which will be described in this chapter.

HYPOTHALAMIC-PITUITARY-ADRENAL FEEDBACK SYSTEM

During stress, plasma ACTH is elevated, and then cortisol is produced and released by the adrenal cortex. ACTH, also called corticotropin or adrenocorticotropin, is secreted by the anterior pituitary gland under the regulatory control of corticotropin-releasing factor (CRF), which is secreted by the hypothalamus. Catecholamines and vasopressin have also been shown to stimulate the release of ACTH (1). In stressful situations (Table 16.1), ACTH secretion increases to many times the basal rate and increases cortisol production and secretion.

The major effect of ACTH on cortisol production is to stimulate the conversion of cholesterol to pregnenolone. This is accomplished by an increase in cholesterol binding to mitochondrial cytochrome P-450 in adrenal cortex cells. Cytochrome P-450 catalyzes the conversion of this rate-limiting step in steroid hormone production. Once cholesterol is converted to pregnenolone, further enzyme-mediated conversions occur before the adrenocortical hormones are produced (Fig. 16.1).

Table 16.1.
Conditions that Stimulate ACTH and Cortisol Secretion

Cold exposure	Hypoglycemia
Pain	Infection
Anxiety	Trauma
Hemorrhage	Toxins
Exercise	Depression
Starvation	Alcoholism

Source: Adapted from Tepperman J, Tepperman HM. ACTH and adrenal glucocorticoids. In Tepperman J, Tepperman HM (eds.): Metabolic and Endocrine Physiology. Chicago: Year Book Publishers, 1987, p. 183.

As cortisol levels increase in response to ACTH stimulation, CRF release from the hypothalamus is turned off. The decrease in CRF then leads to a reduction in further ACTH and cortisol secretion. This complete chain of events is referred to as the hypothalamic-pituitary-adrenal axis.

CIRCADIAN RHYTHM

In addition to stress-induced release of cortisol, another factor influences cortisol secretion: the daily circadian rhythm. This circadian, or diurnal, rhythm is the cyclic release of cortisol occurring throughout a 24-hr period as a result of intrinsic endocrine function.

By the age of 3 an individual's circadian rhythm is usually established. Minimal secretion of cortisol occurs just before and in the initial hours of sleep; maximal secretion of cortisol occurs just before and in the initial hours of wakefulness (Fig. 16.2). During the rest of the day,

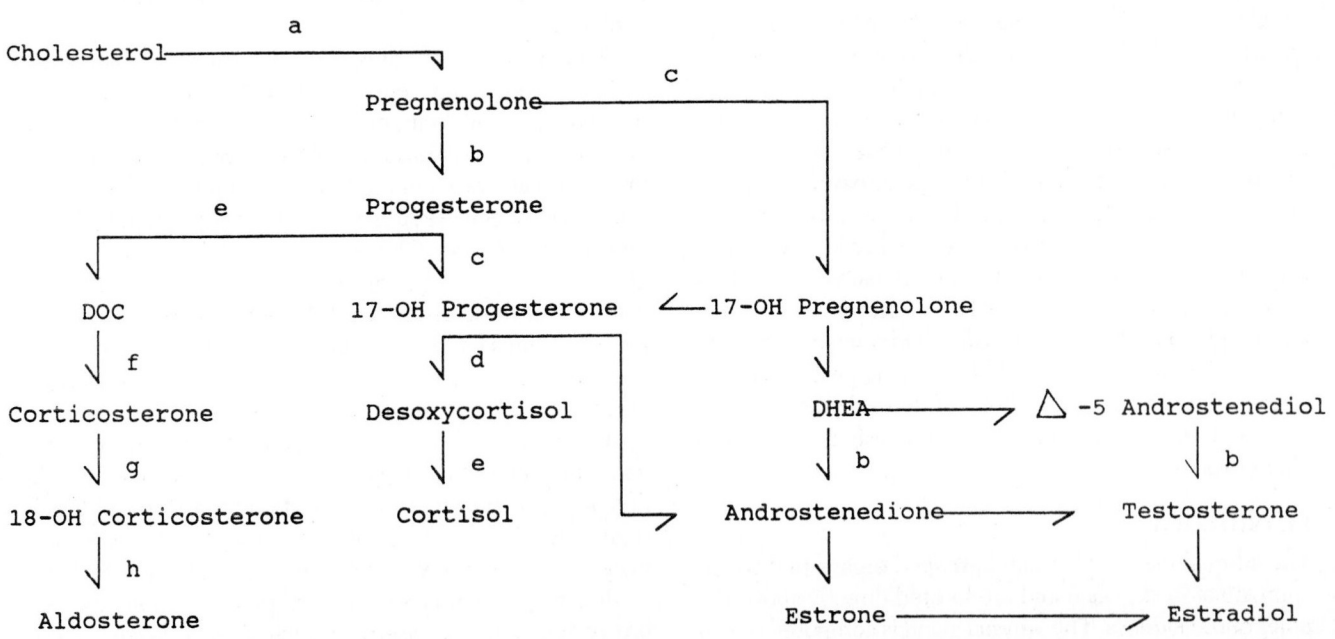

Figure 16.1. Adrenal corticosteroid synthesis. *a*, Cholesterol side-chain cleavage; *b*, 3-β-hydroxysteroid dehydrogenase; *c*, 17-α-hydroxylase; *d*, 21 hydroxylase; *e*, 11-β-hydroxylase; *f*, hydroxylase; *g*, corticosterone methyl oxidase; *h*, 18-OH dehydrogenase. *DHEA*, dehydroepiandrosterone; *DOC*, 11-desoxy-corticosterone.

intermittent secretions of cortisol occur. This cycle is influenced most by feeding habits but can also be affected by changes in sleep patterns of at least 2 to 3 weeks duration (2).

CORTISOL PHARMACOKINETICS

As described above, serum levels of cortisol vary throughout the day owing to the circadian rhythm and a variety of stresses. The basal secretion of cortisol by the adrenal cortex ranges from 8 to 37.5 mg/day in an unstressed individual and can be as high as 200 to 500 mg/day when stress is present (2, 3).

When a serum level of cortisol is measured in an individual patient, it is compared to what would be considered a normal level at that particular time during the circadian rhythm. Highest serum cortisol levels occur early in the morning, around 8:00 A.M., in reaction to peak ACTH levels a few hours earlier. Morning serum cortisol levels are normally within the range of 83 to 552 nmol/L (3 to 20 μg/dL) when measured by radioimmunoassay (RIA) using a competitive-protein-binding technique (2). In using a fluorimetric assay, a slightly higher range of 138 to 690 nmol/L (5 to 25 μg/dL) is considered normal (2). Both serum cortisol and ACTH levels progressively decrease throughout the day, with a nadir around 8:00 to 12:00 P.M. The serum cortisol level at 8:00 P.M. is usually one-half to one-third of the 8:00 A.M. level and is always less than 276 nmol/L (10 μg/dL) (4). Cortisol is 90% protein-bound in the serum, with 75% bound to corticosteroid-binding-globulin (CBG), also known as transcortin, and 15% bound to serum albumin. Unbound cortisol is the active component that provides feedback to the HPA system and regulates the secretion of ACTH.

Cortisol clearance occurs in the liver, where it is conjugated with glucuronide or sulfate groups (2). This increases the water solubility of the compound, which is necessary for renal excretion. The plasma half-life of cortisol is 70 to 90 min, with less than 1% of unchanged cortisol excreted by the kidneys over 24 hr. Clearance of cortisol is decreased in liver disease, hypothyroidism, starvation, pregnancy, infancy, and old age. Clearance is increased in high estrogen states, neonates, and severe chronic illness. Medications that induce hepatic microsomal enzymes also increase the clearance of cortisol. These medications include phenytoin, phenobarbital, secobarbital, aminoglutethimide, and rifampin. On the other hand, cortisol clearance is decreased by ketoconazole, a hepatic enzyme inhibitor.

In analyzing serum cortisol levels, the RIA assay is preferred over the fluorimetric assay. This is because the fluorimetric assay produces false serum cortisol results with concurrent use of certain medications (spironolactone, quinacrine, niacin, quinidine, benzyl alcohol), in uremia, and in hyperbilirubinemia (2, 4). Although medications do not interfere with the RIA method, false serum cortisol results may occur with pregnancy, congenital adrenal hyperplasia, and adrenal cancer.

CUSHING'S SYNDROME

Definition and Etiology

Cushing's syndrome is the clinical manifestation of a chronic and inappropriate elevation of serum cortisol levels. The syndrome was first described by Harvey Cushing in 1932 in the Johns Hopkins Hospital medical journal (5). Dr. Cushing noted that 12 patients with adenomas of the pituitary gland had similar clinical findings: increased adi-

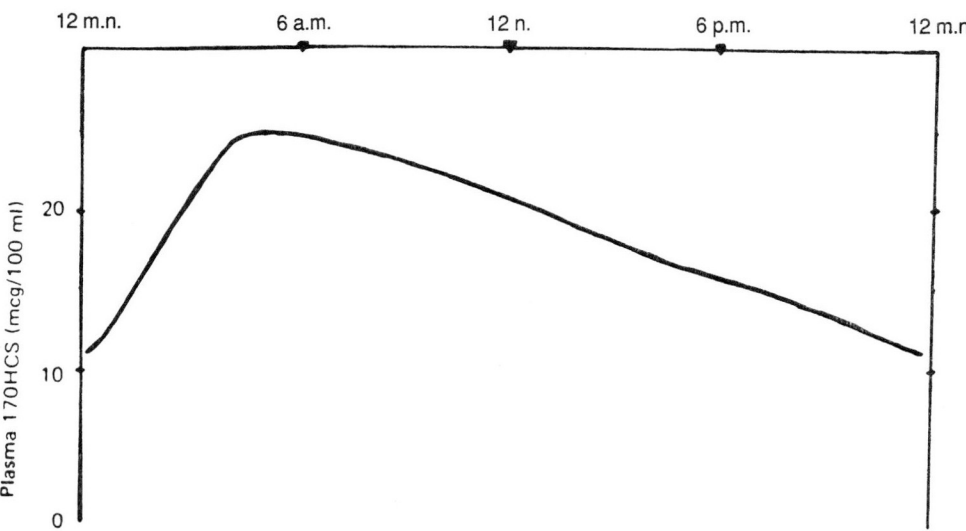

Figure 16.2. Diurnal variation in plasma cortisol. (Reprinted with permission from Pincus G, Nakao T, Tait JF, (eds): Symposium on the Dynamics of Steroid Hormones. New York, Academic Press, 1965, p 387.)

pose tissue in the face, neck, and trunk; hypertrichosis in females and prepubertal males; amenorrhea; striae; hypertension; easy fatigability; weakness; and spinal deformities. Cushing was unable to identify the underlying hormonal imbalance and multiple etiologies of hypercortisolism. This was accomplished later by other endocrinologists who expanded on Cushing's original findings.

Ever since the corticosteroids have been available for therapeutic use, the primary cause of Cushing's syndrome has been iatrogenic. However, spontaneous Cushing's syndrome has many different etiologies, nearly all of which result in excess cortisol secretion by the adrenal gland.

The causes of cortisol hypersecretion are classified as either ACTH-dependent or ACTH-independent (Fig. 16.3). ACTH-dependent etiologies, based on a chronic hypersecretion of ACTH, account for approximately 80% of all cases of spontaneous Cushing's syndrome (6). Elevated ACTH levels lead to overstimulation of the adrenal zona fasciculata and zona reticularis and, therefore, to increased secretion of cortisol and androgens. ACTH-dependent causes include the following:

1. pituitary microadenomas resulting in an increased release of ACTH (Cushing's disease);
2. ectopic, malignant ACTH-secreting tumors (e.g., small-cell carcinoma of the lung, islet-cell tumor, thymoma, and bronchial adenoma); and
3. ectopic CRF-secreting tumors.

Of these etiologies, only Cushing's disease is responsive to the HPA feedback system (7).

ACTH-independent etiologies involve cortisol-secreting tumors, which lead to elevated serum cortisol levels and secondarily to suppressed ACTH release. Accounting for fewer than 20% of patients with Cushing's syndrome, ACTH-independent causes include the following (7):

1. nodular hyperplasia of the adrenal cortex,
2. adrenal cortical tumors, and
3. ectopic production of cortisol.

The overall incidence of Cushing's syndrome is only 1 in 1000, females having a 3.5 times higher risk than males

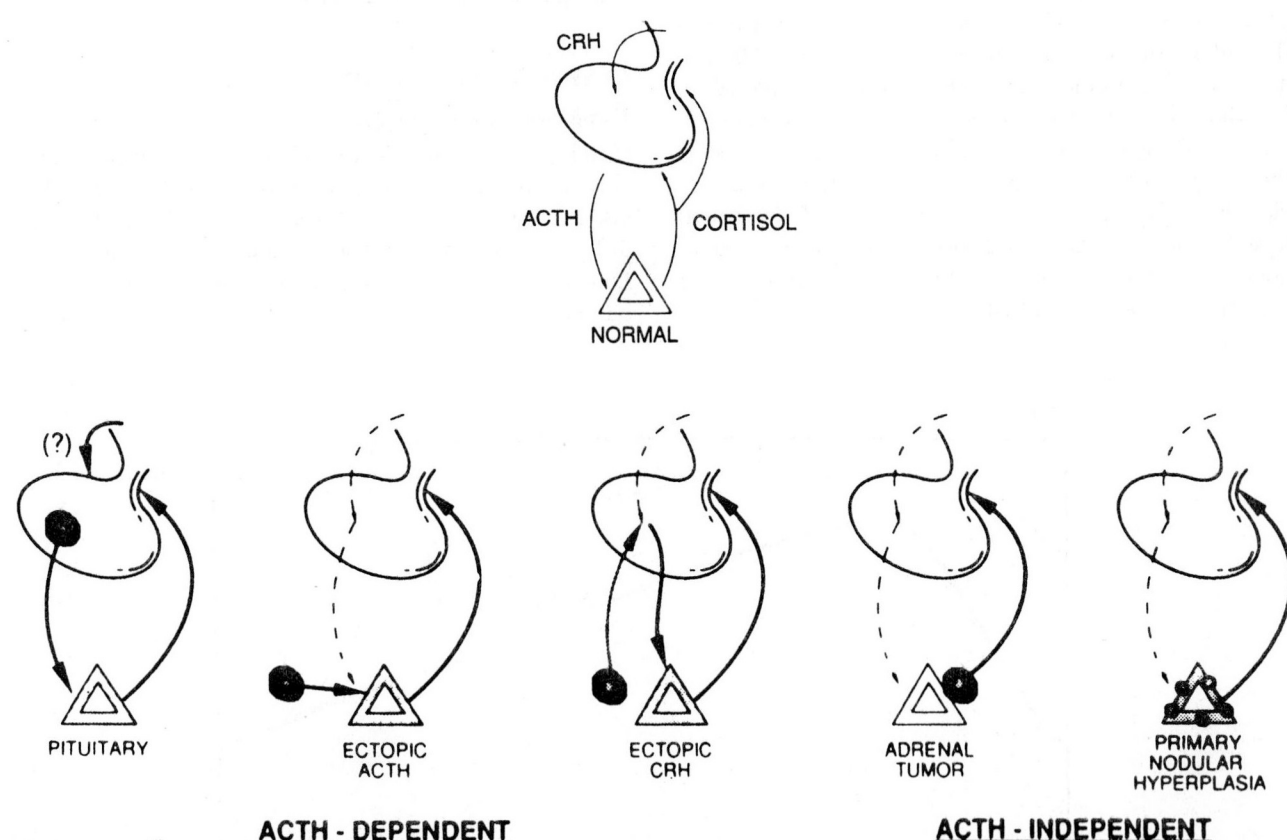

Figure 16.3. Etiologies of Cushing's syndrome. (Reprinted with permission from Schteingart DE: Cushing's syndrome. Endocrinol Metab Clin North Am 18:311–338, 1989.)

and having a propensity to developing pituitary microadenomas (Cushing's disease) as the cause of Cushing's syndrome (8). Over 50% of people who develop spontaneous Cushing's syndrome are between 20 and 40 years of age. The 5-year mortality rate for untreated Cushing's syndrome exceeds 50%.

Clinical Manifestations

The clinical manifestations of Cushing's syndrome are usually insidious in onset and encompass many different organ systems (Table 16.2). Often the clinical signs are vague and the patient will see many different specialists before the syndrome is diagnosed.

An overall change in appearance and increased total body fat are classic initial findings (9). Obesity is common, and fat is redistributed to central areas of the body, resulting in truncal or centripetal obesity with a protuberant abdomen and wasted extremities. Rounding of the face ("moon facies") and increased dorsocervical fat pads ("buffalo hump") are also classic findings.

The skin of a patient with Cushing's syndrome is fine and translucent, because of atrophy of the epidermal layer and connective tissue beneath it (10). A florid complexion, vascular striae, easy bruising, and poor wound healing are results of hypercortisolemic atrophy. Hyperpigmentation from the stimulatory action of cortisol on melanocytes may be seen. The growth of fine lanugo facial hair is also a common result of cortisol hypersecretion.

An increase in androgen levels may accompany hypercortisolism (10). This is manifested in female patients as the abnormal growth of body hair (hirsutism). Androgen excess also contributes to acne, seborrhea, and amenorrhea in women. Male patients with Cushing's syndrome experience a decrease in libido, a decrease in body hair, and testicular atrophy.

Muscle wasting and myopathy are common in Cushing's syndrome because of the catabolic effects of cortisol on muscle tissue. Proximal muscle weakness, primarily of the lower extremities, is often exhibited as difficulty in climbing stairs and standing up from a sitting position.

Hypercortisolism has many effects on the metabolic functions of bone. Inhibition of osteoblasts by cortisol may cause osteopenia and ultimately osteoporosis (11). Hypercalciuria is also promoted by increased cortisol levels and frequently results in kidney stone formation. In adults, bone pain and fractures are commonly seen as a result of hypercortisolism. Children with Cushing's syndrome have premature closure of the long bone epiphyses, leading to stunted growth and short stature (6).

Diastolic hypertension is another frequent finding in Cushing's syndrome. The elevated blood pressure is thought to result from mineralocorticoid excess or a direct inhibitory effect of cortisol on prostacyclin, a potent

Table 16.2.
Presenting Signs and Symptoms in Cushing's Syndrome

Sign or Symptom	(N = 601) %	(N = 50) %
Obesity	88	94
Generalized		60
Truncal		40
Moonface	75	84
Menstrual irregularities	60	76
Muscular weakness	61	58
Bruising	42	36
Psychological difficulties	42	
Acne	45	
Hirsutism	65	82
Backache	40	
Striae		52
Osteoporosis on radiograph		46
Hypertension		
B.P. 140/90		72
B.P. 100 diastolic		54
Renal calculi		16
Cholelithiasis		10

Source: From Kishi DT, Romac DR. Adrenocortical dysfunction. In: Herfindal ET, Gourley DR, Hart LL, eds. Clinical Pharmacy and Therapeutics. Baltimore: Williams & Wilkins, 1988: 114.

vasodilator (10). Mineralocorticoid excess also contributes to the hypokalemia, hypernatremia, and edema that are seen in Cushing's syndrome.

Psychiatric disturbances are common in patients with Cushing's syndrome (10). Manifestations range from mild irritability to mania, depression, and suicide. Common symptoms include mood lability, euphoria, increased anxiety, crying, insomnia, and decreases in memory and concentration.

Immunosuppression occurs with hypercortisolism (9). This leads to a predisposition for bacterial and opportunistic infections ranging in severity from fungal skin infections to *Pneumocystis carinii* pneumonia and cryptococcal meningitis. These complications contribute significantly to the morbidity of Cushing's syndrome. Immunosuppression also results in anergic responses to skin tests in patients with Cushing's syndrome (9).

Certain laboratory test findings are specific to patients with Cushing's syndrome. Electrolyte abnormalities include hypokalemia and alkalosis. Clinically unimportant hypernatremia may be found. Renal function tests may be altered secondary to nephrocalcinosis, hypertension, or repeated infections (9). Hypercalciuria and hypophosphatemia are common. Hyperglycemia and glycosuria are frequent in Cushing's syndrome. Plasma lipoproteins and cholesterol levels are often elevated. Patients may have elevated hemoglobin, hematocrit, and red blood cell counts (polycythemia). The total white blood cell count may be elevated with granulocytosis and lymphopenia.

Diagnosis

A preliminary clinical diagnosis of Cushing's syndrome must be evaluated through various laboratory tests. These are referred to as "dynamic" tests because they test the functional status of the HPA system. Initial tests determine the presence of hypercortisolism and resistance to dexamethasone suppression. Further tests determine the underlying etiology. An algorithm for the diagnosis of Cushing's syndrome can be found in Figure 16.4.

SCREENING TESTS

Screening tests for Cushing's syndrome include measurement of serum cortisol levels and 24-hr urinary free cortisol.

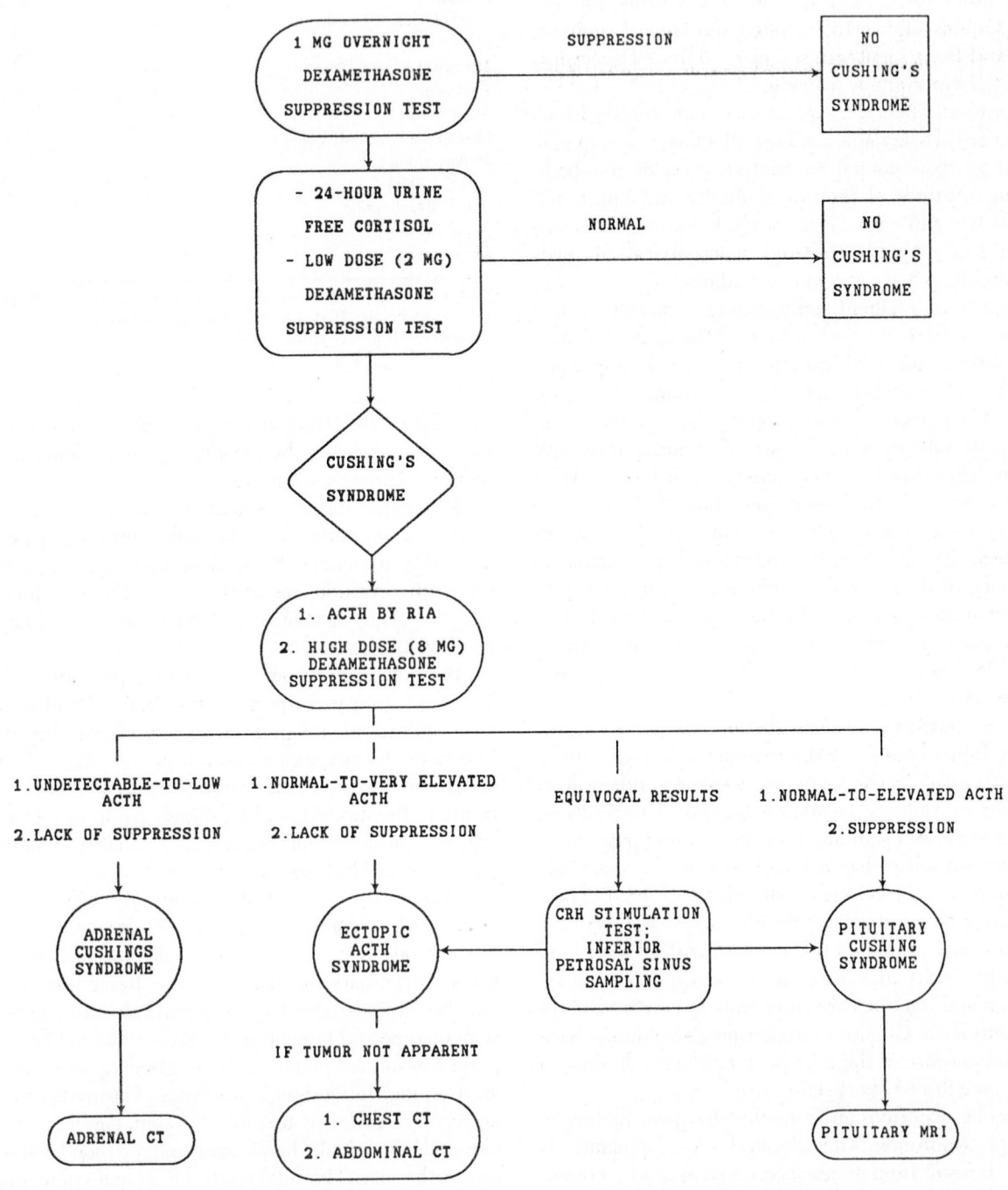

Figure 16.4. An algorithm for the diagnosis of Cushing's syndrome. (Adapted from Kaye TB, Crapo L. The Cushing's syndrome: an update on diagnostic tests. Ann Intern Med 112:434–444, 1990, with permission.)

Sequential serum cortisol levels are often obtained for patients with suspected Cushing's syndrome. These patients typically demonstrate little or no fluctuation in a constantly normal or elevated serum cortisol level. This lack of diurnal variation usually occurs months or years before frank elevation of serum cortisol levels is observed. However, because cortisol is highly bound to corticosteroid-binding globulin (CBG) in the serum, the measurement of serum cortisol levels may lead to misleading and false positive results in patients who have elevated CBG levels. This may occur in pregnancy, diabetes mellitus, hyperthyroidism, estrogen therapy, and obesity (11). In any case, serum cortisol levels are not diagnostic in up to 30% of patients with Cushing's syndrome and are rarely used for diagnosis today.

On the other hand, 24-hr urinary free cortisol is consistently elevated in Cushing's syndrome. This test measures unbound cortisol excreted by the kidney over a 24-hr period of time and is proportional to the unbound fraction of cortisol in the plasma. Normal basal urinary free cortisol ranges from 20 to 100 µg/24 hr; when it is greater than 100 to 125 µg/24 hr, Cushing's syndrome is likely (8). To ensure accuracy of the test, two or three consecutive 24-hr urine collections should be conducted to confirm Cushing's syndrome. At the same time, urinary creatinine should also be measured; urinary creatinine should not vary by more than 10% from day to day (12). When conducted correctly, the sensitivity and specificity of the urinary free cortisol test in identifying true hypercortisolism is close to 96% (13). False positive results are seen in patients who are under major stress (e.g., trauma or infection), have endogenous depression, or are receiving exogeneous hydrocortisone or cortisone acetate (9, 13).

An alternative 24-hr urine test measures the glucocorticoid metabolite, 17-hydroxycorticosteroid (17-OHCS). The urine test for 17-OHCS is associated with a higher false positive rate than is the urinary free cortisol test, particularly in obese patients (8, 10). Currently, the urinary free cortisol test is considered the simplest, most accurate, and most cost-effective assessment of hypercortisolism.

DEXAMETHASONE SUPPRESSION TESTS

After a screening test for hypercortisolism gives positive results, a dexamethasone suppression test (DST) is employed as the next step in the diagnosis of Cushing's syndrome. Dexamethasone, when administered exogenously, inhibits ACTH secretion and suppresses cortisol serum levels in a normal individual. However, dexamethasone does not interfere with laboratory readings of serum cortisol. For this reason, dexamethasone is preferred over other glucocorticoids in testing the HPA feedback system.

Three DST's are commonly used:

1. the overnight test (which may also be used as a screening test),
2. the low-dose 2-day test, and
3. the high-dose 2-day test.

The overnight test and the low-dose 2-day test are most frequently used for patients with mildly elevated urinary cortisol excretion. Only one of the two low-dose tests is used for a single patient. The high-dose 2-day test is used to further define the etiology of the hypercortisolism.

For the overnight test, the patient takes 1 mg of dexamethasone at 11:00 P.M., with serum cortisol measured at 8:00 A.M. the next day. Normal suppression of the HPA feedback system produces a morning cortisol level of less than 138 nmol/L (5 ug/dL) (9, 14).

For the 2-day low-dose DST the patient is given 0.5 mg dexamethasone orally every 6 hr for 2 days (eight doses). Cushing's syndrome is suspected when urinary cortisol values are greater than 10 µg (>28 umol) per 24 hr or urinary 17-hydroxycorticosteroid levels are greater than 2.5 mg (>6.9 umol) per 24 hr (12).

During the 2-day high-dose DST the patient takes 2 mg of dexamethasone orally every 6 hr for 2 days (eight doses). The high-dose DST is conducted by comparing two 24-hr urine collections measuring urinary free cortisol and/or urinary 17-OHCS. The test is also conducted by comparing serum cortisol levels. The serum cortisol level is measured as a baseline before dexamethasone administration and at 4:00 P.M. on the second day (10, 15) or at 8:00 A.M. on the third day (16). At this point, if the serum cortisol level is less than 138 nmol/L (5 µg/dL), or 50% of the baseline value, then a presumptive diagnosis of pituitary microadenoma (Cushing's disease) is made (10). This is because pituitary microadenomas are HPA-responsive at very high glucocorticoid serum levels. Conversely, if the serum cortisol level is greater than 138 nmol/L (5 µg/dL), then Cushing's syndrome is most likely due to an ACTH-independent etiology or to ectopic ACTH production (10).

A variation on this high-dose 2-day DST was described by Tyrrell and colleagues in 1986 (16). Their high-dose DST is conducted by obtaining a baseline serum cortisol at 8:00 A.M., administering a single dose of dexamethasone 8 mg orally at 11:00 P.M., and measuring of serum cortisol at 8:00 A.M. the next day. The predictive power of this test in diagnosing the etiology of Cushing's syndrome is similar to that of the high-dose 2-day DST (12).

False positive results of the DST are common and occur most often with obesity or when CBG levels are elevated because of high estrogen states seen with pregnancy or the use of oral contraceptives. False positive results also occur when serum cortisol levels are elevated because of stresses such as depression, anxiety, alcohol abuse, and uremia (8). In addition, false positives can occur if the metabolism of dexamethasone is increased because of hepatic microsomal enzyme inducers such as phenytoin or phenobarbital. (See Table 16.3 for a complete list of drug interactions with glucocorticoids.)

LOCALIZATION TESTS

Once a diagnosis of Cushing's syndrome has been made, localization studies are conducted to further determine the etiology of the syndrome and the treatment. If a pituitary source is suspected (e.g., Cushing's disease), a computerized axial tomography (CAT) scan or magnetic resonance (MR) scan of the brain is conducted (6, 7, 11).

Measurement of serum ACTH levels using RIA technology may also be conducted. This test will aid in determining whether ACTH is being secreted at a rate that is higher than normal. Plasma ACTH normally ranges between 4 and 22 pmol/L (20 to 100 pg/mL) in the morning (4). With Cushing's syndrome, due to adrenal tumors, ACTH is suppressed to less than 4 pmol/L (20 pg/mL). With Cushing's disease, due to pituitary microadenomas, plasma ACTH is normal or slightly increased to 9 to 44 pmol/L (40 to 200 pg/mL). Ectopic ACTH syndromes lead to highly elevated ACTH levels of 22 to 440 pmol/L (100 to 2000 pg/mL) (4).

Although measurement of plasma ACTH provides valuable information in the diagnosis of Cushing's syndrome, many problems accompany this test. ACTH levels vary significantly during the day, and ACTH has a very short half-life in the serum (approximately 15 to 25 min). In addition, ACTH samples are stable for only 4 hr and require special handling. Samples should be drawn into special tubes, spun down, and frozen as soon as possible. Finally, ACTH assays are not available at many institutions and must be sent out to specialized laboratories for evaluation.

If an adrenal source of Cushing's syndrome is suspected, a CAT scan of the abdomen should be conducted to rule out adrenal adenoma or carcinoma. Alternatively, an adrenal scan using a radioiodinated contrast agent can be used.

Three different tests are conducted to differentiate pituitary Cushing's disease from an ectopic ACTH syndrome:

1. corticotropin-releasing hormone (CRH) stimulation test,
2. metyrapone stimulation test, and
3. inferior petrosal sinus sampling.

The ovine CRH stimulation test is not yet widely available (8, 10, 14). When administered, this test can be used to diagnose pituitary microadenomas (Cushing's disease) as the underlying etiology of hypercortisolism. To conduct this test, 1 µg/kg or 100 µg of CRH is administered. Blood is drawn at baseline and at 15, 30, 60, 90 and 120 min after administration of CRH to measure both ACTH and serum cortisol levels. In Cushing's disease

Table 16.3.
Drug Interactions with Glucocorticoids

Increased metabolism of glucocorticoids
    Barbiturates
    Phenytoin
    Rifampin
    Carbamazepine
    Aminoglutethimide
    Ketoconazole
Decreased metabolism of glucocorticoids
    Cyclosporine
    Troleandomycin
    Erythromycin
    Estrogens
    Oral contraceptives
    Ketoconazole
Exacerbation of glucocorticoid-induced hypokalemia
    Amphotericin B
    Ethacrynic acid
    Furosemide
    Hydrochlorothiazide
Exacerbation of glucocorticoid-induced gastritis
    Aspirin
    Indomethacin
    Other nonsteroidal antiinflammatory agents
    Alcohol
Glucocorticoid-induced reduction in efficacy with
    Insulin
    Oral antidiabetic agents
    Vaccines
    Warfarin
    Salicylates

Source: Adapted from Hansten PD, Horn JR. Drug interactions, 6th ed. Philadelphia: Lea & Febiger, 1989; and Tatro DS. Drug interaction facts. St. Louis: JB Lippincott, 1990.

(pituitary microadenoma), CRH administration elicits an increased release of ACTH and cortisol. ACTH is usually increased by 50% or greater, and cortisol is increased by 20% or greater. With other etiologies, ACTH levels show no response to CRH administration, either because ACTH is maximally suppressed (e.g., primary adrenal tumors) or because there is an ectopic ACTH syndrome. The CRH stimulation test is, therefore, another means of diagnosing Cushing's syndrome due to a pituitary cause.

Metyrapone, when administered as 750 mg every 4 hr for six doses, blocks the last step in the adrenal synthesis of cortisol: the conversion of 11-deoxycortisol to cortisol. This results in a decreased serum cortisol level and a subsequent increase in ACTH secretion. At the same time, 11-deoxycortisol levels increase, as does the 17-OHCS level, which includes metabolites of both cortisol and 11-deoxycortisol. When patients have pituitary Cushing's disease, there is an increase of 24-hr urinary 17-OHCS of more than 70% over the basal value. Patients with ectopic ACTH syndrome have little or no increase in 24-hr urinary 17-OHCS, because pituitary secretion of ACTH is suppressed.

Inferior petrosal sinus sampling has been shown to be highly effective in making the differential diagnosis between pituitary Cushing's syndrome and an ectopic ACTH syndrome. In this test, ACTH secretion from the pituitary gland is measured directly via catheterization. On the down side, this test is highly invasive, is associated with adverse risks to the patient, and is available only in specialized centers (17).

Surgical Treatment

The treatment of Cushing's syndrome depends on the underlying etiology. In most cases, surgery is the treatment of choice. When a pituitary microadenoma is the cause, microsurgery with a transsphenoidal approach is used. This is usually successful in obliterating ACTH hypersecretion. However, in some situations, pituitary irradiation may be necessary, in which case remission is delayed for up to 6 to 18 months (8).

For benign tumors such as adrenal adenoma or adrenocortical nodular hyperplasia, unilateral adrenalectomy is the primary treatment. Malignant adrenal carcinoma and ectopic ACTH-producing tumors are treated by surgical resection whenever possible. If metastases are present, palliative treatment with steroid-inhibiting medications (e.g., mitotane) will decrease the cushingoid symptoms and may even decrease tumor size. However, medical treatment has not been shown to prolong survival of patients with metastasizing tumors.

In rare cases, bilateral adrenalectomy is performed. However, this is used only as a last resort, since both adrenal cortices are removed and the patient will require replacement therapy permanently.

In all cases in which surgery is used to remove the cause of hypercortisolism, high-dose glucocorticoid therapy should be used in the immediate postoperative period, usually with a rapid taper (e.g., total course of less than 10 days) once the patient is stabilized. This is to ensure an adequate replacement therapy while the HPA feedback system is undergoing recovery.

Table 16.4.
Medications That Are Used to Treat Cushing's Syndrome

Name	Mechanism	Dose[a]	Response Time	Hydrocortisone Replacement	Adverse Effects
Cyproheptadine	Inhibits ACTH secretion	Initially: 8 mg p.o. q.d. MD: up to 24 mg p.o. q.d.	4–6 weeks	Not necessary	Appetite stimulation, weight gain, sedation
Bromocriptine	Inhibits ACTH secretion	10–20 mg/day	NA[b]	NA[b]	Nausea, hypotension, headaches
Aminoglutethimide	Inhibits cortisol synthesis by blocking cholesterol conversion to pregnenolone	Initially: 250 mg p.o. q.i.d. MD: 500–2000 mg/ day divided q.i.d.	NA[b]	Necessary	Drowsiness, lethargy, reversible blood dyscrasias, nausea, anorexia, dizziness, headaches, skin rash, hypotension, tachycardia
Metyrapone	Inhibits cortisol by blocking final step in cortisol synthesis	Initially: 250 mg p.o. b.i.d. MD: up to 1000 mg p.o. q.i.d.	4 months	Necessary	Dizziness, sedation, skin rash, hirsutism, hypertension
Mitotane	Destruction of adrenocortical cells that synthesize cortisol	Initially: 500 mg p.o. b.i.d. MD: 3–12 g/day divided t.i.d.–q.i.d. (doses can be tapered with long-term treatment)	2 weeks– 6 months	Necessary	Anorexia, nausea, vomiting, diarrhea, lethargy, impaired memory, hepatotoxicity
Ketoconazole	Inhibits cortisol synthesis by blocking cholesterol conversion to pregnenolone	Initially: 800–1200 mg/day MD: 600–800 mg/ day	4–6 weeks	Not necessary	Nausea, vomiting, fatigue, pruritis, gynecomastia, hepatotoxicity

[a]MD = maintenance dose.
[b]NA = information not available.

Medical Treatment

Medical treatment of Cushing's syndrome is reserved for intractable cases of Cushing's syndrome or situations in which there will be a delay in surgery. Two types of medications are used:

1. medications that inhibit the pituitary secretion of ACTH and
2. medications that inhibit the adrenocortical secretion of cortisol.

ACTH-dependent syndromes will benefit most from the first type of medications, which include cyproheptadine and bromocriptine. The second type of medications includes aminoglutethimide, metyrapone, ketoconazole, and mitotane. Table 16.4 is a summary of medications used in the treatment of Cushing's syndrome.

CYPROHEPTADINE

Cyproheptadine (Periactin), an antihistamine and serotonin-antagonist, was first reported in 1975 by Krieger and colleagues to be effective in the treatment of Cushing's disease in three patients (18). After 4 to 6 weeks of therapy, each patient had a marked improvement in cushingoid symptoms as well as a normalization of response to a low-dose DST. It was noted, however, that serum cortisol levels did not revert back to a normal circadian rhythm. Subsequent reports have been contradictory with regard to the efficacy of cyproheptadine in Cushing's syndrome (19, 20). Krieger reviewed cyproheptadine treatment in 1976 and reported a 60% success rate (21).

The mechanism of action of cyproheptadine is thought to be an antiserotonin effect on the hypothalamus, resulting in the inhibition of ACTH secretion (7). A maximum dose of 24 mg/day is used, with a decrease in cushingoid manifestations as early as 1 month after beginning treatment. The clinical effects usually last as long as the medication is continued. Adverse effects are common and include increased appetite, weight gain, and sedation.

BROMOCRIPTINE

Bromocriptine (Parlodel), an ergot alkaloid derivative, is a dopamine receptor agonist and prolactin inhibitor that has been used experimentally to induce a temporary remission of ACTH-dependent Cushing's syndrome (22, 23). Although inconsistently effective, bromocriptine has been shown to decrease excess ACTH secretion from pituitary microadenomas.

Large doses of 10 to 20 mg/day of bromocriptine have been used in Cushing's syndrome. These are higher than the doses that are used to treat elevated prolactin levels (7.5 to 10 mg/day). In treating Cushing's syndrome, adverse effects included nausea in 50% of patients, headaches, and hypotension during the first few days of treatment.

At this time, the use of bromocriptine in Cushing's syndrome needs to be further evaluated before its use can be generally recommended.

AMINOGLUTETHIMIDE

Aminoglutethimide (Cytadren) was originally marketed as an anticonvulsant when it was noted to significantly inhibit the synthesis of cortisol, aldosterone, and estrogens. Since then, it has been used to treat Cushing's syndrome (ACTH-dependent) and as a secondary agent in estrogen-receptor-positive breast cancer.

In Cushing's syndrome, aminoglutethimide acts by blocking the first step in the synthesis of cortisol: the conversion of cholesterol to pregnenolone. The effects of aminoglutethimide are short-lived, however, because of a compensatory rise in ACTH levels. The pituitary increases the output of ACTH in response to low cortisol levels, which overrides aminoglutethimide's effect to decrease cortisol output. The net effect is a rebound in cortisol synthesis and secretion that can occur as early as a few days after treatment initiation.

Clinical effects of aminoglutethimide are usually longer-acting in patients with cortisol-secreting adrenal carcinoma or when used concomitantly with metyrapone or pituitary irradiation (24). Owing to a complete cessation of cortisol synthesis, exogeneous steroid replacement therapy with hydrocortisone should be prescribed to prevent adrenocortical insufficiency.

Doses of aminoglutethimide in Cushing's syndrome are usually 500 to 2000 mg/day. Aminoglutethimide has many adverse effects, including drowsiness, lethargy, reversible blood dyscrasias (neutropenia, aplastic anemia, etc.), nausea, anorexia, dizziness, headaches, hypotension, and tachycardia. Skin rashes are common and will usually abate over time if therapy is continued. Aminoglutethimide has been shown to increase the hepatic metabolism of dexamethasone and warfarin but not hydrocortisone.

METYRAPONE

Metyrapone (Metopirone) is an 11-β-hydroxylase inhibitor that blocks the final step in the adrenal synthesis of cortisol. Metyrapone is used in Cushing's syndrome as a testing agent to differentiate a pituitary etiology from ectopic ACTH syndrome. It is also used in the treatment of Cushing's syndrome as an adjunctive agent in combination with aminoglutethimide (25). Serum ACTH levels usually increase during metyrapone treatment, but unlike with aminoglutethimide, these levels are insufficient to overcome the adrenal blockade.

The dosing range of metyrapone is 250 mg orally twice a day up to 1000 mg orally four times a day. Because of its high cost, metyrapone is usually prescribed only for short-term treatment. Adverse effects are primarily gastrointestinal but also commonly include dizziness, hypotension, sedation, and skin rash. Owing to the accumulation of adrenal androgens and mineralocorticoid precursors with metyrapone, adverse effects may also include hypertension and hirsutism in women.

MITOTANE

Mitotane (O,p'-DDD, Lysodren) is an antineoplastic agent that was first used to treat adrenal carcinoma and then later used for Cushing's syndrome by Southern and colleagues in 1961 (26). It acts by inhibiting cortisol synthesis and by destroying the adrenocortical cells that secrete cortisol. The zona reticularis is most sensitive to the action of mitotane, and the zona glomerulosa is least sensitive (7, 8, 26). Mitotane also appears to partially suppress ACTH levels (27), and it can be used alone or in conjunction with pituitary irradiation.

The usual dose of mitotane is 3 to 12 g/day orally in three or four divided doses. Treatment is initiated with a dose of 500 mg orally twice a day and increased to 1 g orally four times a day, as required to suppress cortisol. Response to treatment occurs within 4 to 12 months. For a majority of patients, treatment must be continued on a long-term basis or combined with pituitary irradiation because of a high rate of relapse if a single treatment period is used (28). Doses can be tapered to as low as 500 mg orally twice weekly and continue to maintain a state of remission (27). Hydrocortisone replacement therapy should be initiated within 2 to 4 weeks of mitotane therapy and should also include substitutive mineralocorticoid therapy (28).

The most common adverse effects of mitotane include anorexia, nausea, lethargy, and impaired memory. Hepatotoxic effects may lead to increased serum alkaline phosphatase levels. Decreased serum thyroxine levels may also occur, as a function of decreased plasma binding. Intolerable adverse effects can be managed by discontinuing the medication for a few days and restarting at a lower dose.

KETOCONAZOLE

Ketoconazole (Nizoral) is an imidazole derivative that is used primarily as an antifungal agent. It acts by inhibiting the synthesis of ergosterol in fungi and cholesterol in mammalian cell walls. At high doses, ketoconazole has also been shown to inhibit adrenocortical cytochrome P-450, which is where cholesterol side-chain cleavage occurs, blocking the formation of pregnenolone and further cortisol precursors (7, 29). By this mechanism, ketoconazole has been discovered to be a potent, but reversible, inhibitor of abnormal adrenal cortisol synthesis.

Patients with Cushing's syndrome have responded to high-dose ketoconazole treatment within 4 to 6 weeks of treatment (7, 30). In addition, when doses are managed properly, some synthesis of cortisol still occurs and makes it unnecessary to administer replacement hydrocortisone

(29, 30). Usual initial doses are 800 to 1200 mg/day, with maintenance doses slightly lower at 600 to 800 mg/day.

Adverse effects include nausea, vomiting, fatigue, pruritus, gynecomastia in males, and hepatotoxicity. The use of ketoconazole warrants regular monitoring of liver function tests, and the drug should be discontinued if transaminase abnormalities persist or worsen (31). Ketoconazole is highly bound to plasma proteins and is metabolized by hepatic microsomal enzymes.

Many drug interactions with ketoconazole have been identified. Ketoconazole requires an acidic gastric environment for optimal absorption. Antacids and cimetidine decrease the absorption of ketoconazole, and administration should be separated by at least 2 hr. By another mechanism, isoniazid combined with rifampin has been shown to decrease ketoconazole levels during simultaneous administration of all three medications. This decrease in ketoconazole levels is thought to be due to increased hepatic metabolism. It is recommended that ketoconazole be avoided for patients who are on isoniazid and rifampin.

Because of ketoconazole-induced hepatic enzyme inhibition, cyclosporine serum levels have been shown to increase when cyclosporine is given with ketoconazole. An increase in warfarin activity may also be seen with ketoconazole therapy, owing to plasma protein binding displacement. When ketoconazole is used concomitantly with cyclosporine or warfarin, monitoring parameters of these medications (i.e., cyclosporine levels, serum creatinine levels, and prothrombin times with warfarin) should be followed closely.

Conclusion

Cushing's syndrome can lead to significant morbidity and early mortality if it is left untreated. The cause of Cushing's syndrome is most commonly due to excess administration of exogenous corticosteroids. Endogenous, or spontaneous, Cushing's syndrome is usually of pituitary origin but may also be due to an ectopic or adrenal tumor. Regardless of the cause, hypercortisolism leads to a constellation of symptoms, and the 5-year mortality rate for untreated Cushing's syndrome is over 50%. Infections and cardiovascular complications (e.g., stroke, myocardial infarction, and congestive heart failure) are usual causes of death of patients with untreated hypercortisolism.

Surgical removal of the cause of hypercortisolism, without removal of the adrenal glands themselves, is the primary mode of treatment. As a temporary measure, medical treatment with or without irradiation can be palliative. When medical treatment is used, cyproheptadine is the medication of choice in treating ACTH-dependent Cushing's syndrome. For ACTH-independent Cushing's syndrome, ketoconazole provides effective treatment without requiring glucocorticoid replacement. If adverse effects or drug interactions related to ketoconazole are undesirable, mitotane is the next preferred agent. The use of aminoglutethimide in conjunction with metyrapone should be reserved for short-term use only.

Although the mortality rate for patients with treated Cushing's syndrome still remains high at four times that of the normal population, early intervention and treatment can improve the morbidity and prognosis for these patients.

ADDISON'S DISEASE

Definition and Etiology

Adrenocortical insufficiency is an insidious illness that can lead to rapid mortality if untreated. It results from primary or secondary causes. Primary adrenocortical insufficiency, also known as Addison's disease, results from destruction of the adrenal cortex. Secondary adrenocortical insufficiency is due to deficient pituitary ACTH secretion causing atrophy of the adrenal cortex. The signs and symptoms of adrenal insufficiency are easily overlooked in patients who have other underlying disorders.

Tuberculosis used to be the most frequent cause of Addison's disease, but this is much less commonly the case today in developed countries because of the decreased incidence of tuberculosis. Approximately 80% of primary adrenocortical insufficiency is now idiopathic. The remaining 20% of Addison's disease occurs as a complication of tuberculosis or, in rare situations, is due to cancer, infections (bacterial or fungal), trauma, hemorrhagic disorders, congenital adrenal hypoplasia, or autoimmune destruction of the adrenal gland. Adrenal insufficiency in patients with acquired immune deficiency syndrome (AIDS) occurs rarely and is thought to be due to disseminated infection or neoplasm, autoimmune processes, or changes associated with chronic disease or malnutrition (32). The most common cause of secondary adrenocortical insufficiency is steroid withdrawal in a patient with adrenal atrophy due to exogenous glucocorticoid therapy.

Overall, Addison's disease is an uncommon disorder with an incidence of 50 per million of the population (33). It is usually diagnosed in the third to fifth decade of life. A sex-related predisposition is observed, females developing idiopathic Addison's disease two and one-half times more often than males. When adrenocortical insufficiency is due to tuberculosis, it is more common in males over the age of 40 years. Before corticosteroids were introduced in the late 1940s, patients with chronic adrenal insufficiency had a mortality rate of 80% within 3 years of diagnosis. Today, the overall mortality rate is 1.4 per million.

Drug-Induced Addison's Disease

Medications have been implicated as the cause of Addison's disease in certain situations. Enzyme inhibitors used in Cushing's syndrome and adrenal cancers, such as metyrapone and aminoglutethimide, decrease cortisol secretion and may precipitate Addison's disease. The potential for this to occur is greatest when patients are not given exogenous steroid replacement therapy. Ketoconazole and etomidate (an anesthetic agent) also decrease cortisol secretion and have been known to cause adrenocortical insufficiency. Adrenal radiation and mitotane are both adrenocortical toxins that can culminate in adrenocortical insufficiency.

Anticoagulants such as heparin and warfarin have been reported to cause Addison's disease as a result of adrenal hemorrhage. Waterhouse-Friderichsen syndrome develops when adrenocortical hemorrhage occurs because of anticoagulant use, sepsis, or trauma and is accompanied by fulminant septicemia. Finally, rifampin and other hepatic enzyme inducers may increase the metabolism of cortisol and precipitate adrenocortical insufficiency in patients with preexisting partial adrenal insufficiency (34).

Pathogenesis

In addition to primary or secondary causes, adrenocortical insufficiency can also be acute or chronic. When Addison's disease occurs as a result of gradual destruction of the adrenal gland, chronic adrenal insufficiency is manifested. Patients with chronic adrenocortical insufficiency often have normal basal cortisol secretion but may have difficulty in increasing cortisol secretion with stress. Over time, even basal cortisol secretion becomes inadequate, and clinical manifestations of adrenocortical insufficiency become evident. However, without an acute stressful event, chronic adrenal insufficiency will usually go unnoticed because of the vague symptoms of the disease.

Approximately 25% of patients who are diagnosed as having Addison's disease are in active or impending adrenal crisis. Acute adrenocortical insufficiency is manifested when adrenal need, generated by stress of surgery, trauma, or infection, exceeds the gland's capacity for cortisol production. In these patients the acute stressful event precipitates an Addisonian crisis. This generally occurs when 90% or more of the adrenal cortex is nonfunctioning and is usually accompanied by elevated ACTH levels.

Clinical Manifestations

Signs and symptoms of chronic Addison's disease may be present for months to years without being diagnosed. Adrenocortical insufficiency is not manifested until more than 90% of both adrenal cortices are lost. Nonspecific symptoms are seen in most patients with Addison's disease (Table 16.5) (35). Both mineralocorticoid and glucocorticoid deficiencies contribute to symptoms of salt craving, dizziness, and low systolic blood pressure. Hyperpigmentation of the skin and mucous membranes is usually the hallmark characteristic that prompts the physician to test

Table 16.5.
Clinical Manifestations of Adrenal Insufficiency

Isolated hypoaldosteronism
  Usually asymptomatic
  History of diabetes mellitus and/or renal insufficiency; heparin
    therapy
  Postural hypotension
  Laboratory:
    Hyperkalemia
    Hyponatremia
    Metabolic acidosis
Secondary adrenal insufficiency
Primary glucocorticoid deficiency
  Weakess
  Fatigability
  Anorexia
  Nausea and vomiting
  Myalgias
  Personality changes
  Malaise
  Diarrhea
  Hypotension
  Cushingoid features may suggest exogenous glucocorticoid therapy
  Laboratory:
    Hyponatremia
    Hypoglycemia
    Anemia
    Relative lymphocytosis
    Eosinophilia
Primary adrenal insufficiency
Combined glucocorticoid and mineralocorticoid deficiencies
  Weakness
  Fatigability
  Anorexia
  Nausea and vomiting
  Abdominal pain or discomfort
  Malaise
  Personality changes
  Diarrhea
  History of recent surgery
  Coagulopathy
  History of human immunodeficiency virus infection
  Hypotension/shock
  Weight loss
  Fever (in the acute setting)
  Hyperpigmentation
  Vitiligo
  Body hair loss in females
  Laboratory:
    Hypokalemia
    Hyponatremia
    Elevated blood urea nitrogen
    Prolonged coagulation studies
    Anemia
    Relative lymphocytosis
    Eosinophilia
    Lupus anticoagulant
    Hypoglycemia
    Hypercalcemia

Source: Reprinted with permission from Chin R. Adrenal crisis. Crit Care Clin 7(1):23–42, 1991.

for adrenal insufficiency. It is most pronounced in sun-exposed areas of the body and at pressure points but also occurs on palmar creases, nail beds, the tongue, the nipples, the navel, and the perivaginal and perianal mucosa. Hyperpigmentation, present in 92% of patients, is caused by increased melanocyte-stimulating hormone and β-lipotropin serum levels, which accompany increased ACTH levels (36, 37). Areas of unpigmented skin (vitiligo) also occur but at a much lower incidence of approximately 4 to 17%.

Prolonged gastrointestinal symptoms such as nausea, abdominal discomfort, diarrhea, and vomiting are warning signs that may signal progressive adrenal insufficiency and impending crisis (38).

ADDISONIAN CRISIS

Acute addisonian crisis (apoplexy) results when a patient with undiagnosed Addison's disease becomes stressed or is exposed to a stressful event such as trauma, infection, surgery, or hemorrhage. The signs and symptoms of addisonian crisis are more profound than those of chronic insufficiency and demand immediate diagnosis and treatment. Significant anorexia develops and is accompanied by nausea and vomiting. This leads to severe dehydration and hemodynamic instability. Fever, with or without a concurrent infection, is often present. Abdominal pain and tenderness may confuse the diagnosis as one of an acute abdominal event. Weakness, fatigue, and confusion become profound, and without appropriate treatment, coma and shock are likely to develop.

Hyperpigmentation may exist in patients with previous chronic adrenocortical insufficiency and, if present, is again the distinctive finding that suggests the diagnosis. Laboratory abnormalities such as hyponatremia, hyperkalemia, eosinophilia, lymphocytosis, hypoglycemia, and increased blood urea nitrogen levels are all seen in an adrenal crisis. Hypoglycemia, due to a decrease in hepatic gluconeogenesis, is otherwise a rare finding in a patient with shock and is highly suggestive of an addisonian crisis. In secondary adrenal insufficiency the mineralocorticoid deficiency is not seen, and signs and symptoms of volume depletion, dehydration, and electrolyte abnormalities are absent.

Diagnosis

Clinical and laboratory findings should alert the clinician to the possibility of acute adrenocortical insufficiency in a hospitalized, acutely ill patient. Once an addisonian crisis is suspected, treatment should be instituted at the same time as, or before, beginning a series of diagnostic tests. Failure to treat these patients promptly could lead to rapid deterioration of the patient and death. Figure 16.5 provides an algorithm for the diagnosis of chronic or acute Addison's disease.

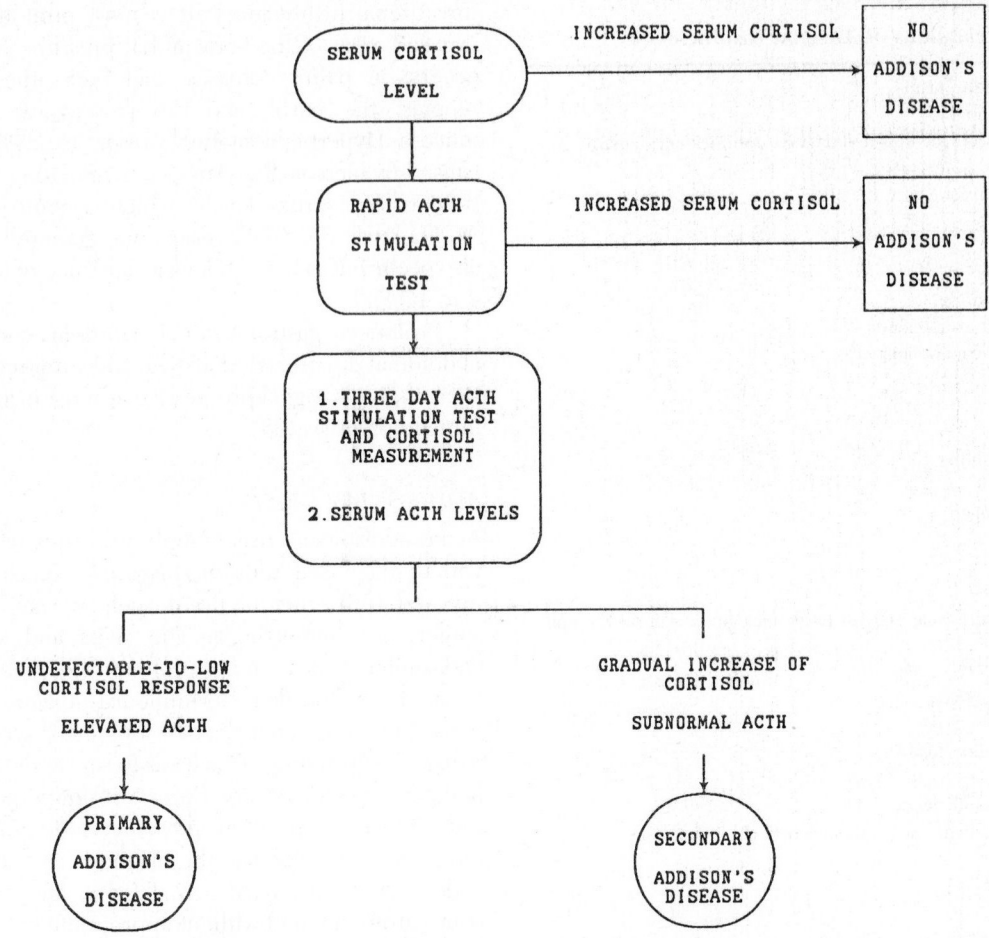

Figure 16.5. An algorithm for the diagnosis of Addison's disease.

SCREENING TESTS

Diagnosis of primary adrenocortical insufficiency is based on dynamic laboratory tests that show a failure of the adrenal cortex to respond to ACTH stimulation. Although plasma cortisol levels are usually low to absent, random measurement of serum cortisol levels rarely provides confirmation of impaired cortisol production. For this reason, measuring serum cortisol levels alone is not recommended as a method of screening for Addison's disease. However, if a serum cortisol level is low (<18 µg/dL) and a simultaneously drawn serum ACTH level is high, a presumptive diagnosis of Addison's disease can be made. Further diagnosis of Addison's disease is based on ACTH stimulation tests that are used to test for adrenal reserve.

ACTH STIMULATION TESTS

The rapid ACTH stimulation test is the method of choice for initial assessment of the patient (2, 37). Either 25 units of ACTH or 0.25 mg of cosyntropin (synthetic ACTH) is administered by the intramuscular or intravenous route. Because of a higher incidence of allergic reactions to natural ACTH, cosyntropin is more commonly used. Serum cortisol levels are obtained just before the injection as a baseline and once or twice at 30 to 120 min after ACTH is given (36, 37). A normal response includes an increase in serum cortisol to ≥ 690 nmol/L (25 µg/dL) at any time during the test or an increase of at least 193 to 276 nmol/L (7 to 10 µg/dL) over the baseline serum cortisol level (37) unless baseline levels are already high as a result of stress. A subnormal response signifies either primary adrenocortical insufficiency or lack of adrenocortical response due to atrophy as a result of secondary adrenocortical insufficiency. A subnormal response may also occur in normal but stressed individuals whose adrenal cortex is already functioning at full capacity.

A 3-day ACTH stimulation test may be conducted to confirm the diagnosis of Addison's disease. This 3-day test is conducted by administering 25 units of ACTH gel (Acthar-gel) intramuscularly or 0.25 mg of cosyntropin in 500 to 1000 mL of normal saline over 6 to 8 hr. This is done once a day in conjunction with 24-hr urine collections for 17-hydroxycorticosteroid (17-OHCS) or urinary free cortisol or by measuring serum cortisol levels. In Addison's

Table 16.6.
Comparison of Glucocorticoid Medications

Name	Biologic Half-Life (HR)	Equivalent Dose (mg)	Relative Potency		Physiologic Replacement Dose (mg)
			Glucocorticoid	Mineralocorticoid	
Short-acting					
Hydrocortisone (cortisol)	8–12	20	1.0	1.0	30
Cortisone Acetate	8–12	25	0.8	0.8	37.5
Intermediate-acting					
Prednisone	18–36	5	3.5–4	0.8	7.5
Prednisolone	18–36	5	4.0	0.8	7.5
Methylprednisolone	18–36	4	5.0	0.5	6
Triamcinolone	18–36	4	5.0	0	6
Long-acting					
Dexamethasone	36–54	0.75	25–30	0	0.75–1.0
Betamethasone	36–54	0.60	25–30	0	0.75–1.0

disease, an increase in serum or urine cortisol or urinary 17-OHCS is absent or minimal. In secondary adrenocortical insufficiency due to reduced ACTH stimulation, cortisol rise is slow but progressive. In normal patients there is an increase in plasma cortisol to 35 to 40 µg/dL by the end of the 3-day infusion and an increase in 17-OHCS to a level above 15 mg/24 hr on the third day. These results can delineate both the diagnosis and cause of the adrenocortical insufficiency.

The ITT (insulin tolerance test) is the most sensitive and accurate test of the HPA axis. Insulin induces hypoglycemia (serum glucose <40 mg/dL), which stimulates ACTH release as a stress response. Plasma cortisol and glucose levels are measured before and at 30, 45, 60, and 90 min after insulin infusion. A normal response is increased plasma cortisol to >18 to 20 mg/dL. This test is rarely used, however, because of relative contraindication for critically ill patients and patients with seizure disorders or cardiovascular or cerebrovascular disease.

PLASMA ACTH LEVELS

Plasma ACTH levels can be measured as an alternative to the cumbersome 3-day ACTH stimulation test. ACTH levels are usually elevated to >55 pmol/L (250 pg/mL) in patients with primary adrenocortical insufficiency. With secondary adrenocortical insufficiency, plasma ACTH levels are between 0 and 11 pmol/L (0 to 50 pg/mL), which is considerably lower than is expected with low serum cortisol levels (2). The difficulty in measuring serum ACTH levels is that specimens must be handled carefully and they must be sent to specialized laboratories for evaluation.

Treatment

ADDISONIAN CRISIS

The treatment of adrenocortical insufficiency is based on glucocorticoid replacement, with or without additional mineralocorticoid replacement. In acute addisonian crisis, high doses of glucocorticoids are required. Hydrocortisone is the preferred corticosteroid, since it has sufficient mineralocorticoid activity (Table 16.6). It is administered initially as 100 mg intravenously every 8 hr. Usually, patients will stabilize within 24 hr, and at that time the dosage can be decreased to 50 mg intravenously every 6 hours. The hydrocortisone dose can be further reduced to a maintenance regimen of 20 to 30 mg/day after approximately 4 or 5 days (2, 4, 36, 39). Patients who are severely ill may require increased doses of hydrocortisone until the other complications (e.g., sepsis) have subsided.

A mineralocorticoid such as fludrocortisone may be added to therapy when the dose of hydrocortisone is ≤ 50 to 60 mg per day (2, 4). Intravenous methylprednisolone or dexamethasone may be used in place of hydrocortisone for patients with congestive heart failure or renal failure to minimize fluid retention.

The administration of intravenous saline and glucose is recommended to treat dehydration, shock, and hypoglycemia. However, the correction of metabolic abnormalities is secondary and will not occur until glucocorticoids are administered (40).

MAINTENANCE THERAPY

Addison's disease is a lifelong illness without a cure and requires chronic corticosteroid replacement. Although hydrocortisone is the most natural replacement corticosteroid, cortisone acetate, prednisone, and prednisolone may also be used. Dexamethasone should be avoided for chronic maintenance therapy, however, because of a higher incidence of adverse effects and a lack of mineralocorticoid effects.

Hydrocortisone is usually administered as 30 to 40 mg/day, divided into a twice- or thrice-daily regimen, with a larger portion of the dose administered in the morning (e.g., 20 to 25 mg hydrocortisone in the morning and 10 to

15 mg in the evening). When cortisone acetate is used in place of hydrocortisone, the dosage is approximately 20% higher. This is due to a need for conversion of cortisone acetate in the liver to hydrocortisone. Prednisone, which is converted in the liver to prednisolone, is another alternative at 5 to 7.5 mg per day.

When a mineralocorticoid is necessary (e.g., with orthostatic hypotension or electrolyte abnormalities), fludrocortisone (Florinef) is used. Dosages should be titrated to the patient's need and often range from 0.05 to 0.1 mg daily or every other day. For patients with cardiac or renal disease the salt and water retention that are related to mineralocorticoid use must be closely monitored.

Surgical Prophylaxis

Any patient being prepared for surgery who had been maintained on corticosteroid treatment within the past 12 months should be considered for perioperative corticosteroid prophylaxis. Regimens for perioperative corticosteroids are discussed in the section below entitled "Clinical Use of Steroids."

Conclusion

Adrenocortical insufficiency can be either primary or secondary and either acute or chronic. Primary adrenal insufficiency, Addison's disease, is usually idiopathic; secondary adrenal insufficiency is largely due to the use of exogeneous corticosteroids. Chronic Addison's disease is very difficult to recognize because of the nonspecific symptoms such as anorexia, weight loss, and fatigue. Acute addisonian crisis is also difficult to recognize but requires prompt treatment, even before laboratory diagnosis is complete.

Before exogeneous corticosteroids were available as a treatment modality, adrenal insufficiency associated with stress was usually fatal. At the same time, chronic adrenal insufficiency was associated with an 80% mortality within 3 years. Today, adrenal insufficiency can be treated effectively with corticosteroids when it is diagnosed on a timely basis.

PATIENT EDUCATION

Patients with Cushing's syndrome or Addison's disease should be advised to always carry an identification card or bracelet that states their need for hydrocortisone in the event of trauma or severe stress. They should also be instructed to maintain a diet with adequate salt and potassium. Patients who are taking oral corticosteroid replacement but are experiencing continuous vomiting or diarrhea or are unable to take their medications should seek parenteral replacement. Finally, if they are experiencing a high fever, they should contact their physician if symptoms do not resolve within 24 to 48 hr.

Table 16.7.
Disease States in Which Glucocorticoids Are Used

Primary or secondary adrenocortical insufficiency
Rheumatic disorders
  Acute gouty arthritis
  Rheumatoid arthritis
  Osteoarthritis
Renal diseases
  Glomerulonephritis
  Nephrotic syndrome
Collagen disorders
  Systemic lupus erythematosus
  Polymyositis
  Wegener's granulomatosis
  Giant-cell arteritis
Allergic disorders
  Angioedema
  Urticaria
  Contact or atopic dermatitis
  Allergic rhinitis
  Erythema multiforme (Stevens-Johnson syndrome)
Respiratory diseases
  Bronchial asthma
  Fulminating or disseminated tuberculosis
  Chronic obstructive pulmonary disease
  Neonatal respiratory distress syndrome
Dermatologic diseases
  Pemphigus
  Bullous dermatitis herpetiformis
  Severe psoriasis
Gastrointestinal diseases
  Ulcerative colitis
  Crohn's disease
  Sprue
Malignancies
  Breast cancer
  Leukemia
  Lymphoma
  Chemotherapy-induced emesis
Hepatic diseases
  Chronic active hepatitis
  Subacute hepatic necrosis
  Alcholic hepatitis
Miscellaneous
  Septic shock
  Hypercalcemia
  Organ transplantation
  Sarcoidosis
  Idiopathic thrombocytopenic purpura (ITP)
  Hemolytic anemia
  Multiple sclerosis
  Cerebral edema

CLINICAL USE OF STEROIDS

Each year, over 5 million people in the United States use corticosteroids. Exogenous corticosteroids have been found to be useful in the treatment of many disease states (Table 16.7). These range from short-term, self-limited conditions such as allergic rhinitis to life-threatening diseases such as leukemia and idiopathic thrombocytopenic purpura. Corticosteroids are used by people in all age groups, for example to treat respiratory distress syndrome in neonates and rheumatoid arthritis in the elderly.

Mechanism of Action

Corticosteroids are composed of 21-carbon molecules. The biologic activity of the corticosteroid depends on the presence of a hydroxyl group at the 11-carbon site. Glucocorticoids that rely on conversion in the liver to the active form do not have biologic activity before this conversion. Examples include cortisone and prednisone, which are converted in the liver to hydrocortisone and prednisolone, respectively. For this reason, cortisone and prednisone are available only for systemic treatment. To have clinical activity, a corticosteroid used for topical treatment must already be in the active, 11-β-hydroxyl form.

The primary pharmacologic actions of glucocorticoids are thought to be due to binding of the steroid to intracellular receptors. Once binding occurs, the steroid associates with the nucleus of the cell and influences the transcription of specific genes (41). This leads to an alteration in protein synthesis. It is thought that glucocorticoids also have various degrees of binding to mineralocorticoid receptors in the kidney and brain (42). This explains the mineralocorticoid activity of some glucocorticoids. Cortisol (hydrocortisone) has equal affinity for both the glucocorticoid and mineralocorticoid receptors. Dexamethasone has the lowest affinity for the mineralocorticoid receptor compared to cortisol, followed by betamethasone and prednisolone. Fludrocortisone, on the other hand, has an affinity almost 12 times higher than that of cortisol (41).

The response of a tissue to a glucocorticoid varies with the type of tissue. In addition, tissues that do not contain glucocorticoid receptors may be affected nonetheless because of mediators produced by primary tissue responses. The primary activity of glucocorticoids is to shield the body from its own defense mechanisms that are activated in stressful situations. If uncontrolled, the body's defense mechanisms can go too far and cause injury. The defense mechanisms that glucocorticoids appear to "dampen" include (a) insulin release; (b) inflammatory processes involving bradykinin, histamine, eicosanoids, serotonin, or plasminogen activator; (c) neurochemical release (CRF, ACTH, β-endorphins); (d) immune reactions (particularly cellular responses); and (e) antidiuretic hormone release. In using a corticosteroid clinically, only one or two of these effects may be desired. For example, glucocorticoids are used in asthma to inhibit cells involved in airway inflammation, including macrophages, T-lymphocytes, eosinophils, and airway epithelial cells (for further information see Chapter 35 on asthma) (43). Unfortunately, at this time, there is no steroid that mediates one system preferentially.

Other effects of glucocorticoids have been observed that do not appear to be related to immunosuppression or antiinflammatory activity. For example, glucocorticoids tend to reverse hypercalcemia associated with sarcoidosis. This is thought to occur because of inhibition of the conversion of 25-hydroxycholecalciferol to 1-α, 25-dihydroxycholecalciferol (44). Another example is the reduction in brain edema by corticosteroids in postoperative or posttraumatic settings.

Pharmacokinetics

The systemic effects of glucocorticoids depend on three factors:

1. the amount of active drug delivered to the systemic circulation,
2. the potency or interaction of the steroid at the receptor site, and
3. the length of time the steroid remains at the receptor site.

Pharmacokinetic principles aid us in understanding these three factors.

BIOAVAILABILITY

The bioavailability of oral corticosteroids depends on the rate of dissolution of the oral preparation in the gastrointestinal tract and its absorption into the systemic circulation. For corticosteroids that are converted in the liver to the active form (e.g., prednisone is converted to prednisolone), bioavailability refers to the active component that is available in the systemic circulation.

When oral prednisone or hydrocortisone is administered to healthy volunteers, bioavailability ranges from 50 to 100%, the time to peak prednisolone levels occurring at approximately 1.3 to 3 hr (45). Fluctuation in availability is seen and is due primarily to variable rates of tablet dissolution. Enteric coating of oral steroid products, such as prednisolone, has been shown to decrease the rate but not the extent of absorption (45). Also, food does not decrease the bioavailability of oral prednisolone. However, when enteric-coated prednisolone tablets are taken with food, a significant decrease in bioavailability is seen (46). For this reason, enteric-coated steroid preparations are not recommended to be taken with food.

Absorption of corticosteroids from other routes of administration has also been studied. Corticosteroids are administered as retention enemas, skin creams and ointments, preparations for inhalation, and ophthalmic liquids. Systemic absorption will occur to some degree with each of these. Approximately 30 to 90% of a hydrocortisone retention enema will be absorbed (46, 47). A daily dose of 400 μg of beclomethasone (two puffs every 6 hr) is therapeutically equivalent to a dose of 7.5 mg of prednisone daily (47). When a spacer is used with an inhaled steroid, less of the medication is systemically absorbed, and suppression of the HPA axis is less likely (43). Newer inhaled steroids, such as fluticasone, have less effect on the HPA axis than beclomethasone does (48).

Absorption of steroid preparations applied to the skin is increased by certain factors. These include young age, administration after a bath (four to five times increased absorption), plastic occlusion (ten times increased absorption), thin skin (e.g., eyelids, scrotum, forehead), and damaged skin (48). High-potency and ointment preparations also have increased absorption.

DISTRIBUTION

Corticosteroids are primarily lipophilic compounds that distribute widely throughout the body. The apparent volume of distribution of prednisolone, however, is only 0.35 to 0.7 L/kg (45). This relatively low volume of distribution is primarily due to high protein binding in the serum. Steroids are bound in the serum to two proteins: albumin and transcortin (corticosteroid-binding globulin). At low concentrations, hydrocortisone and prednisolone are 80 to 90% protein-bound. However, protein binding decreases to approximately 60 to 70% at high steroid concentrations. This is due to a saturation of transcortin binding sites (45, 49). At high concentrations, plasma protein binding is decreased and free drug is available to diffuse more readily into peripheral tissues. This is reflected in a higher volume of distribution of the drug and increased risk for adverse reactions. Similar effects occur in patients with hypoalbuminemia; both serum albumin and transcortin levels are reduced, and the free fraction of corticosteroids is increased. A reduction in corticosteroid dose is recommended for these patients.

CLEARANCE

Clearance of corticosteroids occurs primarily via the liver by metabolic hydroxylation and conjugation. Less than 15% of a corticosteroid dose is eliminated unchanged in the urine. Along with changes in volume of distribution with increasing serum concentrations, total body clearance also increases. After a low dose of prednisolone, the clearance is approximately 7 L/hr. When a higher dose of prednisolone is administered, the mean clearance increases to 12 L/hr (45). This alteration in total body clearance occurs primarily with prednisolone doses that are less than 70 mg/day (46).

Factors that decrease the hepatic clearance of corticosteroids include liver or renal failure, age over 65 years, and concomitant ketoconazole or oral contraceptive use. An increase in clearance occurs with long-term use of corticosteroids (i.e., enzyme induction may occur), in hyperthyroidism, and with enzyme-inducing medications such as phenytoin, rifampin, and barbiturates (Table 16.3).

HALF-LIFE

Half-life is a reflection of both the volume of distribution and clearance of a compound. When these two parameters increase with increasing corticosteroid dose, no change in half-life is expected. This has been shown to be true with prednisolone. The half-life of prednisolone ranges from 2.6 to 5 hr and is constant with increasing doses (45, 49). Hydrocortisone, however, appears to have a dose-dependent increase in half-life. Even when this dose-dependent change is considered, the half-life range for hydrocortisone is only 1.2 to 1.8 hr (45). The clinical significance of this increase in half-life is minimal.

The half-lives of the glucocorticoids are relatively similar; however, marked differences have been observed in the physiologic effects of the different agents. The corticosteroids can be divided into three groups based on their biologic half-life (47, 50, 51). Short-acting agents such as hydrocortisone and cortisone suppress ACTH activity for 8 to 12 hr. Intermediate-acting agents such as prednisone, prednisolone, methylprednisolone, and triamcinolone suppress ACTH activity for 18 to 36 hr. The longest-acting corticosteroids suppress ACTH for 36 to 54 hr and include dexamethasone and betamethasone. The duration of ACTH suppression is also prolonged as the dose of any agent is increased. The pharmacodynamic differences appear to be related to differences in receptor activity and cannot be explained on the basis of the individual agent's pharmacokinetic properties.

Adverse Effects

The adverse effects that are associated with high-dose corticosteroids (see Table 16.8) are similar to those that are exhibited with endogenous hypercortisolism (as was discussed earlier in the section entitled "Cushing's Syndrome"). Endogenous hypercortisolism usually involves an increase in ACTH levels, which leads to increased cortisol, aldosterone, and adrenal androgen production. For this reason, Cushing's syndrome is usually accompanied by edema, hypertension, and hirsutism. However, with iatrogenic hypercortisolism, cortisol levels are elevated but ACTH levels are suppressed and less mineralocorticoid and androgenic effects are seen. This will also depend on the corticosteroid being administered; for example, hydrocortisone has more mineralocorticoid effects than does prednisone or dexamethasone.

In addition to the effects that are seen with endogenous hypercortisolism, certain adverse effects are seen almost exclusively with iatrogenic hypercortisolism. These include euphoria, intracranial hypertension, vasculitis, pancreatitis, gastritis, glaucoma, cataracts, and ischemic bone necrosis. When therapy with corticosteroids is begun, these severe adverse effects should be considered. Prospective monitoring for these complications and correct dosing will help

Table 16.8.
Medical Complications of Glucocorticoid Therapy

Characteristic early in therapy: essentially unavoidable
    Insomnia
    Emotional lability
    Enhanced appetite or weight gain or both
Common in patients with underlying risk factors or other drug toxicities
    Hypertension
    Diabetes mellitus
    Peptic ulcer disease
    Acne vulgaris
Anticipated with use of sustained and intense treatment: minimize risk by conservative dosing regimens and steroid-sparing agents whenever possible
    Cushingoid habitus
    Hypothalamic-pituitary-adrenal suppression
    Infection diathesis
    Osteonecrosis
    Myopathy
    Impaired wound healing
Insidious and delayed: likely dependent on cumulative dose
    Osteonecrosis
    Skin atrophy
    Cataracts
    Atherosclerosis
    Growth retardation
    Fatty liver
Rare and unpredictable
    Psychosis
    Pseudotumor cerebri
    Glaucoma
    Epidural lipomatosis
    Pancreatitis

Source: Reprinted, with permission, from Balow JE. Complications of therapy, pp. 1205–1206. In Boumpas DT (moderator). Glucocorticoid therapy for immune-mediated diseases: basic and clinical correlates. Ann Intern Med 119:1198–1208, 1993.

to reduce morbidity and mortality associated with long-term corticosteroid treatment.

OSTEOPOROSIS

Osteoporosis is a significant obstacle to corticosteroid treatment. Steroids lead to a decrease in bone formation and an increase in bone resorption (52). Bone loss is more prominent in trabecular bones (e.g., ribs and vertebrae) than in the long bones of the body (52). Steroid-induced osteoporosis occurs at a higher rate in postmenopausal women, alcoholics, and patients with altered vitamin D absorption or metabolism.

The cause of steroid-induced bone loss is multifactorial. There are decreased gastrointestinal absorption of calcium and increased renal elimination of calcium. This leads to decreased serum calcium levels, which induce secondary hyperparathyroidism. This further leads to an increase in

osteoclast activity, which increases serum calcium levels and results in osteomalacia.

Information on the treatment of this condition is limited. Although lowering the dose of the glucocorticoid is recommended, alternate-day regimens have not been shown to affect bone loss. Treatment of steroid-induced osteoporosis with exercise, vitamin D, calcium supplements, and sodium fluoride may be helpful (52). Another treatment modality is the use of hydrochlorothiazide when hypercalciuria is present (52). The use of estrogen replacement for postmenopausal women has also been suggested. The efficacy of these treatment regimens in steroid-induced osteoporosis has not yet been adequately studied.

INFECTIONS

Infections are common in steroid-treated patients and include infections of bacterial, fungal, viral, and parasitic origin. Gram-negative bacteria and fungi such as *Candida albicans* and cryptococcus are particularly troublesome for patients who are on long-term corticosteroids. Reactivation of tuberculosis is another concern for patients who have previously had a positive tuberculin skin test. However, the literature does not show an increased incidence of primary tuberculosis in these patients (41).

In addition to being more susceptible to infectious complications, detection of an infectious process in a patient who is being treated with steroids may be difficult. This is due to the immunosuppressant activity of corticosteroids, which blunts the typical manifestations of an infection such as an elevated white blood cell count and inflammation. For this reason, any slight deterioration in well-being should be accompanied by an aggressive search for and treatment of an infectious etiology.

PEPTIC ULCER DISEASE

Gastritis and peptic ulcer disease are controversial complications associated with glucocorticoid administration. The incidence of these complications has been reported as being significantly higher than with placebo but still at a fairly low incidence of 1.8% in a study that pooled data from 71 previously reported trials of 3064 total patients (53). However, steroid-induced peptic ulcer disease may lead to severe complications such as perforation and death, as reported by Dayton and Kleckner in 1987 (54). In their retrospective chart review they found an 85% mortality rate for patients over 50 years of age who developed perforation of a gastric ulcer because of corticosteroid use.

Gastritis and peptic ulcer disease associated with corticosteroids occur as both acute and chronic complications and are more common in the stomach than in the duodenum. This adverse effect tends to be independent of the type of corticosteroid and dose. However, pulse-dosing

Table 16.9.
Adverse Effects of Topical Steroids

Skin atrophy and fibrosis
Icthyosislike changes
Flushing
Telangiectasia
Abnormal pigmentation
Superficial infections (bacterial, fungal, parasitic)
Acne
Rosacealike dermatitis
Perioral dermatitis
Purpura
Delayed skin healing
Glaucoma (associated with ophthalmic use)
Cataracts (associated with ophthalmic use)
Photosensitivity
False scars

Source: Adapted from Takeda K, Arase S, Takahashi S. Side effects of topical corticosteroids and their prevention. Drugs 36(suppl 15):15–23, 1988.

is more highly associated with perforation (54). Monitoring for this complication should include baseline and follow-up endoscopy.

Subjective complaints with steroid-induced peptic ulcer disease are not necessarily correlated with endoscopic findings but should be managed with antacid regimens. The use of prophylactic antacids is also recommended for patients who are on intermittent high doses of corticosteroids (pulse-dosing) and are over the age of 50 years (54). Although prophylactic use of histamine-2 antagonists such as cimetidine and ranitidine is common, this practice should be limited to patients who have additional risk factors for developing peptic ulcer disease (e.g., a previous history of peptic ulcer disease, concomitant use of aspirin or nonsteroidal antiinflammatory agents). For elderly patients the use of nonsteroidal antiinflammatory agents with corticosteroids significantly increases the relative risk of developing peptic ulcer disease (55). In the same study, steroid users who were not receiving nonsteroidal antiinflammatory agents showed no increased risk for ulcer disease, regardless of dose and duration of corticosteroid use.

TOPICAL GLUCOCORTICOIDS

Topical corticosteroids exhibit adverse effects that are unique to their mode of application. Use of fluorinated glucocorticoids (e.g., triamcinolone, betamethasone, dexamethasone) on the face and other areas of thin skin should be avoided because of skin atrophy. A list of this and other complications can be found in Table 16.9. Inhaled corticosteroids are quite safe in low to moderate doses but can cause mild adrenocortical suppression and change in bone density in high doses. The clinical significance of these changes has not been established.

Glucocorticoid Selection

Glucocorticoid preparations differ in their duration of action, mineralocorticoid effects, route of administration, and cost. Hydrocortisone and cortisone acetate are the glucocorticoids that most closely approximate the body's natural glucocorticoid, cortisol. These agents have both glucocorticoid and mineralocorticoid activity and are the preparations of choice for adrenocortical insufficiency. Dexamethasone is a synthetic glucocorticoid that has minimal mineralocorticoid activity and is a particularly useful agent for patients with brain edema, congestive heart failure, or renal failure. Prednisone is an effective, inexpensive glucocorticoid that also needs to be monitored for its mineralocorticoid effects.

Dosing of Corticosteroids

In dosing systemic corticosteroids, the best approach is to use the lowest dose for the shortest time possible and to administer doses in the morning. When corticosteroid therapy is initiated, dosage should be individualized on the basis of the agent being used and the condition being treated. High doses are used initially to achieve antiinflammatory or immunosuppressant effects (e.g., 0.6 to 1 mg/kg/day of prednisone for aggressive disorders) (56). Once the clinical response is achieved, the steroid can be either abruptly discontinued, tapered then discontinued, or tapered for long-term replacement or immunosuppressive treatment. Alternate-day dosing is preferred for chronic corticosteroid treatment, since this is associated with fewer adverse effects and less HPA suppression.

HPA SUPPRESSION

When exogenous corticosteroids are administered, the secretion of CRF (corticotropin-releasing factor) and ACTH (adrenocorticotropic hormone) is suppressed. The degree of HPA suppression is influenced by factors that include dose, dosing interval, time of administration, length of therapy, and route of administration (47, 57). When glucocorticoids with long half-lives are used (e.g., dexamethasone), serum levels are sustained and the circadian rhythm is disrupted. For this reason, dexamethasone produces more HPA suppression than does a short-acting glucocorticoid such as prednisone. Glucocorticoids that are administered as a single morning dose produce less HPA suppression than does a regimen of divided doses throughout the day. This is because the dosing follows the body's natural circadian rhythm, with high cortisol levels in the morning and low levels in the evening. Although the exact time course required for initiation of HPA suppression is not known, the degree of HPA suppression increases as corticosteroid therapy is continued. Whenever possible, the use of adjunctive medications to decrease glucocorticoid dose requirements ("steroid sparing") should be considered. These medications include azathioprine, methotrexate, antimalarial agents, cyclosporin A, and cyclophosphamide (56).

Variations in onset of HPA suppression have been seen between different patients and different studies. Overall, any patient who is receiving long-term oral corticosteroids requires a prolonged taper to discontinue therapy. In addition, such patients will require elevated doses of corticosteroids with surgery or stress for up to 1 year after steroids are discontinued.

ALTERNATE-DAY THERAPY

Dosing of glucocorticoids on an alternate-day basis can minimize HPA suppression and adverse effects while still providing effective treatment of many disease processes. Alternate-day dosing should be considered for any patient who requires corticosteroid therapy that will last longer than several weeks. Conditions that can be managed effectively by alternate-day administration include ulcerative colitis, renal transplant rejection, chronic dermatoses, myasthenia gravis, and asthma (41). Conditions that show a less favorable response to alternate-day dosing include rheumatoid arthritis, systemic lupus erythematosus, and giant-cell arteritis (58).

Short- or intermediate-acting corticosteroids are appropriate for alternate-day dosing. These preparations allow a partial recovery of the HPA axis on the days when the glucocorticoid is not administered. In addition, cushingoid adverse effects such as moon facies, obesity, striae, carbohydrate intolerance, myopathy, infections, and growth inhibition in children are less likely to develop with alternate-day dosing (59).

Daily dosing of glucocorticoids is used initially, and when the disease state is under control, dosing is switched over to alternate days. This change should be made as early in treatment as possible, before the HPA axis has been suppressed significantly. However, a conservative approach should be considered in converting to alternate-day dosing. This is recommended for three reasons (59):

1. HPA suppression may have already occurred.
2. Even with normal HPA function, steroid withdrawal symptoms may occur.
3. The underlying disease may be exacerbated.

The conversion schedule that is chosen depends on the underlying disease, the duration of therapy, the patient's acceptance of alternate-day dosing, and the use of adjunctive therapy (59). First, the daily dose may need to be decreased to 15 to 20 mg/day of prednisone equivalent and then converted to a single morning dose. Next, a very gradual switch to alternate-day dosing can be started. This is accomplished by reducing one day's dose by approximately 10 to 20% and adding the same amount to the next day's dose. This dose should then be continued for at least

Table 16.10.

Scheme for the Conversion to an Alternate-Day Regimen for Glucocorticoids (Initial dose prednisone 60 mg/day)

Day	Dose (mg)	Day	Dose (mg)
A. Reduce dosage by 5 mg every 3 days until a dose of prednisone 20 mg is reached:			
1	55	13	35
2	55	14	35
3	55	15	35
4	50	16	30
5	50	17	30
6	50	18	30
7	45	19	25
8	45	20	25
9	45	21	25
10	40	22	20
11	40	23	20
12	40	24	20
B. Reduce dosage by 2.5 mg on alternate days every 3 cycles until no prednisone on alternate days:			
25	20	49	20
26	17.5	50	7.5
27	20	51	20
28	17.5	52	7.5
29	20	53	20
30	17.5	54	7.5
31	20	55	20
32	15	56	5
33	20	57	20
34	15	58	5
35	20	59	20
36	15	60	5
37	20	61	20
38	12.5	62	2.5
39	20	63	20
40	12.5	64	2.5
41	20	65	20
42	12.5	66	2.5
43	20	67	20
44	10	68	0
45	20	69	20
46	10	70	0
47	20	71	20
48	10	72	0

three cycles before the next reduction in dose is made. An example of a conversion to alternate-day dosing is shown in Table 16.10.

During the conversion period the patient should be monitored closely for adrenocortical insufficiency and exacerbation of the primary disease. Steroid withdrawal may occur and is usually manifested by fatigue, weakness, arthralgia, nausea, hypotension, and dizziness. This is usually managed by restarting small glucocorticoid doses on the off-day or by reinstituting the initial dosing regimen that was used before the tapering process began (41). Exacerbation of the primary disease should be managed with agents other than steroids when possible.

Discontinuation of Glucocorticoids

Short-term, low-dose (i.e., <20 mg of prednisone per day) glucocorticoid treatment of up to approximately 3 weeks' duration can usually be discontinued abruptly with few steroid withdrawal effects (47). The discontinuation of chronic glucocorticoid treatment, however, can be a lengthy and frustrating process. As with the conversion of divided daily doses, exacerbation of the underlying disease can occur with or without steroid withdrawal reactions. One method of tapering chronic glucocorticoid doses for discontinuation of therapy is shown in Table 16.11.

Perioperative or Stress Doses

High-dose, intravenous glucocorticoids are required for surgery or stress in patients with HPA suppression. This includes patients who are maintained on chronic supraphysiologic doses (i.e., >7.5 mg of prednisone per day) and patients who recently (up to 1 year previously) discontinued glucocorticoid treatment. Stress doses are used to replace exogenously the maximum output of cortisol by the adrenal cortex, which is approximately 200 to 500 mg/day.

For major surgical procedures the dose of hydrocortisone used is usually at least 300 mg/day of hydrocortisone or its equivalent. The currently recommended regimen is as follows (35):

1. Preoperative dosing: Either continue the existing dose of glucocorticoid or administer 50 to 100 mg of hydrocortisone for 1 to 2 days before the surgical procedure.
2. On the day of surgery: Administer hydrocortisone 100 mg intravenously early on the morning of surgery, 100 mg constant intravenous infusion during surgery, and/or 100 mg intravenously in the first 8 hr postoperatively.
3. Postoperative day 1: Administer 100 mg for one dose or 300 mg in divided doses every 8 hr.
4. Rapidly taper dose over the next 3 to 4 days as indicated by the patient's recovery.

With minor surgery a similar regimen is used. Hydrocortisone is administered at a dose of 100 mg intravenously every 8 hr for the first 24 hr. After the first day, therapy is converted to oral hydrocortisone and tapered rapidly over a few days.

With other types of stress, such as acute asthmatic attacks, oral or intravenous corticosteroids are administered in moderate to high doses (e.g., prednisone 0.5 mg/kg every 6 hr) (3). (See Chapter 35 on asthma.) The glucocorticoid dose can then be tapered rapidly to the previous maintenance regimen.

In each of these regimens, patient response must be monitored. Perioperative complications may lead to sustained stress after surgery, and intravenous hydrocortisone may need to be continued. The continued use of high-dose corticosteroids may also be deleterious, increasing the patient's susceptibility to infection, altering fluid and electrolyte status, and impairing surgical healing. Patient assessment is essential to optimizing the use of perioperative or stress doses of corticosteroids.

CONCLUSION

Adrenocortical steroid hormones are necessary to maintain metabolic homeostasis of the human body for normal daily living and during times of severe stress. When the normal production and secretion of cortisol, the body's

Table 16.11.

Scheme for the Gradual Reduction and Discontinuation of Glucocorticoids (Initial dose prednisone 40 mg/day)

Day	Dose (mg)	Day	Dose (mg)
A. Reduce dosage by 5 mg on alternate days until a dose of prednisone 10 mg is reached:			
1	40	7	40
2	35	8	20
3	40	9	40
4	30	10	15
5	40	11	40
6	25	12	10
B. Reduce by 2.5 mg on alternate days every 3 cycles until no prednisone is given on alternate days:			
13	40	25	40
14	7.5	26	2.5
15	40	27	40
16	7.5	28	2.5
17	40	29	40
18	7.5	30	2.5
19	40	31	40
20	5	32	0
21	40	33	40
22	5	34	0
23	40	35	40
24	5	36	0
C. If the patient remains stable, reduce by 5 mg on alternate days until a dose of 10 mg every other day is reached:			
37	35	43	20
38	0	44	0
39	30	45	15
40	0	46	0
41	25	47	10
42	0	48	0
D. Reduce by 2.5 mg on alternate days every 3 cycles until a dose of 2.5 mg every other day is reached:			
49	7.5	58	0
50	0	59	5
51	7.5	60	0
52	0	61	2.5
53	7.5	62	0
54	0	63	2.5
55	5	64	0
56	0	65	2.5
57	5	66	0
E. Drop to 1 mg on alternate days for 1 week.			
F. Stop all glucocorticoids.			

Source: Reprinted, with permission, from Helfer EL, Rose LI. Corticosteroids and adrenal suppression: characterizing and avoiding the problem. Drugs 38:838–845, 1989.

major glucocorticoid hormone, are disturbed, serious clinical diseases result. Sustained hypercortisolism produces Cushing's syndrome; chronic adrenocortical insufficiency results in Addison's disease. When cortisol is not available to aid the body in dealing with an acute stressful event, a rapidly fatal addisonian crisis results. Each of these conditions can be managed effectively once the diagnosis is known.

Exogenous corticosteroids have been used to treat a variety of illnesses. Efficacy is greatest in treating illnesses with an inflammatory or immunologic basis. However, the long-term use of systemic corticosteroids is associated with many adverse effects, including electrolyte abnormalities, susceptibility to infections, osteoporosis, gastritis, and peptic ulcer disease. For this reason the smallest dose should be used for the shortest period of time or on alternate days to minimize adrenal atrophy. Discontinuation of corticosteroids must be done very slowly if HPA suppression has occurred. While the drug is being gradually discontinued, the patient should be monitored for disease recurrence or the steroid withdrawal syndrome. Doses of corticosteroids in response to stress (e.g., surgery) will be required for up to 1 year after steroid withdrawal by patients who have HPA suppression.

REFERENCES

1. Axelrod J, Reisine TD. Stress hormones: their interaction and regulation. Science 224:452–459, 1984.
2. Baxter JD, Tyrrell JB. The adrenal cortex. In: Felig P, Baxter JD, Broadus AE, Frohman LA, eds. Endocrinology and metabolism. New York: McGraw-Hill, 1987:511.
3. Byyny BL. Preventing adrenal insufficiency during surgery. Postgrad Med 67(5):219–226, 1980.
4. Tyrrell JB, Forsham PH. Glucocorticoids and adrenal androgens. In: Greenspan FS, Forsham PH, eds. Basic and clinical endocrinology. East Norwalk: Lange, 1986:272.
5. Cushing HC. The basophil adenomas of the pituitary body and their clinical manifestations (pituitary basophilism). Bull Johns Hopkins Hosp 1(3):137–195, 1932.
6. Carpenter PC. Diagnostic evaluation of Cushing's syndrome. Endocrinol Metabol Clin North Am 17(3):445–472, 1988.
7. Schteingart DE. Cushing's syndrome. Endocrinol Metab Clin North Am 18(2):311–338, 1989.
8. Aron DC. Cushing's syndrome: current concepts in diagnosis and treatment. Compr Ther 13(12):37–44, 1987.
9. Aron DC, Findling JW, Tyrrell JB. Cushing's disease. Endocrinol Metab Clin North Am 16(3):705–730, 1987.
10. Felicetta JV. Cushing's syndrome: how to pinpoint and treat the underlying cause. Postgrad Med 86(8):79–90, 1989.
11. Tyrrell JB, Laboratory evaluation of adrenocortical function. In: Wyngaarden JB, Smith LH, eds. Cecil textbook of medicine. Philadelphia: WB Saunders, 1988:1348.
12. Orth DN. Cushing's syndrome. N Engl J Med 332(12):791–803, 1995.
13. Trecan GV, Laudet MH, Thomopoulos P, Luton JP, Bricaire H. Urinary free corticoids: an evaluation of their usefulness in the diagnosis of Cushing's syndrome. Acta Endocrinol 103:110–115, 1983.
14. Kaye TB, Crapo L. The Cushing syndrome: an update on diagnostic tests. Ann Intern Med 112:434–444, 1990.
15. Ashcraft MW, van Herle AJ, Vener SL, Geffner DL. Serum cortisol levels in Cushing's syndrome after low- and high-dose dexamethasone suppression. Ann Intern Med 97:21–26, 1982.
16. Tyrrell JB, Findling JW, Aron DC, Fitzgerald PA, Forsham PH. An overnight high dose dexamethasone suppression test for rapid differential diagnosis of Cushing's syndrome. Ann Intern Med 104:180–186, 1986.
17. Miller J, Crapo L. The biochemical diagnosis of hypercortisolism. Endocrinologist 4:7–16, 1994.
18. Krieger DT, Amorosa L, Linick F. Cyproheptadine-induced remission of Cushing's disease. N Engl J Med 293(18):893–896, 1975.
19. Hsu TH, Gann DS, Tsan KW, Russell RP. Cyproheptadine in the control of Cushing's disease. Johns Hopkins Med J 149:77–83, 1981.
20. Tyrrell JB, Brooks RM, Forsham PH. More on cyproheptadine. N Engl J Med 295(7):1137–1138, 1976.
21. Krieger DT. Cyproheptadine for pituitary disorders. N Engl J Med 295(7):394–395, 1976.
22. McKenna MJ, Linares M, Mellinger RC. Prolonged remission of Cushing's disease following bromocriptine therapy. Henry Ford Hosp Med J 35(4):188–191, 1987.
23. Jeffcoate WJ. Treating Cushing's disease. Br Med J 296(6617):227–228, 1988.
24. Thoren M, Adamson U, Sjoberg HE. Aminoglutethimide and metyrapone in the management of Cushing's syndrome. Acta Endocrinol 109:451–457, 1985.
25. Orth DN. Metyrapone is useful only as adjunctive therapy in Cushing's disease. Ann Intern Med 89(1):128–130, 1978.
26. Southren AL, Weisenfeld S, Laufer A, et al. Effect of O,p'DDD in a patient with Cushing's syndrome. J Clin Endocrinol Metab 21:201–208, 1961.
27. Schteingart DE, Tsao HS, Taylor CI, McKenzie A, Victoria R, Therrien BA. Sustained remission of Cushing's disease with mitotane and pituitary irradiation. Ann Intern Med 92:613–619, 1980.
28. Luton JP, Mahoudeau JA, Bouchard P, et al. Treatment of Cushing's disease by O,p'DDD. N Engl J Med 300(9):459–464, 1979.
29. Oates JA, Wood AJJ. The use of ketoconazole as an inhibitor of steroid production. N Engl J Med 317(13):812–818, 1987.
30. Sonino N, Boscaro M, Merola G, Mantero F. Prolonged treatment of Cushing's disease by ketoconazole. J Clin Endocrinol Metab 61:718–722, 1985.
31. McCance DR, Hadden DR, Kennedy L, Sheridan B, Atkinson AB. Clinical experience with ketoconazole as a therapy for patients with Cushing's syndrome. Clin Endocrinol 27:593–599, 1987.
32. Chin R, Zekan JM. Adrenal insufficiency. Prob Crit Care 4(3):312–324, 1990.
33. Baxter JD, Adrenocortical hypofunction. In: Wyngaarden JB, Smith LH, eds. Cecil textbook of medicine. Philadelphia: WB Saunders, 1988:1351.
34. Wilkins EGL, Hnizdo E, Cope A. Addisonian crisis induced by treatment with rifampicin. Tubercle 70:69–73, 1989.
35. Chin R. Adrenal crisis. Crit Care Clin 7(1):23–42, 1991.
36. Burke CW. Adrenocortical insufficiency. Clin Endocrinol Metab 14(4):947–976, 1985.
37. Kannan CR. Diseases of the adrenal cortex. Dis Mon 34(10):601–674, 1988.
38. Tobin MV, Aldridge SA, Morris AI, Belchetz PE, Gilmore IT. Gastrointestinal manifestations of Addison's disease. Am J Gastroenterol 84(10):1302–1305, 1989.
39. Bayliss RIS. Adrenal cortex. Clin Endocrinol Metab 9(3):477–486, 1980.
40. Waise A, Young RJ. Pitfalls in the management of acute adrenocortical insufficiency: discussion paper. J R Soc Med 82(12):741–742, 1989.
41. Tyrrell JB, Baxter JD. Glucocorticoid therapy. In: Felig P, Baxter JD, Broadus AE, Frohman LA, eds. Endocrinology and metabolism. New York: McGraw-Hill, 1987:787.

42. Munck A, Mendel DB, Smith LI, Orti E. Glucocorticoid receptors and actions. Am Rev Respir Dis 141:S2–S9, 1990.

43. Barnes P. Inhaled glucocorticoids for asthma. N Engl J Med 332(13):868–875, 1995.

44. Frame B, Parfitt AM. Corticosteroid-responsive hypercalcemia with elevated 1-alpha, 25-dihydroxyvitamin D. Ann Intern Med 93:449–451, 1980.

45. Begg EJ, Atkinson HC, Gianarakis N. The pharmacokinetics of corticosteroid agents. Med J Aust 146:37–41, 1987.

46. Frey BM, Frey FJ. Clinical pharmacokinetics of prednisone and prednisolone. Clin Pharmacokinet 19(2):126–146, 1990.

47. Helfer EL, Rose LI. Corticosteroids and adrenal suppression: characterizing and avoiding the problem. Drugs 38(5):838–845, 1989.

48. Giannotti B. Current treatment guidelines for topical corticosteroids. Drugs 36(suppl 5):9–14, 1988.

49. Pickup ME. Clinical pharmacokinetics of prednisone and prednisolone. Clin Pharmacokinet 4:111–128, 1979.

50. Harter JG. Corticosteroids: their physiologic use in allergic disease. NY State J Med 66:827–834, 1966.

51. Haynes RC, Murad F. Adrenocorticotropic hormone: adrenocortical steroids and their synthetic analogs: inhibitors of adrenocortical steroid biosynthesis. In: Gilman AG, Goodman LS, Rall TW, Murad F, eds. Goodman and Gilman's the pharmacological basis of therapeutics. New York: Macmillan 1985:1459.

52. Baylink DJ. Glucocorticoid-induced osteoporosis. N Engl J Med 309(5):306–308, 1983.

53. Messer J, Reitman D, Sacks HS, Smith H, Chalmers TC. Association of adrenocorticosteroid therapy and peptic-ulcer disease. N Engl J Med 309:21–24, 1983.

54. Dayton MT, Kleckner SC, Brown DK. Peptic ulcer perforation associated with steroid use. Arch Surg 122:376–380, 1987.

55. Piper JM, Ray WA, Daugherty JR, Griffen MR. Corticosteroid use and peptic ulcer disease: role of nonsteroidal anti-inflammatory drugs. Ann Intern Med 114:735–740, 1991.

56. Cupps TR. Therapeutic use, pp 1204–1205. In: Boumpas DT, moderator. Glucocorticoid therapy for immune mediated diseases: basic and clinical correlates. Ann Intern Med 119:1198–1208, 1993.

57. Byyny RL. Withdrawal from glucocorticoid therapy. N Engl J Med 295(1):30–32, 1976.

58. Hunder GG, et al. Daily and alternate day corticosteroid regimen in treatment of giant cell arteritis. Ann Intern Med 82:613–618, 1975.

59. Axelrod L. Glucocorticoid therapy. Medicine 55(1):39–65, 1976.

CHAPTER 17

THYROID DISORDERS

BETTY J. DONG

THYROID DISORDERS

Hypothyroidism, hyperthyroidism, and thyroid nodules are common disorders of the thyroid gland that affect 5 to 20% of the population. Because drug therapy is an essential component of medical management, the practitioner should have a basic understanding of thyroid physiology and pathophysiology, the laboratory and clinical manifestations of each disease, and the various medical options available.

Physiology

REGULATION OF THYROID FUNCTION

The thyroid gland, a highly vascular organ lying on top of the trachea, consists of two lobes connected by a middle lobe known as the isthmus. The gland synthesizes, stores, and releases two major metabolically active hormones: triiodothyronine (T_3) and thyroxine (T_4). T_3 is considered more active than T_4 because the thyroid receptor protein within the cell nucleus has about a tenfold higher affinity for T_3 than for T_4. Hormone synthesis and release is achieved by an intricate negative feedback mechanism involving the gland, the hypothalamic-pituitary axis (see Fig. 17.1), and autoregulation of iodide uptake. Physiologic factors (e.g., dopamine, stress) can also influence the hypothalamic-pituitary axis and hormone synthesis.

Low circulating levels of thyroid hormone initiate the release of thyroid-stimulating hormone (TSH) or thyrotropin from the pituitary and the secretion of thyrotropin-releasing factor (TRF) from the hypothalamus. Rising TSH levels increase iodide trapping by the gland, causing a subsequent increase in hormone synthesis and circulating hormone levels that then feed back on the pituitary and hypothalamic centers to shut off TRF, TSH, and further hormone biosynthesis. As the hormone levels drop, the hypothalamic-pituitary centers once again become responsive to release of TSH and TRF.

The gland can also regulate its own uptake of iodide to protect against excessive hormone production if a large iodide load is ingested (i.e., radiographic iodine dye). This autoregulation, known as the "Wolff-Chaikoff" block, is not overcome by TSH stimulation and occurs when a critical intrathyroid iodide concentration effect is established within the gland. The normal gland "escapes" from the block within 7 to 14 days, which prevents subsequent development of hypothyroidism and goiter. "Escape" occurs by a decrease in iodide transport or by an "iodide leak," both of which tend to decrease the intrathyroid iodide concentration and remove the block to further hormone synthesis. In certain thyroid disorders, (e.g., Hashimoto's thyroiditis) the gland cannot escape from the "Wolff-Chaikoff" block, causing hypothyroidism. Conversely, hyperthyroidism results if this critical block does not occur (e.g., multinodular goiter).

HORMONE SYNTHESIS/TRANSPORT/METABOLISM

Both T_4 and T_3 are synthesized within the gland. However, about 80% of the total daily production of T_3 is produced from the peripheral conversion of T_4 to T_3. About 35 to 40% of the secreted T_4 is peripherally monodeiodinated to active T_3, and about 40% is converted to inactive reverse T_3 (rT_3), which has little or no thyroid activity. Many acute conditions, chronic disorders, and drugs can reduce peripheral conversion of T_4 to active T_3 and increase the conversion to inactive rT_3 (see "Euthyroid Sick Syndrome") which can cause diagnostic confusion if such laboratory findings are not properly recognized.

Dietary inorganic iodide trapped by the gland is promptly oxidized by peroxidase to iodine before its incorporation with tyrosine molecules to form monoiodotyrosine (MIT) and diiodotyrosine (DIT). Subsequently, formation of T_4 occurs through the coupling of two diiodotyrosyl residues, and of T_3 by coupling a diiodotyrosyl and monoiodotyrosyl residue. The synthesized hormones are then stored within thyroglobulin until they are released into the circulation through enzymatic cleavage.

In the circulation, the hormones exist in both the active, free (unbound), and the protein-bound, inactive forms. Thyroxine is 99.89% bound; only 0.02% is free. This high affinity for the plasma proteins (thyroxine-binding globulin (TBG), 80%; thyroxine-binding prealbumin (TBPA), 10–15%; and albumin 4–5%) accounts for the high serum concentration and the slow metabolic degradation ($t_{1/2} = 7$ days) of thyroxine. T_3 is three times more potent metabolically than T_4, but its biologic activity is similar because the lower affinity of T_3 for the plasma proteins results in a lower serum concentration and greater clearance ($t_{1/2} = 1.5$ days). About 0.2% of T_3 is free and active.

Overview of Thyroid Assessment

An evaluation of a patient with a thyroid disorder should include:

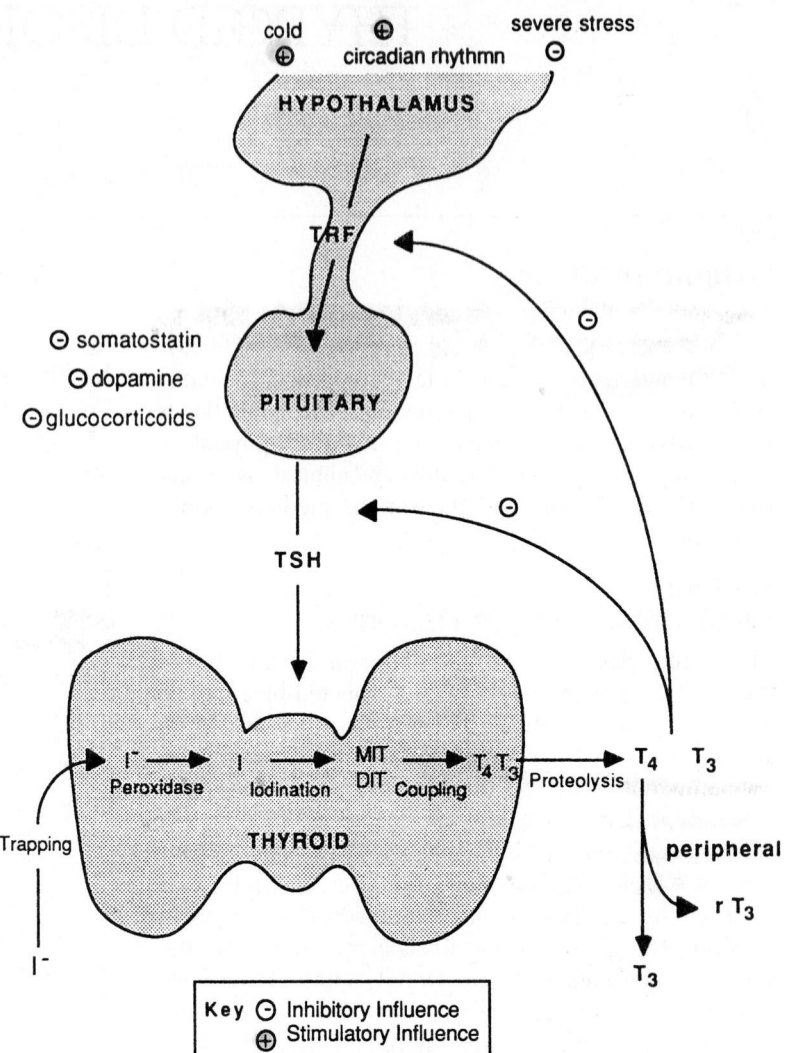

Figure 17.1. Hormone synthesis via negative-feedback control on the hypothalamic-pituitary-thyroid axis.

1. a history of any symptoms of either thyroid excess or deficiency;
2. a history of any neck or thyroid symptoms (e.g., pain, tenderness, difficulty swallowing or breathing);
3. a history of any familial thyroid abnormalities;
4. a history of any upper chest or neck irradiation as a child;
5. an examination of the thyroid for enlargement, consistency, and nodularity;
6. an examination for thyroid hormone effects on target systems;
7. a complete medication history for any use of thyroid or antithyroid drugs, or drugs that can cause thyroid disease; and
8. appropriate thyroid function tests.

THYROID FUNCTION TESTS

Overview

Several laboratory tests are available to assess thyroid homeostasis and metabolic function (1). These tests evaluate circulating hormone levels, glandular activity, hypothalamic-pituitary function, autoimmunity, and various nonspecific metabolic indices (see Table 17.1). The normal range will depend on the laboratory and the assay used. The most cost-effective screening test for thyroid disorders is a TSH level. A free thyroxine level (FT_4) or a free thyroxine index (FT_4I) can be obtained concurrently if the clinical suspicion for thyroid disease is high. If the screening TSH level is abnormal, subsequent determinations of hormone levels are indicated. Thyroid antibodies (ATgA, AMA) confirm the presence of an autoimmune thyroid disorder if a goiter and/or clinical symptoms exist. The thyroid uptake (RAIU) and scan, fine-needle aspiration (FNA), and thyroglobulin offer information in the evaluation of nodular disease and malignancy. The thyrotropin releasing hormone test (TRH) can help identify suspected hypopituitary disease.

Circulating Hormone Levels

Tests of circulating hormone levels measure the free or total (free and protein-bound) concentrations of T_4 and T_3 (see Table 17.1). Direct measurements of circulating

Table 17.1.
Thyroid Function Tests

Test	Normal Values	Measures	Hyperthyroidism	Hypothyroidism	Comments
TT$_4$ (total thyroxine)	64–142 mmol/L (5–11) µg/dL)	Total T$_4$, both free and bound	↑	↓	Affected by changes in thyroxine-binding globulin (TBG)
FT$_4$ (free thyroxine)	12–26 pmol/L (0.8–2.0 ng/dL)	Direct measure of free T$_4$ by equilibrium dialysis or analog method	↑	↓	Levels reflect true thyroid status
FT$_4$I (free thyroxine index)	16–50 mmol/L (1.3–4.2) calculated index using product of RT$_3$U and TT$_4$ 107–118 mmol/L (6.5–12.5) calculated index by dividing TT$_4$ by T$_4$ uptake	Indirect estimate of active free T$_4$ levels	↑	↓	Compensates for changes in TBG concentration; reflects true thyroid status except in euthyroid sick syndrome
RT$_3$U (resin T$_3$ uptake)	0.25–0.37 (25–37%)	Indirect measure of degree of saturation of TBG sites by T$_4$	↑	↓	Affected by changes in TBG
T$_4$U (T$_4$ uptake)	0.6–1.2	Available binding sites on TBG, prealbumin and albumin	↑	↓	Affected by changes in TBG, prealbumin, and albumin
TT$_3$ (total T$_3$)	1.46–2.92 mmol/L (95–190 ng/dL)	Total T$_3$, both free and bound	↑	↓	Affected by changes in TBG
FT$_3$I (free T$_3$ index)	0.37–1.08 mmol/L (24–70 ng/dL)	Product of RT$_3$U and TT$_3$; calculated estimate of active free T$_3$ levels	↑	↓	See comments for FT$_4$I
RAIU (^{131}I radioactive-iodine uptake)	5–15% at 5 hr 10–35% at 24 hr	Iodine trapping ability of gland	↑	↓ or ↑ in subclinical hypothyroidism	Normals vary depending on the degree of dietary iodide intake and on geographic locale; interfered by iodide intake (i.e., constrast dye)
TSH (thyrotropin-stimulating hormone)	0.4–4.8 mIU/L (0.4–4.8 µU/mL)	Pituitary TSH	↓	↑	Most sensitive indicator of adequate circulating hormone levels
Antibodies					
ATgA (thyroglobulin)	0–8%	Autoimmune process, (i.e., Hashimoto's, Graves' disease)	Often +	Often +	Microsomal more sensitive, elevated even with remission
AMA (microsomal)	<1:100 L		Often +	Often +	
TRab	Negative	Thyroid-receptor antibodies	+ (Graves')	−	Indicates Graves' disease, predictive for neonatal Graves' in pregnancy

(continued)

Table 17.1. *(Continued)*

Test	Normal Values	Measures	Hyperthyroidism	Hypothyroidism	Comments
TRH test (thyrotropin-releasing hormone test)	2- to 5-fold rise in serum TSH 30 min after injection 400 μg TRH IV	Ability of pituitary and hypothalamus to respond appropriately to TRH	No response	↓ or no response in pituitary or hypothalmic hypothyroidism	Only useful in the evaluation of secondary hypothyroidism.
Thyroid scan	Isotopes scan with ^{123}I or ^{99}TcO$_4$	Detects hypofunctioning (cold) and hyperfunctioning (hot) nodules and estimates size of gland	Diffusely enlarged; can have hot areas	Cold areas might occur with Hashimoto's disease	Not usually done useless discrete nodules are felt on physical examination

hormone levels include the free unbound thyroxine (FT_4), total T_4 (TT_4), and total T_3 (TT_3). The widely available FT_4 should replace the older and less accurate TT_4. Indirect measurements include the free thyroxine index (FT_4I), the resin T_3 uptake (RT_3U), the T_4 uptake (T_4U), and the free T_3 index (FT_3I).

TOTAL T_3 (TT_3)

The total T_3 (free and bound T_3) is most useful in the evaluation of hyperthyroidism because it can be elevated when the T_4 is normal (e.g., T_3 toxicosis and before the development of elevated T_4 levels). The TT_3 is not reliable in the evaluation of hypothyroidism or euthyroidism because it can be normal or low. Likewise, a low TT_3 does not prove hypothyroidism because multiple factors (e.g., age, acute or chronic disease) can cause a low TT_3 in the euthyroid individual by inhibiting the peripheral conversion of T_4 to T_3.

FREE THYROXINE (FT_4)

The free thyroxine can be directly measured by equilibrium dialysis or by the less accurate analog tests. Similarly, free T_3 (FT_3) can also be measured by equilibrium dialysis; however, this test is not yet readily available.

FREE THYROXINE INDEX (FT_4I), FREE T_3 INDEX (FT_3I)

The FT_4I and the FT_3I are indirectly calculated estimates of the free T_4 and T_3 as derived from TT_4 and TT_3 measurements. Because the TT_4 and the TT_3 depend on TBG, any change in the amount of TBG or the degree of TBG saturation will influence these results (see Table 17.2). These fluctuations in TBG do not accurately reflect the active-free hormone levels, which remain unchanged in a euthyroid state. The FT_4I and FT_3I correct for these TBG changes. An exception is the euthyroid sick syndrome, where the FT_4I or FT_3I can be falsely low. For example, if TBG levels are increased in an euthyroid patient (e.g., pregnancy or estrogen-containing oral contraceptives), the increased number of binding sites will produce a falsely elevated TT_4 and TT_3. However, the free T_4 and T_3 levels remain normal, as indicated by the FT_4I and FT_3I. Conversely, if TBG levels, and therefore TBG binding sites, are decreased in an euthyroid patient (e.g., androgen therapy, nephrosis, cirrhosis), a falsely depressed TT_4 and TT_3 will be seen. Drugs that displace T_4 and T_3 from TBG (e.g., large doses of salicylate [level>15 mg/100 mL]), will also produce a falsely low TT_4 and TT_3, because the binding sites are occupied by salicylates. In these latter situations, both the FT_4I and FT_3I are normal in the euthyroid individual.

Two methods can be used to calculate the index, and the method selected will depend on the laboratory performing the assays. The traditional way to calculate the FT_4I and FT_3I is the product of either the TT_4 or TT_3 and the resin T_3 uptake test (RT_3U). The resin T_3 uptake (RT_3U) is an indirect assessment of the concentration and saturation of TBG by T_4. A newer method uses the T_4 uptake. This method uses T_4 instead of radioactive T_3 and allows not only an estimate of TBG binding sites but also an estimate of prealbumin and albumin sites, without the additional risk of radioactivity. Using this method, the FT_4I and FT_3I are calculated by dividing the TT_4 or TT_3 by the T_4 uptake test. For example, if the TT_4 is 10 μg/dL and RT_3U is 30%, the FT_4I will be 3.0. If the index is calculated using the T_4 uptake of 1.0, a normal FT_4I of 10 will be reported. Most laboratories report only the FT_4I but not the RT_3U or T_4 uptake results.

Glandular Activity

The Radioactive Iodine Uptake (RAIU) measures only the iodine-trapping ability of the gland without regard to the iodine's ultimate fate. After a tracer dose of radioactive iodine, the percentage iodine uptake is measured at 5 and at 24 hours. An elevated uptake >35% at 24 hours) typically occurs in hyperthyroidism, whereas a depressed uptake (<30% in 24 hours) is seen in hypothyroidism. However, an elevated uptake can also occur in early hypothyroidism, indicating an attempt by the failing gland to increase iodine uptake and subsequent hormone synthesis. Difficulty with accurate interpretation of the RAIU dictates that it be used as an adjunct rather than a primary diagnostic tool. Fluctuations in the total iodide pool, through either dietary or therapeutic maneuvers, will falsely alter the true value of the RAIU (see Table 17.2). A thyroid scan is usually obtained concurrently. The scan, a picture of the gland, detects hypofunctioning, non-iodine-concentrating, "cold" areas or hyperfunctioning, hyper-iodine-concentrating, "hot" areas in parts of or the whole gland. An uptake and scan is used to estimate a therapeutic dosage of radioactive iodine therapy. A scan and uptake might also be obtained if discrete thyroid nodules or irregularities are palpable or if there is a history of prior neck irradiation. However, most clinicians prefer to use a fine-needle aspiration rather than an uptake and scan to evaluate a thyroid nodule.

Hypothalamic-Pituitary Function

The integrity of the negative-feedback hypothalamic-pituitary axis is evaluated by the serum thyrotropin (TSH) and the thyrotropin-releasing hormone test (TRH) (see Table 17.1).

TSH LEVELS

The sensitive TSH assay is the most accurate indicator of euthyroidism and thyroid dysfunction. Serum TSH elevations often occur before other overt clinical and laboratory manifestations of hypothyroidism are present. Therefore, the TSH can be elevated despite a normal FT_4, TT_4, and FT_4I, indicating early subclinical hypothyroidism or insufficient hormone replacement. Likewise, in subclinical hyperthyroidism or in overreplacement therapy, the TSH is suppressed into the subnormal range, even though circulating hormone levels are within the normal range. In overt hyperthyroidism, the TSH is often undetectable. The TSH can also be used to differentiate primary thyroid failure (elevated TSH) from secondary pituitary deficiency (absent or low normal TSH). Lastly, the TSH is invaluable in excluding secondary thyroid failure in patients with the euthyroid sick syndrome. The sensitive TSH assays are not perturbed by high levels of human chorionic gonadotropins (HCGs) in pregnancy. However, factors that affect dopamine, which physiologically controls TSH secretion, might alter the TSH level. Dopamine agonists (e.g., dopamine, levodopa, bromocriptine) and high-dose corticosteroids can suppress TSH secretion, and dopamine antagonists (e.g., metoclopramide) can increase TSH secretion (1). These mild drug-induced alterations in TSH levels generally do not interfere with the diagnosis of thyroid dysfunction in patients with true thyroid disease.

THYROTROPIN-RELEASING HORMONE (TRH) TEST

The TRH stimulation test is an easy and safe test that can be performed on an outpatient basis. Rarely, reversible hypotension and shock are reported. In euthyroid individuals, 200 to 400 µg i.v. protirelin (synthetic TRH) should produce a two- to fourfold increase in TSH level from baseline after 30 to 45 minutes. The TRH test is used to diagnose pituitary and hypothalamic hypothyroidism. In hypothalamic hypothyroidism a slow but continuous rise in TSH levels would occur after TRH, whereas in hypopituitary hypothyroidism, no TSH response to TRH would be expected. The sensitive TSH assay obviates the need for TRH testing in hyperthyroidism.

A blunted TSH response (< 2 mIU/L [2 µU/mL]) might also occur in euthyroid patients with renal failure, depression, and starvation; in patients over 40 years old; and in those receiving adequate thyroid hormone suppression therapy, chronic glucocorticoid therapy, dopamine infusions, or L-dopa therapy (1).

Tests of Autoimmunity: Antibodies.

ATgA; AMA

Two main antigens are identified in the thyroid gland: thyroglobulin and the microsomal component. The presence of antithyroglobulin (ATgA) and antimicrosomal (AMA) antibodies suggest an autoimmune process such as Graves' disease and/or Hashimoto's thyroiditis. However, because positive antibodies can occur in patients without thyroid dysfunction or in patients with collagen vascular disorders, their presence is not diagnostic of thyroid illness. The levels of ATgA and AMA are consistently higher during the acute phases of autoimmune thyroid disease and decline during remission and after therapy. The AMA is the more sensitive of the two antibodies because levels remain detectable after remission whereas ATgA titers revert to normal.

THYROID RECEPTOR ANTIBODY (TRab)

An IgG immunoglobulin, capable of stimulating the thyroid gland like TSH, is commonly present in 90% of patients with Graves' disease. There is no need to run a TRab test on a patient with classic symptoms of Graves' disease because the test is expensive (approximately $100) and offers no additional therapeutic or diagnostic information. The TRab will help confirm the diagnosis of Graves' disease in clinically euthyroid patients with an atypical presentation (e.g., ophthalmopathy). The TRab should be done in the pregnant female with a prior history of Graves' disease. A high maternal TRab titer provides predictive information about the risk of neonatal Graves' disease. Lastly, the presence or absence of TRab in patients with Graves' disease may act as a prognostic indicator of the potential for disease relapse and remission.

Nonspecific Indices

A number of nonspecific indices can be abnormal in thyroid dysfunction. Serum cholesterol, carotene, SGOT, creatine phosphokinase (CPK), and LDH levels can be elevated in severe hypothyroidism. The opposite occurs in hyperthyroidism.

Table 17.2.
Summary of Laboratory Alterations by Drug/Disease States[a]

Drugs/Disease	Mechanism	TT_4	RT_3U	FT_4/FT_4I	TT_3	^{131}I Uptake	TSH	Comments
Estrogens, oral contraceptives, pregnancy, heroin, methadone, clofibrate, acute and chronic active hepatitis, familial ↑ TBG.	↑ serum TBG concentrations	↑	↓	No change	↑	No change	No change	FT_4/FT_4I corrects for TBG alterations, TSH indicates true thyroid status
Glucocorticoids (stress dosages)	↓ serum TBG concentrations, ↓ TSH secretion, ↓ T_4 to T_3 conversion	↓	↑	↓	↓	Slight ↓	↓	Evaluate thyroid status after steroids are stopped.
Androgens, anabolic steroids, danazol, L-asparaginase, nephrotic syndrome, cirrhosis, familial ↓TBG.	↓ serum TBG concentrations	↓	↑	No change	↓	No change	No change	FT_4/FT_4I corrects TBG alterations; TSH indicates true thyroid status
Phenytoin in vitro, high dose heparin, furosemide, salicylates (level > 15 mg/100 mL), phenylbutazone, fenoclofenac, halofenate, mitotane, chloral hydrate, 5-fluorouracil	Displacement of T_4 and T_3 from TBG	↓	↑ or little to no change	No change	↓	No change	No change	FT_4/FT_4I corrects for TBG alterations; TSH indicates true thyroid status.

Drug/Condition	Mechanism						Comment
Iodide-containing compounds, contrast media, providone-iodine, kelp, tincture of iodine, saturated solution potassium iodide (SSKI), Lugol's solution	Dilution of total body iodide pools	No change if test not interfered by ioide (i.e., radioimmunoassay)	No change	No change	→	No change	No change in thyroid status
Strong diuresis by furosemide, ethacrynic acid; iodine deficiency	Decrease total body iodide pools	No change	No change	No change	Might be ↑	No change	No change in thyroid status
Phenytoin, carbamazepine, rifampin, phenobarbital	Hepatic enzyme inducer of T_4 metabolism	↑ or no change	↓ or normal	No change	No change	No change in euthyroid patients not on T_4 replacement	No change in thyroid status
Propranolol, old age, fasting, malnutrition, acute and chronic systemic illness (e.g., euthyroid sick syndrome)	Impair peripheral conversion of T_4 to T_3; ↑ rT_3	Normal or →	Normal or →	Usually low	No change	No change	Thyroid replacement not necessary
Dopamine, levodopa, high dose glucocorticoids, bromocriptine	Dopamine suppresses TSH secretion	No change	No change	No change	No change	↓ TSH secretion	Not enough to interfere with diagnosis of hyperthyroidism
Amiodarone, iopodate, iopanoate	Impair pituitary and peripheral conversion of T_4 to T_3	↑	↑	↓	→	Transient ↑	Thyroid abnormalities transient, should be normal within 3 months. Can cause thyroid dysfunction in predisposed patients.

[a]See Table 17.1 for abbreviations.

Euthyroid Sick Syndrome

Many acute and chronic nonthyroid disorders (e.g., starvation, acute depression and other psychiatric disorders, acute infection, chronic cardiac, pulmonary, renal, hepatic, and neoplastic disorders, and AIDS) are associated with impaired peripheral conversion of T_4 to T_3, causing abnormal and confusing thyroid function tests in euthyroid individuals (2). This euthyroid sick syndrome, most common in hospitalized patient, requires appropriate recognition to avoid dangerous and unnecessary hormone replacement. Abnormalities in thyroid function tests vary, but often include a low TT_4, TT_3, a low calculated free T_4 and T_3 index, normal or elevated FT_4, and usually, a normal or slightly elevated TSH <10 mIU/L [10 µU/mL]). The slight elevations in TSH concentrations tend to be transient and indicate a recovery phase. Less frequently, hyperthyroxinemia (e.g., psychiatric illness) occurs. An abnormal binding inhibitor in the sera of sick patients probably accounts for some of the abnormal alterations. Reversal of the abnormal thyroid function test is a good prognostic indicator of recovery and decreased mortality. Thyroid hormone supplementation is dangerous, unnecessary, and might impair normal recovery of thyroid homeostasis (2).

HYPERTHYROIDISM/THYROTOXICOSIS

Symptoms

Hyperthyroidism or thyrotoxicosis is a syndrome caused by excessive production of thyroid hormone and characterized by increased metabolism of all body systems. The clinical symptoms (listed in Table 17.3) reflect increased adrenergic activity, primarily cardiovascular and neurologic. Not all manifestations are present in the same patient. Exogenous ingestion of sympathomimetics or agents with sympathomimeticlike activity will accentuate the hyperthyroid symptoms and should be avoided during active disease.

Thyrotoxicosis-induced increases in heart rate (HR), stroke volume (SV), and cardiac output can cause new-onset or worsening angina, atrial fibrillation, extrasystoles, or congestive heart failure (high output), which are usually resistant to conventional treatment until euthyroidism occurs. Clinically, a rapid bounding pulse, an elevated systolic blood pressure, a wide pulse pressure, cardiomegaly, and a systolic murmur are seen. Tachycardia, increased voltage, and a prolonged P-R interval are seen on an electrocardiogram (ECG). It is important to eliminate thyrotoxicosis as causing or exacerbating the cardiac disease, especially in the elderly, because definitive pharmacologic therapy (i.e., digitalis) is altered (see "Drug Kinetics and Thyroid Function").

Occasionally, a severely toxic patient may have none of the classic hyperthyroid symptoms. This apathetic or masked hyperthyroidism is typical of the elderly patient. Presenting symptoms of fatigue, apathy, listlessness, dull eyes, extreme weakness, congestive heart failure, delayed speech and mentation, and low-grade fever are confusing and obscure the diagnosis. Likewise, premature atrial contractions, atrial fibrillation, or tremor might be the only clue to occult hyperthyroidism in the elderly. Untreated,

Table 17.3.
Signs and Symptoms of Hyperthyroidism and Hypothyroidism

Body System	Hyperthyroidism	Hypothyroidism
General	Heat intolerance; weight loss despite increased appetite; increased sweating; weight gain due to increased appetite.	Cold intolerance; weight gain despite decreased appetite; hoarseness and lowering of the voice pitch; decreased sweating, easy fatigability
Head	Thinning of the hair; fine texture	Dry, brittle, and sparse hair; thinning of the lateral aspects of the eyebrows; puffy facies, large tongue
Eyes	Prominence of the eyes, lid lag, lid retraction, can proceed to loss of visual acuity	Edematous eyelids; ptosis
Neck	Soft diffusely enlarged goiter with or without bruits/thrills	Goiter in primary hypothyrodism; none found in pituitary disorders
Cardiac	Palpitations; high output failure; edema; increased pulse and systolic pressure; wide pulse pressure; presence of systolic murmurs	Cardiac enlargement; poor heart sounds; precordial pain; low output failure; dyspnea
Gastrointestinal	Diarrhea, loose bowels, or hyperdefecation	Constipation
Genitourinary	Amenorrhea or decreased in length of menstrual flow	Menorrhagia, dysmenorrhea
Extremities	Pretibial myxedema; Plummer's nails; hot, flushed and moist skin, palmar erythema	Broad hands and feet, pretibial myxedema; cold and dry skin; brittle nails, yellowish
Neuromuscular	Fatigue, weakness, tremor, rapid deep tendon reflexes	Muscle pain and weakness, paresthesias; delayed deep tendon reflexes
Emotional	Nervousness, irritability, emotional liability; insomnia or shortened sleep cycles	Emotional instability, depression, lethargy, decreased energy and increased sleep requirements; mental sluggishness

Table 17.4.
Etiology of Hyperthyroidism

Graves' disease	Toxic diffuse goiter
Toxic nodules	Single and multinodular
Jod-Basedow disease	Iodine induced
Factitious	Self-administration
Tumors	Secretion of thyroid-stimulating substance
Subacute thyroiditis	Viral inflammatory condition
Hashitoxicosis	Early phase of Hashimoto's disease
T_3-toxicosis	Often precedes onset of T_4-toxicosis

Table 17.5.
Characteristics of Graves' Disease

Hyperthyroidism, goiter, and ophthalmopathy/dermopathy
Positive family history
Females > Males
Elevated FT_4 or FT_4I, T_4, T_3
Suppressed/Undetectable TSH level
Positive ATgA, AMA, TRab
Unknown duration of disease

coma and death are assured. Therefore, the onset of any new or worsening cardiac, neurologic, or "failure-to-thrive" symptoms in the elderly require an evaluation for underlying thyroid disease. Occult thyrotoxicosis is easily confirmed by standard laboratory tests.

Etiology

Thyrotoxicosis has many causes. The primary causes of hyperthyroidism are listed in Table 17.4. Rarely, thyrotoxicosis occurs from thyrotropin-secreting pituitary tumors, from ectopic thyroid tissue (e.g., struma ovarii), from TSH-like substances produced by hydatidiform moles and choriocarcinomas, from self-administration of thyroid (factitious hyperthyroidism), from posttraumatic or radiation injury to the thyroid, and from the initial transient stages of Hashimoto's thyroiditis (Hashitoxicosis).

Graves' Disease

Graves' disease, the most common cause of hyperthyroidism, is characterized by the triad of hyperthyroidism, a diffusely enlarged goiter, and infiltrative ophthalmopathy or dermopathy. Not all of these finding are required for the diagnosis. The diagnosis of Graves' disease is easily made by finding abnormally high levels of FT_4, an undetectable TSH, and positive antibodies (i.e., ATgA and AMA), which occur in 80% of patients with classic symptoms of hyperthyroidism and a diffuse goiter (see Table 17.5). An elevated TT_3 and positive TRab can provide additional confirmatory information in patients with atypical presentations. The RAIU is elevated, and a diffusely enlarged "hot" gland is seen on scan.

The etiology of the disease is unknown. It is predominantly a disease of females (5:1 ratio), with its peak onset occurring between the ages of 30 to 40. It has a strong familial predisposition, although the mode of genetic transmission is unknown. Precipitation of the disease has been reported after trauma, severe emotional stress, weight reduction involving strict diet restriction, stimulants, thyroid hormone, and administration of iodides (Jod-Basedow) (3).

Graves' disease, like Hashimoto's thyroiditis, appears to have an autoimmune basis related to disorders of regula-

tory suppressor T lymphocytes. The major subsets of T lymphocytes are helper and suppressor T lymphocytes. Normally, helper T lymphocytes interact with B lymphocytes to produce appropriate immunoglobulins, while suppressor T lymphocytes exercise immunologic surveillance by preventing T lymphocytes from inappropriately producing immunoglobulins. In Graves' disease, a defect in suppressor T lymphocytes may be responsible for the formation of the abnormal thyroid receptor IgG immunoglobulin (TRab) found in the blood of patients with active disease (4). The presence of lymphocytic infiltration of the thyroid gland, IgG immunoglobulins, and antibodies directed against both thyroglobulin and microsomal tissue strongly support an autoimmune basis for Graves' disease.

The thyroid gland in Graves' disease is usually diffusely enlarged and symmetrical, with a firm and rubbery consistency. Thrills and bruits, indicating high blood flow, might be present in a goiter of a severely toxic individual. A thrill, which is less common, is likely to be felt in the region of the superior thyroid arteries. Bruits are usually audible over the entire thyroid gland. Both will disappear in euthyroidism.

OPHTHALMOPATHY

The ocular manifestations include the noninfiltrative and the characteristic infiltrative ophthalmopathy of Graves' disease (5, 6). The noninfiltrative ocular abnormalities result from hyperactivity of the sympathetic system and can be found in any hyperthyroid condition. Increased sympathetic tone on Muller's superior palpebral muscle causes spasm and retraction of the upper lid, widening the palpebral fissure to give the characteristic stare or frightened expression. On physical examination, lid lag is present when the eyelid movement lags behind eye movement and a narrow white rim of sclera becomes visible between the upper lid and the cornea. These ocular changes can cause symptoms of grittiness, dryness, tearing, itching, redness, and photophobia, which improve with normalization of the hormone levels.

The infiltrative ocular findings are the most striking abnormalities of Graves' disease. Mild eye symptoms are found in 50% of patients; the most severe forms occur in less than 5%. Smokers have higher levels of TRab antibodies and present with more severe and progressive ophthalmopathy than nonsmokers. Various degrees of the following signs and symptoms occur:

1. Edema and swelling of the lids and periorbital tissue, causing chemosis, excessive tearing, photophobia, and conjunctivitis.
2. Proptosis (protrusion of the cornea more than the normal 18 to 20 mm beyond the lateral margin of the orbit) occurs from an increase in the orbital contents. This often produces a wide-eyed staring expression. The globes are firmer and harder than normal. Increased tearing and irritation may occur from the exposed conjunctiva. Cornea scarring and ulceration can occur if the proptosis causes the lid to remain open, exposing and drying out the eye during sleep.
3. Limitation of extraocular eye movements from paralysis of the extraocular muscles, causing loss of upward gaze and loss of convergence to occur. Diplopia may result.
4. Blindness might occur from venous congestion and hemorrhage of the retina and optic nerve.

These infiltrative symptoms can appear before, during, or even years after successful therapy of the hyperthyroidism. The ocular involvement can be unilateral or bilateral, and might not reverse with euthyroidism. The most severe forms are often encountered in patients who are euthyroid or hypothyroid after radioactive iodine ablation. Because worsening of the eye signs can occur abruptly after RAI therapy, prophylaxis with systemic corticosteroids is recommended, particularly in patients who have mild symptoms before RAI therapy (5, 6). It is not known why the eyes and associated muscles are attacked while other organ systems are spared. Histologic examination reveals lymphocytic infiltration and deposition of mucopolysaccharides, fat, and water in all retrobulbar tissues.

DERMOPATHY

The dermopathy of Graves' disease, also known as pretibial myxedema, can occur with the infiltrative ophthalmopathy. Mucopolysaccharide infiltration of the skin causes the cutaneous thickening and hyperpigmentation (orange-peel skin) usually seen over the tibial aspects of the leg. Similar lesions can appear on the dorsa of the feet and hands. Pretibial myxedema is usually asymptomatic, but can be painful or pruritic. Like the infiltrative ocular symptoms, pretibial myxedema can occur at any time in the course of the disease. If necessary, the clinical diagnosis can be confirmed by tissue biopsy. Treatment with topical corticosteroids and plastic wrap is often effective.

Toxic/Multinodular Disease

Toxic nodule (Plummer's disease) is characterized by a single autonomous hyperfunctioning nodule in an otherwise normal gland. The nodule, usually 3 to 5 cm in diameter, is not under TSH regulation and can produce normal or supraphysiologic amounts of thyroid hormone,

causing suppression of existing normal thyroid tissue. Patients can either be euthyroid or toxic. A "hot" nodule appears on the scan as an area of increased iodine concentration, but the rest of the thyroid may not be visible if it is suppressed by the nodule. A toxic nodule is the least common of the three major causes of hyperthyroidism.

Multinodular goiter (multiple nodules) is a common thyroid disorder. New-onset hyperthyroidism in patients in their fifth or sixth decade of life usually results from toxic multinodular goiters. These patients often have a history of a large, firm, multinodular goiter without any symptoms of hypothyroidism or hyperthyroidism for many years. However, many of the nodules function autonomously and activate to produce toxicity in later years, especially if given an iodine load (e.g., iodinated contrast media). This is the most common cause of hyperthyroidism in the elderly patient.

Subacute Thyroiditis

Subacute thyroiditis (deQuervain's thyroiditis) is a spontaneous, remitting, inflammatory thyroid condition that is believed to have a viral cause. Clinical features include the acute onset of diffuse or localized swelling of the gland causing tenderness or pain with swallowing, a recent history of flulike symptoms, fever, malaise, and symptoms of hyper- or hypothyroidism. Laboratory abnormalities include an elevated erythrocyte sedimentation rate (ESR), a low or undetectable RAIU, leukocytosis, and changes in thyroid hormone levels. Elevations in FT_4 levels and clinical hyperthyroidism occur from leakage of hormones and iodoproteins from the inflamed gland in the early stages of the disease. Hypothyroidism occurs if long-standing inflammation of the gland prevents further hormone synthesis after the initial hormone stores are depleted.

The disease is self-limiting, and spontaneous recovery is common. Treatment is symptomatic and consists of heat, rest, analgesics (e.g., nonsteroidals), and β-blockers, if necessary, to control the symptoms of hyperthyroidism. Thioamides are not effective because hormone leakage from the gland rather than increased hormone synthesis causes the elevated hormone levels. Corticosteroids are indicated for severe inflammation if analgesics are ineffective. In the hypothyroid phase, transient thyroid replacement might be necessary to suppress further TSH stimulation to the damaged gland and treat symptoms of hypothyroidism.

T_3-Toxicosis

T_3 thyrotoxicosis is characterized by normal levels of T_4 and elevated levels of T_3. T_3 toxicosis is seen in Graves' disease, toxic goiters, and carcinomas, and is reported in children. Preferential T_3 secretion, producing toxicity, is more prevalent in iodine-deficient areas. Elevated T_3 levels often precede the onset of frank T_4 toxicosis after withdrawal of antithyroid medications in patients with Graves' disease. Therefore, the T_3 level is a good monitoring parameter for relapse in these patients.

Drug-Induced Thyrotoxicosis

Iodine-induced thyrotoxicosis (Jod-Basedow) was first described in the 1800s in residents of iodine-deficient areas who became symptomatic after adequate iodine supplementation. Most cases occurred in patients with multinodular goiters and autonomous functioning nodules that were activated by the increased iodine supplements. Iodides do not cause the underlying thyroid disease; they produce thyrotoxicosis in abnormal thyroid glands that have lost the protective Wolff-Chaikoff block. Hyperthyroidism has also been reported following injections of radiocontrast material or iodinated topical preparations (3).

Paradoxically, lithium is also associated with the development of hyperthyroidism (7). Since lithium acts like iodides in preventing hormone release, lithium is probably suppressing frank hyperthyroidism that became evident after its withdrawal. Lithium has thus been advocated in the treatment of hyperthyroidism if other options are not feasible.

Amiodarone, which contains 37.2% iodine by weight, is implicated in numerous reports of hyperthyroidism (8). The prevalence ranges from 1 to 5% and is more common in areas of endemic iodine deficiency. This complication is probably due to its high iodine content and loss of the protective Wolff-Chaikoff effect in predisposed individuals rather than to a direct pharmacologic effect. A thyroiditis might also be contributory. Because euthyroid patients on amiodarone normally have hyperthyroxinemia, actual thyrotoxicosis must be documented with an elevated serum TT_3 level, a suppressed TSH, and clinical symptoms. Worsening of cardiac symptoms requires investigation of amiodarone-induced hyperthyroidism. Typical laboratory findings in euthyroid individuals on amiodarone include an elevated FT_4 or FT_4I, a subnormal T_3, and an initial transient elevated TSH level that returns to normal after 2 to 3 months of amiodarone therapy.

TREATMENT OF HYPERTHYROIDISM

Overview

The major treatment options for the management of hyperthyroidism include thioamides, radioactive iodine (RAI), and surgery (9, 10) (see Table 17.6). Each has its own advantages and limitations, so treatment must be individualized. In most cases, all three treatment options are appropriate and effective. The cause of the hyperthyroidism, its severity, the patient's age, the size of the goiter, and the presence of thyroid and nonthyroid complications, as well as social and economic issues, should be considered in treatment selection. For example, uncomplicated patients with Graves' disease might be managed medically with thioamides until remission occurs. However, elderly patients with toxic multinodular disease are best managed with definitive treatment such as radioactive iodine or surgery because spontaneous remission is unlikely. Likewise, women with Graves' disease who plan on future pregnancies should have their thyrotoxicosis permanently controlled prior to pregnancy with either surgery or radioactive iodine to prevent disease flares and relapse during pregnancy, during delivery, and postpartum (11, 12). If RAI or surgery is selected, most elderly patients and all severely thyrotoxic patients, should be pretreated with thioamides. Pretreatment depletes the gland of stored hormones, reduces the hypermetabolic rate, and prevents leakage of hormone from the gland after RAI or during surgery, preventing thyroid storm. However, the final decision in the uncomplicated patient is often empiric, depending on available resources, the physician's experience, and the patient's personal preference; and it should be a joint patient-physician decision after discussion of the benefits and risks of each method. Interestingly, a survey of practicing thyroidologists also showed considerable variation in the treatment methods selected (13).

Pharmacologic Management

THIOAMIDES

The thioamides, propylthiouracil (PTU) and methimazole, prevent thyroid hormone synthesis by inhibiting the oxidation binding of iodide and its coupling to tyrosine residue. PTU (but not methimazole) inhibits the peripheral deiodination of T_4 to T_3, so serum T_3 levels decline 20 to 30% more rapidly in severely thyrotoxic patients (i.e., thyroid storm). An immunosuppressive mechanism of action is also postulated (9, 10).

Theoretically, thioamides are preferred over radioactive iodine and surgery to treat the uncomplicated hyperthyroid patient because they do not destroy the gland and control the disease until remission might occur. Therefore, chronic thyroid replacement, which is likely with RAI or surgery, might not be necessary. This advantage of thioamides might be irrelevant because the natural history of Graves' disease appears to be eventual hypothyroidism even if no glandular destruction occurs.

Thioamide selection is based largely on the prescriber's personal preference, although certain pharmacologic differences should dictate the choice. Generally, PTU is preferred over methimazole in patients with thyroid storm or those with severe hyperthyroidism because it blocks the peripheral conversion of T_4 to T_3 and therefore has faster onset. PTU is also the thioamide of choice in pregnancy and in the lactating mother (see "Pregnancy"). Although

Table 17.6.
Management of Hyperthyroidism

Method	Drug	Dose	Mechanism of Action	Toxicity	Comments
Thioamides	Prophylthiouracil (PTU) 50-mg tablets; can be formulated for rectal administration	100–200 mg every 6 hr initially, maintenance of 50–150 mg daily	Blocks organification of hormone synthesis, also inhibits peripheral conversion of T_4 to T_3; immunosuppressive?	Skin rashes, agranulocytosis, gastrointestinal symptoms, hepatitis	Poor remission rate of 20–30%; onset of action approximately 2–4 weeks; DOC in pregnancy and during lactation
	Methimazole (Tapazole) 5- and 10-mg tablets; can be formulated for rectal administration	30–40 mg once daily initially, maintenance of 5–10 mg daily	Blocks organification of hormone synthesis; immunosuppressive?	See PTU; secreted in breast milk; might be tetratogenic (e.g., scalp defects)	DOC for once daily dosing; Appears to have little cross sensitivity to PTU for maculopapular rashes
Iodides	Lugol's solution 8 mg iodide/drop: Saturated solution of potassium iodide (SSKI) 50 mg/drop; IV potassium iodide available	6 mg iodide/day, although larger dosages are given; see surgery for iodide dosages	Blocks hormone release; decreases gland vascularity and increases gland firmness to facilitate surgical removal	Hypersensitivity reactions—rashes, rhinorrhea, parotid and submaxillary swelling	Provides symptomatic relief before onset of thioamides; use in thyroid storm and as a preoperative adjunct; *do not use before RAI*
Adrenergic antagonist	Propranolol (Inderal) Metoprolol (Lopressor) Atenolol (Tenormin) Various tablet strengths; IV propranolol 1 mg/mL; Avoid β-blocker with ISA activity	Propranolol 20–40 mg orally every 6 hr or equivalent β-blocker	Blocks the peripheral action of thyroid hormone, no effect on disease state. Blocks peripheral T_4 to T_3 conversion	Bradycardia, congestive heart failure, asthma, inhibits hyperglycemic response to hypoglycemia	Provides rapid symptomatic relief while awaiting activity of thioamides, RAI, or surgery
	Dilitazem (Cardizem) 30-, 60-, 90-, 120-mg tablets; sustained release tablets might not be as effective	60 mg p.o. q.i.d. or 120 mg t.i.d.	Blocks the peripheral action of thyroid hormone, no effect on disease state	Hypotension, bradycardia, pedal edema	Alternative to patients unable to tolerate β-blockers (e.g, asthma, IDDM)
Radioactive Iodine	^{131}I	80 to 150 μCi/g thyroid tissue; usual dose of 8 to 10 mCi	Destructon of the gland	Hypothyroidism, fear of malignancy, leukemia, and genetic damage	Slow onset of action, approximately 2–4 weeks, full effects seen within 3–4 months
Surgery	Iodides, thioamides or β-blockers preoperatively to prevent storm and facilitate surgery	5–10 drops/day of iodides for 10–14 days before surgery; see β-blockers and thioamides dosing	Removal of the gland; total thyroidectomy might be surgery of choice	Hypothyroidism, hypoparathyroidism, complications of surgery and anesthesia	Incidence of hypothyroidism indirectly proportional to gland remnant left
Iodinated contrast media	Ipodate, Iopanoic acid	500 mg–1 g p.o. q.d. or 3g q 3rd day p.o.	Blocks T_4 to T_3 conversion; release of iodides. See iodides	Similar to iodides	Rapid onset of action; adjunct to thioamides, not for chronic use because effects not sustained

PTU is more commonly prescribed, methimazole is preferable because it can be given as a single daily dose that improves patient acceptance and compliance; is more potent and requires fewer tablets; is cheaper; is better tolerated; and at low doses is less toxic than PTU (9, 14). Therefore, methimazole is the thioamide of choice except in those identified situations where PTU is preferable and in patients unable to tolerate PTU.

Biopharmaceutics

Although methimazole is 10 times more potent than PTU (100 mg of PTU = 10 mg of methimazole), they are equally effective if given in equipotent doses. Both drugs are absorbed rapidly from the gastrointestinal tract, and peak plasma concentrations are reached within 30 minutes of ingestion. The serum half-lives of 4 to 6 hours for methimazole and 1 to 2 hours for PTU do not change as the thyroid status changes. However, the duration of action and frequency of dosing depends on the intrathyroid half-life and not on the short plasma half-lives. The duration of action of methimazole is 24 to 36 hours, allowing once-daily administration (15). The intrathyroid duration of PTU is much shorter, requiring dosing every 6 to 8 hours to be effective.

Dosage Regimens

Initial therapy should begin either with 30 to 40 mg/day orally of methimazole, given as a single daily dose, or in three divided doses to limit gastrointestinal intolerance, or 400 to 600 mg/day of PTU, given in three to four divided doses (9, 10). Although initial single-dose regimens have been used successfully with PTU, the best results are obtained by achieving euthyroidism by multiple dosing, then changing to a maintenance single-dose regimens. Severely toxic or "storm" patients may require dosages as high as 1200 mg/day of PTU or its equivalent, given in divided doses. There are no intravenous preparations, although both drugs can be formulated for rectal administration (16, 17). Once the patient is euthyroid, usually after 4 to 8 weeks (dependent on elimination of existing thyroid stores; $t_{1/2} = 7$ days), the initial dosage can be reduced gradually by one third on a monthly basis until a daily maintenance dose of 5 to 10 mg of methimazole or 50 to 100 mg/day of PTU is reached. Tapering should not start until symptoms are reduced and thyroxine levels are normal. If symptoms do not resolve within the specified time, then patient noncompliance, incomplete blockage of synthesis by insufficient dosage, or an inadequate dosing interval should be considered as causes of failure. A change to methimazole is indicated if PTU was the initial drug because drug failure secondary to noncompliance is more likely to occur with PTU than with methimazole.

A baseline FT_4 or FT_4I, TSH, and white blood cell count (WBC) with differential should be obtained before starting thioamides. A baseline WBC with differential can help ascertain the development of thioamide-induced agranulocytosis because hyperthyroidism per se can be associated with a relative reduction in the neutrophil count. The above thyroid function tests should normalize within 6 to 8 weeks after starting therapy and parallel the clinical response. The FT_4 or FT_4I and TSH should be monitored a minimum of 6 to 8 weeks after the onset of therapy and after any change in the dosing regimen. Once a stable thioamide maintenance dose is reached, thyroid function tests can be routinely monitored every 3 to 6 months.

Duration of Therapy

The duration of thioamide therapy for Graves' disease is empiric, generally 12 to 18 months. Shorter courses of 3 to 6 months have been advocated, but they yielded remission rates of 20 to 40% (18). Several studies suggest that the remission rate might increase with the duration of therapy (19, 20). An 18-month treatment period yielded higher remission rates (61.8%) than therapy for 6 months (41.7%). A study in children noted a 25% increase in the remission rate when the duration was increased by 1 year (21). Therefore, a minimum treatment duration of 12 months is recommended to increase the remission rate. Longer treatment durations can be used if there are no adverse effects and the patient prefers antithyroid therapy over RAI or surgery. Hyperthyroid patients on thioamides can be managed effectively by the pharmacist using a treatment algorithm (see Fig. 17.2).

Prognosis

Disappointing remission rates of 15 to 80% after discontinuation of thioamide therapy has led to progressive disenchantment with the antithyroid drugs as definitive therapy for Graves' disease. Permanent remission is rare except in patients who have concomitant autoimmune thyroiditis. It is unclear why some patients remain in remission while others relapse. No factors have been consistently predictive of successful long-term remission, and most studies have produced conflicting results. Factors associated with poor remission rates have included increased dietary intake of iodides, severe hyperthyroidism, a large goiter that does not regress with thioamide therapy, short duration of thioamide therapy, persistent high titers of TRab after stopping thioamides, recurrent hyperthyroidism, and presence of HLA antigen (10, 19–21).

The best remission rates occur when low or absent TRab titers are reported after therapy. Besides extending the duration of thioamide therapy more than 1 year (as discussed above), high-dose thioamides, and the concomitant administration of thyroxine with thioamides are associated with favorable remission rates. High thioamide blocking doses (i.e., 600 to 800 mg of PTU or 40 to 60 mg of methimazole) given throughout therapy produced better remission rates (75.4%) than conventional therapy (41.6%) but produced greater toxicity (22). Some clinicians advocate the concomitant use of exogenous thyroxine during antithyroid therapy to prevent hypothyroidism and suppress goiter formation from excessive PTU or methimazole administration. However, proper dosing of thioamides should alleviate this problem so concomitant thyroxine therapy has only been recommended when proper titration is difficult. However, recent data suggests that the addition of thyroxine to antithyroid therapy might improve the remission rate by suppressing TSH receptor antibody titers. The recurrence rate was 1.7% in Japanese patients

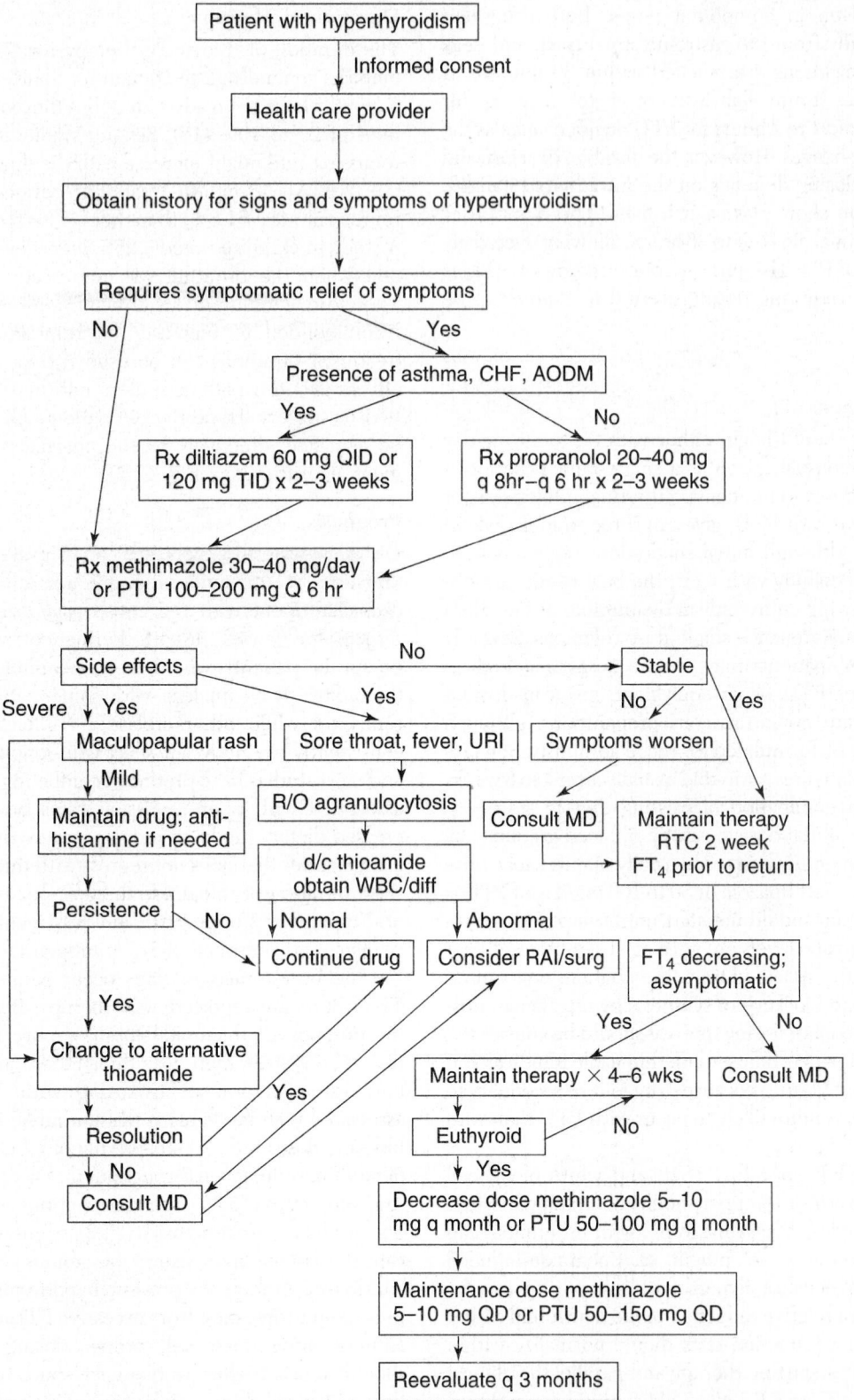

Figure 17.2.   Treatment algorithm for management of hyperthyroidism.

who became euthyroid on methimazole for 6 months, followed by the combination of thyroxine and methimazole for a year, and then thyroxine alone for 3 years, compared with 34.7% in those not given thyroxine (23).

Several factors might indicate a better chance of remission and justify a longer trial of thioamide administration. The best predictor for remission is a reduction in goiter size to normal size during therapy. Patients with small goiters, with mild and short duration of symptoms and illness, and with disappearance of TRab during therapy also have a better chance of remission (10, 19–21). Analysis of HLA specificities (HLA-B8 and DW3) in conjunction with IgG immunoglobulin levels may be highly predictive of remission or relapse after withdrawal of thioamides.

ADVERSE REACTIONS

Toxic reactions to PTU and methimazole occur in 1 to 5% of patients (9, 10). A pruritic maculopapular skin rash, without other systemic manifestations, is the most frequently encountered adverse reaction. Therefore, all patients should be instructed to report symptoms of skin reactions. In ectopic individuals it is also important to distinguish a thioamide rash from a heat rash or hives caused by the hyperthyroidism. In mild cases, the rash might disappear spontaneously despite continued therapy. Antihistamines can provide symptomatic relief of the pruritus. If the rash persists, the alternative thioamide can be substituted because little cross-sensitivity exists. However, if the rash is associated with systemic symptoms (i.e., fever, arthralgias) or if angioneurotic edema, hives, or other anaphylactoid reactions occur, substitution with another thioamide is not recommended because the risks of cross-sensitivity are high.

Hepatitis is more common than previously recognized (22, 24). Approximately 30% of patients on PTU can have asymptomatic elevations in liver transaminases that do not require stopping the drug because they normalize within 3 months when PTU is reduced to maintenance dosages. However, PTU should be immediately stopped in patients with clinical evidence of hepatitis to ensure complete recovery. Hepatocellular and obstructive hepatitis have been reported from both agents; however, hepatocellular damage is most prevalent with PTU and obstructive jaundice with dosages above 40 mg daily of methimazole. Circulating autoantibodies and in vitro peripheral lymphocyte sensitization to PTU indicate a possible autoimmune etiology. These idiosyncratic reactions typically occur during the initial phases of therapy, although delayed reactions have been noted. It is reversible if detected early, although fatalities have been reported. Because of the severity of the reaction and potential for cross-sensitivity, substitution with the alternative thioamide is not recommended. Routine monitoring of liver function tests should be considered in patients with a history of liver disease and risk factors for hepatitis (e.g., alcohol). All patients should be instructed about the symptoms of hepatitis, about avoidance of alcohol, and to immediately report any symptoms of hepatitis to their health care professional.

Rarely, hypoprothrombinemia (PTU), serologic abnormalities (lupus erythematosus [LE], antinuclear antibody [ANA]), lupus, and lupuslike syndromes have also been reported. Recovery occurs after withdrawal of the drug or institution of steroids.

Agranulocytosis (<500 PMNs) is the most serious (but infrequent) adverse reaction to the thioamides. The prevalence is between 0.5 to 6% (9, 10). The onset of fever above 101°F, malaise, gingivitis, and sore throat is so abrupt that routine WBC counts are not usually recommended. Although one study suggests that weekly monitoring of the WBC with differential during the first 3 months of therapy might identify patients with early and asymptomatic agranulocytosis, routine monitoring is not indicated because it might hamper patient compliance and does not appear to be cost-effective (25). All patients should be instructed to immediately report the onset of such symptoms to a health care provider. Older patients (age > 40 years) and those on high-dose methimazole (more than 40 mg/day) therapy appear to be at greater risk for developing this toxic reaction, although it is not necessarily dose related. Low doses (<30 mg/d) of methimazole might be safer than any dose of PTU. Sex is not a predictive factor. This reaction is more likely to occur during the first 6 weeks of therapy, although it can occur at any time in the course of treatment. One study suggests that agranulocytosis might occur earlier with PTU therapy (i.e., 17.7 ± 9.7 days) than with methimazole therapy (36.9 ± 14.5 days) (25). Fortunately, complete resolution of symptoms and recovery of granulocytes is often seen within a few days to 3 weeks after stopping the thioamides. Granulocyte colony-stimulating factors and corticosteroids might shorten the recovery period. If infection occurs, antibiotics, adrenal steroids, and possibly hospitalization (bacteria-free room) are indicated. Rechallenge with the same drug or an alternative thioamide is not recommended because the risk of recurrent agranulocytosis outweighs the benefits of therapy. The degree of cross-sensitivity is not known.

MONOVALENT ANIONS

Potassium perchlorate is the only monovalent anion with sufficient antithyroid activity to be clinically useful. In dosages of 500 mg to 1 g/day, perchlorate is concentrated by the gland where it interferes with iodide binding and causes the discharge of nonorganified iodide from the gland. Because perchlorate is a competitive inhibitor of iodide, it can be used to manage amiodarone or iodide-induced hyperthyroidism, but its antithyroid effect can be overcome by iodine administration. The severe toxicity of irreversible aplastic anemia and nephrotic syndrome has limited the usefulness of the monovalent anions.

IODIDES

Although iodides have been known to relieve the symptoms of thyrotoxicosis since the 1920s, their clinical use has largely been superseded by the thioamides and the β-blockers. Iodides act by several mechanisms of action: inhibiting organification ("Wolff-Chaikoff" effect), inhibiting hormone release, and decreasing vascularity of the gland (3, 9, 10). The rapid relief of thyrotoxic symptoms after 2 to 7 days of iodide administration suggests that inhibition of hormone release is the predominant mechanism of action; a block in organification would not become apparent for several weeks. This rapid response is advantageous for patients in thyroid storm and for those awaiting the onset of thioamide therapy. However, iodides should not be used before RAI therapy (or if RAI might be considered as possible treatment) because iodides can block effective RAI retention by the gland for several weeks after use.

Iodides are routinely given 10 to 14 days before surgery to decrease the vascularity and increase the firmness of the hyperplastic gland which facilitates surgical removal. Preoperatively, the combination of β-blockers and iodides can also be used, although the established regimen of thioamides and iodides is preferable.

Stable iodine is available as either Lugol's solution (5% iodine and 10% potassium iodide), containing 8 mg of iodide per drop, or as the more palatable saturated solution of potassium iodide (SSKI), containing 50 mg/drop. A parental preparation, potassium iodide, is also available (see Table 17.6).

The major adverse effects of iodides are hypersensitivity reactions, including rashes, drug fever, sialoadenitis, conjunctivitis, rhinitis, and collagen vascular disorders. In individuals with underlying thyroid disorders, iodides can produce hyperthyroidism (e.g., multinodular goiter) from failure of the Wolff-Chaikoff block or cause goiter and hypothyroidism (e.g., Hashimoto's thyroiditis) in patients unable to escape from the Wolff-Chaikoff block (3).

Advantages of iodide therapy include simplicity, low cost, low toxicity, and no gland destruction. Limitations of treatment include "escape," treatment relapse, allergic reactions, and interference with subsequent RAI therapy.

LITHIUM

Lithium, which acts like iodides in inhibiting hormone release, has been recommended in doses of 800 to 1200 mg/day for the treatment of thyrotoxicosis (7). Lithium serum levels must be maintained within therapeutic levels to avoid side effects of tremor, ataxia, dizziness, confusion, coma, nausea, vomiting, diarrhea, cardiac arrhythmias, and circulatory collapse. Hyponatremia or sodium depletion from diuretics can potentiate lithium toxicity and should be avoided. Lithium should not be considered a first line agent, but should be reserved for special situations when thioamides, iodides, and β-blockers are contraindicated.

ADRENERGIC ANTAGONISTS

Because many of the signs and symptoms of thyrotoxicosis are mediated through the sympathetic nervous system, drugs that deplete or block the effects of thyroid hormones on tissue catecholamines can provide rapid symptomatic relief before thioamides, RAI, or surgery do. These agents do not affect the underlying disease process, so they should not be used as primary therapy.

Propranolol is the β-blocker most widely used and studied in the treatment of hyperthyroidism, and therefore is the standard against which others are judged (26). When propranolol is given orally in doses of 20 to 40 mg 3 to 4 times a day as necessary, symptomatic relief of palpitations, tachycardia, anxiety, sweating, tremor, and diarrhea occur. Weight loss, however, remains unaffected. Severely toxic patients might require as much as 240 to 480 mg/day to achieve symptomatic relief and maintain the heart rate below 100 beats/min. Propranolol is also surprisingly effective in controlling the neuromuscular manifestations of hyperthyroidism, especially periodic paralysis. It can be used as an adjunct to thioamides and RAI during therapy of neonatal thyrotoxicosis, pregnancy, or thyroid storm, and as a preoperative medication prior to surgery. Although β-blockers have been used successfully as sole agents preoperatively, they are not recommended in the severely toxic patient because inadequate control of severe thyrotoxicosis has resulted in storm. All the selective and nonselective β-blockers (e.g., naldolol, atenolol, metoprolol) appear equally effective in the symptomatic relief of hyperthyroidism. β-Blockers with intrinsic sympathomimetic activity (e.g., pindolol) are not recommended because they do not reduce the heart rate as much as β-blockers without ISA activity.

The kinetics and blood levels of propranolol in toxic patients are subject to large interindividual variation (26). This is attributed to a significant first pass effect seen with oral doses, altered hepatic function in hyperthyroidism, and the presence of an active metabolite, 4-hydroxypropranolol. The clearance of propranolol in thyrotoxicosis might be increased as much as 50% because of enhanced liver blood flow and increased activity of drug-metabolizing enzymes. Because of the increased volume of distribution, the elimination half-life is unchanged. Although the lower propranolol levels reported in hyperthyroidism might be due to individual variations, data suggest that higher propranolol doses are necessary acutely in toxic patients because of the increased clearance rate. Similarly, larger doses of metoprolol are needed because of hyperthyroidism-increased hepatic clearance. The converse is true in hypothyroidism. The clearance of β-blockers such as atenolol and nadolol that are excreted renally is unaltered in hyperthyroidism, and patients can be dosed once daily to improve compliance.

The calcium-channel blockers, particularly diltiazem, might be a useful alternative when β-blockers are contraindicated (e.g., in patients with asthma, congestive heart failure (CHF), or insulin-dependent diabetes). Diltiazem (120 mg t.i.d. or 60 mg q.i.d. orally) is well tolerated and appears to be as effective as propranolol in suppressing the symptoms of thyrotoxicosis (27). However, verapamil has produced detrimental effects in thyrotoxicosis. The potential synergistic benefits of calcium-channel blockers and β-blockers in the management of thyrotoxicosis are unknown.

RADIOACTIVE IODINE (RAI)

Radioactive iodine therapy is indicated for hyperthyroidism in patients past adolescence, those with a history of prior thyroid surgery, those who are poor surgical risks because of complicating nonthyroid illness, those with Graves' ophthalmopathy, and those who fail or experience thioamide toxicity (9, 10). RAI is absolutely contraindicated in pregnancy because the RAI crosses the placenta and destroys the fetal thyroid. It is also the treatment of choice in elderly patients with cardiac disease and in those with toxic multinodular goiters.

^{131}I, which has a half-life of 8 days and delivers high-energy β radiation to a maximal depth of 2 mm, is the isotope commonly used. ^{125}I, which has less tissue penetration and a half-life of 60 days, has not resulted in the lower incidence of hypothyroidism that was initially hoped for. Because ^{125}I emits γ-rays that penetrate only a few microns, larger therapeutic doses are required, which considerably increases the total body radiation without altering the incidence of hypothyroidism.

The dosage of RAI administered is calculated with a formula that incorporates an estimate of the gland size, the uptake of iodine at 24 hours, and the standard microcurie of iodine given per gram of thyroid tissue. At the University of California, patients receive approximately 80 to 150 microcuries per gram of thyroid tissue. Despite the formula, the proper dosage (i.e., one that prevents both recurrent hyperthyroidism and subsequent hypothyroidism) is difficult to calculate or predict.

Millicuries (mCi) of ^{131}I =

$$\frac{\text{estimated gland weight (g)} \times 80{-}150\ \mu\text{Ci/g} \times 100}{\text{24-hour RAI (\%)}}$$

Pretreatment with either thioamides (for approximately 1 month to deplete the gland of stored hormones) or with β-blockers before and after RAI therapy is necessary to prevent exacerbations of thyrotoxicosis in the elderly, in patients with severe heart disease, or in those

with large intraglandular stores of hormones (10). Iodides should not be used before RAI therapy because ^{131}I uptake and efficacy will be significantly impaired for several months. Thioamides should be discontinued 1 week before and after RAI therapy to facilitate optimal ^{131}I uptake and retention. β-Blockers and calcium-channel blockers can be used without compromising RAI therapy.

Resolution of the hyperthyroidism is slow after RAI treatment. Improvement of symptoms might be apparent by 3 to 6 weeks after RAI; however, maximum effects do not occur until 3 to 4 months after an ablative dose. Because of this delayed onset, iodides, ipodate, thioamides, or β-blockers might be necessary for symptomatic control after RAI is given. If a second dose is required, a larger dosage of RAI must be given to optimize gland uptake, exposing the body to greater radiation.

The lowest appropriate age limit for radioactive iodine therapy is controversial. After more than 25 years of extensive clinical experience, RAI is generally accepted as safe for most adult patients under 35 years of age (9, 10). Adolescents have also been safely treated with RAI, although it is not recommended in this age group.

The major concerns about RAI therapy include carcinogenesis, leukemia, and genetic damage. So far, none of these hazards is documented and surveillance is ongoing (9, 10). The radiation dose to the gonads in patients treated with ^{131}I for hyperthyroidism is generally less than 3 rads, which is not significantly different from gonadal irradiation received from commonly used diagnostic tests such as barium enemas or pyelograms. The major complication of RAI is hypothyroidism, which is most common the first year after therapy, and increases at a constant rate of 2.5% a year thereafter, accounting for a 20-year prevalence of 30 to 70%. Immediate side effects of ^{131}I therapy are minimal and might include mild thyroid pain and tenderness, temporary thinning of the hair, and (rarely) dysphagia. Exacerbation of Graves' ophthalmopathy can occur after RAI therapy and prophylactic systemic corticosteroids should be considered in patients with mild eye symptoms (5, 6, 9, 10). Generally, RAI therapy is effective, quick, easy, painless, and relatively nontoxic.

IODINATED CONTRAST MEDIA

An unlabeled use for iodinated contrast dye (e.g., ipodate, iopanoic acid) is in the acute management of hyperthyroidism (9, 28). When ipodate is administered in a daily dose of 500 mg to 1 gram orally or 3 grams every third day to thyrotoxic patients, dramatic improvement in both subjective and objective symptoms parallels the rapid fall in thyroid hormone levels. The changes in serum T_4, serum T_3, and reverse T_3 (rT_3) levels are consistent with the inhibition of the peripheral deiodination of T_4 to T_3. Reductions in serum T_3 levels occur within 6 hours of ipodate administration, declining to 50% of baseline at 24 hours and 70% of baseline (nadir) at 48 hours. T_3 levels remained suppressed for 3 to 5 days after a single administration. Similarly, T_4 levels reached their nadir 3 days after administration and remained depressed for as long as 6 days after the last dose. When compared with propylthiouracil, ipodate produced earlier symptomatic and objective improvement and more rapid declines in T_3 hormone levels. The prolonged suppression of T_3 and T_4 levels suggests that inhibition of hormone secretion, caused by the iodine released, might be an additional ipodate mechanism of action. Although similar inhibition of peripheral T_3 production is seen with most iodinated contrast media, such as iopanoic acid (Telepaque), ipodate (Oragrafin), which contains 61.4% iodine, is the most potent.

Because ipodate is relatively nontoxic, it provides a useful addition to the acute treatment of thyrotoxicosis. Ipodate is recommended as an adjunct to thioamides in the severely toxic or "storm" patient and as an alternative in patients allergic to thioamides. It may also be an effective preoperative preparation in lieu of iodides, but experience is very limited. Another potential use is in patients who may eventually be treated with radioactive iodine therapy because ipodate does not appear to interfere with RAI retention as much as iodides. These agents are not indicated for chronic therapy because the reductions in hormone levels seen within the first month of therapy are not sustained in most hyperthyroid patients (9, 28).

SURGERY

Thyroidectomy is an effective method of therapy for patients in whom RAI or thioamides are contraindicated; for those with large goiters, causing cosmetic disfigurement, respiratory embarrassment, or swallowing difficulties; for those with suspected malignancies; and for selected pregnant and pediatric patients (9, 29). Prior thyroid surgery should be considered a strong deterrent to further surgery because reoperation increases the hazard of vocal cord paralysis and hypoparathyroidism, 10-fold and 30-fold, respectively. Other poor surgical candidates are patients with severe cardiac, respiratory, or debilitating diseases and patients in the third trimester of pregnancy, because spontaneous labor can be precipitated.

The ideal surgical endpoint is a 3- to 8-g remnant of thyroid tissue, left after surgery that produces neither a recurrence of the thyrotoxicosis nor hypothyroidism (29). The risk of recurrent thyrotoxicosis is directly proportional to the amount of thyroid remnant left. Increasing the remnant gland size by 1 gram decreases the risk of postoperative hypothyroidism by 10%; conversely, increasing the remnant size above 10 grams increases the risk of recurrent disease without changing the risk of hypothyroidism. Although euthyroidism might not always be feasible, one series reported a 94% euthyroid success rate

using a modified subtotal thyroidectomy. A subtotal thyroidectomy is the most popular form of surgery performed for hyperthyroidism because it offers the best chance of euthyroidism. Others advocate a total thyroidectomy, despite the risk of hypothyroidism, to prevent recurrence of the hyperthyroidism. Surgery appears to be as safe as nonsurgical treatments for hyperthyroidism if it is performed by experienced hands on patients adequately prepared by the standard combination of thioamides, iodides, or β-blockers. In adequately prepared patients, operative mortality and development of thyroid storm is low. Vocal cord paralysis and permanent hypoparathyroidism occurs in fewer than 1% of patients after a subtotal thyroidectomy. Because of the catastrophic nature of these complications, only surgeons experienced in thyroid surgery should perform such operations.

The major complication is hypothyroidism, which occurs in the first 6 months to 3 years postoperatively, but can develop insidiously as late as 10 years postoperatively. Prevalences of 5 to 75% are reported. The prevalence of hypothyroidism is inversely proportional to the remnant of thyroid tissue left; remnants of 2 to 4 grams result in an prevalence of 70%.

The disadvantages of surgery include expense, need for hospitalization, risks of anesthesia, postoperative complications, and the patient's fear of surgery. These disadvantages may outweigh the advantages of rapid definitive surgical intervention.

SPECIAL TREATMENT CONSIDERATIONS
Pregnancy

The combination of pregnancy and thyrotoxicosis is a rare occurrence (0.02 to 1.4% of the pregnant population) because most hyperthyroid patients are relatively infertile. Usually the thyrotoxicosis and treatment antedate the pregnancy. Nevertheless, because management of hyperthyroidism during pregnancy is difficult, pregnancy is best postponed until the hyperthyroidism is permanently controlled. Hyperthyroidism is difficult to monitor during pregnancy because similar symptoms are common to both conditions. Spontaneous remission of the disease with improvement of symptoms can occur during pregnancy and antithyroid medications are often not necessary (11, 12). This improvement might be related to falls in both the concentrations of thyroid-receptor antibodies (TRab) and titers of thyroid antibodies in pregnancy. However, during delivery, recurrence of hyperthyroidism can be problematic and therapeutically challenging. Untreated maternal thyrotoxicosis can result in abortion, perinatal death, and prematurity, so proper treatment is crucial.

Pregnancy and hyperthyroidism create special management problems because the fetal thyroid, which begins functioning during the 12th to the 14th week, is also at risk.

Radioactive iodine is absolutely contraindicated because transplacental passage of ^{131}I will destroy the fetal thyroid. Chronic iodide administration should also be avoided, because ingestion of as little as 12 mg of iodine throughout pregnancy has caused fetal goiter and asphyxiation. Vaginal povidone or topical iodine can produce high serum concentrations of iodine and should also be avoided (3).

Surgery can be performed safely in the second trimester after suitable preparation with thioamides or short-term administration of iodides or β-blockers. During the last trimester, surgery is not recommended because of the risk of precipitating spontaneous abortion.

Thioamides, which cross the placenta, can be used throughout pregnancy if certain precautions are followed. PTU, and not methimazole, is generally considered the drug of choice in pregnancy because maternal use of methimazole is associated with congenital skin defects (e.g., aplasia cutis) (10–12). However, some have concluded that the association between methimazole and congenital skin defects is not sufficiently supported to preclude the use of these drugs during pregnancy (30). If no other therapeutic options are available, one must balance the dangers of untreated maternal hyperthyroidism against the risks of methimazole toxicity. The dangers of fetal goiter and hypothyroidism are reduced if initial doses of PTU are maintained below 300 mg/day (given in divided doses) and maintenance doses of 50 to 100 mg/day are used throughout pregnancy (10–12). Clinically, the mother should be maintained in a comfortable, mildly hyperthyroid state with the FT$_4$I or FT$_4$D in the upper ranges to prevent fetal thyroid suppression. The appearance of an enlarged maternal goiter during therapy is alarming because it implies the development of maternal and fetal hypothyroidism. The concomitant use of thyroid hormone is not helpful, because thyroid does not cross the placenta, and might make maternal management more difficult.

Fortunately, the intellectual development of offspring exposed to antithyroid drugs in utero appears to be the same as that of siblings not exposed (31). PTU is also preferred over methimazole in the breast-feeding mother because insignificant amounts of PTU are excreted in the milk, whereas 7 to 16% of a methimazole dose is detected in breast milk (11, 12).

Propranolol or another β-blocker is a reasonable short-term adjunct to PTU during pregnancy. Chronic administration of β-blockers should be avoided during pregnancy, particularly in the last trimester, because of the risk of fetal respiratory depression, small placenta, intrauterine growth retardation, impaired responses to anoxic stress, and postnatal bradycardia and hypoglycemia. Propranolol is also excreted in breast milk and should be avoided during lactation. Such findings indicate that propranolol, like iodides, should be used only on a short-term basis in pregnancy.

Exophthalmos/Ophthalmologic Complications

Because the pathogenesis and progression of the ophthalmopathy are not well understood, treatment of the ocular complaints is often symptomatic until euthyroidism occurs.

The preferred therapy of hyperthyroidism in patients with Graves' exophthalmos is controversial. Some clinicians (our preference) favor thyroid ablation with either RAI or surgery to remove the antigen source (i.e., gland) and believe that this method is more effective than thioamides to prevent progression of the ophthalmopathy. However, progression of ocular symptoms has been reported in patients receiving all types of treatment (5, 6). Mild eye symptoms can worsen after RAI therapy, and systemic corticosteroids are recommended after RAI therapy to prevent further progression of the ocular involvement. Hypothyroidism can also aggravate preexisting eye complaints. Regardless of the method of treatment selected, control of the hyperthyroidism and hypothyroidism is essential to prevent deterioration of the ophthalmopathy.

Periorbital edema and chemosis (inflammation of the conjunctiva) respond to elevation of the head of the bed to promote diuresis. Protective glasses, methylcellulose and hydrocortisone drops, and avoidance of smoke and dust might alleviate photophobia and external irritation. With patients whose eyes do not completely close while sleeping, taping the eyelids shut at night is necessary to prevent corneal scarring and drying.

Systemic corticosteroids are indicated for progressive inflammatory exophthalmos and decreasing visual acuity. Prednisone, 60 to 120 mg/day administered in divided doses for 1 to 3 weeks, often produces dramatic resolution of inflammatory eye symptoms. When symptoms resolve, the dose can be tapered over 2 weeks and then gradually withdrawn. In addition to their antiinflammatory action, corticosteroids suppress TRab levels and decrease T$_3$ levels by impairing the peripheral conversion of T$_4$ to T$_3$. Immunosuppressive agents, such as cyclophosphamide and azathioprine, have not been as effective as steroids (5, 6). External orbital radiation therapy, which achieves similar results, can be used in patients with contraindications to steroids. After euthyroidism is achieved, and the eye symptoms are stable, lid or orbital surgery can provide cosmetic or visual corrections.

Atrial Fibrillation

Hyperthyroidism can cause new-onset or worsening atrial fibrillation and congestive heart failure, so routine thyroid function tests should be obtained in all patients presenting with these symptoms. The atrial fibrillation is often difficult to control until euthyroidism occurs. A combination of medications, including β- and calcium-channel blockers, as well as large dosages of digoxin (due to alterations in digoxin kinetics—see "Drug Kinetics and Thyroid Function") might be required to slow the heart rate. Anticoagulation with coumadin is recommended in those with valvular disease and heart failure because of the high incidence of systemic emboli (9). Smaller dosages of coumadin are needed for anticoagulation in hyperthyroidism (see "Drug Kinetics and Thyroid Function"). The dosages of digoxin and warfarin must be adjusted as euthyroidism occurs, to prevent toxicity and maintain maximal therapeutic effects. Spontaneous conversion to normal sinus rhythm after achieving euthyroidism is less likely in patients with underlying heart disease or if the duration of the atrial fibrillation persists after 4 months of euthyroidism.

Neonatal Thyrotoxicosis

Neonatal thyrotoxicosis results from stimulation of the fetal thyroid by transplacental passage of thyroid receptor stimulating antibodies from the maternal circulation. The infants are extremely ill and require supportive measures, including sedation, cooling, oxygen, fluid, and electrolyte replacement, in addition to management of the hyperthyroidism by thioamides, iodides, or β-blockers. Fortunately, the disease is self-limiting and symptoms disappear in 1 to 2 months as the levels of TRab decline. Antithyroid drugs should be withdrawn at this time. High levels of maternal Trab help to predict the risk of neonatal thyrotoxicosis, and Trab should be monitored in all pregnant females with a history of Graves' disease.

Pediatrics

Hyperthyroidism in children is rare, accounting for about 1 to 5% of cases. It is unusual in the first 5 years of life; the peak incidence occurs between the ages of 10 and 12 years. Similarities to the adult form include a preponderance of females over males and a positive history of acute infection, trauma, and stress before the onset of the disease. The signs and symptoms are similar to those seen in the adult (i.e., nervousness, weight loss, tremor, eye signs) but with the notable exception of cardiovascular manifestations. Excessive thirst, behavioral manifestations of restlessness, and inability to concentrate incur difficulties in school and in family relationships, and might be the initial presenting symptoms.

Optimal management of the disease in children is controversial, although all three methods: surgery, RAI, and thioamides have been used (32). Radioactive iodine is usually not recommended because of the high risk of hypothyroidism and the fear of genetic damage, leukemia, and carcinogenesis, although these are unsubstantiated (9, 10). External radiation to the head and neck of children is associated with a high risk of subsequent thyroid carcinoma and dysfunction, although similar results have not been shown with internal RAI radiation (32).

The usual treatment choices include the thioamides and subtotal thyroidectomy. The risks of surgery (mortality, scarring, recurrence of thyrotoxicosis, hypothyroidism, and laryngeal and parathyroid damage) must be weighed against the benefits of speedy correction of the thyrotoxicosis and the lack of need for compliance to the rigid dosing schedules of the thioamides.

Dosage regimens for thioamides in children are similar to those used in adults. Thioamides are the treatment of choice in patients with small goiters and mild disease where a high remission rate is likely. The limitations of medical management include noncompliance, strict parental and physician supervision, the low remission success rates, and the risks of adverse reaction. The advantages of treatment include the potential for remission without damage to the gland. The appropriate method will depend on the circumstances and individuals involved.

Thyroid Storm

Thyroid storm is a medical emergency characterized by (a) acute onset of high fever (sine qua non); (b) cardiovascular symptoms: tachycardia, tachypnea, shock, congestive heart failure, and arrhythmia; (c) gastrointestinal symptoms: diarrhea, vomiting, abdominal pain, and liver enlargement; and (d) central nervous system involvement: agitation and psychosis progressing to apathy, stupor, and coma (33).

The pathogenesis of storm is not well understood but appears to be an exaggerated form of thyrotoxicosis. Storm can be precipitated by childbirth, stress, infection, trauma, diabetic acidosis, inadequate preparation before RAI or surgery, and noncompliance with antithyroid medication.

Prompt recognition and immediate treatment can decrease the 100% mortality rate to 7% or better. Treatment is directed at five major areas:

1. Support of vital functions with sedation, oxygen, fluids, antipyretics, treatment of infection, correction of electrolyte abnormalities, and the routine use of corticosteroids (hydrocortisone 100 to 200 mg i.v. every 6 hours) for unsuspected hypoadrenalism. Peripheral conversion to T_3 is also reduced by corticosteroids.
2. Use of thioamides and iodides to block synthesis and release of hormones. Preferably, large dosages of PTU (200 to 300 mg every 6 hr [600 to 1200 mg/day]) or of methimazole (10 to 20 mg every 6 hr) should be given. Theoretically, iodides should be given 1 hour after thioamide administration to not interfere with the latter's effect and prevent iodizing existing hormone stores, which will aggravate existing storm. Iodides (e.g., Lugol's solution 30 to 60 drops p.o. daily or potassium iodide 1 to 2 g i.v. daily) and the combination of thioamides often control symptoms within 1 day. Lithium can be given in doses of 500 to 1500 mg/day if iodides are contraindicated but offers no advantages over iodides.
3. Blockage of the metabolic effects is accomplished by propranolol (20 to 80 mg p.o. every 6 hr or 0.5 to 2 mg i.v. every 4 hr) or diltiazem (60 to 120 mg p.o. t.i.d.–q.i.d)

4. Eliminate and correct precipitating factors.
5. Remove circulating hormone by plasmapheresis, exchange transfusion, and dialysis when routine measures fail.

HYPOTHYROIDISM

Hypothyroidism or myxedema is a syndrome caused by a deficiency of thyroid hormone and characterized by a slowing down of all body systems. Thyroid hormone stimulates oxygen consumption and is essential for normal growth, maturation, and regulation of all organ systems.

Etiology

Primary hypothyroidism, a disorder of the gland, can be classified as either nongoitrous (no goiter) or goitrous. Goitrous forms include Hashimoto's thyroiditis, drug-induced, dyshormonogenesis, endemic, and multinodular goiters. Nongoitrous forms include cretinism (congenital hypothyroidism), iatrogenic, idiopathic atrophy, and secondary hypothyroidism, either of pituitary or hypothalamic origin.

A goiter (enlargement of the thyroid) should be considered an abnormal finding. Goiters result from TSH stimulation, usually in response to low levels of circulating hormone. However, some patients with a goiter can be euthyroid because the increased TSH secretion causing the goiter also is capable of transiently maintaining normal hormone levels.

SECONDARY HYPOTHYROIDISM

Secondary hypothyroidism can be of either pituitary or hypothalamic cause. Hypothalamic hypothyroidism, caused by inadequate secretion of thyrotropin-releasing factor (TRF), is rare. Low or normal levels of TSH despite abnormally low levels of circulating free thyroid hormones suggest a pituitary cause for the hypothyroidism, such as postpartum hemorrhage (Sheehan's), head injury, pituitary tumors, or idiopathic atrophy of the hypophysis. Concomitant disorders of the adrenals and gonads (Simmond's disease or panhypopituitarism) may also occur. Primary, pituitary, and hypothalamic hypothyroidism can be distinguished by the TRF and TSH tests.

IATROGENIC

Iatrogenic hypothyroidism, caused by radioactive iodine or surgery, is common. Virtually all patients receiving radioactive iodine and about 50 to 75% of patients undergoing total thyroidectomies will develop hypothyroidism (29). Therefore, all patients with a prior history of RAI or surgery should be routinely monitored for development of hypothyroidism.

IDIOPATHIC ATROPHY

Idiopathic atrophy of the thyroid and destruction of the gland represent the end stages of Hashimoto's thyroiditis.

Antibodies, representing a destructive immune process, are frequently found.

CRETINISM (CONGENITAL HYPOTHYROIDISM)

Congenital nongoitrous hypothyroidism, produced by a deficiency of thyroid hormone in utero or in the neonate, may result from defective hormone synthesis, from pituitary or hypothalamic dysfunction, and from incomplete growth of the gland (agenesis). Ectopic thyroid tissue, destruction of the gland by maternal autoantibodies, and destruction by RAI therapy are other possible causes of agenesis. Neonatal goitrous hypothyroidism has been reported after maternal ingestion of iodides and thioamide therapy (12).

The clinical presentation of congenital hypothyroidism depends on the severity of the hypothyroidism, the age of onset, and the cause of the thyroid deficiency. Early recognition of congenital hypothyroidism is now possible by mandatory determination of cord TSH levels at time of delivery. This is extremely important because the clinical symptoms are so subtle that early recognition does not occur until the child is older and irreversible damage results. The earliest manifestations are a heavy expression, a piglike appearance of the eyes, hypothermia, prolonged jaundice, umbilical hernia, hoarseness, thick tongue, protuberant abdomen, constipation, and drooling. Delayed developmental characteristics, failure to thrive, poor appetite, and cretinoid facies might not be recognized until the infant is 3 to 6 months old, when neurologic damage is irreversible (34). Growth retardation, delayed physical development, and hypothyroid symptoms similar to those seen in a adult are of concern. Radiologic evidence of epiphyseal dysgenesis is pathognomonic of neonatal hypothyroidism.

ENDEMIC HYPOTHYROIDISM

Endemic goiter is a descriptive term for thyroid enlargement caused by iodine deficiency during the growth years. Females are affected more often than males, as occurs with other thyroidal disorders. The amount of dietary iodine deficiency determines the degree of nodularity and gland enlargement. Patients may be clinically and chemically euthyroid or hypothyroid. Nevertheless, thyroxine suppression therapy is often indicated to prevent further gland enlargement. Laboratory findings might include a normal or low FT_4D or FT_4I, and a normal or elevated TSH level.

DYSHORMONOGENESIS

Dyshormonogenesis refers to a specific group of familial thyroid disorders resulting from abnormalities in the synthesis, delivery, or peripheral action of thyroid hormones. Impaired hormone synthesis can occur from defects in iodine accumulation, from iodide organification resulting from dehalogenase deficiency, and from a cou-

Table 17.7.
Drug-induced Thyroid Disease

Drug	Mechanism	Drug-Induced Thyroid Effect	Comments
Nitroprusside	Metabolized to thiocyanate, an anion inhibitor	Goiter, hypothyroidism	Increased risk with renal failure and duration of use
Lithium	Inhibits hormone release	Goiter, hypothyroidism; can also cause hyperthyroidism	Usually in patients with untreated thyroid disease (e.g., Hashimoto's thyroiditis)
Iodides and iodine containing compounds (e.g., amiodarone, ipodate; iodinated contrast media)	Inability to escape from Wolff-Chaikoff block	Hypothyroidism, goiter	Usually in patients with untreated Hashimoto's thyroiditis or Graves' disease previously treated with RAI or surgery
	Provides substrate to iodide-deficient autonomous thyroid tissue; loss of Wolff-Chaikoff block	Hyperthyroidism	Usually in patients with multinodular goiters and autonomous nodules (Jod-Basedow disease)
Sulfonylureas, sulfonamides, PAS, resorcinol, phenylbutazone	Inhibits organic binding and organification	Hypothyroidism, goiter	Rare cause of thyroid disease
Immunotherapy (e.g., interferon α, interleukin-2)	Autoimmune process	Hypothyroidism > hyperthyroidism	Generally transient, resolves without treatment
Natural goitrogens cabbage, etc.	Contains thiocyanate and other goitrogens	Hypothyroidism, goiter	Rare, need large consumption of raw vegetables

pling abnormality. Patients with impaired thyroglobulin synthesis, release of abnormal iodopeptides, and peripheral tissue resistance to thyroid have also been described.

Because specific tests are not available, diagnosis depends on elimination of other goitrous causes of hypothyroidism. Diagnostic laboratory abnormalities include low or normal circulating free hormone levels, increased TSH, and absence of antibodies. If necessary, an organification defect in hormone synthesis can be detected by the potassium perchlorate discharge test.

DRUG INDUCED

Goiters can result from the use of certain drugs with antithyroid activity (see Table 17.7). The thioamides and monovalent anions used therapeutically in the treatment of hyperthyroidism can produce goiter if excessive doses are used (goitrogenic).

Iodides and iodide-containing compounds (e.g., povidone iodine, amiodarone, iodinated contrast media) can produce hypothyroidism and goiter in patients with unrecognized thyroid disorders (3, 8). Each 200-mg tablet of amiodarone contains 75 mg of organic iodide. The prevalence of amiodarone-induced hypothyroidism has been reported to range from a low of 1.0% to a high of 9.8% (8). These patients are inordinately sensitive to iodides and unable to normally "escape" from the "Wolff-Chaikoff" block to resume hormone synthesis. High-risk patients include those with cystic fibrosis, untreated Hashimoto's thyroiditis, and Graves' disease previously treated with RAI

or surgery. Older patients and those on long-term amiodarone also appear to be at greater risk of amiodarone-induced hypothyroidism. Unfortunately, the goiter or hypothyroidism may not always be reversible after discontinuation of the iodides or amiodarone. Thyroxine can be given concurrently, if necessary, to treat the hypothyroidism and goiter.

Lithium can also produce hypothyroidism and goiter in up to 10% of patients (7). Although patients without known risk factors can develop lithium-induced hypothyroidism, susceptible patients have a positive family history of thyroid illness, positive thyroid antibodies, abnormal gland findings, and undiagnosed underlying thyroid illness. Lithium's antithyroid effect is similar to that of the iodides and was first demonstrated in patients with bipolar disorder as a side effect of lithium therapy. The onset of a nontender, diffuse goiter with or without hypothyroidism is variable and may appear after 5 months to 2 years of treatment. Discontinuation of lithium does not always cause regression of the goiter and hypothyroidism. However, the goiter and hypothyroidism are responsive to thyroxine therapy, so lithium therapy can be continued if necessary.

Thiocyanate is a well-known inhibitor of iodide trapping, particularly if high blood concentrations are present. Thiocyanate-induced hypothyroidism can occur from long-term use of nitroprusside in patients with renal insufficiency. Plants, such as rutabagas, cabbage, and turnips, contain thioglucosides, which are metabolized in the body to thiocyanates. These dietary goitrogens do not produce any significant degree of hypothyroidism unless large amounts are ingested raw over a long time period.

MULTINODULAR GOITER

Multinodular goiter describes an enlarged thyroid gland containing many hypofunctioning or "cold" and autonomously functioning "hot" nodules. It is a common disorder, affecting women more than men, and occurs in about 5% of all adults beyond age 30. The possibility of malignancy must be eliminated, especially if a history of irradiation is present. Otherwise, cold nodules in a multinodular goiter are rarely malignant. The pathogenesis is not well understood, but is related to iodide deficiency, dietary goitrogens, and enzymatic defects. Clinically, patients can be euthyroid but often develop hyper- or hypothyroidism in later years. Pressure symptoms or a "choking" sensation from compression of the trachea or esophagus, respectively, by the enlarged gland is an indication for surgical removal. Otherwise, thyroxine therapy might be tried to decrease and prevent further growth of the gland. However, therapy usually does not shrink the gland back to normal size. A clinically euthyroid patient with a suppressed TSH should be the goal of therapy.

HASHIMOTO'S THYROIDITIS

Hashimoto's thyroiditis, the most common cause of goiter and/or hypothyroidism, is similar to Graves' disease in prevalence (3–6/10,000/year). Like other thyroid disorders, it is 15 to 20 times more common in females than males and has a strong familial predisposition. Its peak occurrence is in the middle years, although any age group is at risk. It is commonly characterized by diffuse enlargement and lymphocytic infiltration of the gland, an immunologic disturbance, and hypothyroidism. Hashimoto's thyroiditis is a graded disease with many different clinical presentations. Patients can present with thyrotoxicosis in the early stages, (Hashitoxicosis), euthyroidism and goiter, hypothyroidism and goiter, or hypothyroidism without goiter in the late stages of the disease. Euthyroidism occurs if the gland is able to compensate for the inherent block in hormone synthesis by increasing hormone synthesis in response to TSH stimulation. Asymptomatic thyroiditis, characterized by euthyroidism, absence of goiter, normal levels of circulating hormones, and positive antithyroid antibodies, may precede the clinical manifestations of overt goiter and hypothyroidism.

Pathophysiology

An autoimmune process, resulting from defects in suppressor T lymphocytes, is responsible for Hashimoto's thyroiditis. Antibodies directed against thyroglobulin, a microsomal component, and a colloid component, as well as cell-mediated immunity against thyroid antigens are present. Furthermore, Hashimoto's thyroiditis often coexists with other autoimmune disorders including Graves' disease, rheumatoid arthritis, and other collagen vascular diseases. Pernicious anemia, resulting from gastric antibodies directed against intrinsic factor, can be found in about half of the patients with Hashimoto's disease and vice versa. Some postulate that Graves' and Hashimoto's thyroiditis are actually the same disease at different ends of the spectrum because mild thyrotoxicosis may precede the onset of hyperthyroidism; similarly, hypothyroidism is the end result of Graves' disease.

The Hashimoto's gland is unable to bind iodide effectively and is inordinately sensitive to the antithyroid effects of exogenous iodides. This ineffective utilization of iodides results in the formation and release of inactive nonhormonal iodoproteins into the circulation, causing further increases in TSH secretion and goiter formation. If the gland is able to maintain hormone synthesis in response to TSH stimulation, then euthyroidism is maintained. However, the gland eventually fails to keep up with metabolic demands, resulting in goiter and hypothyroidism. Laboratory findings include a low or normal FT_4D or FT_4I, normal or elevated TSH, and positive antithyroglobulin and antimicrosomal antibodies.

Clinical Features

The classic symptoms of hypothyroidism include weakness, fatigue, lethargy, cold intolerance, constipation, and weight gain (see Table 17.3). An exception is the elderly patient, in whom the diagnosis of hypothyroidism might be missed because the symptoms are nonspecific, atypical, or wrongly attributed to the normal aging process. Marked physical changes include a puffy and masklike facies, edematous eyelids, myxedematous skin changes, especially over the pretibial aspects of the leg, loss of hair from the lateral aspects of the eyebrows, a large tongue, cardiomegaly, and a yellowish tint to the skin. Myxedematous cachexia is characterized by intensification of all hypothyroid signs and symptoms, and often precedes the onset of myxedema coma.

The cardiovascular manifestations of hypothyroidism can mimic or exacerbate preexisting low output congestive heart failure. Angina typically becomes quiescent; rarely, the severity and frequency of attacks increase. Hypothyroidism-increased levels of cholesterol might accelerate atherosclerotic changes, although this is speculative (35). Clinical findings include cardiomegaly caused by loss of muscle tone and mucopolysaccharide deposition, dyspnea, edema, and pleural effusions due to impaired cardiac output, decreased stroke volume, and decreased myocardial contractility. Characteristic EKG changes resembling ischemia are seen: slow rate and low voltage, flattened or inverted T waves, and, occasionally, increased PR interval and widened QRS complex. Although glomerular filtration rate (GFR) and renal plasma flow (RPF) are reduced because of decreased cardiac output and blood volume, overt evidence of renal failure does not occur. In severe myxedema, delayed water excretion leading to edema results from changes in GFR or inappropriate antidiuretic hormone (ADH) secretion.

Course

The onset of naturally occurring hypothyroidism (e.g., Hashimoto's thyroiditis) is a gradual, insidious, and nonspecific process, which may go unnoticed by the patient, or in the elderly be attributed to the normal aging process. It is a slow process that may occur with amazing placidity over several months to years before the appearance of a terminal myxedematous state. In contrast, symptoms occurring from iatrogenic causes (e.g., RAI therapy or surgery) occur rapidly and rarely go unrecognized by the patient.

Laboratory Parameters

Pertinent diagnostic laboratory parameters for primary hypothyroidism include a low FT_4I or FT_4D and an elevated TSH level (see Table 17.1). In secondary hypothyroidism, the TSH can be low or normal. The presence of positive antibodies is indicative of an autoimmune cause. An RAIU is not necessary for diagnosis of hypothyroidism; it is usually decreased but an elevated uptake may be present in the early stages of hypothyroidism. Elevations of serum SGOT, LDH, CPK, cholesterol, and triglycerides occur from delayed metabolism of enzymes.

THYROID PREPARATIONS

All of the commercially available preparations of thyroid hormones are effective (see Table 17.8). However, levothyroxine is considered the replacement hormone of choice (36).

Desiccated thyroid (USP) is usually obtained from hog thyroids, although beef and sheep are also used. Because this preparation is standardized only by iodine content (0.17 to 0.23% iodine), the hormone ratio of T_4 to T_3 may vary from a 2:1 (hog) to 3:1 with beef or sheep. Therefore, variability in potency might result from changes in the ratio of the two hormones or from the quantity of organic iodine present. Desiccated thyroid suffers from problems inherent to all T_3-containing preparations (see T_3 below). Improper or prolonged tablet storage, causing a loss of potency, can also contribute to an unpredictable response. Desiccated thyroid tablets appear to be stable for 5 years or longer if kept dry. Inactive preparations, containing small amounts of T_4 and T_3 or iodinated casein, and tablets containing excessive biologic activity have been reported. Allergic reactions to the protein component might also occur. During therapy, the free thyroxine levels (i.e., FT_4I

or FT_4D), TT_3, and TSH should ideally remain within normal limits; however, thyroid function tests are often abnormal, especially if supraphysiologic levels of T_3 occur (36). For these reasons, desiccated thyroid should be an obsolete preparation. However, because this preparation is inexpensive, therapy might be continued if cost is an issue and the patient is reluctant to change. Otherwise, all patients should be changed to levothyroxine. Although 0.1 mg of L-thyroxine is theoretically equivalent to 1 grain or 60 mg of desiccated thyroid, such equivalents might not be valid if dosage titrations were initially based on inactive desiccated thyroid preparations. In one study, only 60 µg of L-thyroxine was equivalent to desiccated thyroid 1 grain (37). This disparity in equivalence should be especially considered when changing to L-thyroxine in patients requiring more than 2 gr/day of desiccated thyroid. A theoretically equivalent dosage of levothyroxine might not be reasonable (e.g., 3 grains of desiccated thyroid equivalent to 300 µg of levothyroxine) because of subpotent desiccated preparations, and dosage retitration is recommended.

Triiodothyronine or T_3 is a chemically pure agent with predictable potency, excellent bioavailability, and a half-life of 1.5 days. T_3 is not recommended for routine thyroid replacement therapy because of its high cost, the need for multiple daily dosing to ensure a uniform response, its greater potential for cardiotoxicity, and greater difficulty in monitoring therapeutic and toxic responses. Because of its rapid absorption, supraphysiologic levels of T_3 occur after ingestion, producing symptoms of mild toxicity in susceptible individuals (36). Furthermore, T_3 administration does not change pretreatment TT_4, FT_4D, or FT_4I levels, which, if not properly recognized, can cause therapeutic confusion and potential overreplacement despite adequate hormone replacement. T_3 administration is best monitored by TSH and TT_3 levels. T_3 is primarily used as a diagnostic agent in the T_3 suppression test and when short-term hormone replacement therapy is indicated. T_3 is used as short-term replacement therapy in patients, following total thyroidectomy for thyroid cancer, who need repeat scans and RAIU. The thyroid hormones must be completely eliminated prior to the scan. Because T_3 has a short half-life, it is rapidly eliminated after discontinuation, producing a short duration of tolerable hypothyroidism prior to RAIU and scan. Intravenous T_3 has also been recommended as the drug of choice for myxedema coma because of its rapid onset of action in 1 to 3 days. However, its routine use in this condition is limited by concerns about its potentially greater cardiotoxicity. Also, mortality has occurred despite the higher T_3 levels achieved after T_3 administration (33, 38). Approximately 25 to 37.5 µg of T_3 is equivalent to 0.1 mg of L-thyroxine. Patients should not receive T_3 as routine hormone replacement therapy.

L-thyroxine, the most commonly prescribed synthetic thyroid preparation, is the preparation of choice for

Table 17.8.

Thyroid Preparations in Treatment of Hypothyroidism

Preparation[a]	Content	Advantages	Disadvantages	Effect on Thyroid Tests	Comments
Desiccated thyroid USP ¼, ½, 1, 1½, 2, 3, 4, 5 grains	Defatted, dried pig thyroid powder, containing 0.17–.23% iodine	Inexpensive	Poor standardizaton with variable hormonal content and T_4/T_3 ratios; deterioration with storage	Normal FT_4/FT_4I, TSH normal or ↑ TT_3	Potency may vary from batch to batch: problems inherent to all T_3 containing products; see T_3 comments. Thyroxine preferable
Sodium L-thyroxine[a], (Synthroid, Levothroid, Levoxyl, Various) 0.025, 0.05, 0.075, 0.088, 0.1, 0.112, 0.125, 0.137, 0.15, 0.175, 0.2, 0.3 mg Inj 200, 500 µg	Synthetic, pure T_4	Stable, smooth action, relatively inexpensive; long half-life ($t_{1/2} = 7$ days); generics and branded products similar in tablet T_4 content	Slow onset of action, cumulative effects;	Normal thyroid function tests; TSH in normal range	Might be more potent than desiccated thyroid, should lower the T_4 dose by 1/2 gr to avoid toxicity when changing from > 2 gr desiccated thyroid to L-thyroxine
Sodium L-thyronine, (Cytomel) 5, 25, 50 µg Inj 10 µg/mL (Triostat)	Synthetic, pure T_3	Uniform absorption, fast onset of action	Expensive, short half-life (1.5 days); requires multiple daily dosing; difficult to monitor—must use T_3 and TSH levels	Low FT_4, normal or ↑ TT_3, normal TSH	Not DOC for hormone replacement; supraphysiologic T_3 levels can produce toxicity
Liotrix ¼, ½, 1, 2, 3 (Thyrolar)	Contains T_4 and T_3 in a ratio of 4:1 (mimics natural secretion of hormone)	Both short- and long-acting effects	Expensive	Normal thyroid function values	No real need for Liotrix since T_4 is peripherally converted to T_3

[a]Approximate dosage equivalence: 1 grain desiccated thyroid = 0.1 mg L-thyroxine = 37.5 µg L-thyronine = Liotrix-1 (see "Comments" column).

hormone replacement. Its popularity stems from its uniform potency, its relatively low cost, and its lack of foreign protein antigenicity. L-thyroxine is relatively stable but does lose about 6% of its potency per year (39). Its long half-life of 7 days makes it amenable to once-a-day dosing, increasing patient compliance and allowing the creation of various convenient dosing schedules (e.g., daily except weekends). The bioavailability of branded thyroxine preparations is 80%; the bioavailability of generic preparations appears similar (40–42). This should be considered when changing from p.o. to i.v. or i.m. dosing regimens. Previous problems with subpotent tablets have been corrected by the 1985 USP requirement that all levothyroxine preparations must be standardized by HPLC assay for tablet levothyroxine content. Adequate replacement therapy is indicated by normalization of TSH and FT_4D or FT_4I levels. L-thyroxine replacement may produce TT_4 levels in the "hyperthyroid ranges" in about 20% of individuals; however, no adjustment in L-thyroxine dosage is necessary if the TSH levels are normal and the patients are clinically euthyroid. T_3 levels are often within the normal range (36, 41).

Liotrix is a combination of synthetic T_4 and T_3 in a 4:1 ratio that mimics the natural secretion of hormones. It is available commercially as Thyrolar. Because this preparation approximates the normal thyroid production, it was once considered the agent of choice, until it was recognized that a significant amount of T_4 is converted peripherally to T_3. Liotrix is stable, is chemically pure, is of predictable potency, and produces laboratory values similar to those seen after T_4 administration. In Thyrolar-1, 50 µg of T_4 and 12.5 µg of T_3 is equivalent to 1 grain of thyroid. Because of its high cost, problems inherent to all T_3-containing preparations, and lack of therapeutic rationale, there is no advantage or need for administration of Liotrix.

TREATMENT OF HYPOTHYROIDISM

Thyroid Dosage Regimens

The administration of thyroid hormones provides adequate replacement therapy for hypothyroidism and shrinkage of any existing goiter through suppression of TSH production (see Fig. 17.1). The average replacement dose is often quoted as 100 to 200 µg daily of thyroxine, which parallels normal thyroid production. However, such a simplistic approach is inappropriate and dangerous. Dosing requirements depend on a multiplicity of factors that include an evaluation of the patient's age and weight, the severity and cause of the illness, the presence or absence of cardiac disease, and the absorption of the hormone.

The average daily maintenance dose for uncomplicated hypothyroidism is 100 to 150 µg/day of levothyroxine, which correlates with a dose of 1.6 to 1.7 µg/kg or about 0.7 to 0.8 µg/lb (36, 41–42). In the elderly, lower levothyroxine doses, 50–100 µg daily (<1.6 µg/kg/day), might be needed to maintain euthyroidism. Patients with iatrogenic hypothyroidism after RAI or surgery might need lower doses initially compared to those with spontaneous hypothyroidism (36, 43). Malabsorption due to short bowel or the concurrent administration of several drugs (see Table 17.9) can affect the daily thyroxine replacement dose (44).

Patients receiving chronic levothyroxine replacement therapy should be evaluated at yearly intervals to ensure that the current levothyroxine dosage is still warranted. Patients placed on chronic levothyroxine replacement therapy before the availability of more potent products and the advent of the sensitive TSH assay will require a reduction in their original dosage. A reduction in levothy-

roxine dosage is also necessary as the patient ages or if there is significant weight loss. Both the FT_4D or FT_4I and TSH should be optimally maintained within the normal range. Suppression of the TSH into the undetectable ranges should be avoided in replacement therapy to minimize overreplacement and subclinical signs of hyperthyroidism (36, 41, 44). Additionally, supraphysiologic doses may predispose patients to decreased bone density and increase the risk of bone loss and osteoporosis (36, 41, 45).

The initial dose of T_4 administered should depend on the patient's age, on the severity and duration of the hypothyroidism, and on the coexistence of underlying cardiac disease. In young, healthy patients with disease of short duration, levothyroxine can be administered in close-to-full replacement doses (e.g., 100–150 µg daily) without fear of precipitating toxicity. This dose can be adjusted as necessary, using the patient's symptoms and laboratory values obtained at steady state (i.e., after 6 to 8 weeks of therapy). However, in patients with long-standing and severe myxedema, in elderly patients, and in patients with cardiac disease (i.e., angina, CHF) who are likely to be extremely sensitive to the metabolic effects of thyroid hormone, therapy must be instituted cautiously with minute doses of thyroxine to avoid cardiovascular compli-

Table 17.9.
Medications and Conditions Affecting Thyroxine Replacement Dosages

Conditions	Mechanism	Recommendation	Comments
Resin Binders (e.g., Cholestyramine, colestipol)	Binds T_4 in gut, $\downarrow T_4$ absorption	Separate time of administration by 4 to 6 hours	↑ dosage of T_4 might be needed
Aluminum containing preparations (e.g., sulcrafate, aluminum hydroxide antacids)	Binds T_4 in gut, $\downarrow T_4$ absorption	Separating time of administration by 4 to 6 hours might not be effective in avoiding this interaction	Avoid aluminum containing products
Iron Sulfate	Binds T_4 in gut, $\downarrow T_4$ absorption	Separating time of administration by 4 to 6 hours might not be effective in avoiding this interaction	↑ dosage of T_4 might be needed if iron cannot be avoided.
Lovastatin	? Binds T_4 in gut, $\downarrow T_4$ absorption	Change to another lipid lowering agents, monitor TFTs and ↑ dosage if needed.	Interaction not well documented and based on one case report
Enzyme Inducers (i.e., phenytoin, carbamazepine, rifampin, phenobarbital)	↑ metabolism and clearance of thyroxine	↑ dosage of thyroxine to normalize TSH level; free T_4 level might remain low.	Not significant in euthyroid individuals not on thyroxine therapy.
Androgens	↓ levels of TBG; higher free T_4 and lower TSH levels might occur	Might need to ↓ dosage of T_4 by 25–50% to normalize TSH	Not significant in euthyroid individuals not on thyroxine therapy.
Pregnancy	↑ levels of TBG and ↑ thyroxine demands	↑ dosage of T_4 by 20–30% to achieve normal TSH level	Not significant in euthyroid individuals on birth control pills or in postmenopausal hormone replacement.
Age	T_4 clearance ↓ with age	Replacement dosages of less than 1.6–1.7µ/kg/day if age > 60 years old	Monitor TFTs yearly and ↓ with advancing age
Malabsorption (i.e., diarrhea, short bowel syndrome)	↓ T_4 absorption	↑ dosage of thyroxine. Monitor TSH to adjust dosage.	High dosage T_4 therapy might be necessary

cations of heart failure, angina, tachycardia, and myocardial infarction. These complications can occur with subtherapeutic doses, so careful monitoring is critical. Control of any angina should occur before attempting thyroxine therapy (36). If necessary, coronary bypass surgery can be performed in hypothyroid patients, with minor complications. Successful and safe replacement of thyroxine is often achieved after coronary bypass. In the high-risk patient, initial doses should not exceed 12.5 to 25.0 μg of T_4 daily. The patient should be told to report any cardiac symptoms immediately. If well tolerated after 1 week, the dose can be increased by similar increments every 1 or 2 weeks until therapeutic levels are achieved. It is not necessary to monitor thyroid function tests until the patient has achieved a therapeutic dosage for a minimum period of 6 to 8 weeks. Complete euthyroidism might never be achieved in high risk individuals without further compromising the cardiac status. Hypothyroid patients on levothyroxine can be managed effectively by using a treatment algorithm (Fig. 17.3).

T_3 has been recommended as the drug of choice in patients with cardiovascular problems because its effects lapse quickly as a result of its short half-life, (3 to 5 days, as opposed to 7 to 10 days for T_4). However, the greater potential of T_3 for cardiotoxicity outweighs its advantage of rapid elimination, so its use cannot be recommended.

Management of Congenital Hypothyroidism

Normal growth and physical and mental development is determined by the age at which treatment is instituted and by how well euthyroidism is maintained (34, 46, 47). The earlier treatment is started, the better the prognosis for normal mental and growth development. Mean IQ is higher in those who receive treatment before 3 months and achieve a serum thyroxine level of 180 nmol/L (14 μg/dL) than in those who do not. If treatment was delayed until 6 months to 1 year, mental development was impaired despite subsequent treatment. Despite early therapy, neurologic deficits also occurred if replacement was inadequate to increase the serum TT_4 to above 103 mmol/L (8 μg/dL) and suppress the TSH into the normal range after 3 to 4 months of therapy. Dwarfism did not occur if therapy was delayed until 5 years old. Because of late detection, infants born athyrotic may have a poorer prognosis for normal mental development than those born with an abnormal or ectopic thyroid gland.

The preparation of choice for hormone replacement is levothyroxine. Thyroxine tablets can be crushed and mixed with either breast milk or formula; suspensions should not be used because of questionable stability. T_3 can be used, but is not recommended for the reasons outlined above (see "Thyroid Preparations"). The appropriate replacement dose of T_4 depends on the age of the infant and the presence of risk factors (see Table 17.10) (34, 47). Full replacement doses can be started in the uncomplicated

infant without cardiac disease. However, the infant with long-standing and severe myxedema will be extremely sensitive to minute doses of thyroid, necessitating initiation with very small doses of thyroxine to prevent toxicity (i.e., hyperactivity and irritability). In these infants, initial doses of T_4 should not exceed 25 to 33% of the normal recommended dose. If no toxicity occurs after 1 or 2 weeks, doses can be gradually increased by similar increments every 1 or 2 weeks until full replacement doses are achieved or until the dose is limited by toxicity.

The optimal replacement dose is determined by normal physical and mental development and reversal of other hypothyroid signs and symptoms. Adequate replacement is achieved when the serum TT_4 level reaches 154 to 180 mmol/L (12–14 μg/dL) (46–47). Normalization of the TSH should not be used as the sole criterion because the hypothalamic-pituitary system is relatively unresponsive to the negative feedback effect of thyroid hormone, causing TSH to remain elevated for months despite proper or excessive hormone replacement. TSH should normalize within 3 or 4 months after the start of therapy; attempts to normalize TSH earlier may result in overreplacement, producing symptoms of overmetabolism, irritability, brain dysfunction, and premature craniosynostosis.

Special Considerations

PREGNANCY

Maternal myxedema is associated with congenital defects, abnormal fetal development resulting from poor placenta maturation, spontaneous abortions, stillbirths, and mental retardation. However, the exact effect of the maternal thyroid function on the fetus is unclear because normal offspring have been reported in women who remained hypothyroid throughout pregnancy. The greatest dangers to the fetus from inadequate maternal replacement therapy are poor placenta development and poor maintenance of the pregnancy. The most critical period is the first trimester. The fetal thyroid begins functioning by the 12th to 14th week of pregnancy and does not depend on the maternal thyroid hormones, which do not cross the placenta. Approximately 75% of pregnant hypothyroid patients receiving adequate replacement doses before pregnancy need a 20 to 30% increase from their baseline replacement dose during the pregnancy to maintain a normal TSH level (48). Therefore, the FT_4I or FT_4D and TSH should be monitored at least every month for the first 3 months to ensure adequate thyroxine replacement. If hormone replacement therapy is adequate and maternal euthyroidism is achieved, as evidenced by a normal TSH and FT_4I or FT_4D level, a normal pregnancy is likely. TT_4 levels will be elevated because of pregnancy-induced TBG levels. After delivery, the prepregnancy dose of levothyroxine can be reinstituted.

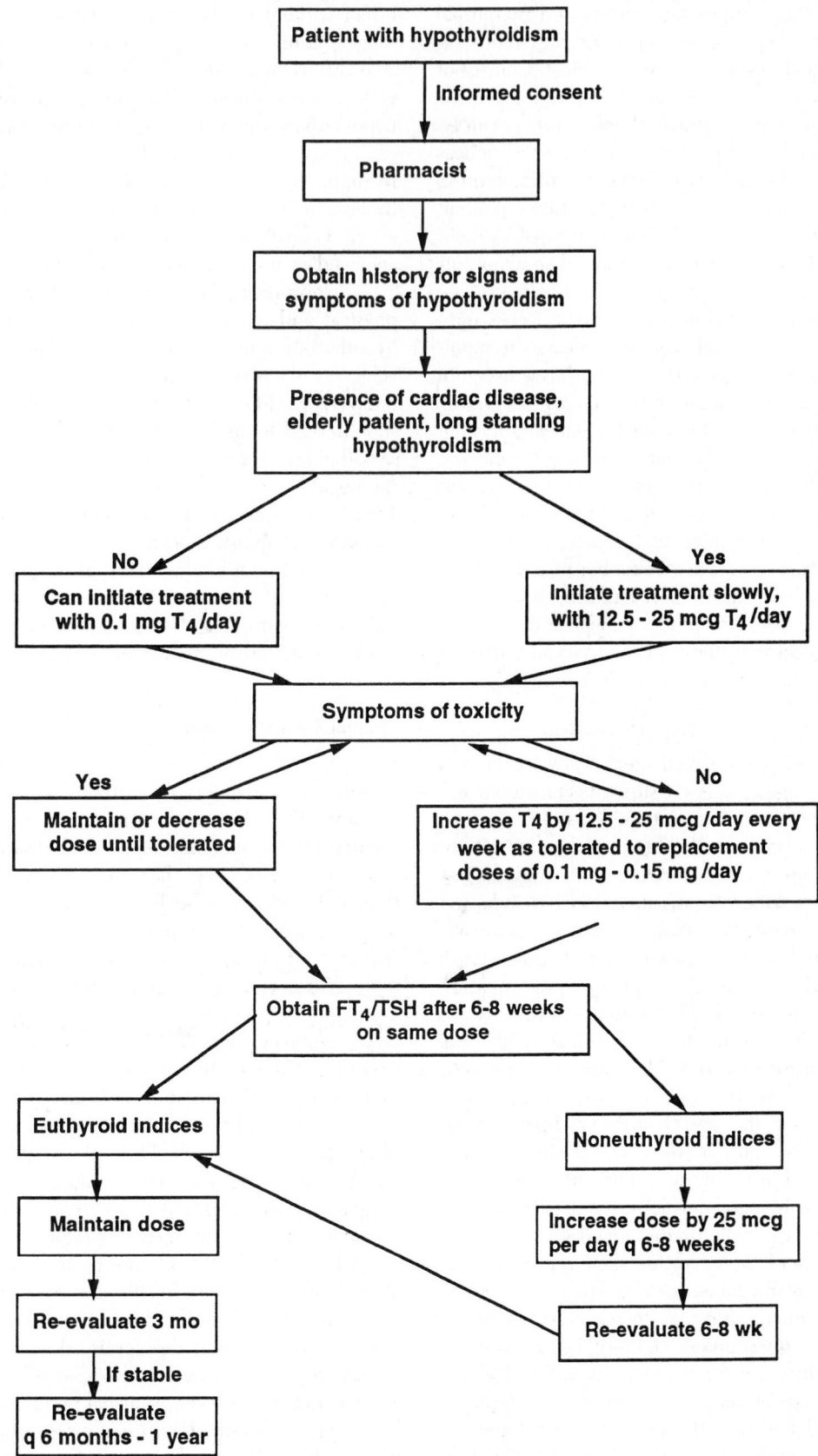

Figure 17.3 Treatment algorithm for management of hypothyroidism.

Table 17.10.
Dose of T$_4$ for Infants and Children (46, 47)

Age	T$_4$ Dosage (µg/kg/day)
0–3 months	10–15
3–6 months	6–8
6–12 months	5–7
1–10 years	3–6
10–16 years	2–4

Postpartum thyroiditis, a transient thyroiditis, can affect approximately 5% of women in the first year postdelivery. High-risk women include those with preexisting autoimmune disorders, including diabetes mellitus, autoimmune thyroiditis, collagen vascular disorders, and women with positive antibodies. In symptomatic women, thyroxine therapy may be necessary for 1 to 3 months, although permanent hypothyroidism can occur.

SUBCLINICAL HYPOTHYROIDISM

Subclinical hypothyroidism is defined as an elevated TSH level in conjunction with normal serum free T$_4$ and T$_3$ concentrations (36, 41, 44). It is controversial whether thyroxine therapy should be started in all patients with subclinical hypothyroidism or whether all patients will develop overt hypothyroidism. Although many patients are elderly and asymptomatic, improvement in cardiac contractility, lipoprotein concentrations, and cognitive function have been reported (44). The decision to start therapy should be based on several considerations, including the risks and benefits of treatment, the likelihood for development of overt hypothyroidism, the degree of TSH elevation, and history of thyroid disease. In patients receiving thyroxine therapy the elevated TSH level indicates either noncompliance or inadequate replacement, and the dosage should be increased to normalize the TSH if noncompliance is not an issue. In patients with a previous history of thyroid disease (e.g., RAI therapy), the potential for progression to overt hypothyroidism is great and replacement therapy is strongly encouraged. In patients with a negative history for thyroid illness, a normal gland, negative thyroid antibodies, and TSH elevation less than 10 mIU/L (10 µU/mL), thyroxine therapy can be withheld, provided close monitoring of the TSH level every 3 to 4 months is feasible. In patients who have an abnormal gland, positive thyroid antibodies, and a TSH level greater than 10 mIU/L (10 µU/mL), thyroxine replacement therapy to normalize the TSH can be considered if the risks and expense of therapy do not outweigh potential benefits of improvement in cardiac contractility, lipoprotein concentrations, and cognitive function.

MYXEDEMA COMA

Myxedema coma is the end stage of long-standing uncorrected hypothyroidism. The clinical symptoms include advanced hypothyroid symptoms, hypothermia, markedly delayed or absent deep tendon reflexes, and altered sensorium, ranging from stupor to coma. Other significant findings include carbon dioxide retention, hyponatremia, hypoglycemia, shock, and paranoid psychosis (33, 38).

Coma can be precipitated by cold weather (hypothermia), stress (surgery), infection, trauma, acid-base disturbances, and unrecognized concomitant illness (i.e., diabetes, arteriosclerotic cardiovascular disease [ASCVD]). Respiratory depressants of any kind (i.e., anesthetics, narcotics, phenothiazines, sedative-hypnotics), which are metabolized slowly in the hypothyroid patient, can precipitate coma by aggravating preexisting hypothermia and carbon dioxide retention. Immediate and aggressive therapy is required to prevent the high mortality rate of 60 to 70%.

Treatment includes hormone replacement and supportive measures. There are no comparative trials in myxedema coma between thyroxine and T$_3$ to indicate which agent is preferable. However, T$_4$ is recommended because there is more clinical experience with its administration than T$_3$ and mortality has been reported after administration of T$_3$ even though higher T$_3$ levels were achieved. Replacement therapy with large doses of L-thyroxine (400 µg i.v. stat) should be given to saturate the TBG. This dose can be reduced, if necessary, if there are existing cardiac risk factors. Alternatively, T$_3$ (20 to 50 µg i.v. every 8 hr) can be administered. Maintenance doses of 50 µg T$_4$ i.v. or 5 µg T$_3$ daily should be started as soon as possible. Hydrocortisone (50 to 100 mg i.v. every 6 hr) must be given concurrently because of the possibility of undetected hypopituitarism masquerading as myxedema.

Supportive measures include assisted ventilation, glucose infusions for hypoglycemia, restriction of fluids because of hyponatremia, and use of plasma expanders for shock and circulatory collapse. Cooling blankets, which may further aggravate shock by vasodilation, are not recommended. Lastly, precipitating factors should be eliminated or corrected. If the proper treatment and support are provided, consciousness, restoration of normal vital functions, and normalization of TSH levels occur within 24 hours.

THYROID NODULES

The discovery of asymptomatic single or multiple nodules in a normal or enlarged thyroid gland is a common occurrence, affecting 4 to 5% of the adult population. Thyroid function tests are often normal and patients are clinically euthyroid. The possibility of malignancy must be eliminated. It is often difficult to determine clinically, if any nodule is cancerous. In general, 10 to 20% of "cold nodules" on thyroid scan may be cancerous whereas "hot nodules" are rarely carcinogenic.

A high index of suspicion for thyroid carcinoma requires surgical intervention. A fine-needle biopsy of the nodule, performed in the outpatient setting, may provide supporting information for or against surgery. Significant risk factors are listed in Table 17.11 (49). In euthyroid patients with no history of thyroid irradiation and a low index of suspicion for cancer, TSH suppression therapy (i.e., TSH level < 0.01 mIU/L [mU/mL]) with thyroxine (0.15 to 0.2 mg daily) can be started to decrease further stimulation and growth of the nodule (36, 49). If significant regression of the nodule(s) occurs after 3 to 6 months of therapy, treatment is continued indefinitely. Any growth of the nodule during thyroid suppression therapy is alarming and requires rebiopsy or surgical removal because of the risk of malignancy.

A significant increase in benign thyroid abnormalities (20 to 33%) and thyroid cancers (6 to 9%) is observed in adults who received external irradiation to the thyroid 20 to 25 years earlier (49). In addition to papillary, mixed papillary-follicular, and follicular malignancies, benign abnormalities, including focal hyperplasia, Hashimoto's thyroiditis, adenomas, Graves' disease, and colloid nodules are reported in radiated glands. Because the malignant tumors are slow growing, the prognosis is good if there are no metastases. Patients with a previous history of external irradiation to the thymus, tonsils, adenoids, or upper head

and neck region might also be at increased risk for multiple thyroid abnormalities and require further thyroid evaluation. Therefore, all patients with a history of childhood irradiation should be evaluated by a physician skilled in thyroid examinations. A physical examination of the thyroid, baseline TSH, FT_4I or FT_4D, and antibodies should be obtained even if the patient is clinically euthyroid and asymptomatic. Unpalpable cancers have been found during surgery. If no abnormalities are found, routine yearly examinations are recommended. The administration of thyroid hormone suppression therapy for patients with a history of irradiation and no detectable thyroid abnormalities, is probably not harmful but does not appear to prevent the appearance of new thyroid abnormalities in the first 4 to 5 years of therapy (49). The presence of any palpable nodules is a strong indication for surgery. A fine-needle biopsy might provide confirmatory evidence for surgery.

Drug Kinetics and Thyroid Function

A number of drugs and disease entities can alter laboratory values and make interpretation of thyroid function tests and thyroid status difficult (see Table 17.2). Conversely, thyroid dysfunction can affect the metabolism and clinical effectiveness of several therapeutic agents (see Table 17.12) (50).

DIGITALIS

Hyperthyroid patients tend to be clinically "resistant" to the glycosides, whereas hypothyroid patients are very sensitive. This observation is consistent with alteration of digitalis kinetics in thyroid dysfunction. Both the volume of distribution (V_d) and clearance are decreased in hypothyroidism; an increased V_d and clearance occurs in hyperthyroidism. The half-life is not changed. Because the V_d determines the loading dose and the clearance maintenance dose, both the loading and maintenance dose should be lower in hypothyroidism. Likewise, larger loading and maintenance digoxin doses are required for thyrotoxicosis. The dosage of digoxin must be adjusted as euthyroidism occurs to prevent toxicity and maintain maximal therapeutic effects.

WARFARIN

Warfarin therapy is also altered by thyroid dysfunction. In thyrotoxicosis, both the synthesis and catabolism of vitamin K-dependent clotting factors are increased, producing no net change in the level of clotting factors. However, an enhanced anticoagulant response occurs because the warfarin-induced decrease in clotting factor synthesis is combined with hyperthyroidism-induced increases in factor catabolism. The opposite occurs in hypothyroidism: the anticoagulant response is less because of delayed catabolism of clotting factors. Therefore, thyrotoxic patients need

Table 17.11.
Factors for Thyroid Cancers

Evidence	Low Index of Suspicion	High Index of Suspicion
History	Familial history of thyroid disease or endemic goiter	Previous history of neck or head irradiation
Patient characteristics	Older women; soft nodule; multinodular goiter	Children, young adults, males; solitary firm dominant nodule; vocal cord paralysis; enlarged lymph nodes; hoarseness
Laboratory characteristics	High levels of antithyroid antibodies; hot nodules on scan; cystic lesion on echo; negative thin-needle biopsy (although does not rule out malignancy)	Elevated thyroglobulin; elevated serum calcitonin; cold nodule on scan; solid lesion on echo; positive thin-needle biopsy
Thyroxine therapy (not recommended in patients with history of irradiation)	Regression after 0.2–0.3 mg/day for 3–6 months	No regression

Adapted from reference 49.

Table 17.12.
Effect of Thyroid Status on Drug Acton

Thyroid Status	Drug	Alterations in Drug Action	Expected Clinical Response
Hyperthyroidism	Sympathomimetics (e.g., asthma and cold preparations)	Increased sensitivity to catecholamines	Exacerbation of thyrotoxic symptoms, especially cardiac
	Digitalis	Increased volume of distribution; ? increased renal clearance of digitalis	More resistant to digitalis effect; might require increased dosages to achieve therapeutic effect
	Insulin	Increased renal clearance/metabolism of insulin	Might require more insulin for glucose control
	Coumadin	Increased metabolism of clotting factors—decreased half-life of clotting factors	Require less coumadin for anticoagulation
	Propranolol, Metoprolol, Atenolol	Increased metabolic clearance	Might require higher dosages for desired clinical response
Hypothyroidism	Digitalis	Decreased volume of distribution; of digitalis, ? decreased renal clearance	Increased sensitivity to digitalis effect; require less digitalis to achieve therapeutic effect
	Insulin	Delayed turnover of insulin	Might need less insulin to control diabetes
	Coumadin	Delayed turnover of clotting factors—increased half-life of clotting factors	Require more coumadin for anticoagulation
	Respiratory depressants (e.g., barbiturates, phenothiazines, narcotics)	Increased sensitivity to the respiratory depressant effects of sedative hypnotic agents	Increased CO_2 retention, might precipitate myxedema coma, use cautiously in hypothyroidism
	Theophylline	Decreased metabolic clearance	Might require less drug for clinical response, monitor for toxicity

less warfarin and myxedematous patients require more warfarin to achieve the same hypoprothrombinemic response. As the thyroid status corrects, appropriate dosage adjustments are necessary to maintain therapeutic effectiveness and prevent toxicity.

ENDOCRINE HORMONES

The kinetics of several hormones, including thyroid, are influenced by changes in thyroid status. This results from alterations in hepatic blood flow and metabolism. T_4 has a normal half-life of 6 to 7 days. In hyperthyroidism the half-life is shortened to 3 to 4 days, and in hypothyroidism the half-life is prolonged to 9 to 10 days. Similar changes are described for T_3.

The half-life, secretion, and metabolism of cortisol are similarly affected. Infused cortisol had a half-life of 110 minutes in euthyroid patients, 155 minutes in hypothyroid patients, and 50 minutes in thyrotoxic patients. Although the clearance of cortisol changes as the thyroid changes, the plasma levels remain constant because of compensatory changes in secretion rates to maintain homeostasis.

The metabolism of the sex hormones in thyroid dysfunction are opposite of that expected. Higher plasma levels of testosterone, estrogens, and androgens are found

in hyperthyroidism; the converse in hypothyroidism. It appears that the higher plasma levels found in thyrotoxic patients result from changes in binding protein and from slower elimination.

Insulin kinetics and glucose metabolism are also affected by changes in thyroid status. Glucose intolerance is often observed because of increased insulin degradation rates in patients with hyperthyroidism. Clinically, hypoglycemia is more common in hypothyroidism, suggesting a delay in insulin degradation rates. Catecholamine levels are unchanged by thyroid dysfunction, although many of the thyrotoxic symptoms mimic catecholamine excess and hypothyroid symptoms mimic catecholamine deficiency.

There is definite evidence of hepatic enzyme induction in thyrotoxicosis and delayed metabolism in hypothyroidism (50). The clearance of antipyrine, a drug widely used as a marker of hepatic microsomal function, is increased in hyperthyroidism and decreased in hypothyroidism. Similar results occur with theophylline. Nevertheless, it is not possible to extrapolate such changes to the metabolism of other drugs cleared hepatically. Phenytoin is one example. Even though phenytoin can induce hepatic microsomal enzyme metabolism of thyroid hormones, changes in thyroid function do not appear to affect its metabolism. On the other hand, hypothyroid patients are inordinately sensitive to the effects of respiratory depressants, such as anesthetics, narcotics, phenothiazines, and sedative hypnotics, all of which undergo hepatic metabolism.

Absorption of agents such as riboflavin, ethanol, and acetaminophen appear to be increased in thyrotoxicosis and delayed in hypothyroidism. The significance of this is unclear because most of the data was obtained through animal studies.

CONCLUSION

Hypothyroidism, hyperthyroidism, and nodular disease are common endocrine problems that affect 15% of females and 5% of men. Practitioners should be alert to drugs that cause thyroid illness, interfere with proper laboratory interpretation, or interact with effective medical management. Thyroid function tests presently recommended for detection, evaluation, and monitoring of thyroid disease in symptomatic individuals and in the elderly patient who might have atypical symptoms are reviewed. Many different treatment options are now available for the management of hyperthyroidism, hypothyroidism, and nodular disease. Practitioners should be able to help select the optimal treatment regimen by integrating several patient and medication considerations in their decision making. An understanding of the detection, evaluation, medical management, and education of a patient with thyroid disease is essential for practitioners involved in the care of these individuals.

REFERENCES

1. Surks MI, Chopra IJ, Mariash CN, et al. American Thyroid Association guidelines for use of laboratory tests in thyroid disorders. JAMA 263:1529–1532, 1990.
2. Wartofsky L, Burman KD. Alterations in thyroid function in patients with systemic illness: the "euthyroid sick syndrome." Endocr Rev 3:164–217, 1982.
3. Woeber KA. Iodine and thyroid disease. Med Clin North Am 75:169–178, 1991.
4. Ishikawa N, Eguchi K, Otsubo T, et al. Reduction in the suppressor-inducer T cell subset and increase in the helper T cell subset in thyroid tissue from patients with Graves' disease. J Clin Endocrinol Metab 65:17–23, 1987.
5. Burch HB, Wartofsky LW. Graves' ophthalmopathy. Current concepts regarding pathogenesis and management. Endocr Rev 14:747–793, 1993.
6. Marcocci C, Bartalena L, Bogazzi F, et al. Relationship between Graves' ophthalmopathy and type of treatment of Graves' hyperthyroidism. Thyroid 2:171–178, 1992.
7. Salata S, Klein I. Effects of lithium on the endocrine system: a review. J Lab Clin Med 110:130–136, 1987.
8. Trip MD, Wiersinga W, Plomp TA. Incidence, predictability, and pathogenesis of amiodarone-induced thyrotoxicosis and hypothyroidism. Am J Med 91:507–511, 1991.
9. Klein I, Becker DV, Levey GS. Treatment of hyperthyroid disease. Ann Intern Med 121:281–288, 1994.
10. Franklyn JA. The management of hyperthyroidism. N Engl J Med 330:1731–1738, 1994.
11. Hamburger JI. Diagnosis and management of Graves' disease in pregnancy. Thyroid 2:219–224, 1991.
12. Burrow GN. Thyroid function and hyperfunction during gestation. Endocr Rev 14:194–202, 1993.
13. Solomon B, Glinoer D, Lagasse R, et al. Current trends in the management of Graves' disease. J Clin Endocrinol Metab 70:1518–1524, 1990.
14. Cooper DS. Which antithyroid drug? Am J Med 80:1165–1168, 1986.
15. Roti E, Gardini E, Minelli R, et al. Methimazole and serum thyroid hormone concentrations in hyperthyroid patients: effects of single and multiple daily doses. Ann Intern Med 111:181–182, 1989.
16. Walter RM, Bartle W. Rectal administration of propylthiouracil in the treatment of Graves' disease. Am J Med 88:69–70, 1990.
17. Nabil N, Miner DJ, Amatruda JM. Methimazole: an alternative route of administration. J Clin Endocrinol Metab 54:180–181, 1982.
18. Bouma DJ, Kammer H, Greer MA. Follow-up comparison of short-term versus 1-year antithyroid drug therapy for the thyrotoxicosis of Graves' disease. J Clin Endocrinol Metab 55:1138–1142, 1982.
19. Allannic H, Fauchet R, Orgiazzi J, et al. Antithyroid drugs and Graves' disease: a prospective randomized evaluation of the efficacy of treatment duration. J Clin Endocrinol Metab 70:675–679, 1990.
20. Feldt-Rasmussen U, Glinoer D, Orgiazzi J. Reassessment of antithyroid drug therapy of Graves' Disease. Annu Rev Med 44:323–334, 1993.
21. Lippe BM, Landaw EM, Kaplan SA. Hyperthyroidism in children treated with long term medical therapy: twenty-five percent remission every two years. J Clin Endocrinol Metab 64:1241–1245, 1987.
22. Romaldini JH, Bromberg N, Werner RS, et al. Comparison of effects of high and low dosage regimens of antithyroid drugs in the management of Graves' hyperthyroidism. J Clin Endocrinol Metab 57:563–570, 1983.
23. Hashizume K, Ichikawa K, Sakurai A, et al. Administration of thyroxine in treated Graves' disease: effects on the level of antibodies to thyroid-stimulating hormone receptors and on the risk of recurrence of hyperthyroidism. N Engl J Med 324:947–953, 1991.
24. Liaw Y-F, Huang M-J, Fan K-D, et al. Hepatic injury during propythiouracil therapy in patients with hyperthyroidism: a cohort study. Ann Intern Med 118:424–428, 1993.
25. Tajiri J, Noguchi S, Murakami T, et al. Antithyroid drug-induced agranulocytosis: the usefulness of routine white blood cell count monitoring. Arch Intern Med 150:621–624, 1990.
26. Geffner DL, Hershman JM. Beta-adrenergic blockade for the treatment of hyperthyroidism. Am J Med. 93:61–68, 1992.
27. Milner MR, Gelman KM, Phillips RA, et al. Double-blind crossover trial of diltiazem versus propranolol in the management of thyrotoxic symptoms. Pharmacotherapy 10:100–106, 1990.
28. Wang YS, Tsou CT, Lin WH, et al. Long term treatment of Graves' disease with iopanoic acid (Telepaque). J Clin Endocrinol Metab 65:679–682, 1987.
29. Weber CA, Clark OH. Surgery for thyroid disease. Med Clin North Am 69:1097–1115, 1985.
30. Van Dijke CP, Heydendael RJ, De Kleine MJ. Methimazole, carbimazole, and congenital skin defects [Letter]. Ann Intern Med 106:60–61, 1987.
31. Eisenstein Z, Weiss M, Katz Y, et al. Intellectual capacity of subjects exposed to methimazole or propylthiouracil in utero. Eur J Pediatr 151:558–559, 1992.
32. Zimmerman D, Gan-Gaisano M. Hyperthyroidism in children and adolescents. Pediatr Clin North Am 37:1273–1295, 1990.
33. Gavin LA. Thyroid crises. Med Clin North Am 75:179–193, 1991.
34. LaFranchi S. Diagnosis and treatment of hypothyroidism in children. Compr Ther 13:20–30, 1987.

35. O'Brien T, Dinneen SF, O'Brien PC, et al. Hyperlipidemia in patients with primary and secondary hypothyroidism. Mayo Clin Proc 68:860–866, 1993.

36. Toft AD. Thyroxine therapy. N Engl J Med. 331:174–180, 1994.

37. Sawin CT, Hershman JM, Fernandez-Garcia R, et al. A comparison of thyroxine and desiccated thyroid in patients with primary hypothyroidism. Metabolism 27:1518–1525, 1978.

38. Nicoloff JT, LoPresti JS. Myxedema coma. A form of decompensated hypothyroidism. Endocrinol Metab Clin North Am 22:279–290, 1993.

39. Stoffer SS, Szpunar WE. Levothyroxine loses potency with age [Letter]. JAMA 255:1881–1882, 1986.

40. Escalante DA, Arem N, Arem R. Assessment of interchangability of two brands of levothyroxine preparations with a third-generation TSH assay. Am J Med 98: 374–378, 1995.

41. Helfand M, Crapo LM. Monitoring therapy in patients taking levothyroxine. Ann Intern Med 113:450–454, 1990.

42. Fish LH, Schwartz HL, Cavanaugh J, et al. Replacement dose, metabolism, and bioavailability of levothyroxine in the treatment of hypothyroidism. N Engl J Med 316:764–770, 1987.

43. Bearcroft CP, Toms GC, Willians SJ, et al. Thyroxine replacement in post-radioiodine hypothyroidism. Clin Endocrinol (Oxf) 34:115–118, 1991.

44. Mandel SJ, Brent GA, Larsen PR. Levothyroxine therapy in patients with thyroid disease. Ann Intern Med 119:492–502, 1993.

45. Stall GM, Harris S, Sokoll LJ, et al. Accelerated bone loss in hypothyroid patients overtreated with L-thyroxine. Ann Intern Med 113:265–269, 1990.

46. Heyerdahl S, Kase BF, Lie SO. Intellectual development in children with congenital hypothyroidism in relation to recommended thyroxine treatment. J Pediatr 118:850–857, 1991.

47. Fisher DA, Foley BL. Early treatment of congenital hypothyroidism. Pediatrics 83:785–789, 1989.

48. Mandel SJ, Larsen PR, Seely EW, et al. Increased need for thyroxine during pregnancy in women with primary hypothyroidism. N Engl J Med 323:91–96, 1990.

49. Greenspan FS. The problem of the nodular goiter. Med Clin North Am 75:195–209, 1991.

50. O'Connor P, Feely J. Clinical pharmacokinetics and endocrine disorders. Therapeutic implications. Clin Pharmacokinet 13:345–364, 1987.

CHAPTER 18

PARATHYROID DISORDERS

BETTY J. DONG and RENU F. SINGH

To understand the treatment of common parathyroid disorders, the effects of parathyroid hormone, the consequences of excessive secretion or lack of end organ response, and their relationship to calcium metabolism must first be understood.

There are four parathyroid glands, located posteriorly on the thyroid gland in the neck. Parathyroid hormone (PTH), the principal regulator of extracellular ionic calcium, is released from the parathyroid glands via a negative feedback system responsive to plasma calcium levels. Normal plasma ionic calcium is maintained through the action of PTH on kidney, bone, and intestine. Most of the total body calcium is found in bone, and only a small fraction of the calcium circulates in the bloodstream as the active (ionized) or inactive (bound) form. Approximately 40% of the total serum calcium is bound, primarily to albumin, 15% is complexed with phosphate or other anions, and 45% is in the ionized active form. Therefore, reductions in serum albumin will alter the concentration of protein-bound calcium and increase the free ionized fraction proportionally. The normal total serum calcium concentration is approximately 2.12 to 2.62 mmol/L (8.5-10.5 mg/dL), depending on the laboratory. In patients with hypoalbuminemia, the serum calcium can be adjusted by adding 0.2 mmol/L (0.8 mg/dL) for each 10 g/L (1 g/dL) of albumin below a normal level of 40 g/L (4 g/dL) to the measured serum calcium. This formula might not completely correct for albumin and direct determination of ionized calcium levels might be useful.

PTH protects against hypocalcemia by the following mechanisms:

1. Increasing release of calcium and phosphate from bone resorption.
2. Increasing reabsorption of calcium and magnesium by the kidney.
3. Increasing intestinal absorption of calcium indirectly via vitamin D.
4. Increasing conversion of the metabolite 25-hydroxycholecalciferol to active vitamin D_3 (1,25-dihydroxycholecalciferol or 1,25-$(OH)_2D_3$ or calcitriol) through stimulating the activity of renal tubular 25-OH-1-α-hydroxylase.
5. Increasing the renal excretion of bicarbonate (bicarbonaturia), producing a metabolic acidosis that decreases the ability of circulating albumin to bind calcium, thus increasing calcium by physiochemical means. PTH also acts on the kidney to increase phosphate excretion (hyperphosphaturia) and pre-

vent elevations in plasma phosphate levels from increased bone resorption.

Thus, a reciprocal relationship between calcium and phosphate exists. In hyperparathyroidism, serum calcium is elevated and hypophosphatemia occurs. Conversely, in hypoparathyroidism, hypocalcemia and hyperphosphatemia are seen.

HYPERPARATHYROIDISM

Primary hyperparathyroidism is an endocrine disorder characterized by excessive uncontrolled release of parathyroid hormone (PTH) from adenomatous (single-gland involvement, 80%), hyperplastic (multiple-gland involvement, 20%), or malignant (<2%) parathyroid glands. Hyperparathyroidism, associated with multiple endocrine neoplasia syndromes (MEN), is almost always due to multiple-gland involvement. The hallmark of this disorder is hypercalcemia because of the failure of the negative feedback cycle to suppress further PTH secretion. The etiology of this disorder is unknown, although inheritance via an autosomal dominant trait is described.

Prevalence

Hyperparathyroidism is more common than previously recognized. Earlier detection of asymptomatic disease has resulted from the widespread use of routine serum calcium measurements. Various studies prior to 1969 indicate a prevalence of 10 to 20 cases per 100,000. In a careful population-based study, an incidence of 7.8 cases per 100,000 jumped to 42 cases/100,000 after the introduction of routine calcium measurements. This subsequently fell to 27.7 cases per 100,000, a figure which is similar to rates reported in England and Sweden. There is an increased incidence of hyperparathyroidism with advanced age and it is 2 to 4 times more common in women than in men. Approximately 100,000 new cases develop each year in the United States (1).

Patient Characteristic	Prevalence
Both sexes ≤ 39 yr	10:100,000
Both sexes ≥ 40 yr	50:100,000
Female ≥ 60 yr	188:100,000
Male ≥ 60 yr	91:100,000

Pathogenesis

Excessive release of PTH causes hypercalcemia and hypophosphatemia via the mechanisms previously described. Mild to moderate hyperchloremic acidosis is caused by PTH-induced bicarbonaturia. Hypercalciuria results when the renal threshold for reabsorbing calcium is exceeded; serum calcium is usually greater than 3.00 mmol/L (12 mg/dL). Complications of nephrolithiasis occur from prolonged hypercalciuria in an alkaline medium (bicarbonaturia). Other extraskeletal metastatic calcifications might produce rheumatologic complaints of calcific tendinitis and chondrocalcinosis. Osteomalacia and osteitis fibrosa cystica result from depletion of vitamin D, because of prolonged PTH renal conversion of 25-OH-vitamin D to active 1,25-(OH)$_2$-vitamin D.

Diagnosis

Because the patient is frequently asymptomatic, the diagnosis is made in 80 to 90% of cases by finding an elevated serum calcium level (usually >2.62 mmol/L [10.5 mg/dL]) and an elevated PTH level. The intact PTH level using an IRMA assay is the more sensitive of the PTH assays and should be obtained to confirm the diagnosis of hyperparathyroidism. Total serum calcium levels should be elevated in three separate measurements before hypercalcemia is established. Ionized serum calcium levels should be used in patients with low serum albumin. Drugs that can increase serum calcium concentrations, such as thiazide diuretics, should be withdrawn for several days.

Other abnormal laboratory findings include hypophosphatemia, hyperphosphaturia, hypercalciuria, low serum bicarbonate concentration, elevated serum chloride levels, and elevations in alkaline phosphatase activity with bony involvements. Serum urea nitrogen or creatinine levels can be helpful in evaluating renal function. Radiographic manifestations of osteitis fibrosa cystica, nephrolithiasis, or other extraskeletal calcifications can be present. Other causes of hypercalcemia should be eliminated (see Table 18.1).

Clinical Presentations; Signs and Symptoms

Before the routine use of serum calcium measurements, patients typically presented with symptoms resulting from severe hypercalcemia and bone and renal involvement. Serum calcium levels > 3.00 mmol/L (12 mg/dL) commonly produce gastrointestinal symptoms (e.g., anorexia, nausea, and vomiting), and neurologic manifestations of weakness, delayed deep tendon reflexes, and altered mental status. Rarely, patients are asymptomatic. The high-risk, elderly female might show confusion and dehydration. However, earlier detection of the disease has changed the clinical presentation. Most patients now are relatively asymptomatic or have nonspecific complaints of weakness and easy fatigability.

Table 18.1.
Some Causes of Hypercalcemia

Hyperparathyroidism
  Primary: parathyroid adenomas, hyperplasia or carcinoma
  Secondary: compensatory increase in PTH due to low calcium levels (renal failure, osteomalacia, intestinal malabsorption)
Granulomatous disease (sarcoidosis, tuberculosis, histoplasmosis, coccidioidomycosis, leprosy)
Drugs
  Vitamin D, vitamin A, or calcium intoxification
  Milk-alkali syndrome
  Lithium
Malignancies
  Nonhematologic (breast, bronchus)
  Hematologic (myeloma, leukemia, lymphoma)
Endocrine (adrenal insufficiency, thyrotoxicosis, acromegaly, pheochromocytoma)
Immobilization
Bone disorders (Paget's osteoporosis)
Idiopathic hypercalcemia of infancy
Familial hypocalciuric hypercalcemia
Miscellaneous: renal transplant, hemodialysis

The clinical spectrum and complications of primary hyperparathyroidism are presented in Table 18.2. The severity of the clinical manifestations, especially the degree of hypercalcemia, is generally proportional to the degree of hyperfunctioning tissue and the level of PTH elevation.

Treatment of Hyperparathyroidism

ASYMPTOMATIC

The National Institutes of Health Consensus Development panel has concluded that the diagnosis of hyperparathyroidism in an asymptomatic patient does not always mandate surgery. In patients who are asymptomatic with only a mildly elevated serum calcium, no previous episodes of life-threatening hypercalcemia, and normal renal and bone status, the indications for surgery are less clear because the true progression of the disease is unknown (1). There are no objective criteria to predict which patients will eventually require surgery and which patients can be managed medically. Generally, long-term follow-up studies indicate a benign course with stable hypercalcemia, and rarely, progressive loss of renal function. In a 10-year retrospective study of 248 patients with mild asymptomatic hyperparathyroidism, 51% ultimately required surgical intervention because of complications of their disease while 49% had no deterioration in their clinical status (2). In this latter group, 22% of patients died during this 10-year period (unrelated to the hyperparathyroidism) or were lost to follow-up. Patients who are unlikely to return for consistent follow-up or whose coexistent illness complicates management should be considered surgical candidates. Surgery is also recommended for young patients (<50 years of age) because the outcome of several decades of primary hyperparathyroidism is unknown. Many studies tend to favor early surgical intervention to normalize serum calcium levels, prevent further bone loss, and increase bone density, even though surgery might be less effective in patients with mild disease and difficult-to-locate PTH abnormalities. If medical observation is selected, then patients should be monitored closely at 3- to 6-month intervals with serum calcium and phosphorus levels, renal function tests, and abdominal radiography for the detection of renal stones. Cortical bone mass measurements should also be obtained every 1 to 2 years to assess bone loss. Patients should be told to restrict dairy products, vitamin D-containing preparations, and excessive sunlight exposure. If progression of the disease occurs, then surgical intervention is indicated.

SURGERY

Surgical exploration of the neck and removal of adenomatous, hyperplastic, or malignant tissue is the definitive treatment of choice for symptomatic primary hyperparathyroidism (3). Surgery is absolutely indicated in patients with (a) sustained serum calcium levels above 2.86 to 3 mmol/L (11.5 to 12 mg/dL); (b) evidence of bony involvement; (c) evidence of renal involvement; (d) complications from hyperparathyroidism; and (e) coexisting disease states that might be exacerbated by elevations in serum calcium levels (e.g., hypertension).

Most critical to the surgical treatment of primary hyperparathyroidism is an experienced and skilled surgeon. In competent hands, the evidence of postoperative complications (e.g., vocal cord paralysis) is minimal and the cure rate high. Neuromuscular symptoms are frequently reversed by successful parathyroidectomy, but somatic symptoms are rarely improved by the operation. Postoperatively, serum calcium levels normalize or fall below normal within 24 to 48 hours. Hypocalcemia is usually mild and transient, although tetany and permanent hypoparathyroidism can occur. Patients at high risk for the latter include those with evidence of bone demineralization, those with renal involvement, those with steatorrhea, those undergoing total parathyroidectomy, and those undergoing multiple neck explorations. Serum calcium levels should be monitored daily until levels stabilize, around the fifth or sixth postoperative day. Symptoms of tetany or pretetany should be treated intravenously with 10 to 20 mL of 10% calcium gluconate, given slowly (not faster than 10 mL/min) until symptoms are relieved. Modest degrees of hypocalcemia postoperatively need not be treated except by ensuring an adequate calcium intake. A small percentage of patients will develop permanent hypoparathyroid-

Table 18.2.
Signs and Symptoms of Hypercalcemia and Hyperparathyroidism

System	Symptoms	Complications	Laboratory Tests
Gastrointestinal	Nausea, vomiting, anorexia, constipation, abdominal pain, weight loss	Peptic ulcer disease 10–15%, chronic pancreatitis, cholelithiasis, fecal impaction/intestinal obstruction	↑ amylase
Genitourinary	Polyuria, nocturia, polydipsia, dehydration, uremia symptoms, renal colic pain	Nephrolithiasis, nephrocalcinosis 20–30%, renal failure, pyelonephritis	Hematuria, inability to concentrate urine, pyuria, ↓ Na, ↓ K, ↓ Mg
Skeletal	Vague aches and pains, arthralgias, localized swellings,	Osteitis fibrosa cystica, chondrocalcinosis, pathologic fractures, bone cysts; calcium depositions leading to gout, pseudogout	Radiologic → subperiosteal bone resorption
Neurologic	Emotional lability, slow mentation, poor memory, weakness, easy fatigability, drowsiness, ataxia, coma	Depression, psychoses; headaches, myopathy (proximal), coma	Hyperactive deep tendon reflexes
Cardiovascular	Bradycardia	Hypertension 20–60%, cardiac arrest, bundle branch block, heart block, enhanced digitalis sensitivity	ECG: ↓ Q-T interval, ↑ P-R, ↑ QRS
Metabolic	Dehydration	Hyperchloremic acidosis, insulin hypersecretion and decreased insulin sensitivity	↓ HCO_3, ↑ Cl
Others	Pruritis due to ectopic calcifications in skin; ectopic calcifications in lungs, kidneys, etc.; red eyes	Anemia, band keratopathy, thrombosis, malignancies in gastrointestinal tract, breast, thyroid	

ism, requiring treatment with vitamin D (see "Hypoparathyroidism"). Parathyroid transplantation might be indicated for the patient with secondary hyperparathyroidism (renal osteodystrophy), primary parathyroid hyperplasia, persistent or recurrent hyperparathyroidism, or radical head and neck surgery including thyroidectomy (4).

MEDICAL MANAGEMENT

There is no pharmacologic substitute for the surgical management of hyperparathyroidism. However, medical management of hypercalcemia is indicated in patients who refuse surgery, in symptomatic patients prior to surgery, in those with life-threatening hypercalcemia, in those with resistant or recurrent hyperparathyroidism despite previous neck surgery, and in poor surgical candidates.

Several therapeutic options are available (see Table 18.3). In general, hypercalcemia is corrected by inhibiting bone resorption, increasing calcium excretion, or decreasing calcium absorption. Many of these options are very effective and should lower serum calcium in virtually all patients. A single agent or a combination of agents might be required, depending on the severity of the hypercalcemia, the extent of dehydration, and the duration and degree of effectiveness of the selected agent. Supportive therapeutic measures should also include restriction of dietary calcium intake and mobilization.

Hydration with normal saline is the initial treatment of choice for hypercalcemia of 3 mmol/L (12 mg/dL) or greater from any cause (5, 6). Because hypercalcemia often causes vomiting and polyuria (resulting in dehydration, hypokalemia, and hypomagnesemia) adequate electrolyte replacement and volume expansion are critical. Rehydration should occur at a rate determined by the degree of volume depletion and sufficient to maintain adequate urine output. Adequate hydration should reverse mild hypercalcemic symptoms, restore the glomerular filtration rate, and increase calcium excretion. Serum calcium levels generally decrease by 0.25 to 0.5 mmol/L (1 to 2 mg/dL) within a few hours. Nevertheless, hydration should be used cautiously in patients who are unable to tolerate large fluid volumes (e.g., in CHF, RF).

Once rehydration has been established, further renal calcium excretion can be promoted by mild diuresis with saline with or without a loop diuretic such as furosemide given as 10 to 20 mg intravenously every 6 to 12 hours (5). The use of diuretic therapy is well tolerated even in patients with moderate renal impairment and might reduce serum calcium levels by 0.75 mmol/L (3 mg/dL) within 24 hours. It is essential that patients be adequately hydrated throughout this diuresis, and repletion of electrolytes such as magnesium and potassium be maintained.

In emergent hypercalcemic crisis, the preceding methods might be used more aggressively. Forced diuresis with up to 6 liters per day of normal saline and furosemide, 80 to 100 mg intravenously every 1 to 2 hours, to maintain urinary flow rates of above 200 mL/hr might be required (7). Such an approach will reduce serum calcium levels by 0.5 to 1 mmol/L (2 to 4 mg/dL) within 24 hours, but will necessitate central venous pressure monitoring of fluid status and bladder catheterization in addition to continuous electrolyte repletion.

The early introduction of an antiresorptive agent in the management of severe hypercalcemia is prudent to avoid the potential complications of prolonged saline diuresis. In addition, normocalcemia is rarely sustained by saline diuresis alone. Bisphosphonates have become one of the primary treatment options for the management of hypercalcemia. Bisphosphonates are stable pyrophosphate analogs that bind to hydroxyapatite in bone and act as potent inhibitors of PTH-mediated osteoclastic bone resorption. The calcium-lowering effect varies between different bisphosphonates, and the effect is significantly weaker in patients with primary hyperparathyroidism compared to patients with tumor-induced hypercalcemia.

Etidronate, a first generation bisphosphonate, is poorly absorbed and, like most bisphosphonates, is more effective when administered intravenously. Etidronate reduces serum calcium levels in 24 to 48 hours after administration of 7.5 mg/kg i.v. daily for 3 to 5 days, and the calcium-lowering effect is maintained for up to 1 week. Repeat dosing of etidronate is not recommended earlier than 7 days after the initial course, as its maximal effect occurs after 3 to 7 days. Oral etidronate can be given after a course of intravenous etidronate to maintain normocalcemia. Etidronate therapy might result in hyperphosphatemia, diarrhea, and nausea. Etidronate should be used cautiously in patients with renal dysfunction.

Pamidronate (APD), a second generation bisphosphonate, is more potent than etidronate and less likely to inhibit bone mineralization or osteoblast activity (8). Clinical studies comparing pamidronate to etidronate have demonstrated a greater reduction in serum calcium levels with pamidronate, although there was no difference in the duration of response or rate of hypercalcemic symptom resolution (9, 10). Its onset of action occurs after 24 to 48 hours. Pamidronate is administered as either a 60- or 90-mg infusion, depending on the severity of the hypercalcemia. The recommended dose in moderate hypercalcemia (corrected serum calcium of approximately 12–13.5 mg/dL) is 60 to 90 mg. In severe hypercalcemia (corrected serum Ca^{++} > 13.5 mg/dL) the recommended dose is 90 mg. Pamidronate is preferable to etidronate, as pamidronate is slightly more effective in lowering serum calcium levels; it can be given as a single dose instead of over several days and is generally better tolerated than etidronate. In addition, the cost for a treatment course with pamidronate is comparable to that of etidronate. Pamidronate doses should not be repeated in less than 7 days, as the full response might not be achieved for up to a week. Pamidronate is well tolerated, with a mild, transient fever being the most common adverse effect. It should be used with caution in patients with renal dysfunction.

Calcitonin inhibits bone resorption and enhances urinary calcium excretion. Synthetic and human calcitonin are available in the United States; most experience is with the more potent and longer-acting salmon calcitonin. Calcitonin, although effective in reducing serum calcium levels, rarely produces normocalcemia. Calcium levels will decrease rapidly within 2 to 4 hours after administration of 4 IU/kg s.q. or i.m. every 12 hours. Doses can be increased up to 8 IU/kg every 6 hours if the lower dose is ineffective. The maximal calcium-lowering effect occurs within 12 to 24 hours of administration, causing a decrease of serum calcium by 2 to 3 mg/dL. The duration of action is transient and variable. Loss of efficacy can occur after 2 to 6 days because of an escape phenomenon, causing serum calcium levels to rise despite continued administration. The concomitant use of glucocorticoids (e.g. prednisone 30–60 mg daily) has been used in the past to antagonize the escape and prolong the action of calcitonin, but this has been replaced by the addition of a bisphosphonate to calcitonin (11). This combination therapy results in a sustained reduction in serum calcium levels for several days and is especially useful in patients with severe hypercalcemia requiring a rapid but sustained fall in serum calcium levels. Calcitonin is well tolerated, with transient nausea and vomiting being the most common toxicity. Because of its potential for anaphylactoid reactions, the manufacturer recommends initial skin testing with 1 IU/0.1 mL cutaneously, especially in atopic individuals or those with a history of hypersensitivity to calcitonin. However, anaphylactoid reactions are rare and treatment should not be withheld awaiting skin test results.

Gallium nitrate, an antitumor agent, is a potent inhibitor of bone resorption and is approved for the treatment of hypercalcemia associated with malignancy. Gallium nitrate does not affect bone mineralization. Gallium nitrate (200 mg/m^2 i.v. daily for 5 days) has been shown to be more effective than salmon calcitonin (8 IU/kg s.q. every 6 hours for 5 days) (12), or etidronate (7.5 mg/kg i.v. daily for 5 days) (13) in achieving normocalcemia in patients with hypercalcemia of malignancy. In addition, the duration of normocalcemia was sustained for a longer period of time (8 days) with gallium nitrate than etidronate (3 days). Gallium nitrate is administered as a 200 mg/m^2, 24-hour infusion for 5 consecutive days. Onset of effect is in 24 to 48 hours after the first dose, with a maximal response observed within 7 to 10 days. The major adverse effect associated with gallium nitrate is nephrotoxicity. It should be avoided in patients with a serum creatinine above 221 mol/L (2.5 mg/dL) or if concomitant nephrotoxic drugs such as aminoglycosides or amphotericin B are given.

Patients should be well hydrated, and renal function tests should be monitored. Other side effects include hypophosphatemia and hypocalcemia.

Plicamycin (mithramycin), an antitumor antibiotic that inhibits bone resorption, is the oldest and least expensive agent for producing a prolonged antihypercalcemic effect. However, due to its high potential for toxicity and the current availability of effective, better tolerated agents, plicamycin is generally reserved for patients who have failed, or who are intolerant to a bisphosphonate. Plicamycin produces normocalcemia within 12 to 72 hours after a single dose of 25 µg/kg/day. Because maximum reductions in calcium levels might not occur for 2 to 5 days, it is advisable to wait at least 48 hours before administering additional doses to avoid hypocalcemia. Repeated doses for 3 to 4 doses might be necessary. The duration of action is highly variable, ranging from 5 to 15 days. Reduced doses of 12.5 µg/kg/day can be tried in patients with preexisting hepatic or renal dysfunction. However, its cumulative toxicity generally limits its repeated usage in patients with renal failure, hepatic disease, bone marrow suppression, or platelet or coagulation disorders.

Chronic oral administration of estrogens (e.g., conjugated estrogens 1.25 mg q.d., ethynyl estradiol 30 µg q.d.) and progestins (e.g., norethindrone 5 mg q.d.) have been shown in numerous studies to reduce serum calcium levels and calciuria, and to decrease bone turnover in postmenopausal women with primary hyperparathyroidism (14, 15). Estrogens and progestins block the PTH-resorptive effects without affecting circulating PTH levels. Normalization of serum calcium levels is more likely with estrogens than with progestins; therefore, estrogens are the agents of choice unless contraindications exist. Contraindications to estrogen therapy include a history of thromboembolic disorders, thrombophlebitis, liver disease, abnormal genital bleeding, and pregnancy. The reductions in serum calcium are variable and modest: some women do not respond, and the decline in others might be less than 0.25 mmol/L (1 mg/dL). Nevertheless, estrogens can control hypercalcemia and hypercalciuria in over half of postmenopausal women with hyperparathyroidism in addition to providing beneficial effects on osteoporosis and cardiovascular risk factors.

Intravenous phosphates are not recommended in the management of acute hypercalcemia because of the risk of metastatic soft tissue calcifications, renal failure, and even death. Their use should be restricted to patients with extreme, life-threatening hypercalcemia and hypophosphatemia for whom other treatment regimens have failed (5, 6). Phosphates lower serum calcium levels by raising the calcium phosphate ion product above the solubility product (approximately 60 to 70 when calculated using mg/dL) and precipitating calcium phosphate complexes within the body, primarily in bone and soft tissues.

Table 18.3.
Treatment of Hypercalcemia Secondary to Hyperparathyroidism

Method	Mechanism of Action	Dose	Onset of Ca-lowering Effect	Maximal Effect	Adverse Effects	Comments
Hydration with saline, replacement of depleted electrolytes	Increases calcium excretion	100–250 mL/hr i.v. Saline	Hours	Decreases serum calcium by 1–2 mg/dL	Volume overload	Cautious administration in patients with CHF, RF; careful monitoring of fluid and electrolytes crucial
Forced diuresis; saline + loop diuretic	Increases calcium excretion	Furosemide 10–20 mg i.v. q6–12hr	Within 4 hr	Decreases serum calcium by 1–3 mg/dL	Volume depletion, hypokalemia, hypomagnesemia	Avoid in dehydration; avoid thiazides which decrease calcium excretion
Calcitonin	Inhibits bone resorption	4 IU/kg s.q. or i.m. q12hr; maximum of 8 IU/kg q6hr	2–4 hr	12–24 hr; Decreases serum calcium by 1–3 mg/dL	Hypersensitivity reactions, nausea, vomiting	Escape phenomenon occurs within 2–6 days; refractoriness decreased with glucocorticoids
Etidronate Disodium	Inhibits bone resorption	7.5 mg/kg/day i.v. q.d. for 3–7 days	24–48 hr	3–7 days	Hyperphosphatemia, diarrhea, nausea, nephrotoxicity	Indicated for Paget's disease and hypercalcemia of malignancy; infuse over minimum of 2 hr; use with caution in renal dysfunction; do not repeat dose in less than 7 days after initial course; for chronic maintenance therapy, may follow i.v. course with etidronate 20 mg/kg/day p.o. for 30–90 days
Pamidronate Disodium	Inhibits bone resorption	60–90 mg i.v. over 24 hr	24–48 hr	3–7 days	Fever	Indicated for Paget's disease and hypercalcemia of malignancy; do not repeat dose earlier than 7 days after initial dose; use with caution in renal dysfunction
Gallium Nitrate	Inhibits bone resorption	200 mg/m² i.v. q.d. (24-hr continuous infusion) for 5 days	24–48 hr	7–10 days	Nephrotoxicity	Indicated for hypercalcemia of malignancy; avoid if serum creatinine > 2.5 mg/dL or if concomitant nephrotoxic drugs

Drug	Mechanism	Dose	Onset	Duration	Adverse effects	Comments
Plicamycin	Inhibits bone resorption	25 μg/kg i.v. q24-48 hr; 12.5 μg/kg if pre-existing renal/hepatic dysfunction	24-48 hr	2-5 days	Nausea, vomiting, ↓ platelets, hemorrhage, hepatotoxicity, nephrotoxicity	Toxicity increases with doses > 30 μg/kg or with consecutive doses; avoid in patients with bleeding disorders; use with caution and reduce dosage in patients with renal or hepatic disease; infuse in 1 liter of fluid over 4-6 hours to reduce gastrointestinal toxicity; Observe extravasation precautions
Estrogens, Progestins	Inhibits bone resorption	Ethinyl estradiol 30-50 μg p.o. q.d.; Premarin 0.625-1.25 mg p.o. q.d.; Norethindrone 5 mg p.o. q.d.		2 months	Nausea, vomiting, risk of estrogen/progestin therapy	Effective in postmenopausal women with hyperparathyroidism
Sodium Phosphates	Precipitates calcium phosphate complexes within bone and soft tissue	p.o./rectal elemental phosphorus 2-3 g/day given in 4 divided doses; i.v.: 25-50 mmol inorganic phosphorus infused over 6-8 hr	i.v.: minutes p.o.: delayed	i.v.: 12-24 hr and may last up to one week	i.v.: tetany, convulsions, metastatic calcifications associated with hypocalcemia, renal failure and death; p.o.: rectal: diarrhea, nausea, vomiting	Useful in chronic management of mild disease (serum calcium < 11 mg/dL) with no renal abnormality; i.v. route not recommended for acute hypercalcemic crisis due to high risk of toxicity
Dialysis	Removal of calcium	Hemodialysis or peritoneal dialysis	Immediately		Complications of dialysis	Temporary hypocalcemic effect with the calcium rebounding rapidly after cessation of dialysis

The primary use of oral phosphates is in the outpatient management of patients with hypophosphatemia and mild hypercalcemia. Normalization of serum calcium levels is not the goal because of the risk of soft tissue calcifications. Oral neutral phosphates in doses of 1 to 3 grams daily (in 4 divided doses) have been used chronically to treat mild hyperparathyroidism. Phosphate doses should be adjusted to prevent increases in the calcium phosphate product and minimize the risk of soft tissue calcification. Sodium or potassium phosphate capsules, containing 8 mmol (250 mg) of phosphate, are administered by emptying the capsules and diluting the contents with 75 to 150 mL of water. Diarrhea is the rate-limiting toxicity. Fleets Phospho-Soda can also be used.

Dialysis should be considered in hypercalcemia complicated by renal failure. Peritoneal dialysis and hemodialysis with calcium-free dialysis fluid are equally effective in rapidly removing large quantities of calcium from the blood. Serum calcium levels might be reduced by 0.7 to 3 mmol/L (3 to 12 mg/dL) over 24 to 48 hours. Since phosphate is also removed in dialysis, serum phosphate levels should be monitored after dialysis and supplemented if necessary.

Corticosteroids are not recommended for the treatment of hypercalcemia from primary hyperparathyroidism because of the poor response (16). Similarly, propranolol and cimetidine have not proven to be effective for hypercalcemia due to hyperparathyroidism.

Summary

In selecting an appropriate approach to managing hypercalcemia secondary to hyperparathyroidism, a patient's serum calcium level and clinical status need to be assessed (see Fig. 18.1). All patients with a serum calcium level ≥ 3 mmol/L (12 mg/dL) should be hydrated immediately with intravenous saline. If both the clinical symptoms and hypercalcemia are mild (serum calcium 2.6 to 2.9 mmol/L [10.5 to 11.9 mg/dL]) hydration alone is often sufficient, without the addition of drug therapy. In moderate hypercalcemia (serum calcium 3 to 3.50 mmol/L [12 to 14 mg/dL]) hydration with saline should be followed by a saline diuresis with or without the addition of furosemide, depending on the patient's fluid status. If subsequent serum calcium levels remain above 3 mmol/L (12 mg/dL), pamidronate should be initiated. If the hypercalcemia is severe (serum calcium > 3.5 mmol/L [14 mg/dL]) or the patient is severely symptomatic, a rapidly acting agent, calcitonin, should be given in 1 or 2 doses along with hydration. Concurrently, pamidronate, a slower-acting agent, should be initiated to provide a longer lasting effect. If there are no contraindications such as renal or hepatic dysfunction, thrombocytopenia, or coagulopathy, plicamycin may be more cost-effective than pamidronate. Gallium nitrate might also be substituted for pamidronate if there is no renal impairment or concomitant nephrotoxic drugs. However, gallium nitrate requires a 5-day treatment course and is considerably more expensive than plicamycin or pamidronate. If the patient has marked hypercalcemia but a less urgent reduction in serum calcium is appropriate (e.g., serum calcium > 3.5 mmol/L [14 mg/dL] with mild to moderate symptoms), pamidronate might be started with saline (with or without furosemide) rather than calcitonin. Postmenopausal women should be considered for chronic estrogen therapy provided there are no contraindications. To minimize the risk of endometrial hyperplasia with unopposed estrogen therapy, women with an intact uterus should periodically receive cyclic progestin therapy.

HYPOPARATHYROIDISM

Hypoparathyroidism is an endocrine disorder characterized by decreased secretion or peripheral action of PTH, resulting in hypocalcemia and hyperphosphatemia.

Etiology/Prevalence

The most common cause of hypoparathyroidism is surgical excision or exploration of the anterior neck. In experienced surgical hands, the prevalence of permanent hypoparathyroidism is less than 1% for all thyroid and parathyroid surgeries (17, 18). This risk is increased significantly after subtotal parathyroidectomy for parathyroid hyperplasia (multiple-gland involvement) or after repeated neck surgery for recurrent disease.

Other rare causes include idiopathic hypoparathyroidism (unknown etiology), neonatal hypoparathyroidism, destruction of the parathyroid glands by radiation or metastatic disease, inactive parathyroid hormone, and target organ resistance to PTH (pseudohypoparathyroidism). Functional hypoparathyroidism occurs from severe hypomagnesemia and reverses with magnesium replacement. Because magnesium is required for normal release of PTH and for the action of PTH peripherally, hypocalcemia might persist until the hypomagnesemia is corrected. Some causes of hypomagnesemia include starvation, prolonged intravenous feeding, malabsorption, chronic alcoholism, diuretics, aminoglycosides, and cisplatinum therapy.

Pathogenesis

Deficiency of PTH hormone produces (a) decreased bone resorption, (b) hyperphosphatemia and hypophosphaturia, (c) decreased intestinal absorption of calcium, (d) decreased levels of active 1,25-$(OH)_2$-vitamin D, (e) hypocalcemia and hypercalciuria, and (f) metabolic alkalosis from decreased bicarbonate excretion.

Diagnosis

Hypoparathyroidism should be suspected in the presence of hypocalcemia, hyperphosphatemia, low or undetectable

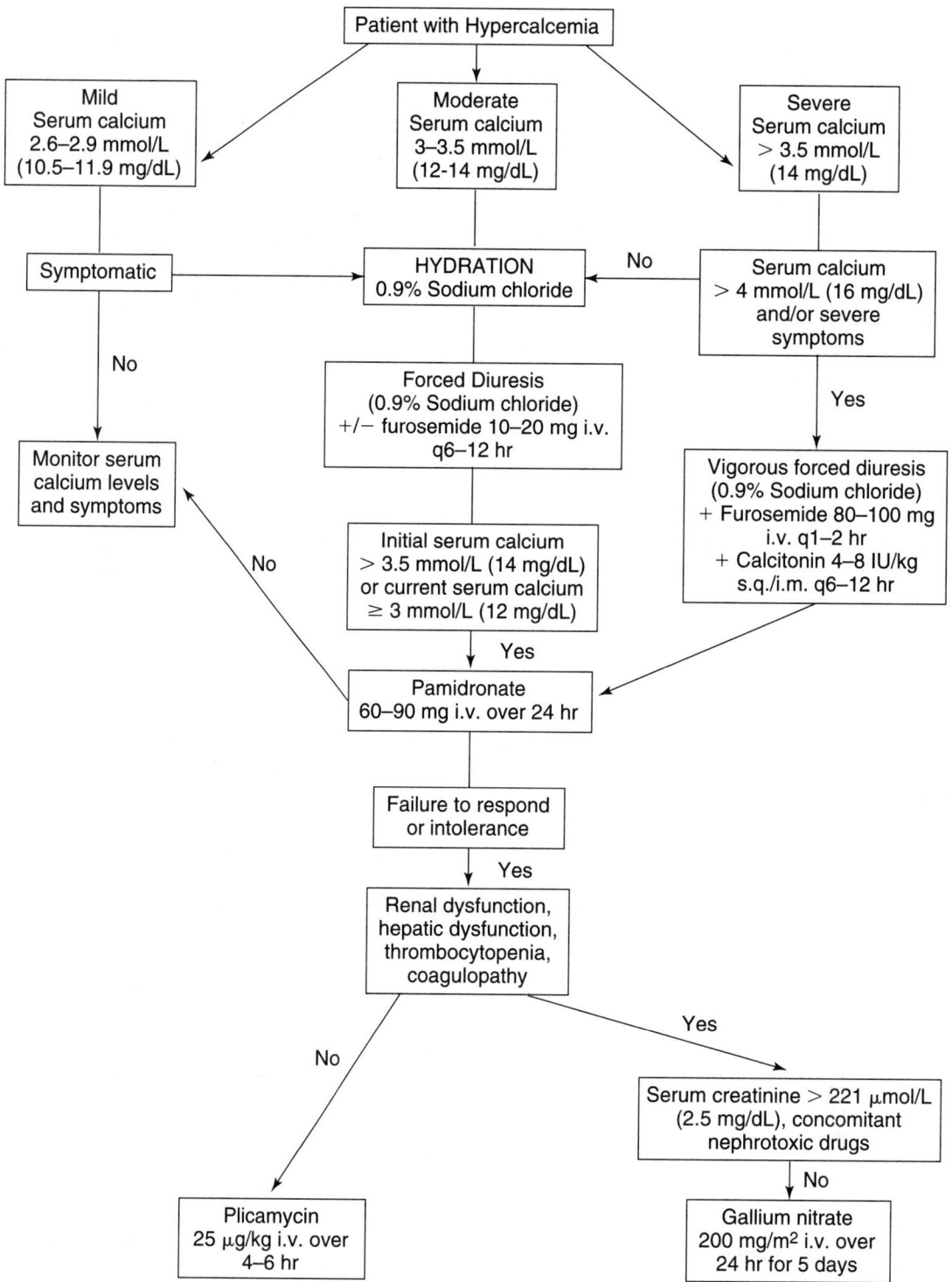

Figure 18.1. Algorithm for the acute medical management of hypercalcemia secondary to hyperparathyroidism.

levels of PTH, and a history of previous neck surgery. However, serum phosphate concentrations might not always be elevated because of dietary restrictions, use of aluminum-containing phosphate binders, or increased mineral uptake by bone. Normal or elevated PTH levels

and hypocalcemia exclude the diagnosis of true hypoparathyroidism and strongly suggest end organ resistance to PTH (pseudohypoparathyroidism) or secretion of inactive PTH hormone. Serum magnesium levels should be checked to exclude the diagnosis of functional hypoparathyroidism. Other causes of hypocalcemia, including drug-induced, should be excluded (see Table 18.4).

The long-term use of anticonvulsants such as phenytoin, phenobarbital, and structurally related compounds increases the hepatic conversion of vitamin D_3 (cholecalciferol) and 25-OH-D_3 (25-hydroxycholecalciferol) to biologically inactive metabolites, causing decreased concentrations of 25-OH-D_3, malabsorption of calcium, hypocalcemia, and osteomalacia. This risk is greater in patients on long-term combination anticonvulsant therapy, in patients with low dietary calcium intake, those with little sunlight exposure, those with diseases predisposing to vitamin D malabsorption, and in blacks because of greater resistance to the irradiating effects of sunlight. Changes in serum calcium, alkaline phosphatase and phosphate levels, and the bony changes of osteomalacia should be closely monitored in these patients.

Another iatrogenic cause of hypocalcemia and osteomalacia is long-term administration of cholestyramine, which binds the bile acids necessary for vitamin D absorption from the intestine. Therapy with higher doses of vitamin D is necessary to overcome the gut inhibitory effects of cholestyramine on vitamin D absorption.

Clinical Findings

The clinical manifestations of hypoparathyroidism are related to the severity and the chronicity of hypocalcemia. Abrupt declines in serum calcium level (e.g., within the first 48 hours after parathyroidectomy) are much more likely to produce hypocalcemic symptoms than gradual reductions of calcium levels. Changes in acid-base status will also affect the symptoms. Alkalosis worsens the hypocalcemia by increasing the plasma protein binding of calcium and decreasing the free ionized fraction. Conversely, acidosis improves the hypocalcemia by increasing

the free, active, ionized calcium levels. The signs and symptoms of hypocalcemia and hypoparathyroidism are presented in Table 18.5.

Treatment of Hypoparathyroidism

Theoretically, the most appropriate therapy for hypoparathyroidism is the administration of PTH. However, no suitable oral preparation is available. An effective alternative to PTH therapy is the administration of calcium supplements and vitamin D in high doses to increase intestinal calcium absorption.

A daily intake of 1 to 2 grams of elemental calcium in 3 or 4 divided doses is usually sufficient to maintain calcium homeostasis in patients with mild hypoparathyroidism. Symptomatic patients with serum calcium levels below 1.87 mmol/L (7.5 mg/dL) often require concomitant therapy with vitamin D to maintain eucalcemia. Therapy directed at reducing serum phosphorus levels is generally not necessary, as normalization of serum calcium levels reduces the renal threshold for phosphorus excretion and lowers serum phosphorus concentrations. However, if serum calcium levels remain low with high serum phosphorus concentrations after a few weeks of calcium supplementation, a phosphate binder such as aluminum hydroxide gel should be added to bind and prevent absorption of dietary phosphorus, in addition to a moderately restricted phosphorus diet to allow increased calcium absorption.

If dietary intake is inadequate, calcium supplementation can be provided effectively through various calcium-containing salts. Calcium gluconate, containing small amounts of calcium, is not very palatable because a large number of tablets must be administered to attain a therapeutic dose. Similarly, calcium chloride is not the best choice because of gastric irritation, occurring from its high calcium content. Calcium carbonate is usually preferred because it is well tolerated, requires fewer tablets to be administered, and is more effective than supplements containing small amounts of calcium (gluconate, lactate). However, calcium carbonate is poorly absorbed in patients with achlorhydria, such as elderly patients, and should be administered with food in this population to facilitate absorption (19). The best-tolerated calcium carbonate preparation (and the most expensive) is Os-Cal, which contains 250 to 500 mg of elemental calcium per tablet. Os-Cal is also available as a combination product of calcium carbonate and cholecalciferol (vitamin D_3). Other calcium carbonate preparations include Tums (200 mg) and Caltrate (600 mg). One gram of calcium is provided by the following salts:

Table 18.4.
Causes of Hypocalcemia

Hypoparathyroidism
    Surgical: postthyroidectomy, postparathyroidectomy, post–neck exploration
    Idiopathic (unknown)
    Neonatal
    Destruction of parathyroids (tumor, radiation)
    Pseudohypoparathyroidism (end-organ resistance to PTH)
    Inactive PTH hormone
Magnesium deficiency (functional hypoparathyroidism)
Acute pancreatitis/malabsorption
Renal failure—secondary hypoparathyroidism
Osteomalacia
Drugs: phenytoin, phenobarbital, cholestyramine (see text); laxative abuse with phosphate enemas; aminoglycoside nephrotoxicity
Hyperphosphatemic states—rhabdomyolysis, EDTA, cytotoxic therapy, malignant hyperthermia
Vitamin D deficiency
Hyperalimentation

Calcium carbonate	2.5 GM (40% calcium)
Calcium chloride	3.7 GM (27% calcium)
Calcium gluconate	11.0 GM (9% calcium)
Calcium lactate	7.7 GM (13% calcium)

Table 18.5.
Clinical Features of Hypocalcemia/Hypoparathyroidism

System	Signs/Symptoms	Complications	Comments
Musculoskeletal	Circumoral and distal numbness and tingling, muscle twitching, hyperreflexia, positive Chvostek's and Trousseau's signs	Tetany: carpopedal spasms, laryngeal stridor, convulsions	Requires emergency treatment with intravenous calcium
Neurologic	Papilledema, increased CSF pressure, basal ganglia calcifications, extrapyramidal symptoms, abnormal EEG	Epilepsy, parkinsonism: complication in 20% of patients with hypoparathyroidism	Improves with eucalcemia, increased sensitivity to dystonic reactions with phenothiazines
Psychiatric	Irritability, paranoia	Depression, psychosis, mental retardation in 20% of children	May improve with eucalcemia
Integument	Dry, scaly skin, coarse, friable dry hair, longitudinal ridges on nails	Exfoliative dermatitis, atopic eczema, psoriasis, increased candida infection	May improve with eucalcemia
Ocular	Visual impairment and opacities of the lens	Lenticular cataracts most common sequelae of hypoparathyroidism	Eucalcemia halts progression of cataracts
Cardiac	Symptoms of heart failure, irregular rhythm, EKG: ↑ Q-T interval, T-wave peaks and inversions	Cardiac dilation	Improves with eucalcemia
Others	Impaired dental development; intestinal malabsorption with steatorrhea		Improves with eucalcemia
Laboratory results	Increased CPK, LDH, ↓ calcium, ↑ phosphate, urinary phosphate low, urinary calcium low to absent, PTH low		

Constipation is a potential problem with all calcium supplements and should be managed.

Vitamin D should be started for hypocalcemic symptoms as soon as possible. The selection of an appropriate vitamin D preparation depends on the cause of the hypocalcemia, cost, onset of action, metabolism, and duration of toxicity after discontinuation (see Table 18.6) (20-21). The newer vitamin D_3 preparations are biologically active and superior to vitamin D_2 in terms of rapidity of onset and offset of action, but they are also more expensive. They should be reserved for difficult-to-manage patients and those with low serum levels of 1,25-$(OH)_2D_3$ (i.e. those with hypoparathyroidism or renal osteodystrophy).

A review of vitamin D metabolism is depicted in Figure 18.2. The generic term *vitamin D* refers to dietary ergocalciferol (vitamin D_2) and cholecalciferol (vitamin D_3). Cholecalciferol is produced in the skin after ultraviolet sunlight exposure. Ergocalciferol is absorbed from the jejunum from dietary sources and undergoes metabolism like cholecalciferol. One milligram of vitamin D_2 is equal to 40,000 IU (20). The active form of vitamin D is 1,25-dihydroxy-vitamin D (1,25-$[OH]_2D$), which is activated in the kidney by the 1-α-hydroxylase enzyme after hepatic 25-hydroxylation. Because parathyroid hormone and hypophosphatemia stimulate activity of this renal

hydroxylase enzyme, a suitable vitamin D preparation in patients with hypoparathyroidism would be one already possessing the 1-α-hydroxyl group (e.g., DHT [dihydrotachysterol] or calcitriol). DHT still requires 25-hydroxylation by the liver and hence should be avoided in hepatic disease. Conversely, in anticonvulsant-induced vitamin D deficiency where there is a decrease in circulating 25-hydroxy-vitamin D (25-[OH]D) but normal levels of active 1,25-dihydroxy-vitamin D, the most appropriate preparation would be calcifediol (25-[OH]D_3).

Vitamin D_2 is commonly used in the treatment of hypoparathyroidism because it is the least expensive of all the preparations. However, because of its slow onset of action, its long duration of action after discontinuation, and the risk of persistent hypercalcemia, DHT or calcitriol might be preferred. Vitamin D_2 therapy can be initiated with 25,000 to 50,000 units/day and then gradually increased to maintenance doses of 50,000 to 200,000 units/day after achieving steady-state levels of serum calcium at each dosage level. Maximal effects on serum calcium are usually achieved in 4 to 6 weeks, but can take up to 12 weeks. DHT is often preferred over vitamin D_2 because the time to maximal effect is faster than with vitamin D_2 (1 to 2 weeks) and it rapidly dissipates in cases of inadvertent overdose. The initial dose of DHT is 0.8 to 2.5 mg daily for several days, then a maintenance dose of

Table 18.6.
Comparison of Vitamin D Preparations

Vitamin D Preparation	Abbreviation	Brand Name	Dose	Characteristics	Activity	Comments
Calciferol Ergocalciferol Caps 10,000 units 25,000 units 50,000 units Liquid 8,000 IU/mL	Vitamin D_2	Calciferol; Drisdol; Deltalin	Initial: 25–50,000 units/day Maint: 50–200,000 units/day 1 mg = 40,000 units 3 mg = 120,000 units	Restores normocalcemia in 4–8 wk; maximal effects in 4–12 wk; long $t_{1/2}$; slow elimination; persists 6–18 wk after cessation	Biologically inactive; requires activation by hepatic 25-hydroxylatin and by renal 1-α-hydroxylase	Least expensive; requires bile salts for complete absorption in gut; poor shelf-life stability
Dihydrotachysterol Tabs/Caps 125 µg Tabs 200 µg 400 µg Solution 0.25 mg/mL or 0.2 mg/mL	DHT	Hytakerol	Initial: 0.8–2.5 mg/day Maint: 0.2–1 mg/day	Restores normocalcemia in 1–2 wk; maximal effect in 1–2 wk; persists 1–3 wk after cessation	Requires only hepatic 25-hydroxylation for activation; contains 1-α-hydroxyl group so no kidney activation necessary	Three times more potent than vitamin D_2; main action is to increase calcium absorption; calcium supplementation recommended; more effective in chronic renal failure and hypoparathyroidism than vitamin D_2
Calcifediol (25-hydroxy-vitamin D_3) Caps 20 µg 50 µg	25(OH)D_3	Calderol	50–100 µg/day	Restores normocalcemia in 2–4 wk; persists 4–12 wk after cessation	Requires kidney for bioactivation	1.5 times as potent as vitamin D_2; preparation of choice in deficiency associated with anticonvulsant therapy, intestinal malabsorption, and hepatobiliary disease; also effective in renal osteodystrophy; therapeutic blood level monitoring available
Calcitriol (1,25-dihydroxy-vitamin D_3) Caps 0.25 µg 0.5 µg	1,25(OH)$_2$$D_3$	Rocaltrol	Initial: 0.25 µg/day Maint: 0.5–3 µg/day	Restores normocalcemia in 3–7 days; $t_{1/2}$ 2–3 hr; persists 3–7 days after cessation	Active	Most potent and most expensive preparation available; requires calcium supplementation in hypoparathyroidism; major advantage is rapid onset/duration of effect

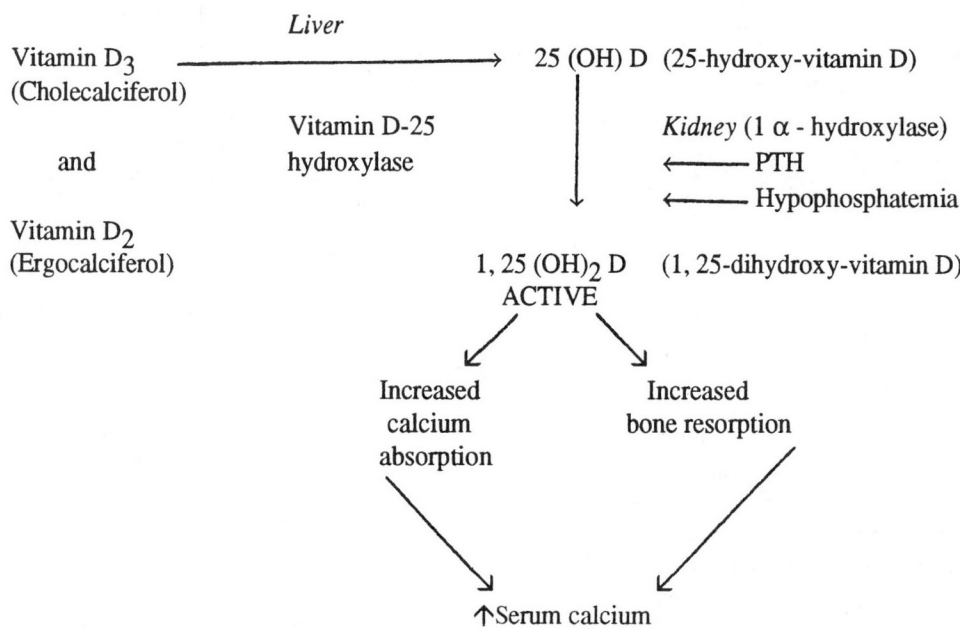

Figure 18.2. Activity and metabolism of vitamin D.

0.2 to 1 mg daily. In order to shorten the time to maximal action, DHT is occasionally initiated with a loading dose of four times the daily maintenance dose for 2 days, followed by twice the daily maintenance dose for 2 days. However, such an approach increases the risk of toxicity, and requires careful monitoring.

Calcitriol is also highly effective in doses of 0.25 μg/day initially, which are then increased as necessary to a maintenance dose of 0.5 to 3 μg daily. Calcitriol exerts its action more rapidly than vitamin D_2, DHT, or calcifediol because it bypasses renal as well as hepatic hydroxylation. Maximal effects with calcitriol are observed within 1 to 3 days, and on discontinuation the effects dissipate over a few days. Doses of all vitamin D preparations should be increased gradually only after maximal effects are achieved to avoid hypercalcemia. Serum calcium levels should ideally be maintained between 2.12 and 2.25 mmol/L (8.5 and 9 mg/dL), leaving a margin for fluctuations. Serum calcium and phosphorus levels should be checked weekly at initiation of vitamin D therapy, then monthly during dosage adjustments and at least every 3 months thereafter. Patients should be monitored carefully for early signs of vitamin D intoxication, which include lassitude, anorexia, thirst, constipation, and bone pain. Frequent adjustments in vitamin D doses might be necessary to prevent vitamin D intoxication. Higher doses of vitamin D are required for patients on anticonvulsants, oral contraceptives, and steroids. The effect of anticonvulsants on vitamin D metabolism is explained above. Estrogens cause a decrease in serum calcium by preventing bone resorption. Glucocorticoids reduce intestinal absorption of calcium by antago-

nizing vitamin D, decrease bone resorption by antagonizing PTH, and reduce renal tubular absorption of calcium. Patients requiring massive blood transfusions might require greater calcium replacements since the excess citrate added to each unit of blood for anticoagulation purposes has a very high affinity for calcium (22).

Toxicities of all preparations of vitamin D include hypercalcemia, hypercalciuria, and nephrolithiasis, which can be prevented by close monthly monitoring of serum calcium, phosphorus, and alkaline phosphatase levels. Availability of $25(OH)D_3$ and $1,25(OH)_2D_3$ assays in more specialized centers might help prevent toxicity from hypercalcemia. Calcitriol has been associated with deterioration of renal function in some patients with previously stable renal function. However, prospective, long-term studies have not confirmed these reports (23).

Thiazide diuretics and sodium restriction have been shown to reduce urinary calcium excretion in patients with mild hypocalcemia, allowing calcium and vitamin D supplementation to be reduced. Serum calcium levels should be carefully monitored. This therapy might also protect against the development of kidney stones, a potential complication of the long-term management of hypoparathyroidism. Long-term studies are necessary to assess the role of this approach. Patients with hypoparathyroidism might be more sensitive to the calciuretic effects of loop diuretics such as furosemide, and these should be avoided.

Parathyroid autografts or allografts have been successfully transplanted in a number of patients when accidental removal or devascularization of the entire parathyroid glands has occurred during thyroid or parathyroid surgery. Parathyroid tissue is transplanted into the forearm muscles or the sternomastoid muscles. Such patients require calcium supplementation for 4 weeks and then can be weaned off (24).

Severe hypocalcemia complicated by tetany requires emergency treatment with intravenous calcium. After assuring the patient's airway, 10 to 20 mL of calcium gluconate 10% is given slowly (not faster than 10 mL/min) until symptoms are relieved or until the serum calcium level increases above 1.87 mmol/L (7.5 mg/dL). A continuous effect can be maintained by infusing 10 to 50 mL of 10% calcium gluconate in 1 liter of normal saline over 24 hours. The plasma calcium level should increase by approximately 0.5 mg/dL/100 mg calcium load per 24 hours. Too-vigorous treatment of the tetany can cause irreversible tissue calcifications. Hypomagnesemia should be corrected and oral calcium and vitamin D supplements started immediately. Drugs that exacerbate hypocalcemia (e.g., loop diuretics) should be avoided. Phenothiazines should be used cautiously because dystonic reactions can occur. Also, inadvertent hypercalcemia can increase the risk of digitalis toxicity in patients receiving digoxin, and such patients require ECG monitoring while receiving intravenous calcium therapy.

Prognosis

The prognosis is excellent. Improvement of most symptoms can be expected with restoration of normal serum calcium levels. In surgery-associated hypoparathyroidism, vitamin D therapy is usually withdrawn after 6 to 8 weeks of treatment to assess whether the patient is able to maintain a normocalcemic state. Such an approach minimizes the risk of vitamin D intoxication.

REFERENCES

1. Consensus Development Conference Panel. Diagnosis and management of asymptomatic primary hyperparathyroidism: consensus development conference statement. Ann Intern Med 114:593–597, 1991.
2. Heath DA, Heath EM. Conservative management of primary hyperparathyroidism. J Bone Min Res 6(suppl 2):S117–S120, 1991.
3. Fischer JA. Asymptomatic and symptomatic primary hyperparathyroidism. Clin Invest 71:505–518, 1993.
4. Baumann DS, Wells SA. Parathyroid autotransplantation. Surgery 113:130–133, 1993.
5. Bilezikian JP. Management of hypercalcemia. J Clin Endocrinol Metab 77:1445–1449, 1993.
6. Nussbaum SR. Pathophysiology and management of severe hypercalcemia. Endocrinol Metab Clin North Am 22:343–362, 1993.
7. Suki WN, Yium JJ, Von Minden M, et al. Acute treatment of hypercalcemia with furosemide. N Engl J Med 283:836–840, 1970.
8. Hall TG, Burns Schaiff RA. Update on the medical management of hypercalcemia of malignancy. Clin Pharm 12:117–125, 1993.
9. Ralston SH, Gallacher SJ, Patel U, et al. Comparison of three intravenous bisphosphonates in cancer-associated hypercalcemia. Lancet 2:1180–1182, 1989.
10. Gucalp R, Ritch P, Wiernik PH, et al. Comparative study of pamidronate disodium in the treatment of cancer-related hypercalcemia. J Clin Oncol 10:134–142, 1992.
11. Fatemi S, Singer FR, Rude RK. Effect of salmon calcitonin and etidronate on hypercalcemia of malignancy. Calcif Tissue Int 292:1549–1550, 1992.
12. Warrell RP Jr, Israel R, Frisone M, et al. Gallium nitrate for acute treatment of cancer-related hypercalcemia: a randomized, double-blind comparison to calcitonin. Ann Intern Med 108:669–674, 1988.
13. Warrell RP Jr, Murphy WK, Schulman P, et al. A randomized double-blind study of gallium nitrate compared with etidronate for acute control of cancer-related hypercalcemia. Clin Oncol 9:1467–1475, 1991.
14. Wishart J, Horowitz M, Need AG, et al. Treatment of postmenopausal hyperparathyroidism with norethindrone. Long term effects on forearm mineral content. Arch Intern Med 150:1951–1953, 1990.
15. Marcus R. Estrogens and progestins in the management of primary hyperparathyroidism. J Bone Min Res 6(suppl 2):S1–S165, 1991.
16. Burns Schaiff RA, Hall TG, Bar RS. Medical treatment of hypercalcemia. Clin Pharm 8:108–121, 1989.
17. Weber CA, Clark OH. Surgery for thyroid disease. Med Clin North Am 69:1097–1115, 1985.
18. Clark OH, Duh QY. Primary hyperparathyroidism. A surgical perspective. Endocrinol Metab Clin North Am 18:701–713, 1989.
19. Recker RR. Calcium absorption and achlorhydria. N Engl J Med 313:70–73, 1985.
20. Kumar R, Riggs BL. Series on pharmacology in practice. Vitamin D in the therapy of disorders of calcium and phosphorus metabolism. Mayo Clin Proc 56:327–333, 1981.
21. Haussler MR, Cordy PE. Metabolites and analogues of vitamin D. Which for what? JAMA 247:841–844, 1982.
22. Netterville JL, Aly A, Ossoff RH. Evaluation and treatment of complications of thyroid and parathyroid surgery. Otolaryngol Clin North Am 23:529–552, 1990.
23. Halabe A, Arie R, Mimran D, et al. Hypoparathyroidism—a long term experience with 1α-vitamin D3 therapy. Clin Endocrin 40:303–307, 1994.
24. Shaha AR, Burnett C, Jaffe BM. Parathyroid autotransplantation during thyroid surgery. J Surg Oncol 46:21–24, 1991.

CHAPTER 19

DIABETES MELLITUS

JOHN R. WHITE, Jr, and R. KEITH CAMPBELL

Diabetes mellitus was recognized as early as 1500 B.C. by Egyptian physicians, who described a disease associated with "the passage of much urine." The term "diabetes" (the Greek word for siphon) was coined by the Greek physician Aretaeus the Cappadocian around A.D. 2. Aretaeus noticed that patients with diabetes had a disease that caused the siphoning of the structural components of the body into the urine ("a melting down of the flesh and limbs into urine"). Although it was known for centuries that the urine of patients with diabetes was sweet, it was not until 1674 that a physician named Willis coined the term "diabetes mellitus" (from the Greek word for honey).

Diabetes mellitus is a complex syndrome that affects multiple organ systems. There is still much to be learned about diabetes mellitus; however, recent pharmacologic and surgical advances have enhanced both the understanding and treatment of this syndrome. The impact of these changes on the diabetic patient has been dramatic. A recent landmark study, The Diabetes Control and Complications Trial, demonstrated conclusively that the level of glycemic control is closely correlated with the appearance and progression of retinopathy, nephropathy, and neuropathy in patients with type I diabetes (1). The process of self-monitoring of blood glucose, in combination with better education programs and new treatment protocols, has allowed strict glycemic control to be realized in many patients. This overall trend toward euglycemic control has been the most significant change in the treatment of diabetes since the discovery of insulin. Other advances in the treatment of the disease include the following:

1. A major research initiative evaluating a method for the prevention of type I diabetes (the National Institutes of Health Study entitled "Diabetes Prevention Trial I" (DPT-1) (2).
2. Funding and initiation of long-term studies to review the benefits of tight control in patients with type II diabetes (3, 4).
3. Novel methods for self-monitoring of blood glucose that are very user-friendly (for example, that require <50 µL of blood, do not require strip wiping or timing).
4. Greater emphasis on patient self-monitoring.
5. The use of extremely pure human insulins.
6. The introduction of novel insulin molecules with improved pharmacokinetic profiles (such as the monomeric insulin LisPro).
7. Food and Drug Administration (FDA) approval of the biguanide metformin, a drug that will offer a new treatment option for patients with type II diabetes.

A thorough, positive education program for the diabetic patient that covers the disease, medication, blood and urine testing, and hygiene is a major component of diabetes management. Studies have demonstrated that poor control of diabetes is often the result of medication error, misinterpretation of test results, and ignorance of the disease (5). Patient education is extremely important for the patient with diabetes. Health care providers must explain the importance of diet control and the food exchange stystem. Patients need to develop a positive attitude, learn how to perform tests to monitor control, learn how to inject insulin, and keep records of the factors that affect diabetic control. Health care providers need to answer patient questions about the disease, blood testing, urine testing, drug therapy, diet products, and foot care and reinforce the information that other members of the team provide. The pharmacist can also monitor the course of diabetic patients. Since diabetic patients see pharmacists more often than they see any other health professional, the pharmacist is in a unique position to have a significant effect on the treatment of diabetic patients. Pharmacists who want to help their diabetic patients not only need to understand pharmacologic facts but also must become competent in selecting, initiating, and individualizing drug therapy for the various types of diabetic patients. Thus, the pharmacist performs three significant functions: referral, monitoring of therapy, and education.

DEFINITION

It is difficult to devise a simple definition of diabetes mellitus because it is a spectrum of conditions that display hyperglycemia as a common symptom. Until recently, diabetes was considered to be a single disease. It is now clear that diabetes is a heterogeneous group of disorders that are elicited secondary to various genetic predispositions and precipitating factors. Not only does insulin-dependent (type I) diabetes mellitus (IDDM) differ from non-insulin-dependent (type II) diabetes mellitus (NIDDM), but there appears to be heterogeneity within each of these two types (6). Diabetes is a chronic disease that is characterized by disorders in carbohydrate (and associated fat and protein) metabolism because of an absolute or relative deficiency in the action of insulin and possibly abnormally high amounts of glucagon and other insulin-antagonizing substances such as growth hormone, sympathomimetic amines, and corticosteroids (the so-called counterregulatory hormones). Insulin secretion in patients with diabetes may be normal or totally deficient.

Properly classifying the patient with diabetes into one of several categories in which hyperglycemia is a clinical finding is critical in developing a patient-specific treatment regimen. In the past, patients with diabetes have been classified in numerous ways, including the degree of glucose tolerance, age of onset (juvenile or adult), body weight, degree of hyperglycemia or glucosuria or both, susceptibility to ketoacidosis, insulin dependency, degree of severity and stability, treatment priority, presence or absence of hypertension, lipid profile variance, and the presence or absence of large and small blood vessel lesions.

A classification of diabetes and other categories of glucose intolerance based on contemporary knowledge of this heterogeneous syndrome was developed by the National Diabetes Data Group in 1980 to ensure consistency in treatment (7). Table 19.1 summarizes the new classification system and compares it to old methods as well

as listing the therapy that is recommended for each classification.

The two major clinical presentations of diabetes are type II maturity-onset and type I juvenile-onset types. Eighty percent of patients with diabetes are identified after the age of 35 and are of the obese, maturity-onset type (8). They retain some pancreatic function, and the diabetes may be controlled by diet or by diet plus an oral hypoglycemic agent. Insulin may be required in 20 to 30% of cases, although this type of patient rarely develops ketoacidosis (8). Many type II diabetic patients have normal or high levels of insulin, and sluggish insulin secretion in response to glucose and a relative tissue resistance to insulin due to a low number of insulin receptors may be responsible for the symptoms. Ten percent of patients with diabetes have a type II stable, nonobese, maturity-onset type; 5% have brittle, adult-onset diabetes, which more closely resembles the juvenile-onset presentation. Insulin-dependent (type I) diabetes accounts

Table 19.1.
Classification and Therapy of Diabetes

Current Terminology	Others	Diet	Exercise	Insulin	Oral Hypoglycemic	Education
Type I: insulin-dependent diabetes mellitus (IDDM)	Juvenile onset (JOD) Youth onset (YOD) Ketosis prone Brittle	1. Regular meal schedule 2. Restrict "simple sugars" 3. No restriction of total carbohydrate (i.e., 50–60% of total calories) 4. Limited fats (i.e., 22% of total calories) 5. Avoid fad diets 6. Increase fiber	Yes	Yes	No	Yes
Type II: non-insulin-dependent diabetes mellitus (NIDDM) A. Obese B. Normal weight	Adult onset (AOD) Maturity onset (MOD) Ketosis resistant	Obese 1. Hypocaloric intake 2. Limit fats Nonobese: 1. Eucaloric intake 2. Restrict "simple sugars" 3. Limit fats 4. Increase fiber 5. Beware of "dietetic"	Yes	Not usually	Individualize	Yes
Diabetes associated with other conditions Secondary diabetes	Hyperglycemia secondary to pancreatic disease, endocrine disease, drug or chemicals, certain genetic syndromes	Change if underlying condition necessitates	Yes	Adjust to correct hyperglycemia	Individualize	Yes
Gestational diabetes (GDM)	Gestational diabetes	1. Avoid simple sugars 2. Avoid excessive weight gain	Yes	Use to tightly control diabetes	No	Yes
Impaired glucose tolerance (IGT)	Asymptomatic diabetes Chemical diabetes Borderline diabetes Latent diabetes	Avoid extra calories; hypocaloric intake if overweight, or usual diabetic diet	Yes	Not usually	No	No

Table 19.2.
Distinguishing Features of Two Major Types of Diabetes Mellitus

	Insulin-Dependent Type I (IDDM)	Non-Insulin-Dependent Type II (NIDDM)
Age of onset	Usually, but not always, during childhood or puberty	Frequently over 35
Type of onset	Abrupt	Usually gradual
Prevalence	0.5%	5–6%
Incidence	<10–15%	>75%
Family history of diabetes	Infrequently positive	Commonly positive
Primary cause	Pancreatic β-cell deficiency	End organ (insulin receptors) unresponsiveness to insulin action
Nutritional status at time of onset	Usually undernourished	Usually obese
Postglucose plasma or serum insulin[a]	Absent	>100 µU/mL at 2 hr
Symptoms	Polydipsia, polyphagia, and polyuria	Maybe none
Hepatomegaly	Rather common	Uncommon
Stability	Blood sugar fluctuates widely in response to small changes in insulin dose, exercise, and infection	Blood sugar fluctuations are less marked
Etiology	Unknown; possible factors include: *Inheritance:* associated with specific HLA tissue types but only 40–50% concordance in twins *Autoimmune disease:* 50–80% circulating islet cell antibodies *Viral infections:* Coxsackie, mumps, influenza	Unknown; possible factors include: *Inheritance:* 95–100% concordance in twins but not associated with specific HLA tissue types *Autoimmune disease:* negative <10% circulating islet cell antibodies No evidence for viral infections
Proneness to ketosis	Frequent, especially if treatment program is insufficient in food and/or insulin	Uncommon except in the presence of unusual stress or moderate to severe sepsis
Insulin defect	Defect in secretion; secretion is impaired early in disease; secretion may be totally absent late in disease	*Insulin deficiency:* Most patients show failure of insulin secretion to keep pace with inordinate demands engendered by obesity; may appear initially as failure to respond to glucose alone, suggesting an impairment in the glucoreceptor of the pancreatic β cell *Insulin resistance:* Some patients have a defect in tissue responsiveness to insulin and evidence of hyperinsulinemia; in such patients, insulin resistance may be mediated by decreased number of insulin receptors in target cells
Plasma insulin (endogenous)	Negligible to zero	Plasma insulin response may be either adequate but delayed, so postprandial hypoglycemia may be present when diabetes is discovered or may be diminished, but not absent
Vascular complications of diabetes and degenerative changes	Infrequent until diabetes has been present for >5 years	Frequent
Usual causes of death	Degenerative complications in target organs (e.g., renal failure due to diabetic nephropathy)	Accelerated atherosclerosis (e.g., myocardial infarction); to a lesser extent, microangiopathic changes in target tissues (e.g., renal failure)
Diet	Mandatory in all patients	If diet is used fully, hypoglycemic drug therapy may not be needed
Insulin	Necessary for all patients	Necessary for 20–30% of patients
Oral agents	Rarely efficacious	Efficacious

[a]Normal response is between 50 and 135 µU/mL at 60 min and less than 100 µU/mL at 120 min after 100 g of oral glucose.

for only 15 to 20% of diabetes cases (8). Patients with this type of diabetes have no pancreatic function and require insulin to sustain life. The blood glucose levels of type I diabetic patients may fluctuate widely despite treatment, and these patients are more prone to ketosis than are the type II diabetic patients. Table 19.2 compares the distinguishing features of the two major clinical types of diabetes.

PREVALENCE

Diabetes mellitus and its complications are now the third leading cause of death in the United States, accounting for 300,000 lives each year (9). Patients who are diagnosed with diabetes include 2.8% of the U.S. population but account for 5.8% of total personal health care expenditures in 1992 (10). Seven to eight percent of hospital admissions are due to diabetes. A new case of diabetes is diagnosed every 60 seconds, and the chance of developing diabetes doubles with every 20% of excess weight and every decade of life.

Diabetes is the leading cause of new cases of blindness; diabetic patients are 25 times more prone to blindness than are nondiabetic patients. Diabetic patients are 17 times more prone to kidney disease, and approximately half of insulin-dependent diabetic patients will succumb to end-stage renal disease (ESRD) (9). Diabetes is the leading cause of ESRD requiring chronic hemodialysis and renal transplantations. Macroangiopathy occurs prematurely and progresses at an accelerated rate in patients with diabetes (responsible for 75% of deaths of patients with non-insulin-dependent diabetes). Diabetic patients are twice as prone to heart disease and stroke as are nondiabetic patients and are 25 times more prone to developing gangrene. Diabetes is the leading cause of nontraumatic amputations in the United States. Up to 50% of men with diabetes of long duration are sexually impotent.

Overall, the economic cost of diabetes more than quadrupled over the 5-year period between 1987 and 1992, increasing from 20 billion dollars to 92 billion dollars (10). As an example of the cost of diabetic complications, approximately one-third of all cases of ESRD in the United States are the result of diabetes (11). The U.S. Renal Data System reported in 1993 that the cost of medical care for patients with ESRD in the United States was about 7.2 billion dollars (12). If we extrapolate from this data, it is reasonable to suggest that the cost of diabetes-induced ESRD in the United States is between 2 and 3 billion dollars per year.

ETIOLOGY

Numerous factors have been associated with the development of diabetes. Table 19.3 summarizes some of the factors that have been linked to the development of diabetes. The etiology of diabetes is far from completely understood.

One factor that seems to be common to all of the types of diabetes is stress. Emotional stress and physiologic stress may contribute as precipitating factors in the development of diabetes. With this in mind, it is interesting to note that more initial presentations of the disease are observed in North America during the winter months.

Table 19.3.
Etiologic Factors Associated with Diabetes Mellitus

Obesity
Increasing age
Heredity
Emotional stress
Autoimmune β cell damage
Endocrine diseases (e.g., Cushing's disease)
Viral stress decreasing β cells
Vasculitis in tissue highly perfused with capillaries (eye, kidney, etc.)
Insulin receptor defects
Drugs (e.g., cortisone, estrogen, thyroid, phenytoin, diazoxide, thiazide diuretics)
Post-insulin-receptor defects

Type I diabetic patients have a defect in pancreatic β-cell function that may be attributed to several causes. Genetic defects in production of certain macromolecules may interfere with proper insulin synthesis, packaging, or release, or the β cells may not recognize glucose signals or replicate normally. Extrinsic factors that affect β-cell function include damage caused by viruses such as mumps or Coxsackie B4, by destructive cytotoxins and antibodies released by sensitized lymphocytes, or by autodigestion in the course of an inflammatory disorder involving the adjacent exocrine pancreas.

Genetic susceptibility to insulin-dependent diabetes appears to be linked to two genes on chromosome 6. These genes control the production of human lymphocyte antigens (HLA) DR3 and DR4 (8, 13). Individuals with either or both of these antigens have a greater chance of developing diabetes than does the individual who lacks the antigen(s). Ninety-five percent of patients with type I diabetes have one or both of these antigens. However, 40% of patients without diabetes possess one or both of these antigens. Conversely, patients who carry HLA-DQA1°0102 or HLA-DQB1°0602 seem to be protected from the development of IDDM (2).

The reaction of these predisposed individuals to certain environmental stimuli (β-cell cytotoxic virus or chemicals) is abnormal and leads to β-cell destruction directly, through "autoimmune mechanisms," or because of lack of regeneration of the β cell after damage (13). This hypothesis is being vigorously studied. In fact the majority of patients who develop IDDM have measurable circulating antibodies, islet cell antibody (ICA), and insulin autoantibodies (IAA) before the development of overt IDDM (14). Additionally, before the development of overt diabetes, patients have an impairment in insulin response to glucose challenge. The insulin response is less than normal but is sufficient to maintain euglycemia until the disease progresses to the overt stage (15).

Many type II diabetic patients have excess insulin and are obese. The hyperinsulinism and insulin resistance may be correlated with a decrease in insulin receptors. Studies have also shown that the tissues of patients with type II diabetes exhibit reduced insulin binding. A reduced number of insulin receptors and the problem of insulin binding are major factors in the etiology of non-insulin-dependent diabetes (15).

Blood glucose levels can be elevated by a variety of mechanisms. Some diabetic patients may have elevated blood glucose because of an excess of glucagon. Others can have a defect in somatostatin or an excess of growth hormone, cortisol, epinephrine, or other hormones that influence the regulation of blood glucose. Numerous drugs have also been implicated in increasing blood glucose levels, including chlorthalidone, corticosteroids, diazoxide, phenytoin, glucagon, caffeine, cyclophosphamide, lithium, epinephrine and other catecholamines, estrogens, ethacrynic acid, furosemide, lithium, nicotinic acid, thiazide diuretics, thyroid preparations, and sugar-containing medications (16). Other drugs may cause lower-than-normal blood glucose levels, including anabolic steroids, sulfonylureas, disopyramide, ethanol, fenfluramine, monoamine oxidase inhibitors, propranolol, and large doses of salicylates (16).

In summary, an individual's blood glucose levels can be elevated via numerous mechanisms. There can be a decrease in the amount of insulin produced or released, a defect in an individual's ability to sense glucose and respond by releasing insulin, and a genetic mutation of the structure of insulin. Insulin antibodies can reduce the effectiveness of insulin. There can be decreased insulin receptor affinity, as well as a decrease in the actual number of receptors, or a post-insulin-receptor defect, and there are numerous hormones and chemicals that can affect blood glucose levels.

PATHOPHYSIOLOGY AND SYMPTOMS

As with the etiology of diabetes, there is still a great deal that must be learned about the specific cellular biochemical mechanisms that are involved in the pathophysiology of diabetes. The consequences of a lack of insulin or a lack of effect of insulin are well known. The consequences of high blood glucose levels may be subcategorized into acute and chronic effects. It should also be noted that the symptoms and consequences differ between patients with type I and type II diabetes. The complex cellular effects of insulin provide numerous clues as to the type of intervention that should be implemented to improve the prognosis of a diabetic patient.

NORMAL INSULIN PRODUCTION AND EFFECTS

Insulin is a protein that is composed of 51 amino acids in two chains (A and B chains) connected by two disulfide bonds. Insulin is synthesized and stored in the β-cells of the islets of Langerhans, which are located in the pancreas. The

pancreas produces a parent protein that is referred to as preproinsulin. Preproinsulin is cleaved to form a smaller protein: proinsulin. Proinsulin is cleaved to form equimolar amounts of C-peptide and insulin (8). The normal human pancreas contains approximately 200 units of insulin. A basal amount of insulin is secreted continuously at a rate of approximately 0.5 to 1.0 unit/hr. Insulin is also released in response to blood glucose levels of 100 mg/dL or greater. The average daily insulin secretory rate in the adult is 25 to 50 units/day. Insulin is cleared metabolically by the liver, peripheral tissues, and the kidney. Insulin follows first-order elimination kinetics. The serum half-life of insulin is approximately 4 to 5 min.

The important metabolic sites that are sensitive to insulin include the liver, where glycogen is synthesized, stored, and broken down; skeletal muscle, where glucose oxidation produces energy; and adipose tissue, where glucose may be converted to fatty acids, glyceryl phosphate, and triglycerides. Insulin affects the metabolism of carbohydrates, protein, and lipids (17).

CARBOHYDRATE METABOLISM

In the nondiabetic patient, insulin acts in concert with glucagon, somatostatin, growth hormone, corticosteroids, epinephrine, and parasympathetic intervention to maintain blood glucose between 40 and 160 mg/dL at all times. At least three types of cells have been identified in the islets of Langerhans of the normal human pancreas. The α cells produce glucagon, which acts to increase blood glucose levels. The β cells are responsible for producing, storing, and releasing insulin. The δ cells produce a tetradecapeptide called somatostatin. Somatostatin inhibits both insulin and glucagon secretion and suppresses growth hormone (17). Its primary effect is to suppress glucagon, resulting in a fall in blood glucose levels. This effect persists for only 60 to 120 min.

These three cell types work in conjunction with each other to maintain euglycemic balance. Ingestion of a carbohydrate load by a person without diabetes results in a prompt increase in the amount of insulin that is released into the blood. At the same time there is a decrease in plasma glucagon. Glucagon is released in response to low blood glucose levels and the ingestion of protein. The release of glucagon stimulates insulin secretion; insulin in turn inhibits the release of glucagon.

The presence of insulin favors the uptake and use of glucose by insulin-sensitive sites. In the skeletal muscle, glucose uptake and subsequent energy production are increased. In the liver, glucose uptake and the formation of glycogen are increased in the presence of insulin.

A minimum blood glucose level of 40 mg/dL is required to provide adequate fuel for the brain, which can use only glucose as fuel and does not depend on the presence of insulin for its utilization. Glucose spills into the urine, resulting in energy and water loss, when blood glucose levels exceed the renal threshold of the kidneys (180 mg/dL).

PROTEIN METABOLISM

The presence of insulin favors the production of structural proteins from constituent amino acids. When glucose is present intracellularly in sufficient quantities for needed energy production, most structural proteins will retain their integrity. In the absence of insulin the production of structural proteins is not favored, and intracellular glucose levels are insufficient to match energy demands. In an attempt to produce energy, skeletal muscle will convert its structural proteins to constituent amino acids. The liberated amino acids are transported to the liver, where they are converted to glucose via gluconeogenesis. Hepatic glucose enters the blood but is not taken up by needed

tissue because of an insulin deficiency. Thus, hyperglycemia is escalated, and structural proteins are wasted.

FAT METABOLISM

The presence of insulin favors the production of triglycerides from free fatty acids. When insulin deficiency causes an energy deficit, free fatty acids are liberated from storage as triglycerides. The free fatty acids are oxidized to form β-hydroxybutyric acid, acetoacetic acid, and acetone. β-Hydroxybutyric acid may be used as an energy source, but in the absence of insulin the production of these keto acids will eventually be greater than their metabolism and excretion. If insulin is not given to the patient, metabolic ketoacidosis will ensue. The keto acids will cause the pH to decline, and diuresis secondary to the elimination of ketones and glucose will cause dehydration. The body's neutralizing factors will eventually be depleted, and the patient will continue to deteriorate to the point of coma and

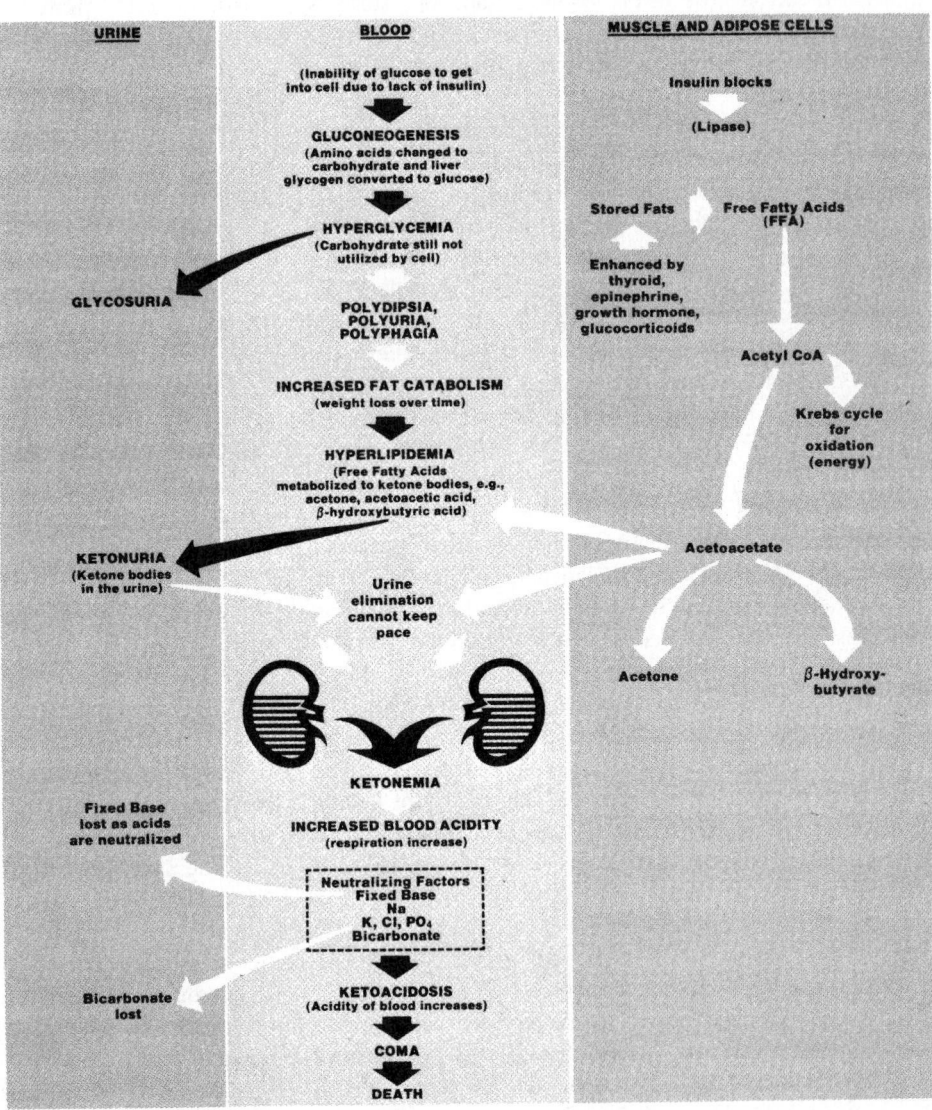

Figure 19.1. Clinical manifestations of a complete lack of insulin.

possibly death. Figure 19.1 shows the clinical manifestations in an untreated type I diabetic who is insulinopenic (completely lacks insulin).

METABOLISM IN TYPE II PATIENTS

In patients with type II diabetes the problem is not due to a lack of insulin but to ineffectiveness of insulin (18). Usually, use of glucose and circulating levels of insulin is sufficient to avoid ketoacidosis. However, glucose does accumulate in the blood and can reach very high levels, resulting in a syndrome called diabetic nonketotic hyperosmolar coma. Both ketoacidosis and hyperosmolar coma are treated by first determining the cause of the problem, then giving fluids and electrolytes and low doses of insulin either intravenously or intramuscularly. Close monitoring of electrolytes, pH, acid-base, and glucose is required to avoid complications.

In summary, in the fed state, a high insulin level is necessary for incorporation of glucose into liver and muscle glycogen, for muscle to consume glucose for energy needs, for both liver and adipose tissue to make fatty acids from glucose, for amino acids to be incorporated into muscle protein, for circulating chylomicrons to discharge their fatty acid into adipose tissue, and for these in turn to be reesterified and incorporated into the triglyceride storage droplet in the middle of the cell (18). Thus, in patients who are insulinopenic (type I), the acute problems affect fat, protein, and carbohydrate metabolism, resulting in high blood glucose and ketone levels. In patients who have ineffective insulin (type II), enough insulin gets into cells to meet the patient's energy requirements, but glucose accumulates in the blood, causing hyperglycemia with relatively minor acute symptoms.

To complicate the picture even further, numerous factors other than a lack of insulin may cause an increase in blood glucose. These include Cushing's disease, pheochromocytoma, aldosteronism, hyperthyroidism, pancreatitis, cirrhosis, pregnancy, emotional stress, infections, and miscellaneous drugs that have been mentioned earlier. One should also keep in mind that there are numerous factors that can decrease blood glucose levels, such as an exogenous insulin excess, nonfasting reactive hypoglycemia, fasting hypoglycemia, and several medications (19).

SYMPTOMS

Type I diabetes usually presents in a rapid fashion, typically with polyuria, polyphagia, polydipsia, weakness, weight loss, dry skin, and often ketoacidosis (30% of all cases of diabetic ketoacidosis occur in previously undiagnosed patients) (20). Type II diabetes is frequently unaccompanied by any symptoms and is often discovered when glucose is found in the urine or when elevated blood sugar is noticed during a routine examination. Careful study of these older, obese diabetic patients sometimes reveals glucosuria, proteinuria, postprandial hyperglycemia, microaneurysms, and even retinal exudates.

Other symptoms of hyperglycemia that are associated with diabetes include blurred vision, tingling, numbness in the feet, slow-healing skin infections, itching, drowsiness, and irritability. Patients with the above symptoms and patients who have a family history of diabetes or are overweight and in the 40- to 65-year-old age group, should be screened closely for hyperglycemia. Monilial infections of the vagina and anus and a history of complications during pregnancy are also warning signs to test for diabetes. The earlier diabetes is diagnosed, the more easily it can be controlled and the better is the long-term prognosis.

LONG-TERM EFFECTS OF HYPERGLYCEMIA

The chronic complications of diabetes include macrovascular disease (peripheral, cerebral, cardiovascular disease), microvascular disease (retinopathy and nephropathy), neuropathy (peripheral and autonomic), foot problems, and others. While the molecular mechanisms leading to chronic complications have not been conclusively delineated, several abnormal pathways have been suggested. Most salient in this list of deleterious biochemical pathways is the production of high concentrations of advanced glycosylation end products (AGE) and sorbitol. While there has been considerable debate about whether the lesions that develop within the diabetic patient's retina, kidneys, nerves, and vascular system are due to a disorder in the structure and function of blood vessels or are a consequence of prolonged hyperglycemia caused by inadequate metabolic control, the bulk of the data suggests that microvascular disease and neuropathy are linked to hyperglycemia.

AGEs and Aminoguanidine

Proteins throughout the body are nonenzymatically glycosylated at a rate that is proportional to the ambient glucose concentration. These glycosylated proteins are highly reactive, forming bonds with other glycosylated proteins, collagen, and other molecules, eventually forming advanced glycosylation end products (AGEs) (see Figure 19.2). Advanced glycosylation end products are very stable and are incorporated into the basement membrane matrix of capillaries. This process causes the thickening of basement membranes and a reduction in the production of active endothelial-derived relaxing factor (and corresponding vasoconstriction) (21, 22). The net result of this process is leakage across the basement membranes, which appears as hard exudates in the patient with diabetic retinopathy and as proteinuria in the patient with diabetic nephropathy. This process is thought to be one of the major pathways leading to the development of microvascular disease.

A new drug, aminoguanidine, has been shown to effectively block the production of AGEs while not altering blood sugar levels. Aminoguanidine has been shown to reduce microvascular disease in diabetic animals and appears to be well tolerated by human subjects. Phase III trials evaluating aminoguanidine are currently underway in the United States.

Sorbitol and Aldose Reductase Inhibition

Another important biochemical pathway leading to the development of chronic complications in patients with diabetes is the sorbitol pathway (23). Many cell lines, such as the Schwann cell in the central nervous system, do not require insulin for uptake of glucose. These cell types will be subject to intracellular hyperglycemia during times of ambient hyperglycemia. During times of intracellular hyperglycemia an inordinately high fraction of glucose is shunted into the sorbitol pathway (see Figure 19.3), leading to the production of high concentrations of sorbitol via the enzyme aldose reductase. High concentrations of sorbitol cause a reduction in the uptake of myoinisotol, which in turn results in the downregulation of the Na^+/K^+ ATPase system, with a reduction in energy production. Additionally, sorbitol creates an intracellular osmotic gradient, resulting in hypervolemia of the cell, probably further compromising the function of the cell. This pathway is thought to be important in the development of neuropathy in patients with diabetes. Aldose reductase

inhibitors, which reduce the production of sorbitol, have been used experimentally in patients with diabetic complications. Aldose reductase inhibitors that have been studied to date include statil, tolrestat, ponalrestat, and others.

The most promising compound at this point in terms of efficacy and likelihood of FDA approval is tolrestat (Alredase). A manuscript that was published recently in the *Annals of Internal Medicine* suggested that tolrestat is significantly more effective than placebo in retarding and even reversing neuropathy in patients with diabetes. During this 1-year trial, patients who were treated with placebo had a significant worsening of signs and symptoms of neuropathy, while those treated with tolrestat had a significant improvement of their neuropathy compared to baseline (24).

The Diabetes Control and Complications Trial

The most significant controversy in the field of diabetes since the discovery of insulin has revolved around the question "Does glycemic control affect the appearance and progression of chronic complications?" In 1993 the results of the Diabetes Control and Complications Trial (DCCT), a long-term, multicenter, randomized, prospective study evaluating this question, were published (1). The study evaluated 1441 patients with IDDM. Two cohorts were studied: a primary prevention cohort (patients with little or no evidence of diabetic complications) and a secondary

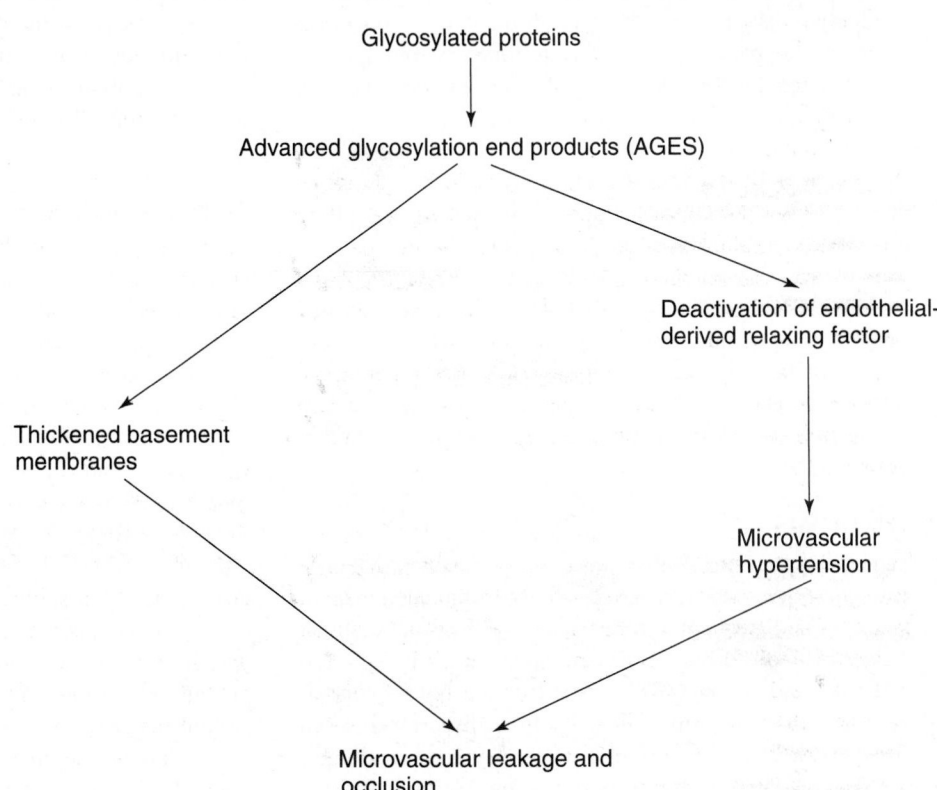

Figure 19.2. AGEs and microvascular disease

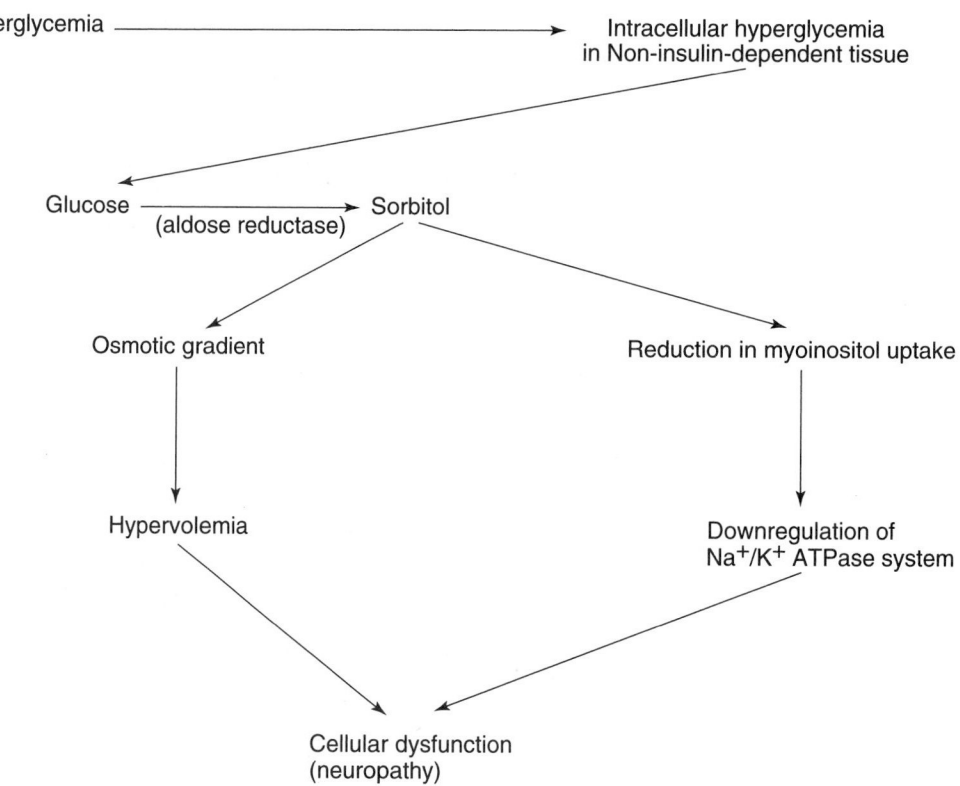

Figure 19.3. The sorbitol pathway

intervention cohort (patients with mild to moderate complications). Patients in both cohorts were randomized to receive either conventional therapy (one to two insulin injections per day and avoidance of acute symptoms of hyperglycemia) or intensive therapy (three or more injections per day or subcutaneous insulin infusion pump therapy and strict glycemic control). The study was discontinued 1 year earlier than had been planned when an interim analysis of the data showed overwhelming support for intensive therapy. Results were reported in terms of relative risk reduction or, simply stated, what level of risk reduction for the appearance or progression of a chronic complication is imparted by intensive therapy versus conventional therapy. The results of the study are shown in Table 19.4. In addition to the significant chronic complication findings, the study also reported a threefold increase in hypoglycemic episodes and more weight gain in the patients who were treated with intensive insulin therapy. Because of the findings of this study, there is a renewed emphasis on strict but reasonable glycemic control to prevent severe chronic diabetic complications. Patients are being educated to normalize their blood glucose levels through multiple daily injections of insulin or the use of insulin infusion pumps in conjunction with self-monitoring of blood glucose levels and a strict diet and exercise program. The acute effects of hyperglycemia are summarized in Table 19.5.

Table 19.4.
Results of Intensive Insulin Therapy versus Conventional Therapy in the Diabetes Control and Complications Trial

60% reduction in the development of clinical neuropathy
35% reduction in the development of microalbuminuria
56% reduction in the development of macroalbuminuria
27% reduction in the initial appearance of retinopathy
34–76% reduction in the clinically significant retinopathy
45% reduction in the progression to severe retinopathy
34% reduction in low-density lipoprotein concentration
41% reduction in the risk of macrovascular disease
Threefold increase in the incidence of severe hypoglycemia

Source: From (1).

Table 19.5.
Harmful Effects of Hyperglycemia

Increased capillary basement membrane thickening
Glucose metabolized via polyol pathway, increased sorbitol
Faulty lipid metabolism, atherosclerosis
Abnormal minor (glycosylated) hemoglobins
Impairment of phagocytosis (ability to fight infection)
Increased platelet adhesiveness
Red blood cell inflexibility
Increased neonatal morbidity and mortality

Table 19.6.
Complications of Diabetes Mellitus and Their Treatment

Body Location	Description	Treatment
Eyes	Retinopathy, cataract formation, glaucoma, and periodic visual disturbances; leading cause of new blindness	Strict control of blood glucose to avoid need for treatment via laser photocoagulation, vitrectomy
Mouth	Gingivitis, increased incidence of dental cavities and periodontal disease	Strict control and daily hygiene; see dentist, floss, brush, and Water-Pik often
Reproductive system (pregnancy)	Increased incidence of large babies, still-births, miscarriages, neonatal deaths, and congenital defects	Strict control before and during pregnancy
Nervous system	Motor, sensory and autonomic neuropathy leading to impotence, neurogenic bladder, parathesias, gangrene	Strict control, daily foot care, surgery, tricyclic antidepressants and phenothiazines
Vascular system	Large vessel disease and microangiopathy	Strict blood glucose control, artery bypass surgery
Skin	Numerous infections and specific lesions due to small vessel disease, increased lipids in blood, and pruritus	Strict control, daily hygiene
Kidneys	Diabetic glomerulosclerosis causing nephropathy	Strict control, eventually diet low in proteins, prednisone, dialysis and renal transplantation
Reticuloendothelial system (infections)	Diabetics have a higher incidence of cystitis, tuberculosis, and skin infections and a more difficult time overcoming infections; moniliasis is common in diabetic women	Strict control and aggressive antiinfective therapy

Data on the link between hyperglycemia and chronic complications is being evaluated. Most diabetologists agree that the better the glycemic control, the more promising the long-term outcome. However, a small percentage of patients may be relatively resistant to long-term complications even with poor glycemic control, while another small subgroup may suffer multiple chronic complications while being treated intensively. Table 19.6 summarizes the complications of diabetes mellitus and the treatment recommendations for each complication.

Major advances have been made in the treatment of some specific complications of diabetes. Retinopathy can be successfully treated by laser photocoagulation. If the patient suffers a retinal vitreous hemorrhage, surgical vitrectomy can be performed to help restore the patient's vision (25). Strict glycemic control before and during pregnancy has greatly reduced the incidence of perinatal mortality in infants of diabetic mothers (18). Neuropathies and diabetic cataracts improve with strict glycemic control and have also recently been treated experimentally with aldose reductase inhibitors. Tolrestat, as was mentioned earlier, is currently undergoing phase III clinical trials. Furthermore, diabetic impotence can be treated surgically by inserting a penile prostheses (26) or by the use of the new ErectAid device. Training the diabetic patient to monitor foot care and vigorously treat any foot problems can reduce the incidence of gangrene in the extremities. Strict metabolic control can also reduce the thickness of basement membranes and improve serum lipid levels in

diabetic patients. Diabetic patients who normalize their blood glucose and glycosylated hemoglobin levels have a decreased frequency of severe infections (18).

Type I diabetic patients are predisposed to the development of diabetic nephropathy. The basement membrane of the capillaries in the glomerulus thickens and progresses to a nodular pattern (Kimmelstiel-Wilson syndrome). Nephropathy usually occurs in diabetic patients 10 to 15 years after diagnosis. Proteinuria is the first clinical manifestation, with progression to hypertension, azotemia, hypoalbuminemia, and edema. Treatment to control the complications of nephropathy and dialysis or transplantation may be necessary for patients who have progressive renal disease. Strict blood glucose control is necessary to reduce, or possibly prevent, pathologic changes due to hyperglycemia. While many antihypertensive drugs have been evaluated for use in the prevention and treatment of diabetic nephropathy, a recent metaanalysis of the studies concluded that angiotensin-converting enzyme inhibitors (ACEIs) had a greater effect on reducing diabetic proteinuria and slowing down reduction of creatinine clearance than did other types of antihypertensive medication (27). Additionally, ACEIs had an effect on proteinuria and creatinine that could not be explained by reductions in blood pressure alone. An ACEI-mediated nephroprotective effect was hypothesized. A landmark manuscript published by Lewis and colleagues demonstrated that captopril 25 mg three times a day significantly reduced the time to doubling of serum creatinine, time until hemodialysis was required, and time until death (28). The Lewis study also reported a nephroprotective effect elicited by ACEIs that could not be explained by changes in systemic blood pressure alone. Currently, many practitioners are treating patients who have diabetic proteinuria, with or without hypertension, with ACEIs in an attempt to slow the progression of nephropathy.

Because of the high incidence of gangrene in diabetic patients, foot care is extremely important in the educational process of patients with diabetes. This complication results from a combination of factors, including atherosclerosis, decreased pain sensation due to neuropathy, decreased responsiveness of leukocytes, and trauma. The reduced blood flow results in ischemic tissue changes. Because of neuropathy, the diabetic patient may not detect areas of injury or infection, and the progression to gangrene can be rapid. Diabetic patients should thus be instructed to monitor foot care daily, never go barefoot, strictly control their blood glucose, and avoid trauma to the feet by properly cutting toenails and selecting shoes that fit properly (19).

DIAGNOSTIC TESTS

Most currently used diagnostic tests measure an individual's ability to handle a glucose load. Type I diabetes is usually easy to diagnose because patients present with all of the classic symptoms of diabetes and high amounts of

Table 19.7.
Criteria for Diagnosis of Diabetes and Impaired Glucose Tolerance

1. Diabetes—adult
   a. Unequivocal elevation of plasma glucose level and classic symptoms (polyuria, polydipsia, weight loss)
   b. Fasting plasma glucose (FPG) 7.8 mmol/L (140 mg/dL) on more than one occasion
   c. Oral glucose tolerance test (OGTT) with FPG 7.8 mmol/L (140 mg/dL), 2-hr PG 11.1 mmol/L (200 mg/dL), one intervening PG 11.1 mmol/L (200 mg/dL).
2. Diabetes—children
   a. Plasma glucose 11.1 mmol/L (200 mg/dL) with classic symptoms
   b. OGTT (1.75 g glucose/kg body weight up to maximum of 75 g) with FPG 7.8 mmol/L (140 mg/dL), 2-hr PG 11.1 mmol/L (200 mg/dL), one intervening PG 11.1 mmol/L (200 mg/dL)
3. Gestational diabetes
   Two or more of the following plasma glucose concentrations exceeded with a 100-g glucose dose: FPG 5.8 mmol/L (105 mg/dL); 1-hr postdose, 10.5 mmol/L (190 mg/dL), 2-hr postdose 9.2 mmol/L (165 mg/dL); 3-hr postdose 8.0 mmol/L (145 mg/dL)
4. Impaired glucose tolerance
   OGTT with FPG 7.8 mmol/L (140 mg/dL), 2-hr PG 7.8 mmol/L (140 mg/dL) and 11.1 mmol/L (200 mg/dL), one intervening value 11.1 mmol/L (200 mg/dL)
5. Normal glucose values—nonpregnant adults OGTT with FPG 6.4 mmol/L (115 mg/dL), 2-hr PG 7.8 mmol/L (140 mg/dL), intervening PG 11.1 mmol/L (200 mg/dL)

glucose in the urine and blood. Type II diabetes is more of a challenge to diagnose because patients often do not present with the classic symptoms. Furthermore, many of these patients have borderline diabetes, and tests do not give a clear indication as to whether or not the patient has diabetes. Table 19.7 summarizes the criteria developed by the National Diabetes Data Group and adopted by the American Diabetes Association. These criteria are now recommended for use in the diagnosis of diabetes and impaired glucose tolerance.

Oral Glucose Tolerance Test (OGTT)

This diagnostic test measures a person's ability to handle a glucose load over a period of time and, although controversial, is a quite reliable test for diabetes. Following an overnight fast, a morning fasting blood sugar is drawn, and the patient ingests a 75-g glucose load. Then blood samples are drawn at half-hour intervals for 2 hours and then at 3 hours (29). Urine samples are often taken at the same time and tested for glucose to estimate the renal threshold for glucose. In normal subjects the blood glucose returns to normal in less than 2 hours. In diabetic patients the glucose peak is higher and occurs much later than in normal subjects; levels also decline at a slower rate. A normal OGTT occurs when the fasting plasma glucose is less than 115 mg/dL, the 2-hour plasma glucose is less than 140 mg/dL, and the intervening glucose values are below 200 mg/dL. Because of criteria that accept random or fasting glucose levels as diagnostic, many clinicians have questioned the need for this test. Several other factors, including infections, stress, pregnancy, metabolic abnormalities, and certain drugs, can impair glucose tolerance and produce abnormal results. One should screen for the possibility of these factors when using the OGTT.

Fasting Plasma Glucose (FPG)

Various blood or plasma tests for glucose are used in establishing the diagnosis of diabetes. The simplest test is the FPG test, in which blood is drawn from the patient after an overnight fast. A normal FPG depends on the particular laboratory, but it is usually set between 65 and 110 mg/dL. The diagnosis of diabetes may be confirmed in the patient with two or more fasting plasma glucose levels that are elevated above 140 mg/dL. However, a normal FPG does not rule out diabetes. This test is used in nonpregnant adult patients who neither are receiving drugs nor have other diseases that could be responsible for the abnormal results (29).

2-Hour Postprandial Blood Glucose (2HPP)

The 2HPP is used as a screening test in which a blood glucose level is drawn 2 hours after the patient ingests a 100-g glucose load. In nondiabetic patients, blood glucose levels return to normal in less than 2 hours following a glucose challenge, whereas hyperglycemia persists in a diabetic patient. Although this test is often used to evaluate diabetes control, it can easily be manipulated by the diabetic patient.

Note that each of the blood glucose tests can be manipulated by the diabetic patient, who can improve his or her blood glucose control for several days before the test. Furthermore, blood glucose tests may be elevated because of emotional stress, physical exertion, and stimulants such as tobacco, coffee, and tea. Other causes of elevated blood glucose include acute stress such as fever, trauma, major operations, myocardial infarction, or cerebral vascular accident (19). Chronic illness that causes prolonged physical inactivity, starvation, and malnutrition can result in abnormally low fasting blood glucose levels. Potassium depletion from any cause can result in fasting hyperglycemia (19). Another cause of pseudohyperglycemia is chronic renal disease with uremia.

Caution should be exercised in using diagnostic tests for diabetes. A patient should not be diagnosed as having diabetes unless it is certain that the disease exists. To inappropriately label a patient with this diagnosis leads to personal frustration, including insurance riders, driver's license limitations in some states, and possible limitations in employment opportunities (19). Health care providers who are monitoring elderly patients should be alert to the fact that, as an individual ages, tolerance to glucose decreases. This results in some elderly patients being labeled as diabetic and being placed on medications that are probably unnecessary.

Glycosylated Hemoglobin (Hemoglobin A1c)

Glycosylation of hemoglobin is a postsynthetic, nonenzymatic chemical reaction between glucose and phosphorylated sugar (glucose-6-phosphate) with the end-terminal valine of the B chain of the hemoglobin molecule (8). Since hemoglobin is exposed to the ambient glucose concentration in the blood, a higher concentration of glucose will result in more glycohemoglobin formation. The result is that this hemoglobin becomes an important index of the long-term control of diabetes and may be a more reliable index than the degree of hyperglycemia or glucosuria. In the nondiabetic patient, glycosylated hemoglobin is between 3 and 8% of all hemoglobin, whereas in patients with poorly controlled diabetes it may range between 8 and 20%. Glycohemoglobin is a clinically useful gauge of glycemic control. Glycohemoglobin concentration correlates with the level of glycemic control for the previous 60 days, or when the red blood cells are about halfway through their 120-day cycle. The major subcategory of the glycohemoglobins is hemoglobin A1c. Some laboratories test specifically for hemoglobin A1c; others test for all of the glycosylated hemoglobins. It is important to know which test a laboratory is using and what its specific normal range

is. Numerous recent studies have shown that when a patient with relatively uncontrolled diabetes brings his or her blood glucose under strict control, there is a dramatic improvement in glycosylated hemoglobins (8, 30). The DCCT confirmed that there is a strong correlation between glycosylated hemoglobin concentrations and the progression of microangiopathy in patients with IDDM. This test is particularly useful for patients who have poor compliance in record keeping or who make an extra effort to achieve acceptable plasma glucose levels only at the time of physician visits. The test has an advantage also in that it can be taken at any time and is not affected by recent meals or physical activities. Note that it is not a test that is done frequently, but rather two or three times a year. Finally, some clinicians are studying this test for use as a screening or diagnostic test. Additional tests are being evaluated to determine whether specific glycoproteins such as glycoalbumin correlate well with diabetes control.

SELF-MONITORING OF BLOOD GLUCOSE

Since 1980 there has been a trend to educate diabetic patients to self-monitor blood glucose. This procedure has received increasing medical acceptance, and annual sales of blood glucose monitoring products have grown rapidly. This movement is continuing to gain momentum and may soon result in blood glucose monitoring by all patients with diabetes. The objective of diabetes treatment is to achieve blood glucose levels that are as close to normal as possible through a program of education, diet, exercise and medications. Achieving the objective requires active and routine patient involvement to ensure that glycemic control is being attained.

Besides possibly decreasing complications, strict blood glucose control can also avoid some of the problems that are inherent in urine testing. Urine tests are inconvenient, messy, and affected by a wide variety of medications and do not reflect the current blood glucose levels because of differences in patients' renal threshold and residual urine left in the bladder (30). Additionally, one cannot verify hypoglycemia with urine testing.

Self-monitoring of blood glucose is feasible, practical, and acceptable to patients. It allows the patient to better understand the factors that affect blood glucose levels; gives an accurate reflection of the blood glucose after exercise, before and after meals, and when the patient is placed on medications or is ill; helps the patient to better understand diabetes and the objectives of therapy; assists in detecting and therefore avoiding hypoglycemia; helps the patient to understand the symptoms of hypoglycemia and hyperglycemia; improves the relationship between the health care professional and the patient; and helps the patient to become a more active, intelligent participant in managing diabetes.

The disadvantages of self-monitoring glucose, which include the increased expense and the annoyance of obtaining a drop of blood, are greatly outweighed by the many advantages. Several devices are now available to assist the patient in obtaining a drop of blood easily and almost painlessly (31).

Several methods of determining blood glucose levels are available to diabetic patients. Selection of a specific product should be made on the basis of cost, ability to perform the test accurately, accuracy of the method, flexibility of the system (is a meter required?), convenience to the patient, and motivation of the patient to achieve strict control. Since maintenance of blood sugar control is impossible without measurement and since it is convenient and less costly for the patient to self-monitor, self-monitoring of blood glucose is highly recommended for all types of diabetic patients. Pregnant diabetic patients, patients with altered or shifting renal threshold, labile patients who have difficulty bringing their diabetes under control, patients with frequent hypoglycemia, patients who have difficulty using a urine test, and patients who prefer monitoring their own blood glucose are all excellent candidates for self-monitoring of blood glucose. Blood glucose monitoring is a necessity for patients who are using continuous subcutaneous insulin infusion.

Most of the tests that are available for use by patients involve the glucose oxidase/peroxidase reaction to detect glucose. Some of the tests use a reflectance photometer to read the strip and give a digital readout of the blood glucose values. Other methods have a color reaction on the strip, which is compared to a chart on the side of the bottle that the patient visually reads.

While the visually read strips have the advantage of being less expensive and very portable, the meter-read monitoring of blood glucose gives the patient a more accurate determination of blood glucose. Both systems greatly improve the patient's ability to understand the factors that affect blood glucose levels and therefore improve blood glucose control.

Recently, the American Diabetes Associations position statement on Self Monitoring of Blood Glucose (SMBG) was revised (32). In this position statement the use of non-brand-name monitoring strips with blood glucose meters was strongly discouraged. Also, the position statement suggests that almost all patients with diabetes would benefit from SMBG.

Urine Tests

Patient-performed tests are available for the evaluation of urine glucose, urine ketones, and urine protein.

Glucosuria is observed in many conditions (e.g., pregnancy or impaired renal function) and is not a persistent finding in diabetes. It does occur when the mean blood glucose level is 180 mg/dL or more but rarely when the level is less than 130 mg/dL. The major exception occurs when the renal threshold for glucose is increased with age; therefore older diabetic patients may "spill" no glucose at all despite a high blood glucose level. Thus, one of the major disadvantages of urine testing to monitor diabetes is the fact that renal thresholds for glucose differ from patient to patient. There is also residual urine left in the bladder, even when the patient double-voids. This means that at any point at which the patient tests his or her urine, the test could be affected by blood glucose levels of the previous 2 to 3 hr. Because of the problems that are inherent in urine glucose monitoring, this method is not recommended unless a patient will not or cannot monitor blood sugar (33).

Urine ketone tests that are available include Acetest, Chemstrip K, Ketostix, and others. Urine ketone testing should be encouraged for the patient with diabetes during acute illness or stress or when blood glucose levels are not well controlled. Patients with IDDM should test for urine ketones when blood sugar readings are greater than 240 mg/dL and should report ketone readings of moderate or greater levels to their practitioner.

Finally, urine tests are available for the evaluation of urine proteins. Constant routine monitoring of urine protein is usually not warranted. Urine protein tests are used primarily as a screening tool for diabetic nephropathy. Diabetic patients who test negative with standard dipstick methods may be further evaluated with an in-office microalbumin screening test (Micro-bumintest) or by 24-hr urine collections analyzed via radioimmunoassay (RIA). These methods are much more sensitive than the standard dipstick method. Patients who have had type I diabetes for more than 5 years should be screened annually; patients with type II diabetes should be screened annually from the time of diagnosis (34).

GENERAL PRINCIPLES IN THE TREATMENT OF DIABETES

The treatment objectives for diabetes are summarized in Table 19.8. In achieving the objectives, one must remember that diabetes is a heterogeneous condition and that there is tremendous variance among patients. The treatment protocol needs to be individualized and can be developed only after the type of diabetes has been categorized. In general, glucose metabolism is normalized in diabetic patients who achieve excellent control. The DCCT verified that strict glycemic control is associated with a reduction in the appearance and progression of chronic complications in patients with IDDM. These benefits may be realized in patients with NIDDM as well. Excellent control will significantly improve the quality of life by producing a relative degree of healthiness. The most challenging diabetic patient is the type I insulin-dependent diabetic who has wide daily fluctuations of blood glucose.

Table 19.8.
Treatment Objectives for Diabetes Mellitus

Normalize glucose metabolism
    Normalize glycosylated hemoglobin
    Urine glucose and ketones negative
    Fasting blood glucose: 3.9–8.3 mmol/L (70–140 mg/dL)
    2-hr postprandial glucose level less than 10 mmol/L (180 mg/dL)
    Urinary excretion of glucose less than 5% in 24 hr
Avoid symptoms of diabetes mellitus
Avoid frequent hypoglycemia
Normalize nutrition and achieve ideal body weight
Achieve normal growth and development
Minimize or prevent complications
Accept diabetes with a realistic but positive attitude
Enjoy normal and flexible lifestyle
Promote emotional well-being; have patient take charge of condition

The formula to achieve these objectives combines a program of weight loss and diet with an individualized exercise program and the use of medications: insulin for patients with type I diabetes and possibly insulin or oral agents for patients with the type II diabetes. Diet, exercise, and medications are greatly enhanced by a program of education and weight reduction.

Education

In the *Guidelines for Diabetes Care* (35) that is published by the American Diabetes Association is a summary of specific guidelines for education of individuals with diabetes in both acute care and ambulatory care facilities. This document specifically lists the steps that should be followed in training the patient with diabetes to care for his or her own condition. The diabetic patient spends 365 days a year caring for the condition and monitoring the results of his or her efforts. It thus becomes essential that each patient with diabetes understand the disease and be able to follow specific steps necessary to care for the condition and to evaluate whether or not the treatment protocol is achieving its objectives.

The educational process requires a health team approach that includes a physician, a nurse, a dietitian, a pharmacist, and possibly a social worker and an exercise physiologist. It is also important that the patient be continually educated and participate with other patients who have diabetes. This can be achieved by active involvement in the Juvenile Diabetes Foundation or the local affiliate of the American Diabetes Association. It is important that the educational process be well organized and that it assess each individual patient's needs. It is also important that patients be periodically evaluated for their competence in performing urine or blood tests, mixing and injecting insulin, rotating injection sites, using the diet exchange system, and following an exercise prescription. Table 19.9 lists some of the statistics that show a strong

need for diabetic patient education (9). The education for a patient with diabetes should be broken down into at least three areas:

1. Initial management of the diabetes, which provides necessary information to bring the patient under control and gives the patient some time to adjust to the condition. This level of education is based on the limitations of the individual and family to accept and/or assimilate all there is to know about diabetes at the time of diagnosis and the limitations of some settings to provide additional education.
2. Home management of diabetes places emphasis on increasing knowledge and flexibility as some experience is gained in living with diabetes. This level is perceived as essential for every individual but must be tailored to each person's needs and capacity. This type of educational experience is preferably offered in a nonhospital environment that is as close to home as possible.
3. Improvement of life-style is the third area in which educational guidelines should be developed. This form of education deals with advanced learning and is viewed as enriching the individual's life with flexibility, insight, and self-determination. Unfortunately, many diabetic patients are forced to discover this information by trial and error.

At each level of education, information is provided about nutrition, medication, self-monitoring, how to treat hypoglycemia, how to handle hyperglycemic episodes and illness, what activities should be practiced on a daily basis, and specific steps in developing good hygiene and a routine schedule. Assessing psychological adjustment is a method of determining whether or not the patient is accepting the educational process.

Exercise

Although physicians nearly always recommend exercise as part of the treatment of diabetes, it is seldom prescribed. Recently, more physicians have begun to understand the improvement that exercise brings to the control of diabetes, and programs are being developed to specifically prescribe daily exercise for diabetic patients (36, 37). Exercise produces an improvement in insulin sensitivity or the ability of insulin to be used to drive glucose into the cell. Exercise lowers blood glucose by allowing glucose to

Table 19.9.
Need for Patient Education

3 of 5 patients make errors in insulin measurement.
65–90% of patients have major deficits in selecting and using foods according to prescribed diet.
Fewer than 10% of diabetics were following a "minimally adequate regimen."
35% of patients lack any formal training.
17% were placed on insulin without instructions.
50% who had been trained could not demonstrate skills in any of the major areas of self-care.

penetrate the muscle cell and be metabolized without the assistance of insulin. Glucose may be used to varying degrees without insulin in all types of cells. Exercise also improves circulatory function, an important factor in the management of diabetes. Exercise also helps to maintain normal body weight and aids in breathing, digestion, and metabolism. An exercise log may help the patient to maintain a regular daily schedule. Patients who monitor their own blood glucose become motivated to exercise because they easily see the beneficial effects of exercise on maintaining good blood sugar and control.

An exercise program should be prescribed for both type I and type II diabetic patients. Diabetic patients should be evaluated before the exercise prescription is determined. The person's health, interests, and motivation to exercise should be taken into consideration in developing a specific method of exercising. If blood glucose is greater than 300 mg/dL, exercise can result in an excessive rise in counterregulatory hormones that, in the presence of inadequate insulin availability, can cause decreased muscle glucose uptake and an increase in liver glucose production, which actually causes blood glucose to increase further. Thus, type I diabetic patients should know their blood glucose level before beginning exercise. If the blood glucose is less than 300, injected insulin that has been absorbed subcutaneously can possibly be absorbed more rapidly, resulting in excessive insulin, which, in combination with the exercise, can cause a serious drop in blood glucose. Diabetic patients over 40 years of age or patients who have had diabetes for more than 25 years should have an exercise stress test and then have an individualized graded exercise program prescribed. Diabetic patients with peripheral sensory neuropathy and/or vascular insufficiency should avoid exercise that may cause trauma to the feet-for example, jogging. Diabetic patients with proliferative diabetic retinopathy should avoid strenuous exercise, which may induce hemorrhage. Another problem that needs to be considered in exercise programs is preventing hypoglycemia during exercise. Hypoglycemia can be prevented by ingesting additional carbohydrates before exercise begins (approximately 15 g 30 min before exercising). Patients should also inject insulin at a nonexercise site-for example, in the abdomen if they are going to be running. The patient should log the exercise and monitor what effect it has on his or her blood glucose control. By doing this, a patient will be encouraged to exercise regularly. If hypoglycemia occurs repeatedly during regularly scheduled exercise, a decrease in the insulin dose may be required. Patients should also be warned to wear an identification bracelet or necklace when exercising in case they do become hypoglycemic. Diabetic patients should also carry a quick source of sugar with them when exercising in case of an insulin reaction.

Table 19.10.
Diabetes Diet Therapy

Diet compliance is critical.
Avoid fad diets and prolonged fasting.
Note that "dietetic" does not equal "diabetic"; read labels carefully.
Avoid quick-acting (simple) sugars.
Decrease consumption of animal (saturated) fats.
Control calories, attempt to achieve an ideal body weight.
Increase amount of fiber in the diet.
Try to avoid alcohol.
Avoid smoking.
Take vitamin-mineral supplements.
Understand and use the diabetic diet system and the glycemic index.

Diet

Diet is the cornerstone of treatment of both type I and type II diabetes. It is the first line of treatment in type II diabetes and, in combination with exercise and insulin, is a necessary component of treatment regimens for type I diabetes. Table 19.10 provides a quick overview of diabetes diet therapy.

Patients should be taught to read labels carefully because many sugarless and dietetic products actually contain a high number of calories and are not effective in helping the diabetic patient to achieve or maintain an ideal body weight. Diabetic patients should also avoid quick-acting simple sugars because they cause a rapid rise in blood glucose levels. The new guidelines from the American Diabetes Association Task Force on Nutrition state that a prudent amount of simple sugar may be ingested. Ingestion of animal (saturated) fats should be minimized because of the increased incidence of atherosclerotic disease in diabetic patients. The main goal in diabetes diet therapy is to control calories. Some excellent studies have been done that show the importance of increasing fiber in the diet of diabetic patients. However, each patient needs to see how he or she responds to the various types of fiber. Some fibers that have a high degree of pectin can cause constipation; other fiber products, because of their bulk nature, can cause flatulence and diarrhea (38). To achieve the objectives of diet therapy, the patient must spend some time with a dietitian to specifically determine the number of calories to be ingested each day and the percentage of those calories that should be carbohydrates, fat, and protein. Patients also need to be educated in the relatively simple diabetic diet exchange system. The diet exchange system allows patients to have a large variety of foods, and if the patient will follow the diet, weight can be lost and ideal body weight can be achieved. Remember, about 80% of diabetic patients are obese and have non-insulin-dependent diabetes. If weight loss can be achieved in this group, often the diabetes will disappear. Table 19.11 shows the dietary recommendations for type I and type II diabetes (39). Diet therapy for

Table 19.11.
Dietary Strategies for Two Types of Patients with Diabetes

Strategy	Obese, Non-Insulin-Dependent	Nonobese, Insulin-Dependent
Decrease calories.	Yes	No
Protect or improve pancreatic β-cell function.	Very urgent priority	Seldom important because β cells are extinct
Increase frequency and number of feedings.	Usually no	Yes
Maintain day-to-day consistency of intake of calories.	Not crucial if average caloric intake remains in low range	Desirable
Maintain day-to-day consistency of ratios of carbohydrates, protein, and fat for each of the feedings.	Not crucial	Desirable
Time meals consistently.	Not crucial	Very important
Allow extra food for unusual exercise.	Not usually appropriate	Usually appropriate
Use food to treat, abort, or prevent hypoglycemia.	Yes	Important
During complicating illness, provide small, frequent feedings or give carbohydrate intravenously to prevent starvation ketosis.	Often not necessary because of resistance to ketosis	Important

patients with type II diabetes has a high degree of failure and often creates feelings of frustration, pessimism, failure, and anger, which in turn result in poorly informed and inadequately motivated patients. The failure rate can also cause frustration and a negative attitude on the part of the physician who treats the patient. Successful diet programs require behavior modification on the part of the patient. Patients should be encouraged to join groups such as Weight Watchers and to keep a diet log that is similar to an exercise log. The patient should write down, for a period of 4 to 10 days, each time he or she eats, how much he or she eats, and why he or she eats-whether because of social pressure, loneliness, depression, nervousness, or the time of day or because the patient truly needed nourishment. By having patients use smaller plates, take only one helping of food, and be conscious of why they eat, it is possible to change dietary behavior. Diet support groups can be of assistance in modifying behavior (29).

One reason for failure of diet therapy in diabetic patients is that physicians or dietitians prescribe changes in diet without first adjusting the dose of insulin or oral agents. The first steps in diet therapy should be to prescribe an exercise program, lower the medication dose, and put the patient on a diet containing fewer calories. Insulin overtreatment is probably one of the most common causes of inadequate diabetic control and weight gain. In one group of diabetic patients, 75% needed a reduction in insulin dose of at least 10%; 35% of the overtreated patients had large appetites, and 30% had hepatomegaly and headaches (37). Diabetic patients should be educated to determine whether or not they have involved themselves in a vicious cycle of taking too much insulin and then eating up to that level of insulin. Note also that type II diabetic patients have too much insulin to begin with and still feel hungry even after eating a large meal, possibly because of their excess insulin levels.

Alcohol Use by the Patient with Diabetes

In general, alcohol use by diabetic patients is discouraged, but each individual diabetic patient should be assessed to determine whether the advantages of alcohol (e.g., reducing emotional tension, relieving anxiety, and stimulating appetite) outweigh the potential effects on blood glucose control.

Either hyperglycemia or hypoglycemia may develop in diabetic patients who ingest alcohol. Hypoglycemia is the most common effect. The hypoglycemic effect of alcohol is believed to be due either to increased early endogenous insulin response to glucose or to inhibition of hepatic gluconeogenesis. Relatively small quantities of alcohol (48 mL of 100-proof alcohol) may cause this effect. Thus, if a diabetic patient is fasting and consumes alcohol, hypoglycemia may be severe, leading to coma or death. If the person has adequate amounts of glucose in the blood, then alcohol has a less clinically significant effect.

Patients who consume alcoholic beverages must consider the caloric content of the beverage and should be encouraged to choose "light" type drinks over standard brews. The sugar content of wines and mixed drinks must also be considered. Alcohol in combination with a sugared mixture in a patient who is fed can add to the hyperglycemic state.

The additive hypoglycemic effects of alcohol with insulin have produced severe hypoglycemia resulting in coma, brain damage, and even death. Tolbutamide and chlorpropamide have been reported to interact with alcohol, resulting in a disulfiramlike reaction. An advantage of the second-generation sulfonylureas is that they do not cause such a reaction when they are taken with alcohol.

Patients who do choose to consume ethanol should be counseled to do so only in small quantities (1 to 2 oz/day) that are taken slowly and in combination with food.

MEDICATIONS IN THE TREATMENT OF DIABETES MELLITUS

The medications that are used to treat diabetes can be categorized into two broad areas: oral antidiabetic agents and insulin. The oral agents, which may be further subcategorized into sulfonylureas and biguanides, are effective only in type II (non-insulin-dependent) diabetes. Insulin is used for type I diabetes and for approximately 30% of patients with type II diabetes. Insulin is also used for all diabetic patients during times of stress, such as infection, surgery, ketoacidosis, or hyperosmolar coma. Other medications that are being evaluated experimentally for the control of hyperglycemia include α-glucosidase inhibitors, insulinotropins, oxirane carboxylic acids, thiozolidindiones, and insulin analogs. Finally, it should be noted that a new sulfonylurea, glimepiride (Amaryl), is likely to be available by the time this text is published.

Sulfonylureas

Drug therapy should never be considered for a patient with mild, well-tolerated type II diabetes until after diet therapy is tried for an appropriate length of time (3 to 4 months). If diet therapy fails, then a trial of sulfonylureas is indicated. Before 1970, when the University Group Diabetes Program (UGDP) published its very controversial report, most patients with non-insulin-dependent diabetes were given sulfonylureas. The UGDP was a prospective study initiated in 1961 to evaluate the effectiveness of antidiabetic therapy in preventing vascular and late complications of diabetes. Eight hundred patients from 12 different diabetes clinics were included in the study. These newly diagnosed type II diabetic patients who should have been treated with diet alone were assigned at random to one of five treatment programs: tolbutamide in fixed doses of 1.5 g, placebo or diet alone, insulin in a fixed dose, insulin in variable doses, and phenformin. The study was interrupted because of an unexpected finding of a higher incidence of cardiovascular deaths in the tolbutamide- and phenformin-treated group. Controversy surrounding the study is still not settled, and many emotional editorials have appeared in the literature about the faults of the study and the conclusions that were made. Even though subsequent studies failed to substantiate the findings of the UGDP (40, 41), the oral hypoglycemic agents were less frequently used until the late 1970s, and the FDA still requires tolbutamide package inserts to contain reference to "an increased risk of cardiovascular mortality."

In 1984, two new, more potent agents were approved for use in the United States. The marketing of these products stimulated the use of oral antidiabetic agents. Currently, oral hypoglycemic agents account for approximately 1% of all prescriptions that are written in the United States (42). Seventy-five percent of this market is controlled by three agents: glyburide, glipizide, and chlorpropamide. It is estimated that 40% of all patients with type II diabetes are treated with oral hypoglycemic agents.

Sulfonylureas have demonstrated both pancreatic and extrapancreatic effects but are useful only in patients who have intact, viable β cells (type II patients) (43, 44). In the absence of other secretagogues, sulfonylureas in vitro directly stimulate the release of insulin. In vivo, sulfonylureas sensitize β cells to glucose, increasing insulin secretion indirectly. Additionally, glucagon release from the pancreas is inhibited by sulfonylureas. Sulfonylureas may affect glucose levels by several extrapancreatic mechanisms such as increasing insulin-receptor-binding affinity, increasing insulin effect by postreceptor action, and decreasing hepatic insulin extraction. The relative clinical importance of each of these mechanisms is still a subject of research and debate.

The following patient characteristics are sometimes predictive of a positive clinical response to sulfonylureas:

1. The patient is not diagnosed with diabetes until after the age of 40.
2. The duration of diabetes is less than 5 years.
3. The patient is close to or above his or her ideal body weight.
4. There has been no prior insulin treatment or the disease has been controlled with less than 40 units of insulin per day.
5. The fasting blood glucose is <180 mg/dL.

Once a firm diagnosis of diabetes has been made, diet has been given an adequate trial, and the criteria for the use of oral hypoglycemic agents have been met, an appropriate drug can then be selected. The products that are available in the United States are summarized in Table 19.12. Efficacy, potency, and toxicity are major factors to consider in the selection of a drug. The differences in metabolism of each sulfonylurea account for clinical differences with reference to the onset, duration of action, and sometimes side effects. Tolbutamide and chlorpropamide are the oldest drugs and have therefore been studied best. Long-term studies of these agents indicate a primary failure rate of 3 to 30%, an overall success rate of 20%, and an incidence of adverse effects of less than 5%. In general, the incidence of adverse effects reported for chlorpropamide is higher than that for the other products: approximately 9% for chlorpropamide versus 1 to 3% for tolbutamide. The severity of many of these side effects can be correlated with the differences in the half-life, metabolism, and excretion of the drugs. Note that chlorpropamide has the longest half-life and also has the highest incidence

Table 19.12.
Biopharmaceutics and Pharmacokinetics of the Oral Hypoglycemic Agents

Drug	Total Daily Dose (mg)	Doses/Day	Half-Life (hr)	Dosage Forms (mg)	Onset of Action (hr)	Duration (hr)	Metabolism and Excretion	Comments
Tolbutamide (Orinase)	500–3000	2–3	5–6	250, 500	1	6–12	Hepatic metabolism to hydroxy- and carboxy-tolbutamide, which are weakly active and inactive, respectively; metabolites are excreted via kidneys	Most benign, least potent, short $t_{1/2}$; good choice in renal failure.
Acetohexamide (Dymelor)	250–1500	1–2	5	250, 500	1	12–18	Metabolized to hydroxyhexamide (greater activity than parent compound) and inactive metabolites; metabolites excreted via kidney	Avoid in patients with renal failure; significant uricosuric effects.
Tolazamide (Tolinase)	100–1000	1–2	7	100, 250, 500	4–6	16–24	Multiple metabolites; hydroxytolazamide moderately active, other metabolites inactive; metabolites excreted via kidney	Absorbed slowly, possible choice in patients with renal failure.
Chlorpropamide (Diabenense)	100–500	1	35	100, 250	1	24–72	80% metabolized to weakly active and inactive metabolites excreted via kidney, 20% of parent compound excreted unchanged	Antabuselike reaction, highest incidence of hypoglycemia; avoid for elderly patients and patients with renal failure.
Glyburide (Diabeta, Micronase)	1.25–20	1–2	3–5	1.25, 2.5, 5.0	1.5	18–24	Metabolized to moderately active and inactive metabolites; metabolites excreted 50% via fecal route, 50% via renal route	Potent agent, dose should be divided if >10 mg/day; may require dosage adjustment if creatine clearance is <30 mL/min.
(Glynase)	0.075–12	1–2	3–5	1.5, 3, 6	1.5	18–24		
Glipizide (Glucotrol)	2.5–40	1–2	3–7	5.0, 10.0	1	16–24	Metabolized to inactive compounds excreted via renal (88%) and fecal (12%) routes	Potent agent, dose should be divided if >15 mg/day; good choice in renal failure patients; patients should be instructed to take on an empty stomach.
(Glucotrol XL)	5–20	1	3–7	5, 10	1–2	24		

From reference 43.

of side effects of a serious nature. For this reason, some clinicians favor tolbutamide because of its short half-life and less toxicity. The side effects of sulfonylureas are summarized in Table 19.13. Patient counseling guidelines for the sulfonylureas are summarized in Table 19.14.

The sulfonylureas that are metabolized to inactive or weakly active metabolites (tolbutamide, tolazamide, glipizide) are safer for use by patients with renal failure. The most common side effect of the sulfonylureas is hypoglycemia. Glyburide and glipizide, the second-generation agents, have been marketed with specific claims differentiating them from the previously marketed first-generation products. The substitutions on the aryl-sulfonylurea nucleus are large nonpolar groups. This results in a marked increase in the hypoglycemic activity. The second-generation drugs are 50 to l00 times more potent on a weight basis than are first-generation agents. Glyburide and glipizide also produce fewer drug interactions because of protein binding displacement when compared to the first-generation agents. This is because they are present physiologically at much lower concentrations than their first-generation counterparts are and because they bind nonionically. Frequent drug-drug interactions between first-generation drugs and alcohol, anabolic steroids, β-adrenergic blocking agents, dicoumarol, monoamine oxidase inhibitors, phenylbutazone, salicylates, and sulfonamides may result in enhanced hypoglycemia (16). Drugs that may interfere with diabetes control by causing hyperglycemia include asparginase, clonidine, corticosteroids, diazoxide, estrogens, ethacrynic acid, furosemide, glucagon, lithium, niacin (high doses), phenytoin, sympathomimetic amines, and thiazide diuretics (16).

Chlorpropamide causes an increased sensitivity to circulating levels of antidiuretic hormone and a resultant hyponatremia in approximately 4 to 5% of patients. The chlorpropamide-induced hyponatremia is three times more common in females who are more than 65 years old who are being treated with a diuretic. The hyponatremia is reversible, improvement being observed within a week after the medication is discontinued.

Conditions in which the sulfonylureas are usually contraindicated include acidosis, severe infections accompanying diabetic onset, major surgery (during and after), sulfa sensitivity, and pregnancy. Sulfonylureas also are possible teratogens. They should not be used early in pregnancy and are absolutely contraindicated late in gestation, since they may cause prolonged and severe hypoglycemia in the newborn.

Approximately 40% of type II diabetic patients do not achieve satisfactory control with the oral agents. Secondary failure occurs in patients who initially respond to oral agents but subsequently fail to be adequately controlled. The secondary failure rate ranges from 3 to 30% The failure rate tends to increase year after year for patients who experience initial satisfactory control. Patients who fail to respond to the first-generation drugs should be started on one of the second-generation products.

DOSING OF SULFONYLUREAS

Sulfonylurea therapy should be initiated with a low dose of the chosen agent. The dose may be increased weekly on the basis of blood glucose control and symptoms. Use of low doses initially is particularly important for the elderly because their poor eating habits and decreased renal function predispose them to hypoglycemic reactions. Low doses are given once daily before breakfast; higher doses are split and given two or more times throughout the day, depending on the half-life of the drug.

Doses of any given agent should be maximized before a decision to abandon therapy is made. Increasing the dose above maximum levels may result in an increased incidence of adverse effects without producing any further decrease in blood glucose and is not recommended. Treatment with any given agent should continue for 1 month before a change in therapy is warranted. Nonresponse to the sulfonylureas after this trial period is referred to as "primary failure." For these patients, either trial of another oral agent or insulin therapy is indicated. Patients who are treated with insulin may at a later time be given a trial of oral agents. Patients who do not respond to either insulin or oral agents or type II patients who are extremely insulin-resistant may be treated with a combination of insulin and oral agents.

Table 19.13.
Side Effects of Sulfonylureas

GI: less than 5%—take with meals (except glipizide)
Skin: less than 2%
Antabuse effect: approximately 4%, especially with chlorpropamide
Hepatotoxicity: rare, greater than 500 mg Diabinese daily
Hematological: Very rare—cause and effect are questionable
SIADH: 4% with chlorpropamide (if on a diuretic, incidence increases)—does not occur with second-generation drugs
Hypoglycemia: especially in elderly and patients with renal insufficiency

Table 19.14.
What Health Care Providers Should Tell the Diabetic Patient Taking Sulfonylureas

Name, purpose, directions for use
Can be taken with food (except glipizide).
Take regularly, exactly as physician prescribed.
Contact M.D. if fever, sore throat, or mouth lesions develop.
Exercise caution when using alcohol.
Use drug in conjunction with diet.
Use of other drugs should be physician or pharmacist approved.
Carry sugar source for hypoglycemia.

Biguanides (Metformin)

In December 1994 a new drug, metformin (Glucophage), was approved by the FDA for treatment of NIDDM. Metformin is chemically related to the drug phenformin, which was removed from the market several years ago because of a high incidence of lactic acidosis (45). Metformin has a much lower (tenfold to 100-fold) incidence of lactic acidosis than phenformin does. In fact, all cases of lactic acidosis with metformin that were reported in the European literature after years of use involved patients who attempted suicide by overdose or patients for whom the drug was inappropriately prescribed. Metformin differs from the sulfonylureas in several regards. Metformin is not a hypoglycemic agent but is instead an anti-hyperglycemic medication. It is not associated with hypoglycemia, as are the sulfonylureas, except in cases of extended fasting or overdose. In contrast to the sulfonylureas, this drug has no effect on insulin, glucagon, or somatostatin concentrations. Metformin's effect on blood glucose is a result of its ability to increase insulin sensitivity at the receptor and/or postreceptor level. In addition to lowering blood glucose concentrations, metformin may also cause a reduction in weight, a reduction in triglycerides (as much as 50%), a reduction in total cholesterol (10%), and reductions in arterial blood pressure (47). Animal studies have suggested that metformin is antiatherosclerotic. Metformin therapy should be initiated at a dose of 500 mg twice a day and titrated upward to 500 mg three or four times a day or 850 mg two or three times a day. Side effects include a metallic taste and abdominal discomfort, which can be minimized by dosing before meals and by titrating doses slowly so that tolerance can develop. Metformin should not be used by patients with renal failure, liver failure, or any hypoxic disease that would increase the likelihood of lactic acid accumulation. Combination therapy with metformin and sulfonylureas can be an effective means of lowering blood sugar levels and may be more effective than monotherapy with either agent (46).

Insulin

Type I diabetic patients who have absolute insulin deficiency must be treated with exogenous insulin. Generally, patients who require insulin initially tend to be younger than 30 years old, lean, prone to developing ketoacidosis, and markedly hyperglycemic even in the fasting state. Insulin is indicated for type II diabetic patients who do not respond to diet therapy, either alone or combined with oral antidiabetic drugs. Insulin therapy is also necessary for some type II diabetic patients who are subjected to the stress of infection, pregnancy, or surgery.

Diabetic children should begin giving their own injections at around ages 8 to 9, although parents should administer one or two injections per week to stay in practice and should inject in areas that are difficult for the child to reach. By combining the appropriate modification of diet, exercise, and variable mixtures of short- and longer-acting insulins, it has been possible to achieve acceptable but not excellent control of blood glucose. All patients who use insulin should be strongly encouraged to self-monitor blood glucose levels.

CHOICE OF INSULINS

Choice of insulin must be governed by several factors, such as time action profile, effects of mixing, species, strength, purity, and others (refer to Table 19.15). There are several manufacturers of insulin in the U.S. market, and they offer about 20 different brands of insulin. All the mentioned factors must be considered in selecting insulin. Choice of an insulin product based purely on cost is inappropriate. Table 19.16 summarizes the insulins that were available in the United States at press time and compares their onset and duration of action as well as the species source and strength.

Time-Activity Profiles

Insulins may be categorized in three groups on the basis of their time action profiles: short-acting, intermediate-acting, and long-acting. General parameters such as time of onset, time to peak, and duration of action of these various groups of insulin are shown in Figure 19.4. However, these numbers are only guidelines and should not be substituted for documentation of individual patient response. A number of factors such as species, site of injection, depth of injection, ambient temperature, individual patient characteristics, and exercise may alter the time-activity profiles of insulins. (Refer to Table 19.17.)

The short-acting insulins include Semi-Lente, Regular, and Regular Buffered insulins (8). Regular and Buffered Regular insulin formulations are clear and contain solubilized crystalline insulin. Regular insulins are the only insulin products that may be administered intravenously; all other insulin formulations are suspensions. Buffered Regular (Velosulin Human R) is the insulin of choice for external insulin infusion pumps. It is buffered with diphosphates rather than acetates; this makes the insulin

---

Table 19.15.
Factors Considered in Comparing Insulins

Kinetic formulation, time-action profile
Species source (human versus pork versus beef)
Strength (U-100 versus U-500)
Methods of achieving long action (e.g., protein, such as protamine; Zn content)
Purity
Mixability
Cost, manufacture dependability, availability

Table 19.16.
Insulins Available in the United States

Product	Manufacturer	Strength
Short-acting		
Pork		
Iletin II Regular	Lilly	U-100, U-500
Purified Pork Regular	Novo-Nordisk	U-100
Beef/Pork		
Iletin I Regular	Lilly	U-100
Human		
Humulin Regular	Lilly	U-100
Novolin R	Novo-Nordisk	U-100
Velosulin Human R	Novo-Nordisk	U-100
Intermediate-acting		
Pork		
Iletin II Lente	Lilly	U-100
Iletin II NPH	Lilly	U-100
Purified Pork Lente	Novo-Nordisk	U-100
Purified Pork NPH	Novo-Nordisk	U-100
Beef/Pork		
Iletin I NPH	Lilly	U-100
Iletin I Lente	Lilly	U-100
Human		
Humulin L (Lente)	Lilly	U-100
Humulin N (NPH)	Lilly	U-100
Novolin L (Lente)	Novo-Nordisk	U-100
Novolin N (NPH)	Novo-Nordisk	U-100
Long-acting		
Human		
Humulin U (Ultralente)	Lilly	U-100
Fixed combinations (all are U-100 insulins)		
Human		NPH/REG
Humulin 70/30	Lilly	70/30
Novolin 70/30	Novo-Nordisk	70/30
Humulin 50/50	Lilly	50/50

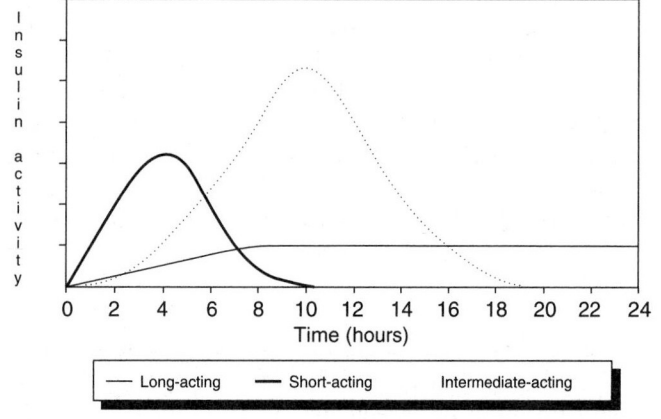

Insulin Time-Activity Profiles
short vs. intermediate vs. long-acting

Insulin Type	Onset	Peak	Duration
Short-acting	0.5–1 hr	2–4 hr	6–8 hr
Intermediate-acting	1–4 hr	6–10 hr	16–24 hr
Long-acting	4–6 hr	18 hr	24–36 hr

Figure 19.4.   Time-activity relationships for insulin

Table 19.17.
Factors Affecting Serum Insulin Concentrations

1. Site of injection—abdominal versus arm versus leg versus thigh
2. Exercise enhances absorption
3. Depth of injection
4. Concentration of insulin
5. Increase in ambient temperature, increased absorption
6. Massage of site increases absorption
7. Insulin antibodies attract and hold insulin
8. Variance in degrading enzymes at site yields day-to-day variation
9. Insulins react with receptors

more stable in insulin catheters, preventing crystallization. Semi-Lente is an amorphous precipitate of insulin and zinc in the form of a suspension, with a slightly delayed onset and peak and a greater duration of action compared to regular insulin.

Intermediate-acting insulins include NPH and Lente insulins. Some clinicians consider Human Ultralente to be an intermediate-acting formulation, since its time-activity profile falls between those observed with classic intermediate-acting insulins and the long-acting insulins. NPH (Neutral Protamine Hagedorn) preparations contain a suspension of zinc-insulin crystals and protamine. Protamine is a protein that is derived from fish sperm, which causes an allergic response in a small number of patients. Lente insulin is a suspension composed of a 30:70 mixture of Semi-Lente and Ultra-Lente. The Lente insulins are produced from various forms of the zinc-insulin complex and are very useful for the patient who has a sensitivity to protamine.

The long-acting insulins include the Ultralente insulins. The long-acting insulins Human Ultralente may be associated with a slight peak effect in some patients. Protamine zinc insulin was discontinued several years ago.

Strength

The FDA decertified U-80 insulin in March 1980 and recently has decertified U-40 insulin. At the present time, two strengths of insulins are available for use: U-100 and U-500. U-500 insulin may be special-ordered from Eli Lilly and Company but is available only with a prescription. In foreign countries, patients are required to have a prescription from a physician to get insulin, and U-40 insulin is often the only strength available.

Species Source

The species source of insulin can influence the effect of insulin on blood glucose control and insulin resistance and sensitivity. Commercially available species sources of insulin include beef, pork, beef/pork mixtures, biosynthetic human, and semisynthetic human. Structurally, beef and pork insulin differ from human insulin by three and one amino acids, respectively (8). The degree of antigenicity parallels the structural similarity, pork being less antigenic than beef but more antigenic than human insulin. About 80% of patients with persistent local allergy to mixed beef-pork insulin improve if they are treated with pure pork insulin or human insulin (8). Initial data indicates that insulin antibody formation occurs at a slower rate in patients who are receiving synthetic human insulin than in those who are using purified pork or beef insulin. It is predicted that purified pork insulin will not be of much use in the future, since it costs more than the human insulin and has no advantages over human insulin.

Human insulin is the least antigenic of the available insulins. However, its solubility is greater than that of the animal source insulins. This increased solubility results in more rapid absorption and a shorter duration of action. Therefore a patient who is being switched from one source of insulin to another should be monitored very closely.

The three forms of human insulin-of biosynthetic-recombinant DNA origin using *Escherichia coli* (Eli Lilly), of biosynthetic-recombinant DNA origin using baker's yeast (Novo, Nordisk), and semisynthetic (Novo-Nordisk)-are therapeutically equivalent. Insulin is produced through recombinant processes by the insertion of the human gene for proinsulin into the *E. coli* or baker's yeast genome. These genetically altered organisms are fermented in an appropriate media that is conducive to the production of proinsulin (or a miniproinsuluin). The proinsulin is harvested, enzymatically altered to form insulin, and purified. Human insulin is also produced via a semisynthetic method by the enzymatic transpeptidation of pork insulin at position 30 of the B chain with the substitution of threonine for alanine.

The recommendations for dosing insulin when changing from beef to human insulin or from conventional to purified insulin are summarized in Table 19.18. Human insulin is indicated for the patient types listed in Table 19.19. Patients who suffer from insulin allergy (local cutaneous reactions, rashes) should definitely be placed on human insulin. A small percentage of patients are allergic to pork insulin and may be treated with human or purified beef insulin. If local reactions continue, however, they may be treated by mixing an antihistamine such as diphenhydramine with the insulin before injection. Often, if the patient continues to use the insulin even though there is a mild local cutaneous reaction, the patient will become desensitized, and the problem will disappear after several weeks. Also, desensitization kits can be obtained from Eli Lilly.

Purity

Another factor that may affect choice of insulin is purity. New analytical techniques that use chromatography and electrophoresis to separate and isolate protein have made purer forms of insulin readily available. The average

Table 19.18.

Recommendations for Dosing Insulin When Changing from Beef to Human or Conventional to Purified Insulin

Highly variable from patient to patient to patient—MONITOR PATIENT CLOSELY

Decrease of 9–20% reported

Recommend 10% dose decrease of normal doses

Recommend 20% decrease if patient receiving more than 50 units/day

Table 19.19.

Patients Who Should Use Human Insulin

Patients with insulin resistance (using more than 100–200 units/day)

Patients with insulin allergy (local cutaneous reactions, rashes, etc.)

Patients with lipoatrophy or lipohypertrophy

All type II diabetics using insulin for a short period of time (e.g., during surgery, infections)

Any patient using insulin intermittently (e.g., gestational diabetics, TPN patients)

All newly diagnosed type I patients

Pregnant diabetics; antibodies are passed to the fetus

content of certain minor components of insulin, such as proinsulin, glucagon, and somatostatin have been decreased, resulting in fewer insulin-sensitivity reactions. All the insulins listed in Table 19.16 are now classified as highly purified insulins, because they have fewer than 10 parts per million of proinsulin. High purification of human insulin is clinically important in that it may result in reduced insulin doses, decreased frequency of lipoatrophy (subcutaneous concavities caused by wasting of the lipid tissue), and a decreased insulin antibody titer.

INSULIN DOSING

A number of dosing regimens are used in the administration of insulin to patients with IDDM (Figure 19.5). Commonly used methods include the following:

1. Single daily injection of intermediate-acting insulin.
2. Two daily injections of intermediate-acting insulin.
3. Two daily injections of 70/30 intermediate/short-acting, premixed insulin.
4. Two daily injections of split and mixed intermediate and short-acting insulin.
5. Three daily injections of short-acting insulin in combination with a single injection of long-acting insulin.
6. Continuous subcutaneous insulin infusion (insulin infusion pump).
7. Sliding scale (multiple daily injections of short-acting insulin).

The choice of regimen depends on the level of patient and practitioner motivation, the patient's ability to monitor control and adjust doses, and the level of control desired. Initial goals at the time of diagnosis are to eliminate the threat of ketoacidosis, obviate overt signs and symptoms of the disease, replete body mass, and rebalance fluid and electrolyte status. Some practitioners prefer to achieve this goal initially with method 1; others believe that the psychological acceptance of two or more injections is greater if this treatment is introduced soon after diagnosis.

Daily Insulin Requirements

Most IDDM patients require between 0.5 and 1.0 unit of insulin per kilogram per day. This total daily dose may be given as one injection (see method 1) or may be divided into several doses to more closely mimic physiologic insulin secretion. Premeal doses of insulin are adjusted; approximately 1 to 2 units of insulin is given for each 50 mg/dL of desired decrease in blood glucose levels.

Comparison of Methods

METHOD 1

A single injection of intermediate-acting insulin is not sufficient to control blood glucose levels for a 24-hr period. This regimen usually results in hyperglycemia before the next dose and may cause hypoglycemia that coincides with peak levels about 8 hr after the dose. A dose that is high enough to cover the patient for 24 hr is usually also high enough to cause hypoglycemia at the peak. This regimen may be sufficient to circumvent ketoacidosis in most patients but results in erratic blood glucose swings. Unfortunately, a large percentage of patients are treated with this regimen. The level of control that this method affords is minimal. Patients who are treated with this regimen can be expected to have HbA$_{1-c}$ levels of approximately 11 to 13%, with blood glucose levels commonly greater than 300 mg%, and sometimes complain of symptoms.

METHOD 2

Glycemic control with method 2 is slightly greater than that with method 1. With method 2, two-thirds of the total daily insulin requirement is injected before breakfast, and one-third is injected just before the evening meal. Both doses are intermediate-acting formulations. There is a decreased chance of experiencing hypoglycemia with this method in comparison with method 1. The level of control afforded by this method is marginal to average, with HbA$_{1-c}$ and blood glucose levels slightly lower than are seen with the above regimen.

METHODS 3 AND 4

These two methods provide average to above-average control with two injections per day. The only difference between the two methods is that with method 3 the patient can only increase or decrease the individual doses but not alter the ratio of short-acting to intermediate-acting insulin. The patient usually takes two-thirds of the total daily dose before breakfast and one-third of the total daily

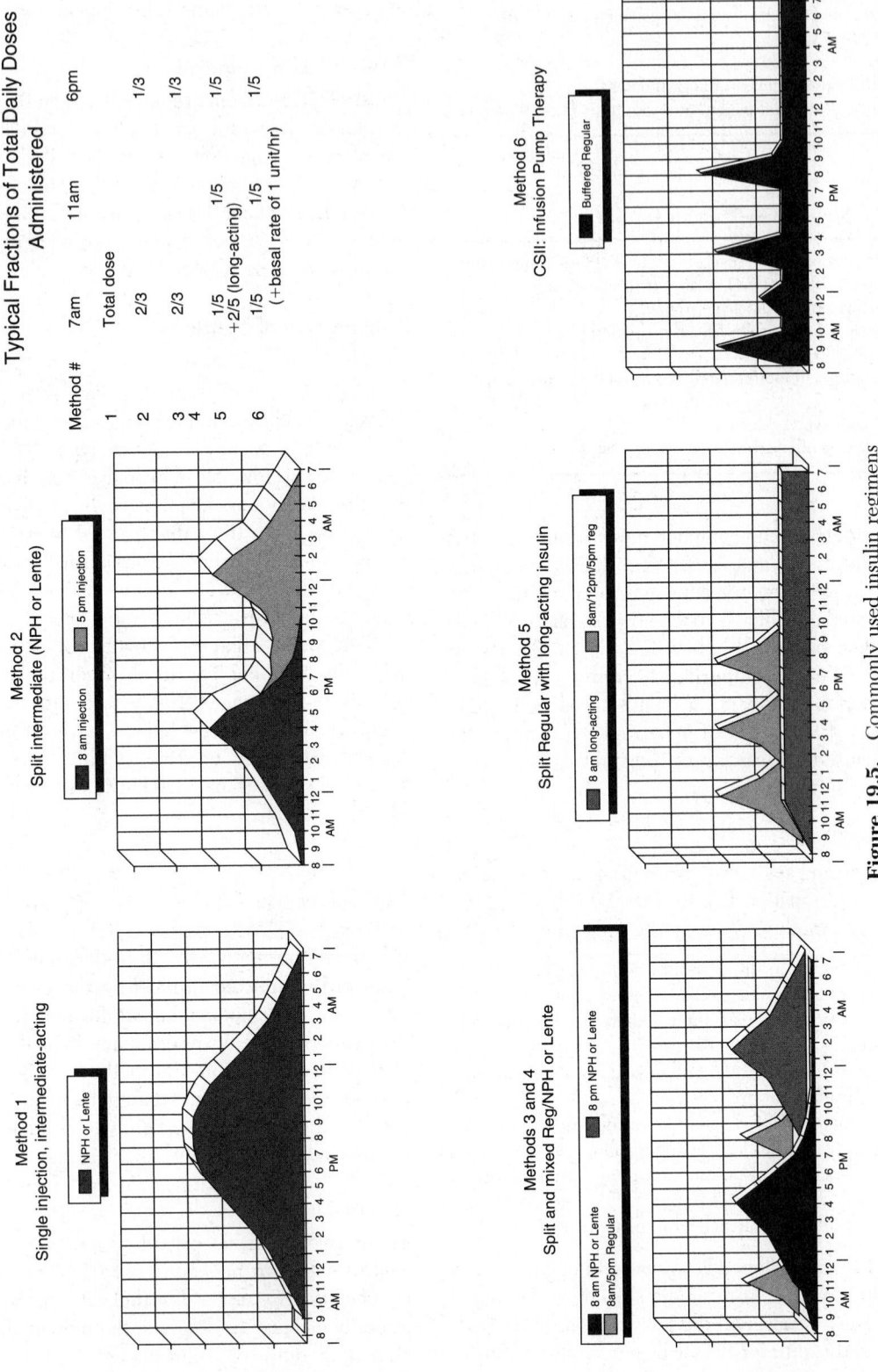

Figure 19.5. Commonly used insulin regimens

dose before the evening meal. The split and mixed regimen is initiated with a 70/30 mixture of intermediate/short-acting insulin, but this ratio may be altered according to insulin needs. With these methods it is recommended that the patient monitor blood glucose levels before meals and at bedtime and alter the appropriate insulin dose accordingly. Of the two methods, method 4 is preferred; however, method 3 is significantly more effective than method 1 or 2. A common variation of method 3 is to administer a mixed (intermediate- and short-acting) dose before breakfast, a dose of short-acting insulin before the evening meal, and a dose of intermediate-acting insulin at bedtime. Glycemic control expected with this method may range from average to good with HbA$_{1-c}$ levels from 7 to 9%, preprandial blood glucose levels from 120 to 160 mg%, and few symptoms.

METHOD 5

This multidose method uses doses of short-acting insulin before each meal in combination with one or two daily doses of long-acting insulin, which provide basal insulin. Variations of this method include the administration of regular insulin before each meal with a dose of intermediate-acting insulin at bedtime. This regimen requires a great deal of patient motivation but provides excellent glycemic coverage and allows the patient a great deal of latitude with regards to meals (the patient may increase or decrease the dose to compensate for anticipated meals).

METHOD 6

Continuous subcutaneous insulin infusion is an excellent method of insulin administration. Initially, this method requires intensive patient training, but the latitude in lifestyle that the pump affords is unparalleled by other dosage regimens. This method provides the patient with a continuous basal amount of insulin (0.5 to 1 unit/hr) in combination with pulsatile doses to cover meals. Pumps that are currently available are about the size of a deck of cards and weigh only a few ounces. Insulin reaches the patient via a small plastic catheter and through a subcutaneous needle. Table 19.20 summarizes the criteria that are used for selecting insulin pump patients (47). Numerous products are in the developmental stage. The pumps can be compared on the basis of insulin dilution requirements, size, ease of use, type and completeness of alarm system, supplemental dose features, whether or not they indicate the total amount of insulin given over a 1-day period, and cost. Patients who use the pumps must purchase numerous auxiliary items. Glycemic control with methods 5 and 6 will in most cases be very good. HbA$_{1-c}$ levels may approach normal (6 to 7%), and preprandial blood glucose levels between 80 and 120 mg%, may be expected.

Table 19.20.
Criteria for Selecting Insulin Pump Patients

1. Pregnant diabetics
2. Diabetics with early complications
3. Diabetics who have had a renal transplant
4. Brittle (difficult-to-control) diabetics
5. Motivated type I diabetics
6. At present, type II and children are not being encouraged
7. All patients must be:
   a. Willing and highly motivated
   b. Capable of being educated
   c. Responsible for keeping records and following specific procedures
   d. Willing to perform and log blood tests daily
   e. Willing to be hospitalized for 2–4 days if necessary

METHOD 7

The sliding scale method described here is reserved for hospitalized patients who undergo frequent blood glucose monitoring. Insulin dosage adjustments with some of the other methods are based on patient-specific sliding scales. The sliding scale method may be used for a patient with diabetes who is acutely ill and requires more insulin than normal or may be used initially after diagnosis to determine daily insulin requirements. Basic sliding scales vary from institution to institution and according to various patient responses. The following is an example of a sliding scale that uses regular insulin for an adult:

Blood Glucose	Subcutaneous Insulin Dose
<140 mg%	0 units
140-200 mg%	2 units
201-300 mg%	5 units
301-400 mg%	10 units
>400 mg%	12 units

The scale is adjusted on the basis of patient response to various doses of insulin.

Interpretation of Blood Glucose Levels

Several problems may be encountered in self-monitoring of blood glucose. Proper patient technique and understanding of a patient's particular method should always be ascertained before insulin dose adjustments. Patients who are being treated with methods 3 through 6 should routinely check blood glucose levels at least four times daily, before meals and at bedtime. Additionally, early morning (3:00 to 4:00 A.M.) and postprandial levels may be checked on a nonroutine basis as needed. Patients who use method 1 should also be instructed to check blood glucose levels. However, it is difficult to target particular out-of-range levels, since only one dose is administered daily.

Generally, an increase in insulin dose of one unit can be expected to decrease the blood glucose level by approximately 50 mg%. Some patients adjust doses daily on the basis of the previous day's response. This approach may be reasonable for some; however, it is probably more prudent to alter doses only after a trend has been identified.

Several problems have been observed with the interpretation of morning fasting blood glucose levels. The first is called the "dawn phenomenon" (48). This effect results from a rise in blood glucose levels that increases insulin need starting at about 5:00 A.M. and continuing until about 9:00 A.M. The early morning glucose rise can be caused by insufficient treatment; but in studies involving patients with continuous subcutaneous insulin infusion, the dawn phenomenon still can occur. Food ingestion is another factor that could influence early morning rise. Yet studies of fasting patients have shown that blood glucose levels can increase in the early morning. Although the condition is not fully understood and the prevalence of the phenomenon is not totally known, it is a cause for concern for patients who are trying to achieve strict control. The most logical mechanism for the dawn phenomenon is an increased glucose production or decreased glucose utilization due to the morning rise of cortisol levels and/or other circadian factors.

Another problem requiring dosage adjustment is the Somogyi phenomenon. This is a condition in which there is early morning hyperglycemia that is secondary to hypoglycemia. In simpler terms, a diabetic patient suffers an episode of hypoglycemia during sleep that results in the release of hormones that increase blood glucose levels such as cortisol, glucagon, and adrenalin. These hormones cause blood glucose levels to increase, and when the patient arises in the morning and tests his or her blood or urine glucose, it is elevated. Since the precipitating problem in the Somogyi phenomenon is hypoglycemia, the necessary step in treatment is to decrease the insulin dose.

The assessment of morning hyperglycemia must include an early morning (3:00 to 4:00 A.M.) blood glucose determination. If hypoglycemia is observed, then the bedtime or evening insulin dose should be decreased. If the level is within normal limits or high, then a slight increase in the evening insulin dose is warranted.

Insulin for Patients with NIDDM

Insulin therapy is useful for patients with NIDDM who are not candidates for oral therapy or patients who do not have an adequate response to oral therapy. Patients with NIDDM will frequently respond to one or two daily doses of intermediate-acting insulin. Recent research has suggested that single injections of intermediate-acting insulin administered in the evening may be more effective than a single dose administered in the morning (49, 50). Theoretically, this regimen is thought to suppress nighttime hepatic glucose production, causing fasting blood sugar levels to be lower, reducing insulin resistance. Some patients with NIDDM will not respond to one injection per day therapy and will require two injections per day of intermediate-acting insulin. Finally, a fraction of NIDDM patients will have progression of disease to the point at which they will require multiple injections of insulin daily to maintain reasonable glycemic control. Since insulin is lipogenic and its use often results in weight gain, NIDDM patients who are being treated with insulin should be reminded of the importance of diet and exercise and not consider insulin a replacement for these key treatment modalities.

Combination Insulin and Sulfonylurea Therapy for Patients with NIDDM

Many studies evaluating the effectiveness of combination insulin sulfonylurea therapy have been reported in the literature. Recently, a metaanalysis of the better-controlled studies was published (51). This study concluded that a marginal reduction in insulin dose may be realized for patients who are being treated with combination therapy and that some patients will have a reduction in blood glucose levels. Overall, the study found that the benefits of combination therapy were minimal for most patients. Nevertheless, combination therapy is a viable regimen for some patients. For patients who are being treated with sulfonylureas who lack adequate response, a small dose (10 units) of intermediate-acting insulin may be added at bedtime (52). The insulin dose should be titrated on the basis of the patient's fasting blood sugar level. Conversely, for the patient who is taking insulin, an intermediate dose of sulfonylurea may be added to the regimen with the monitoring of appropriate blood sugar levels.

MIXING AND STORING OF INSULIN

Because of improved purity, insulins are more stable and may be stored by the user at room temperature for up to 1 month. Insulin should be injected at room temperature. If insulin is purchased in bulk, the vials that are not in use can be kept in the refrigerator. Insulin should be protected from extreme temperatures. Patients should exercise caution when traveling in very hot or very cold climates.

With the increased use of split and mixed regimens there has been much interest in the question of insulin stability in mixtures. Regular and NPH insulin are stable when mixed together in any ratio. This is considered the mixture of choice when a short- and intermediate-acting insulin is required (53). Premixed NPH and Regular insulin are available in Europe in the following ratios: 90:10, 80:20, 70:30, 60:40, and 50:50. Patients should be instructed to adhere to the following sequence when mixing NPH and Regular insulin:

1. Inject the appropriate quantity of air into the NPH insulin vial.
2. Inject the appropriate quantity of air into the Regular insulin vial.
3. Withdraw the dose of Regular insulin.
4. Withdraw the dose of NPH insulin.

Regular and Lente (also Ultra-Lente) insulin interact when mixed, the result being a blunting of the short-acting insulin. Patients should be instructed to either inject immediately after mixing or consistently inject after a measured period of time. The reaction between Lente and Regular insulin continues for 24 hr, so the response from an injection that is taken immediately after mixing may be significantly different from the response from an injection taken 24 hr after mixing. Patients may require a higher ratio of Lente/Regular than would be required with NPH/Regular. Velosulin Regular insulins should not be mixed with Lente insulins. The phosphate buffers will precipitate the zinc from these formulations, the result being an increased activity of short-acting insulin.

Lente insulins may be mixed with each other in any ratio without affecting the time-activity profile of the components. Mixtures of this nature remain stable for up to 18 months.

ADVERSE REACTIONS TO INSULIN

The major complications of insulin therapy (47) are summarized in Table 19.21. These adverse effects may be either immunologically mediated or pharmacologically mediated. Hormones and drugs that influence insulin requirements are listed in Table 19.22.

Hypoglycemia

A special effort should be made to educate the diabetic patient with reference to the symptoms and treatment of hypoglycemia. Factors that predispose the patient to insulin reactions (hypoglycemia) include insufficient food intake (skipping meals, vomiting, or diarrhea), excessive exercise, inaccurate measurement of insulin, concomitant intake of hypoglycemic drugs, termination of diabetogenic conditions, and strict glycemic control. Symptoms include a parasympathetic response (nausea, hunger, or flatulence), diminished cerebral function (confusion, agitation, lethargy, or personality changes), sympathetic responses (tachycardia, sweating, or tremor), coma, and convulsions. Ataxia and blurred vision are also common. In elderly patients with decreased nerve function, diabetic patients with advanced neuropathy, patients with longstanding diabetes (10 years or more), or patients receiving β-blockers, the symptoms of hypoglycemia are sometimes lacking, and the reaction may go undetected and untreated. All manifestations of hypoglycemia are relieved rapidly by glucose administration. In unconscious patients, injections of glucagon or intravenous glucose or dextrose may be required.

Table 19.21.
Complications of Insulin Therapy

Related to insulin purity and/or species source
  Insulin lipoatrophy
  Insulin allergy (local 5–10%; systemic less than 1%)
  Insulin antibody formation (100%, including immunologic resistance)
Unrelated to insulin purity and/or species source
  Hypoglycemia (100%)
  Insulin edema
  Insulin lipohypertrophy
  Complications of diabetes secondary to inadequate control by conventional forms of insulin therapy

Table 19.22.
Hormones and Drugs Influencing the Requirements of Insulin

Increasing Requirement	Decreasing Requirement
Cortisol	Tetracycline
Prednisone	Salicylates
Glucagon	Alcohol
Growth hormone	Biguanides
Catecholamines	Sulfonylureas
Thyroxine	Propranolol
Oral contraceptives	
Diuretics	
Phenytoin	

Because of the potential danger of insulin reactions, the diabetic patient should always carry packets of table sugar or candy for use at the onset of hypoglycemic symptoms. Note also that if a hypoglycemic person is mistakenly thought to be hyperglycemic and is given insulin, severe hypoglycemia and subsequent brain damage may result. Thus, when there is doubt as to whether a diabetic is hypoglycemic or hyperglycemic, sugar should be given initially until the condition can be evaluated accurately. Spouses or caregivers of diabetic patients should be trained to administer glucagon in the event of hypoglycemic-induced unconsciousness. Glucagon should be administered in a dose of 1 mg given subcutaneously or intramuscularly. Glucagon may cause nausea and vomiting; therefore the unconscious patient should be positioned lying on the stomach to avoid aspiration.

Virtually every patient who is treated with insulin will experience hypoglycemia at some time. Ten percent of insulin-treated patients will experience at least one episode of severe hypoglycemia per year requiring assistance. Mortality secondary to hypoglycemia in insulin-treated patients may be as high as 3% (37). Patients in the DCCT who were treated with intensive insulin therapy had a threefold increase in the incidence of hypoglycemia when compared to patients who were treated with conventional therapy (1).

Lipohypertrophy

Lipohypertrophy is a problem that is encountered by patients who do not rotate injection sites. With repeated use of a single injection site, the area becomes anesthetized, which encourages the use of that site. These fatty tumorous formations will usually resolve after the patient begins to rotate injection sites and use proper injection technique. There is no evidence to suggest that this problem is of immunologic origin. Therefore switching to more highly purified products will have little effect.

Insulin Resistance

Insulin resistance, a condition requiring more than 200 units of insulin per day for more than 2 days in the absence of ketoacidosis or acute infection, occurs in only about 0.0001% of diabetic patients. These patients almost invariably have high titers of insulin-neutralizing antibodies or are very obese. These patients should first be switched to a human insulin and, if necessary, placed on glucocorticoids (prednisone in a dose of 5 to 60 or 80 mg/day) (8).

Lipoatrophy

Lipoatrophy, or the wasting away of fatty tissue, appears to be an immunologically mediated phenomenon. The loss of fat is most commonly observed at the injection site but may occur distant from the injection site. This adverse effect is more common in females than in males. The treatment of choice for insulin lipoatrophy is human insulin. Human insulin should be injected directly into the atrophied area until the site has filled in. After resolution the patient should be instructed to continue to inject the area every 2 to 3 weeks to prevent recurrence (54).

DIABETIC KETOACIDOSIS

The physiologic events that lead to diabetic ketoacidosis (DKA) are described in Figure 19.1. DKA is a life-threatening condition that occurs secondary to an insulin deficit. DKA may occur in diabetic patients who also have an active infectious process, in diabetic patients who discontinue insulin therapy, or in diabetic patients who are subjected to other forms of stress (e.g., myocardial infarction, stroke). Twenty to thirty percent of all cases of DKA occur in previously undiagnosed cases of diabetes (20).

Signs and symptoms of DKA include polydipsia, polyuria, weakness, fruity breath, dry mucus membranes, tachycardia, and hypotension. The level of consciousness may range from almost normal to frankly comatose. Laboratory signs include elevated serum glucose, creatinine, and blood urea nitrogen. Hyponatremia is a common finding, along with glucosuria and ketonuria.

Treatment of DKA consists of insulin, fluids, and electrolytes. Insulin is usually administered initially with a bolus intravenous dose between 0.1 and 0.2 unit/kg, followed by a continuous infusion of 0.1 unit/kg/hr. Normal saline is administered at a rate of 0.5 to 1 L/hr until blood pressure and pulse have been stabilized, at which point normal saline may be substituted. Some practitioners recommend the use of either dextran or 5% albumin initially in the presence of shock. When blood glucose levels begin to approach normal, D5 normal saline may be used. If potassium levels are elevated, initially no potassium should be administered until the level reaches the normal range. Patients with potassium levels that are within the normal range should be given potassium 10 to 20 mEq/hr. Hypokalemic patients may be given much larger doses. The use of phosphate in DKA is controversial, but it is usually administered to patients with low levels at a rate of 5 to 10 mmol/hr. Bicarbonate should be administered only to patients whose arterial pH levels are <7.1 and in doses of 44 mEq/hr (20, 55).

PROGNOSIS

The outlook for the diabetic patient has never been more positive. More and more government funds are being allocated for diabetes research to better understand the condition and to develop systems of prevention and treatment that result in normalization of blood glucose levels and, it is hoped, a decrease in the long-term complications. Many states have funds through the Center for Disease Control to develop diabetes control projects with the objective of reducing the morbidity and mortality of diabetes. Research on the efficacy of transplantation of pancreas or of islet tissues is ongoing. Much work is also being done to develop a miniaturized closed-loop system that could be implanted in diabetic patients. Blood glucose could be determined, and insulin would automatically be injected to maintain blood glucose at a preset level. With the massive amount of work being done in the study of diabetes, it is expected that within 20 years, either there will be a device that simplifies the treatment of diabetes to the point at which the patient will be virtually unaware of having diabetes or there will be a surgical transplantation technique that will cure the condition. Additionally, prevention of diabetes may be possible in the future. The new approach to educating patients and giving the patient the responsibility for self-monitoring should also produce positive results and decrease complications while prolonging the diabetic patient's life span and improving the quality of his or her life. The DCCT has proven that strict glycemic control in patients with IDDM reduces the incidence and slows the progression of microvascular disease and neuropathy. The new oral antidiabetic agents, human insulins, and human insulin analogs will probably add further potential flexibility to the diabetic's therapy.

CONCLUSION

Diabetes is a complex, heterogeneous disorder that requires a health team effort if treatment objectives are to be achieved. Through a combination of diet, exercise, medications, and education that result in the patient's taking charge of the condition, the outlook for the diabetic patient is continually improving.

Health care providers must make a special effort to educate diabetic patients about treatment and monitoring. Members of the health care team must communicate and reinforce the information that they provide to the diabetic patient. Health care providers should actively participate in diabetes associations, keep up on the various educational methods and programs relating to diabetes, and become active in the American Association of Diabetes Educators. Health care providers should familiarize themselves with the complete line of diabetes care products that diabetic patients need. The opportunity for specialists in the care of diabetes is great, and those who participate will find that the rewards are even greater.

REFERENCES

1. Diabetes Control and Complications Trial Research Group. The effect of intensive treatment on the development and the progression of long-term complications in insulin-dependent diabetes mellitus. N Engl J Med 329:977–986, 1993.
2. Anonymous. Diabetes prevention trial: type I protocol. Bethesda, MD: National Institutes of Health, 1994.
3. Glycemic control and complications in type II diabetes: design of a feasibility trial. Diabetes Care 5(11):1560–1571, 1993.
4. Anonymous. UK Prospective Diabetes Study. II: reduction in HbA1c with basal insulin supplementation, sulfonylurea, or biguanide therapy in maturity-onset diabetes mellitus. Diabetes 34:793–798, 1985.
5. Watkins JD, Robers DE, Williams TF, et al. Observation of medication errors made by diabetic patients at home. Diabetes 16:883, 1967.
6. Salans LB. Diabetes mellitus, a disease that is coming into focus. JAMA 247:590, 1982.
7. National Diabetes Data Group. Diabetes 28:1039, 1979.
8. Galloway JA, Potvin JH, Shuman CR, eds. Diabetes mellitus. 9th ed. Indianapolis: Lilly Research Laboratories, 1988.
9. Podolsky S. Clinical diabetes: modern management. New York: Appleton-Century-Crofts, 1980:17.
10. Anonymous. Direct and indirect costs of diabetes in the United States in 1992. New York: American Diabetes Association, 1993.
11. Eggers PW. Effect of transportation on the medicare end-stage renal disease program. N Engl J Med 318:223–229, 1988.
12. Anonymous. USRDS 1993 annual report. Bethesda: U.S. Renal Data System, 1993.
13. Zimmet P, King H, Serjeantson S, Kirk R. The genetics of diabetes mellitus. Aust NZ J Med 16:419–424, 1986.
14. Skyler JS, Marks JB. Immune intervention in type I diabetes mellitus. Diabetes Rev 1(1):15–42, 1993.
15. Davidson MB. Pathogenesis of type II diabetes mellitus: an interpretation of current data [Review]. Am J Med Sci 29(7):35–39, 1986.
16. Hansten PD. Drug Interactions. 5th ed. Philadelphia: Lea & Febiger, 1985: 150–169.
17. Cahill GF Jr. Disorders of carbohydrate metabolism: diabetes mellitus. In: Wyngaarden JB, Smith LH Jr., eds. Cecil textbook of medicine. 16th ed. Philadelphia: WB Saunders, 1982, vol 1:1054–1056.
18. Kaplan SA. Diabetes mellitus: UCLA conference. Ann Intern Med 96:635–649, 1982.
19. Olson OC. Diagnosis and management of diabetes mellitus. Philadelphia: Lea & Febiger, 1981:10–17.
20. Sanson TH, Levine SN. Management of diabetic ketoacidosis. Drugs 38(2):89–300, 1989.
21. Brownlee M. Glycosylation of proteins and microangiopathy: hospital practice [Symposium Supplement]. 27(suppl 1):46–50, 1992.
22. Brownlee M. Glycation products and the pathogenesis of diabetic complications. Diabetes Care 15(12):1838, 1992.
23. Kirchain WR, Rendell MS. Aldose reductase inhibitors. Pharmacotherapy 10(5):326–336, 1990.
24. Guigliano D, Marfella R, Quatrato A, De Rosa N, et al. Tolrestat for mild diabetic neuropathy: a 52-week, randomized, placebo-controlled trial. Ann Int Med 118:7–11, 1993.
25. Campbell RK, Klein OG. Eye care for the diabetic patient. JAMA 245:2087, 1981.
26. Bohannon NJ, Zilbergeld B, Bullard DG, et al. Treatable impotence in diabetic patients. West J Med 136:6–10, 1982.
27. Kasiske BL, Kalil RSN, Ma JZ, Liao M, Keane WF. Effect of antihypertensive therapy on the kidney in patients with diabetes: a mega-regression analysis. Ann Int Med 118:129–138, 1993.
28. Lewis EJ, Hunsicker LG, Bain RP, Rohde RD. The effect of angiotensin-converting enzyme inhibition on diabetic nephropathy. N Eng J Med 329:1456–1462, 1993.
29. Anonymous. The physician's guide to type II diabetes (NIDDM): diagnosis and treatment. Alexandria, VA: American Diabetes Association, 1992.
30. Jovanovic L, Peterson CM. The clinical utility of glycosylated hemoglobin. Am J Med 70:331, 1981.
31. Campbell RK. Diabetes and the pharmacist. 2nd ed. Elkhart, IN: The Ames Co., 1986.
32. Anonymous. Self monitoring of blood glucose: American Diabetes Association consensus statement. Diabetes Care 17:81–86, 1994.
33. White J, Campbell RK. Diabetes care products. In: Handbook of nonprescription drugs. 10th ed. Washington, DC: American Pharmaceutical Association, 1992:237–281.
34. Roenstock J. Management of early diabetic nephropathy. Drug Therapy 12:61–68, 1989.
35. Anonymous. Guidelines for diabetes care. Pitman, NJ: American Association of Diabetes Educators/New York: American Diabetes Association, 1981.
36. Brownless, VH. Exercise and the diabetic patient. Drug Ther 12:66, 1982.
37. Richter EA, Ruderman NB, Schneider SH. Diabetes and exercise. Am J Med 70:201, 1981.
38. Kurtzman P. Role of food fiber in health. US Pharmacist 7:63, 1982.
39. West KM. Recent trends in dietary management. In: Podolsky S, ed. Clinical diabetes: modern management. New York: Appleton-Century-Crofts, 1980:70.
40. Paasikivi J, Wahlberg F. Preventative tolbutamide treatment and arterial disease in mild hyperglycemia. Diabetologia 7:323–327, 1971.
41. Ohneda A, Maruhama Y, Itabashi H, et al. Vascular complications and long term administration of oral hypoglycemic agents in patients with dialbetes mellitus. Tohoku J Exp Med 124:205–222, 1978.
42. Kennedy DL, Piper JM, Baum C. Trends in use of oral hypoglycemic agents, 1964-1986. Diabetes Care 11:558–62, 1988.
43. Gerich JE. Oral hypoglycemic agents. New Engl J Med 321:1232–1245, 1989.
44. Skillman TG, Feldman JM. The pharmacology of the sulfonylureas. Am J Med 70:361, 1981.
45. Bailey CJ. Biguanides and MIDDM. Diabetes Care 15:755–772, 1992.
46. Hermann LS, Schersten B, Litzen P, Kjellstrom T, et al. Therapeutic comparison of metformin and sulfonylurea, alone and in various combinations. Diabetes Care 17(10):1100–1109, 1994.

47. Galloway JA, DeShazo RD. The clinical use of insulin and the complications of insulin therapy. In: Ellenberg M, Rifkin H, eds. Diabetes mellitus: theory and practice. 3rd ed. Garden City, NY: Medical Exam Publishing Co., 1982.

48. Schmidt MI. The dawn phenomenon. Infusion 1:1, 1982.

49. Yki-Jarvinen H, Kauppila M, Kujansuu E, Lahti J, et al. Comparison of insulin regimens in patients with non-insulin-dependent diabetes mellitus. 327(20):1426–1433, 1992.

50. Seigler DE, Olsson GM, Skyler JS. Morning vs. bedtime isophane insulin in type II (non-insulin-dependent) diabetes mellitus. Diabetic Medicine 9(9):826–833, 1992.

51. Pugh JA, Wagner ML, Sawyer J, Ramirez G, Tuley M, Friedberg SJ. Is combination sulfonylurea and insulin therapy useful in NIDDM patients?: a meta-analysis. Diabetes Care 15(8):953–959, 1992.

52. Lebovitz HE, ed. Therapy for diabetes mellitus and related disorders. Alexandria, VA: American Diabetes Association, 1991.

53. White J, Campbell RK. The guide to mixing insulins. Hospital Pharmacy 26;12; 1046–1050, 1991.

54. Valenta LJ, Elias AN. Insulin-induced lipodystrophy in diabetic patients resolved by treatment with human insulin. Ann Int Med 102:790–791, 1985.

55. Fish LH. Diabetic ketoacidosis. Postgrad Med 96(3):75–96, 1995.

CHAPTER 20

HYPERLIPIDEMIA

KEVIN M. RODONDI

BACKGROUND

Coronary heart disease (CHD) is one of the leading causes of morbidity, and mortality in the United States and other industrialized nations. Three of the treatable risk factors for CHD are hypertension, cigarette smoking, and hypercholesterolemia (1, 2). Public health efforts, as well as an increasing health consciousness of the average American, has focused attention on these treatable risk factors, and particularly on cholesterol. The consumer is continuously bombarded with information on the dangers of elevated cholesterol levels. Commercial interests have taken advantage of increasing concerns to market the latest food and products to lower cholesterol levels in the blood. The result can lead to misconceptions and an unnecessary concern over cholesterol.

Hyperlipidemia is defined as an abnormal elevation in blood cholesterol, cholesterol esters, triglycerides, or phospholipids. The clinical importance of hyperlipidemia depends on which of these lipids are elevated and to what extent. Studies have demonstrated that elevated cholesterol levels are an independent and significant risk factor for CHD (1, 3, 4). Hypertriglyceridemia has not been established as an independent risk factor for CHD. However, it is considered a potential marker for other underlying lipoprotein disorders (1, 5–7).

Although the association between elevated cholesterol and CHD is established, there is controversy about the potential benefits of interventions to lower cholesterol levels (8–11). Clinical studies conducted to assess the benefits of cholesterol reduction have been criticized for biased reporting methods, which may overemphasize the benefit of lowering cholesterol levels. The extrapolation of benefits in specific study patient populations to the public at large has also been questioned. Consensus statements have been developed by several groups outlining current recommendations for the treatment of hypercholesterolemia and hypertriglyceridemia (1, 2, 4, 7, 12, 13). There is agreement that (a) there is overwhelming evidence that elevated cholesterol increases the risk of CHD; (b) evidence indicates that lowering serum cholesterol levels is beneficial in reducing the risk of CHD in certain patients; (c) a balanced approach to the patient is required that addresses all risk factors for CHD; (d) a sustained commitment on the part of the clinician and the patient is necessary to make any intervention worthwhile in reducing the risk of CHD; (e) dietary intervention is the cornerstone of therapy; and (f) drug therapy should only be considered in patients who fail dietary therapy, have significantly elevated cholesterol levels, or have elevated cholesterol levels in the presence of significant risk factors.

LIPIDS AND LIPID TRANSPORT

Cholesterol is a lipid that serves as a precursor of bile acids and steroid hormones, and is a primary component of cell membranes. Quantities of cholesterol required for normal life functions are manufactured by the body. In the average person, cholesterol levels in the blood reflect about 40 to 60% endogenous cholesterol, with the remainder coming from the diet (14). Triglycerides are composed of free fatty acids which are used as an energy substrate. Triglycerides in the body are provided by fats in the diet, and through the conversion of carbohydrates in the liver.

Cholesterol and triglycerides, as well as other lipids, are transported though the bloodstream in spherical particles called lipoproteins. They have been divided into five major categories depending on their composition: (a) chylomicrons, composed of exogenous or dietary triglycerides; (b) very low density lipoproteins (VLDL), composed primarily of triglycerides; (c) remnant particles or intermediate density lipoproteins (IDL), composed of cholesterol esters and triglycerides; (d) low density lipoproteins (LDL) composed primarily of cholesterol; and (e) high density lipoproteins (HDL) composed of cholesterol. LDL accounts for 60 to 70% of total serum cholesterol and is the major atherogenic class of lipoproteins. HDL is 20 to 30% and VLDL is about 10 to 15% of total serum cholesterol (1, 15, 16).

Cholesterol and triglycerides in the diet enter into the exogenous pathway of lipid transport (Fig. 20.1). Cholesterol and triglycerides form chylomicrons in the intestinal endothelium which then enter the lymphatic system, where they are transported into the general circulation. Once in the bloodstream the chylomicrons interact with the enzyme lipoprotein lipase on the vascular endothelium. Lipase hydrolyzes the triglycerides into free fatty acids and monoglycerides, which are absorbed by muscle and adipose tissue. The fatty acids are oxidized as an energy substrate or converted back into triglycerides. This process converts the chylomicrons into a cholesterol-rich remnant particle. This remnant particle is taken up by the liver,

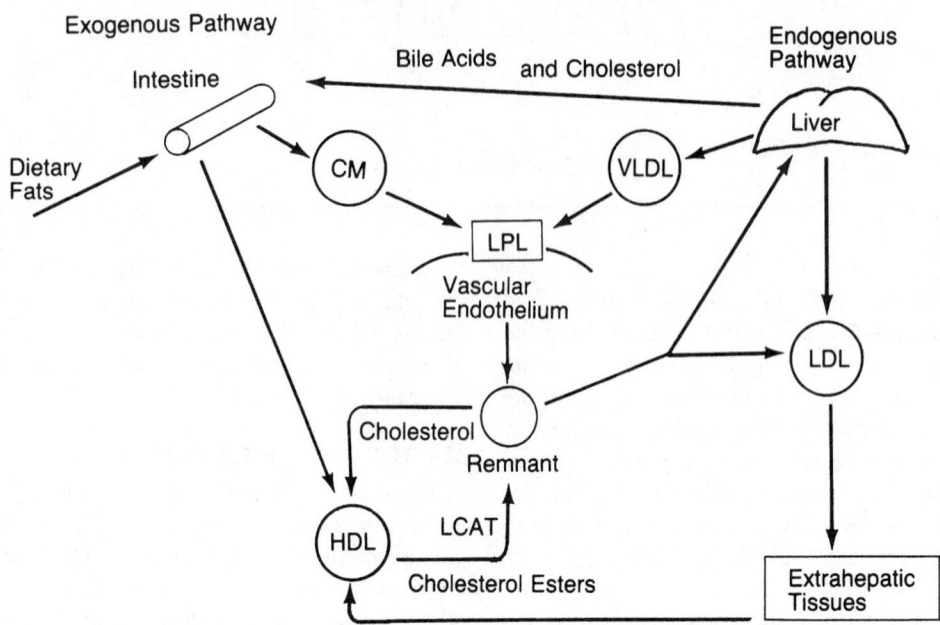

Figure 20.1. Lipid transport. Schematic of exogenous and endogenous lipid pathways. CM, chylomicron; VLDL, very low density lipoprotein; LPL, lipoprotein lipase; LDL, low-density lipoprotein; HDL, high-density lipoprotein; LCAT, lecithin cholesterol acyltransferase.

Table 20.1.
Conversion Table for Lipids

Cholesterol		Triglyceride	
mg/dL	mmol/L	mg/dL	mmol/L
35	0.9	200	2.3
130	3.4	400	4.5
160	4.1	500	5.6
190	4.9	1000	11.3
200	5.2		
240	6.2		

To convert serum cholesterol levels to plasma cholesterol levels multiply by 0.97.
To convert cholesterol level in mg/dL to mmol/L multiply by 0.02586.
To convert triglyceride level in mg/dL to mmol/L multiply by 0.01129.

which converts the cholesterol into bile salts or redistributes it to other body tissues. Bile salts are excreted by the liver into the intestine, where they solubilize dietary fats in the intestine to increase their absorption (15, 16).

Lipids produced by the body are transported through the endogenous pathway. Triglycerides can be synthesized by the liver, especially in the presence of excess carbohydrates. The liver secretes the triglycerides into the bloodstream as VLDL. Like chylomicrons, VLDL is converted into a VLDL remnant by interacting with lipoprotein lipase on the vascular endothelium. Approximately one half of these remnants are metabolized by the liver. The remainder undergo further transformation into LDL where most of the triglycerides are removed and

replaced with cholesterol esters. LDL transports cholesterol to various body tissues where they interact with LDL receptors on cell membranes. The LDL particles are taken up by the cells, where the cholesterol is used for steroid synthesis or as part of cell membranes. Excessive circulating LDL cholesterol will cause cholesterol to be deposited outside of the cell, causing atherogenic plaques to form in the vascular endothelium. Some LDL particles are degraded and eliminated through a scavenger pathway (15, 16).

High density lipoproteins are synthesized by the liver and the intestine. The HDL particle serves as a receptacle for circulating free cholesterol in the tissues and is returned to the liver and kidney to be catabolized. An individual with abnormally low HDL levels (less than 0.9 mmol/L [35 mg/dL]) is at an increased risk of CHD, presumably because of the decreased ability to remove excess circulating cholesterol (1, 4). Table 20.1 provides the conversion of lipids from mg/dL to mmol/L.

ETIOLOGY OF HYPERLIPIDEMIA

Hyperlipidemia can be caused by genetic predisposition, through secondary causes (e.g., underlying disease states, medications, or life-style), or both. The most severe forms of hyperlipidemia occur in individuals with specific inherited traits that result in defects in lipid metabolism or transport (e.g., absence of LDL receptors). Patients with hereditary (primary) disease will usually require medication and intensive intervention to prevent morbidity associated with the condition. Mild or moderate hyperlipidemia is most commonly caused by some degree of inherited predisposition in combination with one or more secondary causes (1).

Diet and life-style have a significant effect on lipid profiles. Body weight is positively correlated with LDL cholesterol and triglycerides, and negatively correlated with HDL cholesterol. Therefore, weight reduction in overweight individuals usually will result in a reduction of LDL cholesterol and triglycerides, and a concomitant increase in HDL cholesterol. Dietary intake is also a key factor in determining the lipid profile, which has led to the specific recommendations for dietary changes in patients with hyperlipidemia described later in this chapter. After dietary causes, hypothyroidism is the most common cause

of secondary hyperlipidemia. Tables 20.2 and 20.3 list examples of secondary causes of lipoprotein abnormalities (17).

Effects of Medications on Plasma Lipids

Selected medications that may cause unintended changes in lipid levels are outlined in Table 20.4. The effects of antihypertensive agents on lipid profiles have received particular attention. Thiazide diuretics, and to a lesser extent loop and potassium sparing diuretics, tend to increase triglyceride and VLDL levels significantly and LDL levels modestly, and have minimal effect on HDL levels. Indapamide, a nonthiazide diuretic, appears to be free of adverse lipoprotein effects. Nonselective β-blocking agents without sympathomimetic activity (e.g., propranolol) may increase serum triglyceride levels, decrease HDL and have little effect on total and LDL cholesterol. β_1-Selective agents (e.g., metoprolol and atenolol) have a similar effect on triglycerides but less effect on HDL levels. Pindolol, a β-blocking agent with intrinsic sympathomimetic activity, has little effect on triglyceride levels and may actually increase HDL cholesterol. Postsynaptic α_1-receptor-blocking agents such as prazosin, doxazosin, and terazosin have favorable lipoprotein effects and may reduce triglyceride levels and increase HDL cholesterol while slightly decreasing total and LDL cholesterol. Angiotensin-converting enzyme inhibitors and calcium channel blockers tend to be lipid neutral. Centrally acting agents (e.g., clonidine, methyldopa) may slightly lower HDL and total cholesterol levels (18–20).

Limited data is available on the lipid altering effects of other medications including: amiodarone, antacids, ascorbic acid, aspirin, biguanides, cimetidine/ranitidine, interferons, high dose ketoconazole, nonsteroidal antiinflammatory drugs, aminosalicylic acid, and sulfonylureas (18).

Table 20.2.
Secondary Causes of Hyperlipidemia

Predominant Lipid Abnormality is Hypertriglyceridemia	Predominant Lipid Abnormality is Hypercholesterolemia
Acromegaly	Amiodarone
Alcohol excess	Anabolic steroids
β-blockers	Anorexia nervosa
Burns	Chlorinated hydrocarbon insecticides
Chronic renal failure	Cholestasis
Diabetes	Cyclosporine therapy
Estrogen therapy	Growth hormone deficiency
Glucocorticoids	Hypothyroidism
Glycogen storage disease	Myelomatosis (IgA, IgG)
Hyperandrogenism in women	Nephrotic syndrome
Isotretinoin	Progestins
Lipodystrophy	Thiazide diuretics
Systemic lupus and polyclonal gammopathy	
Thiazide diuretics	
Weight gain	

From Stone NJ. Secondary causes of hyperlipidemia. Med Clin North Am 78:117–141, 1993.

Table 20.3.
Examples of Secondary Causes of Lipid and Lipoprotein Abnormalities

Lipid/Lipoprotein Patterns	High Cholesterol	TG Excess (200–400 mg/dL)	Low HDL (<35 mg/dL)	Chylomicronemia Syndrome (TG > 1000 mg/dL)
Dietary	Saturated fats, dietary cholesterol	Weight gain	Low-fat diet	Alcohol and fat plus primary disorder
Drugs	Diuretics, prednisone, cyclosporine	Retinoic acid, β-blockers	Anabolic steroids, progestins, β-blockers	Steroids or estrogens added to primary disorder
Disorders of metabolism	Hyperthyroidism, pregnancy, diabetes	Obesity, non-insulin-dependent diabetes, pregnancy	Obesity, non-insulin-dependent diabetes	Diabetes or hypothyroidism plus primary disorder
Diseases	Nephrotic syndrome, obstructive liver disease	Chronic renal failure +/− dialysis	Chronic renal failure +/− dialysis	Rarely systemic lupus erythematosus, lymphoma

HDL, high density lipoprotein; TG, triglyceride.
From Stone NJ. Secondary causes of hyperlipidemia. Med Clin North Am 78:117–141, 1993.

Table 20.4.
Selected Medications Affecting Lipoprotein Levels

Agents	Total Cholesterol	LDL	HDL	VLDL	Triglyceride
Estrogens	↓	↓	↑	↑	↑
Progestins		↑	↓	↓	↓
Anabolic Steroids	—	↑	↓	—	↑
Retinoids	↑	↑	↓	↑	↑
Corticosteroids	↑	↑	↑	↑	↑
Cyclosporin A	↑	↑	—	—	—
Phenothiazines	↑		↓		
Anticonvulsants	—	—	↑		—
Antihypertensive agents					
Thiazides		↑	—	↑	↑
Nonselective β-blockers	—	—	↓	↑	↑
α$_1$-blockers		↓	↑		↓

LDL, low density lipoprotein; HDL, high density lipoprotein; VLDL, very low density lipoprotein; dashes, no substantial change; ↑ increase; ↓ decrease. This provides general effects of drug classes, specific drugs within a class may differ in lipid effects.
From Henkin Y, Como JA, Oberman A. Secondary dyslipidemia; inadvertent effects of drugs in clinical practice. JAMA 267:961–968, 1992.

CLINICAL IMPLICATIONS OF HYPERLIPIDEMIA

Although increased serum cholesterol levels have been directly linked to the risk of CHD, it is LDL cholesterol that is more closely associated with the risk and extent of disease. Low HDL cholesterol has also been identified as a risk factor for CHD. The association of cholesterol levels with the risk of CHD is not a linear relationship. The risk of CHD increases more quickly with total cholesterol levels above 240 mg/dL (6.2 mmol/L), which has been defined as the cutoff for high blood cholesterol. This corresponds to the 80th percentile of the U.S. adult population (1, 4).

A number of clinical trials have studied the effect of dietary or pharmacologic interventions for cholesterol reduction in altering CHD risk. Four major randomized, placebo controlled trials have been conducted evaluating the primary outcomes of death or clinically apparent disease after treatment with diet and pharmacologic intervention. Three of the trials have addressed primary prevention, or the treatment of subjects with no manifestations of cardiovascular disease. These are the World Health Organization (WHO) trial (21), the Lipid Research Clinics Coronary Primary Prevention Trial (LRC-CPPT) (22, 23) and the Helsinki Heart Study (24). The Coronary Drug Project (CDP) evaluated secondary prevention in men with a history of myocardial infarction (25). These studies showed a reduction in CHD morbidity and mortality after cholesterol reduction by dietary and pharmacologic intervention in large populations of middle aged men (Table 20.5). However, these studies have been criticized for stating the benefit of cholesterol reduction on outcomes as a reduction in relative risk instead of absolute risk. Some critics contend that this method of reporting has led professionals and others into believing that there are greater benefits to cholesterol reduction than actually occur (8–11, 26). In addition, the majority of clinical research has been in a narrow study population of middle aged men with elevated cholesterol levels, which yields results that may not be applicable to the population at large.

Despite the controversy surrounding the clinical research, most clinicians agree that the apparent benefit of cholesterol reduction in study patients at risk for CHD warrants interventions in the general population for those at increased risk without evidence of preexisting CHD (primary prevention) or in patients with evidence of CHD (secondary prevention) (4). This position is strengthened by studies in patients with coronary artery disease or previous myocardial infarction where interventions producing lower lipid levels halted progression of coronary lesions, reduced the incidence of cardiac events, and also resulted in the regression of measurable coronary lesions (27–29). Several groups have published position papers outlining recommendations for the treatment of hypercholesterolemia, including the American Heart Association (12) and the National Cholesterol Education Program Adult Treatment Panel II (NCEP-ATP II) (4).

Recent studies have suggested that the benefit of intervention and treatment for hypercholesterolemia to prevent CHD may not be applicable to the elderly (30–32). The correlation of CHD risk and cholesterol declines with age and it is uncertain if cholesterol reduction will decrease the incidence of CHD or death due to CHD. Further, there may be increased risk to drug therapy in the elderly and the benefit may not be significant if there is a high likelihood of death due to other causes. This evidence does call into question guidelines to treat patients over 65 years of age. An alternative recommendation is that for patients 55–65 years of age, screening and treatment may be appropriate for men and women who already have evidence of atherosclerosis or in men who are at higher risk of death due

Table 20.5.
Hypercholesterolemia Trials—Study Characteristics and Clinical Outcomes

Study	Subjects	Drug	Years of Follow-up	Outcomes	Incidence* Placebo	Incidence* Drug	Relative Risk Reduction (%)	Absolute Risk Reduction*
WHO (21) Primary prevention	Men 30–59 yr Avg chol 6.45 mmol/L	Clofibrate	5	Death	19	25	−24	−6
				Nonfatal MI	31	23	26	8
				Death or nonfatal MI	50	48	NS	
LRC-CPPT (22, 23) Primary prevention	Men 33–59 yr Avg chol 7.55 mmol/L	Cholestyramine	7.4	Death	37	36	NS	
				Nonfatal MI	118	102	14	16
				Death or nonfatal MI	149	135	9	14
Helsinki (24) Primary prevention	Men 40–55 yr Avg chol 7 mmol/L	Gemfibrozil	5	Death	21	22	NS	
				Nonfatal MI	35	22	37	13
				Death or nonfatal MI	56	44	20	12
CDP (25)		Niacin	6.2	Death	254	244	NS	
				Nonfatal MI	138	102	26	36
				Death or nonfatal MI	392	346	12	46
Secondary prevention	Men 30–60 yr Avg chol 6.45 mmol/L	Clofibrate	15†	Death	582	520	11	62
			6.2	Death	254	255	NS	
			15†	Nonfatal MI	138	131	NS	
				Death	582	578	NS	

*Incidence and absolute risk reductions are in events per thousand subjects.
†15-year follow-up conducted after completion of treatment phase.
Modified from Grumbach K. How effective is drug treatment of hypercholesterolemia? J Am Board Fam Pract 4:437–445, 1991.

to CHD vs. other causes. Screening and treatment is generally not appropriate for most elderly women. Screening and treatment should only be done in patients who express a desire for treatment and to whom the uncertainties of potential risks and benefits have been explained. In general, elderly people in their late 70s and beyond should not be screened or treated for high blood cholesterol (31).

Although triglycerides have not been linked to CHD risk, hypertriglyceridemia may be a sign of underlying lipid abnormalities since patients in this classification often have elevated LDL cholesterol and decreased HDL cholesterol. The ATP II (4). has defined serum triglyceride levels below 2.3 mmol/L (200 mg/dL) as normal; between 2.3 and 4.5 mmol/L (200–400 mg/dL) as borderline high; 4.5 to 11.3

mmol/L (400–1000 mg/dL) as high; and above 11.3 mmol/L (1000 mg /dL) as very high. Fasting triglyceride levels above 11.3 mmol/L (1000 mg/dL) will require treatment because of associated complications including acute pancreatitis, lipemia retinalis, and eruptive skin xanthomas. There is disagreement on whether high triglyceride levels require treatment for a possible increase in CHD risk, especially if there are no other CHD risk factors. However, there appears to be a relationship between elevated triglyceride levels and low HDL cholesterol levels, which has been identified as a risk factor for CHD. Therefore, reducing triglyceride levels with an associated increase in HDL cholesterol may be beneficial for the patient. Because of the difficulty in assessing risk,

Table 20.6.
Classification of Cholesterol and Triglyceride Levels Based on NCEP (ATP II) Guidelines

	Desirable	Borderline High Risk	High Risk for CHD	High Risk for Pancreatitis
Cholesterol	<200 (5.2)	200–239 (5.2–6.2)	≥240 (6.2)	
LDL Cholesterol	<130 (3.4)	130–159 (3.4–4.1)	≥160 (4.1)	
HDL Cholesterol	≥60 (1.6)		<35 (0.9)	
Triglyceride	<200 (2.3)	200–400 (2.3–4.5)	400–1000 (4.5–11.3)	>1000 (11.3)

Units are reported in mg/dL followed by the corresponding value in mmol/L in brackets. Rounding during conversion from mg/dL to mmol/L causes an apparent overlap between borderline high and high risk categories.
Modified from Schaefer EJ. New recommendations for the diagnosis and treatment of plasma lipid abnormalities. Nutr Rev 51:246–252. 1993.

Table 20.7.
Assessment of Blood Cholesterol Levels for Primary Prevention for Adults Without Evidence of Coronary Heart Disease

Non-Fasting Total Blood Cholesterol and HDL Cholesterol Measurement	
Result	Action
Desirable blood cholesterol with HDL ≥35 mg/dL	Repeat total cholesterol and HDL cholesterol within 5 years, provide general information.
Borderline high cholesterol level with less than two CHD risk factors and HDL ≥35 mg/dL	Provide information on diet, physical activity, and risk factor reduction. Repeat total cholesterol and HDL cholesterol in 1 to 2 years.
HDL cholesterol <35 mg/dL or Borderline high blood cholesterol with two or more risk factors or High blood cholesterol	Do further lipoprotein analysis; treatment decision based on LDL cholesterol.

Lipoprotein Analysis After 9- to 12-Hour Fast	
Result	Action
Desirable LDL cholesterol	Repeat total cholesterol and HDL cholesterol within 5 years; provide general information.
Borderline high-risk LDL cholesterol with fewer than two or more risk factors	Provide information on Step I diet and physical activity. Reevaluate annually including lipoprotein analysis and risk assessment.
Borderline high-risk LDL cholesterol with two or more risk factors (based on 2 or more measurements) or High-risk LDL cholesterol (based on two or more measurements)	Full clinical evaluation, evaluate secondary causes, evaluate familial disorders, consider influences of age, sex, and other CHD risk factors. Initiate dietary therapy.

From reference 4.

nonpharmacologic interventions to reduce triglyceride levels are appropriate and may include dietary intervention, exercise, smoking cessation, reducing alcohol intake, and evaluating medications that may increase triglyceride levels. Patients with borderline hypertriglyceridemia usually do not require treatment unless they have elevated cholesterol levels or significant risk factors for CHD. Triglyceride levels below 2.3 mmol/L (200 mg/dL) can be considered normal in the absence of other CHD risk factors (1, 4, 7).

PATIENT EVALUATION

The ATP II (4) has recently established revised guidelines including a classification scheme for total cholesterol, LDL cholesterol, and triglyceride levels that is outlined in Table 20.6. The ATP II classification scheme of total and LDL cholesterol offers guidelines that can be used in making treatment decisions for the prevention of CHD. The revised ATP II assessment criteria in Table 20.7 include the consideration of total cholesterol, HDL cholesterol and LDL cholesterol in conjunction with established risk factors (Table 20.8) for screening patients for primary prevention of CHD.

ATP II guidelines recommend screening all adults 20 years or older for elevated cholesterol levels every 5 years. Interventions are listed in Table 20.9 and are based on the total, HDL, and fasting LDL cholesterol levels. The fasting LDL cholesterol level can be measured directly or by the following formula: LDL cholesterol = total cholesterol − HDL cholesterol − triglycerides/5. LDL cholesterol levels should be determined on two separate occasions and the results averaged to determine the patients risk category. If the two levels differ by more than 0.7 mmol/L (30 mg/dL) a third level should be taken and all three averaged to make an assessment. Significant interlaboratory variability in cholesterol level determinations has been well documented (33). The clinician should be confident that results used to classify a patient's risk have been determined accurately and the laboratory adheres to established standards for cholesterol measurement (4).

TREATMENT

A comprehensive treatment plan is required that addresses all the risk factors for CHD. Secondary hyperlipidemia may resolve by treating underlying causes, including hypothyroidism, diabetes mellitus, diet, and drugs. Initial treatment should also include smoking cessation and control of hypertension when appropriate. The patient's life-style should be assessed and simple methods of reducing cholesterol levels and risk of coronary heart disease such as moderate exercise and weight control should be part of the overall treatment plan. Patient education should include specific recommendations that are easy for patients to understand and incorporate into their daily routine (Table 20.10).

Diet

Diet is the cornerstone of therapy for the treatment of hyperlipidemia. Three dietary habits can significantly add

Table 20.8.
ATP II Guidelines of CHD Risk Factors Based on Factors Other Than Low Density Lipoprotein Cholesterol

Male ≥ 45 years of age
Female ≥ 55 years of age or premature menopause without estrogen replacement therapy
Family history of premature CHD
   (definite myocardial infarction or sudden death before 55 years of age in father or other male first-degree relative, or before 65 years of age in mother or other female first-degree relative)
Current cigarette smoking
Hypertension
   (confirmed blood pressure ≥ 140/90 mm Hg, or taking antihypertensive medication)
Low HDL cholesterol
   (<35 mg/dL [0.9 mmol/L])
Diabetes mellitus
Subtract 1 risk factor if confirmed high HDL cholesterol
   (≥ 60 mg/dL [1.6 mmol/L])

From reference 4.

Table 20.9.
NCEP ATP II Recommended Interventions Based on LDL Cholesterol Levels

Intervention	Initiate Treatment Based on LDL Levels	Minimal LDL Goal
Dietary Therapy		
Without CHD and fewer than two risk factors	≥160 mg/dL (4.1 mmol/L)	<160 mg/dL (4.1 mmol/L)
Without CHD and with two or more risk factors	≥130 mg/dL (3.4 mmol/L)	<130 mg/dL (3.4 mmol/L)
With CHD	>100 mg/dL (2.6 mmol/L)	≤100 mg/dL (2.6 mmol/L)
Drug Therapy		
Without CHD and fewer than two risk factors	≥190 mg/dL (4.9 mmol/L)	<160 mg/dL (4.1 mmol/L)
Without CHD and with two or more risk factors	≥160 mg/dL (4.1 mmol/L)	<130 mg/dL (3.4 mmol/L)
With CHD	≥130 mg/dL (3.4 mmol/L)	≤100 mg/dL (2.6 mmol/L)

From reference 4.

Table 20.10.
Practical Aspects of CHD Life-style Interventions

Clinical Quotes	Translation into Risk Factor Reduction	Translation into Specific Recommendations
Stay lean	• Reduces total, VLDL, and LDL cholesterol levels • Reduces triglyceride levels, increases HDL levels • Reduces blood pressure • Increases exercise tolerance	• Control portion sizes • Avoid "empty" calories from excess alcohol • Avoid overconsumption of food—even "healthy food" consumed in excess results in weight gain
Adopt a healthy diet	• Reduces total, VLDL, and LDL cholesterol levels • Reduces triglyceride levels, increases HDL levels • Reduces blood pressure • Increases exercise tolerance	• No more than 6 oz. lean meat per day • 2–3 servings low-fat dairy products daily • 4–6 servings fruit, vegetables daily • 8–10 servings grain products daily • This serving distribution not only controls the macronutrient content of the diet (protein, carbohydrates, fat), but also improves the micronutrient content of the diet (vitamins, minerals)

Exercise	• Reduces resting blood pressure
	• Increases HDL cholesterol levels
	• Increases exercise tolerance
		• Regular program of exercise, 30 min 2–3 times per week
		• Take advantage of opportunities:
		  • Stairs
		  • Walk the dog
		  • Park further from the store

From Denke MA. Diet and lifestyle modification and its relationship to atherosclerosis. Med Clin North Am 78:218, 1994.

Table 20.11.
Dietary Recommendations of ATP II for the Treatment of Hypercholesterolemia

Nutrient	Step One Diet	Step Two Diet
Total fat	≤30%	≤30%
Saturated fat	<10%	<7%
Polyunsaturated fat	<10%	<10%
Monounsaturated fat	5–15%	5–15%
Carbohydrate	50–70%	50–70%
Protein	10–20%	10–20%
Cholesterol	<300 mg	<200 mg
Calories	To maintain optimal weight	To maintain optimal weight

Percent indicates percentage of total daily calories.
Modified from Schaefer EJ. New recommendations for the diagnosis and treatment of plasma lipid abnormalities. Nutr Rev 51:246–252, 1993.

to cholesterol levels: (a) a high intake of saturated fats; (b) a high intake of cholesterol; and (c) caloric intake in excess of requirements, leading to obesity (4, 34). Several dietary protocols have been developed, and most follow the recommendations of the American Heart Association (34), and the ATP II (4) recommendations. These diets all have the goal of reducing total fat intake to less than 30% of calories, reducing saturated fat intake while increasing polyunsaturated and monounsaturated fats, reducing cholesterol consumption, keeping daily total caloric intake at levels required to reach and maintain an ideal weight, and providing carbohydrate and protein at appropriate ratios for a balanced diet. Revised NCEP ATP II dietary guidelines are summarized in Table 20.11.

Step one of the NCEP diet is a balanced approach that is recommended for all individuals as a public health effort

and is also part of the initial treatment program of patients being treated for hypercholesterolemia. Step two is used for patients with severe forms of hypercholesterolemia or who do not receive adequate control of cholesterol using the step one diet (Fig. 20.2). Low fat diets are difficult to maintain, since most easily obtained or prepared foods in industrialized nations are high in fats and total calories. Most patients will require intensive and sustained dietary counseling to maintain the dietary plan, since it usually necessitates a change in how they and their families prepare and eat their food. In addition, fats add flavor to the diet and increase satiety, so reducing fat consumption makes the diet less pleasing.

All patients being screened for cholesterol levels should receive dietary information modeled after the NCEP or similar dietary protocols. Patients with CHD risk factors and/or cholesterol levels requiring intervention should be given thorough dietary counseling to help them adhere to the NCEP diet as part of their treatment. Patients usually understand the concept behind a dietary treatment plan, but often do not understand how to apply dietary guidelines to their daily eating habits.

Patients should be instructed on which foods to choose or avoid (Tables 20.12 and 20.13). Increased consumption of fruits and vegetables should be encouraged. In general, packaged, highly processed foods, and most snack products are high in calories and fat and should be avoided. Oils, meat, dairy products, and condiments can also be a significant source of fat in the diet. Patients should be reminded that foods low in cholesterol may not necessarily be low in fats. FDA guidelines now mandate nutritional labeling on most foods which can serve as a check for total

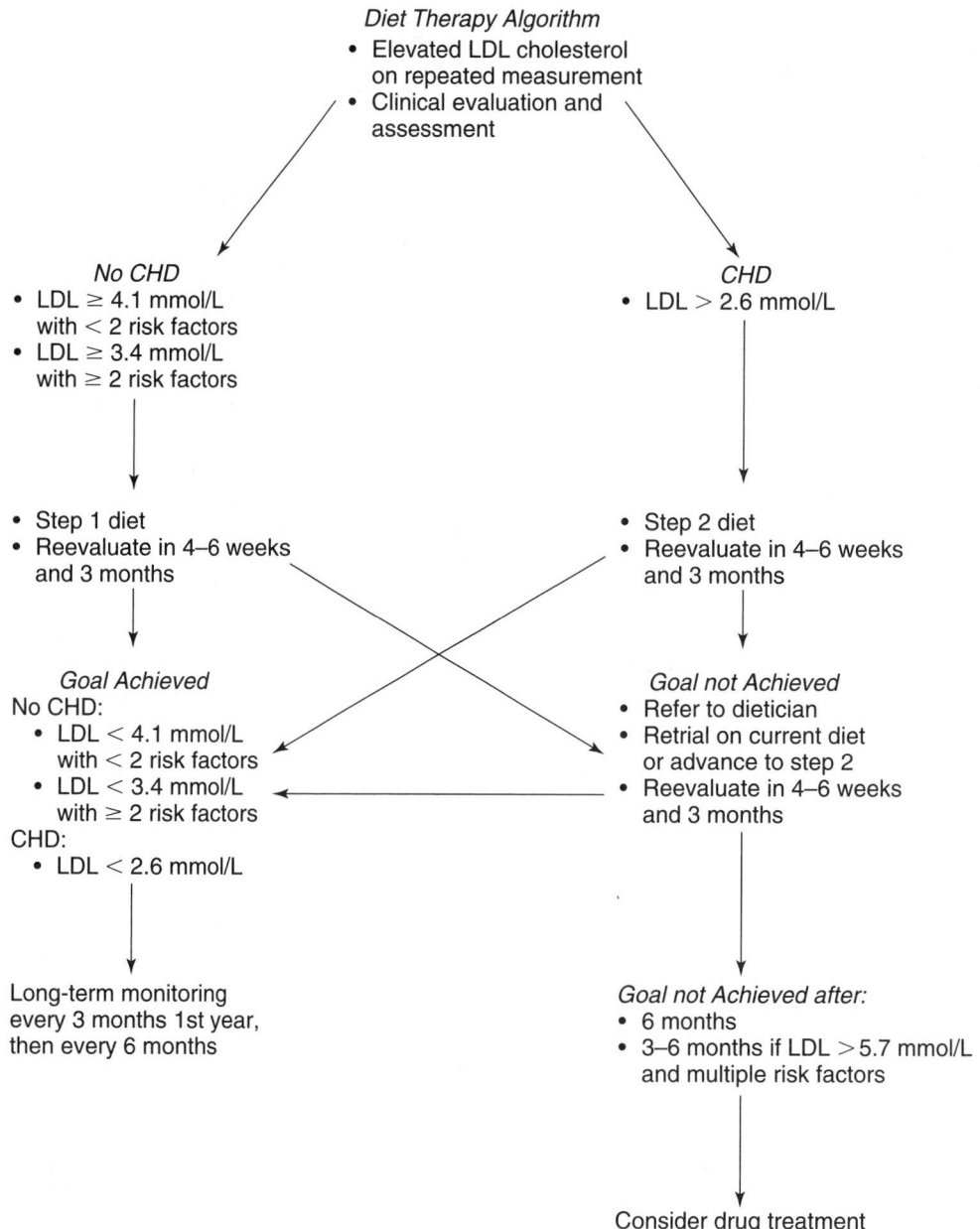

Diet Therapy Algorithm
- Elevated LDL cholesterol on repeated measurement
- Clinical evaluation and assessment

No CHD
- LDL ≥ 4.1 mmol/L with < 2 risk factors
- LDL ≥ 3.4 mmol/L with ≥ 2 risk factors

CHD
- LDL > 2.6 mmol/L

- Step 1 diet
- Reevaluate in 4–6 weeks and 3 months

- Step 2 diet
- Reevaluate in 4–6 weeks and 3 months

Goal Achieved
No CHD:
- LDL < 4.1 mmol/L with < 2 risk factors
- LDL < 3.4 mmol/L with ≥ 2 risk factors
CHD:
- LDL < 2.6 mmol/L

Goal not Achieved
- Refer to dietician
- Retrial on current diet or advance to step 2
- Reevaluate in 4–6 weeks and 3 months

Long-term monitoring every 3 months 1st year, then every 6 months

Goal not Achieved after:
- 6 months
- 3–6 months if LDL >5.7 mmol/L and multiple risk factors

Consider drug treatment

Figure 20.2

calories and fat and cholesterol content of a reasonable serving size (35). A conversion of fat content in grams to calories will determine if it represents over 30% of calories for a product, which is not desirable. Total grams of fat multiplied by 9 kCal/g yields calories from fat.

Evidence has suggested a cholesterol lowering benefit and/or prevention of CHD for several substances including bran, red wine, fish oil, antioxidant vitamins, and others. Commercial interests have capitalized on these findings and sometimes make bold claims regarding the healthful effects of their products. Although these substances may provide some benefit in reducing CHD risk or cholesterol levels, they may also be associated with some adverse effects, or their benefit may remain unproven. For example, since there is no negative effect from moderate increases of bran in the diet, patients should not be discouraged from this practice. However, they should be cautioned regarding commercially available bran products that may be high in sugar or fats to increase their palatability, thereby countering beneficial effects. Further, excessive bran consumption may cause constipation, impaction, or other complications.

Table 20.12.
Recommended Diet Modifications to Lower Blood Cholesterol (The NCEP Step 1 Diet)

Category	Choose	Decrease
Fish, chicken, turkey, and lean meats	Fish, poultry without skin, lean cuts of beef, lamb, pork or veal, shellfish	Fatty cuts of beef, lamb, pork, spare ribs, organ meats, regular cold cuts, sausage, hot dogs, bacon, sardines, roe
Skim and low-fat milk, cheese, yogurt, and dairy substitutes	Skim or 1% fat milk (liquid, powdered, evaporated), buttermilk	Whole milk (4% fat; regular, evaporated, condensed: cream, half-and-half, 2% milk, imitation milk products, most nondairy creamers, whipped toppings)
	Nonfat (0% fat) or low-fat yogurt	Whole-milk yogurt
	Low-fat cottage cheese (1% or 2% fat)	Whole-milk cottage cheese (4% fat)
	Low-fat cheeses, farmer or pot cheeses (all of these should be labeled no more than 2 to 6 g of fat per ounce)	All natural cheeses (e.g., bleu, Roquefort, Camembert, cheddar, Swiss), low-fat or light cream cheese, low-fat or light sour cream, cream cheeses, sour cream
	Sherbet, sorbet	Ice cream
Eggs	Egg whites (2 egg whites equal 1 egg in recipes), cholesterol-free egg substitutes	Egg yolks
Fruits and vegetables	Fresh, frozen, canned, or dried fruits and vegetables	Vegetables prepared in butter, creams, or other sauces
Bread and cereals	Homemade baked goods using unsaturated oils sparingly, angel food cake, low-fat crackers, low-fat cookies	Commercial baked goods: pies, cakes, doughnuts, croissants, pastries, muffins, biscuits, high-fat crackers, high-fat cookies
	Rice, pasta	Egg noodles
	Whole-grain breads and cereals (oatmeal, whole wheat, rye, bran, multigrain, etc.)	Breads in which eggs are a major ingredient
Fats and oils	Baking cocoa	Chocolate
	Unsaturated vegetable oils: corn, olive, rapeseed, (canola oil), safflower, sesame, soybean, sunflower	Butter, coconut oil, palm oil, lard, bacon fat
	Margarine or shortenings made from one of the unsaturated oils listed above, diet margarine	
	Mayonnaise, salad dressings made with unsaturated oils listed above, low-fat dressings	Dressings made with egg yolk
	Seeds and nuts	Coconut

From The Expert Panel: Report of the National Cholesterol Education Program expert panel on detection, evaluation, and treatment of high blood cholesterol in adults. Arch Intern Med 148:36–69, 1988.

Table 20.13.
Fatty Acid Composition of Vegetable Oils and Animal Fats

High in saturated fats
Coconut oil	Palm kernel oil	Butterfat
Cocoa butter	Palm oil	Beef tallow

High in monosaturated fats, low in saturated fats
Olive oil	Peanut oil	Rapeseed (Canola) oil

High in polyunsaturated fats, low in saturated fats
Soybean oil	Corn oil	Sunflower oil
Safflower oil		

Information taken from American Medical Association Council on Scientific Affairs: Saturated fatty acids in vegetable oils. JAMA 263:693–695, 1990.

Confusion over health claims for foods resulted in the U.S. Nutrition Labeling and Education Act of 1990. As required by this Act, the FDA implemented their final rule regarding seven accepted health claims, two of which regard CHD risk reduction. The first is the association between fruits, vegetables, and grain products that contain fiber, particularly soluble fiber, which may reduce the risk of CHD. The second is that diets low in saturated fats and cholesterol may reduce the risk of CHD. The FDA reviewed evidence regarding ω-3 fatty acids and the reduction in CHD risk, but did not authorize any health claim for these products (36).

Diet alone can reduce cholesterol levels by 5 to 10% or more in compliant patients, and intervention should be given a 6-month trial before determining the effectiveness in lowering cholesterol levels. Patients are less likely to succeed on dietary therapy without ongoing counseling and follow-up. Drug therapy must be considered if an adequate trial of dietary therapy does not achieve the desired goal.

Drug Therapy

Drug therapy must be sustained to effectively reduce the risk of CHD. The clinician should be confident that all nondrug approaches to reduce cholesterol or triglycerides have been given an adequate trial before exposing the patient to the risks associated with drug therapy. Drug therapy may be considered earlier in patients with multiple risk factors, for whom diet modification alone will probably not result in sufficient LDL cholesterol reduction to meet goals. Drug therapy may be held or delayed in males under 35 years old, premenopausal women, or the elderly, for

Drug Therapy Algorithm

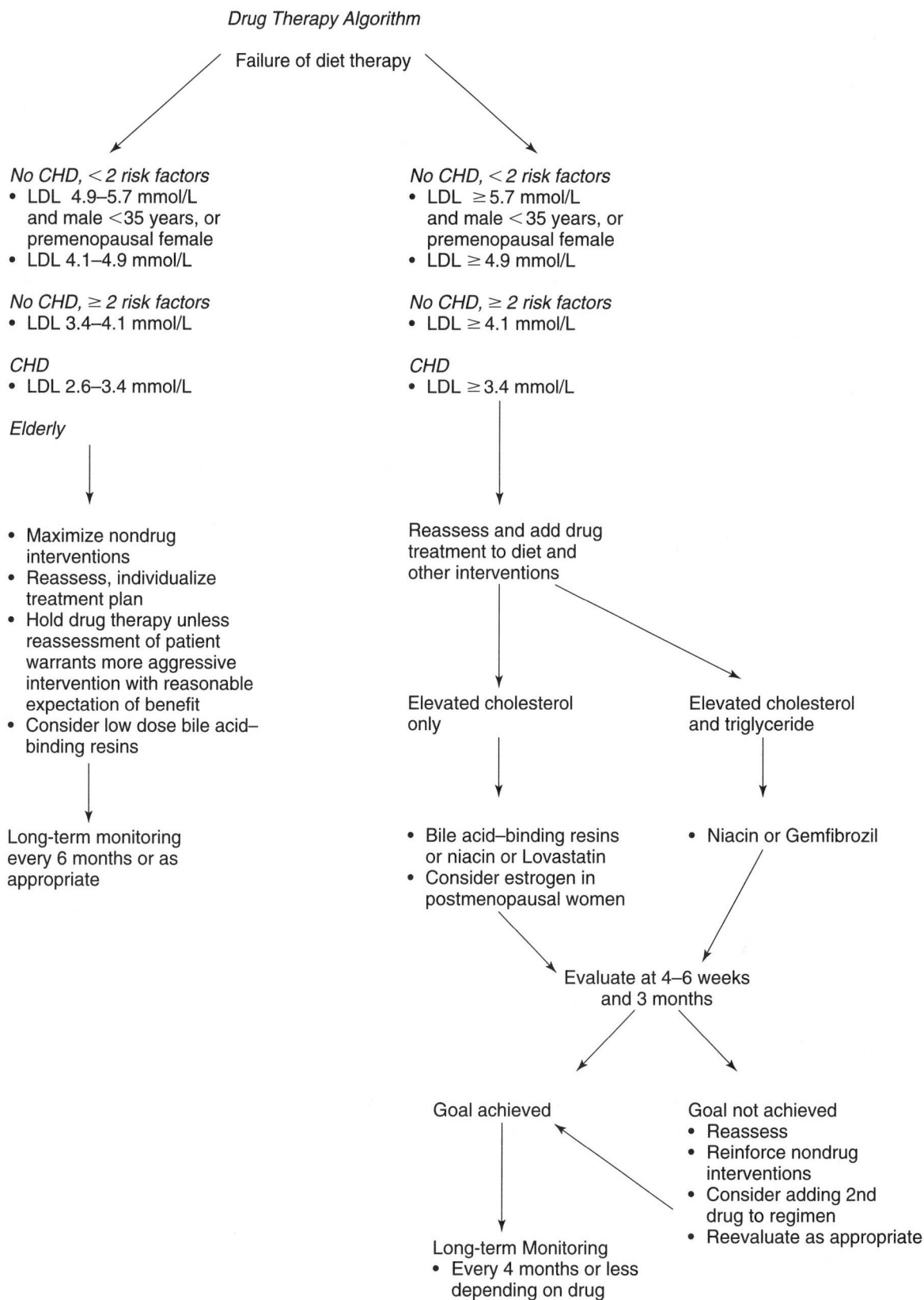

Figure 20.3

Table 20.14.
Drugs Used in the Treatment of Hyperlipidemia

Drug	Effects on Lipids	Mechanism of Action	Usual Daily Dose	Adverse Effects	Comments
Cholestyramine	↓ Cholesterol	↑ LDL metabolism	12–24 g in 2–4 divided doses	Constipation, bloating, abdominal pain, gas	Proven in clinical trials, taste and side effects may limit compliance, binds many drugs
Colestipol	See cholestyramine	See cholestyramine	15–30 g in 2–4 divided doses	Same as cholestyramine	
Niacin	↓ Triglycerides and Cholesterol	↑ LDL catabolism	2–3 g t.i.d.	GI, flushing, pruritus, hepatotoxicity	Inexpensive, proven in clinical trials, side effects may limit compliance
Lovastatin	↓ Cholesterol	↓ Cholesterol synthesis ↑ LDL catabolism	20–40 mg in 1 or 2 doses	GI, myalgias, myositis, lens opacities, elevated liver enzymes	First available HMG-CoA reductase inhibitor, long term adverse effects unknown, prodrug
Pravastatin	See lovastatin	See lovastatin	20–40 mg in 1 or 2 doses	Similar to lovastatin	Newer agent, long term effects unknown, less lipophilic than lovastatin or simvastatin
Simvastatin	See lovastatin	See lovastatin	10–20 mg in 1 or 2 doses	Similar to lovastatin	Newer agent, long-term effects unknown, more potent than lovastatin or simvastatin, prodrug
Fluvastatin	See lovastatin	See lovastatin	20–40 mg in 1 or 2 doses	Similar to lovastatin	Newest agent, least information available, LDL lowering ability slightly less than lovastatin
Gemfibrozil	↓ Triglyceride and cholesterol	↑ VLDL catabolism	600 mg b.i.d.	GI, myalgias, increased liver enzymes	Proven in clinical trials, less toxicity than clofibrate
Probucol	↓ Cholesterol	↑ LDL clearance	500 mg b.i.d.	Diarrhea, abdominal pain, HA, dizziness, parasthesias	No longer widely used, may decrease HDL cholesterol

whom the benefit-to-risk ratio of intervention may be uncertain. However, patients with very high cholesterol levels will probably require drug therapy in addition to dietary interventions. Figure 20.3 provides an algorithm for determining candidates for drug therapy. Table 20.14 summarizes the drugs used in the treatment of hyperlipidemia.

The appropriate drug should be selected by taking into account (a) the type of hyperlipidemia; (b) the effectiveness of the drug; (c) the adverse effect profile of the drug; (d) the patient's compliance history; and (e) the cost of therapy. Nonpharmacologic therapy should be continued while a single drug is added to the treatment plan. The dose should be increased until the goal is achieved, the maximum dose is reached, or the patient cannot tolerate the side effects. If the goal is still not achieved after an ad-

equate trial, a more effective agent should be considered, or a second drug that has a different mechanism of action can be added to the regimen.

BILE ACID–BINDING RESINS

Cholestyramine and colestipol are bile acid–binding resins that are indicated for the treatment of hypercholesterolemia. Following oral administration, bile acid–binding resins form a nonabsorbable complex with bile acids in the intestine that removes the bile acids from the enterohepatic circulation. The resins may also increase LDL catabolism in the liver by causing an increase in LDL receptors, resulting in a decrease of LDL cholesterol of 15 to 20%. There may be a slight, compensatory increase in VLDL production, causing an increase in triglyceride levels. Although the increase is usually small and may be transient, it should be considered in patients with a mixed hyperlipidemia with both cholesterol and triglyceride.

The major side effects of the bile acid–binding resins are constipation, bloating, abdominal pain, gas, and nausea. Constipation, which occurs in about 20% of patients, can be reduced with stool softeners and by increasing dietary fiber. Side effects may become more tolerable with prolonged therapy. Bile acid-binding resins have been reported to interfere with the absorption of fat-soluble vitamins when doses over 24 grams daily are given. Although rare, vitamin A, D, and K deficiencies have been reported with the use of binding resins.

Bile acid–binding resins may bind to numerous drugs and interfere with their absorption when given concomitantly. The binding resins can decrease the absorption of digoxin, warfarin, iron salts, thiazides, antibiotics, thyroid hormones, and phenobarbital. Patients should be instructed to take other medications 1 hour before or 4 hours after taking cholestyramine or colestipol to avoid potential interactions.

The bile acid–binding resins should be given in at least 4 oz of a beverage or soup, or sprinkled on a highly pulpy fruit like applesauce. The dose should be sprinkled on top of the desired liquid to allow hydration before mixing. The drug should not be taken dry in order to reduce the risk of esophageal irritation or blockage. Colestipol beads are odorless and tasteless as compared to cholestyramine powder and may be preferable to some patients. One-gram tablets of cholestyramine and colestipol are also available. The tablets should be taken whole and not crushed.

The usual daily doses of cholestyramine and colestipol are up to 24 grams and 30 grams respectively, given in 4 divided doses. The daily dose can also be given in 2 divided doses without a loss in efficacy. A common regimen is to divide the total daily dose by the number of meals the patient routinely eats in a day. The dose is then given with each of the patient's meals. The taste and side effects make the bile acid–binding resin difficult to tolerate for the lifelong regimen required for the treatment of hypercholesterolemia. This should be considered in patients with a history of noncompliance.

NIACIN (NICOTINIC ACID)

Niacin reduces both triglycerides and cholesterol, and is indicated for the treatment of hypertriglyceridemia, hypercholesterolemia, or mixed hyperlipidemias. Nicotinamide, which shares the vitamin properties of niacin, does not share the lipid-lowering properties. Niacin acts by decreasing VLDL synthesis by the liver with a concomitant drop in LDL production. Niacin may also cause a rise in HDL levels by reducing their catabolism. Niacin generally decreases VLDL triglycerides by 20 to 40%, LDL cholesterol by 20 to 35%, and increases HDL by 10 to 20%.

The most prominent side effect of niacin is a prostaglandin-mediated reaction causing acute flushing and pruritus. This side effect is usually seen at the beginning of therapy, with subsequent dosing changes, and when resuming therapy after missed doses. Tolerance to this adverse effect quickly develops with continued dosing. Flushing and pruritus can be prevented by giving from 80 to 325 mg of aspirin 30 minutes before each dose and by giving niacin with food.

Niacin can cause abdominal pain and discomfort, and some clinicians avoid niacin in patients with a history of peptic ulcer disease (PUD) because of concern over aggravating PUD or interfering with the clinical presentation. The gastrointestinal upset can be reduced by administering all doses with food. Sustained release preparations are available that may reduce GI discomfort, although this is not well documented. Adverse effects include a dose-dependent increase in aspartate aminotransferase and alkaline phosphatase, jaundice, and chronic liver damage. Elevations in liver enzymes usually occur if the niacin dose is increased by more than 2.5 g/month. Although these changes may resolve with continued dosing, liver enzymes should be monitored periodically. Some clinicians believe that the sustained release niacin preparations are associated with a higher incidence of liver function abnormalities (37). Niacin can cause hyperuricemia and glucose intolerance, but this is usually not a problem unless the patient has preexisting gout or diabetes.

The usual dose of niacin ranges from 3 to 6 grams daily in divided doses. Higher doses are usually limited by the adverse effects of niacin. Therapy should be initiated slowly to minimize the risk of liver toxicity and so that the patient can become tolerant to flushing and GI distress associated with the drug. The starting dose is 100 mg given 3 times daily; then the daily dose is gradually increased by 300 mg each week until the desired effect is achieved or the maximum dose is reached.

HMG-COA REDUCTASE INHIBITORS

The HMG-CoA reductase inhibitors are a new class of drugs for the treatment of hyperlipidemia. Lovastatin (mevinolin) was the first commercially available agent in this class and was followed by simvastatin, pravastatin, and more recently fluvastatin. Simvastatin is an analog of lovastatin, and like lovastatin is a prodrug that must be converted to the active metabolite. Pravastatin is administered in its active form and is metabolized to inactive components. Fluvastatin is structurally distinct from the other statins and is administered in its active form. Lovastatin, simvastatin, and fluvastatin are lipophilic with a high degree of protein binding (~95-98%). Pravastatin is hydrophilic and has a lower degree of protein binding then the other statins (~50%). These agents inhibit the enzyme

3-hydroxyl-3-methylglutaryl-coenzyme A (HMG-CoA) reductase, which is responsible for the conversion of HMG-CoA to mevalonate early in the synthetic pathway for endogenous cholesterol production.

Lovastatin causes a significant reduction in serum LDL cholesterol levels, apparently by an increase in LDL receptors in response to decreased cholesterol production. The increased LDL receptors further decrease circulating free cholesterol. In doses of 10 to 80 mg, lovastatin can decrease total and LDL cholesterol as much as 30% and 40%, respectively. Lovastatin may also cause a decrease in triglycerides and an increase in HDL. The cholesterol lowering effect of lovastatin is increased when it is given with another cholesterol lowering agent (14, 38). The cholesterol lowering ability of pravastatin and simvastatin is similar to lovastatin, but that of fluvastatin is slightly lower. In doses tested of 10 to 40 mg, pravastatin and lovastatin have similar effects on cholesterol on a mg per mg basis. Simvastatin is approximately twice as potent as both lovastatin and pravastatin (39, 40).

Adverse effects of lovastatin include diarrhea, abdominal cramps, constipation, and myalgias. Myositis (myalgias with a marked increase in serum creatine phosphokinase) can occur with lovastatin, and the frequency may increase when lovastatin is given in combination with gemfibrozil (5%), cyclosporine (28%), or niacin (2%). Reversible lens opacities that do not impair vision have been reported with lovastatin. For this reason, annual eye examinations are recommended while on lovastatin therapy. Elevations in serum transaminases may require discontinuing therapy in some patients. These elevations can occur 3 to 12 months after therapy begins and usually reverse when therapy is discontinued. Liver function tests should be performed periodically, and lovastatin should be discontinued if liver enzymes are three times normal values.

Adverse effects of pravastatin, simvastatin, and fluvastatin are similar to lovastatin, although these agents are relatively new and there is insufficient information to draw conclusions about long-term effects. Pravastatin may have a lower potential for myositis than lovastatin. An increase in the frequency of skin rash was the only adverse effect reaching statistical significance when compared to placebo in short-term trials of pravastatin (41).

Drug interactions of lovastatin include reduced clearance when given with erythromycin and increased bleeding time or prothrombin time when given with warfarin. Simvastatin also may prolong prothrombin time in patients on warfarin therapy. Simvastatin may also interact with digoxin causing an increased "cardioactive material." Cholestyramine will reduce the bioavailability of pravastatin.

Lovastatin is most effective in lowering cholesterol levels when given in a twice daily dosing regimen. A once daily dosing regimen given at night is also effective, since it takes effect during the peak of cholesterol synthesis in the early morning hours. The least effective dosing regimen is once every morning. Dosing starts at 20 mg given with the evening meal. The dose can be increased every 4 weeks by 20-mg increments until the desired effect is achieved or a maximum dose of 80 mg is reached. Doses of 20 to 40 mg daily are usually sufficient for patients with moderately increased cholesterol. Lovastatin should be administered with meals, since this increases the bioavailability by about 50%.

Although the bioavailability of pravastatin is slightly reduced when given with meals, it does not affect its LDL lowering effect. Therefore, it can be given without regard to meals. Pravastatin should be administered one hour before or after cholestyramine to prevent reduced bioavailability of pravastatin. The initial dose of pravastatin is 10 to 20 mg at bedtime, which can be increased at intervals of at least 4 weeks until goal is achieved or the maximum dose is reached. The usual dosing range is 10 to 40 mg given once daily.

Because of its increased potency, the usual starting dose of simvastatin is 5 to 10 mg once daily in the evening. The dose can be increased at intervals of at least 4 weeks until goal is achieved or a maximum daily dosage of 40 mg is reached. GI absorption of the drug does not appear to be altered when it is administered with food.

The starting dose of fluvastatin is 20 mg once daily at bedtime, with an increase up to 40 mg once daily if required. Doses should be increased at intervals of at least 4 weeks. Dividing a 40-mg daily dose into a twice daily regimen may slightly increase the cholesterol lowering ability. Fluvastatin can be given without regard to meals.

HMG-CoA reductase inhibitors are much easier for patients to tolerate than standard first line drug therapy for hypercholesterolemia and are therefore better accepted. However, since this class of drugs is relatively new, long-term effects have not been well described. Studies with HMG-CoA reductase inhibitors to document the effect on CHD risk are currently underway. It is reasonable to expect a benefit because of their documented ability to reduce cholesterol levels. As more experience is gained with the HMG-CoA reductase inhibitors, they may take the place of current first line agents because of increased patient acceptance.

CLOFIBRATE

Clofibrate was the first drug approved by the FDA for the treatment of hyperlipidemia. Clofibrate increases VLDL catabolism by increasing lipoprotein lipase activity, reduces cholesterol production in the liver, and increases LDL catabolism. The result is a decrease in VLDLs and triglycerides, and a minor decrease in total and LDL cholesterol. Clofibrate is indicated in the treatment of hypertriglyceridemia.

The Coronary Drug Project (25) demonstrated a high incidence of noncardiovascular mortality and a higher incidence of cholelithiasis requiring surgery or causing complications with clofibrate. As a result, clofibrate is no longer considered an agent of first choice. The most frequent adverse effects of the drug are nausea, diarrhea, and gastrointestinal distress, which usually decrease with continued use. Clofibrate can also cause an increase in aspartate aminotransferase levels and has been associated with a flulike syndrome accompanied by an increase in creatine phosphokinase levels. Clofibrate can potentiate the effect of warfarin causing an increase in the prothrombin time. The usual dose is 2 grams given daily in 2 to 4 divided doses.

GEMFIBROZIL

Gemfibrozil is similar to clofibrate and also decreases plasma triglycerides levels by increasing VLDL catabolism via lipoprotein lipase. In addition, gemfibrozil may reduce the synthesis and excretion of VLDL. Gemfibrozil can reduce triglyceride and VLDL concentrations by 40 to 60%. LDL levels may decrease or increase, but HDL levels usually increase by 17 to 31% (24).

Adverse effects of gemfibrozil are similar to those of clofibrate, although less severe. The most common side effects are gastrointestinal, and include abdominal and epigastric pain, diarrhea, nausea, vomiting, and flatulence. Other side effects include rashes, headache, blurred vision, dizziness, leucopenia, muscle pains, and liver function test abnormalities.

The dose of gemfibrozil ranges from 900 to 1500 mg daily in 2 divided doses given 30 minutes before the morning and evening meals. The usual dose is 1200 mg daily. Gemfibrozil can be used to treat hypertriglyceridemia as well as some mixed hyperlipidemias.

PROBUCOL

Probucol can cause a 10 to 21% reduction in total cholesterol, which includes a reduction in both LDL and HDL cholesterol. Its effect on triglycerides is variable. The clinical significance of lowering HDL levels is unclear, but because of the higher incidence of CHD associated with low HDL levels, the effect is undesirable.

The adverse effects of probucol tend to be minor and transient. They include diarrhea in about 10% of patients, flatulence, abdominal pain, nausea, and vomiting. Headache, dizziness and paresthesias have also been reported.

The usual adult dose is 500 mg twice a day given with the morning and evening meals. The total daily dose should not exceed 1 gram.

OTHER AGENTS

Although several studies have documented the cholesterol lowering ability of the aminoglycoside neomycin (42, 43), the drug is not FDA approved for the treatment of hyperlipidemia. The exact mechanism of action is unknown; however, the drug may reduce the absorption of cholesterol from the gut. Neomycin has no role as a lipid-lowering agent because of potential nephro- and ototoxicity and the availability of safer agents.

Levothyroxine can increase the number of LDL receptors and increase LDL catabolism. In addition, it can increase the enzymatic conversion of cholesterol. Dextrothyroxine, the dextro isomer of thyroxine, was synthesized in the hopes of retaining the lipid lowering properties while avoiding the metabolic and cardiac side effects associated with levothyroxine. Because these side effects persist, the usefulness of dextrothyroxine is limited and it no longer should be prescribed as lipid lowering therapy.

Recent evidence suggests that diets that include a large quantity of fish can reduce the incidence of coronary thrombosis and reduce the mortality of CHD. The fat in fish is rich in highly unsaturated ω-3 fatty acids, mainly eicosapentaenoic acid (EPA) and docosahexaenoic acid (DHA). The effect of these fatty acids on lipids is equivocal. Studies have shown both increases and decreases in LDL cholesterol, decreases in triglycerides, and no change or an increase in HDL cholesterol. These studies used diets rich in fish or fish oil, or doses of ω-3 fatty acids of up to 30 g/day (44, 45). Adverse effects include diarrhea, increases in bleeding time, and decreases in platelet aggregation. Fish oil capsules available on the market recommend doses of 3 g/day or less, which may have no substantial effect on serum lipids. There is no acceptable evidence that fish oil can prevent heart disease (44).

There has been recent evidence that the antioxidant vitamins C, E, and β-carotene may possibly be effective in the treatment and prevention of CHD. Much of the evidence is based on epidemiologic data, animal studies, or studies monitoring dietary consumption. Findings from some of these studies have been inconsistent. Several large prospective studies evaluating the protective effects of antioxidants in several disease states are underway based on this promising, preliminary evidence. However, until more definitive information is available, the role of antioxidants is unproven (46, 47).

SUMMARY

The association between hypercholesterolemia and CHD risk has been established, although the link between hypertriglyceridemia and CHD is not apparent. Although there is a need to treat hyperlipidemia in specific patient groups, the benefit of broad interventions in the general public is controversial. Using ATP II guidelines and 1990 population data, it is estimated that 52 million Americans aged 20 years or older would require dietary intervention and 12.7 million of these would require drug therapy (48). The cost of medical therapy is substantial, and cost-benefit models estimate that interventions are most cost-effective in high-risk groups (49). Medical therapy for smoking cessation and the control of hypertension is less costly and can result in a greater reduction in CHD risk than controlling cholesterol levels (50). This emphasizes the need for an individual and balanced approach to each patient at risk for CHD that addresses all risk factors as part of the treatment plan.

A multidisciplinary approach to treatment is required that reinforces life-style changes and compliance to therapy. Nonpharmacologic interventions must be emphasized even after a decision is made to use drug therapy. The decision to begin drug therapy in a hyperlipidemia should be patient specific and should address the potential risks and benefits for that patient.

REFERENCES

1. The Expert Panel. Report of the National Cholesterol Education Program expert panel on detection, evaluation, and treatment of high blood cholesterol in adults. Arch Intern Med 148:36–69, 1988.
2. Working Group on Management of Patients with Hypertension and High Blood Cholesterol. National education programs working group report on the management of patients with hypertension and high blood cholesterol. Ann Intern Med 114:224–237, 1991.
3. Pekkanen J, Linn S, Heiss G, et al. Ten-year mortality from cardiovascular disease in relation to cholesterol level among men with and without pre-existing cardiovascular disease. N Engl J Med 322:1700–1707, 1990.
4. The Expert Panel on Detection, Evaluation, and Treatment of High Blood Cholesterol in Adults. Summary of the second report of the National Cholesterol Education Program (NCEP) expert panel on detection, evaluation, and treatment of high blood cholesterol in adults (adult treatment panel II). JAMA 269:3015–3023, 1993.
5. National Institute of Health Office of Medical Applications of Research. Treatment of hypertriglyceridemia. JAMA 251:1196–1200, 1984.
6. Austin MA, Hokanson JE. Epidemiology of triglycerides, small dense low density lipoprotein, and lipoprotein (a) as risk factors for coronary heart disease. Med Clin North Am 78:99–115:1994.
7. NIH Consensus Conference. Triglyceride, high-density lipoprotein, and coronary heart disease. JAMA 269:505:1993
8. Brett AS. Treating hypercholesterolemia: how should practicing physicians interpret the published data for patients? N Engl J Med 321:676–680, 1989.
9. Labreche DG. Reassessment of the value of lowering serum cholesterol: how should physicians interpret the published data for patients. Clin Pharm 7:592–603, 1988.
10. Leaf A. Management of hypercholesterolemia: are preventive interventions advisable? N Engl J Med 321:680–684, 1989.
11. Olson RE. A critique of the report of the National Institutes of Health expert panel on detection, evaluation, and treatment of high blood cholesterol. Arch Intern Med 149:1501–1503, 1989.
12. Gotto AM, Bierman EL, Connor WE, et al. Recommendations for treatment of hyperlipidemia in adults. Circulation 69:1065A–1090A, 1984.
13. National Institute of Health Office of Medical Research. Lowering blood cholesterol to prevent heart disease. JAMA 253:2080–2086, 1985.
14. McKenny JM. Lovastatin: a new cholesterol lowering agent. Clin Pharm 7:21–36, 1988.

15. Schaefer EJ, Levy R. Pathogenesis and management of lipoprotein disorders. N Engl J Med 312:1300–1310, 1985.
16. Ginsberg HN. Lipoprotein metabolism and its relationship to atherosclerosis. Med Clin North Am 78:1–20, 1994.
17. Stone NG. Secondary causes of hyperlipidemia. Med Clin North Am 78:117–141, 1993.
18. Henkin Y, Como JA, Oberman A. Secondary dyslipidemia: inadvertent effects of drugs in clinical practice. JAMA 267:961–968, 1992.
19. Weinberger MH. Antihypertensive therapy and lipids. Arch Intern Med 145:1102–1105, 1985.
20. Flamenbaum W. Metabolic consequences of antihypertensive therapy. Ann Intern Med 98:875–880, 1983.
21. Oliver MF, Heady JA, Morris JN, Cooper J. A cooperative trial in the primary prevention of ischaemic heart disease using clofibrate. Br Heart J 40:1069–1118:1978.
22. Lipid Research Clinics Program. The lipid research clinics coronary primary preventions trial results. I. Reductions in incidence of coronary heart disease. JAMA 251:351–364, 1984.
23. Lipid Research Clinics Program. The lipid research clinics coronary primary preventions trial results. II. The relationship of reduction in incidence of coronary heart disease to cholesterol lowering. JAMA 251:365–374, 1984.
24. Frick MH, Elo O, Haapa K, et al. Helsinki heart study; primary-prevention trial with gemfibrozil in middle aged men with dyslipidemia. N Engl J Med 317:1237–1245, 1987.
25. Coronary Drug Project Research Group. Clofibrate and niacin in coronary heart disease. JAMA 231:360–381:1975.
26. Grumbach K. How effective is drug treatment of hypercholesterolemia? A guided tour of the major clinical trials for the primary care physician. J Am Board Fam Pract 4:437–445, 1991.
27. Brown G, Albers JJ, Fisher LD, et al. Regressions of coronary artery disease as a result of intensive lipid-lowering therapy in men with high levels of apolipoprotein B. N Engl J Med 323:1289–1298, 1990.
28. Buchwald H, Varco RL, Matts JP, et al. Effect of partial ileal bypass surgery on mortality and morbidity from coronary heart disease in patients with hypercholesterolemia. N Engl J Med 323:946–955, 1990.
29. Rossouw JE, Lewis B, Rifkind BM. The value of lowering cholesterol after myocardial infarction. N Engl J Med 323:1112–1119, 1990.
30. Krumholz HM, Seeman TE, Merrill SS, et al. Lack of association between cholesterol and coronary heart disease mortality and morbidity and all-cause mortality in persons older than 70 years. JAMA 272:1335–1340, 1994.
31. Hulley SB, Newman TB. Cholesterol in the elderly: is it important? [Editorial]. JAMA 272:1372–1374, 1994.
32. La Rosa JC. Dyslipoproteinemia in women and the elderly. Med Clin North Am 78:163–180, 1993.
33. Garber A, Sox HC, Littenberg B. Screening asymptomatic adults for cardiac risk factors: the serum cholesterol level. Ann Intern Med 110:622–639, 1989.
34. American Heart Association Nutrition Committee. Dietary guidelines for healthy American adults. Circulation 77:721A–724A, 1988.
35. Anon. Mandatory Nutrition Labeling--FDA's final rule. Nutr Rev 51:101–105, 1993.
36. Anon. The FDA's final regulations on health claims for foods. Nutr Rev 51:90–93, 1993.
37. Etchason JA. Niacin-induced hepatitis: a potential side effect with low-dose time release niacin. Mayo Clin Proc 66:23–28, 1991.
38. Sitori CR. Pharmacology and mechanism of action of the new HMG-CoA reductase inhibitors. Pharmacol Res 22:555–563, 1990.
39. Larsen ML, Illingworth DR. Drug treatment of dyslipoproteinemia. Med Clin North Am 78:225–245, 1993.
40. Tobert JA. Efficacy and long-term adverse effect pattern of lovastatin. Am J Cardiol 62:28J-34J, 1988.

41. Jungnickel PW, Cantral KA, Maloley PA. Pravastatin--a new drug for the treatment of hypercholesterolemia. Clin Pharm 11:677–689, 1992.

42. Hoeg JM, Schaefer EF, Romano CA, et al. Neomycin and plasma lipoproteins in type II hyperlipoproteinemia. Clin Pharmacol Ther 36:555–565, 1984.

43. Miettenen T. Effects of neomycin alone and in combination with cholestyramine on serum cholesterol and fecal steroids in hypercholesterolemic subjects. J Clin Invest 301:595–597, 1979.

44. Anon. Fish oil for the heart. Med Letter 29:7–9, 1987.

45. Mueller BA, Talbert RL. Biological mechanisms and cardiovascular effects of omega-3 fatty acids. Clin Pharm 7:795–807, 1988.

46. Byers T. Vitamin E supplements and coronary heart disease. Nutr Rev 51:333–336, 1993.

47. Manson JE, Gaziano JM, Jonas MA, Hennekens CH. Anitoxidants and cardiovascular disease--a review. J Am Coll Nutr 12:426–432, 1993.

48. Sempos CT, Cleeman JI, Carroll MD, et al. Prevalence of high blood cholesterol among US adults; and update based on guidelines from the second report of the National Cholesterol Education Program adult treatment panel. JAMA 269:3009–3014, 1993.

49. Kinosian BP, Eisenberg JM. Cutting into cholesterol: cost-effective alternatives for treating hypercholesterolemia. JAMA 259:2249–2254, 1988.

50. Taylor WC, Pass TM, Shepard DS, Komaroff AL. Cholesterol reduction and life expectancy. Ann Intern Med 106:605–614, 1987.

CHAPTER 21

ACUTE AND CHRONIC RENAL DISEASES

JAY F. MOUSER and LAWRENCE J. HAK

Renal failure is a major cause of morbidity and mortality. It is estimated that per million population, between 100 to 200 patients die each year in the United States from diseases of the kidney and urinary tract (1). The number of patients being treated for end stage renal disease (ESRD) is increasing by approximately 9 percent per year (2). If this pace continues, the number of patients with ESRD will double in 7 to 8 years. As reported by the United States Renal Data System, at the end of 1992, there were over 200,000 patients with ESRD in the United States. Estimated charges for direct medical care for ESRD patients were $8.6 billion in 1991, leading to an average annual cost of $47,000 per patient. When treatment costs for acute renal failure (ARF) are added to this, the total amount spent on renal diseases in the United States today is astronomical.

At the end of 1992, there were over 22,000 patients on the kidney transplant list, while only about 8,000 cadaveric kidney transplants were performed that year. The largest increases in newly diagnosed patients are in the elderly population, diabetic patients, and hypertensive patients. At the end of 1991, 31% of ESRD patients were 65 years of age or older. Diabetes accounted for 26%, hypertension accounted for nearly 24%, and glomerulonephritis accounted for about 18% of cases (2).

Patients with renal failure frequently have other major medical problems requiring aggressive drug therapy. In the medical management of these patients, the clinician must be able to assess the degree of renal insufficiency, recognize pharmacologic agents that can worsen renal function, and perform adjustments of drug dosing. This chapter examines the causes, clinical course, and therapeutic management of patients with acute and chronic renal failure.

NORMAL KIDNEY FUNCTIONS

The primary function of the kidney is to maintain the internal environment of the body through regulation of body fluid volume, electrolyte composition, and acid-base balance. The kidneys are also responsible for the production and secretion of various hormones and enzymes. Erythropoietin is produced by the renal cortical cells and stimulates erythrocyte maturation in the bone marrow.

Also, 1,25-dihydroxycholecalciferol (the active form of vitamin D) is formed in the proximal tubule cells and plays an important role in the regulation of body calcium and phosphate balance. As such, complications of renal disease reflect impairment of the normal physiologic functions of the kidney—primarily regulation of water and electrolyte balance, arterial blood pressure, erythrocyte production, vitamin D activity, and excretion of metabolic waste products.

Nephron Function

The nephron is the functional unit of the kidney. Each nephron consists of a glomerular capillary network that is surrounded by Bowman's capsule, a proximal tubule, a loop of Henle, a distal tubule, and a collecting duct (Fig. 21.1). There are about a million nephrons in each kidney and thus a tremendous reserve that allows an active life even when as much as 75% of the tissue has been destroyed.

A plasma ultrafiltrate is formed in the glomerular capillary with collection of the filtered fluid in Bowman's capsule. The filtrate then enters the proximal tubule, where approximately two thirds of the filtered sodium and water is reabsorbed. Over 90% of filtered bicarbonate and nearly all of filtered glucose and amino acids are also reabsorbed in the proximal tubule.

The loop of Henle consists of the terminal portion of the proximal tubule, the thin descending and ascending limbs, and the thick ascending limb. The loop of Henle is responsible for dilution of urine and is also the site of magnesium reabsorption. The distal tubule and collecting duct function for final adjustment in urine composition. Here, antidiuretic hormone (ADH) regulates water reabsorption and aldosterone regulates sodium reabsorption and potassium excretion. An extensive peritubular capillary network nourishes the tubular cells and brings substances to the tubules for secretion. The afferent arterioles supply blood to the glomerulus, and the efferent arterioles carry blood from the glomerulus.

CLINICAL EVALUATION OF RENAL FUNCTION

The kidneys account for only 0.4% of the total body weight, but receive approximately 20 to 25% of the cardiac output (3). This represents the highest blood flow

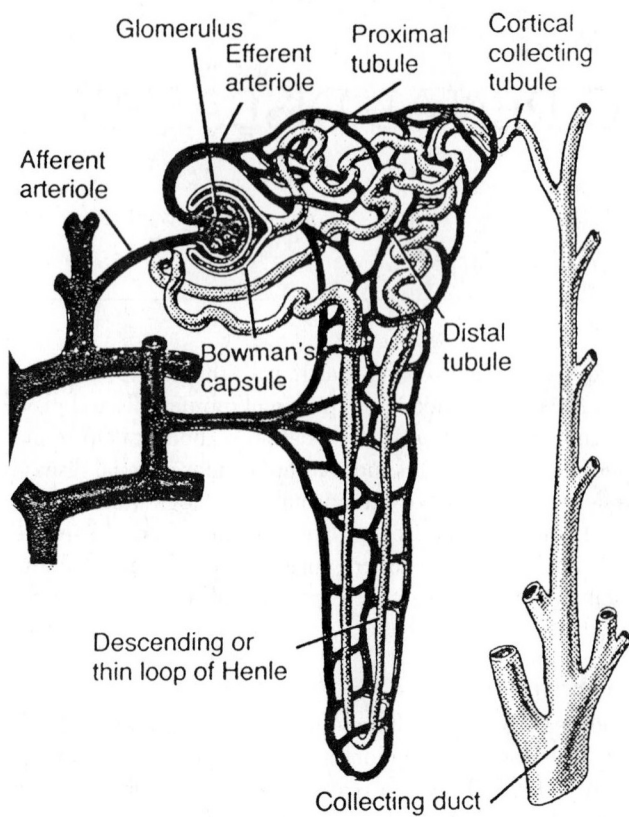

Afferent arteriole
Glomerulus
Efferent arteriole
Proximal tubule
Cortical collecting tubule
Bowman's capsule
Distal tubule
Descending or thin loop of Henle
Collecting duct

Figure 21.1. The nephron. (From Smith: The Kidney: Structure and Functions in Health and Disease. New York, Oxford University Press, 1951.)

per unit of organ weight. Nearly one fourth of the plasma arriving at the glomerulus is filtered to become the glomerular filtrate. Changes in the rate of filtrate formation (GFR) result from changes in glomerular capillary permeability, surface area, or changes in net filtration pressure. Factors influencing the effective filtration pressure are the afferent and efferent arteriole resistance. Increased afferent resistance will decrease glomerular capillary pressure and thus GFR, while increased efferent resistance leads to increases in glomerular capillary pressure and increases in GFR. Tubular obstruction increases the pressure in Bowman's space, which opposes the glomerular capillary filtration pressure; as a result, GFR decreases.

Determination of GFR

GFR is approximated by measuring the urinary excretion rate of a marker substance known to be filtered and excreted in equal amounts. Properties of the ideal marker substance are that it be neither absorbed nor secreted by the renal tubules and be freely filtered across glomerular membranes, not metabolized in renal tubules or produced by the kidneys, and not eliminated by nonrenal routes (4). These critical properties are satisfied ideally by inulin. To

measure inulin clearance, requires a continuous intravenous infusion of inulin, several samples of blood and urine collected at specified times, and assay of these samples for inulin concentrations. Since the filtered amount of inulin is equal to the amount of inulin excreted, then

$$\text{GFR} = \frac{U_{\text{in}} \cdot V}{P_{\text{in}}} \qquad (21.1)$$

where GFR = glomerular filtration rate (mL/min), U_{in} = urine inulin concentration (mg/dL), P_{in} = plasma inulin concentration (mg/dL), measured at the midpoint of the collection period, and V = volume per unit time (i.e., the total urine volume collected divided by the total time of collection, expressed as mL/min). Since GFR varies according to body size, values are typically expressed by standardizing them to body surface area. The average GFR in young male adults is approximately 120 mL/min/1.73 m². This value is usually 10 to 15% lower in women.

Creatinine Clearance

In clinical practice creatinine clearance is the index of GFR most often used. Determination of creatinine clearance is convenient, inexpensive, and easily calculated from a timed urine collection assayed for creatinine and a single measurement of serum creatinine. Measurement is most accurate if the urine collection interval is 24 hours and a blood sample is obtained at the midpoint of this timed collection (5). The calculation for creatinine clearance is similar to GFR (see above), except that urine and serum creatinine concentrations are substituted for inulin concentrations.

Creatinine Production

Creatinine production results from the nonenzymatic hydrolysis of muscle stores of creatine and creatine phosphate. Creatinine is produced at a relatively constant daily rate: Approximately 1 mg of creatinine is produced daily from about 20 g of muscle (6). Therefore, creatinine production depends on muscle mass and is influenced by age and gender. After age twenty, creatinine production decreases by approximately 2 mg/kg/24 hr per decade of life in both males and females (7).

Because creatinine is filtered by the glomerulus and is also secreted in the proximal tubule, its clearance approximates but is always greater than GFR (8). If GFR is greater than 25 mL/min, then creatinine clearance approximates GFR reasonably well. However, creatinine secretion is enhanced in patients with lower GFR, and especially in disease states affecting primarily the glomeruli (i.e., acute glomerulonephritis), leading to overestimation of GFR. In patients with ESRD, nonrenal creatinine elimination (gut metabolism) accounts for significant creatinine elimination (9).

Often it is difficult to obtain accurate 24-hr urine collections. As such, creatinine clearance may be estimated, using the following formula derived by Cockroft and Gault: (10)

$$C_{cr} \text{[men]} = \frac{(140 - \text{age}) \cdot \text{weight}}{72 \cdot S_{cr}} \quad (21.2)$$

where C_{cr} is creatinine clearance (mL/min), age is in years, weight is in kilograms, and S_{cr} is the serum creatinine concentration (mg/dL). In women, Equation (21.2) is multiplied by 0.85. Factors other than a decreased GFR can alter the serum creatinine level and must be considered when assessing renal function. Patients with decreased muscle mass as a result of old age or cachexia will have a decreased creatinine production and therefore a low or normal serum creatinine level, even though their renal function may be impaired (11, 12).

Creatine is the amino acid precursor of creatinine. Synthesis of creatine from glycine, arginine, and methionine occurs in the liver. Thus, individuals with advanced liver disease have decreased creatine production and decreased body pools of creatine. This will result in decreased creatinine production and serum creatinine concentrations below expected values for any given level of renal function. In patients with liver disease, formulas that estimate renal function based on a serum creatinine level should not be used, as they will greatly overestimate renal function (13).

Creatine is also contained in meat. Cooking converts creatine to creatinine, which is absorbed and contributes to the total body creatinine pool (14). Individuals who do not eat meat will have a decreased intake of creatine and creatinine, which will result in a decreased body pool of these substances. This accounts for a lower than usual serum creatinine, even though these individuals may have normal renal function.

Laboratory determination of serum creatinine is based on the alkaline picrate method of Jaffe, modified for increased specificity and to accommodate automation (7). Since this is a colorimetric test, other noncreatinine chromogens can result in overestimation of serum creatinine. Some of these agents are reported in Table 21.1 (15–18). Large elevations in serum creatinine levels without appreciable changes in the blood urea nitrogen (BUN) should alert the clinician to possible laboratory interference. Some drugs (i.e., cimetidine) compete with creatinine for tubular secretion and thus result in elevated serum creatinine concentrations.

Blood Urea Nitrogen

Urea nitrogen is derived from hepatic deamination of amino acids, causing liberation of ammonia, which combines with available carbon dioxide. Urea is eliminated primarily by the kidney through glomerular filtration and

Table 21.1.

Agents that Cause a False Elevation in Serum Creatinine using the Jaffe Method

Acebutolol	Fluorescein
Acetohexamide	Fructose
Acetoacetate	Glucose
Acetone	Levodopa
Aminophippuric acid	Methyldopa
Ascorbic acid	Moxalactam
Cephalothin	Nitrofurantoin
Cefamandole	Phenolsulfonphthalein
Cefoperazone	Pyruvate
Cefoxitin	Sulfobromophthalein

Adapted from Siest G, Galteau MM. Drug Effects on Laboratory Test Results. Analytic Interferences and Pharmacological Effects. St Louis, Yearbook Medical Publishers, 1988; Ross DL, Neely AE. Textbook of Urinalysis and Body Fluids. Norwalk, CT: Appleton-Century-Crofts, 1983: 68–122; and Young DS. Effects of Drugs on Clinical Laboratory Tests, ed. 3. Washington, D.C.: The American Association of Clinical Chemistry, 1990.

undergoes reabsorption in the proximal tubule. The extent of reabsorption depends on the urine flow rate, such that 40% of the filtered urea is reabsorbed with diuresis and 60% is reabsorbed with antidiuresis. Normal BUN concentrations are 10 to 15 mg/dL but may increase to over 150 mg/dL with severe renal failure. In general, BUN concentrations greater than 100 mg/dL are associated with higher risks of complication during renal failure and the need for dialysis to be initiated. The BUN is less accurate than either serum creatinine levels or creatinine clearance in assessing renal function. The major limitations are related to a number of factors that can alter urea generation and urea clearance in the absence of changes in renal function. Urea generation depends on protein catabolism and is therefore altered by changes in dietary intake, liver disease, blood in the gastrointestinal tract, steroid-induced catabolism, and the antianabolic effect of tetracyclines, doxycycline being the only exception (19). Since the amount of urea reabsorbed is inversely proportional to the urine flow rate, low-flow states will elevate BUN disproportionately to changes in serum creatinine concentration. Any factors that lower the absolute or effective blood volume (and hence renal blood flow) will increase BUN. Table 21.2 lists factors responsible for an elevation of BUN in the absence of renal impairment (15, 20).

Sodium Excretion

Renal tubular sodium reabsorption (i.e., the difference between the amount of sodium filtered and the amount excreted) is the predominant mechanism that regulates sodium excretion. Tubule reabsorption accounts for greater than 99% of filtered sodium under normal conditions. As an example, when the GFR is 120 mL/min and the plasma sodium concentration is 145 mEq/L, approximately 17

Table 21.2.
Factors Elevating BUN without Renal Impairment

High protein diet
Febrile illness with catabolism
Gastrointestinal bleeding
Hyperthyroidism
Hypovolemia
    Diuretic induced
    Hemorrhage
    Vomiting and diarrhea
Decreased cardiac output
    Congestive heart failure
    Myocardial infarction
Steroids—catabolic effect
Tetracyclines—antianabolic effect

mEq of sodium is filtered per minute. Over the course of a day this is equivalent to about 25,000 mEq (or 575 grams) of filtered sodium. However, only 100 to 250 mEq of sodium is excreted per day (<1%).

The fractional excretion of sodium (FE_{Na}) is the fraction of filtered sodium excreted in urine using creatinine as an estimate for GFR (1, 21). Thus, FE_{Na} (%) is calculated as follows:

$$FE_{Na} = \frac{U_{Na} \cdot P_{cr}}{U_{cr} \cdot P_{Na}} \cdot 100 \qquad (21.3)$$

where U_{Na} is urine sodium concentration (mEq/L), P_{cr} is plasma creatinine concentration (mg/dL), U_{cr} is urine creatinine concentration (mg/dL), and P_{Na} is plasma sodium concentration (mEq/L).

FE_{Na} is a useful guide to distinguish whether an abrupt rise in BUN is the result of impaired renal perfusion (i.e., prerenal azotemia) or acute tubular necrosis (ATN). During ATN, tubular transport of sodium is impaired and FE_{Na} values usually exceed 2%. FE_{Na} values less than 1% suggest prerenal azotemia. However, values between 1 and 2% may have little predictive value. The FE_{Na} may be elevated in patients receiving diuretics. The renal failure index (RFI) has also been proposed to help differentiate prerenal ARF from ATN (21). The RFI is determined by dividing the urine sodium concentration by the urine to plasma creatinine ratio. RFI values less than 1 suggest prerenal failure and values greater than 4 may indicate ATN (22).

Urinalysis

Examination of urine is an indispensable method for evaluating patients with renal insufficiency. A urinalysis is usually performed on a random sample of urine and provides useful information about the presence of renal disease. A urinalysis consists of the following major components.

PHYSICAL AND CHEMICAL PROPERTIES

The urine should be clear but usually has a faint yellow tinge due to the presence of urochromes. Erythrocytes and white blood cells cause turbid urine. Agents that may cause urine to change color are shown in Table 21.3. Concentrated urine has a deepened color. Increasing amounts of bilirubin produce colors ranging from yellow-brown to deep olive green. Urine containing old blood, hemosiderin, or myoglobin is brown to black. Small amounts of red blood cells produce a characteristic smoky appearance. Patients with porphyria may void a normal-colored urine, but the sample may develop a deep purple or brownish color on standing. Food pigments, such as the pigment in beets, can color the urine red (16, 17, 20).

Table 21.3.
Agents Causing Changes in Urine Color Not Related to Disease

Color	Drug
Darkening on standing	Cascara
	Chloroquine
	Levodopa
	Methocarbamol
	Methyldopa
	Metronidazole
	Nitrofurantoin
	Phenytoin
Red	Anthraquinone
	Daunorubicin
	Deferoxamine
	Doxorubicin
	Ibuprofen
	Phenolsulfonphthalein
Orange-brown	Cascara
	Chloroquine
	Chlorzoxazone
	Furazolidone
	Ibuprofen
	Iron sorbitex
	Phenazopyridine
	Phenytoin
	Primaquine
	Quinine
	Senna
	Sulfamethoxazole
	Sulfasalazine
Blue-green	Amitriptyline
	Doan's Pills
	Indigo blue
	Methylene blue
	Resorcinol
	Triamterene
Deep yellow	Cascara
	Fluorescein
	Quinacrine
	Riboflavin

Table 21.4.
Conditions Associated with Persistent Changes in Urine pH

Persistently acid urine (pH < 7.0)
  Metabolic acidosis
  Respiratory acidosis
  Pyrexia
  Phenylketonuria
  Alkaptonuria
Persistently alkaline urine (pH > 7.0)
  Urinary tract infection with urea-splitting organisms
  Metabolic alkalosis
  Carbonic anhydrase inhibitors
  Hyperaldosteronism
  Cystinosis

Adapted from Siest G, Galteau MM. Drug Effects on Laboratory Test Results. Analytic Interferences and Pharmacological Effects. St Louis, Yearbook Medical Publishers, 1988; Ross DL, Neely AE. Textbook of Urinalysis and Body Fluids. Norwalk, CT: Appleton-Century-Crofts, 1983: 68–122; and Young DS. Effects of Drugs on Clinical Laboratory Tests, ed. 3. Washington, D.C.: The American Association of Clinical Chemistry, 1990.

pH

The pH of the urine varies between 4.5 and 8 in patients with healthy kidneys. The pooled daily urine specimen is usually acidic (pH 6). Decreased pulmonary ventilation during sleep causes respiratory acidosis and the development of a highly acidic urine. Following meals, the urine becomes alkaline for a few hours. Thus, pH varies widely depending on the time of collection. Highly concentrated urine is usually strongly acidic and may be irritating. When urine stands it becomes alkaline, as urea is broken down to ammonia. Tests for pH should therefore always be done on freshly voided urine (16, 17). Urine that is persistently acid or alkaline may suggest the presence of systemic or urinary tract disease. Conditions associated with persistently acid or alkaline urine are listed in Table 21.4 (16, 17, 20). Some agents known to alter urine pH are listed in Table 21.5 (18).

CONCENTRATING ABILITY

Specific gravity is the most convenient way of measuring the amount of dissolved solids in the urine (e.g., urea, sodium, and chloride) and provides an accurate assessment of renal concentrating ability. By definition, the specific gravity of urine is the ratio of urine weight to the weight of an equal volume of distilled water. In health, the specific gravity may range from 1.003 to 1.030. Concentrated and dilute urine refer to specific gravities greater than or less than 1.010, respectively. Specific gravity is a useful tool in differentiating between prerenal azotemia and ATN. Usually in prerenal azotemia, the kidney should conserve sodium and water, leading to a specific gravity greater than 1.030. Conversely, during ATN, the kidney loses its ability to concentrate leading to a lower urine specific gravity.

The measurement of osmolality is more accurate and less influenced by large dense molecules such as protein and radiographic contrast media. To test concentrating ability, the patient is either deprived of water for a number of hours or given vasopressin 10 USP units subcutaneously. Failure to concentrate urine to more than 800 mOsm/kg or 1.020 specific gravity demonstrates decreased concentrating ability. When renal function approaches 20% of normal, the specific gravity and osmolality become fixed and stabilize at 1.010 and 300 mOsm/kg, respectively. The term *isosthenuria* is used to describe urine that is consistently at 1.010 or 300 mOsm/kg (16, 17).

PROTEIN CONTENT

Normally, nearly all filtered protein is reabsorbed or catabolized by the proximal tubular cells, as less than 150 mg of protein is excreted in the urine per day. Proteinuria is an important indicator of renal disease. Its evaluation requires a knowledge of factors that cause proteinuria without renal pathology. Nonpathologic or functional proteinuria is transient in nature and usually occurs in young adults. Proteinuria can occur with excessive exercise, exposure to cold, postural changes, such as standing from a recumbent position, and pregnancy. Proteinuria associated with renal disease occurs as a consequence of numerous disorders (see Table 21.6) (17, 23). Proteinuria is a common characteristic of nearly every form of glomerular disease and contributes to several nephrotic syndrome complications (discussed below).

Protein in the urine is measured by sulfosalicylic acid, heat and acetic acid, or dipstick methods. Because of its simplicity, the dipstick method is frequently used as a screening test for proteinuria. There are various urine dipstick products commercially available to detect and quantitate urine protein. In general, if protein losses are

Table 21.5.
Agents Causing a Change in Urine pH

Increase urine pH
  Acetohexamide
  Amiloride
  Amphotericin B
  Citrates (potassium or sodium)
  Epinephrine
  Niacinamide
  Sodium Bicarbonate
  Triamterene
Decrease urine pH
  Ammonium chloride
  Ascorbic acid
  Corticotropin
  Diazoxide
  Glucose
  Methenamine mandelate
  Metolozone
  Niacin
  Sucrose

greater than 3 g/day, a glomerular origin is suspected. Protein losses of less than 3 g/day are nondiagnostic, and the source is often unclear. The source of protein loss is also evaluated using electrophoresis, which differentiates pre-renal, glomerular, or tubular origin. Drugs may cause false-positive results with the sulfosalicylic acid and the heat and acetic acid methods, but not with the dipstick method (Table 21.7).

CELLS AND CASTS

Normal urine contains a small number of red blood cells, white blood cells, and hyaline casts. Casts are cylindrical elements with parallel sides that derive their shape and size from the tubular segment in which they were formed. Factors favoring cast formation are an acid pH, highly concentrated urine, proteinuria, and stasis within the tubules. The transparent hyaline casts are composed entirely of protein. Cellular casts represent red blood cells, white blood cells, or renal epithelial cells trapped within the protein matrix. Granular casts represent degraded cellular casts and usually indicate renal parenchymal damage. Tables 21.8 and 21.9 list the cells and casts that may be found in urine and their importance (16, 17).

ACUTE RENAL FAILURE

Approximately 5% of hospitalized patients develop ARF (24). The National Kidney and Urological Diseases Advisory Board 1990 Long-Range Plan concluded that ARF is the most costly kidney condition requiring hospitalization and that the number of cases has increased recently (25). Despite recent advances in intensive care medicine and

dialysis technology, the mortality rate remains at 50 to 60% and has not significantly changed over the past several decades (24, 26). Possible explanations for the lack of substantial improvement in survival may be that older, more complex patients, often with multiorgan failure and septicemia, are being hospitalized. Also, an increased number of surgical procedures are being performed in elderly patients, thus contributing to the mortality statistics (27).

Clinical conditions associated with ARF include the use of nephrotoxic drugs, hypotension, hypoxia, and sepsis. Onset of ARF necessitates changes in patient management and drug dosage adjustments. The management of these patients requires an understanding of the underlying pathophysiology and consists of preventive measures, supportive care, and efforts to preserve renal function. In this section, the etiology, pathophysiology, clinical course, and treatment of ARF will be reviewed. Since there are many causes of ARF, only the major causes will be discussed.

ARF is broadly defined as the abrupt deterioration in renal function that results in the inability of the kidney to regulate water and solute balance (27, 28). ARF is classified according to the amount of urine produced per day: anuric ARF (less than 100 mL/day); oliguric ARF (100–400 mL/day); and monoliguric ARF (greater than 400 mL/day) (27). Although ARF is often thought of as a decrease in urine output, nonoliguric ARF accounts for up to 60% of patients with ARF (29). Patients with nonoliguric ARF fail to concentrate the urine that is produced and continue to retain urea, creatinine, and other waste products of metabolism. Mild ARF has been defined as a rise in serum creatinine concentration to greater than 2.0 to 3.0 mg/dL. Severe cases are associated with rises of serum creatinine above 5 mg/dL (29). Clinicians also rely on acute increases of 25% in serum creatinine concentrations or decreases of 25% in creatinine clearance to define ARF (30). However, the rate of creatinine rise will vary depending on the extent of renal injury, dietary intake, and muscle mass of the patient.

Table 21.6.
Diseases Associated with Proteinuria

Infectious disease
  Poststreptococcal glomerulonephritis
  Infective endocarditis
  Syphilis
Neoplastic disease
  Lymphoma
  Leukemia
  Carcinoma: colon, lung, breast, stomach, kidney
Multisystem and connective tissue diseases
  Systemic lupus erythematosus
  Polyarteritis
  Sarcoidosis
  Sjögren's syndrome
  Amyloidosis
  Diabetes mellitus
Miscellaneous conditions
  Allergic reactions: bee stings, serum sickness
  Chronic allograft rejection
  Preeclampsia

Adapted from Kaysen GA. Proteinuria and the nephrotic syndrome. In: Schrier RW, ed. Renal and Electrolyte Disorders, ed. 4. Boston, Little, Brown & Co, 1992: 681–726.

Table 21.7.
Causes of False Reactions in Urine Protein Tests

	Methods		
Conditions or Drugs	Heat and Acetic Acid	Sulfosalicylic Acid	Dipstick Methods
Highly alkaline urine	−	−	−
p-Aminosalicylate	+	+	0
Contrast media	+	+	0
Penicillin (high dose)	+	+	0
Sulfonamides	0	+	0
Tolbutamide metabolites	+	+	0

(+), false-positive; (−), false-negative; (0), not affected

Table 21.8.
Cells Found in Urine

Cell	Normal Values	Clinical Importance
Red blood cell	0–2 per HPF[a]	Genitourinary (GU) tract lesions, acute tubulointerstitial disease, anticoagulants, systemic disease resulting in coagulation disorders
White blood cell	0–5 per HPF	Urinary tract infection, GU inflammation
Renal epithelial cell (nonsquamous)	0–2 per HPF	Tubular damage
Bacteria	None	Urinary tract infection (criteria for infection depends on method of urine collection)
Oval fat bodies[b]	None	Nephrotic syndrome, diabetic glomerulosclerosis, major skeletal trauma

[a]HPF, high-power field
[b]Renal tubular epithelial cells containing fat droplets

Table 21.9.
Casts Found in Urine

Hyaline	Normal finding, particularly in dehydration
Granular	Renal parenchymal disease, dehydration
Fatty	Nephrotic syndrome, diabetic glomerulosclerosis
Red cell	Glomerulonephritis, systemic lupus erythematosus, bacterial endocarditis
White cell	Pyelonephritis
Epithelial cell	Tubular damage

Table 21.10.
Causes of Prerenal Acute Renal Failure

Decreased cardiac output
  Congestive heart failure
  Pericardial tamponade
  Pulmonary embolism
  Cardiomyopathy
  Myocardial infarction
Hypovolemia
  Major trauma
  Burns
  Hemorrhage (surgical, postpartum)
  Volume depletion (renal losses, skin, vomiting, diarrhea)
  Sequestration (hypoalbuminemia, pancreatitis, peritonitis)
Increased renal vascular resistance
  Renal vasoconstriction (norepinephrine, dopamine)
  Systemic vasodilation (sepsis, vasodilatory agents)
  Anesthesia
  Surgery
Systemic vasodilation
  Bacterial sepsis
  Antihypertensives
  Afterload reduction
Renovascular obstruction[a]
  Renal artery (atherosclerosis, thrombosis, embolism)
  Renal vein (thrombosis)

[a]In bilateral renal disease or single functioning kidney
Adapted from Conger JD, Brinner VA, Schrier RW. Acute renal failure: pathogenesis, diagnosis and management. In: Schrier RW, ed. Renal and Electrolyte Disorders, ed. 4. Boston, Little, Brown & Co, 1992: 495–537.

Etiology. The causes of ARF may be divided into three categories: prerenal or hypoperfusion states, intrarenal or intrinsic renal parenchymal injury, and postrenal ARF or urinary obstructive disorders (31).

Prerenal. Prerenal azotemia is the most common cause of ARF (32). It occurs when renal blood flow (RBF) is reduced to a level adequate to sustain cells but inadequate to maintain normal GFR. As such, cellular injury does not occur and the decreased GFR can be rapidly restored once the pathophysiologic state is corrected (33). Reduced RBF may be secondary to any event that results in decreased renal perfusion or intense renal vasoconstriction. Underlying factors include hypovolemia, hypotension, insufficient cardiac output, and vascular obstruction. Causes of prerenal azotemia are listed in Table 21.10 (1). Mild hypoperfusion, caused by volume depletion, leads to prerenal azotemia with a mild decrease in GFR. The kidneys attempt to increase intravascular volume by conserving salt and water through increased proximal and distal reabsorption, as well as increased ADH release. GFR is maintained initially but only small amounts of concentrated urine are produced. This urine is low in sodium, has a high urine creatinine to plasma creatinine ratio, and a low (<1) FE_{Na}. Other factors that may help to differentiate prerenal ARF from intrinsic or postrenal ARF are shown in Table 21.11. Rapid attention and correction of prerenal azotemia can prevent ischemic injury and the associated morbidity and mortality (27).

Postrenal. Postrenal azotemia is simply an accumulation of nitrogenous wastes secondary to obstruction of urine flow.

This disorder accounts for approximately 15% of the patients with ARF (1). Causes of postrenal azotemia are listed in Table 21.12. These causes should be ruled out initially because they are often easily corrected, preventing the progression to intrinsic renal damage.

Intrinsic. Acute intrinsic renal failure refers to a decrease in renal function resulting from more severe or prolonged ischemic, toxic, or immunologic mechanisms (Table 21.13) and is associated with structural damage to glomeruli, tubules, vascular supply, or interstitial tissue (1). Such damage to the renal parenchyma often follows prerenal or postrenal azotemia, and if the degree of insult or duration of hypoperfusion or obstruction is sufficient, it is not

Table 21.11.
Urinary Indices to Differentiate Etiologies of Acute Renal Failure

	Prerenal	Acute Tubular Necrosis	Postrenal Obstruction
Protein	–	2–4+	–
WBC	–	2–4+	1+
RBC	–	2–4+	Variable
Casts	+/– hyaline	RTE, WBC	–
Osmolality (mOsm/kg)	>400	<350	<350
Specific gravity	>1.013	<1.013	–
U_{Na} (mEq/L)	<20	>40	Variable
FE_{Na} (%)	<1	>2	>1
BUN : S_{cr} ratio	>20 : 1	<20 : 1	–
U_{cr} : S_{cr} ratio	>40	<20	<20
RFI	<1	>4	>1.5

WBC, white blood cell; RBC, red blood cell; RTE, renal tubular epithelial cell; U_{Na}, urine sodium concentration; FE_{Na}, fractional excretion of sodium; BUN, blood urea nitrogen; U_{cr}, urine creatinine; S_{cr}, serum creatinine; RFI, renal failure index = $U_{Na}/(U_{cr} : S_{cr})$
Adapted from Mann JH, Fuhs DW, Hemstrom CA. Acute renal failure. Drug Intell Clin Pharm 20:421–38, 1986.

Table 21.12.
Causes of Postrenal Acute Renal Failure

Bilateral ureteral obstruction
  Intraureteral (emboli, stones, crystals)
  Extraureteral (tumor, retroperitoneal fibrosis)
  Papillary necrosis (acute pyelonephritis)
Bladder obstruction
  Mechanical (prostatic hypertrophy, malignancy, infection)
  Functional (anticholinergics, ganglionic blockers, neuropathy)
Urethral obstruction

immediately reversible. Recovery from intrarenal disease commonly takes 10 to 14 days and may require 6 weeks to a year or longer (26).

ARF is commonly used interchangeably with ATN, which denotes a histologic finding signifying necrotic damage to the renal tubules. However, ATN accounts for approximately 75% of the cases of ARF. Numerous surgical and medical insults are associated with the development of ARF. The highest incidence is associated with abdominal aneurysm resection, severe trauma, and open heart surgery (1).

Pathogenesis. Although considerable experimental work using animal models has resulted in several theories, the pathogenesis of ARF remains unclear. Several mechanisms are thought to be involved in the development of renal dysfunction. Acute intrinsic renal damage can be induced by ischemia, nephrotoxins, or, frequently, a combination of both. Reduction in RBF leading to ischemia is recognized as the most frequent mechanism of ARF (33). In response to reduced RBF, the production of vasoactive substances (e.g., the prostaglandins PGI_2 [prostacyclin] and PGE_2)

results in vasodilation, whereby RBF to the kidney can be appropriately maintained (29). The nonsteroidal antiinflammatory agents (NSAIDs) inhibit prostaglandin synthesis and limit the kidney's production of these vasodilatory substances. This appears to be particularly detrimental in patients with congestive heart failure and reduced effective arterial blood volume and in those with actual volume depletion (34).

Clinical situations where diminished RBF may lead to ischemic ARF include volume depletion, systemic hypotension, severe hemorrhage, cardiogenic shock, or surgical procedures in which repair of renal artery lesions requires aortic cross-clamping proximal to the renal arteries. RBF may also become structurally impaired by renal artery lesions or atheromatous disease. In these situations, GFR becomes dependent on angiotensin II for maintaining efferent arteriolar tone. Treatment with angiotensin-converting enzyme (ACE) inhibitors reduces the glomerular capillary filtration pressure because of decreased efferent arteriolar tone, as a result, GFR falls. On discontinuing the ACE inhibitor, GFR rapidly increases.

α-Adrenergic receptor-mediated systemic vasoconstriction associated with norepinephrine or high-dose dopamine can also result in marked reductions in RBF. Severe renal hypoperfusion is also associated with eclamptic complications of pregnancy (35). Nephrotoxic agents, especially aminoglycosides, amphotericin B, and radiocontrast dyes, are commonly associated with the development of ARF. Finally, endotoxin-mediated renal vasoconstriction may occur in sepsis (36).

In response to diminished RBF, the kidney attempts to maintain intravascular volume by conserving sodium and

Table 21.13.
Intrinsic Causes of Acute Renal Failure

Sequelae of prolonged prerenal azotemia
Nephrotoxic agents (drugs and radiocontrast)
Ischemic events
  Massive hemorrhage
  Pregnancy (preeclampsia, postpartum renal failure)
  Crush injury
  Septic shock
  Transfusion reaction
  Venous occlusion
  Arterial thrombosis
Glomerular
  Systemic lupus erythematosus
  Poststreptococcal glomerulonephritis
  Drug-induced vasculitis
  Malignant hypertension
Tubulointerstitial
  Acute tubular necrosis
  Acute interstitial nephritis
  Acute pyelonephritis
  Hyperuricemia
  Hypercalcemia

water through increased reabsorption in the proximal and distal tubules and by increasing ADH release. Despite these autoregulatory mechanisms, ischemia may occur as RBF diminishes to the extent that nutrient and oxygen supplies cannot meet metabolic demands of the renal tubular cells. During the ischemic insult, the lack of oxygen causes cessation of mitochondrial oxidative phosphorylation, leading to depletion of adenosine triphosphate (ATP) stores (37). Thus, cells with the greatest dependence on mitochondrial ATP production, may be most susceptible to oxygen deprivation-induced ATP depletion (38). In experimental models, renal epithelial cell ATP concentrations are decreased shortly after ischemic insult and exogenous administration of ATP results in accelerated recovery of ATP levels and a shortened duration of ARF (39).

Severe depletion of ATP may be expected to disable many energy-dependent processes, including active transport and the maintenance of intracellular homeostasis and cell structure (3). Cellular volume regulation depends on Na,K-ATPase activity, which is limited by decreased ATP during ischemia such that accumulation of intracellular sodium and water leads to osmotic cellular swelling and disruption of cell membranes (40).

Calcium homeostasis is disrupted by reduced calcium ATPase. This may cause increased intracellular calcium concentrations, leading to further mitochondrial injury and exacerbation of ATP depletion (41). A high intracellular calcium concentration may activate phospholipases and proteases, which then alter membrane lipid composition, further contributing to cellular damage (38).

During reperfusion, injury may worsen as oxygen free radicals are produced. This occurs when xanthine oxidase converts hypoxanthine to xanthine while donating an electron to generate superoxide radicals from the products of purine metabolism (e.g., AMP degradation) (38). Experimentally, oxygen free radicals increase membrane permeability via lipid peroxidation and may also cause oxidation of important sulfhydryl groups on proteins, including important renal transporter proteins (42).

Besides intrarenal vasoconstriction, various other explanations for diminished renal function have been postulated (3). These include backleak of glomerular filtrate into peritubular fluid through damaged tubular epithelia, tubular obstruction from cellular debris, and decreased glomerular capillary permeability. Urine flow and tubular capacity to reabsorb can be diminished by sloughing of the brush border membranes and the formation of casts within the tubular lumen. The sloughing of tubular membranes disrupts tubular integrity and allows backleak of glomerular ultrafiltrate via disrupted tubular epithelium into the peritubular circulation. This increased permeability results in the return of urea, creatinine, and other waste products into the systemic circulation. Tubular obstruction also increases intratubular hydraulic pressure, which opposes glomerular filtration pressure, leading to an unfavorable glomerular filtration pressure gradient and reduced GFR (1).

Another theory suggests that GFR declines because of an altered glomerular capillary ultrafiltration coefficient (K_f). Substantial reductions in the effective surface area for filtration cause a decrease in GFR. Experimental data supports that the reduction in K_f may be due to production of angiotensin II (1).

Damage to the glomeruli can also result from immunologic reactions and vascular occlusive diseases (e.g., hemolytic-uremic syndrome, renal-artery thrombosis, or embolic diseases) are thought to cause glomerular damage similar to mechanisms described earlier for ischemic events of the kidney (1, 3).

Clinical Course. The clinical course of ARF is often divided into four sequential phases: initiation or injury, maintenance, diuretic, and recovery (43). Characteristic of the initiation phase is significant change in hemodynamics and markedly decreased renal function. The maintenance phase of ARF usually lasts from several days to weeks and is commonly associated with oliguria. Treatment is focused on minimizing fluids and maintaining electrolyte balance until renal function returns. Impaired renal function may coexist with cellular repair processes. Surviving tubular cells appear to regenerate new tubular cells necessary to restore functional capacity. This process is likely under the influence of a variety of peptide growth factors (44). Renal cells release growth factors, including epidermal growth factor (EGF) and insulinlike growth factor (IGF-1), which may mediate repair of injured cells and recovery of renal function. Also, there appears to be some role for purine nucleotides in stimulating renal epithelial cell growth (45).

Once kidney repair begins, it is typical to see a diuretic phase, which begins prior to measurable reductions in serum creatinine and urea nitrogen. This diuresis is thought to result from the return of glomerular filtration function before complete correction of tubular reabsorption capacity. An osmotic diuretic effect may also occur because of accumulated uremic toxins and fluid during the oliguric phase (43). It is important to provide patients with adequate volume and electrolyte repletion during the diuretic phase of ARF.

Therapeutic Management. Management of ARF consists of preventive measures, removal of underlying causes or complications, supportive care, and proposed treatment modalities. Preventive therapy may be designed to avoid nephrotoxic drugs or maintain an euvolemic state and adequate renal perfusion pressure. Supportive care during the ARF episode is directed at treatment of infectious complications; maintaining adequate fluid, electrolyte and acid-base balance; and providing optimal nutritional support. Specific treatment of ARF is aimed at increasing urine output and RBF, restoring normal fluid and electrolyte balance, removing metabolic wastes, and minimizing further nephrotoxic injury.

Prevention. In the patient who suddenly develops oliguria with rising BUN and serum creatinine concentrations, it is important to distinguish whether the underlying disease process is prerenal or postrenal, since rapid correction of these entities can prevent progression to ischemic injury and development of ARF. Adequate correction of volume deficits can lead to prompt restoration of renal perfusion. Therapeutic agents known to further reduce blood flow must be withdrawn and potential nephrotoxins, such as aminoglycosides, radiocontrast dye, NSAIDs, and ACE inhibitors should be administered cautiously, if at all.

Initial efforts should also be directed at ruling out urinary tract obstruction. Factors suggesting obstruction include a normal urinalysis, rapid changes in urine output, and residual urine on postvoiding catheterization. If renal calculi are present, a radiograph of the abdomen will detect the 90% that are radiopaque. In the absence of obstruction, the urinary indices provide the most reliable method of distinguishing prerenal azotemia from acute tubular necrosis.

Table 21.11 will help in distinguishing reversible prerenal failure from acute tubular necrosis, but its usefulness is limited following the administration of diuretics or in those patients with underlying chronic renal failure. If prerenal azotemia is suspected, aggressive fluid resuscitation should result in an increased urine output. If urine flow does not increase, additional fluids should be given cautiously if at all, as fluid overload is likely to ensue if ARF is already established.

Prevention of associated complications, such as infection and gastrointestinal bleeding are very important. Careful maintenance of intravenous lines, minimal use of indwelling urinary bladder catheters, and early recognition and treatment of wound and other infections is necessary. Surveillance for signs of blood loss, such as testing stools for occult blood, monitoring the hematocrit, and control of gastric pH with H_2-antagonists or antacids, will minimize the morbidity associated with bleeding.

During clinical situations, when exposure to potential nephrotoxic insults is likely to occur, specific preventive measures, such as hydration and volume repletion before and during nephrotoxin exposure, are recommended (43). As an example, when using amphotericin B or aminoglycosides, ensuring that patients are well hydrated may eliminate or reduce the severity of renal damage. Normal saline or mannitol infusion 1 hour prior to amphotericin B administration may reduce the degree of renal injury, possibly related to the maintenance of urinary output with increased solute excretion and prevention of tubular obstruction (46). Other preventive measures to consider

are therapeutic drug monitoring of aminoglycoside concentrations, fluid hydration prior to cisplatin therapy, and the use of allopurinol and urine alkalinization during high-dose chemotherapy to avoid uric acid nephropathy. Combination therapy with more than one nephrotoxic agent carries additional risk and should be avoided if possible. Substitution of less nephrotoxic agents should be considered in elderly patients and others at risk of renal dysfunction. For example, in high-risk patients, it may be possible to avoid radiocontrast agents and use less invasive diagnostic techniques such as ultrasonography.

Supportive Care. ARF often persists for several days or weeks, requiring prolonged supportive care. The minimum daily fluid requirements should include replacement of measurable losses (i.e., urine output, nasogastric suction, vomiting, chest tube drainage, and fistula output) and insensible losses through the skin and lungs (approximately 600 to 900 mL/day). The choice of fluid intake should be determined by the need for colloid or crystalloid, electrolytes, and calories (22).

Electrolyte abnormalities that commonly occur in ARF are hyperkalemia, hyperphosphatemia, and hypermagnesemia. Treatment of hyperkalemia is discussed in Chapter 9. Restriction of dietary phosphate and the administration of phosphate-binding antacids usually maintains serum phosphate within normal ranges. Avoidance of magnesium-containing antacids will decrease the potential for hypermagnesemia.

With renal failure, the kidney can no longer regenerate bicarbonate and metabolic acidosis ensues. This acidosis accelerates proteolysis and branched chain amino acid oxidation, and can be corrected by administering sodium bicarbonate (47). ARF in the setting of multiple organ failure is associated with lean body mass catabolism, malnutrition, and a high rate of mortality (48). Attempting to enhance patient outcomes through the use of adequate nutritional support remains controversial (26). An early clinical study showed improved survival and enhanced recovery of renal function in patients receiving small doses of essential amino acids plus glucose, when compared to glucose alone (49). Subsequent studies suggested that there might be improved recovery of renal function and better patient outcomes; however, these reports have not been conclusively proven. In general, most clinicians agree that patients who are severely ill will do better if they are given adequate caloric intake (20 to 30 kcal/kg/day) to attenuate gluconeogenesis and thwart catabolism. For further discussion on nutrition requirements in ARF, see Chapter 10.

Changes in renal function make it necessary to alter the dose and/or dosing interval for drugs excreted by the kidney. Renal insufficiency influences drug disposition through changes in drug bioavailability, reduced protein binding, altered apparent volume of distribution, and altered renal metabolism (4). Tailoring regimens to within targeted drug concentrations and monitoring free or unbound concentrations may minimize risks of drug toxicity associated with renal failure (50). For more extensive reviews, see Chapter 1 and the comprehensive tables published by Benet (51, 52).

Therapy. Therapeutic modalities for treatment of ARF are designed to increase RBF, increase urine output, maintain fluid and electrolyte balance, remove metabolic wastes, and slow or reverse kidney damage. Because there is evidence to suggest that nonoliguric ARF is associated with less morbidity and mortality, clinicians have often tried to convert oliguric ARF to nonoliguric ARF. The evidence is clear that vasodilators and diuretics are of no value when administered after ARF is established (53). However, in early ARF, there is some evidence in favor of their use.

As soon as possible after a decrease in urine output is noted, a short course of mannitol might be tried. In adults, a sufficient dose of mannitol is needed to expand intravascular volume and increase renal perfusion pressure. A wide range of mannitol doses have been tried (22). In general, 20% mannitol solution dosed at 0.5 g/kg can be infused over 30 to 60 minutes, then repeated in an hour if there is no response. If urine output follows, additional doses are titrated to maintain urine output. Proposed mechanisms of benefit include increased filtration pressure, improved urine flow, reduced tubular cell inflammation, and improved RBF by decreasing renal vascular resistance (26). If a diuresis does not occur and additional doses are given, intravascular volume overload and congestive heart failure may occur.

The beneficial effects of loop diuretics in early ARF are thought to occur from decreased tubule obstruction, reduction of active transport and oxygen demand, or renal vasodilation (3). The loop diuretics (furosemide, ethacrynic acid, and bumetanide) affect the ascending limb of the loop of Henle to increase solute diuresis. Ethacrynic acid is not used in patients with renal failure because of accumulation and ototoxicity. Bumetanide is an effective and potent loop diuretic and can be used in patients with ARF; however, its use in these patients has not been extensively studied. The use of furosemide has been evaluated in both animals and humans. In uncontrolled clinical studies, the use of diuretics in patients with oliguric ARF has been associated with a response rate of 40 to 100% for conversion to a nonoliguric state (53–55). However, studies clearly suggest that if any benefits are to be gained, therapy with diuretics or mannitol should begin during the first 24 hours following an insult (57). When furosemide is administered, an initial dose of 1.5 to 2 mg/kg should be infused intravenously over 15 to 30 minutes. If urine output does not increase within an hour, the dose should be doubled and repeated. Doses greater than 500 mg are unlikely to be of benefit. If urine output increases, additional doses can be given to maintain urine flow.

Dopamine infusions are used to increase cardiac output and cause renal artery vasodilation, increasing RBF and GFR (58). Dopaminergic effects occur at lower doses of 1 to 5 µg/kg/min, and α-adrenergic (vasoconstriction) effects predominate at higher doses (10 to 20 µg/kg/min). Low-dose dopamine administration may benefit those patients unresponsive to diuretics alone by increasing RBF through renal artery vasodilation. The combination of low-dose dopamine with furosemide may increase urine output in early oliguric ARF. It appears helpful in converting oliguric ARF to nonoliguric ARF. Despite the lack of controlled trials, most clinicians would agree that nonoliguric patients are easier to manage than oliguric patients and have a better prognosis, with fewer complications, fewer requirements for dialysis, and shorter hospital courses than those with oliguric renal failure (26). Maintaining a high urine output may prevent volume overload and allow for increased nutritional support.

The early use of dialysis in the management of acute renal failure has been associated with increased survival. A small prospective study of casualties during the Vietnam War demonstrated that patients whose BUN was maintained below 50 mg/dL and whose serum creatinine concentration was maintained below 5 mg/dL had a mortality rate of 37%, whereas those given dialysis for a BUN above 120 mg/dL and serum creatinine concentration above 10 mg/dL had a mortality rate of 80% (59). It is postulated that early dialysis provides a better biochemical environment for fighting infections and for wound healing. Hemodialysis, peritoneal dialysis, and hemofiltration may become indicated in patients with neurologic signs and symptoms of uremia, severe hyperkalemia, volume overload, or severe acidosis. The use of dialysis is further discussed in Chapter 22.

DRUG-INDUCED NEPHROPATHIES

The kidneys are uniquely vulnerable to toxic injury because relative to their weight, they have the largest endothelial surface area and highest blood flow of any organ. Concentration of potential nephrotoxins occurs within the renal tubules, through secretion and reabsorption, thus exposing the tubular lumen and peritubular cells to high concentrations of potential toxins. Renal medullary and papillary tissues are vulnerable to toxic damage because of a combination of low blood flow and extremely high solute concentration. Also, the kidneys are highly active metabolic organs capable of transforming relatively innocuous substances, such as acetaminophen, into highly reactive metabolites (4, 60). The lesions associated with drug-induced nephropathy can be divided into four major categories: acute tubular necrosis (ATN), acute tubulointerstitial disease (ATID), chronic tubulointerstitial disease (CTID), and glomerulonephritis. A list of drugs and chemicals associated with each of these lesions is provided in Table 21.14.

ATN is a nonspecific response to either ischemia or direct toxic insult. ARF may result from cellular by-products of tubular necrosis obstructing the proximal tubule. As intratubular pressure increases and glomerular filtration is reduced, filtered wastes regain access to the circulation by leaking across transtubular membranes (61–63). The type of cellular injury associated with ATN varies with the type of renal insult. In a study of 121 patients who developed ATN, hypotension (27%) and dehydration (27%) were the sole causes of ARF. More than one acute insult was identified in 62% of these patients (64).

ATID, also known as acute interstitial nephritis, is characterized by interstitial edema and renal cellular infiltrates made up of monocytes, large and small lymphocytes, and plasma cells. Eosinophils may or may not be present. Tubular damage is suggested by the presence of cellular infiltrates located along the tubular basement membrane or between tubular epithelial cells (65). Drug-induced ATID appears to be a hypersensitivity reaction and often is associated with systemic signs of an allergic

Table 21.14.
Agents Associated with Nephrotoxicity

Acute tubular necrosis	Acute tubulointerstitial disease
Antibiotics	Penicillins
Aminoglycosides	Ampicillin, Amoxicillin
Amphotericin B	Methicillin
Cephalosporins	Nafcillin
Bacitracin/Polymixins	Oxacillin
Sulfonamides	Penicillin
Metals	Other antibiotics
Mercurials	Cephalosporins
Platinum	Erythromycin
Bismuth	Rifampin
Radiocontrast media	Sulfonamides
Miscellaneous agents	Metals
Acetaminophen	Bismuth, Gold
Cisplatin	Miscellaneous agents
Cyclosporine	NSAIDs
Methotrexate	Captopril
	Furosemide
Glomerulonephritis	Phenytoin
Allopurinol	Thiazides
Ampicillin	
Captopril	**Chronic tubulointerstitial disease**
Cocaine	Acetaminophen
Cyclophosphamide	Aspirin
Daunorubicin	Lithium
Gold	Phenacetin
Hydralazine	
Methicillin	
Penicillamine	
Penicillin	
Rifampin	
Thiazides	

reaction such as fever, skin rash, eosinophilia, and arthralgia. Hypersensitivity is further suggested by the small number of patients developing the reaction, the lack of dose-related effect, and a sudden recurrence with reinstitution of therapy (66, 67).

The renal lesions associated with CTID are deep within the medulla, close to the tip of the renal papilla. Capillary sclerosis and necrosis of these medullary structures can extend to include degeneration of the loops of Henle. Interstitial fibrosis can cause tubular compression, resulting in functional impairment of the tubules. Clinical symptoms consist of progressive renal insufficiency, varying degrees of hypertension, hematuria, leukocyturia, proteinuria, and the inability to concentrate urine. Analgesic nephropathy, the most widely known form of this disease, is responsible for more chronic renal failure worldwide than any other drug-induced nephropathy.

Glomerulonephritis may be caused by several different mechanisms. In some cases there is a direct dose-dependent effect on glomerular structures; in the majority, however, the glomerulus is involved through immunologic reactions. Drugs may act as haptens or antigens that either produce circulating antigen-antibody complexes or cause complex formation within the glomerulus. Damage to or alteration of the glomerular basement membrane produces proteinuria, a hallmark of this disease. The most common drug-induced lesion has been membranous glomerulonephritis with proteinuria and nephrotic syndrome.

Selected Nephrotoxic Drugs
AMINOGLYCOSIDES

Aminoglycosides are avidly concentrated within the renal cortex. Following initial binding to tubular brush border membranes, they are vacuolized and taken up by the proximal tubular cells. Once within the cell, they are transported to the lysosomes. Continued uptake results in lysosomal dysfunction and eventual degeneration, allowing lysosomal enzymes to act on other cell organelles. Tubular cell necrosis may result from continued exposure. The initial manifestations of nephrotoxicity include release of brush border and lysosomal enzymes, glycosuria, aminoaciduria, and tubular proteinuria. Defects in proximal tubular transport may be detected by the presence of β_2-microglobulin. Hypokalemia, hypomagnesemia, and loss of concentrating ability may also be seen. Patients who develop aminoglycoside nephrotoxicity are most often nonoliguric. The occurrence of toxicity is most closely related to treatment duration and is usually seen following 7 to 10 days of therapy. Additional risk factors for the development of nephrotoxicity include age, dose, high trough serum concentrations, and low urine flow rates. Proper patient selection based on culture and sensitivity data, early withdrawal of unnecessary therapy, dose adjustment to ensure therapeutic levels, and maintenance of good urine output during therapy seem to constitute the optimal way to minimize toxicity (68–74).

AMPHOTERICIN B

Interaction of amphotericin B with membrane sterols results in disruption of cell membranes. The possibility of direct vasoconstriction of the renal vasculature has also been suggested. Toxicity is dose related and is seen in up to 80% of patients treated with a cumulative dose of 2 to 3 grams. Early manifestations of amphotericin B nephrotoxicity include renal-concentrating defects, distal renal tubular acidosis with potassium wasting, and modest proteinuria. The occurrence of renal failure is usually associated with proximal tubular necrosis. Since nephrotoxicity often limits a full course of therapy, many attempts to limit toxicity have been tried. To date, no regimen or manipulation in therapy has been found to attenuate the toxicity consistently, although encouraging results have been seen with sodium supplementation of 150 mEq/day. Alternate-day therapy may be used when toxicity is recognized, and discontinuation is recommended when the BUN exceeds 50 mg/dL (68, 75, 76).

CYCLOSPORINE

Cyclosporine has achieved a major role in the prevention of allograft rejection. The most common side effect is a dose-dependent decline in GFR with reversible increases in serum creatinine and BUN concentrations. This toxicity can complicate the management of renal transplant recipients, since distinguishing between graft rejection and cyclosporine toxicity is difficult, even with the use of decision algorithms (77, 78). Enhanced toxicity may occur with the simultaneous use of acyclovir, ketoconazole, amphotericin B, aminoglycosides, and cotrimoxazole. Reduction in toxicity has been attempted by prolonging the infusion time to up to 24 hours and with the administration of transdermal clonidine and thromboxane synthetase inhibitors (79, 80). Attempts have been made to monitor plasma levels of cyclosporine and to maintain trough concentrations of 100 to 250 ng/mL. In vitro data suggest that there is little immunosuppression in mixed lymphocyte cultures at concentrations below 100 ng/mL. The search for a therapeutic window using pharmacokinetic monitoring continues to be an important function at transplantation centers (81–83). (See Chapter 22, "Dialysis and Renal Transplantation.")

RADIOGRAPHIC CONTRAST MEDIA

The increased use of contrast media associated with intravenous pyelography, angiography, and computed tomography has led to greater recognition of this class of agents as an important cause of ARF. The diagnosis must be considered when one of these agents is used in a high-risk patient who subsequently develops any degree of renal failure. Mild nonoliguric renal failure may be transient, with serum creatinine reaching a peak in 3 to 5 days and a return to baseline within 10 to 14 days. Severe oliguric renal failure may occur within 24 hours of the contrast administration, with a return to baseline within 3 weeks, residual renal impairment, or renal failure requiring dialysis. High-risk patients include those with diabetes mellitus, preexisting renal disease, multiple myeloma, advanced age, coexisting liver disease, peripheral vascular disease, hypertension, dehydration, and prior exposure to contrast media. The precise mechanism of nephrotoxicity in unknown, but may include impaired renal perfusion, glomerular injury, tubular injury, and tubular obstruction. Prevention is aimed at avoidance of unnecessary procedures, vigorous hydration (particularly in high-risk patients) using low doses of contrast media, and avoidance of multiple contrast procedures. The use of hyperosmolar (1500 mOsm/kg) or less hyperosmolar (750 mOsm/kg) contrast agents does not seem to influence the risk for developing nephrotoxicity. Extracellular volume expansion with 800 mL/hour of normal saline during the procedure and liberal oral or parenteral fluids both before and after the procedure have significantly reduced toxicity, even in high-risk patients (68, 84–86).

ANGIOTENSIN-CONVERTING ENZYME INHIBITORS

Acute reversible nonoliguric renal failure may occur following initiation of ACE inhibitor therapy in patients with bilateral renal artery stenosis or renal artery stenosis in a solitary kidney. Low renal perfusion stimulates the renin-angiotensin system. Angiotensin II causes renal vasoconstriction and increases efferent arteriolar tone, which acts to maintain glomerular filtration pressure. ACE inhibition leads to dilation of efferent arterioles, which will cause an abrupt decline in renal function in those dependent on efferent tone to maintain GFR (87–89).

CHRONIC ANALGESIC ABUSE

The two renal lesions seen with chronic analgesic abuse are papillary necrosis and cortical interstitial nephritis. Together they represent the syndrome identified as CTID. Ischemia is an important factor in the development of papillary necrosis, since the oxygen tension near the papillae is about 20 mm Hg. Local production of prostaglandins probably promotes dilation of medullary blood vessels and maintains local blood flow. Prostaglandin inhibitors therefore play a role in the development of chronic toxicity. In addition, the kidney is capable of converting phenacetin and acetaminophen, in the presence of salicylates, to highly reactive intermediates. Combination analgesic therapy seems always to be a feature in this disease. Other clinical features of this disease include nocturia, hematuria, renal colic, and the occasional finding of necrotic tissue in the urine. Of patients who develop this form of chronic renal failure, approximately 23% have continued deterioration of renal function and 12% either die or receive maintenance dialysis within 6 months of diagnosis. Health care practitioners can play a critical role in recognizing analgesic abusers. Reformulation of essentially all combination analgesic products that once contained phenacetin has not caused a significant reduction in this disease (90–94).

CISPLATIN

Cisplatin is highly concentrated in the proximal tubular cells. Intracellular transformation of the chloride ligands on the molecule into a highly reactive aquated compound is thought to occur because of the low intracellular chloride concentration. This transformed molecule is then able to alkylate purine and pyrimidine bases of DNA. ATN occurs because cellular degeneration results in a proximal tubular obstruction from cellular debris. The incidence and severity of renal toxicity is both dose and duration dependent. A rise in serum creatinine and BUN levels may be preceded by proteinuria, tubular casts, enzymuria, and the presence of β_2-microglobulin in the urine. Cisplatin nephrotoxicity has been reduced with prehydration with saline. One such approach has been the administration of 5% dextrose in 0.45 to 0.9% sodium chloride at a rate of 250 mL/hr beginning 2 hours prior to cisplatin. The dose of cisplatin is administered in 250 mL of a 3% sodium chloride solution. Mannitol 12.5 g is given immediately prior to cisplatin and then infused at the rate of 10 g/hr for 3 hours. This technique provides adequate chloride to prevent the aquation reaction within the cisplatin container and provides an osmotic diuresis to minimize exposure to proximal tubular cells (68, 95, 96).

CHRONIC RENAL FAILURE

Chronic renal failure (CRF) is defined as a progressive deterioration in renal function. It may take from months to years for ESRD to develop. This progressive deterioration is evidenced by a rise in BUN and serum creatinine levels, a decline in creatinine clearance, and the development of uremic symptoms as ESRD approaches. A list of complications in renal failure is provided in Table 21.15. Although the concentration of urea can be correlated with the degree of renal impairment, no specific uremic toxins have been identified as being responsible for all the complications of the uremic syndrome. Other uremic toxins that have been identified include ammonia, guanidine, guanidinosuccinic acid, methyl guanidine, and myoinositol (97–99).

Etiology

Important causes of chronic renal failure are listed in Tables 21.14 and 21.16. In patients with mild renal failure (serum creatinine less than 2 mg/dL and no microalbuminuria) aggressive treatment of the primary disease is associated with marked slowing or even interruption of the

Table 21.15.
Complications in Renal Failure

Sodium and water imbalance
Acid-base imbalance
Potassium imbalance
Anemia
Hemostatic defects
Calcium and phosphate abnormalities
Hyperuricemia
Carbohydrate intolerance
Hypertension
Gastrointestinal disturbances
Neuromuscular disturbances
Renal osteodystrophy
Dermatological disorders
Psychological disorders

Table 21.16.
Etiology of Chronic Renal Failure

Renal
  Glomerulonephritis
    Acute
    Chronic
    Rapidly progressive
  Interstitial nephritis
  Ischemic renal disease
    Bilateral renal artery stenosis
    Bilateral fibromuscular hyperplasia
    Urinary tract infection (pyelonephritis)
  Congenital anomalies
    Polycystic kidney disease
    Medullary cystic disease
    Hypoplastic kidneys
  Systemic diseases
    Diabetes
    Hypertension
    Systemic lupus erythematosus
    Polyarteritis nodosa
    Amyloidosis
    Chronic hypercalcemia
    Chronic hypokalemia
    Hyperuricemia
  Drugs and chemicals

progression of renal failure. In this respect, control of blood pressure and hyperglycemia is critical. Of concern is that in others with more advanced renal failure and those with microalbuminuria, the deterioration in renal function is predictable and progression to ESRD is inevitable. To this end, extensive research efforts are being directed toward the suggested relationships between dietary protein intake and the presence of hyperlipidemia on the rate of progression of renal disease.

PROTEIN

Brenner et al. (100) proposed that after the initial reduction in the number of functioning nephrons, the remaining nephrons hypertrophy and increase their single nephron glomerular GFR by increasing glomerular capillary pressure and flow. This hyperfiltration ultimately results in a loss of glomerular capillary permselectivity, with proteins leaking into the capillary space, stimulating mesangial cell proliferation and glomerulosclerosis. A high-protein diet also increases RBF and GFR and may possibly add to the already elevated glomerular hemodynamics found in patients with CRF. For this reason, the use of low-protein diets in patients with CRF has been under investigation for the past 10 years. Most of these studies have not controlled for multiple causes of renal failure, so the results are difficult to interpret. Recently, the Modification of Diet in Renal Disease (MDRD) study reported the results of two randomized multicenter trials involving 840 patients with various chronic renal diseases (101). This study was also troubled by enrolling patients with ages ranging from 18 to 70 years. Dietary therapy was initiated at a relatively advanced stage of the disease and antihypertensive regimens varied among the study groups. Results showed that those patients with moderate renal failure (GFR of 25 to 55 mL/min/1.73 m^2) appeared have a small though not statistically significant benefit from a low-protein diet. No benefit was seen in patients with more severe renal insufficiency. This study did point out the value of lowering blood pressure and proposed that specific diseases may respond differently to dietary protein restriction.

LIPIDS

It is now known that patients with diabetes or hypertension who have proteinuria are at greater risk for increased cardiovascular morbidity and mortality (102). A common finding in these patients is increased low-density lipoprotein (LDL) cholesterol, increased lipoprotein A, and reduced levels of high-density lipoprotein (HDL) cholesterol. It is thought that LDL is taken up by mesangial cells, which induces their proliferation and production of macrophage chemotactic factors. The macrophages along with mesangial cells oxidize LDL and form foam cells. This causes mesangial cell injury and leads to an increased mesangial matrix and glomerulosclerosis. Both experimental and clinical data suggest that lipid abnormalities not only contribute to cardiovascular disease but also to the progression of renal disease. The possibility that the use of lipid lowering agents will be effective in slowing the rate of progression of renal dysfunction in CRF patients is currently being investigated.

Complications and Treatment

Of the numerous CRF complications listed in Table 21.15, only the most common and clinically relevant factors are discussed here. Most patients have few symptoms of CRF when greater than 25% of normal renal function still exists. To a great extent, the symptoms of CRF can be explained on the basis of an imbalance between dietary intake and urinary excretion. Furthermore, many of these symptoms can be managed through appropriate dietary and drug therapy. When this therapy is no longer effective, maintenance dialysis treatments or renal transplantation become indicated (see Chapter 22).

SODIUM AND WATER IMBALANCE

When creatinine clearance falls to less than 25 mL/min, the ability of the kidney to handle wide fluctuations in sodium and water intake is lost. Urinary excretion of water and salt tends to be fixed. If intake is below output, then salt and water depletion may occur. More commonly, when intake exceeds output, retention occurs. In these patients, the use of diuretic therapy becomes a mainstay in the maintenance of fluid balance. As GFR falls to 25 mL/min, thiazide diuretics become ineffective and loop diuretics such as furosemide, bumetanide, or torsemide must be used. Furosemide is highly protein bound. As such, in the tubular fluid of patients with nephrotic syndrome, the drug is bound to albumin and resistance to its effects might occur (103). In these situations, higher doses become necessary to overcome protein binding in tubular fluid and achieve desired diuretic responses. Bed rest is also beneficial in mobilizing interstitial fluid to the intravascular compartment. By expanding the central blood volume, renal perfusion improves and delivery of sodium to the site of diuretic activity is enhanced. For this reason, diuretics are best given immediately upon arising from the daily sleep. In patients refractory to loop diuretics, the addition of metolazone, which acts at different sites along nephron, may maximize the diuretic response. Finally, patients with edema should be placed on a salt restricted diet (2 g/day) to assist in reducing positive sodium balance. On a practical basis this means no added salt to the home-cooked diet. It also means restricting intake of processed foods and especially meals from fast food restaurants.

ACID-BASE IMBALANCE

A normal adult consuming a mixed diet generates approximately 1 mEq/kg of metabolic acid daily. This hydrogen is rapidly buffered by circulating bicarbonate and is excreted by the lungs as respiratory acid. The bicarbonate lost in this process is regenerated by the kidney as titratable acidity and ammonia are excreted. With renal failure, this regeneration of bicarbonate is impaired and metabolic acidosis occurs. While this metabolic acidosis appears to be reasonably well tolerated, it does contribute to the catabolic state by stimulating branched-chain amino acid metabolism.

Metabolic acidosis may be corrected by the administration of sodium bicarbonate or sodium citrate. The amount of buffer required varies among individual patients but ranges from 20 to 40 mEq/day. This can be replaced by giving sodium bicarbonate tablets or powder, where each 325-mg tablet provides 4 mEq of bicarbonate. With the oral administration of sodium bicarbonate, the bicarbonate reacts with gastric hydrochloric acid and generates carbon dioxide, which must be eliminated through belching. In patients who find elimination of stomach gas to be painful, the use of Shohls solution (a combination of sodium citrate and citric acid) provides an alternative buffer source. The sodium citrate in this formulation combines with hydrochloric acid to form citric acid, which is then absorbed and metabolized to carbon dioxide and water without the generation of stomach gas. Shohls solution contains 1 mEq of sodium/mL and thus 1 mEq of buffer/mL. The use of potassium citrate solutions in these patients should be avoided because of the potential for hyperkalemia.

POTASSIUM IMBALANCE

Even though potassium is excreted almost exclusively in the urine, hyperkalemia rarely occurs in patients who have GFR above 10 mL/min in the absence of acute changes in potassium intake. This balance is maintained by increased potassium secretion in the distal renal tubule and increased fecal potassium losses. Factors that jeopardize this balance include the administration of potassium-sparing diuretics, increased potassium intake, and acidosis, which shifts potassium extracellularly from the intracellular compartment. Treatment of hyperkalemia is discussed in Chapter 9, "Fluid and Electrolytes Therapy and Acid-Base Balance."

CALCIUM AND PHOSPHORUS ABNORMALITIES

As renal function decreases, urinary phosphorus excretion diminishes slightly. The modest elevation in serum phosphorus suppresses calcitriol production by the kidney and this reduces calcium absorption from the gastrointestinal tract. The resultant reduction in ionized calcium stimulates parathyroid hormone (PTH) secretion. Increased PTH enhances renal tubular phosphorus excretion, stimulates calcium resorption from bone, and increases tubular reabsorption of calcium. The net effect is normalization of serum phosphorus and calcium levels with a slight but significant increase in circulating PTH levels. As renal mass declines, the ability of the kidney to excrete phosphorus in response to the PTH levels is impaired, leading to sustained elevations in serum phosphorus concentration. Phosphorus levels are usually normal until the GFR decreases to approximately 30 mL/min. A sustained elevation in serum phosphorus further inhibits the renal conversion of 25 hydroxycholecalciferol to 1,25 dihydroxycholecalciferol, which results in impaired intestinal calcium absorption and bone resistance to PTH.

Numerous skeletal abnormalities result from disturbances in calcium and phosphorus homeostasis secondary to CRF. These bone abnormalities are collectively referred to as the renal osteodystrophies. Management of renal osteodystrophy is aimed at keeping serum calcium and

phosphorus levels near normal and suppressing PTH secretion. Early conservative management consists of restricting dietary phosphorus through reduction of foods high in phosphorus such as meat, milk, legumes, beer, and colas (Table 21.17). Patients who are placed on a low-protein diet also have reduced phosphate intake such that a 40-gram low-protein diet provides approximately 25 mmol of phosphorus per day (104). As renal failure progresses and GFR becomes less than 30 mL/min, even dietary restriction is insufficient to prevent hyperphosphatemia from occurring. In these patients, phosphorus removal provides an important therapeutic challenge. Previously, the use of aluminum-containing phosphate binding gels were demonstrated to be very effective in maintaining phosphorus levels and in circumventing the development of renal osteodystrophy (105). The difficulty with this therapy is that aluminum is absorbed and there is

Table 21.17.
High-Phosphorus Foods

Dairy
    Cheese, all types
    Cream
    Cream pies or desserts
    Custard
    Ice cream
    Milk, all kinds
    Pudding
    Yogurt
Protein foods
    Braunschweiger
    Eggs
    Liver
    Peanut butter
    Salmon
    Sardines
    Tuna
Vegetables
    Baked beans and pork 'n' beans
    Beans
    Peas
    Lentils
    Mixed vegetables
    Soybeans and soy foods
Breads and cereals
    Barley
    Bran
    Cornbread
    Waffles (from mix)
    Whole-grain breads
Miscellaneous
    Chocolate
    Nuts
Beverages
    Beer
    Colas

From Delmez JA, Slatopolsky E. Hyperphospatemia: its consequences and treatment in patients with chronic renal disease. Am J Kidney Dis 19:303–17, 1992.

Table 21.18.
Oral Calcium Preparations

	% Calcium	Strength	Elemental Calcium Content
Liquid			
Calcium glubionate	6.5	1800 mg/5 mL	115 mg/5mL
Tablets			
Calcium gluconate	9	500 mg	45 mg
		650 mg	58.5 mg
		1000 mg	90 mg
Calcium lactate	13	325 mg	42.3 mg
		650 mg	84.5 mg
Calcium acetate	25	667 mg	169 mg
Calcium carbonate	40	625 mg[a]	250 mg
		650 mg	260 mg
		667 mg	266.8 mg
		750 mg	300 mg
		1250 mg	500 mg
		1500 mg[a]	600 mg

[a]Chewable

clear evidence that aluminum toxicity occurs. This toxicity can result in encephalopathy, osteomalacia, and myopathy. It is now recommended that chronic administration of aluminum-containing phosphate binders should be avoided, if at all possible. These agents are still recommended for binding phosphorus in severely hyperphosphatemic patients, but for acute episodes only. Once serum phosphorus levels decrease, calcium carbonate or calcium acetate may be used to further bind phosphate and to provide elemental calcium. Table 21.18 lists available calcium supplements. Therapy should not be instituted unless serum phosphorus concentration is under 5.5 to 6 mg/dL. A calcium-phosphorus product (multiplying the calcium concentration by the phosphorous concentration) greater than 55 must be prevented to avoid soft tissue calcification.

If serum calcium and PTH cannot be normalized with more conservative regimens, a trial of vitamin D is warranted (106). Of the many vitamin D congeners available, 1,25-dihydroxyvitamin D_3 (calcitriol) offers an advantage over ergocalciferol (vitamin D_2) and cholecalciferol (vitamin D_3) in that it has a shorter onset and duration of action. The potential for vitamin D intoxication and sustained hypercalcemia, which may require weeks for resolution, is a major hazard associated with pharmacologic doses of vitamins D_2 and D_3. If vitamin D intoxication occurs with the use of calcitriol it is rapidly corrected upon discontinuing therapy.

PLATELET AND BLEEDING ABNORMALITIES
(See also Chapter 15, "Clotting Disorders")
Bleeding is a frequent complication of uremia manifested by ecchymosis, purpura, gastrointestinal bleeding, and

epistaxis. Capillary fragility and coagulation factor defects do not appear to play a major role. Quantitative and qualitative platelet abnormalities are presumed to be the etiology in most patients. Although severe thrombocytopenia with platelet counts below 50,000/mL are rare, minor deficiencies where platelet counts below 150,000/L have been noted in over half the patients studied. Platelet factor III is reduced and platelet aggregation is inhibited in advanced renal failure, resulting in prolonged bleeding times and poor clot retraction. Uremic toxins are thought to be responsible for these abnormalities. Improved platelet function can be obtained after adequate dialysis. Treatment for severe bleeding requires red cell transfusion and the administration of fresh platelet concentrates.

The management of bleeding in chronic renal failure has been the subject of recent research. Effective treatments include the blood product, cryoprecipitate; a synthetic derivative of ADH, desmopressin (1-deamino-8-D-arginine vasopressin); and conjugated estrogens (107–111). Janson et al. (107) showed that cryoprecipitate enriched with Factor VIII and von Willebrand Factor (VWF) effectively shortened bleeding times. Desmopressin also shortens bleeding times and causes an increased release of Factor VIII:VWF complex (109). Although the precise mechanism of action has not been established, it is proposed that each may increase plasma concentrations of VWF, a large glycoprotein necessary for primary hemostasis. Cryoprecipitate is a heterogenous blood preparation, associated with an increased risk of blood-borne disease (e.g., transmission of the human immunodeficiency virus and viral hepatitis). Furthermore, both desmopressin and cryoprecipitate have relatively short-lived effects, lasting only a few hours, which limits their clinical utility in management of uremic bleeding. Preliminary evidence suggests that conjugated estrogen infusions shorten bleeding times for longer durations (up to 14 days). Thus, estrogen therapy may become important in the management of uremic bleeding, especially when a longer-lasting hemostatic competency is desired (110–111). Prevention of acute bleeding depends on adequate treatment of the uremic state with hemodialysis or peritoneal dialysis. Patients should be advised to avoid drugs having antiplatelet activity, particularly aspirin.

ANEMIA (See also Chapter 14, "Other Anemias")
Anemia develops in virtually all patients with chronic renal failure. The anemia is normochromic and normocytic, and rarely does the hematocrit fall below 20%. In the absence of congestive heart failure and angina, the anemia is usually well tolerated. The anemia is caused by a number of factors that are listed in Table 21.19. The earliest clinical signs are pallor and fatigue, which occur when serum creatinine exceeds 3 mg/dL (112). The primary cause of the anemia of CRF is a decrease in erythropoietin (EPO) concentration.

Table 21.19.
Causes of Anemia of Chronic Renal Failure

Decreased erythropoietin activity
Shortened red blood cell lifespan
Gastrointestinal blood loss
Dialysis
    Iron deficiency from dialyzer blood loss
    Folic acid deficiency from dialyzer blood loss
    Red cell destruction from hemolysis
    Splenic sequestration

Natural EPO is produced and secreted primarily by the kidney in response to hypoxia. EPO enhances erythropoiesis by stimulating bone marrow production of erythroid cells. In patients with normal renal function, serum EPO levels rise to 10 to 100 times the normal level, in response to anemia. In patients with CRF, EPO production is blunted in response to hypoxia, indicating an impaired ability to produce EPO by the kidneys (113).

A recombinant human erythropoietin (rHuEPO) is now available for the treatment of anemia associated with CRF, reducing the need for red blood cell transfusions or anabolic steroids and their concomitant risks. EPO is administered either intravenously or subcutaneously, with a usual starting dose of 50 to 100 units per kg three times a week. It is important to evaluate and adequately control hypertension prior to initiating therapy. Hypertension occurs in approximately 25% of patients receiving rHuEPO, perhaps related to too fast a rate of rise in the hematocrit. Although rare, seizures have occurred and may also be related to a fast rise in the hematocrit. It is important to monitor the hematocrit and reduce the dose, usually in increments of 25 units/kg/dose, if the hematocrit increases by more than 4% in a 2-week period (114). Iron deficiency will blunt or inhibit responses to rHuEPO therapy. Transferrin saturation should be at least 20% and ferritin concentration at least 100 ng/mL before initiating therapy. Patients may require supplemental iron therapy while receiving epoetin (114). Iron deficiency may also result from chronic blood loss due to uremia, blood loss due to dialysis, or malabsorption of iron. Iron deficiency should be treated with oral ferrous sulfate, 300 mg three times daily, or parenteral iron in patients with gastrointestinal intolerance. Folic acid is removed during dialysis, which can result in folic acid deficiency. Daily supplementation of folic acid is then necessary.

The target hematocrit range is 30 to 33%. Maintenance doses of rHuEPO should be individualized to maintain the hematocrit within the target range. In patients with CRF not on dialysis, the usual maintenance dose needed is around 75 to 150 units per kg administered once weekly. Many patients are able to self-administer the dose at home. CRF patients who are on dialysis often require doses around 75 units/kg three times weekly (114).

Previously, anabolic steroids were used regularly to increase erythropoiesis in the treatment of anemia of CRF. The major disadvantage of these agents is a greater risk for hepatotoxicity and an association with hepatocellular carcinoma from chronic use. The need for anabolic steroids has been reduced greatly by the availability of rHuEPO.

CARBOHYDRATE ABNORMALITIES
Approximately 70% of CRF patients have varying degrees of glucose intolerance, as evidenced by elevated postprandial blood glucose levels, even though fasting glucose levels are often normal. With normal renal function, approximately 40% of circulating insulin is cleared by the kidneys. In renal failure there is decreased clearance and the elimination half-life of insulin is prolonged, but there is peripheral resistance to the insulin (115, 116).

HYPERTENSION (See also Chapter 37, "Hypertension")
Hypertension significantly increases the risk for developing coronary heart disease, stroke, and ESRD. Patients with proteinuria have an increased risk for developing cardiovascular disease. Treatment regimens that reduce proteinuria (low-protein diets, ACE inhibitors, calcium channel blockers, etc.) appear to slow the rate of progression of renal disease. Reductions in blood pressure have added significantly to the positive outcomes of other treatment modalities, such as control of blood sugar and the use of low-protein diets.

Some antihypertensive regimens have not been recommended for use in patients with renal failure because of demonstrated decreases in RBF, but experimental studies have suggested that by reducing renal hemodynamics, a renal protective effect is gained. Thus, moderate reductions in GFR with the initiation of antihypertensive therapy ultimately results in slowing the rate of progression of renal failure and prolonging the time until ESRD occurs.

Several questions remain unanswered concerning the different classes of antihypertensive agents and their effectiveness in slowing the progression of renal insufficiency. Tierney et al. retrospectively assessed hypertensive patients following at least 1 year of various antihypertensive treatments. The number of patients with a serum creatinine greater than 2 mg/dL increased from 15% to 50% as systolic blood pressure increased from less than 150 mm Hg to greater than 180 mm Hg (117). Thus, no specific class of antihypertensives is clearly superior for preventing the progression of renal function deterioration. In another retrospective review, Rostland et al. found that no matter how well blood pressure is controlled, 15% of patients will have a progressive deterioration in renal function (118). It appears that hypertensive patients with tighter control of blood pressure may have a lower incidence of progressive renal insufficiency than those who are poorly controlled. However, in some individuals, progressive declines in renal function occur despite controlling diastolic blood pressure at approximately 90 mm Hg (119). Practitioners are now recommending that systemic blood pressure be controlled to less than 130/85 mm Hg, if possible, in patients with established renal insufficiency (119).

The kidney plays a major role in the control of blood pressure, through regulation of the extracellular fluid volume and the renin-angiotensin system. In most patients with CRF, both renin excess and increased fluid volume contribute to hypertension. Since extracellular volume expansion is a major cause of hypertension, sodium restriction and diuretics are often used as first-line antihypertensive therapy. Questions have been raised about the initial use of diuretics, which lack renal protective effects because of stimulation of the renin-angiotensin system and maintenance of a high glomerular capillary pressure (120).

In general, the thiazides have been shown to be more effective than other diuretics in the treatment of hypertension. Hydrochlorothiazide (12.5 to 25 mg given once daily) is the thiazide often initially chosen. However, when fluid overload occurs and diuresis cannot be accomplished with thiazides because of decreased renal function, furosemide or other loop blocker diuretics should then be used. Furosemide has a short duration of action and usually should be divided and given as two daily doses. The dosage can range from 40 to over 200 mg/day. Although metolazone is a thiazide diuretic, it is effective in conjunction with furosemide in more severe renal impairment because of its inhibition of proximal sodium and chloride reabsorption. Usual doses required are 2.5 to 5 mg daily. The potassium-sparing diuretics should be avoided in renal failure because of the potential for severe hyperkalemia.

β-Blockers lower blood pressure by reducing cardiac output and are useful agents in renal failure because they inhibit renin release and decrease renal vascular hypertension. It is especially appropriate to consider these agents in CRF patients with ischemic heart disease. When used in combination with diuretics, the antihypertensive effects are additive. The higher lipophilic β-blockers (propranolol, metoprolol, timolol, labetalol, and pindolol) are extensively metabolized by the liver and do not require dosage adjustments in patients with renal insufficiency. In contrast, those with low lipophilicity (atenolol, acebutolol, betaxolol, bisoprolol, carteolol, and nadolol) are primarily excreted by the kidney and require dosage modifications when creatinine clearance falls below 50 mL/min (121).

Antihypertensive treatment in patients with renal impairment using ACE inhibitors and calcium antagonists has recently been reviewed (119). It is now thought that these agents have renal protective properties through their effects on renal hemodynamics. The ACE inhibitors preferentially dilate efferent arterioles, decreasing glomerular capillary pressure, which reduces glomerular hypertension. Additionally, studies have shown beneficial effects on reduced proteinuria in patients with chronic glomerular disease and diabetic nephropathy. Experimental models also suggest that ACE inhibitors attenuate proliferation of mesangial cell matrix swelling associated with glomerulosclerosis (122). Typically, ACE inhibitors are initiated at much lower doses today then those doses used when captopril was first marketed, which resulted in proteinuria. Initial dosage suggestions are listed in Table 21.20. Of the ACE inhibitors listed, all are excreted renally except fosinopril and thus require dosage modification in patients with renal impairment (121, 123). In azotemic patients, careful monitoring of potassium levels is necessary to prevent life-threatening hyperkalemia associated with ACE inhibitors.

Calcium antagonists may have both afferent and efferent vasodilatory effects on the renal vasculature, resulting in decreased glomerular pressure and slowing the rate of GFR decline. Following oral administration, most calcium antagonists undergo extensive hepatic first-pass metabolism. Some of these metabolites are active, and the effect of renal impairment on their elimination is unknown. Therefore, while initial dosage adjustments in renal failure patients may be unnecessary, slow titration of maintenance doses should always be considered.

Table 21.20.

Initial Dosage Recommendations of Angiotensin-Converting Enzyme Inhibitors in Renal Insufficiency

Drug	C_{cr} (30–60 mL/min)	C_{cr} (10–30 mL/min)	C_{cr} (<10 mL/min)
Captopril	12.5 mg twice daily	6.25–12.5 mg twice daily	6.25–12.5 mg once daily
Benazepril	5–10 mg once daily	5 mg once daily	?
Enalapril	5 mg once daily	2.5 mg once daily	1.25 mg once daily
Fosinopril	10 mg once daily	10 mg once daily	10 mg once daily
Lisinopril	10 mg once daily	5 mg once daily	2.5 mg once daily
Quinapril	5 mg once daily	2.5 mg once daily	?
Ramipril	1.25–2.5 mg once daily	1.25 mg once daily	?

C_{cr}, creatinine clearance
Adapted from Carter BL. Dosing of antihypertensive medications in patients with renal insufficiency. J Clin Pharmacol 35:81–6, 1995; Hoelscher DD, Weir MR, Bakris GL. Hypertension in diabetic patients: an update of interventional studies to preserve renal function. J Clin Pharmacol 35:73–80, 1995; and Olin B. Cardiovascular agents. In: Drug Facts and Comparisons. St. Louis, MO: Facts and Comparisons, Inc., 1995: 135d–166.

The centrally acting agents, methyldopa and clonidine, are both useful in reducing blood pressure in patients with chronic renal failure. Because methyldopa and its active metabolite accumulate with decreased renal function, dosing adjustments are necessary. Clonidine requires dosing adjustments at creatinine clearances below 50 mL/min.

The peripheral vasodilators, hydralazine and minoxidil, are not used alone in the hypertension of renal failure because of compensatory mechanisms causing increased renin release, sodium retention, and tachycardia, which occur as a result of decreased peripheral vascular resistance. However, in combination with agents that decrease volume and renin, they are effective in the management of uncontrolled hypertension. These agents do not require dosing modifications in renal failure because of their high hepatic clearance.

The α-adrenergic blockers prazosin, terazosin, and doxazosin reduce blood pressure by producing venous and arterial vasodilation. They are useful in treating patients with renal failure and do not require dosing modifications with decreased creatinine clearance.

GASTROINTESTINAL DISORDERS

Patients with advanced renal failure commonly have gastrointestinal complications such as anorexia, nausea, and vomiting. They complain frequently of a metallic or salty taste, and their breath smells of ammonia. They may develop stomatitis, parotitis, erosive gastritis, uremic colitis, and mucosal and submucosal ulcerations. Uremic patients have in their salivary secretions high concentrations of urea, which undergoes conversion to ammonia in the presence of bacterial ureases. Many symptoms are due to the irritative effects of ammonia on the gastrointestinal tract.

Frequently, antacids are administered to patients with gastrointestinal irritation. When the creatinine clearance falls to below 30 mL/min, magnesium-containing antacids should be restricted. If magnesium-containing antacids are given in chronic renal failure, serum magnesium levels may rise above 6 mEq/L, causing depression of the central nervous system, lethargy, somnolence, and loss of deep tendon reflexes. Dialysis removes magnesium effectively and may be indicated if severe toxicity develops.

HYPERURICEMIA (See also Chapter 32, "Gout and Hyperuricemia")

Uric acid is the end product of purine metabolism. It circulates primarily as urate, is filtered at the glomerulus, and is almost completely reabsorbed in the proximal tubules. Elevated serum uric acid levels may occur when creatinine clearance falls below 30 mL/min and renal excretion of uric acid is impaired. Potential complications from hyperuricemia are gouty attacks, uric acid kidney stones, and urate nephropathy. For unknown reasons, chronic renal failure patients rarely develop gout unless there is a previous history of underlying gout. The association between hyperuricemia and progression of renal disease is also unclear.

Nephrotic Syndrome

Nephrotic syndrome is the metabolic and clinical consequence of continued heavy proteinuria, usually greater than 3.5 g of protein per day. In addition to proteinuria, this syndrome is characterized by hypoalbuminemia, edema, hyperlipidemia, and hypercoagulability. A large number of glomerular lesions can be associated with nephrotic syndrome. Factors causing glomerulonephropathies that result in nephrotic syndrome include systemic, metabolic, and endocrine diseases, allergens, microorganisms, drugs, and toxins (Table 21.6).

Increased glomerular permeability to plasma protein leads to each of the clinical and metabolic derangements associated with nephrotic syndrome. Hypoalbuminemia is the direct result of albumin loss in the urine, which accounts for 60 to 90% of urinary protein. Loss of larger molecular weight proteins including immunoglobulins is associated with abnormalities in immune response and increased susceptibility to serious infections. Enhanced hepatic synthesis of lipoproteins appears to result from hypoalbuminemia and a reduction in colloid oncotic pressure. The associated hyperlipidemia may cause an increased risk of ischemic heart disease. Edema is due to sodium retention by the kidney and a reduction in intravascular colloid oncotic pressure. Edema seen with nephrotic syndrome is marked by a distribution pattern that includes the face and periorbital region, particularly in the morning. Edema of the lower extremities can be seen as the day progresses. Numerous defects in clotting factors, the fibrinolytic system, and platelet function are responsible for the hypercoagulable state. Low levels of antithrombin III seem to correlate with the clotting defects.

Treatment is aimed at reducing risk factors and symptoms associated with nephrotic syndrome. In the past, high-protein diets were recommended to compensate for urinary protein losses, but this therapy led to increased glomerular permeability. Currently, a dietary protein intake of about 1 g/kg/day is recommended. Edema calls for dietary sodium restriction to about 2 grams per day. Nonsteroidal antiinflammatory agents (indomethacin 150 mg/day) and ACE inhibitors have been shown to reduce proteinuria and reduce the tendency for edema formation. Hyperlipidemia is treated with dietary control of saturated fat and cholesterol intake. Lipid-lowering agents may be used if LDL-cholesterol levels remain elevated. Efforts should also be directed toward reducing other atherosclerotic risk factors such as smoking and hypertension, and by adding a mild exercise program. Treatment of the hypercoagulable state is directed at prevention of embolic events and avoidance of prolonged immobilization. Prophylactic anticoagulation may be necessary with unavoidable immobilization or in patients with a previous history of thromboembolism (124, 125).

Because of the large variety of glomerular diseases associated with nephrotic syndrome, histologic evaluation is often necessary to determine the specific lesion. Treatment depends on the histologic findings or the presence of signs or symptoms suggestive of a systemic disease. Idiopathic nephrotic syndrome, that arising from an unknown cause, is usually treated with steroids. Steroid therapy with oral prednisone 60 mg/m^2/day in divided doses for 4 to 8 weeks is used to achieve remission, particularly in children. Steroids are then used primarily to minimize the frequency and complications of relapse. Short courses of intermittent steroid therapy, 40 mg/m^2 in a single dose on alternate days for 4 weeks have been used to prevent relapse and minimize steroid toxicity. Cytotoxic therapy has been used in frequently relapsing patients who develop adverse effects from steroids. Cyclophosphamide and chlorambucil have been shown to induce prolonged remission. The reader is referred to disease-specific treatment protocols for other types of glomerulonephropathy (23, 126, 127).

CONCLUSION

The normal kidney is a remarkable organ that functions to maintain the internal environment of the body through regulation of body fluid volume, electrolyte composition, acid-base balance, and production of hormones and enzymes. Although it is highly vulnerable to a variety of toxins, the kidney has the unique ability to regenerate new tubular cells and often recover from the iatrogenic misadventures it encounters. On the other hand, the number of patients being treated for ESRD is rapidly increasing and extensive research efforts are directed toward slowing the progressive deterioration in renal function. Aggressive management of underlying disease processes, including tight control of blood pressure and hyperglycemia can slow or halt progression of renal failure. The goals of successful management are to remove underlying causes, prevent associated complications, provide symptomatic care, and normalize the internal environment through dietary restriction, drugs, and dialysis.

REFERENCES

1. Conger JD, Briner VA, Schrier RW. Acute renal failure: pathogenesis, diagnosis and management. In: Schrier RW, ed. Renal and Electrolyte Disorders, 4th ed. Boston, Little, Brown, 1992: 495–537.
2. Excerpts from the United States Renal Data System. 1994 Annual Data Report. Am J Kidney Dis 24(suppl 2):S1–S181, 1994.
3. Brezis M, Rosen S, Epstein FH. Acute renal failure. In: Brenner BM, Rector FC, eds. The Kidney, 4th ed. Philadelphia, WB Saunders, 1991: 993–1061.

4. Matzke GR, Millikin SP. Influence of renal function and dialysis on drug disposition. In: Evans WE, Schentag JJ, Jusko WJ, eds. Applied Pharmacokinetics: Principles of Therapeutic Drug Monitoring, 3rd ed. Vancouver, WA, Applied Therapeutics, Inc., 1992: 8-1–8-49.
5. Chow MS, Schweizer R. Estimation of renal creatinine clearance in patients with unstable serum creatinine concentrations: comparison of multiple methods. Drug Intell Clin Pharm 19:385–90, 1985.
6. Alleyne GA, Millward DJ, Scullard GH. Total body potassium, muscle electrolytes, and glycogen in malnourished children. J Pediatr 76:75–81, 1970.
7. Bjornsson TD. Use of serum creatinine concentrations to determine renal function. In: Gibaldi M, Prescott L, eds. Handbook of Clinical Pharmacokinetics, New York, ADIS Press, 1983: 277–300.
8. Walser M, Drew HH, LaFrance ND. Creatinine measurements often yield false estimates of progression in chronic renal failure. Kidney Int 34:412–18, 1988.
9. Mitch WE, Collier VU, Walser M. Creatinine metabolism in chronic renal failure. Clin Sci 58:327, 1980.
10. Cockroft DW, Gault MH. Prediction of creatinine clearance from serum creatinine. Nephron 16:31–41, 1976.
11. Goldberg TH, Finklestein MS. Difficulties in estimating glomerular filtration rate in the elderly. Arch Intern Med 147:461–3, 1987.
12. Hatton J, Parr MD, Blouin RA. Estimation of creatinine clearance in patients with Cushing syndrome. Ann Pharmacother 23:974–7, 1989.
13. Hull JH, Hak LJ, Koch GG, et al. Influence of range of renal function and liver disease on predictability of creatinine clearance. Clin Pharmacol Ther 29:516–21, 1981.
14. Jacobson FL, Christensen CK, Morgensen CE, et al. Pronounced increase in serum creatinine concentration after eating cooked meat. Br Med J 21:1049–50, 1979.
15. Siest G, Galteau MM. Drug Effects on Laboratory Test Results. Analytical Interferences and Pharmacological Effects. St. Louis, Year Book Medical Publishers, 1988.
16. Ross DL, Neely AE. Textbook of Urinalysis and Body Fluids. Norwalk, CT, Appleton-Century-Crofts, 1983: 68–122.
17. Kark RM, Lawrence JR, Pollak VE, et al. A Primer of Urinalysis, 2nd ed. New York, Harper & Row, 1963.
18. Young DS. Effects of Drugs on Clinical Laboratory Tests, 3rd ed. Washington D.C., The American Association of Clinical Chemistry, 1990.
19. Neu HC. A symposium on the tetracyclines: a major appraisal. Bull NY Acad Med 54:141–155, 1978.
20. Friedman RB, Young DS. Effects of Disease on Clinical Laboratory Tests, 2nd ed. Washington D.C., The American Association of Clinical Chemistry, 1990.
21. Miller TR, Anderson RJ, Linas SL, et al. Urinary diagnostic indices in acute renal failure: a prospective study. Ann Intern Med 89:47–51, 1978.
22. Mann HJ, Fuhs DW, Hemstrom CA. Acute renal failure. Drug Intell Clin Pharm 20:421–38, 1986.
23. Kaysen GA. Proteinuria and the nephrotic syndrome. In: Schrier RW, ed. Renal and Electrolyte Disorders, 4th ed. Boston, Little, Brown, 1992: 681–726.
24. Hou SH, Bushinsky DA, Wish JB, et al. Hospital-acquired renal insufficiency: a prospective study. Am J Med 74:243–8, 1983.
25. National Kidney and Urologic Diseases Advisory Board 1990 Long Range Plan. NIH publication No. 90–583, 1990:47–8.
26. Finn WF. Recovery from acute renal failure. In: Brenner BM, Lazarus JM, eds. Acute Renal Failure, 2nd ed. New York, Churchill Livingstone Inc., 1988:875–918.
27. Brezis M, Rosen S, Epstein FH. Acute renal failure. In: Brenner BM, Rector FC, eds. The Kidney, 4th ed. Philadelphia, WB Saunders, 1991:993–1061.

28. Valtin H. Renal Dysfunction: Mechanisms Involved in Fluid and Solute Imbalance. Boston, Little, Brown, 1979:227.

29. Anderson RJ, Linas SL, Barns AS, et al. Nonoliguric acute renal failure. N Engl J Med 296:1134–8, 1977.

30. Anto HR, Chou SY, Porush JG, et al. Infusion of intravenous pyelography and renal function. Effects of hypertonic mannitol in patients with chronic renal insufficiency. Arch Intern Med 141: 1652–6, 1981.

31. Harter HR, Martin KJ. Acute renal failure: classification, evaluation, and clinical consequences. Postgrad Med 72:243–8, 1982.

32. Bullock ML, Umen AJ, Finkelstein M, et al. The assessment of risk factors in 462 patients with acute renal failure. Am J Kidney Dis 5:97–103, 1985.

33. Conger JD, Schrier RW. Renal hemodynamics in acute renal failure. Annu Rev Physiol 42:603–14, 1980.

34. Galler M, Folkert VW, Schlondorff D. Reversible acute renal insufficiency and hyperkalemia following indomethacin therapy. JAMA 246:154–5, 1981.

35. Grunfeld JP, Ganeval D, Bournerias F. Acute renal failure in pregnancy. Kidney Int 18:179–91, 1980.

36. Auguste LJ, Stone AM, Wise L. The effects of *Escherichia coli* bacteremia on in vitro perfused kidneys. Ann Surg 192:65–8, 1980.

37. Trifillis AL, Kahng MW, Trump BF. Metabolic studies of glycerol-induced acute renal failure in the rat. Exp Mol Pathol 35:1–13, 1981.

38. Weinberg JM. The cell biology of ischemic renal injury. Kidney Int 39:476–500, 1991.

39. Siegel N, Avison MJ, Reilly HF, et al. Enhanced recovery of renal ATP with postischemic infusion of ATP-MgCl$_2$ determined by ^{31}P-NMR. Am J Physiol 245:F530–4, 1983.

40. Shanley PF, Brezis M, Spokes K, et al. Transport-dependent cell injury in the S3 segment of the proximal tubule. Kidney, Int 29:1033–7, 1986.

41. Brezis M, Shina A, Kidroni G, et al. Calcium and hypoxic injury in the renal medulla of the perfused rat kidney. Kidney Int 34:186–94, 1988.

42. Paller MS, Hoidal JR, Ferris TF. Oxygen free radicals in ischemic acute renal failure in the rat. J Clin Invest 74:1156–64, 1984.

43. Hyneck ML. Current concepts in clinical therapeutics: drug therapy in acute renal failure. Clin Pharm 5:892–910, 1986.

44. Humes HD, Cieslinski DA, Coimbra TM, et al. Epidermal growth factor enhances renal tubule cell regeneration and repair and accelerates the recovery of renal function in postischemic acute renal failure. J Clin Invest 84:1757–61, 1989.

45. Lake EW, Humes HD. Acute renal failure: directed therapy to enhance renal tubular regeneration. Sem Nephrol 14:83–97, 1989.

46. Valdes ME, Landau SE, Shah DM, et al. Increased glomerular filtration rate following mannitol administration in man. J Surg Res 26:473–7, 1979.

47. Hara Y, May RC, Kelly RA, et al. Acidosis, not azotemia, stimulates branched-chain amino acid catabolism in uremic rats. Kidney Int 32:808–14, 1987.

48. Hak LJ. Nutrition in renal failure. In: Torosian MH, ed. Nutrition for the Hospitalized Patient: Basic Science and Principles of Practice, New York, Marcel Dekker Inc., 1995:499–503.

49. Abel RM, Beck CH, Abbott WM, et al. Improved survival from acute renal failure after treatment with intravenous L-amino acids and glucose. N Engl J Med 288:695–9, 1973.

50. Levy RH, Moreland TA. Rationale for monitoring free drug levels. Clin Pharmacokinet 9(suppl 1):1–9, 1984.

51. Benet LZ, Williams RL. Design and optimization of dosage regimens: pharmacokinetic data. In: Gilman AG, Rall TW, Nies AS, Taylor P, eds. The Pharmacologic Basis of Therapeutics, ed. 8. New York, Pergamon Press, 1990:1650–1735.

52. Benet LZ, Massoud N. Pharmacokinetics. In: Benet LZ, Massoud N, Gambertoglio JG, eds. Pharmacokinetic Basis for Drug Treatment. New York, Raven Press, 1984: 1–28.

53. Levinsky NG, Bernard DB, Johnston PA. Enhancement of recovery of acute renal failure: effects of mannitol and diuretics. In: Brenner BM, Stein JH, eds. Contemporary Issues in Nephrology, New York, Churchill Livingstone, 1980: 163–179.

54. Eliahou HE, Bata A. The diagnosis of acute renal failure. Nephron 2:287–295, 1965.

55. Luke RG, Briggs JD, Allison MI, et al. Factors determining response to mannitol in acute renal failure. Am J Med Sci 259:166–174, 1970.

56. Kjellstrand CM. Ethacrynic acid in acute tubular necrosis. Nephron 9:337–340, 1972.

57. Rudnick MR, Bastl CP, Elfinbein IB, et al. The differential diagnosis of acute renal failure. In: Brenner BM, Lazarus JM, eds. Acute Renal Failure, 2nd ed. New York, Churchill Livingstone Inc., 1988: 177–232.

58. Tiller DJ, Mudge GH. Pharmacologic agents used in the management of acute renal failure. Kidney Int 18:700–11, 1980.

59. Lordon RE, Burton JR. Posttraumatic renal failure in military personnel in southeast Asia. Am J Med 53:137–42, 1972.

60. Duggin GG. Mechanisms in the development of analgesic nephropathy. Kidney Int 18:553–61, 1980.

61. Myers BD, Moran SM. Hemodynamically mediated acute renal failure. N Engl J Med 314:97–105, 1986.

62. Stein JH, Fried TA. Experimental models of nephrotoxic acute renal failure. Transplant Proc 17:72–80, 1985.

63. Solez K, Racusen LC, Olsen S. The pathology of drug nephrotoxicity. J Clin Pharmacol 23:484–90, 1983.

64. Rasmussen HH, Ibels LS. Acute renal failure: multivariate analysis of causes and risk factors. Am J Med 73:211–8, 1982.

65. Antonovych TT. Drug-induced nephropathies. In: Sommers SC, Rosen PP, eds. Pathol Annu 19(part 2):165–96, 1984.

66. Laberke HG. Drug-associated nephropathy part II: tubulointerstitial lesions. In: Berry CL, et al. Current Topics in Pathology. New York, Springer-Verlag, 1980: 183–215.

67. Revert L, Montoliu J. Acute interstitial nephritis. Semin Nephrol 8:82–8, 1988.

68. Bennett WM, Elzinga LW, Porter GA. Tubulointerstitial disease and toxic nephropathy. In: Brenner BM, Rector FC, eds. The Kidney, 4th ed. Philadelphia, WB Saunders, 1991: 1430–96.

69. Matzke GR, Lucarotti RL, Shapiro HS. Controlled comparison of gentamicin and tobramycin nephrotoxicity. Am J Nephrol 3:11–7, 1983.

70. Sawyers CL, Moore RD, Lerner SA, et al. A model for predicting nephrotoxicity in patients treated with aminoglycosides. J Infect Dis 153:1062–8, 1986.

71. Williams PJ, Hull JH, Sarubbi FA, et al. Factors associated with nephrotoxicity and clinical outcome in patients receiving amikacin. J Clin Pharmacol 26:79–86, 1986.

72. Johnson MW, Mitch WE, Heller AH, et al. The impact of an educational program on gentamicin use in a teaching hospital. Am J Med 73:9–14, 1982.

73. Garrison MW, Rotschafer JC. Clinical assessment of a published model to predict aminoglycoside-induced nephrotoxicity. Ther Drug Monit 11:171–5, 1989.

74. Contreras AM, Gamba G, Cortes J, et al. Serial trough and peak amikacin levels in plasma as predictors of nephrotoxicity. Antimicrob Agents Chemother 33:973–6, 1989.

75. Heidemann HT, Gerkens JF, Spickard WA, et al. Amphotericin B nephrotoxicity in humans decreased by salt repletion. Am J Med 75:476–81, 1983.

76. Sacks P, Fellner SK. Recurrent reversible acute renal failure from amphotericin. Arch Intern Med 147:593–5, 1987.

77. Kahan BD. Clinical summation. An algorithm for the management of patients with cyclosporine-induced renal dysfunction. Transplant Proc 17:303–8, 1985.

78. Neild GH, Taube HE, Hartley RB, et al. Morphological differentiation between rejection and cyclosporin nephrotoxicity in renal allografts. J Clin Pathol 39:152–9, 1986.

79. Luke J, Luke DR, Williams LA, et al. Prevention of cyclosporine-induced nephrotoxicity with transdermal clonidine. Clin Pharm 9:49–53, 1990.

80. Smeesters C, Chaland P, Giroux L, et al. Prevention of acute cyclosporine A nephrotoxicity by a thromboxane synthetase inhibitor. Transplant Proc 20(suppl 2):663–9, 1988.

81. Luke RG, Greifer I. Posttransplant risks of cyclosporine: nephrotoxicity. Am J Kidney Dis 5:342–3, 1985.

82. Whiting PH, Simpson JG. The enhancement of cyclosporine A included nephrotoxicity by gentamicin. Biochem Pharmacol 32:2025–8, 1983.

83. Burckart GJ, Canafax DM, Yee GC. Cyclosporine monitoring. Drug Intell Clin Pharm 20:649–52, 1986.

84. Mission RT, Cutler RE. Radiocontrast-induced renal failure. West J Med 142:657–64, 1985.

85. Dawson P. Contrast agent nephrotoxicity. An appraisal. Br J Radiol 58:121–4, 1985.

86. Parfrey PS, Griffiths SM, Barrett BJ, et al. Contrast material-induced renal failure in patients with diabetes mellitus, renal insufficiency, or both. N Engl J Med 320:143–9, 1989.

87. Textor SC, Gephardt GN, Bravo EL, et al. Membranous glomerulopathy associated with captopril therapy. Am J Med 74:705–11, 1983.

88. Peirpont GL, Francis GS, Cohn JN. Effect of captopril on renal function in patients with congestive heart failure. Br Heart J 46:522–27, 1981.

89. Packer M. Identification of risk factors predisposing to the development of functional renal insufficiency during treatment with converting-enzyme inhibitors in chronic heart failure. Cardiology 76(suppl 1):50–5, 1989.

90. Knapp M, Avioli LV. Analgesic nephropathy. Arch Intern Med 142:1197–9, 1982.

91. Schreiner GE, McAnally JF, Winchester JF. Clinical analgesic nephropathy. Arch Intern Med 141:349–57, 1981.

92. Nanra RS. Renal effects of antipyretic analgesics. Am J Med 75(suppl):70–81, 1983.

93. Goldberg M. Analgesic nephropathy historical and epidemiological overview. In: Bertani T, ed. Drugs and Kidney. New York, Raven Press, 1986: 193–201.

94. Perneger TV, Whelton PK, Klag MJ. Risk of kidney failure associated with the use of acetaminophen, aspirin, and nonsteroidal antiinflammatory drugs. N Engl J Med 331:1675–9, 1994.

95. Litterst CL. Alterations in the toxicity of cis-dichlorodiamine-platinum-II and in tissue localization of platinum as a function of NaCl concentration in the vehicle of administration. Toxicol Appl Pharmacol 61:99–108, 1981.

96. Finley RS, Fortner CL, Grove WR. Cisplatin nephrotoxicity: a summary of preventative interventions. Drug Intell Clin Pharm 19:362–7, 1985.

97. Alfrey AC, Chan L. Chronic renal failure: manifestations and pathogenesis. In: Schrier RW, ed. Renal and Electrolyte Disorders, 4th ed. Boston, Little, Brown, 1992:539–79.

98. Levey AS, Madaio MP, Perrone RD. Laboratory assessment of renal disease: clearance, urinalysis, and renal biopsy. In: Brenner BM, Rector FC, eds. The Kidney, 4th ed. Philadelphia, WB Saunders, 1991: 919–68.

99. Tsochope W, Ritz E. The management of renal insufficiency. In: Suki WN, Massry SG, eds. Therapy of Renal Diseases and Related Disorders. Boston, Martinus Nijhoff, 1984: 495–504.

100. Brenner BM, Meyer TW, Hostetter TH. Dietary protein intake and the progressive nature of kidney disease. N Engl J Med 307:652–9, 1982.

101. Klahr S, Levy AS, Beck GJ, et al. The effects of dietary protein restriction and blood pressure control on the progression of chronic renal disease. N Engl J Med 330:877–84, 1994.

102. Keane WF. Lipids and the kidney. Kidney Int 46:910–20, 1994.

103. Brater DC. Resistance to diuretics: mechanisms and clinical implications. Adv Nephrol 22:349–369, 1993.

104. Delmez JA, Slatopolsky E. Hyperphosphatemia: its consequences and treatment in patients with chronic renal disease. Am J Kidney Dis 19:303–17, 1992.

105. Balasa RW, Murray RL, Kondelis NP, et al. Phosphate-binding properties and electrolyte content of aluminum hydroxide antacids. Nephron 45:16–21, 1987.

106. Hsu CH, Patel SR, Young EW, et al. The biological action of calcitriol in renal failure. Kidney Int 46:605–12, 1994.

107. Janson PA, Jubelirer SJ, Weinstein MS, et al. Treatment of bleeding tendency in uremia with cryoprecipitate. N Engl J Med 303:1318–22, 1980.

108. Watson AJ, Keogh JA. 1-Deamino-8-D-arginine vasopressin on prolonged bleeding time in chronic renal failure. Nephron 32:49–52, 1982.

109. Mannucci PM, Remuzzi G, Pusiner F, et al. Deamino-8-D-arginine vasopressin shortens the bleeding time in uremia. N Engl J Med 308:8–12, 1983.

110. Vigano G, Gaspari F, Locatelli M, et al. Dose-effect and pharmacokinetics of estrogens given to correct bleeding time in uremia. Kidney Int 34:853–8, 1988.

111. Livio M, Mannucci PM, Vigano G, et al. Conjugated estrogens for the management of bleeding associated with renal failure. N Engl J Med 315:731–5, 1986.

112. Fried W. Hematological aspects of uremia. In: Nissenson AR, Fine RN, Gentile DE, eds. Clinical Dialysis, 2nd ed. Norwalk, CT, Appleton-Crofts, 1990: 391–408.

113. Paganni EP. Overview of anemia associated with chronic renal disease: primary and secondary mechanisms. Semin Nephrol 9(suppl 1):3–8, 1989.

114. Schwenk MA, Halstenson CE. Recombinant human erythropoietin. DICP, Ann Pharmacother 23:528–36, 1989.

115. Rabkin R, Simon NM, Steiner S, Calwell JA. Effect of renal disease on renal uptake and excretion of insulin in man. N Engl J Med 282:182–6, 1970.

116. Smith JD, DeFronzo RA. Endocrine dysfunction in chronic renal failure. In: Nissenson AR, Fine RN, Gentile DE, eds. Clinical Dialysis, 2nd ed. Norwalk, CT, Appleton-Crofts, 1990: 458–93.

117. Tierney WM, McDonald CJ, Luft FC. Renal disease in hypertensive adults: effect of race and type II diabetes mellitus. Am J Kidney Dis 13:485–93, 1989.

118. Rostland SG, Brown G, Kirk KA, et al. Renal insufficiency in treated essential hypertension. N Engl J Med 320:684–8, 1989.

119. Brown TE, Carter BL. Hypertension and end stage renal disease. Ann Pharmacother 28:359–66, 1994.

120. Bauer JH, Reams GP. Antihypertensive drugs. In: Brenner BM, Rector FC, eds. The Kidney, 4th ed. Philadelphia, WB Saunders Co, 1991: 2148–73.

121. Carter BL. Dosing of antihypertensive medications in patients with renal insufficiency. J Clin Pharmacol 35:81–6, 1995.

122. Hoelscher DD, Weir MR, Bakris GL. Hypertension in diabetic patients: an update of interventional studies to preserve renal function. J Clin Pharmacol 35:73–80, 1995.

123. Olin B. Cardiovascular agents. In: Drug Facts and Comparisons. St. Louis, MO: Facts and Comparisons, Inc., 1995: 135d–166.

124. Border WA, Glassock RJ. The management of nephrotic syndrome. In: Suki WN, Massry SG, eds. Therapy of Renal Diseases and Related Disorders. Boston, Martinus Nijhoff, 1984: 195–208.

125. Bernard DB, Salant DJ. Clinical approach to the patient with proteinuria and the nephrotic syndrome. In: Jacobson HR, Striker GE, Klahr S, eds. The Principles and Practice of Nephrology. Philadelphia, B.C. Decker, 1991: 250–61.

126. Sherbotle JR, Hoyer JR. Idiopathic nephrotic syndrome: minimal-change disease and focal segmental glomerulosclerosis. In: Jacobson HR, Striker GE, Klahr S, eds. The Principles and Practice of Nephrology. Philadelphia, B.C. Decker, 1991: 288–292.

127. Eknoyan G. Noninflammatory vascular diseases of the kidney. In: Suki WN, Massry SG, eds. Therapy of Renal Diseases and Related Disorders, Boston. Martinus Nijhoff, 1984: 283–8.

CHAPTER 22

DIALYSIS THERAPY

ARASB ATESHKADI

Chronic renal failure may occur as a result of extensive and prolonged insult to the glomerular or tubular structures. These damages result from exposure to toxic substances (e.g., amphotericin B, aminoglycosides, compound analgesics), intrarenal diseases (e.g., polycystic kidney disease, primary glomerulopathies), or postrenal factors (e.g., ureteral obstruction, neoplasm). Renal failure may also develop secondary to systemic diseases such as hypertension, diabetes mellitus, and certain autoimmune disorders (e.g., systemic lupus erythematosus) (1). As renal function declines, accumulation of nitrogenous wastes and other toxins leads to uremia, which literally means "urine in the blood" but is clinically defined as symptomatic renal failure (2). These uremic signs and symptoms encompass a myriad of complications affecting most major organs and systems, including the cardiovascular, pulmonary, neuromuscular, and central nervous systems (1, 3). If the patient does not receive a kidney transplant, dialysis becomes necessary to sustain life. Patients who are receiving dialysis have end-stage renal disease (ESRD).

End-stage renal disease remains a major cause of morbidity and mortality. In 1991, over 215,000 patients were treated for ESRD under the Medicare program (4), increasing at an annual rate of 8 to 9% (5). In the United States, diabetes mellitus (i.e., diabetic nephropathy) is the most common cause of ESRD, accounting for one-third of the cases, followed by hypertension (28.3%), glomerulonephritis (12.6%), cystic kidney disease (3.0%), and interstitial nephritis (3.0%). Other causes, including drug-induced nephropathies, account for 19.3% of ESRD cases (4).

THE ROLE OF DIALYSIS

The kidneys are involved not only in water and electrolyte homeostasis, but also in the production and/or metabolism of many peptide hormones, including insulin, erythropoietin, parathyroid hormone (PTH), and 1,25-dihydroxyvitamin D_3 (calcitriol). Therefore, dialysis can never completely replace normal renal function nor return the patient to a state of normal health. At best, dialysis provides waste removal that is equivalent to a glomerular filtration rate of 0.6 to 0.9 L/hr (10 to 15 mL/min) (6) without compensating for the endocrine and metabolic activities of the kidney. Dialysis is used to remove toxic metabolites, electrolytes, and large quantities of accumulated fluid in order to avoid volume overload, correct acid-base balance, and prevent congestive heart failure and pulmonary edema. The ultimate goals of dialysis are to improve health-related quality of life and to decrease morbidity and mortality (7). While dialysis therapy prolongs patient survival, morbidity and mortality rates remain high, partly because of a number of complications that are associated with the dialysis modality.

The two forms of renal replacement therapy are renal transplantation and dialysis. Dialysis therapy can be divided into two main types: that done by an extracorporeal machine (i.e., hemodialysis) and that done by the peritoneal cavity (i.e., peritoneal dialysis). Despite its high initial cost (8), transplantation is the treatment of choice because of its favorable patient and economic outcomes; however, the long waiting time for cadaveric organs, the presence of medically disqualifying comorbid conditions, and an overall low transplantation rate indicates that dialysis will remain, within the foreseeable future, the primary mode of renal replacement therapy (9). Of the ESRD patients who were enrolled in Medicare in 1990, 60% received in-center hemodialysis, 28% had a functioning renal transplant, and 20% were maintained on continuous ambulatory peritoneal dialysis (CAPD) or continuous cycling peritoneal dialysis (CCPD) (4). Dialysis therapy is by no means standardized. Choices of vascular access, catheters, heparin dosing, dialyzers, dialysis machines, dialysate, and base buffers may vary from one center to the other. The choice of dialysis modality varies greatly among different countries.

UREMIC TOXINS

The constellation of signs and symptoms that are associated with uremia has been attributed in part to the accumulation of compounds that are collectively labeled "uremic toxins." The search for these uremic toxins has led to the identification of over 100 compounds in the serum and has given rise to the "uremic toxin" theory of uremia (Table 22.1) (10). These toxins include well-known molecules such as hydrogen ion, inorganic phosphorus, potassium, and several small (300 to 500 daltons) and middle-molecular-weight (1500 to 5000 daltons) substances. Nearly all potential uremic toxins are products of protein metabolism (11). Unfortunately, however, a cause-and-effect relationship between these compounds and the clinical manifestations of uremia has not been clearly established (1). Nonetheless, throughout the history of renal replacement therapy, attempts have been made to base the dialysis prescription on the removal of these uremic toxins.

The ideal marker of uremia, and hence the dose of dialysis, has the following characteristics: (a) it is accumulated in renal failure; (b) it is removed by dialysis; (c) it has proven toxicity; (d) it has production and elimination representative of other potential toxins; (e) it has a concentration-dependent clinical outcome; and (f) it is easily measured in blood, urine, and dialysate (10). Not surprisingly, no marker meets all these criteria. Given the lack of an ideal uremic marker, a combination of several markers together with clinical signs and symptoms is used in monitoring patients on dialysis.

Urea

Urea is a product of protein metabolism and is minimally toxic. In addition, urea is present in high concentrations

Table 22.1.
Potential Uremic Toxins

β_2-Microglobulin
Alkaloids
Amines
Amino acids
Ammonia
Atrial natriuretic factor
Benzoates
Calcium
Catecholamines
Cyanides
Cyclic AMP
Endorphins
Furanpropionic acid
Gastrin
Glucagon
Glucuronate
Glycols
Growth hormone
Guanidines
Hippurates
Hydrogen ion
Hypoxanthine
Indoles
Lysozyme
Mannitol
Middle molecules
Myoinositol
Oxalate
Parathyroid hormone
Phenolic acids
Phenols
Phosphorus
Polypeptides
Potassium
Prolactin
Pseudouridine
Sodium
Urea
Uric acid

Source: Adapted with permission from (10).

and is inexpensive and easy to measure. To date, urea is the only solute for which concentration has been correlated with outcome (12). Factors that affect blood urea concentrations include protein intake, protein catabolism, protein elimination (e.g., loss in dialysate), and liver function. Although urea removal by dialysis has been used as a marker for other small solutes (12, 13), its blood concentrations do not accurately predict patients' uremic status. While blood urea concentrations cannot be ignored, they must be interpreted in conjunction with the patient's protein intake. A patient with a low blood urea concentration may be severely undernourished and underdialyzed (i.e., receiving an inadequate dose of dialysis) (14). Nevertheless, since small solute removal is considered an important aspect of prescribing therapy (15), urea may be viewed in dual roles, both as a marker of protein intake and as a surrogate marker for small-solute uremic toxins (13).

Middle Molecules

Middle molecules are a heterogenous group of unrelated compounds that may interfere with peripheral nerve function and appetite (10, 16). In assessing the in vitro clearance of dialyzers, vitamin B_{12} (molecular weight: 1353 daltons) is used as a marker of middle molecular clearance (Table 22.2) (10). Although perhaps not as important as small solutes (15), middle molecules are important in the development of dialysis-related complications, such as arthropathy and malnutrition.

Hippuric Acid

Hippuric acid (molecular weight: 179 daltons) is a protein-bound compound that exerts several toxic metabolic effects. It may be a marker of other toxic organic-acid-like compounds that are excreted by renal tubules (10).

β_2-Microglobulin

β_2-Microglobulin is a globular protein with a molecular weight of 11,800 daltons. As a component of the human Class I major histocompatibility complex, β_2-microglobulin is present on numerous cell types and is continuously shed from these cell membranes. Approximately 95% of circulating β_2-microglobulin is eliminated via glomerular filtration followed by tubular reabsorption and intratubular degradation; the other 5% is metabolized by unknown extrarenal sites (17). Therefore, compared to subjects with normal renal function, patients with renal impairment have significantly higher serum concentrations of β_2-microglobulin. Recently, β_2-microglobulin has been identified as an important modulator in arthropathies that are associated with long-term dialysis treatment (18). Elimination of β_2-microglobulin is increased with the use of larger-pore (high-flux) dialysis membranes. The high-flux dialyzers have pore sizes that allow the passage of compounds with molecular weights greater than 15,000 daltons, which closely resembles the native glomerular pores (6).

Table 22.2.
Characteristics of Frequently Used Dialysis Filters

Manufacturer and Model	Membrane	Surface area (m^2)	Ultrafiltration coefficient (mL/hr/mm Hg)	Clearance (Q_B = 12 L/hr or 200 mL/min)	
				Urea	Vitamin B_{12}
Hollow fiber					
Asahi					
Pan 200	PAN	1.4	44	170	103
PAN 250	PAN	1.8	54	174	115
Baxter					
CF 15	CU	0.9	4.1	168	41
CF 23	CU	1.25	5.2	176	55
CA 50	CA	0.5	2.4	128	26
CA 90	CA	0.9	4.3	169	42
CT 110G	CTA	1.1	22	185	109
CT 190G	CTA	1.9	36	192	137
Fresenius					
Hemoflow F 40	PS	0.7	20	165	75
Hemoflow F 60	PS	1.25	40	185	118
Toray					
BK-1.0U	PMMA	1.0	9	169	85
BK-2.1P	PMMA	2.1	19	194	125
Parallel-plate (flat plate)					
Gambro					
Lundia IC-3H	CU	0.8	5.2	159	43
Lundia IC-6N	CU	1.6	9	182	63
Hospal					
1800-S	AN69	0.7	30	145	55
3000-S	AN69	1.2	50	180	80

Abbreviations: CA = cellulose acetate; CTA = cellulose triacetate; CU = cuprophan; PAN and AN69 = polyacrylonitrile; PMMA = polymethylmethacrylate; PS = polysulfone; Q_B = blood flow rate

PRINCIPLES OF DIALYSIS

Despite continuous modifications in the biotechnology of dialysis, the basic principles of hemodialysis and peritoneal dialysis have remained unchanged since the introduction of these modes of therapy over 50 years ago. The three basic components of a hemodialysis system are a blood compartment, a dialysate compartment, and a semipermeable membrane that separates the blood and dialysate compartments. Fundamentally, hemodialysis consists of the perfusion of heparinized blood and physiologic salt solution (i.e., dialysate) on opposite sides of a semipermeable membrane. The waste products of protein metabolism and other toxins move from the blood compartment into the dialysate by passive diffusion along concentration gradients (19) (Fig. 22.1). Conversely, if a substance is in the dialysate in a higher concentration than that in the blood (e.g., bicarbonate), this solute will diffuse from the dialysate into the systemic circulation.

The second process that occurs during dialysis is ultrafiltration, which is the movement down the hydrostatic pressure gradient of water and nonprotein plasma components from the blood into the dialysate. This is the primary mode for removal of excess body fluids. Ultrafiltration (expressed as mL/hr/mm Hg) can be maximized by increasing the hydrostatic pressure gradient (mm Hg) across the dialysis membrane. The amount of fluid that will be removed during a dialysis session depends on the ultrafiltration coefficient of the dialysis filter (Table 22.2). Through trial and error a postdialysis target weight is determined for every patient, such that 0 to 5 kg will typically be removed during each dialysis session. If a patient requires a large amount of fluid removal during each dialysis session, a dialysis filter with larger ultrafiltration coefficient is most appropriate.

Total separation of diffusion and ultrafiltration does not occur in standard hemodialysis procedures. However, for selected patients these two processes may be performed in sequence, rather than simultaneously. This form of "sequential" hemodialysis therapy is particularly beneficial for patients who have fluid overload between dialysis periods as well as for patients with poor cardiac function who are unable to tolerate simultaneous, extensive ultrafiltration (20). With sequential dialysis, some patients may tolerate removal of as much as 4 L/hr of fluid. The primary problem of long-term sequential dialysis treatment is that the reduced diffusion time may not allow adequate removal of uremic waste products.

The three principles of dialysis also apply to peritoneal dialysis. As with hemodialysis, dialysis across the peritoneal membrane consists of diffusion and ultrafiltration (21). Diffusion occurs from the blood to the dialysate or from the dialysate to the blood, depending on the concentration gradient for the particular substance (Fig. 22.2). The degree of diffusion is critically influenced by (a) the thickness of the peritoneal membrane, (b) the effective surface area of the membrane that is exposed to the dialysate, (c) the peritoneal capillary blood flow, (d) the dialysate flow rate, (e) the volume of instilled dialysate, and (f) the temperature of the dialysate (21, 22).

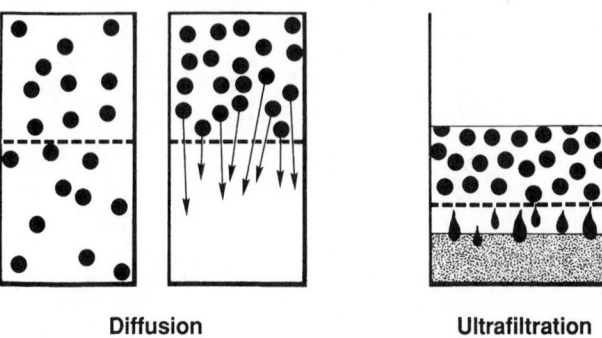

Diffusion   **Ultrafiltration**

Figure 22.1. Diffusion of endogenous solutes from the blood to the dialysate (left panel) is limited by the pore size of the membrane (shown as a dashed line), the molecular size of the solute, and the time that the dialysate fluid is in contact with the blood. Ultrafiltration (right panel) is the removal of plasma water with or without the accompaniment of solute. The limiting processes for water removal are the amount of pressure the membrane can tolerate without rupturing and the pressure difference that is created across the membrane.

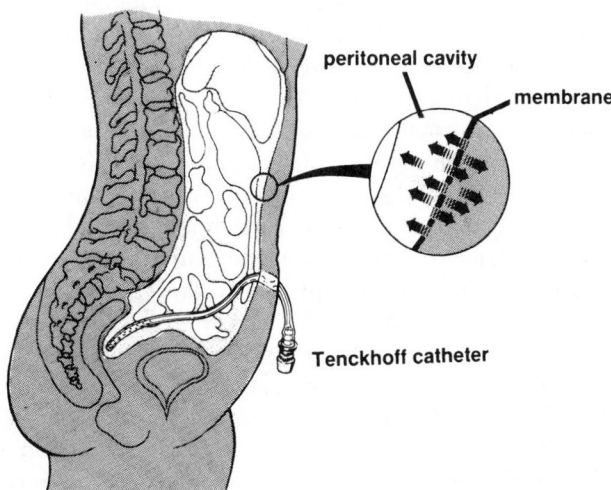

Figure 22.2. Diffusion and ultrafiltration occur across the peritoneal membrane and are depicted in the expanded insert. These processes are bidirectional; that is, solutes and water can be absorbed from the peritoneal cavity or drawn into the cavity. The rate-limiting process is the concentration of a particular solute and dextrose in the dialysis fluid.

Unlike hemodialysis, in which the membrane that separates the blood from the dialysate compartment can be selected to obtain the optimal diffusion and ultrafiltration, with peritoneal dialysis only one membrane is available per patient. Ultrafiltration during peritoneal dialysis can be accomplished by changing the dextrose concentration in the dialysate. An increase in dextrose concentration increases the osmolality of the peritoneal compartment, resulting in increased fluid removal.

INDICATIONS FOR DIALYSIS

Indications for dialysis may be classified as absolute (established), relative, or early (Table 22.3) (5, 6). Certain uremic complications, such as pericarditis, uremic encephalopathy, and intractable pulmonary edema, require immediate dialysis to sustain life. Other conditions that do not require urgent treatment create the dilemma as to when to initiate dialysis. This is an important decision, since a delay in starting renal replacement therapy is associated with increased morbidity and mortality (10). Therefore, it is best not to wait for manifestation of absolute indications but to initiate therapy on the basis of early or relative indications (5). Unfortunately, since patients may have anxieties about starting dialysis, they tend to tolerate and adjust to their increasing incapacitation. With decreasing appetite, patients also spontaneously restrict their protein intake; therefore, their blood urea nitrogen (BUN) level may not reflect the degree of uremia (23). Furthermore, treatment of anemia with erythropoietin may produce a sense of well-being that can mask some of the uremic signs and symptoms. Conversely, centrally acting antihypertensive agents (e.g., clonidine, a-methyldopa) may cause drowsiness and depression, thus mimicking uremic symptoms (6). Given these caveats, for many patients, dialysis is initiated after a 10% weight loss or when mild encephalopathy develops (6).

Numerous economic and medical advantages are associated with early initiation of dialysis. These include (a) lower mortality (10, 23); (b) improved blood pressure and volume control; (c) provision for a more liberal diet, which allows for a higher protein consumption; and (d) decreased use of health care resources (9, 23). Unfortunately, only 20 to 25% of patients with chronic renal failure are referred to a nephrologist at a reasonable time before initiation of dialysis (6, 9). Referral of a patient to a multidisciplinary nephrology team should occur when the serum creatinine concentration has increased to 133 μmol/L (1.5 mg/dL) in women and 177 μmol/L (2.0 mg/dL) in men. Proper early intervention involves the predialysis management of a number of comorbid conditions related to advanced renal failure, such as anemia, hypertension, malnutrition, calcium-phosphate abnormalities, dyslipoproteinemias, and metabolic acidosis (9). It is recommended that dialysis be initiated whenever early indications of dialysis are present, especially malnutrition (Table 22.3).

Table 22.3.
Indications for Initiating Dialysis

Absolute indications
  Pericarditis
  Uremic encephalopathy or neuropathy (e.g., asterixis, seizures, foot
    drop)
  Pulmonary edema that is unresponsive to diuretics
  Hypertension that is unresponsive to treatment
  Severe bleeding diathesis due to uremia
  Persistent nausea
  Serum creatinine > 1061 µmol/L (> 12 mg/dL) and BUN > 35.7
    mM/L (> 100 mg/dL)
  Life-threatening electrolyte abnormalities (e.g., hyperkalemia)
  Severe metabolic acidosis
Relative indications
  Mild encephalopathy (e.g., daytime drowsiness, imprecise memory,
    decreased attentiveness and cognitive tasking)
    Sensorimotor peripheral neuropathy (e.g., dysesthesias, restless
    leg syndrome)
  Severe peripheral edema unresponsive to diuretics
  Anorexia with progressive nausea and vomiting
  Ascites without hepatic disease
  Recurrent gastritis, stomatitis, duodenitis, pancreatitis
  Pruritus
  Anemia refractory to erythropoietin
  Mild bleeding diathesis
  Infectious complications
  Depression
Early indications
  Decrease in ideal body weight by 10%
  Decrease in muscle mass (decreased 24-hr excretion of creatinine)
  Growth retardation in children
  Increased susceptibility to infection
  Anorexia
  Decrease in serum albumin to < 40 g/L (< 4 g/dL)
  Decrease in protein intake to < 0.8 g/kg/day in patients on unre-
    stricted diet
  GFR by iothalamate 0.9 L/hr (< 15 mL/min)
  Serum creatinine > 884 µmol/L (> 10 mg/dL) and BUN > 35.7
    mM/L (> 100 mg/dL)
  Decrease in serum transferrin?
  Decrease in serum prealbumin?
  Serum total cholesterol < 2.6–3.9 mM/L (< 100–150 mg/dL)?
  Immunologic abnormalities associated with malnutrition (e.g., im-
    paired, delayed hypersensitivity to common skin antigens such as
    mumps and *Candida*)?

Source: Adapted with permission from (5).

HEMODIALYSIS

Effective dialysis entails convective bulk fluid removal, ultrafiltration, and diffusion of toxic materials down a concentration gradient from blood to dialysate. Convection is the process by which solutes are lost during ultrafiltration. Ultrafiltration depends on (a) the difference in blood and dialysate transmembrane colloid osmotic pressure, (b) membrane permeability, and (c) blood dilution (10). The use of high dialysate and blood flow rates with high-flux (larger-pore) and high-efficiency (larger surface area) dialyzers has necessitated precise ultrafiltration control systems to avoid uncontrolled fluid loss, dehydration, and hypotension (23, 24).

Vascular Access

Dialysis access can be achieved at the bedside by insertion of a catheter into the femoral or subclavian vein. Significant complications can occur with these initial temporary access devices, including venous thrombosis, emboli, and infection (25). Permanent vascular access for hemodialysis may be accomplished by several techniques (26). The simple arteriovenous fistula has the longest survival of all blood-access devices and the lowest rate of complications. An arteriovenous fistula is formed by the anastomosis of an artery and a vein that allows access to the circulation by skin puncture. Bovine grafts and polytetrafluoroethylene grafts have also been used for chronic dialysis access, especially when fistula placement is unsuccessful or not feasible. The choice of a blood-access device depends primarily on how soon the patient will require dialysis and the adequacy of the patient's vascular system. The access placement must occur weeks to months before the initiation of hemodialysis to allow for proper healing and maturation of the fistula. During this time, a tunneled subcutaneous catheter may be used as a temporary hemodialysis access site (9).

Dialyzers

In recent years, numerous new hemodialysis filters have become available (19, 27). Two basic forms of dialyzers, the hollow fiber dialyzer and the flat plate dialyzer, now predominate (Table 22.2). Most dialysis centers use several types of dialyzers and select the optimal dialysis filter for the individual patient. For stable young patients without cardiac or bleeding problems, the dialyzer that has the highest clearance of urea and creatinine, the two primary uremic waste products, should be selected. For older patients, very small individuals, and those with multiple medical complications, greater attention to individualization is required.

More recently, the interaction of blood with the extracorporeal circuit has been viewed as a significant cause of morbidity and possibly mortality. This has led to the unofficial labeling of dialyzers as either *biocompatible* or *bioincompatible*. Biocompatible membranes have a relative lack of effect on blood constituents (e.g., monocytes, macrophages, lymphocytes, and neutrophils) and do not cause some of the systemic reactions that arise from acute and chronic exposure to dialyzers. Polysulfone, polyacrylonitrile, polymethylmethacrylate, polycarbonate, and polyamide membranes are examples of synthetic biocompatible membranes. Although most biocompatible membranes are also high-flux, such membranes may be also be standard or high-efficiency (28).

A bioincompatible membrane (e.g., cuprophan) activates the complement system, suppresses the immune system, induces cytokine release, enhances production of β_2-microglobulin, and increases the risk of morbidity and,

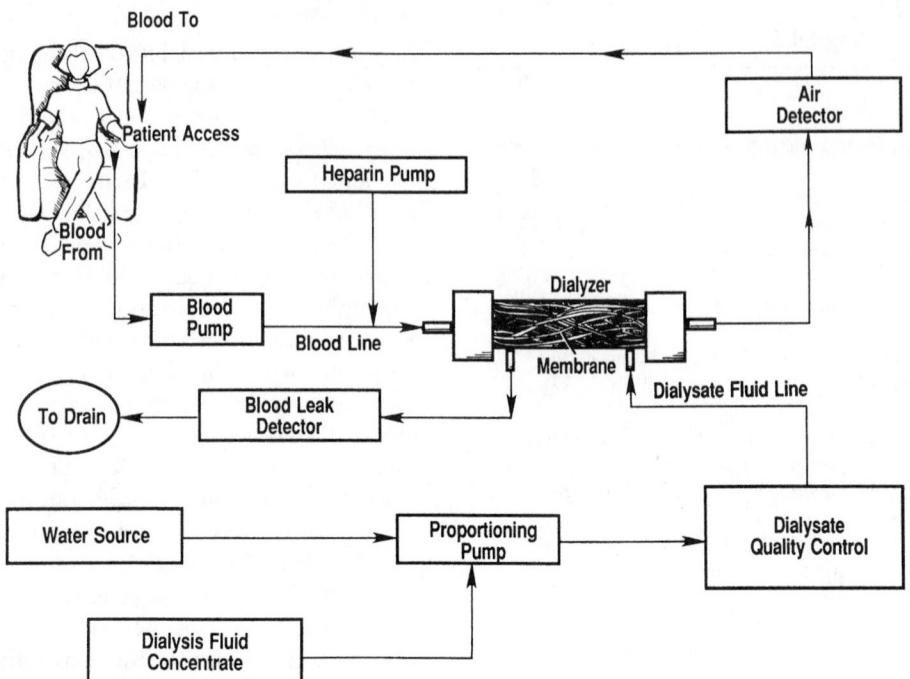

Figure 22.3. Outline of the blood flow and dialysate flow pathways during hemodialysis. Blood flows from the patient via the blood pump at a rate of 200 to 500 mL/min through the dialyzer and back to the patient. Heparin is administered into the blood line to prevent clotting in the dialyzer. The dialysate is prepared via the combination of dialysis fluid concentrate with water and then is pumped at a rate of 500 to 800 mL/min through the dialsate side of the dialyzer.

possibly, mortality (28). As a result, such membranes may increase the risk of infection and malignancy, cause intradialytic cardiovascular instability, increase protein catabolism, and potentiate musculoskeletal effects of long-term hemodialysis (28). These effects are discussed below in the appropriate sections.

Hemodialysis Technique

The process of hemodialysis consists of pumping the patient's heparinized blood through the blood compartment of the dialysis filter at a rate of 12 to 30 L/hr (200 to 500 mL/min) (average 15 L/hr or 250 mL/min) (Fig. 22.3) (19, 29). Generally, anticoagulation is achieved by infusing heparin either continuously or intermittently into the blood line of the dialyzer. The dialysate is prepared from a commercially available concentrated liquid or dried salts and treated water. This fluid is warmed to body temperature and then perfused through the dialysate compartment of the dialysis filter. Although several types of hemodialysis machines may still be available in different clinical settings, most of the current generation of dialysis machines are single-pass systems. That is, the dialysate flows through the system once and is not recycled. This process results in greater efficiency of diffusion, since there is no accumulation of endogenous solutes within the dialysate compartment.

The duration of dialysis therapy has steadily decreased since the 1970s from approximately 12 hours three times a week to 4 hours three times a week (30). Recent advances in dialysis technology, including precise volumetric control systems and dialyzers with larger pores (high flux) and larger surface areas (high efficiency), have allowed the removal of the same amount of small solutes over a shorter period than is possible with cellulosic membranes (23). With these membranes it may be possible to reduce dialysis time by approximately 30 to 40% while maintaining adequate solute and fluid removal. However, inappropriately short dialysis sessions are associated with complications (31, 32).

COMPLICATIONS OF HEMODIALYSIS

Complications of dialysis may be related to the vascular access, to the dialysis procedure itself, or specifically to chronic dialysis.

Cardiovascular Complications

Cardiovascular disease is the most common cause of mortality among the dialysis population, accounting for 50% of the deaths (9, 33). Conditions such as myocardial infarction, coronary artery disease, moderate-to-severe congestive heart failure, vascular stroke, or peripheral vascular disease are present in one-third or more of hemodialysis patients (33). The presence of cardiovascular disease at the initiation of dialysis is an independent predictor of mortality (34).

The hemodialysis procedure per se is associated with both acute (e.g., hypotension, sudden death) and chronic (e.g., left ventricular hypertrophy, heart failure, coronary artery disease) cardiovascular complications. Some of these cardiovascular complications are due to rapid ultrafiltration and the presence of an arteriovenous fistula or prosthetic graft for hemodialysis (35). The presence of a hemodialysis vascular access creates a state of high cardiac output proportional to the intradialytic blood flow rate (33).

Predisposing factors to these cardiovascular complications include hypertension, chronic anemia, hyperparathyroidism, aluminum overload, presence of an arteriovenous fistula, volume overload, high-output cardiac failure, and dyslipoproteinemias (33, 35, 36). Treatment strategies before the initiation of dialysis, such as cessation of smoking, correction of hypertension, and regular aerobic exercise may reduce the cardiovascular morbidity and mortality during dialysis (9). It is unclear whether modifications of the common dyslipoproteinemias (commonly hypertriglyceridemia) in patients with chronic renal failure and ESRD will positively affect mortality rates (37). Since myocardial calcification and fibrosis contribute to one-half of heart failure cases (especially diastolic dysfunction), control of calcium, phosphorus, vitamin D, and PTH abnormalities may help to prevent both cardiovascular and bone diseases (9).

LEFT VENTRICULAR HYPERTROPHY

The majority of hemodialysis patients have left ventricular hypertrophy, which is a risk factor for death for both nonuremic hypertensive patients and ESRD patients (35). For both types of patients, hypertension is the most important pathogenic factor in the development of left ventricular hypertrophy and the ensuing diastolic dysfunction (9). Since left ventricular hypertrophy is frequently associated with left atrial dilation, patients are at risk for development of atrial fibrillation. Indeed, left ventricular hypertrophy may be a risk factor for sudden death of hemodialysis patients (34, 35).

Commonly, left ventricular hypertrophy leads to diastolic dysfunction, which is caused by a reduced left ventricular compliance (35). In contrast, the systolic function is usually normal or high. Hemodialysis patients are often in a state of volume overload. Because of a decreased left ventricular distensibility, the left ventricular pressure will be unusually high, predisposing the patient to pulmonary congestion and edema. During the rapid intradialytic fluid removal, the left ventricular pressure is rapidly reduced, resulting in intradialytic hypotension; therefore, dialysis hypotension may signal the presence of left ventricular hypertrophy and a patient who is at risk for

sudden death (35, 36). In patients with significant vascular disease (e.g., coronary, carotid, or peripheral artery diseases) the prolonged hypotension leads to ischemic symptoms and possibly myocardial infarction and stroke (38). In the absence of atrial fibrillation, positive inotropic drugs are rarely of value. Large and rapid changes in intravascular volume should be avoided during dialysis (35). Ideally, hypertension and anemia should be treated aggressively in the predialysis stage to reduce the degree of left ventricular hypertrophy. Such treatment strategies remain important when the patient starts renal replacement therapy (9).

CORONARY ARTERY DISEASE

The coronary artery disease that is commonly present among the ESRD population can be exacerbated by the intradialytic hypotension, which increases oxygen demand, and anemia of chronic renal failure, which increases myocardial oxygen demand and decreases supply. The balance in oxygen supply and demand may also be affected by the presence of an arteriovenous fistula in hemodialysis patients. Arteriovenous fistulas with high flow rates may precipitate heart failure, even in the absence of coronary artery disease (35).

Treatment of anemia with erythropoietin can reduce the left ventricular hypertrophy (39) and reduce myocardial ischemia, although a higher target hematocrit may be necessary (>33 to 36%) (40). For patients with significant coronary artery disease, CAPD may be preferred because of (a) the absence of an arteriovenous fistula, (b) adequately maintained left ventricular end-diastolic pressure (an important factor for myocardial perfusion), and (c) absence of rapid volume shifts (35).

Infections

Before the age of renal replacement therapy, infections were a major cause of death of patients with chronic renal failure (41). In this era, infection is a major cause of morbidity and the second most common cause of mortality, accounting for 15 to 30% of all deaths among the dialysis patients (9). Dialysis patients in general are at an increased risk of infection for three main reasons: malnutrition, decreased immune function, and invasion of the skin and other integuments for the purpose of placing dialysis catheters and performing hemodialysis. Furthermore, the uremic skin is dry and atrophic and more likely to chafe. Hemodialysis with a bioincompatible membrane can adversely affect the patient's immune system and serve as an additional risk factor for infection (42). The use of biocompatible membranes is associated with as much as a 50% reduction in the incidence of infection (9).

Delayed wound healing and wound dehiscence are common following surgical incisions (41). *Staphylococcus aureus* and *S. epidermidis* are the two most frequently isolated pathogens, usually causing infection at the vascular access site, with or without associated bacteremia. Patients are also at risk for developing pneumonia and urinary tract infection, in addition to infections caused by *Mycobacterium tuberculosis,* hepatitis A, hepatitis B, and hepatitis C (41).

IMMUNE SYSTEM DYSFUNCTION

Patients with uremia manifest a number of immune function abnormalities, some of which are unaffected or even worsened by hemodialysis. These relative abnormalities are part of a multifactorial process that predisposes patients to infection (1). Although neutrophil counts may be normal or modestly elevated, hemodialysis patients have consistent neutrophil defects, including decreased chemotaxis, phagocytosis, and in vitro killing of bacteria (1, 43). This is due to a number of factors, including iron deficiency or iron overload, protein-calorie malnutrition, hyperparathyroidism, and the presence in the uremic serum of a specific granulocyte inhibitory protein (1).

T$_4$ lymphocytes, natural killer cells, monocytes, and macrophages constitute the cell-mediated arm of the immune system. Evidence of defects in cell-mediated immunity in ESRD patients comes from the following observations: (a) prolonged survival of skin allografts, (b) impairment of cutaneous delayed-type hypersensitivity to common antigens (e.g., *Candida*), (c) remission of systemic lupus erythematosus when renal function reaches end-stage, (d) increased incidence of tuberculosis, and (e) an abnormally high incidence of malignant tumors (43, 44). Humoral immunity appears for the most part to be unaffected.

Vascular Access Complications

Complications related to the vascular access (clotting and stenosis) are the leading cause of morbidity among the hemodialysis population (45) and perhaps the major factor limiting continued use of hemodialysis (9). Hemodialysis access problems are related primarily to clotting of the arteriovenous fistula, which frequently requires surgical revision (45). Infection of the access site can also complicate hemodialysis therapy (45). Because of repeated needle sticks, such infections often can lead to bacteremia and sepsis.

The nasal carriage of *S. aureus* is a risk factor for the development of infections (e.g., bacteremia) by this microorganism in hemodialysis patients. At the time of onset of hemodialysis, more than 40% of hemodialysis patients are nasal carriers of *S. aureus.* Administration of mupirocin 2% ointment (a topical antistaphylococcal agent) intranasally once per week is effective in reducing the incidence of *S. aureus* infections and is only rarely associated with the emergence of mupirocin resistance (46).

RECIRCULATION

Expressed as percent of intradialytic blood flow rate, recirculation occurs when an amount of dialyzed blood is recycled through the dialyzer inlet instead of returning to the systemic circulation. The risk and severity of recirculation increases under the following circumstances: (a) high blood flow rates; (b) vascular access problems; (c) stenosis at the access outflow; (d) closely situated, or common, vascular inlet and outlet pathways; (e) incorrect position of the needle in the arteriovenous fistula; and (f) use of small needle and tubing diameter (10, 24). In cases of a vascular access problem, surgical correction may become necessary. The use of high-flux dialyzers at high blood flow rates will increase the extent of recirculation and decrease the effective dialyzer clearance (23).

Intradialytic Symptoms

The exposure during dialysis of large volumes of blood to a foreign surface (i.e., dialyzer), extracorporeal circuit, and substances from manufacturing and sterilization processes is associated with a number of intradialytic symptoms, including muscle cramps, chest or back pain, hypoxemia, fever, nausea, vomiting, seizures, and cardiac arrhythmias. During rapid fluid removal, patients may experience hypotension and muscle cramps. With the advent of newer, more precise ultrafiltration systems and sodium modeling, ultrafiltration is now more precise and gradual. This has resulted in a reduction in many of the nonspecific intradialytic symptoms (23). The replacement of acetate with bicarbonate as the dialysate base buffer has led to a reduction in the incidence of nausea, vomiting, and hypotension (23). In addition, the use of bicarbonate dialysate is associated with improved survival.

DIALYZER REACTIONS

There are two types of dialyzer reactions. Type A is an anaphylactoid or allergic reaction to some component of the hemodialysis circuit that develops within the first 20 min of a dialysis session, often immediately after initiating blood flow. Signs and symptoms are similar to those of a drug-induced anaphylactic reaction and may be due to sensitization to a component of the extracorporeal circuit, such as ethylene oxide (a common sterilizing agent) (Table 22.4). Atopic patients and those receiving angiotensin-converting-enzyme (ACE) inhibitor therapy are at an increased risk of developing Type A dialyzer reactions. Treatment involves immediate discontinuation of dialysis and the institution of standard therapy for anaphylactic reactions, such as epinephrine, antihistamines, corticosteroids, and, if necessary, ventilatory support (47). Type A reactions may be avoided by a more thorough rinsing of the dialyzer and/or allowing a longer

Table 22.4.
Dialyzer Reactions

Type A Reactions	Type B Reactions
Immediate onset	Onset within 40 min
Manifestations:	Manifestations:
Abdominal cramps	Back pain
Angioedema	Chest pain
Flushing of the skin	Dyspnea (if severe)
Hypotension	Fever (low grade)
Laryngeal edema	Mild hypoxemia
Nausea and vomiting	Postdialytic fatigue
Pruritus	Role for complement
Sensation of heat	activation
Urticaria	
Role for ethylene oxide and formaldehyde	
Predisposing factors:	
ACE inhibitors	
Atopy	
Elevated total serum Ig E	
Eosinophilia	

drying period before use. Polyacrylonitrile membranes should be used with caution for patients who are taking ACE inhibitors (28).

Type B reactions occur within 20 to 40 min of initiating dialysis and primarily involve chest and back pain. Usually, symptoms subside with continued dialysis. However, in severe cases, dyspnea may develop, necessitating discontinuation of dialysis. Type B reactions may be due to intradialytic complement activation (Table 22.4) (47).

HYPOXEMIA

An intradialytic reduction in arterial pO_2 is commonly related to the dialysate buffer and the dialyzer type. With the use of an acetate buffer, CO_2 is lost into the dialysate; this results in a compensatory hypoventilation. Bronchoconstriction and increased pulmonary artery constriction may also contribute to the hypoxemia. When the urea clearance is higher than 9 L/hr (150 mL/min), acetate must be replaced with bicarbonate (24). However, the use of excess bicarbonate in the dialysate may cause an intradialytic "metabolic" alkalemia, which also results in a compensatory hypoventilation. In such cases the dialysate bicarbonate concentration must be reduced to ≤35 mM/L (mEq/L). Evidence for dialyzer-induced hypoxemia is less clear; however, the nonsubstituted cellulose membranes may play a role, especially with the use of an acetate buffer (47).

POSTDIALYTIC SYMPTOMS

Often, the patient feels weak and fatigued after a dialysis session. This is most likely due to intradialytic cytokine and complement activation, for which the concentrations are at their highest at the end of the session. Biocompatible polymer membranes (e.g., polysulfone, polyacrylonitrile, polymethylmethacrylate) have permeability and blood interactive characteristics that are different from those of cellulosic membranes. Therefore, complement and cytokine stimulation may not be as amplified with these dialyzers, and the postdialysis symptoms, if any, may be less intense (47).

DIALYSIS DISEQUILIBRIUM SYNDROME

Described since 1962, dialysis disequilibrium syndrome is one of a number of CNS abnormalities that are seen in patients with ESRD (20). It often occurs in patients who are undergoing rapid dialysis or patients who have recently started hemodialysis. Although the exact mechanism is unclear, the signs and symptoms of dialysis disequilibrium syndrome are due to the increased intracranial pressure that results from dialysis-induced cerebral edema (20). Younger patients, especially pediatric patients, and those with a previous neurologic disorder (e.g., head trauma, stroke, malignant hypertension) appear to be at a greater risk for this syndrome (20). The minor disequilibrium symptoms include headache, restlessness, dizziness, nausea, vomiting, and muscular twitching. Major signs and symptoms include disorientation, hypertension, tremors, and seizures (20, 48). The latter is of most clinical concern. Probably because of better patient management, the clinical manifestations of dialysis disequilibrium syndrome have become milder over the past 20 years.

Diagnosis of dialysis disequilibrium syndrome is one of exclusion. The symptoms are usually self-limiting, although complete recovery may take several days (20). Prevention is key to the management of dialysis disequilibrium syndrome. Patients who are started on dialysis before the appearance of uremic encephalopathy are at a lower risk. The sudden rise in intracranial pressure may be prevented by the use of slow dialysis-that is, low blood flow rates at frequent intervals-or by a combination of hemofiltration (ultrafiltration only) and conventional dialysis (i.e., sequential dialysis) (20). High-risk patients or patients who are already having convulsive activity may benefit from predialysis administration of anticonvulsants such as phenytoin. Patients with certain neurologic disorders, such as intracranial lesions (e.g., head trauma, recent stroke, brain tumor, subdural hematoma), or conditions characterized by cerebral edema (hyponatremia, hepatic encephalopathy, malignant hypertension) are at increased risk of dialysis disequilibrium syndrome and subsequent brain damage (20). Such patients should instead be started on peritoneal dialysis (48).

Treatment of dialysis disequilibrium syndrome involves the addition to the dialysate of osmotically active solutes (e.g., glucose, glycerol, albumin, NaCl, mannitol) or the use of sodium bicarbonate instead of sodium lactate or acetate

(20). Mannitol has become a widely used osmotic agent for decreasing intracranial pressure (20).

β_2-Microglobulin Amyloidosis

Patients who receive long-term hemodialysis (typically for 10 or more years) commonly suffer from a syndrome of pain and osteoarthropathy called *dialysis-related amyloidosis,* which with its crippling consequences may limit the duration of long-term dialysis therapy (18, 49). The term "amyloid" refers to substances that consist of rigid and linear aggregated fibrils but appear homogenous under light microscopy. Amyloid may be made primarily of immunoglobulins, β_2-microglobulin, or other proteins. The tissue deposition of these fibrils leads to organ damage (1). In patients with ESRD, β_2-microglobulin and its fragments are the principal components of amyloid fibrils (18). There is little doubt that certain bone and joint disorders that are observed in long-term dialysis patients are most commonly due to β_2-microglobulin amyloidosis. Dialysis-related amyloidosis may lead to the development of carpal-tunnel syndrome, destructive arthropathy of the medium-sized joints (e.g., knees, wrists, shoulders, pelvis, vertebral column), and periarticular cystic bone lesions (17, 33). The signs and symptoms of carpal-tunnel syndrome include diminished sensitivity to stimulation (hypesthesia); abnormally low sensitivity to pain (hypalgesia); tenderness, weakness, and wasting of the lateral (radial) side of the palms; and decreased motor nerve conduction velocity (17). The signs and symptoms of the arthropathy include pain, noninflammatory swelling, joint dysfunction, and pathologic fractures (23).

The risk of carpal-tunnel syndrome relates to the duration of dialysis, such that the incidence is small in patients who are hemodialyzed for less than 8 years, increases to 30 to 50% after 15 years, and reaches 100% after 20 years of regular hemodialysis (17, 18). Patients over the age of 40 appear to be at an increased risk. With progressive amyloidosis the hips become affected, resulting in pathological fractures of the femoral neck. Symptomatic spinal damage may also occur with progressive disease (17).

As was previously stated, β_2-microglobulin is eliminated primarily by the kidneys. Hemodialysis patients have serum β_2-microglobulin concentrations that may reach 60 times the normal values (1 to 3 mg/L) (18). The retention of β_2-microglobulin in ESRD appears to be a necessary, although not sufficient, factor for pathogenesis of dialysis-related amyloidosis; therefore, other as-yet-unidentified factors are also needed for the development of amyloidosis (18). Dialysis-related amyloidosis is especially prevalent in long-term dialysis patients who are dialyzed with cuprophan membranes and less so in patients who are dialyzed with biocompatible or similar synthetic membranes (e.g., polyacrylonitrile) (23). There are two possible reasons for this membrane effect. First, compared with some high-flux membranes, the less permeable cellulosic dialyzers do not adequately remove middle molecules such as β_2-microglobulin. In addition, certain high-flux membranes (e.g., polymethylmethacrylate, polyacrylonitrile) can adsorb β_2-microglobulin and further increase its clearance (18).

Second, the blood-dialyzer interaction during hemodialysis induces an inflammatory response, leading to the release of cytokines and activated complement components. Both the synthesis and release of β_2-microglobulin are mediated by cytokines such as tumor necrosis factor, interleukin-2, interferon-α, and interferon-γ (17). Therefore, it is probable that hemodialysis per se may increase β_2-microglobulin synthesis and release. Biocompatible membranes, such as polyacrylonitrile and polysulfone, cause less inflammatory reaction and cytokine release (27). Therefore, the use of biocompatible high-flux membranes has the advantage of increasing the removal and decreasing the synthesis and release of β_2-microglobulin.

Dialysis-related amyloidosis can also occur in long-term CAPD patients (18). Peritoneal dialysis itself can activate intraperitoneal monocytes and induce the release of inflammatory cytokines (17). With prolonged follow-up, the incidence of carpal-tunnel syndrome in CAPD patients is only slightly less than that in hemodialysis patients (14% versus 18%) (23). However, patients who are on CAPD typically have lower serum β_2-microglobulin concentrations than do patients who are on hemodialysis. This may be due to a longer sustenance of residual renal function (a major determinant of serum β_2-microglobulin concentration) in the CAPD population (50) and/or the greater permeability to middle molecules of the peritoneal membrane compared to a standard cellulosic membrane (10). Nevertheless, CAPD is not considered to be effective for the treatment of dialysis-related amyloidosis (23). In fact, with extended follow-up time, CAPD patients appear to develop complications that are similar to those associated with β_2-microglobulin (33).

The early diagnosis of dialysis-related amyloidosis is difficult, and patients often present with advanced complications. β_2-Microglobulin deposits can be identified radiologically in a sensitive and noninvasive manner (17). The most commonly used diagnostic method involves the presence of cystic findings on roentgenogram. While carpal-tunnel syndrome may be treated surgically, there is no established treatment for the amyloidosis. Attempts should be made to remove as much β_2-microglobulin as possible, since the maintenance of low β_2-microglobulin concentrations may slow the progression of amyloidosis (49). The high-flux (larger-pore), biocompatible membranes (e.g., polysulfone, modified cellulose, polyacrylonitrile, cellulose triacetate, polymethylmethacrylate) are preferred for preventing and slowing the progression dialysis-related amyloidosis (17, 23), especially for patients who are older than 50 years (17). Successful renal transplantation can prevent dialysis-related amyloidosis. In addition, for patients with advanced dialysis-related amyloidosis, renal transplantation can arrest the progression of the disease and effectively reduce osteoarticular pain (17). However, transplantation cannot remove the β_2-microglobulin deposits, nor can it reverse previous damage.

ADEQUACY OF HEMODIALYSIS

In 1992 the gross annual mortality rate in the United States for patients undergoing maintenance dialysis was 23.6%-higher than that in any other Western industrialized nation. Even after adjustment for age and diabetes, the mortality rate remains high. In fact, the U.S. mortality rate is approximately twice and thrice the mortality rates of comparable patients in Europe and Japan, respectively (51). Moreover, over the past decade, this mortality rate has been on the rise (52). This disturbing trend is mostly due to underdialysis (51, 52). Currently, one-half to two-thirds of the ESRD patients in the United States receive an inadequate dialysis dose (52, 53). European hemodialysis patients receive, on the average, 30% higher dialysis doses than U.S. patients do (29). According to one estimate, increasing the amount of delivered dialysis in the United States could save 8000 to 16,000 lives per year (54).

Dialysis Quantification

Clinicians who care for dialysis patients have long struggled with the question "What is an adequate dialysis dose?" Almost any amount of dialysis can potentially sustain life longer than no dialysis (11); and before the advent of dialysis in 1960, uremia was uniformly fatal. In the past, hemodialysis therapy was not individualized and usually consisted of 3- to 4-hr sessions, thrice weekly, using blood flow rates of 12 to 18 L/hr (200 to 300 mL/min) and a dialysate flow rate of 30 L/hr (500 mL/min). Any diversion from this common practice was based more on clinical impression than on quantitative measures. However, in recent years, it has become evident that inadequate dialysis is associated with an exponential increase in the number of adverse clinical outcomes, including increased mortality (11, 23, 55, 56). The subjective and objective findings that are associated with underdialysis are useful; however, they overlap with the clinical manifestations of nonuremic causes (Table 22.5) (10).

In response to the widespread concern about underdialysis, a number of investigators have attempted to quantitatively define "adequate dialysis." Clinically, adequate dialysis is defined as the dose of dialysis below which one observes a significant worsening of morbidity and mortality (11). Identification of underdialysis using clinical parameters is not appropriate, since many of the signs and symptoms of morbid events are the same in adequately dialyzed patients as in underdialyzed patients.

Table 22.5.
Signs and Symptoms of Underdialysis

Nervous system	Skin
Stupor, coma	Pruritus
Polyneuritis	Melanosis
Confusion	Defective wound healing
Fatigue	Endocrinology
Motor weakness	Glucose intolerance
Disturbances in concentration	Growth retardation
Insomnia	Hyperparathyroidism
Headache	Hyperlipidemia
Irritability	Hypogonadism
Reduced sociability	Impotence
Restless legs	Diminished libido
Cramps	Bone disease
Tics	Osteodystrophy, osteomalacia
Electroencephalographic changes	Amyloidosis
Electromyographic changes	Nutritional status
Gastrointestinal system	Weight loss
Hiccup	Wasting
Stomatitis	Miscellaneous
Parotitis	Thirst
Pancreatitis	Hypothermia
Gastritis	Fetor
Colitis	Exercise intolerance
Ulceration	Ascites
Anorexia	Cardiovascular system
Nausea	Pericarditis
Vomiting	Hypertension, hypotension
Hematological system	Atheromatosis
Anemia	Cardiomyopathy
Bleeding	Edema
Immune system	
Susceptibility to infection	
Cancer	
Decreased response to vaccination	
Skin anergy	

Source: Adapted with permission from (10).

Therefore, in 1974 the National Institutes of Health initiated the multicenter National Cooperative Dialysis Study (NCDS) to evaluate quantitative methods for prescribing hemodialysis therapy on an individualized basis while limiting patient morbidity (12). In this study of 151 patients, four treatment groups were divided according to two parameters: dialysis treatment time (2.5 to 3.5 hr versus 4.5 to 5.0 hr) and time-averaged BUN concentration or TAC_{urea} (~20 and 40 mM/L [~50 and 100 mg/dL]). TAC_{urea} is simply the area under the BUN curve divided by time. BUN concentration was considered a surrogate marker for small molecules, while treatment time was considered a marker for middle molecules. However, because removal of middle molecules is also a function of membrane surface area and since different dialyzers were used in the study, treatment time was not an appropriate marker for dialysis of middle molecules (15).

Patients in the high-TAC$_{urea}$ group (~40 mM/L or 100 mg/dL) withdrew from the study for medical reasons at a significantly higher rate than did those in the the the low-TAC$_{urea}$ group (~20 mM/L or 50 mg/dL). Hospitalization was also greater in the the high-TAC$_{urea}$ group. The clinical abnormalities that resulted in drop-outs and hospitalizations were mostly gastrointestinal (anorexia, nausea, vomiting, bleeding), cardiac (pericarditis, pleuritis, sudden death, congestive heart failure), and hematologic (worsening of anemia) (13). Although it was originally believed that dialysis treatment time had no significant effect, a later review of the NCDS's significant findings indicated that reducing the dialysis time increased the hospitalization rate by 181%, especially for patients who had high TAC$_{urea}$ (14). Indeed, the short-time (2.5 to 3.5 hr), high-TAC$_{urea}$ group was discontinued early because a preliminary analysis indicated excessive hospitalization and medical withdrawal in this group. In other words, treatment time influenced the rate of hospitalization.

Further analysis of the NCDS data revealed the following about the high-TAC$_{urea}$ treatment groups: (a) a significantly higher incidence of early (within 3 to 6 weeks) neurologic deterioration, (b) increased severity of sleep abnormalities and muscle cramps, (c) worsening of anemia and increased transfusion requirements, and (d) an increased risk of cardiovascular morbidity, such as hypertension (14).

Although the was no difference in mortality between the groups, the observation period was not long enough. However, the poststudy follow-up demonstrated the highest mortality rates (usually from cardiovascular causes) in the high-TAC$_{urea}$ patients. This suggests that the effects of underdialysis may have long-term consequences (14). All together, the post-NCDS analyses identified four factors that can independently affect outcome. These factors, listed in order of importance, are (14):

1. BUN concentration: A higher TAC$_{urea}$ is associated with greater morbidity.
2. Protein catabolic rate (PCR): In a stable patient the PCR is a marker of dietary protein intake, because most uremic toxins are by-products of protein metabolism, and so the PCR depicts urea kinetics between dialysis sessions. A lower PCR (dietary protein intake) is associated with greater morbidity, indicating the importance of undernutrition in dialysis patients. It must be noted that PCR is an unreliable index of dietary protein intake in overtly catabolic or anabolic patients. Furthermore, since protein intake may vary from day to day, the PCR is not always a reliable indicator of protein intake (10).
3. Comorbid conditions.
4. Dialysis time: A shorter dialysis time is associated with greater morbidity. Inappropriately short dialysis sessions lead to inadequate removal of small and middle molecules such as urea.

In 1985, Gotch and Sargent, in their reanalysis of the NCDS data, developed a means by which dialysis can be quantified. They developed the parameter Kt/V, which is the product of the dialyzer clearance, usually of urea (K, in milliliters per minute), and the treatment time (t, in minutes), normalized to the urea distribution volume (V, in milliliters). Kt/V is a dimensionless parameter that takes into account dialysis intensity (Kt) by the patient's size (V) and describes the prescribed fractional clearance of total body water (13). In other words, Kt/V is the exponent that determines the decrease in BUN during each dialysis session (16):

$$BUN_{postdialysis} = BUN_{predialysis} \times e^{-Kt/V} \qquad (22.1)$$

The Kt/V concept can also be used to determine a dialyzer's fractional clearance of any toxic substance that may be accumulating in the uremic plasma.

The amount of delivered dialysis may also be measured independent of K, t, or V by using predialysis and postdialysis blood urea concentrations:

$$\ln \left(\frac{BUN_{predialysis}}{BUN_{postdialysis}} \right) = Kt/V \qquad (22.2)$$

In using equation (22.2) it is important that postdialysis BUN be measured 30 min after the end of a session, since because of a rebound effect, values may be 5 to 10% higher than BUN concentrations immediately postdialysis. This rebound effect is a result of reequilibration of urea between the intravascular and intracellular pools and is especially noticeable with the use of high-flux dialyzers (11, 23). It may also be due to an increase in intradialytic protein catabolism induced by loss of amino acids and glucose and/or a catabolic effect of the dialyzer as it interacts with blood (10).

According to the mechanistic analysis, an adequate dialysis prescription includes a PCR of 1.0 g/kg/day and a Kt/V of 1.0 for a patient who uses a cellulosic dialyzer thrice weekly, with no added benefit for higher dialysis doses. Furthermore, it was concluded that the relationship between protein intake and dialysis dose and outcome was not continuous and that the risk of failure increases if Kt/V falls to below 0.7 (13). However, it is now believed that there is a continuous inverse correlation between Kt/V and morbidity, such that there is no optimal Kt/V (10).

To avoid the complications of calculating Kt/V, the fractional urea clearance during a single dialysis session may be calculated with the use of the parameter urea reduction ratio (URR):

$$URR = \frac{(BUN_{predialysis} - BUN_{postdialysis})}{BUN_{predialysis}} \times 100 \qquad (22.3)$$

Therefore, URR represents the percent reduction in blood urea concentration during the course of one dialysis session. It offers the advantage of determining dialysis dose independent of patient size, dialysis time, blood and dialysis flow rates, and dialysis clearance. The relationship between Kt/V and URR is curvilinear (53), such that to achieve a Kt/V greater than 1.0, a URR of >50% is required. Without ultrafiltration a URR of 60% or greater is necessary to achieve a Kt/V greater than 1.0 (11).

RELEVANCE OF THE NATIONAL COOPERATIVE DIALYSIS STUDY

The patient selection criteria that were employed in the NCDS resulted in the inclusion of a study population that is different in many respects to the general ESRD population. First, the NCDS cohort were somewhat younger than the current ESRD population. Second, many of the common comorbid conditions (e.g., advanced atherosclerotic cardiovascular disease, pulmonary disease, recurrent infections, and malignancies) were excluded from the study. Furthermore, the NCDS excluded patients with diabetes, who now account for one-third of the U.S. ESRD population. As will be discussed below, these patients benefit from more dialysis than do nondiabetics (57). Finally, even after a relatively healthy cohort was selected, only 50% of randomized subjects were able to complete the study (12, 15). With these restrictions, less than 20% of the ESRD population meets the NCDS criteria (15). Accordingly, the NCDS results apply to, at best, only a minority of dialysis patients. The majority of hemodialysis patients will require higher doses of dialysis. In fact, increasing the Kt/V to 1.4 to 1.6 is associated with a significant decrease in patient morbidity and mortality. These improvements are more pronounced in diabetics than in nondiabetics (15).

POTENTIAL MISAPPLICATION OF Kt/V

The use of the Kt/V model to prescribe a dose of dialysis makes the following potentially invalid assumptions: (a) an absence of residual renal function, (b) no weight change in the interdialytic period, and (c) a constant interdialytic interval (i.e., dialysis every other day rather than thrice weekly). Hence, the use of this model is associated with inaccuracies, leading some investigators to view TAC_{urea} and URR as better markers of dialysis adequacy (11, 23). Like URR, TAC_{urea} accounts for urea removal and accumulation rates, two major components of urea modeling, whereas Kt/V measures only removal rate. In addition, TAC_{urea} takes into account the interdialytic changes in urea nitrogen, from which PCR and dietary protein intake can be calculated. TAC_{urea} is independent of patient size, dialysis schedule, residual renal function, volume of distribution, and other confounding variables. However, a target TAC_{urea} cannot be prescribed, since this parameter depends also on the dietary protein intake the patient (11, 23). TAC_{urea} may be calculated as follows:

Table 22.6.

Reasons Urea Clearance Prescribed Is Less Than Actual Urea Clearance

Patient-related factors
    Effective time on dialysis less than prescribed
    Inadequate effective blood flow rate:
        Recirculation
        Inadequate arterial blood flow in access
        Use of subclavian catheter with blood flow limitation
Staff-related factors
    Blood flow rate less than prescribed during dialysis session
    Error in setting the blood blow flow rate
    Inadequate dialyzer quality control
Mechanically related factors
    In vitro estimation of dialyzer clearance
    Blood pump miscalibration
    Dialysate flow miscalibration
    Clotting of dialyzer

Source: Adapted with permission from (11).

$$TAC_{urea} = \frac{T_d(C_1 + C_2) + I_d(C_2 + C_3)}{2(T_d + I_d)} \quad (22.4)$$

where C_1 is the predialysis BUN concentration, C_2 is the postdialysis BUN concentration, C_3 is the BUN concentration before the next dialysis session, T_d is the dialysis time, and I_d is the interdialysis period (23).

If the delivered dialysis dose is based on equation (22.2), two methods can be used to calculate the adequacy of dialysis: from the right side of the equation, based on K, t, and V, or from the left side of the equation, based on predialysis and postdialysis BUN. Calculations that are based on K, t, and V are estimates of the dose prescribed; using predialysis and postdialysis BUN, one obtains the actual delivered dose of dialysis (11). Ideally, the prescribed dose should be consistent with the delivered dose; however, calculation of the Kt/V parameter increases the chance of compounding errors, since its individual components K, t, and V are all subject to many inaccuracies and imprecisions that most often lead to overestimation of the actual delivered dose of dialysis. First, there are many errors associated with calculating urea clearance (K) (Table 22.6). Often, the dialyzer clearance is estimated in vitro, and since for many dialyzers the in vivo clearances are lower and may vary by up to 99% of the in vitro values, this parameter is often overestimated (24). Second, the urea volume of distribution (V) is commonly assumed to be a fixed and constant ratio of total body weight, which is not the case for all patients. This parameter depends on body size and the time in relation to a dialysis session, when the weight was measured. Finally, the recorded duration of dialysis session (t) is often inaccurate (Table 22.7). Commonly, the dialysis time is recorded from the time of needle insertion until after the end of the session when the needle is removed and hemostasis is obtained. However, since

Table 22.7.

Reasons Dialysis Time Prescribed Is Less Than Actual Dialysis Time

Patient-related factors
  Late going on, patient tardy
  Early sign-off with consent or against advice
  Medical complications
Staff-related factors
  Late going on, staff tardy
  Wrong patient taken off
  Time calculated incorrectly
  Time off read incorrectly
  Written time on earlier than actual time on
  Written time off later than actual time off
Mechanically related factors
  Dialyzer leak
  Clotted dialyzer during dialysis
  Improperly set alarm limits, malfunctioning air detectors, pump failures, etc.

Source: Adapted with permission from (11).

approximately 5 to 10% of this time does not involve effective dialysis, dialysis times are often overestimated (11, 23).

At least one report suggests that the delivered dose of dialysis is typically lower than the prescribed dose by 20% (58). Therefore, it is always preferable to assess the actual amount of dialysis that is delivered and compare it to the prescribed dose because, unless a rigorous quality-monitoring program is in effect, the delivered dialysis dose is often significantly less than the amount prescribed. Discrepancies may reveal in-center sources of error that routinely overestimate the adequacy of dialysis.

Effect of Dialysis Time

An appropriately long dialysis session allows slower ultrafiltration, thus preventing the cardiovascular instability associated with rapid fluid removal and better hypertension control. For a given dialyzer a more prolonged session also provides a higher dialysis dose and reduces the risk of developing certain intradialytic symptoms (which are discussed below). Since the 1970s, several factors have led to a considerable reduction in dialysis time compared to a decade ago (32). Weekly dialysis times have decreased from 15 to 18 hr in the 1970s to 12 to 15 hr in the 1980s to 6 to 12 hr in the 1990s (53).

Alterations in membrane composition and permeability have resulted in the development of high-flux and high-efficiency dialyzers. The use of these dialyzers in the setting of higher blood and dialysate flow rates and improved precision in ultrafiltration control have allowed higher solute clearances in shorter periods of time. In addition, certain fiscal and patient-related factors have led to considerable reductions in dialysis time compared to two decades ago (11, 23). For example, some patients may

pressure the dialysis staff to shorten their dialysis sessions. In addition, the rising costs of labor and other resources, coupled with fixed and reduced Medicare reimbursement rates, may have adversely affected dialysis times (11, 51).

Patients who receive relatively short but adequate dialysis exhibit significantly lower depression scores. However, shortening dialysis times without close monitoring of adequacy via subjective and objective means may have deleterious consequences, since there is less margin of safety in cases in which delivered and prescribed dialysis doses do not match (10). Unfortunately, over the years, the reduction in dialysis times has been correlated with increased mortality rates among the U.S. hemodialysis population (23, 29), which is most likely due to the associated reduction in delivered dose of dialysis (59). Indeed, patients who are dialyzed less than 3.5 hr have a higher mortality rate than do those who are dialyzed for longer periods (23). Some investigators believe that dialysis time may be a predictor of mortality, independent of Kt/V (9). In long-term, uncontrolled studies of patients who receive dialysis for more than 10 years, survivors have consistently had longer dialysis times than did nonsurvivors (23). The lower rates of ESRD morbidity and mortality in Europe and Japan are at least partly due to longer dialysis times. Whereas the average weekly dialysis time in the United States is 9 hr, that in Europe and Japan is 12 hr and 15 hr, respectively (52).

Given the effect of dialysis time, selection of the appropriate dialyzer assumes a much more important role in ensuring adequate delivery of dialysis. The high-flux and high-efficiency membranes are not only more biocompatible than a cellulosic dialyzer, but also have favorable intradialytic and interdialytic effects (23).

Effect of Nutrition and Dietary Protein Intake

Healthy adults require 0.75 g/kg/day of high-quality protein to maintain a neutral or positive nitrogen balance (56). By contrast, hemodialysis patients require 1.2 g/kg/day of primarily high-quality protein and a caloric intake of 35 kcal/kg/day (16, 55, 56). This higher protein requirement is due to a higher protein catabolism as a result of (a) metabolic acidosis, (b) infections, (c) the blood-dialyzer interaction (especially with bioincompatible membranes), and (d) losses of protein and amino acid in the dialysate that ranges from 10 to 13 g per session (55). Unfortunately, most patients have nutritional intakes below the recommended level; this explains the high prevalence of protein-calorie malnutrition among hemodialysis patients (16). Protein-calorie malnutrition is a consequence of (a) disturbances in protein and energy metabolism (hypercatabolism), (b) disturbances in certain hormonal regulations, (c) infections and other comorbid conditions, and (d) poor dietary intake resulting from anorexia and underdialysis (56). There are numerous causes of anorexia and decreased dietary intake in the ESRD population (Table 22.8); however, the most common cause is inadequate dialysis (16, 55, 56).

Protein-calorie malnutrition is an important risk factor for morbidity and mortality in the ESRD population (16). Signs of protein-calorie malnutrition include reduced energy stores (subcutaneous fat stores); reduced muscle mass as indicated by lower serum creatinine concentrations or as measured by anthropometric methods; low total body nitrogen; low serum concentrations of albumin, transferrin, and other visceral proteins; and abnormalities in the plasma and intracellular amino acids profiles (16, 55). The risk of death is inversely related to the predialysis serum concentrations of creatinine (marker of muscle mass), BUN (marker of dietary protein intake), albumin (marker of visceral proteins), and cholesterol (marker of dietary intake) (56, 60, 61). Serum albumin concentration is by far the most potent laboratory predictor of mortality in both hemodialysis and CAPD patients. The risk of death increases exponentially with decreasing serum albumin values. With a reference value of 40 g/L (4 g/dL), a serum albumin value between 35 and 40 g/L (3.5 to 4.0 g/dL), which is still within the normal reference range for most laboratories, is associated with a twofold increase in mortality rate (60). The mortality risk increases nearly sevenfold when the albumin concentration is 30 to 35 g/L (3.0 to 3.5 g/dL), 15-fold when it is 25 to 30 g/L (2.5 to 3.0 g/dL), and nearly 19-fold when it is less than 25 g/L (2.5 g/dL). Furthermore, a low serum albumin is a predictor of arteriovenous graft thrombosis, pulmonary edema, infections such as pneumonia and sepsis, and days of hospitalization (62).

From the NCDS it was not possible to state with certainty that low PCR is a strong predictor of therapy

Table 22.8.
Causes of Malnutrition in Dialysis Patients

Underdialysis (uremic toxicity)
Unpalatable or inadequate diets
Gastropathy (diabetic patients)
Inflammation, infection, sepsis
Medications
Psychosocial and socioeconomic factors
    Loneliness
    Depression
    Ignorance
    Poverty
    Alcohol and drug abuse
Effects of the hemodialysis procedure
    Cardiovascular instability
    Nausea, vomiting
    Postdialysis fatigue
Effects of the peritoneal dialysis procedure
    Abdominal discomfort
    Glucose absorption
    Peritonitis

Source: Adapted with permission from (56).

failure (15). A patient who is underdialyzed suffers from nausea, vomiting, and anorexia such that the patient's nutritional status may over time be compromised. The decreased BUN concentration that follows a decrease in dietary protein intake may falsely indicate that the dose of dialysis is adequate, thus creating a cycle of worsening malnutrition and underdialysis. It is now clear that the dietary protein intake is dependent on the dose of dialysis, such that for a malnourished and underdialyzed patient, an increase in the dialysis dose will in a few weeks result in an increase in dietary protein intake (16, 55). This relationship between PCR and Kt/V is actually curvilinear and plateaus at Kt/V values of 1.6 to 2.7, such that beyond a certain Kt/V value (~1.8), no further increase in PCR is seen (16, 55).

Preliminary evidence indicates a beneficial effect for the administration of intradialytic parenteral nutrition to patients who are malnourished (63).

Effect of Dialysis Membrane

Aside from the difference in delivered dose of dialysis, another potential explanation for the difference in mortality rates between the United States and other Western countries is a more common use of bioincompatible membranes (e.g., cuprophan) in the United States (11, 52). The assessment of dialysis dose may be complicated by dialyzer-related factors, such as membrane thickness, surface area, pore size, biocompatibility, and composition. Because of their large surface areas, the high-efficiency membranes have higher urea clearances and allow for higher doses of dialysis to be delivered with a minor increase in dialysis time. Compared with cellulosic membranes, the high-flux dialyzers have larger pores that allow a higher clearance of middle molecules (e.g., β_2-microglobulin) and are generally more biocompatible (i.e., induce minimal inflammatory-type reactions to contact with blood) (64, 65). Therefore, patients who are dialyzed with biocompatible membranes are less catabolic, have a lower incidence of arthropathy due to β_2-microglobulin accumulation, and have decreased morbid events, such as infectious complications (10, 11). Therefore, to fully assess the adequacy of dialysis, the type of dialyzer membrane that is used must also be considered. Accumulating evidence suggests a lower incidence of morbidity and mortality with high-flux dialyzers; however, no prospective study has yet evaluated the adequate dialysis dose with the use of these newer membranes (53).

The bioincompatible dialysis membranes (e.g., cuprophan) can affect both protein intake and catabolism, thus influencing a patient's overall nutritional status. The high-flux, biocompatible membranes (e.g., polyacrylonitrile, polysufone) have a clear advantage in that they lack an effect or have a significantly reduced effect on protein catabolism. Furthermore, compared to hemodialysis by cellulosic membranes, high-flux dialyzers require a lower dialysis dose to achieve the same dietary protein intake (16, 55, 56, 66). For example, a delivered Kt/V of 0.85 with the use of a polyacrylonitrile membrane provides the patient with a PCR of 1 g/kg/day; however, to achieve the same PCR with a cellulosic membrane, a delivered Kt/V of 1.0 is required (16, 55, 66). This is likely because the high-flux membranes have a higher clearance for middle molecules for the same amount of urea removal (16, 55). If so, then the adequacy of dialysis must ideally be based on removal of both small (e.g., urea) and larger solutes (e.g., β_2-microglobulin). Another explanation for this membrane effect may be that the biocompatible membranes do not stimulate the production of activated complement components, interleukin-1, and tumor necrosis factor, which may suppress appetite and increase muscle catabolism (16,55).

Dialyzer Reuse

A dialyzer may be discarded after a single use. However, a number of centers clean and sterilize their dialyzers for reuse by the same patient. Over the past 20 years in the United States, the number of centers reusing dialyzers increased from 18% to 68% (32). With repeated dialyzer use, fiber bundles are lost owing to obstruction by clotting. Since this reduces the effective clearance, cuprophan dialyzers are currently discarded once the volume loss exceeds 20%. Such a guideline has not been set for other membrane types (10). Although it is believed that dialyzer reuse should not affect the adequacy of dialysis (23), this view has been challenged, with the contention that reuse may actually increase the risk of mortality (32). With reuse, there is a potential risk of death from sepsis due to inadequate sterilization of the dialyzer (32). However, dialysis reuse may be safely performed by following the established sterilization guidelines of the Association for the Advancement of Medical Instrumentation. Hence, the National Kidney Foundation Ad Hoc Committee on Reduction of Morbidity and Mortality in U.S. Maintenance Dialysis Patients has concluded that when appropriately performed, dialyzer reuse is safe and decreases the cost of treatment, thus allowing the delivery of a larger dose of dialysis (51). Furthermore, because of protein film coating of the membrane (28), the reuse of cellulosic membranes is associated with decreased intradialytic complement activation, which may reduce the incidence of certain intradialytic symptoms (53).

Recommendations

There is a great need for long-term trials of dialysis adequacy and optimization. The evaluation of dialysis adequacy must include all three parameters: BUN, PCR, and Kt/V (or URR). It is strongly emphasized that the goal of adequate dialysis is not only high urea removal, but also adequate dietary protein (i.e., at least 1.2 g/kg/day) and

Table 22.9.
Laboratory Tests That Are Used in the Assessment of Dialysis Adequacy

Nonretention products
  Albumin
  Bicarbonate
  Cholesterol
  Coagulation test
  Hemoglobin and hematocrit
  Parathyroid hormone
  pH
  Platelet count
  Red blood cell count
  Total protein
  Transferrin
  Triglycerides
Retention products
  β_2-Microglobulin
  Creatinine
  Hippuric acid
  Phosphate
  Potassium
  Urea
  Uric acid

Source: Adapted with permission from (10).

caloric intake (i.e., at least 35 kcal/kg/day). The adequacy of dialysis must be based on the dose delivered rather than the dose prescribed. In making such an assessment, the patient's residual renal function must be included to provide a more valid estimation of clearance values. Dialysis therapy should aim not at a target BUN, but rather at a high enough Kt/V (or URR) that achieves optimal dietary protein intake and nutritional status (15). A hemodialysis session must provide a minimum Kt/V of 1.2 (or URR of 60%); however, a Kt/V of 1.3 to 1.4 is recommended, since further reductions in morbidity and mortality may be obtained past this threshold (51). Diabetic patients may respond better to even higher doses ≥ 1.4) (57). According to one estimate, for every Kt/V increase of 0.1, there is an associated 7% reduction in mortality (29).

In assessing the adequacy of dialysis, the clinical manifestations of underdialysis should never be ignored (Table 22.5). In addition, certain objective laboratory tests provide useful information regarding the overall health of the dialysis patient (Table 22.9) (10). Patients should be monitored monthly for dialysis adequacy and protein-calorie malnutrition; the monitoring should include edema-free postdialysis body weight, and serum concentrations of albumin and transferrin. In addition, dietary intake should be monitored at least every 6 months (51). One method is to (a) determine the baseline fistula recirculation value when dialysis is initiated or when a new access is being used for the first time; (b) start the patient on 4-hr dialysis sessions, because it is much easier to reduce dialysis time than to increase it; (c) perform kinetic modeling using a three-point system of obtaining predialysis, postdialysis, and again predialysis BUN; (d) determine endogenous residual renal function, if present, within 1 month of initiation of dialysis; and (e) calculate TAC_{urea}, URR, Kt/V, and PCR from these data. These measurements are repeated quarterly to maintain Kt/V at 1.2 and TAC_{urea} at ~20 mM/L (50 mg/dL). These values will usually correspond to a PCR of at least 1.0 g/kg/day. If the patient is underdialyzed without recirculation problems, the dialysis time may be increased; alternatively, the effective dialyzer clearance may be increased by using a dialyzer with a larger surface-area membrane. If recirculation is greater than 20%, correction of the arteriovenous fistula is indicated (23).

Given the high morbidity and mortality in patients with ESRD, the focus must now shift from dialysis adequacy to "optimal" dialysis dose (23). Optimal dialysis may be defined as the dialysis dose "above which no further improvement in the morbidity and mortality of patients can be expected" (11). Although many have tried to define adequate dosage of dialysis, no studies have defined the optimal dialysis dose. A treatment goal of simply keeping the patient alive and out of the hospital for a few months might be questioned as appropriate (11). In the absence of guidelines for optimal dialysis, the dialysis prescription must aim at Kt/V values that are high enough to achieve optimal dietary protein intake and nutritional status. This may involve the use of biocompatible membranes (e.g., polyacrylonitrile, polysulfone) and/or extension of dialysis treatment time. On the basis of reports of increased patient survival, a delivered Kt/V of 1.6 to 1.9 may be reaching toward optimum (67).

PERITONEAL DIALYSIS

Peritoneal dialysis was first attempted in humans in 1923 (68). The broad use of this mode of therapy was limited by the availability of a suitable access device for chronic therapy (68). However, the development of this type of device in the late 1960s did not greatly enhance the use of peritoneal dialysis (69). The principle reasons for this were the high rate of adverse effects, especially peritonitis and bowel perforation, and the lack of patient acceptance. This lack of patient acceptance was in part due to the severe limitations placed on the patient's lifestyle. Specifically, the dialysis process often required 10 to 12 hr per treatment and three or four treatments a week.

Peritoneal dialysis has undergone several modifications over the years. In 1976, CAPD was developed; it freed patients from most of the lifestyle limitations (70). As the name implies, CAPD is a continuous dialysis process that allows the patient a more normal ambulatory lifestyle (which will be discussed later in this chapter).

The Peritoneal Membrane

The peritoneal cavity is formed within the abdomen by a single-layered membrane that lines both the thinner surface of the abdomen and the visceral organs. The side of the peritoneal cavity is either parietal, if it covers the abdominal wall, or visceral, if it covers the visceral organs. The peritoneal surface area approximates the body surface area, thus ranging from 1 to 2 m^2. The adult peritoneal cavity contains approximately 100 mL of lipid-rich fluid that acts as a lubricating agent. The peritoneal space can be enlarged to several liters in the presence of ascites or by instillation of dialysate solution (21,22).

The peritoneal membrane has pores that are large enough to allow the passage of compounds up to 5000 daltons. Therefore, CAPD clears larger substances more effectively than did the older, cellulosic hemodialysis membranes. The routes of absorption from the peritoneal cavity differ for small solutes and macromolecules (molecular weights 20,000 daltons) (e.g., albumin, dextrans). Whereas small solutes diffuse down their concentration gradient into the systemic circulation, macromolecules are absorbed primarily via the subdiaphragmatic lymphatic system (71).

With chronic peritoneal dialysis the character of the mesothelial layer may change, mostly because of the hyperosmolarity of the dialysate solutions (21). These alterations may lead in some patients to peritoneal fibrosis (thickening), decreased permeability, and diminished ultrafiltration (22,72).

Mechanics of Peritoneal Dialysis

Like hemodialysis, peritoneal dialysis has three basic components: a blood compartment (i.e., systemic circulation), a dialysate compartment (i.e., peritoneal cavity), and a semipermeable membrane that separates the blood and dialysate compartments (i.e., the peritoneal membrane). Peritoneal dialysis is a procedure by which the dialysis solution is instilled into the peritoneal cavity via an indwelling catheter. In the presence of dialysate, solute transfer occurs via diffusion and convection bidirectionally across the peritoneal membrane to and from the blood compartment (21). Since the dialysis fluid contains glucose (dextrose) as an osmotic agent, fluid is pulled from the intravascular space into the peritoneal cavity by ultrafiltration. This osmotic effect is lost as the dialysate glucose is absorbed, especially if the duration of dialysate residence, called dwell time, is prolonged.

Peritoneal Access Devices and Placement Techniques

Dialysis access can be achieved at the bedside by insertion of a stylocath (single-use catheter) into the peritoneal cavity; however, significant problems can occur with these initial temporary access devices. Permanent access to the peritoneal cavity for peritoneal dialysis may be accomplished by several techniques. The first catheter developed for long-term peritoneal dialysis was described by Tenckhoff in 1968 (69). The present version of this catheter has a low rate of abdominal discomfort during dialysis. Several other catheters for long-term peritoneal dialysis have been introduced in the last few years (73). The relative advantages and disadvantages of these access devices remain theoretical.

The existing varieties of indwelling catheters and administration sets were designed to prevent contamination and to reduce infectious complications of peritoneal dialysis (73). The chronic (permanent) indwelling catheters are constructed from silicone rubber, polyurethane, and other soft materials. The Tenckhoff cathether is the most commonly used peritoneal catheter (72). The catheter has two sections, intraperitoneal and extraperitoneal, each available in different designs (73). The intraperitoneal portion is placed via a surgical procedure in the left or right lower peritoneum, preferably in one of the pelvic gutters just above the hips (21,73). The extraperitoneal end is passed through subcutaneous layers and placed approximately halfway between the umbilicus and the pubis in the caudal direction (21,73). The indwelling catheter is then immobilized to allow healing, prevent leaks, and serve as a barrier for migration of skin microorganisms. For this purpose, one or preferably two Dacron cuffs are placed above and/or below the abdominal muscle layers, and the patient is allowed to heal before peritoneal dialysis is begun. During this healing period, the patient undergoes training for self-administration of dialysis and care of the catheter using sterile technique. The waiting period between catheter placement and dialysis initiation varies among patients. The healing period is usually 4 to 6 weeks for patients with potentially impaired wound healing, such as diabetic patients and those receiving high-dose steroids. A young and relatively healthy patient can often start dialysis in 2 weeks after catheter placement. Patients who are about to undergo CCPD may start even sooner, since they can use lower initial volumes with no daytime dwell.

Dialysate Solutions

The peritoneal dialysis solution is made hypertonic with hydrous dextrose to create a diffusive gradient between the peritoneal and blood compartments and to augment ultrafiltration. The dialysate contains electrolytes such as sodium, potassium, chloride, magnesium, and calcium in addition to hydrous dextrose in concentrations of 15, 25, or 42.5 g/L (1.5, 2.5, or 4.25 g/dL) (Table 22.10) (22,72). Besides dextrose, other osmotic agents have been used experimentally, including glycerol and amino acids (74). A variety of excipients including potassium, calcium, and lactate may be added to the dialysate to control the balance of electrolytes and to correct the metabolic acidosis that is

Table 22.10.
Commercially Available Peritoneal Dialysis Solutions

Calcium	2.5 or 3.5 mEq/L
Chloride	95, 96, or 102 mEq/L
Dextrose	1.5, 2.5, or 4.25 g/dL
Lactate	35 or 40 mEq/L
Magnesium	0.5 or 1.5 mEq/L
Sodium	132 mEq/L

associated with ESRD.

Continuous Ambulatory Peritoneal Dialysis

In CAPD, as the name implies, patients are dialyzed continuously, 24 hours a day, 7 days a week. Given its demanding and time-consuming nature, CAPD requires a reliable and highly motivated patient. Omission of only a few exchanges per week will reduce the urea clearance, with the potential of increasing morbidity and mortality. A typical CAPD regimen involves four daily exchanges-three with a dialysate dwell time of about 4 to 6 hr and on with an overnight dwell time of about 10 to 12 hr (21,72). Commercial CAPD solutions are available in volumes of 1 to 3 L in flexible polyvinyl chloride plastic bags similar to those of large-volume parenterals. The bags have a port for the connection of an administration set and a port for administration of excipients (e.g., antibiotics).

The fresh dialysate bag is connected to a permanent indwelling catheter via an administration set. A volume of dialysate (commonly 2 L) is warmed to body temperature and infused by gravity into the peritoneal cavity over 10 to 20 min. The warming of the dialysate is intended to prevent pain and cramping during the initial minutes of an exchange. Depending on the catheter and administration set, the empty bag is either removed and retained for drainage or folded and tucked inside the patient's clothing or carried inside a separate belt underneath the clothing while still connected to the catheter (21,72). After the prescribed dwell time, the same bag is connected or unfolded and placed at a level that is lower than the peritoneal cavity to allow drainage by gravity, which also takes 10 to 20 min. When the drainage has ceased, the tubing is again clamped, and using sterile technique (mask and gloves), the patient disconnects the bag of drained fluid. Then a fresh bag of sterile dialysate fluid is connected to the tubing and allowed to infuse into the peritoneal cavity. Fresh unused dialysate is clear and colorless; spent or used dialysate is clear and straw-colored (72). During bouts of peritonitis the spent dialysate becomes cloudy; this is considered a diagnostic sign of infection.

Automated Peritoneal Dialysis

The two main forms of continuous peritoneal dialysis are CCPD and tidal peritoneal dialysis. These procedures involve the use of a dialysate cycling machine, which automatically instills and drains peritoneal dialysate solutions. In CCPD, the most common variation of CAPD, there are, on the average, four 2-L exchanges at night while the patient is sleeping. In the daytime, the patient may carry 0 to 2 L of dialysate in the peritoneal cavity. With tidal peritoneal dialysis, there is a minimal dwell volume (often ⁻1 L) that always remains in the peritoneal cavity. The cycler instills fresh dialysate at regular intervals to achieve three goals: (a) to minimize the amount of drain and fill times during which no effective dialysis takes place, (b) to maintain an optimum transmembrane solute gradient for enhancement of solute removal, and (c) to minimize the stagnant fluid layer that is in contact with the peritoneal membrane (61). Continuous cycling and tidal peritoneal dialysis are not used frequently for long-term therapy of chronic renal failure; however, they are the predominant routes of peritoneal dialysis in the acute care environment.

COMPLICATIONS OF PERITONEAL DIALYSIS

Exit-Site and Tunnel Infections

Exit-site infections and tunnel infections occur at a rate of about 0.5 episode per patient-year (21). An infected exit-site is characterized by redness, induration, and/or purulent discharge. Other symptoms include heat, drainage, odor, tenderness, and pain. Crust formation around the exit site and positive cultures from the exit site in the absence of inflammation do not indicate infection (75). If the infection infiltrates the deeper subcutaneous tissues, the patient is said to have a tunnel infection. Edema, redness, and tenderness over the subcutaneous path of the catheter indicate the presence of tunnel infection. However, it may be difficult to differentiate between exit-site and tunnel infections (21,74). Tunnel infections often precede the development of peritonitis (72).

Treatment of exit-site infection has included the use of systemic and intraperitoneal antibiotics, use of topical antibiotics and disinfectants applied with a variety of dressings, debridement of the infected subcutaneous cuff, and removal of the catheter (21). The presence of erythema alone may be an early sign of infection and requires topical therapy with chlorhexidine, mupirocin, or hydrogen peroxide. When exit-site infection is suspected, the patient must be instructed to cleanse the site frequently with hydrogen peroxide and povidone-iodine. When purulent discharge is present, Gram stain and culture should be obtained (76). The catheter must be immobilized to avoid traumatization of sensitive tissues (45).

Empiric oral antibiotics are used against the common causative organisms (S. aureus and S. epidermidis), starting with either a first-generation cephalosporin (e.g., cephalexin, cephradine), dicloxacillin, or trimethoprim-

sulfamethoxazole (72). Single-dose vancomycin as either 1 g intravenously or 2 g intraperitoneally (half-dose if <40 kg) may also be used (76, 77). Once the culture results are known, they must guide antibiotic treatment. The optimal duration of therapy has not been established; however, it must be noted that prolonged antibiotic use is a predisposing factor for the development of fungal peritonitis (78). If within 1 week of starting treatment for S. aureus infection there is no sign of improvement, rifampin 600 mg daily must be added (76).

For Gram-negative infections, oral ciprofloxacin 500 mg twice daily is recommended (76). To avoid decreased absorption, ciprofloxacin must be dosed several hours before or after phosphate binders. If no improvement is observed within 2 to 3 weeks, the catheter must be removed. Likewise, the catheter must be removed for Pseudomonas or Xanthomonas exit-site infections, since they are unlikely to respond to antimicrobial therapy (76).

Treatment of tunnel infections involves antibiotic treatment and possibly surgical drainage. If response is not obtained, the catheter must be removed (72).

Peritonitis

Peritonitis is the most prevalent infectious complication of CAPD, occurring at a rate of 0.8 episode per patient-year (22). CAPD peritonitis is directly responsible for 7 to 10% of deaths, equivalent to 1.3 to 1.9% of all CAPD patients (79). By worsening the patient's general status, peritonitis may be responsible for further deaths.

Breakdown in aseptic technique during dialysis exchanges is one of the major risk factors for the development of peritonitis (21). The peritonitis-causing organism may directly enter through the catheter lumen or migrate along the catheter through a tunnel. The development of catheter biofilms or exit-site infections may also contribute to peritonitis (45). Rarely, peritonitis is due to intestinal or genitourinary sources or from hematogenous seeding.

Peritoneal dialysis patients have many of the immune deficiencies described above for hemodialysis and undialyzed uremic patients. In addition, the presence of a low-pH, hyperosmolar dialysate solution inhibits phagocytosis, chemotaxis, bactericidal killing, free oxygen radical generation, and leukotriene B_4 synthesis of both peripheral neutrophils and peritoneal macrophages (80). This diminished intraperitoneal immune capacity may contribute to the development of peritonitis. Therefore, the routine use of 4.25% glucose solutions should be avoided. Protein-calorie malnutrition and diabetes may increase the risk of peritonitis (23). Possibly because of socioeconomic factors, black patients and less educated patients also have a higher incidence of peritonitis (21). Bacterial colonization of the nares with S. aureus is a risk factor for both exit-site infection and peritonitis (45). Recurrent peritonitis occurs in up to one-third of the patients and is a major cause of

Table 22.11.
Relative Frequencies of Organisms Causing Peritonitis

Organism	Frequency (%)
Coagulase-negative *Staphylococcus*	30–40
Staphylococcus aureus	15–20
Streptococcus spp.	10–15
Neisseria spp.	1–2
Diphtheroid spp.	1–2
Escherichia coli	5–10
Pseudomonas spp.	5–10
Enterococcus spp.	3–6
Klebsiella spp.	1–3
Proteus spp.	3–6
Acinetobacter spp.	2–5
Anaerobic organisms	2–5
Fungi	2–10
Other (e.g., *Mycobacterium* spp.)	2–5
Culture-negative	0–30

Source: Adapted with permission from (77).

technique failure (i.e., discontinuation of a dialysis modality due to complications) (21).

Peritonitis that is associated with CAPD is typically much less serious than that caused by gastrointestinal (GI) perforation. Most of the cases are of bacterial origin, although other forms, such as chemical, viral, mycobacterial, and fungal, also exist. Up to 60% of peritonitis episodes are caused by *Staphylococcus spp.*, mostly *S. epidermidis* (77). Gram-negative organisms, mostly *Enterobacteriaceae, Pseudomonas* spp., and *Acinetobacter* spp., cause up to 44% of cases (Table 22.11) (77). Polymicrobial peritonitis accounts for 5% of cases, and may be indicative of intraabdominal viscus perforation (21, 72). So-called sterile peritonitis, also termed eosinophilic peritonitis, may be due to transient allergic reaction to some component of the CAPD catheter and usually occurs within the first few weeks after catheter insertion (72).

INITIAL ASSESSMENT OF CAPD PERITONITIS

Peritonitis is diagnosed on the basis of the presence of two of the following three symptoms: (a) abdominal pain and rebound tenderness, (b) the presence of more than 100 white blood cells per cubic millimeter of peritoneal fluid (with 50% neutrophils), and (c) a positive dialysate culture (76). A cloudy effluent is the most common presenting sign of peritonitis (76); however, the effluent may be clear or may remain cloudy after microbiologic cure (21). When peritonitis is suspected, a Gram stain of the dialysate must be obtained. The Gram stain is positive in up to 40% of cases. Culture of the spent dialysate must also be obtained, but therapy should not await the results (76). Although intravenous antibiotics can produce effective drug concentrations within the peritoneal cavity, usually within 2 to 4 hr after dosing (81), intraperitoneal administration of antibiotics rapidly produces high local concentrations due to the

large difference in the volumes of the peritoneal and systemic compartments (81, 82). With intraperitoneal administration the patient is trained to inject the antibiotic directly into the dialysate bag before each exchange.

INITIAL MANAGEMENT OF CAPD PERITONITIS

Since CAPD peritonitis is less severe than other forms of peritonitis, treatment is usually undertaken on an outpatient basis. However, the following circumstances necessitate patient hospitalization: (a) inability or unwillingness to self-administer antibiotics, (b) noncompliance with therapy or follow-up, and (c) presence of significant systemic symptoms, such as fever, vomiting, abdominal pain, or hypotension (72). Once CAPD peritonitis has been diagnosed, two or three rapid dialysis exchanges of 20 min each may provide symptomatic benefit (76). Also, the addition of heparin to the fresh dialysate may help to reduce the number of subsequent peritoneal adhesions and reduce postinfectious complications (77). Heparin 1000 units/L is added to the regular dialysis regimen until the dialysate color is clear again, which usually takes 2 to 3 days (76).

Before the causative organism is determined, empiric broad-spectrum antibiotic therapy must be initiated against common Gram-positive and/or Gram-negative bacteria, which may cause approximately 90% of all CAPD peritonitis cases (21). Table 22.12 provides the antibiotic dosing guidelines for the treatment of CAPD peritonitis (76).

GRAM-POSITIVE ORGANISMS ON GRAM STAIN

Once a Gram-positive organism has been identified, vancomycin must be administered at a dose of 2 g in one 6-hr exchange every 7 days. Since this regimen is associated with a higher incidence of chemical peritonitis, an intermittent regimen of vancomycin 30 to 50 mg/L in every bag may be preferred (76). There is no therapeutic advantage to using intravenous vancomycin. If methicillin resistance is not suspected, a first-generation cephalosporin (e.g., cefazolin) may be administered as an initial intraperitoneal loading dose of 500 mg/L followed by a maintenance dose of 125 mg/L in each subsequent dialysis bag (76).

GRAM STAIN NEGATIVE OR NOT DONE

In more than 60% of cases, the Gram stain may be negative. In such cases, or if a Gram stain was not performed, the patient's past history, intraabdominal pathology, or coexistent catheter infection may help to guide the initial antibiotic selection (76). As empiric therapy, vancomycin is administered in combination with either an aminoglycoside or ceftazidime. Since these combinations are equally effective, ceftazidime may be preferred to avoid the nephrotoxicity and ototoxicity of aminoglycosides. If an aminoglycoside is used, an intermittent dosing regimen

Table 22.12.

Antibiotic Dosing Guidelines For the Treatment of CAPD Peritonitis

	Initial[a] (mg/2 L bag)	Maintenance[a]	
		Intermittent (mg/2 L bag per dosing interval)	Continuous (mg/2 L bag)
Aminoglycosides			
Amikacin	500	150/d	12–15
Gentamicin	70–140	50/d	8–16
Netilmicin	70–140	60/d	8–16
Tobramycin	70–140	50/d	8–16
Cephalosporins			
First-generation			
Cefazolin	500–1000	1000/d	250–500
Cefonicid	250	ND	50
Cephalothin	1000	ND	200
Cephradine	500	ND	250
Cephalexin	1000 PO	500/QID PO	NA
Second-generation			
Cefamandole	1000	1000/d	500
Cefotetan	1000	1000/d	50
Cefoxitin	1000	ND	200
Cefuroxime	1000	ND	150–400
Third-generation			
Cefixime	400 PO	400/d PO	NA
Cefoperazone	2000	ND	400–1000
Cefotaxime	2000	2000/d	500
Ceftazidime	1000	500/d	100–250
Ceftizoxime	1000	1000/d	250
Ceftriaxone	1000	1000/d	250–500
Penicillins			
Azlocillin	500	ND	500
Mezlocillin	3000 IV	3000/BID IV	500
Piperacillin	4000 IV	4000/BID IV	500
Ticarcillin	1000–2000	2000/BID	250
Quinolones			
Ciprofloxacin	750 PO	750/BID PO	50
Fleroxacin	800 PO	400/d PO	NA
Ofloxacin	400 PO	200/d PO	ND
Vancomycin and others			
Vancomycin	1000–2000	1000–2000/7d	30–50
Teicoplanin	400	ND	40[b]
Aztreonam	1000	ND	500
Clindamycin	300	ND	300
Erythromycin	ND	500/QID PO	150
Metronidazole	500 PO/IV	500/TID PO/IV	ND
Rifampin	600 PO	600/d PO	NA
Antifungal agents			
Amphotericin B	1000–2000	1000/BID	100
Flucytosine	1000–2000	1000/BID	100
Ketoconazole	400 PO	200–800/d PO	NA
Miconazole	200	ND	100–200
Combinations			
Ampicillin +	1000–2000	1000/BID	100
Sulbactam	1000–2000	500/BID	100
Imipenem +	500–1000	500/BID	100–200
Cilistatin	500–1000	500/BID	100–200
Sulfamethoxazole +	1600 PO	1600/1–2 d PO	200–400
Trimethoprim	320 PO	320/1–2 d PO	40–80

Source: Adapted with permission from (76).

Abbreviations: NA = not applicable; ND = no data; IV = intravenous; PO = oral; d = once a day; BID = twice a day; TID = three times a day; QID = four times a day.

[a]Doses are for a 70-kg adult. The route of administration is intraperitoneal unless otherwise specified. There is no evidence that mixing different antibiotics in dialysis fluid (except for aminoglycosides and penicillins) is deleterious for the drugs or patients. Do not use the same syringe to mix antibiotics.

[b]This is in each bag × 7 days, then in 2 bags/day × 7 days, and then in 1 bag/day × 7 days.

(e.g., 20 to 25 mg/L/day of gentamicin or 60 mg/L/day of amikacin) is preferred over continuous dosing, since the former provides a more favorable intraperitoneal bactericidal profile (76). Prolonged therapy with aminoglycosides (>2 to 3 weeks) increases the risk of toxicity and should be avoided.

GRAM-NEGATIVE ORGANISMS ON GRAM STAIN

In the rare event that the Gram stain identifies a Gram-negative organism, initial therapy must contain either an aminoglycoside (without a loading dose) or ceftazidime (with a loading dose) (76). A loading dose of aminoglycoside does not increase efficacy and may increase systemic toxicity. The presence of Gram-negative organisms or a polymicrobial infection (Gram-negative and Gram-positive bacteria) may indicate a perforated bowel or viscus, prompting the need for surgical evaluation (76).

GRAM STAIN REVEALS YEAST

Various *Candida* spp. account for 70% of fungal peritonitis cases (78). Aside from rapid sterilization of the peritoneal cavity, the goals of therapy are to prevent peritoneal adhesion formation and to maintain peritoneal membrane permeability. The presence of yeast in the dialysate requires antifungal therapy with oral flucytosine 2 g as a loading dose, followed by 1 g/day, plus intraperitoneal fluconazole 150 mg every 2 days (76).

GRAM-POSITIVE ORGANISMS IN CULTURE

If the culture results indicate the presence of *S. aureus*, *S. epidermidis*, or a streptococcus, treatment with vancomycin is continued for 10 to 14 days (e.g., three weekly doses). If a patient with *S. aureus* or *S. epidermidis* peritonitis does not exhibit clinical improvement within 4 to 5 days, rifampin 600 mg per day should be added to the vancomycin and continued for 3 weeks (76). If the culture reveals *Enterococcus* spp., an aminoglycoside (e.g., gentamicin 20 mg/L x 1 bag/day) must be added to provide synergy. Since *Enterococcus* spp. are usually from a GI source, the possibility of an intraabdominal pathology may need to be pursued (76). For uncomplicated Gram-positive peritonitis, antibiotic treatment may continue for 10 to 14 days, or 7 days after the last positive culture (76,77).

CULTURES ARE NEGATIVE

In 10 to 15% of cases, dialysate cultures may be negative. If within 4 to 5 days the patient is improving with the empiric therapy, with no suggestion of Gram-negative organism on Gram stain, monotherapy with vancomycin for a total of 2 weeks is appropriate. If the empiric antibiotic(s) does not result in clinical improvement, removal of the catheter must be considered (76).

GRAM-NEGATIVE ORGANISMS IN CULTURE

The presence of a Gram-negative organism indicates the possibility of an intraabdominal pathology (e.g., bowel perforation). In such a circumstance, surgical exploration must be considered, especially if a polymicrobial infection is present. With the presence of a single Gram-negative organism (e.g., *Escherichia coli*), the patient should not receive a second vancomycin dose. Instead, depending on the antibiotic sensitivity pattern, therapy should continue for 14 days with either an aminoglycoside, a cephalosporin (e.g., ceftazidime), or an extended-spectrum penicillin (e.g., piperacillin). With the presence of *Pseudomonas* or *Xanthomonas* spp., dual therapy is required (e.g., ceftazidime plus tobramycin) (76). If an extended-spectrum penicillin is to be used with an aminoglycoside, it is best to administer the penicillin intravenously to avoid the intraperitoneal inactivation of the aminoglycoside. Peritonitis caused by *Pseudomonas* or *Xanthomonas* often requires the removal of the peritoneal catheter and 3 to 4 weeks of antibiotic therapy (76).

FUNGAL ORGANISMS IN CULTURE

Previously, catheter removal was uniformly recommended as part of the treatment of fungal peritonitis (83). However, with the availability of the triazole antifungal fluconazole, treatment may commence with the catheter in place, especially for the treatment of nonfilamentous (yeast) peritonitis. Treatment consists of intraperitoneal fluconazole 150 mg every 2 days plus oral or intraperitoneal flucytosine 1 g/day for 4 to 6 weeks. If clinical improvement is not observed within 4 to 7 days, the catheter should be removed. Antifungal treatment should be continued with oral fluconazole 100 mg and flucytosine 1 g daily for 10 days after the catheter is removed (76).

Although amphotericin B has an excellent antifungal spectrum, its intraperitoneal administration is very painful and can cause peritoneal adhesions. Intravenous amphotericin B should be used only to treat nonresponsive cases of fungal peritonitis, especially those caused by filamentous fungi (e.g., *Aspergillus* spp.) (78).

ANAEROBIC ORGANISMS IN CULTURE

The presence of anaerobic organisms is highly suggestive of bowel perforation and requires surgical exploration. In addition, antibiotic therapy is needed in the form of oral or intravenous metronidazole 500 mg every 8 hr plus vancomycin and ceftazidime (76).

Most patients with peritonitis exhibit clinical improvement within 48 hr after the initiation of appropriate treatment. If symptoms persist past 96 hr, the presence of intraabdominal or genitourinary pathology should be suspected. Alternatively, the peritonitis may be due to less-common or fastidious organisms (e.g., mycobacteria) (76).

PREVENTION OF CAPD INFECTIONS

Strategies that are aimed at preventing infections reduce CAPD-related morbidity, method failure, and possibly mortality. Since CAPD requires frequent manipulation of the dialysis catheter through repeated connections and disconnections of the administration set, the patient or caregiver must be trained to observe aseptic techniques. Recent advances in the disconnect systems using the "flush-before-fill" technique (e.g., Y-connector set) has limited the required manipulations during exchanges, thus reducing the incidence of peritonitis and exit-site and tunnel infections caused by touch contamination (75,84–86). This is mainly due to a reduction in *S. epidermidis*, polymicrobial, and other Gram-positive infections (84). Unfortunately, the rates of *S. aureus* and gram-negative infections have not changed (45,84,87).

The nasal carriage of *S. aureus* is an established predisposing factor for peritonitis and tunnel and exit-site infections (85). Up to 60% of dialysis patients are nasal carriers of this organism, compared to 10 to 30% of the general population; the carriage rate is even higher among diabetic patients (9). The nasal eradication of *S. aureus* has the potential to reduce catheter loss after peritonitis or exit-site infection (88). The eradication of nasal *S. aureus* with intranasal mupirocin 2% ointment, administered thrice daily for 7 days, can reduce the incidence of peritonitis and exit-site infection due to *S. aureus* (88); however, the incidence of infections by other Gram-positive and Gram-negative bacteria may simultaneously increase (88). Rifampin administered 300 mg twice daily for 5 consecutive days every 12 weeks can prevent peritonitis and exit-site infections without a significant effect on nasal carriage of *S. aureus* (89). Thus, patients with recurrent CAPD infections may benefit from intermittent treatment with rifampin.

An anti-*S. aureus* vaccine has been developed for reducing the incidence of CAPD infections. It is currently undergoing clinical testing.

Mechanical Complications

Patients who are starting on CAPD often have an arteriovenous fistula placed so that in case the peritoneal dialysis catheter fails, hemodialysis may be started. The vascular access complications that were discussed above also applies to these patients. In addition, defects in the peritoneal catheter, tubing, or dialysate bag may result in leakage of peritoneal fluid from around the exit site and requires immediate replacement of the tubing. Patients with catheter leakage should be treated for peritonitis (72).

Cardiovascular Complications

Because of a slow ultrafiltration rate and the absence of an arteriovenous fistula, many of the cardiovascular compli-

cations that are associated with hemodialysis are less prevalent with CAPD (35). The continuous nature of CAPD prevents the larger and rapid volume shifts of hemodialysis, thus minimizing the risk of rapid reduction in left ventricular pressure and hypotension (35). However, aggressive fluid removal with the use of hypertonic (4.25% hydrous dextrose) solutions can result in hypotension (usually orthostatic) (79). Compared to undialyzed patients, CAPD patients have lower left ventricular end-diastolic and end-systolic volumes, lower stroke index and cardiac index, and a faster myocardial contraction speed (35). Therefore, CAPD is the preferred mode of dialysis for patients with significant cardiovascular disease (e.g., pre-existing left ventricular hypertrophy and coronary artery disease).

Miscellaneous Medical Complications

INCREASED INTRAABDOMINAL PRESSURE

The infusion of peritoneal dialysate increases the intraabdominal pressure by up to fivefold without a significant increase in pressure inside the stomach or at the lower esophageal sphincter (90). This increased intraabdominal pressure can increase the stress on structures of the abdomen and lead to a number of complications, including a sensation of bloating and symptoms of esophageal reflux (72).

ALTERATION OF RESPIRATORY FUNCTION

The dialysate-induced increase in intraabdominal pressure can push against the diaphragm in a manner similar to that observed during pregnancy or obesity. The resulting displacement in diaphragm decreases the functional residual capacity of the lungs. If severe enough, it may lead to small airway collapse, ventilation-perfusion mismatch, and arterial hypoxemia. Paradoxically, a less-severe displacement may actually improve the efficiency of diaphragmatic contraction and improve ventilation (90).

A serious complication of peritoneal dialysis is the leakage of dialysate across the diaphragm, resulting in hydrothorax (i.e., fluid in the pleural cavity) (21). Most patients who develop hydrothorax are female. While mild hydrothorax may be asymptomatic, life-threatening respiratory compromise may occur in severe cases (90). The most common clinical manifestations include dyspnea, chest pain, hypotension, and, in rare instances, atrial fibrillation (91).

The goal of treatment is to resolve the pleural effusion and prevent its recurrence (91). CAPD should be temporarily discontinued until the effusion spontaneously regresses (90). For severe dyspnea or cardiovascular instability a chest tube must be placed to allow draining of fluid (91). If hydrothorax recurs, surgical repair may be necessary. Alternatively, the pleural space can be closed off with talcum powder, iodized talc, triamcinolone acetonide, fibrin adhesive, or autologous blood instillation.

BACK PAIN

The increased intraabdominal pressure places excess stress on the lumbar vertebrae. In the presence of poor abdominal muscle tone, the spinal stress is increased, leading to back pain or sciatica. Treatment involves the use of smaller dialysate volumes (90), although this may compromise dialysis adequacy. The optimal solution may be to start the patient on nighttime intermittent peritoneal dialysis (90).

HERNIAS

Up to one-quarter of CAPD patients may develop a hernia, most commonly at the site of incision for catheter insertion, the inguinal canal, or the umbilicus (90). If the hernia is left untreated, bowel incarceration and strangulation may ensue, requiring emergency surgery. Treatment of hernia involves surgical correction (92).

ABDOMINAL WALL AND GENITAL EDEMA

Although less frequent than hernias, edema of the abdominal wall and genitals is more bothersome for the patient. Edema is caused by tears or defects in the peritoneum and may reach the scrotal or labial area. Treatment involves bed rest and temporary cessation of CAPD (90).

LOSS OF ULTRAFILTRATION

Although rare, a loss of ultrafiltration is troublesome, since, depending on the cause, it may require discontinuation of CAPD. There are two types of ultrafiltration failure. Most cases are Type I failure, in which the permeability of the peritoneal membrane to glucose is increased, resulting in rapid absorption of intraperitoneal glucose and loss of transmembrane osmotic gradient. Although the ability to remove fluid is lost, the clearance of other solutes, such as creatinine or urea, is maintained or even increased, since their removal depends on diffusion. Type I ultrafiltration failure usually occurs in patients who are on long-term CAPD but can also occur during bouts of peritonitis when peritoneal permeability and intraperitoneal glucose absorption are increased. The treatment of Type I ultrafiltration failure involves the use of hypertonic dialysate (4.25%) and more frequent dialysis exchanges (80).

Type II ultrafiltration failure is due to a reduction in effective peritoneal surface area that results from extensive scar tissue formation (fibrosis) and peritoneal adhesions. Permeability to glucose remains normal or is decreased. Type II failure most commonly results from severe and prolonged peritonitis, usually due to *S. aureus* or a fungus, and often necessitates discontinuation of CAPD (80).

ADEQUACY OF PERITONEAL DIALYSIS

Dialysis Quantification

The combined annual mortality and drop-out rates from peritoneal dialysis is 35%, so after 3 years, only 25% of patients remain on peritoneal dialysis. This high attrition rate is similar to the rates of other countries and may be due in part to inadequate dialysis (93); hence, there is a need for a quantitative approach to prescribing CAPD. Currently, there is no established dose-response relationship for CAPD. Until recently, CAPD patients routinely received a standard daily therapy consisting of four 2-L exchanges. For the purpose of quantifying dialysis dose, creatinine rather than BUN was proposed as a marker for quantification of CAPD (93). On the basis of clinical experience, a normalized weekly creatinine clearance of 40 to 50 $L/1.73 m_2$ of body surface area was suggested as providing minimally adequate dialysis (94). On the basis of this estimation, it was determined that the amount of adequate dialysis that is required in CAPD is two-thirds that required in hemodialysis (23, 93). The weekly Kt/V for the standard CAPD regimen of four daily 2-L exchanges is approximately 1.7 (1.5 to 1.8) per week, compared to a weekly Kt/V of 3.0 to 3.6 for hemodialysis (15, 93). The low CAPD Kt/V is similar to the high-TAC_{urea} (i.e., high-failure) groups in the NCDS; however, the mortality rates are similar to those of the general hemodialysis population (15). There are two explanations for this incongruity. First, because of its continuous nature, CAPD is performed 168 hr/week, compared to about 12 hr/week for hemodialysis. Therefore, as is seen in Figure 22.4, the concentrations of blood urea (or other uremic toxins) with CAPD are at a relatively constant steady state, whereas a sawtooth profile is observed with hemodialysis (i.e., peak predialysis concentrations followed by trough postdialysis concentrations) (15). This discrepancy in the minimum dialysis dose between the two modalities led to the development of the "peak concentration hypothesis" (95). This hypothesis states that uremic signs and symptoms may be associated with peak BUN concentrations; therefore, hemodialysis requires a higher dialysis dose to achieve a peak BUN concentration at or below the steady-state concentration with CAPD. On the basis of this hypothesis, the weekly Kt/V required for minimally adequate CAPD was estimated at 1.7, equivalent to a weekly hemodialysis Kt/V of 2.6 (96). This hypothesis has since been supported by clinical studies (15, 93, 96).

The second reason for the discrepant minimum dialysis dose requirements is that residual renal function is better preserved during CAPD than during hemodialysis (10, 50). To illustrate, in calculating Kt/V for urea, K should include both dialyzer and renal clearances. For example, CAPD and hemodialysis may both provide a dialysis dose that is equivalent to a glomerular filtration rate (GFR) of 0.6 L/hr (10 mL/min); however, if the CAPD patient has a native

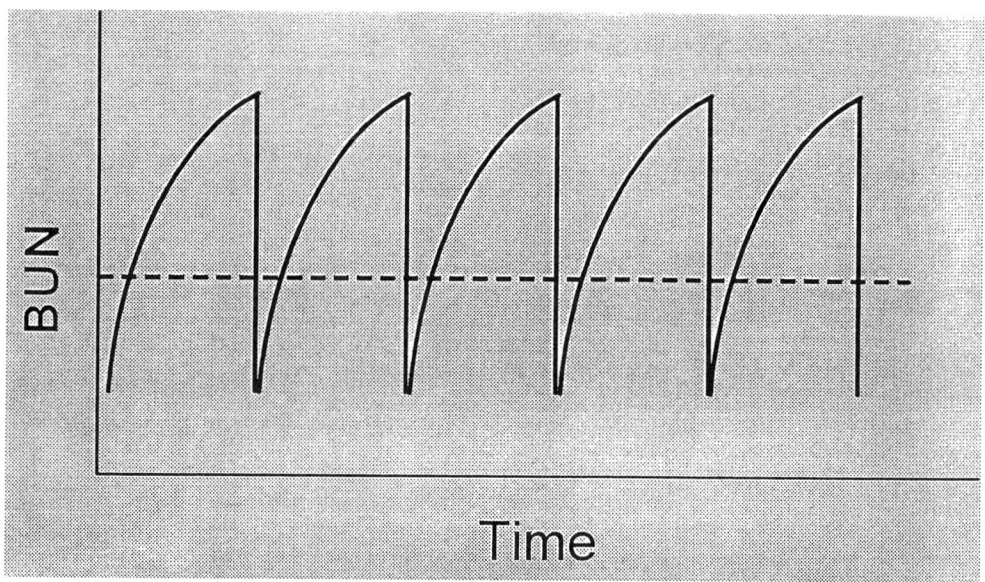

Figure 22.4. The BUN concentration-time profile hemodialysis (solid line) and CAPD (dashed curve).

GFR of 0.3 L/hr (5 mL/min) while the hemodialysis patient has lost all residual renal function, the CAPD patient will have a 50% higher effective urea clearance.

There is a strong correlation between weekly creatinine clearance and Kt/V (15). Recently, urea has been proposed as a marker solute (93). However, both urea and creatinine kinetics can predict clinical outcome in CAPD patients, although creatinine appears to be a more sensitive predictor of outcome (97). The Kt/V method of assessing dialysis adequacy offers two additional advantages: it allows the assessment of dietary protein intake, and it allows for prospective prescription of a dialysis dose, rather than calculating the dose in retrospect (61). The use of urea modeling (Kt/V) together with weekly creatinine clearance values provides a more useful method of assessing the adequacy of dialysis (61). With the scarcity of well-controlled studies assessing the adequacy of peritoneal dialysis, a minimum weekly Kt/V of 2.0 has been recommended on the basis of uncontrolled studies (93).

Effect of Nutrition and Dietary Protein Intake

CAPD patients lose approximately 6 g/day of albumin and 9 g/day of total protein into the dialysate. This amount is increased to 15 g/day during bouts of peritonitis. As in hemodialysis, a low serum albumin concentration (≤35 g/L or 3.5 g/dL) is a strong predictor of morbidity and mortality in the CAPD population (61). The dietary protein intake of CAPD patients depends on the dose of dialysis, such that for a malnourished and underdialyzed patient an increase in the dialysis dose will result within a few weeks in increased dietary protein intake (16, 55). For a given dose of dialysis (Kt/V), CAPD provides a higher dietary protein intake than hemodialysis, possibly because of improved

appetite and well-being associated with CAPD's enhanced removal of middle molecules (93). Since studies assessing the adequacy of peritoneal dialysis on the basis of urea kinetics are lacking, the aim should be a PCR of ≥0.8 g/kg/day and possibly ≥1.2 g/kg/day (56), the number of dialysis exchanges being adjusted to allow the lowest practical BUN concentration in this setting (23). According to these criteria a substantial number of CAPD patients in the United States are currently being underdialyzed (93).

Since in peritoneal dialysis the dialyzer surface area cannot be altered, adjustment of dialysis dose involves alterations in (a) the number of daily exchanges and dwell time, (b) the volume of the dialysate, and/or (c) the osmolarity of the dialysate. Table 22.13 depicts the influence of altering the number of daily exchanges on CAPD weekly clearances of certain solutes (15). Since small solute transport (e.g., for urea, creatinine, hydrogen ion, potassium, and phosphate) is limited by dialysate flow (i.e., dialysate volume/day) and large solutes are limited by the membrane pore size(s), increasing the number of daily exchanges has a more profound effect on small solute removal (15).

Recommendations

Much like hemodialysis, the assessment of dialysis adequacy must be multidimensional and include parameters such as BUN, PCR, Kt/V, and creatinine clearance. Assessment of urea and creatinine clearances must include the contribution from residual renal function. Dialysis therapy should aim not at a target BUN, but rather at a high enough Kt/V that achieves optimal dietary protein intake and nutritional status. In the presence of adequate nutrition (dietary protein intake 1.2 g/kg/day; 35 kcal/kg/

Table 22.13.
Effect of Altering Daily CAPD Exchanges on Solute Clearances[a]

Solute	2 Exchanges	3 Exchanges	4 Exchanges	5 Exchanges
Urea	63%	83%	100%	115%
Creatinine	66%	85%	100%	112%
Vitamin B_{12}	82%	93%	100%	105%
Insulin	89%	96%	100%	103%
β_2-Microglobulin	92%	97%	100%	102%

Source: Adapted with permission from (15).
[a]The standard 4×2 L exchange per day is used as the basis for comparison.

day) the delivered weekly Kt/V should be at least 1.72 (51) and possibly as high as 2.1 (61). Alternatively, a weekly creatinine clearance (CAPD plus renal clearance) of 50 L/1.73 m_2 of body surface area may be used as the target (51). Patients should be monitored monthly for protein-calorie malnutrition; the monitoring should include body weight (measured with an empty peritoneum) and serum concentrations of albumin and transferrin. In addition, dietary intake should be monitored at least every 6 months (51). Adequacy of dialysis should be determined every 3 months (61).

THE CHOICE OF MODALITIES

The choice of one dialysis method over another depends on several personal, medical, economic, and psychosocial factors. However, in certain situations the patient may not have a choice in selecting a mode of renal replacement therapy. For example, if a patient has lost all viable vascular sites for placement of an arteriovenous fistula, CAPD will be the only choice. Similarly, hemodialysis may be the only remaining choice for a CAPD patient who has lost all ultrafiltration capacity owing to peritoneal fibrosis.

Which Method in Which Condition?

The answer to the question "Which method in which condition?" depends on the effect of hemodialysis and CAPD on several aspects of morbidity and mortality. In many clinical situations the use of peritoneal dialysis is preferred to hemodialysis (Table 22.14) (21, 38, 74). Since the hemodialysis procedure routinely requires the use of heparin to prevent fistula clotting, CAPD will be more suitable for a patient with bleeding diathesis. Similarly, the rapid removal of fluid and electrolytes during hemodialysis stresses the heart to an extent that a patient with coronary artery disease may not be able to tolerate. Hence, such patients may benefit from the slow and continuous nature of CAPD (21).

EASE OF BLOOD PRESSURE CONTROL

Treatment of hypertension in ESRD patients is difficult and often requires multiple drugs. Because of its stable control of sodium and water balance, control of hyperten-

Table 22.14.
Potential Advantages and Disadvantages of CAPD Compared to Standard Hemodialysis

Advantages	Disadvantages
Steady-state biochemical parameters	Excessive glucose load
Hemodynamic stability (slow and sustained ultrafiltration)	Continued necessity for sterile exchange
Better removal of larger molecules (e.g., β_2-microglobulin)	Requires patient motivation and compliance
Better preservation of residual renal function	Higher protein loss
No need for heparin	Peritonitis
Lesser degree of anemia	Increased intraabdominal pressure
Lower serum PTH concentration	Higher mortality among older (>40 years) diabetic patients
Lower incidence of high-turnover bone disease	
Higher aluminum clearance	
Lower mortality among younger (≤40 years) diabetic patients	
Possibly better among older non-diabetics	
Easier access for dialysis	
No machine dependence	
Allows long-distance travel	
Allows uninterrupted employment and social activities	
Better glycemic control with intraperitoneal insulin	

sion is easier in CAPD patients than in hemodialysis patients. In fact, a significant number of CAPD patients may not require antihypertensive drugs (38, 74).

SLOW AND SUSTAINED ULTRAFILTRATION

Rapid fluid removal during a typical thrice-weekly hemodialysis session causes intravascular fluid volume depletion leading to hypotension. In predisposed individuals, sustained hypotension may lead to complications of ischemic vascular disease, such as stroke and myocardial infarction (38). Owing to its slower rate of ultrafiltration and its consequent lack of effect on blood pressure during treatment, patients with severe cardiovascular disease (e.g., diabetics) may benefit from CAPD (35, 38).

PRESERVATION OF RENAL RESIDUAL FUNCTION

Residual renal function, even at low levels, has significant clinical importance, including a substantial contribution to the removal of small solutes and middle molecules (Table 22.15) (15,50). In addition, the increased removal of sodium, potassium, phosphate, and hydrogen ions allows for a less restrictive fluid and dietary intake (38, 50). Compared to hemodialysis, CAPD preserves residual renal function for a longer period (50). This may be due to (a) better removal of toxins involved in residual nephron damage, (b) preservation or enhancement of growth factors that are beneficial to the GFR and renal blood flow, (c) less ischemic injury to the kidneys because of a more stable hemodynamic status (10), and (d) lack of membrane-induced inflammatory changes (e.g., production of tumor necrosis factor and interleukin-1), which may cause vascular or immunologic renal injury (38).

Because of better-preserved residual kidney capacity, and perhaps a better chance of later recovery of some renal function, CAPD is recommended for patients who have uncontrolled hypertension, heart failure, severe nephrotic syndrome, rapidly progressive renal failure, analgesic nephropathy, chronic urinary obstruction, and cholesterol emboli (50).

EFFECT ON ANEMIA

Virtually all patients with chronic renal failure develop a normocytic, normochromic anemia. Without treatment the hematocrit stabilizes at between 20 and 25%. Causes include (a) reduced erythropoietin synthesis by the kidneys, (b) decreased red blood cell survival, (c) GI bleeding, (d) presence of inhibitors of erythropoiesis (e.g., aluminum, PTH), and (e) blood loss due to hemodialysis (40). Hemodialysis patients are usually more anemic and have a higher blood transfusion requirement than CAPD patients do, mostly because of lesser availability of endogenous erythropoietin (98). CAPD patients have higher erythropoietin concentrations because of (a) higher clearance of uremic toxins, which may inhibit erythropoietin production; (b) the production of erythropoietin by stimulated peritoneal macrophages (due to infusion of

Table 22.15.
Clinical Importance of Residual Renal Function

Maintenance of endocrine functions of the kidneys
   Erythropoietin synthesis
   Conversion of vitamin D to its active form
   Elimination of the natural β_2-microglobulin
   Insulin metabolism
   PTH metabolism
Increased urea clearance
Better volume control
Improved adequacy of dialysis

dialysate); and (c) better preservation of residual renal function (50,98).

EFFECT ON MINERAL METABOLISM AND RENAL BONE DISEASE

Hypocalcemia associated with hyperphosphatemia, hyperparathyroidism, and vitamin D resistance is frequently encountered in chronic renal failure and can lead to secondary complications such as renal osteodystrophy (i.e., defective bone formation), myocardial calcification, and myocardial fibrosis. Chronic renal failure is associated with two general types of bone disease: high-turnover disease, which is characterized by fibrous tissues in the bone marrow, and low-turnover disease, which is characterized by osteomalacia (gradual softening and bending of the bones) (99, 100). Hyperparathyroidism is the main cause of high-turnover bone disease, although metabolic acidosis may worsen the condition. The major cause of low-turnover bone disease is aluminum intoxication (from aluminum-based phosphate binders) (99).

Although there is controversy about the comparative effectiveness of CAPD versus hemodialysis for aluminum overloading, it is known that the daily clearance of aluminum with CAPD is greater than that with hemodialysis. Furthermore, since most of the plasma aluminum is bound to transferrin, a protein that is lost in significant amounts in the peritoneal dialysate, CAPD may have a higher effective aluminum clearance than standard hemodialysis does (99).

Compared to patients on hemodialysis, CAPD patients have a lower incidence of high-turnover bone disease, mostly for two reasons. First, CAPD has a higher clearance of PTH. Second, with CAPD the serum ionized calcium is increased because of absorption of calcium from the peritoneal dialysate; therefore, the calcium-induced suppression of PTH secretion is significantly higher with CAPD (33). Given the potential cardiotoxicity of PTH (34), a lower serum PTH concentration with CAPD provides a theoretical advantage over hemodialysis.

CHOICE FOR PATIENTS WITH DIABETES

Since diabetic patients who are on dialysis often have a worse prognosis than nondiabetics do (4), kidney transplantation is clearly the preferred mode of renal replacement therapy (38). Nearly half of diabetic ESRD patients do not survive beyond 2 years, and fewer than 20% are capable of any activity beyond personal care (74). These patients often start on dialysis with advanced comorbid conditions (e.g., coronary artery disease), which often progress during the course of dialysis. Furthermore, since younger diabetic patients with minimal comorbid conditions are often selected for transplantation, the remaining dialysis patients have far-advanced coexisting conditions that increase the incidence of mortality (38). Therefore, it is not surprising that diabetic patients require a higher dose of dialysis than do nondiabetics (15).

Among the benefits of CAPD is the ability to use the intraperitoneal route for the administration of insulin. The bioavailability of intraperitoneal insulin is approximately 50% after an 8-hr dwell time. Intraperitoneal insulin diffuses across the visceral peritoneum into the portal venous circulation. Within the liver, insulin inhibits glycogenolysis, gluconeogenesis, and ketogenesis and stimulates the synthesis of glycogen and fatty acids (38, 101). This absorption profile allows for a better glycemic control of patients and a lower risk of hypoglycemia, possibly because of the presence of a basal insulin concentration (38). For a given insulin dose, the intraperitoneal administration produces lower serum insulin concentrations than subcutaneous insulin does; however, the intraperitoneal administration allows a more rapid, consistent, and physiologic absorption of insulin. The lower serum concentrations following intraperitoneal insulin administration may be important in view of the increasing evidence implicating hyperinsulinemia as an atherogenic risk factor (38).

Technique Failure

In CAPD, peritonitis is the most common cause of technique failure, accounting for 40 to 47% of cases. Loss of peritoneal function (15 to 19%), and access-related problems (9 to 15%) are other common causes of drop-outs. The most common causes of technique failure with hemodialysis are cardiovascular instability and loss of vascular access. The rate of method failure rate is higher with CAPD; however, if peritonitis is removed as a cause, the failure rates are similar (79).

Mortality

Mortality rates with CAPD and hemodialysis are similar, cardiovascular causes being responsible for 27 to 43% and 25 to 42% of deaths in CAPD and hemodialysis patients, respectively (79). In general, diabetic patients have a worse prognosis with CAPD; however, it appears that patients who are 40 years of age or younger have better survival on peritoneal dialysis, while patients who are older than 40 years of age have better outcomes on hemodialysis (102). This may be because older diabetic patients, who usually have advanced comorbid conditions such as cardiovascular disease, are preferentially chosen for peritoneal dialysis (38). However, the CAPD mortality rate may be lower for older nondiabetic patients (79). Since the use of biocompatible hemodialysis membranes may result in lower mortality rates, their recent popularity may translate in a few years into a lowered hemodialysis mortality rate.

PHARMACOTHERAPEUTIC CONSIDERATIONS FOR DIALYSIS PATIENTS

Patients who receive chronic dialysis therapy require dose modification for most commonly used drugs (103, 104).

The disposition of drugs that depend largely on the kidney for elimination (i.e., the fraction that is excreted unchanged by the kidney exceeds 60%) may be influenced greatly by changes in renal function. Furthermore, the pharmacokinetics of many drugs that are eliminated predominantly by hepatic routes may also be markedly affected by the development of severe renal insufficiency (105). In addition to these changes in renal and nonrenal clearances, alterations in protein binding and volume of distribution may markedly alter the serum concentration-time profile of a drug relative to that of subjects who have normal renal function (106). Thus, during the development process, all new drugs should be evaluated for patients with renal insufficiency. This information can then form the basis for individualization of drug therapy regimens for dialysis patients.

The effects of the hemodialysis or peritoneal dialysis procedure itself on the pharmacokinetic characteristics of a drug (and thus its serum concentration-time profile) are complex. Since multiple dialysis filters are available and several techniques are currently in use for the delivery of hemodialysis therapy, use of yes-or-no information in terms of dialyzability is inappropriate. Rather, references that provide quantitative estimates of the effect of hemodialysis or peritoneal dialysis on the elimination half-life or total body clearance of a drug should be used (81, 107). A compilation of data for many commonly used antibiotics is given in Table 22.16. This data, coupled with specific information about the type of dialysis procedure used, can be extrapolated to individual patient situations. This clearance information, together with the estimated patient-specific pharmacokinetic parameters, can be used to design a dosing regimen for a given drug for a patient who is receiving dialysis. For the patient who is on dialysis the clearance of the drug from the plasma (Cl_d) can be defined as the sum of the patient's residual renal clearance (Cl_{pt}), the nonrenal clearance (Cl_{nr}), and the dialysis clearance (Cl_{hd} or Cl_{pd}):

$$Cl_d = Cl_{pt} + Cl_{nr} + Cl_{hd} \qquad (22.5)$$

The characteristics of a drug that have the most favorable impact upon its dialyzability include a low molecular weight, low protein binding, a small volume of distribution, a rapid rate of equilibration between tissue binding sites and blood, and a limited amount of nonrenal metabolism and excretion. The additional effect of dialysis clearance is not usually considered important unless the procedure increases overall plasma clearance by at least 30% (107) and/or the fractional drug removal by dialysis exceeds 0.30 (108).

Drug Dosing in Hemodialysis

The actual amount of drug that is removed by hemodialysis is the product of the concentration of the drug in the

Table 22.16.

Effect of Hemodialysis and Intermittent Peritoneal Dialysis on the Clearance and Half-life of Selected Drugs

	$t_{1/2}$ (hr)		Effect of Dialysis			
Drug	Normal	ESRD	$t_{1/2}$ HD	CL_{HD}	$t_{1/2}$ PERITONEAL DIALYSIS	CL_{PD}
Amikacin	1.6	39	3.8–5.5	30–36	18–26	6.7
Ampicillin	1.3	10–20	2.9–5.0	30–154	ND	ND
Azlocillin	0.9	5.1	2.2	ND	2.5	ND
Aztreonam	2.0	7.0	2.7	43	7.0	2.1
Carbenicillin	1.0	18.2	4.3	39.6	ND	ND
Cefaclor	0.7	2.5	1.6	75	ND	ND
Cefamandole	1.0	10.4	4–7	29	7.2	10.2
Cefazolin	2.2	28.0	2.6–5.0	NR	32	NR
Cefmetazole	1.3	29.4	1.5–3.3	86	ND	ND
Cefonicid	4.4	67.0	3.4	NR	ND	ND
Cefotetan	3.0	13.1	9.4/5.7	NR	ND	ND
Cefoxitin	0.8	13–25	4	NR	NR	1.5
Cefoperazone	1.8	2.3	Reduced	NR	ND	ND
Cefotaxime	0.9	2.5	1.9–3.4	14–40	2.9–4.4	NR
Ceftazidime	1.8	26.0	2.8	27–50	8.7	8.5
Ceftizoxime	1.6	28.1	5.3	45	ND	ND
Ceftriaxone	8.0	15.0	16	31	ND	ND
Cefuroxime	1.3	15–22	3.5	NR	11.8	4.7
Cephalexin	0.8	19.0	4.5	25	ND	ND
Chloramphenicol	3.4	5.3	3.2	21–54	ND	ND
Cinoxacin	2.1	9.0	ND	ND	ND	ND
Ciprofloxacin	4.4	8.4–12	3–5.5	29.6–47	ND	ND
Clavulanic acid	1.0	4.3	NR	141	ND	ND
Clindamycin	2.2–3.3	1.9–3.4	1.6–3.1	NR	ND	ND
Cloxacillin	0.6	2.0	NR	NR	ND	ND
Dicloxacillin	0.7	2.2	NR	NR	ND	ND
Erythromycin	2.1	4.0	0.8	28.5	ND	ND
Gentamicin	2.2	53	5.2–11.3	24–47	8.5	12.5
Imipenem	0.9	2.9	1.0	84	ND	ND
Metronidazole	7.9	7.7	2.8	58–125	5.6	15.8
Mezlocillin	1.0	4.3	2.0	28.7	2.1	7.4
Nafcillin	1.0	2.1	NR	0	ND	ND
Netilmicin	2.1	42	3.7–5.2	38–65	ND	ND
Norfloxacin	3.1–7.4	6.5–9.0	ND	ND	ND	ND
Ofloxacin	5–8	28–38	NR	116	ND	ND
Penicillin G	0.7	4.1	2.3	37.5	ND	ND
Piperacillin	1.2	3.9	1.3–2.4	74	ND	ND
Sulfamethoxazole	10	13.3	3.2–11.1	21–84	13–18	1.2
Sulfisoxazole	6.0	11.0	6.0	ND	ND	ND
Ticarcillin	1.2	14.8	3.4	33	10.6	7.2
Tobramycin	2.5	58	4.3–6.7	31–70	25	4.7
Trimethoprim	14	26–40	5–9.4	29–66	17–24	5.1
Vancomycin	6.9	161	NR	16.1	30–43	2.3–14.2

Abbreviations: $t_{1/2}$ = terminal half-life; $t_{1/2}$ HD = half-life during hemodialysis (hr); CL_{HD} = hemodialyzer clearance (mL/min); $t_{1/2}$ HD = half-life during peritoneal dialysis (hr); CL_{PD} = peritoneal dialysis clearance (mL/min); ND = no data; NR = not reported.

recovered dialysate and the dialysate volume. This value divided by the total body stores of the drug before dialysis (product of predialysis concentration and volume of distribution) yields the actual fraction of drug removed by dialysis (FDR). It is often not clinically feasible or analytically practical to measure dialysate drug concentrations. Several methods to predict the FDR have been proposed (108). It is important before using these formulas to differentiate clearance by dialysis (Cl_{hd}) from the clearance during dialysis (Cl_d); the latter equals the sum of the patient's residual endogenous clearance ($Cl_{pt} + Cl_{nr}$) and Cl_{hd}. The fractional drug removal by dialysis may be calculated as follows:

$$FDR = (Cl_{hd} \div Cl_d) \times (1 - e^{-\frac{Cl_d}{V_d}})$$ (22.6)

where V_d is the volume of distribution of the drug and t is the time of dialysis.

Alternatively, FDR may be estimated by using the off-dialysis and during-dialysis elimination rate constants. Again, the overall elimination rate constant, K_d, must be differentiated from the dialysis elimination rate constant, K_{hd}, and the patient's residual elimination rate constant, K_{pt}. The off-dialysis half-life divided into 0.693 yields K_{pt}, and 0.693 divided by the half-life during-dialysis yields K_d. The dialysis elimination rate constant $K_{hd} = K_d - K_{pt}$. Therefore, FDR may also be calculated as follows:

$$FDR = (K_{hd} \div K_d \times (1 - e^{-K_d \times t}) \qquad (22.7)$$

FDR assessment may help to optimize individualized drug therapy for hemodialysis patients. For several drugs the clearance and half-life on and off dialysis have been determined (Table 22.16). If, for example, a dialysis patient received 1 g of cefmetazole intravenously just before 3 hr of dialysis, the FDR, by using literature values for clearance (Table 22.16) and steady-state volume of distribution (14 L or 0.19 L/kg) (109), could be calculated as follows:

Cefmetazole clearance off dialysis, Cl_{pt}, is 0.38 L/hr.
Cefmetazole clearance by dialysis, Cl_{hd}, is 5.17 L/hr.

$$Cl_d = Cl_{pt} + Cl_{hd}$$

$$Cl_d = 0.38 \text{ L/hr} + 5.17 \text{ L/hr}$$

$$= 5.55 \text{ L/hr} \qquad (22.8)$$

$$FDR = (5.17 \text{ L/hr} \div 5.55 \text{ L/hr}) \times (1 - e^{-5.55 \text{ L/hr} + 14L \times 3hr})$$

$$= (0.932)(0.696)$$

$$= 0.648$$

The FDR can also be calculated by using elimination rate constants, as follows:

Cefmetazole half-life off dialysis is 29.4 hr.

$$K_{pt} = \frac{0.693}{t_{1/2}}$$

$$K_{pt} = 0.693/29.4 \text{ hr} \qquad (22.9)$$

$$= 0.0236 \text{ hr}^{-1}$$

Cefmetazole half-life during dialysis is 2.1 hr.

$$K_d = 0.693/2.1 \text{ hr} = 0.33 \text{ hr}^{-1}$$

Thus,

$$K_{hd} = K_d - K_{pt}$$

$$K_{hd} = 0.33 - 0.0236$$

$$= 0.306 \text{ hr}^{-1} \qquad (22.10)$$

$$FDR = (0.306 \text{ hr}^{-1} \div 0.33 \text{ hr}^{-1}) \times (1 - e^{-0.33 \times 3 \text{ hr}})$$

$$= 0.583$$

The FDR can serve as an index of the relative dialyzability of various drugs and can aid in determining whether or not an adjustment must be made to optimize a patient's dosage regimen.

Endogenous clearance of a drug during the period between dialyses may also affect the design of the drug regimen. Knowledge of the amount of drug that is removed both during and between dialysis treatments is often necessary to design an optimal therapeutic regimen. Patients may require postdialytic or interdialytic dosing when the maintenance of serum concentrations within a narrow range is necessary to maximize efficacy or minimize toxicity. Unfortunately, accurate information on the dialysis kinetics of many drugs is not readily available (110). However, if one assumes that drug removal by dialysis and during the interdialytic period follows first-order kinetics-that is, that the drug concentration declines monoexponentially depending on the clearance, the volume of distribution, and the time between observations-then the serum concentration-time profile and dosing regimen for an individual patient may be predicted, as is demonstrated in the following case example.

Case Study

A.L. is a 70-kg nonsmoking female who has been maintained on hemodialysis for 2 years. Because of an acute exacerbation of her asthmatic condition, intravenous theophylline therapy with desired peak and trough concentrations of 19 and 11 mg/L, respectively, is to be initiated.

WHAT IS THE INITIAL LOADING DOSE THAT SHOULD BE ADMINISTERED TO ACHIEVE A PEAK CONCENTRATION OF 19 MG/L?

The first step is to calculate the patient's volume of distribution (V_d):

$$V_d = V_d^* \times \text{total body weight} \qquad (22.11)$$

where V_d^* is the average value for dialysis patients, derived from the literature, expressed in liters per kilogram. The initial loading dose (LD) can then be calculated as

$$LD = C_{max} \times V_d \qquad (22.12)$$

where C_{max} is the desired peak concentration. Pharmacokinetic data from the literature indicates that the mean theophylline volume of distribution is 0.5 L/kg and the desired C_{max} is 19 mg/L. Thus, the V_d is 35 L, and the LD is 665 mg.

WHAT MAINTENANCE DOSE AND DOSING INTERVAL ARE REQUIRED TO MAINTAIN THE DESIRED PEAK AND TROUGH CONCENTRATIONS IF THIS PATIENT IS NOT DIALYZED?

The dosing interval (τ) can be calculated as follows, where C_{min} is the desired trough concentration and Cl_{pt} is the total body clearance (approximately 1.4 L/hr) during the interdialytic period:

$$\tau = \frac{[\ln C_{max} - \ln C_{min}]}{(Cl_{pt} \div V_d)} \quad (22.13)$$

The maintenance dose (MD) can be calculated as:

$$MD = [C_{max} \times V_d][1 - e^{-\frac{Cl_{pt}}{V_d}\tau}] \quad (22.14)$$

The values calculated for τ and MD must be rounded off to clinically feasible values. For this example the calculated τ is 13.7 hr, which should be rounded to 12 hr. This value is used to calculate the MD, which is thus 252.7 mg every 12 hr. This is not feasible clinically; thus 250 mg every 12 hr is the most practical dosing regimen during the interdialytic period. Since τ and MD have been altered from the values that were calculated by using the desired C_{max} and C_{min}, the C_{max} associated with the new regimen (250 mg every 12 hr) can be calculated as

$$C_{max} = \frac{MD}{V_d \times [1 - e^{-\frac{Cl_{pt}}{V_d}\tau}]} \quad (22.15)$$

The C_{min} can be calculated as

$$C_{min} = C_{max} \times e^{-\frac{Cl_{pt}}{V_d}\tau} \quad (22.16)$$

Substitution of this patient's pharmacokinetic parameters into these two equations results in a C_{max} of 18.8 mg/L and a C_{min} of 11.9 mg/L.

WHAT IS THIS PATIENT'S THEOPHYLLINE SERUM CONCENTRATION BEFORE DIALYSIS?

The concentration before dialysis (CbD) depends on the attained C_{max} as well as the Cl_{pt}, V_d, and time from attainment of C_{max} to the start of dialysis (t). If this patient is to start dialysis 4 hr after the administration of theophylline, the CbD is

$$CbD = C_{max} \times e^{-\frac{Cl_{pt}}{V_d}t}$$

$$CbD = (18.8 \text{ mg/L}) \times e^{-(1.4L/hr/35L)4hr}$$

$$= 18.8 \text{ mg/L} \times 0.85 \quad (22.17)$$

$$= 16 \text{ mg/L}$$

whereas if dialysis is initiated at the end of the dosing interval (i.e., 11.5 hr after the attainment of C_{max}), the CbD is approximately 11.9 mg/L.

To know how much drug, if any, to give as a supplemental dose, the effect of dialysis on the plasma concentration-time profile must be determined. The most critical new piece of information that is required to calculate this value is the dialysis clearance of theophylline, which has been reported to vary from approximately 1.2 to 6.0 L/hr (20 to 100 mL/min) (35). Thus, it is critical to know the type of dialysis filter to be used, the clearance of theophylline by this filter, and the duration of dialysis (tD).

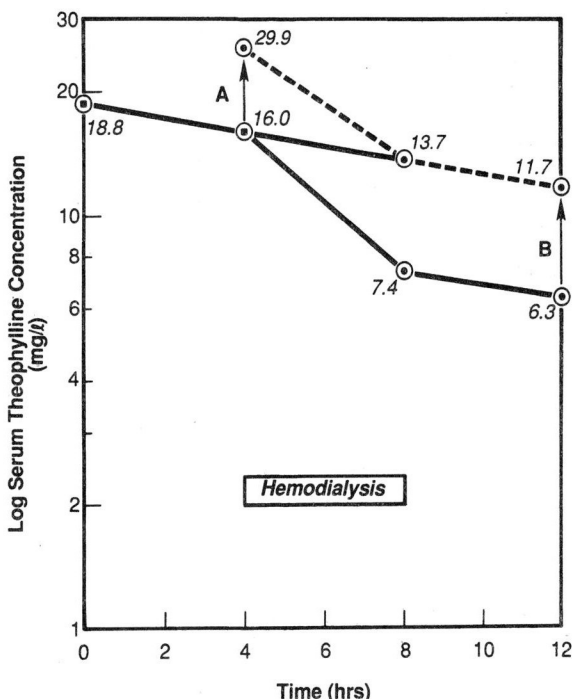

Figure 22.5. The serum concentration time profile of theophylline in the case study patient in the predialysis, dialysis, and postdialysis periods. If it is desired to maintain the same C_{min}, then the serum concentration immediately after administration of the dose bD (A) would increase to 29.9 mg/L. If it is desired to maintain the same C_{max} the serum concentration will decrease to 7.4 mg/L at the end of dialysis, and the C_{min} will thus be 6.3 mg/L. A dose aD of 437 mg would then be required to reachieve the C_{max}, and increase of 187 mg above the usual maintenance dose (B).

WHAT WILL THE POSTDIALYSIS THEOPHYLLINE CONCENTRATION (CaD) BE?

The clearance by dialysis (Cl_{hd}) is approximately 90 mL/min or 5.4 L/hr, and the duration of dialysis is 4 hr. Therefore, the total clearance during dialysis (Cl_d) is approximately 6.8 L/hr. Substitution of this value into equation (22.18) results in the prediction that the serum concentration of theophylline after dialysis will be 46% of the concentration at the start of dialysis:

$$CaD = CbD_{max} \times e^{-(\frac{Cl_{pt}+Cl_{hd}}{V_d})tD}$$

$$CaD = 16 \text{ mg/L} \times e^{-[(5.4L/hr+1.4Lhr)/35L]4hr}$$

$$= 16 \text{ mg/L} \times 0.46 \quad (22.18)$$

$$= 7.4 \text{ mg/L}$$

All the data that is necessary to calculate the supplemental dose needed to maintain the desired serum concentration-time profile is now available. There are three options in terms of the desired concentration-time profile (Fig. 22.5). The optimal choice depends on the patient's clinical status and the relationship of response to specific serum concentrations. The first option is to allow the plasma concentration to decline below the desired C_{min} for the duration of the dialysis procedure and to give a larger dose than the usual maintenance dose (dose aD) to achieve the desired maximum concentration.

HOW IS DOSE AD CALCULATED?

Dose aD is calculated as follows:

$$\text{Dose aD} = V_d \times (C_{max} - C\tau D) \qquad (22.19)$$

where $C\tau D$ is the concentration at the end of the dosing interval on the dialysis day and is calculated as follows:

$$C\tau D = CaD \times e^{-\frac{Cl_{pt}}{V_d}taD} \qquad (22.20)$$

where taD is the time from the end of dialysis to the end of the dosing interval. In this example, taD is 4 hours. Thus,

$$C\tau D = 7.4 \text{ mg/L} \times 0.85$$

$$= 6.3 \text{ mg/L}$$

$$\text{Dose aD} = 35 \text{ L} \times (18.8 \text{ mg/L} - 6.3 \text{ mg/L})$$

$$= 437.5 \text{ mg}$$

This value must be rounded to a clinically useful value of 400 to 450 mg.

Alternatively, a dose can be administered before dialysis (dose bD) to maintain the same minimum serum concentration as on a nondialysis day.

WHAT METHOD ESTIMATES THE DOSE BD?

The dose bD can be estimated as follows:

$$\text{Dose bD} = \frac{[(C_{min} \div e^{-(\frac{Cl_{pt}}{V_d})taD}) \times V_d]}{e^{-(\frac{Cl_{pt} + Cl}{V_d})tD}} - (CbD \times V_d)$$

$$\text{Dose bD} = [\{(11.7/0.85) \times 35L\}/0.46] - 560$$

$$= [480/0.46] - 560 \qquad (22.21)$$

$$= 1045 - 560$$

$$= 485 \text{ mg}$$

To accomplish this, one must accept the potential adverse effects resulting from a higher serum concentration early in dialysis. In this case the C_{max} after this dose would be approximately 30 mg/L.

The last alternative is for individuals receiving a continuous infusion of theophylline. In this situation, one can calculate the continuous infusion rate (dose D) that is needed during the dialysis period to maintain the desired steady-state average serum concentration (C_{ss}).

WHAT IS THE INFUSION RATE THAT WOULD BE REQUIRED TO MAINTAIN A C_{ss} OF 14.9 MG/L IN THIS PATIENT?

The dose D can be estimated as follows:

$$\text{Dose D} = C_{ss} \times (Cl_{pt} + Cl_{hd}) \qquad (22.22)$$

In this example the dose D that is required during dialysis is

$$\text{Dose D} = (14.9 \text{ mg/L}) \times (6.8 \text{ L/hr})$$

$$= 101 \text{ mg/hr}$$

This value is approximately five times the infusion rate of 21 mg/hr that is required to maintain the C_{ss} of 14.9 mg/L during the interdialytic period.

Unfortunately, few clinicians have the patience to endure exercises like this. It is often easier to follow standard general guidelines for dosing, hence the widespread use of tables and nomograms. In the future, however, the availability of therapeutic drug-concentration monitoring coupled with more specific data on the dialyzability of drugs is likely to take clinical drug dosing for the dialysis patient out of the realm of "best guess."

Drug Dosing in CAPD

Factors that increase drug removal by peritoneal dialysis include a low molecular weight, low protein binding, a small volume of distribution, a rapid rate of equilibration between tissue binding sites and blood, and a limited amount of nonrenal metabolism and excretion. Keller and colleagues described several factors that may limit drug removal by CAPD: (a) a low dialysate outflow rate, (b) a low dialysate-to-body ratio of volumes of distribution, (c) a low peritoneal-to-body clearance ratio, and (d) drug protein binding (82). As a general rule, if the amount of drug that is removed by peritoneal dialysis is more than 20 to 30% of the administered dose, supplemental doses are required (81). Lower values are less significant because of the large intersubject variability in the pharmacokinetics of many drugs. Aminoglycosides, most cephalosporins, and probably vancomycin (inconsistent data reported) meet this rule and nearly always require higher doses for patients on CAPD than for nondialyzed patients (81, 82, 111). However, many other commonly used drugs do not require a dosing regimen that is different from those for an anuric patient because of their low clearance by CAPD (82). Many of these agents are not cleared adequately by CAPD because of their pharmacokinetic properties. Drugs with volumes of distribution well above 50% (e.g., digoxin), high nonrenal clearances (e.g., cimetidine), or high protein binding (e.g., tricyclic antidepressants) are not cleared to any significant extent by CAPD.

Table 22.17.

Factors That Influence Solute Movement Across the Peritoneal Membrane

Physicochemical properties of the drug:
    Molecular weight and shape
    Water solubility
    Charge of the compound
Pharmacokinetic properties of the drug:
    Volume of distribution
    Protein binding
Physiology and anatomy of the peritoneal membrane:
    Surface area
    Membrane thickness
    Vascularity
    Blood flow
    Individual peritoneal resistance to drugs
Dialysis regimen:
    Dialysate composition
    Dwell time
    Dialysate volume
    Dialysate outflow rate

PHARMACOKINETICS OF SYSTEMICALLY ADMINISTERED DRUGS

Since pharmacokinetic data on the effect of CAPD is not available for many drugs, consideration of certain general principles allows for a reasonable prediction of whether dosing adjustment is required. This estimation requires the knowledge of several factors that influence drug movement across the peritoneal membrane (Table 22.17) (111). These include the physicochemical and pharmacokinetic properties of the drug, the physiology and anatomy of the dialysis (peritoneal) membrane, and the dialysis regimen.

To assess the amount of drug that is removed by CAPD, both the peritoneal clearance (Cl_{pd}) and the volume of distribution (V_d) of the drug must be known. Similar to calculating the total body clearance, Cl_{pd} can be calculated by dividing the total amount of drug recovered in the spent dialysate from one or more dwell periods (A_{0-t}) by the area under the plasma concentration-time curve during the same period (AUC_{0-t}) (81). Alternatively, if at the end of the each dwell period, equilibrium is reached between the drug concentrations in blood and the peritoneal cavity, and if there is no significant plasma protein binding, the Cl_{pd} is roughly equivalent to the dialysate flow rate. Given the continuous nature of CAPD, the dialysate flow rate rarely exceeds 0.3 to 0.42 L/hr (5 to 7 mL/min), which limits the amount of drug that is removed by CAPD (81, 82). In estimating the supplemental dose of a drug, the amount of drug or the fraction of the dose (f_{pd}) removed by CAPD may be determined from the following formula:

$$f_{pd} = \frac{Cl_{pd}}{Cl_d} \qquad (22.23)$$

where Cl_d is the systemic clearance, which includes the Cl_{pd} and Cl_{pt} of the drug. The Cl_d may be estimated from the literature values for patients with ESRD (Table 22.16). Since plasma protein binding of the drug is the main limiting factor for diffusion of a drug into the peritoneal cavity, the unbound drug fraction (f_u) should be included in equation (22.23):

$$f_{pd} = \frac{Cl_{pd}}{Cl_d} \times f_u \qquad (22.24)$$

Equation (22.24) indicates that the higher the clearance ratio of Cl_{pd} to Cl_d, the higher the fraction of the drug removed by CAPD (81, 111). Compared to actual patient values, this method provides a reasonable estimation of the fraction of a dose that is removed by CAPD (81).

PHARMACOKINETICS OF INTRAPERITONEALLY ADMINISTERED DRUGS

Intraperitoneal administration is the preferred route in at least three clinical situations: (a) for the administration of deferoxamine in the treatment of aluminum overload, (b) for the administration of antibiotics to patients with CAPD peritonitis, and (c) for the administration of insulin (81). The intraperitoneal administration of a low-molecular-weight drug, such as most antibiotics, rapidly achieves high local drug concentrations. This concentration gradient leads to rapid movement (diffusion) of the drug from the peritoneal cavity into the systemic circulation. The reverse movement from the systemic circulation into the peritoneal cavity is much slower and restricted (81, 82). As a result, intraperitoneal antibiotics that are used in the treatment of peritonitis (e.g., cephalosporins, aminoglycosides) are 50 to 80% bioavailable during a 6-hr dwell period (82). Despite this rapid peritoneal absorption, there is insignificant loss of antibacterial activity with penicillins, cephalosporins, aminoglycosides, and vancomycin during a normal dwell period (81). During bouts of peritonitis, because of the higher permeability of the peritoneal membrane, both the rate and the extent of intraperitoneal absorption for certain drugs (e.g., vancomycin, gentamicin, and various β-lactam antibiotics) increase and remain so for days after the episode (81, 82). One concern regarding the intraperitoneal administration of drugs is the potential for irritation of the peritoneal membrane. A combination of imipenem plus cilastatin, high-dose vancomycin, and amphotericin B are three of the better-known causes of chemical peritonitis (81).

CONCLUSION

The advent of dialysis has led to a substantial reduction in the morbidity and mortality of patients with chronic renal failure. Almost any amount of dialysis can sustain life longer than no dialysis. However, despite their benefits, hemodialysis and CAPD are associated with a number of medical and mechanical complications that, by themselves, can affect morbidity and mortality. In recent years, attention has been focused on the adequacy of dialysis. It is now clear that dialysis therapy is not very successful if the patient is malnourished. Therefore, at times the dose of dialysis needs to be increased to affect the patient's nutritional state. Although the nephrologist is ultimately responsible for the management of patients with ESRD, a multidisciplinary approach involving physicians, pharmacists, nurses, and social workers is more likely to result in a positive outcome.

While there is some general consensus about what adequate dialysis consists of, it is not clear what the optimum level of dialysis is. Given the high rate of mortality from ESRD, this issue is of utmost importance and will likely be the focus of research in the future. Among the topics of future research will be the effect of aggressive nutritional support on malnourished predialysis patients; the effect of higher dialysis doses on morbidity and mortality; clinical effects of biocompatible, high-flux, and high-efficiency membranes; modification of cardiovascular risk factors; and immunomodulation with the use of vaccines. Meanwhile, as new drugs and new dialysis membranes are introduced, clinical pharmacokinetics research must continue to provide drug dosing information to aid in ascertaining the best possible outcome for patients on dialysis.

REFERENCES

1. Ateshkadi A, Johnson CA. Chronic renal failure. In: Koda-Kimble MA, Young LY, eds. Applied Therapeutics: The Clinical Use of Drugs, ed. 6. Vancouver: Applied Therapeutics, Inc., 1995:1–29.
2. May RC. Pathophysiology of uremia. In: Brenner BM, Rector FCJ, eds. The Kidney, ed. 4. Philadelphia: WB Saunders, 1991: 1997–2018.
3. Alfrey AC, Chan L. Chronic renal failure: manifestations and pathogenesis. In: Schrier RW, ed. Renal and Electrolyte Disorders, ed. 4. Boston: Little, Brown, 1992: 539–79.
4. National Institute of Diabetes and Digestive and Kidney Disease. USRDS 1994 annual data report. Bethesda, MD: The National Institutes of Health, July 1994.
5. Ismail N, Becker BN. Treatment options and strategies in uremia: current trends and future directions. Semin Nephrol 14:282–99, 1994.
6. Hakim RM. Initiation of dialysis. Adv Nephrol Necker Hosp 23:295–309, 1994.
7. Acchiardo SR. Uremia and adequate dialysis treatment. Semin Nephrol 14:274–81, 1994.
8. Eggers P. Comparison of treatment costs between dialysis and transplantation. Semin Nephrol 12:284–9, 1992.
9. Consensus Development Conference Panel. Morbidity and mortality or renal dialysis: NIH Consensus Conference Statement. Ann Intern Med 121:62–70, 1994.
10. Vanholder RC, Ringoir SM. Adequacy of dialysis: a critical analysis. Kidney Int 42:540–58, 1992.
11. Hakim RM, Depner TA, Parker TF III. Adequacy of hemodialysis. Am J Kidney Dis 20:107–23, 1992.
12. Lowrie EG, Laird NM, Parker TF III, et al. Effect of the hemodialysis on patient morbidity: report from the National Cooperative Dialysis Study. N Engl J Med 305:1176–81, 1981.
13. Gotch FA, Sargent JA. A mechanistic analysis of the National Cooperative Dialysis Study (NCDS). Kidney Int 28:526–34, 1985.
14. Harter HR. Review of significant findings from the National Cooperative Dialysis Study and recommendations. Kidney Int 23(Suppl 13):S107–12, 1983.
15. Keshaviah P. Urea kinetic and middle molecule approaches to assessing the adequacy of hemodialysis and CAPD. Kidney Int 43(Suppl 40):S28–38, 1993.
16. Lindsay RM, Heidenheim AP, Spanner E, et al. Adequacy of hemodialysis and nutrition: important determinants of morbidity and mortality. Kidney Int 45(Suppl 44):S85–91, 1994.
17. Koch KM. Dialysis-related amyloidosis. Kidney Int 41:1416–29, 1992.
18. Gejyo F, Homma N, Arakawa M. Long-term complications of dialysis: pathogenic factors with special reference to amyloidosis. Kidney Int 43(Suppl 41):S78–82, 1993.
19. Cheung AK. Hemodialysis and hemofiltration. In: Greenberg A, Cheung AK, Coffman TM, Falk RJ, Jennette JC, eds. Primer on Kidney Diseases, ed. 1. San Diego: Academic Press, 1994: 258–65.
20. Arieff AI. Dialysis disequilibrium syndrome: current concepts on pathogenesis and prevention. Kidney Int 45:629–35, 1994.
21. Bailie GR, Eisele G. Continuous ambulatory peritoneal dialysis: a review of its mechanics, advantages, complications, and areas of controversy. Ann Pharmacother 26:1409–20, 1992.
22. Piraino B. Peritoneal dialysis. In: Greenberg A, Cheung AK, Coffman TM, Falk RJ, Jennette JC, eds. Primer on Kidney Diseases, ed. 1. San Diego: Academic Press, 1994: 266–71.
23. Hakim RM. Assessing the adequacy of dialysis. Kidney Int 37:822–32, 1990.
24. Parker TF III. Trends and concepts in the prescription and delivery of dialysis in the United States. Semin Nephrol 12:267–75, 1992.
25. Uldall PR. Temporary vascular access for hemodialysis. In: Nissenson AR, Fine RN, eds. Dialysis Therapy, ed. 2. Philadelphia: Hanley & Belfus, 1993: 5–10.
26. Tomasula JR, Delaney V, Butt KMH. Vascular access for chronic hemodialysis. In Nissenson AR, Fine RN, eds. Dialysis Therapy, ed. 2. Philadelphia: Hanley & Belfus, 1993: 10–4.
27. Cheung AK. Dialyzer biocompatibility: practical considerations. In: Nissenson AR, Fine RN, eds. Dialysis Therapy, ed. 2. Philadelphia: Hanley & Belfus, 1993: 75–7.
28. Lazarus JM, Owen WF. Role of biocompatibility in dialysis morbidity and mortality. Am J Kidney Dis 24:1019–32, 1994.
29. Held PJ, Carroll CE, Liska DW, et al. Hemodialysis therapy in the United States: what is the dose and does it matter? Am J Kidney Dis 24:974–80, 1994.
30. Lazarus JM, Hakim RM. Medical aspects of hemodialysis. In: Brenner BM, Rector FC, eds. The Kidney, ed. 4. Philadelphia: WB Saunders, 1991: 2223–99.
31. Held PJ, Levin NW, Boubjerg RR, et al. Mortality and duration of hemodialysis treatment. JAMA 265:871–5, 1991.
32. Shaldon S. Unanswered questions pertaining to dialysis adequacy in 1992. Kidney Int 43(Suppl 41):S274–7, 1993.
33. Churchill DN. Comparative morbidity among hemodialysis and continuous ambulatory peritoneal dialysis patients. Kidney Int 43(Suppl 40):S16–22, 1993.
34. Parfrey PS, Harnett JD. Long-term cardiac morbidity and mortality during dialysis therapy. Adv Nephrol Necker Hosp 23:311–30, 1994.
35. Wizemann V, Timio M, Alpert MA, et al. Options in dialysis therapy: significance of cardiovascular findings. Kidney Int 43(Suppl 40): S85–91, 1993.

36. Ritz E, Deppisch R, Stier E, et al. Atherogenesis and cardiac death: are they related to dialysis procedure and biocompatibility? Nephrol Dial Transplant 9(Suppl 2):165–72, 1994.

37. Cheung AK, Wu LL, Kablitz C, et al. Atherogenic lipids and lipoproteins in hemodialysis patients. Am J Kidney Dis 22:271–6, 1993.

38. Khanna R. Dialysis considerations for diabetic patients. Kidney Int 43(Suppl 40):S58–64, 1993.

39. Silberberg J, Racine N, Barre P, et al. Regression of left ventricular hypertrophy in dialysis patients following correction of anemia with recombinant human erythropoietin. Can J Cardiol 6:1–4, 1990.

40. Ateshkadi A, Johnson CA, Zimmerman SW. Use of recombinant human erythropoietin in patients on peritoneal dialysis. In: Nissenson AR, Fine RN, eds. Dialysis Therapy, ed. 2. Philadelphia: Hanley & Belfus, 1993:228–31.

41. Khan IH, Catto GR. Long-term complications of dialysis: infection. Kidney Int 43(Suppl 41):S143–8, 1993.

42. Himmelfarb J, Hakim RM. Biocompatibility and risk of infection in haemodialysis patients. Nephrol Dial Transplant 9(Suppl 2):138–44, 1994.

43. Descamps-Latscha B, Herbelin A. Long-term dialysis and cellular immunity: a critical survey. Kidney Int 43(Suppl 41):S135–42, 1993.

44. Moran J, Blumenstein M, Gurland HJ. Immunodeficiencies in chronic renal failure. Contrib Nephrol 86:91–110, 1990.

45. Nolph KD. Access problems plague both peritoneal dialysis and hemodialysis. Kidney Int 43(Suppl 40):S81–4, 1993.

46. Boelaert JR. *Staphylococcus aureus* infection in haemodialysis patients. Mupirocin as a topical strategy against nasal carriage: a review. J Chemother 2:19–24, 1994.

47. Salem M, Ivanovich PT, Ing TS, et al. Adverse effects of dialyzers manifesting during the dialysis session. Nephrol Dial Transplant 9(Suppl 2):127–37, 1994.

48. Swartz RD. Hemodialysis-associated seizure activity. In: Nissenson AR, Fine RN, eds. Dialysis Therapy, ed. 2. Philadelphia: Hanley & Belfus, 1993:113–6.

49. Saito A. β_2-microglobulin amyloidosis. Nephrol Dial Transplant 9(Suppl 2):116–9, 1994.

50. Rottembourg J. Residual renal function and recovery of renal function in patients treated by CAPD. Kidney Int 43(Suppl 40):S106–10, 1993.

51. Kopple JD, Hakim RM, Held PJ, et al. Recommendations for reducing the high morbidity and mortality of United States maintenance dialysis patients. Am J Kidney Dis 24:968–73, 1994.

52. Hull AR. Dialysis-related mortality in the United States. Cleve Clin J Med 61:393–7, 1994.

53. Parker TF III. Role of dialysis dose on morbidity and mortality in maintenance hemodialysis patients. Am J Kidney Dis 24:981–9, 1994.

54. Parker TF III, Husni L, Huang W, et al. Survival of hemodialysis patients in the United States is improved with a greater quantity of dialysis. Am J Kidney Dis 23:670–80, 1994.

55. Bergstrom J. Nutrition and adequacy of dialysis in hemodialysis patients. Kidney Int 43(Suppl 41):S261–7, 1993.

56. Bergstrom J, Lindholm B. Nutrition and adequacy of dialysis. How do hemodialysis and CAPD compare? Kidney Int 43(Suppl 40):S39–50, 1993.

57. Collins AJ, Ma JZ, Umen A, et al. Urea index and other predictors of hemodialysis patient survival. Am J Kidney Dis 23:272–82, 1994.

58. Owen WFJ, Lew NL, Liu Y, et al. The urea reduction ratio and serum albumin concentration as predictors of mortality in patients undergoing hemodialysis. N Engl J Med 329:1001–6, 1993.

59. Hakim RM, Breyer J, Ismail N, et al. Effects of dose of dialysis on morbidity and mortality. Am J Kidney Dis 23:661–9, 1994.

60. Lowrie EG, Lew NL. Death risk in hemodialysis patients: the predictive value of commonly measured variables and an evaluation of death rate differences between facilities. Am J Kidney Dis 15:458–82, 1990.

61. Teehan BP, Schleifer CR, Brown J. Adequacy of continuous ambulatory peritoneal dialysis: morbidity and mortality in chronic peritoneal dialysis. Am J Kidney Dis 24:990–1001, 1994.

62. Churchill DN, Taylor DW, Cook RJ, et al. Canadian Hemodialysis Morbidity Study. Am J Kidney Dis 19:214–34, 1992.

63. Kopple JD. Effect of nutrition on morbidity and mortality in maintenance dialysis patients. Am J Kidney Dis 24:1002–9, 1994.

64. Cheung AK. Interactions between plasma proteins and hemodialysis membranes. Adv Nephrol Necker Hosp 22:417–37, 1993.

65. Cheung AK. Quantitation of dialysis: the importance of membrane and middle molecules. Blood Purif 12:42–53, 1994.

66. Lindsay RM, Spanner E, Heidenheim P, et al. PCR, Kt/V and membrane. Kidney Int 43(Suppl 41):S268–73, 1993.

67. Charra B, Calemard E, Ruffet M, et al. Survival as an index of adequacy of dialysis. Kidney Int 41:1286–91, 1992.

68. Drukker W. Hemodialysis: a historical review. In: Maher JF, ed. Replacement of Renal Function by Dialysis, ed. 3. Dordecht, Holland: Kluwer Academic Publishers, 1989:21–86.

69. Oreopoulous DG. Chronic peritoneal dialysis. Clin Nephrol 9:166–73, 1978.

70. Popovich RP, Moncrief JW, Nolph KD, et al. Continuous ambulatory peritoneal dialysis. Ann Intern Med 88:449–56, 1978.

71. Mactier RA. Peritoneal cavity lymphatics. In: Nolph KD, ed. Peritoneal Dialysis, ed. 3. Boston: Kluwer Academic Publishers, 1989:28–47.

72. Niezgoda JA, Wolfson AB. Continuous ambulatory peritoneal dialysis. Emerg Med Clin North Am 12:759–69, 1994.

73. Ash SR. Peritoneal access devices and placement techniques. In: Nissenson AR, Fine RN, eds. Dialysis Therapy, ed. 2. Philadelphia: Hanley & Belfus, 1993:23–8.

74. Khanna R, Oreopoulos DG. Peritoneal dialysis. In: Schrier RW, Gottschalk CW, eds. Diseases of the Kidney, ed. 5. Boston: Little, Brown, 1993:2969–3030.

75. Twardowski ZJ. Peritoneal catheter exit-site and tunnel infections. In Nissenson AR, Fine RN, eds. Dialysis Therapy, ed. 2. Philadelphia: Hanley & Belfus, 1993:165–8.

76. Keane WF, Everett ED, Golper TA, et al. Peritoneal dialysis-related peritonitis treatment recommendations: 1993 update. Perit Dial Int 13:14–28, 1993.

77. Vas SI. Treatment of peritonitis. Perit Dial Int 14(Suppl 3):S49–55, 1994.

78. Michel C, Courdavault L, al Khayat R, et al. Fungal peritonitis in patients on peritoneal dialysis. Am J Nephrol 14:113–20, 1994.

79. Maiorca R, Cancarini GC, Brunori G, et al. Morbidity and mortality of CAPD and hemodialysis. Kidney Int 43(Suppl 40):S4–15, 1993.

80. Chaimovitz C. Peritoneal dialysis. Kidney Int 45:1226–40, 1994.

81. Keller E, Reetze P, Schollmeyer P. Drug therapy in patients undergoing continuous ambulatory peritoneal dialysis: clinical pharmacokinetic considerations. Clin Pharmacokinet 18:104–17, 1990.

82. Keller E. Peritoneal kinetics of different drugs. Clin Nephrol 30(Suppl 1):S24–8, 1988.

83. The Ad Hoc Advisory Committee on Peritonitis Management. Continuous ambulatory peritoneal dialysis (CAPD) peritonitis treatment recommendations: 1989 update. Perit Dial Int 9:247–56, 1989.

84. Holley JL, Bernardini J, Piraino B. Infecting organisms in continuous ambulatory peritoneal dialysis patients on the Y-set. Am J Kidney Dis 23:569–73, 1994.

85. Luzar MA. Exit-site infection in continuous ambulatory peritoneal dialysis: a review. Perit Dial Int 11:333–40, 1991.

86. Piraino B. A review of *Staphylococcus aureus* exit-site and tunnel infection in peritoneal dialysis patients. Am J Kidney Dis 16:89–95, 1990.

87. Nolph KD. What's new in peritoneal dialysis: an overview. Kidney Int 38(Suppl 52):S148–52, 1992.

88. Perez-Fontan M, Garcia-Falcon T, Rosales M, et al. Treatment of *Staphylococcus aureus* nasal carriers in continuous ambulatory peritoneal dialysis with mupirocin: long-term results. Am J Kidney Dis 22:708–12, 1993.

89. Zimmerman SW, Ahrens E, Johnson CA, et al. Randomized controlled trial of prophylactic rifampin for peritoneal dialysis-related infections. Am J Kidney Dis 18:225–31, 1991.

90. Bargman JM. Complications of peritoneal dialysis related to increased intraabdominal pressure. Kidney Int 43(Suppl 40):S75–80, 1993.

91. Spinowitz BS, Charytan C, Gupta B. Hydrothorax and peritoneal dialysis. In: Nissenson AR, Fine RN, eds. Dialysis Therapy, ed. 2. Philadelphia: Hanley & Belfus, 1993:189–91.

92. Spinowitz BS, Charytan C. Abdominal hernias in CAPD. In: Nissenson AR, Fine RN, eds. Dialysis Therapy, ed. 2. Philadelphia: Hanley & Belfus, 1993:187–8.

93. Gotch FA. Adequacy of peritoneal dialysis. Am J Kidney Dis 21:96–8, 1993.

94. Twardowski ZJ, Nolph KD. Peritoneal dialysis: how much is enough. Semin Dial 1:75–6, 1988.

95. Keshaviah PR, Nolph KD, Van Stone JC. The peak concentration hypothesis: a urea kinetic approach to comparing the adequacy of continuous ambulatory peritoneal dialysis (CAPD) and hemodialysis. Perit Dial Int 9:257–60, 1989.

96. Keshaviah P. Adequacy of CAPD: a quantitative approach. Kidney Int 42(Suppl 38):S160–S164, 1992.

97. Brandes JC, Piering WF, Beres JA, et al. Clinical outcome of continuous ambulatory peritoneal dialysis predicted by urea and creatinine kinetics. J Am Soc Nephrol 2:1430–5, 1992.

98. Korbet SM. Anemia and erythropoietin in hemodialysis and continuous ambulatory peritoneal dialysis. Kidney Int 43(Suppl 40):S111–9, 1993.

99. Coburn JW. Mineral metabolism and renal bone disease: effects of CAPD versus hemodialysis. Kidney Int 43(Suppl 40):S92–100, 1993.

100. Delmez JA. Long-term complications of dialysis: pathogenetic factors with special reference to bone. Kidney Int 43(Suppl 41):S116–20, 1993.

101. Chan E, Montgomery PA. Administration of insulin by continuous ambulatory peritoneal dialysis. Pharmacotherapy 13:455–60, 1993.

102. National Institute of Diabetes and Digestive and Kidney Disease. USRDS 1991 annual data report. Bethesda, MD: The National Institutes of Health, August 1991.

103. Schrier RW, Gambertoglio JG, eds. Handbook of Drug Therapy in Liver and Kidney Disease. Boston: Little, Brown, 1991.

104. Bennett WM. Guide to drug dosage in renal failure. Clin Pharmacokinet 15:326–54, 1988.

105. Gibson TP. Renal disease and drug metabolism: an overview. Am J Kidney Dis 8:7–17, 1986.

106. Reidenberg MM. The binding of drugs to plasma proteins from patients with poor renal function. Clin Pharmacokinet 1:121–5, 1976.

107. Lee CC, Marbury TC. Drug therapy in patients undergoing hemodialysis: clinical pharmacokinetic considerations. Clin Pharmacokinet 9:42–66, 1984.

108. Lee CC. The assessment of fractional drug removal by extracorporeal dialysis. Biopharm Drug Dispos 3:163–73, 1982.

109. Halstenson CE, Guay DR, Opsahl JA, et al. Disposition of cefmetazole in healthy volunteers and patients with impaired renal function. Antimicrob Agents Chemother 34(4):519–23, 1990.

110. Gibson TP. Problems in designing hemodialysis drug studies. Pharmacotherapy 5:23–9, 1985.

111. Paton TW, Cornish WR, Manuel MA, et al. Drug therapy in patients undergoing peritoneal dialysis: clinical pharmacokinetic considerations. Clin Pharmacokinet 10:404–25, 1985.

CHAPTER 23

PEPTIC ULCER DISEASE

ROBERT P. HENDERSON and ROGER D. LANDER

Peptic ulcer disease (PUD) is a chronic inflammatory condition involving a group of disorders characterized by ulceration in regions of the upper gastrointestinal tract where parietal cells secrete pepsin and hydrochloric acid. The most common sites are the duodenum and stomach, where the major forms are duodenal and gastric ulceration. Additionally, Barrett ulcer of the esophagus, postbulbar ulcer, some cases of Meckel's diverticulum, and stomal or jejunal ulcers following surgery for peptic ulceration are also classified as peptic ulcer diseases.

Early in the 20th century, PUD was believed to be related to stress and dietary factors. Later, the concept arose that PUD was caused by the injurious effects of digestive secretions such as gastric acid. Peptic ulcer disease results when there is an imbalance between aggressive factors (acid secretion) and protective factors (mucosal defense) (Table 23.1).

Approximately 5 to 10% of the general population will develop a peptic ulcer during their lifetime (1). Peptic ulcer is typically a recurrent disease, with 50 to 90% of patients with duodenal ulcer having a recurrence within 1 year of diagnosis; the relapse rate is lower for gastric ulcer. Recent findings suggest that peptic ulcer disease may have, in part, an infectious component to its etiology (*Helicobacter pylori*) and this may largely account for the recurrent nature of the disease.

Table 23.1.
Factors That Influence Development of Peptic Ulcer Disease

Aggressive Factors	Protective Factors
HCl, pepsin	Secretion of mucus
Alcohol, nicotine	Rapid gastric epithelial cell turnover
Gastric mucosal ischemia	Gastric and duodenal mucosal blood flow
Helicobacter pylori	Normal pyloric function (motility)
Ulcerogenic drugs	Bicarbonate secretion
aspirin,	
NSAIDs	
corticosteroids,	
iron salts	
potassium chloride	
erythromycin	
chemotherapeutic agents	

Duodenal ulcers are approximately four times more common than gastric ulcers. Duodenal ulcers are rarely cancerous, but approximately 5% of gastric ulcers are malignant; therefore, careful evaluation and close follow-up are extremely important in patients with gastric ulcer disease.

Peptic ulcer disease is a dynamic condition, and the incidence varies with age, gender, ulcer type, and geographic location. with duodenal ulcer being more common than gastric ulcer in the United States. Peptic ulcer and its complications tend to occur and recur during autumn and winter months and less so in summer months (1). Duodenal ulcer was previously thought to be more common in men; however, recent trends indicate that the prevalence among women may be similar to men (2). Duodenal ulcer tends to occur between the ages of 25 and 55 years and peaks at 40 years. Gastric ulcer usually does not occur prior to age 40, peaks between 55 and 65 years of age, and is likely influenced by use of ulcerogenic medications.

There has been a decline in the number of peptic ulcer disease-related hospitalizations over the last several decades, with a shift of care to the outpatient setting seen with the introduction of H_2-receptor antagonists and other new therapeutic agents. The incidence of peptic ulcer disease-related surgery has decreased in all ages except the elderly. Mortality from peptic ulcer disease has decreased among persons of all ages and sexes (3). Despite these observations, peptic ulcer disease remains one of the most common gastrointestinal diseases, resulting in substantial human suffering and high economic costs (3, 4).

REGULATION OF GASTRIC SECRETION

The secretion of gastric HCl is intimately related to peptic ulcer disease. A peptic ulcer does not develop when there is no acid secretion. In fact, with few exceptions, therapeutic approaches have largely encompassed Schwarz's dictum, "no acid, no ulcer."

There are three anatomically and functionally distinct regions in the stomach: the cardia (superior region), the body, which accounts for 80 to 90% of the stomach mass, and the antrum (lower prepyloric region). The cardia contains mucus-secreting cells. The body, which includes the fundus, contains parietal cells, responsible for hydrochloric acid and intrinsic factor secretion, and chief cells, responsible for pepsinogen secretion. The antrum contains G cells, responsible for gastrin secretion.

Parietal cells are located in the walls of the oxyntic glands, the secretory units of the gastric mucosa. Hydrochloric acid secretion by parietal cells is the result of the activation of a unique proton pump, hydrogen-potassium ion adenosine triphosphatase (H^+- K^+-ATPase). This magnesium-dependent enzyme is found only on the membranes of parietal cells and exchanges one potassium ion from the canalicular fluid for one hydrogen ion from the cytoplasm. The normal stomach contains approximately a billion parietal cells that can secrete hydrogen ions into the gastric lumen against a 3 million : 1 concentration gradient, producing concentrations as high as 100 to 160 mEq/L. Gastric mucosal integrity is normally maintained by resisting attack from these very high acid concentrations.

Three pathways stimulate gastric acid secretion: (a) the neurocrine pathway, which causes the release of acetylcholine from postganglionic vagal neurons in the stomach; (b) the endocrine pathway, which causes the release of gastrin from antral G cells; and (c) the paracrine pathway, which releases histamine from the mast cells in the lamina propria (5). The neurocrine pathway involves acetylcholine release at parietal and G cells by central mediation of local cholinergic nerves, stimulation of postganglionic branches of the vagus nerve, and distension of the stomach that is mediated through receptors in the gastric wall. These actions result in acid secretion by acting on muscarinic M_3 cholinergic receptors. Acetylcholine also causes G cells to release gastrin, further increasing acid secretion (6–8). These cholinergic actions can be blocked by atropine.

Gastrin is a key factor in the secretion of acid and is secreted by antral G cells in two principal forms: (a) G-34 (big gastrin), a 34 amino acid peptide, is the predominant form in serum, and (b) G-17 (little gastrin), a 17 amino acid peptide that is identical to the C-terminal half of G-34, is the principal form in gastric antral mucosa (6, 9). Both forms of gastrin are equally potent in stimulating gastric acid secretion. Gastrin has several physiologic actions, including stimulation of gastric acid and pepsinogen secretion, hepatic bile flow, insulin release from the pancreas, and pancreatic secretions. In addition, gastrin stimulates gastric and intestinal motility and increases lower esophageal sphincter pressure, which promotes closure of the sphincter.

Gastrin may be measured accurately in the blood by radioimmunoassay, the normal level being less than 200 pg/mL. Gastrin levels are not elevated in chronic peptic ulcer disease; however, these patients may be more sensitive to the effects of gastrin (1). A gastrin assay is necessary for the diagnosis of the gastrin-producing pancreatic adenoma (Zollinger-Ellison syndrome) in which fasting blood gastrin levels are extremely high, typically greater than 200 pg/mL and less than 1000 pg/mL.

Histamine is present in many of the tissues of the body, including the gastric mucosa. In 1971, Sir James Black discovered the H_2 receptor and identified the important physiologic role of histamine in gastric acid secretion. Histamine is contained throughout the stomach in enterochromaffinlike cells in the lamina propria (1, 8). These cells are found in proximity to parietal cells and receive cholinergic innervation. Histamine plays an important role in the process of gastric acid secretion; the role of enterochromaffinlike cells in the pathophysiology of peptic ulcer disease is not well understood.

Gastric acid secretion occurs continuously and is termed interdigestive, or "basal," when no stimuli are present. Basal acid output usually ranges from 0 to 5 mEq/hr, but can rise to 5 to 20 mEq/hr or higher with appropriate stimulation. Acid output is highest between 2:00 P.M. and 1:00 A.M. and lowest between 5:00 A.M. and 11:00 A.M. Gastric secretion can be divided into three phases based on origin: cephalic, gastric, and intestinal.

The cephalic phase represents gastric acid secretion in response to the thought, sight, taste, smell, or chewing of food. Vagal stimulation causes the release of acetylcholine, which causes the parietal cell to secrete hydrochloric acid and antral G cells to release gastrin. The gastric phase begins when food causes distension of the stomach and is mediated by both gastrin and cholinergic nerves, leading to stimulation of the vagus nerve. Amino acids and peptides from protein cause further secretion of acid through the release of gastrin. Gastrin causes release of histamine, which stimulates secretion of acid and pepsinogen. Pepsinogen causes the formation of pepsin, at pH below 4. Pepsins are proteolytic enzymes that exhibit maximal activity at pH 2 to 3.3 and lose their activity above pH 5. The role of pepsin in the pathogenesis of peptic ulcer disease involves its ability to disrupt the mucus-bicarbonate barrier, which normally protects the gastric epithelial surface and mucosa from acid. As the gastric pH decreases, gastrin output in response to amino acids is decreased. The intestinal phase begins when food enters the proximal portion of the small intestine. Gastric secretion can be decreased through negative feedback when the pH in the small intestine becomes too low. A number of other substances are secreted by the stomach, including vasoactive intestinal peptide, cholecystokinin-pancreozymin, serotonin, somatostatin, platelet activating factor, growth factors, and prostaglandins.

The normal gastric mucosa is protected from ulceration by several mechanisms. Gastric epithelial cells secrete mucus and bicarbonate, which helps to protect the mucosa from damage. Mucus and bicarbonate serve as a barrier to hydrogen ion back-diffusion across the gastric mucosa, normally keeping the pH almost neutral at the surface of the mucosa, even when the luminal pH is around 2.0. If ultimately damaged, these mucosal epithelial cells regenerate rapidly and allow the gastric mucosa to heal itself. Rapid gastric mucosal blood flow allows removal of hydrogen ions that cross the gastric mucosa, and if this blood flow is compromised, the risk of mucosal damage is increased. Prostaglandins (e.g., PGE) stimulate secretion of mucus and bicarbonate as well as maintain gastric mucosal blood flow. Normal pyloric function allows stomach emptying and negative feedback mechanisms to reduce acid secretion when acid is excessive. Normally these protective mechanisms counteract aggressive forces on the gastric mucosa. Ulceration typically develops when there is a deficiency in protective factors or an excess in aggressive factors.

DUODENAL ULCER

A duodenal ulcer (DU) is an ulcer in the wall of the duodenum, rarely malignant, extending into the muscularis mucosa. Practically all duodenal ulcers occur in the duodenal bulb. Ulcers that occur beyond the bulb are uncommon and are referred to as postbulbar ulcers. About 10% of patients have multiple duodenal ulcers (10). Duodenal ulcers are usually round or oval and less than 1 cm in diameter, but may be larger and irregular in shape. The true cause of DU is unknown, although it has been assumed for years that they are related to excessive parietal cell HCl acid secretion (9). This could be due to increased parietal cell mass, increased vagal or hormonal drive to secrete acid, increased gastric emptying rate, or defective inhibition of acid secretion (11). Only one third to one half of patients with duodenal ulcers have excessive acid secretory rates, as evidenced by basal gastric hypersecretion and increased peak acid secretion.

Duodenal ulcer disease is both chronic and recurrent. Approximately 60% of healed duodenal ulcers recur within 1 year and 80 to 90% within 2 years (9). Duodenal ulcers probably represent a stage in a dynamic disease process that begins with acute inflammation of the duodenal mucosa and progresses through more severe stages of duodenitis until an ulcer develops. The ulcer usually persists for 4 to 6 weeks but may on occasion heal rapidly. The whole process may repeat itself at some later point. A recurrent ulcer may or may not develop in the same location as the previous one. Certain risk factors such as cigarette smoking, chronic use of aspirin and other nonsteroidal antiinflammatory drugs (NSAIDs), or alcohol contribute to increased risk of ulcer development. Genetic factors appear to be important, with first-degree relatives of DU patients developing ulcers three times as commonly as the general population. Smokers have earlier and more frequent recurrence, with increased mortality. Psychosomatic factors probably do not play an important role in the development of the ulcer. A variety of stress situations appear to be weakly associated with the development of new ulcers. The role of *H. pylori* as an infectious cause of peptic ulcer disease and recurrence is under investigation and is discussed in a later section of this chapter.

GASTRIC ULCER

In the United States, gastric ulcer occurs about one fourth as frequently as duodenal ulcer. Like duodenal ulcer, it is more common in men than in women. The incidence increases after 50 years of age, peaks in the sixth decade, and is unusual in younger ages. Benign gastric ulcer can occur anywhere in the stomach, but is most commonly found at the junction between the antrum and the fundus of the stomach, on the lesser curvature, the so-called "saddle" ulcer. Gastric ulcers are rarely found in the fundus and are usually accompanied by antral gastritis. Benign gastric ulcers are similar to duodenal ulcers histologically, but are deep and usually exhibit more extensive gastritis surrounding the ulcer crater.

Unlike duodenal ulcer, gastric ulcers tend to be associated with lower rates of acid secretion. However, 10 to 20% of patients with gastric ulcer also have duodenal ulcers, with acid secretory rates paralleling those of duodenal ulcer. Gastric ulcers may primarily be caused by the breakdown of the mucosal barrier and subsequent back-diffusion of acid across the gastric mucosa. Normally, less than one tenth of the gastric HCl secreted by the parietal cells is reabsorbed through the gastric mucosa by back-diffusion. In patients with gastric ulcers, the figure tends to be much higher. The healing of gastric ulcer does not result in normalization of the gastric mucosal barrier to back-diffusion. Back-diffusion remains high, even if the ulcer has disappeared. The mucosal barrier defect appears to be generalized, rather than localized, since the ulcer does not necessarily recur at the previous ulcer site. Pyloric sphincter dysfunction and reflux of bile salts appear to also be involved in the genesis of gastric ulceration (12).

The plasma membrane and mucus of surface epithelial cells constitutes the mucosal barrier. The barrier is rendered impermeable to ionized substances due to the high phospholipid content and the tight junctions between these cells. A number of agents can damage the mucosal barrier, allowing rapid back-diffusion of hydrogen ion from the lumen into the mucosa, causing cellular destruction and increased capillary permeability within the damaged mucosa. This in turn results in extravasation of plasma proteins, producing mucosal edema. The rapid cell turnover of the gastric mucosa is also disrupted, leading to desquamation and loss of gastric epithelial cells in the area. NSAIDs are responsible for a significant number of gastric ulcers, presumably due in part to reduced synthesis of cytoprotective prostaglandins.

HELICOBACTER PYLORI (H. PYLORI)

Insight into an important pathogenic factor in PUD was provided over a decade ago when a spiral urease-producing organism, later identified as *H. pylori*, was found in the narrow interface between the gastric epithelial cell surface and the overlying mucus gel layer (mucosal barrier). Early studies found that the presence of this organism was associated with antral gastritis and duodenal and gastric ulcers. *H. pylori* is a common gastric infection affecting more than 50% of the world's population (13) and has become recognized as a major causative factor of gastritis and peptic ulcer disease. Nearly all patients with DU have *H. pylori* gastritis; thus, infection with *H. pylori* may be a prerequisite for the occurrence of almost all duodenal ulcers in the absence of other precipitating factors (such as NSAID use or Zollinger-Ellison syndrome) (14, 15). Evidence supporting these findings are that (a) virtually all *H. pylori*-positive patients demonstrate antral gastritis, (b) eradication of *H. pylori* infection results in resolution of gastritis, and (c) the lesion of chronic superficial gastritis has been reproduced following intragastric administration of *H. pylori* in some animal models and oral administration in humans (14).

It is important to note the emerging role of *H. pylori* in patients with ulcer disease; however, for perspective, the majority of *H. pylori*-infected individuals do not develop duodenal or gastric ulcers. The organism was originally named *Campylobacter pyloridis* and subsequently *Campylobacter pylori*, because of its similarity to other *Campylobacter* species. The name *Helicobacter pylori* was given in 1989 based on functional and enzymatic properties. *H. pylori* is a spiral-shaped gram-negative rod with four to six flagella. It is found below the mucous layer next to the gastric epithelium in the stomach, esophagus, duodenum, and Meckel's diverticulum. It is able to burrow through the mucous layer because of its motility and spiral shape. *H. pylori* produces a urease enzyme that catalyzes urea, forming ammonium and bicarbonate. Current methods of detection rely upon this reaction for positive results. The organism is very sensitive to gastric acid, and the ammonium forms a protective alkaline microenvironment. Transmission at this time appears to occur via human-to-human spread, most likely through the fecal-oral route (15).

Prevalence depends on socioeconomic class, race, and whether the subject resides in a developing country (15). In Western countries, prevalence is low before 20 years of age and increases to 40 to 60% at age 60. In the United States, hispanics and blacks appear to have markedly increased rates compared with that of whites. Lower socioeconomic class and crowding tend to result in higher prevalence rates, with up to 80% prevalence found in family members of infected individuals.

Diagnosis of *H. pylori*

Bicarbonate produced by the urease reaction is largely excreted as carbon dioxide by the lungs and forms the basis of measuring urease activity. Diagnostic tests can be divided into invasive and noninvasive measures and are summarized in Table 23.2. Invasive measures include endoscopy with gastric biopsy and histologic demonstration

Table 23.2.
Diagnostic Tests for *Helicobacter Pylori*

Test	Sensitivity	Comments
Urease Testing		
Breath Testing (nonradioactive ^{13}C) (radioactive ^{14}C)	90–95%	Noninvasive; rapid (60 min); represents the entire mucosa; may be used to monitor therapy
Biopsy	90–98%	Invasive, requires endoscopy to obtain sample for testing (culture, histology, urease); rapid CLO (*Campylobacter-like-organism*) test can provide results within 30 min. with specificity/sensitivity of 80–90%
Histology	70–95%	Invasive, requires endoscopy with 2 or more biopsies (1 or more from the antrum), may require special stains (Giemsa stain, Warthin-Starry silver stain)
Culture	60–95%	Invasive, requires endoscopy; may require 1 week to grow; poor predictive value without histology; may become necessary if antibiotic resistance develops
Serology	90–95%	Noninvasive; does not differentiate active vs. past infection; possible cross-reactivity with similar bacteria, so reliability is questionable; epidemiologic tool; titers decrease with eradication

of organisms, biopsy with direct detection of urease activity in the tissue specimen, and biopsy with culture of the *H. pylori* organism. Noninvasive measures include serological tests for IgG antibodies to *H. pylori* and breath tests of urease activity using orally administered urea labeled with carbon-14 or carbon-13. It is important to note that with the exception of serological assays, all tests may be falsely negative in patients who have taken antibiotics, bismuth compounds, or omeprazole in the recent past. Also, antibody levels decrease slowly following successful eradication of *H. pylori* infection. Currently, there is no readily available, inexpensive, and accurate noninvasive method to monitor eradication of *H. pylori*. Even if there were, it would be questionable if all patients would need testing in view of the high efficacy of treatment and the low reinfection rate.

CLINICAL FINDINGS

The clinical findings of peptic ulcer disease are nonspecific and quite varied. Patients can be asymptomatic or experience any of the following: anorexia, nausea, vomiting, belching and bloating, and heartburn or epigastric pain. DU patients usually describe pain or tenderness between the xiphoid and umbilicus, which is often relieved with food intake. Gastric ulcer typically involves diffuse pain over the midepigastrium and may be worsened by food (9). The differences can be slight, making differentiation difficult based on symptoms alone. Patients may occasionally describe pain that radiates to other areas, such as the back or lower abdomen. The pain is commonly described as sharp, burning, or gnawing. Some patients may perceive abdominal pressure or a hunger sensation. Changes in the character of pain may herald the development of complications, such as penetration, perforation, gastric outlet obstruction, or hemorrhage. It should be emphasized that some patients do not experience pain with active ulcer disease, especially with recurrences, and may not have any ulcer symptoms. Many NSAID-induced ulcers and ulcers in the elderly bleed without any prior symptoms. Therefore, the presence or absence of pain is not reliable in the diagnosis or assessment of healing with therapy in peptic ulcer disease.

RADIOLOGY AND ENDOSCOPY

The diagnosis of PUD depends on radiologic or endoscopic visualization of the ulcer. Radiologic study with barium contrast (upper GI series) is still a common initial method of diagnosis for PUD. At best, single-contrast barium studies with x-rays can detect 70 to 80% of ulcers found with endoscopy, and this rises to approximately 90% with double-contrast barium. Endoscopy is generally not needed when an ulcer is found with barium radiographic study. However, endoscopy is useful for detecting suspected ulcers not found radiographically, for visualizing and performing biopsies of gastric ulcer, and in identifying sources of active gastrointestinal bleeding. Endoscopy permits direct examination of the esophagus, stomach, and duodenum. Thus, most areas in which upper GI disease occurs are readily accessible to direct visualization and biopsy. Equivocal lesions can be easily biopsied, and superficial erosions can be visualized that were not detected radiographically. Endoscopy should be the preferred diagnostic procedure in evaluation of upper GI disorders in pregnant women, in whom radiation is to be avoided. The diagnostic accuracy rate of endoscopy in ulcer disease is in the 95% range.

TREATMENT

The goals of treatment for PUD are to relieve pain, enhance ulcer healing, prevent complications such as GI bleeding or perforation, and prevent recurrence of the ulcer. Although sophisticated drug therapy is available for PUD, other measures involving life-style modifications and avoidance of ulcerogenic drugs are important to optimize therapy. Patients should be advised to stop smoking and avoid alcohol intake, as both can impair ulcer healing. Ulcerogenic drugs, such as aspirin and other NSAIDs should be avoided. Caffeine is a gastric acid stimulant and should be avoided. Foods and beverages that aggravate symptoms should be avoided. Patients should refrain from eating after the evening meal so as not to stimulate acid secretion during the night. Stress management may help in reducing ulcer symptoms. Drug therapy for PUD is primarily oriented toward neutralizing (antacids) or reducing the amount of acid secreted (H_2 antagonists, acid-pump inhibitors) or protecting the gastric mucosa from the effects of acid (sucralfate, prostaglandins). As the role of *H. pylori* is becoming better understood, treatment with antibiotics is becoming an important part of PUD therapy and recurrence prevention.

Antacids

Antacids can provide symptomatic relief and heal peptic ulcers. Although intensive antacid therapy has been shown to be less expensive and as effective as the H_2 antagonists and sucralfate, it is no longer common to find antacids used as sole therapy due to the inconvenience of the regimens used, palatability, and adverse effects. However, antacids are still widely used on an as-needed basis for symptom control. Common antacid preparations include sodium bicarbonate, calcium carbonate, and salts of aluminum and magnesium. Magnesium and aluminum hydroxide are the most commonly used antacids for PUD.

Antacids heal duodenal ulcers by neutralizing gastric acid, which also results in a reduction in the action of pepsin when the gastric pH increases above 4. The acid neutralizing capacity (ANC) is a primary consideration in the selection of an antacid. The ANC varies for commercial preparations and is expressed as mEq/mL; the mEq of acid required to keep an antacid suspension at pH 3 for 2 hours in vitro (see Table 23.3). Antacids with a high ANC are usually more effective in vivo and require less volume for a given ability to neutralize acid. However, the most potent antacids are not necessarily the most useful for chronic therapy. Sodium bicarbonate and calcium carbonate have the greatest ANC, but produce unacceptable side effects when administered chronically. Antacids may provide additional benefit by suppressing the growth of *H. pylori* (16).

Frequent administration of antacid is necessary to buffer the constant secretion of acid produced by the stomach. The stomach in a fasting state empties its contents into the duodenum as often as every 30 minutes to 1 hour, limiting the amount of antacid in the stomach. Acid secretion is greatest in response to a meal and at night. A regimen that administers antacids several times between meals and at bedtime maximizes the buffering ability of the antacid at the times of greatest acid output. The regimen most commonly used is 30 mL of a high-potency antacid 1

Table 23.3.
Comparison of Selected Representative Liquid Antacid Products

Product Name	Ingredients (per 5 mL)	ANC (per 5 mL)	Sodium (mg)
Maalox Suspension	225 mg aluminum hydroxide 200 mg magnesium hydroxide	9	1.4
Maalox TC Suspension	500 mg aluminum hydroxide 300 mg magnesium hydroxide	27.2	0.8
Mylanta Liquid	200 mg aluminum hydroxide 200 mg magnesium hydroxide, 20 mg simethicone	12.7	0.68
Mylanta II Liquid	400 mg aluminum hydroxide 400 mg magnesium hydroxide, 40 mg simethicone	25.4	1.14
Riopan Suspension	540 mg magaldrate (hydroxymagnesium aluminate)	15	<0.1
Riopan Extra Strength	1080 mg magaldrate	30	<0.3
Camalox Suspension	225 mg aluminum hydroxide 200 mg magnesium hydroxide, 250 mg calcium carbonate	18.5	1.2
Titralac Plus Liquid	500 mg calcium carbonate	11	0.0005
Amphojel Suspension	320 mg aluminum hydroxide	10	<2.3
AlternalGEL Liquid	600 mg aluminum hydroxide with simethicone	16	<2.5
Basaljel Suspension	Aluminum carbonate equivalent to 400 mg Aluminum hydroxide	12	2.9

Please consult a comprehensive product reference guide for a complete listing of available products

hour and 3 hours after a meal and at bedtime. Lower dosages of antacids (15 mL, 6 times daily) have proven to be effective and may be more conducive to patient compliance (17–19). Since antacid must be present in the stomach to work, the patient may be awakened at night with pain caused by nocturnal acid secretion. A treatment period of 4 to 6 weeks is necessary to heal 70 to 80% of duodenal ulcers. Treatment for longer than 6 weeks does not offer any additional advantage, except possibly in smokers.

Antacid adverse effects are problematic and contribute to noncompliance. Sodium bicarbonate and calcium carbonate are potent antacids, but have side effects that preclude their use in PUD. Sodium bicarbonate produces gas from CO_2 formation in the stomach, has a tendency to induce systemic alkalosis, and delivers a high sodium load when used chronically. Calcium that is absorbed from calcium carbonate stimulates gastrin release to produce acid rebound. Chronic administration of large doses of calcium carbonate can be associated with the "milk-alkali" syndrome, producing hypercalcemia, hyperphosphatemia, increased blood urea nitrogen (BUN), and systemic alkalosis. This can further cause renal insufficiency and renal calcinosis. Magnesium containing antacids can cause diarrhea, the main dose limiting adverse effect, and are rarely used alone for PUD therapy. Aluminum hydroxide is a weaker antacid than magnesium hydroxide and can cause constipation. Magnesium-aluminum combination products were developed in an attempt to minimize diarrhea. Occasionally, if diarrhea persists, a combination magnesium-aluminum product can be alternated with doses of aluminum hydroxide. Other adverse effects include the development of hypermagnesemia and hyperaluminemia in the presence of renal failure. Phosphorus depletion can occur in patients taking chronic doses of aluminum salts due to binding of phosphate in the intestinal tract, and long-term complications can include osteoporosis.

Antacids can cause drug interactions, usually due to interference with drug absorption or chelation (e.g., tetracycline). Antacids have been reported to significantly reduce the serum concentrations of digoxin, ketoconazole, tetracycline, ferrous sulfate, isoniazid, and fluoroquinolones (e.g., ciprofloxacin) when administered concomitantly. Antacids can increase quinidine serum concentrations by enhancing renal tubular reabsorption of quinidine due to an increase in urine pH.

H₂-Receptor Antagonists

The development and use of H₂-receptor antagonists has significantly changed the management of peptic ulcer disease since their introduction with cimetidine in 1976. Four H₂ antagonists are currently used in this country (cimetidine, ranitidine, famotidine, and nizatidine), and together they are the most frequently prescribed class of drugs for the treatment of PUD (20, 21). All of these agents are useful in the acute and maintenance therapy of duodenal ulcer, benign gastric ulcer, hypersecretory conditions, and gastroesophageal reflux, and in the prevention of upper GI bleeding due to stress ulceration.

H$_2$ antagonists competitively and reversibly bind to the H$_2$-receptor of the parietal cells, causing a dose-dependent inhibition of gastric acid secretion. They differ in potency, chemical structure, adverse effects, and ability to cause drug interactions. Famotidine is the most potent, followed by nizatidine, ranitidine, and cimetidine.

H$_2$ antagonists are more effective than placebo in healing duodenal and gastric ulcers, with 80% of duodenal ulcers healed after 4 weeks and more than 90% healed after 8 weeks. Gastric ulcers usually take longer to heal and often require at least 8 weeks of treatment.

H$_2$ antagonists may be given in divided daily doses or daily as a single dose for acute initial therapy of duodenal and gastric ulcers. The dosage regimens are equivalent and may be administered for up to 8 weeks (Table 23.4). Maintenance therapy for duodenal ulcer should be given as a single daily dose.

Table 23.4.

Dosage Schedule for Drugs Used in the Treatment of Peptic Ulcer Disease

	Initial Therapy	Maintenance Therapy
Cimetidine	300 mg QID	400 mg QHS
	400 mg BID	
	800 mg HS	
Ranitidine	150 mg BID	150 mg HS
	300 mg HS	
Famotidine	20 mg BID	20 mg QHS
	40 mg HS	
Nizatidine	150 mg BID	150 mg HS
	300 mg HS	
Sucralfate	1 g QID	1 g BID
	2 g BID	
Omeprazole	20 mg QD	20 mg HS

Duodenal ulcer recurrence is reported to be approximately 60 to 80% within 12 months following cessation of therapy (9). Risk factors associated with recurrence of peptic ulcers include cigarette smoking, gastric hypersecretion, male sex, presence of *H. pylori* in the original ulcer, low-fiber diet, NSAIDs (including ASA), and poor compliance. Full-dose H$_2$-antagonist therapy (Table 23.4) may be given intermittently to patients at low risk if there is evidence of ulcer recurrence. It may be prudent to screen these patient for *H. pylori* and treat if necessary. Patients with risk factors for recurrence should receive daily maintenance H$_2$-antagonist therapy after the ulcer is initially healed. Treatment may be needed indefinitely in some cases.

CIMETIDINE

Cimetidine is approved for acute and maintenance therapy of DU, active benign gastric ulcer, hypersecretory conditions, and gastroesophageal reflux disease (22). Cimetidine has an oral bioavailability of 60 to 70%, with peak levels produced within an hour of administration. Cimetidine is metabolized in the liver and has an elimination half-life of about 2 hours in patients with normal renal function. The half-life increases as the renal function diminishes, extending to approximately 5 hours in anephric patients.

Cimetidine, like the other H$_2$ antagonists, has very few major side effects. Diarrhea, usually mild and transient, dizziness, and headache have been reported in 2 to 4% of patients. Mental status alteration (confusion, agitation, anxiety, disorientation) may occur, especially in severely ill patients (renal/hepatic impairment) and in the elderly if the dose is not adjusted appropriately. Gynecomastia has been reported in about 4% of patients receiving high-dose cimetidine for long-term treatment of Zollinger-Ellison syndrome. Mild and transient increases in several laboratory test results (AST, ALT, alkaline phosphatase, and

Table 23.5.

Drug Interactions with Antiulcer Drug Medications

Object Drug \ Interacting Drug	Cimetidine	Ranitidine	Famotidine	Nizatidine	Omeprazole	Sucralfate
Fluoroquinolone Antibiotics	N/R°	N/R	N/R	N/R	N/R	Decreased absorption
Ketoconazole	Decreased absorption	Decreased absorption	Decreased absorption	Decreased absorption	Decreased absorption	N/R
Theophylline	Decreased clearance	Decreased clearance	Negligible	Negligible	Negligible	Decreased absorption
Phenytoin	Decreased clearance	Decreased clearance	Negligible	Negligible	Decreased clearance	Decreased absorption
Warfarin	Decreased clearance	Decreased clearance	Negligible	Negligible	Decreased clearance	Decreased absorption
Diazepam	Decreased clearance	Decreased clearance	Negligible	Negligible	Decreased clearance	Negligible
Procainamide	Decreased clearance	Decreased clearance	No effect	No effect	No effect	No effect

°None reported.

serum creatinine levels) have occurred but are not usually clinically important. Cimetidine inhibits the cytochrome P-450 enzyme system in the liver, resulting in several important drug interactions (see Table 23.5).

The oral dosage regimens for cimetidine may be found in Table 23.4. Cimetidine may also be administered IM or IV in doses of 300 mg every 6 to 8 hr. In patients with a creatinine clearance less than 30 mL/min, it is recommended that the dose be decreased by 50%.

RANITIDINE Zantac

Ranitidine is available in oral and parenteral dosage forms. It is well-absorbed after oral administration, with peak serum levels occurring in 2 to 3 hours. Ranitidine undergoes significant first-pass metabolism, with a bioavailability of approximately 50%. The elimination half-life of ranitidine averages 1.7 to 3.2 hours in patients with normal renal function, but is prolonged to 6 to 10 hours in patients with creatinine clearances below 30 mL/min and in the elderly. Ranitidine is metabolized in the liver and excreted in the urine and by the biliary system (22).

Adverse effects of ranitidine are similar to those of cimetidine. It would appear that ranitidine has less effect on endocrine and gonadal function than does cimetidine, but gynecomastia and impotence have occurred rarely.

Ranitidine does not interact with the hepatic cytochrome P-450 system to the same extent as cimetidine and thus appears to produce fewer clinically significant drug interactions (see Table 23.5). It only minimally inhibits hepatic metabolism of drugs such as warfarin, theophylline, diazepam, and propranolol.

Dosing information for ranitidine may be found in Table 23.4. Ranitidine may also be administered intermittently via the IM or IV route in doses of 50 mg every 6 to 8 hours, or it may be given by continuous intravenous infusion at a starting dose of 6.25 mg/hr. Reduction to one third to one half the usual dose should be made in patients with creatinine clearances below 50 mL/min (22).

FAMOTIDINE Pepcid

Famotidine is absorbed incompletely from the GI tract following oral administration, with an oral bioavailability of 40 to 50%. Famotidine has the longest elimination half-life of the currently available H_2 antagonists, an average of 2.5 to 4 hours. The half-life is increased to approximately 12 hours in patients with creatinine clearances below 30 mL/min. Famotidine is metabolized in the liver and excreted in the urine via glomerular filtration and tubular secretion. Side effects of famotidine are similar to those of the other H_2-receptor antagonists, except that it does not appear to exhibit antiandrogenic activity or affect the hepatic clearance of other drugs to the extent that cimetidine does (22, 23).

Oral dosing information for famotidine is given in Table 23.4. Famotidine may also be given by slow IV injection in doses of 20 mg every 12 hours or by continuous IV infusion at a rate of 3.2 to 4.0 mg/hr. Dosage should be reduced to 20 mg/day in patients with creatinine clearances less than 10 mL/min.

NIZATIDINE Axid

Nizatidine is the newest H_2 antagonist to be marketed in the United States and is currently available only in an oral dosage form. Nizatidine is well absorbed orally from the gastrointestinal tract, with a bioavailability of approximately 70%. Peak plasma concentrations occur within about an hour following administration. Nizatidine is approximately one third metabolized in the liver and two thirds excreted unchanged in urine. The elimination half-life ranges from 1 to 2 hours in normal patients and is increased in patients with renal impairment (23).

The adverse effects seen with nizatidine are similar to those of other H_2 antagonists. There is no evidence of antiandrogenic effects, and no serious effects on the central nervous system have been reported. Hepatitis has been reported more frequently than with the other H_2 antagonists. However, more data are needed to confirm the comparative incidence. There is no effect on the cytochrome P-450 enzyme system, making nizatidine a favorable choice when other drugs that might interact with other H_2 antagonists are being administered.

Dosing information for nizatidine is presented in Table 23.4. In patients with creatinine clearances between 20 and 50 mL/min, a 50% reduction in dosage is recommended (22).

Other Agents

SUCRALFATE

Sucralfate is a unique therapeutic agent used for the active and maintenance therapy of duodenal ulcers, treatment of gastric ulcers, and prevention of stress ulceration. It is an aluminum salt of a sulfated disaccharide that exerts its action locally on the GI mucosa. Sucralfate binds to positively charged molecules to form a gelatinous layer at the ulcer site, which protects the ulcer or involved mucosa from the aggressive factors acid, pepsin, and bile salts. It has also been shown to absorb pepsin and bile salts, and it may stimulate the secretion of endogenous cytoprotective prostaglandins (24). Sucralfate undergoes very limited absorption from the GI tract (3 to 5%), although the aluminum ions released by its interaction with gastric acid may be significantly absorbed (25, 26).

Because of its lack of significant systemic bioavailability, sucralfate is generally well tolerated. Its most common adverse effects are constipation (2%), diarrhea, nausea, vomiting, bloating, flatulence, dry mouth or metallic taste, and indigestion (each less than 1% incidence). The small amount of aluminum absorbed from sucralfate is readily excreted by the kidney in patients with normal renal function. However, patients suffering from chronic renal failure or requiring dialysis may accumulate the aluminum systemically, leading to aluminum toxicity. Complications resulting from this include osteomalacia, osteodystrophy, and encephalopathy or seizures. Because of these, it is recommended that sucralfate be given cautiously on a routine basis to patients with renal impairment (22).

The development of gastric bezoars have also been reported (27). Drug interactions with sucralfate have been investigated in recent years, and significant interactions are shown in Table 23.5. The most significant of these is with the fluoroquinolones, where it may be best to place the patient receiving fluoroquinolones on alternate antiulcer medications until the antibiotic course is completed (22). Sucralfate dosing information is given in Table 23.4. No adjustments in renal or hepatic impairment are necessary.

ACID-PUMP INHIBITORS

Omeprazole is a substituted benzimidazole that irreversibly binds to and inhibits the H^+-K^+ ATPase (acid pump) on the apical membrane of parietal cells, the final phase in acid secretion (28). The maximum effect occurs within 2 hours of administration, reducing peak acid output by 80% or more. At 24 hours there is 50% of maximum inhibition, and effects may persist for up to 72 hours after a dose, until new H^+-K^+ ATPase can be synthesized. Mean acid output is suppressed, after administering 20 and 40 mg daily for 7 days, by 79% (range 54 to 98%) and 85% (range 76 to 96%), respectively (29). The antisecretory activity of 20 to 40 mg of omeprazole is greater than that of the H_2 antagonists. Other acid-pump inhibitors under investigation include lansoprazole and pantoprazole.

Omeprazole absorption is variable and increases in an alkaline environment, so more is absorbed as it inhibits acid secretion. It undergoes extensive metabolism in the liver and has an elimination half-life of 0.5 to 1.5 hours. By its potent effect on inhibiting acid secretion, gastrin concentrations can increase by two to four times the normal range. Serum gastrin concentrations return to pretreatment level within 2 weeks of discontinuing the drug.

Omeprazole is as effective as H_2 antagonists for the treatment of peptic ulcers and possibly more effective for gastric ulcer (28, 30, 31). Omeprazole is perhaps most useful for the management of peptic ulcers refractory to conventional therapy with antacids and H_2 antagonists (32). Omeprazole given in doses of 20 to 40 mg daily for 6 to 8 weeks can heal up to 90% of refractory peptic ulcers unresponsive to conventional therapy (6). It is also useful for hypersecretory states such as Zollinger-Ellison syndrome, gastroesophageal reflux disease (GERD), and severe erosive esophagitis, which is typically unresponsive to antacids and H_2 antagonists.

The initial dose of omeprazole is 20 mg daily, given with food, for 4 to 8 weeks. Increasing the dose to 40 mg daily should be considered in patients with an unhealed ulcer after 8 weeks of treatment with 20 mg daily.

Adverse effects of omeprazole include headache, diarrhea, abdominal pain, and nausea in less than 5% of patients. Hyperplasia of enterochromaffinlike cells and gastric carcinoid tumors have been observed in rats given omeprazole, presumably due to marked hypergastrinemia. However, no cases of enterochromaffinlike cell hyperplasia or gastric tumors have been reported in humans. Forty patients with Zollinger-Ellison syndrome were given 82 ± 31 mg per day with no evidence of gastric tumors for up to 4 years (6 to 51 months) (33).

Omeprazole inhibits cytochrome P-450 enzymes and may cause interactions with drugs metabolized by this pathway. Omeprazole has been shown to increase serum concentrations of diazepam, warfarin, and phenytoin (see Table 23.5).

ANTICHOLINERGICS

Anticholinergics are of little importance in the treatment of DU. They can reduce acid secretion by 30 to 35% as compared to 85 to 90% with H_2 antagonists. Anticholinergics have been used with antacids in patients with DU to help reduce stomach emptying and to prolong the buffering activity of antacids. Anticholinergics have no place in the treatment of patients with gastric ulcers. The minor antisecretory activity of this class of drugs is offset by the ability to reduce the motility of the GI tract. This causes retention of acid and pepsin in the stomach.

Treatment of *H. pylori*

Despite the initial efficacy of available therapeutic agents for PUD, the problem of the high recurrence rate after complete healing remains. DUs treated by acid suppression therapy alone, without maintenance, recur in about 80% of patients within 12 months (34, 35). At this time, the major role of therapy directed against *H. pylori* appears to be to reduce or eliminate ulcer recurrence (36–40). As yet unexplained, the combination of an antisecretory agent, such as omeprazole, plus antibiotics are generally necessary for ulcer healing and eradication of *H. pylori* infection. Success rates are poor with antibiotics alone for duodenal ulcer (41), but recent evidence suggests that antibiotics alone may heal gastric ulcers as effectively as omeprazole (42).

H. pylori resides under the mucus gel layer in the highly acidic milieu of the stomach. Data suggest that *H. pylori* eradication therapy depends upon topical, local mucosal delivery of antibiotics. The oral route of antibiotic administration, which produces high transient drug concentrations in the gastric mucosa, is preferred (43–45). In addition, H_2 antagonists have been shown to be effective in increasing antibiotic concentrations in the gastric mucosa, which may explain, in part, the efficacy seen when antisecretory agents are combined with antibiotics versus antibiotics alone (46).

There is no suitable animal model to study therapy, so most of the available information concerning drug selection is based on small trials in humans. A variety of antibiotics have activity against *H. pylori*, including tetracycline, metronidazole, amoxicillin, and clarithromycin. The best combination of agents is currently the subject of debate, but eradication rates of 80 to 90% can be achieved with appropriate therapy. Eradication rates of 90% or higher have been documented with triple therapy regimens with bismuth subsalicylate (2 tablets Q.I.D.), tetracycline (500 mg Q.I.D.), and metronidazole (250 mg T.I.D.) given for 14 days (41, 47–49). Tetracycline is said to have in vitro synergism with metronidazole against 30 to 40% of metronidazole-resistant strains (50). Substitution of oxytetracycline (51) or doxycycline (52) for tetracycline has been shown to reduce eradication to 83% and 65% respectively. Similar eradication rates have been demonstrated with the combination of ranitidine, metronidazole (500 mg T.I.D.) and amoxicillin (750 mg T.I.D.) (53, 54).

Eradication rates of 80 to 90% have been documented with the combination of omeprazole (20 mg B.I.D.) and amoxicillin (1.5–2.0 g/d) (40, 41, 55–57). Omeprazole should be given with the antibiotic and not before, as there is evidence to suggest that pretreatment with omeprazole may reduce the regimen's effectiveness. Two- or three-drug regimens should typically be 2 weeks in duration, although 1-week regimens have been reported to be successful in some patients (58–60). Resistance has been documented, particularly with nitroimidazoles (such as metronidazole), but does not currently appear to be a widespread problem with other agents (14). Single antibiotic regimens without antisecretory drugs do not appear to be effective, have led to enhanced antimicrobial resistance, and are thus discouraged. Generally, antisecretory therapy should continue for a total of 6 weeks if the patient has an active ulcer. If an H$_2$ antagonist was started, then it can be continued; if omeprazole was used, after 2 weeks the dose can be reduced to 20 mg/day or the patient may be switched to a less expensive H$_2$ antagonist.

Summary

The H$_2$ antagonists appear to be equal in effect in their treatment of duodenal and gastric ulcer. Use of these products should be determined by potential for adverse effects, drug interactions, and cost. Sucralfate may be used as an alternative to H$_2$ antagonists, but there is not convincing evidence that the combination of sucralfate with an H$_2$-receptor antagonist is any more beneficial than either agent alone. Omeprazole has demonstrated improved healing of duodenal ulcers compared to conventional therapy and in refractory cases. Treatment of *H. pylori* can reduce peptic ulcer recurrence and has become an important consideration in therapy.

ZOLLINGER-ELLISON SYNDROME (GASTRINOMA)

Zollinger-Ellison (ZE) syndrome is an ulcerogenic neoplasm that occurs in less than 1% of patients with peptic ulcer disease and is one of several hypersecretory syndromes. It is caused by a gastrin-producing adenoma, usually in the pancreas and duodenal wall. The range of basal gastrin concentration in patients with duodenal ulcer disease without gastrinoma is usually under 200 pg/mL. A serum gastrin concentration between 200 and 1000 pg/mL with compatible clinical findings supports the diagnosis of ZE syndrome. Serum gastrin concentrations can exceed 1000 pg/mL (6, 9). In over 70% of patients the basal gastric acid output exceeds 15 mEq/hr (6).

ZE characteristically produces severe, often unremitting, numerous recurrences of peptic ulcers. These may either be single or multiple duodenal or gastric ulcers occurring in unusual locations such as the distal portion of the duodenum or even the jejunum. These patients typically have persistent ulcer pain and diarrhea. ZE syndrome occurs in adults with equal frequency in both sexes and rarely in children.

Treatment

OMEPRAZOLE Prilosec

Until the introduction of omeprazole, many cases of ZE syndrome required combination therapy with H$_2$ antagonists and sucralfate. Omeprazole usually controls acid output with a single daily dose and, other than curative surgery, is considered to be the drug of choice for this disorder at this time. The dose of omeprazole should be adjusted for each patient to produce a basal gastric acid secretion rate under 5 mEq/hr before the next dose (6, 28). The median dosage for patients with ZE syndrome is 60 to 70 mg daily (range 20-360 mg).

H$_2$-RECEPTOR ANTAGONISTS

Prior to the availability of omeprazole, H$_2$ antagonists were the mainstay of therapy for ZE syndrome. To achieve the degree of acid suppression needed they usually must be given in higher doses and/or with greater frequency than is recommended for gastric or duodenal ulcers. However, they offer no advantage over omeprazole.

OCTREOTIDE

Octreotide may suppress gastrin levels and provide symptomatic relief in carefully selected patients with ZE syndrome (61). It inhibits both gastric acid and gastrin production and secondary peptides released by gastrinomas. However, octreotide is expensive, is administered intravenously, and may be impractical in many cases.

Summary

Omeprazole is considered the drug of choice in treating this disorder. Patients have been safely treated for up to 4 years with no major adverse effects; however, further evaluation of long-term safety is essential. A cure rate of 20 to 30% may be possible if the gastrinoma is resectable.

GASTROESOPHAGEAL REFLUX DISEASE (GERD)

Gastroesophageal reflux disease is the syndrome consisting of esophageal mucosal damage produced by retrograde flow of gastric contents into the esophagus. "Heartburn," an epigastric burning sensation, is the most common clinical manifestation of this illness, which is brought about primarily by an ineffective or incompetent lower esophageal sphincter (LES) (9, 62). The LES normally remains closed except during swallowing. It is kept in this closed position because of its inherent muscular tone and through vagal stimulation. As a result of decreased LES tone, gastric contents are refluxed into the esophagus, where the acidity of this material may irritate and damage the mucosa. Increases in intragastric pressure or volume make reflux more likely, but decreased LES tone is necessary for reflux to occur. Symptoms, in addition to heartburn, may include dysphagia, belching, and regurgitation of liquid into the mouth, which may even produce morning hoarseness or result in pulmonary aspiration with resultant pneumonitis or chronic asthma. Though many patients experience heartburn occasionally, severe or recurrent symptoms deserve investigation.

Diagnosis of GERD is based on history, and esophagitis may be demonstrated by barium swallow, esophagoscopy with or without esophageal mucosal biopsy, and esophageal motility and clearance studies. Several things can worsen reflux by altering LES pressures or intragastric pressures. These are listed in Table 23.6.

Table 23.6.
Drugs that Decrease LES Pressure and May Worsen GERD Symptoms

Alpha-adrenergic antagonists
Anticholinergics
Benzodiazepines
Beta-adrenergic antagonists
Calcium channel blockers
Dopamine
Nitrates
Progesterone
Prostaglandins E_1, E_2, A_2
Theophylline

Treatment

The goals of treatment for GERD are useful guides to understanding the rationale for treatment. These goals include decreasing reflux, neutralizing the refluxate, improving esophageal clearance, and protection of the esophageal mucosa (9). Mild, uncomplicated cases of occasional heartburn can be effectively treated with antacids (63). Other straightforward measures that may be adequate in mild cases include dietary avoidance of offensive foods, especially during the evening or at bedtime, weight reduction, and elevation, or "blocking," of the head of the bed. Elevating the head of the bed should be accomplished by placing the bed legs on 6- to 8-in.-high blocks or by employing a wedge under the mattress to achieve a straight incline from foot to head. Each of these measures should be employed in individual patients where particularly applicable, but they should be continued only if they improve symptoms. In addition, the patient should be instructed to avoid certain offending medications when possible (see Table 23.6). If necessary, antacids in a dose necessary to provide 40 to 80 mEq of ANC or a bedtime dose of an H_2 antagonist may be added to these nonpharmacologic measures.

Though most patients can be managed with life-style modifications and antacids, some patients with moderate to severe disease with esophagitis may require additional intervention with prescription medications, including the H_2 antagonists, omeprazole, and prokinetic agents such as metoclopramide or cisapride.

H_2-receptor antagonists must often be given in higher doses to patients with moderate to severe esophagitis. One study that demonstrated the impact of dosage regimen on response rates compared oral ranitidine 150 mg twice a day with ranitidine 300 mg four times a day. At the end of 8 weeks of therapy, the healing rate was significantly better in the high-dose regimen (response rate of 75% versus 54% in the low-dose group) (64). It is sometimes necessary to give doses such as this for long treatment periods (8 weeks) for initial therapy, and 3 to 6 months or longer of high-dose therapy may be required if the patient has a recurrence.

Omeprazole 20 to 40 mg/day can be used in the management of GERD and esophagitis. Ambulatory esophageal pH recordings have shown almost total control of reflux episodes in patients given these regimens (65). Omeprazole has been evaluated in patients who have failed to respond to various H_2 antagonists. In a dose of 40 mg/day, omeprazole treatment for 12 weeks successfully healed almost 90% of such cases (66). However, following discontinuation of therapy, many patients will have clinical recurrences of esophagitis. It is therefore usually recommended to place patients who recur on long-term maintenance therapy. At this point, omeprazole may be considered the most efficacious maintenance therapy, as only 17% of patients receiving omeprazole 20 mg daily developed recurrence (67, 68). Further experience with the long-term use of omeprazole will be helpful in determining its safety during this type treatment. Reglan   propulsid

Prokinetic agents, such as metoclopramide or cisapride, are sometimes used in the management of GERD. These agents both increase LES pressure and hasten gastric emptying. Metoclopramide is usually administered in a regimen of 10 mg four times daily before meals and at bedtime. It is most often combined with an H₂ antagonist or omeprazole. Side effects of metoclopramide include blurred vision, dry mouth, depression and pseudo-parkinsonism.

Cisapride is a newer prokinetic agent that enhances gastrointestinal motility through mechanisms not yet completely elucidated (69). This agent displays some indirect cholinomimetic effects and also appears to cause some serotonergic stimulation. Following oral administration, cisapride is very well absorbed but appears to have a bioavailability of approximately 40 to 50%. Peak serum concentrations are reached within 2 hours of administration, and food causes an increase in bioavailability. It is extensively metabolized by the liver, and has an elimination half-life of 7 to 10 hours. Cisapride is given in an oral dose of 10 mg three to four times daily, 15 minutes before meals and at bedtime, with an increase to 20 mg/dose if necessary. In a number of clinical trials, cisapride appeared to be as effective as H₂ blockers in the acute treatment of symptomatic erosive esophagitis and has proven more effective than placebo for maintenance therapy. Cisapride has not been studied in direct comparison to omeprazole in GERD (69).

Cisapride is generally well tolerated, with gastrointestinal adverse effects such as diarrhea and cramping being the most commonly reported. It appears to cause fewer extrapyramidal effects than metoclopramide.

Summary

Effective management of GERD can often be accomplished by employing life-style changes. When this does not completely alleviate symptoms, drug therapy may be instituted, with first-line therapy being antacids on an as-needed basis. For moderate to severe esophagitis, H₂ antagonists, omeprazole, and prokinetic agents, each used individually or in combination where appropriate, provide healing in the majority of cases. Recurrence rates are high, necessitating long-term maintenance therapy in those patients who suffer recurrence. The long-term safety profile of the chronic therapy does not present long-term risks to this population.

STRESS-RELATED ULCERATION

Stress ulceration can be defined as superficial erosions of the gastric mucosa that develop when severe physiologic demands are placed upon a critically ill individual (9). This type of ulceration differs from traditional peptic ulcer disease in a number of ways. Stress ulcerations are often small and numerous versus the typical single lesion seen in PUD. The lesions are superficial rather than deep or penetrating and are most commonly located in the acid secreting portion of the stomach, but may also occur in the duodenum or gastric antrum. Stress ulceration also tends to be painless, with the major clinical manifestation being bleeding. Approximately 80% of untreated seriously ill patients will develop stress ulcers, with serious hemorrhage occurring in 5 to 20%. The associated mortality with hemorrhage ranges from 50 to 80%. The incidence of stress-related ulceration has declined with the increased use of prophylactic drug therapy and better nutritional and ventilatory support of critically ill patients. However, stress-related ulceration remains a significant and potentially life-threatening complication in the critically ill patient.

Risk Factors

All seriously ill patients are at risk for stress-related ulceration. Severe burns (>35% of body surface), sepsis, hemodynamic shock from a variety of causes, and others with severe illness are at increased risk. The Canadian Critical Care Trials Group study showed that two strong, independent risk factors for the development of GI bleeding among critically ill patients were respiratory failure, defined as a need for mechanical ventilation for over 48 hours, and the presence of coagulopathy (70).

Pathogenesis

The pathogenic mechanisms involved in the formation of stress ulcers include reduced mucosal blood flow, presence of gastric acid, and disruption of mucosal barriers. The gastric mucosal epithelium normally has a very high oxygen requirement, making it particularly susceptible to reductions in mucosal blood flow. Gastric acid output is sometimes, but not always, increased in patients who develop stress ulcerations. It appears, however, that the presence of acid is necessary for the development of these superficial erosions. The presence of gastric acid, in concert with the breakdown in natural mucosal barriers, leads to hydrogen ion back-diffusion into the mucosal cells, causing mucosal damage, which then develops into superficial ulceration. The mucosal damage also leads to a decrease in mucus production, reduced bicarbonate secretion, and inhibition of mucosal prostaglandin synthesis. During long periods of stress and/or the lack of adequate nutrition and oxygenation, the regeneration of gastric epithelium is also impaired. Eventually, the development of these ulcers predisposes the patient to hemorrhage, which may occur in small amounts as quickly as 24 to 48 hours following the onset of injury or severe stress. Larger amounts of blood loss, often leading to hemodynamic compromise and mortality, usually occur 3 or more days after the initial injury or stress event (9, 71).

Diagnosis

Blood loss, as represented by gross examination of gastric contents or positive guaiac of nasogastric (NG) aspirate, is usually the first sign of the occurrence of ulceration. Although not all patients with minor blood loss will progress to clinically important bleeding, upper GI endoscopic examination is the most reliable method for confirming ulceration. Radiographic examination is less reliable than endoscopic examination for detecting acute stress induced mucosal erosion (9).

Treatment

The need for routine prophylactic administration of pharmacologic agents to all patients in intensive care units remains controversial. High-risk patients, as defined previously, are targeted by many institutions and receive prophylactic therapy. Therapeutic goals in these patients include maintenance of gastric pH above 4.0 and/or protection of gastric mucosa and enhancement of mucosal barriers. Antacids, H_2 antagonists, and sucralfate have all been used as prophylactic therapy against stress ulceration.

Antacids were originally used heavily in the prophylaxis of stress ulceration. However, large doses are often necessary to maintain intragastric pH above 4. Monitoring of pH from gastric aspirates is also essential in order to adjust the dose of antacid to achieve this pH goal.

H_2 antagonists are also effective in raising the intragastric pH above 4 and are given either as intermittent bolus therapy or by continuous infusion. Continuous infusion of H_2 antagonists has generally been shown to produce a more consistent elevation of intragastric pH, with dosage ranges of 37.5 to 100 mg/hr (cimetidine), 6.25 to 12.5 mg/hr (ranitidine), and 3.2 to 4.0 mg/hr (famotidine) (72). Continuous infusion cimetidine was shown to be more effective than placebo in preventing GI hemorrhage in critically ill patients (73).

Sucralfate has also been used effectively in the prevention of stress ulceration (71). A recent study compared sucralfate 1 gram every 4 hours to a continuous ranitidine infusion of 6.25 mg/hr and to an antacid suspension with a buffering capacity of 1.2 mEq/mL, given in a starting dose of 20 mL q2h and titrated to maintain intragastric pH above 4 (74). There was no difference found between the groups with respect to occurrence of macroscopic bleeding. Sucralfate can be administered every 4 hours as a suspension either orally or via NG tube.

Currently, a controversy exists regarding the possible causative role that stress ulcer prophylaxis may play in the development of bacterial pneumonia in these critically ill patients. The mechanism for this involves gastric pH changes produced by H_2 antagonists and antacids, since a pH above 4 may create an environment where growth of gram-negative bacteria is enhanced, in that low intragastric pH normally functions as a deterrent to bacterial growth. It is proposed that this increased colonization of the stomach leads to a greater risk of aspiration of these bacteria into the respiratory tract (75). Since sucralfate does not raise intragastric pH significantly, it is currently thought by some clinicians that it may offer an advantage in this regard (74). Further investigation may better delineate any differences between sucralfate, H_2 antagonists, antacids, and other therapies with regard to resultant pneumonia.

DRUG-INDUCED ULCERATION

Drug-induced GI adverse effects are common and can result in significant morbidity. Drugs such as erythromycin, iron salts, corticosteroids, and potassium chloride can cause gastroduodenal damage; however, the drugs most frequently associated with acute and chronic gastroduodenal injury, including ulceration, are NSAIDs. NSAID-induced adverse GI effects may be seen in 2 to 30% of patients (77, 78). Prolonged ingestion of NSAIDs is a major cause of GU, and more than 10% of patients on NSAIDs have endoscopically verified peptic ulcers. Elderly patients with osteo- and rheumatoid arthritis, appear to be at increased risk of ulceration and overt hemorrhage, especially women. In one retrospective study, users of NSAIDs were found to be four times more likely to die from PUD or upper GI bleeding than nonusers (79).

Cigarette smoking can increase the risk of ulceration and its complications in persons taking NSAIDs. Individuals who smoke have impaired healing and greater recurrence of ulcers, as well as an increased likelihood that surgery will be required for ulcer repair.

Pathogenesis

NSAIDs are thought to induce damage of the gastric mucosa via two mechanisms: (a) by direct effects of the acidic agent on the gastric mucosa, and (b) by inhibiting the production of protective prostaglandins (Fig. 23.1). Gastric mucus provides a barrier that protects the stomach epithelium from gastric contents through several mechanisms: (a) the mucosa secretes bicarbonate, via receptor-mediated active transport, which buffers acidic contents, (b) the mucus layer thickens in response to epithelial injury, allowing rapid epithelialization to take place after insults from agents such as aspirin and ethanol, and (c) gastric mucosal blood flow helps to protect the mucosa from injury. If the mucous barrier is disrupted, a compensatory increase in mucosal blood flow helps to remove the H+ ions that can damage the mucosa. When the blood flow does not increase, cell death follows.

Prostaglandins are stimulated by stress or trauma to the cell membranes. These protective substances have an antisecretory effect on gastric acid production and defend the stomach against acid and other noxious substances. Prostaglandins have a variety of GI effects but are thought

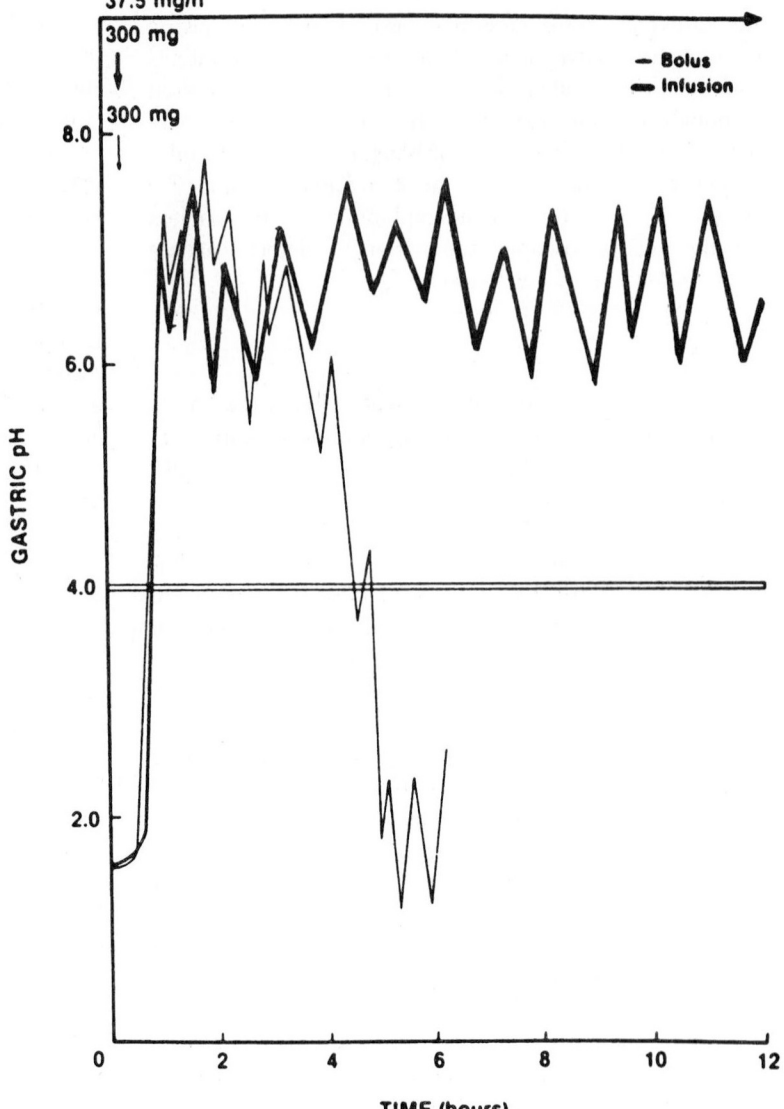

Figure 23.1. Effect of cimetidine bolus (light line) versus primed infusion (bold line) on gastric pH in the "typical patient." (With permission from Ostro MJ, Russell JA, Soldin SJ, et al. Control of gastric pH with cimetidine: boluses versus primed infusions. Gastroenterology 89: 532–537, 1985.)

to primarily aid the gastric mucosal defense by stimulating bicarbonate secretion and synthesis of mucus.

NSAIDs inhibit prostaglandin synthesis, allowing disruption of prostaglandin-mediated mucosal defenses. NSAIDs act as weak organic acids that can increase basal levels of gastric acid secretion and can also alter and disrupt cell membranes, allowing back-diffusion of H^+ ions to occur. Once these weak acids disrupt cell membranes, they become trapped within the mucosal cells, inducing alterations in the morphology in exposed mucosal cells.

Treatment

Discontinuing NSAID use is not always feasible, particularly when NSAIDs are used for the treatment of rheumatoid and osteoarthritis. Consequently, availability of

effective treatment for the prevention and management of NSAID-induced ulceration is important.

Misoprostol and other prostaglandin E1 analogs have been studied for efficacy in protecting the gastric mucosa against ulcerogenic agents (80–82). Other analogs include enprostil, arbaprostil, trimoprostil, rioprostil, enisprostil, and ornoprostil. Prostaglandins appear to facilitate regeneration of the mucosa after injury by NSAIDs and should be effective in the healing and prevention of mucosal damage. Misoprostol aids in mucosal defense by enhancing secretion of mucus and increasing bicarbonate production and mucosal blood flow. Misoprostol has some antisecretory effects, but this likely provides little protective effect, since the more potent antisecretory H_2 antagonists do not appear to be effective in preventing NSAID-induced ulceration.

Prophylactic use of misoprostol has been shown to reduce NSAID-induced GU by 75% and 95% in doses of 100 μg or 200 μg four times daily, respectively. Misoprostol and other prostaglandin analogs have been shown to be comparable to conventional therapy in healing peptic ulcers, but their propensity to cause diarrhea precludes their routine use for therapy at this time.

Currently, misoprostol is the only agent indicated for the *prevention* of NSAID-induced gastric ulceration. Patients who should receive misoprostol prophylaxis include those at high risk of developing ulcers, such as elderly patients, patients with concomitant diseases, and patients with a history of peptic ulceration (83–85). This agent is rapidly and extensively absorbed and exhibits plasma protein binding of 80 to 90%. Plasma concentrations of misoprostol are decreased when the dose is administered with food, and concomitant use of antacids decreases total bioavailability. The recommended dose of misoprostol is 200 μg four times daily with meals. A dosage of 100 μg four times daily with food is suggested for patients who do not tolerate the higher dose. Dosage adjustment is not necessary in the presence of renal or hepatic insufficiency.

Misoprostol produces minor adverse effects including nausea, abdominal discomfort, headache, dizziness, and diarrhea. Diarrhea is the most troublesome adverse effect and has occurred in 14 to 40% of patients. These adverse effects are similar to the symptoms seen with gastric ulceration. The diarrhea may be dose-related, tends to occur early in the course of therapy, and may be self-limited or may require discontinuation of the drug in some patients. In women, menstrual disturbances, spotting, and abdominal cramping may occur. Misoprostol can induce abortions and is contraindicated during pregnancy (FDA pregnancy category X). Women in their child-bearing years *must not* be pregnant when therapy is initiated and should use effective contraception while on misoprostol therapy. If pregnancy occurs while taking misoprostol, the patient should discontinue therapy and contact her physician immediately. Patients should be counseled accordingly as a point of emphasis.

H₂-antagonist prophylaxis with ranitidine has been shown to reduce the incidence of NSAID-induced DU, but no consistent effect on GU has been observed (83, 86, 87). Omeprazole appears to be more effective than H₂ antagonists once an ulcer develops in patients who continue to use NSAIDs (81). Once an ulcer has formed following NSAID therapy, other commonly used therapeutic agents should be used in preference to misoprostol. Any of the commonly used drugs already discussed appear to heal ulcers once NSAID treatment is stopped.

CONCLUSION

Great strides have been made in the treatment of PUD over the last two decades. New therapies continue to be developed. The emergence of *H. pylori* as a cause of peptic ulcers and gastritis adds yet another dimension to the complexity of these disorders. Effective antiulcer and antibiotic therapy may reduce the recurrence of duodenal and gastric ulcers, a major problem with PUD.

It must be stressed, however, that the pathophysiology of PUD is complex, with considerable etiologic diversity. Each patient should be carefully evaluated and therapy individualized to maximize therapeutic and pharmacoeconomic outcomes. Emphasis should not be placed just on healing of the initial ulcer, but also on prevention of recurrence.

REFERENCES

1. Lam SK, Hui WM, Ching CK. Peptic ulcer disease. Part 1: epidemiology, pathogenesis, and etiology. In: Humbrich WS, Schaffner F, Berk JE, eds. Bockus gastroenterology, 5th ed. Philadelphia: WB Saunders, 1995:700–748.
2. Kurata JH. Ulcer epidemiology: an overview and proposed research framework. Gastroenterology 96:569–580, 1989.
3. Bloom BS. Cross national changes in the effects of peptic ulcer disease. Ann Intern Med 114:558–562, 1991.
4. Sonnenburg A. Costs of medical and surgical treatment of duodenal ulcer. Gastroenterology 96:1445–1452, 1989.
5. Wolfe MM, Soll AH. The physiology of gastric acid secretion. N Engl J Med 319:1707–1715, 1988.
6. Gray GM. Peptic ulcer diseases. In: Dale DC, Federman DD, eds. Scientific American medicine. New York: Scientific American, 1993: Section 4–II, 1–15.
7. Guyton AC. Secretory functions of the alimentary tract. In: Guyton AC. Textbook of medical physiology, 8th ed. Philadelphia: WB Saunders, 1991:709–725.
8. Goldschmidt M, Feldman M. Gastric secretion. In: Stein JH, ed. Internal medicine, 4th ed. St. Louis: Mosby-Year Book, 1994:346–351.
9. McGuigan JE. Peptic ulcer and gastritis. In: Isselbacher KJ, Braunwald E, Wilson JD, et al. Harrison's principles of internal medicine, 13th ed. New York: McGraw-Hill, 1994:1362–1382.
10. Hui WM, Lam SK. Multiple duodenal ulcer. Gut 28:1134–1141, 1987.
11. Richardson CT. Pathogenic factors in peptic ulcer disease. Am J Med 71(suppl 2C):1, 1985.
12. Brooks FP. The pathophysiology of peptic ulcer disease. Dig Dis Sci 30(suppl 11):15, 1985.
13. Taylor DN, Blaser MJ. The epidemiology of *Helicobacter pylori* infections. Epidemiol Rev 13:42–49, 1991.
14. NIH consensus development panel on *Helicobacter pylori* in peptic ulcer disease. *Helicobacter pylori* in peptic ulcer disease. J Am Med Assoc 272:65–69, 1994.
15. Fennerty MB. *Helicobacter pylori*. Arch Intern Med 154:721–727, 1994.
16. Berstad A, Alexander B, Weberg R, et al. Antacids reduce *Campylobacter pylori* colonization without healing the gastritis in patients with nonulcer dyspepsia and erosive prepyloric changes. Gastroenterology 95:619–624, 1988.
17. Weberg R, Aubert E, Dahlberg O, et al. Low dose antacids for duodenal ulcer. Gastroenterology 95:1465–1469, 1988.
18. Berstad A, Rydning A, Aadland E, et al. Antacid therapy of duodenal ulcer: effects of smaller doses. Scand J Gastroenterol 17:953, 1982
19. Nauert C, Caspary WF. Duodenal ulcer therapy with low-dose antacids: a multicenter trial. J Clin Gastroenterol 13(suppl 1):5149–54, 1991.

20. Feldman M, Burton ME. Histamine$_2$-receptor antagonists (part one). N Engl J Med 323:1672–1680, 1990.

21. Feldman M, Burton ME. Histamine$_2$-receptor antagonists (part two). N Engl J Med 323:1749–1755, 1990.

22. Anon. Drugs used in disorders of the upper gastrointestinal tract. Section 9: gastrointestinal drugs. In: Bennet DR, eds. Drug evaluations. Chicago: American Medical Association, 1994:1–1–1–31.

23. Anon. 56:40: Miscellaneous GI drugs. In: McEvoy GK, ed. AHFS 95 drug information. Bethesda, American Society of Health-Systems Pharmacists, 1995:2021–2065.

24. Szabo S. Pathways of gastrointestinal protection and repair: mechanisms of action of sucralfate. Am J Med 86(suppl 6A):23–31, 1989.

25. Lauritsen K, Laursen LS, Rask-Madsen J. Clinical pharmacokinetics of drugs used in the treatment of gastrointestinal diseases. Part I. Clin Pharmacokinet 19:11–31, 1990.

26. Lauritsen K, Laursen LS, Rask-Madsen J. Clinical pharmacokinetics of drugs used in the treatment of gastrointestinal diseases. Part II. Clin Pharmacokinet 19:94–125, 1990.

27. Reddy AN. Sucralfate gastric bezoar. Am J Gastroenterol 81:149–150, 1986.

28. Wilde MI, McTavish D. Omeprazole. An update of its pharmacology and therapeutic use in acid-related disorders. Drugs 48:91–132, 1994.

29. Lind T, Cederberg C, Olausson M, et al. Omeprazole in elderly duodenal ulcer patients: relationship between reduction in gastric acid secretion and fasting plasma gastrin. Eur J Clin Pharmacol 40:557–560, 1991.

30. Delchier JC, Isal JP, Eriksson S, et al. Double blind multicentre comparison of omeprazole 20 mg once daily versus 150 mg twice daily in the treatment of cimetidine- or ranitidine-resistant duodenal ulcers. Gut 30:1173–1178, 1989.

31. Cooperative Study Group. Double-blind comparative study of omeprazole and ranitidine in patients with duodenal or gastric ulcer: a multicentre trial: Gut 31:653–656, 1990.

32. Savarino V, Mela G, Sumberaz A, et al. Omeprazole in H$_2$-blocker non-responders [Letter]. Gut 31:584, 1990.

33. Maton PN, Vinayer R, Furcht H, et al. Long-term efficacy and safety of omeprazole in patients with Zollinger-Ellison syndrome: a prospective study. Gastroenterology 97:827–836, 1989.

34. Gudmand-Hoyer E, Jensen KB, Krag E, et al. Prophylactic effect of cimetidine in duodenal ulcer disease. Br Med J 1:1095–1097, 1978.

35. Boyd EJS, Penston JG, Johnston DA, et al. Does maintenance therapy keep duodenal ulcer healed? Lancet 1:1324–1327, 1988.

36. Marshall BJ, Goodwin CS, Warren JR, et al. Prospective double blind trial of duodenal ulcer relapse after eradication of Campylobacter pylori. Lancet 2:1437–1441, 1988.

37. Borody T, Cole P, Noonan S, et al. Long-term Campylobacter recurrence post-eradication . Gastroenterology 94:A43, 1988.

38. Graham DY, Lew GM, Klein PD, et al. Effect of treatment of Helicobacter pylori infection on the long-term recurrence of gastric or duodenal ulcer: a randomized, controlled study. Ann Intern Med 116:705–708, 1992.

39. Coghlan JG, Gilligan D, Humphries H, et al. Campylobacter pylori and recurrence of duodenal ulcers: a 12-month follow-up study. Lancet 2:1109–1111, 1987.

40. Adamek RJ, Wegener M, Labenz J, et al. Medium-term results of oral and intravenous omeprazole/amoxicillin Helicobacter pylori eradication therapy. Am J Gastroenterol 89:39–42, 1994.

41. Chiba N, Babu VR, Rademaker JW, et al. Meta-analysis of the efficacy of antibiotic therapy in eradication of Helicobacter pylori. Am J Gastroenterol 87:1716–1727, 1992.

42. Sung JJY, Chung SCS, Ling TKW, et al. Antibacterial treatment of gastric ulcers associated with Helicobacter pylori. N Engl J Med 332:139–142, 1995.

43. Scembri M, Lambert J, Loncar B, et al. Amoxycillin concentrations in the gastric mucosa are determined by luminal levels. Microbial Ecol Health Dis 4:S182, 1991.

44. Lambert HR, Loncar B, Schembri MA, et al. Luminal amoxicillin determines gastric mucosal concentrations. Gastroenterology 100:A104, 1991.

45. Lamouliatte H, Cayla R, Meyer M, et al. Pharmacokinetics of oral and intravenous amoxicillin in human gastric mucosa. Ital J Gastroenterol 23(suppl 2):109, 1990.

46. Westblom TU, Duriex DE. Enhancement of antibiotic concentrations in gastric mucosa by H$_2$-receptor antagonists: implications for treatment of Helicobacter pylori infection. Dig Dis Sci 36:25–28, 1991.

47. Borody TJ, Brandl S, Andrews P, et al. Use of high efficacy, lower dose triple therapy to reduce side effects of eradicating Helicobacter pylori., Am J Gastroenterol 89:33–38, 1994.

48. Axon ATR. Helicobacter pylori therapy: effect on peptic ulcer disease. J Gastroenterol Hepatol 6:131–137, 1991.

49. Graham DY, Lew GM, Evans DG, et al. Effect of triple therapy (antibiotics plus bismuth) on duodenal ulcer healing. Ann Intern Med 115:266–269, 1991.

50. Xia HX , Daw MA, Sant S, et al. Clinical efficacy of triple therapy in Helicobacter pylori-associated duodenal ulcer. Eur J Gastroenterol Hepatol 5:141–144, 1993.

51. Lynch Daf, Sobala GM, Gallacher B, et al. Effectiveness of a five times daily triple therapy regime for eradicating Helicobacter pylori. Ir J Med Sci 161(suppl 10):92, 1992.

52. Borody TJ, George LL, Brandl S, et al. Helicobacter pylori eradication with doxycycline-metronidazole-bismuth subcitrate triple therapy. Scand J Gastroenterol 305:502–504, 1992.

53. Hentschel E, Brandstatter G, Dragosics B, et al. Effect of ranitidine and amoxicillin plus metronidazole on the eradication of Helicobacter pylori and the recurrence of duodenal ulcer. N Engl J Med 328:308–312, 1993.

54. Goh KL, Peh SC, Parasakthi N, et al. Omeprazole 40 mg o.m. combined with amoxycillin alone or with amoxycillin and metronidazole in the eradication of Helicobacter pylori. Am J Gastroenterol 89:1789–1792, 1994.

55. Bayerdorffer E, Mannes GA, Sommer A, et al. High dose omeprazole treatment combined with amoxicillin eradicates Helicobacter pylori. Gastroenterology 102:A38, 1992.

56. Labenz J, Gyenes E, Ruhl GH, et al. Amoxicillin plus omeprazole versus triple therapy for eradication of Helicobacter pylori in duodenal ulcer disease. Gut 34:1167–1170, 1993.

57. Labenz J, Ruhl GH, Bertrams J, et al. Medium- or high dose omeprazole plus amoxicillin eradicates Helicobacter pylori in gastric ulcer disease. Am J Gastroenterol 89:726–730, 1994.

58. Logan RPH, Gummett PA, Misiewicz JJ, et al. One week eradication regimen for Helicobacter pylori. Lancet 2:1249–1252, 1991.

59. Hosking SW, Ling TKW, Yung MY, et al. Randomized controlled trial of short term treatment to eradicate Helicobacter pylori in patients with duodenal ulcers. Br Med J 305:502–504, 1992.

60. Sung JJY, SC Chung S, Ling TKW, et al. One-year follow-up of duodenal ulcers after 1-wk triple therapy for Helicobacter pylori. Am J Gastroenterol 89:199–202, 1994.

61. Mozell EJ, Cramer AJ, O'Dorsio TM, et al. Long term efficacy of octreotide in the treatment of Zollinger-Ellison syndrome. Arch Surg 127:1019–1026, 1992.

62. Kahrilas PJ, Hogan WJ. Gastroesophageal reflux disease. Schlesinger MH, Fordtran JS, eds. Gastrointestinal disease, Philadelphia: WB Saunders, 1993:385–401.

63. Graham DY, Smith JL, Patterson DJ. Why do apparently healthy people use antacid tablets? Am J Gastroenterol 78:257–260, 1983.

64. Johnson NJ, Boyd EFS, Mills JG, Wood JR. Acute treatment of reflux esophagitis: a multicentre trial to compare 150 mg ranitidine b.d. with 300 mg. q.d.s. Aliment Pharmacol Ther 3:259–66, 1989.

65. Pasqual JC, Henery P, Bruley S, et al. Comparison of the effects of two doses of omeprazole on 24-hour esophageal pH in gastroesophageal reflux disease [Abstract]. Gastroenterology 92:1567, 1987.

66. Sontag SJ. The medical management of reflux esophagitis: role of antacids and acid inhibition. Gastroenterol Clin North Am 19:683–712, 1990.

67. Koelz HR, Birchler R, Bretholz A, et al. Healing and relapse of reflux esophagitis during treatment with ranitidine. Gastroenterology 91:1198–1205, 1986.

68. Klinkenberg-Knol EC, Jansen JBMJ, Lamers CBHW, et al. Use of omeprazole in the management of reflux oesophagitis resistant to H_2 receptor antagonists. Scand J Gastroenterol 24(suppl 166):88, 1989.

69. Barone JA, Jessen LM, Colaizzi JL, et al. Cisapride: a gastrointestinal prokinetic drug. Ann Pharmacother 28:488–500, 1994.

70. Cook DJ, Fuller HD, Guyatt GH, et al. Risk factors for gastrointestinal bleeding in critically ill patients. N Engl J Med 330:377–381, 1994.

71. Kleiman RL, Adair CG, Ephgrave KS. Stress ulcers: current understanding of pathogenesis and prophylaxis. Ann Pharmacother 22:452–460, 1988.

72. Smythe MA, Zarowitz BJ. Changing perspectives of stress gastritis prophylaxis. Ann Pharmacother 28:1073–1085, 1994.

73. Ben-Menachem T, Fogel R, Patel RV, et al. Prophylaxis for stress related gastric hemorrhage in the medical intensive care unit. Ann Intern Med 121:568–575, 1994.

74. Prod'hom G, Leuenberger P, Koerfer J, et al. Nosocomial pneumonia in mechanically ventilated patients receiving antacid, ranitidine or sucralfate as prophylaxis for stress ulcer. A randomized clinical trial. Ann Intern Med 120:653–662;1994.

75. Tryba M. The gastropulmonary route of infection-fact or fiction? Am J Med 91(suppl 2A):135s–146s, 1991.

76. Lewis JH. Gastrointestinal injury due to medicinal agents. Am J Gastroenterol 81:819–834, 1986.

77. Agrawal NM. Anti-inflammatories and gastroduodenal damage: therapeutic options. Eur J Rheumatol Inflamm 13:17–24, 1993.

78. Bianchi PG, Lazzaroni M. Prevention and treatment of non-steroidal gastroduodenal lesions. Eur J Gastroenterol Hepatol 5:420–432, 1993.

79. Griffin MR, Ray WA, Schaffner W. Nonsteroidal antiinflammatory drug use and death from peptic ulcer in elderly persons. Ann Intern Med 109:359–363, 1988.

80. Graham DY, Agrawal NM, Roth SH. Prevention of NSAID-induced gastric ulcer with misoprostol: multicentre, double-blind, placebo controlled trial. Lancet 2:1277–1280, 1988.

81. Walt RP. Misoprostol for the treatment of peptic ulcer and antiinflammatory-drug-induced gastroduodenal ulceration. N Engl J Med 327:1575–1580, 1992.

82. Roth SH: Misoprostol in the prevention of NSAID-induced gastric ulcer: a multicenter, double-blind, placebo-controlled trial. J Rheumatol 17(suppl 20):20–24, 1990.

83. Graham DY. Prevention of gastroduodenal injury induced by chronic nonsteroidal antiinflammatory drug therapy. Gastroenterology 96:675–681, 1989.

84. Jones MP, Schubert ML. What do you recommend for prophylaxis in an elderly woman with arthritis requiring NSAID's for control? Controversies, dilemmas, and dialogues. Am J Gastroenterol 86:264–265, 1991.

85. Smith JL. What do you recommend for prophylaxis in an elderly woman with arthritis requiring NSAID's for control? Am J Gastroenterol 86:266–267, 1991.

86. Ehsanullah RSB, Page MC, Tildesley G, et al. Prevention of gastroduodenal damage induced by nonsteroidal anti-inflammatory drugs: controlled trial of ranitidine. Br Med J 297:1017–1021, 1988.

87. Robinson MG, Griffin JW, Bowers J, et al. Effect of ranitidine on gastroduodenal mucosal damage induced by nonsteroidal anti-inflammatory drugs. Dig Dis Sci 34:424–428, 1989.

CHAPTER 24

INFLAMMATORY BOWEL DISEASE

ROSEMARY R. BERARDI

Inflammatory bowel disease (IBD) is a general term that is used to describe two major chronic, nonspecific inflammatory disorders of the gastrointestinal (GI) tract: ulcerative colitis (UC) and Crohn's disease (CD), the causes of which remain unknown. UC is usually limited to the colon and rectum; it may affect the rectum alone, only the descending and sigmoid colon and rectum, or the entire colon (Fig. 24.1). In contrast, CD may affect any part of the GI tract from mouth to anus. The disease may involve only the terminal ileum, regions of the small intestine (regional enteritis), only the colon, or both the small intestine and colon (Fig. 24.1). The anatomic location is important, since the response to medical therapy may vary, depending on the site of involvement. Both UC and CD are characterized by recurrent acute inflammatory episodes and periods of remission. The pathophysiologic differences and clinical features usually permit an accurate diagnosis in most patients. It is estimated that IBD afflicts approximately 2 million Americans, usually before the age of 40. In the United States, complications of these diseases are believed to claim 1000 lives a year. Despite years of research, cures have not been found.

EPIDEMIOLOGY

The epidemiologies of UC and CD share many features but differ in some respects (Table 24.1). Both diseases are more common in western populations and in urban rather than rural areas (1, 2). There is a higher rate of IBD among Jewish people born in the United States and Europe than in Israeli-born Jews (1–3). In the United States, UC and CD are more prevalent in Caucasians and in females; however, there has been a recent increase of CD in African Americans (3). Ulcerative colitis and CD have been reported in different members of the same family (3). Although IBD can occur at any age, the peak age of incidence is in the teens or early twenties. A second, but controversial, peak may occur later in life (1, 3). The incidence of smoking differs in patients with UC and CD from that of the general population (1, 3).

ETIOLOGY AND PATHOGENESIS

The cause of UC and CD is not known; however, a hypothesis involving immunopathologic alterations has been proposed (3–6). Altered immunologic findings, many of which appear with the active inflammatory process and subside with its quiescence, have been reported in patients with IBD. Treatment with corticosteroids or immunosuppressives is associated with a favorable response, and removal of diseased bowel is often followed by disappearance of immunologic components. Microbial pathogens, dietary antigens, and the patient's own intestinal epithelial cells (autoimmune) have been implicated as antigenic triggers in the intestinal lumen (3–6). The abnormal immune response observed in IBD leads to inflammation and tissue damage, which is generally confined to the GI tract. Chronicity is thought to result from chronic exposure to antigenic triggers. Many of the similarities between UC and CD suggest that they may be heterogeneous disorders with distinctly different antigenic triggers. Genetic and environmental factors such as smoking, medications, and stress may modify disease activity by interacting with the mucosal immune system.

Antigenic Triggers

The chronic inflammatory nature of IBD has always suggested an infectious etiology, but attempts to culture bacterial pathogens have been largely unsuccessful (3, 4). The bacterial overgrowth that is often seen in CD reflects a favorable environment for bacterial growth but is not related to the pathogenesis. The similarity of CD to tuberculosis suggests that the disease might be caused by an atypical mycobacterium; however, this theory remains unproven. It seems unlikely that *Clostridium difficile* or *Helicobacter jejuni* is an etiologic agent in either CD or UC, but a coexisting infection may influence disease exacerbation (4). The role of gut anaerobes, viruses, and defective cell-wall bacterial variants remains uncertain. Although no conclusive evidence implicates a specific pathogen in IBD, it is possible that host immune and genetic factors are required to initiate the infectious hypothesis.

Dietary antigens represent most of the nonpathogenic antigens that are presented to the intestinal mucosa (1, 3). Chronic exposure to dietary luminal antigens produces a low-grade chronic inflammation of the lamina propria in healthy individuals (3). Failure to suppress the inflammatory response to normal dietary antigens could result in the immune activation that is observed in IBD. Although IBD has been linked to chemical food additives, cow's milk, increased consumption of refined sugars, and reduced intake of dietary fiber, evidence supporting a primary causal role for dietary antigens is not compelling (1). It is

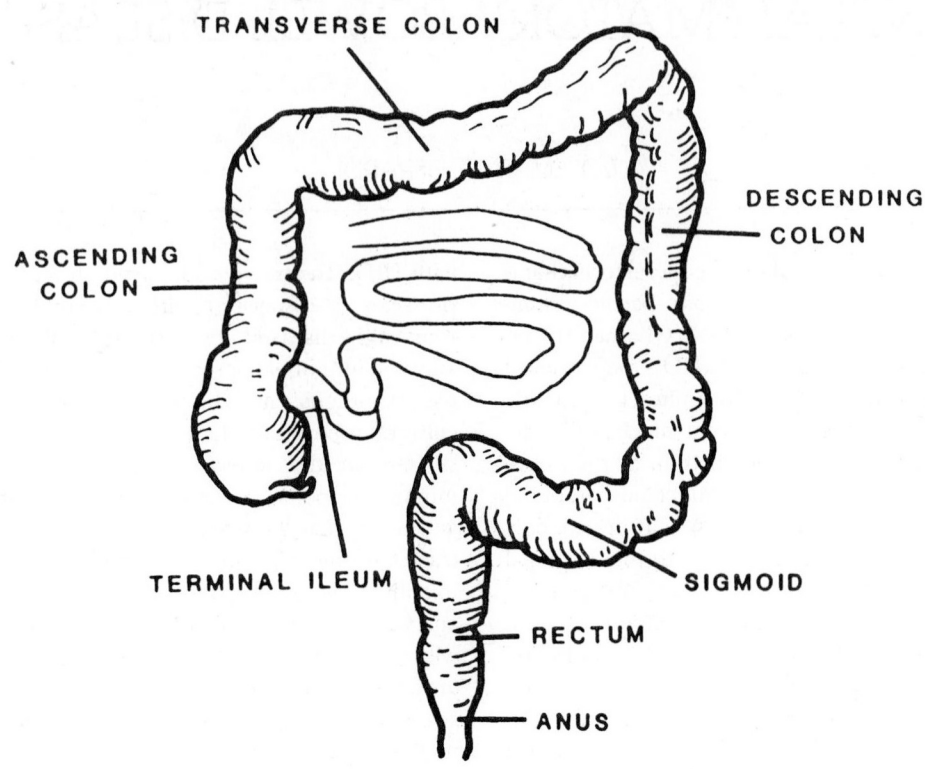

Figure 24.1. Anatomic location of various segments of the bowel.

Table 24.1.
Epidemiology of Ulcerative Colitis and Crohn's Disease

Factor	Ulcerative Colitis	Crohn's Disease
Incidence (per 100,000)	2–10	1–6
Prevalence (per 100,000)	35–100	10–100
Urban-rural	More common in urban	More common in urban
Ethnicity	Higher incidence in Jewish people	Higher incidence in Jewish people
Race	Higher incidence in Caucasians	Higher incidence in Caucasians
Gender	Slightly higher incidence in females	Slightly higher incidence in females
Age of onset	15–25, ?50–80	15–25, ?50–80
Cigarette smoking	Less common in smokers	More common in smokers
Socioeconomic status	More common in high socioeconomic status	More common in high socioeconomic status

Source: (1–3).

possible that dietary antigens play a secondary role that is mediated by genetic factors.

The autoimmune theory for the pathogenesis of IBD is based on similarities between the patient's intestinal epithelial cells and either luminal microbial or dietary antigens (3). Because of similarities between proteins, the patient's immune response is directed at the epithelial cells and the cells are destroyed by one of several cytotoxic mechanisms. Additional evidence is required to support this theory.

Immune Response

Antigenic triggers in the intestinal lumen activate macrophages and T lymphocytes to release numerous endogenous mediators of inflammation in IBD (3–6). Many of the mediators of tissue damage also serve to amplify the immune response and promote further inflammation. Cytokines, prostaglandins, neuropeptides, and various metabolites of arachidonic acid, including leukotrienes and lipoxins, frequently correlate with disease activity and provide a rationale for drug therapy. Increased production of potent proinflammatory cytokines, including interleukin-1 (IL-1), interleukin-6 (IL-6), interferon-γ (IFN-γ), and tissue necrosis factor, stimulate epithelial, endothelial, and mesenchymal cells and activate immune cells. The chemotactic cytokines, interleukin-8 (IL-8), macrophage chemotactic and activating factor, and other chemotactic substances such as leukotriene B_4 serve to increase macrophage and neutrophil migration from the circulation into the inflamed mucosa. This process may be related to ischemic injury involving the release of superoxide and other reactive oxygen species (3, 6). Mucosal and serum prostaglandin concentrations are elevated in IBD, but there is evidence against their role as mediators of inflammation, since nonsteroidal antiinflammatory drugs have failed to induce clinical improvement (3, 5). Alterations in the mucosal immune system are central to the pathogenesis of IBD; however, no consistent immunologic abnormality has been established as the primary defect in UC or CD.

Genetic Influences

The most established risk factor for developing IBD is a positive family history. The incidence of IBD among first-degree relatives of patients with IBD is 30 to 100 times that of the general population (3). Studies with monozygotic twins also support the presence of a genetic influence. Although there is an ongoing search for a subclinical marker to detect an abnormal genotype, no specific genetic marker has been identified for either UC or CD.

Cigarette Smoking

Cigarette smoking increases the risk of CD and decreases the risk of UC (1). There is extensive evidence implicating cigarette smoking as a risk factor for CD and for disease recurrence. Ex-smokers also seem to be at increased risk, but the risk is somewhat less than that for current smokers. In contrast, there appears to be a decreased risk of UC among current cigarette smokers. However, former smokers are at increased risk when compared to those who have never smoked. The mechanism by which smoking protects patients with UC is unknown but probably involves multiple factors. Patients with UC or CD should be advised to stop smoking, given the health hazards of smoking and the uncertainty of its protective effect against UC.

Medications

Nonsteroidal antiinflammatory drugs (NSAIDs) can cause a variety of effects in patients with IBD, including asymptomatic mucosal inflammation, strictures, obstruction, perforation, and hemorrhage (1). NSAIDs have also been linked to colitis in patients without previous IBD and may activate quiescent IBD (1). Because NSAIDs are often used to treat the arthropathy that accompanies IBD, patients who are taking NSAIDs should be monitored

closely for signs of obstruction, perforation, or bleeding. There is conflicting data regarding oral contraceptive use and the risk of developing IBD (1).

Psychological Factors

Emotional and psychological factors have been implicated in the etiology of IBD, but there is no evidence that stress is causative and that psychotherapy is effective (1). However, psychological factors may influence the clinical course of the disease and the patient's response to therapy, since acute flares of activity often occur in association with stressful events. It is possible that the nervous system has a regulatory effect on the immune system. Management of IBD should include the realization that the symptoms of IBD, such as diarrhea, pain, and rectal bleeding, are in themselves likely to cause various psychological responses to the disease.

ANATOMIC, PATHOLOGIC, AND CLINICAL FEATURES

The distinction between the anatomic and pathologic features of UC and CD can assist in understanding the clinical features of the diseases. A summary of the most

Table 24.2.

Important Anatomic, Pathologic, and Clinical Features of Ulcerative Colitis and Crohn's Disease[a]

Feature	Ulcerative Colitis	Crohn's Disease
Anatomic		
Small bowel only	0	++
Small bowel and colon	0	+++
Colon only	+	++
Anorectal only	+++	0
Diffuse, continuous involvement	+++	+
Cobblestoning	0	+++
Pathologic		
Transmural	0	+++
Fissures and fistulas	+	++
Crypt abscesses	+++	+
Strictures	0	++
Shortening of the colon	++	0
Pseudopolyps	++	0
Clinical		
Rectal bleeding	+++	+
Diarrhea	+++	+++
Abdominal pain	+	+++
Malaise, fever	+	+++
Weight loss	++	+++
Extraintestinal manifestations	+	+
Perianal disease	+	++
Intestinal obstruction	0	++
Toxic megacolon	++	+
Risk of malignancy	++	+

[a]Frequencies represent estimates and are categorized as being consistent (+++), frequent (++), infrequent (+), or rare (0). None of the features are always present or always absent.

important anatomic, pathologic, and clinical features is presented in Table 24.2.

Ulcerative Colitis

Ulcerative colitis affects primarily the mucosa and submucosa of the rectum and the left colon, the rectum being involved histologically in more than 90% of the cases. Distal UC may be described as proctitis or proctosigmoiditis, depending on the location of mucosal inflammation. Lesions usually develop in the rectum and spread proximally; however, initial disease may involve the entire colon (Fig. 24.1). The disease extends to the total colon (universal colitis or pancolitis) in 5 to 10% of patients and may involve a minimal portion of the terminal ileum (backwash ileitis). In severe forms of UC, such as toxic megacolon, deeper layers of the colon may be involved.

The inflammatory process in UC is continuous with no intervening areas of normal mucosa; deeper layers of the bowel are not usually involved. Chronic recurrent mucosal inflammation with concomitant tissue repair may lead to characteristic findings such as the formation of crypt abscesses, pseudopolyps, shortening of the colon (foreshortening), and a "lead-pipe" appearance. Dysplasia in colonic biopsies may represent a premalignant change and a risk of carcinoma (3, 7).

The clinical features of UC vary with disease severity (Table 24.3). Determining whether the disease is mild, moderate, or severe is important because treatment and prognosis are related to disease severity. Clinically, mild UC is most common and afflicts about 60% of all patients. In these individuals the disease usually involves only the sigmoid and rectum. Diarrhea and rectal bleeding are mild, and systemic symptoms are usually absent. Moderate disease affects about 25% of all patients. Diarrhea, with

varying degrees of rectal bleeding, is usually the major presenting symptom. Abdominal cramping is more prominent but is often relieved by defecation. Severe UC occurs in 10 to 15% of all patients and is characterized by a sudden onset of profuse diarrhea, rectal bleeding, and severe abdominal cramps. The patient is usually febrile, dehydrated, and profoundly weak. Blood loss can result in a rapid pulse, low blood pressure, and anemia. Death may occur during the acute attack.

Crohn's Disease

The term "Crohn's disease" is preferred to "granulomatous enteritis" or "regional enteritis," since not all patients with CD have accompanying granulomas and the disease can affect any part of the GI tract, not just a specific region. The distal ileum and right colon (ileocolitis) are the most common sites of involvement, accounting for more than two-thirds of cases affecting the small bowel. Although the terminal ileum is generally involved, other areas of the small intestine can be affected either alone or along with the colon. The colon is involved in about two-thirds of patients, about 15 to 20% having only colonic involvement. In the majority of patients with CD of the colon, the rectum is spared. Sections of bowel that appear normal by radiography or colonoscopy can have histological features of CD.

In contrast to UC, CD is characterized by chronic inflammation extending through all layers of the bowel wall as well as the mesentery and regional lymph nodes. Mesenteric nodes are enlarged and are often matted together to form an abdominal mass. The transmural process can lead to the formation of fissures and fistulas and a thickened, edematous bowel, which can result in stenosis with possible obstruction. The disease is distinguished

Table 24.3.
Clinical Features of Ulcerative Colitis Based on Disease Severity

Feature	Mild	Moderate	Severe
Frequency	60%	20–25%	10–15%
Location	Rectum and distal colon	Rectum and $\frac{1}{3}$–$\frac{1}{2}$ of colon	Rectum and entire colon
Weight loss	Uncommon	<10 lb	>10 lb
Fever	Uncommon	Intermittent	Persistent
Abdominal pain	Uncommon	Common	Severe
Bowel sounds	Normal	Normal	Absent
Diarrhea	3–5 stools/day	>5 stools/day	Hourly
Rectal bleeding	Intermittent	Common	Severe
Tachycardia	Uncommon	Frequent	Common
Anemia	Uncommon	Hct > 0..30 (30%)	Hct < 0.30 (30%)
Leukocytosis	Uncommon	Common	Common
Albumin	Normal	Normal	Reduced
Extraintestinal manifestations	Uncommon	Common	Severe
Risk of malignancy	Not increased	Increased after 10 yr	Increased after 10 yr
Mortality (acute attack)	<0.5%	2%	10–25%

Table 24.4.
Clinical Feature of Crohn's Disease Based on Disease Location

Feature	Small Bowel	Ileocolitis	Colitis
Diarrhea	>90%	>90%	>90%
Abdominal pain	Common	Common	Very common
Malnutrition	Common	Common	Less common
Fistula	10–20%	30–50%	10–30%
Obstruction	30–40%	40–50%	10–20%
Perianal disease	Uncommon	Common	Very common

from UC in that it often involves segments of the bowel separated by normal-appearing mucosa (skip lesions). In advanced cases the mucosa has a nodular or "cobble-stoned" appearance. Although certain anatomic and pathologic features enable CD of the colon to be distinguished from UC, this distinction is not possible in about 20% of cases.

The clinical features of CD vary but usually reflect the anatomic location of the disease (Table 24.4). A low-grade fever occurs in more than 50% of patients in the absence of any complications. Malabsorption and nutritional deficiencies result in weight loss in more than 80% of patients. Abdominal pain tends to be steady and localized to the right lower quadrant. A colicky or cramping pain, usually associated with bowel movements, may be superimposed on the steady pain. When CD is confined to the small bowel, diarrhea often occurs without bleeding. With colonic involvement, diarrhea is accompanied by rectal bleeding in about 50% of patients. Most patients have recurrent episodes of diarrhea, abdominal pain, and fever lasting from a few days to several months. Perianal fissures, fistulas or abscesses may be the presenting feature. Acute CD may be mild, moderate, or severe, depending on the extent of mucosal involvement.

NUTRITIONAL ASPECTS

In general, patients with severe UC or CD are prone to extracellular fluid and electrolyte losses, anemia, and hypoalbuminemia. Nutritional deficiencies are frequent and complex in CD because of the problem of food avoidance and the many mechanisms responsible for malabsorption and malnutrition. Mechanisms include: inadequate food intake; inflammatory involvement of the small intestine resulting in decreased absorption of nutrients, lactase deficiency, and protein-losing enteropathy; small bowel bacterial overgrowth with associated malabsorption of cobalamin and altered bile salt metabolism; intestinal surgery; and, the catabolic effects of chronic inflammation (3). Prolonged periods of poor nutrition and underlying disease can result in protein-calorie malnutrition, dehydration, acid-base and electrolyte disturbances, and deficiencies of vitamins D, K, B_{12}, and folic acid. The consequences of these nutritional disorders can be espe-

cially serious for children with CD and may lead to growth retardation and delayed sexual maturation.

EXTRAINTESTINAL MANIFESTATIONS

Many extraintestinal manifestations are associated with IBD and may precede or accompany the underlying intestinal disorder (Table 24.5). Extraintestinal manifestations may be related to the clinical activity of the inflammatory process, its anatomic location, or the disordered physiology of the small intestine (3). The arthritic, skin, and eye manifestations occur more often in patients with UC and Crohn's colitis than in patients with CD of the small intestine. The arthritis is usually asymmetric and affects the joints of the knees, hips, ankles, wrists, and elbows. In most patients it tends to parallel the activity and severity of the bowel disease, often subsiding with therapy, colectomy, or spontaneous remission. In contrast, ankylosing spondylitis may appear years before bowel symptoms and runs a course independent of the intestinal disease.

Minor abnormalities in hepatic transaminases commonly occur in patients with IBD; however, clinically important liver disease is uncommon. Cirrhosis, chronic hepatitis, and sclerosing cholangitis, although infrequent, tend to occur more often in UC (3). Fatty infiltration of the liver is common and may reflect malnutrition and protein depletion. Disturbances in the physiology of the small intestine may give rise to the formation of cholesterol gallstones and calcium oxalate kidney stones. Cholelithiasis occurs in CD with ileal involvement or resection and results from diminished bile salt reabsorption. Nephrolithiasis also occurs in ileal CD and results from increased oxalate absorption secondary to malabsorption of fatty acids. Renal amyloid may cause nephrotic syndrome and renal failure in CD (3).

The most common hematologic complication in IBD is iron-deficiency anemia secondary to blood loss, although chronic anorexia and malabsorption can lead to other complex anemias. A small number of patients may develop an idiopathic hemolytic anemia or a drug-related hemolytic anemia associated with the administration of sulfasalazine. Thromboembolic events resulting from abnormalities of clotting factors during active episodes may complicate the

Table 24.5.
Extraintestinal Manifestations of Inflammatory Bowel Disease[a]

Manifestation	Incidence (%)	Related to Intestinal Disease Activity
Arthritis/arthralgias	25–30	Yes
Aphthous mouth ulcers	5–10	Yes
Episcleritis or uveitis (iritis)	5–10	Yes
Erythema nodosum	1–5	Yes
Pyoderma gangrenosum	1–5	Usually
Sacroilitis	10–15	No
Ankylosing spondylityis	1–2	No
Abnormal liver transaminases	30–50	No
Liver disease	1–3	No
Sclerosing cholangitis	1–4	No
Cholelithiasis[b]	20–30	No
Nephrolithiasis[b]	25–35	No
Renal disease[b]	1–3	No

[a] In general, the extraintestinal manifestations in ulcerative colitis and Crohn's colitis are similar in type and prevalence.
[b]Manifestation seen primarily in Crohn's disease of the small intestine.

course of both diseases (3). Therapy involves the risk of colonic bleeding during anticoagulation. Unfortunately, there is no definitive explanation for many of the extraintestinal manifestations.

COMPLICATIONS

Local complications arise from the intestinal component of IBD and include pseudopolyps, perianal fissures, abscesses, fistulas, intestinal obstruction, colonic perforation, massive hemorrhage, toxic megacolon, and colon cancer (3).

The incidence of abscesses and fistula formation is higher in CD than in UC and may be the initial indication of the disease. Fistulas occur most commonly in the perianal and perirectal areas; enterocutaneous, enterovaginal, and enteroenteric fistulas occur less often. Intestinal obstruction is rarely a problem in UC; however, small bowel obstruction is a common complication of CD and may be due to the inflammation and edema of the involved intestine or to the fixed narrowing of the bowel secondary to scar formation. Colonic perforation is uncommon in CD but may complicate toxic megacolon or occur in UC in the absence of acute dilation. The risk of perforation and peritonitis is greatest during an initial severe attack and is associated with a high mortality rate. Massive hemorrhage occurs infrequently in severe UC. Most patients are managed with blood transfusions, but surgery may be required.

Toxic Megacolon

Toxic megacolon may occur in CD of the colon but is more likely to complicate severe attacks of UC (3). This serious complication is usually preceded by a rapidly deteriorating clinical course and is associated with a high mortality rate.

It is characterized by acute dilation of the transverse colon to a diameter greater than 6 cm with accompanying systemic toxicity. The pathogenesis of the acute dilation is related to the deep inflammatory process, which involves all layers of the colon and results in the inability of the colon to contract. It can occur at any time throughout the natural course of the disease and may be complicated by perforation and peritonitis. Toxic megacolon may be triggered by anticholinergics, opiates, and other antimotility agents used to treat diarrhea or by severe electrolyte abnormalities such as hypokalemia (3). Medications that inhibit the propulsive activity of the colonic musculature are contraindicated in patients with severe UC and should be used cautiously for patients with moderate disease activity. Because the risk of perforation is high, barium enema and colonoscopic examination are contraindicated in severe UC.

Toxic megacolon is considered a medical emergency that requires rapid and intensive therapy. Clinically, the patient is severely ill with a high fever, profound weakness, tachycardia, volume depletion, electrolyte imbalance, leukocytosis, abdominal pain, distention, and tenderness. A decrease in stool frequency may reflect colonic atony rather than improvement of colitis. Medications that decrease intestinal motility should be withdrawn. Nasogastric suction is begun to remove swallowed air and to reduce the passage of fluid into the colon. Medical treatment consists of fluid and electrolyte replacement, blood transfusions if indicated, and intravenous corticosteroids. Although the value of intravenous corticosteroids has not been confirmed in well-controlled clinical trials, most clinicians initiate therapy with divided doses equivalent to at least 40 mg of prednisone per day (3). Because of the fear of perforation and the likelihood of bacteremia, intravenous therapy with broad-spectrum antibiotics directed at enteric Gram-negative, enterococcal, and anaerobic pathogens should be instituted. The initial 24 to 48 hr of treatment are crucial and determine the future management of the patient. If significant improvement does not occur, and if perforation seems imminent, an emergency colectomy should be performed. The overall mortality rate of surgery after perforation is about 50% but can be reduced to less than 5% if surgery is performed before perforation (3). Most patients who are successfully treated medically are likely to undergo colonic resection for intractable disease within a year (3).

Colon Cancer

The risk of colon cancer is greater in patients with IBD than for the general population; a higher incidence is observed with UC than with CD (3, 7). The risk of developing cancer with UC increases when the duration of the disease is more than 8 to 10 years and when the disease involves the entire colon (3, 7). Patients with long-standing UC are at risk for developing cancer even if their symptoms have been mild or their disease is quiescent (3). Because colonic cancer in UC is virulent, various screening methods have been offered to detect patients who are at risk of developing a malignancy. Tests to examine stool occult blood are useless in UC because of colitis-induced bleeding (3). Colonoscopic surveillance with multiple mucosal biopsies for dysplasia is often recommended, but has not been proven to decrease the risk of cancer to a level comparable to that in the general population (7). Most algorithms for surveillance are similar and recommend performing colonoscopy with biopsy every 1 to 2 years for patients with pancolitis of 8 to 10 years' duration (7). More frequent examinations may be required, depending on the degree of risk and histologic findings. Patients with left-sided colitis require less frequent surveillance; patients with ulcerative proctitis should not undergo regular colonoscopic examinations (7). A prophylactic total colectomy can cure UC and prevent colonic cancer. However, the risks of malignancy and severe colitis must be weighed against the risks of surgery and the inconvenience of an ileostomy.

DIAGNOSIS

A diagnosis of IBD should be considered for all patients who present with persistent abdominal pain and diarrhea or bloody diarrhea. Occasionally, fever, weight loss, or one of the extraintestinal manifestations may overshadow the intestinal symptoms. Because UC and CD are "nonspecific" diseases, the diagnosis is usually made by exclusion and relies on the clinical picture, stool findings, sigmoidoscopic or colonoscopic appearances, and histological assessment (3). Once the diagnosis of IBD is established, the distinction between UC and CD of the colon is usually possible.

In general, laboratory tests are nonspecific and do not establish a diagnosis. Leukocytosis and an elevated erythrocyte sedimentation rate may reflect the inflammatory process. Electrolyte abnormalities, particularly hypokalemia, exist when there is severe diarrhea. Hypoalbuminemia may reflect the patient's poor nutritional status and overall clinical condition. Anemia often accompanies chronic blood loss. Indications of malabsorption may be present when CD involves the small intestine.

Sigmoidoscopic or colonoscopic examination of the bowel is most important in establishing mucosal inflammation in both UC and CD. A rectal or colonic biopsy usually confirms the presence of an abnormal and inflamed mucosa. Radiography (with or without contrast) also provides essential information and complements endoscopy. Barium contrast studies are used in diagnosing CD when involvement of the small bowel or fistula is suspected. A plain film of the abdomen may be indicated for patients for whom a barium enema and endoscopy are contraindicated. Computed axial tomography and ultrasonography are useful in diagnosing abscess and fluid collections.

CLINICAL COURSE

The initial attack of UC is usually abrupt with symptoms ranging from nonbloody diarrhea to fulminant diarrhea with colonic hemorrhage. For about 50% of patients the first attack is mild; for about 30% the attacks are of moderate severity; about 20% present with severe disease (3). The majority of patients will have highly variable (mild to severe) intermittent attacks with varying intervals of asymptomatic remissions. A smaller number may be troubled by continuous symptoms with intermittent flares of disease activity. Neither the severity of the first attack nor the extent of colonic involvement can predict the frequency of recurrence. Patients with mild disease have a prognosis similar to that of the general population. Morbidity is greatest when the onset of symptoms is severe and colonic involvement is extensive. About 50% of patients with severe initial disease will require a colectomy within 2 years; the same percentage of patients with pancolitis will require a colectomy in 5 years (3). Older patients (>50 years of age) are least likely to suffer relapse and least likely to undergo colectomy. Disease-related complications and the risk of colon cancer contribute to the clinical course.

Crohn's disease, like UC, follows a clinical course of acute exacerbations and remissions. The disease is characterized by recurrent attacks of diarrhea, abdominal pain, and low-grade fever, resulting in gradual deterioration over a period of years. Blood loss and poor nutrition lead to anemia, weight loss, malnutrition, and fatigue. Approximately 60% of patients with CD will require surgery within 10 years of the initial diagnosis; of these, about 45% will eventually require another operation (3). Partial or complete obstruction constitutes the most frequent indication for surgery and occurs more rapidly in patients with ileocolitis than in those with only small bowel or only colonic involvement. Perianal or perirectal disease develops in about one-half of Crohn's patients with colonic involvement. For patients who develop sclerosing cholangitis or ankylosing spondylitis, the extraintestinal manifestations may be more troublesome than the underlying bowel disease.

NUTRITIONAL MANAGEMENT

Maintenance of adequate nutrition is an important goal for patients with IBD, particularly patients with CD who have extensive intestinal involvement or who have undergone extensive bowel resection. Factors that contribute to malnutrition in CD include diminished oral intake, increased caloric requirements, malabsorption of nutrients resulting from loss of absorptive surface, loss of proteins and electrolytes due to bleeding and mucosal inflammation, and treatment with sulfasalazine or corticosteroids (3, 8). Replacement of vitamins, minerals, and other nutrients is indicated whenever there is clinical or laboratory evidence of deficiency. Specifically, iron, folic acid, and B_{12} deficiencies should be identified and treated appropriately. Because oral iron may aggravate IBD, it may be preferable to give the iron parenterally or as a blood transfusion. Fat malabsorption in patients with CD may contribute to malabsorption of vitamins A, D, and K; replacement of these vitamins may be necessary. Patients with CD involving the small intestine may present with deficiencies of calcium, magnesium, B complex vitamins, and vitamin C.

Most patients with IBD are able to eat adequate amounts of a well-balanced diet. Some patients are lactose intolerant and should avoid dairy products or should use lactase-containing preparations. Frequently, patients will associate specific foods with exacerbation of their disease and exclude these foods from their diet. Patients should be instructed to limit *only* those foods that consistently and reliably produce symptoms.

The use of enteral or parenteral nutrition as adjunct therapy in IBD to restore a balanced nutritional state is well established. Indications for supplemental parenteral nutrition in treating IBD include short bowel syndrome, high output stomas or fistulas, and perioperative support of the severely malnourished patient. Supplemental nutrition must be differentiated from primary therapy, which is intended to improve the disease process itself. The efficacy of nutritional support as primary therapy in IBD patients is not well established (3, 8, 9). While parenteral nutrition is considered to be a valuable adjunct to therapy in treating both severe UC and CD, there is little evidence that the overall course of either of these diseases is altered by bowel rest and nutrition (8). Until more definitive information is obtained, parenteral nutrition should be used to improve the nutritional status of severely ill patients with IBD who cannot be fed enterally and for selected patients with CD in whom bowel rest may be of value.

MEDICAL MANAGEMENT

Medical management of IBD is aimed at terminating the acute attack, inducing remission, maintaining remission, and controlling chronic symptoms. Specific treatment depends on the severity of symptoms; the extent, location, and severity of the inflammatory process; and, the response to previous medications. Acute exacerbations, quiescent symptom-free periods, and chronic symptomatic periods will necessitate different goals of therapy. The approach to management should be individualized.

Therapeutic Agents
ANTIDIARRHEALS, ANTISPASMODICS, AND ANALGESICS
Antidiarrheals, antispasmodics, and analgesics provide symptomatic relief without affecting IBD activity. These agents should be used as supplements to first-line medications and should not replace them. Antidiarrheals, such as diphenoxylate and loperamide, are useful for patients with mild chronic IBD and those who have diarrhea resulting from small bowel resection. Symptomatic treatment of diarrhea may permit a reduction in the dosage of other medications, thereby reducing the incidence of adverse effects. Antidiarrheals are ineffective in treating the severe forms of IBD, since diarrhea results from a loss of colonic absorptive capacity due to widespread destruction of the colonic mucosa. Antidiarrheals are contraindicated in treating severe disease because they may precipitate toxic megacolon.

Cholestyramine is the drug of choice for treating bile salt diarrhea resulting from resection of the terminal ileal (3, 10). Cholestryramine may also prevent the formation of oxalate kidney stones and steatorrhea. Clonidine or octreotide may be effective in enhancing fluid and electrolyte absorption in refractory diarrhea, but their usefulness is limited because of the numerous adverse effects associated with their use (10).

Antispasmodics, including tincture of belladonna or opium and other anticholinergics, may be effective in reducing cramps and rectal urgency. They should be given before meals to decrease peristalsis associated with eating. Antispasmodics should be avoided if obstruction is suspected and are contraindicated in treating severe IBD.

Pain management should be aimed at controlling disease activity. Analgesics may be used to supplement treatment but should not become the mainstay of chronic pain control. Narcotics, when used to relieve severe pain, should be given on a scheduled basis rather than only when needed (11).

SULFASALAZINE
Sulfasalazine (salicylazosulfapyridine, SASP) is the most commonly prescribed medication used to treat IBD (3, 12–17). It is a conjugate of 5-aminosalicylic acid (5-ASA, or mesalamine) and sulfapyridine (SP) linked by a diazo bond (Fig. 24.2). When SASP is administered orally, about 20% of the dose is absorbed, some of which is excreted in the bile. The remainder of the parent drug passes unchanged into the colon, where colonic bacteria cleave the diazo bond to form 5-ASA and SP. Most of the liberated 5-ASA remains in the colon and is excreted in the feces. The SP is absorbed, metabolized in part by acetylation in the liver, and excreted in the urine (12–14). Because 5-ASA and SP are readily absorbed when given orally, the diazo linkage provides a delivery system by which higher concentrations of 5-ASA can reach the diseased intestinal sites. One gram of SASP releases approximately 400 mg of 5-ASA.

The mechanism by which SASP acts in IBD is uncertain. It is unlikely that its antibacterial activity accounts for its clinical efficacy. SASP and 5-ASA, the primary

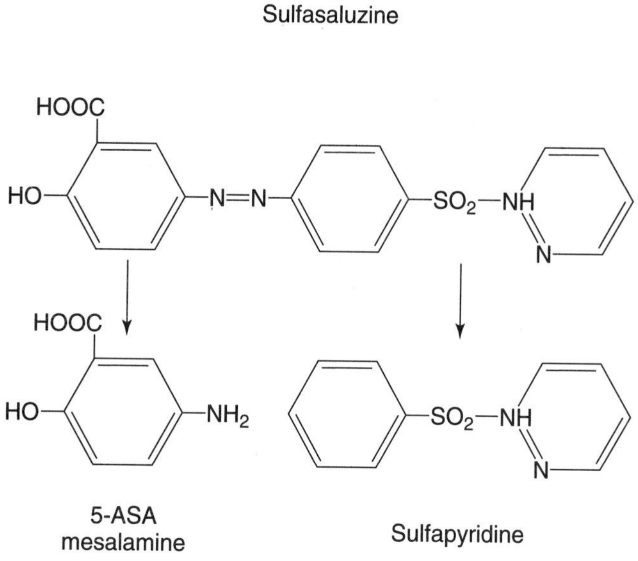

Sulfasaluzine

Figure 24.2. Structures of sulfasalazine, 5-aminosalicylic acid, and sulfapyridine.

active moiety, interfere with arachadonic acid metabolism (3, 12–14). Both agents inhibit the lipoxygenase pathway and decrease the synthesis of chemotactically active leukotrienes in peripheral blood neutrophils and within the intestinal mucosa (Fig. 24.3). SASP and 5-ASA also inhibit the cyclooxygenase pathway and lower intestinal prostaglandin concentrations (3, 12–14). However, it is unlikely that prostaglandins are important mediators of inflammation, as NSAIDs inhibit only the cyclooxygenase pathway and are ineffective in treating IBD (3, 12–14). 5-ASA may act as a free radical scavenger or as an inhibitor of immunoglobulin secretion (3, 12).

Increased intestinal transit (diarrhea) or concomitant antibiotic administration may result in reduced breakdown of SASP and decreased liberation of 5-ASA. In some patients, bacterial overgrowth permits the metabolism of SASP in the small intestine with delivery of 5-ASA to more proximal portions of the bowel.

Use in Ulcerative Colitis. The efficacy of SASP as a sole agent to treat severe acute UC is uncertain; however, SASP is considered to be inferior to glucocorticosteroid (GCS) therapy (3, 12–15). This may be due in part to the diminished metabolism of SASP in the colon as a result of severe diarrhea. Although studies have shown SASP to be effective in mild to moderate UC, GCS produce a more rapid response (3, 13–15). The oral dose of SASP used to treat acute mild or moderate disease is usually 2 to 4 g/day given in four divided doses (3). Although higher SASP doses (6 to 8 g/day) may be given, they are often intolerable. Therapy is sometimes initiated at a lower dose (500 mg twice a day) and gradually increased by 500

mg every 2 to 3 days. Clinical response to SASP usually occurs within 3 to 4 weeks.

Once remission has been induced, 1 to 3 g/day of SASP is usually effective in maintaining remission (3, 12–16). Although the relapse rate tends to vary inversely with the daily dose, higher doses are associated with increased adverse effects. For most patients, the optimum maintenance dose is 2 g/day. If this dose causes troublesome adverse effects, a daily dose of 1 g is better than no maintenance treatment. Alternatively, if flare-ups occur while the patient is taking 2 g/day, a larger dose is worth trying. The duration of maintenance therapy remains unresolved, but most clinicians favor prolonged or indefinite treatment if the drug is well tolerated.

Use in Crohn's Disease. SASP is effective in treating symptomatic mild or moderately active CD. However, patients with small bowel disease respond less favorably to SASP than do those with colonic involvement (3, 12, 13, 16, 17). Release of 5-ASA in the colon is thought to contribute to this difference in efficacy. A dose of SASP 3 to 4 g/day is usually sufficient for induction therapy, but higher daily doses may be necessary (3, 12, 17). As in active UC, response to SASP requires 3 to 4 weeks of treatment. Patients who are unresponsive to GCS tend not to respond to SASP (3).

Nonsurgical patients with quiescent CD and those who have undergone surgery for CD are often treated with SASP in an attempt to maintain remission. However, controlled clinical trials have not confirmed the efficacy of SASP in preventing recurrent attacks in nonsurgical patients (3, 12, 16, 17). Although study results are conflicting, typical maintenance doses of SASP also appear to be ineffective in preventing postoperative recurrence of CD (3, 12, 16, 17). With this in mind, a trial dose of 2 to 3 g/day of SASP may be in order to determine whether a specific patient may benefit from SASP therapy.

SASP is sometimes used in combination with local or systemic GCS on the assumption that the effects of the two drugs are additive and that SASP may produce a steroid-sparing effect. Combining SASP with oral GCS may result in more rapid initial improvement than with SASP alone, but differences in efficacy are usually not apparent with continued therapy. Combination therapy offers no clear steroid-sparing effect (17).

Adverse Effects. The frequency of adverse effects reported with SASP varies from 20 to 50% (3, 12–18). The adverse effects are of two types: dose-dependent and dose-independent. Many patients will complain of one or more dose-dependent symptoms (Table 24.6) during the initial 4 to 6 weeks of therapy. However, most of these symptoms can be relieved by lowering the SASP dose or temporarily discontinuing the drug and restarting it at a lower dose. The frequency of these adverse effects appears to correlate with SP concentrations in the blood, especially

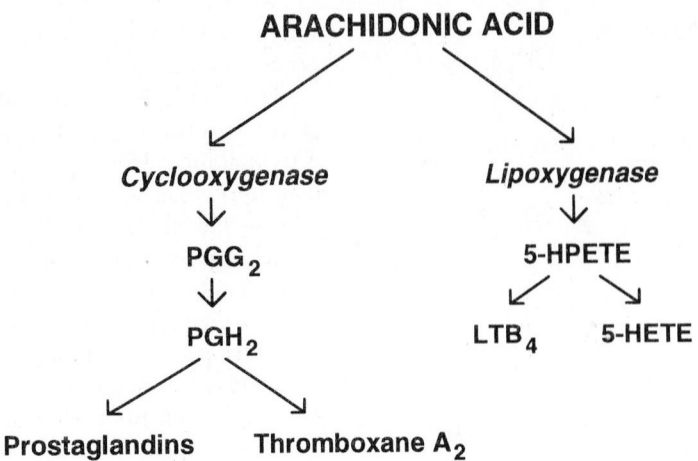

Figure 24.3. Arachidonic acid metabolism.

Table 24.6.
Adverse Effects of Medications Used to Treat Inflammatory Bowel Disease

Sulfasalazine	Glucocorticosteroids	Azathiaprine/6-MP
Dose-dependent	*Major*	Bone marrow depression
Nausea	Infection	Nausea
Vomiting	Hypertension	Diarrhea
Dyspepsia	Psychosis	Fever
Diarrhea	Hypokalemia	Skin rash
Anorexia	Hyperglycemia	Infection
Headache	Osteoporosis	Arthralgias
Malaise	Cataracts	Pancreatitis
Male infertility	Glaucoma	Hepatitis
Dose-independent	*Minor*	**Cyclosporine A**
Fever	Moon face	Tremor
Skin rash	Acne	Paresthesias
Hemolytic anemia	Hirsuitism	Headache
Agranulocytosis	Insomnia	Nausea
Pulmonary complications	Striae	Anorexia
Hepatitis	Weight gain	Hypertrichosis
Pancreatitis	Vascular fragility	Gingival hyperplasia
Neurologic toxicity		Nephrotoxicity
		Hypertension
Mesalamine (5-ASA)	**Metronidazole**	**Methotrexate**
Fever	Dyspepsia	Anorexia
Skin rash	Metallic taste	Nausea
Nausea	Skin rash	Vomiting
Diarrhea	Dark urine	Diarrhea
Pancreatitis	Glossitis	Stomatitis
Hepatitis	Disulfiram-like	Headache
Nephrotoxicity	Peripheral neuropathy	Fever
Headache	Neutropenia	Alopecia
Alopecia	Pancreatitis	Leukopenia
		Pneumonitis
		Nephrotoxicity
		Hepatic fibrosis/cirrhosis

when the dose of SASP exceeds 4 g/day. Intolerance to the GI symptoms may be overcome by beginning with a dose of 500 mg/day and gradually increasing it, administering the drug with meals, or using the enteric-coated tablet.

Dose-related adverse effects tend to be more common in slow acetylators (3, 14). Hemolysis and leukopenia occur infrequently and are also thought to be related to SP blood concentrations and slow acetylator status (3, 14). SASP may alter sperm morphology and decrease sperm counts, resulting in male infertility (3, 14). The incidence is thought to be highest in slow acetylators; the effects are reversible within 3 months of discontinuing SASP.

Dose-independent adverse effects (Table 24.6) include hypersensitivity reactions that are typical of the sulfonamides (3, 12–14). Skin rashes commonly occur and, in 2 to 3% of patients, progress to a point at which discontinuation of the drug is required. Hematologic effects include hemolytic anemia and bone marrow suppression. Fever, pulmonary infiltrates, hepatitis, pancreatitis, polyneuritis, agranulocytosis, thrombocytopenia, and a lupus-like syndrome with polyarthritis and vasculitis have been reported (3, 12).

Desensitization. The hypersensitivity reactions observed with SASP may require permanent withdrawal of the drug for a patient who is otherwise receiving therapeutic benefit. For patients who have less serious reactions (fever and/or rash), a desensitization program can be undertaken by first discontinuing the drug and withholding it until the side effects subside. SASP can be restarted with an extremely low dose, which is progressively increased in small increments over a prolonged time period. However, the availability of 5-ASA products now makes desensitization unnecessary.

Drug Interactions. Broad-spectrum antibiotics may alter the therapeutic activity of SASP because the cleavage of SASP to SP and 5-ASA depends on normal intestinal flora. Folate deficiency may occur in patients receiving long-term SASP therapy, as SASP inhibits folic acid absorption and interferes with folate metabolism in the jejunal brush border (3). Some clinicians recommend folic acid supplementation of 1 mg/day with long-term SASP therapy. The interaction between SASP and other highly protein-bound drugs (e.g., warfarin) may lead to displacement of these drugs from their protein binding sites. Concomitant administration of SASP and digoxin may decrease digoxin bioavailability and reduce digoxin serum concentrations. The administration of iron and SASP may result in chelation and possibly decreased blood levels of both

drugs. The clinical importance of many of these interactions is uncertain.

5-AMINOSALICYLIC ACID PREPARATIONS

5-ASA can be targeted to the small bowel and colon by oral dosage forms that protect it from absorption. Enemas and suppositories permit delivery of 5-ASA to the distal colon and rectum.

Oral Preparations. Several strategies have been used to create a SP-free oral preparation that delivers high concentrations of 5-ASA to the distal small bowel and colon. Second-generation products include azo-bond coupling of 5-ASA with agents other than SP, such as olsalazine; delayed-release pH-dependent enteric-coated tablets such as Asacol; and, sustained-release products such as Pentasa (Table 24.7). All of these preparations are effective in treating active UC and in maintaining remission (14–17, 19-23). Studies indicate that the sustained-release and possibly the delayed-release 5-ASA forms are effective in treating active CD, particularly when the small bowel is involved (17, 19). Results also suggest that these preparations may be effective in maintaining remission in quiescent CD and in preventing postoperative recurrence (16, 17). However, response rates appear to be related to the concentration of 5-ASA delivered to the small bowel and colon (17). Oral preparations under investigation include balsalazide, Rowasa, Salofalk, Claversal, and 4-ASA (14, 17, 19).

In general, the 5-ASA preparations are better tolerated than SASP and permit delivery of higher concentrations of 5-ASA to the inflamed mucosa (14, 17, 23). About 10 to 20% of patients experience a fever or rash indicating a hypersensitivity reaction to 5-ASA (Table 24.6). Patients who are allergic to aspirin should not take 5-ASA. The potential for nephrotoxicity exists in patients receiving high daily doses, concomitant 5-ASA-liberating medications, and those with preexisting renal disease.

Azo-Bond Coupling. Olsalazine consists of two salicylate molecules linked by a diazo bond (Table 24.7). On a molar basis, olsalazine delivers twice as much 5-ASA to the colon

Table 24.7.

Comparison of Aminosalicylate Preparations

Product	Formulation	Delivery of 5-ASA	Urinary Recovery of 5-ASA (%)
Sulfasalazine	5-ASA linked to sulfapyridine carrier by azo-bond	Colon	17–37
Olsalazine	Two 5-ASA linked by azo-bond	Colon	14–27
Balsalazide	5-ASA linked to aminobenzoyl-alanine carrier by azo-bond	Colon	15–25
Asacol	5-ASA coated with Eudragit-S; delayed-release (pH > 7)	Ileum-colon	20–35
Pentasa	5-ASA encapsulated in ethylcellulose microgranules; sustained-release	Pylorus-colon	30–55

as does SASP (20, 21). Its efficacy in treating acute IBD and in maintaining remission is similar to that of SASP when equivalent 5-ASA doses are used. Olsalazine, 500 mg twice daily, is indicated primarily for maintenance of remission in UC when patients are intolerant of SASP. A dose-dependent secretory diarrhea has been reported in up to 17% of patients receiving 1 g/day. Although higher doses (1.5 to 3 g/day) are effective in treating mild to moderate acute UC (20, 21), they are not prescribed because of increased potential for diarrhea. However, a recent study suggests that the incidence of diarrhea may be less than was previously reported (22). Patients should be counseled to report any change in stool frequency or volume after initiation of olsalazine therapy. Preliminary results with balsalazide appear promising (Table 24.7).

Delayed-Release Tablets. Asacol, a delayed-release tablet (Table 24.7), contains 400 mg of 5-ASA coated with an acrylic resin (Eudragit-S). On oral administration, 5-ASA is released in the terminal ileum or colon when the intestinal pH is sufficient (pH > 7) to dissolve the enteric-coating. Because intestinal pH and motility may vary in patients with IBD, Asacol may not provide reliable site-specific release of 5-ASA. In 2 to 3% of patients, intact or partially intact tablets have been found in the stool. Patients should be instructed to observe for intact tablets in the stool. Therapy in UC or CD is usually initiated with 2.4 g/day in three divided doses and may be increased to 4.8 g/day if necessary. Maintenance of remission, especially in CD, may require dosage regimens similar to the regimen used for remission induction. Studies involving UC patients demonstrate efficacy similar to that of SASP when Asacol is used to treat acute mild to moderate disease and to maintain remission (14, 16, 19, 23). Although Asacol offers a theoretical advantage to patients with ileal CD, its efficacy has not been firmly established in well-controlled clinical trials.

Sustained-Release Microgranules. Pentasa, a sustained-release dosage form (Table 24.7), contains 250 mg of 5-ASA microgranules, which slowly and continuously dissolve in the small intestine and colon. Approximately 20 to 50% of the 5-ASA is released in the small bowel; the remainder is released in the colon (19, 24). In contrast to Asacol, Pentasa's release characteristics are primarily time-dependent rather than pH-dependent (19). Patients should be advised that small beads may be left in the stool after the 5-ASA is released. The efficacy of Pentasa (4 g/day in four divided doses) in treating acute mild to moderate UC and in maintaining remission (2 g/day in two divided doses) has been established (14, 16, 19, 23). Recent clinical trials performed with Pentasa also demonstrate the drug's ability to induce and maintain remission in mild to moderate CD, regardless of disease location. A dose-related response appears to be evident for both treatment and maintenance

(16, 17, 19). A recent study revealed that Pentasa, in a dose of 4 g/day for 16 weeks, resulted in significant improvements from baseline in quality-of-life parameters, including ability to sleep, social activities, work/occupation, hobby/recreation, sexual relations, and indoor/outdoor activities (25). Pentasa (3 g/day) has been reported to decrease the rate and severity of endoscopic recurrence after curative surgery for ileal CD (26).

Topical Preparations. Topical administration of 5-ASA exerts a local antiinflammatory effect in the distal colon and rectum (14, 15, 27, 28). Less than 15% of the rectally administered dose is absorbed (27). The 5-ASA rectal enema (4 g/60 mL) is indicated for the treatment of ulcerative proctitis and proctosigmoiditis. It is preferable to administer the enema at bedtime and to retain it for 8 hr. Improvement occurs within a week, but the usual course of therapy is 3 to 6 weeks, depending on symptoms and sigmoidoscopic findings. For patients with mild to moderate disease, the 5-ASA enema is as effective as oral SASP or GCS enema. Additionally, patients who are refractory to oral SASP and oral or rectal GCS may respond to rectal 5-ASA alone or combined with oral therapy (14, 15, 27). Rectal suppositories (500 mg twice a day), which are indicated for distal ulcerative proctitis, should be retained at least 1 to 3 hr or longer to achieve maximum benefit. Lower daily doses of the enema (1 to 2 g/day) and the suppository (250 to 500 mg/day), as well as alternate-day dosing, have been investigated as maintenance therapy, but the optimal regimen has not been determined (14, 15, 27, 28). Topical 5-ASA appears to be less effective in treating CD, but clinical trials have been limited.

Topical 5-ASA preparations are associated with fewer adverse effects than are their oral counterparts, presumably because of lower systemic availability. Adverse effects of rectal 5-ASA occur in 1 to 10% of patients and include headache, flatulence, abdominal pain, diarrhea, dizziness, and fatigue, many of which are indistinguishable from symptoms of the underlying disease. Anal irritation or a hypersensitivity reaction to 5-ASA or the sulfite contained in the rectal suspension may occur. Most patients who are intolerant of SASP will tolerate the 5-ASA enema or suppository. The monthly cost of 5-ASA enemas, as well as patient acceptance and compliance, should be considered when less costly and more convenient treatment alternatives are available.

GLUCOCORTICOSTEROIDS

The glucocorticosteroids (GCS) remain the drugs of choice for treating acute moderate to severe attacks of IBD. When compared to SASP, they provide a more immediate response; clinical improvement usually occurs within a few days to a week. The exact mechanism by which GCS suppress intestinal inflammation is unknown, but theories

Table 24.8.
Glucocorticosteroids Used in the Treatment of Inflammatory Bowel Disease

Glucocorticoid	Antiinflammatory Effect	Mineralocorticoid Effect
Hydrocortisone	1	2
Tixocortol	1	0
Betamethasone	2.5	0
Prednisone	4	1
Prednisolone	4	1
Methylprednisolone	5	0
Fluticasone	?	0
Budesonide	200	0

include interaction with the immune system, inhibition of prostaglandins, stabilization of lysosomal membranes, and blocking of kinin release (3, 29).

The GCS most widely used to treat UC and CD include hydrocortisone, prednisone, prednisolone, and methylprednisolone (Table 24.8). GCS are usually given intravenously to the acutely ill patient and replaced by oral therapy once the disease subsides. A number of oral and rectal preparations are available for use by patients with mild to moderate disease. Recent studies suggests that systemic absorption of GCS may not be required and may even be disadvantageous (29). The potential adverse effects of systemic GCS (Table 24.6) limit their use in the prolonged treatment of IBD.

Use in Ulcerative Colitis. The efficacy of GCS in treating acute UC is well documented (3, 14, 29). The optimal dose and route (parenteral, oral, or topical) of GCS administration vary with disease severity and activity. Once remission occurs, GCS should be gradually tapered. The reduction of the GCS dose should be based on the duration of treatment and the ability to prevent exacerbations. The general consensus is that oral GCS have no value in the maintenance of remission and that prolonged use can be harmful (16). Maintenance of quiescent UC can be accomplished successfully in most patients with oral SASP or 5-ASA and, if necessary, occasional GCS enemas.

Parenteral Administration. The continuous or intermittent intravenous administration of GCS (prednisolone-equivalent 60 mg/24 hr in divided doses) reportedly induces remission in 60 to 80% of patients with acute UC. Although few studies have assessed the relative value of the available GCS and specific dosage regimens, methylprednisolone 40 to 80 mg/24 hr is often preferred for the very ill patient. Equipotent doses of intravenous betamethasone, dexamethasone, or hydrocortisone may also be used; however, hydrocortisone is associated with increased mineralocorticoid activity (Table 24.8). Once clinical improvement occurs, intravenous therapy should be discontinued and

oral GCS should be instituted. If the patient deteriorates or if no progress occurs after 7 to 10 days, colectomy should be considered (14). Pulsed intravenous methylprednisolone therapy of 1 g/24 hr is no more effective than conventional intravenous regimens for the treatment of severe active UC (14, 30).

For most severely ill patients, intravenous GCS are considered superior to ACTH because they do not depend on adrenal responsiveness and have fewer adverse effects. There is evidence to suggest that for patients with new-onset severe UC or those who have not received recent GCS therapy, parenteral ACTH (120 units/24 hr) may be the drug of choice (14). However, ACTH is rarely used in the United States to treat severe IBD.

Oral Administration. Most patients with mild to moderately active UC respond favorably to oral GCS. The optimal GCS dose (prednisolone-equivalent 40 mg/day) produces improvement or remission in several weeks with minimal adverse effects (14, 29). Equipotent doses of prednisone, hydrocortisone, or methylprednisolone may be used. In an attempt to mimic the natural diurnal rhythm of GCS secretion and to minimize side effects, single morning doses and alternate-day dosing are often advocated. For most patients, a single GCS dose is as effective as divided doses; however, a few patients may respond best to multiple daily doses. The daily dose should be taken as a single morning dose, or the largest portion of the dose should be given in the morning. Because a decrease in side effects frequently parallels a diminution in therapeutic effect, alternate-day therapy is generally not recommended for patients with IBD (14). Alternatively, growth-stunted children who require maintenance GCS may benefit from this regimen.

Topical Administration. Patients with mild attacks of UC, especially those with disease limited to the distal colon and rectum, frequently respond to rectal instillation of GCS (14, 15, 29). The beneficial effect of topical GCS appears to result primarily from a local antiinflammatory effect (29). Although rectal preparations may result in up to 50% of the drug being absorbed, the degree of adrenal suppression and adverse effects appear to be less than those observed with oral administration of the equivalent dose of the same drug (14, 29). A number of factors, including the volume and composition of the fluid vehicle, the GCS dose, and the dwell time, probably account for variations in systemic absorption. Whether acute intestinal inflammation alters drug absorption is unclear.

Retention enemas (e.g., hydrocortisone 100 mg or methylprednisolone 40 mg) should be administered at bedtime to permit overnight contact with the inflamed mucosa. An additional dose may be administered in the morning after the first bowel movement. Once remission occurs, usually within 2 to 3 weeks, an alternate-night schedule may be used for an additional 2 weeks. Patients should be instructed to instill the enema in the supine position and then change to the left, right, and prone positions for at least 20 min each to facilitate maximal topical coverage. Although enemas may spread as far proximally as the hepatic flexure, they appear to be most effective for UC patients with left-sided colitis or proctosigmoiditis.

Rectal foams may be useful for patients who are unable to retain enemas because of local inflammation, tenesmus, or diarrhea. A foam is more easily retained than a liquid enema but does not usually spread beyond the sigmoid colon (14). Although foams offer the added advantages of convenience and compliance, their use should be limited to patients whose disease is confined to the sigmoid or rectum.

Use in Treating Crohn's Disease. The use of GCS in the treatment of CD is similar to that described for UC, although the results are not always as dramatic (3, 16, 17, 29). Therapy is usually initiated with a prednisolone-equivalent daily dose of 40 to 60 mg; in severe cases the GCS should be administered intravenously. If improvement occurs, the GCS dose should be tapered and eventually withdrawn. Unfortunately, the response to GCS in CD is often less successful than in UC, and remission is usually more difficult to achieve. Although this is not supported in the literature, most clinicians maintain patients on a minimum GCS dose for about 1 to 2 months before attempting the steroid taper. Patients with ileal or ileocolonic disease appear to respond more favorably to GCS than do those with colonic CD, although GCS enemas are effective in treating left-sided Crohn's colitis. Patients with extensive small bowel resection may have decreased GCS absorption (17). For most patients, continuing GCS therapy after remission induction generally does not alter the frequency of recurrence or the frequency of relapse after surgery (16, 17, 29). When symptoms persist or recur despite surgical resection, other therapeutic options should be considered.

GCS should be used with caution in CD patients with fistula, abscess, and malnutrition, because of the increased risk of infection as well as fluid and electrolyte disturbances. The decision to begin treatment with GCS should be made only after the risks and benefits have been carefully evaluated for an individual patient. Even when the response to GCS therapy appears to be satisfactory, the disease tends to progress despite apparent clinical activity.

Potential New Glucocorticosteroids. The antiinflammatory effects of GCS in treating IBD are unsurpassed by those of any other drug type. However, the beneficial effects are often offset by troublesome adverse effects. Several approaches to this problem include using prodrug conjugates in which conventional GCS are linked to inert molecules such as dextran and then detached by bacterial enzymes in the distal bowel; using delayed-release or sustained-release enteric coatings; and, identifying GCS that have high tissue uptake and affinity for GCS receptors as well as rapid and extensive biotransformation in the liver. Among the new GCS, tixocortol pivalate, fluticasone propionate, and budesonide (Table 24.8) are the principal contenders for use in treating IBD (2, 31, 32). Of these, budesonide has emerged as the most promising. An oral, controlled-release dosage form appears to be efficacious in treating active ileocolonic CD, causing less suppression of endogenous plasma cortisol levels and less adverse effects than oral prednisolone (32). The efficacy of budesonide enema is similar to that of conventional GCS when used to treat active UC, but does not appear to have appreciable effects on adrenal gland function (31). Whether oral or topical budesonide formulations can maintain long-term remission without toxicity requires further investigation. To date, none of the newer GCS have been approved for use in the United States.

IMMUNOSUPPRESSANTS

The evidence that the immune system mediates tissue injury in IBD has led to the use of a number of immunosuppressive agents. Because of their toxic effects and limited efficacy, these medications are usually reserved for patients who are unresponsive or intolerant to SASP, 5-ASA, and GCS.

Azathioprine and 6-Mercaptopurine. Azathioprine (AZA) is metabolized to 6-mercaptopurine (6-MP) and subsequently converted to inactive 6-thiouric acid by xanthine oxidase. The specific mechanism by which AZA and 6-MP act in IBD is uncertain but is probably related to their ability to inhibit nucleotide biosynthesis and purine nucleotide interconversion (33, 34). The effect of 6-MP on T cells and its antiinflammatory effect may contribute to its efficacy in treating IBD. AZA and 6-MP have similar therapeutic and toxic effects (33–37).

Early clinical trials failed to confirm the efficacy of AZA (2 mg/kg/day) and 6-MP (1.5 mg/kg/day) when used as single agents to treat IBD refractory to SASP and GCS. Recent studies, however, confirm their efficacy in inducing and maintaining remission and in reducing or eliminating concurrent GCS therapy in patients with UC or CD (33–35). When AZA or 6-MP is continued after the GCS is withdrawn, remission is usually sustained. Unfortunately, there is a high relapse rate in attempting to taper or stop the immunosuppressive agent (33–35). AZA and 6-MP are also effective in relieving some extraintestinal manifestations and in healing fistulas. The response to AZA or 6-MP may require 3 to 6 months or longer (35). The typical starting dose is 0.5 to 1.5 mg/kg/day; higher doses are often associated with leukopenia. The results from a recent study indicate that low-dose (50 mg/day) 6-MP is associated with minimal hematologic toxicity (36). The daily dose should be reduced by at least 50% for patients who are receiving allopurinol. Because of the concern over toxic effects, treatment with AZA or 6-MP is often prematurely discontinued before beneficial effects have been obtained.

The long-term use of AZA and 6-MP has been associated with a number of toxic adverse effects (Table 24.6). However, recent studies suggest a lower incidence of these adverse effects when AZA and 6-MP are used in lower doses to treat IBD (33–34, 36). The potential for bone marrow suppression requires that blood counts be monitored regularly, especially when therapy is initiated. Drug fever and arthralgias often occur within weeks of beginning treatment. Despite an improved safety profile, patients on long-term AZA or 6-MP therapy should be monitored closely for signs of infection, pancreatitis, and hepatitis. A theoretical risk of developing neoplasia, particularly non-Hodgkin's lymphoma, after long-term treatment with AZA or 6-MP exists, but a recent report found no increase in non-Hodgkin's lymphoma in IBD patients (37).

For patients with refractory UC, a bowel resection can be curative; however, some patients may wish to avoid or delay colectomy. In CD, the use of AZA or 6-MP should be reserved for patients with refractory disease whose clinical condition or extent of intestinal involvement preclude bowel surgery. For these patients, it may be prudent to begin with an initial dose of 50 mg of either AZA or 6-MP, with subsequent increases, if necessary. The maximum dose should not exceed 1.5 mg/kg/day. AZA or 6-MP should be added to the drug regimen, and an attempt should be made to taper or withdraw GCS.

Cyclosporin A. Cyclosporin A (CPA), a potent inhibitor of cell-mediated immunity, may play an important role in the treatment of severe UC or CD that is refractory to GCS therapy (33, 34, 38–40). CPA exerts its immunosuppressant activity by inhibiting T-cell production of cytokines, including IL-2, IL-3, IL-4, and IFN-γ (33, 34, 38). A number of controlled and uncontrolled trials have been conducted involving UC and CD patients using intravenous, oral, or topical dosage forms with various dosage regimens (33, 34, 38–40). The results of these studies suggest that CD low-dose CSA (≤5 mg/kg/day orally) is not effective either for treatment of active CD or for maintenance of remission. Uncontrolled trials at high doses (>5 mg/kg/day orally or 4 mg/kg/day intravenously) suggest that CPA may be effective in treating severe acute CD and fistula. Both controlled and uncontrolled trials indicate that high-dose CPA (10 mg/kg/day orally or 4 mg/kg/day intravenously) is effective in treating severe UC. Improvement appears to be higher among patients who receive CPA and GCS than among those who receive CPA alone. When CPA is used to treat acute disease, the response usually occurs within several weeks, but relapse occurs when the drug is withdrawn. Finally, CPA enemas (≤5

mg/kg/day) for left-sided colitis do not appear to be effective.

The potential advantages of CPA therapy must be balanced against the risk of irreversible nephropathy and other serious adverse effects (Table 24.6). In most cases, the adverse effects are dose-related; the two most frequent are paresthesias (20%) and hypertrichosis (50%). The most important issue is the potential for permanent renal damage. Unfortunately, serum creatinine is not a good monitoring parameter for CPA-associated nephropathy, as it does not always rise with renal impairment (38). Severe infections may complicate CPA therapy in IBD, especially when the patient is on concomitant GCS. The recommended starting dose for CPA is 2 to 4 mg/kg/day intravenously or 8 mg/kg/day orally (33, 34, 38). Because of slow, incomplete, and variable intestinal absorption, careful monitoring of blood levels is required when CPA is given orally. Maintaining an adequate blood level with oral CPA, in patients with severe CD, is often difficult because of inflammation or resection of the small bowel. There appears to be a relatively strong correlation between clinical response and whole blood CSA concentrations in IBD when high-dose therapy (whole blood CPA concentration >400 ng/mL) and low-dose therapy (whole blood CPA concentration <200 ng/mL) are compared (38). It is unclear whether the relationship between clinical response and whole blood CPA concentration between 200 and 400 ng/mL is linear or whether there is a threshold for clinical response. Patients receiving CPA should be monitored for drug interactions when receiving other medications that interact with hepatic cytochrome P-450.

Studies to date indicate that CPA must be used at relatively high and potentially toxic doses to achieve efficacy in IBD. These findings suggest that high-dose CPA should be used as "rescue" therapy, since it is rapid-acting and can serve as a bridge to other agents, such as AZA or 6-MP, that take longer to act but are potentially safer for long-term use. It appears that low-dose CPA is not effective as maintenance therapy in treating IBD and therefore should not be used for this purpose. Although the use of CPA in the treatment of refractory IBD is encouraging, treatment should be limited to formal clinical trials.

Methotrexate. Methotrexate (MTX), a folic acid antagonist, is currently under investigation for the treatment of severe refractory IBD (33, 34, 41). MTX exerts it effect on proliferating cells while sparing resting cells. Among its numerous potential effects, it appears to decrease IL-6 production in a dose-dependent manner (33). Preliminary results suggest that, when given weekly as an intramuscular injection of 25 mg, MTX improves symptoms and reduces the requirements for GCS in patients with severe active CD and UC (33, 41). However, there appears to be a significant relapse rate in patients followed for up to 1 year (33). Of major concern are the potential teratogenic and toxic effects, which limit its usefulness (Table 24.6). Additional well-controlled trials are needed to evaluate the efficacy and safety of MTX in treating IBD patients refractory to GCS.

METRONIDAZOLE

Metronidazole (MTZ) appears to be beneficial in treating active ileocolonic or colonic CD, but is not effective in treating small bowel CD or active UC (16, 17, 42). The mode of action of MTZ in IBD is unclear, but is presumed to be related to its immunosuppressive, rather than its antibacterial, properties. Effective doses range from 10 to 20 mg/kg/day, and response to treatment usually requires several months. Higher doses may be required for patients with refractory fistula or perineal disease (17, 42). Most patients with mild to moderate Crohn's colitis or ileocolitis usually respond to 250 mg of MTZ four times daily. Attempts to reduce or discontinue the MTZ dose have been associated with worsening disease activity. The usefulness of MTZ in maintenance or remission of CD has not been well studied, although a recent report suggests that it may be effective in preventing recurrence after ileal resection (43).

Many adverse effects have been reported with the short-term use of MTZ (Table 24.6). The most troublesome of these is peripheral neuropathy, which has been reported to occur in up to 50% of patients and appears to be dose-dependent (17, 42). Although the drug has not been proven to be mutagenic, teratogenic, or carcinogenic in humans, results of animal and laboratory tests have caused concern about these possibilities. Therefore, MTZ should be discontinued after several months if it is ineffective or should be tapered after 3 to 4 months, if possible, when the disease is controlled. At present, MTZ should be reserved for CD patients with colitis, fistula, or perineal disease who do not respond to SASP or 5-ASA preparations.

POTENTIAL NEW AGENTS

Many new agents are being investigated for use in treating IBD (44–47). Studies with eicosanoid inhibitors, such as eicosapentanoic acid and docosahexanoic acid, members of the omega-3 fatty acid family, suggest that dietary supplementation may be effective in treating UC (44). Zileuton, a specific lipoxygenase inhibitor, has been shown to be superior to placebo in patients with active UC who were not taking SASP (44, 47). The addition of transdermal nicotine to conventional therapy appears to improve symptoms in patients with active UC (45). However, transdermal nicotine does not appear to be effective in maintaining remission of UC, and adverse effects appear to be troublesome (46). The use of reactive oxygen species such as superoxide dismutase looks promising; it is possible that α-tocopherol and penicillamine also work by this mechanism (44, 47). The results of studies evaluating prostaglandin analogs such as misoprostol seem promising

(44, 47). Controlled trials of antituberculous agents are needed to support their role in the treatment of CD (44). Theoretically, inhibitors of complement activation, neuropeptides, such as substance P, and platelet-activating factor may have a role in the treatment of IBD (44, 47). A limited number of trials have been conducted using clonidine, sucralfate, lidocaine, anti-CD$_4$ monoclonal antibody, sodium cromoglycate, and short-chain fatty acids (butyrate). Although results obtained from clinical trials with some of these newer agents appear promising, their efficacy and safety have not been established, and their role, if any, in the management of IBD is unknown.

Recommendations

The goal of medical therapy in treating IBD is to induce and maintain remission. Drug selection, dose, and the route of administration are determined by the location, extent and severity of intestinal involvement. Treatment strategies for managing UC and CD are presented in Figures 24.4 and 24.5. See also Table 24.9.

ULCERATIVE COLITIS

Patients with acute severe UC usually require intravenous GCS equivalent to 40 to 60 mg/day of prednisolone. If the patient progressively improves during the next 7 to 10 days, oral GCS should replace the intravenous drug. Once remission has been induced, GCS should be gradually withdrawn, and maintenance therapy should be instituted with SASP at 1 to 2 g/day. If the patient is unable to tolerate SASP, maintenance therapy with olsalazine, Asacol, or Pentasa may be warranted.

Acute moderate disease may respond to oral doses of 2 to 4 g/day of SASP. Doses may be lower initially and then gradually increased as tolerance to the adverse effects develops. Alternatively, treatment with Asacol (800 mg three times a day) or Pentasa (1 g four times a day) may be useful for patients who do not tolerate SASP. Symptomatic improvement with SASP, Asacol, and Pentasa often takes 3 to 4 weeks. GCS enemas may provide additional therapeutic benefit. If a more immediate response is required, or if the response to SASP or any of the 5-ASA preparations is inadequate, the drug should be discontinued, and oral GCS should be instituted in a prednisolone-equivalent dose of 20 to 40 mg/day. GCS should be tapered over 2 to 3 weeks, and maintenance therapy with either SASP or a 5-ASA preparation should be initiated. If the patient remains GCS-dependent, the addition of AZA or 6-MP may permit withdrawal of the GCS for patients who wish to avoid a colectomy.

Patients with mildly active UC and those in whom the disease involves only the rectum usually respond to either oral SASP, Pentasa, Asacol, or a rectal GCS retention enema. Although 5-ASA enemas and supposi tories are effective, the cost of a course of therapy is many times that of SASP or steroid enemas. Therefore their use is often

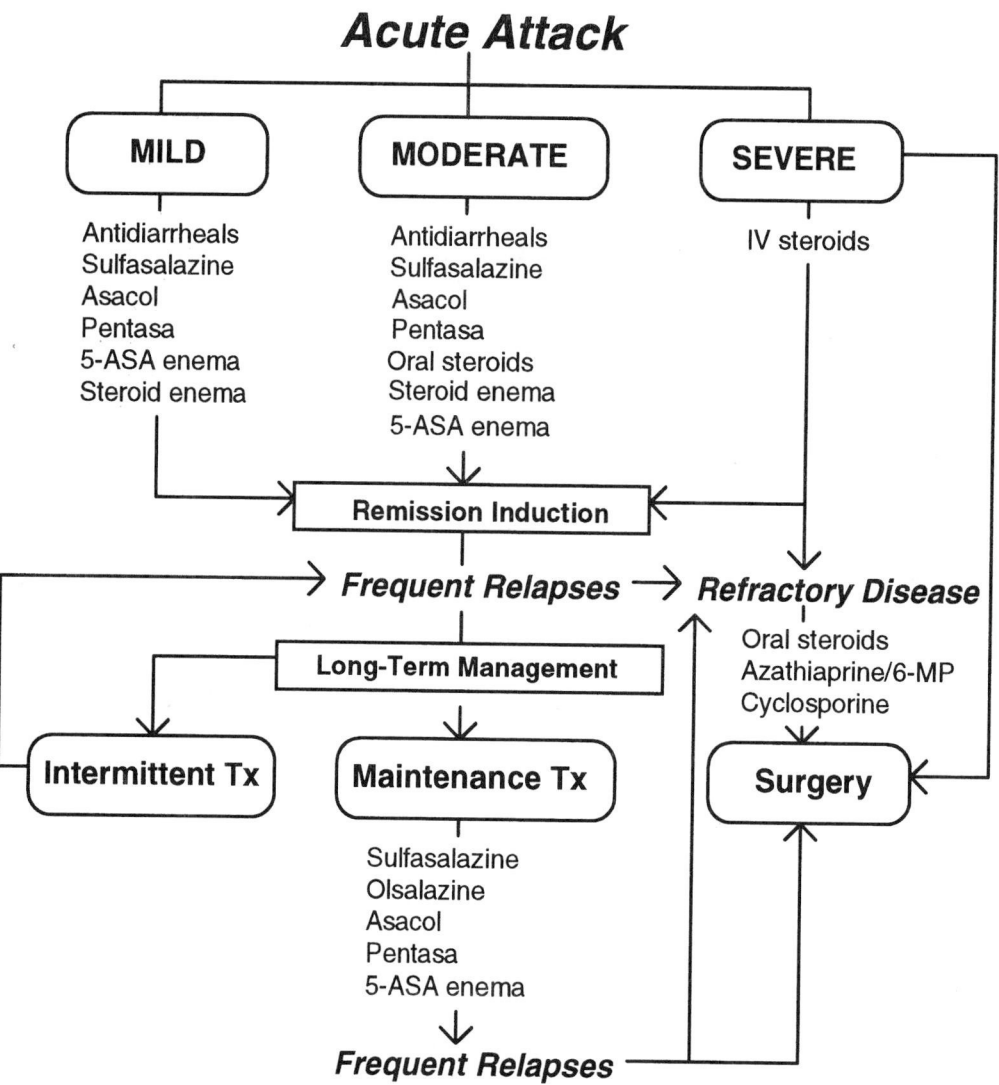

Figure 24.4. Strategies for managing ulcerative colitis.

reserved for individuals with mild to moderate active disease of the distal colon who do not respond to GCS or SASP. Frequent relapses may require maintenance therapy with low-dose SASP. Pentasa, Asacol, and olsalazine should be used for individuals who are intolerant to SASP.

CROHN'S DISEASE

Patients with severe active CD usually require intravenous GCS in doses similar to those used in treating UC. GCS should be continued until symptomatic relief is obtained, and then they should be tapered. For patients whose symptoms worsen when GCS are withdrawn, consideration should be given to the addition of either AZA or 6-MP to the regimen in an attempt to withdraw or reduce the GCS dose.

Therapy for patients with mild to moderate ileitis or ileocolitis should be initiated with 40 to 60 mg/day of oral prednisolone-equivalent. Pentasa or Asacol should be considered for patients with ileal or ileocolonic disease, especially if the patient's clinical condition permits a longer response time. SASP, in doses of 3 to 4 g/day, may be tried for 4 to 6 weeks in mild to moderate active CD that involves the colon. If the response to SASP, Pentasa, or Asacol is inadequate, oral prednisone should be instituted. Metronidazole, in a maximum dose of 20 mg/kg/day, may be useful in treating patients with Crohn's colitis, fistula, or severe perianal disease. Pentasa or Asacol may be useful in maintaining remission in nonsurgical patients and may be of value after surgical resection.

PREGNANCY, LACTATION, AND FERTILITY

The management of IBD in pregnancy is of concern because the disease occurs frequently in young adults and many of the drugs (or their metabolites) used in treatment cross the placental barrier and are secreted into breast milk (48). SASP and GCS do not appear to affect the fetus; there

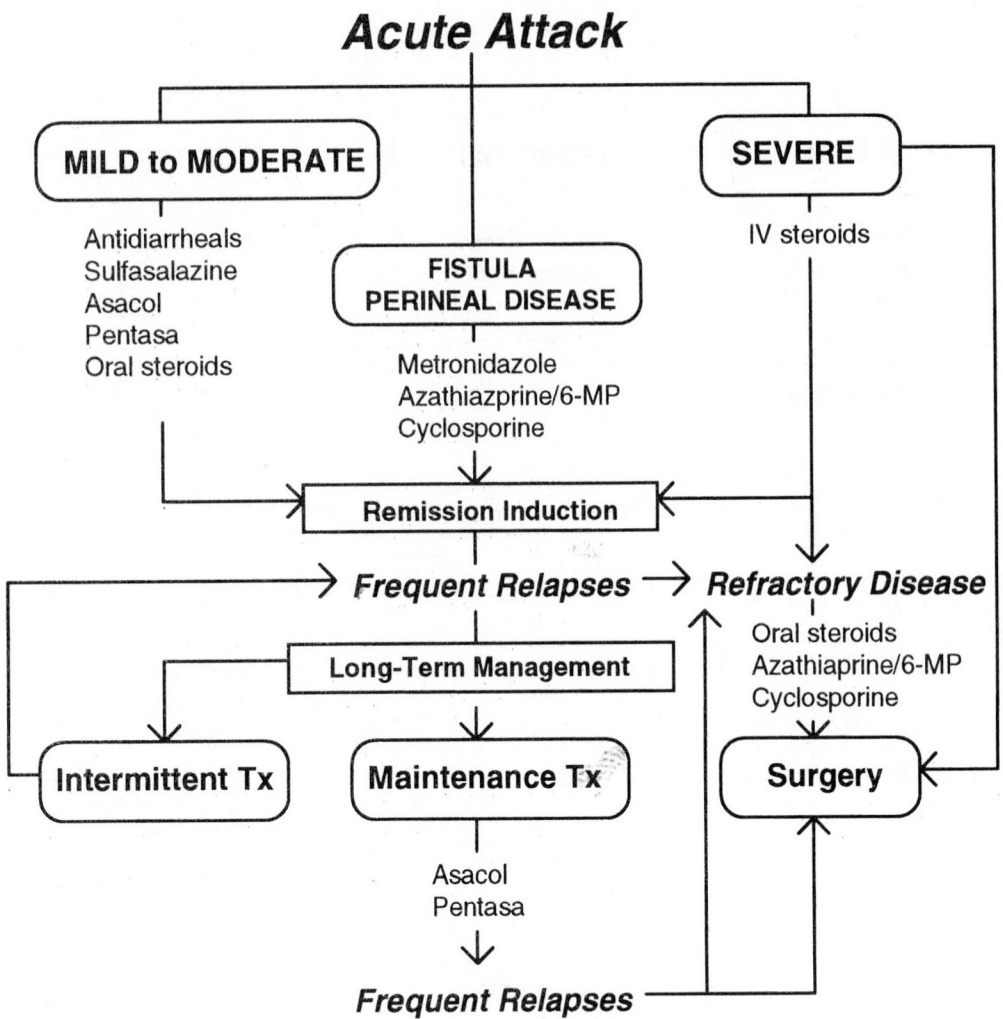

Figure 24.5. Strategies for managing Crohn's disease.

Table 24.9.
Efficacy of Medical Therapy in Ulcerative Colitis and Crohn's Disease[a,b]

Drug	Ulcerative Colitis		Crohn's Disease			
	TX	MTN	TX	MTN	Fistula	Perianal
Sulfasalazine	++	++	++	−	−	−
Olsalazine	++	++	++	−	−	−
Asacol	++	++	++	+	−	−
Pentasa	++	++	++	+	−	−
Steroids	++	−	++	−	−	−
Metronidazole	−	−	++	−	+	+
Azathiaprine/6-MP[c]	+	+	+	+	+	+
Cyclosporine[c]	+	−	+	−	+	+

[a](++) = effective; (+) = likely to be effective; (−) = documented efficacy lacking.
[b]TX = remission induction; MTN = maintenance of remission.
[c] = refractory disease.

is little evidence to suggest that SASP causes kernicterus or is teratogenic. MTZ and the immunosuppressants should be avoided, although there is increasing evidence that AZA may not be harmful to the fetus (48, 49). For the majority of patients, pregnancy does not affect the course of IBD, nor is the outcome of pregnancy affected. In addition, IBD does not adversely affect fertility, but male patients should be informed that SASP may reversibly inhibit spermatogenesis. Folic acid supplementation may be necessary for patients taking SASP. Although it is always best to avoid medication during pregnancy, the potential risks and benefits must be carefully evaluated for each individual.

CHILDREN AND ADOLESCENCE

When IBD begins in childhood, the clinical course is similar to that observed when the onset occurs later in life, except for more severe growth retardation, which is more common in the patient with CD. Because malnutrition contributes to growth failure, nutritional supplementation must be aggressively pursued. Medications used in the treatment of IBD in children are similar to those used to treat adult patients. However, prolonged use of high-dose GCS may suppress growth and cause other steroid-related adverse effects. Although MTZ and the immunosuppressants have been used in children, they should be used with caution because of the potentially serious complications related to these medications (50).

SURGICAL MANAGEMENT

Surgery is indicated only after failure of all reasonable attempts at medical management or to treat actual and impending complications. The decision to operate must be weighed against the disabilities of the disease and the adverse effects of long-term medical therapy.

Surgery is eventually required for 20 to 25% of patients with UC (3). In contrast to CD, removal of the colon in UC removes the primary focus of the disease and usually rids the patient of systemic complications. Generally accepted indications for surgical intervention in UC include failure of medical therapy, toxic megacolon, colonic perforation or hemorrhage, anal complications, and the risk of developing colonic cancer. Although a prophylactic colectomy has been recommended for children and adults with long-standing pancolitis, the most reasonable approach is periodic evaluations that include colonoscopy with accompanying histologic examination of biopsies for precancerous changes. Total proctocolectomy with a permanent ileostomy is the operative procedure of choice. Postoperative mortality is 3% in elective colectomy, 10 to 15% in patients undergoing emergency surgery for acute severe disease, and 50% in those who have had colonic perforation.

The indications for surgery in CD are influenced by the site of involvement and the fact the surgery is not a curative form of therapy. Possible indications include failure of medical management, intestinal obstruction, strictures, fistulas, abscess formation, perforation, and hemorrhage. Approximately 60% of patients will require surgery within 10 years of initial symptoms, and the rate of recurrence after intestinal resection is reported to be as high as 75% after 15 years (3). In view of the high recurrence rate following resection, the procedure of choice is usually conservative intestinal resection of diseased bowel with primary bowel anastomosis. The most controversy occurs when CD involves only the colon. Increasing losses of the small bowel through resection and disease may eventually limit its absorptive surface, resulting in malabsorptive syndromes and malnutrition.

PROGNOSIS

The prognosis for patients with IBD is favorably affected by adequate nutritional support and effective medications. Approximately 90% of patients with acute UC will respond to medical management with successful remission. The overall mortality of an acute attack is increased with pancolitis or when toxic megacolon develops. Left-sided colitis and ulcerative proctitis respond well to medical treatment and have a favorable prognosis. The prognosis of patients with UC, with extensive colonic involvement and long-standing disease, may depend on the development of colon cancer, but total colectomy affords a cure. The long-term prognosis for patients with CD is not as favorable as that for patients with UC because of the variable nature of the disease and the, less-than-optimal, response to medical therapy. A large number of patients will require surgery at some point; unfortunately, surgery is often followed by disease recurrence. Morbidity and mortality, often associated with disease complications such as peritonitis and sepsis, usually increase with the duration of the disease.

SUMMARY

Despite the limitations of medical and surgical treatment, the majority of patients with IBD are able to adjust to their chronic illness and lead productive lives. Management must be individualized and should include emotional support by the family and health care providers. Until the cause of IBD is understood, curative drug therapy is beyond the reach of medicine. Fortunately, a few drugs offer the majority of patients some assistance. Promising new agents offer hope, but we must await confirmation of their efficacy and safety.

REFERENCES

1. Sandler RS. Epidemiology of inflammatory bowel disease. In: Targan SR, Shanahan F, eds. Inflammatory bowel disease: from bench to bedside. Baltimore: Williams & Wilkins, 1994:5.

2. Sonnenberg A, McCarty DJ, Jacobsen SJ. Geographic variation of inflammatory bowel disease within the United States. Gastroenterology 100:143–49, 1991.

3. Stenson W. Inflammatory bowel disease. In: Yamada T, Alpers DH, Owyang C, et al, eds. Textbook of gastroenterology. Philadelphia: JB Lippincott, 1995:1748.

4. Thayer WR, Chitnavis V. Inflammatory bowel disease: the case for an infectious etiology. Med Clin North Am 78:1233–47, 1994.

5. MacDermott RP. Alterations in the mucosal immune system in ulcerative and Crohn's disease. Med Clin North Am 78:1207–31, 1994.

6. Gross V, Arndt H, Andus T, et al. Free radicals in inflammatory bowel diseases: pathophysiology and therapeutic implications. Hepatogastroenterol 41:320–27, 1994.

7. Bachwich DR, Lichtenstein GR, Traber PT. Cancer in inflammatory bowel disease. Med Clin North Am 78:6:1399–1412, 1994.

8. Lewis JD, Fisher RL. Nutrition support in inflammatory bowel disease. Med Clin North Am 78:1443–56, 1994.

9. Griffiths AM, Ohlsson A, Sherman PM. Meta-analysis of enteral nutrition as a primary treatment of active Crohn's disease. Gastroenterology 108:1056–67, 1995.

10. Barrett KE, Dharmsathaphorn K. Pharmacological aspects of therapy in inflammatory bowel diseases: antidiarrheal agents. J Clin Gastroenterol 10:57–63, 1988.

11. Kaplan MA, Korelitz BI. Narcotic dependence in inflammatory bowel disease. J Clin Gastroenterol 10:275–78, 1988.

12. Allgayer H. Sulfasalazine and 5-ASA compounds. Gastroenterol Clin North Am 21:643–58, 1992.

13. Hanauer SB, Baert F. Medical therapy of inflammatory bowel disease. Med Clin North Am 78:1413–26, 1994.

14. Hanauer SB, D'Haens G. Medical management of ulcerative colitis. In: Targan SR, Shanahan F, eds. Inflammatory bowel disease: from bench to bedside. Baltimore: Williams & Wilkins, 1994:545.

15. Bitton A, Peppercorn MA. Medical therapy of ulcerative proctitis and proctosigmoiditis, including refractory disease. Inflammatory Bowel Disease 1:207–19, 1995.

16. Sachar DB. Maintenance therapy in ulcerative colitis and Crohn's disease. J Clin Gastroenterol 20:117–22, 1995.

17. Plevy SE, Targan SR. Specific management of Crohn's disease. In: Targan SR, Shanahan F, eds. Inflammatory bowel disease: from bench to bedside. Baltimore: Williams & Wilkins, 1994:582.

18. Laasila K, Leirisalo-Repo M. Side effects of sulphasalazine in pateints with rheumatic diseases or inflammatory bowel disease. Scand J Rheumatol 23:338–40, 1994.

19. Small RE, Schraa CC. Chemistry, pharmacology, pharmacokinetics, and clinical applications of mesalamine for the treatment of inflammatory bowel disease. Pharmacotherapy 14:385–98, 1994.

20. Segars LW, Gales BJ. Mesalamine and olsalazine: 5-aminosalicylic acid agents for the treatment of inflammatory bowel disease. Clin Pharm 11:514–28, 1992.

21. Wadworth AN, Fitton A. Olsalazine: a review of its pharmacodynamic and pharmacokinetic properties, and therapeutic potential in inflammatory bowel disease. Drugs 41:647–64, 1991.

22. Nilsson A, Danielsson A, Lofberg R, et al. Olsalazine versus sulphasalazine for relapse prevention in ulcerative colitis: a multicenter study. Am J Gastroenterol 90:381–87, 1995.

23. Sutherland LR, May GR, Shaffer EA. Sulfasalazine revisited: a meta-analysis of 5-aminosalicylic acid in the treatment of ulcerative colitis. Ann Intern Med 118:540–49, 1992.

24. Layer PH, Goebell H, Keller, J, et al. Delivery and fate of oral mesalamine microgranules within the human small intestine. Gastroenterology 108:1427–33, 1995.

25. Singleton JW, Hanauer S, Robinson M. Quality-of-life results of double-blind, placebo-controlled trial of mesalamine in pateints with Crohn's disease. Dig Dis Sci 40:931–35, 1995.

26. Brignola, C, Cotton M, Pera A, et al. Mesalamine in the prevention of endoscopic recurrence after intestinal resection for Crohn's disease. Gastroenterology 108:345–49, 1995.

27. Campieri M, Gionchetti P, Belluzzi A, et al. Role of rectal formulations: enemas. Scand J Gastroenterol 25(Suppl 172):63–65, 1990.

28. Williams CN. Role of rectal formulations: suppositories. Scand J Gastroenterol 25(Suppl 172):60–62, 1990.

29. Andus T, Targan S. Glucocorticoids. In: Targan SR, Shanahan F, eds. Inflammatory bowel disease: from bench to bedside. Baltimore: Williams & Wilkins, 1994:487.

30. Rosenberg W, Ireland A, Jewell DP. High-dose methylprednisolone in the treatment of acute ulcerative colitis. J Clin Gastroenterol 12:40–41, 1990.

31. Lofberg R. New steroids for inflammatory bowel disease. Inflammatory Bowel Disease 1:135–41, 1995.

32. Rutgeerts P, Lofberg R, Malchow H, et al. A comparison of budesonide with prednisolone for active Crohn's disease. N Engl J Med 332:842–45, 1994.

33. Berstein CN, Shanahan F. Immunomodulatory therapy in inflammatory bowel disease. In: Targan SR, Shanahan F, eds. Inflammatory bowel disease: from bench to bedside. Baltimore: Williams & Wilkins, 1994:503.

34. Choi PM, Targan SR. Immunomodulator therapy in inflammatory bowel disease. Dig Dis Sci 39:1885–92, 1994.

35. Pearson DC, May GR, Fick GH, et al. Azathioprine and 6-mercaptopurine in Crohn's disease: a meta-analysis. Ann Intern Med 122:132–42, 1995.

36. Bernstein CN, Artinian L, Anton PA, et al. Low-dose 6-mercaptopurine in inflammatory bowel disease is associated with minimal hematologic toxicity. Dig Dis Sci 39:1638–41, 1994.

37. Connell WR, Kamm MA, Dickson M, et al. Long-term neoplasia risk after azathioprine treatment in inflammatory bowel disease. Lancet 343:1249–52, 1994.

38. Sandborn WJ. A critical review of cyclosporine therapy in inflammatory bowel disease. Inflammatory Bowel Disease 1:48–63, 1995.

39. Lichtiger S, Present DH, Dornbluth A, et al. Cyclosporine in severe ulcerative colitis refractory to steroid therapy. N Engl J Med 330:1841–45, 1994.

40. Santos J, Baudet S, Casellas, F et al. Efficacy of intravenous cyclosporine for steroid refractory attacks of ulcerative colitis. J Clin Gastroenterol 20:285–89, 1995.

41. Feagan BG, Rochon J, Fedorak RN, et al. Methotrexate for the treatment of Crohn's disease. N Engl J Med 332:292–97, 1995.

42. Bernstein CN, Shanahan F. Role of antibiotics in the management of inflammatory bowel disease. In: Targan SR, Shanahan F, eds. Inflammatory bowel disease: from bench to bedside. Baltimore: Williams & Wilkins, 1994:524.

43. Rutgeerts P, Hiele M, Geboes K, et al. Controlled trial of metronidazole treatment for prevention of Crohn's recurrence after ileal resection. Gastroenterology 108:1617–21, 1995.

44. Zarling EJ, Sedghi S. Current and promising new therapies for inflammatory bowel disease. Hosp Formul 28:466–85, 1993.

45. Pullan RD, Rhodes J, Ganesh S, et al. Transdermal nicotine for active ulcerative colitis. N Engl J Med 330:811–15, 1995.

46. Thomas GAO, Rhodes J, Mani V, et al. Transdermal nicotine as maintenance therapy for ulceractive colitis. N Engl J Med 332:988–92, 1995.

47. Gaginella TS. Targeting future drugs for inflammatory bowel disease. In: Targan SR, Shanahan F, eds. Inflammatory bowel disease: from bench to bedside. Baltimore: Williams & Wilkins, 1994:531.

48. Hanan IM. Fertility and pregnancy. In: Targan SR, Shanahan F, eds. Inflammatory bowel disease: from bench to bedside. Baltimore: Williams & Wilkins, 1994:695.

49. Alstead EM, Ritchie JK, Lennard-Jones JE, et al. Safety of azathiazoprine in pregnancy in inflammatory bowel disease. Gastroenterology 99:443–46, 1990.

50. Hofley PM, Piccoli DA. Inflammatory bowel disease in childhood. Med Clin North Am 78:1281–302, 1994.

CHAPTER 25

NAUSEA AND VOMITING

BRUCE D. CLAYTON and CARLA B. FRYE

Nausea is the subjectively unpleasant sensation of the awareness of the urge to vomit. It is often preceded or accompanied by a variety of autonomic signs such as pallor, sweating, tachycardia, salivation, and increased respiratory rate.

Vomiting is the reflex expulsion of the stomach contents via the esophagus and mouth and is usually associated with nausea and retching. Nausea and retching can occur without expulsion, and occasionally expulsion occurs without prior nausea and retching. This is known as projectile vomiting.

Retching is the involuntary but unsuccessful effort to vomit. It involves mainly the respiratory muscles of the abdomen, diaphragm, and chest and is often accompanied by bradycardia.

The vomiting reflex is found in many species and probably evolved as a protective mechanism to limit the effects of ingested toxic materials (1). In humans the tendency to experience nausea and vomiting varies greatly. Causes of nausea and vomiting are listed in Table 25.1. The treatment of nausea and vomiting depends on the cause, which should be determined before beginning therapy.

PHYSIOLOGIC BASIS OF VOMITING

The principal anatomic elements involved in vomiting are shown diagrammatically in Figure 25.1. Integration of the vomiting reflex occurs in the vomiting center (VC), which is located in the lateral reticular formation of the medulla. Afferent fibers from sensory receptors in the pharynx, stomach, intestines, and other viscera connect directly with the VC through the vagus and splanchnic nerves and, when stimulated, produce vomiting. The center also responds to stimuli originating in other tissues, such as the cerebral cortex, vestibular apparatus of the inner ear, and blood. These so-called central stimuli are believed to travel first to the chemoreceptor trigger zone (CTZ), which then activates the VC to induce vomiting. The CTZ is located in the medullary region known as the area postrema, which is located on the caudal margin of the fourth ventricle. An important function of the CTZ is to sample blood and spinal fluid for potentially toxic substances and, when these are detected, to initiate vomiting. It is therefore appropriate that the CTZ is located in the area postrema, a region of the brain that is not protected by the blood-brain barrier. The CTZ cannot initiate emesis independently but only through stimulation of the CTZ (2). Both the VC and the CTZ occur bilaterally and are much smaller than shown in Figure 25.1.

The higher centers of the brain can be a source of stimuli for the vomiting center (Fig. 25.1). The reaction to unpleasant sights and smells is a common example of this. Vomiting can occur as a conditioned response (e.g., the pretreatment nausea that occurs in some patients who are about to receive a course of anticancer chemotherapy). The cerebrum can greatly modify the vomiting response to stimuli from other sources such as visceral or vestibular nerve pathways, leading to enhancement or repression of vomiting. The large placebo response that is seen in many trials of antiemetics can be explained in these terms, as can suppression of motion sickness by the patient's concentration on some mental activity. Psychological factors can thus play an important role in nausea

Table 25.1.
Causes of Vomiting

1. Ingestion of certain substances present in food and the environment
2. Administration of certain drugs, particularly opiates, general anesthetics, and antineoplastic drugs
3. Motion or other effects of the vestibular apparatus
4. Infection—part of the prodrome of many infections
5. Respiratory problems such as violent coughing
6. Cardiovascular disease such as infarction
7. Disorders of the gastrointestinal tract:
   a. Gastrointestinal tract obstruction
   b. Mucosal lesions such as ulcers, inflammation, and atrophy
   c. Liver disease
   d. Pancreatic and small intestinal diseases
   e. Diseases of the components of the gut wall (collagen, smooth muscle, nerve)
   f. Peritonitis
8. Renal diseases such as renal failure, pyelonephritis, uremia, and uretic colic
9. Metabolic and endocrine disorders such as diabetic ketoacidosis, uremia, hyperparathyroidism, adrenal insufficiency, and pregnancy
10. Gynecologic disorders such as pelvic inflammation and complications of pregnancy
11. Normal pregnancy
12. Neurologic disorders such as increased cranial pressure, hemorrhage, epilepsy, meningitis, migraine, vertigo, and Meniere's syndrome and brain metastases
13. Psychiatric disorders including bulimia, rumination, and anorexia nervosa
14. Drug withdrawal syndromes
15. Radiation therapy

and vomiting, although they are usually outweighed by physical factors.

There is some confusion in the literature as to whether vestibular and hypermedullary stimuli travel directly to the VC or reach it, as shown in Figure 25.1, via the CTZ. These pathways have not been properly elucidated, but the scheme shown in the figure is supported by recent publications (1, 3). Evidence indicates that in humans the CTZ may even influence the sensory input that the VC receives from the viscera. The variability in the literature is due to research on different species of experimental animals, which vary greatly in their anatomy and physiology of emesis.

Drugs that exert an emetic effect by acting on the CTZ include apomorphine, cardiac glycosides, morphine, the ergot alkaloids, anesthetics, and many antineoplastic agents. There is considerable species difference in the sensitivity of the CTZ to emetic drugs as well as great variation in the extent to which emesis is stimulated by other routes, such as stimulation of the sensory receptors of the viscera. Apomorphine is the only drug that produces vomiting solely by direct action on the CTZ in all species. The complexity of the pharmacology of emetic drugs is illustrated by morphine, which can act on the CTZ directly or indirectly via the vestibular afferent system. It can also antagonize the emetic action of other drugs by direct depression of the VC.

The neurochemical control of vomiting is not completely understood. However, four neurotransmitter systems appear to play significant roles in mediating the emetic response: dopaminergic, histaminic, cholinergic, and 5-hydroxytryptamine₃. *Dopamine* receptors are found in both the CTZ and the gastrointestinal tract. Dopamine agonists, such as apomorphine and L-dopa, produce emesis by acting on the CTZ and peripheral dopamine receptors that stimulate the CTZ, whereas dopamine antagonists, such as the phenothiazines and metoclopramide, block emesis. *Histamine* (H₁ and H₂) receptors are also found in the CTZ, but histamine receptor blockade results in antiemetic activity limited to vestibular causes. The neurotransmitters that are involved in motion sickness are better understood. The sensory disorientation that occurs in motion sickness results in an imbalance in *cholinergic* and adrenergic activity in the region of the medulla near the VC and CTZ. The result is excess acetylcholine that affects the VC either directly or, more likely, through an effect on the CTZ (1). Recent studies indicate that *5-hydroxytryptamine₃* (5-HT₃) or serotonin receptors appear to be principal mediators in the emetic reflex. High concentrations of the 5-HT₃ receptors have

Figure 25.1. Anatomic structures involved in the vomiting reflex, showing the site of action of common antiemetic drugs: 1, site of action of sedative; 2, site of action of antihistamines and anticholinergics; 3, site of action of dopamine antagonists; and 4, proposed sites of action of serotonin antagonists. The vomiting reflex is mediated through the vomiting center. This center receives impulses from afferent fibers from the stomach and intestines and from fibers from the CTZ. It sends out impulses via afferent fibers to the muscles of the throat, epiglottis, and stomach as shown in Figure 25.2.

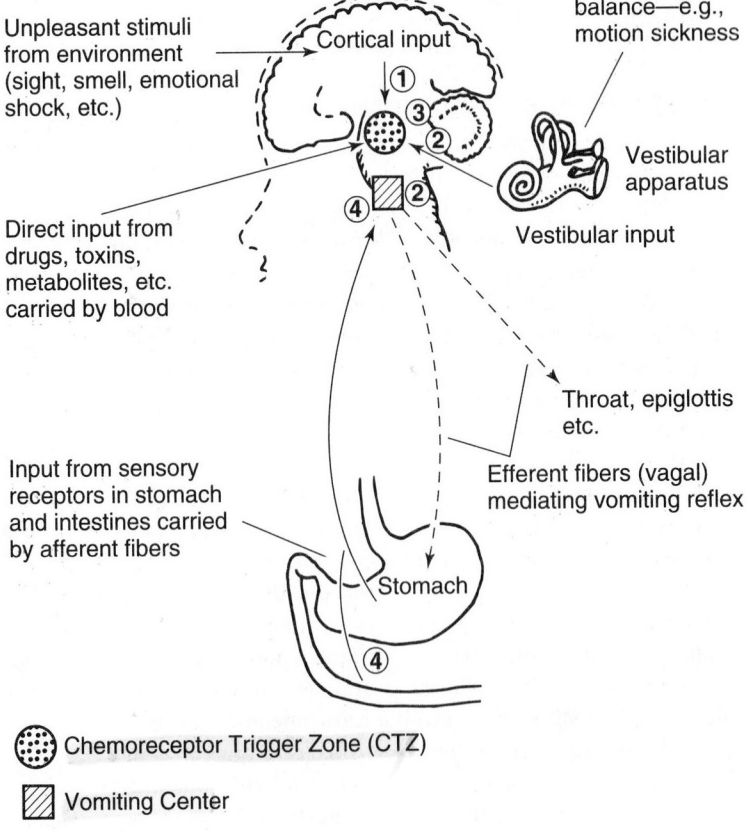

Disturbances of balance—e.g., motion sickness

Unpleasant stimuli from environment (sight, smell, emotional shock, etc.)

Cortical input

Vestibular apparatus

Vestibular input

Direct input from drugs, toxins, metabolites, etc. carried by blood

Throat, epiglottis etc.

Efferent fibers (vagal) mediating vomiting reflex

Input from sensory receptors in stomach and intestines carried by afferent fibers

Stomach

Chemoreceptor Trigger Zone (CTZ)

Vomiting Center

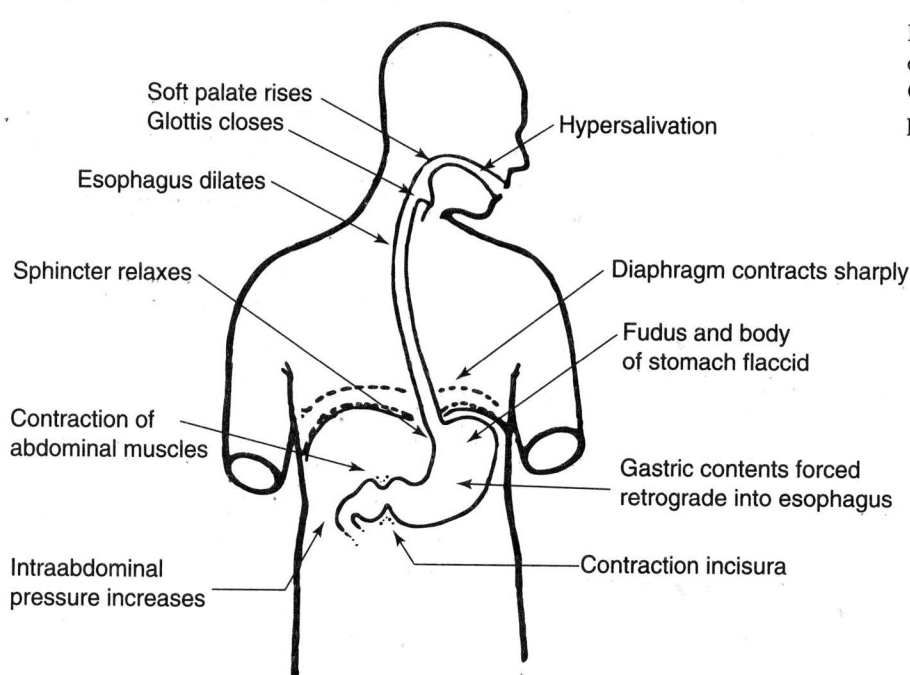

Figure 25.2. The mechanism of the complex act of vomiting. (From Whelan G. Curr Therapeut 26(12):26, 1985, with permission.)

Soft palate rises
Glottis closes

Hypersalivation

Esophagus dilates

Diaphragm contracts sharply

Sphincter relaxes

Fudus and body
of stomach flaccid

Contraction of
abdominal muscles

Gastric contents forced
retrograde into esophagus

Contraction incisura

Intraabdominal
pressure increases

recently been identified in the area postrema-nucleus tractus solitarii region of the medulla (4). About 90% of the 5-HT$_3$ in the adult human body is located in the enterochromaffin cells of the gastrointestinal tract; the remainder is present in the central nervous system and the platelets. The 5-HT$_3$ receptors in the gastrointestinal (GI) tract are thought to be located on visceral afferent nerve terminals within the abdomen (5), sending sensory signals via the vagus and the greater splanchnic nerve to the central nervous system.

There may be other, different receptors that initiate emesis for drugs such as the cardiac glycosides and the opiates. Emesis is thus mediated through a variety of receptor types, and it is possible that more will be discovered.

Anatomically, the VC is well placed to coordinate the various efferent functions associated with vomiting (see Fig. 25.2). When the VC is stimulated, efferent impulses are sent to the salivary, vasomotor, and respiratory centers and to cranial nerves VIII and X. The vomiting reflex begins with a sudden deep inspiration that increases abdominal pressure, which is further increased by contraction of the abdominal muscles. The soft palate rises and the epiglottis closes, thus preventing the aspiration of vomitus into the lungs. The pyloric sphincter contracts and the cardiac sphincter and esophagus relax, allowing stomach contents to be expelled. The flow of saliva increases to aid the expulsion.

ANTIEMETIC DRUGS

Considerable effort has been spent in developing antinausea drugs. Initially, emphasis was on the treatment of motion sickness and nausea of pregnancy, but more recently it has focused on the treatment of nausea and vomiting caused by antineoplastic agents. Nausea and vomiting are common complications of chemotherapeutic regimens, often so severe as to cause the patient not to return for further treatment. Only recently have satisfactory antiemetic therapies begun to emerge.

In selecting drugs for the treatment of nausea and vomiting, it is important to remember that therapy must be individualized. Multiple pathways are available for a variety of stimuli to induce nausea and vomiting, and correlations between serum levels and efficacy have not been established for most antiemetics. For these reasons, treatment regimens should be regarded only as guidelines.

Dopamine Antagonists

The dopamine antagonists include the phenothiazines, the butyrophenones and related compounds, and the substituted benzamides, which include metoclopramide. These compounds inhibit dopamine receptors, and the antiemetic action of the compounds is thought to be, at least in part, due to inhibition of dopamine receptors in the CTZ. Unfortunately, the antiemetics that act as dopamine antagonists may also produce symptoms of dystonia, parkinsonism, akathisia, and tardive dyskinesia, since the extrapyramidal nigrostriatal system is highly innervated by dopaminergic fibers (6).

PHENOTHIAZINES

The phenothiazines have been the most widely used antiemetics since the 1950s. Two key modifications of the phenothiazine heterocyclic structure improve antiemetic activity. Halogenation (prochlorperazine, perphenazine) or thiethylation (thiethylperazine) of position 2 (R1), in combination with the attachment of a piperazine side chain at the 10 position (R2), enhances antiemetic (as well as extrapyramidal) activity. The phenothiazines also have varying amounts of anticholinergic and antihistaminic activity that may inhibit the vestibular pathway and the vomiting center of the brain (7).

Adverse effects of the phenothiazines include orthostatic hypotension and excessive sedation, which may limit use in ambulatory patients. Extrapyramidal effects occur most frequently with perphenazine but are readily controlled with diphenhydramine or benztropine. Other adverse effects of the phenothiazines, such as cholestatic jaundice and blood dyscrasias, are potential complications but rarely occur because of the intermittent and short-term use of these agents as antiemetics. The phenothiazines can be given orally, parenterally, and rectally. The latter routes are useful when vomiting precludes the oral route.

Phenothiazines are used primarily for treatment of mild to moderate nausea and vomiting associated with anesthesia and surgery, radiation therapy, and anticancer chemotherapy. Prochlorperazine has been the phenothiazine most widely used and studied as an antiemetic. Onset of action is 10 to 20 min for intramuscular administration, 30 to 40 min for oral tablet administration, and 60 min for rectal suppository administration. The duration of action is 3 to 4 hr, regardless of the route. Prochlorperazine has routinely been administered in a dose of 10 mg every 4 to 6 hr orally or intramuscularly or 25 mg every 6 hr rectally to provide optimal antiemetic efficacy. At these dosages, comparative studies in cancer chemotherapy patients indicate that it is more effective than placebo, equivalent in potency to low-dose metoclopramide (0.1 to 0.3 mg/kg/dose) and droperidol and less effective than tetrahydrocannabinol (THC), high-dose metoclopramide (1 to 3 mg/kg/dose), and nabilone (6). Recent studies have demonstrated significantly improved antiemetic activity when doses of 30 to 40 mg of prochlorperazine administered by slow intravenous infusion. There was no substantial increase in adverse effects if diphenhydramine was administered prophylactically to prevent extrapyramidal reactions (7–9).

BUTYROPHENONES

The butyrophenones, like the phenothiazines, are dopamine antagonists and are effective antiemetic agents with similar uses and side effects. The main side effect is sedation, although extrapyramidal side effects do occur. The butyrophenones are less likely to produce hypotension than are the phenothiazines. Droperidol is an effective antiemetic for use in cytotoxic therapy and in combination with fentanyl in surgery but is for parenteral administration

only. The onset of pharmacologic action of droperidol occurs within 3 to 10 min, but peak pharmacologic effects may not be apparent until 30 min post-injection. Duration of antiemetic action is 2 to 4 hr, but sedating and tranquilizing effects may persist for up to 12 hr after a single dose.

Haloperidol is also used as an antiemetic. It is usually given in doses of 1 to 3 mg orally or intramuscularly every 3 hr. Oral bioavailability is 60%. Peak plasma concentrations occur within 2 to 6 hr. Haloperidol appears to undergo first-pass metabolism and enterohepatic recirculation. Following intramuscular administration, peak plasma concentrations occur within 10 to 20 min, with peak pharmacologic action within 30 to 45 min.

METOCLOPRAMIDE

Metoclopramide has dual action as an antagonist of both dopamine and 5-HT$_3$ receptors, protecting against the emetic effects of dopamine and serotonin agonists. The action of metoclopramide is more selective than that of the phenothiazines in that it shows neuroleptic activity only at very high doses. Through a peripheral action, possibly as a partial agonist of enteric postsynaptic neurons (10), metoclopramide also increases the motility of the stomach and small intestine and relaxes the pyloric sphincter, increasing the activity of the upper regions on the GI tract. The antidopaminergic and antiserotonergic effects of metoclopramide on the gut complement the central antiemetic effect and are particularly useful in treating nausea and vomiting associated with GI cancer, gastritis, peptic ulcer, radiation sickness, and migraine. Metoclopramide is contraindicated in patients with intestinal obstruction who are at high risk for colonic rupture. It appears to be of little value in the treatment of motion sickness, although it has been widely used for this purpose in Europe.

Early clinical trials of metoclopramide at doses of 0.1 to 0.3 mg/kg showed only minimal antiemetic effect for a variety of antineoplastic agents. In 1981, after extensive animal testing, a trial investigating the use of high-dose (1 to 3 mg/kg) metoclopramide gave very encouraging results (11).

There are no major differences in the pharmacokinetics of conventional- and high-dose metoclopramide (12). Oral doses are rapidly absorbed, but variable first-pass metabolism provides an oral bioavailability of 32 to 100% (13). Peak levels occur in about 1 hr. High lipophilicity results in a large volume of distribution (2.8 to 4.5 L/kg). Approximately 85% of an orally administered dose appears in the urine within 72 hr. Of the 85% eliminated in the urine, about half is present as free or conjugated metoclopramide. The terminal half-life is 4.5 to 8.8 hr. One study to date indicates that there is substantial pharmacokinetic variability between patients with various cancers. The authors attribute this variability primarily to differences in body weight and serum alkaline phosphatase levels (14). Although an early study indicated that serum levels >800 ng/mL were necessary to achieve maximum protection against cisplatin-induced emesis, more recent trials have failed to show that serum metoclopramide concentrations are predictive of antiemetic response or adverse effects.

Several controlled and uncontrolled studies have investigated routes of administration for optimal antiemetic therapy, ease and expense of administration, and frequency of adverse effects. Although optimal doses and time schedules have not been completely delineated, the studies indicate that oral, continuous intravenous, and intermittent intravenous administration routes provide comparable antiemetic activity against a variety of chemotherapeutic agents. Oral therapy tends to be associated with a greater frequency of loose stools than intravenous administration, and scheduled dosing may be difficult if vomiting occurs. Rectal administration shows significant variation in the bioavailability of extemporaneously compounded suppositories (30 to 86%) but is successful in reducing the frequency of emesis as described in a case report of one patient (15). Other points such as legal aspects of compounding, formulation stability, and cost must also be considered (16).

Adverse effects associated with metoclopramide therapy include diarrhea, sedation, dizziness, and extrapyramidal symptoms. Diarrhea occurs in about 50% of patients receiving high-dose metoclopramide and cisplatin, but this may be related to cisplatin therapy. Mild sedation is observed in most patients who receive higher doses. The extrapyramidal symptoms include akathisia, restlessness, and dystonic reactions (including torticollis, oculogyric crisis, and Parkinsonlike symptoms). The overall frequency is 3 to 5%, but as many as 30% of young men under the age of 30 years may suffer from extrapyramidal effects. Extrapyramidal symptoms subside within 5 min of intravenous diphenhydramine administration. Many cancer chemotherapy protocols now include both high-dose metoclopramide and routine doses of diphenhydramine when highly emetogenic cytotoxic agents are used (see the section entitled "Chemotherapy-Induced Emesis").

Serotonin Receptor Antagonists

A new group of compounds known as the serotonin (5-HT$_3$) receptor antagonists have made a major impact in the treatment of emesis associated with cancer chemotherapy, radiation therapy, and postoperative nausea and vomiting. Serotonin receptors of the 5-HT$_3$ type are located centrally in the chemoreceptor trigger zone of the area postrema of the medulla and peripherally in the enterochromaffin cells of the GI tract and the vagal nerve terminals. Two serotonin (5-HT$_3$) receptor antagonists, ondansetron and granisetron, were made available in 1991

Table 25.2.
Pharmacokinetics of Serotonin Antagonists[a]

Variable	Ondansetron		Granisetron
	P.O.[b]	I.V.[c]	I.V.[d]
Bioavailability	56%		
Half-life (hr)			
Cancer patients		4.0	9
Volunteers			
20–40 yr	3.3	3.5	4.9
60–75 yr[e]	4.5	4.7	7.7
>75 yr[e]	5.5	5.5	
Liver impairment			
Moderate		9.2	NA
Severe		20.6	NA
Protein binding	70–76%	70–76%	65%
Volume of distribution (L/kg)			3.97

Source: Cerenex Pharmaceuticals (17); SmithKline Beecham Pharmaceuticals (18).
[a]High intersubject and intrasubject variability was noted in these studies.
[b]Single 8-mg oral dose.
[c]Single 0.15-mg/kg i.v. dose.
[d]Single 40-µg/kg i.v. dose.
[e]No dosage adjustment is required in the elderly.

and 1994, respectively. Table 25.2 compares the pharmacokinetic properties of these agents. Serum concentrations do not correlate with antiemetic efficacy, and there does not appear to be accumulation after multiple dosing. Ondansetron is extensively metabolized, with only 5% recovered in the urine as unchanged drug. The primary metabolic pathway is hydroxylation of the indole ring followed by glucuronide or sulfate conjugation. In vitro measurement of plasma protein binding of ondansetron is 70 to 76% (17). Granisetron metabolism involves N-demethylation and aromatic ring oxidation followed by conjugation. Animal studies suggest that some of the metabolites may also have (5-HT$_3$) receptor antagonist activity. In normal volunteers, approximately 12% is eliminated unchanged in the urine in 48 hours. The remainder is excreted as metabolites, 49% in the urine and 34% in the feces. Both ondansetron and granisetron are metabolized by hepatic cytochrome P-450 drug-metabolizing enzymes; inducers or inhibitors of these enzymes may change the clearance and the half-life of these serotonin antagonists. At this time, no dosage adjustments are recommended. Ondansetron and granisetron do not induce or inhibit the cytochrome P-450 enzyme system (17, 18). Table 25.3 compares the frequency of adverse effects of the serotonin antagonists. Note that the clinical studies that are cited for frequency of adverse effects of granisetron used a dosage of 40 µg/kg. Because no statistical difference in antiemetic efficacy has been demonstrated between 10 µg/kg and 40 µg/kg, the recommended dose in the United States is now 10 µg/kg (18). A particular advantage to this group of serotonin

Table 25.3.
Comparison of Frequency of Adverse Events of Serotonin Antagonists

	Granisetron	Ondansetron		
	40 µg/kg I.V.	8 mg TID P.O.	0.15 mg/kg × 3 I.V.	32 mg × 1 I.V.
Diarrhea	4%	NA	16%	8%
Headache	14%	21%	17%	25%
Fever	8.6%	NA	8%	7%
Akathisia	0%	0%	0%	0%
Extrapyramidal reactions[a]	0%	0%	0%	0%
Somnolence	4%	—	—	—
Constipation	3%	7%	11%	11%

Source: Cerenex Pharmaceuticals (17); SmithKline Beecham Pharmaceuticals (18).
[a]There have been rare reports consistent with, but not diagnostic of, extrapyramidal reactions with both granisetron and ondansetron.

antagonists is that there is no dopaminergic blockade, and thus no extrapyramidal adverse effects have been reported (19). There have, however, been rare reports consistent with, but not diagnostic of, extrapyramidal reactions with both granisetron and ondansetron (17).

Cisplatin, a potent serotonin agonist, is well recognized for its almost 100% emetic potential when it is administered to patients without antiemetic prophylaxis. It is thus the primary agent against which the efficacy of antiemetics are measured. The serotonin antagonists have been shown to actively control nausea and vomiting associated with cisplatin and several other emetogenic chemotherapeutic agents in both animals and humans. Comparative studies between ondansetron and metoclopramide concluded that ondansetron is more effective than metoclopramide in the control of high-dose cisplatin-induced nausea and vomiting (19–21). The first international, multicenter, double-blind, randomized, parallel group study to directly compare the efficacy and safety profile of ondansetron and granisetron in the control of cisplatin-induced acute emesis concluded that no significant differences were observed between any of the treatment groups with respect to emetic control, nausea, or adverse reactions. Headache was the most frequently reported drug-related adverse effect, occurring in 9% of all patients (22).

Anticholinergic Drugs

Antimuscarinic drugs include muscarinic antagonists such as scopolamine and antihistamines of the H_1 receptor antagonist type. These drugs are used in the treatment of motion sickness and, in the case of the antihistamines, for treating nausea and vomiting associated with pregnancy. The antiemetic effects of the antihistamines are due to their anticholinergic activity and not to the blocking of histamine receptors (23). Motion sickness is believed to be mediated by an excess of acetylcholine in the medulla in the region of the VC and CTZ; the anticholinergic antiemetics probably block acetylcholine in this central region and not peripherally.

In spite of the very extensive literature on antimotion sickness drug testing, there is a distinct lack of basic clinical pharmacology such as dose-response relationships and pharmacokinetic parameters. The most commonly used anticholinergic antiemetic drugs include scopolamine (hyoscine) and the antihistamines promethazine, diphenhydramine, cyclizine, and meclizine. The choice of drug depends on the period for which antinausea protection is required and the side effects. Clinical studies indicate that the drug of choice is oral scopolamine (0.2 to 0.6 mg) for short periods of motion and an antihistamine for longer periods (1). Of the antihistamines, promethazine (25 mg) is the drug of choice (23). Although higher doses have a longer duration of action, sedation is usually a problem. Cyclizine (50 mg) has fewer side effects than promethazine but has a shorter duration of action and is less effective for severe conditions. Meclizine (50 mg) is similar to cyclizine, and both drugs are used when nausea is mild and protection is required for short periods. Diphenhydramine has a long duration, but excessive sedation is usually a problem. For very severe conditions, sympathomimetic drugs such as ephedrine are used in combination with scopolamine or antihistamines.

The transdermal delivery system for administering scopolamine ("scopolamine patch") has produced good results (24). The system, a 2-mm-thick patch with a surface area of 2.5 cm^2, contains 1.5 mg of scopolamine. Part of the dose is contained in the hypoallergenic contact adhesive and is released immediately to saturate skin binding sites and to initiate absorption. The remainder of the dose is contained in a reservoir separated from the contact surface by a membrane that releases the drug at a constant rate of about 5 µg/hr for a period of approximately 66 hr. The patch is backed by a water-resistant layer. The manufacturers recommend that the patch be applied to the postauricular skin (a highly permeable skin site of the body) 4 to 6 hr before expecting motion.

About 67% of people using transdermal scopolamine

complain of dryness of the mouth, although this is not a contraindication. Drowsiness occurs in about 17% of patients, and about 12% of users experience blurred vision, which is probably due in some cases to transfer of the drug to the eyes by the fingers. Potential users should be advised to try the patches before using them in a travel situation and to wash their hands after applying the patch. The patches should not be used for pediatric patients, during pregnancy, for patients with glaucoma or a family history of glaucoma, and for patients who have a psychosis.

Corticosteroids

A variety of studies have shown that dexamethasone and, to a lesser extent, methylprednisolone can be effective antiemetics as single agents or in combination with other antiemetics. The mechanism of action by which the corticosteroids act as antiemetics is unknown, but it has been suggested that the drugs act by inhibiting prostaglandin synthesis in the hypothalamus. Other actions of the corticosteroids such as mood elevation, increased appetite, and a sense of well-being may be responsible for patient acceptance and positive outcomes (25).

The antiemetic effects of dexamethasone are comparable to those of metoclopramide (1 to 2 mg/kg) in controlling nausea and vomiting associated with low-dose cisplatin (<60 mg/m^2) therapy and standard doses of chemotherapeutic agents with moderately emetogenic activity. However, metoclopramide appears to be more effective than dexamethasone against high-dose cisplatin (120 mg/m^2) and other highly emetogenic cancer chemotherapy agents. Dexamethasone also appears to be more effective against emesis induced by moderately emetogenic agents than standard doses of oral prochlorperazine (10 mg) (25). Kris and colleagues also demonstrated that the overall antiemetic activity can be improved when dexamethasone is added to metoclopramide and prochlorperazine therapy. A single dose of dexamethasone administered with metoclopramide shortly before administration of chemotherapy significantly reduced the frequency of emesis (26). A more recent study indicates that patients who received a combination of granisetron and dexamethasone reported fewer episodes of nausea and vomiting induced by moderately emetogenic chemotherapy than when either antiemetic agent was used alone (27).

Although few studies have been completed, methylprednisolone may be useful as a single antiemetic agent during chemotherapy with mild to moderately emetogenic agents, but it is not recommended as a single-agent antiemetic with the use of highly emetogenic agents such as cisplatin (25). Further trials are needed to establish the optimum dose regimens for use with the various antineoplastic agents and the advantages of combining corticosteroids with other antiemetics.

The advantage of the steroids, apart from their efficacy, is their relative lack of side effects. Lethargy, weakness, euphoria, a sense of well-being, insomnia, increased appetite, and generalized swelling are more common side effects of corticosteroids when they are used for short-course antiemetic therapy. Other rare effects reported include headache, metallic taste, abdominal discomfort, itchy throat, and a swollen feeling in the mouth (18). Adverse effects associated with the long-term use of corticosteroids are not applicable in this setting. Dexamethasone is also reported to significantly decrease the incidence of diarrhea and sedation associated with metoclopramide therapy (26).

Cannabinoids

Following numerous reports that smoking marijuana reduced nausea, the antiemetic properties of the active ingredient, Δ-9-tetrahydrocannabinol (THC), and synthetic analogs such as nabilone and levonantradol have been studied extensively. Proposed mechanisms of action are that the cannabinoids act in the cerebral cortex to inhibit pathways to the vomiting center, exert an anticholinergic effect on cholinergic terminals in Auerbach's plexus, and possibly mediate the prostaglandin cyclic nucleotide system (28). Other studies indicate that there is no dopaminergic antagonist activity (29).

Pharmacokinetic studies of THC show that absorption from the gastrointestinal tract is slow and erratic, with bioavailability less than 10%, although this may depend on the formulation. THC is highly protein-bound (97%). Peak plasma concentrations are attained in about 1 hour after oral administration, with serum levels in the 5- to 10-ng/mL range producing antiemetic activity. Higher serum levels are associated with greater antiemetic effect but with substantially more adverse effects. The terminal half-life of THC is 20 to 30 hr, but other active metabolites require 1 to 2 days for elimination. Patients report a correlation with the peak serum concentrations and a "euphoric high." The "high" following oral administration usually begins 30 to 60 min after ingestion, peaks in 1 to 3 hr, and lasts for 4 to 6 hr. Smoking THC cigarettes raises bioavailability (about 20%), with onset of action in 6 to 12 min. Peak levels are attained in 30 to 120 min with a duration lasting 3 to 4 hr. Normal behavior is observed 24 hr after administration (28, 29).

THC has been shown to be more effective than placebo and as effective as prochlorperazine in patients receiving moderately emetogenic chemotherapy. It is less effective than metoclopramide and is associated with more side effects when used to prevent emesis secondary to cisplatin therapy. The most common adverse effects associated with THC therapy include dry mouth, sedation, orthostatic hypotension, dizziness, and confusion. Dysphoric effects such as depressed mood, dreaming or fantasizing, distortion of perception, and elated mood are more frequent with dosages >5 mg/m^2. Younger patients appear to tolerate these side effects better than older patients or patients who have not previously used marijuana (30).

Nabilone is rapidly and well absorbed orally (96%) with an elimination half-life of about 2 hr. Studies indicate that nabilone is more effective than placebo and prochlorperazine against moderately emetogenic chemotherapeutic agents. It is not, however, as effective as metoclopramide with vomiting associated with cisplatin therapy. Nabilone has been reported to have fewer euphoric effects than THC (31).

Because of the mind-altering effects of the cannabinoids and the potential for abuse, these agents have served as antiemetics only in patients receiving chemotherapy. The cannabinoids have more utility in younger patients who are refractory to other antiemetic regimens and in whom combination therapy may be more effective.

Benzodiazepines

The benzodiazepines—diazepam, lorazepam, and midazolam—are quite effective in reducing not only the frequency of nausea and vomiting, but also the anxiety that is often associated with chemotherapy (32, 33). This action is probably due to a combination of effects, including sedation, reduction in anxiety, possible depression of the VC, and an amnesic effect. Of these, the amnesic effect appears to be the most important as far as treating cancer patients is concerned, and in this respect, lorazepam and midazolam are superior to diazepam. The sedative and amnesic effects are dose-related, higher doses (≥4 mg) of lorazepam inducing amnesic effects that persist for a longer period of time and occur in a larger percentage of patients. Amnesia does not correlate well with sedation, since sedation may remain high while the amnesic effects decline.

Following intravenous administration of either lorazepam or midazolam, the onset of sedative, anxiolytic, and amnesic action usually occurs within 1 to 5 min. The duration of action following intravenous administration of midazolam is usually less than 2 hr; however, dose-dependent actions may persist for up to 6 hr in some patients. After intramuscuar administration the onset of action of lorazepam is 15 to 30 min, and the duration of action is 12 to 24 hr. Following intramuscular administration of midazolam, onset of action occurs within 5 to 15 min but may not be maximal for 20 to 60 min; the duration of action is about 2 hr, although the range is 1 to 6 hr. The onset of action of orally administered lorazepam is about 30 min, with peak activity occurring within 2 hr. Duration of action is 4 to 6 hr. The elimination half-life of lorazepam is 10 to 20 hr, with no active metabolites, whereas that of midazolam is 1 to 12 hr, with active metabolites.

Clinically, midazolam and lorazepam are most useful in combination with other antiemetics such as metoclopra-

mide and dexamethasone. The anxiolytic and amnesic effects result in marked subjective support by patients (34). The greatest benefit from benzodiazepine therapy is derived by patients who have not received prior chemotherapy and who have not developed negative conditioning by episodes of nausea and vomiting (see the section entitled "Anticipatory Nausea and Vomiting"). Side effects associated with benzodiazepine therapy are drowsiness and dizziness. Patients should not be left unattended in the sedated, amnesic state, since vomiting episodes may still occur. Because of its short half-life and short duration of action, midazolam may be a more appropriate adjunctive antiemetic for outpatient use.

PATIENT ASSESSMENT AND MANAGEMENT

An accurate diagnosis is essential before beginning treatment for nausea and vomiting, since symptomatic therapy may be contraindicated (e.g., in GI obstruction, acute appendicitis, or cerebral edema), or the underlying disease may be serious and require specific measures. The causes of vomiting should be kept in mind (see Table 25.1) in deciding on the treatment plan.

The appearance, frequency, and timing of nausea and vomiting, together with associated specific and nonspecific symptoms such as jaundice, diarrhea, weight loss, pain, and fever, are important in making a diagnosis. Blood in the vomitus, an important sign, can be fresh and bright red, such as that due to an esophageal tear, or altered, having the appearance of coffee grounds, indicating a GI bleed. Bile in the vomitus gives it a green or yellow color and suggests that the pyloric sphincter is open, allowing reflux of duodenal contents into the stomach.

The cause of vomiting is usually obvious (e.g., pregnancy, motion, or the use of certain drugs), but in some cases diagnosis can be difficult, especially if psychogenic factors are involved. With unexplained vomiting, the first step in assessment is elimination of the possibility of upper GI tract lesions or systemic conditions such as meningitis or uremia. The patient should also be assessed for the need to treat the sequelae of prolonged vomiting, such as fluid and electrolyte depletion.

Chronic vomiting, with or without weight loss, can be psychogenic. This is suggested when the vomiting has been occurring for some time (especially if the patient has delayed seeking help), when there is a family history of vomiting, or when the patient is able to suppress vomiting or vomiting rarely occurs in a public place.

The principles involved in treating vomiting are as follows:

1. Treat the cause if it can be identified.
2. Treat for fluid and electrolyte loss. In most cases this involves giving adequate fluids orally, particularly fluids containing glucose. If fluid loss leads to metabolic disturbances, the

patient should be hospitalized and given appropriate intravenous fluids.

3. Give appropriate symptomatic drug treatment, after considering contraindications and adverse drug reactions. The choice of drug and dose must be individualized.
4. For unexplained vomiting, continue with diagnostic examinations (35).

The features of vomiting-induced metabolic disturbances include:

1. Dehydration, suggested by oliguria, weight loss, mental confusion, and reduced tissue turgor.
2. Sodium depletion, suggested by thirst and hypotension.
3. Potassium depletion, suggested by muscle weakness.
4. Alkalosis, which can occur as a result of loss of hydrogen ions in the vomitus, and the concentration of extracellular fluid secondary to fluid loss.

Sodium, potassium, and chloride depletion occur mainly because of loss in the vomitus but also as a consequence of other metabolic disturbances.

TREATMENT OF SELECTED CAUSES OF NAUSEA AND VOMITING

Chemotherapy-Induced Emesis

Chemotherapy-induced emesis (CIE) is the most unpleasant adverse effect associated with the use of antineoplastic agents. Many patients regard it as the most stressful aspect of their disease, more so even than the prospect of dying. Since the object of therapy in many cases is to prolong life for a relatively short period, the effect of CIE on the quality of life must be considered. Also, many patients whose prognosis is good find it difficult to comply and may request that therapy be discontinued because of CIE. In one multicenter survey, as many as 10% of patients refused to continue with chemotherapy because of nausea and vomiting (36).

Three types of emesis have been identified in patients receiving chemotherapy: (a) anticipatory nausea and vomiting, (b) acute chemotherapy-induced emesis, and (c) delayed emesis. Patients may also have emesis for reasons other than chemotherapy, perhaps induced by medications such as analgesics or tumor-related complications such as intestinal obstruction. Addressing these matters is usually more important than selection of antiemetic therapy (37). Apart from distressing the patient, severe vomiting complicates the patient's medical condition, causing dehydration, metabolic alkalosis, electrolyte deficiencies, nutritional impairment including cachexia, and physical injury including esophageal tears and bone fractures.

ANTICIPATORY NAUSEA AND VOMITING

The patient's fear of CIE may lead to anticipatory nausea and/or vomiting (ANV). Anticipatory nausea alone has been reported in up to 44% of patients, and anticipatory vomiting has been reported in up to 38% (38). ANV correlates with the emetic potential of chemotherapy regimens and with the severity of nausea and vomiting after chemotherapy. Although considerable interpatient variability is observed, the onset of ANV usually occurs 2 to 4 hr before treatment and is most severe at the time of drug administration (39).

Patients who experience ANV are more likely to be younger and to have received twice as many courses of chemotherapy with more drugs for about three times longer than patients who do not experience ANV (38, 40). It is believed that ANV is a conditioned response that is triggered by the sight or smell of the clinic or hospital or by the knowledge that treatment is imminent. ANV tends to become more severe as treatments progress unless behavior therapy modifies the conditioned response (41). Such treatments include progressive muscle relaxation, mind diversion, hypnosis, self-hypnosis, and systematic desensitization. People with a negative attitude toward therapy, such as the belief that it will be of no benefit, are more likely to develop ANV than are those with a positive attitude. A positive relationship between the patient and counselor is important in the success of behavioral treatment of CIE. The patient needs to be able to communicate freely with the staff about real and imagined fears concerning therapy and thereby develop positive attitudes toward his or her treatment. The rotation of medical staff that occurs in hospitals and clinics can impede the development of such relationships (41).

Complications associated with ANV underscore the need for accompanying the initial course of emesis-producing chemotherapy with the most effective antiemetic regimen and continuing vigorous therapy with each subsequent cycle of chemotherapy (37). Addition of lorazepam to antiemetic regimens induces an amnesic effect about chemotherapy and emesis in some patients (42) and has received more subjective support from patients (43). If delayed emesis (see the section below) is associated with any of the agents in the chemotherapeutic regimen, effective antiemetic therapy should be continued long enough to reduce the frequency of nausea and emesis, thus minimizing the risk of preconditioning the patient against further chemotherapy and ANV.

ACUTE CHEMOTHERAPY-INDUCED EMESIS

The choice of antiemetic therapy for patients receiving antineoplastic therapy should take into account both patient and drug factors.

Patient Factors. The incidence and severity of CIE are generally greater among people of advanced age, those in poor general health (especially if they are cachexic), and those with metabolic disturbances (i.e., dehydration, uremia, GI tract obstruction, or infection). The patient's age can also influence the response to antiemetic drugs. For example, patients under the age of 30 are more sensitive to the extrapyramidal effects of dopaminergic blockade from phenothiazines or high-dose metoclopramide than older patients are. On the other hand, younger patients tolerate cannabinoids better than older people do. Patients who have a history of chronic heavy alcohol use (more than five mixed drinks per day) tolerate chemotherapy with fewer bouts of emesis than do those without this history (37). Patients who are prone to motion sickness seem to be more sensitive to the emetic effects of cytotoxic agents. Since these two types of emesis are mediated by different mechanisms, this correlation probably reflects a psychogenic component. Finally, the patient's mental outlook and attitude to therapy can influence the frequency and severity of emetic reactions considerably.

Drug Factors. The emetogenic potential of antineoplastic drugs varies greatly, ranging from a rate of 90% or greater in the case of cisplatin to 10% or less with chlorambucil. Table 25.4 classifies chemotherapeutic agents in terms of emetogenicity, although emetogenicity is also influenced by the dose, duration, and frequency of courses. The effects of combinations of chemotherapeutic agents on vomiting are poorly understood.

The extensive literature on the testing of antiemetics for use with antineoplastic agents is often difficult to interpret. Comparisons between trials are difficult because of differences in protocol, cytotoxic drugs, and patient characteristics (32, 45). Some studies rely entirely on objective data alone (i.e., the frequency of vomiting and the volume of vomitus) without investigating patient attitudes, performance capabilities, or quality-of-life issues. A patient who vomits only occasionally but experiences nausea continually may have a poorer quality of life than does someone who vomits more frequently but has little intervening nausea.

However, it is clear that major progress has occurred in treating CIE (46), and some general recommendations can be made. All patients who are being treated with moderate to very high emetogenic chemotherapeutic agents (Table 25.4) should receive prophylactic antiemetic therapy before antineoplastic therapy is initiated. Combinations of high-dose metoclopramide, ondansetron, granisetron, dexamethasone, lorazepam, and/or diphenhydramine are the drugs of choice in treating cisplatin-induced emesis (37, 47–50). Haloperidol may be substituted for metoclopramide if the patient tolerates metoclopramide (32). Antiemetic therapy should be continued for 4 to 7 days to prevent delayed vomiting (see the section entitled "Delayed Emesis"). Emesis that is induced by moderately emetogenic agents such as methotrexate and 5-fluorouracil may be treated prophylactically with metoclopramide and dexamethasone, and therapy should be continued for 24 hr (51). A phenothiazine (prochlorperazine) or dexamethasone alone is

Table 25.4.
Relative Emetic Activity of Chemotherapeutic Agents

Agent	Emetic Time Course (hr)	
	Onset	Duration
1. Very high emetic incidence (90%)		
Cisplatin	1–6	24–120
Dacarbazine	1–3	1–12
Mechlorethamine (Mustine)	½–2	8–24
Streptozocin	1–4	12–24
2. High emetic incidence (60–90%)		
BCNU (carmustine)	2–4	4–24
Cyclophosphamide (prop. to dose)	4–12	4–10
Dactinomycin	2–4	<24
Lomustine	1–6	24–36
Mithramycin	2–6	4–6
Procarbazine (prop. to dose)	24–27	Variable
3. Moderate emetic incidence (30–60%)		
Daunorubicin	2–6	24
5-Fluorouracil	3–6	—
4. Low emetic incidence (10–30%)		
Adriamycin	4–6	—
Bleomycin	3–6	—
Cytarabine	6–12	3–5
Etoposide	3–8	—
Methotrexate	4–12	3–12
6-Mercaptopurine	4–8	—
Tamoxifen	12–24	—
Vinblastine (prop. to dose)	4–8	—
5. Very low emetic incidence (10%)		
Chlorambucil	48–72	—
Corticosteroids	4–8	—
Leuprolide	—	—

Source: Adapted from Borison and McCarthy (44); Craig and Powell (51).

recommended if the chemotherapy is of low emetic potential. An alternative for this group may be a cannabinoid plus a phenothiazine to ameliorate central nervous system side effects (51). The rationale for using combinations of antiemetic agents is based on the assumption that cytotoxic agents produce emesis by multiple mechanisms. Antiemetics also act by multiple mechanisms, and a combination could have a synergistic action. Side effects are also a factor in the choice of an antiemetic, and combinations of drugs acting by different mechanisms are less likely to produce adverse reactions than the highest dose of a single drug. In some cases a second antiemetic agent may reduce the side effects of the first drug (e.g., dexamethasone, diphenhydramine, or lorazepam is added to high-dose metoclopramide). All antiemetics should be administered an adequate time before chemotherapy is initiated and should be continued through the characteristic time associated with vomiting for a particular chemotherapeutic agent (Table 25.4). Efficacies, doses, and adverse effects of some antiemetic drugs are given in Table 25.5. Therapy must be individualized, and the doses and treatment sched-

Table 25.5.

Efficacy, Dose, and Toxicity of Antiemetics Used in the Treatment of Cytotoxic-Induced Emesis (CIE)

Drug	Antiemetic Activity[a]	Dosage Range (Doses Must Be *Individualized*)[b]	Adverse Effects[c]
Phenothiazines			
Prochlorperazine	++	5–10 mg q 2–4 h p.o.; 5–10 mg q 3–6 h i.m./i.v.[d]; 25 mg p.r. q 6 h	+/++
Chlorpromazine	++	25–50 mg q 3–6 h p.o. 25 mg q 4–6 h p.o./i.m./i.v.[d]/p.r.	+/++
Thiethylperazine	++	10 mg q 8 h p.o./i.m./p.r.	+/++
Butyrophenones			
Droperidol	++	1–3 mg q 4–6 h i.v. or 5 mg i.v. 30 min prior to chemotherapy then continuous infusion of 1–1.5 mg/hr for 9–12 hr	+/++
Haloperidol	++	1–3 mg q 4–6 h p.o./i.m./i.v.[d]	+/++
Metoclopramide			
High dose	+++	1–3 mg/kg IVPB over 15 min 0.5 hr before and q 2 h × 3–4 doses after chemotherapy	++
Low dose	0/+	0.1–0.3 mg/kg q 4 h p.o./i.m./i.v.	+
Corticosteroids			
Dexamethasone	+++	4–25 mg p.o./i.v. before chemotherapy and q 4–6 h × 1–2 days	0/+
Methylprednisolone	+++	125–500 mg p.o./i.v. 2 hr before chemotherapy and 2 hr after or as infusion	0/+
Benzodiazepines			
Lorazepam	++/+++	1–4 mg q 4–6 h p.o./i.v.; can commence when patient arrives for chemotherapy	+/++
Cannabinoids			
Δ-9-THC	++[e]	5–10 mg/m² q 4 h p.o.; commence night before chemotherapy	++/+++
Serotonin antagonists			
Granisetron	+++	10 mcg/kg IVPB over 5 min within 30 min before starting chemotherapy	++
Ondansetron	+++	8 mg p.o. q 4 h × 3 doses beginning 30 min before start of emetogenic chemotherapy. Follow chemotherapy with 8 mg q 8 hr for 1–2 days. 32 mg IVPB as a single dose, or 0.15 mg/kg IVPB q 4 h × 3 doses. Infuse dose over 15 min beginning 30 min before start of emetogenic chemotherapy.	++

[a]Antiemetic activity against cisplatin: 0, little or none, to +++, high.
[b]Doses are examples only and represent the ranges given in the references cited in the text. Best results are usually obtained with a combination of antiemetics. Frequently, dosing is begun before chemotherapy. IVPB = i.v. piggy-back, p.r. = per rectum.
[c]0, little or none, to +++, high incidence.
[d]Can be administered by slow (15–20 min) i.v. administration.
[e]May have marked efficacy in young patients.

ules given are meant as guidelines only. All antiemetics except antimuscarinics (anticholinergics and antihistamines) have been found to be useful in the treatment of CIE.

DELAYED EMESIS

Delayed emesis is a distinct syndrome that occurs 24 or more hours after the administration of chemotherapy. It has been reported in as many as 93% of patients receiving high-dose cisplatin. Symptoms may occur 24 to 120 hr after cisplatin administration but are most severe at 48 to 72 hr. Delayed nausea and vomiting are usually less severe than those that may occur acutely but can still be of importance in developing ANV and reducing activity, nutritional state, and hydration. The causes of delayed nausea and vomiting are not known. Symptoms may be caused directly by the action of chemotherapeutic agents or their metabolites on the nervous system or gastrointestinal tract (52). Episodes of delayed vomiting are frequently associated with provocative events such as

brushing teeth, using mouthwash, manipulation of dentures, seeing food, and, in the morning, standing up after getting out of bed.

A combination of prochlorperazine 10 mg, lorazepam 0.5 mg, and diphenhydramine 50 mg all given orally 1 hr before breakfast, lunch, and dinner has been reported to be successful in controlling delayed emesis secondary to cisplatin therapy (53). In a randomized, double-blind trial, the combination of oral dexamethasone and metoclopramide decreased the frequency of delayed vomiting (54). Oral ondansetron has not been any more effective than placebo in controlling delayed emesis (55).

Motion Sickness

Motion sickness is a normal, healthy response to exposure to abnormal forms of motion and occurs in animals as well as in humans. The susceptibility to motion sickness varies greatly, approximately one-third of individuals being very sensitive, one-third reacting only to rough conditions, and one-third reacting only to extreme conditions. While there

Table 25.6.
Doses and Duration of Action of Antimotion Sickness Drugs

Drug	Oral Dose[a]	Duration of Action (hr)	Condition
Scopolamine and dexamphetamine	0.2–0.6 mg scopolamine +5–10 mg dexamphetamine[b]	6	Severe
Promethazine and ephedrine	25 mg promethazine +25 mg TID ephedrine	12	Severe
Scopolamine	0.2–0.6 mg q 6 h[c]	4	Severe
Promethazine	25 mg TID	12	Severe
Dimenhydrinate	50 mg 2–3 × daily	6	Moderate
Cyclizine	50 mg 2–3 × daily	4	Mild
Meclizine	50 mg 2–3 × daily	6	Mild

[a]Antimotion drugs are most effective if therapy is initiated before exposure to motion. Usually, therapy should be initiated about 30 min before departure and repeated if necessary.
[b]Used only under special circumstances (e.g., by service personnel).
[c]Not more than four doses should be taken in 24 hr.

is no question about the physical basis of motion sickness, it is also very clear that psychological factors play an important part in both suppressing and enhancing the tendency to be sick.

Motion sickness usually begins with pallor, yawning, restlessness, and cold sweat, particularly on the brow and upper lip. The person then experiences nausea, which may lead to excessive salivation, vomiting, drowsiness, and depression. If the nausea is not relieved, severe headache, prostration, and dehydration may develop. In very sensitive individuals these symptoms may progress rapidly; in less sensitive people, symptoms may wax and wane.

The stimuli that produce motion sickness arise in the labyrinth of the inner ear. They are carried by afferent fibers that synapse in the vestibular region of the medulla, where they are thought to stimulate the release of an excessive amount of acetylcholine that acts on the CTZ, which then stimulates the VC (1, 56). A proposed theory suggests that motion sickness arises when there is conflict between the sensory information being transmitted by the eyes, vestibular system, and nonvestibular proprioceptors, particularly as it relates to previous experience. As a result of this conflict, an imbalance of cholinergic and sympathetic transmitters occurs in the medulla, which can be corrected by giving anticholinergic drugs or sympathomimetics. The vestibular system plays the central role; individuals with a nonfunctional vestibular system are immune to motion sickness.

The importance of conflicting sensory stimuli as a cause of motion sickness is illustrated in a practical way by the relief that is obtained when the person can establish a satisfactory visual earth reference. For example, looking out of a car window (particularly from the front seat) can give marked relief, whereas reading in a car (particularly in the back seat) can provoke motion sickness.

Tolerance to motion sickness usually develops after a few days of continuous motion of a particular kind (getting one's "sea legs"); this process emphasizes the fact that

motion sickness is a response to unfamiliar motion. If exposure to an emetogenic stimulus is sufficiently prolonged, motion sickness may be experienced after cessation of the motion ("mal de debarquement"). Many people experience motion sickness before commencing a journey.

In accordance with the theory of motion sickness, drugs that are used in the treatment of motion sickness include sympathomimetics and anticholinergics (Table 25.6). The choice of drug or drug combination depends on the expected duration and severity of the reaction. For very severe conditions, such as might be experienced by service personnel in a landing craft, combinations of scopolamine and dexamphetamine are the most effective therapy and have the advantage that the stimulatory effects of the dexamphetamine offset the drowsiness caused by the scopolamine. Unfortunately, the tendency for dexamphetamine to be abused limits its use. However, combinations of ephedrine and promethazine are also very effective and have been ranked just below the dexamphetamine-scopolamine combination (23). Dosages are given in Table 25.6.

Of the single drugs, oral scopolamine (0.2 to 0.6 mg) is the most effective for short periods of exposure (less than 6 hr). At the present time, however, commercially prepared oral dosage form is not available in the United States. For longer periods or for moderate to mild conditions, the antihistamines are the drugs of choice. Of these, promethazine 25 mg appears to be the most effective (23). Transdermal scopolamine was used successfully for the treatment of motion sickness of several days' duration. All anti-motion-sickness drugs are more effective if they are used prophylactically rather than after sickness has developed.

For people with severe motion sickness the oral route is unavailable, and therapy is given by the intramuscular route. Scopolamine (0.2 mg) or promethazine (50 mg) (adult dosages) may be given. Promethazine is probably the preferred therapy for acute motion sickness.

In therapeutic doses, all drugs used for the treatment of motion sickness cause side effects. Anticholinergic drugs produce dry mouth, sedation, and blurred vision, and the sympathomimetics produce tachycardia. In the case of scopolamine the total dose should not exceed 1 mg in 24 hr because of effects on the central nervous system.

Psychogenic Vomiting

Psychogenic vomiting can be self-induced, or it can occur involuntarily in response to situations that the person considers threatening or distasteful (e.g., eating food whose origin is considered repulsive).

When a person presents with chronic or recurrent vomiting, a diagnosis of psychogenic vomiting is made after elimination of all other possible causes (Table 25.1). The person with psychogenic vomiting usually does not lose weight and can control vomiting in certain situations (e.g., in public). The identification of the causes of psychogenic vomiting and the successful resolution of the problem may not be possible. A short course of an antiemetic drug such as metoclopramide or antianxiety drugs may be prescribed, along with counseling to treat psychogenic vomiting.

CONCLUSION

Nausea and vomiting vary from minor inconveniences of a transient GI infection to severe and limiting adverse reaction to drug therapy. The consequences of vomiting can be severe. The cause of the nausea and vomiting should be determined before treatment is begun, and specific therapy should be chosen for each of the causes. Drug regimens that are specifically designed for the patient and the cause of nausea and vomiting and that are based on valid clinical studies have a high success rate for the treatment of this disorder. However, care should be taken to minimize any side effects from the antiemetic drugs.

REFERENCES

1. Barnes JH. The physiology and pharmacology of emesis. Molec Aspects Med 7:397-508, 1984.
2. Grunberg, SM. Control of chemotherapy-induced emesis. N Engl J Med 329:1790-96, 1993.
3. Mitchelson, F. Pharmacological agents affecting emesis. Drugs 43:295-315, 1992.
4. Cubeddu LX, Hoffmann IS, Fuenmayor NT, et al. Efficacy of ondansetron (GR38032F) and the role of serotonin in cisplatin-induced nausea and vomiting. N Engl J Med 322:810-16, 1990.
5. Bermudez J, Boyle EA, Miner WD, et al. The antiemetic potential of the 5-hydroxytryptamine₃ receptor antagonist BRL 43694. Br J Cancer 58:644-50, 1988.
6. Wampler G. Pharmacology and clinical effectiveness of phenothiazines and related drugs for managing chemotherapy-induced emesis. Drugs 25 (suppl 1):35-51, 1983.
7. Carr, B, Doroshow J, Blayney, D, et al. Toxicity and dose-response studies of prochlorperazine for cisplatin-induced emesis [Abstract]. Proc Am Soc Clin Oncol 5:252, 1986.
8. Olver IN, Bishop JF, Hollcoat BL, et al. A phase-I dose finding study for intravenous prochlorperazine as an antiemetic for chemotherapy induced emesis [Abstract]. Proc Am Soc Clin Oncol 7:287, 1988.
9. Carr BI, Somlo G, McDevitt J, et al. Pharmacokinetic profiles of high and low dose prochlorperazine [Abstract]. Proc Am Soc Clin Oncol 7:294, 1988.
10. Fozard JR. Neuronal 5-HT receptors in the periphery. Neuropharmacol 23:1473-86, 1984.
11. Gralla RJ. Metoclopramide: a review of antiemetic trials. Drugs 25:63-73, 1983.
12. McGovern EM, Grevel J, Bryson SM. Pharmacokinetics of high-dose metoclopramide in cancer patients. Clin Pharmacokinetics 11:415-24, 1986.
13. Bateman, DN. Clinical pharmacokinetics of metoclopramide, Clin Pharmacokinetics 8:523-29, 1983.
14. Grevel J, Whiting B, Kelman AW, et al. Population analysis of the pharmacokinetic variability of high-dose metoclopramide in cancer patients. Clin Pharmacokinetics 14:52-63, 1983.
15. Parrish RH, Bonzo SM. Use of metoclopramide suppositories. Clin Pharm 2:395-96, 1983.
16. Tami JA, Waite WW. Metoclopramide suppository considerations. Drug Intell Clin Pharm 22:268-69, 1988.
17. Cerenex Pharmaceuticals. Product Information "Zofran^R", Research Triangle Park, NC, December 1993.
18. SmithKline Beecham Pharmaceuticals. Product information "Kytril^R", Philadelphia, PA, February 1994.
19. Marty M, Pouillart P, Scholl S. Comparison of the 5-hydroxy-tryptamine₃ (serotonin) antagonist ondansetron (GR38032F) with high-dose metoclopramide in the control of cisplatin-induced emesis. N Eng J Med 322:816-21, 1990.
20. De Mulder PHM, Selynaeve C, Vermorken JB, et al. Ondansetron compared with high-dose metoclopramide in prophylaxis of acute and delayed cipplatin-induced nausea and vomiting. Ann Intern Med 113:834-40, 1990.
21. Hesketh PJ. Comparative trials of ondansetron vs metoclopramide in the prevention of acute cisplatin-induced emesis. Sem in Oncol 19 (suppl 10):33-40, 1992.
22. Ruff P, Paska W, Goedhals L., et al. Ondansetron compared with granisetron in the prophylaxis of cisplatin-induced acute emesis: a multicenter double-blind, randomized, parallel-group study. Oncology 51:113-18, 1994.
23. Wood CD. Antimotion sickness and antiemetic drugs. Drugs 17:471-79, 1985.
24. Clissold SP, Heel RC. Transdermal hyoscine (scopolamine): a preliminary review of its pharmacodynamic properties and therapeutic efficacy. Drugs 29:189-207, 1985.
25. Cersosimo RJ, Karp DD. Adrenal corticosteroids as antiemetics during cancer chemotherapy. Pharmacotherapy 6:118-127, 1986.
26. Kris MG, Gralla RJ, Tyson LB, et al. Improved control of cisplatin-induced emesis with high-dose metoclopramide and with combinations of metoclopramide, dexamethasone and diphenhydramine. Cancer 55:527-34, 1985.
27. The Italian Group for Antiemetic Research. Dexamethasone, granisetron, or both for the prevention of nausea and vomiting during chemotherapy for cancer. N Engl J Med 3332:1-5, 1995.
28. Vincent BJ, McQuiston DJ, Einhorn LH, et al. Review of cannabinoids and their antiemetic effectiveness. Drugs 25 (suppl 1):52-62, 1983.
29. Anderson PO, McGuire GG. Delta-9-tetrahydrocannabinol as an antiemetic. Am J Hosp Pharm 38:639-46, 1981.
30. Devine ML, Dow GJ, Greenberg BR, et al. Adverse reactions to delta-9-tetrahydrocannabinol given as an antiemetic in a multicenter study. Clin Pharm 6:319-22, 1987.
31. Ward A, Holmes B. Nabilone. A preliminary review of its pharmacological properties and therapeutic use. Drugs 30: 127-44, 1985.

32. Kearsley JH, Tattersall MHN. Recent advances in the prevention and reduction of cytotoxic-induced emesis. Med J Aust 143:341-46, 1985.

33. Bishop JF, Oliver IN, Wolf MM, et al. Lorazepam: a randomized double-blind crossover study of a new antiemetic in patients receiving cytotoxic chemotherapy and prochlorperazine. J Clin Oncol 2:691-95, 1984.

34. Kris MG, Gralla RJ, Clark RA, et al. Consecutive dose-finding trials adding lorazepam to the combination of metoclopramide plus dexamethasone: improved subjective effectiveness over the combination of diphenhydramine plus metoclopramide plus dexamethasone. Cancer Treatment Reports 69:1257-62, 1985.

35. Malagelada, JR, Camilleri M. Unexplained vomiting: a diagnostic challenge. Ann Int Med 101:211-18, 1984.

36. Penta JS, Poster DS, Bruna S, et al. Cancer chemotherapy induced nausea and vomiting in adult and pediatric patients. Am Soc Clin Oncol 4:396, 1981.

37. Gralla RJ, Tyson LB, Kris MG, et al. The management of chemotherapy-induced nausea and vomiting. Med Clin North Am 70:289-301, 1987.

38. Moher D, Arthur AZ, Pater JL. Anticipatory nausea and/or vomiting. Cancer Treat Rev 11:257-64, 1984.

39. Dolgin, MJ, Katz ER, McGinty K, Siegel, JSE. Anticipatory Nausea and vomiting in pediatric cancer patients. Pediatrics 75:547-52, 1985.

40. Alba E, Roma B, de Andres L, et al. Anticipatory nausea and vomiting: prevalence and predictors in chemotherapy patients. Oncology 46:26-30, 1989.

41. Stoudemire A, Cotanch P, Laszlo J. Recent advances in the pharmacologic and behavioral management of chemotherapy-induced emesis. Arch Intern Med 144:1029-33, 1984.

42. Laszlo J, Clark RA, Hanson DC, et al. Lorazepam in cancer patients treated with cisplatin: a drug having antiemetic, amnesic and anziolytic effects. J Clin Oncol 3:864-69, 1985.

43. Kris MG, Gralla RJ, Clark RA, et al. Consecutive dose-finding trails adding lorazepam to the combination of metoclopramide plus dexamethasone: improved subjective effectiveness over the combination of diphenhydramine plus metoclopramide plus dexamethasone. Cancer Treat Rep 69:1257-62, 1985.

44. Borison HL, McCarthy LE. Neuropharmacology of chemotherapy-induced emesis. Drugs 25 (suppl 1):8-17, 1983.

45. Pater JL, Willian AR. Methodologic issues in trials of antiemetics. J Clin Oncol 2:484-97, 1984.

46. O'Brien, MER, Cullen MH. Are we making progress in the management of cytotoxic drug-induced nausea and vomiting? J Clin Pharm Ther 13:19-31, 1988.

47. Smith DB, Newlands ES, Spruyt OW, et al. Ondansetron (GR380032F) plus dexamethasone: effective antiemetic prophylaxis for patients receiving cytotoxic chemotherapy. Br J Cancer 61:323-24, 1990.

48. Cunningham D, Turner A, Hawthorn J, et al. Ondansetron with and without dexamethasone to treat chemotherapy-induced emesis. Lancet 1:1323, 1989.

49. Italian Group for Antiemetic Research. Ondansetron + dexamethasone vs metoclopramide + dexamethasone + diphenhydramine in prevention of cisplatin-induced emesis. Lancet 340:96-9, 1992.

50. Chevallier B on behalf of the Granisetron Study Group. The control of acute cisplatin-induced emesis: a comparative study of granisetron and a combination regimen of high-dose metoclopramide and dexamethasone. Br J Cancer 68:176-80, 1993.

51. Craig JB, Powell BL. Review: the management of nausea and vomiting in clinical oncology. Am J Med Sci 293:34-44, 1987.

52. Kris MG, Gralla RJ, Clark RA, et al. Incidence, course, and severity of delayed nausea and vomiting following the administration of high dose cisplatin. J Clin Oncol 3:1379-84, 1985.

53. Sridhar KS, Donnelly S. Combination antiemetics for cisplatin chemotherapy. Cancer 61:1508-17, 1988.

54. Kris MG, Gralla RJ, Tyson LB, et al. Controlling delayed vomiting: double blind, randomized trial comparing placebo, dexamethasone alone and metoclopramide plus dexamethasone in patients receiving cisplatin. J Clin Oncol 7:108-14, 1989.

55. Kris MG, Tyson LB, Clark RA, et al. Oral ondansetron for the control of delayed emesis after cisplatin. Cancer (Suppl) 70(4):1012-1016, Aug. 15, 1992.

56. Reason JT, Brand JJ. Motion sickness. New York: Academic Press, 1975.

CHAPTER 26

DIARRHEA AND CONSTIPATION

VALERIE W. HOGUE

Constipation and diarrhea are common disorders of the gastrointestinal system experienced by most of the population at some instance in their lives. Generally, these symptoms are self-limiting and may not require any intervention. However, intervention may be considered necessary by patients because of their beliefs and attitude toward normal bowel function. Constipation and diarrhea can affect the ability to carry out work or school responsibilities, and loss of productivity usually requires prompt and effective intervention.

Symptoms of diarrhea and constipation may result from various disease states, medications, dietary changes, food or water contamination, and even psychological distress. Many over-the-counter (OTC) products are available in the United States for resolving the symptoms. Health care providers must understand proper use of these products for self-treatment. Health care providers must also ascertain the possible cause of these symptoms in an effort to prevent masking a serious medical problem and to deter laxative and antidiarrheal abuse.

The financial impact of constipation and diarrhea in the United States is significant. Currently, an estimated $2 billion is spent on antacids and digestive aids, primarily antidiarrheals and laxatives (1). One factor contributing to increased usage is the rise in patient self-treatment with OTC products. A survey of consumer OTC usage trends revealed that of 1356 household respondents, 26% used products for constipation and 28% used products for diarrhea over a 6-month period (2). Women and persons over the age of 60 years used nonprescription laxatives more often. No correlation was observed in these two populations with the use of antidiarrheals.

The decision to self-medicate for constipation or diarrhea depends largely on the individual's perception of "abnormal" bowel habits. In a survey of public perceptions of digestive health and disease, researchers found that 62% of American respondents believed that a bowel movement each day is necessary for good digestive health (3). This idea may have been influenced by the theory of "autointoxication," which stated that the presence of noxious substances in the colon increases cellular degeneration and promotes the aging process (4). Although this theory is obsolete, the belief appears to be common among the elderly whose concern for regularity of bowel movements is shown by their frequent use and abuse of laxatives.

Normal bowel habits may range between 3 and 21 stools per week (5). This demonstrates a wide variation of bowel habits among healthy individuals. The prevalence of self-reported constipation, diarrhea, and defecation frequency in the United States was reported based on the results of a national, population-based survey (6). Respondents ranged in age from 25 to 74 years. The majority of the respondents reported daily defecation (73.3% whites, 63.7% blacks). The frequency of defecation differed significantly with regard to race and gender, but not age. Regardless of gender or race, self-reported constipation was positively correlated with age. This difference may reflect a difference in the perception of constipation by older persons since the frequency of defecation did not change as age progressed.

DEFINITION

The definitions of diarrhea and constipation have been debated for several years, primarily because of variations in the definition of normal bowel habits. Most clinicians will agree that a single definition does not exist that describes either medical problem effectively.

Clinicians generally incorporate two primary aspects in the definition of constipation: (1) difficulty passing stools and (2) infrequent stools. However, patients may describe constipation as less frequent defecation than is normally observed, lower stool volume, difficulty passing stool, hard or firm stool, straining on defecation, a sensation of incomplete evacuation of bowel, or the lack of an urge to stool. A study of young adults not seeking healthcare asked 568 subjects to define constipation. They emphasized function (straining) and consistency (hard stools) rather than the number of stools in their definition (7). Therefore, determining the patient's definition before management is essential.

Diarrhea has been defined with more consistency than constipation. Generally, it is defined as three or more loose or unformed bowel movements per day accompanied by symptoms of fever, abdominal cramps, or vomiting. It has been further described as a condition of abnormal increases in stool weight and liquidity. An increase in stool water excretion above 150 to 200 ml every 24 hours is an objective parameter for acute diarrhea (8).

NORMAL INTESTINAL PHYSIOLOGY

Understanding the normal physiologic flow rate of fluid and electrolytes and a knowledge of the process of defecation provide the basis for discussing the development of constipation and diarrhea. Three major aspects of bowel function exist: colonic absorption, colonic motility, and defecation reflexes.

The daily volume of fluid transversing the duodenum is 9 liters for persons consuming three meals daily. Approximately 8 liters per day are absorbed by the small bowel, of which 1 to 1.5 liters are presented to the colon. The colon absorbs 0.9 to 1.4 liters per day, or approximately 90% of the fluid presented initially. The absorptive capacity of the colon exceeds that of the small intestine, which absorbs only 75% of the fluid presented initially. Daily fecal output is less than 200 ml, which contains approximately 5 mEq of sodium and 8 mEq of potassium.

Colonic motility involves three patterns of muscle contractions controlled by the autonomic nervous system: (1) nonpropulsive segmental contractions, which churn the contents of the lumen; (2) short segmental propulsive contractions, which move contents forward and backward promoting absorption; and (3) long segmental propulsive contractions, which move contents forward over long distances. The urge to defecate occurs when gastric filling and increased physical activity trigger the gastroenteric reflex to produce massive peristalsis. The feces move from the sigmoid colon to the rectum, producing a sensation to defecate. This occurs most often after breakfast (4).

Defecation is initiated via the distension of the rectum by feces. Normally, the rectum can differentiate distension produced by fluids, flatus, and feces through defecation reflexes. Evacuation occurs after relaxation of the internal and external anal sphincters in conjunction with the contraction of the rectosigmoid segment and increased intraabdominal pressure. Voluntary relaxation of the external anal sphincter allows evacuation of the bowel. Conversely, voluntary contraction of the sphincter inhibits defecation.

ETIOLOGY

Constipation may be secondary to underlying disorders or idiopathic (Table 26.1). Diseases producing constipation may be systemic or localized to the gastrointestinal tract. Drugs, including the chronic use of laxatives, may cause constipation (Table 26.2). In addition, psychological factors may cause changes in bowel habits leading to constipation (e.g., irritable bowel syndrome).

Diarrhea may be caused primarily by inhibition of ion absorption, stimulation of ion secretion, retention of fluid in the intestinal lumen, and disorders of intestinal motility. Retention of fluid in the bowel lumen may be precipitated by carbohydrate malabsorption, disaccharidase deficiency,

Table 26.1.
Medical Problems Associated with Constipation

Endocrine/Metabolic Disorders
  Amyloidosis
  Diabetes mellitus
  Hyperparathyroidism
  Hypothyroidism
  Hypokalemia
  Hypercalcemia
  Porphyria
  Pseudohypoparathyroidism
  Uremia
Gastrointestinal Disorders
  Anorectal disorders (anal fissures, hemorrhoids)
  Carcinoma of colon or rectum
  Colonic pseudo-obstruction
  Cystocele, rectocele
  Diverticular disease
  Hirschsprung's disease
  Hypomotility disorders
  Inflammatory bowel disease
  Irritable bowel syndrome
  Ischemic bowel disease
  Rectal prolapse
Neurologic Disorders
  Autonomic neuropathy
  Cerebrovascular accidents
  Cauda equina tumor
  Chagas's disease
  Multiple sclerosis
  Parkinson's disease
Psychiatric Disorders
  Anxiety
  Depression
  Psychosis

Adapted with permission from: Devroede G. In Sleisenger MH and Fortran JS: Gastrointestinal Disease, 5th ed. Philadelphia, W.B. Saunders, 1993, pp. 837–87.

Table 26.2.
Drug-Induced Constipation

Antacids (e.g., calcium- and aluminum-containing)
Anticholinergics
Barium sulfate
Bismuth
Calcium channel blockers (e.g., verapamil, diltiazem)
Central alpha-adrenergic agonists (e.g., clonidine, guanabenz, guanfacine)
Diuretics
Ganglionic blocking agents
Iron
Laxative (overuse)
MAO inhibitors
Opiates
Phenothiazines
Resins (e.g., cholestyramine, colestipol, polystyrene sulfonate)
Sucralfate
Tricyclic antidepressants
Vincristine

Adapted with permission from: Tedesco FJ and DiPiro JT. Laxative use in constipation. Am J Gastroenterol 80(4):303–309, 1985.

lactulose therapy, presence of poorly absorbable salts (magnesium sulfate, sodium phosphate, sodium citrate, antacids), and ingestion of mannitol and sorbitol. Secretagogues from tumors such as vasoactive intestinal polypeptide (VIP), serotonin, and calcitonin may be mediators of secretory diarrhea. Certain laxatives such as docusates, phenolphthalein, and senna may serve as mediators also. Disorders of motility may lead to symptoms of diarrhea in the irritable bowel syndrome, diabetic neuropathy, or thyrotoxicosis. Bacterial and viral infections cause diarrhea commonly (e.g., travelers' diarrhea). Food intolerance associated with disaccharidase (lactase) deficiency may also result in diarrhea.

PATHOPHYSIOLOGY

Constipation

An intact nervous system is vital for normal defecation. Many patients develop constipation secondary to colonic motility disorders caused by congenital or acquired abnormalities of the nervous system. Outlet obstruction, a mechanism of constipation, may be secondary to a hyperactive rectosigmoid junction, increased storage capacity of the rectum, rectal spasticity, and hypertonicity of the anal canal (9).

Diarrhea

Four physiologic mechanisms may contribute to the development of diarrhea: (1) increased osmolality, (2) intestinal ion secretion, (3) impaired absorption, and (4) inflammatory and ulcerative processes. An understanding of these mechanisms of fluid loss aid in comprehending the mechanism of action of antidiarrheals.

INCREASED OSMOLALITY (OSMOTIC DIARRHEA)

Osmotic diarrhea is generally caused by the retention of fluid by nonabsorbable solutes in the bowel lumen. Peristalsis is stimulated by the increased fluid volume in the lumen, resulting in increased transit of the fecal matter by the colon. Since the colon is very efficient in the reabsorption of NaCl and water, increased transit through the colon promotes diarrhea.

Osmotic diarrhea is also evident when enzymes such as lactase are deficient. Lactase deficiency is common among certain racial groups, such as those of African and Asian descent. Lactase is responsible for the degradation of lactase to glucose and galactose, which are then absorbed by the mucosa. In the absence of this enzyme, lactose retains fluid, thereby increasing the volume of water in the stool.

INTESTINAL ION SECRETION (SECRETORY DIARRHEA)

Two factors contribute to secretory diarrhea: (1) inhibition of ion absorption and (2) intestinal ion secretion. As a result, the stool contains an excess of monovalent ions and water. Enterotoxins produced by certain bacteria stimulate intestinal fluid secretion. Laxatives such as phenolphthalein, senna, and dioctyl sodium sulfosuccinate may also cause this type of diarrhea. Certain hormones such as serotonin, calcitonin, prostaglandin E1, and vasoactive intestinal peptide have been implicated as mediators of secretory diarrhea (8).

ALTERED INTESTINAL MOTILITY

Changes in intestinal motility may affect absorption of fluids and electrolytes within the gut lumen. Increased activity may reduce the surface area and limit the contact time for nutrient absorption.

INFLAMMATORY AND ULCERATIVE PROCESSES

Inflammation and ulceration of the intestinal mucosa often result in the release of mucus, serum proteins, and blood into the lumen. The absorption of water and electrolytes is impaired. This malabsorption of fluid and electrolytes is the presumed cause of diarrhea in patients with ulcerative colitis.

CONSEQUENCES OF DIARRHEA

Although diarrhea may be uncomplicated and self-limiting, if persistent, it may cause serious consequences. Sodium and water deficits secondary to fluid loss are common in persistent diarrhea. Potassium losses of approximately 6 to 7 mEq/kg may be observed in untreated patients, which may place patients at risk of developing paralytic ileus and cardiac arrhythmias if potassium is not appropriately replaced. Fecal loss of bicarbonate and impaired renal excretion of acids may subsequently result in metabolic acidosis.

DIAGNOSIS AND CLINICAL FINDINGS

Constipation

Diagnosis of constipation requires cooperation of the patient with the clinician to provide a complete history. During the interview, the patient's definition of normal bowel function must be ascertained to determine the impact of the change in bowel habit. The onset and duration of constipation, a description of the stool, and the presence of symptoms are necessary information. Medication use should be determined, especially that of OTC laxatives. The physical examination should include an abdominal examination, a digital examination of the rectum, and a proctosigmoidoscopy. A barium enema should be initiated in chronically constipated patients and patients with a recent history of constipation, to determine whether obstruction is present.

Diarrhea

A careful history and physical examination are essential for the diagnosis of diarrhea. Ascertaining from the patient the duration of diarrhea, the description of the stool (consistency, color, odor, presence or absence of melanic stool), the frequency of bowel movements, associated symptoms, and any underlying disorders is essential to obtaining a thorough history. Distinguishing between large-stool and small-stool diarrhea helps determine whether the underlying disorder originates from the small bowel or proximal colon or the left colon and rectum, respectively.

Several signs and symptoms of diarrhea suggest underlying disease states. Generally, the passage of blood may indicate inflammatory, infectious, or neoplastic disease. Inflammation or infection may be detected by pus or exudate in the stool. Infection caused by Shigella has a characteristic blood-tinged mucus without an odor. Salmonella infections and Escherichia coli infections in infants are usually characterized by green "soupy" stools. Passage of nonbloody mucus often suggests irritable bowel syndrome, particularly when it is associated with intermittent diarrhea and constipation. Fecal incontinence and nocturnal diarrhea are associated with rectal sphincter dysfunctions secondary to neurologic problems. Less specific signs of diarrhea associated with a patient's desire to loose weight may suggest laxative abuse.

TREATMENT OF CONSTIPATION

There are primary causes of constipation for which nonpharmacologic intervention may relieve symptoms. Deficient fluid and fiber intake is often a significant factor since the American diet generally lacks sufficient fiber content. The average American consumes less than half the recommended daily amount (20–35 g) of fiber. Fiber is useful in preventing constipation. Fiber increases stool bulk, based on the ability of the polysaccharides to absorb and retain water and the extent of bacterial fermentation of these polysaccharides in the gut. A dietary bulk-forming agent such as bran is appropriate in constipation because it is only partially fermented by bacteria, resulting in increased stool bulk, accelerated transit time, and promotion of normal defecation.

Recommendations for increased fiber should be made cautiously. Rapid increases in dietary roughage may cause abdominal bloating and flatulence. Adequate fluid intake is also necessary in order to prevent fecal impaction. Generally, 240 to 360 ml of fluid with each tablespoon of bran is sufficient.

Immobility, common among debilitated and elderly patients, may possibly contribute to the development of constipation. Regular exercise such as walking or jogging may improve constipation associated with a sedentary lifestyle. Pharmacologic intervention may be necessary if modification in diet, increased fluid intake, and exercise are unsuccessful. The recommendation of laxatives would be appropriate.

The classification of laxatives is controversial. They have been categorized primarily by their mechanism of action though the exact mechanisms are unclear. Most laxatives alter intestinal fluid and electrolyte transport mechanisms, thereby causing defecation. (10) The therapeutic options are many. Agents available for use are varied and include bulk-forming agents, hyperosmotic agents, stool softeners, lubricants, saline laxatives, and stimulant laxatives (Table 26.3).

Bulk-Forming Agents

Bulk-forming agents include nonabsorbable polysaccharide and cellulose derivatives. These agents swell in water, forming an emollient gel, which increases bulk in the intestines. Peristalsis is stimulated by the increased fecal mass, which decreases the transit time. It is proposed that microflora metabolize polysaccharides to osmotically active metabolites. The metabolites may alter intestinal motility and electrolyte transport.

Bulk-forming agents generally produce a laxative effect within 12 to 24 hours, but they may require 2 to 3 days to exert their full effect. They are generally safe products associated with minimal side effects. Flatulence may occur if doses are increased rapidly. Intestinal and esophageal obstruction may occur when insufficient liquid is administered with the dose. Therefore, patients should be cautioned to take each dose with at least one 240 ml glass of liquid. Bulk-forming laxatives should not be recommended for patients with intestinal stenosis, ulceration, or adhesions. Rare reports of allergic reactions to karaya have been noted, characterized by urticaria, rhinitis, dermatitis, and bronchospasm (10).

Hyperosmotic Agents

Glycerin and lactulose are hyperosmotic laxatives. They increase osmotic pressure within the intestinal lumen, which results in luminal retention of water, softening the stool. Lactulose is an unabsorbed disaccharide metabolized by colonic bacteria primarily to lactic acid and formic and acetic acids. It has been proposed that these organic acids may contribute to the osmotic effect.

Glycerin is available only for rectal administration (suppository or enema) for treatment of acute constipation. Its laxative effect occurs within 15 to 30 minutes. Lactulose may require 24 to 48 hours for its effect. It should also be reserved for acute constipation since it is equally effective to other less costly medications.

Side effects of glycerin include rectal irritation and burning; hyperemia of the rectal mucosa may occur. Lactulose is associated with flatulence, abdominal cramps, and diarrhea. Caution should be exercised when administering this agent since it may also cause significant electrolyte imbalances and dehydration (11).

Table 26.3.

Laxatives for the Management of Constipation

Laxative Category	Dose Per Day Adult	Dose Per Day Pediatric	Dosage Form[a]	Onset of Action	Patient Information
Bulk-Forming					
Bran	>12 yr: up to 14 g	6–11 yr: up to 7 g 2–5 yr: up to 3.5 g	O	12–72 hr	Should be administered with 240 ml liquid/dose; additional fluid intake encouraged; recommended laxatives in pregnancy
Karaya	>12 yr: up to 14 g	—	O		
Malt soup extract	>12 yr: up to 64 g	6–11 yr: up to 32 g 2–5 yr: up to 16 g	O		
Methylcellulose and Sodium carboxymethyl-cellulose	>12 yr: up to 6 g	6–11 yr: up to 3 g	O		
Polycarbophil	>12 yr: up to 6 g	6–11 yr: up to 3 g 3-5 yr: up to 1.5 g	O		
Psyllium hydrophilic muciloid	>12 yr: up to 30 g	6–11 yr: up to 15 g	O		
Stimulants					
Bisacodyl	>12 yr: 5–15 mg >12 yr: 10 mg	>3 yr: 0.3 mg/kg 2–11 yr: 5–10 mg <2 yr: 5 mg	O RS	6–12 hr 15 min–2 hr	May cause a pink or red discoloration of the urine. May cause skin rash; discontinue medication and contact pharmacist or physician. Tablets should not be chewed
Casanthranol	>12 yr: 30–90 mg	2–12 yr: 15–45 mg <2 yr: 7.5–22.5 mg	O		
Dehydrocholic acid	>12 yr: 750–1500 mg		O		
Phenolphthalein	>12 yr: 30–270 mg	6–11 yr: 30–60 mg 2–5 yr: 15–30 mg	O		
Sennosides	>12 yr: 12–75 mg	6–11 yr: 6–33 mg 2–6 yr: 3–12.5 mg	O		
	>12 yr: 30–60 mg		RS		
Saline Agents					
Magnesium citrate	>12 yr: 11–25 g	6–11 yr: 5.5–12.5 g 2–5 yr: 2.7–6.25 g	O	30 min–6 hr	
Magnesium hydroxide	>12 yr: 2.4–4.8 g	6–11 yr: 1.2–2.4 g 2–5 yr: 0.4–1.2 g	O		
Magnesium sulfate	>12 yr: 10–30 g	6–11 yr: 5–10 g 2–5 yr: 2.5–5 g	O		
Sodium phosphate, monobasic	>12 yr: 9.1–20.2 g >12 yr: 18.24–20.16 g	10–11 yr: 4.5–10.1 g 5–9 yr: 2.2–5.05 g 2–11 yr: 9.12–10.08 g	O RE	 2–15 min	
Sodium phosphate, dibasic	>12 yr: 3.42–7.5 g >12 yr: 6.84–7.56 g	10–11 yr: 1.71–3.78 g 5–9 yr: 0.86–1.89 g 2–11 yr: 3.42–3.78 g	O RE	 2–15 min	
Hyperosmotic Agents					
Glycerin	>12 yr: 3 g	 >6 yr: 2–3 g 5–15 ml <6 yr: 1–1.7 g 2–5 ml	RS RS RE RS RE	15–30 min	May cause rectal burning or irritation

(continued)

Table 26.3. (*Continued*)

| Laxative Category | Dose Per Day | | Dosage Form[a] | Onset of Action | Patient Information |
	Adult	Pediatric			
Lactulose	>12 yr: 10–20 g, then up to 40 g	<12 yr: 5 g[b]	O, RE		May be mixed in fruit juice to increase palatability. May cause belching, flatulence or abdominal cramps. Pediatric dose should be given after breakfast
Lubricants Mineral oil	>12 yr: 15–45 ml >12 yr: 120 ml	6–11 yr: 5–15 ml 6–11 yr: 30–60 ml	O R	6–8 hr	Should not be administered to children <6 yr, pregnant women, or debilitated persons. Bedtime doses should be avoided. May cause pruritis ani especially when administered rectally
Surfactants Dioctyl sulfosuccinate (calcium, potasium, sodium)	(no official recommendation)		O, RE		Oral solutions may be diluted with 120 ml milk, fruit juice, or infant formula; solutions may cause throat irritation

[a]O = oral, RE = rectal enema; RS = rectal suppository.
[b]Use is not currently included in the FDA-approved labeling.

Stool Softeners

Stool softeners are also referred to as emollient laxatives. They include calcium, potassium, and sodium salts of dioctyl sulfosuccinate. Stool softeners are anionic surfactants that lower the fecal surface tension in vitro allowing water and lipid penetration. It has been proposed that, in vivo, these agents stimulate water and electrolyte secretion into the colon.

Softening of the feces generally occurs after 1 to 3 days. Some products (e.g., docusate sodium with casanthrol) combine a stool softener with a stimulant. Adverse effects are rare with docusates. Mild gastrointestinal cramping may occasionally develop. Throat irritation has occurred following the use of the docusate sodium solution. Docusate has been associated with hepatotoxicity when used in combination with oxyphenisatin or dantrol (12).

Lubricants

The primary lubricant laxative is mineral oil. Its mechanism of action involves lubrication of the feces and hinderance of water reabsorption in the colon. Mineral oil is indigestible, and its absorption is limited considerably in the nonemulsified formulation. Greater absorption from the emulsion formulation has been reported, but the clinical significance is unsubstantiated.

The onset of action of mineral oil when taken orally is 6 to 8 hours. Although adverse effects occur rarely with mineral oil, potentially significant effects may occur.

Chronic use of mineral oil has been reported to cause impaired absorption of fat soluble vitamins (A, D, E, and K). Aspiration of the product may cause a lipoid pneumonia; therefore, its oral use should be avoided in young children (younger than 6 years), the elderly, and debilitated patients. Administration at bedtime should be avoided to prevent aspiration. Foreign-body reactions in the lymphoid tissue of the intestinal tract have resulted from its limited amount of absorption. Seepage of the product from the rectum following high-dose oral or rectal administration may cause pruritus ani, increased infection, and decreased healing of anorectal lesions.

Saline Laxatives

Magnesium, sulfate, phosphate, and citrate salts are employed when rapid bowel evacuation is required. The mechanism of action of these poorly absorbed ions is unclear, but it is believed that they produce an osmotic effect that increases intraluminal volume and stimulates peristalsis. Magnesium may cause cholecystokinin release from the duodenal mucosa promoting increased fluid secretion and motility of the small intestine and colon (13).

The laxative effect of the orally administered magnesium and sodium phosphate salts occurs within 0.5 to 6 hours. Phosphate-containing rectal enemas evacuate the bowel within 2 to 15 minutes.

Saline laxatives are safe when administered for short-term management. They are useful in preparation for endoscopic examinations, elimination of parasites and toxic antihelmintics before and/or after therapy, removal of poisons, and fecal impaction. They may cause significant fluid and electrolyte imbalances when used for prolonged periods or in certain patients. Dehydration may occur from repeated administration without appropriate fluid replacement. The risk of hypermagnesemia in patients with renal dysfunction should be considered when initiating magnesium salts because 10 to 20% of the dose may be absorbed systemically. Caution should be exercised when administering the sodium phosphate salts to patients with congestive heart failure when sodium restriction is necessary. These agents are not recommended for children under 2 years of age because of the potential for hypocalcemia in this population.

Stimulant Laxatives

Anthraquinone (casanthrol, cascara sagrada, danthron, sennosides, and aloe) and diphenylmethane (bisacodyl, phenolphthalein) derivatives, castor oil, and dehydrocholic acid are stimulant laxatives. They are termed "stimulants" because they stimulate peristalsis via mucosal irritation or intramural nerve plexus activity, which results in increased motility. Although these effects have long been regarded as mechanisms of action for these agents, their activity may actually be related to their effect on the colonic mucosal cells. It is proposed that stimulant laxatives modify the permeability of these cells, which results in intraluminal fluid and electrolyte secretion.

Defecation occurs between 6 and 12 hours after oral administration of these agents. Therefore, a single bedtime dose promotes a morning bowel movement. The laxative effects of phenolphthalein may persist for several days because up to 15% of the oral dose is absorbed and undergoes enterohepatic recirculation. Unlike the other stimulant laxatives, dehydrocholic acid is administered at least three times daily. Rectal administration of bisacodyl and senna produces catharsis within 15 minutes to 2 hours.

Adverse effects of these medications include abdominal cramps, nausea, electrolyte disturbances (e.g., hypokalemia, hypocalcemia, metabolic acidosis, or alkalosis), and rectal burning and irritation with suppository use. Anthraquinone derivatives have been noted to cause melanosis coli (discoloring of colonic mucosa), which is harmless and reversible. Hypersensitivity reactions may occur (rarely) with phenolphthalein and dehydrocholic acid causing dermatological manifestations (e.g., skin eruptions, rashes, pigmentation, pruritus). These agents may also cause a pink or red discoloration of the urine.

Chronic use of stimulant laxatives should be discouraged, and use beyond 1 week should be avoided. These agents may produce a "cathartic colon" if used for several years (15 to 40). The colon develops abnormal motor function, and roentgenography resembles ulcerative colitis.

Usually, discontinuation of laxative use restores normal bowel function.

Danthron-containing laxatives were removed from the market in 1987 because of their potential for causing intestinal and hepatic tumors in humans. Chronic administration of danthron at high doses produced tumors in rats (14). Although insignificant amounts distribute into the milk of nursing mothers, stimulant laxatives should be avoided during lactation.

Other Agents

Recent data have suggested a potential role for other agents in the management of constipation. Cisapride and naloxone have been used in the treatment of chronic idiopathic constipation.

PROPULSID Cisapride is a piperidinyl benzamide that is chemically related to metoclopramide. It is a prokinetic agent that enhances gastrointestinal motility throughout the entire length of the gastrointestinal tract. The mechanisms by which cisapride facilitates gastrointestinal motility have not been clearly elucidated. However, a proposed mechanism involves its enhancement of acetylcholine release in the myenteric plexus of the gut (15). Cisapride is devoid of antidopaminergic effects.

Cisapride in oral doses of 5 to 20 mg is absorbed rapidly and almost completely from the gastrointestinal tract. The oral bioavailability is approximately 40 to 50% and is enhanced by food. Its tissue distribution in man is not known; however, it is metabolized extensively to metabolites with minimal pharmacologic activity. Its elimination half-life after oral administration is approximately 7 to 10 hours. Some evidence suggests that the half-life of cisapride may increase in elderly patients and those with hepatic impairment (15).

Cisapride was investigated at a dose of 20 mg twice daily in patients with chronic idiopathic constipation or chronic laxative use. Cisapride increased stool frequency by 50%, and reduced mean laxative intake by half (16). In another study, cisapride was used in the treatment of constipation at doses of 5 mg and 10 mg three times a day for 12 weeks. Stool frequency was increased by approximately 70% with both doses compared to 43% with placebo (17).

The side-effect profile of cisapride is moderate based on current experience. Common side effects include abdominal cramping, borborygmi (intestinal rumbling), and diarrhea. Central nervous system side effects, such as somnolence and fatigue, have been reported less frequently.

Concomitant administration of cisapride with specific agents has caused drug interactions. Cimetidine coadministration may cause a 45% increase in the bioavailability of cisapride (15). Cisapride may enhance the absorption of acenocoumarol; therefore, monitoring coagulation times is advisable with concomitant anticoagulant therapy (15).

Because cisapride may accelerate gastric emptying, monitoring should occur when administering agents concomitantly with narrow therapeutic windows (e.g., digoxin and phenytoin).

It has been postulated that endogenous opiates regulate colonic propulsive activity (18). Consequently, the role of opiate receptor antagonists in the treatment of constipation has been investigated. Naloxone (an opiate receptor antagonist) has reversed chronic idiopathic constipation at intravenous and oral doses of 20 to 30 mg per day (19). In addition, naloxone causes acceleration of colonic transit although it has not been shown to affect the number of bowel movements in 48 hours (20). Further studies are necessary to define the role of this agent in the management of chronic constipation.

PATIENT MEDICATION COUNSELING

Providing patient medication counseling for constipation requires determining the patient's perception of normal bowel habits. Only then can the clinician decide whether nonpharmacologic or pharmacologic treatment is appropriate. A discussion of bowel habits should emphasize that though constipation is often self-limiting, it may be a symptom of a more serious disease. Consequently, counseling should include questions about the onset and duration of constipation, as well as a history of medical illnesses. The patient's medication profile should be reviewed for possible drug-induced constipation and for a history of the patient's laxative use. Diet and lifestyle activities are ascertained because lack of exercise (e.g., walking and jogging) and fiber intake are associated with development of constipation. Finally, educating patients (especially children) to respond to the urge to defecate in order to prevent constipation is essential.

If a recommendation for a laxative is appropriate, the clinician should consider the following guidelines:

1. Laxative use should not exceed 1 week of self-medication.
2. Laxatives are inappropriate in the presence of abdominal pain or cramping, nausea, vomiting, or bloating.
3. Daily administration of bulk-forming agents should be the first choice in uncomplicated chronic constipation.
4. Clinicians may recommend one of the following for 1 week or less: a low-dose saline laxative, stimulant laxative at bedtime, or glycerin suppository.
5. Institutionalized or bedridden patients may require laxatives in addition to daily bulk-forming agents to prevent fecal impaction [e.g., weekly intermittent doses of stimulant laxatives, lactulose (30 ml/day), and milk of magnesia].
6. Mineral oil should be avoided in elderly and young children (younger than 6 years) or debilitated patients because of the risk of aspiration.
7. Patients with histories of myocardial infarction, anal fissures, hernias, and colorectal surgery are candidates for prophylactic laxative therapy to prevent straining. Acceptable agents include docusate, milk of magnesia, glycerin suppository, or bulk-forming products.
8. Pregnant patients should use only bulk-forming agents and stool softeners if a laxative is required.

TREATMENT OF DIARRHEA

For most persons, diarrhea is a transient self-limiting complaint of short duration. This form of diarrhea is often referred to as acute, nonspecific diarrhea that is not caused by underlying diseases or etiologic agents. However, the symptoms may often interfere with lifestyle activities and contribute to loss of productivity. The management of acute, nonspecific diarrhea consists of adequate oral

Table 26.4.
FDA-Recommended OTC Antidiarrheals

Medication	Dose	Maximum Dose per Day
Attapulgite	>12 yr: 1.2 g at onset, then repeat after each loose stool	8.4 g
	6–11 yr: 0.6 g at onset, then repeat after each loose stool	4.2 g
	3–5 yr: 0.3 g at onset, then repeat after each loose stool	2.1 g
Kaolin	>12 yr: 26.2 g after each stool	262.0 g
	<12 yr: consult physician	
Polycarbophil and calcium polycarbophil	>12 yr: 1.2 g TID to QID	4–6 g
	6–11 yr: 0.5–1 g TID	3 g
	3–5 yr: 0.33–0.5 g TID	1.5 g
Loperamide[a]	>12 yr: 4 mg at onset, then 2 mg after each loose stool	8 mg[b]; 16 mg
	9–11 yr: 2 mg at onset, then 1 mg after each loose stool	6 mg
	6–8 yr: 1 mg at onset, then 1 mg after each loose stool	4 mg
	<6 yr[c]: 1 mg at onset, then 1 mg after each loose stool	3 mg

[a]Therapy should not exceed 2 days.
[b]Travelers' diarrhea.
[c]Receive only under medical supervision.
Source: Minutes of the Nonprescription Drugs Advisory Committee and the Gastrointestinal Drugs Advisory Committee Meeting of the FDA, April 9, 1993. Facts and Comparisons, 1993.

Table 26.5.
Commercially Available Oral Rehydration Solutions (ORS)

Product	CHO (g/l)	Na+ (mEq/L)	K+ (mEq/L)	Cl– (mEq/L)	Base (mEq/L)	Calories Kcal
Infalyte[a] (Mead-Johnson)	30 (rice syrup solids)	50	25	45	34 (citrate)	126
Pedialyte[b] (Ross Laboratories)	25 (dextrose)	45	20	35	30 (citrate)	100
Rehydralyte (Ross Laboratories)	25 (dextrose)	75[c]	20	65	30 (citrate)	100
WHO Solution[d] (Jianas Bros. Packaging Co.)	20 (glucose)	90[c]	20	80	10 (citrate)	80

[a]Available in hospitals as 6-ounce nursing bottle.
[b]Available in hospitals as 8-ounce nursing bottle.
[c]The American Academy of Pediatrics recommends these solutions with sodium contents of 75–90 mEq/L for replacement of deficit during initial rehydration (Pediatrics 75:358, 1985).
[d]Must be mixed with 1 liter of boiled or treated water; packets available in stores or pharmacies in all developing countries.
Source: Manufacturer's product information.

rehydration and relief of symptoms. Several nonprescription agents available are effective in managing the associated symptoms (Table 26.4).

Rehydration

Fluid losses in acute, nonspecific diarrhea in adults are generally not severe and require only simple replacement of fluid and electrolytes lost in the stool. Patients should be advised to ingest 2 to 3 liters of clear liquids (e.g., "flat" ginger ale, decaffeinated cola, tea, broth, or gelatin) within the first 24 hours. Diet in the next 24 hours should consist of bland foods, including rice, soup, bread, salted crackers, cooked cereals, baked potatoes, eggs, and applesauce (21). A regular diet may be resumed after 2 to 3 days.

Untreated diarrhea in the pediatric population is a major cause of morbidity and mortality, especially in developing countries. Infants and young children are more susceptible to the acute losses of fluid caused by diarrhea because the intestinal surface area of infants and children is greater, that is, in relation to their body size. Consequently, oral rehydration solutions (ORS) are recommended for acute diarrhea. Infants and children with a 5 to 7.5% weight loss should receive ORS solution at doses of 40 to 50 ml/kg administered in the first 4 to 6 hours. Oral maintenance can be administered at a rate of 150 ml/kg/day once rehydration is achieved (22). The World Health Organization (WHO) provides the standard oral rehydration solution (Table 26.5). It is prepared by mixing one packet with the appropriate volume of boiled or treated water. The solution should be discarded within 12 hours if kept at room temperature and within 24 hours if refrigerated. Other oral rehydration solutions are available commercially as ready-to-use preparations (Table 26.5).

Pharmacologic Agents

Various medications, both prescription and OTC, are available for the symptomatic relief of diarrhea. Recently, the FDA has reevaluated the safety and efficacy of OTC products for diarrhea. The Advisory Review Panel on OTC Laxative, Antidiarrheal, Emetic, and Antiemetic Drug Products reviewed several products in 1975 for their safety and efficacy. The FDA evaluated the recommendations of the panel and published tentative rulings on the products in 1986 (24). Currently, the only OTC products considered safe and effective treatments of diarrhea are attapulgite, kaolin (without pectin), polycarbophil, and loperamide.

Attapulgite is a naturally occurring hydrous magnesium aluminum silicate that adsorbs approximately eight times its weight in water because of its large surface area. This adsorbent property reduces the liquidity of the stool. Side effects are minimal with attapulgite since it is not absorbed systemically. It is administered at the onset of symptoms, followed by smaller doses after each loose stool (Table 26.4).

Kaolin is also a naturally occurring hydrated aluminum silicate with adsorbent properties. It is effective in the treatment of acute nonspecific diarrhea based on its ability to improve stool consistency within 24 to 48 hours. Kaolin is no longer approved for OTC use in combination with pectin for the treatment of diarrhea. Studies have not demonstrated that the "fixed" combination (kaolin and pectin) is more effective than kaolin alone. Like attapulgite, side effects with kaolin are minimal. Recommended dosages for adults and children over 12 years of age are indicated (Table 26.4).

Polycarbophil has been used in the management of diarrhea and constipation. It is a hydrophilic polyacrylic

Table 26.6.
Antiinfective Treatment for Common Causes of Infectious Diarrhea

Organism	Therapy of Choice	Alternative	Duration	Considerations
Salmonella				
Uncomplicated	None	None		
Hyperpyrexia and systemic toxicity	Ampicillin 150 mg/kg/day	TMP/SMX[a] Chloramphenicol Cefotaxime	14 days	
Carrier state	Amoxicillin 6 g/day	Ampicillin	4–6 weeks	Chloramphenicol acceptable but not preferred because of risk of resistance[b]
Shigella	TMP/SMX 160/800 mg BID	Ampicillin Ciprofloxacin	3–5 days	
E. coli (ETEC)	TMP/SMX 160/800 mg BID	Ampicillin Ciprofloxacin[e]	5 days	
Campylobacter jejuni	Erythromycin 500 mg QID	Ciprofloxacin	7 days	Treatment necessary in debilitated or patients with septicemia
Yersinia enterocolitica	Gentamicin 5 mg/kg/day or Chloramphenicol 50 mg/kg/day	Doxycycline	7 days	Most cases remit spontaneously
Vibrio cholera	Tetracycline 500 mg QID	Doxycycline	2–5 days	Ampicillin preferred in pregnant women
Clostridium difficile	Vancomycin 125–500 mg po QID	Metronidazole[f]	10 days	Relapse may occur requiring repeat course of therapy
Giardia lamblia	Quinacrine 100 mg TID	Metronidazole Furazolidone[c]	7 days	Furozolidone available in liquid form and may be administered to children
Entamoeba histolytica	Metronidazole 750 mg TID[d]	Tetracycline and Chloroquine	5–10 days	Should treat in conjunction with diloxanide furoate or iodoquinol when using metronidazole

[a]Trimethoprim/sulfamethoxazole.
[b]In patients with hyperpyrexia and systemic toxicity.
[c]Indicated for cases resistant to tetracycline.
[d]Acute intestinal disease.
[e]Use if resistance is widespread.
[f]Generally recommended as initial therapy.
Source: Mandell GL, Douglas RG, Bennett JE. Principles and Practice of Infectious Diseases. New York: Churchill Livingstone, 1990, 3rd edition, ch 192, 194, 199, 200, 207, 249, 275.
Suarez J, Salamone FR. Management and prevention of bacterial diarrhea. Clin Pharm 7:746–759, 1988.

resin that, like attapulgite, possesses adsorbent properties. It is not absorbed systemically, making it devoid of systemic side effects. Epigastric pain and bloating are common sequelae. Administering smaller doses spaced more evenly throughout the day may provide relief from bloating. Controlled fluid intake is recommended for patients in the treatment of diarrhea (see "Rehydration").

Loperamide is a synthetic congener of meperidine, which decreases gastrointestinal motility through its effect on the circular and longitudinal muscles of the intestines. CNS penetration of the drug is low. It does not elicit the CNS side effects associated with opiate use and lacks potential for abuse.

Loperamide relieves symptoms of acute nonspecific diarrhea, and it is effective in the treatment of nondysenteric travelers' diarrhea (25–27). It has been compared with attapulgite in acute diarrhea (26). In this study, the dose of loperamide was 4 mg initially, then 2 mg after each unformed stool, not exceeding 8 mg in 24 hours. Attapulgite was administered initially as 3 g, followed by up to 6 g after each unformed stool to a maximum dose of 9 g in 24 hours. The mean number of unformed stools was significantly lower in the loperamide group in the first and second 12-hour intervals. However, no significant difference was observed in duration of relief from diarrhea following the initial dose.

Although generally well tolerated, loperamide may cause abdominal pain, constipation, drowsiness, fatigue, dry mouth, or nausea and vomiting. Doses for adults should not exceed 8 mg per day for OTC use; however, maximum daily doses of 16 mg are permitted under medical supervision. Children under 6 years of age should not receive loperamide unless medically supervised. The medication should be discontinued after 48 hours if clinical improvement is not evident.

Opiates (opium powder, tincture, and paregoric) have been used extensively in the treatment of acute, nonspecific diarrhea. Opiates contain morphine, which promotes increased smooth muscle tone of the gastrointestinal tract, inhibits gastrointestinal motility and propulsion, and reduces digestive secretions. Paregoric is commonly used at dosages of 5 to 10 ml one to four times daily for adults and 0.25 to 0.5 ml/kg one to four times daily for children (28). Opium tincture contains 25% more morphine than paregoric; therefore, the dose is 0.3 to 1 ml four times a day with a maximum daily dose of 6 ml. Although these agents are currently considered safe and effective antidiarrheals, they are not recommended in nonprescription combination products (29).

Other derivatives of morphine such as codeine and the meperidine congener, diphenoxylate, may be used for diarrhea. At doses of 15 to 30 mg orally every 6 hours, codeine reduces the frequency of loose stools. However, its use has been limited in favor of the various nonnarcotic alternatives for diarrhea currently available. Diphenoxylate, with activity similar to that of morphine on intestinal smooth muscle, is used in combination with atropine sulfate at doses of 2.5 to 5 mg orally four times a day. Unlike loperamide, diphenoxylate has potential for producing euphoria and suppressing opiate withdrawal symptoms at high doses. Consequently, abuse potential exists with diphenoxylate alone. Atropine sulfate has been added to discourage abuse.

The role of antiperistaltic agents in infectious diarrhea has been questioned. The body normally defends itself from invading bacteria by eliminating these organisms during diarrhea. Antiperistaltic agents such as diphenoxylate and loperamide inhibit this process by increasing gastrointestinal transit time. Therefore, these agents are not recommended for the treatment of diarrhea induced by invasive organisms such as enterotoxigenic E. coli (ETEC), Salmonella, or Shigella (30,31). They should also be avoided in patients with fecal leukocytes, fever, or blood in the stools. The risk of toxic megacolon exists when administering these agents in patients with pseudomembranous colitis or ulcerative colitis (31).

Although infectious diarrhea may be treated with antimicrobial therapy, the use of these agents is controversial. Generally, acute diarrhea is self-limiting and may require only symptomatic relief and fluid replacement. Antimicrobial therapy is indicated in severe cases persisting for more than 48 hours; passing six or more loose stools in 24 hours; and/or associated with fever, blood, or pus in the stools (32). Table 26.6 describes the common organisms and their therapy (33).

TRAVELERS' DIARRHEA

Every year 10% of the American population travels to international countries, and more than 8 million of them travel to developing countries (34). Often their excursion is interrupted by a syndrome known as travelers' diarrhea (TD). TD is defined as an infectious disease of the gastrointestinal tract in persons traveling outside their country, which results in a twofold or greater increase in the frequency of unformed bowel movements with associated symptoms. The risk of TD depends on the destination of the traveler. Approximately 20 to 50% of travelers reportedly develop TD (23). The disease primarily affects individuals traveling from industrialized nations to developing countries. Persons traveling from the United States, Canada, or northern Europe would be at risk of developing TD when traveling to Latin America, Africa, the Middle East, or Asia.

The abrupt onset of diarrhea is generally self-limiting, with a median duration of 3 to 4 days. Although persistent diarrhea is uncommon in TD, 10% of the cases may continue for more than 1 week. Travelers should be aware that TD may occur more than once during a trip, so appropriate precautions should be taken throughout the travel period. TD develops from food or water that is contaminated with fecal material containing bacteria, viruses, parasites, or combinations of microbes. The most common offending organism is enterotoxigenic E. coli, which accounts for more than 40 to 50% of the cases. Salmonella and Shigella spp. as well as Campylobacter jejuni also cause TD. Other potential bacterial pathogens include Aeromonas hydrophila, Yersinia enterolytica, Plesiomonas shigelloides, Vibrio parahaemolyticis, and other Vibrio spp. Viruses such as rotavirus and Norwalk virus often contaminate water, but they are not frequent causes of TD in adults. Parasitic enteric pathogens, including Giardia lamblia, Entamoeba histolytica, and Cryptosporidium, cause fewer cases of TD.

Prevention

Instructions to travelers about safe food and water precautions are the mainstay of TD prevention. Travelers should be advised to avoid drinking or brushing their teeth with tap water. Ice cubes should be avoided because they may have been made with contaminated water. Boiled water (as in hot tea or coffee), carbonated beverages, or beer and wine are generally safe to consume. Two reliable methods of purification are vigorous boiling of water and chemical disinfection with tincture of iodine. However, disinfection with iodine often leaves an unpleasant taste. Foods that should be avoided include undercooked or raw foods, salads, and unpasteurized milk and milk products. Foods generally safe for consumption include bread or crackers, peeled fruit or vegetables, and well-cooked foods (23).

Although there is a consensus in the health community about food and water precautions to prevent TD, chemoprophylaxis for the prevention of TD is controversial. Several studies have provided data that demonstrate efficacy for both antimicrobial and nonantimicrobial agents in decreasing the incidence of diarrhea. The nonantimicrobial agent bismuth subsalicylate has been shown to prevent diarrhea in up to 65% of subjects receiving two tablets (524 mg) four times daily for 21 days beginning on the first day of travel. Lower protection rates (40%) were observed in subjects receiving one tablet (262 mg) four times daily (35). In a previous trial, studying the liquid preparation, 60 ml four times daily for 3 weeks resulted in a 62% reduction in illness (36). Bismuth subsalicylate has side effects, including darkening of the tongue and stool and mild tinnitus. Patients taking aspirin concurrently for arthritis may be at increased risk for developing tinnitus secondary to the salicylate component in bismuth subsalicylate. There is concern about patients with renal insufficiency or allergies to aspirin who may consume large quantities of subsalicylate unsupervised. Patients with the acquired immunodeficiency syndrome (AIDS) may be at greater risk of developing encephalopathy from consuming excessive doses of bismuth subsalicylate (37). Concurrent use of anticoagulants is contraindicated with this agent. Bismuth subsalicylate appears to be effective for TD prophylaxis and is recommended by the CDC for use not longer than 3 weeks.

Several antibiotics have been investigated for the chemoprophylaxis of TD. One of the earliest agents studied was doxycycline. Doses of 100 mg per day for 21 days were effective in areas where enterotoxigenic E. coli were sensitive to the drug (38, 39). However, the protection rate decreased in geographic areas with resistant strains (38). In addition, side effects, including photosensitivity and diarrhea, and contraindications in pregnancy and lactation and in children (younger than 8 years of age), increase its risk–benefit ratio for prophylactic use.

Trimethoprim/sulfamethoxazole (TMP/SMX) at doses of 160 mg/800 mg twice daily for 21 days and daily for 14 days has demonstrated efficacy in preventing TD (40, 41). Trimethoprim alone at doses of 200 mg daily for 14 days is effective for prevention of diarrhea (41). Although significant compared with placebo, the protection rate of TMP alone was less than that of the combination (95 vs. 52%). Side effects noted in the studies were primarily dermatologic, including rashes and skin eruptions. Since TMP/SMX can potentially cause serious skin eruptions such as Stevens–Johnson syndrome, the risk of taking these agents for TD prophylaxis is of concern.

Quinolone carboxylic acid derivatives are useful for chemoprophylaxis of TD (Table 26.7). Norfloxacin and ciprofloxacin have been widely studied. Norfloxacin 400 mg orally once daily for 14 days is effective (42). Fewer patients developed diarrhea on norfloxacin than placebo (7 vs. 61%). Norfloxacin provided an 88% protection rate from the development of TD. Resistance was not evident among aerobic gram-negative bacilli. Adverse reactions were limited to one case of a generalized rash 11 days after therapy with norfloxacin, which resolved on discontinuation. In another study, ciprofloxacin 500 mg daily was compared to placebo in persons traveling to Tunisia (43). Ciprofloxacin provided a 94% protection rate and was well tolerated. One case of serious sunburn was observed that was possibly drug related. Ciprofloxacin did not appear to affect aerobic bacterial flora 5 weeks after travel.

Clinicians should counsel travelers who decide to take prophylactic medications to begin chemoprophylaxis on the first day of arrival in the country, and to continue therapy for 1 to 2 days after leaving. Regardless of the length of the trip, travelers should not take these medications beyond 3 weeks (32).

Although prophylactic management of TD with antimicrobial agents has demonstrated significant benefits, the uncertainty of the risk of widespread use must be evaluated. These agents have the potential for side effects

Table 26.7.
Oral Prophylactic Drugs Used to Prevent Travelers' Diarrhea in Adults

Drug	Dose	Geographic Considerations
Bismuth subsalicylate	2–262 mg tablets chewed well QID (with meals and at bedtime)	Not as effective as antimicrobial drugs, but probably effective in all high-risk areas, fewest side effects
Fluoroquinolone antibiotics		
Norfloxacin	400 mg QD	The most predictably effective agents when susceptibilities are not known
Ciprofloxacin	500 mg QD	
Ofloxacin	300 mg QD	
Fleroxacin	400 mg QD	
Trimethoprim-sulfamethoxazole	160 mg TMP/800 mg SMX QD	Resistance common in tropical areas; effective in inland Mexico during the summer
Doxycycline	100 mg QD	Resistance found in many areas of the world, limiting value

Adapted with permission from: DuPont HL, Ericsson CD. Prevention and treatment of travelers' diarrhea. NEJM 328(25):1821–1827, 1993.

such as skin rashes, photosensitivity reactions, blood disorders, Stevens–Johnson syndrome, and staining of the teeth in children. Therefore, prophylactic antimicrobial agents are not recommended for widespread use by travelers.

Treatment

Approaches to the treatment of travelers' diarrhea include many of the remedies for treating acute nonspecific diarrhea: fluid replacement and symptomatic relief with adsorbents, antimotility agents, and short-term antimicrobial therapy. The self-limiting nature of travelers' diarrhea generally allows for successful management with nonspecific agents. However, antimicrobial agents may be useful in persistent diarrhea.

Bismuth subsalicylate is effective for the relief of symptoms of mild to moderate TD. Doses of 30 ml every 30 minutes for eight doses are generally effective in relief of abdominal pain and cramping and reduction of unformed stools (44, 45). Bismuth subsalicylate has not been shown to improve nausea and vomiting associated with TD.

Loperamide, anantimotility agent, is approved for the symptomatic relief of TD at doses of up to 8 mg per day. Loperamide has been compared with bismuth subsalicylate for the treatment of TD. Doses of loperamide were administered at 4 mg initially then 2 mg after each unformed stool, whereas bismuth subsalicylate was administered at recommended doses. Loperamide demonstrated significantly more relief (resolution) of diarrhea and abdominal pains and cramps, and decreased severity of symptoms than did bismuth subsalicylate. There was no significant difference in the duration of diarrhea. Loperamide-treated patients with shigellosis did not experience prolongation of diarrhea (45). This is consistent with results from a study involving 43 patients with two reported cases of loperamide-treated patients with Shigella spp. without prolongation of diarrhea (46).

Although use of antimicrobial agents in the treatment of TD is controversial, they may be appropriate in patients who develop persistent diarrhea. Travelers with (1) diarrhea unresponsive to conventional therapy, (2) three or more loose stools in an 8-hour period, and (3) associated symptoms of nausea, vomiting, abdominal cramps, fever, or blood in the stools may benefit from a short course of therapy. Selection of an appropriate agent may depend on the traveler's symptoms, the location of travel, the climate, and the type of chemoprophylaxis received prior to treatment (32). The recommended duration of treatment is 3 days (23).

Trimethoprim/sulfamethoxazole (160 mg/800 mg) twice a day or trimethoprim 200 mg alone twice a day for 3 to 5 days is effective in reducing the number of unformed stools and decreasing symptoms, including abdominal cramps or pain and nausea (47). The efficacy of ciprof-loxacin 500 mg twice a day and TMP/SMX (160 mg/800 mg) twice a day each for 5 days was compared with placebo (48). Both agents were equally effective. Ciprofloxacin may offer an alternative for patients with hypersensitivities to TMP/SMX.

Other agents that have been effective include furazolidone 100 mg four times a day. It is a broad spectrum antibiotic that includes coverage for Giardia (49). However, its effectiveness is less than TMP/SMX or TMP alone. Fluoroquinolones such as norfloxacin, ofloxacin, and fleroxacin may be as effective as ciprofloxacin. In general, fluoroquinolones are the drugs of choice for adults when traveling to high-risk areas (e.g., Latin America, Africa, the Middle East, and Asia) (32). Data have suggested the use of combination therapy with antimotility agents (loperamide) and antibiotics (TMP/SMX) initially in patients with moderate to severe diarrhea (50). However, further study on the efficacy and safety is warranted.

Future developments in the prophylaxis and treatment of TD may include the use of poorly absorbed antimicrobial agents such as bicozamycin and oral aztreonam (51, 52). These agents should be safe in pregnant women and children. However, more data about their safety and efficacy are needed.

IRRITABLE BOWEL SYNDROME

One of the most frequently encountered disorders of the gastrointestinal tract among young to middle-aged adults is known as the irritable bowel syndrome (IBS). Although this syndrome composes up to 70% of gastrointestinal consultations, little is known about the pathogenesis of IBS (53). It is believed that IBS results from disordered intestinal motility with stress contributing to its recurrence and exacerbation.

The clinical manifestations of IBS may vary. Common symptoms in the absence of organic disease include abdominal pain (frequently associated with distension), flatus, and alternating constipation and diarrhea. Generally, the abdominal pain is relieved by defecation and exacerbated by food. IBS is usually not associated with blood in the stools or weight loss.

Treatment

Treatment of IBS incorporates dietary interventions, bowel habit changes, and pharmacologic management based on the patient's symptoms. If a patient has symptoms of constipation, then increased fluid intake, high-fiber diet, and exercise should be encouraged before the use of laxatives. If constipation persists, psyllium preparations are appropriate. Patients with symptoms of diarrhea, should avoid foods that may precipitate diarrhea such as dairy products, coffee, alcoholic beverages, sorbitol-containing foods, and highly seasoned foods. If symptoms of bloating and gas persist, avoiding gas-producing foods (e.g., beans, cabbage, certain fruits) may be helpful. Bulk-forming agents may be appropriate for resolving diarrhea after dietary changes.

Several pharmacologic agents have been investigated for the management of IBS. Anticholinergics such as propantheline bromide 15 mg three times daily have been used although no evidence is available to support its efficacy. Neuroleptics, antidepressants, and tranquilizers have been used in IBS patients with a history of psychiatric disorders. The benefit of these agents is questionable. Other agents used include phenytoin, calcium channel antagonists, and cisapride (for constipation-predominant IBS); however, further study on the efficacy of these agents is warranted (54–56).

Recently, data have suggested the use of an opiate agonist, loperamide, in the management of IBS-related diarrhea. Studies indicate that IBS patients taking loperamide experience improvement in diarrhea associated with decreases in stool frequency, passage of unformed stools, and incidence of urgency (57, 58). Caution must be exercised in IBS patients with constipation since loperamide may worsen the symptoms (58). An appropriate dose for loperamide in IBS has not been determined. However, doses ranging from 2 mg twice daily to 4 mg three times daily have been used for relief of symptoms. Although loperamide appears to have a significant role in the management of diarrhea in IBS, it is presently approved only by the FDA for over-the-counter use for relief of symptoms in acute diarrhea, including travelers' diarrhea.

CONCLUSION

Constipation and diarrhea are common among healthy persons. They are self-limiting but may require intervention of short duration. Changes in diet and lifestyle may eliminate the need for laxatives in constipation. If laxatives are appropriate, an agent may be selected that is tailored to individual patient needs. A variety of agents are effective, including bulk-forming, hyperosmotic, surfactant, lubricant, saline, and stimulant laxatives.

Acute diarrhea may require intervention to prevent excessive fluid loss and dehydration. Rehydration and the use of adsorbents or antiperistaltic agents are effective in most patients with acute nonspecific diarrhea. Persistent diarrhea secondary to bacterial organisms may require antiinfective agents in addition to conventional measures.

Counseling patients on the self-management of constipation and diarrhea is essential. As more products become available for OTC use, proper counseling will become increasingly important.

REFERENCES

1. Gannon K. The next five years: the hot and not so hot otc drugs. Drug Topics (May 7):28–32, 1990.

2. Gannon K. Who's buying what in otcs. Drug Topics (Jan. 8):32–48, 1990.

3. Ruben BD. Public perceptions of digestive health and disease. Pract Gastroenterol 10:35–40, 1986.

4. Haubrich WS. Constipation. In Berk JE: Bockus Gastroenterology, ed. 4. Philadelphia, WB Saunders, 1985. p 111.

5. Cohnell AM, Hilton C, Irvine G, et al. Variation of bowel habit in two population samples. Br Med J [Clin Res] 2:1095–1102, 1965.

6. Everhart JE, Liang V, Johannes RS, et al. A longitudinal survey of self-reported bowel habits in the United States. Dig Dis Sci 34:1153–1162, 1989.

7. Sandler RS, Drossman DA. Bowel habits in young adults not seeking health care. Dig Dis Sci 32:841–845, 1987.

8. Binder HJ. Pathophysiology of acute diarrhea. Am J Med 88 (suppl 6A):2S–4S, 1990.

9. Devroede G. Constipation. In Sleisinger MH, Fordtran JS: Gastrointestinal Disease: Pathophysiology, Diagnosis, and Management, ed. 5. Philadelphia, WB Saunders, 1993, pp 837–887.

10. Brunton LL. Agents Effecting Gastrointestinal Water Flux and Motility, Digestants, and Bile Acids. In Gilman AG, Rall TW, Nies AS, Taylor P: Goodman and Gilman's The Pharmacological Basis of Therapeutics, ed. 8. New York, Macmillan, 1990, p 914–932.

11. Tedesco FJ, Dipiro JT. Laxative use in constipation. Am J Gastroenterol 80:303–309, 1985.

12. Anon. Safety of stool softeners. Med Lett 19:45–46, 1977.

13. Donowitz M. Current concepts of laxative action: mechanisms by which laxatives increase stool water. Clin Gastroenterol 1:77–84, 1979.

14. Anon. Laxatives. Replacing danthron. Drug Ther Bull 26:53–56, 1988.

15. Barone JA, Jessen LM, Colaizzi JL, et al. Cisapride: A gastrointestinal prokinetic drug. Ann Pharmacother 28:488–500, 1994.

16. Muller-Lissner SA. Treatment of chronic constipation with cisapride and placebo. Gut 28:1033–1038, 1987.

17. Verheyen K, Vervaeke M, Demyttenaere P, et al. Double-blind comparison of two cisapride dosage regimens with placebo in the treatment of functional constipation. Curr Ther Res 41:978–985, 1987.

18. Hedner T, Cassieto J. Opioids and opioid receptors in peripheral tissues. Scan J Gastroenterol Suppl 130:36–40, 1987.

19. Kreek MJ, Schaefer RA, Hahn EF, et al. Naloxone, a specific opioid antagonist reverses chronic idiopathic constipation. Lancet 1:261–262, 1983.

20. Kaufman PN, Krevsky B, Malmud LS, et al. Role of opiate receptors in the regulation of colonic transit. Gastroenterology 94:1351–1356, 1988.

21. Brownlee HJ. Family practitioner's guide to patient self-treatment of acute diarrhea. Am J Med 88(suppl 6A):27S–29S, 1990.

22. Anon. Oral fluids for dehydration. Med Lett 29:63–64, 1987.

23. U.S. Department of Health and Human Services. Health Information for International Travel 1994. Atlanta: HHS Publication No. (CDC) 94–8280.

24. Anon. Antidiarrheal drug products for over-the-counter human use: tentative final monograph. Federal Register 51:16138–16149, 1986.

25. DuPont HL, Sanchez JF, Ericsson CD, et al. Comparative efficacy of loperamide hydrochloride and bismuth subsalicylate in the management of acute diarrhea. Am J Med 88(suppl 6A):15S–19S, 1990.

26. DuPont HL, Ericsson CD, DuPont MW, et al. A randomized open-label comparison of non-prescription loperamide and attapulgite in the symptomatic treatment of acute diarrhea. Am J Med 88(suppl 6A):20S–23S, 1990.

27. Johnson PC, Ericsson CD, DuPont HL, et al. Comparison of loperamide with bismuth subsalicylate for the treatment of acute travelers' diarrhea. JAMA 255:757–760, 1986.

28. Anon. Opium Preparations. American Hospital Formulary Service Drug Information 1994: American Society of Hospital Pharmacists, Washington, D.C. Section 56:08:08, pp. 1881–1882.

29. Anon. Status of certain over-the-counter drug category II and III ingredients. Federal Register 55:20434–20438, 1990.

30. DuPont HL, Hornick RB. Adverse effect of lomotil therapy in shigellosis. JAMA 226:1525–1528, 1973.

31. Brown JW. Toxic megacolon association with loperamide therapy. JAMA 241:501–502, 1979.

32. DuPont HL, Ericsson CD. Prevention and treatment of travelers' diarrhea. N Eng J Med 328:1821–1827, 1993.

33. Suarez J, Salamone FR. Management and prevention of bacterial diarrhea. Clin Pharm 7:746–759, 1988.

34. Salata RA, Olds GR. Infectious diseases in travelers and immigrants. In Warren KS, Mahmoud AF: Tropical and Geographical Medicine, ed. 2. New York, McGraw-Hill, 1990, p 228.

35. DuPont HL, Ericsson CD, Johnson PC. Prevention of travelers' diarrhea by the tablet formulation of bismuth subsalicylate. JAMA 257:1347–1350, 1987.

36. DuPont HL, Sullivan P, Evans DG, et al. Prevention of travelers' diarrhea (emporiatic enteritis): prophylactic administration of bismuth subsalicylate. JAMA 243:237–241, 1980.

37. Mendelowitz PC, Hoffman RS, Weber S. Bismuth absorption and myoclonic encephalopathy during bismuth subsalicylate therapy. Ann Intern Med 112:140–141, 1990.

38. Sack DA, Kaminsky DC, Sack RB, et al. Prophylactic doxycycline for travelers' diarrhea: results of a prospective double-blind study of Peace Corps volunteers in Kenya. N Engl J Med 298:758–763, 1978.

39. Sack RB, Frochlich JL, Zulich AW, et al. Prophylactic doxycycline for travelers' diarrhea: results of a prospective double-blind study of Peace Corps volunteers in Morocco. Gastroenterology 76:1368–1373, 1979.

40. DuPont HL, Evans DG, Rios N, et al. Prevention of travelers' diarrhea with trimethoprim-sulfamethoxazole. Rev Infect Dis 4:533–539, 1982.

41. DuPont HL, Galindo E, Evans DG, et al. Prevention of travelers' diarrhea with trimethoprim-sulfamethoxazole and trimethoprim alone. Gastroenterology 84:75–80, 1983.

42. Johnson PC, Ericsson CD, Morgan DR, et al. Lack of emergence of resistant fecal flora during successful prophylaxis of travelers' diarrhea with norfloxacin. Antimicrob Agents Chemother 30:671–674, 1986.

43. Rademaker CM, Hoepelman IM, Wolfhagen MJ. Results of a double-blind placebo-controlled study using ciprofloxacin for pre-vention of travelers' diarrhea. Eur J Clin Microbiol Infect Dis 8:690–694, 1989.

44. DuPont HL, Sullivan P, Pickering LK, et al. Symptomatic treatment of diarrhea with bismuth subsalicylate among students attending a Mexican university. Gastroenterology 73:715–718, 1977.

45. Johnson PC, Ericsson CD, DuPont HL. Comparison of loperamide with bismuth subsalicylate for the treatment of acute travelers' diarrhea. JAMA 255:757–760, 1986.

46. Van Loon FP, Bennish ML, Butler C. Double-blind trial of lopermide for treating acute watery diarrhea in expatriates in Bangladesh. Gut 30:492–495, 1989.

47. DuPont HL, Reves RR, Galindo E, et al. Treatment of travelers' diarrhea with trimethoprim/sulfamethoxazole and with trimethorpim alone. N Engl J Med 307:841–844, 1982.

48. Ericsson CD, Johnson PC, DuPont HL, et al. Ciprofloxacin or trimethoprim-sulfamethoxazole as initial therapy for travelers' diarrhea. Ann Intern Med 106:216–220, 1987.

49. DuPont HL. Furazolidone versus ampicillin in the treatment of travelers' diarrhea. Antimicrob Agents Chemother 26:160, 1984.

50. Ericsson CD, DuPont HL, Mathewson JJ, et al. Treatment of travelers' diarrhea with sulfamethoxazole and trimethoprim and lopermide. JAMA 263:257–261, 1990.

51. Ericsson CD, DuPont HL, Sullivan P, et al. Bicozamycin, a poorly absorbable antibiotic, effectively treats travelers' diarrhea. Ann Intern Med 98:20–25, 1983.

52. DuPont HL, Ericsson CD, Mathewson JJ, et al. Oral aztreonam, a poorly absorbed yet effective therapy for bacterial diarrhea in U.S. travelers to Mexico. JAMA 267:1932–1935, 1992.

53. McGill B. Functional diarrhea. Evaluation and management. Pract Gastroenterol 4:16–20, 1980.

54. Dlatorre R, Navarro JL, Aldrete JA, et al. Comparison between phenytoin and conventional treatment for irritable bowel syndrome. Curr Ther Res Clin Exp 38:661, 1985.

55. Prior A, Harris SR, Whorwell PJ. Reduction of colonic motility by intravenous nicardipine in irritable bowel syndrome. Gut 28:1609–1612, 1987.

56. Van Outryve M, Milo R, Toussaint J, et al. "Prokinetic" treatment of constipation-predominant irritable bowel syndrome: A placebo-controlled study of cisapride. Clin Gastroenterol 13:49–57, 1991.

57. Cann PA, Read NW, Holdsworth CD, et al. role of loperamide and placebo in the management of irritable bowel syndrome. Dig Dis Sci 29:239–247, 1984.

58. Hovdenak N. Loperamide treatment of the irritable bowel syndrome. Scand J Gastroenterol (suppl)130:81–84, 1987.

CHAPTER 27

HEPATITIS: VIRAL AND DRUG INDUCED

ARCELIA M. JOHNSON-FANNIN

Hepatitis is an inflammation of the liver that may be caused by viral or bacterial infections, chemical toxicity (primarily drugs), or autoimmune hypersensitivity reactions.

VIRAL HEPATITIS

Viral hepatitis is a major health concern worldwide. When consideration is made for reports from developing countries, the number of viruses that can cause hepatitis increases. The categories of viral agents currently implicated in hepatitis are hepatitis A virus (HAV), hepatitis B virus (HBV), hepatitis D virus (HDV), hepatitis C (HCV), hepatitis E (HEV), and (theoretically) hepatitis F (HFV). The symptoms of hepatitis may be mimicked by other viral infections such as cytomegalovirus, Epstein-Barr virus, and mononucleosis (1–5). There have been recent reports of hepatitis due to disseminated herpes simplex virus (HSV) (6, 7).

Hepatitis is a communicable disease for which mandatory reporting is enforced. In 1985, almost 60,000 cases of hepatitis were reported to the CDC. In 1988, the number was approximately 53,500. In 1990, a total of 56,767 cases were reported. In 1992, the number was 46,132, and in 1994 a total of 36,551 cases were reported (8, 9).

VIRAL ETIOLOGIES

Hepatitis A

VIROLOGY AND ETIOLOGY

Hepatitis A virus is a 27-nm particle, composed of four polypeptides that form a tight protein shell (capsid) around the virion RNA. HAV belongs to the family Picornaviridae and has a replication scheme similar to the polioviruses (enteroviruses). Like the enteroviruses, HAV is stable at low pH, allowing survival in gastric medium. HAV differs significantly from the polioviruses in that HAV is thermally more stable and replication of HAV is not blocked by substances known to block poliovirus replication (5, 10). This ability to withstand extreme conditions helps the virus spread and increases its potential for causing epidemics.

EPIDEMIOLOGY AND TRANSMISSION

Hepatitis A is spread almost exclusively by virus shed in the feces then transmitted to the oral cavity. The vehicle for transmission may be contaminated water, food, shellfish, and even fresh produce (3, 11–13). Transmission is enhanced by poor hand washing, poor personal hygiene, and crowded conditions. Outbreaks in North America are sporadic; however, hepatitis A is endemic to certain areas and outbreaks are more common and last longer (2, 14). Approximately 40 to 50% of urban Americans are seropositive for HAV. At particular risk for HAV are male homosexuals, child-care facility employees, and children in day-care facilities. Transmission of HAV via the parenteral route may occur in drug abuse cases, but documentation of HAV transmitted by transfusion is uncommon (13).

During 1983–1988, the reported cases of hepatitis A increased from approximately 9 to almost 11/100,000 population. This apparent trend in increased incidence of hepatitis A could be due to better detection and/or better reporting (8). In 1990, of the 56,767 cases of hepatitis reported to the CDC, 31,441 were hepatitis A. By the end of 1994, 22,457 cases of hepatitis A had been reported (9). The transmission of HAV appears to be directly related to personal hygiene, overcrowding, and the sophistication with which human waste is handled.

CLINICAL PRESENTATION AND DIAGNOSIS

Hepatitis A (previously called infectious hepatitis) is spread primarily by the fecal-oral route. The incubation period is about 28 days, with a range of 15 to 50 days (2, 13). Fecal shedding of the virus is maximal late during the incubation period, and immediately prior to and immediately following the onset of symptoms. Propagation from person to person occurs during viral shedding. Antibodies to HAV (anti-HAV, or HA-Ab) can be detected in the serum after the onset of symptoms. The initial antibodies are primarily of the IgM class, with detectable levels of IgA in some patients. As the symptoms resolve, anti-HAV antibodies of the IgG class predominate, with levels remaining high indefinitely (Fig. 27.1). With the appearance of high titers of anti-HAV, the patient is no longer infectious and is considered protected from further infection as long as IgG anti-HAV titers remain elevated (15, 16).

Not all persons exposed to HAV will develop the clinical disease. In the person who becomes ill, symptoms appear approximately 1 month after exposure to HAV. The symptoms of the preicteric or prodromal phase may be

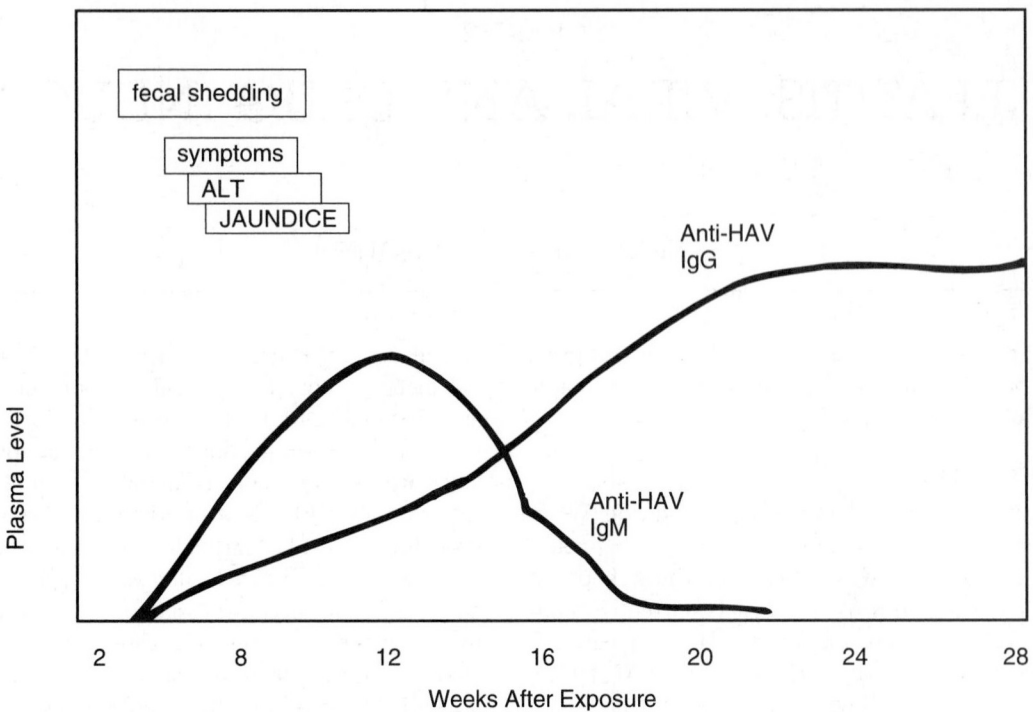

Figure 27.1.   Time course of acute hepatitis A: clinical picture and serologic markers.

mild, mimicking the "flu" or an enteric virus, or may be more pronounced and suggestive of a hepatic problem. Persons older than 18 years may present with jaundice, dark urine, light colored stools, fatigue, fever/chills, and loss of appetite. Children under the age of 2 are often asymptomatic or present with mild fever, malaise, and discomfort. Older children tend to experience diarrhea more often than adults. Other complaints such as joint pain, constipation, and rash can occur but are rare (13, 16, 17). Although the acute illness usually lasts for 10 to 20 days, patients have often begun to feel better by the time the jaundice appears. Recovery is usually complete within 1 or 2 months without progression to chronic hepatitis.

In the majority of HAV hepatitis cases, symptoms are absent or mild and thus of little help in substantiating the diagnosis. Serum aspartate aminotransferase (AST) and alanine aminotransferase (ALT) will be elevated as much as 20 to 100 times the normal. Bilirubin becomes elevated later than AST and ALT. Bilirubin may rise as much as 20 times the normal. However, the amount of rise in bilirubin or enzymes does not indicate degree of injury. The diagnosis of hepatitis A is confirmed by finding anti-HAV (IgM) in the serum (15).

HEPATITIS B
VIROLOGY AND ETIOLOGY

Hepatitis B virus is a 42-nm sphere referred to as the "Dane particle." However, serum known to be HBV positive will contain the intact virion and other material of varying size and shape. One of these is a 22-nm lipoprotein

probably representing excess external viral coating. This material is the hepatitis B surface antigen, HBsAg. It may exist in spherical or filamentous form. There are at least ten major antigenic subtypes of HBsAg and several less important subtypes. The "parent" virion will code for its specific subtypes. However, the "a" specificity appears to be common to all HBsAg subtypes (18, 19). Disruption of the intact virion with mild detergent eludes two other important antigens: the 7-nm polypeptide coat of the nucleocapsid, called hepatitis B core antigen (HBcAg); and the 27-nm soluble protein internal substance of the nucleocapsid, called hepatitis "Be" antigen (HBeAg) (19). The immune competent individual will produce immuno-globulins to each of these antigens.

EPIDEMIOLOGY AND TRANSMISSION

The incidence of reported cases of hepatitis B rose from approximately 18,000 in 1984 to more than 25,000 in 1986 in spite of the availability of a hepatitis B vaccine since 1982. In 1990, 57,767 cases of hepatitis were reported, of which 20,000 were hepatitis B. In 1992, approximately 16,000 cases of hepatitis B were reported. In 1994, a total of 11,400 cases were reported. HBV infections decreased by 59% from 1985 to 1993, perhaps due to safer sex practices among homosexual males (8, 9).

Hepatitis B is transmitted percutaneously. However, hepatitis due to blood transfusions is not likely caused by HBV (1, 13). HBsAg can be found in almost every body fluid of an infected person. The most noted transmission vehicle is contaminated needles. Gaining in importance is transmission of hepatitis B through sexual contact (20) and perinatal inoculation (21). For the U.S. population at large, the risk of hepatitis B infection is estimated to be less than 5%. For intravenous drug users, health-care workers, residents and workers in mental health facilities and prisons, spouses/relatives of infected patients, the sexually promiscuous, the homosexual male, and persons with Down syndrome, the risk factors range from an estimated 12% to 26% (22, 23). It is estimated that more than 200 million persons worldwide carry HBsAg. It is estimated that HBV infects more than 200,000 persons in the United States each year, leading to more than 11,000 hospitalizations (1, 8).

SEROLOGY

Hepatitis B (formerly called "serum hepatitis") infections may be acquired by a number of mechanisms, including close personal contact. However, the primary mode of transmission is percutaneous contact with infected body fluids (i.e., blood, saliva, sputum, semen, or vaginal discharges). Maternal-neonate transfer of HBV can occur either in utero or at the time of delivery if the mother is a "carrier" or has active HBV disease. The incubation period ranges from 30 to 150 days (1, 2). HBsAg is the first serologic marker to appear in the serum, detectable as early as 1 week, but usually evident by the fourth week

after inoculation. HBsAg disappears from the serum within 2 months after onset of jaundice. HBeAg appears concurrently with or within days of HBsAg. This is the stage of intensive viral replication and maximal infectivity. HBeAg and HBsAg decline over the next 4 or 5 weeks, with HBeAG becoming undetectable before HBsAg. After HBeAg disappears, anti-HBe becomes detectable. HBcAg is not usually detectable in sera, but anti-HBc is usually found within 2 weeks of the appearance of HBsAg. The final serologic marker to appear is anti-HBsAg. Anti-HBs can usually be detected before HBsAg completely disappears from the serum (see Fig. 27.2) (15, 16).

CLINICAL PRESENTATION AND DIAGNOSIS

Hepatitis B is a systemic disease. The preicteric symptoms are varied and unpredictable and include flulike complaints, such as loss of appetite, GI distress, fatigue, headache, arthralgia, sore throat, and cough. Most persons infected with the hepatitis B virus do not develop the clinical disease, show no alterations in liver function nor hepatocyte damage, and do not associate the flulike symptoms with liver disease (nonapparent hepatitis). Others may show evidence of mild disease, with minor changes in the liver not progressing to icterus (anicteric symptomatic hepatitis) (3).

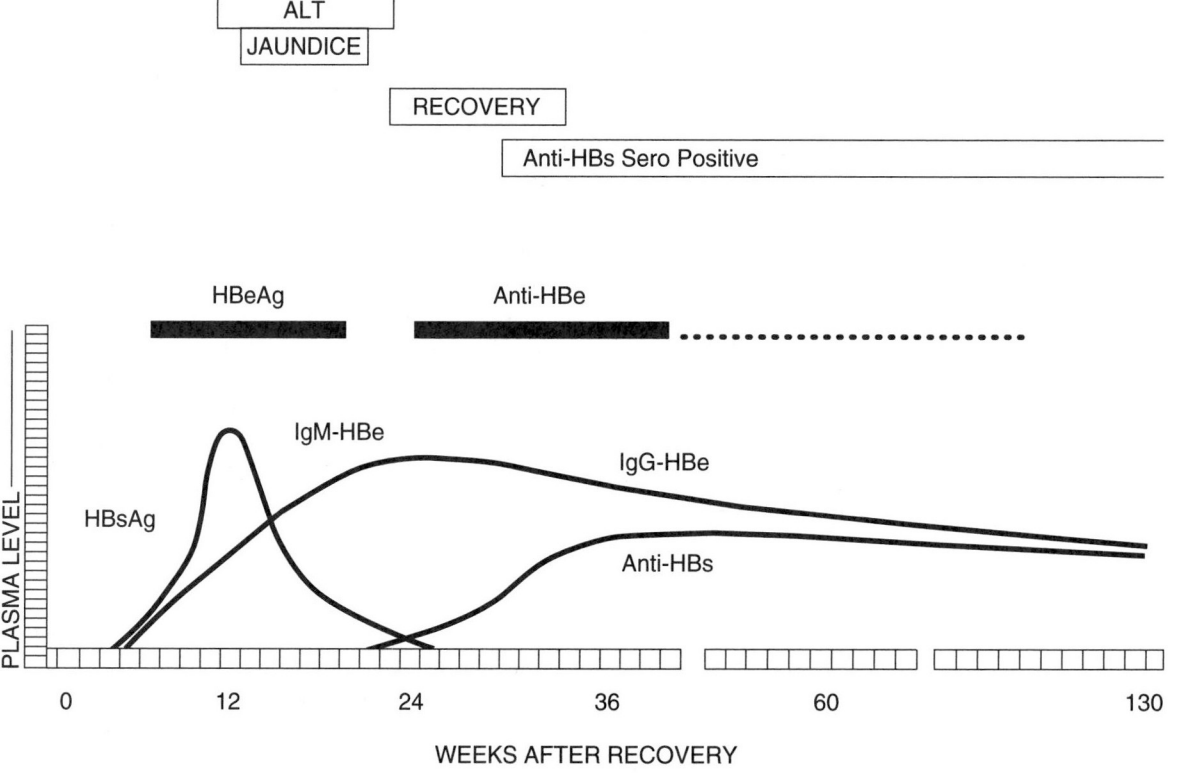

Figure 27.2.   Relative time course of hepatitis B: clinical picture and serologic markers.

In patients with clinical disease (icteric symptomatic hepatitis), the flulike symptoms (prodromal) precede jaundice by 1 to 2 weeks. One to five days before the onset of jaundice, the urine may become dark and the stools appear chalky. With the onset of jaundice, the prodromal symptoms subside. The patient may complain of right upper quadrant pain as the liver enlarges. Splenomegaly is observed in approximately 15% of the patients. Some patients develop transient spider angiomas. In a small percentage of patients biliary obstruction may occur, giving rise to a cholestatic presentation. The liver begins to return to normal, usually within 2 weeks of the onset of jaundice. The duration of icterus is about 6 weeks. In uncomplicated cases of hepatitis B, recovery takes 3 or 4 months after the onset of icterus.

In the patient presenting with jaundice, a diagnosis of hepatitis is a standard suspicion. Serum aspartate aminotransferase (AST) and alanine aminotransferase (ALT), become elevated prior to the onset of jaundice, indicating hepatocyte necrosis (see Fig. 27.2). Alkaline phosphatase levels do not rise unless a biliary obstruction leading to cholestasis is present. Bilirubin levels rise later than AST but are elevated at the onset of jaundice. There is no correlation between the degree of hepatic damage and enzyme or bilirubin levels. In the anicteric symptomatic patient, AST will also be elevated. However, in the absence of jaundice the diagnosis requires a high degree of suspicion. Albumin levels generally remain normal, while globulin levels are predictably elevated. In some patients, prothrombin time is prolonged. This is consistent with extensive hepatocyte necrosis and may signal a poorer prognosis (1–3, 10, 11, 24).

Serologic tests can determine the type of hepatitis virus responsible for the infection. The diagnosis of hepatitis B depends on finding HBsAg in the serum of the patient (see Table 27.1).

Table 27.1.
Significance of Serologic Markers in Hepatitis B

	Serologic Marker					
			Anti-HBc			
Clinical State	HBsAg	HBeAg	IgM	IgG	Anti HBe	Anti HBs
Active disease	+	+	+	+[a]	–	–
Chronic disease						
Active	+	+	–	+	+	+[c]
Persistant		+/–	–	+	+	+
Carrier	+	+	–	–	+[c]	+[c]
Recovered	–	–	–	+[b]	+/–	+[b]

[a]Usually appears during recovery at about 24 weeks.
[b]Titers persist indefinitely in the recovered patient.
[c]Low titers of nonprotective antibody may be present in 10–20% of patients.

Hepatitis D (delta)

Hepatitis delta virus (HDV) is an incomplete or defective RNA virus that requires the hepatitis B virus to replicate. It is a 37-nm virus whose nucleocapsid core is thought to be coated with HBsAg. Although hepatitis delta infections can only occur as a coinfection with hepatitis B, simultaneously, or as a superinfection, the HDV can replicate in cells where HBV is not present (2, 3, 25). The mechanism by which this occurs has not been explained. Hepatitis delta antigen is only occasionally detectable in the serum. Anti-delta IgM is detectable during an acute infection. HDAg and anti-HDAg disappear from the serum when HBsAg is cleared. Delta infections cannot last longer than hepatitis B infections but can alter the severity, chronicity, and morbidity and mortality of hepatitis B infections (15, 24–26).

Hepatitis delta is endemic in hepatitis B patients in Mediterranean countries. In North America, HDV is primarily seen in hepatitis B patients who are drug users or hemophiliacs (27).

Hepatitis non-A, non-B
HEPATITIS C

Hepatitis C virus (HCV) is thought to be the etiology of blood-transmitted non-A, non-B hepatitis. The virus is known to belong to the Flaviviridae family, however the exact structure and size of the virion remain unknown. There is recent evidence to suggest that more than one strain of the virus may exist and be capable of causing hepatitis (28, 29). It is estimated that 5 to 15% of persons transfused with whole blood develop hepatitis. The total number of reported cases of non-A, non-B hepatitis increased since 1990 (9). This apparent increase is thought to occur because blood is now routinely screened for the presence of anti-HCV. HCV is the most likely cause, particularly when pooled blood is the source of the blood product (29). Many persons are testing positive who never had symptoms of the illness. At increased risk are hemophiliacs, dialysis patients, and patients with bleeding disorders requiring blood products (30, 31).

Recently, serologic tests have become available to detect anti-HCV. The tests are based on radioimmune assay and enzyme-linked immunosorbent assay for anti-C100-3 (29). A second generation of assay methods test for proteins of the C22-3 and NS3 region. These assays are more sensitive and can detect the presence of HCV 1 to 3 months earlier during the acute phase of the infection. The most sensitive indicator of an HCV infection is the presence of HCV RNA. The development of a DNA/polymerase chain reaction assay to detect HCV RNA has recently been approved and allows for detection of HCV within days after exposure (32). This assay should allow for the confirmation of HCV in liver and plasma samples.

Table 27.2.
Features of Acute Viral Hepatitis

Indicator	HAV	HBV	HCV	HDV	HEV
Incidence (U.S.A.—1994)	7/100,000	3/100,000	—	—	—
Transmission					
Fecal/oral	yes	no	no	no	yes
Percutaneous	unlikely	yes	yes	yes	unlikely
Intimate contact	yes	yes	yes	yes	unlikely
Serologic marker	anti-HAV	many[a]	anti-HCV	anti-HDV	anti-HEV
Clinical course					
Symptoms	mild	variable	moderate	variable	mild
Complications					
Carrier	no	yes	rare	yes	no
Chronic	no	yes	yes	yes	no
Fulminant	<0.2%	0.2–1%	1%[b]	5–20%	10–15%
Carcinoma	no	yes	yes	yes	no
Recovery	>98%	>95%[c]	50–70%[c]	80–90%[c]	80–90%
Prevention	sanitation	hygiene	hygiene	hygiene	sanitation
Prophylaxis	vaccine Ig	vaccine HBIg	none	none, vaccine[d]	none
Treatment					
Acute	none[e]	none[e]	none[e]	none[e]	none[e]
Chronic	n/a	interferon	interferon	none	none

[a]See Table 27.1.
[b]Could be considerably higher in persons over age 60.
[c]Diminishes with advanced and in the compromised host.
[d]HBV vaccine prevents this dependant infection.
[e]Pallative/supportive measures only.

The clinical features of HCV hepatitis parallel those of the other hepatitis viruses. In many persons, the symptoms of the disease are mild or absent. Elevated serum aminotransferase levels may be the only parameter on which to base a diagnosis of liver disease. In other patients with subclinical infections, AST and ALT may not be elevated. In the symptomatic patient, a preicteric "prodrome" resembling that seen in HBV infections may occur. Symptoms parallel those seen in HBV infections. Some persons with HCV hepatitis develop papular or papular-vesicular lesions on the arms. Fever is not associated with HCV hepatitis. Jaundice does occur, along with a characteristic "peak and valley" pattern of AST and ALT (33). Multiple immune mechanisms appear to be activated during HCV acute infections. Rheumatoid factor may appear in the serum and some patients complain of arthralgias. Finding anti-HCV in the serum confirms the diagnosis. Recovery takes longer than acute HBV hepatitis. The death rate is low from acute HCV, but the progression to chronic (HCV) hepatitis is high (see Table 27.2) (1, 13, 28, 33).

HEPATITIS E

Hepatitis E virus is the waterborne pathogen of non-A, non-B hepatitis. It has been credited with causing epidemics in developing countries where sanitation is a problem. The virus can be recovered from the stool of infected persons 4 to 7 weeks following inoculation. The viral genome has been replicated, revealing a 27- to 34-mn nonenveloped virus designated HEV (34, 35). The detection on anti-HEV has been made possible by the development of an enzyme-linked immunosorbent assay (ELISA) (36). Hepatitis E is thought to be endemic in developing countries. It rarely occurs in North America (37).

HEPATITIS F

Hepatitis F, another distinct non-A, non-B hepatitis virus, is likely to exist. This is supported by the development of hepatitis in persons receiving coagulation factor concentrates from pooled blood who have already recovered from HCV infections. Such persons would be protected from subsequent HCV infections and should be HCV seropositive. A significant portion of these persons are HCV seronegative. Little is known about the virus, suggesting the need for further research (1, 24).

Pathogenesis

During acute viral hepatitis, the liver is described as enlarged, red and glistening, smooth surfaced, and flabby. The morphologic lesions are consistent regardless of which virus is the cause of the hepatitis. The characteristic picture is a combination of hepatocyte necrosis and regeneration, a diffuse mononuclear cell infiltration, hyperplasia of Kupffer cells, and varying degrees of bile stasis. The mononuclear cells are primarily lymphocytes, with some eosinophils noted. Lobular disarray is apparent, probably due to the presence of ballooned hepatic plates, which obliterate the sinusoids, smudging of hepatocyte cell membranes, and the presence of inflammatory cells. Large hepatocytes with a "ground glass" appearance of the cytoplasm due to the presence of HBsAg are characteristic in chronic hepatitis B but are not seen in acute hepatitis B. Although the liver cell plates may be disrupted, leading to focal disruption of the reticulin network, this framework is generally preserved, since the necrosis tends to be limited to single or adjacent group cells. In severe cases of hepatitis, this framework is destroyed, leading to the characteristic pattern of bridging necrosis and a poorer prognosis (1, 2, 13, 38).

Complications

In the majority of hepatitis cases, regardless of the viral cause, resolution of the biochemical changes and complete clinical recovery occurs within 4 months. Mortality is quite low for hepatitis A infections, approximating 0.1%. For hepatitis B the mortality statistic varies. Reports of 5 to 20% mortality in persons with HBV and HDV have been reported during some outbreaks. Current estimates place mortality for hepatitis B at about 1% for hospitalized patients and 10% for the population at large (see Table 27.2) (1, 13). Age (very young or old) and pregnancy are significant risks affecting mortality (17).

For some patients, recovery from hepatitis B is not prompt. Persistent infection may linger for months to years, causing chronic persistent hepatitis, chronic active hepatitis, or chronic lobular hepatitis, or it could lead to the development of the carrier state. A small percentage of those affected by HBV develop fulminant hepatitis (see Fig. 27.3). Chronic persistent hepatitis is characterized by a mild focal lymphocyte infiltration. The lobular structure is retained, there is not fibrosis, and treatment is not usually required. The prognosis is good, with resolution to full recovery in almost all cases. In chronic active hepatitis the liver biopsy shows greater lymphocyte infiltration involving the portal and periportal areas, collapse with bridging necrosis, and often fibrosis. The continuation of the active inflammatory process in CAH is associated with a poor prognosis. The development of cirrhosis is likely (39, 40).

A major reservoir for hepatitis virus is the human carrier. Chronic carriers of the HBsAg harbor the virus without evidence of clinical infection but are a major source of infection for others. This group of patients appears to be at greater risk for developing hepatocellular carcinoma (see Chapter 81, "Liver Tumors"). Approximately 80% of the hepatocellular carcinoma cases have a positive history of hepatitis B (41, 42).

A most interesting hypothesis to explain the differing responses to hepatitis B is related to the type of cellular immune response mounted by the patient to the virus. Theoretically, if the immune response is adequate, the disease follows its usual benign course. If the response is inadequate, the patient develops chronic hepatitis. If the response is absent or severely depressed, the patient becomes a carrier. This theory implies that much of the hepatocellular injury is autoimmune (24, 39). A small percentage (1–5) of recovered hepatitis B patients again

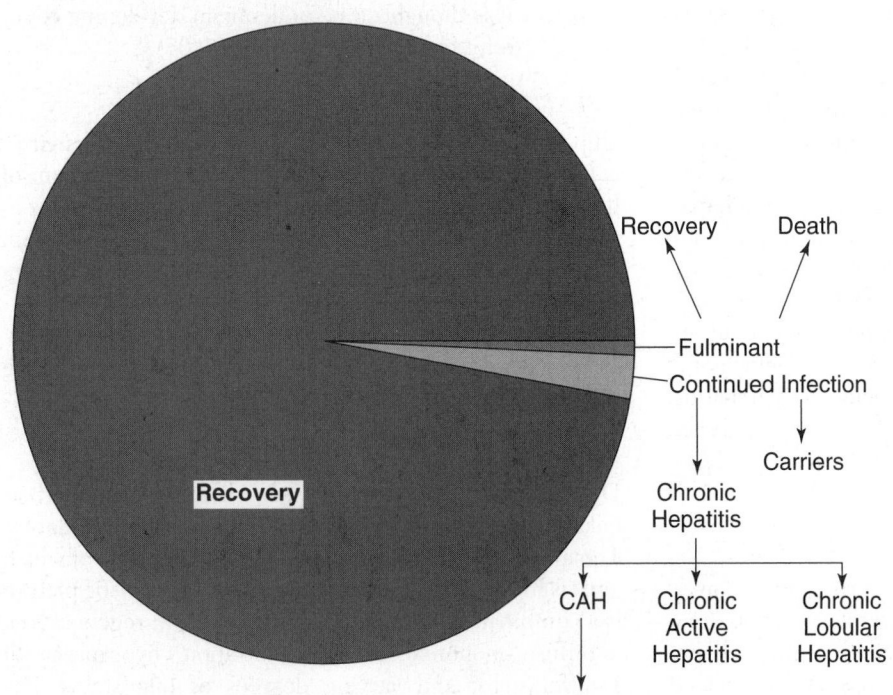

Figure 27.3. Clinical sequelae of acute hepatitis B infection.

develop symptoms of acute hepatitis. In most instances the recurrence will resolve without sequelae. In some cases the relapse progresses to massive hepatic necrosis. The liver shrinks rapidly, bilirubin levels rise rapidly, and the prothrombin time is markedly prolonged. This fulminant hepatic failure progresses to ascites, esophageal bleeding, sepsis, encephalopathy, cardiovascular failure, coma, and death in less than 2 weeks in about 60 to 90% of the patients. The only definitive treatment is liver transplantation (see Table 27.2) (43, 44, 49).

Chronic hepatitis D can develop in a person who has chronic hepatitis B. It is a chronic active hepatitis, usually resulting in increased damage to the liver. Chronic hepatitis C is a common occurrence. It is estimated that as many as 60% of the acute HCV infections progress to chronic infections. The progression to cirrhosis occurs in about 20% of persons infected with HCV. Hepatocellular carcinoma is also associated with HCV infections. There is controversy over the interpretation of this information. Chronic hepatitis following HCV infection is thought to be associated with poor prognosis. However, others consider the 10-year mortality rate in this population to be comparable to persons who did not have an HCV infection (45–47).

Less frequently encountered extrahepatic complications of hepatitis include rashes, cardiac changes, pleural effusions, altered thyroid function, gastritis, steatorrhea, pancreatitis, and aplastic anemia. Rare complications of hepatitis thought to be related to the immune system include: focal glomerulitis, Raynaud's phenomenon, acropapular dermatitis (Gianotti-Crosti disease) in children, arthralgias, and a serum-sickness-like syndrome associated with the prodromal symptoms in hepatitis B infections (2, 13, 49).

Treatment

ACUTE VIRAL HEPATITIS

As with many viral infections, acute viral hepatitis is a self-limiting disorder. The goals of management in hepatitis, regardless of viral cause, are (a) early, accurate diagnosis and virus classification, (b) support and monitoring during the acute illness, (c) recognition of the chronic disease state, and (d) prevention of disease transmission. The patient with uncomplicated disease does not require hospitalization. Hospitalization is indicated for patients who have become dehydrated, are suspected of having a more severe form of hepatitis, or are at particular risk of complications (e.g., pregnancy) (50).

No specific treatment is available. Drugs are of little value and do not alter the severity or time course of the disease. In general, drugs should be avoided if possible to prevent potentiating the liver problem. Drug therapies that must be continued (e.g., antihypertensives) can present therapeutic dosing problems because predictions about liver metabolism are not accurately reflected by levels of liver enzymes. Generally speaking, the capacity of the liver to metabolize drugs is expansive and is not significantly depressed in uncomplicated hepatitis. However, drugs known to cause cholestasis should specifically be avoided.

Bed rest with exercise as tolerated, an appropriate diet, fluids and electrolytes, and education about hepatitis and its transmission are considered basic patient management. In patients for whom nausea/vomiting/diarrhea is a problem, feeding the larger portion of the caloric allowance in the morning may be beneficial. Tube feeding may be required for patients who are too ill to eat. Antihistamines may be used to treat the pruritus. However, normal doses of a drug such as diphenhydramine (25–30 mg q6h prn) may cause more drowsiness than usual due to prolonged hepatic clearance in the acute phase of hepatitis. For the patient complaining of pain, mild analgesics may be prescribed. Acetaminophen, the most often prescribed agent in hospitals, has a wide margin of safety but is implicated in drug-induced liver disease. Doses of 325 to 650 mg q6h should be adequate and appropriate. Aspirin should be avoided because of the potential for gastrointestinal bleeding, the antiplatelet effect, and suppression of the inflammatory response. Antiinflammatory agents (e.g., corticosteroids) should be avoided in acute viral hepatitis. If the prothrombin time is prolonged, 2 or 3 doses of vitamin K given as phytonadione 10 mg/day, PO or SC, may be used. If biliary obstruction is present, the pruritus may be persistent and intense due to the deposition of excess bile acids in the skin. Cholestyramine resin and colestipol HCl are anion-exchange resins capable of binding bile salts into a nonabsorbable, insoluble complex for excretion in the feces. The dose of cholestyramine is 4 grams orally, 3 or 4 times a day before meals. The dose of colestipol is 15 to 30 g/day, divided in 2 to 4 doses. Therapy should continue for 14 to 21 days. Both of these agents are powders that must be mixed with 60 to 90 mL of liquid prior to administration. Because of the poor palatability of the drink, preparing the drug with an appropriate vehicle is important for compliance. Strong fruit juices, pulpy fruit, or cereal may mask the taste and texture sufficiently (1, 13).

The hospitalized patient should be discharged when the symptoms improve and AST, bilirubin, and prothrombin time return to acceptable levels. Follow-up is essential to document biochemical recovery, to ensure clearance of HBsAg, and to recognize chronic or carrier states. The patient who develops fulminant hepatic disease should be treated as a patient with hepatic encephalopathy (see Chapter 28).

CHRONIC HEPATITIS

Chronic hepatitis represents a medical challenge. The goal of any treatment plan is to halt the progression to cirrhosis, liver failure, and death, and to reduce infectivity and transmission. Many treatment options have been proposed with studies aimed primarily at chronic hepatitis B. Two classes of drugs have been most extensively investigated: immunomodulators and antiviral agents. The premise of these approaches is that suppression of viral replication and immune-mediated killing of virus infected cells will lead to a decrease in both infectivity and the severity of the disease (51).

Corticosteroids. The use of corticosteroids in the treatment of chronic hepatitis B grew out of their usefulness in the treatment of autoimmune chronic active hepatitis. These patients have high titers of antinuclear antibodies (ANA), indicating an ongoing immune mechanism as the cause. Several well-controlled, long-term studies have investigated prednisone and prednisolone in doses of 20 to 60 mg/day against nontreated patients. The conclusions are that long-term prednisone or prednisolone is of no benefit in the treatment of chronic active hepatitis B and may, in fact, be deleterious (51). Recent investigations have studied the use of pulse therapy (brief periods of steroids followed by a drug-free period) in the treatment of chronic hepatitis B. Prednisone was given in a high dose, 60 mg/day, and tapered rapidly to 0 mg over a 4-week period. A significant reduction in AST was noted during drug therapy. However, rebound hepatitis occurred between 4 and 10 weeks following cessation of therapy. When compared to similar patients, the nontreated group fared better (53–55). Under 20% of patients with chronic active hepatitis will achieve permanent remission with steroids. The question of whether to use steroids at all, initiate long-term steroid therapy, or use intermittent (pulse) therapy is still raised when considering therapy for chronic hepatitis. However, the current approach is to avoid steroids unless they are used in conjunction with interferon-α therapy (see below).

Antiviral Agents. Vidarabine (ARA-A) is a synthetic nucleoside that inhibits multiplication of DNA viruses. Studies conducted along similar protocol lines have produced varying results. ARA-A has been tried in doses of 5 mg/kg/day for 4 weeks. Some patients showed a loss of HBeAg; others did not. All patients experienced the rather severe side effects of ARA-A, with painful persistent neuropathies the most frequently reported adverse effect. This agent is not considered to be clinically useful in chronic hepatitis (51, 56).

Acyclovir is an antiviral agent that inhibits the replication of varicella viruses. Its selective activity for viral cells over host cells is due to its affinity for viral thymidine kinase over host cellular enzymes. Acyclovir has been given in doses of 45 mg/kg/day to patients with chronic hepatitis, with some evidence of inhibition of viral replication in HBsAg-positive patients. However, since the hepatitis B virus does not make its own thymidine kinase, the usefulness of this drug is questionable (38, 51).

Interferon-α has thus far demonstrated the most promise in the treatment of chronic hepatitis and was approved in 1991 for this indication. The interferons are a family of glycoproteins secreted by monocytes and lymphocytes in response to viral infections. The current marketed agents are from recombinant technology. Interferon-α elicits an antiviral response in cells by binding to specific cell receptors and activating intracellular enzymes. The end result of this enzyme activation is destruction of viral mRNA within the infected cell. Interferon-α has been used with some success in the treatment of chronic hepatitis B and chronic hepatitis C (57, 58). The drug is thought to be as effective in low doses (100,000 U/day) as in high doses. The current trend is to use doses ranging from 1,000,000 U/day to 3,000,000 U/day 3 times a week for 24 weeks. For chronic hepatitis B the recommended adult dose is 3,000,000 U/day 3 times a week for 16 weeks. For nonresponders and in chronic hepatitis C, therapy may be continued for 24 weeks. The response rate is reported to be as high as 85%, with a range of 40 to 85 (57, 58). The response is often transient with as many as 60% of the patients relapsing within 6 to 12 months. Doses up to 5,000,000 U/day 3 times a week for 12 months have produced long-term remission in as many as 40% of treated patients (59–63). Chronic hepatitis D infections may require even higher doses—8 to 9 million units 3 times a week for 12 months. Some population groups (e.g., patients of Mediterranean decent) show a lower response rate to interferon therapy. For those who do respond, the relapse rate is high (60, 61).

Miscellaneous Agents. Other antiviral agents have been studied without much promise. Ribavirin has activity on a variety of RNA and DNA viruses including other Flaviviridae. Oral ribavirin has been tried in chronic hepatitis C infections. The response, similar to interferon-α, is a rapid decrease in AST, breakthrough of disease in some patients despite treatment, and rapid relapse when therapy is discontinued. Investigation into the use of prostaglandin E for fulminant hepatitis has suggested that it may be of benefit (64).

Combination Therapy. The results of single-agent therapy for chronic hepatitis have been disappointing. Since it is likely that most agents studied for the treatment of viral hepatitis act at different stages of viral replication, combination therapy is logical. Azathioprine in combination with prednisone has been used with some success. Prednisone is started at a moderate dose and tapered to a low maintenance dose. The most promising combination therapy is corticosteroids plus interferon-α. Prednisone is given in a regimen of 30 to 60 mg/day for 6 weeks and is followed by 4 to 6 months of interferon-α in doses of 1,000,000 to 3,000,000 units 3 times a week. As many as 60% of patients treated with this regimen have become HBsAg negative. Interferon-α has been tried with zidovudine without much success (65). The most often reported side effects of interferon-α, chills, fever, and neutropenia, are usually mild and well tolerated (61, 62).

Prophylaxis and Prevention

As with all viral infections, prevention of hepatitis is the key to control. Unfortunately, vaccines capable of inducing active immunity to each of the hepatitis viruses are not available. There is a vaccine for hepatitis B and one for hepatitis A. Prophylaxis for other hepatitis infections involves the use of immune globulin, which can at best, provide passive or "passive-active" immunity.

Passive immunity is accomplished when exogenous antibody (as immune globulin) to a particular infectious agent is administered. These antibodies neutralize the infectious agent before extensive colonization can occur, thus preventing the infection and clinical disease. Timing of the administration of the antibodies is important. Active immunization is accomplished by the administration of a vaccine. The noninfectious viral material of the vaccine induces the host to produce antibodies to the specific agent. The vaccine should be administered before exposure so that upon exposure to the pathogen, an anamnestic response will occur, preventing infection and clinical disease. In nonimmunized persons, "passive-active" immunity may be accomplished by administering the vaccine and/or immune globulin. Replication of the infectious agent is not prevented, but the disease may be inapparent with mild symptoms.

Agents used to confer immunity to hepatitis viruses include (a) immune globulin (IGIM), (b) hepatitis B immune globulin (HBIG), (c) hepatitis B virus vaccine, and (d) hepatitis A vaccine. Immune globulin is a sterile, nonpyrogenic solution containing many antibodies common in human serum. The intramuscular preparation is prepared from the pooled venous blood of at least 1000 persons. The donor blood has been tested for HBsAg and HIV. IGIM contains 15 to 18% protein, of which not less than 90% is IgG. The preparation also contains IgA and IgM. IGIM has a cold storage life of 3 years from date of manufacture. Hepatitis B immune globulin (HBIG) is a sterile, nonpyrogenic solution containing 10 to 18% protein, of which not less than 80% is IgG. It is prepared from the serum of persons who have high titers of anti-HBs but do not show evidence of HBsAg. The preparation is free of anti-HIV. HBIG should be refrigerated.

Hepatitis B vaccine is made by recombinant DNA technology. The two recombinant products are sterile suspensions containing HBsAg produced by common baker's yeast (Saccharomyces cerevisiae). The yeast strain has been altered to contain the hepatitis B gene code for HBsAg, subtype adw. Since the specificity is contained in all HBsAg subtypes. The recombinant preparations are free of all human blood products but may contain yeast protein. Strict quality controls have assured products that are consistent from lot to lot. Recombivax HB, marketed by Merck Sharpe Dohme, contains 10 μg/mL HBsAg or 5 μg/mL for pediatric dosing. Engerix-B, marketed by SmithKline Beecham, contains 20 μg/mL HBsAG, or 10 μg/mL for pediatric use. Both preparations are adsorbed on aluminum hydroxide and contain thimerosal as a preservative.

HEPATITIS A

IGIM contains anti-HAV in titers high enough to provide protection in hepatitis A infections. If IGIM is given prior to exposure or within 2 weeks of exposure, it is usually effective in conferring passive immunity and preventing clinically apparent hepatitis A. A dose of 0.02 mL/kg is recommended for persons who have had intimate contact with a hepatitis A patient. Prophylaxis is not recommended for casual contact. In day-care centers for children, identification of hepatitis A cases should be the stimulus for IGIM. For travelers to areas at high risk for hepatitis A, an IGIM dose of 0.06 mL/kg every 4 to 6 months is recommended if the stay is to exceed 3 months. If the visit is for 3 months or less, the standard prophylactic dose is given. Hepatitis A vaccine has been available outside the United States for several years. It is now marketed in the United States. The vaccine is an inactivated whole virus, attenuated by formalin. It is marketed as Havrix by SmithKline Beecham and as Vaqta by Merck.

Havrix contains 1440 ELISA units/mL. Vaqta contains 25 U/0.06 mL (this represents 400 ng of antigen). The vaccine must be given intramuscularly, with the deltoid the preferred site. A single injection produces what are considered to be appropriate immunoglobulin titers. However, a booster dose within 6 to 12 months is recommended for adults. In the pediatric population two doses of Havrix, 360 U/mL are given, intramuscularly, 2 weeks apart. A booster dose within 6 to 12 months is recommended. A single dose of Vaqta 25 U/0.6 mL given intramuscularly has been shown to provide complete protection against hepatitis A (see Table 27.3). However, it

Table 27.3.
Hepatitis A Vaccination Recommendations[a]

Vaccine	Pediatric	Adult
Havrix[b]	360 Elisa U/mL	1440 Elisa U/mL
schedule	two doses, 2 weeks apart	one dose
route[c]	IM	IM
repeat(?)	Booster	Booster
Vaqta[d]	400 ng/0.06 mL	400 ng/0.06 mL
schedule	one dose	one dose
route[c]	IM	IM
repeat(?)	No	No

[a]Duration of protection still questionable pending long term studies. Current estimates range from 6 months to 2 years.
[b]SmithKline Beechman
[c]Vaccination only effective if given IM. Deltoid muscle preferred.
[d]Merck, Sharpe, Dohme

Table 27.4.
Hepatitis B Vaccination Recommendation (μg)

Vaccine[a,b]	Neonate		Child < 10 yr	Adult	
	(+)[c]	(−)[d]		non-Ic[e]	Ic[f]
Recombinant DNA (Recombivax HB) (MSD)	5	2.5	5	10	20
Recombinant DNA (Engerix B) (SmithKline Beecham)	5	2.5	5	10	20

[a]Intramuscular injection
[b]Three doses; initial dose, 1 month after initial, 6 months after initial.
[c]Neonate born to HBsAG/HBeAG-positive mother
[d]Neonate born to HBsAG/HBeAG-negative mother
[e]Non-immunocompromised
[f]Immunocompromised

is still recommended that anyone presenting with known exposure to hepatitis A be given IGIM along with the vaccine to assure adequate prophylaxis (66–70). Side effects associated with the vaccination are mild and transient. Soreness, redness, warmth at the injection site are the most common complaints. Fever is rare (68).

HEPATITIS B

For preexposure prophylaxis of hepatitis B infection in individuals who are at risk, hepatitis B vaccine should be given in three intramuscular injections into the deltoid muscle. The second injection is given 1 month after the first, and the third at 6 months after the first. The adult dose for the vaccine is 10 μg per injection. For children under 10, the dose is 5 μg per injection. For exposure to a known HGsAg-positive person, the nonimmunized person should receive HBIG, 0.06 mL/kg, within 24 hours of exposure and the hepatitis B vaccine series beginning within 7 days of exposure. In neonates born to HBsAg-positive mothers, a 0.5-mL dose of HBIG immediately after birth, along with the hepatitis B vaccine series (5 μg/dose-recombinant), should confer "passive-active" immunity. The child is considered protected if at 1 month after the last vaccination, HBsAg is not detected and anti-HBs is found (see Table 27.4) (50, 71, 72).

Neither IGIM nor HBIG contain immunoglobulins specific for hepatitis C (non-A, non-B in titers high enough to provide immunity. There is no hepatitis C virus vaccine available. Protection against hepatitis B should protect against Hepatitis D.

There is still controversy among the medical community in the United States over the status of vaccination in general. The question is of particular interest in the pediatric population, but with the availability of a cost-effective hepatitis B vaccine and a hepatitis A vaccine, the argument engulfs a larger segment of the population. Who should be vaccinated for hepatitis A and hepatitis B has been addressed by the Centers for Disease Control (CDC),

the Immunization Practices Advisory Committee (ACIP), and the American Academy of Pediatrics (AAP). In the past, these groups agreed that residents of mental retardation facilities and other institutions where carriers are likely, chronic recipients of blood products, dialysis patients, adoptees of countries where HBV is endemic, sexual partners of carriers, homosexual men, heterosexually active persons with multiple partners, intravenous drug users, international travelers, and U.S. populations with endemic hepatitis B should be vaccinated prior to exposure. They agree that postexposure vaccinations should be done in neonates born to HBsAg mothers, accidental percutaneous exposures, sexual partners of HBV-active persons, and household contacts of HBV-active persons. However, this strategy has not significantly lowered the incidence of hepatitis B (22, 73). Integrating hepatitis B vaccine into childhood vaccination schedules has been shown to be effective in halting the transmission of HBV among Alaskan natives and other groups (74). In 1991, the ACIP in collaboration with the National Center for Infectious Diseases, Division of Viral and Rickettsial Diseases, Hepatitis Branch, developed recommendations on HBV vaccinations. This group recommended (a) universal vaccination of all newborn infants regardless of the HBsAg status of the mother and (b) universal vaccination of adolescents in communities where parenteral drug use, teenage pregnancy, and STDs are common (75). The group continues to advocate vaccination of previously mentioned high-risk groups. It is suggested that HBV infections could be all but eliminated in a generation with widespread immunization of infants and adolescents.

Conclusions

Acute viral hepatitis is generally a self-limiting disease, sometimes associated with considerable morbidity but low mortality. Treatment of the mild disease is supportive. Mortality from hepatitis B is greater than from either of the other forms of viral hepatitis. Hepatitis B, C, and D can progress to the chronic active disease, or massive necrosis can develop creating the potential for fulminant hepatic disease. Successful treatment of these more severe illnesses is difficult at best. Therapy with corticosteroids is not recommended except in combination with interferon-α for the treatment of chronic active hepatitis B. The newer antiviral agents may reduce viral replication, thus providing limited benefit in chronic active hepatitis. Interferon-α therapy for chronic active hepatitis B and chronic hepatitis C has shown exceptional results for heretofore untreatable illnesses. The best therapy is aimed at prevention. Proper sanitation, good hygiene, avoiding high-risk situations (drug users, high-risk sexual situations), are of primary importance in controlling the spread of hepatitis. The most significant therapeutic approach is vaccination using recombinant hepatitis B vaccine and inactivated hepatitis A vaccine. The key to cure is prevention. The current vaccination protocol has been expanded to include all infants, adolescents, and high-risk persons. This has reduced the incidence of hepatitis B as evidenced by the declining trend of new cases from 1993 to 1994. With the addition of hepatitis A vaccine for high-risk groups, spread of the two most prevalent hepatitis viruses, A and B, could be controlled.

DRUG-INDUCED HEPATITIS

Etiology

By definition, any agent that induces a "hepatitis" causes necrosis and/or inflammation of hepatocytes. Injury caused by drugs may start out with a picture quite unlike hepatitis, but eventually create necrotic lesions and inflammation. The list of drugs implicated in drug-induced liver disease is extensive. However, it is estimated that fewer than 15 drugs account for more than 80% of the acute hepatic reactions (76). Acetaminophen heads this list. Halothane, methyldopa, isoniazid, oral contraceptives, rifampin, oxyphenisatin, and valproic acid are included. The ingredients in herbal medicines for relaxation have been reported to cause hepatotoxicity (77). Drug-induced hepatic injury is thought to account for 2 to 5% of hospitalizations in the United States and as much as 10% in European countries. In the geriatric population, the incidence is much higher (76).

Patterns of Drug-Induced Injury

Two major types of hepatotoxicity have been noted: (a) direct or toxic, also called predictable, and (b) idiosyncratic, or nonpredictable. Idiosyncratic reactions are sometimes referred to as hypersensitivity reactions. The reaction caused by some drugs cannot be called direct or idiosyncratic even though necrosis and fatty changes may be evident. The oral contraceptives are an example. There are seven basic mechanisms of drug-induced hepatic injury. The characteristic morphologic lesions seen in drug-induced injury can be related to these mechanisms (see Tables 27.5 and 27.6) (78).

Morphologic Changes

NECROSIS

The lesions occur in response to a dose-related, predictable injury. The necrosis is usually localized, but may be massive and diffuse if the response is idiosyncratic rather than toxic. The extent of the necrosis is paralleled by equivalent rises in AST and ALT. Focal necrosis often occurs when a nontoxic parent drug is converted to a toxic metabolite. This process, called bioactivation, is often associated with drugs cleared through the cytochrome P-450 system (78–80). Acetaminophen conversion to a toxic metabolite is an important example. This toxic metabolite is detoxified by conjugation with glutathione. When large amounts of the metabolite are formed, glutathione is depleted. With the sulfhydryl group of glutathione unavailable, the metabolite then binds covalently to the hepatocyte. This is thought to cause the necrosis. A 10-g dose of acetaminophen is likely to produce a toxic necrosis. Acetaminophen blood levels correlate well with liver damage. A blood level of at least 200 μg/mL 4 hours after ingestion or 100 μg/mL at 8 hours after ingestion is an indication for treatment. The goal of treatment is to supply sulfhydryl groups. N-acetylcysteine is given in a dose of 140 mg/kg for 1 dose, followed by 70 mg/kg q4h for a total of 17 doses (see Chapter 4, "Clinical Toxicology"). Damage already done cannot be corrected with treatment; however, survivors usually have adequate liver function (81, 82).

Acetaminophen hepatotoxicity is particularly associated with chronic alcohol abusers and persons who take repeated doses without eating. Even at doses between 7.5 and 12 g/day, liver toxicity in these patient populations have been reported. These patients present with markedly elevated AST (usually above 1200 U/L), and often a high prothrombin time. Because the acetaminophen blood level may not be sufficiently high to suggest toxicity, drug-induced hepatotoxicity often goes undiagnosed (83).

Halothane causes a focal necrosis in some persons and an idiosyncratic necrosis on subsequent exposure in others.

Table 27.5.
Mechanisms of Drug-Induced Hepatic Injury

No.	Description
1[a]	Disruption of metabolic processes
2[a]	Toxic destruction of essential cell structures
3[a]	Induction of immunologic reaction
4	Carcinogenic effect
5	Disruption of hepatocyte blood supply
6	Transmission of infections
7	Exacerbation of underlying disease

[a]Toxic or idiosyncratic reaction.

Table 27.6.
Morphological Changes Induced by Frequently Encountered Drugs

Mechanism	Morphology	Drug Class	Sample Agents
2	necrosis (toxic)	mushrooms	*Amanita phalloides*
		metals	phosphorus
		hydrocarbon	carbon tetrachloride
		analgesics	acetaminophen
		anesthetics	halothane[a]
2	hepatitis	anesthetics	halothane[a]
		antituberculin	isoniazide
		antihypertensive	methyldopa
		chemotherapeutic	nitrofurantoin
			ketoconazole
		anticholesterol	lovastatin[b]
1	steatonecrosis	sedative	alcohol
		chemotherapeutic	methotrexate
			tetracycline
		cardiovascular	animodarone
1	cholestasis	chemotherapeutic	erythromycin
		antipsychotic	chlorpromazine
		anabolic steroids	testosterone
		hormones	oral contraceptives
		cardiovascular	captopril, verapamil
		analgesic	propoxyphene
		anticonvulsant	carbamazepine
3	granulomas	xanthine oxidase inhibitor	allopurinol
		chemotherapeutic	sulfonamides
		antiinflammatory	phenylbutazone

[a]Toxic or idiosyncratic reaction.
[b]Hepatitis and cholestasis.

Obese adults and women appear more susceptible. A genetic predisposition has been postulated. If the necrosis is massive, postmortem pathology shows changes indistinguishable from viral hepatitis (84, 85).

HEPATITIS

The hepatocyte damage is identical to the lesion seen in viral hepatitis. Methyldopa is thought to act a hapten, creating a complex capable of inducing an autoimmune reaction in the hepatocyte. The resulting inflammatory response is responsible for the hepatitis. The immunologic reaction initiated by the methyldopa can be an acute hypersensitivity response—acute hepatitis—or a toxic complex, much like that seen in lupus, can develop, creating a chronic hepatitis. Isoniazid causes hepatocellular necrosis very similar to viral hepatitis in as many as 10% of persons taking the drug. (Refer to Chapter 64, "Tuberculosis.") A severe toxic hepatitis occurs in about 1%. Patients on isoniazid who are rapid acetylators might be at greater risk for developing drug-induced hepatitis (79).

FATTY LIVER (STEATONECROSIS)

Microvesicular (small droplets) fat accumulates in the hepatocyte. Inflammatory cells may be present, especially if necrosis coexists. AST and ALT may be normal or elevated, depending on severity. Alcohol is the most common cause of this type of lesion. Alcohol indirectly increases the synthesis of fatty acids, which are taken up by hepatocytes. If the hepatocyte becomes engorged and breaks open, an inflammatory response occurs leading to necrosis. Valproic acid and intravenous, high-dose tetracycline are thought to produce similar hepatitislike lesions (80).

CHOLESTASIS

Hepatic obstruction of biliary micelle by drugs leads to cholestatic hepatitis. The reaction may be hypersensitivity induced, as with chlorpromazine, erythromycin, and other antibiotics. The cholestasis may appear alone or with hepatocellular necrosis. Mortality is low, but recovery can sometimes take a long time (87, 88).

Diagnosis

Establishing the diagnosis of drug-induced hepatitis is usually difficult because the evidence is circumstantial. The clinical illness and liver function tests may be so like viral hepatitis as to be indistinguishable. Complete serology should be done to rule out viral hepatitis. A thorough drug history, including all nonprescribed and over-the-counter agents is essential. Association of symptoms with the start of a new drug might provide initial evidence. If the drug reactions is idiosyncratic, eosinophilia is frequently evident. Biopsy is not indicated, as it only defines the lesion, not the cause. The decision to call the hepatitis drug induced is to some extent based on what is not found. In chronic active hepatitis, virtually no drug, taken regularly, should be excluded as a possible cause (78).

Treatment and Prognosis

The first line of therapy is to remove the offending agent. The patient may improve rapidly, often within 1 or 2 weeks. Cholestatic hepatitis caused by drugs like chlorpromazine does not show rapid improvement. Alcoholic hepatitis usually resolves rapidly. However, alcoholic hepatitis from a drug such as amiodarone does not. Although the liver is healing, other organs of the body that may have been affected by the drug must be supported. If the hepatitis is severe and fulminant hepatic failure seems possible, corticosteroids may be indicated. With the exception of acetaminophen overdose (discussed earlier), there is no definitive treatment for drug-induced hepatitis (78).

Conclusions

Drug-induced liver disease is not as predictable as other medical problems, but understanding the potential for a hepatocellular injury with certain drugs provides an edge. For patients who are at risk (age, underlying liver disease, renal disease), monitoring for hepatic damage should be routinely performed.

For patients who are not considered at risk, routine monitoring of liver function is of questionable value. The best treatment is prevention or early intervention. Appropriate patient education is probably the best method of providing that treatment.

REFERENCES

1. Zuckerman AJ. Viral hepatitis. Transfus Med 3:7–19, 1993.
2. Lisanti P, Talotta D. An overview of viral hepatitis. A through E. AORN J 59:997–1005, 1994.
3. Anon. Hepatitis knowledge base. Ann Intern Med 93:191–222, 1980.
4. Tabor E. The three viruses of non-A, non-B hepatitis. Lancet 1:743–745, 1985.
5. Bradley DW. Hepatitis non-A, non-B viruses become identified as hepatitis C and hepatitis E viruses. Prog Med Virol 37:101–135, 1990.
6. Mudido P, Marshall GS, Howell RS, et al. Disseminated herpes simplex virus infection during pregnancy. A case report. J Reprod Med 38:964–968, 1993.
7. Fairley I, et al. Herpes hepatitis in pregnancy. J Clin Pathol 47:478, 1994.
8. Anon. Summary of notifiable diseases, United States 1993. MMWR 42(53), 1994.
9. Anon. Summary-cases of selected notifiable diseases through week 52, 1994. MMWR 44(1), 1995.
10. Koff RS. Viral hepatitis. New York: John Wiley & Sons, 1978, ch 1.
11. Bloch AB, Stramer SL, Smith JD, et al. Recovery of hepatitis A virus from a water supply responsible for a common source outbreak of hepatitis A. Am J Pub Health 80:428–431, 1990.
12. Rosenblum LS, Mirkin IR, Allen DT, et al. A multifocal outbreak of hepatitis A traced to commercially distributed lettuce. Am J Pub Health 80:1075–1080, 1990.
13. Ryder SD, Williams R. Liver disease. Postgrad Med J 70:162–184, 1994.
14. Shaw FE, Shapiro CN, Welty TK, et al. Hepatitis transmission among the Sioux Indians of South Dakota. Am J Pub Health 80:1091–1094, 1990.
15. Hoofnagle JH, Di Bisceglie AM. Serologic diagnosis of acute and chronic viral hepatitis. Semin Liver Dis 11:73–83, 1991.
16. Herrera JL. Serologic diagnosis of viral hepatitis. South Med J 87:677–684, 1994.
17. Balistreri WF. Viral hepatitis. Ped Clin North Am 35:637–669, 1988.
18. Holland PV. Hepatitis B surface antigen and antibody (HBsAg/anti-HBs). In: Gerety RJ, ed. Hepatitis B. Orlando, FL: Academic Press, 1985:5–25.
19. Pushko P, et al. Identification of Hepatitis B virus core protein regions exposed or internalized at the surface of HBcAg particles by scanning with monoclonal antibodies. Virology 202:912–920, 1994.
20. Alter MJ, Magolis HS. The emergence of hepatitis B as a sexually transmitted disease. Med Clin North Am 74:1529–1541, 1990.
21. Quint WG, et al. Absence of hepatitis B virus (HBV) DNA in children born after exposure of their mothers to HBV during in vitro fertilization. J Clin Microbiol 32:1099–1100, 1994.
22. Gerberding JL. Incidence and prevalence of Human Immunodeficiency virus, hepatitis B virus, hepatitis C virus, and cytomegalovirus among health care personnel at risk for blood exposure: final report from a longitudinal study. J Infect Dis 170:1410–1417, 1994.
23. Rosenblum LS, Hadler SC, Castro KG, et al. Heterosexual transmission of hepatitis B virus in Belle Glade, Florida. J Infect Dis 161:407–411, 1990.
24. Anon. The A to F of viral hepatitis. Lancet 336:1158–1160, 1990.
25. Nishioka NS, Dienstag JL. Delta hepatitis-a new scourge? N Engl J Med 312:1515–1516, 1985.
26. Sheen IS, et al. Role of hepatitis C and delta viruses in the termination of chronic hepatitis B surface antigen carier state: a multivariate analysis in a longitudinal follow-up study. J Infect Dis 170:358–361, 1994.
27. Hershow RC, Chomel BB, Graham, DR, et al. Hepatitis D virus infection in Illinois state facilities of the developmentally disabled. Ann Intern Med 110:770–785, 1989.
28. Mondelli MU, et al. Immunobioloby and pathogenesis of hepatitis C virus infection. Res Virol 144:269–274, 1993.
29. Chicheportiche C, et al. Analysis of ELISA hepatitis C virus- positive blood donors population by polymerase chain reaction and recombinant immunoblot assay (RIBA). Comparision of second and third generation RIBA. Acta Virol (Praha) 37:123–131, 1993.
30. Verbaan H, et al. Intravenous drug abuse—the major source of hepatitis C virus transmission among alcohol dependant individuals? Scand J Gastroenterol 28:714–718, 1993.
31. Medin C, et al. Seroconversion to hepatitis C virus in dialysis patients: a retrospective and prospective study. Nephron 65:40–45, 1993.
32. Dussol B, et al. Detection of hepatitis C infection by polymerase chain reaction among hemodialysis patients. Am J Kidney Dis 22:574–580, 1993.
33. Brechot C. Hepatitis C virus genetic variability: clinical implications. Am J Gastroenterol 89:s41–s47, 1994.
34. Reyes GR. Hepatitis E virus (HEV): molecular biology and emerging epidemiology. Prog Liver Dis 11:203–213, 1993.
35. Reyes GR, Kim JP, Luk KC, et al. Isolation of a cDNA from the virus responsible for enterically transmitted non-A, non-B hepatitis. Science 247:1335–1339, 1990.
36. Coursaget P, et al. Hepatitis type E in a French population: detection of anti-HEV by a synthetic peptide-based enzyme-linked immunosorbent assay. Res Vir 145:51–57, 1994.

37. Lok AS, Loldevila-Pico C. Epidemiology and serologic diagnosis of hepatitis E. J Hepatol 20:567–569, 1994.

38. Koff RS. Viral hepatitis. New York: John Wiley & Sons, 1978, ch 11.

39. Berry MA, Herrera JL. Diagnosis and treatment of chronic viral hepatitis. Compr Ther 20:16–19, 1994.

40. Maruyama T, et al. Serology of acute exacerbation in chronic hepatitis B virus infection. Gastroenterology 105:1141–1151, 1993.

41. Sherlock, S. Viruses and hepatocellular carcinoma. Gut 35:828–832, 1994.

42. Chen DS. From hepatitis to hepatoma: lessons from type B viral hepatitis. Science 262:369–370, 1994.

43. Katelaris PH, Jones DB. Fulminant hepatic failure. Med Clin North Am 73:955–970, 1989.

44. Hayashi PH, Zeldis JB. Molecular biology of viral ahepatitis hepatocellulur carcinoma. Compr Ther 19:188–196, 1993.

45. Sherlock DS. Chronic Hepatitis C. Dis Mon 40:117–196, 1994.

46. Alter MJ. The detection, transmission, and outcome of hepatitis C virus infection. Infect Agents Dis 2:155–166, 1993.

47. Lee HS, et al. Predominant etiologic association of hepatitis C virus with hepatocellular carcinoma compared with hepatitis B virus in elderly patients in a hepatitis B-endemic area. Cancer 72:2564–2567, 1993.

48. Chu CM, et al. The role of hepatitis C virus in fulminant viral hepatitis in an area with endemic hepatitis A and B. Gastroenterology 107:189–195, 1994.

49. A-Kader HH, Balistreri WF. Hepatitis C virus: implications to pediatric practice. Pediatr Infect Dis J 12:853–866, 1993.

50. Pastorek JG. The ABCs of hepatitis in pregnancy. Clin Obstet Gynecol 36:843–854, 1993.

51. Guillevin L, Lhote F, Leon A, et al. Treatment of polyarteritis nodosa related to hepatitis B virus with short term steroid therapy associated with antiviral agents and plasma exchanges. A prospective trial in 33 patients. J Rheumatol 20:289–298, 1993.

52. Dusheiko GM, et al. Treatment of chronic viral hepatitis. J Antimicrob Chemother 32:107–120, 1993.

53. Hoofnagle J, Davis GI, Pappas C, et al. A short course of prednisolone in chronic type B hepatitis: report of a randomized, double-blind, placebo controlled trial. Ann Intern Med 104:12–17, 1989.

54. Perrilo RP, Regenstein FG, Peters MG, et al. Prednisone withdrawal followed by recombinant alpha interferon in the treatment of chronic type B hepatitis: a randomized controlled trial. Ann Intern Med 109:95–100, 1988.

55. Fong TL, et al. Short term prednisone therapy affects aminotransferase activity and hepatitis C virus RNA level in chronic hepatitis C. Gastroenterology 107:196–199, 1994.

56. Di Bisceglie AM, Hoofnagle JH. Antiviral therapy of chronic viral hepatitis. Am J Gastroenterol 85:650–654, 1990.

57. Tine F, et al. Inteferon treatment in patients with chronic hepatitis B: a meta-analysis of the published literature. J Hepatol 18:154–162, 1993.

58. Romeo R, et al. Eradication of hepatitis C virus RNA after alpha-inteferon therapy. Ann Intern Med 121:276–277, 1994.

59. Di Bisceglie AM, Martin P, Kassianides C, et al. Recombinant inteferon alpha therapy for chronic hepatitis C. N Engl J Med 321:1506–1510, 1989.

60. Hoofnagle JH. Therapy of acute and chronic viral hepatitis. Adv Intern Med 30:241–242, 1994.

61. Gibas Al. Use of interferon in the treatmant of chronic viral hepatitis. Gastroenterologist 1:129–142, 1993.

62. Watson AR. High-dose interferon alfa-2A for the treatment of chronic hepatitis C. Ann Pharmacother 28:341–342, 1994.

63. Negro F, et al. Continuous versus intermittent therapy for chronic hepatitis C with recombinant interferon alfa-2a. Gastroenterology 107:479–485, 1994.

64. Feldman M. Selected summaries: revolutionary lifesaving therapy for acute hepatic failure, or yet another false hope? Gastroenterology 98:1088–1093, 1990.

65. Janssen HL, Berk L, Heijtink RA, et al. Interferon-alpha and zidovudine combination therapy for chronic hepatitis B: results of a randomized, placebo-controlled trial. Hepatology 17:383–388, 1993.

66. Brindle RJ, et al. Inadequate response to intradermal hepatitis A vaccine. Vaccine 12:483–484, 1994.

67. Wiedermann G, et al. Immunogenicity of an inactivated hepatitis A vaccine after exposure at 37 degrees C for 1 week. Vaccine 12:401–402, 1994.

68. Werzberger A, Mensch B, Kuter B, et al. A controlled trial of a formalin-inactivated hepatitis A vaccine in healthy children. N Engl J Med 327:543–557, 1992.

69. Tilzey AJ, Palmer SJ, Barrow S, et al. Clinical trial with inactivated hepatitis A vaccine and recommendations for its use. Br Med J 304:1272–1276, 1992.

70. Innis BL, Snitbhan R, Kunasol P, et al. Protection against hepatitis A by inactivated vacccine. JAMA 271:1328–1334, 1994.

71. Keyserling HL, et al. Antibody responses of healthy infants to recombinant hepatitis B vaccine administered at two, four, and twelve or fifteen months of age. J Pediatr 125:67–69, 1994.

72. Chirico G, et al. Hepatitis B immunization in infants of hepatitis B surface antigen-negative mothers. Pediatrics 92:717–719, 1993.

73. Chung RT, Kaplan LM. Parenterally transmitted hepatitis: viruses, vaccines, and antiviral therapy. Compr Ther 19:163–173, 1993.

74. McMahon BJ, et al. Seroprevalence of hepatitis B viral markers in 52,000 Alaska Natives. Am J Epidemiol 138:544–549, 1993.

75. Centers for Disease Control. Hepatitis B virus: a comprehensive strategy for eliminating transmission in the United States through universal childhood vaccination: recommendations of the Immunization Practices Advisory Committee (ACIP). MMWR 40:RR-13, 1991.

76. Tredger JM, Neuberger JM, Williams R. Drugs in acute hepatic necrosis. In Testa B, Perrissound D, eds. Liver drugs: from experimental pharmacology to therapeutic application. Boca Raton, FL: CRC Press, 1988:67.

77. MacGregor FB, Abernethy VE, Dahabre S, et al. Hepatotoxicity of herbal remedies. Br Med J 299:1156–1158, 1989.

78. Lewis JH, Zimmerman HJ. Drug-induced hepatotoxicity. Med Clin North Am 73:775–792, 1990.

79. Kaplowitz N. Drug-induced hepatotoxicity. Ann Intern Med 104:826–839, 1986.

80. Lee MG, Hanchard B, Williams NP. Drug-induced acute liver disease. Postgrad Med J 65:367–370, 1989.

81. Seeff LB, Cuccherini BA, Zimmerman HJ, et al. Acetaminophen hepatotoxicity in alcoholics: a therapeutic misadventure. Ann Intern Med 104:399–404, 1986.

82. Whitcomb DC, Geoffrey DB. Association of acetaminophen hepatotoxicity with fasting and ethanol use. JAMA 272:1845–1850, 1994.

83. Kumar S, Rex DK. Failure of physicians to recognize acetaminophen hepatotoxicity in chronic alcoholics. Arch Intern Med 151:1189–1191, 1991.

84. Gut J, et al. Mechanisms of halothane toxicity: novel insights. Pharmacol Ther 58:133–155, 1993.

85. Scheider DM, et al. Hepatic dysfunction after repeated isoflurane administration. J Clin Gastroenterol 17:168–170 1993.

86. Lienart F, Morrissens M, et al. Doxycycline and hepatotoxicity. Acta Clin Belg 47:205–208, 1992.

87. Mazuryk H, Kastenberg D, Rubin R, Munoz SJ. Cholestatic hepatitis associated with the use of nafcillin. Am J Gastroenterol 88:1960–1962, 1993.

88. Belknap MK, McClelland KJ. Cholestatic hepatitis associated with amoxicillin-clavulanate. Wis Med J 92:241–242, 1992.

CHAPTER 28

CIRRHOSIS

RICHARD BROWN, KATHY BIRD, and ANGELA PENTECOST

Cirrhosis is characterized by a diffuse increase in the fibrous connective tissue of the liver, with areas of both necrosis and regeneration of parenchymal cells imparting a nodular or glandular texture. In later stages, cirrhosis leads to such deformity of the liver that it interferes with hepatobiliary function and the circulation of blood both to and from the liver. Currently, no specific medical therapy exists for cirrhosis, except prevention. However, drugs are used to treat the complications of this disorder.

ETIOLOGY

Several major types of cirrhosis have been described (Table 28.1), but cirrhosis associated with alcohol abuse, or *Laennec's cirrhosis*, is by far the most commonly encountered form in the United States (1). Alcoholic liver disease usually begins with severe fatty changes in the liver. In the early stages this fatty infiltration is not associated with fibrosis and scarring. Later stages are marked by a prominent inflammation, an increase in fibrous tissue, and a progressive shrinkage, nodularity, and hardening of the liver.

In experimental animals, dietary derangements can induce fatty changes in the liver, with subsequent development of cirrhosis. Therefore, it is often claimed that dietary indiscretion in alcoholics may be an important underlying associated cause of cirrhosis. This concept is supported by the observation that when a chronic alcoholic is hospitalized and placed on an adequate diet, excess fat can be mobilized, and the liver structure and function may return to normal. This reversibility is less clear if fibrosis has already occurred. Other evidence implicates alcohol as a direct hepatotoxin. One group of investigators was able to demonstrate development of cirrhosis in baboons that were maintained on a balanced diet but given large daily doses of alcohol (2).

Biliary cirrhosis refers to cirrhosis following chronic obstruction of bile flow (cholestasis). Primary biliary cirrhosis follows long-standing cholestasis that is generally of unknown etiology, but it may have an underlying immunologic basis with elevated IgM, autoantibodies, and circulating complement-fixing immune complexes. Secondary biliary cirrhosis may be caused by stones or a tumor obstructing bile flow, leading to an inflammatory reaction and scarring.

Less common causes of cirrhosis are related to chronic viral hepatitis, immune-mediated chronic hepatitis, and various metabolic disorders (Table 28.1).

Table 28.1.
Cirrhosis: Incidence and Etiology

Type	Frequency (%)	Etiology
Alcohol-associated (Laennec's)	60–70	Alcohol abuse and protein deficiency inducing fatty changes, inflammation, and scarring liver
Biliary (primary and secondary)	10–15	Obstruction to bile flow, e.g., immune complexes, stones, and carcinoma; often secondary to long-standing bacterial infection
Postnecrotic	10–15	Scarring following massive hepatic necrosis such as that seen in chronic viral hepatitis, after exposure to hepatotoxic drugs, or in immune-mediated hepatitis
Metabolic	5–10	Excessive iron (hemochromatosis) or copper (Wilson's disease) deposition, α-1-antitrypsin deficiency, other inborn errors of metabolism

EPIDEMIOLOGY

It is difficult to cite an incidence of cirrhosis, since patients often do not exhibit any signs or symptoms. Autopsies at various hospitals have shown a frequency ranging from 3% to 15%. Cirrhosis is the ninth leading cause of death in the United States (3). Worldwide, the annual death rate from cirrhosis of all causes is as high as 15 to 40 persons per 100,000 population (4). Death and hospitalization rates of patients with chronic liver disease and cirrhosis are on the decline in the United States. In 1989, chronic liver disease was the underlying cause of death for 26,720 persons and a contributing cause of death for an additional 14,101 persons. From 1980 through 1989 the age-adjusted death rate for chronic liver disease decreased 23%, from 13.5 to 10.4 per 100,000 persons. Chronic liver disease appeared as the first diagnosis in an estimated 72,232 hospitalizations in 1989 and as a secondary diagnosis in an additional 218,156 hospitalizations. From 1980 through 1989 the hospitalization rate attributed to chronic liver disease and cirrhosis declined 44%, from 50.6 to 28.2 per 100,000 persons (5). Table 28.1 lists the relative frequencies of the various types of cirrhosis that are encountered clinically. The largest percentage is Laennec's cirrhosis, which occurs principally in patients between 40 and 60 years of age and is found most often in males. A history of chronic alcoholism can be obtained in 50 to 90% of these patients in the United States. The quantity of ethanol required by an individual to cause cirrhosis is 80 g/day for 5 years. With approximately 11 to 12 grams per average drink, 6 to 7 drinks per day over this period could be considered an etiological factor in cirrhosis. In Third World countries, children are frequently affected following maternally acquired hepatitis B (1, 3, 4).

CLINICAL FINDINGS AND DIAGNOSIS

Cirrhosis is insidious in its development and often produces no clinical manifestations. Up to 50% of all cases are discovered only at the time of postmortem examination. Many patients seek medical help, complaining of vague, nonspecific symptoms such as weight loss, loss of appetite, nausea, vomiting, and ill-defined digestive disturbances. Others enter the hospital acutely ill with the full syndrome of acute *alcoholic hepatitis* (a precursor to cirrhosis). These patients have *jaundice* (bilirubin levels range from 2 mg/dL to more than 40 mg/dL, mildly elevated serum aminotransferase (ALT and AST) and alkaline phosphatase levels, a low serum albumin level, evidence of impaired coagulation (prolonged prothrombin time), and right upper quadrant pain. In the later stages of cirrhosis, patients may have the complications of cirrhosis: ascites, gastrointestinal (GI) bleeding, and mental deterioration. Hepatocellular carcinoma develops in as many as 10% of subjects with long-standing cirrhosis.

COMPLICATIONS

The complications of cirrhosis generally relate to abnormalities in the portal venous system. The portal vein receives blood draining from the arterial and capillary system of the entire GI tract. This system is unique in that while it is a venous system, it has a second set of microvasculature (or sinusoids) that runs throughout the liver and then rejoins to empty into the hepatic veins and eventually the inferior vena cava. The main function of the portal venous network is to act as a pathway for detoxification and metabolism by the liver of substances absorbed from the GI tract. The portal venous system does not provide oxygenated blood to the liver (this is done by the hepatic artery). The anatomy of the portal system allows first-pass (presystemic) metabolism of orally administered drugs such as propranolol, verapamil, and morphine. As scarring and nodularity increase in the liver during cirrhosis, the blood flow through the portal system becomes obstructed, leading to a dramatic rise in the pressure of the portal vein and its tributaries in the GI tract (i.e., *portal hypertension*). Blood may also be shunted around the liver to empty directly into the systemic circulation (inferior vena cava). The clinical problems that arise secondary to portal hypertension include ascites, GI bleeding (varices), and encephalopathy.

Ascites

Ascites, which is characterized by the accumulation of protein-rich fluid in the peritoneal cavity, is one of the most striking features of cirrhosis. Complaints associated with ascites include a rapidly developing inability to fit into one's clothes, abdominal and back pain, gastroesophageal reflux, and shortness of breath secondary to impaired diaphragm movement or pleural effusions. The amount of fluid in the abdomen can vary from a few liters to 20 or more liters, leading to a large protuberant abdomen and an umbilical hernia. Ascitic fluid is a good culture medium for bacterial growth, and infections can occur spontaneously (spontaneous bacterial peritonitis). An unexplained high fever or elevated white blood cell count is an indication for obtaining a culture of an aspirate from the ascitic fluid or initiating appropriate antibiotic therapy.

Several postulates exist to explain the mechanism underlying the formation of ascites (see Fig. 28.1), none of which is fully accepted as the definitive answer (6, 7). Most of the postulates agree that disruption of hepatic architecture and blood flow due to inflammation, cell necrosis, fibrosis, or obstruction lead to hemodynamic alterations, causing an elevated lymphatic pressure within hepatic sinusoids, which eventually causes excessive transudation (weeping) of protein-rich fluid from the surface of the liver into the peritoneal cavity. According to the underfill theory, both the lymphatic leakage and high prehepatic venous pressure (portal hypertension) cause a net flow of volume from the vascular spaces to the third space of the peritoneal cavity via hydrostatic forces. The high protein content of the ascitic fluid may also help to draw volume out of the vasculature. As a result, effective vascular volume throughout the body is decreased, causing secondary sodium and water retention by the kidney. The renin-angiotensin system is a major mediator of the sodium and water retention, ultimately causing release of aldosterone by the adrenal gland. Release of antidiuretic hormone (ADH) may also be increased. Serum levels of aldosterone and ADH remain elevated because of impaired metabolism secondary to liver failure.

A major inconsistency with the underfill theory is that some patients have an increased, not decreased, total blood volume and not all patients have demonstrable hyperaldosteronism. According to another (the overfill) theory, the primary defect in ascites formation is excessive renal reabsorption of sodium and water. As plasma volume expands, ascites results because of overflow of fluid out of the splanchnic circulation and from increased pressure in the portal system. This implies that an unknown primary renal stimulus initiates the volume expansion. Increased sympathetic activity and a variety of hormonal substances

Mechanisms of Ascites Development

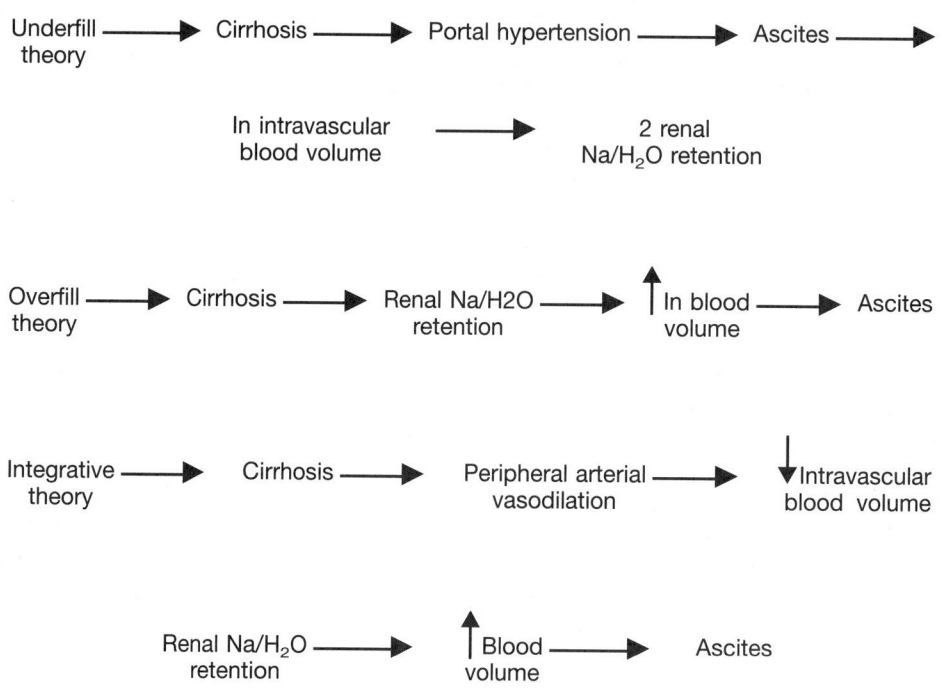

Figure 28.1. Ascites mechanisms.

have been proposed as factors affecting renal function in cirrhotic patients (8).

Schrier and colleagues (6) propose an integration of these two theories, citing a possible systemic intravascular vasodilation that causes a relative decrease in effective plasma volume or pressure, followed by excessive renal retention of sodium and water. Central blood volume has a primary influence on renal circulation. In cirrhotics, measurement of this vascular space reveals a reduced circulating volume even in patients who had not yet developed ascites. This volume reduction results from a vasodilated peripheral vascular system. The kidneys and arterial baroreceptors sense a peripheral vascular shift from the central circulation, activate vasoconstrictive systems, and enhance sodium reabsorption. The renin angiotensin aldosterone system and the release of vasopressin act to increase central vascular filling (9). Rocco and Ware (7) believe that both intrahepatic hypertension and a primary renal defect are responsible for the early stages of ascites.

Hypoalbuminemia, secondary to decreased hepatic synthesis and lymphatic leakage into the peritoneum, may contribute to further accumulation of ascites. A low serum albumin concentration causes a reduced serum osmotic (oncotic) pressure that again favors flow of fluid from the vasculature into the extravascular third space. Not all patients with cirrhosis have hypoalbuminemia, but those

that do may have both ascites and extensive peripheral edema with a relative systemic hypovolemia. Portal hypertension resulting in ascites can be distinguished from other causes (hepatoma, pancreatic ascites, biliary ascites) by evaluation of a serum albumin-ascites gradient. If the value of the gradient (serum albumin–ascites albumin) exceeds 1.1 g/dL, with 97% certainty, portal hypertension is present (10). Patients often have hyponatremia from retention of free water, induced by elevated antidiuretic hormone (ADH) levels. Hypokalemia may develop secondary to hyperaldosteronism and excessive vomiting.

GI Bleeding (Varices)

GI hemorrhage occurs in about one-fourth to one-third of patients. About one-third of these patients die from the initial hemorrhage. Even nonfatal GI hemorrhages tend to be massive. The major cause of GI bleeding associated with cirrhosis is shunting of blood away from the high-pressure portal system to low-pressure systemic collaterals in the esophagus (esophageal varices), rectum (hemorrhoids), and other parts of the GI tract. These veins become enlarged and tortuous and can easily rupture. Bleeding may be increased by an impaired clotting system caused by deficiencies in the vitamin K–dependent clotting factors. *Esophageal varices* account for about 50 to 60% of the GI bleeding observed in cirrhosis, and peptic ulcer disease accounts for another 25%.

Hepatic Encephalopathy

The ultimate result of advanced cirrhosis or severe hepatitis is liver failure and hepatic coma (hepatic encephalopathy). This is characterized by increasing drowsiness, personality changes, and mental confusion, with a characteristic flapping tremor of the fingers and hands when the wrists are hyperextended (liver flap or asterixis). Eventually, a deepening coma and death follow. Neurological complications include incoordination, tremor, nystagmus, and incontinence. As the disease progresses, a characteristic sweet, pungent odor (fetor hepaticus) may be present in the patient's breath. The cause of the odor is unclear but may be related to exhalation of mercaptans.

The diagnosis of hepatic encephalopathy may be complicated by other neurologic disorders including alcohol withdrawal–induced tremors, Wernicke's disease (mental disturbances, ataxia, and nystagmus from acute thiamine deficiency), Korsakoff's syndrome (psychosis and confabulation from chronic thiamine deficiency), and cerebellar damage from chronic alcohol ingestion. The presence of asterixis is a major differentiating factor.

The pathogenesis of hepatic encephalopathy is not well understood, but it may be related in part to increased arterial and central nervous system (CNS) ammonium levels. Although a direct cause-and-effect relationship has not been shown between encephalopathy and blood ammonium concentration, when factors that influence ammonium production are decreased, the patient's sensorium often clears. Dietary ingestion of food or bleeding into the gastrointestinal tract (e.g., esophageal bleeding) introduces a rich source of protein into the intestinal tract. Ammonia is produced in the lower gastrointestinal tract when these proteins and urea are metabolized by bacterial enzymatic action. The ammonia is then absorbed into the bloodstream and converted to ammonium ion. Normally, the liver converts the ammonium into urea for excretion by the kidney, but when the liver is malfunctioning or the blood is being shunted away from it, as in advanced cirrhosis, serum ammonium levels increase, and encephalopathy ensues. It is theorized that the cerebrotoxicity of ammonia is due to inhibition of oxidative metabolism by the citric acid cycle in the brain. α-Ketoglutarate combines with ammonia to produce high CNS levels of *glutamine* (a by-product of ammonium metabolism), while at the same time robbing the citric acid cycle of the α-ketoglutarate that is needed for production of high-energy adenosine triphosphate (ATP). Serum ammonium levels and cerebrospinal fluid (CSF) glutamine are sometimes measured to confirm hepatic encephalopathy.

An alternative explanation for the pathogenesis of hepatic encephalopathy concerns derangements in plasma and brain amino acid patterns (11–13). Characteristically, there is a relative elevation in methionine and *aromatic amino* acid levels (e.g., phenylalanine, tyrosine, and tryptophan) and a corresponding relative deficiency in *branched-chain* amino acids (e.g., valine, leucine, and isoleucine). These derangements lead to an imbalance of brain neurotransmitters, causing elevated levels of serotonin, octopamine, and phenylethanolamine and a decrease in dopamine and possibly norepinephrine. Serotonin is an end product of tryptophan metabolism, while phenylethanolamine and octopamine are by-products of phenylalanine and tyrosine metabolism.

While the exact reason for these derangements in plasma and brain amino acids is unknown, a number of observations have been made (7–9). The normal ratio of branched-chain amino acids (BCAAs) to aromatic amino acids (AAAs) is 4:1 to 6:1. In both sepsis and liver failure, catabolic states lead to a negative nitrogen balance and preferential use of BCAAs as a source of energy. As ammonia levels rise, glucagon secretion is stimulated, which in turn stimulates hepatic gluconeogenesis to convert amino acids into glucose for energy. In response to gluconeogenesis, insulin is secreted, which leads to increased uptake and metabolism of BCAAs by skeletal muscle. As liver failure progresses, the liver can no longer store or release glucose in adequate amounts, and thus greater quantities of BCAAs must be metabolized by skeletal muscle for energy.

Simultaneously, the plasma clearance of AAAs and methionine, which depends on hepatic metabolism, is diminished. The net result is an alteration of the BCAA/AAA ratio. In acute liver failure the AAAs rise dramatically, while BCAAs remain normal. In chronic hepatic disease the AAAs remain abnormally high, while BCAA concentrations drop to low levels, thus further lowering the BCAA/AAA ratio. In addition to alterations in amino acid metabolism, there appears to be a derangement of the blood-brain barrier during chronic liver disease. In people with hepatic encephalopathy, there is a selective increase in transport of AAAs across the blood-brain barrier, possibly via an exchange of CSF glutamine (from ammonia metabolism) for AAAs in the plasma. The arterial concentration of ammonium and other amines may be accentuated by excessive dietary protein consumption, GI hemorrhage (source of protein), overdiuresis leading to dehydration, or other conditions that lead to severe electrolyte imbalance and metabolic alkalosis.

An entirely different avenue of research suggests that the gamma-aminobutyric acid (GABA)–benzodiazepine receptor complex is involved in the pathogenesis of hepatic encephalopathy (14). GABA is the primary inhibitory neurotransmitter in the CNS. According to this theory, an increase in CNS GABA-ergic neurotransmission may partially account for the behavioral and electrophysiologic manifestations of encephalopathy. This hypothesis is based on the observation that an accentuation of CNS inhibitory neurotransmitter tone can cause ataxia, sedation, and coma. While GABA levels do not seem to be elevated in patients with encephalopathy, it is speculated that other endogenous or exogenous GABA-like ligands may be involved. Not surprisingly, these patients also demonstrate unusual sensitivity to benzodiazepinelike drugs that elicit GABA-ergic-like activity.

Other Associated Disorders

Anemia and other hematologic disorders commonly accompany cirrhosis. Chronic alcohol abusers tend to malabsorb *folic acid,* as well as iron. In addition, their diets may be deficient in both iron and folate. *Iron deficiency* may be further aggravated by a blocking of iron uptake into the bone marrow induced by chronic alcoholism and by slow GI bleeding due to gastritis. Thrombocytopenia and leukopenia may occur because of folic acid deficiency and hypersplenism secondary to portal hypertension.

Endocrine disorders are seen in advanced cirrhosis because of the liver's inability to metabolize the steroid hormones of the adrenals and gonads. In the male, increased circulating estrogen levels cause gynecomastia, testicular atrophy, loss of body hair, impotence, spider angiomas, and palmar erythema.

The concurrent impairment of renal function with hepatic failure is termed the *hepatorenal syndrome* (HRS). HRS develops in about 4% of patients with decompensated cirrhosis and is associated with a poor prognosis. More than 95% of these patients die within a few weeks after onset of azotemia. HRS is characterized by increased renal vascular resistance and decreased systemic vascular resistance. The complex hemodynamic changes occur in response to vasoactive agents that produce different effects on the systemic and renal circulation. The vasoactive agents and systems involved in HRS are the renin-angiotensin-aldosterone system, the sympathetic nervous system, antidiuretic hormone, and the renal prostaglandin and kinin systems. HRS may occur acutely or progressively. The acute onset generally occurs in patients with end-stage cirrhosis or in consequence to other complications such as encephalopathy, bacterial infections, or bleeding. Clinical symptoms include oliguria that develops within a few days, along with a rapid increase in plasma urea and creatinine levels, tense ascites, dilutional hyponatremia, hypotension, and jaundice. A slower progressive type involving other chronic types of renal conditions associated with liver disease exhibits a gradual decrease in glomerular filtration rate that may last for several weeks or months. These patients may also demonstrate ascites that is poorly responsive to diuretics (15).

TREATMENT OF CIRRHOSIS

Management of cirrhosis is largely symptomatic (Table 28.2). In Laennec's cirrhosis the primary treatment is to encourage the patient to abstain from alcohol. Fluid and electrolyte balance should be maintained either by parenteral administration or by oral therapy. If the patient is vomiting, antiemetics may be used. However, the phenothiazine-type antiemetics (e.g., prochlorperazine) have been associated with cholostasis and should be used with caution. Analgesics may be cautiously administered for abdominal pain. Aspirin-containing products and nonsteroidal antiinflammatory drugs may worsen gastritis or GI bleeding. Also, acetaminophen hepatotoxicity may be more prevalent in alcoholic patients. Narcotics may lead to profound CNS and respiratory depression if the patient's liver status is severely compromised or if the patient is already obtunded. Sedatives and hypnotics should be avoided if there is any danger of the patient's developing hepatic coma. If there are no signs of impending hepatic coma, the patient should be maintained on a 2000- to 3000-calorie diet with 1 g of protein per kilogram of body weight. If encephalopathy is present, dietary supplements that are rich in branched-chain amino acids and low in aromatic amino acids (e.g., Hepatic Aid) have been used in an attempt to prevent negative nitrogen balance in patients who are intolerant to standard proteins.

Vitamin replacement is essential in most cirrhotic patients, especially those with a recent alcoholic history. Replacement of thiamine at 50 to 100 mg/day along with a good diet may improve mentation, decrease symptoms of nutritional polyneuropathy, and improve gait disorders. Continuation of thiamine therapy beyond 1 or 2 weeks is of questionable value, since it is a water-soluble vitamin whose stores are rapidly replaced. Up to 1 g per day may occasionally be required if the patient displays severe nystagmus, Wernicke's encephalopathy, or oculogyric crisis. Iron replacement or folic acid supplements are required if the patient is anemic. Iron deficiency is confirmed by measurement of serum iron, TIBC, and ferritin concentrations (see Chapter 13, "Iron Deficiency and Megaloblastic Anemias").

Vitamin K, 10 mg subcutaneously daily for 3 or more days, is given if the prothrombin time is elevated. If the prothrombin time is not reversed after 3 to 5 doses, further doses should be avoided, as an occasional patient will demonstrate a paradoxical lengthening of the prothrombin time from excessive vitamin K. This paradoxical effect is theorized to be a result of consumptive processes induced by overstimulation of the production of clotting factors, leading to an eventual depletion of the body stores. Vitamin K_1, or *phytonadione (Aquamephyton),* gives a more rapid response when given parenterally than does either vitamin K_3 (mendadione) or vitamin K_4 (menadiol). In giving vitamin K parenterally, the subcutaneous route is preferred, but it may also be given by very slow intravenous infusion in 50 mL of 5% dextrose in water (D_5W) over 15 to 20 min. Intramuscular injections are contraindicated if the patient has a prolonged prothrombin time or throm-

Table 28.2.
Drugs Used in Cirrhotic Patients

Thiamine
  Reason: reverse mental confusion secondary to thiamine deficiency
    (Wernicke's syndrome) and decrease peripheral neuropathies
  Dose: 100–200 mg/day, occasionally higher
  Monitoring parameters
    Mental status
    Decrease in nystagmus, peripheral neuropathies; more than 10
    days of therapy is unwarranted
Vitamin K (phytonadione) (AquaMethyton preferred)
  Reason: prevent bleeding secondary to decreased production of fac-
    tors II, VII, IX, and X (vitamin K–dependent factors)
  Dose: 10–15 mg/day, not to exceed 3 doses
  Monitoring parameters:
    Hypersensitivity—fever, chills, anaphylaxis, flushing, sweating
    Prothrombin time
Spironolactone
  Reason: diuresis in ascites; specific for antagonism of preexisting
    hyperaldosteronism
  Dose: 200–400 mg/day, occasionally higher; may be given as a single
    daily dose
  Monitoring parameters:
    Weight (avoid more than 1-kg weight loss per day)
    Mental status
    Serum K^+
    Urine Na^+ and K^+ (Na^+ should not exceed K^+ at therapeutic
    doses)
    Abdominal girth
    BUN (increased in dehydration)
    Gynecomastia—prolonged use
    Blood pressure
Loop diuretics
  Reason: diuresis in ascites after failure of high-dose spironolactone
  Dose: start at 40 mg, titrate to 1-kg weight loss per day; occasionally
    very high doses (200–600 mg/day) required
  Monitoring parameters:
    Same as spironolactone except urine electrolytes of no value
    Possible hearing loss with rapid IV bolus
Vasopressin
  Reason: vasoconstrictor for esophageal bleeding
  Dose: 0.2–0.4 u/min i.v. infusion
  Monitoring parameters:
    Rate of GI bleeding
    Signs of ischemia—chest pain, elevated blood pressure, brady-
    cardia
    GI cramping
    Serum Na^+
Sodium tetradecyl sulfate, ethanolamine oleate, or sodium morrhuate
  Reason: sclerosing agent for esophageal bleeding
  Dose: 0.5–2 mL of 1–1.5% tetradecyl, 5% ethanolamine, or 5%
    sodium morrhuate solution in each varix about 2 cm apart
  Monitoring parameters:
    Signs of GI bleeding
    Chest pain, fever, local ulceration
Propranolol
  Reason: prevent GI bleeding
  Dose: 40–320 mg/day titrated to 25% reduction in resting pulse rate
    if tolerated

Monitoring parameters:
  Signs of GI bleeding
  Mental changes
  Vital signs: pulse >60; blood pressure >100/70
  Signs of congestive heart failure, bradycardia
  Signs of bronchospasm
  Renal function
Lactulose
  Reason: hepatic encephalopathy; converted to lactic acid to lower
    bowel pH and prevent absorption of NH_3
  Dose: 20–30 g q.i.d. or 300 cc of 50% lactulose qs to 700–1000 cc
    as rectal enema titrated to 3–4 soft stools per day
  Monitoring parameters:
    Mental status, liver flap
    Diarrhea
Neomycin
  Reason: hepatic encephalopathy; sterilizes gut to prevent bacterial
    breakdown of protein and thus decreases serum NH_3 levels
  Dose: 2–6 g/day, orally or rectally
  Monitoring parameters:
    Mental status, liver flap
    Diarrhea, bacterial overgrowth
    Renal function
    Signs of ototoxicity
Hepatamine and Hepatic-Aid[a]
  Reason: hepatic encephalopathy; replace branched-chain amino
    acids
  Dose: Titrate to caloric and nitrogen needs
  Monitoring parameters:
    Mental status
    Serum ammonia, CSF glutamine
    Serum amino acid levels (BCAA:AAA ratio)
    Electrolyte balance
Dopamine[a]
  Reason: hepatorenal syndrome
  Dose: 1–4 µg kg/min
  Monitoring parameters:
    Mental status, liver flap
    Urine output
    Blood pressure
Cochicine[a]
  Investigational use only; efficacy unclear
  Reason: antiinflammatory and antifibrotic effects
  Dose: 0.6 mg p.o. b.i.d. or 1 mg p.o. q.d. 5 days/week
  Monitoring parameters:
    Nausea, abdominal pain, diarrhea
Norfloxacin[a]
  Reason: prevention of spontaneous bacterial peritonitis (SBP)
  Dose: 400 mg daily or 400 mg b.i.d. Monitoring parameters:
    Reduction in incidence of SBP episodes
Flumazenil[a]
  Investigational use only; efficacy unclear
  Reason: reversal of hepatic encephalopathy
  Dose 0.2–0.4 mg titrated to response
  Monitoring parameters:
    Reversal of mental obtundation

[a]Not recommended for all patients

bocytopenia due to the possibility of hematoma and further complications. Since phytonadione is a colloidal suspension, there is a small risk of development of fever, chills, and even anaphylactic reactions with rapid intravenous injection. If the patient is malabsorbing fats, menadiol is the vitamin K of choice for oral administration, since it is water-soluble and is absorbed independent of bile acids.

Ascites

The reversal of ascites is a time-consuming process requiring weeks and even months of conservative management including bed rest to decrease plasma renin release, salt restriction (500 mg to 2 g/day), and, in some cases, fluid restriction. Approximately 5% of patients will have a spontaneous diuresis with bed rest alone, and another 10 to 25% will respond to salt restriction (7). Fluid restriction is warranted only in cases of hyponatremia, since excessive fluid restriction may lead to decreased renal blood flow and azotemia. Hospitalization is usually recommended for these patients for three reasons: (a) intensive education on medications and diet; (b) close monitoring of serum and urine electrolytes, urea nitrogen, and creatinine; and (c) investigation into the cause of the liver disease.

Diuresis is the cornerstone of drug therapy of ascites, but the diuresis must be slow. If urinary losses exceed the volume of fluid reabsorbed from ascites or peripheral edema, volume depletion with hypotension and renal insufficiency can ensue. In patients who are treated with sodium restriction alone, no more than 300 mL of ascites can be reabsorbed per day. Even with the use of a diuretic, the maximum rate of reabsorption is 750 to 1440 mL per 24 hours (16, 17). Diuresis should be limited to 0.2 to 0.3 kg weight loss per day in those without edema and 0.5 to 1 kg per day in patients with edema (7). Others allow a slightly more liberal diuresis of 0.75 to 2 kg weight loss per day (17). These recommendations assume that each liter of volume lost is equivalent to a 1-kg weight loss. In patients with concurrent peripheral edema, a greater diuresis may be acceptable for the first 1 to 2 days because peripheral edema equilibrates more readily with the vasculature than does ascitic fluid. Other monitoring parameters include volume of urine output, changes in abdominal girth, postural blood pressures, blood urea nitrogen (avoiding prerenal azotemia), increase in urine potassium/sodium ratio from pretreatment baseline, and changes in mental status.

Although slow diuresis with any diuretic is acceptable for the treatment of ascites, the first diuretic given is usually *spironolactone (Aldactone)*. It is a gentle, slow-acting diuretic, specific for antagonizing the effects of the hyperaldosteronism that exists in many of these patients. In contrast to the small doses of spironolactone that are used as an adjunct in hypertension, the dose in ascites is begun at 50 to 100 g per day. A 3- to 5-day lag period exists for the onset and maximum response from spironolactone, so frequent dose adjustments should be avoided. Doses are titrated upward in 50- to 100-mg intervals every 3 to 5 days, 400 mg per day being needed eventually in 75% of patients. Even greater doses, up to 1 g per day, have been used, but this is expensive, and other diuretics such as furosemide are usually added before doses of this magnitude are tried. The delayed onset and long duration of spironolactone are due to the long half-life (approximately 17 hr) of its active metabolite, canrenone. For patients' convenience, once-daily dosing should be recommended. Multiple daily doses are not necessary unless the patient cannot swallow the required number of tablets without gastric distress. Triamterene (Dyrenium) or amiloride (Midamor) may be slightly more rapid in onset, but they are not specific aldosterone inhibitors. Clinically, they are probably equal in effect to spironolactone, although the response of ascites to these drugs in comparison with spironolactone has not been extensively studied.

Besides the general monitoring parameters cited above for diuretic therapy, serum and urine electrolyte levels, especially potassium, must be monitored. If hyperaldosteronism is present, it is not uncommon to see very little or no urinary sodium excretion and exceedingly large urinary potassium losses. One measure of having achieved the desired spironolactone dose is a reversal of the urine electrolyte pattern to normal (i.e., sodium loss greater than potassium loss). Patients with urine sodium-to-potassium ratios greater than 1 tend to respond to lower dosages of spironolactone (100 to 150 mg/day); those with ratios less than 1 often require larger doses, averaging 400 mg/day (7).

Hyperaldosteronism, if present, may also cause a reduction in serum potassium concentration. While the use of spironolactone with potassium supplements is nearly always contraindicated in treatment of other diseases because of a high risk of inducing hyperkalemia, this combination may be necessary early in the treatment of ascites, especially if the patient has GI losses of potassium secondary to vomiting or diarrhea. Serum potassium must be monitored daily to avoid either hypoalkalemia or hyperkalemia. Since these patients are often placed on low-sodium diets, salt substitute use should be discouraged to further limit the complexity of potassium supplementation in this setting. Long-term use of spironolactone can lead to gynecomastia, a problem that is frequently present in cirrhosis independent of diuretic use.

High spironolactone doses may fail to produce the desired diuresis in some patients or may cause hyperkalemia. In these situations the addition of more potent diuretics such as thiazides and loop diuretics may be warranted. The dose should be started low, 50 mg/day of hydrochlorothiazide or 20 to 40 mg/day of furosemide, and gradually increased. Some patients are especially refractory, requiring several hundred milligrams per day of furosemide to obtain the desired 0.5- to 1-kg/day weight loss. One drawback to the use of thiazides and loop diuretics is that they cause a significant natriuresis, which negates the value of monitoring urine electrolytes. Intravenous furosemide should be avoided if possible, since it can decrease glomerular filtration rates (18).

Paracentesis (aspiration of peritoneal fluid with a needle), except for removal of small volumes (250 to 1500 mL) to decrease pain and respiratory distress from abdominal stretching, has traditionally been discouraged because of the risk of abdominal perforation and introduction of infection. Of greater concern was that if large volumes are removed, 15 to 100% (mean 58%) of the fluid reaccumulates over the next 24 to 48 hr, leading to transient hypovolemia and the possibility of shock, encephalopathy, or acute renal failure (16).

Recently, however, the combination of therapeutic paracentesis with intravenous albumin infusions (to hold volume in the vascular space) has become an accepted mode of therapy (19–22). A typical regimen is removal of 4 to 6 L/day via paracentesis, with replacement of 40 to 50 g of albumin after each tap. Paracentesis with albumin replacement is superior to diuretic therapy; it decreases ascites faster and shortens hospital stay without significant worsening of hepatic, renal, or cardiovascular function. Single large-volume (5-L) paracentesis without albumin replacement also appears to be safe in patients with painful, tense ascites (23); but repeated large-volume paracentesis without albumin replacement may result in hyponatremia or renal impairment in some patients (20). One other possible concern over paracentesis is an increased risk of spontaneous bacterial peritonitis secondary to reduced ascitic fluid opsonic activity (24). Arguments about the high cost of albumin are counterbalanced by decreased hospitalization time. The use of Dextran as a volume expander after paracentesis has been looked at as an alternative to albumin (25). It has been shown to help prevent the asymptomatic abnormalities in lab values at a decreased cost (18). Albumin has also been used without paracentesis in an attempt to increase intravascular volume and to induce diuresis. The drawbacks to this treatment are a short duration of response, the risk of inducing variceal hemorrhage, and high cost. Generally, treatment with albumin without paracentesis is to be avoided unless all other therapies have failed. In Europe, ascites recirculation with removal, concentration, and reinfusion of peritional fluid has been found to be safe and effective (26). The possibility of reaccumulation of ascites after paracentesis will require continuation of a low-sodium diet and diuretics.

A *peritoneovenous shunt* (*LeVeen shunt*), in use extensively for the last 18 to 20 years, was devised for use in refractory cases of ascites (27, 28). The shunt consists of a surgically implanted one-way valve in the abdominal wall,

an intraabdominal cannula, and an outflow tube tunneled subcutaneously from the valve to a vein that empties directly into the inferior vena cava. As the diaphragm descends, the pressure in the intrathoracic veins drops, and intraperitoneal pressure rises. This pressure differential pumps the ascitic fluid into the venous system. The results may be dramatic, with urine output as high as 15 L occurring during the first 24 hours. Supplemental diuresis with furosemide may be required to prevent vascular overload. However, use of this procedure is limited by such complications as fever, shunt occlusions, hypokalemia, infection, shunt leaks, disseminated intravascular coagulopathy (DIC), and (less frequently) variceal hemorrhage, bowel obstruction, pulmonary edema, and pneumothorax (27). A Veterans Administration Cooperative study involving 3860 patients demonstrated no improved survival and significant morbidity in patients treated with peritoneovenous shunt compared with diuretic therapy (28). However, shunting alleviated disabling ascites more rapidly than medical management did.

Spontaneous Bacterial Peritonitis

By definition, spontaneous bacterial peritonitis (SBP) is the spontaneous infection of ascitic fluid without any evidence of an intraabdominal or extraabdominal source for the infection. SBP occurs in approximately 30 to 40% of all cirrhotic patients (29). While some patients may be asymptomatic, commonly observed signs and symptoms include fever, chills, vomiting, abdominal pain or tenderness, decreased bowel sounds, and encephalopathy. Diagnosis is made through paracentesis. Positive cultures and/or PMN cell counts of >250/mm^3 are indicative of SBP (30, 31).

The exact pathophysiology for SBP is unclear, but several potential mechanisms have been proposed. One of the most likely routes is through hematogenous spread. Portal blood flow in cirrhotic patients may bypass the liver, permitting circulating bacteria to avoid removal by the hepatic reticuloendothelial filtering system. Second, portal hypertension causes congestion in the lymphatic and splanchnic veins, resulting in inflammation and edema in the bowel wall. A decreased local resistance to bacterial invasion via bowel translocation may occur in these patients (30).

The organisms of primary concern in SBP are the enteric Gram-negative bacilli and some streptococcus strains. Anaerobes and pseudomonal and staphylococcal species are not an issue. Empiric therapy has traditionally been ampicillin or a first-generation cephalosporin in combination with an aminoglycoside. More recently, clinical use of less toxic alternative agents such as cefotaxime, ampicillin/sulbactam, ticarcillin/clavulanate, or second-generation cephalosporins such as cefotetan or cefoxitin have also provided acceptable outcomes. Caution is advised with cefotetan, since the presence of the methylthiotetrazole side chain may further complicate an existing hypoprothrombinemic state. Cefotaxime is generally accepted to be the current drug of choice for SBP (32, 33). Either drug can be used until final culture and sensitivity information is available. Duration of therapy may be shortened to 5 days owing to the relative low innoculum of organisms in the ascitic fluid (34).

Some patients are at greater risk for development of SBP and its complications. These include cirrhotic patients with ascites who have GI hemorrhage, encephalopathy, or a history of previous episodes of SBP; patients with decreased protein levels in their ascitic fluid; and those awaiting liver transplant. Prevention of SBP in these patients has been attempted. Four hundred milligrams of Nofloxacin given once daily has been sucessfully used as prophylactic treatment for high-risk patients. This fluoroquinolone causes a selective intestinal decontamination that eliminates the Gram-negative bacilli yet preserves the remaining normal flora. Norfloxacin was shown to markedly reduce the incidence of SBP in patients with previous SBP episodes and is considered a safe and effective long-term treatment for SBP prophylaxis (35). Twice-daily dosing of the drug may be required in patients who are experiencing gastrointestinal hemorrhage (36). Singh and colleagues have also shown trimethoprim-sulfamethoxazole to be of value in SBP prevention (37).

GI Bleeding

Bleeding from esophageal varices is a grave sign and may be difficult to stop. It often requires multiple transfusions. Even if the bleeding is stopped, the chances of the patient hemorrhaging again are high. One way to control a simple bleed is by direct pressure. Historically, placement of a lumened inflatable balloon tube (Linton, Minnesota, or Sengstaken-Blakemore tube) to slow the bleeding by compression is sometimes tried, with varied results. The balloon inflates, and the varix is compressed between the balloon and esophageal wall, leading to a clotting of the laceration. This procedure is complicated by vomiting and a high rate of aspiration or recurrence of bleeding as soon as the balloon is deflated. Bleeding is stopped in 40 to 80% of patients, but use of this procedure, by current standards, is only a temporary measure.

Injecting sclerosing agents into esophageal varices is receiving increased interest (38–43). This approach is considered by many to be the therapy of choice. Although not a new technique, *sclerotherapy* remained impractical until the widespread availability of the flexible, fiberoptic esophagoscope in the 1970s. Percutaneous transhepatic sclerotherapy or embolization is a major operative procedure involving insertion of a catheter into the gastric and coronary veins via initial entry into the portal vein. Hypertonic glucose or Gel Foam is then injected into the vessels to obliterate them and prevent flow to the esophageal vessels. A less invasive procedure involves direct injection of bleeding varices with a sclerosing agent via an endoscope. The most commonly used sclerosants in the United States are sodium tetradecyl sulfate (Sotradecol), ethanolamine oleate (Ethamolin), and sodium morrhuate (Scleromate). Injection of these agents into a bleeding varix leads to intense inflammatory response, thrombus formation, and cessation of bleeding within 2 to 5 min. A more permanent fibrotic obliteration of the vessel will develop over several days.

Sclerotherapy controls acute variceal bleeding in 90 to 95% of patients, nearly twice the rate of benefit achieved with either balloon tamponade or vasopressin (38). A single treatment controls bleeding in 90% of subjects, the remainder requiring one or more repeated treatments over several weeks. Success rates are lower in patients who are treated while actively bleeding, rather than controlling bleeding initially by more conservative methods. Failure of therapy is defined as continuation of bleeding after two injections of a sclerosing agent during a single admission (44). Compared with portacaval and splenorenal shunt procedures, sclerotherapy is almost equally effective in stopping bleeding, there is no difference in survival, and there is much lower morbidity (40, 41). Prophylactic sclerotherapy in patients with endoscopic evidence of varices, but with no history of past or current bleeding, is of no apparent clinical benefit (42, 43).

A 0.5 to 3% solution of tetradecyl, a premixed solution of ethanolamine 5% or morrhuate 5% for injection is used. After passing the endoscope, approximately 0.5 to 2 mL of sclerosing solution is injected into each varix at points about 2 to 4 cm apart. If bleeding recurs, therapy can be repeated. While it appears that sclerotherapy is effective in stopping acute bleeding and in preventing rebleeding, compared with more conventional therapy, over 50% of patients rebleed, and long-term mortality does not decrease. Side effects associated with sclerotherapy include pericarditis, chest pain, dysphagia, pyrexia, cardiac tamponade, formation of esophagobronchial fistulae, and local ulcerations.

Following sclerotherapy, prophylaxis with antacids, histamine-2 (H$_2$) antagonists, omeprazole, and/or sucralfate may be initiated. Dosing of these drugs is the same as that recommended for treatment of peptic ulcer disease or reflux esophagitis (see Chapter 23, "Peptic Ulcer Disease"). Careful monitoring of mental status in patients who are treated with cimetidine is a must, since cirrhosis may predispose them to the mental confusion associated with this agent (45). The pharmacokinetics of ranitidine may also be altered in cirrhosis, resulting in its accumulation (46). Sucralfate suspension has been used to prevent ulcers at the sclerosis site. Investigators using endoscopy have shown that the drug complex coats the varices and decreases ulcer formation (47). The aluminum component of sucralfate may complex with coadministered norfloxacin, resulting in poor absorption. The importance of this is questionable, since the value of norfloxacin in SBP prevention is probably dependent on a local intestinal, rather than a systemic action.

A newer endoscopic technique for control of variceal bleeds is endoscopic variceal banding therapy (EBT). The success rate of this procedure may be as high as 90% (48). The procedure involves endoscopic placement of a small rubber band over a distal varix. Banding is executed by suction aspiration of a large varix into the end portion of the sleeve with a triggering of the band over the base of the varix. This requires a specially modified endoscope that carries a triggering device and rubber band on a small sleeve over the objective end of the scope. Though not widely used, EBT has a control rate of 86% for acute bleed. It has also been associated with a lower complication rate, although the risk of rebleeding may be slightly higher than that of sclerotherapy (49, 50).

The natural hormone vasopressin (also known as antidiuretic hormone or ADH) was frequently used to treat bleeding varices before the advent of sclerotherapy. Vasopressin significantly decreases portal blood flow and pressure by constricting portal and other splanchnic arterioles. This slows or stops bleeding long enough to allow thrombus formation at the site of bleeding. The use of this drug is declining and remains controversial, since the benefits in morbidity and mortality have never been clearly proven (51). Sclerotherapy has been shown consistently to be more effective than vasopressin, but vasopression may be given first to slow bleeding and make visualization of bleeding varices by endoscope easier.

The major limitation to vasopressin therapy is side effects. The intense vasoconstrictor action decreases cardiac output and may cause coronary ischemia. This is especially a problem in patients who have coronary artery disease or hypertension, but ischemic changes have also been reported in patients with no prior evidence of ischemic disease (51). Bradycardia due to stimulation of the vagus nerve is the most widely observed side effect of vasopressin (51). It also may produce skin blanching, GI cramping, and even bowel necrosis due to stimulation of smooth muscle contraction. Women may experience uterine pain similar to menstrual cramps. Finally, vasopressin may lead to excess water retention and a dilutional hyponatremia (51).

In an attempt to reduce toxicity, continuous intravenous infusions starting at 0.2 to 0.4 unit/min or direct intraarterial infusion via a catheter into the superior mesenteric artery at 0.05 to 0.4 unit/min have been tried (51). The maximum recommended intravenous infusion rate is 0.9 unit/min. Infusions may be continued for up to 72 hr with a slow tapering of the dose over time. The results have been varied, some authors claiming up to 50 to 70% effectiveness (51). Others claim poor response and a high incidence of complications, including bleeding from the site of catheter insertion and septicemia (52).

A combination of vasopressin infusion and intravenous nitroglycerin (40 µg/min titrated according to blood pressure to a maximum of 400 µg/min) (53) or sublingual nitroglycerin (0.6 mg every 30 min for 6 hr) (54) may cause an additional decrease in portal pressure. In the study using intravenous nitroglycerin, there was less bleeding in the combination therapy group; in the trial with sublingual nitroglycerin, the rate of bleeding cessation was equal to that with vasopression alone. In both studies, combination therapy led to a marked reduction in cardiac complications.

The use of somatostatin has also been evaluated in controlling variceal bleed. Somatostatin reduces portal pressure and blood flow with continuous intravenous administration. It offers efficacy equal to that of vasopressin with considerably decreased side effects. Its use is limited by its significantly higher cost; therefore it is not considered as a first-line therapy (55).

Bleeding from other GI sites, especially bleeding due to gastritis and peptic ulcer, is usually treated with nasogastric suction, tap water lavage, H_2 antagonists, omeprazole, or hourly antacids (56). Occasionally, 20 units of vasopressin, 1 to 2 ampules of norepinephrine, or ice is used in a gastric lavage to cause localized vasoconstriction in an attempt to slow bleeding. No evidence documents these latter maneuvers to be any more effective than tap water lavage or H_2 antagonists alone; therefore their use is generally discouraged.

It has been suggested that since propranolol and possibly other beta-adrenergic blockers decrease portal venous pressure, they may prevent gastrointestinal bleeding associated with portal hypertension (57–62). Primary therapy is defined as treatment of patients with known varices but without a history of active bleeding. Secondary intervention involves administration of the drug following resolution of an acute bleeding episode. Although data is still somewhat limited, overall analysis of the benefit of primary therapy is positive (57–59). For example, in the European Cooperative study group, a median dose of 160 mg/day (range 40 to 320 mg) led to a cumulative 74% of patients in the propranolol group who were free of bleeding after 2 years, compared with 39% in the placebo group. Two-year survival was 72% in the treated patients and 37% in the untreated subjects (59).

The results for secondary prophylaxis are also encouraging but somewhat more complex. Lebrec and colleagues (60) showed that oral propranolol in doses that reduced the heart rate by 25% significantly reduced the frequency of rebleeding, compared with placebo, during a 2-year study in chronic alcoholics with a history of prior esophageal bleeding. Only 21% of patients in the propranolol group had recurrence of bleeding, compared with 68% in the placebo group. Cumulative survival was 90% in the propranolol group and 57% in the placebo group. None of the patients showed deterioration of hepatic or renal function while taking propranolol; but because propranolol may decrease cardiac output and liver blood flow, patients should be monitored closely.

A similar study by Burroughs et al. (61) failed to confirm the findings of Lebrec. However, the patients in Burroughs' study had more severe liver disease and included some with cirrhosis from causes other than chronic alcoholism. Selective beta-blockade with atenolol or metoprolol is less effective than sclerotherapy in arresting acute variceal bleeding (57, 58).

A follow-up study by Poynard, Lebrec, and colleagues (62) confirms the benefits of propranolol, with 71% of subjects free of bleeding at 1 year and 57% at 2 years. In this study, five factors were identified that increased the risk of rebleeding: hepatocellular carcinoma, continued alcohol abuse, lack of suppression of pulse rate by propranolol, a previous history of rebleeding, and noncompliance with drug therapy. Of particular concern, 12 of 14 (86%) patients who discontinued beta-blocker therapy abruptly rebled. The time of greatest risk for rebleeding is within the first 3 to 4 days of stopping therapy, but it may occur up to 150 days later (57, 58, 62–64). It is not possible to be certain that drug discontinuation is responsible for rebleeding in the cases in which the occurrence is delayed.

A recent randomized controlled study by Teres et al. in Barcelona (65) compared sclerotherapy with propranolol in prevention of rebleeding for varices. Although rebleeding was less with sclerotherapy (26 of 58 subjects) than with propranolol (37 of 58 subjects) titrated to reduce resting heart rate by 25%, complications were significantly more frequently observed and of greater severity with sclerotherapy. The authors could not recommend either approach on the basis of the study findings.

Surgical treatment may be required for patients who have repeated GI bleeding (especially esophageal varices) or those who have bleeding that cannot be stopped by the more conservative measures already described (38). A *portacaval shunt* involves anastomosis of the portal vein directly to the inferior vena cava, thus bypassing the cirrhotic liver. This decreases portal hypertension and lowers back-pressure on the abdominal venous system. Unfortunately, these patients have a poor prognosis, since the only way to carry toxins to the liver for detoxification is now the hepatic artery. If they survive the initial surgery, patients may die of sepsis or develop hepatic failure and encephalopathy. The Warren shunt decompresses varices by shunting splenic blood flow to the renal vein (splenorenal shunt) and may decrease hepatic perfusion less.

Hepatic Encephalopathy

If the patient develops signs of an impending hepatic coma (e.g., confusion, drowsiness, asterixis), lactulose is indi-

cated, and dietary protein should be decreased to 20 to 30 g/day. Use of CNS depressants should be minimized. Diuretics should be withheld at this stage, since hypovolemia, hypokalemia, and metabolic alkalosis tend to aggravate encephalopathy.

Lactulose is a synthetic disaccharide of galactose and fructose that is neither absorbed nor hydrolyzed in the small bowel. It is degraded by colonic bacteria to lactic, acetic, and formic acids, thus decreasing the pH of the colonic contents to an endpoint of approximately 5.5. The effect of lactulose was originally attributed to replacement of proteolytic bacteria such as *Escherichia coli*, *Proteus*, and *Bacteroides* with organisms such as *Lactobacillus* that thrive in a more acidic medium and lack urease and other enzymes that are used in the production of ammonia. However, most investigators cannot demonstrate a marked change in the colonic flora and attribute the effects of lactulose solely to the pH changes that occur. As the colon becomes more acidic, the ratio of ammonium ion to ammonia increases, and less absorption of the ammonia occurs. There may also be back-diffusion of ammonia from the blood to the intestinal lumen under acidic pH conditions. In any event, lactulose therapy results in a decrease in arterial ammonium levels (66).

Each 15 mL of lactulose oral liquid contains 10 g of lactulose, and it is usually given in a dose of 30 to 40 mL, 3 to 4 times daily. Use of retention enemas (67) of 300 mL of 50% lactulose diluted to 700 to 1000 mL with tap water has also been reported. Onset of effect by either route is 12 to 48 hr. Once improved mental state has been achieved, the dose can be tapered slowly to identify the smallest effective dose. Patient tolerance may be improved by diluting the drug in fruit juice or carbonated beverages. In most patients, lactulose may be discontinued after several days to a few weeks if the patient's mental status improves. In a few patients, prolonged therapy for months or years may be required if discontinuation of the drug causes a recurrence of symptoms.

The most common complaints of patients treated with lactulose are nausea (because of the sweet taste of the drug), gaseous distension, bloating, belching, or diarrhea caused by osmotic effects in the bowel. Diarrhea may account for part of the therapeutic effects of lactulose (68), but compared with sorbitol, lactulose is more effective in overcoming the encephalopathy, indicating that other mechanisms are working. The dose is usually adjusted so that the patient has two to three soft, semiformed stools daily. Watery diarrhea should be avoided. Of course, if the patient's mental state improves at a dose that produces fewer than two to three stools per day, it is not logical to give a larger dose.

The success rate with lactulose has been reported to be around 85%. Unfortunately, a few patients become resistant after prolonged therapy, and others die from complications of the disease, even though their encephalopathy has cleared. Fluid losses secondary to diarrhea should be considered in monitoring lactulose therapy. Serum sodium should be monitored to detect hyponatremia associated with loss of free water from osmotic diarrhea.

An alternative to lactulose is neomycin in doses of 1 to 2 g four times daily. Neomycin destroys colonic bacteria, slowing the degradation of protein to ammonia. If the patient does not respond, the dose of the neomycin should be increased to 8 to 12 g/day, and the protein restriction should be lowered to 0 to 20 g/day. For patients who cannot take medications orally, a retention enema of 2 to 4 g of neomycin in 200 mL of saline thickened with methylcellulose may be used morning and night. When the patient improves, the maintenance dose of neomycin may be lowered to 2 to 4 g per day.

The duration of therapy varies with both lactulose and neomycin and may last for less than 1 week in most cases or up to months and even years in poorly controlled patients. Some degree of protein restriction may be indicated, since an intolerance to protein intake may be observed in select patients. Many patients who look well-compensated can rapidly deteriorate after eating a single high-protein meal.

One well-controlled study (69) failed to show a clear superiority of either neomycin (83% effective) or lactulose (90% effective) in the treatment of acute encephalopathy. For long-term use, lactulose has the potential advantage of less toxicity, but it is considerably more expensive. The possibility that sterilization of the gut by neomycin might decrease the effectiveness of lactulose appears to be of minimal consequence (70); in fact the two drugs have added effectiveness when used together (71).

Neomycin is considered a nonabsorbable antibiotic. However, from 1% to 3% of a dose is absorbed (72), and there are several reported cases of ototoxicity in patients on chronic oral neomycin therapy (73). Most of these patients had been taking neomycin for at least 8 months and had coexisting renal dysfunction. Annual auditory testing should be performed, and the patient should be observed for subjective changes in hearing status if the drug is to be used for prolonged periods.

Neomycin has also been implicated in development of the hepatorenal syndrome. Although neomycin is renal toxic when given parenterally, it is difficult to determine whether the renal changes with oral dosing are drug-induced or a progression of the disease process itself. The consensus is that the latter mechanism prevails.

Another consequence of neomycin therapy is diarrhea from changes in the bowel flora. This may not be a serious problem, since patients are often given cathartics to cleanse the bowel and eliminate excess ammonia. However, cathartics alone are not effective in moderating encephalopathy, and they should always be accompanied by lactulose or neomycin and protein restriction. Since cathartics can cause fluid and electrolyte imbalance, they may worsen encephalopathy. Adequate intravenous infusions of dextrose or saline with potassium supplements should be maintained.

Corticosteroids

Cirrhotic patients with biopsy-proven alcoholic hepatitis may benefit from the antiinflammatory and antifibrotic effects of corticosteroid therapy. The beneficial effect may be related to the corticosteroid's inhibition of cytokine production.

The efficacy of steroids in the treatment of liver disease remains controversial. Clinical trials have shown conflicting results in regard to mortality. A metaanalysis of the randomized trials was completed to determine the efficacy of steroids on short-term mortality in patients with alcoholic hepatitis. The combined data indicated that steroids provide a protective efficacy of 27% in patients with hepatic encephalopathy. This figure increased in patients without active GI bleeding. Among subjects without hepatic encephalopathy, steroids had no protective efficacy. This data suggests that only patients with severe disease would benefit from steroid therapy. Patients with severe disease are defined as those with hepatic encephalopathy or a discriminant function higher than 32 [discriminant function = 4.6 (patient's prothrombin time − control time) + bilirubin]. Patients with severe disease who have active GI bleeding or require treatment for active infection should be excluded from steroid therapy (74).

Prednisolone is the most studied and appears to be the preferred steroid. The dosing regimen is 40 mg/day for 4 weeks and is then tapered over 2 to 4 weeks (75).

Branched-Chain Amino Acids

One of the goals of management of progressive liver disease is to provide adequate nutritional support, including protein and calories. Positive nitrogen balance must be established without exacerbating hepatic encephalopathy caused by giving inappropriate combinations of amino acids. In experimental animals and to a lesser extent in humans, administration of diets that are high in branched-chain amino acids and low in aromatic amino acids and methionine may help to restore normal amino acid balance and reduce encephalopathy (11–13, 76). An 8% amino acid solution (*Hepatamine*) is marketed that contains more branched-chain amino acids than standard parenteral nutrition solutions. The ratio of BCAAs to AAAs in Hepatamine is 37:1, compared with 5:1 in conventional crystalline amino acid solutions. Mixing 500 mL of Hepatamine with 500 mL of 50% dextrose in water yields 40 g/L of amino acids. Indications for use of this therapy and its efficacy are debated. The high cost and questionable efficacy of Hepatamine (compared with more conventional therapy) have led most institutions to limit the use of branched-chain amino acid solutions to patients with life-threatening encephalopathy refractory to conventional therapy and those with documented elevated serum ammonia levels. In most cases an amino acid screen is used to assess the ratio of BCAA:AAA in the patient. The cost of an amino acid screen is approximately equal to one day's therapy with Hepatamine.

For the alert patient without central venous access, enteral therapy has been proposed. One such dietary supplement is *Hepatic-Aid,* a complex of carbohydrate, protein, and fat in a readily digestible form. One package of Hepatic-Aid mixed in a blender with 250 mL of water yields 340 mL of suspension for oral or nasogastric administration, which contains 2.2 g of nitrogen (15 g protein), 98 g of carbohydrate, 12 g of fat, and 560 calories (500 nonprotein calories). One to four packages may be given per day, but the administration rate should be slow at first to prevent glucose overload. Use of oral branched-chain amino acids is discouraged because of questionable efficacy, high cost, and disagreeable taste. A.S.P.E.N. Medical Practice Guidelines for nutritional supplementation of liver-diseased patients with specific recommendations are available (77).

Benzodiazepine Receptor Antagonists

As was introduced in the section on clinical findings and diagnosis, some investigators believe that endogenous or exogenous GABA-ergic-like compounds that stimulate the GABA-benzodiazepine receptor complex in the brain may be responsible for symptoms of encephalopathy (14, 78). Preliminary data suggests that the benzodiazepine antagonist, flumazenil, may be valuable in both short-term and long-term management of encephalopathy.

In a series of 14 subjects, 71% of patients had short-term improvement in symptoms after intravenous administration of flumazenil (79). Arousal was greatest in patients with deeper coma (stage III to IV encephalopathy). Although response was rapid, the duration of effect was only 1 to 2 hr with parenteral therapy. The usual dose was 0.2 to 0.4 mg, some subjects receiving up to ten doses.

A single case report describes long-term use of oral therapy (80). A patient given 25 mg twice daily experienced complete reversal of symptoms for 14 months. Previously, this patient had experienced 12 attacks of coma over a 2-year period. Discontinuation of the drug led to a recurrence of symptoms within 48 hr.

A randomized double-blind placebo-controlled crossover trial from Canada shows a significant clinical improvement in 5 of 11 (45%) hepatic coma patients receiving flumazenil in the initial treatment phase and 1 of 2 (50%) in the crossover phase of the study. The authors conclude that the agent is efficacious and safe for relieving neurological symptoms in cirrhotics with hepatic coma (81). This

trial has been criticized (82). The use of benzodiazepine receptor antagonist therapy in these patients remains investigational and controversial.

Dopamine

Dopamine and norepinephrine are important mediators of normal sympathetic activity in both the CNS and the periphery, especially in the kidney. Some of the neurological manifestations of hepatic failure, as well as the hepatorenal syndrome, may be due to accumulation of other beta-hydroxylated phenylethylamines such as octopamine and serotonin. These compounds may replace normal transmitters and act as false neurotransmitters in sympathetic nerve terminals and granules. Precursors of false neurotransmitters, such as phenylalanine and tyrosine (Fig. 28.2), are produced from protein in the gut by bacterial amino acid decarboxylases. Normally, these precursors are metabolized rapidly in the liver by monoamine oxidase (MAO), allowing norepinephrine that is formed elsewhere in the body to predominate. When hepatic function is impaired or when blood is shunted away from the liver, these false neurotransmitters may replace normal transmitters. Systemically, this may lead to lowered peripheral vascular resistance and shunting of blood away from the kidney. Similarly, asterixis and other signs of hepatic encephalopathy might result from displacement of transmitters such as dopamine and norepinephrine in the basal ganglia and other areas in the brain.

If the displacement of normal central and peripheral transmitters by less active amines can account for hepatic coma and its cardiovascular complications, then the restoration of normal transmitter stores might restore normal function. For hospitalized patients this is accomplished by administering low-dose infusions of dopamine (1 to 4 μg/kg/min). This may increase renal blood flow and help to reverse the hepatorenal syndrome. Unfortunately, the mortality rate of people with the hepatorenal syndrome approaches 100%, even in those who receive dopamine.

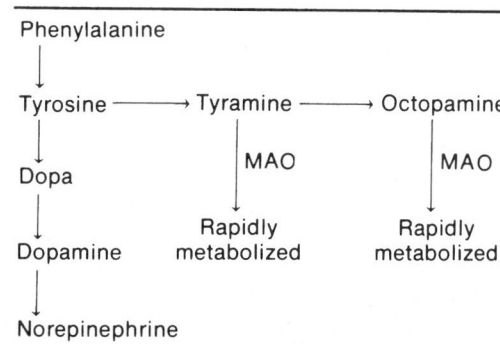

Figure 28.2. Synthetic pathway of neurotransmitters. Monoamine oxidase (MAO) action occurs mainly in the liver and is depressed in hepatic disease and shunting.

Failure to improve urine output or increase blood pressure within the first 24 hours of dopamine treatment is a poor prognostic sign. Since dopamine does not cross the blood-brain barrier, encephalopathy may not be helped. However, by referring to Figure 28.2, it can be seen that dopamine is also a precursor to norepinephrine, which may help to restore natural neurotransmitter balance in a second way.

Primary Biliary Cirrhosis: Colchicine and Other Drugs

Colchicine, a drug with both antiinflammatory and antifibrotic properties has been evaluated as a potential disease-modifying agent for several years. In one study, 57 patients with biopsy-proven primary biliary cirrhosis were treated with either 0.6 mg of colchicine twice daily or placebo (83). The colchicine-treated patients had significant improvement in biochemical parameters (serum bilirubin and transferase levels) but no difference (compared with placebo) in histological progression. A second group of investigators conducted a randomized, double-blind, placebo-controlled trial of colchicine, 1 mg/day, 5 days per week, in 100 patients with cirrhosis caused by alcohol abuse or a prior history of hepatitis (84). Median survival improved from 3.5 years in the placebo group to 11 years in the colchicine-treated patients, and deaths from liver failure were reduced from 24% in the placebo group to 15% in the treatment group. Side effects in both trials were mild, primarily consisting of nausea, abdominal pain, and diarrhea. Although these results are encouraging, flaws in the study design and the relatively small number of subjects treated prevent widespread endorsement of colchicine therapy at this time.

Numerous other drugs have been tried in the treatment of primary biliary cirrhosis, including penicillamine, chlorambucil, azathioprine, cyclosporine, corticosteroids, and methotrexate (85). Each of these therapies is based on the hope that antiinflammatory or immunmodulating effects may alter the disease process. Cyclosporine showed modest improvement in symptoms, enzyme levels, and histologic findings in a controlled trial for the treatment of PBC. However, toxicity with this drug is a limiting factor in therapy. A controlled, multicenter trial with ursodeoxycholic acid also showed improvement in symptoms, enzyme levels, and histologic findings in some patients but showed little effect in patients with advanced disease (86). In addition, sequestration of copper by penicillamine may have a therapeutic effect. Unfortunately, either most of the trials with these drugs have been limited by a small sample size without adequate controls or the improvement obtained has been only marginal. At this time, none of these drugs can be recommended. Ursodiol may be effective in slowing the progresssion of PBC and, additionally, may decrease the need for transplantation (87).

PROGNOSIS

The outlook for patients with cirrhosis depends entirely on the stage of the disease and the presence of complications. If the cause of the cirrhosis is alcoholism and the patient continues to drink, the prognosis is poor. Conversely, discontinuation of drinking increases survival. In one large series of 1155 patients with cirrhosis from a variety of causes, the overall 5-year survival was about 40% (88). The causes of death were liver failure in 49%, hepatocellular carcinoma in 22%, bleeding in 14%, hepatorenal syndrome in 8%, and other causes in the remainder. Patients who entered the study with compensated cirrhosis (mild or absent symptoms) became symptomatic at the rate of 10% per year. Survival was higher in this group of patients: 54% at 6 years. People who entered the study with symptoms already present (ascites, history of bleeding, or encephalopathy) had a survival rate of only 21% at 6 years and a much higher incidence of hepatocellular carcinoma. In the United States, cirrhosis has become one of the five most frequent causes of death in people over the age of 40 (3).

CONCLUSION

Despite extensive investigation of liver function and pathologies, there is no effective therapy for many liver diseases. Discontinuation of alcohol intake in patients with proven cirrhosis is of primary importance. Use of naltrexone in an effort to decrease craving may prove valuable in this setting (89). Although therapy for cirrhosis is focused mainly on symptomatic management, other forms of chronic liver disease such as hepatitis B and autoimmune hepatitis can be treated specifically with modern antiviral therapy (see Chapter 25, "Hepatitis"). Although the lesions of advanced cirrhosis are irreversible, it is estimated that 70% or more of liver tissue must be destroyed before the body is unable to eliminate drugs and toxins via the liver (90). Unfortunately, it is difficult to tell which patients have reached this stage of involvement, so practitioners should always be aware of the potential inability of patients with advanced liver disease to excrete certain drugs and adjust doses accordingly. These dosage reductions are often empiric, since data quantifying the degree of adjustment necessary is generally unavailable.

REFERENCES

1. Cotran R, Kumar V, Robbins S. Pathological basis of disease, 4th ed. Philadelphia: WB Saunders, 1989:941–57.
2. Rubin E, Lieber C. Fatty liver, alcoholic hepatitis, and cirrhosis produced by alcohol in primates. N Engl J Med 290:128, 1974.
3. Anonymous. Trends in mortality from cirrhosis and alcoholism: United States. Morbid Mortal Week Rep 35:703–05, 1983.
4. World Health Statistics Annual. Geneva: World Health Organization, 1985.
5. Anonymous. Deaths and hospitalizations from chronic liver disease: United States. Morbid Mortal Week Rep 41:969–73, 1993.

6. Schrier R, Arroyo V, Bernardi M, et al. Peripheral arterial vasodilation hypothesis: a proposal for the initiation of renal sodium and water retention in cirrhosis. Hepatology 8:1151–57, 1988.

7. Rocco V, Ware A. Cirrhotic ascites: pathophysiology, diagnosis, and management. Ann Intern Med 105:573–85, 1986.

8. Porayko M, Wiesner R. Management of ascites in patients with cirrhosis. Postgrad Med 92(8):156, 1992.

9. Wood LJ, Massie D, McLean AJ, et al. Renal sodium retention in cirrhosis: tubular site and relation to hepatic dysfunction. Hepatology 8(4):831, 1988.

10. Runyon B, Montano A, Akriviadis E, et al. The serum-ascites albumin gradient in the differential diagnosis of ascites is superior to the exudate/transudate concept. Ann Intern Med 117:215, 1992.

11. Fraser C, Arieff A. Hepatic encephalopathy. N Engl J Med 313:869–73, 1985.

12. Bode J, Shafer K. Pathophysiology of chronic hepatic encephalopathy. Hepatogastronenterology 32:259–65, 1985.

13. Sax H, Talamini M, Fischer J. Clinical use of branched-chain amino acids in liver disease, sepsis, trauma and burns. Arch Surg 121:358–66, 1986.

14. Basile A, Gammal S. Evidence for the involvement of benzodiazepine receptor complex in hepatic encephalopathy; implications for treatment with benzodiazepine receptor anatgonists. Clin Neuropharmacol 11:401–22, 1988.

15. Badalamenti S, Graziani G, Salerno F, et al. Hepatorenal syndrome: new perspectives in pathogenesis and treatment. Arch Intern Med 153:1957–67, 1993.

16. Shear L, Ching S, Gabuzda G. Compartmentalization of ascites and edema in patients with hepatic cirrhosis. N Engl J Med 282:1391–96, 1970.

17. Pockros P, Reynolds T. Rapid diuresis in patients with ascites from chronic liver disease: the importance of peripheral edema. Gastroenterology 90:1827–33, 1986.

18. Daskalopoulos G, Laffi G, Morgan T, et al. Immediate effects of furosemide on renal hemodynamics in chronic liver disease with ascites. Gastroenterology 92:1859, 1987.

19. Gines P, Arroyo V, Quintero E, et al. Comparison of paracentesis and diuretics in the treatment of cirrhotics with tense ascites; results of a randomized study. Gastroenterology 93:234–41, 1987.

20. Gines P, Tito L, Arroyo V, et al. Randomized comparative study of therapeutic paracentesis with and without intravenous albumin in cirrhosis. Gastroenterology 94:1493–1502, 1988.

21. Panos MZ, Moore K, Vlavianos P, et al. Single, total paracentesis for tense ascites: sequential hemodynamic changes and right atrial size. Hepatology 11:662, 1990.

22. Tito LI, Gines P, Arroyo V, et al. Total paracentesis associated with intravenous albumin in the management of patients with cirrhosis and ascites. Gastroenterology 98:146, 1990.

23. Pinto P, Amerian J, Reynolds T. Large-volume paracentesis in nonedematous patients with tense ascites: its effect on intravascular volume. Hepatology 8:207–10, 1988.

24. Runyon B, Antillon M, Montano A. Effect of diuresis versus therapeutic paracentesis on ascitic fluid opsonic activity and serum complement. Gastroenterology 97:158–62, 1989.

25. Runyon B. Care of patients with ascites. N Engl J Med 330(5):340, 1994.

26. Smart H, Triger D. A randomised prospective trial comparing daily paracentesis and intravenous albumin with recirculation in diuretic refractory ascites. J Hepatol 10:191–97, 1990.

27. Epstein M. Peritoneovenous shunt in the management of ascites and the hepatorenal syndrome. Gastroenterology 82:790–99, 1980.

28. Stanley M, Ochi S, Lee K, et al. Peritoneovenous shunting as compared with medical treatment in patients with alcoholic cirrhosis and massive asictes. N Engl J Med 321:1632–38, 1989.

29. Gines P, Arrovo V, Rodes J. Pharmacotherapy of ascites associated with cirrhosis. Drugs 43(3):325, 1992.

30. Conn H, Fessell JM. Spontaneous bacterial peritonitis in cirrhosis: variations on a theme. Medicine 50:161, 1991.

31. Wyngaarden J, Smith L, Bennett J. Cecil textbook of medicine, 19th ed. Philadelphia: WB Saunders, 1992:795.

32. Ariza J, Xiol X, Esteve M, et al. Aztreonam vs cefotaxime in the treatment of gram-negative spontaneous bacterial peritonitis in cirrhotic patients. Hepatology 14:91–8, 1991.

33. Felisart J, Rimola A, Arroyo V, et al. Cefotaxime is more effective than is ampicillin-tobramycin in cirrhotics with severe infections. Hepatology 5:457–62, 1985.

34. Fong TL, Akriviadis EA, Runyon BA, et al. Polymorphonuclear cell count response and duration of antibiotic therapy in spontaneous bacterial peritonitis. Hepatology 9:423–26, 1989.

35. Gines P, Rimola A, Planas R, et al. Norfloxacin prevents spontaneous bacterial peritonitis recurrence in cirrhosis: results of a double-blind, placebo-controlled trial. Hepatology 12:716–24, 1990.

36. Soriano G, Guarner C, Tomas A, et al. Norfloxacin prevents bacterial infection in cirrhotics with gastrointestinal hemorrhage. Gastroenterology 103:477, 1991.

37. Singh N, Gayowski T, Yu VL, Wagener MM. Trimethoprim-sulfamethoxazole for the prevention of spontaneous bacterial peritonitis in cirrhosis: a randomized trial. Ann Intern Med 122:595–98, 1995.

38. Terblanche J, Burroughs A, Hobbs K. Controversies in the management of bleeding esophageal varices. N Engl J Med (part 1) 320:1393–97, 1989; (part 2) 320:1469–75, 1989.

39. Cello J, Crass R, Grendell J, et al. Management of the patient with hemorrhaging esophageal varices. JAMA 256:1480–84, 1986.

40. Rice T. Treatment of esophageal varices. Clin Pharm 8:122–31, 1989.

41. Henderson J, Kutner M, Millikan W, et al. Endoscopic variceal sclerosis compared with distal splenorenal shunt to prevent recurrent variceal bleeding in cirrhosis. Ann Intern Med 112:262–69, 1990.

42. Santangelo W, Dueno M, Estes B, et al. Prophylactic sclerotherapy of large esophageal varices. N Engl J Med 318:814–16, 1988.

43. Sauerbruch T, Wotzka R, Kopcke W, et al. Prophylactic sclerotherapy before the first episode of variceal hemorrhage in patients with cirrhosis. N Engl J Med 319:8–15, 1988.

44. Goff J. Gastroesophageal varices: pathogenesis and therapy of acute bleeding. Gastro Clin North Am 22(4):779, 1993.

45. Ziemniak J, Bernhard H, Schentag J. Hepatic encephalopathy and altered cimetidine kinetics. Clin Pharmacol Ther 34(3):375, 1983.

46. Gonzalez-Martin G, Paulos C, Veloso B, et al. Ranitidine disposition in severe hepatic cirrhosis. Int J Clin Pharm 25:139–42, 1987.

47. Roark G. Treatment of postsclerotherapy esophageal ulcers with sucralfate. Gastrointest Endosc 30:9–10, 1984.

48. Stiegmann GV, Goff JS, Sun JH, et al. Endoscopic ligation of esophageal varices. Am J Surg 159:21–26, 1990.

49. Van Stiegmann G, Cambre T, Sun JH. A new endoscopic elastic band ligating device. Gastrointest Endosc 32:230–33, 1986.

50. Stiegmann GV, Goff JS, Michaletz-Onody PA, et al. Endoscopic sclerotherapy as compared with endoscopic ligation for bleeding esophageal varices. N Engl J Med 326:1527–32, 1992.

51. Stump D, Hardin T. The use of vasopressin in the treatment of upper gastrointestinal haemorrhage. Drugs 39:38–53, 1990.

52. Fogel M, Knaver C, Andres L, et al. Continuous intravenous vasopressin in active upper gastrointestinal bleeding: a placebo controlled trial. Ann Intern Med 96:565–69, 1982.

53. Gimson A, Westaby D, Hegarty J, et al. A randomized trial of vasopressin plus nitroglycerin in the control of acute variceal hemorrhage. Hepatol 6:410–13, 1986.

54. Tsai Y, Lay C, Lai K, et al. Controlled trial of vasopressin plus nitroglycerin versus vasopression alone in bleeding esophageal varices. Hepatology 6:406–09, 1982.

55. Rice T. Treatment of esophageal varices. Clin Pharm 8(2):122, 1989.

56. Laine L, Peterson W. Bleeding peptic ulcer. N Engl J Med 331(11):717–27, 1994.

57. Lewis J, Davis J, Allsopp D, et al. Beta-blockers in protal hypertension: an overview. Drugs 37:62–9, 1989.

58. Hayes P, Davis J, Lewis J, et al. Meta-analysis of value of propranolol in prevention of variceal hemorrhage. Lancet 336:153–56, 1990.

59. Pascal J, Cales P, et al. Propranolol in the prevention of first upper gastrointestinal tract hemorrhage in patients with cirrhosis of the liver and esophageal varices. N Engl J Med 317:856–61, 1987.

60. Lebrec O, Poynard T, Bernuau J, et al. A randomized controlled study of propranolol for prevention of recurrent gastrointestinal bleeding in patients with cirrhosis. Hepatology 4:355–84, 1984.

61. Burroughs A, Jenkins W, Sherlock S, et al. Controlled trial of propranolol for the prevention of recurrent gastrointestinal bleeding in patients with cirrhosis. N Engl J Med 309:1539–42, 1983.

62. Poynard T, Lebrec D, Hillon P, et al. Propranolol for prevention of recurrent gastrointestinal bleeding in patients with cirrhosis: a prospective study of factors associated with rebleeding. Hepatol 7:447–51, 1987.

63. Lebrec D, Bemuau J, Rueff B, Benhamou J. Gastrointestinal bleeding after abrupt cessation of propranolol administration in cirrhosis. N Engl J Med 307:560, 1982.

64. Alabaster S, Gogel H, McCarthy D. Propranolol withdrawal and variceal hemorrhage. JAMA 250:3047, 1983.

65. Teres J, Bosch J, Bordas J, et al. Propranolol versus sclerotherapy in preventing variceal rebleeding: a randomized controlled trial. Gastroenterology 105:1508–14, 1993.

66. Avery GS, Davies EF, Brogden RN. Lactulose: a review. Drugs 4:7–48, 1972.

67. Kersh ES, Rifkin H. Lactulose enemas. Ann Intern Med 78:81–4, 1973.

68. Rodgers JB Jr, Kiley JE, Balint JA. Comparison of results of long term treatment of chronic hepatic encephalopathy with lactulose and sorbitol. Am J Gastroenterol 60:459–65, 1973.

69. Conn HO, Leevy CM, Vlahcevic J, et al. Comparison of lactulose and neomycin in the treatment of chronic portal systemic encephalopathy. Gastroenterology 72:573, 1977.

70. Conn HO. Interactions of lactulose and neomycin. Drugs 4:4–6, 1972.

71. Weber F, Fresard K, Lally B. Effects of lactulose and neomycin on urea metabolism in cirrhotic subjects. Gastroenterology 82:213–17, 1982.

72. Breen K, Bryant R, Levinson J, et al. Neomycin absorption in man. Ann Intern Med 76:211–18, 1972.

73. Berk D, Chalmer T. Deafness complicating antibiotic therapy of hepatic encephalopathy. Ann Intern Med 73:393–96, 1970.

74. Imperiale T, McCullough A. Do corticosteroids reduce mortality from alcoholic hepatitis? Ann Intern Med 113:299–307, 1990.

75. Ramond M, Poynard T, Rueff B, et al. A randomized trial of prednisolone in patients with severe alcoholic hepatitis. N Engl J Med 326:507–12, 1992.

76. Horst D, Grace N, Conn H, et al. Comparison of dietary protein with an oral, branched chain-enriched amino acid supplement in chronic portal-systemic encephalopathy: a randomized controlled trial. Hepatology 4:279–87, 1984.

77. Anonymous. Guidelines for the use of parenteral and enteral nutrition in adult and pediatric patients. J Parenteral Enteral Nutr 17 (suppl 4):14–15SA, 1993.

78. Basile AS, Hughes RD, Harrison PM, et al. Elevated brain concentrations of 1,4-benzodiazepines in fulminant hepatic failure. N Engl J Med 325(7):473–78, 1991.

79. Bansky G, Meier P, Riederer E, et al. Effects of the benzodiazepine receptor antagonist flumazenil in hepatic encephalopathy in humans. Gastroenterology 97:744–50, 1989.

80. Ferenci P, Grimm G, Meryn S, et al. Successful long-term treatment of portal-systemic encephalopathy by benzodiazepine antagonist flumazenil. Gastroenterology 96:240–43, 1989.

81. Pomier LG, Giguere JF, Lavoie J, et al. Flumazenil in cirrhotic patients in hepatic coma. Hepatology 19:32–7, 1994.

82. Sterling R, Shiffman M, Schubert M. Flumazenil for hepatic coma: the elusive wake-up call? Gastroenterology 107:1204–05, 1994.

83. Bodenheimer H, Schaffner F, Pezzullo J. Evaluation of colchicine therapy in primary biliary cirrhosis. Gasteroenterology 95:124–29, 1988.

84. Kershenobich D, Vargas F, Barcia-Tsao G, et al. Colchicine in the treatment of cirrhosis of the liver. N Engl J Med 318:1709–13, 1988.

85. Stavinoha M, Soloway R. Current therapy of chronic liver disease. Drugs 39:814–40, 1990.

86. Fennerty MB. Primary sclerosing cholangitis and primary biliary cirrhosis. Postgrad Med 94(6):81, 1993.

87. Poupon R, Poupon R, Balkau B, et al. Ursodiol for the long-term treatment of primary biliary cirrhosis. N Engl J Med 333(19):1342–47, 1994.

88. D'Amico G, Morabito A, Pagliaro L, Marubini E. Survival and prognostic indicators in compensated and decompensated cirrhosis. Dig Dis Sci 31:468–75, 1986.

89. Anonymous. Approval of naltrexone for use in chronic alcoholism. Washington, DC: Food and Drug Administration, Jan. 1995.

90. Bass N, Williams R. Guide to drug dosage in hepatic disease. Clin Pharmacokinet 15:396–420, 1988.

CHAPTER 29

PANCREATITIS

PAULA A. THOMPSON and KATHERINE C. HERNDON

Pancreatic inflammatory disease may be classified as either acute or chronic based on the reversibility of functional and structural changes that arise within the gland. Following clinical resolution of an acute attack of pancreatitis, the pancreas will recover normal exocrine and endocrine function, as well as morphology, once the underlying cause of acute inflammation is eliminated. Although most attacks have a mild, self-limited course, severe disease complicated by multiple organ system failure and life-threatening infection may develop. Though mild scarring and impaired function may persist for a limited time following an acute attack, seldom does acute pancreatitis progress to chronic disease (1–3).

In contrast, the persistent inflammation of chronic pancreatitis is associated with a permanent and often progressive loss of pancreatic exocrine and endocrine function and irreversible structural damage. Recurrent exacerbations of pancreatitis, which frequently complicate chronic disease, are virtually impossible to distinguish clinically from discrete attacks of acute pancreatitis (4).

Reliable incidence and prevalence data are difficult to obtain. The incidence of both acute and chronic forms varies considerably among geographic areas as a consequence of differences in regional, environmental, and genetic factors (2, 4, 5). It does appear, however, that the incidence of pancreatic inflammatory disease has increased tenfold over the past 20 years. This may be due to an increase in alcohol abuse or may only reflect improved diagnostic techniques (6).

ANATOMY

Embryologic Development

The pancreas derives from two separate outpocketings of the endodermal lining of the duodenum, one dorsal and one ventral. These appear at approximately 4 weeks gestation, and each remains connected to the duodenum via a duct. The two pancreatic buds fuse by the 7th week of gestation, with the dorsal component forming the neck, body, and tail, and the ventral component forming the uncinate process. Both dorsal and ventral portions contribute to the region called the head. Also at this time, the dorsal duct of Santorini (accessory duct) combines with the ventral duct of Wirsung (pancreatic duct), which communicates with the duodenum by way of the common bile duct (7).

At approximately the 3rd month of gestation, endocrine and exocrine tissue can be distinguished. The secretory unit of the exocrine pancreas is the acinus (from the Latin for "berries in a cluster"). The acini remain connected to the main pancreatic duct through a network of interconnecting ductules. The islets of Langerhans (pancreatic islets) make up the endocrine pancreas and comprise four major cell types, each apparently secreting a single hormone. Approximately 50 to 80% of the islet cell mass is composed of B cells that secrete insulin. Glucagon, pancreatic polypeptide, and somatostatin are secreted by A cells, PP cells, and D cells, respectively. Insulin and glucagon are critical in the regulation of carbohydrate metabolism (see Chapter 19). Furthermore, in addition to the systemic effects exerted by each of these hormones, they play a role in the regulation of pancreatic exocrine secretion. Insulin may potentiate the actions of stimulatory factors, whereas glucagon, somatostatin, and pancreatic polypeptide exert inhibitory effects (8, 9).

A fairly common developmental abnormality, *pancreas divisum*, occurs when the ducts of the embryonic pancreatic buds fail to fuse. Autopsy studies have suggested an overall incidence of approximately 7%. It has been postulated that this condition can predispose to the development of pancreatitis, but this is controversial and may be only an incidental finding (4, 7, 9).

Anatomy

The adult pancreas is a flattened and elongated gland, usually ranging from 12 to 15 centimeters in length and weighing 70 to 110 grams. It is lobular, rather like the salivary glands, and its lack of a fibrous capsule makes it soft in texture. The pancreas lies in the retroperitoneum, the head nestled within the curve of the duodenum as it exits the stomach, and the tail extending obliquely to the left (Figure 29.1). Approximately 80% by weight is acinar, 18% ductular, and 2% endocrine tissue.

Blood is supplied to the pancreas by the celiac and superior mesenteric arteries, and the blood ultimately drains into the hepatic portal vein. The lymphatic vessels draining the pancreas terminate primarily in the pancreatosplenic and pancreatoduodenal lymph nodes. Sympathetic innervation is predominately through splanchnic neurons synapsing in the celiac plexus, and parasympathetic innervation is derived from the vagal nerve (8, 9).

PHYSIOLOGY

Overview

Pancreatic exocrine function is complex and incompletely understood. (Endocrine function is discussed in Chapter 68.) During the course of a day, the pancreas can secrete 1.5 to 3 liters of isosmotic alkaline fluid containing more than 20 enzymes and proenzymes (zymogens). This fluid is commonly termed "pancreatic juice." Each acinus consists of 20 to 50 pyramid-shaped acinar cells surrounding a central lumen that synthesize and secrete digestive enzymes (Figure 29.1). The lumen is drained by an intralobular ductule. The proximal ductular cells, extending into the lumen of the acinus, are termed centroacinar cells and are primarily responsible for secretion of water and electrolytes. The intralobular ductules coalesce with interlobular ductules, ultimately draining into the main pancreatic duct. This duct, as well as the common bile duct, enters the duodenum at the ampulla of Vater (hepatopancreatic ampulla). The sphincter of Oddi (sphincter of the hepatopancreatic ampulla) regulates flow from both ducts (10–12).

Secretion of Water and Electrolytes

The principle cations of pancreatic juice are sodium and potassium, which are secreted at fixed concentrations similar to their plasma concentrations. The principle anions are bicarbonate and chloride, which vary reciprocally in concentration, maintaining the sum of the two fairly constant at approximately 150 mEq/L (Figure 29.2). Bicarbonate is secreted by centroacinar cells, whereas secretions from the acinar cells are rich in chloride. The relative concentration of each reaching the duodenum depends on the amount secreted and the exchange of bicarbonate for chloride in the ductules. The concentration of bicarbonate, physiologically the most important of the electrolytes, increases with increasing flow rates of pancreatic juice, whereas chloride concentration decreases under these circumstances. Flow rates range from a basal level of 0.2 to 0.3 ml/min to 4 ml/min during stimulation. At maximal rates of secretion, bicarbonate concentration approaches 120 mEq/L, and the pH of the resulting pancreatic juice is approximately 8.3. This alkalinity buffers the acidic chyme delivered to the duodenum from the stomach and main-

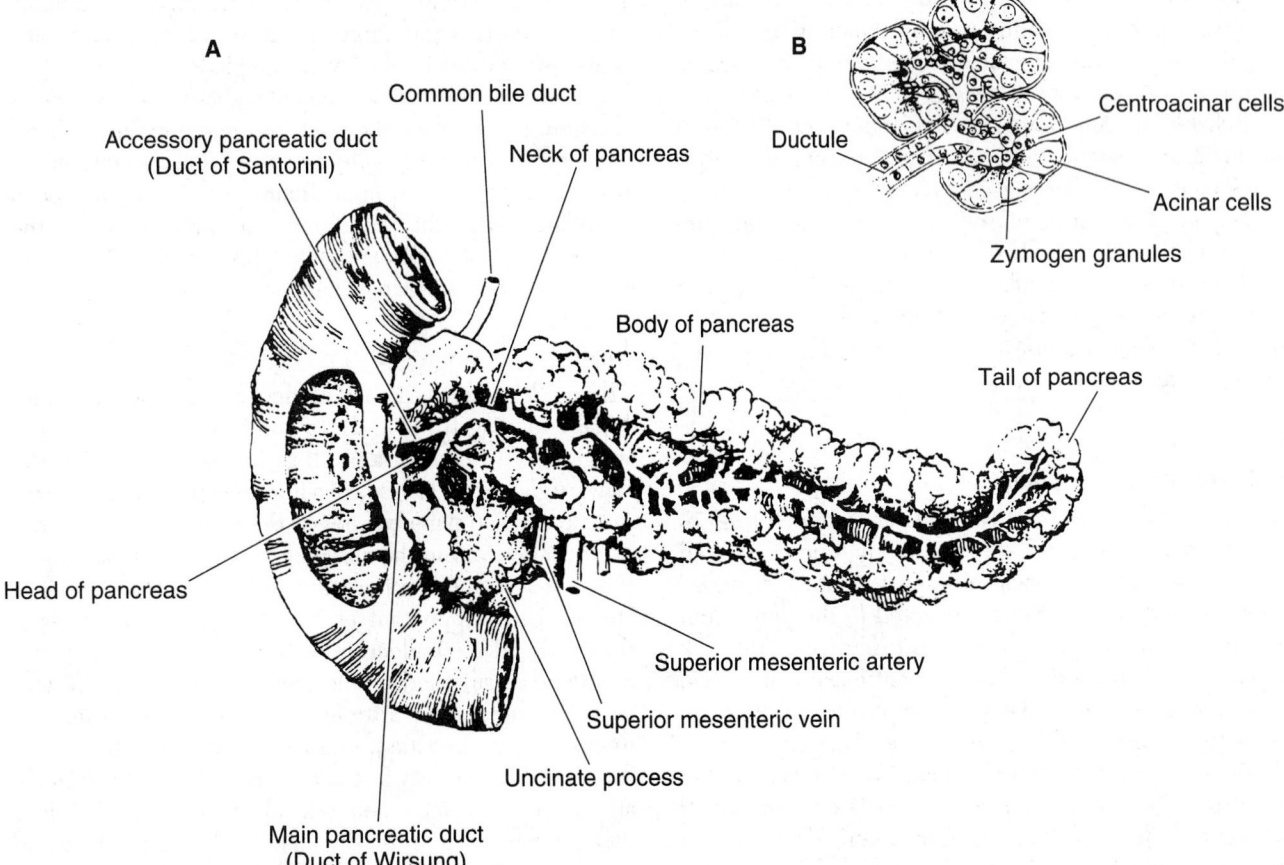

Figure 29-1.   Structure of the pancreas. (A) Dissected to show ductal system. (B) Enlargement of a representative acinus.

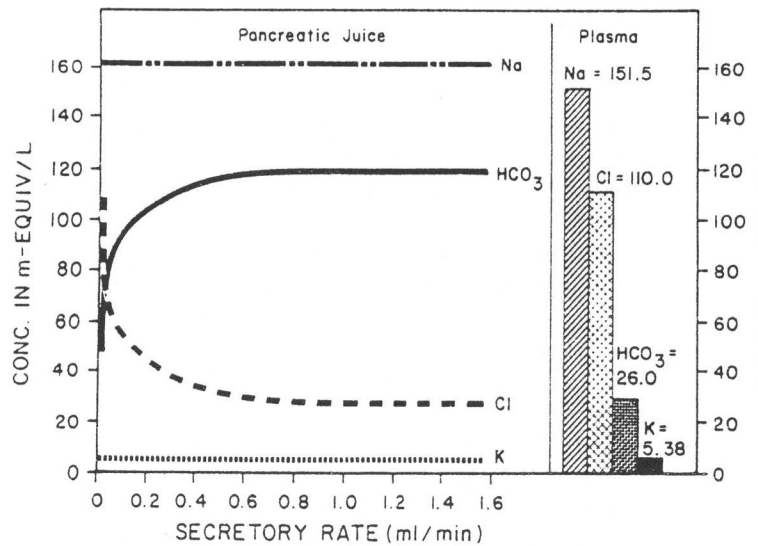

Figure 29-2. Relationship between ion concentration in pancreatic juice and secretory flow rate. Reprinted with permission from: Pandol S. Pancreatic physiology. In Sleisenger MH, Fordtran JS: Gastrointestinal Disease: Pathophysiology/ Diagnosis/ Management, ed 5. Philadelphia, W.B. Saunders Company, 1993, p 1586.

tains a pH that is optimal for the functioning of pancreatic enzymes (11). Other ions present in pancreatic juice include calcium and trace amounts of magnesium, zinc, phosphate, and sulfate. Water enters the ductules passively down the concentration gradient established by the active transport of solute, maintaining isosmolality (10–12).

Enzymes

Protein comprises up to 10% of pancreatic juice, and over 90% of this protein consists of the digestive enzymes and proenzymes (10, 12). These enzymes are synthesized in the rough endoplasmic reticulum of the acinar cells and stored in secretory vesicles (zymogen granules) prior to their release by exocytosis. There are four major categories of enzymes corresponding to the four classes of organic compounds found in food: proteins, carbohydrates, lipids, and nucleic acids (Table 29.1). The proteases and phospholipases are secreted as inactive zymogens that become active in the intestinal lumen through the action of enterokinase produced by the duodenal mucosa. Enterokinase cleaves a small fragment of trypsinogen to form active trypsin that can then activate other zymogens, including additional trypsinogen molecules.

The pancreas is protected from autolysis not only by secretion of proteolytic enzymes in zymogen form, but also by the presence of trypsin inhibitor that binds to trypsin in a 1:1 ratio, rendering it inactive. This protein is present in sufficient quantity to protect against small amounts of trypsin that may become active in the ductules, but its activity is insignificant in the duodenal lumen (10, 11, 13).

Regulation of Exocrine Function

A discussion of all the putative regulatory factors of pancreatic exocrine function, both neural and hormonal, is

Table 29.1.
Major Digestive Enzymes Secreted by the Pancreas

Proteolytic
Trypsinogen (3)[a] $\xrightarrow{\text{Enterokinase, Trypsin}}$ Trypsin
Chymotrypsinogen (2)[a] $\xrightarrow{\text{Trypsin}}$ Chymotrypsin
Proelastase (2)[a] $\xrightarrow{\text{Trypsin}}$ Elastase
Procarboxypeptidase A (2)[a] $\xrightarrow{\text{Trypsin}}$ Carboxypeptidase A
Procarboxypeptidase B (2)[a] $\xrightarrow{\text{Trypsin}}$ Carboxypeptidase B

Amylase
α-Amylase

Lipolytic
Lipase
Procolipase $\xrightarrow{\text{Trypsin}}$ Colipase [cofactor essential for optimum lipase activity]
Prophospholipase A_2 $\xrightarrow{\text{Trypsin}}$ Phospholipase A_2
Esterase

Nucleases
DNAse
RNAse

[a]Number of molecular forms described (12).

beyond the scope of this text. The roles of secretin, cholecystokinin (CCK), and cholinergic neurons in pancreatic secretions have been well established and will be reviewed briefly. Inhibition of secretion will also be addressed.

STIMULATION

Secretin, a peptide hormone released from the mucosa of the duodenum and jejunum, stimulates bicarbonate and water secretion, primarily in response to the presence of acid in the small intestine. The pH threshold for secretin release is 4.5. The presence of bile salts and some fatty acids within the intestinal lumen can also trigger secretin release. In addition to its effect on bicarbonate, secretin may cause a weak stimulation of pancreatic enzyme release (8, 9, 14).

Cholecystokinin, also a peptide hormone secreted by the mucosa of the small bowel, causes the release of an enzyme-rich juice from the pancreas. Production of CCK occurs when amino acids and/or fatty acids enter the duodenum. Intravenous administration of CCK also stimulates enzyme release, whereas pancreatic response is substantially reduced by the administration of CCK antagonists. The combined release of secretin and CCK potentiates the pancreatic response, increasing bicarbonate and volume secretion (8, 9, 14).

Secretin and CCK exert their effects, at least in part, through the binding to specific receptor sites on the pancreatic cell membranes. Vasoactive intestinal peptide (VIP), structurally similar to secretin, increases bicarbonate release by binding to the secretin receptor. Gastrin shares the C-terminal structure of CCK, and its binding triggers a relatively weak release of enzymes. A muscarinic receptor mediates cholinergic stimulation of bicarbonate and enzyme release, and other receptor sites have also been identified. Possibly the most intriguing is a site for bombesin, a tetradecapeptide isolated from amphibian skin. (Gastrin-releasing peptide, or GRP, is the mammalian analog.) It is postulated that bombesin stimulates enzyme-rich secretion through both a direct effect on the acinar cell and indirectly by stimulating CCK release. Finally, substance P receptors can bind substance P-like neurotransmitters released from intrapancreatic neurons, resulting in increased pancreatic secretion. The physiologic importance of the latter two mediators has not been established.

The response of pancreatic cells to the binding of these ligands appears to be mediated by two intracellular transducer systems. The formation of an agonist–receptor complex will stimulate either cAMP synthesis through the activation of adenylate cyclase (secretin/VIP) or formation of other intracellular messengers (including calcium released from intracellular stores) via polyphosphoinositide-specific phospholipase C (CCK/gastrin/bombesin/substance P/acetylcholine) (10–12).

INHIBITION

Inhibitory mechanisms are less well understood than stimulatory ones. Intravenous infusions of amino acids or glucose inhibit pancreatic function, probably due at least in part to the release of glucagon and somatostatin from islet cells. Pancreatic polypeptide may also decrease exocrine function by modulating cholinergic pathways although the physiologic significance of this has not been delineated (8, 9, 10–12, 14). A negative feedback loop has also been postulated whereby trypsin in the intestinal lumen inactivates a CCK-releasing peptide, decreasing CCK release and pancreatic enzyme secretion (13, 15, 16).

PHASES OF PANCREATIC SECRETION

Pancreatic function can best be described in terms of interdigestive (fasting) and digestive (postprandial) periods. Digestive secretion can be further subdivided into cephalic, gastric, and intestinal phases. The pancreas is not quiescent between meals, but rather displays a basal secretion that is cyclical.

Vagal nerves mediate the cephalic phase in which pancreatic secretion can be stimulated by the sight, smell, or taste of food. In sham feeding experiments (patients chew food without swallowing it), pancreatic enzyme secretion increased to approximately 50% of the maximal secretion elicited by intravenous CCK (9, 10). Neurotransmitters in addition to acetylcholine are probably involved since atropine does not completely block this response. VIP and GRP have been implicated. Gastric acid production is also stimulated during this phase, triggering secretin release that increases bicarbonate and enzyme secretion. Gastric distension causes increased pancreatic secretion mediated through a gastropancreatic vagovagal reflex, but the relative contribution of this gastric phase has not been determined in humans.

The most important phase is triggered when chyme enters the small intestine. This intestinal phase is regulated by the hormones secretin and CCK, and by enteropancreatic vagovagal reflexes triggered by volume and/or hyperosmolality in the gut. During all phases of pancreatic secretion, it is the interplay of neural and hormonal factors that results in the coordinated response of the pancreas to feeding (9, 10, 12, 13).

ACUTE PANCREATITIS

The inflammatory process of acute pancreatitis is caused by intrapancreatic activation of proteolytic and lipolytic digestive enzymes resulting in necrosis of pancreatic acinar cells and vascular damage. The clinical course of acute pancreatitis is often difficult to predict, and the factors that govern severity of the disease are largely unknown. Approximately 80% of patients will have a mild form of the disease termed "interstitial pancreatitis," which is characterized by interstitial edema and mild peripancreatic fat necrosis (17–20). The remaining patients develop severe disease with areas of hemorrhage and extensive necrosis of the pancreatic parenchyma and peripancreatic fat (17–20). Although interstitial pancreatitis may be associated with serious systemic toxicity, its course is usually mild and self-limited with a resultant mortality of less than 2%. In contrast, the clinical course of necrotizing pancreatitis is generally more severe, particularly if the necrosis is extensive, and carries a higher risk of local and systemic complications, such as organ failure and infection. The mortality of severe acute pancreatitis remains in the range of 10 to 30% (18, 20).

Etiology

Acute pancreatitis is associated with many other disease processes and events. Biliary tract stone disease and ethanol abuse account for 60 to 80% of acute bouts of pancreatitis, with the frequency of each depending on the patient population being evaluated (2, 17, 20). Female patients and those living in suburban areas tend to have pancreatitis as a result of biliary tract stone disease, whereas ethanol abuse is more frequently associated with pancreatitis in males and inner-city dwellers (2, 20). A number of miscellaneous causes account for 10 to 15% of pancreatitis attacks, with another 10 to 15% of cases classified as idiopathic (2, 17, 20). However, recent studies suggest that up to two-thirds of idiopathic cases may be caused by occult biliary microlithiasis (20).

Although the passage of biliary tract stones into or through the terminal biliopancreatic ductal system can clearly trigger acute pancreatitis, the mechanism by which the passage of stones initiates disease is unclear (2, 17). Biliary pancreatitis may be associated with recurrent episodes of acute disease, but development of chronic pancreatitis is rare. In contrast, most patients with ethanol-associated pancreatitis have consumed large amounts of alcohol for many years prior to the initial onset of symptoms. Since most of these patients have functional and morphologic pancreatic damage prior to their first attack, it appears that most cases of acute alcoholic pancreatitis actually represent acute inflammation of chronic pancreatitis (2, 6, 17, 20). Less commonly, alcohol may cause acute pancreatitis in the absence of chronic disease (6).

Although gallstones are the most common obstructive cause of acute pancreatitis, inflammation may also result from other lesions that interfere with the flow of pancreatic juice through the ductal system. Thus, pancreatitis may occur as a result of ductal strictures, sphincter of Oddi dysfunction, or tumors of the pancreas, ampulla, or duodenum (6, 17). Blunt trauma to the abdomen may also cause pancreatitis as a result of disruption of the pancreatic ductal system. Similarly, pancreatitis can occur as a postoperative complication following procedures that involve manipulation of the pancreas or during endoscopic retrograde cholangiopancreatography (ERCP) in which a side-viewing endoscope is passed into the duodenum, and a catheter introduces a radio-opaque contrast medium into the pancreatic duct. Certain viral, parasitic, and bacterial infections may also precipitate acute attacks. Less frequent causes of acute pancreatitis include penetrating duodenal ulcer, end-stage renal disease, organ transplantation, hypertriglyceridemia, and various toxins (2, 6, 20).

More than 85 drugs have been associated with the development of acute pancreatitis although the frequency of drug-induced disease is generally low (6, 21). Since scattered case reports comprise the bulk of the literature on drug-induced pancreatic disease, it is usually difficult to link drugs with pancreatic inflammation conclusively. Mallory and Kern classified drugs into three categories based on the clinical evidence implicating them in the development of acute pancreatitis: definite, probable, and questionable (22). The association was considered "definite" when drug therapy resulted in the development of abdominal pain combined with hyperamylasemia that resolved when therapy was discontinued or recurred when the drug was reintroduced (Table 29.2).

The pathogenesis of drug-induced pancreatic injury is unknown, but it does not appear to differ substantially from that of acute pancreatitis induced by other causes. Possible mechanisms include pancreatic ductal constriction, immune suppression, arteriolar thromboses, direct cellular toxicity, hepatic production of free radicals, and osmotic or metabolic effects (23). Since drug-induced acute pancreatitis cannot be distinguished clinically from that induced by other causes, it should be considered when other etiologies of disease have been ruled out.

Pathophysiology

The activation of trypsin from trypsinogen appears to play a primary role in the inflammation and necrosis of acute pancreatitis by its direct proteolytic activity and by its activation of zymogens and other bioactive substances that contribute to the pancreatic and systemic sequelae. Activation of the proteolytic enzyme elastase causes the dissolution of the elastic fibers of pancreatic blood vessels, leading to intrapancreatic hemorrhage. Chymotrypsin augments this vascular damage and the resulting edema. In the presence of bile acids, phospholipase A_2 produces pancreatic parenchymal necrosis. Phospholipase A_2 may also contribute to the development of adult respiratory distress syndrome (ARDS), a systemic complication of acute pancreatitis, by degrading pulmonary surfactant (6, 20). Liberation of lipase leads to pancreatic and peripancreatic fat necrosis. The kallikrein–kinin system is also activated by trypsin, leading to the release of vasoactive peptides that cause vasodilation, increased vascular permeability, and accumulation of leukocytes (20). A local and regional cellular necrosis results from the ischemia, inflammation, and edema of the pancreatic tissue and vasculature. A cycle then ensues in which continued enzyme release contributes to further pancreatic injury.

In severe disease, pancreatic enzymes, vasoactive peptides, and other toxic factors extravasate from the pancreas into peripancreatic spaces and the peritoneal cavity, causing a widespread chemical irritation (18). These materials

Table 29.2.
Agents Associated with Acute Pancreatitis

Definite Association
Asparaginase
Azathioprine
Didanosine
Estrogens
Furosemide
Isoniazid
Mercaptopurine
Metronidazole
Pentamidine
Sulfonamides
Sulindac
Tetracycline
Thiazides
Valproic acid

Probable Association
Bumetanide
Chlorthalidone
Cimetidine
Clozapine
Corticosteroids
Ethacrynic acid
Methyldopa
Phenformin
Procainamide
Salicylates
Sulfasalazine
Zalcitabine

Questionable Association

Acetaminophen	Indomethacin
Amiodarone	Interleukin-2
Ampicillin	
Carbamazepine	Isotretinoin
Cholestyramine	Ketoprofen
Cisplatin	Lisinopril
Clonidine	Mefenamic acid
Colchicine	Metolazone
Cyclosporine	Nitrofurantoin
Cyproheptadine	Opiates
Cytarabine	Oxyphenbutazone
Diazoxide	Phenolphthalein
Diphenoxylate	Piroxicam
Enalapril	Propoxyphene
Ergotamine	Ranitidine
Erythromycin	Tryptophan
Gold compounds	

Adapted from references 6, 21, 24.

may also reach the systemic circulation through retroperitoneal lymphatic and venous circulation to contribute to systemic complications, including respiratory and renal failure, encephalopathy, and cardiovascular collapse (18). The complement, coagulation, and fibrinolytic systems may also be activated by the release of trypsin, possibly playing a role in the development of coagulation disorders (6).

The mechanism by which pancreatic enzymes become prematurely activated within the gland to initiate the cascade of events that causes acute pancreatitis is unknown. Proposed mechanisms have focused on biliary tract stone disease, postulating that reflux of hepatic bile or duodenal contents into the pancreatic ductal system or pancreatic ductal hypertension may lead to extravasation of juice into the pancreatic parenchyma (2, 17, 20). More recently, investigators have proposed that activation of trypsin may occur within the pancreatic acinar cell rather than in the ductal or intercellular space (17). Obstruction in the pancreatic duct could disturb the normal events that maintain segregation of lysosomal enzymes, including cathepsin B, from digestive enzymes, thus allowing them to mix intracellularly. Cathepsin B is capable of converting trypsinogen to trypsin, which could then activate the remaining digestive zymogens. Ethanol is thought to exert a direct toxic effect on the pancreas and may also induce obstruction in the pancreatic duct by stimulating contraction of the sphincter of Oddi (2).

Clinical Presentation

The classic presentation of acute pancreatitis consists of abdominal pain, nausea, and vomiting. The abdominal pain is usually epigastric, but may be located anywhere in the abdomen or lower chest (2). Pain is usually sudden in onset and increases in severity over several hours . Pain may be quite severe, and it is most commonly described as a steady, dull, or boring pain that frequently radiates to the back. Patients may move about continually in search of a comfortable position, and partial relief is often found by sitting and leaning forward or lying on the side in the fetal position (2). Pain resolves over 1 to 3 days in mild cases, but may last many days to weeks during severe attacks. Painless pancreatitis has been reported infrequently. Nausea and vomiting are almost invariably present and are usually preceded by the onset of pain. Epigastric tenderness to deep palpation is a consistent finding on abdominal examination, as is mild abdominal distention. Bowel sounds are frequently diminished but not absent. Fever in the range of 100°F to 102°F is seen in most patients as the pyrogenic products of pancreatic injury enter the circulation. Pancreatic encephalopathy characterized by disorientation, delirium, or hallucinations is sometimes observed although most patients present without changes in mental status (2, 17). Tachycardia and hypotension progressing to circulatory shock can occur in severe cases as a result of hypovolemia caused by vomiting, hemorrhage, and fluid sequestration within the retroperitoneal space. Excessive circulating kinins contribute to this circulatory instability through vasodilatory effects and increased vascular permeability (17, 20).

Diagnosis

The diagnosis of acute pancreatitis is based on careful clinical evaluation of the patient, laboratory tests, and radiographic imaging. Mild cases of acute pancreatitis often represent a diagnostic dilemma since symptoms may be nonspecific, and pancreatic enzyme levels and imaging studies are often virtually normal (20). Occasionally, acute pancreatitis must be distinguished from other processes that present with abdominal pain, nausea, vomiting, and hyperamylasemia, such as acute cholecystitis and bowel obstruction (2).

LABORATORY TESTS

Leukocytosis, ranging from 10,000 to 25,000 cells/mm^3, is a frequent finding during routine laboratory evaluation of patients with acute pancreatitis (2, 20). Hyperglycemia, hypertriglyceridemia, and hypoalbuminemia are also common. Liver function tests frequently reveal mild hyperbilirubinemia and elevations in serum alkaline phosphatase and transaminase levels, which tend to be more pronounced with biliary pancreatitis. Hypovolemia may result in hemoconcentration, as evidenced by elevated hematocrit, blood urea nitrogen, and serum creatinine levels.

PANCREATIC ENZYMES

Elevation of serum amylase has remained central to the diagnosis of acute pancreatitis since its first association with the disease in 1929 (6, 20). The serum amylase level typically rises rapidly during the initial 2 to 12 hours of an attack and then declines over the following 3 to 5 days (2). The sensitivity of the test may be compromised if patients fail to present to the emergency room within hours of the onset of symptoms. Furthermore, hyperamylasemia is associated with a variety of nonpancreatic conditions, including diseases of the biliary tract, liver, intestines, female genitourinary tract, lungs, breast, prostate, and salivary glands (25). The magnitude of increase in serum amylase activity has no prognostic value and does not correlate with the severity of the acute attack. Generally, patients with biliary pancreatitis present with a more marked hyperamylasemia than do patients with alcohol-related disease (20, 25). The use of pancreatic isoamylase fractions to confirm a pancreatic origin of hyperamylasemia has been advocated by some clinicians. Unfortunately, most nonpancreatic abdominal diseases that simulate pancreatitis are also associated with increased pancreatic rather than nonpancreatic amylase levels (25). In contrast, serum lipase is derived almost exclusively from the pancreas. However, hyperlipasemia is not specific to pancreatic disease and may also occur in nonpancreatic acute abdominal conditions (2, 25). Although serum lipase typically parallels amylase in onset of elevation, lipase elevation persists longer, thus enhancing its diagnostic utility in patients who present

several days after the onset of symptoms. The use of other pancreatic enzymes such as immunoreactive trypsinogen, chymotrypsin, elastase, and phospholipase A$_2$ as markers for acute pancreatitis does not appear to provide any diagnostic advantage over the determination of serum amylase and lipase activity. Additionally, measurement of the urinary amylase level and the amylase–creatinine clearance ratio offers little benefit in improving diagnostic accuracy (20, 25).

IMAGING

Radiographic studies play an important role in confirming the diagnosis of pancreatitis as well as providing important etiologic and prognostic information. Although the abdominal radiograph is not considered diagnostic, it has several uses in this setting (25). Most important, it may help exclude nonpancreatic diseases that may simulate pancreatitis, including bowel obstruction and perforated viscus. The primary role of ultrasonography is in the evaluation of the biliary tract for stones, dilatation, or obstruction (25). Ultrasound examination is often precluded by excessive bowel gas or ileus that may accompany acute pancreatitis. Computed tomography (CT) and, more recently, dynamic contrast-enhanced CT are valuable tools for identifying the extent of pancreatic necrosis that correlates with the severity of disease and the risk of developing complications (20).

Prognosis

The clinical course of acute pancreatitis is uncomplicated in approximately 80% of attacks. Thus, the majority of patients with acute pancreatitis have mild disease that promptly resolves with conservative therapy (17–20). The remaining patients develop severe disease that is usually the clinical expression of pancreatic necrosis (19). Although the mortality of interstitial pancreatitis remains low (less than 2%), necrotizing pancreatitis has an associated mortality ranging from 10% (sterile necrosis) to 30% (infected necrosis) (18). The most important indicator of severity of acute pancreatitis is the development of organ failure (18, 19).

Multiple clinical criteria systems have been developed to assess the severity and prognosis of pancreatitis. Predictors of severity are necessary to allow more aggressive therapy to be targeted at patients with severe disease and to encourage early detection of complications (17, 20). Ranson and colleagues developed 11 prognostic criteria that can be measured 48 hours after admission to the hospital to indicate the severity of an acute attack (Table 29.3) (2, 17, 26). Although more complex than Ranson's criteria, the Acute Physiology and Chronic Health Evaluation (APACHE) II can also be used to assess patients with acute pancreatitis within hours of admission and at daily

Table 29.3.
Ranson's Prognostic Criteria

	Nonbiliary Pancreatitis	Biliary Pancreatitis
On admission		
Age (yr)	>55	>70
WBC/mL	>16,000	>18,000
Glucose (mg/dL)	>200	>220
LDH (IU/L)	>350	>400
AST (IU/L)	>250	>250
Within 48 hours of admission		
Decrease in Hct (points)	>10	>10
Increase in BUN (mg/dL)	>5	>2
Calcium (mg/dL)	<8	<8
PaO2 (mm Hg)	<60	—
Base deficit (mEq/L)	>4	>5
Fluid deficit (L)[a]	>6	>4

Adapted from reference 26.
Abbreviations: WBC, white blood cells; LDH, lactate dehydrogenase; AST, aspartate transaminase; Hct, hematocrit; BUN, blood urea nitrogen; PaO2, partial pressure of oxygen.
[a]Input minus output.

Table 29.4.
APACHE II Variables[°]

Temperature	Serum sodium
Heart rate	Serum potassium
Mean arterial pressure	Serum creatinine
Respiratory rate	Hematocrit
Oxygenation	White blood count
Arterial pH	Glasgow coma score
Age points	Chronic health assessment points

Adapted from reference 27.

intervals thereafter (2, 6, 27). Table 29.4 lists the variables that are evaluated under the APACHE II system (27). Severe acute pancreatitis is characterized by three or more Ranson criteria or at least eight APACHE II points (19). Systemic complications related to organ failure, including cardiovascular collapse, ARDS, and acute renal failure, are responsible for death early in the course of acute pancreatitis. Infectious complications, accounting for 80% of deaths from acute pancreatitis, develop later in the course of an acute attack (2, 17, 20).

Complications

Acute pancreatitis may be complicated by either local or systemic events (Table 29.5). Local events include the development of acute fluid collections located in or near the pancreas, occurring early in the course of 30 to 50% of attacks (19). Acute fluid collections lack a well-defined wall and regress spontaneously in 50% of cases (18, 19). Fluid collections may also progress to become pseudocysts or abscesses. A pseudocyst is a collection of pancreatic juice

Table 29.5.
Complications of Acute Pancreatitis

Local
Necrosis (sterile or infected)
Pancreatic fluid collection (sterile or infected)
Pseudocyst
Abscess
Pancreatic ascites
Blood vessel rupture or thrombosis
Bowel necrosis, obstruction, perforation
Ileus
Fistula
Systemic
Shock
Renal failure
Pulmonary insufficiency (including adult respiratory distress syndrome)
Coagulopathy
Gastrointestinal hemorrhage
Encephalopathy
Retinopathy
Hypocalcemia
Hyperglycemia

Adapted from references 2 and 6.

enclosed by a well-defined wall of fibrous tissue forming 4 or more weeks after the onset of an acute attack. Approximately 50% of these acute pseudocysts resolve within 6 weeks (18, 19). Pseudocysts may be clinically silent, or they may cause severe abdominal pain and elevation of pancreatic enzymes. Pancreatic abscess, another late-developing complication, is a circumscribed intra-abdominal collection of pus, containing little or no pancreatic necrosis (19). The term *pancreatic abscess* is also used to describe infection within a pseudocyst. In contrast, the development of pancreatic necrosis is an early event appearing within the first 4 days of an acute attack. Necrosis can be found in approximately 20% of acute pancreatitis cases and is necessary for the subsequent development of infection. Pancreatic infection, which occurs in 30 to 50% of patients, usually develops within the first 2 weeks of illness (18).

Severe acute pancreatitis may be complicated by multiple organ system failure, which most commonly involves the cardiovascular, renal, and pulmonary systems (2, 6). Cardiovascular decompensation, the result of hypovolemia and vasodilation caused by circulating vasoactive peptides, has the highest associated mortality. Acute renal failure is a consequence of hypovolemia and decreased renal perfusion. Pulmonary complications vary from mild arterial hypoxemia, usually detected during the first 2 days of an attack, to ARDS, the result of infradiaphragmatic inflammation (2).

Therapy

In the absence of effective specific therapy for the underlying disease process, the treatment of acute pancreatitis remains largely supportive. In patients with mild disease, principles of management include eliminating oral intake, maintaining adequate hydration with intravenous fluid, and providing parenteral analgesia to relieve pain (6, 17). With standard conservative therapy, the majority of cases of acute pancreatitis will subside within 3 to 10 days (20). In contrast, severe acute pancreatitis almost invariably requires management in an intensive care unit. Quantification of attack severity with the APACHE II system or Ranson's criteria and the identification of pancreatic necrosis are important early steps in patient management since patients with severe or necrotizing disease are more likely to incur complications (17, 19). Patients must be reassessed and monitored throughout the attack for the development of complications, particularly organ failure and infection. In addition, elimination of factors that precipitated the acute attack may improve the patient's course and prevent recurrence of disease (6, 20).

GENERAL SUPPORTIVE MEASURES

Acute pancreatitis may be associated with severe intravascular volume contraction and hypovolemia that results from exudation of protein-rich fluid into the inflamed peripancreatic retroperitoneum and peritoneal cavity, as well as sequestration of fluid within the bowel affected by ileus. Additionally, volume losses are incurred through vomiting, hemorrhage, and nasogastric suction. The primary goal of therapy early in the course of acute pancreatitis is to replace intravascular volume, plasma proteins, and electrolytes to avoid cardiovascular compromise of these patients. Volume replacement with crystalloid solutions is adequate for most patients, but intravenous colloids may be required if protein-rich fluid losses are massive. Potassium, calcium, and magnesium losses may also necessitate intravenous replacement. Hyperglycemia should be managed with insulin as required. Clinical status, vital signs, and appropriate laboratory and radiographic studies should be frequently reassessed. Severe acute pancreatitis requiring aggressive fluid resuscitation and maximal supportive care should be managed in the intensive care setting. The complicated course of severe disease often necessitates continuous hemodynamic and arterial blood gas monitoring as well as intensive management of cardiovascular, pulmonary, renal, and septic complications.

It is standard practice to eliminate oral intake of food and liquids early in the course of an acute attack in order to minimize pancreatic exocrine secretion and halt the autodigestive process. Following resolution of abdominal pain, hyperamylasemia, and complications, feeding may be reintroduced with liquids and the diet advanced as tolerated (17). Nasogastric suction has not been shown to improve the clinical course of mild-to-moderate pancreatitis (28, 29). It is appropriate therapy, however, for patients with severe nausea and vomiting or significant abdominal distention and ileus (2, 6, 17, 20). Total parenteral nutrition is an important adjunct to therapy of patients with severe or protracted disease where oral intake may be suspended for an extended period during a time of increased caloric need (30).

ANALGESIA

Narcotic analgesics will usually be required to control the severe abdominal pain that frequently accompanies acute pancreatitis. Transient elevations in serum amylase and lipase that often follow administration of opiates should not preclude their use since these effects do not appear to be detrimental to the disease course. Therapy is commonly initiated with meperidine administered parenterally at regular intervals in doses of 50 to 100 milligrams since it reportedly causes less spasm of the sphincter of Oddi than morphine and its derivatives (17, 20). However, since there is little evidence to suggest a clinically significant difference in the degree of sphincter spasm produced by any particular opiate, it appears that efficacy should serve as the primary guide for analgesic management of these patients (2).

UNPROVEN THERAPIES

Medical therapies designed to decrease pancreatic enzyme secretion, inhibit activity of proteolytic enzymes, or modulate the pancreatic inflammatory response have generally not been successful in preventing complications or improving the course of acute pancreatitis (Table 29.6). Attempts to treat acute pancreatitis by pharmacologically reducing pancreatic exocrine secretion with glucagon, calcitonin, atropine, and somatostatin have been disappointing (2, 6, 20, 31). A recent meta-analysis of six controlled studies evaluating the use of somatostatin in acute pancreatitis suggested a reduction in mortality, but further assessment is needed (32). Additionally, histamine (H_2)-receptor

Table 29.6.
Unproven Therapies for Acute Pancreatitis

Drugs	
Glucagon	$CaNa_2EDTA$
Calcitonin	Indomethacin
Somatostatin	Prostaglandin E_2
Antacids	Corticosteroids
Cimetidine	Fluorouracil
Atropine	Prophylthiouracil
Aprotinin	Dextran
Gabexate mesilate	Heparin
Camostate	Vasopressin
Fresh frozen plasma	ϵ-Aminocaproic acid
Procedures	
Nasogastric suction	Thoracic duct drainage
Peritoneal lavage	Hypothermia

Adapted from references 2, 6, 31, 33.

antagonist therapy with cimetidine, designed to reduce acid delivery to the duodenum and thus duodenal release of secretin, failed to improve patient outcome in controlled clinical trials (6, 20, 31). Inhibition of pancreatic secretion may not prove to be a rational therapeutic approach to the management of acute pancreatitis since exocrine pancreatic secretion is strongly inhibited in animal models of the disease (33).

Inhibition of pancreatic enzymes that are responsible for parenchymal damage and systemic complications has also proven ineffective. Protease inhibitors, including aprotinin, gabexate, and camostate, as well as the phospholipase A_2 inhibitor, $CaNa_2EDTA$, have failed to generate significant reductions in complications or mortality in patients with severe disease (6, 20, 31). Similarly, the administration of fresh frozen plasma to replenish circulating antiprotease activity has met with little success (6, 31). The local and systemic inflammation that accompanies acute pancreatitis may be controlled by nonsteroidal antiinflammatory drugs or prostaglandin E_2 (31). Well-designed, controlled, prospective studies are warranted to establish the value of these medical therapies designed to interrupt the cycle of pancreatic autodigestion.

ANTIBIOTICS

Even though infection has emerged as the most important cause of death in acute pancreatitis, the role of prophylactically administered antibiotics remains to be established. Early studies evaluating the use of antibiotics in patients with relatively mild disease failed to show any clinical benefit (17). Development of secondary pancreatic infection is limited to those patients with necrotizing disease, so the applicability of these studies in clinical practice is unclear. A recent study suggested that imipenem reduced the incidence of pancreatic sepsis in patients with necrosis, but mortality rate was not affected (34). It is certainly appropriate to initiate empiric antibiotic therapy in patients with pancreatic necrosis confirmed by CT scan and clinical evidence of infection or a deteriorating clinical condition. The presence of infected necrosis should be confirmed with CT scan-guided percutaneous needle aspiration of fluid from necrotic areas for gram stain and culture (18, 20). Pathogens most frequently isolated from infected necrosis include *Escherichia coli, Klebsiella pneumoniae, Enterococcus* species, *Staphylococcus aureus, Pseudomonas aeruginosa, Proteus mirabilis, Enterobacter aerogenes,* and *Bacteroides fragilis,* presumably originating in the colon (17). Once infection develops in the necrotic pancreas, surgical debridement is mandatory (18, 20).

CORRECTION OF BILIARY TRACT DISEASE

Virtually all clinicians agree that removal of residual biliary tract stones is necessary to prevent recurrent attacks of biliary pancreatitis. However, the optimal timing of stone removal and the choice between endoscopic and surgical treatment are subjects of continuing debate. Early intervention (within 72 hours of admission) may offer some benefit to the patient with severe biliary pancreatitis and persistent signs and symptoms (6, 20). Otherwise, it appears that either surgical or endoscopic procedures for biliary duct clearance should be performed prior to discharge from the hospital once pancreatic inflammation has resolved (2).

CHRONIC PANCREATITIS

Chronic pancreatitis is an inflammatory process leading to irreversible damage to pancreatic structure and function. All patients experience loss of exocrine tissue and fibrosis, and many lose endocrine function as well. The clinical course may consist of recurrent acute attacks, which are difficult to distinguish from acute pancreatitis, or steady progression of symptoms.

Further subclassification of chronic pancreatitis based on etiologic, pathologic, radiologic, or other criteria has proved elusive. One classification system that has been employed is the Marseilles-Rome system, which distinguishes three types (35):

1. Chronic calcifying pancreatitis, usually resulting from alcohol abuse, is the most common, accounting for more than 95% of cases (3). It is characterized by intraductal protein plugs and, often, calcified stones.
2. Chronic obstructive pancreatitis is relatively uncommon and occurs as a result of obstruction of the main pancreatic duct by tumor, stricture, or congenital abnormalities. This type is notable in that protein plugs and stones are absent, and damage may be reversible in part when obstruction is alleviated.
3. Chronic inflammatory pancreatitis, not well studied, is characterized by fibrosis, infiltration by monocytes, and atrophy of exocrine tissue.

Etiology

Ethanol abuse is by far the most common cause of chronic pancreatitis, particularly in Western countries, accounting for 70 to 80% of reported cases (4, 36, 37). A hereditary form, transmitted by an autosomal dominant gene with incomplete penetrance, has been described. Trauma can precipitate this disease. In addition, a tropical form exists in some Afro–Asian countries in which malnutrition is presumed to play a role. Other etiologic factors that have been proposed include hyperparathyroidism, hyperlipidemia, and *pancreas divisum* although a definitive role in disease initiation and progression has not been delineated for any of these. Up to 30% of cases are classified as idiopathic. Although gallstone disease may coexist with chronic pancreatitis, cholelithiasis does not appear to predispose a patient to this condition (1, 4, 36, 37).

As many as 45% of alcoholics show evidence of chronic pancreatitis at autopsy (approximately 50 times the incidence in nondrinkers) (4, 36). The following scenario summarizes the clinical course of a representative patient. He is a male alcoholic (men are five to ten times more likely to be affected than women) who began to drink heavily at age 25 and who started to experience attacks of pain by age 35. Within five years, abdominal radiographs showed calcification of the pancreas, and he developed symptoms of diabetes. At 45 years of age, pancreatic insufficiency had progressed to the point that steatorrhea was troublesome although attacks of pain were less severe because of increased fibrosis of the pancreas. He was dead at 50, probably from complications of alcoholism rather than pancreatitis, per se (1, 37). Major predictors of mortality appear to be age at diagnosis (the older the patient, the worse the prognosis), smoking, and drinking (38).

Pathophysiology

Although many questions remain to be answered concerning the cellular mechanisms involved in the initiation and progression of chronic pancreatitis, it appears that alcohol changes the nature of pancreatic secretions (3, 36). The absolute amount of protein in secretions increases, facilitating the formation of protein plugs, particularly in the smaller ductules. GP2, a 97-kilodalton protein that is analogous to the protein uromodulin responsible for the formation of renal costs, has been isolated from ductal plugs and may play a role in their formation (39). The resulting obstruction can lead to inflammation and fibrosis. In addition, trypsinogen is secreted in increased concentration, causing shifts in the trypsinogen-to-trypsin inhibitor ratio in pancreatic juice. Thus, a protective mechanism against autolysis may also be compromised (3, 36).

At least one protein, however, appears to be secreted in lower concentrations in the presence of alcohol. Lithostathine, formerly known as pancreatic stone protein, normally inhibits the formation of insoluble calcium salts in the ductules. Hence, a deficiency of this protein may allow increased precipitation of calcium salts, exacerbating obstruction, inflammation, and fibrosis (1, 3, 40).

Clinical Presentation

Pain and malabsorption are the hallmarks of chronic pancreatitis although a significant number of patients may also develop diabetes mellitus, pseudocysts, jaundice, peptic ulceration, or gastrointestinal bleeding (3, 5, 36). The cause(s) of pain have not been delineated, but intraductal hypertension, ischemia, pseudocyst, obstruction of the bile duct, or inflammation, especially in and around the pancreatic nerves, may be involved (42–45). The pain, sometimes accompanied by nausea and vomiting, is similar to that of acute pancreatitis. It is epigastric and often described as steady, boring, and either sharp or dull, with a characteristic radiation to the back in 65% of cases. Relief may be obtained by leaning forward from a sitting position, and pain is usually aggravated by eating. This pain with eating, in addition to malabsorption, contributes to the weight loss often observed in these patients. Up to 15% of patients may be pain free, but this is more commonly the case with idiopathic than with alcoholic pancreatitis (4, 40).

Loss of exocrine function occurs in all cases of chronic pancreatitis, but it may remain subclinical until fairly late in the course of the disease. Malabsorption does not manifest itself until less than 10% of pancreatic secretory function remains. Lipase activity decreases relatively more than protease activity; therefore, steatorrhea (fat in the stool) presents earlier and is usually more severe than azotorrhea (protein in the stool) (4, 36, 46, 47). Although some decrease in absorption of carbohydrates and fat-soluble vitamins does occur, symptoms rarely develop (36, 48). Bicarbonate secretion also declines with disease progression (3, 46).

Diagnosis

A diagnosis of chronic pancreatitis is generally straightforward in an alcoholic patient with recurrent bouts of epigastric pain and evidence of calcification of the pancreas by radiography. Diagnosis is made more difficult, however, if the patient is without pain, or if a distinction is sought between chronic pancreatitis and either recurring acute pancreatitis or pancreatic cancer. Physical examination and routine laboratory tests are of limited utility since they are usually within normal limits. Even serum lipase and amylase are generally normal although they may be elevated during acute exacerbations or decreased late in the course of the disease. Imaging techniques and pancreatic function tests provide the most useful diagnostic tools. They are presented next in approximately the order in which they should be considered based on effectiveness, invasiveness, and expense.

IMAGING

Radiography can reveal calcifications (usually diagnostic) and displacement of the stomach or duodenum indicating the presence of a pseudocyst. Ultrasonography will usually demonstrate pancreatic enlargement and pseudocysts although CT is superior in detecting pseudocysts and can reveal dilated pancreatic ducts as well as pancreatic enlargement and calcifications. ERCP is the most sensitive procedure for viewing changes in the ductal system (4, 36, 37).

PANCREATIC FUNCTION TESTS

These have been reviewed extensively elsewhere and can be classed as direct or indirect, invasive or noninvasive (49, 50). Direct tests, the gold standard for measuring pancreatic secretory function, are invasive, requiring intubation of the duodenum. A patient is given intravenous secretin, CCK, or both, and the increase in secretion of bicarbonate and/or enzymes is measured. Indirect tests, which may be either invasive or noninvasive, measure markers of pancreatic function in the blood or stool. Indirect tests are of limited usefulness, unfortunately, because of their relative lack of sensitivity early in the course of chronic pancreatitis. Examples of indirect tests include measurement of fat or chymotrypsin in stool samples, evaluation of pancreatic secretion after ingestion of a test meal (Lundh test), and measuring urinary excretion of para-aminobenzoic acid (PABA) after hydrolytic cleaving of PABA from NBT-PABA by chymotrypsin in the intestine (bentiromide test).

Therapy

Chronic pancreatitis is progressive and, with the possible exception of the obstructive form, irreversible. Treatment, therefore, is directed at managing the pain, malabsorption, and other complications that arise from this disease. If alcohol use is involved, every effort should be made to convince the patient to abstain. Unfortunately, however, this may not slow the course of the disease (1, 3).

PAIN

Treatable causes of pain such as pseudocyst, peptic ulcer, or bile duct stricture should be identified and addressed as the first step in the management of chronic pancreatic pain. Abstinence from alcohol may reduce pain in up to 50% of patients, but the majority will require some form of analgesia (41, 43). Salicylates, nonsteroidal antiinflammatory drugs, or acetaminophen should be tried initially. Opioid analgesics may be needed for the 20% of patients who suffer from intractable pain even though up to 8% of them can be expected to become addicted (35).

Enzyme replacement therapy, which will also be discussed for the treatment of malabsorption, may also help alleviate pain, especially in patients with nonalcoholic chronic pancreatitis (13, 41, 45, 51). The presence of proteases in the duodenum may suppress pancreatic function through a negative feedback mechanism that inhibits release of CCK (15, 16). Enzymes contained in nonenteric-coated preparations may be more reliably delivered to the duodenum than enzymes from enteric-coated dosage forms. The latter are sometimes released in more distal portions of the small intestine because of the relatively low duodenal pH caused by decreased bicarbonate secretion in chronic pancreatitis (3, 46). As a result, nonenteric preparations may be more effective at suppressing CCK release and reducing pain. Octreotide, a somatostatin analogue, has not consistently demonstrated efficacy in the treatment of pain, but it may have a role in the management of pancreatic pseudocysts (41, 52) and in decreasing complications after pancreatic surgery (53).

Despite maximum medical management, up to 30% of patients will still experience pain. This pain may diminish ("burn out") over time as the pancreas becomes progressively more fibrotic, but some patients will require surgical intervention to control pain. A percutaneous celiac plexus block will provide temporary relief in a majority of patients (41), but most will require a more definitive procedure such as a lateral pancreaticojejunostomy, which facilitates drainage of the main duct, or a partial pancreatectomy. Response rates range from 50 to 90% for these procedures (43, 45). Endoscopic stent placement may provide relief for up to 100% of patients, but long-term efficacy and complications are still being evaluated (51, 54).

MALABSORPTION

Patients with documented weight loss and steatorrhea should receive treatment for malabsorption. Two types of pancreatic enzyme replacement preparations are currently available. Pancreatin is derived from freeze-dried porcine or bovine pancreases and contains at least 2 USP (United States Pharmacopeia) units of lipase and 25 USP units each of protease and amylase per milligram. Pancrelipase, extracted from porcine pancreases, is more potent, containing at least 24, 100, and 100 USP units of lipase, protease, and amylase, respectively, per milligram (Table 29.7) (55).

Rapid-release and enteric-coated dosage forms are also available. Although rapid-release forms more reliably deliver proteases to the upper duodenum where they may exert a negative feedback inhibitory effect, they expose lipase to the acid environment of the stomach. Lipase is pH-labile, maximally active at pH 8, and irreversibly inactivated at pH less than 4. Enteric coatings that dissolve at approximately pH 5.6 to 6.0 better protect lipase from gastric acidity, but enzyme release may be delayed.

Since lipid malabsorption and steatorrhea are the primary clinical problems associated with pancreatic insufficiency, the dose of lipase to be delivered to the duodenum is a paramount concern. Maximal postprandial delivery of lipase from a normal pancreas is 140,000 U/hr for four hours (560,000 U total). Supplying 5 to 10% of this will significantly decrease steatorrhea; therefore, the enzyme supplement should provide at least 28,000 U over a 4-hour period. Up to 92% of conventional rapid-release formulations may be inactivated in passage through the stomach, so large doses are recommended (55).

One approach to enzyme replacement therapy is to start the patient on a rapid release formulation (e.g., eight tablets of Viokase® with meals). Efficacy of therapy can be assessed by monitoring fat content of stools. If steatorrhea persists, another agent can be added to increase gastric pH in an attempt to increase the delivery of active lipase to the duodenum. Agents that may be useful include H_2-receptor antagonists and omeprazole (12, 43, 55–57). Sodium

Table 29.7.

Some Commercial Pancreatic Enzyme Preparations

Product[a]	Formulation[b]	Dosage Form[c]	Enzyme Content (USP Units)		
			Lipase	Protease	Amylase
Rapid Release					
Cotazym	PL	C	8000	30,000	30,000
Ilozyme	PL	T	11,000	30,000	30,000
Pancreatin 5× USP	PC	T	12,000	60,000	60,000
8× USP	PC	T	22,500	180,000	180,000
Viokase	PL	T	8000	30,000	30,000
Viokase	PL	P	16,800	70,000	70,000
Enteric Coated					
Cotazym-S	PL	MS	5000	20,000	20,000
Creon	PC	MS	8000	13,000	30,000
Entolase-HP	PL	MS	8000	40,000	50,000
Festal II	PL	T	6000	20,000	30,000
Ku-Zyme HP	PL	MS	8000	30,000	30,000
Maxamase	PL	MS	16,000	48,000	48,000
Pancrease	PL	MS	4000	25,000	20,000
Pancrease MT-4	PL	MT	4000	12,000	12,000
Pancrease MT-10	PL	MT	10,000	30,000	30,000
Pancrease MT-16	PL	MT	16,000	48,000	48,000
Ultrase MT12	PL	MT	12,000	29,000	29,000
Ultrase MT20	PL	MT	20,000	65,000	65,000
Ultrase MT24	PL	MT	24,000	78,000	78,000
Zymase	PL	MS	12,000	24,000	24,000

[a]These products, available before passage of the 1938 Food, Drug, and Cosmetic Act, are not approved by the FDA and cannot be considered pharmaceutically or therapeutically equivalent (12).
[b]PC, pancreatin, PL, pancrelipase.
[c]C, capsule; MS, microspheres; MT, microtablets; P, powder; T, tablet.

bicarbonate and aluminum-containing antacids may also increase the efficacy of supplements, but calcium- and magnesium-containing antacids worsen steatorrhea (44). Another approach is to give the patient a trial of an enteric-coated preparation. Even with careful management of supplements, however, the elimination of steatorrhea is very difficult (13).

Problems that may be encountered with enzyme-replacement therapy, especially at high doses, include abdominal pain, oral and perianal irritation, nausea, vomiting, diarrhea, and rare hypersensitivity. There have also been reports of hyperuricosuria although this appears to be more common in cystic fibrosis patients receiving pancreatic enzymes. Finally, patient compliance is often less than optimal because of the administration of large numbers of tablets, gastrointestinal distress, and the expense of the regimen (13, 55).

CONCLUSION

Acute and chronic pancreatitis appear to be distinct clinical entities that are often, though not always, alcohol related. Acute pancreatitis is an autodigestive process characterized by inflammation, edema, and necrosis, whereas chronic pancreatitis is associated with intraductal protein plugs and calculi leading to irreversible loss of functional tissue. An acute process may evolve into chronic disease, but this is uncommon and cannot be predicted. In acute pancreatitis, it is important to establish the severity of the attack so that appropriate therapy can be instituted and the patient's risk for developing complications evaluated. With chronic pancreatitis, care is directed toward pain relief and managing declining endocrine and exocrine function. In both, therapy remains almost exclusively supportive. Although there have been recent advances in our understanding of pathophysiology and treatment, much remains unclear. Controlled clinical trials are needed to assess the role of medical therapy directed at the underlying pathogenesis of acute and chronic pancreatic disease.

REFERENCES

1. Steer ML, Waxman I, Freedman S. Chronic pancreatitis. N Engl J Med 332 (22): 1482–1490, 1995.
2. Steer ML. Acute pancreatitis. In: Yamada T. Textbook of Gastroenterology. Philadelphia, J.B. Lippincott Company, 1991, p. 1859.
3. Sarles H, Bernard JP, Johnson C. Pathogenesis and epidemiology of chronic pancreatitis. Ann Rev Med 40:453–468, 1989.
4. Owyang C, Levitt M. Chronic pancreatitis. In: Yamada T. Textbook of Gastroenterology. Philadelphia, J.B. Lippincott Company, 1991, p. 1874.
5. Larsen S. Diabetes mellitus secondary to chronic pancreatitis. Danish Medical Bulletin 40(2):153–162, 1993.

6. Steinberg W, Tenner S. Acute pancreatitis. N Engl J Med 330(17): 1198–2010, 1994.

7. Mitchell CJ. The relationship between pancreas divisum and pancreatitis: medical aspects. In: Burns GP, Bank S. Disorders of the Pancreas: Current Issues in Diagnosis and Management. New York, McGraw-Hill, Inc, 1992, p. 141.

8. Moossa AR, Mulholland M. Pancreas: anatomy and structural anomalies. In: Yamada T. Textbook of Gastroenterology. Philadelphia, J.B. Lippincott Company, 1991, p. 1851.

9. Ermak TH, Grendell JH. Anatomy, histology, embryology, and development anomalies. In: Sleisenger MH, Fordtran JS. Gastrointestinal Disease: Pathophysiology/ Diagnosis/ Management, ed 5. Philadelphia, W.B. Saunders Company, 1993, p. 1654.

10. Owyang C, Williams J. Pancreatic secretion. In: Yamada T. Textbook of Gastroenterology. Philadelphia, J.B. Lippincott Company, 1991, p. 294.

11. Pandol S. Pancreatic physiology. In: Sleisenger MH, Fordtran JS. Gastrointestinal Disease: Pathophysiology/ Diagnosis/ Management, ed 5. Philadelphia, W.B. Saunders Company, 1993, p. 1585.

12. Valenzuela JE. Pancreatic physiology. In: Valenzuela JE, Reber HA, Ribet A. Medical and Surgical Diseases of the Pancreas. New York, Igaku-Shoin, 1991, p. 1.

13. Lebenthal E, Rolston DDK, Holsclaw DS. Enzyme therapy for pancreatic insufficiency: present status and future needs. Pancreas 9(1):1–12, 1994.

14. Chey WY. Regulation of pancreatic exocrine secretion. Int J Pancreatol 9:7–20, 1991.

15. Owyang C, Louie DS, Tatum D. Feedback regulation of pancreatic enzyme secretion: suppression of cholecystokinin release by trypsin. J Clin Invest 77:2042–2047, 1986.

16. Owyang C, May D, Louie DS. Trypsin suppression of pancreatic enzyme secretion: differential effect on cholecystokinin release and the enteropancreatic reflex. Gastroenterol 91:637–643, 1986.

17. Bradley EL. Acute Pancreatitis: Diagnosis and Therapy. New York: Raven Press, 1994, ch 1–4, 9–11, 30–34.

18. Banks PA. Acute pancreatitis: medical and surgical management. Am J Gastroenterol 89(8 Suppl):S78–S85, 1994.

19. Bradley EL. A clinically based classification system for acute pancreatitis. Arch Surg 128(5):586–590, 1993.

20. Marshall JB. Acute pancreatitis: a review with an emphasis on new developments. Arch Intern Med 153(10):1185–1198, 1993.

21. Underwood TW, Frye CB. Drug-induced pancreatitis. Clin Pharmacy 12:440–448, 1993.

22. Mallory A, Kern F. Drug-induced pancreatitis: a critical review. Gastroenterol 78:813–820, 1980.

23. Banerjee AK, Patel KJ, Grainger SL. Drug-induced pancreatitis: a critical review. Med Toxicol Adverse Drug Exp 4:186–198, 1989.

24. Rabassa AA, Trey G, Shukla U, et al. Isoniazid-induced acute pancreatitis. Ann Intern Med 121:433–434, 1994.

25. Agarwal N, Pitchumoni CS, Sivaprasad AV. Evaluating tests for acute pancreatitis. Am J Gastroenterol 85(4):356–365, 1990.

26. Ranson JHC. Etiological and prognostic factors in human acute pancreatitis: a review. Am J Gastroenterol 77:633–638, 1982.

27. Agarwal N, Pitchumoni CS. Assessment of severity in acute pancreatitis. Am J Gastroenterol 86(10):1385–1391, 1991.

28. Levant JA, Secrist DM, Resin H, Studevant RAL, Guth PH. Nasogastric suction in the treatment of alcoholic pancreatitis. JAMA 229(1):51–52, 1974.

29. Sarr MG, Sanfey H, Cameron JL. Prospective, randomized trial of nasogastric suction in patients with acute pancreatitis. Surgery 100(3):500–504, 1986.

30. Pisters PWT, Ranson JHC. Nutritional support for acute pancreatitis. Surg, Gynecol & Obstet 175:275–284, 1992.

31. Niederau C, Schulz HU. Current conservative treatment of acute pancreatitis: evidence from animal and human studies. Hepato-Gastroenterology 40:538–549, 1993.

32. Carballo F, Dominguez E, Fernandez-Calvet L, et al. Is somatostatin useful in the treatment of acute pancreatitis?: a meta-analysis. Digestion 49:12–13, 1991.

33. Loser C, Folsch UR. A concept of treatment in acute pancreatitis: results of controlled trials, and future developments. Hepato-Gastroenterology 40:569–573, 1993.

34. Pederzoli P, Bassi C, Vesentini S, Campedelli A. A randomized multicenter clinical trial of antibiotic prophylaxis of septic complications in acute necrotizing pancreatitis with imipenem. Surg, Gynecol & Obstet 176:480–483, 1993.

35. Sarles H, Adler G, Dani R, et al. The pancreatitis classification of Marseilles-Rome 1988. Scand J Gastroenterol 24:641–642, 1989.

36. Grendel JH, Cello JP. Chronic pancreatitis. In: Sleisenger MH, Fordtran JS. Gastrointestinal Disease: Pathophysiology/ Diagnosis/ Management, ed. 5. Philadelphia, W.B. Saunders Company, 1993, p. 1654.

37. Young HS. V. Diseases of the pancreas. Scientific American, Inc. 1994, Section 4, p. 1–17.

38. Lowenfels AB, Maisonneuve P, Cavallini G, et al. Prognosis of chronic pancreatitis: an international multicenter study. Am J Gastroenterol 89(9):1467–1471, 1994.

39. Freedman SD, Sakamoto K, Venu RP. GP2, the homologue to the renal cast protein uromodulin, is a major component of intraductal plugs in chronic pancreatitis. J Clin Invest 29:83–90, 1993.

40. Yamadera K, Moriyama T, Makino I. Identification of immunoreactive pancreatic stone protein in pancreatic stone, pancreatic tissue, and pancreatic juice. Pancreas 5(3):255–260, 1990.

41. Malfertheiner P, Dominguez-Munoz JE, Buchler MW. Chronic pancreatitis: management of pain. Digestion 55(suppl 1):29–34, 1994.

42. Ebbehoj N. Pancreatic tissue fluid pressure and pain in chronic pancreatitis. Danish Medical Bulletin 39(2):128–133, 1992.

43. Karanjia ND, Rever HA. The cause and management of the pain of chronic pancreatitis. Gastroenterol Clin of N Amer 19(4):895–904, 1990.

44. Tenner S, Levine RS, Steinberg WM. Drug treatment of acute and chronic pancreatitis. In: Lewis JH. A Pharmacologic Approach to Gastrointestinal Disorders. Baltimore, Williams & Wilkins, 1994, p. 311.

45. Banks PA. Management of pancreatic pain. Pancreas 6(Suppl 1) S52–S59, 1991.

46. Beglinger C. Relevant aspects of physiology in chronic pancreatitis. Dig Dis 10:326–329, 1992.

47. Layer P, Holtmann G. Pancreatic enzymes in chronic pancreatitis. Int J Pancreatol 15(1):1–11, 1994.

48. Ladas SD, Giorgiotis K, Raptis SA. Complex carbohydrate malabsorption in exocrine pancreatic insufficiency. Gut 34:984–987, 1993.

49. Goldberg DM, Durie PR. Biochemical tests in the diagnosis of chronic pancreatitis and in the evaluation of pancreatic insufficiency. Clin Biochem 26:253–275, 1993.

50. Ribet A, Moreau J, Valenzuela JE. Diagnosis of chronic pancreatitis. In: Valenzuela JE, Reber HA, Ribet A. Medical and Surgical Diseases of the Pancreas. New York, Igaku-Shoin, p. 113.

51. Ihse I, Andersson R, Axelson J. Pancreatic pain: is there a medical alternative to surgery? Digestion 54(suppl 2):30–34, 1993.

52. Buchler MW, Binder M, Friess H. Role of somatostatin and its analogues in the treatment of acute and chronic pancreatitis. Gut (Suppl 3):S15–S19, 1994.

53. Friess H, Klempa I, Hermanek P, et al. Prophylaxis of complications after pancreatic surgery: results of a multicenter trial in Germany. Digestion 55(suppl 1):35–50, 1994.

54. Geenen JE, Rolny P. Endoscopic therapy of acute and chronic pancreatitis. Gastrointestinal Endoscopy 37(3):377–382, 1991.

55. Kraisinger M, Hochhaus G, Stecenko A, et al. Clinical pharmacology of pancreatic enzymes in patients with cystic fibrosis and *in vitro* performance of microencapsulated formulations. J Clin Pharmacol 34:158–166, 1994.

56. Regan PT, Malagelada JR, DiMagno EP, et al. Comparative effects of antacids, cimetidine and enteric coating on the therapeutic response to oral enzymes in severe pancreatic insufficiency. N Engl J Med 297:854–858, 1977.

57. Bruno MJ, Rauws EAJ, Hoek FJ, et al. Comparative effects of adjuvant cimetidine and omeprazole during pancreatic enzyme replacement therapy. Dig Dis & Sci 39(5):988, 1994.

CHAPTER 30

RHEUMATOID ARTHRITIS AND ITS THERAPY

ERIC G. BOYCE and LAWRENCE J. LEVENTHAL

Rheumatoid arthritis (RA) is a highly variable, chronic inflammatory condition of unknown etiology affecting mostly the joints but often with periarticular and systemic involvement. The word *rheuma* was used by ancient Greek physicians to mean "flowing," which fit well with their humoral theory of disease. The term *rheumatism* was linked to joint ailments in the 1600s by a French physician who used it as an inexact label for a systemic condition, and *rheumatoid arthritis* was coined in 1858 as a label for cases reported earlier in the century. Although many refinements and developments in the understanding of RA have ensued, the pathogenesis of the disease remains unknown, and current therapies are nonspecific and rarely curative. Patients with RA are extensive users of health care systems, with usage rates and costs at rates that are two to three times greater than the general population (1). The goals of drug and nondrug therapy should be to provide safe, effective, and inexpensive treatment that will diminish pain, improve well being, prevent or slow disease progression, and reduce the need for health care and disability services.

ETIOLOGY

The etiology of rheumatoid arthritis is unknown, but theories implicate genetic, hormonal, viral, mycobacterial, autoimmune, atmospheric, environmental, and other etiologies. RA is associated with HLA-DR4 and HLA-DR1 (which are class II major histocompatibility complex antigens), the homozygous C-kappa genotype (constant region of IgG, and so on), and T-cell receptor beta chains (2). These associations imply that immunogenetics play an important role in RA since class II major histocompatibility complex antigens are involved in immune regulation and immunoglobulins, and T-cells are part of the immune response.

A hormonal link is supported by the female preponderance of this disease, decreased risk of developing RA generally associated with a history of pregnancy or possibly oral contraceptive use, and increased risk following breast feeding (3). Less severe RA is found in patients who used oral contraceptives prior to the onset of RA. Despite these data, oral contraceptives are not recommended for prophylaxis.

Infectious etiologies of RA are supported by a number of findings. Sera from RA patients demonstrates hyperre-

activity to Epstein-Barr virus antigens. RANA (rheumatoid arthritis nuclear antigen) is found in patients with RA and may be similar to Epstein-Barr nuclear antigens. White blood cells from patients with RA are hyperreactive to *Mycobacterium tuberculosis*. Antimicrobial agents are of some benefit in RA. In theory, the infection would lead to an autoimmune response.

EPIDEMIOLOGY

RA affects 0.3 to 1.5% of the population and is two to three times more common in women than in men. It can be seen in any culture or race. RA occurs at any age, with the peak incidence in women occurring between 30 and 60 years of age. Children with chronic arthritis that meet certain criteria are given a diagnosis of juvenile rheumatoid arthritis, which is a different diagnosis than RA.

Genetic predisposition is suggested by the increased incidence of RA in certain families, monozygote twins, and individuals with specific genetic markers for HLA-DR4, HLA-DR1, C-kappa, or subtypes of HLA-DR4, HLA-DR1, or HLA-DQ. HLA-DR4, a class II major histocompatibility complex antigen, occurs in 36% of the population as a whole, 58 to 65% of those with RA, 60% of those with rheumatoid factor-negative RA, 69 to 75% of those with rheumatoid factor-positive RA, and more commonly in patients with more severe RA.

PATHOGENESIS

The pathophysiology of the joint changes seen in rheumatoid arthritis has been well described at the tissue level and somewhat at cellular, biochemical, and molecular levels. The chronic inflammation, synovial proliferation, and bone and cartilage destruction seen in RA appear to be associated with abnormalities in immune, inflammatory, and repair responses that involve the direct actions, secretions or regulation of macrophages, lymphocytes, neutrophils, fibroblasts (which may be specialized macrophages), and other cells.

A normal diarthrodial joint is a functional interface that supports and limits the relative movement of two or more bones over defined ranges. The joint capsule surrounds the joint space and connects to the surrounding bones (Figure 30.1). The synovium, or synovial tissue, is the internal structure of the joint capsule that secretes synovial fluid

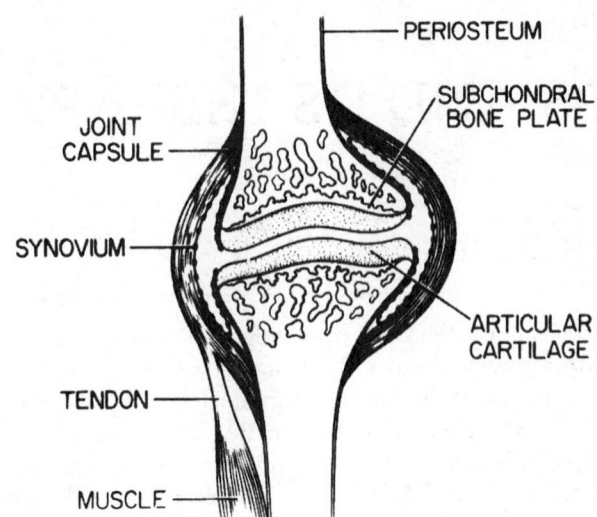

Figure 30.1. Normal diarthrodial joint. The typical diarthrodial joint, such as the knee, is freely movable. The articulating surfaces are covered by a smooth layer of hyaline cartilage and are enclosed in a fibrous capsule. The fibrous capsule merges externally with periosteum, tendons, ligaments, and fascia and internally with the synovial membrane that lines the joint cavity. Articular cartilage is not covered by synovial membrane. A small amount of synovial fluid is normally present within the joint cavity.

and contains many blood vessels and immunologically active cells. Connective tissue surrounds the synovial tissue and provides stability to the joint capsule and the synovial lining membrane. Tendons, ligaments, and muscles also serve to stabilize the joint. Cartilage, which is composed of proteoglycan groups and 70% water, is bathed in synovial fluid and acts to cushion the forces between the opposing bones during movement or compression. Synovial fluid provides nutrients, removes wastes from the cartilage, and helps maintain the structure of the cartilage through hydration. This normal anatomy and physiology are altered in RA by immunologically mediated changes in bone, cartilage, supporting tissues, and synovial tissue and fluid.

The event initiating immunologic abnormalities in RA is unknown, but it may involve an altered reaction to an exogenous or autoantigen. Potential antigens include the Fc (constant) portion of IgG, Type II collagen found in cartilage, Type III collagen found in synovium and blood vessels, chondrocyte membrane, and *Mycobacterium tuberculosis*. The overreactivity to antigens may be linked to the major histocompatibility complex (MHC) class II antigens HLA-DR4 or HLA-DR1 or to adhesion molecules on fibroblasts (4). MHC class II antigens are expressed on the surface of macrophages and other antigen-processing cells in association with processed antigen and regulate the interaction with helper T-cells.

Macrophages are important in the pathogenesis of RA through their release of interleukin-1 (IL-1) and tumor necrosis factor (TNF) in response to antigens, immune complexes, complement, gamma interferon (IFN-gamma), and collagen from cartilage and synovium (Table 30.1) (5). IL-1 stimulates the activation and proliferation of lymphocytes and secretion of a tissue growth factor. IL-1 and TNF are chemotactic and stimulate the release of IL-6, granulocyte-macrophage colony stimulating factor (GM-CSF), prostaglandin E_2 (PGE_2), collagenase, proteinase, and Substance P. IL-1 increases PGE_2 production by inducing phospholipase-A_2 and prostaglandin H synthase. TNF-alpha is secreted with IL-1 but appears less important than IL-1 in inflammation and enzyme release (5). Prostaglandin E_2 (PGE_2) and leukotriene B_4 (LTB_4) are inflammatory mediators that are increased in patients with RA. Levels of IL-1, TNF-alpha, GM-CSF, and soluble IL-2 receptors increase in the blood, synovial fluid, and/or synovial tissue in patients with RA and may correlate with disease activity (5, 6). IL-1 receptor antagonist production by synovial tissue cells from patients with RA is less than expected given the amount of IL-1 produced (7). Expression of MHC class I antigens, which are associated with cytotoxicity, and an adhesion molecule on the surface of rheumatoid synovial fibroblasts are enhanced by IL-1, TNF-alpha, and IFN-gamma (4). IFN-gamma also increases the expression of MHC class II antigens (4) and decreases the IL-1 and TNF mediated release of PGE_2 (8). TNF-alpha levels correlate with rheumatoid cachexia (9). IL-1 and TNF-alpha inhibitors have also been identified (5).

T-cells from patients with RA demonstrate markers for activated (CD3+) and suppressor/cytotoxic (CD8+) T-cells, activation by enhanced HLA-DR antigen expression, hyperreactivity to soluble antigen and chondrocyte membrane, and mature and hyperreactive memory T-cells (10). Natural killer (NK) cells are found in early rheumatoid synovial tissue (11). Patients with RA have gone into remission when infected with the human immunodeficiency virus (12), implicating a key role of helper T-cells in RA. However, patients with RA have small numbers of activated helper (CD4+) T-cells, low levels of activated T-cell products IL-2 and IFN-gamma in synovial fluid, T-cells that are hyporesponsive to mitogenic stimuli, and a low degree of expression of activation receptors on the surface of synovial T-cells (10). These effects may indicate a defect in helper T-cells in patients with RA, leaving the role of T-cells in RA unclear.

IL-6 is increased in inflammatory synovial fluid and increases production of GM-CSF, immunoglobulins, and liver acute-phase reactants following secretion from monocytes, T-cells, and fibroblasts (Table 30.1) (5, 10). GM-CSF is secreted by synovial tissue, macrophages, fibroblasts, endothelial cells, and activated lymphocytes and acts to promote growth of certain bone marrow cell lines, increase MHC class II expression on synovial macrophages, stimu-

Table 30.1.
Actions of Immunological Mediators in Rheumatoid Arthritis[a]

Substance	Source	Stimulates (Inhibits)
IL-1, TNF	Macrophages	MHC-I expression, chemotaxis
		Release of PGE_2, IL-6, GM-CSF, collagenase, proteinase, Substance P
IL-1	Macrophages	Lymphocyte proliferation and activation
		Growth factor release
IL-6	Fibroblasts	T-cell and B-cell function
	T-Lymphocytes	GM-CSF release
IFN-gamma	T-Lymphocytes	MHC-I and MHC-II expression
		(Inhibits Collagenase and PGE_2 release)
GM-CSF	Macrophages	Bone marrow cell formation, IL-1 production
	Lymphocytes	PMN activation, monocyte attraction
PGE_2	Fibroblasts	Growth factor release, cartilage degradation, inflammation, pain
Collagenase	Fibroblasts	Cartilage degradation
Growth factors		Synovial tissue proliferation
Transforming		Synovial tissue proliferation
growth factor		IL-1 production, monocyte chemotaxis
		(Inhibits lymphokine and protease secretion, synoviocyte growth, and HLA-DR expression)

[a]Abbreviations: GM-CSF, granulocyte macrophage colony stimulating factor; IFN, interferon; IL, interleukin; MHC, major histocompatibility complex; PG, prostaglandin; PMN, neutrophils; TNF, tumor necrosis factor.

late IL-1 production, activate neutrophils, and attract monocytes (Table 30.1) (5, 10).

Antibodies, immune complexes, complement, and complement split products also increase in patients with RA. Rheumatoid factor, an autoantibody directed against the Fc portion of IgG, is positive in 80% of patients with RA. Hyaluronic acid, a normal component of synovial fluid, may facilitate the formation of immune complexes of rheumatoid factor and IgG. Other autoantibodies are also be seen.

Synovial tissue proliferates in RA, becomes hypervascular, and develops into an invasive tissue known as the pannus. Platelet-derived growth factor, epidermal growth factor, transforming growth factor, basic fibroblast growth factor, and receptors for these growth factors have been found in synovial fluid and tissue (5). These growth factors may lead to the tumorlike growth of synovial tissue in RA, possibly in an autocrine manner. Platelet-derived growth factor is regulated by IL-1 and PGE_2 (Table 30.1) (5). Migrating circulatory macrophages may also help maintain the hyperplastic synovium. Transforming growth factor decreases lymphokine and protease secretion, synoviocyte growth, and HLA-DR expression, but enhances collagen and fibronectin gene transcription, protease inhibitor and IL-1 production, monocyte chemotaxis, and immunosuppression (5).

The bone resorption and cartilage destruction of RA are due to cellular activities and secretions. Collagenase, PGE_2, plasminogen activator (a neutral proteinase of both tissue and urokinase types that is converted to plasmin), and stromelysin are able to degrade cartilage or collagen and are produced by synovial fibroblasts or chondrocytes after stimulation by IL-1 or TNF (5, 8). The effect of IL-1 and TNF on collagenase and PGE_2 production is diminished by IFN-gamma (Table 30.1) (8). Hyperreactivity of

peripheral blood and synovial T-cells to chondrocyte membrane may also explain the cartilage destruction. Phagocytes from rheumatoid synovial fluid have contained type II collagen, indicating active phagocytosis of cartilage. Plasma parathyroid hormone and calcitriol levels may also correlate with periarticular bone loss in RA patients (13). Plasmin inhibitor-plasmin complexes are slightly elevated in patients with rheumatoid vasculitis and may correlate with prolongation of partial thromboplastin time possibly due to release of plasminogen activator from vessel walls (14). Activated macrophages may secrete a procoagulant that enhances the formation of fibrin or fibrinoid material over synovial lining or within a rheumatoid nodule.

The inflammation, synovial proliferation, and collagen destruction of RA lead to changes in synovial fluid, synovial tissue, cartilage, and bone. The pressure within the joint increases from vacuum or subatmospheric pressures in the normal joint to supraatmospheric pressures when inflamed. Rheumatoid synovial fluid is similar to that seen in other inflammatory joint diseases with respect to leukocytosis (mostly polymorphonuclear cells) and decreased viscosity. The synovial tissue becomes hypervascular and blood flow increases with vasodilation, but this may not be enough to meet the metabolic demands resulting from the inflammation. Lactate levels are high in inflamed synovial fluid. Increased synovial fluid, synovial tissue proliferation, and cartilage destruction lead to limitation of movement and discomfort. Cartilage and bone destruction further destabilize the joint.

DIAGNOSIS AND CLINICAL FINDINGS

The criteria for the classification of rheumatoid arthritis were revised in 1988 by the American College of Rheumatology (15). These criteria (Table 30.2) are intended to serve as the standard in research and to aid in the clinical

Table 30.2.
The Classification of Rheumatoid Arthritis Based on the 1987 Revised "Traditional" Method[a]

The patient must meet four of the following seven criteria to be classified as having rheumatoid arthritis.

1. Morning stiffness of or near joints lasting 1 hour before maximum benefit[b]
2. Arthritis, as demonstrated by soft tissue swelling or fluid, in three or more joint areas, including right or left PIP, MCP, wrist, elbow, MTP, ankle, or knee joints[b,c]
3. Arthritis, as demonstrated by soft tissue swelling or fluid, in the hand joints (PIP, MCP, or wrist)[b,c]
4. Symmetric arthritis in the areas noted in criteria 2. PIP, MCP, and MTP joint area symmetry does not need to be absolute in order to meet this criteria[b,c]
5. Rheumatoid nodules as noted by subcutaneous nodules near bones or joints or on extensor surfaces[c]
6. Positive rheumatoid factor determined by a test positive in less than 5% of normal subjects
7. Radiologic changes of the hands or wrists including erosions or bone decalcification in or next to involved joints

[a]Abbreviations: PIP, proximal interphalangeal joint(s); MCP, metacarpophalangeal joint(s); MTP, metatarsophalangeal joint(s).
[b]Present for at least 6 weeks.
[c]Must be observed by physician.
Source: Adapted from reference 17.

Table 30.3.
Function Class

Functional Class	Description
Class I	Ability to perform daily living activities without restriction
Class II	Moderate restrictions but still able to do normal activities
Class III	Major restriction in performing work or self-care activities
Class IV	Unable to perform self-care or confined to bed or wheelchair

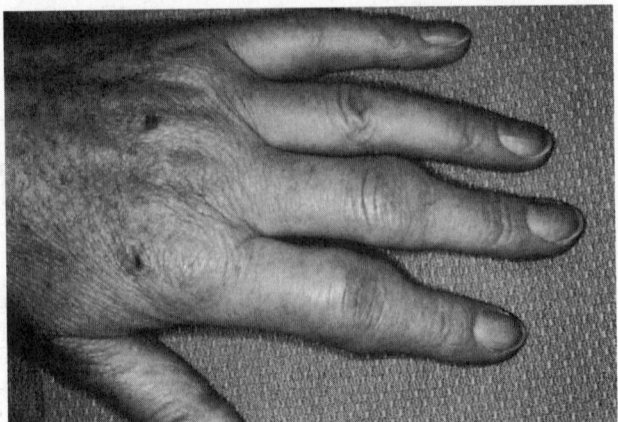

Figure 30.2. Rheumatoid arthritis: hand, fusiform swelling. Soft tissue swelling occurs as an early finding in rheumatoid arthritis and usually appears as typical fusiform or spindle-shaped enlargement of proximal interphalangeal joints. The second and third fingers of this patient are most involved. These proximal interphalangeal joints are tender and have a limited range of motion.

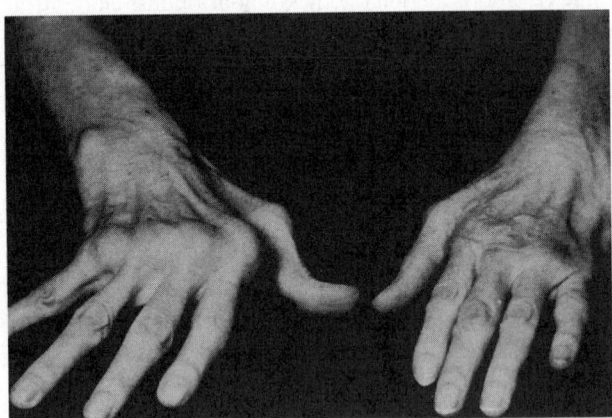

Figure 30.3. Rheumatoid arthritis: hands, ulnar deviation, and muscle atrophy. Ulnar deviation and subluxation of metacarpophalangeal joints have occurred in the patient's right hand. These joints also appear swollen. Muscle atrophy has developed in the dorsal musculature of both hands.

setting but are not intended to impede making a diagnosis of RA based on clinical findings and impressions. These classification criteria emphasize the chronic, symmetric, and small peripheral joint involvement in RA in conjunction with signs of its underlying pathophysiology. Despite these revised criteria and extensive educational efforts, the diagnosis of RA may be delayed 36 weeks (median; range 4 weeks to 10 or more years) after onset of symptoms and 18 weeks after first medical encounter (16).

The onset of RA varies from slow and insidious to rapidly progressive. The course of the disease is also highly variable: 10 to 20% of patients have a relatively short course with subsequent remission; 70 to 80% have mild-to-moderate disease with cyclic exacerbations; 10 to 15% develop progressive, destructive disease. Restricted activity is noted in 70% of patients with RA and 89% of patients with RA and comorbid disorders (1). Proper assessment of the patient's abilities is needed to adequately assess their

disease. Functional classification serves as a means to follow a patient's global ability to perform daily living activities (Table 30.3). More specific activities of daily living questionnaires and quality of life surveys are also useful but not yet widely used clinically.

Joints are the primary area of involvement in RA, ranging from quiescent or mild synovitis to severe synovitis, considerable synovial thickening and/or proliferation, detectable synovial fluid, and obvious bone deformity. RA usually affects diarthrodial joints, including the joints of the hands (Figure 30.2) and feet such as the proximal interphalangeal (PIP) joints, metacarpal-phalangeal (MCP) joints, metatarsal-phalangeal (MTP) joints, wrists and/or ankles.

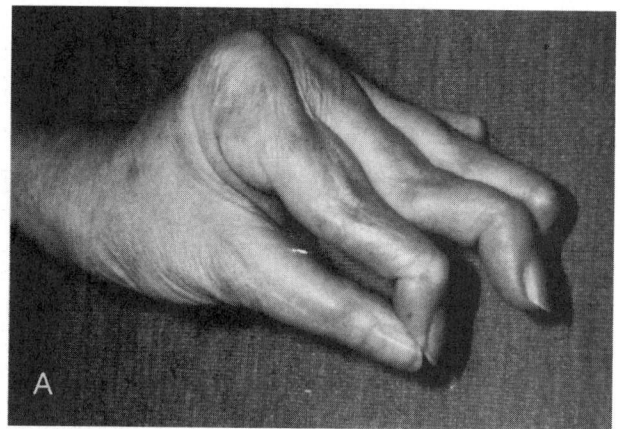

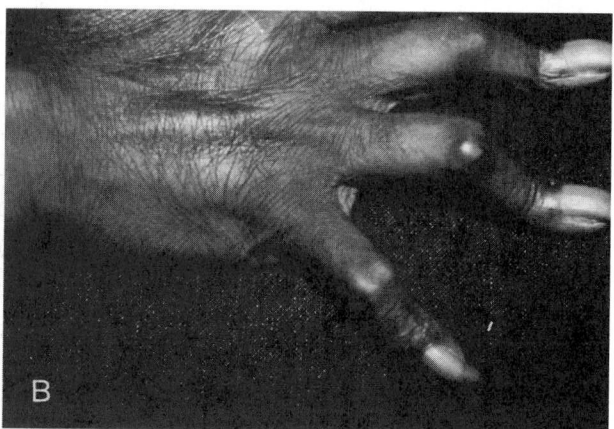

Figure 30.4. **A.** Rheumatoid arthritis: hand, swan-neck deformity. Swan-neck deformities are present in the second and third fingers of this patient with rheumatoid arthritis. This deformity results from contracture of the interosseous and flexor muscles and tendons resulting in a flexion contracture of the metacarpophalangeal joint, hyperextension of the proximal interphalangeal joint, and flexion of the distal interphalangeal joint. There is no rupture of the extensor apparatus, and the metacarpophalangeal joints are not dislocated. When a swan-neck deformity is present, the patient may be unable to flex the proximal interphalangeal joint if the metacarpophalangeal joint of the involved finger is held in extension. **B.** Rheumatoid arthritis: hand, boutonniere deformity. Boutonniere deformities, present in the third, fourth, and fifth fingers, are characterized by persistent flexion of the proximal interphalangeal joint and hyperextension of the distal interphalangeal joint. This deformity is caused by weakening of the central slip of the extrinsic extensor tendon and a palmar displacement of the lateral bands to the flexor side of the joint fulcrum. Since the mechanism of this deformity resembles a knuckle being pushed through a buttonhole, it has become known as the boutonniere deformity.

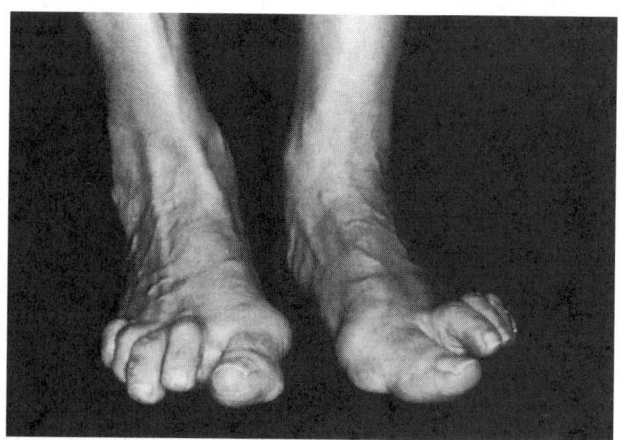

Figure 30.5. Rheumatoid arthritis: foot deformities. The most common foot deformities in rheumatoid arthritis are hallux valgus and hammer toes. The "cock-up" toe deformities in this patient are associated with subluxation of the metatarsophalangeal joints. Superimposed painful corns and bunions result from irritation caused by faulty shoes.

Elbows, shoulders, sternoclavicular joints, temporomandibular joints, knees, and hips are commonly involved. Cervical spine involvement may lead to severe pain and subluxation.

Stiffness is a gel-like sensation experienced in the joints or more generally in patients with RA when attempting to move after waking in the morning or after a period of inactivity. The degree of stiffness diminishes with move-

ment. Plasma levels of keratan sulfate, a large cartilage proteoglycan degradation product, are inversely proportional to the duration of morning stiffness.

Joint deformities in RA are the result of the destruction of periarticular bone caused by inflammatory mediators, enzymes, phagocytosis, and physical stress. Common deformities seen in RA include ulnar deviation, swan-neck deformities, Boutonniere deformities, hammer or cock-up toe formation, and ankylosis (Figures 30.3 to 30.6). Opposing or compensating forces lead to a zigzag pattern of deformity. In the late stages of progressive disease, bony deformities may predominate, and acute inflammation may be absent or minimal. Joints become destabilized due to muscle, tendon, ligament, or joint capsule changes.

General, constitutional symptoms are common in RA. Fatigue, which occurs in many patients particularly during active RA, may be related to abnormal sleep patterns, anemia, depression, muscle weakness, and/or neuropeptides. Depression is commonly seen in patients with RA and may affect their perception of the activity of their arthritis. The association between depression and disease activity is unclear except that depression is associated with loss of valuable activities (17). Anxiety and social problems also occur commonly in patients with RA. The cachexia and muscle weakness that occur in RA are associated with inactivity, catabolic effects of inflammatory mediators, use of corticosteroids, and other factors.

Extraarticular involvement in RA is associated with rheumatoid factor positivity, male gender, circulating immune complexes, and more severe arthritis. Extraarticu-

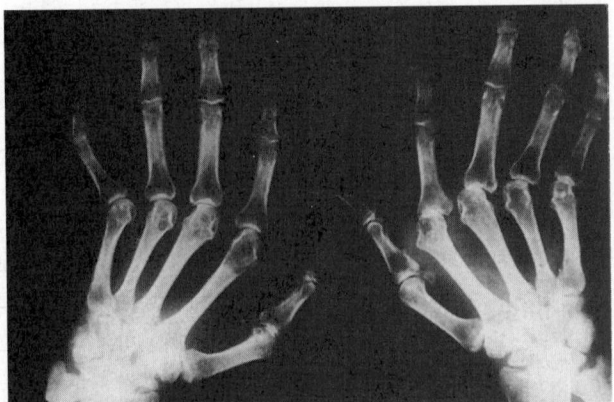

Figure 30.6. Rheumatoid arthritis: hands, advanced deformity (radiograph). The metacarpophalangeal joints demonstrate marked narrowing with subluxation and ulnar deviation. Erosions are seen in the metacarpal heads. The proximal interphalangeal joints are narrowed, but there is no reactive bone change. Demineralization is present in bones adjacent to the metacarpophalangeal and proximal interphalangeal joints. The carpal spaces are narrowed, and the carpal bones and ulnar styloid processes also reveal erosions.

lar features include rheumatoid nodules, vasculitis, vital organ effects, anemia, Felty's syndrome, Sjogren's syndrome, ocular inflammation, and others. Rheumatoid nodules (Figure 30.7), which contain monocytes and macrophages surrounding a necrotic area, occur in 25% of patients with RA, almost all of whom are rheumatoid factor positive. Rheumatoid nodules generally occur subcutaneously over bone in pressure point areas, but may be found in other tissues and organs.

Vasculitis is frequently seen in patients with severe, nodular, sero-positive RA. Clues to the presence of vascular inflammation include the presence of the spectrum of skin manifestations from palpable purpura to digital infarcts, ischemic ulcers, and progression to gangrene and necrosis (Figure 30.8). Larger vessel involvement with major organ compromise is seen on rare occasions.

A mild anemia of chronic disease is seen in patients with RA. This anemia responds poorly to iron therapy but will respond to improvements in the activity of RA and to erythropoietin administration (18). Anemia of chronic disease may occur in conjunction with iron deficiency. Hemolytic anemia is a rare feature of RA.

The combination of RA, splenomegaly, and leukopenia, sometimes in association with thrombocytopenia, lymphadenopathy, leg ulcers and infections defines Felty's syndrome. As with vasculitis, Felty's syndrome is more common in patients with severe, sero-positive, nodular RA. Joint infections may occur more commonly in patients with RA, particularly in those with prosthetic joints.

Vital organs are also affected in RA. Rheumatoid lung disease occurs in up to 20% of RA patients and is

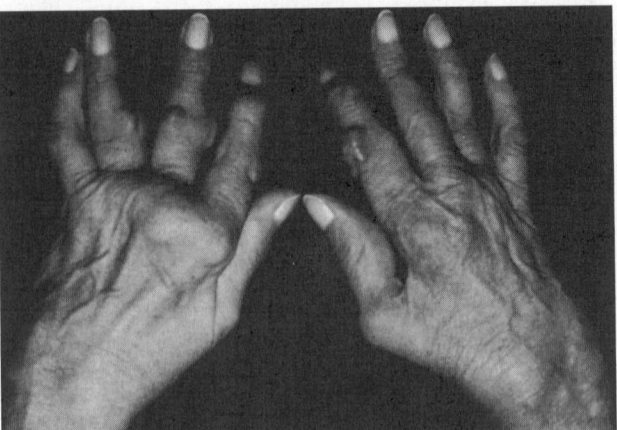

Figure 30.7. Rheumatoid arthritis: subcutaneous nodules, fingers. Multiple subcutaneous nodules can be seen in the fingers of this patient with rheumatoid arthritis. Subcutaneous nodules are most frequently found on the dorsal forearm surface distal to the olecranon process but also may appear in the fingers, over the Achilles tendon, on the occiput, and at other pressure points such as the ischial tuberosity and sacrum. They are most commonly described in rheumatoid arthritis and rheumatic fever but also may occur in other rheumatic diseases like systemic lupus erythematosus and mixed connective tissue disease. This patient also displays marked synovial proliferation with subluxation of metacarpophalangeal joints of the left hand.

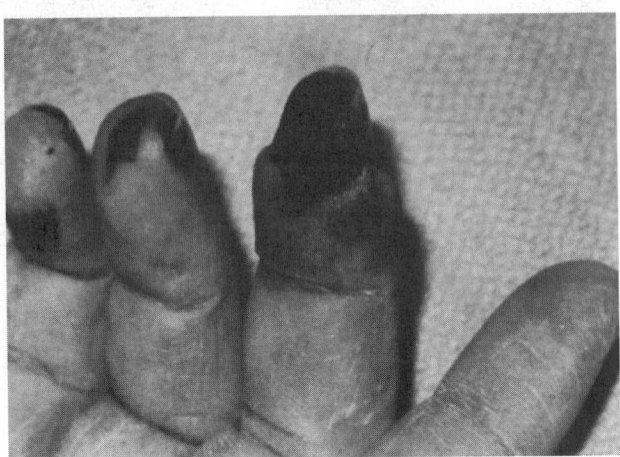

Figure 30.8. Atrophy and gangrene of the tip of the middle finger can be seen. Less extensive necrotic lesions are present at the ends of the fourth and fifth fingers. These digital infarcts are caused by inflammatory occlusion of small arteries. Similar-appearing lesions may occur in polyarteries, other connective tissue diseases, embolic illnesses, diabetes mellitus, and other conditions.

characterized by pulmonary effusions, pleuritis, and possibly fibrosis. It may also be associated with therapy for RA, rheumatoid nodules, genetic or environmental factors. Renal disease secondary to RA is rare, but subclinical renal dysfunction is found, particularly in patients with progressive RA. Renal abnormalities are usually related to medications (NSAIDs, gold salts, penicillamine) or amyloidosis secondary to longstanding inflammation. Cardiac manifestations of RA most commonly involve the pericardium (pericarditis with or without effusions) and are usually asymptomatic. Heart valve dysfunction, embolic phenomena, conduction defects, aortitis, and myocardiopathy occur less frequently.

Keratoconjunctivitis sicca with complaints of dry eyes (xerophthalmia) and dry mouth (xerostomia) are clues to the presence of secondary Sjogren's syndrome. Other ocular abnormalities in RA patients include episcleritis, scleritis, and scleromalacia perforans.

Neurologic complications are frequently seen in RA. Their pathogenesis is usually related to myelopathies associated with cervical spine instability, entrapment of peripheral nerves through confined compartments, or ischemic neuropathies related to vasculitis often presenting as a mononeuritis multiplex.

Rheumatoid factor (RF) is an antibody, usually IgM, but IgG and IgA are also found, which is directed against the Fc portion of IgG. Plasma titers of RF are positive in approximately 80% of patients with RA, and in up to 5% of the population at large. RF is also detected in rheumatoid synovial fluid and in the plasma of patients with other inflammatory or infectious disorders. Higher plasma titers of RF are usually associated with more active RA. Plasma titers are useful in following a sero-positive patient's response to second-line drug therapy and possibly disease activity in individual patients. False-positive hepatitis C antibody tests are found in patients with RA and may be due to a RF directed against hepatitis C.

Other antibodies may be seen in patients with RA. Antinuclear antibodies, which are autoantibodies directed against nuclear proteins and are commonly seen in patients with systemic lupus erythematosus and other disorders, are sometimes found in patients with RA in low titers. Other autoantibodies are also found.

Erythrocyte sedimentation rate (ESR) is a nonspecific indicator of inflammation that correlates with the number of joint effusions in active RA and is useful clinically in diagnosis of and monitoring RA. Measurement of ESR is done by placing whole blood in a small tube for 1 hour, allowing red blood cells to fall to the bottom of the tube and measuring the number of millimeters that the red blood cells have vacated. Normal ESRs are generally 0 to 15 mm per hour, but may vary depending on method and laboratory. C-reactive protein and platelet counts are nonspecific acute phase reactants that are elevated in patients with active RA. Plasma hyaluronic acid levels correlate with the number of tender or swollen joints but are not used clinically.

Joint radiographs are helpful in working-up and following patients with RA. Early radiographic findings include soft tissue swelling. Periarticular bone loss may occur within 3 to 4 months of onset of RA. Bone erosions, bone cysts, and deformities may become evident as the disease progresses (Figure 30.6). Radiographic classification may be useful in following patients over time. Joint scintigraphy may be useful in detecting soft tissue swelling in early RA, but add nothing to the clinical examination. Magnetic resonance imaging (MRI) scans are well suited for evaluating soft tissue, cartilage, ligaments, and changes in bone marrow, but their clinical utility in detecting early bony erosive changes is currently under evaluation.

TREATMENT

The goals of therapy in rheumatoid arthritis are to improve or maintain current function in the patient's daily living activities, diminish progression of the patient's joint and extraarticular disease, and minimize adverse drug effects using beneficial, safe, and cost-effective therapies. Therapy should be individualized for each patient based on the course of RA, degree of articular and extraarticular disease, concurrent diseases and therapies, age, need for relief, and a host of other factors. Early in the course of disease, it may be difficult to predict whether or not a patient's RA will follow a rapidly progressive, slowly progressive, unprogressive, or remitting course. Therapeutic decisions are thus complicated and restricted by the currently available options.

Nonspecific drug and nondrug therapies are used to control acute inflammation and attempt to control the progression of the disease, but very few patients will achieve a cure. Specific measures, such as surgery, are useful in correcting deformities and enhancing the ability to perform certain tasks. Better understanding of the etiology and pathogenesis of RA should lead to better therapy.

Traditionally, the treatment of RA has been described as a pyramid in which education, rest, exercise, proper diet, and nonsteroidal antiinflammatory drugs serve as the base of the pyramid and would be used in most, if not all, patients. The next levels of the pyramid involve the addition of one of the "second-line" or slow-acting agents to patients with progressive disease or sustained severe synovitis. Corticosteroids and orthopedic surgery are used as adjunctive measures at any level of the pyramid. Many investigators promote approaches other than this traditional pyramid, particularly the use of second-line agents earlier in a patient's course.

Nondrug therapies are widely used in all stages of RA. Patients should be well informed of the nature and possible progression of their disease in order to promote self-awareness, self-determination, and self-reliance as well as the knowledge of when to seek help from others. Family support is essential since negative attitudes toward the patient's disease lead to less coping and adaptation and more stress. Rest serves to spare joints, decrease inflammation, and ideally leads to repair of damaged tissues. Patients with RA and fatigue should not diminish activity completely but should be encouraged to rest on a routine basis each day. Prolonged immobility may lead to increased stiffness and diminished mobility of joints and strength. For selected patients, hospitalization with rest and possibly minor revisions in drug therapy may have dramatic results. Intensive hospitalization for 14 days resulted in a threefold improvement in RA at a two-and-a-half-fold increase in cost versus no hospitalization (19). Physical therapists assist in development of an appropriate exercise program that decreases joint inflammation, maintains range of motion, and increases overall well-being through range-of-motion cardiovascular fitness or strength-building programs that do not overstress joints and muscles. Such exercise programs may also diminish the development of osteoporosis in those on corticosteroids or otherwise prone to develop it. Nutrition is important to help patients lose weight if overweight and maintain protein and calcium intake. Fish oils, certain plant seed oils, and a vegetarian diet may be of some benefit in RA. Occupational therapists assist in the design and use of special eating utensils, grooming aids, working aids, and other self-help aids that are useful in maintaining patients' self-reliance. Splints may be useful in stabilizing a weak joint, resting an active joint, or possibly diminishing the rate of joint destruction. Walking aids or wheelchairs may dramatically improve a patient's mobility and stability when mobile. Hot paraffin wax treatments may decrease inflammation and discomfort. Surgery is very useful in RA to repair or replace damaged joints, fuse joints for stability, correct tendon or ligament instability, release carpal tunnel syndrome, or perform synovectomies. These nondrug therapies need to be individualized based on the patient's needs and current disease activity.

Systemic and topical analgesics may benefit selected patients with RA. Systemic analgesics, such as acetaminophen and opioid analgesics, are generally considered to be of limited benefit because of the inflammatory nature of this disease, but they may help occasionally as adjuncts to antiinflammatory medications. Topical ointments, creams, and liniments may provide some local relief. Although designated as topical, systemic absorption is possible and may lead to toxicity or drug interactions such as increased effect of warfarin in patients using topical salicylates (20). Capsaicin cream inhibits Substance P and temporarily relieves the pain associated with joint inflammation, but its effects are not antiinflammatory.

NONSTEROIDAL ANTIINFLAMMATORY DRUGS (NSAIDs)

The efficacy of all nonsteroidal antiinflammatory drugs in RA is equivalent. The impression that nonacetylated salicylates are less effective is not documented by clinical studies (21). Onset of effect is within a few days to a week (longer for agents with longer half-lives) with maximum effects in 1 to 4 weeks. NSAIDs decrease ESR, C-reactive protein, RF, and the number of circulating activated T-cells in RA patients. Hemoglobin levels may not increase possibly due to increased bleeding or limited effects on the underlying disease process.

Adverse effects, cost, and ease of administration are major factors in choosing a NSAID. If a patient does not tolerate or respond to maximum antiinflammatory doses for 2 weeks or loses response, then subsequent selections can be taken from a different or the same chemical class. Less than 50% of those starting an NSAID will be on that agent after 12 months (22). Aspirin is inexpensive and may be safer than previously thought (23). The high doses of NSAIDs needed to treat RA increases the likelihood of toxicity. NSAIDs are currently first-line agents, but long-term toxicity limits their use so that many patients decrease the dose or stop the NSAID when the response to second-line drugs is evident.

NSAIDs are used to treat acute synovitis in all stages of RA because of their inhibition of prostaglandin synthesis, membrane-related enzyme activities, membrane anion transport, arachidonate precursor uptake and insertion into monocyte membranes, collagenase release, and neutrophil function (21). The d-isomer (S(+) isomer) of the propionate derivatives (Table 30.4) possess antiinflammatory activity. Subtherapeutic levels of NSAIDs may enhance the secretion of prostaglandins in vitro; PGE levels in synovial fluid continue to be suppressed even after synovial levels of the NSAID drop to very low levels. NSAIDs enhance cytotoxic and suppressor T-cell activity, which may result in inhibition of B-cell activity. Most currently available NSAIDs increase or do not alter leukotriene levels, but ketoprofen and investigational agents inhibit leukotriene synthesis and bradykinin activity. Glycosaminoglycan synthesis in joint cartilage is inhibited by sodium salicylate, but other NSAIDs are noted to inhibit cartilage destruction. The clinical significance of many of these differences is unclear.

NSAIDs are generally well absorbed following oral administration and highly bound to albumin. Plasma protein binding of salicylates is greater than 95% at low levels but diminishes as the salicylate level increases and binding sites become saturated. The half-lives and dosing of NSAIDs vary considerably (Table 30.4) (21). Synovial fluid levels of NSAIDs rise and fall at rates slower than their serum levels, with synovial fluid levels becoming greater than serum levels at times proportional to their half-life (24). This may explain in part why ibuprofen, which has a half-life of 2.1 hours, is effective when given twice or four times daily (21). Synovial fluid levels of NSAIDs with longer half-lives generally do not exceed serum levels during the dosing interval (24). Most NSAIDs undergo

Table 30.4.
Nonsteroidal Antiinflammatory Drugs Used in Rheumatoid Arthritis

Classes	Drug (Active Metabolite)	Half-Life (hours) Normal	Half-Life (hours) in ESRD[a]	Daily Dose (mg/day)	Doses per Day
Acetic acids	Diclofenac	1–2	1–2	150–200	3–4
	Etodolac	7	NC[b]	800–1200	3–4
	Indomethacin	1–16	NC	100–200	3–4
	IndomethacinSR[c]	1–16	NC	150	1–2
	Nabumetone			1000–2000	1–2
	(acetic acid)	22–30[d]	39		
	Sulindac	8	NC	300–400	2
	(sulfide)	16–18			
	Tolmetin	1–5		1600–2000	3–4
Fenamates	Meclofenamate	1–3		300–400	3–4
Oxicams	Piroxicam	30–86	44	10–20	1
Propionates	Fenoprofen	1.5–4		1600–3200	3–4
	Flurbiprofen	3–6		200–300	2–4
	Ibuprofen	1–2.5	2.5	1600–3200	3–4
	Ketoprofen	1–4	3.2	150–300	3–4
	KetoprofenSR[c]	1–4	3.2	200	1
	Naproxen	9–17	15	500–1500	2–3
	Oxaprozin	42–50		1200–1800	1
Salicylates	Aspirin	0.2–0.3	NC	2400–6500	3–5
	(Salicylate)	2–30	NC		
	Diflunisal	5–20	15–138	500–1500	2–3
	Salsalate	2–30	NC	2000–3000	3–4
	Other salicylates	2–30	NC	2400–6500	3–5

[a]End stage renal disease.
[b]No change in half-life.
[c]SR = sustained-release product.
[d]Longer half-life in elderly patients.

hepatic metabolism, but appreciable amounts are excreted unchanged in urine. Glucuronidation of ketoprofen and possibly other NSAIDs may be reversed in patients with renal failure (21). Aspirin is rapidly deacetylated in plasma to salicylic acid, which then displays nonlinear pharmacokinetics at antiinflammatory plasma levels of 150 to 250 mg/L. Sulindac is metabolized to an inactive renally excreted product and its active product. Nabumetone is metabolized to its active component. Naproxen is unusual in that at high doses its excretion is increased and serum levels are lower than expected from the increase in dose. End stage renal disease prolongs the half-life of diflunisal (Table 30.4). Dosage adjustments may be needed in patients with end stage renal or hepatic disease, depending on the specific drug.

Adverse Effects

Adverse effects from NSAIDs involve many organ systems and demonstrate considerable interpatient variability. Indomethacin, phenylbutazone, and meclofenamate are more frequently associated with severe adverse effects. Older studies demonstrated that aspirin was associated with more adverse effects than other NSAIDs, but recent studies have demonstrated a safer profile for aspirin than for nonaspirin products. This may be due to the current use of lower doses of aspirin (2665 mg/day on average)

compared to previous higher doses (2600 to 5000 mg/day) or to patient selection (23). Nonacetylated salicylates appear to be associated with fewer effects on certain organ systems than other NSAIDs.

Gastrointestinal effects are most common and include abdominal discomfort, distress, nausea, vomiting, diarrhea, bleeding, and ulceration (25). Meclofenamate has a high incidence of diarrhea. Microbleeding from aspirin is greater than from other NSAIDs. Gastric ulceration or bleeding occurs in 0.5 to 3% of patients on NSAIDs, but mucosal damage is found in up to 75% of individuals on chronic NSAIDs (25). Preliminary studies show that nabumetone and etodolac may cause less gastric or duodenal ulceration than other NSAIDs (25). Patients at high risk for peptic ulceration or bleeding include the elderly and those with a history of peptic ulcer disease or gastrointestinal bleeding, liver or renal disease, on high doses of NSAIDs, and receiving corticosteroids chronically. There is no apparent association between NSAID-induced ulceration and *Heliobacter pylori* infection (25, 26). Misoprostol, a PGE$_1$ analog, protects against gastric ulceration associated with chronic NSAID use, but it is also associated with considerable diarrhea and gastrointestinal cramping. Misoprostol is contraindicated in pregnancy because of its ability to induce abortions. The cost effectiveness of misoprostol is limited to very high risk patients if the initial estimates on the rates of ulceration and bleeding are accurate. Histamine-2 receptor antagonists are less effective in preventing NSAID-associated gastric ulceration or bleeding, but are the drugs of choice in preventing duodenal ulceration or bleeding in high risk patients (25). Histamine-2 antagonists are used to diminish dyspepsia associated with NSAIDs. Omeprazole may prove to protect against gastrointestinal damage, but sucralfate has little protective effect. Treatment of NSAID-induced gastric or duodenal ulcers include histamine-2 antagonists. Omeprazole may be preferred in patients who will remain on a NSAID or who smoke.

Nonsteroidal antiinflammatory agents are also associated with cholestatic and/or cellular hepatotoxicity. Diclofenac and sulindac may cause a higher incidence of liver toxicity (21). Aspirin-induced hepatotoxicity has been associated with more active arthritis. NSAID-associated hepatotoxicity is generally reversible but may lead to chronic liver failure, need for a liver transplant, or death.

The most common renal disorder associated with nonsteroidal antiinflammatory agent use is decreased renal blood flow due to prostaglandin inhibition, but interstitial nephritis, tubular necrosis, and papillary necrosis are also seen. Patients with cardiovascular conditions or cirrhosis, or who are elderly, elderly on loop diuretics, on high doses of NSAIDs, or renally insufficient appear to need vasodilatory renal prostaglandins in order to maintain sufficient renal blood flow and subsequent glomerular filtration. Sulindac, nabumetone, and nonacetylated salicylates, plus possibly etodolac, have less of an effect on renal prostaglandins than other NSAIDs and may be preferred in high-risk patients. NSAID-induced prostaglandin-mediated renal dysfunction is generally reversible, but chronic renal failure has been reported.

NSAIDs inhibit platelet aggregation because of concentration-dependent inhibition of platelet thromboxane production. Production of vascular prostacyclin, an antithrombosis prostaglandin, may also be inhibited. Nonacetylated salicylates do not affect thromboxane or prostacyclin production. Aspirin causes irreversible inhibition of platelet aggregation, but the effect is reversible with other NSAIDs. A nonacetylated salicylate or NSAID with a short half-life is preferred in patients about to undergo surgery. The antiplatelet effect will generally disappear within 24 hours of stopping a short half-life NSAID. Severe aspirin toxicity is associated with hypoprothrombinemia. Agranulocytosis and aplastic anemia are rarely associated with NSAIDs.

Commonly occurring central nervous effects include dizziness, fussiness, and headache. These are more common in the elderly. The use of indomethacin is limited due to the high percentage of central nervous system effects, including hallucinations, dizziness, headaches, confusion, disorientation, and nightmares. Aseptic meningitis occurs rarely, mostly in patients with systemic lupus erythematosus taking ibuprofen, but other NSAIDs have also been implicated.

Hypersensitivity reactions to NSAIDs include bronchoconstriction, nasal polyps, urticaria, rhinitis, angioedema, and anaphylaxis. Bronchospasm and nasal polyps may be due to the inhibition of prostaglandin synthesis, which is consistent with the cross-sensitivity among these drugs (27). Nonacetylated salicylates have been suggested as safe alternatives in sensitive patients, but cross-sensitivity with nonacetylated salicylates has occurred (28). Photosensitivity may also be associated with NSAIDs.

Drug Interactions

Drug interactions associated with NSAIDs are generally mediated by pharmacodynamic or pharmacokinetic effects. NSAIDs may diminish the effectiveness of antihypertensives (beta-blockers, ACE inhibitors) and loop diuretics because of effects on renal prostaglandins, but the effect varies from serious to unimportant. Inhibition of renal function may alter the pharmacokinetics of renally excreted drugs. Lithium levels increase after administration of many NSAIDs, but not aspirin or sulindac. Salicylates inhibit the action of uricosurics. Aspirin has a pharmacokinetic interaction with warfarin, but all NSAIDs that exhibit antiplatelet effects increase bleeding potential in patients on warfarin. High-dose methotrexate may be much more toxic when used with NSAIDs, but the low doses of methotrexate used to treat RA are usually safely administered with most NSAIDs. Aspirin plus methotrexate led to a higher incidence of increases in liver enzymes (29). Acetazolamide levels are increased by aspirin by protein-binding displacement and decreased renal clearance.

NSAIDs may be the target of pharmacokinetic or pharmacodynamic interactions. Salicylate levels are decreased by magnesium-aluminum hydroxide combination antacids, which increase urine pH and enhance salicylate renal excretion, and corticosteroids, which increase liver metabolism and renal clearance. Drugs causing gastrointestinal or renal toxicity may increase NSAID toxicity. NSAIDs interact with each other in pharmacokinetic and pharmacodynamic effects, including additive toxicity.

SECOND-LINE ANTIRHEUMATIC DRUGS

Second-line agents, previously referred to as disease-modifying or slow-acting antirheumatic drugs, include antimalarials (chloroquine and hydroxychloroquine), methotrexate, azathioprine, sulfasalazine, injectable gold salts, auranofin (oral gold), cyclosporine A, minocycline, cyclophosphamide, and penicillamine. These drugs have varied activities on the immune system, but their mechanisms of action in RA remain unclear (30). The traditional use of second-line agents has been in patients with potentially reversible progressive disease; rheumatologists are more likely to use them earlier in the disease in an attempt to diminish long-term joint destruction. Beneficial antiinflammatory effects of second-line agents are seen over 1 to 6 months and may lead to remission or decreased progression of the disease in only a few patients (31, 32). However, second-line drugs have not definitively proven to significantly diminish the progression of joint disease.

Choosing among second-line agents is difficult. Recent review (31) and metaanalyses (32) of published data concluded that gold sodium thiomalate and methotrexate were among the most efficacious, but methotrexate was among the least toxic, and injectable gold salts were among the most toxic. Hydroxychloroquine and auranofin were ranked as least effective, with hydroxychloroquine among the least toxic, and auranofin was least to intermediately toxic. Sulfasalazine was ranked as both least and most effective, with intermediate toxicity. Azathioprine was of intermediate efficacy and among the least toxic (31). Penicillamine was ranked as intermediately to mostly efficacious but most toxic. Second-line drug therapy costs (drug, monitoring, toxicity) differed among agents with per patient per month estimates of $155 for auranofin and hydroxychloroquine; $185 to $225 for penicillamine, methotrexate, and azathioprine; and $295 for injectable gold (33). Additionally, patients are generally not able to continue therapy with these agents very long despite the chronic nature of RA. Only 50% of those starting the drug will be on oral gold (auranofin) after 10 months; on hydroxychloroquine, penicillamine, injectable gold, or azathioprine after 20 to 27 months; and on methotrexate after 60 months (22). Other agents were not included in these analyses.

Currently, methotrexate is widely considered the initial second-line drug of choice in severe RA. Antimalarials are also widely used, but in less severe disease or as an adjunct to other second-line agents. Sulfasalazine, azathioprine, and auranofin are used less often, and penicillamine and cyclophosphamide even less because of their smaller benefit-to-toxicity ratio. Cyclosporine A and minocycline are not widely used because of lack of experience. Methotrexate, azathioprine, and cyclophosphamide are useful in treating extraarticular manifestations such as steroid-resistant rheumatoid lung or vasculitis.

In patients with recently diagnosed, early RA, the use of second-line agents is controversial. Auranofin has been shown to retard disease progression in early RA (34), demonstrating that early RA may be reversible or preventable. However, it is difficult to predict which patients will develop progressive, erosive disease and if the toxicity and cost will be offset by the potential benefits.

Second-line agents may be combined with or added to each other to increase efficacy. Combinations have included two, three, and four drugs such as antimalarials, methotrexate, azathioprine, oral and injectable gold, sulfasalazine, penicillamine, cyclophosphamide, chlorambucil, and pulse methylprednisolone (35). Although many regimens were more effective than single second-line drug regimens, toxicity and/or no additional benefit were seen with some regimens (35). The use of cyclophosphamide in combinations is limited by long-term toxicity and has been replaced by either azathioprine or methotrexate. A few regimens have been associated with reversal of bony erosions (36, 37). However, recent reviews and metaanalyses have not supported the general use of combination second-line agents (35).

Antimalarials have been used in RA since a 1951 report of a patient whose RA improved after mepacrine was used to treat the patient's discoid lupus (38). Chloroquine became widely used, but it has been widely replaced by hydroxychloroquine in the treatment of RA though chloroquine may be more effective (32). Hydroxychloroquine diminishes the functions of macrophages (30) but also increases pain threshold (39). Hydroxychloroquine is administered at doses of 2 to 4 mg/kg or 200 to 400 mg per day orally. Chloroquine oral doses are 200 to 300 mg daily of the base.

Hydroxychloroquine is readily absorbed following oral administration with peak levels in 1 to 3 hours. Hydroxychloroquine is 45% bound to serum albumin, distributes into red blood cells and other tissues, and has a half-life of approximately 40 days. Dosage adjustment is not needed in renal dysfunction since only 22 to 34% of hydroxychloroquine is excreted unchanged in urine. Chloroquine pharmacokinetics are similar, with a half-life of 6 to 50 days and lack of appreciable removal by hemodialysis.

Pooled data from clinical studies reveal that chloroquine and hydroxychloroquine are least toxic of second-line drugs. Adverse effects include gastrointestinal tract (4.6%), rash (2.3%), ocular (0.7%), and, less commonly, mucous membrane, leukopenia, central nervous system, neuromuscular, and cardiac effects (32). Corneal deposits occur in at least 20%, and symptomatic retinopathy in 2 to 17% of those receiving chloroquine, with higher frequencies seen in those receiving higher doses or who are elderly. Hydroxychloroquine appears to be rarely discontinued because of retinopathy at the dosage ranges listed, but patients should see an ophthalmologist every 3 to 12 months for a full ophthalmic examination. Hydroxychloroquine may also exacerbate psoriasis and cause allergic reactions. Chloroquine has decreased the normal response to intradermal rabies vaccine in normal subjects (40).

Methotrexate (MTX) is effective in RA at doses ranging from 7.5 to 15 mg weekly orally, intramuscularly, or subcutaneously (41) administered in one dose or in three equal doses every 12 hours. High-dose MTX (500 mg/m^2) followed by leucovorin rescue every 2 weeks has been of some use in refractory patients with RA (42). MTX differs from other second-line agents in its rapid response as early as 4 to 6 weeks, a recurrence in the arthritis flare seen soon after the withdrawal of MTX (43), and an increase in rheumatoid nodules during its use. MTX was most effective in decreasing tender joint counts in a recent metaanalysis of second-line agents (32) but may not alter the bony progression of the disease. It is contraindicated in pregnant women.

MTX absorption is highly variable and is diminished following cholecystectomy. MTX is found in high levels in synovial membrane and bone even after serum levels have diminished (44). MTX is metabolized to an active metabolite, 7-hydroxy-methotrexate. Biliary excretion may account for 9 to 26% of MTX elimination and 2 to 5% of 7-hydroxy metabolite elimination after low doses of MTX. MTX elimination is decreased in patients with end stage renal disease, increased by hemodialysis, and not altered by peritoneal dialysis.

Patients should be monitored every 2 to 6 weeks for adverse effects from MTX. Pooled clinical studies have revealed that withdrawals from MTX are due to hepatic effects (10.3%), mucous membrane effects (2.6%), nausea and/or vomiting (2.1%), gastrointestinal effects (2.1%), leukopenia (1%), blood effects (1.5%), and diarrhea (0.5%) (32). The majority of the liver effects were elevations of liver enzymes rather than abnormalities on liver biopsy. Liver biopsies are the definitive method of detecting hepatoxocity, but are not routinely recommended in patients with RA receiving MTX due to the low incidence of hepatotoxicity and the morbidity, mortality, and costs associated with liver biopsy (45). Preteatment liver biopsy may be indicated in alcoholics and viral or persistent hepatitis patients. Increased incidence of abnormalities in liver enzymes are noted in patients on MTX plus aspirin (29), alcoholism, diabetes, and obesity. Although usually irreversible, severe liver toxicity may be reversible. Sustained elevation of mean corpuscular volume in a patient treated with MTX may indicate folate deficiency and may predict MTX hematologic toxicity. Severe neutropenia may develop at low doses in RA in patients with end stage renal disease. Concurrent folic acid (46) and leucovorin (47) administration may diminish MTX-induced stomatitis and macrocytic anemia, but leucovorin use has diminished MTX efficacy (48). Folic acid is administered 1 mg four days per week, omitting the day before, day of, and day after MTX administration. Severe MTX toxicity is reversed by leucovorin. Allopurinol mouthwashes (5 mg/ml suspension in water) have been useful in the treatment of MTX-induced stomatitis (49), but patients should be discouraged from swallowing the suspension. MTX is also associated with infections, rashes, and pneumonitis that may progress to pulmonary fibrosis.

Drug interactions involving MTX may have serious consequences. As noted, aspirin is associated with increases in MTX hepatotoxicity. Salicylate and probenecid inhibit MTX excretion. Cholestyramine binds to MTX and enhances its excretion. Folinic acid may reverse the efficacy of MTX (48), depending on the dose and timing of administration.

Azathioprine has demonstrated efficacy in treating RA at doses of 1.0 to 2.5 mg/kg or 50 to 200 mg per day. Azathioprine has a half-life of 0.2 to 1 hour, is removed by hemodialysis, and is converted to 6-mercaptopurine, its active form. Allopurinol inhibits the metabolism of azathioprine, requiring the dose of azathioprine to be decreased by 67 to 75%.

The risk of adverse effects from azathioprine has been of concern, but a recent postmarketing surveillance study has revealed a relatively safe adverse effect profile in RA (50). Monitoring complete blood counts, liver function tests, and examination of mucous membranes every 2 to 6 weeks is still necessary to evaluate azathioprine-induced gastrointestinal distress, leukopenia, stomatitis, and liver toxicity. Infections and pulmonary toxicity have also been reported. Severe bone-marrow suppression is rarely seen and may be associated with deficiencies in purine metabolic enzymes (51).

Sulfasalazine was developed in the 1940s to treat RA but only recently has been used widely in the treatment of RA following promising studies (32). Sulfasalazine is broken down to sulfapyridine and aminosalicylate in the gut. Both sulfasalazine and its sulfapyridine metabolite have effects against RA.

Recently, pooled data of studies involving second-line agents found that the adverse effect withdrawal rate from sulfasalazine was less than for gold but similar to that of penicillamine (32). Sulfasalazine was withdrawn for nausea and/or vomiting (12.5%), skin rash (3.8%), liver effects (1.6), leukopenia (1.1%), mucous membranes (1.1%), fever (1.1%), anemia (0.5%), and lung effects (0.5%) (32). Toxic epidermal necrolysis, a potentially life-threatening skin rash, has been reported following sulfasalazine therapy (52). Monitoring for toxicity is mostly based on clinical presentation of the patient.

Injectable gold salts have been used to treat RA since the 1920s, but the initial doses used, 100 to 200 mg per week, were associated with unacceptable toxicity. Currently used doses are more tolerable. Generally, two test doses, one of 10 mg then one of 25 mg, are used for the first two weekly intramuscular injections of the injectable gold salt and followed by 25- to 50-mg maintenance doses. If the patient responds to weekly maintenance doses, the dosage interval may be widened to every 2 weeks, then every 3 weeks, and so on. An oral form of gold, auranofin, became available in the early 1980s and is effective at doses of 3 to 9 mg daily. Auranofin appears to be less effective, but also less toxic, than injectable gold (32).

Injectable gold salts and auranofin, which are 50 and 28% elemental gold, respectively, differ in many aspects of their pharmacokinetics. Two injectable gold salt forms are available: aurothiomalate is a water soluble solution, and aurothioglucose is less water soluble and in a suspension. Auranofin is 20 to 25% absorbed orally. Gold is extensively bound to serum albumin and widely distributed to kidneys, liver, reticuloendothelial system, spleen, synovial membrane, skin, hair, and nails. Skin serves as a large storage site following chronic injectable gold administration. A higher percentage of injectable gold is retained in body tissues compared to auranofin. The half-lives of both forms of gold are at least 1 to 3 weeks. Most of the absorbed gold salt is excreted in urine, but 85% of auranofin is recovered in feces. Gold is removed by peritoneal dialysis, but not hemodialysis.

Injectable gold was discontinued because of adverse effects more than other second-line agents (32). The reasons for withdrawal included skin rash (13%), proteinuria (3.7%), mucous membrane effects (1.8%), leukopenia (1.5%), thrombocytopenia (1.1%), gastrointestinal effects (1.3%), hepatic (0.9%), and blood effects (0.9%), and, less commonly, diarrhea, fever, alopecia, as well as renal, lung, and ocular effects (32). Nitritoid reactions, characterized by flushing and syncope, may occur up to 30 minutes following an injection of gold salts, particularly aurothiomalate. Aurothioglucose may be considered, or the patient may be asked to sit or lay down for 20 to 30 minutes following each injection if such reactions occur. Gold storage in skin can lead to chrysiasis, a bronzelike appearance. Injectable gold-induced proteinuria, but not hematologic or dermatologic toxicity, are associated with HLA-DRw3 or HLA-B8 (53). Safe monitoring of injectable gold salts requires an evaluation of complete blood and platelet count, urinalysis, skin, and mucous membranes just prior to each injection. Auranofin adverse reaction withdrawals were less than other second-line agents and included diarrhea (3.9%), skin rash (3.2%), gastrointestinal (1.1%), proteinuria (0.9%), and, less commonly, thrombocytopenia, leukopenia, anemia, alteration in taste, nausea, vomiting, as well as mucous membrane, hepatic, lung, and central nervous system effects (32). Auranofin monitoring includes an evaluation of complete blood and platelet count, urinalysis, skin, mucous membranes, and the gastrointestinal tract every 2 to 4 weeks. Other organ toxicity, such as lung and liver, also requires monitoring for either type of gold. Severe diarrhea, bloody gastroenteritis, proteinuria, mucositis, rash, hematologic toxicity, or other serious abnormalities usually indicate discontinuation of gold.

Cyclosporine A, which inhibits T-cell function, has been of benefit in RA at initial doses of 2.5 to 10 mg/kg per day (54), and as effective as chloroquine (55). Nephrotoxicity, hypertension, hypertrichosis, fatigue, and gastrointestinal and neurologic complaints (paresthesias) were frequent. Infections may be a problem associated with cyclosporine use, particularly pneumocystis carinii, and other fungal, bacterial, and viral infections. Cyclosporine plus an oral corticosteroid may be beneficial in the treatment of rheumatoid lung (56). The use of cyclosporine in RA is currently limited by adverse effects, cost, monitoring, and unknown proper dosage or target blood levels.

Minocycline is effective in patients with RA in a manner similar to other second-line agents with a slow onset of effect and no loss of effect shortly after discontinuation of the drug (57, 58). The major adverse effects include gastrointestinal effects and dizziness. Metronidazole was effective in those patients who could tolerate it, but the level of toxicity was unacceptable (59).

Cyclophosphamide is effective in RA at doses of 75 to 150 mg (0.68 to 3.4 mg/kg) per day, but carries considerable short- and long-term toxicity even at lower doses. Doses are adjusted to keep the white blood cell count within the normal or low normal range. Intravenous cyclophosphamide at high doses (500 mg/m^2) every 4 to 6 weeks for six cycles may be useful in treating rheumatoid vasculitis but is poorly tolerated and minimally effective in patients with refractory RA (60).

Cyclophosphamide is inactive and converted in the liver to active metabolites, which are 56% plasma protein bound. The half-life of cyclophosphamide increases from 5 to 7 hours in normal renal function to 4 to 12 hours in end stage renal disease. Renal dysfunction decreases the excretion of cyclophosphamide metabolites, leading to increased toxicity and requiring a decrease in dose. Cyclophosphamide is removed by hemodialysis.

Cyclophosphamide is associated with short- and long-term toxicity. Leukopenia, hemorrhagic cystitis, hair loss, gastrointestinal disturbance, infertility, inappropriate secretion of antidiuretic hormone, and immunosuppression are serious effects. Immunosuppression leads to an increased incidence of fungal, viral, and bacterial infections. Cyclophosphamide causes pneumonitis and pulmonary fibrosis. The occurrence of malignancies was four times greater in a group of RA patients who had received cyclophosphamide than in those who had not. Other than physical findings, complete blood counts and urinalyses are used to monitor cyclophosphamide therapy. Cyclophosphamide interacts with other agents that affect bone marrow function.

Penicillamine is effective in the treatment of severe, progressive RA by starting at low doses of 125 to 250 mg per day and increasing every 2 to 4 weeks to a maximum of 500 or 750 mg per day although up to 1500 mg per day has been used. Efficacy and toxicity do not correlate with serum levels.

Peak plasma levels of penicillamine are seen 1 to 3 hours after administration, but only 30 to 70% is absorbed in fasting individuals and less in patients recently fed or given iron tablets or antacids containing aluminum or magnesium hydroxides (61). Penicillamine is 70 to 80% bound to serum albumin. Approximately 2 to 8% of penicillamine is hepatically metabolized to its methyl metabolite, but the major route of elimination is urinary excretion (61). The half-life of penicillamine is 1.5 to 3 hours. In patients with end stage renal disease on hemodialysis three times weekly and RA, penicillamine doses of 250 mg three times weekly yielded serum drug and metabolite levels that were similar to those seen after higher daily doses in patients with normal renal function (62). Penicillamine is removed by hemodialysis (62).

The use of penicillamine is limited by adverse effects that increase as the dose increases. Withdrawals from penicillamine were due to skin rash (7.1%), proteinuria (5%), thrombocytopenia (2.5%), alterations in taste (2.5%), nausea or vomiting (2%), leukopenia (1%), and, less commonly gastrointestinal, fever, hepatic, diarrhea, renal, lung, breast, and mucous membrane effects (32). Patients who undergo poor sulfoxidation are 3.9 times more likely to experience toxicity to penicillamine at comparable doses than those who undergo ample sulfoxidation, but without a difference in efficacy (63). Penicillamine-induced proteinuria, but not dermatologic or hematologic toxicity, are associated with HLA-DRw3 or HLA-B8 (53). Penicillamine induces autoimmune disorders such as myasthenia gravis, systemic lupus erythematosus, Goodpasture's syndrome, polymyositis, hemolytic anemia, and pemphigus. Penicillamine-induced peripheral neuropathy may respond to pyridoxine. Since penicillamine is a metabolic byproduct of penicillin, caution should be used when administering penicillamine to penicillin-allergic patients though it is generally considered safe. Fetal abnormalities may occur when penicillamine is given during pregnancy, including connective tissue defects. At the initiation of therapy, patients should be monitored every 2 to 4 weeks for adverse effects by monitoring urinalysis, taking a complete blood count, and examining skin and mucous membranes. Once stable, every 4- to 6-week monitoring may suffice. Penicillamine may chelate iron salts and lead to malabsorption of both agents from the gastrointestinal tract.

CORTICOSTEROIDS

Corticosteroids have been used to treat RA by low oral daily doses, intraarticular injections, and intravenous pulses of high doses. Corticosteroids inhibit T- and B-cell activity, chemotaxis of leukocytes, number of mast cells in rheumatoid synovium, and release of collagenase and lysosomal enzymes. Low-dose oral corticosteroids, at prednisone-equivalent doses of 2.5 to 15 mg per day, can dramatically decrease swelling and tenderness and improve the sense of well-being in patients treated with NSAIDs or just started on slow-acting antirheumatic drugs. However, the risk of cumulative toxic effects on the skeleton, metabolism, and other organ systems limit the chronic use and dose of corticosteroids. Corticosteroids may increase the incidence of peptic ulcer and gastrointestinal hemorrhage, particularly in patients receiving NSAIDs. Hypothalamic-pituitary-adrenal suppression can be seen even with the use of low-dose corticosteroids. An unconventional use of corticosteroids in RA includes an approach similar to patient-controlled analgesia and may result in lower average daily doses (64). High-dose corticosteroids are the initial drug of choice for severe extraarticular features of RA, such as vasculitis and rheumatoid lung.

Intraarticular injections of corticosteroids should be used judiciously, preferably into only a few joints that are inflamed to the point of considerably limiting the patient's ability to function or rehabilitate. Intraarticular injections of corticosteroids use compounds that are insoluble salts of active corticosteroids. A needle with attached syringe is inserted into a joint space under aseptic conditions. Synovial fluid is removed and should be analyzed further for white blood cells and differential, bacteria, crystals, and other features. With the needle still in place, the syringe is changed, and the corticosteroid is injected. A dose of 2.5 to 10 mg of prednisolone tebutate equivalents would be used in a small joint such as a PIP, MCP, or MTP joint of a hand or foot; 10 to 25 mg in a wrist, ankle, or elbow; and 20 to 50 mg in a shoulder, ankle, knee, or hip. These insoluble corticosteroid salts may also benefit tenosynovitis, bursitis, and carpal tunnel syndrome. Following injection of the joint or other structure, brief passive range of motion or activity can be used to enhance spread of the drug followed by a period of joint rest lasting 24 to 48 hours. Intraarticular corticosteroids may cause a crystal synovitis because of their insoluble nature and may be safe in children, except in hip joint injections (65). Joint infections are rare, but multiple injections to the same joint may result in breakdown of articular cartilage. The effects of this modality can be dramatic and may last for months to years.

Pulse, high-dose methylprednisolone (1 gram daily intravenously for 1 to 3 days) may produce short-term benefits in the treatment of refractory RA or in those with severe extraarticular disease. It does not appear to have long-term effects or retard disease progression. Pulse methylprednisolone has been able to decrease synovial fluid polymorphonuclear cells, lymphocytes, immune complexes, and C-reactive protein. Severe adverse effects to high-dose, pulse corticosteroids include the rare occurrence of seizures, cardiac arrhythmias, and sudden death. Dysgeusia occurs in more than 50% of patients, but less commonly occurring adverse effects requiring intervention include hypotension, gastric ulceration, and infections (66).

EXPERIMENTAL THERAPIES

Experimental therapies continue to be developed in attempts to develop more specific, safer, and more effective agents. These experimental therapies generally target immune and inflammatory system components, including cells (T-cells, B-cells, macrophages) and mediators (immunoglobulins, interleukins, prostaglandins, leukotrienes). Oral type II collagen has been used effectively in RA (67) following the hypothesis that it would desensitize patients to collagen, which is a likely target of the autoimmunity in RA. Lymphocytes are the target of total lymphoid irradiation, thoracic-duct drainage, antilymphocyte globulin (68), antithymocyte globulin (69), anti-CD4 antibody (70), Campath®-1H (humanized rat antihuman CD52 monoclonal antibody that lyses helper T-cells mostly) (71), and a monoclonal antibody to intercellular adhesion molecule 1 (ICAM-1) (72).

Altering the fatty acid precursors of prostanoids and leukotrienes has also shown some benefit through the use of gamma linolenic acid (GLA) (73, 74), eicosapentanoic acid (EPA), and docosahexaenoic acid (DHA) (75), as well as a vegetarian diet (76). GLA (found in borage seed oil, evening primrose oil, and black currant seed oil) and EPA and DHA (omega-3 fatty acids found in fish oil) lead to the formation of antiinflammatory or less inflammatory prostaglandins and leukotrienes than PGE_2 or LTB_4, which are derived from arachidonic acid. Experimental NSAIDs include agents that inhibit inflammatory mediators other than prostaglandins. RA may also respond to other immunologically active compounds such as gamma globulin, IL-1 antagonists, interferon-gamma (77), thymopoietin derivatives, levamisole, ciamexon (78), and amiprilose (79).

Future advances in rheumatology, immunology, and molecular biology may prove useful in designing treatments for RA that may specifically act against possible defects in the HLA-DR4 antigen, macrophages, lymphocytes, mast cells, or other components of the immune system.

Patients must be cautioned regarding use of nonpharmaceutic therapies, including copper bracelets, herbal remedies, megadose vitamins, bee venom, snake venom, and others. Such remedies may provide relief in anecdotal reports, but few stand up to the rigor of controlled clinical study.

PROGNOSIS

The prognosis in most patients with rheumatoid arthritis is expected to be good. Approximately 10 to 20% of patients with RA have a mild single cycle of the disease that remits spontaneously, 70 to 80% have multiple cycles of mild-to-moderate arthritis, and 10 to 15% have multiple cycles of progressive, severe disease. Patients with RA may experience temporary or permanent disability, considerable morbidity from medications or the systemic features of the disease, and some decrease in survival, particularly those with more severe disease. Quality of life, which can be assessed by a number of questionnaires, is affected in many patients at some time during the course of the disease. A very small number of patients will become confined to a wheelchair or bed because of RA.

CONCLUSION

Rheumatoid arthritis is a chronic, autoimmune disease of unknown etiology that affects joints and other tissues and organs. Alterations in the immune, inflammatory, and related systems result in the tumorlike proliferation of synovial tissue and destruction of bone and cartilage. The variable course of rheumatoid arthritis may or may not be altered by the drug and nondrug therapies used.

Nondrug therapies are used to help the patient cope and to maintain or correct the problems associated with rheumatoid arthritis. NSAIDs are used as one of the baseline measures to treat the acute inflammation, but may also have effects on the immune system and on cartilage formation and destruction. Chronic adverse effects may limit their use. In patients with progressive or probable progressive disease, second-line agents are used despite a poor therapeutic ratio, inability to sustain therapy with any one agent, questionable effects on the progression of the disease, and lack of consensus on which agent or agents to use and how early to initiate this type of therapy. Methotrexate and antimalarials appear to be the current second-line drugs of choice, but others are still considered.

Let us hope that research will lead to effective, more specific, and less toxic therapies. Early intervention in patients with unresponsive inflammation, rapidly progressive disease, and/or high rheumatoid factor titers will ideally diminish the relentless progression of the disease in the 10 to 15% of those who will develop severe rheumatoid arthritis.

REFERENCES

1. Yelin EH, Felts WR. A summary of the impact of musculoskeletal conditions in the United States. Arthritis Rheum 33:750–755, 1990.
2. McDermott M, Kastner DL, Holloman JD, et al. The role of T cell receptor β chain genes in susceptibility to rheumatoid arthritis. Arthritis Rheum 38:91–95, 1995.
3. Brennan P, Silman A. Breast-feeding and the onset of rheumatoid arthritis. Arthritis Rheum 37:808–813, 1994.
4. Chin JE, Winterrowd GE, Krzesicki RF, Sanders ME. Role of cytokines in inflammatory synovitis: the coordinate regulation of intercellular adhesion molecule 1 and HLA class I and class II antigens in rheumatoid synovial fibroblasts. Arthritis Rheum 33: 1776–1786, 1990.
5. Arend WP, Dayer JM. Cytokines and cytokine inhibitors or antagonists in rheumatoid arthritis. Arthritis Rheum 33:305–315, 1990.
6. Rubin LA. The soluble interleukin-2 receptor in rheumatic disease [Editorial]. Arthritis Rheum 33:1145–1148, 1990.
7. Firestein GS, Boyle DL, Yu C, et al. Synovial interleukin-1 receptor antagonist and interleukin-1 balance in rheumatoid arthritis. Arthritis Rheum 37:644–652, 1994.
8. Meyer FA, Yaron I, Yaron M. Synergistic, additive, and antagonistic effects of interleukin-1β, tumor necrosis factor α, and δ-interferon on prostaglandin E, hyaluronic acid, and collagenase production by cultured synovial fibroblasts. Arthritis Rheum 33:1518–1525, 1990.

9. Boubenoff R, Roubenoff RA, Selhub J, et al. Abnormal vitamin B_6 status in rheumatoid cachexia: association with spontaneous tumor necrosis factor α production and markers of inflammation. A&R 38:105–109, 1995.

10. Firestein GS, Zvaifler NJ. How important are T cells in chronic rheumatoid synovitis [Editorial]? Arthritis Rheum 33:768–773, 1990.

11. Tak PP, Kummer JA, Hack CE, et al. Granzyme-positive cytotoxic cells are specifically increased in early rheumatoid synovial tissue. Arthritis Rheum 37:1735–1743, 1994.

12. Calabrese LH, Wilke WS, Perkins AD, Tubbs RR. Rheumatoid arthritis complicated by infection with the human immunodeficiency virus and the development of Sjogren's syndrome. Arthritis Rheum 32:1453–1457, 1989.

13. Sambrook PN, Shawe D, Hesp R, et al. Rapid periarticular bone loss in rheumatoid arthritis: possible promotion by normal circulating concentrations of parathyroid hormone or calcitriol (1,25-dihydroxyvitamin D_3). Arthritis Rheum 33:615–622, 1990.

14. Kawakami M, Kawagoe M, Harigai M, et al. Elevated plasma levels of $α_2$-plasmin inhibitor-plasmin complex in patients with rheumatic diseases: possible role of fibrinolytic mechanisms in vasculitis. Arthritis Rheum 32:1427–1433, 1989.

15. Arnett FC, Edworthy SM, Bloch DA, et al. The American Rheumatism Association 1987 revised criteria for the classification of rheumatoid arthritis. Arthritis Rheum 31:315–324, 1988.

16. Chan KA, Felson DT, Yood RA, Walker AM. The lag time between onset of symptoms and diagnosis of rheumatoid arthritis. Arthritis Rheum 37:814–820, 1994.

17. Katz PP, Yelin EH. The development of depressive symptoms among women with rheumatoid arthritis. Arthritis Rheum 38:49–56, 1995.

18. Pincus T, Olsen NJ, Russell IJ, et al. Multicenter study of recombinant human erythropoietin in correction of anemia in rheumatoid arthritis. Am J Med 89:161–168, 1990.

19. Helewa A, Bombardier C, Goldsmith CH, et al. Cost-effectiveness of inpatient and intensive outpatient treatment of rheumatoid arthritis: a randomized, controlled trial. Arthritis Rheum 32:1505–1514, 1989.

20. Yip ASB, Chow WH, Tai YT, Cheung KL. Adverse effect of topical methylsalicylate ointment on warfarin anticoagulation: an unrecognized potential hazard. Postgrad Med J 66:367–369, 1990.

21. Furst DE. Review: are there differences among nonsteroidal antiinflammatory drugs? Comparing acetylated salicylates, nonacetylated salicylates, and nonacetylated nonsteroidal antiinflammatory drugs. Arthritis Rheum 37:1–9, 1994.

22. Pincus T, Callahan LF. Variability in individual responses of 532 patients with rheumatoid arthritis to first-line and second-line drugs. Agents Actions 44(suppl):67–75, 1993.

23. Fries JF, Ramey DR, Singh G, et al. A reevaluation of aspirin therapy in rheumatoid arthritis. Arch Intern Med 153:2465–2471, 1993.

24. Netter P, Bannwarth B, Royer-Morrot MJ. Recent findings on the pharmacokinetics of non-steroidal anti-inflammatory drugs in synovial fluid. Clin Pharmacokin 17:145–162, 1989.

25. Lichtenstein DR, Syngal S, Wolfe MM. Nonsteroidal antiinflammatory drugs and the gastrointestinal tract: a double edged sword. Arthritis Rheum 38:5–18, 1995.

26. Gubbins GP, Schubert TT, Attaasio F, et al. Heliobacter pylori seroprevalence in patients with rheumatoid arthritis: effect of nonsteroidal anti-inflammatory drugs and gold compounds. Am J Med 93:412–418, 1992.

27. Szczeklik A, Gryglewski RJ, Czerniawska-Mysik G. Relationship of inhibition of prostaglandin biosynthesis by analgesics to asthma attacks in aspirin-sensitive patients. Br Med J 1:67–69, 1975.

28. Chudwin DS, Strub M, Golden HE, et al. Sensitivity to non-acetylated salicylates in a patient with asthma, nasal polyps, and rheumatoid arthritis. Ann Allergy 57:133–134, 1986.

29. Fries JF, Singh F, Lenert L, Furst DE. Aspirin, hydroxychloroquine, and hepatic enzyme abnormalities with methotrexate in rheumatoid arthritis. Arthritis Rheum 33:1611–1619, 1990.

30. Boyce EG. Pharmacology of antiarthritic drugs. Clin Podiatric Med Surgery 9:327–348, 1992.

31. Furst DE. Rational use of disease-modifying antirheumatic drugs. Drugs 39:19–37, 1990.

32. Felson DT, Anderson JJ, Meenan RF. The comparative efficacy and toxicity of second-line drugs in rheumatoid arthritis: results of two metaanalyses. Arthritis Rheum 33:1449–1461, 1990.

33. Prashker MJ, Meenan RF. The total costs of drug therapy for rheumatoid arthritis: a model based on costs of drug, monitoring, and toxicity. Arthritis Rheum 38:318–325, 1995.

34. Borg G, Allander E, Lund B, et al. Auranofin improves outcome in early rheumatoid arthritis. Results from a 2-year, double blind, placebo controlled study. J Rheumatol 15:1747–1754, 1988.

35. Felson DT, Anderson JJ, Meenan RF. The efficacy and toxicity of combination therapy in rheumatoid arthritis: a meta-analysis. Arthritis Rheum 37:1487–1491, 1994.

36. Csuka ME, Carrera GF, McCarty DJ. Treatment of intractable rheumatoid arthritis with combined cyclophosphamide, azathioprine, and hydroxychloroquine: a follow-up study. JAMA 255:2315–2319, 1986.

37. Tiliakos NA. Low-dose cytotoxic drug combination therapy in intractable rheumatoid arthritis: two years later [Abstract]. Arthritis Rheum 29(suppl):S79, 1986.

38. Page F. Treatment of lupus erythematosus with mepacrine. Lancet 2:755–758, 1951.

39. Middleton GD, McFarlin JE, Lipsky PE. Hydroxychloroquine and pain thresholds [Letter]. Arthritis Rheum 38:445–446, 1995.

40. Pappaioanou M, Fishbein DB, Dreesen DW, et al. Antibody response to preexposure human diploid-cell rabies vaccine given concurrently with chloroquine. New Engl J Med 314:280–284, 1986.

41. Brooks PJ, Spruill WJ, Parish RC, Birchmore DA. Pharmacokinetics of methotrexate administered by intramuscular and subcutaneous injections in patients with rheumatoid arthritis. Arthritis Rheum 33:91–94, 1990.

42. Shiroky JB, Neville C, Skelton JD. High dose intravenous methotrexate for refractory rheumatoid arthritis. J Rheumatol 19:247–251, 1992.

43. Kremer JM, Rynes RI, Bartholomew LE. Severe flare of rheumatoid arthritis after discontinuation of long-term methotrexate therapy: double-blind study. Am J Med 82:781–786, 1987.

44. Bologna C, Edno L, Anaya JM, et al. Methotrexate concentrations in synovial membrane and trabecular and cortical bone in rheumatoid arthritis patients. Arthritis Rheum 37:1770–1773, 1994.

45. Berquist SR, Felson DT, Prashker MJ, Freedberg KA. The cost-effectiveness of liver biopsy in rheumatoid arthritis patients treated with methotrexate. Arthritis Rheum 38:326–333, 1995.

46. Morgan SL, Baggott JE, Vaughn WH, et al. The effect of folic acid supplementation on the toxicity of low-dose methotrexate in patients with rheumatoid arthritis. Arthritis Rheum 33:9–18, 1990.

47. Shiroky JB, Neville C, Esdaile JM, et al. Low-dose methotrexate with leucovorin (folinic acid) in the management of rheumatoid arthritis: results of a multicenter randomized, double-blind, placebo-controlled trial. Arthritis Rheum 36:795–803, 1993.

48. Joyce DA, Will RK, Hoffman DM, Laing B, Blackbourn SJ. Exacerbation of rheumatoid arthritis in patients treated with methotrexate after administration of folinic acid. Ann Rheum Dis 50:913–914,1991.

49. Montecucco C, Caporali R, Rossi S, Porta C. Allopurinol mouthwashes in methotrexate-induced stomatitis [Letter]. Arthritis Rheum 37:777–778, 1994.

50. Singh G, Fries JF, Spitz P, Williams CA. Toxic effects of azathioprine in rheumatoid arthritis: a national post-marketing perspective. Arthritis Rheum 32:837–843, 1989.

51. Kerstens PJSM, Stolk JN, De Abreu RA, et al. Azathioprine-related bone marrow toxicity and low activities of purine enzymes in patients with rheumatoid arthritis. Arthritis Rheum 38:142–145, 1995.

52. Jullien D, Wolkenstein P, Roupie, et al. Toxic epidermal necrolysis after sulfasalazine treatment of mild psoriatic arthritis: warning on the use of sulfasalazine for a new indication [Letter]. Arthritis Rheum 38:573, 1995.

53. Wooley PH, Griffin J, Panayi GS, et al. HLA-DR antigens and toxic reaction to sodium aurothiomalate and D-penicillamine in patients with rheumatoid arthritis. New Engl J Med 303:300–302, 1980.

54. Tugwell P, Bombardier C, Gent G, et al. Low-dose cyclosporin versus placebo in patients with rheumatoid arthritis. Lancet 335:1051–1055, 1990.

55. Landewé RBM, Goei Thé HS, van Rijthoven AWAM, Breedveld FC, Dijkmans BAC. A randomized, double-blind, 24-week controlled study of low-dose cyclosporine versus chloroquine for early rheumatoid arthritis. Arthritis Rheum 37:637–643, 1994.

56. Alegre J, Teran J, Alvarez B, Viejo JL. Successful use of cyclosporine for the treatment of aggressive pulmonary fibrosis in a patient with rheumatoid arthritis [Letter]. Arthritis Rheum 33:1594–1596, 1990.

57. Tilley BC, Alarcon GS, Heyse SP, et al. Minocycline in rheumatoid arthritis: a 48-week, double-blind, placebo-controlled trial. Ann Intern Med 122:81–89, 1995.

58. Kloppenburg M, Breedveld FC, Terwiel JP, Mallee C, Dijkmans BAC. Minocycline in active rheumatoid arthritis: a double-blind, placebo-controlled trial. Arthritis Rheum 37:629–636, 1994.

59. Marshall DA, Hunter JA, Capell HA. Double blind, placebo controlled study of metronidazole as a disease modifying agent in the treatment of rheumatoid arthritis. Ann Rheum Dis 51:758–760, 1992.

60. Arnold MH, Janssen B, Schrieber L, Brooks PM. Prospective pilot study of intravenous pulse cyclophosphamide therapy for refractory rheumatoid arthritis [Letter]. Arthritis Rheum 32:933–934, 1989.

61. Netter P, Bannwarth B, Pere P, Nicolas A. Clinical pharmacokinetics of D-penicillamine. Clin Pharmacokin 13:317–333, 1987.

62. Matthey F, Perrett D, Greenwood RN, Baker LRI. The use of D-penicillamine in patients with rheumatoid arthritis undergoing hemodialysis. Clin Nephrol 25:268–271, 1986.

63. Madhok R, Zoma A, Torley HI, et al. The relationship of sulfoxidation status to efficacy and toxicity of penicillamine in the treatment of rheumatoid arthritis. Arthritis Rheum 33:574–577, 1990.

64. Wilder RL. Neuroendocrine control of inflammation. Update in Rheumatology, University of Pennsylvania School of Medicine, Philadelphia, September 25, 1990.

65. Sparling M, Malleson P, Wood B, Petty R. Radiographic followup of joints injected with triamcinolone hexacetonide for the management of childhood arthritis. Arthritis Rheum 33:821–826, 1990.

66. Baethge BA, Lidsky MD, Goldberg JW. A study of adverse effects of high-dose intravenous (pulse) methylprednisolone therapy in patients with rheumatic disease. Ann Pharmacotherapy 26:316–320, 1992.

67. Trentham DE, Dynesius-Trentham RA, Orav EJ, et al. Effects of oral administration of type II collagen on rheumatoid arthritis. Science 261:1727–1729, 1993.

68. Binder AI, So A, Ansell BM, Denmam AM. Intensive immunosuppression in intractable rheumatoid arthritis. Br J Rheumatol 25:380–383, 1986.

69. Schmerling RH, Trentham DE. Prolonged improvement in refractory rheumatoid arthritis after antithymocyte globulin therapy of brief duration [Letter]. Arthritis Rheum 32:1495–1514, 1989.

70. Herzog C, Walker C, Pichler W, et al. Monoclonal anti-CD4 in arthritis [Letter]. Lancet 2:1461–1462, 1987.

71. Isaacs JD, Watts RA, Hazelman BL, et al. Humanized monoclonal antibody therapy for rheumatoid arthritis. Lancet 340:748–752, 1992.

72. Kavanaugh AF, Davis LS, Nichols LA, et al. Treatment of refractory rheumatoid arthritis with a monoclonal antibody to intercellular adhesion molecule 1. Arthritis Rheum 37:992–999, 1994.

73. Leventhal LJ, Boyce EG, Zurier RB. Treatment of rheumatoid arthritis with gamma-linolenic acid. Ann Intern Med 119:867–873, 1993.

74. Leventhal LJ, Boyce EG, Zurier RB. Treatment of rheumatoid arthritis with blackcurrant seed oil. Br J Rheumatol 33:847–852, 1994.

75. Kremer JM, Lawrence DA, Jubiz W, et al. Dietary fish oil and olive oil supplementation in patients with rheumatoid arthritis: clinical and immunologic effects. Arthritis Rheum 33:810–820, 1990.

76. Haugen MA, Kjeldsen-Kragh J, Bjerve KS, Hostmark AT, Forre O. Changes in plasma phospholipid fatty acids and their relationship to disease activity in rheumatoid arthritis patients treated with a vegetarian diet. Br J Nutrition 72:555–566, 1994.

77. Cannon GW, Emkey RD, Denes A, et al. Prospective 5-year followup of recombinant interferon-gamma in rheumatoid arthritis. J Rheumatol 20:1867–1873, 1993.

78. Baerwald C, Goebel KM, Krause A, Heymanns J. A randomized controlled trial of ciamexon versus placebo in the immunomodulatory treatment of rheumatoid arthritis. Arthritis Rheum 33:733–738, 1990.

79. Riskin WG, Gillings DB, Scarlett JA. Amiprilose hydrochloride for rheumatoid arthritis. Ann Intern Med 111:455–465, 1989.

CHAPTER 31

OSTEOARTHRITIS

JANELLE M. MAHONEY and MICHAEL L. SCHMITZ

Osteoarthritis (OA), also known as degenerative joint disease (DJD), is a common, progressive disorder initially affecting joint soft tissue with subsequent involvement of underlying bone and secondary inflammation of the contiguous synovium. OA commonly affects the spine, knees, hips, and shoulders and the interphalangeal joints of the hands and feet and is characterized by pain, deformity, and limitation of joint function. In contrast to rheumatoid arthritis and other joint disorders, systemic abnormalities are not present in OA. The disease usually becomes symptomatic between the fourth and sixth decades of life (1).

EPIDEMIOLOGY

OA is the most common arthritis disorder in the United States, although precise prevalence is hard to determine because of diagnostic discrepancies and the low correlation between clinical symptoms and radiologic evidence of the disease. Although age of onset and rate of progression are variable, approximately 30% of people 45 to 64 years of age will demonstrate symptoms or radiologic changes consistent with OA (2). Osteoarthritis increases in prevalence with age but is not necessarily a result of normal aging (3). Sixty-three to eighty-five percent of people over 65 years of age demonstrate signs and/or symptoms of OA, 12% of those affected being unable to perform daily activities, and half of these individuals being totally disabled (4). OA appears to affect different joints at different ages. For example, OA is evident in the first metatarsophalangeal joint after 25 years of age, in the wrist and spine after 35 years of age, in the distal interphalangeal joints after 45 years of age, and in the hip and knee joints after 55 years of age (2, 5). OA symptoms affect approximately 60 million Americans, resulting in more loss of time from work than any other chronic disease (1, 2).

OA does not show a predilection for a particular race, geographic area, climate, or socioeconomic class. Gender differences do exist, male incidence being greater before age 45 and female incidence being greater after age 45 (6–8). Women are also more prone to knee and hand joint involvement than are men (9). Chronic excessive body weight has also been correlated with, but not causative, of OA, as no consistent relationship has been demonstrated between weight bearing and osteoarthritis. This is evidenced by the development of OA in mammals that have skeletons but have no weight-bearing joints (e.g., whales, porpoises, and bats) (1).

NORMAL JOINT FUNCTION

The diarthroidal joints are principally affected by OA; however, the fibrocartilaginous joints of the spine are also frequently involved. Diarthroidal joints consist of hyaline cartilage-covered bone ends that are juxtaposed and united by a fibrous capsule lined with synovial tissue. Typical examples are the knee and hip joints. Fibrocartilaginous joints, such as intervertebral disks, consist of bone united by fibrous tissue. The diarthroidal joints have a greater range of motion than fibrocartilagenous joints at the expense of joint stability.

Articular cartilage covers and protects bone from the forces encountered with normal joint activity. Cartilage is a matrix of hydrophilic proteoglycan complexes enclosed in a collagen fibril structure and is 80% water by weight (10). The proteoglycan molecules confer shock-absorbing and lubricative properties onto cartilage because of their capacity to retain and release great amounts of water. As in a water-filled sponge, compressive forces cause an expulsion of water from the pressure region, resulting in matrix deformation (7).

This deformation increases the contact area under the compressive force and reduces stress on the cartilage and underlying bone. The highly polyanionic proteoglycans retard continued deformity by attracting water and inhibiting further outflow. When the pressure load is relieved, the matrix regains its original form through proteoglycan rehydration. The maintenance of a functional joint depends on the ability of the chondrocytes (cartilage cells) to synthesize and degrade the matrix components (proteoglycans, collagen) in equilibrium (10). A hallmark of OA is the disruption of this balance, with the degradative processes overwhelming the synthetic processes and causing a net loss of proteoglycan matrix.

The synovial tissue of the diarthroidal joints provides lubrication, nutrition, and elimination of waste products for articular hyaline cartilage. The synovial lubrication lowers the hyaline-hyaline coefficient of friction to approximately that of two pieces of wet ice sliding across each other. OA alters the hyaline-hyaline interface and surrounding tissues to increase drastically this coefficient of friction and ultimately reduce joint mobility.

ETIOLOGY

OA is a heterogeneous disorder. Although a number of investigators have proposed pathophysiologic mechanisms for OA, the etiology of OA appears to be multifactorial and, as yet, is incompletely elucidated. A number of factors (genetic, hormonal, nutritional, and environmental) are thought to contribute to the progression of the disorder, although an initiating event leading to the imbalance of reparative processes has not been identified. Evidence suggesting that the development of OA is related to joint overuse remains equivocal (6, 11). It has been well-accepted that the etiology of OA begins in the cartilage and is associated with changes in the proteoglycan and collagen matrix; however, the importance of the relationship between the synovium, cartilage, and subchondral bone cannot be minimized.

PATHOPHYSIOLOGY

OA is marked by concurrent anabolic and catabolic processes (7, 12–16). Articular cartilage, synovial tissue, and subchondral bone are the principal loci for the pathologic changes associated with OA. The effects of OA, unlike those of rheumatoid arthritis, are limited to the joints.

OA results from alterations in the biochemical composition of articular cartilage. Histologically, collagen content may remain stable, but the structure becomes disorganized and weakened. A resultant increase in cartilage hydration associated with proteoglycan swelling dilutes the proteoglycan component of cartilage (17–19). Proteolytic and lysosomal enzyme activity induced by interleukin-1 further degrades the proteoglycan structure (20). A reduction in osmotic pressure causes a loss of cartilage resiliency. Loss of the elastic properties of cartilage results in fibrillation, fissuring, and eventual ulceration of the surface, thus decreasing surface congruity and precipitating further injury.

Subchondral bone proliferates in an attempt to increase the surface area available for load bearing. As subchondral bone proliferates, it becomes more sclerotic and is more susceptible to microfractures and further sclerosis. Osteophytes, a cardinal feature of OA, are osseous outgrowths that appear at the bony margins of the joint (21). These masses may enlarge the joint, compress spinal nerves, and severely limit joint mobility. Subchondral cysts surrounded by sclerotic bone begin to appear in advanced disease and are most evident in the hip joint. The subchondral bone loses elasticity and the ability to absorb shock from continued sclerosis, resulting in increased vascularity and intraosseous venous pressure (22). Continuous destruction of the cartilage may eventually result in the exposure of subchondral bone. Completely denuded bone grinds against the bone of the adjacent joint surface and becomes eburnated, shiny, and smooth. Points of maximum pressure show the most damage.

Proliferation of subchondral bone is accompanied by hypertrophy of all soft tissues (i.e., ligaments, tendons, muscles) in the joint, including the synovium (7). Hyper-

trophic changes are physiologic attempts to repair damage. However, the resultant tissue enlargement and synovial effusions are responsible for joint deformity, further limitation of motion, and pain (23).

Chronic synovitis (inflammation of the synovium) is thought to be caused by the presence of proteoglycan and collagen fragments following proteolytic attack. Neovascularization and focal hemorrhages may be marked in the synovial tissue. Crystals of calcium pyrophosphate dihydrate, calcium hydroxyapatite, or both may or may not be present and appear to be correlated with advanced radiographic disease and greater frequency of intraarticular corticosteroid injections (17).

CLINICAL PRESENTATION

Joint pain is the most common complaint of patients with OA. The pain is exacerbated by increased joint activity, especially weight-bearing activity, and is relieved with rest in the early stages of the disease. Pain is generally characterized as dull and aching with episodes of lancinating pain that are usually related to certain movements. Pain is initially intermittent but eventually becomes constant and disabling.

Patients frequently complain of joint stiffness after rest, which is generally short in duration. Morning stiffness may be present but usually subsides within minutes, compared with the prolonged stiffness associated with rheumatoid arthritis. Affected joints may manifest restricted range of motion, tenderness, bony enlargement, effusion, and crepitus (a frequently audible crackling sensation) (24–26). Erythema and palpable warmth are rare but possible in OA.

Patients with OA of the fingers commonly have firm nodules located on the dorsolateral and dorsomedial aspects of the distal interphalangeal joints. The nodules, called Heberden's nodes, represent cartilage-covered bony spurs. Nodule formation is usually painless and may occur in the thumb as well as the feet (27). Women are 10 times more likely than men to develop Heberden's nodes (9). Hypertrophic bony changes at the proximal interphalangeal joint are called Bouchard's nodes and may be accompanied by intense swelling and erythema. These nodes are also more common in women.

Although OA affecting the hip may be the most incapacitating, because of mobility limitations, spinal OA can be the most painful. Nerve root compression from spinal involvement of facet joints may lead to local or referred pain, paresthesias, muscle spasms, and eventual muscle atrophy. OA of the knee is characterized by tenderness, synovitis, crepitus, palpable osteophytes, limited range of motion, and joint deformity (21, 24).

DIAGNOSIS

The diagnosis of OA is based primarily on clinical symptoms and exclusion of other disease processes.

Table 31.1.
Osteoarthritis Classification Criteria

Presence of osteophytes
Pain
Joint stiffness less than 30 min duration
Crepitus
Bony enlargement and tenderness with no palpable warmth
Age over 50 years

Source: Adapted from Schuomacher HR: Primer on Rheumatic Diseases, 9th ed. Atlanta: National Arthritis Foundation, 1988, pp. 172–177.

Radiographic findings typically include joint-space narrowing, sclerosis of subchondral bone, subchondral cysts, and osteophyte formation, in contrast to the juxtaarticular osteoporosis associated with rheumatoid arthritis. However, radiographic findings without symptomatic complaints are common and do not warrant treatment.

The increased volume of synovial fluid from affected joints shows decreased viscosity, increased protein concentration, and normal hyaluronate concentrations. The cartilage and fibrin fragments and crystal deposition suggest OA but do not constitute a definitive diagnosis. Probably important to the destructive process, increased concentrations of lysosomal enzymes, prostaglandins (PGs), and interleukin-1 are present in the synovial fluid of affected joints, although these findings are not exclusive to OA.

Results of hematologic studies are usually normal, with the exception of a slightly elevated erythrocyte sedimentation rate (ESR) during episodes of inflammation. Rheumatoid factor and antinuclear antibody serology are generally negative.

Most investigators believe OA to result from several diverse causes. If the cause is unknown or thought to be genetic, the term *primary OA* is applicable. Secondary OA refers to all other situations in which a causative factor is known or presumed (e.g., trauma). Regardless of the cause, efforts to standardize reporting have generated several classification criteria including (a) the presence of osteophytes, (b) pain, (c) joint stiffness of less than 30 min duration, (d) crepitus, (e) bony enlargement and tenderness with no palpable warmth, and (f) age over 50 years (Table 31.1). These criteria are not intended to be diagnostic, but the presence of all six is a sensitive and specific indicator for OA (12).

TREATMENT

The treatment of OA is directed primarily toward alleviating pain, the chief reason for patients to seek medical attention (28). Preservation or improvement of joint function, minimization of disability, patient education, and maintenance of a good quality of life are also primary goals of therapy. OA treatment programs include nonpharmacologic therapy (psychosocial counseling, education, and physiotherapy), pharmacologic therapy, and surgical intervention. Treatment modalities may vary, depending on the clinical severity of disease, and must be individualized for each patient.

NONPHARMACOLOGIC THERAPY

Nonpharmacologic modes of therapy are paramount to the management of OA and are usually effective for managing mild-to-moderate OA. The early stages of OA may respond to nonpharmacologic measures alone, and initial attempts to achieve acceptable therapeutic outcomes should reflect this. As in other pain syndromes, the symptoms of OA are magnified and possibly worsened by anxiety. Patients with OA should be assured that the disease is not the rapidly crippling illness that rheumatoid arthritis can be and that several effective treatment options exist (1).

Patient education is aimed at reducing irrational fears and providing accurate information on the course of the disease. Because of joint stiffness associated with rest, patients may fear erroneously that joints will "freeze" if they are not in constant motion. Patients should be taught the principles of joint protection and pain alleviation. Gentle range-of-motion exercises during periods of prolonged inactivity can prevent associated joint stiffness. Patients should be encouraged to comply with prescribed physiotherapeutic regimens and curtail weight-bearing, high-impact exercises to limit excessive joint stress.

Physiotherapy focuses on maintenance of a proper balance between exercise and rest. Short periods of isometric (not isotonic) exercises throughout the day should be encouraged to preserve or improve range of motion, relieve joint stiffness, minimize joint stress, and strengthen periarticular muscle groups. Characteristically, periarticular muscles are atrophied in patients with OA, because of inactivity due to pain (29). Increased pain, lasting for more than 1 hour after exercising, is an indication for reducing but not eliminating exercises. Alternating exercise with non-weight-bearing rest 2 to 4 times daily for an hour or more will allow cartilage rehydration and promote reparative processes. Excessive joint-loading activities (e.g., heavy lifting) should be avoided. The use of walking aids (i.e., canes, crutches, walkers), running shoes for walking, or specifically designed orthopedic shoes may relieve some joint pressure and pain. Application of moderate heat for muscle relaxation or of ice packs for acute inflammation before exercising can reduce joint stiffness and increase exercise tolerance. Weight reduction is imperative in obese patients to reduce excessive joint stress. Patients should be instructed to continue nonpharmacologic therapy to minimize the need for drug therapy (27).

PHARMACOLOGIC THERAPY

Analgesics

Since there is no cure for OA, pharmacologic intervention is palliative and directed toward alleviation of pain and improving joint function. Therapy traditionally includes the use of analgesics and nonsteroidal antiinflammatory drugs (NSAIDs). Analgesics are usually employed early in the disease to minimize NSAID-associated renal and gastrointestinal adverse effects and to decrease the potential for NSAID-induced inhibitory effects on cartilage proteoglycan synthesis. Acetaminophen in doses of 325 to 650 mg 3 to 4 times daily, not to exceed 2.6 g/day with prolonged use, is a useful and effective analgesic regimen. Scheduled dosing is more effective than "as needed" administration for the management of chronic pain. Propoxyphene alone provides no better analgesic effects than acetaminophen alone, but there may be additive effects when the two agents are combined. However, the use of centrally active medications (e.g., propoxyphene) increases the incidence of adverse central nervous system (CNS) effects. These agents should not be used in patients who are particularly susceptible to adverse CNS effects (e.g., the elderly). Codeine and other narcotic analgesics are rarely appropriate and should be used only briefly if required.

NSAIDs

In the early stages of OA there may be no evidence of inflammation. However, advanced disease is commonly associated with synovial inflammation, which may be a source of pain. NSAIDs have both analgesic and antiinflammatory activity and would seem to be a logical choice for the treatment of OA after failure with analgesics alone. However, there is limited evidence that NSAIDs are effective for any other reason than analgesia. A double-blind, placebo-controlled trial of acetaminophen (4 g/day) versus ibuprofen at 1.2 g/day or 2.4 g/day demonstrated no superiority of effect from the NSAID (30). Although the exact mechanism of action is unknown, NSAIDs are thought to inhibit peripheral prostaglandin and endoperoxide synthesis through reversible cyclooxygenase inhibition (31). It has been shown that prostaglandins and endoperoxides are responsible for mediation of inflammation. Inhibition of histamine and kinins and release of free oxygen radicals purportedly prevent pain receptor sensitization and inflammation.

PHARMACOKINETICS

Following oral administration, all NSAIDs are rapidly absorbed. Food and various dosage formulations (e.g., enteric-coated, delayed release) may delay the rate of absorption, but the extent of absorption generally remains unaffected. Salicylate levels can be detected in the serum 5 to 30 min after oral administration, and peak concentrations are usually attained within 0.25 to 2.0 hr, depending on the dosage form and specific formulations. Maximum therapeutic effects may not be attained, however, for 2 to 3 weeks after starting therapy. All NSAIDs are highly protein bound (≥90%), primarily to albumin. These agents are metabolized chiefly by hepatic biotransformation and

are excreted primarily through the kidneys. The half-life of NSAIDs varies from 1 to 8 hr following ingestion of a single oral dose, with the exception of piroxicam($t\frac{1}{2}$ = 50 hr). A half-life of sulindac is 7.8 hr, and that of its active metabolite is 16.4.

SPECIFIC AGENTS

The NSAIDs that are currently available include derivatives of salicylates, propionic acids, indoleacetic acids, pyrroleacetic acids, fenamates, pyrazoles, oxicams, phenylacetic acids, pyranocarboxylic acid, naphylalkanones, and pyrrolizine carboxylic acid; they are listed in Table 31.2. Selection of a particular agent should depend on efficacy, side effect profile, patient preference, and cost.

Caution should be used in giving NSAIDs to patients with a history of hypersensitivity to NSAIDs, including aspirin, as cross-sensitivity may occur among different structural derivatives. NSAIDs are contraindicated in patients with a history of pulmonary or anaphylactoid manifestations of hypersensitivity associated with prior NSAID use.

EFFICACY

All currently approved NSAIDs are equipotent in providing symptomatic relief of OA if taken at the recommended doses (32). The potential for NSAIDs to alter disease progression remains controversial, and research is ongoing. Several NSAIDs have been implicated in the acceleration of joint destruction. Numerous in vitro investigations have shown NSAIDs to effectively reduce hyaluronic acid synthesis (the core of the proteoglycan molecule) and inhibit proteoglycan formation (33–35). Aspirin, indomethacin, sulindac, flurbiprofen, diclofenac, and ketoprofen have been identified as being deleterious to hip joints in human subjects (33). It has been proposed that osteoarthritic joints require adequate perfusion to maintain joint structure reparative processes (34). This perfusion is enhanced by inflammation. Inhibition of PG synthesis may interfere with joint blood flow and cause the already compromised joint to deteriorate more rapidly (34). This hypothesis was tested in 105 patients with OA of the hip who were randomly allocated to receive indomethacin (a *potent* PG inhibitor) 50 to 75 mg/day or azapropazone (a *weak* PG inhibitor) 600 to 900 mg/day (34). The time to reach arthroplasty, the endpoint in the OA process, was 50% longer and cartilage proteoglycan content was substantially higher in the group treated with azapropazone. Finally, overuse of a pain-free joint is another potential mechanism of enhanced joint destruction associated with NSAID use. Therefore, NSAIDs may not be indicated in the long-term treatment of OA.

Conversely, several investigators have demonstrated an NSAID-induced inhibition of proteinase activity, release of collagenase, and proteoglycan degradation in experimental models (35). These effects would seem to protect joint

Table 31.2.
Nonsteroidal Antiinflammatory Agents

Drug	Usual Daily Dose	Maximum Daily Dose	Usual Dosing Interval	Trade Name	Relative Cost[a]
Salicylates					
Aspirin	3.9–5.1 g	5.1 g	4–6 times/day	Various	+
Sodium Salicylate	3.9–5.1 g	5.1 g	4–6 times/day	Uracel 5	+
Choline salicylate	5.2–7.0 g	7.0 g	4–6 times/day	Arthropan	++
Magnesium salicylate	3.9–5.1 g	4.0 g	4–6 times/day	Doan's	++
Salsalate	3.0–4.0 g	1.5 g	b.i.d.–t.i.d.	Disalcid	+++
Diflunisal	0.5–1.5 g		b.i.d.–t.i.d.	Dolobid	++++
Proprionic acids					
Fenoprofen	1200–3200 mg	3200 mg	t.i.d.–q.i.d.	Nalfon	++++
Ibuprofen	1200–3200 mg	3200 mg	t.i.d.–q.i.d.	Motrin	++
Ketoprofen	150–300 mg	300 mg	t.i.d.–q.i.d.	Orudis	++++
Naproxen	500–1000 mg	1200 mg	b.i.d.	Naprosyn	+++
Flurbiprofen	100–200 mg	300 mg	b.i.d.	Ansaid	+++
Oxaprozin	600–1200 mg	1800 mg	q.d.	Daypro	++++
Indoleacetic acids					
Indomethacin	75–150 mg	200 mg	b.i.d.–t.i.d.	Indocin	++
Pyrroleacetic acids					
Sulindac	300–400 mg	400 mg	b.i.d.	Clinoril	+++
Tolmentin sodium	500–1000 mg	1250 mg	t.i.d.–q.i.d.	Tolectin	+++
Fenamates					
Mefenamic acid	750–1000 mg	1000 mg	t.i.d.–q.i.d.	Ponstel	+++
Meclofenamate sodium	200–400 mg	400 mg	t.i.d.–q.i.d.	Meclomen	+++
Pyrazoles					
Phenylbutazone	200–400 mg	400 mg	t.i.d.–q.i.d.	Butazolidin	+
Oxicams					
Piroxicam	20 mg	20 mg	q.d.	Feldene	++
Phenylacetic acids					
Diclofenac	100–150 mg	200 mg	b.i.d.–q.i.d.	Voltaren	+++
Pyranocarboxylic acid					
Etodolac	600–1200 mg	1200 mg	b.i.d.–q.i.d.	Lodine	++++
Naphylalkanones					
Nabumetone	1000–2000 mg	2000 mg	q.d.–b.i.d.	Relafen	++++
Pyrrolizine carboxylic acid					
Ketorolac tromethamine	10 mg	40 mg for 5–14 days only	4–6 times/day	Toradol	++++

[a]Relative costs based on average wholesale price cost of maximum daily dosage.

structure integrity and/or enhance reparative processes. However, valid conclusions on either the deleterious or beneficial effects of NSAIDs on osteoarthritic joints cannot be drawn from comparisons of such diverse experimental systems (36).

Until further research provides definitive answers, simple analgesia is recommended for mild-to-moderate OA. Dosing with NSAIDs during periods of severe pain or inflammation in moderate-to-severe disease should be alternated with analgesics or low-potency NSAIDs during periods of quiescence (35).

ADVERSE EFFECTS

The use of NSAIDs is not without adverse effects, some of which may be severe in certain patient populations. On the basis of the risk for adverse effects, it is recommended that

the smallest dose that provides symptom relief should be used in concordance with constant and careful reevaluation of need by both the prescriber and the patient.

All NSAIDs may produce adverse gastrointestinal (GI) effects including nausea, vomiting, dyspepsia, diarrhea, constipation, and gastritis. Severe effects include GI ulceration, perforation, and hemorrhage. Although the nonacetylated salicylates (i.e., salsalate, choline salicylate) have been associated with a lower incidence of gastric bleeding, no NSAID is completely free of the risk of causing gastric injury when taken on a chronic basis. Gastric ulcers occur in 10 to 15% of chronic NSAID users, one-third of whom are asymptomatic (33). The proposed mechanisms of GI injury include local irritation, inhibition of PG synthesis (prostaglandins inhibit gastric acid secretion), decreased availability of sulfhydryl donors (which are

Table 31.3.
Factors Related to Increased Risk of NSAID-Induced GI Complications

History of peptic ulcer disease
History of GI bleeding
Advanced age
Short duration of exposure
Large NSAID doses
Cigarette smoking
Concurrent corticosteroid therapy
Concurrent anticoagulant therapy

required for PG receptor activation), and inhibition of platelet aggregation (37, 38). Factors related to an increased risk of GI complications include (a) a history of peptic ulcer disease or gastrointestinal bleeding, (b), advanced age, (c) short duration of exposure, (d) cigarette smoking, (e) corticosteroid use, and (f) anticoagulant therapy (Table 31.3) (39, 40). Since the appearance of adverse GI effects is a dose-related phenomenon, initiation with low-dose NSAIDs is warranted in these high-risk patients (40). Instructing patients to take their medication with meals may also prevent or lessen most GI discomfort. Buffered aspirin is associated with the same GI toxicity as regular aspirin and should not be considered safe. However, because of its delayed release, enteric-coated aspirin is a reasonable alternative. The use of topical NSAIDs (e.g., trolamine salicylate, Aspercreme) or rectal suppositories may circumvent GI injury, but extensive studies have not yet demonstrated efficacy in OA. Further investigation of these formulations is warranted (41).

Until recently, no treatment has been proven to prevent NSAID-induced gastric ulcers and bleeding. The addition of H$_2$-antagonists or sucralfate has not been shown to reduce the severity or incidence of NSAID-induced ulcers or bleeding. Misoprostol, a synthetic prostaglandin analog with antisecretory and cytoprotective effects, has been shown to prevent and heal gastric ulcers associated with long-term NSAID therapy (42). Prophylactic misoprostol is indicated in (a) patients who are at high risk of developing gastric ulceration (such as those with a history of upper GI ulcers) and (b) patients who are at high risk of developing complications (i.e., bleeding, perforation, death) from NSAID-induced ulcers, including the elderly and patients with debilitating disease. The most common adverse effects are dose-related and include a self-limiting diarrhea in 5 to 40% of patients, abdominal pain, nausea, and flatulence. Halving the normal dose of 200 µg 4 times daily may decrease the incidence of adverse effects. Misoprostol is contraindicated in pregnant women and women of childbearing potential unless they practice adequate birth control because of its ability to induce uterine contractions and cause expulsion of uterine contents.

The effects of NSAIDs on renal function may be problematic in some patients, particularly those with preexisting renal insufficiency, and are usually detected by increases in serum creatinine and blood urea nitrogen levels. Because normal renal function depends at least partially on PG synthesis, the administration of agents that inhibit PG synthesis (i.e., NSAIDs) may induce renal injury. Vasodilatory PGs are released in response to the vasoconstriction produced by angiotensin II in patients with congestive heart failure or intravascular volume contraction or patients who are on chronic diuretic therapy. When this compensatory mechanism is blocked, renal blood flow and glomerular filtration rate are reduced, and secondary ischemia may occur. Decreased renal blood flow associated with aging puts the elderly population at increased risk for complications. NSAID-induced reduction in renal blood flow may also increase sodium reabsorption, resulting in edema and possible interference with antihypertensive therapy.

NSAIDs have been associated with hypoaldosteronemia and resultant hyperkalemia due to inhibition of aldosterone release secondary to PG inhibition (43). Papillary necrosis has also been reported, but definite drug causation has not been established (43). Interstitial nephritis has been observed and is generally considered to be an allergic manifestation consisting of eosinophilia, rash, arthralgias, fever, proteinuria, and nephrotic syndrome.

Renal function should be evaluated at baseline, 1 week after starting therapy, and every 3 months during chronic therapy with NSAIDs in susceptible patients (i.e., the elderly, patients with preexisting renal disease). Sulindac appears to be the only renal-sparing NSAID and is a reasonable alternative in these patients (44).

All NSAIDs, except the nonacetylated salicylates, inhibit platelet aggregation. Therefore, these agents are relatively contraindicated in patients with coagulation defects and those who are currently receiving anticoagulant therapy. Leukopenia, thrombocytopenia, and agranulocytosis may occur rarely and are generally reversible. Periodic assessment of hematologic indices (i.e., hemoglobin, hematocrit, red blood cell count, white blood cell count, and platelets) will afford early detection and possible prevention of these adverse events.

Some NSAIDs, especially indomethacin, have been associated with altered mental status. Dizziness, tinnitus, headache, vertigo, nervousness, excitation, somnolence, fatigue, confusion, depression, emotional lability, psychiatric disturbances, and syncope may result from NSAID use, particularly in the elderly. Dosage reduction is indicated to ameliorate these signs and symptoms. Confusion, agitation, and/or seizures may represent serious salicylate intoxication in the elderly. Since acid-based disturbances (i.e., respiratory alkalosis followed by metabolic acidosis) often accompany salicylate toxicity, a wide anion gap is generally diagnostic. However, serum salicylate levels should be determined to confirm the diagnosis. Elevated liver function test results have been reported rarely in association with NSAID use and are an indication for discontinuation of therapy (27).

The potential for fetal adverse effects is not clearly defined. The risks of prolonged maternal labor, perinatal mortality, and teratogenicity have not yet been established. Therefore, conservative approaches are recommended, and avoidance of these agents during pregnancy is ideal (45). Although most NSAIDs are excreted in breast milk, toxicology data for nursing infants is not conclusive, and these agents are not recommended in lactating females.

DRUG INTERACTIONS

Although numerous drug interactions involving the NSAIDs have been reported, few are clinically important. Drug interactions of importance are those involving anticoagulants, sulfonylureas, corticosteroids, and uricosuric agents. Because NSAIDs are highly protein-bound, other highly protein-bound drugs, including warfarin, tolbutamide, and phenytoin, may be displaced. As a result, hypoprothrombinemia, hypoglycemia, and other toxicities may develop. GI toxicity may be compounded in combining NSAIDs with corticosteroid therapy because of additive cytotoxic effects. Finally, the uricosuric effects of NSAIDs, probenecid, and sulfinpyrazone are antagonistic when these drugs are used concomitantly.

STEROIDS

Systemic corticosteroids are not indicated for the treatment of OA. Intraarticular administration of corticosteroids, however, appears to be beneficial for the temporary relief of pain and inflammation, while improving joint mobility. Like the NSAIDs, the mechanism of action of steroids is not clearly defined. It is thought that the inhibition of polymorphonuclear leukocyte (inflammatory cell) migration and extravasation along with reduction of vascular permeability results in diminished inflammatory response and secondary pain prevention (46).

Corticosteroids that are available for intraarticular administration include hydrocortisone, betamethasone, methylprednisolone, triamcinolone, and dexamethasone (Table 31.4). Administration is performed with the use of a local anesthetic, usually 1 to 2% lidocaine. Aseptic technique is recommended. Dosages vary with the degree of inflammation and the size and location of the affected joint. Beneficial effects usually occur within 24 hr after an injection, reach a maximum in 1 week and last for 2 to 4 weeks, when the suspension formulations are used. Activity should be limited for 48 hr following injection to avoid exacerbating joint destruction from overuse of the pain-free joint (46).

Long-term use of intraarticular corticosteroids is still controversial because of the potential for serious adverse

Table 31.4.
Corticosteroids Available for Intraarticular Injection

Corticosteroid	Formulation	Dosage Range[a]
Betamethasone sodium Phosphate/acetate	Suspension	1.5–12 mg
Dexamethasone acetate	Suspension	4.0–16 mg
Dexamethasone sodium phosphate	Solution	1.0–4.0 mg
Hydrocortisone acetate	Suspension	10–50 mg
Methylprednisolone acetate	Suspension	4.0–80 mg
Prednisolone acetate	Suspension	2.0–30 mg
Prednisolone tebutate	Suspension	4.0–40 mg
Prednisolone sodium phosphate	Solution	2.0–30 mg
Triamcinolone acetonide	Suspension	2.5–40 mg
Triamcinolone hexacetonide	Suspension	2.0–20 mg
	Suspension	2.0–20 mg

[a]Dosages may vary, depending on the size and location of the affected joint and the degree of inflammation.

effects, including arthropathy, infection, postinjection flare, and tendon rupture. Steroid arthropathy is a condition of accelerated degeneration of articular cartilage, subchondral bone, and surrounding ligaments caused by repeated corticosteroid injections (47). Originally thought to result from overuse of an abnormal joint, steroid arthropathy has been shown to result from a specific effect of the steroids on the metabolism of articular cartilage (46, 47). Since the progression of destruction is proportional to the number of injections administered, conservative use is recommended, and administration should be no more frequent than every 4 to 6 weeks.

Joint infection secondary to intraarticular steroid therapy occurs rarely (<1%) and is usually caused by *Staphylococcus aureus*. Complications due to this infection can be devastating, so early diagnosis and treatment are critical. Immunocompromised individuals, including those taking systemic corticosteroids, are at an increased risk for joint infection and should be closely monitored. Joint aspiration should be performed to differentiate between infection and postinjection flare, a self-limited synovitis caused by deposition of steroid crystals in the joint cavity. Joint infection should be suspected if inflammation persists for 72 hr, even if cultures are negative.

Ruptured tendons may also occur with the use of intraarticular steroids, not only as a result of direct injury during administration, but also as a consequence of overactivity. Several investigators have reported reduced tendon tensile strength and slowed repair processes after repeated intraarticular injections for prolonged periods. Overuse of a pain-free joint can intensify the strain on weakened tendons and result in ruptures.

CHONDROPROTECTIVE AGENTS

In the OA process, a reduced concentration of proteoglycans due to depolymerization of their glycosaminoglycan precursors and decreased synthesis of fully functional proteoglycans has led to the investigation of agents that may boost precursor pools exogenously. Extensive research has produced several agents that appear to be "chondroprotective," in that they can be used as substrate for synthesis of proteoglycans by the chondrocyte and may also retard further progression of cartilage breakdown. These agents, glycosaminoglycan-peptide complex (GP-C, Rumalon), glycosaminoglycan polysuflate (GAGPS, Arteparon), and galactosaminoglycuronoglycan sulfate (GAGGS, Matrix), which are not yet available in the United States, are isolated from bovine lung, tracheal cartilage, and bone marrow.

Long-term studies with GP-C, GAGPS, and GAGGS in Europe have demonstrated significant improvement in OA symptoms, joint status, joint function, quality of life, and ability to work in afflicted patients (48). Surgical interventions and use of NSAIDs were significantly decreased in patients who were treated with GP-C, GAGPS, and GAGGS compared with controls (48). Reports of heparin-related anticoagulant effects associated with GAGPS preclude the use of this agent in patients with coagulopathies, those with a history of gastrointestinal ulcers, or those receiving anticoagulant therapy. Caution is advised in using this agent in elderly patients. Otherwise, adverse effects and contraindications appear to be minimal with GP-C, GAGPS, and GAGGS. These drugs are administered intramuscularly twice weekly at 2- to 6-month intervals. GAGPS may also be administered intraarticularly or periarticularly. GAGGS may be given orally.

Although the exact mechanism of action is unknown, most beneficial effects are believed to result from inhibition of the catabolic and lysosomal enzymes (collagenases, metalloproteinases) that are responsible for structural damage in OA (48, 49). The chondroprotective agents also purportedly stimulate reparative processes in injured articular cartilage (48, 49). Whatever the mechanism, numerous investigations have demonstrated GP-C and GAGPS to be effective in the treatment of OA. These agents may herald a major breakthrough in the therapy of OA. Delineation of the biochemical mechanisms of action and efficacy will be the primary focus of further research with these agents.

Intraarticular injections of orgotein (superoxide dismutase) are also being investigated for the treatment of OA. This novel antiinflammatory agent, isolated from bovine liver, purportedly eliminates the generation of superoxide free radicals and stabilizes the membranes of inflammatory cells (50). Oxygen free radicals are responsible for direct degradation of collagen and proteoglycans. Although orgotein has no central or peripheral analgesic properties, inhibition of inflammatory mediators may reduce or prevent the pain associated with OA. Dosing, dosage intervals, and place in therapy have not been established for this agent.

SURGERY

Surgical intervention may provide the most immediate improvement in patients with OA. Arthroscopic procedures focus on joint debridement to prevent further destruction of joint surfaces and stimulate repair by the remaining healthy tissue. Although osteotomies are rarely performed now, total or partial prosthetic joint replacement remains a treatment option for patients with advanced OA. However, surgery can be very costly and carries the risk of morbidity and mortality, which may not be acceptable in some patients, especially the elderly. Unfortunately, risks and costs are additive in patients with multiple joint disease, and surgery is not always curative. Surgical treatment of OA is generally reserved for patients with severe, debilitating disease for whom the potential benefits outweigh the potential risks.

CONCLUSION

Osteoarthritis is a painful, progressive condition that may cause significant disability and compromised quality of life. Recent therapeutic advances have resulted from progress in understanding the etiology and pathogenesis of OA. Pharmacologic therapy has been aimed primarily at relief of pain and inflammation associated with advanced disease; however, it is now being carefully scrutinized for efficacy and possible deleterious effects to osteoarthritic joints. New developments have revitalized interest in the reversibility of disease progression. Future research will be directed toward the identification of risk factors and specific markers of cartilage destruction in the hope of arresting progression before it is too late and assessing the role of inflammation in the disease process and clinical presentation. Eliciting mechanisms of interleukin-1 regulation, delineating the role of extraarticular structures in the disease process, and stimulating subchondral bone reparative antibody technology and cartilage growth and transformation factors will also play a prominent role in future investigations. If disease progression cannot be altered, the area of cartilage autotransplantation remains an option to be explored.

REFERENCES

1. Howell DS, Altman RD, Brown HE, Gorrlieb NL. A comprehensive regimen for osteoarthritis. Med Clin North Am 55(2):457–69, 1971.
2. Tsang IK. Update on osteoarthritis. Can Fam Physician 6:539–41, 614, 1990.
3. Hamerman D. Current leads in research on the osteoarthritic joint. J Am Geriatr Soc 31:299–304, 1983.
4. Yelin E. Impact of musculoskeletal conditions on the elderly. Geriatr Med Today 8(3):103–18, 1989.
5. Swedberg JA, Steinbauer JR. Osteoarthritis. Am Fam Physician 45(2):557–68, 1992.
6. Lawrence JS. Generalized osteoarthritis in a population sample. Am J Epidemiol 90:381–89, 1969.
7. Bland JH, Cooper SM. Osteoarthritis: a review of the cell biology involved and evidence for reversibility: management rationally

related to known genesis and pathophysiology. Semin Arthritis Rheum 14(2):106–33, 1984.

8. Hartz AJ, Fischer ME, Bril G, Kelber S, Rupley D, Oken B, Rimm AA. The association of obesity with joint pain and osteoarthritis in the HANES data. J Chronic Dis 39:311–19, 1986.

9. Bejelle A. Epidemiological aspects of osteoarthritis. Scand J Rheumatol 43(Suppl):35–48, 1981.

10. Kuettner K, Thonar EJMA, Aydelotte MB. Modern aspects of articular cartilage biochemistry. Verh Dtsch Ges Inn Med 95:436–74, 1989.

11. Puranen J, Ala-Ketola L, Peltokallio J. Running and primary osteoarthrosis of the hip. Br Med J 2:242–45, 1975.

12. Schuomacher HR. Primer on rheumatic diseases, 9th ed. Atlanta: National Arthritis Foundation 1988:171–77.

13. Ehrlich GE. Osteoarthritis beginning with inflammation. JAMA 232(2):157–59, 1975.

14. Johnson L. Kinetics of osteoarthritis. Lab Invest 8(6):1223–41, 1959.

15. Altman RD, Kapila P. Dean DD, Howell DS. Future therapeutic trends in osteoarthritis. Scand J Rheumatol 77 (suppl):37–42, 1989.

16. Mankin H. The response of articular cartilage to mechanical injury. J Bone Joint Surg (Am) 64:460–66, 1982.

17. Schumacher R. The role of inflammation and crystals in the pain of osteoarthritis. Semin Arthritis Rheum 18(suppl 2):81–5, 1989.

18. Redler I, Zimny ML. Scanning electron microscopy of normal and abnormal articular cartilage and synovium. J Bone Joint Surg (Am) 52:1395–1404, 1970.

19. McDevitt CA, Gilbertson EMM, Muir H. An experimental model of osteoarthrosis: early morphological and biochemical changes. J Bone Joint Surg (Br) 59:24–35, 1977.

20. Pujol JP, Loyau G. Interleukin-1 and osteoarthritis. Life Sci 41:1187–98, 1987.

21. Bjelle A. The management of degenerative joint disease. Scand J Rheumatol 42 (suppl):7–67, 1987.

22. Radin EL, Paul IL, Rose RM. Role of mechanical factors in the pathogenesis of primary osteoarthritis. Lancet 1:519–21, 1972.

23. Merritt JL. Soft tissue mechanisms of pain in osteoarthritis. Semin Arthritis Rheum 18(suppl 2):51–6, 1989.

24. Bienstock H, Fernando KR. Arthritis in the elderly: an overview. Med Clin North Am 60:1173–89, 1976.

25. Blechman W. Managing the older arthritic. Geriatrics 39:131–32, 1984.

26. Gross M. Psychosocial aspects of osteoarthritis: helping patients cope. Aging 13:40–3, 1983.

27. Covington TR, Mallow LP, Hendersen RP, Stevenson JG. Degenerative joint disease. Consult Pharm 2:404–12, 1987.

28. Ehrlich GE. Future directions in therapy of pain in osteoarthritis. Semin Arthritis Rheum 18(suppl 2):100–04, 1989.

29. Sirca A, Susec-Michieli M. Selective type II fibre muscular atrophy in patients with osteoarthritis of the hip. J Neurol Sci 44:149–59, 1980.

30. Bradley JD, Brandt KD, Katz BP, Kalasinski LA, Ryan SI. Comparison of an anti-inflammatory dose of ibuprofen, an analgesic dose of ibuprofen, and acetaminophen in the treatment of patients with osteoarthritis of the knee. New Engl J Med 325:87–91, 1991.

31. Trang LE. Prostaglandins and inflammation. Semin Arthritis Rheum 9(3):153–90, 1980.

32. Hart FD, Huskisson EC. Nonsteroidal anti-inflammatory drugs: current status and rational therapeutic use. Drugs 27:232–55, 1984.

33. Newsman NM, Ling RAM. Acetabular bone destruction related to non-steroidal anti-inflammatory drugs. Lancet 2:11–4, 1985.

34. Raced S, Revell P, Hemingway A, Low F, Rainsford K, Walker F. Effect of nonsteroidal anti-inflammatory drugs on the course of osteoarthritis. Lancet 2:519–22, 1989.

35. Furst DE. Comments on possible long-term consequences of non-steroidal anti-inflammatory use. J Clin Pharmacol 28:550–53, 1988.

36. Calin A. Clinical aspects of the effect of NSAID on cartilage. J Rheumatol 16 (suppl 18):43–4, 1989.

37. Seifert CF, Stanaszek WF. Arthritis in the elderly: update 1990. J Geriatr Drug Ther 4(4):7–41, 1990.

38. Soll AH. Mechanisms by which nonsteroidal anti-inflammatory drugs damage the mucosa. In: Soll AH (moderator). Non-steroidal anti-inflammatory drugs and peptic ulcer disease. Ann Intern Med 114:307–19, 1991.

39. Lanza FL. Endoscopic studies of gastric and duodenal injury after use of ibuprofen, aspirin and other nonsteroidal anti-inflammatory agents. Am J Med 77:19–24, 1984.

40. Griffin MR, Piper JM, Daugherty JR. Snowden M, Ray WA. Non-steroidal anti-inflammatory drug use and increased risk for peptic ulcer disease in elderly persons. Ann Intern Med 114:257–63, 1991.

41. Elliott DP. Preventing upper gastrointestinal bleeding in patients receiving nonsteroidal antiinflammatory drugs. Drug Intell Clin Pharm 24:954–58, 1990.

42. Graham DY, Agrawal NM, Roth SH. Prevention of NSAID-induced gastric ulcer with misoprostil: multicentre, double-blind, placebo-controlled trial. Lancet 12:1277–80, 1988.

43. Clive DM, Stoff JS. Renal syndromes associated with nonsteroidal antiinflammatory drugs. N Engl J Med 310:563–72, 1984.

44. Bunnign RD, Barth WF. Sulindac: a potentially renal-sparing non-steroidal anti-inflammatory drug. JAMA 248:2864–67, 1982.

45. Martinez EM, Lopez JR. Use of analgesics during pregnancy. Drug Intell Clin Pharm 20:850–51, 1986.

46. Stefanich RJ. Intraarticular corticosteroids in treatment of osteoarthritis. Orthop Rev 15(2):27–33, 1986.

47. Chandler GN, Jones DT, Wright V, Hartford SJ. Charcot's arthropathy following intraarticular hydrocortisone. Br Med J 1:952, 1959.

48. Rejholec V. Long-term studies of antiosteoarthritic drugs: an assessment. Semin Arthritis Rheum 17 (suppl 1):35–53, 1987.

49. Burkhardt D, Ghosh P. Laboratory evaluation of antiarthritic drugs as potential chondroprotective agents. Semin Arthritis Rheum 17 (suppl 1):3–34, 1987.

50. McIlwain H. Silverfield JC, Cheatum DE, Poiley J, Taborn J, Ignaczak T, Multz CV. Intraarticular orgotein in osteoarthritis of the knee: a placebo-controlled efficacy, safety, and dosage comparison. Am J Med 87:295–300, 1989.

CHAPTER 32

GOUT AND HYPERURICEMIA

PIERRE A. MALOLEY and MARK S. SHAEFER

Gout is a chronic metabolic disease, most commonly afflicting males over 30 years of age. It was recognized as a human malady and treated before the ancient Greeks ruled the Mediterranean world. Gout was associated with wealthy intellectuals who were known to overindulge in food and drink. Despite this long history, no specific cause was identified until 1848, when Sir Alfred Garrod identified uric acid as the cause of gout. One of the major therapeutic advances of the 19th century was the use of colchicine to treat the symptoms of the disease. As the role of purines in the disease process was discovered, specific dietary recommendations were also made for patients with gout. Treatment improved in the 20th century with the development of new drugs. Acute attacks were treated with colchicine and later with indomethacin or phenylbutazone. The use of uricosuric agents closely followed these advances, and since 1965, allopurinol has also been used for the long-term management of gout.

Uric acid is an end product of protein catabolism. In humans it is the final product resulting from the breakdown of purines. DNA and RNA are degraded, yielding the nucleosides adenosine and guanosine. The enzyme xanthine oxidase (XO) converts guanosine directly to xanthine and converts adenosine first to hypoxanthine then to xanthine; finally, xanthine is converted into uric acid. At a physiologic pH of 7.4 the monovalent form of uric acid is the predominant form (1).

Total body content of uric acid ranges from 1.0 to 1.2 g in a normal man, with a daily turnover rate of 600 to 800 mg. These values are slightly lower for women. In a normal person this turnover constitutes 50 to 60% of the urate pool each day. Almost 70% of the uric acid is excreted in the urine; the remainder is secreted into the gastrointestinal (GI) tract by a passive process and is degraded by intestinal microorganisms to ammonia and carbon dioxide (2, 3).

A four-component hypothesis for urate handling by the kidney best explains the actions of drugs to increase or decrease uric acid levels. These four components are filtration, reabsorption, secretion, and postsecretory reabsorption, either in the later part of the proximal tubule, in the distal tubule, or in both. Approximately 95% of the serum uric acid is filtered freely across the glomerulus. The other 5% of plasma urate is protein-bound. Ninety-eight percent to 100% of this filtered urate is reabsorbed in the early part of the proximal tubule. A variable percentage of the filtered load is secreted back into the tubular lumen in

a more distal part of the proximal tubule. The fourth component may occur in the distal part of the proximal tubule, in the distal tubule, or in both (2).

Hyperuricemia is defined as a urate level greater than 480 μmol/L (8.0 mg/dL) in men and 420 μmol/L (7.0 mg/dL) in women. These values are more than two standard deviations above the mean population values. The lower value for females is because of an estrogen-dependent sex difference. This difference, which manifests at puberty and is related to greater urate clearance, diminishes or disappears after menopause (4).

Two laboratory methods are used to measure serum urate concentrations. The colorimetric method is used by most autoanalyzers. It is nonspecific, and false elevations can occur from amino acids in the test sample, uremia, high doses of vitamin C, and other xanthines such as caffeine, theobromine, and theophylline, as well as levodopa.

The uricase method is more specific and yields levels that are lower by 24 to 60 μmol/L (0.4 to 1.0 mg/dL) than the colorimetric values. The clinician must know which method is used to analyze uric acid serum levels. The definitions of hyperuricemia given in the text above are based on colorimetric determinations (1).

ETIOLOGY

Hyperuricemia and gout are traditionally classified as either primary or secondary. Primary gout refers to cases in which the basic metabolic defect is unknown, or if it is known, the main manifestation is that of hyperuricemia and gout. Secondary gout refers to those cases in which hyperuricemia is part of some other acquired disorder or in which the basic metabolic defect underlying the hyperuricemia is known but the main clinical characteristics are not those of gout. The distinctions may not always be clear (2).

Patients with primary hyperuricemia and gout have elevated serum uric acid levels that are caused by either an increased production of uric acid, an impaired clearance of uric acid, or a combination of both. Ten to twenty percent of patients with primary gout and hyperuricemia are overproducers of uric acid. Overproducers of uric acid can be identified with a 24-hr urinary uric acid excretion test. Patients who overproduce uric acid generally have a miscible urate pool that is more than two to three times normal. On a diet that is essentially free of purine-containing foods for more than 5 days, normal men excrete

975 to 3497 mmol (164 to 588 mg) of uric acid per day (5). Patients who excrete more than 3569 mmol (600 mg) of uric acid in 24 hr on a purine-restricted diet or more than 4758 to 5948 mmol (800 mg to 1 g) of uric acid on a normal diet can be classified as overproducers (3). Another method for quantitative analysis of uric acid production involves the use of a spot urine specimen. This method expresses uric acid in terms of excretion per deciliter of glomerular filtrate. With this method a value of 0.4 mg of urinary uric acid/dL (20 μmol/L) of glomerular filtrate is considered normal. Patients who are overproducers have values above 0.7 mg/dL (42 μmol/L) (6).

Primary hyperuricemia and gout may also (rarely) result from one of two identified enzymatic defects. Patients who lack hypoxanthine guanine phosphoribosyl-transferase (HGPRT) activity show one of two phenotypes. Complete HGPRT deficiencies present as the Lesch-Nyhan syndrome. This syndrome is associated with hyperuricemia, hyperuricaciduria, renal calculi, and a neurologic disorder characterized by self-mutilation, mental retardation, choreoathetosis, and spasticity. Patients with partial deficiency may have only gouty arthritis, hyperuricemia, hyperuricosuria, and renal calculi in the second or third decade of life. Patients with phosphoribosyl-1-pyrophosphate (PRPP) synthetase variants have increased de novo purine production. These patients may have gouty arthritis in their teens or early twenties (7).

Secondary hyperuricemia is associated with increased nucleic acid turnover, decreased renal function, increased purine production, or drug-induced decreased elimination of uric acid. A deficiency of glucose-6-phosphatase can also lead to hyperuricemia from infancy. This results from increased purine biosynthesis as well as decreased uric acid clearance from hyperlactacidemia (7).

Drug-induced hyperuricemia is the most common of the secondary hyperuricemias. Of the drugs that are responsible, diuretics are the most frequently implicated. The mechanism of diuretic-induced hyperuricemia is not clear, but it may relate to an increased reabsorption of uric acid in the proximal tubule. Another possible explanation is a decreased tubular secretion or an increased postsecretory reabsorption of uric acid. Spironolactone is the only diuretic that does not cause hyperuricemia.

Aspirin can cause increased serum urate concentrations when it is ingested in doses of less than 2 g/day. Doses of more than 2 g cause a uricosuric effect. Low doses preferentially inhibit tubular secretion, and high doses inhibit reabsorption of uric acid.

Pyrazinamide inhibits urate secretion. It markedly decreases urinary excretion of urate even when there are high levels of filtered urate. Another antitubercular drug, ethambutol, is also associated with decreased renal clearance of uric acid. Other drugs that are known to increase serum levels of uric acid include nicotinic acid, ethanol, cyclosporine, methoxyflurane, levodopa, and epinephrine (2, 8).

Hyperuricemia may be associated with any disorder that causes an increase in the rate of proliferation of cells. This leads to an increase in purine production and an elevation of the urate pool. Hyperuricemia occurs with lymphoid and myeloid proliferative disorders and may also occur with diseases such as psoriasis and dissemination of solid tumors.

Hyperuricemia occurs in up to half of patients with chronic myelogenous leukemia. Patients with chronic lymphocytic leukemia rarely present with hyperuricemia. Hyperuricemia often occurs in myeloid metaplasia and polycythemia vera. Patients with sickle cell anemia, hemolytic anemia with secondary erythrocytosis, and thalassemia may have hyperuricemia, even though it is uncommon in primary red blood cell disorders (2).

Chronic lead ingestion leading to nephropathy is associated with gout and hyperuricemia. Lead presumably causes a defect in the tubular secretion of urate as well as inhibiting guanase, the enzyme that deaminates guanine to xanthine. In these cases of saturnine gout, uric acid clearance is reduced markedly, even though creatinine clearance may be only slightly decreased (2).

Patients who fast for 1 or 2 days have increased levels of serum urate. In most cases these elevations in urate levels result from a decreased urinary output of uric acid because urate excretion is inhibited by elevated ketone levels. Doses of alcohol of 112 to 135 g given with food are associated with an important increase in blood lactate concentration, decreased urinary uric acid output, and overproduction of uric acid. The combination of fasting and ethyl alcohol may have an additive effect on uric acid retention (9).

Hyperuricemia may also result from other causes of increased ketoacids and lactic acid, such as exercise and uncontrolled diabetes. Additionally, hypothyroidism, hyperparathyroidism, and hypoparathyroidism have all been associated with hyperuricemia, presumably because of a reduction in the renal excretion of urate (3).

EPIDEMIOLOGY

Many studies have related gout to racial, geographic, dietary, and other socioeconomic factors. The one consistent marker is the relationship between elevated uric acid levels and gout. The epidemiology of gout was studied as a part of the Heart Disease Epidemiology Study at Framingham, Massachusetts. This study involved a total of 5127 subjects who were of age 30 through 59 on initial evaluation. Thirteen subjects, 0.2% of the total population, had experienced a gouty attack before entry in the study. The mean age of the population at the beginning of the study was 44 years. Fourteen years later, when the mean age of the population was 58, 1.5% of the population (76 subjects) had experienced an attack of gout. Gout had occurred in 2.8% of the men and 0.4% of the women. The prevalence of gouty arthritis was found to increase with increasing uric acid levels. In men with uric acid levels under 360 μmol/L (6 mg/dL), the frequency of gout was 0.6%. The rate progressed to 1.9% with levels of 360 to 410 μmol/L (6 to 6.9 mg/dL); and when levels exceeded 530 μmol/L (9 mg/dL), 90% of the men had gout. The frequency of gout for all men with uric acid levels above 420 μmol/L (7 mg/dL) was 20% (10).

PATHOGENESIS

A combination of factors is most likely responsible for the formation of urate crystals in patients with gout. The degree of hyperuricemia, the location of the joint, abrupt changes (increases or decreases) in serum uric acid levels, the physical state of the joint, resolution of joint effusions, the presence of certain protein polysaccharides, and the temperature of the joint are all involved in urate crystal formation.

Acute attacks of gout develop when monosodium urate crystals deposit in the synovium of joints involved. These crystals are derived from either preformed synovial deposits or de novo synthesis. Characteristically, acute attacks affect the peripheral joints; the most distal joints are more likely to be affected early in the course of a patient's gouty arthritis. A possible explanation for this involves the temperature of the joints, since monosodium urate solubility varies directly with temperature. The solubility of urate in physiologic saline is 400 μmol/L (6.8 mg/dL) at 37°C but only 270 μmol/L (4.5 mg/dL) at 30°C. Joint temperatures decrease distally. The average temperature of the knee is 33°C, and that of the ankle is 29°C. However, this factor alone cannot explain why gout develops in some people and not in others who have similar uric acid levels. Also involved may be the increased solubility of urate in proteoglycans, chondroitin sulfate, and hyaluronic acid, which are all abundant in the synovial fluid and cartilage. Urate solubility may be affected by genetic or environmental alterations in these substances that predispose to, or even initiate, attacks of gout (2).

Another explanation was proposed by Simkin, who was concerned with the predisposition of gout in the first metatarsophalangeal joint. Gout in this joint is referred to as podagra, and more than 50% of first attacks of gout occur in this joint. Ultimately, most patients with gout experience podagra. The base of the big toe is subjected to extreme forces in the normal process of walking. Shoes compound the problem by forcing the joint to endure these forces in an unnatural position. The joint that has experienced degenerative changes or recent trauma, including trauma that may have been unnoticed, is likely to be the site of a synovial effusion. At night while the patient sleeps, the effusion resolves. Water leaves the joint faster than urate

does; the result is a transiently high intraarticular urate concentration that favors crystal formation. This explains the common nocturnal onset of gout in the big toe and may help to explain the occasional attack of gout that develops in a person with a normal urate serum concentration (11).

Urate crystals in the synovial fluid or surrounding tissues and the reaction of the body's defense mechanisms to these crystals cause the typical gouty attack. This reaction begins within 4 to 8 hr of the presence of these crystals in the synovial fluid. Many factors are involved in this acute inflammatory response. Monosodium urate (MSU) crystals have sharp irregular crystal facets with multiple outward projections. These surface irregularities favor the absorption of immunoglobulin G and other polypeptides. Adsorption of these polypeptides increases crystal phagocytosis by polymorphonuclear leukocytes (PMNs). In addition, MSU crystals are electronegative and therefore bind, denature, and cleave Hageman factor (clotting factor XII). This activates the clotting, kininogen, plasminogen, and complement cascades. Prostaglandins play a role in the inflammatory response of gout, causing vasodilation, increased vascular permeability, and release of chemotactic substances that attract PMNs. Although the extent of involvement of these other factors is unclear, the role of PMNs is well established (2).

Synovial fluid from patients with gout has an average leukocyte count of 19.5×10^9/L (19,500 cells/mm^3), 90% or more of which are neutrophils. PMNs, monocytes, and synovial cells phagocytize MSU crystals that are coated with protein. This causes a fusion of lysosomes with a phagosome, producing a phagolysosome that contains enzymes. The protein coat on the crystal is digested by the enzymes, allowing hydrogen bond-mediated membranolysis to occur. Cellular autolysis results when the phagolysosome is lysed and hydrolytic enzymes are released into the cytoplasm. This also leads to increased permeability of the outer membrane of the cell and a subsequent release of enzymes into the extracellular medium. Urate crystals are digested by peroxidases in phagocytic cells, which can also adsorb leukocyte-derived proteins that may terminate the stimulus for further phagocytosis. This series of events causes the clinical findings that mark the beginning and the resolution of an acute attack of gout (12).

DIAGNOSIS AND CLINICAL FINDINGS

Acute attacks of gout are most often characterized by the sudden onset of unbearable pain in one joint of the lower extremities. The first attack is not associated with other symptoms and is usually monoarticular, although polyarticular involvement in a first attack occurs in about 10% of cases. The attack lasts a variable but limited period of time and is followed by a completely asymptomatic period. Over time the periods between attacks become shorter, and the symptoms of the attack fail to resolve completely. This leads to chronic crippling arthritis. The peak age of onset of gout is between 30 and 50 years in men. When women develop gout, it is almost always after menopause. Gout in patients of either sex before the age of 30 should lead to an investigation for possible enzyme defects, purine overproduction, or renal disease. Gout rarely affects patients this young.

Other commonly affected joints, in order of frequency of involvement, are the instep, ankle, heel, knee, wrist, finger, and elbow. Although acute gout initially is predominantly a disease of the joints of the lower extremities, later in the course any joint may be involved. Rare sites of involvement are the shoulder, hip, spine, sacroiliac, sternoclavicular, and temporomandibular joints (11, 13).

Patients may report several trivial episodes of pain in the big toe or ankle before the first attack of gout. Most patients have their initial attack during periods of good health. Attacks commonly occur while the patient is sleeping; many patients are awakened by excruciating pain. Occasionally, patients first detect the symptoms as their feet touch the cold floor when they get up in the morning. Three or four hours after the onset of an attack, the skin over the affected joint becomes red, hot, swollen, and exquisitely painful and tender. Inflammation is slight at first but progresses and can resemble a bacterial cellulitis. The systemic signs of the attack include fever, leukocytosis, and elevation of the erythrocyte sedimentation rate (4, 7). Systemic signs are more likely in patients with polyarticular involvement. Temperatures may reach values as high as 39.4°C. In one study, neither fever nor leukocytosis correlated with the number of joints involved (13). Untreated attacks of gout may last for hours to several weeks. As the patient recovers, the skin over the affected joint often desquamates. Even though an attack may have been severe, with marked swelling and incapacitation, recovery is generally complete with the first attack. Patients return to their preattack state of health until the next attack (7).

The periods between attacks, called intercritical periods, vary in length. Although a rare patient may never experience a reoccurrence, most patients experience a second attack within 6 months to 2 years. As the disease progresses, the intercritical periods become shorter and the attacks become polyarticular, more severe, and longer-lasting. Eventually, patients enter a phase of chronic gout without pain-free intercritical periods.

Modern treatment of gout with allopurinol and uricosurics has all but eliminated the occurrence of chronic tophaceous gout. Before these agents became available, 50 to 70% of patients with gout developed the chronic tophaceous form. It now affects approximately 3% of patients. Tophaceous gout is a consequence of consistently elevated levels of uric acid, and it correlates directly with the levels of urate. In one series the mean serum

urate concentration was 540 μmol/L (9.1 mg/dL) (uricase method) in 722 nontophaceous patients, 590 to 650 μmol/L (10 to 11 mg/dL) in 456 patients with minimal-to-moderate tophaceous deposits, and above 650 μmol/L (11.0 mg/dL) in 111 patients with extensive tophaceous deposits. Tophi are usually firm and movable with thin and reddened overlying skin. They are commonly found on the helix or antihelix of the ear; the finger, hand, knee, foot, or toe; the ulnar surface of the forearm; the olecranon bursa; or the Achilles tendon. The thin skin overlying the tophi may break down and extrude a milky white substance composed mainly of urate crystals. Infection by skin flora may develop in these areas and will heal slowly. Eventually, these deposits lead to the destruction of the articular cartilage and portions of the subchondral bone (7, 14, 15).

Renal involvement in gout is the most serious, and second most common, clinical manifestation. Two forms of renal disease are possible: urate nephropathy or uric acid nephropathy. Urate nephropathy results from the deposition of MSU salt crystals in the renal interstitium and the accompanying inflammation. This progresses slowly but is not thought to decrease life expectancy. It is not known whether the urate deposits cause a deterioration in renal function. Uric acid nephropathy results from the deposition of uric acid crystals in the collecting tubules. Acute renal failure occurs in patients who overproduce and overexcrete uric acid as a result of aggressive chemotherapy, lymphoma, leukemia, or enzymatic defects. This renal failure correlates not with the serum urate concentration but with the amount of uric acid excreted. Before the advent of hemodialysis, renal failure accounted for 17 to 25% of deaths in the gouty population. Kidney damage in gout usually occurs when there is diabetes, hypertension, renal vascular disease, glomerulonephritis, pyelonephritis, renal calculi with urinary tract infection, congenital nephropathy, or some other cause of primary nephropathy that is not directed from gout. It is currently accepted that asymptomatic hyperuricemia does not result in renal destruction until uric acid levels exceed 650 μmol/L (11 mg/dL) for prolonged periods (16–18).

Many criteria have been developed for establishing the diagnosis of gout. A diagnosis of gout must be firmly established before the institution of expensive and potentially toxic therapy. Gout should be considered in a patient with an acute onset of monoarticular or asymmetric polyarticular arthritis of the distal extremities. The diagnosis of acute gouty arthritis may be established by the demonstration of MSU crystals in white cells of synovial fluid or a tophus. The synovial fluid in gouty patients is cloudy and less viscous than normal. Leukocyte counts average 13.5×10^9/L (13,500 cells/mm^3) (range 1.0 to 70.0×10^9/L (1000 to 70,000 cells/mm^3)), with a predominance of PMNs. Total protein is normal, as is the glucose

Table 32.1.
Criteria for Diagnosis of Acute Gout[a]

Definite
   Demonstration of sodium urate crystals in affected joint
Suggestive[b]
  1. More than one attack of arthritis
  2. Development of maximum inflammation within 1 day
  3. Oligoarthritis attack
  4. Redness over joint
  5. Painful or swollen first metatarsophalangeal joint
  6. Unilateral attack on first metatarsophalangeal joint
  7. Unilateral attack on tarsal joint
  8. Tophus
  9. Hyperuricemia
10. Asymptomatic swelling within a joint

[a]Criteria established by the American Rheumatism Association.
[b]A minimum of six criteria should be present to be suggestive of gout.

concentration. The Gram stain and culture of the aspirate should be negative. Needle-shaped crystals 2 to 10 μm long are present. When viewed with a polarized light microscope with a first-order red decompensator, the crystals are negatively birefringent. Urate crystals may not be found in patients with gout, because of the difficulty in aspiration of fluid from involved joints. Acutely inflamed joints have intracellular urate crystals in 85% of patients with gout. A probable diagnosis of gout may be established by using criteria established by the American Rheumatism Association (Table 32.1). In addition to these criteria, complete resolution of synovitis with colchicine treatment may suggest the diagnosis. The clinical findings of pseudogout, acute sarcoidosis, psoriatic arthritis, and acute calcific tendonitis may mimic those of gout. Pseudogout and sarcoidosis may even respond to a trial of colchicine therapy, especially if it is given intravenously. If uric acid levels are normalized in a patient for a prolonged period without resolution of joint symptoms, another diagnosis should be sought (4, 7, 19).

Assessment of the gouty patient should begin with a detailed history and physical examination. A family history may demonstrate a predisposition for gout, and all medications should be checked for their potential to induce hyperuricemia. It is also important to classify the hyperuricemia as a problem with overproduction or underexcretion or possibly both. A 24-hr urine collection should be obtained to measure urine uric acid and creatinine. At the same time, samples for serum creatinine and blood urea nitrogen levels should be obtained, as a measure of kidney function. Uric acid excretion above 3569 mmol (600 mg) in 24 hr in a patient on a low-purine diet for 4 to 5 days should be considered abnormal. In the absence of a purine-free diet, excretion of more than 5948 mmol (1000 mg) per 24 hr is diagnostic of overproduction. Hyperuricemia with a normal 24-hr excretion indicates underexcretion (19).

TREATMENT

Treatment of gout and hyperuricemia has a two-step approach. The first step is to terminate the acute attack and resolve the pain. Once the acute attack is resolved, the goal is to gradually reduce the serum uric acid concentration. Antiinflammatory agents that are useful for acute attacks include colchicine and nonsteroidal antiinflammatory drugs (NSAIDs). Serum uric acid levels should not be reduced until the acute attack has been terminated. The process of lowering uric acid levels should proceed slowly and cautiously, because rapid lowering of uric acid levels may precipitate another acute attack. In some mild cases, patients may be able to control the hyperuricemia by diet modifications and weight reduction. Agents that are available to decrease uric acid levels include the xanthine oxidase inhibitor, allopurinol, and the uricosuric drugs probenecid and sulfinpyrazone. Hypouricemic therapy is used to decrease the body stores of urate in an attempt to prevent or reverse the complications due to deposition of urate.

Acute Gouty Arthritis

The treatment of acute gout is directed at alleviating the pain rapidly and attempting to restore joint mobility. It is often beneficial to immobilize the affected joint and, in severe cases, to use analgesics in addition to antiinflammatory therapy. Antiinflammatory medications should be started as soon after the onset of pain as possible.

COLCHICINE

Extracts of colchicum have been used to treat acute episodes of gout for more than 1200 years. Colchicine, an alkaloid of colchicum, was isolated in 1820, and although it is one of the oldest treatments for gout, it remains useful in certain cases. It is effective in alleviating acute attacks of gout as well as in prophylaxis of future attacks. Colchicine is also effective in the treatment of pseudogout, sarcoid arthritis, and calcific tendonitis. Colchicine may be used to establish a probable diagnosis of gout, since the antiinflammatory action is limited to these conditions (20). This action is particularly useful in cases in which small joints are involved; aspiration of synovial fluid and isolation of uric acid crystals from these joints are often difficult. Response to colchicine is between 75 and 90%. Response rates depend on how quickly therapy is initiated after the onset of an attack. Colchicine is most effective when given within the first 12 to 36 hr of an attack. Signs and symptoms of inflammation abate within 12 to 24 hr; in 90% of patients the pain is gone within 24 to 48 hr. Most patients should be treated first with indomethacin or another of the NSAIDs that tend to be less toxic than colchicine when used for the short term (3, 7, 21–23).

Colchicine has antiinflammatory activity but no analgesic activity. It has no effect on serum levels of urinary excretion of uric acid. The mechanism of action of colchicine is not yet fully understood. Possible mechanisms include diminished PMN chemotaxis, metabolism, and lysosomal enzyme release. The mechanism of decreased chemotaxis is related to the ability of colchicine to impair chemotactic factor. Colchicine also interferes with sodium urate deposition by decreasing lactic acid production by PMNs (24).

After oral administration, colchicine is rapidly absorbed from the GI tract and partially metabolized in the liver. Unchanged drug may be reabsorbed from the intestine after biliary secretion. Concentrations of colchicine and metabolites decrease after 1 to 2 hr and then increase as a result of reabsorption of unchanged drug. The acute GI toxicity related to colchicine is possibly related to this drug recycling. Colchicine is concentrated in leukocytes but also appears in other tissues, including the kidneys, liver, and intestinal tract. The plasma half-life after intravenous dosing is approximately 20 min. The half-life in leukocytes averages 60 hours. Colchicine and its metabolites are excreted primarily in the feces, smaller amounts being excreted in the urine. Colchicine may have a prolonged half-life in patients with severe renal disease as a result of large decreases in renal excretion, and measurable quantities of drug have been found in urine for up to 10 days after therapy has been discontinued in patients with normal renal function (22, 25).

Colchicine has a very narrow therapeutic index. Acute gout attacks are treated with an initial oral dose of 0.5 to 1.2 mg of colchicine. This is followed by a dose of 0.5 to 0.6 mg every hour or 1.0 to 1.2 mg every 2 hr. Therapy is continued until the patient improves, adverse GI effects develop, or a maximum of 8 to 10 mg has been administered. The effective dose is usually between 4 and 8 mg (3, 7, 22). Death has occurred after administration of as little as 7 mg (26). As many as 80% of patients experience some adverse GI effects that require dosage modification. Patients with preexisting Crohn's disease, diverticulitis, peptic ulcer disease, or a history of GI bleeding should not be given oral colchicine. If treatment with colchicine is deemed necessary for these patients, the dose may be given intravenously. Colchicine for intravenous use should be mixed with 0.9% sodium chloride or sterile water for injection, since dextrose 5% in water or bacteriostatic saline may cause precipitation. A dose of 1 to 2 mg should be mixed with 10 to 20 mL of the appropriate diluent and injected slowly over a period of 2 to 5 min or into the line of a flowing intravenous solution. Care should be taken to ensure that the intravenous injection site is patent and not infiltrating. Colchicine causes severe local irritation to the skin and tissues and should never be given subcutaneously or intramuscularly. After an initial dose of 2 mg intravenously, 0.5 mg may be given every 6 hr

until a response occurs. Alternative dosing methods include a one-time dose of 3 mg or 1 mg initially, followed by 0.5 mg once or twice daily if needed. The total daily recommended intravenous dose is 4 mg. A total intravenous dose of more than 5 mg should not be given during any one treatment period. Additional courses of therapy should not be given for at least 3 days because of risk of GI toxicity (3, 25, 26).

Colchicine may cause bone marrow depression with agranulocytosis, thrombocytopenia, leukopenia, and aplastic anemia. These adverse effects are rare and usually occur only in patients who have received excessive doses or who have decreased renal or hepatic function. Other rare adverse effects that may occur with prolonged administration include loss of body and scalp hair, rashes, peripheral neuropathy, myopathy, vesicular dermatitis, anuria, renal damage, or hematuria. Increased serum concentrations of alkaline phosphatase may also occur with colchicine administration (27).

Colchicine may still be considered as primary therapy in patients who have used it successfully in the past. These patients generally know the total dose of colchicine that worked for them previously and should be given half the total dose at one time and the rest in 0.5- to 0.6-mg increments every hour until the total dose is given. Patients who have hypersensitivity reactions to aspirin and the NSAIDs may also be candidates for colchicine therapy. Some patients who are taking warfarin should not take NSAIDs and should use colchicine. Other patients with a relative contraindication to NSAIDs include those with renal failure, congestive heart failure, and hypertension. NSAIDs in these patients can cause decreased renal function and sodium and water retention. If these patients cannot tolerate colchicine, sulindac, which perhaps has a safer renal profile, should be tried cautiously (28).

Gouty patients with alcoholic cirrhosis should also be treated with colchicine. Since these patients may have preexisting GI distress, renal insufficiency, and ascites, the intravenous dose of colchicine should be reduced by one-half (29).

The frequency of recurrent attacks of gout may be reduced by prophylactic treatment with colchicine. Patients who experience fewer than one attack per year may be given 0.5 to 0.6 mg of colchicine one to four times each week. If attacks are more frequent, the dose is usually 0.5 to 0.6 mg each day. Some patients may require as much as three times this dose each day to control the disease. Patients with a history of gout who are undergoing surgical procedures should receive 0.5 to 0.6 mg of colchicine three times daily for 3 days before and 3 days after surgery (30).

INDOMETHACIN

Indomethacin is a potent antiinflammatory drug that also has antipyretic and analgesic properties. It is considered by

Table 32.2.
Nonsteroidal Antiinflammatory Drugs for Gout

Drug (Trade Name)	Dose[a] (mg)	Dosing Interval	Dosage Form (mg)
Piroxicam (Feldene)	40	q.d.	Capsules (10, 20)
Sulindac (Clinoril)	200	b.i.d.	Tablets (150, 200)
Naproxen (Naprosyn)	750 load		Tablets (250, 375, 500)
(Anaprox-Na⁺ salt)[b,c]	then 250	t.i.d.	Tablets (275, 550)
Ketoprofen (Orudis)	100	t.i.d.	Capsules (25, 50, 75)
Ibuprofen (Motrin, Rufen)[c]	800	t.i.d.	Tablets (200, 300, 400, 600, 800)
Indomethacin (Indocin)	50	t.i.d.–q.i.d.	Capsules (10, 25, 50, 75)
			Suspension (25/5mL)
			Suppositories (50)
Tolmetin (Tolectin)	400	t.i.d.–q.i.d.	Tablets (200, 600)
			Capsules (400)
Fenoprofen (Nalfon)	600–800	q.i.d.	Capsules (200, 300)
			Tablets (600)
Phenylbutazone (Butazolidin)	400 load then 100	q4h until relief	Tablets (100)
			Capsules (100)
Flurbiprofen (Ansaid)	400 load then 50–100	b.i.d.–q.i.d.	Tablets (50, 100)
Etodolac (Lodine)	200–400	b.i.d.–q.i.d.	Capsules (200, 300)

[a]Recommended doses for the treatment of acute gouty attacks.
[b]275 mg of naproxen sodium is equivalent to 250 mg of naproxen.
[c]Also available over the counter under various trade names.

many to be the agent of choice for the treatment of acute gouty attacks. Indomethacin should be started as soon as possible after the onset of an acute gouty attack. Unlike colchicine, it is usually effective even when treatment is delayed by several days. The probable mechanism of action of indomethacin is potent inhibition of prostaglandin synthesis. In addition, indomethacin may exert an inhibitory effect on the mobility of PMNs (3, 7, 21, 29).

Indomethacin given by the oral route is rapidly and completely absorbed. Peak plasma concentrations are attained within 30 to 120 min. Absorption of indomethacin that is administered with food is delayed, but the serum concentration-time profile is similar to that observed in fasting subjects. Indomethacin suppositories are available for patients who are unable to take oral doses. Peak concentrations from rectal administration are generally more rapid but lower than those achieved with similar oral doses. Bioavailability from suppositories is approximately 80%. The half-life of indomethacin ranges from 1 to 16 hr. Possibly, this large range results from extensive enterohepatic recycling and unpredictable biliary discharge. Indomethacin is metabolized primarily by the hepatic microsomal enzyme system and extramicrosomal deacylation. All metabolites are inactive (30).

An initial dose of 50 to 75 mg of indomethacin should be given, followed by 50 mg every 6 hr. This dose is continued for 24 to 48 hr, and then it is gradually tapered. Treatment following an acute gouty attack is generally continued for at least 2 weeks. Common adverse effects include headache, dizziness, nausea, and vomiting. These adverse effects are generally better tolerated than those

seen with colchicine. Additionally, sodium and water retention, hyperkalemia, and renal dysfunction may occur in some patients (2, 3, 29). Because it irritates the gastric mucosa, indomethacin should be given with food, milk, or an antacid (29). Indomethacin should be used with caution by elderly patients, patients with congestive heart failure (21), and patients with a history of peptic ulcer disease.

When indomethacin is given concurrently with probenecid, indomethacin serum levels are increased. This is most likely due to decreased biliary secretion (30).

OTHER ANTIINFLAMMATORY AGENTS

There are many other NSAIDs, and most are useful in the treatment of gout. Agents such as sulindac, tolectin, ibuprofen, piroxicam, naproxen, and ketoprofen are just a few of the many drugs that are available. These compounds also inhibit the synthesis of prostaglandins. Many of the newer agents may have a lower overall rate of adverse effects than indomethacin, particularly in the elderly. Doses of the drugs for the treatment of gout are usually the same as or higher than the doses that are used to treat rheumatoid arthritis (Table 32.2). These drugs should not be used by patients who are allergic to aspirin or by asthmatics with nasal polyps. The most common adverse effect with these agents is GI disturbance, and they should all be taken with food or milk to decrease this problem. These drugs should be used with caution by patients who have a history of gastrointestinal bleeding. Gastrointestinal hemorrhage can be life-threatening and has occurred with all of these drugs (31–34).

PHENYLBUTAZONE

Phenylbutazone has been used quite effectively in the past for the treatment of gout. Because of the risk of agranulocytosis and aplastic anemia, phenylbutazone is not recommended as initial therapy for any of its indications. It should be used only after all other NSAIDs have been tried and found unsatisfactory.

Phenylbutazone is a potent antiinflammatory drug that works as well as or better than colchicine for acute attacks of gout. It is absorbed rapidly and completely from the GI tract. Peak plasma levels are achieved within 2 hr of ingestion. The half-life of phenylbutazone ranges from 48 to 72 hr. It is highly protein-bound and is almost completely metabolized. In addition to its antiinflammatory and antipyretic activity, phenylbutazone has a paradoxical effect on urate excretion. At doses of 600 mg/24 hr or more it increases uric acid excretion; at lower doses it can decrease the rate of renal urate clearance (22).

In the extremely rare case in which all other therapy fails and the decision is made to use phenylbutazone, a dose of 600 to 800 mg, divided into three or four doses, can be given initially; thereafter the dose should be reduced to a maximum of 400 mg/day divided into four doses. The dose should be tapered over the next few days and then discontinued (29). The rate of taper should be dictated by the clinical signs of the disease. Patients should not be given this drug for longer than 7 days because of the potential toxicity. Adverse effects are similar to those experienced with indomethacin. GI discomfort, reactivation of peptic ulcer disease, and fluid and salt retention are common and sometimes extreme. This drug should be used with extreme caution for patients with congestive heart failure or preexisting renal dysfunction. Hypersensitivity reactions such as rashes and, less commonly, hepatitis or nephritis may occur (2, 3, 21, 29).

Asymptomatic Hyperuricemia

Hyperuricemia exists when the serum concentration of urate exceeds the solubility limits. This level is generally considered to be 420 μmol/L (7 mg/dL) with the uricase method or 480 μmol/L (8 mg/dL) with the less specific colorimetric method (4). Once hyperuricemia is diagnosed, the decision to treat must be based on careful evaluation of the patient's clinical condition. If treatment is begun, it requires lifelong therapy and therefore includes the risk of adverse reactions and a substantial cost to the patient. Controversy exists as to when asymptomatic hyperuricemia should be treated. It is impractical and perhaps imprudent to treat every person who has mild hyperuricemia, since the risks of gout and its sequelae are small (16, 35). Some clinicians believe that drug therapy is not warranted unless uric acid levels exceed 720 to 780 μmol/L (12 to 13 mg/dL) in the truly asymptomatic patient. These concentrations may be associated with joint changes and renal complications. Patients who have developed hyperuricemia as a result of other medications may require treatment if the causative agent must be continued. Hypouricemic agents should also be used for patients with recurrent episodes of gout. Patients who have developed tophi or other complications of gout should be candidates for treatment with urate-lowering drugs, even in the absence of clinical disease.

Once the decision to treat has been made, two options are available: xanthine oxidase (XO) inhibitors and uricosurics (Fig. 32.1). Two uricosuric agents, probenecid and sulfinpyrazone, are available to increase renal elimination of uric acid. Allopurinol is the XO inhibitor (Table 32.3). Therapy is generally based on the etiology of the hyperuricemia and overall physical condition of the patient. Uricosuric agents are considered the logical choice for patients who are underexcreters of uric acid. Overproducers should be started on therapy with allopurinol. Allopu-

Table 32.3.
Drugs for Acute and Chronic Gout and Hyperuricemia

Drug	Dosage Form (mg)	Initial Dose (Average Maintenance)	Comments
Probenecid (Benemid)	Tablets (500)	250 mg b.i.d. (500 mg b.i.d.)	Hydrate well; avoid salicylates; caution in peptic ulcer disease and renal impairment; take with meals.
Sulfinpyrazone (Anturane)	Tablets (100) Capsules (200)	50 mg b.i.d. (100–200 mg b.i.d.)	Same as probenecid.
Allopurinol (Zyloprim, Lopurin)	Tablets (100, 300)	100 mg q.d. (300 mg q.d.)	Hydrate well; adjust dose in renal impairment; report any rash; take with meals.
Colchicine	Tablets (0.5, 0.6) Injection (1 mg/2 mL)	p.o. 0.5–1.2 mg followed by 0.5–1.2 mg q1–2h i.v. Refer to text.	Caution in GI, renal, and hepatic disorders; bone marrow depression with long-term use.
Probenecid/colchicine (ColBenemid)	Tablets (500/0.5)	1 tablet q.d. (1 tablet b.i.d.)	

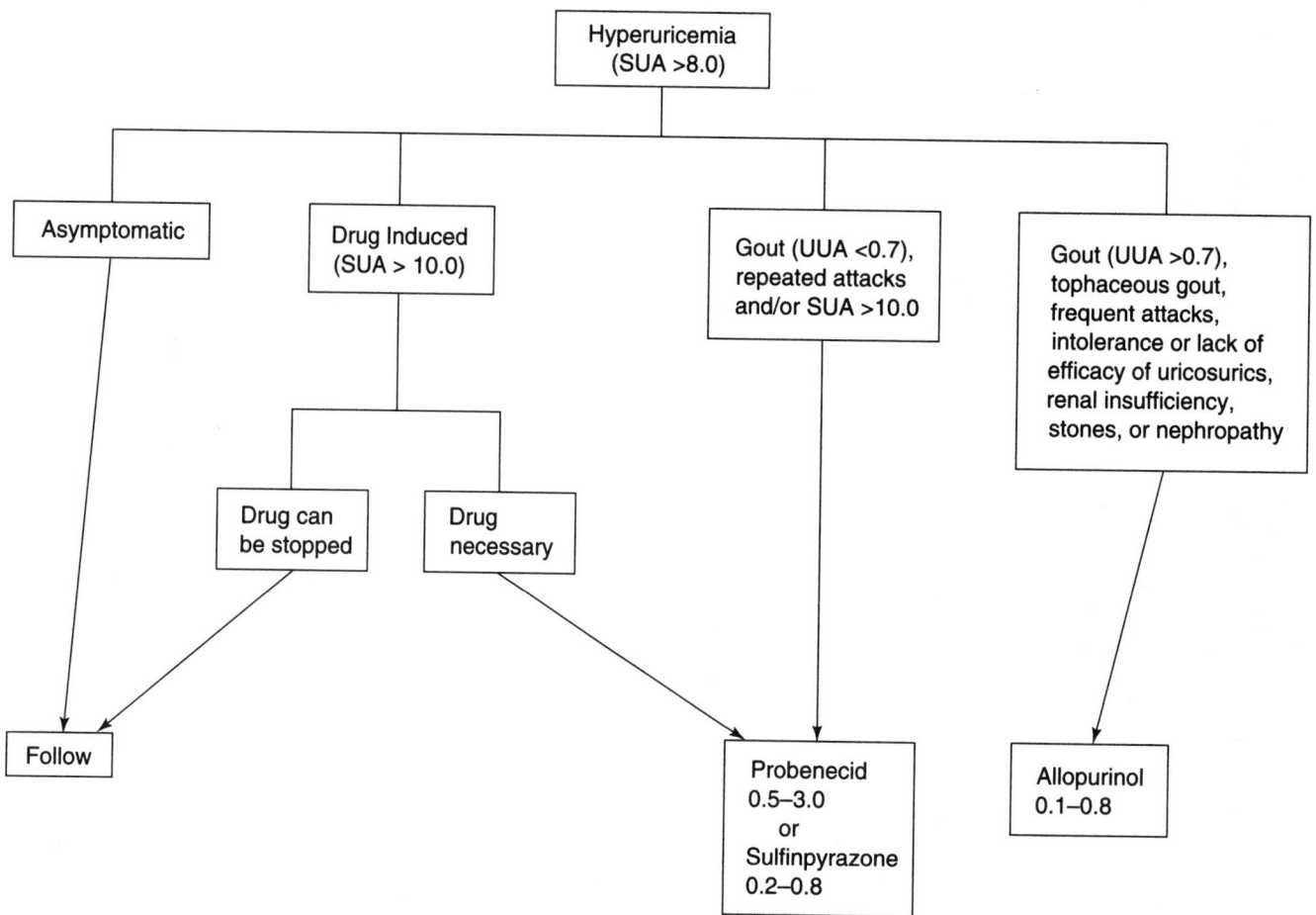

Figure 32.1. The management of hyperuricemia. Serum urate (SUA) is in milligrams per deciliter, measured by the colorimetric method. The excretion rate of urinary uric acid (UUA) is in milligrams per deciliter of glomerular filtrate. Doses of hypouricemic drugs (probenecid, sulfinpyrazone, and allopurinol) are in grams, with values indicating the starting dose on the left progressing toward a maximal dosage on the right. Most patients' hyperuricemia is well controlled by intermediate doses. (Source: Adapted from Nashel DJ, Chandra M. Acute gouty arthritis: special management considerations in alcoholic patients. JAMA 247;58–59, 1982.)

rinol is also a rational choice for patients with tophi, renal stones, or moderate-to-severe renal dysfunction. All forms of hyperuricemia may be treated with allopurinol, but the toxicity profiles of the agents must be taken into consideration.

PROBENECID

Probenecid competitively inhibits the active reabsorption of uric acid at the proximal convoluted tubule. This tubular blocking action promotes the urinary excretion of uric acid, thereby decreasing serum urate concentrations (36). Absorption of probenecid is rapid and complete; peak levels are achieved in 1 to 5 hr. The peak action of the drug occurs at about 2 hr and lasts for about 8 hr. Probenecid is highly protein-bound, primarily to albumin. The drug accumulates in the kidney but not in other organs. Probenecid is metabolized by oxidation of the alkyl side chains and glucuronide conjugation. These processes account for about 90% of the metabolism. The elimination half-life is

dose-dependent, approximately 2 to 6 hr with 0.5- to 1-g doses and 4 to 12 hr with a 2-g dose. Renal elimination is dose-independent but does depend on the pH and rate of urine formation. Alkalinization of the urine results in an increased elimination of probenecid (37).

Doses of 1 to 2 g of probenecid can cause a fourfold to sixfold increase in the elimination of uric acid (21). Active metabolites of probenecid contribute little to the elimination of uric acid (37). Probenecid therapy should not be started during an acute attack of gout because it may exacerbate and prolong the inflammatory phase. Therapy should begin with 250 mg twice a day during the first week of therapy and then increase gradually in increments of 250 to 500 mg/week. A dose of 1 g/day will result in adequate urate lowering in approximately 60% of patients (3). Doses should be adjusted to maintain serum uric acid levels below 420 μmol/L (7 mg/dL). The dose may also be increased if the 24-hr urine uric acid excretion is not above 4160 mmol (700 mg) (7). The drug may increase the frequency of acute attacks during the first year of therapy, even if urate concentrations are maintained at or below normal.

Patients should be advised to drink large quantities of fluid, at least 2 L/day, while taking probenecid. This decreases the risk of formation of uric acid stones (3). Alkalinization of the urine to a pH > 6 greatly increases the solubility of uric acid; the resulting increased elimination of probenecid is not therapeutically important (37). Probenecid may not be effective and should not be used by patients with renal impairment who have a creatinine clearance of less than 0.83 mL/sec (50 mL/min) (22).

Probenecid is usually well tolerated; the adverse effects that are most commonly associated with probenecid are GI discomfort in 8 to 18% of patients, hypersensitivity reactions in 5%, precipitation of uric acid stones in 10%, and precipitation of acute gouty attacks in 10%. Gastrointestinal complaints may be decreased by taking each dose with food (3, 36).

Probenecid should be used cautiously by patients with a history of peptic ulcer disease, and it should not be used by patients with a blood dyscrasia or uric acid kidney stones. The drug should never be used to treat hyperuricemia caused by cancer chemotherapy, myeloproliferative neoplastic diseases, or radiation because of greatly increased risks of uric acid nephropathy.

Because probenecid inhibits renal tubular secretion of many weak organic acids, it causes many interesting drug interactions. Probenecid inhibits the secretion of the penicillins, cephalosporins, nalidixic acid, rifampicin, and nitrofurantoin. This leads to higher levels of antibiotics for prolonged periods. This drug interaction has been used therapeutically to increase the duration and plasma concentrations of the penicillins and cephalosporins. The efficacy of nitrofurantoin is decreased by this interaction, and the toxicity is increased. The renal elimination of naproxen, indomethacin, and sulfinpyrazone is also decreased. The doses of naproxen and indomethacin must be decreased, but the concomitant use of probenecid and sulfinpyrazone does not cause increased adverse reactions. In contrast, the clearance of allopurinol is increased in the presence of probenecid, but the effects of the two drugs are additive, and the combination may be used to therapeutic advantage.

The diuresis produced by furosemide and the thiazides is increased because their renal elimination is decreased when they are given with probenecid. Concomitant administration with heparin has been reported to increase clotting time. Patients who are receiving chlorpropamide should have their blood sugar levels monitored closely at the start of probenecid therapy, since the half-life of chlorpropamide may be increased and may result in hypoglycemia. Interactions with other sulfonylureas may occur but are controversial. Low-dose aspirin is an absolute contraindication with probenecid or sulfinpyrazone

therapy, because the aspirin will block the excretion of uric acid and therefore block the therapeutic effect of these uricosuric agents.

SULFINPYRAZONE

Like probenecid, sulfinpyrazone competitively inhibits active reabsorption of uric acid at the proximal convoluted tubule, thereby promoting the urinary excretion of uric acid and reducing serum urate concentrations. Sulfinpyrazone is a potent uricosuric agent that is chemically related to phenylbutazone. In addition, it reduces platelet adhesiveness and can result in prolonged platelet survival (22).

Oral administration of sulfinpyrazone results in rapid and complete absorption. Peak plasma levels are usually obtained within 1 hr. The half-life is relatively short, ranging from 1 to 3 hr. Approximately 98% of plasma sulfinpyrazone is bound to proteins. Twenty to forty-five percent of a dose is excreted unchanged in the urine, most of the excretion occurring within 6 hr. The uricosuric action of the drug results from inhibition of the tubular reabsorption of uric acid in the nephron (36).

On a weight-for-weight basis, sulfinpyrazone is three to six times as potent as probenecid as a uricosuric. Therapy should be started with a daily dose of 100 mg, given as 50 mg twice a day, for about the first week. The dose is then increased by 100-mg increments each week until an effective dose is reached. A typical regimen might be 50 mg twice a day for 1 week, 100 mg twice a day for 1 week, 150 mg twice a day for 1 week, and so on, until a maintenance dose of 200 to 400 mg/day is achieved. The drug may increase the frequency of acute attacks during the first year of therapy, even if urate concentrations are maintained at or below normal. There is evidence that the administration of prophylactic doses of colchicine, 1 mg/day or less, during the first 6 months will decrease the frequency of subsequent attacks. Most clinicians agree with the prophylactic use of colchicine and/or NSAIDs for patients taking uricosuric agents during this phase (7, 21, 22).

As with probenecid, this drug should not be used when creatinine clearance is less than 0.83 mL/sec (50 mL/min). Periodic blood counts should be performed during sulfinpyrazone therapy because of the rare occurrence of anemia, leukopenia, thrombocytopenia, and agranulocytosis. No uricosuric should be used by patients who are overproducers of uric acid.

When used in recommended doses, sulfinpyrazone is usually well tolerated, with a low rate of adverse effects. The most common adverse effects are those affecting the GI tract (nausea or peptic ulcer reactivation). These may occur in as many as 10 to 15% of patients. As with probenecid, there is the risk of inducing uric acid crystalluria; therefore patients who are on this therapy should consume large quantities of fluid (36). Bronchoconstriction may occur in some patients who are aspirin-

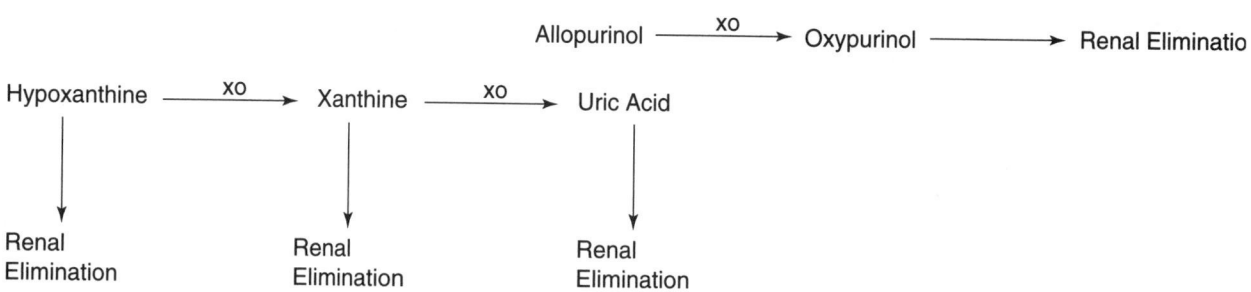

Figure 32.2. Inhibition of xanthine oxidase (XO) by allopurinol and oxypurinol. Note that both allopurinol and oxypurinol inhibit every XO-catalyzed reaction. Further note that the solubilities of renally eliminated products are independent of one another, increasing the body's ability to eliminate products of purine metabolism.

sensitive. In addition to these adverse effects, sulfinpyrazone has been noted to cause an immunoallergic acute interstitial nephritis. These changes are for the most part reversible.

Although sulfinpyrazone inhibits the renal tubular secretion of many weak organic acids, the elevation in plasma concentrations of penicillins and cephalosporins is not clinically useful. Sulfinpyrazone decreases the antiinfective action of nitrofurantoin and increases its toxicity. Salicylates should not be used with sulfinpyrazone because they block the uricosuric action.

ALLOPURINOL

Allopurinol is the most commonly used agent for the long-term control of chronic gout. Allopurinol inhibits XO, the enzyme that catalyzes the conversion of xanthine to uric acid and hypoxanthine to xanthine. Allopurinol itself is metabolized by XO to oxypurinol, which also inhibits XO (Fig. 32.2). The inhibition of XO by allopurinol and oxypurinol decreases the concentrations of serum and urinary uric acid. The decrease in uric acid concentrations is accompanied by an increase in urinary concentrations of xanthine and hypoxanthine. The solubilities of uric acid, xanthine, and hypoxanthine are independent, thus greatly reducing the chances of crystalluria (38–40).

These actions are due not only to XO inhibition but also to a decrease in de novo purine biosynthesis. Allopurinol is converted to a ribonucleotide by HGPRT. The critical rate-limiting enzyme in purine biosynthesis, PRPP amidotransferase, is inhibited by the allopurinol ribonucleotide. Patients who are deficient in HGPRT activity, such as those with Lesch-Nyhan syndrome, do not demonstrate this decrease in purine biosynthesis (2, 41).

Allopurinol is well absorbed from the intestinal tract and has a short half-life of only 2 to 3 hr. The half-life of oxypurinol is much longer than that of allopurinol (18 to 30 hr). The long half-life of the active metabolite allows once-daily dosing in chronic therapy (25).

Allopurinol is the drug of choice for overproducers of uric acid, but it is also efficacious for patients who are underexcreters. Many clinicians prescribe allopurinol be-

cause of the decreased risk of nephrolithiases. However, because of uncommon but potentially dangerous adverse effects associated with allopurinol, it should be recommended only in the following cases: tophaceous gout, major uric acid overproduction (urinary excretion of > 5350 mmol (900 mg) of uric acid per 24 hours on a diet with rigid purine restriction), frequent gouty attacks that are unresponsive to prophylactic colchicine, intolerance or lack of efficacy of uricosuric agents, recurrent uric acid calculi, renal insufficiency, recurrent calcium oxalate, renal calculi when associated with hyperuricosuria, and prevention of acute urate nephropathy in patients receiving cytotoxic therapy for malignancies. Asymptomatic hyperuricemia, uncomplicated gout, and acute gouty attacks are not considered proper indications for the use of allopurinol (42).

Allopurinol is effective in doses of 100 to 300 mg/day. The average adult dose for a patient with gout and normal renal function is 300 mg once a day. For cases of moderately severe tophaceous gout, doses of 400 to 600 mg/day in divided doses may be required. A single daily dose is possible for normal patients because of the prolonged half-life of the active allopurinol metabolite, oxypurinol. In patients with impaired renal function, allopurinol and oxypurinol may accumulate, and the dose should be reduced. The usual dose of 300 mg/day should be reduced to 200 mg when the creatinine clearance is 0.17 to 0.33 mL/sec (10 to 20 mL/min) and to 100 mg when the creatinine clearance is less than 0.17 mL/sec (10 mL/min). For patients with a creatinine clearance less than 0.05 mL/sec (3 mL/min), a 300-mg dose twice a week should be adequate to reduce serum urate concentrations. To reduce the risk of an acute gouty attack when initiating therapy, the dose should begin at 100 mg/day and be increased by 100 mg weekly until serum urate levels fall below 360 μmol/L (6 mg/dL) or the maximum recommended dose of 800 mg/day is reached. When begun after an acute gouty attack, prophylactic NSAIDs and/or colchicine 0.5 to 1.2 mg/day may be administered with allopurinol to decrease the risk of another acute attack. When at all possible, let the acute gouty attack resolve before initiating therapy to lower uric acid. If the acute attacks occur after therapy has been started, doses should not be adjusted. Allopurinol therapy should be continued indefinitely; intermittent therapy is of little benefit and may place the patient at risk of an acute attack (7, 21, 22).

Allopurinol is also used to treat or prevent hyperuricemia associated with tissue breakdown resulting from cancer chemotherapy or radiation. It also reduces the chances of the patient developing secondary uric acid nephropathy from myeloproliferative neoplastic diseases.

Allopurinol is generally well tolerated, with an overall adverse effect rate less than 1%. The frequency of adverse effects increases in the presence of renal insufficiency. The most frequently occurring adverse effect is a pruritic maculopapular rash. Exfoliative, urticarial, erythematosus, hemorrhagic, and purpuric skin eruptions also occur. Stevens-Johnson syndrome has rarely been reported. Skin reactions may be delayed and have been reported as occurring as long as 2 years after therapy is started. These reactions are sometimes severe and associated with a hypersensitivity reaction that can be fatal. Symptoms include a variety of skin eruptions, fever, lymphadenopathy, eosinophilia, and generalized vasculitis. Renal and hepatic damage may occur if the reaction is severe and generalized. Other, less common adverse effects include alopecia, exfoliative dermatitis, leukopenia and neutropenia, hepatitis as part of a generalized hypersensitivity reaction, and nephrolithiases (41–46).

Drug Interactions

Allopurinol and oxypurinol inhibit the metabolism of azathioprine and 6-mercaptopurine, increasing their potential toxicity. When administered concomitantly, the doses of these drugs should be reduced by 25 to 33%. Patients who are receiving allopurinol with either ampicillin or amoxicillin have an increased frequency of rash. In addition, patients who are receiving uricosuric therapy with allopurinol have an increased excretion of oxypurinol. This effect can reduce the inhibition of XO. Even though this occurs, the combination of allopurinol and a uricosuric is generally additive, and no dosage adjustments are necessary (21, 22).

PROGNOSIS AND CONCLUSIONS

Gout is characterized by hyperuricemia that results from an overproduction or an underexcretion of uric acid, or both. It is an acute inflammatory joint disease with deposition of uric acid crystals in the affected joints. Progression of the disease is variable and patient-dependent. The risk of progression to a debilitating chronic disease is decreased today as a result of effective treatments. Treatment with hypouricemic agents for long-term control should be based on careful patient assessment. When this therapy is deemed necessary, treatment is lifelong. Occasional gout or asymptomatic hyperuricemia may not require drug treatment. In these cases, alterations in diet and lifestyle may be enough to keep a patient symptom-free.

REFERENCES

1. Bell JE. Uric acid. Hosp Pharm 7:356–357, 1972.
2. Boss GR, Seegmiller JE. Hyperuricemia and gout: classification, complications and management. N Engl J Med 300:1459–1468, 1979.
3. Mangini RJ. Drug therapy reviews: pathogenesis and clinical management of hyperuricemia and gout. Am J Hosp Pharm 36:497–504, 1979.
4. Lo B. Hyperuricemia and gout [topics in primary care medicine]. West J Med 142:104–107, 1985.
5. Seegmiller JE, Grayzel AI, Laster L, et al. Uric acid production in gout. J Clin Invest 40:1094–2098, 1962.
6. Simkin PA, Hoover PL, Paxson CS, et al. Uric acid excretion: quantitative assessment from spot, midmorning serum and urine samples. Ann Intern Med 91:44–47, 1979.
7. German DC, Holmes EW. Hyperuricemia and gout. Med Clin North Am 70:419–436, 1986.
8. Demartine FE. Hyperuricemia induced by drugs. Arthritis Rheum 8:823–829, 1965.
9. Maclachlan MJ, Rodnan GP. Effects of food, fast and alcohol on serum uric acid and acute attacks of gout. Am J Med 42:38–57, 1967.
10. Hall AP, Barry PE, Dawber TR, et al. Epidemiology of gout and hyperuricemia: a long term population study. N Engl J Med 42:27–37, 1967.
11. Simkin PA. The pathogenesis of podagra. Ann Intern Med 86:230–233, 1977.
12. McCarty DJ. Pathogenesis and treatment of crystal-induced inflammation. In: McCarty DJ, ed. Arthritis and Allied Conditions. 10th ed. Philadelphia: Lea & Febiger, 1985:1494–1514.
13. Hadler NM, Franck WA, Bress NM, et al. Acute polyarticular gout. Am J Med 56:715–719, 1974.
14. Krane SM. Crystal-induced joint disease. In: Rubenstein E, Federman DD, eds. Medicine. Vol. 2, Sect. IX. New York: Scientific American, 1982:1–15.
15. Holmes EW. Clinical gout and the pathogenesis of hyperuricemia. In: McCarty DJ, ed. Arthritis and allied conditions. 10th ed. Philadelphia: Lea & Febiger, 1985:1445–1480.
16. Liang MH, Fries JF. Asymptomatic hyperuricemia: the case for conservative management. Ann Intern Med 88:666–670, 1978.
17. Yu TF, Berger L. Impaired renal function in gout, its association with hypertensive vascular disease and intrinsic renal disease. Am J Med 72:95–100, 1982.
18. Yu TF, Berger L. Renal function in gout. IV: An analysis of 524 gouty subjects including long-term follow-up studies. Am J Med 59:605–613, 1975.
19. Palella TD, Kelley WN. An approach to hyperuricemia and gout. Geriatrics 39:89–102, 1984.
20. Wallace SL, Bernstein D, Diamond H. Diagnostic value of the colchicine therapeutic trial. JAMA 199:525–528, 1967.
21. Bergman HD. Drug therapy in gout. US Pharm Jan, Vol 2, pp 58–64, 1977.
22. Emmerson BT. Drug control of gout and hyperuricemia. Drugs 16:158–166, 1978.
23. Lomen PL. Flurbiprofen in the treatment of acute gout. Am J Med 80(3A):134, 1986.
24. Spilberg I, Mandell B, Mehta J, et al. Mechanism of action of colchicine in acute urate crystal-induced arthritis. J Clin Invest 64:775–780, 1979.
25. Flower RJ, Moncada S, Vane JR. Analgesic-antipyretics and anti-inflammatory agents: drugs employed in the treatment of gout. In:

Gilman GA, Goodman LS, Rall TW, Murad F., eds. The pharmacological basis of therapeutics. 7th ed. New York: Macmillan, 1985: 674–715.

26. Freeman DL. Frequent doses of intravenous colchicine can be lethal [Letter]. N Engl J Med 309:310, 1983.

27. Naidus RM, Rodvien R, Mielke CH. Colchicine toxicity: a multisystem disease. Arch Intern Med 137:394–396, 1977.

28. Ciabattoni G, Cinotti GA, Pierucci A, et al. Effects of sulindac and ibuprofen in patients with chronic glomerular disease. N Engl J Med 310:279–283, 1984.

29. Nashel DJ, Chandra M. Acute gouty arthritis, special management considerations in alcoholic patients. JAMA 247:58–59, 1982.

30. Simkin PA. Management of gout. Ann Intern Med 90:812–816, 1979.

31. Helleberg L. Clinical pharmacokinetics of indomethacin. Clin Pharmacokinet 6:245–258, 1981.

32. Brogden RN, Heel RC, Speight TM, et al. Piroxicam: a reappraisal of its pharmacology and therapeutic efficacy. Drugs 28:292–323, 1984.

33. Widmark PH. Piroxicam: its safety and efficacy in the treatment of acute gout. Am J Med 72(2A):63–65, 1982.

34. Schweitz MC, Nashel DJ, Alpea P. Ibuprofen in the treatment of acute gouty arthritis. JAMA 239:34–35, 1978.

35. Warnock DG. Treatment of hyperuricemia and gout [Letter]. N Engl J Med 301:1240, 1979.

36. Kantor T. Ketoprofen: a review of its pharmacologic and clinical properties. Pharmacotherapy 6(3):93–103, 1986.

37. Gutman AB. Uricosuric drugs, with special reference to probenecid and sulfinpyrazone. Adv Pharmacol 4:91–136, 1966.

38. Cunningham RF, Israili ZH, Dayton PG. Clinical pharmacokinetics of probenecid. Clin Pharmacokinet 6:135–151, 1981.

39. Yu TF. The effect of allopurinol in primary and secondary gout. Arthritis Rheum 8:905–906, 1965.

40. Houpt JB. The effect of allopurinol (HPP) in the treatment of gout. Arthritis Rheum 8:899–904, 1965.

41. Klineberg JR. The effectiveness of allopurinol in the treatment of gout. Arthritis Rheum 8:891–895, 1965.

42. Rundles RW. The development of allopurinol. Arch Intern Med 145:1492–1502, 1985.

43. Singer JZ, Wallace SL. The allopurinol hypersensitivity syndrome: unnecessary morbidity and mortality. Arthritis Rheum 29:82–87, 1986.

44. Vincent PC. Drug-induced aplastic anemia and agranulocytosis: incidence and mechanisms. Drugs 31:52–63, 1986.

45. Ohsawa T, Ohtsubo M. Hepatitis associated with allopurinol. Drug Intell Clin Pharm 19:431–433, 1985.

46. Worth CT, Hussein SM. Peripheral neuropathy due to long term ingestion of allopurinol. Br Med J 291:1688, 1985.

CHAPTER 33

SYSTEMIC LUPUS ERYTHEMATOUS

STEPHEN H. FULLER and THOMAS H. WISER

Systemic lupus erythematous (SLE) is a multisystem inflammatory disorder of unknown etiology that is characterized by autoantibody production. In recent years, advances in immunology and immunopharmacology have led to increased recognition of the disease, insight into its pathogenesis, and improved therapeutic interventions. These events have allowed for better application of scientific knowledge to the disease, which has resulted in a decrease in morbidity and mortality from SLE.

Lupus is the latin word for "wolf" and has been used since at least A.D. 230 to describe the cutaneous lesions that resemble the malar erythema of a wolf. It was not until 1875 that the rash was noted to resemble a butterfly. Clinical recognition of the disease was greatly enhanced when the lupus erythematous (LE) cell was discovered in 1948 and the immunofluorescent antinuclear factor test was started in 1957 (1). Since the 1960s, advances have occurred through increased practitioner recognition of the disease (recent revision of diagnostic criteria), expanded diversity and refinement of diagnostic tests, and an enhanced understanding of disease mechanisms. Also, the increased use of immunosuppressant drug therapy has improved the prognosis of patients with major organ (central nervous system and renal) involvement (2–5).

Most of the symptoms of SLE relate to the key pathology: inflammation. Clinically distressing symptoms, including heat, swelling, pain, tenderness, and local tissue destruction, all relate to the inflammatory process. However, no single theory can completely explain the pathological process, so researchers suspect multifactorial etiologies and triggering mechanisms (e.g., one defect to trigger the immune response and another to permit a significant antibody reaction). Other etiological factors include genetic predisposition, drugs, viral infections, ultraviolet rays, hormones, environmental pollutants, and emotional stress. Hence, SLE may not be a single disease but rather a constellation of signs and symptoms that are produced by a variety of etiologies.

There is no known cure for SLE, so therapy is primarily palliative. However, newer therapies aim to relieve symptoms, prevent the inflammatory response and subsequent tissue destruction, and prolong survival.

EPIDEMIOLOGY

SLE is estimated to have a prevalence of 14.6 to 50.8 per 100,000 of the U.S. population with an annual incidence of 2.2 to 7.6 new cases per 100,000 reported each year. These figures are slightly higher than international figures reporting a prevalence of 2 to 36 per 100,000 with an annual incidence of 3.3 to 4.8 cases per 100,000 people. SLE can occur in all races but is observed two to three times more often in Blacks, Hispanics, and Asians compared to Caucasians. Sexual differences in SLE suggest an underlying hormonal role in the development of the disease, since it is seen primarily in women of childbearing ages (5–8:1) versus men. However, this sexual predominance fades in older patients, the sex ratio being 2:1 (female: male) in SLE patients who are diagnosed after 65 years of age. In terms of age, 65 percent of patients are diagnosed between the ages of 15 and 55, 20 percent of patients before the age of 15, and 15 percent of patients after the age of 55. A hereditary component also appears to be involved in the development of SLE, multiple genes being emphasized as affecting regulation of the immune system and the sex hormones. The genetic link appears evident, since first-degree family members have SLE rates of 5 to 12%, with a rate of 14 to 57% in monozygotic twins and rates of 5 to 9% in dizygotic twins. Although SLE occurs primarily in women of childbearing age, there are many etiological factors that are still not understood concerning this disease (1, 6–10).

PATHOPHYSIOLOGY

Although the etiology of SLE remains an enigma, it is evident that much of the tissue damage that occurs is caused by the inflammatory reactions of the antigen-antibody complexes that are formed during the disease processes. SLE is thought to be primarily the result of a variety of defects in regulation of the immune system, including lymphocyte (B and T cell) function abnormalities, antilymphocyte antibodies, and abnormalities in the complement system. Antilymphocyte antibodies are thought to be responsible for destruction of T suppressor cells, which inhibit T cytotoxic cells. In addition, antilymphocyte antibodies decrease interleukin-2 production, further decreasing immune function. There is also strong evidence supporting the excessive activation of B cells and exaggerated production of autoantibodies, which react with the host's cellular (cell membrane) and subcellular (nuclear and cytoplasmic) antigens to form destructive immune complexes (1, 11). These complexes are composed of immunoglobulin M, G, and A (IgM, IgG, IgA) and may be seen in the circulation or may form on the cell or tissue surfaces and correlate with the clinical manifestations. It is also postulated that patients with SLE have a defect in removing these immune complexes (1, 11).

During the immune complex formation and deposition the complement system is activated; fixation occurs, resulting in low complement levels (C1, C7, C4). These low levels also serve as an indirect measure of immune complex formation, since complement is responsible for clearing the immune complexes. The degree of hypocomplementemia relates directly to the severity of disease activity, extreme hypocomplementemia occurring in patients with renal and central nervous system (CNS) disease. During immune complex formation, chemotactic factors are released, attracting phagocytic cells. This results in the production of lysosomal enzymes, causing tissue destruction. The characteristic SLE pathologic changes include three histologic lesions: (a) hematoxylin bodies (bluish, globular masses that are suspected of being the inclusion bodies of LE cells), (b) onion-skin lesions (characteristic concentric perivascular fibrosis found in central and penicillary arteries of the spleen), and (c) Libman-Sacks verrucous endocarditis (characteristic lesions consisting of nonbacterial vegetations on heart valves, especially the mitral valve, chordae tendineae, and endocardium of the papillary muscle). Other pathologic involvement in most other organs relates to vasculitis or mononuclear cell infiltrates (1).

The theory of an immunoregulatory defect is considered to be the result of a combination of factors, including genetic, viral, hormonal, or environmental; however, the exact mechanism is unknown. Further, patient susceptibility or predisposition must also be present for the disease to manifest itself. Many of these variables that are implicated in the development of the disease are discussed here.

Genetic factors play a significant role in the formation of the disease. SLE occurs in relatives of patients who have the disease at a frequency of about 5 to 12%, which is a several-hundred-fold increased frequency compared to the general population (9, 10). Immunologic abnormalities are found more often in family members of SLE patients than in the general population, and there is a 14 to 57% prevalence of the trait in monozygotic twins compared to approximately a 5 to 9% frequency in dizygotic twins and other first-degree relatives. In addition, certain ethnic groups have a high prevalence of SLE; for example, blacks develop the disease at a rate that is three times higher than that of the general population (1, 10). Numerous other genetic relationships that also implicate genetic causality include an increased prevalence in certain HLA phenotypes (DR2, DR3 and certain subtypes), patients with reduced CR1 receptors on erythrocytes, and patients with decreased C4A genes (11).

Viral etiologies and other transmissible infectious agents have received a lot of attention because electron microscopic observations in SLE tissues resemble tubuloreticular structures and the nucleoprotein core of paramyxoviruses. Serologic studies of antiviral antibodies in patients with SLE are often elevated; however, they are usually directed toward several unrelated viruses. This suggests a nonspecific B-lymphocyte activation rather than a unique antigenic exposure. Although direct viral isolation from tissue of SLE patients has been attempted, the conventional or cocultivation techniques have not been successful in identifying specific viruses (11). Hence, although viral etiologies are suspected in SLE, it still remains to be determined whether virus expression is the result or cause of SLE, so ultrasensitive research techniques and continued research are needed in this area of discovery.

The high incidence of SLE in women of reproductive age suggests that hormonal factors may play an important role in the development of the disorder. Selected animal model studies with mice indicate that females have an earlier appearance of dsDNA antibodies, more severe complications (e.g., nephritis), and a shorter life span. The administration of androgens appears to improve survival and reduce the nephritis complications in the female animals (11). Furthermore, estrogen hormones enhance immune reactivity, and androgen hormones suppress it. The mechanisms are unknown for these effects, but it is thought that estrogens depress T-cell-mediated immunity (the natural killer cell function) and allow B-cell antibody proliferation. By contrast, androgens inhibit both B-cell and T-cell maturation and depress the reactivity of passively transferred lymphocytes and, therefore, depressed immune reactivity (12).

Environmental influences may also contribute to the development of SLE. Sunlight, thermal burns, and other physical stress (e.g., infection, pregnancy, or surgery) have been implicated in modifying the disease process. Drug-induced SLE, the presence of antibodies in laboratory workers exposed to SLE sera and household contacts of SLE patients, and dietary effects on clinical symptoms also support environmental influences in SLE (11).

CLINICAL FEATURES

The diagnosis of SLE is based upon the presence of clinical features as outlined in the Revised Criteria for the Classification of SLE (Table 33.1) combined with laboratory values that help to confirm the diagnosis (13). The most common complaints of SLE patients are fatigue, fever, and weight loss, which occur in 80 to 100% of patients. Fatigue is often a patient's initial and most common complaint, and it often responds to exercise and/or medication. However, fatigue may be present when no other clinical symptoms are obvious, and it becomes

Table 33.1.
The 1982 Revised Criteria for the Classification of Systemic Lupus Erythematosus

Criterion	Definition
Malar rash	Fixed erythema, flat or raised, over the malar eminences, tending to spare the nasolabial folds
Discoid rash	Erythematous raised plaques with adherent keratotic scaling and follicular plugging; atrophic scarring may occur in older lesions
Photosensitivity	Skin rash as a result of an unusual reaction to sunlight by patient history or physician observation
Oral ulcers	Oral or nasopharyngeal ulceration, usually painless, observed by a physician
Arthritis	Nonerosive arthritis involving two or more peripheral joints characterized by swelling, tenderness, or effusion
Serositis	Pleuritis (convincing history of pleuritic pain or rub heard by physician or evidence of pleural effusion OR pericarditis) documented by ECG, rub, or evidence of pericardial effusion
Renal disorder	Persistent proteinuria > 0.5 g/day or > 3+ if quantitation not performed OR cellular casts (red cell, hemoglobin, granular, tubular, or mixed)
Neurologic disorder	Seizures OR psychosis in the absence of offending drugs or known metabolic problems (uremia, ketoacidosis, or electrolyte imbalance)
Hematologic disorder	Hemolytic anemia with reticulocytosis, OR leukopenia, < 4000/mm^3 total on two or more occasions, OR lymphopenia, < 1500/mm^3 on two or more occasions, OR thrombocytopenia, < 100,000/mm^3 in the absence of offending drugs
Immunologic disorder	Positive LE cell preparation OR anti-DNA antibodies OR anti-Sm antibodies OR false-positive serologic test for syphilis known to be positive for at least 6 months and confirmed by *Treponema pallidum* immobilization or fluorescent treponemal antibody absorption test
Antinuclear antibody	An abnormal titer of antinuclear antibody by immunofluorescence or an equivalent assay at any point in time and in the absence of drugs known to cause "drug-induced lupus" syndrome

The proposed classification is based upon 11 criteria. For the purpose of identifying patients in clinical studies, a person shall be said to have systemic erythematous lupus if any 4 or more of the 11 criteria are present, serially or simultaneously, during any interval of observation.

worse with acute exacerbations of the disease. Episodic fevers (>101°F) occur in 80% of patients with SLE; however, infectious disease processes must be ruled out. Weight loss (>5 lb) often occurs before the actual diagnosis of SLE and is thought to be related to the loss of appetite from SLE-induced gastrointestinal inflammation. This results in dyspepsia, difficulty swallowing, and gastroesophageal reflux disease. However, these gastrointestinal symptoms as well as peptic ulcer disease can also occur from the medications that patients receive for the treatment of SLE (nonsteroidal antiinflammatory drugs, (NSAIDs), steroids, and immunosuppressants) (14, 15).

Musculoskeletal manifestations are found in 95% of SLE patients and often precede the diagnosis by several months. Joint involvement is symmetrical and primarily involves the wrists, small joints of the hand, and knees and less frequently the ankles, elbows, hips, and shoulders. The arthritis of SLE is migratory in nature, symptoms moving between the affected joints over 24 to 48 hr (14). In contrast to rheumatoid arthritis, morning stiffness and joint involvement tend to be nonerosive and nondeforming. However, patients with chronic disease may experience subcutaneous nodules (5 to 7%), arthritic deformities (3 to 50%), and tenosynovitis (10 to 13%) (11, 13). Patients receiving high-dose steroids therapy on a chronic basis may suffer from avascular necrosis (osteonecrosis) or steroid-induced osteoporosis, which can result in demineralization of trabecular bone, resulting in fractures of the hip or spine. In addition, steroids may cause patients to experience joint pain and swelling due to fluid retention or muscle tenderness (steroid myopathy) in addition to the symptoms that are already present (14–16).

Skin lesions are present in 80% of SLE patients and occur with systemic flares of lupus or on exposure to sunlight (usually ultraviolet B rays) or other sources of ultraviolet light (fluorescent light). Fair-skinned, blond-haired, blue-eyed individuals tend to be more photosensitive, as are patients with anti-Ro antibodies present. In addition, an individual's degree of photosensitivity can vary throughout the SLE disease and with each type of skin lesion. Fifty percent of patients experience the classic "butterfly" or malar rash, which derives its name from the butterfly-shaped erythema covering the cheeks and bridge of the nose (2). The malar rash is acute in onset and may last for hours to days and is often accompanied by other SLE symptoms. Other patients develop maculopapular rashes that are distributed in areas exposed to ultraviolet light; these patients are considered to be photosensitive.

Subacute cutaneous lupus erythematosus (SCLE) and chronic discoid lupus erythematosus (DLE) lesions develop in 10% to 20% of SLE patients, respectively. Conversely, 10 to 50% of patients with SCLE or DLE can go on to develop mild SLE. Patients who experience SCLE or DLE will often have antibodies to Ro but none to dsDNA, complement levels being normal. SCLE lesions are small, erythematous, scaly papules that are typically located on the shoulders, neck, forearms, and upper torso areas. SLCE lesions tend to join together to form confluent areas, in contrast to the discrete, well-defined discoid lesions. Discoid lesions are the one of the most common dermatologic manifestations of lupus and appear as round, well-defined, red-purple, scaly plaques that occur primarily on the head, neck, and upper torso. The severity of the rash often depends on the intensity of the ultraviolet exposure, and rashes tend to last only hours to days if the aggravating source is removed. These rashes can be confused with psoriasis, so biopsies are often helpful for the appropriate diagnosis. The SCLE rashes usually heal without scarring; however, discoid lesions may result in scarring and depigmentation. Vascular lesions can occur in up to 50% of patients and are believed to form from leukocyte infiltration resulting in vascular damage. These lesions affect different vessel locations and can result in urticaria, purpura, and petechiae on the hands or feet. Mucous membranes are involved in over 25% of patients, and discoid lesions often appear on the lips or mouth (2).

Almost all SLE patients will demonstrate some renal abnormalities at a cellular level within 36 months of being diagnosed with SLE; however, clinical signs and symptoms of lupus nephritis do not correlate well with the extent of renal damage. Clinical nephritis occurs in over 50% of patients, the staging of the nephritis being correlated with progression of kidney disease and complications such as hypertension, nephrotic syndrome, and renal failure if not treated adequately. The most common renal abnormalities are proteinuria (in 78% of patients) and hematuria, pyuria, and casts in the urine of more than 40% of patients (14, 17). Glomerular damage induced by SLE may not result in clinical symptoms until later. The World Health Organization (WHO) classifications of the stages of lupus glomerulonephritis are often used to help determine the renal prognosis for an individual patient (Table 33.2) (3–4, 17–19).

Mesangial glomerulonephritis (Type II) is characteristic of most initial lupus nephritis and has a milder clinical presentation (minimal proteinuria and hematuria, normal creatinine clearance). Because of minimal involvement of the glomerulus and lack of involvement of the tubules, interstitium, and vascular areas, these patients have an excellent renal prognosis (Table 33.2). Patients with proliferative lupus nephritis are characterized as focal proliferative (Type III) and diffuse proliferative (Type IV). Proliferative forms of nephritis display irregularities such as glomerular capillary wall thickening, necrotic changes of the glomeruli, leukocyte and immunoglobulin infiltration, fibrinoid changes, and tubular degeneration and interstitial inflammation. In addition, the clotting system is activated in some of these patients, resulting in glomerular thrombi and fibrin-related antigens being deposited in the glomerulus, which are prognostic for severe renal disease (17). Focal proliferative nephritis involves fewer than 50% of the glomerular tufts, so these patients have some clinical abnormalities, but their prognosis is good unless transition occurs to a diffuse proliferative nephritis, which is more widespread and severe. Membranous glomerulonephritis (Type V) can also affect glomerular function, cause interstitial inflammation, and produce slight tubule changes. However, it is difficult to determine which patients will progress to more severe stages of lupus nephritis; therefore, it is important to determine whether

Table 33.2.
Clinical, Laboratory, and Pathological Findings in Lupus Nephritis Patients[a]

| Parameter | Class | | | | |
	Normal Glomeruli (I)	Mesangial GN (II)	Focal Proliferative GN (III)	Diffuse Proliferative GN (IV)	Membranous GN (V)
Incidence	Rare	≈25%	≈20%	≈40%	≈15%
Hypertension	None	None	Occasional	Common	Late onset
Proteinuria (g/day)	None	<1	<2	1–20	3.5–20
Hematuria (RBC/HPF)	None	5–15	5–15	Many	None
Pyuria (WBC/HPF)	None	5–15	5–15	Many	None
Casts	None	Occasional	Many	Many	None
GFR (mL/min)	Normal	Normal	60–80	<60	Normal
CH_{50}	Normal	Normal to decreased	Decreased	Greatly decreased	Normal
Anti-DNA	Normal	Normal to increased	Increased	Greatly increased	Normal
Immune complexes	Normal	Normal to increased	Increased	Greatly increased	Normal
Renal prognosis	Excellent	No progression unless transition occurs	Insufficiency usually does not develop. 5-year mortality <10%	Progression to death in 2 years in 50% if not treated. 5-year mortality <25% overall	Slowly progressing renal insufficiency. 5-year mortality <25%
Transition	To class II or IV 15–20%	To class IV 20–40%	To class V 2–5%	To class III or V 5–10%	

[a]Adapted from (7, 13, 15).

Table 33.3.
Renal Pathology Scoring System[a,b]

	Activity Index	Chronicity Index
Glomerular changes		
	Fibrinoid changes[c]	Glomerular sclerosis
	Cellular proliferative	Fibrous crescents
	Cellular crescents[c]	
	Hyaline thrombi, wire loops	
	Leukocyte infiltration	
Tubulointerstitial changes		
	Mononuclear cell infiltration	Interstitial fibrosis
		Tubular atrophy

[a] Adapted from (27).
[b] Each factor is scored from 0 to 3.
[c] Fibrinoid necrosis and cellular crescents are weighted by a factor of 2 because such lesions are more ominous than the other active lesions.

the lesions represent active inflammation or chronic sclerosis and fibrosis. This can be determined only by renal biopsy, active lesions predicting continued injury to the glomerulus (which may be responsive to aggressive therapy) and chronic lesions suggesting irreversible fibrotic lesions and sclerosis, which usually do not respond to therapy (Table 33.3). In summary, patients presenting with renal clearance or urinary abnormalities (Table 33.2) would be suspected of lupus nephritis if immune function markers (C3, CH50, anti-dsDNA antibodies) were abnormal. Although a renal biopsy may not be needed in patients who appear to have renal disease, a biopsy can provide information regarding the type of lesion(s) and activity of the lesions(s), which can help to guide the clinician in selecting the best treatment (3, 17, 18).

Pulmonary manifestations occur in over 50% of lupus patients, symptoms of pleurisy, coughing, and dyspnea being the most frequently reported patient complaints and usually the first clue of lung involvement. Pleurisy, or chest wall pain, is often the only patient complaint and occurs on moving or changing position and frequently disturbs the patient's sleep. Since many patients suffer benign chest wall pain due to muscle inflammation, patients should be evaluated by listening (via stethoscope) to inspirations for pleural friction rubs. This rough sound of the pleural membranes rubbing together along with the radiographic presence of a pleural effusion usually indicates pleuritis as a sign of lupus lung involvement (14).

Atelectasis (progressive shrinking of lungs with decreased lung volumes) is seen in many SLE patients, causing basal infiltrates and diaphragmatic elevation leading to dyspnea. Acute lupus pneumonitis occurs less frequently (5 to 12%) but has a short-term mortality rate of 50%. Patients experience high fevers, dyspnea, tachycardia, and pulmonary infiltrates and can become cyanotic. This fatal pulmonary manifestation is thought to be due to an acute alveolar damage from immune complexes. Other

pulmonary manifestations include chronic lupus pneumonitis, pulmonary hypertension, and pulmonary hemorrhage. Most pulmonary manifestations of SLE show restrictive lung disease patterns on pulmonary function tests with reductions of carbon monoxide diffusion capacity and fibrosis of the lungs (20).

Many patients (10 to 80%) with SLE will experience some type of neuropsychiatric manifestation within two years of SLE diagnosis. Central nervous system events are considered to be functional (psychiatric) or organic (neurologic). However, it is often difficult for a clinician to determine whether symptoms are functional or organic in origin. There are no specific tests to diagnosis CNS lupus, and although computed tomography (CT) scans have not shown structural changes in the brain, magnetic resonance imaging (MRI) has shown some focal lesions and atrophy. More practically, patients with CNS symptoms often demonstrate other presentations of active lupus with the presence of Sm, antilymphocyte, and antiribosomal P antibodies. The psychiatric manifestations include depression, anxiety, and mania and are believed to indicate how individuals react to the stress of being diagnosed with SLE. Depression or anxiety is diagnosed in a majority of patients and is often seen soon after the diagnosis of SLE because of the uncertainties associated with the diagnosis of SLE. Many patients recover through the support of family and SLE support groups and with the use of medications; however, some patients will continue to suffer from psychosomatic complaints (insomnia, constipation, fatigue). Psychoses occur in approximately 25% of patients and are thought to be caused by functional and/or organic abnormalities as well as medications that the patients may be receiving (steroids, NSAIDs, sedatives, narcotics). Ironically, high doses of steroids often improve psychotic manifestations (21, 22).

Other neurologic disorders that are seen in lupus patients include headaches, seizures, and neuropathies. Headaches are usually due to muscle tension, and virtually 100% of patients complain of having headaches sometime during progression of their lupus. Seizures occur in 15 to 20% of patients and are usually generalized tonoclonic seizures, but patients have been reported to experience petit mal and temporal seizures. Seizures may be secondary to other organic disorders (metabolic abnormalities, uremia) and should be considered a part of CNS lupus only if other symptoms of organic brain disease or lupus develop concomitantly. Ten to fifteen percent of patients experience other neurologic manifestations such as cranial or peripheral neuropathies and stroke. These disorders can result in diplopia, nystagmus, visual field deficits, hallucinations, weakness of the lower extremities, and loss of rectal and bladder continence (21, 22).

Up to 50 percent of SLE patients have cardiac manifestations, the most predominant area affected being

Table 33.4.
Antinuclear Antibodies in Several Diseases[a]

Condition	ANA (% positive)	Antibodies[b]						
		dsDNA	Sm	ssDNA	Histone	U_1RNP	Ro	La
Normal	<5	0	0	0	0	0	0	0
SLE	>95	75	25	>75	25–70	40	25–50	15
RA	25–50	70	Rare	50–60	—	47	—	—
Scleroderma	75	0	Rare	—	—	20	95	—
Sjögren's	68	Rare	Rare	14	—	5–60	—	14–87
DIL	95	Rare	Rare	80	90	—	—	—

[a]Adapted from (1, 7, 21).
[b]Percent of patients having specific antibodies in each condition. Antibodies: dsDNA = double-stranded DNA, SMA = antismith, ssDNA = single-stranded DNA, RA = Rheumatoid arthritis, DIL = Drug-induced lupus, U_1RNP = U_1Ribonucleoprotein, Ro = anti-Ro, La = anti-La.

the pericardium. Pericardial SLE is suspected if a patient suffers from substernal chest pain and/or an audible pericardial rub with electrocardiogram (ECG) abnormalities or detection of fluid on the echocardiogram. Myocarditis (which can lead to congestive heart failure (CHF)) is suspected when patients present with resting tachycardia, unexplained cardiomegaly, and ECG (ST-T wave) abnormalities. Patients with SLE also have a high incidence of coronary artery disease and hypertension, the latter being associated with chronic lupus nephritis. SLE patients also frequently present with systolic murmurs that are secondary to anemia, cardiomegaly, and tachycardia (23).

Anemia occurs in approximately half of SLE patients and is thought to be due to a combination of the chronic inflammatory process of lupus, the decrease of erythropoiesis from renal insufficiency, and the adverse effects of medications (i.e., intestinal blood loss and bone marrow suppression). Therefore, most patients present with a normochromic, normocytic anemia with a decrease in the number of reticulocytes. In addition, 10 to 50% of lupus patients suffer from hemolytic anemia, leukopenia (WBC < 4500/mm3), and/or thrombocytopenia (<150,000/mm3). This alone usually does not appear to expose lupus patients to infection or bleeding abnormalities, since only 17% and 10% of patients have WBC <4000/mm3 or platelets < 50,000, respectively. However, several patients (25%) have antibodies to several clotting factors (lupus anticoagulant). The result is a prolonged partial thromboplastin time (PTT) with a normal prothrombin time (PT) and INR, which can enhance the chances of bleeding if thrombocytopenia also coexists. Patients have also been reported to have antiphospholipid (anticardiolipin) antibodies, which have resulted in thrombus formation and thrombocytopenia (24).

Since many of the symptoms described are present with other connective tissue conditions, patients with SLE could initially be misdiagnosed as having rheumatoid arthritis, scleroderma, Sjögren's syndrome, or other connective tissue diseases. Therefore, clinicians should use the 1982 ARA criteria (Table 33.1) for the diagnosis and classification of SLE. These clinical symptoms combined with laboratory findings will confirm the diagnosis of systemic lupus erythematosus. The best lab screening test for SLE is the fluorescent antinuclear antibody (ANA) test, which should be used when anyone is suspected of having SLE. Most patients with SLE will exhibit a positive ANA and have very high titers (antibody concentrations much greater than a dilution of 1:320). The ANA test is positive in up to 95% of patients with SLE; however, 5% of patients with clinical lupus will be ANA negative. Therefore, patients with negative ANAs usually do not have further antibody tests performed unless their symptoms strongly suggest a connective tissue disorder. In addition, 5% of patients without lupus will have slightly positive ANA tests, but titers are usually less than 1:320 with a homogeneous pattern.

Although the ANA is a sensitive test, it is not completely specific, since up to 50% of patients with rheumatoid arthritis, scleroderma, and Sjögren's syndrome will have a positive ANA titer. Therefore, the pattern of the fluorescence of the ANA test is observed to increase the specificity of the diagnosis. Four ANA fluorescence patterns are observed: homogeneous, nuclear rim (peripheral), speckled, and nucleolar; rim and speckled patterns are more specific for SLE. However, most clinicians decide to use laboratory tests evaluating the presence of more specific antibodies. Each antibody test should be used discriminately, since many are not specifically diagnostic for SLE (Table 33.4).

There are several different autoantibody tests, which are characterized according to whether the antibodies bind nucleic acids (DNA), nucleic-acid-binding proteins (histones, ribonucleoproteins, RNPs), or cell membrane antigens (antiphospholipids). Some DNA tests include the double-stranded DNA (ds-DNA) and the single-stranded DNA (ss-DNA) tests. Ribonucleoprotein (or RNA) tests include the U_1RNP, Sm, Ro, and La antibody tests. If patients have the presence of dsDNA and Sm antibodies and decreasing levels of complement (C3, CH50), it is considered highly specific for SLE. However, only 75% and 25% of patients with SLE will produce antibodies to dsDNA and Sm, respectively. Other antibodies that are less specific for SLE include ssDNA (single-stranded DNA) and nucleoproteins (NP), which are also found in rheumatoid arthritis patients; ribonucleoproteins (U_1RNP), which are also found in scleroderma patients; and Ro and La antibodies, which are found in patients with Sjögren's syndrome. Several antibodies are found together and have different prognostic implications. The Sm and U_1RNP antibodies are often found together and have been reported to predict less severe renal disease. The Ro and LA antibodies are often found together in patients with "ANA negative lupus" or with subacute cutaneous lupus. The presence of histone antibodies (antibodies that form to drug-nuclear protein complexes) are found in 90% of patients experiencing drug-induced lupus. All antibodies tend to decrease within normal limits when patients are successfully treated and in remission (1, 14, 25).

DRUG-RELATED LUPUS SYNDROME

The first drug-related lupus (DRL) syndromes involved sulfonamides and penicillins in the late 1940s and early 1950s. Anticonvulsants and cardiovascular medications were implicated in the late 1950s and 1960s. Since then, more than 50 drugs have been implicated as causing a positive ANA, and at least five have been associated with DRL syndrome, procainamide and hydralazine being the most common culprits (Table 33.5).

Although several theories have been proposed to explain DRL, the exact etiology cannot be explained. Originally, several medications (e.g., oral contraceptives) were thought only to exacerbate symptoms in patients with existing lupus conditions; however, some medications (hydralazine, procainamide) produce lupuslike symptoms in patients who were not previously diagnosed with idiopathic SLE. A popular hypothesis associates drug-related lupus with patients who are genetically slow acetylators (linked to HLA-DR4), a feature that results in a slow rate of drug acetylation by the N-acetyltransferase enzyme. This causes an accumulation of drug, which forms a complex with nuclear proteins (DNA, histones). Antinuclear antibodies are then formed against the complexes, resulting in a stimulation of T and B cells, the formation of antibodies, and an inflammatory response. Further evidence shows that a slow acetylation phenotype may predispose a patient to becoming ANA positive and developing lupus symptoms sooner than a fast acetylator. However, patients who have a fast acetylator phenotype can develop a positive ANA and DRL symptoms. Experts also agree that DRL is related to the medication dose, the duration of therapy that a patient receives, and probably other unidentifiable factors that will determine whether a patient develops DRL (14, 26–28).

Patients who are experiencing DRL differ vastly from patients with idiopathic SLE (Table 33.6). Drug-related lupus occurs most often in older patients (averaging 53 years for hydralazine and 62 years for procainamide) compared to the average age of onset of 20 to 40 years for idiopathic SLE. This is probably reflective of the older population of patients using procainamide and hydralazine. Women make up approximately 90% of patients with idiopathic SLE, compared to 40 to 60, of patients with DRL. Racial differences show Caucasian patients representing 90 to 95% of DRL versus only approximately 65% of patients with idiopathic SLE. Although there are differences in which populations acquire DRL and SLE, many of the clinical presentations are similar (26–28).

In differentiating between idiopathic SLE and DRL, evaluation of the clinical presentation and laboratory values can be helpful (Table 33.6). Patients with DRL typically

Table 33.5.
Drug-Related Lupus: Implicated Medications[a]

Definite	Possible		Unlikely
Hydralazine	Anticonvulsants	Antithyroid	Griseofulvin
Procainamide	Phenytoin	Propylthiouracil	Phenylbutazone
Isoniazid	Carbamazepine	Methimazole	Oral contraceptives
Chlorpromazine	Valproic acid	Miscellaneous	Gold salts
Methyldopa	Ethosuximide	Penicillamine	Penicillin
	Trimethadine	Sulfasalazine	
	Beta-blockers	Sulfonamides	
	Propranolol	Nitrofurantoin	
	Metoprolol	Levodopa	
	Labetalol	Lithium	
	Pindolol	Cimetidine	
	Oxprenolol	Quinidine	
	Acebutolol	Captopril	

[a]Developed from (23).

Table 33.6.
Drug-Related Versus Idiopathic SLE[a]

	Idiopathic SLE	Drug-Related Lupus
Clinical features		
Age	20–40	53–62
Sex (F : M)	9 : 1	6 : 4
Race	All	Not blacks
Acetylation type	Slow-fast	Slow
Onset of symptoms	Gradual	Abrupt
Constitutional symptoms (fever, malaise)	83%	50%
Arthralgia and arthritis	90%	95%
Pleuropericarditis	50%	50%
Hepatomegaly	25%	25%
Skin rash (all types)	74%	10–20%
Discoid lesions	20%	0%
Malar erythema	42%	2%
Renal disease	53%	5%
CNS disease	32%	0%
Hematologic disease	Common	Unusual
Immune abnormalities		
ANA	95%	95%
LE cells	90%	90%
Anti-RNP	40–50%	20%
Anti-Sm	20–30%	Rare
Anti-dsDNA	80%	Rare
Antihistone	25%	90%
Complement	Reduced	Normal
Immune complexes	Elevated	Normal

[a]Adapted from (7, 22–24)

have a milder clinical presentation with less organ involvement. Predominating clinical features include arthralgias, myalgias, weight loss, and malaise. Joint involvement tends to be nondeforming, migratory, and similar to that in idiopathic SLE, involving the smaller joints of the hands, elbows, knees, shoulders, and feet. Cardiopulmonary lesions can result in dyspnea, hemoptysis, pleuritis, pleural effusion, and pericarditis in 30 to 50% of patients. Renal and CNS findings are not common (<5%) in DRL, dermatologic manifestations (urticaria, purpura, malar rash) being found less often in DRL (2 to 20%) than in idiopathic SLE. Hematological abnormalities (leukopenia, thrombocytopenia) can occur, but they are much less severe than in idiopathic SLE. Signs and symptoms of drug-induced lupus usually occur within 3 months to 2 years after drug therapy is initiated. However, a few cases of DRL have occurred as early as 2 weeks and as late as 4 years after initiation of drug therapy. Drug-related lupus is also different from idiopathic SLE because it is reversible and signs and symptoms fade within days to weeks after discontinuation of the medication (14, 26–28).

Several laboratory tests are commonly used to help clinicians diagnose drug-related lupus in patients presenting with clinical signs and symptoms; these include ANA, dsDNA, and histone antibody tests. The commonly used ANA will be positive in 95% of DRL and idiopathic SLE patients, so a positive ANA may not differentiate between DRL and idiopathic SLE. However, if the ANA test is negative, DRL can be ruled out. Since many patients will develop a positive ANA test before having signs and symptoms of DRL, the combination of an ANA and clinical features are necessary for a a diagnosis of DRL to be considered. A positive dsDNA antibody test is indicative of idiopathic SLE (but not DRL), whereas a positive antihistone test is very common (90%) with DRL and less common (25%) with idiopathic SLE (Table 33.6) (26–28).

Procainamide

Procainamide-induced SLE is the most common drug-induced lupus, 90 percent of patients having positive ANA titers within 1 year of starting therapy. Approximately 30% of these patients will develop clinical signs of lupus within 3 months to 2 years (26–28). There appears to be a total dose relationship to procainamide-induced lupus, most patients having received ≥14 g (total dose) or a daily dose of >1600 mg. In addition, patients who have a slow acetylator phenotype will develop a positive ANA and DRL symptoms sooner than fast acetylators will. The most common signs and symptoms of procainamide-induced lupus are arthritis, pleuritis, and pleural effusions (26–28).

Hydralazine

The number of patients reported to have a positive ANA on hydralazine varies from 24 to 54%, with 2 to 21% of patients developing symptoms of DRL. The incidence of hydralazine-induced lupus is directly related to the dose, no cases having been reported in patients receiving less than 50 mg/day. Incidence rates increased from 4% to 12% as patients receive 100 mg/day and 200 mg/day, respectively. Hydralazine-induced symptoms are characterized as early and late onset. Patients suffering from early onset hydralazine-induced lupus complain primarily of fever and malaise that usually occur within the first 30 days of hydralazine therapy. Patients complaining of late onset hydralazine-induced lupus have signs and symptoms that usually start 2 years after initiation of therapy and include arthritis, myalgias, and rash. A few patients have been reported to have renal manifestations (27, 28).

Other medications that cause positive ANA tests include isoniazid (25%), chlorpromazine (20 to 50%), β-blockers (10 to 30%), and methyldopa (14 to 18%); however, few patients develop clinical features (27, 28). Treatment of drug-induced lupus consists of discontinuing the medication if symptoms of DRL are present and observation for resolution of signs and symptoms of lupus. Medical symptoms usually resolve in days to weeks; however, patients may have a positive ANA for months to years after discontinuation of the medication. Medications are often used to treat the signs and symptoms of drug-induced lupus based on the severity of the clinical features. Aspirin and other NSAIDs are used for patients complaining of arthralgias and myalgias. Patients suffering from more severe signs and symptoms may receive glucocorticoids (prednisone 0.5 to 1.0 mg/kg) for several weeks to resolve the drug-induced lupus more quickly (26, 28).

PROGNOSIS

The prognosis of SLE patients has improved over the last 30 years; 80 to 90% of patients survive at least 10 years, compared to earlier survival rates of 55 to 60%. This is believed to be a result of earlier detection, improved treatment modalities, and the availability of renal dialysis and transplantation. Several factors have been related to a poor outcome in SLE patients, and many of these prognostic indicators are used along with clinical signs and symptoms to monitor progression of the disease. Non-SLE factors that are thought to be related to a poorer prognosis include age at onset (early diagnosis, 15 to 30 years of age, being poor), female gender, and black race. Of these factors, the data is conflicting concerning age and gender, so these factors are considered to be very controversial. However, black patients are considered to have a worse prognosis than Caucasian patients. Lupus-specific factors that predict a poor prognosis include overall disease activity and involvement of major organs. In terms of overall disease activity, patients who have several flares that are unresponsive to high-dose steroid therapy usually have a worse prognosis. Patients with major organ involvement include patients who have renal and CNS manifestations. Patients with renal disease have a worse prognosis if they are noted to have proliferative nephritis (especially diffuse), a high activity index, and chronic sclerotic lesions on biopsy; smoking and hypertension severely worsen the prognosis. Patients with neurological involvement (psychoses, seizures, stroke, cognitive impairment) are also at increased risk of morbidity and mortality. Laboratory values that are associated with a poor prognosis and active disease include azotemia, elevated serum creatinine, increased urinary protein excretion, high levels of dsDNA antibodies, low levels of complement, the presence of complement fixation by the dsDNA antibodies, and prolonged and severe anemia. Since many of these laboratory values change with acute and active disease, they are used along with clinical symptoms to monitor the progression of SLE. High levels of dsDNA antibodies and low levels of C3 or CH_{50} are associated with active renal disease; these laboratory values normalize as the disease is successfully treated (3, 14, 17–18, 25).

TREATMENT

General Principles

SLE is an inflammatory disease that results in acute and chronic complications; therefore, treatment is aimed at relieving acute symptoms and preventing chronic complications. Specific goals of therapy must be tailored to the clinical manifestations of each patient. These include minimization of the signs and symptoms of active disease and normalization of laboratory values that are used to monitor SLE disease activity. These goals are achieved through the use of treatment (nonpharmacologic and pharmacologic) and the discriminate use of laboratory tests (Table 33.7).

Nonpharmacologic therapy includes education of the patient and his or her family; development of proper exercise, diet, and rest habits; and psychological and

Table 33.7.
Specific Goals of Therapy in Treating SLE

Minimize Signs/Symptoms	Treatment	
	Nonpharmacologic	Pharmacologic
Fatigue	Rest, minimize	
Arthralgias/myalgias	Rest	NSAIDs, steroids (if severe)
Fever	Watch for	Acetaminophen, antibiotics
Rash	Avoid sun, use sunscreen	Antimalarials, steroids
Pulmonary signs	Avoid smoking	NSAIDs, steroids, antimalarials,
Nephritis		Steroids, immunosuppressants
CNS signs	Psychotherapy	Antidepressants, antipsychotics, steroids, therapy for anemia type
Hematologic		
Normalize Laboratory	Desired goal	
Antibody levels (ANA, dsDNA, Sm, histone)	Decrease	
Complement levels (C4, CH50)	Increase	
Immunecomplexes	Decrease	
GFR (mL/min)	Increase	
Proteinuria (g/day)	Decrease	
Hematuria (RBC/hpf)	Decrease	

supportive therapies. Lupus patient education and support groups can be reached through the Lupus Foundation of America (1-800-558-0121) or the American Lupus Society (1-213-373-1335). Patients should be educated about the severity of their SLE, acute symptoms, the need for compliance with medications, and the adverse effects of their medications (5, 14). Patients should be instructed to minimize their exposure to direct sunlight, especially if they have a history of photosensitivity on exposure to ultraviolet light. These patients should never sunbathe, should apply sunscreen (SPF ≥15) to exposed body parts, and should wear long-sleeved shirts and broad-brimmed hats to minimize sun exposure when outdoors during the summer (5, 29).

Pharmacologic treatment varies with the severity of the disease. Nonmajor organ involvement usually requires short-term symptomatic treatment, since clinical features are not life-threatening. This includes arthritis/arthralgias, rashes, pleurisy, pericarditis, myositis, and constitutional symptoms such as fever, fatigue, and alopecia. These patients can often be managed with NSAIDs, antimalarial drugs, or low-dose glucocorticoids (15 to 30 mg/day of oral prednisone) to relieve symptoms. Rashes often do not require therapy, but when medication is necessary, the lesions often respond to potent topical steroids or antimalarial therapy. If patients experience a rash during tapering of oral steroid therapy, the rash will usually resolve on increasing the steroid dose. Myositis usually resolves as systemic symptoms dissipate; however, high-dose glucocorticoids (prednisone >40 mg/day) may be useful to decrease fatigue, muscle weakness, and enzyme abnormalities. Although fever is often seen in lupus patients and does respond to NSAID therapy, infection must be considered in all lupus patients as a source of the fever (5, 29).

Major organ involvement can include renal, CNS, pulmonary, vascular, and hematologic manifestations. In general, if SLE manifestations are life-threatening or major organs are at risk for irreversible damage, aggressive therapy (high-dose glucocorticoids, immunosuppressants) is considered. SLE major organ manifestations that respond to steroid therapy include myocarditis, pneumonitis, hematologic disease, CNS manifestations, and active forms of lupus nephritis. After therapy is initiated, patient signs and symptoms and laboratory values are monitored. Most patients respond within 3 to 4 weeks; some severe manifestations require longer to respond. Patients with mesangial (mild) nephritis are initially treated with prednisone (0.5 mg/kg/day); renal (proteinuria, hematuria, creatinine clearance) and immune abnormalities (serum complement, dsDNA antibodies) reverse in 2 to 4 weeks. If a response is not seen after 4 weeks, steroid doses can be increased or another medication can be added. (5, 14). Patients with severe

proliferative renal disease will usually display high levels of proteinuria and hematuria, have a creatinine clearance less than 50 mL/min, and have large increases and decreases of dsDNA antibodies and complement, respectively. Treatment must be more aggressive with oral prednisone 1 to 2 mg/kg/day for 6 to 10 weeks or pulse steroid therapy consisting of intravenous methylprednisolone (10 to 30 mg/kg/day or 500 to 1000 mg for 3 to 6 days) followed by high-dose (40 to 60 mg/day) oral prednisone. Most patients (75%) with severe disease (active nephritis, CNS, pneumonitis, vasculitis) begin to respond in a few days. Pulse doses of methylprednisolone for 1 to 3 days each month can be used to control some lupus patients without the addition of immunosuppressant agents (azathioprine, cyclophosphamide) (5, 14).

Although short-term trials of azathioprine compared to steroids do not show that it provides any additional benefits in treating lupus nephritis, long-term trials do suggest that azathioprine results in a better renal prognosis (fewer sclerotic changes on biopsy, overall improved renal function). Cyclophosphamide does provide additional benefit to steroid therapy in severe SLE nephritis, as is evidenced by fewer sclerotic lesions on biopsy and improved renal function. For patients with refractory nephritis who have active disease, some clinicians will use a combination of high-dose steroids, azathioprine, and cyclophosphamide, which can cause severe toxicity. For some patients, clinicians will try plasmapheresis.

Plasmapheresis (plasma exchange to reduce the concentration of circulating antibodies in the bloodstream) has been performed 2 to 4 times a week for 4 weeks along with immunosuppressive drugs to treat acute, severe glomerulonephritis. However, recent data from the Lupus Nephritis Collaborative Study Group suggests that plasmapheresis is not useful for the treatment of lupus nephritis (30). If all of these therapeutic modalities fail, the patients will progress to end-stage renal disease and require dialysis or renal transplantation (3, 5). Diagnosis of lupus involvement in the CNS is difficult, since the clinical presentation can be caused by other factors. There are no laboratory tests that are specific for CNS involvement in lupus patients, and high dsDNA antibodies and low serum complement do not correlate with CNS manifestations. Therefore, CNS involvement in lupus is a diagnosis of exclusion, and therapy consists of medications to treat each manifestation. Patients suffering from strokes may have a hypercoagulable state, which can be confirmed by the presence of antiphospholipid antibodies. These patients should be considered for long-term anticoagulation therapy with warfarin. Patients suffering from depressive or psychotic disorders should receive antidepressants or antipsychotics, respectively. Patients with seizures disorders secondary to CNS lupus are treated with anticonvulsant therapy (5, 21).

Many of the pulmonary manifestations in lupus (such as pulmonary edema) may be secondary to other problems associated with lupus (renal failure, CHF) and are treated by controlling the primary problems. Two serious pulmonary complications that are seen in patients with SLE include diffuse pneumonitis and bacterial pneumonia. The problem may be diagnosed by clinical presentation and the occasional use of a lung biopsy. Antibiotics should be used to treat the pneumonia, and steroid therapy should be used for the pneumonitis (5, 20, 29). Patients with active SLE often develop severe anemia of chronic disease (anemias caused by a chronic disease, e.g. renal disease, etc.), which reverses occasionally with NSAID therapy but most frequently with low-dose steroid therapy. Some patients suffer from a mild and transient thrombocytopenia, which usually does not require therapy. If platelet levels are less than 100,000/mm^3, patients will often respond to oral prednisone in doses of 30 to 50 mg/day. Patients should receive prednisone therapy until the platelet count rises to within the normal limits (5, 24). If this is unsuccessful, other therapies include intravenous gamma globulin (6 to 15 mg/kg/day for 4 to 7 days) or danazol (400 to 800 mg/day). Patients usually begin to respond in a few weeks.

Nonsteroidal Antiinflammatory Drugs (NSAIDS)

The first line of therapy for mild manifestations of SLE includes aspirin (salicylates) or other NSAIDs (Table 33.8). Salicylates and NSAIDs both have antipyretic, analgesic, and antiinflammatory effects, making them good for the signs and symptoms of lupus. These agents work primarily by inhibition of the cyclooxygenase enzyme, which is responsible for converting arachidonic acid to prostaglandins, which mediate inflammation. Other postulated mechanisms include inhibition of lipoxygenase and leukotriene

formation, decreasing chemotaxis, T- and B-cell proliferation, and inhibition of free radical formation. Selection of the most appropriate NSAID for the patient should be based on efficacy, toxicity, dosing convenience, and costs. Most clinical trials show that there are little if any differences in efficacy among aspirin and the NSAIDs, with slight differences among their adverse effect profiles. Therefore, selection of an NSAID for SLE is often based upon factors such as physician/patient preference, patient's tolerance to side effects, frequency of administration, and cost of therapy (31, 32). The information on NSAIDs pertaining to the pharmacokinetics, dose and administration, adverse effects and drug interactions, and patients who are at risk for them is outlined in Chapter 30.

Upon selection of NSAID therapy for treatment of lupus, patients should receive therapy for 2 to 4 weeks to evaluate the efficacy of the NSAID. If a particular NSAID is found to be ineffective or causes adverse effects, another NSAID should be selected and used for another 2- to 4-week trial period. No more than one NSAID should be used at a time, since no increase in efficacy has been demonstrated but increased side effects are possible (31, 32). If NSAID therapy fails, immunosuppressive agents such as glucocorticoids or antimalarials are often tried, depending on the lupus manifestation (Table 33.9).

Antimalarials

Patients presenting with lupus-induced rashes (from SLE or discoid lupus) are candidates for antimalarial treatment. The efficacy of antimalarial treatment has been well documented in patients with dermatologic manifestations (DLE, SCLE), 60 to 90% of patients responding to treatment (33). Although antimalarials are not considered to be effective for the major organ manifestations of SLE,

Table 33.8.
Nonsteroidal Antiinflammatory Drugs (NSAIDs)[a]

Drug	Trade Name	Half-life (h)	Daily Dose	Dosing Schedule
Diclofenac	Voltaren, Cataflam	2–3	100–200 mg	B.I.D.–Q.I.D.
Diflunisal	Dolobid	7–15	500–1000 mg	B.I.D.
Etodolac	Lodine	7–8	400–900 mg	B.I.D.–T.I.D.
Fenoprofen	Nalfon	2–3	1.2–3.2 g	T.I.D.–Q.I.D.
Flurbiprofen	Ansaid	3–4	200–300 mg	B.I.D.–T.I.D.
Ibuprofen	Motrin, Rufen	1–3	1.2–3.2 g	T.I.D.–Q.I.D.
Indomethacin	Indocin	3–4	50–200 mg	B.I.D.–Q.I.D.
Ketoprofen	Orudis, Oruvail	2–4	150–300 mg	T.I.D.–Q.I.D.
Ketorolac	Toradol	4–9	20–40 mg	T.I.D.–Q.I.D.
Meclofenamate	Meclomen	2–3	200–400 mg	Q.I.D.
Nabumetone	Relafen	22–30	500–2000 mg	Q.D.
Naproxen	Naprosyn, Anaprox	12–15	0.5–1.1 g	B.I.D.
Oxaprozin	Daypro	42–50	600–1800 mg	Q.D.
Piroxicam	Feldene	14–158	20 mg	Q.D.
Sulindac	Clinoril	16–18	200–400 mg	B.I.D.
Tolmetin	Tolectin	2–7	0.6–2.0 g	Q.I.D.

[a]Adapted from reference 30.

Table 33.9.
Corticosteroids and Immunosuppressive Agents

Drug	Trade Name	Dose/Schedule	Indications
Hydroxychloroquine	Plaquenil	200–600 mg P.O. divided B.I.D.	Mild disease rashes, arthritis, serositis
Chloroquine	Aralen	125–500 mg P.O. divided B.I.D.	
Prednisone	Various	0.5–1.0 mg/kg P.O. daily	Mild disease
		1.0–2.0 mg/kg P.O. daily	Moderate–severe disease, renal, CNS, refractory symptoms
Methylprednisolone	Various	10–30 mg/kg daily OR 0.5–1 g I.V. daily × 3–6 days	Severe disease
Azathioprine	Imuran	1–4 mg/kg P.O. daily	Severe disease
Cyclophosphamide	Cytoxan	1–4 mg/kg P.O. daily	Severe disease
		0.5–1.0 g/m² every 1–3 months	
Methotrexate	Rheumatrex	7.5–15 mg P.O. each week	Mild–moderate disease
Cyclosporin	Sandimmune	5 mg/kg daily	Not defined yet

antimalarials have been shown to have some beneficial effects for the treatment and prevention of mild or nonmajor organ involvement (arthritis, fever, fatigue, serositis, thromboembolic events). In addition, antimalarial therapy has allowed clinicians to reduce steroid doses in some patients when treating mild to moderate SLE conditions (33, 34). Several mechanisms of action have been proposed for antimalarial medications. These include stabilization of lysosomal membranes, inhibiting lysosomal enzyme release; binding to DNA substrates, thus interfering with DNA antibody attacks; a decrease in prostaglandin and leukotriene production; and inhibition of chemotaxis and phagocytosis by neutrophils (33, 34).

The antimalarials that are most frequently used to treat SLE manifestations are chloroquine and hydroxychloroquine. Patients initially receive chloroquine (250 mg/day) or hydroxychloroquine (400 to 600 mg/day) for the first 1 to 2 weeks of therapy, most patients showing regression of erythematous skin lesions during the first 2 weeks. Patients should continue to receive maintenance doses of chloroquine (125 to 250 mg/day) or hydroxychloroquine (200 mg/day) for several months until the SLE manifestations have been completely resolved. The optimal duration of therapy is not well established, but attempts should be made to taper antimalarial therapy by administrating very low doses 2 to 3 times weekly before discontinuation of therapy. Unfortunately, in the majority of patients (90%), symptoms will return within 3 years of stopping therapy (33).

The antimalarials are rapidly and almost completely absorbed from the gastrointestinal tract on oral administration; food enhances absorption. These drugs are widely distributed; this explains adverse effects such as mild neurotoxicity, retinal deposits, and drug-induced rashes. Antimalarials are eliminated primarily by renal excretion (70 to 75%), the remainder being metabolized. Little information exists on alteration of doses in hepatic or renal impairment (33, 34).

Antimalarial medications cause several adverse effects but are generally considered to be safe, and hydroxychloroquine is reported to have fewer adverse effects than chloroquine has. The most common adverse effects are gastrointestinal (epigastric burning, abdominal bloating, nausea, vomiting), which usually begin shortly after initiation of therapy. These and other adverse effects appear to be dose-related and can be minimized by splitting the total daily dose (200 mg twice a day instead of 400 mg every morning) administrating antimalarials with food, and using small maintenance doses after the initial treatment period (33).

Since antimalarial medications are well distributed to the skin, patients may experience cutaneous lesions or pigmentary changes. Rashes tend to be morbilliform, maculopapular, or urticarial in presentation. Pigmentation changes include graying of the hair or blue-black discoloration of the skin. Neurologic side effects include headache, insomnia, and nervousness, which are usually mild and can be minimized by using lower doses. Muscle weakness in the proximal lower extremities has been reported after patients have received several months of antimalarial therapy and is often confused with glucocorticoid-induced muscle weakness (33).

Antimalarials can cause three types of ocular toxicity, two of which-accommodation changes causing blurred or double vision and corneal deposits associated with halos around lights-are benign and reversible. The most serious and publicized adverse effect of antimalarials is retinal toxicity, which can lead to irreversible changes in vision. Early manifestations (premaculopathy) include changes in color vision with a loss of visual field tests to red objects due to destruction of rods and cones because of deposition of these medications in the pigment layers of the retina. These patients usually have mild pigmentary changes, and the visual changes are reversible if the medication is discontinued. Patients who have extensive pigmentary changes will develop a bull's eye retinal lesion, which leads to permanent visual field defects (33, 34). The risk of retinal toxicity is related to total daily dose and not the duration of therapy or cumulative dose. Patients who are at risk for retinal toxicity are usually more than 65 years of age and have received daily doses greater than 6.5 mg/kg of hydroxychloroquine or 4 mg/kg of chloroquine. If a patient is discovered to have retinal lesions (even if they are asymptomatic), therapy should be discontinued. If these doses are not exceeded, retinal toxicity is not common. Although many of the retinal lesions will reverse upon discontinuation of antimalarial therapy, patients should have ophthalmic examinations (funduscopy, visual acuity, color tests) performed before initiation of therapy and every 6 months while receiving antimalarial therapy (33, 34).

Corticosteroids

Corticosteroid therapy is considered a mainstay in the treatment of SLE for reducing mild to severe inflammatory signs and symptoms during the first or acute episodes of the disease. The therapeutic effect is thought to be due to the antiinflammatory and immunosuppressive actions of corticosteroids. Steroid therapy should not be automatically initiated for mild SLE manifestations but should be reserved for clinical manifestations that are serious or life-threatening or in circumstances in which the patient is not responsive to NSAIDs or antimalarial therapy. Specific indications for corticosteroid use include severe serositis (pleuritis or pericarditis), immune-mediated hematologic abnormalities (thrombocytopenia or hemolytic anemia), renal disease, severe CNS disease, or severe constitutional symptoms. Topical steroids are indicated for dermatologic manifestations of SLE.

The goals of treatment with corticosteroids are: (1) to relieve the symptoms; (2) to sustain improvement in the clinical manifestations; (3) to normalize laboratory abnormalities (Table 33.2); and (4) to decrease antibody concentrations which may be elevated (Table 33.4). Intravenous infusions commonly result in prompt relief of fulminant disease and can be lifesaving. Prednisone is the oral corticosteroid that is used more frequently than others (e.g., dexamethasone) because of its shorter biologic half-life and subsequent ease in switching to alternate-day therapy. Prednisone doses vary from 0.5 to 1.0 mg/kg/day in mild SLE to 1 to 2 mg/kg/day in acute, severe SLE. Methylprednisolone is the most common intravenous form (15 mg/kg over 30 min) of corticosteroid used (29, 35).

Once the therapeutic goals are achieved, treatment decisions are based on controlling signs and symptoms and minimizing drug toxicity. After the disease has been controlled for at least 2 weeks, the steroid regimen should be changed to once-daily dosing. After the patient has been asymptomatic for another 2 weeks, the dose should be tapered, the ultimate goal being alternate-day dosing

and possibly discontinuation. Special precautions are warranted in tapering prednisone doses of 20 mg/day or less and transferring to alternate-day dosing, since adrenal insufficiency due to hypothalamic-pituitary-adrenal (HPA) suppression from steroid use can occur. An example of a tapering schedule is as follows: 20 mg/day for 2 weeks, 17.5 mg/day for 3 weeks, 15 mg/day for 4 weeks, then 15 mg/day alternating with 12.5 mg/day for 2 to 4 weeks, 15 mg/day alternating with 10 mg/day for 2 to 4 weeks, 15 mg/day alternating with 7.5 mg/day for 2 to 4 weeks, 15 mg/day alternating with 5 mg/day for 2 to 4 weeks, 15 mg/day alternating with 2.5 mg/day for 2 to 4 weeks, then 20 mg alternating with 0 mg every other day for 4 weeks, then 17.5 mg alternating with 0 mg every other day for 4 weeks, and so on until the patient is off the prednisone therapy. This schedule may take 6 months to a year or even longer if disease exacerbations occur. A patient with non-major organ involvement may allow a faster tapering schedule, and patients with severe disease may require slower tapering schedules. Flares without major organ involvement (e.g., fatigue, fever, arthralgias, or serositis) may simply respond to reverting back to the previous dose until the symptoms resolve or adding NSAIDs or hydroxychloroquine. Major organ involvement during a flare (e.g., nephritis) may not be controlled by reverting to the previous dose; it may be necessary to use very high doses to control these signs and symptoms, which will subsequently require a new, slower tapering schedule.

Recent studies suggest that high-dose oral prednisone and/or low-dose oral cyclophosphamide or pulse intravenous cyclophosphamide reduces lupus nephritis morbidity, maintains renal function, and stabilizes serologic markers. The Lupus Nephritis Collaborative Study Group also documented two important issues: (a) the utility of initial serum creatinine values in predicting renal failure and (b) the concept that plasmapheresis most likely has no role in treatment protocols (30, 36, 37).

In addition to the previously described HPA suppression with chronic steroid use, other complications that result from prolonged steroid therapy include fluid and electrolyte disturbances, hypertension, peptic ulceration, osteoporosis, myopathy, increased susceptibility to infections including tuberculosis, cataracts, growth arrest, hyperglycemia, and Cushing's habitus. All of these are elaborated in Chapter 30, which covers systemic corticosteroid therapy.

Cyclophosphamide

A group of medications that are used frequently for moderate-to-severe SLE manifestations are the alkylating agents, which fundamentally disturb cell growth, mitotic activity, differentiation, and cell function. These cytotoxic agents inhibit DNA formation in a nonspecific manner, unrelated to cell cycle. This results in the death of cells that contribute to the inflammatory response (neutrophils, T and B lymphocytes). Suppression of B lymphocytes results in a direct suppression of antibody (IgG) formation, which additionally reduces the inflammatory response. Unfortunately, if high doses of these medications are given, the death of these cells results in immunosuppression and places patients at risk for neutropenia and infection (38). Cyclophosphamide is currently the most widely used and studied alkylating agent in the treatment of SLE and is usually reserved for patients with lupus nephritis, CNS manifestations of lupus, and resistance to other, less toxic therapies.

Cyclophosphamide is well-absorbed, so it can be administered either orally or intravenously. Approximately 70% of cyclophosphamide is metabolized with metabolites, and 30% of unchanged drug is excreted by the kidney; therefore, dosages must be adjusted in renally impaired patients (39). Despite the fact that cyclophosphamide is metabolized by the cytochrome oxidase pathways, medications that are known to effect microsomal enzymes (cimetidine and barbiturates) do not usually cause clinically significant drug interactions (38).

Both low oral doses and high intravenous doses of cyclophosphamide are used. The oral dosages range between 1 and 4 mg/kg/day for 4 to 8 weeks, and the intravenous dosages range between 500 and 1000 mg/M^2 every 4 weeks for variable lengths of time determined by the patient response (38–40). Clinical effects are usually seen within 2 to 3 weeks of therapy; white blood cell counts (primarily neutrophils) also reach nadirs at this point. Immunosuppressive effects are thought to be worse in using daily oral cyclophosphamide compared to intermittent monthly intravenous boluses. Regardless, patients must have their granulocyte counts monitored on a frequent basis to maintain cell counts that are not less than 1000 to 300/mm3. If granulocyte levels fall below 300/mm^3, doses should be adjusted appropriately (38, 39).

Hemorrhagic cystitis can occur in 20 to 30% of patients receiving chronic cyclophosphamide therapy. In most patients the cystitis resolves on a dose reduction or discontinuation of cyclophosphamide; however, chronic administration can result in further hemorrhage and bladder carcinomas. This may be minimized by using intravenous bolus doses (rather than oral administration) and by increasing fluid intake to maintain adequate hydration of the bladder 24 hours before, during, and after administration of the drug. This enhances excretion of the cyclophosphamide and decreases contact with the bladder, which is the cause of the hemorrhagic cystitis (29, 38). Other adverse effects to cyclophosphamide include dose-related nausea and vomiting (which are prevented with antiemetics) and alopecia, which is reversible. In addition to the adverse drug reactions (ADRs)

listed previously, other ADRs that occur from chronic administration include gonadal suppression (temporary or permanent decreases in sperm or ova production) and pulmonary and cardiac inflammatory complications (29, 38, 39).

Cyclophosphamide has been shown to decrease proteinuria, DNA antibodies, and serum creatinine (slightly) and to increase complement (C3) levels when the lupus nephritis is resolving. Studies have shown that the addition of cyclophosphamide to the drug therapy of patients with lupus nephritis who are refractory to high-dose steroid therapy decreases the progression to end-stage renal disease and lowers the daily requirements of glucocorticoids (36–38, 40–43). Because recent studies have evaluated the long-term efficacy and safety of low-dose and/or intermittent boluses of cyclophosphamide with oral steroids, future studies need to concentrate on comparing and contrasting therapies to determine the most efficacious approach to the treatment and prevention of renal deterioration.

Azathioprine

Azathioprine is used alone and in combination for the treatment of SLE. Like other cytotoxic agents (e.g., cyclophosphamide), azathioprine is not as effective as corticosteroids in the treatment of symptomatic, multisystem SLE when used alone. However, azathioprine augments glucocorticoid therapy in SLE patients who have renal disease and during acute, severe episodes of SLE that are not fully controlled with prednisone alone or prednisone and cyclophosphamide. Azathioprine is most effective in patients with resistant discoid lupus and SLE patients with minimal renal involvement (38, 40). Austin and colleagues demonstrated that patients had better outcomes when they were treated with either azathioprine or cyclophosphamide at low doses along with low-dose prednisone than in patients who are given prednisone alone (36). Azathioprine is generally considered to be well tolerated by patients and possibly less toxic than cyclophosphamide except for the oncogenic properties. Serious adverse effects may occur with its use, including herpes zoster, sterility, cancer, hepatic toxicity, and hematologic/lymphoreticular toxicity (leukopenia, non-Hodgkin's lymphoma, leukemia, and thrombocytopenia) (29, 36, 40, 45).

Azathioprine is given orally in doses starting at 0.5 mg/kg/day and titrated upward to doses of 4 mg/kg/day. Patients on azathioprine should be monitored for hematopoietic or lymphoreticular toxicity every 2 weeks during the first 3 months of therapy while doses are being adjusted, then monthly while patients are receiving therapy. Baseline liver functions tests should be performed, and liver function should be monitored every 6 months during therapy (5, 38).

Methotrexate

Limited studies have been performed using methotrexate to treat SLE and/or its manifestations (5, 29). Rothenberg and co-workers suggest that methotrexate is a rational therapeutic alternative to antimalarials or low-dose corticosteroids and may be particularly useful in the management of SLE in the presence of arthritis, skin rashes, serositis, or fever (44). The usual dosages that are used in SLE treatment are 7.5 to 15 mg orally once a week, which are comparable to dosage regimens that are used in rheumatoid arthritis. Adverse effects include leukopenia, thrombocytopenia, hepatotoxicity, gastrointestinal disturbances, oral mucositis, teratogencity, and renal impairment. Therefore, patients should be monitored like patients receiving methotrexate for rheumatoid arthritis (Chapter 30) with dosage adjustments for patients with renal impairment (5, 29, 38).

Cyclosporine

Cyclosporine is considered an experimental or investigational drug in the treatment of SLE, and few clinical trials have been performed involving SLE patients (5, 29, 46). Most patients who are treated with cyclosporine develop increased high blood pressure or elevated serum creatinine, which can be particularly harmful in patients with SLE (5). Recently, Hussein and colleagues studied and recommended consideration for cyclosporine use in treating lupus nephritis during pregnancy because of its established safety concerning teratogenicity in renal transplant recipients (47). Further study is highly recommended because the majority of their patients developed hypertension. Additional adverse drug effects include hirsutism and tremor. This agent should be considered only in patients with severe, steroid-resistant SLE who cannot be considered as candidates for cytotoxic agents. Doses that have been used are low (e.g., 5 mg/kg/day).

PREGNANCY AND LUPUS

There are several important issues regarding the relationship between pregnancy and SLE. These issues include increased lupus activity (flares) during pregnancy, the impact of SLE on fetal outcome and premature delivery, and the use of medications for SLE in pregnant patients. Most resources report that 50 to 60% of pregnant patients with lupus will experience a flare of their lupus, usually during the third trimester of their pregnancies. Over 85% of these flares are mild to moderate and require little or no increase of the patients' medications (prednisone) or the addition of medications to treat these flares, and few result in renal failure. Laboratory values that are consistent with an increase in lupus activity usually reveal a decrease in CH_{50} levels and worsening renal values.

Although many pregnant SLE patients reach full-term pregnancy and most infants are normal upon delivery, SLE activity during pregnancy can cause up to 12 to 30% more fetal loss (miscarriage, stillbirth) and 20 to 50% more premature deliveries compared to pregnant patients without lupus. Fetal loss and premature delivery have been directly related to the following exacerbations during pregnancy: worsening renal disease and hypertension, elevations of anti-dsDNA and phospholipid antibodies (e.g., lupus anticoagulant and cardiolipin antibodies), and possibly decreased levels of serum complement (CH_{50}). Therefore, clinicians should consider monitoring pregnant patients closely (especially as they enter the third trimester), including monitoring of serum creatinine, complete blood cell count, urinalysis for protein, and serological tests for CH_{50}, anti-dsDNA, and antiphospholipid antibodies (48).

Most pregnant patients will need to maintain their lupus medication treatment during pregnancy to prevent maternal and fetal adverse outcomes. Corticosteroids are considered the drugs of choice in pregnant patients because of their efficacy and relative few adverse effects compared to other medications. Although corticosteroids cross the placenta, much is metabolized by placental hydroxygenase before it reaches the fetus. Few problems are noted in the mother or fetus when patients have received prednisone or other steroids for the treatment of SLE. In addition, steroids may actually be beneficial in causing fetal lung maturation. NSAIDs and aspirin are relatively safe (pregnancy category B) during the first trimester but are considered harmful (pregnancy category D) during the second and third trimesters because of their effects on premature closure of the ductus arteriosus. Ironically, low-dose aspirin (81 mg/day) is often used during lupus pregnancies that are complicated by antiphospholipid antibodies (lupus anticoagulant, anticardiolipin antibodies) to decrease fetal complications. If NSAIDs or aspirin is used during pregnancy, use should be restricted to the lowest possible dose, and these medications should be restricted for use in the first trimester. Although the data on use of antimalarial drugs in pregnant humans is sparse, the information that is available does not indicate that these medications are teratogenic. Although doses that are used for prophylaxis of malaria do not seem to predispose the fetus to risk of teratogenic abnormalities, doses of antimalarials that are used for SLE have been associated with congenital abnormalities in a few case reports. Despite the possible risk of antimalarials, most experts agree that a patient with uncontrolled (active) lupus has a greater chance of experiencing spontaneous abortion or neonatal death than an improbable teratogenic risk. Therefore, if patients are on antimalarial medications when they become pregnant, they should remain on these medications throughout pregnancy. Immunosuppressant medications (azathioprine, cyclophosphamide) have been associated with teratogenicity (pregnancy category D) and should be avoided if possible (48).

CONCLUSION

Systemic lupus erythematosus is a multisystem disease consisting primarily of abnormal autoantibody production. The disease course and prognosis are highly variable among patients, but marked improvement in survival and quality of life provides hope to the patients. Today, health care providers have greater opportunities in disease identification, prognosis indicators, refined therapies, and improved guidelines for drug therapy use.

REFERENCES

1. Pisetsky DS. Systemic lupus erythematosus: epidemiology, pathology, and pathogenesis. In: Schumacher HR, ed. Primer on rheumatic diseases. 10th ed. Atlanta: Arthritis Foundation, 1993:100–105.
2. Sontheimer RD, Gilliam, JN. Systemic lupus erythematous and the skin. In: Lahita, RG, ed. Systemic lupus erythematous. 2nd ed. New York: Churchill-Livingston, 1992:657–681.
3. Ponticelli C. Current treatment recommendations for lupus nephritis. Drugs 40(1):19–30, 1990.
4. Gladman DD. Indicators of disease activity, prognosis, and treatment of systemic lupus erythematosus. Curr Opin Rheumatol 5:587–595, 1993.
5. Hahn, BH. Management of systemic lupus erythematous. In: Kelley WN, Harris ED, Ruddy S, Sledge CB, eds. Textbook of rheumatology. 4th ed. Philadelphia: WB Saunders, 1993:1043–1056.
6. Hochberg MC. Epidemiology of systemic lupus erythematosus. In: Lahita, RG, ed. Systemic lupus erythematosus. 2nd ed. New York: Churchill-Livingston, 1992:103–116.
7. Fessel WJ. Systemic lupus erythematous in the community: incidence, prevalence, outcome and first symptoms; the high prevalence in black woman. Arch Intern Med 134:1027–1035, 1974.
8. Michet CJ Jr, McKenna CH, Elvaback LR. Epidemiology of systemic lupus erythematous and other connective diseases in Rochester, Minnesota, 1950 through 1979. Mayo Clin Proc 60:105–113, 1985.
9. Hochberg MC. The incidence of systemic lupus erythematous in Baltimore, Maryland, 1970–1977. Arthritis Rheum 28:80–86, 1985.
10. Hopkinson N. Epidemiology of systemic lupus erythematosus. Ann Rheum Dis 51:1292–94, 1992.
11. Woods, VL. Pathogenesis of systemic lupus erythematosus. In: Kelley WN, Harris ED, Ruddy S, Sledge CB, eds. Textbook of rheumatology, 4th ed. Philadelphia: WB Saunders, 1993:999–1016.
12. McCruden, AB, Stimson, WH. Sex hormones and immune function. In: Ader, R, Felton, DL and Cohen, N (eds). Psychoneuroimmunology. San Diego: Academic Press, 1991:475–493.
13. Tan EM, Cohen AS, Fries JF, et al. The 1982 revised criteria for the classification of systemic lupus erythematous. Arthritis Rheum 25:1271–1277, 1982.
14. Schur PH. Clinical features of SLE. In: Kelley WN, Harris ED, Ruddy S, Sledge CB (eds.). Textbook of Rheumatology. 4th ed. Philadelphia, WB Saunders Co., 1993:1017–1042.
15. Venables PJ. Diagnosis and treatment of systemic lupus erythematosus. Br Med J 307:663–667, 1993.
16. Feldman DS, Zuckerman JD, Buyon JP. Articular manifestations of systemic lupus erythematosus. In: Lahita, RG, ed. Systemic lupus erythematosus. 2nd ed. New York: Churchill-Livingston, 1992:823–844.

17. Pollack VE, Kant KS. Systemic lupus erythematous and the kidney. In: Lahita, RG, ed. Systemic lupus erythematous. 2nd ed. New York: Churchill-Livingston, 1992:683–706.
18. Appel GB, Cohen DJ, Pirani CL, et al. Long-term follow of patients with lupus nephritis: a study based on the classification of the World Health Organization. Am J Med 83:877–885, 1987.
19. Ginzler EM, Antoniadis I. Clinical manifestations of systemic lupus erythematosus, measures of disease activity, and long-term complications. Curr Opin Rheumatol 4:672–680, 1992.
20. Lawrence EC. Systemic lupus erythematosus and the lung. In: Lahita, RG, ed. Systemic lupus erythematous. 2nd ed. New York: Churchill-Livingston, 1992:731–745.
21. West SG. Neuropsychiatric lupus. Rheum Disease Clin North Am 20(1):129–158, 1994.
22. Iverson GL. Psychology associated with systemic lupus erythematosus: a methodological review. Semin Arthritis Rheum 22(4):242–251, 1993.
23. Stevens, MB. Systemic lupus erythematous and the cardiovascular system. In: Lahita, RG., ed. Systemic lupus erythematous. 2nd ed. New York: Churchill-Livingston, 1992:707–717.
24. Laurence J, Wing JL, and Nachman R. The cellular hematology of systemic lupus erythematosus. In: Lahita, RG., ed. Systemic lupus erythematous. 2nd ed. New York: Churchill-Livingston, 1992:771–805.
25. Craft J, Hardin JA. Antinuclear antibodies. In: Kelley WN, Harris ED, Ruddy S, Sledge CB, eds. Textbook of rheumatology, 4th ed. Philadelphia: WB Saunders, 1993:164–187.
26. Hess EV, Mongey AB. Drug related lupus: the same or different from idiopathic disease? In: Lahita, RG, ed. Systemic lupus erythematous. New York: Churchill-Livingston, 1992:893–904.
27. Stratton MA Drug-induced systemic lupus erythematous. Clin Pharm 4:657–663, 1985.
28. Skaer TL Medication-induced systemic lupus erythematosus. Clin Therapeut 14(4):497–506, 1992.
29. Klippel JH. Systemic lupus erythematous: treatment. In: Schumacher HR, ed. Primer on rheumatic diseases. 10th ed. Atlanta: Arthritis Foundation, 1993:112–115.
30. Lewis EJ, Hunsicker LG, Lan S-P, et al. for The Lupus Nephritis Collaborative Study Group. A controlled trial of plasmapheresis therapy in severe lupus nephritis. N Engl J Med 326:1373–1379, 1992.
31. Clements PJ, Paulus HE. Nonsteroidal anti-inflammatory drugs (NSAIDs). In: Kelley WN, Harris ED, Ruddy S, Sledge CB, eds. Textbook of rheumatology. 4th ed. Philadelphia: WB Saunders, 1993:700–730.
32. Furst DE. Are there dfferences among nonsteroidal antiinflammatory drugs? Arthritis Rheum 37(1):1–9, 1994.
33. Rynes RI. Antimalarial drugs. In: Kelley WN, Harris ED, Ruddy S, Sledge CB, eds. Textbook of rheumatology. 4th ed. Philadelphia: WB Saunders, 1993:731–742.
34. Wallace DJ. Antimalarial agents and lupus. Rheumat Disease Clin North Am 20(1):243–263, 1994.
35. Haynes RC. Adrenocorticotropic hormone: adrenocortical steroids and their synthetic analogs; inhibitors of the synthesis and actions of adrenocortical hormones. In: Gilman AG et al., eds. The pharmacological basis of therapeutics. 8th ed. New York: Pergamon Press, 1990:1431–1462.
36. Austin HA, Klippel JH, Balow JE, et al. Therapy of lupus nephritis: controlled trial of prednisone and cytotoxic drugs. N Engl J Med 314:614–619, 1986.
37. Levey AS, Lan S-P, Corwin HL, et al. and the Lupus Nephritis Collaborative Study Group. Progression and remission of renal disease in the lupus nephritis collaborative study. Ann Intern Med 116:114–123, 1992.

38. Fauci AS, Young KR Jr. Immunoregulatory agents. In: Kelley WN, Harris ED, Ruddy S, Sledge CB. Textbook of rheumatology. 4th ed. Philadelphia: WB Saunders, 1993:797–821.

39. Calabresi P, Chabner BA. Antineoplastic agents. In: Gilman AG, et al., eds. The pharmacological basis of therapeutics. 8th ed. New York: Pergamon Press, 1990:1209–1263.

40. Dinant HT, Decker JL, Klippel JH, et al. Alternate modes of cyclophosphamide and azathioprine therapy in lupus nephritis. Ann Intern Med 96:728–736, 1982.

41. McCune WJ, Golbus J, Zeldes W, et al. Clinical and immunologic effects of monthly administration of intravenous cyclophosphamide in severe systemic lupus erythematous. N Engl J Med 318(22):1423–1431, 1988.

42. Boumpas DT, Austin HA, Balow JE, et al. Therapy of lupus nephritis: controlled trial of pulse methylprednisolone versus two different regimens of pulse cyclophosphamide. Lancet 340:741–744, 1992.

43. Moroni G, Banfi G, Ponticelli C. Clinical status of patients after 10 years of lupus nephritis. Quart J Med 84:681–689, 1992.

44. Rothenberg RJ, Graziano FM, Grandone JT, et al. The use of methotrexate in steroid-resistant systemic lupus erythematosus. Arthritis Rheum 31:612–615, 1988.

45. Balow JE: Lupus nephritis: natural history, prognosis and treatment. Clin Immunol Allergy 6:353–366, 1986.

46. Favre H, Miescher PA, Huang YP, et al. Cyclosporin in the treatment of lupus nephritis. Am J Nephrol 9(suppl 1):57–60, 1989.

47. Hussein MM, Mooij JM, Roujouleh H. Cyclosporine in the treatment of lupus nephritis including two patients treated during pregnancy. Clin Nephrol 40(3):160–163, 1993.

48. Petri M. Systemic lupus erythematosus and pregnancy. Rheum Disease Clin North Am 20(1):87–118, 1994.

CHAPTER 34

OSTEOPOROSIS AND OSTEOMALACIA

REBECCA ROGERS PREVOST

Osteoporosis and osteomalacia are two diseases of the calcified connective tissue, bone. They differ from each other etiologically, but the primary pathologic difference is that though both disorders cause deficient mineralization of bone, osteoporosis also results in loss of bone matrix. These disorders may be silent for an extended period, which results in a delay of diagnosis. It is possible for patients to suffer from both disorders concomitantly, but they may present independent of one another. Typically, osteomalacia is diagnosed in children visually by the bending of long bones. Osteoporosis is confirmed after a fracture or multiple fractures have occurred, which leads to significant morbidity and loss of independence for many, particularly the elderly. As the population ages, osteoporosis and osteomalacia will become increasingly prevalent. Billions of health care dollars are spent yearly on treatment after diagnosis of these potentially preventable disorders. Therefore, prevention must become the cornerstone of therapy. This chapter will address the pathophysiology and etiology of osteoporosis and osteomalacia, then focus on the various diagnostic, therapeutic, and preventive modalities in current use.

OSTEOPOROSIS

Osteoporosis can be divided into several types. Type I is associated with accelerated bone loss (2 to 3% of total bone per year) beginning with the onset of menopause and lasting approximately 10 years if no intervention is implemented. This results in an increased risk of vertebral compression and distal forearm fractures approximately 20 years after onset. Type II is more insidious, causing slow, progressive bone loss (approximately 0.5 to 1% per year) over many years, resulting in hip and vertebral fractures in both men and women over the age of 70 (1). Therefore, osteoporosis is primarily a disease of the aged. It is estimated that 3500 American women enter menopause every day, and that during the next decade, this population will grow to between 40 and 60 million women (2).

A third type is known as secondary osteoporosis. Medical therapies that can cause drug-induced osteoporosis are glucocorticoids, gonadotropin-releasing hormone (GnRH) agonists, and heparin. Immobilization due to accidents or serious illness can also result in bone loss. Secondary osteoporosis can occur at any age.

Physiology

Skeletal formation begins during the 6th week of embryologic development, when mesenchymal cells differentiate into chondrocytes, which form a cartilagenous skeleton. Shortly thereafter, calcification begins, and growth plates are formed on the bone ends (3). The skeletal mass of infants doubles in the first year of life, and 37% of the total skeletal mass is accumulated during adolescence. Skeletal growth continues until genetic height is attained, but mineralization of bone continues until the third decade (4, 5). Infants, children, and adolescents have a greater ability to retain ingested calcium than adults, which aids in attainment of desired peak bone mass. Adequate calcium intake during the years of skeletal growth and mineralization is obviously vital. Exercise to produce dense bone is also very important. Several growth factors are also involved in optimal bone production, but their exact roles have not been elucidated.

Bone loss (resorption) and formation is a dynamic process that occurs throughout life. These two opposing processes are usually coupled in bone-remodeling units (BRU); there are greater than 1 million active BRUs, involving 15 to 20% of the bone surface, at any given time (6). This is shown schematically in Figure 34.1 (7). The importance of BRUs lies in two goals: (1) to provide the serum with a readily available source of calcium for maintenance of physiologic processes such as muscle contraction and nerve conduction, and (2) to strengthen, revitalize, and rehydrate the bone matrix.

One of the first signals to bone matrix for the initiation of bone resorption is a decrease in serum calcium below the normal values of 9 to 11 mg/dL. Hypocalcemia causes secretion of parathyroid hormone (PTH) from the four parathyroid glands located in the neck adjacent to the thyroid gland. PTH not only initiates bone resorption but also causes three additional actions aimed at increasing serum calcium: inhibition of renal phosphorus reabsorption, increased renal calcium reabsorption, increased renal production of 1,25 hydroxyvitamin D [1,25 $(OH)_2$-D)], which increases dietary calcium absorption from the gastrointestinal tract. Gut absorption of calcium is by active transport in the distal duodenum and proximal jejunum. 1,25 (OH)-D induces calcium-binding proteins to carry calcium through the gut cell wall. If gastrointestinal concentrations of phosphorus, dietary phytates or oxalates, or free fatty acids is high, this process is impaired. Calcium

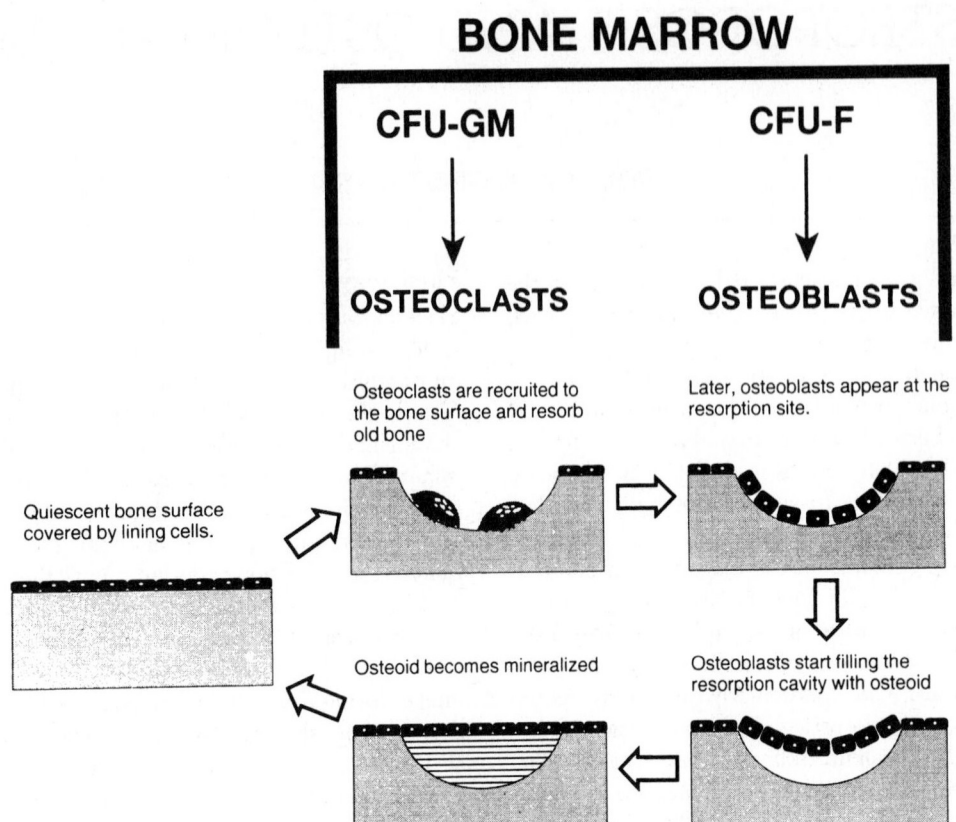

Figure 34.1. The relation between bone marrow and the bone-remodeling process. Replenishment of osteoclasts and osteoblasts from their respective hematopoietic progenitors (granulocyte-macrophage colony-forming units [CFU-GM]) and mesenchymal progenitors (fibroblast colony-forming units [CFU-F]) in the bone marrow is critical for remodeling, which is accomplished by cycles involving the resorption of old bone by osteoclasts and the subsequent formation of new bone by osteoblasts. Reprinted by permission.

can also undergo passive absorption if gastrointestinal concentrations are very high and an acidic medium is present.

When bone resorption begins, evidence suggests that surface osteocytes (inactive osteoblasts) contract to allow osteoclasts exposure to mineralized bone matrix (Figure 34.1). Osteoclasts secrete collagenases and proteinases that solubilize the bone matrix to a depth of approximately 1 mm^3. The goal of calcium release is therefore accomplished. This is followed in several days by the influx of osteoblasts to begin new bone synthesis. Osteoblasts promote collagen synthesis into new bone matrix, also known as osteoid, over a period of about 10 days. Next, the new bone must become mineralized with hydroxypapatite, a compound primarily consisting of calcium and phosphorus, having the chemical structure $Ca_{10}(PO_4)_6(OH)_2$. The bone matrix also contains sodium, potassium, magnesium, and carbonate. The complete mineralization and hardening process takes several months. The now inactive osteoblasts become sequestered in bone tissue and also lie as flattened lining cells (surface osteocytes) on the new bone.

Bone resorption occurs on bone surface, and the type of bone with the greatest surface area is trabecular, or cancellous bone. Trabecular bone is found primarily in the vertebrae and the metaphyses of long bones. The long bone shafts are primarily cortical (compact) in structure. Approximately 25% of trabecular bone is remodeled each year, compared to approximately 2 to 3% of cortical bone (8).

Pathogenesis

MENOPAUSE-ASSOCIATED OSTEOPOROSIS

Menopause is defined as the loss of ovarian function. The ovaries no longer respond to the hypothalamic secretion of GnRH, or the anterior pituitary secretion of follicle-stimulating hormone (FSH) and leutinizing hormone (LH). Endogenous estrogen production from the ovaries is therefore lost. Women still have some endogenous estrogen production that results from the conversion of androstenedione to estrone in peripheral fat tissue. As a general rule, obese women have greater estrone production than thin women. This loss of estrogen is accompanied by a loss of bone. Several theories describe this relationship. Estrogen may be responsible for stimulating calcitonin secretion, thus inhibiting bone resorption. However, estrogen receptors are known to exist on osteoblasts, and estrogen may be integral to optimal osteoblast function. Furthermore, estrogen appears to inhibit the release of interleukins 1 and 6. Interleukins are known to stimulate bone resorption. In Type I or menopausal osteoporosis, there is an uncoupling of resorption and formation in favor of resorption. Bone loss is greater from trabecular sites than cortical sites.

Drug-Induced Osteoporosis

GLUCOCORTICOIDS

Corticosteroid-induced bone loss has been recognized since Dr. Cushing first described hypercortisolism in the 1930s, but the incidence of osteoporosis in patients receiving steroids is not known. The estimated rate is 30 to 50%, which approximates the incidence of osteoporosis in patients with true Cushing's disease (hypercortisolism) (9). Proposed mechanisms for this drug-induced side effect include a steroid-induced secondary hyperparathyroidism, inhibition of osteoblast function, direct effect on the ovaries and testes to decrease sex hormone production, and impaired active transport of dietary calcium in the gastrointestinal tract. A review of studies documenting corticosteroid-induced bone loss correlated risk for developing osteoporosis to prednisone dose and duration of therapy. The studies indicated that patients who ingested greater than 7.5 mg of prednisone per day for more than 6 months were at risk for developing osteoporosis (9). Losses of trabecular bone are greater than cortical. Men are equally affected, and no protection appears to be offered by race. Certainly, a patient who elicits concern is the patient with a condition subject to exacerbations who is prescribed repeated courses of

Table 34.1.
Means to Minimize Risk for Corticosteroid-Induced Osteoporosis

- Use corticosteroids with caution in patients wth the following conditions:
  Underlying debilitating disease
  Immobilization
  Post-menopausal
  Therapy anticipated for greater than 2 months
- Use lowest effective dose
- Use topical or inhaled products
- Supplement therapy with calcium and vitamin D, particularly in patients with low dietary intake
- Minimize use of other medications that adversely affect bone mineralization
- Use estrogen replacement therapy in postmenopausal women, provided prevailing medical condition allows

corticosteroids at relatively short intervals. Some suggestions for minimizing bone loss associated with corticosteroid therapy are listed in Table 34.1. Recent evidence shows that inhaled corticosteroids do not decrease bone density at low doses but may have some effect at higher doses. Inhaled corticosteroids should be employed if clinical condition allows (10).

HEPARIN

Heparin was first reported to cause osteoporosis in 1965 (11, 12). Since that time, evidence has increased, but the number of actual cases identified is still small. The risk of developing osteoporosis with heparin appears to depend on dose and duration (i.e., 20,000 units per day for more than 20 weeks) (13). Potential mechanisms include an increase in PTH activity, leading to increased osteoclast activity, decreased osteoblast activity, heparin-induced increase in collagenase activity, and a decrease in the production of 1,25 hydroxyvitamin D due to decreased renal conversion enzyme activity. This bone loss has been shown to reverse on discontinuation of heparin. One population particularly at risk are pregnant women requiring anticoagulation, in whom warfarin therapy is contraindicated. Whether calcium and vitamin D supplementation during heparin therapy is beneficial is not known, but it is considered prudent. It is likely that this risk also exists with low molecular weight heparin, but to date this has not been described.

GONADOTROPIN-RELEASING HORMONE (GNRH) AGONISTS

A group of medications recently marketed (leuprolide, nafarelin, goserelin) are associated with bone loss in women (14) and men (15). The GnRH agonists are used for conditions such as precocious puberty, endometriosis, leiomyomata (benign fibroid tumors), infertility, and prostatic cancer. Initial stimulation of the hypothalamic-pituitary-ovarian or hypothalamic-pituitary-testicular axis is followed by shutdown of these axes because of downregulation of receptors. The net result is a hypoestrogenic or hypotestosterone state. Trabecular bone loss can be rapid, varying from 2 to 6% over one year. It is currently recommended that use of these agents be limited to 6 months (16). Some research has suggested longer use is safe in females if estrogen is administered concomitantly; however, this may limit the therapeutic effects of the GnRH agonist if regression of endometriosis or shrinkage of leiomyomata is the goal. Further, the effective "add-back" dose of estrogen needed to prevent bone loss is in question.

OTHER MEDICATIONS AND SOCIAL HABITS

Furosemide and other loop diuretics are known to cause calciuria, as are caffeine and phosphorus-containing sodas. High phosphorus content in the gastrointestinal tract inhibits calcium absorption, as does alcohol. Cigarette smoking appears to have an antiestrogenic effect (17). Although these compounds are not known to result in overt bone loss, they are often prescribed or ingested by those at risk for osteoporosis. Minimizing ingestion of these compounds is most prudent.

Other Causes of Osteoporosis

Anorexia nervosa can decrease bone density by two mechanisms: deficiency of dietary calcium and vitamin D, and by inducing pseudomenopause. Many women suffering from anorexia have estrogen deficiency and cease to have menstrual cycles. The bone loss associated with anorexia resembles that of menopause. Likewise, premature ovarian failure and premenopausal surgical castration (oophorectomy) result in estrogen deficiency that will lead to accelerated bone loss unless hormone replacement therapy is initiated.

Patients who suffer quadriplegia or paraplegia, as well as posttraumatic immobilization resulting in traction or prolonged bed rest, are at risk for bone loss. Daily weight-bearing improves bone density and is essential to good skeletal health (18).

Men may be protected from osteoporosis by several factors, including a higher peak bone mass than women and no distinct cessation of sex hormone production equivalent to female menopause. However, approximately 14% of all vertebral compression fractures and almost 25% of all hip fractures do occur in men. Secondary causes assume a much greater role, but hypogonadism resulting in low testosterone is a primary cause. In many cases, sexual function will not be affected by low serum testosterone. Other causes of osteoporosis in men are diseases such as Cushing Syndrome, hyperthyroidism, cancer, glucocorticoid therapy, chronic alcohol ingestion and other dietary factors, smoking, and prolonged immobilization. Treatment options are the same as those for women, except for the use of exogenous testosterone instead of estrogen if a deficiency is identified (19).

Signs and Symptoms of Osteoporosis

An early symptom of osteoporosis is back pain in the lumbar or thoracic spinal region; however, many patients may not identify this as early disease. The pain is precipitated by usual activity that in the individual's past would not have been considered stressful. Spinal movement may be restricted. The patient may notice a loss in height of several inches, or this may be identified during yearly physical examinations. Progressive kyphosis, or curvature of the spine, may develop as compression fractures worsen. This may result in the classic dowager's hump. The abdomen protrudes as the ribs eventually rest on the iliac crest of the pelvis because of the loss of truncal space.

Table 34.2.
Factors That Increase or Minimize Risks for Development of Osteoporosis

Risk Factors for Development of Osteoporosis	Protective Factors for Development of Osteoporosis
General	High normal body mass
Slender build (thin, small frame)	African or Mediterranean race
Caucasian or Asian race	Weight-bearing exercise
Female	Estrogen replacement therapy
Menopause	Adequate lifetime calcium
Oophorectomy during reproductive years	intake
Positive family history	Avoidance of risk factors
Medical therapy	
Glucocorticoids	
Loop diuretics	
GnRH agonists	
Heparin	
Diet	
Chronic low-calcium intake	
Chronic high-phosphorus intake	
Personal habits	
Smoking	
Heavy consumption of caffeine	
Heavy consumption of alcohol	
Inactivity	

Wrist fractures, primarily of the distal radius, may occur if the individual suffers a fall and instinctively catches on an outstretched hand. Falls are also associated with fractures of the proximal femur, proximal humerus, and pelvis. Fractures of this type are associated with significant morbidity, particularly as the individual ages. Fractures resulting in surgery or prolonged hospitalization place the individual at risk for thromboembolic sequelae, pneumonia, worsening of disease due to immobilization.

Diagnosis and Clinical Findings

As noted, most victims of osteoporosis are identified after fractures have occurred. However, patients can be screened for osteoporotic risk factors and potentially diagnosed early enough for intervention to produce a beneficial effect. Risk factors are listed in Table 34.2. Although Caucasian or Asian race has long been considered a risk factor, recent evidence shows that black women with the same body habitus and other risk factors listed in Table 34.2 are at equal risk for osteoporosis (20).

Serum or urine chemistry is generally not helpful in osteoporosis diagnosis. Serum calcium, phosphorus, alkaline phosphatase, PTH, 25-hydroxyvitamin D and 1,25-hydroxyvitamin D are all usually within normal limits. Urinary calcium and byproducts of collagen catabolism such as hydroxyproline or deoxypyridinoline may be measured. Baseline measurements may find urine concentrations of these substances to be within normal limits or slightly elevated. But decreases in these urinary values from baseline can be used as indicators of a positive response to antiresorptive drug therapy, such as estrogen or calcitonin.

Elevated bone alkaline phosphatase may be of value in the diagnosis of osteoporosis. Serum bone GLA-protein, also known as osteocalcin, is the only protein known to be specific for bone tissue and dentin. It is synthesized by osteoblasts and incorporated into bone matrix. Serum concentrations are detectable by radio-immunoassay (21). High rates of bone turnover are manifested by higher serum concentrations of osteocalcin. Several radiographic techniques may be considered for diagnosing osteoporosis, but authorities differ regarding their recommendations for widespread use of these techniques. A routine spinal radiograph, often performed in symptomatic patients, will not detect osteoporosis until 20 to 50% of spinal bone has been lost (22). This technique is not useful to follow progression of bone loss or assess efficacy of medical intervention. Single-photon absorptiometry (SPA) is a relatively inexpensive measurer of cortical bone mineral density at one discrete site. The site (usually the distal forearm) is exposed to a beam of photons, and the transmitted fraction is measured in gm/cm^2. The greater the bone density, the lower the transmitted fraction. Unfortunately, SPA information is not applicable to the entire skeleton. Dual photon absorptiometry (DPA), dual energy x-ray absorptiometry (DXA), and quantitative computed tomography (QCT) are better indicators of trabecular bone density, such as the vertebrae. QCT is the most expensive and exposes the patient to the greatest amount of radiation. Excellent reviews of these techniques are available (23). Clinical use of these measurements is evolving at this time, but acceptable uses with regard to osteoporosis include early screening for osteoporosis to implement intervention, diagnosis of osteoporosis, and response assessment to dietary and pharmacologic therapy.

Treatment of Osteoporosis

Figure 34.2 provides the practitioner with a decision algorithm for osteoporosis treatment and prevention in postmenopausal women.

ESTROGEN

The data in support of estrogen replacement therapy for women at menopause onset is unequivocal. The rapid bone loss observed in unsupplemented women is attenuated in those prescribed estrogen, resulting in a reduced fracture rate of at least 50% (24, 25). There is increasing evidence that estrogen is beneficial for women greater than 10 years postmenopausal for attenuation of further bone loss (26). However, not all women entering menopause will develop osteoporosis, so screening for osteoporotic risk factors (Table 34.2) and screening for contraindications to estrogen therapy are vital. Contraindications to estrogen therapy

have traditionally included history of endometrial and breast cancer, but there may be exceptions to this rule (27). Other contraindications include liver disease, undiagnosed genital bleeding, active thromboembolic disorder, history of thromboembolic disorder due to hormonal therapy, and known or suspected pregnancy.

Estrogens are available as several different compounds and by various routes of administration. The two routes proved to provide osteoporosis prevention at this time are oral and transdermal. The daily dose of estrogen shown to preserve bone mineral density is equivalent to 0.625 mg conjugated estrogens (28). See Table 34.3 for marketed estrogens and equivalent osteoporotic therapeutic doses. Although prices vary among individual products, therapy can be achieved at a cost of approximately 30 to 50 cents per day, or about $100 per year, making preventive therapy very cost effective.

Benefits Other Than Prevention of Osteoporosis. Estrogen also brings relief from other conditions associated with menopause, such as vasomotor symptoms (hot flushes) and urogenital atrophy manifesting as vaginal itching and dryness. Although not FDA approved for prevention of heart disease, estrogens are known to favorably affect the lipid profile by increasing high-density lipoproteins (HDL) and decreasing low-density lipoproteins (LDL). This effect is greater with oral products than transdermal; however, transdermal estrogens do provide some benefit, as well as dramatically decreasing triglycerides (29). It is estimated that estrogen therapy can reduce a woman's risk of cardiovascular mortality by 50% (30). Several long-term clinical trials such as the Women's Health Initiative, which will not be completed until the turn of the century, are aimed at assessment of cardiovascular protection afforded by estrogen therapy.

Risks. Prolonged exposure to estrogen at high doses is associated with endometrial hyperplasia and endometrial cancer in women with intact uteri. Concomitant progestin therapy can prevent endometrial tissue buildup (31). While many regimens have been employed, the most commonly advocated are described in Table 34.4. Women posthysterectomy do not require concomitant progesterone.

Other concerns include increased risk of coagulation defects, hypertension, and cholecystitis reported in younger women prescribed oral contraceptives. These concerns may not be valid with the lower estrogen doses prescribed for menopausal replacement. The incidence of cholecystitis does appear to be two- to threefold higher (32) and might be prevented by use of transdermal estrogen. All underlying risk factors should be addressed before initiating estrogen replacement therapy.

The data connecting estrogens to breast cancer is also equivocal. The Nurses' Health Study (33) found an increased incidence of breast cancer in older women (60 to 69 years of age) who had taken estrogen for more than 5 years. However, the dose of estrogen ingested was not con-

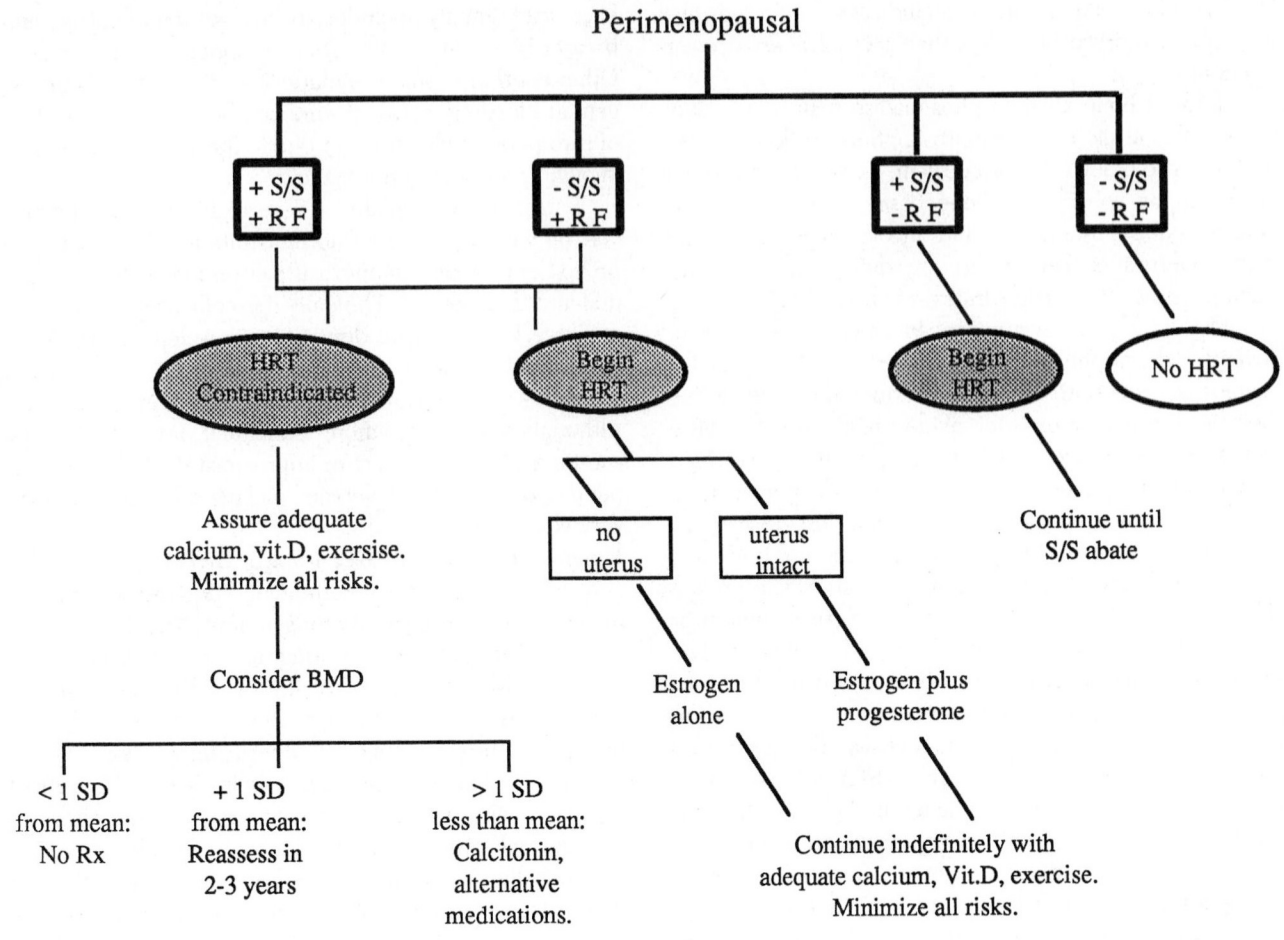

Figure 34.2. Decision algorithm for osteoporosis treatment and prevention in perimenopausal women.

trolled for, and no information regarding additional underlying risk factors for breast cancer was provided. Self-breast examination and yearly physical examination as well as mammograms should be employed for women on estrogen replacement, as in all women more than 50 years of age.

The most common side effects of estrogen therapy include breast tenderness, peripheral edema, and headaches. Cyclic administration may be effective in relieving these side effects. Enzyme inducers such as rifampin and phenobarbital may increase hepatic metabolism of estrogen; therefore, response to estrogen should be monitored and estrogen dosage increased if indicated. Estrogens may increase the effects of both corticosteroids and tricyclic antidepressants; monitor patients prescribed these combinations closely.

Table 34.3.
Estrogen Equivalencies for Osteoporosis Therapy

Component	Osteoporosis Dose (mg)	Available Strengths (mg)
Conjugated estrogens	0.625	0.3, 0.625, 0.9, 1.25, 2.5
Esterified estrogens	0.625	0.3, 0.625, 1.25, 2.5
Estradiol, micronized	0.5	0.5, 1, 2
Piperazine estrone sulfate	1.25	0.625, 1.25, 2.5, 5.0
17 β-estradiol	0.05	0.05, 0.1-mg patches

CALCITONIN

Calcitonin is an endogenous hormone secreted by the thyroid gland in response to dietary or elevated serum calcium. Females have been shown to have less endog-

Table 34.4.
Hormone Replacement Regimens in Osteoporosis[a]

Patients with intact uteri	
Estrogen oral (equivalent to 0.625-mg conjugated estrogen)	
Estradiol transdermal patch 0.05 mg	Calendar days 1–25
plus	
Progestin (equivalent to 5–10-mg medroxyprogesterone)	Calendar days 1–12 or 16–25 (at least 10 days per month)
or,	
Estrogen (equivalent to 0.625-mg conjugated estrogen)	
Estradiol transdermal patch 0.05 mg	Every day
plus	
Progestin (equivalent to 2.5-mg medroxyprogesterone)	Every day
Patients posthysterectomy	
Estrogen (equivalent to 0.625-mg conjugated estrogen)	
Estradiol transdermal patch 0.05 mg	Every day

[a]Dosage adjustments may be necessary based on individualized patient response and combination therapies.

enous calcitonin secretion in response to dietary calcium than males, which implies a basis for reduced bone density in females. Salmon calcitonin is the only compound other than estrogen currently approved in the United States for prevention and treatment of osteoporosis. Calcitonin prevents bone resorption by inhibiting osteoclast activity. Diminution of osteoclast activity is rapid, based on observations in tissue culture. Calcitonin also has an analgesic effect: Women with osteoporotic vertebral fractures report symptomatic pain improvement after therapy with intranasal salmon calcitonin (34).

Current administration routes include injectable and intranasal. For prevention of osteoporosis in menopausal and surgically castrated women, the dose of calcitonin is 100 units subcutaneously every day, but doses of 50 to 100 units every other day are effective also. In the presence of established vertebral fractures, a dose of 200 units daily is recommended (35). Patients should ingest adequate calcium and Vitamin D also. Therapy duration has not been defined; studies of 1 to 3 years duration show evidence of continued benefit.

Side effects with calcitonin include nausea and gastrointestinal discomfort in approximately 8 to 10% of patients; this may be minimized by bedtime administration. Initially, facial flushing and dermatitis may occur in 2 to 5% of patients, but this usually abates with continued therapy. Pruritis at the injection site is also problematic. Patients should be instructed to administer calcitonin subcutaneously as opposed to intramuscularly to minimize these side effects. Desensitization, due to formation of neutralizing antibodies to salmon calcitonin, reported with higher doses, does not appear to occur with doses recommended for osteoporosis (36).

Calcitonin is a viable therapeutic option for patients in whom estrogens are contraindicated or for patients intolerant to estrogen side effects or regimens. It may also be considered in patients with glucocorticoid-induced osteoporosis, bone loss due to immobilization, and hypoestrogenic states resulting from therapy with GnRH agonists. It has an excellent safety profile and few additional metabolic effects. One barrier to its widespread acceptance is administration route; the marketing of intranasal calcitonin may improve patient compliance. Further, it does not compare favorably with other therapy options in regard to price, with yearly therapy costs of approximately $4000 to $15,000.

CALCIUM

Calcium is vital as adjunct therapy for osteoporosis. However, calcium alone will not retard the rapid bone loss occurring at menopause. A recent consensus statement by the National Institutes of Health (37) has recommended higher calcium intakes for some age groups than the currently established recommended daily allowances (RDA) (Table 34.5). Adequate calcium intake throughout life is essential for attaining peak bone mass, and may affect the rate at which bone is lost later in life. Calcium is a threshold nutrient. The daily calcium intake below which the body must obtain calcium from bone is approximately 400 mg. Women with optimal calcium intake are not likely to receive additional benefit from calcium supplements, whereas women with very low intake will receive additional

Table 34.5.
Optimal Calcium Requirements

Group	Optimal Daily Intake (in mg of elemental calcium)
Infant	
Birth–6 months	400
6–12 months	600
Children	
1–5 years	800
6–10 years	800–1200
Adolescents	
11–24 years	1200–1500
Men	
25–65 years	1000
Over 65 years	1500
Women	
25–50 years	1000
Over 50 years (postmenopausal)	1500
On estrogens	1000
Not on estrogens	1500
Over 65 years	1500
Pregnant and nursing	1200

Source: National Institutes of Health Consensus Development Conference Statement, June 6–8, 1994.

Table 34.6.
Vitamin D Preparations[a]

Product	Component	Units	Mg	Available Products
Ergocalciferol	D_2	8000 IU/ml	0.2 mg/ml	OTC 60 ml dropper
		50,000 IU	1.25 mg	Tablets, capsules
		500,000 IU	12.5 mg	1-ml ampules for injection
Cholecalciferol	D_3	400 IU	0.01 mg	OTC tablets, component in infant feedings and multivitamins
Calcifediol	25(OH)-D_3	800, 2000 IU	20, 50 mcg	Capsules
Calcitriol	1,25(OH)$_2$-D_3	0.25, 0.5 mg		Capsules
		1 mg/ml, 2 mg/ml		Ampules
Dihydrotachysterol	synthetic D_2	0.125, 0.2, 0.4 mg		Tablets
		0.2 mg/ml		Intensol liquid
		0.2 mg/5 ml		Liquid
		0.125 mg		Capsules
		0.25 mg/ml		Liquid

[a]1 IU of Vitamin D activity is equal to 0.025 mcg of Vitamin D_3. 40,000 IU of Vitamin D activity is equal to 1mg.

benefit (38). The sources of calcium, dietary or pharmaceutic supplements, are equally efficacious, provided ingestion is equal in milligrams of elemental calcium. Calcium carbonate and tribasic calcium phosphate have the greatest percentage elemental calcium, 40 and 39%, respectively. As a general rule when calculating calcium intake, one can estimate 250 mg from each full serving of a dietary source known to be high in calcium. These include dairy products, canned fish including bones, and some green vegetables such as collard greens, broccoli, and rhubarb.

The elderly may have decreased calcium absorption either due to lower vitamin D concentrations, resulting in less active transport of calcium, or due to achlorhydria. Ingestion of supplements with meals will enhance passive absorption. Calcium citrate is not dependent on gastric pH for absorption and may be a good choice in the elderly although limited marketing increases the cost for this calcium salt. This product contains 21% elemental calcium.

Concern exists regarding patient self-overmedication due to zealous support for calcium therapy. However, homeostatic mechanisms decrease intestinal fractional absorption when intake is great. The use of supplements is rarely associated with hypercalciuria or renal calcium stones. The primary side effect from calcium supplements is constipation. Fiber will impair absorption, as will iron therapy. Separate ingestion of tetracycline compounds and calcium by at least 2 hours to avoid intestinal chelation.

VITAMIN D

Vitamin D is a fat soluble vitamin that might be more appropriately considered a hormone, based on its physiologic function. The two exogenous sources of vitamin D are ergosterol (Vitamin D_2) from plant sources and cholecalciferol (Vitamin D_3) from animal sources such as fish liver oils. Endogenous production of Vitamin D_3 in the skin requires ultraviolet light exposure. These compounds first undergo hydroxylation in the liver to 25-hydroxyvitamin D [25 (OH)-D], then are further hydroxylated in the kidney to result in the physiologically active compound 1,25 hydroxyvitamin D [1,25 (OH)$_2$-D]. The production of 1,25(OH)$_2$-D is under the influence of PTH, calcium, and phosphorus. Its presence enhances gastrointestinal absorption of calcium. Therefore, a confounding factor in impaired calcium absorption may be inadequate vitamin D status. Optimal serum 25 OH-D serum concentrations range from 20 to 30 ng/mL. Many elderly are known to have decreased dietary intake of Vitamin D, and their exposure to sunlight may be minimal, especially if institutionalized. Production of 1,25 (OH)$_2$-D is usually within normal limits until serum 25-OH-D concentrations decrease below 7 ng/mL. Several studies have verified that osteoporotic patients have deficient 25-OH-D serum concentrations. The combination of vitamin D_3 and calcium has been shown to decrease the incidence of hip fractures in elderly women (39). In patients with preexisting vertebral compression fractures, calcitriol [1,25(OH)$_2$-D] proved to be more effective than calcium alone in preventing further vertebral fractures (40). When calcium and Vitamin D are used concomitantly, the calcium dose required may be decreased since intestinal calcium absorption should be enhanced. One therapeutic recommendation for elderly patients is Vitamin D 800 units per day to achieve 25-OH-D serum concentrations of 20 to 25 ng/mL, with calcium 600 to 800 mg per day. Twenty-four-hour urinary calcium concentrations are measured every 3 months, with the desired concentration less than 350 mg per 24 hours (41). For a comparison of vitamin D supplements, see Table 34.6.

FLUORIDE

It has long been recognized that people living in areas with high-fluoride water content have very dense bone, but those exposed to fluoride toxicity (fluorosis) have brittle bone. Dental programs employing fluoridated water, rinses, and toothpastes are known to prevent carie development. Sodium fluoride is not FDA approved for osteoporosis treatment in the United States but is approved in eight European countries.

Fluoride increases bone mineral density in several ways (42). In the presence of therapeutic amounts of fluoride, fluoride substitutes for the hydroxyl ion in the crystal lattice, resulting in fluoroapatite instead of the physiologic compound, hydroxyapatite. Second, an increased number of osteoblasts appear on bone surfaces, thus uncoupling the bone-remodeling unit in favor of anabolism. At low rates of bone turnover, this new bone is lamellar, or normal in appearance, but at high bone turnover rates, this bone may be abnormal. Fluoride also stimulates collagen synthesis and calcium deposition. Fluoride exerts most of its effect on trabecular bone, which has a higher turnover rate than cortical. For appropriate mineralization to occur, it is vital that therapeutic amounts of calcium also be administered during fluoride therapy. If adequate calcium is not provided, calcium is acquired from cortical bone.

Side effects of fluoride therapy include gastrointestinal complaints in 10 to 40% of patients and painful lower extremity syndrome in 50%. The cause of this peripheral pain is not known but is thought to be due to cortical bone stress fractures. Several studies have shown an increase in nonverterbral fractures. Tooth mottling may occur in children. Case reports of rheumatoid arthritis exacerbations limit sodium fluoride's use in this population (43). The biggest concern limiting sodium fluoride is that though it may decrease the incidence of vertebral fractures, this may be at the expense of cortical fractures, which would offer an unacceptable risk–benefit ratio. Only 55 to 75% of patients will respond to fluoride therapy; at this time, no tool is available to predict who will have a positive response. Before response assessment is made, 2 to 6 months of therapy are necessary.

At this time, sodium fluoride therapy cannot be recommended for routine use, but moderate doses in combination with calcium may produce optimal bone. It should be used with caution in patients with rheumatoid arthritis, those with renal compromise, and patients with gastrointestinal bleeds. Impaired bioavailability occurs when ingested concomitantly with antacids, milk or dairy products, calcium, iron, or magnesium. Ingestion of these substances and fluoride should be spaced by at least 2 hours.

BISPHOSPHONATES

The bisphosphonates are compounds which adsorb onto hydroxyapatite crystals at sites of active bone resorption. Three bisphosphonates are marketed in the U.S. Etidronate and pamidronate are FDA approved for treatment of hypercalcemia of malignancy. However, etidronate has been evaluated in patients with osteoporosis. Regimens with etidronate administered 400 mg orally daily for 2 weeks followed by 10 to 14 weeks of calcium were designed to mimic the bone remodeling cycle. Improved bone mineral density and decreased fracture rates were observed in women with osteoporosis (44, 45).

The compound alendronate (Fosamax™) is FDA approved for treatment of osteoporosis. Placebo controlled studies show progressive increases in hip, spine and total bone mineral density of approximately 5% over three years. Alendronate is not cycled; patients take 10 mg orally once daily. Oral bioavailability is approximately 0.78% in women. To optimize absorption, alendronate should be taken upon arising in the morning. Patients should be instructed to ingest the 10 mg tablet with 6 to 8 ounces of water, at least 30 minutes prior to ingestion of other foods, beverages, or other medications. They should not lie down for 30 minutes after ingestion. Adequate calcium and vitamin D through dietary sources or supplements is also necessary to assure optimal increases in bone mineral density.

Alendronate is not metabolized; drug not adsorbed onto bone is excreted unchanged in urine and feces. It is contraindicated in patients with creatinine clearances less than 35 mL/minute. The side effect profile of alendronate is limited primarily to gastrointestinal complaints such as abdominal pain or distension, nausea, dyspepsia, constipation, flatulence, and dysphagia.

Alendronate should be considered in patients with established osteoporosis in whom estrogen is contraindicated. Further studies are needed on combined estrogen and alendronate therapy. Further studies are also needed in patients with drug-induced osteoporosis or that due to immobilization. Alendronate therapy is estimated to cost the patient approximately $700.00 per year.

PATIENT EDUCATION

Patient counseling and education is the key to successful preventive therapy. Teenage women should be advised to increase their calcium intake and exercise so that they meet menopausal years with optimal bone mass. Perimenopausal and postmenopausal women likewise should be encouraged to ingest adequate calcium, participate in weight-bearing exercise, and have adequate exposure to sunlight for Vitamin D production, as well as minimize the risk factors listed in Table 34.2. Compliance with hormone replacement therapy not only will minimize the menopausal symptoms of urogenital atrophy, night sweats, hot flushes, and so on, but will enhance the lipid profile and protect from bone loss. Since effects diminish on therapy discontinuation, patients should be encourage to continue therapy indefinitely. Estrogen and progesterone doses em-

Table 34.7.
Osteomalacia Etiologies and Therapies

Type of Osteomalacia	Cause	Treatment
Vitamin-D-deficient rickets (VDDR)	Inadequate sunlight Inadequate dietary intake	Vitamin D
Inadequate calcium absorption	Chelators in diet: phytates, oxalates, excess phosphate	Change diet Calcium supplements
Phosphorus deficiency	Aluminum ingestion prematurity with prolonged feeding of low-phosphorus formula or TPN	Avoid aluminum antacids, contaminated sources; increase phosphorus intake
Gastric rickets	Gastrectomy Achlorhydria	Calcium citrate or other highly soluble calcium salt
Biliary rickets	Abnormal fat metabolism	Injectable vitamin D
Enteric rickets	Injury to small bowel by diseases such as Crohn's, coeliac sprue, short bowel syndrome	Injectable vitamin D
Hypophosphatemic rickets (Albright's syndrome)	Genetic or acquired fault of phosphorus Reabsorption in proximal tubule	Phosphate, $1,25(OH)_2D$
Type I Vitamin-D-dependent rickets	Genetic or acquired deficiency of 25-hydroxyvitamin D-1-hydrolase	$1,25(OH)_2D$
Type II Vitamin-D-dependent rickets	Gut cells fail to recognize autogenous 1,25 (OH) D	$1,25(OH)_2D$ and calcium
Renal tubular acidosis	Varied, results in renal calcium wasting	Alkalinization with sodium bicarbonate
Oncogenic osteomalacia	Bone/soft tissue neoplasia	Biphosphonates, vitamin D
Anticonvulsant-induced osteomalacia	Alterations in cytochrome P-450 enzyme pathway resulting in deficient 25(OH)D	$1,25(OH)_2D$
TPN-induced rickets in premature infants	Inadequate calcium/phosphorus in TPN solution	Increase calcium and phosphorus to maximum solubility

ployed in menopause have few associated side effects and are lower than doses employed for contraception. HRT regimens employed vary widely; instructions should be reinforced during counseling sessions. Women should have annual physical exams, including mammography after the age of 50, and they should be competent in self-breast examination. They should be encouraged to seek additional counseling if concerns exist regarding therapy rather than to self-discontinue.

OSTEOMALACIA

Osteomalacia is an osteopenia manifested by inadequate bone mineralization that usually results in bone deformities. Generally, when this disorder appears in childhood, it is referred to as rickets, and as osteomalacia when occurring in adulthood. Osteomalacia was first described in 1645 during the Northern Europe industrial revolution, when many children and adults worked long hours with very little exposure to sunlight. However, it was not until the 1800s that an association with lack of sunlight was suggested. The identification of vitamin D and its sources has prevented most cases of vitamin-D-deficient rickets, but several circumstances may put patients at risk for osteomalacia today.

Pathogenesis

When phosphorus and calcium are not available for production of hydroxyapatite, the mineralized compound

of bone matrix, osteomalacia may develop. The causes may vary and include inadequate dietary intake of calcium, phosphorus, or vitamin D; genetic or acquired deficiencies of enzymes; and neoplasia (47, 48). A unique group at risk are premature infants being fed by total parenteral nutrition (TPN). These infants missed the greatest opportunity for in-utero accretion of calcium and phosphorus, the third trimester of pregnancy. It is difficult to solubilize adequate calcium and phosphorus in TPN, but the development of pediatric amino acid solutions has allowed an increased capability (49). Table 34.7 lists types of osteomalacia, causes, and general treatment guidelines.

Diagnosis, Signs, and Symptoms

Although there are varied and multiple pathogenic causes, patient manifestations are much the same with all causes. Infants and young children may have marked growth stunting, and they may be apathetic, irritable, and hypokinetic. Frequently, they have an enlarged abdomen, referred to as rachitic potbelly. They may have impaired dentition, resulting in extensive caries. Joint enlargement at the ankles, knees, and elbows may be present. Kyphosis and bowing of long bones is evident. The child may present with fractures.

Adult osteomalacia manifests similarly; patients complain of easy fatigue and malaise, and often of diffuse, nonspecific bone pain. Pressing on long bones elicits pain.

Adults may also present with bone deformities depending on the length of time the disease has been present.

Radiographic observation reveals abnormalities of the epiphyseal plate in children since bone growth is rendered abnormal. In both children and adults, cortical and trabecular mineralized bone will be covered by a large osteoid seam, or area of unmineralized bone. Looser's lines, also known as pseudofractures, are a prominent finding, especially on bone scan. They may progress to frank fractures easily under minimal stress.

On serum chemistry analysis, PTH and alkaline phosphatase are elevated. Serum calcium, phosphorus, and 25 (OH) D are usually depressed. Urinary calcium is typically decreased unless the patient has phosphorus deficiency. These findings can differentiate osteoporosis and osteomalacia since these values are within normal limits in osteoporosis.

Another diagnostic test used in adults is an assessment of tetracycline uptake in bone. Typically, a tetracycline is administered for 3 days. Eleven days later, a tetracycline is administered for 3 days. Three days later, bone biopsy of the iliac crest is performed. This site is used since it contains both cortical and trabecular bone. The distance between the two tetracycline bands is observed and measured via fluorescent microscopy. It can be used as an assessment of the rate of bone mineralization and can also differentiate osteoporosis from osteomalacia (50).

Treatment

The treatment of osteomalacia depends on the underlying disorder identified, as seen in Table 34.7. If the cause is due to vitamin D deficiency, large doses may be needed for 4 to 6 weeks but can be reduced as healing ensues. Therapy with vitamin D can be monitored with serum alkaline phosphatase, which will decrease as body stores of vitamin D are replete and therapeutic action occurs. Table 34.6 lists the vitamin D preparations available and the typical doses employed for various underlying disorders. The success of treatment depends on the underlying disorder.

CONCLUSION

Research shows that a combination of vitamin D, calcium, and estrogen and progesterone results in an overall increase in total body calcium and improved bone mineral density in women with a propensity for osteoporotic fracture, as compared to calcium plus vitamin D or vitamin D alone (46). Fortunately, women can adhere to this regimen at a total cost of less than $1 per day, making prevention truly cost effective. The best prognosis for patients at risk for osteoporotic fractures is prevention through early intervention. A decision algorithm such as the one in Figure 34.2 may be used for therapeutic decision making. Reaching menopause or facing potentially drug-induced osteoporosis with the greatest bone mineral density may decrease the risk of fractures. Minimizing alcohol, caffeine, and high-phosphorus intake, and ceasing smoking may also decrease risks. Therapy for osteoporosis is still in evolution, and it will take several generations to define the optimal protocol.

As with osteoporosis, the best prognosis for osteomalacia is obtained by preventive measures. Early identification and treatment can prevent bone deformities, so patients at risk, such as premature infants on TPN, patients on phenytoin therapy, and patients postgastrectomy, as well as others listed in Table 34.7, should be monitored closely. After resolution of acute disease, dietary therapy may be adequate to prevent relapse depending on the underlying cause.

This chapter is dedicated to the memory of Myrtle Byrd Carter.

REFERENCES

1. Riggs BL, Melton LJ III. Involutional osteoporosis. N Engl J Med 314:1676–1686, 1986.
2. Young RL, Kumar NS, Goldzieher JW. Management of menopause when estrogen cannot be used. Drugs 40:220–230, 1990.
3. Iannotti JP. Growth plate physiology and pathology. Orthoped Clin North Am 21:1–17, 1990.
4. Matkovic V. Calcium intake and peak bone mass. N Engl J Med 327:119–120, 1992.
5. Ettinger B. Role of calcium in preserving the skeletal health of aging women. So Med J 85(suppl 2):22S–30S, 1992.
6. Kanis JA. The restoration of skeletal mass: a theoretic overview. Am J Med 91(suppl 5B):29S–36S, 1991.
7. Manolagas SC, Jilka RL. Bone marrow, cytokines, and bone remodeling. Emerging insights into the pathophysiology of osteoporosis. N Engl J Med 332:305–311, 1995.
8. Silverberg SJ, Lindsay R. Postmenopausal osteoporosis. Med Clin North Am 71:41–57, 1987.
9. Lukert BP. Glucocorticoid-induced osteoporosis: pathogenesis and management. Ann Intern Med 112:352–364, 1990.
10. Ip M, Lam K, Yam L, et al. Decreased bone mineral density in premenopausal asthma patients receiving long-term inhaled steroids. Chest 105:1722–1727, 1994.
11. Griffith GC, Nichols G, Asher JD, Hanagan B. Heparin osteoporosis. J Am Med Assoc 193:91–94, 1965.
12. Jaffe MD, Willis PW. Multiple fractures associated with long-term sodium heparin therapy. J Am Med Assoc 193:152–154, 1965.
13. De Swiet M, Ward PD, Fidler J, et al. Prolonged heparin therapy in pregnancy cases bone demineralization. Br J Obstet Gynecol 90:1129–1134, 1983.
14. Uemura T, Mohri J, Osada H, et al. Effect of gonadotropin-releasing hormone agonist on the bone mineral density of patients with endometriosis. Fertil Steril 62:246–250, 1994.
15. Goldray D, Weisman Y, Jaccard N, et al. Decreased bone density in elderly men treated with the gonadotropin-releasing hormone agonist decapeptyl (D-Trp⁶-GnRH). J Clin Endocrinol Metab 76:288–290, 1993.
16. Comite F. GnRH analogs and safety. Obstet Gynecol Surv 44:319–325, 1989.
17. Kiel DP, Baron JA, Anderson JJ, et al. Smoking eliminates the protective effect of oral estrogens on the risk for hip fracture among women. Ann Intern Med 116:716–721, 1992.

18. Eisman JA, Sambrook PH, Kelly PJ, Pocock NA. Exercise and its interaction with genetic influences in the determination of bone mineral density. Am J Med 91(suppl 5B):5S–9S, 1991.

19. Jackson JA, Kleerekoper M. Osteoporosis in men: diagnosis, pathophysiology, and prevention. Medicine 69:137–152, 1990.

20. Grisso JA, Kelsey JL, Strom BL. Risk factors for hip fracture in black women. N Engl J Med 330:1555–1559, 1994.

21. Price PA, Parathemore JG, Deftos LJ. New biochemical marker for bone metabolism. J Clin Invest 66:878–883, 1980.

22. Hall FM, Davis MA, Baran DT. Bone mineral screening for osteoporosis. N Engl J Med 316:212–214, 1986.

23. Genant HK, Faulkner KG, Gluer CC. Measurement of bone mineral density: current status. Am J Med 91(suppl 5B):49S–53S, 1991.

24. Kiel DP, Felson DT, Anderson JJ, et al. Hip fracture and the use of estrogens in postmenopausal women. The Framingham study. N Engl J Med 317:1169–1174, 1987.

25. Ettinger B, Genant HK, Conn CE. Long-term estrogen replacement therapy prevents bone loss and fractures. Ann Intern Med 102:319–324, 1985.

26. Felson DT, Zhang Y, Hannan MT, et al. The effect of postmenopausal estrogen therapy on bone density in elderly women. N Engl J Med 329:1141–1146, 1993.

27. ACOG Committee Opinion. Estrogen replacement therapy in women with previously treated breast cancer. American College of Obstetricians and Gynecologists (ACOG) Technical Bulletin. No. 135. Washington, DC, 1994.

28. Lindsay R, Hart DM, Clark DM. The minimum effective dose of estrogen for prevention of postmenopausal bone loss. Obstet Gynecol 63:759–763, 1984.

29. Whitcoft SI, Crook D, Marsh MS, et al. Long-term effects of oral and transdermal hormone replacement therapies on serum lipid and lipoprotein concentrations. Obstet Gynecol 84:222–226, 1994.

30. Stampfer MJ, Colditz GA. Estrogen replacement therapy and coronary heart disease: a quantitative assessment of the epidemiologic evidence. Prev Med 20:47–63, 1991.

31. Woodruff JD, Picker JH. Incidence of endometrial hyperplasia in postmenopausal women taking conjugated estrogens (Premarin) with medroxyprogesterone acetate or conjugated estrogens alone. Am J Obstet Gynecol 170:1213–1223, 1994.

32. Boston Collaborative Drug Surveillance Program. Surgically confirmed gall bladder disease, venous thromboembolism, and breast tumors in relation to postmenopausal estrogen therapy. N Engl J Med 290:15–19, 1974.

33. Colditz GA, Hankinson SE, Hunter DJ, et al. The use of estrogens and progestins and the risk of breast cancer in postmenopausal women. New Engl J Med 332:1589–1593, 1995.

34. Pun KK, Chan LWL. Analgesic effect of intranasal salmon calcitonin in the treatment of osteoporotic vertebral fractures. Clin Ther 11:205–209, 1989.

35. Civitelli R, Gonnelli S, Zacchei F, et al. Bone turnover in postmenopausal osteoporosis. Effect of calcitonin treatment. J Clin Invest 82:1268–1274, 1988.

36. Reginister JY. Effect of calcitonin on bone mass and fracture rates. Am J Med 91(suppl 5B):19S–22S. 1991.

37. National Institutes of Health Consensus Development Conference Statement: Optimal Calcium Intake. Bethesda, MD. June 6–8, 1994.

38. Dawson-Hughes B, Dallal GE, Krall EA, et al. A controlled trial of the effect of calcium supplementation on bone density in postmenopausal women. N Engl J Med 323:878–883, 1990.

39. Chapuy MC, Arlot ME, Duboef F, et al. Vitamin D_3 and calcium to prevent hip fractures in elderly women. N Engl J Med 327:1637–1642, 1992.

40. Tilyard MW, Spears GFS, Thomson J, Doveay S. Treatment of postmenopausal osteoporosis with calcitriol or calcium. N Engl J Med 326:357–362, 1992.

41. Gallagher JC. Vitamin D metabolism and therapy in elderly subjects. So Med J 85(suppl 2):S43–S47, 1992.

42. Riggs BL, Hodgson SF, O'Fallon WM, et al. Effect of fluoride treatment on the fracture rate in postmenopausal women with osteoporosis. N Engl J Med 322:802–809, 1990.

43. Duell B, Chesnut CH. Exacerbation of rheumatoid arthritis by sodium fluoride treatment of osteoporosis. Arch Intern Med 151:783–784, 1991.

44. Storm T, Thamsborg G, Steiniche T, et al. Effect of intermittent cyclical etidronate therapy on bone mass and fracture rate in postmenopausal women with osteoporosis. N Engl J Med 322:1265–1271, 1990.

45. Watts NB, Harris ST, Genant HK, et al. Intermittent cyclical etidronate treatment of postmenopausal osteoporosis. N Engl J Med 323:73–79, 1990.

46. Aloia JF, Vaswani A, Yeh JK, et al. Calcium supplementation with and without hormone replacement therapy to prevent postmenopausal bone loss. Ann Intern Med 120:97–103, 1994.

47. Mankin HJ. Rickets, osteomalacia, and renal osteodystrophy. An update. Orthoped Clin North America 21:81–96, 1990.

48. Econs MJ, Drezner MK. Tumor-induced osteomalacia—unveiling a new hormone. N Engl J Med 330:1679–1681, 1994.

49. Koo WWK, Tsang RC. Calcium, magnesium, phosphorus, and vitam D. In Tsang, Lucas, Uauy, Zlotkin: Nutritional Needs of the Preterm Infant, ed. 1. Baltimore, Williams and Wilkins, 135–155, 1993.

50. Frost HM. Tetracycline based histological analysis of bone remodeling. Calcif Tissue Res 15:671–686, 1969.

CHAPTER 35

ASTHMA

KATHRYN BLAKE and ALAN K. KAMADA

DEFINITION

In recent years asthma has been redefined as an inflammatory disease rather than a disease of merely bronchoconstriction. Currently, asthma is recognized as a chronic lung disease with the following characteristics:

1. Airway obstruction that is reversible either spontaneously or with treatment (although some patients may not reverse completely).
2. Airway inflammation.
3. Increased airway responsiveness (bronchial hyperresponsiveness) to a variety of stimuli (1, 2).

There is also increasing evidence that a "fixed" or irreversible component may be present with advanced disease. Based on these features, asthma research has been refocused from its bronchoconstrictor to its immunologic aspects. Treatment recommendations have also changed and now emphasize the earlier institution of antiinflammatory therapy to reflect the inflammatory processes present in the disease.

EPIDEMIOLOGY

An estimated 12 million persons in the United States have asthma. The prevalence of asthma increased by 29 percent from 1980 to 1987, and this is reflected in greater utilization of health care resources for treatment of the disease. One percent or 6.5 million outpatient visits were for asthma in 1985, and from 1970 to 1987 hospital discharge rates with asthma as the first-listed diagnosis increased approximately threefold. This increase was most dramatic in children, as the discharge rate rose by 43 percent from 19.8 to 28.4 discharges per 10,000 from 1979 to 1987 (1).

Asthma also accounts for considerable health care expenditures. Inpatient hospital services were estimated to be $1.5 billion in 1990, with another $1.1 billion spent on prescription drugs. Total expenditures for asthma care in 1990 was estimated to be a staggering $6.2 billion. Asthma is also costly in other ways. An estimated 10 million school days were missed by children with asthma in 1990, resulting in $900 million lost by parents required to stay home from work and care for their children. Work absences due to asthma accounted for another $850 million in lost productivity (3).

Of greatest concern is the increasing mortality due to asthma, despite advances in the diagnosis and treatment of the disease. In 1989 for example, 5150 persons died from asthma in the United States. Risk factors associated with asthma deaths include increased age; African-American race, especially in the 15- to 44-year-old age group (five times higher than Caucasians as compared to threefold higher for all ages); previous episode of respiratory failure with intubation; and hospitalization within the past year. However, a recent study suggests that risk of death may be due less to race than to issues linked to urban poverty (4). Other contributing factors include psychologic and psychosocial problems such as depression, denial, alcohol abuse, recent family loss and disruption, unemployment, and schizophrenia. Inadequate general medical management and lack of access to health care have also been implicated as increasing the risk for death due to asthma (1).

PATHOPHYSIOLOGY

Asthma is a complex disease. Airway obstruction is responsible for its clinical manifestations; however, bronchial hyperresponsiveness and underlying airway inflammation are also characteristic features.

HISTOLOGIC CHANGES

Histologic changes occur in the airways and lungs of patients with asthma. Airway inflammation and epithelial damage have been observed in all severities of asthma, including newly diagnosed cases (5). Typical airway changes include epithelial shedding, smooth muscle hypertrophy and constriction, mucosal edema, mucus secretion and plugging, and influx of inflammatory cells such as eosinophils, macrophages, mast cells, neutrophils, and T-lymphocytes (Fig. 35.1) (1, 6, 7). Many of these inflammatory features contribute to the airway narrowing, which results in the clinical manifestations of asthma. Also present in some cases may be subepithelial fibrosis or collagen deposition in the basement membrane, which may or may not be a reversible process.

Bronchial Hyperresponsiveness

Bronchial hyperresponsiveness is an exaggerated bronchoconstrictive response to physical and pharmacologic

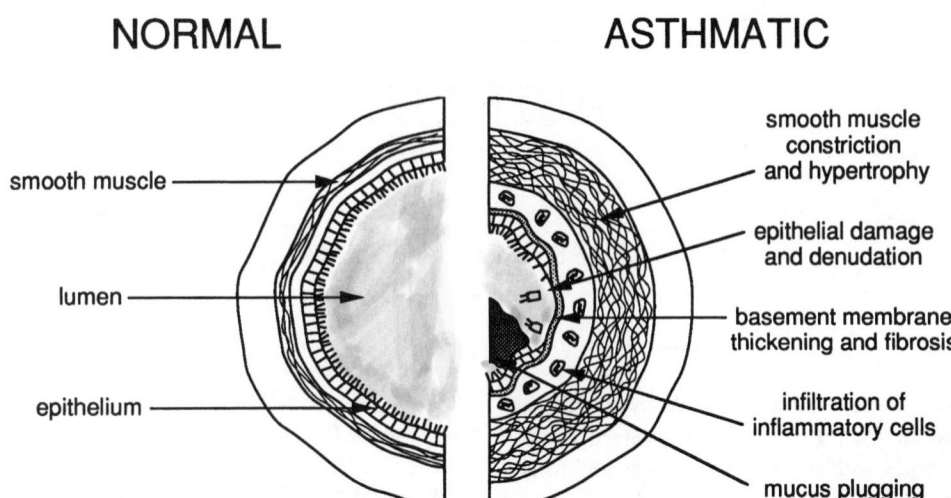

Figure 35.1.   Diagram illustrating the histologic changes present in the airways of an asthmatic patient as compared to normal.

stimuli such as cold air, exercise, allergens, viral infection, and certain chemicals. The degree of hyperresponsiveness can be measured by inhalation challenge testing with histamine or methacholine and is thought to correlate with severity of disease and medication requirements. Bronchial hyperresponsiveness may be a result of airway inflammation, but the mechanisms are unclear (6). An alternative hypothesis proposes that airway inflammation and bronchial hyperresponsiveness are not sequential, but parallel events.

Airway Inflammation

Airway inflammation is a complex interaction of various cells and mediators that results in the bronchial hyperresponsiveness and airway obstruction, as well as ongoing inflammation (Fig. 35.2). Our understanding of these interactions, while vastly increased in recent years, is still not complete.

INFLAMMATORY CELLS

A variety of cells are important in the inflammatory response, as they produce and liberate mediators, which in turn recruit other cells and/or have direct toxic effects, resulting in perpetuation of this vicious cycle.

Mast cells are important in the initiation of inflammatory responses following exposure to allergens and the resulting immediate bronchoconstriction. Following binding of allergen to immune globulin E (IgE)-bound high-affinity receptors on the surfaces of mast cells, various mediators such as histamine, eosinophil and neutrophil chemotactic factors, leukotrienes, prostaglandins, and platelet-activating factor (PAF) are released. Further evidence for the importance of the mast cell is the finding of increased numbers of degranulated mast cells in the airways of asthmatics who died from fatal attacks. Also, the number of mast cells in bronchoalveolar lavage fluid has been corre-

lated to the degree of bronchial hyperresponsiveness (5–7).

The importance of eosinophils in the pathogenesis of asthma has been known for many years, primarily due to the association between asthma and peripheral blood eosinophilia. Eosinophils are present in the peripheral blood, bronchial mucosa, and bronchoalveolar lavage fluid of patients with asthma, and the number of cells has been correlated with the degree of bronchial hyperresponsiveness. Eosinophils may be a source of lipid-derived mediators, and eosinophil granules contain major basic protein (MBP), eosinophil cationic protein (ECP), eosinophil-derived neurotoxin (EDN), and eosinophil peroxidase (EPO). Major basic protein and ECP are detectable in the sputum of asthmatic patients and may be responsible for much of the damage to airway epithelium, which may in turn contribute to bronchial hyperresponsiveness (5, 7).

Alveolar macrophages, normally present within the lumen of large and small airways, produce and release a number of mediators thought to be involved in the initiation and amplification of the inflammatory process. These include leukotrienes, PAF, and eosinophil and neutrophil chemotactic factors. Additionally, macrophages may be activated by IgE-dependent mechanisms. The contribution of macrophages to the pathophysiology of asthma is unclear, but they may be involved in the development of the late response and bronchial hyperresponsiveness (6, 7).

Neutrophils may also be a source of lipid-derived mediators, specifically platelet-activating factor, prostaglandins, leukotrienes, and thromboxanes, which contribute to bronchial hyperresponsiveness and inflammatory changes. However, their role in the pathogenesis of asthma in unclear (7). High numbers of neutrophils found in the airways of patients who died from sudden-onset asthma suggest a role for this cell type in sudden-onset fatal asthma, with perhaps a lesser role in chronic asthma (8). A

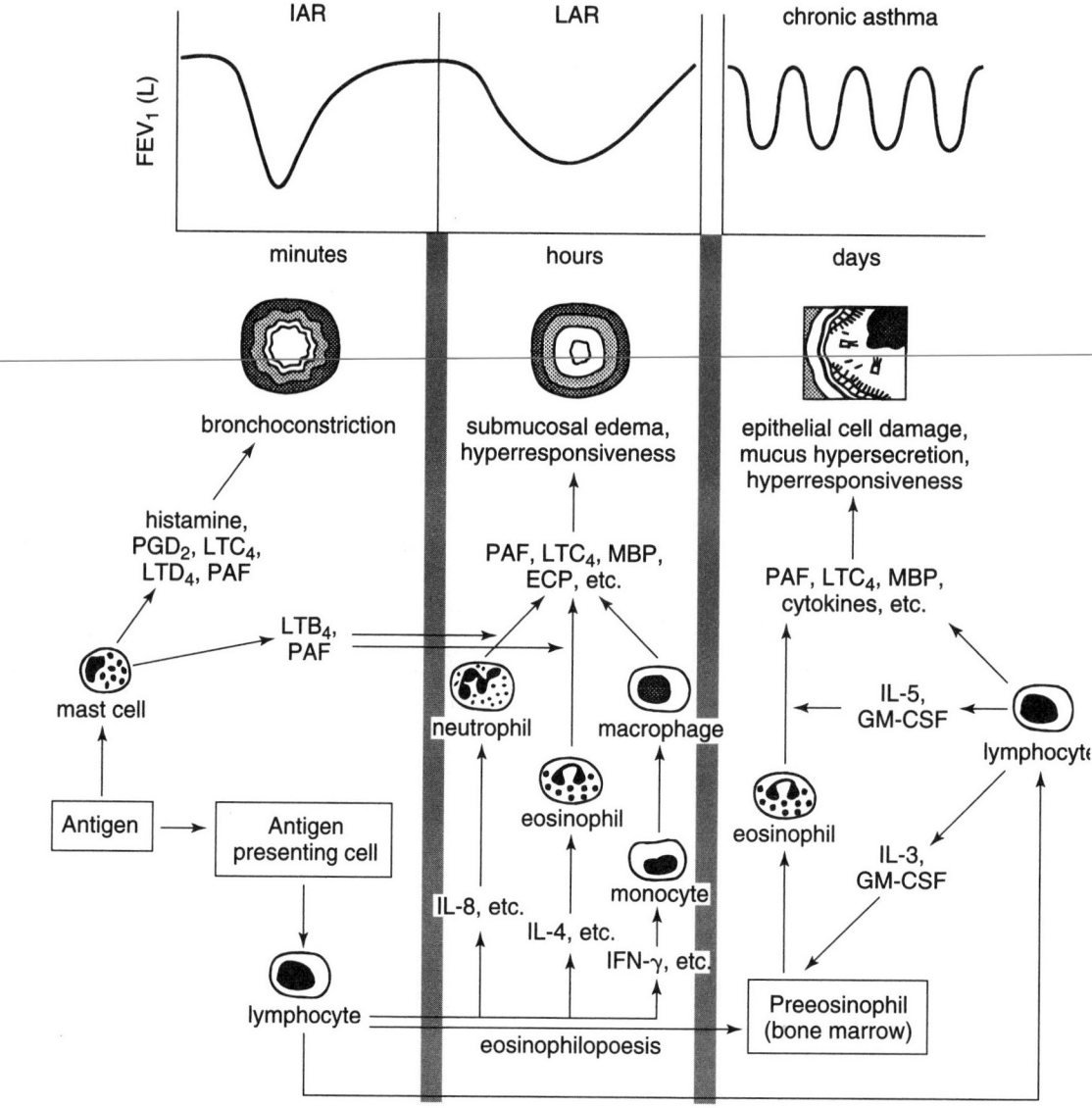

Figure 35.2. Greatly simplified diagram illustrating the relationships between immediate asthmatic response (IAR), late asthmatic response (LAR), and chronic asthma, and inflammatory cells, cytokines, and mediators. From reference 7, with permission.

role for the neutrophil in occupational asthma has also been proposed (6).

T-lymphocytes have received much attention in recent years, as their role in the pathogenesis of asthma is thought to be increasingly important. While B-lymphocytes are involved in IgE production, T-lymphocytes produce cytokines such as interleukin (IL)-4, IL-5, and interferon-γ (IFN-γ), which are intimately involved in the regulation of IgE production. T-lymphocytes play a major role in regulating the immune response as other cytokines control eosinophil production, mast cell differentiation, cell chemotaxis activation, and degranulation. The Th2-like subset, producing IL-3, IL-4, IL-5, IL 6, IL-10, granulocyte macrophage-colony-stimulating factor (GM-CSF), and tumor necrosis factor-α (TNF-α), but not IL-2 or

IFN-γ, is thought to be of particular importance due to this cytokine milieu (6, 7).

MEDIATORS

The cells involved in inflammatory processes present in asthma produce and release numerous mediators responsible for many of the pathophysiologic changes. It has been proposed that for a substance to be defined as a mediator, three criteria must be fulfilled:

1. It must be capable of producing the pathologic changes observed in asthma or physiologic changes that define asthma.
2. It must be produced in the lung during an asthmatic episode and measurable in body fluids.
3. Removal by specific inhibition or antagonism must result in amelioration or attenuation of the asthmatic response (9).

Table 35.1.
Mediators, Their Sources, and Their Actions Relevant to Asthma

Mediator	Source	Action
major basic protein (MBP)	eosinophils	epithelial damage
histamine	mast cells	smooth muscle constriction, mucosal edema, mucus secretion
leukotrienes (LTB_4, LTC_4, LTD_4, LTE_4)	mast cells, basophils, eosinophils, neutrophils, macrophages, monocytes	smooth muscle constriction, mucosal edema and inflammation
prostaglandins (PGD_2, PGE_2, $PGF_{2,\alpha}$, PGI_2)	mast cells, endothelial cells	smooth muscle constriction, mucosal edema, mucus secretion
thromboxanes (TXA_2)	macrophages, monocytes, platelets	smooth muscle constriction, mucus secretion
platelet-activating factor (PAF)	mast cells, basophils, eosinophils, neutrophils, macrophages, monocytes, platelets, endothelial cells	smooth muscle constriction, mucosal edema and inflammation, mucus secretion, bronchial hyperresponsiveness

A number of substances have been implicated as mediators of asthma. These may be preformed or may be rapidly produced by cells following activation or stimulation. Those thought to be important in the pathogenesis of asthma include histamine and the many products of arachidonic acid metabolism such as leukotrienes, prostaglandins, thromboxanes, and PAF. Actions of mediators that are pertinent to the pathophysiology of asthma include epithelial damage, smooth muscle contraction, mucosal edema and inflammation, and mucus secretion (Table 35.1). Specific antagonists of mediators and inhibitors of enzymes involved in their production have shed light on the importance of the various mediators in the pathophysiology of asthma, and are under investigation as potential antiinflammatory therapies for the future.

ADHESION MOLECULES

Adhesion of inflammatory cells to surfaces of the vasculature is an important early step in the inflammatory response, as it allows for the infiltration and migration of relevant cells to sites of inflammation. To facilitate this process, glycoproteins or adhesion molecules are expressed by cell membranes of basophils, granulocytes, lymphocytes, neutrophils, monocytes, platelets, as well as endothelial and epithelial cells after their activation by mediators or other cells. Adhesion molecules have other functions such as promoting activation of cells and cell-cell communication and promoting migration and infiltration of cells. Complex interactions whereby mediators affect the expression of adhesion molecules, which in turn result in production of mediators, also exist (10, 11).

Adhesion molecules are divided into families based on their chemical structures, and those thought to be of particular importance in inflammation include the integrins, the immunoglobulin supergene family, selectins, and carbohydrate ligands. A major role of adhesion molecules in inflammation is the recruitment of leukocytes from the vascular lumen to tissue sites. To facilitate this process, transient and reversible binding of the adhesion molecules to specific ligands on endothelial cells occurs after expression, resulting in slowing or rolling of the circulating leukocyte along the surfaces of the vasculature. In response to the initial adhesion event or mediators, activation of the leukocyte or endothelial cell follows. Finally, firm adhesion occurs, which anchors the leukocyte to the endothelial cell surface and allows for diapedesis between endothelial cells and migration into the extracellular matrix and site of inflammation (11).

Studies addressing further mechanisms of leukocyte adhesion and infiltration in the airways are now in progress. Monoclonal antibodies to the functional epitopes of adhesion molecules will facilitate a better understanding of the cells and their interactions, and ultimately the roles of adhesion molecules in the pathophysiology of asthma and other inflammatory diseases. Specific blocking of relevant adhesion molecules has already been proposed as a novel therapeutic approach or a complement to existing antiinflammatory asthma therapy.

Neural Mechanisms

Neural regulation of the airways is complex, with increased responsiveness to cholinergic stimuli seen in asthmatic patients. Changes in the muscarinic receptor or increases in cholinergic sensitivity might cause increased parasympathetic tone and reflex bronchoconstriction in asthmatics; however, these mechanisms appear to be only partially responsible for the bronchospasm following inhalation of relevant agents. Further evidence is the apparent lack of usefulness of anticholinergic therapies in the treatment of chronic asthma.

There is increasing evidence that neural mechanisms via the nonadrenergic, noncholinergic (NANC) system interlinked with the sympathetic and parasympathetic systems, may contribute to the bronchoconstriction and airway inflammation present in asthma. Sensory neuropeptides, substance P and neurokinin A, present in human airway nerves, are bronchoconstrictive to asthmatics. Neural endopeptidase, the enzyme that degrades the neuropeptides, has been shown to increase neurokinin-induced bronchospasm in an animal model. Protection from neurokinin A-induced bronchoconstriction by nedocromil sodium provides further evidence for the role of the NANC system in airway obstruction (12).

There are also data supporting a role for neuropeptides in inflammation. Mucus secretion, plasma extravasation, and other proinflammatory effects such as eosinophil and neutrophil chemotaxis, adhesion of neutrophils, and stimulation of lymphocytes and other cells are proasthma effects of the neuropeptides. Their ability to cause inflammation and bronchial hyperresponsiveness characteristic of asthma and their presence in the airways suggest that neurokinin A and substance P may be important mediators of the disease (12).

CLINICAL PRESENTATION AND DIAGNOSIS

Symptoms of asthma include shortness of breath or dyspnea, wheezing, cough, and sputum production. Chest "tightness" is a common complaint among asthmatic patients. Objective signs of the disease are reduced airflow, increased airway resistance and reduced conductance, hyperinflation of the lungs, and bronchial hyperresponsiveness. In acutely obstructed patients, tachypnea, tachycardia, retractions, cyanosis, and hypoxemia may also be present. The National Asthma Education Program (NAEP) Guidelines for the Diagnosis and Management of Asthma (1) base treatment recommendations on the classification of asthma as mild, moderate, or severe (Table 35.2).

Airflow is easily measured, and while reduced airflow is a characteristic feature of asthma, other diseases may present with similar obstruction. Airflow is typically measured by spirometry or peak expiratory flow (Figs. 35.3A and B), and normal (predicted) values based on height, age, gender, and race are established. Forced expiratory volume in one second (FEV_1) is the most commonly used spirometric evaluation of pulmonary function and consists of the volume of air expelled within the first second of forced expiration after maximal inhalation. It is normally over 70 percent of the total volume of expired air or the forced vital capacity (FVC); however, in obstructive processes such as asthma, FEV_1 is reduced, as is FVC and the FEV_1/FVC ratio. Peak expiratory flow (PEF) is the maximal rate at which air is exhaled from the lungs with a forced expiratory maneuver and correlates fairly well with FEV_1 (although for some patients it does not correlate well with symptoms). Peak flow meters are simple, portable, and relatively inexpensive devices, which facilitate accurate and objective self-monitoring of pulmonary function. A disadvantage of both FEV_1 and PEF is their dependence on patient effort (1, 13).

Asthma often occurs with a predominance of nocturnal symptoms, and this is reflected as a typical pattern of lower pulmonary function in the morning. Allergies, atopic dermatitis, rhinitis, and sinusitis are commonly associated with asthma. Because asthma is a chronic disease with the potential for acute exacerbations, symptoms may be continuous, episodic, or continuous with episodic exacerbations. Symptoms can occur seasonally, perennially, or perennially with seasonal exacerbations. Exacerbations may be slowly progressing or have rapid onset. A number of factors may trigger asthma symptoms or exacerbations, such as allergens (pollens, molds, mites, animal danders), viral respiratory tract infections, environmental irritants (smoke, strong odors, cold dry air), exercise, food additives (sulfites, tartrazine), and medications (aspirin, NSAIDs, β-blockers). While the psychologic effect of emotions do not induce asthma, the physiologic response to certain emotions (hard laughter, crying, fear, anger, anxiety) may precipitate asthma symptoms. Following exposure to a relevant allergen, an immediate asthmatic response (IAR), a drop in pulmonary function occurring within minutes, and a late asthmatic response (LAR), a second drop in pulmonary function occurring after several hours of exposure, may be observed (Fig. 35.3C). While isolated IAR or LAR may occur, a dual response following exposure is also common.

Bronchial hyperresponsiveness, another characteristic feature of the disease, is the exaggerated bronchoconstrictor response following exposure to physical and chemical stimuli. It may persist for weeks to months following exposure to stimuli such as viral respiratory infections. Bronchial hyperresponsiveness can be measured by inhalation of increasing doses of histamine or methacholine, with the end point being the dose required to elicit a ≥ 20 percent fall in pulmonary function, typically FEV_1. The provocative concentration or dose required for a ≥ 20 percent fall in FEV_1 (PC_{20} or PD_{20}) is inversely proportional to bronchial hyperresponsiveness; thus, a lower PD_{20} is indicative of more reactivity (Fig. 35.3D). Not only can measures of bronchial hyperresponsiveness be used for the diagnosis of asthma, but changes in PD_{20} over time can be useful for gauging response to treatment.

The diagnosis of asthma is usually made based on clinical history and objective measures of pulmonary function. It can be elusive, as a number of other diagnoses, including foreign body aspiration, laryngotracheomalacia, bronchiolitis, and cystic fibrosis, may also present with wheezing (Table 35.3). Recurrent exacerbations, provoking factors such as allergens, irritants, exercise, or viral respiratory infections, and a history of nocturnal symptoms are particularly characteristic of asthma. While the history is of great importance and is helpful in narrowing the diagnosis of the disease, it is not diagnostic. Of note, the physical examination may be normal when no symptoms are present. Chest radiographs (posterior-anterior) may be normal in mild disease, but signs of air trapping are more often present with severe, chronic asthma. Rhinitis,

Table 35.2.

Classification of Asthma by Severity of Disease[a]

Characteristics	Mild	Moderate	Severe
A. Pretreatment			
Frequency of exacerbations	Exacerbations of cough and wheezing no more often than 1 or 2 times/week.	Exacerbation of cough and wheezing on a more frequent basis than 1 or 2 times/week. Could have history of severe exacerbations, but infrequent. Urgent care treatment in hospital emergency department or doctor's office < 3 times/year.	Virtually daily wheezing. Exacerbations frequent, often severe. Tendency to have sudden severe exacerbations. Urgent visits to hospital emergency departments or doctor's office > 3 times/year. Hospitalization > 2 times/year, perhaps with respiratory insufficiency or, rarely, respiratory failure and history of intubation. May have had cough syncope or hypoxic seizures.
Frequency of symptoms	Few clinical signs or symptoms of asthma between exacerbations.	Cough and low-grade wheezing between acute exacerbations often present.	Continuous albeit low-grade cough and wheezing almost always present.
Degree of exercise tolerance	Good exercise tolerance but may not tolerate vigorous exercise, especially prolonged running.	Exercise tolerance diminished.	Very poor exercise tolerance with marked limitation of activity.
Frequency of nocturnal asthma	Symptoms of nocturnal asthma occur no more often than 1 or 2 times/month.	Symptoms of nocturnal asthma present 2 or 3 times/week.	Considerable, almost nightly sleep interruption due to asthma. Chest tight in early morning.
School or work attendance	Good school or work attendance.	School or work attendance may be affected.	Poor school or work attendance.
Pulmonary function			
• Peak Expiratory Flow Rate (PEFR)	PEFR > 80% predicted. Variability[b] < 20%	PEFR 60–80% predicted. Variability 20–30%	PEFR < 60% predicted. Variability > 30%.
• Spirometry	Minimal or no evidence of airway obstruction on spirometry. Normal expiratory flow volume curve; lung volumes not increased. Usually a > 15% response to acute aerosol bronchodilator administration, even though baseline near normal.	Signs of airway obstruction on spirometry are evident. Flow volume curve shows reduced expiratory flow at low lung volumes. Lung volumes often increased. Usually a > 15% response to acute aerosol bronchodilator administration.	Substantial degree of airway obstruction on spirometry. Flow volume curve marked concavity. Spirometry may not be normalized even with high dose steroids. May have substantial increase in lung volumes and marked unevenness of ventilation. Incomplete reversibility to acute aerosol bronchodilator administration.
• Methacholine sensitivity	Methacholine PC_{20} > 20 mg/mL[c]	Methacholine PC_{20} between 2 and 20 mg/mL	Methacholine PC_{20} < 2 mg/mL
B. After optimal treatment is established			
Response to and duration of therapy	Exacerbations respond to bronchodilators without the use of systemic corticosteroids in 12 to 24 hours. Regular drug therapy not usually required except for short periods of time.	Periodic use of bronchodilators required during exacerbations for a week or more. Systemic steroids also usually required for exacerbations. Continuous around-the-clock drug therapy required. Regular use of anti-inflammatory agents may be required for prolonged periods of time.	Requires continuous, multiple around-the-clock drug therapy including daily corticosteroids, either aerosol or systemic, often in high doses.

[a]Characteristics are general; because asthma is highly variable, these characteristics may overlap. Furthermore, an individual may switch into different categories over time.

[b]Variability means the difference either between a morning and evening measure or among morning peak flow measurements each day for a week.

[c]While the degree of methacholine/histamine sensitivity generally correlates with severity of symptoms and medication requirements, there are exceptions.

From reference 1.

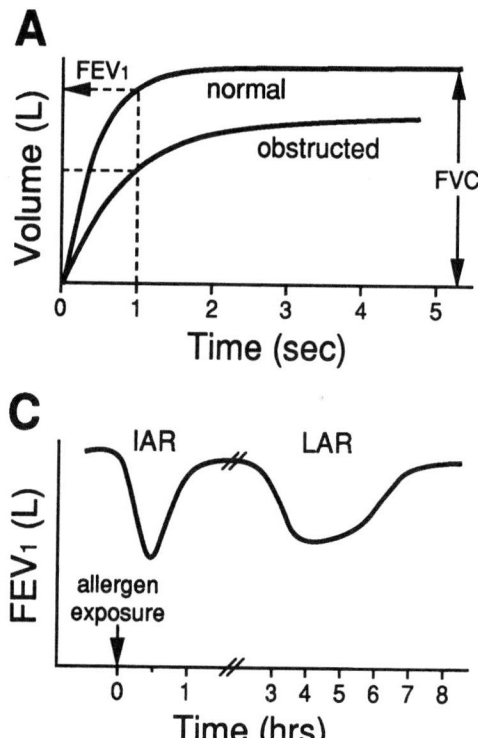

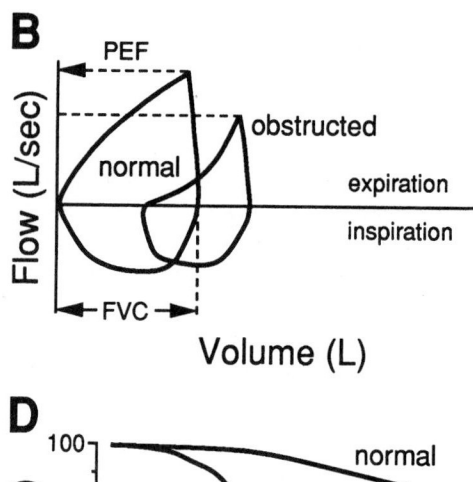

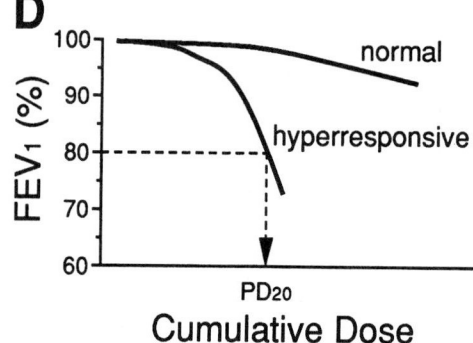

Figure 35.3. A, Typical spirometry of normal and obstructed patients. Note the lower FEV_1, FVC, and FEV_1/FVC ratio in the obstructed patient. B, Typical flow-volume loops of a normal and obstructed patient. Note the lower peak expiratory flow, increased lung volume, and typical "scooped out" expiratory curve in the obstructed patient. C, Typical immediate and late asthmatic responses seen following exposure to relevant allergen. IAR

occurs within minutes, while LAR occurs several hours after exposure. Patients may demonstrate isolated IAR, isolated LAR, or dual responses; D, Typical pulmonary function seen with histamine or methacholine challenge testing in normal and hyperresponsive patients. Concentration or dose of histamine or methacholine required to elicit a drop of FEV_1 of 20% (PC_{20} or PD_{20}) is inversely proportional to bronchial hyperresponsiveness.

sinusitis, eczema, blood eosinophilia, and nasal secretion and sputum eosinophilia may also be present (1, 14, 15).

Objective measures of pulmonary function showing reversible airflow obstruction (either spontaneously or with treatment) are critical in establishing the diagnosis of asthma. Demonstrating bronchial hyperresponsiveness by inhalation challenge testing with histamine, methacholine, or exercise can also be helpful in making the diagnosis; however, these tests can pose some danger and require sufficient precautions. Due to safety reasons, provocation with specific allergens is rarely recommended (14, 15). A number of other techniques have been implemented in the diagnosis of asthma, such as IgE antibody testing, allergen skin testing, examination of spontaneously produced or induced sputum, and direct investigative methods (bronchoalveolar brushings, lavage, and biopsy); however, the latter are limited by low specificity, their experimental nature, and potential safety risks (1, 2).

NONPHARMACOLOGIC THERAPY

Patient education and environmental controls along with pharmacotherapy are all integral components of successful

Table 35.3.
Differential Diagnosis of Asthma

Children:	Adults:
foreign body aspiration	mechanical obstruction
vascular rings	laryngeal dysfunction
laryngotracheomalacia	chronic bronchitis
enlarged lymph node or tumor	emphysema
laryngeal webs	congestive heart failure
stenosis of the trachea or bronchus	pulmonary embolism
bronchiolitis	pulmonary infiltration
cystic fibrosis	with eosinophilia
chlamydia tracheomatous	cough secondary to drugs
bronchiolitis obliterans	
bronchopulmonary dysplasia	
aspiration from dysfunctions of swallowing mechanism or gastroesophageal reflux	
vascular engorgement	
pulmonary edema	

asthma therapy. Patient education is a major component of asthma care and is emphasized in the NAEP guidelines. Education consists of assisting the patient and family members in understanding the disease and the goals of treatment, facilitating close self-monitoring and early recognition of symptoms, and understanding asthma medications (appropriate use and potential untoward effects) as well as encouraging good compliance. This is an area where clinicians can have a major impact on quality of care. Environmental controls include allergen and trigger avoidance measures, and in some cases when the number of sensitivities is limited, immunotherapy (allergy shots) (1).

PHARMACOTHERAPY

As outlined by the National Asthma Education Program's Guidelines for the Diagnosis and Management of Asthma (1), treatment should have the following goals:

1. Maintain normal activity levels, including exercise.
2. Maintain normal or near normal pulmonary function.
3. Prevent chronic and troublesome symptoms.
4. Prevent recurrent exacerbations.
5. Avoid adverse effects from medications.

Maintaining an affordable cost of care and reasonable medication regimens (facilitating better compliance) could also be included in this list of treatment goals. As asthma is a chronic condition with periodic exacerbations, therapy requires continuous attention with efforts at preventing or minimizing acute symptoms.

The medications used to treat asthma can be divided into the general categories of bronchodilators and antiin-flammatory agents (Fig. 35.4). Bronchodilators can be further subclassified into those that reverse acute bronchoconstriction and those that prevent bronchospasm from occurring. Not only must the symptoms of bronchoconstriction be treated, but the underlying inflammation must be addressed as well.

Bronchodilators
β-ADRENERGIC AGONISTS

β-Adrenergic agonists are potent bronchodilators. Two classes of β-adrenergic agonists exist: short-acting (albuterol, bitolterol, metaproterenol, pirbuterol, terbutaline) and long-acting (salmeterol, formoterol-investigational), which have very different roles in the treatment of asthma. Currently available β-adrenergic agonists stimulate the α, β_1, and β_2 receptors, but it is the action on the β_2 receptors that produces the therapeutic response in asthma (Table 35.4). Drugs with modifications of the catecholamine ring and side chains have been developed to prolong the duration of effect, enhance β_2-receptor selectivity, and confer oral bioavailability over the catecholamines (Fig. 35.5). A different modification exists for bitolterol mesylate, which is a prodrug slowly hydrolyzed in the lung to colterol; colterol has a duration of action similar to isoproterenol.

When a β_2-adrenergic agonist binds to the receptor on the cell membrane, a conformational change occurs in the part of the receptor adjacent to the G protein. Activation of adenylate cyclase occurs, leading to increased intracellular levels of cyclic AMP and a reduction in cytosolic calcium ion concentration resulting in smooth muscle

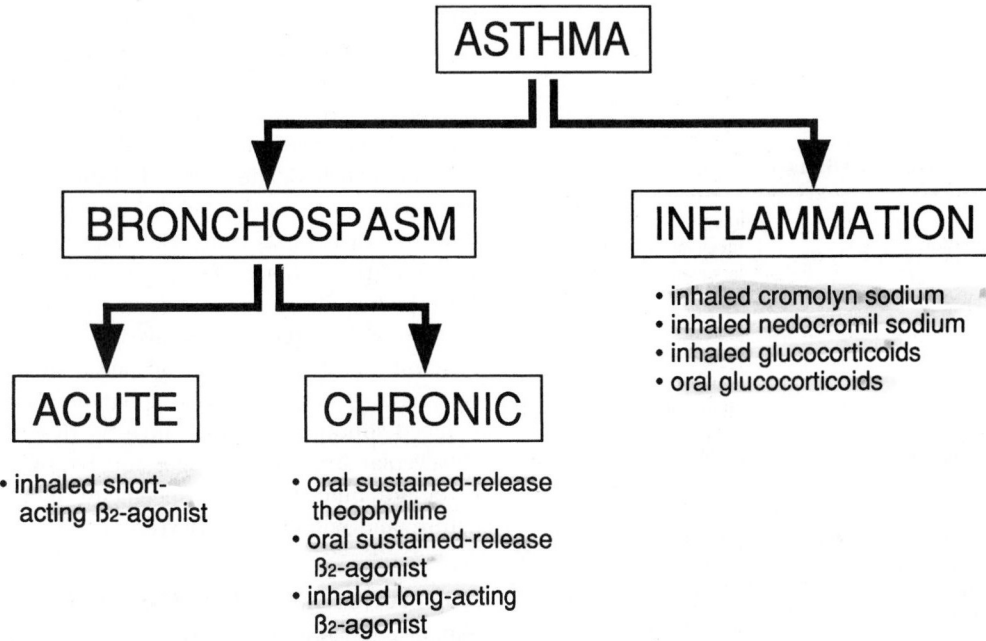

Figure 35.4.   Scheme of the bronchodilator and antiinflammatory medications used in the treatment of asthma.

Table 35.4.
Adrenergic Stimulants Used in the Treatment of Obstructive Airways Disease[a]

Agent	Route of Administration[a]			Relative potency	Duration (hr)		Receptor Stimulation		
	Injected	Inhaled	Oral	(Scale of 4)	Bronchodilation	Bronchoprotection	β_2	β_1	α
Catecholamines									
Ephedrine	−	−	+	1	2–3		+	+	+
Epinephrine	+	+	−	3(injected[d])	1–2	0.5–1.0	+	+	+
Isoproterenol	+	+	−	4	1–2	0.5–1.0	+	+	−
Isoethraine	+	+	−	2+	2–3	0.5–1.0	++	+	−
Rimiterol[b]	+	+	−	2+	2–3		++	+	−
Hexoprenaline[b]	+	+	+	2+	2–3		++	+	−
Bitolterol[c]	−	+	−	3+	4–6	2–4	+++	±	−
Resorcinols									
Metaproterenol	+[b]	+	+	3	3–4	1–2	++	+	−
Terbutaline	+	+	+	4	4	2–4	+++	±	−
Fenoterol[b]	+	+	+	4	4–6	2–4	+++	±	−
Saligenins									
Albuterol	+[b]	+	+	4	4–6	2–4	+++	±	−
Salmeterol	−	+	−	4	8–12	8–12	+++	±	−
Other									
Pirbuterol	−	+	+	4	4–6	2–4	+++	±	−
Procaterol	−	+	+	4	4–6	2–4	+++	±	−
Carbuterol[b]	−	+	+	3	4	2–4	+++	±	−
Formoterol[b]	−	+	+	4	8–12	8–12	+++	±	−

[a]Not all dosage forms are marketed in the United States.
[b]Drug not available in United States.
[c]Active moiety is colterol.
[d]By the inhaled route, epinephrine is the least potent β-agonist, with the shortest duration of action. Available O.T.C. (Primatene-Mist, others).

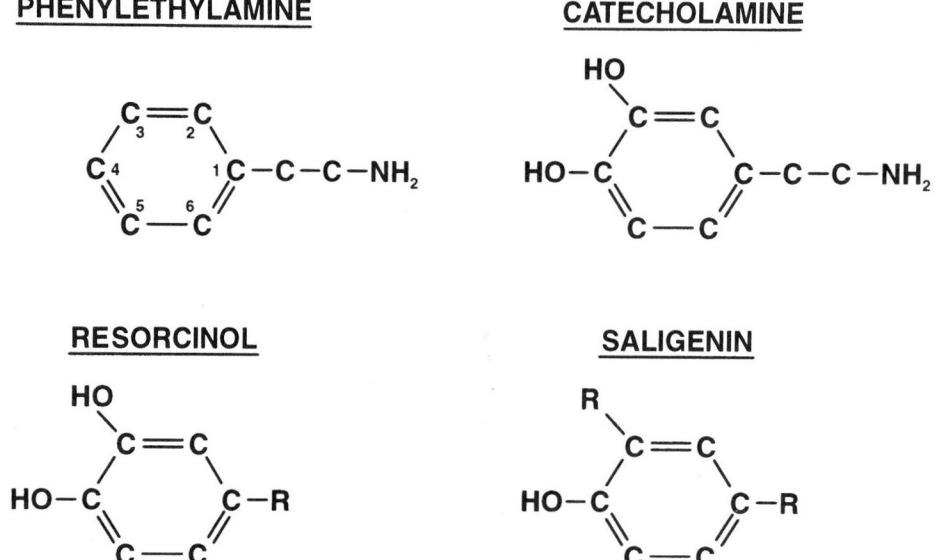

Figure 35.5. Basic structure of the sympathomimetic amines. The carbon atoms of the basic phenylethylamine structure are labeled in the conventional manner, with numbers used to identify the positions in the benzene ring. R represents various carbon moities.

relaxation (16). There is evidence indicating that β-adrenergic agonists may open Ca^{2+}-activated K^+ channels by direct linking to the G protein, which may occur at very low β-adrenergic concentrations and be independent of cyclic AMP (17). The long duration of effect for salmeterol is believed to be due to the binding of the lipophilic side chain to an exoreceptor, which is adjacent to the active portion of the β receptor. The exoreceptor anchors the agonist and permits nearly continuous stimulation of the β receptor. The mechanism for the long duration of activity of formoterol is less clear but is believed due to its extreme lipophilicity and high affinity for the β receptor (18). β-Adrenergic agonists have certain antiinflammatory effects including inhibition of preformed and newly generated mediators released from mast cells, reduction of microvascular leakage, and enhancement of mucociliary clearance, but the clinical significance is yet to be determined. However, neither short-acting nor long-acting drugs affect inflammation when evaluated by lung biopsy (19, 20).

β-Adrenergic agonists may be administered orally, subcutaneously, or by inhalation. When given orally, much larger doses must be used compared with the inhaled route due to high first-pass metabolism. Although included in several guidelines for the management of acute asthma (1, 2), the subcutaneous route is less often used, since highly potent, $β_2$-selective drugs are available that may be given via inhalation. In addition, administration to the lung by the inhaled route provides for a more rapid onset of action and fewer systemic adverse effects. Inhaled β-adrenergic agonists may be administered via a number of ancillary devices, which are described in detail below. β-Adrenergic agonists also can be administered intravenously in patients with impending respiratory failure; however, potentially life-threatening adverse effects greatly limit the safety of this route of administration (21). It is believed that the intravenous route allows drug to reach airways poorly accessed by the inhaled route when diminished tidal volumes and small airway obstruction with mucous plugs and edema are present in patients with severe bronchoconstriction. Interestingly, the intravenous route has been advocated for rapid reduction of serum potassium in patients with severe hyperkalemia due to other causes (22).

$β_2$-Adrenergic agonists have both bronchodilator and bronchoprotective effects, and differences in these effects can distinguish between the drugs and dosages. All are functional antagonists and can reverse smooth muscle constriction due to any stimulus. Irrespective of device or drug administered, equipotent doses at the β receptor produce equivalent responses, but the duration of effect and magnitude of adverse effects will vary between drugs. Short-acting agents have an onset of effect within minutes and peak effect in 30 to 90 minutes. In contrast, long-acting agents have a much slower onset of effect (10 to 20 minutes) and a longer time to peak effect (2 to 4 hours). Formoterol may have a more rapid onset than salmeterol. Short-acting β-adrenergic agonists provide bronchodilation for about 4 to 6 hours and protection from provocateurs for about 2 to 4 hours. In contrast, long-acting agents provide bronchodilation and bronchoprotection up to 12 hours and possibly 24 hours after a single dose.

Clear dose-response relationships for peak effect and duration of effect are apparent for inhaled β-adrenergic agonists. This is particularly important in severe acute asthma, when repeated dosing with as much as a five- to tenfold increase in dose is needed to reverse bronchoconstriction. This dose-response relationship is not relevant to the long-acting β-adrenergic agonists, as use of these agents is confined to the management of chronic asthma. Both short-and long-acting agents protect against exercise-induced asthma, but the latter sustain this effect for at least 12 hours after a dose. Both short- and long-acting agents protect against the early fall in pulmonary function after exposure to allergen, but only the long-acting agents inhibit bronchoconstriction during the LAR (23). This effect on the LAR is believed to be due to a combination of functional antagonism and antiinflammatory effects.

Adverse effects may occur after acute use (minutes to hours) or chronic regular use (weeks to years) (Table 35.5). Acute adverse effects are seen following oral and inhaled administration and are principally due to $β_2$-receptor stimulation in skeletal muscle and vascular smooth muscle, producing tremors, reflex tachycardia, and headache, and $β_1$ and $β_2$ stimulation in the heart, resulting in tachycardia and palpitations. Other acute effects include activation of Na^+, K^+ ATPase in skeletal muscle (which may result in hypokalemia), gluconeogenesis, and increased insulin secretion (possibly enhancing hypokalemia). Tachyphylaxis to systemic effects usually occurs within 2 weeks with continued therapy (16).

There has been considerable concern in recent years regarding the potential for β-adrenergic agonists to cause worsening asthma with regular or excessive use. The package insert for these drugs states the maximum daily dose as two inhalations four to six times daily. In one study, patients treated with fenoterol, two inhalations four times daily for 6 months, had worsening of their asthma symptoms compared to as-needed therapy (24), and a follow-up study with this same drug has supported this finding (25). In another study, patients who used excessive amounts of albuterol or fenoterol were found to have an increased risk of death or near death from asthma (26). The cause for worsening asthma in these studies is not clear, but some experts have suggested that the increased need for β-adrenergic therapy over days or months is an indication of worsening asthma rather than toxicity due to the drugs themselves. In addition, long-term regular administration of β-adrenergic agonists can increase bronchial hyperreactivity (27), diminish the duration of bronchoprotective effects (28), and decrease the bronchodilator duration but not peak (29). However, other studies have not shown tolerance or tachyphylaxis to the bronchoprotective or bronchodilator effects with regular use (30). Since few studies report data on individual subjects, it is not known if contributing factors are present that protect against or predispose certain asthmatics to this effect.

Short-acting $β_2$-selective adrenergic agonists are the drug of choice for the treatment of acute exacerbations of

Table 35.5.
Principal Locations of Adrenergic Receptors and Responses to Their Activation

Site	Receptor Type	Response
Lung		
Tracheobronchial smooth muscle	Mainly β_2	Relaxation
Bronchial glands	β_2	Increased secretion
Heart		
Sinoatrial node	β_1	Increased heart rate
Atria	β_1 (β_2)	Faster conduction
Bundle of His-Purkinje fibers	β_1	Faster conduction and automaticity
Ventricles	β_1 (β_2)	Faster conduction, increased contractility, increased tendency for automaticity and pacemaker activity
Arterioles		
Abdominal viscera, renal arterioles	Alpha, β_2	Alpha: vasoconstriction β_2: vasodilation
Cerebral	Alpha	Mild vasoconstriction
Coronary	Alpha, β_2	Alpha: vasoconstriction β_2: vasodilation
Mucosal	Alpha	Vasoconstriction
Pulmonary	Alpha, β_2	Alpha: vasoconstriction β_2: vasodilation
Salivary glands	Alpha	Vasoconstriction
Skeletal muscle	Alpha, β_2	Alpha: vasoconstriction β_2: vasodilation
Skin	Alpha	Vasoconstriction
Systemic Veins	Alpha	Vasoconstriction
Uterine Smooth Muscle	Alpha, β_2	Alpha: contraction in pregnancy β_2: relaxation (nonpregnant)
Stomach	Alpha, β_2	Alpha: sphincter constriction β_2: decreased motility and tone
Intestine	Alpha, β_2	Alpha: sphincter contraction β_2: decreased motility and tone
Liver	β_2	Gluconeogenesis Glycogenolysis
Pancreas		
Acini	Alpha	Decreased secretion
Beta cell (islets)	Alpha, β_2	Alpha: secretion β_2: increased secretion
Skin		
Sweat glands	Alpha	Increased secretion
Pilomotor muscles	Alpha	Contraction
Fat cells	β_2	Lipolysis
Mast cells	Alpha, β_2	Alpha: increased mediator release β_2: decreased mediator release
Eye		
Radial muscle of iris	Alpha	Contraction

From reference 48, with permission.

asthma according to the NAEP guidelines (1). High doses at frequent intervals (every 20 minutes or continuously) should be administered initially by jet nebulization. Several studies indicate that high doses of β-adrenergic agonists from a metered-dose inhaler (4 inhalations and higher) with a spacer at frequent intervals may be given with similar effect (16). High dosages are limited only by the occurrence of cardiac adverse effects, principally tachycardia, which is unlikely to pose a problem in otherwise healthy children or adults. Patients with preexisting cardiovascular disease, however, should be observed

closely when administered high dosages. As patients begin to improve, the dose should be initially decreased, then the dosing interval extended. Nebulized β-adrenergic agonists can be administered by compressed air at home and can avoid costly emergency room treatment. However, patient education is essential so that patients do not delay seeking medical care if symptoms fail to improve or worsen.

The consensus from the recent literature is that short-acting β-adrenergic agonists should be used on demand rather than regularly scheduled in the chronic treatment of asthma symptoms. This will avoid the worsening of asthma symptoms described in several studies and provides a means of evaluating asthma control and the need for additional therapy. The therapeutic role of long-acting β_2-adrenergic agonists is currently being defined.

In contrast to the short-acting agents, long-acting β_2-adrenergic agonists are not to be used on demand but rather are prescribed on a twice daily basis. Due to their prolonged onset of action, these agents are not appropriate for use in the treatment of acute symptoms. The misconception that salmeterol has a rapid onset of action may have contributed to the approximately 20 deaths that occurred within 8 months after the release of salmeterol in the Unites States. It is not known if regular administration of long-acting β_2-adrenergic agonists will cause the worsening of asthma symptoms seen with some of the shorter-acting agents. The long-acting agents may be used prophylactically for exercise-induced asthma or as a replacement for other oral bronchodilators (theophylline or oral β_2-adrenergic agonists). They should only be used in patients who are already taking an inhaled glucocorticoid and continue to be symptomatic (nocturnal symptoms or requirement for a short-acting β_2-adrenergic agonist more than three times daily). Whether it is more appropriate to increase the dose of inhaled glucocorticoid or add a long-acting β_2-adrenergic agonist is being evaluated (31). Long-acting β_2-adrenergic drugs will likely replace other oral bronchodilators in most asthma treatment plans. However, syrup formulations of β_2-adrenergic agonists will continue to have a place in the treatment of asthma in young children who cannot yet effectively use these drugs by the inhaled route.

THEOPHYLLINE

Methylxanthines, of which theophylline is the primary drug, have been used in the treatment of acute and chronic asthma for over 50 years. Dyphylline, caffeine, and theobromine (found in chocolate) are methylxanthines with much weaker bronchodilator properties than theophylline, and enprofylline, though more potent, has unacceptable cardiovascular effects. Salts of theophylline have been developed to improve solubility and absorption. Since theophylline absorption is related to lipophilic characteristics rather than water solubility, only the ethylenediamine salt (aminophylline), used for intravenous administration, is of clinical importance. Oral salt formulations (choline, calcium salicylate, sodium glycinate) simply contain less anhydrous theophylline by weight, and thus, it is the fraction of theophylline in these dosage forms that will determine the prescribed dose.

Although theophylline has long been used in the treatment of asthma, its mechanism of action is still largely unknown. Its bronchodilatory effects are well known, but theophylline is now believed to have antiinflammatory or immunomodulatory effects as well. The bronchodilator effects are believed to be due in part to phosphodiesterase inhibition, which results in increased levels of cyclic AMP, promoting smooth muscle relaxation. However, theophylline levels above the therapeutic range for asthma are needed to raise levels of cyclic AMP, which has cast doubt on this mechanism for bronchodilation. The discovery of over twenty isoenzymes of phosphodiesterase with differential expression in different cells and evaluation of selective inhibitors of these enzymes will likely clarify the importance of this mechanism for its therapeutic effect. Theophylline is also an adenosine receptor antagonist. The effects of adenosine, a potent bronchoconstrictor, can be inhibited by therapeutic concentrations of theophylline. However, enprofylline, which has about five times the bronchodilator effects of theophylline, does not inhibit adenosine. Additional effects include prostaglandin inhibition and catecholamine release, although the clinical relevance has not been established.

In addition to its ability to stabilize mast cells, other antiinflammatory and immunomodulatory effects of theophylline have been observed. Adenosine-stimulated release of mediators from mast cells, neutrophil activation, induction of IL-1β by IL-1α, synthesis and release of TNF-α, and cytokine release from T-lymphocytes are inhibited by theophylline (32). Observed immunomodulatory effects on T-lymphocytes suggest that theophylline may inhibit the movement of T-lymphocytes from the peripheral circulation into the airways; these effects have been observed to occur at serum concentrations less than 55 μmol/liter (10 μg/mL) (32). The clinical relevance of these properties remains to be established, as the antiinflammatory effects are weaker than those achieved with inhaled glucocorticoids.

Other related pharmacologic actions of theophylline include increased right and left ventricular ejection fraction, reduced fatigue of the diaphragmatic muscles, which may decrease work of breathing, decreased vascular permeability, and enhanced mucociliary clearance (32), though some of these effects have not been consistently observed in all studies (32).

Theophylline is administered orally, intravenously, and rectally, although the latter is rarely used because of unpredictable absorption. Theophylline has no antiasthma effects when given by the inhaled route. Familiarity with the pharmacokinetics of theophylline is essential to safe and effective use of this drug. In addition, recognition that differences in the formulations of slow release products can result in significant differences in the rate and extent of absorption is also important. A thorough discussion on the latter may be found in reference 33. Clinicians who use this drug must stay abreast of new information relating to therapeutic efficacy and toxicity (pharmacokinetics of slow-release formulations, drug interactions, combination therapy with other antiasthma therapy). Inappropriate use leading to toxicity can have dire consequences for the patient.

The therapeutic range has been defined as 55 to 110 µmol/liter (10 to 20 µg/mL), although a lower range of 27.5 to 82.5 µmol/liter (5 to 15 µg/mL) has been proposed (32). Recent evidence indicates some immunomodulatory and antiinflammatory effects occur at relatively low concentrations 27.5 to 55 µmol/liter (5 to 10 µg/mL). Toxic effects may be seen at concentrations above 82.5 µmol/liter (15 µg/mL).

Theophylline pharmacokinetics largely depend on factors influencing hepatic metabolism after 1 year of age, when approximately 90 percent of a dose is metabolized in the liver. Below 1 year of age, nearly half a dose is excreted as unchanged theophylline in the urine. N-demethylation and hydroxylation are the major metabolic pathways and are regulated by several P-450 enzymes including 1A2, 2E1, and 3A3. Both pathways are saturable within the therapeutic range, and persons with high initial clearance rates may be at greatest risk. Factors influencing hepatic metabolism of theophylline include age, concurrent diseases, and drug interactions. Hyperthyroidism, cystic fibrosis, smoking, and ingestion of a high-protein/low-carbohydrate diet are common conditions known to increase theophylline clearance, whereas age less than 1 year or over 60 years, congestive heart failure, prolonged fever (greater than 102°F), hypothyroidism, and liver disease are some conditions known to decrease theophylline clearance. Nearly 80 drugs have been evaluated with respect to their effect on theophylline clearance, and approximately half have clinically important interactions (Tables 35.6 and 35.7) (34). Theophylline rarely affects the pharmacokinetics of other drugs.

Dosing schemes and monitoring guidelines for theophylline administration in acute and chronic asthma are presented in Figure 35.6 (16, 35) and Figure 35.7 (34), respectively. However, the dosages listed are merely guidelines for attaining serum concentrations within the therapeutic range and should be confirmed with serum concentration measurement.

Adverse effects to theophylline are generally mild and temporary when serum concentrations are less than 110 µmol/liter (20 µg/mL) and include caffeinelike effects such as nausea and vomiting, headache, and insomnia. The severity of adverse effects worsen as the serum concentration exceeds 110 µmol/liter (20 µg/mL) (Fig. 35.8) (36). However, minor symptoms of toxicity such as nausea and vomiting may not precede more severe toxicity and cannot be relied upon as a dosing end point. Only serum concentration measurement can reliably predict the potential for severe or life-threatening toxicity. Nonserum concentration-related adverse effects reported include learning and concentration difficulties in school children

and behavior problems. However, controlled studies have failed to confirm a relationship to theophylline.

In general, severe toxicity from theophylline use is rare. However, when severe toxicity occurs, it is often life-threatening. In one study of 35,000 theophylline users over 9 years in a health maintenance organization, the risk of being hospitalized for theophylline toxicity was only 8 per 10,000 person-years' exposure (37). The manifestations and severity of toxicity after theophylline overdosing differs between acute single ingestion and chronic repeated dosing and will determine management and outcome. Patients with acute single overdosing have hypotension, hypokalemia, low serum bicarbonate, and higher serum concentrations of theophylline, and are less likely to suffer seizures or death than those with chronic overdosing. Generalized seizures and arrhythmias frequently develop in patients with chronic overdosing at serum concentrations of 220 to 385 µmol/liter (40 to 70 µg/mL); patients over the age of 60 years are at greatest risk (38). In contrast, life-threatening events usually do not occur in cases of acute overdose unless the serum concentration exceeds 550 µmol/liter (100 µg/mL) (38). Treatments for toxicity include oral activated charcoal, phenobarbital, or diazepam for seizures, antiarrhythmics for life-threatening arrhythmias, and charcoal hemoperfusion.

Theophylline is a relatively weak bronchodilator compared with inhaled β₂-adrenergic agonists. However, a log-linear dose-response relationship is observed at serum concentrations between 27.5 to 110 µmol/liter (5 to 20 µg/mL), although less benefit is seen for increases between 82.5 to 110 µmol/liter (15 and 20 µg/mL). Like the β-adrenergic agonists, theophylline is a functional antagonist and can inhibit bronchospasm induced by various stimuli including histamine, methacholine, exercise, and distilled water in a serum concentration-related manner (32). Protection has been noted at serum concentrations less than 55 µmol/liter (10 µg/mL) for exercise and methacholine-induced bronchoconstriction. However, studies examining the long-term effects of theophylline in reducing bronchial hyperresponsiveness measured by bronchoprovocation with histamine or methacholine have been conflicting (32). It appears that theophylline is effective in preventing the fall in airway function during both the IAR and LAR after inhaled allergen and in inhibiting the subsequent increase in airway responsiveness to histamine (39). The effect seen with theophylline is similar to that after inhaled cromolyn from a MDI (39).

Until inhaled β-adrenergic agonists were introduced in the late 1970s and 1980s, theophylline had a well-established role in the treatment of acute asthma. With the recognition that early intervention with systemic glucocorticoids prevented relapse in acute asthma and the introduction of inhaled glucocorticoids for chronic asthma, further questions were raised concerning the value of

Table 35.6.
Clinically Significant Drug Interactions with Theophylline

Drug	Type of Interaction	Effect[a]
Adenosine	Theophylline blocks adenosine receptors.	Higher doses of adenosine may be required to achieve desired effect.
Alcohol	A single large dose of alcohol (3 mL/kg of whiskey) decreases theophylline clearance for up to 24 hours.	30% increase
Allopurinol	Decreases theophylline clearance at allopurinol doses ≥ 600 mg/day.	25% increase
Aminoglutethimide	Increases theophylline clearance by induction of microsomal enzyme activity.	25% decrease
Carbamazepine	Similar to aminoglutethimide.	30% decrease
Cimetidine	Decreases theophylline clearance by inhibiting cytochrome P450 1A2.	70% increase
Ciprofloxacin	Similar to cimetidine.	40% increase
Clarithromycin	Similar to erythromycin.	25% increase
Diazepam	Benzodiazepines increase CNS concentrations of adenosine, a potent CNS depressant, while theophylline blocks adenosine receptors.	Larger benzodiazepine doses may be required to produce desired level of sedation. Discontinuation of theophylline without reduction of diazepam dose may result in respiratory depression.
Disulfiram	Decreases theophylline clearance by inhibiting hydroxylation and demethylation.	50% increase
Enoxacin	Similar to cimetidine.	300% increase
Ephedrine	Synergistic CNS effects.	Increased frequency of nausea, nervousness, and insomnia.
Erythromycin	Erythromycin metabolite decreases theophylline clearance by inhibiting cytochrome P450 3A3.	35% increase. Erythromycin steady-state serum concentrations decrease by a similar amount.
Estrogen	Estrogen containing oral contraceptives decrease theophylline clearance in a dose-dependent fashion. The effect of progesterone on theophylline clearance is unkown.	30% increase
Flurazepam	Similar to diazepam.	Similar to diazepam.
Fluvoxamine	Similar to cimetidine.	Similar to cimetidine.
Halothane	Halothane sensitizes the myocardium to endogenous catecholamines, theophylline increases the release of endogenous catecholamines.	Increased risk of ventricular arrhythmias.
Interferon, human recombinant α A	Decreases theophylline clearance.	100% increase.
Isoproterenol (IV)	Increases theophylline clearance.	20% decrease.
Ketamine	Pharmacologic.	May lower theophylline seizure threshold.
Lithium	Theophylline increases renal lithium clearance.	Lithium dose required to achieve a therapeutic serum concentration increased an average of 60%.
Lorazepam	Similar to diazepam.	Similar to diazepam.
Methotrexate (MTX)	Decreases theophylline clearance.	20% increase after low dose MTX, higher dose MTX may have a greater effect.
Mexiletine	Similar to disulfiram.	80% increase.
Midazolam	Similar to diazepam.	Similar to diazepam.
Moricizine	Increases theophylline clearance.	25% decrease.
Pancuronium	Theophylline may antagonize nondepolarizing neuromuscular blocking effects; possibly due to phosphodiesterase inhibition.	Larger dose of pancuronium may be required to achieve neuromuscular blockade.
Pentoxifylline	Decreases theophylline clearance.	30% increase
Phenobarbital (PB)	Similar to aminoglutethimide.	25% decrease after two weeks of concurrent PB.
Phenytoin	Phenytoin increases theophylline clearance by increasing microsomal enzyme activity. Theophylline decreases phenytoin absorption.	Serum theophylline *and* phenytoin concentrations decrease about 40%.
Propafenone	Decreases theophylline clearance, and pharmacologic interaction.	40% increase. β_2-Blocking effect may decrease the efficacy of theophylline.

(continued)

Table 35.6. *(Continued)*

Drug	Type of Interaction	Effect[a]
Propranolol	Similar to cimetidine, and pharmacologic interaction.	100% increase. β_2-blocking effect may decrease efficacy of theophylline
Rifampin	Increases theophylline clearance by increasing cytochrome P450, 1A2 and 3A3 activity.	20–40% decrease
Sulfinpyrazone	Increases theophylline clearance by increasing demethylation and hydroxylation. Decreases renal clearance of theophylline.	20% decrease
Tacrine	Similar to cimetidine, also increases renal clearance theophylline.	90% increase
Thiabendazole	Decreases theophylline clearance.	190% increase
Ticlopidine	Decreases theophylline clearance.	60% increase
Troleandomycin	Similar to erythromycin.	33–100% increase depending on troleandomycin dose.
Verapamil	Similar to disulfiram.	20% increase
Zileuton	Similar to cimetidine.	75% increase

[a]Average effect on steady-state theophylline concentration or other clinical effect for pharmacologic interactions. Individual patients may experience larger changes in serum theophylline concentration than the value listed.
From reference 34 with permission.

Table 35.7.

Drugs That Have Been Documented Not to Interact with Theophylline or Drugs That Produce No Clinically Significant Interaction with Theophylline

albuterol, systemic and inhaled	lomefloxacin
amoxicillin	mebendazole
ampicillin, with or without sulbactam	medroxyprogesterone
atenolol	methylprednisolone
azithromycin	metronidazole
caffeine, dietary ingestion	metoprolol
cefaclor	nadolol
co-trimoxazole (trimethoprim and sulfamethoxazole)	nifedipine
diltiazem	nizatidine
dirithromycin	norfloxacin
enflurane	ofloxacin
famotidine	omeprazole
felodipine	pinacidil
finasteride	prednisone, prednisolone
hydrocortisone	ranitidine
isoflurane	rifabutin
isoniazid	roxithromycin
isradipine	sorbitol (purgative doses do not inhibit theophylline absorption)
influenza vaccine	sucralfate
ketoconazole	terbutaline, systemic
	terfenadine
	tetracycline
	tocainide

From reference 34, with permission.

theophylline. There have now been many well-designed studies published evaluating the addition of theophylline to optimal inhaled β_2-adrenergic agonists plus systemic glucocorticoids in both the emergency department and in hospitalized patients being treated for acute severe asthma. In all but two studies, one in the emergency department

(40) and one in hospitalized patients (41), no difference was noted when theophylline was added to optimal inhaled β_2-adrenergic agonists and systemic glucocorticoids. However, no studies have evaluated the effectiveness of theophylline in patients with impending respiratory failure. In most studies, the addition of theophylline significantly increased the incidence of adverse effects. These studies indicate that in the treatment of acute asthma, intravenous theophylline should be reserved for those patients who fail to respond to high-dose inhaled β_2-adrenergic agonists and systemic glucocorticoids (42–47).

In contrast, theophylline continues to be important in the management of chronic asthma, but its role is being redefined. There are patients who, despite the regular use of inhaled glucocorticoids, have fewer symptoms, less inhaled β-adrenergic agonist use, and fewer exacerbations requiring systemic glucocorticoids, with the addition of theophylline (32). Some steroid-dependent asthmatics are unable to tolerate the withdrawal of theophylline even with subsequent additional glucocorticoid (32). Theophylline is as effective as cromolyn in the treatment of mild to moderate pediatric patients with asthma, although there is no additive effect when the two drugs are combined (16). Adverse effects occur more frequently with theophylline compared with cromolyn. Theophylline is also effective for the treatment of nocturnal asthma, and a single dose of a slow-release formulation may provide control of symptoms throughout the night. However, the long-acting inhaled β_2-adrenergic agonists can provide better control of daytime and nocturnal symptoms with fewer adverse effects compared with theophylline (32).

ANTICHOLINERGICS

Anticholinergic drugs have been used in the treatment of asthmalike symptoms for over 400 years. Until the

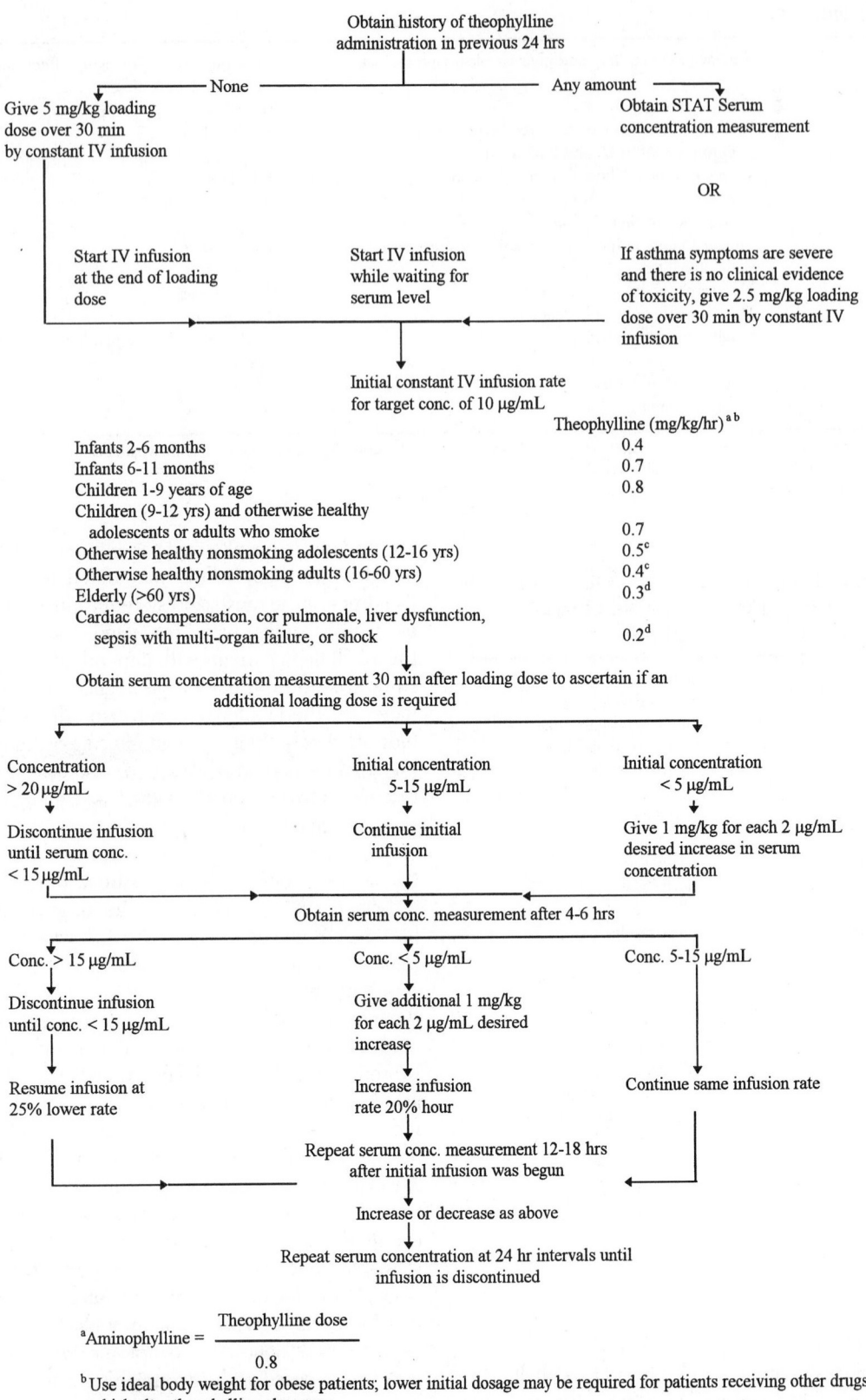

Obtain history of theophylline
administration in previous 24 hrs

——————— None   Any amount ———————

Give 5 mg/kg loading   Obtain STAT Serum
dose over 30 min   concentration measurement
by constant IV infusion

                                                                           OR

Start IV infusion   Start IV infusion   If asthma symptoms are severe
at the end of loading   while waiting for   and there is no clinical evidence
dose   serum level   of toxicity, give 2.5 mg/kg loading
                                                         dose over 30 min by constant IV
                                                         infusion

                           Initial constant IV infusion rate
                           for target conc. of 10 µg/mL

                                                         Theophylline (mg/kg/hr)[a][b]
Infants 2-6 months   0.4
Infants 6-11 months   0.7
Children 1-9 years of age   0.8
Children (9-12 yrs) and otherwise healthy
   adolescents or adults who smoke   0.7
Otherwise healthy nonsmoking adolescents (12-16 yrs)   0.5[c]
Otherwise healthy nonsmoking adults (16-60 yrs)   0.4[c]
Elderly (>60 yrs)   0.3[d]
Cardiac decompensation, cor pulmonale, liver dysfunction,
   sepsis with multi-organ failure, or shock   0.2[d]

Obtain serum concentration measurement 30 min after loading dose to ascertain if an
                           additional loading dose is required

Concentration   Initial concentration   Initial concentration
> 20 µg/mL   5-15 µg/mL   < 5 µg/mL

Discontinue infusion   Continue initial   Give 1 mg/kg for each 2 µg/mL
until serum conc.   infusion   desired increase in serum
< 15 µg/mL   concentration

                           Obtain serum conc. measurement after 4-6 hrs

Conc. > 15 µg/mL   Conc. < 5 µg/mL   Conc. 5-15 µg/mL

Discontinue infusion   Give additional 1 mg/kg
until conc. < 15 µg/mL   for each 2 µg/mL desired
                           increase

Resume infusion at   Increase infusion   Continue same infusion rate
25% lower rate   rate 20% hour

                           Repeat serum conc. measurement 12-18 hrs
                           after initial infusion was begun

                           Increase or decrease as above

                           Repeat serum concentration at 24 hr intervals until
                           infusion is discontinued

[a]Aminophylline = $\dfrac{\text{Theophylline dose}}{0.8}$

[b] Use ideal body weight for obese patients; lower initial dosage may be required for patients receiving other drugs
    which alter theophylline clearance.
[c] Not to exceed 900 mg/day, unless serum concentration levels indicate the need for a larger dose.
[d] Not to exceed 400 mg/day, unless serum concentration levels indicate the need for a larger dose.

Figure 35.6.   Algorithm for intravenous theophylline use in acute asthma. Adapted from references 16 and 35.

Titration Step 1
Starting Dosage
Children < 45kg: 12-14 mg/kg/day up to a maximum of 300 mg/day divided Q4-6 hrs[a]
Children > 45 kg and adults: 300 mg/day divided Q6-8 hrs[a]

↓

after 3 days

Titration Step 2
If tolerated, increase dose to:
Children < 45kg: 16 mg/kg/day up to a maximum of 400 mg/day divided Q4-6 hrs[a]
Children > 45 kg and adults: 400 mg/day divided Q6-8 hrs[a]

↓

after 3 more days

Titration Step 3
If tolerated, increase dose to:
Children < 45kg: 20 mg/kg/day up to a maximum of 600 mg/day divided Q4-6 hrs[a]
Children > 45 kg and adults: 600 mg/day divided Q6-8 hrs[a]

↓

Peak Serum Concentration	Dosage Adjustment
>9.9 µg/mL	If symptoms are not controlled and current dosage is tolerated, increase dose about 25%. Recheck serum concentration after three days for further dosage adjustment.
10 to 14.9 µg/mL	If symptoms are controlled and current dosage is tolerated, maintain dose, and recheck serum concentration at 6-12 month intervals.[b] If symptoms are not controlled and current dosage is tolerated consider adding additional medication(s) to treatment regimen.
15-19.9 µg/mL	Consider 10% decrease in dose to provide greater margin of safety even if current dosage is tolerated.[b]
20-24.9 µg/mL	Decrease dose by 25% even if no adverse effects are present. Recheck serum concentration after 3 days to guide further dosage adjustment.
25-30 µg/mL	Skip next dose and decrease subsequent doses at least 25% even if no adverse effects are present. Recheck serum concentration after 3 days to guide further dosage adjustment. If symptomatic, consider whether overdose treatment is indicated .
>30 µg/mL	Treat overdose as indicated. If theophylline is subsequently resumed, decrease dose by at least 50% and recheck serum concentration after 3 days to guide further dosage adjustment.

[a] Patients with more rapid metabolism, clinically identified by higher than average dose requirements, should receive a smaller dose more frequently to prevent breakthrough symptoms resulting from low trough concentrations before the next dose. A reliably absorbed slow-release formulation will decrease fluctuations and permit longer dosing intervals. For products containing theophylline salts, the appropriate dose of the theophylline salt should be substituted for the anhydrous theophylline dose. To calculate the equivalent dose for theophylline salts, divide the anhydrous theophylline dose listed below by 0.8 for aminophylline, by 0.65 for oxtriphylline, and by 0.5 for the calcium salicylate and sodium glycinate salts.

[b] Dose reduction and/or serum theophylline concentration measurement is indicated whenever adverse effects are present, physiologic abnormalities that can reduce theophylline clearance occur (e.g., sustained fever), or a drug that interacts with theophylline is added or discontinued.

Figure 35.7. Algorithm for immediate-release oral theophylline use in chronic asthma. From reference 34, with permission.

Figure 35.8. Relationship of serum concentration and symptoms of toxicity among 50 adults monitored consecutively in the Medical Intensive Care Unit of the University of Iowa during constant intravenous infusions of theophylline averaging 0.9 mg/kg/hr as aminophylline. Symptoms of toxicity were recorded by a pulmonary physician before the result of the serum concentration measurement became available. Mild toxicity included nausea, vomiting, headache, nervousness, and insomnia. Moderate toxicity consisted of mild symptoms in conjunction with sinus tachycardia and occasional premature ventricular contractions (PVCs). Patients in the severe category experienced serious arrhythmias such as multiple PVCs or ventricular tachycardia and/or grand mal seizures that occurred in two patients, one of whom died. Previous symptoms of nausea and vomiting or other minor symptoms of toxicity were absent in half of the patients in the moderate and severe categories. From reference 36, with permission.

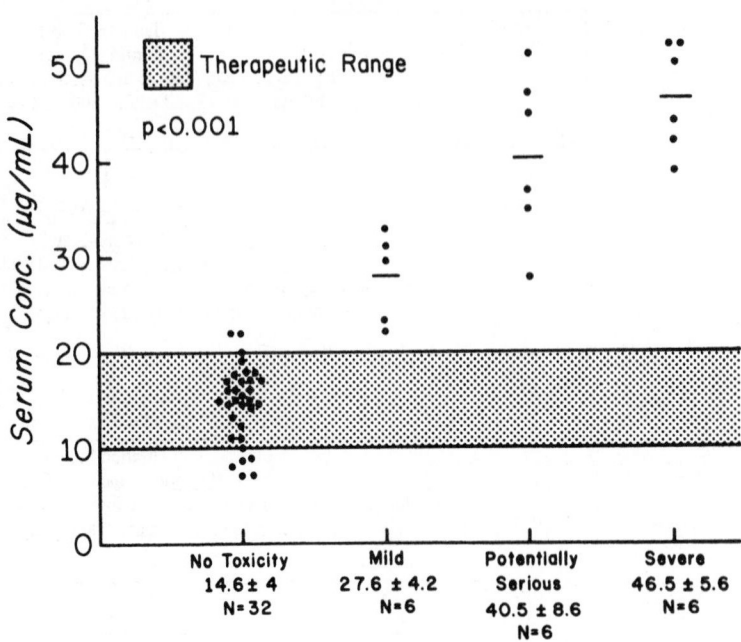

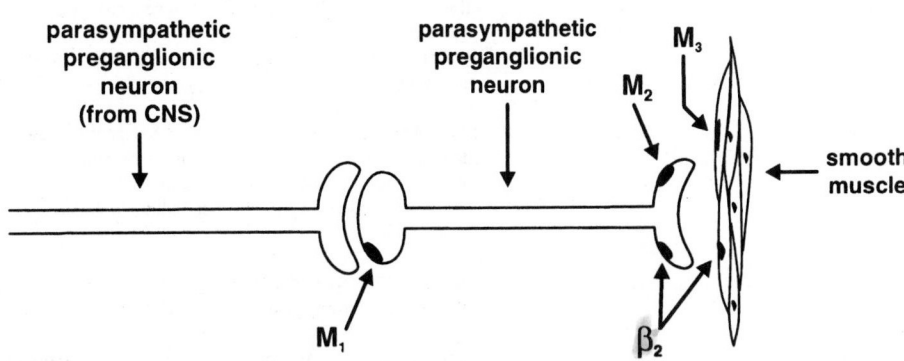

Figure 35.9. Diagram of parasympathetic nervous system illustrating location of M_1, M_2, M_3, and β_2 receptors.

introduction of quaternary ammonium derivatives such as ipratropium, glycopyrrolate, atropine methonitrate, and oxitropium, central nervous system adverse effects limited their use. Traditionally it has been believed that acetylcholine stimulation of the muscarinic receptor on bronchial smooth muscle induces the formation of cyclic GMP, which releases intracellular calcium, causing smooth muscle contraction. Recent information suggests that stimulation of the muscarinic receptor may activate an inhibitory G protein and decrease the activity of adenylate cyclase, resulting in decreased cAMP, causing smooth muscle contraction. Two other mechanisms include activation of phospholipase C via a different G protein, which releases stores of intracellular calcium producing smooth muscle contraction, and formation of a second messenger, diacylglycerol, which activates protein kinase C and causes a slow and prolonged contraction (48).

The parasympathetic (versus the sympathetic) nervous system is largely responsible for the control of baseline airway caliber. Therefore, anticholinergic drugs, which are competitive antagonists rather than functional antagonists, will be most useful in those patients whose symptoms are due to excessive cholinergic stimulation. Unfortunately, it is not possible to predict those patients whose asthma symptoms may be caused by excessive cholinergic stimulation. Since most mediators, such as histamine, allergens, and exercise, cause bronchoconstriction only partially through cholinergic stimulation, anticholinergics will be less effective than β_2-adrenergic agonists and theophylline, which are functional antagonists.

Currently available anticholinergics are nonselective competitive antagonists at the muscarinic receptor. Recently, five muscarinic receptor subtypes have been discovered; three receptors have been characterized pharmacologically (Fig. 35.9) (48, 49). Stimulation of M_1 receptors on the terminal of parasympathetic preganglionic neurons facilitates cholinergic transmission. M_2 receptors, located on the postganglionic terminal, inhibit acetylcholine release when stimulated and thus function as inhibitory feedback receptors. It is believed that abnormal functioning or absence of the M_2 receptors is responsible for asthma induced by β-blocker drugs (48). Blockade of the β_2-adrenergic receptor on cholinergic nerves stimulates release of acetylcholine, which is normally turned off by the M_2 receptor. Dysfunction of the M_2 receptor allows continued release of acetylcholine, resulting in exaggerated bronchoconstriction. M_3 receptors located on airway smooth muscle also facilitate cholinergic transmission. Therefore, selective blockers at the M_1 and M_3 receptors would likely have enhanced benefit over nonselective muscarinic receptor blockers. Antagonism of M_3 receptors, also located on mucus glands, will cause drying of secretions; therefore, drugs will need to be developed for inhalation use to avoid unwanted systemic adverse effects (49).

With the availability of ipratropium bromide for nebulization, a quaternary amine, there is no longer any reason to use nebulized atropine. Atropine is rapidly absorbed when given by the inhaled route, resulting in dose-related adverse effects including tachycardia, meiosis causing blurred vision, difficulty swallowing, and flushing. Ipratropium is remarkably free of unwanted adverse effects because of its minimal systemic absorption. Adverse effects may include dry mouth, irritated throat, or bitter taste.

Anticholinergics do not produce maximal bronchodilation when compared with β-adrenergic agonists in asthmatics but do have a longer duration of effect. Maximum bronchodilation occurs in 1.5 to 2 hours; however, 50 percent of the eventual maximum occurs within 3 to 5 minutes and 80 percent within 30 minutes (50), which is comparable clinically to the time of peak effect (30 minutes) with inhaled β_2-adrenergic agonists. At usual doses, the duration of bronchodilation is 4 to 6 hours. Ipratropium bromide incompletely protects against bronchoconstriction induced by histamine, cold air, allergen, exercise, prostaglandins, bradykinin, serotonin, and other mediators that have effects only partially mediated through vagal reflex mechanisms. Dose-response relationships exist for ipratropium bromide when delivered by metered-dose inhaler and nebulization (16).

The role of anticholinergics in the treatment of asthma is being redefined. The development of selective muscarinic receptor antagonists may change how anticholinergics are used in asthma management. Inhaled anticholinergics may be used in the treatment of severe acute asthma, but clinical studies indicate a wide variability in response. These drugs are not considered first-line therapy but may provide additional bronchodilation when added to optimal dosages of β_2-adrenergic agonists in patients who fail to adequately respond to the latter or patients who present with severe airways obstruction (2). Little information exists on the use of anticholinergics in combination with high-dose intermittent or continuously nebulized β_2-adrenergic agonists in severe acute asthma.

One study suggests that like the β_2-adrenergic agonists, anticholinergics should not be used on a regularly scheduled basis without concomitant antiinflammatory therapy in the treatment of chronic asthma, as an accelerated decline in pulmonary function can occur (51). The combination of theophylline or β-adrenergic agonists with ipratropium can produce additive effects in chronic asthma; however, the long-term effects on airway inflammation are unknown (16). There is little information on the use of anticholinergics in combination with inhaled glucocorticoids, cromolyn, or nedocromil in chronic asthma. Currently, anticholinergics may be indicated in those persons who continue to be symptomatic despite therapy with inhaled glucocorticoids. However, it would be reasonable to document bronchodilator responsiveness prior to initiating chronic therapy with inhaled anticholinergics, as only a small percentage of asthmatics may be expected to respond. Limited data indicate that anticholinergics may be effective in psychogenic asthma.

Antiinflammatory Agents
CROMOLYN/NEDOCROMIL

Cromolyn sodium has been available for the treatment of asthma for approximately two decades, and nedocromil sodium has been available for the last few years. Though structurally distinct and possibly pharmacologically distinct, these two drugs are often discussed together. Neither drug has acute bronchodilator effects. The exact mechanisms of action for each are largely unknown, but both are capable of inhibiting the IgE-mediated release of mediators from mast cells. However, this effect seems to vary depending on the species and the cell type tested. Other drugs with greater mast cell stabilizing activity do not have therapeutic efficacy (48). Cromolyn is also effective in preventing mast cell degranulation induced by nonimmunolgic stimuli such as phospholipase A, dextran, and polymyxin B. The mechanism by which cromolyn and nedocromil inhibit mediator release at the cellular level is unclear but likely involves regulation of intracellular calcium probably by phosphorylation of a specific membrane protein that inhibits calcium influx into the cell. Cromolyn and nedocromil also inhibit the release of mediators from eosinophils, alveolar macrophages, neutrophils, and monocytes (52). Other effects regulated by cromolyn include inhibition of phosphodiesterase, modification of the vagal reflex, and inhibition of irritant receptors. Cromolyn and nedocromil also inhibit chemotaxis of inflammatory mediators and may inhibit release of inflammatory neuropeptides that induce bronchoconstriction through efferent cholinergic pathways (48, 52).

Neither cromolyn nor nedocromil is effective orally or intravenously. Cromolyn or nedocromil that is systemically absorbed is largely excreted unchanged in the urine or the bile. The half-life for clinical effectiveness is short (less than 4 hours); thus, these drugs require dosing three to four times daily (52). In some patients, particularly children, twice daily dosing may also be effective. Symptoms should be brought under control with three to four times daily dosing before attempting to reduce the dose further. Adverse effects from cromolyn and nedocromil are rare and most often include transient bronchospasm, cough, and dry throat. Bronchospasm is quickly relieved with administration of an inhaled β_2-adrenergic agonist. Infrequent adverse effects include anaphylaxis, generalized or facial dermatitis, myositis, gastroenteritis, and immunologic reactions in the lung. Because of the lack of systemic effects, cromolyn is often regarded as the safest antiinflammatory therapy for asthma for use in children and during pregnancy.

Both cromolyn and nedocromil inhibit the early and late response to inhaled allergen. They also prevent exercise induced asthma (though to a much lesser extent than inhaled β_2-adrenergic agonists). Dose-response relationships have been observed in both circumstances. Both drugs modify bronchoconstriction induced by sulfur dioxide, aspirin, and cold air, and nedocromil has additional effects on substance P-, bradykinin-, and neurokinin A-induced bronchoconstriction (48, 52). Despite the variety of effects, cromolyn and nedocromil are most valued for their ability to decrease airway responsiveness measured by histamine or methacholine-induced bronchoconstriction when given for at least 12 weeks. Cromolyn and nedocromil have effects similar in magnitude to that of low dose inhaled glucocorticoids (<400 µg/day) on airway reactivity, although their effects have not been found to be uniformly consistent. This variability may indicate that patients may be responders or nonresponders to these drugs. There appears to be no benefit to adding cromolyn or nedocromil to high dose inhaled glucocorticoids (>1000 µg/day) or oral glucocorticoids. However, some patients on moderate doses of inhaled glucocorticoids may achieve a reduction in glucocorticoid dose with added cromolyn or nedocromil (16, 52).

Numerous studies have compared the combination of cromolyn or nedocromil with theophylline versus each drug alone. Both classes of drugs are indicated for the treatment of mild to moderate chronic asthma, and both appear to provide similar control of symptoms. Cromolyn and nedocromil, however, are more effective in reducing airway responsiveness than theophylline. The combination of cromolyn or nedocromil with theophylline in general is no more effective than either drug alone (16, 52). However, cromolyn and nedocromil may have to be administered three to four times daily, which would likely result in decreased compliance compared with oral theophylline. In comparison with each other, nedocromil may be slightly more effective than cromolyn, particularly in younger patients (52).

Cromolyn and nedocromil are not indicated for the relief of acute symptoms of asthma as neither has bronchodilator effects. Neither is the first choice for the prevention of exercise-induced asthma, as inhaled β_2-adrenergic agonists are markedly more effective. Both are indicated for the treatment of mild to moderate asthma, and although clinical effects may be noted within 1 week of starting therapy, 4 weeks is generally required to determine if an individual has a response to therapy. The NAEP guidelines (1) but not the International guidelines (2) also list cromolyn as an alternative for severe asthma, although inhaled glucocorticoids are likely to be more effective. In general, cromolyn and nedocromil are most effective in patients with seasonal asthma and are effective when used immediately prior to exposure to an allergen. Given the unpredictable response to therapy, attempts have been made to characterize those patients most likely to respond. Such patients have an age less than 17 years, positive history of atopy, positive skin tests, high serum measurements of IgE, eosinophilia, and mild to moderate disease (48).

GLUCOCORTICOIDS

With the new emphasis on antiinflammatory therapy, glucocorticoids, particularly inhaled, are now a cornerstone in the treatment of asthma. Inhaled antiinflammatory agents are recommended in all asthmatic patients requiring regular inhaled bronchodilator treatments. Systemic glucocorticoids are reserved for severe chronic asthma and acute exacerbations.

Systemic. Glucocorticoids have been used in the treatment of asthma for over 40 years. Structural changes to cortisone have resulted in synthetic glucocorticoids with enhanced potencies and prolonged duration of action. Cortisone itself is inactive and must be interconverted at the 11-ketone group to a hydroxy molecule via metabolic pathways to its active form, cortisol or hydrocortisone, just as prednisone requires interconversion to prednisolone. The specific mechanism of action of glucocorticoids is not well established despite their long history in the treatment of asthma; however, many of their biochemical actions are known.

Glucocorticoids have many actions that may contribute to their effectiveness in controlling inflammation. After penetrating the cell wall, a number of complex steps involving activation and binding of the glucocorticoid receptor and its subunits are necessary. Ultimately, binding to a specific sequence of DNA within the nucleus, termed the *glucocorticoid responsive element* (GRE), occurs, resulting in transcriptional regulation of primary target genes and biochemical effects (53).

Glucocorticoids are known to prevent and reverse down regulation of β_2-receptors and induce increases of receptor density. Production of various cytokines and mediators thought to be important in the inflammation of asthma are inhibited by glucocorticoids. These include IL-1, IL-2, IL-3, IL-4, GM-CSF, IFN-γ, TNF-α, histamine, bradykinin, leukotrienes, prostaglandins, thromboxanes, and other arachidonic acid metabolites. The cells involved in inflammation are also affected by glucocorticoids. Lymphocyte, eosinophil, monocyte, and basophil circulating cell counts are reduced, cytokine-mediated eosinophil survival is inhibited, and eosinophil and neutrophil chemotaxis are reduced. Physiologic effects of glucocorticoids include inhibition of microvascular leakage and, of particular relevance to asthma, reduction of bronchial hyperresponsiveness (53).

A slow onset of action and slow dissipation of effects, consistent with clinical responses by patients with asthma, is a characteristic feature of glucocorticoid pharmacodynamics. This was demonstrated in an early study. Following administration of a single dose of 40 mg prednisolone, the onset of improvements of pulmonary function in stable asthmatics occurred 3 hours after administration. Maximal effects were seen 9 to 12 hours following the dose, with a gradual return to baseline values after 36 hours (16).

Due to their structural modifications, the various glucocorticoids differ in their potencies and durations of action (Table 35.8). These effects in turn influence their recommended doses, as well as the risk for adverse effects, as do their pharmacokinetic parameters (Table 35.9) (54).

Glucocorticoids are generally well absorbed following oral administration. One exception is with concomitant antacids, which can inhibit absorption of prednisone. Liver disease has the potential for reducing glucocorticoid clearance; however, it is not a significant factor in individualizing prednisolone doses as it is extensively metabolized in other organs. Other drugs can, however, affect glucocorticoid clearance. Most notable are macrolide antibiotics, which reduce clearance, and anticonvulsants and rifampin, which enhance clearance (Table 35.10) (54).

Prolonged use of systemically administered glucocorticoids is limited by adverse effects (Table 35.11). These can be severe and debilitating, and necessitate use of the lowest possible doses. Limited short courses may be necessary, however, for treatment of acute exacerbations. Typically, 30 to 80 mg/day of prednisolone (or equivalent) is administered for 3 to 10 days depending on response, with tapering of the dose required only after approximately

Table 35.8.
Relative Potencies and Equivalent Doses of Glucocorticoids Commonly Used in the Treatment of Asthma

Glucocorticoid	Relative Antiinflammatory Potency	Equivalent Dose (mg)
hydrocortisone	1	20
prednisolone	4	5
methylprednisolone	5	4
dexamethasone	25	0.75

Table 35.9.
Pharmacokinetic Parameters of Glucocorticoids Commonly Used in the Treatment of Asthma (mean or mean ± SD)

Glucocorticoid	Clearance (mL/min/1.73m²)	Half-life (hours)	Volume of Distribution (L/1.73 m²)
hydrocortisone	425.5	1.9 ± 1.1	70
prednisolone	198 ± 38	3.25 ± 0.58	53.5 ± 13.5
methylprednisolone	384 ± 56.2	2.58 ± 0.19	91.0 ± 9.9
dexamethasone	216 ± 21.5	4.37 ± 1.16	33.4 ± 4.2

From reference 54, with permission.

Table 35.10.
Potential Drug Interactions with Glucocorticoids

Interacting Medication, Disease State, or Factor	Effect on Glucocorticoids
antacids	decreased bioavailability
ketoconazole	impaired elimination
erythromycin, troleandomycin	impaired methylprednisolone elimination
oral contraceptives	impaired elimination
hypothyroidism	possibly impaired elimination
aminoglutethimide	enhanced elimination
carbamazepine	enhanced elimination
ephedrine	enhanced elimination
phenobarbital	enhanced elimination
phenytoin	enhanced elimination
rifampin	enhanced elimination
hyperthyroidism	possibly enhanced elimination

From reference 54, with permission

Table 35.11.
Adverse Reactions of Systemic Glucocorticoid Therapy

adrenal suppression and insufficiency
fluid and electrolyte imbalances
hypertension
hyperglycemia
increased susceptibility to infection
peptic ulcers
osteoporosis
myopathy
behavioral disturbances
posterior subcapsular cataracts
growth suppression
Cushingoid habitus (moon facies, buffalo hump, central obesity)
striae
ecchymosis
acne
hirsutism

Table 35.12.
Manufacturer's Maximum Recommended Doses of Inhaled Glucocorticoids

| Glucocorticoid | µg/inhalation | Children[a] | | Adults | |
		Inhalations/day	µg/day	Inhalations/day	µg/day
beclomethasone dipropionate	42	10	420	20	840
flunisolide	250	4	1000	8	2000
triamcinolone acetonide	100[b]	12	1200	16	1600

[a]Ages 6–12 years for beclomethasone dipropionate and triamcinolone acetonide, ages 6–15 years for flunisolide.
[b]According to manufacturer 200 µg from metering valve, but 100 µg retained in spacer.
From reference 54, with permission.

2 weeks or more of therapy. For more severe acute cases, intravenous therapy consisting of methylprednisolone sodium succinate 1 mg/kg every 6 hours, followed by oral prednisone 1 to 2 mg/kg/day for 3 to 7 days may be required. If maintenance oral glucocorticoids are needed for control of chronic symptoms, it is important that the lowest effective doses be given and that therapy be periodically reevaluated to minimize the patient's risk for severe adverse effects. Alternate day regimens, as compared to daily doses, pose a somewhat reduced risk for glucocorticoid adverse effects (54).

Inhaled. Inhaled glucocorticoids, created by a further modification of the basic glucocorticoid molecule, represent a potent therapy in the treatment of asthma. Those available in the United States are administered by inhalation via metered-dose inhalers, and include beclomethasone dipropionate, flunisolide, and triamcinolone acetonide. These antiinflammatory agents have also been shown to improve the inflammation and bronchial hyperresponsiveness characteristic of asthma, but with a greatly reduced potential for systemic toxicities as compared to systemic administration. As antiinflammatory therapy is recommended for all but the mildest asthmatics, those receiving inhaled glucocorticoids should also receive concomitant short-acting inhaled β_2-adrenergic agonists for symptomatic relief. Explicit maximum doses are recommended by the manufacturers of inhaled glucocorticoids for both children and adults (Table 35.12) (54). These agents are not approved for use in children ≤ 6 years of age, and although currently unavailable in the United States, glucocorticoids for nebulized administration are under investigation.

Dosing of inhaled glucocorticoids is typically four times a day, although flunisolide dosing recommendations call for twice daily administration. Twice daily treatments have been compared to four-times-a-day dosing regimens with other inhaled glucocorticoids (with the same total daily dose). While twice daily administration may allow for improved compliance, deterioration of asthma control was observed with this regimen (55, 56). In contrast, two studies of patients with mild asthma demonstrated no difference in their responses to four-times-a-day or twice daily

dosing of beclomethasone dipropionate (57, 58). Thus, at least in more severe asthmatic patients, frequency of dosing inhaled glucocorticoids may be a more important determinant of their efficacy than the total daily dose administered. In patients with moderate disease, a trial of twice daily dosing is warranted; dosing may be increased to three to four times daily if symptoms are not controlled (59).

Local adverse effects with inhaled glucocorticoid therapy include oropharyngeal candidiasis (thrush), coughing, dysphonia, and hoarseness. Myopathy of the vocal cords may be the mechanism for development of dysphonia. These effects appear to be dose dependent, so treatment should consist of the lowest possible dose that allows for control of asthma symptoms. Auxiliary spacer devices used with metered-dose inhalers reduce oropharyngeal deposition of the glucocorticoid and reduce the incidence and severity of these effects, and are therefore recommended. Mouth rinsing with water or mouthwash following treatments can also reduce the risk for topical adverse effects (2).

The risk for systemic adverse effects with inhaled glucocorticoids has received increasing attention in recent years due to the use of these agents as first-line antiinflammatory therapy. While this remains an area of controversy, most would agree that the risk for such effects is increased with higher doses, especially upward of 1000 µg/day. Adrenal suppression, growth suppression in children, and osteoporosis are of greatest concern. The potential for these effects appears to have considerable interpatient variability but can be reduced by using spacers with metered-dose inhalers and mouth rinsing following inhalation treatments. Monitoring for these adverse effects, particularly with high-dose treatment, is appropriate (60).

Limited data are available regarding the equivalence of inhaled glucocorticoids either to each other or to a reference standard such as prednisolone. Budesonide, available internationally but not approved in the United States, has been reported to have the equivalence of 35 to 58 mg prednisone daily, in terms of controlling asthma symptoms, at the 2000-µg/day dosage. At 1840 µg daily, systemic effects (suppression of blood eosinophils and plasma cortisol concentrations) comparable to 15 mg prednisone were demonstrated (61). No similar data are available for beclomethasone dipropionate, flunisolide, or triamcinolone acetonide; however, these glucocorticoids are believed to be less potent than budesonide based on studies performed in animal models (60).

Newer inhaled glucocorticoids, such as budesonide and fluticasone propionate, are currently in development in the United States. These agents are thought to be more potent than the available agents and to have a reduced risk for systemic glucocorticoid adverse effects. Properties of newer glucocorticoids that may contribute to these claims include a higher affinity to the glucocorticoid receptor, increased topical-to-systemic potency ratio, reduced oral bioavailability, higher degree of first-pass metabolism, more rapid clearance, lack of active metabolites, and availability for administration via dry powder inhaler devices.

INHALED DRUG DELIVERY

Administration of medications by the inhaled route offers the advantage of delivery directly to the site of action. Inherent to this is a reduced dosage requirement, less risk for systemic adverse effects, and potential for improved efficacy and a faster onset of action. Unfortunately, inhaled drug delivery can be affected immensely by a number of factors, such as the aerosol particle size, the inhalation technique, and the delivery device used for administration.

Deposition of inhaled aerosol particles occurs primarily by inertial impaction, sedimentation, and diffusion. Inertial impaction is the means by which larger particles, those unable to flow in the airstream with changes in direction, are deposited. This typically occurs with particles over 5 μm in aerodynamic diameter and results in oropharyngeal deposition as well as deposition into the bifurcations of the larger airways. Smaller particles, those that do not impact and flow in the slower airstream in conducting airways, are deposited by gravitational sedimentation, especially with breath-holding maneuvers. Finally, particles under 0.5 μm in diameter deposit by random Brownian diffusion; however, since these contain an extremely small proportion of the total aerosol and drug mass, they are less important for inhaled drug delivery. Thus, the ideal or "respirable range" of aerosol particles for deposition in the lower respiratory

Table 35.13.
Advantages and Disadvantages of the Various Inhalation Delivery Systems

Device	Advantages	Disadvantages
Nebulizer	Simple to use (requires minimal coordination) Can use in mechanically ventilated patients	Requires water-soluble drug Inefficient delivery Significant drug wasted (residual volume) Numerous factors can affect delivery Device variability (brand to brand, lot to lot) Inconvenient, bulky, costly, and time-consuming Requires electric power source Need to clean nebulizer (potential for infection) Potential for breakdown of drug (ultrasonic) Costly
Metered-dose inhaler	Requires minimal time for treatments Small, portable Can use in mechanically ventilated patients	Requires significant coordination Chlorofluorocarbon propellants to be phased out Difficulty in determining number of doses remaining Numerous excipients
MDI with spacer	Significantly reduces coordination required Improves pulmonary drug deposition Reduces risk for adverse effects	Bulky, costly
Breath-actuated MDI	Requires minimal coordination Potential for improved pulmonary drug deposition	No additional benefit if good inhaler technique used Cannot use with spacer (potential for adverse effects) Difficulty in determining number of doses remaining Cannot use in mechanically ventilated patients Chorofluorocarbon propellants to be phased out
Dry powder inhaler	Breath-actuated, requires minimal coordination Improves pulmonary drug deposition Lacks excipients Some are single-dose units that require assembly.	Young children and acutely obstructed may not generate adequate inspiratory flow to actuate Requires change in inhalation technique Increased oropharyngeal drug deposition and systemic absorption increases risk for systemic adverse effects Potential for drug to aggregate Potential to provoke cough (not widely reported) Cannot use in mechanically ventilated patients

tract is 0.5 to 5 µm in aerodynamic diameter (48, 62).

Generation of therapeutic aerosols is made by nebulizers, metered-dose inhalers (MDIs), and new dry powder inhaler (DPI) devices. Factors that can affect the deposition of aerosols include the aerosol particle size, density, and shape, dispersion (monodispersing vs. heterodispersing), the hygroscopic nature of the drug, and the effects of electric charges. Patient factors include inspiratory flow rate, inspiratory volume, breath-holding, breathing frequency, lung volume at which inhalation commences, anatomic variations of the airways, and airway narrowing. The use of auxiliary devices such as spacers with MDIs can also affect drug delivery via the inhaled route (48, 62). Each type of delivery device, nebulizers, MDIs, and DPIs, has distinct advantages and disadvantages (Table 35.13).

Nebulizers

Two types of nebulizer are available, those driven by compressed air ("jet") and ultrasonic ones. Aerosols from ultrasonic nebulizers are produced by a piezoelectric transducer vibrating at a high frequency (1 to 3 MHz). Most nebulizers have a "dead" or residual volume, the amount of liquid that is not aerosolized, and up to 75 percent of the aerosol output is not available to the patient. Hence, nebulizers are inefficient methods for delivering medications and require higher "doses" in comparison to other inhaled delivery methods. Aerosol generation and drug delivery via nebulizers depends on the choice of nebulizer (considerable brand to brand and lot to lot differences exist), use of vents and triggers, driving gas flow rate and humidity, temperature, volume fill, and characteristics of the solution to be nebulized. Advantages of nebulizers are that little coordination is required and they can be used by infants and young children and in ventilator circuits. The major disadvantages of nebulizers relate to their inefficiency and inconvenience. Nebulizers are expensive, require an electric power source, are time-consuming to use, and require cleaning following treatments to avoid contamination and possible infection. Also, a water-soluble medication is required and there is potential for mechanical difficulties and chemical breakdown of the drug (due to the heat and vibrations produced by ultrasonic nebulizers) (48, 62).

Metered-Dose Inhalers

Metered-dose inhalers have become the standard of treatment; however, their continued use may be in jeopardy, as the chlorofluorocarbons used as propellants are slated to be phased out of production (although alternative propellants are undergoing development). Nevertheless, the MDI has simplified delivery of inhaled medications as they are more convenient, portable, and require little time for treatments. Unfortunately, technique is extremely important for the proper use of MDIs, as

Table 35.14.
Recommended Technique for the Proper Use of a Metered-Dose Inhaler

1. Remove cap
2. Shake canister
3. Exhale (to functional residual capacity or fully if *slow* exhalation)
4. Hold MDI upright and
   a. place lips around mouthpiece, or
   b. place mouthpiece ~ 2 inches or 2 fingerwidths from mouth, or
   c. place lips around spacer mouthpiece (if using a spacer device)
5. Start to inhale slowly (≤ 30 L/minute)
6. Actuate MDI while continuing to inhale
7. Inhale completely and hold breath for 10 seconds (or at least 4 to 5 seconds)
8. Wait one minute
9. Repeat treatment (steps 2–7), if more than one inhalation prescribed
10. For inhaled steroids, rinse mouth with water or mouthwash and expel contents

significant hand-lung coordination is required (Table 35.14). Breath-actuated devices have further simplified use of MDIs by significantly lessening the degree of coordination needed; however, these provide no advantage in patients with good inhaler technique and cannot be used with spacer devices, which have many advantages of their own. Spacers (Fig. 35.10) reduce the amount of coordination required to properly use MDIs, allowing them to be used in younger children. Use can also result in improved pulmonary drug deposition and reduce the risks for topical as well as systemic adverse effects from medications. Thus, the use of spacer devices is often worth the extra cost and bulkiness (48, 62).

Dry Powder Inhalers

Development of dry powder inhalers such as the Rotahaler, Turbuhaler, and Diskhaler (Fig. 35.11) has been facilitated, in part, because of the impending ban on the chlorofluorocarbon propellants used in MDIs. Dry powder inhalers are breath-actuated devices that allow for inhalation of medication in the form of a dry micronized powder. Because they are breath actuated, minimal coordination is needed; however, a change in inhalation technique (as compared to the MDI) is necessary. With DPIs, deep and forceful inspiration of over 60 L/min (>30 L/min with Turbuhaler and ≤30 L/min for MDIs) is required for optimal pulmonary drug delivery (48, 62). One advantage, noted specifically with the Turbuhaler device in particular, is that they appear to provide for twice the pulmonary drug deposition in comparison to the conventional MDI (without a spacer) (63). However, the increased inspiratory flow required with DPIs and their inability to be used with spacers likely increases oropharyngeal drug deposition. This along with increased pulmonary drug deposition and absorption may increase the risks for topical and systemic

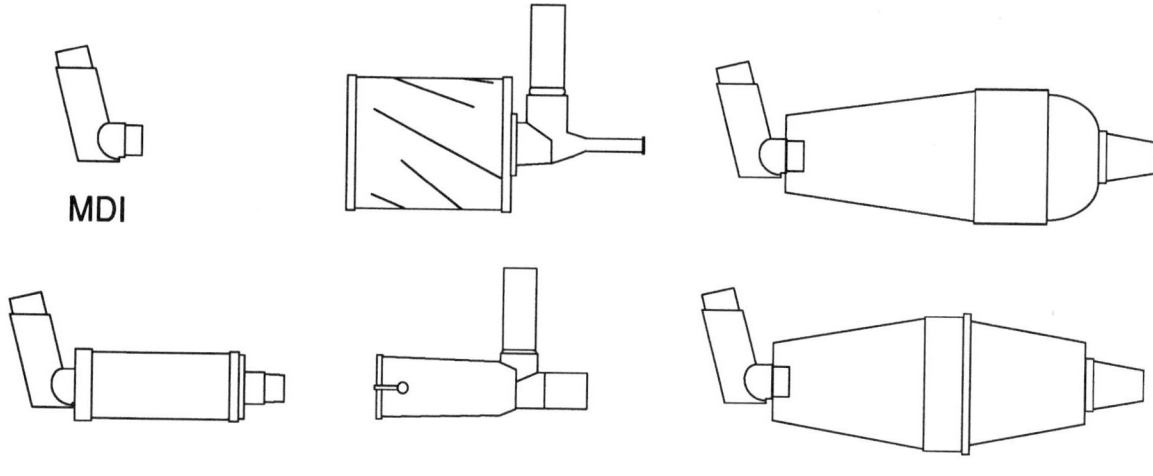

MDI

MDIs with various spacer devices

Figure 35.10. Diagram of a metered-dose inhaler and some of the various spacer devices.

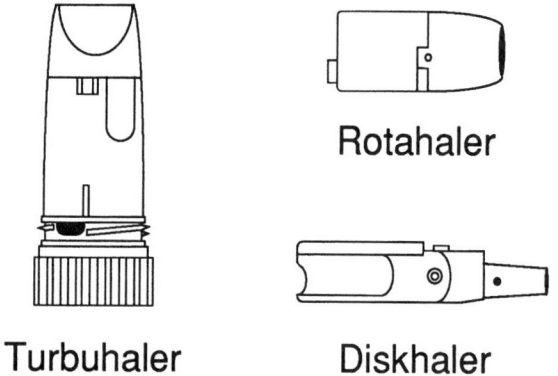

Rotahaler

Turbuhaler   Diskhaler

Figure 35.11. Diagram of some of the new breath-actuated dry powder inhaler devices.

adverse effects from medications, particularly glucocorticoids. Drug aggregation due to high humidity has largely been overcome by use of lactose fillers, and the potential for provoking cough has not been widely reported. A continuing concern is whether young children or acutely obstructed asthmatics can generate enough inspiratory flow to actuate DPIs (60).

TREATMENT GUIDELINES

The increased prevalence and morbidity due to asthma, along with the new emphasis on the inflammatory components of the disease and antiinflammatory therapy, have led to the development of a number of asthma treatment guidelines and consensus statements. The first formal treatment guidelines were published in 1989, to provide conformity in the management of asthma in children (64). These were followed by published guidelines from Australia, Britain, Canada, and the United States (NAEP) (1, 65–67). In an attempt to consolidate these regionally

specific guidelines, the International Consensus on the Diagnosis and Management on Asthma was published in March 1992 (2). The discussion below on chronic and acute management of asthma reviews the treatments outlined in the NAEP and International guidelines and emphasizes any new trends that may be present. Both reports outline the treatment of chronic and acute asthma in children and adults, as recommended by panels of nationally and internationally recognized experts. These treatment guidelines will certainly be revised further as new classes of drugs enter the market.

The International Consensus Report on Diagnosis and Management of Asthma recommends establishing a six-part program for the effective management of asthma (2):

1. Educate patients to develop a partnership in asthma management.
2. Assess and monitor asthma severity with objective measures of lung function.
3. Avoid or control asthma triggers.
4. Establish medication plans for chronic management.
5. Establish plans for managing exacerbations.
6. Provide regular follow-up care.

Figures 35.12 to 35.14 (1, 2) present selected algorithms for the management of chronic and acute asthma.

Chronic Asthma

As inflammation in asthma is believed to cause most of the chronic symptoms and pathologic changes observed, much of the current treatment emphasizes the use of antiinflammatory drugs. However, prior to initiation of any therapy, an assessment must be made of the severity of asthma symptoms as all guidelines base treatment on whether asthma is mild, moderate, or severe.

Chronic Management of Asthma: Stepwise Approach to Asthma Therapy

Step up: Progression to the next higher step is indicated when control cannot be achieved at the current step and there is assurance that medication is used correctly. If PEFR ≤ 60% predicted or personal best, consider a burst of oral corticosteroids and then proceed.

Step down: Reduction in therapy is considered when the outcome for therapy has been achieved and sustained for several weeks or even months at the current step. Reduction in therapy is also needed to identify the minimum therapy required to maintain control.

Outcome: Control of Asthma

- Minimal (ideally no) chronic symptoms, including nocturnal symptoms
- Minimal (infrequent) episodes
- No emergency visits
- Minimal need for p.r.n. β_2-agonist
- No limitations on activities, including exercise
- PEF circadian variation < 20%
- (Near) normal PEF
- Minimal (or no) adverse effects from medicine

Outcome: Best Possible Results

- Least symptoms
- Least need for p.r.n. β_2-agonist
- Least limitation of activity
- Least PEFR circadian variation
- Best PEFR
- Least adverse effects from medicine

Therapy[b]

- Inhaled corticosteroid 800–1000 µg daily (>1000 µg under specialist's supervision)

and

- Sustained release theophylline and/or oral β_2-agonist, or long acting inhaled β_2-agonist, especially for nocturnal symptoms with or without
- Short acting inhaled β_2-agonist once a day; may consider inhaled anticholinergic

and

- Oral corticosteroids (alternate day or single daily dose)

and

- Short acting inhaled β_2-agonist p.r.n., up to 3–4 times a day

Therapy[b]

- Inhaled corticosteroids daily 800–1000 µg (>1000 µg under specialist's supervision)

and

- Sustained release theophylline, oral β_2-agonist, or long acting inhaled β_2-agonist, especially for nocturnal symptoms; may consider inhaled anticholinergics

and

- Short acting inhaled β_2-agonist p.r.n., not to exceed 3–4 times a day

Therapy[b]

- Inhaled antiinflammatory daily
  — Initially: Inhaled corticosteroid 200–500 µg or cromolyn or nedocromil (Children begin with a trial of cromolyn)
  — If necessary: inhaled corticosteroid 400–750 µg (Alternatively, particularly for nocturnal symptoms, proceed to Step 3 with additional long acting bronchodilator)

and

- Short acting inhaled β_2-agonist p.r.n., not to exceed 3–4 times a day

Step Down

- Once control is reached at any step, and sustained, a step down— reduction in therapy— may be carefully considered and is needed to identify the minimum therapy required to maintain control.
- Advise patients of signs of worsening actions to control it.

Therapy[b]

- Short acting inhaled β_2-agonist p.r.n., not more than 3 times a week
- Short acting inhaled β_2-agonist or cromolyn before exercise or exposure to antigen

Clinical Features Pretreatment[a]

- Intermittent, brief symptoms < 1–2 times a week
- Nocturnal asthma symptoms < 1–2 times a month
- Asymptomatic between exacerbations
- PEFR or FEV$_1$ > 80% predicted variability < 20%

Clinical Features Pretreatment[a]

- Exacerbations > 1–2 times a week
- Exacerbations may affect activity and sleep
- Nocturnal asthma symptoms > 2 times a month
- Chronic symptoms requiring short acting β_2-agonist almost daily
- PEFR or FEV$_1$ 60–80% predicted variability 20–30%

Clinical Features Pretreatment[a]

- Frequent exacerbations
- Continuous symptoms
- Frequent nocturnal asthma symptoms
- Physical activities limited by asthma
- PEFR or FEV$_1$ < 60% predicted variability > 30%

STEP 1: MILD   **STEP 2: MODERATE**   **STEP 3: MODERATE**   **STEP 4: SEVERE**

[a] One or more features may be present to be assigned a grade of severity; an individual should usually be assigned to the most severe grade in which any feature occurs.
[b] All therapy must include education about prevention (including environmental control appropriate) as well as control of symptoms.

Figure 35.12.   Algorithm of the stepwise approach for the treatment of chronic asthma. From reference 2.

Mild asthma can be managed with inhaled β_2-adrenergic agonists in most persons. Children under the age of 5 years, however, who are unable to use an inhaled bronchodilator effectively, will usually need treatment with an oral β_2-adrenergic agonist. Some young children can be taught to use an MDI with a spacer; however, the child's technique should be checked frequently. In addition, treatment with an inhaled β_2-adrenergic agonist prior to exercise or exposure to allergens and irritants is also effective.

When symptoms become more frequent and exacerbations affect activity or sleep, patients are classified as

Acute Exacerbations of Asthma in Adults[a]
Emergency Department Management

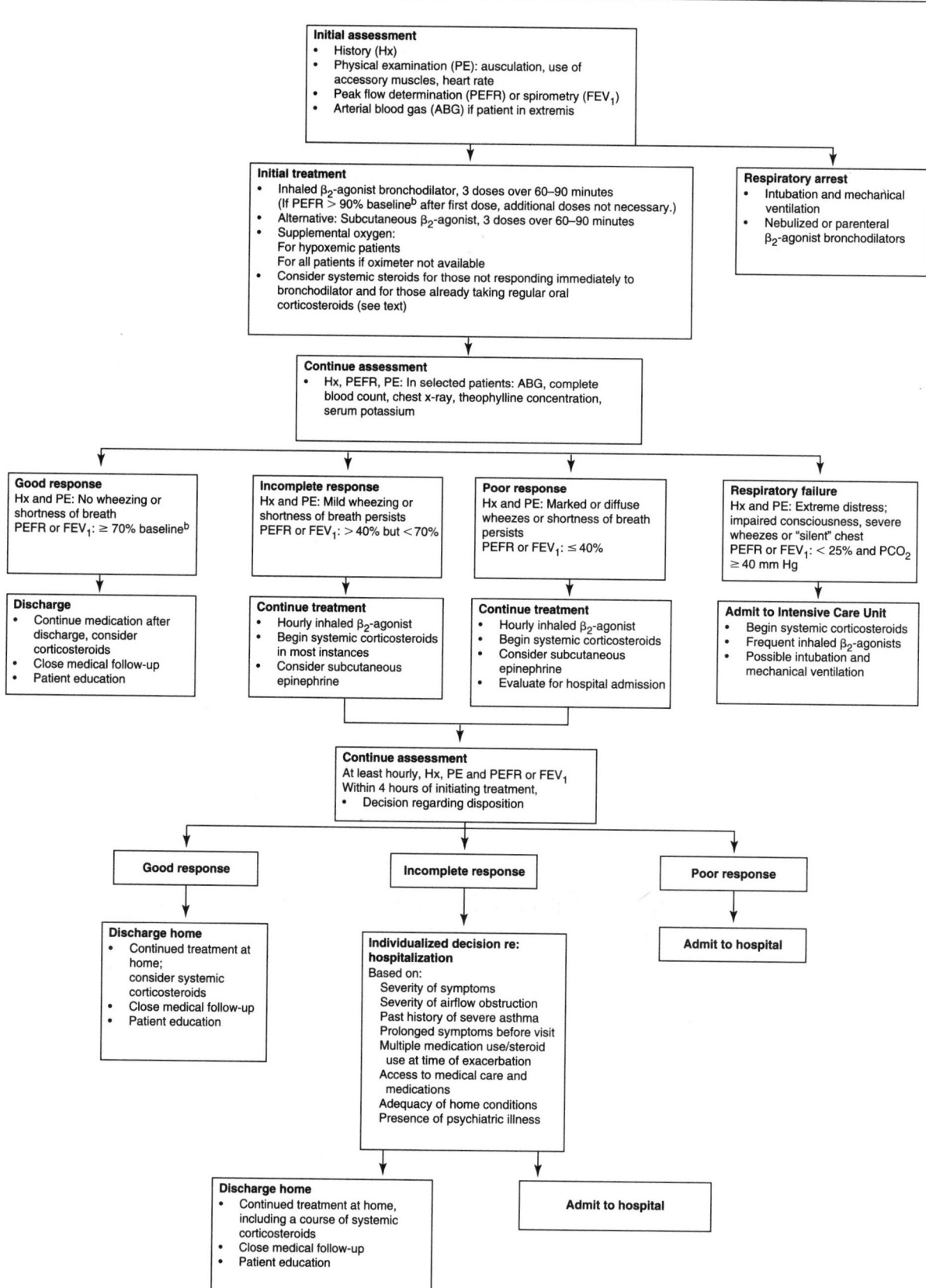

Figure 35.13. Algorithm of the management of acute exacerbations of asthma in adults treated in the Emergency Department. From reference 1.

having moderate asthma. Low dose inhaled glucocorticoids (200 to 500 µg/day), cromolyn, or nedocromil are indicated. Cromolyn and nedocromil are preferred as initial therapy in children, as these drugs are quite effective in this age group and adverse effects are minimal. If symptoms persist, children may need to be switched to an inhaled glucocorticoid, or the inhaled glucocorticoid dose may be increased. In some patients, particularly children, cromolyn may be combined with an inhaled glucocorticoid in order to keep the dose of the inhaled glucocorticoid as low as possible, thereby minimizing adverse effects. Alternatively, sustained-release theophylline or a long-acting inhaled β_2-adrenergic agonist may be added before increasing the dose of inhaled glucocorticoids. The serum concentration of theophylline should be maintained between 27.5 and 87.5 µmol/liter (5 to 15 µg/mL), although recent data indicated that serum concentrations less than 55 µmol/liter (10 µg/mL) may be sufficient to provide supplementary antiinflammatory effects in addition to mild bronchodilator effects. Some patients, however, may require a dosage increase of the inhaled glucocorticoid along with an added bronchodilator. The international guidelines (2) describe a somewhat more vigorous approach than those developed by the NAEP.(1) In general, the international guidelines emphasize an aggressive use of inhaled glucocorticoids before adding a long-acting bronchodilator to a regimen. The NAEP guidelines do not mention long-acting inhaled β_2-adrenergic agonist therapy (as these drugs were not available in the United States at the time the guidelines were developed) but do suggest oral β_2-adrenergic agonist therapy as an alternative. In addition, the NAEP guidelines suggest the addition of short-acting β_2-adrenergic agonist therapy given three to four times daily. Short-acting β_2-adrenergic therapy is now recommended for use only on an as-needed basis. If symptoms become more frequent, a short course of oral glucocorticoids is indicated with a subsequent evaluation of therapy. In children with frequent exacerbations requiring glucocorticoid intervention, evidence exists that increasing the dose of inhaled glucocorticoids (to 2.25 mg/day) for several days may control symptoms and avoid treatment with oral glucocorticoids (68).

The hallmark of treatment in the severe asthmatic is the use of high dose inhaled glucocorticoids (over 800 µg/day), possibly in combination with a long-acting bronchodilator to provide added control of nocturnal symptoms. The NAEP guidelines but not the International guidelines include the possibility of adding cromolyn to the high dose inhaled glucocorticoids, although clinical studies suggest only minimal added benefit. If theophylline is used, the serum concentration should still be maintained between 27.5 and 87.5 µmol/liter (5 to 15 µg/mL) as in the treatment of moderate asthma. Again,

oral or long-acting inhaled β_2-adrenergic agonists may be added, but in young children frequent nebulized β_2-adrenergic agonists may be used. The addition of inhaled anticholinergic drugs to a short-acting inhaled β_2-adrenergic is described in the International guidelines. In patients with symptoms that are particularly difficult to control, oral prednisone given on alternate days may be added. The lowest effective dose should be used to minimize adverse effects that are likely to occur when combined with inhaled glucocorticoids.

In the treatment of asthma, consideration must be given to the management of other diseases or provoking stimuli that may precipitate asthma symptoms, especially when asthma symptoms persist despite optimal pharmacotherapy and compliance (69). Allergic rhinitis and asthma are closely related pathophysiologically, and allergic rhinitis symptoms may require treatment in some patients if asthma symptoms are to be controlled. Similarly, acute or chronic sinusitis may aggravate asthma symptoms even in the absence of a bacterial infection. Gastroesophageal reflux may cause nocturnal coughing in some infants and may be mistaken for asthma symptoms.

A key to the outpatient management of asthma is the self-monitoring of asthma signs and symptoms by the patient. Home monitoring of peak expiratory flow rate (PEFR) provides an objective means to assess severity of symptoms and response to therapy (1). Airway obstruction can be detected and treated even before wheezing is audible or symptoms are experienced by the patient. Patients should be instructed to determine their personal best value from which green, yellow, and red zones are calculated. The green zone indicates "all clear"; symptoms are not present and medications are to be taken as usual. The green zone is usually 80 to 100 percent of predicted or their personal best. The yellow zone, 50 to 80 percent predicted or personal best, indicates "caution," and that the usual medication regimen may need to be modified. The red zone, below 50 percent predicted or personal best, indicates "medical alert," and patients are to use inhaled β_2-adrenergic agonist medication immediately and follow up with medical personnel. Additional information on peak flow monitoring and examples of peak flow diaries may be obtained by writing to the address at the end of the chapter and requesting the *Asthma Management Kit for Clinicians*.

Consideration for the cost of therapy is essential in the management plan for any chronic illness. If patients are unable to afford the medications prescribed, compliance will be poor and symptom reoccurrence will be common. Compliance is especially important in the treatment of asthma, a life-threatening disease in which death can occur within minutes of an acute severe exacerbation. In addition, many asthmatics are atopic and may require costly therapy for treatment of allergic rhinitis, allergic

Acute Exacerbations of Asthma in Adults
Hospital Management

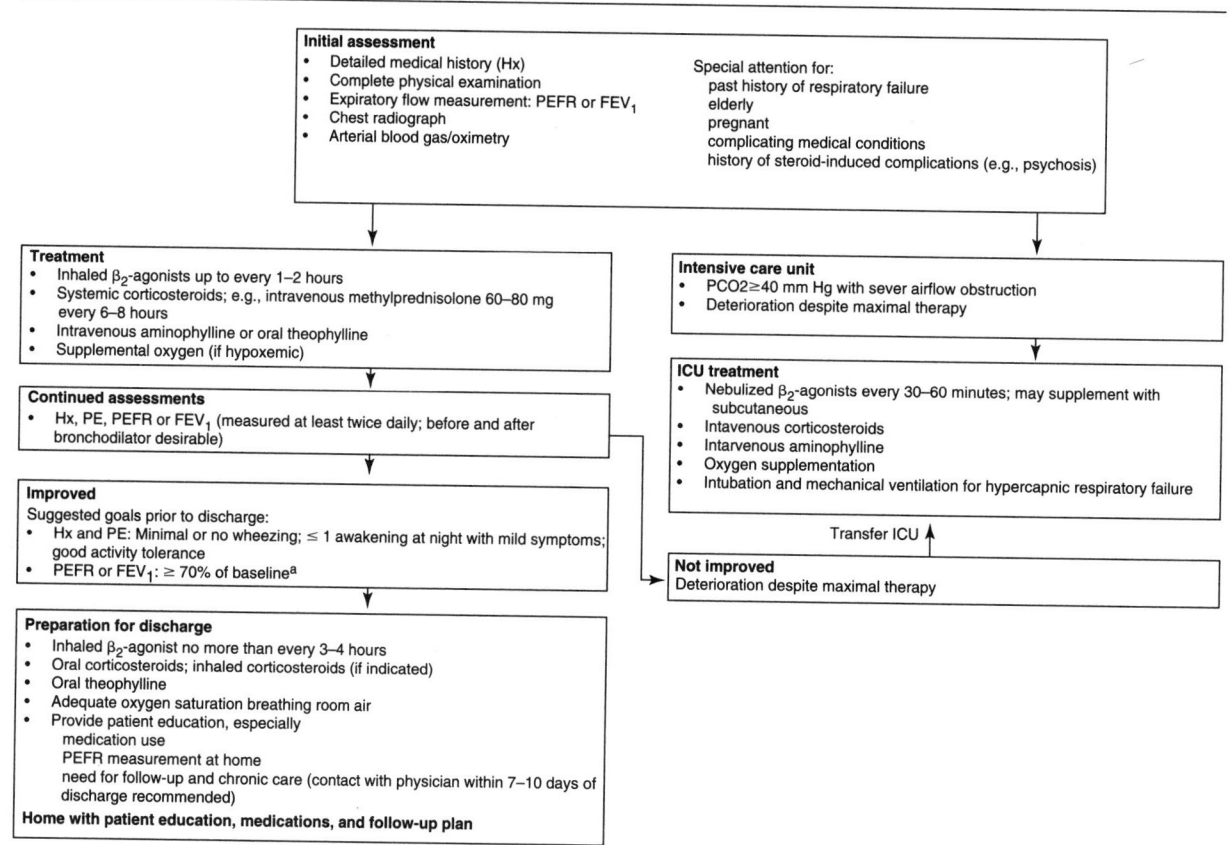

Initial assessment
- Detailed medical history (Hx)
- Complete physical examination
- Expiratory flow measurement: PEFR or FEV₁
- Chest radiograph
- Arterial blood gas/oximetry

Special attention for:
 past history of respiratory failure
 elderly
 pregnant
 complicating medical conditions
 history of steroid-induced complications (e.g., psychosis)

Treatment
- Inhaled β₂-agonists up to every 1–2 hours
- Systemic corticosteroids; e.g., intravenous methylprednisolone 60–80 mg every 6–8 hours
- Intravenous aminophylline or oral theophylline
- Supplemental oxygen (if hypoxemic)

Continued assessments
- Hx, PE, PEFR or FEV₁ (measured at least twice daily; before and after bronchodilator desirable)

Improved
Suggested goals prior to discharge:
- Hx and PE: Minimal or no wheezing; ≤ 1 awakening at night with mild symptoms; good activity tolerance
- PEFR or FEV₁: ≥ 70% of baseline[a]

Preparation for discharge
- Inhaled β₂-agonist no more than every 3–4 hours
- Oral corticosteroids; inhaled corticosteroids (if indicated)
- Oral theophylline
- Adequate oxygen saturation breathing room air
- Provide patient education, especially
   medication use
   PEFR measurement at home
   need for follow-up and chronic care (contact with physician within 7–10 days of discharge recommended)

Home with patient education, medications, and follow-up plan

Intensive care unit
- PCO2 ≥ 40 mm Hg with sever airflow obstruction
- Deterioration despite maximal therapy

ICU treatment
- Nebulized β₂-agonists every 30–60 minutes; may supplement with subcutaneous
- Intavenous corticosteroids
- Intarvenous aminophylline
- Oxygen supplementation
- Intubation and mechanical ventilation for hypercapnic respiratory failure

Transfer ICU ↑

Not improved
Deterioration despite maximal therapy

[a] PEFR % baseline refers to the norm for the individual, established by the clinician. This may be % predicted based on standardized norms or % patient's personal best.

Figure 35.14. Algorithm of the management of acute exacerbations of asthma in adults treated in the hospital. From reference 1.

conjunctivitis, or eczema. Presented in Table 35.15 are the approximate average wholesale prices in 1995. Before recommending treatment, health care providers should obtain detailed information on payment methods.

Acute Exacerbations

Over the last decade, the management of acute asthma symptoms has moved from emergency department to the home treatment as patients have been able to acquire compressors and nebulizers through insurance and medicaid coverage or have been taught to use high doses (2 to 4 inhalations every 20 minutes for 3 doses) of an MDI with a spacer device. The at-home use of oral glucocorticoids by selected patients has also contributed significantly to this trend. In teaching patients home management of acute symptoms, it is critically important that patients recognize signs of deterioration that will require professional medical intervention. As in the management of chronic asthma, an assessment of the severity of symptoms must be performed prior to treatment recommendations. Patients who are at

risk for life-threatening events should always seek professional intervention rather than self-management at home. As outlined in the NAEP guidelines (1), these include patients who

1. have ever been intubated or admitted to the intensive care unit for asthma;
2. had 3 emergency visits or 2 hospitalizations for asthma in the past year or one of either in the last month;
3. currently use or have recently been withdrawn from systemic glucocorticoids;
4. have had a syncope/hypoxic seizure due to asthma; and
5. have psychiatric or psychosocial problems (which may result in noncompliance).

If symptoms are mild to moderate in severity, patients may be initially managed at home. Inhaled β₂-adrenergic agonists are the initial treatment and may be administered as 2 to 4 inhalations from a MDI with a spacer device or doses from a nebulizer every 20 minutes for 3 doses to treat more moderate symptoms. If symptoms do not improve,

Table 35.15.
Approximate List Price (1995) for Drugs Commonly Used in the Treatment of Asthma

Drug (Generic Name)	Dose/day	Approximate Cost/month (list price)
Albuterol MDI	2 inh PRN	$25
Albuterol Nebulizer Solution (20 mL)	2.5 mg PRN	$15
Albuterol Nebulizer Solution (unit dose, #25)	2.5 mg PRN	$25
Beclomethasone MDI	4 inh BID	$35
Cromolyn MDI (200 inhalations)	2 inh QID	$60
Cromolyn Nebulizer Solution (20-mg ampule)	20 mg QID	$90
Flunisolide MDI	2 inh BID	$45
Nedocromil MDI (112 inhalations)	2 inh QID	$60
Salmeterol MDI	2 inh BID	$50
Triamcinolone MDI	4 inh BID	$40

inhaled or nebulized β_2-adrenergic agonists may be administered hourly and oral glucocorticoids may be started at home. Children whose asthma is precipitated by an upper respiratory tract infection may begin a short course of oral glucocorticoids at the first symptom of an upper respiratory tract infection even in the absence of wheezing. This can reduce the number of wheezing days, emergency department visits, and hospitalizations (70). Contact with a medical professional is necessary at this time for children, although adults may continue with self-observation and seek medical care if symptoms do not improve over the next few hours. Patients with symptoms of severe asthma such as the inability to speak in complete sentences or walk 100 feet without stopping, severe wheezing or breathlessness, or peak expiratory flow less than 50 percent predicted require professional medical intervention. Children should be taken to an emergency department, but adults may continue home management under the supervision of a medical professional. The dose of inhaled or nebulized β_2-adrenergic agonists should be increased and oral glucocorticoids begun if not previously started. If symptoms do not improve over the next few hours, adults should receive additional care in an emergency department. It is essential that patients be taught signs of worsening asthma that indicate emergency department care is needed.

In the emergency department, treatment begins with nebulized β_2-adrenergic agonists administered three times during the first hour. Some studies have advocated high doses of β_2-adrenergic agonists from a metered-dose inhaler attached to a spacer in the emergency department, but this is not currently considered standard care. Alternatively, β_2-adrenergic agonists may be administered subcutaneously, although adverse effects are more common and efficacy is generally less than by the inhaled route. Laboratory assessments may include arterial blood gas measurement, complete blood count, chest radiographs, and theophylline and serum potassium concentration measurement. Supplemental oxygen is indicated for all patients who are hypoxemic. If symptoms persist after 1 hour, frequent or continuous nebulized β_2-adrenergic are begun and systemic glucocorticoids are generally indicated. However, systemic glucocorticoids may be started concurrently with nebulized β_2-adrenergic treatment if symptoms are severe (2). Intravenous aminophylline is no longer indicated in the treatment of asthma in the emergency department except in those patients who take theophylline for treatment of chronic symptoms. If symptoms do not improve within 4 hours or signs of respiratory failure are present, the patient will require hospitalization. Patients who are discharged from the emergency department should receive a course of oral glucocorticoids in most instances.

Patients who are admitted to the hospital continue treatment with frequent inhaled β_2-adrenergic agonists and systemic glucocorticoids. Most studies of intravenous aminophylline in the hospitalized patient have failed to show an improved benefit over optimal doses of inhaled β_2-adrenergic agonists and systemic glucocorticoids. However, patients who fail to improve and those admitted to the intensive care unit should received intravenous aminophylline. Although data are limited, inhaled anticholinergics may be added to β_2-adrenergic therapy. Intensive care unit patients may benefit from subcutaneous, intramuscular, or intravenous β-adrenergic agonists.

Patient education about discharge medications, peak expiratory flow rate monitoring, and the importance of a follow-up visit is an essential component of discharge procedures. Inhaled glucocorticoids may be initiated at discharge while the patient continues treatment with oral glucocorticoids. Initiating inhaled glucocorticoid therapy at this time with patient education will reinforce to the patient the importance of this therapy in achieving long-term control. Oral theophylline may be initiated in some patients and should be continued in those who received theophylline treatment in the hospital. All patients should be taught correct techniques for inhaled β_2-adrenergic therapy whether administered by nebulizer, metered-dose inhaler with or without a spacer, or dry powder inhaler, as this therapy is essential for maintaining optimal lung function.

ALTERNATIVE TREATMENTS

Because of the many toxicities and adverse effects associated with chronic oral glucocorticoid use, a number of "alternative" asthma therapies have been investigated. These include methotrexate, troleandomycin (TAO), gold, intravenous gamma globulin (IVIG), and cyclosporine. Consideration and institution of alternative treatments are reserved for severe, steroid-dependent asthmatics. Not all patients respond to treatment, and each treatment has risks for adverse effects of its own (Table 35.16). While the goal of therapy is usually reduction of systemic glucocorticoid doses, some studies have demonstrated improvements in pulmonary function (although none are bronchodilators in the traditional sense) and bronchial hyperresponsiveness (71). For alternative treatments it is particularly important to define the goal of therapy, as improving pulmonary function may not be realistic in the severe asthmatic with concomitant glucocorticoid dose reductions.

Methotrexate is effective in treating psoriasis and rheumatoid arthritis, two other inflammatory diseases, and has been used in the treatment of severe asthma. Studies have shown that some patients will respond by maintaining their pulmonary function while allowing reduction of oral glucocorticoid requirements. Unfortunately, efficacy is not universal and no reduction of bronchial hyperresponsiveness has been observed. Major limitations of treatment include gastrointestinal adverse effects and hepatotoxicity (71).

Troleandomycin inhibits methylprednisolone elimination; thus, its mechanism has been postulated to be via inhibition of glucocorticoid metabolism. Efficacy has also been seen when used in combination with prednisone, a glucocorticoid whose metabolism is not affected by troleandomycin, and in some patients bronchial hyperresponsiveness has improved. This suggests that troleandomycin may have other beneficial effects in treating asthma, independent of its pharmacokinetic interaction with meth-

ylprednisolone. Adverse effects of troleandomycin include enhanced glucocorticoid adverse effects (if methylprednisolone is not tapered sufficiently), gastrointestinal upset, and mild and transient elevations of liver enzymes. Theophylline clearance is reduced with concomitant troleandomycin; therefore, serum levels must be monitored and dosages adjusted accordingly (71).

Gold, another medication useful in treating rheumatoid arthritis, may also represent a beneficial therapy in steroid-dependent asthma. Glucocorticoid dose reduction as well as improvements in bronchial hyperresponsiveness have been observed in some studies. Adverse effects of gold include gastrointestinal adverse effects, dermatitis, and proteinuria. As with other alternative therapies, its mechanism of action remains unclear. A marked steroid-sparing effect with maintenance of pulmonary function has been observed in one study of steroid-dependent asthmatics following treatment with intravenous gamma globulin. While relatively free of severe adverse effects in comparison to other alternative asthma treatments, therapy is often prohibited by the high cost (71).

The immunosuppressant cyclosporine also has a potential role in severe asthma, as activated T-lymphocytes are thought to play an important role in the disease process. A steroid-sparing effect and improved pulmonary function (without glucocorticoid tapering) have been observed with treatment in separate studies; however, major limitations are renal toxicity and hypertension as well as the other adverse effects common with cyclosporine (71). Immunosuppression when cyclosporine is used in conjunction with high doses of oral glucocorticoids is also a concern.

FUTURE THERAPIES

With increased research and knowledge of the pathophysiology of asthma, many novel treatment modalities may be on the horizon. A number of specific mediator antagonists and inhibitors of enzymes important in their synthesis are undergoing clinical trials. Those with particular promise include leukotriene receptor antagonists and inhibitors of

Table 35.16.
Properties of Alternative Asthma Treatments

Treatment	Bronchodilator	Steroid-Sparing	Hyperresponsiveness	Major Adverse Effects and Limitations
Methotrexate	−	+	−	liver toxicity, gastrointestinal upset
Troleandomycin	−	+	±	potential for increased steroid adverse effects, increased liver enzymes, gastrointestinal upset, reduces theophylline clearance
Gold	−	+	±	renal toxicity, rash, gastrointestinal upset
IVIG	−	+	−	intravenous administration, costly
Cyclosporine	−	+	?	renal toxicity, hypertension, paresthesias, potential for immunosuppression

+, benefit reported; −, no benefit reported; ±, variable effects reported; ?, effects unknown

5-lipoxygenase, the enzyme involved in the production of many arachidonic acid-derived mediators. Inhibitors of phosphodiesterase isoenzymes, which may have both bronchodilator and antiinflammatory action, are also being investigated for their use in the treatment of asthma (49).

Leukotrienes have a number of proinflammatory actions as well as bronchoconstrictive properties and appear to be important mediators of the inflammation of asthma. Two approaches to blocking the effects of leukotrienes have been developed: competitive antagonists of leukotriene receptors and inhibitors of leukotrienes synthesis. Inhibitors of leukotriene production, 5-lipoxygenase inhibitors, consist of direct enzyme inhibitors and inhibitors of 5-lipoxygenase activating protein (FLAP), necessary for arachidonic acid metabolism. While still undergoing development, both approaches (receptor antagonists and enzyme inhibitors) have demonstrated efficacy (improved pulmonary function) with chronic therapy, and thus appear to be promising future treatments for asthma. In addition, receptor antagonists have shown efficacy in protection against allergen- and exercise-induced bronchoconstriction, and the ability to improve bronchial hyperresponsiveness. Adverse effects of these agents appear to be mild and limited to headache and gastrointestinal disturbances (72).

Phosphodiesterase (PDE) isoenzymes regulate the breakdown of cyclic AMP and cyclic GMP within cells. Data from animal models and in vitro studies have shown the ability of isoenzymes III, IV, and V to relax precontracted smooth muscle as well as inhibit contraction. Inhibitors of PDE IV (and possibly III) are thought to suppress the infiltration and activation of inflammatory cells, as well as their release of cytokines. While a number of agents, both selective isoenzyme and dual PDE III/IV inhibitors, are undergoing development, limited data from clinical trials are available. There is evidence for bronchodilator (antibronchoconstrictor) activity with PDE III inhibitors; however, these agents cannot considered potential replacements for β-agonists. The proposed antiinflammatory effects of dual PDE III/IV inhibitors along with bronchodilator activity make for an intriguing potential new asthma therapy. Adverse effects of these agents, however, may limit their usefulness (73).

A number of other agents are early in stages of development or clinical trials. Those being studied as potential antiinflammatory agents include phospholipase A_2 and cyclooxygenase inhibitors; antagonists of cytokines, thromboxane, bradykinin, and PAF; cell adhesion blockers; inhibitors of neurogenic inflammation; immunomodulators; and suppressors of IgE. Potassium channel activators, calcium antagonists, and selective anticholinergics may represent novel bronchodilators (49).

IMPROVING OUTCOMES

Outcome studies comparing the effects of different interventions on the morbidity, mortality, and quality of life of patients with asthma have recently received increased interest. Such studies are likely to become more important in the future for guiding treatment of patients covered by HMOs and other health insurers, and as part of the FDA drug approval process.

It is expected that patient education will result in improved outcomes of patients with asthma, and this has been supported in a clinical trial (74). In this study, patients who received care from an intensive outpatient treatment clinic with emphasis on teaching aggressive self-management strategies during an asthma exacerbation had a reduced hospital admission rate and hospital day use rate. Another study demonstrated that use of a spacer device with a MDI resulted in fewer symptoms and missed school days in comparison to a group of children who did not use a spacer (75). Comparative studies of the medications used to treat asthma and their effects on quality of life are underway; however, data at this time must be considered preliminary.

CONCLUSION

Asthma is now recognized as much more than bronchoconstriction and may well represent a number of defects with similar clinical presentations. Therapy must target not only the symptoms resulting from bronchospasm but also the underlying inflammation and characteristic bronchial hyperresponsiveness. While the pathophysiology of the disease remains complex, increased understanding has led to improved use of the currently available medications and facilitated the development of entirely new treatment modalities. These new therapies along with an increased knowledge of the disease pathophysiology and the improved use of the currently available medications will undoubtedly require the future reassessment and reevaluation of the many asthma treatment guidelines.

Asthma Management Resources may be obtained by writing to

National Heart, Lung, and Blood Institute Information Center
P.O. Box 30105
Bethesda, MD 20824-0105

and asking for

International Consensus Report on the Diagnosis and Treatment of Asthma. Publication No. 92-3091. March 1992.
Guidelines for the Diagnosis and Management of Asthma. National Asthma Education Program. Publication No. 91-3042. August 1991.

REFERENCES

1. Office of Prevention, Education, and Control, National Asthma Education Program. Guidelines for the diagnosis and management of asthma. Bethesda, MD: United States Department of Health and Human Services, Public Health Service, National Institutes of Health, National Heart, Lung, and Blood Institute, August 1991.
2. International consensus report on diagnosis and management of asthma. Bethesda, MD: United States Department of Health and

Human Services, Public Health Service, National Institutes of Health, National Heart, Lung, and Blood Institute, August 1992.

3. Weiss KB, Gergen PJ, Hodgson TA. An economic evaluation of asthma in the United States. N Engl J Med 326:862–868, 1992.

4. Lang DM, Polansky M. Patterns of asthma mortality in Philadelphia from 1969 to 1991. N Engl J Med 331:1542–1546, 1994.

5. Holgate ST. Asthma: past, present and future. Eur Respir J 6:1507–1520, 1993.

6. Barnes PJ. New concepts in the pathogenesis of bronchial hyperresponsiveness and asthma. J Allergy Clin Immunol 83:1013–1026, 1989.

7. Kay AB. Asthma and inflammation. J Allergy Clin Immunol 87:893–910, 1991.

8. Sur S, Crotty TB, Kephart GM, Hyma BA, Colby TV, Reed CE, Hunt LW, Gleich GJ. Sudden onset fatal asthma. A distinct entity with few eosinophils and relatively more neutrophils in the airway submucosa? Am Rev Respir Dis 148:713–719, 1993.

9. Smith HR, Henson PM. Mediators of asthma. Semin Respir Med 8:287–301, 1987.

10. Calderón E, Lockey RF. A possible role for adhesion molecules in asthma. J Allergy Clin Immunol 90:852–865, 1992.

11. Integrins and other adhesion molecules. Am Rev Respir Dis 148:S27–S87, 1993.

12. Joos GF, Germonpre PR, Kips JC, Peleman RA, Pauwels RA. Sensory neuropeptides and the human lower airways: present state and future directions. Eur Respir J 7:1161–1171, 1994.

13. Siefkin AD. Using pulmonary function testing in the diagnosis and treatment of asthma. Clin Rev Allergy 8:179–197, 1990.

14. Ellis EF. Asthma in infancy and childhood. In: Middleton E Jr, Reed CE, Ellis EF, Adkinson NF Jr, Yuninger JW, Busse WW, eds. Allergy: principles and practice, 4th ed. St. Louis: Mosby-Year Book, 1993:1225–1262.

15. Mathison DA. Asthma in adults: diagnosis and management. In: Middleton E Jr. Reed CE, Ellis EF, Adkinson EF Jr, Yuninger JW, Busse WW, eds. Allergy: principles and practice, 4th ed. St. Louis: Mosby–Year Book, 1993:1263–1299.

16. Jenne JS, Murphy SA. Drug therapy for asthma: research and clinical practice. New York: Marcel Dekker, 1987.

17. Kume H, Graziano MP, Kotlikoff MI. Stimulatory and inhibitory regulation of calcium-activated potassium channels by guanine nucleotide binding proteins. Proc Natl Acad Sci U S A 89:11051–11055, 1992.

18. Lofdahl CG, Chung KF. Long acting β_2 adrenoceptor agonists: a new perspective in the treatment of asthma. Eur Resp J 4:218–226, 1991.

19. Laitinen LA, Laitinen A, Haahtela T. A comparative study of the effects of an inhaled corticosteroid, budesonide, and of a β_2-agonist, terbutaline, on airway inflammation in newly diagnosed asthma. J Allergy Clin Immunol 90:32–42, 1992.

20. Roberts JA, Bradding P, Walls AF, Britten KM, Wilson S, Holgate ST, Howarth PH. The influence of salmeterol zinafoate on mucosal inflammation in asthma. Am Rev Respir Dis 145:A418.1992.

21. Cheong B, Reynolds SR, Rajan G, Ward MJ. Intravenous β agonist in severe acute asthma. Br Med J 297:448–450, 1988.

22. Murdock IA, Anjos RD, Haycock GB. Treatment of hyperkalemia with intravenous salbutamol. Arch Dis Child 66:527–528, 1991.

23. Twentyman OP, Finnerty JP, Harris A, Palmer J, Holgate ST. Protection against allergen-induced asthma by salmeterol. Lancet 336:1338–1342, 1990.

24. Sears MR, Taylor DR, Print CG, Lake DC, Li Q, Flannery RM, Yates DM, Lucas MK, Herbison GP. Regular inhaled beta-agonist treatment in bronchial asthma. Lancet 336:1391–1396, 1990.

25. Taylor DR, Sears MR, Herbison GP, Flannery EM, Print CG, Lake DC, Yates DM, Lucas MK, Li Q. Regular inhaled beta agonist in asthma: effects on exacerbations and lung function. Thorax 48:134–138, 1993.

26. Spitzer WO, Suissa S, Ernst P, Horwitz RI, Habbick B, Cockcroft D, Boivin JF, McNutt M, Buist AS, Rebuck AS. The use of beta-agonists and the risk of death and near death from asthma. N Engl J Med 326:501–506, 1992.

27. van Schayck CP, Graafsma SJ, Visch MB, Dompeling E, van Weel C, van Herwaarden CLA. Increased bronchial hyperresponsiveness after inhaling salbutamol during 1 year is not caused by subsensitization to salbutamol. J Allergy Clin Immunol 86:793–800, 1990.

28. Ramage L, Lipworth BJ, Ingram CG, Cree IA, Dhillon DP. Reduced protection against exercise induced bronchoconstriction after chronic dosing with salmeterol. Respir Med 88:363–368, 1994.

29. Repsher LH, Anderson JA, Bush RK, Falliers CJ, Kass I, Kemp JP, Reed C, Siegel S, Webb DR. Assessment of tachyphylaxis following prolonged therapy of asthma with inhaled albuterol aerosol. Chest 85:34–38, 1984.

30. Booth H, Fishwick K, Harkawat R, Devereux G, Hendrick DJ, Walters EH. Changes in methacholine induced bronchoconstriction with the long acting β_2 agonist salmeterol in mild to moderate asthmatic patients. Thorax 48:1121–1124, 1993.

31. Greening AP, Ind PW, Northfield M, Shaw G. Added salmeterol versus higher-dose corticosteroid in asthma patients with symptoms on existing inhaled corticosteroid. Lancet 344:219–224, 1994.

32. Barnes PJ, Pauwels RA. Theophylline in the management of asthma: Time for reappraisal? Eur Resp J 7:579–591, 1994.

33. Glynn-Barnhart A, Hill M, Szefler SJ. Sustained release theophylline preparations. Practical recommendations for prescribing and therapeutic drug monitoring. Drugs 35:711–726, 1988.

34. Hendeles L, Jenkins J, Temple R. Theophylline immediate-release oral dosage forms: FDA Labeling Guidelines. Pharmacotherapy 15(4):409–427, 1995.

35. Weinberger M, Hendeles L, Theophylline. Middleton E Jr, Reed CE, Ellis EF, Adkinson NF Jr, Yunginger JW, Busse WW. Allergy: principles and practice, 4th ed. St. Louis: Mosby-Year Book, 1993:816–855.

36. Hendeles L, Bighley L, Richardson RH, Hepler CD, Carmichael J. Frequent toxicity from IV aminophylline infusions in critically ill patients. Drug Intell Clin Pharm 11:12–17, 1977.

37. Derby LE, Jick SS, Langlois JC, Johnson LE, Jick H. Hospital admission for xanthine toxicity. Pharmacotherapy 10:112–114, 1990.

38. Shannon M. Predictors of major toxicity after theophylline overdose. Ann Intern Med 119:1161–1167, 1993.

39. Hendeles L, Harman E, Huang D, O'Brien R, Blake K, Delafuente J. Theophylline attenuation of airway responses to allergen: comparison with cromolyn metered-dose inhaler. J Allergy Clin Immunol 95:505–514, 1995.

40. Wrenn K, Slovis CM, Murphy F, Greenberg RS. Aminophylline therapy for acute bronchospastic disease in the emergency room. Ann Intern Med 115:241–247, 1991.

41. Huang D, O'Brien RG, Harman E, Aull L, Reents S, Visser J, Shieh G, Hendeles L. Does aminophylline benefit adults admitted to the hospital for an acute exacerbation of asthma? Ann Intern Med 119:1155–1160, 1993.

42. Rodrigo C, Rodrigo G. Treatment of acute asthma. Lack of therapeutic benefit and increase of the toxicity from aninophylline given in addition to high doses of salbutamol delivered by metered-dose inhaler with a spacer. Chest 106:1071–1076, 1994.

43. Strauss RE, Wertheim DL, Bonagura VR, Valacer DJ. Aminophylline therapy does not improve outcome and increases adverse effects in children hospitalized with acute asthmatic exacerbations. Pediatrics 93:205–210, 1994.

44. Murphy DG, McDermott MF, Rydman RJ, Sloan EP, Zalenski RJ. Aminophylline in the treatment of acute asthma when β_2-adrenergics and steroids are provided. Arch Intern Med 153:1784–1788, 1993.

45. DiGiulio GA, Kercsmar CM, Krug SE, Alpert SE, Marx CM. Hospital treatment of asthma: lack of benefit from theophylline given in addition to nebulized albuterol and intravenously administered corticosteroid. J Pediatr 122:464–469, 1993.

46. Carter E, Cruz M, Chesrown S, Shieh G, Reilly K, Hendeles L. Efficacy of intravenously administered theophylline in children hospitalized with severe asthma. J Pediatr 122:470–476, 1993.

47. Self TH, Abou-Shala N, Burns R, Stewart CF, Ellis RF, Tsiu SJ, Kellermann AL. Inhaled albuterol and oral prednisone therapy in hospitalized adult asthmatics. Does aminophylline add any benefit? Chest 98:1317–1321, 1990.

48. Witek TJ, Schachter EN. Pharmacology and therapeutics in respiratory care. Philadelphia: WB Saunders, 1994.

49. Barnes PJ. New drugs for asthma. Eur Respir J 5:1126–1136, 1992.

50. Pakes GE, Brogden RN, Heel RC, Speight TM, Avery GS. Ipratropium bromide: a review of its pharmacological properties and therapeutic efficacy in asthma and chronic bronchitis. Drugs 20:237–266, 1980.

51. van Schayck CP, Dompeling E, van Herwaarden CL, Folgering H, Verbeek AL, van der Hoogen HJ, van Weel C. Bronchodilator treatment in moderate asthma or chronic bronchitis: continuous or on demand? A randomised controlled study. Br Med J 303:1426–1431, 1991.

52. Brogden RN, Sorkin EM. Nedocromil sodium: an updated review of its pharmacological properties and therapeutic efficacy in asthma. Drugs 45:693–715, 1993.

53. Taylor IK, Shaw RJ. The mechanism of action of corticosteroids in asthma. Respir Med 87:261–277, 1993.

54. Szefler SJ. Glucocorticoid therapy for asthma: clinical pharmacology. J Allergy Clin Immunol 88:147–165, 1991.

55. Toogood JH, Baskerville JC, Jennings B, Lefcoe NM, Johansson SA. Influence of dosing frequency and schedule on the response of chronic asthmatics to the aerosol steroid, budesonide. J Allergy Clin Immunol 70:288–298, 1982.

56. Malo JL, Cartier A, Merland N, Ghezzo H, Burek A, Morris J, Jennings BH. Four-times-a-day dosing frequency is better than twice-a-day regimen in subjects requiring a high-dose inhaled steroid, budesonide, to control moderate to severe asthma. Am Rev Respir Dis 140:624–628, 1989.

57. Boyd G, Abdallah S, Clark R. Twice or four times daily beclomethasone dipropionate in mild stable asthma. Clin Allergy 15:383–389, 1985.

58. Meltzer EO, Kemp JP, Welch MJ, Orgel HA. Effect of dosing schedule on efficacy of beclomethasone dipropionate aerosol in chronic asthma. Am Rev Respir Dis 131:732–736, 1985.

59. Barnes PJ. Inhaled glucocorticoids for asthma. N Engl J Med 332:868–875, 1995.

60. Kamada AK. Therapeutic controversies in the treatment of asthma. Ann Pharmacother 28:904–914, 1994.

61. Toogood JH, Baskerville J, Jennings B, Lefcoe NM, Johansson SA. Bioequivalent doses of budesonide and prednisone in moderate and severe asthma. J Allergy Clin Immunol 84:688–700, 1989.

62. Newman SP, Delivery of drugs from the respiratory tract. In: Chung KF, Barnes PJ, eds. Pharmacology of the respiratory tract: experimental and clinical research. New York: Marcel Dekker, 1993.

63. Thorsson L, Edsbacker S, Conradson TB. Lung deposition of budesonide from Turbuhaler is twice that from a pressurized metered-dose inhaler P-MDI. Eur Respir J 7:1839–1844, 1994.

64. Warner GO, Götz M, Landau LI, Levison H, Milner AD, Pedersen S, Silverman M. Management of asthma: a consensus statement. Arch Dis Child 64:1065–1079, 1989.

65. Woolcock A, Rubinfeld AR, Seale JP, Landau LL, Antic R, Mitchell C, Rea H, Zimmerman P. Thoracic society of Australia and New Zealand. Asthma management plan. Med J Aust 151:650–653, 1989.

66. British Thoracic Society, Research Unit of the Royal College of Physicians of London, King's Fund Center, National Asthma Campaign. Guidelines for management of asthma, I-chronic persistent asthma and II-acute severe asthma. Br Med J 201:651–653, 1990.

67. Hargreave FE, Dolovich J, Newhouse MT, eds. The assessment and treatment of asthma: a conference report. J Allergy Clin Immunol 85:1098–1111, 1990.

68. Wilson NM, Siverman M. Treatment of acute, episodic asthma in preschool children using intermittent high dose inhaled glucocorticoids at home. Arch Dis Child 65:407–410, 1990.

69. Woolcock AJ. Steroid resistant asthma: what is the clinical definition? Eur Respir J 6:743–747, 1993.

70. Brunette MG, Lands L, Thibodeau LP. Childhood asthma: prevention of attacks with short-term corticosteroid treatment of upper respiratory tract infection. Pediatrics 81:624–629, 1988.

71. Szefler SJ, Alternative therapy in severe asthma: rationale and guidelines for applications. In: Middleton E Jr, Reed CE, Ellis EF, Adkinson NF Jr, Yuninger JW, Busse WW. Allergy: principles and practice, 3rd. ed. St. Louis, Mosby-Year Book, 1991:1–14.

72. Chanarin N, Johnston SL. Leukotrienes as a target in asthma therapy. Drugs 47:12–24, 1994.

73. Nicholson CD, Shahid M. Inhibitors of cyclic nucleotide phosphodiesterase isoenzymes–their potential utility in the treatment of asthma. Pulm Pharmacol 7:1–17, 1994.

74. Mayo PH, Richman J, Harris HW. Results of a program to reduce admissions for adult asthma. Ann Intern Med 112:864–871, 1990.

75. Cunningham SJ, Crain EF. Reduction of morbidity in asthmatic children given a spacer device. Chest 106:753–757, 1994.

CHAPTER 36

CHRONIC OBSTRUCTIVE PULMONARY DISEASE

TRACEY L. GOLDSMITH and JEFFREY J. WEBER

The term *obstructive pulmonary disease* encompasses several separate and distinct sets of pathologic changes, including asthma, chronic bronchitis, and emphysema. Interference with ventilation from an obstruction to airflow is the common element, in contrast to restrictive lung disease where the defect is reduced capability for lung expansion. Asthma is discussed in detail in Chapter 35, but it can be summarized as a clinical syndrome characterized by narrowing of the airways as a result of bronchial hyperreactivity, excessive bronchial secretions, and inflammatory changes of the airways. The resulting obstruction to airflow is usually reversible.

Chronic obstructive pulmonary disease (COPD) includes chronic bronchitis and emphysema. Airflow obstruction in these patients may respond to various therapeutic efforts, but these diseases are largely irreversible. Chronic bronchitis is defined by chronic or recurrent excess mucus secretion into the bronchial tree that occurs on most days during a period of at least 3 months of the year for at least 2 consecutive year (1). Emphysema is described as a condition of the lung characterized by abnormal permanent enlargement of the air spaces distal to the terminal bronchiole, accompanied by destruction of their walls, and without obvious fibrosis (1). Chronic bronchitis and emphysema are frequently indistinguishable on clinical examination, and many patients have components of both diseases.

INCIDENCE

Chronic obstructive pulmonary disease is the fourth leading cause of mortality in the United States (2). In 1993, over 95,000 deaths were attributed to COPD (2). Current best estimates suggest that 82% of COPD deaths are attributable to smoking. COPD mortality currently is higher in whites than blacks and higher in males than females. This latter trend is changing, however, with predictions that within 10 to 20 years there will be an equal number of deaths of men and women related to cigarette consumption (3). The mortality from COPD is increasing, particularly among older patients (4). Various estimates of the number of people in the United States affected by COPD range as high as 20 million (5), but these numbers are likely underestimates of the prevalence of the disease because of the number of undiagnosed patients with mild to moderate disease and no clinical symptoms.

PATHOPHYSIOLOGY

The normal function of the respiratory system is to exchange oxygen (O_2) and carbon dioxide (CO_2) so that oxygen is delivered to and carbon dioxide is removed from the blood. CO_2 is the major stimulus for the respiratory center, which is located in the medulla of the brain. When $PaCO_2$ levels increase, ventilation is stimulated, resulting in increased removal of CO_2. Anatomically, the respiratory tract has three components that support this process: a conducting system, respiratory exchange units, and a vascular supply. The conducting system is composed of the nose, pharynx, larynx, trachea, and bronchi. Obstructions of the upper airway can result from foreign objects, tumors, and so on. The lower respiratory tract, or the respiratory exchange units, include the bronchioles, alveolar ducts, alveolar sacs, and alveoli. Exchange of O_2 and CO_2 occurs between the alveoli and the vascular supply (capillaries). Normal airway integrity is maintained through the relationship of pressures in and around the airway and the elasticity of the airway.

With obstructive pulmonary disease, changes in these normal processes occur. If airway integrity is compromised through diseases such as chronic bronchitis or emphysema, obstruction of the lower airway results. Changes in pulmonary vasculature result from hypoxia. Pulmonary hypertension may develop and is seen as elevated mean pulmonary artery pressures and pulmonary vascular resistance. Cor pulmonale, or hypertrophy of the right ventricle due to primary lung disease, may then develop and progress to heart failure. These alterations in normal lung structure and function may occur in the course of chronic bronchitis and emphysema.

In contrast to the normal patient, the respiratory drive in patients with COPD becomes less responsive to changes in arterial pH and $PaCO_2$. Hypoxic drive begins to play a larger role. A patient with respiratory failure who receives oxygen administration will have an increase in $PaCO_2$. This increase may be due to an effect on hypoxic drive, but may also be due to changes in ventilation/perfusion caused by the alleviation of hypoxic-induced vasoconstriction. Stable

COPD patients rarely experience significant $PaCO_2$ increases during oxygen therapy, but during acute exacerbations leading to respiratory failure, larger increases (10–13 mm Hg) in $PaCO_2$ can occur, leading to further alterations in mental status and acidosis. However, concerns about oxygen supplementation causing narcosis should not prohibit its administration (6).

High $PaCO_2$ levels are not as ominous as once thought. Adaptive changes with chronic COPD allow patients to tolerate high $PaCO_2$ levels. In mechanically ventilated patients, the concept of permissive hypercapnia (allowing the $PaCO_2$ to climb) is felt to be less harmful than the mechanical ventilation that is required to keep values "normal." The patient compensates by retaining bicarbonate, and a pH as low as 7.25 may be fairly well tolerated. Occasionally, additional bicarbonate can be administered if needed.

Chronic bronchitis and emphysema can be described on the basis of type and area of lung involvement. The chronic or recurrent nature of excessive mucus secretion in chronic bronchitis, accompanied with inflammation, interferes with normal mechanisms to maintain airway integrity. Excessive mucus production is the result of irritation of the airway by smoke or other irritants. With chronic irritation, the mucus glands increase in number and size, and their ducts dilate within the bronchial mucosa. Airway obstruction results from narrowing of the airway by thick, tenacious mucus and from bronchiolar inflammation and edema. Excess mucus secretion results in plugs or consolidations. Occlusion of the respiratory exchange units, primarily the small peripheral airways, occurs from these plugs, reducing the functional air exchange area and causing destruction of the alveoli. It is important to note that airway obstruction is not necessarily always present in chronic bronchitis and may occur only during acute exacerbations. In addition to mucus hypersecretion and inflammation, chronic or recurrent bacterial infection is common in chronic bronchitis.

In contrast to chronic bronchitis, actual destruction of distal air spaces, including the bronchioles, alveolar ducts, and alveolar sacs, is the primary culprit in emphysema. The result is loss of elastic recoil. Elastic recoil contributes to the force of expiration; if decreased, distal airways will collapse during expiration and trap air. Pathologically there are three types of emphysema. Centriacinar (centrilobular) emphysema is characterized by involvement of the proximal regions of the acinus, with distal alveoli left intact (1). This form is most common in emphysema due to cigarette smoking. Panacina (panlobular) emphysema is characterized by destruction of all areas of the pulmonary lobule and is more commonly associated with hereditary emphysema (α_1-antitrypsin deficiency) (1). The last form of emphysema is distal acinar emphysema. It is characterized by involvement of the distal acinus, alveolar ducts, and alveo-

lar sacs (1). This distinction is made at postmortem examination of lung tissue.

ETIOLOGY

Chronic bronchitis is associated strongly with cigarette smoking but can occur in persons who have never smoked. Other factors such as pollution or occupational exposures have also been associated with bronchitis. Emphysema is also associated with smoking, although other environmental factors may be important. Cigarette smoking causes increased bronchial reactivity and inflammation. Ciliary function is depressed, resulting in decreased clearance of mucus and particles. Macrophage function is similarly inhibited. Release of lysosomal enzymes destroys the connective tissue in the lung. Other factors such as increasing age, male sex, and existing impairment of lung function are also associated risks for COPD.

A history of chronic bronchitis can often be elicited in patients with centriacinar emphysema. Inborn errors resulting in enzyme deficiencies are rare causes of emphysema. If an imbalance occurs between elastase (enzymes that degrades elastin in the lung parenchyma) and elastase inhibitors, alveolar destruction results. A deficiency of α_1-antitrypsin (or α_1-proteinase inhibitor), an elastase inhibitor, has been demonstrated in some patients with panacinar emphysema, indicating a genetic basis for alveolar wall destruction.

CLINICAL PRESENTATION AND DIAGNOSIS

By the time they seek medical attention, patients are usually far advanced in their disease, with symptoms of airway obstruction. This delay is medical intervention occurs because the pathologic changes have been progressing for years, but overt clinical symptoms occur later. The usual presentation of COPD begins with cough and increased sputum production, reminiscent of chronic bronchitis. The patient may have noticed a decline in exercise tolerance. Weight loss (sometimes profound) may be reported by the patient with primary emphysema; however, the patient with chronic bronchitis is typically obese. Dyspnea, or breathlessness, is the sensation of labored or difficult breathing. It occurs later in the course of COPD and may be worsened by exposure to cold, dampness, pollution, and/or acute infection. Considerable interpatient variation exists in the subjective perception of dyspnea. There is a close intrapatient correlation between dyspnea and worsening degree of airway obstruction in patients with advanced COPD (7).

Respiratory infections of bacterial, viral, and mycoplasmal etiology can trigger an acute COPD exacerbation, especially in the patient with chronic bronchitis (8). Alternatively, bacteria can be secondary invaders following viral or mycoplasmal infections (8). Most of these bacterial respiratory infections are caused by pathogens offenders including *Haemophilus influenzae, Streptococcus pneumoniae,* and *Branhamella catarrhalis.* Patients with mucus hypersecretion are predisposed to repeated infections. Decreased removal of bronchial secretions physically impairs the defenses of the lungs against infection, and the mucus provides a good growth medium for bacteria. Colonization of the airways by these organisms has been clearly demonstrated. It remains unclear whether colonization or recurrent infection contributes to the progression of COPD by accentuating the rate of decline of pulmonary function.

Certain characteristic signs of COPD may be noted on physical examination. A prolonged expiratory effort may be seen as a sign of airway obstruction in primary emphysema. These patients may also exhale through pursed lips in an attempt to control the rate of expiration. Grunting may be heard on inspiration. The patient may be using the accessory respiratory muscles to aid in breathing. An overall increase in respiratory rate is common. Wheezes may be heard during bouts of airway obstruction in both chronic bronchitis and emphysema. An increase in the anteroposterior diameter of the chest and the classic "barrel chest" may occur in both diseases. These signs and symptoms do not correlate well with severity of illness. The chest x-ray may be helpful if emphysematous bullae or marked vascular changes are present.

Pulmonary function tests provide good information on the degree of airway obstruction and also help assess the efficacy of drug therapy. Lung volumes and rates of flow can be measured by spirometry. Several important parameters should be reviewed. Vital capacity (VC) is a measure of the volume of air moved during a forced respiratory cycle (i.e., forced inspiration and expiration). The volume of air moved with a normal inspiration or expiration is termed tidal volume (TV). After a maximal expiration, the volume of air left in the lungs is called the residual volume (RV). The same volume of air remaining in the lungs after a normal expiration is then called functional residual

capacity (FRC). The sum of the VC plus the RV equals the total lung capacity (TLC). In COPD, RV is increased because of obstruction to airflow, while TLC can be either normal (as in chronic bronchitis) or increased (as in emphysema). Vital capacity is reduced in COPD.

Other pulmonary function parameters that should be understood are forced expiratory volume (FEV_1), forced vital capacity (FVC) and FEV_1/FVC ratio. FEV_1 is the volume of air exhaled during forced exhalation in the first second. This parameter is decreased in the patient with an obstruction to outflow, such as COPD. FEV_1 above 2 liters is usually not associated with dyspnea with normal activity. With a 50% decrease in FEV_1, dyspnea on exertion is present, while a 75% decrease will be associated with dyspnea at rest. There can be considerable day-to-day variability in FEV_1, with most stable COPD patients showing up to 20% fluctuation (9). Therefore, evidence of response to therapy is generally viewed as greater than a 20% increase in FEV_1. FVC denotes the volume of gas expelled from the lungs during rapid and complete exhalation, and is reduced in COPD. In a patient without lung disease, the FEV_1/FVC ratio is normally 0.8 or greater. Therefore, a patient with chronic or acute airway obstruction would have a FEV_1/FVC ratio less than 0.8. Because of the significant overlap in these parameters between chronic bronchitis and emphysema, these tests are of limited value in distinguishing between them for diagnostic purposes.

No specific laboratory information is useful in differentiating the various forms of COPD, with the exception of emphysema due to α_1-antitrypsin deficiency. This diagnosis is made by a serum protein electrophoretic study. Sputum and blood eosinophilia, usually associated with asthma, may be present if the COPD patient also has an asthma component. This information could be useful in determining the role of bronchodilator therapy, and possibly the use of corticosteroids.

As COPD progresses, other acute and chronic complications may develop. Patients in whom chronic bronchitis

Table 36.1.
Clinical Presentation of COPD

	Chronic Bronchitis ("Blue Bloater")	Emphysema ("Pink Puffer")
Symptoms	Chronic cough, heavy sputum production	Dyspnea, minimal cough, minimal sputum production
Weight	Obesity common	Marked weight loss
Smoking History	Common	Common
Blood Gases	Low PaO_2	Normal or slightly low PaO_2
	Elevated $PaCO_2$	Normal or slightly high $PaCO_2$
	Respiratory acidosis	Normal pH or mild respiratory acidosis
Cor Pulmonale	Early development	Late development
Respiratory Failure	Repeated episodes	Rare until end stage
Pulmonary Function Tests	Decreased FEV_1	Decreased FEV_1
	Decreased FVC	Decreased FVC
	Increased residual volume	Greatly increased residual volume

is the predominant feature of COPD may undergo repeated episodes of acute respiratory failure. These patients may develop cor pulmonale and right-sided congestive heart failure. The term *blue-bloater* has been associated with this type of COPD patient. Hypoxemia and respiratory acidosis are common findings. In patients with predominant emphysema, acute respiratory failure is rare until the end stages of the disease. These patients are referred to as *pink-puffers*, since alveolar ventilation is maintained until the terminal stages of the disease. Table 36.1 summarizes the pertinent clinical features distinguishing chronic bronchitis and emphysema.

GOALS OF THERAPY

The treatments for chronic bronchitis and emphysema are very similar. Therefore, the therapy of COPD will be discussed, with areas of particular benefit in primary chronic bronchitis or primary emphysema highlighted. There are no clearly agreed upon standards for the goals of therapy in COPD. Goals can include symptomatic relief, objective evidence of improvement in airflow limitation, limiting the progressive decline in pulmonary function, and/or decreasing morbidity and mortality (10). Until definitive standards are established and more is known about the pathogenesis of COPD, therapy should be minimally aimed at halting or slowing the progression of the pathologic changes, improving the patients' quality of life, and preventing acute exacerbations of the disease. An individualized approach to therapy will be necessary but general recommendations can be summarized as follows.

Alter Environmental Influences. A normal decline in FEV_1 occurs with aging; however, environmental influences can accelerate that decline. Since cigarette smoking is involved in most COPD cases, the patient must be persuaded to stop smoking. Many of the changes seen in COPD are reversible with cessation of smoking, although some damage will remain. Exposure to other pollutants such as environmental or industrial pollutants should also be limited as much as possible. Humidification of inspired gases may be beneficial during use of artificial airways (either endotracheal tubes or tracheostomies), even in the patient not on mechanical ventilation (1).

Smoking constitutes the primary environmental risk factor that the patient can control. Increased emphasis on efforts to decrease smoking-related deaths has resulted in new research developments in smoking cessation. The majority of people who successfully quit smoking still do it on their own (unassisted "cold turkey"). The overall success rate of this approach, defined as those able to abstain for 6 months or longer, is probably less than 5% (11). Recognition of nicotine as a cause of drug dependence with a significant withdrawal syndrome has led to the development of numerous nicotine replacement products. Choices include nicotine polacrilex gum and a transdermal nicotine

patch. Nicotine nasal spray and inhaler are under development.

The most successful smoking cessation programs used a combined approach of behavioral and pharmacologic interventions. The overall success rate (commonly defined as the percentage who maintain abstinence for a 1-year period) of this approach is approximately 35% (11). Some of these studies have been criticized because they were felt to recruit highly motivated people, thereby increasing their success rates. A recent analysis of smoking cessation trials concluded that success with nicotine therapy was "largely independent of the intensity of additional support provided" (12). Methods such as acupuncture and hypnosis are sometimes used but little evidence exists to justify the high cost of these therapies. Frequent feedback and support from health care professionals and various forms of group therapy currently offer the best approach.

Pharmacologic therapy is indicated only in those patients who are identified as having significant physical withdrawal. Studies utilizing nicotine patches (with minimal behavioral intervention) have success rates in the neighborhood of 15% (13). Transdermal nicotine has advantages over nicotine delivery systems. These offer once daily dosing and a smoother nicotine delivery. The gum may be chewed slowly over 30 minutes to assure absorption, and at least 6 pieces per day are needed to obtain adequate plasma levels. Plasma levels associated with the patch are slow to rise and therefore do not resemble the fast peak levels seen after smoking and with faster delivery systems. Therefore there is less dependence potential, but the patch will not totally provide the "satisfaction" smokers may seek. For this reason, some smokers may find that use of the gum with the patch works best.

Correct Air Flow Obstruction. Several therapeutic modalities have been studied, including inhaled and oral bronchodilators, corticosteroids, and mucolytics. Individual agents or combinations of agents have met with varying rates of success.

Improve Patient's Functional Status. Many attempts to demonstrate objective improvement in pulmonary function tests with drug therapy have resulted in varying degrees of improvement. Significant subjective improvement noted by the patient has varied between studies. However, if the patient's outlook improves, subjective improvement should not be taken lightly. A percentage of increasing dyspnea and decreasing exercise tolerance can be detrimental to the patient's outlook and therefore detrimental to the treatment program. Since both maximum exercise and excercise endurance are decreased with COPD, effective programs aimed at improving overall conditioning and respiratory muscle performance can be very helpful in managing dyspnea and respiratory fatigue (7). Not only are programs aimed at overall conditioning potentially beneficial, exercise regimens targeting the upper extremities and respiratory muscles may improve dyspnea and overall fatigue.

Prevent Acute Disease Exacerbations. Since acute respiratory decompensations are frequently associated wtih respiratory infections, vaccination against common sources of infection is warranted. The long-term use of prophylactic antibiotics is controversial and certainly not without risk of adverse effects; therefore, this practice is usually not recommended in the United States. The patient should be protected from rapid environmental changes including cold, dampness, or heavy pollution, because these frequently trigger acute deterioration.

Optimize Drug Therapy Regimens. Although no specific drug or combination of drugs will reverse the damage already done to the respiratory tract, drug therapy is very important in controlling symptoms and managing progression of the disease. The patient may be exposed to any number of drugs with additive adverse effect profiles, and close monitoring is essential to ensure compliance and limit adverse effects. Concomitant drug therapy that could reduce ventilatory drive should be avoided whenever possible. Drugs that aggravate sequelae of COPD (such as arrhythmias), should also be used with caution.

Maintain Adequate Nutrition. COPD is often associated wtih significant loss of weight and muscle mass. Decreased caloric intake, increased energy expenditure due to the increased work of breathing, and declining pulmonary function measures are possible explanations (14). The suggestion that weight loss may be the result of the same destructive processes responsible for emphysema is worthy of additional study (14). Many patients have a body weight less than 90% of ideal. The degree of weight loss affects time of survival—patients with less than 90% of ideal body weight have a survival rate of under 70% at 3 years.(14) There is some suggestion that COPD patients who develop acute respiratory failure may have a poorer nutritional status than those with stable COPD (15). Substantial weight loss has been noted in both hospitalized and nonhospitalized (16) COPD patients. Malnutrition can result in decreased respiratory muscle function and depressed immune function, which may predispose the patient to infection. Hypophosphatemia also contributes to poor respiratory muscle function, so supplementation should provide adequate phosphates to avoid this complication.

SPECIFIC THERAPY

A summary of the drug therapy of COPD can be found in Table 36.2.

Anticholinergics

Anticholinergic therapy is gaining greater acceptance as a first-line therapy in both stable and acute exacerbations of COPD (17). Cholinergic stimulation increases the activity

Table 36.2.
Drug Therapy of Stable COPD

Step 1	**Ipratropium** MDI (with spacer*) or nebulizer for those patients who cannot master the proper technique; instruct patient on proper administration technique; 2–6† inhalations 4 times a day; instruct patient about importance of regular use; side effects of dry mouth and bitter taste. If drug trial results in < 20% improvement in FEV_1, go to step 2.
Step 2	Add a **β₂-agonist** MDI (with spacer*) or nebulizer for those patients who cannot master the proper technique; instruct patient on proper administration technique; dose based upon product selected; instruct patient about importance of regular use; side effects of tachycardia and tremor. If follow-up spirometry fails to demonstrate improvement, discontinue the β_2-agonist. If improvement is noted but overall outcome is still suboptimal, go to step 3.
Step 3	Add **theophylline** beginning with up to 400 mg/day as a long-acting dosage form; adjust dose at 3 day intervals by 25% to maintain serum level between 10–15 µg/mL; monitor for side effects of tachycardia, tremor, nervousness, GI side effects. If no objective or subjective improvement noted and outcome is still suboptimal discontinue theophylline and go to step 4.
Step 4	Trial of **corticosteroids: prednisone** 30–40 mg/day for 2–4 weeks; assess objective response with spirometry (i.e. improvement in FEV_1 of at least 20%); titrate dose to the lowest effective dose (< 10 mg/day); consider trial of inhaled corticosteroids; patients unable to maintain a similar response with inhaled corticosteroids can be placed back on the oral dosage form.

*Spacers are preferred for most patients who use MDIs.
†Few controlled studies show benefits from doses greater than 2 puffs every 6 hours.

of guanyl cyclase, the enzyme responsible for catalyzing the formation of cyclic GMP. Cyclic GMP stimulates bronchoconstriction; therefore, administration of an anticholinergic agent will prevent the formation of cyclic GMP. The result is inhibition of bronchoconstriction.

The anticholinergic drugs atropine and ipratropium have been used in COPD. Atropine by nebulization is effective and is associated with a decreased incidence of systemic adverse effects compared to parenteral atropine. Some systemic absorption does occur, so the patient should be closely monitored for signs of systemic adverse effects, such as dry mouth, blurred vision, or tachycardia. Because of potentially additive adverse cardiovascular and β-agonists or theophylline. The dose of atropine by nebulization is 0.025 mg/kg three to four times a day, with a range of 1 to 2.5 mg/dose. Because of safer alternatives with quaternary compounds, any experts prefer to avoid atropine sulfate.

Ipratropium bromide is an analog of atropine. It acts as a bronchodilator by the same mechanisms as atropine; however, because it is a quaternary compound, little systemic absorption occurs. Studies comparing ipratropium to β-agonists in stable COPD patients show that ipratropium bromide produces equal or greater bronchodilation at usual doses (18, 19). At maximal doses, the bronchodilation produced by β-agonists probably equals that of ipratropium in COPD (20), but adverse effects are more frequent. Ipratropium bromide produces a response within 15 minutes when inhaled, with effects seen for 4 to 6 hours (18). Because of its slower onset compared to β-agonists, patients may prefer β-agonists for acute bronchospasm, with ipratropium being used on a scheduled basis. Ipratropium bromide is administered as 2 inhalations 4 times a day, increasing to 6 inhalations if needed. Adverse effects occur infrequently and consist of dryness of the mouth and throat, bitter taste, cough, and nausea.

When prescribed therapy with ipratropium or other inhaled aerosol, the patient should be instructed on the proper use of metered-dose inhalers (MDIs). Metered-dose inhalers are a convenient way to deliver aerosolized drugs. However, many patients find it difficult to actuate the inhaler properly and synchronize inhalation and exhalation for maximum drug deposition. It is estimated that up to 89% of adults are unable to correctly use MDIs (21). Aerosol deposition within the airways is decreased in these cases. Patients have also been known to exhale during actuation of the inhaler, preventing any airway deposition of drug. Pharmacologic activity occurs only when sufficient drug is deposited at bronchial receptors. Many authorities have made recommendations on the optimal use of MDIs. One group recommends inhalation of the aerosol during a slow, deep inhalation with breathholding for 10 seconds (22). Actuation of the MDI between tightly closed lips and actuation up to 2 inches in front of widely opened lips are both recommended, and study results disagree on the optimal technique. However, properly performed closed mouth technique is as efficacious as using an add-on auxiliary device (spacer) (23). Therefore, either open or closed mouth technique is acceptable.

Thorough, repeated instructions, involving observation of the patient's technique whenever possible, should be given with each patient visit. Instructions to the patient for appropriate use of MDIs should include

1. Use the inhaler only in the frequency and dose prescribed. If symptoms worsen, seek medical attention before routinely increasing the dose.
2. Shake the MDI canister thoroughly immediately prior to use.
3. Exhale slowly and completely.
4. Inhale slowly and deeply while depressing the MDI canister.
5. Hold breath for 10 seconds (or as long as possible if not able to do so for 10 seconds).
6. Wait at least 1 minute between multiple doses.
7. Clean MDI case and cap thoroughly with water at least once per day.

Many experts prefer to use spacers routinely. Spacers decrease particle size, resulting in decreased particle deposition in the upper airway and greater delivery of drug to the more distal airways. In doing so, these devices protect against deposition of aerosols in the oral mucosa and systemic absorption. These auxiliary systems may be useful in patients who fail to properly use MDIs despite education, although many patients may benefit equally from proper explanation and reinforcement of correct MDI use. Because the incidence of inappropriate technique is so high (21), spacers should be routinely offered to patients.

Ipratropium may also be administerd by nebulizer. For nebulization, a dose of 0.5 mg every 4 to 6 hours as needed is used. Because of their expense, size, and lack of increased efficacy, nebulizers may be useful for patients unable to use MDIs with spacers, seriously ill patients who are not fully alert, and patients who psychologically would benefit from the use of a nebulizer (24). Considerable debate still exists about the role of nebulizers in inhalational therapy.

Sympathomimetics

Sympathomimetics, or β-agonists, are frequently used in COPD to control dyspnea and improve exercise tolerance. These drugs work by activating adenyl cyclase and increasing levels of cAMP, resulting in airway smooth muscle relaxation. There is also some evidence that these drugs may increase diaphragmatic contractility (25) and improve cor pulmonale (26). β-Agonists were considered by many to be first-line therapy in COPD patients. This is currently controversial, since anticholinergic inhalers are equally or more efficacious.

The earliest β-agonists included drugs such as epinephrine, ephedrine, and isoproterenol. Although inhaled β-agonists are more efficacious, epinephrine remains useful in acute reversal of bronchospasm for some patients. However, its short duration of action, nonselectivity, development of refractoriness, and lack of an oral dosage form obviously limit chronic use. Ephedrine and isoproterenol use has been replaced by newer, safer β-agonists.

The most commonly used β-agonists are inhaled β$_2$-agonists administered via inhalation, although oral and parenteral products are also used. Systemic therapy is associated with more frequent adverse effects and lower efficacy. Rapid airway response is seen with inhaled β-agonists, whereas the onset of action with oral therapy in acute airway obstruction is delayed. Therefore, inhaled β-agonists are preferred in patients capable of using the devices. Table 36.3 reviews the currently available β-agonists, dosage forms, and dosing recommendations (27, 28). Standard dosing recommendations are usually applied to the COPD patient, but have not been well studied for optimum response in these patients.

Table 36.3.
β-Adrenergic Agonists

Drug (Generic/Trade)	Receptor Activity	Routes of Administration	Usual Dose	Onset of Action	Duration of Action
Epinephrine	α, β$_1$, β$_2$	SC	Varies with product	5–10 min	1–4 hr
		IM			1–4 hr
		Inhalation		1–5 min	1–3 hr
Ephedrine	α, β$_1$, β$_2$	PO	25–50 mg q 3–4 hr	15–60 min	2–4 hr
		SC	25–50 mg	1 hr	
		IM	25–50 mg	10–20 min	1 hr
Isoproterenol	β$_1$, β$_2$	Inhalation	Varies with product	2–5 min	0.5–1 hr
Isoetharine	Primarily β$_2$	Inhalation	Varies with product	1–5 min	1–2 hr
Metaproterenol (Alupent, Metaprel)	Primarily β$_2$	PO	20 mg tqid	15 min	4 hr
		Inhalation	2–3 inhalations q 3–4 hr	1 min	3–4 hr
Terbutaline (Brethane, Brethine, Bricanyl)	Primarily β$_2$	PO	2.5–5 mg tid	30 min	4–8 hr
		SC	0.25–0.5 mg q 4 hr	6–15 min	1.5–4 hr
		Inhalation	2 inhalations q 4–6 hr	5–30 min	4–6 hr
Albuterol (Proventil, Ventolin)	Primarily β$_2$	PO	2–4 mg tqid	30 min	4–6 hr
		Inhalation	2 inhalations q 4–6 hr	5–15 min	4–6 hr
Bitolterol (Tornalate)	Primarily β$_2$	Inhalation	2–3 inhalations q 8 hr	3–5 min	4–8 hr
Pirbuterol (Maxair)	Primarily β$_2$	Inhalation	1–2 inhalations q 4–6 hr	within 5 min	5 hr
Salmeterol/12 hr (Seravent)	Primarily β$_2$	Inhalation	1–2 inhalations q 12 hr	within 20 min	

Prefer inhaled route whenever possible.
Prefer primarily β$_2$ agents.
From Olin (27), and McEvoy (28).

β-Agonists should be compared on the basis of selectivity for β$_2$-receptors, available dosage forms, onset and duration of action, and cost. Metaproterenol, terbutaline, albuterol, bitolterol, salmeterol, and pirbuterol are all relatively β$_2$-specific agents. β$_2$ selectivity results in a decreased rate of systemic adverse effects, particular adverse cardiovascular effects, compared wtih the nonselective agents. Because of this specificity, these drugs are frequently prescribed. Metaproterenol, terbutaline, albuterol, bitolterol, salmeterol, and pirbuterol are all available for inhalation. They vary in onset and duration of action, with salmeterol having the longest onset and duration of action at up to 20 minutes and 12 hours, respectively. Because of the prolonged onset of action, salmeterol is not appropriate for treatment of acute bronchospasm. Salmeterol has been studied extensively in asthma, but studies in COPD patients are ongoing. The side-effect profiles are similar in nature, but vary in frequency. Minimal cardiovascular adverse effects are seen with the β$_2$ selective agents. Tremor is common to all the agents and is the primary adverse effect of albuterol and bitolterol. Transient hypokalemia may be induced by high doses of these agents. Combined therapy with inhaled and oral β-agonists may be seen, but additive adverse effects are likely to occur.

Appropriate instruction for MDI use should accompany β-agonist inhaler therapy, just as with ipratropium. β-Agonists may also be delivered via nebulization, but this practice is subject to the same concerns as the ipratropium. The relative doses of β-agonists for nebulization are similar to doses used in asthma and are higher than those for MDI inhalation because of the reduced efficiency of nebulizers in delivering the drug. However, patients who are severely dyspneic may benefit from nebulizer therapy if the MDI has not proven effective. Part of this improved response may relate to delivery of the drug as a wet aerosol.

Use of Aerosol Bronchodilators in Ventilated Patients

Aerosols are routinely used in the treatment of critically ill intubated patients. Very little information exists regarding the most effective method of delivery, proper dose, and optimum ventilator settings to assure delivery. Recommendations based on current knowledge include the following:

1. When using MDIs in the ventilated patient, the clinician should be aware that adequate amounts of medication may not reach the patient's airways. Physiologic parameters such as airway mechanics and close observation for systemic effects should be used to titrate and determine optimal dosing. MDIs administered through an in-line spacing device has been shown to have greater efficiency of aerosol deposition to lung tissue when compared to jet nebulization (29).
2. For jet nebulizers, it is reommended to use the largest possible volume of fill.
3. Ventilators should be set at reduced inspiratory flows (40–50 mL/min) to prolong inspiratory time, although caution is advised for those patients with excessive amounts of intrinsic peak end-expiratory pressure (PEEP) (30).

Recently, continuous β-agonist nebulization has been tried in many intensive care units. Tachycardia and hypokalemia have been observed, so careful titration according to physiologic effect is necessary (31). Further research needs to be done on this mode of delivery.

Combination β-Agonist/Anticholinergic Regimens

Data regarding the effects of using an anticholinergic medication with a β-agonist have been conflicting. The overall weight of the evidence favors an additive effect with chronic use but not acute use. Additive effects during chronic use have been recently supported by a large multicenter trial called COMBIVENT (32). The study found an additional bronchodilation of 20 to 40% for the combination over single agents. Despite this finding, clinical COPD symptoms scores were not significantly different. A stepwise approach to the selection of a bronchodilator based on objective measurements such as peak flow or spirometry is felt to be more useful than using only symptomatic end points. Patients can be started on a single bronchodilator initially and the combination tried if objective tests indicate a suboptimal response. The increased effectiveness of the combination is not surprising, since the two classes of drugs have different mechanisms and sites of action. Anticholinergic drugs are felt to act primarily in the central airways where cholinergic receptors are abundant, whereas the β-agonists' site of action includes peripheral as well as central airways (33).

Several studies conducted in emergency rooms examined the effect of combination therapy during acute exacerbations. Results demonstrated significant benefit with either ipratropium or sympathomimetics as the initial agent, but were unable to demonstrate significant improvement with the combination (34–36). If the combination is used during the acute treatment of COPD, an attempt should be made to determine whether a single agent will be sufficient once the patient is stable. The following step-care approach has been suggested: (a) obtain baseline spirometry; (b) administer ipratropium; (c) repeat spirometry 30 minutes later; (d) administered inhaled β-agonist; and (e) repeat spirometry (37).

Methylxanthines

At one time, theophylline was the mainstay of bronchodilator therapy in the COPD patient. With more effective bronchodilators now available, theophylline's role in COPD has declined. However, theophylline may still be beneficial in the management of chronic COPD, especially if a bronchoconstrictive component can be identified. When added to regimens of inhaled anticholinergics or β-agonists, theophylline produces additive bronchodilation (5, 38, 39). Once therapy is maximized with inhaled bronchodilators with suboptimal response, patients may be given a trial of theophylline followed by pulmonary function testing to assess response to therapy. Significant improvement can be demonstrated through pulmonary function testing (39–41), as well as through decreased dyspnea (39, 41) and quality of life measures (39). Theophylline may also reduce overnight declines in FEV_1 and resultant morning respiratory symptoms when administered as an evening dose (42), and may still have an important role in this setting.

As intravenous aminophylline, theophylline has been evaluated in acute exacerbations of COPD (43). In addition to a regimen consisting of β-agonists, corticosteroids, antibiotics, and oxygen (when needed), patients received either intravenous aminophylline or placebo. The results were not promising, with no significant improvement seen with the addition of theophylline. Because study numbers were small, questions still remain about the role of theophylline in acute COPD exacerbations.

In addition to questions regarding the overall efficacy of theophylline in COPD, the mechanisms by which it may produce beneficial effects is unclear. Several proposed effects on the cardiac and respiratory systems include (a) bronchodilation, (b) improved respiratory muscle contractility and reserve, (c) stimulation of central ventilatory drive, (d) increased mucociliary clearance, (e) decreased mean pulmonary artery pressure and pulmonary vascular resistance, (f) increased collateral ventilation, and (g) improved biventricular cardiac performance (41, 44). Although demonstrated in several small trials, the significance of these effects has not been fully examined in COPD patients on a large scale. Indeed, it is likely that a combination of these effects is responsible for any positive benefit seen. Theophylline does not possess the bronchodilatory potency of β-agonists. Improved respiratory muscle reserve appears to account for improvement in dyspnea in patients with stable, severe COPD (41). The ability to lower pulmonary artery pressure and decrease pulmonary vascular resistance has been demonstrated in both acute and long-term studies of theophylline, although study populations have been small (45). Infusion of intravenous theophylline results in a significant decrease in these parameters as well as a direct inotropic action; both are advantageous in the patient who has progressed to cor pulmonale and heart failure. Ventricular afterload is reduced and biventricular cardiac function is improved as a result.

Theophylline probably produces these effects through a number of actions, including inhibition of phosphodiesterase, alteration in calcium movement, blockade of adenosine receptors, prostaglandin antagonism, and alteration of cyclic AMP binding to the binding protein (44). Phosphodiesterase inhibition has traditionally been accepted as the mechanism of action of theophylline, but it is questionable whether this accounts for its effects at clinically used doses. The other effects have been noted at clinically useful levels and thus may be responsible for the efficacy of the drug (46).

When initiating therapy, the clinician must address several issues related to theophylline. A multitude of dosage forms and salts of theophylline are available. The acuity of the situation will dictate choice of dosage form (e.g., the patient in acute respiratory failure who cannot take oral medication is best managed by parenteral therapy). However, chronic therapy decisions must include an assessment of patient compliance, dosage form preference, factors that influence the clearance of theophylline, and cost. Chapter 35, "Asthma," provides a detailed discussion of theophylline, including dosage form comparisons, detailed pharmacokinetics, and drug interactions.

Recommendations for dosing of theophylline in COPD are similar to those for asthma. Continuous infusions for acute therapy are generally in the range of 0.2 to 0.7 mg/kg/hr (47), whereas oral dosages for chronic therapy start at up to 400 mg/day and increase by 25% at 3-day intervals until the desired dose is achieved (47). Serum concentrations up to 20 µg/mL show a linear correlation with improvement in FEV_1 in the COPD patient (48). However, as serum concentration exceeds 15 µg/mL (47). when used in COPD, theophylline therapy should be monitored closely to assess the degree of benefit the patient is receiving (primarily symptomatic control). Careful monitoring is also warranted to prevent or limit adverse effects that may be more common in these patients (e.g., they may be particularly sensitive to the arrhythmogenic effects of theophylline) (49). Many COPD patients continue to smoke, thereby increasing theophylline clearance. The clearance of theophylline may be reduced in advanced stages of COPD or in the presence of cor pulmonale with or without heart failure (47).

Given the adverse effect profile of the theophylline, evidence of significant benefit should be obtained before subjecting the patient to long-term therapy. Preferably, pre- and posttheophylline pulmonary function testing should be used, as well as dyspnea scoring. The clinician must be able to monitor the patient for side effects and toxicity such as nausea, vomiting, tremors, headaches, confusion, arrhythmias, and seizures. Further evidence of objective benefits on diaphragmatic contractility, stimulation of hypoxic drive, and improved cardiac performance may define the role of theophylline in COPD more clearly.

Corticosteroids

The role of corticosteroids in COPD has been the subject of much debate. A recent analysis summarized studies performed in more stable COPD patients and concluded that oral corticosteroids improve baseline FEV_1 by 20% or greater, approximately 10% more often than patients receiving placebo (50). Subjective improvements in exercise tolerance and dyspnea have been reported (51). Subjective improvement can occur without actual improvement in pulmonary function tests, exercise tolerance, or

arterial oxygen saturation (52, 53). Since corticosteroids can result in euphoria, especially in higher doses, reports of subjective improvement may reflect a side effect of corticosteroid therapy. Recently, the effect of corticosteroids on quality of life measures has been reported in COPD patients (54). Although improvement in quality of life measures was reported, it was postulated that longer-term studies would be needed to fully measure the extent of improvement. Only with longer periods of observation would measures such as exercise tolerance be evaluable, due to the lag time in muscle recovery following renewed or increased use.

Since bronchodilator therapy alone has been associated with increasing mortality and an accelerated rate of decline in FEV_1 in patients with asthma and COPD (55), interest has been growing regarding the addition of corticosteroids to reverse this trend. Recent studies (56, 57) designed to examine the spectrum of obstructive airway disease have shown improvement in morbidity, hyperresponsiveness, and rate of decline of FEV_1 with the combination of corticosteroids and bronchodilators. Subgroup analysis demonstrates that the greatest benefit is seen in patients with an asthmatic clinical presentation, but suggests that some benefit may also be achieved in some patients with COPD and some hyperresponsivity. This may be difficult to apply clinically, however, since in practice it can be very difficult to categorize a patient at the extremes of asthma versus COPD because many patients have overlapping characteristics. More studies need to be done to better address this issue.

Patients wih severe airway obstruction secondary to COPD seem to respond better to corticosteroids than do the more stable patients. A demonstrable increase in FEV_1 has been shown in patients hospitalized for acute exacerbations of COPD given corticosteroids (58). Patients who have not responded to corticosteroids during stable periods of their disease may benefit in acute exacerbations or respiratory insufficiency. High corticosteroid doses are usually recommended, although the effects of lower doses have not been adequately studied. A small clinical trial of parenteral methylprednisolone versus placebo in patients with COPD undergoing abdominal surgery indicated that methylprednisolone hastened recovery of pulmonary function following surgery (59).

Corticosteroids should be tried in patients uncontrolled on bronchodilators. The optimal period for determination of responders to therapy and administration route remain unclear. Hudson et al. (60) recommended a trial of oral corticosteroids for 1 to 2 weeks in patients with significant airflow obstruction. Weir et al. (61) demonstrated that some responders do not show maximum response for at least 2 weeks and recommended a longer corticosteroid trial. Studies evaluating oral versus inhaled corticosteroids have demonstrated efficacy differences, with fewer patients responding to inhaled corticosteroids than to an oral regimen (62). However, in a recent study in which a spacer device was used to deliver inhaled beclomethasone, this mode of therapy was as effective as oral prednisolone (54).

Several different corticosteroid regimens can be selected. When oral therapy is selected, methylprednisolone 20 to 40 mg daily or prednisone equivalent may be initiated. Improvements in FEV_1 of 20% or more indicate a positive response, and therapy with corticosteroids should be continued. Subjective improvements in dyspnea and exercise tolerance should also be noted. If the patient responds, the dose of corticosteroid should be tapered to the lowest effective dose. Therapy can be continued with oral corticosteroids, but inhaled corticosteroids should be tried to minimize the risk of systemic adverse effects. Inhaled products can also be selected initially to determine if the patient is a corticosteroid responder. Several inhaled corticosteroid products are available, although beclomethasone is commonly used. A beclomethasone dose of 2 puffs 3 to 4 times daily is recommended, although some clinicians prefer a regimen of 10 puffs twice daily. Inhaled triamcinolone, 2 puffs 3 to 4 times daily, and flunisolide, 2 to 4 puffs daily, are alternatives. If inhalers cannot be used, alternate-day oral corticosteroid use in severe COPD appears to be an effective alternative. Studies comparing daily to alternate-day therapy in equivalent doses have shown a similar degree of improvement in pulmonary symptoms (63). Both inhaled and alternate-day oral corticosteroids produce fewer systemic side effects than daily oral corticosteroids. The use of inhaled corticosteroids or alternate-day therapy can also significantly reduce dependence on oral corticosteroids. During acute exacerbations or respiratory insufficiency, parenteral courses of corticosteroids may be needed. Methylprednisolone 0.5 mg/kg intravenously every 6 hours or hydrocortisone 100 to 250 mg intravenously every 6 hours for 72 hours can be used in acute respiratory insufficiency. Tapering over several days should be done to avoid precipitation of another episode of acute respiratory insufficiency.

If inhaled corticosteroids are to be used, the patient should receive adequate instructions on the use of the MDI. Instructions like those discussed under the anticholinergic MDIs should be provided. A spacer should be used with steroid MDIs; they reduce the risk of oropharyngeal candidiasis and increase the efficacy of inhaled steroids (54, 64). Additional counseling to rinse the mouth thoroughly after use of the corticosteroid inhaler is necessary, since this may decrease the risk of oral candidiasis associated with corticosteroid deposition in the oral cavity. The patient should be instructed to seek medical attention at the first sign of oral candidiasis. Oral candidiasis is characterized by a sore throat, patchy white exudates, and an underlying erythematous mucosa. This usually responds easily to temporarily discontinuing the corticosteroid inhaler and

treating with local antifungal therapy. The patient should also be told to use the β-agonist inhaler first if combination inhaler therapy is prescribed, so that maximal deposition of corticosteroid in the lower airway will occur. The patient should be informed about the differences in response between inhaled corticosteroids and β-agonists. In contrast to β-agonists, inhaled corticosteroids do not produce an immediate effect in acute dyspnea.

Recent evidence demonstrates that clinically used corticosteroid doses can produce muscle weakness (65). Regimens that averaged 1.4 to 21.3 mg/day methylprednisolone equivalent, either as continuous therapy or in repeated short-course regimens over a 6-month period, produced this effect (65). Both respiratory and peripheral muscles are affected. Respiratory muscle involvement may enhance dyspnea, thereby appearing as though COPD is worsening. The mechanism behind this finding has not been elucidated, and the overall significance of steroid-induced muscle weakness for the use of corticosteroids in COPD remains unclear.

Antibiotics and Vaccines

Certain organisms, particularly *S. pneumoniae*, *H. influenzae*, and *B. catarrhalis* are often cultured from the respiratory tract of COPD patients. Frequently this represents colonization of the airway and is not associated with infection. Although widely used in COPD, the role of antibiotics in the absence of signs of infection is clearly debatable. Studies evaluating the prophylactic use of antibiotics during high-risk months (i.e., winter) in chronic bronchitis patients have not shown a difference in the frequency of acute exacerbations. Antibiotic use at the onset of purulent sputum production, symptoms consistent with a head cold, increased cough, fever, or other subjective symptoms is a common practice that has not been associated with a decreased number of acute exacerbations. However, some evidence indicates that duration of illness may be decreased (66). In patients with only a mild exacerbation of COPD due to respiratory infection, antibiotic therapy is not recommended unless the patient deteriorates or fails to resolve (8). Moderate to severe exacerbations should probably be treated with oral antibiotics. The most commonly prescribed antibiotics include tetracycline, ampicillin, amoxicillin, amoxicillin/clavulanate, and cotrimoxazole. Erythromycin is generally not preferred for empiric therapy because of its lack of *H. influenzae* coverage. If these agents fail, other options include oral quinolones, clarithromycin, or azithromycin. Pneumonia complicating acute respiratory failure may be best managed with parenteral therapy, although oral options such as the quinolones may be considered. Cost and local susceptibility patterns should govern the final selection of the antibiotic regimen. Duration of antibiotic therapy is usually 7 to 10 days.

Vaccination with pneumococcal and influenza virus vaccines has been recommended in high-risk patient groups. Pneumococcal vaccine is formulated to provide prophylaxis against the most common strains of *S. pneumoniae*. Clear evidence that COPD patients are at an increased risk of infection by *S. pneumoniae* and thus increased mortality has not been presented (67). Antibody titers to the organisms may be elevated in COPD, probably as a result of chronic upper airway colonization. When given the vaccine, these patients respond by further increasing their antibody titers. Therefore, many clinicians recommend giving the vaccine to individuals with COPD. The most current dosing recommendation for adults is 0.5 mL by subcutaneous or intramuscular injection. Since antibody titers decline with time, the question of revaccination has been posed. An increased frequency of adverse effects with revaccination has been reported in the literature. At this time, revaccination should only be considered for those patients at highest risk of infection who received the vaccine 6 years or more ago. Those patients include asplenic, nephrotic syndrome, renal failure, or transplant recipient patients (68).

Influenza virus vaccine provides active immunity to the virus. As opposed to pneumococcal vaccine, influenza virus vaccine should be given annually. It is recommended in high-risk groups such as patients with COPD. The vaccine is reformulated periodically to cover the most common strains. The clinician must remember that transient increases in theophylline levels had occurred with use of the vaccine, so the patient should be monitored for signs of theophylline toxicity for 24 hours after vaccination. The usual adult dose is 0.5 mL intramuscularly. Amantadine 100 mg twice daily for 14 days may be given during outbreaks of Influenza A to high-risk patients who have not been immunized, or during acute influenza if started within the first 48 hours.

Oxygen Therapy

Oxygen therapy is an option for patients with severe chronic hypoxemia, cor pulmonale, or nocturnal or exercise-induced hypoxemia. In the setting of severe COPD, long-term oxygen therapy improves the survival rate in these patients (69–71). It is usually considered when the baseline PaO$_2$ drops below 55 mm Hg or below 60 mm Hg with concomitant right heart failure, polycythemia, or impaired mentation. Oxygen can be administered by devices that allow for ambulation or by fixed devices. Devices which allow the patient to ambulate are preferable. It can be administered continuously, during exercise, or nocturnally. The number of hours per day the patient uses oxygen continuously seems to relate to the effectiveness of this therapy, with those patients who use oxygen for at least 15 hours per day showing the greatest benefit (69). Patients may be reluctant to use continuous oxygen therapy, so nocturnal use may be more attractive. Oxygen use in combination with a structured exercise program may improve exercise tolerance. One to four liters of oxygen by nasal cannulae is usually required. The goal of therapy is to maintain oxygen saturation above 90%.

Mucolytic/Expectorant Agents

Agents that reduce the viscosity of mucus will aid in its expectoration, although the absolute value of such treatments has not been demonstrated in large-scale trials. Many agents, including acetylcysteine, oral iodinated glycerol, guaifenesin, terpin hydrate, and saturated potassium iodide solution, have been used. Although these agents may improve some symptoms, they do not improve dyspnea or objective measures of long function. Side effects can include coughing, chest discomfort, bronchospasm, and thyroid dysfunction. The latter has been reported with iodinated glycerol and is a possible adverse result of chronic therapy with any agent containing iodine (72).

Of the mucolytics, acetylcysteine and oral iodinated glycerol have been studied in COPD. Acetylcysteine, with its free sulfhydryl group, works by interfering with disulfide linkages. With the disulfide bonds broken, mucus becomes less viscous and more amenable to removal. Although acetylcysteine may be effective in lowering mucus viscosity, the efficacy of chronic administration in reducing the frequency of exacerbation of airway obstruction has not been demonstrated (73). It may be administered orally or via inhalation, nebulization, or intratracheal instillation. After administration, mucus liquefies and the patient must cough or use other measures to remove it. Acetylcysteine can induce airway irritation and bronchospasm, requiring bronchodilator use. In addition, the drug has a strong, foul odor that many patients find intolerable. It may also cause nausea.

Oral iodinated glycerol has been shown to be effective in improving symptoms in patients with stable, chronic bronchitis. Patients reported decreases in cough frequency and severity and chest discomfort with doses of 60 mg 4 times daily (74).

The patient type most likely to respond to mucolytic therapy is the patient with a major bronchitic component, where increased secretions are a more common problem. If a 4- to 6-week trial of the mucolytic/expectorant does not produce improvement, therapy should be discontinued. Adequate hydration and effective cough can do much to remove mucus from the airway and are preferable to the expectorants.

Respiratory Stimulants

Chronic hypercapnia in the COPD patient is usually well tolerated and may be compensatory to reduce respiratory muscle fatigue (75). It is best managed by proper muscle conditioning and bronchodilators. Only during acute respiratory failure should respiratory stimulants be considered.

Doxapram is a central nervous system stimulant that increases the rate and depth of respiration by stimulating central medullary respiratory centers. It has been used in short-term infusions in acute respiratory failure secondary to COPD in an attempt to prevent or reverse hypercapnia and respiratory depression. The benefit of this therapy is questionable, since arterial oxygenation is usually not improved due to the increased work of breathing induced by the drug. Carbon dioxide concentrations usually do not improve for the same reason. When used to avoid mechanical ventilation, doxapram therapy is usually unsuccessful. Adverse effects include hypertension, tachycardia, dyspnea, seizures, and muscle hyperreflexia. With its narrow margin of safety, overdosage may occur if therapy is not managed carefully.

If doxapram is used in acute respiratory failure, a continuous infusion of 1 to 2 mg/min to a maximum of 3 mg/min should be administered. The recommended duration of therapy is not to exceed 2 hours. Vital signs and arterial blood gases should be monitored in addition to observing the patient for signs of toxicity.

Other respiratory stimulants that have been tried in COPD include medroxyprogesterone and acetazolamide. Medroxyprogesterone 20 mg orally 3 times daily has been shown in small clinical trials to improve carbon dioxide elimination and alveolar ventilation (76, 77). Acetazolamide, although potentially useful in acute respiratory failure to increase alveolar ventilation and correct metabolic alkalosis, does not appear to be beneficial in the chronic management of COPD. Further large-scale studies are required before routine use of these agents can be recommended.

α_1-Proteinase Inhibitor

Approximately 1 to 13% of patients with emphysema have a deficiency of α_1-antitrypsin (AAT)(78). This deficiency leads to progressive destruction of elastin tissues and alveolar destruction caused by unopposed neutrophil elastase activity. An α_1-proteinase inhibitor obtained from pooled human plasma is available as chronic replacement therapy for patients with this congenital disorder who have demonstrable panacinar emphysema. Maintenance of AAT serum concentrations above 80 mg/dL should slow the rate of lung destruction. α_1-Proteinase inhibitor is not indicated for patients who have not developed signs and symptoms of emphysema, those with other forms of emphysema, or patients with FEV_1 below 20% of predicted. Although it is found to be nonreactive for the HIV antibody and hepatitis B surface antigen, hepatitis B immunization is still recommended with hepatitis B vaccine. Hepatitis B immune globulin, 0.06 mL/kg intra-

muscularly, may be given with the fist dose of vaccine if therapy with α_1-proteinase inhibitor is indicated before the vaccination regimen can be administered. Treatment with α_1-proteinase inhibitor requires weekly therapy. A dose of 60 mg/kg/week intravenously appears to maintain the inhibitor at an appropriate level within the lungs (79). The drug is well tolerated without adverse cardiovascular, respiratory, or hematologic effects.

Lung Transplantation

Lung transplantation for COPD has been a viable surgical treatment for COPD since the 1980s. Initially, double-lung and heart-lung transplantations were considered preferable to single-lung transplantations because of perceived ventilation/perfusion mismatches between the emphysematous lung and the transplanted lung. Subsequent work demonstrated that single-lung transplantation is effective, although FEV_1 returns to only 50 to 60% of predicted within the first 2 years (80). Although this is less than the improvement noted with double-lung or heart-lung transplantation, acceptable return of functional capability of the patient is noted. Survival rates are 67% at the end of 2 years with single-lung transplantation (80). Because single-lung transplantation allows a greater number of patients to benefit from lung transplantation compared to double-lung or heart-lung transplantation, some centers are performing the single-lung procedure preferentially. Bronchiolitis obliterans, probably related to chronic rejection, remains a major reason for progressive loss of graft function. Work in the surgical management of COPD is continuing. The absolute number of potential recipients compared to donor lung availability may limit the utility of this treatment.

MANAGEMENT OF OTHER COMPLICATIONS

Breathlessness

This discomfort of breathlessness is one of the major factors affecting quality of life for many patients with COPD. It may significantly restrict the patient's ability for any level of exercise. Breathlessness does worsen as pulmonary function declines, but there is a great deal of interpatient variability in the relationship between this symptom and commonly measured physiologic lung parameters. Factors contributing to breathlessness include mechanical, sensory, and behavioral components (81).

Because the primary mechanical abnormality involves expiratory flow limitation, the onset of inspiration occurs before expiratory flow is complete. With each breath, inspiratory muscles must overcome the elastic recoil associated with expiration, placing more demand on already compromised respiratory muscles, including the diaphragm. The resultant lung hyperinflation is felt to cause negative mechanical and sensory stimuli that contribute to the feeling of breathlessness. Anxiety also accompanies the feeling of breathlessnes and may itself contribute to the symptom (81).

Bronchodilators can relieve feelings of breathlessness even with the achievement of only small changes in FEV_1 (41). Anticholinergic medications may also reduce breathlessness. The mechanism for both medications is likely a reduction in gas trapping and lung hyperinflation, which results in a reduction in motor and sensory stimulation of breathlessness.

Supplemental oxygen has been shown to relieve breathlessness. This is likely related to decreased ventilatory demand due to altered peripheral chemoreceptor sensitivity. It is also possible that oxygen has central effects on the perceived discomfort of breathlessness. Beneficial effects of supplemental oxygen have been observed in patients who do not meet current American Thoracic Society criteria for long-term oxygen therapy (82).

Opiates have been shown to substantially increase the exercise capacity of patients with COPD. Mechanisms include both a reduction in ventilatory drive and an altered central perception of inspiratory effort. Improvements in workload and duration of exercise during opiate therapy have been found to be greater than those seen with anticholinergics and β-adrenergic stimulants. Special precautions are necessary due to the possible respiratory depression that may occur. Current use is primarily restricted to palliative care patients due to adverse effects such as sedation and the problem of physical tolerance (83, 84).

Benzodiazepines have not been shown to provide consistent beneficial effects when compared to placebo. They may be used in a patient whose breathlessness has a significant anxiety component (81).

Pulmonary Hypertension and Cor Pulmonale

Pulmonary hypertension develops in response to chronic hypoxemia. Cor pulmonale, or hypertrophy of the right ventricle, is a subsequent result. Right ventricular or biventricular failure may develop. Since sustained hypoxemia is postulated to be the major stimulus behind increased pulmonary vascular resistance and pulmonary hypertension, oxygen therapy is one of the primary therapies used in cor pulmonale. Diuretics have been used to manage dyspnea and edema. Digoxin may be beneficial in the patient with biventricular failure resulting from cor pulmonale, but its usefulness in isolated right ventricular failure is limited. Vasodilators reduce right ventricular afterload and may be used in patients with resistant pulmonary hypertension or right ventricular failure. Aggressive management of the underlying pulmonary disease, prevention of sustained hypoxemia, and patient education are the best means to reduce the incidence of this complication.

Acute Respiratory Failure

Acute respiratory failure may be precipitated by infection, use of central nervous system depressant drugs, bronchospasm, mucus plugging, or changes in environmental pollutants. Other stresses (e.g., surgery) may precipitate acute respiratory failure. The patient may have signs of diaphragmatic fatigue noted as asynchronous breathing. The PaO_2 is usually below 50 mm Hg, the $PaCO_2$ above 45 mm Hg, and the pH acidotic. Oxygen therapy and possible mechanical ventilation will be required. Mechanical ventilation is reserved until absolutely necessary, because it is difficult and slow to wean the COPD patient from ventilatory support. Physiotherapy aimed at improving drainage of secretions and relieving obstruction is beneficial. Supportive drug therapy, including β-agonists, corticosteroids, anticholinergics, theophylline, and/or respiratory stimulants may be instituted based on clinical symptoms (see Table 36.4). Antibiotic therapy should be initiated in the patient with signs of infection. Cardiac failure or arrhythmias should be treated by appropriate measures. Invasive cardiopulmonary monitoring should be instituted at this time. Nutritional support should be instituted early to prevent further loss of muscle mass.

PROGNOSIS

The best indicators of prognosis are degree of obstructon and age (85). Development of complications such as cor pulmonale and hypoxia are negative indicators for survival. FEV_1 obtained after bronchodilators is a good predictor of survival (85). Once FEV_1 decreases below 0.75 liters, severe airway obstruction is present and is associated with increased 5-year mortality. When the patient has dyspnea, the rate of mortality increases; up to 50% of patients die within 5 years. Their course will likely be characterized by multiple exacerbations, hospitalizations, and multiple drug therapies to treat symptoms or prevent progression. Poor nutrition and exercise intolerance frequently develop, and patients undergo important alterations in life-styles in severe disease.

CONCLUSIONS

Chronic obstructive pulmonary disease is a potentially preventable disease. Recognition that smoking contributes to the majority of COPD cases logically leads to the conclusion that cessaton of smoking would dramatically decrease the incidence of COPD. Public education about the hazards of smoking should continue. Obviously, health care professionals should model wellness by not smoking and should make concerted efforts to have patients stop smoking. Once COPD develops, those affected with moderate-to-severe disease are faced with a multitude of drug therapies with clearly debatable efficacy. The pro-

Table 36.4.
Drug Therapy of Acute Respiratory Failure

Oxygenation

Relief of hypoxemia with nasal cannula at 2–4 L/min or Venturi mask of 24–28%. Goal is to achieve 90% saturation of a normal hemoglobin level. If oxygenation is adequate and mental status deteriorates (secondary to increased $PaCO_2$) oxygen can be decreased.

Bronchodilators

β_2-agonists are preferred in the ER due to faster onset of action and peak effect. Evidence of a significant clinical benefit is lacking for the combined use with ipratropium in the acute setting.* Monitor for common side effects such as tremor, tachycardia, exacerbation of arrhythmias such as atrial fibrillation/flutter, multifocal atrial tachycardia, and premature ventricular contractions.

Ipratropium 4–6 inhalations (or 0.5 mg by nebulization which is preferred for acute respiratory failure) 4–6 times per day. May be preferred over β_2-agonists in COPD for cardiac patients due to fewer systemic adverse effects.

Corticosteroids

Methylprednisolone 0.5 mg/kg IV every 6 hours or hydrocortisone 100–250 mg IV every 6 hours. Begin to taper by the third day. The rate of tapering of the corticosteroid dose is based upon severity of disease and clinical response.

Antibiotics

Assess likelihood of infection. Institute appropriate antibiotics, if necessary.

Theophylline

While there are no data supporting use, in a life-threatening situation, use is warranted until benefits are disproven. Benefit/risk ratio must be carefully assessed due to adverse effects of nervousness, tremor, tachycardia, worsening arrhythmias, and gastrointestinal side effects. A loading dose of 5 mg/kg IV should be given if the patient was not previously on theophylline; maintenance infusion rates should range between 0.2–0.7 mg/kg/hr individualized based on patient history, concomitant drugs, and target blood levels of 10–15 µg/mL.

Fluids and Electrolytes

Ensure adequate fluid intake with appropriate electrolyte replacement including phosphates.

Nutrition

Initiate nutrition as soon as possible. Overfeeding should be avoided due to increased CO_2 production associated with excess caloric intake.

Mucolytics

Acetylcysteine may be used, especially for patients on mechanical ventilation with excessive secretions resulting in mucus plugging. They are not recommended for routine use since they are bronchial irritants and may promote bronchospasm.

Respiratory Stimulants

Use is controversial and cannot be routinely recommended.

Physiotherapy

Although commonly employed, the value of physiotherapy in acute respiratory failure is not determined.

*While many clinicians use anticholinergics concurrently, there is no evidence of additive effect in COPD (as there is in asthma).

gressive nature of the disease means the costs to the patient, both personally and financially, and to society are high. Ongoing evaluation of the benefit of screening for early diagnosis and intervention in patients at risk for COPD holds future promise. It is hoped that results of current and future investigations will improve the outlook for those patients affected by COPD.

REFERENCES

1. American Thoracic Society. Standards for the diagnosis and care of patients with chronic obstructive pulmonary disease (COPD) and asthma. Am Rev Respir Dis 136:225–244, 1987.
2. National center for Health Statistics. Monthly Vital Statistics Report 42(12):19, 1994.
3. Peto R, Lopez AD, Boreham J, et al. Mortality from tobacco in developed countries: indirect estimation from national vital statistics. Lancet 339:1269–1278, 1992.
4. Thom TJ. International comparisions in COPD mortality. Am Rev Respir Dis 140:S27–S34, 1989.
5. Bleecker ER. Acute bronchodilating effects of ipratropium bromide and theophylline in chronic obstructive pulmonary disease. Am J Med 91(4A):24S–27S, 1991.
6. Carroll GC, Rothenberg DM. Carbon dioxide narcosis. Chest 102:986, 1992.
7. Altose MD. Assessment and management of breathlessness. Chest 88 (suppl 2):77S–83S, 1985.
8. Murphy TF, Sethi S. Bacterial infection in chronic obstructive pulmonary disease. Am Rev Respir Dis 146:1067–1083, 1992.
9. Mendella LA, Manfreda J, Warren CPW, Anthonisen NR. Steroid response in stable chronic obstructive pulmonary disease. Ann Int Med 96:17–21, 1982.
10. Chapman KR. Therapeutic algorithm for chronic obstructive pulmonary disease. Am J Med 91(4A):17S–23S, 1991.
11. Gritz ER. Reaching toward and beyond the year 2000 goals for cigarette smoking: research and public health priorities. Cancer 74:1423–1432, 1994.
12. Silagy C, Mant D, Fowler G, et al. Meta-analysis on efficacy of nicotine replacement therapies in smoking cessation. Lancet 343: 139–142, 1994.
13. Gourlay S. The pros and cons of transdermal nicotine therapy. Med J Aust 160:152–159, 1994.
14. Wilson DO, Rogers RM, Wright EC, Anthonisen NR. Body weight in chronic obstructive pulmonary disease—the National Institutes of Health intermittent positive-pressure breathing trial. Am Rev Respir Dis 139:1435–1438, 1989.
15. Driver AG, McAlvey MT, Smith VL. Nutritional assessment of patients with COPD and acute respiratory failure. Chest 82:568–571, 1982.
16. Braun SR, Keim NL, Dixon RM, et al. The prevalence and determinants of nutritional changes in chronic obstructive pulmonary disease. Chest 86(4):558–563, 1984.
17. Braun SR, Levy SF. Comparison of ipratropium bromide and albuterol in chronic obstructive pulmonary disease: a three-center study. Am J Med 91(4A):28S–32S, 1991.

18. Tashkin DP, Ashutosh K, Bleecker ER, et al. Comparison of the anticholinergic bronchdilator ipratropium bromide with metaproterenol in chronic pulmonary disease. Am J Med 81(5A):81–90, 1986.

19. Ashutosh K, Lang H. Comparison between long-term treatment of chronic bronchitic airway obstruction with ipratropium bromide and metaproterenol. Ann Allergy 53(5):401–406, 1984.

20. Easton PA, Jadue C, Dhingra S, Anthonisen NR. A comparison of the bronchodilating effects of a beta-2 adrenergic agent (albuterol) and an anticholinergic agent (ipratropium bromide), given by aerosol alone or in sequence. N Engl J Med 315:735–739, 1986.

21. Epstein SW, Manning CP, Ashley MJ, et al. Survey of the clinical use of pressurized aerosol inhalers. Can Med Assoc 120(7):813–816,1979.

22. Newman SP, Clark SN. Inhalation technique with aerosol bronchodilators: does it matter? Pract Cardiol 9:157–164, 1983.

23. Rachelefsky GS, Rohr AS, Wo J, et al. Use of a tube spacer to improve the efficacy of a metered-dose inhaler in asthmatic children. Am J Dis Child 140(11):1191–1193, 1986.

24. Self TH, Rumbak MJ, Kelso TM. Correct use of metered-dose inhalers and spacer devices. Postgrad Med 92(3):95–106, 1992.

25. Aubier M, Vires N, Murciano D, et al. Effects and mechanism of action of terbutaline on diaphragmatic contractility and fatigue. J Appl Physiol 56:922–929, 1984.

26. Brent BN, Mahler D, Bueger HJ, et al. Augmentation of right ventricular performance in chronic obstructive pulmonary disease by terbutaline: a combined radionuclide and hemodynamic study. Am J Cardiol 50:313–319, 1982.

27. Olin BR, ed. Bronchodilators (sympathomimetics). Facts and comparisons. St. Louis, MO: JB Lippincott, 1995: 173a–177b.

28. McEvoy GK, ed. Sympathomimetic agents. AHFS drug information 95. Bethesda, MD: American Society of Health-System Pharmacists, 1995:804–854.

29. Fuller HD, Dolovich MB, Posmituck G, Pack WW, Newhouse MT. Pressurized aerosol versus jet aerosol delivery to mechanically ventilated patients: comparison of dose to the lungs. Am Rev Respir Dis. 141:440–444, 1990.

30. Manthous CA, Hall JB, Administration of therapeutic aerosols to mechanically ventilated patients. Chest 106:560–571, 1994.

31. Lin RY, Smith AJ, Hergenroeder P. High serum albuterol levels and tachycardia in adult asthmatics treated with high-dose continuously aerosolized albuterol. Chest 103:221–225, 1993.

32. COMBIVENT Inhalation Aerosol Study Group. In chronic obstructive pulmonary disease, a combination of ipratropium and albuterol is more effective than either agent alone: an 85-day multicenter trial. Chest 105:1411–1419, 1994.

33. Ohrui T, Yanai M, Sekizawa K, et al. Effective site of bronchodilation by beta-adrenergic and anti-cholinergic agents in patients with chronic obstructive pulmonary disease: direct measurement of intrabronchial pressure with a new catheter. Am Rev Respir Dis 146:88–91, 1992.

34. O'Driscoll BR, Taylor RJ, Horsley MG, Chambers DK, Bernstein A. Nebulised salbutamol with and without ipratropium bromide in acute airflow obstruction. Lancet 2:1418–1420, 1989.

35. Patrick DM, Dales RE, Stark RM, Laliberte G, Dickinson G. Severe exacerbations of COPD and asthma: incremental benefit of adding ipratropium to usual therapy. Chest 98(2):295–297, 1990.

36. Rebuck AS, Chapman KR, Abboud R, et al. Nebulized anticholinergic and sympathomimetic treatment of asthma and chronic obstructive airways disease in the emergency room. Am J Med 82:59–64, 1987.

37. LeDoux EJ, Morris JF, Temple WP, Duncan C. Standard and double dose ipratropium bromide and combined ipratropium bromide and inhaled metaproterenol in COPD. Chest 95:1013–1016, 1989.

38. Filuk RB, Easton PA, Anthonisen NR. Responses to large doses of salbutamol and theophylline in patients with chronic obstructive pulmonary disease. Am Rev Respir Dis 132:871–874, 1985.

39. Guyatt GH, Townsend M, Pugsley SO, et al. Bronchodilators in chronic air-flow limitation: effects on airway function, exercise capacity, and quality of life. Am Rev Respir Dis 135:1069–1074, 1987.

40. Eaton ML, MacDonald FM, Church TR, Niewoehner DE. Effects of theophylline on breathlessness and exercise tolerance in patients with chronic airflow obstruction. Chest 82:538–542, 1982.

41. Murciano D, Auclair MH, Pariente R, Aubier M. A randomized, controlled trial of theophylline in patients with severe chronic obstructive pulmonary disease. N Engl J Med 320(23):1521–1525, 1989.

42. Martin RJ, Park J. Overnight theophylline concentrations and effects on sleep and lung function in chronic obstructive pulmonary disease. Am Rev Respir Dis 145:540–544, 1992.

43. Rice KL, Leatherman JW, Duane PG, et al. Aminophylline for acute exacerbations of chronic obstructive pulmonary disease–a controlled trial. Ann Intern Med 107:305–309, 1987.

44. Aubier M, Roussos C. Effect of theophylline on respiratory muscle function. Chest 88(suppl 2):91S–97S, 1985.

45. Matthay RA. Effects of theophylline on cardiovascular performance in chronic obstructive pulmonary disease. Chest 88(suppl 2):112S–117S, 1985.

46. Lakshminarayan S, Sahn SA, Weil JV. Effect of aminophylline on ventilatory responses in normal man. Am Rev Respir Dis 117:33–38, 1978.

47. Edwards DJ, Zarowitz BJ, Slaughter RL. Theophylline. In: Evans WE, Schentag JJ, Jusko WJ, eds. Applied pharmacokinetics—principles of therapeutic drug monitoring, 3rd ed. Vancouver, WA: Applied Therapeutics, 1992: Ch 13.

48. Whiting B, Kelman AW, Barclay J, Addis GJ. Modelling theophylline response in individual patients with chronic bronchitis. Br J Clin Pharmacol 12:481–487, 1981.

49. Levine JH, Michael JR, Guarnieri T. Multifocal atrial tachycardia: a toxic effect of theophylline. Lancet 1:12–14, 1985.

50. Callahan CM, Dittus RS, Katz BP. Oral corticosteroid therapy for patients with stable chronic obstructive pulmonary disease: a meta-analysis. Ann Intern Med 114:216–223, 1991.

51. Strain D, Kinazewitz GT, Franco DS, George RB. Effect of steroid therapy on exercise performance in patients with irreversible chronic obstructive pulmonary disease. Am Rev Respir Dis 129:A65, 1984.

52. Strain DS, Kinasewitz GT, Franco DS, George RB. Effect of steroid therapy on exercise performance in patients with irreversible chronic obstructive pulmonary disease. Chest 88(5):718–721, 1985.

53. Evans JA, Morrison IM, Saunders KB. A controlled trial of prednisone, in low dosage, in patients with chronic airflow obstruction. Thorax 29:401–406, 1974.

54. Weir DC, Burge PS. Effects of high dose inhaled beclomethasone dipropionate, 750 μcg and 1500 μcg twice daily, and 40 mg per day oral prednisolone on lung function, symptoms, and bronchial hyperresponsiveness in patients with non-asthmatic chronic airflow obstruction. Thorax 48:309–316, 1993.

55. van Schayck CP, Dompeling E, Van Herwaarden CL, et al. Bronchodilator treatment in moderate asthma or chronic bronchitis: continuous or on demand? A randomised controlled study. Br Med J 303:1426–1431, 1991.

56. Dompeling E, van Schayck CP, van Grunsven PM, et al. Slowing the deterioration of asthma and chronic obstructive pulmonary disease observed during bronchodilator therapy by adding inhaled corticosteroids. Ann Int Med 118:770–778, 1993.

57. Kerstjens HAM, Brand PLP, Hughes MD, et al. A comparison of bronchodilator therapy with or without inhaled corticosteroid therapy for obstructive airways disease. N Engl J Med 327(20):1413, 1992.

58. Albert RK, Martin TR, Lewis SW. Controlled clinical trial of methylprednisolone in patients with chronic bronchitis and acute respiratory insufficiency. Ann Intern Med 92:753–758, 1980.

59. Fraser IM, Hyland RH, Hutcheon MA, et al. Preliminary study of the effects of postoperative methylprednisolone therapy on lung function recovery in patients with chronic obstructive pulmonary disease. Clin Pharm 8:214–219, 1989.

60. Hudson LD, Monti CM. Rationale and use of corticosteroids in chronic obstructive pulmonary disease. Med Clin North Am 74(3): 661–690, 1990.

61. Weir DC, Robertson AS, Gove RI, Burge PS. Time course of response to oral and inhaled corticosteroids in non-asthmatic chronic airflow obstruction. Thorax 45:118–121, 1990.

62. Weir DC, Gove RI, Robertson AS, Burge PS. Corticosteroid trials in non-asthmatic chronic airflow obstruction: a comparison of oral prednisolone and inhaled beclomethasone dipropionate. Thorax 45:112–117, 1990.

63. Blair GP, Light RW. Treatment of chronic obstructive pulmonary disease with corticosteroids—comparison of daily versus alternate-day therapy. Chest 86(4):524–528, 1984.

64. Salzman GA, Pyszczynski DR. Oropharyngeal candidiasis in patients treated with beclomethasone dipropionate delivered by metered-dose inhaler alone and with Aerochamber. J Allergy Clin Immunol 81(2):424–428, 1988.

65. Decramer M, Lacquet LM, Fagard R, Rogiers P. Corticosteroids contribute to muscle weakness in chronic airflow obstruction. Am J Respir Crit Care Med 150:11–16, 1994.

66. Anthonisen NR, Manfreda J, Warren CPW, et al. Antibiotic therapy in exacerbations of chronic obstructive pulmonary disease. Ann Int Med 106:196–204, 1987.

67. Williams JH, Moser KM. Pneumococcal vaccine and patients with chronic lung disease. Ann Int Med 104:106–109, 1986.

68. Spike JS, Fedson DS, Facklam RR. Pneumococcal vaccination: controversies and opportunities. Inf Dis Clin North Am 4(1):11–27, 1990.

69. Nocturnal Oxygen Therapy Trial Group. Continuous or nocturnal oxygen therapy in hypoxemic chronic obstructive lung disease. Ann Int Med 93:391–398, 1980.

70. Report of the Medical Research Council Working Party. Long-term oxygen therapy in chronic hypoxic cor pulmonale complicating chronic bronchitis and emphysema. Lancet 1:681–686, 1981.

71. Cooper CB, Waterhouse J, Howard P. Twelve-year clinical study of patients with hypoxic or cor pulmonale given long-term domiciliary oxygen therapy. Thorax 42:105–110, 1987.

72. Becker CB, Gordon JM. Iodinated glycerol and thyroid dysfunction. Four cases and a review of the literature. Chest 103(1):188–192, 1993.

73. British Thoracic Society Research Committee. Oral N-acetylcysteine and exacerbation rates in patients with chronic bronchitis and severe airways obstruction. Thorax 40:832–835, 1985.

74. Morgan EJ, Petty TL. Summary of the National Mucolytic Study. Chest 97(2):24S–27S, 1990.

75. Begin P, Grassino A. Inspiratory muscle dysfunction and chronic hypercapnia in chronic obstructive pulmonary disease. Am Rev Respir Dis 143:905–912, 1991.

76. Dolly ER, Block AJ. Medroxyprogesterone acetate and COPD: effect on breathing and oxygenation in sleeping and awake patients. Chest 84:394–398, 1983.

77. Skatrud JB, Dempsey JA. Determinants of chronic carbon dioxide retention and its correction in humans. J Clin Invest 65:813–821, 1980.

78. Hutchison DCS, Barter CE, Cook PJL, et al. Severe pulmonary emphysema: a comparison of patients with and without alpha-1-antitrypsin deficiency. O J Med 41:301–315, 1972.

79. Olin BR, ed. Alpha$_1$-proteinase inhibitor. Facts and comparisons. St. Louis, MO: JB Lippincott, 1995:187c–187d.

80. Levine SM, Anzueto A, Peters JI, et al. Medium term functional results of single-lung transplantation for endstage obstructive lung disease. Am J Respir Crit Care Med 150:398–402, 1994.

81. O'Donnell DE. Breathlessness in patients with chronic airflow limitation: mechanisms and management. Chest 106:904–912, 1994.

82. Dean NC, Brown KJ, Himelman RB, et al. Oxygen may improve dyspnea and endurance in patients with chronic obstructive pulmonary disease and only mild hypoxia. Am Rev Respir Dis 146:941–945, 1992.

83. Light RW, Muro JR, Sato RI, et al. Effects of oral morphine on breathlessness and exercise tolerance in patients with chronic obstructive pulmonary disease. Am Rev Respir Dis 139:126–133, 1989.

84. Johnson MA, Woodcock AA, Geddes DM. Dihydrocodeine for breathlessness in pink puffers. Br Med J 286:675–677, 1993.

85. Anthonisen NR, Wright EC, Hodgkin JE, and the IPPB Trial Group. Prognosis in chronic obstructive pulmonary disease. Am Rev Respir Dis 133:14–20, 1986.

CHAPTER 37

HYPERTENSION

ROBERT T. WEIBERT

Blood pressure control continues to be an important component in reducing cardiovascular risk, along with the modification of other cardiovascular risk factors, especially the lowering of cholesterol. Lifestyle modification to reduce blood pressure may control Stage 1 hypertension and is important adjunctive therapy in treating all hypertension. Drug treatment continues to be an individualized approach, treatment being tailored to individual patients on the basis of considerations of age, race, other disease states, effect on quality of life, drug costs, and patient compliance. The adverse consequences of antihypertensive drugs should be minimized, and step-down drug therapy can be attempted after a sustained period of controlled blood pressure.

The majority of hypertensive patients will require long-term antihypertensive drug treatment, and more pharmacologic agents are available for the treatment of hypertension than for any other condition. Clinicians can provide information about the pharmacology, pharmacokinetics, drug interactions, and adverse effects of these agents. In addition, maintaining patients on long-term drug treatment is an opportunity for pharmacists to cooperatively participate in providing follow-up care. Although there has been a reduction in cardiovascular deaths over the past 20 years, achieving long-term control of hypertension in millions of patients remains an important objective.

DEFINITION

Blood pressure varies from minute to minute and is influenced by measurement technique, time of day, emotion, pain, discomfort, hydration, temperature, exercise, posture, and drugs. The dividing line between normal blood pressure and hypertension is arbitrary. Early insurance industry actuarial data showed a continuum; the higher the blood pressure, the greater risk of developing complications. The 1993 Report of the Joint National Committee on Detection, Evaluation and Treatment of High Blood Pressure (JNC V) criteria for establishing a diagnosis of hypertension are as follows:

After screening, the diagnosis of hypertension is confirmed when the average of two or more diastolic blood pressure (DBP) measurements visits are 90 mm Hg or

Table 37.1.
Classification of Blood Pressure

Classification	Systolic Pressure (mm Hg)	Diastolic Pressure (mm Hg)
Normal blood pressure	<130	<85
High normal blood pressure	130–139	85–89
Stage 1 (mild)	140–159	90–99
Stage 2 (moderate)	160–179	100–109
Stage 3 (severe)	180–209	110–119
Stage 4 (very severe)	≥210	≥120

Source: From (1).

higher or the average of two or more systolic blood pressure measurements (SBP) is consistently greater than 140 mm Hg. JNC V classifies blood pressures as shown in Table 37.1. Single, casual measurements of blood pressure may inaccurately classify individuals as having hypertension and cause unnecessary emotional, social and financial problems (1).

ETIOLOGY

More than 90% of patients with sustained elevation of arterial blood pressure have essential hypertension with no identifiable cause. The term "essential hypertension" evolved from the mistaken concept that high blood pressure was "essential" for adequate tissue perfusion. A small percentage of patients may have potentially curable hypertension caused by renal disease, adrenal disease, coarctation of the aorta, or another rare condition (1). Renovascular hypertension, which is considered the most prevalent remediable cause of hypertension, is estimated to cause hypertension in less than 0.5% of the hypertensive population (2).

Drug-Induced Hypertension

Hypertension may occur in up to 5% of patients who take oral contraceptives. However, most women show small but measurable increases (9/5 mm Hg) in blood pressure during the first 2 years on the pill (3). Factors that may increase the likelihood of oral contraceptive hypertension include age greater than 35 years, smoking, obesity, and a family history of hypertension. Although the estrogen is the most important component, the amount and type of progestin may further influence the effect on blood pressure. Proposed mechanisms for contraceptive-induced hypertension include stimulation of the renin-angiotensin-aldosterone system and sodium and fluid retention. Oral contraceptive-hypertension may develop gradually over 1 to 2 years and is usually reversible within 1 to 8 months after therapy is stopped. However, if blood pressure does not normalize within 3 months, further evaluation and therapy are appropriate. Oral contraceptive-induced hypertension is best prevented by checking blood pressure every 6 months and using the agent that has the lowest effective estrogen dose (<30 μg) and a progestin content of 1 mg or less (3). Women who are at higher risk or who actually develop hypertension may need alternative forms of contraception (see Section 18).

Other drugs may also significantly increase blood pressure. A double dose of the sympathomimetic diet drug phenylpropanolamine (PPA) causes a significant increase in blood pressure to a peak of 173/103 mm Hg (4). There are reports of intracranial hemorrhage following PPA use. A metaanalysis of the effect of nonsteroidal antiinflammatory drugs (NSAIDs) on blood pressure demonstrated that NSAIDs elevate supine mean blood pressure by 5.0 mm Hg (5). NSAIDs antagonized the antihypertensive effects of β-blockers (6.2 mm Hg increase) to a greater extent than they antogonized vasodilators or diuretics (5). Cyclosporine causes vasoconstriction and sodium retention, inducing hypertension in a high percentage of patients. Recombinant human erythropoietin (rHuEPO) causes hypertension that is not responsive to antihypertensive therapy and must be managed by a dose reduction or discontinuation of rHuEPO (1). Also, corticosteroids, monoamine oxidase inhibitors, and products that contain large quantities of sodium, such as effervescent solutions, may increase blood pressure.

INCIDENCE

The NHANES III survey found that more than 50 million Americans have blood pressure of ≥140/90 mm Hg or are taking antihypertensive medications (1). The majority have mild hypertension with diastolic blood pressures ranging from 90 to 104 mm Hg. The prevalence of hypertension increases with age and is greater among blacks than whites and is greater in less educated people. Men and women of the same race are affected approximately equally. Massive public health efforts have increased the awareness of patients and the medical community of the need to identify and treat hypertension (6). Most hypertensive patients are now aware of their condition. The major challenge for health care providers is to maintain long-term treatment.

PATHOGENESIS

Blood pressure is maintained within a relatively constant range, despite changes in posture and wide variations in the demand for blood supply. While much is known about the complex system that regulates blood pressure, the pathogenesis of essential hypertension remains mysterious. Early theories suggested that renal sodium retention expanded vascular volume, increasing cardiac output. The increased cardiac output was believed to have led to increased vascular resistance (7). Further investigations suggest that natriuretic hormones may initiate sodium retention (7). Another theory suggests that inherited cellular defects cause increased intracellular sodium, leading to increases in ionic calcium and increased vascular tone and reactivity (7). A possible primary role of the sympathetic nervous system has also been suggested (7). It is likely that several interrelated mechanisms, rather than a single causative defect, control blood pressure in essential hypertension. A relationship between hypertension and obesity, insulin resistance, hyperinsulinemia, glucose intolerance, and hypertriglyceridemia has been reported (8, 9). This relationship has been termed "the deadly quartet" or "syndrome X" (10). This has led to the theory that hyperinsulinemia is a cause of hypertension (10). However, even with continued insights into the regulation of blood pressure, essential hypertension remains a process that must be controlled rather than a curable disorder.

DIAGNOSIS, SYMPTOMS, AND CLINICAL FINDINGS

Hypertension is usually an asymptomatic disease and is most often detected by screening. Because hypertension is easily detected and effective therapy is available, screening is recommended for all adults (5). Although headache, epistaxis, and tinnitus were once thought to be symptoms of high blood pressure, no relationship has been demonstrated between these symptoms and either systolic or diastolic blood pressure (11). It now appears that worksite screening programs produce minimal psychosocial consequences (12). Increased absenteeism following a diagnosis of hypertension is associated with higher baseline anxiety levels, and reassurance may be beneficial for these patients (12).

The initial evaluation of patients with possible hypertension is an important process with several objectives (13):

1. *Establishing a Diagnosis of Hypertension* (1). The average of two or more measurements of blood pressure with the subject seated and the diastolic pressure reported as the disappearance of sound (Phase V) on two subsequent visits after an elevated blood pressure at screening confirms the diagnosis of hypertension. JNC V classifications are shown in Table 37.1.

   Correct measurement techniques are crucial in determining whether a casual screening or office blood pressure reflects a true increase in blood pressure. Accurate measurement of blood pressure requires correct cuff width (two-thirds of the length between the shoulder and elbow), correct arm position, a bared arm, and the lightest possible pressure on the stethoscope head. Patients should be comfortably seated and relaxed with the arm held passively at the level of the heart. They should not have smoked or ingested caffeine within the prior 30 min. Ideally, both phase 4 (muffling) and phase 5 (disappearance) Korotkoff's sounds should be recorded. Twenty-one percent of patients with untreated borderline hypertension were shown to have "white coat hypertension" based on ambulatory monitoring of blood pressure (14). This exaggerated pressor response is more pronounced when blood pressure is measured by a physician than by a technician and may be specific to the physician's office. White coat or office hypertension occurs more often in females, younger patients, and patients who were recently diagnosed as hypertensive (14).

Ambulatory blood pressure monitoring (ABPM) for 24 hr or longer is possible by using portable monitoring devices (1, 15). ABPM is not cost-effective for all patients but may be useful in evaluating patients with high normal blood pressure who have target organ damage, drug-resistant hypertension, episodic hypertension, transient hypotension, office hyperten-

Table 37.2.
Evaluation of Hypertensive Patients

A. Medical History
1. Family history of hypertension and hypertensive complications
2. History of cardiovascular, cerebrovascular or renal disease or diabetes mellitus
3. Duration and level of elevated blood pressure
4. Effectiveness and side effects of previous drug treatment
5. Medication history for drugs that elevate blood pressure
6. Lifestyle and health habits:
   a. Smoking
   b. Ethanol excess
   c. Sodium intake
   d. Caffeine
   e. Exercise
   f. Emotional stress
B. Physical examination
1. Two or more blood pressure measurements with patient supine or seated and standing
2. Verification of blood pressure in the contralateral arm
3. Height and weight
4. Fundoscopic examination for arteriolar narrowing, arteriovenous compression, hemorrhages, exudates, and papilledema
5. Neck examination for carotid bruits, distended veins, and enlarged thyroid
6. Cardiac examination for increased rate, size, precordial heave, murmurs, arrhythmias and S3, S4 heart sounds
7. Abdominal examination for bruits, enlarged kidneys, and aortic dilation
8. Extremity examination for edema and decreased or absent pulses
9. Neurologic assessment
C. Laboratory tests
1. Hemoglobin and hematocrit
2. Urinalysis
3. Serum potassium
4. Serum creatinine
5. Fasting plasma glucose
6. Total and HDL cholesterol
7. Serum uric acid

Source: From (1).

Table 37.3.
Clinical Findings Suggestive of Secondary Hypertension

Finding	Secondary Cause
Abdominal bruit	Renovascular disease
Abdominal or flank mass	Polycystic kidney disease
Hypokalemia	Hyperaldosteronism
Headache, palpitations, sweating, "spells"	Pheochromocytoma
Delayed or absent femoral pulse	Aortic coarctation
Truncal obesity	Cushing's syndrome

sion, or syncope. Damage to target organs appears to correlate best with data from ABPM.

2. *Avoiding Early Dropout.* The problem of early dropout from hypertension treatment programs is well documented. The rate of dropout from care during the first year of treatment frequently approaches 50% (16). The most important part of the initial visit is to ensure that the patient will return for further follow-up.

3. *Evaluation for the Presence of Cardiovascular Risk Factors and Quantitation of Hypertensive Vascular Disease.* The medical history, physical examination, and laboratory testing are directed toward identifying risk factors, the extent of any existing vascular damage, and the presence of concurrent diseases. The Joint National Committee has provided guidelines for evaluating patients (Table 37.2) (1).

4. *Screening for Secondary Causes of Hypertension.* Most patients with elevated blood pressure have essential hypertension. Any patient whose medical history or physical examination suggests a possible cause of secondary hypertension warrants additional diagnostic evaluation (Table 37.3) (1).

5. *Explanation of Findings.* To avoid early dropout and to work toward long-term control of hypertension, patients need to become active participants in their own care. To do so requires that patients understand:

   a. the potential benefits and risks of therapy,
   b. that their blood pressure exceeds normal limits,
   c. the possible consequences of uncontrolled hypertension,
   d. that hypertension is usually asymptomatic and symptoms do not reliably indicate the level of blood pressure,
   e. that prolonged follow-up and therapy are needed,
   f. that treatment will control but not cure high blood pressure,
   g. their target goal blood pressure,
   h. the presence of any other cardiovascular risk factors and how these indicate their own probability of developing cardiovascular disease.

The initial evaluation documents the presence of hypertension, begins to establish long-term compliance, and establishes the extent of target organ damage and the existence of other risk factors (15, 16). This allows a rational basis for planning treatment.

COMPLICATIONS

Target organ disease (TOD) from arterial hypertension can be cardiac, cerebrovascular, peripheral vascular, renal, and ocular. The risk of complications and premature death is related to the degree of elevation of blood pressure. Hypertension is additive with other risk factors in the development of coronary heart disease (CHD) and stroke. Data from the MRFIT study describe the combined effects of cardiovascular risk factors (17). In men less than 46 years of age a DBP greater than 90 mm Hg increased deaths to a rate 1.6 times the rate for men without risks; having two risk factors increased the rate 3 to 4 times, and having all three major risk factors increased the death rate sixfold (Table 37.4). The major correctable and noncorrectable risk factors are shown in Table 37.5.

Left ventricular hypertrophy (LVH) and left vzezntricular dysfunction are important complications related to hypertension (18). Echocardiography demonstrates that left ventricular muscle mass is increased in 15 to 20% of patients with hypertension. Cardiovascular events occur more than twice as frequently in hypertensive patients with LVH (26%) than in patients without LVH (12%). Patients with LVH have a 5 to 6 times higher risk of sudden death or other cardiovascular mortality than do those without LVH.

The major complications associated with hypertension are stroke and coronary heart disease. A metaanalysis of nine prospective observational studies of 420,000 patients with a mean 10-year follow-up provided an assessment of these risks (19). The combined data demonstrated a positive, continuous increase in risk within the range of

DBP 70 to 110 mm Hg. There was no evidence of a threshold DBP, and lower blood pressures were always associated with less risk. Higher blood pressures even within the range that is considered to be normotensive are associated with increasing cardiovascular risks. A prolonged difference in DBP of 10 mm Hg was associated with 56% less stroke and 37% less coronary heart disease (19).

TREATMENT

Information from observational studies has clearly demonstrated that a lower DBP is associated with a lower risk of stroke and CHD. However, the effects of differences in blood pressure may develop over decades. Whether maintaining blood pressure reductions over a few years will decrease these cardiovascular risks is a question that randomized trials have attempted to answer. A detailed epidemiologic analysis has recently summarized the findings from 14 unconfounded randomized trials of antihypertensive drugs that were reported between 1965 and 1986 (20). There were a total of 37,000 patients, 30,000 of whom were treated for mild hypertension (20). Most trials used a "stepped-care" approach starting with a diuretic. Two trials started with a β-blocker. The usual goal of treatment was to reduce DPB to 90 mm Hg or less, and the mean time of follow-up was 5 years. The average difference in blood pressure between the treatment and control groups was 6 mm Hg. This reduction in blood pressure produced a highly significant reduction in stroke, a decrease of 42%. This benefit of stroke reduction appears soon after the lowering of blood pressure. The effect of blood pressure reduction on CHD was much smaller (14%), and the reduction in fatal CHD (11%) was not significant. The reduction in the odds of stroke was 33 to 50% in the clinical trials, which corresponds to the 35 to 40% predicted from observational studies. The reduction in the odds of CHD was 4 to 22% in the clinical trials, which was less than the 20 to 25% predicted from observational studies. The shortfall in CHD reduction could be due to chance, the influence of chronic atherosclerotic processes that were not reversed by BP reduction, or cardiotoxic adverse effects of the treatments that limited CHD reduction. An analysis that included the SHEP, STOP-Hypertension, and MRC trials found that the benefit of drug therapy on CHD rises to 16% and stroke reduction was similar (45%) (21).

In summary, a 5 to 6 mm Hg reduction of DBP with diuretic-based regimens produced risk reductions of 45% for stroke and 16% for CHD. Improved compliance with antihypertensive therapy and an 8 to 10 mm Hg reduction in DBP should reduce stroke by 50% and CHD by 20%. Because CHD occurs more frequently, the absolute benefit of a 20% decrease in CHD could exceed the benefit of a 50% decrease in stroke. But other therapies for CHD (smoking cessation, cholesterol reduction, as-

Table 37.4.
Effect of Combined Risk Factors in Total Deaths/1000 in MRFIT

Risk factor	Men Age 35–45 Years		Men Age 46–57 Years	
	Deaths/1000	Increase°	Deaths/1000	Increase°
None	5.4		19.3	
DBP > 90	8.4	1.6	25.8	1.3
Cholesterol > 250 mg/dL	10.0	1.9	25.4	1.3
Smoker	12.8	2.4	38.8	2.0
DBP + cholesterol	15.8	2.9	37.9	2.0
DBP + smoker	23.2	4.3	56.4	2.9
DBP/cholesterol/ smoker	33.2	6.1	70.7	3.7

°Increased risk = deaths for men with risk factor/deaths for men with no risks.

Table 37.5.
Risk Factors for Cardiovascular Disease

Correctable	Noncorrectable
• Hypertension	• Family history of heart disease or stroke
• Cigarette smoking	• Older age
• Elevated cholesterol	• Male
• Reduced HDL cholesterol	• Target organ damage
• Diabetes mellitus	
• Obesity	

pirin, and β-blockers) show stronger evidence of cardiac benefit and should be emphasized for high-risk patients. A high risk of stroke is a clearer indication for antihypertensive therapy than is an increased risk of CHD. Elderly patients have a 2% annual incidence of stroke, and patients with a prior transient ischemic attack have a 5% incidence.

Antihypertensive Therapy Trials

VETERANS ADMINISTRATION COOPERATIVE STUDY

The Veterans Administration Cooperative Study clearly demonstrated that reducing blood pressure to normal or near-normal levels decreases the occurrence of complications and provided the early evidence of the benefits of drug treatment (22–24). Complications developed three times as frequently in untreated patients. The treatment of moderate hypertension (DBP > 104 mm Hg) abolished hypertensive complications (congestive heart failure, accelerated hypertension, renal failure) and reduced cerebrovascular accidents by 75%. However, treatment did not decrease the incidence of myocardial infarction. Finally, the VA study has shown that even partial reduction of blood pressure (DBP 90 to 104 mm Hg) decreases cardiovascular complications (25).

HYPERTENSION DETECTION AND FOLLOW-UP PROGRAM COOPERATIVE STUDY

The Hypertension Detection and Follow-up Program (HDFP) randomized almost 11,000 patients to referred-care (RC) or stepped-care (SC) groups (26–28). Seventy percent of the patients had "mild hypertension" (DBP 90 to 104 mm Hg). The treatment goal for HDFP patients was the lesser of a 10 mm Hg decrease from entry blood pressure or a DBP < 90 mm Hg. The 5-year DBP averaged 84 mm Hg for the SC group and 89 mm Hg for the RC group, a difference of only 5 mm Hg. Strokes were reduced by 45%, and death from myocardial infarction was decreased 26%. The 5-year mortality was 16.9% lower for the SC group than for the RC group. Mortality was 20.3% lower for the SC subgroup with entry DBP of 90 to 104 mm Hg (5.9 versus 7.4 per 100). The subgroup with DBP 90 to 140 mm Hg and no evidence of end organ damage at entry had 28.6% fewer deaths at 5 years. The HDFP did not demonstrate a significant reduction in mortality for white women or for patients who were less than 50 years of age, as the death rate was low in both groups. A posttrial surveillance study followed HDFP participants for an additional 2 years, providing 6.7-year mortality data. Mortality differences increased further to 95.1 per 1000 SC patients compared to 116.3 per 1000 RC patients (29).

MULTIPLE RISK FACTOR INTERVENTION TRIAL (MRFIT)

The MRFIT trial followed 12,800 men over 7 years (25). A special intervention group (SI), which received stepped-

care treatment for hypertension, counseling for cigarette smoking, and dietary advice to lower cholesterol, was compared to a usual-care (UC) group. Risk factors in the SI group decreased in comparison to the UC group. However, the SI group showed only a nonsignificant 7% lower rate of CHD mortality. The possibility that antihypertensive drug therapy had an adverse effect on some patients has been raised as a potential explanation for the similar mortality despite the reduction of risk factors. Follow-up analysis has described a 3.34 increased risk of CHD death in men with baseline electrocardiogram (ECG) abnormalities who were given diuretic drugs compared to men who were not treated with diuretics (30). Men without ECG changes had a risk of 0.95. However, no relationship was demonstrated between CHD mortality and hypokalemia or diuretic dose.

EUROPEAN WORKING PARTY ON HIGH BLOOD PRESSURE IN THE ELDERLY TRIAL (EWPHE)

The EWPHE trial assessed the effects of antihypertensive drug therapy on patients over 60 years of age (31). In this trial, 840 patients were randomized as to treatment or placebo with entry DBP of 90 to 119 mm Hg and followed over 12 years. Treatment reduced total mortality (9%) and cardiovascular mortality (27%). Therapy with combined hydrochlorothiazide/triamterene adversely affected glucose tolerance, serum uric acid, and creatinine. Subanalysis shows little or no benefit from the treatment of patients over 80 years of age, most of whom were women (32).

SYSTOLIC HYPERTENSION IN THE ELDERLY PROGRAM (SHEP)

The SHEP trial assessed the effects of antihypertensive drug therapy on the risk of nonfatal and fatal stroke in patients over 60 years of age with isolated systolic hypertension (33). In this trial, 4736 patients were randomized to treatment with chlorthalidone or placebo with entry SBP of 160 to 219 mm Hg and DBP < 90 mm Hg over an average 4.5-year follow-up. The 5-year incidence of total stroke was 5.2 per 100 treated patients and 8.2 per 100 placebo patients. Treatment of isolated systolic hypertension reduced stroke by 37% and reduced all cardiovascular events by 32%.

SWEDISH TRIAL IN OLD PATIENTS WITH HYPERTENSION (STOP-HYPERTENSION)

The STOP-Hypertension trial assessed the effects of antihypertensive drug therapy on the risk of nonfatal and fatal stroke, myocardial infarction, and other cardiovascular complications in patients over 70 years of age with diastolic hypertension (34). In this trial, 1627 patients were randomized as to treatment with β-blockers, a diuretic, or placebo with entry SBP of 180 to 230 mm Hg and DBP > 90 mm Hg over an average 2-year follow-up. Treatment reduced primary endpoints (94 versus 58 events) and total stroke (53 versus 29 events), and benefits were discernible up to age 84. There was a significant reduction in total mortality of 43%.

MEDICAL RESEARCH COUNCIL (MRC) TRIAL IN OLDER ADULTS

The MRC trial assessed the effects of diuretics or a β-blocker on the risk of stroke, CHD, and death in 4396 adults ages 65 to 74 years over a mean 5.8-year period (35). Treated patients had a 25% reduction in stroke and a 19% reduction in coronary events compared to patients given a placebo. The β-blocker group showed no significant reduction in endpoints. The reduction in stroke was greatest in nonsmokers taking diuretics.

TREATMENT OF MILD HYPERTENSION STUDY (TOMHS)

The TOMHS trial assessed the effects of five antihypertensive drug therapies and a sustained lifestyle modification program on the risk of developing LVH, the effect on quality of life, and the risk of clinical cardiovascular events over a 4-year period (36). In this trial, 902 patients with an entry DBP of 90 to 99 mm Hg were randomized as to placebo or one of five antihypertensive agents in addition to nutritional and hygienic intervention. Greater reduction in blood pressure was achieved with drug treatment (−15.9/−9.1 mm Hg) than with nutritional invention plus placebo (−12.2/−8.6 mm Hg). Drug treatment reduced nonfatal cardiovascular events and reduced progression to LVH by ECG compared to nutritional intervention. Drug treatment also improved quality of life, though differences between the treatment groups were modest and inconsistent. In these mild hypertensive patients without a history of cardiovascular disease, no evidence of a J-shaped curve relationship was found. Nutritional intervention resulted in substantial reductions in blood pressure. However, if a target blood pressure of <140/90 mm Hg is not reached after 3 to 6 months, an antihypertensive drug should be added.

SUMMARY OF TREATMENT STUDIES

Early studies clearly demonstrated the benefit of treating moderate and severe hypertension. The JNC recommends that patients with DBP of 90 to 94 mm Hg first attempt to lower blood pressure by nonpharmacologic methods for 3 to 6 months (1). If this fails to lower blood pressure, then drug treatment should be started in all patients with TOD or other cardiovascular risk factors. Trials of antihypertensive drugs in mild hypertension have shown a reduction in stroke, LVH, CHF, and accelerated hypertension. Drug treatment for DBP ≥ 95 mm Hg is recommended if nondrug methods fail. The goal of therapy is a SBP < 140 mm Hg and a DBP < 90 mm Hg.

Lifestyle Modification

Lifestyle modification to reduce blood pressure should be the initial approach for young patients with mild hypertension and no other cardiovascular risk factors. Lifestyle modification is also continued to augment drug therapy.

SODIUM RESTRICTION

Restriction of sodium chloride to less than 6 g (2.3 g sodium) daily is achievable and may control hypertension in some patients with Stage 1 hypertension (1). The TOHP-I study demonstrated only a modest (−1.7/−0.9 mm Hg) reduction in blood pressure with sodium reduction (37). Modest dietary sodium restriction has also been shown to have adjunctive benefit with most antihypertensive drug therapy (38). This degree of sodium restriction can be achieved by refraining from adding salt at the table and avoiding highly salted processed foods.

WEIGHT REDUCTION

The prevalence of hypertension is 50% greater in overweight adults than in normal-weight adults (39). The TOHP-I study also found that a weight loss of 3.9 kg led to a reduction in blood pressure of −2.9/−2.3 mm Hg (37). Weight reduction is the most effective nonpharmacologic intervention to lower blood pressure. The JNC recommends that all hypertensive patients who are above their ideal weight should attempt to control blood pressure with weight loss. Reductions in blood pressure can occur with a weight loss as small as 10 pounds. A goal body weight of within 10% of desirable weight will minimize weight effects of blood pressure. It is well-recognized that weight reduction is difficult to achieve and sustain.

EXERCISE

Exercise training decreases blood pressure in hypertensive patients an average of 11/8 mm Hg (40). Exercise training is also beneficial in weight reduction, lowers plasma triglycerides, and improves insulin sensitivity (40). The addition of either diltiazem or propranolol did not produce additive benefit to exercise training (41). Exercise training lowered blood pressure and total and LDL cholesterol while increasing HDL cholesterol. Propranolol limited the exercise increase in HDL cholesterol. (41). A regular physical activity program should be started gradually and may control blood pressure without drug therapy in patients with mild hypertension.

Dynamic endurance exercises (walking, running, cycling, and swimming) are recommended; isometric exercises (rowing and competitive sports) are not suitable (42). Because hypertensive patients may show exaggerated blood pressures during exercise, intensive training should not be started until diastolic blood pressures are below 105 mm Hg (42). Drugs that are effective in treating superelevated blood pressures (SBP > 200 mm Hg) during exercise include cardioselective β_1-blockers, verapamil, clonidine, and converting-enzyme inhibitors (42).

TOBACCO AVOIDANCE

Smoking increases the risks of cancer and pulmonary disease and more than doubles the risk of cardiovascular disease (1). Cigarette smoking acutely raises blood pressure from 3/5 to 12/10 mm Hg (43). While office blood pressures do not differ for smokers, 24-hour ambulatory blood pressure monitoring has shown higher daytime blood pressures in smokers, particularly in Caucasians above the age of 50 (43). Also, smoking was shown to interfere with the reduction of blood pressure by propranolol in black patients (44). Finally, the reduction of cardiovascular risk by antihypertensive treatment is not as great in smokers as in nonsmokers (1). The JNC recommends that a smoking cessation program is a key component of the treatment of hypertension.

ALCOHOL

Moderate to heavy alcohol intake increases the incidence of hypertension (1, 45). The JNC recommendations are to limit alcohol consumption to 30 mL of ethanol daily (2 oz whiskey, 8 oz wine, or 24 oz beer) (1). Alcohol also interferes with antihypertensive drug treatment independently of noncompliance (46). Alcohol use should be evaluated in patients with resistant hypertension.

CAFFEINE

Caffeine increases blood pressure in people who do not regularly consume methylxanthines, while habitual consumption of caffeine is believed to be associated with the development of complete tolerance to its pressor effect (47). However, ambulatory blood pressure monitoring of habitual coffee drinkers demonstrated a consistent 4/4 mm Hg worksite increase in blood pressure and a 12/9 mm Hg increase during formal stress testing (48). Because of the potential to increase blood pressure, hypertensive patients should be advised to limit coffee to two cups daily and to avoid coffee consumption before blood pressure measurement. JNC V places no limitations on consumption of caffeine-containing beverages.

CATION SUPPLEMENTATION AND STRESS REDUCTION

Both calcium and potassium supplementation have been used for possible modest blood pressure lowering effects (1). The role of these cations in treating hypertension is still under investigation. The use of relaxation and biofeedback therapy to reduce behavioral stress and lower reduce blood pressure was ineffective in the TOHP-I study (37).

SUMMARY OF LIFESTYLE MODIFICATIONS

The JNC has concluded that weight control and sodium restriction have been shown to independently reduce blood pressure and are additive with pharmacologic agents (1). Alcohol restriction is also recommended. A nutritional program to lose weight and restrict sodium and alcohol achieved a 39% success in normalizing blood pressure without drug therapy (49). Smoking cessation and exercise programs are recommended for all hypertensive patients. Lifestyle modification alone should be tried for all patients with DBPs between 90 and 94 mm Hg if they are without target organ damage or other cardiovascular risk factors. Patients who do not normalize blood pressure after 3 to 6 months of lifestyle modification should start drug treatment.

DRUG THERAPY

Drug therapy should be initiated if blood pressure remains at or above 140/90 mm Hg during 3 to 6 months of lifestyle modification. Antihypertensive drug therapy may be started sooner in patients with TOD or other known cardiovascular risk factors of smoking, diabetes, or hypercholesterolemia (1). In initiating drug therapy it is important to remember that hypertension is a disease of decades. Unless hypertension is severe, it is important to start a simple drug regimen that minimizes side effects and encourages long-term compliance.

Understanding the site and mechanism of action of the various antihypertensive drugs is important in planning therapy. All current drugs impair normal homeostatic mechanisms, and most reduce peripheral vascular resistance. Pharmacologic classification and dosage information are presented in Table 37.6. Common adverse effects and special precautions for antihypertensive drugs are given in Table 37.7. The hemodynamic and hormonal effects are shown in Table 37.8. Drug interactions are listed in Table 37.9.

Diuretics

Thiazide and related diuretics were the mainstay of therapy in most antihypertensive drug trials. Thiazide-type diuretics are effective in small doses, equivalent to 12.5 to 25 mg of hydrochlorothiazide. Using these lower doses may reduce the incidence and severity of the metabolic abnormalities of hypokalemia, hyperglycemia, and hyperuricemia. Reducing hydrochlorothiazide from 50 mg/day to 25 mg/day resulted in a 5 mm Hg increase in SBP with no change in DBP (50). This dose reduction led to a decrease in uric acid and an increase in serum potassium, but fasting and postprandial glucose, hemoglobin A_1C, and serum lipids were unchanged (50). Serum lipids and hemoglobin A_1C decreased significantly after discontinuation of diuretics. Diuretics add to the effectiveness of most other

Table 37.6.
Antihypertensive Drugs

Drug	Class	Dosage Size (mg)	Dose Range (mg)
Diuretics			
Chlorothiazide	Diuretic	250/500	500–2000
Hydrochlorothiazide	Diuretic	25/50/100	12.5–50
Chlorthalidone	Diuretic	25/50/100	12.5–50
Indapamide	Diuretic	2.5	2.5–5.0
Metolazone	Diuretic	2.5/5/10	2.5–5.0
Bumetanide	Loop diuretic	0.5/1.0/2.0	0.5–10.0
Ethacrynic acid	Loop diuretic	25/50	25–400
Furosemide	Loop diuretic	20/40/80	20–600
Torsemide	Loop diuretic		
Potassium-sparing diuretics			
Amiloride	Potassium-sparing diuretic	5	5–20
Spironolactone	Potassium-sparing diuretic	25/50/100	25–100
Triamterene	Potassium-sparing diuretic	50/100	50–300
Beta-blockers			
Acebutolol	Beta-blocker	200/400	200–1200
Atenolol	Beta-blocker	25/50/100	50–100
Betaxolol	Beta-blocker	10/20	10–40
Bisoprolol	Beta-blocker	5/10	2.5–20
Carteolol	Beta-blocker	2.5/5	2.5–10
Metoprolol	Beta-blocker	50/100	100–450
Nadolol	Beta-blocker	20/40/80/120/160	40–320
Penbutolol	Beta-blocker	20	20–80
Pindolol	Beta-blocker	5/10	10–60
Propranolol	Beta-blocker	10/20/40/60/80/90 SR: 80/120/160	40–320
Timolol	Beta-blocker	5/10/20	10–40
Alpha-beta-blocker			
Labetalol	Alpha-beta blocker	100/200/300	200–2400
Central adrenergic agonists			
Clonidine	Central antiadrenergic	0.1/0.2/0.3	0.1–0.6
Clonidine TTS	Central antiadrenergic	TTS 1/2/3	0.1–0.3
Guanabenz	Central antiadrenergic	4/8	8–32
Guanfacine	Central antiadrenergic	1	1–3
Methyldopa	Central antiadrenergic	125/250/500	500–2000
Peripheral adrenergic blockers			
Guanadrel	Peripheral antiadrenergic	10/25	10–75
Guanethidine	Peripheral antiadrenergic	10/25	10–50
Reserpine	Peripheral antiadrenergic	0.1/0.25/0.5/1.0	0.1–0.25
Alpha$_1$-adrenergic blockers			
Prazosin	Alpha$_1$-blocker	1/2/5	1–20
Terazosin	Alpha$_1$-blocker	1/2/5/10	1–20
Doxazosin	Alpha$_1$-blocker	1/2/4/8	1–16
Vasodilators			
Hydralazine	Vasodilator	10/25/50/100	40–200
Minoxidil	Vasodilator	2.5/10	10–40
Angiotensin-converting-enzyme inhibitors			
Benazepril HCl	CEI	5/10/20/40	20–80
Captopril	CEI	12.5/25/50/100	50–450
Enalapril maleate	CEI	2.5/5/10/20	2.5–40
Fosinopril sodium	CEI	10/20	10–80
Lisinopril	CEI	5/10/20	5–40
Quinapril HCl	CEI	5/10/20/40	10–80
Ramipril	CEI	1.25/2.5/5/10	2.5–20

(continued)

Table 37.6. *(Continued)*

Drug	Class	Dosage Size (mg)	Dose Range (mg)
Calcium channel blockers			
Amlodipine	Calcium entry blocker	2.5/5/10	5–10
Diltiazem	Calcium entry blocker	30/60/90/120 SR: 90/120	120–240
Felodipine	Calcium entry blocker	2.5/5/10	5–10
Nifedipine	Calcium entry blocker	10/20 SR: 20/60/90	10–120
Nicardipine	Calcium entry blocker	20/30	20–40
Isradipine	Calcium entry blocker	2.5/5	5–20
Verapamil	Calcium entry blocker	80/120/240 SR: 120/180/240	240–480

Table 37.7.
Adverse Antihypertensive Drug Effects

Drug	Adverse Effects	Special Precautions
Thiazide diuretics	Hypokalemia, hyperuricemia, glucose intolerance, increased serum cholesterol, triglycerides, sexual dysfunction, dehydration, hyponatremia, hypomagnesemia	LVH, CHD, diabetes mellitus/gout Renal failure Digitalis
Loop diuretics	Same as thiazide diuretics	Effective in renal failure
Beta-blockers	Fatigue, insomnia, nightmares, depression, sexual dysfunction, bronchospasm, bradycardia, increased triglycerides, decreased HDL cholesterol, dermatitis, GI upset, withdrawal rebound, psoriasis	Asthma, COPD CHF, heart block Diabetes mellitus, hyperlipidemia Peripheral vascular disease
Alpha-beta blocker	Asthma, nausea, fatigue, dizziness, headache, orthostatic hypotension, fever, hepatotoxicity	Asthma, COPD CHF, heart block Diabetes mellitus
Angiotensin-converting enzyme inhibitors	Hyperkalemia, cough, hypotension, angioedema, rash, loss of taste, proteinuria, renal failure, neutropenia, cholestasis	Renal failure Pregnancy
Calcium entry blockers	Headache, flushing, hypotension, dizziness, palpitations, nausea	Caution in CHF/heart block
Dihydropyridine CEB	Edema, tachycardia	
Verapamil	Constipation, conduction defects, CHF bradycardia	Caution with digitalis
Central antiadrenergics	Sedation, dry mouth, fatigue, sexual dysfunction, postural hypotension, impaired concentration, withdrawal rebound hypertension, contact dermatitis from patch	Depression Caution when discontinue to avoid rebound
Methyldopa	Hepatitis, Coombs' positive hemolytic anemia, colitis, lupuslike syndrome	Caution in elderly
Peripheral antiadrenergics	Sexual dysfunction, nasal congestion, orthostatic hypotension, diarrhea, sodium/fluid retention	Asthma, CHF Caution in elderly
Alpha$_1$-blockers	First-dose syncope, orthostatic hypotension headache, dizziness, drowsiness, tachycardia, sodium/fluid retention, priapism	Caution with first dose
Vasodilators	Headache, tachycardia, dizziness, sodium/fluid retention	Angina pectoris, CHF
Hydralazine	Positive ANA, lupuslike syndrome, hepatitis, nasal congestion, GI disturbances	
Minoxidil	Hypertrichosis, facial coarsening, pleural/pericardial effusion	

antihypertensive drugs and can reverse the fluid retention that is associated with some antihypertensive drugs. Hydrochlorothiazide has proven efficacy, can be administered once daily, and is inexpensive.

Hypokalemia is dose related, and moderate hypokalemia (between 3.0 and 3.5 mEq/L) occurs in 2% of patients who are treated with HCTZ 25 mg/day compared to 11% of patients treated with HCTZ 50 mg/day (51). Hypokalemia is worsened by high-sodium diets and can be minimized by sodium restriction. The risk of ventricular arrhythmias and sudden death may be increased by hypokalemia in patients with baseline ECG abnormalities (30). The risk of primary cardiac arrest is increased by high-dose thiazide diuretic therapy (52). Hypokalemia should be minimized by using low-dose thiazide therapy, restricting sodium intake, using potassium supplements,

Table 37.8.
Hemodynamic and Hormonal Effects of Antihypertensive Agents

Drug	PVR	CO	HR	PRA	GFR
Converting-enzyme inhibitors					
Alpha$_2$-agonists					
Beta-blockers					0/–
Calcium blockers	–	–/0/+			0/+
Labetalol					
Loop diuretics					
Peripheral antiadrenergics				–/0	
Alpha$_1$-blockers		0/+		–/0	
Thiazide diuretics					
Vasodilators					+/0

PVR = peripheral vascular resistance; CO = cardiac output; HR = heart rate; PRA = plasma renin activity; GFR = glomerular filtration rate.
Note: Some effects vary between specific agents within each group.
+ = increase; – = decrease; 0 = no change.

and adding potassium-sparing drugs. In trials using thiazide diuretics alone (MRFIT and the Oslo Study), patients with baseline ECG abnormalities had worse outcomes. In the EWPHE trial, which used a potassium-sparing combination agent, there was a reduction in total cardiac mortality.

Thiazide diuretics may produce other metabolic abnormalities, including an increase in total cholesterol, LDL-cholesterol, and triglycerides. A low-fat diet decreases the thiazide-induced changes. Thiazide-induced glucose intolerance is related to the degree of hypokalemia and is minimized by preventing potassium depletion. In the VA Cooperative studies, an average increase in fasting glucose was 6 mg/dL, and 3% of patients developed a fasting glucose greater than 140 mg/dL. Thiazides increase serum uric acid of approximately 1 mg/dL, which is not associated with adverse effects on renal function and does not require uric acid-lowering drugs unless the patient has symptomatic gout (53).

Diuretics were associated with impotence at a frequency of 19.6 per 1000 patient-years in the MRC trial. Male patients taking thiazide diuretics reported significantly greater sexual dysfunction than did control subjects; diuretic therapy did not adversely affect other aspects of quality of life (54).

Thiazide diuretics are particularly effective for patients with low-renin hypertension, which is often seen in the elderly and blacks (55). Finally, thiazide diuretics may slow the rate of bone loss in the elderly and reduce the incidence of hip fractures (56).

LOOP DIURETICS

Furosemide has a shorter duration of action than do the thiazide diuretics and causes less blood pressure reduction. Newer loop diuretics, torsemide and bumetanide, have longer duration of action. Loop diuretics are often used for patients with fluid retention who are unresponsive to thiazide diuretics or patients with decreased renal function. Thiazide diuretics are ineffective for patients with impaired renal function (creatinine clearance < 50 mL/min). These patients can be treated with the loop diuretics metolazone or indapamide. Furosemide (40 mg/day) has also been shown to produce less hypokalemia than does hydrochlorothiazide (50 mg/day) in hypertensive patients (51).

THIAZIDELIKE DIURETICS

Chlorthalidone is a long-acting diuretic similar to thiazides that produces greater hypokalemia and was the primary therapy in the SHEP trial. Metolazone is a thiazidelike diuretic that is effective for patients with renal impairment and is markedly effective in producing diuresis when combined with furosemide. Indapamide is a sulfonamide diuretic with antihypertensive effects that does not appear to elevate serum lipids.

POTASSIUM-SPARING DIURETICS

The potassium-sparing diuretics amiloride, spironolactone, and triamterene are used mainly to prevent or correct hypokalemia from other diuretics. Neither amiloride or triamterene has a significant antihypertensive effect.

AMILORIDE

Amiloride is a potassium-sparing diuretic that acts in the distal tubule. Amiloride is excreted in the urine as unchanged drug and has natriuretic and antikaliuretic effects for approximately 24 hr. The primary adverse effect is hyperkalemia. The presence of diabetes mellitus, cirrhosis, renal insufficiency, concomitant angiotensin-converting-enzyme inhibitors therapy, or potassium supplements increases the risk of hyperkalemia.

SPIRONOLACTONE

Spironolactone is a competitive aldosterone antagonist that is used in combination with thiazide diuretics to prevent or correct hypokalemia or as an alternative diuretic for patients with gout or diabetes (57). Food enhances the absorption of spironolactone, which is rapidly metabolized to pharmacologically active metabolites, including canrenone. Spironolactone may be superior to potassium supplements in correcting diuretic-induced hypokalemia and also corrects coexisting magnesium deficiency. Hyperkalemia occurs in 3% of spironolactone-treated patients who have normal renal function and are not taking potassium supplements (57). In contrast, 25% of patients with renal insufficiency who are taking potassium supplements can develop hyperkalemia. Gynecomastia is related to dosage and duration of treatment and has occurred in more than 50% of male patients (57). Impotence, hirsutism, menstrual irregularities, and gastrointestinal symptoms are adverse effects that can limit therapy. Limiting spironolactone dosage to ≤100 mg/day appears to reduce the incidence of adverse effects.

TRIAMTERENE

Triamterene is used principally in combination products to reduce the potassium loss with thiazide diuretics. Triamterene-hydrochlorothiazide combinations can produce hypokalemia or hyperkalemia. The risk of hyperkalemia is increased by the presence of other risks including renal impairment, potassium supplementation, converting-enzyme inhibitors, and diabetes mellitus. A triamterene urinary sediment (triamterene crystals) has developed in over 50% of patients. This has caused nephrolithiasis and may be a risk factor for interstitial nephritis (58). Triamterene-hydrochlorothiazide decreases production of renal PGE_2, a renoprotective prostaglandin, while amiloride-hydrochlorothiazide increases renal PGE_2 production (59). Finally, the combination of indomethacin and triamterene may cause reversible acute renal failure (60). In high-risk patients or when hypokalemia develops, potassium-sparing agents are effective in preventing or reversing hypokalemia.

Beta-Blockers

Beta-blockers are effective antihypertensive agents, particularly for young white patients (hyperkinetic circulation), and have additive benefit for patients with coronary artery disease.

PHARMACOLOGY

Beta-blockers competitively inhibit catecholamine neurotransmitters at both cardiac receptors (β_1) and noncardiac receptors (β_2) (61). Cardiac effects include reductions in heart rate, venous return, cardiac output, and cardiac work. In addition, β-blockers reduce plasma renin activity, reduce norepinephrine release, and prevent the pressor response to exercise or stress catecholamine release.

EFFECTIVENESS

In the VA Cooperative Study Group, β-blockers were equivalent to hydrochlorothiazide in white patients, but hydrochlorothiazide was more effective in black and elderly patients (23). Beta-blockers may provide primary protection from CHD, and they reduce the secondary risk following myocardial infarction (61). Beta-blockers are effective in producing LVH regression.

COMPARISON OF β-BLOCKERS

While the available β-blockers are similar in both efficacy and safety, there are two important differences in pharmacology (Table 37.10). Cardioselective (β_1-selective) agents produce fewer negative effects on the heart in patients with congestive heart failure or conduction system disease. Cardioselective β-blockers may be better

tolerated by patients with chronic obstructive pulmonary disease and peripheral vascular disease. Cardioselective (β_1-selective) agents produce less impairment in response to hypoglycemia in diabetic patients. Unfortunately cardioselectivity is reduced or lost at higher doses. Drugs with β-agonist activity or intrinsic sympathomimetic activity (ISA) may avoid the decrease in cardiac output and heart rate. ISA β-blockers are preferred for patients who experience bradycardia with other β-blockers. ISA β-blockers may also produce fewer problems for patients with peripheral vascular disease, lipid disorders, or diabetes mellitus. However, ISA β-blockers are not cardioprotective.

Beta-blockers can also be classified into two groups on the basis of their pharmacokinetic properties. The β-blockers that are eliminated by hepatic metabolism are highly lipophilic, absorbed in the small intestine, undergo extensive "first-pass" metabolism, have variable bioavailability, have relatively short plasma half-lives, and more readily penetrate the blood-brain barrier. Beta-blockers that are eliminated unchanged by the kidney are hydrophilic, are incompletely absorbed throughout the gut, have longer plasma half-lives, and are less able to penetrate the central nervous system. Because the antihypertensive effect of β-blockers appears to outlast the presence of the drug in plasma, all agents can be used on a twice-daily schedule, and the longer-acting drugs can be given once daily. The bioavailability of propranolol and metoprolol is increased approximately 60% when the drugs are taken with food. Propranolol has a wide dose range, and plasma concentrations from a fixed dose may vary 20-fold between patients. The hydrophilic agents (atenolol and nadolol) have relatively flat dose-response curves but will accumulate in renal failure.

Several disease states contraindicate the use of β-blockers or influence the selection of a β-blocker, and the choice of agents should be individualized for patients. Although pregnancy was once considered a contraindication, studies indicate that β-blockers improve fetal outcome when they are used to treat hypertension in pregnancy.

ADVERSE EFFECTS

Many adverse effects are related to β-adrenergic blockade in predisposed patients. Adverse effects from β_1-blockade include bradycardia, conduction abnormalities, and left ventricular failure (61). Adverse effects from β_2-blockade include bronchospasm, cold extremities, and worsening claudication. A metaanalysis concluded that β-blocker therapy did not worsen claudication in patients with mild to moderate peripheral vascular disease (PVD) (62). These adverse effects tend to occur early in therapy even at low doses. Central nervous system (CNS) effects may be most common with propranolol, and frank depression or vivid visual hallucinations can occur. However a large case

Table 37.9.
Anithypertensive Drug Interactions

	Alpha$_1$-Blockers	Alpha$_2$-Agonists	Beta-Blockers	Calcium Entry Blockers	Converting-Enzyme Inhibitors
Antacids			Decreased effect		Decreased effect (captopril)
Antinflammatory drugs	Decreased effect	Decreased effect	Decreased effect		Decreased effect/ nephrotoxicity
Antipsychotics	Postural hypotension	Postural hypotension	Increased effect of both drugs	Postural hypotension	Postural hypotension
Barbiturates		Additive CNS depression, decreased guanfacine	Decreased effect (hepatic β-blockers)	Decreased effect (verapamil)	
Beta-blockers	First-dose syncope	Rebound hypertension/ bradycardia		Additive cardiac depression	
Carbamazepine			Decreased effect (hepatic β-blockers)	Decreased effect (verapamil)	
Calcium blockers	First-dose syncope		Additive cardiac depression		
Cholestyramine/ colestipol					
Cimetidine			Increased effect (hepatic β-blockers)	Increased effect	
CNS depressants		Additive CNS depression			
Corticosteroids					
Cyclosporine				Increased cyclosporine	
Digitalis			Additive cardiac depression	Increased digitalis	
Diuretics	First-dose syncope	Additive effect	Additive effect	Additive effect	Postural hypotension/ additive effect
Epinephrine			Severe increase in blood pressure (nonselective)		
Ergot alkaloids			Vasoconstriction		
Ethanol	Postural hypotension	Postural hypotension	Postural hypotension	Postural hypotension	Postural hypotension
Indomethacin	Decreased effect	Decreased effect	Decreased effect		Decreased effect
Insulin			Hypoglycemia, masked symptoms, hypertension	Decreased insulin (diltiazem)	Possible hypoglycemia
Levodopa		Levodopa toxicity			
Lidocaine			Increased lidocaine		
Lithium		Lithium toxicity with methyldopa			Lithium toxicity
Monoamine oxidase inhibitors		Markedly increased BP/CNS toxicity			
Phenothiazines		Increased BP with methyldopa			
Phenytoin				Decreased effect	
Potassium/potassium- retaining drugs					Hyperkalemia
Probenecid					
Propafenone			Increased effect (hepatic β-blockers)		
Quinidine			Increased effect (hepatic β-blockers)	Hypotension, bradycardia (verapamil)	
Rifampin			Decreased effect (hepatic β-blockers)	Decreased effect	
Salicylates					Decreased effect

Loop Diuretics	Peripheral Adrenergic Blockers	Reserpine	Thiazide Diuretics	Triamterene	Vasodilators
Decreased effect	Decreased effect	Decreased effect	Decreased effect	Decreased effect	Decreased effect
Postural hypotension	Decreased effect	Decreased effect	Postural hypotension	Postural hypotension	Postural hypotension
Additive effect		Hypotension/ bradycardia	Additive effect		Additive effect
Additive effect			Additive effect		
			Decreased effect		
Potassium loss		Additive CNS depression	Potassium loss		
Digitalis toxicity		Arrhythmias	Digitalis toxicity		
Additive effect	Additive effects	Additive effect		Decreased potassium loss	
Postural hypotension Decreased effect	Postural hypotension	Postural hypotension	Postural hypotension Decreased effect	Postural hypotension Decreased renal function	Postural hypotension
Hyperglycemia			Hyperglycemia		
	Postural hypotension	Decreased levodopa			
Lithium toxicity			Lithium toxicity		
	Decreased effect	CNS excitation			
				Hyperkalemia	
Decreased effect					
Decreased effect			Decreased effect		

(continued)

Table 37.9. *(Continued)*

	Alpha$_1$-Blockers	Alpha$_2$-Agonists	Beta-Blockers	Calcium Entry Blockers	Converting-Enzyme Inhibitors
Sulfonylureas			Hypoglycemia/ hypertension		
Sympathomimetics	Decreased effect	Decreased effect	Decreased effect 1	Decreased effect	
Theophylline			Pharmacologic antagonism/increased theophylline		
Tricyclic antidepressants		Decreased effect	Increased depression		

control analysis did not demonstrate that β-blockers were causally related to depression (63). Some patients have a pressor response to propranolol with worsening hypertension. Dermatologic reactions have included marked exacerbation of psoriasis. The addition of propranolol doubled the hydrochlorothiazide-induced increase in fasting glucose and glycosylated hemoglobin levels (64). Beta-blockers decrease HDL cholesterol, increase triglycerides, and blunt the effectiveness of dietary modification to lower cholesterol. Lipid changes are not associated with ISA β-blockers. Treatment with glucose tolerance factor-chromium reversed the adverse effects of β-blockers on HDL cholesterol (65).

The withdrawal of β-blockers may produce β-adrenergic supersensitivity. Both abrupt cessation and gradual withdrawal over 4 to 8 days have caused overshoot hypertension and cardiovascular complications within 48 to 72 hr after the last β-blocker dose (66). Symptoms of the withdrawal syndrome are nervousness, restlessness, anxiety, malaise, fatigue, headaches, insomnia, vivid dreams, tachycardia, palpitations, tremors, diaphoresis, excessive salivation, abdominal cramps and pain, anorexia, nausea, and vomiting. Cardiovascular morbidity has included encephalopathy, cerebrovascular accidents, unstable angina, myocardial infarction, and sudden death. Beta-blocker withdrawal syndrome can be reversed by readministration of small doses of the β-blocker. To prevent β-adrenergic supersensitivity, the β-blocker dose should be reduced over 7 to 10 days to the equivalent of 30 mg/day of propranolol and then maintained at this low dose for 2 additional weeks. The risk of β-blocker withdrawal is not only for patients with known ischemic heart disease. The withdrawal of β-blockers in patients who are free of coronary heart disease resulted in a fourfold increase in new onset of coronary heart disease (66). ISA β-blockers do not cause a withdrawal syndrome and are not cardioprotective (66).

Alpha-Beta-Blocker

Labetalol is a nonselective β-blocker and an α-blocker that reduces the β$_2$-blockade increase in peripheral vascular resistance (PVR) and sustains blood flow to the extremities and kidney. Labetalol does not reduce HDL cholesterol but may cause orthostatic hypotension and sexual dysfunction. Labetalol may be more effective than other β-blockers for elderly or black patients and has been used by patients with pulmonary disease.

Angiotensin-Converting-Enzyme Inhibitors

Angiotensin-converting-enzyme (ACE) inhibitors block the generation of angiotensin II, which is a potent vasoconstrictor and a stimulator of aldosterone secretion. The antihypertensive efficacy of ACE inhibitors is comparable to that of diuretics and β-blockers as monotherapy for hypertension. ACE inhibitors are more effective in younger and white patients and less effective in black patients unless higher doses are used or they are combined with diuretics (67). The combination of low-dose diuretic therapy and ACE inhibitors may control up to 85% of patients (67). ACE inhibitors are also synergistic with calcium entry blockers and additive with β-blockers. ACE inhibitors prolong the survival of patients with severe congestive heart failure and produce regression of left ventricular hypertrophy. ACE inhibitors also improve insulin sensitivity. They are also used to treat renovascular hypertension. Another unique benefit of ACE inhibitors is the reduction of angiotensin II-mediated intraglomerular capillary pressure. This effect appears to retard the progression of diabetic renal disease, stabilize renal function, and decrease proteinuria (67). ACE inhibitors avoid many of the adverse effects that were common to earlier antihypertensive drugs. They do not alter plasma lipids, glucose, or uric acid, nor do they aggravate bronchospastic or peripheral vascular disease. ACE inhibitors also do not cause CNS depression or sexual dysfunction. They may increase alertness and produce mood elevation, which may have contributed to the positive effect on the quality of life seen with captopril (67).

ACE inhibitor therapy has been suggested as initial antihypertensive therapy because it will control about 50% of patients and has few side effects. Initial ACE inhibitor

Loop Diuretics	Peripheral Adrenergic Blockers	Reserpine	Thiazide Diuretics	Triamterene	Vasodilators
Hyperglycemia			Hyperglycemia		
Decreased effect	Decreased effect/ increased effect of direct SANS	Decreased effect/ increased effect of direct SANS			
	Decreased effect	CNS excitation			

therapy is also an indirect means of classification of renin status. Patients with a poor decrease in blood pressure from ACE inhibitors are likely to have low-renin hypertension. For patients who do not respond to initial ACE inhibitor therapy, addition of low doses of a thiazide diuretic controls blood pressure in up to 85% of patients by working synergistically with ACE inhibitor treatment.

COMPARISON OF ACE INHIBITORS

The available ACE inhibitors differ in pharmacokinetics. Captopril binds to angiotensin-converting enzyme by a sulfhydryl, and the other ACE inhibitors do not (67). Benazepril, enalapril, fosinopril, perindopril, quinapril, and ramipril are administered as pro-drugs; this delays their onset of action and prolongs the effect. Captopril should be taken without food and requires twice daily dosing. Some clinicians use captopril three times a day, but twice a day is preferable for most patients. All the other agents are given once daily. The primary route of elimination is the kidney, and doses should be reduced in renal insufficiency. Benazepril and fosinopril are eliminated by both renal excretion and hepatic metabolism, and dose reductions are not needed for patients with renal dysfunction.

ADVERSE EFFECTS

Adverse effects that are common to all ACE inhibitors are hypotension, hyperkalemia, cough, angioedema, and renal insufficiency (67). Hypotension occurs when patients are sodium depleted or have high renin and is more common with captopril because of its rapid onset of action. To reduce this risk, diuretics should be discontinued for 3 days before the initial ACE inhibitor dose. The risk of hyperkalemia is greater for patients with diabetes or renal insufficiency; if sodium intake is restricted; and if potassium-sparing diuretics, potassium supplements, or NSAIDs are given. Intractable, dry cough, requiring discontinuation of ACE inhibitor therapy, may develop in more than 20% of patients. Inhaled sodium cromoglycate may be effective in treating ACE inhibitor-induced cough

(68). Cough develops more frequently with enalapril than with captopril and is believed to be due to an effect of ACE inhibitor on vagal C fibers (67). Adverse effects of captopril have also included neutropenia, skin rash, proteinuria, and taste disturbances (67). Using lower doses of captopril has dramatically reduced the incidence of these complications. ACE inhibitors may also increase the risk of hypoglycemia (69).

A new pharmacologic class of drugs is the angiotensin II (AII) type 1 receptor antagonists, which displace AII from the type 1 receptor subtype, antagonizing smooth muscle contraction, sympathetic pressor response, and aldosterone release (70). These agents will likely be as effective as ACE inhibitors in treating hypertension and do not produce the cough that is associated with ACE inhibitors. The first of the AT_1 receptor antagonists is losartan.

Calcium Entry Blockers

Calcium entry blockers (CEBs) are a fourth class of drugs that are considered to be effective monotherapy for the initial treatment of hypertension. CEBs impair the transport of calcium through the voltage-sensitive calcium channels in vascular smooth muscle cells; this decreases contractile force, vascular smooth muscle tone, and peripheral resistance. The CEBs are particularly effective for patients with low-renin hypertension (i.e., elderly and black hypertensives) and have greater antihypertensive efficacy with higher pretreatment blood pressures. Verapamil is equally effective for black or white hypertensive patients (71). CEBs are also used to treat angina, variant angina, certain arrhythmias, and migraine headaches; this makes them attractive antihypertensive agents for patients with those conditions. CEBs also do not adversely affect asthma, gout, peripheral vascular disease, lipids, and diabetes mellitus. However, recent controversy has arisen regarding the possible increased risk of myocardial infarction associated with calcium channel blockers (72).

COMPARISON OF CALCIUM ENTRY BLOCKERS

The calcium entry blockers have three chemical classes. Verapamil is a phenylalkylamine; diltiazem is a benzothi-

Table 37.10.
Pharmacologic Properties of β-Blockers

Property	Acebutolol	Atenolol	Labetalol	Metoprolol	Nadolol
β_1-Selectivity	+	+	−	+	−
Intrinsic sympathomimetic activity	+	−	−	−	−
Lipid solubility	Low	Low-moderate	Moderate	Low	
Metabolism/excretion	Hepatic/renal	Renal hepatic/renal	Hepatic/renal	Renal	

azepine; and amlodipine, felodipine, isradipine, nicarda-pine, and nifedipine are dihydropyridines. All CEBs that are used for hypertension have comparable efficacy but differ in their adverse effect profiles. The CEBs have limited oral bioavailability because of first-pass hepatic metabolism. Only diltiazem (35%) has significant renal elimination. Because of short plasma half-lives, extended-release products are available for verapamil, diltiazem, and nifedipine, allowing once or twice daily administration. Extended-release products may also decrease dose-related adverse effects. However, postinfarction trials of CEBs have not demonstrated cardioprotection. Addition of a diuretic to a CEB usually has only minimal additive effect; this may be due in part to the natriuretic effect of the CEBs.

ADVERSE EFFECTS

The adverse effects of the calcium entry blockers are primarily extensions of their pharmacologic actions and can be categorized as vasodilation, negative inotropic effects, conduction disturbances, gastrointestinal effects, and metabolic effects. Vasodilatory side effects include head-aches, flushing, palpitations, hypotension, and peripheral edema. Vasodilation is more common with dihydropyridine CEBs. Negative inotropic effects are least with the dihydropyridines and greatest with verapamil. While diltiazem has an intermediate negative inotropic effect, it can produce or worsen congestive heart failure in patients with preexisting left ventricular dysfunction. Conduction disturbances are also greatest with verapamil, intermediate with diltiazem, and infrequent with dihydropyridines. Verapamil often causes constipation, which may be re-lieved with stool softeners. Verapamil decreases digoxin elimination and can increase serum digoxin levels by 50 to 75%. Other calcium entry blockers may also interact with digoxin, but usually to a lesser degree. If a CEB is used in combination with a β-blocker, a dihydropyridine agent is preferred to reduce the additive cardioinhibitory and cardiodepressive effects.

Sympathetic Inhibitors

Many antihypertensive drugs interfere with the sym-pathetic nervous system. These agents may act in the central nervous system, the peripheral nervous system, or both.

ALPHA₁-ADRENERGIC BLOCKING AGENTS

These drugs produce a selective postsynaptic α_1-adreno-ceptor inhibition, causing decreased peripheral resistance and vasodilation without reducing cardiac output or inducing a reflex tachycardia. These agents produce a slightly greater decrease in standing blood pressure than in supine blood pressure. They have additive effects with β-blockers and diuretics. While the JNC does not cur-rently recommend α_1-adrenergic inhibitors as initial therapy for hypertension, their advantages include a favorable lipid profile effect, equal efficacy in all age and race groups, and a favorable effect on plasma glucose (1). Doxazosin, in contrast to enalapril, reduced total cho-lesterol and triglycerides and increased HDL cholesterol while resulting in a similar reduction in blood pressure (73). This resulted in a greater reduction in calculated coronary heart disease risk than occurs in treatment with enalapril (73). Alpha₁-adrenergic inhibitors may also re-duce preload and afterload in severe chronic congestive heart failure. Another potential group that may benefit from α_1-adrenergic inhibitors are patients with benign prostatic hypertrophy (BPH). Alpha₁-adrenergic inhibi-tors increase urine flow and decrease urinary frequency in patients with BPH by inhibition of norepinephrine-induced contraction of prostate smooth muscle.

Comparison of α_1-Adrenergic Blockers. The three α_1-adrenergic inhibitors appear to have similar antihyperten-sive effects and adverse effects. The α_1-adrenergic inhibi-tors undergo substantial hepatic first-pass metabolism. The newer agents, doxazosin and terazosin, have a longer duration of action than does prazosin and can be dosed once daily.

Adverse Effects. The most striking adverse effect of the α_1-adrenergic inhibitors is the first-dose syncope. Pro-found orthostatic hypotension with syncope can occur 1 to 3 hr after the first dose in patients with a low plasma volume from diuretic therapy or patients who are taking other antihypertensive drugs that blunt their response to the acute decrease in blood pressure. To avoid this problem, the initial dose should be limited to the equivalent of 1 mg of prazosin and should be taken at bedtime or when the patient can be observed.

Pindolol	Propranolol	Timolol	Betaxolol	Bisoprolol	Carteolol	Penbutolol
–	–	–	+	+	–	–
+++	–	–	–	–	++	+
Moderate	High	Low	Low	Low	Low	High
Hepatic/renal	Hepatic	Hepatic	Hepatic (80%)	Hepatic/renal	Renal (70%)	Hepatic

CENTRAL α₂ AGONISTS

Central α_2-adrenergic agonists stimulate α_2-adrenergic receptors in the lower brainstem, which decreases sympathetic outflow to the cardiovascular system. Some agents also block peripheral α_2-adrenergic receptors. The combined sympatholytic effects cause a decrease in peripheral vascular resistance (74). The central α_2-adrenergic agonists are equally effective in all age and race subgroups and can be used for patients with renal insufficiency, diabetes mellitus, bronchospastic disease, and ischemic heart disease. The efficacy of these drugs is similar to that of other antihypertensives when used as monotherapy for the initial treatment of hypertension. Unlike peripheral sympatholytics, the central α_2-adrenergic agonists do not cause significant sodium and fluid retention. The central α_2-adrenergic agonists do not adversely effect glucose metabolism and have neutral or favorable effects on plasma lipids (74). These agents also produce a regression in left ventricular hypertrophy. In addition to its use in hypertension, clonidine has increased the success of smoking cessation, particularly for women, and decreasing craving as well as withdrawal symptoms.

Comparison of α₂-Adrenergic Agonists. Newer formulations of the central α_2-adrenergic agonists provide sustained antihypertensive efficacy with less frequent dosing and have reduced the occurrence of symptomatic side effects. Clonidine can be given twice daily; often a daily bedtime dose is effective and lessens sedation. A clonidine suppression test has been used to assess the contribution of increased sympathetic outflow in patients with essential hypertension. Clonidine is also available as a transdermal therapeutic system (TTS) that is applied once weekly. Transdermal clonidine controls blood pressure in 60 to 80% of patients with mild hypertension (75). Severe withdrawal rebound hypertension is less likely to occur with transdermal therapy than with oral clonidine (75). The transdermal system is a convenient form of treatment with equal efficacy and fewer adverse effects than oral clonidine, the principle adverse effect being a contact dermatitis that develops in 10 to 15% of patients.

Guanfacine is a long-acting central α_2-adrenergic agonist that is metabolized by the liver (70%) and excreted unchanged by the kidneys (30%) with a prolonged elimination half-life of 16 to 23 hr. The long duration of action allows once-daily dosing and reduces adverse effects. Guanfacine also has a relatively flat dose-response curve with little increase in antihypertensive effect from doses greater than 1 mg.

Guanabenz is a guanidine derivative that blocks central sympathetic vasomotor impulses and also produces a guanethidinelike postganglionic blockage. Guanabenz decreases cholesterol and triglycerides without changing HDL cholesterol. Guanabenz is used on a twice-daily dosing schedule.

Methyldopa, the first central α_2-adrenergic agonist, has largely been replaced by the newer agents. A methyldopa metabolite, α-methyl norepinephrine, is the active agonist that reduces CNS sympathetic outflow. Methyldopa has an orthostatic effect that is greater than that of clonidine, but both cardiac output and renal function are usually preserved. Because sodium/water retention can produce a "pseudotolerance," methyldopa is normally combined with a diuretic. Methyldopa can be used on a twice-daily dosing schedule.

Adverse Effects. Sedation and dry mouth are the most frequent adverse effects of central α_2-adrenergic agonists. These symptoms often disappear after the first few weeks. Saliva substitutes or sugarless gum or candy can provide relief from the dry mouth. Sedation is additive to other sedating drugs including alcohol; patients should be cautioned about these combinations and driving. Serious hypersensitivity reactions have occurred with methyldopa, including drug fever, colitis, hepatotoxicity, a positive Coombs' test, and hemolytic anemia. The risk of serious toxicity and impaired mental function make alternative antihypertensive drugs preferable to methyldopa.

Abrupt discontinuation of clonidine has caused an acute withdrawal syndrome (AWS) that is characterized by a rapid increase in blood pressure, headaches, palpitations, tremor, restlessness, diaphoresis, and nausea. AWS appears to be rare with transdermal clonidine and guanfacine. The risk of AWS is higher in younger patients with severe hypertension who are treated with high doses and multiple antihypertensive agents. Combination with β-blockers increases the risk of a hypertensive episode on discontinuation of clonidine (76). This combination should be avoided; if it is used, the β-blocker should be tapered and stopped before decreasing the clonidine. Avoiding excessive doses, encouraging patient compliance, and tapering clonidine slowly may help to prevent AWS. However, patients should be warned to seek immediate medical help if they develop signs and symptoms of AWS. Treatment by restarting medications required is usually effective in reversing AWS, and labetalol has been effective for combined central agonist/β-blocker AWS (77).

PERIPHERAL SYMPATHOLYTICS

Guanethidine is actively transported into the peripheral adrenergic neuron, where it depletes norpinephrine and produces a postural hypotension. Guanethidine decreases venous return to the heart, decreases cardiac output, and interferes with the sympathetic reflexes that control the resistance (arteriolar) and capacitance (venous) vessels. Because guanethidine depletes myocardial catecholamines, it can worsen congestive heart failure. Guanethidine is slowly and variably absorbed, undergoing partial first-pass hepatic metabolism. With chronic administration the half-life of guanethidine is 5 days with 50% of the drug excreted unchanged in the urine. Because of the long half-life, guanethidine can be taken once daily, and dosage adjustments should be made only after 2 to 3 weeks. Prolonged standing, exercise, and heat increase postural hypotension. The dose of guanethidine should be adjusted on the basis of standing blood pressure, and blocks can be used to elevate the head of the bed to sustain a nighttime postural effect. Guanadrel is an adrendergic blocking agent that also depletes norepinephrine from peripheral neurons. Guanadrel has a more rapid onset and shorter duration of action than guanethidine. Because of the postural effect, standing blood pressure must always be measured. These agents are reserved for treating resistant hypertension.

Adverse Effects. The major problem with both guanethidine and guanadrel is postural and exercise hypotension. Patients should be warned to rise slowly from supine or sitting positions, to flex their arms and legs before arising, and to avoid additive vasodilating factors such as prolonged standing, hot showers, and drinking alcohol. Postural effects are most pronounced in the morning on arising. Other dose-related problems include sexual dysfunction and diarrhea, which may require discontinuation of therapy. A pseudotolerance due to fluid retention may develop unless diuretic therapy is adequate. Because guanethidine diffuses poorly into the CNS, sedation and depression are infrequent problems. Several drugs can interfere with the uptake of the sympatholytics into the adrenergic neuron and rapidly block the antihypertensive effects. Guanadrel may cause less sexual dysfunction and orthostasis than does guanethidine. However, patients should be given similar precautions to minimize the risks of postural hypotension. Diuretics are needed to reduce sodium/water retention and weight gain.

Reserpine. Reserpine acts in both the central and peripheral sympathetic nervous systems, depleting norepinephrine and serotonin stores in the brain and peripheral

adrenergic nerve endings. Reserpine also increases vagal tone; this contributes to the reduced heart rate and increased gastric acid secretions. The onset of action of reserpine may take several days; maximal hypotensive effects may take weeks. Adverse effects are frequent with high doses and include nasal congestion from cholinergic stimulation. CNS changes include drowsiness, sedation, dizziness, sleep disturbances, difficulty in concentration, poor memory, and depression. Other antihypertensive agents are preferred because of greater efficacy and fewer adverse effects.

Vasodilators

Vasodilators directly relax arteriolar smooth muscle and decrease peripheral vascular resistance. They do not interfere with autonomic reflexes or produce postural hypotension. This stimulates carotid sinus baroreceptors, producing reflex increases in heart rate, renin release, and sodium and water retention. These drugs have usually been used in combination with a diuretic and a β-blocker or sympatholytic agent to prevent the reflex increases in cardiac output and fluid retention that blunt the effect of vasodilators when they are used alone. The elderly develop less reflex tachycardia.

COMPARISON OF VASODILATORS

Hydralazine is metabolized by hepatic acetylation with substantial first-pass elimination. Hydralazine is effective when taken twice daily; food increases bioavailability. The acetylation rate is genetically determined; slow acetylators experience greater hypotensive effects and usually should not receive more than 200 mg of hydralazine daily.

Minoxidil is a potent vasodilator that markedly reduces peripheral vascular resistance and is reserved for the treatment of severe hypertension. It can produce blood pressure reductions of 30 to 40 mm Hg when combined with diuretics and β-blockers. Minoxidil is well absorbed and undergoes hepatic metabolism. Despite a relatively short half-life, the antihypertensive effect persists for 12 to 24 hr, and minoxidil is dosed twice daily. Minoxidil produces marked sodium/water retention, and large doses of loop diuretics are often needed to control the edema. Reflex tachycardia and increased cardiac output are prevented by adequate β-blocker therapy.

Diazoxide is a nondiuretic thiazide that dilates peripheral arterioles and is used to treat hypertensive emergencies. Intravenous injection produces a profound decrease in both systolic and diastolic blood pressure that does not require continuous infusion and infrequently causes hypotension. Diazoxide is metabolized in the liver and excreted in urine with a duration of action of 2 to 24 hr. Diazoxide is administered as a minibolus (1 to 3 mg/kg) every 10 min with a maximum of 150 mg or as a 15 mg/min infusion. Diazoxide produces sodium and water retention, and diuretic therapy is necessary to maintain blood pressure control. Hyperglycemia is a problem with prolonged use. Patients with renal failure or myocardial ischemia are predisposed to the adverse effects of diazoxide.

Nitroprusside is an instant-acting vasodilator that is useful in virtually all hypertensive emergencies. Nitroprusside relaxes both arteriolar and venous smooth muscles. Nitroprusside reacts with cysteine, forming nitrocysteine, which activates guanylate cyclase, leading to increased cyclic GMP, which relaxes vascular smooth muscle. Controlled intravenous infusions of nitroprusside are highly effective in treating hypertensive emergencies. The onset and cessation of the hypotensive action are immediate. Nitroprusside is unstable and must be protected from light. The nitroprusside metabolite thiocyanate may rapidly accumulate with impaired renal function, and plasma thiocyanate concentrations greater than 10 mg/dL are toxic. Nitroprusside decreases peripheral resistance and can improve left ventricular function in patients with congestive heart failure or with impaired cardiac output after a myocardial infarction.

ADVERSE EFFECTS

Adverse effects from reflex sympathetic stimulation or direct vasodilation include headache, dizziness, postural hypotension, tachycardia, and palpitations (78). The reflex tachycardia can precipitate or aggravate angina pectoris. Hydralazine commonly causes throbbing headaches and also causes a pyridoxine-deficiency-induced peripheral neuropathy. A positive antinuclear antibody (ANA) develops in 15 to 20% of hydralazine-treated patients, which can lead to a lupuslike syndrome, particularly if doses greater than 200 mg/day are used. Symptoms can include arthalgia, arthritis, fever, malaise, rash, and weight loss. Symptoms can resolve rapidly and often disappear within 6 months; however, rheumatoid symptoms and a positive ANA can persist for years.

Minoxidil causes marked sodium and water retention. leading to weight gain, peripheral edema, cardiac enlargement, pulmonary hypertension, and pericardial effusion (78). Minoxidil causes hypertrichosis in nearly all patients. This can be partly controlled with dipilatories but limits its use by women. Coarsening of facial features can also occur.

CLINICAL USE OF ANTIHYPERTENSIVE DRUGS

Drug treatment remains empiric because the fundamental cause of essential hypertension remains unknown. JNC V recommends initial antihypertensive drug therapy as monotherapy with either a diuretic or β-blocker because these drugs have been shown to reduce cardiovascular morbidity and mortality in controlled clinical trials. While these two classes are preferred for initial drug therapy,

angiotensin-converting-enzyme inhibitors, calcium entry blockers, and α_1-blockers are alternatives for patients with special considerations. If the response is not adequate, one approach is to gradually increase the dose of the initial drug to the recommended maximum (79). For many patients it may be appropriate to use sequential individualized monotherapy by discontinuing the initial drug and substituting an agent from a different class before combining two drugs. An alternative concept is to use synergistic combinations in very low doses as initial therapy. Patients with Stage 3 and Stage 4 hypertension often need two or three antihypertensive drugs, and agents should be added at shorter intervals (80).

Two trials have compared drug therapy using agents from several classes of antihypertensive drugs. A VA Cooperative study used a goal DBP < 90 mm Hg (81). Diltiazem was the most effective therapy, with a 59% success rate. Diltiazem also ranked first for black patients (64%). Captopril and prazosin were least successful (42%). Hydrochlorothiazide (46%), clonidine (50%), and atenolol (51%) were intermediate in success rates. Drug intolerance was most frequent with clonidine (14%) and prazosin (12%). The fewest number of dropouts was with diuretics (3%).

The TOMHS study found that all drug classes except ACE inhibitors were equally effective in reducing blood pressure (82, 83). All drugs were well tolerated, and 72% of patients continued their initial treatment, most not requiring any dose increase. An unexpected finding was that the greatest improvment in the quality of life was for patients taking a diuretic or β-blocker. Chlorthalidone was most effective in reducing LVH.

For hypertension that is not controlled by two drugs, the JNC V recommendations are to substitute for one of the drugs or add a third drug from a different class. Additional drugs should be added or substituted in gradually increasing doses until blood pressure is controlled, side effects are intolerable, or maximal recommended doses are reached. Usually, an interval of 1 to 2 months will allow maximal antihypertensive action before changes are made. In many instances, using smaller doses of drugs with different sites of action is preferred to maximal doses of a single drug. This has the advantage of having additive effects of drugs while minimizing side effects.

Refractory Hypertension

Patients with blood pressure that is not controlled (≥160/ 100 mm Hg) by a triple drug regimen are considered resistant. Several potential causes should be evaluated including:

- Patient noncompliance
- Inadequate drug doses

- Drug combinations that act at the same site
- Volume overload (excess sodium intake, inadequate diuretic therapy, renal insufficiency)
- Obesity
- Renovascular hypertension
- Excess alcohol intake
- Drug interactions
- Drug-induced hypertension

Step-Down Therapy

For patients who have maintained control of their blood pressure (DBP ≤ 85 mm Hg) for 6 months to 1 year, a stepwise reduction in antihypertensive medications may be attempted (1). Short-term studies described a relatively high success rate (40 to 50%) of discontinuation of drug treatment, but a long-term evaluation found only 8% of previously treated patients who remained normotensive off medications (84). Virtually all hypertensive patients who are off medication can be expected to relapse unless effective nonpharmacologic treatments are implemented. A reasonable approach is to step down to one medication after blood pressure control for 6 months to 1 year on multiple drugs. Cessation of drug therapy should be reserved only for patients with no medical complications and mild hypertension who have demonstrated weight loss, sodium reduction, and/or increased exercise. Patients who are off drugs should have their blood pressure measured every 3 to 6 months. They should be informed that permanent remission is rare and that eventual reinstitution of drug treatment is likely.

Hypertensive Emergencies and Urgencies

A hypertensive emergency is a severe elevation of blood pressure, usually a diastolic blood pressure above 120 to 130 mm Hg, with acute or progressive end-organ damage (1, 77). If end-organ damage is absent, it is a hypertensive urgency. Hypertensive crises may involve an abrupt increase in vascular resistance secondary to increased circulating vasoconstrictor substances, leading to ischemia, which triggers the further release of vasoconstrictors (1, 77). Therapy should interrupt this cycle and decrease blood pressure to lower levels while avoiding an abrupt decrease to normotensive or hypotensive blood pressures, which may cause ischemia or infarction. For a hypertensive emergency the target is usually to lower blood pressure 25% to a DBP of 100 to 110 mm Hg. Sodium nitroprusside infusion is the current therapy of choice (77). Other treatment options include intravenous nicardapine and intravenous labetalol (77). Hypertensive urgency is encountered more commonly than emergencies and can be effectively managed with oral or sublingual therapy. Both oral nifedipine and oral clonidine are effective for urgent hypertension, but nifedipine acts more rapidly and controls 96% of patients within 2 hr (85). Sublingual or buccal

Table 37.11.
Complicated Hypertension

Condition	Drugs to Avoid	Alternative Drugs
Heart failure	Beta-blockers, reserpine	ACE inhibitors, diuretics, prazosin
Renal failure	Thiazide diuretics, guanethidine	Furosemide, clonidine, hydralazine, ACE inhibitors, prazosin, minoxidil
Angina pectoris/ myocardial infarction	Hydralazine	Beta-blockers
Diabetes mellitus	Beta-blockers	ACE inhibitors, clonidine
Cerebrovascular disease	Furosemide, guanethidine	Clonidine

nifedipine has an onset of action of 5 to 10 min. Oral therapy can be administered quickly, rarely causes hypotension, and facilitates the transition to long-term treatment. Overly aggressive treatment can cause myocardial ischemia and cerebral hypoperfusion.

Complicated Hypertension

The presence of hypertensive complications or coexisting disease states can influence the selection of antihypertensive drugs. See Table 37.11.

Congestive Heart Failure and LVH

The presence of left ventricular hypertrophy (LVH) is an independent risk factor for cardiac dysrhythmias and sudden death. Premature ventricular contractions are 40 to 50 times more prevalent in hypertensive patients, and the risk of sudden death is increased 5 to 6 times by their presence (18). Many antihypertensive drugs reduce LVH, including β-blockers, calcium entry blockers, ACE inhibitors, and central adrenergic agonists (1). Diuretics may be less effective in reversing LVH and can increase cardiac risk by causing electrolyte disturbances. Vasodilators increase left ventricular mass and should not be used as monotherapy. For patients with overt congestive heart failure the ACE inhibitors in combination with diuretics can reduce mortality (8).

Renal Insufficiency

Treatment of hypertension can slow the progression of renal disease (1, 9). If the serum creatinine is greater than 2 mg/dL, furosemide, bumetanide, or metolazone is needed, as thiazide diuretics are ineffective (1, 9). Sodium retention becomes a major factor in treating patients with renal insufficiency; larger doses of loop diuretics may be added to most regimens. Other drugs that are effective for patients with renal disease and do not adversely effect renal blood flow or glomerular filtration are ACE inhibitors, calcium entry blockers, central antiadrenergics, and vasodilators (86, 87). ACE inhibitors and calcium entry blockers appear to have unique benefits for patients with renal disease. These agents increase renal blood flow and glomerular filtration rate, prevent tubular sodium reabsorption, and may limit the progression of renal disease (86, 87). Dosage reductions are needed for antihypertensive drugs that are excreted by the kidney, and patients with chronic renal failure may exhibit an increased sensitivity to some drugs, including alpha blockers and ACE inhibitors.

Coronary Artery Disease

The benefits of antihypertensive treatment in preventing the complications of coronary artery disease have been less than were predicted. To prevent the development of the complications of coronary artery disease, emphasis should be given to correcting other cardiovascular risk factors, especially smoking, hyperlipidemia, and diabetes mellitus (1). Calculating an individual coronary risk profile can aid in the management of patients (50). Patients with angina pectoris or a previous myocardial infarction can be treated with β-blockers or calcium blockers, which reduce angina. Beta-blockers are also shown to reduce mortality following myocardial infarction, at least in men. ACE inhibitors also reduce mortality following myocardial infarction. (See Chapter 41 on myocardial infarction.) Because of the increased of arrhythmias, caution must be exercised to avoid diuretic-induced hypokalemia and hypomagnesemia. Drugs that cause reflex tachycardia, such as hydralazine, should be avoided.

Cerebrovascular Disease

Antihypertensive therapy can reduce the risk of recurrent stroke by 42% and is an important component of therapy for patients with cerebrovascular disease (20). It is important to avoid orthostatic hypotension. Therapy should be started cautiously, as elderly patients with cerebrovascular disease are more likely to develop hypotension from these drugs.

Diabetes Mellitus

Hypertension is twice as frequent in diabetic patients than in nondiabetics (88). Eventually, 50% of diabetic patients become hypertensive. Insulin resistance and hyperinsulinemia may contribute to the pathogenesis of hypertension in these patients (10, 88). Diabetic vascular disease and associated serum lipid abnormalities compound the cardiovascular risks. Nephropathy develops in up to 50% of patients with insulin-dependent diabetes mellitus (IDDM) and 40% of patients with non-insulin-dependent diabetes mellitus (NIDDM) (88).

Treatment of hypertension should lower blood pressure without worsening diabetic control, serum lipids, or diabetic complications. Thiazide diuretics worsen glucose control and increase cholesterol, and these effects may not reverse with dosage reduction (88, 89). Loop diuretics may produce less impairment of glucose control (89). The mechanism of diuretic glucose elevation is likely hypokalemia, which suppresses insulin secretion (88). Patients with IDDM whose glycemic control is from exogenous insulin do not have this complication. Beta-blockers also adversely affect glucose by blocking insulin release and glycogenolysis (64, 88). Beta-blockers also abolish catecholamine-mediated symptoms of hypoglycemia, such as tremor and tachycardia (88). These agents can also worsen peripheral vascular disease, which is 30 times more common in diabetics. Beta-blockers that are cardioselective and not lipophilic are preferred for patients with NIDDM (89). ACE inhibitors do not adversely effect glycemic control or lipid metabolism and have the potential to decrease proteinuria and slow the progression of diabetic renal disease (90, 91). Information regarding the effect of calcium entry blockers on glycemic control is conflicting. Nifedipine has increased serum glucose; verapamil has improved glycemic control (88). Diltiazem can decrease proteinuria in diabetic patients as effectively as lisinopril (92). Guanfacine may improve glycemic control, and α-blockers can blunt the deterioration in glucose tolerance caused by β-blockers (90). Autonomic neuropathy and orthostatic hypotension are 30 times more common in diabetic patients than in nondiabetics, and drugs that produce postural hypotension should be used cautiously. Finally, sexual dysfunction is a common problem in male diabetics; drugs that cause sexual dysfunction should be avoided.

Elderly

Nearly two-thirds of the 29 million people in the United States who are 65 years of age or older have some elevation of blood pressure (1). The HDFP and EWPHE trials have demonstrated benefit for elderly patients (up to age 80) who are treated for diastolic hypertension (DBP ≥ 90 mm Hg) (93). Isolated systolic hypertension (ISH), which is defined as SBP > 160 mm Hg and DBP < 90 mm Hg, is more prevalent above age 60 (94). ISH is associated with an increased risk of stroke and cardiovascular disease that is independent of other risk factors (93). The Systolic Hypertension in the Elderly Program (SHEP) trial demonstrated a 36% reduction in stroke from the treatment of ISH for 4.5 years in patients age 60 years and older (94). Drug treatment in SHEP was low-dose chlorthalidone (12.5 to 25 mg) and atenolol 25 mg with potassium supplements if required (95). An important further analysis found that this drug treatment of ISH did not cause deterioration in measures of cognition, emotional state, physical function, or leisure activities (96). A metaanalysis of antihypertensive trials involving elderly patients concluded that treatment reduced both stroke and CHD mortality without evidence of a J-curve phenomenon (94).

The selection of drug therapy for the elderly may be complicated by physiologic changes. Elderly hypertensives usually have a reduced cardiac output, intravascular volume, and heart rate and an increased peripheral vascular resistance (97). The elderly often have developed LVH, which impairs coronary reserve and is associated with a possible increased risk of ventricular ectopy and sudden death (97). Diminished baroreflexes increase the risk of postural hypotension, and renal function may be reduced. Alpha$_1$-blockers, labetalol, guanethidine, and guanadrel can increase orthostatic hypotension; this limits their use by the elderly. Calcium entry blockers are effective, are physiologically appropriate, and do not adversely affect renal function. Their adverse effects are similar to those seen in younger patients. Although plasma renin activity decreases with age, the ACE inhibitors are effective in the elderly. The ACE inhibitors do not have adverse metabolic effects and reduce the incidence of arrhythmias in cardiac failure (97). The elderly should be treated with an individualized approach to drug therapy, and initial treatment should be guided by the axiom "start low and go slow."

Pregnancy

Hypertension complicates 10% of pregnancies and is more frequent in nulliparous women and women who have had multiple pregnancies (98). Hypertension during pregnancy can be due to chronic hypertension, preeclampsia, preeclampsia plus chronic hypertension, or transient hypertension. Chronic hypertension is well tolerated during pregnancy if DBP remains < 100 mm Hg. Preeclampsia can be life threatening to both the fetus and the mother. Preeclampsia develops most often in nulliparous women, occulting near term with a pathophysiology of a marked increase in peripheral resistance (99). Signs of preeclampsia include proteinuria, edema, hemoconcentration, hypoalbuminemia, increased urate, and hepatic or coagulation abnormalities (99). Life-threatening complications are hemolytic anemia and marked hepatic dysfunction. Progression to seizures is termed eclampsia, which is a major cause of maternal death.

Methyldopa has a long history of safe use in pregnancy with normal follow-up evaluations in children up to 10 years after treatment (99). Beta-blockers, labetalol, thiazide diuretics, and hydralazine have also been used to treat hypertension during pregnancy with apparent success. Limited information is available about the use of calcium entry blockers in pregnancy. ACE inhibitors and atenolol are avoided because they reduce uterine blood flow (98, 99). For the treatment of severe hypertension during pregnancy, intravenous hydralazine is commonly used (100). Diazoxide is used for refractory patients. Parenteral labetalol may become the second-choice agent. Calcium entry blockers are also effective, but concurrent magnesium sulfate may potentiate their effect and cause a precipitous fall in blood pressure. Calcium entry blockers also reduce uterine blood flow (99).

Racial Differences

The prevalence of hypertension among blacks is substantially higher than among whites (38% versus 29%), and hypertension-related morbidity and mortality is threefold to fivefold higher than in Caucasians. (95, 101, 102). Hypertension is often poorly controlled in black patients. Environmental factors, particularly dietary excess, high sodium consumption, and low dietary potassium, calcium, and magnesium, contribute to these differences (95, 102). The development of obesity and insulin resistance may be an important mechanism in black hypertensives. Approximately 50% of black hypertensives show salt sensitivity, and hypertension is often associated with low plasma renin and volume dependence (102). Thiazide diuretics are effective therapy for black hypertensive patients. In addition, for the socioeconomically depressed segment of the black population, thiazides offer cost-effective treatment. However, approximately 50% of black hypertensives will require two or more drugs (95). Blacks have a lower response rate to β-blockers and ACE inhibitors than do white hypertensives. This difference may be less if higher drug doses are used or β-blockers and ACE inhibitors are used in combination with diuretics. A comparison of different antihypertensive drugs in black hypertensives demonstrated blood pressure control of 60% with atenolol, 57% with captopril, and 73% with verapamil (103).

The prevalence of hypertension in Hispanics appears to be higher than in Caucasians but less than in blacks (100). Mexican Americans are likely to be obese and to have diabetes mellitus. Hypertension in Hispanics is often unrecognized or poorly controlled (100).

Asians and Pacific Islanders also have a lower incidence of hypertension than Caucasians do, but this appears to be modified by socioeconomic factors. Racial differences in drug response may be particularly important in the Asian population. Men of Chinese descent have a twofold greater sensitivity to the β-blocking effects of propranolol (104) than Caucasians. Men of Chinese descent had a greater decrease in both heart rate and blood pressure, despite a significantly higher metabolic clearance of propranolol than white subjects (104). Asian patients also have a reduced metabolism of nifedipine and frequently develop palpitations (105). Because of possible racial differences in drug response and metabolism, antihypertensive drugs should be started with reduced doses in treating Asian patients.

Adverse Drug Effects

Because of the long-term treatment of hypertension, it is important that the drug therapy have minimal adverse effects. Adverse drug effects are listed in Table 37.7.

Quality of Life and Cost of Care

The cost of treatment and the adverse effects of antihypertensive drugs on the quality of life are important concerns. Drug therapy may produce subtle changes in emotion, behavior, and physical and cognitive function (1). In an early study, physicians thought that all patients had improved, but only 48% of the patients agreed (106). However, 99% of relatives thought that the patient had gotten worse since starting antihypertensive treatment. Problems observed included decreased memory, irritability, depression, hypochondria, and decreased sexual interest (106). Captopril improved general well-being, caused fewer side effects, and had higher quality-of-life scores compared to methyldopa or propranolol (107). Addition of a diuretic worsened outcome for all drug treatment groups. For black hypertensives there was no difference in quality of life with atenolol, captopril, or verapamil (108). However, verapamil produced a significantly greater decrease in blood pressure. The Trial of Antihypertensive Interventions and Management (TAIM) evaluated the effects of a low-sodium and high-potassium diet, a weight loss diet, a placebo, chlorthalidone, or atenolol on sexual function and quality of life (109). Few drug-related side effects were found. Chlorthalidone produced erection problems in 28% of men on a usual diet, but a weight loss diet removed this effect. The weight loss diet reduced physical complaints and increased health satisfaction. The TAIM findings emphasize the importance of weight reduction in addition to drug regimens for overweight hypertensives (109). A comparison of captopril and enalapril found higher quality-of-life scores with captopril, with similar blood pressure control and adverse effects (110).

The assessment of cost-benefit issues is needed to reduce medical costs while providing quality patient care. The costs of antihypertensive medications are widely variable. Combination diuretic products cost three or more times as much as hydrochlorothiazide. Beta-blockers and calcium entry blockers also show a wide cost variation (111). ACE inhibitors and calcium entry blockers are four to twenty times more expensive than generic diuretics or generic β-blockers (106). With the increasing cost of antihypertensive medications, some patients are not compliant because they cannot afford expensive drugs. Estimates of the long-term cost-effectiveness projected that the cost per year of life saved was $10,900 for propranolol, $16,400 for hydrochlorothiazide, $31,600 for nifedipine, $61,900 for prazosin, and $72,100 for captopril (112). Lowering DBP by 1 mm Hg was estimated to be equivalent to lowering cholesterol by 6% (112). However, these cost estimates have been severely criticized because of the multiple assumptions and wide differences in the patient populations between the many studies that were compared (113). A cost-minimization analysis attempted to compare the total costs of antihypertensive therapy including drug acquisition cost, laboratory monitoring, supplemental drug acquisition costs, clinic visits, and treatment of side effects (114). Mean total costs for antihypertensive drug classes were $895 for β-blockers, $1043 for diuretics, $1165 for central α-agonists, $1243 for ACE inhibitors, $1288 for α₁-blockers, and $1425 for calcium channel blockers.

The choice of antihypertensive agent should still be based on patient characteristics, concomitant diseases, and the cost of drug therapy.

Sexual Dysfunction

Antihypertensive drugs can cause impotence, ejaculation difficulties, and decreased libido (115). Sexual dysfunction is reported by 4 to 7% of normotensive controls. The incidence of antihypertensive-induced sexual dysfunction is difficult to quantitate. Reports frequently range from 9 to 25% or higher, with increased frequency when multiple drug therapy is used and with advancing age (115). The MRC trial reported an increased frequency of impotence with both bendrofluazide and propranolol. Sexual symptoms distress scores were worsened by methyldopa and propranolol but not by captopril either alone or combined with a diuretic (116). The risk of sexual dysfunction is greatest with peripheral adrenergic inhibitors and less with central α-agonists and diuretics. Lower incidences of sexual problems are also described with β-blockers. (115). The drugs that are least likely to cause sexual problems are the ACE inhibitors, calcium entry blockers, α₁-blockers, and direct vasodilators (115).

Depression

Depletion of biogenic amines may be pathogenic in depression. Antihypertensive medications that interfere with the sympathetic nervous system and neurotransmitter concentrations may induce depression (117). There is substantial evidence that reserpine and methyldopa can induce or worsen depression. Beta-blockers may produce CNS effects, and an increased use of antidepressant drugs has been seen in patients treated with β-blockers (117). Diuretics, calcium entry blockers, and ACE inhibitors have the lowest association with depression and are the preferred agents for patients who are at risk for depression. (117).

J-Curve

There is controversy regarding a "J-shaped curve" relationship between treated DBP and cardiac mortality in which lowering blood pressure below a critical point leads to an increase in mortality. The J-curve appeared to cause an increase in mortality in patients with preexisting ischemic heart disease whose DBP was lowered to less than 85 mm Hg (118). In the EWPHE trial a U-shaped relation was described in which total mortality was increased in patients with the lowest thirds of treated SBP and DBP (119). A review of 13 studies with a combined total of 48,000 patients found a consistent J-shaped relationship between cardiac events and treated DBP (120). There was no increase in stroke at lower treated blood pressures. A proposed mechanism is increased myocardial ischemia in hypertensive patients with left ventricular hypertrophy when DBP is lowered below 85 mm Hg. A suggested compromise is to "be cautious in lowering blood pressure levels below 85 mm Hg in patients with known ischemic heart disease" (120). The risk of myocardial infarction was increased among treated hypertensive patients who achieved diastolic pressures of less than 80 mm Hg (121).

Serum Lipids

The combination of elevated blood pressure and elevated blood cholesterol creates a synergistic increase in the risk of cardiovascular disease (122). Nonpharmacologic interventions of diet, exercise, weight reduction, and smoking cessation are the foundation for the management of both hypertension and high blood cholesterol. The potential effects of antihypertensive drugs on serum lipids must be considered in treated patients who are hypertensive and dyslipidemic (122, 123). Thiazide-type diuretics produce a modest (5 to 10 mg/dL) increase in total cholesterol, LDL cholesterol, and triglycerides. Diuretic increases in cholesterol are greater with higher doses and worse in blacks than in nonblacks (123). Beta-blockers, except those with ISA or α-blocking properties, reduce HDL cholesterol and increase serum triglycerides. Drugs that have minimal effects on serum lipids include calcium entry blockers, converting-enzyme inhibitors, ISA β-blockers, labetalol, hydralazine, minoxidil, and possibly indapamide. The α_1-adrenergic blockers and the central α_2-adrenergic agonists may slightly decrease total and LDL cholesterol. In the Coronary Primary Prevention Trial the thiazide diuretics reduced the effect of lipid-lowering drugs on LDL cholesterol (122). However, not all patients who are taking diuretics experience adverse lipid alterations, and a low-fat, low-cholesterol diet may minimize lipid changes. Some studies have suggested that the hyperlipemic effects of diuretics may not persist more than 1 year (122, 123). Patients with coronary heart disease (CHD) and hypertension need agressive cholesterol-lowering therapy and careful lowering of blood pressure. Beta-blockers may be needed for patients with CHD for antianginal effects and secondary prevention of myocardial infarction despite their adverse effects on serum triglycerides and HDL cholesterol. Antihyperlipidemic treatment may slow the progression of atherosclerosis and possibly induce plaque regression. The Primary Prevention Trial demonstrated that a reduction of both blood pressure and cholesterol is needed to reduce cardiovascular morbidity (124).

Drug Interactions

The effect of many antihypertensive drugs can be increased or decreased by the concurrent use of other drugs (125, 126). In addition, antihypertensive drugs can interact with other drugs. Often, potentially interacting drugs can be successfully used in combination if the possibility of the interaction is recognized, the effects are monitored, and drug doses are adjusted if needed. Common interactions are listed in Table 37.9.

Compliance

The single most important factor in the successful treatment of hypertension is patient compliance. Untreated and uncontrolled hypertension in aware hypertensive patients remains an important problem (127, 128). Public awareness programs have identified the marjority of people with hypertension, but the problems of patient dropout and noncompliance with treatment still result in fewer than 50% of hypertensive patients having controlled blood pressure. Continuous effort is needed to prevent patient dropout, encourage lifestyle changes, and improve medication compliance.

Noncompliance is a complex problem, and prediction of compliance by clinicians is poor. A systematic procedure to screen for medication noncompliance can help to identify patients who need extra attention to acheive blood pressure control. A patient-tracking system and a missed-apppointment follow-up program are needed to achieve long-term attendance and blood pressure control. Failure to achieve blood pressure control is twice as great in nonattenders (no appointment in 6 months) as in attenders (67% versus 30%) (128).

Several important areas must be considered in attempting to overcome noncompliance. Combinations of techniques are usually needed.

- Education about the consequences of untreated hypertension and the role of drug and nondrug treatments serves as a foundation for compliance.
- The patient must understand and believe that hypertension is a serious condition that needs treatment.
- Simplification of the drug regimen can improve compliance.
- Avoid side effects by starting with low doses and individually selected drugs.
- Schedule drug doses once or twice daily.
- Label prescriptions with clear, explicit directions, and indicate the purpose of the drug.
- Tailor medication times to coincide with existing daily habits.
- Provide written schedules or pillbox organizers for patients who are taking multiple drugs.
- Encourage the use of prompting cues such as stickers or calendars to remind patients to take medications.
- Discuss potential problems such as drug costs, confusion with other drugs, and previous problems with drug therapy.
- Activate the patient by providing feedback of blood pressure response or self-monitoring of blood pressure.

- Encourage or reward patients for keeping appointments, taking medications, and reducing blood pressure.
- Screen for noncompliance by monitoring attendance, patient self-reports, blood pressure response, and changes in biochemical or physical parameters (e.g., pulse or serum potassium).
- Provide close professional supervision, and establish a positive relationship with patients.

PHARMACISTS AND HYPERTENSION

The major opportunity for pharmacists is to cooperatively assist in acheiving long-term control of blood pressure. Pharmacists can provide patient education, monitor prescription drug use for noncompliance, implement medication refill reminder systems, screen for drug interactions and adverse drug reactions, and monitor blood pressure response (127–132). In specialized settings, clinical pharmacists have managed hypertensive patients with improved compliance and blood pressure control (131, 132).

CONCLUSION

Hypertension continues to be a national health problem. However, hypertension must be viewed as one of several major cardiovascular risk factors. Treatment must address all cardiovascular risks. The greatest patient benefit may be from controlling blood pressure by nonpharmacologic interventions. For patients who are unable to control blood pressure, drug therapy can effectively reduce risks if long-term control of hypertension is achieved.

REFERENCES

1. The Fifth Report of the Joint National Committee on Detection, Evaluation and Treatment of High Blood Pressure (JNC V). Arch Intern Med 153:154–83, 1993.
2. Working Group on Renovascular Hypertension. Detection, evaluation and treatment of renovascular hypertension. Arch Intern Med 147:820–24, 1987.
3. Woods JW. Oral contraceptives and hypertension. Hypertension 11(suppl I):11–14, 1988.
4. Lake CR, Zaloga G, Bray J, et al. Transient hypertension after two phenylpropanolamine diet aids and the effects of caffeine: a placebo-controlled follow-up study. Am J Med 86:427–32, 1989.
5. Johnson AG, Nguyen TV, et al. Do nonsteroidal anti-inflammatory drugs affect blood pressure? A meta-analysis. Ann Intern Med 121:289–300, 1994.
6. Littenberg B, Garber AM, Sox, HC Jr. Screening for hypertension. Ann Intern Med 112:192–202, 1990.
7. Zachariah PK. Hypertension: an overview. Mayo Clin Proc 64:1403–15, 1989.
8. Yusus S, Pepine CJ, Garces C, et al. Effect of enalapril on myocardial infarction and unstable angina in patients with low ejection fractions. Lancet 240:1173–78, 1992.
9. National High Blood Pressure Education Program. National High Blood Pressure Program Working Group report on hypertension and chronic renal failure. Arch Intern Med 151:1280–86, 1991.
10. Reaven GM. Insulin resistance, hyperinsulinemia, and hypertriglyceridemia in the etiology and clinical course of hypertension. Am J Med 90(suppl 2A):7S–11S, 1991.
11. Weiss NS. Relation of high blood pressure to headache, epistaxis and selected other symptoms. N Engl J Med 287:631–33, 1972.
12. Rudd P, Price MG, Graham LE, et al. Consequences of worksite hypertension screening: differential changes in pyschosocial function. Am J Med 80:853–60, 1986.
13. Williams Larson AW, Strong CG. Initial assessment of the patient with hypertension. Mayo Clin Proc 64:1533–42, 1989.
14. Pickering TG, James GD, Boddie C, Harshfield GA, Blank S, Laragh JH. How common is white coat hypertension? JAMA 259:225–28, 1988.
15. National High Blood Pressure Education Program Coordinating Committee. National High Blood Pressure Education Program Working Group Report on Ambulatory Blood Pressure Monitoring. Arch Intern Med 150:2270–80, 1990.
16. Klein LE. Compliance and blood pressure control. Hypertension 11(suppl II):61–4, 1988.
17. Kannel WB, et al. Overall and coronary heart disease mortality rates in relation to major risk factors in 325,348 men screened for MRFIT. Am Heart J 112:825–36, 1986.
18. Lavie CJ, Venture HO, Messerli FH. Regression on increased left ventricular mass by antihypertensives. Drugs 42:945–61, 1991.
19. MacMahon S, Peto R, Cutler J, et al. Blood pressure, stroke, and coronary heart disease. 1: prolonged differences in blood pressure: prospective observational studies corrected for regression dilution bias. Lancet 335:765–74, 1990.
20. Collins R, Peto R, MacMahon S, et al. Blood pressure, stroke, and coronary heart disease. 2: short-term reductions in blood pressure: overview of the randomised drug trials in their epidemiological context. Lancet 335:827–38, 1990.
21. Herbert PR, Moser M, Mayer J, et al. Recent evidence on drug therapy of mild to moderate hypertension and decreased risk of coronary heart disease. Arch Intern Med 153:578–81, 1993.
22. Veterans Administration Cooperative Study Group on Antihypertensive Agents. Effects of treatment on morbidity in hypertension: results in patients with diastolic blood pressure averaging 115 through 129 mm Hg. JAMA 202:1028–34, 1967.
23. Veterans Administration Cooperative Study Group on Antihypertensive Agents. Effects of treatment on morbidity in hypertension: results in patients with diastolic blood pressure averaging 90 through 104 mmHg. JAMA 213:1143–52, 1970.
24. Taguchi J, Freis ED. Partial reduction of blood pressure and prevention of complications in hypertension. N Engl J Med 291:329–31, 1974.
25. Multiple Risk Factor Intervention Trial Group. Risk factors changes and mortality results. JAMA 248:1465–77, 1982.
26. Hypertension Detection and Follow-up Program Cooperative Group. Five year findings of the hypertension detection and follow-up program. I: reduction in mortality of persons with high blood pressure, including mild hypertension. JAMA 242:2562–71, 1979.
27. Hypertension Detection and Follow-up Program Cooperative Group. Five year findings of the hypertension detection and follow-up program. II: mortality by race, sex and age. JAMA 242:2572–77, 1979.
28. Hypertension Detection and Follow-up Program Cooperative Group. The effect of treatment on mortality in mild hypertension. N Engl J Med 307:976–80, 1982.
29. Hypertension Detection and Follow-up Program Cooperative Group. Persistence of reduction in blood pressure and mortality of participants in the Hypertension Detection and Follow-up Program. JAMA 259:2113–22, 1988.
30. Multiple Risk Factor Intervention Trial Group. Baseline rest electrocardiographic abnormalities, antihypertensive treatment, and mortality in the Multiple Risk Factor Intervention Trial. Am J Cardiol 55:1–14, 1985.

31. European Working Party on High Blood Pressure in the Elderly Trial (EWPHE). Mortality and morbidity results from the European Working Party on High Blood Pressure in the Elderly Trial. Lancet 1:1349–54, 1985.

32. European Working Party on High Blood Pressure in the Elderly Trial (EWPHE). Efficacy of antihypertensive drug treatment according to age, sex, blood pressure, and previous cardiovascular disease in patients over the age of 60. Lancet 2:589–92, 1986.

33. SHEP Cooperative Research Group. Prevention of stroke by antihypertensive drug treatment in older persons with isolated systolic hypertension: final results of the Systolic Hypertension in the Elderly Program (SHEP). JAMA 265:3255–64, 1991.

34. Dahlof B, Lindholm LH, Hannson L, et al. Morbidity and mortality in the Swedish Trial in Old Patients with Hypertension (STOP-Hypertension). Lancet 338:1281–85, 1991.

35. MRC Working Party. Medical Research Council trial of treatment of hypertension in older adults: principal results. Br Med J 304:405–11, 1992.

36. Neston JD, Grimm RH Jr, Prineas RJ, et al. Treatment of mild hypertension study: final results. JAMA 270:713–24, 1993.

37. MacGregor GA, Sagnella GA, Markandu ND, et al. Double-blind study of three sodium intakes and long-term effects of sodium restriction in essential hypertension. Lancet 2:1244–47, 1989.

38. Weinberger MH. Is salt restriction relevant and feasible as adjunctive treatment of hypertension? Drugs 39:809–13, 1990.

39. Schotte D, Stunkard AJ. The effect of weight reduction on blood pressure in 301 obese patients. Arch Intern Med 150:1701–04, 1990.

40. Hagberg JM, Seals DR. Exercise training and hypertension. Acta Med Scand Suppl 711:131–36, 1990.

41. Kelemen MH, Effron MB, Valenti SA, et al. Exercise training combined with antihypertensive drug therapy: effects on lipids, blood pressure and left ventricular mass. JAMA 263:2766–71, 1990.

42. Klaus D. Management of hypertension in actively exercising patients: implications of drug selection. Drugs 37:212–18, 1989.

43. Mann SJ, James GD, Wang RS, et al. Elevation of ambulatory systolic blood pressure in hypertensive smokers: a case control study. JAMA 265:2226–28, 1991.

44. Materson BJ, Reda D, Freis ED, et al. Cigarette smoking interferes with treatment of hypertension. Arch Intern Med 148:2116–19, 1988.

45. Beevers DG, Maheswaran R, Potter JF. Alcohol, blood pressure and antihypertensive drugs. J Clin Pharm Ther 15:395–97, 1990.

46. Puddy JB, Beilin LJ, Vandongen R. Regular alcohol use raises blood pressure in treated hypertensive subjects: a randomised controlled trial. Lancet 1:647–51, 1987.

47. Sharp DS, Bentowitz NL. Pharmacoepidemiology of the effect of caffeine on blood pressure. Clin Pharmacol Ther 47:57–60, 1990.

48. Jeong D-U, Dimsdale JE. The effects of caffeine on blood pressure in the work environment. Am J Hypertens 3:749–53, 1990.

49. Stamler R, Stamler J, Grimm R, et al. Nutritional therapy for high blood pressure: final report of a four-year randomized controlled trial-the hypertension control program. JAMA 257:1484–91, 1987.

50. Anderson KM, Wilson WF, Odell PM, Kannel WB. An updated coronary risk profile: a statement for health professionals. Circulation 83:356–61, 1991.

51. Licht JH, Haley RJ, Pugh B, Lewis SB. Diuretic regimens in essential hypertension: a comparison of hypokalemic effects, BP control, and cost. Arch Intern Med 143:1694–99, 1983.

52. Siscovick DS, Psaty BM, Koepsell TD, et al. Diuretic therapy for hypertension and the risk of primary cardiac arrest. N Engl J Med 330:1852–57, 1994.

53. Langford HG, Blaufox D, Borhani NO, et al. Is thiazide-produced uric acid elevation harmful? analysis of data from the Hypertension Detection and Follow-up Program. Arch Intern Med 147:645–49, 1987.

54. Chang SW, Fine R, Siegel D, et al. The impact of diuretic therapy on reported sexual function. Arch Intern Med 151:2402–08, 1991.

55. Bravo EL. Individualizing drug therapy for the hypertensive patient. Hosp Pract 30:97–108, 1995.

56. Wasnich R, Davis J, Ross P, Vogel J. Effect of thiazide on rates of bone mineral loss: a longitudinal study. Br Med J 301:303–05, 1990.

57. Skluth HA, Gums JG. Spironolactone: a re-examination. DICP 24:52–9, 1990.

58. Spence JD, Wong DG, Lindsay RM. Effects of triamterene and amiloride on urinary sediment in hypertensive patients taking hydrochlorothiazide. Lancet 2:73–5, 1985.

59. Zawada ET. Antihypertensive therapy with triamterene-hydrochlorothiazide vs amiloride-hydrochlorothiazide: comparison of effects on urinary prostaglandin E2 excretion. Arch Intern Med 146:1312–14, 1986.

60. Favre L, Glasson P, Valloton MB. Reversible acute renal failure from combined triamterene and indomethacin: a study in healthy subjects. Ann Intern Med 96:317–18, 1982.

61. Hampton JR. Choosing the right β-blocker: a guide to selection. Drugs 48:549–68, 1994.

62. Radack K, Deck C. β-adrenergic blocker therapy does not worsen intermittent claudication in subjects with peripheral arterial disease: a meta-analysis of randomized controlled trials. Arch Intern Med 151:1769–76, 1991.

63. Bright RA, Everitt DE. β-blockers and depression: evidence against an association. JAMA 267:1783–87, 1992.

64. Dornhorst A, Powell SH, Pensky J. Aggravation by propranolol of hyperglycaemic effect of hydrochlorothiazide in type II diabetics without alteration of insulin secretion. Lancet 1:123–26, 1985.

65. Roeback JR Jr, Hla KM, Chambless LE, Fletcher RH. Effects of chromium supplementation on serum high-density lipoprotein cholesterol levels in men taking beta-blockers. Ann Intern Med 115:917–24, 1991.

66. Psaty BM, Koepsell TD, Wagner EH, et al. The relative risk of incident coronary heart disease associated with recently stopping the use of β-blockers. JAMA 263:1653–57, 1990.

67. Leonetti G, Cuspidi C. Choosing the right ACE inhibitor: a guide to selection. Drugs 49:516–35, 1995.

68. Hargreaves MR, Benson MK. Inhaled sodium cromoglycate in angiotensin-converting enzyme inhibitor cough. Lancet 345:13–16, 1995.

69. Herings RMC, de Boer A, Stricker BHC, Leufkens HGM, Porsius A. Hypoglycaemia associated with use of inhibitors of angiotensin converting enzyme. Lancet 345:1195–98, 1995.

70. Baauer JH, Reams GP. The angiotension II type 1 receptor antagonists: a new class of antihypertensive drugs. Arch Intern Med 155:1361, 1995.

71. Cubeddu LX, Aramda K. Somgj B, et al. A comparison of verapamil and propranolol for the intital treatment of hypertension: racial differences in response. JAMA 256:2214–21, 1986.

72. Phillips BG, MacFarlane LL, Carson DS. Calcium-channel blockers and risk of myocardial infarction: more hype than harm. Circulation 92:1074, 1079, 1326, 1995.

73. Khoury AF, Kaplan NM. Alpha-blocker therapy of hypertension: an unfulfilled promise. JAMA 266:394–98, 1991.

74. Weber MA. Clinical pharmacology of centrally acting antihypertensive agents. J Clin Pharmacol 29:598–602, 1989.

75. Langley MS, Heel RC. Transdermal clonidine: a preliminary review of its pharmacodynamic properties and therapeutic efficacy. Drugs 35:123–42, 1988.

76. Mehta JL, Lopez LM. Rebound hypertension following abrupt cessation of clonidine and metoprolol: treatment with labetalol. Arch Intern Med 147:389–90, 1987.

77. Kaplan NM. Management of hypertensive emergencies. Lancet 344:1335–38, 1994.

78. Pettinger WA, Mitchell HC. Side effects of vasodilator therapy. Hypertension 11(suppl II):II–34–36, 1988.

79. Schoenberger JA. Epidemiology and evaluation: steps toward hypertension treatment in the 1990s. Am J Med 90(suppl 4B):4S-7S, 1991.

80. Fneichel RR, Lipicky RJ. Combination products as first-line pharmacotherapy. Arch Intern Med 154:1429–30, 1994.

81. Matterson BJ, Reda DJ, Cushman WC, et al. Single-drug therapy for hypertension in men: a comparison of six antihypertensive agents with placebo. N Engl J Med 328:914–21, 1993.

82. Neaton JD, Grimm RH, Prineas RJ, et al. Treatment of mild hypertension study: final results. JAMA 270:713–24, 1993.

83. Black HR. Treatment of mild hypertension study: the more things change ... [Editorial]. JAMA 270:757–59, 1993.

84. Dannenberg AL, Kannel WB. Remission of hypertension: the "natural" history of blood pressure treatment in the Framingham study. JAMA 257:1477–83, 1987.

85. Jaker M, Atkin S, Soto M, et al. Oral nifedipine vs oral clonidine in the treatment of urgent hypertension. Arch Intern Med 149:260–65, 1991.

86. Schlueter WA, Batle DC. Renal effects of antihypertensive drugs. Drugs 37:900–25, 1989.

87. Inman SR, Stowe NT, Vidt DG. Role of the renal microcirculation in antihypertensive therapy. Cleve Clin J Med 61:356–61, 1994.

88. Christlieb AR. Treatment selection considerations for the hypertensive diabetic patient. Arch Intern Med 150:1167–74, 1990.

89. O'Bryne S, Feely J. Effects of drugs on glucose tolerance in non-insulin dependent diabetics (part I). Drugs 40:6–18, 1990.

90. O'Bryne S, Feely J. Effects of drugs on glucose tolerance in non-insulin dependent diabetics (part II). Drugs 40:203–19, 1990.

91. Kasiske BL, Kalil RSN, Ma JZ, et al. Effect of antihypertensive therapy on the kidney in patients with diabetes: a meta-regression analysis. Ann Intern Med 118:129–38, 1993.

92. Slataper R, Vicknair N, Sadler R, Bakris GL. Comparative effects of different antihypertensive treatments on the progression of diabetic renal disease. Arch Intern Med 153:973–80, 1993.

93. Bennet NE. Hypertension in the elderly. Lancet 344:447–49, 1994.

94. Applegate WB, Pressel S, Wittes J, et al. Impact of the treatment of isolated systemic hypertension on behavioral variables: results from the Systolic Hypertension in the Elderly Program. Arch Intern Med 154:2154–60, 1994.

95. Cooper ES, Kuller LH, Saunders E, et al. Cardiovascular diseases and stroke in African-Americans and other racial minorities in the United States: a statement for health professionals. Circulation 83:1462–80, 1991.

96. Insua JT, Sacks HS, Lau TS, et al. Drug treatment of hypertension in the elderly: a meta-analysis. Ann Intern Med 121:355–62, 1994.

97. O'Malley K, Cox JP, O'Brien E. Choice of drug treatment for elderly hypertensive patients. Am J Med 90(suppl 3A):27S–33S, 1991.

98. National High Blood Pressure Education Program Working Group Report on High Blood Pressure in Pregnancy. Am J Obstet Gynecol 163:1691–1712, 1990.

99. Galley EDM. Hypertension in pregnancy: practical management recommendations. Drugs 49:555–62, 1995.

100. Cangiano JL. Hypertension in Hispanic Americans. Cleve Clin J Med 61:345–50, 1994.

101. Eisner GM. Hypertension: racial differences. Am J Kidney Dis 16(suppl 1):35–40, 1990.

102. Rutledge DR. Race and hypertension: what is clinically relevant. Drugs 47:914–32, 1994.

103. Saunders E, Weir MR, Kong W, et al. A comparison of the efficacy and safety of a β-blocker, a calcium channel blocker, and a converting enzyme inhibitor in hypertensive blacks. Arch Intern Med 150:1707–13, 1990.

104. Zhou H-H, Koshakji RP, Silbertein DJ, et al. Racial differences in drug response: altered sensitivity to and clearance of propranolol in men of Chinese descent as compared to American whites. N Engl J Med 320:565–70, 1989.

105. Ahsan CH, Macklin RB, Challenor VF, et al. Ethnic differences in the pharmacokinetics of oral nifedipine. Br J Clin Pharmacol 31:399-403, 1991.

106. Perez-Stable EJ. Management of mild hypertension: selecting an antihypertensive regimen. West J Med 154:78–87, 1991.

107. Croog SH, Levine S, Testa MA, et al. The effects of antihypertensive therapy on the quality of life. N Engl J Med 314:1657–64, 1986.

108. Croog SH, Kong W, Levine S, et al. Hypertensive black men and women: quality of life and effects of antihypertensive medications. Arch Intern Med 150:1733–41, 1990.

109. Wassertheil-Smoller S, Blaufox D, Oberman A, et al. Effect of antihypertensives on sexual function and quality of life: the TAIM study. Ann Intern Med 114:613–20, 1991.

110. Testa MA, Anderson RB, Nackley JF, Hollenberg NK, the Quality of Life Hypertension Study Group. Quality of life and antihypertension therapy in men: a comparions of captopril and enalapril. N Engl J Med 328:907–13, 1993.

111. Friedman RB, Katt JA. Cost-benefit issues in the practice of internal medicine. Arch Intern Med 151:1165–68, 1991.

112. Edelson JT, Weinstein MC, Tosteson ANA, et al. Long-term cost-effectiveness of various initial monotherapies for mild to moderate hypertension. JAMA 263:407–13, 1990.

113. Kaplan NM. Cost-effectiveness of antihypertensive drugs: fact or fancy? Am J Hypertens 4:478–80, 1991.

114. Hilleman DE, Mohiuddin SM, Lucas D Jr, et al. Cost-minimization analysis of initial antihypertensive therapy in patients with mild-to-moderate essential diastolic hypertension. Clin Ther 16:88-102, 1994.

115. Materson BJ. Sexual dysfunction during antihypertensive treatment. Prog Pharmacol 6:117–24, 1985.

116. Croog SH, Levine S, Sudilovsky A, et al. Sexual symptoms in hypertensive patients. Arch Intern Med 148:788–94, 1988.

117. Beers MH, Passman LJ. Antihypertensive medications and depression. Drugs 40:792–99, 1990.

118. Cruickshank JM, Thorp JM, Zacharias FJ. Benefits and potential harm of lowering high blood pressure. Lancet 1:581–83, 1987.

119. Staessen J, Bulpitt C, Clement D, et al. Relation between mortality and treated blood pressure in elderly patients with hypertension: report of the European Working Party on High Blood Pressure in the Elderly. Br Med J 298:1552–56, 1989.

120. Farnett L, Mulrow CD, Linn WD, et al. The J-curve phenomenon and the treatment of hypertension: is there a point beyond which pressure reduction is dangerous? JAMA 265:489–95, 1991.

121. McCloskey LW, Psaty BM, Koepsell, Aagaard GN. Level of blood pressure and risk of myocardial infarction among treated hypertensive patients. Arch Intern Med 152:513–20, 1992.

122. Working Group on Management of Patients with Hypertension and High Blood Cholesterol. National education programs working group report on the management of patients with hypertension and high blood cholesterol. Ann Intern Med 114:224–37, 1991.

123. Kasiske BL, Ma JZ, Kalil RSN, Louis TA. Effects of antihypertensive therapy on serum lipids. Ann Intern Med 122:133–41, 1995.

124. Samuelsson O, Wilhelmsen L, Andersson OK, et al. Cardiovascular morbidity in relation to change in blood pressure and serum cholesterol levels in treated hypertension: results from the Primary Prevention Trial in Goteborg, Sweden. JAMA 258:1768–76, 1987.

125. Francis Lam YW, Shepherd MM. Drug interactions in hypertensive patients: pharmacokinetic, pharmacodynamic and genetic considerations. Clin Pharmacokinet 18:295–317, 1990.

126. Brown J, Dollery C, Valdes G. Interaction of nonsteroidal anti-inflammatory drugs with antihypertensive and diuretic agents: control of vascular reactivity by endogenous prostanoids. Am J Med 81(suppl 2B):43–57, 1986.

127. Winickoff RN, Murphy PK. The persistent problem of poor blood pressure control. Arch Intern Med 147:1393–96, 1987.

128. McClellan WM, Hall W, Brogan D, et al. Continuity of care in hypertension: an important correlate of blood pressure control among aware hypertensives. Arch Intern Med 148:525–28, 1988.

129. Lachman BE. Increasing patient compliance through tracking systems. Calif Pharm 34:54–8, 1987.

130. Oto-Kent DS. Controlling hypertension: pharmacists can make a difference. Calif Pharm 36:42–3, 1989.

131. McKenney JM, Slining JM, Henderson HR, et al. The effect of clinical pharmacy services on patients with essential hypertension. Circulation 48:1104–11, 1973.

132. Hawkins DW, Fiedler FP, Douglas HL, Eschbach RE. Evaluation of a clinical pharmacist in caring for hypertensive and diabetic patients. Am J Hosp Pharm 36:1321–26, 1979.

CHAPTER 38

CONGESTIVE HEART FAILURE

PAUL E. NOLAN, Jr, CYNTHIA L. RAEHL, and DAWN G. ZAREMBSKI

DEFINITION OF THE DISEASE

Although a precise definition of congestive heart failure (CHF) remains elusive (1), CHF can be defined as a clinical syndrome characterized by dyspnea and fatigue (2). These symptoms are caused by left ventricular (LV) dysfunction and resultant activation of cardiac and peripheral neurohormonal maladaptive mechanisms that promote fluid retention. However, there is a subgroup of patients with LV dysfunction who are asymptomatic. This subgroup is considered to have heart failure (HF) but without symptoms. The primary cardiac mechanisms that underlie the clinical syndrome of CHF and asymptomatic HF are systolic (i.e., contracting) dysfunction and diastolic (i.e., filling) dysfunction, either alone or in combination.

ETIOLOGY

In 1971 the Framingham Study, a community-based epidemiologic investigation, reported that hypertension (HTN) preceded CHF in 75% of all cases; coronary artery disease (CAD) was implicated in 39% of cases; 29% of all patients had CAD with accompanying HTN; rheumatic heart disease (RHD) was observed in 21% of cases; and both RHD and HTN were seen in 11% of all patients (3). Miscellaneous causes accounted for 5% of the cases and included congenital heart disease, thyrotoxicosis, atrial fibrillation, and idiopathic dilated cardiomyopathy. These can ultimately cause decreases either in the contractile performance of the heart (i.e., systolic dysfunction) or in the ability of the heart to adequately fill during diastole (i.e., diastolic dysfunction) (Table 38.1). A more recent report from the Framingham Study indicates that the percentage of patients with CAD as an attributable cause of CHF has risen to 54% of all cases, and CAD is found with accompanying HTN 31% of the time (4). These results are consistent with those from some hospital-based studies of CHF, which have reported CAD as the most common cause of CHF (5). Despite these findings, an antecedent diagnosis of HTN, either alone or in conjunction with other causes, remains the most common risk factor for CHF in the community, occurring in 74% of patients (4).

Drugs are a relatively uncommon cause of CHF. They are generally implicated as causes of dilated cardiomyopathies (6). The anthracycline antineoplastic agent doxoru-

bicin is a well-described cause of CHF. Other anthracycline antineoplastics as well as bleomycin and cocaine also may cause CHF. In some series, excessive ethanol ingestion may cause up to 40% of the cases of idiopathic dilated cardiomyopathy (5).

INCIDENCE/PREVALENCE

Heart failure is becoming an increasingly prevalent health care problem with notable socioeconomic consequences (7). Approximately 3.5 million Americans are afflicted with HF. These patients account for nearly 2.3 million hospital discharges and about 11.4 million outpatient visits. The estimated total (i.e., including cardiac transplantation) health care cost for treating HF is $38.1 billion.

Approximately 700,000 new cases are diagnosed yearly, with about 280,000 deaths (7). Therefore there is a net increase of over 400,000 patients with HF per year. Although HF can occur at any age, there is a remarkable increase with advancing age. According to data obtained from the Framingham study, CHF occurs in 1% of the U.S. population aged 50 to 59 years and doubles with each subsequent decade (8).

PATHOGENESIS

Several generalized pathophysiologic conditions can lead to the development of HF (9). These include pressure

Table 38.1.
Etiology of Heart Failure

A. *Systolic Dysfunction*
   Decreased EF and increased LVEDV and increased LVEDP
   Hypertension
   Coronary artery disease
   Idiopathic
   Valvular disease (e.g., mitral or aortic regurgitation)
   Drug-induced (e.g., doxorubicin, ethanol)
B. *Diastolic Dysfunction*
   Normal or increased EF and increased LVEDP, but with normal or decreased LVEDV
   Hypertension
   Coronary artery disease
   Restrictive cardiomyopathies (e.g., amyloidosis)
   Valvular heart disease (e.g., aortic stenosis)
   Hypertrophic cardiomyopathy (e.g., IHSS)

EF = ejection fraction; LVEDV = left ventricular end-diastolic volume; LVEDP = left ventricular end-diastolic pressure; IHSS = idiopathic hypertrophic subaortic stenosis.

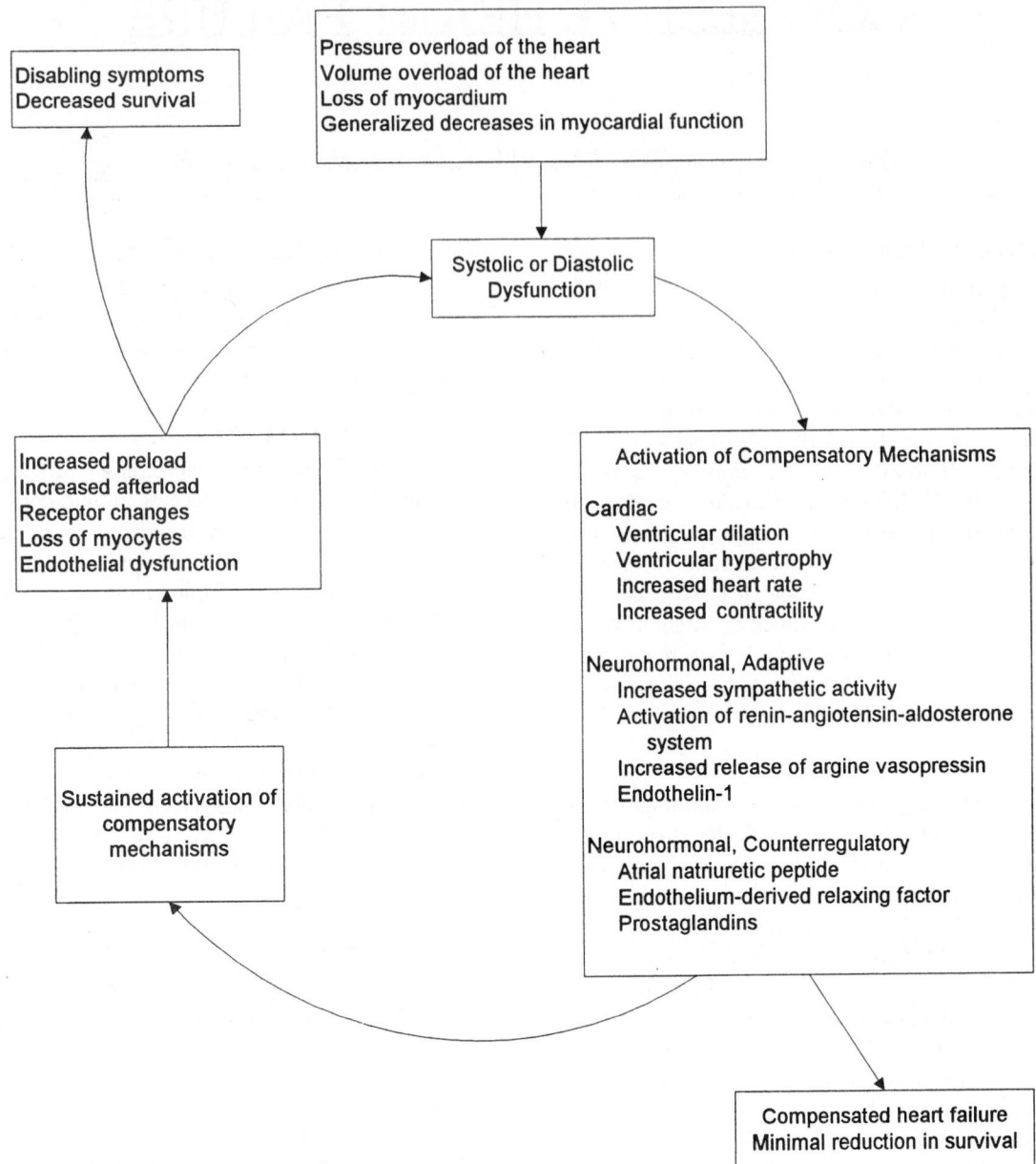

Figure 38.1. Pathogenesis of congestive heart failure.

overload of the heart (e.g., HTN or aortic stenosis), volume overload (e.g., mitral or aortic valve regurgitation), loss of functional myocardial tissue (e.g., acute myocardial infarction), a generalized decrease in myocardial contractility (e.g., several types of dilated cardiomyopathies) or restricted filling (e.g., constrictive pericarditis or amyloidosis). These conditions can manifest as a reduction in systolic emptying (i.e., systolic dysfunction) or diastolic relaxation and filling (i.e., diastolic dysfunction). Systolic and diastolic dysfunction in turn can lead to a decrease in stroke volume and cardiac output. The decrease in cardiac output is sensed as a decrease in end-organ perfusion pressure by arterial baroreceptors (1).

In response to decreased cardiac output, a number of compensatory (i.e., adaptive) responses, many of which are neurohormonally mediated, become activated (Figure 38.1) (9–12). Within the heart, ventricular dilation and hypertrophy (i.e., ventricular remodeling) occur. The former develops in response to an elevated end-diastolic pressure, a consequence of either systolic or diastolic dysfunction. An elevated end-diastolic pressure produces mechanical stretch, which stimulates myocyte lengthening through replication of sarcomeres in series (i.e., ventricular dilation) (10). Ventricular dilation is an attempt to increase preload or end-diastolic volume to increase cardiac output (9, 12). As the ventricular chamber increases in size, it can fill to a greater extent during diastole, and consequently stroke volume will increase during systole. This response is often depicted by the Frank-Starling relationship between systolic performance and diastolic filling. Preload is determined largely by the extracellular fluid volume and venous return. However, an increase in preload may raise systolic wall tension. According to the LaPlace relationship, systolic wall tension equals the product of aortic pressure (P) times the internal radius of the ventricle (R) divided by 2 times the wall thickness (2h), that is, $[T = (P \times R)/2h]$. Preload is a component of wall tension in that it corresponds to the internal radius of the ventricular chamber. Therefore increases in preload will increase wall tension.

Cardiac myocyte hypertrophy or an increase in wall thickness also occurs, especially in response to pressure overload, and is the result of an increase in the diameter of myocytes through the parallel addition of new sarcomeres (9–12). This response is analogous to a weightlifter's increase in skeletal muscle size in response to lifting heavier weights. According to the LaPlace equation, the increase in wall thickness should result in a reduction in wall tension (or afterload) imposed on individual myocytes. Afterload refers to the hemodynamic load against which the ventricle must contract to deliver its stroke volume. Afterload corresponds to the systolic wall tension defined previously. A major peripheral component of afterload is the systemic arteriolar tone or systemic vascular resistance, which is also a component of blood pressure (i.e., P in the LaPlace equation).

The increases in preload and cardiac hypertrophy are mediated largely by initial activation of the sympathetic nervous system (SNS) and secondary activation of the renin-angiotensin-aldosterone (RAA) system (9–12). Mechanical stretch can also stimulate hypertrophy. Norepinephrine (NE) stimulates the release of renin by the kidney. Renin, both locally and systemically, first acts on angiotensinogen to convert it to angiotensin I (AI). AI is then converted to angiotensin II (AII) by angiotensin-converting enzyme (ACE). AII also can be synthesized via ACE-independent pathways (13). NE and AII serve as mitogens for cardiac myocytes to increase the number of sarcomeres (i.e., cardiac hypertrophy) (10–13). AII stimulates the release of aldosterone from the adrenals and facilitates secretion of arginine vasopressin (AVP) (9, 12). Aldosterone and AVP trigger renal sodium and water retention, respectively. Blood volume is expanded, and therefore preload is augmented. AII also enhances the formation of preproendothelin by endothelial cells (10). Preproendothelin is cleaved to form endothelin-1, which can stimulate release of renin and aldosterone as well as conversion of AI to AII in endothelial cells. Therefore endothelin-1 also promotes sodium retention. In addition, myocardial contractility is enhanced because NE and AII are positive inotropic agents, the former via stimulation of

β_1 receptors (9, 12, 13). NE also increases heart rate via β-receptor stimulation. Increases in contractility and heart rate coupled with the increases in preload and myocardial hypertrophy serve to maintain cardiac output (9, 12).

In the peripheral circulation, NE, AII, and endothelin-1 also promote systemic vasoconstriction via stimulation of vascular α, AII, and endothelin receptors, respectively, to maintain perfusion pressure (10, 12). However, systemic vasoconstriction causes an increase in afterload. Sustained increases in afterload can lead to a decreased stroke volume and cardiac output, especially in advanced CHF. This increase in afterload can be compensated by release of atrial natriuretic peptide (ANP) in response to atrial stretch, which occurs as a consequence of increased preload (12). ANP inhibits the release of NE and produces vasodilatory and natriuretic effects to reduce the hemodynamic load on the heart. Endothelium-derived relaxing factor (EDRF or nitric oxide) and selected prostaglandins may also promote vasodilation.

Thus in the beginning, a balance appears to exist between vasoconstrictor and vasodilator systems (9, 12). However, with time, the initial adaptive responses can overshoot (i.e., become maladaptive) (9), and there is a progressive, vicious cycle in the disease process, leading to a manifestation of the symptoms of CHF and usually death. Within the heart, sustained ventricular remodeling results in side-to-side slippage of myocytes and further ventricular dilation to increase preload; deposition of collagen among myocytes, which increases tissue stiffness, decreases compliance, and elevates end-diastolic pressure; continued myocyte hypertrophy, which produces myocyte energy starvation from decreases in capillary density coupled with increases both in the distance between perfusing capillaries and in ATP-consuming myofibrils and contributes to myocyte cell death; and increases in wall tension on surviving myocytes (9–12).

Continuous activation of neurohormonal responses also occurs to maintain an effective cardiac output (9, 12). However, these sustained neurohormonal responses are ultimately deleterious. Sustained increased concentrations of NE subsequently results in a diminished contractile response due to down-regulation of β (predominantly β_1) receptors and uncoupling of β receptors (12). In addition, increased, persistent activation of the SNS is directly cardiotoxic, impairs parasympathetic influence on the heart, diminishes the normal arterial baroreceptor response, and is proarrhythmic (9, 14). Peripheral vasoconstriction is further augmented by NE, AII, and endothelin-1 (9, 12). Vasodilator capacity is also impaired, perhaps because of increased sodium content of peripheral vessels (12). In addition, circulating cytokines such as tumor necrosis factor alpha (TNF-α) (15) and interleukin-1 (IL-1) (16) may diminish endothelial-mediated vasorelaxation as well as produce negative inotropic effects (15).

Counterregulatory vasodilator responses to ANP, EDRF, and prostaglandins become overwhelmed (9, 12). Enhanced sodium and water retention override counterbalancing salt-excreting systems (ANP and prostaglandins) and further expand intravascular volume and pressure, resulting in circulatory congestion and edema. Alterations in skeletal muscle structure and function produce fatigue and exercise intolerance (10).

In summary, heart failure begins when myocardial and peripheral adaptive responses are activated to maintain an effective perfusion pressure. Heart failure progresses when these compensatory, chiefly neurohormonally mediated responses persist. This leads to a series of deleterious effects on the heart, circulation, and end-organs and results in the manifestation of disabling symptoms and ultimately death.

DIAGNOSIS AND CLINICAL FINDINGS

Knowledge of the pathophysiology of CHF easily predicts the expected signs, symptoms, and associated laboratory findings (17). However, many patients with impaired left ventricular ejection fractions may exhibit no signs of symptoms of CHF. Up to 20% of individuals with ejection fractions less than 40% may not meet clinical criteria diagnostic for CHF (18). Nonetheless, most patients with diminished ejection fractions (<40%) will exhibit signs and symptoms characteristic of CHF. Characteristic symptoms of CHF include weight gain and pulmonary congestion. Weight gain secondary to salt and water retention is common in heart failure patients. Increases in extracellular and plasma volume lead to congested pulmonary and systemic circulations. Pulmonary congestion is manifest by varying degrees of breathlessness: dyspnea on exertion (DOE), orthopnea (dyspnea that occurs in the supine position), paroxysmal nocturnal dyspnea (PND, an exaggerated form of orthopnea, which occurs when the patient is awakened abruptly at night with a feeling of suffocation), dyspnea at rest, and pulmonary edema (fluid accumulation within the alveoli). Some patients complain of cough or asthma symptoms.

Typically, dyspnea on exertion is the first symptom of CHF that develops (19). As the disease progresses, the degree of physical activity that produces dyspnea is reduced. Patients with severe CHF will complain of dyspnea at rest. Orthopnea occurs within minutes after assumption of a supine position. A supine position will place the lower extremities on the same vertical plane as the heart. Venous pooling, which occurs while standing will be reduced, and the fluid will be reintroduced into the circulatory system, leading to pulmonary congestion. Sitting upright will relieve orthopnea once it occurs. Orthopnea is often circumvented by increasing the number of pillows the patient uses when sleeping. Paroxysmal nocturnal dyspnea awakens the patient after 2 to 4 hr of sleep with the feeling of suffocation. Relief is obtained by maintaining an upright position and may take up to 30 min to occur. Severe pulmonary congestion, with accumulation of fluid in the alveoli, can occur, producing pulmonary edema. Patients may experience severe shortness of breath and anxiety as a result. Often, patients with pulmonary edema will expectorate a pink, frothy sputum.

Systemically, inadequate perfusion of the skeletal muscles often leads to easy fatigability and weakness. Exercise tolerance is diminished, and patients adjust their lifestyle accordingly, such as no longer walking up a flight of steps. Nocturia (increased urine formation at night), which results from redistribution of blood flow to the kidney during recumbency, often occurs early in the course of CHF. Oliguria may become manifest later as the patient's heart failure worsens. A host of cerebral symptoms may also be observed and can include impairment of memory, confusion, and insomnia.

A number of cardiac and systemic physical findings are observed with varying frequencies. An early diastolic third heart sound, S3 (i.e., Ken-tuc'-ky", where "Ken," "tuc," and "ky," represent S_1, S_2, and S_3, respectively), is believed to be related to impaired diastolic relaxation of the ventricle and suggests an elevated end-diastolic pressure. An S_3 is a hallmark of moderate-to-severe heart failure (20). A resting sinus tachycardia is often present. Objective cardiac findings often include an enlarged heart (palpable as a cardiac heave) and increased cardiothoracic ratio (>0.50) as determined by chest radiograph; a diminished ejection fraction as determined by echocardiography, coronary arteriography, or radionuclide techniques; and an enlarged left ventricular chamber size as evidenced by echocardiography or radionuclide techniques.

Systemic venous congestion may manifest as dependent peripheral edema, jugular venous distention (JVD), and congestive hepatomegaly. A minimal gain of approximately 10 pounds of extracellular fluid volume is necessary before peripheral edema is noted. This edema usually develops in the gravity-dependent areas of the body such as in the ankles, in the feet, or above the shinbone (i.e., pretibial) in ambulatory patients and in the sacral area when the patient is supine. Peripheral edema may be physically uncomfortable as well as cosmetically unattractive. Central venous pressure (CVP) is estimated by elevating the patient's head to a 45 degree angle and observing the peak of the maximal venous pulsation within the internal jugular vein. In this position the CVP does not normally exceed 2 cm of vertical distance above the sternal angle. Because the sternal angle usually lies about 5 cm above the right atrium, the CVP can be estimated by noting the vertical distance and adding 5 cm to the value. The liver is also characteristically congested in CHF and is generally palpable several centimeters below the right costal margin. Pressure placed on the abdomen will further increase the jugular venous pressure (as the right ventricle is unable to accept the increased blood returned to the heart) and produce a positive hepatojugular reflex. Hepatic edema may cause right upper quadrant pain. Generalized visceral edema may also occur and cause abdominal distention and anorexia.

The presence of any single symptom warrants further diagnostic examination with consideration of CHF as a possible cause. It is important to remember that symptoms alone are not indicative or exclusive for CHF and that proper evaluation will include consideration of the clinical presentation and potential underlying causes. Past medical history is important to elicit the presence of prior myocardial infarction, hypertension, and valvular disease.

An understanding of the previously described cardio-vascular physical examination is essential to monitoring the efficacy of heart failure therapy. Along with medical history and chest radiograph, clinicians have relied on the presence of an S_3, pulmonary rales, an abnormal jugular venous pressure, and peripheral edema to monitor CHF. However, in chronic heart failure, cardiocirculatory compensatory mechanisms make these physical signs less reliable. Patients can have very high left ventricular filling pressures but no detectable rales because the lymphatic drainage has increased proportionately (21). Third heart sounds are commonly present and therefore are nonspecific in filling pressures. Signs of venous congestion are often absent, given the effects of diuretics and vasodilators. However, the blood pressure measurement can provide information that helps to assess the adequacy of heart failure therapy. Neither systolic blood pressure (SBP) nor diastolic blood pressure (DBP) alone is an adequate measure. Rather, the proportional pulse pressure [(SBP – DBP)/SBP] can be used because it represents the activation of compensatory mechanisms and cardiac output. The proportional pulse pressure can identify patients with a low cardiac index. Because most patients with severe chronic heart failure have a SBP of 100 mm Hg or less, the pulse pressure as a proportion of total systolic pressure is useful. Stevenson and colleagues found a proportional pulse pressure <25% in 91% of patients with cardiac index of ≤2.2 L/min/m (2, 21).

Numerous laboratory abnormalities are observed in patients with CHF. Simple laboratory tests (e.g., serum electrolytes, serum creatinine and blood urea nitrogen chest, and serum digoxin concentrations), body weight, and chest radiograph are used most frequently in monitoring ambulatory patients with congestive heart failure (22). The patient can monitor body weight at home every several days, and serum electrolytes and markers of renal function are checked about every 1 to 2 months, provided that there are no changes in therapy. Total body sodium is frequently increased. However, a dilutional hyponatremia is frequently seen, owing to a diminished ability to excrete free

Table 38.2.
Classification Systems for Congestive Heart Failure

New York Heart Association Functional Classification

Class I: No limitation; ordinary physical activity does not cause symptoms

Class II: Slight limitation of physical activity; ordinary activity results in symptoms

Class III: Marked limitation of physical activity; less than ordinary activity leads to symptoms

Class IV: Inability to carry on any activity without symptoms; symptoms are present at rest

Classification of Heart Failure Based on Maximal Exercise Tolerance

Class A: No impairment; VO_{2max} ≥ 20 mL/min/kg

Class B: Mild to moderate impairment; VO_{2max} = 16–20 mL/min/kg

Class C: Moderate to severe impairment; VO_{2max} = 10–15 mL/min/kg

Class D: Severe impairment; VO_{2max} ≤ 10 mL/min/kg

*VO_{2max} = maximal oxygen uptake. It is a function of the maximum cardiac output that the heart can generate and the maximal amount of oxygen (O_2) that the exercising tissues can extract.

water. Hyponatremia may worsen with diuretic treatment. Patients with CHF generally have deficits of both total body and intracellular potassium and magnesium, which may or may not be reflected in the serum concentrations of these cations (23). Potentially lethal ventricular arrhythmias may occur as secondary consequences of electrolyte imbalances. Impaired hepatic function may occur secondary to venous congestion and may be characterized by elevations in plasma concentrations of hepatic enzymes. Reductions in renal blood flow and glomerular filtration rate will be reflected by increases in both serum creatinine and blood urea nitrogen (BUN) levels. The urine is usually concentrated, with a high urine specific gravity, and there may be associated proteinuria. More sophisticated measures of cardiac function, such as echocardiography, radionuclide ventriculography, or exercise testing, are used less frequently and at longer intervals (usually every 12 to 24 months).

To evaluate both the severity of heart failure and the responses to therapy, two classification systems have been developed: the New York Heart Association (NYHA) Functional Classification (24) and a classification based on exercise tolerance (25) (Table 38.2). Unfortunately, these classification systems do not correlate well. The NYHA classification, despite its reliance on subjective findings during exertion, is commonly used to classify the severity of CHF (24). Because patients often downgrade their expectations for exercise tolerance as their failure progresses, they may underestimate the impact of their disease. Most likely, the NYHA classification will remain popular among practitioners because of its simplicity and convenience. Other measures of quality of life in heart failure include the Chronic Heart Failure Questionnaire, the Specific Activity Scale, the Minnesota Living with

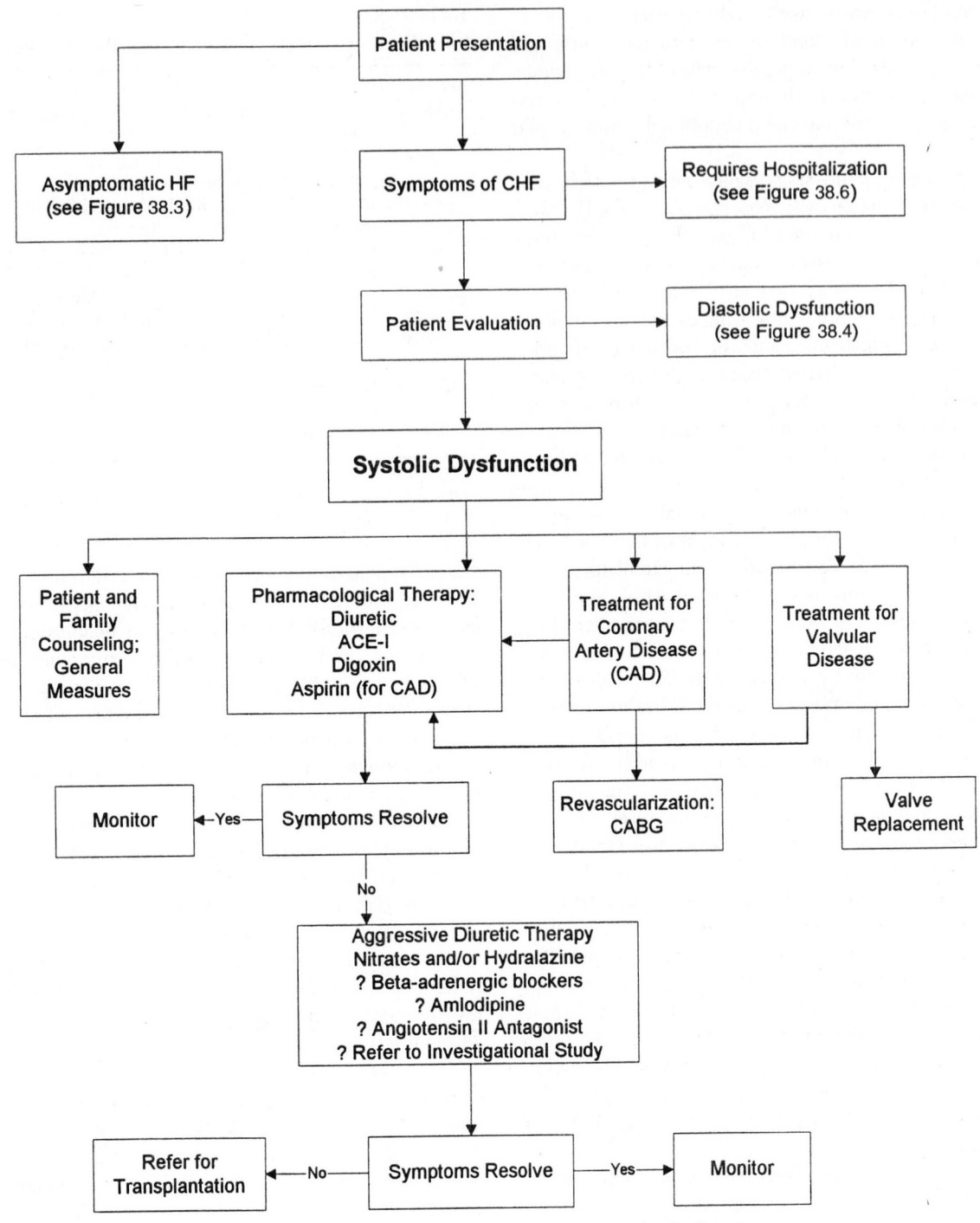

Figure 38.2.   Treatment of symptomatic systolic dysfunction.

Heart Failure Questionnaire, the Yale Scale, and the Quality of Life Questionnaire in Severe Heart Failure (26).

The exercise tolerance classification system uses an incremental treadmill exercise protocol and noninvasive monitoring of respiratory gas exchange, heart rate, and blood pressure to grade the severity of chronic CHF (25). Maximal oxygen uptake (VO$_{2max}$, expressed in milliliters per minute per kilogram) is determined by maximal cardiac output and by maximal oxygen extraction by the exercising muscles. Despite its relative objectivity and prognostic usefulness, it is a more complex, costly, and time-consuming method for evaluating levels of CHF and responses to therapy. Furthermore, it is effort-dependent and may not be representative of the usual degree of physical activity of the typical patient. An alternative

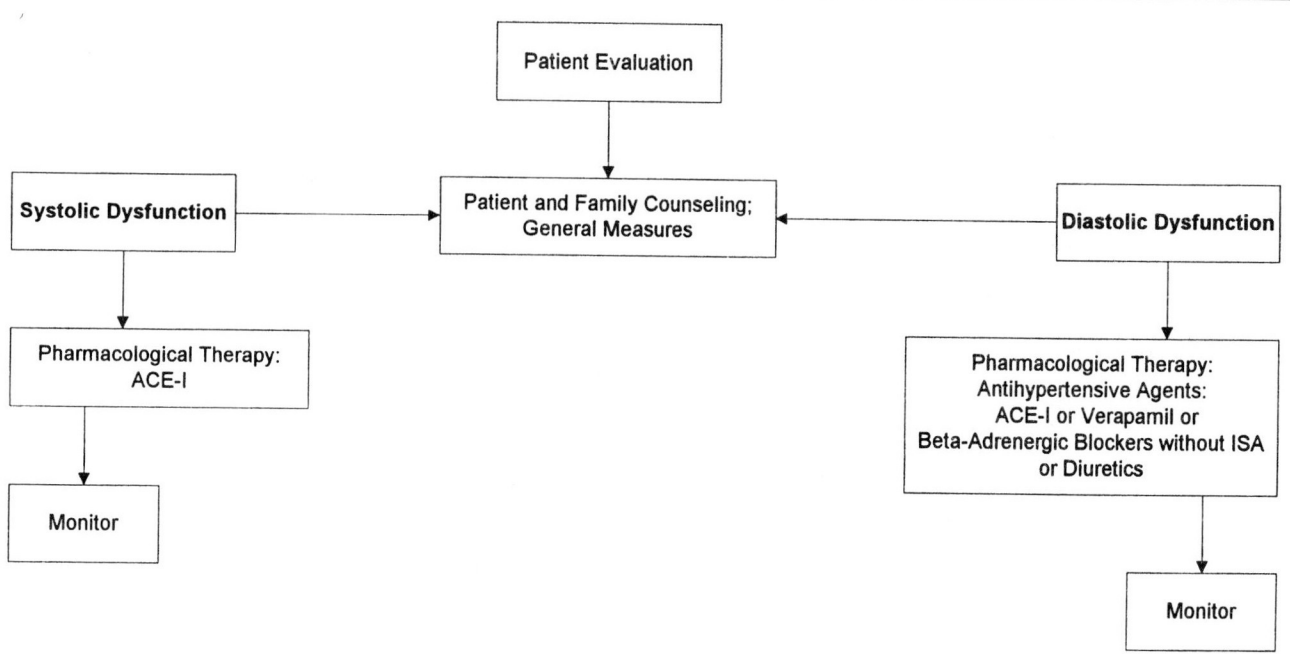

Figure 38.3. Treatment of asymptomatic heart failure.

measure of quantifying exercise capacity in patients with CHF is the 6-minute walk (27).

TREATMENT OF CHRONIC CHF SECONDARY TO SYSTOLIC DYSFUNCTION

The basic goals in the treatment of CHF are (a) to relieve the symptoms due to central and circulatory congestion and to improve quality of life, (b) to prevent occurrence or progression of the disease, and (c) to prolong life (28). New therapies should neither worsen symptoms nor shorten life. Therapeutic goals are achieved by using a combination of patient education (29), nonpharmacologic interventions (30), and pharmacologic interventions (30, 31). Nonpharmacologic treatment consists of salt restriction, initial reduction of the heart's workload with abbreviated rest followed by exercise training on recovery, lifestyle changes, and identification and treatment of precipitating causes (29, 30). Currently, pharmacologic therapy of CHF consists of vasodilators (usually angiotensin-converting enzyme inhibitors, ACE-I), diuretics, and mild inotropic enhancement with digitalis glycosides (30, 31).

The majority of this chapter is devoted to the treatment of symptomatic and asymptomatic heart failure due to systolic dysfunction (Figures 38.2 and 38.3, respectively). Heart failure secondary to diastolic dysfunction is treated much differently and is therefore discussed in a separate section (Figures 38.3 and 38.4).

GENERAL MEASURES

Ideally, initial measures in the management of CHF should focus on preventing development of the disease (29, 30). For example, alteration of correctable risk factors for CAD,

a major etiologic factor for the development of CHF, should be attempted. Proper prevention should include attempts to normalize serum lipids, blood pressure, and body weight. Patient education should also emphasize the importance of smoking cessation and moderate exercise.

Proper management of CHF should include attempts to modify or correct systemic diseases causing or precipitating CHF exacerbations (30). Coronary artery disease, if present, may impair ventricular function through ongoing myocardial ischemia. Attempts at revascularization in appropriate patients may help in enhancing both ventricular function and survival. Patients with valvular disease may benefit from attempts to surgically repair or replace defective myocardial valves. In patients with symptomatic bradycardia, optimal cardiac output can be ensured through the maintenance of sinus rhythm with the placement of a pacemaker. Additional precipitating factors include systemic infection, pulmonary embolism, hypocalcemia, anemia, and endocrine disorders (e.g., hyperthyroidism).

Initial restriction of physical activity to some degree has been a therapeutic maneuver used in the management of virtually any patient with CHF (29). However, severe restrictions on physical activity may worsen a patient's exercise tolerance and lead to additional psychological problems. Current recommendations limit physical activity to that which the patient tolerates. In addition, many patients with CHF will benefit from a prescribed cardiac rehabilitation program. Strenuous physical activity may not be tolerated even by individuals with compensated CHF. However, regular aerobic exercise can enhance the cardiovascular system and improve exercise tolerance (32, 33). General improvement in physical condition can be accom-

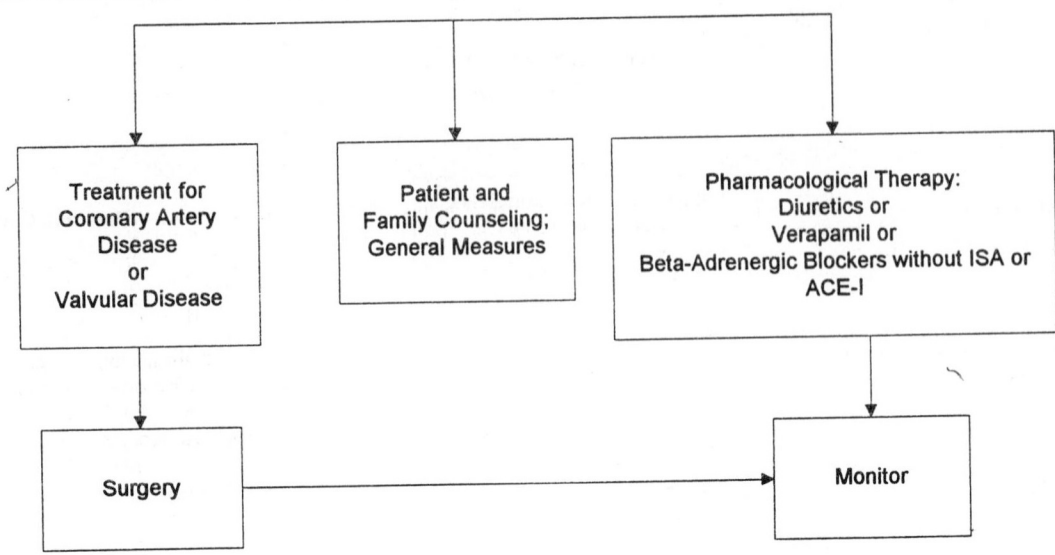

Figure 38.4. Treatment of symptomatic diastolic dysfunction.

panied by hemodynamic benefits, including reduction of the resting heart rate, reduction of exercise associated peak systolic blood pressure, and an improvement in the tissue extraction of oxygen. Patients' capacity to exercise will vary widely. Therefore each patient should receive individualized instruction. It is not possible to predict exercise tolerance from either the LVEF or other clinical parameters. However, patients who cannot increase their cardiac output with exercise will probably do poorly. These patients will often drop their systolic pressure while exercising, a finding that suggests that no cardiac reserve remains. Such patients may not tolerate any exercise program. Similarly, patients who have recently experienced a myocardial infarction should begin exercising only under the direction of a health care practitioner. Heart failure patients should "begin low and go slow," thereby avoiding overexertion. Many patients prefer walking programs. Such programs may improve mental health and combat some of the psychological dilemmas that CHF patients typically have.

Patient education should also focus on proper nutrition, with special attention to the potential harm of excess sodium intake (29). Limiting a patient's salt intake helps to counteract the exaggerated renal retention of sodium. Elimination of added salt and the removal of high-sodium foods (e.g., salted nuts, pretzels, salt-cured meats, potato chips, pickles, olives, processed meats, some canned vegetables and soups) will decrease daily sodium intake to about 1.5 to 3.0 g (3.75 to 7.5 g of sodium chloride, since 1.0 g Na = 2.5 g NaCl). The typical U.S. diet contains twice this amount of sodium. Exclusion of all salt from cooking will further reduce the patient's sodium intake to between 1.2 and 1.5 g. However, excessive sodium restriction may reduce the palatability of food and may secondarily compromise adequate nutrition. The use of spices to flavor various foods should be encouraged and may enhance patient compliance with a low-sodium diet. Note that over-the-counter medications may be a hidden source of sodium intake.

Patient noncompliance with prescribed medical and pharmacologic regimens often precipitates worsening of CHF. In a study of patients admitted to a Chicago hospital for heart failure treatment, 64% were noncompliant with their medical regimens (34). Almost one-half of the patients in this study had uncontrolled hypertension as a precipitating factor for heart failure. Hospital admissions may be reduced through proper attention to patient education (35).

Some prescription medications may also precipitate exacerbations of CHF. Beta-adrenergic blocking therapy initiated at the usual antihypertensive doses and "first-generation" calcium channel-blocking agents (e.g., verapamil, diltiazem, and nifedipine) are representative examples. Furthermore, the addition of antiarrhythmic agents with negative inotropic properties can worsen preexisting heart failure. Stricter attention to these precipitating factors could significantly reduce the number of hospitalizations and ease the clinical and economic burden of CHF on both patients and society.

VASODILATORS

Vasodilator therapy has provided new promise for the treatment of CHF (36). These agents have been shown to alter the capacitance (preload) and resistance (afterload) vessels either directly or indirectly. The net result is that vasodilators enhance physiologic performance of the diseased left ventricle; they relieve symptoms of dyspnea; and they improve exercise tolerance. Since investigations of the early 1970s, vasodilator therapy has become an integral component in the treatment of patients with chronic CHF.

Most important, current evidence strongly suggests that vasodilator therapy, when added to digoxin and diuretics, is the only drug treatment modality that favorably alters mortality in patients with CHF (37–41). In general, the selection and dose of a vasodilating agent for chronic CHF management should be based on studies that have evaluated the long-term beneficial and adverse effects of an agent (Table 38.3). The following section describes several vasodilators that are used in the treatment of CHF from an historic perspective. However, unless a patient is unable to tolerate ACE-I, vasodilator therapy should begin with ACE-I.

Nitrates

Nitrates are one of the initial groups of vasodilating agents used in the management of CHF (42). These agents predominantly decrease preload through vasodilation of venous capacitance vessels. Nitrates may also improve cardiac function by decreasing afterload via dilatation of large arteries and arterioles, especially following acute administration and when used in high doses in the management of patients with CHF. However, the afterload-reducing effects of nitrates are generally minimal, and they are therefore combined with other vasodilators that have greater afterload-reducing effects, such as hydralazine. However, nitrates alone are often effective in relieving pulmonary congestion associated with CHF. In a study using nitrate monotherapy (i.e., isosorbide dinitrate) for patients with CHF, clinical status was improved, treadmill exercise time increased, and cardiac dimensions were reduced after 3 months of therapy. Therefore nitrates may be added to other therapeutic regimens (37, 38, 43).

Of the available nitrate formulations that are used in treating chronic CHF, oral isosorbide dinitrate (ISDN) is the most frequently prescribed and well-studied agent. Although many large clinical trials have used a four-times-daily dosing strategy, ISDN is most frequently prescribed in doses of 10 to 80 mg three times a day, retaining about a 12-hr nitrate-free dosing interval. It no longer seems important to give the highest dose that an individual patient tolerates. Rather, it is more important to use a dosing regimen that allows nitroglycerin levels to fluctuate, thereby better avoiding the problem of nitrate tolerance induced by constant nitrate plasma levels (44).

Nitrate tolerance has been consistently demonstrated when the vascular endothelium is constantly exposed to nitroglycerin (44). Investigation into this issue has revealed that tolerance appears to be mediated by depletion of sulfhydryl groups at the cellular level and is associated with undesirable reflex neurohormonal stimulation, producing fluid retention. A variety of agents have been used to attempt to prevent the development of nitrate tolerance, including the use sulfhydryl-containing compounds, ACE

inhibitors, and diuretics. All of these strategies have produced mixed results. Intermittent three-times-daily (administration at 7:00 A.M., 12:00 noon, and 5:00 P.M.) dosing of nitrates appears to be the most pragmatic and perhaps effective mechanism to minimize the development of tolerance. If nitroglycerin patches are prescribed, they should be applied for 12 hr and then removed for 12 hr. Because most patients experience dyspnea on exertion during the waking hours, the nitrate-free interval is usually at night. These intermittent dosage regimens do not preclude the administration of short-acting sublingual tablets or lingual spray nitroglycerin for episodes of either acute dyspnea or angina.

The most frequently encountered adverse nitrate effect is headache, which often responds to mild analgesics such as acetaminophen. Headaches usually disappear after several days of nitrate administration. Some patients will continue to experience severe headaches with nitrates and therefore may not tolerate any nitrate administration. Dizziness, flushing, postural hypotension, weakness, and occasionally skin rash are also reported. In summary, nitrates are safe and effective vasodilators that are useful as adjunctive therapy to hydralazine (37, 38) or ACE-I (43) in the treatment of CHF.

Hydralazine

Hydralazine is a direct-acting arteriolar dilator that principally reduces afterload. Reductions in afterload by hydralazine may also result in moderate reductions in preload because of the dependence of left ventricular filling pressure on the resistance to ventricular emptying during systole. Hydralazine can markedly reduce left ventricular filling pressure in patients with either mitral or aortic valve regurgitation. Clinically, hydralazine is most commonly used together with other vasodilators that possess greater preload-reducing properties such as nitrates (37, 38).

Two investigations have evaluated the long-term clinical effects of hydralazine monotherapy in CHF (45, 46). The first study was a double-blind, randomized trial comparing hydralazine, approximately 50 mg every 6 hr, with placebo for up to 26 weeks (45). There were no differences between the two groups in assessment of clinical status, in maximal treadmill exercise duration, or in mortality. The second trial was of similar design and compared hydralazine at an average dose of 50 mg every 8 hr with placebo for 1 year (46). The hydralazine group improved both in exercise duration and in symptomatic status. However, almost one-half of the patients who were originally enrolled in the hydralazine group withdrew from the study (compared to 40% in the placebo group), and the 1-year mortality rate was approximately 30% for both groups. Thus, when administered as a single vasodilator at maximal doses of up to 225 mg/day, hydralazine may

Table 38.3.
Vasodilator Drugs

Drug	Principal Site of Action	General Mechanism(s) of Action	Initial Dose	Target Dose	Recommended Maximal Dose	Adverse Effects	Drug Interactions
Isosorbide dinitrate[a] (ISDN)	Venous vasodilator	Direct-acting vasodilator	10 mg t.i.d.[b]	40 mg t.i.d.	80 mg t.i.d.	Headache, dizziness, flushing, postural hypotension	Other vasodilators (increased risk of hypotension)
Hydralazine[c]	Arteriolar vasodilator	Direct-acting vasodilator	10–25 mg t.i.d.	75 mg t.i.d.	100 mg t.i.d.	Headache, palpitations, postural hypotension, nausea, vomiting, systemic lupus erythematosus, increases in heart rate, myocardial ischemia, fluid retention	Same as for ISDN
Angiotensin-converting enzyme inhibitors (ACE-I)	Balanced vasodilators	Neurohormonal antagonism				Hypotension, dizziness, increased serum creatinine, hyperkalemia, cough, maculopapular rash, dysgeusia, leukopenia, proteinuria	K+-sparing diuretics and K+ supplements (increased risk of hyperkalemia); lithium (increased lithium concentrations); aspirin and NSAID (may antagonize hemodynamic effects of ACE-I); other vasodilators (increased risk of hypotension)
Captopril			6.25–12.5 mg q 8 hr	50 mg q 8 hr	100 mg q 8 hr		
Enalapril			2.5 mg q 12 hr	10 mg q 12 hr	20 mg q 12 hr		
Lisinopril			5 mg q 24 hr	20 mg q 24 hr	40 mg q 24 hr		
Quinapril			5 mg q 12 hr	20 mg q 12 hr	20 mg q 12 hr		
Ramipril			1.25–2.5 mg q 12 hr	5–10 mg q 12 hr	10 mg q 12 hr		

[a]Used alone for symptom relief or with hydralazine to improve survival; has also been used with ACE-I.
[b]Maintain 12-hr nitrate-free interval.
[c]Used in combination with oral ISDN to improve survival.
[*]Adapted from (31).

possibly improve the quality of life but does not appear to improve survival.

The first study to demonstrate that drug regimens can reduce mortality in CHF used a combination of oral ISDN and hydralazine (37). The Veterans Administrative Cooperative Study on Vasodilator Therapy of Heart Failure-I (V-HeFT-I) demonstrated that the ISDN-hydralazine combination, when added to digoxin and diuretics, reduced the 2-year CHF mortality by 34% among symptomatic patients with ejection fractions less than 45%. The improvement in mortality was associated with an increase in left ventricular ejection fraction that was not evidenced in the placebo group. The average ISDN and hydralazine doses for patients receiving both agents were 136 mg/day and 270 mg/day, respectively. Another vasodilator, prazosin, at an average daily dose of 19 mg, did not affect mortality. Interestingly, even though the ISDN-hydralazine combination improved overall mortality, it did not improve exercise tolerance. Unfortunately, this combination was often associated with adverse effects. Side effects forced the discontinuation of therapy in 19% of patients who were assigned to the ISDN-hydralazine treatment arm.

Hydralazine doses for treating patients with chronic CHF are exceedingly variable, even though the placebo-controlled trials used relatively fixed dosage regimens (47). Baseline estimates of a patient's systolic blood pressure (SBP), resting heart rate (HR), and renal function should be determined before the initiation of therapy. Single doses less than 75 mg of oral hydralazine are often ineffective in patients with CHF. Many patients respond favorably to 300 mg/day, as evidenced from data obtained in the V-HeFT trials (37, 38). Total daily dose can be divided into equal doses administered every 6, 8, or 12 hr. Unfortunately, side effects increase with increasing daily doses. Current data suggests that the dose should be titrated from approximately 300 mg/day while monitoring SBP (not less than 95 mm Hg), HR (avoidance of a resting tachycardia), improvements in pulmonary and systemic symptoms, and the appearance of adverse effects. Patients with the highest elevations in CVP have required doses as large as 2400 mg/day, and those with creatinine clearances less than 35 mL/min may exhibit the longest duration of action (at least 12 hr). The most common adverse effects, which are generally dose related, include headache, palpitations, postural hypotension, nausea, vomiting, and systemic lupus erythematosus (seen particularly in doses greater than 200 mg/day). Salt and water retention may occur during long-term therapy with hydralazine. Mild-to-moderate increases in resting heart rate and myocardial ischemic events in patients with CHF have also been reported following the administration of hydralazine.

Prazosin

Prazosin is a specific, competitive antagonist of postsynaptic α_1 receptors located in the walls of precapillary arteriolar resistance vessels and postcapillary venous capacitance vessels. Prazosin is therefore considered to be a balanced vasodilator in that it reduces both preload and afterload to approximately the same degree. Prazosin therapy was one of the treatment arms in the V-HeFT-I trial (37). However, prazosin therapy did not improve mortality rates relative to placebo. Therefore little enthusiasm remains for using prazosin as a primary vasodilator in the treatment of CHF. However, it remains unknown whether prazocin confers benefit when added to either the combination of ISDN-hydralazine or angiotensin-converting-enzyme inhibitors.

Angiotensin-Converting-Enzyme Inhibitors

The angiotensin-converting-enzyme (ACE) inhibitors, such as captopril, enalapril, lisinopril, quinapril, and ramipril, competitively block the conversion of angiotensin I (AI) to angiotensin II (AII). AII is a potent peripheral arteriolar vasoconstrictor. AII also stimulates the release of aldosterone and AVP and facilitates both central and peripheral activity of the sympathetic nervous system. In addition, the enzyme that converts AI to AII is identical to the enzyme that degrades a number of endogenous vasodilator substances (e.g., bradykinin). Therefore the vasorelaxant effects of these substances may be accentuated in the presence of ACE-I. Thus the reductions in both preload and afterload that are seen after the administration of an ACE-I may potentially result from a number of different but interrelated mechanisms. Captopril and lisinopril bind directly to the converting enzyme. Enalapril is a prodrug, which is hydrolyzed to the active ACE-inhibitor, enalaprilat. The ACE inhibitors have emerged as the cornerstone in the medical management of CHF (36). Currently, only captopril, enalapril, lisinopril, quinapril, and ramipril are approved for this indication.

Captopril and enalapril have been prospectively evaluated in randomized, double-blind, placebo-controlled trials, each of 3 months duration (48, 49). Captopril, administered as an average dose of almost 75 mg three times daily (over 50% of the patients received 100 mg three times daily), improved clinical signs and symptoms, treadmill exercise duration, and NYHA functional class compared with placebo (48). There were also fewer deaths and treatment failures in the captopril group. For patients with mild-to-moderate heart failure who were receiving diuretic maintenance therapy, captopril treatment was a suitable alternative to digoxin therapy. Exercise tolerance improved significantly, as did NYHA classification, in the captopril-treated patients but not the digoxin-treated patients. At doses of 5 mg twice daily, enalapril improved NYHA functional class, treadmill exercise duration, patients' feeling of well-being, and hemodynamic findings compared to placebo (49). There were fewer deaths in the enalapril group. Similar findings have been reported for lisinopril, quinapril, and ramipril.

Several landmark clinical trials related to the treatment of CHF have been conducted using ACE-I. One of these trials was the Cooperative North Scandinavian Enalapril Survival Study (CONSENSUS) (39). This study compared enalapril with placebo in terms of the mortality of severe CHF (NYHA Class IV). CAD was the most frequent cause of CHF (73% of patients). All patients were optimally treated with digoxin and diuretics at the start of the trial; they could also receive other vasodilators (i.e., nitrates, hydralazine, prazosin). Enalapril and placebo treatments were assigned in a randomized, double-blind fashion. Enalapril therapy started with 5 mg twice daily and was increased to 10 mg twice daily after 1 week if no adverse effects were observed. The dose was titrated upward to a maximum of 20 mg twice daily. The overall 6-month mortality rate in the enalapril group was 26%, compared with 44% in the placebo group, a 40% reduction (p = 0.002). Mortality at 1 year was significantly reduced by 31% in the enalapril group (p = 0.001). The reduction in total mortality was primarily a result of a reduction in progression of heart failure. No difference was observed in the incidence of sudden death between the two groups. A striking improvement in NYHA classification was also observed in the enalapril group and was accompanied by a decrease in the heart size and the number of required medications. The proportion of patients who were withdrawn from both the placebo and enalapril groups was the same, substantiating the excellent tolerance of enalapril.

Following the beneficial effects observed in the CONSENSUS study, additional clinical trials were designed to assesses the use of ACE-I in treating patients with mild-to-moderate CHF. The Veterans Administration Cooperative Study II (V-HeFT-II) was undertaken to compare the use of ACE-I with combined ISDN-hydralazine in treating patients with NYHA Class II to III heart failure who also were receiving digoxin and diuretics (38). Enalapril proved to be superior to the ISDN-hydralazine combination, since it significantly reduced the 2-year mortality by 28% (p = 0.016). Interestingly, the reduction in mortality was due primarily to a reduction in sudden cardiac death. Enalapril prevented the emergence of new ventricular tachycardia at 1 and 2 years of follow-up. This reduction in sudden cardiac death was more likely to occur in patients who had less severe heart failure (NYHA class I or II). There was no difference in mortality due to progressive pump failure between the two groups. In addition, no difference in the number of patients hospitalized between the two groups was observed. However, treatment with the combination of ISDN-hydralazine resulted in a significant improvement in exercise tolerance. These findings hold important implications with regards to the mechanism through which ACE inhibitors exert their beneficial effects. Given the greater survival benefit observed with ACE-I compared with other vasodilators, it is possible that the effect on mortality is mediated by a localized vasodilator mechanism. The antagonism of angiotensin and additional vasoconstrictor neurohormones as well as direct protective effects on the myocardium and/or coronary vasculature have been postulated as potential mechanisms through which ACE inhibitors affect mortality.

The data obtained from the V-HeFT-II trial was supported by the results obtained from the Studies of Left Ventricular Dysfunction (SOLVD) treatment trial (40). The SOLVD trial evaluated individuals with NYHA functional Class II and III heart failure who were receiving conventional heart failure treatment (digoxin, diuretics, and non-ACE-I vasodilators). No comparison was made between ACE-I and other vasodilator regimens. Patients were randomized to receive either placebo or enalapril at doses of 2.5 to 20 mg/day. Enalapril significantly reduced mortality by 16% throughout the follow-up period. The major effect was observed within the first 6 months and was most evident in patients with more severely depressed ejection fractions. Total mortality at 2 years was similar to that seen in the V-HeFT-II trial. However, unlike the results obtained from the VHeFT-II trial, the reduction in mortality was due primarily to a reduction in the progression of heart failure. No significant difference was observed in deaths classified as arrhythmic. Fewer hospitalizations were observed in the group receiving enalapril (21% versus 25% percent, respectively).

In an extension of the SOLVD trial, relatively asymptomatic patients (i.e., NYHA Class I and II) with ejection fractions less than 35% who were not yet receiving conventional heart failure therapy (digoxin, diuretics, non-ACE-I vasodilators) were studied in a double-blind, placebo-controlled fashion (50). Although no impact on mortality was observed, the frequency of hospitalizations for new or worsening heart failure was 20% lower for individuals receiving ACE-I therapy. In addition, enalapril reduced the frequency of myocardial infarction by 23% and unstable angina by 20%.

Another large-scale multicenter trial was conducted to evaluate the preventative use of ACE-I in treating post-myocardial infarction patients with asymptomatic left ventricular dysfunction (51). This trial was based on the ability of ACE-I to diminish the progressive ventricular dilatation that is observed in the postinfarction period of large myocardial infarctions. The Survival and Ventricular Enlargement (SAVE) trial demonstrated a significant 19% reduction in mortality in individuals with diminished ejection fractions (<40%) who are treated with captopril, 150 mg daily given in divided doses. Therapy was begun 3 to 16 days postinfarction in asymptomatic individuals. Captopril also reduced the frequency of hospitalizations and supported the data obtained from SOLVD by demonstrating a 25% reduction in acute myocardial infarction.

ACE inhibitors appear consistently to improve both the clinical status of patients with CHF and their longevity. On the basis of data obtained in the aforementioned clinical trials, vasodilator therapy with ACE-I should begin when signs and symptoms of CHF are absent or mild (i.e., NYHA class I and II). In addition, current guidelines recommend the use of ACE-I as first-line therapy (i.e., before digoxin and/or diuretics) (31). Alternative, non-ACE-I, vasodilator therapy (i.e., ISDN-hydralazine) should be reserved for individuals who are unable to tolerate ACE-I. At present, it is not precisely known whether the benefit observed with enalapril, captopril, lisinopril, quinapril, and ramipril is a class effect, which can be attributed to all ACE inhibitors. Further study is needed before additional ACE-I can be recommended for use in treating patients with CHF.

The doses of ACE-I are variable but should be titrated upward from relatively small doses and targeted to the doses that were shown to be beneficial in large clinical trials. Clinical observations, which can be used to guide the dosing of these agents, include a decrease in systolic blood pressure (to levels not less than 80 to 90 mm Hg), the relief of signs and symptoms, improvements in physical activity, and the appearance of other adverse effects. The initial dose of captopril can range from 6.25 to 25 mg every 8 hr, depending on the patient's baseline clinical status. A typical maintenance dose ranges from 12.5 to 50 mg every 8 hr. The initial dose of enalapril that many U.S. investigators frequently use is 2.5 to 5 mg every 12 hr. The maintenance dose usually ranges from 5 to 20 mg every 12 hr. The usual doses for these and the other ACE-I can be found in Table 38.3. The lowest possible starting dose for these agents should be used for patients who are hypotensive, who are hyponatremic (serum Na^+ <130 mEq/L), who have an elevated serum creatinine (>1.7 to 2 mg%), or who are taking either K^+-sparing diuretics or large doses of Na^+-wasting diuretics. Daily maintenance doses can probably be reduced and the dosing interval extended (i.e., every 12 hr for captopril; every 24 hr for enalapril, quinapril, and ramipril; and every other day for lisinopril) for patients with diminished renal function (i.e., estimated creatinine clearance <30 to 40 mL/min).

The most common adverse effect of an ACE-I is hypotension. The peak hypotensive response to captopril generally occurs within 30 to 90 min postdose, whereas this effect frequently occurs within 2 to 4 hr following a dose of enalapril and 7 hr following a dose of lisinopril. A single studied showed that hypotension was often more severe and prolonged after a dose of enalapril than after a dose of captopril (52). However, this investigation used large fixed doses of both drugs rather than optimizing the dose of each agent to either hemodynamic or clinical effects as well as fixed doses of diuretics. It is best to administer the first ACE-I dose under the watchful eye of a clinician so that first-dose syncope or presyncope can be treated

appropriately. Patients who are dehydrated or have low intravascular fluid volume or a low serum sodium are particularly susceptible to ACE-I-induced orthostasis and syncope. Therefore diuretic dosages can be held the day of first dose administration or perhaps for 24 hr before administering the first ACE-inhibitor test dose.

Increases in BUN and serum creatinine can occur after the administration of an ACE-I and may be related to the degree and duration of observed hypotension and secondary renal hypoperfusion. Serum potassium, sodium, and magnesium tend to normalize with chronic administration of ACE-I, regardless of changes in blood pressure or renal function. Consequently, oral potassium supplementation or the administration of potassium-sparing diuretics is generally unnecessary for patients with CHF who are taking ACE inhibitors. All diuretic and electrolyte therapy should be assessed before initiating ACE-I therapy. Two weeks after beginning the ACE-I, the following laboratory tests should be repeated: serum BUN, serum electrolytes including both potassium and magnesium, and urinalysis. Maculopapular rash, cough, taste disturbances, leukopenia, and proteinuria have occurred secondary to the administration of ACE-I. Therefore it is prudent to check a baseline complete blood count (CBC) with differential and repeat it 2 weeks after beginning ACE-I therapy and again every 6 months. Captopril has also been demonstrated to decrease the clearance of digoxin.

Special attention is needed to detect patients who may have both CHF and bilateral renal artery stenosis (single renal artery stenosis in patients with only one kidney). Because many patients with CHF have severe coronary artery disease, atherosclerosis of other arteries is expected. In a study of 89 patients referred to a heart failure unit, six (7%) had renal artery stenosis (53). The suspicion of renal artery stenosis is usually raised after the serum creatinine abruptly increases after beginning ACE-I vasodilator therapy. Another clue to renal artery stenosis is late onset (>50 years of age) hypertension. Once renal artery stenosis is confirmed (usually with digital subtraction angiography), either angioplasty or surgery can correct the stenosis. The patient can then safely receive ACE-I therapy for CHF. However, if surgical or mechanical correction of the renal artery stenosis is not possible, the ACE-I is contraindicated and will need to be discontinued.

DIGITALIS GLYCOSIDES

Classically, digitalis glycosides have been used as inotropic drugs for the treatment of CHF and other congestive states. However, some controversy still remains over the true benefit of cardiac glycosides in the management of CHF, particularly with respect to their effect on survival. In the discussion that follows, digoxin will be the only cardiac glycoside that is extensively reviewed because of its predominant use in clinical medicine.

Mechanism of Action

The inotropic effects of digoxin are produced indirectly, through inhibition of the transport enzyme sodium-potassium adenosine triphosphatase (Na^+-K^+ ATPase) (54). This enzyme complex catalyzes Na^+ efflux from the myocardial cell in exchange for K^+. When Na^+ efflux is inhibited, relatively high intracellular concentrations of Na^+ result. Sodium is subsequently exchanged for calcium (Ca^{+2}) via a Na^+–Ca^{+2} exchange carrier. The increased intracellular concentrations of Ca^{+2} ultimately enhance myocardial contractility through a complex series of intracellular Ca^{+2} movements.

Digoxin also has effects on the autonomic nervous system, such that with nontoxic doses there is a slowing both in heart rate and in atrioventricular conduction (55). These parasympathomimetic effects are maintained with chronic digoxin therapy (56). The increases in parasympathetic activity may result in increases in diastolic filling time, decreases in myocardial oxygen consumption, and perhaps a more favorable clinical outcome.

More recently, digoxin has been shown to have beneficial neurohormonal effects (56, 57). With continued dosing, digoxin decreases sympathetic activity as estimated by plasma norepinephrine concentrations (56). In addition, acute dosing with digoxin decreases plasma renin activity (57). Collectively, these effects may have long-term beneficial effects for patients with CHF.

Pharmacokinetics

A vast amount of literature describes the absorption, distribution, metabolism, and elimination of digoxin (58). Digoxin is available as a parenteral product and as a tablet, elixir, and capsule. The systemic availability of the tablet, elixir, and capsule are 70 to 80%, 75 to 85%, and 90 to 100%, respectively. The upper portion of the small intestine is the major site of absorption. Digoxin undergoes very little first-pass effect. The extent of digoxin absorption appears to be independent of the dose that is administered.

Digoxin is distributed into a number of tissues (58). On a milligram-per-gram basis the highest concentrations of digoxin are found in the kidneys, heart, liver, adrenal glands, diaphragm, and intestinal tract. However, approximately 50% of the apparent total body stores of digoxin are found in the skeletal muscles. As a result of this extensive distribution to lean tissue, digoxin should generally be dosed by using an estimate of the patient's ideal body weight. The plasma protein binding of digoxin is independent of concentration and averages 20 to 30%. Albumin is the principal binding protein. In patients with normal renal function, the volume of distribution at steady state (V_{ss}) averages 6 to 7 L/kg with a standard deviation of 1.4 L/kg.

Digoxin undergoes metabolism primarily by two different pathways (58). One of these pathways involves sequential hydrolysis of digitoxose sugar moieties; the other route results in the formation of reduced metabolites. The reduced (i.e., dihydro) metabolites are inactive. In contrast, the hydrolysis products, digoxigenin bis-digitoxosides and mono-digitoxosides, have potencies that approach that of the parent compound. However, the contribution of these two metabolites to the overall activity of digoxin in humans is unknown at this time. In adults with normal renal and hepatic function, the systemic clearance (CL_s) of digoxin averages approximately 180 mL/min/l.73 m^2. Renal clearance (CL_R), which exceeds both creatinine and insulin clearances, generally accounts for about 70% of the CL_s. The nonrenal clearance (CL_{NR}) of digoxin includes metabolism, biliary excretion, and possibly intestinal secretion and resultant fecal elimination. The CL_s of digoxin is linearly correlated with creatinine clearance (CL_{cr}). The apparent terminal elimination half-life ($t_{1/2}$) of digoxin in young adults with normal renal and hepatic function averages 36 hr.

A number of clinical conditions (Table 38.4) can alter the pharmacokinetics of digoxin (58, 59). The bioavailability of digoxin tablets can be reduced by abdominal radiation and by various malabsorption syndromes such as hypermotility, diarrhea, and subtotal villus atrophy. Cholesterol-binding resins (cholestyramine and colestipol), kaolin-pectin, large doses of antacids, oral metoclopramide, sulfasalazine, activated charcoal, oral neomycin, and sucralfate also decrease the absorption of digoxin tablets. In contrast, the absorption of digoxin may be enhanced by propantheline (and perhaps other anticholinergic drugs) and oral antibiotics such as tetracycline or erythromycin. These antibiotics decrease the number of colonic bacteria that metabolize digoxin to the inactive reduced metabolites. The V_{ss} of digoxin is reduced in the setting of chronic renal failure, whereas it is increased by physical activity. Chronic renal failure also increases the elimination $t_{1/2}$. Drugs that have consistently reduced the CL_s of digoxin include quinidine, verapamil, spironolactone, amiodarone, and propafenone. Captopril, hypothyroidism, and advanced CHF have also been demonstrated to decrease CL_s of digoxin. Hyperthyroidism, rifampin, and orally administered activated charcoal increase the CL_s of digoxin. In addition to the pharmacokinetic interactions between the above drugs and digoxin, β-adrenergic blocking drugs, amiodarone, and the calcium channel–blocking agents verapamil and diltiazem enhance the effects of digoxin on slowing atrioventricular (AV) nodal conduction and on decreasing sinoatrial (SA) nodal rate.

Serum Concentration-Response Relationship

Despite the abundance of knowledge about digoxin's pharmacokinetics, a relationship between the intensity of the inotropic response, the development of toxicity, and the apparent serum concentration of digoxin is difficult to

Table 38.4.
Conditions of Altered Digoxin Pharmacokinetics or Pharmacodynamics

Condition	Clinical Management
A. Reduced bioavailability	
1. Abdominal radiation	1. Consider administering digoxin as elixir or capsule.
2. Malabsorption syndromes	2. As in 1.
a. Hypermotility	
b. Diarrhea	
c. Subtotal villus atrophy	
3. Drugs	3. Consider administering digoxin 1 to 2 hr before or 2 to 3 hr after a, b, c, e, f, and g; consider administering digoxin as capsule or elixir for d.
a. Cholesterol-binding resins	
b. Kaolin-pectin	
c. Large doses (e.g., 30 mL) of antacids	
d. Metoclopramide (oral)	
e. Sulfasalazine	
f. Neomycin (oral)	
g. Sucralfate	
B. Enhanced bioavailability	
1. Propantheline (and perhaps other anticholinergics)	1. Be alert for possible occurrence of digoxin toxicity.
2. Oral antibiotics	2. Thought to be a problem in 10% of population who extensively metabolize digoxin to inactive reduction products by colonic bacteria; avoid antibiotics if possible. If antibiotics must be administered, be alert for possible occurrence of digoxin toxicity.
a. Erythromycin	
b. Tetracycline	
C. Reduced systemic clearance	
1. Renal failure	1. Adjust doses of digoxin to the reductions in creatinine clearance.
2. Drugs	
a. Quinidine	a. Reduce digoxin dose by 50% upon start of quinidine; monitor serum digoxin levels (SDGs).
b. Verapamil	b. Consider reducing digoxin dose by about 50% on initiation of verapamil; monitor serum digoxin levels and look for additive effects on SA and AV nodes.
c. Spironolactone	c. Consider reducing digoxin dose by about 50%; monitor SDCs, and be alert for signs and symptoms of toxicity.
d. Amiodarone	d. Consider reducing digoxin dose by about 50%; monitor SDCs, and look for additive effects on SA and AV nodes.
e. Captopril	e. Routine reduction of digoxin appears to be unnecessary; monitor SDCs, and be alert for signs and symptoms of toxicity.
f. Propafenone	f. Consider reducing digoxin dose by about 25%, or monitor SDCs and be alert for signs and symptoms of toxicity.

define (58, 60, 61). This lack of a definitive therapeutic range is in part reflective both of digoxin's rather modest inotropic effects and of the overlap that exists between therapeutic and toxic serum concentrations. In addition, many of the commercially available assays that are used to determine apparent serum digoxin concentrations (SDCs) are relatively nonspecific. Both active and inactive metabolites as well as endogenous digoxinlike substances can cross-react with many of these assays. A radioimmunoassay using a double antibody system and a newer monoclonal antibody assay may be the most specific laboratory test (62). Nonetheless, many clinical laboratories and reference texts list the therapeutic range for digoxin as 0.5 or 0.8 to 2.0 ng/mL. In a review of about 50 studies, which attempted to correlate the SDC to both nontoxic effects, a mean level of 1.4 ng/mL was observed in patients without toxicity, whereas patients with overt toxicity demonstrated serum levels that were two to three times greater (60). Even though statistical significance was achieved in most of these studies, the overlap between therapeutic and toxic concentrations was considerable. This overlap may have been related to any one of the many factors that tend to predispose patients to the development of digoxin toxicity. Nonetheless, two recent digoxin withdrawal studies, the RADIANCE (63) and PROVED (64) trials, have suggested a therapeutic range for digoxin between 0.9 and 2.0 ng/mL (mean concentration: 1.2 ng/mL) in patients with CHF.

Dosing Guidelines

Several pharmacokinetic equations provide prospective dosing guidelines for digoxin. One study compared several of these equations and demonstrated universally a poor correlation between predicted and measured SDC (65). Because the equations tended to overestimate the measured SDC, any one of them should provide safe initial approximations of a patient's digoxin dose. However, the method of Koup and colleagues, using a CL_{NR} of 20 mL/min/1.73 m^2, provided the best correlation between the predicted and measured steady-state SDC (66).

To use the method developed by Koup and his colleagues, the patient's ideal body weight (IBW) must first be estimated:

$$IBW_{male} = 50 \text{ kg} + 2.3 \times (\text{height in inches above 5 feet})$$
$$IBW_{female} = 45 \text{ kg} + 2.3 \times (\text{height in inches above 5 feet})$$

If the patient's actual weight is less than the estimated IBW, use the actual weight. An estimate of the patient's body surface area (BSA) in square meters using the patient's IBW is then needed:

$$BSA \text{ (m}^2) = IBW \text{ (kg)}^{0.425} \times \text{height (cm)}^{0.725} \times 0.007184$$

Thereafter, the patient's creatinine clearance (CL_{cr}) can be estimated by using the Cockcroft and Gault equation (67):

$$CL_{cr} = \frac{(140 - \text{Age}) \times ABW}{72 \times SrCr} \times \frac{1.73 \text{ m}^2}{BSA}$$

where Age is the patient's age in years, ABW is the patient's actual body weight, and SrCr is the patient's serum creatinine. If the patient is female, multiply the above result by 0.85.

Next the CL_s for digoxin must be estimated:

$$CL_s = (1.303 \times CL_{cr}) + 20 \text{ mL/min/1.73 m}^2$$

The initial estimate of the patient's daily digoxin dose can now be calculated by using the steady-state equation and a target SDC (i.e., 1.2 ng/mL):

$$CSS = \frac{F \times D}{CL_s \times \tau}$$

where:

D = dose (ng)
C_{ss} = steady-state digoxin level (ng/mL)
CL_s = systemic clearance (mL/min/1.73 m^2)
τ = dosing interval (1440 min/day)
F = fraction absorbed (0.75 for tablets)

The above equation provides initial dosing guidelines for patients with CHF so that there is a low probability of achieving a potentially toxic SDC. A trough SDC can be obtained either after a few days, to verify that a serious overprediction or underprediction of the measured SDC has not occurred, or at the attainment of steady-state (usually 7 to 10 days for most adult patients) (58). General indications for determinations of SDCs in an individual patient are (a) establishing an initial relationship between the maintenance dose of digoxin and the corresponding serum level; (b) after the addition of a drug that is known or suspected to interact pharmacokinetically with digoxin; (c) during a change in physiologic parameter that is known

or suspected to alter the pharmacokinetics of digoxin, such as renal function; (d) after a substitution in the dosage form of digoxin; (e) to confirm the suspicion of the occurrence of digoxin toxicity; (f) to evaluate either a poor response to initial therapy or a decline in response following early therapeutic success; and (g) to assess patient compliance (68). In addition, elderly patients may represent a subgroup in whom routine measurement of SDCs may be indicated because of the difficulty in predicting digoxin doses. It must be reemphasized that SDCs are not predictive of efficacy and toxicity and should therefore be used only to supplement clinical judgment. Strict attention should be given to the timing of blood collection for serum digoxin assay and its relationship to the time of last dose. Collecting blood during the distribution phase (lasting up to 12 hr after an oral dose) may cause the SDC to be falsely elevated and potentially useless in evaluating possible toxicity.

Digoxin Toxicity

Despite the objective means used to develop rational dosing guidelines for digoxin, digoxin toxicity has remained a worrisome clinical problem. Previous estimates of the frequency of digitalis toxicity in hospitalized patients taking digoxin have ranged from 4 to 35%, accompanied by a high mortality rate of up to 41% (60). The incidence in ambulatory settings is unknown. A more recent retrospective review of the medical records of 563 patients who were taking digoxin and who were admitted to a large urban teaching hospital for heart failure has provided contemporary insight into the pattern of digoxin intoxication (69). On the basis of predetermined clinical and laboratory criteria, digoxin toxicity was definitely diagnosed in only four (0.8%) patients and could not be excluded in another 16 (4%). None of the patients died. This shows that the incidence of digoxin intoxication and its associated mortality in hospitalized patients has been declining.

The diagnosis of digoxin intoxication remains a challenge (60, 61). It can be acute or chronic, and it generally results from either excessive ingestion, a change in disposition, or an increased sensitivity to digoxin. Digoxin intoxication can manifest as a number of noncardiac and cardiac symptoms (Table 38.5). Anorexia, nausea, and vomiting are the most common but nonspecific symptoms of digoxin toxicity. Dizziness, fatigue, and malaise are common neurologic findings, whereas headache, delirium, acute psychoses, and neuralgic pain (including trigeminal neuralgia) are uncommon ones. Seeing halos around lights and perceiving greens (chloropsia) or yellows (xanthopsia) more prominently are classically reported visual disturbances associated with digitalis intoxication, but in reality patients rarely report these. Gynecomastia and sexual dysfunction have been reported occasionally in males and

Table 38.5.
Signs and Symptoms of Digoxin Intoxication

Noncardiac
  Gastrointestinal: anorexia, nausea, vomiting
  Neurologic: fatigue, malaise, delirium, acute psychosis, neuralgic
    pain
  Ocular: halo vision, green or yellow vision
  Miscellaneous: gynecomastia and sexual dysfunction (males)
Common cardiac arrhythmias[a]
  Ventricular premature depolarizations (VPDs), including multifocal
    VPDs and bigeminy or trigeminy
  First-degree AV block
  Mobitz type I AV block
  Nonparoxysmal junctional tachycardia
  Supraventricular tachycardia with block
  Ventricular tachycardia (including bidirectional ventricular tachy-
    cardia)

[a]Virtually every known cardiac arrhythmia has occurred secondary to digitalis intoxication.

may be the result of digitalis-induced increases in estradiol levels. True digoxin allergy is rarely reported.

Virtually any cardiac arrhythmia or conduction disturbance can be associated with digoxin toxicity (60, 61). Digoxin-induced arrhythmias are generally classified as (a) decreases in impulse conduction, (b) enhancement of automaticity, or (c) combinations of these. In patients with definite digoxin toxicity, the most common arrhythmias that are observed are atrioventricular block and sinus bradycardia (66% and 26%, respectively) (69). Junctional arrhythmias are probably the next most common rhythm at time of presentation with digoxin toxicity followed by sinus pauses. Ventricular premature depolarizations (VPDs), especially multifocal or those that occur in a bigeminal pattern, are common. Atrial fibrillation with a ventricular response rate less than 50 beats per minute suggests digoxin toxicity. Ventricular tachycardia and ventricular fibrillation can occur and mandate the use of digoxin-specific Fab fragments (Digibind). However, it should also be recalled that ventricular rhythm disturbances are common findings in patients with left ventricular dysfunction. Finally, some patients may present with paroxysmal supraventricular tachycardia, often with a 2:1 block. In short, rhythm disturbances are common outcomes and may be the first sign of digoxin toxicity.

A number of factors predispose patients to digoxin toxicity (Table 38.6), most commonly, such patients are elderly and have reduced renal function (60, 61). Hypokalemia and hypomagnesemia are associated with an increased incidence of digitalis-induced arrhythmias. Hypokalemia appears to increase myocardial uptake of digoxin. Magnesium (Mg^{2+}) serves as a cofactor for the enzyme, Na^+–K^+–ATPase, and therefore hypomagnesemia may decrease intracellular potassium. Acid-base disturbances such as alkalosis can alter the serum concentration and total body stores of potassium and subsequently may

increase the sensitivity to digitalis. Diuretic-induced alkalosis, even in the setting of normal serum potassium, increases the frequency of digitalis-associated arrhythmias. Elderly patients are at greater risk for developing digoxin toxicity either as a result of age-related decreases in renal function or perhaps secondary to increased sensitivity of Na^+–K^+-ATPase to the inhibitory effects of digoxin. Renal dysfunction alone predisposes patients to digoxin toxicity because of decreases in both the volume of distribution and elimination of digoxin. Hypothyroidism and hypoxia, through unidentified mechanisms, increase a patient's sensitivity to digoxin. Finally, the development of digoxin toxicity may be enhanced by drugs that either diminish the CL_s of digoxin or increase its absorption or share similar pharmacodynamic properties as digoxin.

Treatment of Digoxin Toxicity

The severity of digoxin toxicity should be considered before initiating a treatment plan (60, 61). In general, blood should be obtained for determination of serum K^+, Mg^+, and digoxin levels. Efforts should be made to identify and remove any factors that may predispose the patient to digoxin toxicity. Discontinuance of the digoxin and supportive treatment may be all that is necessary to manage the noncardiac symptoms such as nausea, vomiting, and anorexia. Withdrawal of digoxin may also be sufficient in treating asymptomatic cardiac manifestations such as first-degree AV block or Mobitz Type I second-degree AV block.

In the management of many of the digoxin-induced ectopic arrhythmias (e.g., nonparoxysmal AV junctional tachycardia, atrial tachycardia with block, VPDs, and ventricular tachycardia), potassium can be administered, unless serum K^+ is elevated ($\geq$5.0 mEq/mL or greater), the patient is ingesting K^+-conserving drugs, severe renal insufficiency is present, markedly delayed AV conduction is observed (i.e., greater than first-degree AV block), or the patient has ingested a massive overdose of digoxin (60, 61). Potassium chloride salts are used, as many digoxin patients

Table 38.6.
Factors That May Predispose Patients to the Development of Digoxin Intoxication

Electrolyte abnormalities
  Hypokalemia
  Hypomagnesemia
  Hypercalcemia
Advanced age
Acid-base disturbances
  Alkalosis
Hypoxia
Renal dysfunction
Hypothyroidism
Drug interactions (see Table 38.4)

may be hypochloremic secondary to concomitant diuretic therapy. If possible, potassium should be given orally at doses of up to 40 mEq every 1 to 4 hr. Alternatively, potassium can be administered intravenously at rates not exceeding 10 to 20 mEq/hr. The concentration of the potassium solution should not exceed 40 to 60 mEq/L, since higher concentrations may produce pain and venous sclerosis. Normal saline may be a better choice than 5% dextrose solution for diluting the potassium, to avoid the occasional paradoxical worsening of the hypokalemia sometimes observed in the severely K^+-depleted patient.

Magnesium can suppress digitalis-induced ectopic rhythms, especially those of ventricular origin (70). Ten milliliters of 20% (2 g) magnesium sulfate solution can be administered intravenously over 1 to 2 min followed by 0.5 to 1.0 mEq/kg intramuscularly every 4 hr for five doses. Daily replacement therapy may be required thereafter. Lymphocyte Mg^{2+} content could be monitored to guide repletion of this cation because serum Mg^{+2} does not reflect total body magnesium stores. Magnesium supplementation should be avoided in treating patients with severe renal insufficiency, a greater than first-degree AV block, or hypermagnesemia.

The Class IB antiarrhythmic drugs, lidocaine and rarely phenytoin, are most useful in treating digitalis-induced ventricular arrhythmias (60, 61). Lidocaine is administered intravenously as a dose of 1 to 2 mg/kg at a rate of 50 mg/min. Within 20 to 30 min a second bolus dose, at half of the initial dose, should be given. An infusion of 15 to 50 µg/kg/min should be started at the time of first bolus dose. The most common adverse effects of lidocaine involve the central nervous system and can include drowsiness, parasthesias, feelings of dissociation, agitation, muscle twitching, or generalized convulsions. These adverse effects appear to be dose-dependent and serum level–dependent. Alternatively, 15 to 20 mg/kg of intravenous phenytoin at a rate not to exceed 25 mg/min can be given. Hypotension and myocardial depression, which can occur secondary to phenytoin administration, appear to be related to the rate of drug administration. Phenytoin can be diluted in normal saline at concentrations ranging from 1 to 10 mg/mL. Other antiarrhythmic drugs that have been used in treating digitalis-induced ectopic rhythms include β-blockers, bretylium, procainamide, quinidine, mexiletine, tocainide, and amiodarone. The use of quinidine and amiodarone for digitalis-induced arrhythmias may not be the optimal choice since they both share the potential for increasing SDC. Other antiarrhythmics discussed are probably safer to use. For reversing symptomatic digoxin-induced bradycardia or SA or AV conduction delays, atropine administered in intravenous doses of 0.5 to 2.0 mg may be useful. If the bradycardia or conduction delays are hemodynamically significant and refractory to atropine, temporary intravenous pacing is indicated.

In the setting of an accidental or suicidal ingestion of large amounts of digoxin, syrup of ipecac can decrease absorption if it is administered within an hour of ingestion (60, 61). Gastric lavage can also be used. Orally administered activated charcoal, cholestyramine, or colestipol can also minimize absorption.

If attempts to remove digoxin are delayed or unsuccessful and the patient is experiencing potentially life-threatening ventricular arrhythmias, refractory hyperkalemia, or conduction deficits that are resistant to conventional therapy, digoxin-specific antibodies (Fab fragments, Digibind®) are indicated (61). The Fab antibodies bind to both intravascular and interstitial digoxin. An initial response, consisting of an increase in total serum digoxin, a decrease in serum potassium, and a reversal of the adverse electrophysiologic effects of digoxin, is frequently observed within 1/2 to 1 hour after the Fab infusion. These digoxin-specific antibodies often completely reverse the toxic effects of digoxin (and digitoxin) within a few hours. A treatment response is expected in at least 90% of patients with definitive life-threatening digoxin toxicity (71). Caution must be exercised in administering Fab fragments to patients with digoxin toxicity and concomitant severe renal impairment.

Digoxin Controversy

Over the past 10 to 15 years, several studies have attempted to determine the role of digoxin in the management of patients with chronic CHF who are also in normal sinus rhythm (72). Some studies suggest that patients with poorly compensated CHF (i.e., patients with an S_3 gallop rhythm, a greater left ventricular end-diastolic dimension, a lower ejection fraction, or previously unknown episodes of atrial fibrillation) may benefit from the chronic administration of digoxin. Recent trials have shown beneficial effects of digoxin with respect to relief of symptoms, exercise performance, frequency of decompensation, and improvement in ejection fraction. Recently, patients with NYHA Class II to III CHF and ejection fractions less than 35% who were clinically stable on a regimen of digoxin, diuretics, and ACE-I were randomized to continuous digoxin therapy or withdrawal of digoxin (63). Morbidity and recurrent symptoms were six times more likely to occur in patients who were withdrawn from digoxin therapy. Similar results were observed in patients who were stabilized on a regimen of diuretics but not receiving ACE-I (64). Given small sample sizes in these studies, the effect of digoxin on mortality could not be evaluated. Individuals who appear to benefit most from digoxin are heart failure patients with left ventricular systolic dysfunction and cardiomegaly. Conclusive data from an ongoing U.S. National Heart, Lung and Blood Institute trial in conjunction with the Department of Veteran Affairs Cooperative Studies Program is being awaited to determine the effects of digoxin on survival. However, given that the trial has not been prematurely terminated, it can be inferred that digoxin does not confer an increase in mortality in patients with CHF due to systolic dysfunction.

DIURETICS

Diuretics remain an integral component of the treatment of patients with chronic CHF because these agents diminish the characteristic pulmonary and systemic circulatory congestion of this clinical syndrome through the excretion of sodium and water (73). Therefore even though diuretics as monotherapy have not been shown to prolong life, their effect in relieving symptoms justifies their widespread use. Most patients with clinically diagnosed CHF will be maintained on some diuretic regimen. Diuretics may also indirectly provide favorable hemodynamic effects by decreasing intraventricular wall tension. This occurs principally through a reduction in preload that is secondary, in part, to venodilation. Preload reduction can sometimes slightly improve systolic function. Nevertheless, the major effect of chronically administered diuretics in the management of CHF remains the relief of pulmonary and systemic congestive symptoms.

Principles of Diuretic Usage

Before the initiation of a diuretic regimen for a patient with chronic CHF, a number of general principles of diuretic usage should be considered:

1. Therapy to rid patients of all traces of peripheral edema is often unnecessary and may potentially be harmful.
2. Begin therapy with the smallest effective dose and titrate upward to minimize a patient's weight loss to 0.5 to 1.0 kg/day except in extreme cases of pulmonary edema.
3. The more proximally a diuretic acts within the nephron, the greater will be the loss of both fluid and electrolytes.
4. Diuretics, which act proximally to the terminal portion within the distal tubule where sodium is exchanged for both potassium and hydrogen, will likely produce both hypokalemia and metabolic alkalosis.
5. Diuretics that produce hypokalemia frequently also cause hypomagnesemia.
6. Diuretics should be administered as frequently (or infrequently) as necessary.
7. Combination diuretic therapy is often required as a patient's CHF worsens.
8. Osmotic diuretics are not generally useful in the management of CHF.

CLASSIFICATION OF DIURETICS

Thiazides

The major site of diuretic action of the thiazides is the distal convoluted tubule, where they induce a maximal fractional excretion of sodium of approximately 3 to 6 percent (Table 38.7) (74). Therefore these compounds are considered moderately potent diuretics. In addition, the efficacy of thiazide diuretics depends on the glomerular filtration rate for delivery to the site of action. The individual thiazide agents are essentially interchangeable in terms of diuretic effectiveness. Therefore hydrochlorothiazide (HCTZ) is generally prescribed because of its relative low cost. HCTZ or another thiazide is usually the initial diuretic for CHF, unless the patient has either impaired renal function (estimated creatinine clearance of less than 40 mL/min) or severe congestive symptoms. In each of these instances a loop diuretic would represent a more logical initial choice. Adverse effects that may occur secondary to thiazide administration include hypokalemia, hyponatremia, hypomagnesemia, hyperuricemia, hyperlipoproteinemia (i.e., increases in total cholesterol, LDL cholesterol, and triglycerides and decreases in HDL cholesterol), and impaired carbohydrate tolerance. The latter adverse effect is probably of concern only for insulin-dependent diabetics. Mild heart failure is usually responsive to low thiazide doses such as 12.5 mg to 25 mg of HCTZ. Hydrochlorothiazide doses greater than 50 mg provide little further symptom relief and are more likely to cause electrolyte imbalances.

Metolazone

Metolazone is a thiazide-type drug in that its principal site of action is the distal convoluted tubule of the nephron (Table 38.7) (74). This drug has also been demonstrated to have proximal tubular effects to reduce sodium reabsorption. Major differences between metolazone and the thiazides are that metolazone retains its effectiveness even when renal function is markedly reduced and that metolazone has a duration of action much longer than that of most thiazides. Metolazone and the thiazides produce similar adverse effects. Metolazone can be used as a single diuretic in doses such as 2.5 mg daily. However, it is often used in combination with loop diuretics (sequential diuresis) and therefore may be prescribed as 2.5 mg every 1 to 4 days. When metolazone is administered in conjunction with loop diuretics, it is important to administer metolazone ½ to 1 hr before the administration of the loop diuretics to achieve maximal diuresis.

Loop Diuretics

These drugs act principally at the thick ascending limb of the loop of Henle, where they may increase the fractional excretion of sodium up to 25% (Table 38.7), and are the most potent class of diuretics (74). Loop diuretics also increase renal blood flow by enhancing production of the renal vasodilatory prostaglandin (PGE) (73). This effect contributes to the natriuretic effects of the loop diuretics. Loop diuretics remain effective despite reductions in glomerular filtration rate.

Furosemide, ethacrynic acid, bumetanide, and torsemide represent this most potent subgroup of diuretics

Table 38.7.
Diuretics That Are Commonly Used in the Management of CHF

Class	Principal Site of Action Within Nephron	Initial Oral Dose Range	Target Dose	Recommended Maximal Dose	Adverse Effects	Drug Interactions
Thiazides Hydrochlorothiazide Many others	Distal convoluted tubule	25 mg q 24 hr	As needed	50 mg q 24 hr	Hypokalemia, hyponatremia, hypomagnesemia, azotemia, hyperlipoproteinema, hyperglycemia, rash, pancreatitis, cholestatic jaundice	Loop diuretics (excessive hypokalemia)
Metolazone	Distal convoluted tubule	2.5 mg q 24 hr	As needed	10 mg q 24 hr	As for thiazides	As for thiazides
Loop diuretics Furosemide Ethacrynic acid Bumetanide	Thick ascending limb of the loop of Henle	20 to 40 mg q 24 hr 25–50 mg q 24 hr 0.5 to 1.0 mg q 12–24 hr	As needed	240 mg q 12 hr	As for thiazides except for hypocalemia and deafness	Thiazides or metolazone (excessive hypokalemia)
Potassium-sparing Spironolactone	Distal convoluted tubule, aldosterone-dependent Na⁺/K⁺ exchange site	25 mg q 24 hr	As needed	200 mg q 12 hr	Hyperkalemia, gynecomastia	ACE-I or K⁺ supplements (increased risk of hyperkalemia) Digoxin (increase in digoxin level)
Triamterene	Distal convoluted tubule, Na⁺/K⁺/H⁺ exchange site, not aldosterone-dependent	50 mg q 24 hr	As needed	100 mg q 12 hr	Hyperkalemia, azotemia, renal stones	ACE-I or K⁺-supplements (increased risk of hyperkalemia)
Amiloride	Same as triamterene	5 mg q 24 hr	As needed	40 mg q 24 hr	Hyperkalemia, azotemia	ACE-I or K⁺-supplements (increased risk of hyperkalemia)

Source: Adapted from (31).

available for the treatment of CHF (73, 74). Furosemide is the most commonly prescribed agent within this subgroup. Adverse effects that occur secondary to the administration of loop diuretics are similar to those caused by the thiazide diuretics. However, the loop diuretics may produce adverse effects such as hypocalcemia and deafness, which are not shared with either the thiazide compounds or metolazone. Initial doses of furosemide (20 to 40 mg/day) and bumetanide (0.5 to 1.0 mg/day) can promote a prompt diuresis. However, as heart failure progresses, increasingly larger doses will be needed. Although doses vary widely, patients suffering from end-stage heart failure may require twice-daily doses ranging from 20 to 320 mg or more. A good rule of thumb for estimating the dose of furosemide is 40 mg multiplied by the patient's serum creatinine (73).

Potassium-Sparing Diuretics

Spironolactone, triamterene, and amiloride exert their diuretic effects at the terminal portion of the distal convoluted tubule (Table 38.7) (74). Spironolactone, which is converted primarily to the active metabolite, canrenone, acts at an aldosterone-sensitive site, whereas triamterene and amiloride act at a site that is not under the control of aldosterone. These compounds are considered weak diuretics, since they induce a fractional excretion of sodium of only 2 to 5 percent. Potassium-sparing diuretics are principally useful as adjuncts with thiazides, metolazone, and loop diuretics to counteract the hypokalemia and hypomagnesemia that are frequently induced or exacerbated by these other drugs. Hypokalemia and hypomagnesemia are directly arrhythmogenic, and they may potentiate arrhythmias secondary to either digoxin or circulating catecholamines. These combined electrolyte disturbances appear to be best prevented by the administration of potassium-sparing diuretics. However, therapy with potassium-sparing agents should be individualized.

In selecting a potassium-sparing diuretic, it should be noted that spironolactone is effective only in relative hyperaldosteronemic states (74). Triamterene and amiloride are effective even when levels of aldosterone are not increased. Elevated levels of aldosterone are frequently observed in patients with CHF. Spironolactone's effects do not become maximal for several days because it takes 3 to 4 days for canrenone to attain steady-state concentrations. Likewise, the effects of spironolactone persist for several days following cessation of therapy because of the presence of the active metabolite. Spironolactone is currently being investigated in the RALES trial as a means of further antagonizing the RAA system to produce an enhanced clinical benefit. Both triamterene and amiloride attain steady-state effects in about 1 to 1.5 days. A potential consequence of prescribing any of the potassium-sparing diuretics is hyperkalemia. However, this is more likely to occur in patients with severe renal dysfunction or in patients receiving concomitant potassium supplements or

ACE-I. Spironolactone may cause gynecomastia, and triamterene-containing renal stones have occasionally been reported. Heart failure patients who are taking a potassium-sparing diuretic should be advised not to use a salt substitute (which contains potassium) without first seeking the advice of their physician. In addition, potassium-sparing diuretics and ACE-inhibitors generally should not be concomitantly administered.

Diuretic Resistance

To optimize diuretic therapy for patients with CHF, a practitioner must be familiar with the physiologic and pharmacologic factors that mediate a diminished clinical response to diuretics (i.e., diuretic resistance) (73, 74). Patient noncompliance with the prescribed diuretic regimen will minimize the effectiveness of the drug. Also, an increased sodium intake can offset the natriuretic effects of the diuretic. Therefore a reduction in sodium consumption must usually accompany the institution of diuretic therapy.

Uremia may diminish the response to loop diuretics, which chemically are organic acids. Therefore to reach their site of action within the nephron, these drugs depend on the organic acid secretory pump, which can be blocked by the increased circulating concentrations of endogenous organic acids seen in uremia. This example of diuretic resistance may be overcome by either using much higher doses of the loop diuretic or combining the loop diuretic with another diuretic that has a different site of action within the nephron, such as a thiazide or metolazone.

Nonsteroidal antiinflammatory drugs (NSAIDs) lessen the natriuretic effect of loop diuretics. NSAIDs block the renal hemodynamic effects of these agents by inhibiting prostaglandin synthesis. This effect was initially reported with indomethacin and has subsequently been shown to occur with ibuprofen, sulindac, naproxen, and aspirin. NSAID-induced diuretic resistance can be counteracted by discontinuing the offending agent if possible, by using larger or more frequent doses of loop diuretics, or by combining the loop diuretic with a thiazide or metolazone.

CHF can also partially attenuate the response to loop diuretics by a number of mechanisms. The rate of gastrointestinal absorption and the corresponding peak serum concentrations of oral doses of loop diuretics are decreased in the setting of CHF, especially for patients in the decompensated state. These effects will slow the rate of delivery of the drug to its site of action within the nephron, which will result in a diminished maximal response. The administration of an intravenous dose of the loop diuretic with a thiazide or metolazone may result in a more effective diuresis. Individual patients with CHF will even become resistant to intravenous doses of a loop diuretic because of unexplained alteration in the patient's pharmacodynamic response to the drug. Larger single intravenous doses, more frequent and smaller intravenous doses, and a short-term intravenous infusion of the loop diuretic are useful initial strategies to overcome the diminished response. However, if a patient with relatively good renal function does not respond to approximately 400 to 500 mg of intravenous furosemide (or the equivalent dose of another loop diuretic), then a second diuretic such as a thiazide or metolazone or an afterload reducing agent such as hydralazine or captopril should be added produce a satisfactory diuretic response. Some patients may be able to assume responsibility for making minor adjustments in their own diuretic regimen based on weight, dyspnea, and peripheral edema. A simple but useful monitoring tool is a daily log of a patient's weight.

Adverse Effects

When using diuretics, clinicians must be attuned to the potential development of adverse reactions (73, 74). Electrolyte disturbances, mainly hypokalemia and hypo-magnesemia, are commonly associated with diuretic use and may potentiate digoxin intoxication and arrhythmic complications. Sodium loss resulting in hyponatremia will stimulate the RAA system and further stimulate potentially deleterious compensatory mechanisms. Dehydration may occur with excessive diuretic administration. Close attention to changes in body weight are warranted, and patients should be instructed to monitor and record daily weights. In addition, through strict patient education, some patients may be permitted to alter the diuretic regimen as necessary on the basis of changes in weight, fluid intake, and edema. Careful attention to clinical parameters at home with concomitant adjustments in the diuretic regimen may lead to reductions in the frequency of heart failure exacerbations and resultant hospital admissions.

In summary, the current medical management of symptomatic CHF due to systolic dysfunction should include an ACE-I unless contraindications exist. These compounds almost uniformly reduce mortality, hospital-ization, and symptoms. In addition, most patients will require a diuretic and digoxin for additive symptomatic relief. For asymptomatic HF due to systolic dysfunction, ACE-inhibitors also should serve as first-line agents.

MISCELLANEOUS PHARMACOLOGIC TREATMENTS

Calcium Channel Blockers

Several theoretical reasons exist for considering calcium channel–blocking drugs in the treatment of CHF:

1. These agents are powerful arteriolar dilators and thus reduce left ventricular afterload.
2. These drugs produce hemodynamic effects similar to those of hydralazine, which has improved survival in patients with mild-to-moderate CHF.
3. These agents have antiischemic effects that make them an attractive therapeutic option for treating CHF due to coronary artery disease.

4. These drugs improve diastolic dysfunction, a significant cause of heart failure symptoms, due to their beneficial effects on left ventricular relaxation (75).

However, the first-generation calcium channel antagonists, verapamil, diltiazem, and nifedipine, have universally produced hemodynamic and clinical deterioration in patients with heart failure due to systolic dysfunction. Possible explanations for these detrimental effects include direct negative inotropic properties, further activation of deleterious neurohormonal responses, and an increase in blood volume, which may increase afterload. Nonetheless, in patients with severe asymptomatic aortic regurgitation and normal left ventricular systolic function, nifedipine significantly reduces and delays the need for aortic valve replacement (76). In addition, nifedipine may have a role in the treatment of CHF due to chronic severe mitral regurgitation (77).

The second-generation dihydropyridines (i.e., nitren-dipine, nicardipine, felodipine, and amlodipine) may be less likely to worsen heart failure and may be beneficial in the treatment of CHF. A recent placebo-controlled trial evaluated the effect of amlodipine when added to ACE inhibitors, digoxin, and diuretics (78). Amlodipine signifi-cantly reduced combined morbidity/mortality by 31% and all-cause mortality by 45% in patients with CHF due to nonischemic causes. No beneficial effect was observed in patients with CHF secondary to ischemic cardiomyopathy. V-HeFT III is evaluating the effects of felodipine versus placebo, when added to diuretics and ACE-I with and without digoxin, with respect to mortality and morbidity in patients with mild-to-moderate CHF. A recent small-scale, 16-week trial compared felodipine with enalapril and showed equivalent beneficial effects with respect to neurohormonal activation and exercise tolerance but greater quality-of-life scores in the felodipine group (79). However, larger comparative trials are needed to investi-gate the effects of these agents on survival.

Angiotensin II Antagonists

Despite continuous treatment with ACE-I, a subgroup of patients with CHF may remain symptomatic and demon-strate a progressive decline in LVEF (80). These patients manifest persistent formation of AII. In addition, some patients with CHF treated with ACE-I may exhibit increases in plasma AII concentrations in response to exercise (81). The formation of AII is not completely blocked by ACE-I within certain tissues. These observa-tions collectively suggest a potential additive benefit of AII receptor antagonists to ACE-I in the treatment of CHF. Furthermore, AII antagonists may offer a therapeutic alternative to patients who are not able to tolerate ACE-I.

Losarten is the first orally available AII (i.e., AT$_1$ receptor) antagonist. Compared to placebo, losarten demonstrates favorable neurohormonal and hemodynamic effects in patients with CHF treated with digoxin and diuretics (82). Symptomatic hypotension can be minimized with dose titration. Excess cough does not compromise treatment. Effective doses range between 25 and 50 mg/day. Nonetheless, the effect of AII antagonists on survival of patients with CHF remains to be determined.

β-Adrenergic Blocking Agents

Despite the often assumed risk of precipitating an acute episode of heart failure when using β-adrenergic blocking agents in treating patients with CHF, emerging evidence has suggested that heart failure patients can significantly benefit from carefully up-titrated β-blocker therapy (83). Treatment with β-blockers has been examined in several small, randomized studies incorporating over 2000 patients with either ischemic or nonischemic cardiomyopathy and using either β_1-specific antagonists (e.g., metoprolol) or nonspecific β-blockers with additional vasodilatory properties (e.g., bucindolol and carvedilol). A recent metaanalysis of these investigations demonstrated improvements in NYHA functional class and left ventricular EF after 3 months of therapy (84). A second metaanalysis has shown that β-blockers significantly reduce both the need for hospitalization and the frequency of heart transplantation (85). Additional benefits conferred by β-blocker therapy include an improvement in contractility and reductions in systolic wall stress and end-diastolic pressure (83). Possible mechanisms underlying these beneficial effects consist of (a) direct antagonism of the sympathetic nervous system, (b) a reduction in plasma norepinephrine, and (c) up-regulation of β receptors.

Despite these favorable improvements, several questions remain with respect to β-blocker therapy:

1. Which agent(s) afford(s) the greatest clinical benefit?
2. Which patient population is most likely to benefit?
3. When should β blocker therapy be instituted?
4. Do β blockers improve survival?

Several of these questions are being answered by ongoing clinical studies.

Newer Inotropic Drugs

A number of inotropic drugs have been or are being investigated in the management of chronic CHF (86). Mechanistically, each of these agents somehow elevates intracellular concentrations of calcium in myocardial cells that consequently results in increases in contractility. Some of these agents also have peripheral vasodilatory effects. So far, the major pharmacologic categories investigated are (a) orally active β-adrenergic receptor agonists such as xamoterol, pirbuterol, and prenalterol; (b) dopaminergic receptor agonists such as levodopa and ibopamine; (c) phosphodiesterase inhibitors such as am-

rinone, milrinone, and enoximone; and (d) agents with multiple modes of action such as pimobendan and vesnarinone.

Beta-agonists appear to be limited principally by the development of β-receptor down-regulation and increased mortality (86). Initial enthusiasm for β-adrenergic agonists has waned, since most long-term studies failed to demonstrate improvement in symptoms or mortality. Xamoterol, a β_1-selective adrenergic partial agonist, appeared to offer potential in patients with mild-to-moderate failure. However, it increased the mortality of patients with severe heart failure. These mixed findings have resulted in little enthusiasm for the promotion of xamoterol in the treatment of CHF.

With respect to dopaminergic receptor agonists, ibopamine appears to be promising for the treatment of CHF (86). Ibopamine is a prodrug that exerts its positive inotropic effect through β_1-agonism and vasodilation via dopamine agonism. In prospective controlled studies, ibopamine improves exercise tolerance and provides clinical benefits similar to those of ACE inhibitors. Ibopamine also produces favorable neurohormonal effects such as reductions in plasma NE, renin, and aldosterone concentrations. However, long-term mortality studies are needed before serious consideration can be given to its potential therapeutic role in heart failure.

Milrinone and enoximone inhibit the activity of the phosphodiesterase isozyme (PDE III) in both the myocardium and the peripheral vasculature (86). Although these agents improve hemodynamics and anaerobic threshold, their long-term use results in a significant increase in mortality.

Vesnarinone

Vesnarinone is a novel oral inotropic agent that increases myocardial contractility with minimal effects on heart rate and myocardial oxygen consumption. Vesnarinone has a complex mechanism of action that produces increased intracellular calcium concentrations via mild inhibition of PDE III (87). Vesnarinone also inhibits production of the cardiodepressant cytokines, TNF-α, and IFN-γ (88).

A large clinical trial assessed the use of two different doses of vesnarinone (60 mg/day and 120 mg/day) versus placebo in patients with NYHA Class III heart failure and EF less than 30% (87). The majority of patients were receiving diuretics and ACE inhibitors. The 120-mg arm was terminated early because of an observed twofold increase in mortality in this group compared with placebo. However, the 60-mg arm demonstrated a 50% reduction in the risk of worsening heart failure or death compared with the placebo group. Unfortunately, the use of vesnarinone was also associated with a 2.5% incidence of reversible neutropenia. Currently, vesnarinone continues to be studied in Phase III clinical trials.

ARRHYTHMIA MANAGEMENT IN HEART FAILURE PATIENTS

Prevention of sudden cardiac death in heart failure patients remains an unmet therapeutic challenge. Although heart failure is a progressive disease, defined often by a slow deterioration in ventricular function, mortality in patients with heart failure is classified as sudden or "unexpected" in up to 80% of all patients in some studies and in 28 to 68% of patients treated with ACE inhibitors (89). Sudden death is generally defined as death preceded by a short duration of acute symptoms (<1 hr). Ventricular tachycardia degenerating to ventricular fibrillation and ventricular fibrillation itself are the most common causes of sudden death in individuals with coronary artery disease. Heart failure is an independent predictor of sudden death, and almost all heart failure patients exhibit asymptomatic ventricular arrhythmias on 24-hr electrocardiographic recordings. Despite the knowledge that sudden death is common among heart failure patients, no clear consensus on the treatment of asymptomatic ventricular arrhythmias in patients with heart failure has emerged. The risks predisposing heart failure patients to sudden death are multifactorial. Structural changes in the myocardium such as enhanced protein deposition and stretching of tissues may enhance arrhythmogenesis. Neurohormonal activation with elevated circulating catecholamines coupled with parasympathetic withdrawal may stimulate arrhythmia development, as can hemodynamic derangements. Electrolyte disturbances (e.g., hypokalemia or hypomagnesemia), often induced by diuretic therapy, are common predisposing factors to arrhythmia development. Even the inotropic agents that are used to enhance myocardial contractility (such as digoxin and the experimental newer inotropes) are known to produce arrhythmias. Finally, antiarrhythmic drugs themselves are known to produce proarrhythmic results, most markedly in patients with depressed EF.

Although antianginal drugs are not usually considered antiarrhythmic agents, they may decrease the risk of arrhythmias by reducing myocardial ischemia. Optimization of nitrate, ACE-I, and antiplatelet therapy is especially important for patients with heart failure. VHeFT-II demonstrated a reduction in sudden death rates for patients with mild-to-moderate CHF (NYHA Class II to III) treated with enalapril (90).

The Cardiac Arrhythmia Suppression Trial (CAST) demonstrated the danger of trying to suppress asymptomatic ventricular arrhythmias in postmyocardial infarction patients who had mild-to-moderate left ventricular dysfunction but no overt CHF (91). Two class IC antiarrhythmic agents (encainide and flecainide) increased the mortality in all patients and particularly in patients with ejection fractions less than 30%. A third arm of this trial using moricizine also demonstrated a deleterious effect on

mortality (92). Therefore mere suppression of premature ventricular complexes in at least this patient population is not a desirable therapeutic goal.

Treatment of patients with a history of life-threatening ventricular arrhythmias is warranted. The risk of recurrent cardiac arrest in the these individuals may be as high as 15 to 50% over a 2- to 3-year period (89). Current treatment options include electrophysiologic-guided drug testing, amiodarone, and the use of an implantable cardioverter defibrillator. If antiarrhythmic agents are selected, the patients should be carefully monitored for drug-induced exacerbations of heart failure. The agents that are most likely to lead to CHF exacerbations include quinidine, procainamide, disopyramide, and Class IC agents.

Amiodarone currently appears to offer the greatest potential benefit in reducing the risk of sudden death in patients with CHF (89). A metaanalysis has suggested that empirical treatment with amiodarone significantly decreases total mortality and sudden death in postmyocardial infarction patients, many of whom had left ventricular dysfunction (93). In addition, two recent studies have investigated the prophylactic use of amiodarone in patients with heart failure and asymptomatic, non-life-threatening ventricular arrhythmias. The GESICA trial reported a nearly 30% reduction in total mortality in the group of patients with CHF treated with amiodarone (94). However, the Veterans Affairs Survival Trial of Antiarrhythmic Therapy in Congestive Heart Failure study showed a trend of improved survival only in patients with CHF secondary to nonischemic causes (95). In both studies, about 90% of the patients also were receiving ACE inhibitors, and there were no differences in severe adverse effects between the amiodarone and placebo groups. Thus if ventricular arrhythmias must be treated in patients with CHF, it appears that amiodarone should be the antiarrhythmic drug of choice (89).

PREVENTION OF THROMBOEMBOLIC COMPLICATIONS

In CHF, diminished cardiac output, abnormal flow through dilated cardiac chambers, and perhaps decreased contractility may predispose the patient to the development of mural thrombi and consequent emboli (96). However, the annual incidence of either aterial thromboembolism or stroke approximates 1.9%. Furthermore, it is generally unknown what percentage of these events are secondary to cormorbid conditions such as atrial fibrillation or atherosclerotic cerebrovascular disease. Furthermore, although patients with more severe CHF (i.e., NYHA Class IV) appear to have an increased incidence of embolic events, they also are more likely to have coexistant atrial fibrillation. In addition, patients with CHF secondary to idopathic dilated cardiomyopathy do not have an increased risk for thromboembolism when compared with a more heterogenous group of patients with CHF. Therefore until a randomized controlled trial is performed to assess the routine use of warfarin anticoagulation and antiplatelet therapy for patients with CHF in normal sinus rhythm, therapy is not warranted. For patients with coexisting atrial fibrillation or other predisposing conditions, warfarin anticoagulation targeted to an INR of 1.5 to 3.5 is generally indicated. Antiplatelet therapy may be indicated for patients with concurrent CAD.

CORONARY ARTERY REVASCULARIZATION IN THE MANAGEMENT OF CHF

Because of the prevalence of CAD as a cause for CHF, coronary artery revascularization may be an important therapeutic strategy for selected patients (97). It is relatively clear that coronary artery bypass graft (CABG) surgery confers an improved survival benefit on patients with moderate to severe LV systolic dysfunction and concurrent symptom-limiting angina pectoris. It remains unknown, however, whether patients with LV systolic dysfunction due to CAD, but without symptom-limiting angina, will benefit from CABG surgery. This uncertainty of benefit suggests that perhaps only patients with moderate or large ischemic areas should be revascularized. Furthermore, it is also unclear whether percutaneous transluminal coronary angioplasty is a suitable alternative to CABG surgery. Studies are needed to compare these methods of coronary revascularization.

CARDIAC TRANSPLANTATION

During the past three decades, cardiac transplantation has become a vital therapeutic option for patients with CHF (98). The 1- and 5-year posttransplant survival rates approach 85% (99) and 65% to 75%, (98) respectively. However, the limited availability of donor hearts restricts the number of actual transplants to about 2200 per year, despite the fact that nearly 4000 patients are currently or will soon be listed as transplant candidates (98) and that there is a potential need for 16,000 transplants per year for patients up to 55 years of age and up to 40,000 per year for patients under age 65 (99).

Because of the shortage of available donor hearts, patients who are referred for cardiac transplantation undergo a specific evaluation to prioritize the individuals who are most likely to benefit (99). Most patients who are referred for transplantation are adults up to 55 or 65 years of age. Patients usually have a resting ejection fraction under 20 to 25%. The cause of CHF is determined for each patient; potentially reversible and precipitating factors are corrected; and medical therapy, if possible, should be maximally tailored to delay the need for transplantation. Other coexistent systemic illness with a poor prognosis (e.g., cancer or a life-threatening infectious disease) that could decrease posttransplant survival should be identified. These diagnostic and therapeutic efforts are used to categorize potential recipients as critical, unstable, stable, or ineligible with respect to the urgency for transplantation. Some patients who are awaiting transplantation may require bridges to transplantation either for life-threatening ventricular arrhythmias, which may be treated with empirical amiodarone or implantable cardio-defibrillators, or for severe hemodynamic instability, which can be managed with parenteral inotropes such as dobutamine, ventricular assist devices, or the total artificial heart.

Proper selection and management of donor hearts and donor-recipient matching are essential to transplant success (99). Donors are usually considered up to 45 and 50 years of age for males and females, respectively. Cerebral blood flow imaging or an electroencephalogram (EEG) may be required to certify brain death, and echocardiography can identify cardiac dysfunction in the donor heart. ABO-identical blood type donors are generally preferred to ABO-compatible donors. In addition, recent data suggests that minimization of histocompatibility lymphocyte A (HLA) mismatches improves graft survival following transplantation (100). Recipients also undergo screening to detect selected IgG circulating antibodies that are likely to trigger hyperacute rejection during the immediate posttransplant period (99).

The impressive survival following orthotopic cardiac allograft transplantation can be traced largely to improved immunosuppression and perhaps most specifically to the introduction of cyclosporine (101). Cyclosporine is most commonly coprescribed with corticosteroids (usually prednisone) and azathioprine (i.e., triple drug therapy) following transplantation. Immunosuppressive therapy must be tailored for each patient, with careful monitoring for potential adverse effects, cyclosporine whole blood concentrations, drug-drug interactions, signs and symptoms of rejection, and infectious complications. Induction therapy with antilymphocyte antibodies (usually either rabbit or equine polyclonal antithymocyte globulin or the monoclonal antibody OKT3) is still used at several centers to facilitate earlier corticosteroid tapering or withdrawal and to delay mean time to initial allograft rejection. In addition, antilymphocyte antibodies are used to treat corticosteroid-resistant or hemodynamically severe allograft rejection.

Posttransplant complications may include a variety of bacterial, viral, fungal, or protozoal infections (99). Posttransplant hypertension remains a common complication. Accelerated allograft coronary artery atherosclerosis is the principal cause of death in long-term cardiac transplant survivors.

Newer medical therapies are emerging for the management of the cardiac transplant patient (101). These include new immunosuppressive drugs such as tacrolimus (previously known as FK 506), myclophenolate mofetil, and sirolimus (previously known as rapamycin). Whether these agents can improve on the cyclosporine-based regimens remains to be determined. Calcium channel blockers such as diltiazem and inhibitors of 3-hydroxy-3-methylglutaryl coenzyme A (HMG–C$_O$A) reductase inhibitors such as pravastatin may decrease the rate of development of allograft coronary artery atherosclerosis. In addition, the coadministration of ketoconazole, an inhibitor of cyclosporine metabolism, decreases the cost of cyclosporine therapy and may reduce the incidence of rejection.

TREATMENT OF HEART FAILURE DUE TO DIASTOLIC DYSFUNCTION

Diastolic dysfunction, an inadequacy of ventricular relaxation and impaired LV filling, can present with the same signs and symptoms of CHF as those associated with systolic dysfunction, or it can be asymptomatic (2). However, diastolic dysfunction can be differentiated from systolic dysfunction by objective measures of LV function (i.e., ejection fraction) such as radionuclide angiography or scanning or echocardiography (2, 102). In diastolic dysfunction, patients have a normal or near-normal LVEF (i.e., >40%) (2). Typical causes of diastolic dysfunction include systemic HTN, aortic stenosis, and hypertrophic cardiomyopathies, each of which produces significant left ventricular hypertrophy, and CAD, in which impaired diastolic relaxation results from associated myocardial ischemia (102). In some series of patients with CHF, diastolic dysfunction may account for 30 to 40% of the cases (103). The prognosis of patients with symptomatic diastolic dysfunction appears to be more favorable than that of patients with symptomatic systolic dysfunction: an 8% annual mortality rate versus a 15 to 20% annual mortality rate, respectively (2). However, older, more severely ill patients with diastolic dysfunction may have a prognosis similar to that of patients with systolic dysfunction (103).

With respect to treatment of either symptomatic or asymptomatic diastolic dysfunction, no large-scale, prospective, controlled investigations exist. Nonetheless, the goals of therapy should parallel those of the treatment of systolic dysfunction. However, positive inotropic drugs, even digitalis glycosides, should be avoided unless there is accompanying systolic dysfunction (2). For symptomatic patients (Figure 38.4), diuretics in conjunction with salt restriction are initially indicated to relieve congestive symptoms (2). Thereafter, β-adrenergic blockers, calcium channel blockers (i.e., verapamil), or ACE-I may be beneficial. The former two are negative inotropic and negative chronotropic agents. In addition, both agents possess antiischemic effects that would be beneficial for patients with symptomatic diastolic dysfunction secondary to CAD. All of these agents, especially ACE inhibitors, may promote regression of LV hypertrophy. ACE inhibitors also possess other benefits that are mediated via antagonism of neurohormonal maladaptive responses. Surgical therapy

may be indicated for symptomatic diastolic dysfunction secondary to either CAD or aortic stenosis. For asymptomatic patients (Figure 38.3), antihypertensive agents in general effect a reduction in LV hypertrophy, the greatest mean reduction occurring in patients treated with ACE inhibitors (2).

TREATMENT OF ACUTE HEART FAILURE

Acute heart failure is a common medical emergency that generally occurs in one of two clinical settings. Patients with chronic failure may acutely decompensate. This condition is either a natural progression of heart failure or may be precipitated by factors such as infection, onset of arrhythmias, or medication noncompliance. Acute heart failure may also occur in association with acute myocardial infarction. Although similar agents are used to treat acutely decompensated chronic heart failure caused by myocardial infarction, selection of specific drugs depends on which compensatory mechanisms have been activated. The following discussion is limited to acute decompensation of chronic heart failure.

Pathophysiology Overview

Acute decompensation of chronic severe heart failure is characterized by failure of compensatory mechanisms to maintain adequate perfusion to the vital organs. Most patients will exhibit some or all of the following: (a) increased afterload or impedence to left ventricular ejection, (b) increased preload or elevated left ventricular filling pressures and secondary pulmonary congestion, (c) myocardial hypertrophy, (d) sodium retention, (e) peripheral edema, (f) myocardial ischemia, (g) neurohumoral activation, including the sympathetic nervous system, the RAA system, and vasopressin-antidiuretic hormone. Excessive activity of each of these mechanisms contributes to the vicious circle of congestive heart failure ultimately leading to death. Therapy for patients with acutely depressed LV function will be aimed at reducing elevated left ventricular filling pressure and augmenting cardiac output through the use of intravenous fluids and parenteral administered diuretics, vasodilator therapy, or inotropic agents. Because clinical examination alone is incapable of identifying and quantifying the compensatory mechanisms, therapeutic decisions are frequently guided by the intelligent use of hemodynamic monitoring in conjunction with a patient's clinical signs and symptoms.

Unlike the earlier stages of heart failure, which may require a multitude of tests for diagnosis, the patient with severe decompensation is easily recognized. Classically, hypotension occurs, but blood pressure may be maintained by peripheral vasoconstriction. Compensatory tachycardia is often observed and is especially ominous if it persists. The patient's skin may appear cool and pale due to vasoconstriction. However, diaphoresis may occasionally be observed. Skin mottling and cyanosis indicate shunting of blood from the periphery in an effort to maintain perfusion to the heart and brain. Urine output decreases; and in severe failure states, inadequate cerebral perfusion alters mental status. Dyspnea and tachycardia are often present. Systemic venous and pulmonary congestion may manifest as elevated central venous pressure, peripheral edema, and pulmonary edema.

Acute cardiogenic pulmonary edema is the most dramatic sign of left ventricular failure (104). The terrified patient is sitting bolt upright and expectorating pink, frothy sputum. The patient feels as if he or she is drowning. Diaphoresis may be accompanied by cool, ashen skin. Respiratory rate is rapid, and accessory muscles are used for respiration. Pulmonary auscultation reveals rhonchi, wheezes, and rales. Although heart sounds may be difficult to hear, an S_3 is usually present. Overt signs of venous congestion are usually evident. The strategy for treating this emergency involves (a) immediate institution of nonspecific measures, (b) identification and removal of precipitating causes, (c) initiation of invasive hemodynamic monitoring, and (d) implementation of patient-specific drug treatment based on clinical and hemodynamic findings.

Hemodynamic Monitoring

The use of bedside hemodynamic monitoring with flow-directed pulmonary artery (i.e., Swan-Ganz) catheters and systemic arterial catheters has revolutionized critical care medicine. Although some experts contend that this procedure is overused, there is little disagreement about its value in managing patients with acutely decompensated chronic CHF (105).

Insertion of the pulmonary artery catheter is performed by a physician at the bedside, usually with the aid of fluoroscopy. A balloon is attached to the tip of the catheter and, when inflated, allows the catheter to follow the blood flow (106). Right heart catheterization entails antegrade passage of the catheter into the internal jugular vein, superior vena cava, and right atrium, across the tricuspid valve, and into the right ventricle (Figure 38.5). The catheter is advanced into the pulmonary artery until the inflated balloon is as large as the pulmonary artery. The catheter is then wedged, yielding the pulmonary capillary wedge pressure (PCWP). Potential complications of right heart catheterization (pulmonary infarction, arrhythmias, thromboembolism, perforation, balloon rupture, and catheter knotting) are usually minimized in the hands of experienced physicians.

Hemodynamic Data

The systemic arterial pressure (via arterial line) is continuously monitored, but in severe heart failure states, this will not provide a reliable indicator of tissue perfusion. The PCWP is extremely important, as it indicates pulmonary venous pressure and correlates with signs of pulmonary

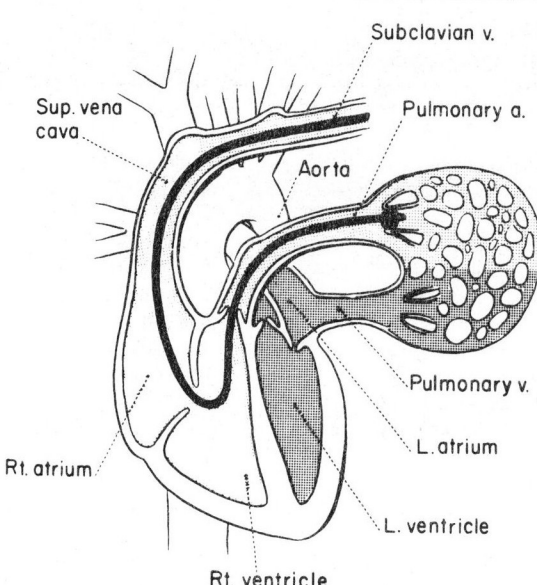

Figure 38.5. Final anatomic positioning of the Swan-Ganz cathether, depicting balloon inflation in the pulmonary artery. (Source: From (106), with permission.)

congestion (Table 38.8). It also indirectly measures the filling pressure of the left ventricle or preload. The pulmonary artery diastolic pressure is also a valuable index of left ventricular filling pressure. Systemic vascular resistance (SVR) is the most common measure of ventricular afterload. Even though SVR does not accurately reflect the interaction of factors both internal and external to the myocardium, it remains the best indirect estimate of left ventricular afterload. Stroke volume is the volume of blood ejected with each heartbeat. Cardiac output is the amount of blood ejected by the heart per unit time and is usually expressed as liters per minute. Cardiac output (CO) varies with body size and is therefore normalized by dividing by the patient's body surface area, yielding cardiac index (CI). Estimates of cardiac output are generally obtained by thermodilution technique. A thermal indicator (usually cooled sterile D5W or normal saline) is injected into the right atrium. A thermistor at the end of the catheter measures the change in blood temperature downstream. The CO is then computer-calculated by using a modification of the Fick principle.

Even though it is not widely used, the ateriovenous oxygen difference is a better indicator of blood flow than is CI (105). It is fairly constant and independent of body surface area, metabolic rate, or oxygen uptake. The arteriovenous oxygen difference assesses the adequacy of CO in relation to the metabolic needs of the tissues. It requires withdrawal of blood samples from the pulmonary and radial arteries. If the patient is not hypoxemic, the mixed venous oxygen content (or saturation) is a good predictor of clinical outcome. A mixed venous oxygen

Table 38.8.
Normal Hemodynamic Values

Systemic arterial pressure (systolic/ diastolic)	120/80 mm Hg
Mean arterial pressure	70–80 mm Hg
Pulmonary artery pressure (systolic/ diastolic)	30/15 mm Hg
Pulmonary capillary wedge pressure	<10–12 mm Hg
Left atrial pressure	5–12 mm Hg (mean)
Left-ventricular end-diastolic pressure	5–12 mm Hg (mean)
Pulmonary vascular resistance	150–250 dynes/sec/cm^5
Systemic vascular resistance	900–1200 dynes/sec/cm^5
Stroke volume	70–130 mL
Right ventricular stroke work	10–15 g·m
Left ventricular stroke work	60–80 g·m
Cardiac output	4–8 L/min
Cardiac index	2.0–4.0 L/min/m^2
Mixed venous oxygen content	13–16 mL/dL
Arterial oxygen content	18–20 mL/dL
Pulmonary capillary oxygen content	20 mL/dL
Arterial–mixed venous oxygen difference	5.0–5.5 mL/dL
Oxygen consumption	22 ± 40 mL/min

Source: Adapted from (105).

saturation of less than 40% is associated with a very poor prognosis.

Therapy of Decompensated Heart Failure

Nonspecific measures designed to decrease pulmonary congestion and improve oxygenation are indicated for all patients with acute failure (104). Supplemental oxygen, perhaps facilitated by mechanical ventilation, improves oxygen delivery. The patient should be in the sitting position to minimize respiratory distress. Morphine sulfate administration is beneficial, owing to its potent venodilatory effect and anxiolytic action. Small doses (2 to 4 mg) are repeated often until acute pulmonary congestion is relieved or alternative parenteral vasodilator therapy is begun. Respiratory depression and systemic hypotension may limit morphine use. Intravenous furosemide exerts an almost immediate venodilatory effect and should not be delayed because hemodynamic monitoring capability is not yet available (107, 108). Blood pressure support may be safely achieved with dopamine infusions before hemodynamic monitoring. Once the Swan-Ganz catheter and arterial line are inserted, patient-specific regimens may be tailored on the basis of the hemodynamic profile and the clinical signs and symptoms.

Diuretics

A mainstay of treatment for acute decompensation and pulmonary edema, intravenous furosemide, causes venodilation and reduces PCWP and pulmonary artery pressure (Figure 38.6) (108). The venodilatory action of intravenous furosemide is observed within several minutes of administration and precedes its natruretic effect (73). Intrave-

nous furosemide (initial dose 20 to 40 mg) may dramatically relieve the signs and symptoms of pulmonary congestion. Oral furosemide generally does not exert an acute venodilatory activity. Until recently, investigators thought that diuretics had little effect on cardiac output. This concept has now been challenged, so less concern prevails for furosemide-induced decreases in cardiac output secondary to overaggressive lowering of elevated filling pressures (107). Bumetanide is an alternative potent loop diuretic, although furosemide is usually given first. The initial intravenous bumetanide dose is 0.5 to 1.0 mg administered over 1 to 2 min. Like furosemide, frequency of repeat doses is governed by hemodynamic data, urine output, and relief of pulmonary congestion.

Vasodilators

By blocking the vicious positive feedback mechanisms of severe heart failure, parenteral vasodilators may abruptly improve cardiac output and relieve pulmonary congestion (104). The patient's hemodynamic profile guides selection of specific vasodilators relative to effects on preload and afterload (Figure 38.6). Sodium nitroprusside is often the first vasodilator used, since it acts on both preload and afterload. It exhibits a fast onset of action and short duration of action; thus sodium nitroprusside is easily titrated. In many patients it will lower pulmonary artery pressure, PCWP, and SVR, resulting in increased cardiac output. The initial infusion rate is 0.25 to 0.5 µg/kg/min and is titrated upward on the basis of clinical response and hemodynamics. Generally, BP, pulmonary artery pressures, and urine output are monitored continuously. Cardiac output and SVR are determined every 2 to 6 hr to aid in dosage adjustment. The most common hazard of nitroprusside in treating severe heart failure is hypotension. Combination nitroprusside and dopamine therapy is common. Dopamine maintains blood pressure and, depending on dose, may improve renal and coronary blood flows.

Intravenous nitroglycerin is especially useful in acute decompensation, since it is easily titrated. Because it predominantly increases venous capacitance (i.e., decreases preload), its effect is primarily to decrease PCWP and pulmonary artery pressures (104, 109). Thus it provides dramatic relief for patients with severe pulmonary congestion. It may also moderately decrease SVR and thus improve cardiac output. Intravenous nitroglycerin doses vary widely; however, initial therapy may begin at 5 to 10 µg/min. Dangers of nitroglycerin represent an extension of its pharmacologic action and are usually limited to hypotension.

Amrinone and milrinone are phosphodiesterase inhibitors that have both positive inotropic actions and significant vasodilator activity (86, 104). The vasodilatory actions may be more prominent than their inotropic effects. Therefore their indications overlap those for the intravenous vasodi-

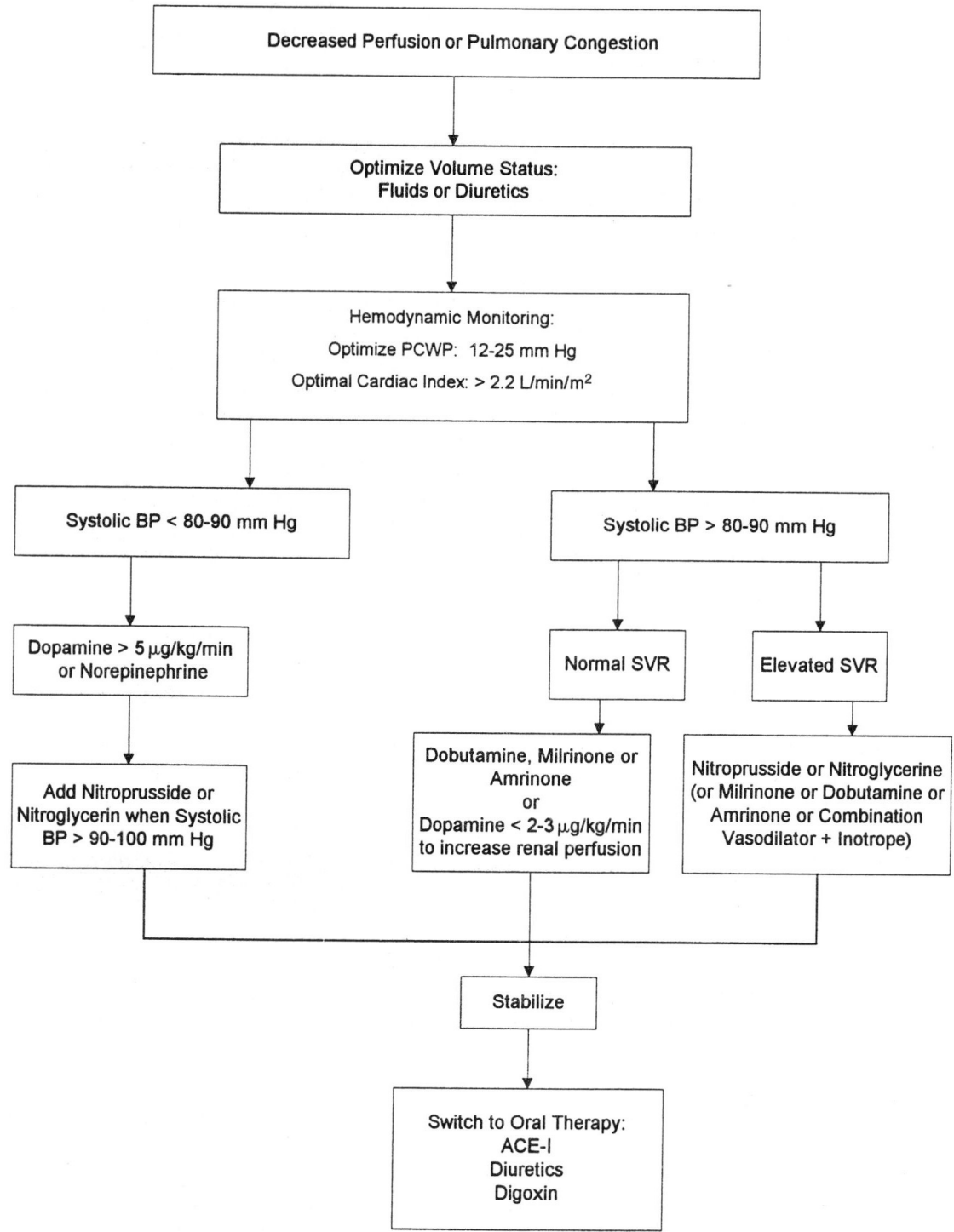

Figure 38.6. Hospitalization for CHF with acute decompensation.

lators, nitroglycerin and nitroprusside, and the parenteral sympathomimetics, dopamine and dobutamine (Figure 38.6). In contrast to nitroglycerin and nitroprusside, amrinone and milrinone have relatively long terminal half-lives. They may also accumulate in renal failure. Dose- and duration-dependent thrombocytopenia is of special concern with amrinone but not with milrinone. Other side effects reflect vasodilation and inotropic effect: hypotension and arrhythmias. For amrinone, therapy is usually begun with a 0.75-mg/kg intravenous bolus given slowly over 2 to 3 min. Maintenance infusions vary between 5 and 10 μg/kg/min. For milrinone, dosing guidelines incorporate loading doses of 37.5 to 75 μg/kg followed by maintenance infusions of 0.375 to 0.75 μg/kg/min. Combination dobutamine and either milrinone or amrinone therapy may provide greater improvement in left ventricular performance than either agent alone.

Sympathomimetic Amines

Because severe chronic congestive failure is complicated by overstimulation of the sympathetic nervous system, administration of exogenous catecholamines is generally reserved for acute decompensatory episodes. Dopamine may be especially useful in treating patients with mild-to-moderate hypotension (Figure 38.6) (86, 104). The initial dose is 0.5 to 1.0 μg/kg/min and is titrated upward according to filling pressures, cardiac output, and urine output. If hypotension is severe, dopamine doses in the range of 10 to 20 μg/kg/min will provide the alpha stimulation that is necessary to maintain perfusion to the vital organs and improve cardiac output. Dopamine side effects include tachycardia, ventricular arrhythmias, and excessive vasoconstriction, especially at higher doses. Nevertheless, it remains a valuable agent, especially when it is used in combination with nitroprusside.

Dobutamine is a synthetic catecholamine that is a selective β_1 agonist (86, 104). The improvement in cardiac output may then cause a reflex decrease in both filling pressures and SVR (Figure 38.6). Dobutamine infusions are begun at 1 to 2 μg/kg/min and titrated upward every 10 to 30 min, with optimal maintenance infusions generally between 5 and 15 μg/kg/min. Side effects are usually limited but may include tachycardia, arrhythmias, headaches, anxiety, and tremor.

PROGNOSIS

Despite the lack of published information describing the natural history of heart failure in the absence of treatment, several studies of patients receiving treatment have revealed that their overall prognosis is grim. In the initial report from the Framingham Study, the probability of death within 5 years of the diagnosis of CHF was 62% for men and 42% for women (3). More recently, the Framingham Study reported median surivial rates for men at 1, 2, 5, and 10 years after the onset of CHF to be 57%, 46%, 25%, and 11%, respectively. Corresponding rates in women were 64%, 56%, 38%, and 21% (4). In addition, median survival for males and females was 1.7 years and 3.2 years, respectively. These survival statistics are worse than those reported for the placebo group in the V-HeFT I treatment trial. However, when only the patients in the Framingham Study who survived the initial 90 days after the diagnosis of CHF are included, their suvival rates parallel those reported for the placebo patients in V-HeFT I.

Several clinical variables have been shown to be predictive of prognosis in patients with CHF (110).

Decreases either in left ventricular EF (especially below 20%) or in VO_{2max} (principally ≤14 mL/min/kg) predict a poor prognosis. Increases in cardiothoracic ratio on chest roentgenogram, severity of symptoms (i.e., higher NYHA Class), plasma NE (>600 pg/mL), and plasma ANP also predict a poor prognosis. The presence of arrhythmias (i.e., couplets and triplets or nonsustained ventricular tachycardia) is an independent predictor of a diminished survival (111). The cause of a patient's CHF may be predictive of prognosis. For example, in the Framingham Study, men with CHF due to valvular disease had a worse prognosis than did men with CHF due to CAD (4). For women the worst prognosis occurred in those with a history of diabetes mellitus. Older patients also exhibited a worse prognosis than younger patients. Even patients who are treated with "life-saving" pharmacologic therapy have an unsatisfactory prognosis. In V-HeFT II, for example, the 5-year survival rate in the enalapril group was approximately 55%. Thus CHF remains a highly lethal clinical syndrome, despite medical intervention.

CONCLUSIONS

Congestive heart failure remains a commonly occurring clinical syndrome whose prevalence is increasing as the general population ages. Although many different treatment modalities are currently available for managing these increasing numbers of patients, ACE inhibitors now serve as the cornerstone of medical therapy for the majority of these patients. A sound working knowledge of the pathophysiology and how to implement, monitor, and integrate these varying therapies is essential to achieve the therapeutic goals of prevention of initiation and progression of CHF and improvement in symptoms, the quality of life, and the longevity of patients with CHF.

REFERENCES

1. Harris P. The problem of defining heart failure. Cardiovasc Drug Ther 8:447–452, 1994.
2. Gaasch WH. Diagnosis and treatment of heart failure based on left ventricular systolic or diastolic dysfunction. JAMA 271:1276–1280, 1994.
3. McKee PA, Castelli WP, McNamara PM, Kannel WB. The natural history of congestive heart failure: The Framingham Study. N Engl J Med 285:1441–1446, 1971.
4. Kalon KLH, Anderson KM, Kannel WB, Grossman W, Levy D. Survival after onset of congestive heart failure in Framingham Heart Study subjects. Circulation 88:107–115, 1993.
5. Yusuf S, Them T, Abbott RD. Changes in hypertension treatment and in congestive heart failure mortality in the United States. Hypertension 13(suppl I):I-74–I-79, 1989.
6. Dec GW, Fuster V. Idiopathic dilated cardiomyopathy. N Engl J Med 331:1564–1575, 1994.
7. O'Connell JB, Bristow MR. Economic impact of heart failure in the United States: time for a different approach. J Heart Lung Transplant 13:S107–112, 1994.
8. Kannel WB, Belanger AJ. Epidemiology in heart failure. Am Heart J 121:951–957, 1991.

9. Parmley WW. Pathophysiology of congestive heart failure. Clin Cardiol 15(suppl I):I-5–I-12, 1992.

10. Weber KT, Anversa P, Armstrong PW, Brilla CG, et al. Remodeling and reparation of the cardiovascular system. J Am Coll Cardiol 20:3–16, 1992.

11. Katz AM. The cardiomyopathy of overload: an unnatural growth response in the hypertrophied heart. Ann Intern Med 121:363–371, 1994.

12. Packer M. Pathophysiology of chronic heart failure. Lancet 340:88–92, 1992.

13. Dzau VJ. Autocrine and paracrine mechanisms in the pathophysiology of heart failure. Am J Cardiol 70:4C–11C, 1992.

14. Floras JS. Clinical aspects of sympathetic activation and parasympathetic withdrawal in heart failure. J Am Coll Cardiol 22(suppl A):72A–84A, 1993.

15. Ferrari R, Corti A, Bachetti T. Tumor necrosis factor alpha in heart failure. Heart Failure 11:142–149, 1995.

16. Tedgui A, Bernard C. Cytokines and vascular reactivity. Heart Failure 11:159–165, 1995.

17. Braunwald E, Grossman W. Clinical aspects of heart failure. In: Braunwald E, ed. Heart disease: a textbook of cardiovascular medicine. 4th ed. Philadelphia: WB Saunders, 1992:444–463.

18. Marantz PR, Tobin JN, Wassertheil-Smoller S, et al. The relationship between left-ventricular systolic function and congestive heart failure diagnosed by clinical criteria. Circulation 77:607–612, 1988.

19. Harlan WRI, Oberman A, Grimm R, et al. Chronic congestive heart failure in coronary artery disease: clinical criteria. Ann Intern Med 86:133–138, 1977.

20. Mattelman SJ, Hakki A, Iskandrian AS, et al. Reliability of bedside evaluation in determining left ventricular function: correlation with left-ventricular ejection fraction determined by radionuclide ventriculography. J Am Coll Cardiol 1:417–420, 1983.

21. Stevenson LW, Perloff JK. The limited reliability of physical signs for estimating hemodynamics in chronic heart failure. JAMA 261:884–888, 1989.

22. Fleg JL, Hinton PC, Lakatta EG, Marcus FI, et al. Physician utilization of laboratory procedures to monitor outpatients with congestive heart failure. Arch Intern Med 149:393–396, 1989.

23. Packer M, Gottlieb SS, Kessler PD. Hormone-electrolyte interactions in the pathogenesis of lethal cardiac arrhythmias in patients with congestive heart failure. Am J Med 80(Suppl 4A):23–29, 1986.

24. Criteria Committee, New York Heart Association, Inc. Diseases of the Heart and Blood Vessels: Nomenclature and Criteria for Diagnosis, 6th ed. Boston: Little, Brown, 1964:114.

25. Weber KT, Janicki JS. Cardiopulmonary exercise testing for evaluation of chronic cardiac failure. Am J Cardiol 55:22A–31A, 1985.

26. Guyatt GH. Measurement of health-related quality of life in heart failure. J Am Coll Cardiol 22(suppl A):185A–191A, 1993.

27. Guyatt GH, Sullivan MJ, Thompson PF, Fallen EL, Pugsley SO, Taylor DW, Berman LB. The 6-minute walk: a new measure of exercise capacity in patients with chronic heart failure. Can Med Assoc J 132:919–923, 1985.

28. Poole-Wilson PA. Relation of pathophysiologic mechanisms to outcome in heart failure. J Am Coll Cardiol 22(suppl A):22A–29A, 1993.

29. Dracup K, Baker DW, Dunbar SB, Dacey RA, et al. Management of heart failure. II: Counseling, education, and lifestyle modifications. JAMA 272:1442–1446, 1994.

30. Armstrong PW, Moe GW. Medical advances in the treatment of congestive heart failure. Circulation 88:2941–2952, 1993.

31. Baker DW, Konstam MA, Bottorff M, Pitt B. Management of heart failure. I: Pharmacologic treatment. JAMA 272:1361–1366, 1994.

32. Sullivan MJ, Higginbotham M, Cobb FR. Exercise training in patients with chronic heart failure delays ventilatory anaerobic threshold and improves submaximal exercise performance. Circulation 79:324–329, 1989.

33. Coats AJ, Adamopoulos S, Meyer TE, et al. Effects of physical training in chronic heart failure. Lancet 335(8681):63–66, 1990.

34. Ghali JK, Kadakia S, Cooper R, Ferlinz J. Precipitating factors leading to decompensation of heart failure: trait among urban blacks. Arch Intern Med 148:2013–2016, 1988.

35. Rosenberg S. Patient education leads to better care for heart patients. HSMHA Health Rep 86:793–802, 1971.

36. Braunwald E. ACE-inhibitors: a cornerstone of the treatment of heart failure. N Engl J Med 325:351–353, 1991.

37. Cohn JN, Archibald DG, Ziesche S, Franciosa JA, et al. Effect of vasodilator therapy on mortality in chronic congestive heart failure. N Engl J Med 314:1547–1552, 1986.

38. Cohn JN, Johnson G, Ziesche S, Cobb FR, et al. A comparison of enalapril with hydralazine-isosorbide dinitrate in the treatment of congestive heart failure. N Engl J Med 325:303–310, 1991.

39. The CONSENSUS Trial Study Group. Effects of enalapril on mortality in severe congestive heart failure: results of the Cooperative North Scandinavian Enalapril Survival Study. N Engl J Med 316:691–695, 1987.

40. The SOLVD investigators. Effect of enalapril on survival in patients with reduced left ventricular ejection fractions and congestive heart failure. N Engl J Med 325:293–302, 1991.

41. Garg R, Yusuf S, for the Collaborative Group on ACE Inhibitor Trials. Overview of randomized trials of angiotensin-converting enzyme inhibitors on mortality and morbidity in patients with heart failure. JAMA 273:1450–1456, 1995.

42. Cohn JN. Nitrates for congestive heart failure. Am J Cardiol 56:19A–23A, 1985.

43. Fonarow GC, Chelimsky-Fallick C, Stevenson LW, Luu M, et al. Effect of direct vasodilation with hydralazine versus angiotensin-converting enzyme inhibition with captopril on mortality in advanced heart failure: the Hy-C trial. J Am Coll Cardiol 19:842–850, 1992.

44. Elkayam U. Tolerance to organic nitrates: evidence, mechanisms, clinical relevance, and strategies for prevention. Ann Intern Med 114:667–677, 1991.

45. Franciosa JA, Weber KT, Levine TB, Kinasewitz GT, et al. Hydralazine in the long-term treatment of chronic heart failure: lack of a difference from placebo. Am Heart J 104:587–594, 1982.

46. Conradson T-B, Ryden L, Ahlmark G, Saetre H, et al. Clinical efficacy of hydralazine in chronic heart failure: one-year, double-blind, placebo-controlled study. Am Heart J 108:1001–1006, 1984.

47. Packer M, Meller J, Medina N, Gorlin R, et al. Hemodynamic evaluation of hydralazine dosage in refractory heart failure. Clin Pharmacol Ther 27:337–346, 1980.

48. The Captopril Multicenter Research Group. A placebo-controlled trial of captopril in refractory chronic congestive heart failure. J Am Coll Cardiol 2:755–763, 1983.

49. Sharpe DN, Murphy J, Coxon R, Hannan SF. Enalapril in patients with chronic congestive heart failure: a placebo-controlled, randomized, double-blind study. Circulation 70:271–278, 1984.

50. The SOLVD Investigators. Effect of enalapril on mortality and the development of heart failure in asymptomatic patients with reduced left ventricular ejection fractions. N Engl J Med 327:685–691, 1992.

51. Pfeffer MA, Braunwald E, Moye LA, et al. The effect of captopril on mortality and morbidity in patients with left ventricular dysfunction after myocardial infarction: results of the survival and ventricular enlargement trial. N Engl J Med 327:667–669, 1992.

52. Packer M, Lee WH, Yushak M, Medina N. Comparison of captopril and enalapril in patients with severe chronic heart failure. N Engl J Med 315:847–853, 1986.

53. Meissner MD, Wilson AR, Jessup M. Renal artery stenosis in heart failure. Am J Cardiol 62:1307–1308, 1988.

54. Smith TW. Digitalis. Mechanisms of action and clinical use. N Engl J Med 318:358–365, 1988.

55. Watanabe AM. Digitalis and the autonomic nervous system. J Am Coll Cardiol 5:35A–42A, 1985.

56. Krum H, Bigger JT, Goldsmith RL, Packer M. Effect of longterm digoxin therapy on autonomic function in patients chronic heart failure. J Am Coll Cardiol 25:289–294, 1995.

57. Gheorghiade M, Ferguson D. Digoxin: a neurohormonal modulator in heart failure? Circulation 84:2181–2186, 1991.

58. Reuning RH, Geraets DR, Rocci ML, Vlasses PH. Digoxin. In: Evans WE, Shentag JJ, Jusko WJ, eds. Applied pharmacokinetics: principles of therapeutic drug monitoring. 3rd ed. Vancouver, WA: Applied Therapeutics, Inc., 1992:20-1–20-28.

59. Rey AM, Gums JG. Altered absorption of digoxin, sustained-release quinidine, and warfarin with sucralfate administration. DICP Ann Pharmacother 25:745–746, 1991.

60. Smith TW, Antman EM, Friedman PL, Blatt CM, et al. Digitalis glycosides: mechanisms and manifestations of toxicity. Prog Cardio-vasc Dis 26:413–458, 495–540; 27:21–56, 1984.

61. Kelly RA, Smith TW. Recognition and management of digitalis toxicity. Am J Cardiol 69:108G–119G, 1992.

62. Mojaverian P, Green PJ, Jhangiania RK, Chase GD. Digoxinlike immunoreactive substance: monoclonal and polyclonal RIA and FPLA compared. J Pharm Biomed Anal 7:585–592, 1989.

63. Packer M, Gheorghiade M, Young JB, Constantini PJ, et al. for the RADIANCE Study. Withdrawal of digoxin from patients with, chronic heart failure treated with angiotensin-converting enzyme inhibitors. N Engl J Med 329:1–7, 1993.

64. Uretsky BF, Young JB, Shahidi FE, Yellen LG, et al. on behalf of the PROVED Investigative Group. Randomized study assessing the effect of digoxin withdrawal in patients with mild to moderate chronic congestive heart failure: results of the PROVED Trial. J Am Coll Cardiol 22:955–962, 1993.

65. Jones WN, Perrier D, Trinca CE, Hager WD, et al. Evaluation of various methods of digoxin dosing. J Clin Pharmacol 22:543–550, 1982.

66. Koup JR, Jusko WJ, Elwood CM, Kohli RK. Digoxin pharmacoki-netics: role of renal failure in dosage regimen design. Clin Pharmacol Ther 18:9–21, 1975.

67. Luke DR, Halstenson EC, Opsahl JA, Matzke GR. Validity of creatinine clearance estimates in the assessment of renal function. Clin Pharmacol Ther 48:503–508, 1990.

68. Nolan PE, Mooradian AD. Digoxin. In: Bressler R, Katz MD, eds. Geriatric Pharmacology, 1st ed. New York: McGraw-Hill, 1993:151–164.

69. Mahdyoon H, Battilana G, Rosman H, Goldstein S, et al. The evolving pattern of digoxin intoxication: observations at a large urban hospital from 1980 to 1988. Am Heart J 120:1189–1194, 1990.

70. Cohen L, Kitzes R. Magnesium sulfate and digitalis-toxic arrhyth-mias. JAMA 249:2808–2810, 1983.

71. Antman EM, Wenger TL, Butler VP, Haber E, et al. Treatment of 150 cases of life-threatening digitalis intoxication with digoxin-specific Fab antibody fragments. Circulation 81:1744–1752, 1990.

72. Jaeschke R, Oxman AD, Guyatt GH. To what extent do congestive heart failure patients in sinus rhythm benefit from digoxin therapy? A systematic overview and metaanalysis. Am J Med 88:279–286, 1990.

73. Mokrzycki MH. Diuretic treatment of heart failure. Heart Failure. 10:181–191, 1994.

74. Ellison DH. The physiologic basis of diuretic synergism: its role in treating diuretic resistance. Ann Intern Med 114:886–894, 1991.

75. Elkayam U, Shotan A, Mehra A, Ostrzega E. Calcium channel blockers in heart failure. J Am Coll Cardiol 22(suppl A):139A–144A, 1993.

76. Scognamiglio R, Rahimtoola SH, Fasoli G, Nistri S, Volta SD. Nifedipine in asymptomatic patients with severe aortic regurgitation and normal left ventricular function. N Engl J Med 331:689–694, 1994.

77. Rothlisberger C, Sareli P, Wisenbaugh T. Comparison of single dose nifedipine and captopril for chronic severe mitral regurgitation. Am J Cardiol 73:978–981, 1994.

78. Packer M. Prospective randomized amlodipine survival evaluation (PRAISE). Presented at the Annual Meeting of the American College of Cardiology, New Orleans, March 19–22, 1995.

79. De Vries RJ, Quere M, Lok DJ, Sijbring P, Bucx JJ, Dunselman PH. Felodipine versus enalapril in heart failure: results on peak oxygen consumption, Holter recordings, hemodynamics, neurohormones, and quality of life. J Am Coll Cardiol 25:416A–417A, 1995.

80. Pouleur H, Konstam MA, Benedict CR, Donckier J, Galanti L, Melin J, Kinan D, Ahn S, Rousseau MF. Progression of left ventricular dysfunction during enalapril therapy: relationship with neuro-hormonal reactivation. Circulation 88(suppl I):1–293, 1993.

81. Aldigier JC, Huang H, Dalmay F, Lartigue M, Baussant T, Chassain AP, Leroux-Robert C, Galen FX. Angiotensin converting enzyme inhibition does not suppress plasma angiotensin II increase during exercise in humans. J Cardiovasc Pharmacol 21:289–295, 1993.

82. Crozier I, Ikram H, Awan N, Cleland J, Stephen N, Dickstein K, Frey M, Young J, Klinger G. Makris L, Rucinska E. Losartan in heart failure. Hemodynamic effects and tolerability. Circulation 91:691–697, 1995.

83. Eichhorn EJ, Hjalmarson A. β-blocker treatment for chronic heart failure: the frog prince. Circulation 90:2153–2156, 1994.

84. Zarembski DG, Nolan PE, Slack MK, Lui CY. Meta-analysis of the use of low-dose–adrenergic blocking therapy in idiopathic and ischemic cardiomyopathy. Am J Cardiol (in press).

85. Tsuyuki RT, Avezum A, Yusuf S. Beta blocker therapy for congestive heart failure: a systematic overview (updated abstract). Paper presented at the Annual Meeting of the American College of Clinical Pharmacy, Washington, DC, August 6–9, 1995.

86. Chatterjee K, Wolfe CL, DeMarco T. Nonglycoside inotropes in congestive heart failure: are they beneficial of harmful? Cardiol Clin 12:63–72, 1994.

87. Feldman AM, Bristow MR, Parmley WW, Carson PE, et al. Effects of vesnarinone on morbidity and mortality in patients with heart failure. N Engl J Med 329:149–155, 1993.

88. Matsumori A, Shioi T, Yamada T, Matsui S, Sasayama S. Ves-narinone, a new inotropic agent, inhibits cytokine production by stimulated human blood from patients with heart failure. Circulation 89:955–958, 1994.

89. Stevenson WG, Stevenson LW, Middlekauff HR, Saxon LA. Sudden death prevention in patients with advanced ventricular dysfunction. Circulation 88:2953–2961, 1993.

90. Fletcher RD, Cintron GB, Johnson G, Orndorff J, et al. Enalapril decreases prevalence of ventricular tachycardia in patients with chronic congestive heart failure. Circulation 87(suppl VI):VI-49–VI-55, 1993.

91. Echt DS, Liebson PR, Mitchell LB, et al. Mortality and morbid-ity in patients receiving encainide, flecainide, or placebo: the Cardiac Arrhythmias Suppression Trial. N Engl J Med 324:781–788, 1991.

92. The Cardiac Arrhythmia Suppression Trial II Investigators. Effect of the antiarrhythmic agent moricizine on survival after myocardial infarction. N Engl J Med 27:27–33, 1992.

93. Zarembski DG, Nolan PE, Slack MK, Caruso AC. Empiric longterm amiodarone prophylaxis following myocardial infarction. Arch Intern Med 153:2661–2667, 1993.

94. Doval HC, Nul DR, Grancelli HO, Perrone SV, Bortman GR, Curiel R. Randomized trial of low-dose amiodarone in severe congestive heart failure. Lancet 344:493–498, 1994.

95. Singh SN, Fletcher RD, Fisher SG, Singh BN, Lewis HD, Deedwania PC, Massie BM, Colling C, Lazzeri D. Amiodarone in patients with congestive heart failure and asymptomatic ventricular arrhythmia. N Engl J Med 333:77–82, 1995.

96. Baker DW, Wright RF. Management of heart failure. IV: Anticoagulation for patients with heart failure due to left ventricular systolic dysfunction. JAMA 272:1614–1618, 1994.

97. Baker DW, Jones R, Hodges J, Massie BM, et al. Management of heart failure. III: The role of revascularization in the treatment of patients with moderate or severe left ventricular systolic dysfunction. JAMA 272:1528–1534, 1994.

98. Stevenson LW, Warner SL, Steimie AE, et al. The impending crisis awaiting cardiac transplantation: modeling a solution based on selection. Circulation 89:450–457, 1994.

99. Hunt SA, Chairman. 24th Bethesda Conference: Cardiac Transplantation. J Am Coll Cardiol 22:1–64, 1993.

100. Opelz G, Wujciak T, for the Collaborative Transplant Study. The influence of HLA compatibility on graft survival after heart transplantation. N Engl J Med 330:816–819, 1994.

101. Valentine HA, Schroeder JS. Recent advances in cardiac transplantation. N Engl J Med 333:660–661, 1995.

102. Lenihan DJ, Gerson MC, Hoit BD, Walsh RA. Mechanisms, diagnosis, and treatment of diastolic heart failure. Am Heart J 130:153–166, 1995.

103. Setaro JF, Soufer R, Remetz MS, Perlmutter RA, Zaret BL. Long-term outcome in patients with congestive heart failure and intact systolic left ventricular performance. Am J Cardiol 69:1212–1216, 1992.

104. Smith TW, Braunwald E, Kelly RA. The management of heart failure. In: Braunwald E, ed. Heart disease: A Textbook of Cardiovascular Medicine, 4th ed. Philadelphia: WB Saunders, 1992:464–519.

105. McGrath RB. Invasive bedside hemodynamic monitoring. Prog Cardiovasc Dis 29:129–144, 1986.

106. Bollish SJ, Foster TJ. Swan-Ganz catheter: an important tool for monitoring drug therapy in the critically ill. Hosp Formul 16:99–103, 1980.

107. Stevenson LW, Tillisch JH. Maintenance of cardiac output with normal filling pressures in patients with dilated heart failure. Circulation 74:1303–1308, 1986.

108. Nairns RG, Chusid P. Diuretic use in critical care. Am J Cardiol 10:139–145, 1984.

109. Bayley S, Valentine H, Bennett ED. The hemodynamic responses to incremental doses of intravenous nitroglycerin in left ventricular failure. Intens Care Med 10:139–145, 1984.

110. Francis GS. Determinants of prognosis in patients with heart failure. J Heart Lung Transplant 13:S113–S116, 1994.

111. Cohn JN, Johnson GR, Shabetai R, Leob H, et al. Ejection fraction, peak exercise oxygen consumption, cardiothoracic ratio, ventricular arrhythmias, and plasma norepinephrine as determinants of prognosis in heart failure. Circulation 87(suppl VI):VI-6–VI-16, 1993.

CHAPTER 39

CARDIAC ARRHYTHMIAS

FRANK M. POMPILIO and MARK A. GILL

The appropriate selection of treatment for any arrhythmia is aided by an understanding of cardiac anatomy and electrophysiology. This chapter reviews the aspects of anatomy and electrophysiology that support an understanding of antiarrhythmic agents. The frequency of serious adverse reactions from antiarrhythmic drugs should be compared to the morbidity associated with the particular disturbance under consideration. This balance, when known, is presented under each type of arrhythmia. Once a drug is chosen, the principles of pharmacokinetics may be applied to tailor the regimen to each patient. This chapter provides examples of equations used to calculate drug dosage regimens.

ELECTROPHYSIOLOGY

The electrical system of the heart consists of intrinsic pacemakers and conduction tissues. It is convenient to conceptualize the progression of normal cardiac rhythm in terms of anatomical basis (Fig. 39.1). Figure 39.2 correlates the standard electrocardiogram with this normal electrical pathway.

The rate of electrical firing of the heart depends on the most rapid pacemaker. Spontaneous electrical firing or automaticity can occur anywhere in the heart under certain conditions. Normally, the sinoatrial node (SA node), which is located where the superior vena cava meets the right atrium, has the most rapid intrinsic rate (60 to 100 beats/min). Therefore, any electrical activity not initiated by a normal impulse generated by the SA node is considered an arrhythmia. Most arrhythmias are labeled as to the anatomical location and rate.

Firing of the SA node initiates contraction of the atria. The electrical impulse is conducted through the atria via the internodal tracts to the atrioventricular (AV) node near the coronary sinus, between the two atria. The AV node has pacemaker properties but normally serves to coordinate atrial and ventricular contraction. The AV node normally limits excessively rapid atrial rates from activating the ventricles.

The conduction system in the ventricles is more elaborate than that in the atria since the muscle mass is larger. Rapid and effective excitation is critical because the ventricles contribute the most to cardiac output.

Fibers leaving the AV node are called the Bundle of His. They separate into the bundle branches, which traverse the septum between the ventricles. Conduction between the AV node and the Bundle of His is measured by the PR interval (Fig. 39.2). The final conducting components of the ventricles are the Purkinje fibers, which emanate from the bundle branches to stimulate the ventricular cardiac muscle to contract. The QRS complex measures depolarization of the ventricles. The QT interval reflects repolarization of the ventricles.

THE ACTION POTENTIAL

Conduction and electrical firing in myocardial cells may be analyzed by measuring the membrane potential of various tissues. The electrical potential of these membranes is established by the flow of ions. When electrodes are placed into these tissues, a characteristic repetitive pattern is seen called an action potential (Fig. 39.3). This action potential may be divided into five phases. Phase 0 is the period of depolarization. It is mediated by two ionic currents. The initial event is the rapid influx of sodium ions into the cardiac cell. As the sodium depolarizes the tissues, the threshold for the slow response is reached. The slow response depends on the transfer of calcium. Phase 1, the rapid repolarization of the tissue, may depend on inactivation of the sodium current and activation of chloride flow. Phase 2 is a plateau phase maintained primarily by calcium flow. Phase 3 is the repolarization of the cells initially begun by inhibition of calcium flow. Repolarization is accelerated by potassium flow outward. The rate of fall of phase 3 and its depth will determine the membrane responsiveness. Tissues may depolarize only after reaching a particular level of repolarization, at least −50 to −55 mV for normal Purkinje fibers. The tissue cannot be reactivated regardless of the stimulus until falling below the threshold potential (x in Fig. 39.3). This level of repolarization will therefore determine the end of the absolute refractory period (ARP). The ARP varies in length depending on the action potential duration (APD). Phase 4 is the depolarization of the cells. In Purkinje fibers, it is brought on by stimulation from the sinus node. Phase 4 may develop spontaneously if the slope is increased. The action potential of pacemaker tissue, such as the sinus node, differs from that of Purkinje fibers. The depth of depolarization is less dramatic, and phase 4 has a steeper slope that determines the rate of sinus firing and its automaticity. The precise ionic currents responsible for pacemaker cells are not entirely known.

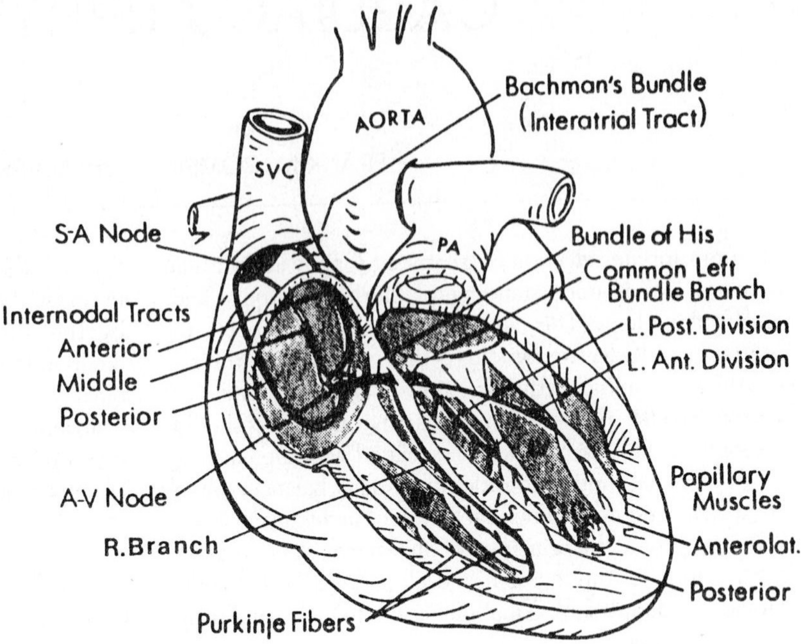

Figure 39-1. Anatomy of the electrical system of the heart. The impulse is generated by the sinoatrial (S-A node) and is conducted through the atria to the atrioventricular (A-V) node, which directs the current to the Bundle of His, into the bundle branches, and finally to the Purkinje fibers.

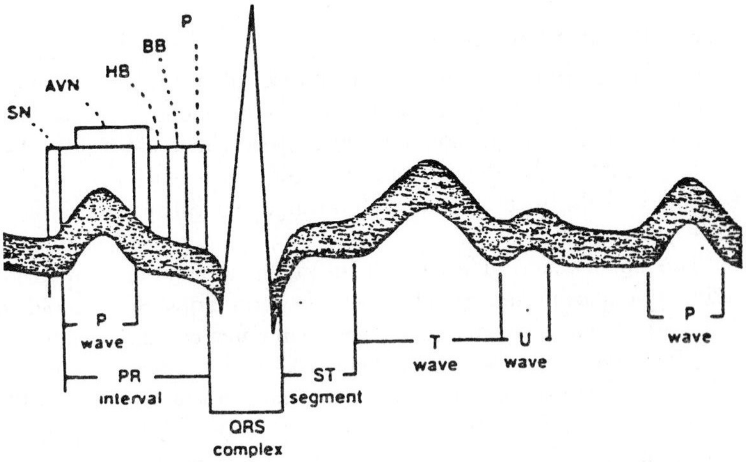

Figure 39-2. The normal electrocardiogram. The P wave is atrial depolarization. The PR interval (0.12 to 0.20 sec) is formed from the firing of the S-A node (SN) and conduction through the A-V node (AVN), Bundle of His (HB), the Bundle branches (BB), and Purkinje fibers (P). The QRS complex (0.05 to 0.10 sec) is ventricular depolarization. The S-T segment is the refractory period. The T wave is ventricular repolarization. The QT interval is 0.35 to 0.44 sec in duration.

ARRHYTHMIA GENESIS

In general, arrhythmias may be described as abnormalities in electrical development, as in ectopic tachyarrhythmias; in electrical conduction, as in reentry arrhythmias; or in a combination of both mechanisms.

Abnormalities in electrical development result from automaticity or triggered activity producing ectopic beats (1). Ectopic beats may develop as pacemaking cells emerge when anoxia, stretch, catecholamine excess, or edema increase the slope of phase 4. Abnormal automaticity may develop at any site in the heart. Generally, the fastest firing tissue drives the heart. In the normal heart, atrial pacemakers have faster intrinsic rates than ventricular pacemakers. When the sinus node rate falls below the intrinsic rate of another tissue, that tissue then drives the heart. Triggered activity is caused by early after-depolarizations requiring a preceding action potential for

their induction. After-depolarizations can occur with oscillations in the plateau phase of the action potential leading to a second depolarization before the first is completed. Hypoxia, fiber stretch, catecholamines, high pCO_2, and overdose of digitalis can lead to triggered activity.

Reentry arrhythmias depend on different velocities along adjacent fibers and unidirectional block in electrical conduction (Fig. 39.4). This allows for continued excitation in a repetitive manner. This circus rhythm may develop as areas of infarcted tissue block or delay conduction. A single circuit of the fibers may induce a premature contraction, whereas continuous cycling of impulses might produce sustained tachycardia. This process may occur in both atrial and ventricular tissue.

Antiarrhythmics have varying effects on reentry mechanics. One effect might be to inhibit membrane responsiveness in fiber 2 such that block is produced in

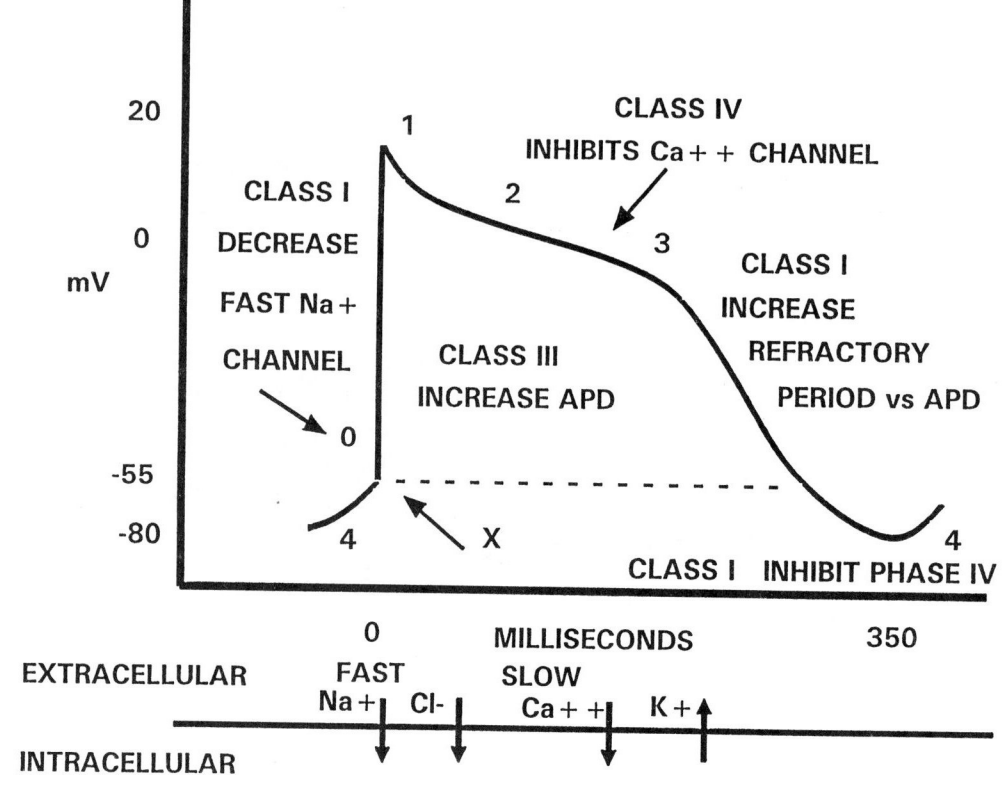

Figure 39-3. The action potential of a cardiac conduction cell correlated with electrolyte shifts. X is the threshold potential. The effects of the antiarrhythmic drug classes (see Table 39.1) are noted for the phases of the action potential.

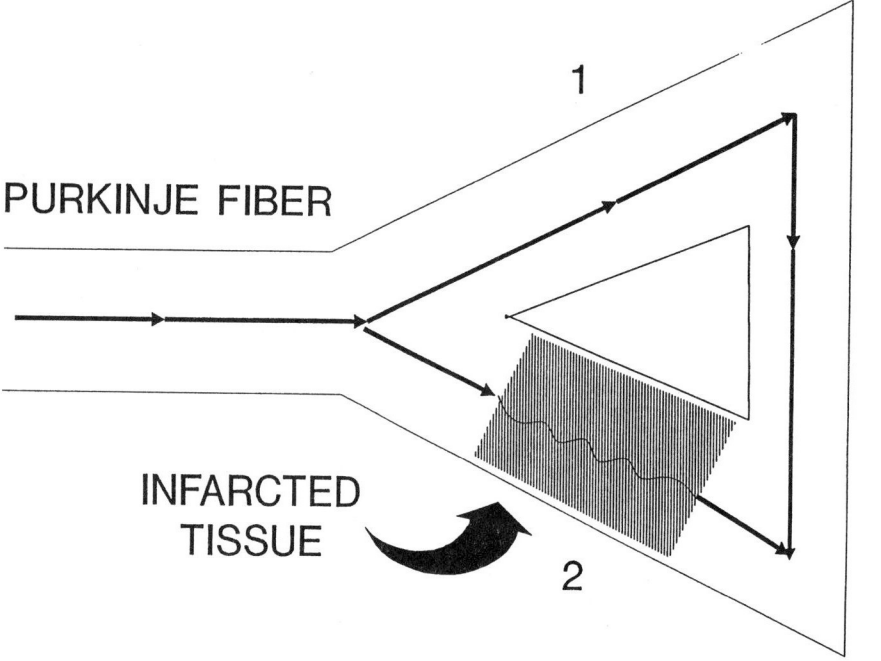

Figure 39-4. Reentry. A conduction fiber that bifurcates into fibers 1 and 2 to stimulate ventricular tissues. The normal pattern is for conduction through fibers 1 and 2 at similar rates. In this figure, fiber 2 was infarcted, which slows conduction until it is blocked by refractory cells. The impulse is impeded along fiber 1. Fiber 2 is activated by the impulse crossing the ventricular muscle tissue. The retrograde impulse finds fiber 2 repolarized and crosses, but at a slow rate. This circuit may be repeated or may terminate if fiber 1 is depolarized.

both directions (Fig. 39.5). Another effect might be to enhance conduction in the damaged portion of fiber 2 such that the impulse down fiber 1 finds depolarized fiber and cannot maintain the circuit (Fig. 39.6).

Conduction velocity may decrease by blocking the fast response and allowing emergence of the slow response as in infarction or digoxin toxicity. In addition, since ARP depends on the APD, if repolarization is accelerated, cardiac tissue may be more excitable. A measure of this is the maximum upstroke velocity of phase 0, referred to as

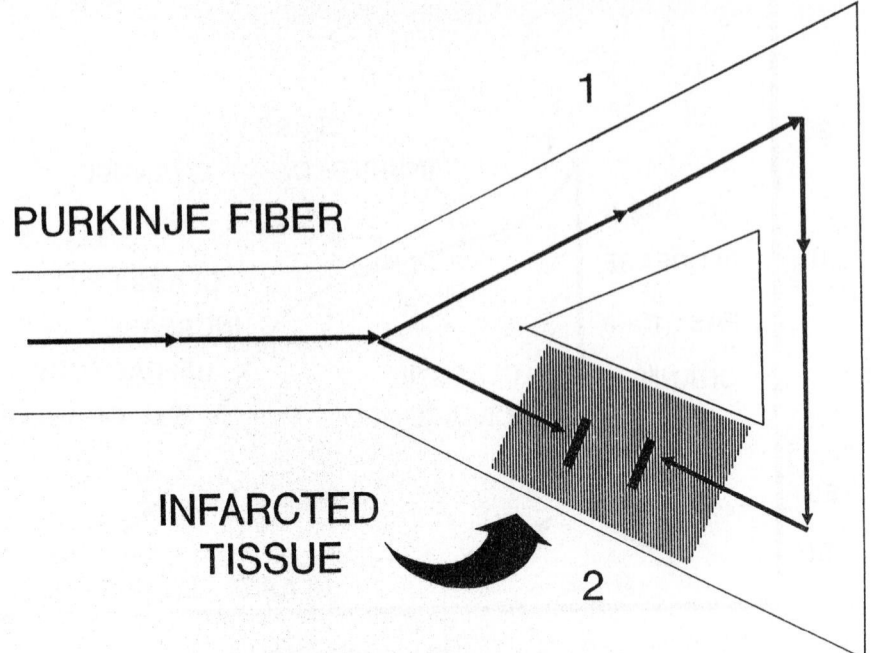

Figure 39-5. Antiarrhythmic drug effect on reentry. Antiarrhythmics may inhibit reentry by slowing conduction in both directions in fiber 2 so that the cells are still refractory when the impulses arrive.

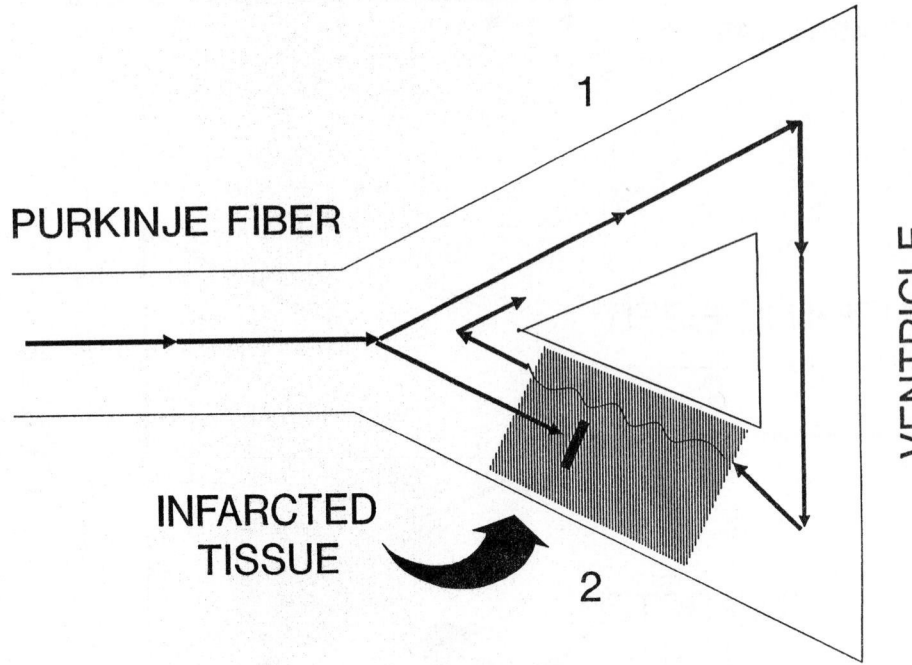

Figure 39-6. Antiarrhythmic drug effect. Another effect enhances conduction in the damaged portion of fiber 2 so that the impulse down fiber 1 finds depolarized fiber and cannot maintain the circuit.

$\dot{V}_{max}$. Mechanisms (primarily drugs) that prolong the APD also lengthen the ARP and thereby reduce excitability. This prolongation of repolarization is associated with lengthening of the QT interval (called QTc when corrected for heart rate) (Fig. 39.2). Prolongation of depolarization also serves to lengthen the QRS duration.

DRUG ACTION

Antiarrhythmic drugs are classified according to their electrophysiologic properties (Table 39.1). Class I drugs depress myocardial membranes with varying ability to slow dV/dt of phase 0 through inhibition of sodium transport. This class is further separated into three groups based on

Table 39.1.
Classification of Antiarrhythmic Agents

Class	PR Interval	QRS Duration	Q-Tc Duration	Agent
Ia	0, +[a]	+++	+++	Quinidine Procainamide Disopyramide Moricizine[b]
Ib	0	0	0,−	Lidocaine Tocainide Phenytoin Mexiletine
Ic	+	+++	+++	Flecainide Encainide Propafenone
II	+++	0	0,−	β-Blockers
III	+	+	+++	Bretylium Amiodarone[c] Sotalo[d] NAPA
IV	+++	0	0	Calcium-channel Blockers

[a]Symbols: 0, no activity; −, slight shortening; +, slight prolongation; +++, significant prolongation.
[b]Moricizine has been placed in various categories, e.g., Ia, Ib, and I without any subgroup.
[c]Amiodarone also has properties of Class I, II, and IV.
[d]Sotalol also has β-blocking properties of Class II.

differing effects on repolarization and conduction (2). Class Ia drugs (quinidine, procainamide, and disopyramide) lengthen refractory periods and the duration of action potentials. Prolongation of the PR and QT intervals and widening of the QRS is expected. In contrast, Ib agents (lidocaine, tocainide, mexiletine, and phenytoin) shorten repolarization and the QT interval. Conduction and the QRS interval are altered minimally. Lastly, Ic antiarrhythmics are the most potent depressants of phase 0 in Class I. Class Ic (flecainide and propafenone) is noted for slowing of conduction as seen by widening of PR and QRS intervals with minimal effect on APD or QT interval.

Class II includes the β-blocking drugs. Many arrhythmias are produced or exacerbated by hyperactivity of the sympathetic nervous system. Elevated sympathetic tone results in an increase in automaticity and a reduction in refractory period that could induce the activity of reentrant circuits. The clinical effects of Class II agents depend on several variables, including the presence or absence of membrane stabilizing effects (i.e., propranolol, pindolol, and acebutolol act like Class I with a decrease in dV/dt of phase 0), intrinsic sympathomimetic activity (pindolol or acebutolol), which in theory would counter the bradycardia and AV conduction depression of β-blockade. The effects

of Class II drugs depend on the ambient sympathetic tone. In states of increased adrenergic activity, such as myocardial infarction, Class II drugs will decrease the resting membrane potential, decrease dV/dt of phase 0, and slow conduction velocity, whereas in normal sympathetic tone, these three parameters are unchanged.

Class III agents include bretylium, N-acetylprocainamide (NAPA), amiodarone, and sotalol. These drugs prolong the action potential duration from phase 2 lengthening, and to a similar degree, prolong the refractory period. Bretylium, amiodarone, and sotalol have other differing electrophysiologic effects. For example, bretylium initially increases sympathetic tone followed by a decrease, whereas amiodarone and sotalol are both sympatholytic. In addition, some effects of amiodarone are felt to be from a decrease in thyroid hormone activity. NAPA does not alter QRS duration but does prolong QTc intervals.

Class IV includes the calcium channel blockers verapamil, diltiazem, and bepridil. These agents block the calcium-mediated current passing through the slow channel. The predominant effect is to prolong the action potential duration. They also decrease phase 4 depolarization and increase the threshold potential. The result is a slowing of A-V conduction. Bepridil can also depress phase 0 and prolong APD, giving it properties of Class I and Class III antiarrhythmics (2). Because of the broad spectrum of effects bepridil has on cardiovascular electrophysiology, it has been evaluated for treatment in supraventricular and ventricular arrhythmias; however, its use for the treatment of arrhythmias has been limited because of reported cases of agranulocytosis and *torsade de pointes*.

Some have questioned the utility of this classification system because arrhythmia suppression by an agent within a subclass (e.g., Ic) may not predict positive response from another Ic antiarrhythmic (3). There is evidence that this disparity exists for other classes (e.g., Ia and Ib) (4,5). In addition, this classification system does not support agents with multiple antiarrhythmic properties, such as moricizine, amiodarone, and sotalol. A more practical approach of characterizing agents by antiarrhythmic action could alleviate difficulties with the current classification system (2,6,7).

SINUS BRADYCARDIA

Sinus bradycardia is defined in adults as a heart rate below 60 beats/min, with each impulse originating in the SA node, followed by normal conduction through the AV node and His–Purkinje system. The normal range in children varies according to age. In most cases, sinus bradycardia is a normal physiologic variant. It usually reflects diminished SA node automaticity though it may also be caused by improper impulse propagation out of the SA node.

SA node automaticity is regulated by underlying autonomic tone (sympathetic and vagal), and is lower during sleep and in trained athletes. Sinus rates as low as 30 beats/min as well as sinus pauses of up to 2.8 sec with first and second-degree AV block have been observed in completely asymptomatic individuals (8). The slow heart rate results in a longer ventricular filling time and a larger end-diastolic volume. Ventricular wall stretching produces an increased force of contraction by the Frank-Starling mechanism. The higher stroke volume results in an unchanged cardiac output despite the bradycardia. As long as the heart rate increases appropriately in response to elevations in sympathetic tone (e.g., exercise), many patients with resting sinus bradycardia remain asymptomatic. Asymptomatic sinus bradycardia is a benign condition that does not require treatment, aside from elimination of underlying factors that may worsen the bradycardia. These include drugs (e.g., β-blockers, digitalis, calcium channel blockers, or cholinergic agents), hypothyroidism, increased intracranial pressure, and certain electrolyte abnormalities.

Sinus bradycardia is seen in 10 to 41% of patients with acute myocardial infarctions, especially the inferior type (9). It is most often caused by increased vagal tone associated with inferior ischemia or infarction. Ischemic sinus node dysfunction may also occur but is less common. Sinus bradycardia is usually seen in the early hours after infarction and is frequently asymptomatic. Uncomplicated asymptomatic sinus bradycardia does not require treatment aside from careful observation.

Therapy is indicated when hypotension, heart failure, chest pain, shortness of breath, ventricular irritability, or decreased level of consciousness is present (10). Initial treatment should include lower extremity elevation and infusion of volume expanders. Drugs that may further worsen hypotension (e.g., morphine, nitroglycerin) or bradycardia (e.g., β-blockers, calcium channel blockers) should be titrated carefully. Severe bradycardia may increase ventricular irritability and result in arrhythmias such as premature ventricular contractions (PVCs). These often resolve after correction of the bradycardia and do not require conventional antiarrhythmics.

Atropine

The direct vagolytic action of atropine increases sinus node automaticity and accelerates conduction, usually producing a prompt increase in heart rate and blood pressure. The initial recommended dose is 0.5 to 1 mg intravenously, repeated as needed to a maximum of 0.04 mg/kg or 3 mg (10). Lower doses should be avoided since they may produce a vagal *stimulation* with worsened bradycardia, or a biphasic response of slowing followed by acceleration in 2 to 3 min. Total atropine doses of 3 mg produce full vagal blockade and may induce unwanted effects (10). Adverse cardiovascular effects include excessive tachycardia with increased myocardial oxygen consumption, ventricular irritability, and the potential for increasing infarct size (11).

This mandates cautious use in patients with acute myocardial infarction. Noncardiac effects include urinary retention, blurred vision, dry mouth, mydriasis, and toxic psychosis. Adverse reactions are minimized by using the lowest effective dose. Patients with sinus node disease may exhibit an inadequate response to atropine, whereas patients with denervated hearts after transplantation will have no response to atropine; both will require pacemakers.

Isoproterenol

Isoproterenol, a β-adrenergic agonist, is a second line drug that should be used with extreme caution in an acute myocardial infarction because it increases heart rate, ventricular irritability, and myocardial oxygen consumption. Peripheral vasodilation may exacerbate hypotension, which further limits use. It may be temporarily useful for refractory *torsade de pointes* and hemodynamically unstable bradycardia in the denervated heart of cardiac transplant patients until pacemaker therapy can be initiated (10).

Pacemakers

Patients not responding to atropine or those with persistent symptoms require pacemakers. Either the transvenous or transcutaneous route may be used. Transvenous pacing is the most reliable, with ventricular pacing the traditional mode. Atrial pacing gives the best hemodynamic response but requires intact and reliable AV conduction. Dual chamber pacemakers that sequentially pace the atrium and ventricle may be preferred in patients with severe heart failure. In transcutaneous cardiac pacing, a low-density current is passed between two self-adhesive pads located anteriorly and posteriorly over the apex of the heart. This gives a hemodynamic response comparable to that of transvenous pacing and has the advantages of faster, easier, and less invasive implementation (12). Its primary limitation is a lower reliability, with successful pacing in 40 to 80% of patients.

Sinus bradycardia associated with an acute myocardial infarction is usually transient, therefore temporary pacemakers generally suffice. It is not associated with a higher incidence of complications or mortality. With proper management, this arrhythmia carries a good to excellent prognosis.

SICK SINUS SYNDROME

The sick sinus syndrome (SSS) encompasses a wide spectrum of impulse formation or conduction abnormalities in the SA node, perinodal tissues, atria, and AV node. It may be idiopathic or seen in patients with cardiac or other diseases such as amyloidosis, collagen vascular diseases, or endocrine imbalances. SSS is more common in the elderly and is thought to be caused by a degenerative process associated with an increase in conducting system fibrous tissue (13). Its many ECG and electrophysiologic manifestations include (a) sinus bradycardia with an inadequate chronotropic response to exercise, (b) sinus pauses or arrest, (c) SA node exit block, (d) paroxysmal supraventricular tachyarrhythmias (usually atrial fibrillation or flutter), alternating with sinus bradycardia, called the *tachycardia–bradycardia syndrome*, (e) prolonged suppression of SA node activity after conversion from supraventricular tachycardia, or (f) carotid hypersensitivity, seen as abnormal sinus slowing or pauses after carotid sinus massage.

Some patients with ECG or electrophysiologic evidence of SSS are asymptomatic, have a good prognosis, and do not require treatment (14). Others develop a broad spectrum of central nervous system or hemodynamic symptoms, ranging from brief periods of fatigue, irritability, dizziness, and confusion, to syncope (Stokes–Adams attacks), seizures, and congestive heart failure. Angina and palpitations may also be seen in patients with the tachycardia–bradycardia syndrome.

Before initiating treatment, reversible or transient causes of sinus node dysfunction should be excluded or minimized. Drug-induced causes include digitalis, β-blockers, calcium channel blockers (especially verapamil), Class Ia and Ic antiarrhythmics, and certain antihypertensives. Treatment is indicated in *symptomatic* patients with a documented correlation between inadequate sinus node activity and symptoms. Pharmacologic attempts to increase SA node automaticity (e.g., chronic administration of atropine) are not effective. Antiarrhythmic drugs are likewise not useful, with the exception of the tachycardia–bradycardia syndrome, where they may be used in the management of the tachycardic component. Many tachycardia–bradycardia patients require concomitant pacemakers because of prolonged pauses when converting from the tachyarrhythmia to sinus rhythm, or an exacerbation of the bradycardic episodes caused by the antiarrhythmic. Those with intermittent atrial fibrillation may also benefit from anticoagulants (discussed under "Atrial Fibrillation").

Pacemakers

Permanent pacemakers are the therapy of choice. SSS is the most common indication for permanent pacemakers, accounting for 40 to 50% of the pacemaker population. Several pacing options are available. Atrial, ventricular, or dual demand pacemakers sense and pace the atria, ventricle, or both chambers, respectively. Rate-responsive pacemakers respond to various signals (motion sensors, respiratory rate, oxygen saturation, or lactate levels) with a faster pacing rate, thereby simulating a more physiologic response to exercise. Recent evidence has shown an association between traditional ventricular-demand pace-

makers and adverse events, including chronic atrial fibrillation, congestive heart failure, and thromboembolism (15). Causes include a lack of AV synchrony and abnormal retrograde ventriculoatrial conduction. Atrial demand pacemakers are therefore preferable, however patients must first be carefully screened to exclude AV node and His–Purkinje system conduction defects. Drugs with negative AV chronotropic or dromotropic effects must be administered carefully.

Pacing relieves symptoms and is generally well tolerated. Previous studies in SSS patients did not demonstrate improved morbidity or mortality (50% at 5 years) (13,16), possibly because of underlying poor cardiac function. Recognition of the deleterious effects of ventricular-demand pacemakers now raises the question of whether they may have offset a trend toward higher survival. Recent studies have shown an improved short-term survival in elderly patients with atrial pacemakers (15). Long-term studies in large populations should also be performed.

ATRIOVENTRICULAR BLOCK

Abnormalities of atrioventricular conduction are classified into three types, based on the extent of impulse transmission across the AV node. The anatomic location of the conduction block determines the clinical significance, prognosis, and therapy.

First-Degree AV Block

First-degree AV block is defined as a prolongation of the PR interval to ≥0.20 sec, with 1:1 atrioventricular conduction of all impulses. This is a relatively common ECG finding, with a prevalence of 0.5 to 10%. Conduction delay in the AV node is the most common cause. Both cardiac (AV nodal disease, acute myocardial infarction, myocarditis) and noncardiac (enhanced vagal tone) etiologies have been identified. Patients are rarely symptomatic, and treatment is not generally required (14). Digitalis, β-blockers, calcium channel blockers, and potassium may cause or worsen this pattern. First-degree AV block is not an absolute contraindication to these drugs, but close observation is necessary because they may produce higher-grade block.

Second-Degree AV Block

In second-degree AV block, there is intermittent failure of atrioventricular impulse conduction. The anatomic site of block may be the AV node, His bundle, or bundle branch system. This type of block is subdivided into Mobitz Types I and II.

Mobitz Type I, or Wenckebach block, is characterized by a gradual prolongation of atrioventricular conduction (PR interval on ECG) until a sinus impulse (P-wave) is not conducted to the ventricles. The cycle then begins anew with a short followed by progressively longer PR intervals and a nonconducted P-wave. Electrophysiologic studies usually implicate a conduction abnormality in the AV node proximal to the bundle of His. The presence and extent of Mobitz Type I AV block is influenced by underlying autonomic tone. It may be seen in normal individuals (especially trained athletes) or may be caused by drugs (e.g., digitalis, β-blockers, or verapamil), electrolyte abnormalities, or inflammation. This pattern is also seen in acute inferior myocardial infarction. It usually appears within the first 72 hr after infarction, is transient, and infrequently progresses to higher-grade block (9).

Many patients with Mobitz Type I AV block are asymptomatic, in which case drugs or pacemakers are not required (14). Close observation of patients with acute myocardial infarction or digitalis toxicity is warranted. Treatment is indicated when the patient exhibits symptoms (central nervous system or hemodynamic), ventricular irritability, or the ventricular rate persists at <40 beats/min (12). Atropine facilitates AV nodal conduction by decreasing the effective and functional refractory periods of the AV node. It frequently restores 1:1 conduction in patients with Mobitz Type I block and normal AV nodes (11) and may be useful in managing digitalis toxicity. However, this effect is unpredictable in patients with acute myocardial infarction, and temporary pacemakers are therefore indicated. β-blockers, verapamil, and digoxin should be dosed with caution in these patients.

Mobitz Type II block is present when the PR interval of conducted beats remains constant, with unpredicted intermittent nonconduction of atrial impulse(s). It reflects a conduction abnormality distal to the bundle of His and is frequently associated with a wide QRS (bundle branch block) pattern on ECG. This type of block is seen in acute anterior or anteroseptal myocardial infarction, usually during the first 72 hr after infarction. It reflects extensive ischemia and necrosis of the septum, bundle branches, and Purkinje fibers. Almost all patients are symptomatic. Mobitz Type II AV block with bundle branch block is an unstable rhythm with an ominous prognosis, often progressing abruptly to complete heart block, severe bradycardia, or asystole. Atropine is generally ineffective. Pacemakers are therefore mandatory and usually permanent (14).

Third-Degree AV Block

Third-degree AV block occurs when no P-waves are conducted to the ventricles. Also known as complete heart block, it reflects a total absence of atrioventricular conduction. This results in an escape rhythm with the AV junction, His bundle, or Purkinje cells serving as the pacemaker. The site of block is related to the symptoms, prognosis, and therapy. When conduction is blocked within the AV node (proximal conducting system), the AV junction or proximal His bundle cells function as the pacemaker. Normal-appearing QRS complexes are seen, reflecting

normal ventricular impulse conduction. The physiologic escape rate for the AV junctional cells is 40 to 60 beats/min, which increases in response to elevated sympathetic tone. Complete heart block with AV junctional escape may be a congenital rhythm or be seen (usually transiently) in acute inferior myocardial infarction. This is a relatively stable rhythm. Normal ventricular conduction along with the ability to increase the rate with exercise allows some patients to remain asymptomatic. Infants and children with congenital proximal complete heart block may tolerate this rhythm well for long periods, requiring close observation but no intervention (8,14). Treatment is indicated in patients with (a) symptoms (hypotension, syncope, persistent chest pain, heart failure), (b) inadequate chronotropic response to exercise, or (c) ventricular arrhythmias. Atropine may be used in the emergent situations but is of limited value and without long-term effectiveness. Permanent pacemakers are the therapy of choice. Pacemakers are reliable and well tolerated in infants and children with the congenital form of this rhythm. The role of pacemakers in myocardial infarction patients remains unclear.

Complete heart block in the distal His bundle or Purkinje system (distal conducting system) results in an idioventricular escape rhythm with wide QRS complexes occurring at a rate of 30 to 40 beats/min. This reflects abnormal impulse conduction through the ventricles and the slow intrinsic rate of ventricular pacemaker tissues. This pattern may be seen in acute myocardial infarction as well as other diseases such as myocarditis, cardiomyopathy, and sarcoidosis. The slow rate coupled with abnormal ventricular conduction usually causes hemodynamic or central nervous system symptoms. In patients with acute anterior or anteroseptal myocardial infarction, this is an unstable rhythm with abrupt progression to asystole or ventricular arrhythmias. Atropine is not effective (11). Patients with third-degree AV block and an idioventricular rhythm require permanent pacemakers (12,14) regardless of symptoms. The abrupt occurrence of this type of block in the setting of an acute myocardial infarction carries an ominous prognosis and a high risk of sudden death.

SINUS TACHYCARDIA

Sinus tachycardia is characterized by a rate of more than 100 and usually less than 180 beats/min, with impulses originating in the SA node and conducted normally to the AV node and His–Purkinje system. In most cases, it reflects increased SA node automaticity. A gradual acceleration and deceleration may allow differentiation from other supraventricular tachycardias. The rate varies with sleep or changes in posture. Sinus tachycardia is a normal physiologic response to a myriad of conditions, including exercise, anxiety, pain, stress, fright, fever, hypoxia, anemia, hypovolemia, hypotension, early congestive heart failure, hyperthyroidism, and pheochromocytoma. It is seen in about one-third of patients with acute myocardial infarction and is attributed to sympathetic overactivity. Drugs with direct or indirect sympathomimetic or vagolytic activity may cause or contribute to sinus tachycardia. Common causes include sympathomimetics, catecholamines, β-agonists, methylxanthines, and anticholinergics.

Most individuals with sinus tachycardia are asymptomatic, except perhaps for palpitations. Patients with coronary artery disease may experience angina due to increased myocardial oxygen demand. Those with poor cardiac reserve and sustained episodes of tachycardia may develop congestive heart failure.

The treatment of sinus tachycardia consists of management of the underlying condition. Treatment of the tachycardia itself is not necessary and may have deleterious effects since decreasing the heart rate will decrease the cardiac output and oxygen delivery to the tissues. In the rare instance (e.g., hyperthyroidism) where sinus tachycardia is sustained and symptomatic, propranolol or another β-blocker may be given provided the patient is not in congestive heart failure.

AV NODAL REENTRY

Paroxysmal supraventricular tachycardias are a group of common arrhythmias frequently seen in healthy individuals with otherwise normal cardiovascular systems. Reentry (sometimes called circus movement tachycardia) is the mechanism for more than 90% of cases. Several variants may be seen. AV nodal reentry is sometimes known as paroxysmal supraventricular tachycardia (PSVT) and accounts for 50 to 60% of cases. Reentry using an accessory atrioventricular pathway (AV reentry, Wolff–Parkinson–White syndrome or concealed bypass tract conduction—discussed in a separate section) causes 30% of cases. Finally, reentry within the SA node (4%) or atria (4 to 8%)

may also occur, primarily in patients with underlying heart disease. Typical features of reentry include (a) abrupt initiation and termination, (b) a regular rate of 150 to 250 beats/min (up to 325 in infants), (c) narrow QRS complexes of normal morphology, and (d) 1:1 AV conduction. Abrupt initiation and ventricular rate regularity are specific characteristics of AV nodal reentry, often used as clues in differentiating it from ectopic atrial tachycardia, atrial fibrillation, or atrial flutter.

An understanding of the electrophysiology of reentry is useful in the evaluation of therapeutic modalities. Under normal conditions, impulses begin in the SA node and terminate in the Purkinje fibers where the surrounding tissue is refractory. In reentry, the impulse is able to reactivate the conducting system by "hiding" in the heart long enough for the surrounding tissue to regain excitability. Slow conduction in the AV node makes this a likely site for reentry. In AV nodal reentry, there are at least two functional pathways in the AV conducting system, sharing common proximal and distal limbs (Fig. 39.7). The α-pathway has slow conduction velocity and a short refractory period, whereas the β-pathway has fast conduction velocity and a long refractory period. During sinus rhythm, each impulse arrives at the AV junction, travels antegrade (toward the ventricles) down both pathways, reaches the His bundle via the fast β-pathway, and terminates in the His–Purkinje system. Conduction down the slow α-pathway ceases at the His bundle, where the tissue is refractory (Fig. 39.7A). The relatively long cycle length in sinus rhythm allows both pathways to recover excitability before the next sinus impulse arrives at the AV junction.

In reentry (Fig. 39.7B), a premature impulse enters the AV node at a time when the slow α-path will conduct, but the fast β-path is refractory. The impulse travels through

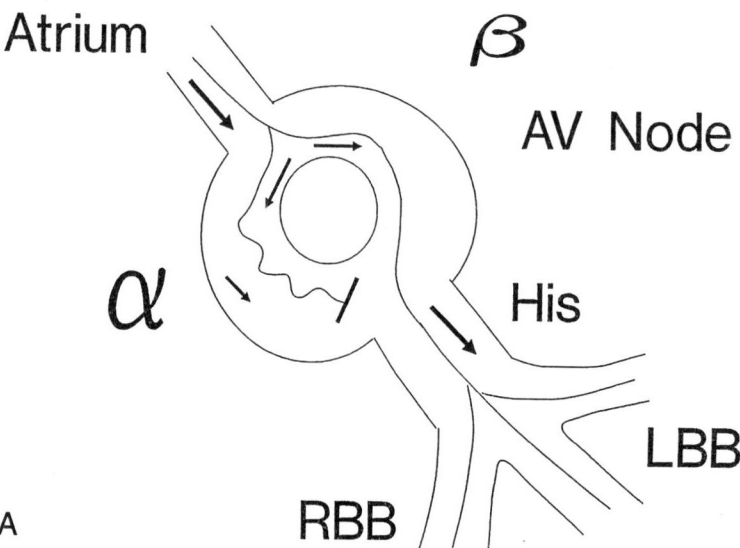

A

Figure 39-7A. AV Nodal Reentry. Sinus rhythm. The impulse is blocked in the α-pathway and reaches the ventricles via the β-pathway.

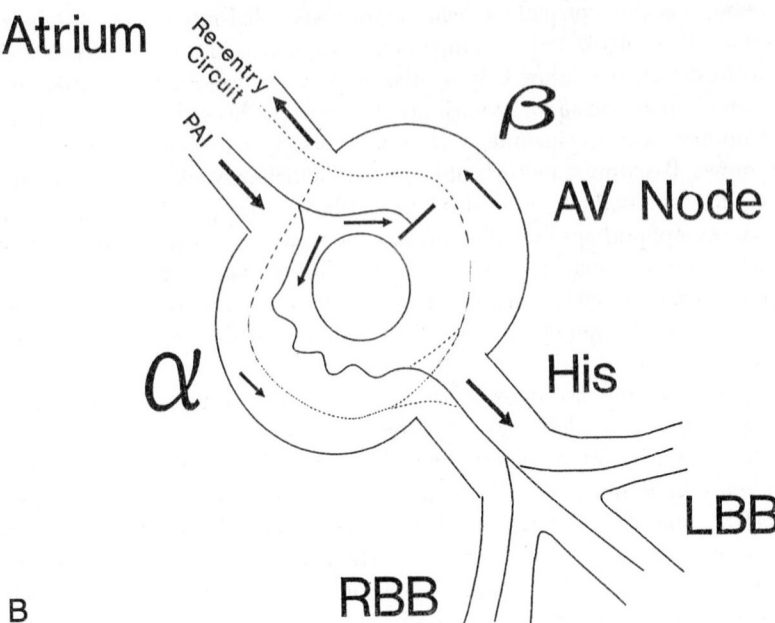

Figure 39-7B. AV Nodal Reentry. PAI, premature atrial impulse; His, bundle of His; RBB, right bundle branch; LBB, left bundle branches; solid line, PAI. The premature impulse is blocked in the β-pathway and reaches the ventricles via the α-pathway. If the β-pathway is recovered, AV nodal reentry may be initiated. Dotted line is a reentry circuit.

the AV junction via the α-pathway. The His–Purkinje system and ventricles are then activated in normal fashion. Additionally, retrograde transmission (toward the atria) occurs up the now recovered β-pathway, creating an atrial echo. Should the α-pathway be recovered, the impulse will travel antegrade (toward the ventricles), and a reentry circuit is created. The impulse travels antegrade down the slow α-pathway and retrograde up the fast β-pathway, with the atria and ventricles as "innocent bystanders" (1). In AV nodal reentry, the entire circuit is located in the AV junction. Clearly, to induce and sustain reentry, the premature impulse must be critically timed, and a fine balance must exist between conductivity and refractoriness. The impulse must always find excitable tissue in the direction in which it is propagating. If refractory tissue is encountered, the circuit is broken, and the rhythm terminates abruptly. On ECG, the premature atrial beat has a prolonged PR-interval. Subsequent P-waves are frequently buried in the QRS complex, reflecting simultaneous activation of the atria and ventricles. QRS morphology is normal unless there is aberrant conduction or antegrade preexcitation down an anomalous AV connection (Wolff–Parkinson–White syndrome).

AV nodal reentry may be seen at any age from infancy to adulthood. It is a common arrhythmia in infants, children, and young adults. Approximately 50% of patients have no underlying heart disease. Brief runs are often detected on 24-hr ECG monitors of asymptomatic persons. Many cases are idiopathic. Noncardiac causes such as fever, infection or drugs (sympathomimetics, catecholamines, β-agonists) may be seen in a minority of patients.

The clinical manifestations depend on the heart rate, the duration of the arrhythmia, and the presence of underlying heart disease. Reentrant rhythms are not usually life-threatening, except in patients with the Wolff–Parkinson–White syndrome. Most patients will notice the fast heart rate almost immediately and may complain of dizziness, lightheadedness, weakness, or nonspecific chest discomfort. Less common symptoms include dyspnea, syncope, and angina. Congestive heart failure is uncommon because ventricular (His–Purkinje) conduction remains normal in most patients. However, the shortened ventricular filling time lowers stroke volume and may induce congestive heart failure in patients with a tenuous cardiovascular reserve. Infants often have nonspecific symptoms such as fussiness, lethargy, poor feeding, or rapid breathing, yet may present with severe congestive heart failure and shock.

Acute Treatment

The goal of treatment for AV nodal reentry is to interrupt the circuit by slowing conduction or prolonging refractoriness in either AV junctional pathway. When the impulse encounters refractory tissue, the tachycardia will terminate abruptly. Correctable contributing factors such as fever, infection, hypoxia, anemia, or hyperthyroidism should be treated. The arrhythmia may be terminated using pharmacologic, electrical, or other measures. The immediate treatment is dictated by the hemodynamic status of the patient.

DC CARDIOVERSION

In patients with hemodynamic instability (severe hypotension or heart failure, pulmonary edema, myocardial ischemia, acute alteration in mental status), electrical cardioversion is the therapy of choice. Direct current (DC) cardioversion depolarizes a critical number of myocardial cells simultaneously, allowing the sinus node to reestablish dominance as the pacemaker. For conversion of supraventricular tachycardias, lower energies (10 to 50 joules, or 0.5 joules/kg) are often adequate. This is a uniformly effective, immediate method of termination with minimal adverse effects. The only major adverse effect is the induction of ventricular arrhythmias, which can be avoided by synchronizing the electrical discharge to the QRS complex. Myocardial damage is rare with lower energies. Short-acting sedatives may be given before the procedure in older children and adults. Electroconversion is not advised in patients with stable cardiovascular status because other measures are considered less invasive and safer. Moreover, DC cardioversion precludes a direct assessment of the efficacy of various other maneuvers and drugs on the arrhythmia. This information is useful in managing recurrent episodes.

VAGAL MANEUVERS

In hemodynamically stable patients, interventions to increase vagal tone are performed first. These measures decrease conductivity and increase refractoriness in the AV node and decrease automaticity in the SA node by increasing parasympathetic tone. Used either alone or in conjunction with antiarrhythmic drugs, vagotonic maneuvers will terminate 50 to 80% of cases of AV nodal reentrant tachycardia.

The most common vagal measures are carotid sinus massage (or pressure) and the Valsalva maneuver. Carotid sinus massage stimulates the baroreceptors of the carotid artery, which slows the sinus rate, prolongs AV conduction, lowers cardiac output, decreases venous return, and decreases peripheral vascular resistance (17). Alteration in the critical balance between conduction and refractoriness disrupts the cycle and terminates the rhythm. The Valsalva maneuver (prolonged forced expiration against a closed glottis) may be induced by blowing into a blood pressure manometer tube to maintain a pressure of 30 to 60 mm Hg for 10 to 30 sec. Conversion to sinus rhythm occurs during the relaxation phase, when a parasympathetic surge induces antegrade AV nodal block. Other vagotonic procedures include deep breathing, gagging, coughing, eyeball pressure, and squatting.

Carotid sinus massage and Valsalva maneuver may not be successful in infants and young children. In these patients, the diving reflex may be initiated by immersing the face in a pan of ice water for 10 to 15 sec, or placing a washcloth soaked in ice water on the face. This causes an acute vagal surge that is more prominent and clinically effective in young patients. A slowing of the tachycardia rate is followed by abrupt conversion to sinus rhythm. The diving reflex may induce asystole and should be used only under monitored conditions.

Background increases in sympathetic tone may attenuate the effectiveness of vagal maneuvers (18). This may explain the lower efficacy when standing, as compared with the supine position. These measures are generally more effective in the young, probably relating to a reduction in overall autonomic tone associated with aging. Vagal maneuvers should be performed as early as possible after arrhythmia initiation, before elevated sympathetic tone reduces efficacy (18).

Vagotonic procedures of all types should not be used in patients with a history of sinus node dysfunction since prolonged sinus node recovery time may cause sinus arrest after the reentry circuit is terminated. Carotid sinus massage or pressure may cause carotid artery ischemia in patients with preexisting atherosclerotic narrowing or (rarely) ventricular tachyarrhythmias (17). Pressure to the carotid arteries should never be applied bilaterally. Both carotid arteries should be examined *before* the procedure, and it should not be attempted in patients with evidence of cerebrovascular insufficiency (e.g., carotid bruits). Because of the prevalence of sinus node and cerebrovascular disease in the elderly, vagotonic stimuli should be avoided or used with great caution in this population.

ADENOSINE

If vagal maneuvers are unsuccessful, adenosine is the drug of choice for terminating AV nodal reentry (10). Adenosine is an ubiquitous endogenous purine nucleoside. Its myriad biologic effects include regulation of coronary, cerebral, renal, and skeletal blood flow, modulation of neurotransmission and immune response, inhibition of platelet aggregation, stimulation of gastrin secretion, inhibition of lipolysis, and induction of bronchoconstriction. The actions of adenosine on cardiac tissues include a very transient powerful negative dromotropic effect on the AV node and a similar negative chronotropic effect in the sinus node, AV junction, and ventricles. In electrophysiologic studies, the primary effects are a lengthening of sinus cycle and a prolongation of the AH-interval, followed by complete or partial AV nodal block (19). Adenosine has no effect on the His–Purkinje interval. Cardiac activity is thought to be related to alterations in calcium and potassium ion currents, but the precise mechanisms are unclear (20). Adenosine exerts minimal effect on vagal tone.

Adenosine is produced in many tissues and organs, but plasma concentrations are low because of rapid transport and metabolism. Local effects are mediated through interactions with intracellular and extracellular receptors, which may be up-regulated, down-regulated, supersensitized, and desensitized under different conditions. Analogs with agonist and antagonist activity and variable receptor affinity further modulate the effect. The effects of adenosine depend primarily on binding to the cell surface receptors; therefore, the concentration in the extracellular

Table 39.2.
Sites of Primary Drug Action in AV Nodal Reentry

Av node antegrade slow conduction pathway
  Calcium-channel blockers (verapamil, diltiazem)
  Digoxin
  Adenosine
  β-blockers
  Amiodarone
AV node retrograde fast conduction pathway
  Class Ia drugs (quinidine, procainamide, disopyramide)
  Class Ic drugs (flecainide, encainide, propafenone)
  Class III drugs (amiodarone, sotalol)
Suppression of atrial ectopy
  Class Ia drugs (quinidine, procainamide, disopyramide)
  Class Ic drugs (flecainide, encainide, propafenone)
  β-blockers
  Class III drugs (amiodarone, sotalol)

space correlates directly with the magnitude of the effect. Extracellular fluid concentrations are linked to adenosine production and elimination via multiple pathways.

Adenosine is continuously produced and released by erythrocytes and cells in the liver, heart, skeletal muscle, and endothelium. At physiologic concentrations (0.1 to 1 μM), it is taken up avidly by erythrocytes and phosphorylated into adenosine monophosphate by adenosine kinase. At higher concentrations, it is deaminated by adenosine deaminase to inosine, which is further metabolized to hypoxanthine and uric acid. These metabolites have no antiarrhythmic effect. The balance between production and elimination is tightly regulated at the local level.

Adenosine is closely related to another endogenous compound, adenosine-5′-triphosphate (ATP). ATP and adenosine share similar biologic actions but have different potencies at the various receptors. Exogenous ATP is rapidly dephosphorylated to adenosine in vivo, and most of its cardiac effect is caused by adenosine formation. ATP also has vagal stimulant properties that contribute minimally to the antiarrhythmic effect (21). ATP has been used as an antiarrhythmic for many years in Europe, but is not available in the United States.

Adenosine restores sinus rhythm within 10 to 20 sec in 85 to 100% of adults and children with spontaneous or induced AV nodal reentrant tachycardias (20,22–25). Antegrade pathway conduction block occurs in the majority of patients (Table 39.2) (20,21,24,25). In patients with sinus node or intraatrial reentry, atrial fibrillation or flutter, ectopic atrial tachycardia, or ventricular tachycardia adenosine induces a higher grade AV block (20,26)—the transiently (<20 sec) slower ventricular rate may allow visualization of P-waves and therefore aid in diagnosis, but atrial activity is unchanged, and these arrhythmias are rarely terminated.

In randomized (22,25) and nonrandomized (24,27) comparative trials of adenosine and verapamil, conversion rates are comparable or favor adenosine for patients with AV nodal reentry or AV reentry involving an accessory pathway. Termination of the tachycardia is generally more rapid with adenosine than verapamil, but the clinical importance of this is unclear. Repetitive administration results in consistent conversion at a similar dosage each time or repeated failures.

Adenosine is not absorbed by the oral route. After intravenous injection, it is rapidly distributed into intracellular, extracellular, and interstitial spaces. It crosses the blood–brain barrier, and a vasodilatory effect on the cerebral vessels may account for the common occurrence of headache. In vitro studies have measured a half-life of <10 sec (28). Traditional pharmacokinetic studies are hampered by rapid clearance, with ongoing metabolism as specimens are collected. Parameters such as distribution volume and clearance have therefore not been reported.

Noncardiac adverse effects occur in 15 to 81% of patients (19,21,22,24,25). The most common are flushing, dyspnea or a feeling of suffocation, and headache. Chest pain or pressure may mimic angina. Cough, malaise, and nausea have also been observed. Inhaled adenosine has been reported to induce bronchoconstriction in asthmatics.(19) The effect of intravenous adenosine in patients with preexisting obstructive airway disease is not known since most clinical trials have excluded asthmatics. Adenosine should therefore be used with caution in these patients. Adverse effects after intravenous adenosine abate within 1 to 2 min and are therefore limited in most patients.

Despite the action of adenosine to reduce systemic vascular resistance, intravenous boluses are well tolerated hemodynamically. Blood pressure remains unchanged or may even increase at the time of conversion to sinus rhythm. Masking of peripheral vasodilation in conscious subjects receiving bolus doses may be the result of autonomic reflexes. The lack of negative inotropic effect gives a theoretic advantage for adenosine in patients with severe heart failure; however, trials in this population are lacking.

Postconversion arrhythmias or conduction disorders occur in up to 60% of patients receiving adenosine. Sinus bradycardia, sinus tachycardia, sinus arrest, and various degrees of AV block last less than 1 to 2 min and do not require intervention in most patients. However caution should be exercised in patients with sinus node disease since sinus arrest for up to 4 sec has been observed (22). Premature atrial or ventricular impulses after conversion to sinus rhythm occur in 33 to 60% of patients (21,22). This may reinitiate reentry, an effect that is more common after adenosine than after verapamil.

Drug interactions with adenosine may involve alterations in extra- and intracellular transport as well as receptor affinity. Although many drugs have in vitro or theoretic mechanisms for interaction, systematic clinical trials are lacking. Interactions with dipyridamole and theophylline have the strongest documentation. Dipyridamole blocks the cellular uptake of adenosine, thereby inhibiting its metabolism (28). This may enhance the negative chronotropic and dromotropic effects of adenosine. Very limited evidence suggests a similar effect with diazepam. Aminophylline and theophylline bind to the extracellular adenosine receptor sites and therefore act as competitive antagonists (19). Patients receiving these drugs (and possibly caffeine) may exhibit a blunted response to adenosine. Carbamazepine can suppress AV conduction at therapeutic or mildly elevated blood levels. In the presence of carbamazepine, conduction inhibition through the AV node by adenosine can be enhanced producing a higher degree of heart block (10,26). When treating patients with adenosine, caution should be taken with those patients who are on carbamazepine. The possible role of calcium in the pharmacologic effect of adenosine suggests potential interactions with calcium channel blockers and digoxin, but these have not been well studied. The clinical implications of these interactions have not been established. The ultra-short duration of action of adenosine should minimize long-term effects of any drug interactions observed.

The standard adult dose of adenosine is 6 mg given by rapid intravenous bolus over 1 to 2 sec, followed by a normal saline flush. If no response is observed in 2 min, 12 mg intravenously may be given. A second 12 mg dose may be given in 1 to 2 min if needed. Clinical trials of adenosine in infants and children have used doses of 0.0375 to 0.25 mg/kg (23), but the drug is not FDA-approved for pediatric use. Despite the lack of FDA approval, adenosine is considered by some clinicians the drug of choice (after vagal maneuvers fail) for the acute management of AV nodal reentrant tachycardia in children (29). The ultra-short half-life of the drug mandates careful attention to the site and rate of administration. The pharmacologic effect depends on the amount of drug delivered to the heart. A slow administration rate or slow rate of blood flow (e.g., heart failure) may result in significant metabolism before the drug reaches the heart and therefore attenuate the effect of the drug. Conversely, administration into central veins (e.g., femoral vein during electrophysiologic studies) may result in a more marked response. Reflex tachycardia due to vasodilation has been reported after slow administration. Individual variation in underlying autonomic tone as well as the administration of other antiarrhythmics may enhance or attenuate adenosine's effect.

The very high efficacy rate of adenosine is comparable to or perhaps even better than that of verapamil. It can restore sinus rhythm more rapidly than verapamil although the clinical importance of this is unclear. The lack of negative inotropic and hypotensive effects makes it especially useful in patients with heart failure or hypotension. However DC cardioversion remains the treatment of choice in severe hemodynamic instability. The very short half-life allows rapid titration of individual doses, reduces concern for long-lasting or cumulative adverse effects, and minimizes the importance of drug interactions. Adenosine is an ideal drug for studying arrhythmias in the electrophysiology laboratory. However, the short half-life may also be a limitation because of the recurrence of reentry and lack of utility for long-term prophylaxis. Moreover, the prevalence of adverse reactions is high compared with verapamil. Verapamil and adenosine share the need for cautious use in patients with sinus node dysfunction, conduction system disease, or Wolff–Parkinson–White syndrome. Adenosine is preferred in patients with hypotension or heart failure, whereas verapamil is favored in patients with obstructive airway disease or those taking dipyridamole or methylxanthines (and possibly benzodiazepines, β-blockers, digoxin, and carbamazepine).

Monitoring parameters include heart rate and rhythm and blood pressure. Patient's subjective assessment of adverse effects can be a major limitation in treatment—some clinical trial participants have refused to complete studies because of adverse effects. The pharmacist should inform the patient of the likelihood and nature of noncardiac adverse effects, as well as their duration and lack of cardiac significance.

VERAPAMIL

Verapamil inhibits channel-mediated entry of calcium into the cell. Effects are most evident in the SA node, AV node, and the cardiac and peripheral vascular smooth muscles since these tissues depend on calcium flux for action potential generation. In contrast, atrial and ventricular myocardium and the His–Purkinje system are normally fast-channel (sodium flux dependent) tissues. This explains the lack of efficacy of verapamil in ventricular arrhythmias.

The net effect of verapamil results from an interplay between direct and indirect effects. Direct actions include a depression of automaticity in the SA and AV nodes (negative chronotropic effect), a reduction in conduction velocity in the AV node (negative dromotropic effect), a reduction in myocardial contractility (negative inotropic effect), and a dilation of coronary and peripheral arteries. These effects are modified by reflex sympathetic stimulation evoked by the peripheral arterial dilation. Increased cardiac automaticity and contractility largely offset the negative chronotropic and inotropic effects. The net cardiac effect is a negative dromotropic effect on antegrade conduction through the AV node (Table 39.2). Other effects become important only in diseased hearts (e.g., sinus node disease or congestive heart failure).

Among the calcium channel blocking agents, verapamil has the lowest degree of peripheral arterial dilation relative to its effects on the heart. This characteristic is advantageous in treating arrhythmias, but the relatively prominent negative inotropic effect may be a limitation in some patients. In contrast, nifedipine is a much more potent vasodilator, causing marked hemodynamic alteration before conduction effects are seen. Therefore nifedipine is not useful as an antiarrhythmic. Diltiazem has electrophysiologic and hemodynamic effects comparable to those of verapamil, and has demonstrated efficacy and safety in clinical trials (30,31).

Intravenous verapamil doses of 5 to 10 mg or 0.075 to 0.15 mg/kg over 2 min (3 min in elderly patients) will convert 60 to 90% of adult patients with AV nodal reentry to normal sinus rhythm within 5 to 10 min. If there is no response, a second dose of 0.15 mg/kg intravenously may be given 15 to 30 min later. Vagal maneuvers should be performed before the second dose.

After oral administration, ≥90% of the dose is absorbed, but extensive first-pass metabolism limits systemic availability to 20 to 35% (32,33). Food prolongs the time to peak concentration but not the extent of absorption. Large inter- and intrapatient variability exists, with serum levels after administration of the same dose varying by as much as 10-fold. Verapamil is approximately 90% protein bound to albumin and α-1-acid glycoprotein (33). The volume of distribution of 4.5 to 7 liters/kg in healthy adults is increased in cirrhosis. It is converted rapidly and extensively in the liver to multiple metabolites that are largely inactive. The only active metabolite, norverapamil (the N-demethylated derivative), has approximately 20% of the potency of the parent drug. Verapamil undergoes bi- or triexponential decline with an elimination phase half-life of 3 to 5 hr after a single dose (32,33). Long-term administration may result in nonlinear accumulation with a decreased clearance and prolonged half-life (33). Seventy percent of an oral or intravenous dose is recovered in the urine in 5 days, almost exclusively as metabolites, with 10 to 15% found in the feces (34).

Patients with cirrhosis demonstrate a significantly higher bioavailability (52.3% versus 22% for normals) due to a less marked first-pass effect, as well as a longer half-life and lower clearance (32,35). Those with arrhythmias or congestive heart failure may have altered hepatic clearance related to hepatic blood flow.

After single intravenous doses, verapamil displays a good relationship between serum levels and electrophysiologic effects. Studies of oral administration have, however, yielded a poor correlation of serum levels with clinical efficacy. This is explained in part by stereoselective differences in its pharmacodynamics and pharmacokinetics. Commercially available preparations of verapamil are racemic mixtures of the d- and l-isomers. The l-isomer has more potent negative chronotropic, inotropic, and dromotropic effects (36). Stereoselective first-pass metabolism after oral dosing results in preferential extraction of the l-isomer. Bioavailability of the l-isomer (20%) is therefore

lower than the d-isomer (50%) (35). The l-isomer has a distribution volume, clearance, and unbound fraction approximately twice that of the d-isomer (35). The relative ratios of l- and d-isomers after intravenous and oral administrations are therefore different, with intravenous dosing giving a larger fraction of total verapamil concentration as the more active l-isomer. Serum levels required for a given PR-interval prolongation after intravenous doses are 2 to 3 times lower than those after oral administration (33). This may explain the higher efficacy after acute intravenous versus chronic oral administration and wide inter- and intrapatient variability in response to a fixed serum level. Another explanation for the discrepancy in clinical effect of intravenous versus oral dosing is preferential myocardial uptake after intravenous administration (33). Alteration of response by underlying sympathetic tone further disrupts the relationship between serum level and drug effect. Conventional assays measuring total verapamil concentration are not useful in assessment of efficacy. Analytic methods to isolate the individual enantiomers are not widely available.

Adverse reactions occur in 10 to 14% (34) of patients receiving verapamil but require discontinuation in only 1 to 5%. Adverse effects after intravenous administration are an extension of the pharmacologic effect and include hypotension, disturbances in AV conduction, bradycardia or sinus arrest, and congestive heart failure. These reflect calcium channel blockade in the vascular smooth muscle, AV node, SA node, and myocardium, respectively. Mild, transient hypotension is the most common adverse reaction. Most patients do not require treatment; in some, the reduction in afterload may even allow an *increase* in the cardiac output. In symptomatic patients, placement in Trendelenburg's position with intravenous fluid administration is usually adequate treatment. Patients with borderline blood pressures before verapamil (systolic pressure ≤90 to 100 mm Hg) may develop severe hypotension. These patients should receive adenosine. Alternatively, pretreatment with 1 g of intravenous calcium chloride or gluconate is thought to block the peripheral but not the cardiac receptors (37,38). Calcium therefore blunts or abolishes the hypotensive effect while preserving AV nodal effect when given either before or after verapamil. Sudden cardiovascular collapse with profound hypotension, bradycardia, apnea, and death has been reported after verapamil administration in neonates and infants (39). Although verapamil is an excellent drug in older children, it should be avoided in children less than 1 year of age (29,40).

Verapamil is not thought to have a significant proarrhythmic effect but requires cautious use in patients with preexisting conduction disorders. Premature atrial or ventricular impulses occasionally reactivate reentry. Atrial fibrillation and serious ventricular arrhythmias are uncommon. Bradycardia or heart block caused by excessive AV nodal effect may require treatment with isoproterenol, atropine, calcium, or pacemakers. Verapamil is contraindicated in patients with preexisting SA nodal disease (sick sinus syndrome) because of high risk for prolonged sinus arrest after termination of the arrhythmia. Verapamil is a first-line drug in most patients, but it is contraindicated in sinus node disease, marked hypotension, heart failure, and neonates. Adenosine is preferred in these patients.

An important drug interaction occurs between verapamil and β-blockers. Concomitant administration of these drugs results in AV blocking and negative inotropic effects by independent mechanisms. This increases the risk of serious cardiovascular effects such as congestive heart failure (41), high-degree AV block, or hypotension. Serum levels of digoxin may be increased by verapamil (42) via an increase in half-life and reduction in distribution volume and total clearance. Furthermore, verapamil should be used with caution in suspected digoxin toxicity because of its additive effects on the AV node.

Monitoring parameters for intravenous verapamil in arrhythmias include cardiac rhythm and rate and blood pressure. Continuous ECG monitoring is strongly advised. Routine serum level assessment is not recommended.

PHARMACOLOGIC VAGAL STIMULATION

If vagal maneuvers, adenosine, or verapamil is unsuccessful, pharmacologic vagal stimulation may be attempted. Edrophonium (5 to 10 mg IV) inhibits acetylcholinesterase, resulting in a direct vagal effect. Metaraminol (0.5 to 2 mg IV), phenylephrine (0.5 mg IV) or methoxamine (5 to 15 mg IV) will transiently raise blood pressure (to a goal of systolic 160 to 170 mm Hg), stimulate the carotid baroreceptors, and induce a reflex increase in vagal tone. These drugs should be preceded and followed by vagotonic maneuvers. They should be used with caution in patients with baseline sinus node dysfunction. Further caution is advised when using edrophonium in patients receiving digoxin, and with pressor agents in patients with severe congestive heart failure. Although their use in adults has been largely surpassed by adenosine and verapamil, these drugs maintain their usefulness in infants and children.

OTHER DRUGS

Diltiazem, digoxin, propranolol, quinidine, procainamide, amiodarone, and sotalol may also be used to terminate AV nodal or AV reentry. Diltiazem inhibits antegrade AV nodal conduction with comparable effectiveness to verapamil. Doses of 0.15 to 0.25 mg/kg intravenously over 2 min will restore sinus rhythm within 2 to 10 min in 60 to 100% of patients (31,43). Repeat doses of 0.35 mg/kg intravenously over 2 min, 15 min after initial dose, is associated with additional success in initial nonresponders (31). A potential advantage of diltiazem is a mild negative inotropic effect compared to verapamil (44), which may allow its use in patients with severe left ventricular impairment (45).

Digoxin has a lower response rate and a longer onset of action for conversion to sinus rhythm (several hours) than verapamil. It produces direct slowing of AV conduction by a different mechanism (vagal and antiadrenergic effect blocks AV nodal conduction) (Table 39.2). Patients who fail to respond to other drugs or maneuvers may respond to digoxin, especially children without accessory pathway conduction. Digoxin is also useful in patients with severe left ventricular dysfunction. Specific aspects of digoxin therapy are discussed under "Atrial Fibrillation."

Propranolol prolongs antegrade AV conduction and refractoriness and also depresses automaticity at the SA node, AV junction, and His–Purkinje fibers (Table 39.2). Propranolol is not a first-line drug because it is less efficacious than adenosine and verapamil, and is contraindicated in patients who have received verapamil because of the additive effects on cardiac conduction and contractility. It is primarily used in infants and children who have not received verapamil and when digoxin is not desirable (e.g., accessory pathway conduction). Metoprolol and esmolol have the advantages of cardioselectivity and ultra-short half-life, respectively.

Quinidine, procainamide, encainide (no longer commercially available), flecainide, and propafenone block conduction in the fast (usually retrograde) pathway (Table 39.2). They are not as effective in AV nodal or AV reentry and are reserved for refractory cases. They may be useful in cases where supraventricular and ventricular tachyarrhythmias cannot be distinguished. Class I antiarrhythmic agents should be used with caution because of their potential for proarrhythmias.

Amiodarone and sotalol suppress ectopic atrial activity. In addition, amiodarone prolongs antegrade and retrograde AV conduction, whereas sotalol primarily prolongs retrograde conduction only (Table 39.2). Both agents are highly effective in terminating supraventricular tachyarrhythmias; however, their use is limited by unfamiliarity with dosing and serious adverse effects.

PACEMAKERS

Patients who fail to respond to pharmacologic strategies should receive electrical therapy, which may include DC cardioversion (as above) or specialized pacing techniques. Pacing techniques include 1 to 2 critically timed extra stimuli or a rapid sequence of impulses (burst overdrive pacing) (46). As a rule, burst-pacing techniques are more effective. The goal of pacing is to create a strategically timed region of refractoriness. The paced impulse enters the circuit, collides with the advancing wavefront, blocks the succeeding wavefront, and stops the reentry circuit. Proximity of pacing site to the anatomic origin of the arrhythmia enhances the likelihood of success. Though highly effective, pacing is an invasive technique requiring transvenous or transesophageal catheter placement and electrophysiologic studies for application. Complications include tachycardia acceleration and fibrillation of the paced chamber(s).

Chronic Treatment

The need for prophylaxis is dictated by the frequency of episodes, the tachycardia rate, and its hemodynamic effects. In general, the presence and extent of symptoms are related to the rate and duration of the arrhythmia. The benefits of arrhythmia suppression must be balanced carefully against the risks and inconveniences of long-term antiarrhythmic therapy. In the absence of heart disease, most patients have infrequent attacks of short duration without cardiovascular compromise and do not require chronic suppression. Patients with underlying heart disease, frequent attacks, or debilitating symptoms (syncope, angina, hypotension, heart failure) may benefit from prophylaxis.

The goal of chronic prophylaxis is to prevent or minimize the frequency of attacks and their hemodynamic consequences. Complete abolition is not necessary and may be worse than no therapy because of proarrhythmic or other adverse drug effects. Precipitating factors such as sympathomimetics, β-agonists, caffeine, tobacco, or ethanol should be limited or discontinued. Patients with arrhythmias responsive to physical maneuvers such as carotid sinus pressure should be instructed in their proper application. This may obviate pharmacologic prophylaxis.

Ideally, treatment should be guided by electrophysiologic studies (EPS). Percutaneously inserted catheters are positioned in the heart to permit repetitive initiation and termination of arrhythmias, to identify the site of origin and mechanism of the arrhythmia, and to evaluate the efficacy of drugs and other maneuvers. Suppression of induced arrhythmias in the laboratory is often a valuable predictor of efficacy for subsequent episodes. EPS, therefore, serve the following functions:

1. To rapidly achieve a therapeutic regimen in patients with hemodynamically serious consequences such as syncope, hypotension, or heart failure. EPS permit expeditious trials of multiple antiarrhythmic drugs or techniques. Identification of serum level-antiarrhythmic effect relationships may allow individualized targeting of drug doses.
2. To accurately characterize the electrophysiologic mechanism of the arrhythmia. This allows more rational drug or technique selection.
3. To identify the underlying mechanism prior to the institution of nonpharmacologic options such as pacemakers, surgery, or catheter ablation.
4. To identify symptomatic patients with Wolff–Parkinson–White syndrome who are at risk for developing life-threatening arrhythmias.

EPS are limited by poor predictability of response in as many as one-third of patients. This is sometimes explained by alterations in autonomic tone at the time of spontaneous arrhythmia recurrence—EPS are performed in the resting, supine state, whereas arrhythmias recur in ambulatory patients. These differences in sympathetic tone alter the electrophysiologic characteristics and response to drugs. Furthermore, EPS are costly and uncomfortable. Some practitioners therefore prefer to treat patients with well-tolerated arrhythmias empirically, reserving EPS for patients who fail initial strategies.

Strategies for the pharmacologic prophylaxis of AV nodal reentry are not as well established as those for managing acute episodes. Many therapeutic options exist, some or all of which may give a satisfactory outcome. As a rule, patient response is not as predictable and efficacy rates are lower than for acute episodes, with no one drug emerging as the treatment of choice. Initial selections are based on specific patient considerations, dosing intervals, adverse effect profile, cost of drugs and monitoring tests, and physician preference or experience. Treatment may be directed at either the antegrade or retrograde pathway. Calcium channel blockers, digoxin, or β-blockers are common initial choices. Quinidine is also efficacious but requires hospitalization for the first few days of therapy because of potential proarrhythmic events. Nondrug therapies include antitachycardia pacemakers and surgery to ablate or modify the AV node.

VERAPAMIL

Despite its excellent intravenous efficacy for acute episodes of AV nodal reentry, oral verapamil has been less successful in the prophylaxis of recurrent arrhythmias. Efficacy varies widely between 40 and 90%. Successful termination with intravenous verapamil does not predict long-term efficacy with oral treatment. Serum levels required for specific AV node conduction effects are higher after oral (in comparison to IV) administration (32,35). The lower potency of oral dosing may result from stereospecific presystemic metabolism of racemic verapamil, which causes preferential hepatic extraction of the more active l-isomer (35,36). Since the l-isomer accounts for most of the AV nodal effect, this may explain both the more frequent therapeutic failures and the wide variability in serum level-response data (36). Alterations in autonomic tone at the time of arrhythmia recurrence further modulate the efficacy of verapamil.

Initial daily doses of 120 to 240 mg are titrated to average maintenance doses of 240 to 480 mg. The sustained-release preparations offer comparable bioavailability, slower absorption with less fluctuation, and more sustained serum levels, permitting once- or twice-daily dosing. Observations of significant nonlinear accumulation with a prolonged half-life after chronic oral dosing may permit a longer dosing interval for the conventional tablets as well (33).

Oral verapamil is very well tolerated in most patients. Smooth muscle relaxation in the gastrointestinal tract may cause constipation. Peripheral edema and headache may also be seen. Verapamil does not aggravate bronchospastic or vasospastic disorders and so is safer in patients unable to take β-blockers.

The effectiveness of oral diltiazem for prophylaxis of recurrent reentrant supraventricular arrhythmias is not well defined. Daily doses of 180 to 360 mg were thought to be effective; however, a recent placebo-controlled trial failed to demonstrate a beneficial effect of diltiazem over placebo for suppression of supraventricular tachycardia (47). Larger clinical trials are necessary to establish the role of oral diltiazem for this indication.

Monitoring parameters for oral verapamil therapy include cardiac rhythm and rate, constipation, and peripheral edema. Routine serum-level monitoring is not advised.

DIGOXIN

The suppressant effect of digoxin on AV nodal conduction occurs via a mechanism different from that of verapamil. It is particularly useful in infants and children, often as a single agent, after Wolff–Parkinson–White syndrome with antegrade accessory pathway conduction has been excluded. Its positive inotropic effect is unique among the common antiarrhythmics and permits its use in patients with heart failure. The ideal digoxin dose is one that controls the ventricular rate during the tachyarrhythmia yet does not cause bradycardia while in sinus rhythm. Specific aspects of digoxin therapy are discussed under "Atrial Fibrillation."

QUINIDINE

Quinidine is the leading antiarrhythmic drug in the United States in terms of frequency of use. During one recent period (1989–90), it comprised 44% of the market for antiarrhythmic agents(38a). Quinidine is a prototype Class Ia drug that differs from digoxin and verapamil by its action on the fast (sodium) channel. Its net effect reflects a modification of its direct action by an indirect vagolytic effect. The direct action is a generalized slowing of both automaticity and conduction velocity in the SA node, AV node, and His–Purkinje systems. Vagolysis overrides many of these effects, resulting in a *net increase* in sinus rate and AV nodal conduction velocity. His–Purkinje conduction time remains delayed, reflecting minimal autonomic influence in these tissues. The effects of quinidine are minimal in healthy well-polarized tissues and most marked at rapid heart rates, in ectopic pacemakers, and in hypoxic or ischemic tissues. Peripheral α-adrenergic blockade and relaxation of vascular smooth muscle associated with intravenous administration may further influence cardiac action. Alteration of baseline susceptibility to the direct or indirect action of quinidine may explain interpatient variation in net effect.

The efficacy of quinidine in supraventricular tachycardias results from a decrease in atrial ectopy, thus suppressing the inciting premature impulses, as well as a slowing of conduction in the retrograde fast path (Table 39.2). It is not useful after reentry has begun and may even be deleterious because of an increase in AV nodal conduction velocity. Patients should therefore be "digitalized" before initiation of quinidine therapy for supraventricular tachyarrhythmias. Interestingly, controlled studies of quinidine in AV nodal reentry are lacking despite widespread clinical use.

After oral administration, quinidine demonstrates variable absorption and first-pass effect, resulting in about 70% bioavailability (range 45 to 100%) (48). Peak serum concentrations are seen at 1 to 2 hr for the standard formulation of the sulfate salt and 3 to 5 hr with the sustained-release formulations of the sulfate and gluconate salts. The rate and extent of absorption is reduced in patients with heart failure (49). Quinidine is 80 to 89% protein-bound to albumin and α-1 acid glycoprotein. It demonstrates two-compartment kinetics, with average distribution and elimination phase half-lives of 7 min and 6 to 7 hr, respectively (48). The steady-state distribution volume in normals is 3 liters/kg (48). About 85% is metabolized to several active and inactive forms, including 3-hydroxyquinidine, 2-oxoquinidinone, and quinidine-N-oxide. Ten to 20% is eliminated unchanged in the urine in 24 hr, primarily by glomerular filtration. Total clearance averaging 4.5 ml/min/kg is widely variable and may be dose- and route-of-administration-dependent (48,50).

Quinidine metabolites may contribute to both the antiarrhythmic and proarrhythmic effects (51). Total serum levels of 3-hydroxyquinidine are lower than those of the parent compound, but a higher unbound fraction results in free metabolite levels comparable to those of the parent drug (50). Both quinidine and 3-hydroxyquinidine may accumulate with multiple dosing, resulting in higher serum levels as well as an increase in QTc interval prolongation (50).

Patients with congestive heart failure have a decreased volume of distribution and total clearance, without alteration in half-life (49). Increased levels of α-1 acid glycoprotein concentration commonly observed after acute myocardial infarction may result in diminished drug effect because of more extensive protein binding (52). Patients with cirrhosis demonstrate decreased protein binding, an increased half-life and volume of distribution, and no change in total clearance (48). A diminished volume of distribution and renal clearance without change in half-life are seen with renal failure.

Quinidine is available in several salts: quinidine sulfate (83% base), quinidine gluconate (62% base), and quinidine polygalacturonate (60% base). Since dosages are expressed as the salt rather than the base, it is important to account for the different potencies when switching forms. The usual daily dose is 200 to 400 mg of the sulfate salt or its equivalent 3 to 4 times daily for the conventional tablets. Dosage should be decreased in congestive heart failure and (possibly) cirrhosis. Children and young adults (<30 years) may require higher doses. Dosage adjustment in renal insufficiency is controversial.

Intravenous administration has traditionally been discouraged because of dose- and rate-related hypotension caused by α-adrenergic blockade and a direct peripheral venodilation. Reports suggest that intravenous administration is safe when given no faster than 0.5 mg/kg/min to a total dosage of 10 mg/kg of quinidine gluconate, with careful blood pressure monitoring (53). Administration intramuscularly is not advised since it gives erratic absorption, is painful, and may result in sterile abscess formation.

The utility of serum-level monitoring is hindered by the nonspecificity of common analytic methods. The parent drug, its metabolites, and dihydroquinidine (a known impurity in commercial grade drug) may all be detected to varying degrees. The different pharmacokinetic and pharmacodynamic profiles of these compounds obscure the relationship between serum levels and therapeutic or adverse effects. Assays of total (bound and unbound) quinidine are further limited in diseases such as acute myocardial infarction, where the extent of protein binding can vary from day to day. High-performance liquid chromatography (HPLC) is considered the most specific and therefore the reference procedure, with a therapeutic range of 1 to 3 to 4 µg/ml (52). The double extraction photofluorometric and enzyme immunoassay (EMIT) assays have therapeutic ranges of 2 to 5 µg/ml. Individualized "target serum level" goals based on clinical or EPS response may be more useful than values based on population parameters. It is also important to recognize that "therapeutic range" estimates derived from trials of ventricular arrhythmias may not be applicable to supraventricular tachycardias. Serum level measurement is therefore useful in suspected noncompliance or toxicity but may not be necessary in well-controlled patients without clinical toxicity.

Adverse effects occur in 18 to 50% of patients taking quinidine, with 9 to 14% patients requiring drug discontinuation (54,55). In the Boston Collaborative Drug Surveillance Program (54) gastrointestinal reactions, primarily diarrhea with or without nausea, were particularly troublesome and the most common reason for discontinuing therapy, accounting for 7.8%. Fever was seen in 1.7%. Various dermatologic reactions, cinchonism (tinnitus, dizziness, hearing and visual disturbances) and hematologic reactions (thrombocytopenia, hemolytic anemia) each

occurred in less than 1% of patients. As a rule, patients who do not have disabling gastrointestinal effects have excellent long-term tolerance of quinidine.

The most serious cardiac reaction is exacerbation of arrhythmias. This may manifest as the induction of a new arrhythmia or conversion of an existing stable arrhythmia to an unstable one. Paroxysmal syncope or presyncope is correlated on ECG with intermittent pleomorphic ventricular tachycardia or fibrillation, often of the *torsade de pointes* pattern. It typically follows a pause or abrupt decrease in ventricular rate. The first tachycardic QRS complex occurs as a triggered response, emerging from a large postpause U-wave. The intervening sinus beats often demonstrate a markedly prolonged QTc interval. *Torsade de pointes* occurs in 2 to 3% of patients begun on quinidine (51). Patients with pretreatment QT prolongation, bradycardia, hypokalemia, hypomagnesemia, heart block, and heart failure (or possibly those taking digoxin) (42) are at increased risk. Proarrhythmic effects can appear at any time, generally within 3 to 5 days after initiation of therapy or dosage increase. As many as 50% will have serum levels <2 µg/ml, reflecting the idiosyncratic rather than toxic nature of the reaction (51). In vitro testing suggests that quinidine metabolites or impurities may also contribute to the proarrhythmic effect (51). Proarrhythmic events are less common in patients with SVTs than are ventricular arrhythmias, possibly because SVT patients are more likely to have structurally normal hearts. Most episodes are self-limiting and usually abate 12 to 24 hr after discontinuing the drug. Some patients develop cardiovascular insufficiency or collapse. Treatment is limited to discontinuation of the drug, maintaining serum potassium levels at or above normal, DC cardioversion, or overdrive pacing; most antiarrhythmic drugs are ineffective.

Other cardiovascular reactions include bradyarrhythmias or an increased ventricular rate in patients with atrial fibrillation. Hypotension following intravenous administration of quinidine is minimized by slow infusion rates. Symptomatic hypotension is treated by administration of fluids and a reduction in infusion rate.

A recent meta-analysis evaluating the safety and efficacy of quinidine revealed a disturbing threefold increase in death rate for patients on maintenance therapy compared to placebo over a 1-year period (55). The percentage of patients dying in the quinidine group was 2.9% versus 0.8% in the placebo group; however, the causes of death were not well characterized and included causes other than cardiovascular. Death related to chronic quinidine therapy is thought to result from proarrhythmia, a belief that has not yet been clinically documented. Some cardiologists are recommending against using Class 1 agents in favor of low-dose amiodarone (55a).

The interaction of quinidine with digoxin is particularly important in the management of supraventricular tachycardias since the concomitant use of digoxin is important to protect the AV node from the vagolytic effects of quinidine. Reduction of digoxin dose is often necessary. Other drug interactions of quinidine include those with hepatic enzyme inducers (phenobarbital, phenytoin, rifampin) or inhibitors (cimetidine) and warfarin.

Monitoring guidelines for quinidine in AV nodal reentry prophylaxis include heart rate and rhythm, QRS and QTc intervals, and gastrointestinal symptoms. Patients with intolerable gastrointestinal reactions should be evaluated on a different salt or a sustained-release preparation (at equivalent dosage) before switching to another drug. Administration with food may also lessen symptoms. Serum levels may be monitored, but the laboratory should be contacted to determine assay methodology, its limitations, and the recommended therapeutic range. To facilitate detection and treatment of proarrhythmic events, some recommend that patients should be hospitalized for the first 3 to 5 days of therapy. Others point out that the proarrhythmia onset may be delayed despite these precautions.

β-BLOCKERS

Propranolol and the other β-blocking agents have many effects on cardiac conduction and contractility. Their efficacy in supraventricular tachycardias results from a slowing of automaticity in sinus and ectopic pacemakers, a decrease in conduction velocity through the AV node, and an increase in the refractory period of the AV node (Table 39.2). "Quinidinelike" membrane-stabilizing properties are seen only at very high doses and do not contribute to arrhythmia control. When successful during EPS evaluation, long-term efficacy is very good. Despite their numerous adverse effects and contraindications, these agents retain their usefulness in the prophylaxis of AV nodal reentry because their mechanism of action differs from that of the other commonly used drugs. They are especially useful in supraventricular tachycardias associated with excessive catecholamine release as in hyperthyroidism, pheochromocytoma, exercise, or emotional upset. A reduction in exercise tolerance may be bothersome in young patients. In theory, most of the currently available β-blocking drugs should be effective in supraventricular tachycardias, but large-scale studies are lacking. Dosage requirements for propranolol and the other β-blockers are difficult to predict because of variation in the response of individual patients to fixed concentrations of drug. Underlying sympathetic tone and variations in pharmacokinetics further modify patient response. Other aspects of β-blockers are discussed under "Sudden Death."

OTHER DRUGS

Procainamide, disopyramide, flecainide, encainide, sotalol, and amiodarone all have good efficacy in controlling AV nodal reentry. Unfortunately, adverse effects relegate them to a secondary role. The proarrhythmic effects of flecainide and encainide are major limitations. These drugs should be used with careful observation, especially in patients with structural heart disease.

NONPHARMACOLOGIC THERAPIES

Nonpharmacologic therapies for AV nodal reentry include pacemakers, surgical interruption of the reentry circuit, and percutaneous catheter ablation or modification. They are indicated when medical therapy is ineffective or not tolerated. Since these modalities allow patients to remain drug-free, noncompliant patients, younger patients unwilling to comply with lifelong drug treatment, elderly patients in which symptoms of the arrhythmia or adverse effects of antiarrhythmic medication may be intolerable, or females desiring pregnancy may also be candidates. Extensive EPS and cardiac-mapping studies are important in maximizing success.

Pacemakers. Permanent pacemakers have been used in the chronic management of AV nodal reentry for many years. They either minimize arrhythmia genesis or terminate tachycardias after they occur. Overdrive pacing at a rate slightly faster than the sinus rate, or programmed atrial and ventricular stimulation, will alter refractoriness in the limbs of the reentrant circuit and therefore prevent the arrhythmia. Techniques for terminating the tachycardia are the same as those discussed under "Acute Management" (46). The most sophisticated devices are activated automatically by a sensing function, may be programmed both before and after insertion, and have a memory function that remembers and delivers an algorithm of previously successful terminating sequences. Unfortunately, reliable termination of AV nodal reentry requires concomitant antiarrhythmic drug therapy in as many as 50% of patients receiving pacemakers (46). Adverse effects include precipitation of tachyarrhythmias, syncope, and sudden death, especially in patients with accessory pathways. Additionally, pacemakers require regular checks and reprogramming, may not eliminate symptoms, and are not curative. This last limitation has become more meaningful as surgical methods offering complete cure have evolved. Patients with sinus node disease are ideal candidates since the pacemaker can manage both tachycardic and bradycardic episodes. They are also useful in those who are not candidates for surgery or refuse surgery.

Surgery. Surgical techniques include (a) careful dissection of the perinodal tissue to alter intranodal or accessory pathway conduction, which is especially useful in the Wolff–Parkinson–White syndrome or (b) cryoablation of atrial fibers around the AV node to abolish extranodal retrograde pathways while preserving antegrade conduction (56). These procedures have been studied in both adults and children, primarily with AV nodal reentry or AV reentry using an accessory pathway. They are highly successful on short-term evaluation but incur the typical risks and limitations of open chest procedures.

Percutaneous Catheter Modification of the AV Node. Recent refinements in technique have allowed the sophisticated goal of selective modification of the AV node using percutaneously placed catheters. Either the antegrade (slow) or retrograde (fast) pathway can be abolished or impaired. Modification of the AV node or surrounding tissues is achieved by applying direct current, laser, or most commonly radiofrequency energy sources. Antegrade pathway conduction modification has become the preferred method over retrograde conduction because of greater efficacy, more than 90% versus 50 to 90%, respectively, and minimal risk for AV block, less than 2% versus 2 to 8%, respectively (57,58). Complications other than AV block include thromboembolism, arrhythmias (including inappropriate sinus tachycardia), and valvular damage. Intravenous heparin is infused during the procedure to prevent thomboemboli formation. Postmodification therapy may include 3 to 6 months of aspirin or warfarin therapy and β-blockers for the control of inappropriate sinus tachycardia if it occurs. The benefit of short-term antiplatelet or anticoagulation therapy following the modification procedure has not yet been determined. The percutaneous approach has the advantage of avoiding an open chest procedure with cardiopulmonary bypass. Because of the curative properties, high efficacy, and low potential for adverse effects, percutaneous modification is fast becoming a preferred method of treatment. However, long-term follow-up data regarding cardiac effects and safety for this treatment modality is needed.

Nonpharmacologic strategies for the management of AV nodal reentry and AV reentry associated with an accessory pathway are evolving rapidly. Their primary use at present is limited to patients who are resistant or intolerant to antiarrhythmic drug therapy. Their expeditious, cost-effective, and curative features are major attributes. As technologies are developed and refined, nonpharmacologic therapy is likely to be useful in a wide spectrum of populations.

ECTOPIC ATRIAL

Enhanced automaticity (ability to generate spontaneous impulses) of an ectopic atrial focus may result in an arrhythmia known as ectopic atrial tachycardia. Like reentry, it is initiated by a premature atrial impulse. Unlike reentry, this arrhythmia is characterized by a "warm-up period" with gradual acceleration, and termination via a gradual deceleration. The ventricular rate ranges from 100 to 280 beats/min. Periods of AV block are common. This arrhythmia is important because ectopic atrial tachycardia with block in a patient taking digitalis is highly suspicious

for toxicity. Other acute causes include acute myocardial infarction, trauma, chronic lung disease, or certain metabolic abnormalities.

Multifocal atrial tachycardia (MAT) is a form of ectopic atrial tachycardia thought to be caused by either enhanced automaticity or triggered activity (59). On ECG, at least three different ectopic P-wave morphologies are seen, representing ≥3 ectopic foci, with irregular PR- and PP-intervals. The ventricular rate of 130 to 220 beats/min is variable ("irregularly irregular") during the tachycardic episodes. This allows differentiation from AV nodal or AV reentry but may result in confusion with atrial fibrillation. MAT is seen in 0.3 to 0.4% of hospitalized patients. It occurs typically in elderly patients with chronic lung or heart disease who are critically ill with acute pulmonary or cardiac failure or sepsis. It is associated with an elevation in circulating catecholamines and may be precipitated by hypoxia, electrolyte disturbances, acid–base disorders, or drugs such as methylxanthines or β-agonists.

Ectopic atrial tachycardia is often nonresponsive to standard antiarrhythmics or pacing. Vagal maneuvers, verapamil, adenosine, and digoxin commonly initiate or increase AV block, thereby slowing the ventricular rate. However, the atrial rate remains unchanged and the arrhythmia persists. Special care must be exercised in treatment with digoxin since this drug may *induce* ectopic atrial tachycardia. In cases of suspected digitalis-induced arrhythmia, potassium is the agent of choice since it will counteract the action of digitalis at the cellular level. Phenytoin, lidocaine, propranolol, or digoxin-immune Fab fragments may also be used. DC cardioversion is dangerous in digitalis toxicity since it may precipitate intractable ventricular arrhythmias.

MAT is often difficult to manage. Pharmacologic attempts to block the AV node or decrease ectopic activity are rarely successful. Trials of digoxin, quinidine, procainamide, phenytoin, and lidocaine have been disappointing. Surgery to resect or ablate the ectopic foci, as well as electrical modalities (pacing or DC countershock), are also ineffective. Treatment of the underlying disease is the only reliable therapy. Correction of predisposing factors will terminate the arrhythmia in most patients though recurrence is common. Verapamil (60) and metoprolol (61) have been reported to slow the ventricular rate, reduce atrial ectopy, and/or reduce abnormal atrial or AV junctional-triggered activity. In one trial, metoprolol was associated with a larger reduction in ventricular rate and higher rate of conversion to sinus rhythm (62) than verapamil. However, the hypotensive and adverse pulmonary effects of these drugs limit their utility. They should be reserved for patients with symptoms of hypoperfusion. The high mortality rate of patients with MAT (40 to 50%) is due to the underlying condition, not the arrhythmia. Antiarrhythmics have not been shown to reduce mortality.

ATRIAL FIBRILLATION

Atrial fibrillation (AF) is characterized by rapid, chaotic atrial firing at a rate of 350 to 600 beats/min ("auricular delirium"). The AV node blocks most impulses, resulting in random, irregular ventricular conduction averaging 100 to 180 impulses/min in untreated cases. Ventricular (His–Purkinje) conduction is usually normal. AF is thought to be caused by intraatrial reentry. Uneven refractoriness of adjacent atrial tissues allows the formation of multiple reentrant wavelets. These wavelets become wandering reentry circuits completely dissociated from one another. AF may be chronic, paroxysmal, or a single, isolated occurrence. Transition from paroxysmal to chronic AF depends on the underlying etiology and the duration of paroxysmal episodes. AF is the most common *sustained* arrhythmia and the second most common overall.

The prevalence of AF is about 0.4% in individuals under 60 years old, and 2 to 4% for those over 60 years (63). Paroxysmal or single isolated episodes of AF are seen with cardiac surgery, fever, infection, pulmonary embolism, ethanol intoxication, or drug toxicity (sympathomimetics, β-agonists, methylxanthines). AF is also seen in 10 to 15% of patients with acute myocardial infarction (9), usually lasting less than 24 hr. Chronic AF is associated with congestive heart failure, coronary artery disease, rheumatic heart disease, dilated or hypertrophic cardiomyopathy, hypertensive heart disease, hyperthyroidism and certain congenital heart diseases. AF without associated cardiovascular disease ("lone AF") occurs in 0.5 to 30%, with the wide range reflecting different definitions and populations (64).

The principal hemodynamic effects of AF result from (a) a shortened diastolic filling time, leading to decreased left ventricular end-diastolic volume and stroke volume and (b) a loss of synchronized atrial contraction, resulting in increased mean left atrial pressure in addition to the preceding two effects. Loss of atrial systole causes a 20 to 30% reduction in stroke volume in normals, which is increased in patients with heart disease. When coupled with incomplete ventricular filling, the net effect is a decrease in cardiac reserve. Elevations in heart rate are initially associated with an increased cardiac output. Once a critical rate is exceeded, ventricular filling time becomes a limiting factor, and further increases in heart rate result in reduced cardiac output.

The nonhemodynamic consequence of AF is embolism resulting from turbulent blood flow through the atria with mural thrombus formation. Embolic risk is highest in the first 2 to 4 weeks after the onset of AF and at the time of transition from paroxysmal to chronic AF. In some patients, the embolic event is the presenting manifestation of previously undetected AF. Embolism to arteries in the cerebral circulation is most common and accounts for about 7% of all strokes (65). Other locations include the extremity, mesenteric, coronary, and renal circulations. Framingham study patients with chronic AF due to rheumatic mitral valve disease were found to have a 17.6-fold increase in stroke risk, with a 5.6-fold increase for AF of other causes (66). Risk factors for embolism in chronic AF include a history of previous emboli or an association with advanced age, congestive heart failure, ventricular dysfunction, and left atrial enlargement (64,67). In patients with lone AF, stroke risk is low in young but probably higher in older patients and those with hypertension.

The clinical manifestations of AF include the signs and symptoms of congestive heart failure, most commonly in the pulmonary system, and exacerbated with exercise. Some patients may develop angina or symptoms of cerebral insufficiency such as confusion, fatigue, or syncope. Palpitations may be especially troublesome in patients with paroxysmal AF. Elderly patients with diseased AV nodes may have slow ventricular rates at rest but will nonetheless have reduced cardiac reserve with exercise or stress. As many as 30% are asymptomatic at the time of diagnosis (68). Irregular apical and radial pulses result from random impulse transmission through the AV node and are the classic physical signs of AF. ECG findings include a lack of discrete atrial activity, variable R-R intervals, normal-appearing QRS complexes (unless aberrant conduction or bundle branch block are present), and an irregular baseline between QRS complexes.

Acute Treatment

The primary goal of the acute management of AF is to correct the hemodynamic manifestations by increasing cardiac output. This is usually accomplished by pharmacologic slowing of the ventricular rate, which lengthens diastolic filling time and increases stroke volume. Electrical or chemical conversion to sinus rhythm in the acute phase is reserved for patients with hemodynamic instability or ventricular rate more than 150 beats/min (10). The optimal ventricular rate for maximizing cardiac output is unknown. An arbitrary ventricular rate of less than 100 beats/min is often chosen as a therapeutic goal. However, the following therapeutic aspects must be emphasized: (a) Strict attention to ventricular rate should not be at the expense of objective and symptomatic relief or of drug intoxication. (b) Underlying factors favoring tachycardia should be considered, especially excess catecholamine release as in infection, hyperthyroidism, or sympathomimetic drug overdose. In these patients, a rate of 100 to 120 beats/min may be acceptable as long as the signs and symptoms are controlled. Strict adherence to a goal of a rate less than 100 beats/min may result in bradycardia when the underlying problem is corrected. Rate titration should consider the clinical appearance of the patient as well as the anticipated rapidity of catecholamine correction. (c) Aggressive treatment of coexisting conditions such as fever, infection, hypoxia, anemia, or hyperthyroidism is essential.

A review of the role of the AV node in AF is useful in understanding the pharmacologic management. The AV node is not involved in the initiation and perpetuation of AF per se but plays a critical role as a "filter" of atrial impulses. The AV node is the primary determinant of ventricular rate in AF. In contrast, the SA node determines the rate in sinus rhythm. The intrinsic conductivity of AV nodal tissues as well as extracardiac factors that may alter conduction (autonomic tone, drugs) have a critical influence on ventricular rate. Vagal stimulation results in increased filtering and less conduction across the AV node. Increased sympathetic tone enhances AV nodal conduction, resulting in an inappropriate excessive increase in ventricular rate with exercise or stress. Control of ventricular rate both at rest and during exercise is important in maintaining the function of the patient. However, changes in AV nodal conductivity *will not* terminate the arrhythmia.

DIGOXIN

Digitalis is generally considered the drug of choice for the acute control of ventricular rate. Digitalis has positive inotropic and negative chronotropic and dromotropic properties. The last effect accounts for its efficacy in AF, is seen only at higher doses, and occurs via a variety of mechanisms. The predominant effect is indirect via vagal stimulation, with direct AV nodal action having a minor role. This vagotonic effect is largely attenuated by catecholamines, explaining the limited ability to control ventricular rates during exercise or stress (69–71). Digitalis does not suppress ectopy; most patients remain in AF. In fact, digoxin does not prevent recurrence of paroxysmal atrial fibrillation in those patients in sinus rhythm. The effect of digitalis on accessory pathways differs from that on the AV node, and it should not be used in patients with AF and the Wolff–Parkinson–White syndrome (referred to in a separate section).

Optimally, individual digoxin-loading doses are determined based on the observed response to initial therapy. Doses of 0.5 mg intravenously are followed by 0.125 to 0.25 mg intravenously or orally every 4 to 8 hr until the desired response is seen. The dose and interval should take into account the time for tissue distribution of 6 to 8 hr. This regimen will usually result in rate control in 12 to 24 hr. In a recent prospective observational study, the average total dose of digoxin needed for initial control of ventricular rate was 0.8 mg (range 0.125 to 6.125 mg), and the average time to initial ventricular rate control was 9.5 hr (72). Administration intramuscularly is not advised because of erratic absorption and excessive pain at the injection site. Infants, children, and patients with hyperthyroidism may require higher than estimated doses, whereas those with coronary artery disease or obstructive airway disease may be

especially sensitive to digitalis. Oral maintenance doses for AF average 0.25 to 0.375 mg daily in adult patients with normal renal function. Calculated doses may be used as a guideline, but the clinical response of the patient is a better criterion of efficacy.

Monitoring parameters for digoxin use in AF include ventricular rate (apical pulse) and the signs and symptoms of congestive heart failure. The radial (peripheral) pulse is *not* an appropriate monitoring criterion since it may not reflect efficacy in patients with very high apical rates. In these patients, some ventricular contractions may not elicit detectable peripheral pulses, causing a "pulse deficit." Renal function and serum electrolytes (especially potassium and magnesium) should also be monitored, along with observation for signs and symptoms of toxicity. The use of serum levels as a guide to dosage requirements is not advised in the management of supraventricular tachycardias such as AV nodal reentry and AF. Correlation between therapeutic response (i.e., ventricular rate) and serum levels is poor (73,74). This is probably because other factors (underlying autonomic tone, exogenous catecholamines, electrolyte concentrations) alter cardiac sensitivity to digitalis, independent of serum levels. Despite this limitation, serum levels may be useful in evaluating patient compliance, suspected toxicity, or drug interactions. Levels should be drawn at least 6 to 8 hr after dosage administration to allow for tissue distribution.

Two drug interactions of digoxin are relevant to the management of supraventricular tachyarrhythmias. An elevation of serum digoxin levels to 2 to 3 times baseline occurs in most patients taking digoxin and quinidine concomitantly. Digoxin levels increase within hours after quinidine administration, reaching a new steady state in several days. This interaction depends on the serum level of quinidine but not that of digoxin and is caused by a decrease in volume of distribution and renal and nonrenal clearance of digoxin by quinidine. Since there is no evidence for an alteration of digoxin receptor site activity or sensitivity, digoxin toxicity may ensue. Reducing the dose by 50% as well as careful serum level monitoring are advised (42). Serum digoxin levels may be increased by a similar mechanism in patients receiving verapamil or diltiazem, with new steady-state digoxin levels achieved in 7 to 14 days. The clinical importance of this reaction is not well established although some have recommended a digoxin dosage reduction by 50% (42).

The subjective evaluation of patients for digoxin toxicity is difficult because of the nonspecific nature of the symptoms. Anorexia, nausea, vomiting, weakness, and lethargy are the most common symptoms. Vision changes, disorientation, and hallucinations are less common. Elevated serum levels may assist in the diagnosis; however, there is overlap between toxic and therapeutic values. Moreover, electrolyte abnormalities (hypokalemia, metabolic alkalosis, hypomagnesemia, or hypercalcemia) or hypoxia may contribute to clinical toxicity even at "nontoxic" serum levels. Toxic cardiac effects result from enhanced automaticity, promotion of triggered activity, and/or a depression of AV nodal conduction. A useful monitoring tool for toxicity in AF patients is the ECG. The excessive effects of digoxin result in an exaggerated AV nodal block, seen initially as occasional long equal pauses (intermittent junctional escape). Eventually, the ventricular rate becomes *regular* at 35 to 30 beats/min, reflecting complete junctional escape. At higher levels, junctional pacemaker firing may accelerate, causing a junctional tachycardia. PVCs caused by enhanced firing of ectopic ventricular foci are also common. As toxicity progresses, essentially all arrhythmias may be seen. Toxicity is managed by discontinuation of the drug, potassium unless contraindicated, antiarrhythmics, and/or digoxin-immune Fab fragments. Refer to the section on "Digitalis-Induced PVCs" for management details.

Other aspects of digoxin therapy may be found in Chapter 38, "Congestive Heart Failure."

VERAPAMIL

Verapamil exerts a direct effect on the AV node that is not mediated by the autonomic nervous system. Thus, in contrast to digoxin, verapamil retains its usefulness during exercise or stress. Some patients may demonstrate regularization of ventricular rate while remaining in AF; however, this does not augment hemodynamic function (75). A lack of suppressant effect on ectopic foci results in conversion to sinus rhythm in only 10 to 15%, probably through improved hemodynamic function. Verapamil is prompt, reliable, effective, and relatively safe. The dose for AF is the same as that for AV nodal reentry: 5 to 10 mg (0.075 to 0.15 mg/kg) intravenously over 2 to 3 min, repeated in 30 min if needed. It has an onset of action of 5 to 10 min and duration of about 30 min after a bolus injection. Constant infusions of 5 mg/hr initially, titrated to a ventricular rate <100 beats/min, a systolic blood pressure ≥90 mm Hg, and a maximum dose of about 10 mg/hr for up to 7 days have been reported (76) although this is not an FDA-labeled method of administration. Infusions should be preceded by bolus doses as above. Because of its rapid onset of action and more predictable effect in patients with high circulating catecholamine levels, some practitioners consider verapamil the drug of choice over digoxin in AF (77). The primary limitation of verapamil is its negative inotropic effect. Downward dosage adjustment should be considered in patients with heart or liver failure because of impaired drug elimination. It should be used cautiously in patients receiving digoxin (because of the previously discussed drug interaction) and patients with Wolff–Parkinson–White syndrome. Monitoring parameters include the ECG, ventricular rate, blood pressure,

and the signs and symptoms of heart failure. Other aspects of verapamil are discussed in the section "AV Nodal Reentry."

DILTIAZEM

Successful treatment of AF and atrial flutter can also be achieved with intravenous diltiazem (78). Diltiazem exerts a direct effect on the AV node similar to verapamil. Restoration of sinus rhythm with diltiazem occurs infrequently, similar to verapamil. The potential advantages of diltiazem over verapamil are its low incidence of hypotension and minimal negative inotropic effect (78). The doses of diltiazem for AF is 0.25 mg/kg intravenously over 2 min followed by 0.35 mg/kg in 15 min if the initial response was inadequate. Diltiazem controls ventricular rate in about 5 min with continued control for 3 to 10 hr after 1 or 2 bolus doses (43,78). In patients requiring ventricular rate control until other methods of arrhythmia suppression can be employed (long-term antiarrhythmic therapy or cardioversion) a 24-hr intravenous infusion can be administered at a rate of 10 to 15 mg/hr (79). The dose of diltiazem should be reduced in patients with heart or liver failure because of its reliance on hepatic elimination. It should be used cautiously in patients receiving digoxin and patients with Wolff–Parkinson–White syndrome. Diltiazem should not be given in close temporal proximity with intravenous β-blockers. Monitoring parameters include the ECG, ventricular rate, blood pressure, and the signs and symptoms of heart failure.

ESMOLOL

The β-blocker esmolol demonstrates the typical effects of a cardioselective β-blocker without intrinsic sympathomimetic activity or membrane-stabilizing effects and demonstrates the additional unique property of an ultra-short duration of action. This permits its use to slow AV nodal conduction directly, with minimal concern for long-lasting adverse effects. Esmolol is rapidly hydrolyzed by red cell esterases, with distribution and elimination half-lives of 2 and 9 min, respectively (80). The total clearance of 17 to 20 liters/kg/hr reflects the largely hepatic elimination to methanol and a metabolite with minimal β-blocking activity (80,81). Esmolol is initiated with a loading dose of 500 μg/kg for 1 min, followed by maintenance infusions of 50 to 300 μg/kg/min. If control is not established, the loading dose is repeated and the infusion rate increased. Dosage adjustments may be made as often as every 5 to 15 min. Most patients respond at 100 μg/kg/min.

Clinical trials have shown esmolol to be comparable to propranolol in reducing the ventricular rate in supraventricular tachycardias, with an overall response rate of 64 to 72%, including 6 to 14% who converted to sinus rhythm (80–82). Comparative studies with verapamil have shown similar reductions in ventricular rate with a higher number of patients converting to sinus rhythm after esmolol (83). The onset of action is less than 5 min, with a return to baseline heart rate 10 to 20 min after discontinuation. Esmolol therefore offers the flexibility to continually and rapidly titrate the dosage to the desired effect. Further, there is an added element of safety should adverse effects occur.

The primary adverse effect is hypotension, occurring in 33 to 44% of patients (80,82). Hypotension is most common at doses ≥200 µg/kg/min, in postoperative or elderly patients over 65 years old, or those with baseline hypotension (82). Most patients remain asymptomatic and are managed by a reduction in dosage. Severe hypotension may require discontinuation, with blood pressure returning to normal in 20 to 30 min. Local injection-site irritation is concentration- and duration-related and occurs in up to 8% of patients. This effect is minimized by diluting infusions to <10 mg/ml, which may hamper use in volume-restricted patients. Limited data supports the safety of esmolol in patients with traditional contraindications to β-blockers, such as diabetes mellitus or obstructive airway disease (80,82). In general, however, it should be avoided or used with caution in these patients.

β-blockers are particularly useful in AF caused by high circulating catecholamine levels, including hyperthyroidism or sympathomimetic overdose, because they pharmacologically attenuate the underlying cause of the arrhythmia. Critically ill perioperative and cardiac patients should be managed with esmolol. β-blockers may be necessary for only a short time in these patients since correction of the precipitating cause may "restore" digoxin sensitivity or even allow conversion to sinus rhythm.

PACING

At the present time, cardiac pacemakers or other devices are not considered first-line treatments in the acute management of AF.

Chronic Treatment

After initial control of ventricular rate, pharmacologic or electrical methods may be used for conversion to sinus rhythm. If successful, maintenance therapy (generally with the same antiarrhythmic used for conversion) is begun in an attempt to sustain sinus rhythm. Patients who remain in AF or revert shortly after conversion are given drugs to slow the ventricular rate and maximize cardiac output. Chronic AF patients may also be candidates for long-term anticoagulation. Therapeutic goals in chronic AF include relief of symptoms, reduction in embolic risk, and improvement in overall cardiac function and exercise tolerance.

Conversion to sinus rhythm is desirable since it will improve cardiac performance, relieve clinical symptoms, and decrease the risk of embolism markedly. Patients with AF of recent onset may convert spontaneously to sinus rhythm during initial drug treatment or after the inciting stress is eliminated. Unfortunately, not all patients will remain in sinus rhythm. Although conversion to sinus rhythm is crucial for some patients (e.g., those with hemodynamic instability), in others it may be neither practical nor useful. Ideally, an assessment of the likelihood of sustained sinus rhythm should be made before attempted conversion. Higher success rates are seen in patients with a corrected or controlled underlying cause and those with recent arrhythmia onset. Patients likely to revert to AF include those with cardiomegaly (particularly left atrial enlargement), mitral valve disease, AF of more than 3 to 6 months duration, and moderate-to-severe heart failure (84). A curious finding has been a lack of atrial mechanical function (systole) for several days or weeks after cardioversion despite a return of normal electrical activity (85). This may account for the lack of improvement in exercise tolerance and cardiac output, as well as the continued risk for embolism in the period immediately following conversion.

DC COUNTERSHOCK

Cardioversion may be accomplished either electrically or pharmacologically. Direct current (DC) countershock depolarizes a critical number of myocardial cells simultaneously, allowing the SA node to reestablish control as the pacemaker. The current should be synchronized with the QRS complex on ECG to avoid delivery during the vulnerable period of ventricular recovery. Lower initial energies are often used though as many as 300 to 400 Joules may ultimately be required. An antiarrhythmic (usually quinidine) is initiated 1 to 2 days before cardioversion to help maintain sinus rhythm. Short-acting sedatives or anesthetics are given immediately before the procedure. DC countershock is initially successful in 80 to 95% of patients (68,84,86,87). Data compiled from 824 patients demonstrated a 2.4% frequency of complications, including emboli in 1.3%, ventricular arrhythmias in 0.4%, and miscellaneous complications in 0.6% (84). DC cardioversion should be performed with caution in patients with digitalis toxicity because of the higher risk of ventricular arrhythmias. It is generally not necessary to withhold digoxin immediately before countershock in *nontoxic* patients (88). Patients with known or suspected sick sinus syndrome should be evaluated carefully for possible pacemaker insertion before attempted cardioversion, especially if receiving drugs that exacerbate bradycardia such as calcium channel or β-blockers. Short-term anticoagulation is appropriate to decrease the embolic risk. See "Anticoagulants."

DRUGS FOR CONVERSION TO SINUS RHYTHM

Pharmacologic conversion to sinus rhythm, though less invasive than DC countershock, is also less successful.

Digitalis, verapamil, and diltiazem rarely convert patients with AF to sinus rhythm, probably because of their minimal effects on atrial automaticity.

Quinidine. Quinidine is the most commonly used agent for pharmacologic cardioversion and is also used to maintain sinus rhythm postconversion. Quinidine may have both beneficial and deleterious effects in AF. A decrease in atrial ectopy accounts for its efficacy, whereas its vagolytic effect at the AV node may *enhance* impulse transmission resulting in a very rapid ventricular rate. Therefore, patients with AF should be digitalized before administration of quinidine. Because of the possibility of quinidine-induced long QT syndrome or *torsade de pointes*, all patients should be hospitalized with cardiac monitoring for attempted conversion. A typical therapeutic strategy is to administer quinidine for several days, then proceed to DC countershock if conversion does not occur with quinidine alone. Common dosage regimens for conversion are 300 to 400 mg of the sulfate salt orally q6h. Intravenous quinidine may also be given with close hemodynamic monitoring, as discussed under "AV Nodal Reentry." The reported success rate with quinidine conversion averages 71% (84).

After the first successful conversion, the risks and cost of prophylactic antiarrhythmics to sustain sinus rhythm must be weighed against the likelihood of reversion to AF. Patients thought to be at low risk for reversion to AF may be observed off antiarrhythmics, with the proviso that only about 30% (68,86) of untreated patients will maintain sinus rhythm for 1 year. If AF recurs, prophylactic antiarrhythmic therapy is initiated. There is no superior drug for maintaining sinus rhythm. Strategies are often influenced by personal experience, local tradition, and theoretical considerations. Quinidine has the strongest literature evidence for efficacy, but adverse effects, including death from proarrhythmic events, are severe limitations. Daily maintenance doses of 800 to 1600 mg of the sulfate salt (or its equivalent) have yielded success rates of 40 to 60% after 1 year (54). Subtherapeutic serum concentrations, poor compliance, and inappropriate initial selection of patients for conversion contribute to the lower long-term success.

Other Drugs. Patients who do not convert or fail to sustain sinus rhythm with quinidine may be given procainamide or disopyramide in standard doses. Flecainide is also effective but reports of proarrhythmic effects in AF patients (89,90) limit use. Trials of amiodarone for induction and maintenance of sinus rhythm have demonstrated efficacy in maintaining sinus rhythm as well as controlling ventricular rate if AF recurs. However, the high response rate must be balanced against its toxicity, which is common and may be severe. Sotalol has also been shown effective in terminating AF and maintaining sinus rhythm and serves as an alternative in AF resistant to other agents. The use of sotalol is limited by proarrhythmia, which has been reported in 2% of patients treated for supraventricular

tachycardia (91). Flecainide, amiodarone, and sotalol therapy are discussed later in this chapter.

DRUGS TO CONTROL VENTRICULAR RATE

In some patients, conversion is not attempted because the likelihood of sustained sinus rhythm is thought to be low. Others convert initially but revert to AF shortly thereafter. Therapy in these patients is directed at regulation of the ventricular rate. The optimal rate for maximizing cardiac output has not been established. A reasonable goal is a ventricular rate of less than 80 to 90 beats/min at rest and 100 to 110/min with mild exercise. Most are given digoxin, with or without other agents. As reviewed earlier, sympathetic stimulation may override the effect of digoxin resulting in unacceptably high rate. Trials comparing digoxin with either verapamil or diltiazem have yielded conflicting results. Although all have noted better rate control with the calcium channel blocker, some have shown an associated improvement in exercise capacity (71,92), whereas others have observed no change (69,70). Therefore, better control of the ventricular rate may not improve cardiac output or exercise tolerance, thus negating any major advantage of calcium channel blockers over digoxin. β-blockers may be used in patients with excess catecholamine effect but can worsen heart failure and decrease exercise tolerance (41). Quinidine is not useful in patients with chronic AF and may even be detrimental because of its vagolytic effect.

Monitoring parameters for chronic AF patients include subjective symptoms such as dyspnea, fatigue, angina, and palpitations, as well as objective criteria such as ventricular (or apical) rate. Objective measurements of exercise tolerance and cardiac output may be performed, but they do not always correlate with a subjective sense of improvement.

ANTICOAGULANTS

Anticoagulants are used to reduce the embolic risk associated with AF. Recent data from five randomized multicenter trials has refined antithrombotic treatment for stroke prevention in patients with AF (93–97). The decision to anticoagulate an individual patient with AF is based on the presence of risk factors associated with stroke risk. Cerebral embolism commonly results in large neurologic deficits with severe residual disability, occurs without warning symptoms, is recurrent in about 11% of patients, and carries a mortality of up to 25% (98). On the other hand, the incidence of major bleeding with anticoagulants at conventional intensities has been estimated at 2 to 5% yearly, with 1% per year suffering intracranial hemorrhage (98). These values may be even higher in the elderly, who comprise the majority of patients with AF.

After the onset of AF, several days are required for thrombus formation. Anticoagulants are therefore not

Table 39.3.
Stratification of Thromboembolic Risk in Atrial Fibrillation[a,b]

	Thromboembolic Risk (per Year)			
	High (>6%)	Medium–High (4–6%)	Medium–Low (2–4%)	Low (<2%)
Underlying heart disease	Prior embolism Old mechanical prostheses	Mitral stenosis Thyrotoxicosis Coronary disease Modern mechanical pros- theses History of stroke/TIA	Mitral regurgitation Aortic valve disease Heart failure Increasing age Hypertension Diabetes Bioprostheses	Lone AF (age 60) Isolated mitral valve pro- lapse
Long-term A/C therapy	A/C (INR = 2.5–3.5)[c]	A/C (INR = 2.0–3.0)[d]	A/C (INR = 2.0–3.0)[e]	No therapy

[a]Adapted from Stein B, Halperin JL, Fuster V: Should patients with atrial fibrillation be anticoagulated prior to and chronically following cardioversion? Cardiovasc Clin 21(1):231–247, 1990.
[b]Abbreviations: AF, atrial fibrillation; A/C, anticoagulant; INR, international normalized ratio of prothrombin suppression.
[c]In high-risk patients with old mechanical prostheses, dipyridamole may be added to warfarin.
[d]In patients with mechanical prostheses, INR range should be 2.5–3.5.
[e]The decision for anticoagulation in this group should be individualized.

indicated for AF of less than 2-days duration. Once thrombi are formed, however, several weeks are necessary to allow fibrotic organization and adherence to the atrial wall. Moreover, atrial mechanical function (i.e., atrial systole) may be delayed for several weeks after ECG-documented conversion to sinus rhythm (85). The embolic risk in the Framingham study was 14% within the first year after onset and 5% per year thereafter (66). Risk is similar after pharmacologic or electric cardioversion. The American College of Chest Physicians (ACCP) recommendations for anticoagulants at the time of cardioversion include (99): (a) for AF of more than 2 days duration, anticoagulate with warfarin to an international normalized ratio (INR) intensity of 2.0 to 3.0 for 3 weeks before and 4 weeks after cardioversion; (b) no anticoagulants for AF of <2 days duration, unless other risk factors for embolism are present; (c) for patients requiring emergent cardioversion, anticoagulate with heparin on the day of cardioversion if AF is of several days duration, there is a high risk of recurrence, or other risk factors are present.

Assessment of embolic risk in chronic AF patients remains an enigmatic clinical problem. Table 39.3 is a simplified assessment of embolic risk with suggested management strategies. Consensus exists regarding the high embolic risk in patients with documented recent embolism, AF associated with older mechanical heart valve prostheses, and mitral valve disease. Patients with history of stroke, coronary disease, thyrotoxicosis, and modern mechanical valves are at a high but somewhat lower risk. The medium-to-low risk group comprises the largest number of patients, including those with mitral regurgitation, aortic valve disease, heart failure, hypertension, diabetes, advanced age and bioprostheses. Data regarding risk–benefit aspects of anticoagulants in this group are somewhat limited. Several recent large trials in patients

with chronic nonvalvular AF (93–97) have demonstrated efficacy of warfarin therapy, to an international normalized ratio (INR) of 1.4 to 4.5, compared to placebo. The overall risk reduction for stroke has been reported to be 68% from pooled data of five of these trials (100). Aspirin 325 mg/day was also found to be beneficial for preventing stroke associated with AF (95) and is recommended by the ACCP in patients who are poor candidates for anticoagulation (99). Compared to warfarin, aspirin is less effective but is associated with less hemorrhagic complications (95,101). Careful assessment of bleeding risk is a critical element in the decision for or against anticoagulant use in individual patients. Underlying risk factors for bleeding associated with warfarin therapy include age ≥65 years, history of gastrointestinal bleeding, stroke, cancer, recent surgery, and hypertension (102). Patients unable to comply with medication regimens or laboratory follow-up, as well as those with dementia or alcohol abuse, may be poor candidates for anticoagulation regardless of embolic risk. Bleeding risk is also reduced by maintaining anticoagulants in the less intense range (INR 2.0 to 3.0) whenever possible (102). Scrupulous monitoring is essential and can lower bleeding risk substantially. In the Stroke Prevention in Atrial Fibrillation trial, the annual rate of major hemorrhage for patients anticoagulated with warfarin to an INR of 2.0 to 3.5 was limited to 1.7% by meticulous supervision (versus 0.9% for aspirin 325 mg orally daily and 1.2% for placebo) (95).

NONPHARMACOLOGIC THERAPY

Patients with intolerable symptoms who are resistant to other therapies can be treated by surgical or catheter ablation of the AV node with permanent pacemaker placement. Ventricular rate is controlled, but fibrillation of

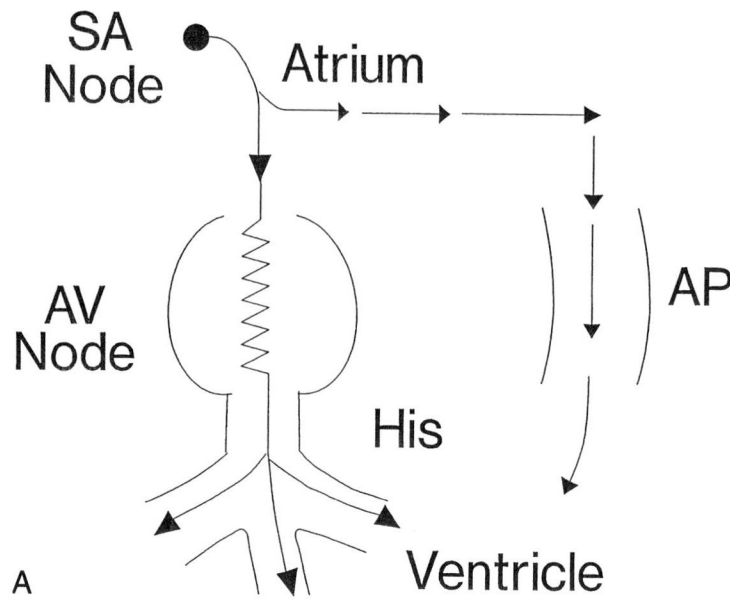

Figure 39-8A. Wolff–Parkinson–White Syndrome. Sinus Rhythm. The impulse reaches the ventricles via the AV node-His–Purkinje system with simultaneous preexcitation via the accessory pathway.

the atria continues. The "corridor procedure" is a surgical procedure that isolates a corridor of tissue that conducts impulses directly from the SA node to the AV node (103). This procedure will control the ventricular rate, but the atria will continue to fibrillate in most patients. An innovative surgical technique known as the maze procedure involves multiple small incisions in the atrium that disrupt the pathways that conduct the reentrant impulses (103). This surgical technique terminates atrial fibrillation, restores AV synchrony, and preserves atrial transport function with a high success rate (104). Nonpharmacologic therapy is reserved for patients with serious symptoms of atrial fibrillation that cannot be controlled by other methods.

PROGNOSIS

The long-term prognosis in patients with chronic AF is poor, with a twofold increase in yearly cardiovascular mortality (10%) over age-matched controls (5%) (65). Mortality is related to age at onset, as well as the presence and extent of coexisting heart disease.

WOLFF–PARKINSON–WHITE

Wolff–Parkinson–White (WPW) syndrome is a congenital heart disease characterized by the presence of an anatomically distinct atrioventricular connection in addition to the AV nodal tissue. This anomalous pathway, called the accessory AV pathway (or Kent bundle), can be located anywhere in the heart and consists of working myocardium that forms an "electrical bridge" connecting the atrium and the ventricle. Impulse conduction may occur both antegrade and retrograde. Patients with WPW typically have sinus rhythm at baseline, with paroxysmal episodes of supraventricular tachycardias (SVTs). While

in sinus rhythm, antegrade conduction is over both the AV node and accessory pathway; ventricular activation is thus a fusion of the two impulses. Since the accessory pathway can activate ventricular muscle directly (bypassing all or part of the AV node and His–Purkinje system), early or "preexcitation" of part of the ventricle occurs (Fig. 39.8A).

The accessory pathway and AV node may form reentry circuits that allow SVTs, most commonly AV reentry or AF (105). AV reentry is distinguished from AV nodal reentry by the use of the accessory pathway as part of the circuit. Accessory pathway conduction in the reentry circuit may be antegrade (called antidromic reentry) or retrograde (orthodromic reentry). Orthodromic reentry is 15 times more common than antidromic. In this form, impulses travel antegrade from the atrium to the ventricle via the AV node and retrograde from the ventricle to the atrium via the accessory pathway (Fig. 39.8B). Multiple accessory pathways are seen in 5 to 15% of patients, usually associated with antidromic reentry.

WPW syndrome is often seen in otherwise healthy infants, children, and young adults. The clinical importance of the arrhythmias varies from relatively benign to life-threatening, depending on the electrophysiologic properties of the accessory pathway and the AV node. Arrhythmias seen in infancy may persist, disappear, or disappear then recur many years later (106). This is thought to reflect a change in the conduction properties of the accessory pathway over time. Orthodromic AV reentry is the most common SVT. The most feared arrhythmia in WPW is AF with antegrade conduction down an accessory pathway with a short refractory period. In this case, the protective effect of the AV node against very rapid ventricular rates is lost. Extremely rapid impulse transmission directly from

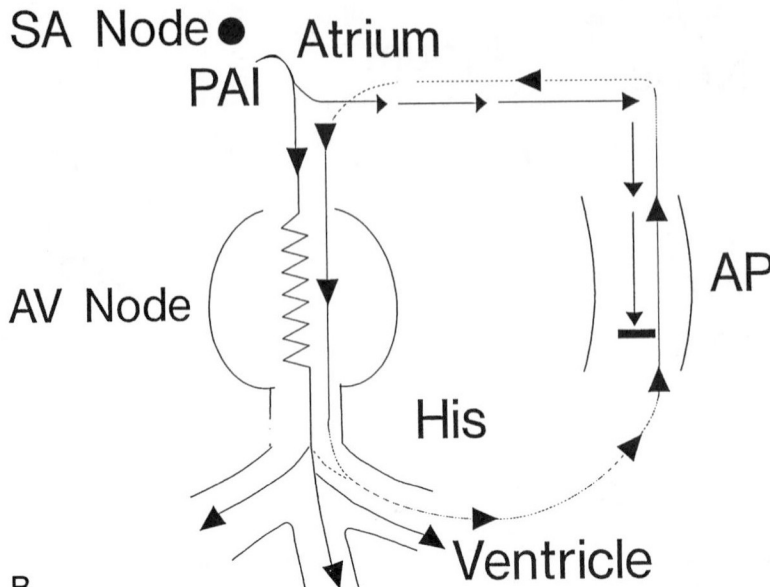

Figure 39-8B. Orthodromic AV Reentry. PAI, premature atrial impulse; AP, accessory pathway; His, bundle of His; solid line, PAI. The premature impulse is blocked in the AP and reaches the ventricles via the AV node-His–Purkinje system. If the AP is recovered, AV reentry may be initiated. Dotted line is a reentry circuit.

B

the atrium to the ventricle may lead to ventricular flutter or fibrillation and sudden death.

The classic ECG in sinus rhythm includes a short PR-interval with a delta wave preceding the QRS complex representing preexcitation. The QRS complex has abnormal morphology due to the fusion of normal conduction down the AV node-His bundle system and preexcitation of the left ventricular free wall. The initiating arrhythmic event is usually a critically timed premature atrial or ventricular impulse. Ventricular rates average 100 to 280/min in AV reentry (higher in children) and 140 to 320/min in AF. The direction of the reentry circuit (orthodromic or antidromic), variation in mode of ventricular activation, and different accessory pathway anatomies all contribute to marked inter- and intrapatient ECG variation during SVTs. Detection of WPW syndrome and differentiation of its associated arrhythmias require an experienced ECG interpreter.

The clinical manifestations and hemodynamic consequences of AV reentry and AF are the same in patients with or without WPW syndrome, ranging from palpitations to syncope and sudden death. WPW patients may be difficult to manage because the effect of the drug on the accessory pathway is not predicted by effect on the AV node. Moreover, drug action on antegrade conduction may differ from that on retrograde. Underlying autonomic tone may alter conduction independent of drug effect. A drug may therefore be beneficial for one patient yet deleterious for another. Management should be individualized by electrophysiologic studies. These studies locate and characterize the accessory pathway, identify the mechanism of the arrhythmia, and evaluate the effects of them on each anatomic component. Other termination techniques such as atrial pacing may also be evaluated.

As a rule, AV *reentry* associated with WPW syndrome is readily terminated using traditional maneuvers and drugs as discussed in the section "AV Nodal Reentry." In patients with AF, however, great care must be exercised to avoid enhanced atrioventricular conduction with subsequent acceleration of ventricular rate and degeneration into ventricular fibrillation. This is a primary consideration in only a small minority (with a short antegrade accessory pathway refractory period). Unfortunately, it is not possible to identify susceptible patients on clinical grounds alone. Some may be entirely asymptomatic, yet have electrophysiologic risk for sudden cardiac death. Moreover, the population at risk based on electrophysiologic studies is much larger than that which will ultimately have a fatal arrhythmia. Little is known about the natural history of asymptomatic WPW syndrome. Extensive testing and treatment to prevent sudden death in asymptomatic individuals remains controversial.

After conversion to sinus rhythm, patients with recurrent symptomatic attacks may receive prophylactic therapy to minimize further episodes of SVT. Regimens commonly include Class Ia or Ic drugs, sotalol, amiodarone, or β-blockers. Controlled comparative trials have not been performed, and no drug has demonstrated superiority. Drug treatment is often suboptimal due to limited efficacy and excessive toxicity. Preventive therapy is reserved for patients with recurrent disabling arrhythmias.

Drug effect on AV nodal and accessory pathway conduction is summarized in Table 39.4. The type Ia drugs quinidine, procainamide, and disopyramide slow or block antegrade accessory pathway conduction, with a lesser and more variable effect on retrograde conduction. These drugs also block retrograde AV nodal conduction and suppress atrial and ventricular ectopy. The effects of drugs

Table 39.4.
Sites of Primary Drug Action in Wolff–Parkinson–White Syndrome

AV node antegrade conduction
    Calcium-channel blockers (verapamil,[a] diltiazem)
    Digoxin[a]
    Adenosine
    β-blockers
AV node retrograde conduction, accessory pathway antegrade
    conduction
    Class Ia drugs (quinidine, procainamide, disopyramide)
AV node and accessory pathway, antegrade and retrograde conduction
    Class Ic drugs (flecainide, encainide, propafenone)
    Class III (amiodarone, sotalol)
Suppression of atrial ectopy
    Class Ia drugs (quinidine, procainamide, disopyramide)
    Class Ic drugs (flecainide, encainide, propafenone)
    β-blockers
    Class III (amiodarone, sotalol)

[a]Digoxin and verapamil may *decrease* the accessory pathway antegrade refractory period, a dangerous effect in WPW with atrial fibrillation. See text for explanation.

may vary with different accessory pathway refractory periods, emphasizing the importance of electrophysiologic studies.

Digitalis and verapamil maintain their AV nodal effects. Digitalis, however, may *shorten* the accessory pathway refractory period. Verapamil generally has minimal effect on the accessory pathway but may also produce a refractory period shortening. These drugs are very effective first-line agents for terminating and preventing the recurrence of AV reentry. However, in AF or flutter, they may accentuate conduction and accelerate ventricular rate in those (unusual) patients with antegrade accessory pathway conduction. Potentially lethal ventricular tachycardia or fibrillation may ensue. Digitalis and verapamil should therefore not be used in AF with documented or suspected preexcitation unless previous electrophysiologic studies have shown them to be safe.

Most trials of adenosine in AV reentry have shown its primary site of action to be the AV nodal loop of the reentrant circuit, with a lesser or no effect on accessory pathway conduction. Coupled with its lack of hypotensive properties, some investigators believe adenosine is safer than verapamil or digitalis in documented or suspected WPW syndrome (29,107).

Propranolol and the other β-blockers alter AV nodal conduction but have minimal effect on accessory pathway conduction in either direction. They are not often used as single agents in WPW but are sometimes combined with other drugs such as digoxin or quinidine.

Amiodarone, sotalol, flecainide, encainide, and propafenone have additional unique antiarrhythmic mechanisms compared to the older agents. These drugs slow AV nodal *and* accessory pathway conduction in *both directions*,

and lengthen atrial and ventricular refractory periods. They can therefore be expected to terminate or control SVTs associated with WPW and also prevent their recurrence by suppressing ectopy. These drugs offer the best antiarrhythmic profile for SVTs associated with accessory pathways. Studies have demonstrated promising results. Unfortunately, the proarrhythmic effects of the Class Ic drugs (69) and sotalol (91) and the toxicities of amiodarone limit use.

Because of the unpredictable and often inadequate response to drugs, nonpharmacologic therapy is an important component of the treatment of WPW syndrome. DC countershock retains its near-uniform reliability and efficacy, and is the treatment of choice in patients with hemodynamic instability. Atrial pacing may be used in AV reentry though it may induce transient AF with rapid ventricular rate in patients with rapid antegrade accessory pathway conduction. Permanent ventricular pacing may be necessary in patients requiring large doses of antiarrhythmics or those with sinus node disease (pacing will eliminate excessive bradycardia while the patient is in sinus rhythm).

Surgical interruption of the accessory pathway is an effective, usually curative, treatment. Following detailed electrophysiologic and cardiac mapping studies, the accessory pathway is transected or ablated using either an endocardial or epicardial approach (106). AV nodal conduction is preserved. Surgical division of accessory pathways is 90 to 100% effective in experienced centers, with <1% mortality in uncomplicated cases and rare early or late recurrences (56).

A less invasive technique, percutaneous catheter ablation, uses DC countershock, lasers, or radiofrequency to modify the AV node or destroy accessory pathways. The success rate and mortality of this procedure is similar to surgical ablation; however, this procedure does not require an open chest or general anesthesia.

Because these procedures are curative, they may be considered the treatment of choice in (a) patients unresponsive or intolerant to antiarrhythmics, (b) those with arrhythmias associated with marked adverse hemodynamic effects, (c) patients with AF with rapid antegrade accessory pathway conduction, (d) young patients who would otherwise require lifelong drug therapy, or (e) females desiring pregnancy.

PREMATURE VENTRICULAR CONTRACTIONS

Premature ventricular contractions (PVCs) are ectopic beats originating in the ventricular muscle. These beats are not initiated by the SA node but are stimulated by the spontaneous electrical firing of the local tissue. PVCs are the most common arrhythmia. Depending on the length of the observation, the frequency of PVCs in otherwise healthy subjects is variable. One-half of young males have PVCs with 24-hr monitoring (108). The frequency of PVCs increases with advancing age and the presence of cardiac disease. In most patients, this arrhythmia produces no symptoms whatsoever. However, it is also the most common arrhythmia (40 to 80%) seen with myocardial infarctions, where it may adversely affect survival.

PVCs may be separated into simple and complex arrhythmias. PVCs seen in asymptomatic, noncardiac disease subjects are usually simple, in that they are isolated beats, occurring singly, with a wave pattern on the ECG that repeats itself, indicating that the beat originates from the same site (unifocal). These appear to be well tolerated until their frequency compromises ventricular filling. Complex PVCs are uncommon in noncardiac disease subjects but are frequent in patients with coronary artery disease. They may be subclassified as multiform or multifocal, which means that the ECG wave form is different between ectopies, suggesting more than one site in the ventricles is showing automaticity. Another complex classification refers to paired PVCs or runs of PVCs. These are consecutive PVCs without intervening sinus beats. The final type of complex PVC is one that is termed early R-on-T, referring to the R wave of the PVC interrupting the T wave of the sinus beat. Complex PVCs are highly correlated with sudden death.

Several classes of drugs may induce PVCs. These include the sympathomimetic amines (epinephrine, pseudoephedrine, phenylephrine, phenylpropanolamine, amphetamine); the methylxanthines (caffeine, theophylline); digitalis; cocaine; and certain general anesthetics (cyclopropane and halothane). Type Ia antiarrhythmics, flecainide, and sotalol may also induce PVCs and ventricular tachycardia. These drugs should be discontinued, or their doses should be reduced.

A variety of noncardiac conditions may induce PVCs, such as anemia, surgery, hypoxia, stress, hypokalemia, and hypomagnesemia. Elimination of the precipitating condition should resolve the PVCs and obviate any potential toxicity of antiarrhythmics.

The approach to treating PVCs has changed in recent years as a result of the Cardiac Arrhythmia Suppression Trials (CAST I and CAST II) (109,110). These trials attempted to compare the use of encainide, flecainide, moricizine, and placebo to suppress asymptomatic or mildly symptomatic premature ventricular contractions in order to reduce mortality after a myocardial infarction. The trial with encainide and flecainide was suspended after a preliminary analysis when excessive mortality was observed with these agents in contrast to placebo (114). The use of moricizine yielded similar results to encainide and flecainide when compared to placebo (113). The results of these trials indicate that the suppression of PVCs does not decrease sudden cardiac death after a myocardial infarction. Therefore, in an otherwise healthy person, asymptomatic PVCs do not require suppression. Some patients may complain of palpitations that, if intolerable, can be treated with a β-blocker. Suppression of PVCs in the presence of other comorbid conditions to reduce sudden death must be balanced against the risk of increased mortality associated with antiarrhythmic therapy and is discussed in the section "Sudden Death."

PVCs are an independent risk factor for sudden death; however, even though they may predispose to sudden death, the cause of death is not known. It may be a random event precipitated by the unfortunate timing of PVCs. Procainamide, lidocaine, and quinidine reduce the frequency of, though they do not totally eliminate, PVCs. However, studies evaluating the response to these drugs do not demonstrate a significant decrease in mortality rate. On the other hand, death may be a result of acute ischemia, which is not altered by antiarrhythmic drugs. The agents shown to improve survival rate may act on ischemia not on the basis of their antiarrhythmic effects.

DIGITALIS-INDUCED PVCS

PVCs are the most common arrhythmia produced by digitalis. Generally this arrhythmia resolves when the digitalis is discontinued. For frequent or symptomatic PVCs, potassium replacement in hypo- or normokalemic patients may suppress the arrhythmia. For sustained PVCs induced by digitalis, lidocaine or phenytoin has been used successfully. Phenytoin is considered an ideal agent to treat digitalis-induced arrhythmias since it improves AV conduction while it suppresses ventricular irritability. Unfortunately, phenytoin is not nearly as effective in PVCs of different etiology. For refractory arrhythmias that are life-threatening, especially when an overdose of digitalis has produced hyperkalemia, digoxin immune Fab (antigen binding fragments from antibodies to digoxin in sheep) can be administered intravenously over 30 min or IVP if an arrest is imminent (115). The amount of antibody depends on the quantity of digitalis to be bound based on the formula (116):

$$\text{Dose Fab (in \# of vials)} = \text{Digoxin stores (in mg) } 0.5 \text{ mg/vial} \quad (39.1)$$

Phenytoin

For the treatment of digitalis-induced PVCs, phenytoin would most likely be given parenterally, yet its hypotensive effects via this route are particularly troublesome. Phenytoin may lower blood pressure in 2 to 8% of patients given intravenous doses through vasodilation and myocardial depression. Parahydroxylation by the liver accounts for 50 to 76% of an administered dose of phenytoin, whereas 5% is eliminated unchanged in the urine. Phenytoin is 93% protein-bound, primarily to albumin. The degree of binding may be reduced in renal or hepatic disease, where serum albumin concentrations may be reduced. In addition, in uremia and cirrhosis, the extent of binding to albumin is reduced. In such situations, the free drug concentration may be adequate, whereas the total measured phenytoin concentration may not be within the therapeutic range despite adequate arrhythmia suppression. Most arrhythmias are controlled by phenytoin plasma levels of 10 to 20 µg/ml.

In most situations, phenytoin should be initiated with a loading dose. The diluent in the parenteral product may cause cardiovascular collapse and central nervous system depression. These complications may be reduced or avoided with rates of administration of 50 mg/min or less. Intramuscular injection may obviate this problem, but absorption is erratic and slow as a result of precipitation of phenytoin in the muscle. Phenytoin distributes into a volume (Vd) that approaches total body water (0.7 liter/kg), which may be used to estimate loading dose (LD), based on the desired plasma concentration (Cp) of 15 µg/ml as follows:

$$LD = Cp \times Vd \qquad (39.2)$$
$$= 15 \text{ µg/ml} \times 0.7 \text{ liter/kg}$$
$$= 10.5 \text{ mg/kg}$$

The entire dose may be infused intravenously no faster than 50 mg/min or by intermittent bolus infusions of 100 mg over 2 min given every 5 min until arrhythmia suppression, a maximum dose of 1 g, or toxicity occurs. Digitalis-induced PVCs may be eliminated by the loading dose of phenytoin and not require a maintenance dose. Sustained PVCs require maintenance doses of phenytoin that are influenced by the capacity-limited metabolism of the drug. With therapeutic concentrations, the rate of metabolism is often near saturation. The Michaelis–Menton kinetics of phenytoin suggest that changes in dose lead to exponentially greater increases in serum concentration. Therefore, the typical patient should be given 300 to 400 mg/day as a single dose or divided into two doses. Subsequent adjustments should be made in 100 mg/day increments at approximately 2-week intervals. Additional bolus doses may be given to treat ectopic beats to avoid the delay to steady-state conditions. (For further information refer to Chapter 50 "Seizure Disorders.")

Parenteral therapy with phenytoin may produce bradycardia, hypotension, and prolonged Q-Tc interval and QRS complex duration related to rate of administration. Central nervous system toxicity may be related to blood concentrations. Nystagmus may be the initial sign of toxicity when levels exceed 20 µg/ml. Phenytoin levels above 30 µg/ml may produce ataxia. Mental changes are common with concentrations above 40 µg/ml. Toxic responses such as gingival hyperplasia, folate deficiency, peripheral neurop-

athy, hypertrichosis, and osteoporosis are seen with chronic therapy.

Other than for digitalis-induced arrhythmias, phenytoin has limited usefulness as an antiarrhythmic. Phenytoin does appear to be particularly effective in suppressing PVCs in pediatric patients, especially in those with arrhythmia after surgery for congenital heart disease (117).

VENTRICULAR TACHYCARDIA

Ventricular tachycardia (VT) is a rapid (100 to 250 beats/min), regular, ectopic rhythm of three or more consecutive ventricular complexes. VT is more serious than PVCs, producing more marked hemodynamic deterioration as a result of decreased diastolic filling and loss of coordinated ventricular contraction with atrial kick. VT is also ominous since it often degenerates into ventricular fibrillation. VT may be seen in the prehospital phase of an AMI, as a result of enhanced automaticity. At this stage, the rhythm is somewhat more stable. The third phase of VT seen in ischemic heart disease is noted after several days to weeks.

There are two general types of VT. Nonsustained VT is three or more coupled PVCs occurring at rates greater than 100 beats/min and terminating spontaneously in <30 sec. These may require only close observation if they are asymptomatic. VT present beyond 30 sec is considered to be sustained VT. Sustained VT is often associated with hemodynamic instability. The drug therapy of sustained VT may be defined by laboratory-programmed electrical stimulation of the rhythm to determine the most efficacious drug, dose, and plasma concentration. This laboratory model is reported to reflect clinical VT and predict appropriate therapy. The successful drug concentration in the acute laboratory situation correlates well with the therapeutic level observed chronically for drugs such as quinidine and procainamide but not for propranolol, which depends on prevailing sympathetic tone (118). Patients whose arrhythmia is not controlled during laboratory-programmed electrical stimulation usually have a relapse of their VT while on chronic suppression therapy.

In the patient with VT and hemodynamic instability, the therapy of choice is electrical cardioversion. In patients without a pulse, the rhythm should be treated as with ventricular fibrillation. VT with a pulse but in an unstable patient may be cardioverted with synchronized shock of 100 joules (10). VT in the late hospital phase of an AMI is often asymptomatic, but it is a highly important risk since patients with VT are five times more likely to die within 1 year than those without the arrhythmia (119). However, whether antiarrhythmics influence the mortality rate is not known. In drug-refractory VT, options include surgical or radiofrequency ablative techniques and implantable cardioverter defibrillator (120,121).

Lidocaine

Lidocaine is the drug of choice for rapid control of VT and suppression of PVCs when indicated. The therapeutic serum concentration for lidocaine is 1 to 5 μg/ml. Lidocaine is usually initiated with an intravenous loading dose to produce rapid arrhythmia control. Any loading dose must account for the small central compartment, 0.5 liter/kg in normal subjects, reduced to 0.3 liter/kg with congestive heart failure, and increased to 0.6 liter/kg in liver disease (122). A minimum concentration in the central compartment must be reached, since the heart acts as if it belongs in this compartment, while limiting the maximum concentration since the brain also is present in this compartment. The loading dose (LD) may be calculated to produce a plasma concentration (Cp) of 3 μg/ml using the central volume (Vc) of 0.5 liter/kg as follows and administered over 1 to 2 min:

$$LD = Cp \times Vc \qquad (39.3)$$

$$= 3 \ \mu g/ml \times 0.5 \ liter/kg$$

$$= 1.5 \ mg/kg$$

Since the loading dose will be rapidly distributed away from the heart and the central compartment with an alpha phase half-life of about 10 min, arrhythmias may recur after the initial dose. Additional boluses, using one-half the initial dose, may be given after 10 to 20 min or when ectopy recurs. Unfortunately, all bolus doses are effective only transiently because of the rapid distribution.

An alternative is to give the initial load, followed by a high-dose infusion of 120 μg/kg/min for 25 min, followed by an appropriate maintenance infusion. The high-dose infusion is intended to avoid the subtherapeutic levels produced on a constant infusion of lidocaine for arrhythmia suppression. This constant infusion may be calculated based on the steady-state serum level of about 3 μg/ml (Cpss), and the clearance of lidocaine (Cl), which is 15.6 ml/min/kg in normal males, 20.2 ml/min/kg in normal females, 5.5 ml/min/kg in congestive heart failure, and 6.0 ml/min/kg for chronic liver disease (122), as follows:

$$R = Cpss \times Cl \qquad (39.4)$$

$$= 3 \ \mu g/ml \times 6 \ ml/min/kg$$

$$= 18 \ \mu g/kg/min \ (with \ liver \ failure)$$

Other factors that may reduce lidocaine clearance include advanced age, propranolol, and cimetidine. Only 5% of lidocaine is eliminated unchanged in the urine, and renal failure does not decrease the clearance of lidocaine. Certain metabolites of lidocaine such as monoethylglycinexylide (MEGX) and glycinexylidide (GX) are active compounds. GX is cleared by the kidneys and may accumulate in renal impairment. MEGX and GX may

contribute to the toxicity of lidocaine when it is administered for extended periods.

Lidocaine blood concentrations may be obtained at any point during the first 12 hr of therapy. There are advocates for early (1 to 2 hr after the start of the infusion) and late (2 to 4 hr) sampling followed by a delayed sample at 8, 12, or 24 hr (123). Levels of 1 to 2 μg/ml are only rarely effective. Many patients have control of their arrhythmia with concentrations of 3 to 5 μg/ml, and neurologic toxicity may limit any further dose increases. Paresthesias, dizziness, drowsiness, and euphoria may be seen. Resistant arrhythmias may require concentrations of 6 to 8 μg/ml at the risk of further confusion, nausea, vomiting, dysarthria, and psychoses. Pushing lidocaine beyond 9 μg/ml is rarely justified. Sweating, tremors, and muscle fasciculation may precede seizures, respiratory arrest, and coma. Lidocaine metabolites may contribute to the neurologic toxicity.

A downward adjustment in lidocaine dose may be required after 24 hr or at the onset of signs and symptoms of toxicity. Steady-state concentrations should be expected by approximately four times the normal lidocaine half-life of 100 min. In patients with liver disease, steady state may be delayed because of the half-life of 300 min (122). Patients with uncomplicated myocardial infarction (AMI) receiving constant infusions of lidocaine have developed progressive accumulation after 30 hr. Such patients have prolonged elimination half-lives for lidocaine of 3 to 4 hr after discontinuing their infusions. A partial explanation for this phenomenon has derived from changing aspects of plasma protein binding of lidocaine. In normal subjects, lidocaine is 60 to 80% plasma protein-bound (30% to albumin and 70% to α_1-acid glycoprotein or AAG). The magnitude of the binding correlates closely with concentrations of AAG. As total lidocaine blood concentrations rise in these AMI patients, AAG accumulates. The drug redistributes out of red blood cells into AAG, decreasing free lidocaine concentration. Free lidocaine clearance does not change with the AMI (124). It is probable that it is the free concentration of lidocaine that is responsible for toxicity. A therapeutic range for the free lidocaine concentration has not been established. To avoid the accumulation of lidocaine with prolonged administration, it has been suggested that the infusion rate be reduced by one-half after the first 24 hr of dosing (125).

Procainamide

Procainamide is an alternative when lidocaine toxicity or arrhythmias resistant to lidocaine develop. Procainamide is a versatile drug that can be administered orally and parenterally, but toxicity, not therapeutic inadequacy, has relegated procainamide to a secondary role.

After oral administration, procainamide averages 75% bioavailability, but certain patients may absorb as little as 10%. In addition, the rate of absorption and time to peak serum concentration varies considerably. First-pass hepatic metabolism may account for some of the reduced bioavailability. Food may delay the absorption. There are various manufacturers of both immediate-release and sustained-release procainamide. Switching between generic and proprietary immediate-release procainamide may result in arrhythmia recurrence (126). Similarly, interchange of the sustained-release procainamide may also result in arrhythmia relapse in certain patients, yet mean data suggest bioequivalence for at least two products (127). Sustained release of procainamide is accomplished by either a wax matrix or a nondisintegrating core. Generally, the areas under the curve, maximum to minimum serum procainamide concentrations, and steady-state procainamide concentrations for the two types of products are similar; however, the time to maximum serum concentration is delayed for the nondisintegrating matrix (128). Patients may complain of whole or partial tablets appearing in the stool, but this may not reflect incomplete absorption. Patients should be cautioned not to chew or crush the sustained-release tablets. Drug interactions and altered procainamide concentrations may be observed when procainamide is given along with trimethoprim, quinidine, cimetidine, and ranitidine.

Intravenous procainamide displays two-compartment kinetics similar to lidocaine. A rapid distribution phase with a half-life of 5 min occurs, with the drug binding extensively to tissues. There is evidence that procainamide does not penetrate well into fat. Thus total weight should not be used in calculating doses; ideal weight is preferred. Rapid arrhythmia control may require intravenous bolus doses. The negative inotropic and hypotensive effects of procainamide limit the rate at which the drug may be given. Even in emergency situations, procainamide should not be given at a rate exceeding 30 mg/min to avoid hypotension. The loading dose (LD) will be influenced by the therapeutic range for procainamide (Cp) of 4 to 8 μg/ml, the distribution volume (Vdss) of 2 liters/kg, and the procainamide content (S) of the hydrochloride salt, 0.82, as follows:

$$LD = Cp \times Vdss/0.82 \qquad (39.5)$$

$$= 6 \text{ } \mu g/ml \times 2 \text{ liters/kg}/0.82$$

$$= 14.6 \text{ mg/kg}$$

In renal impairment and congestive heart failure, the volume of distribution may be decreased by 25%. Loading doses have been given as small boluses of 50 to 100 mg every 5 min until arrhythmia control is seen or toxicity develops. An alternative is a loading infusion of 17 mg/kg over 1 hr, followed by the maintenance dose (see below). The generally accepted therapeutic range for procainamide is 4 to 8 μg/ml. However, the indication for the drug may influence the therapeutic range. This range of 4 to 8 μg/ml may be appropriate for patients with acute or chronic

coronary artery disease with the intent of suppressing PVCs. On the other hand, suppression of ventricular tachycardia may require higher doses, producing concentrations in the range of 10 to 20 μg/ml.

The selection of procainamide maintenance doses is intimately related to its metabolic fate. Procainamide may be excreted unchanged in the urine to the extent of 50%. The liver and other sites will transform 7 to 24% of procainamide to its major metabolite, N-acetyl-procainamide (NAPA). The rate of acetylation varies between patients, who may be grouped as fast or slow. Fast acetylators convert a higher percentage of procainamide to NAPA than slow acetylators. About 85% of NAPA is excreted unchanged by the kidneys; thus NAPA accumulates more than procainamide as renal function deteriorates. It seems that procainamide and NAPA compete for renal tubular secretion. NAPA may thus prolong the procainamide half-life (129).

The typical patient receiving intravenous procainamide is placed on a dose of 2 to 4 mg/min. This may be tailored to the patient, using 2.8 mg/kg/hr as a standard, reduced in cardiac or renal impairment by one-third for moderate impairment and two-thirds for severe impairment (130). Calculations using population averages of kinetic variables for oral procainamide have not been particularly accurate. In general, patients may be started on 50 mg/kg/day and titrated to response or toxicity. The dose should be reduced in cardiac or renal impairment by one-third for moderate impairment and two-thirds for severe impairment. In renal impairment, the procainamide half-life may be increased from a normal of 2 to 4 hr to 5 to 10 hr, whereas the NAPA half-life is greatly increased from a normal of 6 hr to as much as 42 hr. Age, independent of renal function, may also affect procainamide clearance (Cl) as follows:

$$Cl \text{ (ml/min/kg)} = 11.9 - (0.143 \times age) + \qquad (39.6)$$

$$(0.0321 \times ClCr) - (1.11 \times CHF)$$

where CHF is a constant of 1 if moderate heart failure is present (128).

Although the metabolite NAPA has some antiarrhythmic activity, the two drugs do not have the same electrophysiologic effects, and in patients, they may be additive or antagonistic. Thus the use of ratios or sums of the two serum concentrations has met with mixed results. Some clinicians use a minimum sum of 10 μg/ml and a maximum of 25 to 30 μg/ml (130,132). There is probably more benefit to the use of NAPA concentrations in monitoring for toxicity than for predicting efficacy.

A limiting factor in the compliance with procainamide is the dosing interval for the immediate-release product. With normal renal function, the maintenance dose of 50 mg/kg/day must be given at 3- to 4-hr intervals. The sustained-release formulations allow a 6-hr dosing interval. There is evidence than an 8-hr interval may be appropriate in some cases although the FDA indication is for 6 hr (133,134). It is suggested that patients receive the immediate-release product first, for titration, then be converted to a sustained-release product if necessary. The total daily dose of the immediate release product should be the initial daily dose of the sustained-release product. It has been suggested that sustained-release procainamide preparations should be avoided in patients with colostomies (135) or in other rapid gastrointestinal transit states.

Adverse effects commonly seen with procainamide include gastrointestinal distress, weakness, dizziness, nervousness, and blurred vision. These symptoms resolve if the dose is reduced, but many patients develop tolerance to these effects with continued procainamide use without a dose reduction. Cardiac toxicity seen with procainamide concentrations exceeding 12 µg/ml may include progressive lengthening of the Q-Tc interval and QRS complex duration, hypotension, and myocardial depression. However, procainamide may be less likely to produce an exacerbation of heart failure than other agents such as encainide or tocainide (136). A lupuslike syndrome may develop in more than 20% of patients taking procainamide. Procainamide lupus differs from systemic lupus erythematosus in that arthritic features are more prominent, whereas dermatologic, hematologic, and renal changes are rare. Symptoms may develop as early as 2 weeks after initiating procainamide or as long as 2 years later. Risk factors include high doses, high serum concentrations, and slow acetylation status. Recently, a hepatic-mixed function oxidase metabolite, procainamide-hydroxylamine, has been implicated in causing the lupus (137). Common signs and symptoms for monitoring include fever, rash, myalgias, arthralgias, pericarditis, pleuritis, hepatosplenomegaly, and rarely pericardial tamponade. Many more patients will have positive serologic tests for lupus than will have symptoms. (See Chapter 33, "Systemic Lupus Erythematosus.") Originally, the sustained-release product was reported to produce neutropenia more frequently than immediate-release procainamide (138). More recent data suggest that the rate of neutropenia is less than 1% and the risk is independent of formulation (139). All patients should be monitored for this hematologic complication with frequent white blood cell counts at the beginning of therapy. Patients should be followed for unexplained fevers because of the risk of infection related to the neutropenia.

Disopyramide

Disopyramide currently is available for oral use in the treatment of ventricular arrhythmias. It may also be as effective as quinidine in the management of atrial fibrillation. Parenteral disopyramide is as effective as lidocaine in the treatment of ventricular arrhythmias, but it is not yet available in the United States (140).

Disopyramide is well absorbed (F = 0.83). With the immediate-release product, peak serum concentrations occur in 2 hr. Disopyramide is 50 to 65% protein-bound, with the majority bound to AAG and a small amount (5 to 10%) to albumin. The degree of binding is nonlinear, with higher disopyramide concentrations a greater amount of the drug is free (141). It is assumed that the free drug is active (142). The volume of distribution in normal persons is 0.8 liter/kg. Variable amounts of disopyramide (36 to 71%) have been reported to be cleared by the kidney as unchanged drug. The remainder is an N-dealkylated metabolite with some antiarrhythmic activity. Healthy subjects have half-lives ranging from 4.4 to 8.2 hr. Renal impairment may prolong the half-life from 8.4 to 53 hr. The half-life may also be prolonged in patients with AMI. There appears to be an interaction with phenytoin and disopyramide where phenytoin increases the metabolism of disopyramide (143). Other interactions include erythromycin and rifampin, which can increase or decrease disopyramide serum levels respectively.

The therapeutic range for disopyramide appears to be 3 to 6 µg/ml. This therapeutic range may not apply in certain diseases, using the conventional assay measuring total disopyramide. In cirrhosis, the AAG content decreases, and the free disopyramide concentration increases in comparison to normal subjects (144). Postmyocardial infarction patients, have the opposite problem, a rise in AAG with decrease in free disopyramide concentration (145). In some studies, atrial arrhythmias responded to lower concentrations than ventricular ectopies. Although steadily increasing the plasma concentration of disopyramide progressively reduces the frequency of ectopy, responders and nonresponders have similar mean levels. Therefore, patients should be titrated to response rather than selecting an arbitrary drug serum level.

Oral disopyramide may be initiated with a loading dose of 300 mg of the immediate-release product (200 mg for moderate renal impairment, moderate liver dysfunction, or decompensated heart failure). Maintenance doses of 100 to 150 mg may be given at 6-hr intervals; the lower dose is indicated for renal, liver, and cardiac insufficiency. The recommended maximum daily dose is 800 mg, yet up to 1600 mg has been used with close monitoring. For patients with severe renal impairment, the dosing interval may be prolonged to 12, 24, or 36 hours for creatinine clearances of 15 to 40, 5 to 15, or 1 to 5 ml/min, respectively.

A sustained-release preparation of disopyramide has been marketed. It has been studied in both normal volunteers and patients with arrhythmias (146). The dosing interval may be prolonged from 6 hr with the immediate-release to 12 hr with the sustained-release product. A proposed theoretical advantage of the sustained-release product is the avoidance of a transient high-peak serum disopyramide concentration. This, coupled with the potential for higher free drug concentration as a result of the nonlinear protein-binding characteristics of disopyramide, may lead to fewer adverse effects, yet this has not been proved.

Common adverse reactions observed with disopyramide have been anticholinergic symptoms of dry mouth, blurred vision, constipation, and urinary retention. Anticholinergic reactions may occur in as many as 45% of patients receiving disopyramide, and 25% may require cessation of therapy (147). Acetylcholinesterase inhibitors, such as pyridostigmine, may effectively prevent the anticholinergic effects of disopyramide (148). Hypoglycemia has been associated with disopyramide with risk factors of advanced age, chronic renal impairment, and malnutrition. Death has resulted from persistent hypoglycemia (149). Like quinidine, disopyramide may prolong the Q-Tc interval and QRS complex duration. Initial reports on disopyramide were encouraging, indicating that quinidine produced more frequent adverse effects, yet the reports of acute heart failure developing during chronic disopyramide have dampened enthusiasm for this drug. Disopyramide has a negative inotropic effect. The risk of developing symptomatic heart failure may be as high as 16% (150). The drug has been used without complications in patients with heart failure, but such patients are at a much greater risk for decompensation. The onset of symptoms is variable, and there is no apparent correlation with the dose. Patients developing signs and symptoms of heart failure should have disopyramide discontinued. Symptoms usually resolve over a few days, but some patients may require diuretics or digitalis. As with other antiarrhythmics that prolong the Q-Tc interval, disopyramide may cause ventricular arrhythmias, at times with symptoms similar to quinidine syncope. Many patients revert after discontinuing the disopyramide; others may require suppression with lidocaine.

Encainide

Encainide is a Class Ic antiarrhythmic agent that is structurally dissimilar to other currently available drugs. In 1991, encainide was voluntarily withdrawn from the market in the United States because of the implications of the Cardiac Arrhythmia Suppression Trials (109,111). It is currently available through the manufacturer for patients who were receiving encainide prior to its removal and who cannot be switched to another agent.

Electrophysiology studies of encainide must be interpreted with care since the effects of encainide differ between single-dose and multiple-dose studies because of the presence of active metabolites [O-desmethylencainide (ODE), 3-methoxy-O-desmethylencainide (3-MODE), N-desmethylencainide (NDE), and N-O-didesmethylencainide (DDE)] that accumulate with multiple dosing.

ODE is more potent than the parent compound. The effects observed are believed to be due to metabolites and include increases in effective atrial refractory period, ventricular refractoriness, and prolongation of the atrial, AV nodal, and His–Purkinje conduction, with little change in repolarization. Encainide is classed as Ic because it produces a decrease in the rate of rise of phase 0 with little effect on APD.

Absorption of encainide after oral dosing is rapid, with peak blood concentrations in 1.5 hr, but the extent of absorption varies from 7 to 82% (148). Encainide is oxidized extensively with a genetically determined rate, showing polymorphism. Most subjects are extensive metabolizers (EM), with ODE and MODE higher than encainide, and NDE absent in plasma. In slow or poor metabolizers (PM, 7 to 10% of population) ODE is lower, and NDE is the major metabolite. In EM subjects, encainide undergoes a substantial first-pass effect with a short half-life of 1.5 hr, whereas ODE has a half-life of 13 hr. In PM subjects, the bioavailability is greater, with concentrations of parent drug some 20 times higher than in EMs. The major metabolite that is present in PM is NDE, which has little activity; thus the antiarrhythmic effects are due to encainide. Renal impairment in EMs produces slower clearance of ODE and MODE metabolites (149). Cirrhosis in EMs produces higher oral availability and higher serum encainide concentrations but equivalent concentrations of ODE and MODE (149). Quinidine may interact with encainide particularly in EM (150). Quinidine is a potent inhibitor of the enzyme responsible for encainide polymorphism, cytochrome $P = 450_{dbl}$. Quinidine prolongs the half-life of encainide, decreases nonrenal encainide clearance, and reverses encainide EKG changes but only in EM. In PM, quinidine has no effect on encainide pharmacokinetics. Diltiazem also interacts with encainide and with ODE and MODE in EM. Diltiazem is a hepatic enzyme inhibitor that decreases the first-pass metabolism of encainide, but electrophysiologic changes do not occur (151).

Encainide appears to be effective in suppressing VT and PVCs. It is superior to quinidine in the suppression of PVCs with fewer adverse effects (152). The therapeutic range for encainide is not established although in PMs concentrations of more than 265 ng/ml may be necessary. The daily dose of encainide has been 100 to 250 mg given in three to four doses. Higher doses may be proarrhythmic. QRS complex prolongation may predict arrhythmia suppression. With a baseline of <0.12 sec, a prolongation of 40 to 50% is suggested, whereas a QRS more than 0.12 sec should be prolonged only by 25 to 30%.

Minor toxicity may occur in as many as 60% of patients and includes dizziness, lightheadedness, visual disturbances, tremor, headache, gastrointestinal intolerance, or metallic taste. More serious are the proarrhythmic effects not seen in normal persons or in SVT but in VT or ventricular fibrillation (VF). Marked hypotension and progressive VF have occurred without associated QRS or Q-Tc prolongation as with other agents. It is unclear whether these cardiovascular effects were related to the increased mortality rate in encainide-treated patients reported in the Cardiac Arrhythmia Suppression Trial (109,111).

Propafenone

Propafenone has recently been marketed in the United States after originating in West Germany in 1977. It is currently the most widely used antiarrhythmic in Germany (153). Propafenone is a type Ic antiarrhythmic that blocks the fast inward sodium channel, producing a slowed rate of rise of phase 0 of the action potential. Propafenone also has weak β-blocking and calcium channel blocking effects (154). There is a dose-related increase in PR interval and QRS duration.

Currently, propafenone is marketed only in an oral dosage form in the United States. Absorption is complete (>95%) with time to maximal concentration in 1 to 3 hr. The drug is highly protein bound (77 to 95%) and undergoes saturable metabolism leading to variable bioavailability of 11 to 39%. Propafenone is almost completely cleared by the liver with polymorphic oxidative metabolism via cytochrome $P-450_{dbl}$ (155). Extensive metabolizers (EM) have a half-life of 5.5 hr, whereas poor metabolizers (approximately 7% of the U.S. population) have a half-life of 17.2 hr. The major metabolite of propafenone is 5-hydroxypropafenone, which is active and only detectable in EM. Patients that are poor metabolizers exhibit greater β-blocking effects, possibly because of higher blood concentrations of the parent compound, which tends to accumulate with chronic dosing.

Propafenone is indicated for use in life-threatening arrhythmias, such as sustained ventricular tachycardia and ventricular fibrillation. Although not FDA approved, propafenone has shown efficacy in supraventricular arrhythmias, including AF and reentrant tachycardia, and is considered by some clinicians to be the antiarrhythmic of choice in Wolff–Parkinson–White syndrome (107). In light of the CAST results, the use of propafenone in the suppression of ventricular arrhythmias should be restricted to patients in which the benefit outweighs the risk.

The most common adverse reaction to propafenone is a metallic or bitter taste that may resolve without changing the dose. Propafenone may cause central nervous system effects such as dizziness, headache, paresthesias, and fatigue or gastrointestinal effects such as nausea, vomiting, anorexia, and constipation, which can be minimized by decreasing the dose or increasing the dosing interval (156). Despite the β-blocking properties of propafenone, the risk

of bronchospasm seems low. Propafenone has rarely been associated with liver injury and agranulocytosis. Cardiac adverse effects of propafenone include proarrhythmia, worsening of congestive heart failure, and conduction disturbances (156).

Drug interactions with propafenone are likely because of its extensive hepatic metabolism and high protein binding. Cimetidine and quinidine increase serum propafenone serum levels through altered hepatic metabolism. Rifampin increases the hepatic metabolism of propafenone, resulting in decreased serum levels. Propafenone inhibits the metabolism of warfarin, resulting in a prolonged anticoagulant response. Propafenone may increase serum digoxin levels requiring dosage adjustment of the latter drug. Similarly, propafenone may increase serum propranolol levels; however, the dosage adjustment may not be required since the therapeutic range for propranolol is very wide.

The starting dose of propafenone is 150 mg three times a day. The dose may be increased to a maximum of 300 mg three times a day with a minimum of 3 to 4 days between increases. The elderly and patients with hepatic dysfunction or renal impairment may require lower doses. Severe liver dysfunction may lead to greatly increased bioavailability from lessened first-pass metabolism. Use of 20 to 30% of the normal dose of propafenone may be appropriate in patients with liver impairment. Patients treated chronically require careful monitoring because of the potential for propafenone to accumulate over time.

TORSADE DE POINTES

Torsade de pointes is a proarrhythmia characterized by rapid series of ventricular tachycardia with varying axis on the EKG. *Torsade de pointes* may or may not be associated with the prolonged Q-T interval. *Torsade de pointes* may be a result of type Ia antiarrhythmics, sotalol, metabolic derangements, or idiopathic mechanisms. Type Ia antiarrhythmics should be monitored closely for Q-Tc prolongation to avoid episodes of *torsade de pointes* that may impair hemodynamics or lead to malignant ventricular arrhythmias. In the absence of the prolonged Q-T interval syndrome, *torsade* can be managed as VT. On the other hand, the prolonged Q-T interval syndrome is commonly caused by quinidine and in the past was termed "quinidine syncope." The syncope most frequently occurs within 1 to 3 days of initiation of quinidine although occasionally patients may be receiving the drug for longer than a year when symptoms develop. However, this delayed syndrome is typically at or below the therapeutic range. When the syndrome develops in patients receiving quinidine for atrial fibrillation, the VT occurs typically after conversion to sinus rhythm. The frequency of the long QT syndrome is higher for quinidine than for the other Class Ia agents disopyramide or procainamide (157). Unlike the Class Ia agents, the frequency of *torsade de pointes* induced by sotalol increases with increasing dose (158). The therapy of choice for *torsade* is intravenous magnesium (10) 2 g over 1 min. Magnesium administration is effective even in normo-magnesemic patients. Magnesium may cause hypotension and hypokalemia (159). An alternative therapy is rapid pacing. Bretylium has also been used in quinidine induce VT (160).

Flecainide

Flecainide is a fluorinated analogue of procainamide currently available in oral form only. Since CAST reports FDA indications for flecainide are limited to documented life-threatening arrhythmias, such as sustained VT, and VF. It is also indicated for paroxysmal AF and reentrant tachycardia associated with disabling symptoms. Flecainide should not be used for chronic AF because of an excess development of VT and VF. In addition, flecainide should not be used in patients with a recent myocardial infarction.

Absorption after oral dosing of flecainide is fairly rapid, with peak serum concentrations occurring in 3 to 4 hr. The bioavailability is nearly 100%. There is no apparent first-pass effect. Food does not affect the absorption of flecainide. Flecainide has a large volume of distribution, 8 to 10 liters/kg, reflecting substantial tissue distribution. The protein binding of flecainide is 37 to 58%. The free fraction of flecainide is proportional to serum albumin and AAG concentrations. The binding of flecainide is loose however, and in a situation such as immediately post-AMI where AAG levels rise, flecainide is displaced, producing higher free flecainide concentrations. About one-quarter of flecainide is excreted unchanged by the kidneys, and the remainder is primarily conjugated by the liver as inactive metabolites. The normal half-life of flecainide is about 14 hr and is prolonged by ventricular arrhythmias, heart failure, and renal impairment (161). Flecainide is marketed as a racemic mixture. The enantiomers of flecainide are metabolized with a genetically determined rate showing polymorphism. Patients are termed poor metabolizers (PM) and extensive metabolizers (EM) (162). Significantly longer half-lives may be expected in patients with liver cirrhosis (163). It is recommended that initial dosing should be low, 50 to 100 mg orally twice daily, and increased at 4-day intervals as needed and tolerated. The usual maintenance dose is 100 to 200 mg twice daily. The therapeutic range for flecainide is 318 ng/ml (with a reported 50% probability of efficacy) to 710 ng/ml (with <10% probability of cardiovascular toxicity) (164).

Interactions with flecainide have been observed with digoxin, cimetidine, and propranolol. Cimetidine may reduce the clearance of flecainide. Propranolol and flecainide may be additive in terms of negative inotropism.

Flecainide may raise serum digoxin concentrations by an apparent decrease in distribution volume.

Unlike other Class I drugs, flecainide does not produce frequent gastrointestinal toxicity. Dizziness and blurred vision may occur. A prolongation of P-R interval and QRS complex duration should be expected, and up to 30% is well tolerated. Flecainide may induce serious arrhythmias that may not be preceded by conduction changes. A history of sustained ventricular tachycardia, daily doses of flecainide over 400 mg, high flecainide concentrations (>1 μg/ml), and reduced ejection fractions may contribute to drug-induced arrhythmias. This proarrhythmic effect of flecainide may occur in 6.6% of patients with sustained VT but only 0.9% with nonsustained VT (165). The mortality rate of the proarrhythmic events was also higher in sustained VT. Structural heart disease may also predict higher proarrhythmias from flecainide. The results of the CAST trial suggest that flecainide and perhaps any Class Ic agent should not be used in anything but a life-threatening arrhythmia. Even in such a situation, flecainide may be considered after Class Ia and Class Ib drugs.

Moricizine

Moricizine is a Class I agent that was developed in the Soviet Union and used there since 1971. Moricizine structurally resembles phenothiazines, but the antiarrhythmic does not possess antidopaminergic effects. Moricizine cannot be assigned to a subgroup of Class I because it has properties of all three. Moricizine prolongs QRS duration like Class Ia, shortens APD-like Class Ib agents, and prolongs the PR-interval-like agents in Class Ic. Moricizine has been described as a membrane-stabilizer with anticholinergic properties and the ability to suppress both normal and abnormal automaticity (166).

Moricizine is completely absorbed after oral administration, with peak blood levels occurring at 1 to 3 hr, but bioavailability is limited to 34 to 38% by pronounced first-pass metabolism. Food may lower peak moricizine levels, but the extent of absorption is not decreased (167). Moricizine has a large apparent volume of distribution (300 liters) and is highly protein bound (~95%) to albumin and α_1-acid glycoprotein. Moricizine is metabolized by sulfooxidation, ring hydroxylation, N-dealkylation, and glucuronide and sulfate conjugation to at least 26 metabolites. The drug induces cytochrome P-450 activity, causing a decrease in its own elimination half-life with chronic dosing from 1.9 hr (single dose) to 1.4 hr. Drug blood levels do not predict response, and in fact the onset of antiarrhythmic action is substantially delayed (~16 hr) beyond the time to peak level of the drug (168).

Moricizine may be as effective as quinidine or disopyramide with fewer adverse effects in treating patients with ventricular arrhythmias (167). In the Cardiac Arrhythmia

Pilot Study (CAPS) trial, moricizine was less effective than encainide and flecainide in suppressing PVCs and nonsustained VT (169). However, in patients with depressed left ventricular function (ejection fraction <0.45), the agents were similar. In contrast, moricizine continued to be studied in the CAST trial, whereas encainide and flecainide were withdrawn from randomization because of excessive mortality compared to moricizine or placebo (170). Subsequently, moricizine was found to produce excess mortality relative to placebo, and the trial was stopped (110). The current FDA-approved indication for moricizine is life-threatening, sustained VT.

Adverse effects due to moricizine are infrequent and include dizziness, nausea, headache, perioral paresthesia. Moricizine has proarrhythmic effects observed in 3.2 to 15% of patients (166). The rate of proarrhythmia has been reported up to 27 to 45% in patients with ejection fractions <40% (171). Cimetidine may reduce the clearance of moricizine, and moricizine may reduce the clearance of theophylline.

The starting dose of moricizine is 200 mg three times a day. There is evidence that twice-a-day dosing is equivalent to three-times-a-day dosing. The dose may be increased to 300 mg three times a day with small incremental adjustments at 3-day intervals. Reduced dosages are recommended in renal or liver impairment.

Mexiletine

Mexiletine is classified as a Class Ib agent with a structure and mechanism of action similar to those of lidocaine. At the present time, mexiletine is available in an oral dosage form only, with FDA approval for life-threatening ventricular arrhythmias, such as sustained VT.

Mexiletine is well absorbed orally, with a bioavailability of 80 to 90% in healthy volunteers and peak concentrations occurring at 2 to 4 hr. Absorption may be delayed and incomplete in patients with AMI. Antacids, narcotics, cimetidine, and atropine delay the time to peak concentration but not the serum concentration-time profile for mexiletine. On the other hand, metoclopramide increases the rate of absorption with no effect on serum concentration-time profile. Mexiletine after intravenous administration is thought to exhibit three-compartment kinetics. It has a large volume of distribution, about 5 liters/kg, extensive tissue protein binding, and <1% of the drug remains in the blood (172). Mexiletine is primarily metabolized by the liver, with about 8% of the drug recovered unchanged in the urine in healthy volunteers. Urine excretion is pH-dependent, with a more rapid clearance as pH decreases (172). The elimination half-life of mexiletine is 9.4, 12.1, and 16.7 hr after oral dosing to healthy subjects, patients with arrhythmia, and AMI patients, respectively. Cigarette smoking may induce the conjugation of mexiletine, reducing the half-life from 11.1

to 7.2 hr (173). Phenytoin enhances the metabolism of mexiletine, with a decrease in mexiletine half-life of about 50% (172). Renal function does not appear to affect the clearance of mexiletine, and the drug does not seem to be dialyzable (174).

The therapeutic range for mexiletine is 0.75 to 2.0 µg/ml. Because of the slow clearance of mexiletine, a loading dose may be required, but full loading doses are rarely tolerated. A compromise is to give a starting dose of 400 mg once, followed by 200 mg every 8 hr, or 10 to 15 mg/kg/day. There is evidence that a 12-hr regimen with same total daily dose is as effective as the 8-hr regimen (175).

There is a high frequency of adverse reactions in the induction phase of mexiletine, but with chronic use, it is considered to be comparable to quinidine or procainamide (176). Adverse effects frequently limit the dose of mexiletine and reduce the ability to suppress arrhythmias. When this occurs, it may be possible to add other drugs to a tolerated but ineffective dose of mexiletine. In fact, the combination of quinidine and mexiletine has been more effective than quinidine alone with fewer adverse effects (177). A side benefit is that mexiletine may block the increase in Q-Tc interval produced by quinidine (178). The additive antiarrhythmic effect is also demonstrated with mexiletine and disopyramide (179), and mexiletine and sotalol (180). Mexiletine effectively reduces the frequency of PVCs in most patients, even those who have failed to respond to other agents. Chronic, sustained recurrent VT does not respond well to mexiletine, but if electrophysiologic studies show mexiletine to control induced VT, it is usually effective chronically (181). The frequency of adverse effects may be as high as 54% of patients receiving chronic mexiletine, usually involving neurologic or gastrointestinal effects. Tremor, dizziness, vertigo, paresthesias, nystagmus, diplopia, ataxia, and confusion may occur. Nausea, vomiting, and dyspepsia are common. Cardiovascular effects include hypotension, sinus bradycardia, AV dissociation, and in overdosage, widened QRS complex. In usual doses, mexiletine does not reduce left ventricular function.

Tocainide

Tocainide, an amine analogue of lidocaine, is indicated for the suppression of life-threatening ventricular arrhythmias. It is especially useful if the arrhythmias responded first to lidocaine. It currently is available only in an oral dosage form. It appears to be absorbed rapidly and completely, but food may decrease the peak plasma concentration without altering the extent of absorption. About one-half the tocainide is cleared unchanged by the kidneys; the rest is glucuronidated by the liver. The normal elimination half-life of 11 hr may be prolonged in patients with chronic arrhythmias, ventricular dysfunction, and renal impairment (182). The therapeutic range for tocainide concentrations is 3 to 9 μg/ml. Toxicity may occur with concentrations above 10 μg/ml. Rifampin may induce metabolism of tocainide leading to shortened tocainide half-life (183). Cimetidine, on the other hand, decreases the bioavailability of tocainide (184).

Tocainide is indicated for the suppression of ventricular arrhythmias. It has very limited utility in atrial arrhythmias. Although tocainide may reduce the frequency of PVCs, it may not be as effective or as well tolerated as older drugs such as quinidine (185). Tocainide may be effective when Class Ia drugs have failed.

The utility of tocainide chronically is limited by the high frequency of adverse reactions (up to 70%). Ataxia, tremor, dizziness, paresthesias, night sweats, nausea, and vomiting are common toxicities. As with lidocaine and procainamide, tocainide may produce confusion, psychoses, and seizures. Symptoms may resolve if the drug is administered with meals, by reducing the magnitude of the peak serum concentration without altering the extent of absorption. There are case reports of an association between the use of tocainide and the development of pulmonary fibrosis and interstitial pneumonitis. The pulmonary toxicity may resolve after discontinuing tocainide (186). Agranulocytosis has been reported with tocainide. Although neutropenia is rare, it may be life threatening. It is suggested that white blood cell counts be monitored frequently, particularly early in therapy. Rash and fever have also been reported. Cross-reactivity may occur in patients allergic to lidocaine or procainamide.

Sotalol

Sotalol is the most recent antiarrhythmic agent to be marketed. It was FDA approved in 1992 for use in life-threatening ventricular arrhythmias. Sotalol is categorized as a Class III agent that also has properties of Class II (β-blockade). The marketed product is a racemic mixture of d- and l-sotalol, both with equal effect on lengthening the APD and refractory period. The main difference between the two compounds is the relative lack of β-blocking activity of d-sotalol.

Oral absorption of sotalol is virtually complete with a bioavailability of 90 to 100% and no first-pass metabolism. Food and antacids can reduce the bioavailability by about 20%, however this is probably not clinically significant (187). Peak plasma concentrations occur within 2 to 4 hr of an oral dose. The hydrophilic nature of sotalol prevents much distribution into tissue or protein binding. It has a volume of distribution of 0.9 to 2.4 liters/kg. Hepatic metabolism of sotalol is minimal with no active metabolite formation. The primary route of elimination is renal. The elimination half-life of sotalol depends on renal function and varies as follows: 6 to 18 hr in normal renal function, 24 to 64 hr in moderate renal failure, and 34 to 98 hr in

end-stage renal failure (187). Sotalol is removed by hemodialysis (188).

The adverse effects of sotalol can be attributed to its β-blocking and QT prolongation properties. Fatigue, dyspnea, and bradycardia are the most common reasons for discontinuing sotalol (91). Other adverse effects include dizziness, headache, bronchospasm, and exacerbation of congestive heart failure. Proarrhythmia is the most serious adverse effect attributed to sotalol with an overall occurrence of 4.3% (91). The most common arrhythmias induced are *torsade de pointes* and sustained VT/VF. The incidence of proarrhythmia increases with increasing doses of sotalol, most occur at doses more than 320 mg/day (91). Proarrhythmias are most likely to occur within 7 days of sotalol initiation or dose increase.

Initial dosing of sotalol should begin with 80 mg twice a day and titrated every 2 to 3 days to the desired therapeutic effect. Most patients respond to doses between 160 and 320 mg/day; however, some patients may require doses up to 640 mg/day for arrhythmia suppression (189). Doses above 320 mg/day should be used only when the therapeutic benefit outweighs the risk of proarrhythmia.

The Class II and III properties of sotalol allow for this drug to be effective in a variety of arrhythmias. Sotalol can suppress atrial and ventricular ectopy, depress reentrant conduction, and block the ventricular response to AF. A trial comparing sotalol to quinidine has shown equal efficacy in maintaining sinus rhythm after DC cardioversion for chronic AF with better tolerance (190). In a study comparing seven drugs with antiarrhythmic properties (imipramine, mexiletine, pirmenol, procainamide, propafenone, quinidine, and sotalol) in patients with ventricular tachycardia, sotalol was more effective at suppressing arrhythmias and had the least probability of discontinuance because of adverse effects (191).

VENTRICULAR FLUTTER AND FIBRILLATION

Some consider ventricular flutter a separate entity from ventricular fibrillation (VF). Ventricular flutter is a rapid ectopic firing at one or more sites in the ventricles at a fairly regular rate of 150 to 300 beats/min. QRS complexes appear to run into each other, obliterating S-T segments and P waves, but the wave appears "saw-toothed." Classically, VF was a rapid (150 to 500 beats/min), disorganized ventricular rhythm. In VF, the ectopic beat does not develop from a single area; instead, the firing is random and changing. Individual fibers or groups of fibers contract independently. When observed, the heart shows areas of twitching. Consequently, there is no effective net contraction and no pumping of blood.

Almost 50% of patients who develop VF do not have warning arrhythmias (see under "Premature Ventricular Contractions"), especially during the early phase of AMI. Often the period between warning arrhythmias and VF is very short (measured in seconds). In the setting of an AMI, 88% of patients with VF will develop it within the first 6 hr of the infarct. If resuscitated, such patients in general have a good prognosis. VF associated with or caused by heart failure may occur at any time after an infarct and is associated with a higher mortality rate because myocardial damage is more extensive.

Since the criteria for predicting VF are not very accurate, some centers use prophylactic antiarrhythmics to prevent fatal VF. This therapy is highly controversial. Some studies, using relatively low-dose infusions (2 mg/min), report that lidocaine does not prevent VF, particularly in the first few hours of the infarct (192). Higher doses of lidocaine (3 mg/min) have been shown to prevent VF at the expense of frequent toxicity (15%) in patients under 70 years old without heart failure or block (193). This regimen is recommended for the first 24 hr only. Recently, prophylactic lidocaine has come under intense criticism because of unacceptable toxicity (in 51% of patients) and questionable efficacy (194). Unfortunately, serum lidocaine concentrations provided little help in preventing these adverse reactions. This lack of efficacy was confirmed by meta-analysis of multiple trial suggesting that prehospital mortality was not decreased with lidocaine and the in-hospital mortality was actually increased by lidocaine (195).

Electrical Cardioversion

The primary treatment of VF is electrical cardioversion. The likelihood of successful conversion is increased if coronary artery perfusion is maintained. In 80% of patients, a single shock is adequate to convert to a more stable rhythm. Nonresponders should receive cardiopulmonary resuscitation with repeated shock therapy, epinephrine, and lidocaine. Lidocaine has been the preferred pharmacologic agent for VF. Bretylium is an effective alternative.

Bretylium

Bretylium is considered by some to be an alternative for patients resistant to lidocaine although there are others who advocate bretylium before lidocaine in the management of DC conversion-resistant VF. Clearly, a distinction should be drawn in indications for these agents. The prevention of VF is different from the suppression of active PVC. To complicate matters further, VF in sudden death syndrome may respond differently than VF in ischemia. Bretylium may have poor-to-adequate activity in PVC suppression, but it has excellent antifibrillatory activity. Bretylium is taken up by the amine pump in the adrenergic neuron. It displaces norepinephrine, then blocks subsequent release of catecholamines. The temporary period of sympathetic excess may produce hypertension and arrhythmias, particularly in patients with digitalis toxicity. The antiarrhythmic action of bretylium may be independent of

its sympatholytic effects. The hypertension observed with bretylium, however, correlates well with changes in norepinephrine plasma concentration (196). The ability of bretylium to reduce the disparity in refractory periods between normal and infarcted tissues may indicate why it is effective in VF, which is felt to be sustained by reentry between these two tissues. Since bretylium does not depress automaticity, PVC frequency is largely unaffected.

Bretylium exhibits two-compartment kinetics. Elimination of bretylium is primarily 70 to 80% via the kidneys. In normal volunteers, the half-life is 7.8 hr, compared with 33.4 hr in patients with impaired renal function. The relationship between total body clearance of bretylium (TBC) and creatinine clearance (CC) may be defined by the following: (197)

$$TBC = 0.362\ CC + 3.242\ (r = 0.93) \qquad (39.7)$$

This equation may be useful if infusions of bretylium are administered. The antiarrhythmic concentration is not well established; a range of 0.5 to 1.5 μg/ml has been suggested.

Bretylium may produce chemical defibrillation without electric shock when it is given undiluted by rapid injection of 5 mg/kg. Rapid administration should be reserved for emergency use, as in cardiopulmonary resuscitation. The average time to reversion after bretylium is 9 to 10 min. If after 5 to 10 min there is no response, another 10 mg/kg may be given up to a maximum of 30 to 35 mg/kg. For less serious arrhythmias, bretylium can be given over 8 to 10 min, with 5 to 10 mg/kg as the loading dose. If the arrhythmia persists, the dose may be repeated at 1-hr intervals up to 30 mg/kg. For chronic suppression, bretylium may be given intramuscularly or by intermittent infusions (over 8 to 10 min), every 6 to 8 hr. Bretylium has also been given by constant infusion at 1 to 2 mg/min.

The common adverse effects of bretylium are related to its adrenergic-blocking actions producing transient hypertension followed by hypotension, worsened arrhythmias, and angina. Rapid intravenous injection often produces nausea and vomiting. Hyperthermia is an unusual reaction to bretylium. A reported temperature of 108.2°F was ascribed to bretylium infusion (198). The febrile illness resolved when the infusion was stopped.

Amiodarone

Amiodarone is a Class III agent with properties of Class I, II, and IV. Its use is generally restricted to the treatment of drug-resistant arrhythmias because of serious adverse effects. Amiodarone at this time has a restricted indication from the FDA for recurrent ventricular fibrillation or recurrent hemodynamically unstable ventricular tachycardia where other agents have failed through ineffectiveness or toxicity. Amiodarone structurally resembles thyroxine.

Amiodarone is currently available in an oral dosage form. (The intravenous preparation is pending a 1995 release.) Bioavailability is poor and erratic with 22 to 86% absorption (199). The time to peak absorption is about 6 hr. After absorption, the drug is widely distributed to fat, lung, liver, muscle, and spleen with a very large volume of distribution, approximately 5000 liters. The elimination half-life varies from 26 to 107 days and appears biphasic. Amiodarone is metabolized to its major active metabolite desethyamiodarone (DEA). The utility of monitoring serum concentrations of amiodarone is controversial because of the extensive distribution to tissues and apparent role of DEA in arrhythmia suppression. There is some evidence that arrhythmias may recur if concentrations fall below 1.0 μg/ml. Toxicity may occur if serum concentrations exceed 2.5 μg/ml. Variable correlations have been made with red cell concentrations of amiodarone. Various dosing schemes have been suggested to avoid the delay in reaching steady-state serum amiodarone concentrations. Up to 1600 mg daily for a week, then 800 mg daily for 2 to 4 weeks, and finally the dose is reduced to the minimally tolerable dose, usually 200 to 600 mg daily in two divided doses.

A wide range of adverse effects may be encountered with the long-term use of amiodarone. Corneal deposits are a frequent occurrence. In one series, 79% of patients developed microdeposits but no change in visual acuity (200). Some cardiologists suggest observing only for visual symptoms such as photophobia or blurring, which develop less frequently than the microdeposits (201). Abnormal liver enzymes may be encountered in 10 to 20% of patients (202). The drug appears to concentrate in liver tissue. Although enzymes may rise typically two to three times normal, hepatic function may not change, and the drug may be continued with ultimate resolution of the problem. Alternatively, severe liver damage and death has been associated with amiodarone (202). Dermatologic reactions to amiodarone may occur in up to 11.6% of patients (201) and have been described as photosensitivity or blue-gray skin discoloration. Pulmonary abnormalities associated with amiodarone are considered to be a justification for discontinuing therapy. Pulmonary fibrosis, the most severe abnormality, is usually symptomatic and may be reversible on discontinuation with or without the administration of glucocorticoids. However, pulmonary fibrosis due to amiodarone may also be fatal. Amiodarone-induced pulmonary abnormalities rarely occur at doses <400 mg/day (202). The iodine content of amiodarone is 37%, which is thought to be responsible for the occurrence of hypo- or hyperthyroidism. Amiodarone interferes with the metabolism of thyroxine (T_4), resulting in increased serum concentrations of T_4 and decreased serum concentrations of triiodothyronine (T_3). Patients typically are not symptomatic of hyperthyroidism; in fact, TSH levels may be increased, which suggests insensitivity to thyroid hormone effect. If symptomatic, patients may notice tremor, myopathy, and

sleep disturbance (202). There is controversy over the predictability of antiarrhythmic response and toxicity with the use of the serum reverse T3 concentrations (rT3). Very high rT3 levels (in excess of 130 ng/dl) have been associated with the development of pulmonary fibrosis, arrhythmogenicity, and sudden cardiac death (203). Amiodarone-induced hyperthyroidism may require dose reduction or withdrawal, and antithyroid therapy. Amiodarone-induced hypothyroidism may present with signs of sinus bradycardia, which can reduce cardiac output and/or constipation. Treatment of hypothyroidism includes amiodarone dosage reduction or withdrawal, and thyroid hormone replacement therapy. Proarrhythmia associated with amiodarone is infrequent. A recent evaluation of pooled data from multiple trials of patients treated with amiodarone reported an overall proarrhythmia incidence of 2% and an incidence of <1% for *torsade de pointes* (205).

Amiodarone may produce drug interactions with warfarin, digoxin, procainamide, and quinidine (204). It has been suggested that the dose of quinidine or procainamide be reduced by 30 to 50% when amiodarone is added and that QT and QRS intervals should be monitored for excessive prolongation. Amiodarone inhibits the metabolism of warfarin. It is suggested that the warfarin maintenance dose be decreased by one-half when amiodarone is added, and prothrombin times should be monitored carefully. When amiodarone is given to patients receiving digoxin, it is suggested that the digoxin maintenance dose should be halved and adjusted according to serum digoxin concentrations.

A wide variety of arrhythmias respond to therapy with amiodarone. It is effective in the maintenance of sinus rhythm after DC cardioversion in patients with AF (206) and in the termination of reentrant arrhythmias, including the Wolff–Parkinson–White syndrome. Amiodarone is also effective in the suppression of ventricular arrhythmias (207–209) and appears to decrease cardiac mortality in postmyocardial infarction patients (209–212). Trials are currently underway that will help define the role of amiodarone use in postmyocardial infarction patients (213,214). One other area where amiodarone may be effective is the treatment of patients who developed *torsade de pointes* on other antiarrhythmics (215).

SUDDEN DEATH

The predominant cause of sudden death is ventricular fibrillation usually preceded by sustained VT and/or PVCs. In approximately 25% of cases, sudden death (presumably via VF) is not preceded by a prior history of cardiac symptoms. Thus the prevention of VF with chronic antiarrhythmics becomes a question of patient selection. Sudden cardiac collapse via VF in ambulatory patients often (55%) is not associated with an AMI. These patients after resuscitation have a very high (three times greater than primary VF with an AMI) mortality rate. Chronic antiarrhythmics have produced mixed results in sudden death.

In the recent years, antiarrhythmic use in the prevention of sudden death has changed significantly, especially in light of the results from CAST I and II. Drug use has become more conservative and is based on patient risk of sudden death determined by the degree of underlying heart disease and the type of presenting arrhythmia. One system of classifying arrhythmias based on risk of sudden death has been proposed by Morganroth and Bigger (216). They classify ventricular arrhythmias as benign, potentially lethal, or lethal based on the type of arrhythmia that is present and the degree of underlying heart disease.

Patients with benign ventricular arrhythmias are characterized as having PVCs or nonsustained VT (NSVT) as the presenting arrhythmia, no hemodynamic symptoms, and no structural heart disease. About 30% of patients with ventricular arrhythmias are classified as having benign arrhythmias. The risk of sudden death in these patients is minimal, therefore, no therapy is recommended. Some patients have intolerable symptoms from the arrhythmia (i.e., palpitations), which, if necessary, can be treated with β-blockers.

Potentially lethal arrhythmias comprise about 65% of patients with ventricular arrhythmias and carry a moderate to high probability for sudden death. They are further categorized into two types for treatment purposes. The first type of potentially lethal arrhythmias occurs in patients with PVCs or NSVT, no hemodynamic symptoms, and a moderate degree of structural heart disease (left ventricular ejection fraction ≥40% no late potentials on signal averaged ECG). Because of the moderate risk of sudden death in this group, antiarrhythmics are not considered beneficial, and treatment is the same as with benign ventricular arrhythmias.

The second type of potentially lethal ventricular arrhythmia includes patients who have asymptomatic or mildly symptomatic PVCs and/or NSVT and a moderate to severe degree of structural heart disease (≥10 PVCs per hour, LVEF <40%, late potentials on signal averaged ECG, and decreased heart rate variability). Because the risk of sudden death in these patients is high, treatment is recommended and should include antiarrhythmics guided by electrophysiologic studies.

About 5% of ventricular arrhythmias are considered lethal. These patients have sustained VT and VF with hemodynamic symptoms, and have severe underlying cardiac disease (previous MI, LVEF <40%, cardiomyopathy, and/or coronary artery disease). The risk of sudden death is highest in patients with lethal ventricular arrhythmias. The recommended sequence of therapy includes EPS-guided Class Ia antiarrhythmics followed by either a Class Ib or a combination of Ia and Ib. If the Class I agents fail, then amiodarone or sotalol can be considered, with

ablative techniques, surgical intervention, or implantable cardiac defibrillators as alternatives.

When considering the choices for chronic management of VF and prevention of sudden death, β-blockers also deserve consideration. Unfortunately, a variety of conditions may preclude patients from the potential benefit of β-blockade, such as uncontrolled heart failure, bradycardia, second- or third-degree heart block, sinoatrial block, insulin-dependent diabetes mellitus, peripheral vascular disease, and chronic obstructive pulmonary disease. The remaining discussion is limited to β-blockers with substantial literature supporting their use in sudden death, AMI, or arrhythmias.

Propranolol has not met with exceptional results in ventricular ectopic suppression. It may not be effective in preventing ectopy after an AMI. In the treatment of VT, propranolol has been disappointing. However, it may be useful in exercise-induced arrhythmias, ventricular arrhythmias associated with mitral valve prolapse, digitalis-induced arrhythmias, and arrhythmias associated with a long QT interval.

Propranolol has been studied in post-AMI with mixed results in lowering the risk of sudden death. The report from the National Heart, Lung and Blood Institute revealed a 26% lower mortality rate for propranolol compared to placebo (167). The site of the infarct, age, and sex had no influence on the response to propranolol. The initial dose of propranolol, 40 mg three times daily, was adjusted to 60 or 80 mg three times daily depending on the serum propranolol concentrations.

Propranolol is felt to have the highest membrane-stabilizing potency of the β-blockers. Called a "quinidinelike" action, it is manifest however only in overdose situations. Propranolol is a nonselective antagonist to β_1 (cardiac) and β_2 (lungs and blood vessels) receptors. It is well absorbed (more than 90%), but first-pass hepatic extraction may reduce bioavailability to about 30%. Protein binding is of the order of 90%. Propranolol is cleared rapidly by hepatic metabolism, with a half-life of 3.5 to 6 hr.

Propranolol may be given intravenously under rare situations, as 0.5 to 0.75 mg repeated every 2 min up to a maximum of 0.1 mg/kg. The effective dose may be repeated at 6- to 8-hr intervals. The oral propranolol dose is much higher but variable. A typical starting dose is 10 mg every 6 hr. The dosing interval may not correlate with the short half-life; a twice-daily regimen has been effective.

The most common adverse reactions seen with propranolol involve the central nervous system and include fatigue, hallucinations, weakness, insomnia, and nightmares. These effects may not be related to β-blockade, and differences between the various β-blockers have not been demonstrated. Since it is nonselective, propranolol may exacerbate bronchospasm. Although propranolol may precipitate or worsen congestive heart failure, if the arrhythmia is felt to have induced symptoms, propranolol may relieve the symptoms because it suppresses the arrhythmia. The β-blockers with intrinsic sympathomimetic activity may produce less cardiac depression and may be indicated in patients prone to heart failure. Propranolol (by β-blockade) may allow α-vasoconstriction, producing cold or painful extremities. Gangrene, skin necrosis, and claudication have been observed. Nonselective agents should be avoided after such symptoms develop; cardioselective or high intrinsic sympathomimetic agents are preferred.

Timolol is a nonselective antagonist with good absorption (over 90%) and bioavailability (75%). Protein binding is low at 10%. Timolol is cleared primarily by the liver, with slight (20%) renal excretion. The half-life is short, 3 to 4 hr. Adverse effects are similar to propranolol.

Timolol has been compared to placebo in the chronic prophylaxis of post-AMI (218). Placebo patients had nearly three times as many arrhythmias requiring treatment as the timolol group. Besides a decrease in overall mortality rate with timolol, the incidence of sudden death and presumably fatal VF was reduced by approximately one-half. The study utilized a fixed-dose regimen (5 mg twice daily for two days, then 10 mg twice daily), which was associated with a significant reduction in resting heart rate. Whether beneficial effects in mortality might be seen without bradycardia is not known.

Metoprolol may be considered an alternative to propranolol for arrhythmias because it is somewhat selective for β₁-receptors, and it may be preferred over propranolol for patients with chronic or acute obstructive pulmonary disease. Metoprolol should be used with caution because in high doses it may also block β₂-receptors.

Metoprolol is well absorbed, over 95%, with greater bioavailability than propranolol, about 50%. Protein binding is slight, 12%. Metoprolol is cleared hepatically with a half-life of 3 to 4 hr. The typical patient is started at 20 mg four times daily. Metoprolol has adverse effects similar to those of propranolol, with less risk for patients with asthma or peripheral vascular disease.

Metoprolol has been compared with placebo in patients with AMI treated for 90 days (219). Metoprolol was initiated as 15 mg intravenously, followed by an oral dose of 100 mg twice daily. It reduced mortality by 36%, with beneficial effects in all age groups.

Other β-blockers of potential usefulness in ventricular arrhythmias include acebutolol, atenolol, bisoprolol, nadolol, and pindolol.

As a class, β-blockers appear to be beneficial in the management of post-AMI patients. The efficacy seems to be independent of intrinsic sympathomimetic activity, β₂ receptor blockade, and membrane-stabilizing properties. However, these properties may aid with individual drug selection in certain patients. The duration of therapy has not been established. The onset of therapy has varied

between studies, yet some evidence exists that immediate β-blockade (e.g., within 12 hr after the onset of pain) may limit the enzyme-estimated infarct size.

CONCLUSION

Cardiac arrhythmias are complex, have various etiologies and alterations in electrophysiology, differ in severity and prognosis, and require individualized treatment with potentially toxic drugs. A thorough understanding of the pharmacology, pharmacodynamics, pharmacokinetics, and adverse reactions for each antiarrhythmic drug is required for safe and effective treatment of patients with arrhythmias. No one drug is effective for any arrhythmia in all patients although certain drugs are clearly first-line agents. Doses of many antiarrhythmics should be calculated using known values for the pharmacokinetic variables. However, these doses are usually only estimates of the required dose for a patient, and adjustments may be required. Patients must be monitored carefully, which frequently involves drug-level monitoring. Many new antiarrhythmics have been marketed. The ultimate question still remains unresolved for most arrhythmias—will these drugs improve mortality?

REFERENCES

1. Wit AL. Cellular electrophysiologic mechanisms of cardiac arrhythmias. Cardiol Clin 8:393–409;1990.
2. Nattel S. Antiarrhythmic drug classifications: a critical appraisal of their history, present status, and clinical relevance. Drugs 41(5):672–701, 1991.
3. Saini V, Podrid PJ, Slater W. Encainide and flecainide: are they interchangeable. Amer Heart J 117:1253–1258, 1989.
4. Wyse DG, Mitchell LB, Duff HJ. Procainamide, disopyramide, and quinidine: discordant antiarrhythmic effects during crossover comparison in patients with inducible ventricular tachycardia. J Am Coll Cardiol 9:882–889, 1987.
5. Hession M, Blum R, Podrid PJ, Lampert S, Stein J, Lown B. Mexiletine and tocainide—does response to one predict response to the other? J Am Coll Cardiol 7:338–343,1986.
6. Task Force of the Working Group on Arrhythmias of the European Society of Cardiology. The Sicilian Gambit: A new approach to the classification of antiarrhythmic drugs based on their actions on arrhythmogenic mechanisms. Circ 84:1831–1851, 1991.
7. Wyse DG. Pharmacologic therapy in patients with ventricular tachyarrhythmias. Cardiol Clin 11(1):65–83, 1993.
8. Dreifus LS, Michelson EL, Kaplinsky E. Bradyarrhythmias: clinical significance and management. J Am Coll Cardiol 1:327–338, 1983.
9. Hindman MC, Wagner GS. Arrhythmias during myocardial infarction: mechanisms, significance, and therapy. Cardiovasc Clin 11(1):81–102, 1980.
10. Emergency Cardiac Care Committee and Subcommittees, American Heart Association. Adult advanced cardiac life support. JAMA 268(16):2199–2241, 1992.
11. Schweitzer P, Mark H. The effect of atropine on cardiac arrhythmias and conduction (Parts 1 and 2). Am Heart J 100:119-127, 251–261, 1980.
12. Wood M, Ellenbogen, KA. Bradyarrhythmias, emergency pacing, and implantable defibrillation devices. Crit Care Clin 5(3):551–568, 1989.
13. Rodriguez RD, Schocken DD. Update on sick sinus syndrome, a cardiac disorder of aging. Geriatrics 45(1):26–36, 1990.

14. ACC/AHA Committee on Pacemaker Implantation. Guidelines for implantation of cardiac pacemakers and antiarrhythmia devices: a report of the American College of Cardiology/American Heart Association Task Force on assessment of diagnostic and therapeutic cardiovascular procedures. J Am Coll Cardiol 18(1):1–13, 1991.

15. Santini M, Alexidou G, Ansalone G, Cacciatore G, Cini R, Turitto G. Relation of prognosis in sick sinus syndrome to age, conduction defects and modes of permanent cardiac pacing. Am J Cardiol 65:729–735, 1990.

16. Sgarbossa EB, Pinski SL, Maloney JD. The role of pacing modality in determining long-term survival in the Sick Sinus Syndrome. Ann Intern Med 119(5):359–365, 1993.

17. Schweitzer P, Teichholz LE. Carotid sinus massage: Its diagnostic and therapeutic value in arrhythmias. Am J Med 78:645–654, 1985.

18. Mehta D, Ward DE, Wafa S, Camm AJ. Relative efficacy of various physical manoeuvres in the termination of junctional tachycardia. Lancet 1:1181–1185, 1988.

19. Parker RB, McCollam PL. Adenosine in the episodic treatment of paroxysmal supraventricular tachycardia. Clin Pharm 9(4):261–271, 1990.

20. DiMarco JP, Sellers TD, Lerman BB, Greenberg ML, Berne RM, Belardinelli L. Diagnostic and therapeutic use of adenosine in patients with supraventricular tachyarrhythmias. J Am Coll Cardiol 6(2):417–425, 1985.

21. Rankin AC, Oldroyd KG, Chong E, Dow JW, Rae AP, Cobbe SM. Adenosine or adenosine triphosphate for supraventricular tachycardias? Comparative double-blind randomized study in patients with spontaneous or inducible arrhythmias. Am Heart J 119(2Pt1):316–323, 1990.

22. DiMarco JP, Miles W, Akhtar M, et al. Adenosine for paroxysmal supraventricular tachycardia: Dose ranging and comparison with verapamil. Ann Intern Med 113(2):104–110, 1990.

23. Till J, Shinebourne EA, Rigby ML, Clarke B, Ward DE, Rowland E. Efficacy and safety of adenosine in the treatment of supraventricular tachycardia in infants and children. Br Heart J 62:204–211, 1989.

24. Rankin AC, Rae AP, Oldroyd KG, Cobbe SM. Verapamil or adenosine for the immediate treatment of supraventricular tachycardia. Q J Med 74(274):203–208, 1990.

25. Hood MA, Smith WM. Adenosine versus verapamil in the treatment of supraventricular tachycardia: a randomized double-crossover trial. Am Heart J 123:1543–1549, 1992.

26. Chronister C. Clinical management of supraventricular tachycardia with adenosine. Am J Crit Care 2:41–47, 1993.

27. Garratt C, Linker N, Griffith M, Ward D, Camm AJ. Comparison of adenosine and verapamil for termination of paroxysmal junctional tachycardia. Am J Cardiol 64(19):1310–1316, 1989.

28. Klabunde RE. Dipyridamole inhibition of adenosine metabolism in human blood. Eur J Pharmacol 93:21–26, 1983.

29. Till JA, Shinebourne EA. Supraventricular tachycardia: diagnosis and current acute management. Arch Dis Child 66:647–652, 1991.

30. Huycke EC, Sung RJ, Dias VC, et al. Intravenous diltiazem for termination of reentrant supraventricular tachycardia: a placebo-controlled, randomized, double-blind, multicenter study. J Am Coll Cardiol 13(3):538–544, 1989.

31. Dougherty AH, Jackman WM, Naccarelli GV, et al. Acute conversion of paroxysmal supraventricular tachycardia with intravenous diltiazem. Am J Cardiol 70:587–592, 1992.

32. McAllister RG, Kirsten EB. The pharmacology of verapamil. IV. Kinetic and dynamic effects after single intravenous and oral doses. Clin Pharmacol Ther 31(4):418–426, 1982.

33. Hamann SR, Blouin RA, McAllister RG. Clinical Pharmacokinetics of verapamil. Clin Pharmacokinet 9:26–41, 1984.

34. McCall D, Walsh RA, Frohlich ED, O'Rourke RA. Calcium entry blocking drugs: Mechanisms of action, experimental studies and clinical uses. Curr Probl Cardiol 10(8):2–80, 1985.

35. Hoon TJ, Bauman JL, Rodvold KA, Gallestegui J, Hariman RJ. The pharmacodynamic and pharmacokinetic differences of the D- and L-isomers of verapamil: Implications in the treatment of paroxysmal supraventricular tachycardia. Am Heart J 112(2):396–403, 1986.

36. Echizen H, Vogelgesang B, Eichelbaum M. Effects of d,l-verapamil on atrioventricular conduction in relation to its stereoselective first-pass metabolism. Clin Pharmacol Ther 38(1):71–76, 1985.

37. Weiss AT, Lewis BS, Halon DA, Hasin Y, Gotsman MS. The use of calcium with verapamil in the management of supraventricular tachyarrhythmias. Int J Cardiol 4:275–280, 1983.

38. Haft JI, Habbab MA. Treatment of atrial arrhythmias: effectiveness of verapamil when preceded by calcium infusion. Arch Intern Med 146:1085–1089, 1986.

38a. Salerno DM. Quinidine. Worse than adverse? Circulation; 84(5): 2196–2198, 1991.

39. Epstein ML, Kiel EA, Victorica BE. Cardiac decompensation following verapamil therapy in infants with supraventricular tachycardia. Pediatrics 75(4):737–740, 1985.

40. Garson A. Jr Medicolegal problems in the management of cardiac arrhythmias in children. Pediatrics 79(1):84–88, 1987.

41. Packer M, Meller J, Medina N, et al. Hemodynamic consequences of combined beta-adrenergic and slow calcium channel blockade in man. Circulation 65(4):660–668, 1982.

42. Bussey HI. The influence of quinidine and other agents on digitalis glycosides. Am Heart J 104(2 Pt 1):289–302, 1982.

43. Buckley MM-T, Grant SM, Goa KL, et al. Diltiazem: a reappraisal of its pharmacological properties and therapeutic use. Drugs 39(5):757–806, 1990.

44. Bohm M, Schwinger RHG, Erdmann E. Different cardiodepressant potency of various calcium antagonists in human myocardium. Am J Cardiol 65:1039–1041, 1990.

45. Heywood JT, Graham B, Marais GE, Jutzy KR. Effects of intravenous diltiazem on rapid atrial fibrillation accompanied by congestive heart failure. Am J Cardiol 67:1150–1152, 1991.

46. De Belder MA, Malik M, Ward DE, Camm AJ. Pacing modalities for tachycardia termination. PACE 13:231–248, 1990.

47. Clair WK, Wilkinson WE, McCarthy EA, Pritchett ELC. Treatment of paroxysmal supraventricular tachycardia with oral diltiazem. Clin Pharmacol Ther 51:562–565, 1992.

48. Ueda C. Quinidine. In Evans WE, Schentag JJ, Jusko WJ, eds.: Applied Pharmacokinetics, ed 3. Spokane, Applied Therapeutics, Inc, 1992;23:1–22.

49. Woosley RL, Echt DS, Roden DM. Effects of congestive heart failure on the pharmacokinetics and pharmacodynamics of antiarrhythmic agents. Am J Cardiol 57:25B–33B, 1986.

50. Wooding-Scott RA, Smalley J, Visco J, Slaughter RL. The pharmacokinetics and pharmacodynamics of quinidine and 3-hydroxyquinidine. Br J Clin Pharmacol 26:415–421, 1988.

51. Roden DM, Thompson KA, Hoffman BF, Woosley RL. Clinical features and basic mechanisms of quinidine-induced arrhythmias. J Am Coll Cardiol 8(1):73A–78A, 1986.

52. Wooding-Scott RA, Darling IM, Slaughter RL. Comparison of assay procedures used to measure total and unbound concentrations of quinidine. Drug Intell Clin Pharm 23:999–1004, 1989.

53. Swerdlow CD, Yu JO, Jacobson E, et al. Safety and efficacy of intravenous quinidine. Am J Med 75:36–42, 1983.

54. Cohen IS, Jick H, Cohen SI. Adverse reactions to quinidine in hospitalized patients: Findings based on data from the Boston Collaborative Drug Surveillance Program. Prog Cardiovasc Dis 20(2):151–163, 1977.

55. Coplen SE, Antman EM, Berlin JA, Hewitt P, Chalmers TC. Efficacy and safety of quinidine therapy for maintenance of sinus rhythm after cardioversion: a meta-analysis of randomized control trials. Circulation 82:1106–1116, 1990.

55a. Zehender M, Hohnloser S, Muller B, Meinertz T, Just H. Effects of amiodarone versus quinidine and verapamil in patients with chronic atrial fibrillation: results of a comparative study and a 2-year follow-up. J Am Coll Cardiol 1992 Apr;19(5):1054–1059.

56. Ferguson B Jr, Cox JL. Surgical therapy for patients with supraventricular tachycardia. Cardiol Clin 8(3):535–555, 1990.

57. Manolis AS, Wang PJ, Estes NAM 3rd. Radiofrequency catheter ablation for cardiac tachyarrhythmias. Ann Intern Med 121:452–461, 1994.

58. Akhtar M, Jazayeri MR, Sra J, et al. Atrioventricular nodal reentry: clinical, electrophysiological, and therapeutic considerations. Circulation 88:282–295, 1993.

59. Scher DL, Arsura EL. Multifocal atrial tachycardia: mechanisms, clinical correlates, and treatment. Am Heart J 118(3):574–580, 1989.

60. Hazard PB, Burnett CR. Verapamil in multifocal atrial tachycardia: hemodynamic and respiratory changes. Chest 91(1):68–70, 1987.

61. Hazard PB, Burnett CR. Treatment of multifocal atrial tachycardia with metoprolol. Crit Care Med 15(1):20–25,1987.

62. Arsura E, Lefkin AS, Scher DL, Solar M, Tessler S. A randomized, double-blind, placebo-controlled study of verapamil and metoprolol in treatment of multifocal atrial tachycardia. Am J Med 85:519–524, 1988.

63. Alpert JS, Petersen P, Godtfredsen JG. Atrial fibrillation: natural history, complications, and management. Annu Rev Med 39:41–52, 1988.

64. Petersen P. Thromboembolic complications in atrial fibrillation. Stroke 21(1):4–13, 1990.

65. Stein B, Halperin JL, Fuster V. Should patients with atrial fibrillation be anticoagulated prior to and chronically following cardioversion? Cardiovasc Clin 21(1):231–247, 1990.

66. Wolf PA, Kannel WB, McGee DL, Meeks SL, Bharucha NE, McNamara PM. Duration of atrial fibrillation and imminence of stroke: the Framingham study. Stroke 14(5):664–667, 1983.

67. Stroke Prevention in Atrial Fibrillation Investigators. Predictors of thromboembolism in atrial fibrillation: II. echocardiographic features of patients at risk. Ann Int Med 116:6–12, 1992.

68. Lundström T, Rydén L. Chronic atrial fibrillation: long-term results of direct current conversion. Acta Med Scand 223:53–59, 1988.

69. Lewis RV, Irvine N, McDevitt DG. Relationships between heart rate, exercise tolerance and cardiac output in atrial fibrillation: the effects of treatment with digoxin, verapamil and diltiazem. Eur Heart J 9:777–781, 1988.

70. Lewis RV, Laing E, Moreland TA, Service E, McDevitt DG. A comparison of digoxin, diltiazem and their combination in the treatment of atrial fibrillation. Eur Heart J 9:279–283, 1988.

71. Lang R, Klein HO, Di Segni E, et al. Verapamil improves exercise capacity in chronic atrial fibrillation: double-blind crossover study. Am Heart J 105(5):820–825, 1983.

72. Roberts SA, Diaz C, Nolan PE, et al. Effectiveness and costs of digoxin treatment for atrial fibrillation and flutter. Am J Cardiol 72:567–573, 1993.

73. Beasley R, Smith DA, McHaffie DJ. Exercise heart rates at different serum digoxin concentrations in patients with atrial fibrillation. Br Med J 290:9–11, 1985.

74. Goldman S, Probst P, Selzer A, et al. Inefficiency of "therapeutic" serum levels of digoxin in controlling the ventricular rate in atrial fibrillation. Am J Cardiol 35:651–655, 1975.

75. Klein GJ, Twum-Barima Y, Gulamhusein S, Carruthers SG, Donner AP. Verapamil in chronic atrial fibrillation: Variable patterns of response in ventricular rate. Clin Cardiol 7(4):474–483, 1984.

76. Frisolone JA. Continuous verapamil infusion. DICP 23(12):1005–1006, 1989.

77. Klein HO, Kaplinsky E. Digitalis and verapamil in atrial fibrillation and flutter: Is verapamil now the preferred agent? Drugs 31:185–197, 1986.

78. Salerno DM, Dias VC, Kleiger RE, et al. Efficacy and safety of intravenous diltiazem for treatment of atrial fibrillation and atrial flutter. Am J Cardiol 63:1046–1051, 1989.

79. Ellenbogen KA, Dias VC, Plumb VJ, et al. A placebo-controlled trial of continuous intravenous diltiazem infusion for 24-hour heart rate control during atrial fibrillation and atrial flutter: A multicenter study. J Am Coll Cardiol 18(4):891–897, 1991.

80. The Esmolol Multicenter Study Research Group. Efficacy and safety of esmolol vs propranolol in the treatment of supraventricular tachyarrhythmias: A multicenter double-blind clinical trial. Am Heart J 110(5):913–922, 1985.

81. The Esmolol vs Placebo Multicenter Study Group. Comparison of the efficacy and safety of esmolol, a short-acting beta blocker, with placebo in the treatment of supraventricular tachyarrhythmias. Am Heart J 111:42, 1986.

82. Sung RJ, Blanski L, Kirshenbaum J, et al. Clinical experience with esmolol, a short-acting beta-adrenergic blocker in cardiac arrhythmias and myocardial ischemia. J Clin Pharmacol 26(suppl A):A15–A26, 1986.

83. Platia EV, Michelson EL, Porterfield JK, Das G. Esmolol versus verapamil in the acute treatment of atrial fibrillation or atrial flutter. Am J Cardiol 63:925–929, 1989.

84. Morris DC, Hurst JW. Atrial fibrillation. Curr Probl Cardiol 5(1):1–50, 1980.

85. Lewis RV. Atrial fibrillation: the therapeutic options. Drugs 40(6): 841–853, 1990.

86. Karlson BW, Herlitz J, Edvardsson N, Olsson SB. Prophylactic treatment after electroconversion of atrial fibrillation. Clin Cardiol 13(4):279–286, 1990.

87. Dalzell G, Anderson J, Adgey A. Factors determining success and energy requirements for cardioversion of atrial fibrillation: Revised version. Q J Med 78(285):85–95, 1991.

88. Mann DL, Maisel AS, Atwood JE, et al. Absence of cardioversion-induced ventricular arrhythmias in patients with therapeutic digoxin levels. J Am Coll Cardiol 5:882–888, 1985.

89. Feld GK, Chen P-S, Nicod P, Fleck RP, Meyer D. Possible atrial proarrhythmic effects of class 1C antiarrhythmic drugs. Am J Cardiol 66:366–367, 378–383, 1990.

90. Sihm I, Hansen FA, Rasmussen J, Pedersen AK, Thygesen K. Flecainide acetate in atrial flutter and fibrillation. Eur Heart J 11:145–148, 1990.

91. MacNeil DJ, Davies RO, Deitchman D. Clinical safety profile of sotalol in the treatment of arrhythmias Am J Cardiol 72:44A–50A, 1993.

92. Roth A, Harrison E, Mitani G, Cohen J, Rahimtoola SH, Elkayam U. Efficacy and safety of medium- and high-dose diltiazem alone and in combination with digoxin for control of heart rate at rest and during exercise in patients with chronic atrial fibrillation. Circulation 73(2):316–324, 1986.

93. Petersen P, Godtfredsen J, Boysen G, Andersen ED, Andersen B. Placebo-controlled, randomized trial of warfarin and aspirin for prevention of thromboembolic complications in chronic atrial fibrillation: The Copenhagen AFASAK study. Lancet 1(8631):175–179, 28 Jan 1989.

94. The Boston Area Anticoagulation Trial for Atrial Fibrillation Investigators. The effect of low-dose warfarin on the risk of stroke in patients with nonrheumatic atrial fibrillation. N Engl J Med 323(22):1505–1511, 1990.

95. The Stroke Prevention in Atrial Fibrillation Investigators. The stroke prevention in atrial fibrillation study: final results. Circulation 84:527–539, 1991.

96. Connolly SJ, Laupacis A, Gent M, et al. Canadian atrial fibrillation anticoagulation study. J Am Coll Cardiol 18(2):349–355, 1991.

97. Ezekowitz MD, Bridgers SL, James KE, et al. Warfarin in the prevention of stroke associated with nonrheumatic atrial fibrillation. N Engl J Med 327(20):1406–1412, 1992.

98. Asplund K, Beermann B, Bergfeldt L, et al. Treatment of atrial fibrillation: Recommendations from a workshop arranged by the

Medical Products Agency (Uppsala, Sweden) and the Swedish Society of Cardiology. Eur Heart J 14:1427–1433, 1993.

99. Laupacis A, Albers G, Dunn M, Feinberg W. Antithrombotic therapy in atrial fibrillation. Chest 102(Suppl 4):426S–433S, 1992.

100. Atrial Fibrillation Investigators. Risk factors for stroke and efficacy of antithrombotic therapy in atrial fibrillation: analysis of pooled data from five randomized controlled trials. Arch Intern Med 154:1449–1457, 1994.

101. Stroke Prevention in Atrial Fibrillation Investigators. Warfarin versus aspirin for prevention of thromboembolism in atrial fibrillation: stroke prevention in atrial fibrillation II study. Lancet 343:687–691, 1994.

102. Levine MN, Hirsh J, Landefeld S, Raskob G. Hemorrhagic complications of anticoagulant treatment. Chest 102(Suppl 4):352S–363S, 1992.

103. Pritchett ELC. Management of atrial fibrillation. N Engl J Med 326(19):1264–1271, 1992.

104. Cox JL, Boineau JP, Schuessler RB, et al. Five-year experience with the maze procedure for atrial fibrillation. Ann Thorac Surg 56:814–824, 1993.

105. Berry VA. Wolff-Parkinson-White syndrome and the use of radiofrequency catheter ablation. Heart Lung 22:15–25, 1993.

106. Prystowsky EN. Diagnosis and management of the preexcitation syndromes. Curr Probl Cardiol 13(4):225–310, 1988.

107. Porter RS. Adenosine: Supplementary considerations about activity and use. Clin Pharm 9(4):271–274, 1990.

108. Brodsky M, Wu D, Denes P, Kanakis C, Rosen KM. Arrhythmias documented by 24 hour continuous electrocardiography in 50 male medical students without apparent heart disease. Am J Cardiol 39:390–395, 1977.

109. The Cardiac Arrhythmia Suppression Trial (CAST) Investigators. Mortality and morbidity in patients receiving encainide, flecainide, or placebo: the Cardiac Arrhythmia Suppression Trial. N Engl J Med 324(12):781–788, 1991.

110. The Cardiac Arrhythmia Suppression Trial II Investigators. Effect of the antiarrhythmic agent moricizine on survival after myocardial infarction. N Engl J Med 327(4):227–233, 1992.

111. The Cardiac Arrhythmia Suppression Trial (CAST) Investigators. Preliminary report: Effect of encainide and flecainide on mortality in a randomized trial of arrhythmia suppression after myocardial infarction. N Engl J Med 321:406–412, 1989.

112. Lee AJ. Digibind: emergency treatment for digitalis toxicity. J Emergency Nursing 15:266–268, 1989.

113. Boucher BA, Lalonde RL. Digoxin-specific antibody fragments for the treatment of digoxin intoxication. Clin Pharm 5:826–827, 1986.

114. Huang SK, Marcus FI. Antiarrhythmic drug therapy of ventricular arrhythmias. Curr Prob Cardiol 11:178–240, 1986.

115. Horowitz LN, Josephson ME, Farshidi A, Spielman SR, Michelson EL, Greenspan AM. Recurrent sustained ventricular tachycardia. Circulation 58:986–997, 1978.

116. Bigger JT, Weld FM, Rolnitzky LM. Prevalence, characteristics, and significance of ventricular tachycardia detected with ambulatory electrocardiographic recording in the late hospital phase of acute myocardial infarction. Am J Cardiol 48:815–823, 1981.

117. Manolis AS, Linzer M, Salem D, Estes NA 3rd. Syncope: current diagnostic evaluation and management. Ann Intern Med 112:850–863, 1990.

118. Blanck Z, Dhala A, Deshpande S, et al. Catheter ablation of ventricular tachycardia. Am Heart J 127(4 part 2):1126–1133, 1994.

119. Pieper JA, Johnson KE. Lidocaine. In Evans WE, Schentag JJ, Jusko WJ, eds: Applied Pharmacokinetics, ed. 3. Spokane, WA, Applied Therapeutics, Inc, 1992, 21:1–37.

120. Vozeh S, Berger M, Wenk M, Ritz R, Follath F. Rapid prediction of individual dosage requirements of lidocaine. Clin Pharmacokinet 9:354–363, 1984.

121. Shand DG. Alpha-1-acid glycoprotein and plasma lidocaine binding. Clin Pharmacokinet 9:27–31, 1984.

122. LeLorier J, Grenon D, Latour Y, et al. Pharmacokinetics of lidocaine after prolonged intravenous infusions in uncomplicated myocardial infarctions. Ann Intern Med 87:700–702, 1977.

123. Grubb BP. Recurrence of ventricular tachycardia after conversion from proprietary to generic procainamide. Am J Cardiol 63:1532–1533, 1989.

124. Hilleman DE, Patterson AJ, Mohiuddin SM, Ortmeier BG, Destache CJ. Comparative bioequivalence and efficacy of two sustained-release procainamide formulations in patients with cardiac arrhythmias. Drug Intell Clin Pharm 22:554–558, 1988.

125. Baker BA, Reynolds JR, Gleckel L, A'Zary E, Bodenheimer MM. Comparative bioavailability of two oral sustained-release procainamide products. Clin Pharm 7:135–138, 1988.

126. Funck-Brentano C, Light RT, Lineberry MD, Wright GM, Roden DM, Woosley RL. Pharmacokinetic and pharmacodynamic interaction of N-acetylprocainamide and procainamide in humans. J Cardiovascular Pharmacology 14:364–373, 1989.

127. Coyle JD, Lima JJ. Procainamide. In Evans WE, Schentag JJ, Jusko WJ, eds: Applied Pharmacokinetics, ed. 3. Spokane, WA, Applied Therapeutics, Inc, 1992;22:1–33.

128. Bauer LA, Black D, Gensler A, Sprinkle J. Influence of age, renal function and heart failure on procainamide clearance and n-acetylprocainamide serum concentrations. Int J Clin Pharmacol Ther Toxicol 27:213–216, 1989.

129. Lima JJ, Goldfarb AL, Conti DR et al. Safety and efficacy of procainamide infusions. Am J Cardiol 43:98–105, 1979.

130. Kuehl P, Arquin P, Fridahl J. Steady state bioavailability of a sustained release procainamide preparation. Drug Intell Clin Pharm 16:475–476, 1982.

131. Giardina EG, Fenster PE, Bigger JT Jr, Mayersohn M, Perrier D, Marcus FI. Efficacy, plasma concentrations and adverse effects of a new sustained release procainamide preparation. Am J Cardiol 46:855–862, 1980.

132. Flanagan AD. Pharmacokinetics of a sustained release procainamide preparation. Angiology 33:71–77, 1982.

133. Gottlieb SS, Kukin ML, Medina N, Yushak M, Packer M. Comparative hemodynamic effects of procainamide, tocainide, encainide in severe chronic heart failure. Circulation 81:860–864, 1990.

134. Rubin RL, Curnutte JT. Metabolism of procainamide to the cytotoxic hydroxylamine by neutrophils activated in vitro. J Clin Invest 83:1336–1343, 1989.

135. Ellrodt AG, Murata GH, Riedinger MS, Stewart ME, Mochizuki C, Gray R. Severe neutropenia associated with sustained release procainamide. Ann Internal Med 100:197–201, 1984.

136. Meyers DG, Gonzalez ER, Peters LL, Davis RB, Feagler JR, Egan JD, Nair CK. Severe neutropenia associated with procainamide: comparison of sustained release and conventional preparations. Am Heart J 109:1393–1395, 1985.

137. Sparboro JA, Rawling DA, Fozzard HA. Suppression of ventricular arrhythmias with intravenous disopyramide and lidocaine: efficacy comparison in a randomized trial. Am J Cardiol 44:513–520, 1979.

138. Lima JJ, Boudoulas H, Blanford M. Concentration dependence of disopyramide binding to plasma protein and its influence on kinetics and dynamics. J Pharmacol Exp Ther 219:741–747, 1981.

139. Whiting B, Holford NHG, Sheiner LB. Quantitative analysis of the disopyramide concentration-effect relationship. Br J Clin Pharmacol 9:67–75, 1980.

140. Nightingale J, Nappi JM. Effect of phenytoin on serum disopyramide concentrations. Clin Pharm 6:46–50, 1987.

141. Pedersen LE, Bonde J, Graudal NA, Backer NV, Hansen JE, Kampmann JP. Quantitative and qualitative binding characteristics of disopyramide in serum from patients with decreased renal and hepatic function. Br J Clin Pharmacol 23:41–46, 1987.

142. Caplin JL, Johnston A, Hamer J, Camm AJ. The acute changes in serum binding of disopyramide and flecainide after myocardial infarction. Eur J Clin Pharmacol 28:253–255, 1985.

143. Capparelli EV, DiPersio DM, Zhao H, Kluger J, Chow MS. Clinical pharmacokinetics of controlled-release disopyramide in patients with cardiac arrhythmias. J Clin Pharmacol 28:306–311, 1988.

144. Zema MJ. Serum drug concentrations and adverse effects in cardiac patients after administration of a new controlled-release disopyramide preparation. Ther Drug Monit 6:192–198, 1984.

145. Teichman S. The anticholinergic side effects of disopyramide and controlled release disopyramide. Angiology 36:767–771, 1985.

146. Cacoub P, Deray G, Balou A, Grimaldi A, Soubrie C, Jacobs C. Disopyramide-induced hypoglycemia: case report and review of the literature. Fundam Clin Pharmacol 3(5):527–535, 1989.

147. Podrid PJ, Shoenberger A, Lown B. Congestive heart failure caused by oral disopyramide. N Engl J Med 302:614–617, 1980.

148. Wehmeyer AE, Thomas RL. Encainide: a new antiarrhythmic agent. Drug Intell Clin Pharm 20:9–13, 1986.

149. Bergstrand RH, Wang T, Roden DM et al. Encainide disposition in patients with renal failure. Clin Pharmacol Ther 40:148–154, 1986.

150. Funck-Brentano C, Turgeon J, Woosley RL, et al. Effect of low dose quinidine on encainide pharmacokinetics and pharmacodynamics. Influence of genetic polymorphism. J Pharmacol Exp Ther 249:134–142, 1989.

151. Kazierad DJ, Lalonde RL, Hoon TJ, Mirvis DM, Bottorff MB. The effect of diltiazem on the disposition of encainide and its active metabolites. Clin Pharmacol Ther 46:668–673, 1989.

152. Morganroth J, Somberg JC, Pool PE, et al. Comparative study of encainide and quinidine in the treatment of ventricular arrhythmias. J Am Coll Cardiol 7:9–16, 1986.

153. Luderitz B, Manz M. Pharmacolgic treatment of supraventricular tachycardia: the German experience. Am J Cardiol 70:66A–74A, 1992.

154. Parker RB, McCollam PL, Bauman JL. Propafenone: A novel type Ic antiarrhythmic agent. Drug Intell Clin Pharm 23:196–203, 1989.

155. Lee JT, Kroemer HK, Silberstein DJ, et al. The role of genetically determined polymorphic drug metabolism in the β-blockade produced by propafenone. N Engl J Med 322:1764–1768, 1990.

156. Bryson HM, Palmer KJ, Langtry HD, Fitton A. Propafenone: a reappraisal of its pharmacology, pharmacokinetics and therapeutic use in cardiac arrhythmias. Drugs 45(1):85–130, 1993.

157. Roden DM. Torsade de Pointes. Clin Cardiol 16:683–686, 1993.

158. Lazzara R. Antiarrhythmic drugs and torsade de pointes. Eur Heart J 14(Supp 4):88–92, 1993.

159. Iseri LT, Allen BJ, Brodsky MA. Magnesium therapy of cardiac arrhythmias in critical-care medicine. Magnesium 8:299–306, 1989.

160. Manolis AS, Linzer M, Salem D, et al. Syncope: current diagnostic evaluation and management. Ann Intern Med 112:850–863, 1990.

161. Roden DM, Woosley RL. Drug therapy: flecainide. N Engl J Med 315:36–40, 1986.

162. Gross AS, Mikus G, Fischer C, Hertrampf R, Gundert-Remy U, Eichelbaum M. Stereoselective disposition of flecainide in relation to the sparteine/debrisoquine metaboliser phenotype. Br J Clin Pharmacol 28:555–566, 1989.

163. McQuinn RL, Pentikainen PJ, Chang SF, Conard GJ. Pharmacokinetics of flecainide in patients with cirrhosis of the liver. Clin Pharmacol Ther 44:566–572, 1988.

164. Salerno DM, Granrud G, Sharkey P, et al. Pharmacodynamic and side effects of flecainide acetate. Clin Pharmacol Ther. 40:101–107, 1986.

165. Morganroth J, Anderson JL, Gentzkow GD. Classification by type of ventricular arrhythmia predicts frequency of adverse cardiac events from flecainide. J Am Coll Cardiol 8:607–615, 1986.

166. Fitton A, Buckley MMT. Moricizine: A review of its pharmacological properties, and therapeutic efficacy in cardiac arrhythmias. Drugs 40:138–167, 1990.

167. Mann HJ. Moricizine: a new Class I antiarrhythmic. Clin Pharm 9:842–852, 1990.

168. Nestico PF, Morganroth J, Horowitz LN. New antiarrhythmic drugs. Drugs 35:286–319, 1988.

169. CAPS Investigators. Effects of encainide, flecainide, imipramine, and moricizine on ventricular arrhythmias during the. year after acute myocardial infarction. Am J Cardiol 61:501–509, 1988.

170. Bigger JT. The events surrounding the removal of encainide and flecainide from the CAST and why CAST is continuing with moricizine. J Am Coll Cardiol 15:243–245, 1990.

171. Clyne CA, Estes NAM 3rd, Wang PJ. Moricizine. N Engl J Med 327(4):255–260, 1992.

172. Gillis AM, Kates RE. Clinical pharmacokinetics of the newer antiarrhythmic agents. Clin Pharmacokinet 9:375–403, 1984.

173. Grech-Belanger O, Gilbert M, Turgeon J, LeBlanc PP. Effect of cigarette smoking on mexiletine kinetics. Clin Pharmacol Ther 37:638–643, 1985.

174. Wang T, Wuellner D, Woosley RL, Stone WJ. Pharmacokinetics and nondialyzability of mexiletine in renal failure. Clin Pharmacol Ther 37:649–653, 1985.

175. Steen SN, Hughes EM, Sharon G, MacGregor TR. Efficacy of oral mexiletine therapy at a 12-h dosage interval. Chest 97:358–363, 1990.

176. Singh JB, Rasul AM, Shah A, Adams E, Flessas A, Kocot SL. Efficacy of mexiletine in chronic ventricular arrhythmias compared with quinidine: a single blind randomized trial. Am J Cardiol 53:84–87, 1984.

177. Giardina EG, Wechsler ME. Low dose quinidine-mexiletine combination therapy versus quinidine monotherapy for treatment of ventricular arrhythmias. J Am Coll Cardiol 15:1–45, 1990.

178. Duff HJ, Roden D, Primm RK, Oates JA, Woosley RL. Mexiletine in the treatment of resistant ventricular arrhythmias: enhancement of efficacy and reduction of dose-related side effects by combination with quinidine. Circulation 67:1124–1128, 1983.

179. Kim SG, Mercando AD, Tam S, Fisher JD. Combination of disopyramide and mexiletine for better tolerance and additive effects for treatment of ventricular arrhythmias. J Am Coll Cardiol 13:659–664, 1989.

180. Luderitz B, Mletzko R, Jung W, Manz M. Combination of antiarrhythmic drugs. J Cardiovasc Pharmacol 17(suppl 6):S48–S52, 1991.

181. DiMarco JP, Garan H, Ruskin JN. Mexiletine for refractory ventricular arrhythmias: results using serial electrophysiologic testing. Am J Cardiol 47:131–138, 1981.

182. Roden DM, Woosley RL. Drug therapy: tocainide. N Engl J Med 315:41–45, 1986.

183. Rice TL, Patterson JH, Celestin C, Foster JR, Powell JR. Influence of rifampin on tocainide pharmacokinetics in humans. Clin Pharm 8:200–205, 1989.

184. North DS, Mattern AL, Kapil RP, Lalonde RL. The effect of histamine-2 receptor antagonists on tocainide pharmacokinetics. J Clin Pharmacol 28:640–643, 1988.

185. Wassenmiller JE, Aronow WS. Effect of tocainide and quinidine on premature ventricular contractions. Clin Pharmacol Ther 28:431–435, 1980.

186. Feinberg L, Travis WD, Ferrans V, Sato N, Bernton HF. Pulmonary fibrosis associated with tocainide: report of a case with literature review. Am Rev Respir Dis 141:505–508, 1990.

187. Nappi JM, McCollam PL. Sotalol: a breakthrough antiarrhythmic? Ann Pharmacother 27:1359–1368, 1993.

188. Blair AD, Burgess ED, Maxwell BM, Cutler RE. Sotalol kinetics in renal insufficiency. Clin Pharmacol Ther 29:457–463, 1981.

189. Hohnloser SH, Woosley RL. Sotalol. N Engl J Med 331(1):31–38, 1994.

190. Juul-Moller S, Edvardsson N, Rehnqvist-Ahlberg N. Sotalol versus quinidine for the maintenance of sinus rhythm after direct current

cardioversion of atrial fibrillation. Circulation 82:1932–1939, 1990.

191. Mason JW (for the ESVEM Investigators). A comparison of seven antiarrhythmic drugs in patients with ventricular tachyarrhythmias. N Engl J Med 329(7):452–458, 1993.

192. Chopra MP, Thadani U, Portal RW, Aber CP. Lignocaine therapy for ventricular ectopic activity after acute myocardial infarction: a double-blind trial. Br Med J 3(776):668–670, 1971.

193. Lie KI, Wellens HJ, van Capelle FJ, Durrer D. Lidocaine in the prevention of primary ventricular fibrillation. A double-blind, randomized study of 212 consecutive patients. N Engl J Med 291(25):1324–1326, 1974.

194. Rademaker AW, Kellen J, Tam YK, Wyse DG. Character of adverse effects of prophylactic lidocaine in the coronary care unit. Clin Pharmacol Ther 40:73–80, 1986.

195. Hine LK, Laird N, Hewitt P, Chalmers TC. Meta-analytic evidence against prophylactic use of lidocaine in acute myocardial infarction. Arch Intern Med 149:2694–2698, 1989.

196. Duff HJ, Roden DM, Yacobi A, et al. Bretylium: relations between plasma concentrations and pharmacologic actions in high-frequency ventricular arrhythmias. Am J Cardiol 55:395–401, 1985.

197. Adir J, Narang PK, Josselson, J. Nomogram for bretylium dosing in renal impairment. Ther Drug Monit 7:265–268, 1985.

198. Perlman PE, Adams WG Jr, Ridgeway NA. Extreme pyrexia during bretylium administration. Postgrad Med 85:111–114, 1989.

199. Naccarelli GV, Rinkenberger RL, Dougherty AH, Giebel RA. Amiodarone: pharmacology and antiarrhythmic and adverse effects. Pharmacotherapy 5:298–313, 1985.

200. Heger JJ, Prytowsky EN, Jackman WM, et al. Amiodarone, clinical efficacy and electrophysiology during long term therapy for recurrent ventricular tachycardia or ventricular fibrillation. NEJM 305:539–545, 1981.

201. Peter T, Hamer A, Mandel WJ. Evaluation of amiodarone therapy in the treatment of drug resistant cardiac arrhythmias: long term follow up. Eur Heart J. 6:151–162, 1985.

202. Gill J, Heel RC, Fitton A. Amiodarone: an overview of its pharmacological properties, and review of its therapeutic use in cardiac arrhythmias. Drugs 43(1):69–110, 1992.

203. Kerin NZ, Blevins RD, Benaderet D, et al. Relation of serum reverse T3 to amiodarone antiarrhythmic efficacy and toxicity. Am J Cardiol. 57:128–130, 1986.

204. Saal KA, Werner JA, Greene HL, Sears GK, Graham EL. Effect of amiodarone on serum quinidine and procainamide levels. Am J Cardiol. 53:1264–1267, 1984.

205. Hohnloser SH, Klingenheben T, Singh BN. Amiodarone-associated proarrhythmic effects: a review with special reference to torsade de pointes tachycardia. Ann Intern Med 121:529–535, 1994.

206. Gosselink AT, Crijns HJ, Van Gelder IC, et al. Low-dose amiodarone for maintenance of sinus rhythm after cardioversion of atrial fibrillation or flutter. JAMA 267(24):3289–3293, 1992.

207. Herre JM, Suave MJ, Malone P, et al. Long-term results of amiodarone therapy in patients with recurrent sustained ventricular tachycardia or ventricular fibrillation. J Am Coll Cardiol 13:442–449, 1989.

208. Weinberg BA, Miles WM, Klein LS, et al. Five-year follow-up of 589 patients treated with amiodarone. Am Heart J 125(1):109–120, 1993.

209. The CASCADE Investigators. Randomized antiarrhythmic drug therapy in survivors of cardiac arrest (the CASCADE study). Am J Cardol 72:280–287, 1993.

210. Cairns JA, Connolly SJ, Gent M, Roberts R. Post-myocardial infarction mortality in patients with ventricular premature depolarization: Canadian amiodarone myocardial infarction arrhythmia trial pilot study. Circulation 84:550–557, 1991.

211. Ceremuzynski Y, Kleczar E, Krzeminska-Pakula M, et al. Effect of amiodarone on mortality after myocardial infarction. J Am Coll Cardiol 20:1056–1062, 1992.

212. Pfisterer ME, Kiowski W, Brunner H, Burckhardt D, Burkart F. Long-term benefit of 1-year amiodarone treatment for persistent complex ventricular arrhythmias after myocardial infarction. Circulation 87:309–311, 1993.

213. Cairns JA, Connolly SJ, Roberts R, Gent M. Canadian amiodarone myocardial infarction arrhythmia trial (CAMIAT): rationale and protocol. Am J Cardiol 72:87F–94F, 1993.

214. Camm AJ, Julian D, Janse G, et al. The European myocardial infarct amiodarone trial (EMIAT). Am J Cardiol 72:95F–98F, 1993.

215. Mattioni TA, Zheutlin TA, Sarmiento JJ, et al. Amiodarone in patients with previous drug-mediated torsade de pointes: long term safety and efficacy. Ann Intern Med 111(7):547–580, 1989.

216. Morganroth J, Bigger JT. Pharmacologic management of ventricular arrhythmias after the Cardiac Arrhythmia Suppression Trial. Am J Cardiol 65:1497–1503, 1990.

217. National Heart, Lung, and Blood Institute. The β-blocker heart attack trial. JAMA 246:2073–2074, 1981.

218. Norwegian Multicenter Study Group. Timolol induced reduction in mortality and reinfarction in patients surviving acute myocardial infarction. New Engl J Med 304:801–807, 1981.

219. Hjalmarson A, Elmfeldt D, Herlitz J, et al. Effect on mortality of metoprolol in acute myocardial infarction. A double-blind randomized trial. Lancet 17;2(8251):823–827, 1981.

CHAPTER 40

ANGINA PECTORIS

KEVIN M. SOWINSKI and JULIE A. JOHNSON

Angina pectoris is a clinical syndrome of chest discomfort. Caused by reversible myocardial ischemia, it produces disturbances in myocardial function without causing myocardial necrosis. Myocardial ischemia is a result of increased myocardial work and/or decreased myocardial oxygen supply. The specific causes of increased demand or decreased supply will be discussed in depth. A number of types of angina may be referred to as reversible syndromes of myocardial ischemia. These include stable angina, variant or Prinzmetal's angina, silent myocardial ischemia, and unstable angina. Discussion of these syndromes will be the focus of this chapter.

EPIDEMIOLOGY

Angina pectoris is a usually a manifestation of atherosclerotic coronary artery disease, the leading cause of death in the United States. Coronary artery disease results in an estimated 27.7 million physician office visits and causes approximately .5 million deaths annually (1). It is difficult to estimate the prevalence of angina in the population as a whole because it is affected by age, gender, and risk factor profile. Prevalence increases with age, is greater in males, and depends on the number of cardiovascular risk factors. The average annual mortality rate from angina is approximately 4%, based on the Framingham data (2), but is highly variable and related to coronary artery anatomy, age, gender, cardiovascular risk factors, anginal functional class, and the ischemic syndrome with which the patient presents (2).

ETIOLOGY/PATHOPHYSIOLOGY

Angina pectoris is usually associated with large single- to multivessel atherosclerotic coronary artery disease, coronary artery vasospasm, or both. Approximately 85% of patients with angina pectoris have significant coronary artery disease (defined as greater than 75% atherosclerotic reduction) in a major epicardial coronary vessel (3). Numerous risk factors place individuals at higher risk for developing atherosclerosis, including dyslipidemia, family history of premature myocardial infarction or sudden death, cigarette smoking, hypertension, diabetes mellitus, males older than 45 years of age, and females greater than 55 years of age not receiving estrogen replacement therapy (4).

Although most patients with angina have significant occlusions in one of the major coronary arteries, there is a lack of correlation between the extent of atherosclerotic coronary artery disease and the severity of anginal symptoms (5). Usually, the severity of anginal symptoms tends to be more significant in patients with multivessel disease than in patients with single-vessel disease, but, in any given patient, the extent of underlying atherosclerotic coronary artery disease cannot be predicted from the severity, nature, duration, or quality of discomfort. Two examples of a lack of clinical-pathologic correlation are (1) patient with advanced three-vessel coronary artery disease who experiences only silent myocardial ischemia and (2) patient with Prinzmetal's (variant) angina with episodes of excruciating angina yet minimal or no coronary atherosclerosis. In addition, the severity and duration of anginal symptoms are not related to prognosis. Prognosis is mainly determined by the extent and severity of underlying atherosclerotic coronary artery disease, extent of left ventricular systolic dysfunction, and the presence and severity of ischemia during exercise (5).

Myocardial ischemia is caused by an imbalance between coronary blood flow (supply) and the metabolic needs of the myocardium (demand). Myocardial ischemia occurs when myocardial oxygen demand exceeds myocardial oxygen supply. It is useful to describe the determinants of myocardial oxygen supply and demand since drug therapy is designed to affect the balance between these two variables (Figure 40.1). The major determinants of myocardial oxygen demand are heart rate, contractility, and left ventricular systolic wall tension. Of the three determinants, heart rate is likely to be the most important, the one most easily adjusted with current drug therapies and the easiest to assess clinically. Myocardial contractility refers to the rate of rise in the intraventricular pressure during isovolumetric contraction and is influenced by a number of variables, including, but not limited to, autonomic nervous system, heart rate, blood calcium level, and temperature. A number of antianginal agents decrease myocardial contractility and reduce myocardial oxygen demand. Clinical assessment of the beneficial effects of drugs on myocardial contractility is much more difficult. Systolic wall tension is directly related to the ventricular systolic pressure and ventricular wall radius and is inversely related to wall thickness. Preload and afterload are important components of these factors. Reducing systolic blood pressure reduces afterload, which ultimately deceases oxygen demand. Reductions in preload reduce left ventricular dimension

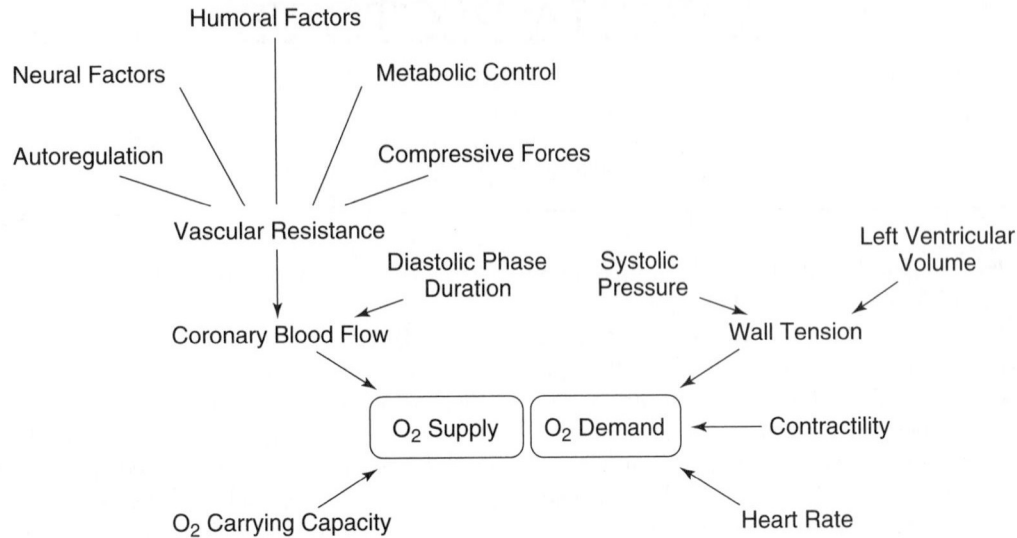

Figure 40.1. Factors effecting myocardial oxygen supply and demand. Adapted from reference 6.

and ultimately reduce myocardial oxygen demand. One may clinically estimate myocardial oxygen demand by using the double-product (product of heart rate and systolic blood pressure). Although the double-product provides a useful estimate of myocardial oxygen demand, it does neglect to consider contractility as an important factor.

Myocardial oxygen supply is determined by two factors: coronary blood flow and the oxygen-carrying capacity of blood (6). Although the oxygen-carrying capacity can be affected by certain conditions (e.g., anemia), the most important determinant of myocardial oxygen supply is clearly coronary blood flow. Normally, the arteriolar resistance vessels are the most important regulators of coronary blood flow, whereas large epicardial vessels are low-resistance vessels. Myocardial ischemia develops when narrowing of the epicardial vessels by vasospasm or atherosclerosis results in high enough resistances to restrict coronary blood flow. A number of complex factors determine coronary blood flow, including duration of diastole and coronary vascular resistance, the latter of which is determined by metabolic control, autoregulation, extravascular compressive forces, and humoral and neural factors.

CHRONIC STABLE ANGINA

Chronic stable angina pectoris is termed "stable" because the characteristics of an anginal episode (frequency, severity, duration of symptoms, time of day, and so on) have not changed over the previous two months. Typical exertional angina is usually caused by increased myocardial oxygen demand and is usually associated with fixed-obstruction of a coronary artery by an atherosclerotic plaque. During periods of increased metabolic demand (e.g., physical exertion), delivery of oxygen-carrying blood through the atherosclerotic vessel is insufficient to meet the myocardium's oxygen requirements, resulting in myocardial ischemia. It is becoming increasingly appreciated, however, that angina in some individuals is related to decreased supply, likely caused by coronary artery vasoconstriction. Although it is easy to separate angina into that which is caused by increased demand and decreased supply, most patients fall somewhere in between these two extremes.

Patients experiencing angina may be classified as having either mainly fixed-threshold angina or mainly variable-threshold angina. Anginal syndromes in patients with fixed-threshold angina are precipitated by increased myocardial oxygen demand and tend to occur at some reproducible level of myocardial work. Typically, an individual can predict what level of physical activity is likely to produce an anginal attack (e.g., walking up two flights of stairs, walking around the block). On any given day, this is fairly reproducible. On the other hand, patients with variable-threshold angina have difficulty predicting when or with what level of exertion they will experience an anginal attack. On any given day, the anginal threshold is extremely variable causing these patients to have good and bad days. The reason for the somewhat variable threshold for causing angina is likely related to a predominance of a vasoconstrictive component leading to decreased oxygen supply and subsequent myocardial ischemia. Although most individuals with variable-threshold angina have some degree of fixed atherosclerosis, dynamic narrowing of the coronary vasculature by coronary vasoconstriction is important in the genesis of anginal symptoms.

CLINICAL PRESENTATION

Classically, angina presents as substernal, retrosternal, or transsternal discomfort that radiates, usually, to the neck and left arm. Some patients may experience radiation to other areas of the body, including the right arm. The quality of discomfort varies from patient to patient, which reflects wide variability in the way in which patients perceive pain and discomfort. The discomfort is usually a dull, rather than sharp, stabbing pain, and patients may describe it as a strangling or constricting sensation. The following descriptors may also be used: pressure, heaviness, fullness, squeezing, burning, aching, gas, "viselike" or anxiety. The severity of discomfort may range from slight discomfort to disabling pain. Anginal discomfort usually has a gradual onset and lasts only a few minutes if the precipitating factor is removed. Relief is usually afforded by rest and/or sublingual nitroglycerin. A long duration of anginal discomfort implies severe ischemia, coronary spasm, unstable angina, or impending myocardial infarction. Symptoms lasting for several days are unlikely to be angina. The frequency of anginal attacks ranges from several per day to one per week or month and determines the specific need for therapy; this will be discussed in more detail later in the chapter. The New York Heart Association or the Canadian Cardiovascular Society's functional classification (Table 40.1) for angina may be used to assess the frequency and patterns of patient's angina. In addition, patient diaries documenting times of anginal discomfort and consumption of sublingual nitroglycerin may be used to classify anginal patterns.

Certain patients may not experience typical symptoms of anginal pain when myocardial ischemia is present, but rather have what are termed "anginal equivalents." Anginal equivalents may be episodes of myocardial ischemia that result in symptoms of systolic or diastolic left ventricular dysfunction but are not necessarily associated with chest pain or other symptoms characteristic of anginal discomfort. Anginal equivalents are usually caused by exertion and are relieved by rest or nitroglycerin. Common symptoms of anginal equivalents include exertional dyspnea, fatigue, and exhaustion.

Many patients also have myocardial ischemia in the absence of any objective signs of angina (pain, anginal equivalents, and so on), which is termed "silent myocardial ischemia." Silent myocardial ischemia can be detected by exercise ECG testing (as asymptomatic ST-segment depression), by portable ECG testing, or both. Silent myocardial ischemia can be categorized into three types: type I, which is totally asymptomatic; type II, which occurs in patients after having suffered a myocardial infarction; and type III, which occurs in patients who have objective evidence of coronary artery disease (e.g., stable angina, unstable angina, postmyocardial infarction, variant angina). Type III patients have both asymptomatic and symptomatic ischemic episodes. The incidence of silent myocardial ischemia varies from 2 to 4% in totally asymptomatic patients, 20 to 30% in patients after a myocardial infarction, and 44 to 88% in patients with symptomatic ischemia (7). The prognosis of silent myocardial ischemia also varies depending on the type of silent myocardial ischemia the patient has. Patients with type I silent myocardial ischemia, who have abnormal stress ECG tests, have an increased incidence of coronary events, including myocardial infarction and angina. The prognosis in patients with type II silent myocardial ischemia appears to be similar to other survivors of myocardial infarction who have symptomatic ischemia. Finally, patients with type III silent myocardial ischemia have increased risk for myocardial infarction and death, but are not at a higher risk than those patients with only symptomatic angina.

An important topic that relates to the frequency of anginal attacks is the circadian pattern of anginal occur-

Table 40.1.
Classification of Angina Pectoris

Class	New York Heart Association Functional Classification	Canadian Cardiovascular Society Classification
I	Symptoms occur with unusual activity; minimal or no functional impairment	*Angina does not occur with ordinary physical activity* (walking, climbing stairs) but may occur with strenuous, rapid or prolonged exertion (work, recreation)
II	Symptoms occur with prolonged or slightly more than usual activity; mild functional impairment	*Slight limitation of ordinary activity.* Angina may occur with walking or climbing stairs rapidly, after meals, in the cold, in the wind or under emotional stress, walking uphill, walking more than two blocks on the level, and climbing one flight of stairs at a normal pace under normal conditions
III	Symptoms occur with usual activities of daily living; moderate functional impairment	*Marked limitation of ordinary physical activity.* Angina may occur after walking one or two blocks on the level or climbing one flight of stairs in normal conditions at a normal pace
IV	Symptoms occur at rest; severe functional impairment	*Inability to carry on any physical activity without discomfort.* Angina may be present at rest

Adapted from Chub C. Angina pectoris and coronary disease. In Brandenburg RO, Fuster V, Giuliani ER, McGoon DC (eds): Cardiology: Fundamentals and Practice, ed 2. Chicago, Year Book Medical Publishers, 1987, pp 1073–1104.

rence. The incidence of myocardial infarction, sudden cardiac death, Prinzmetal's angina, and myocardial ischemia associated with stable angina is higher in the morning hours (8). In addition, the threshold for precipitation of anginal attacks tends to be lower in the morning. This phenomenon may lead to patients experiencing anginal attacks in the morning at lower levels of exertion than would be necessary at other times of day. Patients should be instructed to perform morning activities at a somewhat slower pace to minimize the possibility of provoking myocardial ischemia.

A number of factors have been associated with provocation of anginal episodes, including physical exertion; emotions (anger, excitation, frustration, anxiety); exposure to cold, heat, and humidity; meals; and sexual intercourse. Patients with variable-threshold angina tend to complain of angina evoked by a number of these provocative factors, including temperatures, emotion, and meals. As described earlier, those factors that tend to increase myocardial oxygen demand (exertion, sexual intercourse) precipitate angina in those patients with fixed obstructions.

CARDIAC EVALUATION AND DIAGNOSIS
Clinical Findings

The physical examination may be normal in patients with ischemic heart disease, or it may reveal the presence of other risk factors for development of atherosclerotic coronary artery disease. Resting electrocardiography is normal in approximately one-third of patients with chronic stable angina. Abnormal ECG findings include ST-segment depression, T-wave inversion, and in patients with Prinzmetal's angina, ST-segment elevation (1). Ambulatory ECG monitoring may be useful in determining the "total ischemic burden," which quantifies both asymptomatic and symptomatic ischemic episodes. This is important in assessing patients with silent myocardial ischemia.

Exercise Testing

Treadmill or bicycle exercise testing provides a method to study the relationship between myocardial oxygen supply and myocardial oxygen demand. Exercise testing is usually conducted using a specific protocol, such as the Bruce or Naughton protocol (1). These protocols allow for incremental increases in workload of exercise in stages by increasing the speed and incline of the treadmill. Endpoints that are measured during exercise testing include duration of exercise, workload achieved, ECG changes, blood pressure, and HR responses and symptoms. As described earlier, the product of heart rate and systolic blood pressure (i.e., the "double product") is used as an index of myocardial oxygen consumption. In patients with known ischemic heart disease (i.e., presence of angina symptoms, previous myocardial infarction), exercise electrocardiography provides important prognostic informa-

tion (11). In addition, exercise testing with concomitant ECG monitoring may be useful in patients with an equivocal history of chest pain, for risk stratification, to determine whether medical or surgical treatment is appropriate and for assessment of drug efficacy. Exercise electrocardiography may also provide prognostic information for certain patients. Short exercise duration with anginal symptoms, exercise-induced hypotension, and early onset of angina with ST-segment depression are all poor prognostic signs for development of cardiovascular events. It should be noted that exercise testing in the presence of drug therapy, notably β-blockers and calcium channel blockers, may complicate the interpretation of exercise testing by reducing the maximum heart rate achieved during exercise (9, 10).

Radionuclide Imaging

Other techniques are also useful in the diagnosis and classification of angina both at rest and during exercise. Thallium-201 myocardial perfusion scanning can be used in conjunction with exercise testing to provide additional information regarding reversible and irreversible defects in blood flow to the myocardium. Thallium is a potassium analog that is transported into normal cardiac cells. Thallium is injected at peak exercise, then the patient undergoes a myocardial scanning procedure. Perfusion defects that are detected at this point can represent either infarcted tissue or stress induced ischemic tissues; 2 to 3 hours later, the patient undergoes repeat myocardial scanning. Perfusion defects that are no longer present represent areas of reversible ischemia rather than infarction. Thallium myocardial perfusion scanning in conjunction with exercise testing appears to be more sensitive and specific in the diagnosis of coronary artery disease. It is more expensive than exercise testing alone, cannot usually be performed in a physician's office, and requires the injection of a radionuclide. It should be reserved for special cases, and almost always a regular exercise test should be used first (1). In patients who are unable to exercise because of certain medical conditions, alternative tests are available that use pharmacologic agents to simulate the stress of exercise. Dipyridamole or adenosine-induced vasodilation in conjunction with thallium myocardial scanning offers sensitivity and specificity for the diagnosis of coronary artery disease that is similar to exercise testing with thallium myocardial scanning (12–14).

Other Diagnostic Techniques

Echocardiography may be useful in the detection of myocardial wall motion abnormalities at rest and ischemic-induced wall motion abnormalities during exercise. Echocardiography in conjunction with exercise testing may provide additional information about left ventricular function that would not be provided by exercise testing alone.

Although each of the tests described yields important diagnostic and prognostic information in patients with coronary artery disease, definitive diagnosis and assessment of prognosis can be attained only by cardiac catheterization with left ventricular angiography. These methods allow assessment of the severity of coronary anatomy obstruction and assessment of ventricular function. Cardiac catheterization is accomplished by inserting a catheter into the brachial or femoral artery and advancing it into the left ventricle and coronary arteries. During coronary angiography, injections of radiocontrast dye are made into the coronary arteries. The coronary artery anatomy is visualized, and the extent of coronary obstruction is assessed. Because of the cost of this procedure and the risk associated with it, it has been suggested that coronary angiography should be considered only under certain circumstances. Patients who may benefit from this procedure include (1) those whose angina is unresponsive to maximal medical therapy and who are being considered for revascularization procedures (discussed later in the chapter) and (2) those in which the definitive diagnosis of coronary artery disease cannot be made by less invasive means.

PHARMACOLOGY OF AGENTS USED FOR TREATMENT OF ANGINA

Nitrates

MECHANISM OF ACTION

The intracellular mechanism of action of organic nitrates is complex. Organic nitrates enter blood vessel walls and are converted intracellularly to inorganic nitrates, which are cleaved to form nitrous oxide. Nitrous oxide reacts further with sulfhydryl groups to form S-nitrosothiols. The presence of sulfhydryl groups is necessary for the formation of nitrous oxide and S-nitrosothiols and subsequent stimulation of guanalyte cyclase (15, 16). Nitrous oxide and/or S-nitrosothiols can then activate smooth muscle guanylate cyclase, resulting in formation of intracellular cyclic guanosine monophosphate (cGMP). Cyclic guanosine monophosphate causes decreased intracellular calcium concentrations by increasing calcium extrusion from the cell.

Nitrates act as vasodilators in virtually all vascular beds, including veins, arteries, and arterioles. However, higher concentrations are required for vasodilatory effects in arteries and arterioles than in veins. This is especially true for arterioles, which require concentrations that may not be achieved clinically (17). Nitrates cause venodilation at low concentrations, thus reducing venous tone, venous return, and preload, and resulting in reductions in myocardial oxygen demand. Additionally, at higher doses, nitrates may cause arterial vasodilation, thus decreasing systolic blood pressure and afterload, and leading to reductions in myocardial oxygen demand. Because nitrates are such potent vasodilators, there may be reflex sympathetic discharge, attenuating some of the beneficial effects seen by nitrates (17).

Nitrates may also have several effects on the coronary circulation, including enhancement of coronary collateral blood flow, dilation of normal coronary arteries in patients with atherosclerosis, and dilation of coronary stenotic vessels. Lastly, nitrates may reverse coronary vasospasm, making them particularly useful in treatment of vasospastic angina. These effects may potentially lead to increases in myocardial oxygen supply.

NITRATE TOLERANCE

A decreased pharmacologic response in the presence of continuously or frequently administered nitrates is well documented and is termed "nitrate tolerance." Examples of regimens showing the development of tolerance are 24-hour ("round the clock") applications of transdermal nitroglycerin, continuous infusions of intravenous nitroglycerin, and isosorbide dinitrate (ISDN) administered four times daily. It is likely that all nitrates cause some degree of tolerance and attenuation of pharmacologic effect if used continuously (18). It appears that both the hemodynamic and antianginal effects are attenuated with continuous administration. The mechanism for nitrate tolerance is complicated, and a variety of mechanisms have been proposed, including (1) depletion of sulfhydryl donors impairing the intracellular formation of nitrous oxide and S-nitrosothiols, resulting in decreased formation of cGMP, (2) sympathetic activation following vasodilation, producing reflex vasoconstriction and sodium retention, (3) decreased hematocrit, caused by hemodilution, and increased intravascular volume, minimizing the ability of nitrates to decrease left ventricular filling pressures (18).

Prevention of nitrate tolerance clinically involves the provision of a daily nitrate-free interval. Nitrate-free intervals of at least 10 to 12 hours per day with chronic dosing have been shown to reduce occurrence of nitrate tolerance (19–21). The time of day for provision of a nitrate-free interval is usually at night; however, in patients who have nocturnal angina (i.e., most of their attacks at night), it would be prudent to move their nitrate-free interval to the daytime hours. Although nitrate-free intervals may benefit those who have angina that occurs predictably, those patients with severe or unpredictable (occurs day and night) angina would be left unprotected during the nitrate-free interval. In such patients, use of either β-blockers (alone or in combination with nitrates) or calcium channel blockers (alone or in combination with nitrates) would be appropriate.

NITRATE PRODUCTS

A number of nitrates are available for use clinically, as shown in Table 40.2. Sublingual nitroglycerin is used in the

Table 40.2.
Pharmacologic Characteristics of Currently Available Nitrates

	Dosage	Dosing Interval	Onset of Action	Duration of Action
Nitroglycerin				
Sublingual	0.15–0.6 mg	prn	1–5 min	10–30 min
Sublingual spray	0.4 mg/spray	prn	2–5 min	10–30 min
Buccal	1–3 mg	prn or q 4–5 hr (while awake)	2–5 min	3–5 hr
Oral SR	2.6–13 mg	tid, qid[a]	30–45 min	2–8 hr
Transdermal patches	2.5–15 mg/24 hr	qd (12 hr on/12 hr off)[a]	30–60 min	8–14 hr
2% ointment	½–2 in	q6h (daytime)[a]	20–60 min	3–8 hr
ISDN				
Sublingual	2.5–10 mg	prn	3–15 min	1–2 hr
Chewable	5–10 mg	prn	3–15 min	1–2 hr
Oral	5–40 mg	bid,[a] tid[a]	15–30 min	3–6 hr
Oral SR	40 mg	qd,[a] bid[a]	30–60 min	6–10 hr
ISMN				
Oral	10–20 mg	bid[a]	30 min	6–8 hr
Oral SR	60 mg	qd[a]	30 min	6–10 hr

[a]Needs nitrate-free interval when used chronically to prevent development of tolerance.

management of acute episodes of angina and for prophylaxis against an expected anginal episode. It has been shown to be effective at increasing exercise time and at relieving anginal symptoms and is available as sublingual tablets and aerosol spray. The patient should be instructed, in the event of an acute attack, to sit down, place the dose (spray or tablet) under his or her tongue, and not to swallow the tablet. Relief of pain should occur within 5 minutes. If the pain is not relieved within this time, the process may be repeated until a total of three doses have been given (approximately 15 minutes), after which time the patient should contact his or her physician or go to an emergency room. Failure of nitroglycerin to control the pain may indicate a more serious ischemia or infarction. Adverse effects seen with the sublingual form of nitroglycerin include lightheadedness, dizziness, tachycardia, and headache. Patients may or may not experience burning under the tongue after taking the sublingual dose; the absence of a burning sensation is not necessarily an indication of a lack of potency.

Nitroglycerin is a labile compound that requires special storage and handling. Sublingual tablets should be dispensed in the original, unopened, manufacturer's brown bottle. When the bottle is opened, the patient should remove the cotton plug and discard it. The tablets should be stored in the manufacturer's brown bottle, in a cool, dry place to avoid degradation of the tablets. Patients should be instructed to refill their prescriptions frequently (approximately every 6 months) to ensure adequate potency of the tablets. Because of these storage problems associated with the sublingual nitroglycerin, the aerosol spray dosage form has some distinct advantages. Each canister has a shelf life of 3 years, has 200 metered doses, and does not require the

same rigid storage conditions as the tablets. The adverse effects and efficacy of each product are similar (22).

A buccal tablet formulation of nitroglycerin is available that provides for both immediate and long-term delivery of nitroglycerin. The tablet is placed on the gum between the upper teeth and inner lip. A gel forms around the tablet, which contains nitroglycerin impregnated in a cellulose matrix. The tablet can stay in place for hours and provides both immediate and sustained delivery of nitroglycerin as long as the tablet remains intact, which may be as long as 6 hours in some patients. This is advantageous in that the tablet can provide both acute and prophylactic treatment of anginal episodes. Tolerance to the effects of buccal nitroglycerin is minimal, mainly because the tablet is not in place while the patient sleeps, allowing for a nitrate-free interval.

Nitroglycerin 2% ointment has been documented to have efficacy in patients with angina (23). It is easy to use but rather inconvenient for patients because of the messiness that is involved with application of the ointment. Patients should be instructed to apply the specified dose (a 1/2- to 2-inch line of ointment) to the chest, back or upper limbs. Patients should rotate the site where the application is made in an attempt to reduce skin irritation. Family members or other persons applying the ointment to the patient should be instructed to use gloves during the application because of the chance for nitroglycerin absorption. The ointment can be removed easily by removing the paper containing the ointment and wiping the skin clean of any residual ointment. There will continue to be absorption of nitroglycerin for a short time because the skin acts as a reservoir for the drug.

Another form of topically available nitroglycerin, which

has become enormously popular since its introduction in 1982, is nitroglycerin transdermal patches. These patches were designed to deliver a constant amount of nitroglycerin per hour over a specific period, maintaining nitroglycerin concentrations at steady state. Patients should be instructed to apply a new patch each day to a hairless area of the chest, back, or upper limbs. The site should be rotated daily to prevent local skin irritation. Various factors may increase the absorption of the drug, including physical exercise and high temperatures (e.g., saunas). The ease of administration compared to nitroglycerin ointment has made these patches very popular with patients; however, the issue of tolerance necessitates that patients wear the patch for no more than 12 to 14 hours per day.

Two oral organic nitrates are available in the United States: isosorbide dinitrate (ISDN) and isosorbide 5-mononitrate (5-ISMN). Both are available as immediate release and sustained release preparations. ISDN is also available as a sublingual and chewable tablet, which can be used for treatment and prophylaxis of acute anginal episodes. The sublingual tablet has a somewhat slower onset and a longer duration of action than sublingual nitroglycerin. The chewable tablet also has a longer duration of action than sublingual nitroglycerin. When patients chew the tablet, whatever particles remain in the mouth will result in continued absorption.

ISDN is metabolized to two metabolites, 2-ISMN and 5-ISMN, the latter of which is marketed as a separate entity. ISDN has widely variable bioavailability and a plasma half-life of 1 to 2 hours, whereas 5-ISMN has nearly complete bioavailability and a longer plasma half-life (24), resulting in more predictable concentrations after oral dosing and allowing for once or twice daily dosing. Tolerance to the pharmacologic effects of ISDN and 5-ISMN have been described for both agents (20, 25). Avoidance of tolerance with ISDN may be attained by administration of the immediate release compound three times daily, with the last dose taken with the evening meal (20). This provides a nitrate-free interval during the nighttime period. Twice daily dosing schedules of immediate release 5-ISMN, administered at 8:00 AM and 3:00 PM, enhanced exercise performance for 7 hours after the morning dose and for 5 hours after the afternoon dose (21).

ADVERSE EFFECTS

Adverse effects caused by all nitrates are an extension of their pharmacologic actions. Headache occurs in most patients and may be described as a throbbing or pulsating sensation. Most patients can take over-the-counter analgesics (aspirin, acetaminophen, and so on) to alleviate this problem. Other adverse effects related to vasodilation include hypotension, dizziness, lightheadedness, and facial flushing. Reflex tachycardia may also occur because of their

potent peripheral vasodilating effects, which causes sympathetic nervous system activation.

β-Blockers

MECHANISM OF ACTION

β-adrenergic receptor blockers competitively inhibit the binding of circulating and neurally released catecholamines to the β-adrenergic receptor. β-receptor blockade attenuates the cardiac responses to adrenergic stimulation by catecholamines and exerts a beneficial effect in angina, mainly because of its effect on heart rate and contractility at high levels of sympathetic stimulation. The beneficial effects provided by β-blockers in angina are several-fold. First, β-blockers reduce heart rate mainly during times of sympathetic stimulation, which results in reduced cardiac work and thus myocardial oxygen demand. In addition, by slowing heart rate, β-blockers increase diastolic filling time, resulting in improved oxygen supply. Second, β-blockers reduce myocardial contractility and arterial blood pressure and, as a result, reduce myocardial oxygen demand. A potential problem with β-blockers is that they may increase coronary vasoconstriction. In the presence of blockade of β_2-receptors, which mediate vasodilation, there is unopposed α-receptor-mediated vasoconstriction. This is a particular concern in patients with rest or variant angina, where β-blockers could potentially precipitate an anginal episode (26, 27).

PHARMACOLOGIC CHARACTERISTICS

The β-blockers differ in their pharmacologic characteristics, including receptor selectivity, pharmacokinetics, lipophilicity, and intrinsic sympathomimetic activity (Table 40.3) (26, 27).

β-adrenergic receptors can be divided into at least two subtypes (β_1 and β_2-adrenoceptors) based on the physiologic responses they mediate. β_1-receptors predominately reside in the myocardium, and their stimulation results in increased heart rate, myocardial contractility, and atrioventricular nodal conduction. β_2-receptors also reside in the heart but are the predominant receptors in pulmonary and vascular tissue, where they are responsible for bronchodilation and vasodilation. β-blockers can be classified as "nonselective" or "cardioselective." Cardioselective agents (atenolol, metoprolol, and acebutolol) are relatively more selective toward binding to β_1 receptors than β_2 receptors. Theoretically, β_1-selective agents would be more effective at antagonizing the effects of catecholamines at β_1-receptors while causing minimal β_2-receptor blockade. β_1-selective antagonists have a theoretical advantage in patients with pulmonary disease (e.g., chronic obstructive pulmonary disease, asthma) or when blockade of β_2-receptor is clearly undesirable, such as in patients with peripheral vascular disease or insulin-dependent diabetes mellitus. However, it is important to remember that

Table 40.3.
Pharmacologic Characteristics of the Currently Available β-Blockers

Agent	Receptor Selectivity	ISA	Lipid Solubility	Primary Route of Elimination	Half-Life (hr)	Usual Maintenance Dose
Acebutolol	β_1	+	Moderate	Renal/Hepatic	3–4	200–600 mg BID
Atenolol[a]	β_1	0	Low	Renal	6–9	50–100 mg QD
Betaxolol	β_1	0	Low	Hepatic	14–22	10–20 mg QD
Bisoprolol	β_1	0	Low	Renal	9–12	5–10 mg QD
Carteolol	$\beta_1\ \beta_2$	++	Low	Renal	5–6	2.5–10 mg QD
Metoprolol[a]	β_1	0	Moderate	Hepatic	3–7	50–100 mg BID
Nadolol[a]	$\beta_1\ \beta_2$	0	Low	Renal	14–24	40–80 mg QD
Penbutol	$\beta_1\ \beta_2$	+	High	Hepatic	5	20 mg QD
Pindolol	$\beta_1\ \beta_2$	+++	Moderate	Renal/Hepatic	3–4	5–20 mg BID
Propranolol[a]	$\beta_1\ \beta_2$	0	High	Hepatic	3–5	Variable
Timolol	$\beta_1\ \beta_2$	0	Moderate	Hepatic	4–5	10–20 mg BID
Labetalol	$\beta_1\ \beta_2\ \alpha_1$	0	Moderate	Hepatic	6–8	200–400 mg BID

Abbreviations: ISA, intrinsic sympathomimetic activity; BID; twice daily; QD, once daily.
[a]Agents approved by the Food and Drug Administration for the treatment of chronic stable angina.
Note: Nadolol t½. Author has published paper on healthy volunteers with mean nadolol t½ of 11.6 hours. 20 hours is certainly not the low end of nadolol t½ (Am Heart J1990;120:572) 14-24 hrs is cited in numerous β-blocker reviews, including Med Clin N Am 1988;72:37 Acebutolol- 3 different sources cite lipid solubility of acebutolol as *moderate*.

cardioselectivity is relative, and achievement of high enough concentrations, which can occur within the clinically used dosage range, will result in the loss of cardioselectivity.

Several β-blockers possess intrinsic sympathomimetic activity (ISA). These compounds produce some degree of β-receptor stimulation at low states of sympathetic activation. However, at higher levels of sympathetic activation (e.g., during exercise), these agents act as antagonists. Few data suggest that drugs with ISA are more beneficial than agents without ISA in the treatment of angina. Because these drugs tend not to affect resting heart rate or cardiac output, they may have theoretical advantages in a patient with already low resting heart rate and cardiac output. Finally, these agents may be detrimental in patients with rest angina or postmyocardial infarction.

Given the differences in pharmacologic characteristics that have been described, it should be emphasized that it appears as if all β-blockers, regardless of differing pharmacologic characteristics, are effective in treating angina (28).

The pharmacokinetic properties of β-blockers are extremely variable and are related to the drug's lipophilicity or hydrophilicity. In general, drugs that are highly lipid soluble tend to be well absorbed from the gastrointestinal tract, hepatically metabolized, have highly variable bioavailability, undergo extensive hepatic "first pass" metabolism, and have short plasma terminal elimination half-lives. Table 40.3 lists the lipid solubility of a number of β-blockers ranging from low to high lipid solubility. β-blockers that are more water soluble tend to be incompletely absorbed from the gastrointestinal tract, are eliminated mainly unchanged in the urine, have less variable bioavailability, negligible first pass hepatic metabo-

lism, and longer plasma terminal elimination half-lives. Although the pharmacokinetics of β-blockers are highly variable, most of these compounds can be dosed once or twice daily for the treatment of angina. The pharmacokinetic properties of a drug and individual patient characteristics should guide the selection of the appropriate agent. For example, if atenolol were to be used in a patient with angina and impaired renal function, a lengthening of the dosing interval may be necessary since atenolol is eliminated mainly by the kidneys.

ADVERSE EFFECTS

The adverse effects associated with β-blockers are an extension of their pharmacologic effects and include sinus bradycardia, sinus arrest, atrioventricular (AV) block, reduced left ventricular function, bronchoconstriction, fatigue, depression, nightmares, sexual dysfunction, and intensification of insulin-induced hypoglycemia. Because of these effects, β-blockers should be avoided or used with caution in patients with bradyarrhythmias, AV conduction disturbances, asthma or chronic obstructive pulmonary disease, congestive heart failure, diabetes mellitus, or peripheral vascular disease.

A final issue of clinical importance is the β-blocker withdrawal syndrome. Prolonged therapy with β-receptor antagonists results in an increase in the number of β-receptors. Abrupt withdrawal of β-blockers in these patients may result in an increased number of sensitized receptors available for adrenergic stimulation and possible precipitation of anginal syndromes, unstable angina, and possibly myocardial infarction. Because of this, it is prudent, when discontinuing the use of β-blockers, to decrease the dose gradually over a 1- to 2-week period.

Calcium Channel Blockers

MECHANISM OF ACTION

Calcium channel blockers are a chemically heterogeneous group of agents that block the transmembrane flux of calcium into cardiac and vascular smooth muscle cells, thus reducing intracellular calcium concentrations. This reduction in intracellular calcium concentrations results in a reduction of the excitation-contraction-coupling mechanism responsible for myocardial and smooth muscle contraction (29).

PHARMACOLOGIC CHARACTERISTICS

Because of the chemical heterogeneity of calcium channel blockers and the existence of at least two receptor binding sites (30), these agents exert different pharmacologic effects that depend on the pharmacologic classification of the agent. Calcium channel blockers can be placed into one of three distinct pharmacologic classes that are based on chemical structure, as shown in Table 40.4: dihydropyridines, phenylalkylamines, and benzothiazepines. Calcium channel blockers have five major physiologic effects: decreased systemic vascular resistance, decreased coronary vascular resistance, increased epicardial coronary artery size, decreased myocardial contractility, and slowing of sinus and AV nodal conduction. Reductions in systemic vascular resistance, heart rate, and myocardial contractility will result in decreased myocardial oxygen demand, whereas decreased coronary vascular resistance and increased epicardial coronary artery size will increase myocardial oxygen supply.

As described earlier for the β-blockers, selection of the most appropriate calcium channel blocker should be based on both the characteristics of the drug and the characteristics of the patient being treated.

ADVERSE EFFECTS

Calcium channel blockers are relatively well tolerated. Most of the adverse effects associated with their use are related to their pharmacologic effects. The degree or significance of each adverse effect depends on the individual agents. Flushing, headache, and dizziness are related to the vasodilatory effects of calcium channel blockers. Dihydropyridines, which are the most potent peripheral vasodilators, tend to cause these adverse effects to the greatest extent. Peripheral edema, likely related to arteriolar vasodilation, is also most commonly seen in patients treated with dihydropyridines. Depression of myocardial contractility occurs most commonly in patients treated with verapamil and, to a lesser extent, with diltiazem. These two agents should be used with caution in patients with congestive heart failure or in combination with β-blockers. Bradycardia and atrioventricular block can be seen in patients receiving verapamil and, to a lesser extent, diltiazem. These two adverse effects would occur most commonly in patients with baseline sinus bradycardia or AV nodal dysfunction. Because nifedepine is such a potent peripheral vasodilator, reflex sympathetic activation may actually increase heart rate, leading to increased myocardial oxygen demand and precipitation of angina. Calcium channel blockers may also cause gastrointestinal adverse effects such as nausea and constipation. The latter is caused most commonly by verapamil and may be particularly problematic in the elderly. Bepridil has been associated with

Table 40.4.
Pharmacologic Characteristics of Currently Available Calcium Channel Blockers

	Heart Rate	Myocardial Contractility	AV Nodal Conduction	Vasodilation		Half-Life	Usual Maintenance Dose[a]
				Peripheral	Coronary		
Dihydropyridines							
Amlodipine[b]	Reflex ↑	−	−	+++	++	30–50 hr	5–10 mg qd
Felodipine	Reflex ↑	−	−	+++	++	11–16 hr	5–10 md qd
Isradapine	−	−	−	+++	++	8 hr	5–10 mg bid
Nicardipine[c]	Reflex ↑	−	−	+++	++	2–4 hr	20–40 mg tid
Nifedipine[b]	Reflex ↑	↓ −	−	+++	++	2–5 hr	10–20 mg tid
Phenylalkylamines							
Verapamil[b]	↓	↓↓	↓↓	++	+	3–7 hr	80–120 mg tid
Bepridil[c]	↓	↓	↓	+	+	24 hr	300 mg qd
Benzothiazepines							
Diltiazem[b]	↓	↓	↓	+	++	4–6 hr	60–90 mg tid–qid

↑ increase, ↓ decrease, − no change
[a]Maintenance dosages represent those of immediate release preparations. Some but not all of sustained release preparations of calcium channel blockers are approved for treatment of angina; see manufacturer's literature regarding the approved indications and usual dosage regimens for sustained release preparations.
[b]Approved by the Food and Drug Administration for the treatment of chronic stable angina and angina associated with coronary artery spasm.
[c]Approved by the Food and Drug Administration for the treatment of chronic stable angina.

Class I antiarrhythmics. It can induce new arrhythmias, including ventricular fibrillation. In addition, because of its ability to prolong the QT interval, bepridil can cause torsade de pointes type ventricular tachycardia. Because bepridil can cause serious ventricular arrhythmias and agranulocytosis, its use should be reserved for patients failing to respond optimally to other antianginal drugs.

MANAGEMENT OF CHRONIC STABLE ANGINA PECTORIS

The goals of treatment for chronic stable angina are to minimize the frequency and severity of angina and increase patients' functional capacity while causing as few adverse effects as possible. The management of chronic stable angina involves four areas: correction of concomitant cardiovascular risk factors, lifestyle modifications, medical treatment, and revascularization techniques.

General Management

Correction and treatment of all modifiable cardiovascular risk factors is important for multiple reasons. Cardiac rehabilitation and efforts targeted at exercise, lipid management, hypertension control, and smoking cessation can reduce cardiovascular mortality, improve functional capacity, and attenuate myocardial ischemia. Correction of lipid disorders may also retard the progression and foster the reversal of coronary atherosclerosis and reduce the risk of further coronary events (31). Other cardiovascular risk factor reductions should include weight loss if overweight and alcohol consumption only in moderation (31). Smoking cessation is especially important in patients with ischemic heart disease. Smoking is associated with increased morbidity and mortality, silent ischemia, arrhythmias, and coronary vasospasm in patients with coronary artery disease (31). A number of different techniques are available for assisting in smoking cessation, including pharmacologic and nonpharmacologic approaches. Although risk factor reductions may not reverse existing ischemic heart disease, they may aid in the secondary prevention of cardiovascular events. As with any disease or syndrome that increases cardiovascular risk (e.g., hypertension), the first goal of therapy is to decrease this risk. Health care providers can play an important role in educating the patients about cardiovascular risk factor reduction.

Alterations in lifestyle are also important in patients with coronary artery disease because of the many factors that may provoke anginal episodes. Inclusion of the patient's family in discussions regarding lifestyle modifications may help patient compliance regarding these changes, but more important, it fosters an understanding of certain limitations that may be placed on the patient. Patients should be counseled to modify their participation in strenuous activities in an attempt to avoid excessive fatigue and exhaustion; an example of this would be the use of a golf cart rather than walking while playing golf. Another lifestyle modification would be the reduction or elimination of factors known to precipitate an anginal episode. Some patients may know exactly how much exertion they can tolerate before having an anginal attack; other patients may need to "learn" what their threshold is. In general, patients should perform morning activities at a slower pace and avoid sudden bursts of activity. Patients who are particularly susceptible to heat precipitating an anginal attack should be in an air conditioned environment. Patients who develop angina when going outside when it is very cold may cover their mouth and face with a scarf. Eating small meals or napping after meals may help avoid postprandial anginal attacks. Lastly, emotional outbursts (e.g., anger, anxiety, frustration) should be avoided.

Exercise training programs are also an important lifestyle modification. Exercise programs should adhere to accepted guidelines (32) for patients with heart diseases. Exercise programs are useful as adjuncts to reducing other coronary risk factors, including obesity, diabetes, and hypertension. Exercise has a beneficial conditioning effect both on skeletal and cardiac muscle and may decrease oxygen demand in muscle for any given level of exercise. Exercise also favorably affects fat and carbohydrate metabolism, which may aid in the management of other cardiovascular risk factors.

Drug Therapy of Stable Angina

Decisions about when to initiate drug therapy in a particular patient depend on the frequency and severity of anginal attacks. If angina occurs less than once weekly, institution of nitroglycerin tablets or spray for treatment of acute attacks is usually indicated. The specific dose administered depends on the patient's hemodynamic response. Sublingual nitroglycerin tablets are available over a wide dosing range from 0.15 to 0.6 mg, whereas the spray delivers 0.4 mg with each actuation. These products are also useful for the prevention of angina when taken just prior to the initiation of exertion or some other event that precipitates angina.

If angina occurs more frequently than one episode per week, the use of chronic prophylactic therapy is necessary. Three drug classes can be used for this purpose: nitrates, β-blockers, and calcium channel blockers. The selection of an initial drug for chronic treatment of angina should be based on the patient's characteristics and concomitant conditions (see Table 40.5). The initial selection is usually a long-acting nitrate product, which includes oral nitroglycerin capsules, transdermal nitroglycerin patches, nitroglycerin ointment, ISDN, or ISMN. The selection of one product over another should be based on patient preference and ease of administration. A 10- to 12-hour nitrate-free period is necessary with all these products to avoid development of tolerance. Regardless of which drug is selected, it should be started at a low dose in order to

Table 40.5.

Recommended Drug Therapy in Patients Who Have Angina in Conjunction with Other Medical Conditions

Clinical Condition	Preferred Drug	Drugs to Avoid or Use with Caution
Cardiac Arrhythmias/Conduction Disturbances		
Sinus bradycardia	Nitrate, nifedipine	Diltiazem, verapamil, β-blockers
Sinus tachycardia (no CHF)	β-blocker, verapamil, diltiazem	Nifedepine, nitrates
Supraventricular tachycardia	Verapamil or β-blocker	
Atrioventricular block	Nifedipine, nitrate	β-blockers, diltiazem, verapamil
Atrial fibrillation	Verapamil, β-blocker, diltiazem	
Ventricular arrhythmias	β-blocker	
Left Ventricular Dysfunction	ISDN + CHF therapy	β-blockers, diltiazem, verapamil
Miscellaneous Conditions		
Postmyocardial infarction	Non-ISA β-blockers	ISA β-blockers
Systemic hypertension	β-blockers or CCBs	
Severe preexisting headaches	β-blockers	Nitrates, dihydropyridines
COPD/asthma	Nitrates, CCBs	β-blockers
Hyperthyroidism	β-blockers	
Raynaud's syndrome	Nitrates, CCBs	β-blockers
Claudication	Nitrates, CCBs	β-blockers
Depression	Nitrates, CCBs	β-blockers
IDDM	Nitrates, CCBs	β-blockers

Abbreviations: COPD, chronic obstructive pulmonary disease; ISA, intrinsic sympathomimetic activity; IDDM, insulin-dependent diabetes mellitus; ISDN, isosorbide dinitrate; CCB, calcium channel blocker

Adapted from Shub C, Vlietstra RE, McGoon MD. Selection of optimal drug therapy for the patient with angina pectoris. Mayo Clin Proc 1985;60:539–548.

reduce the incidence of adverse effects early in therapy. Subsequent dosage adjustments can be based on incidence of the adverse effects, headache, dizziness, and hypotension. Effectiveness can be assessed by decreased use of sublingual nitroglycerin for acute attacks, improvement in patient's quality of life (i.e., ability to have normal activities without experiencing angina), and objective assessment by exercise testing.

β-blockers may also be selected as initial therapy for angina in those patients with concomitant hypertension, previous history of myocardial infarction, or migraine headaches. This allows treatment of two conditions with single drug therapy. In addition, β-blockers may be selected in those patients who cannot tolerate nitrate therapy because of adverse effects or failure to suppress angina, especially if the patient has mainly fixed-threshold angina. All β-blockers appear to be effective in the management of stable angina though all are not approved by the FDA for this purpose (see Table 40.3 for approved agents). Selection of the initial agent should be based on the pharmacologic characteristics discussed earlier.

Calcium channel blockers are also effective and can be used as initial therapy for angina. They are particularly useful in patients with contraindications to β-blockers or patients with mainly variable-threshold angina. All calcium channel blockers appear to be effective in the management of stable angina though all are not approved by the FDA for this purpose (see Table 40.4 for approved agents). The initial agent selected should be based on the pharmacologic characteristics discussed earlier.

Combination drug therapy is frequently used when monotherapy is unsuccessful in the management of anginal episodes. It should be emphasized that combination drug therapy should be reserved for those patients who do not benefit or who have intolerable adverse effects at maximal doses of a single drug. Because tolerance develops to chronic therapy with nitrates, β-blockers and calcium channel blockers are frequently used in combination with nitrates to prevent angina occurrence during nitrate-free intervals.

The combination of β-blockers and nitrates is used commonly and has a therapeutic rationale based on the pharmacology of each drug class. Nitrates offset the β-blockers' potential deleterious increase in left ventricular diastolic pressures and volumes by reducing preload, whereas the β-blockers inhibit the nitrate-induced sympathetically mediated reflex tachycardia. Combination therapy with calcium channel blockers and nitrates also offers the same therapeutic rationale although the combination of dihydropyridines and nitrates may cause excessive hypotension, rebound tachycardia, and headaches.

Therapy with a β-blocker and calcium channel blocker should theoretically reduce myocardial oxygen demand further than could each agent alone. In addition, since β-blockers may increase coronary artery tone, the addition of a calcium channel blocker may attenuate this potentially detrimental effect. A number of studies have documented the efficacy of these two drug classes in combination (33). The concern regarding the use of these drugs is the potential for additive adverse effects; specifically, slowing of AV and sinus nodal conduction, hypotension, and impairment of systolic function. These concerns may be minimized by selection of patients who are least likely to experience these adverse effects. Patients who are normotensive, have little or minimal systolic dysfunction, and have no conduction disturbances are the best candidates for this therapy. The most dangerous combination, with regard to potentiated adverse effects, is likely to be the combination of a β-blocker and verapamil, because verapamil is the most potent calcium channel blocker at slowing AV nodal conduction and decreasing contractility.

Lastly, with regard to combination therapy, calcium channel blockers have been used in combination. Each class of calcium channel blockers has distinct differences in their effects on cardiac contractility, coronary artery blood flow, AV nodal conduction, and peripheral vascular resistance. Given these differences, it is possible that interactions may occur at the receptor level if they are used in combination. In fact, the binding of dihydropyridine compounds to their receptor is enhanced by diltiazem. The opposite is also true. Conversely, verapamil and dihydropyridines antagonize each other's binding. This suggests that some rationale exists for the use of a combination such as nifedipine and diltiazem to produce beneficial pharmacologic effects. A number of small clinical studies have evaluated the combination of various calcium channel blockers in the treatment of ischemic heart disease and found the combination to be effective but associated with frequent adverse effects. With the limited research experience collected to date on this topic, the routine use of combination calcium channel blockers cannot be recommended.

Platelet aggregation is important in the pathogenesis of the acute coronary syndromes, but less important in the pathogenesis of stable angina. Data from two studies in patients with chronic stable angina, (34, 35) show that aspirin reduced the incidence of first myocardial infarction. The mechanism of aspirin's benefit appears to be an inhibition of platelet aggregation and thrombi formation at the site of atherosclerotic plaque disruption. Although the lowest effective dose is controversial, it is recommended that all patients with angina or clinical or laboratory evidence of ischemic heart disease receive chronic aspirin (160 to 325 mg/day) therapy indefinitely (36).

In those patients in which medical therapy is not effective in reducing the number of anginal syndromes or where the underlying coronary artery disease is severe, revascularization therapy with either percutaneous transluminal coronary angioplasty or coronary artery bypass surgery may be an alternative.

MANAGEMENT OF SILENT MYOCARDIAL ISCHEMIA

Therapies used for treatment of silent myocardial ischemia are similar to those used to treat other types of chronic angina, including nitrates, β-blockers, and calcium channel blockers. There is, however, a great deal of controversy regarding whether or not to treat silent myocardial ischemia. The agents described do reduce the number of ischemic episodes that patients experience (37), but there is a lack of evidence that suppression of nonsymptomatic ischemic episodes will improve long-term prognosis. A recent trial (38) has shown atenolol to be effective at reducing ischemic episodes in asymptomatic and mildly symptomatic patients and at reducing cardiovascular events. The question remains whether or not suppression of ischemic episodes in these types of patients will translate into reductions in long-term mortality. Additional studies in this area are currently being conducted and are being planned for the future (37, 39). For now, it appears that the routine treatment of silent myocardial ischemia cannot be recommended, but should be reserved for those patients who are at high risk for other cardiovascular events or those patients who have other conditions (e.g., hypertension) that require drug therapy with antianginal drugs (e.g., β-blockers or calcium channel blockers).

VARIANT ANGINA

Variant angina or Prinzmetal's angina is myocardial ischemia that is associated with coronary artery vasospasm and is not necessarily associated with atherosclerotic coronary artery disease. Imbalance between myocardial oxygen supply and demand is caused by reduced myocardial oxygen supply due to a critical narrowing of a large coronary vessel. The clinical manifestations of variant angina are similar to those seen with stable angina though the pain may be somewhat more intense. The patient's history of angina is usually quite different since pain usually occurs at rest most frequently between midnight and 8:00 AM (40).

Sublingual nitroglycerin therapy should be used for acute anginal episodes, as discussed for chronic stable angina. Calcium channel blockers are effective in the chronic prophylactic management of patients with variant angina. The selection of a particular drug depends mainly on patient characteristics. Nitrates are also effective in these patients, but the scheduling of a nitrate-free period may not necessarily be best during the sleeping hours. Because most episodes occur in the nighttime or morning hours, the nitrate-free interval should be scheduled during the day. Nitrate therapy should be reserved for patients with continued symptoms on maximized therapy with calcium channel blockers. Combination therapy with two calcium channel blockers (diltiazem and nifedipine) has been shown to reduce frequency of angina episodes in patients not receiving full benefit from either agent alone. This drug combination was associated with frequent adverse effects (41). Finally, as described earlier, β-blockers should not be used in the treatment of variant angina since they may exacerbate coronary artery vasospasm.

UNSTABLE ANGINA

Unstable angina is a syndrome that is intermediate between chronic stable angina and acute myocardial infarction. The quality of the chest pain is similar to that of chronic stable angina though the intensity and duration may be greater. Unstable angina has three primary modes of presentation (1, 42). The first, and usually most severe presentation of unstable angina, is rest angina, which is greater than 20 minutes in duration. New onset angina (usually within the previous 1 to 2 months), which occurs with minimal exertion, is also classified as unstable angina. Finally, a patient with previously diagnosed chronic stable angina whose angina is increasing in frequency or duration or who has a lower threshold for symptom onset is also described as having unstable angina. The electrocardiographic changes typically observed in patients with unstable angina are ST segment changes (either elevation or depression) and T-wave inversion. These ECG changes are commonly observed only during the ischemic episode and reverse with relief of chest pain (1).

A working diagnosis of unstable angina is typically based on the patient's history and chief complaints. Acute myocardial infarction is ruled out by measurement of serial cardiac isoenzymes (e.g., creatine kinase—MB, lactate dehydrogenase 1 and 2). Once the patient's condition is stabilized, evaluation of the degree of ischemia and underlying atherosclerotic disease can usually be assessed by exercise testing and/or cardiac catheterization.

Pathophysiology

As with chronic stable angina, unstable angina can be caused by increases in myocardial oxygen demand or decreased myocardial oxygen supply. However, in most patients, unstable angina is due to a decrease in myocardial oxygen supply. Three processes contribute to the decreased myocardial oxygen supply in most patients with unstable angina: progression of atherosclerosis, platelet aggregation,

and thrombus formation. In some patients, coronary vasospasm or increases in vasomotor tone may also contribute to the decrease in myocardial oxygen supply.

In patients who have either new onset angina or worsening of previously stable angina, the most likely cause is rapid progression of atherosclerosis. Rapid progression of atherosclerosis is likely due to fissuring or disruption of the atherosclerotic plaque, leading to platelet aggregation and thrombus formation. As the plaque heals, the thrombus is incorporated, and the size of the atherosclerotic plaque increases (43). This process is depicted in the lower portion of Figure 40.2. Pathologic studies suggest that this is a common, recurrent series of events in most patients with unstable angina. The more common and most severe presentation of unstable angina is rest angina for greater than 20 minutes. Like the patients described earlier, plaque disruption, platelet aggregation, and thrombus formation are important pathophysiologic events in the development of this form of unstable angina. In this case, the thrombus is causing a partial to nearly complete occlusion of the coronary artery and is responsible for the symptoms. This differs from the pathophysiology of acute myocardial infarction in that acute myocardial infarction is usually associated with total occlusion of the coronary artery.

Treatment of Unstable Angina

Treatment approaches for patients with unstable angina are based on their risk of nonfatal myocardial infarction or death. Patients with new onset angina or worsening angina are considered low risk. Patients with rest pain for longer than 20 minutes are considered intermediate or high risk, depending on several other factors (42). Treatment guidelines for patients with unstable angina were developed and

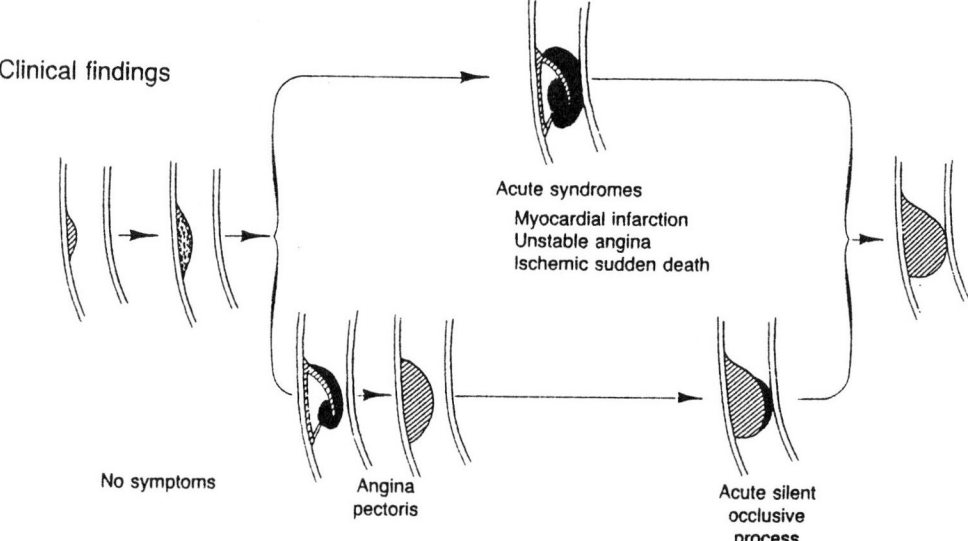

Figure 40.2. Progression of coronary atherosclerosis according to clinical findings. Adapted from reference 43.

published by the U.S. Public Health Service and the National Heart Lung and Blood Institute in 1994. These guidelines can be obtained from the U.S. Department of Health and Human Services (AHCPR Publication No. 94-0602). A summary of the recommendations has also been published (44). The treatment recommendations that follow are based on these guidelines.

There are two general goals of therapy in the management of patients with unstable angina (42). The primary goal is to prevent myocardial infarction by inhibiting extension of the thrombus. The second goal is to reverse the ischemia and relieve the chest pain by either increasing myocardial oxygen supply or decreasing myocardial oxygen demand.

ASPIRIN

Patients suspected of having unstable angina or acute myocardial infarction should immediately be given aspirin 160 to 325 mg to chew and swallow, except in the case of a definite contraindication (e.g., documented hypersensitivity, active bleeding). This recommendation is based on data showing that early administration of aspirin is superior to placebo in preventing progression of unstable angina to acute myocardial infarction (45). Meta-analysis of the trials lasting greater than 3 months suggest that aspirin therapy reduces the risk of acute myocardial infarction by 48% and the risk of death by 51% (46). Therefore, it is recommended that patients with unstable angina be placed on life-long aspirin therapy unless there are clear contraindications. The appropriate dosage of aspirin in these patients is the subject of some debate. The data suggest that dosages greater than 325 mg per day are no more effective than 325 mg per day though the higher dosages are associated with more adverse effects (46). Doses of 75 to 160 mg per day seem to have efficacy similar to 325 mg per day (46). Therefore, it is recommended that all unstable angina patients take aspirin 75 to 325 mg daily; with selection of the dose based on clinician and/or patient preference. Because the lower dosage forms of aspirin ("baby aspirin") tend to be more expensive, many clinicians choose to use the regular strength (325-mg) aspirin.

HEPARIN

Heparin therapy is indicated in patients with intermediate- to high-risk unstable angina. In this patient group, the primary goal of therapy is to prevent extension of the thrombus and thus prevent acute myocardial infarction. Although aspirin is superior to placebo in these patients, data suggest that heparin alone may be superior to aspirin alone (45, 47). In a study of 484 unstable angina patients, myocardial infarction occurred in 3.7% of aspirin-treated patients and 0.8% of heparin-treated patients (47). Interestingly, some studies have not shown heparin to be superior to aspirin or placebo (48, 49). Nonetheless, the

expert panel that developed the clinical practice guidelines recommend that heparin be administered immediately when a diagnosis of intermediate- to high-risk unstable angina is made (42). In most patients, heparin will be given along with aspirin as described. The recommended dosage regimen is 80 units/kg intravenous bolus followed by a constant rate infusion of 18 units/kg per hour adjusted to an activated partial thromboplastin time (aPTT) of 1.5 to 2 times control. In institutions not equipped to administer heparin by continuous infusion, the recommended regimen is 5000 units intravenous bolus every 4 hours (42). Heparin therapy should be continued for 2 to 5 days or until a revascularization procedure, such as coronary artery bypass grafting or angioplasty, is performed (42).

OTHER ANTIPLATELET AND ANTICOAGULANT DRUGS

The effects of several other antiplatelet agents on acute myocardial infarction and death have been studied in patients with unstable angina. Dipyridamole plus aspirin has been shown to have efficacy similar to aspirin, suggesting that dipyridamole is an unnecessary addition (46). Dipyridamole alone has been studied only on a limited basis, and meta-analysis suggests that it is not significantly better than placebo (46). Sulfinpyrazone may be more effective than placebo (46) but is inferior to aspirin (50). Ticlopidine has been shown to be superior to placebo, but it appears to offer no greater effect than aspirin (46). The higher cost of ticlopidine and more significant adverse effect profile, notably neutropenia, makes aspirin the preferred agent over ticlopidine. Ticlopidine would, however, be a reasonable alternative in patients with hypersensitivity to aspirin. In summary, several antiplatelet agents have been studied, but none have proved to be superior to aspirin.

Intense investigation surrounds the use of anticoagulants, such as hirudin, which directly inhibit thrombin. It is thought these agents may be more efficacious than heparin and may require less intensive monitoring. However, several comparative studies of hirudin versus heparin in patients with unstable angina and/or acute myocardial infarction were stopped prematurely because the rate of intracranial hemorrhage was higher with hirudin than heparin (51). Thus, the future role, if any, of these agents in treatment of patients with unstable angina remains to be clarified.

THROMBOLYTICS

Thrombolytic agents lyse existing clots through activation of plasminogen and have been proved to significantly reduce mortality in patients with acute myocardial infarction. Since the primary pathophysiologic abnormality in unstable angina is thrombus formation, and since unstable angina can be a precursor to acute myocardial infarction, it seemed reasonable that thrombolytic agents would be beneficial in patients with unstable angina. However, multiple clinical studies have been conducted with thrombolytic agents in unstable angina and have consistently shown they provide no beneficial effect (52). In fact, some studies suggest thrombolytics may be detrimental in patients with unstable angina (52, 53). Thus, use of thrombolytic therapy in patients with unstable angina is not recommended.

β-BLOCKERS

β-blockers are effective antiischemic and antianginal agents that act to decrease myocardial oxygen demand by decreasing heart rate and contractility. It is recommended that, unless there are contraindications, all patients with unstable angina should receive β-blocker therapy (42). Meta-analysis of randomized, placebo-controlled β-blocker trials in unstable angina suggest that β-blockers decrease the risk of acute myocardial infarction by 13% (42). Use of β-blockers in unstable angina has not been clearly shown to reduce mortality. However, the mortality-reducing effects of β-blockers in acute myocardial infarction and postmyocardial infarction patients are clear, and these data help form the basis of the recommendation for β-blockers in patients with unstable angina.

β-blockers should not be given to patients with marked first-degree AV block (ECG PR interval greater than 0.24 second), second- or third-degree AV block, a history of asthma, or severe left ventricular dysfunction with congestive heart failure or cardiogenic shock. In patients with bradycardia (heart rate less than 60 beats per minute) or hypotension (SBP less than 90 mm Hg), β-blockers should be withheld until heart rate or blood pressure increases. In patients with COPD (who may have a component of reactive airways disease), or diabetes mellitus, β-blockers should be used cautiously at first, and a β_1-selective agent may be preferable in these patients over a nonselective agent.

Intravenous β-blocker therapy should be instituted in high-risk patients and oral therapy initiated in intermediate-and low-risk patients. Examples of the most commonly employed intravenous β-blocker protocols are (1) metoprolol 5 mg intravenous every 5 minutes times three doses, followed immediately by initiation of metoprolol 50 mg orally every 6 hours; (2) atenolol 5 mg intravenous, repeated again in 5 minutes, with subsequent initiation of 50 to 100 mg oral atenolol daily. The target resting heart rate for angina patients treated with β-blockers is 50 to 60 beats per minute. Oral dosages should be adjusted to achieve this heart rate. There are no data to suggest that β_1-selective agents are more effective than nonselective agents, thus selection of the specific drug can be based on other issues such as route of elimination, half-life, and cost. It may be prudent to avoid β-blockers

with intrinsic sympathomimetic activity during the acute phase of unstable angina since these agents have been shown to be less effective than other β-blockers in the setting of acute myocardial infarction.

NITRATES

There are few controlled clinical trials on the use of intravenous nitroglycerin (NTG) in patients with unstable angina. Nonetheless, intravenous NTG is widely used in clinical practice, and it is recommended that it be given to any patient with unstable angina who continues to have chest pain following administration of three sublingual NTG and initiation of β-blockers (42). Additionally, intravenous NTG is recommended for all nonhypotensive high-risk unstable angina patients. Therapy should be initiated at a dose of 5 to 10 µg/min with 10 µ/min dosage increases every 5 minutes until chest pain is relieved or the patient develops dose-limiting side effects such as headache or hypotension (SBP less than 90 mm Hg or greater than 30% drop in mean blood pressure). Patients should be converted from intravenous to oral nitrate therapy once they have been symptom free for 24 hours.

CALCIUM CHANNEL BLOCKERS

Calcium channel blockers should be reserved for patients in whom angina is not controlled with optimal doses of β-blockers and nitrates or in patients unable to tolerate either nitrates or β-blockers (42). Additionally, calcium channel blockers are recommended for use in patients with a known vasospastic component to their angina. Neither individual studies nor meta-analysis of calcium channel blockers in unstable angina shows any beneficial effects on mortality or incidence of myocardial infarction (54). Nifedipine has been shown in several studies to increase the risk of myocardial infarction and/or death when used without concomitant β-blocker therapy in patients with unstable angina (55,56). Therefore, nifedipine (and probably other dihydropyridine calcium channel blockers) should be avoided in patients with unstable angina; if they must be used, they should be administered only in combination with a β-blocker (42).

Revascularization Procedures

Two revascularization procedures, coronary artery bypass grafting (CABG) and percutaneous transluminal coronary angioplasty (PTCA), are widely available for the treatment of ischemic heart disease. These procedures have become widely used in the United States for the management of ischemic heart disease, with more than 300,000 of each performed in 1991. Because of the risk of morbidity and mortality associated with each procedure, it must be evaluated in each patient whether the potential benefits of the procedure outweigh the risks. Extensive guidelines for each of these procedures have been published (57, 58).

Atherectomy and stent placement used in conjunction with PTCA are other techniques that are currently under investigation.

CORONARY ARTERY BYPASS GRAFTING

Coronary artery bypass grafting is a surgical procedure in which the affected stenosed coronary artery or arteries is bypassed in an attempt to reinstitute "normal" coronary blood flow; one of two techniques can be used to accomplish this. The first technique involves removal the saphenous vein from the leg, which is then used to bypass the affected vessel. The distal end of the vessel is connected to the aorta, and the proximal end is connected to the coronary artery at a point distal to the obstruction. The second technique involves connecting the distal end of the internal mammary artery beyond the narrowing of the coronary vessel. A number of studies have been performed to investigate which types of patients may benefit from CABG rather than continued medical management. From these trials, it appears as though the following patient types will obtain greater benefit from CABG than from medical therapy: patients with significant left main coronary artery disease, patients with multivessel coronary artery disease and impaired left ventricular function, patients with three-vessel coronary artery disease or two-vessel disease (one vessel involvement being the left anterior descending coronary artery). Currently, no data suggest improved outcome with CABG versus medical therapy in patients with two-vessel (no left anterior descending coronary artery involvement) or single-vessel disease. In these patients, PTCA may be a treatment option (1).

In patients who have had CABG, stenosis of the bypass graft may occur. Coronary disease of the saphenous vein grafts are thought to occur in three stages, early (within 1 month), intermediate (within 1 year), and late (greater than 1 year). Occlusion rates of 5 to 15%, 15 to 25%, and up to 50% have been reported for early, intermediate, and late phases, respectively (59). The role of thrombosis in each of the phases has been documented. The use of antiplatelet therapy with aspirin or ticlopidine (if aspirin sensitive) may reduce rates of occlusion. The late phase of vein graft occlusion is likely related to atherosclerosis of the graft. Prevention of late-phase occlusion may be afforded by reducing risks for development of atherosclerosis (lipid-lowering drugs, diet modification, smoking cessation, and so on). However, antiplatelet therapy should also be continued given its role in the management of ischemic heart disease.

PERCUTANEOUS TRANSLUMINAL CORONARY ANGIOPLASTY

Percutaneous transluminal coronary angioplasty is an extension of cardiac catheterization that involves passing a balloon-tipped catheter over a guidewire into the coronary artery. The guidewire is slipped past the obstruction, and the balloon-tipped catheter is passed over the wire and positioned at the level of the lesion. The balloon is then inflated, causing dilation of the stenosed vessel. The beneficial actions of PTCA are probably related to arterial intimal disruption, plaque fissuring, and stretching of the arterial wall. Short-term complications from PTCA include abrupt closure of the vessel, ischemia, extensive dissection, platelet deposition, thrombosis formation, myocardial infarction, and death. PTCA is effective (defined as less than 50% obstruction after the procedure) in approximately 90% of patients with nonoccluded, single-vessel disease (60). The success rate may be lower in patients with unstable angina, advanced age, women, and patients with totally occluded vessels. In those patients who have undergone successful PTCA, the major concern involves long-term restenosis, which occurs in 40 to 60% of patients usually within 6 months of the procedure. No interventions have been shown to reduce the risk of restenosis, but given the role of antiplatelet therapy in the long-term management of ischemic heart disease, it should be continued long term.

CONCLUSION

Angina pectoris is a manifestation of atherosclerotic coronary artery disease, the leading cause of death in the United States. Risk factor modification and elimination of precipitating factors may help reduce the frequency of anginal attacks. Drug therapy with nitrates, β-blockers, and calcium channel blockers, alone or in combination, are effective at reducing anginal episodes and reducing the frequency of anginal attacks. CABG and PTCA are effective alternatives to medical therapy in certain patients with angina pectoris poorly controlled with medical therapy. Unstable angina is a syndrome intermediate to chronic stable angina and acute myocardial infarction. Unstable angina requires more intensive management than stable angina. The primary goal of treatment for unstable angina is to prevent myocardial infarction. Drug therapy with aspirin, heparin, β-blockers, and NTG are used in patients with unstable angina.

REFERENCES

1. Rutherford JD, Braunwald E. Chronic ischemic heart disease. In: Braunwald E, ed. Heart Disease A textbook of cardiovascular medicine. 4th ed. Philadelphia, W.B. Saunders, 1992, pp 1292–1364.
2. Kannel WB, Feinleib M. Natural history of angina pectoris in the Framingham study: prognosis and survival. Am J Cardiol 29:154–158, 1972.
3. Lambert CR. Pathophysiology of stable angina pectoris. Cardiol Clin 9:1–10, 1991.
4. Detection, evaluation and treatment of high blood cholesterol in adults (Adult Treatment Panel II). Circulation 89:1329–1445, 1994.
5. Shub C. Stable angina pectoris 1. Clinical patterns. Mayo Clin Proc 64:233–242, 1990.

6. Ardehali A, Ports TA. Myocardial oxygen supply and demand. Chest 98:699–705, 1990.

7. Bleske BE, Shea MJ. Current concepts of silent myocardial ischemia. Clin Pharm 9:339–357, 1990.

8. Muller JE, Tofler GH, Stone PH. Circadian variation and triggers of onset of acute cardiovascular disease. Circulation 79:733–743, 1989.

9. Chaitman B. Exercise stress testing. In Braunwald E (ed.): Heart Disease A textbook of cardiovascular medicine. 4th ed. Philadelphia, W.B. Saunders, 1992, pp 161–179.

10. Schlant RC, Blomquist CG, Brandenburg RO, et al. Guidelines for exercise testing: a report of the joint American College of Cardiology/American Heart Association task force on assessment of cardiovascular procedures (subcommittee on exercise testing). Circulation 74:653A–667A, 1986.

11. Goldman L, Cook EF, Mitchell N, et al. Incremental value of the exercise test for diagnosing the presence or absence of coronary artery disease. Circulation 66:945–953, 1982.

12. Zaret BL, Wackers FJT, Soufer R. Nuclear Cardiology. In Braunwald E (ed.): Heart Disease A textbook of cardiovascular medicine. 4th ed. Philadelphia, W.B. Saunders, 1992, pp 276–311.

13. Ritchie JL, Bateman TM, Bonow RO, et al. Guidelines for clinical use of cardiac radionuclide imaging: A report of the American Heart Association/American College of Cardiology Task Force on assessment of diagnostic and therapeutic cardiovascular procedures, committee on radionuclide imaging, developed in collaboration with the American Society of Nuclear Cardiology. Circulation 91:1278–1303, 1995.

14. Beller GA. Pharmacologic stress testing. JAMA 265:633–638, 1991.

15. Ignarro LJ, Lippton H, Edwards JC, et al. Mechanism of vascular smooth muscle relaxation by organic nitrates, nitrites, nitroprusside and nitric oxide: Evidence for involvement of S-nitrosothiols as active intermediates. J Pharmacol Exp Ther 218:739–749, 1981.

16. Parker JO. Nitrate therapy in stable angina pectoris. N Engl J Med 316:1635–1642, 1987.

17. Abrams J. Nitrates. Med Clin N Amer 72:1–35, 1988.

18. Elkayam U. Tolerance to organic nitrates: Evidence, mechanisms, clinical relevance, and strategies for prevention. Ann Intern Med 114:667–677, 1991.

19. DeMots H, Glasser SP. Intermittent transdermal nitroglycerin therapy in the treatment of chronic stable angina. J Am Coll Cardiol 13:789–793, 1989.

20. Parker JO, Farrell B, Lahey KA, Moe G. Effect of intervals between doses on the development of tolerance to isosorbide dinitrate. N Engl J Med 316:1440–1444, 1987.

21. Thadani U, Maranda CR, Amsterdam E, et al., Lack of pharmacologic tolerance and rebound angina pectoris during twice-daily therapy with isosorbide-5-mononitrate. Ann Intern Med 120:353–359, 1994.

22. Parker JO, Vankoughnett KA, Farrell B. Nitroglycerin lingual spray: clinical efficacy and dose response relation. Am J Cardiol 57:1–5, 1986.

23. Reichek N, Goldstein RE, Redwood DR, Epstein SE. Sustained effects of nitroglycerin ointment in patients with angina pectoris. Circulation 50:348–352, 1974.

24. Fung H-L. Pharmacokinetics and pharmacodynamics of organic nitrates. Am J Cardiol 60:4H–9H, 1987.

25. Thadani U, Prasad R, Hamilton S, Karpow S, Reder R, Teague S. Isosorbide-5-mononitrate in angina pectoris: does BID dosing schedule prevent development of tolerance? Circulation 74:suppl 2:II-137 (abstract), 1986.

26. Frishman WH. β-Adrenergic blockers. Med Clin N Amer 72:37–81, 1988.

27. Sproat TT, Lopez LM. Around the β-blockers, one more time. DICP, Ann Pharmacother 25:962–971, 1991.

28. Thadani U, Davidson C, Singleton W, Taylor SH. Comparison of the immediate effects of five β-adrenoceptor-blocking drugs with differ-

ent ancillary properties in angina pectoris. N Engl J Med 300:750–755, 1979.

29. Weiner DA. Calcium channel blockers Med Clin N Amer 72:83–115, 1988.

30. Snyder SH, Reynolds IJ. Calcium-antagonist drugs receptor interactions that clarify therapeutic effects. N Engl J Med 313:995–1002, 1985.

31. Balady GJ, Fletcher BJ, Froelicher ES, et al. Cardiac rehabilitation programs: A statement for healthcare professionals from the American Heart Association. Circulation 90:1602–1610, 1994.

32. Fletcher GF, Balady G, Froelicher VF, Hartley LH, Haskell WL, Pollock ML. Exercise standards: a statement for health professionals from the American Heart Association Circulation 91:580–615, 1995.

33. Strauss WE, Paraisi AF. Combined use of calcium-channel and beta-adrenergic blockers for the treatment of chronic stable angina: rationale, efficacy and adverse effects. Ann Intern Med 109:570–581, 1988.

34. Ridker PM, Manson JE, Gaziano M, Buring JE, Hennekens CH. Low-dose aspirin therapy for chronic stable angina: A randomized, placebo-controlled clinical trial. Ann Intern Med 114:835–839, 1991.

35. Iuul-Moller S, Edvardsson N, Jahnmatz B, Rosen A, Sorensen S, Omblus R. Double-blind trial of aspirin in primary prevention of myocardial infarction in patients with stable chronic angina pectoris. The Swedish Angina Pectoris Aspirin Trial (SAPAT) Lancet 340: 1421–1425, 1992.

36. Cairns JA, Hirsh J, Lewis HD, Resnekov L, Theroux P. Antithrombotic agents in coronary artery disease. Chest 102:456S–481S, 1992.

37. Deedwania PC. Is there evidence in support of the ischemia suppression hypotheses? J Am Coll Cardiol 24:21–24, 1994.

38. Pepine CJ, Cohn PF, Deedwania PC, et al. Effects of treatment on outcome in mildly symptomatic patients with ischemia during daily life: the atenolol silent ischemia study (ASIST). Circulation 90:762–768, 1994.

39. Knatterud GL, Bourassa MG, Pepine CJ, et al. Effects of treatment strategies to suppress ischemia in patients with coronary artery disease: 12-week results of the asymptomatic cardiac ischemia pilot (ACIP) study. J Am Coll Cardiol 24:11–20, 1994.

40. Ogawa H, Yasue H, Oshima S. Circadian variation of plasma fibrinopeptide A level in patients with variant angina. Circulation 80:1617–1626, 1989.

41. Prida XE, Gelman JS, Feldman R, Hill JA, Pepine CJ, Scott E. Comparison of diltiazem and nifedipine alone and in combination in patients with coronary artery spasm. J Am Coll Cardiol 9:412–419, 1987.

42. Clinical Practice Guideline Number 10. Unstable Angina: Diagnosis and Management. U.S. Department of Health and Human Services. AHCPR Publication No. 94-0602.

43. Fuster V, Badimon L, Badimon JJ, et al. The pathogenesis of coronary artery disease and the acute coronary syndromes. N Engl J Med 326:242–250, 310–317, 1992.

44. Braunwald E, Jones RH, Mark DB, et al. Diagnosing and managing unstable angina. Circulation 90:613–622, 1994.

45. Theroux P, Ouimet H, McCams J, et al. Aspirin, heparin or both to treat acute unstable angina. N Engl J Med 319:1105–1011, 1988.

46. Antiplatelet Trialists' Collaboration. Collaborative overview of randomised trials of antiplatelet therapy — I: Prevention of death, myocardial infarction and stroke by prolonged antiplatelet therapy in various categories of patients. Br Med J 308:81–106, 1994.

47. Theroux P, Waters D, Qui S, et al. Aspirin versus heparin to prevent myocardial infarction during the acute phase of unstable angina. Circulation 88:2045–2048, 1993.

48. Holdright D, Patel D, Cunningham D, et al. Comparison of the effect of heparin and aspirin versus aspirin alone on transient myocardial ischemia and in-hospital prognosis in patients with unstable angina. J Am Coll Cardiol 24:39–45, 1994.

49. RISC group. Risk of myocardial infarction and death during treatment with low dose aspirin and intravenous heparin in men with unstable coronary artery disease. Lancet 336:827–830, 1990.

50. Cairns JA, Gent M, Singer J, et al. Aspirin, sulfinpyrazone or both in unstable angina. N Engl J Med 313:1369–1375, 1985.

51. Sobel BE. Intracranial bleeding, fibrinolysis, and anticoagulation. Causal connections and clinical implications (Editorial). Circulation 90:2147–2152, 1994.

52. Waters D, Lan JY. Is thrombolytic therapy striking out in unstable angina? Circulation 86:1642–1644, 1992.

53. The TIMI IIIB Investigators. Effects of tissue plasminogen activator and a comparison of early invasive and conservative strategies in unstable angina and non-Q-wave myocardial infarction. Results of the TIMI IIIB Trial. Circulation 89:1545–1556, 1994.

54. Held PH, Yusuf S, Furberg C. Calcium channel blockers in acute myocardial infarction and unstable angina: an overview. Br Med J 299:1187–1192, 1989.

55. Muller JE, Morrison J, Stone PH, et al. Nifedipine therapy for patients with threatened and acute myocardial infarction: a randomized, double-blind, placebo-controlled comparison. Circulation 69:740–747, 1984.

56. Lubsen J, Tijssen JG. Efficacy of nifedipine and metoprolol in the early treatment of unstable angina in the coronary care unit: findings from the Holland Interuniversity Nifedipine/Metoprolol Trial (HINT). Am J Cardiol 60:18A–25A, 1987.

57. Kirklin JW, Akins CW, Blackstone EH, et al. ACC/AHA guidelines and indications for coronary artery bypass graft surgery, a report of the American College of Cardiology/American Heart Association task force on assessment of diagnostic and therapeutic cardiovascular procedures (subcommittee on coronary artery bypass graft surgery). Circulation 83:1125–1173, 1991.

58. Ryan TJ, Faxon DP, Gunnar RM, et al. Guidelines for percutaneous transluminal coronary angioplasty, a report of the American College of Cardiology/American Heart Association task force on assessment of diagnostic and therapeutic cardiovascular procedures (subcommittee on percutaneous transluminal coronary angioplasty). Circulation 78:486–502, 1988.

59. Pearson T, Rapaport E, Criqui M, et al. Optimal risk factor management in the patient after coronary revascularization, a statement for healthcare professionals from an American Heart Association writing group. Circulation 90:3125–3133, 1994.

60. Landau C, Lange RA, Hillis LD. Percutaneous transluminal coronary angioplasty. N Engl J Med 330:981–993, 1994.

CHAPTER 41

ACUTE MYOCARDIAL INFARCTION

EDGAR R. GONZALEZ

Acute myocardial infarction (AMI) is a common manifestation of ischemic heart disease and a leading cause of admission to both community and university hospitals. In the United States, more than 500,000 people die each year from AMI (1). Approximately 50% of patients with AMI die within the first few hours as a result of ventricular fibrillation. Mortality among AMI victims ranges from 10 to 15% in the first year and is 3 to 4% per year thereafter (2). Survival after myocardial infarction (MI) is determined by the extent of viable myocardium and by the occurrence of post-MI complications. Modern coronary care has decreased the mortality from fatal arrhythmias, but it has not significantly changed the number of deaths from other post-MI complications such as reinfarction or cardiogenic shock (3).

PATHOGENESIS

Infarcted myocardium is dead muscle, usually resulting from an occluded coronary artery. The involved area can be divided into three zones: the zone of infarction, the zone of injury, and the zone of ischemia (Fig. 41.1). The infarct may be confined to the interior of the myocardium (subendocardial) or may involve the full thickness of the myocardium (transmural).

The most common cause of myocardial infarction is atherosclerosis of the coronary arteries, which narrows the coronary lumen and reduces myocardial blood supply. Below a certain critical level of blood flow, myocardial cells develop ischemic injury. Irreversible damage (i.e., myocardial infarction) results from prolonged ischemic injury to a region of cardiac muscle (4). Patients with significant disease (equal to or greater than 70% luminal diameter narrowing) of one or more of the major coronary arteries (right, left main, left anterior descending, or left circumflex) are at greatest risk of ischemic insult (Fig. 41.2). The atherosclerotic plaque is usually not solely responsible for totally occluding a coronary artery (5). A thrombus is frequently superimposed on the plaque lesion in the coronary. The precipitants of thrombosis are not well understood, but they may relate to ulceration of the plaque or to regional changes in blood flow that trigger platelet aggregation (4). Less frequently, coronary vasospasm may precipitate clot formation and complete coronary occlusion (5). Rarely, myocardial infarction can occur in the absence of coronary narrowing if there is a marked disparity between myocardial oxygen supply and demand. Cocaine abuse has been implicated as a possible cause of such a disparity. Myocardial infarction may occur in various locations in the left ventricle, or in the right ventricle, depending on which coronary artery is occluded.

SIGNS AND SYMPTOMS

Time is a crucial factor in the identification and treatment of patients with AMI because of the demonstrated benefits of early treatment with thrombolytic therapy in the first 1 to 2 hours after the onset of symptoms and because of the ever-present threat of sudden death. A recent report from the GISSI multicenter study group sought reasons for delayed presentations (6). Investigators compared 590 patients who presented more than 12 hours after symptom onset with 600 patients treated within 2 hours and 603 patients treated between 6 and 12 hours. Sixty percent of patients seen within 2 hours received thrombolytic therapy, versus 18% of patients admitted more than 12 hours after the onset of symptoms. Factors associated with delayed hospital admission included age over 65, living alone, diabetes mellitus, mild-to-moderate rather than severe pain, onset of pain at night or at home. Health care practitioners must educate patients about when and how to seek care for chest pain.

The patient's chief complaint and history are invaluable in establishing a diagnosis of MI. Discomfort is the most common presenting complaint. The discomfort is described as oppressive, burning, a tightness, squeezing, choking, expanding, or indigestion-like. There may be a sense of "impending doom." The discomfort is typically substernal and may radiate to the neck, throat, jaw, shoulders, and arms. The discomfort is similar to angina pectoris in location and quality, but discomfort in angina is brief, whereas the discomfort of AMI lasts from 30 minutes to several hours and is more severe. It usually begins while the patient is at rest, does not subside, and is only partially relieved by nitroglycerin. At least 15 to 20% of MIs are not accompanied by any symptoms ("silent MI"). "Silent" infarction is seen most commonly in diabetic and elderly patients.

Most patients admit to prodromal symptoms: vague chest discomfort, weakness, fatigue, nausea, vomiting, and diaphoresis prior to the acute attack (1). Less commonly, an episode of light-headedness or syncope heralds the onset of AMI.

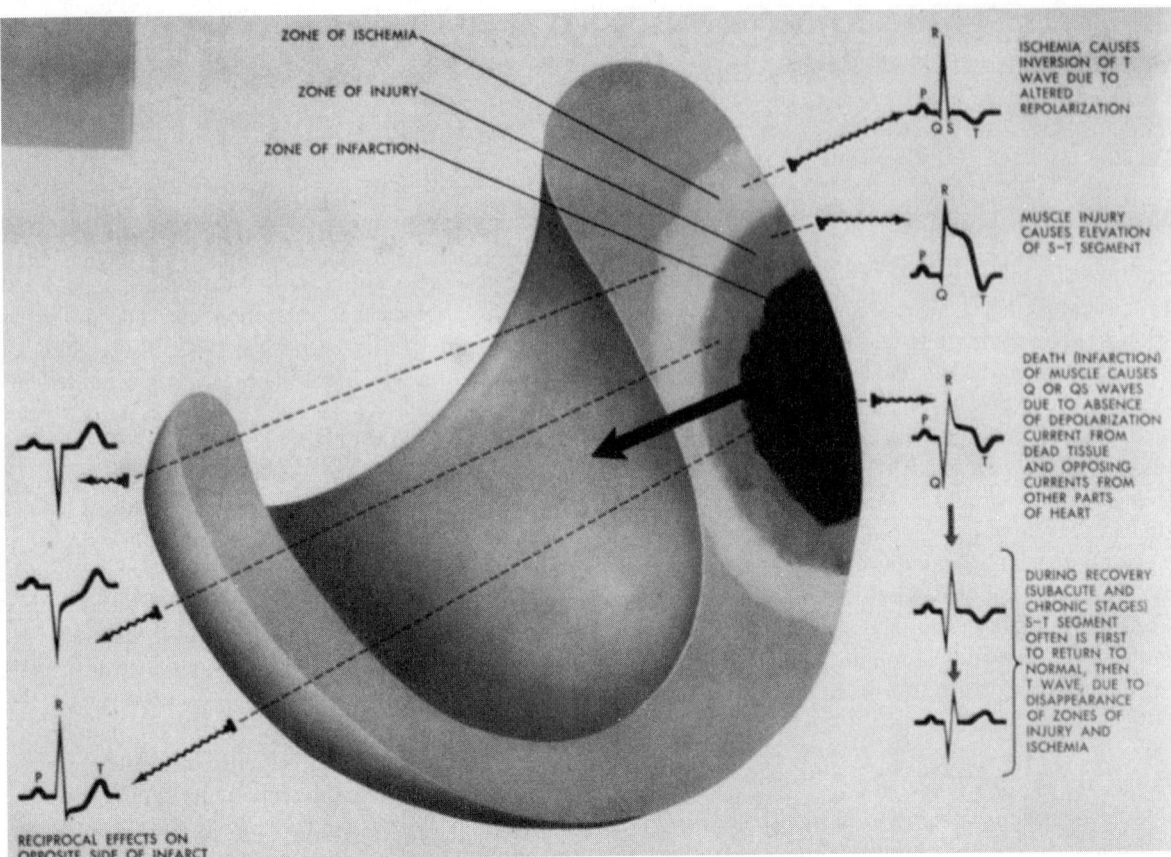

Figure 41.1. Effects of cardiac infarction, injury, and ischemia. (With permission. From Yonkman FF, ed. The Ciba Collection of Medical Illustrations: Heart. New York, Ciba Pharmaceutical Company, 1969:62.)

Numerous factors associated with myocardial infarction include vasospasm, severe exertion, emotional stress, hemorrhage, trauma, respiratory dysfunction, hypoglycemia, administration of catecholamines or ergot alkaloids, and hypersensitivity reactions (1).

DIAGNOSIS AND CLINICAL FINDINGS

A detailed history may help differentiate ischemic myocardial pain from noncardiac chest pain. Precipitating factors should be identified, and the patient's medication history and compliance should be assessed.

The patient is often anxious, restless, cool, sweaty, and pale. Heart rate varies widely; sinus tachycardia and mild fever are commonly observed. Sinus bradycardia is more common with an inferior myocardial infarction. Blood pressure varies widely from patient to patient. Temporally in a given patient, hypertension may accompany pain. Hypotension may result from the vasodilating effect of morphine, left ventricular dysfunction, and/or hypovolemia. The respiratory rate is often rapid, and respiratory effort may be shallow. Heart sounds may be normal or faint. A fourth heart sound (atrial gallop) is common. Low-grade fever up to 38°C and leukocytosis may be observed during the first few days following AMI. Evidence of coronary risk

factors may be present, such as retinopathy from hypertension and/or diabetes, and xanthomas due to hyperlipidemia.

ELECTROCARDIOGRAPHIC FINDINGS

The electrocardiogram (ECG) permits detection of the three pathophysiologic events occurring during an AMI: ischemia (T-wave inversion), injury (S-T segment elevation), and infarction (pathologic Q waves) (Fig. 41.1). The diagnostic feature of MI is the deep, wide Q wave, or Q-S pattern (i.e., an initial slight upward deflection followed by a pronounced downward deflection) in the ECG leads corresponding to the area of injury. Transmural infarction (through and through, full thickness) is diagnosed if the ECG shows Q waves or loss of R waves. Nontransmural infarction (subendocardial or epicardial) is present if the ECG shows only S-T segment elevation and T-wave inversion. Nontransmural infarction may be less frequently associated with thrombosis. Although Q waves are seen more commonly in transmural than in nontransmural infarction, both types of infarcts may occur with or without Q waves. Therefore, it is more appropriate to use the terms *Q-wave infarction* and *non-Q-wave infarction* (7).

SERUM ENZYME STUDIES

Intracellular enzymes are released into the systemic circulation from infarcted myocardium. The three enzymes most frequently assayed are creatine kinase (CK), lactate dehydrogenase (LDH), and aspartate aminotransferase (AST). Each enzyme has a particular time course for appearance in the systemic circulation following an AMI (Fig. 41.3). The temporal pattern of peak enzyme concentrations is of diagnostic importance. Standard practice is to obtain serial cardiac enzyme concentrations every 8 hours for the first 24 hours in patients with a suspected AMI. CK activity can be used to estimate infarct size. Blood CK concentrations peak (two to three times normal) within 24 hours and

return to normal in 3 to 4 days. Serial CK measurements following infarction result in excellent clinical sensitivity. The major criticism of CK is its poor specificity. CK activity can be elevated following skeletal muscle trauma related to surgery, exercise, or intramuscular injections.

LDH is the slowest rising enzyme activity following AMI. When assessed within the second and third days postinfarction, LDH has a relatively high specificity (94%) and good clinical sensitivity (85%) for AMI (1,2). The ubiquitous nature of AST makes it a relatively nonspecific indicator of myocardial cell damage. Therefore, AST activity is rarely used today for the purpose of assessing the presence or absence of an AMI.

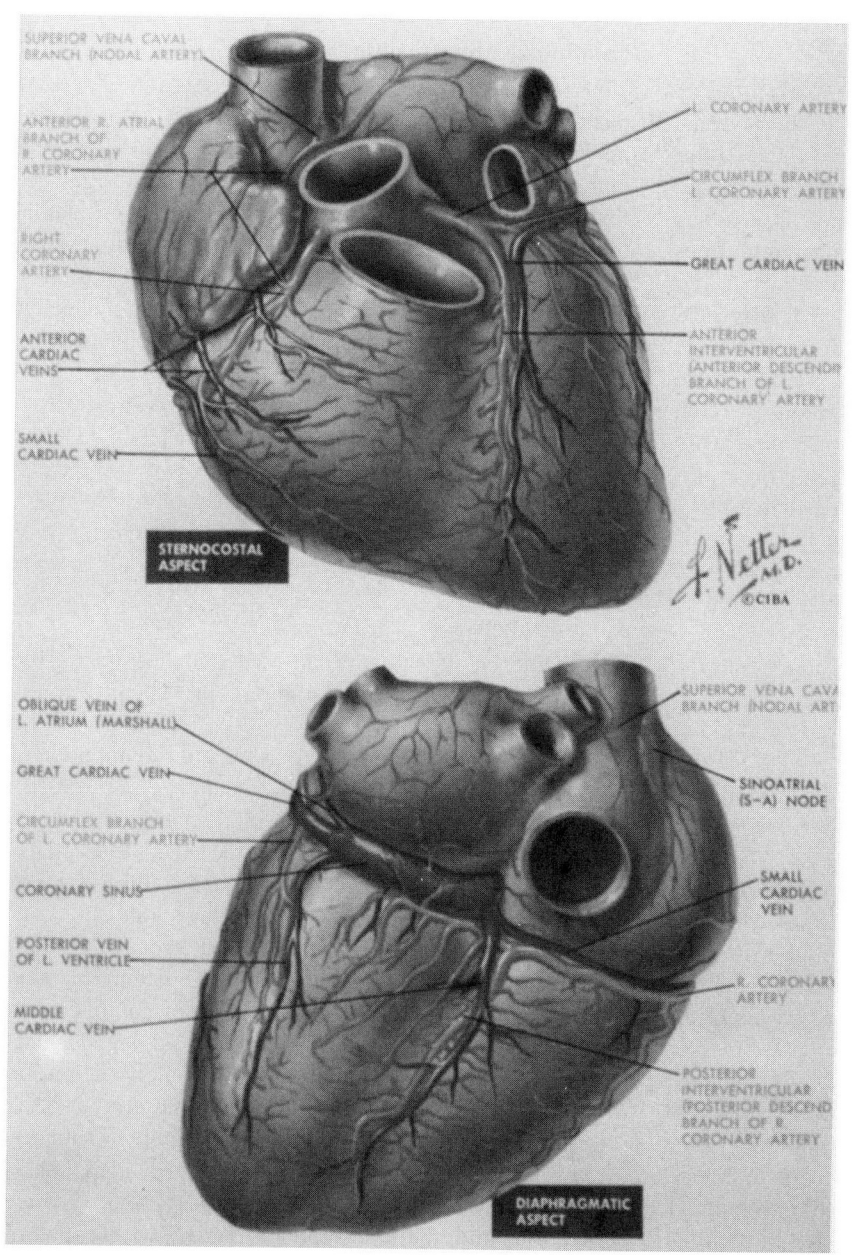

Figure 41.2. Coronary arteries and veins: blood supply of the heart. (With permission, from Yonkman FF, ed. The Ciba Collection of Medical Illustrations: Heart. New York, Ciba Pharmaceutical Company, 1969:16.)

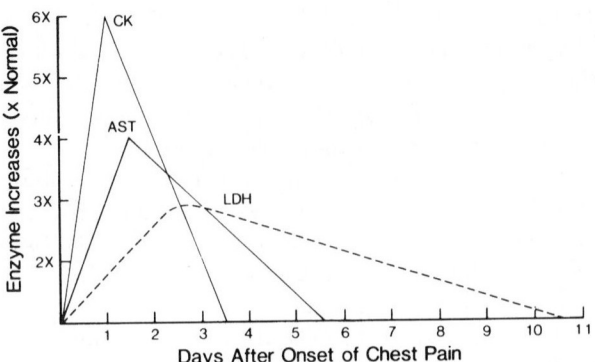

Figure 41.3. The time course of cardiac enzyme release during acute myocardial infarction. (With permission, from Zeller FP, Bauman JL. Current concepts in clinical therapeutics: acute myocardial infarction. Clin Pharm 5:556, 1986.)

CK-MB and LDH-1 are the respective isoenzymes of CK and LDH with highest concentrations in the myocardium. The use of isoenzyme increases the specificity of the test for AMI. Within 48 hours after infarct, the sensitivity and specificity of CK-MB for myocardial injury approaches 100%. However, CK-MB is less specific for infarction because it can be elevated following traumatic injury to the heart due to cardiopulmonary resuscitation or electrical countershock. Since LDH_2 is normally the major LDH isoenzyme in blood, the usual serum pattern is LDH_2 more than LDH_1. A change in this relationship is seen after MI, renal necrosis, and hemolysis. Within 48 hours post-acute episode, 80% of AMI patients will have flipped their normal LDH isoenzyme pattern to LDH_1 more than LDH_2.

Serum myoglobin (S-Mgb) is an intracellular muscle protein that can serve as another marker for AMI. Because of S-Mgb's small size compared with CK, S-Mgb is able to diffuse faster through injured cell membranes. S-Mgb appears at abnormal levels as early as 1 to 3 hours after the onset of AMI and peaks much more rapidly than either CK or LDH (8). S-Mgb is of value in the early evaluation of potential AMI patients. A rapid rise in S-Mgb, and a doubling of the S-Mgb concentration within the first 2 hours of treatment, even if the second level is within normal limits, is highly specific for AMI (8). Because elevated S-Mgb levels usually return to normal within 12 to 24 hours after the onset of symptoms, an isolated normal S-Mgb or a serial S-Mgb level that does not double does not necessarily rule out AMI (8).

Early reports suggest that an assay based on monoclonal antibodies against troponin-1 may be a better marker for acute myocardial infarction than the CK-MB study (9). Troponin is part of the contractile apparatus of the myocardium. It appears that elevations in troponin-1 occur rarely or not at all in patients without cardiac injury. Clinical studies show that when an elevated troponin-1 level is detected, the patient is likely to have myocardial injury. Many centers are now evaluating the value of troponin assays in the diagnosis of acute myocardial infarction.

Radionuclide Imaging

Radionuclide imaging techniques are valuable in assessing myocardial ischemic injury. Acute infarct scintigraphy (hot-spot imaging) with infarct-avid Tc99m pyrophosphate aids in localizing and measuring the necrotic area. Scans are usually positive 2 to 5 days after infarction. Myocardial perfusion imaging with thallium 201, which is taken up and concentrated by viable myocardium, reveals a defect ("cold spot") within 6 hours after AMI. Radionuclide ventriculography frequently reveals wall motion abnormalities and reduced ventricular ejection fraction in patients with AMI.

Laboratory Abnormalities

Nonspecific laboratory abnormalities associated with AMI include polymorphonuclear leukocytosis (12,000 to 15,000 per mm^3), which persists for 3 to 7 days, and an elevated erythrocyte sedimentation rate, which peaks during the first week. Electrolyte abnormalities include hypokalemia and hypomagnesemia. Hypokalemia and hypomagnesemia occur commonly in patients being treated with diuretics. These electrolyte abnormalities can precipitate malignant ventricular arrhythmias in patients with ischemic, hypertrophied, or dilated hearts.

Summary

In summary, AMI is diagnosed when any two of the three clinical features discussed are present: ischemic chest pain, new abnormal Q waves or S-T segment changes, or abnormally elevated cardiac enzymes.

Complications

The incidence of death after an AMI is highest during the first several hours after onset of symptoms. The probability of a successful outcome is inversely proportional to the elapsed time between symptom onset and the initiation of therapy. If the infarction occurs outside the hospital setting, immediate transport to a hospital emergency department for management is essential. Once acute therapy has been instituted and the patient has been stabilized, he or she should be transferred to the coronary intensive care unit (CICU) for further observation and care.

Approximately 50% of hospitalized MI patients develop complications (10). Two general classes of complications have been defined: electrical (arrhythmias) and mechanical (heart failure). ECG monitoring and prompt recognition and treatment of electrical complications have reduced the in-hospital mortality from MI. Unfortunately, a similarly favorable trend has not been observed with AMI-associated heart failure despite advances in hemodynamic monitoring and inotropic support. Left ventricular failure with subsequent pulmonary congestion is the primary cause of in-hospital death from MI.

Of the 500,000 patients hospitalized yearly for acute MI, 400,000 patients survive to hospital discharge (11). The major mortality risk is within the first 6 months of hospitalization; death is equally distributed between sudden and nonsudden cardiac events (11,12). Approximately 10% of patients die within the first year of their MI, 5% die within the second year, and 3 to 4% die each year thereafter (11). The major determinants of death in post-MI patients are the extent of jeopardized myocardium and the degree of electrical instability. Anterior infarction, early left ventricular failure, late significant arrhythmias, and poor left ventricular ejection fraction are major predictors of poor prognosis during the peri-infarction period (11). Although Q-wave infarct patients have twice the initial mortality compared with non-Q-wave infarctions, their 1-year mortality rates are comparable (13). Factors associated with late mortality post-MI include advancing age (13), history of prior infarction or chronic angina (14), female gender (15), hypertension (16), diabetes mellitus (16), and continued cigarette smoking (11).

Treatment

Reduction in mortality is the major goal of therapy in patients with AMI. The management of AMI is designed to relieve pain and anxiety, to recognize and control life-threatening arrhythmias, to limit infarct size, and to prevent complications.

General

Patients with suspected AMI are treated in the intensive care or coronary care unit to allow for monitoring and prompt response to emergencies. The ECG is continuously monitored. Peripheral venous access for intravenous drug administration is obtained. Intramuscular drug administration is avoided because of possible interference with cardiac enzyme determinations, unpredictable drug absorption during episodes of hypoperfusion, and bleeding during anticoagulation. Vital signs, pain relief, body weight, bowel habits, and diet are closely monitored.

Critical to limiting myocardial ischemic damage is reducing the oxygen demand of the heart, which is the product of heart rate, contractility, and myocardial wall tension. During the first 24 hours, patients with AMI are confined to bed rest so as to reduce myocardial oxygen demand. Early ambulation is feasible in patients with uncomplicated MI (i.e., absence of electrical instability or power failure) and may lessen the need for anticoagulation in these patients.

Hypoxemia usually results from ventilation perfusion abnormalities, commonly due to left ventricular dysfunction. Administration of oxygen reduces hypoxemia and increases oxygen delivery to ischemic tissues. Oxygen is administered for the first 24 to 48 hours. In patients with chronic obstructive lung disease, low flow rates of oxygen are appropriate to avoid carbon dioxide retention. Endotracheal intubation and positive airway pressure mechanical ventilation should be used if adequate oxygenation (oxygen saturation ≥90%) cannot be maintained by mask. High-level, continuous positive airway pressure will improve tissue oxygenation and reduce the spontaneous respiratory effort without producing circulatory depression in AMI patients with left ventricular dysfunction (17). Arterial puncture for arterial blood gas determinations should be avoided shortly after the administration of thrombolytic therapy to minimize the risk of arterial bleeding.

Bed Rest

Patients should limit their activities to bed rest during the first 24 hours after the acute event. This is done to decrease myocardial oxygen consumption during the healing process after an acute MI and to prevent extension or reinfarction. Activities over the next few days should begin gradually, starting with personal hygiene and in-bed range-of-motion exercises. Patients may begin ambulating 4 to 5 days post-MI. The gradual introduction of activities may decrease the requirement for anticoagulation in this patient population.

Analgesia

Pain relief is an initial therapeutic objective. Prompt pain relief attenuates the autonomic hyperactivity that increases myocardial oxygen demand and predisposes to tachyarrhythmias (18). Sublingual nitroglycerin is tried first unless the patient's systolic blood pressure is less than 90 mm Hg. In the presence of persistent ischemia and hypotension, a small amount of nitroglycerin paste may be applied and promptly removed if hypotension worsens. Nitroglycerin must be used with caution in patients with right ventricular infarction because precipitous hypotension may ensue since nitroglycerin increases venous capacitance and decreases venous return to the right atrium. Intravenous access should be obtained for fluid resuscitation. Vasopressor agents should be avoided and are seldom required. If hypotension with bradycardia develops, intravenous atropine (0.5 to 1.0 mg) should be administered.

Numerous analgesic drugs (morphine, meperidine, pentazocine, and nalbuphine) have been used in AMI. Morphine is the agent of choice except in patients with well-documented morphine hypersensitivity. In addition to relieving pain and anxiety, the hemodynamic effects of morphine are invaluable in patients with pulmonary edema. Morphine is a potent vasodilator. It increases venous capacitance and decreases systemic vascular resistance (19). These effects are most pronounced in patients with heightened sympathetic tone. Four to 8 mg should be administered by slow intravenous injection, and doses of 2 to 8 mg repeated at 5- to 15-minute intervals until the pain is relieved or evident toxicity (i.e., hypotension, respiratory depression, or vomiting) precludes further administration. Morphine-induced hypotension can be minimized by maintaining the patient in a supine position.

Concomitant administration of atropine 0.5 to 1.0 mg intravenously may help reverse the vagomimetic effects of morphine on blood pressure and heart rate. Meperidine 25 to 75 mg by slow intravenous injection every 2 to 3 hours as needed for pain control is a suitable alternative in morphine-intolerant patients. The anticholinergic effects of meperidine will counteract the heightened vagal tone in AMI patients with either bradycardia or nausea. Tachycardia is a potential adverse effect of meperidine administration. Patients should be monitored for the respiratory depressant effects of narcotic analgesics. Naloxone, 0.4 mg intravenously, may be administered at 5-minute intervals as needed to reverse narcotic-induced respiratory depression.

Nalbuphine hydrochloride (Nubain) is a synthetic opioid analgesic with mixed narcotic agonist and antagonist effects. Results of one study comparing the hemodynamic effects of nalbuphine and morphine in patients with acute MI indicate that nalbuphine relieves pain and reduces myocardial oxygen demand without producing hypotension. Nalbuphine is a useful agent in patients with AMI because it produces less respiratory depression, less hypotension, and less vagal stimulation than morphine. Nalbuphine 10 mg is administered intravenously every 3 to 6 hours as needed for pain relief. Although butorphanol (Stadol), a synthetic opioid agonist-antagonist, does not appear to significantly alter systemic hemodynamics, it should be avoided in patients with AMI because of concerns that this agent may increase systemic vascular resistance and myocardial oxygen demand (20).

The persistence of pain over several hours is a bad prognostic sign, usually indicative of continued myocardial ischemia and necrosis. In this setting, nitroglycerin may effectively relieve refractory chest pain. Nitroglycerin decreases myocardial oxygen demand by reducing intramyocardial wall tension. Patients with signs and symptoms of pulmonary edema derive the most benefit from intravenous nitroglycerin administration. In addition, intravenous nitroglycerin may limit infarct size. This agent will be discussed in greater detail later in this chapter.

Sedation

Anxiety may have deleterious effects on the cardiovascular system, especially in patients with acute MI. The treatment of anxiety should aim to reduce not only the somatic complaints but also the adrenergic hyperactivity often present in MI patients. Three groups of medications can be used to treat cardiac symptoms and anxiety disorders. Antidepressant drugs lower anxiety, but do not suppress adrenergic response and should be avoided in AMI patients during acute recovery. In contrast, β-blockers blunt the adrenergic response but do not affect anxiety. Benzodiazepines can be used to relax the patient and theoretically decrease catecholamine outpouring secondary to stress (11,12). Alprazolam (Xanax) and diazepam (Valium) have shown to be effective in decreasing anxiety and catecholamine levels in acute MI patients (11).

Diet

A clear liquid diet is instituted for the first day during the convalescence period (1,2). This diet may require less shunting of blood to the gastrointestinal tract and lower the overall metabolic requirements of the body. Afterward, an appropriate diet (e.g., a low-cholesterol, low-sodium, diabetic diet) may be started.

Stool Softeners

Once patients are on an appropriate diet, stool softeners are often employed to decrease isometric stress associated with defecation. Either docusate sodium (Colace) 100 mg or docusate calcium (Surfak) 240 mg once or twice a day is satisfactory in softening the stool.

Antiplatelet Agents

The use of aspirin 160 to 325 mg per day in AMI patients is highly recommended unless the patient has contraindications to aspirin therapy (see "Thrombolytic Agents"). Two chewable aspirins (total of 160 mg) should be administered when the patient is first seen in the emergency department.

Anticoagulation

Although anticoagulants in AMI remain controversial, they may be used to prevent systemic and pulmonary embolus formation as well as to halt the progression of the infarction. Most patients with uncomplicated AMI do not require full anticoagulation because the low incidence of deep venous thrombosis and pulmonary embolism outweighs the risks of anticoagulation.

The incidence of hemorrhagic side effects from anticoagulation in patients with AMI ranges from 3 to 7%. The mortality rate as a result of hemorrhage is 2 to 4% in warfarin-treated patients and less than 1% in patients receiving heparin (21). Cerebrovascular accidents (CVA) occur in 2 to 3% and pulmonary embolus in 1 to 2% of post-MI patients. On the basis of these observations, only those patients at high risk (i.e., left ventricular hypokinesia and/or mucal thrombin), as described earlier, should be fully anticoagulated (21).

Full dose heparin is administered following thrombolytic therapy to prevent coronary artery reocclusion after successful thrombolysis. The risk of reocclusion is high immediately after thrombolysis because blood flowing through the newly opened coronary artery is exposed to thrombin bound to fibrin in the residual thrombus.

Clinical studies of patients with venous thrombosis and acute myocardial infarction indicate that there is a relation between the anticoagulant response to heparin and clinical efficacy (22). Patients treated with streptokinase benefit from heparin therapy at relatively small doses (e.g., 12,500 units subcutaneously every 12 hours). Whereas, this subcutaneous regimen of heparin failed to produce benefit in AMI patients treated with t-PA. Full-dose heparin (e.g., 5000-unit bolus followed by 30,000 units per 24 hours by continuous infusion) improves patency after coronary thrombolysis with t-PA. A plausible explanation for these apparently contradictory findings is that the lack of systemic lytic effect seen with t-PA requires that heparin be administered early and in high doses when compared with heparin requirements following thrombolysis with strep-tokinase.

An intravenous loading dose of 5000 units (approximately 70 units/kg) followed by a continuous infusion of approximately 1000 units (approximately 15 to 25 units/kg/hr) is usually employed. The partial thrombo-plastin time (PTT) should be checked no earlier than 4 hours after the initial bolus. Earlier evaluation of PTT may yield extremely high values because of the effect of the initial 5000-unit bolus. The infusion rate may be titrated by increments of 100 to 200 units per hour so that PTT is maintained 1.5 to 2 times the control. Side effects include hemorrhage (intracranial, gastrointestinal) and thrombocytopenia. Contraindications are a history of hemorrhage, uncontrolled hypertension, vasculitis, and blood dyscrasias.

Acute MI patients, who do not have contraindications to heparin, should receive heparin 5000 units subcutaneously every 12 hours to decrease the risk of clot formation. Patients with obesity, ventricular aneurysm, cardiogenic shock, a history of thrombophlebitis, or a history of arterial or venous embolism are predisposed to thrombus formation and should be fully anticoagulated. Patients with transmural anterior myocardial infarction have a 30 to 40% incidence of developing left ventricular thrombi. Anticoagulation of these patients early in the course of therapy will prevent cerebrovascular accidents (CVAs). Anticoagulation with warfarin for 3 months is recommended following an anterior transmural MI. Patients with acute MI and who are at increased risk of systemic thromboembolic events should be anticoagulated with warfarin for at least 3 months. A prothrombin time of 1.5 to 2.5 times control (INR 2 to 3) should be the goal of oral anticoagulation (21,23).

Patients with inferior wall myocardial infarction do not usually exhibit left ventricular thrombus formation with resultant CVA. Only those patients with accompanying heart failure, atrial arrhythmias, large acute MI, old anterior wall infarction, or apical dyskinesis or akinesis should be anticoagulated. A two-dimensional echocardiogram can be used to assess the presence of a left ventricular thrombus (21,23).

The Warfarin Re-Infarction Study group (23) randomized 1214 acute MI patients within 27 days from onset of symptoms to receive either warfarin to attain a prothrombin time of 1.5 to 2.0 times control or placebo for a mean duration of 37 months (range, 24 to 63 months). Warfarin reduced mortality by 24%, the incidence of reinfarction fell by 34%, and there was a 55% decrease in the incidence of CVA. All differences reached statistical significance. The risk of major bleed was 0.6% per year. The authors concluded that warfarin therapy after an MI is safe and can significantly affect mortality and morbidity.

In summary, it is not justifiable to anticoagulate all patients after an MI because the risk of anticoagulation exceeds the potential benefit. The use of full-dose anticoagulation in AMI patients must be based on the relative risk and potential benefit derived from treatment. In patients with an absolute contraindication to anticoagulation (e.g., recent subarachnoid bleed or active gastrointestinal tract bleeding), the potential benefits of anticoagulation do not justify the risk. In patients with relative contraindications to anticoagulation (history of peptic ulcer disease, recent surgery), the risk of bleeding must be weighed against the risk of embolization.

Treatment and Prophylaxis of Arrhythmias

The most common post-MI complication is disturbance of the normal cardiac rhythm. Pharmacologic manipulation of the cardiac conduction system and the autonomic nervous system, and correction of electrolyte abnormalities reduce the morbidity and mortality associated with cardiac arrhythmias in AMI patients. Arrhythmias occurring in patients with AMI require vigorous treatment when they produce hemodynamic compromise, increase in myocardial oxygen demand, or predispose to malignant ventricular arrhythmias.

Ventricular fibrillation (VF) is the most common cause of death in the early hours post-MI and may occur without prior evidence of ventricular premature complexes (24). Ventricular fibrillation occurs in approximately 11% of patients with AMI and carries a 46% mortality rate. Approximately 60% of episodes occur within 4 hours and 80% within 12 hours of symptoms. Although there was no consensus regarding a reduction in morbidity and mortality, routine prophylactic antiarrhythmic therapy was once advocated during the initial 24 hours post-AMI (23). Today, the routine use of prophylatic antiarrhytmics in patients with AMI is disputed. Treatment with antiarrhythmics is commonly instituted in patients with warning arrhythmias (i.e., couplets, multifocal PVCs, runs of three or more consecutive PVCs). Lidocaine hydrochloride is the prophylactic antiarrhythmic agent of choice in AMI. This agent suppresses ventricular arrhythmogenicity by decreasing automaticity, blocking reentry pathways, and elevating the fibrillatory threshold. Prompt administration of lidocaine can reduce the incidence of malignant ventricular arrhythmias during the early phase of AMI. However, no data support that mortality is reduced with prophylactic lidocaine therapy in patients with AMI (24). Lidocaine may produce asystole to aggravate myocardial dysfunction. Therefore, lidocaine is now reserved for AMI patients with warning arrhythmias, young patients presenting within 6 hours of symptoms, and patients treated with thrombolytic therapy.

Lidocaine 1.0 mg/kg is administered by intravenous injection over 2 minutes followed immediately by an intravenous infusion of 1 to 4 mg per minute (20 to 50 µg/kg/min). Because of the short distribution half-life (6 to 8 minutes) of lidocaine, an additional 0.5 mg/kg bolus should be given 10 minutes after the initial bolus to prevent the occurrence of subtherapeutic plasma lidocaine concentrations. If ventricular arrhythmias persist, 50-mg bolus injections can be repeated to a maximum of 250 mg of lidocaine over a 20-minute period.

Lidocaine is metabolized by the liver and has a half-life of approximately 90 minutes. The metabolism of lidocaine is impaired in the presence of AMI, circulatory shock, hepatic failure, cimetidine, and β-adrenergic blockers. Accumulation of the metabolites of lidocaine may occur in elderly patients and in patients with hepatic and/or renal dysfunction. The dose of lidocaine should be reduced and individualized in such cases.

Excessive doses of lidocaine can produce central nervous system toxicity and possibly cardiovascular depression. The toxicity of lidocaine is directly related to its concentration in blood. Plasma lidocaine concentrations should be maintained between 1.5 and 5 mcg/ml. Patients with AMI may tolerate higher plasma concentrations (8 µg/ml). This may be related to increased binding of lidocaine to alpha-1-acid glycoprotein, which is released into the systemic circulation in large concentrations after AMI.

Procainamide and bretylium are alternatives to lidocaine in AMI patients with refractory arrhythmias. These drugs are discussed in Chapter 39.

β-adrenergic receptor blocking agents reverse the arrhythmogenic effect of circulating catecholamines and reduce electrical instability during ischemic insult to the myocardium (25). Both propranolol and metoprolol effectively reduce the incidence of ventricular fibrillation associated with AMI (26,27). This effect is most noticeable in patients with hypertension or tachycardia (27). The recommended dosage of propranolol for intravenous administration during AMI is 0.1 mg/kg in three divided

doses given slowly at 5-minute intervals, followed by a maintenance oral regimen of 180 to 320 mg per day (25). Intravenous metoprolol (15 mg) is administered in three equal doses at 5-minute intervals, followed by a maintenance oral regimen of 100 to 200 mg per day. Patients should be monitored for signs and symptoms of excessive β-adrenergic blockade (bradycardia, atrioventricular conduction delay, hypotension). Circulatory collapse is a rare complication of β-adrenergic blockade in patients with AMI; patients with left ventricular impairment show only a modest fall in mean arterial pressure, heart rate, and cardiac output (25,28,29). These agents are contraindicated in patients with bradycardia, hypotension, or bronchospastic airway disease, or overt congestive heart failure.

Sinus bradycardia is a common finding in patients with inferior wall MI. Transient episodes of bradycardia are often observed during the initial hours post-MI and may exert a protective function (30). If the bradycardia is associated with hypotension or a ventricular arrhythmia, atropine 0.5 to 1.0 mg should be administered by rapid intravenous injection. Atropine may be repeated at 2- to 4-hour intervals as needed to maintain a heart rate above 60 beats per minute. Asymptomatic bradycardia should not be treated because the risk of increased myocardial oxygen demand outweighs any potential benefit from treatment. Atropine should not be administered in doses less than 0.5 mg because a paradoxical slowing of the heart rate may occur. Electrical pacing is used to manage atropine-refractory bradycardia. Intravenous isoproterenol (0.5 to 2.0 µg/min) should be used, if at all, only until a pacemaker can be placed because of the risks of tachyarrhythmias or hypotension.

Sinus tachycardia occurs in 30% of AMI patients during the first few days postinfarction (31). Anxiety, pain, fever, and ventricular dysfunction commonly cause this arrhythmia. Young patients with a first anterior wall myocardial infarction may present in a hyperdynamic state with sinus tachycardia, hypertension, and ventricular ectopy. These patients may benefit from acute therapy with β-adrenergic blockers (25–30).

Atrial fibrillation or flutter occurs in up to 20% of AMI patients and is often associated with left ventricular dysfunction (31). Because of this association, these rhythms are seen more often with anterior wall myocardial infarction and are associated with increased mortality. Therapy is indicated if the arrhythmia produces a rapid ventricular response and/or hemodynamic compromise. Restoration of normal sinus rhythm by electrical cardioversion is an immediate priority in the setting of acute hemodynamic instability. Patients may develop hemodynamic instability from supraventricular tachycardia. Intravenous verapamil 5 mg over 2 minutes and repeated in 30 minutes to a total of 20 mg may be used for conversion to normal sinus rhythm or for control of ventricular response rate. Verapamil should be used with caution, if at all, in patients with left ventricular dysfunction, hypotension, Wolff-Parkinson-White syndrome, or wide complex tachycardias. Adenosine has the advantage of a shorter half-life and has less propensity to produce hypotension than verapamil. The usual dose of adenosine is 6 mg, followed by 12 mg in 3 to 5 minutes if a response is not observed. Total doses above 18 mg increase the risk of atrioventricular block, flushing, chest pain, and bronchospasm.

Electrolyte abnormalities, most notably hypokalemia and hypomagnesemia, should be identified and corrected. These electrolyte abnormalities can precipitate malignant ventricular arrhythmias in patients with ischemia, hypertrophied or dilated hearts, or hypoxemia.

Hypokalemia is the most common electrolyte abnormality encountered in clinical practice, occurring in 23 to 40% of patients treated with thiazide diuretics (32). When loop and thiazide diuretics are used in combination, the incidence increases to approximately 100% (33). Hypokalemia is present in 9 to 25% of patients with acute MI and may predispose these patients to VF (34). Ornato and colleagues (35) found a 49% incidence of hypokalemia in their out-of-hospital cardiac arrest victims. Fifty-five percent of all hypokalemic sudden death victims were receiving diuretics without potassium supplementation; hypokalemia occurred in 13% of victims receiving diuretics plus potassium supplementation. Fortunately, hypokalemia is significantly (p less than 0.001) less common in uncomplicated acute MI patients (11%) compared with sudden death victims (50%) (36). Nonetheless, hypokalemia should be identified and corrected in the acute MI setting.

The effect of hypomagnesemia in cardiac disease is well known (38,39). Magnesium deficiency is associated with a high frequency of cardiac arrhythmias, symptoms of cardiac insufficiency, and sudden cardiac death (33,38–40). Experimental and clinical studies show that magnesium and potassium metabolism are closely linked (38,41).

Hypomagnesemia, often accompanied by hypokalemia, is usually caused by diuretics (41,42). Transient hypomagnesemia not induced by renal magnesium loss has been observed in patients with acute myocardial infarction (43). Because hypomagnesemia can precipitate refractory ventricular fibrillation and can hinder the replenishment of intracellular potassium, it must be corrected if present. One or two grams of magnesium sulfate (2 to 4 mL of a 50% solution) is diluted in 100 mL of D_5W and administered over 60 minutes (37). A 24-hour magnesium infusion (8 Gms $MgSO_4$ in 500 mL D_5W) started on admission to the CICU can significantly lower the incidence of ventricular tachycardia (43). Magnesium supplementation is a relatively safe method of reducing the incidence of postinfarction ventricular arrhythmias (40,43).

Magnesium toxicity is rare, but side effects from too rapid administration include flushing, sweating, mild bradycardia, and hypotension. Hypermagnesemia may produce depressed reflexes, flaccid paralysis, circulatory collapse, respiratory paralysis, and diarrhea.

Clinical studies on the use of magnesium in AMI have yielded contradictory results. Studies, such as the Leicester Intravenous Magnesium Intervention Trial (LIMIT II), conducted prior to the Fourth International Study of Infarct Survival (ISIS-4), suggested that magnesium was highly effective in reducing the odds of death and capable of producing survival benefits comparable to those produced by aspirin and thrombolytic therapy in AMI patients (44). Whereas, the ISIS-4 trial failed to show any benefit from magnesium with respect to post-AMI mortality reduction (44). Important differences in methodologic design between LIMIT-II and ISIS-4 may explain the disparity in response produced by magnesium in AMI patients. The primary difference is that although in the trials preceding ISIS-4, magnesium was usually administered before or at the time of reperfusion of the infarct-related artery, in ISIS-4, reperfusion was likely to occur in many patients before the administration of magnesium (44). Considering the proposed mechanisms by which magnesium could improve survival in AMI, administration prior to reperfusion seems to be of obvious importance. This applies to the postulated preservation of high-energy phosphates and reduction in mitochondrial calcium overload during acute ischemia as well as to a possible role in arrhythmia reduction and reduction in reperfusion injury and stunning (44). Furthermore, the low mortality associated with the combined use of thrombolytics, anticoagulants, and antiplatelet drugs may mask the true benefit produced by magnesium (45). Although further studies are needed to better define the role of early administration of magnesium in AMI patients receiving thrombolytic therapy, magnesium improves left ventricular function and reduces mortality in post-AMI patients, especially those who are not candidates for thrombolytic therapy (45).

Cardiogenic Shock
HEART FAILURE

Cardiogenic shock develops in 10 to 15% of hospitalized AMI patients (18). If untreated, cardiogenic shock follows a rapid downward spiral of progressive circulatory failure and impaired cellular metabolism leading to organ dysfunction and death (46). Despite aggressive pharmacologic and surgical intervention, 80 to 100% of cardiogenic shock victims do not survive to hospital discharge (47). This near-universal mortality reflects the self-perpetuating cycle of myocardial ischemia and heart failure. Early therapeutic interventions aimed at increasing coronary perfusion pressure and decreasing myocardial oxygen demand should, at least theoretically, produce improved survival.

CLINICAL ASSESSMENT

The classic physical findings in cardiogenic shock are hypotension, tachycardia, diminished peripheral pulses, decreased urine output, clouded sensorium, and pulmonary edema. These are indicative of heart failure and circulatory insufficiency. Restlessness, agitation, and confusion are seen with mild-to-moderate impairment in cerebral blood flow while lethargy and obtundation may indicate severe cerebral hypoperfusion. The clinical features of pulmonary edema include rales over the lower lung fields, bronchospasm, dyspnea, copious pulmonary secretions, and profound cyanosis with rapid shallow breathing. If cardiogenic shock occurs with relative hypovolemia, the lung fields may appear clear. Arterial blood gases allow prompt assessment of the patient's respiratory function and acid–base status. Ventilatory adequacy can be determined by measuring the carbon dioxide tension in arterial blood ($PaCO_2$). A $PaCO_2$ above 50 Torr in the presence of a low arterial pH suggests hypoventilation.

The arterial oxygen tension (PaO_2 reflects the adequacy of oxygenation. Adequate arterial oxygenation ($PaO_2 \geq 70$ Torr) in cardiogenic shock usually requires supplemental oxygen administration. Although sinus tachycardia is generally present, sinus bradycardia, supraventricular tachycardia, ventricular tachycardia, or complete heart block may also be present in the cardiogenic shock. Diminished intensity of heart sounds reflecting the reduced myocardial contractility may be present. A systolic apical murmur may indicate mitral regurgitation due to papillary muscle dysfunction. With progressive loss of cardiac output, blood pressure will fall despite compensatory sympathoadrenal reflexes. Weak, thready, or absent peripheral pulses result from both a reduction in arterial blood pressure and an increase in peripheral resistance with reduced peripheral blood flow. This leads to the cold, damp, mottled skin commonly seen in patients with cardiogenic shock. A urine output of less than 20 mL per hour with a spot urine sodium of less than 10 mcg per liter suggests the presence

of a reduced glomerular filtration rate and subsequent stimulation of the renin angiotensin system.

HEMODYNAMICS

Cardiogenic shock is best defined in hemodynamic terms: systolic arterial pressure less than 80 mm Hg, cardiac index less than 1.8 L/min/m², and pulmonary capillary wedge pressure more than 18 mm Hg with urine output less than 20 mL per hour. Because not only accurate diagnosis but proper treatment requires hemodynamic guidance, it is almost always necessary to place a pulmonary artery (Swan-Ganz) catheter when signs of systemic hypoperfusion or severe pulmonary congestion are present. The Swan-Ganz catheter is designed to negotiate through the right atrium, right ventricle, and pulmonary artery without radiographic guidance. This is performed by inflation of a small air-filled balloon that is carried along by blood flow into proper position at a point where the balloon wedges into a pulmonary artery of similar diameter. A lumen beginning at the distal end of the catheter is connected to a transducer for continuous pressure monitoring. During insertion, central venous, right atrial, systolic right ventricular, and pulmonary arterial pressures may be recorded (Table 41.1). Additionally, this catheter provides infusion ports for administration of drugs.

The Swan-Ganz catheter has become an important tool in differentiating the causes of peripheral hypoperfusion and pulmonary congestion. In the presence of an AMI, the hemodynamic parameters define four subsets based on the presence or absence of hypoperfusion and/or pulmonary congestion (Table 41.2). These subsets are useful diagnostically and therapeutically (48). Hemodynamic parameters are all normal in subset I; the predicted mortality is 3%. Subset II clinically consists of pulmonary congestion without peripheral hypoperfusion and is defined hemodynamically by a cardiac index (CI) more than 2.2 L/min/m² and a pulmonary capillary wedge pressure (PCWP) more

Table 41.1.
Hemodynamic Parameters

	RAP	RVP	PAP	PCWP
Normal range (mm Hg)	0–8	15–30	15–30 / 5–12	5–12
Increased in:	RVF, RVI, PE, COPD, PCT		Systolic: PE, COPD, VSD Diastolic: PE, COPD, LVI, MS	LVI, MS, PCT
Comments:	RAP = LVEDP in PE, COPD, MS	RVP not useful	PAD = PCWP (>5 mm Hg) in PE, COPD	PCWP ≤ 20–25 pulm. edema In AMI optimal PCWP: 14–18 mm Hg

Abbreviations: RAP, right atrial pressure; RVP, right ventricular pressure; PAP, pulmonary artery pressure; PAD, pulmonary artery diastolic pressure; PCWP, pulmonary capillary wedge pressure; RVI, right ventricular infarction; PE, pulmonary embolus; COPD, chronic obstructive pulmonary disease; PCT, pericardial tamponade; LVI, left ventricular infarction; MS, mitral stenosis; AMI, acute myocardial infarction; RVF, right ventricular failure; LVEDP, left ventricular end-diastolic pressure.

Table 41.2.
Hemodynamic Classification and Relationship to Clinical Presentation and Percent Mortality Based on Hemodynamic Signs

	Subset I	Subset II
>2.2	Normal hemodynamics Mortality = 3%	Pulmonary congestion Rales present Mortality = 9%
CI[a]		
	Subset III	Subset IV
<2.2	Peripheral hypoperfusion Rales absent Mortality = 23%	Pulmonary congestion Rales present Peripheral hypoperfusion Mortality = 51%
	<18	<18
	PCWP	

With permission from Ornato JP, ed. Cardiovascular Emergencies. Churchill Livingstone, New York, 1986:123.
[a]Abbreviations: CI, cardiac index (liters/min/m); PCWP, pulmonary capillary wedge pressure (mm Hg).

than 18 mm Hg. The group mortality is 9%. Treatment generally includes diuretics and venodilators. Patients with peripheral hypoperfusion without pulmonary congestion constitute subset III and have a mortality rate of 23%. In this group, either relative volume depletion or slow heart rate cause a CI less than 2.2 L/min/m^2 with PCWP less than 18 mm Hg. Lastly, cardiogenic shock from either myocardial failure or mechanical lesions constitutes subset IV. Coexistent pulmonary congestion and peripheral hypoperfusion hemodynamically manifest as a CI less than 2.2 L/min/m^2 and a PCWP more than 18 mm Hg. Systemic blood pressure cannot be maintained despite reflex vasoconstriction that elevates the systemic vascular resistance (SVR) more than 1400 dyne-cm-sec^{-5}. Expected mortality in subset IV is 51%.

MEDICAL INTERVENTION

The goals of medical management of cardiogenic shock are to (1) optimize left ventricular filling pressure, (2) minimize the impedance to left ventricular ejection, and (3) maximize contractility without excessively increasing myocardial oxygen demand. Therapeutic agents used to remedy acute heart failure include diuretics, positive inotropic agents, and vasodilators.

Treatment of subset II is directed primarily at reducing PCWP. Diuretics are the cornerstone of therapy because they can be given by rapid intravenous administration with few adverse effects. In the patient with cardiogenic shock, intravenous diuretics exert two distinctly important effects. The immediate effect is an increase in venous capacitance redistributing blood away from the lungs and decreasing pulmonary capillary pressures (49). The second effect is to increase sodium and water excretion by the kidneys. Loop

diuretics produce renal vasodilation that may increase their diuretic effect (50). The resultant diuresis decreases both intravascular volume and left ventricular volume and filling pressure.

Overzealous diuresis should be avoided because excessive reductions in left ventricular filling pressure may worsen cardiac output. Diuretic-induced electrolyte abnormalities should be identified and promptly corrected. To minimize electrolyte abnormalities and to prevent the risk of suboptimal cardiac filling pressures, the smallest effective dose of the diuretic should be employed. The patient's hemodynamic parameters and urine output should guide subsequent diuretic administration. If diuretics are ineffective and acute ischemia is present, topical or intravenous nitroglycerin might provide added preload reduction.

The finding of isolated peripheral hypoperfusion (subset III) is of major prognostic importance because of the high mortality associated with it. These patients present with hypovolemia and/or bradycardia. The goal of therapy is to improve the cardiac index and to reverse the hypoperfusion while minimizing myocardial oxygen expenditure.

Hypovolemia will abnormally reduce left ventricular filling pressure, which may contribute to hypotension and vascular collapse. Fluid loss may be due to chronic diuretic therapy, vomiting, diarrhea, diaphoresis, or internal hemorrhage. Hypovolemia should be identified, and if present, should be corrected before more aggressive circulatory support is initiated. The majority of these patients demonstrate a reduction in stroke volume and a compensatory tachycardia. In general, cardiac output will increase with fluid resuscitation until the PCWP reaches approximately 15 to 18 mm Hg, above which point further increases in cardiac output are minimal (51).

Initial fluid resuscitation should consist of 50 to 100 mL of normal saline or 5% albumin administered intravenously over 5 to 10 minutes with appropriate hemodynamic assessment, and volume status monitoring. Table 41.3 lists

Table 41.3.
Comparative Prices of Volume-Expanding Agents

Type	Amount (mL)	Agerage Cost ($)	Cost per 500 mL IV Expansion ($)
Albumin 5%	500	122.00	122.00
Albumin 25%	100	150.00	150.00
Hydroxyethyl starch (hetastarch)	500	24.79	25.00
Dextran 40	500	33.00	30.00
Dextran 70	500	21.00	20.00
Ringer's lactate	1000	1.50	4.00
Normal saline	1000	1.50	4.00

Adapted from Chernow B, ed. The Pharmacologic Approach to the Critically Ill Patient. Baltimore: Williams & Wilkins, 1983:185.

Table 41.4.
Inotropes and Vasoactive Agents

Drug Usual Dose	Receptor Specificity					Pharmacologic Effect				
	α	β$_1$	β$_2$	Dop	Sm Msc	VD	VC	INT	CHT	RBF
Norepinephrine (Levophed) IV 2–12 μg/min	++++	++					++++	+	++	↓
Dopamine (Inotropin)										
2–5 μg/kg/min		+		++++		+		++	+	↕
6–10 μg/kg/min		++++	++	+		+		++++	++	
10–20 μg/kg/min	+++	++++	+				+++	+++	+++	
Dobutamine (Dobutrex)			++			++	+	++++	++	↑
2.0–15.0 μg/kg/min	+	++++								
Amrinone (Inocor)		?				++		+++	+++	
0.75 mg/kg										
5–10 μg/kg/min										↑
Nitroprusside (Nipride)					++++ A = V					
0.5–10 μg/kg/min										↕
Nitroglycerin 5–300 μg/min					++++ A < V					↕
Hydralazine (Apresoline)					A					↑
5–20 mg IV bolus					++++					

(continued)

the commercially available volume-expanding agents. No ideal agent for volume expansion has been identified. Crystalloids are less expensive but produce relatively short-lived volume expansion. Colloids increase plasma oncotic pressure and produce sustained volume expansion but are more expensive. There is no conclusive evidence that the type of fluid used in volume resuscitation influences the development of pulmonary complications.

A small group of patients in subset III have a normal stroke volume but a slow heart rate. Temporary transvenous pacing may restore cardiac output, but the increase in myocardial oxygen demand outweighs the marginal increase in cardiac output at rates beyond 90 to 100 beats per minute (46). The most substantial rise in CI is observed in patients with resting heart rates of 50 to 70 beats per minute (51).

Subset IV carries the highest mortality. The goal of therapy is the simultaneous improvement in CI and PCWP (47). The choice of therapies lies between inotropic agents and peripheral vasodilators (51). Vasodilators are usually better because they have a more favorable impact on myocardial oxygen demand. However, when severe hypotension is present, a positive inotropic effect will prevent further circulatory collapse. The ideal inotropic agent must maintain or improve myocardial contractility while mini-

mizing oxygen demand. Because no such agent exists, this is best accomplished by careful titration of combined therapy with inotropic and vasodilator drugs (Table 41.4).

INOTROPIC AGENTS

Inotropic agents increase the peak tension produced by the myocardium during systole and shorten the time spent in systole (52). All inotropes in clinical use have important effects on the peripheral arterial and venous vasculature as well as on myocardial oxygen demand. Sympathomimetic amines are the most commonly used inotropes. They stimulate both α- and β-adrenergic and dopaminergic receptors to varying degrees (52). α-adrenergic stimulation mediates peripheral vasoconstriction. β$_1$-adrenergic stimulation exerts positive chronotropic, dromotropic, and inotropic effects. β$_2$-adrenergic stimulation produces vasodilation and bronchodilation. Stimulation of dopaminergic receptors mediates vasodilation of renal, adrenal, mesenteric, coronary, and cerebral vascular beds.

Norepinephrine. Norepinephrine increases myocardial contractility and causes vasoconstriction of arterial and venous vascular beds by stimulating β$_1$- and α-adrenergic receptors. In cardiogenic shock, it may increase cardiac output and redistribute blood flow to the heart and brain. The average adult dose is 2 to 12 mcg per minute although

Table 41.4. *(Continued)*

Hemodynamic Effect					
MAP	PCWP	CO	SVR	UO	Comments
↑	↑	↕	↑	↓	Decreased peripheral perfusion, painful extravasation, arrhythmias, angina
↑	↑	↕	↕	↕	Arrhythmias, headache, hypertension, decreased peripheral perfusion, painful extravasation
↕	↓	↑	→↓	↑	Headache, palpitation, hypotension
↕	↓	↑	↕	↑	Thrombocytopenia, nausea, flulike syndrome, arrhythmias, hypotension
↓	↓	↕	↓	↕	Hypotension, nausea, abdominal pain, tremor, headache, confusion
↓	↓	↕	→↓	↕	Headache, tachycardia, hypotension, nausea
↓	→	↑	↓	↑	Hypotension, headache, reflex tachycardia, angina

With permission, from Ornato JP, ed. Cardiovascular Emergencies. Churchill Livingstone: New York, 1986:123.
Key: α, α-adrenergic; β_1, β_1-adrenergic; β_2, β_2-adrenergic; DOP, dopaminergic; Sm Msc, smooth muscle; VD, vasodilation; VC, vasoconstriction; INT, inotropic; CHT, chronotropic; RBF, renal blood flow; MAP, mean arterial pressure; PCWP, pulmonary capillary wedge pressure; CO, cardiac output; SVR, systemic vascular resistance; UO, urine output; +, low; ++++, high; A, arterial; V, venous; ↑, increase; ↓, decrease; →, no change.

higher doses may be needed to achieve what is believed to be an optimal mean arterial pressure of 75 mm Hg. Norepinephrine should be infused through a central venous line to minimize the risk of extravasation. If this should occur, 10 to 15 mL of sodium chloride solution containing 5 to 10 mg of phentolamine mesylate should be infiltrated liberally throughout the affected area, which is identified by a cold, hard, and pale appearance. Norepinephrine infusions require careful monitoring of arterial blood pressure. With increasing doses, the α-adrenergic effect becomes more pronounced resulting in renal vasoconstriction, oliguria, and a marked increase in systemic vascular resistance. High doses will also increase the risk of tachyarrhythmias and myocardial ischemia. Anxiety, respiratory difficulty, angina, headaches, peripheral vasoconstriction, and metabolic acidosis can also be observed.

Dopamine. Dopamine is a precursor of norepinephrine. It stimulates dopaminergic, β_1- and α-adrenergic receptors in a dose-dependent fashion (53,54). Dopamine also releases endogenous norepinephrine (53). In low doses (2 to 5 mcg/kg/min), dopamine produces vasodilation of renal, mesenteric, coronary, and cerebral arteries. In the dosage range of 6 to 10 mcg/kg/min, it increases cardiac output through β-adrenergic stimulation. At progressively higher infusion rates (10 to 20 mcg/kg/min), the α-adrenergic effects of dopamine become most prominent, producing peripheral vasoconstriction (53). Because there is a large interpatient variation in sensitivity to dopamine, infusions should be slowly titrated until the desired effect is seen (54). Dopamine infusions should not be discontinued abruptly; a gradual taper is recommended when the drug is no longer required. The ECG should be monitored for tachyarrhythmias. Dopamine may produce or exacerbate nausea, vomiting, and angina. The risk of extravasation is the same as with norepinephrine and should be managed accordingly.

Comparative studies have shown that dopamine is more effective and less arrhythmogenic than isoproterenol in patients with cardiogenic shock (54). Dopamine appears to produce a greater increase in cardiac output and urine flow than does norepinephrine (54). Dopamine may not be a desirable agent in patients with elevated PCWP and SVR. However, it is invaluable when low SVR and profound hypotension compromise coronary perfusion pressure (56).

Dobutamine. Dobutamine is a relatively selective positive inotrope. It was synthesized to minimize the arrhythmogenic side effects of isoproterenol (56). Dobutamine is a potent β_1-adrenergic agonist with mild β_2- and α-adrenergic activity. Experimental data suggest that dobutamine exerts a positive inotropic effect by stimulating α-

and β-adrenergic receptors in the myocardium (57). Dobutamine produces a dose-related increase in cardiac output, which is accompanied by a significant reduction in left ventricular filling pressure (55). Dobutamine may often decrease the systemic vascular resistance (18). This effect and the lack of drug-mediated endogenous catecholamine release explain why dobutamine has a more favorable impact than either norepinephrine or dopamine on myocardial oxygen demand (56).

Dobutamine is administered as a continuous intravenous infusion starting at 2 to 3 mcg/kg/min and increased by 1 to 2 mcg/kg/min every 10 to 30 minutes until optimal hemodynamic effects are achieved or side effects develop. The usual maintenance dose ranges from 7.5 to 20 mcg/kg/min. Doses above 30 mcg/kg/min frequently lead to side effects (56). Sinus tachycardia is the most frequent toxic effect of dobutamine although it occurs less commonly than with dopamine or isoproterenol. Other side effects include nausea, headaches, anxiety, angina, tremors, hypotension, or hypertension.

Several studies have shown that the clinical and hemodynamic responses of dobutamine and dopamine are different and complimentary (55,58,59). Dopamine exerts a greater increase in systemic blood pressure and an increase or no change in left ventricular filling pressure when compared to equal doses of dobutamine. Dobutamine is indicated in clinical situations where pulmonary congestion and circulatory collapse are due to loss of ventricular contractility with no significant loss of vascular tone (55). The combination of dobutamine and dopamine may show more favorable results than either agent alone, especially in cardiogenic shock patients requiring mechanical ventilation (59).

The ability of dobutamine to increase cardiac output without increasing oxygen demand, or reducing coronary blood flow through tachycardia, has led to its use in heart failure associated with an AMI. However, additional studies are needed to establish its role as the inotrope of choice in cardiogenic shock.

Amrinone. Amrinone, a nonglycosidic, noncatecholamine intravenous inotropic vasodilatory agent, is indicated for use in severe heart failure (60). Its positive inotropic effect develops within minutes and persists for 60 to 90 minutes following a single intravenous administration. This action is not impaired by β- or α-adrenoceptor blocking agents (52). Initial therapy with amrinone 0.75 mg/kg by intravenous injection over 2 to 3 minutes followed by an infusion of 5 to 10 mcg/kg/min will increase cardiac contractility and decrease SVR. Improvements in CI, PCWP, and SVR average 50%, but greater benefits have been observed in some patients (61–63).

Amrinone is promoted as a "major advance" in inotropic therapy because of its sustained hemodynamic improvements and its reduction in myocardial oxygen demand (60). Few studies have compared amrinone with other inotropes in patients with severe fractory heart failure (64). Klein and coworkers reported that initial improvements in CI and SVR were greater with dobutamine than with amrinone. However, the hemodynamic effects of amrinone were maintained for the 24 hours, whereas deterioration from initial response was noted to occur with dobutamine. These results are in conflict with those of other studies (60). Overall, amrinone does not appear to be superior to any other currently available inotropic agent and may actually be more prone to toxicity. Thrombocytopenia is reported to occur in up to 50% of patients treated with amrinone (65). The thrombocytopenia is rapidly reversible on drug withdrawal. Short-term intravenous infusions may produce nausea, vomiting, liver function test abnormalities, a flulike syndrome, dysrhythmias, and hypotension (60). Intravenous amrinone should be an agent reserved for cases of severe and refractory heart failure.

Vasodilators

Generalized sympathetic vasoconstriction is a useful compensatory mechanism for maintaining systemic pressure and coronary perfusion in cardiogenic shock. However, excessive vasoconstriction decreases cardiac output and increases myocardial oxygen demand. By decreasing this reflex vasoconstriction, vasodilator drugs can reduce ventricular wall stress and produce an improvement in cardiac output similar to that observed with inotropic drugs. The primary effects of these agents appear to be related to their peripheral actions on arterial and venous beds. By dilating the arterial resistance bed, vasodilators reduce impedance with a resultant increase in stroke volume. Vasodilating drugs that also reduce venous tone will decrease venous return to the heart, which will lower the filling pressure in both ventricles. These actions correct the combined hemodynamic abnormalities present in cardiogenic shock and may improve the balance between myocardial oxygen supply and demand.

The use of vasodilators is limited by their potential to produce hypotension in patients with heart failure. These agents produce a triphasic response: (1) at low doses, cardiac output increases and PCWP decreases with little change in arterial pressure; (2) at moderate doses, cardiac output increases, PCWP decreases, and arterial pressures decrease or remain unchanged; and (3) at high doses, cardiac output, PCWP, and arterial pressure all decrease (41). Vasodilators should be avoided in patients without high filling pressures. Hemodynamic measurements should be followed closely in all patients receiving vasodilator therapy, particularly when concomitant diuretic therapy is employed.

Sodium Nitroprusside. Sodium nitroprusside is the most widely used vasodilator in the management of cardiogenic shock. Its rapid onset and short duration of action make it a suitable agent in hemodynamically unstable situations. Numerous studies have reported improvement in left ventricular function, tissue perfusion, coronary output, and clinical status in patients with low output states and high SVR refractory to dopamine (67). However, nitroprusside should not be routinely used in patients who develop high left ventricular filling pressures within the first few hours after acute myocardial infarction since it may produce a "coronary steal" phenomenon (i.e., decrease coronary blood flow away from ischemic areas) (68).

The recommended dosing range is 0.5 to 5 mcg/kg/min, but higher doses (up to 10 mcg/kg/min) may be needed. The major complication of nitroprusside is hypotension. Patients should be monitored for signs of cyanide or thiocyanate toxicity. Cyanide toxicity is detected by the presence of metabolic acidosis; thiocyanate toxicity is manifested by confusion, hyperreflexia, and convulsions. Thiocyanate levels above 12 mg/dl suggest thiocyanate toxicity (69). Low-dose infusions (less than 3 mcg/kg/min) for less than 72 hours rarely lead to toxicity.

Nitroglycerin. Nitroglycerin reduces intramyocardial wall tension, improves myocardial blood flow, and lowers systemic vascular resistance. Intravenous nitroglycerin is an effective adjunct in the management of heart failure associated with myocardial infarction. It is administered by continuous intravenous infusion at 10 to 20 mcg per minute and increased by 5 to 10 mcg per minute every 5 to 10 minutes until the desired hemodynamic or clinical response occurs. Low doses (30 to 40 mcg/min) produce predominantly venodilation; high doses (250 mcg/min) lead to arteriolar dilation as well (70).

In cardiogenic shock, the beneficial effects of nitroglycerin are due to systemic vasodilation, which increases cardiac output and lowers oxygen consumption, and to direct vasodilation of the coronary circulation, which increases blood supply to ischemic areas compared to nitroprusside (71). The combination of nitroglycerin and an inotrope (dopamine or dobutamine), although not extensively studied, appears to produce marked hemodynamic improvements while reducing the risk of ischemia damage (72). Overall, patients with the most severe degree of left ventricular failure have the most beneficial hemodynamic effects.

Recent studies have suggested a difference between nitroglycerin and nitroprusside relative to their effect on myocardial blood flow (73). Nitroglycerin has a greater vasodilatory effect on collateral capacitance vessels. Nitroprusside has a greater vasodilatory effect on arteriolar resistance vessels. Therefore, nitroglycerin is less likely to produce coronary steal. Furthermore, nitroprusside has a greater propensity to lower coronary perfusion pressure than does nitroglycerin (74). The risk reduction in mortality in trials with nitroglycerin in AMI is 45%; this is greater

than the 23% reduction in mortality observed with nitroprusside in AMI (75). These data suggest that intravenous nitroglycerin reduces mortality in AMI.

Nitroglycerin is generally well tolerated. Potential complications of intravenous nitroglycerin include reversible hypotension and bradycardia, hypoxemia due to increased pulmonary ventilation–perfusion mismatch, methemoglobinemia, and headache. In general, the drug has been well tolerated.

Mechanical Circulatory Support

The near universal mortality among patients with cardiogenic shock despite medical management has identified the need for other modalities to augment left ventricular function and reverse circulatory collapse. Mechanical circulatory support attempts to meet these needs while favorably affecting the balance between myocardial oxygen supply and demand. The decision to institute mechanical circulatory support is based on the presence of a low cardiac index (less than 1.8 L/min) and an elevated PCWP (more than 20 mm Hg) despite maximal inotropic, vasodilator, and vasopressor support (76–78). The major uses of mechanical circulatory assist devices are in those patients who are potential transplant recipients and in patients with medically refractory unstable angina unamenable to invasive procedures.

The intraaortic balloon pump (IABP) was the first mechanical assist device used for improving aortic and coronary blood flow while reducing left ventricular workload in cardiogenic shock (76). The IABP is a balloon-tipped arterial catheter that is placed just below the aortic arch via the femoral artery. Balloon inflation increases diastolic perfusion pressure and coronary blood flow; balloon deflation improves cardiac output by reducing afterload. The net effect of intraaortic balloon counterpulsation (IABC) is to improve the balance between myocardial oxygen supply and demand (5). Serious complications from IABC are common and include damage to or perforation of the aortic wall, limb ischemia, thrombocytopenia and hemolysis, systemic embolization, wound infection, and failure due to balloon rupture (77). Cardiac arrhythmias are a relative contraindication to IABC and must be corrected for effective counterpulsation.

IABC can provide temporary hemodynamic improvement in patients with cardiogenic shock (18,76), but it minimally affects long-term survival. The failure to permanently reverse the shock syndrome following AMI is probably the result of preexisting irreversible tissue necrosis. Contraindications to IABC include aortic regurgitation, aortic dissection or aneurysm, near terminal or untreatable medical conditions, ventricular fibrillation, or asystole (4,5,21).

The IABP is not considered a true ventricular assist device (VAD) because the term *VAD* is usually reserved for those devices that are able to totally support the circulation (78). There are two types of VADs: nonpulsatile devices used for cardiopulmonary resuscitation and pulsatile devices used for long-term support. As the number of patients awaiting cardiac transplantation continues to increase, so will the need for VADs as a bridge to heart transplantation. The reader is referred to an excellent review on this topic by Miller (78).

Prognosis

Even under optimal conditions, the prognosis of the AMI patient with cardiogenic shock is grave. Of the 10 to 30% who do survive to hospital discharge, 50% will die within the following 24 months (2).

LIMITATION OF INFARCT SIZE

Irreversible myocardial ischemic injury in humans takes up to 6 hours to develop. If reperfusion of the ischemic zone is instituted within 3 to 4 hours, the area of infarction may be reduced. Although direct measure of infarct size in human hearts can be made only at autopsy, infarct size can be assessed indirectly by trends in the ECG, by the pattern of myocardial enzyme release, or by radionuclide techniques. Because infarct size correlates with mortality, interventions capable of reducing MI size might be expected to reduce the rate of postinfarction death. Results obtained in animal models of AMI indicate that interventions designed to reduce myocardial oxygen demand, to enhance oxygen supply, or to reduce the acute inflammatory response can salvage ischemic myocardium (79). This section examines pharmacologic intervention that may limit infarct size by decreasing myocardial oxygen consumption or by improving myocardial oxygen demand.

β-Adrenergic Blocking Agents

β-adrenergic blockade reduces myocardial oxygen consumption by reducing heart rate, contractility, and blood pressure. β-adrenergic blockers can also reduce catecholamine levels in the ischemic heart and produce favorable redistribution of coronary blood flow (80–82).

Clinical trials with these agents can be divided into two groups: (1) those in which treatment was begun early and endpoints such as enzyme levels, ECG changes, and reinfarction rates are investigated, and (2) those in which treatment was begun later after resolution of the infarct, with mortality rate reduction as the endpoint. There is evidence that intravenous therapy followed by oral administration with atenolol, propranolol, metoprolol, sotalol, or timolol reduces serum CK concentrations. Reduction in ECG abnormalities post-AMI has been reported following acute intervention with propranolol, practolol, and metoprolol. Studies show that β-blockers limit infarct size, reduce the incidence of malignant ventricular arrhythmia,

and reduce mortality following acute administration in patients with AMI (83).

The Metoprolol in Acute Myocardial Infarction (MI-AMI) trial was a multicenter, double-blind, placebo-controlled randomized study in which 2877 patients with suspected or definite myocardial infarction received 5 mg of metoprolol (Lopressor) intravenously every 2 minutes for a total of 15 mg within 24 hours of onset of symptoms (84). Patients were randomized into the study after arrival at the coronary care unit. After intravenous dosing, patients received oral metoprolol 100 mg every 6 hours for the first 2 days beginning 15 minutes after the last intravenous injection. The dose was then decreased to 100 mg every 12 hours for the remaining 13 days of the study. The cumulative mortality for all patients at the conclusion of the 15-day trial was 123 (4.3%) deaths in the treatment group compared with 142 (4.9%) deaths in the placebo group. This difference did not reach statistical significance. Mortality in patients with definite MI was 120 of 2028 in the metoprolol group versus 137 of 2099 in the placebo group. High-risk patients in MIAMI were found to benefit, whereas other subgroups did not benefit.

In the First International Study of Infarct Survival (ISIS-1), a total of 16,207 patients were randomized to receive 5 to 10 mg of atenolol (Tenormin), in 5-mg intravenous doses, or placebo within a mean of 5 hours of onset of suspected MI. Oral dosing in the treatment group followed, with 100 mg of atenolol per day as either a single dose or divided every 12 hours for a total of 7 days. Vascular mortality occurred in 313 of 8037 (3.89%) atenolol-treated patients and 365 of 7990 (4.57%) control patients. The beneficial effect of atenolol in decreasing the incidence of mortality was statistically significant (2p less than 0.04) (85).

The Thrombolysis in Myocardial Infarction—Phase II (TIMI II) study addressed the use of early and late β-adrenergic blocker therapy following recombinant tissue plasminogen activator (rt-PA) administration (86). Patients were randomly assigned to receive immediate β-adrenergic blocker administration (three doses of metoprolol 5 mg intravenously at 2-minute intervals followed by 50 mg orally twice a day for 24 hours, then 100 mg twice a day) or delayed administration (starting on day 6 post-MI) consisting of metoprolol 50 mg twice a day for 24 hours, then 100 mg twice daily. The time of enter into the study was less than 4 hours since onset of AMI (mean 2.6 hours). Ejection fraction and early mortality were found to be similar between the two groups, however at day 6, 16 patients in the immediate metroprolol intervention group and 31 patients in the delayed group had nonfatal reinfarctions (p = 0.02). Recurrent ischemic episodes totaled 107 patients in the early metroprolol intervention group compared to 147 patients in the delayed intervention group (p = 0.005). Mortality at the end of the 6-week study was 5.0% in immediate metoprolol therapy versus 12.1% in delayed intervention (p = 0.001).

Based on TIMI II data, intravenous β-blocker therapy reduces mortality and reinfarction rate when administered within 2 hours of the onset of symptoms in AMI patients receiving thrombolytic therapy (86). If intravenous β-blocker therapy is initiated within 4 hours of symptom onset, there is a reduction in nonfatal reinfarction and recurrent ischemia (86). β-blockers may also reduce the risk of intracranial bleeding in AMI patients treated with thrombolytics.

β-adrenergic blockers are also valuable in AMI patients with atrial tachyarrhythmias or rapid ventricular response rates in atrial fibrillation (30). Well-designed trials with large numbers of patients show that timolol, metoprolol, and propranolol significantly reduce long-term mortality of AMI. Because these agents were administered after resolution of the MI, the reduction in mortality is likely due to a decrease in the incidence of arrhythmias or reinfarction and not related to infarct size reduction.

Although β-adrenergic blockers are contraindicated in patients with serious myocardial dysfunction, cardiac conduction abnormalities, hypotension, peripheral hypoperfusion, or bronchospastic airway disease, it is reasonable to consider their use in AMI patients without contraindications, irrespective of concomitant thrombolytic therapy (83). Recent studies suggest that esmolol infusions, at a reduced dosage, may be used safely and effectively in thrombolytic-treated AMI patients with relative contraindications to β-blocker therapy (e.g., congestive heart failure, pulmonary disease, peripheral vascular disease, bradycardia, or systolic blood pressure less than 100 mm Hg) (87).

Calcium Channel Blockers

Experimental data in animals suggest that calcium channel blockers may prevent the progression of ischemia and subsequent necrosis by decreasing myocardial oxygen demand without compromising cardiac output (1). Recent clinical trials indicate that these agents do not alter outcome in AMI patients. Verapamil may reduce infarct size but does not alter acute mortality (88). The Danish Multicenter Study Group randomized 100 patients to receive verapamil 0.1 mg/kg intravenously followed by 120 mg orally three times a day or placebo for 6 months (89). Patients were randomized within 4 hours of onset of symptoms of acute MI. Verapamil failed to alter acute mortality, long-term mortality, or reinfarction rate when compared with placebo (89).

Studies with nifedipine (20 mg orally every 4 hours for 14 days) failed to show a significant reduction in enzymatically assessed infarct size compared with placebo (90). A slight trend for higher mortality was observed in the nifedipine group. The Nifedipine Angina Myocardial

Infarction Study (NAMIS) was the first multicenter placebo-controlled trial to assess nifedipine (Procardia) 20 mg every 4 hours, starting 4.6 ± 0.1 hours after the onset of chest pain for 14 days. A total of 171 patients with either threatened MI or early acute MI were admitted into the study. No significant difference in size of infarction, as assessed by CK-MB serum levels, between the two groups was noted. A startling observation was that the nifedipine-treated group exhibited a higher incidence of mortality (7.9 versus 0% in the control group) during the 2-week study period. Long-term mortality at 6-month follow-up was not statistically significant between the nifedipine and placebo groups (90).

The Norwegian Nifedipine Multicenter Trial randomized 277 patients to receive either nifedipine 10 mg five times a day or placebo (91). Unlike the NAMIS trial, randomization occurred within 12 hours of onset of symptoms. Treatment on the average was initiated within 5.5 ± 2.9 hours of symptoms, and nifedipine was administered for 6 weeks. Results showed no difference in CK-MB release or 6-week mortality between the two groups.

A placebo-controlled trial of diltiazem in AMI reported a reduction in early recurrent infarction (one-tailed, P = .03, two-tailed, P = .06) in patients with a non-Q wave myocardial infarction (92). This multicenter, double-blinded study consisted of 576 patients who were randomized to receive either drug treatment or placebo within 24 to 72 hours of onset of infarction.

Diltiazem 90 mg every 6 hours or placebo was continued for 14 days. Reinfarction, defined as a secondary increase in CK-MB during the study period, was observed in 15 of 287 (5.2%) diltiazem-treated patients compared with 27 of 289 (9.3%) control patients (p = 0.0297); however, 61% of the diltiazem patients and 64% of the placebo group were receiving concurrent β-adrenergic blocker therapy, and 80% were also receiving long-acting nitrates. Side effects such as heart block, bradycardia (HR less than 40 bpm), and hypotension (SBP less than 90 mm Hg) were more pronounced in the diltiazem group compared with placebo. Although the study concluded that diltiazem was effective in preventing early reinfarction in non-Q-wave MI, no difference in mortality between the two groups was observed during the 14-day study period (93).

The Multicenter Diltiazem Post-Infarction Trial (MD-PIT) evaluated 2466 patients with acute MI in a randomized, double-blind, placebo controlled trial (94). Patients received either placebo or diltiazem 60 mg orally four times a day. Therapy was initiated between 3 and 15 days post-MI. There was no difference in mortality between groups; however, there were 11% fewer recurrent cardiac events (e.g., nonfatal reinfarction, death from cardiac cause) in the diltiazem group. Further analysis of the MDPIT data indicates that diltiazem-treated patients with left ventricular dysfunction (ejection fraction less than 40%), pulmonary congestion, and acute anterolateral Q-wave MI at baseline had a predictable higher incidence of cardiac death and nonfatal reinfarction (94). Long-term diltiazem therapy in AMI patients failed to demonstrate any significant benefit and produced detrimental side effects in patients with left ventricular dysfunction.

Although there is laboratory evidence that calcium channel blockers reduce infarct size, these results are not observed under clinical conditions. Currently, there is no reason to recommend general treatment with calcium channel blockers to reduce infarct size. However, patients with documented or suspected vasospastic angina and AMI patients undergoing emergent angioplasty may benefit from the use of calcium channel blockers as long as left ventricular function is relatively well preserved (83).

Nitrates

Oganic nitrates, such as nitroglycerin and nitroprusside, reduce preload and afterload by their veno- and arteriolar-dilatory effects. Nitrates reduce myocardial oxygen demand and dilate the epicardial coronary vasculature. Nitroglycerin infusion decreases both enzymatically assessed infarct size and hospital mortality in patients with left ventricular dysfunction (95). Intravenous nitroglycerin is preferred because it minimizes the risks of hypotension and tachycardia observed with oral nitrates and is less likely to produce "coronary steal" than is nitroprusside. Prompt initiation of intravenous nitroglycerin therapy can reduce infarct size and reduce the incidence of congestive heart failure in patients with AMI. Nitroglycerin is most useful in patients with ongoing ischemia or heart failure.

Angiotensin Converting Enzyme (ACE) Inhibitors

Patients with an anterior wall MI and reduced left ventricular function may benefit from therapy with an ACE inhibitor if it is initiated within the first 2 weeks after the AMI (96). In patients with left ventricular dysfunction, the use of long-term ACE inhibitor therapy may reduce mortality. ACE inhibitors may produce several benefits in the post-MI patient. Early therapy with an ACE inhibitor may inhibit early infarct expansion, ventricular thinning, and dilation. Long-term ACE inhibitor therapy may inhibit the progression of late global dilation of the uninfarcted tissue. These benefits are additive to those observed with thrombolytic therapy

The initiation of ACE inhibitor therapy within the first 2 weeks post-AMI may save the lives of 5 patients for every 1000 patients with left ventricular dysfunction (96). Ideal candidates for ACE inhibitor therapy include patients with anterior wall infarcts and AMI patients with congestive heart failure, hypertension, or unsuccessful thrombolysis. To achieve the greatest amount of benefit

from the ACE inhibitors in the post-MI patient, therapy should be started during the first week after the AMI.

Recent studies by Pfeffer and colleagues show that early and continued use of captopril in patients with asymptomatic left ventricular dysfunction after acute myocardial infarction improved survival and reduced morbidity and mortality due to major cardiovascular events (SAVE Trial). Patients (n = 2231) with ejection fractions ≤40% but without overt heart failure or recurrent ischemia were randomly assigned to receive either captopril 50 mg three times daily or placebo within 3 to 16 days after their acute myocardial infarction. Patients were followed for an average of 42 months. Captopril reduced all cause mortality by 19%, the risk of cardiovascular death was reduced by 21%, the risk of congestive heart failure requiring hospitalization was reduced by 22%, and the risk of recurrent myocardial infarction was reduced by 25%. These benefits were seen in patients who received thrombolytic therapy, aspirin, and/or β-adrenergic blockers, and in those who did not (97).

In contrast, the Second Cooperative New Scandinavian Enalapril Survival Study (CONSENSUS II) failed to demonstrate a benefit from the administration of enalapril (up to 20 mg per day) in patients placed on this therapy within 24 hours after their acute myocardial infarction. A total of 6090 patients were randomized to receive either enalapril or placebo along with conventional therapy (i.e., thrombolytics, nitrates, aspirin, β-blockers, diuretics, analgesics, and calcium antagonists). The trial was prematurely stopped because of the high probability that enalapril was no more effective than placebo in improving 6-month survival (98).

The Studies of Left Ventricular Dysfunction (SOLVD) Prevention Trial showed that long-term enalapril significantly reduced the incidence of heart failure and the need for hospitalization when compared with placebo in patients with asymptomatic left ventricular dysfunction (ejection fraction ≤35%). Approximately 80% of patients in the SOLVD Prevention Trial had suffered an acute myocardial infarction prior to enrollment in the study. The efficacy of enalapril in preventing the development of heart failure was evident as early as 3 months after the start of treatment (99).

THROMBOLYTIC AGENTS

Thrombolytic therapy has assumed a central role in the management of patients with AMI. The interest in thrombolytic therapy stems from four clinical findings: (1) approximately 85% of transmural myocardial infarctions (evaluated within 4 hours of onset of symptoms) are caused by a coronary thrombus; (2) thrombolytic agents can lyse clots effectively; (3) myocardial salvage can occur if therapy is begun within 6 hours after the onset of symptoms; and (4) a reduction in mortality can be

Table 41.5.
Comparison of Thrombolytic Agents

Agent	Half-Life (min)	Dose	Advantages	Disadvantages
APSAC	105	30-unit bolus	Long-acting bolus dose	Antigenicity, "lytic" effect
Streptokinase	90	1.5 million units over 1 hr	Proven value, inexpensive	Antigenicity, "lytic" effect
rt-PA	36	100 mg over 3 hr	Proven value, clot-selective, nonantigenic	Expensive, inconvenient regimen
r-Pro-urokinase	7	70 mg over 1 hr	Clot-selective, nonantigenic	Short half-life, investigational
Urokinase	16	2-million-unit bolus	Effective, nonantigenic	Expensive, "lytic" effect

With permission, from Monk JP, Heel RC. Anisoylated plasminogen streptokinase activator complex (APSAC). A review of its mechanisms of action, clinical pharmacology and its therapeutic use in acute myocardial infarction. Drugs 34:25–49, 1987.
Legend: anisoylated plasminogen-streptokinase activator complex (APSAC), recombinant tissue-type plasminogen activator (rt-PA).

achieved in some patients who receive thrombolytic agents (83,100,101).

Pharmacologic Thrombolysis

Thrombolytic agents activate both soluble plasminogen and surface-bound plasminogen to plasmin. Pharmacologic thrombolysis occurs when surface-bound plasminogen is converted to surface-bound plasmin. Plasmin, generated in proximity to the fibrin clot, lyses fibrin and dissolves the clot. Streptokinase, urokinase, and anisoylated plasminogen-streptokinase-activator complex (APSAC) are non-fibrin-selective thrombolytic agents. Recombinant tissue-type plasminogen activator (rt-PA) and recombinant single-chain urokinase plasminogen activator (r-scu-PA) are fibrin-selective agents because they activate plasma plasminogen to a lesser extent than surface-bound plasminogen. However, fibrin-selectivity is relatively dose dependent, and all agents will activate circulating plasminogen to different degrees (streptokinase more than APSAC more than urokinase more than r-scu-PA more than rt-PA) (102). Table 41.5 lists the half-life, dose, advantages, and disadvantages for each of these agents (102).

The goals of thrombolytic therapy are to lyse coronary thrombi during the early phase of AMI, to limit infarct size by reperfusing jeopardized myocardium, and to reduce morbidity and mortality. Thrombolytic agents can be infused by either the intracoronary or the intravenous route. Patients with recent onset of chest pain (usually less than 6 hours), with persistent ECG abnormalities indicating an evolving transmural AMI, are candidates for thrombolytic therapy (100). Patients with recent CVA, surgery, cardiopulmonary resuscitation, active bleeding, or bleeding diathesis should not receive thrombolytic therapy.

Intracoronary streptokinase is initiated with a 10,000- to 30,000-unit bolus, followed by an infusion of 2000 to 4000 units per minute. Clot lysis generally occurs within 30 minutes after initiation of the infusion and requires an average of 65,000 units of streptokinase. The infusion is

continued for 30 to 60 minutes after successful reperfusion or until a predetermined maximal dose of streptokinase (150,000 to 500,000 units). Intravenous streptokinase is administered at a dose of 750,000 to 1.5 million units over 30 to 60 minutes. After streptokinase, patients receive full-dose, intravenous heparin for 24 to 72 hours. Early treatment reestablishes flow in the infarct-related coronary artery in 60 to 90% of patients treated with intracoronary and 35 to 62% of patients treated with intravenous streptokinase (101).

Urokinase may be used in patients with hypersensitivity to streptokinase or with high streptococcal antibody titers. Patients who have received streptokinase within 1 to 2 months of a repeat course may require larger doses or treatment with urokinase because streptokinase antibodies can be found in high concentrations for up to 3 months (95,102). Three units of urokinase are approximately equivalent to 1 unit of streptokinase. Urokinase is most commonly used by intracoronary administration to prevent acute closure in patients undergoing balloon dilatation of the right coronary artery or in patients requiring emergent coronary angioplasty after failed therapy with an intravenous thrombolytic.

Anisoylated human plasminogen-streptokinase-activator complex (APSAC) is a direct plasminogen-activator complex formed when streptokinase and human plasminogen are acylated with a p-anisoyl derivative. This renders the activator inactive, but the acylation of the catalytic site of the plasminogen molecule is reversible over time. The streptokinase-plasminogen complex of APSAC dissociates at a rate slower than the deacylation rate, ensuring that the fibrinolytic activity of the drug is controlled by the latter. The deacylation half-life is about 105 minutes in human plasma or whole blood in vitro, and the plasma clearance half-life of fibrinolytic activity has been reported at 90 to 112 minutes in patients with AMI. The extended half-life of APSAC allows it to be administered as a single intravenous injection over 4 to 5 minutes.

The main advantages of APSAC over alternative thrombolytic drugs is its ease of administration by the intravenous route in patients with AMI (82). At the recommended dose of 30 units injected intravenously over a period of 4 to 5 minutes in patients with AMI of less than 6-hours duration, reperfusion of occluded coronary arteries occurs in about 72% of patients at 90 minutes (range 53 to 91% in individual studies) (103–105). Subsequent reocclusion has been reported in 0 to 20% of patients in most studies, with an average reocclusion rate around 10% (102). Thrombolytic therapy with intravenous APSAC improves left ventricular function and survival in patients with AMI (83).

Unlike streptokinase, APSAC, and urokinase, tissue-type plasminogen activators (t-PA) have minimal affinity for free, circulating plasminogen. Tissue-type plasminogen activator produces clot-selective thrombolysis by activating fibrin-bound plasminogen; the activity of t-PA is dose dependent. Pharmacologic doses of t-PA activate circulating plasminogen, resulting in systemic fibrinogenolysis and a modest systemic lytic state (106,107). The short half-life of t-PA, approximately 5 minutes, does not assure prompt reversal of hemostatic abnormalities. This process depends on the replenishment of fibrinogen and the elimination of fibrinogen breakdown products.

Various dosing regimens for t-PA have been explored in an attempt to increase patency and reduce the risk of bleeding. Recent studies suggest that an accelerated (front-loaded) 90-minute infusion of t-PA produces more rapid reperfusion without any change in safety. Patients with acute myocardial infarction (n = 281) were randomized to receive 100 mg of t-PA over 3 hours (i.e., a 10-mg bolus followed by 50 mg for 1 hour, then 20 mg per hour for 2 hours) or 100 mg of t-PA over 90 minutes (a 15-mg bolus followed by 50 mg over 30 minutes, then 35 mg over 60 minutes). The 60-minute patency rates were significantly higher (p less than 0.03) with front-loaded t-PA. Both groups experienced similar rates of recurrent ischemia, reinfarction, angiographic reocclusion, stroke, major bleeding complications, and death. These findings suggest that speed of reperfusion is linked to the rate of administration of t-PA (108).

Successful reperfusion is indicated by the sudden relief of chest pain, resolution of S-T segment elevation, or the onset of reperfusion tachyarrhythmias. These occur in 15% of patients but do not usually require treatment.

Bleeding complications are the major concern with thrombolytic agents as a result of their general interference with hemostatic mechanisms. Thrombolytics do not differentiate between pathologic clots and hemostatic plugs. Lysis of hemostatic plugs can lead to bleeding complications following pharmacologic thrombolysis. Clinical studies show a 5% risk of major bleeding complications from thrombolytic therapy (83,101). Bleeding complications are minimized by avoiding drugs that affect hemostasis and by avoiding excessive venipuncture. Compared with streptoki-

nase, t-PA appears to be associated with a slightly higher risk of stroke in patients who present with an acute myocardial infarction (109). Data from the GISSI-2 trial suggest that there are four additional strokes per 1000 patients treated with t-PA when compared with streptokinase. Logistic regression analysis on the data from the GISSI-2 trial revealed a significant association between the risk of stroke and older age, female gender, anterior infarction, and more extensive left ventricular dysfunction at the time of admission. In the ISIS-3 study, streptokinase was associated with significantly fewer noncerebral bleeds, total strokes, and intracranial bleeds compared with either t-PA or APSAC (110). When GISSI-2 and ISIS-3 data are combined, t-PA was associated with significantly higher total stroke rates (1.4 versus 1%) (0.6 versus 0.3%) when compared with streptokinase (109). The GUSTO trial showed that t-PA was associated with a significant excess of hemorrhagic strokes (p = 0.03) when compared with streptokinase (111).

Data produced by the SAVE and SOLVD trials suggest a possible benefit from the early administration of ACE-inhibitors to patients with left ventricular dysfunction and who are recovering from an acute myocardial infarction. The negative findings of the CONSENSUS II trial may have resulted from too early initiation of ACE-inhibitor therapy and the inadequate follow-up period (112).

Allergic reactions are more common with streptokinase and APSAC. Intravenous diphenhydramine may be required in some cases. Hypotension occurs in approximately 10% of patients treated with streptokinase or APSAC. Once the patient receives streptokinase, the patient is sensitized to the drug and should not receive it again for at least 6 months (95,102). Other side effects with thrombolytics include angina, flushing, dyspnea, mild febrile reactions, nausea and vomiting, and occasionally, rash, all of which may be symptoms of mild allergic reactions. Allergic reactions and hypotension are rare in patients treated with t-PA.

Successful thrombolytic therapy in AMI depends on more than just the ability to reperfuse the occluded coronary artery. Prevention of reocclusion and subsequent salvage of infarcted myocardium should reduce morbidity and mortality following thrombolytic therapy. Results of early studies that compared reperfusion rates achieved by t-PA and streptokinase suggested that t-PA was twice as effective as streptokinase in establishing reperfusion of acutely occluded coronary arteries (106,107). In recent trials, myocardial salvage, mortality reduction, or bleeding complications have not differed in patients treated with t-PA versus streptokinase (113). Clinical experience provides little evidence for the superiority of t-PA over other thrombolytic agents in acute myocardial infarction. The largest trials measuring myocardial function after thrombolytic therapy failed to show that t-PA is more effective than streptokinase (114,115), urokinase (116), or APSAC (117). Additionally, t-PA is no safer than other thrombolytics (115,118). The International Study of 20,749 AMI patients showed no difference in mortality rate between t-PA (8.9%) and streptokinase (8.5%) (119). There was also no difference in the incidence of ventricular fibrillation, reinfarction, or shock between treatment groups. The echocardiographically measured ejection fraction, and the incidence of congestive heart failure also did not differ between treatment groups (115,119).

The ISIS-3 assessed the relative efficacy of streptokinase, APSAC, and t-PA. The mortality in all groups was the same (120). The GUSTO Trial randomized more than 40,000 patients to treatment with t-PA or streptokinase or the combination of these two agents (111). Overall, the 30-day mortality with streptokinase was 7.3%, whereas the mortality with t-PA was 6.3% (111). Furthermore, if the patient had an AMI with a relatively high risk of mortality, the benefit of t-PA was magnified. For example, patients with anterior wall AMI had an 8.6% mortality rate when treated with t-PA and a 10.5% mortality rate when treated with streptokinase. Similar difference were not observed with inferior wall AMI patients or elderly patients in the GUSTO Trial (111).

Although cost is an important consideration in the selection of thrombolytic therapy, a more sound approach would be to have both t-PA and streptokinase available and use the agents selectively. For example, young patients with anterior wall infarctions would be best treated with t-PA, whereas patients over age 75 and those at increased risk of hemorrhagic CVAs should receive streptokinase. The most important issue to ensure is that therapy is initiated as promptly as possible, preferably within 30 minutes after the patient arrives in the emergency department (96).

POSTREPERFUSION MANAGEMENT

After successful thrombolysis, the stenotic vessel may reocclude. The rate of reocclusion varies but may be as high as 30% (100). The likelihood of reocclusion and recovery of regional ventricular function depends on the severity of residual stenosis. After successful thrombolysis, anticoagulation is advocated although there is no consensus on the type, dosage, or duration of therapy. Most often, full-dose heparin is used for 24 to 72 hours. Aspirin (160 mg per day or 325 mg per day) is administered for 3 months or longer (100). There is no role for dipyridamole as an adjunctive antiplatelet agent after thrombolytic therapy (129,130).

Percutaneous transluminal coronary angioplasty (PTCA) provides a viable therapeutic alternative in those patients who present to a hospital that is capable of performing emergency PTCA (Table 41.6). A major limitation of PTCA is that it requires a skilled team, a fully

Table 41.6.

Proposed Indications for Peructaneous Transluminal Coronary Angioplasty in Patients with Acute Myocardial Infarction

1. Unstable angina
2. Acute myocardial infarction
3. Peri-infarction angina
4. Symptomatic coronary artery disease

staffed catheterization laboratory, and a surgical team on stand-by. Potential complications of PTCA include catheter-induced occlusions caused by dissection, spasm, or subintimal hematoma and residula stenosis. PTCA involves the passing of a balloon-tipped catheter along the venous circulation into the coronary tree to the site of coronary occlusion. Once at this site, the balloon is inflated causing the occlusive plaque to regress against the vessel wall. Balloon is deflated and reinflated several times until the plaque is reduced and approximately 70% of the arterial caliber is restored. Although routine angioplasty performed within 24 hours of thrombolytic therapy offers no clinical benefit and is associated with an increased incidence of reocclusion and complications (83). Angioplasty is recommended in patients with ongoing ischemia or pump failure. The application of emergent angioplasty to patients who present with acute myocardial infarction may offer several advantages over thrombolytic therapy. PTCA is more effective than thrombolytic therapy in restoring patency and preventing reocclusion, and in reducing the risk of death and reinfarction (121). Angioplasty is associated with significantly less (p = 0.05) risk of hemorrhagic strokes when compared with t-PA (121). The benefits of angioplasty are especially apparent in patients with advanced age, anterior infarctions, or present tachycardia (122). Angioplasty is also recommended in patients with ongoing ischemia or heart failure.

The safety and efficacy of coronary artery bypass-graft (CABG) surgery in AMI patients are well established (100). The systemic lytic state after thrombolysis may increase the morbidity of the surgical procedure if it is performed within 24 hours after infusion. Although the indications and timing for CABG surgery in AMI patients are controversial, most clinicians agree that surgery can alter the natural history of AMI if reperfusion of the ischemic area can occur within 6 hours of symptoms (123). Emergency CABG surgery for AMI is successful in a few centers set up to perform cardiopulmonary bypass within 6 hours of symptoms, but this is not feasible in most hospitals.

Summary

The most important factor for successfully limiting infarct size is the prompt institution of therapy that salvages viable myocardium. The ability of any drug or intervention to reduce infarct size in humans is optimal when therapy can be started less than 4 hours after the onset of symptoms. Intravenous administration of a clot-specific thrombolytic agent may prove to be the initial therapy of choice. Because thrombolytic therapy dissolves only existing thrombi and does not affect the underlying causes of coronary artery occlusion, further study and therapy to reduce the risk of reinfarction and death should be initiated. Percutaneous transluminal coronary angioplasty may reduce the reocclusion rate after thrombolysis. β-blockers and possibly nitroglycerin can provide valuable alternatives when thrombolysis is unavailable.

Prognosis

Considerable effort has been spent on the search for predictors of survival and factors determining the occurrence of reinfarction after AMI (124). Most patients who survive AMI initially have an uncomplicated event; the pain subsides and there is no evidence of heart failure or arrhythmias. Mortality after MI in unselected groups of patients ranges from 4 to 6% per year (124). Mortality is higher in patients with moderate impairment of left ventricular function and three-vessel coronary disease. These patients may benefit from elective CABG after AMI.

Survival after MI relates to the extent and location of the coronary obstructive lesion and to the adequacy of residual myocardial function. To prevent or retard the progression of atherosclerotic coronary heart disease, conventional coronary risk-factor reduction is necessary (125). Continued cigarette smoking after MI increases the likelihood of reinfarction and coronary death in men and women of all ages. Reduction of excess caloric and cholesterol intake is advisable. Control of systemic hypertension decreases both myocardial oxygen demand and the risk of stroke. Medical management with antianginal drugs reduces myocardial oxygen demand and decreases myocardial ischemia. Chronic therapy with β-adrenergic blockers decreases myocardial ischemia. Chronic therapy with β-adrenergic blockers reduces both the recurrence of MI and the incidence of sudden death for up to 2 years after AMI (126). Exercise training improves physical work capacity and favorably affects weight control and psychologic status.

In the absence of contraindications, one 325-mg tablet of aspirin should be taken after an AMI to prevent reinfarction (127). Aspirin in a daily dose of 325 mg reduces the rate of reinfarction by 21% (128) and mortality by 10% (129). The FDA approved aspirin for this indication in 1985. Higher doses of aspirin are no more effective, and lower doses have not been investigated. Neither dipyridamole nor sulfinpyrazone can be recommended for the prevention of recurrent myocardial infarction. The combination of aspirin and dipyridamole is no more effective than aspirin alone (129,

130), and the efficacy of sulfinpyrazone has not been proved (131).

CONCLUSION

Myocardial infarction is one of the most common reasons for hospitalization in the western world. The acute mortality rate is about 15%; approximately 10% of patients will die during the first year after their AMI. Short- and long-term survival depends on the extent and location of the coronary obstructive lesions and the prompt correction of post-MI complications. The presence or absence of mechanical, electrical, ischemic, and vascular abnormalities provides the necessary information to institute appropriate medical and/or surgical treatment.

REFERENCES

1. Zeller FP, Bauman JL. Current concepts in clinical therapeutics: acute myocardial infarction. Clin Pharm 5:553–572, 1986.
2. Alpert JS, Braunwald E. Acute myocardial infarction: pathological, pathophysiological, and clinical manifestations. In: Braunwald E. Heart Disease, 2nd ed. Philadelphia: WB Saunders, 1984:1262–1270.
3. Sobel BE, Braunwald E. The management of acute myocardial infarction. In: Braunwald E. Heart Disease, 2nd ed. Philadelphia: WB Saunders, 1984:1301–1321.
4. Epstein SE, Palmeri ST. Mechanisms contributing to precipitation of unstable angina and acute myocardial infarction: implications regarding therapy. Am J Cardiol 54:1245–1252, 1984.
5. Moseri A, L'Abbate A, Baroldi G, et al. Coronary vasospasm as a possible cause of myocardial infarction. A conclusion derived from the study of "preinfarction" angina. N Engl J Med 299:1271–1277, 1978.
6. GISSI Investigators Avoidable Delay Study Group. Epidemiology of avoidable delay in the care of patients with acute myocardial infarction in Italy. Arch Intern Med 155:1481–1488, 1995.
7. Zelma MJ. Q wave, S-T segment, and T wave myocardial infarction. Am J Med 78:391–398, 1985.
8. Tucker JF, Collins RA, Anderson AJ, et al. Value of serial myoglobin levels in the early diagnosis of patients admitted for acute myocardial infarction. Ann Emerg Med 24:704–708, 1994.
9. Adams JE III, Bodor GS, Davilla-Roman VG, et al. Cardiac troponin-1: a marker with high specificity for cardiac injury. Circulation 88;101–106, 1993.
10. Rude RE. Acute myocardial infarction and its complications. Cardiol Clin 2:163–171, 1984.
11. Hoehn-Saric R, McLeod DR. Cardiac symptoms and anxiety disorders: Contributing factors and pharmacologic. Am J Cardiol 60:68J–73J, 1987.
12. Barker PH, Clanachan AS. Inhibition of adenosine accumulation into guinea pig ventricle by benzodiazepines. Eur J Pharmacol 78:241–244, 1982.
13. Forrester JS, Waters DD. Hospital treatment of congestive heart failure: Management according to hemodynamic profile. Am J Med 65:173, 1978.
14. Herling IM. Intravenous nitroglycerin: Clinical pharmacology and therapeutic considerations. Am Heart J 108:141, 1984.
15. Swan NA, Evenson MK, Needham KE, et al. Effect of combined nitroglycerin and dobutamine infusion in left ventricular dysfunction. Am Heart J 106:35, 1983.
16. Parmley WW, Chatterjee K, Charuzi Y, et al. Hemodynamic effects of noninvasive systolic unloading (nitroprusside) and diastolic

augmentation (external counterpulsation) in patients with acute myocardial infarction. Am J Cardiol 33:810, 1974.

17. Rasanen J, Vaisanen IT, Heikkila J, et al. Acute myocardial infarction complicated by left ventricular dysfunction and respiratory failure: the effects of continuous positive airway pressure. Chest 87:278–360, 1985.

18. Dole WP, O'Rourke RA. Pathophysiology and management of cardiogenic shock. Circ Probl Cardiol 8:1, 1983.

19. Lee G, DeMaria AN, Amsterdam EA, et al. Comparative effect of morphine, meperidine, and pentazocine on cardiopulmonary dynamics in patients with acute myocardial infarction. Am J Med 60:341–355, 1976.

20. Stadol. In: Physicians Desk Reference. Montvale, NJ: Medical Economics Publishing Company, 49:739–742, 1995.

21. Kaplan K. Prophylactic anticoagulation following acute myocardial infarction. Arch Intern Med 146:595–597, 1986.

22. Prins MH, Hirsh J. Heparin as an adjunctive treatment for thrombolytic therapy for acute myocardial infarction. Am J Cardiol 67:3A–11A, 1991.

23. Smith P, Arnesen H, Holme I. The effect of warfarin on mortality and reinfarction after myocardial infarction. N Engl J Med 323:147–152, 1990.

24. Wyman MG, Gore S. Lidocaine prophylaxis in myocardial infarction: a concept whose time has come. Heart Lung 12:358–361, 1983.

25. Singh BN, Venkatesh N. Prevention of myocardial reinfarction and of sudden death in survivors of acute myocardial infarction: role of prophylactic beta-adrenoceptor blockade. Am Heart J 108:450–455, 1984.

26. Norris RM, Brown MA, Clarke ED, et al. Prevention of ventricular fibrillation during acute myocardial infarction by intravenous propranolol. Lancet 2:883–886, 1984.

27. Ryden L, Arniego R, Arnman K, et al. A double-blind trial of metoprolol in acute myocardial infarction: effects on ventricular tachyarrhythmias. N Engl J Med 308:614–618, 1983.

28. Mueller H, Ayres SM, Religi A, et al. Propranolol in the treatment of acute myocardial infarction. Circulation 49:1078–1081, 1974.

29. Chadda K, Goldstein S, Byington R, et al. Effect of propranolol after acute myocardial infarction in patients with congestive heart failure. Circulation 73:503–510, 1986.

30. Wagner GS. Arrhythmias in acute myocardial infarction. Med Clin North Am 68:1061–1068, 1984.

31. Cristal N, Szwarcberg J, Gueron M. Supraventricular arrhythmias in acute myocardial infarction: prognostic importance of clinical setting; mechanisms of production. Ann Intern Med 82:35–39, 1975.

32. Morgan DB, Davidson C. Hypokalemia and diuretics: an analysis of publications. Br Med J 280:905–909, 1980.

33. Hollifield JW. Potassium and magnesium abnormalities: diuretics and arrhythmias in hypertension. Am J Med 77:28–32, 1984.

34. Kafka S, Langevin L, Armstrong PW. Serum magnesium and potassium in acute myocardial infarction. Arch Intern Med 147:465–469, 1987.

35. Ornato JP, Gonzalez ER, Starke H, et al. Incidence and causes of hypokalemia associated with cardiac resuscitation. Am J Emerg Med 3:503–506, 1985.

36. Salerno DM, Asinger RW, Elsperger J, et al. Frequency of hypokalemia after successfully resuscitated out-of-hospital cardiac arrest compared with that in transmural acute myocardial infarction. Am J Cardiol 59:84–88, 1987.

37. Ornato JP, Gonzalez ER. Refractory ventricular fibrillation. Emergency Decisions 4:35–41, 1986.

38. Dyckner T, Wester PO. Magnesium in cardiology. Acta Med Scand 661(suppl):27–31, 1982.

39. Ebel H, Gunther T. Role of magnesium in cardiac disease. J Clin Chem Clin Biochem 21:249–265, 1983.

40. Rasmussen HS, Norregard P, Lindeneg O, et al. Intravenous magnesium in acute myocardial in acute myocardial infarction. Lancet 1:234–235, 1986.

41. Whang R, Flink EB, Dyckner T, et al. Magnesium depletion as a cause of refractory potassium repletion. Arch Intern Med 145:1686–1689, 1985.

42. Whang R, Oei TO, Aikawa JK, et al. Predictors of clinical hypomagnesemia. Arch Intern Med 144:1794–1796, 1984.

43. Rasmussen HS, Aurup P, Hojberg S, Jensen K, McNair P. Magnesium and acute myocardial infarction. Arch Intern Med 146:872–874, 1986.

44. Heesch C, Eichhorn EJ. Magnesium in acute myocardial infarction. Ann Emerg Med 24:1154–1160, 1994.

45. Antman E. Randomized trials of magnesium in acute myocardial infarction: when big numbers do not tell the whole story (editorial). Am J Cardiol 75:391–393, 1995.

46. Swan HJ, Forrester JS, Danzig R, et al. Power failure in acute myocardial infarction. Progr Cardiovasc Dis 12:508, 1970.

47. Berkley CE, Russell RO, Mantle JA, et al. Cardiogenic shock. Recognition and management. Cardiovasc Clin 7:251, 1975.

48. Forrester JS, Diamond G, Chartterjee K, et al. Medical therapy of acute myocardial infarction by application of hemodynamic subsets. N Engl J Med 295:1356, 1976.

49. Biddle TL, Paul NY. Effect of furosemide on hemodynamic and lung water in acute pulmonary edema secondary to myocardial infarction. Am J Cardiol 43:86, 1979.

50. Kilcoyne MM, Schmidt DH, Cannon PJ. Intrarenal blood flow in congestive heart failure. Postgrad Med J 51(suppl 6):54, 1975.

51. Gunnar RM, Leab HS, Scanlon PJ, et al. Management of acute myocardial infarction and accelerating angina. Prog Cardiovasc Dis 22:1, 1979.

52. Scholz H. Inotropic drugs and their mechanisms of action. J Am Coll Cardiol 4:389, 1984.

53. Goldberg LI. Dopamine: clinical uses of an endogenous catecholamine. N Engl J Med 291:707, 1974.

54. Holzer J, Karliner JS, O'Rourke RA, et al. Effectiveness of dopamine in patients with cardiogenic shock. Am J Cardiol 32:79, 1973.

55. Francis GS, Sharma B, Hodges M. Comparative hemodynamic effects of dopamine and dobutamine in patients with acute cardiogenic circulation collapse. Am Heart J 103:995, 1982.

56. Leier CV, Unverferth DV. Drugs five years later: dobutamine. Ann Intern Med 99:490, 1983.

57. Ruffolo RR. The mechanism of action of dobutamine. Ann Intern Med 100:313, 1984.

58. Maekawa K, Liang CS, Hood WB. Comparison of dobutamine and dopamine in acute myocardial infarction: effects of systemic hemodynamics, plasma catecholamines, blood flows, and infarct size. Circulation 67:750, 1983.

59. Richard C, Ricome JL, Rimailho A, et al. Combined hemodynamic effects of dopamine and dobutamine in cardiogenic shock. Circulation 67:620, 1983.

60. Franciosa JA. Intravenous amrinone: an advance or wrong step (editorial)? Ann Intern Med 102:399, 1985.

61. LeJemtel TJ, Keung E, Ribner JS, et al. Sustained beneficial effects of oral amrinone on cardiac and renal function in patients with severe congestive heart failure. Am J Cardiol 45:123, 1980.

62. Wynne J, Malacoff RF, Benotti JR, et al. Oral amrinone in refractory congestive heart failure. Am J Cardiol 45:1245, 1980.

63. Naccarelli GV, Gray EL, Dougherty AH, et al. Amrinone: acute electrophysiologic and hemodynamic effects in patients with congestive heart failure. Am J Cardiol 54:600, 1984.

64. Klein NA, Siskind SJ, Frishman WH, et al. Hemodynamic comparison of intravenous amrinone and dobutamine in patients with chronic congestive heart failure. Am J Cardiol 48:170, 1981.

65. Chesebro JH, Foster V, Robertson JS, et al. Shortened platelet survival in cardiac failure: predisposition to amrinone-induced platelet reduction. Circulation 66:II-382, 1982.

66. Forrester JS, Waters DD. Hospital treatment of congestive heart failure: management according to hemodynamic profile. Am J Med 65:173, 1978.

67. Parmley WW, Chatterjee K, Charuzi Y, et al. Hemodynamic effects of noninvasive systolic unloading (nitroprusside) and diastolic augmentation (external counterpulsation) in patients with acute myocardial infarction. Am J Cardiol 33:810, 1974.

68. Cohn JN, Franciosa JA, Francis GS, et al. Effect of short-term infusion of sodium nitroprusside on mortality rate in acute myocardial infarction complicated by left ventricular failure. N Engl J Med 306:1129, 1982.

69. Cohn JN, Burke LP. Drugs five years later: nitroprusside. Ann Intern Med 91:752, 1979.

70. Herling IM. Intravenous nitroglycerin: clinical pharmacology and therapeutic considerations. Am Heart J 108:141, 1984.

71. Roberts R. Intravenous nitroglycerin in acute myocardial infarction. Am J Med 74(6B):45, 1983.

72. Swan NA, Evenson MK, Needham KE, et al. Effect of combined nitroglycerin and dobutamine infusion in left ventricular dysfunction. Am Heart J 106:35, 1983.

73. Chiarello M, Gold HK, Leinbach RC, et al. Comparison between the effects of nitroprusside and nitroglycerin on ischemic injury during acute myocardial infarction. Circulation 54:766, 1976.

74. Flaherty JT. Comparison of intravenous nitroglycerin and sodium nitroprusside in acute myocardial infarction. Am J Med 74(6B):53, 1983.

75. Yusuf S, Wittes J, Friedman L. Overview of results of randomized clinical trials in heart disease. I. Treatments following myocardial infarction. JAMA 260:2088, 1988.

76. Weiss WR. Intra-aortic balloon pumping. Ann Thorac Surg 21:571, 1976.

77. Isner JM, Cohen SR, Virman R, et al. Complications of the intra-aortic balloon counterpulsation device: clinical and morphologic observations in 45 necropsy patients. Am J Cardiol 45:260, 1980.

78. Miller LW. Mechanical assist devices in intensive care. Am Heart J 121:1887–1892, 1991.

79. Campbell CA, Przylenk K, Kloner RA. Infarct size reduction: a review of the clinical trials. J Clin Pharmacol 26:317–329, 1986.

80. May GS, Furbery CD, Eberlein KA, et al. Secondary prevention after myocardial infarction. A review of short-term acute phase trials. Prog Cardiovasc Dis 25:335–359, 1985.

81. Mueller HS, Ayres SM. Propranolol decreases sympathetic necrosis activity reflected by plasma catecholamines during evolution of myocardial infarction in man. J Clin Invest 65:338–346, 1980.

82. Pitt B, Crown P. Effect of propranolol in regional myocardial blood flow in acute ischemia. Cardiovasc Res 4:176–179, 1970.

83. Gunnar RM, Bourdillon PD, Dixon DW, et al. Guidelines for the early management of patients with acute myocardial infarction. J Am Coll Cardiol 16:249, 1990.

84. The MIAMI Trial Research Group. Metoprolol in acute myocardial infarction (MIAMI). A randomised placebo-controlled international trial. Eur Heart J 6:199–226, 1985.

85. ISIS-1 (First International Study of Infarct Survival) Collaborative Group. Randomized trial of intravenous atenolol among 16,027 cases of suspected acute myocardial infarction: ISIS-1. Lancet 2:57–66, 1986.

86. The TIMI Study Group. Comparison of invasive and conservative strategies after treatment with intravenous tissue plasminogen activator in acute myocardial infarction: results of the Thrombolysis in Myocardial Infarction (TIMI) Phase II trial. N Engl J Med 320:618–627, 1989.

87. Moos AN, Hilleman DE, Mohiudin SM, Hunter CB. Safety of esmolol in patients with acute myocardial infarction treated with thrombolytic therapy who have relative contraindications to beta blocker therapy. Ann Pharmacother 28:701–703, 1994.

88. Bussman WD, Seher W, Gresengrus M. Reduction of creatinine kinase and creatinine kinase-MB indexes of infarct size by intravenous verapamil. Am J Cardiol 54:1224–1230, 1984.

89. Danish Multicenter Study Group. Verapamil in acute myocardial infarction. Eur Heart J 5:516–528, 1984.

90. Mueller JE, Morrison J, Stone PH, et al. Nifedipine therapy for patients with threatened and acute myocardial infarction: A randomized double-blind, placebo-controlled comparison. Circulation 69:740–747, 1984.

91. Sirnes PA, Overskeid K, Pedersen TR. Evolution of infarct size during the early use of nifedipine in patients with acute myocardial infarction: The Norwegian Nifedipine Multicenter Trial. Circulation 70:638–644, 1984.

92. Gibson RS, Boden WE, Theroux P, et al. Diltiazem and reinfarction in patients with non Q wave MI. N Engl J Med 315:423, 1986.

93. Gibson RS, Young OM, Boden WE, et al. Prognostic significance and beneficial effect of diltiazem on the incidence of early recurrent ischemia after non-Q-wave myocardial infarction: Results from the multicenter diltiazem reinfarction study. Am J Cardiol 60:203–209, 1987.

94. The Multicenter Diltiazem Postinfarction Trial Research Group. The effect of diltiazem on mortality and reinfarction after myocardial infarction. N Engl J Med 319:385, 1988.

95. Mueller JE, Braumwald E. Can infarct size be limited in patients with acute myocardial infarction? Cardiovas Clin 13:147–161, 1983.

96. Hochman J. Modern treatment of acute myocardial infarction. Cardiovascular Reviews and Reports 16:23–35, 1995.

97. Pfeffer M, et al. Effects of captopril on mortality and morbidity in patients with left ventricular dysfunction after myocardial infarction. N Engl J Med 327:669–677, 1992.

98. Swedberg K, et al. Effects of the early administration of enalapril on mortality in patients with acute myocardial infarction. N Engl J Med 327:678–684, 1992.

99. The SOLVD Investigators. Effect of enalapril on mortality and the development of heart failure in asymptomatic patients with reduced left ventricular ejection fractions. N Engl J Med 327:685–691, 1992.

100. Gersh BJ. Role of thrombolytic therapy in evolving myocardial infarction. Modern Concepts Cardiovas Dis 54:13–17, 1985.

101. Schwartz DE, Yamaga CC. Thrombolysis for evolving myocardial infarction. Ann Intern Med 103:463–469, 1985.

102. Sherry S. Appraisal of various thrombolytic agents in the treatment of acute myocardial infarction. Am J Med 83(suppl 2A):31, 1987.

103. Monk JP, Heel RC. Anisoylated plasminogen streptokinase activator complex (APSAC). A review of its mechanisms of action, clinical pharmacology and its therapeutic use in acute myocardial infarction. Drugs 34:25, 1987.

104. Meinertz T, Kasper W, Schumacher M, et al. The German multicenter trial of anisoylated plasminogen streptokinase activator complex versus heparin for acute myocardial infarction. Am J Cardiol 62:347, 1988.

105. AIMS Trial Study Group. Effect of intravenous APSAC on mortality after acute myocardial infarction: preliminary report of a placebo-controlled clinical trial. Lancet 1:545–549, 1988.

106. Crabbe SJ, Cloninger CC. Tissue plasminogen activator: A new thrombolytic agent. Clin Pharm 6:373–386, 1987.

107. Sherry S. Recombinant tissue plasminogen activator (rt-PA): is it the thrombolytic agent of choice for an evolving acute myocardial infarction. Am J Cardiol 59:984–989, 1987.

108. Carney R. Randomized angiographic trial of recombinant tissue-type plasminogen activator in myocardial infarction. J Am Coll Cardiol 20:17–23, 1992.

109. Maggioni A. The risk of stroke in patients with acute myocardial infarction after thrombolytic and antithrombotic treatment. N Engl J Med 327:1–6, 1992.

110. Ridker P. Large scale trials of thrombolytic therapy for acute myocardial infarction: GISSI-2, ISSI-3, and GUSTO-1. Ann Intern Med 119:530–532, 1993.

111. GUSTO Investigators. An international randomized trial comparing four thrombolytic strategies for acute myocardial infarction. N Engl J Med 329:673–682, 1993.

112. Cohn J. The prevention of heart failure—a new agenda (editorial). N Engl J Med 327:725–727, 1992.

113. Sherry S, Marder VJ. Streptokinase and recombinant tissue plasminogen activator (rt-PA) are equally effective in treating acute myocardial infarction. Ann Intern Med 114:417–423, 1991.

114. White HD, Rivers JT, Maslowski AH, et al. Effect of intravenous streptokinase as compared with that of tissue plasminogen activator on left ventricular function after first myocardial infarction. N Engl J Med 320:817–821, 1989.

115. Gruppo Italiano por lo Studio della Sopravvivenza nell'Infarcto Miocardico. GISSI-2: a factorial randomized trial of alteplase versus streptokinase and heparin versus no heparin among 12,490 patients with acute myocardial infarction. Lancet 336:65–71, 1990.

116. Neuhaus KL, Tebbe U, Gotwik M, et al. Intravenous recombinant tissue plasminogen activator and urokinase in acute myocardial infarction: results of the German Activator Urokinase Study (GAUS). J Am Coll Cardiol 12:581–587, 1988.

117. Bassand JP, Cassagnes J, Machecourt T, et al. A multicenter trial of intravenous APSAC versus rt-PA in acute myocardial infarction: assessment of efficacy and safety (Abstract). J Am Coll Cardiol 15(suppl A):214A, 1990.

118. Rao AK, Pratt C, Berke A, et al. Thrombolysis in acute myocardial infarction (TIMI) Trial, Phase I: hemorrhagic manifestations and changes in plasma fibrinogen and the fibrinolytic system in patients treated with recombinant tissue plasminogen activator and streptokinase. J Am Coll Cardiol 11:1–11, 1988.

119. The International Study Group. In-hospital mortality and clinical course of 20,891 patients with suspected acute myocardial infarction randomised between alteplase and streptokinase with or without heparin. Lancet 336:71–75, 1990.

120. ISIS-3. A randomized comparison of streptokinase vs tissue plasminogen activator vs anistreplase and aspirin plus heparin vs aspirin alone among 41,299 cases of suspected acute myocardial infarction. Lancet 339:753–770, 1992.

121. Gibbons R. Immediate angioplasty compared with the administration of a thrombolytic agent followed by conservative treatment for myocardial infarction. N Engl J Med 328:685–691, 1993.

122. Lange R, Hillis L. Immediate angioplasty for acute myocardial infarction (editorial). N Engl J Med 328:726–728, 1993.

123. Robinson L. Surgical interventions for acute cardiothoric emergencies. In: Ornato JP. Cardiovascular Emergencies. New York: Churchill Livingstone, 1986:43.

124. Sanz G, Castaner A, Betrice A, et al. Determinants of prognosis in survivors of myocardial infarction. N Engl J Med 306:1065–1070, 1982.

125. Wenger NK. Uncomplicated acute myocardial infarction: long-term management. Am J Cardiol 52:658–660, 1983.

126. Turi ZG, Braumwald E. The use of beta blockers after myocardial infarction. JAMA 249:2512–2516, 1983.

127. Anon. Aspirin after myocardial infarction. Lancet 1:1172–1173, 1980.

128. Canner PL. Aspirin in coronary disease. Comparison of six clinical trials. Isr J Med Sci 19:413–423, 1983.

129. Klimt DR, Knatterud GL, Stamler J, Meier P. Persantine-aspirin reinfarction study. Part II. Secondary coronary prevention with persantine and aspirin. J Am Coll Cardiol 7:251–269, 1986.

130. Oates JA, Wood AJ. Dipyridamole. N Engl J Med 316:1247–1257, 1987.

131. Temple R, Pledger GW. The FDA's critique of the antueane reinfarction trial. N Engl J Med 303:1488–1492, 1980.

CHAPTER 42

THROMBOEMBOLIC DISEASE

STEVEN R. KAYSER

A rational clinical approach to the management of thromboembolic disease depends on a thorough understanding of and familiarity with the pharmacology of antithrombotic drugs and with the pathophysiology of the underlying thrombotic process. Many disorders that are associated with clotting today require the use of combination antithrombotic agents. To appreciate the rationale for this approach, practitioners must integrate their knowledge and not focus too heavily on one aspect exclusively. A large national consensus conference on antithrombotic therapy that was sponsored by the American College of Chest Physicians reevaluated many aspects of antithrombotic therapy, and these guidelines as well as others should lead to more effective and safer use of antithrombotic drugs (1, 2).

Despite advances in the prevention and management of thromboembolic disease, hospitalizations for conditions associated with arterial and venous thromboembolism account for a large share of the health care dollar. Deep venous thrombosis and pulmonary embolism have been estimated to account for up to 600,000 hospital admissions per year. Arterial embolism associated with myocardial infarction and stroke accounts for many additional hospitalizations.

ETIOLOGY

Many conditions may contribute to the development of thromboembolic disease (Table 42.1) (3–5). In general, any condition or combination of conditions that leads to activation of blood coagulation (hypercoagulability), venous stasis, or damage to the vascular wall puts a patient at risk for the development of a clot. This combination of events is also known as Virchow's triad.

Immobilization and bed rest, with resultant stasis, frequently contribute to thrombosis, especially in elderly and obese people. Prolonged partial occlusion of the veins in any person sitting for prolonged periods may also lead to stasis. A hypercoagulable state existing during the operative period may contribute to clotting. Trauma may initiate clotting; this is a particular problem in patients who have suffered fractures of the hips and pelvis, who may also require prolonged bed rest. Congestive heart failure, ulcerative colitis, myocardial infarction, and other high-risk medical illnesses (e.g., systemic lupus erythematosus) are associated with an increased risk of thrombosis. Carcinomas, particularly pancreatic, bronchogenic, gastric, and prostatic cancers, may produce procoagulant substances that initiate clotting. The increased activity of many clotting factors during pregnancy contributes to an increased risk of thrombosis. Oral contraceptives have been associated with an increased risk of clotting. Less frequently, some unusual blood diseases and hereditary causes have been associated with thrombosis. Deficiencies in protein C, protein S, or antithrombin III have been demonstrated in susceptible patients to be associated with thromboembolic complications. Most recently, a genetic mutation in factor V, factor V Leiden, has been discovered to be one of the most common reasons for the hereditary development of venous thrombosis. A rare circulating antiphospholipid antibody has been described in patients with immunologic diseases such as systemic lupus erythematosus. This is associated mostly with arterial thrombosis (Table 42.1).

PATHOGENESIS

When injury occurs to the vascular endothelium, platelets adhere to exposed collagen as well as to other exposed subendothelial tissue. Following platelet adhesion, release of adenosine diphosphate (ADP) by the injured platelets leads to platelet aggregation (Fig. 42.1). Transformation of this temporary platelet plug to a permanent platelet fibrin clot is achieved through activation of the extrinsic and/or intrinsic blood-clotting system (Fig. 42.2).

Throughout the process of platelet aggregation, a balance is maintained between certain prostaglandins that occur naturally and may be synthesized in vivo. Thromboxane A2 is found in platelets and is a potent stimulant for platelet aggregation as well as a potent vasoconstrictor. Prostacyclin, in contrast, is found in vessel walls and is an inhibitor of platelet aggregation, as well as a vasodilator. The balance between prostacyclin and thromboxane may be altered physiologically but also by various drugs (e.g., aspirin) and even by different doses of these drugs.

Each of the clotting factors circulates in the blood as an inactive protein. Before clotting can occur, each clotting factor must be converted to an active or enzymatic form. Exposure of subendothelial collagen, in addition to interaction with platelets, initiates the intrinsic pathway by stimulating the activation of factor XII. Activated factor XII then stimulates the conversion of factor XI to the active form, which then stimulates activation of factor IX. Activated factor IX, in the presence of calcium, phospholipids (platelet factor 3), and factor VIII, stimulates the

Table 42.1.
Conditions Associated with Venous Thrombosis

- Immobilization
- Stasis
- Surgery and the postoperative period
- Trauma to affected area
- High-risk medical illnesses (e.g., congestive heart failure, myocardial infarction)
- Malignancies
- Pregnancy, oral contraceptives
- Heredity
- Blood disorders (e.g., protein C or S deficiency, antithrombin III deficiency, factor V Leiden, antiphospholipid antibody syndrome)

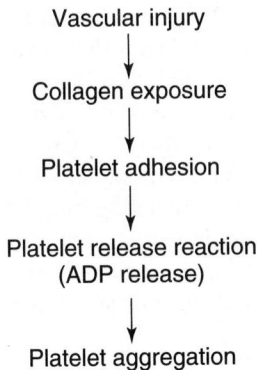

Figure 42.1. Formation of platelet plug.

conversion of factor X to its active form. Activated factor X, in the presence of calcium, phospholipid (platelet factor 3), and factor V, stimulates the conversion of prothrombin to thrombin.

The extrinsic clotting pathway may also stimulate the conversion of prothrombin to thrombin. The release of material that is extrinsic to the blood, such as tissue extract or tissue thromboplastin, activates factor VII, which stimulates the activation of factor X. Factor X thus occupies a central position at the junction of the extrinsic and intrinsic systems; the pathway at this point becomes the common pathway. These two systems act in concert during the evolution of a clot; rarely is one independent of the other (6).

Thrombin, which is generated by both pathways, stimulates the conversion of fibrinogen to fibrin in the presence of ionized calcium. The initial soluble fibrin clot is further converted to an insoluble fibrin polymer when factor XIII is activated by thrombin. In addition to stimulating the conversion of fibrinogen to fibrin, thrombin stimulates platelet aggregation and potentiates the activity of factors V, VIIa, VII, and Xa.

Once thrombin is formed, it is partly removed by absorption into fibrin. This, plus other naturally occurring inhibitors of clotting factors, plays a role in localizing fibrin formation to the sites of injury and in maintaining the fluidity of circulating blood. Agents in normal blood inhibit the activated forms of factors II, X, XI, and XII. Deposition

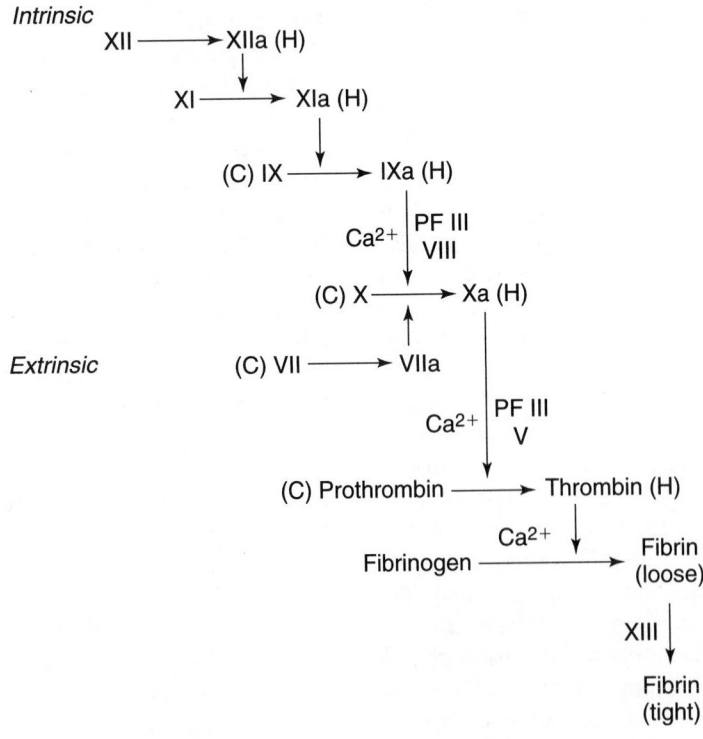

Figure 42.2. Soluble clotting cascade.

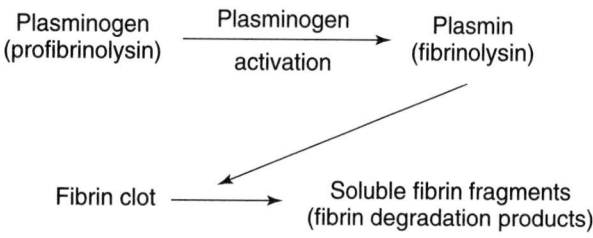

Figure 42.3. Fibrinolysis.

of fibrin also activates plasmin or fibrinolysin, a fibrinolytic enzyme that prevents excessive coagulation (Fig. 42.3).

Two types of thrombi may be formed. "White thrombi," or arterial thrombi, are composed primarily of platelets, although they also contain fibrin and occasional leukocytes. They generally occur in areas of rapid blood flow and are formed in response to an injured or abnormal vessel wall. "Red thrombi," or venous thrombi, are found primarily in areas of relative stasis, where dilution of activated clotting factors by blood flow is prevented. They are almost completely composed of fibrin and erythrocytes, with a small number of platelets.

The choice of an antithrombotic drug is influenced by the type of thrombus. Heparin and the coumarins are used in the treatment of both red and white thrombi. Drugs that affect platelet behavior are most useful for their effects in preventing and treating white thrombi. Fibrinolytic agents dissolve both types of thrombi.

INDICATIONS FOR THERAPY

Antithrombotic therapy has demonstrated a marked benefit in the management of deep venous thrombosis, pulmonary embolism, acute coronary syndromes (unstable angina, acute myocardial infarction), cerebral embolism, and peripheral arterial embolism (see Table 42.2). Therapy is also indicated for the prophylaxis of cerebral embolism associated with atrial fibrillation, prophylaxis of thromboembolism following cardiac valve replacement, the prophylaxis of deep venous thrombosis following hip fractures and other high-risk surgeries, as well as other patients at risk for thrombosis. Other conditions in which antithrombotic therapy may be useful include congestive heart failure, transient ischemic attacks, and disseminated intravascular coagulation (consumption coagulopathy). The selection of an antiplatelet, anticoagulant, or fibrinolytic agent depends on the pathology of the disorder.

DEEP VENOUS THROMBOSIS AND PULMONARY EMBOLISM

The clinical diagnosis of deep venous thrombosis (DVT) is difficult and frequently misleading, most venous clots occurring without prominent findings. Nevertheless, certain clinical signs are helpful. In 80% of cases of DVT reviewed, unilateral ankle edema was present, followed by

Table 42.2.
Indications for Anticoagulant Therapy

Established benefit
  Venous thromboembolism (DVT, PE)
  Post cardiac valve replacement
  Prophylaxis of venous thromboembolism
  Acute coronary syndromes (unstable angina, acute myocardial infarction)
  Atrial fibrillation
  Stroke associated with thromboembolism
  Acute peripheral arterial embolism
Other possible indications
  Post angioplasty
  Disseminated intravascular coagulation
  Transient ischemic attacks

calf tenderness in 50% and a positive Homans' sign (pain on dorsiflexion of the foot) in only 8%. Increased warmth and calf swelling are also consistent with DVT (4, 5, 7, 8).

Deep venous thrombi occur most frequently in the lower extremities, in association with one or more of the previously discussed risk factors. The progression of thrombosis in the calf veins to the iliofemoral system in the thigh is associated with a greater risk of pulmonary embolism. Early recognition and documentation of lower leg thrombosis are necessary to reduce the risk of pulmonary embolism.

The most commom clinical manifestations of pulmonary embolism are sudden onset of unexplained dyspnea, pleuritic chest pain, tachypnea, and sinus tachycardia. Some patients may have hemoptysis or diaphoresis. Electrocardiographic manifestations may include changes in the ST segment and T waves. Chest radiographs are usually not very helpful. Arterial blood gases generally show a reduced pO_2 as well as a decreased pCO_2 caused by hyperventilation.

Objectively, the diagnosis of DVT may be confirmed by phlebography, impedance plethysmography, or Doppler ultrasound. Phlebography (venography) is the most reliable for detecting the presence of DVT (4). Pulmonary embolism may be detected more specifically with the aid of pulmonary perfusion and ventilation scans and pulmonary angiography.

The effectiveness of anticoagulant therapy in proximal vein thrombosis is well established (9). The choice of heparin or fibrinolytic therapy depends on the severity of symptoms and is discussed later in this chapter. Treatment of distal (calf) vein thrombosis is more controversial; while most clinicians treat with heparin, this practice is not supported by all authors. The use of support stockings that are properly fitted for the patient, heat and elevation, and nonsteroidal antiinflammatory drugs (NSAIDs) may be just as helpful for the treatment of calf vein thrombosis. In either case, if heparin is used, NSAIDs must be used cautiously, because they are potentially ulcerogenic and also influence platelet function. Prompt treatment of pulmonary embolism is essential with heparin and/or fibrinolytics because of the morbidity and mortality associated with it (9).

CEREBRAL EMBOLISM

Acute vascular events leading to stroke may be embolic or hemorrhagic. Embolic events account for 85% of strokes, and hemorrhagic events account for the remaining 15%. An accurate diagnosis is essential before therapy is initiated (10).

Anticoagulant therapy may be useful in preventing the recurrence of emboli that are responsible for strokes or in the treatment of evolving strokes or transient ischemic attacks. There is no place for anticoagulant therapy in the treatment of a completed stroke because of the risk of hemorrhage into the infarcted area, which could then lead to extension of neurologic damage (11–13).

Atrial Fibrillation

The prevention of stroke in patients with atrial fibrillation is important because the first stroke may be very debilitating. The primary source of cardioembolism is nonvalvular atrial fibrillation, which accounts for 45% of all cases. This is followed by ischemic heart disease, which accounts for 15%; ventricular aneurysm, 10%; rheumatic heart disease, 10%; prosthetic heart valves, 10%; and idiopathic sources, 10%. The overall incidence of arterial thromboembolism varies on the basis of several criteria, the most important being the presence of comorbid conditions. The patients who are at highest risk include those with anterior wall myocardial infarction, pedunculated thrombi located in the cardiac chamber, congestive heart failure, history of prior embolism, mitral stenosis, prosthetic heart valves, or bacterial endocarditis. Patients who are at less risk include those without a history of any of the above conditions and those with lone atrial fibrillation, mitral valve prolapse, or mild annular calcifications.

Anticoagulant treatment of patients who are at high risk is indicated. Treatment of patients with atrial fibrillation associated with nonvalvular heart disease has been more controversial. Recently, three studies have provided convincing evidence for the efficacy of anticoagulant therapy in these patients (10–12). The first trial to be published was the Atrial Fibrillation, Aspirin, Anticoagulation Study, which investigated the role of aspirin, placebo, or high-dose warfarin therapy (international normalized ratio (INR) of 2.8 to 4.2) in the prevention of stroke in patients with nonrheumatic valvular heart disease. The results strongly suggested that warfarin, but not aspirin (75 mg/day) or placebo, was effective in the prevention of stroke. The results were not statistically significant, however. The Stroke Prevention in Atrial Fibrillation (SPAF I and II) studies (14, 15) and the Boston Area Anticoagulation Trial

for Atrial Fibrillation (BAATAF) study (16) have provided statistically significant data that demonstrate the efficacy of warfarin in prevention of stroke in patients with nonvalvular heart disease. The SPAF-I study investigated the use of aspirin (325 mg/day) and wafarin (INR 1.7 to 4.6) individually versus placebo. Patients who were followed up to a mean of 1.3 years demonstrated a 41% reduction in primary events (ischemic stroke and systemic embolism) with aspirin and a 67% reduction with warfarin. Aspirin did not appear to work in a subgroup of patients over 75 years of age. The incidence of bleeding requiring hospital admission and transfusion was greater in the warfarin group (1.7% compared to 8.9% with aspirin and 1.2% with placebo), and the incidence of cerebral bleeding was greater (0.4% compared to 0.2% in both groups). The BAATAF study investigated the use of warfarin (adjusted to an INR of 1.5 to 2.7) compared to controls who were not given warfarin but who could take aspirin. The results demonstrated an 86% reduction in the risk of stroke for patients taking warfarin over the average 2.2 years of follow-up. Patients who received warfarin had a higher incidence of minor bleeding, but the incidence of major bleeding was the same in both groups. The SPAF-II study continued to follow patients who were randomized in the SPAF-I study to aspirin or warfarin. Additional patients were recruited and randomized also to aspirin or warfarin. Warfarin had an apparent greater benefit in all patients. Unfortunately, it was associated with a higher incidence of intracranial bleeding, which was more common in patients over the age of 75. Patients less than 75 years of age without associated comorbid conditions such as heart failure, hypertension, or prior thromboembolism had a very low incidence of embolism (0.5%/year) on aspirin and would potentially do well on aspirin alone.

Review and analysis of the results from five trials that were completed in the last few years have clearly documented the efficacy of warfarin in decreasing the incidence of thromboembolism associated with atrial fibrillation (14–19). The results with aspirin have been more disappointing. There is a group of patients who do appear to benefit from aspirin alone. Patients with lone atrial fibrillation, without associated risk factors, who are less than 60 years of age are at low risk without any therapy. In patients who are older than 60 years with lone atrial fibrillation without risk factors, aspirin alone appears to offer adequate protection. Despite the greater risk, warfarin offers greater benefit to patients of all ages when atrial fibrillation is associated with concomitant risk factors (20). The optimal level of anticoagulation is an INR of 2.0 to 3.0 (21). Future evaluation of less intense therapy and of antiplatelet therapy is warranted.

MYOCARDIAL INFARCTION

As early as 1948, the American Heart Association recommended anticoagulant therapy for patients who suffered a myocardial infarction. This has not been accepted universally as a treatment regimen. Inconsistent trial results, statistically significant but small clinical reductions in outcome, the availability of newer treatment regimens, the overall reduction in control group mortality, and the fear of bleeding may explain this reluctance.

The rationale for treating acute myocardial infarction with anticoagulants is to decrease mortality and to decrease reinfarction, systemic emboli, and venous thromboembolism. The overall frequency of cerebral emboli in acute myocardial infarction is approximately 4%. The incidence of serious sequelae following stroke may be very significant, with severe deficiency or death occurring in over half of patients.

Several recent publications have provided stronger evidence favoring the use of anticoagulants in the treatment of acute myocardial infarction. Yusuf and colleagues pooled the results from previous studies, subjected them to rigorous review, and concluded that there is, on average, a 22% reduction in mortality in patients who receive anticoagulant therapy (22). Smith and colleagues randomized patients to warfarin (INR 2.8 to 4.8) or placebo within an average of 2.7 days following acute myocardial infarction regardless of site (anterior 47%, inferior 44%) and followed them for an average of 37 months. Overall, there was a risk reduction of 24% for death, 34% for reinfarction, and 55% for cerebrovascular accident in the warfarin group, compared with placebo. No treatment arm, including aspirin alone, was included in this study. The incidence of major bleeding was higher in the warfarin group, but it was often associated with underlying lesions (e.g., malignancy) or the use of unauthorized antiplatelet drug therapy (23). The FDA has recently expanded the approved labeling and indications for warfarin to include myocardial infarction on the basis of this trial (WARIS) as well as the ASPECT study (24). Two new trials are currently enrolling patients to evaluate the efficacy of aspirin compared to the combination of low doses of aspirin and fixed doses of low-dose warfarin.

Antithrombotic agents are also useful in the management of unstable angina (see the discussion in later sections) and in the acute stage of myocardial infarction. Aspirin and heparin decrease the incidence of subsequent infarction and death when they are used in unstable angina. Fibrinolytic therapy with streptokinase, anisoylated plasminogen-streptokinase-activator complex (APSAC or anistreplase), or recombinant tissue plasminogen activator (rtPA or alteplase) in the acute phase of myocardial infarction decreases mortality and preserves myocardial function. (See also further discussion in later sections.)

HEART VALVE PROSTHESIS

Thromboembolism is one of the most frequent complications in survivors of prosthetic valve replacements. The greatest risk of embolism is to the brain. Patients with mechanical heart-valve prostheses should receive lifelong anticoagulation with oral agents such as warfarin. Bioprosthetic valves may offer some patients the option of not requiring long-term anticoagulation. For those who receive bioprosthetic valves in the aortic position, treatment with heparin for 7 to 10 days, followed by low-dose aspirin, may be adequate. Patients with bioprosthetic valves in the mitral position should receive oral anticoagulants for 3 months and then receive aspirin (25).

The addition of an antiplatelet agent to an oral anticoagulant regimen may protect against clotting in patients who develop systemic embolism despite therapeutic INRs. Both aspirin and dipyridamole may be useful adjuncts to oral anticoagulants in this setting.

Patients who receive anticoagulants should be followed closely to ensure adequate intensity and control, since patients receiving anticoagulants who sustain an embolus are likely to have had inadequate anticoagulation (26).

NONPHARMACOLOGIC MANAGEMENT OF THROMBOEMBOLIC DISEASE

Nonpharmacologic measures that contribute to the successful prevention or treatment of thromboembolic disease include proper education, use of support garments, and (infrequently) surgery.

Individualized patient education is important in an overall treatment plan. Prevention of stasis by avoiding prolonged sitting, leg crossing, or wearing constricting garments is extremely important. Properly fitted and prescribed support stockings are helpful. Embolectomy or surgical placement of an inferior vena cava filter (e.g., Greenfield filter) is occasionally performed.

PHARMACOLOGIC MANAGEMENT OF THROMBOEMBOLIC DISEASE

Heparin and the oral anticoagulants (primarily coumarins in the United States) are the major pharmacologic agents that are used in the treatment of clotting disorders.

Prevention of the interaction of platelets with the arterial wall and subsequent microthrombosis and microembolization from these sites with antiplatelet agents is useful. Drugs that accelerate fibrinolysis increase the rate of resolution of emboli.

Laboratory Assessment

Since the response to a given dose of heparin or warfarin is highly variable, laboratory assessment is considered essential. Recurrence of thromboembolism is much greater when therapeutic anticoagulation is not rapidly achieved. Maintaining the appropriate laboratory test in the therapeutic range helps to prevent hemorrhage as well as the development of recurrent thrombosis.

Among the various tests that are available, the most commonly used ones are the prothrombin time (PT), the activated partial thromboplastin time (APTT), and the

Table 42.3.
Clotting Tests Used in the Management of Anticoagulant Therapy

Test	Factors Measured	Normal Value[a]	Drug Monitored
Prothrombin time (PT)[b]	II, V, VII, X	11 sec	Warfarin[c]
Activated partial thromboplastin time (APTT)[d]	All except VII	24–36 sec	Heparin (warfarin)
Activated coagulation time (ACT)[e]	All except VII	80–130 sec	Heparin

[a]University of California, San Francisco.
[b]May also be prolonged by heparin bolus or excessive maintenance dose.
[c]Prefer INR to monitor warfarin. See text.
[d]May also be prolonged by warfarin.
[e]Also known as activated clotting time.

activated coagulation time (ACT), which is also called activated clotting time (Table 42.3).

The PT of Quick is prolonged by deficiencies of factors V, VII, X, and II; by low levels of fibrinogen; and by high levels of heparin. The PT thus reflects alterations in the extrinsic and common pathways. A normal PT is approximately 11 sec. The PT is used to assess warfarin therapy. Because of the variability in sensitivity of the thromboplastin reagent that is used in determining the PT, results from different laboratories may differ. The ratio of the patient's PT to the laboratory control will subsequently differ among laboratories. To standardize interpretation of the intensity of anticoagulation, European investigators adopted the INR in 1983. A World Health Organization primary international reference preparation of thromboplastin is used to standardize the commercial source of thromboplastin that is used by a given laboratory. Acceptance by U.S. laboratories has been slow, but it is apparent now that most laboratories are providing this information, and the antithrombotic literature is now requiring this as a standard. The INR is calculated by raising the calculated PT ratio, PT of the patient/PT control from the laboratory, to the power of the international sensitivity index (ISI), which is assigned to each batch of thromboplastin. (INR = (PT patient/PT control) raised to the ISI.) For example, patient PT of 22 sec and control PT time of 11 sec, equaling a ratio of 2 when raised to an ISI of 2, is equal to an INR of 4 (i.e., 22/11 raised to the power of 2 = 4). Thromboplastin sources that are less sensitive have lower ISIs. This relationship not only has standardized interpretation of laboratory results but also has led to the appreciation that less intense anticoagulation is often as effective as more intense treatment and is associated with a lower incidence of bleeding (27). (See Table 42.4 for recommendations for the intensity of anticoagulation for various indications.) There are several problems with the INR; however, overall it allows for standardization of reporting (28, 29).

The APTT is primarily a measure of the competence of the intrinsic and common clotting pathways. It is insensitive to factor VII and XIII. It is used in screening for deficiencies of the intrinsic clotting system in patients who are considered to be candidates for oral anticoagulation

Table 42.4.
Relative Intensity of Anticoagulant Therapy*

INR 2.0–3.0
  Prophlaxis of venous thrombosis (high risk)
  Treatment of venous thrombosis/pulmonary embolism
  Prevention of systemic embolism associated with:
    Tissue heart valves
    Acute myocardial infarction
    Atrial fibrillation
    Valvular heart disease
INR 2.5–3.5
  Mechanical heart valves (high risk)
  Recurrent systemic embolism (INR 2.0–3.0 may also be effective)

*At present there are two recommended ranges of intensity for anticoagulant therapy: an international normalized ratio of 2.0–3.0 and 2.5–3.5. See text for discussion of more recent experience.
Source: Adapted from (27).

and in monitoring the response to heparin therapy. The APTT is performed with platelet-poor plasma and so does not reflect the activity of platelets. Normal values for the APTT are between 24 and 36 sec. Therapeutic heparinization is considered to be an APTT of 1.5 to 2.5 times control. Finger-stick methods are available for the rapid determination of the APTT at the patient's bedside.

The ACT of whole blood is sensitive to all clotting factors except factor VII, with undetermined sensitivity to factors V and II. The major advantage of this test is that it is a whole blood test; it does reflect the contribution of platelets in coagulation. The ACT can be performed rapidly at the bedside and is frequently used in dialysis suites, catheterization laboratories, and the operating room to evaluate the degree of heparinization. Normal values are 80 to 130 sec.

Disadvantages that are associated with the ACT include limited experience and correlation with monitoring for treatment and lack of correlation with the APTT. The APTT remains the standard for the therapeutic management of heparin.

Duration of Therapy

Little agreement exists regarding the optimal duration of antithrombotic therapy in the treatment of acute thromboembolic events such as deep venous thrombosis or pulmonary embolism. The greatest risk for reembolization is immediately after an initial event. The risk decreases over the next 6 to 8 weeks, and it is during this period that adequate therapy is essential. After acute events, most clinicians continue anticoagulants for 6 weeks to 3 months. Most evidence supports treatment for 3 to 6 months following an initial event. Evidence from a recent trial that randomized patients to 6 weeks versus 6 months of treatment provides some additional insight into this issue. Patients who had reversible risk factors (e.g., surgery) did well with 6 weeks of therapy. Patients with idiopathic venous thromboembolism, however, had a higher recurrence when treatment was discontinued at 6 weeks. These patients should receive treatment for 6 months. Long-term treatment should be reserved for patients with recurrent disease and one or more episodes of unprovoked thromboembolism (30–32).

Treatment of recurrent embolic events or prophylaxis of emboli in patients with prosthetic valves continues longer, frequently for life.

Heparin

MECHANISM OF ACTION

Heparin, a rapid-acting anticoagulant, exerts its antithrombotic effect by accelerating the action of a naturally occurring inhibitor of thrombin, an α_2-globulin, antithrombin III (ATIII). Antithrombin III inhibits activated clotting factors that have a reactive serine residue at their enzymatically active center. Heparin, by binding at the lysine group of ATIII (Fig. 42.4), induces a conformational change in ATIII that allows more ready access of the arginine residue to the serine group on the activated clotting factors (33–35).

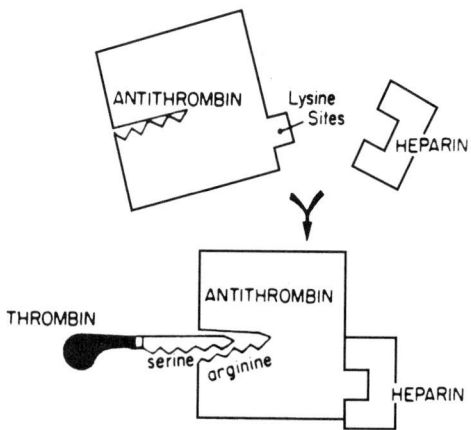

Figure 42.4. Model of heparin-induced conformation change in antithrombin, resulting in rapid inhibition of thrombin. (Source: Reprinted by permission of the New England Journal of Medicine from Rosenberg RD. Actions and interactions of antithrombin and heparin. N Engl J Med 292:146, 1975.)

Commercial heparin is obtained from hog mucosa or bovine lung. The anticoagulant activity of heparin from both sources appears to be equivalent. Differences may exist in the rate of thrombocytopenia, which appears to be greater with heparin from bovine lung. Because of this difference, the heparin source within an institution should be standardized.

Standard or unfractionated heparin is a heterogeneous mixture of molecules with an average molecular weight of 12,000 to 15,000 daltons. Depolymerization of standard unfractionated heparin results in more homogeneous chains of low-molecular-weight heparin (LMWH) with an average molecular weight of 4500 daltons. These LMWHs retain their ability to bind to ATIII and to inactivate factor X, but binding to factor II is markedly decreased. There are a number of other advantages to LMWH as listed in Table 42.5. It is important to acknowledge that LMWH refers to a class of compounds, not to an individual agent, and that one LMWH is not necessarily equivalent to another. Relative activity of these new agents is determined by their ability to neutralize activated factor X, their anti-Xa activity. No clear-cut standard currently exists to compare agents. Two products, enoxaparin and dalteparin, are currently approved in the United States. Several potential and clinically useful advantages of LMWH appear to be a lower incidence of heparin-induced thrombocytopenia, more predictable dose response, lack of need for laboratory monitoring, and a possibly lower incidence of bleeding.

PHARMACOKINETICS

Heparin must be administered parenterally and is effective following intravenous and subcutaneous administration. It should never be administered intramuscularly because of the risk of hematoma formation.

Standard unfractionated heparin is bound to a number of plasma proteins following administration. This binding in part accounts for the variability in response between patients and the resistance that is occasionally observed. LMWHs bind less to proteins, and the anticoagulant response is more predictable. Heparin is metabolized primarily in the liver and reticuloendothelial system and is partly eliminated by excretion into the urine.

The half-life of the anticoagulant effect of heparin in normal individuals and in patients with venous throm-

Table 42.5.
Benefits of Low-Molecular-Weight Heparin

Rapid and predictable antithrombotic effect
Good bioavailability
Effective for postoperative prophylaxis
Resists the inhibitory effect of platelet factor IV
No significant adverse effect on platelets
Long half-life, which allows infrequent dosing

Table 42.6.
Part 1: Intravenous Heparin Administration in Adults

Patient weight: _____ kg (Total body weight)
INTRAVENOUS HEPARIN ADMINISTRATION IN ADULTS
(√ in box activates order)

1. Indication for heparin: _____
2. No IM injections are to be administered during therapeutic heparin.
3. Prior to initiation of heparin obtain:
   APTT   PT   Platelets   Urinalysis   Stool guaiac
4. Loading dose: Note: Usual total body weight.
   Pulmonary embolism (100 units/kg: dose _____ units.
   Other indications (75 units/kg):   dose _____ units.
5. Continuous infusion: Range is 15–25 units/kg/hour depending upon the risk for bleeding (see Part 2 of the table for risk factors).
   Dose:_____ units/hour.
6. Laboratory:
   Obtain APTT 4 hours after loading dose.
   If first APTT > 100 seconds after loading dose, **DO NOT CHANGE THE INFUSION RATE** unless there is evidence of bleeding.
   Continue to check APTT every 4 hours until two consecutive APTT values are 60–80 seconds.
   Daily APTT when dosage no longer requires adjusting.
   Daily CBC, platelets.
   Stool guaiac QOD.
7. Adjustments to continuous intravenous infusion of heparin:

APTT (sec)	Bolus (units)	Hold (minutes)	Rate (units/hr)	Repeat APTT
<50	70 units/kg	0	+200 units/hr	4 hours
	(70 × _____ kg = _____ units)			
50–59	0		+100 units/hr	4 hours
60–80	0	0	0	next A.M.
81–99	0	0	−100 units/hr	4 hours
>100	0	60	−200 units/hr	4 hours

8. If long-term anticoagulation is desired, warfarin should be initiated on day 1 of heparin. The recommended starting dose of warfarin is 7.5–10 mg. For possible exceptions, see Part 2 of the table.
   Dose of warfarin __ mg. Warfarin dose must be written daily.
   Monitor with daily PT/INR. (For therapeutic warfarin guidelines, see Part 2 of the table.)

(continued)

boembolism, as measured by changes in the APTT, is approximately 1.5 hr. The half-life, when plasma heparin activity is measured, depends on the dose and increases with an increased dose. Limited studies show that patients with pulmonary embolism have a greater heparin clearance and shorter half-life than do those with venous thrombosis. This may be due to the continuing thrombin formation on the surface of the embolus, leading to an increased rate of heparin clearance (36, 37).

DOSING AND ADMINISTRATION

Intravenous administration of a large bolus dose of heparin ensures that therapeutic anticoagulation is achieved without delay. Initial doses of 100 to 150 units per kilogram may be required to overcome the initial resistance that is seen and to ensure prolongation of the APTT into the therapeutic range. There is an unacceptable risk of recurrent thrombosis in patients in whom there is a delay in achieving therapeutic levels of anticoagulation. Conversely, there is

no relationship between supratherapeutic APTT response and the risk of bleeding (38).

Numerous approaches have been developed to guide the dosing of heparin. These have shown that the development of guidelines achieves more rapid therapeutic levels more quickly and with a lower incidence of recurrent thrombosis and bleeding. General dosing guidelines can be applied to subsequent changes in the APTT (Table 42.6).

Before the initiation of heparin, baseline clotting studies must be performed and should include at least the prothrombin time (in anticipation of oral anticoagulant therapy) and the APTT.

The initial resistance to heparin therapy returns to normal within several days, and reductions in dose should be anticipated. Laboratory tests should be performed frequently in the beginning and at least daily thereafter.

Heparin therapy has generally been continued for 7 to 10 days following a thromboembolic event, since it is during this time that the incidence of recurrence is the

Table 42.6. *(Continued)*
Part 2: Anticoagulation in Adults, General Information

1. *Selection of initial heparin infusion rate based on bleeding risk:* The initial continuous infusion dose (15–25 units/kg/hr) should be adjusted according to whether the patient is at low or high risk for bleeding. Patients at high risk should receive 15–18 units/kg/hr, and patients at low risk should receive 22–25 units/kg/hr.
   Risk factors for bleeding on heparin:
   a. Surgery, trauma, or stroke within the previous 14 days.
   b. History of peptic ulcer disease, GI bleeding, or GU bleeding.
   c. Platelet count less than 150,000.
   d. Miscellaneous factors such as hepatic failure, uremia, brain metastases.
   e. Age > 70 years.
2. *Duration of heparin:* Patients with deep venous thrombi or pulmonary embolism should receive a minimum of 5 days of heparin. Heparin may be discontinued when warfarin is therapeutic.
3. *Considerations of oral anticoagulation with warfarin:*
   a. Medications that **increase** warfarin effect and may require a reduction in dose include cimetidine, erythromycin, sulfa drugs (e.g., TMP/SMX), metronidazole, ciprofloxacin, and sulfinpyrazone), among others.
   b. Medications that **decrease** warfarin effect and may require an increase in warfarin dose include rifampin, barbiturates, griseofulvin, and bile acid resins, among others.
   c. Factors that may influence warfarin response include the presence of underlying coagulopathies (e.g., congestive heart failure, hepatic disease, nutritional vitamin K deficiency), hyperthyroidism, and febrile illness.
   d. Warfarin should not be administered during pregnancy.
   e. Prothrombin times should be ordered daily, and any increase in the INR of greater than 0.3–0.4 unit per day should result in a dose reduction.
   f. *Therapeutic range for warfarin:* INR of 2.5–3.5 for mechanical prosthetic valves or recurrent systemic embolism; INR of 2.0–3.0 for all other indications.
   g. *Follow-up anticoagulation* may be arranged with the anticoagulation clinic. Please fill out a patient consult form and include the following information: indication, expected duration of therapy, warfarin dosing history, list of medications, primary care provider, and relevant laboratory results.

NOTE: These guidelines are recommendations. They are not intended to replace an individual clinician's judgment.

---

greatest. Shorter-course therapy is as efficacious in the treatment of proximal vein thrombosis and probably pulmonary embolism. Treatment for 5 days versus 10 days was compared in patients with proximal vein thrombosis, and a similar incidence of recurrent venous thromboembolism was noted (7.1% versus 7.0%). Both therapies were followed with warfarin therapy for 12 weeks. In evaluating a patient for shorter-course therapy, it must be understood that if shorter therapy is accepted, this time period must include rigorous attention to maintaining therapeutic levels of anticoagulation (39).

Subcutaneous heparin administration is useful in a number of clinical circumstances. "Low-dose" or "mini-dose" therapy is useful in the prevention of thromboembolism in certain patients who are at risk. (See Table 42.7.) Adjusted-dose subcutaneous heparin can be used as an alternative prophylactic heparin regimen or as an alternative to oral anticoagulant therapy. This involves the twice-daily administration of subcutaneous doses that are adequate to prolong the APTT into the upper range of normal at the midinterval or 6-hour time period. (See the further discussion below of adjusted-dose heparin as a therapeutic treatment.)

The rationale for the use of fixed low doses of heparin is that small amounts of the initial coagulation enzymes (activated factors XII, XI, and IX) eventually lead to large amounts of thrombin being generated. Heparin in relatively low concentrations can prevent this initiation of clotting, while much higher levels of heparin are required to inhibit fibrin formation after thrombin has been generated. Heparin in low subcutaneous doses especially augments the activity of an inhibitor of activated factor X. This inhibitor of factor Xa is probably AT III.

Most experience in the use of low-dose heparin has been accumulated in the prophylaxis of venous thromboembolism and pulmonary embolism during the surgical period and provides the strongest evidence for the efficacy of this route (40). The results show clinically significant benefits in the reduction of venous thrombosis and pulmonary embolism. The newer low-molecular-weight heparins are also effective, and mounting evidence suggests that they are more efficacious in the prevention of venous thromboembolism following orthopedic surgery. The general recommendations for prophylaxis of thromboembolism are included in Table 42.8.

Heparin prophylaxis is most effective in elective gynecologic and abdominothoracic surgery. The administration of fixed-dose, low-dose heparin results in a reduction of thromboembolism of 60 to 70%. Despite this improvement, the overall incidence remains high. Prevention of venous thromboembolism in patients who are undergoing orthopedic surgery is less successful. A

Table 42.7.
Risk Factors for Venous Thromboembolic Disease

	THRIFT	ACCP
Low	Minor surgery (< 30 min), no risk other than age	Uncomplicated minor surgery age < 40 with no clinical risks
	Major surgery (> 30 min), age < 40 no other risks	
	Minor trauma or medical illness	
Moderate	Major general, urologic, gynecologic, cardiothoracic, vascular, or neurologic surgery, age > 40 or other risks	Major surgery in patients age > 40 with no other risks
	Major medical illness, heart or lung disease, cancer, inflammatory bowel disease	
	Major trauma or burns	
	Major surgery, trauma, or illness in patients with previous VTE	
High	Fracture or major orthopedic surgery of pelvis, hip, or lower limb	Major surgery in patients age > 40 or who have additional risks or myocardial infarction
	Major pelvic or abdominal surgery for cancer	
	Major surgery, trauma, or illness in patients with previous VTE	
	Lower limb paralysis or amputation	
Very high	No classification	Major surgery in patients age > 40 plus previous VTE or malignancy, orthopedic surgery, hip fracture, stroke, or spinal cord injury

metaanalysis of various prophylactic procedures revealed an overall incidence of 50% in patients who receive no prophylaxis. This incidence declined with the application of various interventions. Aspirin decreased the incidence to 47%, graduated compression stockings to 37%, dextran to 30%, low-dose heparin to 24%, intermittent pneumatic compression stockings to 22%, warfarin to 19%, adjusted-dose heparin to 17%, and low-molecular-weight heparin to 12%.

Certain high-risk medical patients such as those with congestive heart failure, myocardial infarction, or malignancy may also benefit, with a decrease in pulmonary embolism and subsequent mortality (40).

Administration regimens for low-dose standard heparin generally include 5,000 to 10,000 units subcutaneously from 12 to 2 hr preoperatively, followed by 5,000 to 10,000 units every 8 to 12 hr postoperatively or until the patient is ambulatory. The dose of enoxaparin is 30 mg subcutaneously every 12 hr and is approved for orthopedic surgery. Dalteparin is approved for general surgery patients, and the dose is 2500 units subcutaneously 1 to 2 hr preoperatively and then once daily for 5 to 10 days following surgery. (See Table 42.8.) Although the APTT may be moderately elevated for several hours following administration of standard heparin, laboratory monitoring is not necessary after initial assessment of clotting status. Low-molecular-weight heparins do not influence the APTT.

Low-dose warfarin has been investigated for its role in preventing venous thrombosis after elective total hip or knee replacement. Doses of warfarin that are sufficient to prolong the PT by 1 to 3 sec were started 1 to 2 weeks preoperatively. This regimen was followed by doses that

Table 42.8.
Recommendations for Prevention of Venous Thromboembolism

Indication	Risk Category	Intervention*
General Surgery	Low	Early ambulation
	Moderate	ES, LDH (q12h), IPC
	High	LDH (q8h), LMWH
IPC is alternative for patients at risk for wound complications		
	Very high	LDH, LMWH, dextran plus IPC, warfarin
Orthopedic Surgery	Total hip replacement	Postoperative LMWH ADH, low-intensity warfarin
ES or IPC may be used as adjuvant therapy for > benefit		
	Total knee replacement	Postoperative LMWH or IPC
	Hip fracture surgery	Preoperative LMWH or low-intensity warfarin
Neurosurgery		IPC +/- ES, LDH Combination in high risk
Acute spinal cord injury with paralysis		ADH, LMWH, warfarin
Multiple trauma patients		IPC, warfarin or LMWH when feasible
Medical patients	Myocardial infarction	LDH, full-dose heparin
	Ischemic stroke	LDH, LMWH
	General patients with risk factors	LDH, LMWH
Long-term central vein catheters		Warfarin 1 mg/day

*ES = elastic stockings, LDH = low-dose heparin, IPC = intermittent pneumatic compression, ADH = adjusted-dose heparin, LMWH = low-molecular-weight heparin.
Source: From (2).

were increased to prolong the PT 1.5 times control (no INR reported) immediately after surgery. A decrease in the incidence of venous thrombosis to 21% was observed. Further study with an appropriate control group is required to confirm this observation (41).

In a group of medical and surgical patients, more traditional low-dose heparin (5,000 to 10,000 units every 12 hr) without laboratory adjustment was as effective as warfarin in the prevention of recurrent calf vein thrombosis, but it was not as effective as warfarin in the prevention of recurrent proximal vein thrombosis (41).

Adjusted-dose subcutaneous heparin therapy has been compared to warfarin therapy in the treatment of DVT and pulmonary embolus. Heparin in doses that are adequate to prolong the midinterval APTT to at least 1.5 times the control value was administered to one group of patients, while another group received warfarin in traditional doses. Both groups initially received high-dose intravenous heparin for 14 days. Recurrent proximal vein thromboembolism was prevented in both groups. The frequency of bleeding was greater in patients who were treated with warfarin (42). This type of adjusted dose must be distinguished from prophylactic therapy, and laboratory assessment is essential.

Treatment with LMWH is also promising (43–45). Subcutaneous administration in fixed doses appear to be as safe and effective as standard heparin administered intravenously, if not more so. One major advantage of LMWH is that laboratory monitoring is not required. In fact, the APTT is not affected by these agents. No LMWHs are currently approved for the treatment of venous thromboembolism.

ADVERSE REACTIONS

Hemorrhage is the most frequent adverse reaction to heparin and is generally, but not always, associated with clotting tests outside the recognized therapeutic range. Spontaneous bleeding is rare.

Minor hemorrhage occurs in approximately 4% of courses of anticoagulant therapy, usually into the skin or urine or from the nose. Major hemorrhagic events occur in approximately 2% of courses, usually in the gastrointestinal tract or the central nervous system.

Other adverse effects include thrombocytopenia (46), osteoporosis, hypoaldosteronism, and generalized hypersensitivity reactions. The most common type of thrombocytopenia secondary to heparin appears during the first 3 to 12 days of therapy, is unrelated to dose, and reverses within 3 to 5 days after discontinuation. It may occur in 5 to 10% of patients and can occur with therapeutic intravenous or prophylactic subcutaneous administration. The incidence is less with LMWH. A recent report observed that none of 333 patients and 9 of 332 patients receiving low-molecular-weight heparin and standard hep-

arin, respectively, developed thrombocytopenia (47). The exact mechanism has not been established, but it appears to be immunologically mediated. Osteoporosis occurs with therapy of more than 10,000 units per day for 6 months or longer. Hypoaldosteronism with resultant hyperkalemia and sodium diuresis is uncommonly associated with heparin therapy.

DRUG INTERACTIONS

A direct interaction between heparin and nitroglycerin has been proposed as a mechanism for increasing heparin requirements as is seen in some patients who receive both drugs concomitantly. This has not been a universal observation, however, and a recent controlled trial provides evidence that there is no interference with nitroglycerin doses below 350 µg/min. At doses of nitroglycerin above 350 µg/min, a higher dose of heparin was required to achieve the same prolongation of the APTT. The proposed mechanism is a qualitative antithrombin III abnormality induced by nitroglycerin (48). Close patient monitoring is required, and any resistance can be overcome with appropriate dosage adjustments. Heparin is physically incompatible with many other drugs, and appropriate sources should be consulted before heparin is mixed with other solutions.

The concomitant administration of heparin along with antiplatelet agents must be directed by the clinical indication. There may be an increased risk of bleeding; however, there may be additional efficacy as well. (See the discussion in Chapter 41 on myocardial infarction.)

TREATMENT OF OVERDOSE

Protamine sulfate, a strongly basic molecule, is a specific antidote that combines with and inactivates heparin. The appropriate dose of protamine depends on the dose of heparin, the time since administration, and the route of administration. If administered immediately after intravenous heparin, 1 mg of protamine is given for every 100 units of heparin. If treatment is delayed, the dose of protamine must be decreased. Response can be assessed with the APTT or ACT.

Although protamine has been reported to exert an anticoagulant effect if it is administered in excessive dosages, this is unlikely to be a problem clinically. Of greater concern are the cardiovascular complications that may be associated with protamine. A decrease in blood pressure and systemic vascular resistance has been observed in humans. This appears to be associated most often with too-rapid administration. Anaphylactoid reactions may occur in 2 to 5% of patients (49).

In the event of a major hemorrhage, whole blood or fresh frozen plasma should replace lost volume and clotting factors.

Oral Anticoagulants

Oral anticoagulants exert their pharmacologic effect by interfering with the synthesis of the vitamin K–dependent clotting factors in the liver. These factors are II, VII, IX, and X. Early investigators assumed a competitive antagonism to explain the relationship between warfarin and vitamin K. This has since been disproven. It is now believed that warfarin inhibits the effect of vitamin K at a postribosomal step in the hepatic synthesis of the vitamin K–dependent clotting factors. Vitamin K is required in the conversion of nonactive precursor proteins (precursors of active clotting factors) that lack calcium-binding capacity to active precursor proteins (e.g., prothrombin) that have calcium-binding capacity. This calcium-binding capacity is needed to hold prothrombin onto phospholipid surfaces during its activation to thrombin. Vitamin K accomplishes this activation by carboxylation of glutamyl residues on the precursor protein to form γ-carboxyglutamic acid, which allows for calcium binding. Vitamin K probably carboxylates the glutamyl residues of factors VII, IX, and X as well. During the carboxylation of precursor proteins, vitamin K is converted to vitamin K epoxide. Vitamin K epoxide is then converted back to vitamin K. Warfarin prevents this reaction and thus produces a buildup of inactive precursor proteins. This effect of warfarin can be overcome by the administration of vitamin K (50–52).

The onset of anticoagulant effect of warfarin depends not only on this interaction with vitamin K, but also on the metabolic clearance of clotting factors that are already present in the blood.

PHARMACOKINETICS

The pharmacokinetics of warfarin has been the most extensively studied of coumarin pharmacokinetics (27). Warfarin is completely absorbed in the upper gastrointestinal tract, with peak blood levels occurring in 60 to 120 min. The volume of distribution of warfarin is 12.5% of body weight. This small volume is consistent with the extensive binding of warfarin to albumin, since it is equivalent to the volume of albumin, 2.6 times the plasma volume.

The mean half-life of warfarin is independent of dose and is 42 hr. Warfarin is 99.5% bound to albumin. No apparent relationship exists between the extent of protein binding of wafarin and the concentration of albumin or total protein in the serum. Furthermore, there appears to be no direct correlation between the effect on PT/INR and the dose of warfarin, since so many variables influence dosing (53).

Warfarin is metabolized in the hepatic microsomes by mixed-function oxidase enzymes. It is administered as a racemate that contains equal parts of the R and S isomers. The S isomer is approximately five times more potent than the R isomer. The reason why the R and S isomers differ in potency is unclear. The half-life of the R isomer is 45 hr, and the half-life of the S isomer is 33 hr; they have the same volume of distribution. It has been proposed that differences in permeability or affinity to the receptor site account for the differing potencies.

Knowledge of these two isomers is important because drugs may interact with warfarin stereoselectively. For example, metronidazole inhibits the metabolism of the S isomer but has no effect on the R isomer (51).

DOSING

Oral anticoagulant therapy should be initiated without a loading dose (9, 50, 51, 54). Before the 1980s, clinicians traditionally started therapy with a large initial dose followed by smaller doses over subsequent days. The belief was that therapeutic anticoagulation would be achieved more quickly. Unfortunately, a few clinicians may still initiate warfarin with a loading dose.

The onset of the warfarin effect depends not only on the half-life of the parent drug but also on the half-life of catabolism of the vitamin K–dependent clotting factors. These factors have half-lives of 5 hr for factor VII, 20 to 40 hr for factors IX and X, and up to 60 hr for factor II. Depression of any factor may predispose the patient to bleeding. O'Reilly and Aggeler compared a loading dose of warfarin, 1.5 mg/kg, with two schedules without a loading dose, of 10 mg/day and 15 mg/day. No significant difference was found in the rate of fall of factors II, IX, and X in the different schedules. However, there was a significantly faster decline in factor VII activity with the loading dose compared to the other two regimens. Because the PT is most sensitive to factor VII, a more rapid prolongation of the PT with the loading dose led many to consider this to be proof that loading doses achieve more rapid anticoagulation. Intrinsic coagulation depends most on factors IX and X and less on factor VII. In summary, depression of factor VII offers little if any protection against thromboembolism, and a rapid depression may lead to hemorrhage. Because of the many factors contributing to anticoagulant response, PTs should be obtained daily until therapy is stabilized (54). In addition, loading doses are dangerous for patients with protein C deficiency or protein S deficiency because of increased risk of warfarin-induced skin necrosis.

To achieve a safe and rapid conversion from heparin to warfarin, it is recommended that both anticoagulants be administered concurrently, beginning from the first day of therapy (9). Since evidence exists that 5 days of therapeutic heparinization are as effective as 10 days for the treatment of proximal vein thrombosis, this technique may help to decrease the hospital stay (37). Heparin therapy must be sufficient to prolong the APTT into the therapeutic range throughout this shortened period. Once a stable therapeutic PT response is achieved, heparin may be discontinued.

It has generally been recommended that the degree of oral anticoagulant–induced prolongation of the laboratory test should be the same as for heparin, that is, prolongation to 1.5 to 2.5 times normal. The INR is the preferred standard for assessing the adequacy of anticoagulation with warfarin. The ranges of therapeutic anticoagulation fall within two ranges: an INR of 2.0 to 3.0 and an INR of 2.5 to 3.5 (Table 42.4). As more experience accumulates, even less intense therapy may be possible and may lead to an even lower incidence of bleeding.

TERMINATION OF THERAPY

When a therapeutic course is concluded, warfarin may be discontinued abruptly with little risk of rebound activation of clotting. Since the half-life of warfarin is prolonged, a tapering effect occurs. A recent report suggests that in certain patients there is a rebound hypercoagulable state following abrupt discontinuation, but this observation in a small group of patients requires further confirmation (55).

DETERMINANTS OF ANTICOAGULANT RESPONSE

Many factors may alter the response to warfarin. See Table 42.9 (56, 57).

Diet. Excessive intake of food that is rich in vitamin K may theoretically induce a relative resistance to warfarin. Clinically, this is rarely a problem, and patients may still eat foods such as spinach, kale, cabbage, cauliflower, peas, cereals, and fish. Patients may occasionally be given supplements to improve their nutrition. Although some of these (e.g., Ensure) contain vitamin K, reformulation of these products to decrease the amount of vitamin K minimizes the chance of interference with the warfarin response. Some over-the-counter vitamin supplements (e.g., Centrum) contain small amounts of vitamin K, and infrequent or only occasional use must be considered as a possible cause of variability in response to warfarin. Patients should be instructed to avoid these products or to take them all the time.

Conversely, poor nutrition may lead to an increased hypoprothrombinemic response. Fasting or malabsorption may lead to decreased vitamin K absorption and increased

Table 42.9.
Determinants of Warfarin Response

Diet
Compliance
Drugs
Liver function
Thyroid function
Acute illnesses, particularly febrile
Hereditary resistance
Other

Table 42.10.
Examples of Well-Documented Drug Interactions with Warfarin[a]

Drugs that enhance warfarin effect
  Amiodarone
  Ciprofloxacin
  Cotrimoxazole
  Disulfiram
  Fluconazole
  Cimetidine
  Clofibrate
  Erythromycin
  Metronidazole
  Sulfinpyrazone
Drugs that decrease warfarin effect
  Barbiturates
  Cholestyramine
  Nafcillin
  Carbamazepine
  Griseofulvin
  Rifampin
  Vitamin K

[a]See drug interaction texts and primary literature as well as Chapter 3 in this text for further information. Knowledge of mechanism, clinical significance, and management is essential.

warfarin response. Any acute illness that is associated with diarrhea may quickly induce vitamin K deficiency and result in potentiation of warfarin response.

Drugs. Many drugs may increase or decrease the effect of warfarin. Examples of drugs that can cause important drug interactions with warfarin are listed in Table 42.10. Despite the relatively small number of drugs that have been very well documented to interfere with warfarin, it is necessary to assume that all drugs have the potential for interaction unless proven otherwise (27, 57). An extraordinarily large number of possible interactions have been reported in the literature. With further study, some of the potential interactions may be proven to be clinically relevant.

Liver Function. Since the vitamin K–dependent clotting factors are synthesized in the liver, any disruption of normal liver function may lead to an increased PT, even without warfarin therapy. In the presence of warfarin, this prolongation will be exaggerated.

Hypermetabolic States. Fever or hyperthyroidism may result in increased sensitivity to warfarin because of the increased catabolism of the vitamin K–dependent clotting factors. This is the predominant effect, since the kinetics of warfarin appear to be unchanged. The response to warfarin in myxedema is conversely diminished.

Hereditary Resistance. A hereditary resistance has been identified in animals and humans. Findings that are consistent with an altered affinity of the receptor for oral anticoagulants or for vitamin K have been reported. This is apparently mediated by a single autosomal gene and is very rare.

Other. Many other, less well-documented determinants have been proposed, including climatic changes, smoking, race, age, plasma lipids, congestive heart failure, and renal function.

ADVERSE REACTIONS

Hemorrhage, the most important adverse effect of warfarin, is one of the most frequent reasons for admission to the hospital because of adverse drug reactions. Patients should be informed of the most common sites of bleeding and should look routinely for any signs of bleeding from the gums, nose, throat, skin, gastrointestinal tract, or genitourinary tract.

Cutaneous. Warfarin-induced skin necrosis is most likely to be seen in the buttocks, breasts, and thighs. It occurs within the first 10 days of therapy and usually resolves with discontinuation of warfarin but occasionally requires surgical intervention (50, 51). This adverse effect may be due to microvascular thrombosis secondary to protein C deficiency or protein S deficiency. Adequate heparin therapy may help to prevent its occurrence in some patients. Other skin lesions that have been reported include urticaria, dermatitis, and the "purple toes" syndrome, a nonhemorrhagic reaction that occurs shortly after initiation of therapy.

Teratogenic. Warfarin crosses into the placental circulation and has been reported to cause chondromylasia punctata or stippling of the bones. Nasal bone deformities have been attributed to maternal consumption of warfarin during the first trimester (58).

Although heparin does not cross the placenta and may be safer during pregnancy, it is not without maternal risk, and it has also been associated with increased fetal risk (58).

It appears from limited studies that warfarin does not cross into breast milk (59).

TREATMENT OF OVERDOSE

Excessive hypoprothrombinemia may be reversed with the administration of vitamin K or, if associated with bleeding, with fresh frozen plasma or whole blood. Prolongation of the PT without evidence of hemorrhage may require no more than withholding further warfarin therapy until the PT returns to the therapeutic range. An alternative approach is to administer small doses of oral vitamin K (2.5 mg). This results in a more rapid return to the therapeutic range with little risk of normalization of the PT. If there is evidence of minor bleeding or if the patient is at risk for bleeding, then administration of vitamin K is indicated. Vitamin K1, or phytonadione, is the only vitamin K preparation that should be used, because of its more rapid onset of action. It can be administered intravenously, subcutaneously, or orally; intramuscular administration should be avoided because of the risk of hematoma formation. It should be administered slowly intravenously to prevent cardiorespiratory collapse. Administration of 5 to 10 mg results in a return of the PT to normal in 6 hr after intravenous and in 24 hr after oral administration (60).

Patients who require continued anticoagulation may manifest resistance to subsequent warfarin administration for up to several weeks after vitamin K reversal of warfarin effect.

MANAGEMENT OF MINOR SURGICAL PROCEDURES

Patients who are on warfarin or prolonged therapeutic anticoagulation frequently require minor surgical procedures. Therapy may not need to be interrupted for the performance of many minor procedures, and every patient should be evaluated carefully. Holding the dose of anticoagulant for 1 to 2 days before the procedure may be all that is required (61, 62). To decrease the INR to less than 1.2 before surgical intervention may require withholding up to four doses of warfarin (63). The primary goal should to be to minimize the duration of subtherapeutic anticoagulation.

DRUG INTERACTIONS

Drugs may interact with warfarin by different mechanisms. Pharmacodynamically, drugs may interfere by antagonizing warfarin at the site of action (e.g., vitamin K) and by altering the synthesis of clotting factors (oral contraceptives), clotting factor catabolism (thyroxine), and the hemostatic process (by inhibiting platelet function).

Pharmacokinetically, drugs may interfere with warfarin by altering bioavailability, protein binding, metabolism, and excretion.

It has been proposed for many years that the administration of antibiotics, by suppressing intestinal synthesis of vitamin K by bacteria, would result in enhanced hyprothrombinemia. It is most likely, however, that dietary sources of vitamin K are more important and the gut production is negligible.

The interaction of broad-spectrum antibiotics via suppression of vitamin K and warfarin is clinically unimportant except in debilitated patients or those receiving prolonged parenteral nutrition. Cholestyramine may decrease not only the absorption of warfarin but also the absorption of vitamin K.

Many drugs have been reported to interfere with warfarin absorption, protein binding, and biotransformation. Few drugs actually interact importantly via these mechanisms. Cholestyramine and sucralfate impair warfarin absorption, and sulfonamides may potentiate the effect of warfarin by protein displacement. The influence of protein displacement should be transient, since the increased free level of drug will be metabolized and the levels will return to the predisplacement level.

Amiodarone, cimetidine, ciprofloxacin, cotrimoxazole, disulfiram, erythromycin, fluconazole, metronidazole, and sulfinpyrazone most commonly inhibit the metabolism of warfarin, resulting in an enhanced anticoagulant effect. Allopurinol less significantly interferes via this mechanism.

Barbiturates, carbamazepine, griseofulvin, nafcillin, and rifampin reduce the effect of warfarin by increasing its metabolism via induction of microsomal enzymes (57).

Drugs that affect prothrombin complex concentration may do so by depressing clotting factor synthesis or by increasing the rate of catabolism of clotting factors. Hepatotoxic drugs may potentiate coumarin-induced hypoprothrombinemia by damaging the liver, resulting in decreased synthesis of the vitamin K–dependent clotting factors. Thyroid drugs may increase the response to warfarin secondary to a hypermetabolic state.

Any drug that interferes with hemostasis may increase the risk of therapy with warfarin. Drugs that interfere with platelet function by further impairing hemostasis potentiate the hemorrhagic risk of warfarin and should be avoided. Occasionally, the combination of warfarin with an antiplatelet agent may be useful therapeutically. In these situations, close monitoring is essential.

The selection of a nonsteroidal antiinflammatory drug (NSAID) is a particularly difficult one because not only may these agents interfere with platelet function and cause gastric irritation, but some (such as phenylbutazone) may interact pharmacokinetically with warfarin as well. Of the available NSAIDs, ibuprofen and naproxen appear to be the safest.

Antiplatelet Agents

The role of platelets in thrombogenesis was discussed in the section on the pathogenesis of thromboembolism. Drugs may affect platelet behavior by various mechanisms. They may reduce platelet adhesiveness, decrease or inhibit platelet aggregation, alter platelet membranes, prolong platelet survival, interfere with platelet factor 3 availability, or inhibit glycoprotein IIb/IIIa receptors. Inhibition of glycoprotein IIb/IIIa receptors prevents the binding of fibrinogen to these receptors with subsequent inhibition of platelet aggregation (64).

The importance of drugs that affect platelet function in the clinical management of cardiovascular diseases has become more evident as a result of a number of recent trials. The primary benefits of antiplatelet drug therapy are in the maintenance of graft patency following coronary artery bypass graft surgery, as an adjunct to oral anticoagulants for some patients with atrial fibrillation or mechanical heart valves who develop systemic embolization despite therapeutic anticoagulation, and in the management of patients with unstable angina or myocardial

infarction. A trend toward benefit in preventing reinfarction after a myocardial infarction has been shown.

ASPIRIN

Aspirin produces a detectable inhibitory effect on platelet aggregation that persists for 7 to 10 days after administration of a single dose. The inhibition of platelet aggregation occurs secondary to an irreversible inhibition of cyclooxygenase in the arachidonate pathway. The subsequent effect is to prevent thromboxane A2 formation. (See the previous discussion.) The inhibitory effect of aspirin on cyclooxygenase is more pronounced on platelets and less so on the vessel wall (65). There has been considerable discussion about the optimal dose of aspirin in the prevention of thrombosis. No clear consensus exists. As little as 80 mg/day of aspirin and up to 1 g/day have shown benefit. To minimize adverse effects, the lowest effective dose should be prescribed. For cardiovascular diseases, 81 to 325 mg/day is recommended. For cerebrovascular disease, for example, transient ischemic attacks, 325 mg/day is advised (12). There is a presumed advantage for enteric-coated aspirin as a mechanism to minimize adverse gastrointestinal effects. Other salicylates such as sodium salicylate or choline salicylate do not affect platelets.

Aspirin treatment of unstable angina can decrease the incidence of subsequent infarction and is an accepted therapeutic approach. It is also used along with heparin and thrombolytic agents in the treatment of acute myocardial infarction. The mechanisms for the benefit of aspirin in unstable angina may be severalfold. Inhibition of platelet aggregation, which is frequently associated with arterial vasospasm (particularly in susceptible individuals), may help to maintain adequate flow to the myocardium and prevent ischemia (66).

Primary prevention of myocardial infarction with aspirin has been a topic of considerable interest and debate for years. The Physicians Health Study Research Group reports an overall 47% reduction in the risk of total (fatal and nonfatal) myocardial infarction in male physicians 40 to 84 years of age who were randomized to receive aspirin 325 mg every other day or placebo (67). These results are not supported by a randomized trial of aspirin 500 mg/day that was undertaken involving British male physicians (59). In this study, no difference in fatal and nonfatal myocardial infarctions was shown. In both the U.S. and British studies, there was an increased incidence of strokes in the active treatment groups. In the U.S. trial, the incidence of fatal and disabling hemorrhagic strokes was five times higher in the aspirin group (overall increase 0.02% per year), and in the British trial, disabling or fatal strokes were increased 75% (0.35% per year compared with 0.2% per year in controls). The overall risk of ulcer was 1.22 times greater in the U.S. trial for patients taking aspirin, and the relative risk for bleeding was 1.32 times higher. The incidence of adverse reactions with aspirin in these trials is worrisome. Experience with aspirin in secondary prevention of myocardial infarction, as well as in primary prevention, does not reflect a higher incidence of stroke (66), and recent evaluation of all studies has demonstrated an overall benefit for aspirin (69). The decision to advise the use of aspirin in asymptomatic low-risk patients must be made on an individual basis, and considerable attention must be given not only to the possible benefits and risks but also to alternative risk factor reduction such as controlling hyperlipidemia, hypertension, and obesity. Patients who are older than 50 years of age should receive aspirin 325 mg/day for primary prevention (70). Patients under the age of 50 without a history of stroke, transient ischemic attacks, or acute myocardial infarction should generally not be treated with aspirin.

The role of aspirin in the secondary prevention of myocardial infarction is becoming clearer. Early trials failed to show clear evidence of benefit. Nonfatal reinfarction decreased from 12% to 57%, and the mortality rate decreased 5% to 42%. The shortcomings of these studies were primarily insufficient sample size and power. Pooled analysis of the best-controlled studies did show an average reduction of vascular mortality of 13%, nonfatal infarction of 31%, and nonfatal stroke of 42% with antiplatelet therapy. Two of these trials included sulfinpyrazone (65). Review of studies with aspirin alone has demonstrated a 21 to 26% reduction in myocardial infarction, stroke, or vascular death (69). In the absence of contraindications to aspirin therapy, it should be recommended for all patients after myocardial infarction.

Aspirin is very effective in the acute setting of myocardial infarction. Results of the International Survival in Infarct Study II (ISIS-2), which randomized patients to streptokinase, aspirin, both, or placebo, did show a statistically decreased vascular morbidity in patients receiving either streptokinase, aspirin, or both; the greatest benefit was seen in patients receiving both. The 5-week difference was a 23% reduction with streptokinase, a 21% reduction with aspirin, and a 40% reduction with the combination. Aspirin reduced the incidence of nonfatal reinfarction by 51%, and this effect persisted for 15 months (71). All patients should be treated with aspirin postinfarction.

A Canadian Cooperative Study showed that aspirin in doses of 325 mg four times a day reduced the incidence of stroke and death in men with a previous history of transient ischemic attacks. Dipyridamole has not been shown to be effective (12). Aspirin prophylaxis of venous thromboembolism following total hip replacement is little better than placebo and should not be recommended for routine use.

Aspirin is effective in maintaining both early and late graft patency following coronary artery bypass grafting (CABG). Doses as low as 100 mg/day have been shown to be effective. Dipyridamole has not been shown to be effective individually, nor does it improve outcome when added to aspirin. Ideally, aspirin should be initiated preoperatively, but it is associated with increased incidence of chest tube drainage and reoperation for bleeding. A suggested alternative regimen is to treat with dipyridamole (300 to 400 mg/day) 24 to 48 hr preoperatively, start aspirin 6 hr postoperatively, discontinue the dipyridamole at 48 hr, and continue the aspirin indefinitely (71). Despite the lack of evidence for the role of dipyridamole, its use in this setting is to inhibit platelet deposition immediately without increasing the risk of bleeding, but then it should be discontinued because it has not been shown to prevent reocclusion.

DIPYRIDAMOLE

Dipyridamole may exert an antiplatelet effect by one of several mechanisms. It increases the concentration of cyclic-AMP in platelets, thus potentiating prostacyclin-mediated platelet inhibition. It also increases uptake of adenosine and may stimulate the vascular endothelium to release eicosanoid. Dipyridamole is frequently administered in combination with aspirin; a potentiation of effect has been suggested but remains unproven. Clinically, dipyridamole has been investigated, almost always in combination with aspirin, for the prevention of a second myocardial infarction, prevention of transient cerebral ischemia and stroke, preservation of patency after CABG surgery, and prevention of venous thrombosis and the thromboembolic complications of cardiac valve disease. Very few studies used dipyridamole alone. In the studies in which aspirin was used in combination with dipyridamole and compared with aspirin alone, there appeared to be no benefit from the addition of dipyridamole (72).

The combination of dipyridamole and warfarin in the management of patients with mechanical prosthetic cardiac valves is approved by the Food and Drug Administration. This combination should probably be reserved for patients who develop systemic emboli despite documented therapeutic anticoagulant therapy. No evidence exists to support the use of dipyridamole alone for this indication.

In summary, there is little if any conclusive evidence to document the efficacy of dipyridamole as a single antiplatelet agent, and its widespread use is not justified.

TICLOPIDINE

Ticlopidine is a nonsalicylate antiplatelet drug that may be useful as an alternative to aspirin in the management of stroke and unstable angina after CABG and is useful following coronary stent placement as an aid in preventing restenosis. The effects of ticlopidine are dosage- and time-related, with an onset of action of 24 to 48 hr after oral dosing and a maximal effect seen in 5 to 6 days. It has a half-life of 24 to 34 hr. Ticlopidine exerts its antiplatelet effect via several mechanisms. They generally involve inhibition of ADP induced aggregation. It has also been proposed to interact with the glycoprotein IIb/IIIa receptor, resulting in an inhibition of fibrinogen binding to platelets. This second mechanism is less clear, but the result is a significant antiplatelet effect (73–75).

The efficacy of ticlopidine in the treatment of stroke has been established as a result of two major clinical trials performed in the late 1980s. The Canadian American Ticlopidine Study (CATS) compared ticlopidine 250 mg twice daily with placebo and demonstrated after 3 years an event rate for stroke, myocardial infarction, or vascular death of 15.3% in the placebo group compared with 10.8% in the treatment group (76). The Ticlopidine Aspirin Stroke Study (TASS) compared aspirin 1300 mg/day with ticlopidine 250 mg twice daily. Follow-up ranged from 2 to 6 years. The overall event rate at 3 years was 10% in the ticlopidine group and 13% in the aspirin group. Side effects in the two groups were similar and consisted mainly of diarrhea, rash, and neutropenia (77). Neutropenia secondary to ticlopidine must be monitored closely, and the drug must be discontinued promptly if a reduction in white blood cell count is observed. There was a reported incidence of 0.9% in the TASS study, and one death was reported. Ticlopidine appears to be slightly more effective than aspirin, although it is associated with a higher incidence of side effects. It is a promising alternative to aspirin, but it should be reserved for patients who are intolerant to aspirin.

Fibrinolytic Agents

Fibrinolytic agents play an active role in the dissolution of clots in contrast to heparin and warfarin, which only prevent their occurrence or propagation. Four agents are currently available for clinical use: streptokinase, anistreptlase (APSAC), urokinase, and alteplase (rtPA).

These agents activate plasminogen (Fig. 42.3). Urokinase does this by a direct mechanism, streptokinase by first complexing with plasminogen and further activating plasminogen, and alteplase by catalyzing the conversion of plasminogen to plasmin. APSAC is streptokinase bound to plasminogen and protected from subsequent hydrolysis until it is in the bloodstream. Once hydrolyzed, streptokinase is the active agent.

Fibrinolysis that is induced by these drugs can induce widespread bleeding because they will lyse not only pathologic thrombi but also hemostatic plugs. Careful patient selection is thus important. Fibrinolytic agents should be considered to be contraindicated for patients who have a history of active internal bleeding, a history of cerebrovascular accident or trauma within the last 2 months, known bleeding diathesis, severe uncontrolled hypertension, or any intracranial process such as a neo-

plasm. Care should be taken, and patients should be evaluated on an individual basis if there is a recent (within 10 days to 2 weeks) history of surgery, organ biopsy, bacterial endocarditis, puncture of noncompressible vessel, pregnancy, minor trauma, acute pericarditis, or severe renal and/or hepatic disease. There are other conditions in which they may be contraindicated, and the patient must be evaluated to weigh the risks versus the benefits. Adverse reactions in addition to bleeding include hypotension, allergy, and fever.

The use of fibrinolytic agents in the treatment of pulmonary embolism is indicated for life-threatening symptoms associated with massive pulmonary embolism. This is usually the case when pulmonary embolectomy is being considered. Treatment with streptokinase is initiated with a loading dose of 250,000 units administered over 30 min, followed by an infusion of 100,000 units per hour for 24 to 72 hr. Urokinase is administered as a loading dose of 4400 units per kilogram over 10 min, followed by 4400 units per kilogram per hour for 12 to 24 hr. Tissue plasminogen activator is administered at a dosage of 100 mg over 2 hr. Heparin therapy is started following streptokinase and urokinase and is given simultaneously with rtPA.

The dose of streptokinase and urokinase for the treatment of deep venous thrombosis is the same as for pulmonary embolism. Treatment should be continued for 72 hr with both agents.

The hematologic status of the patient should be evaluated before administration of fibrinolytic agents. The thrombin time, PT, APTT, complete blood count, and platelets should be measured. Once it has been established that the patient's baseline coagulation profile is normal, clotting tests are performed to document that a "lytic" state has been achieved. If the thrombin time is prolonged two to five times the normal value, the dosage should not be increased. On the other hand, if there is no prolongation of the thrombin time, especially with streptokinase, one should consider that there is a high concentration of circulating, neutralizing antibodies. This rarely, if ever, occurs with urokinase or alteplase, and they should be used alternatively if there no response to streptokinase.

The greatest impact of fibrinolytic therapy has been in the treatment of acute myocardial infarction. The three major goals of intervention with these agents in the treatment of acute myocardial infarction are to (a) recanalize the infarct-related artery, (b) preserve left ventricular function, and (c) decrease both short-term and long-term mortality. Many studies have been performed to establish the efficacy of fibrinolytic therapy and to define the differences between the agents (78). (For a more extensive discussion, see Chapter 41 on acute myocardial infarction.)

The percentage of successful recanalization of the infarct-related artery varies significantly from trial to trial. Tissue plasminogen activator achieves the highest patency rate (average approximately 75%), followed by APSAC and streptokinase (average 40 to 70%). A more aggressive regimen of alteplase has been shown to result in a higher patency rate at 90 min (81%) than streptokinase (54%), but they are the same at 180 min, 76 versus 73%, respectively (79). Despite these differences in recanalization rate, there is little difference between the agents in their ability to decrease mortality. The Italian Group for the Study of Streptokinase in Myocardial Infarction (GISSI-2) trial (80), which compared streptokinase and rtPA, and the International Study of Infarct Survival III (ISIS-3) trial, which compared streptokinase, rtPA (duteplase-rtPA manufactured by Burroughs-Wellcome), and APSAC (81), demonstrated no difference in mortality.

The overall impact on mortality from comparative trials of thrombolytic agents is very similar. The ISIS-3 trial showed a 5-week mortality of 10.5% for streptokinase, 10.3% for duteplase, and 10.6% for APSAC (81). The reinfarction rate for the three drugs was 3.6%, 3.1%. and 3.8%, respectively, while the incidence of hemorrhagic stroke was 0.3%, 0.7%, and 0.6%, respectively. The results of the GISSI-2 trial are similar; there was no difference in mortality between the treatment groups (streptokinase and rtPA) (80). The Global Utilization of Streptokinase and Tissue Plasminogen Activator for Occluded Arteries (GUSTO) compared a front-loaded weight-adjusted regimen of rtPA to streptokinase and to a combination of rtPA and streptokinase (82). The mortality rate for front-loaded rtPA was 6.3%, that for streptokinase was 7.3%, and that for the combination was 7.0%. All patients received heparin. The benefit from the front-loaded regimen of rtPA for patients presenting with an anterior wall myocardial infarction within 4 hr of symptom onset in comparison to streptokinse and the combination (82).

Preservation of left ventricular function after fibrinolytic therapy has also been demonstrated and is similar with all of the available agents, the greatest benefit being shown when therapy is administered within 4 hr of on set of symptoms.

Timing of administration of fibrinolytic therapy is important. Early (less than 3 hr from the onset of symptoms) administration results in the greatest decrease in mortality, although benefit has been shown when therapy is given up to 24 hours after symptom onset (83).

Adjunctive therapy with aspirin is important in the treatment of myocardial infarction. The lSlS-2 trial compared streptokinase, aspirin, and streptokinase and aspirin together. The greatest decrease in mortality was seen with the combination; aspirin alone and streptokinase alone were equally effective. Heparin is another helpful adjunct, and the timing of administration and the intensity of treatment have become areas of controversy. Because the half-life of rtPA is so short, heparin administration immediately following the conclusion of the rtPA infusion is important. Heparin therapy following streptokinase and APSAC

therapy may not be as important, and some evidence suggests that it offers no additional benefit (84). The general practice is to use it for several days after infarction. Other adjuncts such as β-blockers and angiotensin-converting-enzyme inhibitors may further decrease mortality in selected patients.

The most serious complication following fibrinolytic therapy is hemorrhage. Despite the reputed greater clot selectivity of rtPA, the incidence of bleeding following all agents is similar. The incidence of stroke was greater with rtPA in both the ISIS-3 trial and GUSTO than it was with streptokinase.

Follow-up of patients receiving fibrinolytic therapy is important, because these agents dissolve the clot but do not affect the underlying coronary lesion. Many patients will ultimately undergo percutaneous transluminal coronary angioplasty or CABG, but until then, they generally receive treatment with antiplatelet agents such as aspirin.

In conclusion, fibrinolytic therapy is an important advance in the management of patients with acute myocardial infarction and selected patients with deep venous thrombosis and pulmonary embolism. On the basis of the published experience, efficacy, and cost, streptokinase is the best deal. There is a slight mortality benefit with rtPA in a specific population of patients; however, there is also a slightly higher incidence of hemorrhagic stroke. What has become most clear from all of the fibrinolytic trials of myocardial infarction is that the earlier the treatment, the better the outcome.

An intriguing new role for fibrinolytic agents may be in the urgent treatment of stroke associated with ischemic cerebral infarction. Several uncontrolled pilot studies of the use of alteplase in the early (within 90 min) and later (91 to 180 min) stages of acute stroke have been reported. The results are very preliminary and inconclusive. They demonstrate that the incidence of intracranial hemorrhage is related to the dose of alteplase. The overall incidence may be as high as 15%. This approaches the approximately 30% benefit that is observed in a small number of patients (85–87).

CONCLUSION

The appropriate use of antithrombotic agents depends on establishing well-defined therapeutic objectives. These objectives are determined to a large extent by the underlying pathophysiology of the thromboembolic event. For example, the patient with an acute myocardial infarction represents a different problem from the patient with a deep venous thrombosis or pulmonary embolism. For the patient with acute myocardial infarction there is a role for aggressive therapy with antithrombotic agents affecting acute fibrinolysis, platelet function, and fibrin deposition. This requires the use of a fibrinolytic agent such as streptokinase, as well as aspirin and heparin. It is thus important to be familiar with the pharmacology, dosing, and laboratory management of these agents to optimize the therapeutic outcome while minimizing the risk of adverse effects, particularly bleeding. Advances in antithrombotic therapy will most likely be in the area of developing even more specific antithrombotic agents or regimens of agents in the treatment of thromboembolic disease.

REFERENCES

1. Anonymous Third ACCP Consensus Conference on Antithrombotic Therapy. Chest 102(Suppl):303S–549S, 1992.

2. Becker RC, Ansell J. Antithrombotic therapy: an abbreviated reference for clinicians. Arch Intern Med 155:149–61, 1995.

3. Goldhaber SZ. Venous thrombosis: prevention, treatment, and relationship to paradoxical embolization. Cardiol Clin 12:505–16, 1994.

4. Weinmann EE, Salzman EW. Deep-venous thrombosis. N Engl J Med 331:1630–41, 1994.

5. Baker WF, Bick RL. Deep venous thrombosis: diagnosis and management. Med Clin North Am 78:685–712, 1994.

6. Furie B, Furie BC. Molecular and cellular biology of blood coagulation. N Engl J Med 326:800–06, 1992.

7. Hirsh J. Diagnosis of venous thrombosis and pulmonary embolism. Am J Cardiol 65:45C–49C, 1990.

8. Moser KM. Venous thromboembolism. Am Rev Resp Dis 151:235–49, 1990.

9. Hyers TM, Hull RD, Weg JG. Antithrombotic therapy for venous thromboembolic disease. Chest 102(Suppl):408S–425S, 1992.

10. Rothrock JF, Hart RG. Antithrombotic therapy in cerebrovascular disease. Ann Intern Med 115:885–95, 1991.

11. Adams HP, Brott TG, Crowell RM, et al. Guidelines for the management of patients with acute ischemic stroke. Stroke 25:1901–14, 1994.

12. Feinberg WM, Albers GW, Barnett HJM, et al. Guidelines for the management of transient ischemic attacks. Stroke 25:1320–35, 1994.

13. Matchar DB, McCrory DC, Barnett HJM, et al. Medical treatment for stroke prevention. Ann Intern Med. 121:41–53, 1994.

14. Stroke Prevention in Atrial Fibrillation Investigators. Stroke prevention in atrial fibrillation: final results. Circulation 84:527–39, 1991.

15. Stroke Prevention in Atrial Fibrillation Investigators. Warfarin versus aspirin for prevention of thromboembolism in atrial fibrillation: stroke prevention in atrial fibrillation II study. Lancet 343:687–91, 1994.

16. Boston Area Anticoagulation Trial for Atrial Fibrillation Investigators. The effects of low-dose warfarin on the risk of stroke in patients with nonrheumatic atrial fibrillation. N Engl J Med 323:1505–11, 1990.

17. Ezekowitz MD, Bridgers SL, James KE, et al. Warfarin in the prevention of stroke associated with nonrheumatic atrial fibrillation. N Engl J Med 327:1406–12, 1992.

18. Connolly SJ, Laupacis A, Gent M, et al. Canadian Atrial Fibrillation (CAFA) Study. J Am Coll Cardiol 18:349–55, 1991.

19. Atrial Fibrillation Investigators. Risk factors for stroke and efficacy of antithrombotic therapy in atrial fibrillation: analysis of pooled data from five randomized controlled trials. Arch Intern Med 154:1449–57, 1994.

20. Albers GW. Atrial fibrillation and stroke: three new studies, three remaining questions. Arch Intern Med 154:1443–48, 1994.

21. The European Atrial Fibrillation Trial Study Group. Optimal oral anticoagulation in patients with nonrheumatic atrial fibrillation and recent cerebral ischemia. N Engl J Med 333:5–10, 1995.

22. Yusuf S, Wittes J, Friedman L. Overview of results of randomized clinical trials in heart disease. I: treatment following myocardial infarction. JAMA 260:2088–93, 1988.

23. Smith P, Arnesen H, Holme I. The effect of warfarin on mortality and reinfarction after myocardial infarction. N Engl J Med 323:147–52, 1990.

24. Anticoagulants in the Secondary Prevention of Events in Coronary Thrombosis (ASPECT) Research Group. Effect of long-term oral anticoagulant treatment on mortality and cardiovascular morbidity after myocardial infarction. Lancet 343:499–503, 1994.

25. Stein PD, Alpert JS, Copeland J, et al. Antithrombotic therapy in patients with mechanical and biological prosthetic heart valves. Chest 102(Suppl):445S–455S, 1992.

26. Cannegieter SC, Rosendaal FR, Wintzen AR, et al. Optimal oral anticoagulant therapy in patients with mechanical heart valves. N Engl J Med 333:11–17, 1995.

27. Hirsh J, Dalen JE, Deykin D, et al. Oral anticoagulants: mechanism of action, clinical effectiveness, and optimal therapeutic range. Chest 102(Suppl):312S–326S, 1992.

28. Le DT, Weibert RT, Sevilla BK, et al. The internationalized ratio (INR) for monitoring warfarin therapy: reliability and relation to other monitoring methods. Ann Intern Med 120:552–558, 1994.

29. Hirsh J, Poller L. The international normalized ratio: a guide to understanding and correcting its problems. Arch Intern Med 154:282–88, 1994.

30. Research Committee of the British Thoracic Society. Optimum duration of anticoagulation for deep-vein thrombosis and pulmonary embolism. Lancet 340:873–76, 1992.

31. Schulman S, Rhedin AS, Lindmarker P, et al. A comparison of six weeks with six months of oral anticoagulant therapy after a first episode of venous thromboembolism. N Engl J Med 332:1661–65, 1995.

32. Sarasin FP, Bounameaux H. Duration of oral anticoagulant therapy after proximal vein thrombosis: a decision analysis. Thromb Haemost 71:286–91, 1994.

33. Hirsh J, Dalen JE, Deykin, et al. Heparin: mechanism of action, pharmacokinetics, dosing considerations, monitoring, efficacy, and safety. Chest 102(Suppl)337S-351S, 1992.

34. Hirsh J, Fuster V. Guide to anticoagulant therapy. Part 1: heparin. Circulation 89:1449–68, 1994.

35. Hirsh J. Heparin. N Engl J Med 324:1565–74, 1991.

36. Pineo GF, Hull RD. Classical anticoagulant therapy for venous thrombo-embolism. Prog Cardiovasc Dis 37:59 –70, 1994.

37. Hirsch J, Van Aken WG, Gallus AS, et al. Heparin kinetics in venous thrombosis and pulmonary embolism. Circulation 53:691–695: 1976.

38. Hull RD, Raskob GE, Rosenbloom D, et al. Optimal therapeutic levels of heparin therapy in patients with venous thrombosis. Arch Int Med 152:1589–1595, 1992.

39. Hull RD, Raskob GE, Rosenbloom D, et al. Heparin for 5 days as compared with 10 days in the initial treatment of proximal vein thrombosis. N. Engl J Med 322:1260–64, 1990.

40. Clagett GP, Anderson FA, Levine MN, et al. Prevention of venous thromboembolism. Chest 102(Suppl):391S–407S, 1992.

41. Francis CW, Marder VJ, Evarts CM, et al. Two-step warfarin therapy: prevention of postoperative venous thrombosis without excessive bleeding. JAMA 249:374–78, 1983.

42. Hull RD, Delmore T, Carter C, et al. Adjusted subcutaneous heparin vs. warfarin sodium in the long-term treatment of venous thrombosis. N Engl J Med 306:189–94, 1982.

43. Lensing AWA, Prins MH, Davidson BL. Treatment of deep venous thrombosis with low-molecular-weight heparins: a meta-analysis. Arch Intern Med 155:601–07, 1995.

44. Hull RD, Raskob GE, Pineo GF, et al. Subcutaneous low-molecular weight heparin compared with continuous intravenous heparin in the treatment of proximal-vein thrombosis. N Engl J Med 326:975–82, 1992.

45. Hull RD, Pineo GF. Low molecular weight heparin treatment of venousthromboembolism. Prog Cardiovasc Dis 37:71–8, 1994.

46. Warkentin TE, Lelton JG. Heparin-induced thrombocytopenia. Prog Hemost Thromb 10:1–34, 1991.

47. Warkentin TE, Levine MN, Hirsh J, et al. Heparin-induced

thrombocytopenia in patients treated with low-molecular-weight heparin or unfractionated heparin. N Engl J Med 332:1330–35, 1995.

48. Becker RC, Corrao JM, Bovill EG, et al. Intravenous nitroglycerin induced heparin resistance: a qualitative antithrombin III abnormality. Am Heart J 119:1254–61, 1990.

49. Horrow JC. Protamine: a review of its toxicity. Anesth Analg 64:348–61, 1985.

50. Hirsh J. Oral anticoagulant drugs. N Engl J Med 324:1865–75, 1991.

51. Hirsh J, Fuster V. Guide to anticoagulant therapy. Part 2: oral anticoagulants. Circulation 89:1469–79, 1994.

52. Sheareer MJ. Vitamin K. Lancet 345:229–34, 1995.

53. Holford NH. Clinical pharmacokinetics and pharmacodynamics of warfarin: understanding the dose-effect relationship. Clin Pharmacokinet 11:483–504, 1986.

54. O'Reilly RA, Aggeler PM. Studies on coumarin anticoagulant drugs: initiation of therapy without a loading dose. Circulation 38:169–77, 1968.

55. Palareti G, Legnani C, Guazzaloca G, et al. Activation of blood coagulation after abrupt or stepwise withdrawl of oral anticoagulants: a prospective study. Thromb Haemost 72:222–26, 1994.

56. O'Reilly RA, Aggeler PM. Determinants of the response to oral anticoagulant drugs in man. Pharmacol Rev 22:35, 1970.

57. Wells PS, Holbrook AM, Crowther NR, et al. Interactions of warfarin with drugs and food. Ann Int Med 121:676–83, 1994.

58. Hall JG, Pauli RM, Wilson KM, et al. Maternal and fetal sequelae of anti-coagulation during pregnancy. Am J Med 68:122–40, 1980.

59. Orme ML, Lewis PJ, deSwiet MS, et al. May mothers given warfarin breast-feed their infants? Br Med J 1:1564–65, 1977.

60. Udall J. Don't use the wrong vitamin K. Calif Med 112:65, 1966.

61. Weibert RT. Oral anticoagulant therapy in patients undergoing dental surgery. Clin Pharm 11:857–64, 1992.

62. Moll AC, Rij GV, Van Der Loos TLJM. Anticoagulant therapy and cataract surgery. Doc Ophthalmol 72:367–73, 1989.

63. White RH, McKittrick T, Hutchinson R, et al. Temporary discontinuation of warfarin therapy: changes in the international normalized ratio. Ann Intern Med 122:40–2, 1995.

64. Lefkovits J, Plow EF, Topol EJ. Platelet glycoprotein IIb/IIIa receptors in cardiovascular medicine. N Engl J Med 332:1553–59, 1995.

65. Special writing group. Aspirin as a therapeutic agent in cardiovascular disease. Circulation 87:659–75, 1993.

66. Hirsh J, Dalen JE, Fuster V, et al. Aspirin and other antiplatelet-active drugs: the relationship between dose, effectiveness, and side effects. Chest 102(Suppl):327S–337S, 1992.

67. Steering Committee of the Physicians Health Research Group. Final report on the aspirin component of the Ongoing Physicians Health Study. N Engl J Med 321:129–35, 1989.

68. Peto R, Gray R, Collins R, et al. Randomized trial of daily aspirin in British male doctors. Br Med J 295:313–16, 1988.

69. Antiplatelet Trialists' Collaboration. Collaborative overview of randomized trials of antiplatelet therapy. I: prevention of death, myocardial infarction, and stroke by prolonged antiplatelet therapy in various categories of patients. Br Med J 308:81–106, 1994.

70. Cairns JA, Hirsh J, Lewis HD, et al. Antithrombotic drugs in coronary artery disease. Chest 102(Suppl):456S–481S, 1992.

71. ISIS-2 (Second International Study of Infarct Survival) Collaborative Group. Randomized trial of intravenous streptokinase, oral aspirin, both, or neither among 17,187 cases of suspected acute myocardial infarction. Lancet 2:349–60, 1988.

72. Fitzgerald GA. Dipyridamole. N Engl J Med 316:1247–57, 1987.

73. Robert S, Miller AJ, Fagan SC. Ticlopidine: a new antiplatelet agent for cerebrovascular disease. Pharmacotherapy 11:317–25, 1991.

74. Ito MK, Smith AR, Lee ML. Ticlopidine: a new platelet aggregation inhibitor. Clin Pharm 11:603–17, 1992.

75. Flores-Runk P, Raasch RH. Ticlopidine and antiplatelet therapy. Ann Pharmacother 27:1090–8, 1993.

76. Gent M, Easton JD, Hachinski VC, et al. The Canadian American Ticlopidine Study (CATS) in thromboembolic stroke. Lancet 1:1215–29, 1989.

77. Haas WK, Easton JD, Adams HP, et al. A randomized trial comparing ticlopidinehydrochloride with aspirin for the prevention of stroke in high risk patients. N Engl J Med 321:501–08, 1989.

78. Ridker PM, Marder VJ, Hennekens CH. Large-scale trials of thrombolytic therapy for acute myocardial infarction. Ann Intern Med 119:530–32, 1993.

79. The GUSTO Angiographic Investigators. The effects of tissue plasminogen activator, streptokinase, or both on coronary artery patency, ventricular function, and survival after acute myocardial infarction. N Engl J Med 329:1615–22, 1993.

80. Italian Group for the Study of Streptokinase in Myocardial Infarction (GISSI-2). A factorial randomized trial of alteplase versus streptokinase and heparin vs no heparin among 12,490 patients with acute myocardial infarction. Lancet 336:65–71, 1990.

81. The International Study Group. In-hospital mortality and clinical course of 20,891 patients with suspected acute myocardial infarction randomized between alteplase and streptokinase with or without heparin. Lancet 336:71–75, 1990.

82. The GUSTO Investigators. An international randomized trial comparing four thrombolytic strategies for acute myocardial infarction. N Engl J Med 329:673–82, 1993.

83. Fibrinolytic Therapy Trialist (FTT) Collaborative Group. Indications for fibrinolytic therapy in suspected acute myocardial infarction: collaborative overview of early mortality and major morbidity results from all randomized trials of more than 1000 patients. Lancet 343:311–22, 1994.

84. Ridker PM, Hebert PR, Fuster V, et al. Are both aspirin and heparin justified as adjunct to thrombolytic therapy for acute myocardial infarction? Lancet 341:1574–77, 1993.

85. Brott TG, Haley EC, Levy DE, et al. Urgent therapy for stroke. Part I: pilot study of tissue plasminogen activator administered within 90 minutes. Stroke 23:632–40, 1992.

86. Haley EC, Levy DE, Brott TG, et al. Urgent therapy for stroke. Part II: pilot study of tissue plasminogen activator administered 91–180 minutes from onset. Stroke 23:641–45, 1992.

87. VonKummer R, Kaeke W. Safety and efficacy of intravenous tissue plasminogen activator and heparin in acute middle cerebral artery stroke. Stroke 23:646–52, 1992.

CHAPTER 43

ALLERGIC AND DRUG-INDUCED SKIN DISEASE

ANN B. AMERSON

Allergic and drug-induced skin diseases encompass a wide variety of conditions, both acute and chronic, with varying morphology. The most commonly encountered allergic skin diseases are atopic dermatitis, contact dermatitis, and urticaria. In addition, ingestion of a number of drugs can produce varied dermatologic reactions. A brief review of skin structure and function is provided as a basis for the discussion of the individual conditions. The etiology, pathogenesis, therapeutic interventions, and management of each condition will be discussed. A glossary of common skin manifestations is included in Table 43.1.

SKIN STRUCTURE AND FUNCTION

The skin, the largest organ of the body, is divided into three (main) distinct layers—the epidermis, the dermis, and the hypodermis (subcutaneous tissue)—as indicated in Figure 43.1 (1, 2). The epidermis is nonvascular and consists of stratified squamous epithelial cells that are of two distinct types: keratinocytes and dendritic cells (2). The dendritic cells are further classified into three types: melanocytes, Langerhans cells, and indeterminate dendritic cells. The epidermis consists of five distinct layers from inside out:

1. Stratum germinativum (basal)
2. Stratum spinosum (prickle)
3. Stratum granulosum (granular)
4. Stratum lucidum (lucid)
5. Stratum corneum (horny)

The keratinocytes are located in the basal layer and serve as stem cells that differentiate into other cells in the upper layers of the epidermis. As the keratinocytes migrate toward the surface, they undergo gradual transformation from living cells to dead, thick-walled flat cells that contain keratin. The basal layer also contains melanocytes, which are the pigment-forming cells (1, 2).

The prickle layer also contains both keratinocytes and melanocytes. The layer is so named because of the cytoplasmic threads called prickles appearing prominently in this layer. The granular layer consists of several thicknesses of flattened cells with protein granules con-

taining keratohyaline. These granules are changed to keratin, a fibrous substance in the outermost layers.

The lucid layer, which appears as a translucent line, is present only in thicker skin such as on the palms and soles. The outermost horny layer or the stratum corneum consists of flat, scaly dead tissue layers that are constantly shedding. The horny layer is the dead end product, whereas the other four layers are considered the living epidermis. A continual process occurs throughout the sublayers of the epidermis in that new cells from the lower layers push older cells toward the top where they eventually become filled with keratin and die. The epidermis under normal conditions can replicate itself in 3 to 4 weeks.

The dermis or corium consists of connective tissue, cellular elements, and ground substance with a rich blood and nerve supply. The sebaceous glands and shorter hair follicles originate in the dermis, which can be divided into two distinct sublayers: the papillary and reticular units. The papillary layer is adjacent to the epidermis and has a rich supply of blood vessels. The reticular sublayer contains coarser tissue that connects the dermis and subcutaneous tissue (hypodermis).

The connective tissue of the dermis comprises collagen fibers, elastic fibers, and reticular fibers that provide support and elasticity of the skin. The cellular elements consist of three types of mesodermal cell groups: reticulohistiocytes, myeloid, and lymphoid. The reticulohistocyte group consists of fibroblasts, histiocytes, and mast cells with immature cells called reticulum cells. Intracytoplasmic granules containing heparin and histamine are present in mast cells. These cells, normally few in number, are increased in itching dermatoses, such as contact or atopic dermatitis. Histiocytes normally are present in small numbers around blood vessels. In pathologic conditions, they migrate in the dermis as monocytes. They may phagocytize bacteria and particulate matter and then are known as macrophages. Fibroblasts form collagen fibers and may serve as precursors for the other connective tissue cells. Polymorphonuclear leukocytes and eosinophils, members of the myeloid group, are quite common in

Table 43.1.
Terms Associated with Allergic and Drug-induced Skin Diseases

angioedema	an allergic skin disease characterized by patches of circumscribed swelling involving the skin and its subcutaneous layers, the mucous membranes, and sometimes the viscera. Also called angioneurotic edema, giant urticaria.
bullae	large vesicles or blisters.
dermographism	pressure or friction on the skin gives rise to a transient, raised usually reddish mark, sometimes white, so that a word traced on the skin becomes visible.
desquamation	peeling of skin in the form of scales.
eczema	inflammation of the skin characterized by redness, itching, and oozing vesicular lesions that become scaly, crusted, or hardened.
erythema	abnormal redness of the skin due to capillary congestion.
exanthem	an eruptive disease (as measles) or its (exanthematous) symptomatic eruption.
excoriation	a raw irritated lesion; the act of abrading or wearing off the skin.
exfoliation	the peeling of the horny layer of the (exfoliative) skin.
lichenoid	resembling lichen, which is characterized by the eruption of flat papules.
macule	a patch of skin that is altered in color but usually not elevated.
maculopapular	combining the characteristics of macules and papules.
morbilliform	resembling the eruption of measles.
papule	a small solid usually conical elevation of the skin caused by inflammation, accumulated secretion, or hypertrophy of tissue elements.
plaque	a localized abnormal patch on a body part or surface and especially on the skin.
pruritus	localized or generalized itching due to irritation of sensory nerve endings from organic or psychogenic causes.
urticaria	an allergic disorder marked by raised edematous patches (wheals) of skin or mucous membrane and usually intense itching. Also called hives.
vesicle	a small abnormal elevation of the outer layer of skin enclosing a watery liquid; blister.
wheal	temporary, small, raised area of the skin usually accompanied by itching or burning.

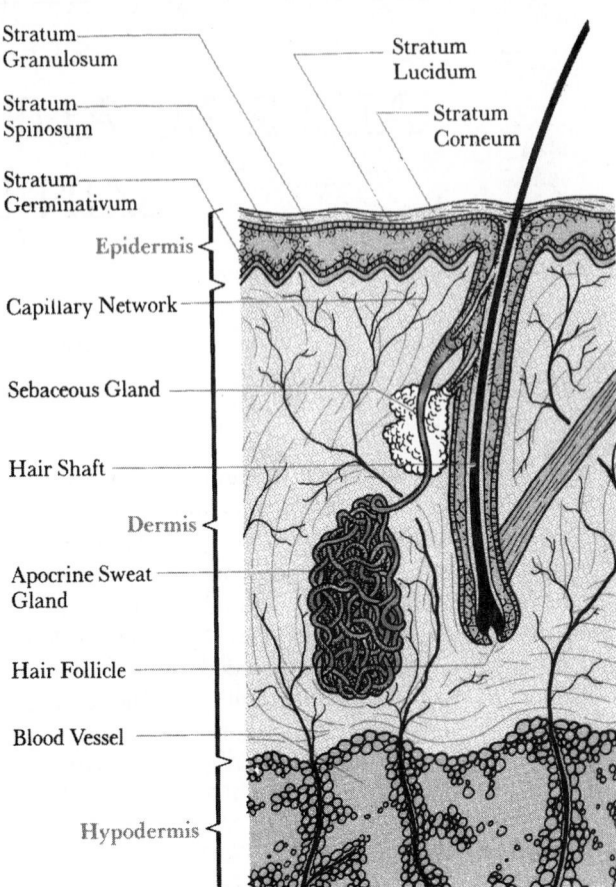

Figure 43.1. Cross-section of human skin. (Reprinted with permission from Handbook of Nonprescription Drugs. Washington D.C., American Pharmaceutical Association, 1990.)

tissues beneath to the dermis. Deeper hair follicles and sweat glands originate in the hypodermis (1, 2).

The skin confines underlying tissue and provides a barrier between the body and environment. It prevents harm from external agents such as ultraviolet radiation, pathogenic organisms, and chemicals. Various factors can alter the effectiveness of the barrier, including age, underlying disease states, use of medications (topical or systemic), and the integrity of the stratum corneum. Other skin functions involve sensation, temperature control, development of pigment, and synthesis of some vitamins. Moisture regulation is another important function (1).

Skin appendages are of two types: cornified and glandular (1, 2). Cornified appendages are hair and nails. Glandular appendages are the sebaceous glands and sweat glands, both eccrine and apocrine. Since these appendages are not usually involved in allergic and drug-induced disease, they will not be discussed further.

MECHANISMS

Although many of the conditions discussed in this chapter are believed to result from allergy, nonimmunologic

dermatoses, particularly where an allergic component is involved. Lymphocytes from the lymphoid group are common in inflammatory lesions of the skin (1, 2).

The hypodermis comprises relatively loose connective tissue. This layer provides pliability to the skin, and its thickness varies. In most areas, it contains a unit for formation and storage of fat. The fat layer functions in thermal control, food reserve, and cushioning. The hypodermis supports the blood vessels and nerves that pass from mechanisms also are postulated to play a role (3, 4). For example, contact dermatitis may be caused through immunologic mechanisms or result from direct irritant properties. The clinical presentation is essentially identical (4).

The basic immunologic mechanisms of allergic reactions include four types (5). Immediate or anaphylactic reactions (Type I) result from the production of IgE antibodies that attach to the surface of basophils or mast cells. With reexposure, the offending substance binds to the antibodies on the cell surface causing release of chemical mediators. These substances may include histamine, serotonin, peptides, leukotrienes, and prostaglandins (5, 6). The clinical effects seen are determined by the interaction of the mediators with the various target organs and may include pruritus, urticaria, bronchospasm, laryngeal edema, and hypotension.

Type II reactions result in antibody-dependent cytotoxicity. The offending substance interacts with surface components of a cell, thus making it appear foreign. Antibodies are produced that react with the cell-bound substance. The antigen–antibody reaction may trigger the complement system or permit attack by mononuclear killer cells resulting in cell death as with drug-induced hemolysis (5).

Type III reactions involve immune complexes. The antigen–antibody complex forms in blood or tissue spaces. IgG or IgM antibodies are usually involved (6). Inflammation or complement activation may result if these complexes deposit on blood vessel walls or basement membranes. Serum sickness and allergic arteritis are examples of Type III reactions (5).

Type IV reactions are termed cell mediated, delayed, or tuberculin type reactions. The offending substance interacts with skin proteins evoking a cell-mediated immune response. Sensitized T lymphocytes release lymphokines in response that cause local edema and inflammation (5).

Type I (immediate or anaphylactic reaction) and Type IV (cell-mediated reaction) are most commonly involved in allergic skin manifestations. In some cases, skin manifestations may occur from circulating immune complexes (Type III—serum sickness). Type II reactions (antibody-dependent cytotoxicity) are unlikely to produce cutaneous manifestations (5, 6). Some cases of drug-induced urticaria are an example of a Type I reaction, and allergic contact dermatitis is an example of a Type IV reaction.

The role of immunologic mechanisms in drug-associated rash is supported by certain clinical features described by Bigby (3). The reaction:

1. Occurs in a small percentage of patients
2. Is not dose dependent
3. (Onset of rash) occurs within 1 to 2 weeks after initiation of therapy

4. Is accompanied by other signs and symptoms (e.g., fever, pruritus, eosinophilia)
5. Resolves on withdrawal of agent and recurs if patient is rechallenged

The immunologic mechanisms involved will be discussed as well as identifying the role of nonimmunologic mechanisms for each condition.

ATOPIC DERMATITIS

Atopic dermatitis, frequently referred to as eczema, is a chronic pruritic skin disorder that occurs in individuals with a personal or family history of allergic diseases such as rhinitis, asthma, or conjunctivitis (7–10). The disorder occurs in infants, children, and adults. The prevalence is higher in children (3 to 4% in the 1960s compared to 10% in the 1990s) (9, 10). Estimated cumulative incidence is 10 to 15% in children up to 14 years of age, and the incidence seems to be increasing (9). Heredity plays a role with a possible inherited defect in some bone-marrow-derived cells (9).

Etiology

The exact cause of atopic dermatitis is unknown. Abnormalities in both immunologic and pharmacophysiologic characteristics occur (7, 8). Several factors support the involvement of immunologic functions: (1) the frequent association of atopic dermatitis with other allergic disorders; (2) substantial elevations of serum IgE; (3) positive wheal and flare reactions to a wide variety of scratch tests; (4) increased susceptibility to viral and fungal infections; and (5) association with immunodeficiency disorders. Pharmacophysiologic abnormalities include evidence of altered adrenergic and cholinergic responses (7–9).

Pathogenesis

Immunologic mechanisms receive the most investigation, but the primary event that initiates the reaction is yet to be identified (7–10). Abnormalities of both humoral and cell-mediated immunity are present. Two of the most important immunologic alterations identified are an impairment of the delayed hypersensitivity response and an increased production of IgE. Identification of cytokines (interferons and interleukins) has allowed further delineation of possible mechanisms. For example, evidence indicates that the mononuclear leukocytes in patients with atopic dermatitis produce lower levels of interferon gamma (IFN-γ) and higher levels of interleukin-4 (IL-4). IFN-γ mediates delayed hypersensitivity reactions, and IL-4 stimulates IgE synthesis (8). IgE apparently is stimulated by specific antigens, attaches to mast cells, and triggers release of mast cell inflammatory mediators (including histamine), which are released on reexposure to the antigens (7). Other factors, however, must play a role since atopic dermatitis occurs in patients with a deficiency of immunoglobulins (e.g., agammaglobulinemia or Weskott–Aldrich syndrome).

Evidence of cell-mediated factors relates to susceptibility and recurrence of viral infections, including herpes simplex, molluscum contagiosum, and warts (7–9). Patients are frequently resistant to sensitization to poison ivy and dinitrochlorobenzene (DNCB) (9). The demonstration of decreased numbers of T lymphocytes may indicate lack of sufficient T cells to control B cell production of immunoglobulin; thus, high levels of IgE are produced (7, 8). Furthermore, phagocytic capacity is decreased, and chemotaxis of neutrophils and monocytes is impaired (7, 9).

Another factor supporting an immunologic basis is the demonstration of significant numbers of Staphylococcus aureus bacteria on both the diseased and normal skin of atopic patients (8, 9). Exacerbations of eczema have developed secondary to Staph aureus skin infections (9).

Pharmacophysiologic responses in atopic patients involve a number of abnormal cutaneous responses. Exaggerated constrictor response of cutaneous vessels, white dermographism (white line is produced when skin is stroked), delayed blanch to cholinergic stimuli, and paradoxical response to application of nicotinic acid are examples (9). A defect in the beta adrenergic receptor was once theorized when it was demonstrated that cyclic AMP responses in atopic patients were subnormal to isoproterenol, prostaglandin E_1, and histamine agents that would normally activate cyclic AMP (7–9). Decreased cyclic AMP levels have accentuated release of inflammatory mediators from mast cells and basophils (7). Evidence suggests cyclic AMP phosphodiesterase activity (responsible for degradation of cyclic AMP) is increased, accounting for cyclic AMP-diminished responsiveness on challenge. This enzymatic abnormality might be a primary defect in patients with atopic dermatitis and does not depend on the beta receptor. Chan and Hanifen have reviewed the extensive work in this area, but further study is necessary to unravel the puzzle of atopic dermatitis (8).

Diagnosis and Clinical Findings

The diagnostic hallmark is pruritis often accompanied by erythema and dry skin. The cutaneous features vary greatly depending on age and chronicity of disease. Environmental factors termed flare factors, which may induce or exacerbate atopic dermatitis, are listed in Table 43.2. Laboratory tests and histologic analysis of biopsy do not provide confirmatory information. IgE levels may be helpful (7, 8). Conditions that should be considered in the differential diagnosis include seborrheic dermatitis, contact dermatitis, nummular dermatitis, scabies, and psoriasis (7).

Atopic dermatitis is divided into three stages based on age: infantile, childhood, and adolescent/adult. In infants, atopic dermatitis is most likely to occur around 3 months

Table 43.2.
Flare Factors in Atopic Dermatitis

Dry skin (xerosis)
Sweating
Exercise
Infection
Anxiety
Scratching
Light touch
Prickly clothes (wool and acrylic)
Heat
Cold
Temperature change
Allergic contact dermatitis
Allergies to foods or inhalants
Coexisting diseases (e.g., scabies)
Greasy ointments

of age. It frequently coincides with the introduction of foods that have been blamed for its occurrence. However, a causal relationship is not well established (7, 10).

The eruption generally begins as erythematous patches on the cheeks and spreads to the extensor surfaces of the extremities. The diaper area is usually spared. Intense itching is evident since the infant scratches constantly and rubs against garments and bedding. Many infantile cases clear over a period of months to years. Some cases continue into the childhood stage or may recur years after resolution of the infantile form.

In the childhood stage, the flexor surfaces are usually involved rather than extensor areas. The eruption is usually either lichenoid, consisting of small, discrete, brown or red-brown papules, or papular, consisting of larger papules with a central crust. Such lesions tend to be chronic, may disappear around the age of 10 to 12, or may continue into adolescence (7, 9).

In the adolescent/adult phase, papules tend to become confluent, forming large lichenified areas. Crusts result from scratching due to intense itching. The lichenoid plaques are poorly marginated and vary in color from bright pink-red to brown or gray-brown. Areas commonly involved are the neck, eyelids, forehead/scalp, anterior chest, and wrists. Dorsal areas of the fingers, toes, and feet may be affected as well (7).

The course of atopic dermatitis is quite variable and generally is marked by remissions and exacerbations (7, 9). Most cases begin in infancy, but onset may not occur until childhood or after puberty. Reported frequency of persistence varies widely, from 10 to 83% (9). Part of the variability can be explained by the imprecise diagnostic criteria available. Some factors that suggest an unfavorable prognosis are severe, widespread dermatitis in childhood, family history of atopic disease, presence of allergic rhinitis and/or asthma, female sex, and early age of onset (less than 1 year of age) (9).

Treatment

Strategies involve a variety of nondrug and drug treatment measures depending on the acuteness or chronicity of the condition. The most common measures include environmental change, skin maintenance care techniques, use of topical corticosteroids, systemic antihistamines, topical or systemic antibiotics, and, selectively, systemic corticosteroids.

Where environmental factors are identified as contributory, avoidance is advised. This might include avoiding extremes of temperature and humidity, strenuous exercise, rough scratchy clothing, bathing with harsh soaps and hot water, irritant chemicals, and allergens (7, 8). These factors and others can precipitate or perpetuate the itch–scratch cycle. Stress, anger, or anxiety may contribute to exacerbations of atopic dermatitis in some patients.

Dry skin and itch are the two problems that are addressed in managing atopic dermatitis. The stratum corneum is inadequately hydrated, and attempts at rehydration can use either a "lubricating" method or a "dry" method. Many patients find relief from the application of greasy ointments such as petrolatum, whereas others find that such substances worsen their condition (7). Various types of topical therapy are described next.

Topical Therapy. Several forms of topical therapy are available. Patients with mild or localized atopic dermatitis may require treatment only with a topical corticosteroid ointment or cream. For patients with extensive disease, a combination of topical measures may be necessary.

Baths. Itching can be relieved at least temporarily by tepid baths containing oatmeal (Aveeno, plain or oilated), bath oils, or tar preparations. Bathing assists with rehydration of the skin but should not be frequent. Strong soaps should be avoided although mild soaps can be used. A lubricating lotion (Cetaphil, Lubriderm, or Nutraderm) can be used instead of soap. To aid dry skin, soaking in lukewarm water then applying of a water-in-oil emulsion (e.g., Eucerin) while the skin is still wet assists in rehydrating the keratin layers (10, 11).

Wet Dressings. When lesions are oozing, acute, and possibly infected, use of wet dressings such as Burow's solution 1 : 20 or tap water are appropriate. Compresses are applied generally for 20 to 60 minutes three to six times a day. The dressings cool and dry by evaporation, thus stimulating vasoconstriction. In very acute situations, compresses can be applied continuously (7).

Topical Corticosteroids. These agents are effective in treating many cases of atopic dermatitis. In an acute phase, high-potency topical steroids can be used for 7 to 10 days. Therapy should then be switched to less potent products for up to several more weeks (10, 11). Patients with severe conditions may require chronic use along with lubricants. Nonfluorinated (hydrocortisone 1% or desonide 0.05%) or low-potency fluorinated preparations (triamcinolone

0.025%) are preferred for long-term use (7, 10, 11). Use of fluorinated corticosteroids should be minimized by application only during acute flares, only to the most problematic areas, or once daily or on alternate days (7). Long-term use of fluorinated corticosteroids, particularly high-potency agents, causes thinning of the skin and can lead to atrophy and telangiectasia, particularly on the face and skinfold areas (groin, armpits) (7, 10).

Topical Antibacterial Agents. Secondary infection frequently due to Staphylococcus aureus can be treated with topical antibiotics if the skin involvement is somewhat limited (7, 10, 11). Preparations containing erythromycin or bacitracin are preferred because of less sensitization than with agents such as neomycin (7). Mupirocin is another agent shown effective, but the relative cost of various agents should be evaluated.

Wet and dry methods have been suggested that combine some of the topical approaches (7). The wet, or lubricating, method includes the following: short baths or showers in tepid water (hot water stimulates pruritis). Mild soaps can be used but sparingly. Following bathing, the skin is lubricated while still wet to help hold water in the stratum corneum. Bath oil, petrolatum, hydrophilic ointment, or topical corticosteroids may be used (10).

The dry method uses either short showers in tepid water or short baths with oilated oatmeal. Bathing with soap and water is not allowed except for use of a moist cloth to cleanse the arms, groin, and axillae. A nonlipid cleanser is applied to the skin surface twice a day and gently wiped off. Oily or greasy lubricants are not used. Topical corticosteroids can be applied using products that are in a water/propylene glycol emollient base (Synalar solution) (7). Obviously with either method, a great deal of patient effort and cooperation is necessary.

SYSTEMIC THERAPY

Agents such as antihistamines, corticosteroids, and antibiotics may be useful under certain circumstances. Two possible benefits from oral administration of antihistamines include relief of pruritis and sedation. Histamine plays some role in atopic dermatitis but probably is not the only mediator involved in pruritis (1). Mixed opinions exist on the benefits of antihistamines in relieving pruritis (7, 10, 11, 12). Studies show conflicting results and often suffer from insufficient numbers of patients (12). Use of antihistamines may relieve pruritis in some patients (7, 12), at least initially (11), but sedation is seen as the primary benefit by some investigators (11, 13). If sedation is the desired goal, then patients should benefit more from the traditional H_1-blockers rather than the newer, less sedating antihistamines (13).

Oral corticosteroids may be used for acute flares to break the itch–scratch cycle (7, 10, 11). Duration of use should be short term in the range of 5 to 7 days. Oral corticosteroid therapy generally is discouraged except in the case of very refractory episodes (7).

Systemic antibiotic therapy may be indicated to treat secondary bacterial infections (e.g., folliculitis) that can develop (7, 10, 11). Therapy is directed toward Gram-positive cocci, particularly Staph aureus. A 7-day course of an antistaphylococcal agent (e.g., dicloxacillin, erythromycin, or cephalexin) often is used (7, 10).

Many patients with atopic dermatitis continue to suffer and may be told by their dermatologists that little more can be done. In patients who are suffering despite "state-of-the-art" therapies, the first step is to break the cycle of scratching. To help achieve this goal, one approach is a major intervention of a "simulated hospitalization" (14). That is, the patient is required to stop the usual routine of school or work, have complete bed rest in a semidarkened room for a few days (e.g., Friday P.M. to Monday A.M.), given light sedation, and a short course (1 week or less) of an oral corticosteroid to reduce inflammation. In addition, if the patient has folliculitis, a course of antibiotics is given.

After this intense few days of therapy to break the cycle of scratching, the major challenge is to keep the skin clear by eliminating the urge to scratch. If the worst scratching is during sleep, a higher dose of a sedating antihistamine may be adequate. For instance, if diphenhydramine 25 mg is not adequate, try 50 mg, or if hydroxyzine 25 mg is not adequate, try 50 mg or higher if needed. If sedating antihistamines are not sufficient, other sedating therapies may be considered for a few days or weeks in the most severe cases where quality of life is being affected to a great degree.

Concurrently with a major intervention with medication, another critically important step should be initiated. That intervention involves dealing with the psychology of atopic dermatitis. Details regarding the techniques used to stop scratching are beyond the scope of this chapter. Some options reported (14, 15) are as follows:

- Habit reversal (scratching can become a habit)
- Behavioral and cognitive interventions
- Relaxation training
- Learning to express anger and to be assertive

Clearly, emotional stress is a major trigger to scratching in some patients with atopic dermatitis. In children, hostility from a parent or discord between parents can trigger the itch–scratch cycle. Dealing with these factors can obviously be very helpful.

Some patients will remain refractory to these treatments and their various combinations. Other therapies being evaluated in atopic dermatitis include phototherapy with ultraviolet (UV) radiation and agents affecting the immune system (e.g., cyclosporin, thymopentin, interferon gamma) (10, 11, 16).

Both pruritis and inflammation may be aided by phototherapy with ultraviolet light in all wave lengths

(bands A and B) (10, 11, 16). Studies have shown benefit with UVA, UVB, and PUVA (oral psoralen plus UVA radiation), but potential risks with long-term use include accelerated photoaging and increased risk of skin cancer (10). This therapy may be best used short term during periods of severe dermatitis.

Oral cyclosporin in doses of 2.5 to 5.0 mg/kg per day has provided benefit to patients with atopic dermatitis, but long-term safety and efficacy remains to be established (10, 16). Cooper (16) has reviewed other agents affecting the immune system, including thymopentin and interferon gamma, which show promise in treating atopic dermatitis.

CONTACT DERMATITIS

Contact dermatitis is an inflammatory response of the skin and is divided into two categories based on origin: allergic contact dermatitis and irritant contact dermatitis. Allergic contact dermatitis is a delayed hypersensitivity reaction with an immunologic basis, whereas irritant contact dermatitis results from a substance that has a toxic effect on tissue with no immunologic basis (4, 17).

The occurrence of contact dermatitis is widespread partly because of the wide variety of substances implicated as causes (see Table 43.3). The prevalence within the general population is not well documented. Some studies have attempted to determine prevalence of allergy to

Table 43.3.
Common Causes of Contact Dermatitis

Pharmaceutical Agents	Rubber Materials
Corticosteroids	Gloves
Neomycin	Finger protectors
"Caine" anesthetics	**Hobby Materials**
Merbromin	Epoxy glues
Thimerosal	Paints
Transdermal patches	Solvents
Lubricants	**Occupational Contactants**
Lotions	Chrome
Hand creams	Epoxy glues
Face creams	Other glues
Bath oils	Formaldehyde
Cosmetics and Fragrances	Nickel
Deodorants	Cobalt
Hair dyes	Solvents
Make-up	Resins
Perfumes	Dyes
Surfactants	Oils and greases
Hand, bath and shower soaps	Solvents and waterless
Soaps used at work	cleaners
Kitchen and laundry soaps	**Metals**
Waterless cleaners	Jewelry
	Plants
	Poison oak or ivy
	Algerian ivy
	Chrysanthemums
	House plants

Adapted from (17, 18, 19).

specific substances in the normal population, and positive patch tests have occurred in the following percentages: nickel (5.8%), neomycin (1.1%), ethylenediamine (0.43%), and benzocaine (0.17%) (18). Gender differences are observed regarding specific allergies. For example, nickel allergy is more frequent in women than in men, but this likely is explained by a higher rate of contact through jewelry and clothing (18). Irritant contact dermatitis is considered more common than allergic contact dermatitis, particularly in the industrial setting (10, 18, 19).

Etiology

Causes of allergic contact dermatitis are varied and commonly include plants, rubber compounds, preservatives, and fragrances (17). Soaps, detergents, petrolatum solvents, acids, and alkalis are frequent offenders in irritant contact dermatitis. Often the dermatitis is related to occupational exposure (19). The origin, allergic or irritant, usually cannot be differentiated by the clinical presentation (4, 19, 20). Irritants may also be allergens (18).

Pathogenesis

In allergic contact dermatitis, certain physiologic events must occur, including (4):

1. Penetration of the stratum corneum by the allergen
2. Interaction with epidermal or dermal cells
3. Interaction with the immune system
4. The inflammatory response

The development of contact hypersensitivity involves combination of the chemical (hapten) and skin protein to form an antigen. The antigen is carried to the regional lymph nodes by epidermal Langerhans cells and probably interacts at these sites to produce specifically sensitized T cells (17, 18). In addition, secretion of interleukin-1 by macrophages is required to initiate the response. Interleukin-1, which enhances many types of immunologic responses, is also produced by epidermal keratinocytes and Langerhans cells. Helper T cells then differentiate into effector cells that release lymphokines producing local inflammation (17). A period of 8 to 10 days is generally required for allergy presentation once sensitization has begun (18).

The histopathologic features include perivascular infiltrates of lymphocytes and monocytes in the upper dermis. Edema is usually present and may involve intracellular and intercellular edema in the epidermis with a condition called spongiosis. Basophils and mast cells are present in the cellular infiltrate that occurs and may participate in the inflammatory reaction. Chronically, hyperkeratosis, acanthosis, and a cellular infiltrate in the superficial dermis containing basophils are present (17).

Patients may report no problem associated with the previous handling of a material sometimes for prolonged periods (years). The latest exposure termed the elicitation dose results in an eruption (20). An earlier exposure resulted in the initial sensitization. Generally, a latent period can be identified.

In the case of irritant contact dermatitis, direct cellular damage occurs with no latent period. Damage is proportional to the toxic properties of the irritant but may depend on repeated exposure for some substances that are mild irritants. With irritant contact dermatitis, those exposed to the same dose under the same conditions for the same length of time would be expected to react. Reduction of the irritant dose (exposure) often has a good prognosis (19).

Diagnosis and Clinical Findings

Contact dermatitis is classified as acute, subacute, or chronic (10, 18). Acute contact dermatitis involves erythema, edema, and formation of papules and vesicles and bullae. The subacute form presents with erythema, tiny superficial vesicles, and less severe symptomatology. In chronic forms, the skin may be cracked and scaly with excoriations and plaque formations (10, 20). Severe itching in the acute phase is prominent and may persist into the other phases. The history and physical examination can provide critical information to establish the diagnosis. An acute dermatitis of the extremities that is of a patchy and streaky nature, coupled with a recent history of outdoor plant exposure, might lead to a diagnosis of poison ivy or oak dermatitis. A dermatitis occurring on the eyelids or face of a woman might be associated with the use of cosmetics, perfumes, or hair sprays. A thorough history regarding general activities, occupation, hobbies, known allergies, previous skin disorders, and family history, along with careful examination of the distribution and extent of the lesions may suggest possible causes (10). A listing of common causes of contact dermatitis is provided in Table 43.3, and the substances most likely involved with reactions in certain body areas are indicated in Table 43.4. In many patients, the diagnosis remains unclear, and the use of patch testing may be indicated, particularly in conditions that become chronic or relatively resistant to treatment or that are suspected to be occupationally related.

Patch testing may assist in diagnosis of delayed hypersensitivity contact dermatitis. Standardized methods and concentrations for testing for a variety of substances have been recommended (18). Even with standardized approaches, both false positive and false negative reactions may occur (19, 20). For example, an irritant reaction may be difficult to differentiate from a weak allergic reaction.

Treatment

Successful treatment requires the identification and/or removal of the allergen (irritant). This may be accom-

Table 43.4.
Causes of Contact Dermatitis by Body Region

Scalp:	Hair dyes (paraphenylenediamine, a permanent dye), hair lotions, permanents (glyceryl thioglycolate), nickel in hair pins, wig attachments and adhesives
Face:	Cosmetics, topical medicaments, plants, preshave and aftershave lotions, airborne allergens
Forehead:	Hatbands, any hair products
Eyes:	Eyelids affected by cosmetics, face creams, lubricants, hair spray, nail polish. Conjunctivitis: thimerosal
Lips and perioral areas:	Lipstck, lip protectants, toothpastes, mouthwashes, mangos
Ears:	Nickel (earrings), perfume, earplugs, earphones, telephone receiver
Neck:	Perfume, nickel (necklace), hair cosmetics, clothing; clothing labels, buttons and zippers
Armpits:	Deodorants, depilatories, clothing, perfumes
Hands:	Materials encountered at work and/or home (e.g., foods, chemicals, topical medicaments, hand lotions and lubricants, rubber gloves, rubber bands, jewelry, plants)
Body (trunk, chest, waist):	Dyes, formaldehyde (fabric finisher), resins, rubber in elastic of clothing, perfumes, scarves
Genitalia:	Bubble bath, antiseptic cleansers, condoms, contraceptive creams or jellies, deodorant douches, scented menstrual pads or tampons
Feet:	Shoes, shower sandals, fabrics, metal eye holes, sole inserts, adhesives, colorants, athlete's foot remedies

Adapted from (18, 20).

plished more easily in the case of poison ivy dermatitis than in the case of dermatitis due to industrial exposure.

Specific drug therapy depends more on the stage and the extent of the dermatitis than on the cause (18). Severe, acute reactions characterized by blistering, swelling, and oozing may require systemic corticosteroids. Various regimens are recommended (10, 18, 20). An initial dose of 60 mg is common (40 to 100 mg) with treatment recommended for periods of 7 to 14 days. Most authors recommend tapering the dose during the treatment period. Specific doses and duration of treatment are probably best determined by the presentation of the patient. Topical corticosteroids are of little benefit in acute edematous blistering dermatitis because of inadequate penetration. Soothing compresses or baths with water, aluminum acetate, or saline may be beneficial in providing relief at this stage (10, 18). Topical steroid therapy once or twice a day can be instituted once the acute symptoms are controlled and continued after oral therapy is stopped. Ointments are usually preferred because cream preparations have a greater variety of ingredients, including fragrances and preservatives, to which the patients may be allergic (20). Oral antihistamines provide little if any benefit other than sedating properties since they do not suppress contact allergy (10, 18). Calamine and other shake lotions, topical antihistamines, and topical anesthetics are best avoided because of lack of benefit and/or potential sensitization (10, 18).

For subacute (moderate) or chronic dermatitis, topical corticosteroid therapy is used rather than systemic therapy. A high-potency agent may be applied twice daily in subacute conditions. Often the skin may be dry so that ointment or cream preparations of corticosteroids are preferred over solutions. Compresses and soaks are usually not indicated, and other lotions (e.g., Calamine) should be avoided because of a drying effect. In chronic situations, low-, medium-, or high-potency corticosteroid preparations are selected based on the degree of skin thickening (lichenification). Overnight occlusion with plastic enhances penetration of the steroid. Caution should be exercised with high-potency agents because of the potential problem mentioned previously, particularly on the face and in skinfold areas. Lubrication generally is needed with frequent application in a thin layer. White petrolatum is a good choice. If secondary infection is present, systemic antibiotic therapy is usually preferred (17).

URTICARIA

Urticaria and angioedema are edematous vascular reactions of the skin (10, 21). Another name for urticaria is hives. When edema extends into the dermis and hypodermis, it is termed angioedema. Urticaria is estimated to occur in about 15% of the population at some time in life with women more frequently afflicted. All age groups can be affected with peak incidence in the second through fourth decades of life (10). Urticaria and angioedema occur concurrently in almost half of the patients, another 40% experience only urticaria, and around 10% experience angioedema only (10). Most cases of urticaria are acute, but if the episodes continue for longer than 6 weeks, the urticaria is termed chronic (10).

Etiology

The etiology of urticaria is varied and often obscure. Urticaria may be associated with or caused by drugs, serums, foods, inhalants, insect bites/stings, contact substances, connective tissue diseases, neoplasms, infections, endocrine disorders, and physical agents (10, 21). The physical agents often include cold, heat, sunlight, pressure, and dermographism (10, 21). The urticaria may be linked to cholinergic or adrenergic factors (21, 22). With adrenergic urticaria, stress was a factor in the development of attacks and elevated plasma concentrations of norepinephrine, epinephrine, and dopamine in a reported case (22). Hereditary angioedema, characterized by recurrent, self-limited attacks, is transmitted by autosomal-dominant inheritance with incomplete penetrance (10). In addition to childhood onset and family history, a specific test for C1-esterase inhibitor, a complement component can be used to confirm the condition. A cause cannot be specifically identified in 70 to 80% of cases and thus the urticaria is termed idiopathic (10, 21).

Pathogenesis

Five pathophysiologic mechanisms have been proposed for urticaria and/or angioedema: IgE mediated, complement mediated, direct mast cell-releasing agents, alteration of arachidonic acid metabolism, and idiopathic (10). Skin biopsies of urticarial lesions show edema in the upper dermis, vascular dilation, and cellular infiltrates in the dermis around the small vessels due to leakage. The infiltrate is lymphocytic and in chronic urticaria comprises primarily T lymphocytes. Cutaneous mast cells are increased (10).

Histamine has been identified as a mediator in the urticarial response. The dermal mast cells produce and store histamine. When activated, the mast cells release histamine as well as other vasoactive substances, including kinins, leukotrienes, and prostaglandins. Kinins are vasoactive peptides, which may be an important factor in the development of urticaria. They slow smooth muscle contraction, cause vasodilation, and increase vascular permeability. Antibodies of the IgE class can interact with antigen on the mast cell surface producing histamine release. Complement-fixing antibodies can also react with antigens on the mast cell surface producing histamine release. Direct histamine release may be caused by certain drugs (e.g., radiocontrast media, opiates) and chemicals (10).

Diagnosis and Clinical Findings

A careful history that describes the pattern of attacks, precipitating cause, duration of wheals, associated symptoms, and atopic background should be taken. As a result, the presence or absence of the following can be established: relationship to any ingested, inhaled, or injected substance; a contact reaction; a systemic disease; a hormonal influence; an emotional cause; or an infection. Although the basic mechanism may still be unknown, these factors can serve as triggers. For example, half of the patients with idiopathic urticaria are made worse by aspirin or nonsteroidal antiinflammatory drugs. Thyroid disease, lymphoma, and systemic lupus erythematous (SLE) have all been linked with urticaria (10, 21).

The skin lesions are circumscribed, elevated, erythematous areas (wheals) of edema that are pruritic (10, 21, 23).

The size of the wheal can vary from 1 to 2 mm to many centimeters, and groups of lesions may be either localized or generalized. Individual lesions tend to resolve in 24 to 48 hours, but new lesions will appear (10). Some patients also develop angioedema that involves deeper dermal swelling but is not pruritic (21). Some patients may experience respiratory, gastrointestinal, or cardiovascular symptoms (23). Laboratory and skin testing is of limited value in establishing a diagnosis or cause (21).

Treatment

The best treatment is identification and removal of the cause. As indicated, in the large majority of cases, this approach is unsuccessful because either the cause cannot be identified or multiple factors are involved (10, 23). Treatment then is directed toward the effector cells and inflammatory mediators to either block release or effect. Therapy also may be directed toward receptor sites on target tissues, such as the cutaneous microvasculature and cells (23).

Antihistamines, which are H_1-receptor antagonists, provide relief in about 65 to 70% of patients with urticaria or angioedema (13, 21). They should be administered on a scheduled basis rather than as needed. Antihistamines are more effective in preventing the actions of histamine than in reversing the effects (10, 24). Other mediators are likely to be involved in patients not responding. Of the available H_1 antagonists, they would be expected to be nearly equal in efficacy. Choice can be based on side effects (e.g., is sedation desirable or undesirable) or pharmacokinetic considerations (see the section "Antihistamines") (13, 23). If one agent is ineffective or not tolerated, a second agent from a different chemical group can be tried. On occasion, a combination of H_1-receptor antagonists can be used (e.g., a nonsedating agent during the day and a sedating agent at night) (13, 23). If treatment with H_1 antagonists is successful, the agent should be tapered to prevent flares (23).

H_2 receptor antagonists like cimetidine may be combined with H_1-receptor antagonists in treating urticaria (23–25). Administered alone, the H_2-receptor blockers have little if any demonstrated benefit. Several studies have claimed greater benefit with the combination, but this has not been a consistent observation (25). The H_2 receptor antagonists may be useful only in certain types of urticaria (e.g., cold, dermographism) and angioedema (25). If a case is refractory, a trial of the combination may be appropriate (13). Doses of cimetidine have ranged from 400 to 1600 mg per day. Ranitidine has been used in standard oral doses (24).

Other potential treatments include tricyclic antidepressants (e.g., doxepin), beta-adrenergic agonists (e.g., terbutaline), and calcium channel blockers (e.g., nifedipine) (23–25). Patients with chronic idiopathic urticaria have benefited from these treatments, but studies with these agents are limited. Use of these alternative therapies should be limited to refractory cases until further data are available.

Drug-Induced Skin Diseases

Cutaneous reactions to drugs result from immunologic or nonimmunologic mechanisms. Immunologic mechanisms require activation of host pathways, and their presence is supported by the clinical features identified by Bigby, which were noted earlier (3, 6). Cutaneous reactions caused by nonimmunologic mechanisms are more common than allergic reactions (6). Nonimmunologic mechanisms associated with cutaneous drug reactions include activation of effector pathways, overdosage, cumulative toxicity, side effects, drug interactions, metabolic changes, and exacerbation of existing dermatologic conditions (6). The most relevant of these, the activation of effector pathways, is not antibody dependent and actually involves at least three different mechanisms. The first involves direct release of mediators from mast cells with presentation as urticaria or angioedema. Drugs implicated in this mechanism are opiates, polymyxin B, and radiographic contrast media. Radiographic contrast media also have activated complement in the absence of antibody, again resulting in urticaria. The third mechanism involves alteration of arachidonic acid metabolism, the most notable example being anaphylacticlike responses to aspirin and nonsteroidal antiinflammatory drugs. The other nonimmunologic mechanisms for the most part produce other skin manifestations that are not the focus of this discussion (e.g., bruising with excess warfarin, color changes due to phenothiazines) (6). Drug-induced skin diseases present through a variety of clinical manifestations, as indicated in Table 43.5. Each of these will be reviewed briefly regarding clinical presentation, diagnostic considerations, and time course.

DRUG EXANTHEM

Drug exanthem is the most common cutaneous reaction, composing almost half of the skin reactions due to drugs (5). It is usually described as a morbilliform or maculopapular eruption, often generalized, but starting usually on the trunk or in areas where pressure and/or trauma occur.

Table 43.5.
Dermatologic Manifestations of Drug-Induced Disease

Exanthematous rashes
Urticaria/angioedema
Fixed drug eruption
Erythema multiforme
Exfoliative dermatitis
Photosensitivity (toxicity and allergy)
Toxic epidermal necrolysis
Vasculitis

The rash is frequently pruritic and symmetric, and consists of erythematous macules and papules that may become confluent (3, 6). Fever and eosinophilia may be present. A drug-induced exanthem must be differentiated from exanthems of viral origin although this is difficult since definitive diagnostic tests are lacking. Occurrence usually is within the first week of starting therapy with the offending agent, frequently within the first 3 days. Some antibiotics and allopurinol are considered exceptions. For penicillin, cephalosporins, and cotrimoxazole, exanthems may appear within the first 2 weeks or sometimes later or even after therapy is stopped. With allopurinol, rashes can occur for 3 weeks or more. Most exanthems can be expected to disappear within 1 to 2 weeks after discontinuing the offending agent.

Some characteristics contribute to a higher risk of drug exanthem. Women have a 35 to 50% higher risk than men. Although estimates have varied from as much as 50 to 100%, clearly a high percentage of patients with infectious mononucleosis taking ampicillin (amoxicillin is also implicated) experience a rash (3, 26). The combination of ampicillin and allopurinol produces a higher frequency of rashes than with either agent alone. Patients with acquired immunodeficiency disease (AIDs) taking cotrimoxazole experience more drug exanthems (3, 26).

URTICARIA

Urticaria is responsible for about one-quarter of drug-induced skin reactions, is described as pruritic, red wheals or as firm erythematous, round, or oval plaques of varying sizes. The epidermis overlying appears normal, and no scaling is evident. A lesion generally is present for less than 24 hours but is replaced by new lesions at other sites. Edema of the reticular dermis is a prominent pathologic feature. The term *angioedema* is used to indicate swelling in deep dermal and subcutaneous tissues often with mucous membrane involvement (3, 6).

If the reaction is IgE dependent, onset can be within minutes but is usually within 36 hours. Other systemic signs and symptoms of the immediate-type hypersensitivity may occur, including bronchospasm, diaphoresis, hypotension, and eosinophilia. A classic example is urticaria associated with an anaphylactic reaction to penicillin. Urticaria as a component of a serum sickness reaction will occur 4 to 12 days after challenge and will include systemic symptoms such as fever, arthralgias, hematuria, and possibly liver or neurologic symptoms. In some cases, the urticaria results from nonimmunologic mechanisms, but it is difficult to differentiate because the time course and presentation resemble the immediate hypersensitivity reaction (3, 6). This reaction is termed pseudoallergic (3).

Discontinuation of the offending agent, if recognized, often results in prompt resolution although some cases may persist for several weeks after presentation (3).

FIXED DRUG ERUPTION

Fixed drug eruption is responsible for about 10% of drug-induced skin disorders. It involves the development of a lesion, often solitary, that appears as erythematous macule and subsequently becomes an edematous plaque (3, 6, 27). Vesicles and bullae with desquamation may occur later (3, 27). After resolution of these acute phases, hyperpigmentation remains with colors varying from brown to violet-brown or even black (27). Lesions most often occur on the face, lip, facial region, and genitalia. Pruritus and burning may accompany the reaction, and their severity reflects the intensity of the inflammatory response.

Also rare, systemic symptoms may range from malaise to severe prostration (27). As the name implies, lesions recur in the same place, with rechallenge by the offending substance. Symptoms recur usually between ½ hour and 8 hours on reexposure. With repeated exposure, the number of lesions may gradually increase. Drugs most often implicated are phenolphthalein (used in over-the-counter laxatives), tetracycline, and oxyphenbutazone (27, 28).

ERYTHEMA MULTIFORME

Erythema multiforme is usually considered an acute, self-limited inflammatory disorder involving skin and mucous membranes although the spectrum can vary widely (3, 6). A prodrome, consisting of malaise, sore throat, and possibly fever with skin lesions developing over 2 to 7 days, may occur. Lesions have a distinctive iris or target appearance and are erythematous plaques with dusky centers with a surrounding ring of edema and a darker erythematous outer border. The plaques are most perfuse peripherally and develop in groups over a period of a few days, fading after 1 to 2 weeks. Sites most commonly involved are the backs of the hands, palms, wrists, forearms, feet, elbows, and knees. Bullous or vesicular lesions accompanied by mucosal involvement and systemic symptoms is termed Stevens–Johnson syndrome. Usually, two or more mucosal surfaces are involved (3, 28).

TOXIC EPIDERMAL NECROLYSIS (TEN)

Toxic epidermal necrolysis, though uncommon, is a serious skin disorder with significant morbidity and mortality. It is somewhat similar to erythema multiforme but is more acute and catastrophic. A brief prodrome of sore throat, malaise, fever, and chills occurs with skin involvement within 24 hours. Lesions are small, dusky, necrotic macules with early and extensive involvement of periorificial areas and mucous membranes. The lesions progressively enlarge to produce large confluent areas of necrosis with extensive epidermal sloughing within 2 to 5 days. Patients are quite ill with mortality ranging from 15 to 60% in reported series (3).

Staphylococcal scaled skin syndrome (SSSS), which usually occurs in children or immunocompromised patients, must be considered in the differential diagnosis. Some differentiating factors for SSSS are that epidermal separation is superficial (e.g., intraepidermal, usually the granular layer), periorificial and mucous membrane involvement is absent or mild, and skin pain is absent. Drug-induced TEN generally involves subepidermal separation (3, 28).

Drugs are the most common cause, particularly in adults. Nonsteroidal antiinflammatory agents, particularly the butazolodins, sulindac and piroxicam, sulfonamides (cotrimoxazole), phenytoin, barbiturates, and allopurinol, are frequently implicated drugs (6, 28). With allopurinol, TEN with concomitant renal/hepatic failure often involves patients with renal insufficiency receiving normal doses. Allopurinol doses should be reduced in patients with renal insufficiency to avoid this reaction (29).

EXFOLIATIVE DERMATITIS

Exfoliative dermatitis involves redness of the entire skin with widespread scaling due to exfoliation. Other than in cases of psoriasis, the condition is eczematous. Severe systemic symptoms may accompany and involve hypovolemia, heart failure, intestinal malabsorption, hypoprothrombinemia, and hypothermia (28). Some drugs reported to cause this reaction include gold, carbamazepine, phenytoin, and captopril (28).

PHOTOSENSITIVITY

Photosensitivity consists of two types: photoallergy and phototoxicity. Most reactions fall into the category of phototoxicity, with photoallergy being uncommon (6, 28). Phototoxic reactions can occur with the first exposure to a drug even within a few hours and are dose related. The reaction resembles sunburn and can in some cases progress to blister (6, 28). Removal of the offending agent usually brings resolution. Such reactions will occur in most patients given adequate amounts of drug and adequate exposure to ultraviolet (UV) light. Chlorpromazine, amiodarone, and doxycycline are examples of drugs implicated in this type of reaction.

Photoallergy involves the combination of the drug, immune system, and light. A delayed hypersensitivity reaction is suspected since the onset is usually delayed and recovery is slow. Such reactions occur in only a small percentage of exposed patients (3). The rash is usually eczematous but may involve lichenoid, urticarial, bullous, or purpuric lesions. The reaction typically occurs in sun-exposed areas but in severe cases may involve areas that are normally protected. Photoallergic reactions may persist for some time after the drug is withdrawn. Drugs that may cause photoallergic reactions are tetracyclines, thiazide diuretics, sulfonamides, phenothiazines, nalidixic acid, and antihistamines (3, 6, 28).

CUTANOUS VASCULITIS

Cutanous vasculitis commonly presents as palpable purpura and usually involves the lower extremities although the reaction may be generalized. Other organs such as the liver, kidney, joints, and gastrointestinal tract may become involved. The cutaneous lesions at various times may be macules, papules, urticarial lesions, and, in the most severe cases, hemorrhagic blisters. The origin of the reaction is thought to involve immune mechanisms, but the precise explanation is unknown (3, 6, 28). Drugs implicated in causing this reaction include sulfonamides, phenytoin, and phenylbutazone (3).

ANTIHISTAMINES

The antihistamines (H_1-receptor antagonists) traditionally have been grouped according to chemical structure: ethanolamines, ethylenediamines, alkylamines, piperazines, piperidines, and phenothiazines (30, 31). However, this classification generally provides little information regarding the expected pharmacodynamic and pharmacokinetic properties. A more useful classification involves the terminology of first-generation (classic) and second-generation (nonsedating) H_1-receptor antagonists. Comparison in this fashion more clearly distinguishes differences in pharmacodynamic properties. Each group can be examined for desirable pharmacokinetic properties (13, 30, 31). Table 43.6 summarizes many of the properties of the H_1-receptor antagonists, including some agents still under investigation.

H_1-receptor antagonists are reversible competitive inhibitors of the actions of histamine on H_1-receptors. The antihistamines block the bronchopulmonary and vasoactive effects of histamine, resulting in decreased vascular permeability, decreased pruritis, and relaxation of smooth muscle (30, 31). Although differences in potency exist, the antihistaminic activity of the various agents is considered similar when equipotent doses are given (31). This effect is demonstrated by suppression of the wheal–flare reactions induced by histamine or allergens. The duration of effect varies among agents (Table 43.6) (28, 30). In addition, second-generation agents also prevent release of inflammatory mediators from IgE-sensitized mast cells and basophils (30, 31). An effect on calcium either by inhibiting influx across the cell membrane or inhibiting intracellular release is probably responsible. These agents may inhibit

Table 43.6.
Anthistamine Activity and Pharmacokinetics

Generic Name (Trade Name)	Chemical Class	T max (h)	T½ (h)	Wheal/fare suppression (hr)	Sedative Activity #	Anticholinergic Activity #
1st Generation						
Azatadine (Optimine)	Piperidine	4	9–12	NF	++	++
Brompheniramine (Dimetane)	Alkylamine	3.1 ± 1.1	24.9 ± 9.3	3–9	+	++
Chlorpheniramine (Chlortrimeton)	Alkylamine	2.5–3.4	24.4	24	+	++
Clemastine (Tavist)	Ethanolamine	3–5	4–6	12–24	++	+++
Cyproheptadine (Periactin)	Piperidine	6–9	a	NF	+	++
Diphenydramine (Benadryl)	Ethanolamine	2–3	3–5	NF	+++	+++
Hydroxyzine (Atavas, Vistaril)	Piperazine	2.0	20.0	2–36	++	++
Promethazine (Phenergan)	Phenothiazine	2.7	12.2	NF	+++	+++
Triprolidine (Actidil)	Alkylamine	2.0	2.1	NF	+	++
Tripelennamine (PBZ)	Ethylenediamine	2–3	a	NF	++	±
2nd Generation						
Astemizole (Hismanal)	—	1–2	10 days	Weeks	±	±
Loratadine (Claritin)	—	1–2	11.0	24	±	±
Cetirizine[b] (Zyrtec)	Piperazine	0.5–1	7.4	24	±	±
Terfenadine (Seldane)	Butyrophenone	1–2	4.5	12–24	±	±

Abbreviations: +++ high, ++ moderate, + low, ± low to none, NF, not found.
[a]Metabolic and excretory fate not fully elucidated.
[b]Not available in the United States.
Adapted from (30, 31, 36, 37).

late phase allergic reactions by effects on leukotrienes or prostaglandins (31).

Classic H_1-receptor antagonists possess anticholinergic activity and produce a central nervous system (CNS) depressant effect. Although sedation is generally undesirable, in many patients with some type of skin disorder (e.g., atopic dermatitis), sedation can be helpful in reducing nocturnal scratching. These effects are clinically apparent at doses used therapeutically. In general, second-generation agents are devoid of clinically apparent anticholinergic activity or CNS effects at therapeutic doses. These agent penetrate poorly into the CNS, and levels are insufficient to block central H_1 or cholinergic receptors. Binding is preferential for peripheral H_1-receptors (13, 30, 31).

Pharmacokinetics

All the agents are generally well absorbed after oral administration with peak serum levels reached at around 2 hours (23, 30, 32). Most agents undergo metabolism through the cytochrome P_{450} system in the liver with clearance and elimination half-lives varying substantially. Active metabolites are formed for some agents like terfenadine and astemizole. The duration of wheal–flare suppression is related to both dose and the serum elimination half-life. Children usually exhibit shorter half-lives than adults (e.g., chlorpheniramine's half-life is a mean of about 11 hours in children compared to about 24 hours in adults, and hydroxyzine's half-life is about 7 hours in children compared to 20 hours in adults). Serum half-lives are expected to be prolonged in elderly patients and those with liver disease (30).

The pharmacokinetic profile of astemizole differs considerably from other agents (30, 31). Astemizole and the primary active metabolite, desmethylastemizole, have a half-life of approximately 9 to 10 days after a single dose (31, 33). With once-daily administration of 10 mg, steady-state levels are achieved after 4 to 6 weeks of administration (31, 33). After continued administration, the half-life for astemizole and its metabolites is 18 to 20 days (31). Inhibition of the wheal–flare response may not be apparent until the second day of administration or later. Initially, use of a loading dose (30 mg) was recommended to decrease the time to onset of effect, but this is no longer recommended. Suppression of the wheal–flare response may be seen for weeks to months compared to a duration of 24 hours or less for most other agents (31, 33).

Adverse Effects and Drug Interactions

The adverse effect profile of first-generation agents includes CNS and anticholinergic effects. The primary effects due to CNS depression include sedation, impaired cognitive function, diminished alertness, difficulty in concentrating, confusion, dizziness, and tinnitus (30, 31). Sedation or drowsiness occurs in 10 to 25% of antihista-

mine users. These effects may result in impaired performance, as reviewed by Meltzer (34). Some first-generation agents, like diphenhydramine, also cause dystonic reactions (30, 34). The common anticholinergic effects include dry mouth, blurred vision, and urinary retention. Some first-generation agents, like tripelennamine, cause gastrointestinal symptoms, including nausea, vomiting, epigastric distress, diarrhea, or constipation (30).

The second-generation agents generally are devoid of sedative and anticholinergic effects. The incidence of sedation is similar to that seen with placebo (30). In some of the skin diseases discussed, sedation may be a desired property and the only benefit in the opinions of some experts.

Drug interactions would be expected with the first-generation agents and other agents that have CNS depressant effects (alcohol, hypnotics, antianxiety agents, antipsychotics, analgesics) or anticholinergic activity (antispasmodics, tricyclic antidepressants, antipsychotics, antiparkinson drugs) (13). These interactions do not occur with second-generation agents.

Since the marketing of second-generation agents, cardiovascular toxicity has become a concern with terfenadine and astemizole (35). Both agents have been associated with the rare occurrence of the ventricular arrhythmia, torsades de pointes (TDP). A prolonged QT interval on electrocardiogram often precedes TDP, which apparently results from abnormal cardiac repolarization. A prolonged QT interval can be caused by (1) overdoses of terfenadine or astemizole (two to three times usual daily dose), (2) liver dysfunction, (3) electrolyte imbalance (hypokalemia or hypomagnesemia), (4) congenital long QT syndrome (rare), or (5) factors that increase the serum levels of unmetabolized terfenadine or astemizole. (These factors involve drugs that inhibit the cytochrome P-450 enzyme system or are due to liver dysfunction.)

To avoid potential problems, patients receiving terfenadine or astemizole should be counseled to avoid increasing their doses above the recommended dosage. They also should be cautioned about avoiding concurrent treatment with ketoconazole, itraconazole, erythromycin, clarithromycin, troleandomycin, and drugs that prolong QT interval (e.g., quinidine). Other imidazole antifungal agents and other macrolides antibiotics should be used cautiously though azithromycin apparently does not affect levels. Patients with significant liver dysfunction or who are receiving concurrent treatment with inhibitors of cytochrome P-450 are probably better treated with loratidine or cetirizine.

CONCLUSION

Allergic and drug-induced skin diseases encompass a varied spectrum of diseases. Although allergy is suspected in many cases, the specific allergen may be difficult to identify. Other mechanisms operate in some diseases, but the clinical presentation does not distinguish the etiology. Drug-induced conditions tend to be acute and resolve, particularly when the offending agent is removed. Atopic dermatitis, contact dermatitis, and idiopathic urticaria tend to be more chronic with exacerbations and remissions. Topical corticosteroids, occasional short-term systemic corticosteroids in severe conditions, and antihistamines are the mainstay of drug therapy in addition to other nonspecific topical treatments.

REFERENCES

1. Jacobs MR, Zanowiak P. Topical antiinfective products in: Feldmann EG, Blockstein WL, eds. Handbook of Nonprescription Drugs. 9th edition. Washington: American Pharmaceutical Association, 1990: 771–773.
2. Sauer GC. Manual of Skin Diseases. 6th edition. Philadelphia: JB Lippincott Co., 1991:1–8.
3. Bigby M, Stern RS, Arndt KA. Allergic cutaneous reactions to drugs. Primary Care 16:713–727, 1989.
4. Thestrup-Pedersen K, Larsen CG, Ronnevig J. The immunology of contact dermatitis. Contact Dermatitis 20:81–92, 1989.
5. Pratt WB. Drug allergy in Pratt WB, Taylor P, editors. Principles of Drug Action: The basis of pharmacology. New York: Churchhill Livingstone, 1990:533–548.
6. Wintroub BU, Stern R. Cutaneous drug reactions: Pathogenesis and clinical classification. J Am Acad Dermatol 13:167–179, 1985.
7. Oakes RC, Cox AD, Burgdorf WHC. Atopic dermatitis. A review of diagnosis, pathogenesis and management. Clin Pediatrics 22:467–475, 1983.
8. Chan SC, Hanifin JM. Immunologic aspects of atopic dermatitis. Clin Reviews Allergy 11:523–541, 1993.
9. Sampson HA. Pathogenesis of eczema. Clin Experimental Allergy 20:459–467, 1990.
10. Horan RF, Schneider LC, Sheffer AL. Allergic skin disorders and mastocytosis. JAMA 268:2858–2868, 1992.
11. Rasmussen JE. Management of atopic dermatitis. Allergy 44:(Suppl 9):108–113, 1989.
12. Hanifin JM. The role of antihistamines in atopic dermatitis. J Allergy Clin Immunol 86(4, part 2):666–669, 1990.
13. Advenier C, Queille-Roussel C. Rational use of antihistamines in allergic dermatological conditions. Drugs 38:634–644, 1984.
14. Hanifin JM. Atopic dermatitis. In Middleton E, et al. Allergy. Principles and Practice. 4th edition, Mosby, St. Louis 1993: 1595–1600.
15. Noren P, Melin L. The effect of combined topical steroids and habit-reversal treatment in patients with atopic dermatitis. Brit J Dermatol 121:359–366, 1989.
16. Cooper KD. New therapeutic approaches in atopic dermatitis. Clin Reviews Allergy 11:543–559, 1993.
17. Mozzanica N. Pathogenic aspects of allergic and irritant contact dermatitis. Clinics in Dermatology 10:115–121, 1992.
18. Maibach H, Epstein E. Allergic contact dermatitis. In Demis DJ. Clinical Dermatology Volume 3. Philadelphia: JB Lippincott Company, 1988: Unit 13-1:1–46.
19. Nethercott JR, Holness DL. Occupational allergic contact dermatitis. Clin Reviews Allergy 7:399–415, 1989.
20. Whittington C. Clinical aspects of contact dermatitis. Primary Care 16:729–738, 1989.
21. Lehach JG, Rosenstreich DL. Clinical aspects of chronic urticaria. Clin Reviews Allergy 10:281–301, 1992.
22. Haustein U. Adrenergic urticaria and adrenergic pruritis. Acta Derm Venereol 70:82–84, 1990.
23. Soter NA. Urticaria: Current therapy. J Allergy Clin Immunol 86(6, part 2):1009–1014, 1990.
24. Kennard CD, Ellis CN. Pharmacologic therapy for urticaria. J Amer Acad Dermatol 25(No. 1, part 2):176–187, 1991.
25. Ormerod AD. Urticaria: Recognition, causes and treatment. Drugs 48:717–730, 1994.
26. Anderson JA. Allergic reactions to drugs and biological agents. JAMA 268:2845–2857, 1992.
27. Korkij W, Soltani K. Fixed drug eruption. A brief review. Arch Dermatol 120:520–524, 1984.
28. Felix RH, Smith AG. Skin Disorders. In Davies DM, ed. 4th edition. Textbook of Adverse Drug Reactions Oxford University Press, Oxford 1991: 514–534.
29. Hande KR, Noone RM, Stone WJ. Severe allopurinol toxicity. Amer J Med 76:47–56, 1984.
30. Simons FER. H_1-receptor antagonists: Clinical pharmacology and therapeutics. J Allergy Clin Immunol 84(6, part 1):845–861, 1989.
31. Simons FER, Simons KJ. The pharmacology and use of H_1-receptor-antagonist drugs. New Eng J Med 330:1663–1670, 1994.
32. Paton DM, Webster DR. Clinical pharmacokinetics of H_1-receptor antagonists (The antihistamines). Clin Pharmacokinetics 10:477–497, 1985.
33. Simons FER. Recent advances in H_1-receptor antagonist treatment. J Allergy Clin Immunol 86(6, part 2):995–999, 1990.
34. Meltzer EO. Performance effects of antihistamines. J Allergy Clin Immunol 86(4, part 2):613–619, 1990.
35. Smith SJ. Cardiovascular toxicity of antihistamines. Otolaryngol Head Neck Surg 111:348–354, 1994.
36. Olin BR, ed. Facts and Comparisons. St. Louis: JB Lippincott Company 1993:188–194a.
37. Antihistamine Drugs. AHFS Drug Information 94. Washington, American Society of Hospital Pharmacists. 1994:1–34.

CHAPTER 44

COMMON SKIN DISORDERS

MADHAVI MENON, ASHKAN GHORBANI, LUKE SLOAN, PETER SANTALUCIA, and ALAN H. TANENBAUM

The skin is the largest organ of the body. Its primary functions are as a protective barrier from the external environment and the maintenance of the homeostatic milieu of the internal environment. As such, the proper function and integrity of the skin is essential to life.

Many disease processes can attack this organ system alone. In addition, skin manifestations can give important clues to underlying systemic pathology, many of which we discuss elsewhere. In this chapter, we describe some common skin dermatoses that pose therapeutic challenges.

ACNE

Acne vulgaris is a chronic, but usually self-limited, disorder occurring within the pilosebaceous units of the face, neck, and upper trunk. It is the most common skin disorder and is estimated to occur to some degree in 85% of adolescents(1). The incidence of acne is the same in both sexes, with peak occurrence between the ages of 16 and 19. It resolves in the vast majority of patients by the age of 25. Females tend to develop the disorder at an earlier age secondarily to the earlier onset of puberty (2). Acne persists more commonly into the 3rd and 4th decades in females in comparison to males (3). Males, however, tend to develop a more severe form of the disease. Genetic factors play a role, particularly for the more severe forms of acne. The high prevalence and the multifactorial origin of the disorder make genetic factors difficult to assess.

Clinical Features

Acne lesions occur within the specialized sebaceous hair follicular units found principally on the face, and to a lesser degree the chest, shoulders, and back. The two basic lesions are noninflammatory and inflammatory. Noninflammatory lesions consist of open comedones (blackheads) and closed comedones (whiteheads). Comedones develop because of an impaction of keratin and sebum within a dilated follicle and are considered the primary lesions in acne. Mild acne consists of only noninflammatory lesions, but unfortunately, most progress beyond this point.

Inflammatory lesions are derived from closed comedones. Papules and pustules represent superficial inflammatory lesions, and a preponderance of these lesions constitutes at least moderate acne. Deeper inflammatory lesions include nodules and cysts and are present in the more severe cases of acne. Patients with nodulocystic acne will often have extensive involvement of the chest and back. See Table 44.1 for a summary of acne lesions.

Scarring can occur, particularly in the deeper inflammatory forms of acne. It is the most devastating clinical feature prompting early aggressive therapy. The most common scar is the atrophic (ice-pick) form, which is permanent. Hypertrophic, keloidlike scars also occur and are more commonly seen on the trunk. These tend to flatten in time.

Often overlooked is the residual pigmentary alteration seen following resolution of inflammatory lesions. This is particularly noticeable in black patients where hyperpigmentation predominates and is often what prompts a visit to the physician. There is no effective treatment for the pigmentary alteration beyond preventing further inflammatory lesions from developing. The majority of the pigmented lesions will fade, but it can take 6 months to 1 year for this to occur.

Pathogenesis

The pathogenesis of acne is multifactorial; however, active sebaceous glands are a prerequisite. The development of acne corresponds with the maturing of these glands under hormonal control at puberty. The only hormone known to stimulate the sebaceous gland directly is androgen (2). This is derived from the testes in males and the ovaries and adrenal glands in females. Circulating testosterone is converted at the tissue level by 5 alpha-reductase to dihydrotestosterone, a potent stimulator of sebum production. Sebum is composed of different lipids, including triglycerides and waxes that assist with hydration of the skin. On the average both male and female acne patients secrete more sebum than nonacne patients, and the level of secretion does correlate with the severity of acne. Acne-prone skin has shown an abnormally high 5 alpha-reductase activity in vitro. In addition, women with more severe acne frequently have biochemical androgen excess.

Excess sebum plays an important role, through a variety of mechanisms, in the development of an acne lesion. The earliest pathologic change in acne is an alteration in the pattern of keratinization within the follicle, which results in the keratinous material becoming more dense (4). Sebum accumulates within this keratin and in fact may cause the abnormal follicular keratinization (2). This mass of material plugs the follicle, causing it to dilate below the surface of the skin. If the follicular opening dilates enough to extrude

Table 44.1.
Acne Lesions

Noninflammatory
   Open comedones (blackheads)
   Closed comedones (whiteheads) precursor to inflammatory lesions
Inflammatory
   Superficial
      Papules
      Pustules
   Deep
      Nodules
      Cysts

this material, an open comedo results. The black color is attributed to the impacted keratinous material present, and is not dirt, nor is it likely due to oxidized sebum or melanin as once thought (5). An open comedo is actually a mature lesion, not capable of becoming inflammatory. If the follicular opening does not dilate sufficiently, the resultant lesion is a closed comedo. This is the principal site for inflammatory lesion development.

Once the follicle has been occluded, an inflammatory lesion is initiated through an interaction between trapped bacteria, principally *Propionibacterium acnes,* and the retained contents. *P. acnes* is an anaerobe found in high levels in adolescents with acne but in significantly lower concentrations in nonacne patients. *P. acnes* secretes chemotactic factors for polymorphonuclear leukocytes that can then invade the follicular wall leading to its disruption and eventual collapse. This results in spillage of its contents into the surrounding dermis with a subsequent increase of inflammatory response. In addition, *P. acnes* produces lipases that hydrolyze the triglycerides of sebum into glycerol and free fatty acids (FFA). It uses the glycerol for growth, and the free fatty acids can further contribute to the inflammatory response. The depth and magnitude of the inflammatory response corresponds with the clinical development of pustules, papules, nodules, and cysts. Figure 44.1 demonstrates the three important pathogenic factors in the development of an acne lesion.

Immune response does play an associated role. Patients with acne have a much higher antibody titer to *P. acnes* than do controls. Both the classical and alternative complement pathways are activated in acne lesions by *P. acnes,* which produces C5a neutrophilic chemotactic factor (6). Small amounts of *P. acnes* can produce profound inflammation in patients with high antibody titers to this organism. Finally, severe acne occurs rarely in females, and this may be due to their exhibiting a better defense mechanism to *P. acnes* than males (7).

A number of exogenous factors can make existing acne worse. Oil-based makeups, pomades, and oily soaps and hair products can occlude the follicle initiating a comedo. Physical pressure from a headband or hat can induce

localized acne. Exposure to excessive heat and humidity can exacerbate acne, but the mechanism is not clear. The ingestion of certain drugs can aggravate acne. Danazol and birth control pills with a high progesterone component do this presumably through increased androgenic activity. Table 44.2 lists other medications that can do this. The mechanism for most of these is not understood. Diet and stress are frequently implicated, but controlled studies are lacking. Unless a patient implicitly believes a food is aggravating the condition, no food, including chocolate, need be eliminated from the diet.

Treatment

The treatment of acne can sometimes be difficult and disappointing. Acne is a chronic condition at times requiring many months to years of individualized treatment in order to achieve control. Nevertheless, if the patient is committed and compliant, it is certainly a treatable disease, and acne control should be expected. Compliance is enhanced if the patient understands both the nature of the disease and the rationale behind the therapy. Virtually all therapy is preventive, with little or no effect on the inflammatory lesions present at the outset. For that reason, maximal efficacy is not reached for several months even with the most effective of treatments. Once acne control is achieved, the patient should understand that maintenance therapy will be required for as long as the tendency to acne persists.

As previously stated, important factors in the pathogenesis of acne are pilosebaceous obstruction by sebum and keratin, androgen-stimulated sebum production, and proliferation of *P. acnes*. Acne therapy is directed at correcting each of these factors. As in other diseases without a single best treatment, a good many therapies exist, each with specific merits. Many topical therapies are readily available over the counter, and, although effective in some patients when used properly, are subject to misuse by uninformed patients. Compliance with a single regimen, whether it be self-medicated or while under a physician's care, should be stressed for optimal results. A summary of therapeutic agents in acne with their principal mode of activity is shown in Table 44.3.

GENERAL SKIN CARE

There is no evidence that excessive cleansing offers therapeutic benefit; in fact, overcleansing can be an irritant. Additionally, surface sebum and bacteria do not play a role in the development of lesions. When choosing a soap, a patient should avoid one with a high oil content. These are usually reserved for dry, sensitive skin, and can be counterproductive in acne. Expensive medicated soaps are usually not indicated as a supplement to other treatment plans. In noninflammatory acne, a mildly abrasive cleanser may be of some benefit by inducing a

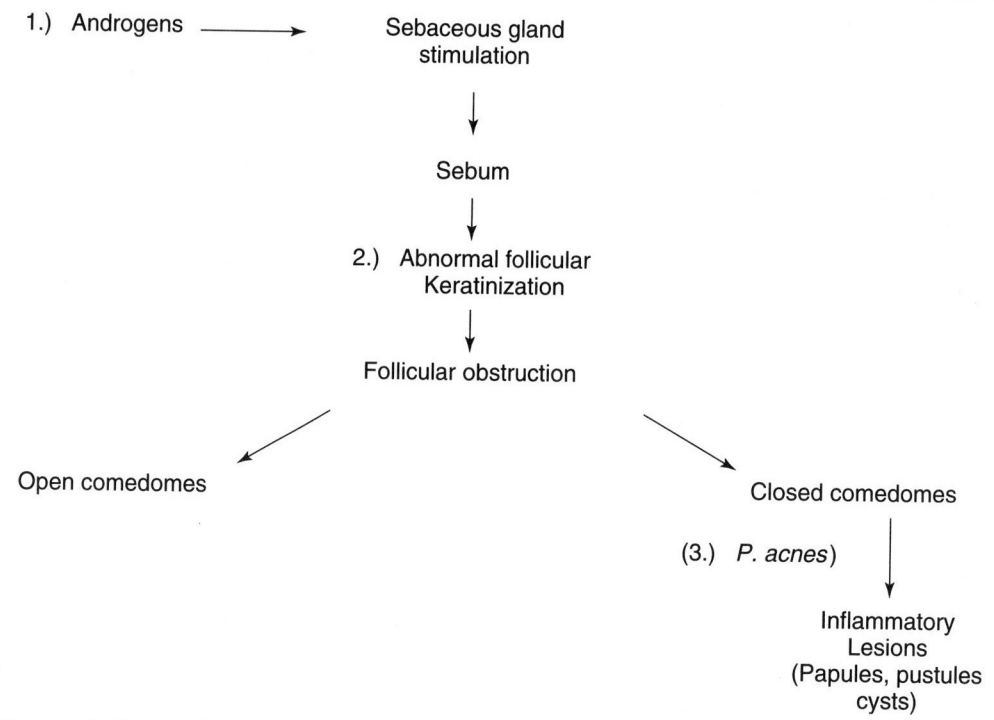

Figure 44.1. Treatment of acne is based on reversing the three primary factors in development of acne lesions, as numbered here.

Table 44.2.
Medications That Aggravate Acne

Hormonal
  Danazol *CYCLOMEN/DANOCRINE – ANDROGEN*
  High progesterone-containing OCP
  Anabolic steroids
  Gonadotropins
  Prednisone
Nonhormonal
  Azathioprine *– IMMUNOSUPPRESSANT – IMURAN*
  Bromides
  Cyanocobalamin *– B vitamin*
  Disulfuram *– ANTABUSE – enzyme inhibitor*
  Gold
  Hydantoin drugs *–*
  Iodides
  Lithium
  Maprotiline *Ludiomil – Antidepressant*
  Quinidine *– ANTI Arrhythmic*
  Quinine *– ANTIMALARIAL, Leg CRAMPS*
  Rifampin *– ANTI TB*
  Thiouracil

Table 44.3.
Summary of Therapeutic Agents in Acne and Principal Mode of Activity

Topical Therapy	Oral Therapy
Antimicrobial (*P. acnes*)	Antimicrobial
Benzoyl peroxide	Antibiotics
Antibiotics	Tetracycline
Clindamycin	Minocycline
Erythromycin	Erythromycin
Meclocycline	Trimethoprim sulfamethoxazole
Tetracycline	Isotretinoin *– ACCUTANE*
Azelaic acid	Comedolytic
Sulfur—minor	Isotretinoin
Salicylic acid—minor	Decreased sebaceous gland activity
Comedolytic	Isotretinoin (principal action)
Tretinoin *> retinoic Acid*	Hormonal therapy
Azelaic acid	Estrogen
Benzoyl peroxide—minor	Cyproterone acetate
Salicylic acid—minor	Spironolactone
Resorcin—minor	
Decreased sebaceous gland activity	
None	

superficial exfoliation of the skin. In inflammatory acne, or in the patient with dry skin from previous acne therapy, a gentle soap is indicated. Avoidance of all cosmetics is best; however, complete avoidance may be an unrealistic expectation. If cosmetics are to be used, they should be water based. Cosmetics should be removed by soap and water and not by cleansing creams.

Astringents are alcohol-based cleansers that are easy to use and leave the face feeling cool and refreshed. Unfortunately, they are of limited value in the treatment of acne.

TOPICAL THERAPY

Topically applied medications remain the cornerstone of acne therapy. They are often effective alone in mild-to-moderate acne and are important adjuncts to oral antibiotics in more severe acne. The most widely used topical preparations are benzoyl peroxide and antibiotics, which inhibit the growth of *P. acnes*, and tretinoin, which reverses the abnormal keratinization in the follicles.

Benzoyl Peroxide. Benzoyl peroxide was first formulated for dermatologic use in 1905, and the compound was recognized as useful for acne in 1934. However, the original ointment vehicle was unsuitable for acne therapy. It was not until the mid-1960s that a stable preparation of benzoyl peroxide in a hydrous media was formulated. Since that time, it has become the most frequently used topical medication in acne because of its effectiveness and ready availability, both over the counter and by prescription. When used properly, it can be effective alone in mild acne, but it is used as an adjunct to other therapies in more severe disease.

The principal mode of action of benzoyl peroxide is thought to be its bactericidal activity against *P. acnes*. It is metabolized to benzoic acid in the skin, and its lipophilic properties allow it to penetrate better than other topical antimicrobials (8). Once it penetrates the follicle, the release of nascent oxygen from the peroxide exerts its effect on the bacteria. Studies have shown a twofold greater reduction of *P. acnes* counts at 4 weeks with 5% benzoyl peroxide than with topical erythromycin or oral tetracycline (9).

Benzoyl peroxide has also been thought to exert comedolytic and exfoliative properties. However, reports of these effects are contradictory, and these actions are considered minor. Benzoyl peroxide has no effect on sebum production or concentration. By reducing the *P. acnes* counts, free fatty acids, which contribute to the comedonal plug and inflammation, are also reduced. Benzoyl peroxide can be irritating to the skin, leading to increased blood flow. Increased blood flow is felt to speed resolution of inflammatory lesions through a "counter irritant" mechanism (10).

Benzoyl peroxide is available over the counter as 2.5, 5.0, and 10.0% creams, lotions, washes, and soaps. It is available in the same concentrations by prescription, usually in various gel vehicles. A 4% formulation in a hydrous media with good activity, but a lower side effect profile, has also been introduced. The selection of the appropriate vehicle is important in the individual patient setting. Gels are considered more effective vehicles for release of the active substance, but they can be more irritating. Although less effective, a wash or lotion may be all that is tolerated in a patient with more sensitive skin. During the winter months, when dry skin can be a problem, switching from the gels to a cream or lotion may be necessary.

There is no difference among the three available concentrations in reducing *P. acnes* numbers in the skin (1). Therefore, when initiating therapy with benzoyl peroxide, it is reasonable to begin with a low concentration (2.5 to 5.0%) to decrease irritation. Initial therapy should be applied once daily. The patient should apply this sparingly, being careful to avoid the periorbital, perinasal, and perioral skin. Often patients will experience mild erythema, burning, or stinging on initial application, and they should be instructed to expect this. By applying the medication at night, the erythema should be minimal by morning. If irritation persists, switching to every-other-night therapy is appropriate.

Tolerance to these side effects is usually achieved as therapy continues. Once tolerance is achieved, the patient should increase the frequency of application to twice a day. Switching to a more potent vehicle, or a higher concentration, should be done only after tolerance is achieved to the lower concentrations without significant improvement in the acne at 4 to 8 weeks. As a general rule, the side effect profile increases more than the efficacy with increasing concentration of benzoyl peroxide.

The most frequent side effect of benzoyl peroxide is the capacity to irritate the skin, which may in part be responsible for its efficacy. It is known that 1 to 2% of people are allergic to this compound. If patients continue to experience erythema and scaling at low concentrations applied on alternate days, they may have an allergic contact dermatitis. In these cases, stopping the medication is all that is required, and an alternative therapy will be necessary. Patients should be warned that benzoyl peroxide can bleach hair and clothes. Allowing the preparation to completely dry before coming in contact with fabrics can minimize this problem. The question whether benzoyl peroxide is carcinogenic has been raised. Two earlier studies on rodents supported this, but case-controlled studies in humans have been negative. To date, it is considered completely safe for use in humans (11).

Tretinoin. Since being introduced for acne in 1969, this derivative of vitamin A has probably become the most effective agent in treatment of the disorder. It was originally thought that its mode of action was related to its ability to promote erythema and peeling of the skin. It is now known that its activity is directed at reducing the cohesiveness of keratinocytes within the sebaceous follicle independent of clinical peeling (1). This inhibition of the retention hyperkeratosis prevents microcomedo formation. For that reason, tretinoin is superior to all other topical or oral therapies for comedonal acne. As inflammatory lesions are derived from comedones, tretinoin is an important adjunct to therapy in more severe acne.

The patient should understand that tretinoin can cause anywhere from mild to severe irritation of the skin, which is more common at initiation of therapy. This is manifested by erythema, dryness, and peeling and is influenced by the formulation used. Tretinoin is now available in a .025, .05, and 0.1% cream, a .01 and .025% gel, and a .05% lotion. Therapy is usually initiated with the .025% cream since the irritation can be much less while the efficacy only slightly so (8). Tretinoin should not be applied more than once daily initially. It should be applied to completely dry skin since moisture increases the permeability of tretinoin and, therefore, its irritant potential. The patient should avoid the periorbital, perinasal, and perioral skin. The erythema and dryness are not required for effectiveness, so if side effects continue to be a problem, using tretinoin every other, or every third night, is recommended. As tolerance develops, the frequency can then be increased.

Many patients will offset the side effects of tretinoin with heavy emollients, but this is counterproductive in the treatment of acne and should be discouraged. The use of other harsh skin care products such as astringents can increase the irritant potential of tretinoin and should be eliminated if possible. A gentle soap should be used, and only if necessary a mild lotion.

Patients can experience a modest exacerbation of their acne on initiation of therapy. This is secondary to the ability of tretinoin to release the retained products of comedones to the skin surface. Patients should understand this so that they will not become discouraged and possibly discontinue this therapy unnecessarily. This flare should resolve in 3 to 6 weeks.

Tretinoin decreases the thickness of the stratum corneum, the most superficial layer of the skin (9). This layer helps protect the skin from damage from the sun. Patients should be counseled to apply the medication around bedtime and to avoid long exposure to UV radiation. If exposure is unavoidable, however, patients should use a sunscreen with an SPF of at least 15. The thinned stratum corneum also allows better permeability of other topical agents, which is an advantage when used in conjunction with topical antibiotics. Systemic toxicity, as potentially seen with oral retinoids, is not a problem with topical tretinoin even when applied in high concentrations.

The small amount that is absorbed is rapidly metabolized by the liver. Although tretinoin has anecdotally been reported in association with congenital birth defects, larger studies have not revealed an increased risk (12). Therefore, though generally considered safe for use even in pregnancy, tretinoin is not often used for medicolegal reasons during this time.

TOPICAL ANTIBIOTICS

Topical antibiotics are used in mild-to-moderate inflammatory acne and as an adjunct in more severe nodulocystic acne. They are not comedolytic, so are not useful alone in noninflammatory acne. The topical antibiotics most commonly used are clindamycin and erythromycin in a variety of vehicles. Meclocycline, a derivative of oxytetracycline, and topical tetracycline are also available. Studies have

consistently shown topical antibiotics to be equally efficacious as low-dose oral tetracycline in moderate inflammatory disease (13). Topical antibiotics are especially useful when tapering oral therapy.

The principal action of topical antibiotics is their antibacterial effect against *P. acnes*. Clindamycin is more lipophilic and appears to be more effective than erythromycin at reducing *P. acnes* counts (8). However, when examining clinical efficacy of the different agents, similar results are obtained, implying that other factors play a role. Topical antibiotics may inhibit *P. acnes* metabolism without killing the organism. This would result in decreased lipase activity, FFAs, and chemotactic factors. Both oral and topical tetracycline have known antiinflammatory activities (14).

Topical antibiotics are usually applied twice a day to moist skin after washing with soap and water. As with other topical products, the vehicle is important. Vehicles with a high alcohol content allow better absorption, but can be more drying. A cream or ointment may be tolerated better initially in patients with more sensitive skin or during winter months.

A response to topical antibiotics is often evident earlier than that seen with other topical therapies. Improvement is often noted within 2 weeks though maximal efficacy cannot be determined for at least 12 weeks.

The most common side effect of topical antibiotics is mild erythema and stinging secondary to the vehicle used. The development of resistant organisms to these antibiotics can occur; however, this has not proved to be a clinical problem. Recolonization of susceptible strains of *P. acnes* is quickly seen on discontinuation of therapy (15). Commercially available topical clindamycin preparations are in the phosphate form and are less readily absorbed through the skin. However, 10% of a daily application does reach the bloodstream, and cases of pseudomembranous colitis (PMC) have now been described with topical use (16). This must be considered a rare but potential side effect, particularly when applied to large surface areas of skin. Topical meclocycline can impart a faint yellow tint to the skin, which will wash off.

COMBINED TOPICAL THERAPIES

Combining two topical therapies that are directed at different factors in the pathogenesis of acne makes sense from a practical standpoint. The most commonly used combination is that of tretinoin, with its comedolytic activity, with topical antibiotics or benzoyl peroxide. As stated previously, by thinning the stratum corneum, tretinoin allows better absorption of the antimicrobials.

The combination of tretinoin and benzoyl peroxide appears to be less irritating than tretinoin alone and is more effective than each used individually. Therapy is initiated with low concentrations of each on an alternate day basis. When tolerance to the irritant effect is acquired, they can each be used daily. The patient is usually instructed to use benzoyl peroxide in the morning, and tretinoin at night. This should be strictly adhered to since the irritant potential is additive when used concurrently. If the patient is unable to tolerate benzoyl peroxide, one of the other topical antibiotics can be used.

A commercially available combination of benzoyl peroxide and erythromycin is now considered more effective than either alone. Erythromycin is more active than benzoyl peroxide against *P. acnes,* but is not lipid soluble. It is thought that benzoyl peroxide somehow carries the more active erythromycin to the target tissue (8).

OTHER TOPICAL THERAPIES

Traditional therapies using salicylic acid (0.5 to 3.0%), sulfur (2 to 10%), or resorcin (2.0 to 6.0%) are not used frequently now. Their effectiveness correlated with their ability to induce erythema and desquamation. Salicylic acid is a keratolytic and has some comedolytic activity, but tretinoin is more effective. Sulfur is not comedolytic but appears to hasten the resolution of inflammatory pustular lesions. The combination of sulfur and salicylic acid is synergistic, so they are frequently compounded together. Each also has a weak antimicrobial activity. Resorcin, another keratolytic, has been shown to be relatively ineffective in acne in the most recent studies (17). If used extensively, systemic absorption can rarely cause methemoglobinemia, cyanosis, and convulsions. These treatments are best reserved for the patient with mild-to-moderate acne who is intolerant of other topical medications. The combination of erythromycin 4.0% and zinc acetate 1.2% was more effective than clindamycin 1% and erythromycin 2% in controlled studies (18). The combination provided enhanced absorption of both products, and the zinc is thought to be antiinflammatory. Side effects include facial burning and redness in a minority of patients.

Some newer topical therapies have been promising in studies and may soon be available commercially. Azelaic acid, a naturally occurring dicarboxylic acid molecule, has been effective for both noninflammatory and inflammatory acne. The dicarboxylic acids were initially found to have a beneficial effect on hyperpigmentary disorders. When patients reported a coincidental improvement in their acne, studies were initiated to investigate this further. A 20% azelaic acid cream was as effective as 0.05% tretinoin cream in reducing comedones with less irritant side effects (19). The best results with azelaic acid cream were seen in papulo-pustular acne. Its efficacy is explained by both a strong comedolytic property and a bacteriostatic effect on *P. acnes.* No side effects beyond a low rate of local irritation were reported.

There have been a number of attempts to employ topical antiandrogens in the treatment of acne. Topical

cyproterone acetate was found to be ineffective, and the results of studies with spironolactone cream have been equivocal. Decreased sebum production and a marked reduction of comedones were reported with the use of topical 17 alpha-propylmesterolone though no formulation is yet commercially available (20). A nonsteroidal antiandrogen, inocoterone acetate (RU882), in a 10% solution exerted a statistically significant, though modest (26%), reduction in the number of inflammatory papules and pustules in treated men (21). However, this compares unfavorably with results expected using established preparations like benzoyl peroxides or topical antibiotics (50 to 75% reduction in lesions at 2 months) (22). Another topically active antiandrogen named RU58841 has recently been synthesized. It has been shown to have high affinity for androgen receptors and minimal systemic effects in hamsters (23). More detailed evaluation is now proceeding.

SYSTEMIC THERAPY ANTIBIOTICS

Oral antibiotics are used at the outset of therapy for patients with moderate-to-severe inflammatory acne. They should be used in conjunction with topical benzoyl peroxide, tretinoin, or occasionally, topical antibiotics. Tetracycline and its derivative minocycline are usually the drugs of first choice. Erythromycin is a frequent alternative and trimethoprim-sulfamethoxazole is rarely prescribed as a third line of therapy. They exert their effect principally by inhibiting *P. acnes,* resulting in decreased chemotactic factor and lipase production. They also exert a direct antiinflammatory response independent of bacteria. This is true more so of tetracycline than the other antibiotics.

Tetracycline in doses of 1 gram a day in two to four divided doses is usually employed first. Occasionally, doses up to 2 grams are necessary in nodulocystic acne. It is best absorbed if not taken with food, dairy products, iron, or antacids. The patients should be instructed to take the medication 1 hour before or 2 hours after a meal. Tetracycline on an empty stomach can cause nausea in some patients and, in these instances, can be taken with a small amount of food.

Clinical improvement is usually noted within 2 to 4 weeks of therapy. The optimal time course for oral antibiotic therapy is not known. Frequently, maximal efficacy is not reached for 4 to 5 months, so continuing therapy for this time should be expected (14). If a good response is achieved, continuing oral antibiotics for an additional 6 months offered no advantages over topical therapy alone (24). Once an adequate response is noted, tapering the dose by 250-mg increments over several weeks is recommended. The goal is to ultimately discontinue oral therapy while maintaining control with topical therapy alone.

A common side effect of tetracycline is vaginal yeast infection, which can be controlled by oral and topical nystatin or other topical antiyeast preparations. Tetracycline can also cause photosensitivity eruptions, so patients should wear a sunscreen with an SPF of at least 15 if planning to spend an extended time in the sun. Tetracycline and its derivatives should never be administered in pregnancy since they may cause liver toxicity in the mother, and bone and teeth abnormalities in the fetus.

If cost were not a factor, minocycline would be the antibiotic of first choice in acne. It is more lipophilic than tetracycline, allowing it to accumulate more readily in the sebaceous follicle, and its clinical efficacy has proven better than tetracycline (25). It is better absorbed with food and is less likely to cause nausea than tetracycline. It is also less likely to cause photosensitivity reactions. The usual initial dose is 50 mg twice a day, so patient compliance is improved.

Minocyline can more frequently cause esophagitis secondary to reflux, so it should not be taken just prior to retiring. A dose-dependent vestibular dysfunction can occur leading to vertigo, ataxia, and nausea and vomiting. Lowering the dose can circumvent this, but often the medication will need to be discontinued. A blue-gray pigmentation of both skin and mucous membranes is reported with minocycline use. This is more prominent in sun-exposed areas and can take up to 7 months to resolve. Doxycycline, another derivative of tetracycline, has shown therapeutic equivalence to minocycline, but is less frequently used in the treatment of acne because of a much higher incidence of photosensitivity reactions.

If a patient is unable to take tetracycline for any reason, erythromycin is an effective alternative. It is equally effective to tetracycline, but a higher incidence of gastrointestinal problems, and the more frequent development of resistant strains of P. acnes make it the second choice. Advantages of erythromycin include the lower rate of monilial overgrowth, the lack of photosensitivity, and that it can be taken with food. It is one antibiotic that is considered safe in pregnancy; however, consulting with the obstetrician is wise before initiating long-term therapy with any medication during pregnancy. The same dosing recommendations are made as for tetracycline.

The safety of long-term antibiotics in the treatment of acne is well established (26). A concern over possible serious superinfections has not been warranted clinically. There is also concern that broad spectrum antibiotics can decrease the effectiveness of oral contraceptives (27). Although this remains controversial, discussion of this possibility should be done with these patients and additional forms of birth control suggested.

Isotretinoin. Oral isotretinoin (13 cis-retinoic acid) is the most effective agent in the treatment of acne. This synthetic derivative of vitamin A was introduced in 1982. Formerly indicated primarily for the treatment of the patient with resistant nodulocystic acne, the majority of treated patients today have therapy-resistant moderate

acne. It should also be considered early in the therapy of patients who exhibit scarring. Dramatic improvement can be seen with isotretinoin, and in contrast to other acne therapies, prolonged remission can be expected. The teratogenicity and multiple potential side effects associated with isotretinoin preclude its use in less severe acne.

The mechanism of action of isotretinoin is multifactorial. It is the only known therapeutic agent that affects all the major factors associated in the pathogenesis of acne (28). Its most profound effect is on reduction of sebaceous gland size and sebum production. A 50 to 90% sebaceous gland size reduction can be expected. This inhibition continues in most patients for more than a year after discontinuing therapy. Isotretinoin also normalizes the keratinization process within the follicle. It has no direct antibacterial properties, but isotretinoin reduces P. acnes counts indirectly by the reduction of sebum. Isotretinoin also has direct antiinflammatory properties by inhibiting chemotaxis of neutrophils and monocytes.

The usual starting dose of isotretinoin is 0.5 to 1.0 mg/kg orally per day. The lower dose is usually initiated and then gradually increased based on clinical response and tolerance of side effects after 4 to 8 weeks. Therapy is continued for 16 to 20 weeks. Oral antibiotics and topical medications that can further dry the skin should be discontinued prior to isotretinoin therapy. Improvement is usually noted within 2 months, and continued improvement can be seen for up to 6 months following therapy. Some patients can have relapses after a course of isotretinoin, but they are usually much milder than the initial disease. This is seen more frequently in those treated with lower doses. If relapse occurs, a second course can be given, but this is not recommended until a 6-month period has elapsed because of the delayed improvement that can be seen.

Nearly all patients who receive isotretinoin will experience mucocutaneous side effects. These consist primarily of dryness of the skin, eyes, nose, and mouth. Moisturizers can be used to combat the dry skin and cheilitis. An antibiotic ointment is recommended for the nasal passages to prevent cracking, bleeding, and potential colonization by S. aureus (10). Conjunctivitis is common, and corneal opacities can occur, but they usually resolve within 6 weeks after therapy. During this period, patients may be intolerant of contact lenses. Artificial tears can be used to offset this problem.

The most common laboratory abnormality in patients on isotretinoin is a dose-related elevation of serum triglyceride levels. Twenty-five percent of patients will have a 10% or greater elevation (28). Less frequently seen is a decrease in high-density lipoprotein levels (15%) and an increase in cholesterol (8%). This is usually not a problem in the young patient treated for acne, but precautions should be taken. Previous recommendations included a baseline lipid profile with repeat samples obtained after 1 week of therapy and every 2 weeks until levels stabilize. More recently, large retrospective studies have suggested that less frequent monitoring may be sufficient (29). A low-fat diet and avoidance of alcohol is necessary in mild-to-moderate elevations. Close monitoring should be done in an obese or diabetic patient. Hyperlipidemia is reversible, with lipid levels returning to baseline within 8 weeks after discontinuing therapy. Less frequently seen is an elevation of hepatic enzymes. These usually return to normal with continued therapy or a reduction in dose (28). Rarely, a decreased white blood cell count or hypercalcemia are seen. The need for laboratory monitoring of these parameters should be discussed with patients prior to therapy with isotretinoin.

Synthetic retinoid therapy has been associated with skeletal changes in a small percentage of patients. In acne patients treated for 20 weeks, significant abnormalities are rare. Most commonly seen are muscle and bone discomfort, which respond to mild analgesic therapy. Skeletal hyperostosis, manifested by small spurs along the vertebral bodies, has been noted in 26% of acne patients in one study. However, 23% of patients had these prior to therapy, and the significance of this finding during short-term therapy is not known (30).

Less than 10% of patients will notice some hair loss during therapy, usually late in the course. Regrowth is to be expected. Photosensitivity can occur, and patients should wear an SPF 15 sunscreen prior to prolonged exposure to the sun. Benign intracranial hypertension is a rare side effect of isotretinoin administration. This is manifested by headache, nausea, vomiting, and visual disturbances. If this occurs, the patient should see his or her physician immediately.

The most serious side effect of isotretinoin is its teratogenicity. Miscarriage and stillbirth are common and a 25-fold increase in major congenital anomalies is seen (2). These involve the cranium, face, heart, brain, and thymus during the period of organogenesis. The female patient must understand the teratogenic potential and the consequences of becoming pregnant while on this medication. A pregnancy test should be performed within 2 weeks of beginning therapy. Treatment should start on the 2nd or 3rd day of the next menstrual cycle. An effective method of birth control must be initiated at least 1 month prior to therapy and continued until 1 month after cessation. Although teratogenic, isotretinoin is not mutagenic, and future pregnancies should not be affected (2). The drug has no known effect on spermatogenesis.

HORMONAL THERAPY

Estrogen therapy has long been noted to improve acne in women. This hormone acts to counteract the androgenic stimulation of the sebaceous gland, decreasing sebum production. Estrogen is usually given in the form of the oral contraceptive pill. The most notable results were obtained using doses of 50 micrograms or greater of ethinyl estradiol or mestranol daily. These have largely been withdrawn from the market now, and OCPs containing 30 micrograms of ethinyl estradiol or less are not as effective (2). However, estrogen therapy with or without antiandrogen therapy continues to be used with some success in the subset of female patients with other signs of hyperandrogenemia (hirsutism, obesity, and laboratory elevations of testosterone). Androgen-dominant OCPs containing norgestral can actually worsen acne and should be avoided (14).

Side effects of this therapy are common and include nausea, weight gain, spotting, breast tenderness, and amenorrhea. Less commonly seen are a brown pigmentation of the skin (chloasma), telangiectasias, allergic reactions, and alopecia. A disadvantage is that it can take several months before noticeable improvement is obtained. Gynecomastia and decreased libido prevent its use in males.

Antiandrogens are a class of drugs that prevent androgen activity at the target sites by competing with dihydrotestosterone for the receptor. This therapy is used most commonly in women with hyperandrogenism secondary to polycystic ovarian disease and adrenal hyperactivity manifested by hirsutism and acne. Cyproterone acetate and spironolactone are two antiandrogens that have been used successfully to treat acne (31).

Excellent results are obtained in women using a combination of low-dose cyproterone acetate (2 mg per day) combined with ethinyl estradiol (35 micrograms per day). This combination was twice as effective in reducing acne lesions than OCP alone. The seborrhea improves first, but by the end of 3 months, acne lesions also regress. Beneficial effects are maintained for many months after withdrawing therapy. A higher dose of cyproterone acetate (25 to 50 mg per day) may be needed in the resistant patient who also has hirsutism. Side effects of cyproterone are uncommon but include a low frequency of headache, dizziness, nausea, and menstrual irregularity. These tend to improve with continued therapy. To date, cyproterone acetate is not available in the United States.

Spironolactone is a weak potassium-sparing aldosterone antagonist diuretic with antiandrogenic properties. It has been used alone in doses of 100 to 200 mg per day, with excellent results achieved in acne regression at 4 to 6 months. Forty percent of cases relapse 6 to 12 months after therapy. It has been used in males without development of gynecomastia and decreased libido at these doses; however, this has been seen in spironolactone therapy for other disorders. Potassium levels were not altered at this dose in subjects of one study; however, spironolactone should be reserved for patients with normal renal function. Periodic evaluation of electrolytes should be done in any patient on long-term spironolactone therapy.

Table 44.4.
Parts of the Electromagnetic Spectrum

Radiation		Wavelength (nm)
X rays		0.01–10
Ultraviolet	UVC	200–290
	UVB	290–320
	UVA	320–400
Visible	Violet	
	Blue	
	Green	400–760
	Yellow	
	Red	
Infrared	Near	
	Middle	760–1,000,000
	Far	
Microwave, radiowave		> 1,000,000

CONCLUSION

Frequently, optimal therapy of acne requires use of a combination of the topical and systemic medications discussed in this chapter. The patient may become confused about the proper use of the different therapeutic agents. When improperly used, the side effect profile increases, and optimal results are not achieved. After evaluating the patients' understanding of their treatment program, addressing any questions they may have is important to ensure compliance.

PHOTODERMATOSES

Exposure to sunlight plays an essential part in many dermatologic diseases. These effects range from acute damage, including sunburn and photosensitive skin disorders, to chronic skin damage, including photoaging and carcinogenesis.

SOLAR RADIATION

The sun emits a broad spectrum of electromagnetic radiation, but at the earth's surface, the solar spectrum consists of wavelengths between 290 and 3000 nm. These are divided into ultraviolet radiation (290 to 400 nm), visible radiation (400 to 760 nm), and near infrared radiation (wavelengths greater than 760 nm), as shown in Table 44.4. Ultraviolet radiation (UVR) is the spectrum that most frequently affects the skin and is divided into three main categories, UVC (200 to 290 nm), UVB (290 to 320 nm), and UVA (320 to 400 nm) (32).

Ultraviolet C

Wavelengths between 200 and 290 nm are referred to as UVC or germicidal radiation, and they are lethal to microorganisms. Mercury vapor lights and xenon lamps are artificial light sources that produce UVC for bacterial sterilization (32). UVC is attenuated during its passage through the atmosphere where it is largely absorbed by the

ozone layer. Increased UVC radiation has been detected at various monitoring stations due to ozone depletion. Freons (chlorofluromethanes) have been targeted as a major cause of ozone depletion; however, numerous pollutants can destroy ozone. Minor changes in the ozone and the loss of its protective effects could be damaging to plant and animal life.

Ultraviolet B

UVB radiation is often referred to as the sunburn spectrum and includes wavelengths between 290 and 300 nm. This spectrum reaches the earth's surface, and on the skin, it is largely absorbed within the epidermis. UVB is a strong inducer of erythema or sunburn and can also produce delayed pigmentation or tanning. UVB contributes to chronic sundamaged skin and skin carcinogenesis. A positive effect of UVB is its importance as a mediator of vitamin D_3 synthesis in the skin. UVB is produced by many artificial light sources for therapeutic purposes and can be blocked by window glass (33).

Ultraviolet A

Although the amount of UVA (315 to 400 nm) reaching the earth is about 10 times greater than that of UVB, it is 1000-fold less potent than UVB in producing erythema (34). In artificially high doses, it can produce erythema and immediate pigment darkening of the skin. UVA is the solar spectrum that most frequently evokes drug photoallergy, phototoxicity, and other photosensitive disorders. It is emitted by numerous therapeutic appliances used to treat dermatologic diseases and is not blocked by untinted window glass. Tanning beds, which emit UVA radiation, have been popular for many years. It has been shown that UVA can be damaging to the skin. In fact, UVA may have carcinogenic and photoaging potential similar to UVB radiation.

Acute Effects of Ultraviolet Radiation

The acute effects of UVR on the skin include sunburn, pigmentation, phototoxicity, and photoallergy.

SUNBURN

Symptoms. Erythema is the first visible sign of sunburn and may be associated with soreness, swelling, and in severe cases, blistering, nausea, and vomiting. Erythema produced by UVB occurs 12 to 24 hours after exposure, whereas UVA-induced erythema is more immediate, within the first 6 hours after exposure (34).

Etiology. UVB is the major cause of sunburn and is much more erythemogenic than UVA. Factors that may modify the effects of UVR on the skin include (1) time of day, (2) season, (3) geographic latitude, (4) clouds, (5) surface reflection, and (6) altitude. The skin type of the person is also important in the effects of UVR on the skin (35, 36).

Pathogenesis. Damage to DNA and cell membranes with

resulting elaboration of inflammatory mediators is thought to be involved in the skin's response to sun damage. Elevated histamine levels have been detected in blisters, and prostaglandins have been elevated in the skin after UVB irradiation (34).

Treatment. Generally, a sunburn patient must suffer through the course of the sunburn. Palliative therapy includes wet dressings, soothing zinc lotions, and spray formulations of topical steroids. Prostaglandin inhibitors, such as indomethacin or aspirin have been found to block the earlier phases of erythema when prostaglandin levels are elevated, but have been of little use for the more delayed effects (37).

TANNING

There are two components of tanning: (1) an immediate pigment darkening produced by UVA, which occurs immediately after radiation, and (2) delayed pigmentation, stimulated by UVB, which occurs 24 to 72 hours after exposure. Delayed pigmentation results in the formation of new melanin, which can be photoprotective (38).

PHOTOSENSITIVE DERMATOSES

Photosensitivity refers to an abnormal reaction in the skin exposed to sun. This may be provoked by a number of substances that come in contact with the skin or are taken internally, see Table 44.5. These are divided into phototoxic, photoallergic, and miscellaneous disorders.

Phototoxic and photoallergic reactions both require the presence of a photosensitizer and ultraviolet radiation to the skin. Phototoxic reactions are nonimmunologic and occur 2 to 6 hours after sun exposure, causing a sunburn type of reaction. Photoallergic reactions occur only in people previously sensitized by a photoallergen and typically occur 24 to 48 hours after sun exposure, producing an eczematoid reaction confined to sun-exposed areas, usually the face, neck, and dorsum of hands. The porphyrias represent a class of skin diseases thought to be a photoreaction to a porphyrin product of the host.

CHRONIC EFFECTS OF ULTRAVIOLET RADIATION

The chronic effects of UVR on the skin include photoaging and cancer.

PHOTOAGING

It is clear that chronic sun exposure changes the appearance of the skin. Photoaged skin is deeply wrinkled, inelastic, coarse, and leathery with associated pigment changes, freckling, telangiectasias, easy bruising, and ultimately, premalignant and malignant skin lesions. Actinic keratoses (solar keratoses) are common sun-induced lesions usually seen in patients with fair complexions who have had excessive sun exposure. They are most prominent in sun-exposed areas of the skin, especially the face and

Table 44.5.
Common Photosensitizers

Oral Photosensitizers	
Antidiabetics (sulfonylureas)	Antimicrobials
Chlorpropamide	Sulfanamides
Tolbutamide	Demeclocycline
Antihistamines	Doxycycline
Diphenhydramine *Benadryl*	Tetracycline
Diuretics	Nalidixic acid
Chlorothiazide	Furocoumarins (drugs)
Hydrochlothiazide	Methoxpsoralen
Furosemide	Trimethylpsoralen
Phenothiazines	Antineoplastic
Chlorpromazine	Dacarbazine
Perchlorperazine	Vinblastine
Promethazine	Nonsteroidals
Trifluperazine	Feldene
Thioridazine	Benoxyprofen
Laxatives	Naproxen
Bisacodyl	Ibupofen
Sweetener	Miscellaneous
Cyclamate	Amantadine
Antifungals	Quinidine
Griseofulvin	Quinine
	Amiodarone

Topical Photosensitizers	
Antiseptics, deodorants, soaps	Coal tar derivatives
Halogenated salicylanilides	Furocoumarins (plants)
Hexachlorophene	Lime, figs, celery, dill, lemon,
Antifungals	bergamot, rye, anise, mustard,
Buclosamide	parsnip, carrot, cow parsley,
Fenticlor	fennel, masterwort, angelica,
Sunscreens	buttercup
p-Aminobenzoic acid (PABA)	
Fragrances	
Musk ambrette	

hands. However, the location of actinic keratoses will vary according to the location of the sun exposure, and individuals who sun bathe can develop lesions anywhere. They are small, rough, ill-defined erythematous lesions covered by adherent scales. When these lesions are present on the lip, they are called actinic cheilitis. Actinic keratoses and actinic cheilitis may develop into squamous cell carcinoma in a small percentage of patients.

PHOTOCARCINOGENESIS

It is well documented that chronic sun exposure may lead to squamous cell and basal cell skin cancers. These are found more frequently in sun-exposed areas and are enhanced by the total exposure to UVR. Squamous cell cancers are most commonly shallow ulcers with a raised border, but they may be red, raised, scaling lesions. Basal cell carcinomas are more often nodules on the skin with a pearly, rolled border with prominent telangiectatic vessels on the surface, and they may ulcerate.

The risk of malignant melanoma appears to be

Table 44.6.
Sunscreen Chemicals Used in the United States

Chemical
  UVA Absorbers
    Benzophenones (UVA and UVB)
      Oxybenzone
      Dioxybenzone
      Sulisobenzone
    Avobenzone (Parsol 1789)
      Butylmethoxydibenzoylmethane
    Anthranilates
  UVB Absorbers
    PABA
      p-Aminobenzoic acid
    PABA esters
      Octyldimethyl PABA (Padimate-O)
      Glyceryl PABA
    Cinnamates
    Salicylates
Physical (UVA and UVB)
  Red Petrolatum
  Titanium dioxide
  Magnesium oxide
  Zinc oxide
  Magnesium salicate
  Ferric chloride

---

increased by intermittent severe sunburn, especially if this occurs during childhood (39). Malignant melanomas may have different clinical presentations, but any mole that appears to have a blue-black color or variations in color, irregular borders, or a rapid change in size, should be evaluated by a dermatologist because these skin cancers can have a grave prognosis if not adequately and promptly treated. The best treatment for most skin cancers is surgical excision.

Photoprotection. The goal of treatment of the photodermatotoses is to block one or more steps in their pathogenesis. Although avoidance of sun is an obvious solution, this is not always feasible. Protective clothing, including a broad-brimmed hat, will reduce UV exposure. Sunscreens are advocated to prevent sunburn and protect against acute and chronic photodamage.

Sunscreens. Sunscreens are topical preparations that block the effect of ultraviolet radiation on the skin by absorbing, reflecting, or scattering UVR. They are divided into physical sunscreens, which are usually opaque products that reflect and scatter UVR, and chemical sunscreens, which contain agents that absorb UVR, as shown in Table 44.6.

Physical Sunscreens. Physical sunscreens are usually opaque and reflect or scatter UVR. They contain iron oxide, titanium dioxide, talc, zinc oxide, ferric chloride, or ichthamnol. They are advantageous in that they absorb a broad spectrum of UVR; however, many people find them cosmetically unacceptable. The recent addition of coloring

agents has made them more pleasing, but they can discolor clothes. They are not easily washed off, but they may melt with prolonged heat, requiring repeated application (40).

Chemical Sunscreens. The chemical sunscreens contain agents that absorb ultraviolet radiation. They may contain agents that absorb UVA or UVB or a combination of agents to give a broad spectrum of coverage.

UVB Absorbers.. *PABA Agents* One of the most widely used chemical agents that absorbs UVB is para-amino benzoic acid (PABA) and its esters. PABA penetrates the stratum corneum of the skin where it attaches to proteins, and thus it is not easily washed off after swimming or bathing. It should be applied at least 1 hour before sun exposure to allow adequate time for PABA binding to the skin.

PABA can cause irritation and hypersensitivity reactions. The PABA esters have a lower potential for allergic or irritant reactions and staining. Currently, the most frequently used ester is octyl-dimethyl-paba, also known as padimate −0 (41).

Cross-reactivity between PABA and sulfonylureas, sulfonamides, thiazides, and parapheneldiamine has been shown, and patients with sensitivity to these medications should avoid PABA-containing sunscreens (42).

Cinnamates. The cinnamates have been increasingly used in the United States for UVB absorption. They have a lower potential for hypersensitivity than the PABA agents and are nonstaining. However, they do not bind the stratum corneum and are easily removed with water.

Salicylates. The salicylates are UVB absorbers and have been ingredients of sunscreens since the 1920s.

UVA Absorbers. The most widely used UVA absorbers are the benzophenone products such as oxybenzone and dioxybenzone. A new compound butylmethoxydibenzoylmethane (Parsol–1789) has been found to be a more effective UVA sunscreen than oxybenzone and has been approved in one sunscreen in the United States (40).

Sun Protection Factor. The concept of sun protection factor (SPF) was developed by Greiter of Austria (43) and was adopted by the FDA in 1978 (44). Currently, manufacturers specify the SPF on the labels of sunscreens. The SPF is a quantitative measure of the product to absorb UVB only. The SPF is the ratio of the dose of UVB energy required to produce minimal erythema (MED) on sunscreen-protected skin compared to the dose of energy required to produce minimal erythema on skin without sunscreen protection (44).

$$SPF = \frac{MED \text{ of sunscreen-protected skin}}{MED \text{ of nonprotected skin}}$$

SPF ranges from 2 (minimal protection) to 40 or more, for ultra protection. Most of the sunscreens with SPFs greater than 30 contain at least three different sunscreen agents or greater concentrations of the agents to achieve increased photoprotection; however, this gives them an increased risk of allergic and irritant reactions (41).

There is controversy concerning whether superpotent sunscreens are needed. In a study by Kaidbey, sunscreens with SPF of 30 prevented sunburn cell induction in the epidermis when compared with SPF of 15, thus suggesting an advantage of 30 in preventing photodamage (45). The SPFs of sunscreens are tested indoors and may vary when used outdoors.

Currently, there are no standardized guidelines for labeling the effectiveness of products in UVA protection. *Quick Tanning Lotions.* Sunless tanning lotions are becoming more popular to obtain color without sun exposure. These products contain 3 to 5% dihydroxyacetone (DHA) or 0.25% 1–4–dihydroxynaphthoquinone (lawsone). These compounds have no effect on melanocytes, do not stimulate melanin production, and do not give photoprotection unless combined with a traditional sunscreen. DHA becomes oxidized and polymerized to an orange-brown color that adheres to the skin and gives a tan appearance for 7 to 10 days.

Substantivity. The substantivity of a sunscreen is a measure of the ability of a sunscreen to adhere to the skin and remain effective despite swimming, bathing, or sweating. A sunscreen is water resistant if it maintains SPF after two 20-minute immersions in a swimming pool, and it is waterproof if it withstands four such immersions (46).

Recommendations. There is strong evidence that sun exposure leads to photoaging and skin cancers, and sun protection should be stressed in the young, in people with fair skin, and in people prone to sun-sensitive disorders. Although the simplest and cheapest way to avoid sun exposure would be to avoid outdoor exposure during hours of intense sunlight (10:00 AM to 3:00 PM) and to wear protective clothing and hats, this is not always feasible, and in these circumstances, sunscreens that provide maximal protection need to be recommended (40).

In elderly people, it had been thought that the use of sunscreen is more questionable because sunscreens block ultraviolet-induced vitamin D synthesis in the skin and may cause an elderly person to be more prone to vitamin D deficiency and thus bone fractures. Recent studies have shown this to be false. Marks and colleagues found that sufficient sunlight is received, most likely through both the sunscreen itself and the lack of total skin coverage at all times, to allow adequate vitamin D production (47).

Systemic Photoprotective Agents. There is currently no effective, safe systemic photoprotective agent that would circumvent the shortcomings of topical sunscreens. Several agents have shown improvement in specific photosensitive diseases, but they are not as effective as general photoprotectors.

Antimalarials. The aminoquinolines (chloroquine, hydroxychloroquine, quinacrine) are occasionally used to treat several light-sensitive diseases, including systemic lupus erythematosus, polymorphous light eruption, solar urticaria, and porphyria cutanea tarda.

Chloroquine has been shown to have many diverse effects, including enzyme inhibition; protein, DNA, and melanin binding; and antihistaminic and antiinflammatory effects. It is also an effective absorber of UV light; however, the exact mechanisms of action in the photosensitive disorders are not known (48). The toxicities of the antimalarials are multiple, and they are not considered the first choice for treatment of the photosensitive disorders. They should be used only after other therapies have failed, and they should be used with close supervision.

Ocular toxicity is the greatest problem with the aminoquinolines. They can cause an irreversible retinopathy that is dose related. To minimize the risk of ocular toxicity, the dose of chloroquine should not exceed 250 mg per day or hydroxychloroquine 400 mg per day (in a patient weighing more than 100 pounds). An ophthalmologic examination should be required before therapy and every 4 to 6 months during therapy. If any changes in vision occur, such as blurred vision or flashes of light, the drug should be stopped until the patient can be examined by an ophthalmologist (49).

Other reported side effects include headache, irritability, toxic psychosis, worsening of psoriasis, and leukopenia. They can cause a blue-black pigmentation of the skin, and quinacrine can give a yellow discoloration to the skin. The antimalarials are regarded as teratogenic and should be avoided during pregnancy (50).

Carotenoids. The carotenoids can exert a photoprotective effect in humans and chlorophyl-containing organisms. Beta-carotene has been found to absorb light in the visible spectrum (360 to 500 nm); however, some think its photoprotective effect is due to its ability to quench single oxygen-derived photochemical reactions (48).

Beta-carotene has been effective in the treatment of erythropoietic protoporphyria, a rare hereditary photosensitive disease due to a defect in porphyrin metabolism; however, its usefulness in other photosensitive diseases has been marginal. Oral ingestion should be regulated to keep a blood level between 600 and 800 µg/ml, which usually corresponds to an adult dose of 150 mg (48). The main side effect of beta-carotene is a slight orange discoloration of the skin, most notable on the palms and soles. Results are not expected until 1 or 2 months of therapy.

Treatment of Photodamage. Although sunscreens and sun avoidance are important to prevent photodamage, once chronic photodamage has occurred, treatment that may obviate future surgical intervention may be needed. Recently, several products have been used to treat photodamaged skin.

Topical Tretinoin. Although topical tretinoin is currently not approved by the FDA to treat photodamaged skin, several studies have supported its beneficial effects. Weiss and colleagues (51) and Leyden and colleagues (52) have reported improvement in fine wrinkling, coarse wrinkling, and hyperpigmented lesions in patients treated with topical tretinoin.

For treatment of photodamaged skin or precancerous lesions, topical tretinoin is usually initiated at a low strength (.025% cream or .1% cream) and applied at bedtime, avoiding areas close to the eyes. The most significant side effect is irritation, which is readily treated by withholding treatment for 1 to 2 days and decreasing the dose or changing to alternate-day therapy. The patient should use sunscreens during the day (53). This treatment should be avoided in pregnancy since it is considered nonessential.

Remember that experience with topical tretinoids is limited, and their long-term effects are unknown. Whether their effects will persist past treatment is unanswered. Their use should be only in motivated patients who are committed to future sun protection and sun avoidance.

Alpha Hydroxyacids. Alpha hydroxyacids and alpha keto acids, including glycolic, pyruvic, and lactic acids, are powerful keratolytic agents and have been used to treat actinic keratosis and wrinkles with some success (54). There are many differing strengths of these acids and differing combinations that produce varying degrees of epidermal damage.

Topical Fluorouracil. Topical 5-fluorouracil is an anticancer agent that has been used to treat many precancerous lesions and dermatoses. It is most often used to treat severe actinic keratoses.

5-fluorouracil (FU) is a structural analog of thiamine and blocks the synthesis of DNA. Cells that are rapidly growing, such as actinic keratoses, require more DNA and thus accumulate larger amounts of lethal FU, resulting in their death (22). Normal skin is much less affected by the fluorouracil (55).

Fluorouracil is available as a 1% cream or solution, 2% solution, and 5% cream or solution. It is usually applied twice daily for 2 to 4 weeks depending on the response. The response includes an inflammatory phase, followed by redness, burning, and oozing, followed by erosion or ulceration that occurs over 1 to 3 weeks depending on the site and strength used. Treatment is stopped when ulceration and crusting appear. The patient must be well informed of this expected response, or there will be many phone calls. Oozing and erosion are expected, and information pamphlets with pictures, which are provided by pharmaceutical companies, should be given to the patient. If applied with the fingers, the hands should be washed immediately afterward, or gloves can be used during application. Fluorouracil should not be applied too close to the eyes.

Topical 5-fluorouracil is a very effective treatment of actinic keratoses, gives good cosmetic results, and may eliminate the need for surgery. Side effects include an irritant dermatitis, which is difficult to distinguish from the desired effect of 5-FU. If severe, the treatment may have to be interrupted and lubricants or topical steroids used. During therapy, the redness and oozing may be a cosmetic embarrassment, and patients should be forewarned of this.

The most frequently encountered local reactions are pain, pruritus, hyperpigmentation, and burning at the site of application. Other rare side effects include photosensitivity, concealing a cancer, nail changes, telangiectasias, and scarring (55). Actinic keratoses that do not respond to treatment should be biopsied.

Overall, when used with discretion and with consistent follow-up examinations, 5-fluorouracil is an effective and economic treatment for actinic keratoses and gives good cosmetic results.

Masoprocol. Topical masoprocol cream comes in a 10% formulation that has antiproliferative activity against keratinocytes and is reported to be effective in the treatment of solar keratosis. It has not been on the market as long as 5-FU. It should be applied twice a day to the area of solar damage for 28 days. There is a high incidence (10%) of allergic contact dermatitis to this product.

CONCLUSION

In summary, a broad range of skin disorders are induced or aggravated by the sun. These include sunburn, tanning, phototoxic reactions, photoallergic drug reactions, cutaneous changes in lupus erythematosus, photoaging, precancerous lesions, and skin cancers. These usually occur on sun-exposed skin, which should be a clue to their recognition by the clinician, who can then proceed with an evaluation to determine the exact etiology and appropriate treatment.

WARTS

Clinical Features

Warts, also known as verrucae, are caused by human papillomaviruses (HPV). They are commonly classified by their clinical appearance and location. This classification includes verruca vulgaris or common wart; myrmecia wart or deep palmoplantar wart; superficial, mosaic-type palmoplantar wart; verruca plana or flat wart; anogenital wart or condyloma acuminata and epidermodysplasia verruciformis. Applying 5% acetic acid for 5 minutes may help reveal inapparent lesions (56).

VERRUCA VULGARIS (COMMON WART)

Approximately 70% of warts are verruca vulgares, or common warts, which are circumscribed, firm, rough, hyperkeratotic papules that may appear singly or grouped on any skin surface. They occur most commonly on the dorsum of hands and fingers and on knees of children. Warts can form at sites of trauma, a property known as the Koebner phenomenon. Although they are generally asymptomatic, periungual warts may become fissured, inflamed, tender, and cause local dystrophic nails. Occasionally, warts consist of threadlike, thin, horny projections. This variant, called verruca filiformis, or filiform wart, occurs commonly on the face and scalp.

MYRMECIA WART (DEEP PALMOPLANTAR WART)

Myrmecia, meaning anthill, are deep, dome-shaped nodules often covered with a thick callus and occur most commonly on the palms and soles. They are usually associated with inflammation such as swelling, redness,and considerable tenderness. Although they can be multiple, they generally do not coalesce. Approximately 24% of warts occur on the plantar surfaces, including both the deep and superficial plantar warts.

SUPERFICIAL, MOSAIC-TYPE PALMOPLANTAR WART

Superficial palmoplantar warts commonly form at points of pressure, especially the heel and the midmetatarsal area, causing pain with weight bearing. They have a rough, hyperkeratotic surface usually studded with punctate black dots ("seeds"), representing thrombosed capillaries, and a firm, horny peripheral rim. Several lesions may coalesce to form a large plaque, known as a mosaic wart.

Superficial palmoplantar warts may be difficult to distinguish from corns and calluses. Shaving off the keratotic surface may aid in differentiating the two entities; warts have a soft central core with black or bleeding points instead of a horny central core of corn.

VERRUCA PLANA (FLAT WART)

Flat warts, also known as juvenile warts, are smooth, slightly elevated, flat-topped papules that are usually less than 5 mm in diameter. They may be flesh-colored, gray, or brown and are usually multiple on the face, hands, and legs of children. Occasionally, men who shave their beards and women who shave their legs may develop numerous flat warts in the respective areas as a result of autoinoculation. Verruca plana make up approximately 35% of warts.

ANOGENITAL WARTS (CONDYLOMA ACUMINATA)

Condyloma acuminata consist of soft, verrucous or flat papules that can coalesce as cauliflowerlike masses. Malignant degeneration can occur, especially on mucosal surfaces such as the cervix. Prior to treating external warts in the anogenital region, it is important to find and treat internal adjacent condyloma (do complete vaginal exam or proctoscopy if indicated).

EPIDERMODYSPLASIA VERRUCIFORMIS

Epidermodysplasia verruciformis is a rare, lifelong, persistent disorder characterized by widespread flat warts with a tendency to coalesce into plaques and tinea versicolorlike lesions. An autosomal recessive inheritance pattern has been suggested, and the disease usually begins in childhood. Lesions almost never regress spontaneously, and

Table 44.7.
HPV Types and Their Clinical Associations

HPV Types	Most Common Clinical Lesions	Less Common Lesions	Oncogenic Potential
1	Deep palmoplantar warts	Common warts	
2, 4	Common warts	Superficial, mosaic-type palmoplantar warts, anogenital warts	
3, 10	Flat warts		
5, 8, 9	Epidermodysplasia verruciformis		Yes
6, 11	Anogenital warts, cervical condyloma	Common warts	Yes
7	Common warts in butchers		
16, 18	Cervical condyloma	Anogenital warts	Yes

approximately one-third of patients develop skin cancers in sun-exposed lesions (57). The lifelong HPV infection in these patients is thought to be due to an altered immunity. A depressed cell-mediated immunity is found in 90% of these patients (58). This immune defect may be primary, perhaps leading to the predisposition of HPV infection and oncogenic transformation by these viruses, or it may be secondary to an overwhelming disseminated, chronic infection.

Extracutaneous, mucosal HPV infections are also recognized. Common warts and condyloma acuminata may occur on other mucosal surfaces such as the oral cavity and the larynx, which may lead to respiratory distress.

Human papillomaviruses have been found in other entities such as focal oral hyperplasia in American Indian children and oral hairy leukoplakia.

Etiology

The papillomaviruses, which are members of the family Papovaviridae, contain double-stranded, circular, supercoiled DNA enclosed in an icosahedral capsid of 72 capsomers without an envelope. The viral particle has a molecular weight of approximately 5×10^6 and is 55 nm in diameter. With the use of DNA hybridization, it became possible to classify the papillomaviruses into different types. The criteria is that if two isolates have less than 50% homology by DNA hybridization, they are considered two different types and are designated numerically. To date, 55 HPV types have been isolated, and each type tends to be associated with different clinical variants. Table 44.7 illustrates different HPV types correlated with common clinical lesions. Potential oncogenic transformation usually occurs in HPV types 5, 8, and 9 associated with epidermodysplasia verruciformis, and HPV types 6, 11, 16, and 18 associated with anogenital and cervical condyloma. The incubation period of HPV is variable and ranges from 1 to 20 months. The mode of transmission of cutaneous warts is most likely by both direct contact and via fomites. It is thought that HPV infection is acquired by inoculation of the epidermis via breaks in the skin. Trauma thus plays a role and may explain the usual distribution of common warts on the hands, fingers, and knees of children. Autoinoculation of the virus may result in new lesions by direct contact. Anogenital warts are generally sexually transmitted with an approximately 60% chance of infectivity within 9 months in a single sexual contact (59). The immunologic state of the exposed individuals is also an important predisposing factor. More than 40% of kidney transplant patients with impaired cell-mediated immunity may develop warts (58).

Epidemiology

The prevalence of warts in the general population is unknown. However, they occur most frequently in children and young adults, in whom the incidence approaches 10% (57). In 1982, it was estimated that approximately 4 million people presented to physicians for nonvenereal warts (56). The peak incidence of warts is between the ages of 12 and 16. Anogenital warts, on the other hand, are the most common viral sexually transmitted disease diagnosed in the United States. The annual incidence of these warts is 0.5 to 1.0% in young adults, with the age of onset ranging from late teens to early thirties (60). From 1966 to 1981, there has been a fivefold increase in the number of reported cases of anogenital warts in the United States (57). The figures from a study covering between 1975 and 1978 estimated an annual incidence rate of 106.5 per 100,000 (57). HPV infection is also increased in patients with impaired cell-mediated immunity as previously mentioned.

Histopathology

The histopathologic features of warts generally consist of acanthosis (thickening of the stratum malpighii), papillomatosis (irregular undulation of the epidermis), hyperkeratosis (thickening of the horny layer), intranuclear inclusions, and parakeratosis (retention of nuclei in the horny layer). The distinguishing features of verruca vulgaris include large keratinocytes with a pyknotic nucleus surrounded by a perinuclear clear halo, referred to as koilocytes, located in the upper stratum malpighii; vertical tiers of parakeratosis overlying the crests of papillomatous elevations; and foci of clumped keratohyalin granules in the intervening valleys. Anogenital warts have similar features but lack a granular layer since they occur on or near a mucosal surface. Although flat warts have diffuse koilocytes in the upper epidermis, they tend to lack papillomatosis and parakeratosis. Immunocytochemical studies have detected viral DNA, antigens, and mature virions in keratinocytes at and above the stratum granulosum. Southern

Table 44.8.
Treatment Modalities for Warts

Chemical destruction
  Acids
  Formalin
  Glutaraldehyde
  Cantharidin
Physical destruction
  Cryotherapy
  Electrosurgery
  Surgical excision
  CO_2 laser
Chemotherapeutic agents
  Podophyllin
  Podophyllotoxin
  5-Fluorouracil
  Bleomycin
  Interferons
  Retinoids
Immunotherapy
  Dinitrochlorobenzene (DNCB)
  Squaric acid dibutylester (SADBE)
  Diphenylcyclopropenone
  Inosine pranobex

Blot hybridization may be used to identify specific HPV types.

Treatment

The approach to the treatment of warts depends on the patient's age, cooperation, immunologic status, previous treatments, and the location, number, size, duration, and type of the lesions. Studies have shown spontaneous regression of warts in two-thirds of children within two years although new warts may continue to appear (58). All warts should be treated to prevent spreading to others and on the patients themselves. Sexual partners of patients with anogenital warts should be examined and treated appropriately. During the treatment process, the patient should be instructed to avoid sexual contact or use condoms. Therapeutic options can be divided into broad categories: chemical destructive therapy, including acids, formalin, glutaraldehyde, and cantharidin; physical destructive therapy, including cryotherapy, electrosurgery, surgical excision, and CO_2 laser; chemotherapeutic agents, including podophyllin, podophyllotoxin, 5-fluorouracil, bleomycin, interferons, and retinoids; and immunotherapy (see Table 44.8). In general, most forms of wart treatment can be expected to have a 60 to 70% cure rate. Patients should be told that warts may need several treatments, often over a period of several weeks to months. It is often useful to pare the wart down prior to using many of the aforementioned modalities. In rare instances, a biopsy should be done to help distinguish benign warts from other verrucous-appearing lesions, such as squamous cell carcinoma, deep fungal infections, and verrucous carcinoma.

ACIDS

Salicylic acid in concentrations ranging from 10 to 60% can be used in paints, pastes, gels, or plasters. It is frequently used for common and palmoplantar warts, including periungual warts. Salicylic acid preparations can be used on all sites of the skin except the face and anogenital area. Other acids are frequently used in combination with salicylic acid. A popular preparation is equal parts of salicylic acid and lactic acid in four parts of flexible collodion. Monochloroacetic acid crystals compounded with 60% salicylic acid has been found to be effective for plantar warts (61). Weekly applications of 50 to 85% trichloroacetic acid and, less commonly, bichloroacetic acid may be effective for anogenital warts when podophyllin is contraindicated; this acid does not need to be washed off, as does podophyllin. Trichloroacetic acid may be compounded with salicylic acid for the treatment of common and palmoplantar warts.

In general, the acids act as keratolytic agents by physically destroying the keratin layer. Paints are most commonly used and are usually a collodion-based liquid. Treatment consists of soaking the wart in warm water for at least 5 minutes, after which the wart is pared down as far as possible without causing bleeding. A pumice stone may be used if necessary. Next, a drop of the acid solution is applied to just cover the wart and allowed to dry to a white film. The wart is then kept covered for 24 hours, and the procedure is repeated daily until the wart is gone. Salicylic acid plasters are especially suited for the treatment of multiple, mosaic plantar warts. After the lesion is pared and moistened with a drop of warm water, the plaster is cut to the size of the wart and applied for 24 to 48 hours, followed by repeated cycles until resolution of the wart. A 40% salicylic acid adhesive plaster is a commonly used preparation. Recently, a topical transdermal 15% salicylic acid patch has been developed to provide continuous passive diffusion of the acid under occlusion (62). The acid is suspended in a karaya gum patch, which acts as a self-adhesive and enhances absorption. Nightly application of this transdermal patch is repeated until the wart is gone.

Recently, the FDA has issued a monograph mandating that all salicylic acid-based wart therapy products be changed to nonprescription status with the maximum of 17% concentration of salicylic acid (63). Lactic acid is no longer allowed as an active agent in over-the-counter products. Pharmacists, however, may compound these acids using a higher concentration as necessary.

FORMALIN

Formalin preparations can be used for plantar or multiple warts. This chemical acts on the affected tissue by its destructive properties. Three to 10% of formalin in aqueous solution can be used to soak the pared wart for 10 to 30 minutes daily. The surrounding normal skin can be protected with petroleum jelly. Formalin 25% in hydrophilic petrolatum has also been used as a daily application. A potential complication of formalin treatment is the development of allergic contact dermatitis.

GLUTARALDEHYDE

Topical application of 10% glutaraldehyde may be less irritating for palmoplantar warts than formalin preparations. A recent study in Japan (64) found a 20% aqueous solution of unbuffered glutaraldehyde to be effective in patients with resistant warts. Glutaraldehyde was applied once a day for 12 weeks. Results showed 18 of 25 (72%) were cured, 5 of which responded after only 4 weeks of treatment. Pigmentary changes were noted immediately after application; however, after healing, no evidence of scarring or permanent pigmentary changes were noted.

CANTHARIDIN

Cantharidin is an extract of the green blister beetle that acts by destroying the epidermis and has the ability to dissociate oxidative phosphorylation. A solution containing 0.7% cantharidin in acetone or flexible collodion may be effective in treating common and plantar warts. The vehicle is applied to the pared wart, allowed to dry, and then covered with adhesive tape for 24 hours, after which the process may be repeated weekly. It is not unusual for warts to recur in a doughnut-shaped ring around the original treated wart. It is best used for plantar warts.

CRYOTHERAPY

Although topical medications have the advantage of being painless, cryotherapy is considered more effective, particularly for anogenital warts, with cure rates up to 90% (65). It is a popular treatment for many types of warts, including common, palmoplantar, flat, and anogenital warts, especially in pregnant women. Recently, the Centers of Disease Control stated that cryotherapy is first-line treatment for condyloma acuminata (65). Cure rates are similar to those of electrosurgery, but cryosurgery is preferred since it requires no local anesthesia. Liquid nitrogen (boiling point −196° Celsius) is the most commonly used vehicle, but solid carbon dioxide may also be effective. Cryotherapy causes cell injury by intracellular ice formation, cell shrinkage, and anoxia by intravascular thrombosis (67).

Before treatment, the wart should be pared down. A cotton-tipped applicator with liquid nitrogen is applied to the wart to create a white "ice ball" extending 1 to 2 mm beyond the visible wart. This process usually takes about 20 to 30 seconds, after which the lesion is allowed to thaw. The procedure is then repeated a few times depending on the size and site of the wart. The object is to produce epidermal necrosis with the subsequent formation of a small blister. The lesion then dries and peels off together with the wart. This regimen may require multiple treatments at 1- to

3-week intervals. A common method is a liquid nitrogen spray that delivers liquid nitrogen via a spray canister rather than a cotton applicator. Carbon dioxide can be obtained from sparklet cylinders and mixed with acetone to form a slush. Freezing techniques using a cotton-tipped applicator are similar to those of liquid nitrogen.

ELECTROSURGERY

Electosurgery is fairly common, but disadvantages include the need for local anesthesia, pain, and greater risk of scarring and infection. Cure rates are generally similar to those of cryotherapy (68). The treatment consists of low-current electrodesiccation followed by gentle curettage of the wart to minimize scarring. It should be used only on small warts.

SURGICAL EXCISION

In some series, simple surgical excision of anogenital warts has been reported to be more effective than podophyllin application (69). However, recurrence rates have been reported to be 20 to 30% in other series (67).

CO₂ LASER

Cure rates with the carbon dioxide laser are up to 90%, but disadvantages include the high expense and the possible necessity for general anesthesia and presence of HPV in the laser smoke (70). It is generally reserved for treating multiple, large, treatment-resistant anogenital, meatal, urethral, or vaginal condylomas.

PODOPHYLLIN

For many years, podophyllin or podophyllum resin has been used in the treatment of anogenital warts. It is a nonhomogeneous, unstable extract obtained from the plants Podophyllum peltatum (found in North America) and Podophyllum emodi (found in India, Tibet, and Afghanistan). The resin has four active agents, or lignans, including podophyllotoxin, 4-dimethylpodophyllotoxin, alpha-peltatin, and beta-peltatin. The maximal active content is about 40% in P. emodi, which consists predominantly of podophyllotoxin and trace amounts of 4-dimethylpodophyllotoxin. P. peltatum has a maximal lignan content of approximately 20% and consists of varying quantities of podophyllotoxin and the two peltatins. Podophyllin is most frequently used as a 20 to 25% solution in compound tincture of benzoin although other vehicles have been used such as mineral oil or ethanol. The resin should be stored at room temperature and be replaced at least every 2 years or earlier if it contains precipitates.

Available studies indicate a variable cure rate ranging from 22 to 98% (66). Podophyllin provides the best results in patients with external, moist condylomas that are relatively new, small, and few in numbers. Before treatment, warts should be wiped dry. Podophyllin is then applied to the wart with a sterile cotton-tipped applicator, from which the excess solution is first wrung out. It is recommended that the area of treatment should not exceed 3 cm in diameter and the chemical be kept off the normal surrounding skin to avoid local and systemic side effects (56). Patients are instructed to wash off the podophyllin 4 hours after application with rubbing alcohol or soap and water. The treatment can be repeated at intervals of 1 to 2 weeks and should not exceed 1.0 ml per week (71).

Podophyllin acts as a strong irritant and arrests mitoses in metaphase by interfering with microtubule formation and causing subsequent epithelial cell death (72). After the application, an acute inflammatory reaction followed by necrosis usually develops over the treated area. Local irritation may range from erythema, burning, edema, pain, and ulceration. Uncircumcised men may occasionally develop balanitis and phimosis (72). Severe chemical burns, necrosis, scarring, and fistula formation have been reported with improper use of podophyllin. Thus, podophyllin should not be used as a home remedy but should be applied only by physicians since local as well as systemic side effects can potentially be severe.

Systemic toxicity of podophyllin has been reported in the literature and usually occurs when the chemical has been applied in large volumes over an extensive area of the skin or has been allowed to be in contact with the skin for a long period. Although podophyllin toxicity is multisystemic, neurologic manifestations are the hallmark features and may include mental status change, peripheral neuropathy, seizures, psychosis, and coma. Other clinical presentations include fever, nausea, vomiting, respiratory stimulation, tachycardia, renal failure, ileus, pancytopenia, leukocytosis, marrow suppression, and death (73). Podophyllin is contraindicated in pregnancy. It is teratogenic in experimental animals, and intrauterine death has been reported following topical application of podophyllin in women (72). To minimize systemic absorption, podophyllin should not be used in the oral mucosa, vagina, cervix, rectum, urethra, or in infants. Alcohol consumption should be avoided for several hours after treatment since alcohol may facilitate absorption of podophyllin.

PODOPHYLLOTOXIN

Podophyllotoxin, a new treatment modality for anogenital warts, is the purified and most biologically active agent of podophyllin. Several clinical studies have reported the effectiveness of 0.5% podophyllotoxin on penile warts by self-application. Von Krogh reported a regimen of 0.5% podophyllotoxin applied by the patient twice daily for 3 consecutive days, resulting in a cure rate of 49% (74). In a subsequent study in which the same preparation was applied by the patient twice daily for 4 and 5 days, he found no significant improvement in efficacy, but an increase in local irritation (74). Edwards and colleagues compared

0.5% podophyllotoxin applied to penile warts by the patient for 3 consecutive days with a 4-day drug-free interval versus 20% podophyllin treatment by a physician once a week (75). Each of these regimens was repeated for up to 6 weeks or cycles. He found an 88% cure rate in the self-treated patients versus 63% in the podophyllin-treated patients. Beutner and colleagues reported a placebo-controlled trial with two to four treatment cycles of 0.5% podophyllotoxin twice daily for 3 days; he noted an 82% clearance in the treated patients versus 13% in the placebo group (74). In these trials, no systemic reactions were reported, and local irritation was considerably less than that induced by podophyllin. Therefore, topical podophyllotoxin is a new, relatively safe, efficacious, cost-effective treatment for anogenital warts that can be used as a home remedy.

5-FLUOROURACIL

5-fluorouracil is a fluorinated pyrimidine antimetabolite that interferes with the synthesis of DNA and to a lesser degree inhibits the formation of RNA. When applied topically, it has a better penetration in abnormal skin than in normal skin and has a direct immunostimulatory effect on the affected epidermis (76). It is used most frequently for the management of urethral and vaginal condylomas, but reports of its effectiveness have also been observed in common, plantar, flat, and external genital warts. It has been used as a topical 1 to 5% cream. The patient can apply 5% 5-fluorouracil cream to the distal urethra with a cotton applicator after urination. Treatment of proximal urethral warts should be performed by a urologist. Applications four times a day for up to 2 weeks may be necessary (65). Intraurethral suppositories can be made by a pharmacist (70). Application of 5% 5-fluorouracil cream to penile warts for 8 weeks has resulted in an 84% response rate (76). Daily 5% 5-fluorouracil cream application at bedtime for 5 days may be effective for vaginal warts. Gynecologists use 5-fluorouracil cream prophylactically to minimize recurrences after laser surgery (77). A topical 1% solution of 5-fluorouracil in 70% alcohol applied twice daily for several weeks has also been used for condylomas (78). Because 5-fluorouracil can cause local inflammation, the vulva and urethra can be protected with zinc oxide or petrolatum.

For common, plantar, and flat warts, 1 to 5% 5-fluorouracil cream or ointment can be used as a single agent daily on a wart covered with a waterproof plaster, or it may be compounded with other acids (79). Five percent 5-fluorouracil compounded with salicylic acid has been reported to be effective (56). Alpha hydroxyacids, particularly pyruvic and glycolic acids, have been combined with 5-fluorouracil (54). 5-fluorouracil powder dissolved in pyruvic acid to achieve a 1 to 2% solution can be applied to the pared wart with an artist camel hair brush until the patient feels a burning sensation. Adhesive tape is then applied over the wart for a few hours, after which the chemical is washed off. The procedure may be repeated in 2 to 3 weeks if necessary. A 0.5% 5-fluorouracil in pyruvic acid:ethanol 1:1 preparation can be used as a home remedy. The patient applies the solution two to three times daily for 2 consecutive days, after which the cycle may be repeated in 1 week if needed.

BLEOMYCIN

Bleomycin is an antibiotic produced by Streptomyces verticillis with antiviral, antibacterial, and antitumor activity. It binds to DNA and prevents thymidine incorporation and single-stranded scission in DNA. Intralesional bleomycin has been reported to be effective as an alternative form of therapy, particularly for recalcitrant palmoplantar and periungual warts (80). A tuberculin syringe with a #30 gauge needle is used to inject 0.1 ml to 1.0 ml of 1 U/ml solution of bleomycin in saline, depending on the size of the wart. The object is to inject intralesionally so that the entire wart blanches. Local pain, erythema, and swelling may persist for 1 to 2 days after treatment. The wart usually blackens, thromboses, forms a eschar, and sloughs off several days after the injection. Cure rates of one or two treatments with a 2-week interval have been reported to be greater than 80% (80). Complications usually from intralesional or perilesional infiltration of bleomycin may include extensive necrosis, permanent nail dystrophy, sclerodermoid changes, joint destruction, and subcutaneous abscesses (67).

Recently, intralesional bleomycin sulfate therapy using a bifurcated needle puncture technique resulted in a 90% cure rate with a single treatment (81). The procedure consists of soaking the wart for 10 minutes in warm water, after which the lesion is anesthetized with 2% lidocaine without epinephrine. Bleomycin sulfate solution (1 U/ml in normal saline) is placed onto the wart surface (0.02 ml/5 mm^2). A sterile, stainless-steel, bifurcated needle, originally made for small pox vaccination, is punctured rapidly through the base of the wart about 40 times per 5 mm^2 area of the lesion. The warts usually resolve in about 3 weeks. In reducing the amount of bleomycin introduced into the skin, this bifurcated needle carries only 0.001 of a unit and minimizes bleomycin from penetrating into the dermis. This type of treatment can be performed on many types of warts, except large condylomas, filiform warts, and warts on the loose skin of the penis and eyelid. It is especially suitable for paronychial warts.

INTERFERONS

Interferons are glycoproteins with antiviral activity made by most cells. Current studies show that interferons used alone or in combination with other conventional therapy are effective (82–89). All three types of interferons, alpha, beta, and gamma, have been shown to be effective intralesionally, subcutaneously, and intramuscularly. Topical treatment has been studied, but with disappointing results (82). Interferon has an antiproliferative activity that may slow the rapidly dividing keratinocytes in warts, and its immunomodulatory effect may enhance the host's response to HPV infection (57). Most of the studies have indicated its effectiveness in condyloma acuminata. Intralesional injection of condyloma with 1×10^6 IU of recombinant alfa-2b interferon three times weekly for 3 weeks resulted in a 36% cure rate in one study (83) and 53% in another (84). A similar study achieved a higher response rate of 62% with intralesional injection of 1×10^6 IU of interferon-alfa weekly for up to 8 weeks (85). Systemic administration of interferon either subcutaneously or intramuscularly in the treatment of genital warts has also been shown to be effective. Dose comparison studies of systemic interferon have shown that intramuscular injection of 5×10^6 IU/mm^2 of interferon-alfa for 28 days followed by three times weekly for 2 weeks is highly effective, but the high incidence of systemic side effects make this dose unacceptable; low-dose intramuscular injection of 1×10^6 IU/mm^2 for 14 days followed by three times weekly for 1 month appears to be the best tolerated and yet effective regimen (86).

Interferon-beta 1×10^6 IU intralesional injections three times weekly for 4 weeks have been shown to have similar efficacy when compared to recombinant alfa-2b and lymphoblastoid interferons (87). In a review of recombinant interferon-gamma for the treatment of recalcitrant warts, the optimal dose of 50 to 100 µg/d subcutaneously resulted in an overall response rate of 50% (88).

Side effects of interferons are flulike symptoms, including fatigue, malaise, fever, chills, nausea, vomiting, headaches, and transient leukopenia, even with intralesional injections. Relapse rates of interferon therapy are up to 25% (89). Together with the high cost of this form of treatment, interferon should be used only for very recalcitrant warts.

RETINOIDS

Retinoids are another mode of therapy for warts under recent investigation. Although the mechanism is unknown, vitamin A derivatives theoretically may block the production of viral particles since these compounds affect cellular differentiation and keratinization while HPV replication appears to be related to keratinocyte differentiation (57). Retinoids may be capable of preventing malignant transformation, which may be crucial in HPV-induced neoplasia. There are several anecdotal reports of topical and oral retinoids being effective in recalcitrant warts, particularly in immunosuppressive patients. Etretinate 1 mg/kg per day for 2 months improved a patient with epidermodysplasia verruciformis with widespread flat wartlike lesions and plaques (90). Other reports state its effectiveness in

recalcitrant plantar warts, but relapses are common and results are not consistent (91). Topical retinoic acid has been used for flat warts, particularly on the face to minimize scarring (92).

IMMUNOTHERAPY

The use of topical sensitizing agents such as dinitrochlorobenzene (DNCB), squaric acid dibutylester (SADBE), and diphenylcyclopropenone is also popular for recalcitrant large nongenital warts. Immunotherapy usually involves initial sensitization of the patient to an agent, followed by applications of the same chemical to the wart to elicit a contact dermatitis at the base of the wart. The mechanism of contact immunotherapy may be related to induction of type IV hypersensitivity or cell-mediated immunity in the wart-infected tissue, resulting in wart destruction (93). It probably involves a nonwart-antigen-specific cell-mediated process. Further, complement-binding wart antibodies in 15% of patients before treatment rose to 43% after therapy (94).

DNCB has been used frequently in the past. Two percent of DNCB in acetone can be applied to an inconspicuous area on the body for 24 to 48 hours covered with a bandage to sensitize the patient (95). The area then usually becomes erythematous with blister formation. In 2 weeks after sensitivity develops, 0.1% DNCB in petrolatum is applied to the wart with a cotton-tipped applicator two to three times a week (95). This procedure may be repeated for an average of 3 to 6 weeks. DNCB therapy has about an 80% cure rate with low recurrence rates and low incidence of scarring. It is particularly effective for large, recurrent, recalcitrant, periungual, plantar, mosaic, and flat warts. Complications may include localized or severe generalized dermatitis and urticaria, pruritis, blistering, and rarely, secondary infection. DNCB is no longer used in industry, but cross-reaction with other chemicals may occur. There are concerns of the mutagenicity of DNCB in the Ames test although it has been used safely in the past for wart treatment.

SADBE and diphenylcyclopropenone may be used without the concern of mutagenicity although they are both unstable compounds. SADBE must be refrigerated because of its tendency to undergo hydrolysis, and diphenylcyclopropenone must be stored in a dark glass and in a dark place to prevent photodecomposition (93). A 0.1% diphenylcyclopropenone solution in acetone may be used to sensitize the patient, followed by applications to the wart with a sequence of increasing strengths at weekly intervals. A 0.01% concentration is initiated and followed by 0.025%, 0.1%, 0.5%, and finally, 1.0% (93).

Cimetidine has been demonstrated to possess immunomodulatory activity and has been reported to be useful in treating warts in children. The mechanism is believed to be due to increased mitogen-induced lymphocyte proliferation and inhibition of T-suppressor cells. Dosage has ranged from 25 to 40 mg/kg per day divided into three or four doses. In most, little change is seen at 1 month, but it has been reported that at 6 to 7 weeks, warts suddenly start to disappear in most patients (96). In this study, warts entirely cleared after 2 months in 26 of 30 (81%) children. Cimetidine is not specifically approved for use in children less than 16 years old; nevertheless, no untoward reactions were seen in the study mentioned. Physicians should be aware that interactions with drugs such as Dilantin and Theophylline can occur. A trial of cimetidine for condyloma acuminata in 12 adults at 400 mg four times a day did not find this drug to be efficacious.

Preliminary studies of systemic immunotherapy with inosine pranobex indicate that it may have an additive effect in treating genital warts when combined with other conventional treatments such as podophyllin, trichloroacetic acid, and CO_2 laser. A 4-week course of 1 g three times a day of inosine pranobex as an adjunctive treatment resulted in a cure rate of more than 80% (97, 98).

SEBORRHEIC DERMATITIS

Seborrheic dermatitis is a chronic, inflammatory, erythematous, and scaling eruption recognized by its characteristic distribution on the body. These seborrheic areas include the scalp, eyebrows, glabella, eyelid margins (often with marginal blepharitis and conjunctivitis), cheeks, paranasal areas, nasolabial folds, beard area, presternal area, central back, retroaricular creases, and in and about the external ear canal. Other less commonly involved areas include the axillae, inframammary areas, umbilicus, groin, and intergluteal cleft. Seborrheic dermatitis in the intertriginous areas may exist alone or in conjunction with other seborrheic areas. Similarly, psoriasis may occasionally have an intertriginous distribution, called inverse psoriasis, along with scalp involvement. In this form, it has been designated as seborriasis.

The scales of seborrheic dermatitis vary from a dry to thick powdery form with little to no erythema to an oily form with greasy or oily scales and crusts on an erythematous base. The former is usually located on the scalp and is referred to as simple dandruff. The greasier scales are found more commonly on the ears and central face such as the glabella, eyebrows, and nasolabial folds.

Etiology and Pathogenesis

Seborrheic dermatitis is a common problem, and the onset is correlated with sebaceous gland activity. During infancy, it is commonly called cradle cap, and spontaneous remission tends to occur by age 1 year, after which the disease is rare until puberty. In these infants, seborrheic dermatitis may become generalized to form an exfoliative erythroderma known as erythroderma desquamativum or Leiner's disease. Infants often have diarrhea, infection, and a failure

to thrive. A small subset of infants with Leiner's disease have been reported with a dysfunction of the fifth component of complement, resulting in decreased opsonic activity. In adults, seborrheic dermatitis has a predilection for males and is more severe in the winter. The disorder is often asymptomatic, but pruritus is not uncommon and at times can be intense.

Seborrheic dermatitis is characterized by an increased epidermal cell turnover. The active ingredient of many antiseborrheic agents, such as coal tar, zinc pyrithione, and selenium sulfide, inhibits mitotic activity. It was once thought that this cytostatic effect was responsible for alleviating the scaling. Although no evidence establishes increased cell turnover as the primary defect, zinc pyrithione, selenium sulfide, and sulfur/salicylic acid preparations all kill yeast. Evidence now suggests that the hyperproliferative state may be secondary to the presence of a lipophilic, pleomorphic fungus, Pityrosporum ovale (99). When oral and topical ketoconazole, an imidazole derivative effective against Pityrosporum, is used in seborrheic dermatitis, the condition improves (100, 101). The primary mechanism of action is thought to be inhibition of ergosterol formation in the cell membrane of fungi. Improvement was correlated with a reduction in the number of yeast organisms. This was recently confirmed using a precipitated sulfur/salicylic acid preparation (102). These observations fulfill all the requirements to implicate the organisms as the etiologic agent (Koch's postulates), but some investigators have demonstrated P. ovale on scalps of patients without the disease. This can be easily explained by the observation that patients with clinical disease inherit a heightened immune responsiveness to the alternate complement pathway, which overreacts to the cell walls of the Pityrosporum yeast (103). How can one explain the parallel occurrence of the disease with the onset of sebaceous gland activity? Recently, it was shown that when the sebum excretion rate was reduced by 70% with isotretinoin, the magnitude of rash improvement varied according the body site. It was concluded that the residual pool of sebum was important for the growth of P. ovale and that, within the physiologic range, sebum had a permissive effect on the growth of this yeast. This observation explains variations in disease activity at certain body sites and the greater prevalence in males since androgens stimulate sebum production. Finally, the pathologic increase in the residual pool of sebum due to immobility could explain the frequent occurrence of seborrheic dermatitis in patients with a variety of neurologic disorders such as idiopathic and neuroleptic-induced Parkinson's disease (104).

Treatment

The mainstay of treatment of seborrheic dermatitis of the scalp is shampoos. As mentioned, sulfur/salicylic acid, coal tar, and zinc pyrithione are available over the counter, but the most effective antifungal agents are 2.5% selenium sulfide and 2% ketoconazole, which can be obtained by prescription (105). The choice of shampoos depends on several factors, including physician and patient preference, cost, and cosmetic appeal to the patient. Depending on the severity of the disease, shampoos can be applied daily to twice weekly. Patients should be reminded that the scalp (not the hair) is being treated, so the patient should allow the shampoo to penetrate for at least 5 minutes before rinsing.

With the exception of accidental oral ingestion, systemic adverse reactions are minimal. Local adverse reactions include skin irritation (usually from the vehicle), occasionally reports of hair loss, and discoloration of hair, especially from selenium sulfide and coal tar. As with other shampoos, oiliness or dryness of the hair and scalp may occur. Topical corticosteroid lotions can be added if lesions are very inflammatory and pruritic. A 1% hydrocortisone lotion, applied one to three times daily, is usually safe and effective. Stronger preparations such as 0.025% triamcinolone lotion, 0.01% fluocinolone acetonide solution, 0.05% clobetasol solution, or 0.1% betamethasone valerate lotion may be required for more severe instances, but they should be used only for very short periods to prevent hypothalamic-pituitary-adrenal (HPA) axis suppression or steroid rosacea. For thick, crusted, and scaly lesions, a mixture of liquid petrolatum, sodium chloride, and phenol can be applied overnight and rinsed off in the morning. Other preparations that use a similar application schedule include various concentrations of sulfur/salicylic acid in an ointment base.

Therapy for other seborrheic areas of the body, including the scalp line, eyebrows, glabella, ears, and nasolabial, can be successfully accomplished with 2% ketoconazole cream applied twice a day. Other alternatives include 1 to 2.5% hydrocortisone cream or 0.5% desonide applied two to three times a day. If there is scaling in the auditory meatus, a polymyxin B-hydrocortisone suspension, or 0.5% desonide and 2% acetic acid, four drops three to four times a day, is effective. The pruritus that sometimes accompanies the scaling is also relieved. Topical steroids should not be used for seborrheic blepharitis because of the potential to induce glaucoma and cataracts. Hot compresses and gentle debridement and a cotton-tipped applicator and 2% ketoconazole shampoo one or more times daily are usually effective. If the lid margins are severely inflamed, 10% sodium sulfacetamide ointment may be added (106).

Special considerations must be made for infants with seborrheic dermatitis. Tar preparations should be avoided for fear they will rub it into their eyes. Topical corticosteroids should be limited to 0.5 to 1% hydrocortisone so as to avoid HPA axis suppression. However, 2% ketoconazole cream should be the treatment of choice for infantile seborrheic dermatitis because of its minimal percutaneous absorption and lack of accumulation in the plasma (107).

PSORIASIS

Psoriasis is an inflammatory disorder characterized by erythematous scaling plaques on virtually any area of the skin surface. The disease affects 1 to 2% of the general population in the United States. It ranks third after acne and warts as the reason for the most office visits to a dermatologist. Psoriasis occurs with equal frequency in both sexes. It may be symptomatic throughout life and be progressive with age or wax and wane in severity. The condition can be present at birth, and an onset was reported at age 108 years. Most patients develop the initial lesions of psoriasis in the third decade of life. Symptoms appear in males at a mean age of 29, and in females at a mean age of 27. With earlier onset, there is a greater probability of a positive family history of psoriasis. Although psoriasis does not follow classic mendelian inheritance, studies of HLA phenotypes suggest a polygenic inheritance that requires environmental factors to induce the clinical expression of the disease. These include cutaneous or systemic microbial infection or colonization, trauma, drugs such as lithium, β-blockers, antimalarials, and nonsteroidal antiinflammatory agents, and corticosteroid withdrawal. Various HLA phenotypes have been reported to be associated with psoriasis, but the strongest association is with the HLA-cw 6 antigen. Presence of this antigen increases the relative risk for development of psoriasis to 13 times that of the population without the antigen.

The morbidity associated with this disease is great. Psoriasis can cause functional impairment, skin disfigurement, and emotional distress. Severe involvement of the hands, feet, and nails may make even routine activities, such as walking or dressing, difficult to perform, particularly in patients with severe psoriatic arthritis. As many as 30% of patients with psoriasis may have arthritis, and 5 to 10% of those patients may experience functional disability. Therefore, psoriasis directly affects the quality of life and may cause difficulty in work performance, problems with social rejection, sexual dysfunction, and depression.

Psoriatic lesions are observed most commonly on the scalp, elbows, knees, trunk, and nails. The primary lesion is an erythematous plaque covered with silvery scales. Scale removal may show punctate bleeding points, termed Auspitz sign, which help differentiate psoriasis from other chronic dermatoses. Several well-recognized clinical variants require particular treatment modalities.

Plaque-type psoriasis is usually located on the extensor surfaces of elbows and knees, the lumbar region of the back, and the scalp. Guttate psoriasis, with small, scaly tear-drop-shaped lesions, classically follows group A streptococcal pharyngitis. Psoriasis can also follow a seborrheic distribution called seborrhiasis. Inverse psoriasis is a form

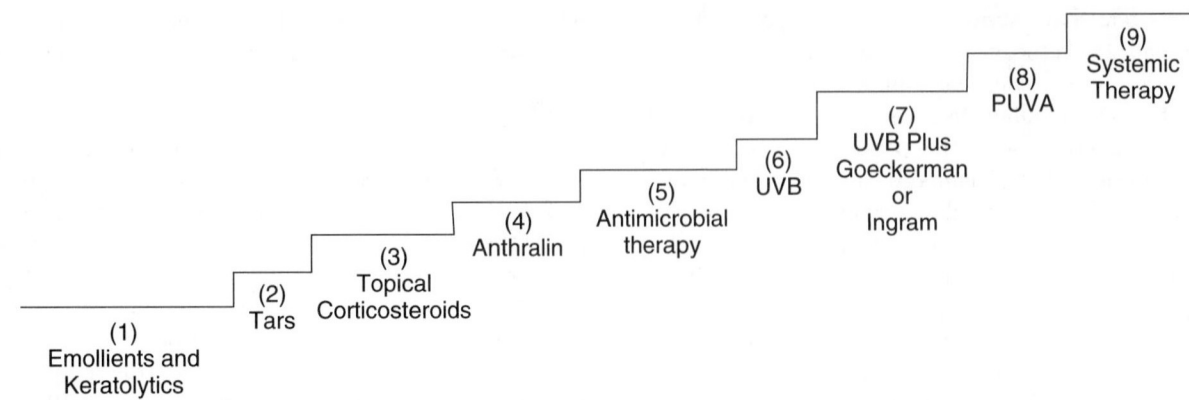

Figure 44.2. Stepped-care approach to psoriasis. Note that as one ascends each level of therapy there is an increased risk for more serious side effects.

of psoriasis that often involves exclusively body folds such as the axillae, groin, inframammary folds, navel, intergluteal crease, and glans penis. Palmoplantar differs from plaque-type psoriasis in the variability of erythema, the loss of sharply marginated plaques, and replacement of the characteristic silvery scales by thickened fissured hyperkeratosis. Erythrodermic psoriasis is an acute inflammatory, erythematous, scaling disorder involving the entire skin surface. This is usually brought on by ingestion of concomitant medications, as mentioned previously, or as a reaction to provoking factors (e.g., infections, chronic topical steroid use, or phototoxic erythema). These patients usually have difficulty in controlling body temperatures. Pustular psoriasis can be localized to the palms and soles or be generalized and may appear after withdrawal of corticosteroid therapy given inappropriately for plaque-type psoriasis. Erythrodermic and generalized pustular psoriasis may be life-threatening because of systemic infections, or cardiovascular or pulmonary complications. For example, in patients with preexisting cardiovascular disease, the erythroderma may precipitate high-output congestive heart failure or arrhthymia (108).

Etiology

There is no agreement about the etiology of psoriasis, but increased epidermal cell proliferation and inflammation have been observed. In psoriatic lesions, cell proliferation is 12 times the normal rate, with a twofold increase in proliferation in uninvolved skin. The increased rate found in uninvolved skin suggests a generalized skin abnormality in psoriasis. As a result of the hyperproliferative state, epidermal turnover and transit times are greatly reduced.

A key feature of newly formed psoriatic lesions is the attraction and migration of inflammatory cells, especially neutrophils. The neutrophils themselves are not abnormal; they are attracted to the epidermis by chemotactic mediators such as microbial products (peptides), complement components (C3a, C5), and the arachidonic acid products leukotriene B4 (LTB4) and hydroxyicosatetraenoic acids (HETEs).

Cytokines have also been implicated in the pathogenesis of psoriasis. These low-molecular-weight glycoproteins are regulatory molecules that mediate cell communication in both normal and pathologic conditions. When cytokines are released from inflammatory cells (T lymphocytes and monocytes) and keratinocytes, they stimulate epidermal proliferation. Cytokine mediators that may be important in the pathogenesis of psoriasis include the interleukins, interferons, and growth factors, including epidermal growth factor. Although many of these cytokines are multifunctional, some have shown stimulation of epidermal proliferation (IL-6, and EGF) and attraction and mediation of neutrophils (IL-8) (109, 110).

The interrelationship between environmental influences, genetic predisposition, and the two pathologic features of psoriasis is best explained by the microbial association with psoriasis. Psoriatic lesions develop from microbial products that activate the alternate complement pathway to produce neutrophil migration and epidermal hyperplasia. The heightened responsiveness to the alternate complement pathway may be a phenotypic expression of a genetic predisposition to psoriasis (111).

Treatment

The hyperproliferative and inflammatory basis of the disease offer two different therapeutic approaches. Most pharmacologic interventions act by modifying one or both of these processes. Therapeutic consideration must also be given to the type of psoriasis, the extent and location of involvement, and the psychological impact of the disease on the patient. Since psoriasis varies in its severity, its management can be similar to the stepped-care program used in the treatment of hypertension (Fig. 44.2). In the first step, side effects are minimal. If treatment resistance is encountered or if the disease is more severe, the second step includes the addition or a change to another form of therapy. Each step in the level of care carries an increased risk of side effects. Therefore, the risk-to-benefit ratio must be assessed before proceeding to the next program. When a patient reaches the highest step in the program, the

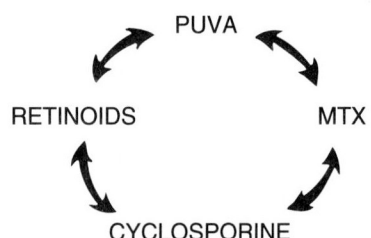

Figure 44.3. Rotation among higher levels of therapy to reduce the incidence of life-threatening side effects.

therapy can be rotated for certain periods of time to minimize life-threatening side effects (Fig. 44.3).

EMOLLIENTS AND KERATOLYTICS

Emollient agents hydrate the stratum corneum and prevent the increased transepidermal water loss observed in psoriasis patients. The hydrating effect softens the stratum corneum and assists in desquamation; the overall effect is moisturizing the skin. An occlusive oily film delivered to the skin surface seals the transepidermal water into the stratum corneum. With water retained in the skin, the stratum corneum becomes more pliable or softer, preventing fissuring and scaling in hyperkeratotic areas. Skin hydration also decreases the binding forces within the stratum corneum and facilitates desquamation.

Most emollient agents are mineral oils and paraffins in an oil-in-water emulsion with emulsifiers, stabilizers, and antimicrobial preservatives. Humectants may be added to the emollient to enhance its water-retaining qualities. These include glycerin, urea, or pyrrolidone carboxylic acid, which hold water within the stratum corneum hygroscopically. Emollients in oil-in-water emulsion can be cosmetically acceptable, but the more "oily" or occlusive the preparation, the more effective the moisturizer. Some patients may find the oily feel to the skin unacceptable. Therefore, patients should be allowed input into the selection of emollients.

Patients should be instructed to apply the emollients three or more times a day. Side effects from frequent application may be acneiform folliculitis or an exacerbation of existing acne from occlusion of the follicular openings. Occlusion of the sweat ducts may produce miliaria, especially in hot and humid climates. The addition of urea or lactic acid may produce a stinging sensation unrelated to any toxic reaction to the skin, whose cause is not known. An occasional problem (as with any topical agent) is allergic contact dermatitis from the contents of the emulsifying agent or its antimicrobial preservatives.

Keratolytic agents promote desquamation of scales. Salicylic acid is the most frequently used keratolytic agent. Concentrations ranging from 2 to 20% are formulated in a variety of ways. For smaller, thinner scaling plaques or for healing patches, a 2% concentration in an ointment base is used. A lotion base, which is excellent for scalp applica-

tions, may have up to 6% salicylic acid. Higher concentrations are used for thicker and hyperkeratotic plaques, and concentrations above 6% show marked keratolytic activity. Lactic acid in concentrations of 5 to 12% can also be used to reduce scaling. A popular combination of keratolytics is 6% salicylic acid in 60% propylene glycol with 20% ethyl alcohol. The preparation is applied under occlusion at night to hydrate the skin to remove thick, adherent scales. During the day, topical steroids can be applied to enhance percutaneous penetration and healing. Salicylic acid at concentrations of 2 to 6% is used with tar in creams, ointments, and shampoos. The combination is very efficacious, but preparations are dark gray or brown, may stain clothing, and have an unpleasant smell, causing problems with patient compliance.

Side effects include allergic contact dermatitis to the vehicle and soreness of the treated area. The latter condition can be alleviated by discontinuing the treatment. Potential side effects of salicylic acid are tinnitus, nausea, and hyperventilation. These systemic side effects are more likely to occur when large areas of damaged skin are exposed to higher concentrations(112, 113).

TARS

The mechanism of action of coal tar is not known. It is currently believed to have antimitotic effects. The initial application of coal tars to normal skin transiently increases epidermal proliferation for the first 2 weeks of treatment. If the coal tar is continued for up to 40 days, a cytostatic effect eventually produces epidermal thinning. Coal tars in combination with ultraviolet-A (UVA) light produce photoadducts that inhibit DNA synthesis.

Coal tar is effective monotherapy, and although it takes longer to clear the psoriasis than other treatments, prolonged remission can be expected. Compliance is difficult because of odor, staining, and irritation. To reduce these problems, extracts or refined products of crude coal tar in a 10% concentration with alcohol may be used. This preparation, called liquor carbonis detergens (LCD), is incorporated into various cream-based vehicles and bath additives. Coal tar preparations can be applied once or twice a day, but patients should be warned of irritation to the groin, axillae, and periorbital region. Side effects include photosensitivity, acneiform eruptions, and folliculitis (114). There is a potential for an increased risk of skin cancer and internal malignancies with the chronic use of topical coal tars. Mutagenic substances in coal tars are absorbed percutaneously and excreted in urine (115). However, to date, no study has clearly shown that chronic use of coal tar alone increases the risk of carcinoma (116).

TOPICAL CORTICOSTEROIDS

Topical corticosteroids are the most frequently prescribed medication for psoriasis. They can be used alone or in combination with other agents. Several modes of action are

Table 44.9.
Potency Ranking of Topical Corticosteroids by Generic Names

Superpotent	Clobetasol propionate 0.05% cream and ointment
	Betamethasone diproprionate[a] 0.05% cream and ointment
	Diflorasone diacetate[a] 0.05% ointment
	Halobetasol propionate 0.5% cream and ointment
Potent	Amcinonide 0.1% cream and ointment
	Halcinonide 0.1% cream
	Fluocinonide 0.5% cream, ointment, and gel
	Desoximetasone 0.25–0.05% cream, ointment, and gel
	Triamcinolone acetonide 0.1% ointment
	Mometasone 0.1% lotion, cream, and ointment
	Betamethasone valerate 0.1% ointment
	Diflorasone diacetate 0.05% cream
Midstrength	Flurandrenolide 0.05% cream and ointment
	Triamcinolone acetonide 0.1% lotion and cream
	Fluocinolone acetonide 0.025% ointment and cream
	Desoximetasone 0.05% cream
	Hydrocortisone valerate 0.2% cream and ointment
	Hydrocortisone butyrate 0.1% cream and ointment
	Betamethasone dipropionate 0.02% lotion
	Betamethasone valerate 0.1% cream
	Fluticasone propionate 0.05% cream
Mild	Alclometasone dipropionate 0.05% cream and ointment
	Desonide 0.05% cream and ointment
	Fluocinolone acetonide 0.01% solution
	Betamethasone valerate 0.05% lotion
	Hydrocortisone, dexamethasone, flumethalone, prednisolone, methylprenisolone in all vehicles.

[a]Some preparations have been placed in the potent category.

probably important in explaining their antipsoriatic activity. The hyperproliferative response is altered by a reduction in DNA synthesis and epidermal mitoses. There is a reduction in phospholipase A activity, which decreases arachidonic acid production and ultimately affects the production of inflammatory mediators LTB 4 and HETE.

Topical corticosteroids also cause vasoconstriction, and the vasoconstrictive properties correlate well with clinical efficacy and are used to rank preparations in order of antiinflammatory potency (Table 44.9). The broad range of potency results, in part, from chemical modifications of hydrocortisone. When the molecule is esterified with valerate, dipropionate, or acetonide groups, the potency increases dramatically from increased penetration to the skin. Penetration can also be increased between 10- and 100-fold by an occlusive dressing. However, HPA-axis suppression is more prevalent when a potent preparation is used. The potency of a corticosteroid preparation can be altered by its vehicle. Gels are generally more effective than ointments, and ointments have greater biological activity than the same corticosteroid in creams or lotions. Creams are generally more effective than lotions.

Ointments can be used on thick scaly plaques, but they should be avoided in the axilla and groin, where folliculitis may develop secondary to rubbing and maceration. In the intertriginous areas, creams are a better choice. For the scalp and other hairy areas, gels, lotions, or sprays are preferable to ointments and creams.

Topical corticosteroids are usually applied twice a day. Applications once or twice a day are as effective as multiple applications, and less frequent applications prevent the development of tachyphylaxis and other side effects.

The incidence of side effects is increased by use of high-potency preparations; application to areas of thin skin such as the face, scrotum, vulva, or intertriginous areas; application to areas where the skin barrier is compromised; and the use of occlusive dressings. Children and patients with renal failure are more susceptible to side effects. To lessen both local and systemic side effects, a weaker potency should be used on the face or in intertriginous areas. On areas of the body requiring higher potency corticosteroids, the preparation should be reduced to a lower strength after clearing of the plaques begins. Local side effects include striae and atrophy, skin fragility producing bruising, poor wound healing, telangiectasia, acneiform eruptions, pigmentary abnormalities, and allergic contact dermatitis to the vehicle.

Topical steroids can mask clinically inapparent dermatophyte infections. Fluorinated corticosteroids and hydrocortisone butyrate and acetate used on the face commonly result in perioral dermatitis and acne rosacealike eruptions. As in the systemic administration of corticosteroids, withdrawal of potent topical preparations can change a stable plaque-type psoriasis to a pustular form. On the other hand, chronic use can precipitate an erythrodermic flare, especially if topical steroids have been applied to extensive areas of the body surface.

Applications to large areas are more likely to produce systemic side effects, including HPA-axis suppression on doses as small as 2 g per day, glucose intolerance, and (rarely) Cushing's syndrome. HPA-axis suppression is reversible after short-term use of potent preparations. Topical corticosteroids should be used with caution around the eyes. Systemic absorption at this site can produce glaucoma, cataracts, or an exacerbation of an ocular infection (117).

ANTHRALIN

Anthralin, or dithranol, is a topical treatment that has not achieved the popularity in the United States that it has in Britain and Europe. The compound, 1,8-trihydroxyanthracene, has several modes of action, but inhibition of mitochondrial DNA synthesis and various cellular enzymes may be the main reasons for its clinical effectiveness. The overall effect is antiproliferative on the epidermis, which decreases mitoses to normalize the epidermal architecture (114).

Commercial preparations of anthralin ointment and creams are available in concentrations of 0.1 to 1%. Anthralin is oxidized easily by exposure to air. Salicylic acid in concentrations ranging from 0.2 to 0.4% is often added to a preparation called Lassar's paste to increase its shelf life. Lassar's paste consists of anthralin in concentrations ranging from 0.1 to 5% mixed into zinc oxide paste with paraffin as a hardener and salicylic acid. This stiff paste is used in the Ingram method for treating large, chronic, plaque-type psoriasis. The treatment program begins with a tar bath and UVB phototherapy, followed by Lassar's paste–anthralin application to the plaques. Talc or cornstarch is applied to the paste, which sets the paste and absorbs excess moisture, to prevent smearing. This is to prevent local irritation when anthralin comes in contact with normal skin. A soft loose garment such as pajamas or a sweatsuit can be worn over the paste. The paste is left on for 4 to 12 hours and often can be left on overnight. It is removed with a cloth and light mineral oil or baby oil, and the excess is washed off in a shower or bath with soap. Lower concentrations of anthralin from 0.1 to 1% are used initially, but higher concentrations of up to 5% are needed as the psoriasis improves.

As the skin barrier is restored with clinical improvement, higher concentrations of anthralin are needed to provide adequate levels in the epidermis for continued therapeutic efficacy. This clinical observation and the fact that anthralin penetrates more rapidly through the altered stratum corneum of psoriasis led to short-contact therapy. Low concentrations of anthralin ointment (0.1 to 0.5%) are left on for 60 minutes or more, whereas higher concentrations (1%) may be left on for only 10 to 20 minutes. Anthralin is then removed with mineral oil, followed by a shower with soap and water. Short-contact anthralin therapy requires a well-motivated intelligent patient and can be used daily on an outpatient basis. Improvement is expected to occur in approximately 3 weeks. The advantages of short-contact therapy over the Ingram method are reductions in both irritation and staining of clothing because earlier washings reduce penetration and irritation in nonlesional skin. Penetration of anthralin through the plaques is far greater and peaks much earlier than in normal skin, maintaining clinical efficacy (118). The inflammation and staining of clothing can be eliminated by the application of 10% triethanolamine in an aqueous cream. This is applied immediately after short-contact therapy, without interfering with the therapeutic effect (119).

Anthralin should not be used on the face because of the potential for eye irritation. Intertriginous areas, especially the antecubital and popliteal fossae, axillae, retroaricular, and inguinal folds, as well as the inner thighs should be avoided. Hair and nails may show discoloration, but low anthralin concentrations, short exposure time, and pre-treatment with neutral henna to coat the hair prevent anthralin penetration into the hair shaft. Nail polish can prevent anthralin penetration of the nail plate. No systemic toxic effects are associated with topical anthralin use, and contact allergy is rare (113).

ANTIMICROBIAL THERAPY

Antimicrobial therapy has been included in the American Academy of Dermatology revised guidelines for the care of psoriasis patients (120). Antimicrobial treatment of psoriasis includes oral and topical antifungals and antibacterials. This therapy is based on accumulating evidence suggesting that psoriasis is aggravated by cutaneous or systemic microbial infections or colonization and that the inflammatory and hyperproliferative response is a direct result of microbial products activating the alternate complement pathway. Psoriasis patients are believed to inherit a heightened immune responsiveness to the alternate complement pathway to produce their disease (111). Over the years, the literature has cited frequent associations of psoriasis with streptococcal infections. The most common association is the guttate variant seen in children and young adults. Patients with either throat culture or serologic evidence of group A streptococcus have good-to-excellent clearing of their disease when treated with rifampin in combination with either penicillin or erythromycin orally (121).

Other indications for antimicrobial treatment include various topical imidazole and nystatin antifungal agents for Candida albicans-associated "napkin" (or diaper) psoriasis in infants, oral ketoconazole for scalp psoriasis, and topical 2% erythromycin ointment for inverse psoriasis, especially in the gluteal fold. Detailed accounts of the approach to antimicrobial treatment of psoriasis are outlined in another text (122).

PHOTOTHERAPY

Phototherapy, either alone or in combination with other treatments, can be used for moderate-to-severe psoriasis. The ultraviolet spectrum is of interest in psoriasis. Within the ultraviolet spectrum, UVB, defined between 290 and 320 nm, and in particular 313 nm, is beneficial in the healing of psoriasis. The UVA spectrum between 320 and 400 nm, by itself, is not effective, but when used with psoralen (PUVA), either orally or topically, it is effective. This combination is referred to as photochemotherapy.

Some general comments can be made about its mode of action. In addition to its antiproliferative effect, ultraviolet radiation suppresses cell-mediated immunity, but the significance of the latter observation remains uncertain.

Phototherapy is indicated in patients who have failed to respond to topical therapy or when psoriasis is widespread. Patients should be selected carefully for phototherapy and excluded if they have psoriasis that is worsened by sunlight, a history of photosensitizing disorder, or are currently taking drugs that are known to photosensitize. Phototherapy can be used on an outpatient basis to produce comparatively long-lasting remission. UVB can also be used at home, but PUVA therapy should be supervised by a dermatologist familiar with photochemotherapy.(123)

ULTRAVIOLET B

If UVB is used as monotherapy, the best results are obtained when erythemogenic doses are used on nonlesional skin. In calculating the initial dose, the patient's skin type is considered. This is estimated on the individual's ability to sunburn and tan and is called the minimal erythema dose (MED), expressed in m_j/cm^2. A test grid is performed on the back using the initial dose, and the skin is examined 24 hours later. If the skin does not show a pink outline of the grid, the dose of light is increased by 15 to 20% of the initial dose. The dose that causes minimal erythema at 24 hours produces the optimal effect in clearing psoriasis. From the MED, time spent in the UVB cabinet can be calculated. In addition to time spent exposed to UVB, the dosage is determined by the intensity of radiation. Intensity varies as the inverse square of the distance from the radiation source, so the distance between the patient and the light source must be considered. Although this may not be a problem in UVB cabinets because of physical constraints, some patients use UVB fluorescent tubes at home where the light-source-to-patient distance will affect the therapeutic response. Various protocols have been developed, but the most common outpatient protocol is three times a week using variable exposure increments of MED with the application of emollients. Most patients will clear with 18 treatments using this protocol (123).

UVB combined with crude coal tar is more effective than either agent alone. This combination, known as the Goeckerman regimen, uses crude coal tar at concentrations of 1 to 5% applied during the evening. Since the tar layer prevents the ultraviolet light from reaching the skin, it should be removed in the morning using mineral oil, before exposure to a suberythemogenic dose of UVB. It was once thought that the UVB would act on the tar to produce photoadducts, but (as previously stated) the photosensitizing wavelength of tar is in the UVB spectrum. Further, UVB does not enhance the tar-induced suppression of DNA synthesis by epidermal cells, so the reason for its synergy is not known.

A more popular treatment regimen used in the United Kingdom and in continental Europe is the Ingram method, where the tar bath and UVB radiation are followed by the application of anthralin in Lassar's paste directly onto the plaques. There are no advantages to adding anthralin to the UVB therapy, and with the potential for irritation and staining of clothing, this may be a reason the Goeckerman regimen is used more frequently in the United States.

A major side effect of UVB therapy is burning from excessive exposure. Sunscreen, zinc oxide, or cloth can be applied to the affected areas to prevent further burning. To prevent ultraviolet-induced conjunctival erosions, protective goggles are worn during treatment. Although premature aging of the skin is dose dependent, tar and UVB used in the described manner seem to show no increase in skin cancers (124).

PHOTOCHEMOTHERAPY

Photochemotherapy consists of an oral administration of a photoactive drug (a psoralen), followed 2 hours later by exposure to UVA. The psoralens are thought to produce photoadducts from the absorption of UVA. The photochemically induced covalent binding of the psoralen to the pyrimidine bases in DNA inhibits its synthesis and cell replication. Psoralen belongs to the furocoumarin class of compounds. The two derivatives currently available in the United States are 8-methoxypsoralen (methoxsalen, 8-MOP) and 4,5′,8-trimethylpsoralen (trioxsalen, TMP). The third psoralen, 5-methoxypsoralen (bergapten, 5-MOP), is currently being investigated for clinical use in the United States but is available in Europe.

8-MOP, however, is more potent in causing suppression of DNA synthesis than the other compounds and is the main psoralen in dermatologic use at this time. 8-MOP is administered in a dose of 0.3 to 0.6 mg/kg. When 8-MOP is administered orally, the blood levels peak at 2 hours, producing maximum sensitivity to UVA. Blood levels can be increased by a low-fat meal. The highest tissue concentrations are found in the gastrointestinal tract, liver, blood, and skin. In the blood, 84% is bound to serum albumin, and tolbutamide can displace the drug from the binding sites to increase the free fraction of 8-MOP. As a result of the displacement, the free fraction of 8-MOP can produce a photosensitivity. 8-MOP is metabolized through the liver by several pathways, including hydroxylation, glucuronide formation, epoxidation, and hydrolysis.

Like PUVA therapy, the patient's skin type guides selection of the starting dose of UVA. Treatment is administered once every other day because the erythema induced by PUVA may not be evident for up to 48 hours after exposure. In general, the dose of UVA is increased by $1.5_j/cm^2$ for each consecutive treatment. Unlike UVB therapy, the time to produce clearing with UVA is longer, usually after 10 to 20 treatments over 4 to 8 weeks. Once clearing has been achieved, the dosage of UVA is held constant. Maintenance therapy must be used because PUVA is only a palliative treatment. The same dose of UVA that induced clearing is used, but the frequency of treatment is reduced gradually to twice a month (125).

Topical psoralens with UVA, known as bath-water PUVA, is a very popular method in Scandinavia. It can be effective for both extensive plaque-type psoriasis and selected parts of the body, such as the hands and feet. This method avoids the gastric side effects of oral psoralens and is ideal for patients with hepatic impairment. The patient soaks in a bath containing a very low concentration of psoralen before exposure to UVA. TMP is usually used because it has less percutaneous absorption than 8-MOP, but this method carries a greater risk of photosensitivity. To reduce the amount of UVA exposure and the number of treatments, oral retinoid agents, such as etretinate, can be used along with PUVA (Re-PUVA). Although the mechanism of synergism is not known, it does not seem to involve the increased photosensitivity seen with the retinoid agents (125). Aside from the erythema and blistering, other acute side effects include pruritus and nausea. Shielding with a drape or sunscreens during subsequent UVA exposure prevents further erythema, and the duration of UVA exposure can be reduced. Pruritus can be controlled with emollients or topical steroids. Dividing the psoralen into two doses given an hour apart can reduce the incidence of nausea. A less desirable alternative, especially for severe refractory nausea, is to reduce the dosage and increase the UVA exposure. A potential chronic complication of PUVA therapy is the development of cataracts. The renal excretion of psoralens usually is completed within 8 hours, but the elimination of a psoralen from the lens of the eye takes about 24 hours. When UVA from natural sunlight reaches psoralens in the lens, there is a theoretical possibility of binding to the protein and DNA of the lens. Although the risk is small, this complication can be nearly eliminated by wearing UVA-blocking wraparound glasses for 12 to 24 hours after ingesting psoralen. Other more common chronic side effects include a dose-dependent increased incidence of squamous cell carcinoma and lentigines (125, 126).

SYSTEMIC CORTICOSTEROID THERAPY

Systemic corticosteroid therapy for psoriasis is included here to emphasize that it is not the treatment of choice because of the many side effects associated with prolonged administration and because of the potential severe rebound side effect. There is a potential for conversion of stable plaque-type psoriasis into a pustular flare after withdrawal of corticosteroid therapy (109).

RETINOIDS

Two synthetic analogs of vitamin A, etretinate and acitretin, have been used in the treatment of psoriasis. Etretinate, an aromatic retinoid, has been available for clinical use in the United States since 1986. Acitretin is an acid metabolite of etretinate with different pharmacokinetics than etretinate. Acitretin has a shorter half-life and is not stored in subcutaneous fat like etretinate. Although its efficacy is similar to that of its parent compound, etretinate, acitretin as of 1995 remains under investigation in the United States

and Canada. The exact mechanism of action on psoriasis is not known, but its various effects on cellular differentiation may cause normalization of keratinization and proliferation. Retinoids also have an antiinflammatory effect by reducing the levels of leukotriene and HETE. Since adverse side effects are greater than those from topical therapies, UVB, and PUVA, retinoids should be reserved for psoriasis recalcitrant to these treatments. The usual starting dose is 0.75 to 1.0 mg/kg per day in divided doses. Maximum dosage of 1.5 mg/kg per day is recommended, and after 8 to 16 weeks of therapy, a maintenance dosage of 0.5 to 0.75 mg/kg per day is required (127). Side effects are similar to those seen with hypervitaminosis A syndrome. Among the major side effects are the embryotoxic and teratogenic effects on animal models and humans. Women of childbearing years are required to use contraception, which should be continued for 2 years after completing treatment. Acitretin may be of more benefit than etretinate in these patients. Other side effects include elevation of triglyceride or cholesterol levels, mucocutaneous changes such as cheilitis, hepatoxicity, and musculoskeletal changes (128).

METHOTREXATE

Methotrexate (MTX) is a folic acid antagonist that inhibits dihydrofolate reductase, blocking key steps in DNA and RNA synthesis. The overall effect is inhibition of cell division and a subsequent decrease of epidermal hyperproliferation, a characteristic pathophysiologic feature of psoriasis. MTX also has some immunosuppressive activity. It probably inhibits DNA synthesis in immunologically competent cells. It affects both cell- and humoral-mediated immunity and decreases the levels of LTB4. MTX taken orally is rapidly absorbed through the gastrointestinal tract, but peak levels occur more slowly than in intramuscular or intravenous routes. It is excreted through the kidneys almost unchanged, and the clearance of MTX correlates with endogenous creatinine clearance. A small amount, however, is excreted by active tubular secretion. MTX is 50 to 70% bound to albumin and may be displaced by acidic drugs such as phenylbutazone, sulfonamides, salicylates, tetracycline, chloramphenicol, and phenytoin. A potential for toxicity exists when these are used in combination with MTX, especially if renal excretion is impaired. Weak organic acids such as salicylates, probenecid, ketoprofen, and phenylbutazone can compete with MTX to prolong its active tubular secretion. Further, direct renal toxicity occurs with the concomitant use of MTX and indomethacin. Therefore, both agents should be used cautiously in psoriatic arthritis patients who have poor renal function (129).

The Food and Drug Administration (FDA) has approved MTX for use in severe, recalcitrant psoriasis. However, patient selection for MTX should take into account not only the characteristics of the disease, but also the socioeconomic impact to the patient and absolute and relative contraindications. The only absolute contraindications are pregnancy and lactation. Relative contraindications can be waived only when the probable benefits of therapy outweigh the potential risks. One relative contraindication that needs further elaboration is alcohol abuse. With chronic administration of MTX, hepatotoxicity resulting in fibrosis and cirrhosis is a serious concern. Alcoholism significantly increases the risk of hepatotoxicity, and MTX should not be used in patients who abuse alcohol.

The usual oral dose of MTX is 10 to 20 mg in either a single weekly dose or divided into three doses given 12 hours apart once weekly. A test dose of 5 to 10 mg is given, and a CBC and liver function test are done 7 days later. In general, 75 to 80% of psoriasis patients will respond within 4 weeks. If no response occurs, the dose is increased by 2.5 to 5.0 mg per week. Although the most common route of administration is oral, it may be given intramuscularly at doses of 10 to 25 mg per week. The total dose rarely exceeds 30 mg. Higher intramuscular doses are allowed because of the more rapid renal clearance. When the psoriasis is in control, MTX may be tapered by 2.5 mg per week until the lowest possible dose is found that provides disease control (130).

Common acute side effects of MTX are nausea and gastrointestinal upset related to dosing. MTX can also produce a phototoxic reaction similar to sunburn. If MTX is used with phototherapy, patients should omit their phototherapy treatments on the days MTX is administered. More serious long-term side effects include hepatotoxicity and bone marrow suppression. The hepatotoxicity seems to be related to the cumulative dose of MTX. Liver function tests are unreliable screening methods for MTX-induced hepatotoxicity, so liver biopsy is currently the only means of monitoring changes attributed to MTX. This has been recommended after a 1.5-g cumulative dose, and subsequent biopsies should be performed following further 1.0- to 1.5-g cumulative doses. Guidelines for monitoring MTX toxicity have been published elsewhere (131). Folinic acid is the treatment of choice for accidental overdose. Leucovorin rescue, as this is called, bypasses the step in folic acid reduction that is blocked by MTX (129).

HYDROXYUREA

Hydroxyurea is a hydroxylated molecule of urea that affects cell proliferation by inhibiting DNA synthesis. The exact mode of action is incompletely understood in psoriasis. Although not approved by the FDA for treatment of psoriasis, it has been reported to be effective. It is less effective than MTX; the response is slower (6 to 8 weeks), and the response is not as complete (the annular areas of psoriasis persist). A good and rapid response can be achieved with pustular psoriasis. Response to the drug ranges from a favorable response in 45 to 63% of patients

to an excellent response in 18 to 38% of patients. This variation may reflect different doses, varying time intervals, and different criteria for evaluating disease activity. Although this medication is not a first-line agent, it may benefit patients with high alcohol intake because of the low prevalence of hepatotoxicity. A major disadvantage is the frequent occurrence of bone marrow suppression (132).

CYCLOSPORINE

Cyclosporine is an 11-amino acid cyclic peptide frequently used to facilitate organ transplantation. Although the precise mechanism of action is not known, the inhibition of lymphokine secretion by activated T cells may play a central role. Because of the cost and toxicity associated with the drug, it is currently recommended only in patients with severe psoriasis that is unresponsive to more conventional therapies. Cyclosporine appears to be as effective as PUVA, UVB, MTX, or retinoid therapy in the treatment of chronic severe plaque psoriasis, but less effective in pustular psoriasis. Clearing with cyclosporine occurs more rapidly than with other systemic modalities, but relapse is common after therapy is withdrawn. A rebound phenomenon, such as those seen in systemic corticosteroid withdrawal, is usually not seen. Dosages required for transplantation (15 mg/kg per day) are not appropriate, but lower doses (2.5 to 5 mg/kg per day) lead to a good response within 4 to 8 weeks. Therapeutic response is faster and more complete with higher doses, but there is a dose-dependent increased incidence of nephrotoxicity and hypertension. These side effects are reported to be reversed after lowering the dose. Other side effects include hepatotoxicity, neurologic abnormalities, gingival hyperplasia, hypertrichosis, and an increased incidence of lymphoma. Because of the many potentially life-threatening side effects, it has been recommended that patients with hypertension, evidence of compromised renal function, concurrent immunosuppression, or history of malignancy, pregnancy, or infection be excluded from taking this medication. To date, little is known about the safety and efficacy of long-term maintenance therapy. One study showed hypertension and renal dysfunction to be a problem, but this was corrected with dose reduction, therapeutic intervention, or both. To reduce the daily dose, combination with UVB, PUVA, or etretinate has been suggested. Phototherapy may not be a desirable combination in view of cyclosporine's immunosuppression and the potential for carcinogenic effects with phototherapy. High-dose etretinate showed only a modest reduction in cyclosporine dose (133, 134).

In conclusion, although systemic cyclosporine is efficacious in clearing psoriasis, several life-threatening side effects limit its use. Because of the toxicity of systemically administered cyclosporine, current investigations are focusing on topical preparations and intralesional cyclosporine.

VITAMIN D₃

VITAMIN D₃

Calcitriol (1,25-dihydroxycholecalciferol) is the active form of vitamin D₃. The skin has receptors for circulating calcitriol, and when bound, keratinocyte proliferation is inhibited, and basal cells are induced to differentiate to squamous cells. In vitro, cultured cells from psoriatic skin exhibit a partial resistance to these effects of calcitriol, which is overcome by large increases in calcitriol concentrations. Clinical studies have confirmed the effectiveness of both topical and systemic calcitriol. Unfortunately, the limiting factor is hypercalcemia from systemic administration. Topical therapy, however, has been well tolerated with little or no side effects in the treatment of localized psoriasis (135).

A synthetic analog of calcitriol, calcipotriol, is an effective topical therapy for psoriasis, without changes in serum levels of ionized calcium. Like calcitriol, calcipotriol shows receptor binding and effects on cell differentiation, but calciptriol is 100 times less potent in its effect on calcium metabolism (136). A thin layer of the ointment preparation is applied to the affected areas twice daily for 8 weeks; improvement usually begins after 2 weeks. Patients should be instructed to use no more than 100 g per week. Adverse reactions include burning, itching, and skin irritation in 10 to 15% of patients. Erythema, dry skin, and worsening of psoriasis, including development of face and scalp psoriasis, has been reported in 1 to 10% of patients. Less than 1% of patients develop hypercalcemia.

Evolving Treatments

The following discussion focuses on systemic therapies that have been designated as evolving treatments by the American Academy of Dermatology guidelines of care for psoriasis.

SULFASALAZINE

SULFASALAZINE

Sulfasalazine contains a sulfapyridine moiety attached to 5-aminosalicylate. This drug has been used commonly in the treatment of ulcerative colitis and Crohn's disease. About one-third of a given dose of sulfasalazine is absorbed from the small intestine. The remaining two-thirds pass to the colon where the compound is split, possibly by intestinal bacteria, into its two components. Most of the sulfapyridine is absorbed in the colon, but only one-third of the 5-aminosalicylate is absorbed. The remainder of the two components is excreted into the feces. There are several proposed mechanisms of action since the drug may act as a whole or in parts. Sulfasalazine has been reported to inhibit folic acid, and the salicylate moiety affects the arachidonic acid pathway by inhibiting cyclooxygenase. It also has antimicrobial effects on the gut microflora.

A double-blind trial has recently found it to be effective in moderate-to-severe, stable, plaque-type psoriasis. Marked improvement was found in 41% of these patients.

Common side effects are related to the gastrointestinal tract, such as nausea and diarrhea. With the low incidence of severe side effects, it may be used in patients whose disease severity may not justify the use of PUVA, etretinate, or MTX. Further studies are needed to clarify its use with other forms of therapy (137–139).

FISH OIL AND FUMARIC ACID

FISH OIL AND FUMARIC ACID

Deep-sea fish oil contains significant quantities of the fatty acids eicosapentaenoic acid and docosahexanenoic acid. These fatty acids have a variety of effects on arachidonic acid metabolism. Eicosapentaenoic acid competes with arachidonic acid as a substrate for cyclooxygenase and lipoxygenase to form biologically less potent prostaglandins and leukotrienes, respectively. Docosahexaenoic acid inhibits prostaglandin production and weakly inhibits leukotriene production. Since elevated levels of leukotrienes are found in the lesions of psoriasis, modifying the levels may influence the course. However, fish oils given orally slightly reduced the redness, scaling, and itching. Although it may not be used as monotherapy, it may be useful as an adjuvant treatment (140).

Fumaric acid therapy for psoriasis has recently been investigated in placebo-controlled studies by Dutch investigators. It consists of an oral treatment with monoethyl and dimethyl esters of fumaric acids. Its mechanism of action against psoriasis is currently not known. Considerable improvement was found in 50% of the patients. The drawback of this medication has been its significant side effects such as flushing, nausea, diarrhea, and fatigue. This may limit future use in psoriasis patients (141, 142).

CLINICAL VARIANTS AND SPECIFIC TREATMENT MODALITIES

CLINICAL VARIANTS AND SPECIFIC TREATMENT MODALITIES

As mentioned previously, several clinical variants of psoriasis have been recognized that will determine the type of treatment modality. The following discussion summarizes specific treatment modalities for these clinical variants. Children and adults with guttate psoriasis are usually given systemic antimicrobial treatment, based on either cultures or antibody titers showing group A streptococcal infection. For both erythrodermic and generalized pustular psoriasis, MTX and etretinate have been successful monotherapies in controlling these eruptions. Localized psoriasis of the palms and soles responds well to PUVA treatments concentrated in these areas, and the addition of etretinate to PUVA (RE-PUVA) is reported to be more effective than PUVA alone. Seborriasis distributed over the scalp, central chest, and groin may respond to oral ketoconazole. Localized psoriasis of the scalp can be treated with 2% ketoconazole shampoo or other antiseborrheic preparations. Inverse psoriasis of the body folds with associated group B streptococcus colonization has been reported to respond to 2% erythromycin ointment. Finally, the choice of treatment for plaque-type psoriasis depends on the extent of body surface involvement. For more localized disease, topical corticosteroids or anthralin may be used. If more than 50% of the body surface is involved, then phototherapy, photochemotherapy, or systemic therapy should be considered. The two most commonly used forms of systemic monotherapies for plaque-type psoriasis are MTX and retinoids, but the latter is less effective and is usually used in combination with other treatments (109, 143).

CONCLUSION

In summary, seborrheic dermatitis and psoriasis are cutaneous eruptions in which disease expression is based on genetic and environmental factors. The pathophysiology of both diseases involves epidermal cell proliferation and inflammation. Therapies for seborrheic dermatitis and psoriasis are directed at these two pathologic features. Seborrheic dermatitis can be treated with shampoos or with topical antifungals and corticosteroids in areas not involving the scalp. The treatment of psoriasis, however, depends not only on the location, but also on its clinical presentation. Since a wide range of therapies are available for psoriasis, consideration must be given to side effects. Ideally, the choice is a regimen that provides adequate therapeutic efficacy without compromising the patient's quality of life.

ROSACEA

Rosacea, also called middle-age acne or acne-rosacea, is a chronic inflammatory disease. It is most common after the age of 30 and more prevalent in people of Celtic and northern European heritage.

Clinical Features

The disease begins with a gradual onset of transient flushing and erythema. Patients may notice flares secondary to emotional stress, alcoholic or hot drinks, and hot or spicy foods. This occurs mainly over the forehead, nose, and cheeks although other areas of the face and neck may be involved. Over a period of months to years, persistent erythema with telangiectasias and eventually erythematous papules and pustules, resembling acne, may develop. Unlike acne, open comedones are never seen in rosacea. The final stage of rosacea, which occurs in severe, chronic cases, is rhinophyma. This is the irreversible soft tissue hypertrophy of the nose, producing the "W.C. Fields nose," which is more common in males (144).

Pathogenesis and Etiology

Pathologic findings in rosacea include dilatation of blood vessels in the papillary dermis and sebaceous hyperplasia. The etiology of rosacea has remained elusive for many years. Recent studies have pointed to Helicobacter pylori, a bacteria that may inhabit the stomach. H. pylori secretes a capsule of ammonia that neutralizes the stomach's acidity, causing the stomach to increase production of gastrin, the hormone responsible for gastric acidity. Elevated gastrin levels may cause the vascular dilatation responsible for many of the clinical manifestations of rosacea.

Treatment

Patients should be instructed to avoid stimuli that may provoke rosacea. The standard treatment for rosacea involves 4 to 6 weeks or oral antibiotics, including tetracycline 250 mg four times a day, or alternatively, minocycline 100 mg twice a day, flagyl 200 twice a day, or erythromycin 250 mg four times a day. Antibiotic therapy is effective, but the disease, nonetheless, often recurs. Topical treatment, including metronidazole twice a day or a mixture of sodium sulfacetamide 10% and sulfur 5% twice a day is effective in controlling recurrences of rosacea following oral antibiotics (145).

The use of "triple therapy" for Helicobacter pylori is a promising treatment for rosacea. This includes oral tetracycline 250 mg four times a day, oral metronidazole 250 mg three times a day, and bismuth subsalicylate one-half ounce four times a day for 3 weeks.

The only effective treatments for rhinophyma include cold steel or laser surgery or dermabrasion (146).

ACKNOWLEDGMENT

We would like to thank our departmental secretary, Sheila F. Short, for her secretarial assistance.

REFERENCES

1. Leyden JJ, Shalita AR. Rationale therapy for acne vulgaris: An update on topical treatment. J Am Acad Dermatol 15:907–914, 1986.
2. Pochi PE. The pathogenesis and treatment of acne. Annu Rev Med 41:187–198, 1990.
3. Ebling FJG, Cunliffe WJ. The sebaceous glands. In: Rook A, Wilkinson DS, Ebling FJG, Champion RH, Burton JL, eds. Textbook of dermatology, 4th ed. Oxford, England, Blackwell Scientific Publications, 1986:1914.
4. Arnold HL, Odom RB, James WD. Acne. Andrews Diseases of the Skin, 8th ed, Philadelphia, PA, WB Saunders Co., 1990: 250–267.
5. Puissegur-Lupo ML. Acne vulgaris: Treatments and their rationale. Postgrad Med 78:76–84, 1985.
6. Webster GF, Leyden JJ, Norman ME et al. Compliment activation in acne vulgaris: In vitro studies with Propionibacterium acnes and Propionibacterium granulosum. Infect Immun 22:523, 1978.
7. Holland DB et al. Lymphocyte subpopulations in patients with acne vulgaris. Br J Derm 109:199–203, 1983.
8. Shalita AR, Leyden JJ. New insights into pathogenesis of acne. 15 Symposium Digest Vol 3 (4):25–32, 1991.
9. Cunliffe WJ. Evolution of a strategy for the treatment of acne. J Am Acad Dermatol 16:591–599, 1987.
10. Wilson BB. Acne vulgaris. Prim Care 16(3):695–712, 1989.
11. Liden S, Lindelof B. Is benzoyl peroxide carcinogenic? Br J Dermatol 123:129–130, 1990.

12. Jick SS, Tenis BZ, Jick H. First trimester topical tretinoin and congenital disorders. Lancet 341:1181–1182, 1993.

13. Katsambas A, Towarky AA, Stratigos J. Topical clindamycin phosphate compared with oral tetracycline in the treatment of acne vulgaris. Br J Dermatol 116:387–391, 1987.

14. Lever L, Marks R. Current views on the aetiology, pathogenesis and treatment of acne vulgaris. Drugs 39(5):681–692, 1990.

15. Hirschmann JV. Topical antibiotics in dermatology. Arch Derm 124:1691–1700, 1989.

16. Parry MF, Chan-Kook R. Pseudomembranous colitis caused by topical clindamycin phosphate. Arch Derm 122:583–584, 1986.

17. Mills OH, Kligman AM. Drugs that are ineffective in the treatment of acne vulgaris. Br J Dermatol 108:371–374, 1983.

18. Schachner L, Pestana A, Kittles C. A clinical trial comparing the safety and efficacy of a topical erythromycin zinc formulation with a topical clindamycin formulation. J Am Acad Dermatol 22:489–495, 1990.

19. Katsambas A, Graups K, Stratigos J. Clinical studies of 20% azelaic acid cream in the treatment of acne vulgaris. Acta Derm Venerol (Stockh) 143(suppl):35–39, 1989.

20. Schmidt JB, Spora J. Efficacy of topically applied 17 alpha-propylmesterolone in acne patients. Endocrinol Experiment 21:71–78, 1987.

21. Lookingbill DP, et al. Inocoterone and acne. Arch Dermatol 128:1197–1200, 1992.

22. Burke B, Early EA, Cunliffe WJ. Benzoyl peroxide versus topical erythromycin in the treatment of acne vulgaris. Br J Dermatol 108:199–204, 1983.

23. Bathman T, Bonfils A, Branck C, et al. RU58841, a new specific topical antiandrogen. J Steroid Biochem Molec Biol 48:55–60, 1994.

24. Hughes BR, et al. Strategy of acne therapy with long-term antibiotics. Br J Dermatol. 121:623–628, 1989.

25. Eady EA, et al. Superior antibacterial action and reduced incidence of bacterial resistance in minocycline compared to tetracycline treated acne patients. Br J Dermatol 122:233–244, 1990.

26. Driscoll MS, et al. Longterm oral antibiotics for acne; Is laboratory monitoring necessary? JAAD 28:595–602, 1993.

27. Hugh BR, Cunliffe WJ. Interactions between the oral contraceptive pill and antibiotics. Br J Dermatol 122:717, 1990.

28. Shalita AR, et al. Isotretinoin revisited. Cutis 42:1–19, Dec., 1988.

29. Barth JH, Macdonald SP, Mark J, et al. Isotretinoin therapy for acne vulgaris: a re-evaluation of the need for measurements of plasma lipids and liver function tests. Br J Dermatol 129:704–707, 1993.

30. Killoyne RF. Effects of retinoids in bone. J Am Acad Dermatol 19(suppl):212–216, 1988.

31. Sciarra F, et al. Antiandrogens: clinical applications. J Steroid Biochem Molec Biol 37(3):349–362, 1990.

32. Pathak MA, Fitzpatrick TB, Greiter F, Kraus EW. Preventive treatment of sunburn, dermatoheliosis, and skin cancer with sunprotective agents. In: Fitzpatrick TB, Eisen AZ, Wolff K, Freedberg IM, Austen KF, eds. Dermatology in General Medicine, 3rd ed. New York, McGraw-Hill, Inc., 1987:1507–1522.

33. Braun-Falco O, Plewig G, Wolff HH, Winkelmann RK. Dermatology, 3rd ed. Berlin, Heidelberg, Springer-Verlag, 1991:ch 13.

34. Soter NA. Acute effects of ultraviolet radiation on the skin. In: Maibach HI. Seminars in Dermatology. Philadelphia, WB Saunders Co., 1990;9(1):11–15.

35. Young AR. Cumulative effects of ultraviolet radiation on the skin. Cancer and photoaging. In: Maibach HI. Seminars in Dermatology. Philadelphia, WB Saunders Co., 1990;9(1):25–31.

36. Diffey BL. Human exposure to ultraviolet radiation. In: Maibach HI. Seminars in Dermatology. Philadelphia, WB Saunders Co., 1990;9(1): 2–10.

37. Morrison WL, et al. The effects of indomethacin on ultraviolet-induced delayed erythema. J Invest Dermatol 68:130, 1971.

38. Arnold HL, Odom RB, James WD. Diseases of the Skin: Clinical Dermatology, 8th ed. Philadelphia, WB Saunders Co., 1990:ch 3.

39. Green A. Sun exposure and the risk of melanoma. Australas J Dermatol 25:99–102, 1984.

40. Taylor CR, Stern RS, Leyden JJ, Gilchrest BA. Photoaging/photodamage and photoprotection. J Am Acad Dermatol 22:1–15, 1990.

41. Lowe NJ. Sunscreens and the prevention of skin aging. J Dermatol Surg Oncol 16:936–938, 1990.

42. Boger J, Araugo OE, Flowers F. Sunscreen efficacy, use, and misuse. South Med J 77:1421–1427, 1984.

43. Pathak MA. Sunscreens: topical and systemic approaches for protection of human skin against harmful effects of solar radiation. J Am Acad Dermatol 7:285–312, 1982.

44. Federal Register. Sunscreen drug products for over-the-counter human drugs: proposed safety, effective, and labeling conditions. Washington, DC, Dept of Health, Education and Welfare, Food and Drug Administration: Aug 25, 1978;43(166):38206–38269.

45. Kaidbey RH. The photoprotective potential of the new superpotent sunscreens. J Am Acad Dermatol 22:449–452, 1990.

46. Lowe NJ. Photoprotection. In: Maibach HI. Seminars in Dermatology. Philadelphia, WB Saunders Co., 1990;9(1):78–83.

47. Marks R, et al. The effect of regular sunscreen use on vitamin D levels in a Australian population. Archives of Dermatology 131:415–421, 1995.

48. Black HS. Systemic photoprotective agents. Photodermatology 4:187–195, 1987.

49. Dubois EL. Antimalarials in the management of discoid and systemic lupus erythematosus. Semin Arthritis Rheum 8:33–51, 1978.

50. Swanbeck G. Aminoquinolones. In: Fitzpatrick TB, Eisen AZ, Wolff K, Freedberg IM, Austen KF, eds. Dermatology in General Medicine, 3rd ed. New York, McGraw-Hill, Inc, 1987:2574–2582.

51. Weiss JS, Ellis CN, Headington JT, et al. Topical tretinoin improves photoaged skin: A double blind, vehicle-controlled study. JAMA 259:527–532, 1988.

52. Leyden JJ, Grove GL, Grove MJ, et al. Treatment of photodamage skin with topical tretinoin. J Am Acad Dermatol 21:638–644, 1989.

53. Gardner SS, Weiss JS. Clinical features of photodamage and treatment with topical tretinoin. J Dermatol Surg Oncol 16:925–931, 1990.

54. Van Scott EJ, Yu RJ. Alpha hydroxyacids. Can J Dermatol 1:108–112, 1989.

55. Goette DR. Topical chemotherapy with 5-fluorouracil. J Am Acad Dermatol 4:663–649, 1981.

56. Arnold HL, Odom RB, James WD. Warts. In: Andrews' Diseases of the Skin, 8th ed. Philadelphia, PA, WB Saunders Co., 1990: 468–475.

57. Cobb MW. Human papillomaviruses infection. J Am Acad Dermatol 22:547–566, 1990.

58. Lowy DR, Androphy EJ. Warts. In: Fitzpatrick TB, et al, eds. Dermatology in General Medicine, 3rd ed. New York, NY, McGraw-Hill Inc., 1987, pp 2355–2372.

59. Highet AS. Viral warts. Semin Dermatol 7(1):53–57, 1988.

60. Beutner KR. Human papillomavirus infection. J Am Acad Dermatol 20(1):114–123, 1989.

61. Steele KS, et al. Monochloroacetic acid and 60% salicylic acid as a treatment for simple plantar warts: effectiveness and mode of action. Br J Dermatol 118:537–544, 1988.

62. Bart BJ, et al. Salicylic acid in karaya gum patch as a treatment for verruca vulgaris. J Am Acad Dermatol 20 (1):74–76, 1989.

63. Food and Drug Administration Health and Human Services. Wart removal drug products for over the counter human use: final monograph. 21 CFR, part 358, 1991.

64. Hirose R. Topical treatment of resistant warts with glutaraldehyde. J Dermatol 21:248–253, 1994.

65. Silva PD, et al. Management of condyloma acuminatum. J Am Acad Dermatol 13:457–463, 1985.

66. Marcus J, Camisa C. Podophyllin therapy for condyloma acuminatum. Int J Dermatol 29 (10):693–698, 1990.

67. Mroczkowski TF, McEwen C. Warts and other human papillomavirus infections. Postgrad Med 78 (7):91–98, 1985.

68. Stone KM, et al. Treatment of external genital warts: a randomized clinical trial comparing podophyllin, cryotherapy, and electrodesiccation. Genitourin Med 66:16–19, 1990.

69. Jensen SL. Comparison of podophyllin application with simple surgical excision in clearance and recurrence of perianal condyloma acuminata. Lancet 2:1146–1148, 1985.

70. Rapini RP. Venereal warts. Primary Care 17(1):127–144, 1990.

71. Campbell BJ. The treatment of warts. Primary Care 13 (3):465–476, 1986.

72. Miller RA. Podophyllin. Int J Dermatol 24:491–498, 1985.

73. Cassidy DE, et al. Podophyllum toxicity: a report of a fatal case and a review of the literature. J Toxicol Clin Toxicol 19(1):35–44, 1982.

74. Beutner KR, von Krogh G. Current status of podophyllin for the treatment of genital warts. Semin Dermatol 9(2):148–151, 1990.

75. Edwards A, et al. Podophyllotoxin 0.5% vs podophyllin 20% to treat penile warts. Genitourin Med 64:263–265, 1988.

76. Rosemberg SK. Sexually transmitted papillomaviral infections: v. prophylactic use of topical 5-fluorouracil in refractory infection in the male. Urology 34 (2):86–88, 1989.

77. Ferenczy A. Comparison of 5-fluorouracil and CO_2 laser for treatment of vaginal condyloma. Obstet Gynecol 64:773–778, 1984.

78. Boyd S. Condyloma acuminata in the pediatric population. AJDC 144:817–824, 1990.

79. Hursthouse MW. A controlled trial on the use of topical 5-fluorouracil on viral warts. Br J Dermatol 92:93–99, 1975.

80. Shumer SM, et al. Bleomycin in the treatment of recalcitrant warts. J Am Acad Dermatol 9:91–96, 1983.

81. Shelley WB, Shelley ED. Intralesional bleomycin sulfate therapy for warts. Arch Dermatol 127:234–236, 1991.

82. Keay S, et al. Topical interferon for treating condyloma acuminata in women. J Infect Dis 158(5):934–939, 1988.

83. Eron LJ, et al. Interferon therapy for condyloma acuminata. N Engl J Med 315(17):1059–1063, 1986.

84. Vance JC, et al. Intralesional recombinant alpha-2 interferon for the treatment of patients with condyloma acuminatum or verruca plantaris. Arch Dermatol 122:272–276, 1986.

85. Friedman-Kien AE, et al. Natural interferon alfa for treatment of condyloma acuminata. JAMA 259(4):533–538, 1988.

86. Weck PK, et al. Interferons in the treatment of genital human papillomavirus infections. Am J Med 85(suppl 2A):159–164, 1988.

87. Reichman RC. Treatment of condyloma acuminatum with three interferons administered intralesionally. Ann Int Med 108:675–679, 1988.

88. Mahrle G, et al. Recombinant interferon-gamma in dermatology. J Invest Dermatol 95(6 suppl):132s–137s, 1990.

89. Kirby P. Interferon and genital warts: much potential, modest progress. JAMA 259(4):570–572, 1988.

90. Lutzner MA. Oral retinoid treatment of human papillomavirus type 5-induced epidermodysplasia verruciformis. N Engl J Med 302(19): 1091, 1980.

91. Gross G, et al. Effect of oral aromatic retinoid (Ro 10-9359) on human papillomavirus–2 induced common warts. Dermatologica 166:48–53, 1983.

92. Bolton RA. Nongenital warts: classification and treatment options. AFP 43(6):2049–2056, 1991.

93. Naylor MF, et al. Contact immunotherapy of resistant warts. J Am Acad Dermatol 19:679–683, 1988.

94. Eriksen K. Treatment of the common wart by induced allergic inflammation. Dermatologica 160:161–166, 1980.

95. Sanders BB, et al. Dinitrochlorobenzene immunotherapy of human warts. Cutis 27:389–392, 1981.

96. Orlow S. Cimetidine therapy for multiple viral warts in children. J Am Acad Dermatol 28(5):794–796, 1993.

97. Taylor MB. Successful treatment of warts. Postgrad Med 84(8):126–136, 1988.

98. Davidson-Parker J, et al. Immunotherapy of genital warts with inosine pranobex and conventional treatment: double blind placebo controlled study. Genitourin Med 64:383–386, 1988.

99. Shuster S. The etiology of dandruff and the mode of action of therapeutic agents. Br J Dermatol 1:235–242, 1984.

100. Skinner RBJR, Noah PW, Taylor RM, et al. Double-blind treatment of seborrheic dermatitis with 2% ketoconazole cream. J Am Acad Dermatol 12:852–856, 1985.

101. Ford GP, Farr PM, Ive FA, et al. The response of seborrhoeic dermatitis to ketoconazole. Br J Dermatol 111:603–607, 1984.

102. Heng MC, Henderson BA, Barker BA, et al. Correlation of Pityrosporum ovale density with clinical severity of seborrheic dermatitis as assessed by a simplified technique. J Am Acad Dermatol 23:82–86, 1990.

103. Belew PW, Rosenberg EW, Jennings BR. Activation of the alternative pathway of complement by Malassezia ovalis (Pityrosporum ovale). Mycopathologia 70:187–191, 1980.

104. Cowley NC, Farr PM, Shuster S. The permissive effect of sebum in seborrhoeic dermatitis: an explanation of the rash in neurological disorders. Br J Dermatol 122:71–76, 1990.

105. Brown M, Evans TW, Tooley PJH. The role of ketoconazole 2% shampoo in the treatment and prophylactic management of dandruff. J Dermatol Treat 1:177–179, 1990.

106. White JW. Localized eczematous disease. In: Sams WM, Lynch PJ, eds. Principles and Practice of Dermatology, New York, Churchill Livingstone, 1990:403.

107. Taieb A, Legrain V, Palmier C, et al. Topical ketoconazole for infantile seborrhoeic dermatitis. Dermatologica 181:26–32, 1990.

108. Christophers E, Krueger GG. Psoriasis. In: Fitzpatrick TB, Eisen AZ, Wolff K, et al, eds. Dermatology in General Medicine, 3rd ed. Philadelphia, WB Saunders, 1987:461.

109. Zanolli MD. Psoriasis and Reiter's disease. In: Sams WM, Lynch PJ, eds. Principles and Practice of Dermatology. New York, Churchill Livingstone, 1990:307.

110. Karasek MA. New developments in our understanding of the biology of psoriasis. Cutis 45:307–310, 1990.

111. Rosenberg EW, Belew PW. Microbial factors in psoriasis. Arch Dermatol 118:143–144, 1982.

112. Felscher Z, Rothman S. The insensible perspiration of the skin in hyperkeratotic conditions. J Invest Dermatol 6:271–278, 1945.

113. Marks R. Topical therapy for psoriasis: general principles. Dermatol Clin 2:383–388, 1984.

114. Lowe NJ, Ashton R. Anthralin and coal tar therapy for psoriasis. Dermatol Clin 2:389–396, 1984.

115. Wheeler L, Lowe NJ. Mutagenicity of urines from patients undergoing coal tar therapy for psoriasis. J Int Dermatol 77:181–185, 1981.

116. Jones SK, Mackie RM, Hole DJ, et al. Further evidence of safety of tar in the management of psoriasis. Br J Dermatol 113:97–101, 1985.

117. Trozak DJ. Topical corticosteroid therapy in psoriasis vulgaris. Cutis 46:341–349, 1990.

118. Fiore M. Practical aspects of anthralin therapy. Cutis 46:351–354, 1990.

119. Ramsay B, Lawrence CM, Bruse JM, et al. The effect of triethanolamine application on anthralin-induced inflammation and therapeutic effect on psoriasis. J Am Acad Dermatol 23:73–76, 1990.

120. Guidelines of care for psoriasis. AAD Bulletin 9:10–15, 1991.

121. Rosenberg EW, Noah PW, Zanolli ME, et al. Use of rifampin with penicillin and erythromycin in the treatment of psoriasis. J Am Acad Dermatol 14:761–764, 1986.

122. Rosenberg EW, Skinner RB Jr, Noah PW. Antimicrobial treatment of psoriasis. In Roenigk H, Maibach HA: Psoriasis, 2nd ed. New York, Marcel Dekker, 1990:815.

123. Paul BS, Diette KM, Parrish JA. Therapeutic photomedicine. In: Fitzpatrick TB, Eisen AZ, Wolff K, et al. Dermatology in General Medicine, 3rd ed. Philadelphia, WB Saunders, 1987:1522.

124. Stern RS, Thibodeau LA, Kleinerman RA, et al. Psoriasis and susceptibility of nonmelanoma skin cancer. J Am Acad Dermatol 12:67–73, 1985.

125. Skinner RB Jr. Psoralens. In: Wolverton SE, Wilkins JK. Systemic drugs for skin diseases. Philadelphia, WB Saunders, 1991:219.

126. Wolff K. Side-effects of psoralen photochemotherapy (PUVA). Br J Dermatol 122(suppl 36):117–125, 1990.

127. Wolverton SE. Retinoids. In: Wolverton SE, Wilkins JK. Systemic Drug for Skin Diseases. Philadelphia, WB Saunders, 1991:187.

128. Ellis CN, Voorhees JJ. Etretinate therapy. J Am Acad Dermatol 12:267–291, 1987.

129. Olsen EA. The pharmacology of methotrexate. J Am Acad Dermatol 25:306–318, 1991.

130. Tung JP, Maibach HI. The practical use of methotrexate in psoriasis. Drugs 40:697–712, 1990.

131. Roenigk HH, Auerbach R, Maibach HI, et al. Methotrexate in psoriasis: revised guidelines. J Am Acad Dermatol 19:145–156, 1988.

132. Boyd AS, Neldner KH. Hydroxyurea therapy. J Am Acad Dermatol 25:518–524, 1991.

133. Griffiths CE. Systemic and local administration of cyclosporine in the treatment of psoriasis. J Am Acad Dermatol 23:1242–1246, 1990.

134. Guenther L. Cyclosporine. In: Wolverton SE, Wilkins JK. Systemic Drugs for Skin Diseases. Philadelphia, WB Saunders, 1991:167.

135. Kragballe K. Treatment of psoriasis by the topical application of the novel cholecalciferol analogue calcipotriol (MC 901). Arch Dermatol 125:1647–1652, 1989.

136. Kragballe K, Wildfang IL. Calcipotriol (MC903), a novel vitamin D3 analogue simulates terminal differentiation and inhibits proliferation of cultured human lymphocytes. Archives of Dermatological Research 282:164–167, 1990.

137. Gupta AK, et al. Sulfasalazine improves psoriasis. A double-blind analysis. Arch Dermatol 126:487–493, 1990.

138. Halasz CI. Sulfasalazine as folic acid inhibitor in psoriasis. Arch Dermatol 126:1516–1517, 1990.

139. Neumann VC, Shinebaum R, Cooke EM, et al. Effects of sulphasalazine on faecal flora in patients with rheumatoid arthritis: a comparison with penicillamine. Br J Rheumatol 26:334–337, 1987.

140. Bittner SB, Tucker WF, Cartwright I, et al. A double-blind, randomized, placebo-controlled trial of fish oil in psoriasis. Lancet 1:378–380, 1988.

141. Nugteren-Huying WM, van der Schroeff JG, Hermans J, et al. Fumaric acid therapy for psoriasis: a randomized, double-blind, placebo-controlled study. J Am Acad Dermatol 22:311–312, 1990.

142. Nieboer C, de Hoop D, Langendijk PN, et al. Fumaric acid therapy in psoriasis: a double-blind comparison between fumaric acid compound therapy and monotherapy with dimethylfumaric acid ester. Dermatologica 181:33–37, 1990.

143. Matsunami E, Takashima A, Mizumo N, et al. Topical PUVA, etretinate, and combined PUVA and etretinate for palmoplantar pustulosis: comparison of therapeutic efficacy and the influences of tonsillar and dental focal infections. J Dermatol 17:92–96, 1990.

144. Fitzpatrick, Thomas B, et al. Dermatology in General Medicine. New York, McGraw-Hill, Inc., 1993:727–735.

145. Bleicher PA, Charles JH, Sober AJ. Topical metronidazole for rosacea. Arch of Dermatol 123:609–614, 1987.

146. Greenbaum SS, Krull EA, Watnick K. Comparison of CO_2 laser and electrosurgery treatment of rhinophyma. JAAD 18:363–368, 1988.

CHAPTER 45

BURNS

TED L. RICE

Skin, the largest organ of the body, performs five major functions. It provides protection from the environment, sensory perception, vitamin production, excretion of water and some wastes, and regulation of body temperature. When the skin is damaged, bacteria are no longer prevented from invading, pain is produced (unless superficial sensory nerves are destroyed), and both fluid and heat are lost through the damaged area.

Extensive skin loss or damage requiring hospitalization can be caused by many different mechanisms that produce similar effects: thermal injury from hot liquids (scalds), flames, or extreme cold (frostbite) and injury from chemicals, radiation (sunburn), electricity, or trauma (abrasion). Patients with extensive exfoliative dermatoses (e.g., the Stevens-Johnson syndrome or toxic epidermal necrolysis) are treated in burn centers.

Fire victims can suffer severe injury or death without significant body surface burns. A classic demonstration of this was the 1942 Coconut Grove Nightclub fire, in which 75 of the 114 deaths were due to smoke inhalation. Carbon monoxide (CO) poisoning is a frequent cause of death. CO binds preferentially to hemoglobin, displacing oxygen and shifting the oxyhemoglobin dissociation curve to the left, resulting in tissue hypoxia. Depending on the material that is burning, smoke contains toxins other than CO, such as cyanide, acrolein, benzine, and phosgene (1, 2).

Outcome following thermal injury is determined by a combination of patient and burn factors. The very young, very old, and previously ill have a poorer prognosis than do healthy, young adults following a similar injury. Scoring systems for injury severity include the Thermal Injury Organ Failure Score, which correlates with outcome, and the Burn Specific Health Scale to accurately assess the impact of nonfatal burn injury (3, 4).

Burn factors that determine patient outcome include depth, extent, and body surface location (5). A list of burn severity criteria is provided in Table 45.1. The important distinction in depth of burn is that partial-thickness injuries heal by cell regeneration, whereas full-thickness injuries, unless very small, require skin-grafting. Small full-thickness burns heal by contraction and reepithelialization from progenitor cells at the edges of the wound.

WOUND ASSESSMENT

Traditionally, the depth of burns is described in degrees of injury as listed in Figure 45.1. As the depth of injury increases, the number for degree of injury increases. A first-degree burn is very shallow and involves only the epidermis. A second-degree burn involves complete destruction of the epidermis and variable portions of the underlying dermis. When destruction to the dermis is limited to the upper third or less, it is called a superficial second-degree burn. Conversely, a deep second-degree burn has tissue destruction below the top one-third but not completely through the dermis. A third-degree, or full-thickness, burn has destruction of the entire epidermis and dermis. The terms "fourth-degree burn" and "fifth-degree burn" have been used to describe tissue destruction through subcutaneous fat and through muscle, respectively (6).

The typical first-degree burn is easily identified. It is painful and erythematous and blanches to pressure. A superficial second-degree burn is painful, forms blisters, and blanches to pressure. A third-degree burn is usually not painful because, superficial nerve endings are destroyed; can appear white, leatherlike, or black (charred); and contains thrombosed blood vessels. This dead tissue is called eschar (pronounced "es'kar"). Unfortunately, sometimes even the most experienced clinician cannot differentiate a partial-thickness from a full-thickness injury. In addition, flame injuries are typically mixtures of full- and partial-thickness injuries. This classic presentation as depicted in Figure 45.2 was described as a target or bulls-eye in which the deepest injury is in the center, with increasingly superficial injury at increasing distance from the center. Early attempts to improve the accurate assessment of injury depth included histologic staining, injection of radioactive compounds or dyes such as bromphenol blue, and fiberoptic perfusion fluorometry. These methods suffered from being invasive, cumbersome, labor-intensive, and inaccurate. Although sensitive to variations in positioning and temperature, the recently developed laser Doppler has better than 90% accuracy of correlation compared with histologic analysis of burn wound depth. The laser Doppler documents a reduction in blood cell velocity in a burn wound, establishing the necessity for surgical removal and grafting. Clinicians must remain cognizant of the need for confirmation of initial assessments of burn depth. Reassessment is necessary because of the changing nature of deep partial-thickness injuries, which may become full-thickness because of inadequate resuscitation or infection (7).

A number of systems are used to calculate the relative percentage of total body surface area (TBSA) burned. The rule of nines is a simple system that can be used to estimate the extent of burn in adults. It represents regions of the body surface as 9% or multiples of 9%; for example, the head and arms represent approximately 9% TBSA each, the torso 36%, each leg 18%, and the perineum 1%. For burns with an uneven distribution the patient's hand is a useful measuring tool. One side of the patient's hand is about 1% TBSA. The rule of nines does not hold for infants and children because their heads represent a larger TBSA than those of adults. A more accurate assessment of TBSA can be made by using the Lund-Browder chart. The chart used at the University of Michigan Burn Center is reproduced in Figure 45.3.

WOUND CLOSURE

When a large portion of the skin sustains full-thickness damage or destruction, the current surgical approach is staged eschar excision (debridement) and placement of autologous skin grafts (8). Split-thickness skin grafts (STSG) approximately 0.06 mm thick are harvested (using a dermatome), expanded by a ratio of 1.5:1 (using a meshing device), and applied to the wound after removal of devitalized tissue and achievement of hemostasis. Once adherent and vascularized, this STSG from the patient's own noninjured skin (autograft or isograft) permanently closes the wound (9).

Unfortunately, the amount of noninjured skin that is available for STSGs often cannot completely cover the open wound. A number of skin substitutes can be used to over the open wound temporarily while waiting for donor site healing and reharvesting of autograft. Commonly used biologic skin substitutes include cadaver skin (allograft or homograft) and animal skin (xenograft or heterograft). Less frequently used biologic skin substitutes are amniotic membranes and tissue-derived collagen. Synthetic skin substitutes include polyurethane films (e.g., OpSite) and petrolatum-impregnated fine mesh gauze (e.g., scarlet red

and Xeroform). Biosynthetic skin substitutes have been developed that are combinations of biologic and synthetic materials, such as Biobrane, which combines collagen with a synthetic membrane (10).

Skin substitutes adhere to the wound; minimize pain; decrease protein, water, and electrolyte loss; and simulate many important skin functions such as providing a barrier to bacteria. Although these skin substitutes provide important functions, they must eventually be replaced by autologous skin. An alternative to reharvesting STSG donor sites is the in vitro production of new skin by culture of autologous epidermis. Since the first successful transplantation of cultured autologous epidermis in 1981, keratinocyte growth techniques have been so improved that current methods allow a several thousandfold expansion of skin specimens within 3 to 4 weeks (11).

PAIN MANAGEMENT

Effective pain management in burn patients requires an understanding of both the physiologic responses to injury and the interrelationships between anxiety, depression, and pain. The extent of the burn is a significant predictor of pain but only in the first week after the injury. Pain varies greatly from patient to patient and undergoes wide fluctuations over time in each patient; the greatest pain is usually experienced during therapeutic procedures such as hydrotherapy with wound debridement and dressing changes (12). Patients with high levels of anxiety or depression tend to report more pain when at rest.

Historically, pain management practices for burn patients have not been optimal, with some centers reporting that no analgesics or psychotropics were administered to children during wound debridement (13). To the observant clinician, careful evaluation of signs such as heart rate, blood pressure, facial expressions, body movement and position, and the quality of an infant's cries is sufficient to evaluate the intensity of pain and guide the need for, and administration of, analgesics. In addition, maintaining analgesic plasma levels within the ranges established for good

Table 45.1.
Burn Injury Severity Classification[a]

	Percent of Body Surface Affected (TBSA)[b]					
	Minor Injury		Moderate Injury		Major Injury	
Depth of Burn	Adult	Child	Adult	Child	Adult	Child
Partial-thickness						
First-degree	<50	<10	50–75	10–20	>75	>20
Second-degree	<15	<10	15–25	10–20	>25	>20
Full-thickness						
Third-degree	<2	<2	2–10	2–10	>10	>10

[a]Irrespective of burn extent, injuries are classified as major when they involve areas of special importance such as the eyes, ears, hands, feet, or genitals. Injuries are major when burns occur in conjunction with other major trauma (e.g., fractures) or inhalation injury.
[b]TBS = total body surface area.

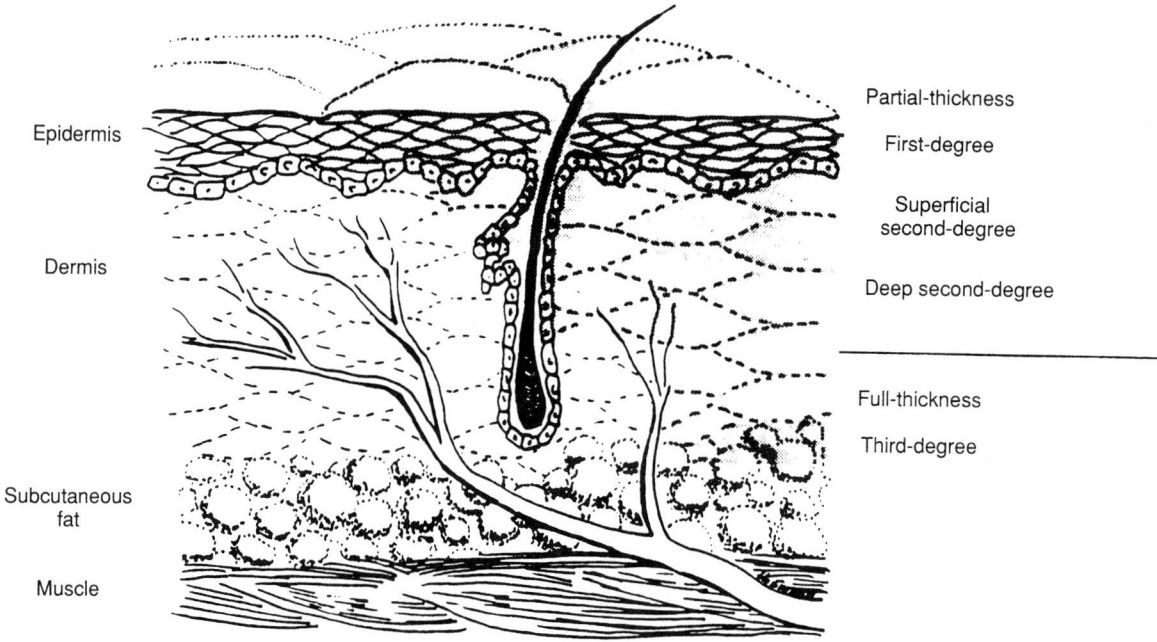

Figure 45.1. Diagram of burn depth in gross skin histology.

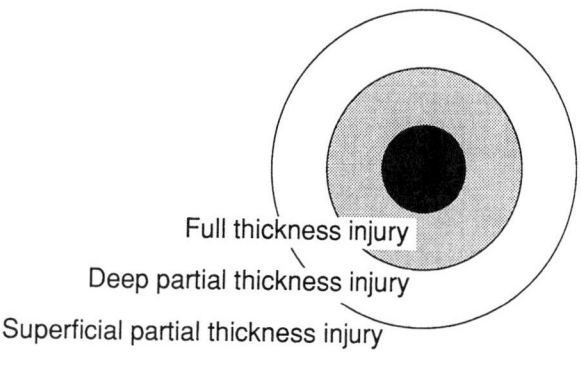

Figure 45.2. Typical pattern of injury following flame burn.

analgesia may be beneficial in centers with rapid access to drug analysis laboratories (14). Currently, a variety of pharmacotherapeutic agents are utilized in pain management, such as ketamine, propofol, and nitrous oxide.

The amount of opioid necessary to achieve pain control in burn patients can be substantial, with morphine sulfate self-administered rates of 108 mg per hour reported (15). This also demonstrates that large doses of morphine sulfate can be administered safely without undue fear of hypoventilation; indeed a dose of 1650 mg per hour has been reported (16). Another important contribution to the improved utilization of opioid analgesics is the allaying of unrealistic fears of producing narcotic addiction in hospitalized patients. The Boston Collaborative Drug Surveillance Program reported only

four cases of reasonably well-documented addiction out of 11,882 patients who received at least one narcotic preparation (17).

Rather than conventional analgesic therapy, such as intermittent intravenous morphine injections, the use of patient-controlled analgesia in both adult and pediatric burn patients is gaining popularity (18,19). However, because of situations such as the need for neuromuscular blockade, many patients with acute burns are not suitable candidates for patient-controlled analgesia (20).

Non-pharmacologic methods or adjuncts to pain management include hypnotherapeutic intervention; distraction therapy, in which video programs of scenic beauty accompanied by music are used in conjunction with analgesics; and cognitive-behavioral therapies such as explanation, personal control, altering the meaning of pain, relaxation, imagery, distraction, and self-hypnosis (21–23).

FLUID RESUSCITATION

Damaged skin loses the ability to serve as a barrier to percutaneous water loss. Evaporative water loss can be substantial (24). In contrast to the normal vapor pressure of approximately 3 mm Hg, the vapor pressure of full-thickness burns is about 30 mm Hg. The amount of water loss in milliliters per hour can be estimated by using the following formula:

$$\text{Evaporative loss (mL/hr)} = (25 + \text{TBSA}) \times \text{BSA}$$

where BSA is body surface area in square meters. In addition, injury to capillaries in the burn wound causes them to leak a protein-rich fluid into the interstitial space,

UNIVERSITY OF MICHIGAN HOSPITALS

BURN CENTER

ESTIMATION OF SIZE OF BURN BY PERCENT

LOCATION DATE SERVICE

Reg. No. Class

Name

Address

1 COLOR IN THE BURN

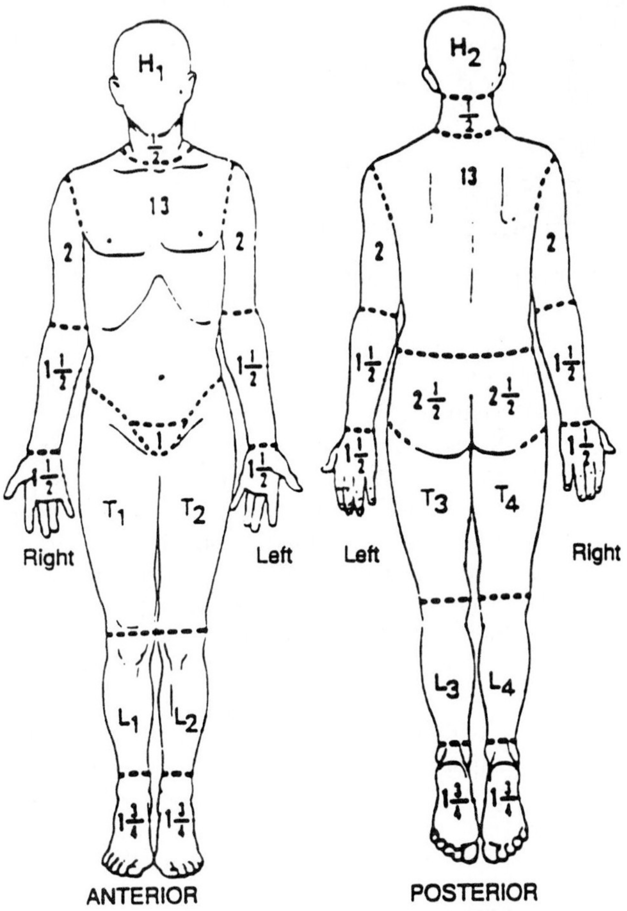

3 CALCULATE EXTENT BURN

	ANTERIOR	POSTERIOR
Head	H_1 ______	H_2 ______
Neck	______	______
Rt. Arm	______	______
Rt. Forearm	______	______
Rt. Hand	______	______
Lt. Arm	______	______
Lt. Forearm	______	______
Lt. Hand	______	______
Trunk	______	______
Buttock	______	______
Perineum	______	______
Rt. Thigh	T_1 ______	T_4 ______
Rt. Leg	L_1 ______	L_4 ______
Rt. Foot	______	______
Lt. Thigh	T_2 ______	T_3 ______
Lt. Leg	L_2 ______	L_3 ______
Lt. Foot	______	______
SUB TOTAL	______	______

% PARTIAL THICKNESS ______ %

& FULL THICKNESS ______ %

% TOTAL AREA BURNED ______ %

2 CIRCLE AGE FACTOR

PERCENT OF AREAS AFFECTED BY GROWTH

AGE	0	1	5	10	15	ADULT
H (1 or 2) = 1/2 of the head	9 1/2	8 1/2	6 1/2	5 1/2	4 1/2	3 1/2
T (1,2,3, or 4) = 1/2 of a thigh	2 3/4	3 1/4	4	4 1/4	4 1/2	4 3/4
L (1,2,3, or 4) = 1/2 of a leg	2 1/2	2 1/2	2 3/4	3	3 1/4	3 1/2

H-2053949-DS Rev. 3/89 | **MEDICAL RECORD** | University of Michigan Medical Center | **ESTIMATION OF SIZE OF BURN BY PERCENT**

Figure 45.3. University of Michigan Hospital's Burn Center estimation of size of burn by percentage.

producing edema and blisters. Blood vessels are generally thought of as solid-walled tubes like plumbing, when in fact they are made of individual cells. When injured or under the influence of cytokines or inflammatory mediators, these cells swell apart and produce small "holes" in the vessel wall. The problem resolves within 24 hr, but until then, large macromolecules (molecular weights up to 80,000) can leak out of the intravascular space. When the TBSA burned exceeds 25%, a generalized "capillary leak" is produced throughout the body, and fluid exudes from unburned vessels into tissue and organs. The exact pathophysiology of this phenomenon is not clear, but the effects of leukotrienes, prostaglandins, arachidonic acid, and oxygen-derived free radicals have been implicated.

Fluid Requirements

The treatment or resuscitation of the burned patient in shock has been the subject of much interest, research, and controversy. Focused interest was generated in the 1940s because hypovolemic shock was the leading cause of death in burned patients who survived their initial injury. The goal of initial fluid resuscitation is to restore and maintain tissue perfusion while minimizing edema formation (25, 26). The success of fluid administration is judged primarily by urine production at a rate of 0.5 to 1.0 mL/kg/hr. In addition, clinical observation of the adequately resuscitated patient should reveal a pulse rate less than 120 (in adults) and a clear sensorium (27). Use of a physiologic salt solution (crystalloid) such as lactated Ringer's is recommended.

The major controversy regarding fluid resuscitation of the burn victim is the necessity of colloid infusion (28–32). Colloid is a general descriptive term for non-diffusible, large-molecular-weight molecules that affect osmotic pressure. Available colloid suspensions include fresh frozen plasma, plasma protein fraction, albumin, dextrans, hetastarch, and pentastarch. Clinicians who routinely use colloids suggest that they are more physiologic and can reduce nonburned tissue edema. Proponents of crystalloids caution that administered colloids can escape from the intravascular space until the capillary leak is sealed. Although no definitive answer is available, it seems reasonable to exclude colloid infusion from resuscitation fluids for the first 12 hr. Representative resuscitation guidelines are listed in Table 45.2. Fluid requirements after the first 24-hr postburn period are determined in the usual fashion, with consideration of fluids lost through the burn wound and nasogastric suction. (See Chapter 9, "Fluid and Electrolyte Therapy and Acid/Base Balance.")

The main benefit of published guidelines is to alert the clinician who is unfamiliar with burn care that unusually large volumes of fluids and rates of administration are required for severely injured patients (33). Almost every author has acknowledged that patient variability prohibits development of a strictly calculated volume of resuscitative fluid and rate of administration.

In severe injuries, release of free hemoglobin from destroyed red cells and myoglobin from damaged muscle (especially following electrical injury) leads to destruction of renal tubules and acute renal failure. Binding of the free pigments to the renal tubules can be prevented by establishing a brisk urine flow (using mannitol if necessary) and alkalinizing the urine (pH $\geq$ 6.5) with parenteral sodium bicarbonate.

PHARMACOKINETIC CONSIDERATIONS IN BURN PATIENTS

The characteristic biphasic metabolic response to injury of an initial short ebb or shock phase (hypometabolic) followed by a flow phase (hypermetabolic) was described by Cuthbertson in 1930. A burn injury that exceeds 10 to 15% TBSA causes pathophysiologic alterations in the cardiovascular, gastrointestinal, renal, and hepatic systems. The plasma proteins that are responsible for drug binding ei-

Table 45.2.
Resuscitation Formulas for Postburn Fluid Requirements During the First 24 Hours Postburn[a]

Formula	Crystalloid	Colloid	Free Water
Adults			
Parkland	Lactated Ringer's 4 mL/kg/TBSA (%) ½ in first 8 hr ¼ in next 8 hr ¼ in last 8 hr	None	None
Evans	Lactated Ringer's 1 mL/kg/TBSA	1 mL/kg/TBSA	2000 mL/m²
Brooke	Lactated Ringer's 1.5 mL/kg/TBSA	1 mL/kg/TBSA	2000 mL/m²
Modified Brooke	Lactated Ringer's 2 mL/kg/TBSA	None	None
Children			
Graves	Lactated Ringer's 3 mL/kg/TBSA	None	Maintenance

[a]TBSA = total body surface area. Maintenance fluid requirements are 100 mL/kg/day for the first 10 kg body weight, 50 mL/kg/day for the second 10 kg body weight, and 20 mL/kg/day for weight in excess of 20 kg.

ther increase or decrease in concentration, resulting in decreased or increased unbound drug concentrations, respectively. Finally, the movement of drugs into and out of the circulatory system is increased through the burn wound. The pharmacokinetics and pharmacodynamics of many drugs are changed after thermal trauma.

Cardiovascular Changes

Cardiac output has been demonstrated to decrease as much as 50% within 6 hr of severe thermal injury. This reduction in output has been attributed to hypovolemia, increased blood viscosity, increased peripheral vascular resistance, and the presence of a cardiotoxic protein termed "myocardial depressant factor" (34). Theoretically, intravenous drugs have a slower rate of distribution and elimination during this initial 48-hr period.

Following resuscitation the hyperdynamic or recovery phase of injury is associated with increases of cardiac output to one and one-half to three times normal. This may not occur in the patient with preexisting myocardial disease. This increase in tissue perfusion is associated with an increased rate of drug distribution and elimination following intravenous administration (35).

Gastrointestinal Considerations

Acute stress-related mucosal damage (SRMD) of the stomach and duodenum following severe burns is extemely common and is presumably related to increased acid secretion (36). The first case of acute gastroduodenal ulcer associated with thermal injury was reported by Swan in 1823. Following the 1842 report on a series of 12 patients by Curling, the syndrome was established and named Curling's ulcer. Prophylaxis and treatment of SRMD include enteral feeding and administration of sucralfate, antacids, or H_2-receptor antagonists (H_2RAs) (37). Cimetidine appears to be unique among the H_2RAs in that following burns, it reduces resuscitative fluid requirements and has increased clearance. A study of burned children demonstrated a reduced cimetidine pharmacodynamic response in addition to an altered pharmacokinetic profile. The absorption of orally administered drugs may be either increased or decreased, depending on the drug pKa and whether intragastric pH has been modified by antacids or H2RAs. (See Chapter 23, "Peptic Ulcer Disease.")

Renal Function

The initial renal insults following a severe burn injury are general hypoxia and reduced perfusion. Following severe injury, liberation of free hemoglobin or myoglobin may result in acute renal failure. These problems can be reversed rapidly with resuscitative efforts and establishment of adequate urine flow. During the postburn hypermetabolic phase, renal blood flow and glomerular filtration rate

(GFR) are increased, although tubular secretion may be impaired. This suggests that the elimination of freely filterable drugs such as the aminoglycosides and vancomycin will increase after burn injury. This effect was demonstrated in a study of 20 burn patients, which reported abnormal increases in both GFR and tobramycin elimination in 13 of 20 patients (38). The need for increased dosage of gentamicin for burn patients has been demonstrated in numerous studies of both adults and children (39–43). There are conflicting results about increased renal elimination of vancomycin following burn injury, but a need for increased dosing is commonly observed (44, 45).

Hepatic Function

The hepatocyte is the most important site for drug metabolism, and in general it produces a metabolite that is more water-soluble (facilitates urinary excretion) and of greater molecular weight (facilitates biliary secretion). The chemical reactions are classified into phase I and phase II biotransformations, which may occur in series. Phase I reactions include addition of a polar group (hydroxylation) or deletion of a nonpolar group (N-demethylation). Phase II conjugation with endogenous compounds such as glucuronic acid may follow phase I reactions. The most important enzymes catalyzing these reactions make up the microsomal enzyme oxidation system and include cytochrome P-450 and cytochrome P-450 reductase.

Although the mechanism is not completely clear, burn injury is associated with a marked depression of phase I reactions, while phase II reactions are unaffected. There is some evidence that decreased enzyme activity is due to oxygen-derived free radical damage to the hepatocyte. This discrepancy is evident in the postburn metabolism of diazepam and lorazepam (34). The phase I metabolism of diazepam is impaired, while the phase II metabolism of lorazepam (glucuronidation) does not differ from normal (46).

Plasma Protein Binding

Although problems associated with changes in unbound drug concentration associated with inverse changes in plasma protein concentrations are theoretically possible, clinically important examples are few. The two proteins that account for most drug serum protein binding are albumin and α-1 acid glycoprotein (AAG) (47).

Albumin is a large molecule (approximately 69,000 daltons) that is capable of binding acidic, neutral, and basic drugs. Despite its large molecular weight, albumin is not confined to the intravascular space, 30% of total exchangeable albumin is in extravascular fluid. Postburn serum albumin concentration is commonly reduced by 50% and often reaches critical levels of 10 g/L (1 g/dL) (normal is 3.5 to 4.9 g/dL for adults). The free fractions of diazepam, phenytoin, and salicylic acid increase after burn injury; this increase has been attributed to a decreased serum albumin concentration.

AAG is an acute-phase reactant that has a high affinity but low capacity for basic drugs and may be saturated at therapeutic concentrations (e.g., lidocaine). The concentration of AAG may increase to as much as 300% of normal during the first postburn week and may not return to normal for 4 to 6 weeks. The free fractions of imipramine, lidocaine, meperidine, and propranolol decrease after the first postburn week, presumably in response to an increased AAG concentration.

The critically important breakpoint for drug serum protein binding is approximately 90%. When binding is less than 90%, the pharmacokinetic parameters change little following pathophysiologic changes in binding. Oral administration of drugs with a high hepatic extraction ratio (such as propranolol) would be affected little by changes in plasma protein binding, because of the first-pass effect. Although the potential for problems is low, the clinician who is monitoring a patient receiving agents that have low therapeutic indices or steep dose-response curves should consider the effect of altered protein binding when evaluating drug toxicity or suboptimal response.

The efficacies of the nondepolarizing neuromuscular blocking agents tubocurarine chloride, metocurine iodide, pancuronium bromide, and atracurium besylate are reduced after the first postburn week, a finding that implies that increased plasma protein binding to AAG is responsible (48, 49). Although increased binding does occur, the relatively small increase cannot explain the sometimes dramatic decrease in response. Investigations of the mechanism for this resistance have ruled out changes in drug clearance or volume of distribution. The decreased potency of these agents may be due to an unidentified substance in the plasma of burn patients.

Drug Movement Through Burn Wounds

Destruction of the normal barriers to percutaneous absorption occurs with burn injury. The diffusion resistance to water movement through injured skin can be less than one-tenth that of normal skin. Gentamicin is absorbed readily following topical application of a 0.1% cream and is absorbed to a smaller extent with a 0.1% ointment (50). Eschar penetration has also been demonstrated in vitro for mafenide acetate, nitrofurazone, povidone-iodine, silver nitrate, and silver sulfadiazine (51).

Drug penetration of the burn wound is not unidirectional. Historically, it has been assumed that eschar penetration by systemically administered drugs was prevented by the avascular nature of the wound. However, systemically administered gentamicin and tobramycin both penetrate burn eschar (52). Drug loss through the burn wound may add substantially to total drug clearance.

INFECTION AND ANTIMICROBIALS

Despite therapeutic advances, infection remains the most important cause of death of burned patients who survive initial resuscitation (53–55). Administration of tetanus immune globulin and/or tetanus toxoid when the patient's tetanus immunization history is not known should be based on the American College of Surgeons guidelines. Colonization of the burn wound has been demonstrated even when the patient is cared for in a laminar-flow room. Explanations for this phenomenon are that endogenous bacteria translocate from the gastrointestinal tract, that bacteria are iatrogenically transmitted, and that normal skin flora proliferate (56). In 15 patients with ≥20% TBSA evaluated within 24 hr of burn injury, the gastrointestinal barrier was compromised, as evidenced by increased absorption of lactulose and mannitol (57). However, the potential consequences of bacterial translocation are still debated (58).

Burn Wound Infection

The methods and materials used in the treatment of burn wound infection have undergone significant changes (59). Although the importance of bacteria in the burn wound has been recognized, the terminology describing the association between wound bacteria and systemic manifestations of infection is confusing. Moncrief and Teplitz suggested that the term "burn wound sepsis" be used to describe the events associated with bacterial proliferation to 100,000 colony-forming units per gram of burn wound tissue and subsequent invasion of adjacent nonburned tissue (60). Unfortunately, this number of bacteria per gram of tissue is not diagnostic of an invasive burn wound infection, and a complex classification scheme ranging from surface contamination to microvascular invasion (I, II, III, IV, V, VIa, VIb, VIc) has been suggested by Pruitt (61).

Whether or not the bacteria are localized to the burn or are disseminated, a rational method for selecting from the available topical antimicrobials is necessary. Similar to the Kirby-Bauer method of determining bacterial susceptibility to systemic agents is the agar-well diffusion method for determining susceptibilities to topical antimicrobials, first reported by Nathan and colleagues (62). Support for this method was supplied by Heggers and colleagues, who demonstrated that the agar-well diffusion test was more reliable than minimum inhibitory concentration determination for predicting bacterial susceptibility (63).

Topical Antimicrobials
SILVER NITRATE

The "modern" use of silver nitrate began in the late 1800s with the prevention of opthalmia neonatorum. Substantial improvement in the treatment of large burns by the use of continuously applied 0.5% silver nitrate solution was

930

reported in 1965 (64). The characteristics that make 0.5% silver nitrate a useful topical antibacterial agent are its safety, water solubility, prolonged antibacterial action, lack of toxicity to viable skin, lack of antigenicity, and ease of preparation. Problems associated with its use include hypochloremia from formation of silver chloride salts, water intoxication because of the hypotonicity of the solution, and hyponatremia or hypokalemia from diffusion into the wet dressings. Other problems are a requirement for bulky dressings that restrict joint motion and ambulation and black staining of everything that comes into contact with the solution.

SILVER SULFADIAZINE

The use of silver sulfadiazine (SSD) in burns was first reported in both a murine burn model and 16 patients (65). SSD is unique among the usual topical antibacterial agents in effectively inhibiting *Candida albicans.* The exact antimicrobial mechanism of action of SSD has not been clearly elucidated, but it is attributed to silver inhibition of DNA replication or cell membrane modification. Two studies imply that the sulfadiazine component is not necessary for in vitro bacterial sensitivity. In addition, clinical efficacy may be associated with a reversal of injury-induced suppression of lymphocyte natural killer cell cytotoxicity rather than strict antibacterial effects.

SSD is the topical agent of choice worldwide because of its safety and efficacy (66–68). Toxicity associated with SSD application is infrequent and associated predominantly with the propylene glycol component of the cream base. The potential for allergic hypersensitivity is shown by circulating sulfadiazine antibodies (predominantly immunoglobulin G) in the serum of treated patients. Although SSD-associated leukopenia has been reported, it is probably an artifact of the physiologic response to burn injury of WBC margination and/or diapedesis (movement through vessels) from the intravascular space (69). Clinicians continue to apply SSD to patients who develop leukopenia.

Because of its demonstrated efficacy, SSD has been incorporated into a number of biologic and synthetic dressings or skin substitutes, to take advantage of its benefits and eliminate the inconvenience of dressing changes with reapplication of cream. Another method that is used to improve on SSD is the addition of other agents such as nitrofurazone, gentamicin, fluoroquinolones, and cerium nitrate. The most successful combination is with chlorhexidine; Silvazine (Smith & Nephew, Clayton, Australia), a commercially available combination, has been used in Australia for over 10 years.

MAFENIDE ACETATE AND NITROFURAZONE

Although it causes pain on application, mafenide acetate is a useful topical antimicrobial for the treatment of subeschar burn wound infections because of its ability to penetrate the burn wound. Mafenide is often used on burned ears to prevent chondritis. Although closely related chemically, mafenide is not a sulfonamide. The primary metabolite (p-carboxybenzene sulfonamide) is a sulfonamide, and it may cause allergic reactions in patients who have sulfonamide hypersensitivity. When applied to large TBSA burns, mafenide can produce systemic metabolic acidosis secondary to carbonic anhydrase inhibition (70). Another disadvantage of mafenide is its high cost, approximately four times that of SSD. The antimicrobial usefulness of nitrofurazone has been demonstrated since the mid-1940s (71). Its primary use has been in prophylaxis of infection following skin grafting.

Systemic Antimicrobials

The use of prophylactic penicillin during the first postburn week was common during the 1950s and 1960s because of a justified concern about infection by *Streptococcus pyogenes.* This organism produced rapid conversion of partial-thickness to full-thickness wounds and fatalities. However, current laboratory methods for monitoring the burn wound and close clinical monitoring of patients allow the rapid recognition of infection. Recent prospective clinical trials have demonstrated no benefit from prophylactic penicillin. Indeed, subsequent wound cultures from penicillin-treated patients have a greater incidence of resistant organisms.

The choice of antibiotics for systemic infections in burn patients should be the same as for other patients (72). However, because the pathophysiologic changes following burn trauma are dynamic, the dosing of systemic antimicrobials must be individualized when possible (73). Increased requirements for aminoglycosides and vancomycin have been demonstrated in burn patients (as was discussed in the section on pharmacokinetics).

NUTRITION SUPPORT

A recent review article explores the intimate relationship between nutrition and wound healing (74). The injury-associated hypermetabolic response with altered nutritional requirements, including vitamins and micronutrients, is discussed. (See also Chapter 12, "Parenteral and Enteral Nutrition.")

Metabolic Response to Trauma

The hypermetabolism following trauma was initially explained as a physiologic response to increased heat loss. The rationale was that burned skin allows increased water loss that lowers the skin/wound temperature when the water evaporates. However, the precise relationship between evaporative water loss and postburn hypermetabolism is unclear, since conflicting results have been reported from similar investigations.

Similarly, it has been assumed that increased thermogenesis was necessary to compensate for heat loss in a cold environment, since damaged skin cannot respond with decreased perspiration and cutaneous vasoconstriction. However, postburn hypermetabolism is not attenuated, even when the environmental temperature is increased above thermal neutrality. A resetting of the hypothalamic thermal regulatory setpoint is suggested by a study comparing burned patients to normal controls, in which the burn patients selected a significantly higher environmental temperature when they were placed in a metabolic chamber.

Metabolic rate may be reduced after relief of pain, although the degree of reduction is not well defined (75). Historically, pain management of hospitalized patients with opioids has been suboptimal because of unnecessary fears of addiction. Morphine requirements of burn patients can be substantial, exceeding 60 mg/hr before development of tolerance (76).

Other contributors to postburn hypermetabolism are prostaglandins, interleukins, components of the complement cascade, and the catabolic neurohumoral milieu of elevated serum cortisol, growth hormone, catecholamines, and glucagon levels (77, 78). Initial insulin secretion inhibition is usually followed by normal or supranormal plasma insulin levels. Despite this insulin recovery, hyperglycemia persists, secondary to insulin resistance at the tissue insulin receptor.

The fuel stores that are mobilized to sustain postburn hypermetabolism include hepatic and muscle glycogen; visceral, plasma, and muscle protein; and fat. Because the major metabolic source of ATP provided to the burn wound is anaerobic glycolysis, the obligatory glucose requirement is increased. Production of glucose from glycogenolysis is relatively short-lived because stores approximate only 100 to 200 g and endogenous glucose production exceeds 400 g per day. Significant endogenous glucose is provided by efficient recycling of pyruvate and lactate via the Cori cycle and the glucose-alanine cycle. Catabolism of muscle protein and direct oxidation of amino acids provide approximately 15 to 20% of the total caloric expenditure in the fasting injured patient. The body adapts to using fat as its main energy source and can mobilize abundant energy from the typical fat stores of approximately 160,000 kcal.

The specific cause of postburn hypermetabolism is not clear but appears to be multifactorial. Completely arresting postburn hypermetabolism is not currently possible. A reasonable approach is to provide the patient with a warm environment, adequate pain relief, early enteral nutrition, and aggressive wound coverage. In addition, an attempt should be made to minimize endogenous protein catabolism by providing exogenous protein and nonprotein calories.

Method of Nutrient Administration

Patients with less than 20% TBSA burns can usually be maintained on a normal diet, unless there is an associated condition such as severe preburn malnutrition or an injury that prevents mastication. Patients with larger burns are often unwilling or unable to consume enough high-protein and caloric-dense food to fulfill requirements. For these patients, nutritional requirements can be met by insertion of a small-bore nasoenteric feeding tube and administration of commercially available enteral feeding formulations such as Osmolite-HN, TwoCal-HN, Traumacal, and Replete. Enteral nutrition is preferred to parenteral nutrition because it is more physiologic, is less costly, and avoids complications associated with parenteral nutrition such as catheter-related sepsis.

In contrast to historical recommendations that focused on parenteral nutrition, current guidelines call for early enteral feeding (79). Even in severely burned patients with absent bowel sounds, feeding into the small intestine through a nasoenteric tube is still possible, because postburn ileus is confined primarily to the stomach (80). In these severely injured patients a nasogastric tube is inserted and connected to suction for 2 to 3 days until gastric function returns. Experimental evidence favoring early enteral feeding demonstrated a reduction in catabolism and the hypermetabolic response in a guinea pig burn model. Another beneficial effect of early enteral feeding is the maintenance of gut mucosal mass. Improved gut wall homeostasis may prevent the increased intestinal permeability that allows translocation of enteric bacteria.

Macronutrient Needs

The metabolic demands associated with severe burns exceed those of any other hospitalized patient. The postburn energy expenditure increases with increasing burn size. However, there is an upper limit to required calories. This upper limit is approximately twice the calculated basal energy expenditure using the Harris-Benedict equation. Numerous methods are available to calculate the burn patient's daily energy requirement, and representative formulas are listed in Table 45.3.

Although mathematical calculation to predict energy requirements is convenient, determination of the patient's specific caloric needs is desirable (81). A complex metabolic chamber is necessary to specifically measure energy expenditure, but a reasonably accurate estimation can be performed at the bedside by using indirect calorimetry (82). Metabolic carts measure the respiratory gas exchange of oxygen (VO_2) and carbon dioxide (VCO_2) to indirectly measure energy expenditure (via the reverse Fick equation).

CARBOHYDRATE REQUIREMENTS

Energy liberated by oxidation of enterally administered carbohydrate is approximately 4 kcal/g. The carbohydrate that is commonly administered parenterally is hydrous dextrose, which liberates 3.4 kcal/g when completely oxidized. The optimal amount of administered carbohy-

Table 45.3.
Various Formulas Used to Estimate Energy Requirements in Burn Patients[a]

Adults
(1) Harris-Benedict equation [estimates basal energy expenditure (BEE)]:
   Male: BEE (kcal) = 66 + (13.7 × W) + (5 × H) − (6.8 × A)
   Female: BEE (kcal) = 665 + (9.6 × W) + (1.7 × H) − (4.7 × A)
(2) Burke and Wolfe:
   kcal per day = 2 × BEE
(3) Curreri:
   kcal per day = 25 × W + (40 × TBSA)
(4) Davies and Liljedahl:
   kcal per day = 20 × W + (70 × TBSA)

Children
(1) Wolfe:
   kcal per day = 2 × BEE
(2) Curreri Junior:
   kcal per day = {0–1 years} BEE + (15 × TBSA)
               {1–3 years} BEE + (25 × TBSA)
               {3–15 years} BEE + (40 × TBSA)

[a]W = weight in kg; H = height in cm; A = age in years. TBSA = total body surface area burned (%).

drate will minimize gluconeogenesis without exceeding energy requirements and being stored as triglycerides.

The utilization of glucose for energy by burned patients has limits. When glucose is oxidized to liberate energy, equimolar concentrations of oxygen are consumed and carbon dioxide is produced (respiratory quotient (RQ) = 1). The normal, fed RQ is approximately 0.84, and it rises when the rate of administered glucose exceeds the maximum rate of utilization. When glucose is converted into fat, more than eight times as much carbon dioxide is released for each mole of oxygen (RQ > 1). Excretion of this extra carbon dioxide could be difficult for a burned patient with an associated inhalation injury. An additional negative aspect of lipogenesis is that it is an energy-consuming process. An elegant study of intravenous glucose, using isotopic tracers, demonstrated that the maximum rate of oxidation is approximately 5 mg/kg/min. At faster rates of glucose administration the RQ rapidly increased above 1.0, suggesting lipogenesis. For a 70-kg patient this maximum rate of glucose utilization translates into 2 L of 25% dextrose-containing total parenteral nutrition solution (500 g) per day (83).

FAT REQUIREMENTS

Fat is an efficient provider of energy at 9 kcal/g, but it is vital only for supplying essential fatty acids to prevent essential fatty acid deficiency syndrome. The amount of fat that burned patients need is not known, but fat should provide a minimum 2% of total calories. Fat is an essential component of cell membranes, functions as a carrier for the fat-soluble vitamins, and is important for wound healing.

Patients with severe thermal injury may have reduced lipolytic capacity, especially after parenteral administration

of fat emulsion. It appears that parenteral administration of long-chain triglycerides is associated with hepatomegaly, impaired clotting, and decreased resistance to infection. Preliminary evidence indicates that lipids that are high in linoleic acid (e.g., safflower or soybean oil) are associated with immunosuppression, presumably because linoleic acid is the precursor of arachidonic acid, which is the principle substrate for prostaglandins (PGE1 and PGE2) and certain leukotrienes. Another advantage of enteral administration is that medium-chain triglycerides are absorbed without the need for bile, and at the cellular level they are transported into mitochondria without the need for carnitine.

Because of the constraint on the rate of carbohydrate administration, fat must usually be provided in substantial quantities as an energy source. Although fat is not often important clinically, it has a specific advantage over glucose for patients with pulmonary dysfunction, when a reduced carbon dioxide production for an equivalent amount of oxygen consumed is useful. The optimal fatty acid chain length and exact dietary fat requirements for burn patients remain to be determined.

PROTEIN REQUIREMENTS

Protein loss across burn wounds is considerable and is greatest in the first 3 postburn days. Although early protein loss across full-thickness burns is greater than that in partial-thickness burns, the rates become approximately the same after postburn day 3. The rate of protein loss is reduced by application of either antimicrobial creams or skin substitutes. By using the average protein loss during the first postburn week (0.5 mg/cm²/hr) a formula that estimates the daily protein loss (g) across the burn wound can be devised: 1.2 × body surface area (m²) × total body surface area burn (%). Protein loss across the burn wound during the second postburn week occurs at approximately half this rate.

The recommended daily allowance of protein for healthy adults is 0.8 g/kg. The optimal amount of protein required by burned patients to prevent catabolism of protein stores and promote wound healing is not well defined. The importance of protein-sparing by providing energy must be considered, but some clinicians advocate a high-protein diet aimed at achieving a 100:1 nonprotein calorie to nitrogen ratio in contrast to the standard 150:1 ratio. In clinical practice, approximately 1.5 to 2 g/kg/day (using lean body weight) of protein is provided initially. Nitrogen-balance studies then determine the adequacy of this regimen. Although the nitrogen balance calculation appears simple:

$$\text{Nitrogen balance} = N(in) - N(out)$$

there is potential error in assessment of both N(in) and N(out). N(in) is the number of grams of nitrogen ingested or infused, and it is common practice to multiply the number of grams of protein or amino acid by 0.16 to estimate grams of nitrogen. This calculation assumes that the protein is made up of 16% nitrogen, but the percentage of nitrogen in available parenteral amino acid products varies from 11.1% to 16.9% (84). The N(out) is calculated by adding the urinary urea nitrogen (UUN) from a 24-hr urine collection to an estimate of nitrogen excretion other than that measured as urine urea. This estimate is comprised of nonurea urinary nitrogen (ammonia, uric acid, creatinine) and nonurinary nitrogen loss (fecal and skin). A commonly used estimate for non-UUN losses is 4 g. One group advocates the measurement of total urinary nitrogen rather than using an inaccurate estimate (85). As was described above, significant quantities of protein (nitrogen) are lost through open burn wounds and must be included in using an estimate.

The branched-chain amino acids (BCAAs) leucine, isoleucine, and valine are unique in that skeletal muscle can oxidize them directly for energy. In contrast, the other amino acids are metabolized almost wholly by the liver. Under ordinary circumstances, only 6 to 7% of the daily energy expenditure is provided through BCAA oxidation by skeletal muscle. The administration of supplemental BCAAs, especially leucine, to burn patients should (theoretically) reduce protein catabolism in skeletal muscle and increase protein synthesis. However, conclusive evidence of beneficial effects of BCAA-enriched solutions in burn patients has not been demonstrated, and further studies are needed (86).

Measurement of serum proteins such as albumin, prealbumin, transferrin, and retinol-binding protein is often regarded as a reliable index of nutritional status. However, because of surgical excision and grafting of wounds, associated blood loss and transfusions, and administration of exogenous albumin, changes in serum protein concentrations as an indication of nutrition regimen adequacy must be viewed with caution. Nitrogen-balance studies are probably the best assessment of protein status, despite the limitations described previously.

Micronutrient Needs

In contrast to the extensive information about macronutrient requirements, little information is available about the micronutrient needs of burn patients. There is evidence that micronutrient needs increase after burns, although the exact amounts have not been defined (87, 88).

VITAMINS

At a minimum, burn patients should receive vitamin supplements based on the Recommended Dietary Allowances (RDA) for enteral administration or the American Medical Association Nutrition Advisory Group (AMA) for parenteral administration. In the absence of preexisting deficiency there is little indication to administer increased amounts of fat-soluble vitamins. Vitamin C is often

supplemented to five times RDA because it has little inherent toxic potential and has an important role in collagen deposition and wound healing. Because of their role as cofactors in metabolism and potential increased losses through the wound and urine, the B vitamin group is supplemented to two times RDA.

TRACE ELEMENTS

In the acute-phase reaction to trauma, plasma concentrations of zinc, iron, and copper are markedly diminished (89). Like vitamin C, zinc is thought to promote wound healing, and it is supplemented to two times RDA. Aggressive iron supplementation must be undertaken with some caution because of the potential for increased bacterial growth due to plasma unbound iron. Deficiency syndromes of copper, selenium, chromium, iodine, manganese, and molybdenum occur in patients on long-term total parenteral nutrition, but no cases of deficiency appear to have been reported as a direct result of burn trauma. These trace elements are administered according to RDA or AMA guidelines.

CONCLUSION

The complex clinical management and rehabilitation of a severely burned patient requires a multidisciplinary team including surgeons, nurses, a pharmacist, a dietitian, a physical therapist, an occupational therapist, a respiratory therapist, and a social worker. A large TBSA full-thickness burn requires surgical excision and split-thickness skin grafting. Fluid requirements during the initial postburn period are surprisingly large, and experienced clinicians have devised guidelines for fluid resuscitation. The pharmacist must be aware that the postburn hyperdynamic and hypermetabolic phase produces multiple pharmacokinetic and pharmacodynamic changes. The nutritional requirements of burn patients can be substantial, with energy needs often approaching twice those of other hospitalized patients. A number of methods are available for estimating energy requirements by mathematical calculation, but determination of the patient's specific caloric needs by indirect calorimetry is desirable. The amount of dietary protein that is required by burn patients to promote wound healing, replace losses, and prevent catabolism of protein stores is not well defined. Usually, intravenous amino acids or enteral protein at 1.5 to 2 g/kg/day is provided, and nitrogen-balance studies are performed. Current guidelines call for the preferential use of enteral (rather than parenteral) nutrition.

Prevention and treatment of infection in the burned patient are of paramount importance, since infection is the most common cause of death of patients who survive initial resuscitation. Treatment of systemic infection in burned patients is similar to methods used for other patients, with dose individualization by antimicrobial serum concentration monitoring when possible. Microbial growth in the burn wound can be substantial after colonization by endogenous or exogenous organisms. The availability of topical antimicrobial agents has dramatically improved the control of burn wound infections.

REFERENCES

1. Arturson MG. The pathophysiology of severe thermal injury. J Burn Care Rehabil 6:129–146, 1985.
2. Silverman SH, Purdue GF, Hunt JL, et al. Cyanide toxicity in burned patients. J Trauma 28:171–176, 1988.
3. Blalock SJ, Bunker BJ, DeVellis RF. Measuring health status among survivors of burn injury: revisions of the burn specific health scale. J Trauma 36:508–515, 1994.
4. Saffle JR, Sullivan JJ, Tuohig GM, et al. Multiple organ failure in patients with thermal injury. Crit Care Med 21:1673–1683, 1993.
5. Punch JD, Smith DJ, Robson MC. Hospital care of major burns. Postgrad Med 85:205–215, 1989.
6. Wachtel TL. Major burns. Postgrad Med 85:178–196, 1989.
7. Robson MC, Smith DJ, Heggers JP. Innovations in burn wound management. Adv Plast Reconstr Surg 4:149–176, 1987.
8. Wong L, Munster AM. New techniques in burn wound management. Surg Clin North Amer 73:363–371, 1993.
9. Demling RH. Burns. N Engl J Med 313:1389–1398, 1985.
10. Nowicki CR, Sprenger CK. Temporary skin substitutes for burn patients: a nursing perspective. J Burn Care Rehabil 9:209–215, 1988.
11. Teepe RGC, Kreis RW, Koebrugge EJ, et al. The use of cultured autologous epidermis in the treatment of extensive burn wounds. J Trauma 30:269–275, 1990.
12. Choiniere M, Melzack R, Rondeau J, Girard N, Paquin MJ. The pain of burns: characteristics and correlates. J Trauma 29:1531–1539, 1989.
13. Perry S, Heidrich G. Management of pain during debridement: a survey of U.S. burn units. Pain 13:267–280, 1982.
14. Osgood PF, Szyfelbein SK. Management of burn pain in children. Pediatr Clin North Am 36:1001–1013, 1989.
15. Wermeling DP, Record KE, Foster TS. Patient-controlled high-dose morphine therapy in a patient with electrical burns. Clin Pharm 5:832–835, 1986.
16. Donahue SR. Morphine sulfate intravenous dose of 1650 mg per hour. Hosp Pharm 24:311, 1989.
17. Porter J, Jick H. Addiction rare in patients treated with narcotics. N Engl J Med 302:123, 1980.
18. Choiniere M, Grenier R, Paquette C. Patient-controlled analgesia: a double-blind study in burn patients. Anaesthesia 47:467–472, 1992.
19. Gaukroger PB, Chapman MJ, Davey RB. Pain control in paediatric burns—the use of patient-controlled analgesia. Burns 17:396–399, 1991.
20. Rovers J, Knighton J, Neligan P. Patient-controlled analgesia in burn patients: a critical review of the literature and case report. Hosp Pharm 29:106, 108–111, 1994.
21. Patterson DR, Questad KA, de Lateur BJ. Hypnotherapy as an adjunct to narcotic analgesia for the treatment of pain for burn debridement. Am J Clin Hypn 31:156–163, 1989.
22. Miller AC, Hickman LC, Lemasters GK. A distraction technique for control of burn pain. J Burn Care Rehabil 13:576–580, 1992.
23. Beyer JE, Levin CR. Issues and advances in pain control in children. Nurs Clin North Am 22(3):661–676, 1987.
24. Rubin WD, Mani MM, Hiebert JM. Fluid resuscitation of the thermally injured patient: current concepts with definition of clinical subsets and their specialized treatment. Clin Plast Surg 13:9–20, 1986.

25. Demling RH. Fluid replacement in burned patients. Surg Clin North Am 67:15–30, 1987.
26. Graves TA, Cioffi WG, McManus WF, et al. Fluid resuscitation of infants and children with massive thermal injury. J Trauma 28:1656–1659, 1988.
27. Aikawa N, Ishibiki K, Naito C, et al. Individualized fluid resuscitation based on haemodynamic monitoring in the management of extensive burns. Burns 8:249–255, 1982.
28. Horton JW, White DJ, Baxter CR. Hypertonic saline dextran resuscitation of thermal injury. Ann Surg 211:301–311, 1990.
29. Gunn ML, Hansbrough JF, Davis JW, et al. Prospective, randomized trial of hypertonic sodium lactate versus lactated Ringer's solution for burn shock resuscitation. J Trauma 29:1261–1267, 1989.
30. Ross AD, Angaran DM. Colloids vs. crystalloids: a continuing controversy. Drug Intell Clin Pharm 18:202–212, 1984.
31. Waters LM, Christensen MA, Sato RM. Hetastarch: an alternative colloid in burn shock management. J Burn Care Rehabil 10:11–16, 1989.
32. Bowser BH, Caldwell FT. The effects of resuscitation with hypertonic vs. hypotonic vs. colloid on wound and urine fluid and electrolyte losses in severely burned children. J Trauma 23:916–923, 1983.
33. Milner SM, Hodgetts TJ, Rylah LA. The burns calculator: a simple proposed guide for fluid resuscitation. Lancet 342:1089–1091, 1993.
34. Martyn J. Clinical pharmacology and drug therapy in the burned patient. Anesthesiology 65:67–75, 1986.
35. Bonate PL. Pathophysiology and pharmacokinetics following burn injury. Clin Pharmacokinet 18:118–130, 1990.
36. Czaja AJ, McAlhany JC, Pruitt BA. Acute duodenitis and duodenal ulceration after burns: clinical and pathological characteristics. JAMA 232:621–624, 1975.
37. Cioffi WG, McManus AT, Rue LW, et al. Comparison of acid neutralizing and non-acid neutralizing stress ulcer prophylaxis in thermally injured patients. J Trauma 36:541–547, 1994.
38. Loirat P, Rohan J, Baillet A, et al. Increased glomerular filtration rate in patients with major burns and its effect on the pharmacokinetics of tobramycin. N Engl J Med 299:915–919, 1978.
39. Zaske DE, Sawchuk RJ, Gerding DN, et al. Increased dosage requirements of gentamicin in burn patients. J Trauma 16:824–828, 1976.
40. Glew RH, Moellering RC, Burke JF. Gentamicin dosage in children with extensive burns. J Trauma 16:819–823, 1976.
41. Zaske DE, Bootman JL, Solem LB, et al. Increased burn patient survival with individualized dosages of gentamicin. Surgery 91:142–149, 1982.
42. Zaske DE, Chin T, Kohls PR, et al. Initial dosage regimens of gentamicin in patients with burns. J Burn Care Rehabil 12:46–50, 1991.
43. Hollingsed TC, Harper DJ, Jennings JP. Aminoglycoside dosing in burn patients using first dose pharmacokinetics. J Trauma 35:394–398, 1993.
44. Garrelts JC, Peterie JD. Altered vancomycin dose vs. serum concentration relationship in burn patients. Clin Pharmacol Ther 44:9–13, 1988.
45. Brater DC, Bawdon RE, Anderson SA, et al. Vancomycin elimination in patients with burn injury. Clin Pharmacol Ther 39:631–634, 1986.
46. Martyn J, Greenblatt DJ. Lorazepam conjugation is unimpaired in burn trauma. Clin Pharmacol Ther 43:250–255, 1987.
47. Bloedow DC, Hansbrough JF, Hardin T, et al. Postburn serum drug binding and serum protein concentrations. J Clin Pharmacol 26:147–151, 1986.
48. Thompson DF. Neuromuscular blocking agents in burn patients. DICP 23:1006–1008, 1989.
49. Dwersteg JF, Pavlin EG, Heimbach DM. Patients with burns are resistant to atracurium. Anesthesiology 65:517–520, 1986.

50. Stone HH, Kolb LD, Pettit J, et al. The systemic absorption of an antibiotic from the burn wound surface. Am Surg 34:639–643, 1968.

51. Stefanides MM, Copeland CE, Kominos SD, et al. In vitro penetration of topical antiseptics through eschar of burn patients. Ann Surg 183:358–364, 1976.

52. Polk RE, Mayhall CG, Smith J, et al. Gentamicin and tobramycin penetration into burn eschar. Arch Surg 118:295–302, 1983.

53. McManus WF. Patterns of infection over the past ten years: historical patterns. J Burn Care Rehabil 8:32–35, 1987.

54. Gelfand JA. Infections in burn patients: a paradigm for cutaneous infection in the patient at risk. Am J Med 76(suppl 5A):158–165, 1984.

55. Luterman A, Dacso CC, Curreri PW. Infections in burn patients. Am J Med 81(suppl 1A):45–52, 1986.

56. Ziegler TR, Smith RJ, O'Dwyer RT, et al. Increased intestinal permeability associated with infection in burn patients. Arch Surg 123:1313–1319, 1988.

57. Deitch EA. Intestinal permeability is increased in burn patients shortly after injury. Surgery 107:411–416, 1990.

58. Barber A, Inner H, Shires GT. Bacterial translocation in burn injury. Semin Nephrol 13:416–419, 1993.

59. Ryan CM, Tompkins RG. Topical therapy. II: burns. In: Chernow B, ed. The pharmacologic approach to the critically ill patient. 3rd ed. Baltimore: Williams & Wilkins, 1994:830–843.

60. Moncrief JA, Teplitz C. Changing concepts in burn sepsis. J Trauma 4:233–245, 1964.

61. Pruitt BA. The diagnosis and treatment of infection in the burn patient. Burns Incl Therm Inj 11:79–91, 1984.

62. Nathan P, Law EJ, Murphy DF, et al. A laboratory method for selection of topical antimicrobial agents to treat infected burn wounds. Burns Incl Therm Inj 4:177–187, 1978.

63. Heggers JP, Velanovich V, Robson MC, et al. Control of burn wound sepsis: a comparison of in vitro topical antimicrobial assays. J Trauma 27:176–179, 1987.

64. Moyer CA, Brentano L, Gravens DL, et al. Treatment of large human burns with 0.5% silver nitrate solution. Arch Surg 90:812–867, 1965.

65. Fox CL. Silver sulfadiazine: a new topical therapy for *Pseudomonas* in burns. Arch Surg 96:184–188, 1968.

66. Monafo WW, West MA. Current treatment recommendations for topical burn therapy. Drugs 40:364–373, 1990.

67. Rice TL. Topical antibacterials. Hosp Pharm 27:1099–1108, 1992.

68. Sawhney CP, Sharma RK, Rao KR, et al. Long-term experience with 1 per cent topical silver sulphadiazine cream in the management of burn wounds. Burns Incl Therm Inj 15:403–406, 1989.

69. Thomson PD, Moore NP, Rice TL, et al. Leukopenia in acute thermal injury: evidence against silver sulfadiazine as the causative agent. J Burn Care Rehabil 10:418–420, 1989.

70. Liebman PR, Kennelly MM, Hirsch EF. Hypercarbia and acidosis associated with carbonic anhydrase inhibition: a hazard of topical mafenide acetate use in renal failure. Burns 8:395–398, 1982.

71. Hooper G, Covarrubias J. Clinical use and efficacy of furacin: a historical perspective. J Intern Med Res 11:289–293, 1983.

72. Dacso CC, Luterman A, Curreri PW. Systemic antibiotic treatment in burned patients. Surg Clin North Am 67:57–68, 1987.

73. Mason AD, McManus AT, Pruitt BA. Association of burn mortality and bacteremia. A 25-year review. Arch Surg 121:1027–1031, 1986.

74. Meyer NA, Muller MJ, Herndon DN. Nutrient support of the healing wound. New Horizons 2:202–14, 1994.

75. Mackersie RC, Karagianes TG. Pain management following trauma and burns. Anesthesiol Clin North Am 7:211–227, 1989.

76. Wermeling DP, Record KE, Foster TS. Patient-controlled high-dose morphine therapy in a patient with electrical burns. Clin Pharm 5:832–835, 1986.

77. Drost AC, Burleson DG, Cioffi WG. Plasma cytokines following thermal injury and their relationship with patient mortality, burn size and time post burn. J Trauma 35:335–339, 1993.

78. DeBrandt JP, Chollet-Martin S, Hernvann A, et al. Cytokine response to burn injury: relationship with protein metabolism. J Trauma 36:624–628, 1994.

79. Enzi G, Casadei A, Sergi G, et al. Metabolic and hormonal effects of early nutritional supplementation after surgery in burn patients. Crit Care Med 18:719–721, 1990.

80. Garrel DR, Davignon I, Lopez D. Length of care in patients with severe burns with or without early enteral nutritional support: a retrospective study. J Burn Care Rehabil 12:85–90, 1991.

81. Cunningham JJ, Hegarty MT, Meara PA, et al. Measured and predicted calorie requirements of adults during recovery from severe burn trauma. Am J Clin Nutr 49:404–408, 1989.

82. Saffle JR, Medina E, Raymond J, et al. Use of indirect calorimetry in the nutritional management of burned patients. J Trauma 25:32–39, 1985.

83. Bell SJ, Blackburn GL. Nutritional support of the burn patient. In: Martyn JAJ, ed. Acute management of the burned patient. Philadelphia: WB Saunders, 1990:138–158.

84. Miller SJ. The nitrogen balance revisited. Hosp Pharm 25:61–65, 1990.

85. Konstantinides FN, Radmer WJ, Becker WK, et al. Inaccuracy of nitrogen balance determinations in thermal injury with calculated total urinary nitrogen. J Burn Care Rehabil 13:254–260, 1992.

86. Oki JC, Cuddy PG. Branched-chain amino acid support of stressed patients. DICP, 23:399–408, 1989.

87. Pasulka PS, Wachtel TL. Nutritional considerations for the burned patient. Surg Clin North Am 67:109–131, 1987.

88. O'Neil CE, Hutsler D, Hildreth MA. Basic nutritional guidelines for pediatric burn patients. J Burn Care Rehabil 10:278–284, 1989.

89. Shewmake KB, Talbert GE, Bowser-Wallace BH, et al. Alterations in plasma copper, zinc, and ceruloplasmin levels in patients with thermal trauma. J Burn Care Rehabil 9:13–17, 1988.

CHAPTER 46

COMMON EYE DISORDERS

ANTON C. DREYER, ANDRIES G. GOUS, and HERMIEN GOUS

A variety of disorders commonly affect the eye. These vary in severity from mild but annoying allergic conjunctivitis or dry eyes to sight-threatening infections. Some of these disorders may be treated with over-the-counter preparations, but the more serious disorders require aggressive therapy, frequently with multiple drugs and often by more than one route of administration. This chapter discusses the common ocular disorders and their treatment, as well as general principles of ophthalmic medications.

Figure 46.1 depicts the various structures of the eye that may be affected by commonly occurring disorders.

OPHTHALMIC MEDICINES USED IN COMMON EYE DISORDERS

There are numerous ophthalmic preparations for topical application to the eye. For an enhanced effect, a systemic form of the same medications may be added to the therapeutic regimen. In such cases and for susceptible patients who are treated with topical medications, systemic side effects may occur. The following text summarizes the ophthalmic products that are used and provides some general considerations about therapy. The tables provide a partial list of available ophthalmic products.

Antimicrobial Preparations

Eye infections are usually caused by bacteria, sometimes by viruses, and much less commonly by fungi. Superficial infections such as conjunctivitis and blepharitis are generally treated adequately with agents that are applied topically. More serious infections may require subconjunctival injections and/or other routes of administration. The precautions that apply to systemic antibiotic use also apply to topical use. Indiscriminate use may lead to the emergence of resistance or hypersensitivity. This holds true especially for the use of the aminoglycosides for trivial conditions (1, 2).

For serious infections or those extending beyond the conjunctiva, cornea, and eyelids, culture and sensitivity tests are essential. In the absence of such tests, broad antiinfective coverage may be obtained (for serious infections) from the combination of an aminoglycoside and a cephalosporin injected subconjunctivally plus appropriate topical therapy (3). Table 46.1 provides a partial list of ophthalmic antimicrobial agents.

Antivirals

The topical antivirals (3) are listed in Table 46.2.

Glucocorticosteroid-Containing Preparations

The topical glucocorticosteroid-containing preparations are listed in Table 46.3. Steroids are available in drop and ointment form and are used for a variety of inflammatory eye conditions. Applied topically, they are ineffective against inflammation of the optic nerve, choroid, and retina. In these cases, systemic steroids are required (2, 4, 5).

The inflammatory process may cause permanent tissue damage. Correctly applied, steroids may save eye structures and preserve sight by suppressing inflammation. Certain infections are absolute contraindications to the use of steroids (e.g., herpes simplex viral infections). The main dangers associated with the use of ocular steroids are given in Table 46.4.

Decongestants (Vasoconstrictors)

Commonly used sympathomimetics are listed in Table 46.5. These agents stimulate α_1-adrenergic receptors on small blood vessels, causing them to constrict. This reduces blood flow in the affected area of the eye, clearing red eyes and shrinking (decongesting) the engorged tissue. Sympathomimetics also cause the radial muscle of the pupil to contract, leading to mydriasis. This effect is less pronounced and of shorter duration than the mydriasis that is produced by the application of parasympatholytics (anticholinergics) such as atropine. These sympathomimetics are nevertheless used for their mydriatic effect. The dose that is required for clinically significant mydriasis is much higher than that needed for decongestion. For some patients, such as patients with diabetic retinopathy, a combination of an α_1-sympathomimetic eye drop and an anticholinergic provides optimal mydriasis (6, 7).

Mydriasis (whether produced by topical application or systemic use of anticholinergics or sympathomimetics) generally leads to obstruction of the trabecular meshwork-canal of Schlemm drainage system for aqueous humor, leading to an increased intraocular pressure in angle-closure glaucoma. The side effects and precautions that are associated with the use of α-sympathomimetic eye drops are listed in Table 46.6.

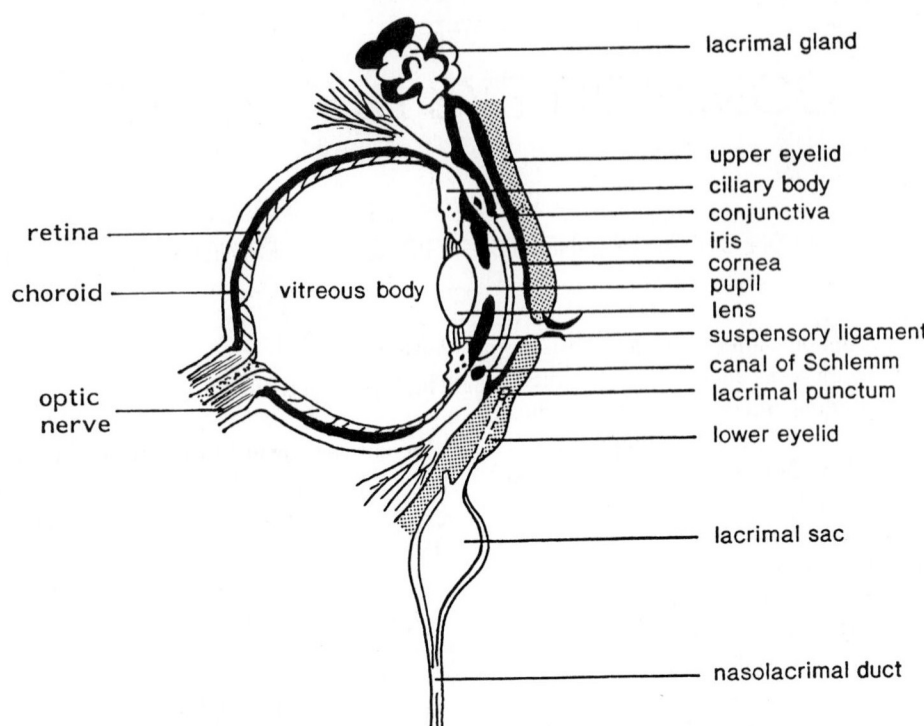

Figure 46.1. Cross-section of the eyeball and lacrimal passages.

Table 46.1.
Ophthalmic Antimicrobials

Drug	Dosage Form/Strength
Bacitracin	Ointment (500 units/g)
Chloramphenicol	Ointment (1%), solution (0.05%, 0.16%, 0.5%, 1.0%)
Ciprofloxacin	Solution (0.3%)
Erythromycin	Ointment (0.5%)
Gentamicin	Ointment or solution (0.3%)
Norfloxacin	Solution (0.3%)
Sulfacetamide	Solution (10.0%, 15.0%, 30.0%), ointment (10.0%)
Sulfisoxazole	Solution (4.0%), ointment (4.0%)
Tetracycline	Ointment (1.0%)
Chlortetracycline	Ointment (1.0%)
Tobramycin	Solution (0.3%), ointment (0.3%)
Combination products	

Neomycin 0.35%; polymyxin B 10,000 units/g, bacitracin 500 units/g in ointment

Polymyxin B 10,000 units/g; bacitracin 500 units/g in ointment

Polymyxin B 10,000 units/g or mL; neomycin 0.35% in ointment or solution

Oxytetracycline 0.5% and polymyxin B 10,000 units/g in ointment

Trimethoprim 0.1% and polymyxin B 10,000 units/g in ointment

Mydriatics (Cycloplegics)

Mydriatic agents are listed in Table 46.7. When applied topically, these anticholinergics produce a dilation of the pupil (mydriasis) and paralysis of accommodation (cycloplegia). They vary in their relative potencies and

Table 46.2.
Ophthalmic Antiviral and Antifungal Agents

Drug	Dosage Form/Strength	Usual Dose
Antiviral		
Acyclovir	Ointment (3%)	5 times a day for 14 days
Idoxuridine	Solution (0.1%), ointment (0.5%)	Solution: q.h. during the day, q. 2 hr at night for 10–21 days; Ointment: 5 × day for 10–21 days
Vidarabine	Ointment (3.0%)	5 × day for 14–21 days
Trifluorothymidine	Solution (1.0%)	9 × day for 14 days
Antifungal		
Natamycin	Suspension (5%)	q. 1–2 hr for 3–4 days, then 8 times per day for 14–21 days

durations of action, atropine being the most potent and having the longest duration of activity (mydriasis lasting 2 to 3 weeks in some patients and cycloplegia for up to 6 days). Tropicamide and cyclopentolate are used when a short-duration effect is required (3).

The mydriatics are used primarily as follows:

1. To dilate the pupil, for easier examination of the fundus, tropicamide is the anticholinergic of choice.
2. To produce cycloplegia for refraction, cyclopentolate or homatropine is used. (Atropine may be more suitable for children under 6 years of age.)

Table 46.3.
Ophthalmic Corticosteroids

Drug	Dosage Form/Strength
Prednisolone acetate	Suspension (0.12% or 1.0%)
Sodium phosphate	Solution (0.12%, 0.5%, or 1.0%)
Dexamethasone phosphate	Solution (0.1%), Suspension (0.1%)
	Phosphate ointment (0.05%)
Medrysone	Solution (1.0%)
Fluorometholone	Suspension (0.1% and 1.0%)

Combination products
  Prednisolone acetate 0.25% and atropine sulfate 1.0%—Solution
  Hydrocortisone 0.5% and chloromycetin 2.5%—Solution
  Hydrocortisone 0.5%, Chloramphenicol 0.1%, and polymyxin B 10,000 units/g—Ointment
  Hydrocortisone 0.5% and neomycin 0.35%—Solution
  Hydrocortisone 1.0%; polymyxin 10,000 units/g; bacitracin 400 units/g and neomycin 0.35%—Ointment and suspension
  Prednisolone 0.2% and sulfacetamide 10%—Solution and ointment
  Prednisolone 0.5% and sulfacetamide 10%—Solution and ointment
  Prednisolone 0.5%, neomycin 0.35%, and polymyxin B 10,000 units/ mL—Suspension
  Prednisolone 1% and gentamicin 0.3%—Suspension
  Dexamethasone 0.1% and neomycin 0.35%—Suspension or ointment
  Dexamethasone 0.1%, neomycin 0.35%, and polymyxin 10,000 units/ mL—Suspension or ointment
  Dexamethasone 0.1% and tobramycin 0.3%—Suspension

Table 46.4.
Dangers Associated with the Use of Ocular Steroids

Aggravation of unrecognized herpes simplex corneal ulceration, which may lead to corneal perforation.
Steroid glaucoma may be produced after a week or more of treatment in patients who are predisposed to chronic simplex glaucoma.
Aggravation of fungal or bacterial infection by decreasing the immune response.
The production of cataracts. (One drop of tropical steroid three times a day for 1 year is potentially cataractogenic.)
Masking of serious hypersensitivity reactions as well as the signs and symptoms of infections.
Occasionally, amounts sufficient to cause systemic effect (such as growth retardation in children) may be absorbed.

Source: Adapted from Lavin MJ, Rose GE: Use of steroid eye drops in general practice. Br Med J 292:1448–1450, 1986; Jones BR, Coster DJ, Falcon MG: Prospects of prevention of recurrent herpetic eye disease. Trans Ophthalmol Soc UK 97:350–355, 1977; and Conradie EA, Straughan JL (eds.): South African Medicines Formulary. Cape Town: Medical Association of South Africa 1988, p. 223.

3. To produce cycloplegia and mydriasis before, during, and after intraocular surgery.
4. To treat inflammation of the anterior segment of the eye. Paralysis of the ciliary muscle relieves the pain and congestion associated with this condition. A longer-acting anticholinergic (atropine or homatropine) is more suitable.

Mydriasis causes the pupil to crowd and block the trabecular meshwork and the canal of Schlemm. This may impair drainage of the aqueous humor, precipitating an attack of acute angle-closure glaucoma in susceptible patients. (See Chapter 48.)

Local Anesthetics

The ophthalmic anesthetics are listed in Table 46.8. The opththalmic use of local anesthetics is reserved for eye surgery and for minor procedures such as the removal of a foreign body. *They should never be given for the relief of symptoms* (6, 8).

Side effects of local anesthetics are usually the consequence of overdose or protracted use. These include the following:

1. Systemic effects such as central nervous system stimulation followed by central nervous system depression, hypertension, and tachydysrhythmias. Systemic side effects are also more likely to occur if the eye is red (increased blood flow will lead to increased absorption) or the patient has impaired kidney or liver function.
2. Minor local allergic reactions may occur, especially in patients who are prone to allergic reactions.
3. Mild, reversible corneal damage may occur. Severe damage and loss of vision have occurred in some cases. Because of possible corneal damage and retarded healing, local anesthetics should not be applied repeatedly to the eye as ongoing therapy in painful conditions.

Cocaine is no longer used as a local anesthetic in ophthalmology because it causes severe damage to the cornea. Systemic side effects and addiction liability further justify not using cocaine.

Artificial Tears

A list of the artificial tear products is provided in Table 45.9. Artificial tears are specially formulated to replace the deficient or incomplete normal tear, so they completely "wet" the eye and resist breaking up into dry spots. The resulting ophthalmic preparations generally have a greater viscosity than do tears (which are much like water). Excessive viscosity leads to poor lid lubrication, corneal injury, crusting on the lid margins, and blockage of tear drainage. Vehicles that are used for artifical tear preparations today are less viscous. They are applied to improve the survival time of the natural tear film as well as to providing an artifical layer. Artifical tear solutions should not contain chemicals that disrupt this basic film (6, 7).

Lubricating ointments (containing an oily substance such as lanolin or mineral oil) are usually used at night to provide lubrication during sleep. The drops should be used during the day and, depending on the severity of the deficiency, may be used hourly or even more frequently if required.

Pharmaceutics and Kinetics of Ophthalmic Medicines

The kinetic properties (rates and extents of absorption, distribution, metabolism, and excretion) of a medicine

Table 46.5.
Ophthalmic Decongestant Products

Product (Manufacturer)	Viscosity Agent	Vasoconstrictor	Preservative
Absorbonac (Alcon)	Povidone		EDTA 0.1%; thimerosal 0.004%
AK-Nefrin (Akorn)	Hydroxyethylcellulose 0.5%	Phenylephrine HCl 0.12%	Benzalkonium Cl 0.01%; EDTA
Allerest eye drops (Pharmacraft)		Naphazolone HCl 0.012%	
Clear Eyes (Ross)		Naphazoline HCl 0.012%	Benzalkonium Cl, EDTA
Collyrium w/tetrahydrozoline (Wyeth-Ayerst)		Tetrahydrozoline HCl 0.05%	Benzalkonium Cl 0.01%; EDTA 0.1%
Comfort eye drops (Sola/ Barnes-Hind)	Hydroxyethylcellulose; polyvinyl alcohol[b]	Naphazoline HCl 0.03%	Benzalkonium Cl 0.005%; EDTA 0.02%
Degest 2 (Sola/Barnes-Hind)	Hydroxyethylcellulose	Naphazoline HCl 0.012%	Benzalkonium Cl 0.0067%; EDTA 0.02%
Eye-Zine (Ocumed)		Tetrahydrozoline HCl 0.05%	
Isopto-Frin (Alcon)	Hydroxypropylmethylcellulose 0.5%	Phenylephrine HCl 0.12%	Benzalkonium Cl 0.01%
Mallazine (Hauck)		Tetrahydrozoline HCl 0.05%	Benzalkonium Cl 0.01
Murine Plus		Tetrahydrozoline HCl 0.05%	Benzalkonium Cl 0.01%; EDTA 0.1%
Naphcon		Naphazoline HCl 0.012%	Benzalkonium Cl 0.01%
OcuClear (Schering)		Oxymetazoline HCl 0.025%	Benzalkonium Cl 0.01%; EDTA
Ocu-Phrin (Ocumed)		Phenylephrine HCl 0..12%	
Optigene III (Pfeiffer)	Povidone	Tetrahydrozoline HCl 0.05%	Benzalkonium Cl 0.004%; EDTA 0.1%
Optised (Various Mfgr)		Phenylephrine HCl 0.12%	
Phenylzin (Cooper Vision)	Hydroxypropylmethylcellulose	Phenylephrine HCl 0.12%	Benzalkonium
Prefrin Liquifilm (Allergan)	Polyvinyl alcohol 1.4%	Phenylephrine HCl 0.12%	Benzalkonium
Relief (Allergan)	Polyvinyl alcohol 1.4%	Phenylephrine HCl 0.12%	
Soothe (Alcon)	Povidone	Tetrahydrozoline HCl 0.05%	Benzalkonium Cl 0.004%; EDTA 0.1%
Tetrahydrozoline hydrchloride (various mfgr.)		Tetrahydrozoline HCl 0.05%	
20/20 Eye drops (S.S.S.)		Naphazoline HCl 0.12%	Thimerosal 0.005%
VasoClear (Iolab)	Polyvinyl alcohol	Naphazoline HCl 0.02%	Benzalkonium Cl 0.01%; EDTA
VasoClear A (Iolab)	Polyvinyl alcohol 0.25%	Naphazoline HCl 0.02%	Benzalkonium Cl 0.005%; EDTA
Visine (Leeming)		Tetrahydrozoline HCl 0.05%	Benzalkonium Cl 0.01%; EDTA 0.1%
Visine A. C.[a] (Leeming)		Tetrahydrozoline HCl 0.05%	Benzalkonium Cl 0.1%; EDTA 0.1%
Visine Extra[b] (Leeming)		Tetrahydrozoline HCl 0.05%	Benzalkonium Cl 0.013%; EDTA 0.1%
Zincfrin (Alcon)		Phenylephrine HCl 0.12%	Benzalkonium Cl 0.01%

[a]Includes zinc sulfate 0.25%.
[b]Includes PEG-400 1%.
Source: Adapted from (7).

influence its local effects on the eye and its possible systemic effects (7).

Drug molecules generally move from one eye structure to another (or into the bloodstream and thus into the system) by means of passive diffusion. The ease of movement from one area of the eye to another or into the bloodstream is determined by, among other things:

1. The condition of the eye tissue. Damage to tissue permits the passage of drug molecules that would not normally penetrate healthy tissue. Inflammation, for example, generally promotes drug penetration into the affected areas.
2. The increased perfusion that occurs when eyes are red. This leads to increased systemic absorption of ophthalmic preparations and a greater likelihood of systemic side effects.
3. Age, which affects tear production. Decreased tear production, sagging lacrimal sacs, and other effects of old age are

believed to affect drug absorption and distribution. The very young and very old tend to absorb topically applied ophthalmic drugs more readily and may consequently manifest systemic side effects.

The ophthalmic structures that lie in front of the lens (i.e., the conjunctiva, sclera, cornea, iris, and aqueous humor; see Fig. 46.1) are readily penetrated by topically applied drugs. However, these drugs rarely pass through anterior structures sufficiently to reach posterior structures (vitreous humor and retina) in therapeutic quantities.

Systemically administered medicines reach the eye via the bloodstream. The choroid and retina, being the most vascular structures, receive the greatest supply. However, systemic drugs may reach other areas of the eye by diffusing from other periocular vessels.

Table 46.6.
Side Effects and Precautions Associated with
α-Sympathomimetic Eye Drops

These eye drops should not be used in greater quantities or more often than prescribed, nor should they be used unnecessarily, because rebound vasodilation may lead to chronic congestion and red eyes. The chronic vasoconstriction that results from the excessive use of decongestant eye drops leads to the formation of new blood vessels as a means of compensation by the eye. The "neovascularization" adds to the chronic congestion and red eye.

Patients should be cautioned against the habitual use of over-the-counter decongestant eye drops

These eye drops should not be used on young children, as absorption may cause marked CNS stimulation and serious hypertension.

These agents should not be used by patients who may suffer attacks of angle-closure glaucoma. Note that many over-the-counter preparations contain sympathomimetic decongestants.

Susceptible adults may absorb sufficient quantities to suffer cardiac tachyarrhythmias and hypertension. Patients who are known to have vascular problems, are eldery, are debilitated, or are taking monoamine oxidase inhibitors or tricyclics should use these eye drops only under supervision. These patients should avoid ophthalmic solutions that contain high concentrations of sympathomimetics.

Source: Adapted from (6, 7).

Table 46.7.
Mydriatic-Cycloplegic Agents

Drug	Dosage Form/Strength
Atropine sulfate	Ointment (0.5%, 1.0%) and solution (0.5%, 1%, 2%, 3%)
Cyclopentolate	Solution (0.5%, 1%, 2%)
Homatropine	Solution (2%, 5%)
Phenylephrine	Solution (2.5%, 10%)
Scopolamine	Solution (0.25%)
Tropicamide	Solution (0.5% or 1%)

Table 46.8.
Ophthalmic Topical Anesthetics

Drug	Dosage Form	Strength
Cocaine	Solution	1.0–4.0%
Benoxinate with fluorescein	Solution	0.4%
Proparacaine HCl with fluorescein	Solution	0.5%
Tetracaine HCl	Solution	0.5%

Note: One or two drops used for temporary anesthesia (lasts for 15–20 min) during examinations and procedures

The formulation of the ophthalmic preparations largely determines their durations of action. Active ingredients in eye drops are more readily absorbed when in solution rather than in suspension. Eye ointments have the most prolonged action. The drug particles that are found in aqueous or oily suspensions are released gradually as they dissolve in the tears. Contact time and frequency of installation affect absorption.

INJURIES

Foreign Bodies in the Eye

Foreign bodies are a common occurrence, with symptoms ranging from little or no discomfort to severe pain. Failure to remove the foreign material may result in physical damage to the eye, development of a secondary infection, or eventual blindness. Objects such as dust particles or small insects can usually be removed by flushing the eye with sterile normal saline, any natural tears product, or, if nothing else is available, tap water. If the object is not removed by flushing the eye, the patient should be referred to an emergency room or an ophthalmologist.

Foreign bodies that are visibly lodged in the conjunctival area may be gently lifted out with a moist sterile cotton applicator. Removal of corneal foreign bodies requires proper instrumentation and should be done by a physician. Foreign bodies that are not readily seen with the naked eye may be made visible by fluorescein staining. If the foreign body is deeply embedded or has penetrated the eye, it will probably require surgical removal. If wood splinters or metal shavings may have become lodged in the eye, patients should be referred immediately to the emergency room (E.R.), an ophthalmologist, or an available physician.

Topical anesthetic eye drops *should not* be used to relieve the painful irritation caused by a foreign body but only to facilitate its removal. The local analgesia that is produced may mask the presence of residual foreign material, which in turn may lead to severe corneal abrasions. Furthermore, chronic ophthalmic use of topical anesthesia can permanently damage the corneal epithelium (8).

After removal of the foreign body, a broad-spectrum antibiotic ophthalmic ointment such as tobramycin or gentamicin (Table 46.1) and a short-acting cycloplegic agent (e.g., 1 drop of cyclopentolate 1%) should be instilled in the lower cul-de-sac, and a moderate pressure patch should be placed over the closed lids for 24 to 48 hr (9). The cyclopentolate should be instilled before the antibiotic. If there was a penetrating injury to the eye, antibiotic ointment should not be used because the injury may allow access to the anterior chamber of the eye (9). Ophthalmic corticosteroid preparations are contraindicated in eye injuries, as they may delay healing and promote the development and spread of infection (4, 5) (Table 46.4).

Table 46.9.
Artificial Tear Products

Product	Viscosity Agent	Preservative
Absorbotear	Hydroxyethylcellulose; povidone 1.67%	Edetate disodium 0.1%; thimerosal 0.004%
Akwa Tears	Polyvinyl alcohol	Benzalkonium Cl 0.01%; edetate disodium
Artificial Tears solution	Polyvinyl alcohol 1.4%	Edetate disodium, chlorobutanol
Celluvisc	Carboxymethylcellulose sodium 1%	
Comfort Tears	Hydroxyethylcellulose; polyvinyl alcohol	Edetate disodium 0.005%; benzalkonium Cl 0.02%
Hypotears	Polyvinyl alcohol 1%	Benzalkonium Cl 0.01%
Isopto Alkaline	Hydroxypropyl methylcellulose 1%	Benzalkonium Cl 0.01%
Isopto Plain	Hydroxypropyl methylcellulose 0.05%	Benzalkonium Cl 0.01%
Just Tears	Hydroxypropyl methylcellulose	Benzalkonium Cl 0.01%; edetate disodium 0.025%
Lacril	Hydroxypropyl methylcellulose 0.5%; geltain A 0.01%	Chlorobutanol 0.5%
Liquifilm Forte	Polyvinyl alcohol 3%	Edetate disodium; thimerosal 0.002%
Liquifilm Tears	Polyvinyl alcohol 1.4%	Chlorobutanol 0.5%
Moisture Drops	Hydroxypropyl methylcellulose 0.5%; dextran 40, 0.1%	Edetate disodium; benzalkonium Cl 0.01%
Murine	Polyvinyl alcohol 1.4%; povidone 0.6%	Benzalkonium Cl; edetate disodium
Muro Tears	Hydroxypropyl methylcellulose; dextran 40	Benzalkonium Cl 0.01%; edetate disodium
Murocel	Methylcellulose 1%	
Refresh	Polyvinyl alcohol 1.4%; povidone 0.6%	
TearGard	Hydroxyethylcellulose	Edetate disodium 0.1%
Teargel	Polyacrylic acid 0.2% and cetrimide 0.01% (as preservative)	
Tearisol	Hydroxypropyl methylcellulose 0.5%	Benzalkonium Cl 0.01%
Tears Naturale	Hydroxypropyl methylcellulose; dextran 70	Benzalkonium Cl 0.01%; edetate disodium 0.05%
Tears Naturale II	Hydroxypropyl methylcellulose 0.3%; dextran 70, 0.1%	Edetate disodium
Tears Plus	Polyvinyl alcohol 1.4%; povidone 0.6%	Chlorobutanol 0.5%
Tears Renewed	Hydroxypropyl methylcellulose; dextran 70	Benzalkonium Cl 0.01; edetate disodium 0.05%
Ultra Tears	Hydroxypropyl methylcellulose 1%	Benzalkonium Cl 0.01%

Source: Adapted from (7).

Contusion Injuries of the Anterior Segment ("Black Eye")

A direct blow to the eye by an object such as a fist, racket ball, tennis ball, or the like can produce a combination of injuries, including a dislocation of the crystalline lens, iridodialysis, traumatic iritis, and hyphema (blood in the anterior chamber). The patient should be checked in the E.R. to make sure that no serious damage has occurred. A "black eye" is usually self-limiting. A "black eye" that was caused by trauma should be treated with cold compresses during the first 24 hr to inhibit swelling. The second day, hot compresses may aid absorption of the hematoma (9).

Chemical Burns

Chemical burns of the cornea and the conjunctiva must be treated immediately by extensive irrigation with sterile water or saline for 5 to 30 min to dilute and remove the offending agent. If sterile water is not available, any source of water should be used (e.g., shower, faucet, drinking fountain, hose). The eyelids should be held apart, and water should be irrigated continuously for at least 5 min. The patient should be referred immediately to an ophthalmologist or the E.R. En route, the eye should be kept irrigated. A wet towel will help to maintain the irrigation. Once the patients is in the E.R., irrigation with at least 2000 mL of normal saline 0.9% for a minimum of 1 hr is

necessary. Instillation of topical anesthetics every 20 min to relieve the pain is recommended. Irrigation should be continued until pH paper reveals that the conjunctival pH has returned to normal (pH between 7.3 and 7.7). Once a normal pH has been attained, a second reading should be done in 5 to 10 min to ensure that the pH has not shifted to a more alkaline or acid range (9).

After the irrigation, topical antibiotics (e.g., gentamicin, tobramycin, or erythromycin) should be started to prevent a secondary infection. If there is an increase in the intraocular pressure due to the trauma, then a carbonic anhydrase inhibitor should be given. To prevent iris adhesions to the lens (posterior synechiae), a mydriatic-cycloplegic agent should be used (1 drop of cyclopentolate 1% or 1 drop of phenylephrine 2.5%). After the emergency haas been controlled, the eye should be patched, and the antibiotic should be continued for 2 to 3 days.

Flash Burns ("Arc-Eye" and Snow-Blindness)

"Arc-eye" results from direct exposure of the eye to ultraviolet irradiation, such as radiation from an arc-flame used for welding, reflection, or sun rays in the snow. Symptoms usually start a few hours after exposure and cause severe pain, lacrimation, and photophobia.

Although the pain associated with "arc-eye" may be quite severe, symptoms normally resolve within 24 hr.

Emergency treatment should include application of cold compresses to the eye and administration of oral analgesics to relieve pain (ASA with codeine). Severe cases of "arc-eye" may require a topical anesthetic such as proparacaine HCl 0.5% and a decongestant such as epinephrine 0.5 to 1.0% to reduce congestion. Patients should not be given a topical anesthetic for routine use, since it may mask the symptoms of other problems (e.g., a welding burn may also involve a foreign body that, if not detected, could lead to further damage). A topical antibiotic ointment such as gentamicin, tobramycin, or neomycin may be needed to prevent infection. Chloramphenicol should be avoided because safer alternatives are available.

DISORDERS OF THE EYELIDS

Lid Edema

This condition manifests as swelling and itching of one or both eyelids in atopic individuals in response to certain allergens. Various ophthalmic medications, cosmetics, insect stings or bites on the eyelid, or plant allergens may act as contact allergens. Systemic allergens include certain foods (e.g., seafood, nuts, eggs, milk products), inhalants (e.g., pollens, hair sprays, deodorant sprays), and drugs (e.g., penicillin, sulfonamides, salicylates).

Signs and symptoms include urticaria of the eyelids in a circumscribed area of subepidermal and epidermal edema with an erythematous margin and blanched center, which may disappear after a few hours (10, 11).

Treatment includes identification and removal of the offending allergen. This may be the only treatment required. Cold compresses over the closed lids may speed resolution, but desensitization, cromolyn sodium, or oral antihistamine therapy is indicated when the responsible allergen(s) cannot be identified or avoided. Topical corticosteroid creams (e.g., triamcinolone 0.1%) may be required if swelling persists for longer than 24 hr.

Blepharitis

Blepharitis is a condition that is characterized by chronic redness of the lid margins, thickening, and often formation of scales sticking to the base of the eyelashes, presenting as either squamous or ulcerative blepharitis, depending on the cause.

Nonulcerative (squamous or seborrheic) blepharitis may be associated with seborrheic dermatitis of the scalp or eyebrows or may be an allergic response to an ophthalmic medication (the medication, the vehicle, or the preservatives and/or buffers). Ulcerative blepharitis is caused by bacterial infection (usually *Staphylococcus*) of the lash follicles and meibomian glands.

Signs and symptoms of squamous blepharitis include redness of the lid margins, lid edema, loss of lashes, and a foreign-body sensation. Excessive itching may indicate an allergic component in the etiology. In ulcerative blepharitis, small pustules develop in the lash follicles and eventually break down to form shallow ulcers. A purulent discharge produces unsightly crusting on the lid margin.

The standard treatment of blepharitis consists of meticulous lid hygiene, with cleansing and debridement of the crusts on the eyelids. Diluted baby shampoo on cotton swabs should be used to cleanse the eyelids. Moist warm compresses will help to reduce the symptoms and increase blood flow (12).

Regular use of a dandruff shampoo may be helpful as well. *Pityrosporum* yeasts have been implicated in seborrheic dermatitis, and these organisms have been identified on the lid margin in patients with blepharitis. The antifungal agent ketoconazole may have some advantages over conventional antidandruff preparations in the treatment of blepharitis (13). Bacterial blepharitis requires antimicrobial therapy such as gentamicin, tobramycin, or erythromycin applied as an ointment three to four times a day for 3 days. Short-term topical steroids have been used concurrently in persistent cases (e.g., prednisolone acetate suspension 0.12%, 1 drop, 3 times a day). The nonprescription preparation 1% mercuric oxide (yellow) ophthalmic ointment has been reported to offer a safe and effective alternative to topical antibiotics (14).

Hordeolum (Stye) and Chalazion

An external hordeolum or stye is a small abscess at the root of an eyelash in the glands of Zeis or Moll. It is very painful but not serious. An internal hordeolum is an infection of a meibomian gland on the conjunctival side of the lid. It may be more serious and painful than an external stye. A chalazion is a chronic enlargement of a meibomian gland from occlusion of its duct. It is painless and may disappear after a few months.

Infection of these glands is usually caused by *Staphylococcus*. Styes may sometimes develop secondary to blepharitis. An external hordeolum (stye) begins with redness and painful swelling of the lid margin, followed by a small, round area of induration. The patient suffers from a foreign-body sensation, photophobia, and lacrimation. A small spot, indicative of suppuration, forms in the center of the induration ("pointing"), and this little abscess ruptures spontaneously with relief of pain.

An internal hordeolum (stye) is more severe, and the area of inflammation is away from the lid margin on the conjunctival side of the lid. A small yellow area can be seen at the site of the affected gland, but it seldom points through the skin and does not rupture spontaneously. A chalazion starts like a stye with lid edema, swelling, and irritation. After a few days it resolves, leaving a painless, slowly enlarging round mass in the lid. It can be seen subconjunctivally as a red or grey mass, and it may disappear after a few months. If not, it should be treated surgically.

Suppuration may be terminated in the early stages by antimicrobials (e.g., erythromycin, bacitracin, or sulfacetamide ophthalmic ointment used every 2 hr). Pointing of a stye may be enhanced by using hot compresses and then draining the stye by pulling the lash or incising with a fine-tipped blade to be able to express the contents of the abscess. If styes must be excised, patients should be advised to seek medical assistance and not to try it themselves. Pus should be removed carefully, and antimicrobial solutions or ointments should be used to prevent spreading of the infection (three times a day for 3 days). Internal meibomian abscesses and chalazions should be referred to a physician for incision and curettage under local anesthesia.

Entropion

Entropion is a common condition that occurs mainly in the elderly (over 65 years of age). The lower eyelids turn inward, causing the eyelashes to abrade the cornea and conjunctiva. This causes a painful, red, watery eye. Surgical repair is the only permanent cure for this condition. Micropore tape is useful as a temporary measure in keeping the lid everted (15).

DISORDERS OF THE CONJUNCTIVA

The conjunctiva lines the back of the eyelid and extends into the space between the lid and the globe as well as over the sclera to the cornea. Dilation of the blood vessels in the conjunctiva and sclera results in a "red eye," which may be caused by various stimuli. Identifying the cause of a "red eye" has often proven difficult. One condition may be easily mistaken for another. Table 46.10 compares conditions that cause "red eye."

Conjunctivitis

Conjunctivitis is a common eye disease that may be acute or chronic. The causes include various conditions that all have inflammation of the conjunctiva as a common symptom. Conjunctivitis is usually bilateral, the eyes are uncomfortable rather than painful, and vision is not affected. Acute conjunctivitis is usually caused by bacteria, viruses, or allergy and by sometimes chemical or mechanical irritants. Chronic conjunctivitis, characterized by exacerbations and remissions over long periods, even years, is also caused by bacteria, viruses, or allergens as well as disorders such as blepharitis and chronic dacryocystitis. Because the conjunctiva contains many small blood vessels, spontaneous subconjunctival hemorrhage sometimes occurs on sneezing or straining on defecation. The condition is painless, does not affect vision, and is localized to one area of the conjunctiva. The situation should resolve spontaneously within 10 to 14 days without treatment. Recurrence warrants exclusion of hypertension and bleeding disorders. Most cases of conjunctivitis are treated on the basis of clinical diagnosis, without the aid of culture and

sensitivity tests. For infections that do not respond to therapy in 2 to 3 days or those extending beyond the conjunctiva, cornea, and eyelids, a culture and a sensitivity test are essential. In the absence of such tests, broad-spectrum antibiotic coverage may be obtained from the combination of an aminoglycoside and a cephalosporin injected subconjunctivally plus appropriate topical therapy (16–19).

BACTERIAL CONJUNCTIVITIS

Infection by various bacteria causes inflammation of the conjunctiva with dilatation of its blood vessels (1, 12, 16, 20). The goblet cells (mucus-secreting cells) and tiny lacrimal glands of the conjunctiva become overactive; the result is watering and a discharge containing many inflammatory white cells. *Staphylococcus aureus* (the most common causative agent), *Staphylococcus epidermidis*, *Streptococus pneumoniae* (pneumococcus), *Streptococcus pyogenes*, and *Haemophilus influenzae* are common causative organisms. Newborn babies sometimes suffer from acute purulent conjunctivitis (ophthalmia neonatorum) caused by *Neisseria gonorrhoeae* or *Chlamydia trachomatis*. The eyes are red and itch, and the purulent discharge tends to accumulate on the lashes, causing them to stick together. The lids may be moderately swollen.

Although the condition can be self-limiting, it often requires treatment with a topical broad-spectrum antibiotic in solution or ointment form. If the diagnosis is based on clinical diagnosis alone (no culture), then erythromycin or bacitracin ointment or sodium sulfacetamide 10 to 15% solution is usually effective. These agents cover the most common Gram-positive microorganisms that normally cause bacterial conjunctivitis. However, since about 50% of staphylococci are resistant to the sulfonamides, a product such as neomycin-polymyxin-bacitracin is effective. Approximately 6 to 8% of patients who are treated with this combination have a sensitivity reaction to the neomycin. If the offending microorganism is *Haemophilus* or *Moraxella*, chloramphenicol is very effective. Other useful broad-spectrum antibiotics include polymyxin B-bacitracin ointment, polymyxin B-trimethoprim, and gentamicin; tobramycin drops or ointment is used as well. Tobramycin and gentamicin are usually used for conjunctivitis caused by Gram-negative microorganisms (16). Topical therapy with ciprofloxacin for as little as 3 days has been shown to effectively control the great majority of pathogenic bacteria associated with bacterial conjunctivitis (20).

A poor clinical response after 2 or 3 days indicates resistant bacteria or a misdiagnosis. Culture and sensitivity tests should be done to determine the causative agent. Proper eye hygiene should be maintained to avoid transmitting the infection. Warm, wet compresses improve the circulation and help to cleanse the discharge. If the eyelids become crusted, the use of a dilute baby shampoo

Table 46.10.

Comparison of a Number of Conditions That Cause Red Eyes

Condition	Appearance of the Eye(s)	Lids and Lashes	Discharge	Other Features	Basic Treatment
Blepharitis	Eyes are moderately red	Lid margins inflamed, swollen, scaly, loss of lashes, pustules in lash follicles	Purulent discharge from pustules on lashes	Seborrheic dermatitis of scalp or eyebrows in nonulcerative type; vision unaffected	Antidandruff shampoo, topical antibiotic and steroid therapy where indicated
Conjunctivitis Bacterial	Conjunctiva red	Lids moderately swollen, lashes sticky and matted on wakening	Mucopurulent	Vision not affected	Topical antibiotic
Viral	Conjunctiva red	Lymphoid follicles inside upper lid	Profuse, clear, watery	Occasionally associated with sore throat and fever; preaudicular adenopathy; vision unaffected	None
Allergic	Conjunctiva red	Lids inflamed, upper inner lid lumpy	Stringy, clear mucoid	Intense itching; usually part of larger allergic syndrome; vision unaffected	Cromolyn Na, lodoxamide, levocabastine, antihistamine
Chlamydial (trachoma)	Conjunctiva red	Lids very swollen, upper inner lid lumpy	Watery	Corneal damage can occur; vision loss may ensue	Topical and oral tetracycline
Dry eyes	Eyes are moderately red and lusterless		Stringy, deficient	Corneal damage may occur, photophobia may exist, and impaired vision may occur	Tear solution, treat underlying cause
Entropion	Eyes red	Lashes turned inwards, chafing cornea and conjunctiva	Watery		Surgery
Keratitis Bacterial	Red rim around cornea, ulcer, and pus visible in cornea		Mucopurulent	Very painful; occasionally visual disturbance	Topical/oral antibiotic; mydriatic to relieve painful iris spasm
Viral (herpes simplex)	Red rim around cornea, dentritic ulcer on cornea		Watery	Usually only one eye affected; painful, eye damage and loss of vision may occur	Topical antiviral; mydriatic to relieve painful iris spasm
Uveitis (iritis)	Red eyes, especially around corneal rim, (circumciliary injection of vessels)		No discharge or excessive tearing	Pain, photophobia, loss of visual acuity, miosis in affected eye	Topical steroids; mydriatic to relieve painful iris spasm and to prevent iris from adhering to lens

Source: Adapted from (6).

solution applied with a cotton swab is effective. Corticosteroids, either separately or with antibiotics, should not be used until a viral etiology has been positively excluded.

The World Health Organization (WHO) recommends the use of a 1% silver nitrate solution in the eyes of newborns to prevent *Neisseriae gonorrhoeae* infection. The use of tetracycline or erythromycin ophthalmic ointment is preferred, as it will prevent both chlamydial and *N. gonorrhoeae* conjunctivitis.

VIRAL CONJUNCTIVITIS

The pathophysiology of viral conjunctivitis is the same as that of bacterial conjunctivitis (10, 21). The most common virus is the adenovirus type 3 and 8 in populations with satisfactory hygiene. The herpes simplex virus may cause serious sight-threatening eye infections. It is often associated with other viral infections such as colds, sore throats, or influenzae.

The patient may feel generally ill and complain of red, watery, and gritty eyes. Lymphoid follicles are usually present on the upper lid conjunctiva, and swollen lymph nodes can often be detected in front of the ear (preauricular node). The discharge is profuse and watery, with minimal lid edema.

Viral infections are usually self-limiting, and because the antiviral agents that are currently available are effective only against the herpes viruses, treatment is often unsatisfactory. The antiviral agents that are effective against DNA herpesvirus are useful in the treatment of herpes simplex eye infections. A 14- to 21-day treatment regimen of either ophthalmic vidarabine 3% or idoxuridine 0.5% ointment administered five times a day or trifluridine 1% solution, 1 drop in the affected eye nine times a day stops viral replication until the infected cells slough from the eye (16). Acyclovir 3% ointment administered five times a day for 14 days or at least 3 days after healing is complete, whichever is shorter, is indicated for the treatment of herpes simplex keratitis (22). Antibacterial ophthalmic preparations may prevent secondary bacterial infections and may be used in conjunction with the antiviral agents. Corticosteroids should be avoided in treating viral infections (16).

ALLERGIC CONJUNCTIVITIS

Allergic conjunctivitis, either acute or chronic, is usually part of a larger allergic syndrome such as hay fever (19, 21). Patients with atopic diseases have an inherited predisposition to develop hypersensitivity to specific inhaled and ingested allergens, which is characterized by development of specific antibodies of the IgE immunoglobulin class. Symptoms of allergic conjunctivitis can be evoked by direct contact with airborne allergens such as pollen, fungal spores, dust, and animal danders, or systemic allergens such as certain foods can stimulate an attack. The eye irritation due to indoor pollutants, as experienced by sufferers of the "sick-building syndrome," is also a form of allergic conjunctivitis (22).

The most commonly occuring types of allergic conjunctivitis are seasonal allergies and the acute allergic response. The seasonal type is characterized by transient attacks of severe itching, watery or mucoid discharge, and a pink eye. The patient may also suffer from asthma or another atopic disease. On examination the lids and conjunctiva are swollen, and papillae can be seen lining the lid conjunctiva, particularly on the upper lids. Symptoms of acute allergic conjunctivitis are similar to the seasonal type but are more severe, often involving only one eye. Neither condition causes visual disturbance.

In allergic conjunctivitis, cold compresses are extremely useful in relieving the symptoms and reducing the swelling. The most effective treatment is removal of the allergen. The use of topical ophthalmic decongestants, antihistamines, or both will provide symptomatic relief. The treatment of allergic conjunctivitis resembles that of lid edema (Table 46.10). Cromolyn sodium 4% and lodoxamide 0.1% administered four to six times a day are safe and effective agents in the treatment of allergic conjunctivitis in patients with a history of atopy, hay fever, eczema, or other systemic allergies and especially in the treatment of children. Lodoxamide 0.1% ophthalmic solution has been shown to provide more rapid relief of symptoms and greater reduction of major signs and symptoms associated with allergic conjunctivitis than does cromolyn sodium 2% (23). Topical use of levocabastine, an H_1-antihistamine, was shown to be an effective and well-tolerated drug in the treatment of allergic conjunctivitis (24–26). Note that patients who suffer from chronic allergic conjunctivitis should be warned against habitual use of over-the-counter sympathomimetic decongestant eye drops because of possible rebound vasodilatation. Precipitation of an attack of angle-closure glaucoma is a danger with the use of sympathomimetic-containing eye drops.

VERNAL CONJUNCTIVITIS

Vernal conjunctivitis is a seasonally recurrent, bilateral inflammation of the conjunctiva (16). It produces itching, watery eyes, photophobia, and a foreign-body sensation in the eye. Positive diagnosis requires the scraping of the conjunctiva to show prominent eosinophils. The inflammation usually occurs the spring and early summer and may occur in the fall. A thick, ropy, mucous discharge is a prominent characteristic of vernal conjunctivitis.

The primary treatment is topical steriods, but since this requires prolonged therapy in most cases, the sequelae of cataract formation from the topical steriod or elevation of intraocular pressure are major complications. When used, prednisolone 1/8% to 1% administered two or three times a day is effective. Cromolyn sodium solution 4% administered four to six times a day (or the ointment at night), a 0.1% solution of lodoxamide administered four to six times a day (or the ointment at night), or a 0.1% solution of lodoxamide administered four times a day may control the symptoms (23).

CHLAMYDIAL KERATOCONJUNCTIVITIS (TRACHOMA)

A chronic form of conjunctivitis is caused by *Chlamydia trachomatis*. It is characterized by subconjunctival hyperplasia and vascularization of the cornea (18, 22) and occurs mainly in hot, dry, underdeveloped countries. It is also common among American Indians and in mountainous areas of the southern United States. It is a most contagious condition in its early stages and is transmitted by direct contact or possibly by handling contaminated articles. Flies are well-known vectors. Another strain of *Chlamydia* is sexually transmitted and is a fairly common cause of neonatal conjunctivitis.

After an incubation period of about a week, swelling of the eyelids, photophobia, and lacrimation occur. Small follicles (appearing as bumps) appear on the inner surface of the upper lid. Exacerbations and remissions are a feature of this disease. Pannus formation with invasion of the cornea develops over time, and corneal scarring and blindness may ensue.

WHO recommendations for the prophylaxis and therapy for trachoma are as follows:

1. Improved hygiene and prevention of spread.
2. Mass prophylactic treatment with tetracycline hydrochloride ointment to both eyes, twice daily for 5 days.
3. Treatment of active trachoma in the individual: tetracycline ointment three times daily for 6 weeks combined with oral sulfonamides for adults and erythromycin for children for 2 weeks.

Other authorities suggest that chloramphenicol be used topically instead of tetracycline, accompanied by trimethoprin/sulfamethoxazole by mouth (adults and children), a tetracycline derivative (adults only), or erythromycin (adults and children).

KERATOCONJUNCTIVITIS SICCA (DRY EYE)

Dry eye is a condition that is characterized by chronic dryness of the conjunctiva and cornea, which may lead to desiccation of the ocular surface (11, 16). Most people who complain of "dry eyes" are seen, on examination, to have a perfectly normal supply of tears. The normal tear film consists of three distinct layers. The inner layer, which overlies the corneal and conjunctival epithelial cells and is produced by the goblet cells, is composed of mucin. This layer acts as a surfactant so that the cornea becomes hydrophilic. The middle layer is the saline layer produced by the accessory lacrimal glands in the conjunctiva. The outer, oily layer comes from the meibomian glands. The main purpose of this outer layer is to retard evaporation of the saline.

Tear film deficiency can be due to a shortage of any of these three constituents. A number of pathologic or environmental conditions can cause such an imbalance. Diseases that are associated with the dry eye syndrome include rheumatoid arthritis, Sjögren's syndrome, Stevens-Johnson syndrome, the menopause, mumps, and vitamin A deficiency. The use of certain medications, such as anticholinergics, diuretics, and oral contraceptives, has been reported to contribute to dryness of the eyes.

Chronic eye discomfort and conjunctival redness accompanied by photophobia are common symptoms of the dry eye syndrome. In advanced cases, corneal damage and various degrees of impaired vision can occur. Frequent use of artifical tears containing methylcellulose or polyvinyl alcohol may produce better results than hypotonic solutions because of their increased viscosity. The number of different natural tears products that are on the market indicates a great deal of variability in patient response from product to product. If tear replacement is not successful, other therapeutic measures such as ocular inserts or a lubricant eye ointment may be effective. A topical antibiotic is required if secondary bacterial infections occur. Sometimes the unrecognized dry eye syndrome is treated with vasoconstrictors and local antihistamines. However, treatment with these medications is ineffective and may only worsen the condition (Table 46.6).

DISORDERS OF THE LACRIMAL SYSTEM (THE WATERING EYE)

The watering eye may be a result of either excess tear production (lacrimation) or deficient tear drainage (epiphora) (12, 27). Causes of lacrimation include corneal irritation by a foreign body or trauma. Causes of poor drainage include the following:

1. Stricture of the nasolacrimal duct (dacryostenosis) is often seen in newborn babies as a result of blockage by debris in the duct. In adults, dacryostenosis may result from inflammatory obstruction of the duct due to chronic nasal infection or from severe or chronic conjunctivitis.
2. Infection of the lacrimal sac (dacryocystitis) is usually secondary to obstruction of the nasolacrimal duct.
3. In senile ectropion the lower lid of the eye sags away from the globe as a result of weakening of the muscles surrounding the eye. The opening (puncti) to the lacrimal drain is thus displaced, resulting in epiphora.

A chronic overflow of tears and moderate edema of the lacrimal sac as well as redness are seen in dacryocystitis. Watery eyes are present in the dry eye syndrome when the tear composition lacks sufficient mucin.

Congenital obstruction resolves spontaneously, although fingertip massage of the lacrimal sac may speed resolution. Surgery may be necessary to correct epiphora due to ectropion. Antibiotic ointments (erythromycin or tobramycin four times a day) may be required in cases of secondary infection.

DISORDERS OF THE CORNEA (KERATITIS)

Keratitis is a condition that is characterized by inflammation of the cornea. Because the cornea does not contain blood vessels, inflammation takes the form of edema, infiltration by white blood cells, and redness around the rim of the cornea. The abundant nerve endings in the cornea make the condition painful. Keratitis most commonly results from infection (by bacteria, viruses, or fungi) or is due to noninfectious causes such as corneal oxygen deprivation brought about by excessive wearing of hard contact lenses, exposure to ultraviolet light, or an inability of the lids to close over the eye. The two most commonly occurring types of keratitis are bacterial and viral keratitis (3, 16).

Bacterial Keratitis

Bacterial keratitis occurs when organisms such as *Staphylococcus aureus*, *Streptococcus pneumoniae*, *Pseudomonas*, and enterobacterial species invade a small erosion on the corneal surface (1, 16, 19, 24). The patient with a bacterial corneal ulcer complains of discomfort and a foreign-body sensation, photophobia, and a mucopurulent discharge. The condition is painful, with redness around the rim of the cornea and a white corneal ulcer visible on examination. Visual disturbance occurs if the ulcer is in the center of the cornea.

Topical and/or oral antibiotic treatment is indicated. Initial therapy should be aggressive and should be based on the results of corneal scraping (culture and sensitivity reports). Therapy should not be started until these results are in hand. The scraping requires the use of a topical anesthetic such as proparacaine 0.5%. The eye should not be covered with a patch; this might encourage further bacterial growth. All corneal ulcers should be referred directly to an ophthalmologist.

VIRAL KERATITIS

Viral keratitis is caused by herpes simplex or herpes zoster (10, 21). The herpes simplex virus is the most common cause of viral keratitis. The eye is red, gritty, photophobic, and painful. Usually, only one eye is involved. Staining with fluorescein may reveal a branching corneal ulcer that may heal without damage but may result in serious corneal scarring.

The herpes zoster virus may attack neuronal tissue, causing a painful condition known as shingles. The ophthalmic neurons may also become involved, in which case an extremely painful condition involving the cornea, tip of the nose, and forehead develops. Corneal scarring may occur, and secondary glaucoma may develop.

Topical antivirals such as acyclovir, idoxuridine, trifluridine, and vidarabine are indicated to treat herpes simplex keratitis. (See the discussion above of the treatment of viral conjunctivitis.) If the 0.1% solution of idoxuridine is used, the regimen is 1 drop in the affected eye hourly during the day and every 2 hr at night (unless the ointment is used at night) (16). Steroid-containing preparations are contraindicated, as they may accelerate corneal damage (4, 5, 15) (Table 46.4). The oral and intravenous antivirals are not as effective as are topical agents in treating viral keratitis.

Unlike herpes simplex, herpes zoster is an indication for the use of topical steroids. This prevents prolonged inflammation and nerve pain. Steroids should be used only after herpes simplex has been excluded. A 0.1% dexamethasone solution, instilled every 2 hr, may be used concomitantly with a mydriatic such as 1% atropine or 0.5% to 1% cyclopentolate solution, one drop three times a day. Intraocular pressure (IOP) must be monitored in these patients, because the infection may cause an increase in IOP. Systemic corticosteroids and recently cimetidine have been used to prevent postherpetic neuralgia (28). Cimetidine (300 mg orally four times a day) is used for 2 to 3 weeks, and when therapy is begun 48 to 72 hr after onset of the disease, it has been shown to reduce pain and pruritus in acute herpes zoster (10, 22). Oral acyclovir (200 to 800 mg five times a day with a maximum dosage of 4000 mg/day) for 10 days in the immunosuppressed patient has been effective, especially if therapy is started within 72 hr of onset of the disease.

DISORDERS OF THE UVEAL TRACT

The uveal tract consists of the iris, ciliary body, and choroid. Uveitis is the generic term for inflammatory conditions of the uveal tract (1, 29). One or all three parts of the uveal tract may be affected simultaneously. Anterior uveitis is an inflammation of the iris (iritis) and/or the ciliary body (iridocyclitis). Posterior uveitis is inflammation of the choroid (choroiditis) and/or the retina (retinitis).

The cause of uveitis is as yet unknown. However, it has been associated with other inflammatory conditions such as arthritis, Crohn's disease, ankylosing spondylitis, and sarcoidosis. Chronic infection, trauma, and anatomical abnormalities such as cataracts have also been implicated. Patients are usually 20 to 50 years of age, and there is a decrease in occurrence in patients over the age of 70 (29).

A patient who is suffering from uveitis can easily be misdiagnosed as having conjunctivitis. Initially, the patient will complain of a red, tender eye that feels bruised to the touch. There may be some photophobia, with no discharge or excessive tearing, and initially the visual acuity is not affected. Uveitis may be unilateral or bilateral, and there may be isolated attacks or repeated episodes (29). Gradually, the eye becomes redder and more painful, and vision becomes disturbed. Careful examination of the eye will show that the pupil on the affected side is smaller than the other and possibly irregular.

No specific therapy is available for uveitis, since the cause is not known. Nonspecific measures include mydriatics, corticosteroids, nonsteroidal antiinflammatory agents, immunosuppressive drugs, and photocoagulation (10, 29). Treatment should be instituted immediately on positive diagnosis to prevent the iris from adhering to the front surface of the lens. The pupil should be dilated by using mydriatic drops to prevent adhesions and scarring between the pupillary border and the anterior lens capsule and to provide relief from photophobia. The mydriatic-cycloplegics that are used include atropine (1 to 4%, 1 drop, one to four times a day) for moderately severe to severe uveitis and homatropine (5%, 1 drop once or twice a day) for mild to moderate uveitis. Cyclopentolate is not used in treating uveitis, since it may further aggravate iritis (29).

Corticosteroids reduce the inflammation and are very effective. Table 46.3 lists the topical steroids and their relative potencies. Drops or ointments are effective in treating with anterior uveitis but not in treating posterior uveitis. The dosage and frequency of the corticosteroids depend on the severity of the disease and can vary from 1 drop every 2 to 4 hr to 1 drop every other day (29). If the patient does not respond to the topical agents, then systemic corticosteroids may be used. (Note: For further information on treatment regimens for uveitis, please refer to reference 29.)

CATARACTS

A cataract is a developmental or degenerative opacity of the crystalline lens. Developmental or congenital cataracts are present at birth; the degenerative type develops slowly with age, leading to a gradual, painless loss of vision. Congenital cataracts are probably caused by chromosomal abnormalities. The degenerative type may be the result of senile degeneration, radiographs, systemic disease (e.g., diabetes), uveitis, or certain drugs (e.g., corticosteroids). The patient experiences a progressive loss of vision, the degree of which depends on the location and extent of the opacity. No medications that are currently available reduce the effect of a cataract once it has formed. The treatment of cataracts involves the surgical removal of the opacity (17).

OPTIC NEURITIS (PAPILLITIS)

Inflammation of the part of the optic nerve that is ophthalmoscopically visible is optic neuritis (papillitis) (18). The precise cause remains obscure. Optic neuritis has been found to develop after viral illnesses, multiple sclerosis, ingestion of certain chemicals (e.g., lead, methanol), bee stings, meningitis, and syphilis. In patients over 60 years of age, an important cause may be temporal arteritis. Vision loss, which may develop within days, is the only symptom.

Removal of the cause in the early stages may restore vision. Otherwise, postneuritic optic atrophy develops with varying degrees of vision loss. Corticosteroids administered systemically (e.g., prednisone 60 mg/day orally) or retrobulbarly (e.g., methylprednisolone acetate 20 mg) may help. Nonsteroidal antiinflammatory agents have also been used orally with some effectiveness (18).

CONCLUSION

The treatment of ocular disorders is dictated by the structure of the eye that is involved, the cause, and the severity. Ophthalmic administration of drugs requires special patient education as well as precautions, and patients who overuse corticosteroid or decongestant ophthalmic preparations may develop adverse effects. Therefore the appropriate drug and dosage form must be selected, and it must be administered correctly for the successful treatment of common eye disorders.

REFERENCES

1. Riley GJ, Baker AS. Eye infections. In: Reese RE, Gordon DR Jr, eds. A practical approach to infection diseases. 2nd ed. Boston: Little, Brown, 1986:156.
2. Vale J, Cox B. Drugs and the eye. Durban, South Africa: Butterworth, 1978:17.
3. Youngson RM. Common eye disorders: lid problems. S Afr Retail Pharmacist 38:25-9, 1989.
4. Lavin MJ, Rose GE. Use of steroid eye drops in general practice. Br Med J 292:1448-50, 1986.
5. Jones BR, Coster DJ, Falcon MG. Prospects of prevention of recurrent herpetic eye disease. Trans Ophthalmol Soc UK 97:350-55, 1977.
6. Plus Continuing Pharmacy Education Programme. Eye conditions and the pharmacists. Published by Pharmaceutical Society of South Africa, compiled by TPS Drug Information Center Johannesburg, 5:141, 1988.
7. Gourley DR. Ophthalmic products. In: Handbook of nonprescription drugs. 9th ed. Washington, DC: American Pharmaceutical Association, 1990:Chap 20.
8. Burns RP, Gipson I. Toxic effects of local anesthetics. JAMA 240:347, 1978.
9. Pavan-Langston D. Burns and trauma. In: Pavan-Langston D, ed. Manual of ocular diagnosis and therapy. 3rd ed. Boston: Little, Brown, 1991:31-46.
10. Fedukowixz HG. External infections of the eye. New York: Appleton-Century-Crofts, 1978:117.
11. Galloway NR. Common eye diseases and their management. Berlin: Springer-Verlag, 1985:44.
12. Grove AS Jr. Eyelids and lacrimal system. In: Pavan-Langston D, ed. Manual of ocular diagnosis and therapy. 3rd ed. Boston: Little, Brown, 1991:47-56.
13. Nelson ME, Midgley G, Blatchford NR. Ketoconazole in the treatment of blepharitis. Eye 4:151-59, 1990.
14. Hyndiuk RA, Burd EM, Hartz A. Efficacy and safety of mercuric oxide in the treatment of bacterial blepharitis. Antimicrob Agents Chemother 34:610-13, 1990.
15. Mars S, Keightley S. The aging eye. Practitioner 233:1560-64, 1989.
16. Pavan-Langston D, Foulks GN. Cornea and external disease. In: Pavan-Langston D, ed. Manual of ocular diagnosis and therapy. 3rd ed. Boston: Little, Brown, 1991:67-124.
17. Bankes JLK. Clinical ophthalmology. Edinburgh: Churchill Livingstone, 1982:33.
18. Berkow R, Fletcher AJ, eds. The Merck manual of diagnosis and therapy. 15th ed. Rahway, NJ: Merck & Co, 1987:Chap 18.
19. Fox J. Conjunctivitis, keratitis and iritis. Nursing 3(45):20-3, 1989.
20. Leibowitz HM. Antibacterial effectiveness of ciprofloxacin 0.3% ophthalmic solution in the treatment of bacterial conjunctivitis. Am J Ophthalmol 112:295-335, 1991.
21. Allansmith MR. The eye and immunology. St. Louis: CV Mosby, 1982:113.
22. Holderness M, Straughan JL, eds. South African medicines formulary. 2nd ed. Cape Town, South Africa: Medical Association of South Africa, 1991:416.
23. Fahy G, Easty DL, Collum L, Lumbroso P, Ober M, Verin P, Mackie I, Verstappen A. Double masked efficacy and safety evaluation of

lodoxamide 0.1% ophthalmic solution versus opticrom 2%: a multicentre study. Ophthalmology Today 341-42, 1988.

24. Leibowitz HM. Clinical evaluation of ciprofloxacin 0.3% ophthalmic solution for treatment of bacterial keratitis. Am J Ophthalmol 112:345-475, 1991.

25. Ciprandi G, Cerqueti PM, Sacca S, Cilli P, Canonica GW. Levocabastine versus cromolyn sodium in the treatment of pollen-induced conjunctivitis. Ann Allergy 65(2):156–58, 1990.

26. Davies BH, Mullins J. Levocabastine eye drops in the treatment of seasonal allergic conjunctivitis under high- and low-pollen conditions: parallel double-blind comparison with placebo and sodium cromoglycate. Allergy 48:519-24, 1993.

27. Klopfer J. Effects of environmental air pollution on the eye. J Am Optometric Assoc 60(10):773-78, 1989.

28. Miller A, Harel D, Laor A, Lahat N. Cimetidine as an immunomodulator in the treatment of herpes zoster. J Neuroimmunol 22(1):69-76, 1989.

29. Pavan-Langston D. Uveal tract: iris, ciliary body, and choroid. In: Pavan-Langston D, ed. Manual of ocular diagnosis and therapy. 3rd ed. Boston: Little, Brown, 1991:173-218.

CHAPTER 47

COMMON EAR DISEASES

MICHAEL A. OSZKO and RICHARD D. LEFF

The ear is a complex structure consisting of bone and cartilage, sensory and nervous tissue, and fluid. In addition to facilitating the sense of hearing, the structures of the ear are intimately involved in the maintenance of balance and equilibrium.

Because of its anatomic complexity, there are a wide range of conditions that can alter normal ear function. This chapter describes four of the most common disease states that are likely to be encountered by the pharmacist: (1) otitis media, (2) otitis externa, (3) vertigo, and (4) tinnitus.

ANATOMY OF THE EAR

The ear can be divided anatomically into three sections: the outer (or external), middle, and inner (or internal) ear (Figure 47.1). The external ear consists of two structures: the auricle and the external auditory canal. The purpose of these structures is to collect and transmit sound waves to the middle ear.

The middle ear consists of the tympanic membrane (ear drum) and an air-filled tympanic cavity that houses three tiny bones known collectively as ossicles (Figure 47.1). Incoming sound waves cause the tympanic membrane to vibrate. The first of the ossicles, the malleus, is attached at one end to the tympanic membrane and at the other to the second bone in the series, the incus. The incus, in turn, is attached to the third bone, the stapes, which sits against a membrane-covered aperture known as the oval window. The ossicles are designed so that the vibrations received from the tympanic membrane are amplified and transmitted to the sensory receptors located in the inner ear.

The middle ear is a relatively closed system, with a pressure approximately equal to atmospheric pressure. Pressure in the middle ear is maintained by the eustachian tube, which connects the tympanic cavity with the nasopharynx.

The inner ear consists of a complex series of canals containing two fluids known as endolymph and perilymph. These canals include the cochlea, which is involved with hearing, and the labyrinth, which is involved with maintaining equilibrium (Figure 47.1). The movement of endolymph in the cochlea, which is caused by vibrations received from the middle ear, results in displacement of tiny hairs projecting from specialized sensory cells. Such displacement transmits impulses to the cochlear (auditory)

branch of the vestibulocochlear nerve (also known as the eighth cranial nerve).

Another series of fluid-filled canals in the inner ear (the labyrinth) functions to maintain balance. Movement of the head results in movement of endolymph in these canals. Like the movement of endolymph in the cochlea, movement of tiny hairs projecting from specialized vestibular sensory cells transmits impulses to the vestibular branch of the vestibulocochlear nerve.

COMMON EAR DISORDERS

Otitis Media

Inflammation of the middle ear, otitis media, is one of the most frequent infectious diseases seen in pediatric patients. As many as 80% of children have had at least one episode by the time they are 3 years old (1). In the United States, otitis media is responsible for at least one in eight visits to office-based pediatricians (2) and accounts for 25 to 30 million prescriptions for oral antibiotics and more than $3.5 billion annually in direct and indirect health care costs (3, 4).

The term *otitis media* commonly denotes an inflammation of the middle ear. It can be more precisely described by its duration, presence or absence of infection, and presence or absence of an effusion (5). Acute suppurative otitis media refers to a clinically identifiable infection of the middle ear in which the symptoms appear suddenly (over several hours) and resolve completely within 3 weeks. If the inflammatory process persists for more than 3 weeks but less than 3 months, it is termed subacute. A middle ear discharge that persists for more than 3 months is termed chronic otitis media. If middle ear inflammation occurs in the absence of an identifiable infectious etiology, it is considered to be nonsuppurative.

Otitis media is frequently associated with an effusion in the tympanic cavity. Secretory otitis media (also known as otitis media with effusion) is the term used if the effusion is located behind an intact tympanic membrane. The effusion may be further characterized as bloody, serous (i.e., serumlike, thin), mucoid (mucuslike, thick), or purulent (puslike). A patient with secretory otitis media may be either symptomatic or asymptomatic.

Myringitis refers to an inflammation of the tympanic membrane and is not necessarily indicative of the presence of otitis media.

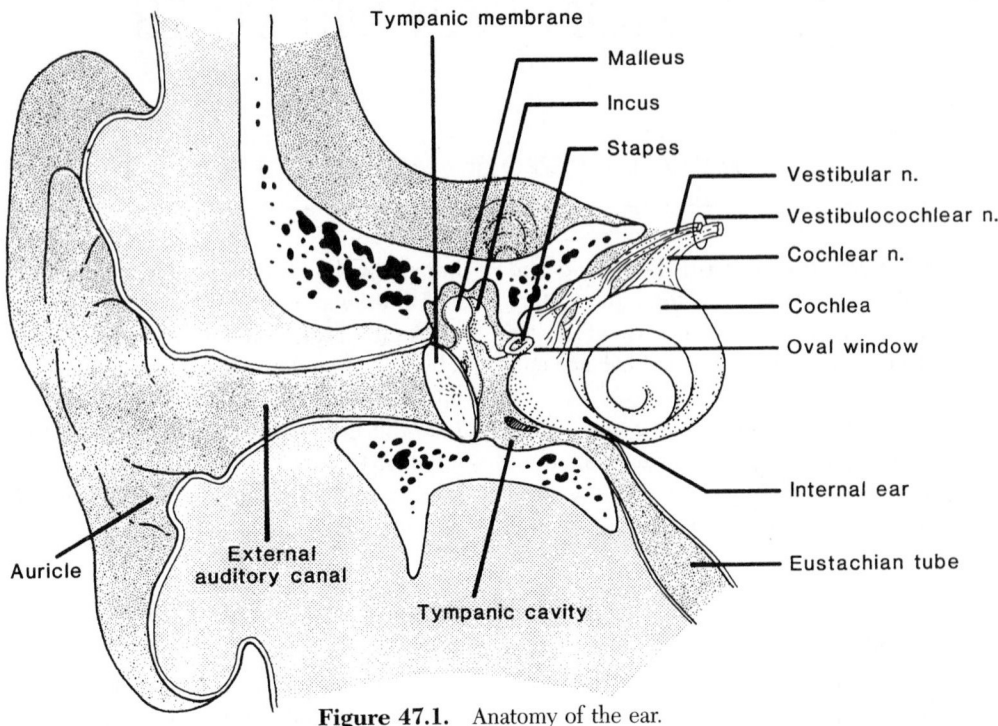

Figure 47.1.   Anatomy of the ear.

PATHOGENESIS

The pathogenesis of otitis media is not completely understood but is thought to be the result of two primary factors (6, 7): (1) eustachian tube dysfunction and (2) introduction of infectious material (i.e., viruses and/or bacteria) into the middle ear.

The eustachian tube equalizes the pressure between the tympanic cavity and the atmosphere. Cilia located in the eustachian tube continuously sweep mucus and debris toward the nasopharynx and away from the middle ear. Obstruction of the eustachian tube may result from either mucous membrane edema (secondary to allergy or an upper respiratory tract infection) or blockage by a foreign body, tumor, or lymphatic (e.g., adenoid) tissue. In addition, developmental differences between children and adults with respect to anatomic positioning, length, and functional patency of the eustachian tube may predispose children, but not adults, to eustachian tube dysfunction (7).

Once an obstruction occurs, a negative pressure (relative to the atmosphere) develops in the tympanic cavity. This negative pressure is caused by the absorption of gases through the epithelial lining of the eustachian tube and tympanic cavity. If the obstruction is suddenly relieved, nasopharyngeal mucus and bacteria may be insufflated into the tympanic cavity. Alternatively, a strong positive pressure originating in the nasopharynx (e.g., nose blowing) may also force nasopharyngeal contents into the middle ear.

Table 47.1.
Risk Factors for the Development of Otitis Media

First episode <18 months of age
Male gender
Previous episode of otitis media
Exposure to second-hand smoke
Sibling history of recurrent otitis media
Bottle feeding
Attendance at large day-care centers

Adapted from (1, 4).

The role of viruses in the pathogenesis of otitis media is becoming increasingly recognized. In one study, viruses were identified in 42% of patients with otitis media, with rhinoviruses and respiratory syncytial viruses most commonly detected (8). Moreover, viruses appear to be strongly associated with "failures" to antimicrobial therapy (9).

Other etiologic factors of otitis media include trauma, immunoglobulin deficiencies (particularly secretory IgA and IgG_2 (6, 10), human immunodeficiency virus infection, and, possibly, a genetic predisposition (11). A number of risk factors for otitis media have been identified (Table 47.1).

MICROBIOLOGY

Although viruses appear to play a concomitant role in the development of otitis media, the major etiologic pathogens are bacteria. In acute otitis media, the organisms most commonly isolated from the middle ear fluid are *Streptococcus pneumoniae, Hemophilus influenzae,* and *Moraxella catarrhalis* (formerly *Branhamella catarrhalis*) (12). These organisms commonly colonize the nasopharynx of young children, but are less frequently found in older children (13). In infants less than 6 weeks old, *Escherichia coli* and group B streptococci are common pathogens. Other less common organisms include staphylococci (both coagulase positive and negative), *Streptococcus pyogenes,* group A streptococci, other Gram-negative rods, *Chlamydia trachomatis,* and anaerobes. In chronic suppurative otitis media, the predominant organisms are staphylococci, *Pseudomonas,* and *Klebsiella* (14).

Up to 34% of *H. influenzae* and 90% of *M. catarrhalis* strains produce beta-lactamases (12). The prevalence of beta-lactamase-producing strains is highly variable and appears to depend on geographic location (15). Recently, resistant strains of *Streptococcus pneumoniae* (an organism that was once exquisitely sensitive to penicillins) are now appearing with increasing frequency in the United States (16).

SIGNS AND SYMPTOMS

The classical presentation of acute suppurative otitis media is that of an acute (within hours) onset of unilateral otalgia (ear pain), fever, and nasal discharge. Symptoms of otitis media displayed by neonates and small children include excessive fussiness, irritability, and/or tugging at the affected ear. Older children may complain of a sore throat and/or a sense of "fullness" or "pressure" in the ear. These symptoms may be associated with a decrease in hearing acuity. Seventy to 80% of patients with otitis media have a recent history of an upper respiratory tract infection, and approximately 50% have had a previous episode of otitis media (2). Less frequent symptoms include dizziness, lethargy, headache, anorexia (or reduced feeding in neonates), nausea, vomiting, diarrhea, and otorrhea.

DIAGNOSIS

The clinical diagnosis of otitis media is based largely on the patient's signs and symptoms. Otoscopic examination of the ear may reveal an erythematous tympanic membrane that is opaque or dull in appearance. The membrane is frequently bulging, and infrequently, it may be perforated and draining pus. Tympanometric testing of the eardrum may reveal reduced compliance, but its diagnostic usefulness is limited in that up to 25% of healthy children will have asymptomatic middle ear effusions (17).

Isolation of the causative organism may be accomplished by aspirating fluid from the middle ear (tympanocentesis). Unfortunately, cultures may be negative in one-third of patients with acute otitis media and two-thirds of patients with recurrent or secretory otitis media (18, 19). Although colonization of the nasopharynx by the responsible bacteria appears to be a prerequisite for infection of the middle ear (20), cultures of the nasopharynx are a poor predictor of the causative organism (21).

TREATMENT

Antibiotic Therapy. Despite the consensus that acute otitis media is primarily of bacterial etiology, there is disagreement on three issues: (1) whether or not this condition should be treated with oral antibiotics, (2) duration of antibiotic therapy, and (3) the endpoint by which antibiotic efficacy should be assessed. In most patients, the symptoms of acute otitis media resolve spontaneously without treatment within 24 to 72 hours with resolution of the effusion within 2 weeks. Thus, it has been suggested that antibiotic therapy should be reserved for those who do not improve within this time (22). Unfortunately, it is impossible to identify a priori patients who will not improve spontaneously, and antimicrobial therapy is generally recommended to reduce the risk of suppurative complications (23, 24).

Table 47.2.
Oral Antibiotics Used in the Treatment of Acute Otitis Media

Antibiotic	Pediatric Dose	Comments
Amoxicillin	40 mg/kg/day in 3 divided doses	
Amoxicillin/Potassium Clavulanate (Augmentin)	40 mg/kg/day in 3 divided doses	Dose based on amoxacillin content
Cefaclor (Ceclor)	40 mg/kg/day in 3 divided doses	
Cefixime (Suprax)	8 mg/kg/day in 1–2 divided doses	
Cefpodoxime proxetil (Vantin)	10 mg/kg/day in 2 divided doses	
Cefprozil (Cefzil)	30 mg/kg/day in 2 divided doses	
Cefuroxime axetil (Ceftin)	500 mg/d in 2 divided doses	
Erythromycin/Sulfisoxazole (Pediazole)	200 mg/kg/day in 4 divided doses	Dose based on erythromycin content
Loracarbef (Lorabid)	30 mg/kg/day in 2 divided doses	
Trimethoprim/Sulfamethoxazole (Bactrim, Septra)	8 mg/kg/day in 2 divided doses	Dose based on trimethoprim content

Adapted from (44).

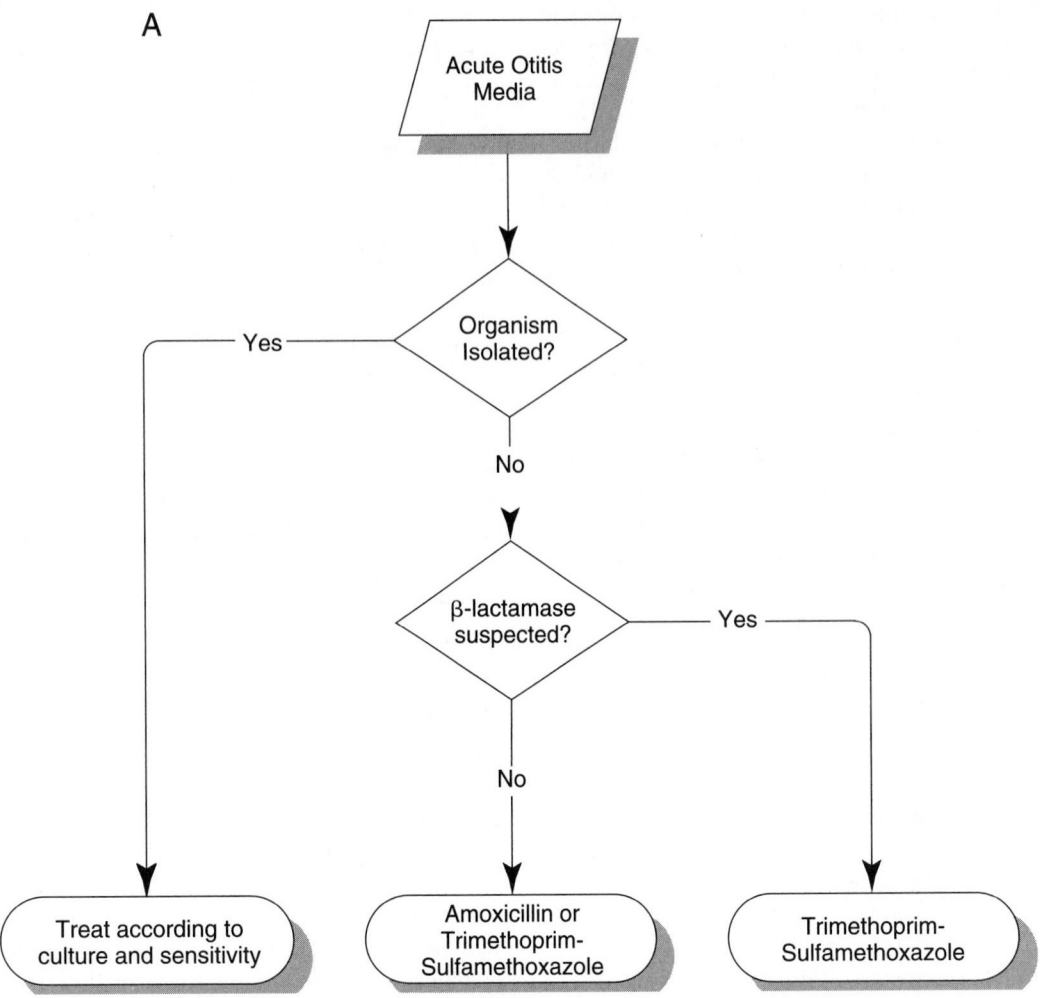

Figure 47.2. 2 Systematic approach to the treatment of otitis media: (A) Acute otitis media, (B) Recurrent otitis media with effusion.

Since, in most cases, the causative organism is not isolated prior to initiating treatment, the choice of antibiotic is based on its efficacy against the most common pathogens. Table 47.2 lists antibiotics that are commonly used to treat otitis media.

Figure 47.2 presents a systematic approach to treating acute otitis media. For most patients, oral amoxicillin is an appropriate first choice. It is effective against the most likely causative organisms, relatively free of serious side effects (rash and diarrhea are the most common), and inexpensive. If a patient is allergic to penicillin, either trimethoprim-sulfamethoxazole or erythromycin-sulfisoxazole is an effective alternative. Both of these contain a sulfonamide, but the incidence of side effects is low (less than 5%), and hematologic toxicity is rare (25).

Because both *H. influenzae* and *M. catarrhalis* are capable of producing beta-lactamases, an antibiotic that is stable against these enzymes should be considered if therapy with amoxicillin appears to be ineffective or if the prevalence of these organisms in a particular geographic

area is high. Amoxicillin combined with potassium clavulanate (a beta-lactamase inhibitor), second-or third-generation cephalosporins (cefaclor, cefixime, cefpodoxime, cefprozil, cefuroxime), trimethoprim-sulfamethisoxazole, and erythromycin-sulfisoxazole are equally effective. The use of broad-spectrum, beta-lactamase-stable antibiotics as initial empiric therapy is unwarranted since they do not improve efficacy rates or reduce the incidence of suppurative complications (26). Furthermore, the newer agents are considerably more expensive than amoxicillin or trimethoprim-sulfamethoxazole, and their broad spectrum contributes to the development of resistant strains of bacteria (27).

The usual length of antibiotic therapy in acute otitis media is 10 days. If the patient's clinical response is unsatisfactory, an additional course of therapy with another antibiotic may be tried. This is unnecessary in most patients. However, middle ear effusion will persist for several days to several months in a small number of patients. Shorter courses of therapy (2 to 5 days) appear to

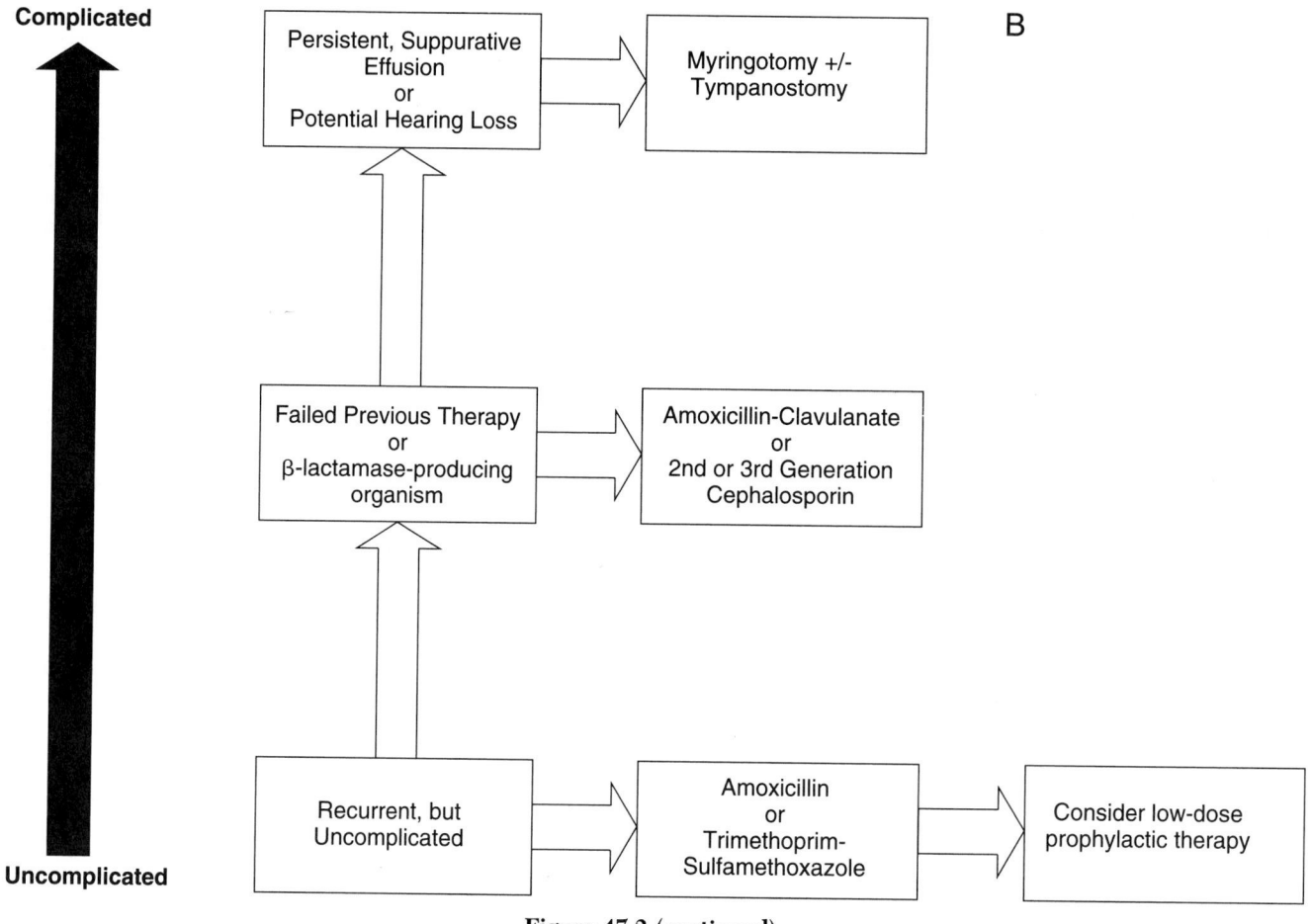

Figure 47.2 (continued).

be as effective as 7- to 10-day courses (28, 29). Recently, a single intramuscular dose of ceftriaxone was as effective as 10 days of oral amoxicillin in uncomplicated acute otitis media in children (30). However, because of potential limitations in the design of these studies and the small number of patients who were studied, further research is necessary before short courses of antibiotic therapy for acute otitis media can be recommended. Antibiotic therapy for otitis media with effusion appears to provide short-term improvement, but long-term benefits have not been shown (31).

Many children experience several episodes of otitis media during their childhood. Recurrent otitis media is defined as three episodes within a 6-month period or four episodes within a 12-month period. Because of the discomfort and the risk of suppurative complications that are associated with each episode, low-dose, prophylactic antibiotic therapy has been advocated and has been shown to be modestly effective (31). In patients with chronic suppurative otitis media, topical application of antibacterial agents (e.g., dilute acetic acid) or antibiotics may be used (14). Topical ciprofloxaxin appears to be effective, but it is

available only for opthalmic use, and its safety and efficacy have not been established. Recurrent episodes of otitis media despite prophylactic therapy necessitate surgical intervention (discussed later).

Adjunctive Therapy. In addition to antibiotics, decongestants, antihistamines, mucolytics, surfactants, immunoglobulins, and bacterial vaccines have been used to treat otitis media (10, 32, 33). None of these agents have been shown to improve the outcome of otitis media. Corticosteroids have been shown in some studies, but not in others, to positively improve the treatment of otitis media when used with antibiotics. However, relapse rates are high when the corticosteroid is discontinued, and the potential toxicities associated with corticosteroids outweigh any potential short-term benefit; their use in the treatment of otitis media is not recommended (34, 35)

If antibiotic therapy fails and otitis media becomes chronic or recurrent, it may be necessary to perform a myringotomy to place tympanostomy tubes. This allows the effusion to drain and the middle ear to be ventilated. This procedure is invasive (often requiring general anesthesia) and is associated with a number of complications (10).

PROGNOSIS

For most children, otitis media is a self-limiting condition that does not recur once adolescence is reached. In a small number of patients, however, otitis media becomes chronic. Intracranial (e.g., meningitis) or extracranial (e.g., labyrinthitis or chronic hearing loss) are rare but potentially serious complications of otitis media (6).

Otitis Externa

Otitis externa is an infectious condition of the external ear canal. Although it may be associated with chronic otitis media, it is more frequently an independent condition that affects patients of all ages. It is characterized by pain, swelling, maceration, and breakdown of the skin and subcutaneous tissues of the external ear canal. Two conditions produce an environment that is favorable for the development of otitis externa: (1) the introduction of a sharp object (e.g., toothpick, hairpin) into the external auditory canal, which disrupts the integrity of the lining of the canal and permits the growth of bacteria or fungi, and (2) the introduction and accumulation of moisture in the canal. Moisture not only softens the lining of the canal but also provides a medium for the growth of bacteria or fungi. Otitis externa commonly occurs when the ear is frequently exposed to water (e.g., swimming) and for this reason is sometimes referred to as "swimmer's ear."

The two most common organisms that are isolated in otitis externa are *Pseudomonas aeruginosa* and *Staphylococcus aureus*. Together, these bacteria account for three-fourths of the organisms that are isolated (36). Fungi, primarily *Aspergillus* and *Candida*, are found in about 10% of cases. Normally, the focus of infection is limited to the external ear. However, it can spread to the surrounding soft tissue or bone. Signs and symptoms of otitis externa include pain, itching, edema, and "weeping" of the ear canal.

TREATMENT

The goal of treatment of otitis externa is to produce an environment in the external ear canal that promotes healing of the inflamed, infected tissue. This includes drying the ear canal and treating the infection. Table 47.3 lists those drugs commonly found in otic preparations used to treat otitis externa.

Antibiotics. Although antibiotics are found in many otic preparations, they may cause contact dermatitis, permit the overgrowth of resistant organisms (including fungi), and result in local (e.g., neomycin) or systemic (e.g., chloramphenicol) toxicities; they are generally not recommended (37). Topical ciprofloxacin has been used to treat otitis externa, but it is available in the United States only as an ophthalmic solution. Until its safety and efficacy have been established, its use is not recommended (38). Oral antibiotics are indicated only if the infection has spread to the surrounding soft tissue. In malignant otitis externa (discussed later), parenteral antibiotics may be necessary.

Other Agents. Corticosteroids possess antiinflammatory, antipruritic, and vasoconstrictive activity and, when applied topically, may be useful in reducing swelling and inflammation in the external ear canal. A few drops of isopropyl alcohol 70% can serve as an excellent drying agent, but it should be used sparingly to prevent excessive drying and subsequent pruritus.

Administration of Otic Drops. In treating otitis externa, three to four drops of the desired solution should be instilled into the ear canal four times daily. To prevent the solution from escaping from the ear canal, the otic drops may be placed on a cotton or gauze wick, which is then inserted into the ear canal and left in place. In addition to keeping the solution in contact with the affected tissues, the wick prevents occlusion of the ear canal due to swelling.

With proper attention to aural hygiene, most cases of otitis externa will resolve in 5 to 7 days. In a small number of patients, the condition becomes chronic and is characterized by dry, scaly, sometimes weeping skin covering the auricle and external ear canal. Again, meticulous aural hygiene, combined with the application of a topical steroid cream (e.g., hydrocortisone) three to four times daily, will manage the patient's symptoms.

Table 47.3.
Selected Otic Preparations for the Treatment of Otitis Externa

Drug Product	Antibiotic	Antibacterial, Antifungal	Corticosteroid	Analgesic	Local Anesthetic
Auralgan Otic				Antipyrine 5.4%	Benzocaine 1.4%
Colymycin S Otic	Neomycin SO$_4$ 3.3 mg/ml, Colistin SO$_4$3 mg/ml		Hydrocortisone 1%		
Cortisporin Otic	Neomycin SO$_4$5 mg/ml, Polymyxin B SO$_4$ 100KU/ml		Hydrocortisone 1%		
Otic Tridesilon		Acetic acid 2%	Desonide 0.05%		
Tympagesic[a]				Antipyrine 5%	Benzocaine 5%
Vosol HC Otic	Acetic acid 2%	Hydrocortisone 1%			

[a]Also contains phenylephrine 0.25%.

Malignant Otitis Externa. Rarely, the superficial infection will spread to the underlying soft tissues and bone. Malignant otitis externa is a potentially life-threatening condition caused by *Pseudomonas aeruginosa*, predominantly in patients with underlying diseases (e.g., diabetes mellitus) (39, 40).

Patients with this condition are usually hospitalized and treated with parenteral antipseudomonal penicillins (e.g., piperacillin), cephalosporins (e.g., ceftazidime), aminoglycosides, or fluoroquinolones (e.g., ciprofloxacin) (39, 40).

Vertigo

Most people have experienced dizziness at some point in their lives. Four classes of conditions have been associated with dizziness: vertigo, syncope, gait disturbances, and miscellaneous head sensations. Vertigo is the most common of these.

Vertigo is the sensation of head motion when, in fact, there is none. This is an important point since other conditions in which the head is moving (e.g., motion sickness) can produce sensations that are similar to vertigo. In most patients, vertigo is the result of vestibular dysfunction (peripheral vertigo), though it may also be due to disease of the central nervous system (central vertigo). The type of spinning sensation experienced by the patient may also be used to classify vertigo. In objective vertigo, the environment appears to be spinning about the patient, whereas in subjective vertigo, the patient himself or herself appears to be turning in place. Vertigo may also be caused by cochlear dysfunction (e.g., Menière's disease), viruses, labyrinth abnormalities, and drugs (e.g., aminoglycosides, loop diuretics) (41).

DIAGNOSIS

The subjective nature of dizziness makes it difficult to diagnose vertigo. Vertigo is often diagnosed without a clear etiology because of the inaccessibility of the inner ear structures to examination. Thus, a careful history is essential to rule out unrelated conditions (e.g., orthostatic hypotension, gait disturbances).

The most objective sign of vertigo obtained on physical examination is nystagmus. Whether nystagmus is spontaneous or positional can provide important clues to the etiology of vertigo (42).

Caloric stimulation is used to test vestibular function. In this procedure, irrigation of the ear canal with cold or warm water will induce vertigo and nystagmus in patients with normal vestibular function. An abnormal response (i.e., the inability to induce vertigo) to caloric stimulation can be helpful in establishing an etiology. Other tests include audiometry, electronystagmography, and radiologic or magnetic resonance imaging of the affected structures (42).

TREATMENT

The treatment of vertigo involves both pharmacologic and nonpharmacologic therapy. Unfortunately, no drugs are specific for treating vertigo although a wide variety of drugs (ranging from anxiolytics to vasodilators) have been tried (43). Table 47.4 lists those drugs that are commonly used to manage the symptoms associated with vertigo. All these drugs can produce significant adverse effects that may outweigh the clinical benefits; therefore, careful patient monitoring is recommended.

Tinnitus

Tinnitus is an unnatural, often bothersome, noise that appears to originate from within the ears themselves. Although it is commonly described as a "ringing" in the ears, the noise may also be hissing, blowing, roaring, screaming, or clicking; the tone may be either high or low pitched. Though nearly everyone has experienced tinnitus at some point in his or her life, it is a chronic problem for 36 million people in the United States, one-fourth of whom suffer from severe symptoms (45). Tinnitus may precede or

Table 47.4.
Drugs Used to Treat Vertigo

Drug Class	Drug	Adult Dose[a]
Antimuscarinic	Scopolamine	Topical: 1 patch (0.5 mg) q 72 hr
H₁ antagonists	Cyclizine	50 mg q 4–6 hr
	Meclizine	12.5–25 mg tid–qid
	Dimenhydrinate	50–100 mg q 4–6 hr
Phenothiazines	Promethazine	25 mg q 8–12 hr
Antiemetics	Trimethobenzamide	Oral: 250 mg tid–qid Rectal: 200 mg tid–qid

[a]Oral route of administration unless otherwise specified.

Table 47.5.
Drugs That Can Cause Tinnitus

Antibiotics
  Aminoglycosides
  Erythromycin
  Minocycline
  Vancomycin
Antimalarial agents
  Chloroquine
  Quinine
Antineoplastic agents
  Cisplatin
Loop diuretics
  Bumetanide
  Ethacrynic acid
  Furosemide
Nonsteroidal antiinflammatory drugs
Salicylates
Tricyclic antidepressants

exist concomitantly with hearing loss and can mask an underlying hearing disorder. The precise etiology of tinnitus is unknown, but it has been associated with numerous vascular, mechanical, metabolic, neurologic, pharmacologic, dental, and psychologic conditions (45).

A number of medications are capable of causing tinnitus with or without hearing loss. The most commonly implicated agents are listed in Table 47.5. Drug therapy has been identified by 10% of patients as the cause of tinnitus (45). High serum concentrations of drugs are most frequently associated with the development of tinnitus although duration of therapy, rate of administration, concomitant administration of other ototoxic drugs, and preexisting medical conditions (e.g., dehydration, renal failure) may also be important (45–48).

In most cases, tinnitus and any associated hearing loss may be reversed by discontinuing the suspected drug or reducing its dose. In a small number of cases, permanent impairment of hearing occurs. In patients suffering from tinnitus that is not due to drugs, pharmacologic treatment using drugs like lidocaine and carbamazepine has been largely unsuccessful, and the long-term toxicities of the drugs outweigh any short-term benefit.

CONCLUSION

Four common ear disorders are frequently encountered by the pharmacist: otitis media, otitis externa, vertigo, and tinnitus. Advancements in our understanding of the pathophysiology and treatment strategies of these diseases will require continual reassessment of the drugs used to treat these disorders.

REFERENCES

1. Teele DW, Klein JO, Rosner B, et al. Epidemiology of otitis media during the first seven years of life in children in greater Boston: A prospective cohort study. J Infect Dis 160:83–94, 1989.
2. Froom J, Culpepper L, Grob P, et al. Diagnosis and antibiotic treatment of acute otitis media: report from the International Primary Care Network. Br Med J 300:582–586, 1990.
3. Bluestone CD. Management of otitis media in infants and children: current role of old and new antimicrobial agents. Pediatr Infect Dis J 7:S129–S136, 1988.
4. Stool SE, Field MJ. The impact of otitis media. Pediatr Infect Dis J 1989; 8:S11–S14.
5. Klein JO, Tos M, Hussl B, et al. Recent advanced in otitis media: definition and classification. Ann Otol Rhinol Laryngol 139(suppl):10, 1989.
6. Lisby-Sutch SM, Nemec-Dwyer MA, Deeter RG, Gaur SM. Therapy of otitis media. Clin Pharm 9:15–34, 1990.
7. Bluestone CD, Ostfeld EJ, Bakaletz LO, et al. Eustachian tube and middle ear physiology and pathophysiology. In: Recent advances in otitis media: Report of the fifth research conference. Ann Otol Rhinol Laryngol 103(suppl 164):13–19, 1994.
8. Arola M, Ruuskanen O, Ziegler T, et al. Clinical role of respiratory virus infection in acute otitis media. Pediatrics 86:848–855, 1990.
9. Chonmaitree T, Owen MJ, Howie VM. Respiratory viruses interfere with bacteriologic response to antibiotic in children with acute otitis media. J Infect Dis 162:546–549, 1990.
10. Kemp ED. Otitis media. Prim Care 17:267–287, 1990.
11. Klein JO, Tos M, Casselbrant ML. Epidemiology and natural history. In: Recent advances in otitis media: Report of the fifth research conference. Ann Otol Rhinol Laryngol 103(suppl 164):9–12, 1994.
12. Stephenson JS, Martin D, Kardatzke D, Bluestone CD. Prevalence of bacteria in middle ear effusion for the 80's. In: Lim DJ, Bluestone CD, Klein JO, et al., eds: Recent Advances in Otitis Media. Proceedings of the Fifth International Symposium. Hamilton, Canada:Decker Periodicals, 1993; 389–392.
13. Stenfors LE, Räisänen S. Occurrence of middle ear pathogens in the nasopharynx of young individuals: a quantitative study in four age groups. Acta Otolaryngol 109:142–148, 1990.
14. Wintermeyer SM, Nahata MC. Chronic suppurative otitis media. Ann Pharmacotherapy 28:1089–1099, 1994.
15. Marchant CD. Spectrum of disease due to *Branhamella catarrhalis* in children with particular reference to acute otitis media. Am J Med 88(Suppl 5A):15S–19S, 1990.
16. Friedland IR, McCracken GH. Management of infections caused by antibiotic-resistant *Streptococcus pneumoniae*. N Engl J Med 331: 377–382, 1994.
17. Klein JO. Persistant middle ear effusions: Natural history and morbidity. Pediatr Infect Dis J 1:S1–S11, 1982.
18. Qvarnberg Y, Kantola O, Valtonen H, et al. Bacterial findings in middle ear effusion in children. Otolaryngol Head Neck Surg 102:118–121, 1990.
19. Karma P: Secretory otitis media. infectious background and its implications for treatment. Acta Otolaryngol 449(Suppl):47–48, 1988.
20. Ogra PL, Barenkamp SJ, Mogi, et al. Microbiology, immunology, biochemistry, vaccination. In: Recent advances in otitis media: Report of the fifth research conference. Ann Otol Rhinol Laryngol 103(suppl 164):27–43, 1994.
21. Groothuis JR, Thompson J, Wright PF. Correlation of nasopharyngeal and conjunctival cultures with middle ear fluid cultures in otitis media. Clin Pediatr 25:85–88, 1986.
22. Browning GG. Childhood otalgia: acute otitis media—antibiotics not necessary in most cases. Br Med J 300:1005–1006, 1990.
23. Bain J. Childhood otalgia: acute otitis media—justification for antibiotic use in general practice. Br Med J 300:1006–1007, 1990.
24. Hamrick HJ, Garfunkel JM. Therapy for acute otitis media: applicability of metaanalysis to the individual patient. J Pediatr 124:431, 1994.
25. Cunningham MJ. Chemoprophylaxis with oral trimethoprim-sulfamethoxazolein otitis media. Clin Pediatr 29:273–277, 1990.
26. Rosenfeld RM, Vertrees JE, Carr J, et al. Clinical efficacy of antimicrobial drugs for acute otitis media: Metaanalysis of 5400 children from thirty-three randomized trials. J Pediatr 124:355–367, 1994.
27. Jacoby GA, Archer GL. New mechanisms of bacterial resistance to antimicrobial agents. N Engl J Med 324:601–612, 1994.
28. Bain J, Murphy E, Ross F. Acute otitis media: clinical course among children who received a short course of high dose antibiotic. Br Med J 291:1243–1246, 1985.
29. Hendrickse WA, Kusmiesz, Shelton S, Nelson JD. Five vs. ten days of therapy for acute otitis media. Pediatr Infect Dis J 7:14–23, 1988.
30. Green SM, Rothrock SG. Single-dose intramuscular ceftriaxone for acute otitis media in children. Pediatrics 91:23–30, 1993.
31. Williams RL, Chalmers TC, Stange KC, et al. Use of antibiotics in preventing recurrent otitis media and in treating otitis media with effusion: A meta-analytic attempt to resolve the brouhaha. JAMA 270:1344–1351, 1993.
32. Mandel EM, Rockette HE, Bluestone CD, et al. Efficacy of amoxicillin with and without decongestant-antihistamine for otitis media in children. N Engl J Med 316:432–437, 1987.
33. Jørgensen F, Andersson B, Hanson LÅ, et al. Gamma globulin treatment of recurrent otitis media in children. Pediatr Infect Dis J 9:389–394, 1990.

34. Parparella MM, Schachern P. New developments in treating otitis media. Ann Otol Rhinol Laryngol 103:7–10, 1994.

35. Agency for Health Care Policy and Research. Otitis media with effusion in young children. AHCPR Publication No. 94-0620, 1994.

36. Farmer HS. A guide for the treatment of external otitis. Am Fam Physician 21(6):96–101, 1980.

37. Rutks J, Alberti PW. Toxic and drug-induced drug disorders in otolaryngology. Otolaryngol Clin North Am 17:761–774, 1984.

38. Årnes E, Dibb WL. Otitis externa: clinical comparison of local ciprofloxacin versus local oxytetracycline, polymyxin B, hydrocortisone combination treatment. Curr Med Res Opin 13:182–186, 1993.

39. Rubin J, Yu VL. Malignant external otitis: insights into pathogenesis, clinical manifestations, diagnosis, and therapy. Am J Med 85:391–398, 1988.

40. Giamarellou H. Malignant otitis externa: the therapeutic evolution of a lethal infection. J Antimicrob Chemother 30:745–751, 1992.

41. Huy PTB. Pathophysiology of peripheral non-Meniere's vestibular disorders. Ann Otolaryngol (Stockh) Suppl. 513, pp. 5–10, 1994.

42. Barker LR, Moses H, Rothman W. Dizziness, vertigo, motion sickness, near syncope, syncope, and disequilibrium. In: Barker LR, Burton JR, Zieve PD. eds. Principles of Ambulatory Medicine. ed. 2. Baltimore, Williams & Wilkins, 1986, pp.1153–1163.

43. Timmerman H. Pharmacotherapy of vertigo: any news to be expected? Ann Otolaryngol (Stockh) Suppl. 513, pp. 28–32, 1994.

44. Sanford JP, Gilbert DN, Gerberding JL, Dande MA. Guide to Antimicrobial Therapy. 1994; Dallas: Antimicrobial Therapy, Inc.

45. Schleuning AJ. Management of the patient with tinnitus. Med Clin North Am 75:1225–1237, 1991.

46. Ryback LP. Drug ototoxicity. Ann Rev Pharmacol Toxicol 26:79–99, 1986.

47. Norris CH. Drugs affecting the inner ear: A review of their clinical efficacy, mechanisms of action, toxicity, and place in therapy. Drugs 36:754–772, 1988.

48. Miller JJ. Handbook of Ototoxicity, CRC Press, Boca Raton, 1985.

CHAPTER 48

GLAUCOMA

DICK R. GOURLEY and CONSTANCE McKENZIE

Glaucoma is a disease of the eye that is characterized by an increase in intraocular pressure (IOP). More than 2 million Americans have glaucoma (one-half of whom are undiagnosed), and approximately 80,000 of them have varying degrees of blindness caused by damage to the optic disk and visual field loss. There may be as many as 10 million Americans who have elevated IOP without clinical signs and symptoms. Glaucoma is the leading cause of legal blindness in the United States. Glaucoma usually manifests itself after age 35, but can occur in younger people as well. Two percent of the population over 40 years of age and 5 to 9% over 65 years of age suffer from glaucoma. The older the patient, the greater the need for evaluation for glaucoma (1, 2). Patients with glaucoma are at a high risk of not adhering to drug therapy regimens. It is estimated that 43% of diagnosed and treated patients do not adhere to drug therapy regimens (3).

Glaucoma is insidious in onset and often produces only minor symptoms of discomfort, such as headache or "tired eyes." Many patients do not seek medical attention until the disorder is well established because of this lack of symptoms. Some patients have a very high IOP but still have no symptoms. Fortunately, optic nerve and retinal damage are late findings of end-stage disease. Symptoms such as persistent headache and eye pain usually cause patients to seek medical assistance before these serious consequences develop (4).

PATHOGENESIS

IOP is physiologically determined by the relative production and elimination of aqueous humor. Increased IOP can result from either increased production of aqueous humor, decreased elimination, or both. The major cause of increased IOP is decreased elimination.

There are more than 40 different types of glaucoma (Table 48.1), but the two major types of glaucoma are angle closure and open angle. The more acute type is angle-closure glaucoma. It occurs in only 5 to 10% of all cases, compared to 90% for open angle. Both types can be further classified into primary and secondary glaucoma. A third type is congenital glaucoma, which results from developmental ocular abnormalities and occurs in less than 2% of cases.

The familial relationship of glaucoma has been well established; whether the hereditary pattern is one consistent with a dominant or recessive autosomal trait remains

equivocal. Patients with a familial history of glaucoma should have routine yearly eye examinations because of this increased risk. Although there are more males with primary open-angle glaucoma, sex predilections for the disease are not clinically apparent. Primary open-angle glaucoma is relatively more common in Caucasians and blacks than in American Indians and Asians. Although many patients may have unilateral involvement initially, it can be anticipated that the other eye will become involved within 5 years. Myopia may be a high-risk factor for glaucoma especially in younger patients (2, 4, 5). A summary of risk factors associated with an increase in probability of primary glaucoma is listed in Table 48.2.

PATHOPHYSIOLOGY

Anatomic factors associated with acute angle-closure glaucoma include small hyperopic (farsighted) eyes, tautness of the iris and large pupils, anterior lens dislocations, swollen hypermature lens, and posterior or anterior synechiae (fibrous scars).

Farsighted individuals are particularly at risk for angle closure since the tissues of their eyeballs are relatively compacted and the lens is shifted anteriorly. In individuals with a lack of tautness of the iris diaphragm (usually in large pupils), a bulging iris (bombe) may occur because of increased iridotrabecular contact.

Two conditions that lead to anterior lens dislocation are ocular trauma or a severe blow to the eye, both of which may lead to pupillary blockage or direct obstruction of the angle. Similarly, a swollen lens, as in inflammatory conditions (uveitis), produces pupillary blockage.

Posterior synechiae can form in the eyes of patients with uveitis and, if present in sufficient numbers, occlude the pupil. An increase in IOP may then result. Anterior synechiae can form after long-standing iritis and produce adhesion of the anterior portion of the iris to the trabecular meshwork. The outflow of aqueous humor is further obstructed, increasing IOP.

The damage from either type of glaucoma is primarily due to the inhibition of aqueous humor outflow. Aqueous humor formation occurs at a rapid rate (approximately 1 ml/min) and depends on several interacting mechanisms within the ciliary processes. Aqueous humor is secreted by the ciliary processes into the posterior chamber (Fig. 48.1), where it flows to the trabecular meshwork and finally out through the canal of Schlemm. Since a decrease in the

Table 48.1.
Classification of Glaucomas[a]

Primary glaucoma
  Primary open-angle glaucoma; synonyms: chronic open-angle glaucoma, chronic simple glaucoma, glaucoma simplex
  Low tension glaucoma
  Primary closed-angle glaucoma; synonyms: primary angle-closure glaucoma, narrow-angle glaucoma, iris-blocking glaucoma, acute congestive glaucoma
  Acute angle-closure glaucoma
  Chronic angle-closure (may also be secondary to other ocular diseases)
  Intermittent angle-closure glaucoma
  Superimposed on chronic open-angle glaucoma (combined mechanism)
Variants of primary glaucoma
  Pigmentary glaucoma
  Exfoliation glaucoma; synonyms: pseudoexfoliation of the lens capsule, glaucoma capsulare
Developmental glaucoma
  Primary congenital glaucoma
  Infantile glaucoma with associated defects such as Axenfeld's and Reiger's anomalies
  Glaucoma associated with hereditary or familial diseases such as aniridia, encephalotrigeminalhemangiomatosis (Sturge-Weber syndrome), neurofibromatosis, oculocerebrorenal (Lowe's) syndrome
Secondary glaucoma
  Inflammatory glaucoma
  Uveitis of all types
  Fuchs's heterochromic iridocyclitis
  Phacogenic glaucoma
  Angle-closure glaucoma with mature cataract
  Phacoanaphylactic glaucoma secondary to rupture of lens capsule
  Phacolytic glaucoma caused by phacotoxic meshwork blockage
  Subluxation of lens
  Glaucoma secondary to intraocular hemorrhage
  Hyphyema
  Hemolytic glaucoma (erthroclastic glaucoma)
  Traumatic glaucoma
  Traumatic recession of chamber angle
  Postsurgical glaucomas: aphakic pupillary block and ciliary block (malignant) glaucoma
  Neovascular glaucoma (especially in diabetic patients)
  Drug-induced glaucoma
    Corticosteroid-induced glaucoma
    Postoperative ocular hypertension from use of alpha-chymotrypsin
  Glaucomas of miscellaneous origin
    Associated with intraocular tumors; retinal detachments (rare); secondary to severe chemical burns of the eye associated with essential iris atrophy
Absolute glaucoma

[a] Reprinted with permission from Paton D, Craig JA. Glaucomas: diagnosis and management. Clin Symp 28:20, 1976.

outflow facility of aqueous humor is the primary mechanism for producing an increase in IOP, the anatomic changes in open-angle and angle-closure glaucoma are important (4, 5).

In open-angle glaucoma, a physical blockage occurs within the trabecular meshwork that retards elimination of aqueous humor. The obstruction is presumed to be between the trabecular sheet and the episcleral veins, into which the aqueous humor ultimately flows.

The impairment of aqueous drainage elevates the IOP to between 25 and 35 mm Hg (normal is 10 to 20 mm Hg), indicating that the obstruction is usually partial. This increase in IOP is sufficient to cause progressive cupping of the optic disk and eventually visual field defects. As the trabecular spaces become more involved, detachment of the cornea and formation of bullae may develop. Since visual acuity remains largely unaffected until late in the disease, scotomata must be regarded as a major indication for medical therapy.

In angle-closure glaucoma, increased IOP is caused by pupillary blockage of aqueous humor outflow and is more severe. The basic requirements leading to an acute attack of angle closure are a pupillary block, a narrowed anterior chamber angle, and a convex iris (iris bombe). The sequence of events leading to increased IOP is depicted in Figure 48.2. When a patient has a narrow anterior chamber (Fig. 48.2A) or a pupil that dilates to a degree where the iris comes in greater contact with the lens (Fig. 48.2B), there is interference with the flow of aqueous humor from the posterior to the anterior chamber. Since aqueous humor is continually secreted, pressure from within the posterior chamber forces the iris to bulge forward (Fig. 48.2C). This may progress to complete blockage (Fig. 48.2D).

The pathologic complications of angle-closure and open-angle glaucoma include the formation of cataracts, peripheral anterior synechiae, atrophy of the optic nerve and retina, and absolute glaucoma (complete blockage of aqueous outflow). The development of cataracts can increase existing pupillary block and the degree of angle closure.

Table 48.2.
Risk Factors Associated with Glaucoma

Age
Familial history
African ancestry
Sex
Hypertension
Diabetes mellitus
Vascular disease
Myopia

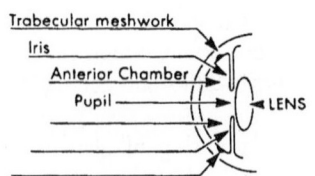

Figure 48.1. Normal eye anatomy.

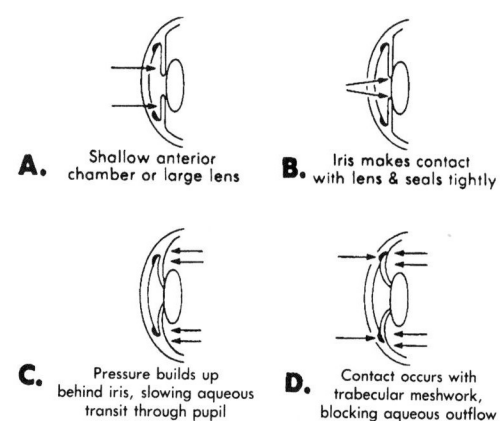

A. Shallow anterior chamber or large lens

B. Iris makes contact with lens & seals tightly

C. Pressure builds up behind iris, slowing aqueous transit through pupil

D. Contact occurs with trabecular meshwork, blocking aqueous outflow

Figure 48.2 Abnormal eye with development of pupillary block.

ETIOLOGY

Drugs that have autonomic effects produce several types of ocular changes. Of great importance is the effect of anticholinergic agents on angle-closure glaucoma. Several factors appear to be associated with drug-induced glaucoma (Table 48.3).

In addition to drugs, glaucoma can occur as a secondary manifestation of systemic disorders or trauma. A list of systemic diseases associated with increased IOP is shown in Table 48.4.

Congenital glaucoma is a rare disorder in which the IOP is increased as a result of developmental abnormalities of the ocular structures in the newborn. It may occur in association with other congenital abnormalities and anomalies such as homocystinuria and Marfan's syndrome. Congenital glaucoma should be considered in newborns who have sensitivity to light, excessive tearing, or spasm of the eyelids.

DIAGNOSIS AND CLINICAL FINDINGS

Open-Angle Glaucoma

The common signs of open-angle glaucoma may be minimal and do not appear immediately. As time progresses, the signs become more marked until they finally restrict vision. In some cases, there may be a total absence of signs. The common signs are increased IOP, visual field loss, optic disk changes, decreased outflow facility, gonioscopically open angles, and positive provocative tests (2, 4, 5).

An increased IOP can have several interpretations. Most normal individuals have pressures of 21 mm Hg or less. However, a small group of patients may sustain glaucomatous damage even with pressures under 20 mm Hg, "low tension glaucoma" (5, 6). In general, pressure readings in the high 20s are suspicious, and those above 30 are cause for serious concern. Patients between the ages of 50 and 75 with pressures above 30 mm Hg as the only sign

of glaucoma should be treated medically because decreased vascular perfusion in older people can endanger the optic nerve. The younger patient with similar readings may require assessment for changes in the optic disk or visual fields at less frequent intervals (2, 4, 5).

In the early stage of chronic open-angle glaucoma, symptoms of pain or visual field loss are usually not present (Table 48.5).

Angle-Closure Glaucoma

Acute angle-closure glaucoma usually presents with signs and symptoms of blurred vision (often with colored halos around light), severe ocular pain, and nausea with occasional vomiting. The eye appears red, the cornea is cloudy, the pupil is middilated, the anterior chamber is narrow, and the IOP is frequently above 50 mm Hg. Visual acuity is reduced by corneal changes or edema. Bullae may be present on the cornea if the acute attack is prolonged. Colored halos result from diffraction of light by the edematous cornea (4, 5).

Ocular pain may vary from moderate to severe. The oculovagal reflex is thought to produce the nausea,

Table 48.3.
Factors Implicated in Potential Drug-Induction of Angle-Closure Glaucoma

Age—usually over 30
History—familial, genetic basis
Race—usually Caucasian
Sex—usually female
Anterior chamber angle—shallow and narrow
Vision—hyperopia, hypermetropia
Convexity of the iris—flattened
Dose and duration of the offending drug used
Duration of effect on eye—longer duration
Route of administration—topical more than systemic

Table 48.4.
Systemic Conditions Associated with Glaucoma (Secondary)[a]

Congenital rubella
Diabetes mellitus
Down's syndrome
Hallerman–Streiff syndrome
Homocystinuria
Hypertension
Idiopathic infantile hypoglycemia
Lowe's syndrome
Marfan's syndrome
Melanoma (intraocular tumors)
Neurofibromatosis (von Recklinghausen's)
Turner's syndrome
Uveitis (secondary)

[a]Modified from Scheie HG, Edwards DL, Yanoff MC. Clinical and experimental observations using alpha chymotrypsin. Am J Ophthalmol 59:469, 1965.

Table 48.5.
Clinical Findings and Symptoms of Primary Glaucoma

Glaucoma	Onset	Early Findings and Symptoms	Late Findings and Symptoms
Open-angle	Insidious	Asymptomatic slight rise in IOP: decreased rate of aqueous humor outflow, optic disk changes (symptoms may be marginal or even at times absent)	Gradual loss of peripheral vision (over months–years); persistent elevation of IOP; optic nerve degenerations; retinal nerve atrophy; edema of the cornea; cataracts; trabecular meshwork degeneration
Angle-closure	Sudden	Blurred vision; severe ocular pain and congestion; conjunctival redness; cloudy cornea; moderately dilated pupil; poor pupil response to light; IOP markedly elevated; nausea and vomiting	Complete blindness in 2–5 days if not treated

Table 48.6.
Diagnostic Studies for Glaucoma

Procedures	Comments
Tonometry	Measures intraocular tension; routinely used for glaucoma should be considered; repeated readings should be done before definite diagnosis; between acute attacks of angle-closure glaucoma, the intraocular tension may be normal; applanation tonometry measures the force applied per unit area, whereas indentation tonometry uses a plunger to produce a pit in the cornea, which serves as a measure of intraocular pressure.
Gonioscopy	Differentiates the type of glaucoma; gonioscopic appearance of narrowed anterior chamber angle is usually diagnostic of angle-closure glaucoma.
Tonography	May reveal impaired facility of aqueous humor outflow; early open-angle glaucoma can be detected by this technique; tonometer is applied to the eye and the resultant reduction in the intraocular tension is measured as an indicator of outflow facility.
Water-drinking test	Rise in intraocular tension after rapid ingestion of a quart of water is significant indication of glaucoma; positive result occurs in 30% of open-angle glaucoma cases; negative result does not rule out glaucoma; tonography and water-drinking test will reveal open-angle glaucoma with 90% reliability.
Ophthalmoscopy	Glaucomatous excavation or cupping of the optic disk is found in chronic primary open-angle and congenital glaucomas; glaucomatous changes of optic disk and/or occlusion of the central retinal vein in absence of elevated intraocular tension should arouse suspicion of glaucoma in early stage.
Visual field examination	Isolated areas of impaired vision surrounded by normal areas in a visual field is indicative of open-angle glaucoma; visual field changes are irreversible; parallel optic disk changes.
Corticosteroid instillation	Striking differences in ocular tension between primary open-angle glaucoma patients and normal subjects are produced by topically instilled corticosteroids; steroid provocative test is used to evaluate genetic predisposition of glaucoma; response of primary angle-closure glaucoma to corticosteroid instillation is much more similar to normal subjects.
Dark room test	Intraocular tension is assessed in patient before and after being placed in a dark room; in chronic angle-closure glaucoma, a considerable rise in the intraocular tension is observed after being in the dark.

vomiting, bradycardia, and sweating that may accompany an acute attack. With very high IOPs, the pupil may become fixed in middilation and eventually damaged. In severe cases, the pupil changes from a round to an oval shape and may resist constriction by topical parasympathomimetic agents.

Chronic angle closure is a less severe form of glaucoma than acute angle closure; the symptoms may range from none to intermittent and severe ocular pain along with halo formation and ocular congestion. Synechiae do not form without ocular congestion, which may be evident only with a moderately high pressure reading.

Diagnostic Procedures

With both major types of glaucoma, several diagnostic procedures (Table 48.6) are available to IOP: evaluate visual field loss, optic disk changes, outflow facility, angle measurements, and provocative tests (1, 2, 4, 5).

DRUGS CONTRAINDICATED IN GLAUCOMA

Specific classes of drugs, such as anticholinergic, adrenergic, and corticosteroid, have been implicated in inducing glaucoma. Any drug with atropinelike side effects can produce pupillary dilation and paralysis of accommodation for near vision. Concern for this iatrogenic complication has prompted Food and Drug Administration (FDA) requirements for warnings on the systemic use of anticholinergics in the presence of glaucoma.

One must distinguish between open-angle and angle-closure glaucoma in arriving at a therapeutic decision about this warning because drug effects differ in the two cases. Drugs that dilate the pupil, for instance, may precipitate an acute attack of angle-closure glaucoma but usually do not produce harmful effects in open-angle cases. Dilation of the pupil in angle-closure glaucoma may cause the peripheral iris to bulge forward, blocking the trabecular meshwork. The aqueous humor is prevented from reaching the outflow channels, which results in an increased IOP. Since excessive resistance to outflow in open-angle glaucoma is caused primarily by changes within the trabecular outflow channels, dilation of the pupil usually will not exacerbate the IOP.

Topical administration of some drugs (Table 48.7) is known to elevate IOP in various patients with glaucoma, and it has been assumed that systemic administration of such medications will have a similar effect. In patients with mild or controlled open-angle glaucoma, it is unwarranted to prohibit the use of systemic sympathomimetic, anticholinergic, and other atropinelike drugs because the evidence that they exacerbate the condition is not well documented (4, 5).

Anticholinergics

In patients with normal eyes, topically instilled anticholinergics such as atropine, scopolamine, and cyclopentolate produce no significant elevation in IOP. However, in patients more than 30 years of age who have abnormally shallow anterior chambers, there is a risk of precipitating acute attacks of angle-closure glaucoma. The incidence has been estimated to be nearly 1 in 4000 (7). Atropine and

scopolamine have a profound effect on the eye because of their longer durations of action than other agents with anticholinergic effects (i.e., phenothiazine, tricyclic antidepressants, and antihistamines). These locally instilled agents cause mydriasis and cycloplegia that may persist for as long as 2 weeks. In some open-angle patients, they produce a slight rise of IOP (less than 6 mm Hg) when instilled into the eyes. Other mydriatics, however, do not appear to have this effect (8).

Conventional doses of atropine systemically administered for preanesthesia have little ocular effect; in contrast, equivalent therapeutic doses of scopolamine can cause definite pupillary dilation (9). Prolonged use of anticholinergics can exacerbate open-angle glaucoma to some extent, but studies have shown that oral atropine at a dose of 0.6 mg every 4 hours for 1 week produces only slight elevations of IOP (10). In another study, the administration of proprietary cold remedies containing 0.2 mg of belladonna alkaloids (given twice daily for 4 days) caused no changes in IOP in 27 normal volunteers and 37 patients with glaucoma (including 18 patients with chronic angle closure) (11).

Propantheline, a commonly used anticholinergic, produces no significant elevation in IOP in either normal or

Table 48.7.
Ability of Drugs to Induce Glaucoma

Drug	Route	Glaucoma Type	
		Open Angle	Angle Closure
Anticholinergics			
Atropine	Topical	Rare	Frequent
Scopolamine	Topical	Rare	Frequent
Belladonna	Topical	Rare	Frequent
Propantheline	Systemic	Rare	Rare
Adrenergics			
Phenylephrine 10%	Topical	Never	Occasional
Epinephrine	Systemic	Never	Rare
Miotics			
Pilocarpine 4–8%	Topical	Never	Occasional
Echothiophate	Topical	Never	Occasional
Isoflurophate	Topical	Never	Occasional
Carbonicanhydrase inhibitors			
Acetazolamide	Systemic	Never	Rare
Antihypertensives	Systemic	Never	Never
Beta-Chymotrypsin	Topical	Rare	Occasional
Prochlorperazine	Systemic	Never	Never
Promethazine (high doses)	Systemic	Never	Rare
Ganglionic blocking agents	Systemic	Rare	Occasional
Amphetamines	Systemic	Rare	Occasional
Tricyclic antidepressants	Systemic	Rare	Occasional
Corticosteroids (at equipotent doses)			
Betamethasone	Topical	Frequent	Never
Dexamethasone	Topical	Frequent	Never
Hydrocortisone	Topical	Occasional	Never
Prednisolone	Topical	Occasional	Never
Triamcinolone	Topical	Occasional	Never
Dexamethasone	Systemic	Occasional	Never
Hydrocortisone	Systemic	Occasional	Never
Prednisolone	Systemic	Occasional	Never

angle-closure patients. Anticholinergics, in fact, can deepen the anterior chamber by inhibiting the contraction of the ciliary body and produce cycloplegia, which widens rather than narrows the anterior chamber angle, making angle closure less likely to occur. No recent reports of exacerbations of glaucoma with diazepam or amitriptyline have appeared in the literature although the manufacturers of these drugs contraindicate their use in patients with this disorder. Very high doses of phenothiazines given for schizophrenia have produced slight elevations of IOP (6). Treatment with miotics easily overcame the effect.

In summary, withholding systemic anticholinergics for fear of inducing open-angle glaucoma is not justified. This is true especially with parenteral atropine or scopolamine given preoperatively prior to general anesthesia. Sensitivity of the eye to systemic drugs is relatively low (1, 6). Although these agents can induce angle-closure in rare instances, the concomitant use of parasympathomimetic miotics will prevent any of the IOP effects. However, ocularly instilled potent anticholinergics, such as atropine, scopolamine, cyclopentolate, and homatropine, should not be used in patients diagnosed with or predisposed to angle-closure glaucoma.

Sympathomimetics

Adrenergic agents commonly found in appetite suppressants, bronchodilators, central nervous stimulants, and vasoconstrictors produce slight pupillary dilation. No adverse effects on open-angle glaucoma have been reported. After systemic administration of these agents, the frequency of deleterious effects on angle-closure glaucoma has been extremely small (12). Adrenergic agents such as epinephrine and phenylephrine have been used ocularly to treat open-angle-glaucoma. These agents *will* elevate the IOP by narrowing the anterior chamber angle when instilled into the eyes of angle-closure patients (6).

General anesthetics producing parasympathetic and sympathetic imbalance may cause pupillary block. Topical pilocarpine 1% may be instilled into the eye prior to inducing anesthesia to prevent this complication (6).

Cardiovascular Drugs

There is no convincing evidence that vasodilators significantly aggravate glaucoma even though subconjunctival injection of strong vasodilators such as isoxsuprine and tolazoline can induce transient elevations in IOP, particularly in chronic open-angle glaucoma. Nitrates, nitrites, aminophylline, nylidirin, and cyclandelate can be used safely in glaucoma (6, 7). Antihypertensives will decrease intraocular blood flow, which can lead to loss of small visual fields in patients with a high IOP. Therefore, it is best to decrease blood pressure gradually in angle-closure patients. If it is necessary to decrease blood pressure rapidly,

one should either increase the patient's miotic medication or simultaneously lower the IOP rapidly with an agent such as acetazolamide.

Miscellaneous Agents

Amphetamines, tricyclic antidepressants, monamine oxidase inhibitors, indomethacin, and cocaine produce slight degrees of mydriasis, but the likelihood of inducing angle closure with these drugs is very low (6, 13). Strong miotics such as pilocarpine 4 to 8% and the indirect-acting nonreversible clolinesterase inhibitors may lead to pupillary block and inhibition of aqueous humor outflow and increase vascular congestion of the peripheral part of the iris so that the swollen iris blocks the canal of Schlemm and prevents the outflow of aqueous humor (6, 13, 14).

Polarizing neuromuscular blocking agents, such as succinylcholine, used as adjuvants to general anesthesia can cause a marked rise in IOP if the patient is not adequately anesthetized. They should not be used in glaucomatous patients. A nondepolarizing neuromuscular blocking agent, such as atracurium, is effective in preventing the rise in IOP.

An acute transient myopia has occurred following vaginal absorption of AVC cream, which contains sulfanilamide, complicated by retinal edema, shallowing anterior chambers, and acute angle closure (15). Similar reactions have occurred with carbonic anhydrase inhibitors (16), tetracycline (17), prochloperazine, and promethazine (18). A few of these may be responsible for ocular hypertension, but more commonly they increase retinal fluid production. These reactions can be classified as idiosyncratic phenomena.

Corticosteroid-Induced Glaucoma

Corticosteroid-induced glaucoma is well documented (6, 12, 19–24). This form of glaucoma is usually without pain, physical findings in the eye, or visual field defects. The lesion probably occurs in the trabecular meshwork and severely decreases the outflow facility. Systematically or topically administered corticosteroids produce decreased outflow facility accompanied by a corresponding increase of IOP. After topical therapy, the glaucomatous change occurs in the eye instilled with the drug. This ocular hypertensive effect is usually fully reversible within 1 month after the discontinuation of the steroid.

The increase in IOP is approximately 10 mm Hg for patients with preglaucomatous anterior chambers and 5 mm Hg in normal persons. In some cases, irreversible eye damage occurs if ocular tension persists for 1 to 2 months or even longer. In addition, cupping of the optic disk and defects of the visual field may develop a few months after topical administration of corticosteroids is begun. Patients

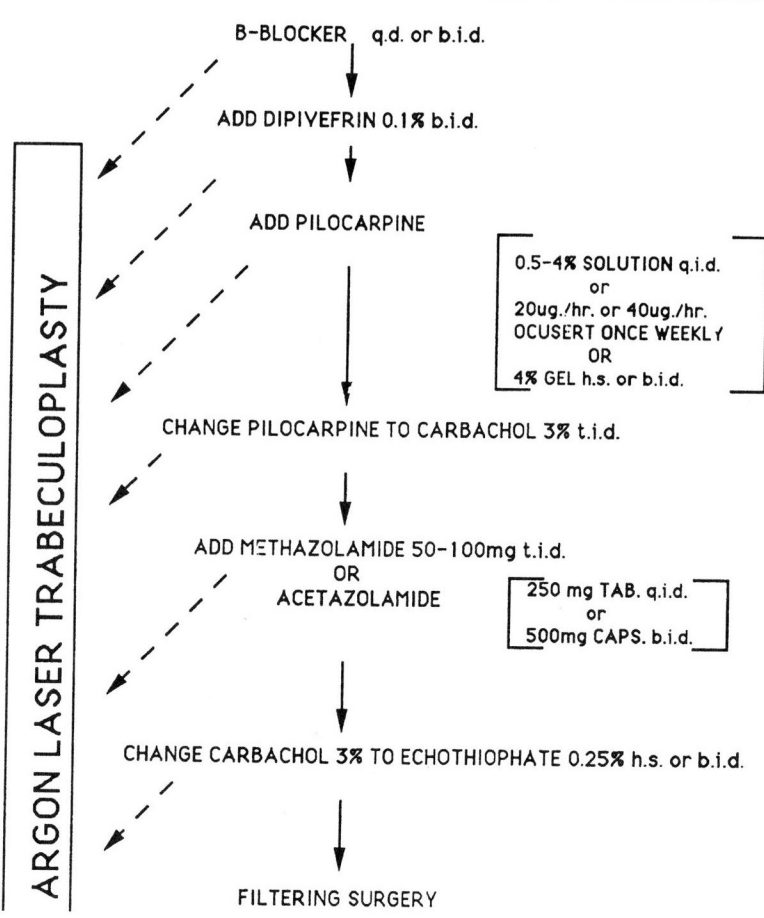

B-BLOCKER q.d. or b.i.d.

ADD DIPIVEFRIN 0.1% b.i.d.

ADD PILOCARPINE

0.5-4% SOLUTION q.i.d.
or
20ug./hr. or 40ug./hr.
OCUSERT ONCE WEEKLY
OR
4% GEL h.s. or b.i.d.

CHANGE PILOCARPINE TO CARBACHOL 3% t.i.d.

ADD METHAZOLAMIDE 50-100mg t.i.d.
OR
ACETAZOLAMIDE

250 mg TAB. q.i.d.
or
500mg CAPS. b.i.d.

CHANGE CARBACHOL 3% TO ECHOTHIOPHATE 0.25% h.s. or b.i.d.

FILTERING SURGERY

ARGON LASER TRABECULOPLASTY

Figure 48.3. Flowchart for the medical management of primary open-angle glaucoma. Argon laser trabeculoplasty is used as an adjunct to drug therapy. (Adapted from Eskridge JB, Bartlett JD. The glaucomas. In Bartlett JD, Jaanus SD (eds): Clinical Ocular Pharmacology. Boston, Butterworths, 1988, p 766.)

on chronic topical steroid therapy should therefore have tonometric examinations every 2 months.

The degree of rise in pressure appears to be associated with the antiinflammatory potency of the agents involved and is most marked with dexamethasone (23) and betamethasone. Equivalent doses of ophthalmic prednisolone and triamcinolone used four times daily gave elevations of IOP similar to those of betamethasone instilled only once daily. The duration of corticosteroid treatment and the age of the patient influenced the degree of ocular hypertension experienced. In some instances, topical epinephrine or systemic carbonic anhydrase inhibitors can maintain the ocular tension within normal limits. On other occasions, it may be necessary to reduce the frequency of administration or substitute a less potent steroid. Withdrawal of the drug may be necessary to return ocular tension to normal levels.

Steroids administered systemically can make preexisting open-angle glaucoma more difficult to control, but their effect on IOP is much smaller than that of topically applied steroids (21). Ocular hypertension may occur during prolonged systemic corticosteroid therapy, usually over a period of 1 year or more, in patients with such conditions as rheumatoid arthritis or systemic lupus erythematosus.

However, this complication should not deter one from using systemic corticosteroid in situations where they are appropriate.

The ocular hypertension effect induced by topical steroids can be categorized for three groups of patients in the general population who do not have diagnosed glaucoma. Two-thirds of the general population (group 1) respond with an average rise in pressure of 1.6 mm Hg after 4 weeks of 0.1% dexamethasone three times daily (24). A second group (29%) responds with an average rise of 10 mm Hg. Finally, a third group (5%) responds with a rise greater than 16 mm Hg. For each group, the rate of IOP increase differs significantly. The clinical implication is that patients who are receiving corticosteroid for at least 1 month and who have tonometric pressures below 21 mm Hg are unlikely to have glaucomatous complications. In addition, since approximately one-third of the general population will have a group 2 or group 3 response to topical steroids, tonometric monitoring should be performed monthly.

Summary of Drug-Induced Glaucoma

Table 48.7 lists drugs that can induce glaucoma. The following factors must be considered in assessing the problem of drug-induced glaucoma. Topically administered drugs induce glaucoma more frequency than those given systemically. Conditions under which any drugs are contraindicated are specific about type of glaucoma and method of treatment for it. Seldom, if ever, does the warning against the use of a particular agent in glaucoma specify the type of glaucoma. Acute angle-closure glaucoma is an emergency, and any agent that might precipitate an attack must be used cautiously. Unfortunately, patients who are predisposed to angle-closure glaucoma are not accurately identified without a gonioscopic examination of the anterior angle. Patients with diagnosed angle-closure glaucoma who have had a corrective surgical procedure are not at risk for another episode of angle-closure glaucoma (25). Patients with chronic open-angle glaucoma that is

adequately controlled by therapy are not at risk when treated with either systemic anticholinergics or sympathomimetics. In general, remarkably few drugs, except ophthalmic preparations, worsen existing or potential glaucoma (6).

Therapy

The goal of glaucoma therapy is the immediate and sustained reduction of IOP to prevent deterioration of the optic nerve and loss of vision. Drugs used in the treatment of glaucoma may be divided conveniently into those that increase the elimination of aqueous humor and those that decrease its formation. Parasympathomimetic miotic agents increase the rate of outflow, thereby facilitating the elimination of aqueous humor. Sympathomimetic mydri-

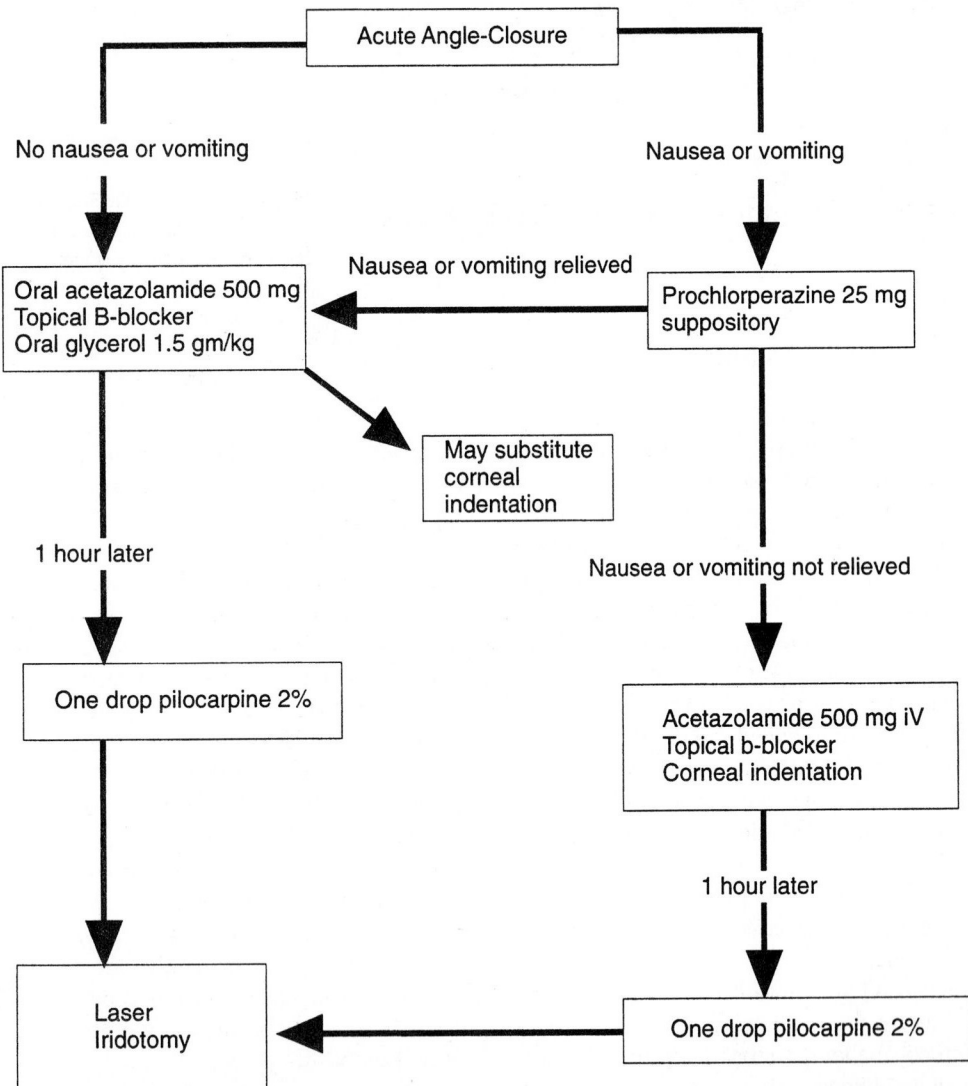

Figure 48.4.   Flowchart for the management of acute angle-closure glaucoma. (Reprinted with permission from Eskridge JB, Bartlett JD. The glaucomas. In Bartlett JD, Jaanus SD (eds): Clinical Ocular Pharmacology. Boston, Butterworths, 1988, p 743.)

atic agents lower elevated IOP by decreasing the rate of aqueous humor formation (2). Beta-blockers such as timolol decrease the rate of formation of aqueous humor but have no effect on outflow (2, 5, 25, 26). The mechanism of action is not clearly understood but thought to be due

Table 48.8.
Basis of Medical Treatment for Glaucoma[a]

Because elevated intraocular pressure is responsible for glaucomatous damage in the majority of patients, therapeutic measures are directed at:
1. Increasing the rate of outflow of aqueous humor via the drainage system

    Drugs: Parasympathomimetics

    Sympathomimetics

    Beta-blockers
2. Decreasing formation of aqueous humor by the ciliary processes

    Drugs: Sympathomimetics

    Carbonic anhydrase inhibitors
3. Reducing volume of aqueous humor in anterior chamber

    Drugs: Hyperosmotics

[a]Adapted from Leopold IH: Glaucoma Drug Therapy. Monograph IV-New Developments in Clinical Practice. Laguna Beach, CA: Allergan Pharmaceuticals, 1981.

to blockade of beta adrenoreceptors in the ciliary body (25–40). Secretion and inflow of aqueous humor are decreased most effectively by the carbonic anhydrase inhibitors (41). Hyperosmotic agents reduce IOP by increasing the osmolarity of the plasma relative to the aqueous and vitreous humor. Ocularly instilled parasympathomimetic miotics, sympathomimetic mydriatics, and orally administered carbonic anhydrase inhibitors find their greatest clinical application in primary open-angle glaucoma (Fig. 48.3 schematically shows the medical management of open-angle glaucoma) (42). Management of acute angle-closure glaucoma and congenital glaucoma is essentially surgical. Medical treatment is limited to preparing the patient for surgery (Fig. 48.4 contains a flowchart of the management of acute angle-closure glaucoma) (42). Treatment of secondary glaucoma should be directed at correcting the underlying cause as will as the elevation of IOP. Table 48.8 summarizes the basis of medical treatment of glaucoma.

Miotics

Miotics are cholinergic agents that facilitate the outflow of aqueous humor from the anterior chamber of the eye

Table 48.9.
Miotic Drugs Used in the Management of Glaucoma

Drug	Dosage[a]	Comments
Parasympathomimetics		
Pilocarpine hydrochloride		
Pilocarpine nitrate	0.25–10%	Instilled 1 or 2 drops in affected eye from q 6–8 hr to as often as q 4 hr. Onset of IOP-lowering effect is rapid with a 4–6 hr duration; although strengths above 4% are available, there is little advantage to using any strength above 4%
Pilocarpine gel	4% gel	Applied to affected eye hs. The gel dosage form is used as an adjunct to daytime medications
Ocuserts	P-20 and P-40	Placed into the affected eye once a week. Ocusert P-20 is generally used in patients controlled by a 2% solution or less; those requiring a greater strength use P-40
Carbachol	0.75–3%	Instilled 1 or 2 drops in affected eye from q 8–10 hr to as often as q 4 hr. Response varied with dose; may require frequent administration for weaker solutions than usually suggested; a suitable alternative when other miotics cannot be used because of allergy or side effects; poor corneal penetration; contraindicated in presence of corneal injury; longer acting than pilocarpine
Short-acting anticholinesterases		
Physostigmine salicylate		
Physostigmine sulfate	0.25–0.5%	Instilled 1 or 2 drops in affected eye q 6–12 hr; 0.25% ointment applied at bedtime. Onset of IOP-lowering effect similar to pilocarpine; considered to be stronger miotic than pilocarpine; aqueous solutions unstable; decomposition on exposure to light
Neostigmine bromide	3–5%	Instilled 1 or 2 drops in affected eye q 4–6 hr. More stable and less irritating than physostigmine; less effective because of poor corneal permeability
Long-acting anticholinesterases		
Echothiophate Iodide	0.03–0.25%	Instilled 1 drop in affected eye no more frequently than q 12 hr. Potent, long-acting; maximum effects in 10–20 hr and may persist for several days; unstable in solution; should be used when shorter-acting miotics are inadequate; contraindicated prior to filtering surgery; not used prior to cataract extraction
Demecarium bromide	0.125–0.25%	Instilled 1 or 2 drops in affected eye q 12 hr. Potent, long-acting; should be used only when shorter-acting miotics do not give desired result; duration of miosis is prolonged
Isoflurophate	0.025%	Instilled 1 or 2 drops in affected eye q 12–24 hr or longer weekly. Potent irritating; blurring of vision common complaint with ointment

[a]For open-angle glaucoma.

(Table 48.9). This is accomplished primarily by their action on the musculature of the iris and the ciliary body. The exact mechanism of improved fluid drainage remains poorly understood. The contraction of the ciliary muscle appears to be a primary mechanism by which the IOP is reduced. The trabecular meshwork and veins peripheral to the canal of Schlemm also may be dilated, thereby facilitating the outflow of aqueous humor. This action is independent of the pupillary constriction or miosis produced by the cholinergic miotic since outflow is unaffected in the absence of miosis. Miotics can lower IOP directly by stimulating the postfunctional effector cells innervated by the cholinergic fibers. Structurally these agents are similar to acetylcholine. Cholinergic miotics are therapeutically beneficial for treatment of open-angle glaucoma and for preoperative preparation for surgery in angle-closure glaucoma. Their disadvantage is their short duration of action, requiring frequent administration.

PARASYMPATHOMIMETICS

Acetylcholine is not used in glaucoma therapy because of its poor corneal penetration upon ocular instillation and rapid inactivation by cholinesterase. Intraocular acetylcholine is used in ophthalmic surgery. Pilocarpine is the most common miotic used for initial and maintenance therapy of chronic primary open-angle glaucoma (2, 4, 5, 25, 42). Pilocarpine penetrates the cornea after ocular instillation, with miosis and decreases in IOP, reaching their maximum levels in 30 to 40 minutes (5, 41–43). It is used in strengths varying from 0.5 to 10% though there appears to be little if any therapeutic advantage in the use of concentrations above 4%. The duration of IOP lowering is 4 to 8 hours. The usual frequency of instillation is two or three times daily, but pilocarpine may be given as often as every 2 hours. The Ocusert system is an innovative method of pilocarpine administration. Slightly larger than a contact lens and containing pilocarpine solution in its core, it is worn in the conjunctival sac of the eye where the drug diffuses out at a constant rate. It is available as Pilo-20 or Pilo-40 and releases 20 and 40 µg of pilocarpine per hour, respectively. Patients previously using 0.5 or 1% drops are controlled with Pilo-20; those using 2 to 4% drops require Pilo-40. The Ocusert is replaced every 7 days. Advantages of the Ocusert include a constant rate of drug released and improved compliance. Disadvantages of the Ocusert include expense and irritation (foreign body sensation), which occasionally results in the patient having to return to pilocarpine drops (43–45).

A pilocarpine HCl gel presoaked system is also available. Goldberg and colleagues compared 4% pilocarpine gel with 4% pilocarpine drops in 15 patients. The gel was applied only once a day in one eye, and the drops were used four times a day in the other eye. IOP and pupil diameters were similar with both forms of pilocarpine

except in the evening, when the eye treated with the gel showed no significant difference, compared to pretreatment values (46).

Carbachol is an unsubstituted carbamylester with a direct action like that of pilocarpine on parasympathetic receptors. It is totally resistant to hydrolysis by cholinesterase or acetylcholinesterase and therefore has a longer duration of action than pilocarpine in comparable strengths for IOP control. Solutions are available in strengths of 0.75 to 3%. In the treatment of open-angle glaucoma, one drop is instilled, usually two or three times daily. Response varies with the dose, and the weaker strength solutions require more frequent administration than usually suggested. When pilocarpine and other miotics cannot be used because of either allergy or intolerable side effects, carbachol may be a suitable alternative. However, if the glaucoma is uncontrollable with pilocarpine, it is doubtful that carbachol would yield much, if any, therapeutic improvement.

Diurnal fluctuations of IOP are diminished more effectively by carbachol than by pilocarpine. The major disadvantage of carbachol is its poor corneal penetration. In addition, it must be prepared in a vehicle such as methylcellulose to ensure prolonged contact with cornea, or with a wetting agent such as benzalkonium chloride to enhance corneal penetration. In the treatment of non-edematous glaucoma, an ointment of carbachol applied locally twice daily causes blurring of vision, a disadvantage of any ophthalmic ointment.

Methacholine bromide is very similar pharmacologically to acetylcholine, except that it is hydrolyzed more slowly by acetylcholinesterase and is almost totally resistant to cholinesterase. However, poor corneal penetration and instability in solution make it an unsuitable miotic for clinical use in glaucoma.

ANTICHOLINESTERASE

The anticholinesterase miotics act by inhibiting the cholinesterase enzyme, thereby permitting the accumulation of acetylcholine and prolonging the parasympathetic activity on the effector end organs of the eye. Physostigmine and neostigmine are reversible agents with short durations of effect. Organophosphate compounds, such as demecarium, echothiophate, and isoflurophate, have long durations of action and are irreversible anticholinesterases. The essential pharmacologic difference between these compounds is the relative irreversibility or permanency of their parasympathomimetic activity. Although the direct- and indirect-acting parasympathomimetic miotics act pharmacologically on different sites, their clinical effects on lowering elevated IOP in glaucoma are quite similar (41, 47).

Anticholinesterase miotics are therapeutically beneficial for the treatment of primary open-angle glaucoma; they are not indicated for the treatment of angle-closure glaucoma or congenital glaucoma. Since these agents act indirectly by inhibiting cholinesterase activity and prolonging the effects of endogenous acetylcholine, parasympathetic fibers to the pupil must be functional. The anticholinesterases are not effective if given after retrobulbar injections of anesthesia such as during cataract extration since liberation of acetylcholine is impaired.

Physostigmine lowers IOP by facilitating the outflow of aqueous humor. It has a longer duration of action and is considered to be a stronger miotic than pilocarpine. Physostigmine can be given in strengths of 0.25 to 1.0% every 4 to 6 hours. The onset of reduction in IOP usually occurs within 10 to 30 minutes, reaching its maximal effect within 1 to 2 hours and lasting 4 hours or more after instillation. The miotic effects may persist much longer. Aqueous solutions of physostigmine are unstable. Decomposition occurring with pH changes and on exposure to light is detected by progressive darkening of the solution. Decomposition products of physostigmine are unstable, quite irritating, and therapeutically ineffective. Physostigmine ointment should be reserved for bedtime use because the intense miosis produced soon after application is less discomforting for the patient while asleep. The prolonged duration of increased aqueous humor outflow facilitation is ideal and convenient because the patient need not be interrupted from sleeping to administer miotics (43, 44).

Neostigmine is more stable but less effective than physostigmine because of poorer corneal penetration. It is less irritating and has fewer unpleasant side effects than physostigmine. Ocular instillation of 3 to 5% aqueous solutions of neostigmine can be given every 4 to 6 hours alone or with pilocarpine on an alternating schedule. Demecarium is chemically similar to neostigmine, with miotic and IOP-lowering activity comparable to that of echothiophate and isoflurophate. In contrast to the organophosphates, the inhibition of cholinesterase activity by demecarium 0.06 to 0.25% instilled every 12 to 48 hours gives beneficial effects on IOP lasting from 12 hours to several days. In open-angle glaucoma, maximal reduction of IOP with demecarium is seen in 24 to 36 hours. The rapidity of the onset and duration of miosis is directly related to the concentrations used. Tolerance and refractoriness to demecarium occur earlier than with echothiophate and isoflurophate.

Echothiophate has a slow onset but is a long-acting cholinesterase inhibitor (47). Aqueous solutions of 0.06 to 0.25% instilled 1 drop every 12 to 24 hours for open-angle glaucoma can produce miosis within 10 to 15 minutes though maximal effect on lowering IOP is not seen until 10 to 20 hours later and may persist as long as 96 hours. Instillation of the 0.25% solution more often than twice daily does not appear to enhance the reduction if IOP (48).

The advantage of echothiophate is its long duration of action, requiring fewer installations and better control of the IOP on a daily basis. The intense miosis can produce a pupillary block and resultant shallowing of the anterior chamber of the eye. Therefore, in the presence of subacute narrow angles or angle-closure glaucoma, echothiophate should not be used. Aqueous solutions of echothiophate are unstable and must be prepared just before dispensing. Storage under refrigeration for no more than 6 months should be recommended to the patient.

Isoflurophate possesses the longest duration of action and is more potent than other anticholinestenases or parasympathomimetic miotics. A drop of 0.01 to 0.1% concentration once or twice daily produces effects on IOP similar to those of echothiophate in open-angle glaucoma. Miosis is maximal within 15 to 20 minutes. IOP is maximally reduced within 24 hours after instillation. Instillation of 0.1% solution more than twice daily yields very minimal additional therapeutic benefit.

ADVERSE SIDE EFFECTS

A direct and short-acting miotic such as pilocarpine can produce local conjunctival irritation as a result of frequent instillations. Allergic sensitivity or refractoriness to pilocarpine develops after prolonged use. Frequent instillation of the short-acting miotics can exacerbate chronic allergic conjunctivitis or blepharitis. Miosis itself can produce decreased night vision (48).

Discontinuation of the offending agent will most often eliminate the symptoms, or another miotic can be tried. Miotics may stimulate progressive deterioration of the visual field defect associated with glaucoma. Poor vision in dim light and blurring of vision from pupillary constriction and accommodative myopia are particularly troublesome for some patients. It is likely that the elderly patient already has diminished visual acuity and therefore should be made aware of the effect of the drug. This problem can be further complicated in aged patients who have cataracts in addition to impairment of vision.

Miotics can produce annoying side effects such as transient headaches, ocular and periorbital pain, twitching of the eyelids, ciliary congestion, and spasms. The direct long-acting anticholinesterase miotics produce the most severe symptoms, including discomfort associated with bright lights and close-up work. The affected eye is extremely myopic. This is particularly intense in younger patients who have active accommodation and are initially myopic. Patients should be reassured that these difficulties will usually diminish within a week or so. Severe fibrinous iritis can be induced by miotics and is most likely to occur with the long- and indirect-acting cholinesterase inhibitors. After intense and prolonged administration of the stronger miotics, pupillary cysts occur (50). These are seen more commonly in children, but the reason is not known.

Anticholinesterase miotics may also produce vitreous hemorrhaging, contact dermatitis, and allergic conjunctivitis. Retinal detachment and cataracts have been associated with the use of anticholinesterase miotics; however, their role is probably as a contributing factor secondary to underlying retinal pathology.

Glaucoma secondary to ocular inflammation may be exacerbated by these agents as a result of further vascular disruption. Lens opacities have been reported in patients treated with anticholinesterase miotics (51–56). Cataractogenic lens changes appear to be related to the drug, the concentration the patient is receiving, and the duration of treatment. Cataract formation does not appear to be directly associated with glaucomatous eyes; patients treated with miotics other than the anticholinesterase miotics are less likely to develop lens opacity. The lens changes may be partly reversible when the drug is discontinued. Progressive worsening of the cataract may occur, however, necessitating surgical extraction.

Systemic absorption of antiglaucoma drugs following ocular instillation may result in undesirable effects (56–62). These are seen more commonly after administration of the indirect- and longer-acting anticholinesterase agents. Gastrointestinal disturbances (i.e., nausea, diarrhea, abdominal pain, muscle spasm and weakness, sweating, lacrimation, salivation, hypotension, bradycardia, bronchial constriction, and respiratory failure) have been experienced (58). Most systemic effects reverse rapidly after discontinuation of the drug. In severe cholinergic toxicity, atropine sulfate 2 mg or pralidoxine chloride 25 mg/kg intravenously or subcutaneously can be given without affecting the control of the glaucoma.

Any potent long-acting miotic agent should be used with caution when a patient has bronchial asthma, parkinsonism, peptic ulcer, or other gastrointestinal disease since anticholinesterase systemic effects can exacerbate their clinical course. There is evidence that echothiophate and other organophosphates can traverse the placenta; therefore, the potential risks and benefits must be considered during pregnancy (60).

When known sensitivities to these agents exist, they should not be used. Considerable inhibition of plasma cholinesterase can be produced by prolonged topical anticholinesterase therapy (61). A patient receiving these agents must be monitored closely for prolongation of apnea when given succinylcholine chloride during surgery (61).

Patients who may be exposed to organophosphate pesticides should be made aware of the potential problems and risks associated with prolonged topical anticholinesterase exposure. There is an additive and cumulative effect on the parasympathetic nervous system. Systemically administered cholinergic agents such as ambenomium, neostigmine, or physostigmine used in disorders such as myasthenia gravis can potentiate the action of the anticholinesterase miotics.

The long-acting, irreversible anticholinesterase miotics should be reserved for use in chronic primary noncongestive glaucoma and secondary glaucoma when the shorter-acting miotics or beta-blockers have not successfully reduced the IOP. Undesirable side effects from these agents can also be minimized by instillation of their lowest effective concentrations at reasonable intervals.

Beta-Blockers

The use of beta-blockers in the treatment of glaucoma has been investigated for several years, and they are now the most widely prescribed drugs for the treatment of glaucoma (26). The reason for the initial clinical trials with these agents was the reduction of beta-adrenergic activity, which seems to be beneficial in the reduction of IOP. These agents reduce or abolish beta-adrenoreceptor stimulation caused by either catecholamine release from sympathetic nerve endings or the adrenal medulla or by injected sympathomimetic agents (26–40). Several beta-blockers have been and are being used in the treatment of open-angle glaucoma, including timolol maleate (26–40, 66–71, 77), propranolol (63), pindolol (64), atenolol (65), levobunolol HCl (26, 72–74), betaxolol HCl (26, 29, 36–38, 67, 75–77), carteolol (26, 39, 67, 78), and metipranolol (26) (see Tables 48.10 and 48.11).

Timolol is a potent, short-acting, nonselective beta-blocker. The ocular hypotensive effect is probably due to suppression of aqueous humor formation by blockage of the beta adrenoceptors in the ciliary body (26, 66). Timolol is available as 0.25 and 0.5% solutions. The usual starting dose is one drop of 0.25% in the affected eye(s) twice a day. If this does not control the glaucoma, the dose may be increased to 0.5% solution, one drop twice a day (27). Timolol may be used alone or in combination with agents such as epinephrine, pilocarpine, carbachol, or acetazolamide (27, 31, 34, 35, 69, 70). The addition of timolol to the therapy of patients on these agents significantly reduced IOP. Conflicting reports about the reduction of IOP when timolol and epinephrine are combined have been clarified. The recommendation is that epinephrine be administered 3 hours after timolol (31, 34, 35).

Studies suggest that the effects of acetazolamide and timolol are similar in reducing IOP. However, the combination of these two agents may be more effective than either drug alone (70).

When adding timolol to a patient's therapy, the other agent should be continued as well. The other agents may be discontinued on the following day or doses adjusted, depending on the therapeutic response of the patient. Stabilization of timolol therapy may take several weeks. A reevaluation should take place 2 and 4 weeks after therapy is begun. If the IOP is maintained, the schedule may be decreased to one drop once a day because of the daily variations in IOP. Tonometer readings should be done at

Table 48.10.

Blockers Used in the Management of Glaucoma

Drug (Year Approved)	Dosage[a]	Comment
Timolol (1978)	0.25 and 0.5% drops	Instill 1 drop in affected eye qd or q 12 hr. Beta-blockers may be used in combination with other miotic agents or carbonic anhydrase inhibitors; may also be used with epinephrine, best results are obtained by administering the epinephrine about 4 hr after the timolol as the latter is releasing the receptors to which the epinephrine must bind
Betaxolol (1985)	0.50% drops	Instill 1 drop qd or q 12 hr. Only cardioselective beta-blocking agent, it maybe advantageous over other beta-blockers in patients with respiratory diseases due to generally good bronchopulmonary tolerability
Levobunolol (1986)	0.50% drops	Instill 1 drop qd or q 12 hr. A nonselective beta$_1$- and beta$_2$-agent, it may in a number of patients be administered once a day
Metipranolol (1990)	0.3% drops	Instill 1 drop qd or q 12 hr. A nonselective beta$_1$-blocking agent, similar in side effect profile to timolol
Caretolol (1992)	1% drops	Instill 1 drop qd or q 12 hr. Use of caretolol may avoid addition of miotic agents in patients who are refractory to beta-blockers alone. Only beta-blocker with intrinsic sympathomimetic activity (ISA). Most potent beta-blockade activity.

[a]For open-angle glaucoma.

Table 48.11.

Selected Pharmacodynamic and Pharmacokinetic Properties of Ocular Beta-Adrenergic Blockers[a]

Property	Timolol	Carteolol	Betaxolol	Levobunolol	Metipranolol
Relative beta-blockade potency (propranolol = 1)	6	10	4	6	2
Beta$_1$ selectivity	0	0	++	0	0
Intrinsic sympathomimetic activity (ISA)	0	++	0	0	0
Local anesthetic effect	0	0	+	0	±
Stinging, burning	++	±	+++	++	+
Heart rate decrease	++	+	±	++	++
Bronchoconstriction	++	+	±	++	++
Dyslipidemia	+	0	?	?	?
Ocular perfusion	±	±	±	?	?
Serum half-life (hr)	3–5	3–7	12–20	6	2

[a]Reprinted with permission from Zimmerman TJ. Topical ophthalmic beta blockers: A comparative review. J Ocular Pharmacology 9(4):373–384, 1993.

different times of the day (27–30, 32, 33). If one drop of timolol (0.5% solution) twice a day is not effective (27), concomitant therapy with other agents is warranted.

Contraindications of timolol include use in patients with bronchospasm (including bronchial asthma or severe chronic obstructive pulmonary disease) and in those with congestive cardiac failure; also beta-blockers should not be used alone in patients with angle-closure glaucoma (use with pilocarpine) (27–29, 37, 71).

Levobunolol, betaxolol, metipranolol and carteolol are additional beta-blockers now on the U.S. market. Levobunolol, a nonselective beta$_1$- and beta$_2$-blocking agent, successfully decreases IOP. It is available as a 0.5% solution and is recommended to be instilled once or twice a day. Wandel and colleagues (72) compared once-a-day dosing of levobunolol 0.5 or 1.0% and timolol 0.5% in 92 patients. Both levobunolol 0.5 and 1.0% were found to have an overall greater effect on IOP than timolol. This once-daily dosing of levobunolol improves patient compli-

ance. If IOP is not controlled with a single dose of levobunolol, the frequency of administration should be increased to twice a day. In this case, levobunolol offers no advantage over timolol (26, 72–74).

Betaxolol, a beta$_1$-adrenergic blocking agent, is available as a 0.25% solution that is instilled into the eye every 12 hours. In a double-blind randomized study, betaxolol (0.5%) was compared with timolol (0.5%). The most frequently reported side effects were mild discomfort and tearing on administration, but side effects were not sufficient to cause discontinuation of therapy. Both drugs had similar efficacy in reducing IOP (26, 67, 75–77). Betaxolol, unlike timolol, offers the advantage of little or no effect on pulmonary disease, but it should still be used with caution. In concentrations ranging from 0.125 to 1%, betaxolol has reduced IOP by as much as 10.1% (76). Because of its selective beta-adrenergic activity, betaxolol produces a greater additive effect than timolol when administered concomitantly with epinephrine. However, betaxolol, like other beta-blockers, should not be administered to patients with heart failure (75–77).

Metipranolol is also a beta₁-adrenergic blocking agent available as a 0.3% solution. Its relative beta blockage potency is the lowest of the beta-blockers. It is reported to have a lower stinging or burning effect on administration than other beta-blockers; otherwise, it has no advantages over other agents (26).

Carteolol is a nonselective beta-adrenergic blocker with intrinsic sympathomimetic activity (ISA) that is available as a 1% solution. It is the most potent of the beta-blockers. It is the only beta-blocker with ISA, and this may prove to be a significant clinical advantage since it may reduce the incidence of systemic adverse effects (26). Although studies are still being conducted, carteolol exhibits reduced cardiovascular and bronchopulmonary side effects.

Side effects of timolol and other beta-blockers include burning or pain after instillation (most common), blurring of vision, and dilated pupils with epinephrine combination. Systemic side effects include cardiovascular problems (bradycardia, palpitations, hypertension, congestive heart failure), central nervous system disturbances (headaches, dizziness, drowsiness, anxiety, and depression), and pulmonary system side effects, including deaths due to precipitation or exacerbation of existing brochospasm (26, 27–29, 32, 33). Patients with diabetes should also use beta-blockers with caution.

Sympathomimetics

Reduction of IOP in open-angle glaucoma may be accomplished successfully by ocular instillation of sympathomimetics. Their mechanism of action is not fully understood, but the main effects appear to be decreasing the rate of aqueous humor production due to vasoconstriction and increasing its outflow.

Epinephrine, 1 to 2% solution instilled every 8 to 24 hours, can reduce IOP in open-angle glaucoma. The rate of aqueous secretion is initially decreased, probably by adrenergic stimulation at receptor sites in the ciliary epithelium. Improved facility of outflow is not immediate but may be seen after several months of epinephrine therapy. The probable mechanism suggested is alpha-adrenergic response to epinephrine at the trabecular meshwork. The pressure lowering by epinephrine of 3 to 15 mm Hg occurs in 6 to 8 hours and lasts from several hours to days. Patient response appears to be highly variable. Epinephrine is seldom used alone for open-angle glaucoma but is usually used with miotics (79–83, 85). Epinephrine does not disturb accommodation and is especially beneficial in overcoming the disabling miosis induced by the parasympathomimetic. When used in combination, it should be given 5 to 10 minutes after the miotic has been instilled. Comparative effects of epinephrine bitartrate 2% and epinephrine borate 1% have been

studied, and no statistical difference in ability to reduce IOP in glaucomatous eyes can be found between individual preparations (69). The commercial borate salt is buffered to enhance corneal penetration and is perhaps better tolerated than the others.

Dipivalyl HCl, a prodrug for epinephrine, is produced by the addition of two pivalyl side chains to epinephrine. Dipivalyl has better lipid solubility than epinephrine, and thus corneal penetration is better (approximately 17 times better). Studies have shown no significant difference in 0.1% dipivalyl (when compared with 2% epinephrine) in lowering IOP. Kass and colleagues (81) as well as Kohn and colleagues (82) compared 0.1% dipivalyl with 2% epinephrine in terms of their effect on lowering IOP, increasing pupil size, and the frequency of side effects. Both investigators found that these agents lowered IOP significantly. Although dipivalyl was less effective in lowering IOP than epinephrine, fewer side effects were reported in patients receiving dipivalyl (82).

Phenylephrine has not proved to be any more effective than epinephrine in lowering IOP. A 10% solution of phenylephrine is used primarily in assisting with ophthalmoscopic examination because it has disturbing cycloplegic effects. Propranolol is an alpha-adrenergic blocker used in the management of angina and cardiac arrhythmias. It has been demonstrated that 20 mg given orally is able to reduce IOP in open-angle glaucoma quite effectively. However, in many cases, the dose had to be increased with time so as to maintain effective reduction of IOP. The fall in systemic blood pressure and the potential for cardiac difficulties associated with propranolol argue against its widespread use for the treatment of glaucoma.

Isoproterenol in a 5% solution produces comparable effects to those of epinephrine, with maximal reduction of IOP in 6 hours and persisting decreases for 12 to 60 hours. Widespread use of isoproterenol for ocular instillation is prevented by the common occurrence of systemic side effects such as tachycardia and palpitations (84).

Appreciable local and systemic side effects are experienced by patients who use ocular sympathomimetics for long periods (82). Local side effects include melanin deposits on the conjunctiva and cornea, hyperemia and corneal edema, and allergic blepharoconjunctivitis (82). Headache, periorbital pain, and lacrimation with intermittent visual blurring and distortion are common complaints. Although the frequency is relatively low, cardiac irregularities and elevations of blood pressure after ocular administration of epinephrine have been reported (83). Side effects, both local and systemic, are promptly relieved after the epinephrine is discontinued. Closer supervision and caution should be exercised for patients who are receiving anesthetics in preparation for surgery because the reported rate of systemic side effects of the ocular sympathomimetic is higher in such cases. Sympathomimetics are contraindicated in angle-closure glaucoma prior to peripheral iridectomy. Gonioscopic examinations are advised before the ocular instillation of a sympathomimetic mydriatic so as to rule out asymptomatic or subacute angle-closure glaucoma. After the iridectomy is performed, ocular epinephrine can be useful, especially if aqueous humor outflow is impaired. It should not be used if IOP can be adequately managed by miotics alone.

Carbonic Anhydrase Inhibitors

The lowering of IOP can be achieved by systemic administration of carbonic anhydrase inhibitors (Table 48.12) (70, 86–93). These agents are of particular value where control of glaucoma is unobtainable with parasympathomimetic miotics. Carbonic anhydrase, a widely distributed enzyme in the body, catalyzes the reversible reaction of water and carbon dioxide to form carbonic acid and subsequently the bicarbonate ion. In the eye, large concentrations of carbonic anhydrase are found in the ciliary process and retina. The mechanism of action of the carbonic anhydrase inhibitor on IOP is not clearly understood. Acetazolamide increases the outflow of aqueous fluid in some glaucoma patients, whereas a decrease in outflow occurs in normal eyes and in eyes with very early glaucoma. The lowering of the intraocular volume does not depend on the diuretic effect of carbonic anhydrase inhibitors and cannot be explained simply as a depletion of the bicarbonate ion content. The buffer system necessary for maintaining secretory functions in the ciliary epithelium is probably impaired or inhibited, thus reducing

aqueous humor formation. Only slight changes in IOP are experienced in normotensive eyes when carbonic anhydrase inhibitors are administered. There is no effect on the IOP when carbonic anhydrase inhibitors are instilled locally. These drugs are used concomitantly with cholinergic miotics and hyperosmotic agents for the emergency treatment of primary angle-closure glaucoma. Prompt and vigorous reduction of IOP to normal levels before peripheral iridectomy gives a better postoperative prognosis.

A single dose of oral or intravenous acetazolamide can reduce IOP for 4 to 6 hours. The maximum effect is seen about 2 hours after oral administration. Following intravenous administration, the maximum effect is attained within 20 minutes. Hypersecretion glaucoma that is infrequent can respond to treatment with carbonic anhydrase inhibitors alone. In chronic primary glaucoma where control has been difficult to obtain with miotics or during acute exacerbations, addition of a carbonic anhydrase inhibitor to cholinergic and sympathomimetic agents may produce satisfactory ocular tension control. Carbonic anhydrase inhibitors are useful in the short-term management of glaucoma secondary to trauma or uveitis and in the preoperative management of congenital glaucoma. Their use in chronic angle-closure glaucoma should be discouraged because symptoms of progressive angle narrowing can easily be obscured.

Long-term use of carbonic anhydrase inhibitors is frequently unsuccessful because of their side effects. Patients differ in their ability to tolerate the various carbonic anhydrase inhibitors, and some may be better tolerated.

Table 48.12.
Carbonic Anhydrase Inhibitors Used to Manage Glaucoma[a]

Drug and Dosage Form	Dose	Onset	Duration	Comment
Acetazolamide tablets 125 and 250 mg	125–250 mg qid	½–1 hr	4–6 hr	Used in short therapy for primary and secondary glaucoma especially if refractory or uncontrollable by miotics; used with miotics and hyperosmotics in emergency treatment of primary angle-closure glaucoma; fair success with long-term use in open-angle glaucoma; failures frequently due to side effects; carbonic anhydrase inhibitor of choice in management of glaucoma
Acetazolamide sequels 500 mg	500 mg bid	1–2 hr	10–18 hr	
Acetazolamide 500 mg vials	500 mg IV	1 min	4 hr	
Methazolamide tablets 25 and 50 mg	25–100 mg	1 hr	10–14 hr	50 mg is equivalent to 250 mg of acetazolamide; few significant differences from acetazolamide with exception of side effects and slower onset of action; drowsiness, fatigue, malaise with minimal gastrointestinal disturbance are common; main indication for chronic glaucoma insufficiently controlled by miotics or acetazolamide
Dichlorphenamide tablets 50 mg	25–50 mg bid, tid, or qd	½ hr	6–12 hr	Metabolic acidosis occurs less frequently with dichlorphenamide than with other carbonic anhydrase inhibitors; used with patient intolerance or refractory to acetazolamide; anorexia nausea, paresthesias, dizziness, or ataxia and tremor should alert one of the possibility of toxicity

[a]Adapted from Flach AJ. Topical acetazolamide and other carbonic anhydrase inhibitors in the current medical therapy of the glaucomas. Glaucoma 8:20–27, 1986.

The drug of choice is usually acetazolamide tablets. However, more than 50% of patients are unable to tolerate this therapy. Acetazolamide sustained-release capsules are somewhat better tolerated, but approximately 40% of patients cannot tolerate acetazolamide in this dosage form. Between 25 and 50% of patients who are intolerant of acetazolamide will be able to take methazolamide. Therefore, patients suffering considerable adverse effects of acetazolamide can be tried on the sustained-release capsules or switched to methazolamide. A reduction in dose also may decrease the side effects. Other ways of minimizing the side effects of carbonic anhydrase inhibitors have not been substantiated. Dichlorphenamide and ethoxozolamide have a greater propensity to cause side effects leading to discontinuation of therapy and are rarely used. Older patients appear to be more intolerant to the carbonic anhydrase inhibitors than younger patients (86–93).

The gastrointestinal effects are a common cause of discomfort for the patient and often become so severe that the drug is discontinued. Nausea, vomiting, intestinal colic, diarrhea, anorexia, and paresthesia of the face and extremities are common side effects. Transient myopia is an unusual and rare occurrence. Long-term treatment with a carbonic anhydrase inhibitor does not appear to deplete intracellular potassium. Since there may be marked depletion of electrolytes, including potassium (88), when treatment with the agent is begun, serum potassium levels and clinical manifestations of cellular potassium depletion should be monitored. However, the routine supplementation of potassium for glaucoma patients receiving carbonic anhydrase inhibitors is not encouraged and is of doubtful value in the absence of depletion.

Acetazolamide produces hyperglycemia in prediabetics and diabetics receiving oral hypoglycemic agents. Hyperuricemia has occurred following treatment with carbonic anhydrase inhibitors. Prolonged use of these drugs can lead to urinary and renal colic secondary to formation of calcium calculi (92, 93). Alkalinization of the urine by acetazolamide results in an enhanced renal tubular reabsorption of drugs such as quinidine, amphetamine, and the tricyclic antidepressants. Alkalinization of the urine can also decrease the acid-dependent antibacterial activity of methenamine. Exfoliative dermatitis secondary to these agents is similar to dermatologic reactions encountered with the sulfonamides. Rare occurrences of idiosyncratic reactions such as cholestatic jaundice, drug fever, and blood dyscrasias, including thrombocytopenia, agranulocytosis, and aplastic anemia, have been reported. Carbonic anhydrase inhibitors are not recommended in patients with hemorrhagic glaucoma, hepatic or renal dysfunction, and renocortical hypofunction or a history of prior sensitivities to the drug.

Hyperosmotic Agents

Hyperosmotic agents lower the IOP by creating an osmotic gradient between the plasma and aqueous humor from the anterior chamber of the eye (Table 48.13) (94). Given systemically, these agents draw fluids from the anterior chamber of the eye into the plasma. Hyperosmotic agents are most useful in the preoperative management of primary acute angle-closure glaucoma. The degree of IOP lowering depends on the tension elevation and the osmotic gradient induced. The greatest effect of rapid changes in plasma osmolarity is on the eye, with very profound pressure elevations. The most commonly used hyperosmotics are mannitol, urea, and glycerol (94, 95).

Mannitol can effectively reduce acutely elevated IOPs when given slowly by the intravenous route as a 20% solution to adults and a 10% solution to children (96, 97). The ocular hypotensive effect is produced in 30 to 60 minutes and lasts from 4 to 6 hours. The effectiveness of the hyperosmotic agents depends on the rate of administration. Mannitol is preferred in the management of secondary glaucoma accompanied by hyperemia or uveitis because it penetrates the eye less readily, which is an advantage when inflammatory processes are active. Agents that enter the eye rapidly produce a lower osmotic gradient and a shorter duration of action than those that do so slowly or not at all. Inflammation greatly increases the ocular permeability of agents such as urea. Therefore, it is less desirable under those circumstances. There is relatively less local tissue irritation, thrombophlebitis, and necrosis occurring with mannitol than with urea when given intravenously. Renal disease does not contraindicate the use of mannitol.

Excessive thirst is a common sensation experienced by patients following infusion of hyperosmotic agents. However, these patients should not be given fluids during the period of osmotic dehydration. Secondary rises in IOP occur after administration of fluids, diminishing the therapeutic effects of the hyperosmotics. Headache is also a common complaint but can be minimized simply by bed rest. Symptoms of cellular dehydration, hypokalemia, and cardiac irregularities secondary to mannitol therapy should be monitored. On rare occasions, disorientation and severe agitation may be observed. Pulmonary edema and congestive heart failure may be precipitated in the elderly, especially with mannitol infusions. Potassium deficiency can accompany diuresis following hyperosmotic infusion, and cardiac patients and patients with hepatic or renal disorders should be cautiously monitored. Since mannitol is not absorbed orally, it is not effective when given by that route.

Urea given by the intravenous route as a 30% solution will reduce elevated IOP within 30 to 40 minutes (98). Miotics and carbonic anhydrase inhibitors are used concomitantly with urea in the management of acute glau-

Table 48.13.

Hyperosmotic Agents Used in the Management of Glaucomas

Drug	Dosage (g/kg body wt)	Route	Comments
Ascorbic acid	0.4–1.0	IV/oral	Gastric distress and diarrhea oral administration; seldom used since more effective agents are available
Glycerin (50% solution)	1.0–1.5	Oral	Nausea, vomiting, hyperglycemia can occur; caution in diabetic patients; as effective as produced
Isosorbide	1–2	Oral	Can be given to diabetic; tension comparable to those of intravenous hyperosmotics; diarrhea, frequently experienced
Mannitol (20% solution)	1.0–2.0	IV	Requires larger volumes than other hyperosmotics; used in diabetics; less irritating and free of tissue necrosis when solution extravasates; not contraindicated in patients with renal disease; monitor for cellular dehydration, hypokalemia, cardiac irregularities, urinary output, and chest pain; more effective for glaucoma with inflammation than urea or glycerol; avoid excessive
Urea (30% solution)	1.0–1.5	IV	Given IV over 30 min; unstable; side effects are sloughing, phlebitis, headaches, nausea, vomiting hemolysis "rebound diuresis"; contraindicated in nephrotic patients; caution in hepatic impairment; use freshly made solution only; maximal effect 1 hr

coma prior to surgery. Nausea, vomiting, confusion, disorientation, and anxiety are seen. Severe headache, a common complaint, can begin soon after the initiation and continue for the duration of the intravenous infusion. The patient's head should not be elevated during this time.

Although urea produces less cellular dehydration because of its ease of penetrability into the cell, a "rebound phenomenon" can occur as the plasma level of the hyperosmotic agent drops below that of the vitreous fluid. As the urea is cleared from the circulation rapidly with diuresis, the osmolality of the blood will decline. The hyperosmotic vitreous in turn draws fluid into the eye, resulting in an increased IOP or pressure "rebound" effect.

Ascorbic acid successfully reduces IOP in rabbits with glaucoma (99). In cases of refractoriness to acetazolamide and miotics, ascorbic acid given intravenously can lower the ocular hypertension. A 20% solution of sodium ascorbate at a pH of 7.2 to 7.4 can produce normal ocular tension in 60 to 90 minutes.

Oral hyperosmotic agents effectively reduce elevated IOP and are useful where the rapid-action infused preparations are not required. Glycerol is a convenient hyperosmotic agent when given as a 50 or 75% solution (100, 101). The ocular penetration of glycerol is poor; therefore, a substantial osmotic gradient can be produced between the plasma and aqueous humor. IOP reduction is as effective as with hyperosmotic agents given by intravenous infusion. IOPs normally return to pretreatment levels within 5 to 6 hours. Hyperglycemia and glycosuria can occur following glycerol and should be used with particular caution in labile diabetics (100, 101). Acute diabetic ketoacidosis has been reported following treatment with glycerol. Nausea, diarrhea, and headache are also common complaints following oral glycerol (100).

The reduction of IOP with isosorbide is comparable to that of intravenous mannitol, urea, or oral glycerol.

Given as a 50% solution orally, its absorption is rapid, and it is primarily unchanged on excretion in the urine. Effective reduction in IOP occurs within 30 minutes after ingestion and remains for 1 to 2 hours or more depending on the dose. Side effects include transient headaches and diarrhea. Other gastrointestinal disturbances such as nausea are usually less of a problem with isosorbide than glycerol (102).

MEDICAL MANAGEMENT

Conservative medical treatment can successfully control most cases of chronic open-angle glaucoma. The stage or severity of the disease as evidenced by the condition of the optic disk and the quality of the visual field should be the major factors in choosing the treatment. Mild elevations of IOP (less than 30 mm Hg) in the presence of a normal optic disk and visual field is not an absolute indication for therapy. These patients should have routine periodic examinations to detect any optic changes because such changes can be detected long before permanent visual field impairment. There is no absolute level of IOP that must be maintained to assure therapeutic success. The IOP should be maintained at a level that prevents further deterioration of the optic disk and impairment of visual field. If the disk is normal on gonioscopic examination, an IOP in the high 20s is not as important clinically as one with concurrent disk involvement or abnormal visual field. The former situation may warrant only close periodic follow-up, whereas in the latter appropriate medical treatment should be started. If there is the slightest indication of disk pathology, the IOP should be maintained at 20 mm Hg or even lower by medical management. In cases of considerable disk degeneration and visual field loss, vigorous treatment should be undertaken to obtain a level of 15 mm Hg or lower.

In situations where advanced cupping of the optic disk and visual loss is not apparent in the presence of high IOP (greater than 30 mm Hg), medical therapy should be initiated. The aim of therapy is to lower the IOP enough to interrupt the course of the disease. Problems common to antiglaucoma therapy must be considered before reducing IOP with drugs. The expense and inconvenience of the medications should be considered as well as whether the side effects and toxicities of the drugs constitute a greater risk to the patient than the increased level of IOP.

For primary open-angle glaucoma, a miotic agent should be given at its lowest effective concentration and at intervals no more frequent than necessary to maintain a satisfactory level of IOP. The IOP should be measured before beginning therapy. The effects of therapy on the IOP can be determined within 1 week or more. If the reduction of IOP is not satisfactory, the concentration of the miotic agent should be increased, keeping in mind, however, that there is little advantage to using concentrations of pilocarpine solutions greater than 4% or its equivalent.

Refractoriness often occurs following prolonged use of cholinergic miotics. Rather than increase the frequency of instillation or strength used, an alternative agent should be selected. Responsiveness to the cholinergic miotics often is restored after their replacement for a brief period by an anticholinesterase miotic. Various combinations of glaucoma medications are often given together to potentiate their therapeutic effects. However, not all combinations produce an additive pharmacologic response.

Epinephrine or phenylephrine may be added to miotic therapy if IOP control is inadequate, provided that gonioscopic examination has failed to demonstrate excessive narrowing of the anterior chamber angle (79). Evidence suggests that greater activity is produced when pilocarpine and epinephrine are applied separately rather than in combination (79–83). Combinations of anticholinesterase miotics can reduce rather than potentiate the effectiveness of each other. Prior installations of physostigmine or demecarium will reduce the activity of subsequently instilled echothiophate or isoflurophate by competitive inhibition of the acetylcholinesterase. Pretreatment with either echothiophate or isoflurophate will enhance only slightly the activity of physostigmine or demecarium. However, the actions of physostigmine on demecarium are additive rather than competitive, regardless of their order of instillation. Differences in the duration of action and type of cholinesterase-inhibiting activity inherent with each miotic given in combination contribute to these predictable responses. Concomitant instillation of miotics, particularly those that act indirectly, offers very few advantages and should not be used in attempts to treat difficult-to-control open-angle glaucoma.

Beta-blocker therapy is the most widely prescribed drug therapy for the treatment of glaucoma (timolol is the most widely used drug) (2, 26). Combinations of beta-blocker with pilocarpine, epinephrine, or acetazolamide have also been used effectively. Other agents may be used when glaucoma is refractory to the cholinergic miotics; however, a beta-blocker should be selected first because it has fewer side effects and is more effective.

Addition of an agent from another class of antiglaucoma drugs is preferred to substitution or addition of an agent from the same group. Deterioration of the glaucoma should always be ruled out. The storage condition of the medication, expiration date, and method of administration should be assessed when a patient experiences diminished effects from the eye drops.

SURGICAL MANAGEMENT

Surgical management of open-angle glaucoma should be reserved for situations in which maximal efforts using miotics, sympathomimetics, beta-blockers, and carbonic anhydrase inhibitors have been unsuccessful in maintaining an acceptable level of IOP and preventing progressive changes of the optic disk or the visual field. The surgical procedure involves creating a collateral drainage from the anterior chamber. An acute-closure glaucoma attack must receive prompt and intensive attention to avoid irreparable damage to the eye. Pilocarpine 1 to 4% or an equivalent cholinergic miotic is instilled into the affected eye at frequent intervals (every 15 minutes for 1 hour, then every hour for 4 to 6 hours) until the IOP is reduced to levels at which surgery can be performed. The surgical procedure is a peripheral iridectomy, which allows the anterior chamber to communicate with the posterior chamber.

Table 48.14 summarizes the basis of surgical treatment of glaucoma. Cholinesterase-inhibiting miotics should be avoided. Intravenous or oral carbonic anhydrase inhibitors or hyperosmotic agents may be required in a patient with an acutely dilated pupil not responsive to the miotic agent.

Control of an attack should be established within 1 to 2 hours following the initiation of this intensive treatment. The subsequent involvement in the unaffected eye is greatly reduced when pilocarpine is given as a prophylactic

Table 48.14.
Basis of Surgical Treatment for Glaucomas

Reestablish circulation between posterior and anterior chamber
    Procedure—Peripheral iridectomy
Create new outflow channels
    Procedures—Iridencleisis
Trephine with iridectomy
Sclerectomy
Cyclodialysis
Cyclodiathermy
Cyclocryosurgery
Goniotomy

measure. Instillation of pilocarpine at normal intervals into the unaffected eye following an episode of acute angle-closure glaucoma is considered appropriate. Treatment of secondary glaucoma should be directed by the underlying and contributory factors. Medical treatment of congenital glaucoma may lower IOP levels, but this disorder can be successfully corrected only by surgery.

LASER THERAPY

Laser trabeculoplasty, an alternative to surgery, is now the most often used nonpharmacologic means of treating chronic open-angle glaucoma. Laser iridotomy, in most cases, is recommended over traditional surgery in angle-closure glaucoma (103–107). Remis and colleagues reported that laser surgery can reduce the IOP by 7 to 13 mm Hg in more than 80% of patients (103).

Argon Laser Trabeculoplasty (ALT)

At least 1 hour before laser trabeculoplasty, apraclonidine hydrochloride 1% is instilled into the operated eye for control of IOP. Apraclonidine hydrochloride is an alpha-adrenergic agonist that is used in a sterile isotonic solution. Ophthalmic apraclonidine when instilled into the eye has minimal cardiovascular effects and reduces IOP (108, 109). It does not have any significant local anesthetic activity and has minimal effect on cardiovascular parameters when instilled into the eye. It is used in conjunction with trabeculoplasty to prevent an acute elevation in IOP, which can occur after ALT. An elevated IOP is a risk factor in the pathogenesis of visual field loss. The mechanism of action of apraclonidine HCl has not been established, but it is postulated that its action may be related to a reduction in aqueous formation. Its onset of action is seen within 1 hour of instillation, and maximal effect is seen within 3 to 5 hours. It is used 1 hour prior to ALT, and a second drop is instilled immediately after completion of the laser surgical procedure (108,109). Apraclonidine hydrochloride has replaced pilocarpine as the agent of choice prior to ALT. A topical anesthetic is instilled prior to the procedure, and then the patient is seated at the slit lamp laser photocoagulator.

Using the argon laser coupled to a high-magnification biomicroscope, the surgeon places approximately 50 to 100 lesions in an evenly spaced sequence on the inner surface of the trabecular meshwork. Histopathologic studies have shown by scanning electron microscopy that laser light energy produces fibrosis at the treatment site. It is theorized that these laser "burns" cause localized shrinkage, which in turn produces tension on the adjacent, untreated trabecular beams. The previously collapsed spaces between the beams are then pulled open, allowing aqueous humor to pass more easily and resulting in a reduction in IOP (103–107).

Laser Iridotomy

Laser iridotomy is the treatment of choice for pupil block or angle-closure glaucoma. In most cases, surgery is recommended over traditional surgery. performed on an outpatient basis. One hour prior to la iridotomy surgery, topical apraclonidine hydrochloride (Iopidine) is instilled in the eye, along with pilocarpi drops. The pilocarpine causes pupillary constriction, whic thins the iris, making laser puncture much easier. At the time of laser surgery, a topical anesthetic is instilled. Using either the Nd:YAG laser or the Argon laser, an opening measuring approximately 50 to 100 microns in diameter is created in the peripheral iris. This iridotomy releases the pupillary block component of angle-closure glaucoma, thus breaking the attack of glaucoma or serving as prophylaxis against subsequent attacks (110).

Complications of laser treatment of glaucoma include intraocular inflammation in the form of uveitis, intraocular bleeding, elevated IOP, diplopia, pigment dissemination, and lens injury (27, 106, 110).

CONCLUSION

The successful outcome of glaucoma treatment depends greatly on the patient's proper use of medications. An asymptomatic patient who does not understand why expensive and inconvenient eyedrops are required will be less inclined to use them according to prescribed instructions. The blurring of vision and occasional discomfort associated with the use of these medications further enhance noncompliance. As a consequence, visual function is often irreversibly impaired, and drugs no longer influence the clinical course of the disease. The patient with glaucoma should understand the nature of the disorder and appropriate expectations for the drugs being used against it. Optimal therapeutic results can occur only in an environment of mutual cooperation and understanding between patients and the health care providers responsible for their care.

REFERENCES

1. Sommer A. Glaucoma screening: too little, too late? J Gen Intern Med 5:533, 1990.
2. Danyluk AW and Paton D. Diagnosis and Management of Glaucoma. Clin Symp 43(4):2–9, 1991.
3. Levy RA. Improving compliance with prescription medications: an important strategy for containing health-care costs. Medical Interface. Mar: 34–41, 1989.
4. Newell FW. The glaucomas. In: Ophthalmology: Principles and Concepts. St. Louis, CV Mosby, 1992, Ch 20.
5. Vaughan D. Glaucoma. In Vaughn D, Asbury T, and Tabbaka KF (eds): General Ophthalmology, ed. 14 Los Altos, CA, Lange Medical Publications, 1995, pp 190–205.
6. Fraunfelder FT. Drug-Induced Ocular Side Effects and Drug Interactions, ed. 2. Philadelphia: Lea & Febiger, 1982.
7. Grant WM. Ocular complications of drugs-glaucoma. JAMA 207: 2089, 1969.

8. Harris LS. Cycloplegic-induced intraocular pressure elevations. Arch Ophthalmol 79:242, 1968.

9. Mehra KS, Chandra P, Khare BB. Ocular manifestations of parenteral administration of scopolamine (hyoscine). Br J Ophthalmol 49:557, 1965.

10. Lazenby GW, Reed JW, Grant WM. Anticholinergic medications in open-angle glaucoma. Arch Ophthalmol 84:719, 1970.

11. Mulberger RD. Effect of a common cold product containing belladonna on intraocular pressure. Eye Ear Nose Throat Mouth 47:61–64, 1968.

12. Grant WM. Systemic drugs and adverse influence on ocular pressure. In Leopold IH (ed): Symposium on Ocular Therapy. St. Louis, CV Mosby, 1968, vol 3, p 57.

13. Willets GS. Ocular side effects of drugs. Br J Ophthalmol 53:252, 1969.

14. Drance SM. The effects of phospholine iodide on the lens and anterior chamber depth. In Liopold IH (ed): Symposium on Ocular Therapy. St. Louis, CV Mosby, 1969, vol 4, p 25.

15. Maddalena MA. Transient myopia associated with acute glaucoma and retinal edema following vaginal administration of sulfanilamide. Arch Ophthalmol 80:186, 1986.

16. Galin MA, Baras I, Zweifach P. Diamox-induced myopia. Am J Ophthalmol 54:237, 1962.

17. Edwards TS. Transient myopia due to tetracycline, JAMA 186:69, 1963.

18. Bard LA. Transient myopia associated with promethazine therapy. Am J Ophthalmol 58:682, 1964.

19. Armaly MF. Inheritance of dexamethasone hypertension and glaucoma. Arch Ophthalmol 77:747, 1967.

20. Becker B, Hahn KA. Topical corticosteroids and heredity in primary open-angle glaucoma. Am J Ophthalmol 57:543, 1964.

21. Bernstein HN, Schwartz B. Effects of long-term systemic steroids on ocular pressure and tonographic values. Arch Ophthalmol 68:742, 1962.

22. Burde RM, Becker B. Steroid-induced glaucoma and cataracts in contact lens wearers. JAMA 213:2075, 1970.

23. Smith CL. Corticosteroid glaucoma—a summary and review of the literature. AM J Med Sci 252:239, 1966.

24. Pappa KS. Corticosteroid drugs. In Mauger TF and Craig EL (eds): Havener's Ocular Pharmacology, ed. 6, St. Louis, CV Mosby, 1994, p 364–428.

25. Hiatt RL, Fuller JB, Smith L, et al. Systemically administered anticholinergic drugs and introcular pressure. Arch Ophthalmol 84:735–740, 1970.

26. Zimmerman TJ. Topical ophthalmic beta-blockers: A comparative review. J Ocular Pharmaco. 9:373–384, 1993.

27. Anon. Timoptic in the Management of Chronic Open-Angle Glaucoma, vol. II, West Point, PA: Merck Sharp and Dohme Publishers, 1979.

28. Wilcockson J, Wilcockson T. Long-term use of timolol in open-angle glaucoma. Curr Ther Res 27:545, 1980.

29. Anon. Beta blockers for glaucoma. Lancet 1:1064, 1979.

30. Boger WP III, Steinert RF, Puliafito CA, et al. Clinical trial comparing timolol ophthalmic solution to pilocarpine in open-angle glaucoma. Am J Ophthalmol 86(1):8–18, 1978.

31. Korey MS, Hodapp E, Kass MA, et al. Timolol and epinephrine, Long-term evaluation of concurrent administration. Arch Ophthalmol 100:742, 1982.

32. Phillips CI, et al. Penetration of timolol eye drops into human aqueous humor. Br J Ophthalmol 65:593, 1981.

33. LeBlanc RP, Krip G. Timolol. Canadian multicenter study. Ophthalmology 88:244, 1981.

34. Kass MA. Efficacy of combining timolol with other antiglaucoma medications. Surv Ophthalmol 28(suppl):274, 1983.

35. Keates EU, Stone RA. Safety and effectiveness of concomitant administration of dipivefrin and timolol maleate. Am J Ophthalmol 91:243, 1981.

36. Levy NS, Boone L, Ellis E. A controlled comparison of betaxolol and timolol with long-term evaluation of safety and efficacy. Glaucoma 7(2):54, 1985.

37. Berry DP, Van Buskirk EM, Shields MB. Betaxolol and timolol. A comparison of efficacy and side effects. Arch Ophthalmol 102:42, 1984.

38. Stewart RH, Kimbrough RL, Ward RL. Betaxolol vs timolol. A six-month double-blind comparison. Arch Ophthalmol 104:46, 1986.

39. Steward WC, Shields MB, Allen RC, et al. A 3-month comparsion of 1% and 2% carteolol and 0.5% timolol in open-angle glaucoma. Graefe's Arch Clin Exp Ophthalmol. 229:258–261, 1991.

40. Kitazawa Y. Multicenter double-blind comparsion of carteolol and timolol in primary open-angle glaucoma and ocular hypertension. Advances in Therapy. 10:95–131, 1993.

41. Derick RJ. Carbonic anhydrase inhibitors. In: Mauger TF and Craig EL (eds): Havener's Ocular Pharmacology, ed. 6, St. Louis, CV Mosby, 1994, p 177–179.

42. Eskridge JB, Bartlett JD. The glaucomas. In Bartlett JD, (ed): Clinical Ocular Pharmacology. Boston, Butterworths, 1995, pp 733–779.

43. Drance SM. Comparison of action of cholinergic and anticholinesterase agents in glaucoma. Invest Ophthalmol 5:130, 1966.

44. Sugrue MF. The pharmacology of antiglaucoma drugs. Pharmacol Ther 43:91, 1989.

45. Pearson D. Complications with the use of Ocusert (letter). Arch Ophthalmol 94:168, 1976.

46. Goldberg I, Ashburn FB, Kass MA, Becker B. Efficacy and patient acceptance of pilocarpine gel. Am J Ophthalmol 88:843, 1979.

47. Leopold IH. Ocular cholinesterase and cholinesterase inhibitors: The Friedenwald Memorial Lecture. Am J Ophthalmol 51:885, 1961.

48. Kellerman L, King AC. Echothiophate iodide in glaucoma. Am J Ophthalmol 62:278, 1966.

49. Harris LS. Dose response analysis of echothiophate iodide. Arch Ophthalmol 86:502, 1971.

50. Everitt DE, Avorn J. Systemic effects of medications used to treat glaucoma. 112:120, 1990.

51. Chin NB, Gold AA, Breinin GM. Iris cysts and miotics. Arch Ophthalmol 71:611, 1964.

52. Axelsson J, Holmberg A. The frequency of cataracts after miotic therapy, Acta Ophthalmol 44:421, 1966.

53. DeRoetth A Jr. Lens opacities in glaucoma patients on phospholine iodide therapy. Am J Ophthalmol 62:619, 1966.

54. Drance SM. The effects of phospholine iodide on the lens and anterior chamber depth. In Liopold IH (ed): Symposium on Ocular Therapy. St. Louis, CV Mosby, 1969, vol 4, p 25.

55. Levene RZ. Echothiophate iodide and lens changes. In Leopold IH (ed): Symposium on Ocular Therapy, St. Louis, CV Mosby. 1969, vol 4, p 45.

56. Shaffer RN, Hetherington J. Anticholinesterase and cataracts. Am J Ophthalmol 62:613, 1966.

57. Ellis PP. Systemic effects of locally applied anticholinesterase agents. Invest Ophthalmol 5:146, 1966.

58. Leopold IH. Cholinesterases and the effects and side effects of drugs affecting cholinergic systemic. Am J Ophthalmol 60:425, 1965.

59. Hiscox PEA, McCulloch C. Cardiac arrest occurring in a patient on echothiophate iodide therapy. Am J Ophthalmol 60:425, 1965.

60. Birks DA, Prior VJ, Silk E. Echothiophate iodide treatment of glaucoma in pregnancy. Arch Ophthalmol 79:283, 1968.

61. Eilderton TE, Farmati O, Zsigmond EK. Reduction in plasma cholinesterase levels after prolonged administration of echothiophate iodide eyedrops. Can Anaesth Soc J 15:291, 1968.

62. Gesztes T. Prolonged apnea after suxamethonium injection associated with eyedrops containing an anticholinesterase agent. Br J Anesth 38:408, 1966.

63. Ohrstrom A, Pandolfi M. Long-term treatment of glaucoma with systemic propranolol. Am J Ophthalmol 86:340, 1978.

64. Smith SE, Smith SA, Reynolds F, Whitmarsh VB. Ocular and cardiovascular effects of local and systemic pindolol. Br J Ophthalmol 63:63, 1979.

65. Elliot MJ, Cullen PM, Phillips CI. Ocular hypertensive effect of atenolol (Tenormin, I.C.I.). Br J Ophthalmol 59:296, 1975.

66. Coakes RL, Brubaker R. The mechanism of timolol in lowering introcular pressure. Arch Ophthalmol 96:2045, 1978.

67. Lesar TS. Comparison of ophthalmic beta-blocking agents. Clin Pharm 6:451–463, 1987.

68. Keates EJ. Evaluation of timolol malcate combination therapy in chronic open-angle glaucoma. Am J Ophthalmol 88:565, 1979.

69. Cyrlin MN, Thomas JV, Epstein DL. Additive effect of epinephrine to timolol therapy in primary open-angle glaucoma. Arch Ophthalmol 100:414, 1982.

70. Daily RA, Brubaker RF, Bourne WM. The effects of timolol maleate and acetazolamide on the rate of aqueous formation in normal human subjects. Am J Ophthalmol 93:232, 1982.

71. Anon. Additions to timoptic contraindictions. FDD Drug Bull 11:1, 1981.

72. Wandel T, Charap AD, Lewis RA, et al. Glaucoma treatment with once-daily levobunolol. Am J Ophthalmol 101:298, 1986.

73. Bersinger RE, Keates EJ, Gotman JD, Novack GD, Duzman E. Levbunolol. A three-month efficacy study in the treatment of glaucoma and ocular hypertension. Arch Ophthalmol 103:375, 1985.

74. Berson FG, Howard BC, Foerster RJ, Lass JH, Novack GD, Duzman E. Levobunolol compared with timolol for the long-term control of elevated introcular pressure. Arch Ophthalmol 103:379, 1985.

75. Stewart RH, Kimbrough RL, Ward RL. Betaxolol vs timolol. Arch Ophthalmol 104:46, 1986.

76. Goldberg I. Betaxolol. Aust NZ J Ophthalmol 17:9, 1989.

77. Allen RC, Hertzmark E, Walker AM, Epstein DL. A double-masked comparison of betazolol vs timolol in the treatment of open-angle glaucoma. Am J Ophthalmol 101:535, 1986.

78. Berrospi AR, Leibowitz HM. A new β-adrenergic blocking agent for treatment of glaucoma, Arch Ophthalmol 100:943, 1982.

79. Becker B, Petitt TH, Gay AJ. Topical epinephrine therapy in open-angle glaucoma. Arch Ophthalmol 66:219, 1961.

80. Briswick VG, Drance SM. Epinephrine salts and introcular pressure. Arch Ophthalmol 75:768, 1966.

81. Kass MA, Mandell AL, Goldberg I, Paine JM, Becker B. Dipivefrin and epinephrine treatment of elevated introcular pressure. Arch Ophthalmol 97:1865, 1979.

82. Kohn AN, Moss AP, Hargett NA, Ritch R, Smith H, Rodos SM. Clinical comparisons of divalyl epinephrine and epinephrine in the treatment of glaucoma. Am J Ophthalmol 87:196, 1979.

83. Carlstedt BC, Stanaszek WF. Glaucoma. US Pharmacist 12(4):7690, 1987.

84. Ross RA, Drance SM. Effects of topically applied isoproterenol on aqueous dynamics in man. Arch Ophthalmol 83:39, 1970.

85. Ballin N, Becker B, Goldman ML. Sustemic effects of epinephrine applied topically to the eye. Invest Ophthalmol 5:125, 1966.

86. Gallin MA, Harris LS. Acetazolamide and outflow facility. Arch Ophthalmol 76:493, 1966.

87. Maren TH. Carbonic anhydrase: chemistry, physiology and inhibition. Physiol Rev 47:595, 1967.

88. Shrader CE, Thomas JV, Simmons RJ. Relationship of patient age and tolerance to carbonic anhydrase inhibitors. Am J Ophthalmol 96:730, 1983.

89. Lichter PR, Newman LP, Wheeler NC, Beall OV. Patient tolerance to carbonic anhydrase inhibitors. Am J Ophthalmol 85:495–502, 1978.

90. Lichter PR. Reducing side effects of carbonic anhydrase inhibitors. Ophthalmology 88:266, 1981.

91. Draeger J, Guttner R, Theilmann W. Avoidance of side-reactions and loss of drug efficacy during long-term administration of carbonic anhydrase inhibitors by concomitant supplement electrolyte administration. Br J Ophthalmol 47:467, 1961.

92. Parfitt AM. Acetazolamide and sodium bicarbonate induced nephrocalcinosis and nephrolithiasis. Arch Intern Med 124:736, 1969.

93. Peyes MB. Acetazolamide and renal stone formation. Lancet 1:837, 1970.

94. Becker B, Kolker AR, Kupin T. Hyperosmotic agents. In Leopold IH (ed): Symposium on Ocular Therapy. St. Louis, CV Mosby, 1968, vol 3, p 42.

95. Kronfeld PC. The efficacy of combinations of ocular hypotensive drugs. Arch Ophthalmol 78:140, 1967.

96. Adams RE, Kirschner RJ, Leopold IH. Ocular hypotensive effect of intravenously administered mannitol. Arch Ophthalmol 69:55, 1963.

97. Weiss DI, Shaffer RN, Harrington DD. Treatment of malignant glaucoma with intravenous mannitol infusion. Arch Ophthalmol 69:154, 1963.

98. Davis M, Duehr P, Javid M. The clinical use of urea for reduction of introcular pressure. Arch Ophthalmol 65:526, 1961.

99. Suzuki Y. Studies on the effect of ascorbic acid on the introcular pressure of rabbits. Acta Ophthalmol 75:201, 1966.

100. D'Alena P, Ferguson W. Adverse effects after glycerol orally and mannital parenterally. Arch Ophthalmol 75:210, 1966.

101. McCurdy DK, Schneider B, Scheic HG. Oral glycerol: the mechanism of introcular hypotension. Am J Ophthalmol 61:373, 1970.

102. Krupin T, Kolker AE, Becker B. A comparison of isosorbide and glycerol for cataract surgery. Am J Ophthalmol 69:373, 1970.

103. Remis LL, Epstein DL. Treatment of glaucoma, Annu Rev Med. 35:195, 1984.

104. Epstein DL. Laser methods in glaucoma. In Grant WM, Chandler PA (eds): Glaucoma. Philadelphia, Lea & Febiger, 1986, p 104.

105. Heuer DK. Glaucoma update. Ophthalmology 95:282, 1988.

106. Wise JB. Ten year results of laser trabeculoplasty. Does the laser avoid glaucoma surgery or merely defer it? Eye 45:1(part 1):4550, 1987.

107. Scheie HG, Edwards DL, Yanoff MC. Clinical and experimental observations using alpha chymotrypsin. Am J Ophthalmol 59:469, 1965.

108. Package insert. Iodipine (apraclonidine hydrochloride 1%). Fort worth: Alcon Surgical, 1991.

109. Pollack IP, Brown RH, Crandall AS, Steward RH, White GL. Prevention of the rise in intraocular pressure following neodymium-YAG posterior capsulotomy using topical 1% apraclonidine. Arch Ophthalmol 106:754–757, 1988.

110. Reid FR. Personal communication. Sept 17, 1991.

CHAPTER 49

HEADACHE

MARY L. WAGNER and STEPHEN D. SILBERSTEIN

The International Headache Society (IHS) now divides headaches into two broad categories and further divides these into 13 subcategories (Table 49.1). The two main categories are primary headache disorders and secondary headache disorders. Headaches that are a symptom of another disease are known as secondary headaches. The primary headache disorders include migraine headache, tension-type headache (TTH), and cluster headache. Migraine is further subdivided into two groups: migraine without aura (formerly common migraine) and migraine with aura (formerly classic migraine). TTH is subclassified as either episodic TTH (ETTH) or chronic TTH (CTTH). Cluster headache is similarly divided into the episodic and chronic varieties. Chronic daily headache (CDH) is a term in common use but not recognized by the IHS as a separate entity. This is confusing because CDH may be due to CTTH or a combination of migraine and TTH, and is often associated with abortive medication overuse (1). The IHS categorizes CDH as part of CTTH, but it has been called a variety of names, including *migraine with interparoxysmal headache, transformed migraine, evolutive migraine, mixed headache syndrome,* and *tension-vascular headache* (1, 2).

Changing concepts of headache pathogenesis have helped develop new headache treatments. The vascular theory of migraine and the muscle contraction theory of TTH are no longer tenable. Migraine and TTH may be part of a continuum of headache disorders involving the pain control system and amplified by neurovascular mechanisms, while cluster headache is a distinct entity that may use similar neurovascular mechanisms.

Headache diagnosis may be difficult, since many disorders have overlapping characteristics. It is based mainly on a complete medical history and general physical and neurologic examinations. Awareness of the presence of comorbid conditions is important, since patients with depression, anxiety, epilepsy, and stroke have a higher prevalence of migraine and the existence of these comorbid conditions influences headache treatment. This chapter discusses the primary headache disorders and their related comorbid conditions.

EPIDEMIOLOGY OF HEADACHES

Migraine Headaches

Migraine occurs in 18% of women, 6% of men, and 4% of children in the United States (3, 4). The American Migraine Study estimated that 23 million Americans suffer from severe migraine headaches (5). Migraine usually begins in the first three decades of life, and prevalence peaks in the fifth decade (4, 6). When headaches begin after age 50, a secondary organic cause must be considered. The prognosis for migraine sufferers is good, since migraine prevalence decreases with increasing age (6, 7). Most migraineurs have a positive family history of migraine. Sixty-two percent of migraineurs also have TTH (4). Contrary to the findings of clinic-based studies, the American Migraine Study found that migraine was more prevalent in families of lower socioeconomic class (3). The annual cost of headaches in terms of absenteeism from work, decreased worker productivity, and the cost of diagnostic tests and treatment ranges from 5 to 17 billion dollars (3, 8). Despite 10 million physician visits each year, migraine is still underdiagnosed and undertreated. Most migraineurs do not see a physician. Only about one third of headache sufferers are prescribed medications, and about half of these will discontinue their medications due to dissatisfaction (3).

Table 49.1.
New International Headache Society Classification of Headache (4,19)

1. Migraine
2. Tension-type headache
3. Cluster headache and chronic paroxysmal hemicrania
4. Miscellaneous headaches not associated with structural lesions
5. Headache associated with head trauma
6. Headache associated with vascular disorders
7. Headache associated with nonvascular intracranial disorders
8. Headache associated with substances or their withdrawal
9. Headache associated with noncephalic infections
10. Headache associated with metabolic disorders
11. Headache or facial pain associated with disorders of the cranium, neck, eyes, ears, nose, sinuses, teeth, mouth, or other facial or cranial structures
12. Cranial neuralgias, nerve trunk pain, and deafferentation pain
13. Headache not classifiable

Tension-Type Headaches

TTH is the most common headache type, with a lifetime prevalence of 69% in men and 88% in women. TTH can begin at any age, but onset during adolescence or young adulthood is most common. About 40% of patients evaluated in headache clinics suffer from CDH (2). Forty percent of patients exhibit a positive family history of TTH (4). Headache prevalence declines with increasing age; severity decreases in the women who continue to report headaches but does not change in men (7). Usually only patients with more severe or chronic headache, unresponsive to over-the-counter preparations, seek medical attention. Twenty-five percent of TTH patients also have migraine. Patients with ETTH are no different from controls in terms of stress, depression, anxiety, emotional conflicts, sleeping problems, and fatigue. Patients with CTTH are often depressed (4). The prognosis of CTTH is controversial, since many studies include more severe patients with coexisting conditions such as migraine and drug overuse.

Cluster Headaches

Cluster headache prevalence is lower than that of migraine or TTH, with a rate of 0.01 to 1.5% in various populations. Prevalence is higher in men than in women and in black versus white patients. Male to female ratio is about 5.6:1. A family history of cluster headache is rare. The most common form of cluster headache is episodic cluster; only about 10% of cluster patients have chronic cluster headache. Cluster headaches can begin at any age, but they most commonly begin in the late 20s. They rarely begin in childhood, and only about 10% of patients develop cluster in their 60s (4, 7, 9, 10).

Cluster events may be associated with high altitudes, sleep apnea, seasonal changes, or rapid eye movement (REM) sleep. Patients with cluster, despite the outward appearance of strength, often have feelings of inadequacy or dependency. The prognosis of cluster headaches is guarded; it is a chronic headache that may last for the patient's life. Drug therapy may help convert patients from chronic to episodic cluster (4, 7, 10).

PATHOPHYSIOLOGY OF HEADACHES

General Pain Theory

Peripheral pain receptors transmit sharp, localized pain via myelinated A-fibers and aching, burning pain via unmyelinated C-fibers to the dorsal horn of the spinal cord. Substance P (SP) and the excitatory amino acids are believed to be the neurotransmitters for the peripheral pain transmission system. In the spinal cord, enkephalins and γ-aminobutyric acid (GABA) modulate pain transmission. From the dorsal horn, two ascending pathways carry pain sensations to the somatosensory cortex (neothalamic pathway) and to the limbic forebrain and other areas (paleothalamic pathway) (11).

The central nervous system (CNS) modulates pain, in part, by the serotonergic and adrenergic pain-control systems. The descending serotonergic system originates in the periaqueductal gray area of the midbrain and, via the raphe magnus in the medulla, connects with the dorsal horn of the spinal cord. Analgesia is produced, in part, by serotonin (5-hydroxytryptamine or 5-HT) interacting with enkephalin-containing neurons. The ascending serotonergic system innervates the cerebral blood vessels, thalamus, hypothalamus, and cortex, and is involved in the regulation of cerebral blood flow (CBF), sleep, and neuroendocrine control. Ascending and descending noradrenergic pathways originate in the locus ceruleus of the pons. The ascending pathway innervates the microcirculation and the cerebral cortex. The descending pathway terminates in the dorsal horn of the spinal cord. Analgesia may be produced by interaction with GABA-containing interneurons (11).

The brain itself is insensitive to pain, but other structures, such as the skin of the scalp, the head and neck muscles, the great venous sinuses, the meningeal and cerebral arteries, parts of the 5th, 9th, and 10th cranial nerves, and parts of the dura mater, are pain sensitive. Pain impulses from these sites are transmitted to the spinal cord and brain stem. Direct connections between the primary sensory neurons (e.g., the trigeminal nerve) and the cerebral blood vessels have been detected (11). The trigeminal nerve contains SP, calcitonin gene related peptide (CGRP), and neurokinin A (NKA).

Stimulation of the trigeminal nerve leads to release of SP, NKA, and CGRP from unmyelinated sensory fibers in the dural vasculature. CGRP mediates vasodilation, whereas SP and NKA induce vascular leakage with extravasation of plasma proteins, platelet aggregation, and mast cell degranulation, resulting in neurogenic inflammation (inflammation and dilation of cephalic vessels) and pain. Drugs such as ergotamine, dihydroergotamine (DHE), and sumatriptan block the release of these substances by stimulating $5-HT_{1B/D}$ heteroreceptors on trigeminal nerve endings. The trigeminal nerve probably plays an important role in the generation of painful impulses in vascular headaches by producing neurogenic inflammation (4).

Migraine Headaches

Any theory of migraine must explain the prodrome, aura, headache, and associated symptoms. Theories of migraine pathogenesis include Wolff's vascular theory, Heyck's theory of open arteriovenous anastomoses (AVAs), and the neurovascular theory.

Wolff's classic vascular migraine theory proposed that the migraine aura was caused by intracerebral vasoconstriction and the headache by painful reactive vasodilation. Local mediators (histamine, 5-HT, vasoactive peptides, kinins, prostaglandins, thromboxane A_2, prostacyclin, and

ADP) serve to produce changes in vasomotor tone. This theory has not been substantiated by CBF studies, which show a decrease in CBF during migraine with aura (classic migraine) but not during migraine without aura (common migraine). It does not explain the prodromal features of migraine or why some antimigraine drugs have no effect on the cerebral vasculature (4).

Heyck's theory of open AVAs, based on reduced arteriovenous oxygen content differences on the headache side, suggests that the sudden opening of these shunts would bypass capillary beds and produce tissue ischemia and pain. However, subsequent microsphere studies have suggested that the increase in venous oxygen content is not due to shunting of blood but rather to increased tissue perfusion (7).

The comprehensive neurovascular theory has replaced these previous theories and is based on CBF studies, magnetic resonance spectroscopy, and magnetoencephalography research. It states that neuronal dysfunction with subsequent vascular changes is responsible for the onset and propagation of migraine.

The hypothalamus and limbic system affect afferent and efferent 5-HT and adrenergic pathways. Disturbances in these areas may precipitate the onset of a migraine headache with prodromal symptoms. Subsequently, the nucleus caudalis trigeminalis, a major relay nucleus for pain in the brainstem may be activated. It is unclear how the nucleus caudalis trigeminalis is stimulated, but it may be due to cortical spreading depression (a short-lasting wave of neuronal depolarization) and/or biochemical dysfunction which may stimulate trigeminal nerve endings. Cortical spreading depression, mediated in part by the N-methyl-D-aspartate (NMDA) receptor, may be caused by an intracellular magnesium deficiency and is further modulated by hypothalamic and limbic 5-HT and adrenergic pathways. An imbalance between facilitary and inhibitory neurons to the nucleus caudalis trigeminalis may render it more sensitive to input that normally would not trigger firing. This may explain why migraine sufferers have an increased susceptibility to head pain even during migraine-free periods. Stimulation of the trigeminal nerve results in release of SP and NKA that cause neurogenic inflammation and may further enhance neuronal sensitivity. Release of CGRP and nitric oxide promote blood flow fluctuations in adjacent microcirculatory blood vessels (4, 7, 12, 13).

A wave of decreased CBF spreading forward from the occipital cortex precedes the symptoms of aura in classic migraine and persists into the headache phase. This change in CBF, occurring only in classic migraine, is associated with neuronal depolarization (cortical spreading depression) that is thought to cause the aura symptoms. Following the aura phase, regional CBF increases and eventually returns to normal. Since the headache begins while CBF is decreased and ends while CBF is elevated, the headache cannot be due to reactive vasodilation as suggested in Wolff's classic hypothesis. The pain of migraine headaches with aura may be caused and propagated by cortical spreading depression, activation of the nucleus caudalis, and subsequent neurogenic inflammation. A hypothalamic/limbic disturbance involving serotonergic and adrenergic pathways or a direct effect on the trigeminal nucleus caudalis may similarly induce neurogenic inflammation in migraine without aura (4, 7, 12, 13).

Serotonin plays an important role in the pathogenesis of migraine headaches. Reserpine, a potent CNS 5-HT-depleting agent, precipitates migraine headaches. Migraine headaches generally improve with age possibly due to deceases in 5-HT receptors in the brain. Sleep reduces CNS 5-HT neuronal firing and aborts migraine attacks. In addition, plasma 5-HT concentrations decrease during a migraine attack and urinary excretion of 5-hydroxy-indoleacetic acid, the main 5-HT metabolite, increase. At least seven 5-HT receptors (5-HT_1, 5-HT_2, 5-HT_3, 5-HT_4, 5-HT_5, 5-HT_6, 5-HT_7), many with subtypes (5-HT_1 [A,B,D,E,F], 5-HT_2 [A,B,C], and 5-HT_5 [A,B]) have been identified. 5-HT receptor distribution and function is not uniform in the brain. Some receptors modulate CBF, whereas others modulate pain, sleep, thermoregulation, motor activity, emotional behavior, and sensory responsiveness. Activation of 5-HT_{1D} receptors decreases the release of 5-HT norepinephrine, acetylcholine, and SP. The inhibitory $5\text{-HT}_{1B/D}$ heteroreceptor on trigeminal nerve terminals blocks neurogenic inflammation and most drugs used to treat acute migraine are agonists at this receptor. 5-HT_2 stimulation results in bronchoconstriction, platelet aggregation, gastrointestinal smooth muscle contraction, and neural depolarization in the CNS. The majority of drugs used in the prevention of migraine are 5-HT_2 antagonists. 5-HT_3 stimulation causes nausea, vomiting, and activation of autonomic reflexes. Metoclopramide, a 5-HT_3 antagonist, is useful in the treatment of migraine-induced nausea (4, 7, 13, 14).

Other neurotransmitters and mediators, such as catecholamines, histamine, vasoactive peptides, endogenous opioids, prostaglandins, free fatty acids, and steroid hormones are also implicated in the pathogenesis of migraine. Migraineurs have an increase in plasma catecholamines before and during the migraine attack. Norepinephrine produces vasoconstriction via the postsynaptic $alpha_1$ receptors and promotes release of serotonin from platelets. Increased dopamine concentrations may be partially responsible for the nausea and vomiting observed during a migraine attack. Cerebrospinal fluid (CSF) concentrations of endogenous opioids have been reported to be both increased and decreased. Estrogens modulate 5-HT_1 and 5-HT_2 receptors and are implicated in the development of menstrual migraine. A rapid fall in estrogen, with resultant increases in prostaglandins and enhanced prolactin release, may be responsible for the initiation of the migraine attack.

Migraine often worsens during the first trimester of pregnancy, but often remits thereafter due to sustained high estrogen levels (4, 16).

In summary, the comprehensive neurogenic theory attempts to explain the complex events leading to a migraine attack. Disturbances of serotonin and related neurotransmitters at the hypothalamic/limbic level in concert with nucleus caudalis trigeminalis hypersensitivity promotes the release of pro-inflammatory and vasoactive substances that induce aura, painful headaches, and related symptoms.

Tension-Type Headaches

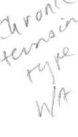

CTTH may be associated with a perceived increase in stressful life events. Depression is common in patients with CTTH. Neurotransmitter abnormalities in 5-HT, norepinephrine, dopamine, and enkephalins have been proposed as causes for depression and headache (4).

Although many patients with TTH have muscle tenderness, TTH is not the result of sustained contraction of the pericranial muscles with subsequent ischemic pain in response to emotion or stress. Muscle ischemia is not present during headache, and muscle blood flow is normal. EMG activity is increased in some muscles, independent of tenderness. A decreased hypothalamic opioid tone was previously thought to explain the patients' increased sensitivity to pain, but recent evidence has shown that CSF β-endorphin concentrations were similar to controls (16). Diminished sympathetic activity, decreased concentrations of 5-HT, and elevated concentrations of SP have been observed in the plasma of some patients (12). Reduced CNS 5-HT levels may be responsible for abnormal pain modulation, producing the decreased pain thresholds observed in most patients with CTTH. A "myofascial-supraspinal-vascular" model has been proposed for TTH (17). In the presence of the pain facilitation, normal subthreshold stimuli may produce significant pain even if myofascial nociceptor hypersensitivity is not present. The cranial muscle ache of a TTH attack may therefore be due to increased neuronal sensitivity and pain facilitation due to chronic or intermittent dysfunction of the monoaminergic or serotonergic function in the hypothalamus, brain stem, and spinal cord.

Cluster Headaches

The pathogenesis of cluster headaches has not been well defined. Cluster events may be related to alterations in the circadian pacemaker. Attacks increase following the beginning and end of daylight savings time, and there is a loss of circadian rhythm for blood pressure, temperature, and hormones, including prolactin, melatonin, cortisol, and endorphins. Hypothalamic dysfunction causes the loss of circadian rhythm. Neurogenic inflammation, carotid body chemoreceptor dysfunction, imbalance of central parasym-

pathetic and sympathetic tone, and increased responsiveness to histamine have been proposed as the cause of cluster pain (4).

DIAGNOSIS AND CLINICAL DESCRIPTION OF HEADACHES

Formal criteria for headache diagnosis were established by the IHS in 1988. A distinction has been made between primary headache disorders and those due to a secondary cause. There are both medical and pharmacologic causes of headache (Table 49.2). A complete history is needed for diagnosis and should include the following information: the age at headache onset, the time of onset (day, season), the location of the pain, the severity and type of pain, the attack frequency (including any change in frequency), the associated symptoms, the precipitating factors, the methods of palliation used, the patient's sleep habits, and the family history. In addition, a complete medication history should be taken to evaluate the dose, duration of use, and effectiveness of previous headache medications as well as to determine if any medications that could exacerbate headaches are being used.

The patient should keep a diary to record any changes between office visits and especially after medication changes. This will make the patient more aware of the disease process as well as help the physician evaluate the effectiveness and adverse effects of treatment. The physician should have patients bring in their medications to periodically check for compliance and any additional medications that other physicians may have prescribed.

Table 49.2.
Medical and Pharmacological Causes of Headache (3,4,75)

Medical	Pharmacological
Angiogram	Alcohol
Stroke	β-Blockers (atenolol)
Infection	Barbiturates
Inflammation	Caffeine and withdrawal
Tumors	Cannabis
Trigeminal neuralgia	Corticosteroids and withdrawal
Diseases of eyes, ears, nose, or throat	Digitalis
	Ergotamine and withdrawal
Menstruation and pregnancy	Estrogens and oral contraceptives
	Fluoxetine
Trauma	Foods (nitrites, glutamate, tyramine, or theobromine)
	Histamine-H₂-antagonists (cimetidine)
	Nonsteroidal Antiinflammatory Drugs (indomethacin)
	Sympathomimetics (amphetamines, dopamine, fenfluramine, theophylline)
	Vasodilators (captopril, dipyridamole, hydralazine, nifedipine, nitrates, prazosin, reserpine)

The pharmacist should also assess for compliance and ask questions to help evaluate potential adverse effects or poor efficacy.

Migraine Headaches

A diagnosis of migraine without aura (common migraine) requires the patient to have at least 5 headache attacks lasting 4 to 72 hours each and two of the following characteristics: unilateral location, pulsating quality, moderate or severe intensity, or aggravation by routine physical activity. During the attack, at least one of the following should occur: nausea/vomiting or photophobia and phonophobia. An organic disorder must be ruled out. If an organic disorder is present, the migraine attacks must not occur for the first time in close temporal relation to the organic disorder (4).

A diagnosis of migraine with aura (classic migraine) requires the patient to have at least two attacks with at least three of the following characteristics: (a) one or more fully reversible aura symptoms; (b) at least one aura symptom develops gradually over more than 4 minutes or two or more symptoms occur in succession; (c) no single aura symptom lasts more than 60 minutes; and (d) headache follows aura with a free interval of less than 60 minutes. In addition, secondary causes of the headache should be ruled out. If the aura lasts longer than an hour but less than a week, the migraine is called migraine with prolonged aura (4).

Migraine is more than just an aura and a headache. Some patients have four phases: the prodrome, the aura, the headache, and the postdrome (Table 49.3) (5, 18). The prodrome occurs hours to days before the headache and in about 60% of patients. During this time, patients may have various psychologic, sensory, constitutional, or autonomic symptoms. Not all patients experience a prodrome, but if they do, their prodromal symptoms are usually the same each time. The symptoms can continue into the aura and headache phases.

The aura develops over 5 to 20 minutes, lasts 20 to 30 minutes, and consists of focal neurologic symptoms that accompany the headache or occur up to an hour before the headache (19). About 20% of migraineurs experience an aura, which may be visual, sensory, or motor, or involve speech. Visual symptoms are the most common and include scintillations (fluorescent flashes of light in the visual field), fortification spectra or teichopsia (alternating light and dark lines in the visual field), photopsia (flashing lights), positive scotomata (bright geometric lights in the visual field), and negative scotomata (blind spots that may move across the visual field). Sensory symptoms include numbness, tingling, or paresthesias of the face or hand. Motor symptoms are usually hemiparetic, while language disturbances consist of difficulty understanding or speaking (aphasia) (5).

Table 49.3.
Migraine Headache Symptoms (4)

Prodrome Phase	
Mental	*General*
Depression	Stiff neck
Euphoria and hyperactivity	Cold feeling
Irritability	Sluggishness
Restlessness	Polydipsia
Mental slowness	Polyuria
Fatigue and drowsiness	Anorexia
Neurologic	Diarrhea
Photophobia	Constipation
Phonophobia	Fluid retention
Hyperosmia	Food cravings

Aura Phase	
Visual (20–35%)	*Sensory (33%)*
Photopsia (flashing lights)	Paresthesias (extremities and
Scotomata (partial loss of sight)	face)
Teichopsia (colors and tran-	*Motor disturbance and aphasia*
sient scotomata)	Monoparesis or hemiparesis
Visual distortions	Difficulty speaking
Hallucinations	Difficulty understanding lan-
	guage

Headache Phase	
Headache	*Neuropsychological*
Location (bilateral, 40%; uni-	Persistence of prodromal symp-
lateral, 60%)	toms
Throbbing quality (40–60%)	Photophobia
Scalp tenderness (66%)	Phonophobia
Short-lived "ice-pick" pain jabs	Osmophobia
(40%)	Lightheadedness
Gastrointestinal	Mood and mental changes
Anorexia	*Other*
Food cravings	Edema and polyuria
Nausea and vomiting (86%)	Nasal stuffiness (10–20%)
Constipation	Rhinorrhea
Diarrhea (16%)	

Postdrome Phase	
Neuropsychologic	*Others*
Fatigue	Mucle weakness and aching
Irritability	Anorexia
Impaired concentration	Food cravings

The headache can begin at any time during the day (20). The pain usually develops gradually and then subsides after 4 to 72 hours in adults and 2 to 48 hours in children. If the headache lasts longer than 72 hours, it is labeled *status migrainosus* (19). The pain is usually located in the temples but can occur anywhere in the face or head and may radiate down the neck and shoulder. The pain is moderate to severe in intensity and usually described as throbbing or pulsating with a unilateral distribution; however, the symptoms may begin as or become bilateral (20). Accompanying symptoms are common. Most patients are anorectic and have nausea; some vomit or have diarrhea. Photophobia and phonophobia cause patients to seek relief in a dark, quiet room to decrease sensory stimulation. Most patients experience between 1 and 4 headaches a month (7).

After the headache phase, some patients experience a postdrome, or recovery, phase that may last up to 24 hours. During this phase, some patients say they feel tired and others say they feel alert, some feel depressed and others feel euphoric, some feel worn out and others feel refreshed. Patients may complain of poor concentration, food intolerance, or scalp tenderness (5).

Tension-Type Headaches

The diagnosis of TTH requires that patients experience at least 10 previous headaches, each lasting 30 minutes to 7 days, with at least two of the following characteristics: a pressing/tightening (nonpulsating) quality, mild to moderate intensity, bilateral location, and no aggravation with physical activity. In addition, the patient should not have nausea/vomiting or a combination of photophobia and phonophobia. ETTH occurs less than 15 days a month, whereas CTTH occurs 15 or more days a month for at least 6 months (4, 7).

Patients describe the onset of the headache as gradual, often occurring after or during stress. Headaches last 30 minutes to a week, with a median duration of 12 hours. The headache is typically worse later in the day. The pain is usually bilateral and may be located in the forehead, the temples, or the back of the head, and may radiate to the neck and shoulders. Patients describe the steady, nagging, persistent, dull, aching pain as a tightness, a soreness, a squeezing sensation, or a constricting viselike pressure. They may say "it's as if a band were wrapped around my head" (4) or complain of scalp tenderness, rigid neck muscles, and jaw discomfort. The pain is mild to moderate in severity and is not aggravated by routine physical activity. Unlike migraine, there is no prodrome or associated autonomic or gastrointestinal symptoms. Some patients complain of anorexia. The frequency of episodic headaches ranges from 2 to 12 days a month, with a median of 6 days a month. The headaches may be precipitated by menstruation (1, 4).

Cluster Headaches

The diagnosis of cluster headaches requires the patient to have at least 5 untreated attacks of severe, unilateral, orbital, supraorbital, and/or temporal pain lasting 15 to 180 minutes. At least one of the following associated symptoms must occur: conjunctival injection, lacrimation, nasal congestion, rhinorrhea, facial sweating, miosis, ptosis, or eyelid edema. Episodic cluster headaches are distinguished by headache periods of 1 week to a year with remission periods lasting at least 14 days, whereas chronic cluster headaches have no remission periods or remissions that last

less than 14 days. Episodic cluster can evolve into chronic cluster headaches (9).

Cluster attacks may begin with slight discomfort that rapidly increases (within 15 minutes) to excruciating pain. The attacks often occur at the same time each day and frequently awaken patients from sleep. Untreated, the attacks generally last for 30 to 90 minutes, but they may last up to 180 minutes. The pain is described as unilateral, deep, constant, boring, pressing, piercing, or burning in nature, located behind or around the eye. It may radiate to the forehead, temples, jaws, nostrils, ears, neck, or shoulder. Patients may say "it's like driving a hot poker into my eye" (4). Some patients cannot describe the pain, and 30% describe it as throbbing or pulsating. Patients are usually pain-free between cluster periods, with remissions lasting 6 months to 2 years; however, isolated, mild, brief attacks may occur between cluster periods. During an attack, patients often feel agitated or restless and feel the need to isolate themselves and move around. Unlike migraine, cluster headaches are not associated with an aura but have, by definition, one or more associated symptoms of autonomic dysfunction. Lacrimation, the most common symptom, is reported by about 83% of patients. Gastrointestinal symptoms are uncommon. The attack frequency varies from one every other day to 8 a day, occurring in cluster periods that last a week to a year. Most patients have one or two cluster periods a year that last 2 to 3 months, with 1 to 2 attacks per day (7, 9, 21).

HEADACHE TREATMENT

General Treatment Guidelines

Headache treatment is divided into nonpharmacologic and pharmacologic therapy, which is further divided into acute and preventive treatment. The goal of acute treatment is to quickly relieve the headache pain as well as any associated symptoms. The goal of preventive treatment is to reduce the frequency and severity of attacks (22).

Drug choice depends on several factors, including the patient's headache type, comorbid conditions, and medication history, as well as each drug's adverse effect profile, pharmacokinetics, mechanism of action, and drug interaction potential. For preventive treatment, the medication selected should be started at a low dose and gradually increased, after ascertaining its effectiveness and lack of adverse effects or drug interactions, to the maximum dose necessary to achieve headache control. An adequate trial may take 1 to 2 months. Once headache control has been achieved, attempts should be made to taper and discontinue drug therapy (22).

Nonpharmacologic treatments for migraine and TTH include relaxation techniques, hypnosis, psychotherapy, biofeedback, physical therapy, and acupuncture (1, 22–24). These techniques may be useful either alone or combined with drug therapy. Physical therapy helps patients relieve stress and muscle tension via massage, stretching exercises, aerobic exercises, ultrasound treatments, electric stimulation, and hot or cold pack therapy (22, 24). Cold compresses to the affected area provided relief in 65 to 70% of TTH patients (24). Marcus established that relaxation therapy decreased headache frequency roughly 65% and allowed 70% of TTH patients and 58% of migraine patients to reduce their medication use (25). Biofeedback was found to decrease migraine headache in 65 to 84% of people when administered by psychologists (26). Physicians may do dry needling or inject trigger points with local anesthetics or corticosteroids (22).

Migraine Headaches

Most migraineurs describe headache-provoking (trigger) factors (Table 49.4), with alcohol, stress, menstruation, and diet being the most common (4). Patients should avoid these triggers and keep regular exercise, mealtime, and sleep patterns. Medications are the mainstay of treatment, but some patients complain of significant adverse effects from the preventive medications, and only 60 to 80% respond to treatment with a 50% reduction in headache frequency (27). Most placebo-controlled trials show an average placebo response (≥50% improvement) of approximately 30% over the first 4 weeks of therapy (28).

Medications are used acutely to abort attacks and chronically to prevent attacks. Some drugs, such as domperidone (30 mg) (29) or metoclopramide (10 mg) (30), work before the attack begins; these medications may prevent the headache if they are administered during the prodrome. Drugs used for acute treatment include: analgesics (aspirin, acetaminophen), nonsteroidal antiinflammatory drugs (NSAIDs), serotonin agonists, ergot alkaloids, neuroleptics, steroids, and narcotics. The sooner treatment is begun, the more effective the medications are. Caffeine, butalbital, isometheptene, and dichloralphenazone are adjunctive medications that are included in combination preparations to improve efficacy (7, 31–33).

Unless patients are prone to stomach ulcers, simple analgesics and NSAIDs are first-line therapy in mild to moderate headache attacks. If these fail, combination analgesics can be used. More severe attacks should be treated with ergotamine, dihydroergotamine (DHE), or

sumatriptan. Ergotamine tartrate should be limited to twice a week because of the risk of rebound headaches caused by more frequent dosing. Sumatriptan is effective but expensive, and up to 52% of patients have recurrent headaches (8). Some clinicians believe that patient-administered sumatriptan and DHE have the best efficacy-to-adverse effect ratio of all the acute-treatment medications (5, 7) and are the most cost-effective, since their use results in a decreased number of emergency visits (8). Since nausea and vomiting are symptoms that are commonly associated with migraine headaches, oral medications may be unsuitable and alternative formulations, as well as antiemetics, may be needed.

Preventive (prophylactic) treatment should be considered when (a) acute symptomatic treatment is required more often than two to three times a week; (b) two or more attacks occur per month that produce disability for more than 3 days; (c) drugs used for acute treatment are ineffective, intolerable, or contraindicated; (d) headaches are severely disabling or are associated with significant neurologic symptoms or signs; and (e) attacks occur in a predictable pattern (5, 27). Preventive treatment includes antidepressants, β-blockers, calcium channel blockers, NSAIDs, serotonin antagonists (methysergide, cyproheptadine), and anticonvulsants (valproic acid). Other, less commonly used, prophylactic treatments include clonidine, calcitonin, captopril, and lithium carbonate. Some clinicians feel that β-blockers and antidepressants have the best efficacy–to–adverse effect ratio of the prophylactic medications (5, 7). Antidepressants may be a good choice for patients with asthma, bradycardia, or comorbid depression, whereas β-blockers may be a good choice for those who have comorbid hypertension or cannot tolerate the anticholinergic effects of antidepressants. Valproic acid is the drug of choice for patients with coexistent mania or epilepsy (4). Preventive treatment should be started at a low dose and increased slowly until headache severity or frequency decreases, the maximum recommended dose is reached, or adverse effects develop. The dose titrations may take several months (5). Once the headaches have been controlled for about 6 months, attempts can be made to taper and discontinue therapy. Patients should be monitored for acute medication overuse, which may result in chronic refractory headaches and withdrawal symptoms when the medication is discontinued.

The pregnant headache patient should be treated conservatively. Nonpharmacologic treatment should be attempted, and if the patient does not respond to this therapy, acetaminophen (alone or with narcotics) can be used. Very severe attacks should be treated in the hospital with intravenous fluids and narcotics. Prednisone has occasionally been used, but aspirin, barbiturates, and benzodiazepines should be limited and ergotamine and sumatriptan should be avoided completely. In the breast-

Table 49.4.
Trigger Factors of Migraine (4)

Psychologic:	stress, tension, anxiety
Neurologic:	bright lights or glare, odors, changes in sleep patterns, hormonal changes, changes in weather or temperature
Physical:	exercise, fatigue, sexual activity, high altitude
Dietary:	missed or delayed meals, food additives, alcohol

feeding migraineur, bromocriptine, ergotamine, and lithium should be avoided, since these drugs readily transfer to the baby via breast milk and can cause significant toxicity. Benzodiazepines, antidepressants, and neuroleptics may be used cautiously. Acetaminophen is preferable to aspirin (34).

Tension-Type Headaches

EPISODIC TENSION-TYPE HEADACHE

TTH patients usually self-medicate with over-the-counter analgesics (aspirin, acetaminophen, ibuprofen, naproxen), with or without caffeine, and rarely seek medical attention. In an effort to decrease the incidence of analgesic overuse, patients should be educated about the effectiveness of nonpharmacologic treatment. If these measures are not effective, prescription NSAIDs or combination analgesic preparations can be used. Combination analgesics contain sedatives, narcotics, or caffeine, and their use should be limited, as overuse may cause dependence. Overusing symptomatic medications, including tranquilizers and analgesics, can cause ETTH to convert to CTTH. Patients with combination migraine/TTH may benefit from parenteral sumatriptan or DHE therapy (1, 24).

Preventive therapy is rarely needed but should be administered when a patient has frequent headaches that produce disability or requires frequent use of symptomatic therapy that may lead to medication overuse. Medications used for TTH prevention include antidepressants, β-blockers, and anticonvulsants. Antidepressants, often the medication of choice, should be started at a low dose and increased slowly every 3 to 7 days. As with other drug therapies, an adequate trial period of at least 1 to 2 months must be allowed. The addition of biofeedback therapy or β-blocking agents may improve the therapeutic benefit derived from antidepressants (35).

CHRONIC TENSION-TYPE HEADACHE (CTTH)

CTTH is often caused by abortive medication overuse by patients with ETTH. Tricyclic antidepressants are most commonly used to treat CTTH due to the high incidence of concurrent depression. Nonpharmacological treatments may also be helpful. Analgesics, tranquilizers, ergot alkaloids, and β-blockers are either ineffective or contraindicated due to their abuse potential or risk of worsening depression (7).

Chronic Daily Headache (CDH)

CDH is often confused with CTTH but they are not identical. CDH may be due to CTTH or combined migraine and TTH, and is often associated with abortive medication overuse. It is important to determine the cause of the chronic headache so that the appropriate treatment can be chosen. When concurrent depression and medica-

tion dependence accompany CDH, treatment is difficult and detoxification may be required. Refractory rebound headaches may occur when aspirin, acetaminophen, or opiate-containing analgesics are overused, or when analgesics are taken more frequently than 3 days a week or ergotamine tartrate more often than 2 days a week (1). To avoid this situation, specific limits should be made known to the patient regarding the quantity and frequency of use of analgesics and ergots (4).

Patients overusing analgesics or ergotamine must be detoxified. This can be done as an outpatient by slowly tapering the offending medication if there are no risk factors and the patient can tolerate it. If the patient cannot tolerate the taper, NSAIDs (7) or a short course (about 2 weeks) of corticosteroids may be useful (36). Clonidine (0.1 to 0.3 mg bid-tid) has been helpful for treating opiate withdrawal symptoms and phenobarbital for short-acting barbiturate withdrawal symptoms (7, 36). Refractory patients often require hospitalization for repetitive intravenous (IV) DHE and an antiemetic to control their refractory headaches (36). Detoxification with IV DHE relieves headaches in about 90% of patients (37), although some patients require fluid and electrolyte replacement as well as phenothiazines (7).

Cluster Headaches

Patients with cluster headaches should avoid alcohol, histamine, and nitroglycerin. Other dietary and drug restrictions have little effect on cluster headaches. Pharmacologic treatment for cluster headaches is divided into acute and preventive therapy, and recommendations are mainly based on uncontrolled trials.

Oral preparations are absorbed slowly and are not recommended for the treatment of acute attacks. Effective abortive treatments that provide rapid onset of action include oxygen, sumatriptan, DHE mesylate, and (perhaps) topical local anesthetics. Inhaled oxygen, 7 to 10 L/min for 10 minutes following the headache onset is 70% effective and is often the drug of first choice. The major limitation is the availability of oxygen. Hyperbaric oxygen (202.6 kPa) for 30 minutes has been reported to provide rapid and long-lasting relief. Parenteral injections of sumatriptan or DHE mesylate provide significant relief for about 80% of patients. Intranasal local anesthetic may provide relief for some patients. Narcotics are not indicated in the acute treatment of cluster headache, since their efficacy is limited and frequent use can lead to overuse and addiction (9).

Most cluster headache patients require preventive treatment because each attack is too short in duration and too severe in intensity to treat with only abortive medication. In addition, ergotamine, DHE, sumatriptan, and oxygen may just postpone, rather than abort, the attack. Preventive therapy for episodic cluster, in order of preference, includes ergotamine or calcium channel blockers, methysergide, lithium or valproic acid, and capsaicin. Corticosteroids are used to break a cluster cycle or to treat severe attacks. Verapamil may be used in combination with ergotamine, lithium or valproic acid (7, 9). Occasionally the NSAID indomethacin is effective. Chlorpromazine, β-blockers, and antidepressants are ineffective for cluster prophylaxis. Some patients may become resistant to therapy and require polypharmacy (9). Resetting the circadian pacemaker with light-exposure therapy may reduce the number of cluster headache attacks (4, 10).

Prophylactic therapy for chronic cluster includes lithium, valproic acid, calcium channel blockers, pizotifen, and methysergide. If medical therapy fails completely, surgical intervention may be beneficial for the psychologically stable patient with strictly unilateral chronic cluster. Surgery consists of neuronal ablation procedures directed toward the sensory input of the trigeminal nerve and autonomic pathways. It is generally 75% effective (4, 7, 10).

Chronic paroxysmal hemicrania, a rare variant of cluster headache usually unresponsive to cluster prophylaxis is treatable with indomethacin (4).

Headaches in Children

When children present with headaches they are usually migraine headaches. Acute treatment begins with simple analgesics and family assurance. Acetaminophen should be used instead of aspirin due to the risk for Reye's syndrome. Since sudden changes in daily routine may precipitate headaches in children, an attempt should be made to maintain a regular daily schedule. Generally ergot derivatives should be avoided in young children; however, DHE can be used alone or in combination with metoclopramide or promethazine. Combination theory can achieve an 80 to 90% improvement in intractable headaches. Pediatric prophylactic drug therapy is the same as that used in adults. The most commonly used medications include propranolol (1 to 3 mg/kg/day) and cyproheptadine (0.2 to 0.4 mg/kg/day). Tricyclic antidepressants may be used as adjunctive therapy or in difficult-to-control patients. A drug taper or holiday should be considered if a child has been headache-free for 3 or more months (4).

PHARMACOTHERAPY OF HEADACHES

Drugs used for the acute (abortive) treatment of headache include simple analgesics (aspirin, acetaminophen, NSAIDs), alone or in combination with caffeine or barbiturates, narcotics (alone or in combination with other drugs), isometheptene combinations, ergotamine, DHE, sumatriptan, neuroleptics, and corticosteroids. Drugs used for preventive (prophylactic) headache treatment include β-blockers, calcium channel blockers, antidepressants, anticonvulsants, lithium, and serotonin agonists. Dosing

and indication for the following agents are described in Tables 49.5 and 49.6.

Nonnarcotic Analgesics

The mechanism of action of nonnarcotic analgesics is not clear, but they probably decrease inflammation by inhibiting the enzyme cyclo-oxygenase, thus inhibiting prostaglandin synthesis. Aspirin concentrations peak within 30 minutes following oral absorption, and peak levels of other NSAIDs are generally achieved within 2 hours (7). The delayed gastrointestinal emptying that commonly occurs in migraineurs may interfere with drug absorption (38). Indomethacin and aspirin are available in suppository form, and ketorolac can be administered parenterally, routes of administration that may be useful for patients with nausea or vomiting. The more lipid-soluble NSAIDs, such as indomethacin or ketoprofen, may be more efficacious, since they have greater CNS penetration (39). These agents should not be taken continuously for more than a week (ketorolac must be limited to 5 days) for menstrual migraine, and otherwise they should be limited to 3 times per week. The dose of aspirin or acetaminophen should be limited to 1000 mg per attack or 4000 mg daily (4). Caffeine has been shown to enhance the analgesic activity of nonnarcotic analgesics (40). Administering metoclopramide prior to analgesics enhances gastric emptying and promotes their absorption.

Aspirin, acetaminophen, and NSAIDs are used for acute (and prophylactic) treatment of migraine and TTH. NSAIDs are particularly useful in menstrual migraineurs. Ketorolac was not as effective as DHE with intravenous (IV) metoclopramide in relieving acute migraine (41). However, naproxen sodium was shown to be as effective as ergotamine in aborting acute migraine headaches (38). To date, other NSAIDs have not been shown to be superior to aspirin (7); however, long-acting NSAIDs may not be associated with rebound headaches (27) and may be useful in treating patients who are abusing ergotamine (7). A 650-mg aspirin and a 1000-mg acetaminophen dose will provide similar pain relief (42). Because of the association between aspirin use and Reye's syndrome in children under the age of 15, acetaminophen should be used in this population. Patients not responding to one agent may respond to another. Generally, prophylactic use of aspirin should be avoided in order to prevent rebound headaches, but the Physician's Health Study reported that 325 mg of aspirin administered every other day to 22,000 men decreased migraine headache frequency by approximately 20% (38).

Adverse reactions to nonnarcotic analgesics include gastrointestinal upset, gastrointestinal bleeding, peptic ulcers, abdominal pain, dizziness, fluid retention, sedation, and tinnitus. NSAIDs are relatively contraindicated in patients with gastritis, peptic ulcer disease, or kidney

Table 49.5.
Abortive Pharmacotherapy (4, 5, 7, 9, 24)

Agent	Usual Adult Dose	Maximum Daily Dose	Time to Onset of Action	Headache	Comments
Ergot alkaloids					
Dihydroergotamine (DHE)	0.25–1 mg (IM/IV) stat; repeat every 1 hr	2 mg (IV)	<10 min (IV) 15–30 min (IM)	M, C	Fewer adverse effects than ergotamine. Total parenteral dose should not exceed 6 mg per week. Intranasal dosage form awaiting FDA approval.
	1 mg (SC) stat; repeat in 1 hr	3 mg (SC/IM)	30 min (SC) 30–60 min (IN)		
	2–3 mg (IN) stat; repeat in 1 hr	6 mg (IN)			
Ergotamine	1–2 mg PO/SL/PR stat; repeat every 30 min prn	6 mg (PO/SL/PR)	30 min (PO)	M, C	Do not use in patients with ischemic heart disease, uncontrolled hypertension, or cerebrovascular disease. Inhalation no longer available.
Serotonin agonists					
Sumatriptan	6 mg SC stat; repeat > 1 hr	12 mg (SC)	10–15 min (SC)	M, C	Should not be used in patients with ischemic heart disease or uncontrolled hypertension. Intranasal dosage form awaiting FDA approval.
	25-100 mg PO stat	300 mg (PO)	30–60 min (PO)		
Narcotic analgesics					
Butorphanol	1 mg IN stat; repeat 60–90 min	8 mg (IN)	15 min	M	Less abuse potential.
	2 mg IM stat; repeat 3–4 hr	4 mg (IM)			
Hydromorphone	2–4 mg (PO) stat	16 mg	15–30 mn	M	Abuse potential.
Meperidine	75–100 mg (PO, PR, IM, IV) stat	400 mg	Peak analgesia 60 min (PO) 20–60 min (PR) 30–50 min (IM) 20 min (IV)	M	Abuse potential.
Morphine	5–10 mg (PO, PR, IM, IV) stat	60 mg	Peak analgesia 60 min (PO) 20–60 min (PR) 30–60 min (IM) 20 min (IV)	M	Abuse potential.
Nonnarcotic analgesics					
Aspirin	325–650 mg PO stat; repeat every 4 hr prn	2600 mg	60 min	M, T	Available rectally.
Acetaminophen	325–650 mg PO stat; repeat every 4 hr prn	2600 mg	60 min	M, T	Available rectally.
Ibuprofen	400–600 mg PO stat; repeat every 6 hr prn	2400 mg	60 min	M, T	Ibuprofen may have fewer gastrointestinal side effects than other NSAIDs.
Ketolorac	10 mg PO stat; repeat every 6 hr prn, or 30–60 mg IM stat	40 mg PO 120 mg IM	60 min	M, T	Pain relief equal to morphine. No sedation or addiction. Need to monitor renal function.
Naproxen	250–750 mg PO stat; repeat every 8 hr prn	1500 mg	60 min	M, T	Naproxen may cause drowsiness.
Naproxen sodium	275–825 mg PO stat; repeat every 8 hr prn	1,650 mg		M, T	
Neuroleptics					
Chlorpromazine	25–50 mg IV/IM stat; repeat every 4 hr prn	400 mg	10–20 min (IV/IM)	M, T	Antiemetic effect.
	25–100 mg PR stat; repeat every 6–8 hr prn		60 min (PR)		
Prochlorperazine	5–10 mg IV/IM stat; repeat every 4 hr prn	40 mg (IV/IM) 75 mg (PR)	10–20 min (IV/IM)	M, T	Antiemetic effect.
	25 mg PR stat; repeat every 8–12 hr prn		60 min (PR)		

(continued)

Table 49.5. *(Continued)*

Agent	Usual Adult Dose	Maximum Daily Dose	Time to Onset of Action	Headache	Comments
Neuroleptics—cont'd.					
Thiothixene	5 mg PO/IM stat	20 mg		M	
Corticosteroids					
Dexamethasone	4–8 mg PO stat; repeat in 60 min	32 mg (PO)		M, C	
Prednisone	40–100 mg PO	200 mg PO		M, C	Short course then rapidly taper over 2–3 weeks. Higher doses needed for episodic cluster.
Miscellaneous agents					
Lidocaine	1 ml of 4% solution IN every 15 min		15–30 min (IN)	C	
Oxygen	7–10 L/min for 15 min		5–10 min (IH)	C	More effective when given at maximum pain intensity.

IM, intramuscular; IV, intravenous; IN, intranasal; PO, oral; PR, rectal; SC, subcutaneous; M, migraine headaches; C, cluster headaches; T, tension-type headaches

disease. Large quantities (more than 50 g/month) of simple analgesics may cause migraine headaches to transform into CDH (3).

Patients should be told to take NSAIDs with meals to minimize their GI adverse effects. They should be monitored for potential gastrointestinal blood loss, renal dysfunction, worsening of hypertension, and aggravation of colitis.

Narcotic Analgesics

The analgesic action of the opioids is related to their action at the μ, κ, and δ opioid receptors located on neurons at supraspinal and spinal levels. Opioids may also produce peripheral analgesia by modulating neuropeptide release from receptor endings. Morphine, meperidine, and their derivatives are nonspecific agonists with a predominant effect at the μ receptor, whereas pentazocine, butorphanol, nalbuphine, and nalorphine exhibit agonist activity at the κ receptor and antagonistic activity at the μ receptor. Buprenorphine is a partial agonist at the μ receptor. Stimulation of the μ receptor results in respiratory depression, miosis, gastroparesis, and euphoria. κ-Receptor agonists produce feelings of disorientation and depersonalization. The δ receptors are also thought to mediate dysphoric effects of opioids (43).

Opioids are useful for patients with intractable menstrual migraine, those who fail or have contraindications to other migraine medications, and patients who require rescue medication, especially in the middle of the night. These agents are less frequently prescribed than other medications, due to the fear of abuse. Dependence and risk for rebound headaches following abrupt opioid discontinuation occurs within 2 to 3 weeks of regular use, but combination preparations that contain a nonnarcotic analgesic, caffeine, and intermediate-acting barbiturates possess a similar potential for abuse and rebound (36).

The efficacy of opioid analgesics is poorly documented in the literature. In a retrospective trial, only 29% of patients with an acute migraine attack experienced relief from an intramuscular meperidine and promethazine combination. An open-label trial with meperidine/hydroxyzine, butorphanol, and DHE/metoclopramide showed that complete relief of vascular headache was achieved in 0%, 27%, and 73% of patients respectively. A double-blind trial with intramuscular butorphanol showed a dose-dependent relief of acute migraine, but 21% and 42% of patients required pain and antiemetic relief medication respectively. A nasal dosage form of butorphanol was shown to be more effective than placebo and to possess a faster onset of action than intramuscular methadone in moderate to severe migraine headaches (7, 44).

Most opioids are absorbed well from the gastrointestinal tract, but bioavailability is often low due to extensive first-pass hepatic metabolism. Opioids are widely distributed; they enter the placenta and in addition are excreted into breast milk. The analgesic duration of action of most opioids is approximately 4 to 6 hours and is independent of their plasma half-life. Two active metabolites, morphine-6-glucuronide and normeperidine, exhibit analgesic and neuroexcitatory properties, respectively (43). The plasma butorphanol concentrations following intranasal administration are similar to those resulting from a parenteral dose, with the exception that peak concentrations are lower and slightly delayed. However, the onset of action with both the parenteral and intranasal formulations occurs within 15 minutes. The most common adverse effects of opioids are sedation, nausea, and vomiting, however, psychiatric reactions have been reported (38). Butorphanol has an adverse effect profile similar to that of most other opioids, and sedation may occur in 43% of patients (45).

Table 49.6.
Preventive Pharmacotherapy (4, 5, 7, 9, 22, 24)

Drug	Starting Dose (mg/day)	Maximum Dose (mg/day)	Headache	Comments
β-*Blockers*				
Atenolol	50	200	M, T	β$_1$-specific at lower doses. Dosed once daily.
Metoprolol	50	300	M, T	β$_1$-specific at lower doses. Long acting dosed once daily.
Nadolol	20	240	M, T	Dosed once daily.
Propranolol	40	320	M, T	More CNS effects. Long acting dosed once daily.
Timolol	10	60	M, T	
Calcium channel blockers				
Diltiazem	120	360	M, C	
Nifedipine	30	180	C	
Verapamil	120	720	M, T, C	The high doses, often used in cluster, need careful monitoring.
Serotonin antagonists-agonists				
Cyproheptadine	4	36	M	Antihistamine activity. Used in children, but may inhibit growth.
Methysergide	2	14	M, T, C	Risk for fibrotic changes. Requires drug holidays.
Antidepressants				
Amitriptyline	10	300	M, T	Strong sedative and anticholinergic effects.
Doxepin	10	150	M, T	
Fluoxetine	10	80	M, T	Fewer anticholinergic effects. Increased risk for insomnia.
Imipramine	10	200	M, T	
Nortriptyline	10	125	M, T	
Phenelzine	30	90	M, T	Requires close medical supervision. Inform patient of dietary restrictions.
Anticonvulsants				
Phenytoin	200	400	M	C_p = 10–20 μg/mL, often used in children.
Valproic acid	250	60 mg kg	M, T, C	C_p = 50–120 μg/mL, use with caution in children.
Nonnarcotic Analgesics				
Ibuprofen	800	2400	M	Menstrual migraine.
Naproxen	500	1500	M	Menstrual migraine.
Corticosteroids				
Prednisone	40	100	C	For episodic cluster. Taper over 1–2 weeks.
Ergot Alkaloids				
Ergotamine	2	4	C	Maximum dose 10 mg/week and may skip doses 1–2 times/week. Do not use in patients with cardiovascular disease. For episodic cluster.
Methylergonovine	0.6	1.6	M, C	Do not use in patients with cardiovascular disease. Replaced ergonovine.
Miscellaneous Agents				
Calcitonin	100 IU IM 200 IU IN		M	
Captopril	25	150	M	
Clonidine	0.2	0.6	M	
Lithium	600	1800	M, C	C_p = 0.4–1.2 mEq/L
Papaverine	300	600	M	Use with caution in patients with glaucoma.

IM, intramuscular; IN, intranasal; M, migraine headaches; C, cluster headaches; T, tension-type headaches

Antiemetics

The associated symptoms of a migraine attack are often very disabling. Metoclopramide, (a 5-HT$_3$ antagonist and 5-HT$_4$ agonist) promethazine, and ondansetron all have been used as adjunctive therapy to improve the accompanying nausea and vomiting. Metoclopramide decreases nausea and vomiting but also enhances drug absorption by decreasing gastric stasis. Their effect is best when administered as soon as symptoms begin (7, 38, 46). Drowsiness and dizziness are the most common adverse effects, but dystonic reactions may occur rarely (38).

Combination Preparations

When patients do not respond to simple analgesics, combination products may have synergistic activity and allow lower doses, minimizing adverse effects. Butalbital helps reduce anxiety and aids in sleep, while caffeine enhances absorption and may aid pain reduction. Adverse effects include drowsiness and dizziness. More than 200 mg of caffeine per day may lead to caffeine withdrawal headaches when the preparations are not taken (24).

There are various combinations of acetaminophen (325 mg, 500 mg, 650 mg) with butalbital (50 mg) that may include caffeine or codeine. These preparations are available in tablet or capsule formulations; some examples include Fioricet, Esgic, Isocet, Bancap, Endolor, Amaphen, Two-Dyne, Phrenilin, and Sedapap. Adults should start with 1 or 2 pills as soon as symptoms begin and repeat every 4 to 6 hours, with a maximum of 6 pills per attack. Acute use of acetaminophen should be limited to 4 g/day for less than 10 days, and chronic use should be limited to less than 2.6 g/day. Some clinicians limit acetaminophen use to less than 2 to 3 times per week.

Acetaminophen is also combined with isometheptene, a sympathomimetic amine with vasoconstrictor properties, and dichloralphenazone, a mild sedative (Midrin). Studies indicate that it is superior to placebo and of similar efficacy to ergotamine with caffeine (Cafergot). It is used in acute migraine in patients who cannot tolerate NSAIDs or ergotamine. Patients should start with 2 capsules and then take 1 capsule every hour, up to a maximum of 5 capsules per attack. Adverse effects include transient dizziness or a skin rash. Rebound headaches may occur with frequent use. Midrin is contraindicated in patients with glaucoma, renal failure, significant hypertension, heart or liver disease or patients using MAOIs within the last 2 weeks (7).

There are also various combinations of aspirin (325 mg or 650 mg) with butalbital (50 mg) that may include caffeine or codeine. These preparations are available in tablet or capsule formulations; some examples include Fiorinal, Fiorgen, Fortabs, Idenal, Isollyl, Lanorinal, Marnal, and other generic preparations.

Aspirin and acetaminophen are also combined with other narcotics such as propoxyphene, dihydrocodeine, hydrocodone, or oxycodone. Again, caution should be used in patients with risk of addiction. Since the bioavailabilities of the oral and IV forms are not equivalent, dosage adjustment will be necessary.

Serotonin Agonists

Animal data suggest that serotonin agonists decrease headache symptoms by decreasing inflammation in the dura mater of the brain by activating prejunctional 5-HT_1 heteroreceptors on the trigeminal nerve. Activation blocks the release of neurokinin such as SP, CGRP, and neuropeptide A (5, 7). These agents are relatively contraindicated and should be used cautiously in patients with coronary artery disease (CAD), peripheral vascular disease (PVD), or uncontrolled hypertension (HTN).

SUMATRIPTAN

Sumatriptan, a serotonin analog that selectively binds to 5-HT_{1A}, 5-HT_{1B}, and 5-HT_{1D} receptors, has been studied in the acute treatment of migraine, TTH, and cluster headaches. Significant pain relief begins within 10 minutes following injection, and migraine headache pain was reduced or completely relieved in 70% of patients within

1 hour and 86% of patients within 2 hours. If the first dose of sumatriptan is not effective, a second injection after an hour usually provides little added benefit. Sumatriptan is especially useful when nausea or vomiting is present, since it also ameliorates associated symptoms such as nausea, vomiting, photophobia, and phonophobia (5, 47). Other studies have noted similar improvement in perioperative migraine, menstrual migraine, and early morning migraine (5). Administering sumatriptan during the aura phase may not delay or prevent the migraine (38). The use of sumatriptan in patients with TTH is poorly documented; smaller (2 to 4 mg) doses may provide relief in 70% of patients with this disorder, although a slower onset of action (60 minutes) has been observed (48). About 75% of cluster headache patients who were given sumatriptan 6 mg subcutaneously (SC) reported headache relief within 15 minutes. The need for rescue with 100% oxygen inhalation at 15 minutes was lower after sumatriptan than with placebo (47).

Orally administered sumatriptan is as effective as SC injection but has a later onset of action. Sumatriptan 100 mg results in greater pain relief and less use of rescue medications than do comparative regimens of ergotamine 2 mg with caffeine (Cafergot) and aspirin 900 mg with metoclopramide 10 mg. Four hours after administration 75% of patients reported headache relief (5, 47).

About 40% of patients initially responding to sumatriptan report a return of headache symptoms 24 to 48 hours after the oral dose or injection, presumably due to sumatriptan's short half-life. Sumatriptan should be readministered when headaches recur, with a limit of 26 mg injections (spaced by at least 1 hour) or 300 mg orally within a 24-hour period (38, 47). It is unclear whether concomitant therapy with sumatriptan would decrease the headache recurrence rate (3). Patients generally prefer the slightly more efficacious injectable form to the tablet (7).

Prior to use, the patient should be instructed on how to load the autoinjector and how to discard the empty syringes. When using the autoinjector syringe, the patient should inject the contents into the deltoid muscle or the lateral part of the thigh. Sumatriptan is expensive, and since it is equally effective whether patient-administered or physician-administered (47), cost-effectiveness studies need to be performed to see if patient administration of sumatriptan decreases emergency visits or improves poor work performance.

Sumatriptan undergoes linear pharmacokinetics. Bioavailability is 14% with oral administration and 96% with SC administration. The plasma half-life is 2 hours, and peak blood concentrations occur within 20 minutes after SC injection (47). The drug has a large volume of distribution (170 L), has low protein binding (14 to 21%), and does not penetrate well into the CNS, but it crosses the placenta and also enters breast milk. Sumatriptan is metabolized primarily to inactive metabolites that are excreted into the urine and feces. Increased plasma concentrations may occur in patients with hepatic failure. Renal clearance is only 20%, and dosage adjustment in renal failure is not necessary. The pharmacokinetics of oral sumatriptan are not affected by food or other antimigraine drugs (47). The maximum single oral dose is 100 mg, as adverse effects (but not efficacy) increase with doses over 100 mg (7). Orally administered sumatriptan is almost equivalent in efficacy to SC, but it has a longer onset time (5). Oral tablets became available in the U.S. September 1995 and an intranasal formulation is under investigation.

Sumatriptan's adverse effects include pain upon injection, tingling, flushing, burning, dizziness, heaviness, neck pain, dysphoria, noncardiac chest pressure, and warm or hot sensations. These effects usually dissipate within 45 minutes. Sumatriptan is contraindicated in ischemic heart disease, as patients may experience coronary vasospasms with symptoms of angina (3, 5). Postmarketing surveillance reports of coronary and neurologic events have prompted revised labeling. Physicians are now required to confirm the diagnosis of migraine, administer the first dose in the office, and perform an electrocardiogram if angina symptoms occur (4). To decrease the risk of additive vasoconstriction, patients should wait at least 24 hours after ergotamine administration before starting sumatriptan (38).

ERGOT ALKALOIDS: ERGOTAMINE AND DIHYDROERGOTAMINE (DHE)

Ergotamine tartrate and DHE are ergot alkaloids that are nonspecific serotonergic ($5\text{-}HT_{1A}$, $5\text{-}HT_{1B}$, $5\text{-}HT_{1D}$, $5\text{-}HT_{1F}$, $5\text{-}HT_{2C}$), adrenergic (α-agonist and antagonist), and dopaminergic receptor agonists (3,5). Stimulation of α-adrenergic and serotonergic receptors constricts arterial smooth muscle. Ergots also cause venoconstriction, decrease platelet aggregation, and decrease neurogenic inflammation (7). Ergots are used as both prophylactic and acute treatment of migraine and cluster headaches. Prophylactic use, however, should be reserved for patients with menstrual migraine and for cluster patients at the beginning of a cycle. DHE, an ergotamine derivative, is a less potent arterial vasoconstrictor but a stronger α-adrenergic blocker than ergotamine. DHE also inhibits the baroreceptor circulatory reflex and has a greater effect on venous capacitance vessels than on resistance vessels (4).

Ergotamine effectively reduces the intensity and duration of attacks and is used to treat moderate to severe migraines when simple analgesics fail (4). It can be administered using sublingual, oral, or suppository dosage forms. The sublingual form is the least effective and the suppository is the most effective (7).

Because ergotamine is an old drug, there are not many well-designed studies; however, it is now the standard drug in many of the controlled trials testing the efficacy of newer agents. One of the first efficacy studies reported headache relief in 41% of patients taking 2 mg orally every hour up to 8 mg and 89% in patients taking 0.5 mg IV ergotamine. Ergotamine (1 to 6 mg) was superior to placebo, aspirin (500 mg), and isometheptene (130 to 390 mg) in several studies; however, two other studies found that ergotamine was not superior to placebo or isometheptene (130 to 390 mg). Ergotamine (1 to 6 mg) was equivalent to tolfenamic acid (200 mg), dextropropoxyphene (65 to 200 mg), naproxen (825 to 1, 375 mg), and pirprofen (200 to 500 mg), but not as good as sumatriptan (100 mg oral). More comparative trials using different dosage forms of ergotamine or DHE are needed. It is not clear whether ergotamine should be avoided during the aura phase of migraine (7).

Since the oral absorption of ergotamine is erratic and poor, it is best administered rectally (49). Due to extensive first-pass metabolism, the bioavailability of orally administered ergotamine is less than 1% (7). Peak plasma concentrations are reached 1 to 2 hours after oral or rectal administration and 20 minutes after IM administration. It is primarily metabolized in the liver, with a clearance about equal to hepatic blood flow. Dosage schemes are individualized for each patient, starting with the lowest dose and increasing to the highest dose that does not cause nausea (4, 7). DHE is available as SC, IM, or IV injection, and an intranasal dosage form is awaiting FDA approval (38). Bioavailability of DHE is best with IV injection and most erratic with SC injection (4, 50, 51). Bioavailability is 43% after intranasal DHE (13 to 100%) and 1% after oral DHE, due to extensive first-pass metabolism through the liver. Peak plasma concentrations occur 30 minutes after IM injection and 45 minutes after subcutaneous injection and intranasal administration. Plasma concentrations do not correlate with effect on blood vessels. DHE half-life is 13 hours, and it has an active metabolite that occurs in concentrations 5 to 7 times higher than itself (4, 7).

Open label trials indicate that parenteral DHE aborts 75% of migraine attacks. Blinded studies found that IV DHE with metoclopramide was superior to placebo, meperidine with hydroxyzine, or butorphanol. Another study found that DHE was superior to lidocaine but inferior to chlorpromazine (7). Unlike ergotamine, DHE has not been shown to produce rebound headaches (38). DHE is effective in patients with menstrual migraine, CDH, and status migrainosus (5). A double-blind study found that SC DHE was as effective as SC sumatriptan with less headache recurrence with DHE (38).

Repetitive IV DHE is 90% effective in treating daily headache, status migrainosus, and cluster headache (52). DHE can also be self-administered via SC injection, (27) and 45% of patients interviewed after 2 to 3 years of self-administered IM DHE had at least a 50% response

(53). Intranasal DHE is as effective as ergotamine tartrate with caffeine in relieving migraine attacks; however, DHE nasal spray did not change the duration or frequency of cluster attacks, while IV DHE relieved acute cluster headache in less than 10 minutes (9). Placebo-controlled double-blind trials of intranasal DHE reported that headache abated within 2 hours in about 35 to 71% of patients (7).

The adverse effects of ergotamine include nausea, vomiting, abdominal discomfort, peripheral vasoconstriction, thirst, pruritus, vertigo, muscle cramps, and paresthesias (7, 27). Chronic ergotamine use can lead to vasospasm, anorectal ulcers, ischemic neuropathy, fibrotic disorders, and drug-induced headache (7). Oral or rectal administration of antiemetics 15 to 30 minutes prior to ergotamine administration decreases the associated nausea (27). Since ergotamine overuse can cause rebound headaches, some clinicians restrict its use to fewer than 2 doses a week (27). Patients with cluster headache, however, may use ergots nightly at the beginning of a cycle as a preventive measure (4, 22). Overdose or prolonged use can cause ergotism and cyanosis, claudication, or gangrene of limbs. Symptoms of ergotism include nausea, confusion, drowsiness, postural hypotension, vasospasm, distal paresthesias, and coldness of the extremities. Ergotism should be treated with a vasodilator for 24 hours (7). Both ergotamine and DHE are relatively contraindicated and should be used with caution in patients with coronary artery disease (CAD), peripheral vascular disease (PVD), or uncontrolled hypertension (HTN). They are contraindicated for use in patients who are pregnant, or who have sepsis, renal failure, or hepatic failure (54). Adverse effects of DHE include burning at the injection site, dizziness, paresthesias, abdominal cramps, and chest tightness. Intranasal DHE may cause nausea, a bitter taste, and local irritation of the nose and throat. DHE has less risk of adverse effects than ergotamine and may not produce rebound headaches after chronic use (4, 27, 38).

Metoclopramide and caffeine enhance the absorption of oral ergotamine. Erythromycin decrease the metabolism of ergotamine and should be avoided. Due to the potential, but not proven, increased risk of adverse events, concomitant methysergide, β-blockers, dopamine, erythromycins and sumatriptan should be used with caution (7, 38). To avoid vasoconstriction, patients should wait 6 or more hours after taking sumatriptan before taking ergotamine preparations (38).

Ergotamine is also available in combination products such as Cafergot (ergotamine tartrate and caffeine) and Wigraine (ergotamine tartrate, caffeine, and tartaric acid).

Corticosteroids

Corticosteroids are thought to decrease perivascular inflammation and are used in status migrainosus and episodic and chronic cluster headaches. In combination with neuroleptics, narcotics, metoclopramide, or DHE, intravenous corticosteroids may be used to treat refractory migraine headaches. Steroids are effective even when patients have had symptoms for a few days and have not responded to other migraine medications (27).

Corticosteroids are the fastest acting of the cluster headache prophylactic therapies, with responses occurring in 1 to 2 days. The most commonly used steroids for episodic cluster headaches are prednisone (starting doses up to 100 mg/day) and dexamethasone (4 mg twice daily). Prednisone produces marked relief in 77% of episodic cluster headache patients and partial improvement in another 12%. Prednisone may decrease cluster headaches in patients under 30 years of age who failed methysergide and patients over 40 years of age who failed therapy with verapamil, ergotamine, and lithium. Steroids help chronic cluster headaches in 40% of patients. These agents are only used as initial therapy for less than a month to break the cycle while waiting for other medications to take effect. Episodic and chronic cluster headaches may recur when steroids are discontinued. Adverse effects include insomnia, mood changes, hyponatremia, hyperglycemia, osteoporosis, and gastric ulcers. Steroids are relatively contraindicated in patients with hypertension, peptic ulcer disease, diabetes, and diverticulosis (4, 7, 9, 27). Additional information regarding corticosteroid pharmacotherapy and monitoring is in Chapter 30, "Rheumatoid Arthritis."

Neuroleptics

Phenothiazines are the neuroleptics most commonly used to treat acute migraine, TTH, and status migrainosus. These agents antagonize dopamine, decrease 5-HT reuptake, produce anticholinergic effects, and block α-adrenergic receptors (which induces orthostatic hypotension). The dopaminergic blockade is responsible for the drugs' beneficial antiemetic effect and undesirable extrapyramidal symptoms (7).

The pharmacokinetics of neuroleptic agents are very similar to those of the antidepressants, and some (chlorpromazine, thioridazine, haloperidol) also have active metabolites. Neuroleptic use should be limited in pregnant or lactating patients (55).

Intravenous injections of chlorpromazine or prochlorperazine are 70 to 90% effective in relieving migraine headaches (7). Although this route of administration is more effective than intramuscular or rectal doses, it carries a greater risk for orthostatic hypotension (56). Up to 80% of patients may experience adverse effects following parenteral injections of phenothiazines, with drowsiness being the most common. Akathisia is seen less frequently, and dystonic reactions are rare. A controlled trial with sulpiride, a substituted benzamide similar to metoclopramide, was superior to paroxetine and showed a moderate decrease in global headache score over an 8-week period in patients with TTH. However, 38% of patients experienced adverse effects and 11% discontinued the medication due to adverse effects (57). Additional information regarding neuroleptic pharmacotherapy and monitoring is in Chapter 55, "Schizophrenia."

β-Blockers

The mechanism of action of β-blockers in the preventive treatment of migraine is not clear, but it is most likely related to the inhibition of β_1-receptors with secondary effects on serotonin. However, β_1-selective agents will exhibit β-nonselectivity at higher doses (58). β-Blockers with intrinsic sympathomimetic activity (ISA) such as practolol, pindolol, and acebutolol are less effective in the treatment of migraine (7, 38). β-Blockers are not useful in the acute treatment of migraine (59). However, when given prophylactically, β-blockers are 60 to 80% effective in producing a 50% reduction in attack frequency and severity of migraine episodes. Within this drug class, the agents are equally effective, and the choice should be based on β_1-selectivity, lack of ISA, and idiosyncratic adverse effects. If one agent does not work the patient may respond to a different β-blocker (5). However, propranolol and timolol are the only β-blockers that have a FDA indication for migraine headaches (38). These drugs do not need to be given more than twice a day (7). Long-acting formulations of propranolol and metoprolol are also effective. Patients with both migraine and TTH may benefit from a combination of a β-blocker and a tricyclic antidepressant (60).

These highly lipid soluble compounds are well absorbed from the gastrointestinal tract, with peak plasma concentrations occurring within 2 hours. However, due to extensive first-pass hepatic metabolism, only 50% of the dose reaches the systemic circulation. The low bioavailability of atenolol and nadolol, which are eliminated renally as unchanged drug, can be explained by their more hydrophilic nature. Penbutolol, pindolol, and timolol do not exhibit first-pass metabolism and are almost completely absorbed. Food does not significantly effect their absorption. Most, if not all, β-blockers enter the CNS. Most β-blockers are also extensively metabolized by the liver to one or more active metabolites. However, the contribution of these metabolites to the overall pharmacologic action of the drug is low. β-Blockers undergo polymorphic drug metabolism, and less than 5% of patients will exhibit exaggerated blood pressure responses to the drug due to poor metabolizing capacity. The plasma half-life of most β-blockers is short, less than 10 hours; however, penbutolol and nadolol exhibit half-lives of 18 to 27 hours and should therefore be dosed once daily (58).

β-Blockers are relatively contraindicated in patients with asthma, depression, hypotension, congestive heart failure, Raynaud's disease, or diabetes. These agents exhibit a wide therapeutic range; drug efficacy and adverse effects are patient specific rather than concentration dependent. Approximately 10 to 15% of patients experience adverse effects; the most common involve the CNS (fatigue, sedation, sleep abnormalities, depression, memory impairment, hallucinations), but patients may also complain of gastrointestinal upset, impotence, and cardiac effects (orthostasis, bradycardia, and decreased exercise tolerance) (7, 38). β-Blockers and ergotamine should be used with caution, as symptoms of ergotism may occur (61). Additional information regarding β-blocker pharmacotherapy and monitoring is in Section 10, "Cardiovascular Disorders."

Antidepressants

Tricyclic antidepressants (TCAs) increase the availability of synaptic norepinephrine or serotonin by inhibiting reuptake. The newer atypical antidepressants (fluoxetine, fluvoxamine, sertraline, paroxetine) are selective serotonin reuptake inhibitors (SSRIs). The monoamine oxidase inhibitors (MAOIs) block the degradation of catecholamines. The lack of a temporal relationship between reuptake inhibition (occurs within hours), prophylactic headache response (3 to 10 days), and antidepressant action (2 to 3 weeks) shows that antinociceptive efficacy is unrelated to antidepressant action. Plausible explanations for the antinociceptive activity of antidepressants include decreases in β-receptor density and norepinephrine-mediated cAMP response, up-regulation of $GABA_B$-receptors, and down-regulation of $5-HT_2$-receptors. Of these, inhibition of the $5-HT_2$-receptors and 5-HT reuptake inhibition may be most crucial (4).

Antidepressants are useful in patients with concurrent depression, anxiety, insomnia, or pain disorders and are 40 to 70% effective in reducing migraine and TTH frequency. The efficacy of TCAS is superior to placebo but similar to propranol (4, 7). Low doses of these agents 1 hour before bedtime are usually sufficient (27). Phenelzine, an MAOI often used in refractory cases, was shown in an open-label trial to be 80% effective for migraine (62). Trazodone, a serotonin-specific antidepressant, is metabolized to m-chlorophenylpiperazine, a migraine precipitant, and should be used with caution (63). Amitriptyline, nortriptyline, and doxepin are the most commonly used (38).

Antidepressants are well absorbed, and food does not affect the extent of absorption. They are highly lipid soluble, widely distributed, and strongly bound to plasma proteins. Due to placental transfer and accumulation in breast milk, antidepressants should be avoided by pregnant or lactating women. Antidepressants are primarily metabolized by oxidative hepatic enzymes, and some drugs (imipramine, amitriptyline, doxepin, fluoxetine) have active metabolites that contribute to drug efficacy and the potential for adverse effects. The half-life of antidepressants generally exceed 24 hours with multiple dosing and allows for once-daily dosing (55). A consistent relationship between antidepressant plasma concentrations and antinociceptive efficacy has not been established.

Adverse effects of TCAs occur in 10 to 20% of patients and include anticholinergic effects (dry mouth, constipation, urinary retention, blurred vision, sedation, memory impairment), cardiovascular effects (hypotension, arrhythmias), sexual dysfunction, and weight gain. These agents are contraindicated in patients with narrow-angle glaucoma and urinary retention, and should be used with caution in patients with cardiac disease or seizure disorders. Although SSRIs are less likely to produce sedation, weight gain, and cardiovascular toxicity, they have been associated with the development of headaches and insomnia. The adverse effect profile of the MAOIs is similar to that of the TCAs, but concurrent ingestion of tyramine-containing foods or use of meperidine and sympathomimetic agents, including Midrin, may precipitate a hypertensive crisis. The concurrent use of fluoxetine and MAOIs has resulted in fatalities, and several weeks must elapse before one agent can be initiated following discontinuation of the other (4). Additional information regarding antidepressant pharmacotherapy and monitoring is in Chapter 54, "Mood Disorders."

Calcium Channel Blockers

Excessive levels of intracellular calcium under ischemic conditions can produce neuronal damage and cell death. Calcium enters the cell primarily by slow voltage–sensitive channels and NMDA-linked receptor channels. Calcium channel blockers affect slow voltage–sensitive calcium channels, of which there are three subtypes, L, T, and N. L-type calcium channels mediate electromechanical coupling of activity in cardiovascular smooth muscle as well as endocrine cells and some neurons. T-type channels are also found in cardiac tissue and are responsible for repetitive spikes in neurons and endocrine cells. N-type channels only affect neurons and mediate system neurotransmitter release. Most calcium channel blockers used in the treatment of headaches affect the L-type channel only. Vascular specificity of calcium channel blockers is determined by differential binding characteristics to L-type channel subunits (64). Flunarizine, a novel calcium channel blocking agent with antiepileptic properties, exhibits nonspecific antagonism to sodium as well as type T and N slow voltage–sensitive calcium channels, and may therefore have significant advantages in terms of cerebral cell protection and lack of cardiovascular effects (65). The antimigraine effect of flunarizine does not appear to correlate with its dopaminergic blockade (66). Calcium channel blockers, in particular nicardipine, are highly lipid-soluble compounds, which is important for drug penetration into the lipid bilayer of neuronal cells and the site of action (27).

These agents, although not FDA approved, are used primarily in the prophylaxis of migraine and cluster headaches and probably exhibit the lowest risk of adverse effects, but they also are not as effective as other treatments (5,7). Studies with calcium channel blockers in headache have focused primarily on three agents: verapamil, nimodipine, and flunarizine. Parenteral (20 mg) or sublingual (10 mg) flunarizine, but not verapamil (10 mg), nimodipine (40 mg), or nifedipine (60 mg), may be useful in treating acute migraine attacks (4, 67). Verapamil prophylaxis is only 40% effective in reducing migraine frequency by 50% (68). Nifedipine is not considered effective in migraine prophylaxis, and nimodipine shows limited efficacy only in the prevention of migraine with aura (7). Small uncontrolled studies with diltiazem and nicardipine support their use in the prophylactic treatment of migraine (7, 69). Flunarizine, not available in the United States, appears to be the most efficacious and is comparable to β-blockers (7). Nimodipine and verapamil are 50 to 80% effective in reducing cluster headache symptoms (9). Therapy with calcium channel blocking agents is initiated at low doses and titrated to response or maximum dose. An adequate trial may require at least 2 months due to a delayed onset of action (27). Verapamil (9), and probably other calcium channel blockers, may be safely taken together with ergotamine.

Calcium channel blockers are well absorbed, but extensive first-pass hepatic metabolism reduces the systemic absorption to less than 50%. Food does not interfere with the absorption of these agents. Following oral administration, peak plasma concentrations are reached within 2 to 3 hours for diltiazem, 1 to 2 hours for verapamil, and less than 1 hour for nimodipine and nicardipine. Peak plasma concentrations of flunarizine occur between 2 to 4 hours after the dose. Calcium channel blockers are widely distributed, enter the placenta, and are excreted into breast milk. With the exception of flunarizine (18 days), most exhibit a terminal half-life of less than 10 hours (55, 70, 71).

The most common adverse effects include dizziness, depression, tremor, constipation, peripheral edema, hypotension, and bradycardia. Flunarizine may cause weight gain, sedation, extrapyramidal symptoms, and depression. Additional information regarding calcium channel blocker pharmacotherapy and monitoring is in Section 10, "Cardiovascular Disorders."

Serotonin Antagonists

METHYSERGIDE

Methysergide is a semisynthetic ergot 5-HT$_{1D}$ receptor agonist and 5-HT$_{2A}$ and 5-HT$_{2C}$ receptor antagonist. It has an active metabolite, methylergometrine, that has dopamine agonist activity. The drug decreases platelet aggregation, inhibits neurogenic plasma extravasation and inflammation, and produces vasoconstriction in the carotid vascular bed (4, 7, 14).

Methysergide is not useful in the treatment of acute cluster headache and migraine attacks; it is primarily used as a preventive agent. In open label trials, methysergide (6–16 mg/day) decreased headache frequency by more than 50% in 64% of migraineurs. Methysergide may be less effective in migraine with aura (53%) than without aura (76%). Several controlled trials have shown methysergide (3–6 mg/day) to be superior to placebo and cyproheptadine, but comparable to pizotifen, lisuride, propranolol, and flunarizine in the prophylaxis of migraine (4, 7). Methysergide is 65 to 70% effective in the prevention of cluster headaches and may be the drug of choice for prophylaxis of episodic type cluster headaches in patients under 30 years of age. Cluster cycles are usually less than 3 months in duration, and the development of long-term adverse effects is less of a concern. However, tachyphylaxis with chronic use may be seen (4, 9).

Due to extensive hepatic first pass metabolism, the oral bioavailability of methysergide is only 13%. Peak blood concentrations occur within an hour, and the drug crosses the blood-brain barrier. It distributes into breast milk. The elimination half-life of methysergide and methylergometrine are 60 and 220 minutes, respectively (7).

Initial dose titration from 1 mg/day by 1 mg/day every 3 days may decrease the risk of acute adverse effects. Administering methysergide with food or antacids or dividing the daily dose decreases gastrointestinal effects. Rarely, methysergide combined with ergotamine or sumatriptan can result in severe vasoconstriction. In order to initiate a drug holiday, the dose should also be tapered down over at least a week to minimize increased headaches (7).

Methysergide is more likely to cause adverse effects than other agents used for headache and results in 20% of patients discontinuing therapy (7). Initial adverse effects, which often decrease with time, include muscle aches, hallucinations, abdominal discomfort, and nausea/vomiting. Other adverse effects include peripheral arterial insufficiency, peripheral edema, and weight gain. Of most concern is the rare chronic event (1:2,500), retroperitoneal, pulmonary, or endocardial fibrosis. This can be minimized by initiating a 1-month drug holiday every 6 months (4, 7). During this holiday, patients will require other prophylactic treatment. Detection of fibrotic changes is possible with chest X-ray, echocardiogram, or magnetic resonance imaging of the abdomen (9). Patients should be told to contact their doctor if they experience any coldness or pain in their fingers or toes, flank pain, chest pain, or dysuria. Fortunately, in most cases these fibrotic changes regress after drug discontinuation. Methysergide is contraindicated in cardiovascular disease, cerebrovascular disease, severe hypertension, peripheral vascular disease, peptic ulcer disease, pregnancy, and familial fibrotic disorders.

CYPROHEPTADINE

Cyproheptadine is a 5-HT$_{2A}$ and 5-HT$_{2C}$ antagonist with antihistaminic and anticholinergic activity. It also blocks calcium channels in dogs. It is often used for migraine prophylaxis in childhood migraine or hormonally mediated migraines. Open label studies indicate that cyproheptadine improves migraine in 43 to 65% of patients, but several comparative trials indicate that it is superior to placebo but inferior to methysergide. Start with 2 mg/day and increase by 2 mg/day every 3 days until efficacy or adverse effects develop, usually with daily divided doses of 12 to 36 mg/day. Administering the majority of the dose at bedtime may minimize daytime drowsiness. Adverse drug reactions are considered to be less than methysergide and include drowsiness, dizziness, dry mouth, increased appetite, and weight gain. Cyproheptadine is contraindicated in patients with glaucoma (4, 5, 7).

Other Serotonin Receptor Antagonists

Investigational or unavailable antiserotonin agents include lisuride, pizotifen, mianserin, sergolexole, and tropisetron.

ANTICONVULSANTS

Anticonvulsants are particularly useful in children and in patients with concurrent manic-depressive disorders, epilepsy, paroxysmal EEGs, or anxiety disorders (5, 27). Valproic acid, carbamazepine, and phenytoin have all shown some effectiveness in decreasing headache pain. However, valproic acid is the most commonly used preparation and is effective in patients with migraine, CDH or cluster headaches (4).

Valproic acid is effective for the prophylactic treatment of migraine (4). Its efficacy is comparable to that of the β-blockers and flunarizine (72). Double-blind studies indicate that prophylactic use of valproic acid is superior to placebo in decreasing the frequency of migraine attacks by 42 to over 50% in 48 to 86% of patients (72–74). One study also reported decreased severity and duration (73). Cluster headaches also improved with valproic acid (600–2000 mg/day) in one small open-label study (9). The frequency, duration, and intensity of TTH was no different with valproic acid versus placebo (72).

The most common adverse effects reported in these trials were nausea, dyspepsia, tiredness, increased appetite and weight gain (72, 74). Other adverse effects include sedation, tremor, transient hair loss, increased bleeding time, and thrombocytopenia. Hepatotoxicity is rare, but baseline liver function tests should be obtained. Nausea may be minimized by using the enteric coated preparation, Depakote. Valproic acid is relatively contraindicated in patients with liver disease or bleeding disorders.

Valproic acid inhibits liver enzymes, decreasing the metabolism of many drugs. Phenytoin and carbamazepine induce liver enzymes, increasing the metabolism of many drugs. Anticonvulsants are also highly bound to albumin and are subject to protein binding displacement interactions with other drugs. Thus, the efficacy and toxicity of any concomitant therapy should be evaluated when these antiepileptic drugs are added or discontinued. Blood samples may be needed to check plasma drug concentrations, liver function, or hematologic function. Valproic acid is teratogenic and should be discontinued 1 to 2 months prior to planned conception and alternate therapies initiated (72). Additional information regarding anticonvulsant pharmacotherapy and monitoring is in Chapter 50, "Seizure Disorder."

LITHIUM CARBONATE

The mechanism of action of lithium is unclear, but it may alter circadian rhythms, reduce rapid eye movement sleep, or decrease neuronal activity by depleting inositol. Lithium improves cyclic migraine and cluster headaches. More patients with chronic (78%) than episodic cluster (63%) headache respond to prophylactic lithium. Nearly 20% of patients receiving lithium for chronic cluster convert to episodic cluster. Lithium improves headaches by 60 to 90% in 42% of patients with episodic cluster headaches and by more than 90% in 54% of patients. Triple therapy with the addition of verapamil and ergotamine has improved episodic cluster in 90% of cases. The starting dose is usually 300 mg twice a day. Since it has a half-life of around 24 hours, it may take 1 to 2 weeks to develop a therapeutic response. Some patients may develop tolerance to lithium effects. Serum concentrations should be monitored weekly during the titration phase and every 3 months thereafter (4, 7, 9).

Common adverse effects include tremor, polyuria, nausea, muscle weakness, and ankle edema. Since long-term effects include hypothyroidism, renal failure, electrocardiogram changes, leukocytosis, and diabetes insipidus, baseline monitoring should include thyroid function, urinalysis, electrocardiogram, leucocyte measurements, and electrolytes. Adverse effects can be minimized by maintaining serum concentrations below 1 mEq/L. Caution should be used when lithium is used in conjunction with verapamil, and lithium doses will most likely need to be reduced. Since lithium has teratagenic risks, it should be avoided in pregnancy. Patients should not alter the salt intake of their diet or take diuretics, because they affect renal lithium elimination (4). Additional information on lithium pharmacotherapy and monitoring is in Chapter 54, "Mood Disorders."

CAPTOPRIL

Captopril inhibits enkephalinase and the angiotensin-converting enzyme and thus the breakdown of endogenous opioids. In an open-label study, captopril decreased migrain related headaches in 50% of patients and was superior to placebo in a small double-blind study. Adverse effects include hypotension, proteinuria, angioedema, rash, and cough (4).

CLONIDINE

The majority of trials indicate that clonidine is no better than placebo in relieving migraine headaches. Clonidine may help decrease the autonomic withdrawal symptoms in patients who discontinue chronic or high-dose narcotics. The patch formulation may be helpful as adjunctive therapy for detoxifying patients who have headaches from excess analgesics or ergotamine use (4, 7).

CAPSAICIN

Intranasal capsaicin may decrease pain by depleting SP in peripheral sensory neurons. When administered on the same side as the headache, it has reduced the number of cluster headaches by 67%, with complete relief in over half of the patients. Patients with episodic cluster headaches respond better than those with chronic cluster headaches. The major limiting factor is the initial painful burning sensation and nasal secretion; however, these complaints usually dissipate after 5 days (44).

CALCITONIN

Calcitonin, a polypeptide hormone secreted by the thyroid, may be effective in preventing migraine headaches and treating other chronic pain states (4). Calcitonin is extracted from salmon or synthesized to resemble human calcitonin. The salmon formulation appears to be identical to the mammalian form but has a greater potency, duration, and antibody formation. The human formulation shares the same linear amino acid sequence as human calcitonin, but is temporarily only available by compassionate plea. The salmon form is available as an injectable dosage form, and an intranasal formulation was approved August 1995. Patients should be monitored for allergic reactions or loss of efficacy. Adverse effects include nausea, flushing, pedal edema, rash, and inflammation at the injection site. The nasal formulation may cause nasal irritation but may have less systemic effects.

CONCLUSIONS

Headaches are very common, but many headache sufferers do not seek medical attention. Patients need an adequate evaluation to rule out medical and medication causes of headaches. Treatment involves both pharmacologic and nonpharmacologic measures, and their effects may be synergistic. Pharmacologic treatment can be abortive and preventative. The goal of abortive treatment is to relieve headache pain and associated symptoms with minimal drug-related adverse effects. Complete remission is an unreasonable expectation, as headaches will recur. Thus, end points for preventative treatment include decreased severity, duration, and frequency of headaches with minimal drug-related adverse effects. There is a delicate balance between headache improvement and adverse effects. Some patients prefer the balance to lean toward less headache improvement because they are unable to tolerate the adverse effects, while others are willing to tolerate more adverse effects in order to achieve better headache relief. Patients also need to be well informed about their therapy and take an active part in their management by avoiding headache trigger factors and evaluating the effects of their therapy.

REFERENCES

1. Silberstein SD. Tension-type and chronic daily headache. Neurology 43:1644–1649, 1993.
2. Mathew NT. Transformed migraine. Cephalagia 13:78–83, 1993.
3. Cady RK, Shealy CN. Recent advances in migraine management. J Fam Pract 36:85–91, 1993.
4. Dalessio DJ, Silberstein SD. Wolff's headache and other head pain, 6th ed. New York: Oxford University Press, 1993.
5. Silberstein SD, Lipton RB. Overview of diagnosis and treatment of migraine. Neurology 44(suppl 7):S6–S16, 1994.
6. Lipton RB, Silberstein SD, Stewart WF. An update on the epidemiology of migraine. Headache 34:319–328, 1994.
7. Olesen J, Tfelt-Hansen P, Welch KMA. The headaches. New York: Raven Press, 1993.
8. Rapoport AM. Recurrent migraine: cost-effective care. Neurology 44(suppl 3):S25–S28, 1994.
9. Silberstein SD. Pharmacological management of cluster headache. CNS Drugs 2:199–207, 1994.
10. Mathew NT. Cluster headache. Neurology 42(suppl 2):22–31, 1992.
11. Bonica JJ. The management of pain, 2nd ed. Philadelphia: Lea & Febiger, 1990.
12. Zagami AS. Pathophysiology of migraine and tension-type headache. Curr Opin Neurol 7:272–277, 1994.
13. Silberstein SD, Silberstein MM. New concepts in the pathogenesis of headache. Pain Management 3:334–342, 1990.
14. Silberstein SD. Serotonin (5-HT) and migraine. Headache 34:408–417, 1994.
15. Silberstein SD, Merriam GR. Sex hormones and headache. J Pain Symptom Manage 8:98–114, 1993.
16. Bach FW, Langemark M, Secher NH, Olesen J. Plasma and cerebrospinal fluid β-endorphin in chronic tension-type headache. Pain 51:163–168, 1992.
17. Olesen J. Clinical and pathophysiological observations in migraine and tension-type headache explained by integration of vascular, supraspinal, and myofascial inputs. Pain 46:125–132, 1991.
18. Blau JN. Migraine prodromes separated from the aura: complete migraine. Br Med J 281:658–660, 1980.
19. Olesen J. Headache Classification Committee of the International Headache Society. Classification and diagnostic criteria for headache disorders, cranial neuralgia, and facial pain. Cephalagia 8(suppl 7):1–96, 1988.
20. Selby G, Lance JW. Observations on 500 cases of migraine and allied vascular headache. J Neurol Neurosurg Psychiatry 23:23–32, 1960.
21. Goadsby PJ. The clinical profile of sumatriptan: cluster headache. Eur Neurol 34(suppl 2):35–39, 1994.
22. Schulman EA, Silberstein SD. Symptomatic and prophylactic treatment of migraine and tension-type headache. Neurology 42(suppl 2):16–21, 1992.
23. Tavola T, Gala C, Conte G, Invernizzi G. Traditional Chinese acupuncture in tension-type headache: a controlled study. Pain 48:325–329, 1992.
24. Trachtenberg DE. Tension headaches. Postgrad Med 95:44–56, 1994.

25. Marcus DA. Migraine and tension-type headache: the questionable validity of current classification systems. Clin J Pain 8:28–36, 1992.
26. Adler CS, Adler SM. Biofeedback-psychotherapy for the treatment of headache. Headache 16:189–191, 1976.
27. Baumel B. Migraine: a pharmacological review with newer options and delivery modalities. Neurology 44(suppl 3):S13–S17, 1994.
28. Couch JR. Placebo effect and clinical trials in migraine therapy. Neuroepidemiology 6:178–185, 1987.
29. Waelkens J, Caers I, Amery WK. Effects of therapeutic measures taken during the premonitory phase. In: Amery WK, Wauquier A, eds. The prelude to the migraine attack. London: Balliere Tindall, 1986:78–83.
30. Spierings ELH. Treatment of the migraine attack. In: Ferrari MD, Lataste X, eds. Migraine and other headaches, Park Ridge, IL: Parthenon, 1989:241–248.
31. Sawynok J, Yaksh TL. Caffeine as analgesic adjuvant: a review of pharmacology and mechanisms of action. Pharmacol Rev 45:43–85, 1993.
32. Yuill GM, Sinburn WR, Liversedge LA. A double-blind crossover trial of isometheptene mucate compound and ergotamine in migraine. Br J Clin Pract 26:76–79, 1972.
33. Ryan RE. A study of Midrin in the symptomatic relief of migraine headache. Headache 14:33–42, 1974.
34. Silberstein SD. Headaches and women: treatment of the pregnant and lactating migraineur. Headache 33:533–540, 1993.
35. Mathew NT. Prophylaxis of migraine and mixed headache. A randomized controlled study. Headache 21:105–109, 1981.
36. Markley HG. Chronic headache: appropriate use of opiate analgesics. Neurology 44(suppl 3):S18–S24, 1994.
37. Silberstein SD, Silberstein JR. Chronic daily headache: long-term prognosis following inpatient treatment with repetitive IV DHE. Headache 32:439–445, 1992.
38. Anonymous. Drugs for migraine. Med Lett Drugs Ther 37:17–20, 1995.
39. Bannwarth B, Netter P, Pourel J, Royer RJ, Gaucher A. Clinical pharmacokinetics of nonsteroidal anti-inflammatory drugs in the cerebrospinal fluid. Biomed Pharmacother 43:121–126, 1989.
40. Migliardi JR, Armellino JJ, Friedman M, Gillings DB, Beaver WT. Caffeine as an analgesic adjuvant in tension headache. Clin Pharmacol Ther 56:576–586, 1994.
41. Klapper JA, Stanton JS. Ketorolac versus DHE and metoclopramide in the treatment of migraine headaches. Headache 31:523–524, 1991.
42. Peters BH, Fraim CJ, Masel BE. Comparison of 650 mg aspirin and 1,000 mg acetaminophen with each other, and with placebo in moderately severe headache. Am J Med 74(suppl 6A):36–42, 1983.
43. Jaffe JH, Martin WR. Opioid analgesics and antagonists. In: Goodman Gilman A, Rall TW, Nies AS, Taylor P, eds. Goodman and Gilman's The pharmacological basis of therapeutics, 8th ed. New York: Pergamon Press Inc., 1990:485–521.
44. Kumar KL. Recent advances in the acute management of migraine and cluster headaches. J Gen Intern Med 9:339–348, 1994.
45. Upmalis DH, Stadol NS. Headache 33:394, 1993.
46. Albibi R, McCallum RW. Metoclopramide: pharmacology and clinical application. Ann Intern Med 98:86–95, 1983.
47. Plosker GL, McTavish D. Sumatriptan. A reappraisal of its pharmacology and therapeutic efficacy in the acute treatment of migraine and cluster headache. Drugs 47:622–651, 1994.
48. Brennum J, Kjeldsen M, Olesen J. The 5-HT$_1$-like agonist sumatriptan has a significant effect in chronic tension–type headache. Cephalalgia 12:375–379, 1992.
49. Sanders SW, Haering N, Mosberg H, et al. Pharmacokinetics of ergotamine in healthy volunteers following oral and rectal dosing. Eur J Clin Pharmacol 39:331–334, 1986.

50. Kanto J, Allonen H, Koski K, et al. Pharmacokinetics of dihydroer-gotamine in healthy volunteers and neurological patients after a single intravenous injection. Int J Clin Pharmacol Ther Toxicol 19:127–130, 1981.

51. Schran HF, Tse FLS. Pharmacokinetics of dihydroergotamine following subcutaneous administration in humans. Int J Clin Pharmacol Ther Toxicol 23:1–4, 1985.

52. Silberstein SD, Schulman EA, Hopkins MM. Repetitive intravenous DHE in the treatment of refractory headache. Headache 30:334–339, 1990.

53. Weisz MA, El-Raheb M, Blumenthal HJ. Home administration of intramuscular DHE for the treatment of acute migraine headache. Headache 34:371–373, 1994.

54. Rall TW. Drugs affecting uterine motility. In: Goodman Gilman A, Rall TW, Nies AS, Taylor P, eds. Goodman and Gilman's The pharmacological basis of therapeutics, 8th ed. New York: Pergamon Press Inc., 1990:933–953.

55. Anon. Drug information, 37th ed. Bethesda: American Society of Hospital Pharmacists, 1995.

56. Thomas SH, Stone CK, Ray VG, Whitley TW. Intravenous versus rectal prochlorperazine in the treatment of benign vascular or tension headache: a randomized, prospective, double-blind trial. Ann Emerg Med 24:923–927, 1994.

57. Langemark M, Olesen J. Sulpiride and paroxetine in the treatment of chronic tension-type headache. An explanatory double-blind trial. Headache 34:20–24, 1994.

58. Kazierad DJ, Schlanz KD, Bottorf MB. Beta blockers. In: Evans WE, Schentag JJ, Jusko WJ, eds. Applied pharmacokinetics, 3rd ed. Vancouver, WA: Applied Therapeutics, 1992, 24–1–24–41.

59. Banerjeee M, Findley LJ. Propranolol in the treatment of acute migraine attacks. Cephalalgia 11:193–196, 1991.

60. Pfaffenrath V, Kellhammer U, Pöllmann W. Combination headache: practical experience with a combination of a β-blocker and an antidepressive. Cephalalgia 6(suppl 5):25–32, 1986.

61. Venter CP, Joubert PH, Buys AC. Severe peripheral ischaemia during concommitant use of beta blockers and ergot alkaloids. Br Med J 289:288–289, 1984.

62. Anthony M, Lance JW. Monoamine oxidase inhibition in the treatment of migraine. Arch Neurol 21:263–268, 1969.

63. Brewerton TD, Murphy DL, Mueller EA, Jimerson DC. Induction of migraine like headaches by the serotonin agonist μ-chlorophenylpiperazine. Clin Pharmacol Ther 43:605–609, 1988.

64. Triggle DJ. Calcium antagonists. History and perspective. Stroke 21(suppl 12):IV49–IV58, 1990.

65. Pauwels PJ, Leysen JE, Janssen PA. Ca^{++} and Na^{+} channels involved in neuronal cell death. Protection by flunarizine. Life Sci 48:1881–1893, 1991.

66. Wober C, Brucke T, Wober-Bingol C, Asenbaum S, Wessely P, Podreka I. Dopamine D$_2$ receptor blockade and antimigraine action of flunarizine. Cephalalgia 14:235–240, 1994.

67. Hoffert MJ, Scholz MJ, Kanter R. A double-blind controlled study of nifedipine as an abortive treatment in acute attacks of migraine with aura. Cephalalgia 12:323–324, 1992.

68. Solomon GD. Verapamil in migraine prophylaxis–a five-year review. Headache 29:425–427, 1989.

69. Roumeau BJ. Nicardipine in the prevention of migraine headaches. Clin Ther 14:672–677, 1992.

70. Bebin M, Bleck TP. New anticonvulsant drugs. Focus on flunarizine, fosphenytoin, midazolam, and stiripentol. Drugs 48:153–171, 1994.

71. Singh BN, Josephson MA. Clinical pharmacology, pharmacokinetics, and hemodynamic effects of nicardipine. Am Heart J 119:427–434, 1990.

72. Jensen R, Brinck T, Olesen J. Sodium valproate has a prophylactic effect in migraine without aura: a triple-blind, placebo-controlled, crossover study. Neurology 44:647–651, 1994.

73. Hering R, Kuritzky A. Sodium valproate has a prophylactic effect in migraine: a double-blind study vs placebo. Cephalalgia 12:81–84, 1992.

74. Rothrock JF, Kelly NM, Brody ML, Golbeck A. A differential response to treatment with divalproex sodium in patients with intractable headache. Cephalalgia 14:241–244, 1994.

75. Askmark H, Lundberg PO, Olson S. Drug-related headache. Headache 29:441–444, 1989.

CHAPTER 50

SEIZURE DISORDERS

BRIAN K. ALLDREDGE

Epilepsy affects approximately 1% of the worldwide population and is the second most common neurologic disorder after stroke. The incidence is highest in the first 10 years of life and declines thereafter through the age of 50 until the elderly years, when the incidence increases again. Epilepsy begins before the age of 18 in over 75% of patients (1). The word "epilepsy" comes from the Greek word meaning "to seize" and is used to characterize *self-sustained, spontaneously recurring seizure disorder*. It is important to note that this definition specifically excludes isolated seizures that have an identifiable cause, such as drug toxicity or metabolic abnormalities.

A *seizure* is defined as the clinical manifestation of excessive or hypersynchronous activity of neurons within the cerebral cortex (2). Though the term often connotes an event characterized by an abrupt loss of consciousness, with generalized muscle contraction and jerking (i.e., a generalized tonic-clonic or grand mal seizure), the clinical manifestations of various seizure types are quite heterogeneous. The specific signs and symptoms that accompany the event depend on the functional area of the brain that is involved and may include various degrees of motor, sensory, or cognitive dysfunction. It is estimated that one of every 11 people in the United States will experience a seizure at some time during life (3).

ETIOLOGY

Seizures may result from primary or acquired disturbances of central nervous system (CNS) function, metabolic derangements, or a variety of systemic diseases. Some of the common causes of new-onset seizures are listed in Table 50.1. Identification of the cause of seizures is of primary importance in the determination of subsequent management. If precipitating factors are identified that are amenable to therapeutic intervention, (e.g., metabolic disorders, hypertensive encephalopathy, or drug overdose), then specific treatment modalities should be instituted to correct the underlying cause. Rarely is there a need for chronic antiepileptic drug (AED) therapy. Conversely, when no cause of seizures can be identified by history, physical examination, laboratory investigation, or neuroimaging studies, the seizure disorder is termed *idiopathic*, and if seizures recur, long-term AED therapy is warranted.

Drugs are a particularly common cause of new-onset seizures. In most instances, drug-induced seizures are dose-related and are more likely to occur in patients who have a history of seizures or impaired drug elimination capacity (4). Table 50.2 lists drugs that have been implicated in causing seizures.

CLASSIFICATION AND CLINICAL MANIFESTATIONS

Whereas an etiologic diagnosis of seizures is needed to establish whether chronic AED therapy is necessary, the classification of epileptic seizures by their clinical and electrophysiologic manifestations is necessary to determine which AED is most likely to be effective. In most circumstances the seizure can be classified after a complete patient history in which the patient describes the events that occurred during the attack. This should include questions about any symptoms that warn the patient of an impending seizure (i.e., the *aura*), the specific ictal manifestations, and any postictal abnormalities. Throughout this process, the patient should be discouraged from labeling the attacks, but rather should be guided to relate the events as they were experienced or as they were described by observers. The current scheme that is used for the classification of epileptic seizures and syndromes was established by the International League Against Epilepsy (5, 6). A modified version of this classification is presented in Table 50.3.

Seizures are classified as being either *generalized* or *partial* on the basis of their clinical and electroencephalographic features. *Generalized seizures* are those that appear to begin in both hemispheres of the brain. Previously, these seizures were subdivided into *convulsive* and *nonconvulsive* generalized seizures according to the severity of associated motor disturbances. Nonconvulsive generalized seizures included absence (*petit mal*), myoclonic, and atonic seizures. Clonic and tonic-clonic seizures were previously referred to as *grand mal* seizures.

Generalized tonic-clonic seizures are characteristic of maximal involvement of neurons of both hemispheres of the brain. Typically, these seizures begin with tonic (rigid) flexion of the extremities followed by extension. During this phase, air is forced from the larynx to produce an audible cry. The tonic phase of the seizure usually lasts 15 to 20 sec and is quickly followed by the clonic (jerking) phase, during which there are spasms of the trunk and extremities and often biting of the tongue. The clonic phase usually lasts 20 to 30 sec and is followed by a postictal state, during which the patient may sleep or awaken confused and disoriented. There is then a gradual return of

Table 50.1.
Common Causes of New-Onset Seizures[a]

Cause	Comment
Primary and Acquired CNS Disorders	
Benign febrile convulsions of childhood	Do not occur after age 5; always consider other causes first.
Idiopathic epilepsy	Onset less common after age 25.
Head trauma	Especially when associated with depressed skull fracture or intracerebral or subdural hematoma.
Stroke	Embolic, or hemorrhage; thrombotic.
CNS mass lesion	Primary or metastatic tumor; brain abscess; arteriovenous malformation.
Metabolic or systemic disorders	
Cerebral hypoperfusion or hypoxia	Cardiopulmonary arrest; cardiac dysrhythmia; severe hypotension.
Meningitis, encephalitis	Acute or chronic; bacterial, viral, fungal, tuberculous, or parasitic.
Hyponatremia	Usually with serum sodium level of 104–118 mEq/L but rapid fall better correlated with seizures than actual level.
Hypoglycemia	Usually with serum glucose level of 20–30 mg/dL but little correlation between hypoglycemic symptoms and glucose levels.
Hypernatremia or hyperosmolar, nonketotic hyperglycemia	Serum osmolality usually greater than 330 mOsm/L.
Hypocalcemia	Convulsant range 4.3–9.2 mg/dL. Common presentation of hypoparathyroidism and pseudohypoparathyroidism. Tetany need not be present.
Hypertensive encephalopathy	Blood pressure usually greater than 250/150 mm Hg or, when acutely elevated from normal BP, above 160/100.
Uremic encephalopathy	Rapid development of uremia more closely associated with seizures than is absolute serum urea nitrogen.
Hepatic encephalopathy	Respiratory alkalosis nearly always present.
Eclampsia	$MgSO_4$ treatment is preferable to phenytoin.
Porphyria	Most anticonvulsants can exacerbate porphyric symptoms. Anticonvulsants of choice are gabapentin and triple bromides.
Drug overdose	See Table 50.2.
Drug withdrawal	Anticonvulsants, ethanol, or sedative-hypnotic drugs (with habituation to daily doses of 600–800 mg secobarbital or its equivalent).
Hyperthermia	Temperature usually above 42°C (107°F); immediate reduction of body temperature to 39°C (102°F) mandatory.

[a]Adapted with permission from Simon RP, Aminoff MJ, Greenberg DA. Clinical neurology. Norwalk, CT: Appleton-Lange, 1989, Chapter 9.

consciousness and orientation over a period of 15 to 30 min, after which the patient has no recall of the event. Increases in blood pressure and heart rate, incontinence of urine or feces, and brief interruption of normal breathing with cyanosis commonly accompany this type of seizure. Generalized tonic-clonic seizures often result from the progression of some other fundamental type of seizure (e.g., simple partial or complex partial seizures), in which case they are termed *secondarily generalized tonic-clonic seizures*. *Primary generalized* seizures are those in which there is no evidence of progression from another seizure type.

Absence (petit mal) seizures occur primarily during childhood and are characterized by an abrupt interruption of consciousness followed by a fixed stare and automatisms (e.g., lip smacking, chewing, grimacing) or mild clonic movements. During the seizure there is no loss of postural tone. The seizure usually lasts less than 45 sec and ends as abruptly as it begins, the patient immediately regaining full alertness. Absence seizures may occur as often as hundreds of times a day and are often initially perceived by family or teachers as daydreaming. This seizure type is characterized by a classic pattern on the electroencephalogram of bilateral 3-Hz spike-wave discharges. Absence seizures usually have their onset between the ages of 4 and 12 years. Rarely does this seizure type persist beyond the age of 20 years. *Atypical absence* seizures differ from traditional absence seizures in having a longer duration, focal motor manifestations, and a greater association with developmental delay.

Atonic seizures are characterized by a sudden loss of muscle tone. Since the patient may fall abruptly, injuries are common, and it is often necessary to protect the patient's head by prescribing the use of a helmet during the daytime. *Myoclonic* seizures are characterized by jerking movements of a single or multiple muscle groups. *Tonic* seizures are similar to generalized tonic-clonic seizures except that they lack the usual clonic phase.

Partial seizures begin in an area of the brain that is limited to one hemisphere and are often indicative of some underlying focal brain lesion (e.g., perinatal injury, trauma, stroke, or CNS tumor). Partial seizures are differentiated according to whether or not consciousness is impaired during the event. *Complex partial seizures* are associated with impairment of consciousness; *simple partial* seizures are not.

Simple partial seizures are characterized by either motor manifestations (e.g., clonic jerking of one arm) or sensory symptoms (e.g., a foul odor or visual distortions). In some patients with motor symptoms the seizure may spread to contiguous areas of the cortex, resulting in the recruitment of additional muscle groups ("jacksonian march"). Autonomic symptoms such as piloerection or pupillary dilatation or psychic symptoms such as feelings of déjà vu or fear may also accompany simple partial seizures;

Table 50.2.
Drugs That Can Cause Seizures[a]

Antimicrobials	*Theophylline*
β-Lactam and related compounds	*Anesthetic and antiarrhythmic agents*
Cephalosporins	Class 1B
Imipenem/cilastatin	Lidocaine
Penicillin and its derivatives	Tocainide
Quinolones	β-Adrenergic blockers
Ciprofloxacin	Esmolol
Enoxacin	Metoprolol
Nalidixic acid	Propranolol
Norfloxacin	Local anesthetics
Isoniazid	Bupivicaine
Psychotropic agents	Chlorprocaine
Antidepressants	Lidocaine
Amitriptyline	Procaine
Bupropion	*Radiographic contrast agents*
Desipramine	Diatrizoate meglumine
Doxepin	Iohexol
Fluoxetine	Iopamidol
Imipramine	Ioxaglate sodium
Maprotiline	Meglumine metrizoate
Nortriptyline	Sodium iothalamate
Paroxetine	*Drugs of abuse*
Protriptyline	Amphetamine
Sertraline	Cocaine
Antipsychotics	Phencyclidine
Chlorpromazine	Methylphenidate
Clozapine	*Sedative-hypnotic drug withdrawal*
Haloperidol	Alcohol
Perphenazine	Barbiturates
Promazine	Benzodiazepines
Thioridazine	Ethchlorvynol
Trifluoperazine	Glutethimide
Lithium	Meprobamate
	Methaqualone
	Methyprylon
	Miscellaneous
	Cyclosporine
	Flumazenil
	Ganciclovir

[a]Adapted from Alldredge BK, Simon RP. Drugs that can precipitate seizures. In: Resor SR, Kutt H, eds. The medical treatment of epilepsy. New York: Marcel Dekker, 1992: 497–523.

Table 50.3.
International Classification of Epileptic Seizures and Syndromes[a]

Partial seizures (focal, local)
  Simple partial seizures (consciousness preserved)
    With motor signs (jacksonian)
    With somatosensory or special sensory symptoms
    With autonomic symptoms or signs
    With psychic symptoms
  Complex partial seizures (consciousness impaired)
    Simple partial onset followed by impaired consciousness
    Impaired consciousness at onset
  Secondarily generalized seizures
    Simple partial seizures evolving to generalized tonic-clonic seizures
    Complex partial seizures evolving to generalized tonic-clonic seizures
    Simple partial seizures evolving to complex partial seizures evolving to generalized tonic-clonic seizures
Generalized-onset seizures (convulsive or nonconvulsive)
  Tonic-clonic seizures
  Absence seizures
    Typical absence seizures
    Atypical absence seizures
  Myoclonic seizures
  Tonic seizures
  Atonic seizures
Localization-related (focal) epilepsies
  Idiopathic
    Benign epilepsy of childhood
  Symptomatic
    Temporal lobe epilepsy
    Extratemporal epilepsy
Generalized epilepsy
  Idiopathic
    Benign neonatal convulsions
    Childhood absence epilepsy
    Juvenile myoclonic epilepsy
    Other
  Idiopathic and/or symptomatic
    Infantile spasms (West syndrome)
    Lennox-Gastaut syndrome
    Myoclonic epilepsies
Special syndromes
  Febrile seizures

[a]Adapted from Commission on Classification and Terminology of the International League Against Epilepsy. Proposal for revised clinical and electroencephalographic classification of epileptic seizures. Epilepsia 22:489–501, 1981; and Proposal for classification of epilepsies and epileptic syndromes. Epilepsia 26:268–278, 1985.

however, they are less common. In all cases, patients can respond to their environment throughout the attack.

Complex partial seizures (*psychomotor* or *temporal lobe* seizures) are characterized by impaired consciousness and a heterogeneous group of abnormal symptoms. Although the variety of symptoms associated with complex partial seizures is wide, each individual usually reports stereotypical attacks. Auras precede complex partial seizures in many patients. Unusual epigastric sensations are most common, although various motor, sensory, or psychic symptoms (as described for simple partial seizures) may occur. Consciousness is then impaired for an average of about 2 min. During this time, patients may exhibit coordinated involuntary movements (automatisms) such as lip smacking, buttoning or unbuttoning of clothing, or wandering behavior. Less often, the behavioral abnormalities include violent outbursts, crying, or sexual actions. For some patients there is diagnostic confusion between the symptoms of absence seizures and those of complex partial seizures. Table 50.4 compares the usual (clinical) features of these two seizure types. Either simple or partial complex seizures may spread to involve both hemispheres of the brain (usually as a generalized tonic-clonic seizure). These events are termed *partial seizures with secondary generalization.*

In some cases the seizure classification, etiologic diagnosis, patient age, and coexistent medical conditions can be used to define a specific *epileptic syndrome.* An epileptic syndrome is a constellation of signs and symptoms that tend to occur together. Identification of epileptic syndromes may provide useful information that is not necessarily implied by either the etiologic diagnosis or the seizure classification, such as a specific choice of AED, the anticipated duration of AED therapy, and patient prognosis. Not all patients who have epilepsy can be classified as having an epileptic syndrome. Examples of epileptic syndromes include childhood absence epilepsy, juvenile myoclonic epilepsy, and Lennox-Gastaut syndrome.

Febrile Seizures

Febrile seizures are defined as generalized tonic-clonic seizures associated with temperatures above 38°C that occur in the absence of other identifiable causes. Febrile seizures are the most common form of epilepsy in children, occurring in 2 to 5% of the population. Affected children are usually between the ages of 3 months and 5 years and are otherwise neurologically and developmentally normal. Febrile seizures are classified as either *simple* or *complex.* *Complex febrile seizures* are prolonged (>15 min), occur in series (2 or more seizures in 24 hr), or have associated focal features. The remainder are classified as simple febrile seizures. *Simple febrile seizures* are usually benign, self-limited, and associated with only a 3% risk of recurrent, nonfebrile seizures in later life (7). The risk of epilepsy is increased to 4 to 11% in children who are affected by complex febrile seizures.

Because most febrile seizures are self-limited and not associated with acute or long-term neurologic sequelae, aggressive treatment is not required. Most febrile seizures occur within 24 hr of a febrile episode and can be prevented by promptly instituting antipyretic measures as soon as the fever is evident. Parents should be instructed to sponge the child with tepid water for 10 to 15 min and to administer acetaminophen every 4 hr for a temperature above 38°C. Acute treatment with AEDs is usually not necessary unless the seizure continues for longer than 10 or 15 min. In this case, either phenobarbital or diazepam is effective. Chronic administration of AEDs to children with a history of simple febrile seizures is not indicated.

Children with complex febrile seizures, preexisting neurologic abnormalities, or a family history of nonfebrile epilepsy are at greater risk for the development of epilepsy in later life. Drug therapy for the prevention of febrile seizures should be considered for these patients, although there is no evidence that the risk of nonfebrile epilepsy is reduced. Phenobarbital is effective for the treatment of febrile seizures; however, it must be administered continuously to ensure adequate drug levels at the onset of a febrile episode. Initiating oral phenobarbital at the onset of febrile illness is not appropriate. Rectal administration of diazepam (using the parenteral solution) results in rapid absorption and provides immediate protection from febrile seizures (7). Many clinicians prefer this treatment, since it does not require continuous administration.

DIAGNOSIS

Table 50.5 outlines the features of a comprehensive evaluation for patients with new-onset seizures. The diagnosis of epilepsy and proper classification of epileptic seizures are based primarily on the patient's history and witnessed accounts of the events. Although a complete evaluation usually includes other laboratory and diagnostic studies, a diagnosis of epilepsy can be clearly established only when an accurate and unambiguous history is obtained. Most patients and witnesses can give a clear

Table 50.4.
Comparison of the Clinical Features of Absence and Complex Partial Seizures

Feature	Absence Seizures	Complex Partial Seizures
Patients affected	Children	Children and adults
Preictal symptoms	No aura; abrupt interruption of consciousness	Aura common
Ictal phenomena	Automatisms common Average duration 10 sec	Automatisms common though more complex than in absence; average duration 2 min
Postictal symptoms	None; abrupt return of consciousness	Fatigue, confusion, drowsiness; gradual return of consciousness
Prognosis	Complete seizure control common	Less favorable response to drug therapy

Table 50.5.
Workup for the Patient with New-Onset Seizures

Patient history
  Seizure description
    Preictal phenomena (aura)
    Ictal manifestations
    Postictal state
    Provocative factors
  Perinatal and developmental history
  History of febrile seizures
  History of head trauma
  History of CNS infection
  Family history of epilepsy
Physical examination
Laboratory evaluation
  CBC
  Electrolytes
  Glucose
  Cerebrospinal fluid
  BUN
  Osmolality
Electroencephalogram
Computed tomographic scanning
Magnetic resonance imaging

account of generalized tonic-clonic seizures. However, more careful questioning is often necessary to elicit the subtle manifestations that accompany partial, absence, and other less dramatic seizure types.

Once it is apparent that a seizure has occurred, subsequent efforts should be directed toward establishing the cause. A thorough evaluation including a medical history and physical and laboratory examinations should be directed toward the variety of primary, metabolic, and systemic factors that may cause new-onset seizures (Table 50.1). Seizures that are due to an acute metabolic or systemic disorder must be differentiated from those that are related to a primary CNS disorder. Even with extensive workup, the etiology of epilepsy remains unidentified in 60 to 70% of patients. A genetic cause is suggested when the age at seizure onset is less than 25 years and there is a family history of epilepsy (8).

The electroencephalogram (EEG) is useful as a tool for both the diagnosis and classification of seizures. Spike and wave discharges on the EEG in conjunction with a clinical history of spontaneously recurring seizures can usually establish the diagnosis of epilepsy. While epileptiform abnormalities on the EEG are usually seen during a seizure, most EEG recordings are made between seizures (interictal EEG). Absence of EEG abnormalities on an interictal recording can rarely rule out the diagnosis of epilepsy. Epileptiform abnormalities are found in only about 50% of epileptic patients after a single interictal recording. Although the yield can be improved with repeated recordings, in 15% of epileptic patients no EEG abnormalities are ever found (8). Just as the

diagnosis of epilepsy is rarely excluded on the basis of a normal interictal EEG, the presence of EEG abnormalities, in and of itself, is not diagnostic for epilepsy. EEG abnormalities are seen in 10 to 15% of the nonepileptic population and are not indicative of epilepsy unless strong evidence from the patient history supports the diagnosis (8).

Computer-assisted tomography (CT) and magnetic resonance imaging (MRI) scans are particularly useful when evidence from the history or neurologic examination suggests a structural lesion of the brain (e.g., focal neurologic abnormalities or a history that is suggestive of partial seizures), although they are often employed in the initial evaluation of patients with new-onset seizures, regardless of the seizure type. MRI is more likely to detect lesions that are associated with partial epilepsy and is preferred over CT (1). Positron emission tomography (PET), an advanced imaging technique that allows more precise localization of areas of abnormal blood flow or metabolism, is useful for evaluation of patients for whom surgical intervention is considered. However, its availability is limited by high equipment costs.

Finally, in some patients, seizurelike activity may be a manifestation of some other nonepileptic condition (Table 50.6). The misdiagnosis of these events as seizures can result in unnecessary and potentially harmful therapy. Accordingly, the diagnosis of epilepsy should be reevaluated whenever the seizurelike events fail to respond to the usual treatments.

Table 50.6.
Disorders That May Mimic Epilepsy[a]

Gastroesophageal reflux
Breath-holding spells
Migraine
  Confusional
  Basilar
  With recurrent abdominal pain and cyclic vomiting
Sleep disorders (especially parainsomnias)
Cardiovascular events
  Pallid infantile syncope
  Vasovagal attacks
  Vasomotor syncope
  Cardiac arrhythmias
Movement disorders
  Shuddering attacks
  Paroxysmal choreoathetosis
  Nonepileptic myoclonus
  Tics and habit spasms
Psychological disorders
  Panic disorder
  Hyperventilation attacks
  Pseudoseizures
  Rage attacks

[a]Reprinted with permission from Scheuer ML, Pedley TA. The evaluation and treatment of seizures. N Engl J Med 323:1468–1474, 1990.

TREATMENT OVERVIEW

Lifestyle Adjustment and Social Issues

Although lifestyle adjustments may be required for patients with epilepsy, most patients respond well to medical therapy and can lead a life that is not severely restricted by their disorder. Nonetheless, some alteration of the patient's usual activities may be required, depending on the timing and clinical manifestation of their seizures. For example, patients who are affected by seizures associated with loss of consciousness or normal muscle control should restrict activities that place them or others at risk of injury. This may include partial or complete restriction of driving privileges and avoidance of activities such as swimming unattended, working at heights, and operating potentially dangerous machinery. Common sense should be the ultimate guide in the determination of specific lifestyle limitations that the patient's epileptic condition necessitates.

Certain changes in daily activities may reduce the occurrence of seizures by avoiding patient-specific risk factors. Conditions that are occasionally identified by patients as seizure precipitants include stress, exercise, alcohol or caffeine consumption, altered sleep schedules, and missed meals. When these or other precipitating conditions are identified, the patient and health provider should work cooperatively to establish guidelines that minimize these risks yet do not unnecessarily encumber the patient's daily routine.

In addition to the lifestyle limitations imposed by their condition, many people who have epilepsy also deal with problems of self-image and the social stigma that is attached to this disorder. Many patient concerns can be dealt with effectively by proper education. The clinician should take care to explain the disorder and its implications and to establish an atmosphere in which the patient is encouraged to voice his or her questions and concerns. The Epilepsy Foundation of American and its local affiliates also have available a wide range of client services and brochures to help patients (and their families) deal with their condition and its psychosocial implications.

Drug Therapy

AED therapy is the mainstay of epilepsy treatment. The goals are to reduce the frequency of recurrent seizures and to minimize the adverse effects associated with AED therapy. Specific therapeutic endpoints must be individualized for each patient. The choice of AED should be based on the seizure classification, the age and sex of the patient, concurrent medical conditions, potential adverse effects, and the pharmacokinetic features of the individual drugs. When these factors are considered and the guiding principles of AED therapy (discussed below) are followed, good to excellent seizure control can be attained in most patients. Nonetheless, some patients may continue to suffer from frequent seizures despite appropriate drug treatment.

PRINCIPLES OF ANTIEPILEPTIC DRUG SELECTION AND USAGE

Preference for Monotherapy with Nonsedating Agents

Monotherapy is preferred to polytherapy with AEDs because of the lower cost associated with the medication and blood level monitoring, reduced potential for adverse reactions and undesirable drug interactions, and improved medication compliance with a more simplified drug administration schedule. Furthermore, a growing body of evidence indicates that polytherapy offers no advantage over monotherapy for about 90% of patients with epilepsy (9). For patients for whom single drug therapy does not provide sufficient seizure control, polytherapy may be necessary to achieve the goals of treatment.

In addition to selecting the minimum effective number of AEDs, it is important to choose agents on the basis of their adverse-effect profile. The specific adverse effects of each drug are discussed below; however, sedating AEDs should be minimized or avoided. Phenobarbital and benzodiazepine AEDs are sedating; phenytoin, carbamazepine, valproate, ethosuximide, felbamate, gabapentin, lamotrigine, and vigabatrin are not. Sedation and decreased mentation are particularly common on initiation of barbiturate and benzodiazepine agents. Over time, however, an adaptive process occurs during which these effects become less noticeable. Despite the development of tolerance to the overt sedative effect of these drugs, evidence suggests that subtle effects on intelligence, memory, complex motor skills, and behavior often persist during treatment. In some cases these changes are noted by patients or their families only after the drug is discontinued (10). In this regard, therapy with nonsedating agents is preferred when possible, and the relative place of sedating AEDs has been reconsidered. For example, phenobarbital is as effective as phenytoin and carbamazepine for the treatment of generalized tonic-clonic seizures, but the latter agents are preferred because of their relative lack of CNS-depressant effects.

When possible, therapy should begin with one of the nonsedating AEDs such as phenytoin, carbamazepine, valproate, or ethosuximide. Except in some of the less common epilepsies (e.g., myoclonic epilepsy), phenobarbital and benzodiazepine agents should be reserved until nonsedating alternatives have failed. Nitrazepam and clobazam are benzodiazepine agents, which may have advantages over clonazepam in terms of sedation-related adverse effects. However, these drugs are not available for use in the United States. In summary, sedating AEDs should be avoided when possible, and in many cases, the

Table 50.7.

Antiepileptic Drugs of Choice Based on Seizure Classification[a]

	Partial Seizures[b]	Generalized Tonic-Clonic Seizures	Absence Seizures	Myoclonic Seizures
Drugs of choice	Carbamazepine Phenytoin	Valproate[c] Carbamazepine Phenytoin	Ethosuximide Valproate	Valproate
Alternatives				
Primary	Valproate Gabapentin[d] Lamotrigine[d] Vigabatrin[e] Phenobarbital Primidone	Phenobarbital Primidone	Clonazepam	Clonazepam
Secondary	Clorazepate[d] Felbamate		Acetazolamide	

[a]Information from (1, 3, 8, 11, 14).
[b]Includes simple partial seizures, complex partial seizures, and partial seizures that secondarily generalize.
[c]Probably the drug of choice for primary (generalized-onset) tonic-clonic seizures.
[d]Approved for use as adjunctive therapy only.
[e]FDA approval pending.

Table 50.8.

Cost Comparison of Innovator-Brand Antiepileptic Drug Therapy

Drug	Sample High-Dose Regimen	Cost/Month[a]
Tegretol (carbamazepine)	600 mg t.i.d.	$97
Felbatol (felbamate)	1200 mg t.i.d.	$119
Neurontin (gabapentin)	600 mg t.i.d.	$162
Lamictal (lamotrigine)	250 mg b.i.d.	$159
Dilantin (phenytoin)	400 mg q.d.	$23
Depakote (valproate)	750 mg t.i.d.	$150

[a]Cost for 30 days of treatment (rounded to nearest dollar) according to wholesale price (AWP) listings, February 1995.

substitution of nonsedating alternatives can result in noticeable improvement in cognitive, motor, and behavioral function.

Drug Selection

Once the diagnosis of epilepsy has been made, the choice of AED therapy is guided by considering the relative efficacy and toxicity of each agent. Proper classification of the patient's seizure type or epileptic syndrome is the most important step in choosing the appropriate agent. Table 50.7 lists the preferred AEDs for the treatment of different seizure types. Table 50.8 offers a cost comparison of some of the common first-line AEDs as well as newer agents that are marketed for the treatment of medically refractory epilepsy.

PARTIAL SEIZURES

Carbamazepine, phenytoin, phenobarbital, and primidone are equally effective for the treatment of partial seizures, including secondarily generalized partial seizures (11).

However, carbamazepine and phenytoin are usually tolerated better. Phenytoin has a long half-life that allows for once-daily dosing; therefore, this agent is preferred for patients who are unlikely to comply with a chronic regimen requiring multiple daily doses. However, phenytoin is associated with cosmetic changes that make it less desirable for the treatment of epilepsy in children, adolescents, and women. Valproate is also useful for the treatment of partial seizures, but carbamazepine provides better seizure control and fewer long-term adverse effects (12). Gabapentin, lamotrigine, vigabatrin, and felbamate are new AEDs that are effective for treating partial seizures. Currently, these agents are most useful for patients who have failed, or are intolerant of, other AEDs (e.g., carbamazepine, phenytoin, and valproate). The relative efficacy of these new agents has yet to be determined. Overall, partial seizures do not respond to treatment as well as do seizures that are generalized from their onset. Indeed, the prognosis for complete control of complex partial seizures in adults is often poor.

GENERALIZED TONIC-CLONIC SEIZURES

Carbamazepine, phenytoin, and valproate are the drugs of choice for the treatment of generalized tonic-clonic seizures. Evidence from some studies suggest that valproate is the drug of choice for the treatment of primary generalized tonic-clonic seizures. Approximately 75 to 85% of patients achieve complete seizure control during monotherapy with this agent (3). Carbamazepine or phenytoin is preferred for the treatment of children under the age of 2 years because of the higher risk of valproate-associated hepatotoxicity in these patients. Phenobarbital and primidone are also effective against generalized tonic-clonic seizures, but because of their adverse effects, they are usually reserved for use as second-line agents.

ABSENCE SEIZURES

Ethosuximide and valproate are equally effective for the treatment of absence seizures. Ethosuximide is preferred over valproate when only absence seizures are involved because it is associated with fewer serious adverse effects. Valproate is preferred if generalized tonic-clonic seizures also occur (1). The response to these agents is dramatic. In controlled trials, 70 to 90% of patients who were treated with ethosuximide or valproate experienced cessation or a dramatic reduction in absence seizures (13, 14). The combination of ethosuximide and valproate is often effective when monotherapy fails to yield adequate results. Clonazepam is also effective against absence seizures. However, because of frequent dose-related adverse effects and the development of tolerance to the antiepileptic effect of this drug, it should be reserved for patients in whom ethosuximide and valproate fail. Carbamazepine is ineffective for the treatment of absence seizures and may even exacerbate these and other seizure types when used for the treatment of children with mixed seizure disorders (15).

MYOCLONIC SEIZURES

Valproate effectively controls myoclonic seizures in 75 to 90% of patients with generalized idiopathic and juvenile myoclonic epilepsy (14). Myoclonic seizures after anoxic encephalopathy are more resistant to treatment. Clonazepam is also effective as monotherapy or in combination with valproate when either drug alone does not provide adequate seizure control.

Initiating Antiepileptic Drug Therapy

Phenytoin and phenobarbital are usually tolerated well when they are initiated at maintenance doses (e.g., 300 mg and 90 mg daily, respectively, in adults). The other AEDs are frequently associated with acute adverse effects, so therapy should begin with low doses and be titrated gradually according to the patient's clinical status. Patients who experience uncomfortable adverse effects at the initiation of therapy may be unwilling to continue treatment with that agent despite a reduction in dosage. Patients should be told to report adverse effects immediately so that an adjustment in therapy can be made as soon as possible. Patients should also know the goal of treatment and the time course over which seizure control is anticipated. The importance of strict compliance with the prescribed regimen should also be emphasized.

Adjusting and Monitoring Antiepileptic Drug Therapy

There is great interpatient variability in the dose-response relationship for all of the AEDs that are in common use. Therefore, after therapy is initiated, the optimal drug dose for each patient should be determined. This necessitates the titration of therapy until the desired clinical response is achieved or the patient experiences unacceptable dose-related adverse effects.

The determination of acceptable seizure control requires input from both patient and clinician. Though complete control of seizures is always desirable, patients may choose to continue therapy that allows minimal interruption of their lifestyle even though seizures occasionally recur. The clinician must assess the temporary disability and potential for harm (to both the patient and others) that may accompany a seizure and use this information, with input from the patient, to determine whether dosage adjustments should be made.

If the first agent does not achieve the desired therapeutic goal, then an alternative AED that is appropriate for the patient's seizure type should be gradually substituted rather than added. Tapering of the first drug should begin once a therapeutic effect (or blood level) of the new agent is attained. The rate of drug tapering is empiric. In this instance, most practitioners prefer to gradually discontinue therapy over a period of several days to weeks (also see the section below entitled "Withdrawal of Antiepileptic Drug Therapy"). Only after monotherapy has failed should multiple AED treatment be tried.

AED therapy fails for many reasons. Although various drugs may demonstrate equal efficacy in large populations of patients, an individual may respond better to one agent than to others. Additional factors that should be considered include poor medication compliance, erroneous diagnosis or seizure classification, progressive neurologic disease, and lifestyle factors that compromise the efficacy of treatment (e.g., recreational drug or alcohol abuse). Noncompliance with treatment is probably the most common cause of AED therapy failure, and this possibility should be carefully investigated. Patients who report a change in the character of their seizures (e.g., seizures are now preceded by an aura, whereas previously there was no warning) or frequent seizures after a long period of complete control should be referred for a thorough medical evaluation to rule out other neurologic disease (e.g., brain tumor).

Blood Levels

The widespread availability of blood level monitoring of AED therapy has had a dramatic effect on the use of these agents. For example, patients were frequently begun on combination AED regimens (e.g., phenytoin and phenobarbital) before clinicians had the capacity to individualize the doses for either agent. On the basis of past experience in which a single drug was occasionally ineffective and above-average doses sometimes led to toxicity, it was assumed that most patients would benefit if multiple drugs were used. Blood level monitoring, in addition to the pharmacokinetic properties of AEDs, is now used to maximize efficacy and minimize adverse effects.

The therapeutic range of plasma concentrations is a useful guide for titrating therapy. Within this range, many patients achieve seizure control without unacceptable side effects. However, it is also common to observe an adequate therapeutic response at concentrations below the usual therapeutic range, and some patients tolerate and indeed require blood levels above the upper limit of the therapeutic range to maintain seizure control. Thus, although these limits are useful as guides to therapy, the clinician should strive to determine the optimum AED plasma concentration for each individual patient (16).

Plasma-concentration monitoring of AEDs is most useful under the following conditions: (a) to document therapeutic failures, (b) to evaluate noncompliance or drug malabsorption, (c) to guide subsequent dosage adjustments that are required on a clinical basis, and (d) to evaluate possible drug-related adverse effects. The timing of blood sampling for drug level determination is important, particularly during therapy with AEDs that have a short half-life (e.g., carbamazepine and valproate). For these agents, blood levels can fluctuate significantly over the course of the dosing interval. Comparisons between drug levels may be inaccurate unless the blood is sampled at a consistent time relative to the dose. For most patients it is recommended that blood samples be taken in the morning, before the first daily dose of medication. An exception is patients with repeated, transient symptoms that are suggestive of dose-related drug toxicity. For these patients, blood sampling should coincide with the adverse experience so that the contribution of the drug level can be assessed.

Plasma-level monitoring of AEDs is often both overused and misused (9). It is common (and arguably appropriate) to document drug levels on an occasional basis in patients whose epileptic condition is well-controlled (e.g., every 12 months). However, other drug-level determinations should not be done unless there is clinical indication of their necessity. Likewise, there is often a tendency to adjust AED therapy on the basis of the level without taking into account the patient's clinical status. For example, it may be tempting to decrease the drug dose when the reported blood level is above the usual therapeutic range. However, some patients require higher concentrations than usual to achieve the desired therapeutic effect. Likewise, patients whose seizures are controlled with levels below the therapeutic range neither need a dose increase nor should be assumed to no longer require AED treatment. In his editorial regarding the use of AED blood level monitoring, W. Edwin Dodson wrote that "[c]hanging an antiepileptic drug dose based only on the drug level is like driving a car looking only at the speedometer and not out the window. Wrecks are inevitable and frequent" (16).

ANTIEPILEPTIC DRUGS

Clinical pharmacokinetic features of the common antiepileptic drugs are summarized in Table 50.9.

Carbamazepine

Carbamazepine is a highly lipophilic iminostilbene compound that is structurally related to the tricyclic antidepressant agent imipramine. Carbamazepine is very effective for the treatment of generalized tonic-clonic and partial seizures, but it is not effective against myoclonic or absence seizures. The antiepileptic effect of carbamazepine may be related to its effects on sodium channels to limit sustained, repetitive firing and alter synaptic transmission.

Carbamazepine (Tegretol and generic) is available as oral (200 mg) and chewable (100 mg) tablets and as a suspension (100 mg/5 mL). A controlled-release dosage form of Tegretol is currently under investigation in the United States. No parenteral formulation of the drug is available. Therapy with carbamazepine is usually initiated at a dose of 100 to 200 mg twice daily with gradual dose titration, in 200 mg increments, every 3 to 7 days. Although the manufacturer recommends that daily doses of carbamazepine not exceed 1200 mg, daily doses of 2000 mg and above are occasionally required for optimal therapy. Because of frequent gastric disturbances, loading doses of carbamazepine are not recommended for usual outpatient therapy. However, single carbamazepine doses of 8 to 10 mg/kg by the nasogastric route are useful for critically ill patients for whom rapid attainment of a therapeutic level is desired (17).

Absorption of carbamazepine from the gastrointestinal tract is slow and erratic and often does not follow first-order kinetics. The time to peak plasma levels after oral administration may vary from an average of 4 to 8 hr to as long as 24 hr. Although prolonged absorption of the drug may be due to slow dissolution of the drug from tablet form, the suspension is also absorbed erratically. Food has no consistent effect on the bioavailability of carbamazepine.

Carbamazepine is almost exclusively cleared by hepatic metabolism. Oxidation of the parent drug to carbamazepine 10,11-epoxide (CBZ-E) is the major metabolic pathway for elimination. The remainder is glucuronidated, sulfur-conjugated, or oxidatively metabolized by other routes. Only 2% of the dose is recovered unchanged in the urine. The half-life of the drug after a single dose may range from 24 to 45 hr. With chronic administration the half-life of carbamazepine is reduced, and interindividual differences in clearance are enhanced. Increased clearance of carbamazepine occurs during the first few weeks of therapy because of autoinduction of cytochrome P-450 activity leading to an increase in oxidation to CBZ-E. This

Table 50.9.
Clinical Pharmacokinetics of Antiepileptic Drugs[a]

	Carbamazepine	Phenytoin	Valproate	Ethosuximide
Adult daily dose	600–2400 mg	300–400 mg	750–2250 mg	1000–2000 mg[b]
Initial dose	100–200 mg b.i.d.	300 mg q.d.	125–250 mg b.i.d.–t.i.d.	500 mg q.d.
Dosage schedule	b.i.d.–q.i.d.	q.d.–b.i.d.	b.i.d.–t.i.d.	q.d.–b.i.d.
Bioavailability (%)	75–85	85–95	100	90–95
Time to peak absorption (hr)	4–8	4–8	2–8	1–7
Volume of distribution (L/kg)	0.8–1.6	0.5–0.7	0.09–0.17	0.6–0.9
Protein binding (%)	75–78	90–93	88–92	0
Plasma half-life (hr)	24–45 (single dose) 8–24 (chronic therapy)	9–40	6–16	20–60
Therapeutic plasma levels				
(µg/mL)	4–12	10–20	50–150	40–100
(µmol/L)	16–48	40–80	200–400	283–708

	Gabapentin	Lamotrigine	Felbamate	Vigabatrin[e]
Adult daily dose	900–3600 mg	200–500 mg	3600 mg	1000–4000 mg
Initial dose	300 mg q.d.	25 mg q.d.[c] or 50 mg q.o.d.[d]	400 mg t.i.d.	500 mg b.i.d.
Dosage schedule	t.i.d.	b.i.d.	t.i.d.–q.i.d.	b.i.d.
Bioavailability (%)	60	98	90	≥80
Time to peak absorption (hr)	2–3	2–4	2–4	1–2
Volume of distribution (L/kg)	0.7–0.8	0.9–1.2	0.75–0.85	0.8
Protein binding (%)	0	55	25	0
Plasma half-life (hr)	5–7	14–27	14–23	5–7[f]
Therapeutic plasma levels				
(µg/mL)	Not determined	Not determined	Not determined	Not determined
(µmol/L)				

	Phenobarbital	Primidone	Clonazepam	Clorazepate
Adult daily dose	100–200 mg	750–1500 mg	6–18 mg	22.5–90 mg
Initial dose	90 mg q.d.	125–250 mg b.i.d.	0.5–1 mg q.d.	7.5 mg t.i.d.
Dosage schedule	q.d.–b.i.d.	b.i.d.–q.i.d.	q.d.–t.i.d.	q.d.–t.i.d.
Bioavailability (%)	95–100	90–100	80–90	–
Time to peak absorption (hr)	1–4	1–3	1–4	0.5–2[g]
Volume of distribution (L/kg)	0.51–0.57	0.4–0.8	2.1–4.3	1–1.8[g]
Protein binding (%)	48–54	20–30	80–90	95–98[g]
Plasma half-life (hr)	72–144	5–18	30–40	55–100[g]
Therapeutic plasma levels				
(µg/mL)	10–40	5–15	5–70 ng/mL	Not determined
(µmol/L)	43–172	23–69	16–220 nmol/mL	

[a]Adapted from Brodie MJ. Established anticonvulsants and treatment of refractory epilepsy. Lancet 336:350–354, 1990; and Levy RH, Dreifuss FE, Mattson RH, Meldrum BS, Penry JK, eds. Antiepileptic drugs, 3rd ed. New York: Raven Press, 1989.
[b]The daily dose for children is 20–40 mg/kg.
[c]Starting dose for patients taking enzyme-inducing AEDs only.
[d]Starting dose for patients taking enzyme-inducing AEDs in combination with valproate.
[e]FDA approval pending.
[f]Plasma half-life does not correlate with duration of pharmacologic effect.
[g]Pharmacokinetic values for N-desmethyldiazepam, the active metabolite of clorazepate.

metabolic conversion is also enhanced by other enzyme-inducing drugs, such as phenytoin, phenobarbital, and primidone. Thus, the metabolic clearance and half-life may vary significantly, depending on the duration of treatment and concomitant drug therapy. It is not uncommon to observe a reduction in the half-life of carbamazepine from 30 hr after a single dose to 12 hr with chronic therapy and a further reduction to 8 hr during polytherapy with other AEDs. Larger daily doses (>1200 mg) and more frequent administration (three or four times a day) of carbamazepine are often necessary to minimize plasma level fluctuations and the attendant risk of breakthrough seizures or transient adverse effects.

Because of the large interindividual variability in carbamazepine absorption and clearance, the time-dependent alterations in metabolism, and the potential for fluctuations in drug concentrations over a dosage interval, careful plasma-level monitoring is often needed to determine optimal therapy. Steady-state concentrations of carbamazepine are reached within several days after therapy is initiated, although levels may decline by as much as 50% during the first month of therapy because of autoinduction of metabolism. After 1 month, autoinduction is complete, and plasma levels vary predictably with changes in dosage.

ADVERSE EFFECTS

Initial, dose-related adverse effects of carbamazepine are common and include dizziness, drowsiness, anorexia, and nausea. Although tolerance to these effects develops within the first few weeks of therapy, their occurrence can be minimized or avoided by gradual dose titration. Persistent gastrointestinal upset may be relieved by giving the drug with meals. Reversible, dose-related symptoms of carbamazepine toxicity include diplopia (commonly the initial manifestation of toxicity), nausea, headache, dizziness, and ataxia. Because of large fluctuations in the blood level of carbamazepine over the course of a usual dosage interval, dose-related toxicities may occur transiently at times of peak drug plasma concentrations.

Other dose-related neuropsychiatric adverse effects of carbamazepine include depression, irritability, mental sluggishness, and impairment of concentration and short-term memory. However, these adverse effects are less common than with phenobarbital and primidone. Furthermore, in several clinical epilepsy trials, patients with personality and behavioral disorders who were treated with carbamazepine had significant improvement during therapy (18). When dose-related adverse effects persist throughout the day, the total daily dose of carbamazepine should be decreased; when they are transient and occur 2 to 4 hr after a dose, an adjustment in the dosing schedule may suffice. Unusual movement disorders and carbamazepine-induced seizures can occur acutely following an overdose.

Rash occurs in approximately 5% of patients treated with carbamazepine, usually between the first and second week of therapy. Benign, maculopapular, urticarial, and morbilliform reactions are most common, but exfoliative dermatitis and Stevens-Johnson syndrome may also occur. In some cases, rash may be accompanied by fever, generalized lymphadenopathy, hepatomegaly, splenomegaly, and, less commonly, nephritis and vasculitis. Symptoms are reversible on drug discontinuation, and corticosteroids may hasten recovery. Cross-reactivity between carbamazepine and other aromatic antiepileptic drugs (e.g., phenytoin, phenobarbital) may complicate the subsequent management of these patients. In such cases, valproate is usually well tolerated (19). Other idiosyncratic adverse reactions include hepatitis and systemic lupus erythematosus (SLE). Hepatitis usually occurs within the first few

weeks of therapy and may coincide with eosinophilia and other symptoms of drug hypersensitivity. Carbamazepine may also cause a mild elevation of liver enzyme levels in fewer than 10% of patients, which appears to have no adverse clinical consequence. Carbamazepine-induced SLE is delayed, usually occurring after 6 to 12 months of therapy.

Among the most worrisome of idiosyncratic adverse reactions associated with carbamazepine is aplastic anemia. Although rare, this condition is fatal in about one-half of patients. The incidence of carbamazepine-associated aplastic anemia is estimated to be 0.5 per 100,000 treatment-years (20). Neither patient age nor daily or total dosage significantly affects this risk. Carbamazepine is also associated with a dose-independent transient leukopenia, which occurs in about 10% of patients. In most cases the leukopenia is mild and resolves, despite continuation of treatment. However, in about 2% of patients, leukopenia persists until the drug is removed (20). Carbamazepine-induced leukopenia does not appear to be a risk factor for aplastic anemia. While aplastic anemia can develop at any time during the first year of carbamazepine treatment, leukopenia is most common within the first month. The risk of serious hematologic reactions to carbamazepine can be minimized by patient education and laboratory monitoring. When therapy is initiated, patients should be counseled to seek immediate medical attention for abrupt onset of high fever, infection, petechiae, or unusual fatigue. If the diagnosis of aplastic anemia is confirmed, carbamazepine should be discontinued immediately, and the patient should not be rechallenged. Laboratory monitoring should include complete blood counts before initiation of treatment and every 2 weeks for the first 2 months of therapy. If no abnormalities are detected, hematologic monitoring should continue either at intervals of 3 months or when the patient develops signs or symptoms of myelosuppression. If mild leukopenia develops, complete blood counts should be evaluated at 2-week intervals until they return to baseline values. Therapy should be discontinued if the absolute neutrophil count drops below 1500/mm^3 or if infection occurs.

Carbamazepine may also cause hyponatremia and water retention, probably by increasing antidiuretic hormone secretion. This effect appears to be dose-related, as it is most often associated with blood levels of carbamazepine above the therapeutic range and often responds to a reduction in dose. At low serum sodium concentrations (<120 mEq/L), patients may report headache, confusion, dizziness, or loss of seizure control. Treatment consists of water restriction and/or reduction or discontinuation of carbamazepine therapy. Treatment with demeclocycline may be effective for patients who require continued carbamazepine therapy. Carbamazepine can cause cardiac conduction disturbances, primarily in older patients. Cardiotoxicity may be more common with higher doses and in patients with an underlying cardiac abnormality. A thorough history and baseline electrocardiogram should precede the initiation of carbamazepine in elderly patients.

DRUG INTERACTIONS

Carbamazepine, a potent inducer of drug metabolism, has been shown to increase the clearance of theophylline, doxycycline, haloperidol, warfarin, corticosteroids, valproate, clonazepam, ethosuximide, lamotrigine, felbamate, and various hormones. Thus, the potential for reduced effectiveness of these agents should be considered when carbamazepine therapy is begun. Because the failure rate of oral contraceptives is increased during coadministration with carbamazepine and other enzyme-inducing AEDs (e.g., phenytoin, phenobarbital, primidone), an alternative form of birth control should be considered. The effect of carbamazepine on plasma levels of phenytoin, phenobarbital, and primidone is inconsistent and probably reflects various degrees of enzyme induction and inhibition. Routine monitoring of blood levels is recommended when carbamazepine is added to the regimen of any patient who is receiving AED therapy.

Drug interactions that affect the blood level and response to carbamazepine are common. Danazol, dextropropoxyphene, erythromycin, isoniazid, verapamil, and diltiazem can inhibit carbamazepine metabolism and induce clinical symptoms of toxicity. Cimetidine may inhibit the metabolism of carbamazepine, but ranitidine has no effect. Carbamazepine levels can also be affected by concomitant therapy with other AEDs. Phenytoin, phenobarbital, and primidone may increase the metabolism of carbamazepine and lead to a reduction in the steady-state plasma concentration. Carbamazepine blood levels may increase, decrease, or remain the same when valproate is added. This may reflect the variable effects of valproate displacement of carbamazepine from protein-binding sites and valproate-mediated inhibition of carbamazepine metabolism.

Phenytoin

Phenytoin, a diphenyl-substituted hydantoin derivative, was introduced for the treatment of epilepsy in 1938. It soon became one of the most widely prescribed antiepileptic drugs because it possessed anticonvulsant activity at nonsedative doses. Phenytoin is effective for the treatment of partial and generalized tonic-clonic seizures, but it has no activity against absence and febrile seizures. Other hydantoin derivatives, including ethotoin and mephenytoin, also have anticonvulsant activity, but their clinical utility is limited. Phenytoin blocks neuronal sodium and calcium conductance, as well as blocking calcium-mediated excitatory neurotransmission, which probably is involved in its ability to regulate neuronal excitability under abnormal

conditions. The specific mechanism of the anticonvulsant effect of phenytoin is unknown.

Phenytoin (Dilantin and generic) is available as the free acid in suspension (30 mg/5 mL and 125 mg/5 mL) and 50-mg chewable tablets. The sodium salt of phenytoin is contained in phenytoin capsules (30 and 100 mg) and phenytoin injectable (50 mg/mL); for these dosage forms, phenytoin content is expressed in milligrams of sodium phenytoin. Because of the difference in molecular weight between the acid and salt forms of the drug, the capsule and parenteral dosage forms contain 8% fewer phenytoin acid equivalents than the suspension and chewable tablets do. This difference in drug content should be accounted for in changing products.

In adults, phenytoin can be initiated at a dose of 300 mg daily. The usual effective maintenance dose is 300 to 400 mg daily. Only Dilantin Kapseals, extended-release phenytoin capsules, are approved for once-daily maintenance dosing. The suspension and parenteral dosage forms should be given in divided daily doses. Loading doses of phenytoin help patients who require rapid attainment of a therapeutic level. The usual loading dose of phenytoin is 15 mg/kg. Oral loading doses of phenytoin can be given as a single dose or divided into individual increments of 200 to 400 mg separated by 2 to 4 hr. Previously, it was recommended that phenytoin loading doses be administered in small increments separated by several hours to enhance the rate of drug absorption (21). However, recent evidence suggests that single-dose loading with phenytoin is well tolerated and results in a shorter delay to the attainment of a therapeutic plasma level than the split-dose technique (22). By either method, phenytoin is absorbed slowly after oral administration, and the resultant peak plasma concentration is approximately half that achieved after an equivalent intravenous loading dose. When given by the intravenous route, phenytoin should be administered at a maximal rate of 50 mg/min to reduce the risk of hypotension and cardiac arrhythmias. These adverse effects are likely related to the 40% propylene glycol diluent that is used in the parenteral formulation of the drug. Blood pressure and heart rate should be measured periodically when large doses of phenytoin are administered intravenously.

Phenytoin is poorly water-soluble at acidic pH. Very little drug exists in solution in the stomach, and phenytoin absorption takes place primarily in the proximal part of the small intestine. Because the rate of drug dissolution in intestinal fluid is dose-dependent, the time to peak drug concentration after an oral loading dose of phenytoin may be delayed. The bioavailability of phenytoin approaches 100% for most well-formulated products, but it is prudent to avoid changing dosage forms and products because small changes in bioavailability can result in large changes in seizure control.

Additional complications of the low water solubility of phenytoin are evident after intramuscular administration. Phenytoin crystallizes when it is injected into muscle, resulting in a depot of drug that is both potentially damaging to local tissue and slowly and erratically absorbed from the injection site. Phenytoin should not be given intramuscularly. When oral administration is not feasible, the nasogastric or intravenous route is preferred.

Fosphenytoin (Cerebyx), a water-soluble prodrug of phenytoin for parenteral administration, is currently under investigation in the United States. The drug does not require propylene glycol as a diluent and is rapidly converted to phenytoin by circulating phosphatases. Fosphenytoin has advantages over phenytoin, including less venous irritation after intravenous administration and more reliable absorption after intramuscular administration. Infusion rates of 150-mg phenytoin equivalents/min have been administered safely in several studies (23).

Under normal conditions, phenytoin is approximately 90% bound to plasma proteins, primarily albumin. Conditions that can alter protein binding including renal failure, a lowered plasma albumin concentration, and the presence of displacing drugs. In each case these factors result in a decrease in phenytoin binding and an increase in the free fraction and volume of distribution. However, despite alterations in the free fraction, the free concentration of phenytoin is not changed significantly. Since the free drug exerts the therapeutic and toxic effects at receptor sites, the clinical response to a given dose of phenytoin is unchanged by altered protein binding. However, careful interpretation of the total (bound and unbound) phenytoin concentration is warranted. Equation 50.1 approximates the concentration of phenytoin that would be observed if the albumin concentration were normal (C_{normal}) from the total (bound and unbound) concentration ($C_{observed}$) and the patient's albumin concentration (Alb) in grams per decaliter (21):

$$C_{normal} = \frac{C_{observed}}{0.2 \cdot Alb + 0.1} \quad (50.1)$$

In patients with end-stage renal disease (creatinine clearance < 10 mL min), the affinity of albumin for phenytoin is reduced by approximately 50%, and Equation 50.2 should be used (21):

$$C_{normal} = \frac{C_{observed}}{0.1 \cdot Alb + 0.1} \quad (50.2)$$

Free (unbound) concentrations are also available from many clinical laboratories.

Phenytoin is eliminated primarily by hepatic metabolism. The major metabolic route involves *para*-hydroxylation of the parent compound to yield 5-(p-hydroxyphenyl)-5-phenylhydantoin. This metabolite is then glucuronidated and excreted primarily in the urine. Other hydroxylated metabolites are also generated during phenytoin metabolism, and all metabolites are inactive. Less than 5% of the drug is eliminated unchanged in the urine.

Unlike many drugs that are cleared from the body by a first-order elimination process, the clearance of phenytoin varies over the range of plasma levels that are clinically useful for the treatment of seizures. At very low plasma levels, phenytoin clearance is first-order, and small dosage changes result in a proportional change in the level. However, as the phenytoin concentration approaches the therapeutic range, the maximal capacity for phenytoin metabolism is approached, and a change in dosage can result in a disproportionately large change in the steady-state level. Thus, phenytoin dosage adjustments must be made cautiously. The Michaelis-Menten model of saturable enzyme kinetics has been used to characterize the relationship between phenytoin dose and plasma level at steady state. By using Equation 50.3, the rate of phenytoin administration (in milligrams per day) can be calculated from the desired steady state plasma level. Population estimates of V_{max} (maximal rate of phenytoin metabolism = 7 mg/kg/day in adults) and K_m (phenytoin concentration at which V_{max} is half-maximum = 4 mg/L in adults) can be used if patient-specific data is not available (21):

$$R_i = \frac{V_{max} \cdot Cp_{ss}}{K_m + Cp_{ss}} \quad (50.3)$$

ADVERSE EFFECTS

Acute, dose-related adverse effects of phenytoin include ataxia, diplopia, dizziness, drowsiness, encephalopathy, and involuntary movements. These symptoms usually occur at phenytoin levels above 30 mg/mL and are reversible when phenytoin is discontinued or the dose is reduced. Involuntary movements during phenytoin intoxication may include dyskinesias of the limbs, trunk, or face and are similar to those encountered with long-term antipsychotic drug therapy. Phenytoin has also been reported to exacerbate seizures at toxic levels, but this is rare. Nystagmus is a dose-related effect that may occur at plasma levels within the therapeutic range and does not necessitate a reduction in dosage.

Adverse effects associated with long-term therapy include gingival hyperplasia, facial coarsening, peripheral neuropathy, and vitamin deficiencies. Gingival hyperplasia is a dose-related effect that occurs in over 40% of adult patients taking phenytoin. It usually begins within the first 3 months and may progress during the first year of phenytoin therapy. Patients who are at risk for gingival hyperplasia include children and those with poor oral hygiene. Patients taking phenytoin should be counseled to brush and floss their teeth regularly and to have regular dental checkups. Mild gingival hyperplasia may respond to improved dental and periodontal care or a reduction in phenytoin dosage. In advanced cases, gum resection surgery may be required.

Alternative AED therapy should be considered for these patients. Chronic phenytoin therapy is also associated with dysmorphic changes in the lips, nose, brow, and other facial structures as well as other cosmetic changes, including hirsiutism and acne. These adverse effects are a major limitation to the use of phenytoin for the treatment of children, adolescents, and young women.

Peripheral neuropathy with decreased deep tendon reflexes and sensory deficits may also occur during long-term phenytoin therapy. These symptoms are probably most common during polytherapy with phenytoin and phenobarbital and are not reversible. Phenytoin-induced megaloblastic anemia with folic acid deficiency occurs in fewer than 1% of patients and responds to folic acid supplementation. Prophylactic folic acid supplementation is unnecessary and may alter phenytoin metabolism. Alterations of bone density, mass, and mineral content have been associated with phenytoin, usually when it is given in combination with other enzyme-inducing AEDs. Although most patients with AED-related bone disease are asymptomatic, clinically apparent osteomalacia and osteporosis may also occur and requires appropriate treatment. Whether patients without clinical evidence of bone disease should receive prophylactic vitamin D and calcium supplementation is not known. Certainly, patients with known risk factors for metabolic bone disease (e.g., inadequate diet, sunlight, or exercise) should be monitored closely. AED-induced alterations in vitamin D metabolism to less active products and impaired absorption of calcium may be related to this complication of chronic therapy.

Idiosyncratic adverse reactions usually occur within the first 8 weeks of phenytoin therapy, including rash, hepatitis, lymphadenopathy, and hematologic alterations. Skin rashes, which occur in fewer than 10% of patients, usually manifest within the first 14 days of phenytoin therapy and may be accompanied by hepatitis, lymphadenopathy, and fever. The rash is usually morbilliform but may progress to Stevens-Johnson syndrome, erythema multiforme, or toxic epidermal necrolysis. Phenytoin should be discontinued if the rash involves mucous membranes or is accompanied by fever. Hepatitis usually occurs in the presence of fever, rash, and lymphadenopathy during the first 3 weeks of therapy and necessitates the immediate discontinuation of phenytoin. Although drug discontinuation optimizes the chance of recovery, some patients continue to deteriorate, and (rarely) phenytoin-induced hepatic injury leads to encephalopathy, coma, and death. Hematologic adverse reactions during phenytoin therapy include a modest, transient depression in leukocytes and (very rarely) aplastic anemia or agranulocytosis. Patients with severe idiosyncratic reactions to phenytoin should not be rechallenged. Also, the potential for cross-reactivity with other aromatic AEDs should be considered (see the discussion above on the adverse effects of carbamazepine).

DRUG INTERACTIONS

Phenytoin, a potent inducer of hepatic microsomal enzymes, can enhance the metabolism of other drugs that are eliminated by similar enzyme systems, including oral contraceptives, warfarin, corticosteroids, cyclosporine, theophylline, and other AEDs. Phenytoin increases the metabolism of carbamazepine, valproate, felbamate, lamotrigine, and clonazepam, resulting in a decrease in plasma concentrations and concomitant reduction in the clinical anticonvulsant effect. Phenytoin also may increase the ratio of primidone to phenobarbital when it is administered to patients who are stabilized on primidone. Although phenytoin may enhance warfarin metabolism, the effect is unpredictable and may even be manifested by a transient increase in the anticoagulant effect of warfarin. Thus, warfarin therapy should be monitored closely during phenytoin coadministration.

Drug interactions affecting phenytoin may involve alterations in phenytoin absorption, metabolism, or protein binding. Antacids and nutritional formulas have been shown to reduce plasma levels of phenytoin, but in neither case is the interaction predictable. Steady-state phenytoin levels may fall during coadministration with aluminum- and magnesium-containing antacids, but the magnitude of the effect is variable. Given the potential for an interaction, it is reasonable to space antacid and phenytoin doses by 2 to 3 hr. Phenytoin levels drop after institution of nasogastric feedings, but the mechanism of this interaction is unclear. With flushing of the nasogastric tube, phenytoin adsorption to the apparatus is probably minimal. Concurrent administration with Isocal and Osmolite, but not Ensure, may reduce phenytoin levels (24). Patients' phenytoin levels should be monitored closely when enteral feedings are initiated or stopped and if the formula is changed. Heparin, phenylbutazone, tolbutamide, and valproate displace phenytoin from plasma protein-binding sites. Many drugs alter the metabolism of phenytoin. It is important to be aware of drugs that can alter phenytoin metabolism, because small changes in phenytoin clearance can have a large effect on the steady-state plasma level. Folic acid, alcohol, and rifampin can increase the metabolism of phenytoin. Drugs that can reduce the metabolism of phenytoin include valproate, isoniazid, amiodarone, cimetidine, omeprazole, phenylbutazone, disulfiram, sulfonamides, and chloramphenicol.

Valproate

Valproate is a unique AED because of its chemical structure and its broad activity against both partial and generalized seizures. Unlike most other AEDs, which have a substituted heterocyclic ring structure, valproate is a short, branched-chain fatty acid. Many clinicians consider valproate to be the drug of choice for the treatment of primary generalized epilepsies including tonic-clonic and absence seizures (14). Ethosuximide and valproate are equally effective against absence seizures. Valproate is as effective as carbamazepine for the treatment of secondarily generalized tonic-clonic seizures, but carbamazepine is more effective against complex partial seizures (12). Valproate is also effective as monotherapy for treating patients who have a combination of generalized tonic-clonic seizures and absence of myoclonic seizures. The mechanism of action of valproate is not completely characterized but probably involves potentiation of γ-aminobutyric acid (GABA), the primary inhibitory neurotransmitter within the CNS.

Valproate is available as valproic acid (Depakene) in soft gelatin capsules (250 mg) and syrup form (250 mg/5 mL) and as divalproex sodium (Depakote) in enteric-coated tablets (125 mg, 250 mg, and 500 mg) and sprinkle capsules (125 mg) that may be emptied onto food. Divalproex sodium dissociates into valproate in the gastrointestinal tract. An intravenous dosage form is currently under investigation. In adults, valproate should be initiated at a dose of 125 to 250 mg two or three times a day with gradual dose titration in 250-mg increments every 3 to 7 days. The usual effective dose of valproate is 750 to 1500 mg divided into three or four daily doses.

The bioavailability of valproate is close to 100% for all oral dosage forms, but the rate of absorption may vary. Peak levels occur within 2 hr after administration of valproate syrup and capsules. Enteric-coated tablets were developed to minimize the gastric distress associated with the plain capsule by prolonging the rate of drug dissolution. Consequently, the time to peak levels is delayed and may vary from 3 to 8 hr (25). Although food has no significant effect on the absorption of the soft gelatin capsules, the rate of valproate absorption from enteric-coated tablets is delayed.

Valproate is highly bound to plasma proteins, so the volume of distribution is small. The extent of protein binding varies and depends highly on the dose and plasma level of the drug. At concentrations below 75 mg/mL, valproate is approximately 90% bound to plasma proteins, primarily albumin. As the total concentration of valproate increases above 100 mg/mL, albumin binding sites become saturated, and the free fraction of the drug may increase by up to 50% (25). The distribution and protein binding of valproate can be affected by a variety of other factors, including albumin and free fatty acid concentrations, pregnancy, age, and the presence of displacing drugs (e.g. phenytoin).

The relationship between the dose and steady-state plasma levels of valproate is curvilinear. Thus, with increasing dosage a less-than-proportional change in the plasma concentration occurs. Since only the unbound fraction of drug is available for metabolic transformation,

this curvilinear relationship may be explained by the increase in valproate clearance that would be expected when free valproate concentrations rise as a consequence of saturable protein binding. Valproate is eliminated almost exclusively by hepatic metabolism with a half-life of 12 to 16 hr in healthy volunteers. The half-life may be reduced during concomitant therapy with other AEDs. Oxidation of valproate at the β and γ positions and glucuronide conjugation of the parent and metabolites are the primary routes of metabolism. The major metabolites of valproate are eliminated slowly and may also be active. This may explain the fact that maximal response to valproate can be delayed by several weeks beyond the time required to achieve steady-state plasma levels of the parent drug. Also, the anticonvulsant effect during valproate therapy outlasts its presence in plasma, further supporting the hypothesis that metabolites contribute to the antiepileptic effect of the drug.

ADVERSE EFFECTS

Valproate is generally well-tolerated, and for this reason it is often preferred over other AEDs. Gastrointestinal adverse effects are most common during valproate therapy. As many as 35% of patients who are treated with either capsules or syrup report nausea, vomiting, anorexia, or other symptoms of gastrointestinal discomfort. Patient tolerance can be improved by using the the enteric-coated products (tablets or sprinkles), and most patients prefer them.

The dose-related neurologic adverse effects that are seen with valproate are like those seen with other AEDs. Fine tremor, a reversible, dose-related adverse effect, occurs frequently. When tremor occurs transiently during the day, adjustment of the drug regimen to minimize plasma level fluctuations may alleviate the problem. Otherwise, a reduction in the total daily dose of valproate or concomitant treatment with a β-adrenergic blocking agent (e.g., propranolol) may be necessary. Behavioral and cognitive adverse effects are less common with valproate than with phenytoin, phenobarbital, and primidone (26).

Other dose-related adverse effects include weight gain, loss or thinning of hair, altered platelet function, and increases in hepatic enzyme levels. Weight gain occurs in up to 50% of patients (26) and probably reflects a reduction in energy use. Hair thinning or alopecia is transient and usually occurs on initiation of therapy. Reduction of valproate dosage may help. Valproate causes a dose-related reduction in platelet count and impairment of platelet function leading to an increase in bleeding time (27). These effects may be significant for patients with high plasma levels of valproate or those undergoing surgical procedures. Approximately 40% of patients will experience a dose-related increase in hepatic enzymes during valproate therapy. This abnormality is usually asymptomatic and rapidly responds to a reduction in dose or discontinuation of the drug. Practitioners should discontinue valproate in the following instances: (a) an elevation in hepatic enzymes three times above baseline, (b) abnormalities in laboratory tests of hepatic synthesis or metabolism (e.g., elevated bilirubin or prothrombin time or decreased serum albumin concentration), or (c) the development of clinical signs or symptoms of hepatitis. Baseline laboratory values, including liver enzymes and hepatic function tests, should be determined before initiating valproate.

Valproate has also been associated with fulminant hepatotoxicity leading to coma and death. Although the overall incidence of hepatic fatalities is very low (1 in 49,000 treated patients), certain patients are particularly at risk. Specific risk factors include age less than 2 years, AED polytherapy, and developmental delay (28). The risk of fatal hepatotoxicity is exceedingly low in patients over the age of 10 years who are on monotherapy. When it occurs, fulminant hepatotoxicity is usually seen during the first 6 months of therapy. Gastrointestinal distress, anorexia, or sudden loss of seizure control may precede the development of fulminant hepatic failure, so patients should be counseled at the start of therapy to report these or other clinical signs or symptoms of hepatitis as soon as they develop. The prognosis may be improved if therapy is discontinued quickly.

Dreifuss and colleagues suggest the following guidelines for minimizing the risk of fatal valproate hepatotoxicity (28):

(a) avoid administering valproate as part of anticonvulsant polytherapy in children under age 3 years, unless monotherapy has failed or the potential benefits of polypharmacy outweigh the risks; (b) avoid administering valproate to patients with preexisting liver disease or a family history of childhood hepatic disease; (c) administer valproate in the lowest possible dose that is consistent with seizure control; (d) avoid concomitant administration of valproate and salicylates, and avoid fasting in children with intercurrent illnesses; (e) monitor clinically for such symptoms as nausea, vomiting, headache, lethargy, edema, jaundice, or seizure breakthrough, especially after febrile illness.

Greater recognition of patients who are at risk for valproate hepatotoxicity is probably responsible for the significant decrease in the number of hepatic fatalities despite the overall increased use of the drug (1).

DRUG INTERACTIONS

Metabolic interactions between valproate and other AEDs are common. Unlike phenytoin, carbamazepine, phenobarbital, and primidone, valproate is not an enzyme-inducing drug. Conversely, valproate may inhibit hepatic drug metabolism. This enzyme inhibition has been implicated in valproate interactions with phenobarbital, phenytoin, and carbamazepine. Valproate inhibits the oxidative metabolism of phenobarbital, leading to an average increase of phenobarbital levels of 80% (29). However, because of variability in this increase (0 to 200%), routine adjustment of the dose of phenobarbital is not recommended. Rather, blood levels of phenobarbital should be monitored, with appropriate adjustment of the dose if necessary. The interaction between phenytoin and valproate is complex and probably involves both enzyme inhibition and protein binding displacement. Phenytoin levels commonly fall after initiation of valproate, probably owing to displacement of phenytoin from protein-binding sites and an attendant increase in phenytoin clearance and volume of distribution. The free fraction of phenytoin may increase further with subsequent increases in valproate dosage. During continued therapy with valproate, phenytoin levels may remain low or rise to the preadministration level or above. Regardless of the subsequent change in phenytoin levels, the free fraction of phenytoin likely remains elevated during polytherapy and may increase further with increasing doses of valproate. Thus, total plasma levels of phenytoin should be interpreted cautiously. Valproate has been reported to induce clinical symptoms of carbamazepine toxicity. However, this interaction is not well characterized.

The metabolism of valproate is susceptible to induction by other AEDs, including phenobarbital, carbamazepine, phenytoin, and primidone. Serum levels of valproate decrease by an average of 30 to 40% (29), and the half-life is reduced to 6 to 9 hr. Because of the difficulty of maintaining consistent, therapeutic concentrations of valproate in patients who are taking other AEDs, monotherapy with valproate is highly recommended.

Antipyretic doses of aspirin may displace valproate from protein-binding sites and competitively inhibit β-oxidation. Unlike other AEDs, valproate does not increase the failure rate of oral contraceptives (29). However, because of the potential teratogenic effects, women of childbearing age should use this agent cautiously.

Ethosuximide

Ethosuximide is a member of the succinimide class of antiepileptic agents, which includes phensuximide and methsuximide. The latter agents share similar antiepileptic effects with ethosuximide, but they are rarely used in the treatment of seizures because they are less effective and their use is associated with more significant adverse effects. Ethosuximide is as effective as valproate for the treatment of absence seizures, but ethosuximide is often preferred for young children because of the potential for valproate-associated hepatotoxicity. Ethosuximide has no activity against partial and generalized tonic-clonic seizures. Although the mechanism of ethosuximide's antiepileptic effect is unknown, the drug may suppress seizures by alteration of calcium flux in the thalamus or by the depletion of excitatory neurotransmitter stores within the CNS.

Ethosuximide (Zarontin) is available as capsules (250 mg) and syrup (250 mg/5 mL) for oral use. The initial dose of ethosuximide is 250 mg daily for children 3 to 6 years of age and 500 mg for children 6 years and older. The dose should be increased at weekly intervals in 250-mg increments as necessary. Infants require larger doses on a weight basis than adolescents and adults do. Despite the long half-life of ethosuximide, the drug is often given in divided doses to minimize gastrointestinal distress.

Ethosuximide is metabolized hepatically to inactive hydroxylated products that are then excreted. Approximately 20% of a given dose is excreted in the urine unchanged. Serum level monitoring helps to guide therapy, but the upper end of the therapeutic range is loosely defined. Many patients tolerate levels above 100 mg/mL, and plasma concentrations of 150 mg/mL or greater are occasionally required for optimal treatment.

ADVERSE EFFECTS

Sedation, nausea, anorexia, and headache are the most common adverse effects reported on initiation of ethosuximide. Tolerance to these symptoms usually develops within the first weeks of treatment, and they can be minimized by reducing the dose or by introducing the drug gradually as outlined above. Behavioral disturbances, including irritability, depression, and frank psychosis, occur independent of the drug dose. These symptoms are rare and usually occur in children or adolescents who have a history of behavioral or psychiatric problems. Discontinuation of the drug is usually required. In most patients, ethosuximide has no detrimental effect on intellectual function. Idiosyncratic reactions during ethosuximide therapy include mild, transient leukopenia, rare pancytopenia, rash, and SLE. Periodic complete blood counts should be performed during the first 6 to 12 months of therapy, and the patient should be observed for the development of clinical symptoms, suggesting serious bone marrow suppression.

DRUG INTERACTIONS

Ethosuximide is not an enzyme inducer or inhibitor and has no important effect on the disposition of most other AEDs. Ethosuximide levels may be reduced by carbamazepine and increased by valproate, presumably by enzyme induction and inhibition, respectively. Phenytoin, phenobarbital, and primidone have no clinical effect on ethosuximide levels.

Gabapentin

Gabapentin is a chemically unique cyclohexane derivative of GABA that was synthesized to cross the blood-brain barrier and mimic the inhibitory effects of this neurotransmitter on the CNS. Gabapentin is effective as adjunctive (add-on) therapy for patients with partial and secondarily generalized tonic-clonic seizures. In clinical trials, gabapentin reduces the frequency of these seizures by 50% or more in 25% of patients. By comparison, only 10% of placebo-treated patients experienced a similar reduction in seizures. The drug is not currently approved for children or as monotherapy, although studies are ongoing to support these indications. The drug has little or no activity against primary generalized tonic-clonic and absence seizures. Although gabapentin was designed to enhance GABA neurotransmission within the CNS, the drug does not alter GABA synthesis, degradation, or uptake or interact with GABA receptors (30). The mechanism of action is unknown.

Gabapentin (Neurontin) is available as oral capsules in 100-mg, 300-mg, and 400-mg strengths. Therapy with gabapentin can be titrated to an effective dose rapidly, giving 300 mg on the first day, 300 mg twice on the second day, and 300 mg three times on the third day. Thereafter, therapy should be titrated according to patient response. Daily doses up to 3600 mg (divided three times a day) have been well tolerated and are sometimes required.

The bioavailability of gabapentin is approximately 60% after oral administration of doses between 900 and 1800 mg daily, but further dosage increases result in less than proportional increases in plasma concentrations. This lack of dose proportionality appears to be caused by saturation of the large neutral amino acid transport mechanism (system L transporter) that is responsible for gabapentin absorption across the intestinal membrane (31). The time to peak absorption of gabapentin is 2 to 3 hr. Food has no effect on the rate and extent of absorption.

Unlike other AEDs, gabapentin is neither metabolized nor bound to plasma proteins. The drug is excreted unchanged in the urine at a rate that is directly proportional to creatinine clearance. Reduction of gabapentin dosage is indicated when creatinine clearance is less than 60 mL/min. The half-life of gabapentin is 5 to 7 hr and does not change with chronic dosing. Although some studies have suggested that gabapentin is more effective at higher plasma concentrations, a therapeutic range of plasma concentrations has not yet been defined.

ADVERSE EFFECTS

Overall, gabapentin is well tolerated and is associated with mild adverse effects, primarily affecting the CNS. In premarketing studies of gabapentin as adjunctive therapy, adverse effects included somnolence (19%), dizziness (17%), ataxia (12%), and fatigue (11%). These adverse effects appear to be dose-related and can be managed by adjustments of gabapentin dosage or the doses of concomitant agents. Rash appears in fewer than 1% of patients, a rate that compares favorably with those of other AEDs. Current evidence does not support the need for routine laboratory monitoring other than baseline laboratory studies.

DRUG INTERACTIONS

Because gabapentin is neither metabolized nor bound to plasma proteins, it has a much lower potential than do other AEDs to interact with other drugs. Indeed, gabapentin does not affect the plasma levels of carbamazepine (including its epoxide metabolite), phenytoin, phenobarbital, or valproate. Likewise, these AEDs do not alter the disposition of gabapentin. Aluminum/magnesium hydroxide antacids (given concomitantly or 2 hr after gabapentin) and cimetidine have been shown to reduce gabapentin plasma levels by 12 to 20%, but these interactions are not likely to be clinically significant.

Lamotrigine

Lamotrigine was originally synthesized in a drug development program to exploit the antiepileptic effect of novel antifolate agents. Lamotrigine has weak antifolate properties, but its efficacy as an AED is unrelated to this property. Rather, lamotrigine inhibits voltage-dependent sodium channels, resulting in a decreased release of excitatory neurotransmitters such as aspartate and glutamate. Lamotrigine is approved as adjunctive therapy for partial and secondarily generalized tonic-clonic seizures in adults. Approximately 25% of patients experience a 50% or greater reduction in partial-onset seizures when lamotrigine is added to existing AED therapy. Preliminary evidence suggests that lamotrigine also has activity against primary generalized epilepsies (including juvenile myoclonic epilepsy) and the Lennox-Gastaut syndrome and that it is effective as monotherapy (30). However, these uses require further study.

Lamotrigine (Lamictal) is available as oral tablets in 25-mg, 100-mg, 150-mg, and 200-mg strengths. Because lamotrigine disposition is significantly affected by other AEDs, the dosage of this agent needs to be adjusted according to concomitant therapy. When administered with enzyme-inducing AEDs (carbamazepine, phenytoin, phenobarbital, and primidone), lamotrigine should be initiated at a dose of 50 mg daily for 2 weeks and increased to 50 mg twice a day for 2 more weeks. Thereafter, the lamotrigine dose may be increased weekly in increments of 100 mg/day to a maintenance dose of 300 to 500 mg daily (divided twice a day). Some patients may benefit from doses up to 700 mg/day. For patients who are receiving enzyme-inducing AEDs with valproate, lamotrigine should be initiated at a dose of 25 mg every other day for 2 weeks and increased to 25 mg/day for 2 more weeks. Thereafter, the lamotrigine dose can be increased every 1 to 2 weeks in increments of 25 mg/day to a maintenance dose of 100 to 200 mg/day (divided twice a day). When given with valproate alone, lamotrigine doses should be reduced further, but more specific recommendations are not available.

The oral bioavailability of lamotrigine is 98%, and peak plasma levels occur 2 to 4 hr after administration. Food has no significant effect on absorption. Lamotrigine is 55% bound to plasma proteins, making clinically significant protein-binding interactions unlikely. Lamotrigine is metabolized by glucuronic acid conjugation to an inactive product. The half-life of lamotrigine is approximately 24 hr during monotherapy, but other AEDs significantly affect the rate of elimination. Concomitant therapy with enzyme-inducing AEDs enhances lamotrigine metabolism and reduces the half-life to approximately 14 hr. The half-life is approximately 27 hr in patients who are taking valproate and enzyme-inducing AEDs. The half-life is increased to 59 hr in patients who are taking valproate without enzyme-inducing AEDs. No clear relationship exists between plasma concentrations of lamotrigine and clinical effect.

ADVERSE EFFECTS

Adverse effects during lamotrigine therapy are usually mild or moderate and resolve with dosage reduction. Pooled data from placebo-controlled add-on studies found that the most common side effects involved the CNS and included dizziness (38%), headache (29%), diplopia (28%), ataxia (22%), and somnolence (14%). Approximately 10% of patients who received lamotrigine developed a skin rash, and it was the most common reason for drug discontinuation (3%) (32). The rash usually develops in the first 4 to 6 weeks of therapy and may be more common in patients who are on an AED regimen that includes valproate. The incidence of rash also increases with higher starting doses and a faster rate of dosage escalation. Stevens-Johnson syndrome, toxic epidermal necrolysis, and other symptoms of the antiepileptic drug hypersensitivity syndrome (e.g., fever, lymphadenopathy, and hematologic and hepatic abnormalities) have also been reported. Patients should be counseled to report the occurrence of a skin rash immediately to their health care provider, and withdrawal of lamotrigine should be considered, particularly if the rash is painful, involves mucous membranes, or is associated with other systemic manifestations.

DRUG INTERACTIONS

As was indicated above, lamotrigine metabolism can be significantly affected by other AEDs. These interactions are clinically significant and should be considered during the initiation and titration of lamotrigine therapy. Lamotrigine does not have a significant effect on the elimination of carbamazepine, phenytoin, phenobarbital, primidone, or oral contraceptives. There are conflicting reports on the effect of lamotrigine on CBZ-E concentrations. One study reported that lamotrigine had no effect on CBZ-E concentrations; however, another study reported that CBZ-E concentrations increased by a mean of 45% during lamotrigine administration (33). Lamotrigine has been shown to increase valproate concentrations by 25% in healthy volunteers (32).

Felbamate

Felbamate is a chemically unique carbamate derivative that is structurally related to the sedative-hypnotic meprobamate. It was approved by the U.S. Food and Drug Administration (FDA) in August 1993 and rapidly became a popular agent for several reasons: (a) it was the first new AED that had been marketed in the United States since valproate in 1978; (b) it was the first drug that was brought to the market through the Antiepileptic Drug Development Program, a program established by the National Institutes for Neurological Disease and Stroke to facilitate the preclinical and clinical evaluation of new chemical entities for the treatment of epilepsy; (c) the drug was shown to be effective as monotherapy and adjunctive therapy for adults with partial seizures (with and without secondary generalization) and as adjunctive therapy for children with partial or generalized seizures associated with the Lennox-Gastaut syndrome; and (d) the drug seemed to be very well tolerated in clinical trials. In other preliminary studies, felbamate also was shown to have activity against absence, atypical absence, and juvenile myoclonic seizures. The mechanism of felbamate's antiepileptic effects is unknown.

More recently, however, felbamate has been associated with potentially life-threatening hematologic and hepatic adverse effects (see the discussion below on adverse effects). These reports have caused reconsideration of the relative risks and benefits of felbamate therapy, and the drug is currently recommended only for "patients who respond inadequately to alternative treatments and whose epilepsy is so severe that a substantial risk of aplastic anemia and/or liver failure is deemed acceptable in light of the benefits conferred by its use" (34).

Felbamate (Felbatol) is available as oral tablets in 400-mg and 600-mg strengths and as an oral suspension (600 mg/5 mL). Therapy with felbamate can be initiated at 1200 mg/day (given three or four times a day) and increased at weekly intervals by 1200 mg/day to a dose of 3600 mg/day. Some patients may require higher doses for maximal benefit. The dosages of concomitant AEDs should be reduced by 20 to 30% on initiation of felbamate, and further reductions may be required during titration of therapy (see the discussion below on drug interactions).

Felbamate is at least 90% absorbed after oral administration, and its bioavailability is unaffected by food or antacids. The drug is 25% bound to plasma proteins (primarily to albumin), so clinically significant protein-binding interactions are unlikely. Felbamate is eliminated by cytochrome P-450-mediated metabolism to inactive products (50%) and by renal excretion of unchanged drug (50%). The half-life is 20.5 hr and is not affected by chronic administration. Plasma concentrations of felbamate have not been correlated with clinical efficacy.

ADVERSE EFFECTS

At the time of FDA approval in 1993, felbamate was shown to be well tolerated in many premarketing clinical trials. When administered as adjunctive therapy to adults with partial seizures, felbamate was associated with headache (37%), nausea (34%), somnolence (19%), anorexia (19%), dizziness (18%), insomnia (17%), and fatigue (17%). The incidence of these adverse effects was reduced by approximately one-half when felbamate was used as monotherapy, a finding suggesting that concomitant AEDs were at least partly responsible for these symptoms. Weight loss was reported in 4% of adults and 6% of children receiving felbamate.

Felbamate had been evaluated in approximately 1700 patients in controlled clinical trials at the time of its introduction to the U.S. market. As is the case with rare idiosyncratic reactions, it was not until felbamate was used in a much larger population that the risks of the drug became known. On August 1, 1994 (after approximately 100,000 patient exposures), Wallace Laboratories announced that felbamate had been associated with 10 cases of aplastic anemia, and the FDA recommended the immediate withdrawal of patients from the drug unless drug discontinuation would pose a more serious risk to the patient. Subsequently, additional cases have been reported, and it is estimated that the risk of felbamate-associated aplastic anemia is more than 100-fold greater than that seen in the untreated population. The estimated incidence is approximately 1/4000. For comparison, the risk of aplastic anemia due to chloramphenicol is estimated to be approximately 1/40,000. The risk of aplastic anemia appears to be highest within the first year of therapy and does not appear to be related to felbamate dosage. The mortality has been approximately 30%.

Felbamate has also been associated with at least 14 cases of acute hepatic failure among approximately 100,000 patient exposures. The period of highest risk appears to be during the first year of therapy, and there is no clear correlation with felbamate dosage. The estimated mortality among these cases is 57%.

In addition to amending the prescribing information for felbamate, the manufacturer has included a patient information/consent form with the package insert. The use of this or some other consent form and the interpretation of the appropriate criteria for felbamate use vary widely among different centers and individual prescribers. The use of laboratory monitoring of hematologic and hepatic function also varies. The manufacturer recommends that liver function tests be performed at baseline and at 1- to

2-week intervals while treatment continues. No guidelines for hematologic monitoring are given. At the Northern California Comprehensive Epilepsy Center we order a complete blood count with differential, platelet count, serum iron, reticulocyte count, alanine transaminase, aspartate transaminase, and bilirubin concentrations at baseline, every 2 weeks for months 1 and 2 of felbamate therapy, every month for months 3 through 12, and every 6 months thereafter. However, the value of these monitoring guidelines has not been established. Felbamate should probably be avoided for patients with a history of hematologic or hepatic abnormalities.

DRUG INTERACTIONS

In animals, felbamate is a weak inducer of cytochrome P-450 activity. However, in clinical use, the drug has variable interactions with other AEDs. The addition of felbamate requires a reduction in the dosage of concomitant AED therapy. Felbamate causes a dose-related increase in steady-state phenytoin plasma concentrations. At felbamate doses of 1200 mg/day, phenytoin concentrations increase by an average of 23%. Felbamate doses of 1800 mg/day increase phenytoin concentrations by an average of 47% above baseline. An initial reduction in phenytoin dosage of 20 to 30% on initiation of felbamate is usually sufficient to prevent symptoms of phenytoin toxicity. However, further phenytoin dosage reductions may be required as the dosage of felbamate is increased. The mechanism of this interaction may involve competition inhibition of phenytoin metabolism.

Felbamate decreases mean carbamazepine concentrations by 20 to 30%; however, CBZ-E concentrations increase by 30 to 55% (35). To prevent dose-related symptoms of toxicity such as diplopia, drowsiness, and ataxia, carbamazepine doses should be reduced by approximately 30% when felbamate therapy is begun. A possible mechanism for this interaction may involve felbamate induction of carbamazepine metabolism to the epoxide metabolite or inhibition of the enzyme that is responsible for the inactivation of CBZ-E. Preliminary evidence suggests that felbamate can also raise plasma concentrations of phenobarbital.

Felbamate causes a dose-related increase in steady-state concentrations of valproate that ranges from 20 to 50%. Felbamate has no effect on the protein binding of valproate, and the interaction is likely the result of felbamate inhibition of valproate metabolism. Valproate dosages should be reduced by approximately 30% on initiation of felbamate, and further dose reductions may be required during the titration of felbamate therapy.

Felbamate concentrations can also be affected by other AEDs. Phenytoin and carbamazepine reduce steady-state concentrations of felbamate by 40 to 50%. However, since there is no consistent correlation between felbamate levels and clinical effect, no adjustment in felbamate dosage is required. Valproate does not have a significant effect on plasma concentrations of felbamate.

Vigabatrin

Vigabatrin is an irreversible inhibitor of GABA-transaminase, the enzyme that is responsible for degradation of GABA. An increase in brain and cerebrospinal fluid concentrations of GABA has been demonstrated in animals during vigabatrin administration; this is presumably the mechanism of the drug's antiepileptic effect (30). Vigabatrin has been used in several European countries, and a new drug application (NDA) is pending approval in the United States. Vigabatrin (Sabril) is likely to be marketed in the United States as adjunctive therapy for refractory partial and secondarily generalized tonic-clonic seizures. In clinical trials, vigabatrin reduces the frequency of these seizures by 50% or more in 33 to 58% of patients at doses of 1 to 4 g/day (36). Vigabatrin has demonstrated activity in the treatment of children with partial seizures, generalized seizures, Lennox-Gastaut syndrome, and West syndrome.

Vigabatrin is at least 80% absorbed after oral administration, peak concentrations occurring within the first 2 hours. Food has no clinically significant effect on the rate and extent of absorption. Vigabatrin is not bound to plasma proteins, and its volume of distribution approaches that of total body water. Elimination is by renal excretion (≥80%), and no metabolites have been identified in humans. Vigabatrin elimination kinetics are first-order, and the elimination half-life is 5 to 7 hr. Although this half-life is short in relation to those of other AEDs, the duration of action of vigabatrin is prolonged because of its irreversible effect on GABA-transaminase. After withdrawal of vigabatrin, enzyme concentrations return to normal over 4 to 6 days, corresponding to new protein synthesis (30). This prolonged effect allows for once- or twice-daily dosing. As expected, there is no correlation between plasma concentrations of vigabatrin and clinical effect.

ADVERSE EFFECTS

Adverse effects during vigabatrin therapy are generally mild and primarily affect the CNS or gastrointestinal tract. These include drowsiness (27%), fatigue (8%), depression (4%), confusion (3%), and gastrointestinal upset (3%). No clinically significant abnormalities in hematologic, hepatic, or renal function have been detected. The most troubling adverse effect that is reported during vigabatrin therapy is psychosis, which may occur in as many as 4 to 6% of patients. Symptoms may include hallucinations, agitation, paranoia, depression, and confusion. These symptoms usually have their onset from 5 to 32 weeks after vigabatrin therapy is begun and are more common in patients with a history of psychiatric disturbances. Psychiatric symptoms resolve completely after vigabatrin withdrawal.

Clinical trials with vigabatrin were suspended in the United States in 1983 because of reports of microscopic vacuoles in the white matter of rats, mice, and dogs. These animals had been exposed to doses of 100 to 500 mg/kg/day for periods ranging from 1 to 12 months. Subsequent evidence suggested that no such changes occur in humans, and clinical trials were restarted. Neuropathologic and autopsy studies have found no evidence of either vacuolization or prolonged sensory-evoked potentials in humans. Furthermore, no other clinical evidence of white matter dysfunction has been found in association with vigabatrin use. Thus, vigabatrin appears to be safe for chronic use in humans.

DRUG INTERACTIONS

Because vigabatrin is neither metabolized nor bound to plasma proteins, it is unlikely to interact with most AEDs. However, vigabatrin has been reported to decrease phenytoin concentrations by 20 to 30% (40). Thus, an increase in phenytoin dosage may be required to maintain a consistent phenytoin effect. The mechanism of this interaction is unknown. No significant alterations in carbamazepine, valproate, phenobarbital, and primidone concentrations have been reported during vigabatrin therapy.

Phenobarbital

All barbiturates have anticonvulsant activity, but only phenobarbital and primidone are used commonly for the chronic treatment of epilepsy, because they are effective at subhypnotic doses. Phenobarbital was first used for the treatment of seizures in 1912, and it continues to be prescribed widely. However, because of adverse effects on the CNS, this agent is now used primarily as an alternative when monotherapy with first-line agents has failed. Phenobarbital is most useful for the treatment of partial and generalized tonic-clonic seizures. Phenobarbital elevates the seizure threshold and prevents the spread of electrical seizure activity. Although the precise mechanism of action is unknown, these effects may be related to the ability of phenobarbital to modulate the inhibitory action of GABA or to attenuate the postsynaptic effects of excitatory neurotransmitters such as glutamate.

Phenobarbital is available as the sodium salt in a variety of dosage forms, including oral capsules and tablets (various strengths), elixir (20 mg/5 mL), and injectable preparations (various concentrations). The usual maintenance dose of phenobarbital for adults is 1 to 3 mg/kg/day. In neonates and children the usual daily dose is 3 to 4 mg/kg. Phenobarbital is usually given as a single daily dose at bedtime to avoid peak sedative effects during the day. Although food may delay absorption, the absolute bioavailability of phenobarbital is unchanged. The long half-life of phenobarbital (approximately 4 days) may cause a delay of 2 to 3 weeks until steady-state levels are achieved.

Therefore, a loading dose should be administered when a prompt therapeutic effect is needed. The usual loading dose of phenobarbital is 15 mg/kg. When it is given intravenously, the rate of administration should not exceed 100 mg/min. Oral loading doses may also be used. The oral loading doses of phenobarbital should be divided into three equal increments and separated by 24 hr. Patients should be monitored for the attendant sedation and incoordination that may occur.

Phenobarbital is nearly completely absorbed after oral and intramuscular administration, peak concentrations occurring in less than 4 hr. Phenobarbital is not highly bound to plasma proteins, and for this reason, clinically significant protein binding interactions are rare. Phenobarbital is eliminated by a first-order process. Thirty to fifty percent of phenobarbital is metabolized by the liver to inactive products that are glucuronidated or sulfated and excreted in the urine. Approximately 25% of the dose is excreted in the urine unchanged. Excretion of phenobarbital is enhanced significantly in alkaline urine and during forced diuresis.

ADVERSE EFFECTS

CNS adverse effects during phenobarbital therapy are generally dose-related and include sedation, nystagmus, dizziness, and ataxia. Mild drowsiness is common on initiation of therapy, but tolerance of this effect usually develops within the first several weeks. Occasionally, sedation will persist during chronic treatment, and for these patients the dose should be reduced. Of greater concern are the subtle effects of phenobarbital on behavior, mood, and cognition. Reversible hyperactivity and insomnia occur in up to 40% of children who are treated with phenobarbital, and paradoxical excitation has been reported in elderly patients as well. These behavioral changes usually occur within the first few months of therapy and are more prevalent in patients with organic brain disease. A noticeable improvement in behavior may be seen when phenobarbital is replaced with valproate or carbamazepine (37). Phenobarbital may also cause depression and lack of interest or ambition that are recognized by others or appreciated only after discontinuation of the drug. Although the cognitive effects of phenobarbital are not well characterized, several investigations have found a dose-related impairment of memory, performance on intelligence and vigilance tests, work performance, and performance of complex verbal and nonverbal tasks. These changes likely persist despite the development of tolerance to the sedative effects of the drug.

Serious adverse effects of phenobarbital are uncommon, and in general, this drug is associated with fewer idiosyncratic adverse effects than are phenytoin or carbamazepine (11). Morbilliform rash is the most common idiosyncratic reaction, occurring in 1 to 3% of patients.

Rarely, the rash may progress to Stevens-Johnson syndrome or exfoliative dermatitis or may occur in conjunction with symptoms of hepatitis or bone marrow suppression. The potential for cross-reactivity between phenobarbital and other aromatic AEDs (e.g., carbamazepine and phenytoin) should be considered in changing therapy for these patients. Megaloblastic anemia with folic acid deficiency occurs in fewer than 1% of phenobarbital-treated patients and responds to folic acid supplementation. Like phenytoin, phenobarbital is associated with bone disorders (e.g., osteomalacia) during chronic therapy.

DRUG INTERACTIONS

Most drug interactions with phenobarbital are characterized by alterations of metabolism. By increasing the synthesis and retarding the degradation of hepatic enzymes, phenobarbital accelerates the metabolism of many agents that are metabolized by the mixed-function oxidase system, including theophylline, warfarin, cyclosporine, chloramphenicol, valproate, felbamate, lamotrigine, chlorpromazine, haloperidol, and tricyclic antidepressants. The degree of enzyme induction and alteration of drug metabolism varies greatly among patients and is to some extent under genetic control. Enzyme induction may last for days to weeks after phenobarbital is discontinued. Carbamazepine levels may remain unchanged or decline during phenobarbital coadministration. Phenobarbital can also inhibit the metabolism of some drugs, presumably by competition for similar metabolic pathways. The effect of phenobarbital on plasma levels of phenytoin is unpredictable; levels may modestly rise, decline, or (as in most cases) show no change. Valproate often causes a clinically important reduction in the metabolism of phenobarbital, with resultant symptoms of phenobarbital toxicity (see the discussion of drug interactions in the section above on valproate). The effect of phenytoin on phenobarbital plasma levels is unpredictable, and in most cases, clinically important alterations are not seen.

Primidone

Primidone is structurally related to the barbiturates, and like phenobarbital, it is effective for the treatment of partial and generalized tonic-clonic seizures. Primidone is an active anticonvulsant agent, as are its two major metabolites, phenobarbital and phenylethylmalonamide (PEMA). Although the clinical use of primidone is similar to that of phenobarbital, adverse effects are more commonly a limiting factor during long-term primidone therapy. Some patients may respond to primidone therapy despite the failure of phenobarbital to control seizures.

Primidone (Mysoline and generic) is available as oral tablets (50 and 250 mg) and as an oral suspension (250 mg/5 mL). Primidone should be initiated slowly, to allow the development of tolerance to the acute gastrointestinal and sedative effects of the parent drug. For adults, therapy can be started at a dose of 125 to 250 mg twice a day with gradual dosage increases every 4 to 7 days in 125- to 250-mg increments until the effective dose is reached.

Metabolic transformation of primidone to phenobarbital and PEMA occurs by oxidative metabolism and pyrimidine ring cleavage, respectively. Primidone and its metabolites are also excreted by the kidney to a significant extent. Because the half-life of primidone is relatively short, the drug is usually given in divided doses to maintain more consistent plasma levels of the parent drug and reduce the likelihood of transient side effects at times of peak primidone levels. Pharmacokinetic monitoring of primidone therapy includes routine assessment of both primidone and phenobarbital levels. Samples should be drawn at a consistent time relative to the dose. Whereas primidone reaches steady-state concentrations quickly, there is usually a delay of 2 to 3 weeks before plateau concentrations of phenobarbital are attained. During chronic treatment, plasma concentrations of phenobarbital are approximately one to three times higher than those of primidone. This fact is sometimes useful in monitoring compliance.

ADVERSE EFFECTS

The adverse effects of primidone are similar to those of phenobarbital. Thus, the potential for primidone-related neurotoxicity is of concern during long-term therapy. In addition, primidone itself is frequently associated with initial dose-related adverse effects, including sedation, dizziness, and nausea. Decreased libido and impotence appear to be more common during primidone therapy than with other AEDs. Serious adverse effects during primidone therapy are rare.

DRUG INTERACTIONS

The metabolism of primidone or its metabolites can be affected by other AEDs, including phenytoin and valproate. Phenytoin increases phenobarbital levels during coadministration with primidone. The result is an approximate doubling of the phenobarbital:primidone concentration ratio. Primidone levels do not appear to be significantly affected during phenytoin therapy. Valproate can reduce the metabolic clearance of metabolically derived phenobarbital and produce signs of barbiturate intoxication during primidone therapy. Valproate has a negligible effect on the plasma concentrations of primidone. Carbamazepine may increase the metabolism of primidone, although in many patients this interaction is not clinically important.

Benzodiazepines

Diazepam, clonazepam, and clorazepate are the only benzodiazepine agents that are FDA-approved for the treatment of seizures. Diazepam and lorazepam have little utility in the chronic treatment of epilepsy, but they are frequently used intravenously for the termination of status epilepticus. In general, benzodiazepines are more effective in suppressing generalized epileptiform activity than focal discharges, and these agents limit the spread of epileptic discharges without suppressing the primary seizure focus. Nonetheless, clinical use of clonazepam and clorazepate for the chronic treatment of epilepsy includes both generalized and partial seizure types. Although the precise mechanism of the anticonvulsant effect of these agents is unknown, the benzodiazepines are thought to facilitate inhibitory neurotransmission in the CNS by enhancing the postsynaptic effects of GABA.

Clonazepam

Clonazepam is useful, alone or as an adjunct to other agents, for the treatment of Lennox-Gastaut syndrome and akinetic and myoclonic seizures. The drug is also useful for the treatment of absence seizures that fail to respond to valproate or ethosuximide. Clonazepam is not approved for the treatment of partial or generalized tonic-clonic seizures, and experience in its use for the treatment of these seizure types is limited.

Clonazepam (Klonopin) is available as oral tablets in strengths of 0.5, 1, and 2 mg. An intravenous preparation is available for use in Europe, but it is not available in the United States. Clonazepam should be initiated at low doses (0.5 mg three times a day for adults, 0.01 to 0.03 mg/kg divided twice or three times a day for infants and children) and gradually titrated upward at 3- to 7-day intervals. The maximum recommended daily dose is 20 mg for adults and 0.1 to 0.2 mg/kg for infants and children. Although the half-life of clonazepam is long enough to allow once-daily dosing for many patients, the drug is often administered in divided doses. This is particularly important for patients who are intolerant of the transient sedative effects that occur after peak absorption and for infants and children, in whom the drug's half-life may be shortened.

Clonazepam is eliminated primarily by reduction of the nitro group to form 7-amino clonazepam, an inactive metabolite. Although loss of efficacy may occur during chronic therapy (see the discussion below of adverse effects), clonazepam does not induce its own metabolism. There is wide variation in the relationship between the dose and plasma levels of clonazepam. There is also significant overlap between the plasma levels that are associated with the antiepileptic effect of the drug and those that are associated with dose-related adverse effects. For these reasons the therapeutic range of clonazepam levels is imprecisely defined, and therapeutic monitoring of clonazepam concentrations is not routinely done.

ADVERSE EFFECTS

Adverse effects are common during clonazepam treatment and necessitate drug discontinuation in up to one-third of patients (38). Dose-related adverse effects are particularly common and include drowsiness and ataxia. Although tolerance of the overt sedative effects of clonazepam and other benzodiazepines usually develops during the first few weeks of therapy, mild impairment of cognitive and motor skills may persist throughout treatment. In other patients, dose-related adverse effects are not tolerable, and clonazepam therapy must be discontinued. Clonazepam can also cause behavioral disturbances, including hyperactivity, irritability, restlessness, and aggressive or violent behavior. Children are affected more frequently than adults are. Dosage reduction may be attempted, but it does not always alleviate behavioral changes. Other noteworthy adverse effects include excessive salivation, bronchial hypersecretion, weight gain, and, rarely, exacerbation of seizures. Abrupt discontinuation of clonazepam may precipitate seizures or status epilepticus. Therefore, clonazepam should be gradually withdrawn when treatment is to be terminated.

The long-term clinical utility of clonazepam is limited by the development of tolerance to the antiepileptic effect. Approximately one-third of patients who initially benefit from clonazepam therapy experience some loss of efficacy, usually within the first 6 months of treatment (38). Although the antiepileptic effect may be restored by increasing the dose, as many as 30% of patients who develop tolerance do not regain adequate seizure control (38).

DRUG INTERACTIONS

Clinically important drug interactions with clonazepam are uncommon. Clonazepam has no significant effect on the pharmacokinetic disposition of phenytoin, carbamazepine, or primidone. However, phenytoin, carbamazepine, and phenobarbital can reduce the steady-state concentrations of clonazepam, presumably by the induction of hepatic metabolism. The combined use of clonazepam and valproate has been reported to exacerbate absence seizures. Although the simultaneous use of these agents is not a strict contraindication, caution should be observed.

Clorazepate

Clorazepate dipotassium is approved for use as an adjunct to other agents for the treatment of partial seizures. Clorazepate is a prodrug that is rapidly decarboxylated in the acidic medium of the stomach to yield N-desmethyldiazepam (DMD), the primary active metabolite. This metabolite is responsible for the antiepileptic effect of the parent compound.

Clorazepate (Tranxene) is available as a prompt-release oral tablet (3.75, 7.5, and 15 mg) and as an extended-release oral tablet (11.5 and 22.5 mg) for once-daily dosing. Therapy with clorazepate should be initiated with the prompt-release form at a dose of 7.5 mg three times a day for adults and 7.5 mg twice a day for children (ages 9 to 12 years). The dose should be increased at 7-day intervals, in increments of 7.5 mg or less, to a maximum daily dose of 90 mg for adults and 60 mg for children. Transient dose-related adverse effects may be minimized and compliance may be improved by switching patients who are stabilized on clorazepate to the extended-release dosage form.

DMD and its hydroxylated metabolites (including oxazepam) are conjugated and excreted in the urine. Plasma level monitoring is of little use in the management of patients who are taking clorazepate.

ADVERSE EFFECTS

Adverse effects of clorazepate are similar to those of clonazepam and include sedation, dizziness, hypersalivation, and behavioral changes. Tolerance to the antiepileptic effect of clorazepate has been reported, but it does not seem to be as common, or to develop as quickly, as with clonazepam.

DRUG INTERACTIONS

Concurrent antacid administration may significantly slow the rate of conversion from clorazepate to DMD, as can other disease states that are characterized by an increase in gastric pH. However, during prolonged administration, steady-state DMD levels are not significantly reduced. Smoking and concurrent AED therapy with enzyme-inducing agents can accelerate the metabolism of clorazepate. Clorazepate has no known effect on the disposition of other AEDs.

TREATING THE PREGNANT WOMAN WHO HAS EPILEPSY

There is much controversy about the treatment of pregnant women who have epilepsy. Central issues are the risk of fetal malformations that are attributable to individual seizures and to the epileptic diathesis, the degree of additional risk that is attributable to AED therapy, and the antiepileptic agent of choice for minimizing the risk of fetal malformations. Although a detailed discussion of these topics is beyond the scope of this chapter, several important principles should be considered. The reader is referred to other reviews for additional discussion of this topic (39, 40) and to Chapter 92, "Drugs in Pregnancy and Lactation."

Therapeutic considerations that are unique during pregnancy include (a) changes in maternal seizure control, (b) the choice of antiepileptic agents, (c) alteration of AED pharmacokinetics, and (d) the potential for AED-associated coagulopathy in the newborn. Approximately 50% of women with epilepsy will have no change in seizure frequency during pregnancy (1). Among the remaining patients, worsening of seizures occurs in approximately 40%, and only 10% experience a reduction in seizures (41). This may be attributable to several factors, including reduced medication compliance caused by maternal fears

that the medication may injure the developing fetus, pharmacokinetic changes in AED disposition, and sleep deprivation.

Overall, the incidence of fetal abnormalities in children of epileptic mothers is approximately 6%, roughly twice that found in the general population. Although there is considerable controversy about which AED has the lowest teratogenic risk, there is a clear association between some AEDs and fetal malformations. Trimethadione is clearly associated with a syndrome of anomalies, and this drug should be avoided during pregnancy. Affected infants may have craniofacial abnormalities, including microcephaly, and ocular defects, cardiac abnormalities, intrauterine growth retardation, short stature, and developmental delay. Currently, there is no conclusive evidence on which to base a preference for the use of carbamazepine, phenobarbital, phenytoin, or valproate during pregnancy (40), and the safety of newer AEDs (gabapentin, lamotrigine, felbamate, and vigabatrin) has yet to be established. Valproate has been associated with neural tube, cardiovascular, and urogenital malformations that some authors suggest are unique to this agent. On this basis, some neurologists prefer to avoid valproate and favor the use of phenytoin or carbamazepine during pregnancy. However, both of these agents have also been associated with major and minor malformations. Phenytoin has been associated with a constellation of anomalies including craniofacial malformations, retardation, deficiencies in growth and mental or motor performance, and limb defects that have been grouped as the *fetal hydantoin syndrome*. However, similar abnormalities have been associated with other AEDs. It is hypothesized that the arene oxide intermediates that are generated during the metabolism of aromatic AEDs may be responsible for these teratogenic effects, but this hypothesis requires further study. Carbamazepine has also been associated with major malformations, including spina bifida (40). Since no AED is clearly less teratogenic than the others, it is recommended that the preferred AED during pregnancy is the drug that best controls the patient's seizures. Also, it is clear that AED polytherapy is associated with a greater risk of fetal malformations. Correspondingly, it is recommended that monotherapy (with the lowest effective dose) be used whenever possible. Folate supplements should also be given daily.

Pregnancy is associated with significant changes in the pharmacokinetic properties of AEDs. These changes include acceleration of hepatic drug metabolism, increased apparent volume of distribution, and alterations in plasma protein binding. The result is a decline in plasma AED concentrations and, in some patients, loss of seizure control. Consequently, AED plasma levels and the clinical status of the patient should be monitored at least monthly during pregnancy. Monitoring of unbound plasma concentrations of phenytoin and valproate is recommended for patients whose clinical response does not appear to correlate with the total plasma concentration. After delivery, AED plasma concentrations should be determined weekly, and appropriate dosage adjustments should be made.

Approximately 50% of the infants who are born to mothers taking phenytoin, phenobarbital, and primidone during pregnancy are deficient in vitamin K-dependent clotting factors at birth. Although neonatal hemorrhage is uncommon, infants should be treated with vitamin K 1 mg intramuscularly immediately at birth. Clotting should then be monitored every 2 to 4 hr, and repeat doses of vitamin K should be administered as needed. Alternatively, coagulopathy can be prevented by treating the mother with vitamin K 20 mg orally each day for 2 weeks before delivery or 10 mg intramuscularly 4 hr before delivery. The effect of maternal carbamazepine and valproate therapy on neonatal hemostasis is unknown.

All AEDs are excreted in breast milk to some degree. The ratio of breast milk to serum concentration is 80% for ethosuximide, 40 to 60% for phenobarbital, 40% for carbamazepine, 15% for phenytoin, and 3% for valproic acid (39). Although most epileptic mothers may safely breast-feed their infants, the potential effect of drug transfer to the baby should be considered, especially if the infant appears to be lethargic or feeds poorly.

Despite the concern of parents and clinicians about the risks of epilepsy and AED therapy during pregnancy, it is important to realize that over 90% of epileptic women have normal children. However, epileptic women of childbearing age must understand the value of prepregnancy planning and, once pregnant, be made aware of the risks for fetal abnormalities, the potential consequences of medication noncompliance, and the need for close therapeutic monitoring during pregnancy and for several weeks following childbirth.

WITHDRAWAL OF ANTIEPILEPTIC DRUG THERAPY

Several community-based studies have shown that, among patients with epilepsy who are followed for more than 10 years, over half will attain a 2- to 5-year remission from seizures during drug therapy. Remission rates tend to be highest for patients who have primary generalized seizures and range from 60% for those with tonic-clonic seizures to 80% for children with typical absence attacks.

In general, patients who remain free of seizures for 2 years or more may be considered candidates for AED withdrawal. The potential benefits of drug withdrawal include avoidance of the cognitive and behavioral adverse effects of AED therapy, reduction in the risk of adverse drug reactions and drug interactions, and a return by the patient to a lifestyle that is unencumbered by the need for chronic medication. However, the decision to withdraw

AED therapy is complex, both medically and socially, and requires clear explanation to the patient of both the risks and benefits.

Medical factors that appear to affect the risk of seizure recurrence after AED drug withdrawal are summarized in Table 50.10. In particular, it is important to consider the age at onset of epilepsy, seizure type, EEG abnormalities, and rate of drug withdrawal in assessing the risk of seizure recurrence. Relapse rates after AED withdrawal in patients who have been free of seizures for 2 years or more are approximately 20% for childhood-onset epilepsy and 40% for adult-onset epilepsy (8, 42). Thus, 60 to 80% of patients will remain free of seizures when AED therapy is withdrawn after a 2-year remission. The risk of seizure recurrence is highest during the period of AED reduction and within the first year after drug withdrawal.

The rate of drug withdrawal may also affect seizure recurrence. Most authors agree that a gradual taper is preferred. Recently, no difference in seizure recurrence rates was found when children were randomly assigned to a 6-week or a 9-month taper period (43). Abrupt withdrawal is a risk factor for status epilepticus. Furthermore, rapid removal of AED therapy itself may precipitate seizures due to drug withdrawal (as distinct from a recurrence of seizures due to the underlying epileptic condition). Seizures during withdrawal are most common with benzodiazepine or barbiturate AEDs. Since there are no means to determine reliably whether recurrent seizures are truly epileptic in origin, the need for continued drug therapy is unclear unless the rate of taper is long enough to effectively rule out a drug-withdrawal phenomenon.

Any decision to withdraw AED therapy on the basis of a favorable medical prognosis must also include a careful assessment of the patient's work and social environments. Not only should patients clearly understand the risks and benefits of drug withdrawal, they must also be encouraged to participate actively in the decision. Patients who have been seizure-free for long intervals often have valid

Table 50.10.

Factors That Affect the Risk of Seizure Recurrence After Antiepileptic Drug Withdrawal

Favorable Prognosis	Unfavorable Prognosis
Childhood-onset epilepsy	Adult-onset epilepsy
Longer seizure-free interval before drug withdrawal	Frequent, severe seizures before remission
Absence seizures	Partial seizures (with and without secondary generalization)
Primary generalized tonic-clonic seizures	EEG abnormalities at time of drug withdrawal
Normal or improved EEG at time of drug withdrawal	Abrupt withdrawal of benzodiazepine or barbiturate antiepileptic drugs
	Atypical febrile seizures

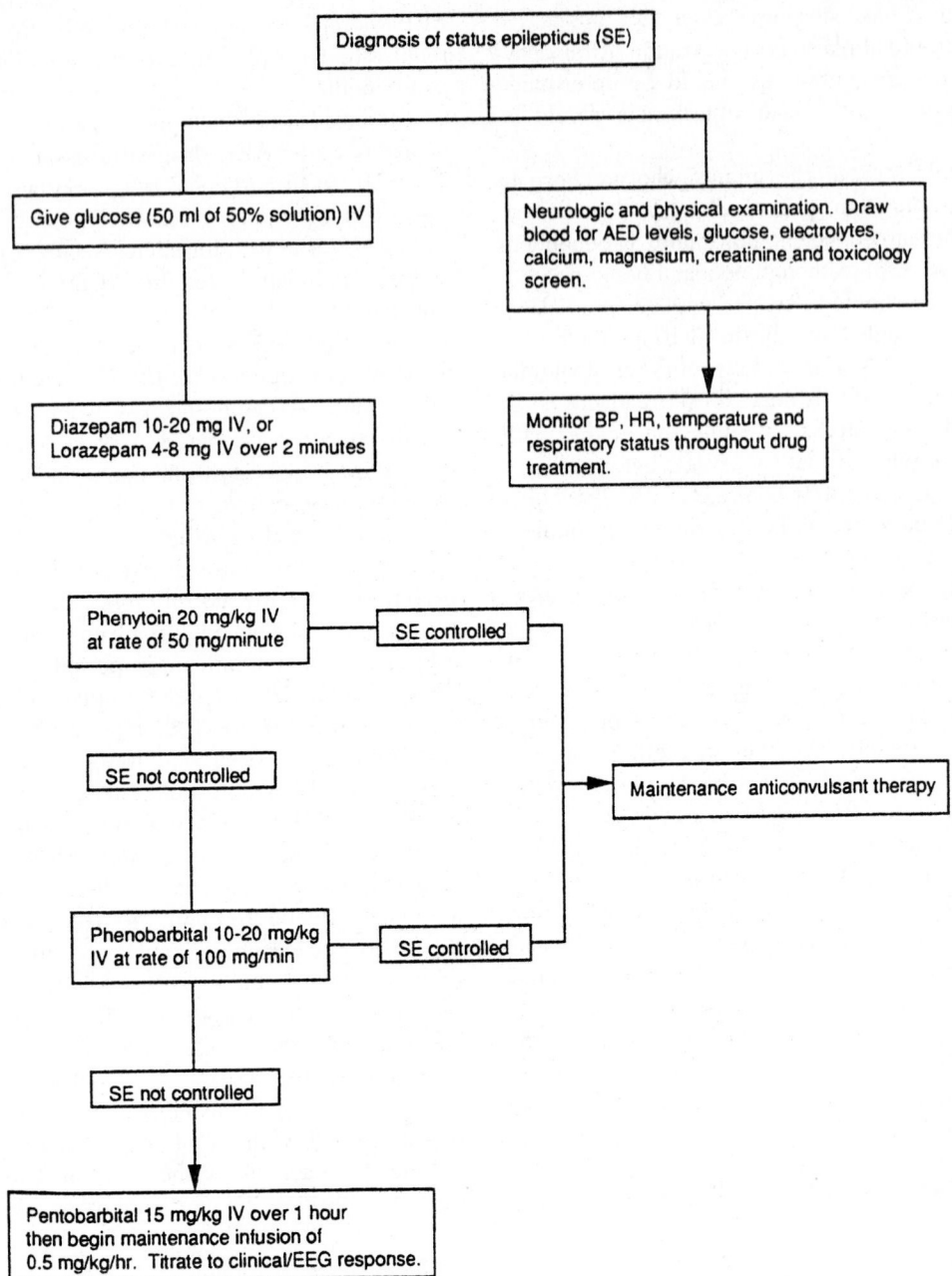

Figure 50.1 Treatment algorithm for status epilepticus in adults.

concerns about the possible recurrence of seizures at home, at work, or while driving. During AED withdrawal it is often recommended that the patient not drive for several months. Furthermore, in some areas a recurrent seizure during this period may result in the suspension of driving privileges until AED therapy is restarted and adequate control is demonstrated. These and other patient-specific social factors should be discussed with each individual for whom AED withdrawal is considered.

NONDRUG THERAPIES

Surgical Treatment

Approximately 300,000 patients in the United States have uncontrolled seizures despite medical therapy (1). For approximately 15% of these patients, surgical intervention may be a viable option. Patients who are most likely to benefit from surgery are those with partial seizures whose symptoms remain intractable despite optimal medical therapy. The degree to which seizures and drug toxicity impair the functional abilities of the patient must also

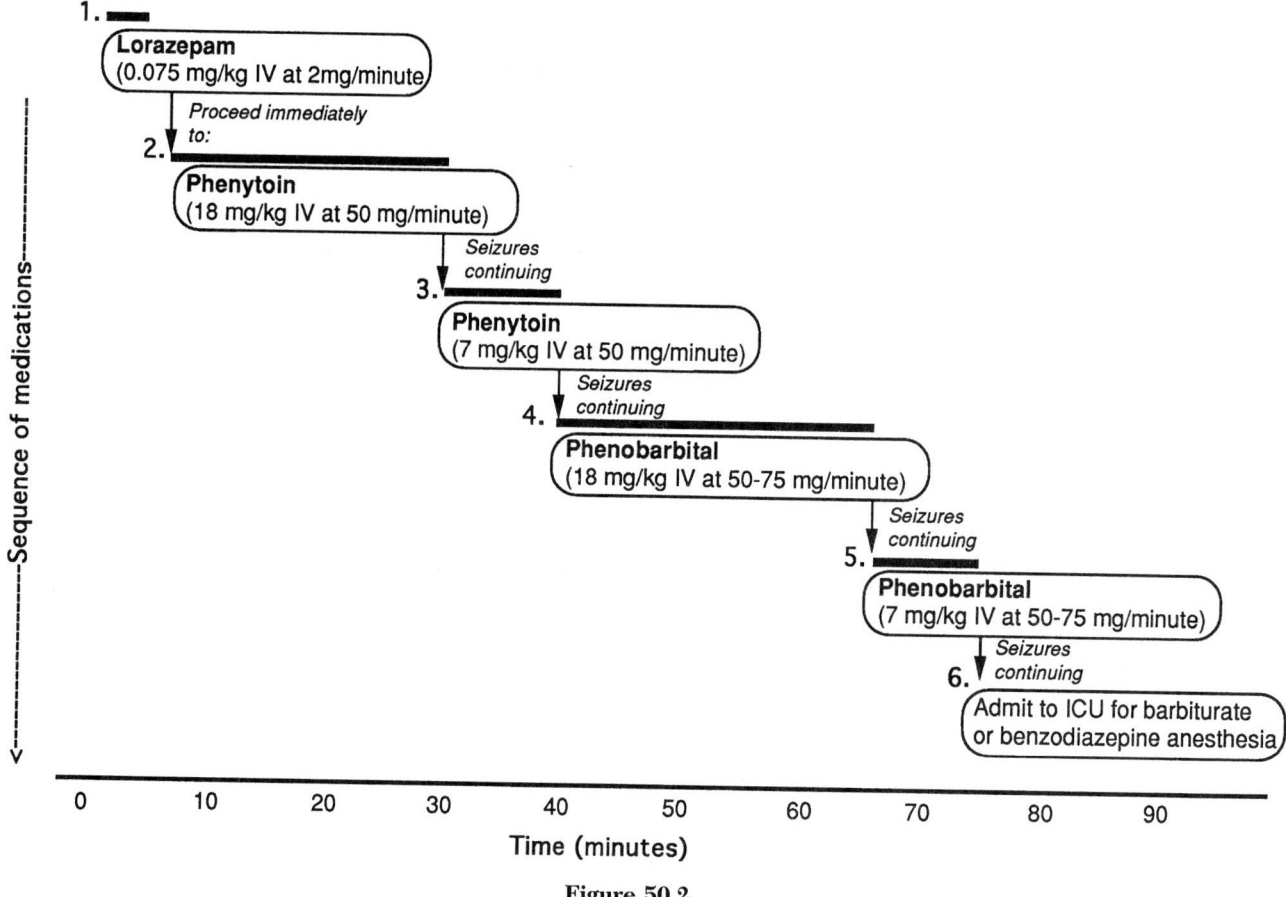

Figure 50.2

be considered. Presurgical evaluation includes intensive medical and neurological testing to localize the lesion. MRI, PET, and single-photon emission computed tomography scans, as well as simultaneous EEG and video telemetry monitoring, are very useful in this regard. Resection of a seizure focus from the anterior temporal lobe is the most common surgery performed. After temporal lobectomy, approximately one-half of patients are rendered free of seizures and one-third experience a significant reduction.

Behavioral Therapies

Psychological techniques for control of epileptic seizures are often successful for patients with seizures triggered by flashing lights or visual patterns, reading, or listening to music (referred to as *reflex epilepsies*). In these cases, behavioral conditioning has been used with success. The role of behavioral therapies in other types of epilepsy remains limited.

STATUS EPILEPTICUS

Status epilepticus (SE) is a medical emergency that requires prompt, effective treatment to minimize permanent neurologic damage and death. SE is defined as repetitive clinical convulsions without recovery of consciousness between attacks or repeated electrographic seizure activity in a comatose patient, usually lasting 30 min or more. However, in most clinical care situations, aggressive anticonvulsant therapy is initiated when seizures last 10 min or longer. Morbidity and mortality after SE are caused primarily by CNS injury due to the condition that precipitated the episode and neuronal injury from continuous electrical and convulsive seizure activity. Even with aggressive medical therapy, SE is fatal in 10 to 12% of patients.

The most common cause of SE in patients with a history of epilepsy is noncompliance with AED therapy. Additionally, the variety of factors listed in Table 50.10 that can cause seizures are also potential causes of SE. The initial workup for patients should include a thorough evaluation to identify potentially treatable causes of SE.

Figure 50.1 is an algorithm that outlines the treatment of SE in adults. The goals of treatment are to (a) terminate seizures as quickly as possible but within at least 90 to 120 min after onset, (b) identify and treat any potentially reversible causes, and (c) medically manage systemic complications that arise from prolonged convulsive seizures (e.g., hyperpyrexia or hypoxia).

Benzodiazepines (diazepam or lorazepam) are the agents of choice for the initial treatment of SE. Diazepam and lorazepam terminate SE in 80 to 90% of patients, usually within 2 to 3 min after intravenous administration. The usefulness of diazepam is limited by its short duration of anticonvulsant effect (15 min to 2 hr). This drug is highly lipophilic and quickly redistributes out of the brain to other fat stores in the body. Lorazepam has a longer duration of action and is often preferred over diazepam for this reason. Phenytoin and phenobarbital are usually administered after benzodiazepines because they have a longer duration of anticonvulsant effect. Use of high-dose barbiturates (e.g., pentobarbital) or benzodiazepines (e.g., midazolam or lorazepam) offer definitive therapy of SE when other treatments are ineffective or when the duration of continuous seizure activity threatens to cause permanent neurologic damage (Fig. 50.2).

CONCLUSION

The effective treatment of epilepsy requires the mutual participation of both patient and clinician. The goal of epilepsy treatment is to reduce the frequency of recurrent seizures while avoiding adverse effects of drug therapy. The specific means by which this goal is attained must be individualized and must take into account the seizure classification, age, sex, and concurrent medical problems of the patient. Monotherapy with nonsedating AEDs is both effective and well tolerated by most patients. Patients and their families also require education and support regarding their condition and its effect, if any, on daily activities.

REFERENCES

1. Porter RJ. Epilepsy: 100 elementary principles. 2nd ed. London: WB Saunders, 1989.
2. Engel J. Seizures and epilepsy. Philadelphia: FA Davis, 1989.
3. Scheuer ML, Pedley TA. The evaluation and treatment of seizures. N Engl J Med 323:1468–1474, 1990.
4. Alldredge BK, Simon RP. Drugs that can precipitate seizures. In: Resor SR, Kutt H, eds. The medical treatment of epilepsy. New York: Marcel Dekker, 1992:497–523.
5. Commission on Classification and Terminology of the International League Against Epilepsy. Proposal for revised clinical and electroencephalographic classification of epileptic seizures. Epilepsia 22:489–501, 1981.
6. Commision on Classification and Terminology of the International League Against Epilepsy. Proposal for classification of epilepsies and epileptic syndromes. Epilepsia 26:268–278, 1985.
7. Knudsen FU. Optimum management of febrile seizures in childhood. Drugs 36:111–120, 1988.
8. Chadwick D. Diagnosis of epilepsy. Lancet 336:291–295, 1990.
9. Brodie MJ. Established anticonvulsants and treatment of refractory epilepsy. Lancet 336:350–354, 1990.
10. Theodore WH, Porter RJ. Removal of sedative-hypnotic antiepileptic drugs from the regimens of patients with intractable epilepsy. Ann Neurol 13:320–324, 1983.
11. Mattson RH, Cramer JA, Collins JF, et al. Comparison of carbamazepine, phenobarbital, phenytoin, and primidone in partial and secondarily generalized tonic-clonic seizures. N Engl J Med 313:145–151, 1985.
12. Mattson RH, Cramer JA, Collins JF, et al. A comparison of valproate with carbamazepine for the treatment of complex partial seizures and secondarily generalized tonic-clonic seizures in adults. N Engl J Med 327:765–771, 1992.
13. Sato S, White BG, Penry JK, et al. Valproic acid versus ethosuximide in the treatment of absence seizures. Neurology 32:157–163, 1982.
14. Mattson RH. General principles: selection of antiepileptic drug therapy. In: Levy RH, Dreifuss FE, Mattson RH, Meldrum BS, Penry JK, eds. Antiepileptic drugs. 3rd ed. New York: Raven Press, 1989:103–115.
15. Snead OC, Hosey LC. Exacerbation of seizures in children by carbamazepine. N Engl J Med 313:916–921, 1985.
16. Dodson WE. Level off. Neurology 39:1009–1010, 1989.
17. Miles MV, Lawless ST, Tennison MB, Zaritsky AL, Greenwood RS. Rapid loading of critically ill patients with carbamazepine suspension. Pediatrics 86:263–266, 1990.
18. Dalby MA. Behavioral effects of carbamazepine. In: Penry JK, Dalby DD, eds. Advances in neurology, vol 11. New York: Raven Press, 1975:331–343.
19. Alldredge BK, Knutsen AP, Ferriero D. Antiepileptic drug hypersensitivity syndrome: in vitro and clinical observations. Pediatr Neurol 10:169–171, 1994.
20. Hart RG, Easton JD. Carbamazepine and hematological monitoring. Ann Neurol 11:309–312, 1982.
21. Winter ME, Tozer TN. Phenytoin. In: Evans WE, Schentag JJ, Jusko WJ, eds. Applied pharmacokinetics: principles of therapeutic drug monitoring. 2nd ed. Spokane: Applied Therapeutics, 1986:493–539.
22. Tuchman AJ, Zisfein J, Paccione M, Rodeos M, Osborn H. Single- versus divided-dose oral phenytoin loading: a controlled study [Abstract]. Neurology 44(suppl 2):A295, 1994.
23. Leppik IE, Boucher BA, Wilder BJ, Murthy VS, Watridge C, Graves NM, Rangel RJ, Rask CA, Turlapaty P. Pharmacokinetics and safety of a phenytoin prodrug given IV or IM in patients. Neurology 40:456–460, 1990.
24. Nation RL, Evans AM, Milne RW. Pharmacokinetic drug interactions with phenytoin (Part II). Clin Pharmacokinet 18:131–150, 1990.
25. Zaccara B, Messori A, Moroni F. Clinical pharmacokinetics of valproic acid-1988. Clin Pharmacokinet 15:367–389, 1988.
26. Dreifuss FE, Langer DH. Side effects of valproate. Am J Med 84(suppl 1A):34–41, 1988.
27. Gidal B, Spencer N, Maly M, Pitterle M, Williams E, Collins M, Jones J. Valproate-mediated disturbances of hemostasis: relationship to dose and plasma concentration. Neurology 44:1418–1422, 1994.
28. Dreifuss FE, Langer DH, Moline KA, Maxwell JE. Valproic acid hepatic fatalities. II: US experience since 1984. Neurology 39:201–207, 1989.
29. Bourgeois BFD. Pharmacologic interactions between valproate and other drugs. Am J Med 84(suppl 1A):29–33, 1988.
30. Harden CL. New antiepileptic drugs. Neurology 44:787–795, 1994.
31. McLean MJ. Clinical pharmacokinetics of gabapentin. Neurology 44(suppl 5):S17–S22, 1994.
32. Lamictal product information. Research Triangle Park, NC: Burroughs Wellcome Co., December 1994.
33. Burstein AH. Lamotrigine. Pharmacotherapy 15:129–143, 1995.
34. Felbatol product information. Cranbury, NJ: Wallace Laboratories, October 1994.
35. Wagner ML. Felbamate: a new antiepileptic drug. Am J Hosp Pharm 51:1657–1666, 1994.

36. Connelly JF. Vigabatrin. Ann Pharmacother 27:197–204, 1993.

37. Mattson RH, Kramer JA. Phenobarbital: toxicity. In: Levy RH, Dreifuss FE, Mattson RH, Meldrum BS, Penry JK, eds. Antiepileptic drugs. 3rd ed. New York: Raven Press, 1989:341–355.

38. Browne TR. Benzodiazepines. In: Browne TR, Feldman RG, eds. Epilepsy: diagnosis and management. Boston: Little, Brown 1983: 235–245.

39. Donaldson JO, Epilepsy. In: Donaldson JO. Neurology of Pregnancy. London: WB Saunders, 1989:229.

40. Delgado-Escueta A, Janz D. Consensus guidelines: preconception counseling, management, and care of the pregnant woman with epilepsy. Neurology 42(suppl 5):149–160, 1992.

41. Dalessio DJ. Seizure disorders and pregnancy. N Engl J Med 312:559–563, 1985

42. Chadwick D. The discontinuation of antiepileptic therapy. In: Pedley TA, Meldrum BS, eds. Recent advances in epilepsy. 2nd ed. New York: Churchill Livingstone, 1985:111–124.

43. Tennison M, Greenwood R, Lewis D, Thorn M. Discontinuing antiepileptic drugs in children with epilepsy: a comparison of a six-week and a nine-month taper period. N Engl J Med 330:1407–1410, 1994.

CHAPTER 51

PARKINSONISM

SAM K. SHIMOMURA and DARLENE FUJIMOTO

In 1817 a general practitioner in London, Dr. James Parkinson, described a disease that he called the "shaking palsy" or "paralysis agitans." It has since been known as Parkinson's disease, parkinsonism, or Parkinson's syndrome. Even today, very little can be added to his description of the signs and symptoms of this disease. A brief excerpt from "An Essay on the Shaking Palsy" characterizes this disease as follows:

Involuntary tremulous motion, with lessened muscular power, in parts not in action and even when supported; with a propensity to bend the trunk forward and to pass from a walking to a running pace; the senses and the intellects being uninjured (1).

Unfortunately, Dr. Parkinson was wrong about the "the intellect being uninjured." Cognitive decline occurs in a higher percentage of parkinsonism patients than in age-matched controls, approximately 15 to 20% having dementia (2).

Until the 1960s, anticholinergics were the mainstay of treatment for Parkinson's disease. The approval of levodopa in 1970 for the treatment of parkinsonism was hailed by an editorial in the *New England Journal of Medicine* as "the most important contribution to medical therapy of a neurological disease in the past 50 years because of its usefulness in one of the prevalent and disabling neurologic illnesses of man" (3). Traditional surgical treatment has benefited a few patients, but it has not been proven to ameliorate the signs and symptoms of the vast majority of patients. However, newer surgical procedures involving transplantation of dopamine-producing fetal cells are sparking renewed interest as well as controversy as a surgical solution to parkinsonism.

BIOCHEMICAL BASIS OF PARKINSONISM

In recent years, much has been elucidated about the biochemical basis of parkinsonism, but not all the information is in. A cholinergic component appears to be involved, since anticholinergics have been found to be useful in the treatment of Parkinson's disease for over 100 years. This cholinergic overactivity has been confirmed by studies that show that centrally acting cholinesterase inhibitors such as physostigmine aggravate parkinsonian tremor, while centrally acting anticholinergics such as benztropine reverse the effects.

Acetylcholine has predominantly excitatory effects on the central nervous system and is responsible for the positive signs of parkinsonism, such as tremor. However, the primary defect in Parkinson's disease appears to be a state of dopamine deficiency. It is estimated that symptoms of the disease do not appear until there is approximately 80% cell loss. In the normal state, there is a balance between the effects of excitatory acetylcholine and the inhibitory effects of dopamine. Although the concentration of acetylcholine seems to be unchanged in parkinsonism, the deficiency of dopamine disturbs the balance, and the cholinergic activity predominates. Other neurotransmitters, such as serotonin, norepinephrine, and γ-aminobutyric acid, substance P, cholecystokinin, glycine, and somatostatin may also be involved in producing the symptoms of parkinsonism. Parkinsonism may be caused by any degenerative, toxic, infective, traumatic, or neoplastic pathology that alters the balance between acetylcholine and dopamine in favor of cholinergic overactivity or dopaminalgic underactivity. On the basis of this hypothesis, anticholinergics are given to decrease central cholinergic activity, and dopamine, as its precursor, levodopa, is given to increase dopaminergic activity (4).

EPIDEMIOLOGY

Approximately 1 million patients in the United States are estimated to suffer from the symptoms of parkinsonism. Each year there are another 20 new cases per 100,000 population. The risk of developing parkinsonism sometime during one's lifetime is 2 to 3%. At least 66% of all those afflicted have onset of signs and symptoms between 50 and 69 years of age. Only about 30% develop the disease before the age of 50 (5). The ages of onset and incidence are the same for men and women (6).

ETIOLOGY

The signs and symptoms of parkinsonism have many different causes (7). Before a diagnosis of primary or idiopathic parkinsonism is established, secondary causes of parkinsonism must be ruled out. Unlike idiopathic parkinsonism, many of the secondary forms of parkinsonism can be cured. Secondary forms of parkinsonism can be caused by arteriosclerosis, trauma, tumors, numerous chemicals such as carbon monoxide, heavy metals, carbon disulfide, cyanide, methylchloride, and some photographic dyes as well a by various infections such as syphilis, poliomyelitis, malaria, typhoid, herpes zoster, coxsackie virus, measles, and encephalitis.

Drugs are another cause of secondary parkinsonism. (Table 51.1). Phenothiazines produce extrapyramidal side effects that may ultimately manifest themselves as a parkinsonismlike syndrome (Table 51.2). Other antipsychotics such as haloperidol, thiothixeneg or loxapine can also produce these symptoms. Early in the treatment with phenothiazine derivatives, a dystonic syndrome may develop. This side effect consists of torsional movements involving most of the muscles of the body, especially those of the tongue and face. Stiff neck (torticollis), facial grimacing, and retrocollis are often seen. Dystonic reactions occur twice as frequently in males as in females and most often between 5 and 45 years of age. The parenteral administration of diphenhydramine 50 mg or benztropine 2 mg will produce a dramatic response within 10 to 30 min. Akathisia may occur after a few weeks of antipsychotic therapy. Patients with akathisia appear jittery and very anxious. They may pace the floor, tap their fingers, and generally give the impression of restlessness. The true parkinsonismlike syndrome usually becomes apparent 2 to 3 months after initiation of drug therapy. It consists of the usual symptoms associated with idiopathic parkinsonism and occurs most frequently in patients over 50 years of age.

Even antipsychotics that are thought to have fewer extrapyramidal side effects, such as thioridazine and chlorpromazine, may cause or unmask parkinsonismlike signs and symptoms in low doses. Parkinsonism caused by these drugs may persist for a considerable time after discontinuation of the drug (up to 2 years in some cases). Therefore, all newly diagnosed parkinsonism patients should be questioned carefully about their prior use of neuroleptic agents (8).

Reserpine depletes the brain of dopamine and in high doses can produce a parkinsonismlike syndrome. Methyldopa is a decarboxylase inhibitor that can also produce parkinsonismlike symptoms when given in large doses. Metoclopramide blocks dopamine receptors and has been shown to worsen parkinsonism symptoms despite Sinemet treatment. Metoclopramide-induced parkinsonism is rare and is usually associated with renal failure. Carbamazepine has also been reported to produce extrapyramidal symptoms, though occurrences are rare.

In 1983, parkinsonism was reported in several young drug users after the intravenous administration of the meperidine analog 1-methyl-4-phenyl-1,2,3,6-tetrahydropyridine (MPTP) (9). MPTP itself eventually turned out to be nontoxic, but its oxidation product, 1-methyl-4-phenylpyridinium ion (MPP^+), was determined to be highly toxic to melanin-containing neurons in the substantia nigra. MPP^+ is formed by the oxidation of MPTP by monoamine oxidase type B (MAO B). In studies involving monkeys, pretreatment with selegiline (a MAO B inhibitor) prevented the oxidation of MPTP to its toxic metabolite and prevented the signs and symptoms of parkinsonism. Selegiline has also been found to slow or perhaps even reverse the progression of idopathic parkinsonism in humans. This fascinating research has caused many researchers to speculate that some environmental contaminant resembling MPTP may be the cause of parkinsonism. The other side benefit of research with MPTP has been the development of an animal model for parkinsonism. Monkeys that are treated with MPTP appear to develop the same clinical, pathologic, and chemical changes that are in human parkinsonism (10).

DIAGNOSIS AND CLINICAL FINDINGS

The signs of advanced parkinsonism are so striking and unique that it hardly ever poses a diagnostic challenge. The patient presents with rigidity, bradykinesia, seborrhea, festinating gait, flexed posture, drooling (the result of difficulty in swallowing), and a characteristic "pill-rolling" tremor. With further observation, the clinician notices a "reptilian stare" consisting of a frozen, masklike face, infrequent blinking of the eyes, and the tendency to sit for long periods of time in a stationary position. The voice may initially be hoarse and harsh; with time, it decreases in volume and resonance into a low monotone.

Most of the clinical features of parkinsonism fall into four general categories: bradykinesia, rigidity, tremor, and postural abnormalities. Bradykinesia is a slowing down of

Table 51.1.
Drugs That May Produce a Parkinsonlike Syndrome

Amitriptyline and other tricyclic antidepressants
Carbamazepine
Chlopromazine and other phenothiazines
Chlorprothixene and thiothixene
Haloperidol and other butyrophenones
Methyldopa
Metoclopramide
MPTP (1-methyl-4-plenyl-1.2.3.6-Tetrahydropyridine)
Reserpine

Table 51.2.
Examples of Phenothiazines that Produce Extrapyramidal Effects

Drug	Relative Degree
Trifluoroperazine	High
Perphenazine	High
Fluphenazine	High
Prochlorperazine	High
Promazine	Moderate
Chlorpromazine	Moderate
Thioridazine	Low

Table 51.3.
Staging Parkinson's Disease

Stage I	Unilateral involvement only.
	Functional impairment usually minimal or absent.
Stage II	Bilateral or midline involvement.
	No impairment of balance.
Stage III	Bilateral involvement.
	First sign of impaired righting reflexes.
Stage IV	Fully developed, severely disabling disease.
	Unassisted standing and walking but markedly incapacitated.
Stage V	Confined to bed or chair unless aided.

voluntary actions with apparent difficulty in initiating movement. When this is severe enough to cause the patient to "freeze" into immobility, it is called akinesia. This can be tested for by assessing the patient's ability to perform rapid, alternating movements. Rigidity is the tendency to move "en bloc." There is an increased hypertonicity with resistance to passive and active movements of muscles. Muscle control and normal associated movements are hampered. Cogwheel rigidity is seen on applying force to bend the limbs; the muscles yield jerkily, giving the impression of cogwheels moving one upon another. The tremor of parkinsonism is generally coarser, slower, and of wider amplitude than that associated with alcoholism, hyperthyroidism, or nervousness. A resting tremor is seen in a relaxed patient and is a slow, rhythmic tremor.

Although moderately advanced to advanced parkinsonism is easily diagnosed, early features and findings of the disease can frequently be confused with those of many other diseases. Hoehn and Yahr have described a staging of Parkinson's disease (see Table 51.3) (11).

The masking of facial expression is often an early feature of parkinsonism, appearing long before more overt signs such as the festinating gait. A friendly, outgoing, and smiling individual may slowly appear to become more restrained, emotionless, and depressed. There is a subtle restraint of smile, a drawing down of the lips and lower face into an unchanging and worried expression. A slight bulging of the eyes and the barely noticeable tremulousness of early parkinsonism can easily mislead the physician into a diagnosis of anxiety, nervousness, or depression. Not only can this diagnosis destroy the patient's confidence and self-esteem, but it may set in motion a self-fulfilling prophecy, and the patient may actually become depressed, anxious, and nervous. The patient may be referred for psychiatric therapy, in which treatment with an antipsychotic may exacerbate the extrapyramidal signs of the disease.

Another patient may present with weakness and stiffness of one hand. There may be no tremor or other

signs of parkinsonism. The patient may also complain of stiff joints, difficulty in turning over in bed or getting up out of a chair, and the inability to perform activities of daily living such as buttoning a shirt or putting on earrings. These presenting signs can often be misdiagnosed as arthritis, or, when unilateral involvement is apparent, the possibility of a stroke may be raised.

Early features of parkinsonism frequently involve only one of the four cardinal signs of rigidity, bradykinesia, tremor, and postural instability. The signs are often unilateral and almost imperceptible at first and slowly progress in severity and spread from one area of involvement such as one finger, hand, or shoulder to the whole body. The upper part of the body is usually affected first; involvement of the lower part of the body, such as a shuffling gait, is usually a later finding.

Dementia and impairment of intellectual function are encountered in a significantly higher percentage of parkinsonism patients than in age-matched controls (12). However, there is continuing debate over whether the dementia is a part of the disease process or due to concurrent drug therapy, Alzheimer's disease, or other factors (13).

TREATMENT

Treatment is aimed primarily at providing maximal relief of symptoms and maintaining the patient's independence and movement. At present, there is no cure for this disease, but significant improvement in drug therapy in the form of selegiline, levodopa, and other dopamine agonists has greatly improved the prognosis of parkinsonism. Surgical treatment with transplanted fetal tissue looks very promising but is still in the experimental stage. Successful treatment currently involves drug therapy as well as nonpharmacologic treatment consisting of education, exercise, and good nutrition. An algorithm for the management of Parkinson's disease was developed at a consensus conference held in Keystone, Colorado, on February 4–5, 1994 and was published in a supplement to the December 1994 issue of *Neurology* (see Figure 51.1) (2).

Drug Treatment

ANTICHOLINERGICS

Anticholinergic drugs have been the mainstay of therapy for parkinsonism for over a century. However, may neurologists are now avoiding the use of anticholinergic agents because the modest benefits of the drugs are outweighed by their many side effects, especially in patients over 60 years of age or those with dementia. Anticholinergics should be considered for younger patients with tremors-predominant parkinsonism. Anticholinergics that do not cross the blood-brain barrier, for example, quaternary ammonium compounds such as propantheline,

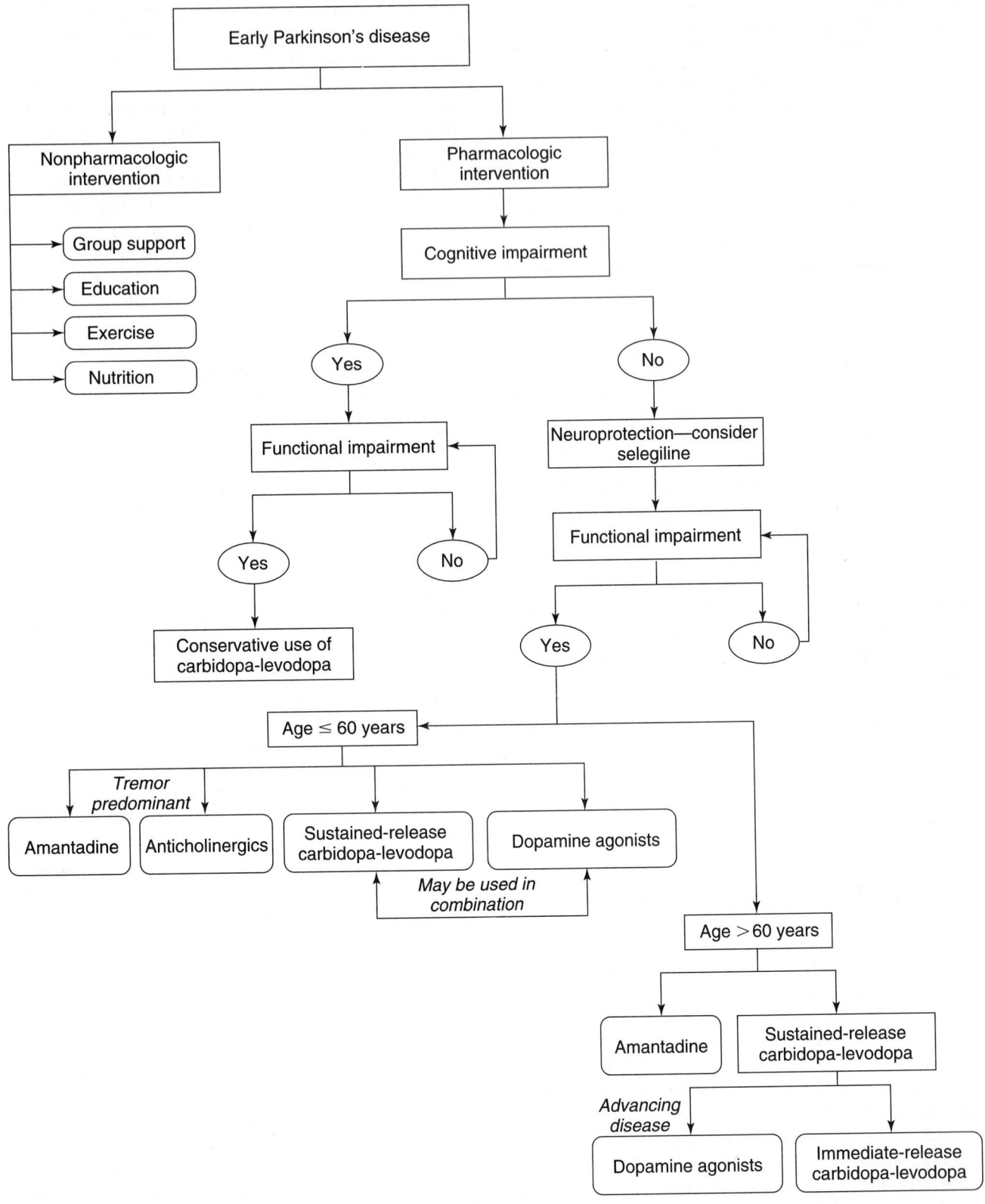

Figure 51.1. An algorithm for the management of Parkinson's disease. (Source: Koller WC, et al. An algorithm for the management of Parkinson's disease. Neurology 44(suppl 10):S6, 1994.)

are ineffective in treating parkinsonism except to lessen the drooling that occurs in some patients. Centrally acting anticholinergics produce moderate improvement in tremor, rigidity, and akinesia in one-third to one-half of patients.

All of the anticholinergics have these side effects: blurred vision, dry mouth, drowsiness, mental confusion, constipation, and urinary retention. In toxic doses they may produce hallucinations, agitation, and elevation of body temperature. The older population in whom parkinsonism usually occurs is particularly susceptible to these anticholinergic side effects.

While the synthetic anticholinergic trihexyphenidyl is frequently prescribed, a number of congeners such as procyclidine, cycrimine, and biperiden are also available. There is no clinically apparent difference among these agents. Any one of them is suitable for initial therapy. The clinician should begin with low doses and gradually increase the dose, weighing satisfactory response against undesirable side effects. Benztropine is used widely because of its long duration of action. A dose of 1 to 2 mg at bedtime will allow most patients mobility on arising during the night or getting out of bed in the morning. Diphenhydramine provides mild anticholinergic and antiparkinsonism effects. Diphenhydramine is also useful as a hypnotic in parkinsonism patients who have difficulty going to sleep or staying asleep.

AMANTADINE

Amantadine is an antiviral agent that produces moderate improvement in parkinsonism. The mechanism of action is currently unknown, although it is postulated that amantadine may release dopamine from intact dopaminergic terminals. Side effects include slurred speech, ataxia, depression, hyperexcitability, insomnia, dizziness, livedo reticularis, and, in extremely large doses, convulsions and hallucinations. In general, the side effects are mild, transient, and reversible. The usual dose is 100 mg/day with breakfast for the first week and then 100 mg with breakfast and lunch. The dose may be increased to a maximum of 400 mg/day. Approximately 90% of amantadine is excreted unchanged in the urine; therefore the dose may be reduced for patients with renal impairment (14). Early studies demonstrated that tachyphylaxis occurs after 4 to 8 weeks in about one-half of patients. A few patients may receive benefits for a much longer term. Therefore, amantadine is often used for short-term, intermittent therapeutic assistance, since its effect is enhanced by concurrent use of levodopa. It has a rapid onset of action, effects being seen within a few days. Amantadine is not a first-line drug, but it may be useful as an adjunct to therapy with anticholinergics and levodopa.

LEVODOPA

Cotzias and colleagues (15) first demonstrated the efficacy of levodopa in treating parkinsonism in 1967. Although small doses of dopa were tried as early as 1961 in treating parkinsonism, most investigators reported transient or no improvement. By switching to the levo isomer of dopa and gradually increasing the dose of the drug, Cotzias and associates were able to push the dose high enough to achieve therapeutic results while keeping the gastrointestinal side effects at a tolerable level.

The next major breakthrough in the use of levodopa was the addition of carbidopa, a decarboxylase inhibitor, to levodopa therapy. High doses of levodopa, 4 to 8 g/day, are generally needed because much of the levodopa is wasted through extracerebral metabolism. Decarboxylase inhibitors, which do not cross the blood-brain barrier, are useful in preventing the conversion of levodopa to dopamine outside the brain. This enables the dose of levodopa to be reduced to one-fourth of the original dose with a concomitant decrease in nausea, vomiting, and cardiac arrhythmias (16). Because this combination reduces the nausea caused by levodopa alone, it was named Sinemet for "without emesis."

Akinesia is generally the first symptom to improve, followed by improvements in rigidity and tremors. Overall, therapy with levodopa can be expected to produce 50% or greater improvement in symptoms in about two-thirds of patients. Levodopa is approximately 3.5 times more effective than anticholinergic therapy in treating parkinsonism.

The rationale for the use of levodopa is based on the finding that parkinsonism may be caused by the depletion of dopamine in the basal ganglia. Dopamine seems to act as a specific transmitter at certain dopaminergic synapses. Dopamine itself was tried in the treatment of parkinsonism, but it does not cross the blood-brain barrier to any appreciable extent. However, the immediate precursor of dopamine, levodopa, does so easily and is therefore effective in restoring dopamine levels in the brain.

Dosage and Administration. The careful titration of dosage for each individual patient is of the utmost importance to achieving successful levodopa therapy. With the introduction of the levodopa/carbidopa combination (Sinemet and Sinemet CR) it is no longer necessary to use such high doses. When the levodopa/carbidopa combination (Sinemet) is used, the dose of levodopa can be reduced by 75%. The patient may be started on 1 tablet of 25 mg carbidopa and 100 mg levodopa (Sinemet 25/100) 3 times a day. About 75 to 100 mg/day of carbidopa are needed to reach the optimal saturation point for carbidopa. The dose may be rapidly increased to effective levels, since the necessity to develop tolerance to the peripheral effects of dopamine is minimized. As the dose is increased, the patient may be switched to tablets containing 25 mg carbidopa and 250 mg levodopa (Sinemet 25/250). The maximum recommended dose of levodopa in such a combination is 2 g/day. In switching a patient from levodopa to the combination, wait at least 8 hr after the last dose of levodopa to prevent toxic effects.

A controlled-release formulation of Sinemet called Sinemet Cr, which contains 50 mg carbidopa and 200 mg levodopa (Sinemet CR 50/200) and 25 mg carbidopa and 100 mg levodopa (Sinemet CR 25/100), decreases fluctuations in response that are seen after prolonged use of levodopa. Sinemet CR is less bioavailable than Sinemet. In converting a patient to the sustained-release formulation, an additional 20 to 25% more levodopa may be required to achieve the same therapeutic effect. The dosing interval for Sinemet CR should be 4 to 8 hr during waking hours. A guideline for converting a patient from Sinemet to Sinemet CR is included in Table 51.4.

Sinemet and Sinemet CR offer several advantages over levodopa alone. In addition to being able to reduce the dose by 75%, there are generally fewer peripheral side effects, a more rapid onset, and a greater degree of improvement, since larger doses can be given before limited by toxic effects. Pyridoxine can be given with this combination without conteracting the effects of levodopa. On the other hand, central nervous system toxicities may increase in onset and severity, since more levodopa is available to the brain.

Initiating Therapy with Levodopa. There has been significant controversy among clinicians about when to initiate levodopa therapy. There is no question that the effectiveness of levodopa diminishes over time. If levodopa is effective for only a limited period of time, advocates of late initiation argue that it is most reasonable to save levodopa until there is significant disability. The proponents of early

Table 51.4.
Antiparkinsonism Drugs

Drug	Dose
Anticholinergics	
Trihexyphenidyl (Artane)	1–5 mg t.i.d., start with low doses. Doses over 20 mg/day are rarely tolerated.
2- and 5-mg tablets. 5-mg time-released capsules	
Benztropine (Cogentin)	Initially 0.5–1 mg/day with slow increase to 1–2 mg/day. Maximum dose 6 mg in divided doses.
0.5-, 1-, 2-mg tablets	
Diphenhydramine (Benadryl)	Usual dose is 75–150 mg/day in divided doses with a maximum of 300 mg.
25- and 50-mg capsules; 12.5 mg/5 mg elixir	
Biperiden (Akineton)	2 mg 3 or 4 times a day.
2-mg tablets	
Cycrimine (Pagitane)	1.25 mg 2 or 3 times a day. Usual range 3.75–15 mg/day in divided doses.
1.25- and 2.5-mg tablets	
Procyclidine (Kemadrin)	2.5 mg 2 or 3 times a day. Usual dosage range 10–20 mg/day in 3 or 4 doses.
5-mg tablets	
Dopaminergic Drugs	
Levodopa (Larodopa, Dopar, Levopa)	Initially 300–500 mg/day with slow increase to 2–8 g/day in divided doses.
100-, 250-, and 500-mg capsules	
Carbidopa (Lodosyn)	75–100 mg/day.
25-mg tablets	
Levodopa/carbidopa (Sinemet)	300/75 to 1500/150 mg/day in 3 or 4 divided doses. Maximum dose 2000/200 mg/day.
10 mg/100 mg, 25 mg/100 mg and 25 mg/250 mg	
Levodopa/carbidopa sustained-release (Sinemet CR)	1 tablet b.i.d. = 300–400 mg Sinemet.
50 mg/200 mg	1½ tablet b.i.d. or 1 tablet t.i.d. = 500–600 mg Sinemet.
	4 tablets in 3 or more divided doses = 700–800 mg Sinemet.
	5 tablets in 3 or more divided doses = 900–1000 mg Sinemet.
Now also available as 25 mg/100 mg	
Amantidine (Symmetrel)	100 mg with breakfast for 5–7 days and then 100 mg with breakfast and lunch.
100-mg capsules, 50 mg/5 mL syrup	
Bromocriptine (Parlodel)	Start with 1.25 mg b.i.d. with meals. If necessary, the dosage may be increased every 14–28 days by 2.5 mg with meals. Maximum dose 100 mg/day.
2.5-mg tablet and 5-mg capsule	
Pergolide (Permax)	Initiate with 0.05 mg for first 2 days. Gradually increase the dosage by 0.1–0.15 mg/day every third day over the next 12 days of therapy. The dosage may then be increased by 0.25 mg/day every third day until an optimal therapeutic dose is achieved. The average dose is 3 mg/day. The maximum dose is 5 mg/day.
0.05-, 0.25- and 1-mg tablets	
Selegiline (Eldepryl)	5 mg at breakfast and 5 mg at lunch.
5-mg tablets	

initiation argue that is is the progession of the disease that makes levodopa less effective over time and that levodopa should be used early to obtain the maximum benefits of the drug.

Studies by Markham and Diamond (17, 18) provide persuasive data to show that the loss of effectiveness of levodopa is due to the progression of the disease and not the duration of time on levodopa. They found that if groups who had equal duration of symptoms—for example, 8 years—but different duration of levodopa therapy (3 years versus 6 years) were compared, their disability scores were similar. On the other hand, patients who had equal duration of levodopa therapy but different duration of symptoms had significantly different disability scores. This data supports the proponents of early initiation of levodopa who implicate duration of disease rather than duration of levodopa as the cause of the loss of effectiveness.

There is also convincing evidence that long-term levodopa therapy can alter the responsiveness of dopamine receptors. Only after prolonged therapy with levodopa do we see a significant number of patients with the "on-off" effect and the "end-of-dose" or "wearing-off" effect. This may be due to the decreased sensitivity of dopamine receptors with prolonged therapy or to a decrease in dopamine receptors caused by levodopa therapy.

Most neurologists will initiate levodopa therapy as soon as the disease interferes with the patient's occupational or social functioning. This may be much earlier for a painter or a surgeon than for someone who is not dependent on fine motor skills. The optimal time to initiate levodopa therapy, therefore, depends heavily on the wishes and needs of the individual patient.

Side Effects. Nausea and vomiting are seen at one time or another in almost all patients taking levodopa. Anorexia may also occur in conjunction with the nausea and vomiting but occasionally may occur alone. The nausea and vomiting are probably a result of both the local and central effects of levodopa. To prevent the gastrointestinal (GI) side effects, levodopa should be initiated with low doses and then slowly increased as tolerated by the patient. Administering the drug with food or antacid will decrease the nausea. If nausea and vomiting become severe despite slow increases in dose and administration with food, symptomatic treatment may be required. Phenothiazine derivatives, such as prochlorperazine (Compazine), should be avoided, since they may counteract the therapeutic effects of levodopa.

Nausea and vomiting are significantly decreased when carbidopa is used in conjunction with levodopa. Other GI side effects include abdominal pain, diarrhea, constipation, peptic ulcer, and GI bleeding.

Cardiac arrhythmias, most commonly sinus tachycardia, and premature ventricular contractions occur in a small number of patients. This side effect can be attributed to the stimulation of β-adrenergic receptors in the heart by dopamine and its metabolites, such as norepinephrine. Treatment consists of discontinuing the levodopa and starting an antiarrhythmic agent. Propranolol is the logical agent, since it has primarily β-blocking actions. Decarboxylase inhibitors such as carbidopa may decrease the prevalence of cardiac arryhthmias.

The orthostatic hypotension that frequently occurs in patients with parkinsonism can be aggravated by levodopa. Several different mechanisms have been proposed, including direct β-effects of dopamine on blood vessels producing vasodilation, α blockade of the peripheral vascular system and depletion of norepinephrine from adrenergic nerve endings by dopamine. Whatever the mechanism, it occurs in at least 25 to 35% of patients early in treatment. Fortunately, the blood pressure usually returns to normal within 2 to 3 months after initiation of therapy. If symptoms are severe, treatment with elastic stockings, an increased salt intake, or sympathomimetic drugs such as ephedrine is indicated.

Levodopa causes behavioral changes manifested as hallucinations, depression, paranoia, agitation, delusions, and loss of judgment. The magnitude of these behavioral changes is difficult to determine, since parkinsonism occurs primarily in older patients who may develop impairment of memory, dementia, and other personality changes independent of levodopa therapy.

Abnormal involuntary movements are related to high doses and prolonged therapy with levodopa. After 6 months or more of therapy, over one-half of the patients show symptoms of grimacing, chewing, active tongue movements, bobbing of the head and neck, and rocking movements of the trunk. When the carbidopa/levodopa combination is used, the onset of abnormal involuntary movements and other central nervous system reactions may be shortened to a few weeks, since more levodopa is available to enter the brain.

The "on-off" effect is a complication of levodopa therapy that often occurs after 2 to 3 years of treatment. There is an abrupt fluctuation in the patient's response to levodopa from being symptoms-free "on" to experiencing full-blown parkinsonism signs and symptoms "off." It may occur at any time and persist in either phase for minutes to hours. In about half of the cases of the "on-off" effect, the "off" phase occurs 3 to 4 hr after the last dose of levodopa and is called "end-of-dose deterioration." Improvement "on" begins about 1 hr after the next dose. The exact mechanism of the "on-off" effect is unknown but may be due to factors that cause fluctuation in the blood level of levodopa or alter the sensitivity of dopamine receptors. The treatment of the "on-off" effect includes more frequent administration of levodopa, the use of the levodopa/carbidopa sustained-release combination, the substitution of a direct-acting dopamine agonist such as bromocriptine or the addition of selegiline.

Drug Interactions. A number of drugs have a potential for interacting with levodopa. The clinical significance of these interactions is largely unknown, because most reports of the interactions are either theoretical or only anecdotal.

Even small amounts of pyridoxine (vitamin B6) can antagonize the effect of levodopa because of an enhancement of the peripheral metabolism of levodopa. A pyridoxine-dependent enzyme catalyzes the conversion of levodopa to dopamine. For this reason, pyridoxine was initially administered to potentiate the effect of levodopa but instead completely reversed it. By catalyzing the conversion of levodopa to dopamine in the intestines, liver, and kidneys, pyridoxine decreases the amount of levodopa available to cross the blood-brain barrier. Although even 5 to 10 mg may antagonize the therapeutic effects of levodopa, for some patients such doses may be given to overcome the torsion dystonia produced by levodopa. However, reducing the dose slowly will usually produce the same effect and is the preferred method for treating this side effect. Small doses of pyridoxine may be given to overcome pyridoxine deficiency resulting from the large amount used in levodopa metabolism or to prevent the peripheral neuropathy that is associated with isoniazid or hydralazine therapy. Since most parkinsonism patients now receive carbidopa, a decarboxylase inhibitor, with their levodopa, even large doses of pyradoxine will not counteract the effects of levodopa. Therefore, pyridoxine restriction is unnecessary in patients receiving Sinemet.

Phenothiazines, butyrophenones, and metoclopramide apparently produce extrapyramidal signs by their ability to block dopamine receptors in the brain. Although low doses of phenothiazines for short periods of time do not significantly reverse levodopa effects, it is best to avoid this combination if possible. An additive hypotensive effect may also complicate therapy with this combination. Clinicians who are unaware of this interaction may try to treat the nausea produced by levodopa with prochlorperazine or metoclopramide. Haloperidol, a butyrophenone, has actions similar to those of the phenothiazines and also produces considerable extrapyramidal effects.

Reserpine can also antagonize the "dopa effect." In fact, the discovery that reserpine depletes the brain of dopamine and produces a parkinsonismlike syndrome was an important clue in determining the biochemical defect in parkinsonism. Reserpine should be avoided for parkinsonism patients whether or not they are on levodopa.

Levodopa may interact with monoamine oxidase type A inhibitors to produce a hypertensive reactions. This is due to a buildup of dopa metabolites, such as norepinephrine, which have vasopressor activity. This combination is potentially dangerous and should be avoided. On the other hand, monoamine oxidase type B inhibitors such as selegiline have a beneficial interaction with levodopa, allowing a 30% reduction of the levodopa dose without causing a hypertensive reaction when it is given in its usual dose (19).

Therapeutic doses of phenytoin (300 to 500 mg/day) have been reported to produce a return of hypokinesia, rigidity, and postural instability in five patients who were previously well controlled on levodopa or levodopa/carbidopa. When the phenytoin was discontinued, the patients slowly returned to their previous level of control over a 2-week period. While the mechanism for this interaction is unknown, it has been postulated that phenytoin may interfere with either the binding of dopamine or the reactivity of the brain to the dopamine.

Laboratory Test Interference. Very few laboratory abnormalities have been noted thus far with levodopa therapy. There is no significant interference with hematologic, renal, endocrine, or liver tests. There have been reports of slight, transient elevations of aspartate aminotransterase and alanine aminotransterase and interference with determination of serum uric acid by the colorimetric method but not by the more specific uricase test. Levodopa also produces an excess excretion of catecholamine metabolites in the urine. Certain metabolites of levodopa cause false positive reactions for ketoacidosis by the dipstick method. The urine, saliva, and sweat may turn reddish and then black because of levodopa metabolites. A positive Coombs' test without frank hemolysis may also be noted. Phenistix, which is used to test for phenylketonuria, is relatively sensitive to levodopa. In fact, it can be used as a screening test for consumption of levodopa for patients who may not respond to levodopa therapy as expected.

Drug Holidays. The term "drug holiday" refers to the complete withdrawal of levodopa after chronic high-dose therapy. It is used when reducing the dose or altering the frequency of dosage does not relieve the adverse effects of long-term therapy or the patient has become increasingly refractory to the therapeutic effects of levodopa. If the patient can tolerate the "drug holiday" of from 1 to 2 days to up to 2 weeks, the dose may be reduced up to 50% when the levodopa is restarted. During the "drug holiday" the signs and symptoms may become very severe, and it is therefore imperative that the patient be hospitalized and kept under close supervision. Thrombophlebitis, pulmonary embolus, depression, and other complications have been reported during the "drug holiday." Improvement is not immediate but comes gradually over a period of a few months and rarely lasts more than a year. Most neurologists believe that it is too dangerous and that the benefits do not outweigh the risks to the patient (20).

BROMOCRIPTINE

Although levodopa has helped the large majority of patients with Parkinson's disease, an increasing number of patients fail to maintain this beneficial response as their disease progresses. For levodopa to be active in the brain, it must be converted to dopamine by pigmented neurons in the substantia nigra. As parkinsonism progresses, the brain loses its ability to convert levodopa to dopamine, and the patient becomes more and more refractory to the beneficial effects of the agent. A drug that stimulates intact postsynaptic receptors directly would solve this problem. There are two distinct dopamine receptors, known as D1 and D2; the main receptor of importance in Parkinson's disease is the D2 receptor.

Bromocriptine (Parlodel) is a direct-acting D2 dopamine agonist that originally was approved by the FDA for endocrine disorders such as amenorrhea/galactorrhea associated with hyperprolactinemia (21). Since late 1981 it has been approved for the treatment of parkinsonism. Bromocriptine acts directly in the brain to stimulate intact postsynaptic receptors. Bromocriptine appears to be about as effective as levodopa and is reserved predominantly for severely disabled Parkinson patients who no longer respond adequately to levodopa alone. It has the advantage of a longer half-life (6 to 8 hr versus about 3 hr for levodopa), greater efficacy against tremors, and a reduction of the "on-off" effect caused by levodopa. Adverse reactions to bromocriptine are qualitatively similar to those to levodopa. Orthostatic hypotension and mental changes are more frequent with bromocriptine, and involuntary abnormal movements and the "on-off" effect are decreased compared to levodopa (22).

While most studies indicate that the optimal dose of bromocriptine for parkinsonism patients who are not taking levodopa is 30 to 90 mg in three divided doses, one study gives hope that low-dose therapy (average dose 15 mg/day) may be just as effective. In this study (23), the patients were started on 1 mg/day of bromocriptine and slowly increased by not more than 1 mg/day at intervals of 1 week or more. At four "dose-stage points" (4, 7.5, 10, and 12.5 mg/day) the dose was not increased for 2 weeks to determine the status of the patients. In their study of 25 patients (14 levodopa-treated patients and 11 not on levodopa), there was a significant improvement (39%) in the combined scores of tremor, rigidity, and bradykinesia while the patients were on bromocriptine therapy. Another study corroborates the efficacy of low-dose bromocriptine therapy (24). Because optimum response to low-dose bromocriptine is delayed for several weeks, rapid increases in drug doses may place the patient on a larger dose than is necessary. The dosage recommendation in Table 51.4 is the FDA-approved dose from the package insert. Currently, most neurologists use bromocriptine primarily for parkinsonism patients who no longer respond to levodopa or who experience severe "on-off" phenomena or other intolerable adverse effects from levodopa.

PERGOLIDE

Pergolide (Permax) is a long-acting dopamine agonist that has been approved as an adjunctive treatment to levodopa/carbidopa in parkinsonism. Pergolide stimulates both D1 and D2 receptors. When pergolide is combined with levodopa, the dosage of levodopa may be reduced by 5 to 30%. Both "on" time and motor function are increased, and the total disability score improves. However, after 6 months the degree of improvement has been shown to decline. The reason for this loss of efficacy with time is unknown. Pergolide has a longer duration of activity than the other direct-acting agonists, 4 to 8 hr, and appears to have fewer pscyhiatric side effects. Side effects are similar to those seen with bromocriptine and include nausea, somnolence, and dyskinesias. The manufacturer recommends taking a single 0.05-mg tablet daily for 2 days and then increasing the dosage over the next 12 days by 0.1mg or 0.15 mg every third day. Further increases are made in 0.25-mg increments at 3-day intervals until the patient has a satisfactory response or experiences an adverse reaction. The dosage should be divided into three daily doses with a maximum of 5 mg/day. The average dose is 3 mg/day combined with an average of 650 mg of levodopa in the form of Sinemet (25, 26).

SELEGILINE

Selegiline (Eldepryl) is a monoamine oxidase B (MAO B) inhibitor that is used primarily as an adjunct to levodopa/carbidopa therapy. Two isoenzymes have been isolated that oxidize monamines and are referred to as MAO A and MAO B. Both are present in the periphery; MAO B predominates in certain areas of the central nervous system, dopamine being one of its major substrates. Selegiline (1-deprenyl) is a specific MAO B inhibitor that allows a patient to eat tyramine-rich foods or take levodopa simultaneously without suffering side effects. When combined with Sinemet, it allows for a reduction in the dose of levodopa by preventing its conversion in the brain by MAO B. It appears to be most useful for patients in the early stages of the disease or when the effectiveness of levodopa is greatly diminished and wide oscillations in motor performance are evident. About 10 to 20% of patients do not respond at all to the addition of selegiline, and it appears to be of little use in advanced stages of the disease.

There have been reports that suggest that selegiline may slow the progression of parkinsonism and thereby increase life expectancy for these patients. Birkmayer and colleagues (27) reported that their patients who received selegiline in addition to levodopa survived 12% longer than those who received levodopa alone. In another study of 54 patients with early Parkinson's disease not receiving levodopa, those who received selegiline were able to function without requiring levodopa for 549 days versus 312 days for those who received placebo (28). The largest study to date to look at this issue involved 800 patients with early untreated Parkinsonism who were given selegiline alone, tocopherol (vitamin E) alone, selegiline and tocopherol, or double placebo for 12 months. Of the 399 patients who received selegiline, 302 were able to function without levodopa compared to only 225 of 401 patients who did not receive selegiline (29). In a follow-up study, the same authors concluded that selegiline (10 mg/day) but not tocopherol (2000 IU/day) delays the onset of disability associated with early Parkinson's disease (30).

Side effects of selegiline include nausea, dizziness, abdominal pain, confusion, hallucinations, dry mouth, vivid dreams, headache, and dyskinesias. Selegiline is metabolized to amphetamine and methamphetamine, so insomnia may occur if evening doses are administered. The usual dose is 10 mg/day given 5 mg with breakfast and 5 mg with lunch. At higher doses, selegiline loses its MAO B selectivity and has the potential to interact with products containing tyramine or other sympathomimetic amines. At the recommended dose, selegiline has very few side effects (31).

General Comfort Medications

Many of the minor signs and symptoms of parkinsonism can be corrected easily with simple over-the-counter medications. For example, constipation is a common finding in parkinsonism. It is frequently aggravated by anticholinergic drugs and levodopa. A stool softener such as docusate sodium or a mild laxative such as milk of magnesia is usually effective. However, a high-fiber diet, plenty of water, and exercise will aid in reducing the need for laxatives. Another common complaint in parkinsonism patients is blurred vision, especially while watching television or movies. This can be attributed to the infrequent blinking of the eyes in parkinsonism. The lubricating action of "artificial tears" eye drops often gives relief. The blurred vision may also be due to anticholinergic drug therapy, and reduction of dosage may be necessary in this case. Parkinsonism patients often have difficulty falling asleep and staying asleep. The drug of choice in this situation is diphenhydramine, because it is an effective hypnotic and also possesses significant antiparkinsonism effects.

Diet

No particular diet has been found to be beneficial for parkinsonism patients. The best diet is one that is well-balanced and high in fiber, since many of these patients have problems with constipation. Some parkinsonism patients have difficulty swallowing and may require cutting up their food and a soft diet.

High protein intake has also been implicated as a factor in decreasing the beneficial effects of levodopa. Since levodopa is absorbed and transported like other amino acids, it has been suggested that high-protein diets may interfere with the absorption of levodopa or other common pathways. For patients who are taking high doses of levodopa and experience the "on-off" effect, it may be worthwhile to reduce the protein intake to the minimum required and consume it with the evening meal.

Psychotherapy

The signs and symptoms of parkinsonism can frequently be aggravated by psychologic factors. The patient may have suffered humiliation from the readily obvious signs of the disease and can become defensive, uncommunicative, and introverted. Since the patient's outlook and motivation can seriously influence the disease, it is important for members of the health care team to provide reassurance, empathy, and encouragement. To add to the problem, many of the drugs that are used to treat parkinsonism produce hallucinations, paranoia delusions, and changes in mood and behavior. Since the antipsychotics that are used to treat these symptoms may aggravate parkinsonism, the best course of action is to start by reducing the doses of the antiparkinson agents.

Physical Therapy

The purely neurological signs, such as tremor and rigidity, do not respond to physical therapy. However, certain secondary disabling manifestations, such as bradykinesia, festinating gait, and freezing of motion, can be lessened, although sometimes only temporarily. The goal is to turn a normally unconscious, automatic movement such as walking into a conscious, voluntary movement in which the patient attempts to place undivided attention on performing a series of small, sequential acts. Activities such as getting up from a chair and walking are broken down into prearranged units so that the patient can practice performing these acts in a flowing, coordinated motion.

Heat and massage are helpful in alleviating painful muscle cramps, and frequent walking and stretching exercises are very valuable in maintaining muscle tone and control. As a patient becomes more bedridden, a water or foam mattress will help to prevent the occurrence of pressure sores. A program of physical therapy may slow the progression of the disabling features of parkinsonism and allow these patients added years of independence.

Speech Therapy

Often, with the advance of the disease, the patient's voice becomes very soft, making it very difficult for them to be heard or understood. Voice exercises along with socialization aid in relieving this problem.

PROGNOSIS

Parkinsonism is a slow, progressive disease. Transplantation of fetal or adrenal tissue has decreased in the akinesia and rigidity in some cases, but these experimental surgical procedures are still unproven and controversial (32, 33). Drugs may relieve many of the signs and symptoms of parkinsonism but do not cure the disease.

Before the introduction of levodopa, a study found that parkinsonism significantly shortened life, mortality being 2.9 times that of the general population of the same age, sex, and race. The average patient died about 9.4 years after onset of the disease, but some have survived for 30 years of more. The most common cause of death was cardiovascular complications, bronchopneumonia, and cancer.

Several studies indicate that the introduction of levodopa may have decreased the mortality rate of parkinsonism almost to that of the general population. A multicenter study of 1,625 parkinsonism patients followed for 4,358 patient-years found a mortality rate of 1.03. When their data was adjusted for the mortality rate of the dropouts, the adjusted mortality rate was 1.33 (34). Another group investigated 349 patients who were treated with either levodopa or levodopa combined with a decarboxylase inhibitor during 1969 to 1975 inclusuve and found that the ratio of actual to expected deaths was 1.85 (35). The excess mortality was accounted for by patients with severe disease at entry in the study.

CONCLUSION

The parkinsonism patient must be closely monitored to achieve maximum benefit from drug therapy. The complex combination of drugs that are often used for these patients must be frequently adjusted because they have a high potential for adverse reactions, drug-drug interactions, and laboratory test interferences. With proper therapy the signs and symptoms of parkinsonism may be controlled for many years, and the life span of these patients may approach that of the general population.

REFERENCES

1. Parkinson J. An essay on the shaking palsy (1817). Reprinted in: Critchley M, ed. James Parkinson. New York: Macmillan, 1955.
2. Koller WC, Silver D, Lieberman A. An algorithm for the management of Parkinson's disease. Neurology 44 (suppl 10):S1–S52, 1994.
3. Poskanzer CC: Editorial. NEJ Med 280;383, 1969.
4. Hoehn MM. Recent advances in the treatment of parkinsonism. Drug Ther Hosp 7:81, 1982.
5. Hoehn MM. The natural history of Parkinson's disease in the pre-levodopa and post-levodopa eras. Neurol Clin 10:331–39, 1992.
6. Rajput AH. Epidemiology of Parkinson's disease. Can J Neurol Scien 11:156, 1984.
7. Calne DB, Duvoisin RC, McGeer E. Speculations on the etiology of Parkinson's disease. Adv Neurol 40:353, 1984.
8. Murdoch PS, Williamson J. A danger in making the diagnosis of Parkinson's Disease. Lancet 1:1212, 1982.
9. Langston JW, Ballard P, Tetrud JW, et al. Chronic parkinsonism in

10. Snyder SH, D'Amato RJ. MPTP: a neurotoxin relevant to the pathophysiology of Parkinson's disease. Neurology 36:250, 1986.
11. Hoehn MM, Yahr MD. Parkinsonism: onset, progression, and mortality. Neurology 17:427, 1967.
12. El-Awar M, Becker JT, Hammond KM, et al. Learning deficit in Parkinson's disease. Arch Neurol 44:180, 1987.
13. Korczyn AD, Inzelberg R, Treves T, et al. Dementia in Parkinson's disease. Adv Neurol 45:399, 1987.
14. Horadam VW, Sharp JG, Smilack JD, et al. Pharmacokinetics of amantadine hydrochloride in subjects with normal and impaired renal function. Ann Intern Med 94:454, 1981.
15. Cotzias GC, et al. Aromatic amino acid and modification of parkinsonism. N Engl J Med 276:374–79, 1967.
16. Boshes B. Sinemet® and the treatment of parkinsonism. Ann Intern Med 94:364, 1981.
17. Markham CH, Diamond SG. Evidence to support early levodopa in Parkinson's disease. Neurology 31:125, 1981.
18. Markham CH, Diamond SG. Long-term follow-up of early dopa treatment in Parkinson's disease. Ann Neurol 19:365, 1986.
19. Robertson DRC, George CF. Drug therapy for Parkinson's disease in the elderly. Br Med Bull 46:124–46, 1990.
20. Mayeux R, Stern Y, Mulvey K, Cote L. Reappraisal of termporary levodopa withdrawal ("drug holiday") in Parkinson's disease. New Engl J Med 313:724, 1985.
21. Vance ML, Evan WS, Thorner MO. Bromocriptine. Ann Intern Med 100:78, 1984.
22. Parkes JD. Bromocriptine in the treatment of parkinsonism. Drugs 17:365, 1979.
23. Teychenne PF, et al. Bromocriptine: low-dose therapy in Parkinson's disease. Neurology 32:577, 1982.
24. Staal-Schreinemachers AL, Wesseling H, Kamphuis DJ, et al. Low-dose bromocriptine therapy in Parkinson's disease: double-blind, placebo-controlled study. Neurology 36:291, 1986.
25. Jankovic J. Long-term study of pergolide in Parkinson's disease. Neurology 35:296, 1985.
26. Langtry HD, et al. Pergolide. Drugs 39:491, 1990.
27. Birkmayer W, et al. Increased life expectancy resulting from addition of 1-deprenyl to Madopar treatment in Parkinson's disease: a longterm study. J Neural Trans M 64:113, 1985.
28. Tetrud JW, et al. The effect of deprenyl (selegiline) on the natural history of Parkinson's disease. Science 245:519, 1989.
29. Parkinson Study Group. Effect of deprenyl on the progression of disability in early Parkinson's disease. N Engl J Med 321:1364, 1989.
30. Parkinson Study Group. Effect of tocopherol and deprenyl on the progression of disability in early Parkinson's disease. N Engl J Med 328:176, 1993.
31. Golbe LI, et al. Selegiline and Parkinson's disease. Drugs 39(5):646, 1990.
32. Freed CR, Breeze RE, Rosenberg NL, et al. Transplantation of human fetal dopamine cells for Parkinson's disease. Arch Neurol 47:505–12, 1990.
33. Takeuchi J, Takebe Y, Sakakura T, et al. Adrenal meducalla transplantation into the putamen in Parkinson's disease. Neurosurgery 26:499–503, 1990.
34. Joseph C, et al. Levodopa in Parkinson's disease: a long-term appraisal of mortality. Ann Neurol 3:116, 1978.
35. Martilla FJ, et al. Mortality of patients with Parkinson's disease treated with levodopa. J Neruol 216:14, 1977.

CHAPTER 52

PAIN MANAGEMENT

LORI A. REISNER-KELLER

Divinum est opus sedare dolorem (Divine is the effort to conquer pain).

—Hippocrates

HISTORY OF PAIN RESEARCH

Pain has plagued humanity since its earliest days. Throughout time, various remedies—some with scientific merit—have attempted to relieve this curse. Documentation of suffering wrought by pain is found in Babylonian tablets and Egyptian papyrus writings. Humans have always sought to understand and control pain–a noble venture, as evidence exists linking pain with consciousness. Earliest treatments included massage, pressure over certain regions, and exposure to cold water, solar heat, or later the heat of fire. Egyptians, Greeks, and Romans used shocks from electric fish to treat painful disorders, and primitive cultures relied on witches, sorcerers, and medicine men to relieve their suffering.

In the early nineteenth century the study of pain emerged as part of experimental science (1). Important advances were also made in pain therapy, most notably the isolation of morphine from crude opium in 1806 and of codeine in 1832 (2). By the mid-1800s, acetylsalicylic acid was introduced, followed by development of ether as an anesthetic. Hypnosis, neurosurgery, electrotherapy, mechanotherapy, hydrotherapy, thermotherapy, and radiation therapy then joined pharmacologic treatments for both surgical and nonsurgical pain (3). Two theories of pain were formulated and expanded during this period. The first was the specificity theory, proposed in 1894 (4). It was based on works of ancient Romans, Arabs, and Europeans and proposed that pain was a specific sensation with its own peripheral and central mechanisms, independent of the other five senses (3). Specific receptors (free nerve endings) that would cause pain when stimulated were thought to exist. Support for this theory came by way of experiments conducted from the late 1800s through the mid-twentieth century: A specific and unique experience was observed to originate from the skin when an appropriate stimulus was applied (5).

The second theory of pain to evolve was known as the intensive, pattern, or summation theory. It was believed that pain resulted from excessive stimulation of the sense of touch. Pain signals were thought to originate as nerve impulses from a peripheral site and to be coded at that distant location instead of within the central nervous system (CNS). The theory also suggested that damage to the body would cause a reverberating circuit between the injured peripheral site and the spinal cord and that the reverberations would summate, or intensify in their effects. Observations that repeated pinpricks could cause intense pain showed that the stimulus-to-response relationship was not proportional, that is, each successive pinprick overlapped the effect of the previous one, rather than being transmitted as a distinct and separate impulse (6). Furthermore, skin receptors were shown to have unique physiologic properties by which they could transmit different degrees of stimulation in the form of impulse patterns (1).

Debate and controversy surrounded each theory, so a third postulate was introduced. Pain was regarded as an original physiologic sensation *and* the psychic reaction produced by that sensation. This marked the first time that an individual's *response* to pain-eliciting phenomena was considered in pain research.

By the 1940s, consolidation of these three theories led to a proposal that pain could be separated into two components: perception and reaction to pain (2). Finally, in the 1960s, Melzack and Wall proposed the gate control theory of pain, which posited that a painful stimulus acted on pain-sensitive receptors and caused an electrochemical nerve impulse to travel to the brain, which then initiated the physical and psychological responses to pain. Though certain key details of the gate control theory have since been revised, it is still widely accepted to explain the way pain signals are collected, transmitted, and interpreted within the CNS. It is useful because it allows for the existence of specific pain receptors as well as for the role of the nervous system in pain mediation. Essentially, the gate control mechanism occurs as follows: Afferent C fibers and A-δ (A-delta) nerve fibers transmit pain signals to an area known as the substantia gelatinosa, which is located in the dorsal horn of the spinal cord (refer to Figure 52.1). Cells within the dorsal horn collect and interpret these signals and send them to transmission cells with terminals projecting to distant sites outside of the dorsal horn. Some of the C fibers and the A-δ fibers terminate in the dorsal root horn, whereas others form a complex known as the lateral spinothalamic tract. Pain impulses travel up along this tract to the thalamus and from there to the cerebral

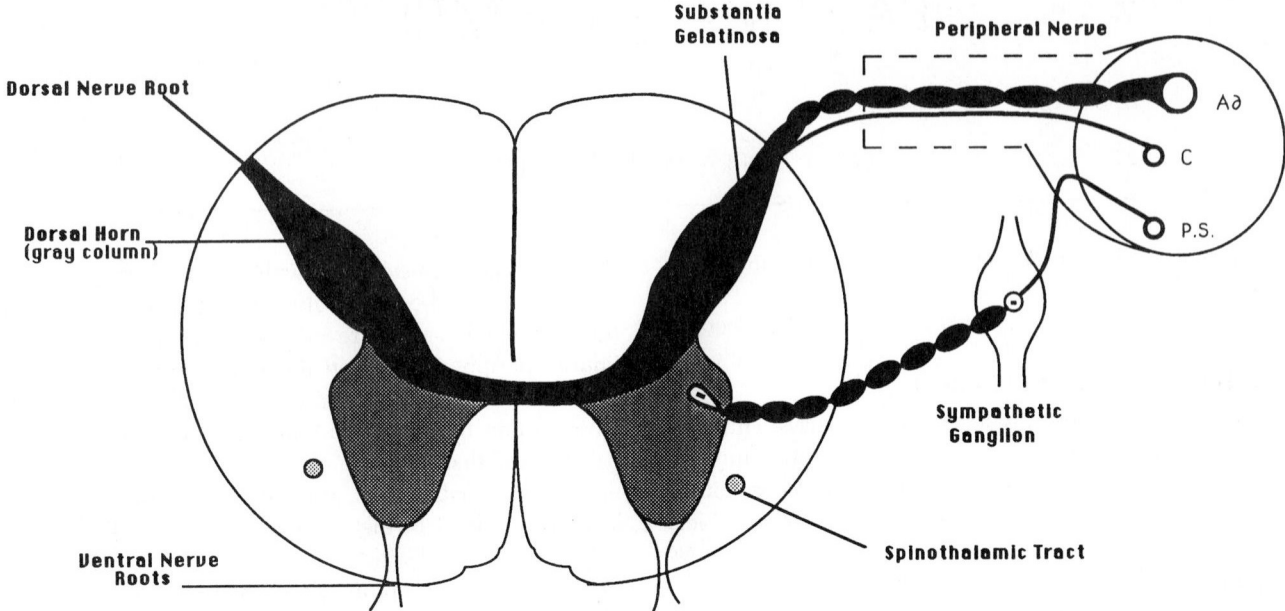

Figure 52.1. Transverse section of the spinal cord with peripheral nerve section illustrating two different types of axons: A-δ fibers and C fibers with cell bodies in the dorsal root and sympathetic fibers with cell bodies in the sympathetic ganglion. A-δ fibers and sympathetic preganglionic fibers are myelinated, while both C fibers and postganglionic sympathetic (P.S.) fibers are unmyelinated. The myelinated fibers carry impulses at a faster rate. Sympathetic fibers are thought to mediate some of the body's response to pain signals traveling along the peripheral nerve to the spinal cord. (Source: Adapted from Fields HL. Pain. New York: McGraw-Hill, 1987; and Clemente CD. Gray's Anatomy, 30th ed. Philadelphia: Lea & Febiger, 1985.)

cortex of the brain (7). Competing nerve impulses can block pain signals at the nervous system "gates," diminishing the intensity of the pain-relaying messages. Other controls exist that descend from the brain to inhibit firing of responsive neurons in the dorsal horn and therefore blunt or halt pain signals (8).

Some researchers believe that humans can be separated into two categories, depending on their pain response. Pain-sensitive (PS) subjects experience pain with qualitative differences, which depend more on psychological variables than is the case with pain-tolerant (PT) subjects. These experiences can be measured by electroencephalographic devices. Because of the role stress plays in pain responsivity and their higher observed stress level, PS subjects demonstrate a lower pain threshold (9). Further research will determine additional criteria for classifying pain response and whether these two categories can be generalized to include a broad range of painful stimuli.

Modern concepts of pain have been derived from these theories, and current therapy is directed at the emotional (psychological) components as well as the sensory or physiologic components of pain. Such interventions as counseling, biofeedback, and stress management training are used to treat the emotional components, and medications, physical therapy, or surgical procedures are used to treat the latter components.

PHYSIOLOGY OF PAIN

The Peripheral Pain Sensory System

When a painful (noxious) stimulus is applied to a sensitive area such as the skin, a series of events occur that are ultimately identified as a painful sensation. Sensitive tissues are those that contain pain receptors, also called nociceptors. Nociceptors are primary afferent nerves with terminals outside of the spinal cord that respond to noxious stimuli. Two phenomena occur via the nociceptors (10). The first is receptor activation or transduction, in which chemical, thermal, or mechanical energy is translated to an electrochemical nerve impulse in the primary afferent nerve. The second event is transmission of the impulse as coded electrochemical information to structures in the CNS that interpret the signal as pain. Transmission occurs initially in the spinal cord, where neurons relay messages from the nociceptors to the brain. The messages elicit many responses, such as a withdrawal reflex or a subjective perceptual event (exclaiming, "Ouch!"). The majority of nociceptors conduct their signals in two velocity ranges. Larger-diameter, myelinated A-δ, or rapid-firing fibers include muscle receptors, among other primary afferents, and constitute most of the known myelinated nociceptors. These A-δ fibers are most sensitive to stimulation by heat and by sharp, pointed instruments; hence they are known as mechanothermal or mechanical nociceptors. A third type of A-δ fiber may exist that is sensitive to irritant

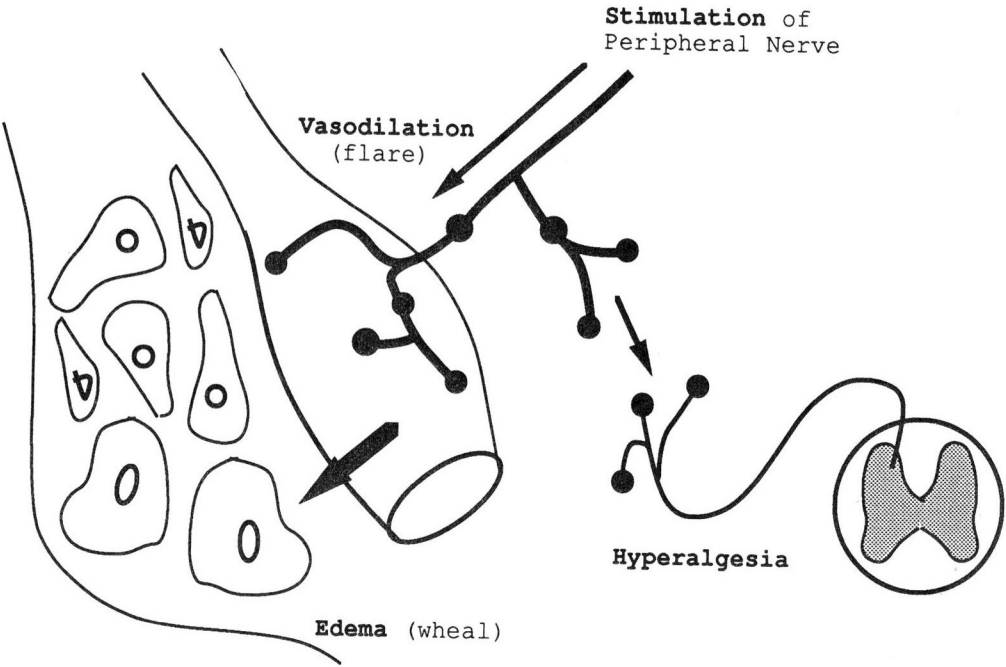

Figure 52.2. Events occurring after an insult to a peripheral nerve. Stimulation of the nerve ending produces a stimulus to vessel walls at the site of injury or trauma. Histamine, bradykinin, and other chemical mediators lead to vasodilation, then edema. Electrochemical signals across nociceptive synapses transmit the pain sensation to pathways in the spinal cord and ultimately to the brain (thalamus). (Source: From Fields HL. Pain. New York: McGraw-Hill, 1987.)

chemicals. A-δ fibers have the property of *sensitization*; that is, repeated application of a noxious stimulus produces increased sensitivity of these receptors (11).

The unmyelinated axons are known as C fibers or slow-firing fibers and make up about 75% of the primary afferents in peripheral nerves. They have a smaller diameter than their fast-conducting counterparts and are sensitive to noxious thermal, mechanical, and chemical stimuli. Like the A-δ fibers, C fibers sensitize with repeated application of painful stimuli, although they may be less sensitive immediately after a stimulus (10).

Evidence of the role of both A-δ and C fibers in pain perception is found in observations that brief, intense stimuli applied to a limb produce two distinct sensations: an early sharp, localized "pricking" pain of brief duration followed by a dull, diffuse, and prolonged unpleasant sensation (12). By using compression to selectively block A-δ fibers, the initial sharp pain is abolished. Likewise, blockade of the C fibers by local anesthetics such as lidocaine will lead to the abolition of dull prolonged pain (13, 14).

How a pain sensation is perceived depends on the size of the area stimulated, the frequency of stimulus application, and the duration and location of the stimulus (15). Although pain is a definite and singular experience based on activity in specific receptors, any single nociceptor's activity is influenced by simultaneous activity at nearby nociceptors. Thus the pain experience is a composite of concurrent inputs at multiple receptors (10).

When tissue injury occurs, the nociceptors undergo depolarization, leading to generation (transduction) of a nerve impulse. Depolarization is followed by pain and hypersensitivity lasting from minutes to days. Persistent pain can result from ongoing tissue damage or lingering chemical irritants released by cells during the initial insult. Other possibilities include a lasting change in the integrity of the receptor itself or even in the CNS (10). Such changes are examples of neuroplasticity, which has garnered great interest in recent pain research. Neuroplasticity may explain the transformation of acute to more chronic pain states following some injuries or traumatic events. A combination of these factors is also possible.

Stimuli above a nociceptor's pain threshold will result in visible signs of tissue damage. More extensive injuries lead to local increased sensitivity to mild stimuli, or hyperesthesia. Hyperesthesia causes injured tissues to develop tenderness, so normally innocuous stimuli produce pain. This hyperalgesia is paralleled by changes in the activity of the nociceptors, including sensitization. After superficial injury to the skin, an intense vasodilation occurs at the injury site (see Figure 52.2). This is rapidly followed by edema (a wheal) and secondary vasodilation that produces reddening (a flare), which spreads to adjacent, uninjured skin. The hypersensitive region enlarges progressively with time and depends mainly on the activity of the C fibers, as both the flare and remote sensitization are blocked by local anesthetics. Thus, activity in C fibers causes vasodilation and sensitizes adjacent C fibers. The long-lasting changes that occur *after* the injurious stimulus may play a major role in determining both the intensity and quality of clinically important pain (10).

Central Pain Transmission

The cell bodies of the nociceptors are located in the dorsal root ganglion, and most of their axons terminate in the dorsal horn of the spinal cord. Some afferents project to the spinal cord through a ventral root as well, and both roots are thought to be important for pain transmission.

Different pain-transmitting pathways may exist, including the spinothalamic, spinoreticular, spinocervical, and dorsal column tracts. Animal models of pain transmission have failed to precisely define the human pain pathways because of species differences, but it is understood that the various nociceptive pathways of the human, primate, cat, and rat reach their destination in the thalamus of the brain (16).

The lateral spinothalamic tract is thought to be the dominant spinal cord pathway for signaling pain in humans, as lesions of this tract result in the absence of pain below the lesion. In addition, stimulation of this tract will induce pain in humans (17). The termination zone of the spinothalamic tract and that of some dorsal column nuclei appear to overlap in the thalamus, and low-threshold stimulation of the dorsal column by either electrical or chemical means can interrupt the flow of pain signal transmission. This "gating" provides the basis for the use of transcutaneous electrical nerve stimulation and dorsal column electrical stimulators in the treatment of chronic pain (18).

CNS opioid receptors have been identified in high concentration in the dorsal horn. They have also been localized in the brainstem, medulla, pons, amygdala, and cerebrum, including the limbic system. In humans, administration of morphine into the brain's ventricles produces potent pain relief in terminal cancer patients (19). The mechanism of opioid analgesia is detailed later in this chapter.

Pain-Producing Substances

Several chemical compounds accumulate near nociceptors after tissue injury. They may arise from cell leakage, synthesis by local substrates released via enzymes induced by damage, or release by the nociceptor itself (10). (Refer to Table 52.1.)

Histamine from mast cells and potassium are among the substances that are released by tissue damage. Both excite nociceptors and produce pain on injection into human skin. Adenosine triphosphate (ATP) may also have this effect. These compounds act either alone or in combination to sensitize nociceptors (20).

One substance that is known to produce pain is bradykinin, a polypeptide that is produced by cleavage of plasma proteins following tissue injury. Actions of bradykinin include both low-concentration indirect production of hyperalgesia and high-concentration direct stimulation of nociceptors (21).

Other compounds that are synthesized in the area of tissue damage are the by-products of arachidonic acid metabolism, including prostaglandins and leukotrienes. These chemicals are present in high concentrations in inflammatory fluids and are potent mediators of inflammation. Prostaglandins are formed from arachidonic acid via the enzyme cyclooxygenase; of these, prostaglandin E_2 is the most potent. Prostacyclin (PGI_2) is also a potent inducer of pain and hyperalgesia. PGE_2 is thought to produce hyperalgesia by direct action on the nociceptors, but prostaglandins may also sensitize nociceptors via coupling to a cyclic AMP system (22). Other prostaglandins contribute to nociceptor activation by their interaction with additional chemical mediators. For example, prostaglandin E_1 produces pain only when it is injected with either bradykinin or histamine. Similarly, norepinephrine may produce peripheral hyperalgesia via enhanced production of prostacyclin. Aspirin and other nonsteroidal antiinflammatory drugs (NSAIDs) have analgesic activity due to their inhibition of cyclooxygenase (23). Bradykinin-induced hyperalgesia may occur by

Table 52.1.
Chemicals That Are Active in Nociceptive Transduction

Substance	Source	Enzyme Mediator	Potency in Producing Pain
Nociceptor Activators			
Histamine	Released from mast cells	None known	+
Potassium	Released from damaged cells	None known	++
Bradykinin	Plasma proteins	Kallikrein	+++
Nociceptor Sensitizers			
Prostaglandins	Arachidonic acid released by damaged cells	Cyclooxygenase	+/-
Leukotrienes	Arachidonic acid released by damaged cells	Lipooxygenase	+/-
Substance P	Primary afferent	None known	+/-

Source: Adapted from Fields HL. Pain. New York: McGraw-Hill, 1987, p. 32.

stimulation of specific PGE$_2$ production and can be blocked by the NSAIDs (24).

Leukotrienes are produced from the enzyme arachidonic acid by lipooxygenase. Like prostaglandins, these agents produce hyperalgesia. However, leukotrienes are not notably blocked by cyclooxygenase inhibitors but are blocked by depletion of polymorphonuclear leukocytes (PMNs). Both prostaglandins and leukotrienes may exert their hyperalgesic effects by mediation of other pain-eliciting compounds (25).

In contrast to substrates that are released in the region of injury, nociceptors themselves discharge pain-enhancing substances. Substance P, a polypeptide, is liberated from some C fibers and excites pain transmission pathways in the dorsal horn. In experimental arthritis, intramuscular gold sodium thiomalate, a neurotoxin, causes substance P depletion by decreasing the number of C fibers in adjacent peripheral nerves. Substance P is a potent vasodilator and leads to release of histamine from mast cells; this explains its role in the immunomodulation as well as the pain of arthritis. Histamine itself also activates nociceptors and produces vasodilation (26).

MODULATION AND INTERRUPTION OF CENTRAL PAIN PROCESSING

Opioid Receptors

Opioids, also called narcotics, that are administered into the spinal fluid reduce nearly all manifestations of clinical pain in humans. Subpopulations of these receptors are characterized by their sensitivity to selective opioid agonists (27). Specific receptors in the CNS and peripheral tissues are responsible for modulating the effects of opioids; they are subdivided into four types: the mu (μ), delta (δ), kappa (κ), and epsilon (ϵ) receptors. Sigma (σ) receptors were once considered part of the class of opioid receptors but are now classified as a distinct receptor type. The μ and κ receptors both produce analgesia; the μ receptor is responsible for the habituating and withdrawal effects of the opioids. μ receptors, located primarily in pain-modulating areas of the CNS, induce central analgesia and respiratory depression (28). κ receptors are responsible for analgesia at the levels of the spinal cord and the brain and are found in greatest concentration in the cerebral cortex and in the substantia gelatinosa of the dorsal horn. Because they are thought to produce analgesia without inducing opioid habituation, there is great interest in the development of κ-specific receptor agonists. Though experimental κ agonists such as spiradoline have shown low dependence and abuse liability, they are not ideal analgesics because of their psychotomimetic (hallucinogenic) and dysphoric effects. δ receptors are located in the limbic area of the brain and in the spinal cord and may play a role in the euphoria that selected opioids produce. Evidence also

exists implicating them in analgesia at the spinal cord level. Some researchers consider δ receptors to be a subpopulation of the μ receptors or as mediators of μ receptors. The function of ϵ receptors has not yet been elucidated; δ receptors, though not true opioid receptors, are believed to produce the psychotomimetic and dysphoric effects of some opioid agonists and partial agonists such as butorphanol and pentazocine (29).

Endogenous opioids known as endorphins, enkephalins, and dynorphins are found in varying concentrations in the CNS (30). Their roles are not completely understood, but dynorphins and enkephalins appear to be responsible for intrinsic regulation of pain perception within the medulla, while endorphins and enkephalins probably serve this function within the substantia gelatinosa. Each of the endogenous opioids has greater preference for a particular receptor type: β-endorphin and enkephalins are potent at μ and δ receptors, and the κ receptor is the target site for the dynorphins (31).

The site of action of opioids depends on the method of administration. Systemically injected or ingested opioids will produce high brain opioid concentrations with relatively low spinal concentrations. The reverse occurs with spinal administration of the drug, that is, intrathecal (into the subarachnoid space) or epidural injection. At the spinal level, opioids are thought to inhibit pain signals carried by the A-δ and C fibers at their synapses in the substantia gelatinosa.

Opioids exert at least part of their analgesic action by inhibiting release of substance P in the central and peripheral nervous systems. They also interfere with the actions of prostaglandins at peripheral sites, particularly μ receptor-specific opioids, which inhibit PGE$_2$ hyperalgesia in a dose-dependent fashion (32). It is speculated that opioids produce analgesia by causing adenosine release, since methylxanthines such as caffeine can antagonize the effects of morphine (33, 34).

Opioids may exert their inhibitory actions via hyperpolarization of neurons through altered conductance of potassium or calcium. However, evidence exists that they also cause in vitro excitatory actions at the nerve terminals. This bimodal action is dose-dependent and helps to explain the mechanisms of opioid tolerance and dependence (35).

Tolerance and tachyphylaxis probably result from repeated exposure of receptors to high doses of opioid analgesics (28). Continuously administered low-dose opioids can slow the development of tolerance. Patient-controlled analgesia, in which a controlled amount of drug is infused continuously, with bolus or "rescue" doses for breakthrough pain, produces less tolerance than do intermittent high doses of an opioid. A second potential approach to delay tolerance is the use of agents that are analgesic at a specific receptor; thus far, however, κ- or δ-specific agents are investigational only. Because of varying degrees of affinity for different receptors, narcotics do not produce complete cross-tolerance to each other. In general, cross-tolerance exists among opioids with high affinity to the same receptor, but less cross-tolerance is seen between opioids acting at different receptors. Since most available opioids have some affinity for each receptor type, the extent of cross-tolerance is variable and unpredictable (36). In changing from one opioid agonist to another, half the calculated equianalgesic dose may be used initially, and then the dose may be titrated upward as required (37).

Beside their analgesic effects, opioids produce drowsiness, sedation, mood changes, disorientation, and memory impairment. Respiratory depression occurs by a direct action on the medullary respiratory and ventilation centers to reduce their responsiveness to carbon dioxide tension and by depression of brain centers that are responsible for the rate and rhythm of respirations. Studies comparing morphine to other opioids have shown that equianalgesic doses of these agents do not differ significantly in their ability to depress respiration. Nausea and vomiting occur by opioid stimulation of dopamine release in the chemoreceptor trigger zone of the medulla. Opioid-induced emesis is treated with antiemetics that exert dopamine-blocking action, for example, droperidol or prochlorperazine. Dopaminergic actions are also involved in the euphoria that is experienced with opioids (38). Miosis occurs through a stimulatory effect on the oculomotor nerve, and pinpoint pupils are pathognomonic for opioid toxicity. Central stimulation by opioids can also induce skeletal muscle rigidity or convulsions, which may not be suppressed by anticonvulsant agents (39).

Opioid receptors have been localized outside of the nervous system. In the gastrointestinal tract, opioids increase smooth muscle tone in portions of the stomach, duodenum, ileum, and large intestine, leading to decreased motility and spasm. Morphine reduces secretion of hydrochloric acid and pancreatic enzymes and inhibits mucosal transfer of fluids and electrolytes across the intestinal epithelium. Digestion and propulsion of food is delayed, and absorption of oral drugs may be slowed. These properties have led to the development of the piperidine opioid congeners diphenoxylate and loperamide to treat hypersecretory diarrhea.

Therapeutic doses of meperidine, morphine, codeine, or their analogs can lead to increased pressure in the common bile duct with elevations of serum lipase or amylase. Spasm and constriction of the sphincter of Oddi are probably responsible for this effect. Methadone, fentanyl, or narcotic agonist-antagonist combinations do not raise biliary pressure to the same degree as do other opioids and can be used to treat pain from biliary colic or pancreatitis (40).

In the cardiovascular system, opioids produce orthostatic hypotension by peripheral arteriolar and venous dilation. This is either a direct effect or the result of opioid-stimulated histamine release. Vasodilation can be reversed partially by histamine-receptor (H_1) blocking agents and completely by opioid antagonists such as naloxone. Patients with coronary artery disease or evolving myocardial infarction may experience reduced myocardial oxygen consumption, but effects on the normal heart are insignificant. Opioid-induced respiratory depression can result in cerebrovascular dilation and increased cerebrospinal fluid (CSF) pressure, effects that are hazardous in patients with cor pulmonale or individuals with cerebrovascular compromise who may suffer further damage from increased CSF pressure. A second factor that discourages the use of opioids is depression of cognitive function and masking of cerebral damage secondary to pathophysiologies such as stroke.

In the smooth muscle of the bladder and ureter, opioids increase the tone of the ureter and the vesical sphincter, leading to urinary hesitancy or retention. Such bladder effects can be reduced by administration of prazosin or similar α_1 adrenergic antagonists. In the uterus, morphine reverses oxytocin-stimulated hyperactivity, leading to prolonged labor. Opiates also depress respiration in the infant, as all narcotics cross the placenta. Epidurally administered opioids are often used during parturition to reduce systemic effects. Preferred intravenous agents in obstetrics are the opioid agonist-antagonists butorphanol and nalbuphine because of their "ceiling effect" on respiration; that is, higher doses do not increase the degree of neonatal respiratory depression (41).

Cutaneous blood vessels dilate with opioids, making the skin flushed and warm. Histamine release is partly responsible for these effects and for the pruritus and sweating that often follow narcotic administration. Urticaria is particularly problematic after spinal administration of opioids but can be relieved by naloxone (39).

Other Pain-Responsive Receptors

Table 52.2 lists the receptors that are involved in modulation of pain pathways. The adrenergic agonists norepinephrine and clonidine, an α_2 agonist, produce significant analgesia in humans when they are administered into the spinal fluid, highlighting the role of adrenergic modulation of pain. Although it can produce peripheral hyperalgesia by enhancing prostacyclin production, norepinephrine acts centrally on the dorsal horn via descending impulses from the brain to inhibit pain. The antinociceptive actions of both clonidine and norepinephrine can be reversed in a dose-dependent manner with adrenergic antagonists such as yohimbine (42, 43).

Serotonin receptors are found along the spinothalamic tract. Serotonin appears to reduce pain centrally by modulating descending impulses from the brain. This forms the basis of treatment of neuropathic pain syn-

Table 52.2.
Receptors That Are Involved in Modulation of Pain Pathways

Receptor	Subtypes	Agonist	Action	Location	Antagonist
Opioid	μ, ∂, κ	Morphine	Analgesia	Brain and spinal cord	Naloxone
Adrenergic	α-1		Reduction in sympathetic	Dorsal column	Prazosin
	α-2	Clonidine	nervous system output	Dorsal column	Yohimbine
	α & β	Norepinephrine		Dorsal column	Yohimbine
Serotonergic		Tricyclic antidepressants	Modulation	Spinothalamic tract	
Cholinergic		Acetylcholine	Antinociception	Dorsal horn	Atropine
GABA-ergic	A		Inhibits firing of nociceptors	Peripheral	
	B	Baclofen		Dorsal horn	

Source: Adapted from Fields HL. Pain. New York: McGraw-Hill, 1987.

dromes with antidepressants that block presynaptic reuptake of serotonin (44). However, noradrenergic systems are probably also involved in this phenomenon, since selective serotonin reuptake inhibitors (e.g., fluoxetine) do not appear to be as effective in treating neurogenic pain as are the tricyclic antidepressants, which block reuptake of both serotonin and norepinephrine (45).

Cholinergic binding sites have been discovered in the dorsal horn. Application of the muscarinic agonist acetylcholine will produce analgesia, which can be reversed by atropine. Such antinociceptive effects are not reduced by opioid antagonists (46).

GABA-ergic receptors are divided into two types: $GABA_A$ receptors are sensitive to muscimol, and $GABA_B$ receptors are sensitive to baclofen. Of known GABA-ergic compounds, only baclofen has been shown to produce analgesia. $GABA_B$ agonists inhibit firing of the nociceptors, particularly the C fibers. Unlike opioids, baclofen does not inhibit substance P release in the spinal column. Baclofen is administered orally or intrathecally to treat central pain syndromes resulting from injury to the spinal cord, especially if consequent muscle spasms are involved (47, 48).

ACUTE VERSUS CHRONIC PAIN

Pain is defined as "an unpleasant sensory and emotional experience associated with actual or potential tissue damage, or described in terms of such damage" (49). Pain is always subjective, and there are no specific tests that can measure pain quantitatively or qualitatively. The clinician can use tests such as a visual analog scale in an attempt to measure pain objectively, as well as observations of grimacing, limping, and tachycardia, but these are crude methods at best and can be used only to support rather than identify a patient's report of pain.

Acute pain arises from an injury, trauma, spasm, or disease to the skin, muscles, somatic structures, or viscera of the body. It is perceived and communicated via the peripheral mechanisms identified as classic pain pathways, that is, the A-δ and C fibers. The intensity of pain is usually proportional to the degree of damage. Acute pain may be

accompanied by signs of autonomic nervous system activity—tachycardia, hypertension, diaphoresis, mydriasis, and pallor—that mimic those of anxiety, which often coexists with acute pain. Acute pain is characterized by limited duration, and diagnosis is not difficult. Acute pain decreases in intensity as the damaged area heals and tissue repair takes place (50).

Superficial pain is derived from the skin or underlying subcutaneous and mucous tissues. It is characterized by local throbbing, burning, or pricking. It may be associated with tenderness, allodynia (pain from a stimulus that normally does not provoke pain), or hyperalgesia. Visceral pain presents as diffuse, dull, aching pain that is poorly localized and is noticed at the onset or early stages of disease. It may be associated with nausea and other autonomic symptoms. Deep somatic pain is dull and aching and can be localized, though there may be radiating components. Injury or disease of deep somatic structures produces the same response as does injury to the skin or viscera (3).

Treatment of acute pain focuses on superficial or deep location of pain and its origin and is directed toward the underlying etiology. Effective management involves the use of agents that target short-term symptomatic relief, and the goal is to mollify pain impulses during the period of tissue healing. Opiates such as morphine and hydromorphone are employed acutely in postsurgical pain treatment, but other important agents are the NSAIDs, since they can limit pain, swelling, and erythema at the site of trauma, enhancing patient comfort and possibly shortening the duration of the pain syndrome.

Chronic pain persists beyond what would be expected from a precipitating injury or tissue insult and is separated into cancer pain and nonmalignant pain, or benign pain. The term "benign" is a misnomer, however, as people with nonmalignant pain often suffer a great deal of physical and psychological damage. Chronic pain is rarely accompanied by autonomic symptoms. Individuals who report chronic pain often fail to show objective evidence of an underlying pathophysiology on physical or radiologic examination, although patients who have undergone multiple surgeries can develop fibrotic (scar) tissue that may be apparent in imaging studies. Chronic pain is further characterized by its location: it may arise from visceral or myofascial (muscle and connective tissue) locations or from neurologic causes such as herpes zoster infection or diabetic neuropathy. Treatment is directed not only toward symptoms, but also toward the suffering and disability that are produced. Symptoms of depression–hopelessness, helplessness, weight loss, and sleep disturbance–may accompany chronic pain and must be treated concomitantly (50). Pain arising from cancer or other malignant disease exhibits characteristics of both acute and chronic pain. It may be constant or intermittent. A definable cause such as tumor recurrence is usually present. As with chronic nonmalignant pain, therapy is composed of psychological and disability interventions along with analgesics in effective and tolerable doses.

In treating chronic pain, narcotic or nonopioid analgesics should be dosed on an around-the-clock basis, as there is no evidence that such pain will abate abruptly. Pain that is initially perceived as minor can proceed to intolerable levels within a few hours. Once this occurs, a larger dose of analgesic will be required to overcome pain-associated anxiety and bring the pain below the threshold of patient tolerance. For malignant pain, habituation is not a concern, as pain modulates the body's response to opioids and tolerance is slow to develop.

FACTORS INFLUENCING PAIN PERCEPTION

Intensity of pain varies with each individual, pain perception being determined by a person's psychological background in addition to physiologic factors. Since pain is multifactorial, it can be classified into emotional, social, spiritual, and physical spheres (Figure 52.3). Emotional pain consists of isolation, depression, and fear, factors that can reinforce each other. Social pain is comprised of strained or broken relationships as well as financial problems resulting from disability. Spiritual pain includes feelings of guilt, regret, or worthlessness. Physical pain encompasses disease and debilitation. Chronic pain can dull normal autonomic responses to stress such as hypertension and sweating. Signs of depression are most often manifested as sleep disturbances and irritability. Delayed sleep onset and frequent waking may occur, and patients may report exhaustion from lack of sleep and from inability

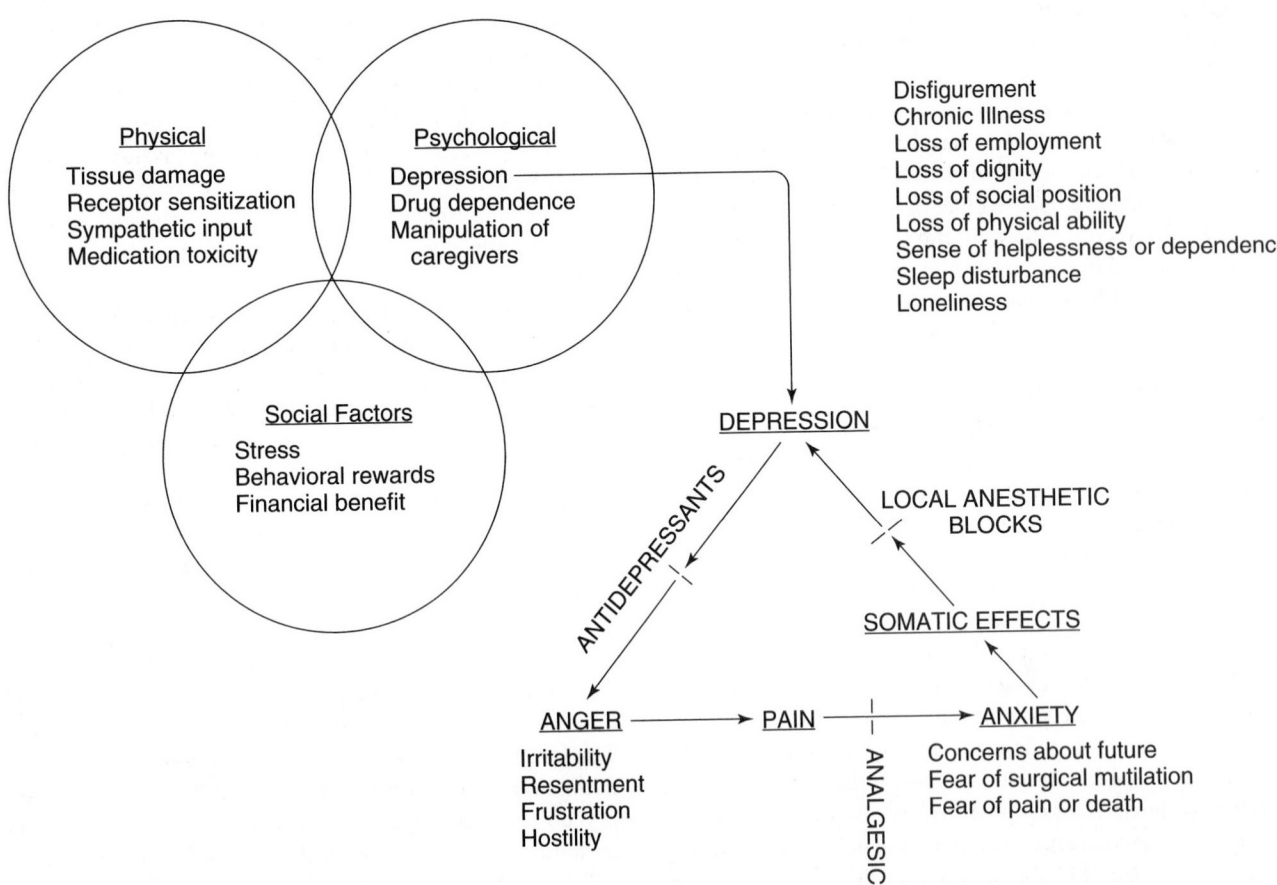

Figure 52.3. Determinants and modifiers of pain response and behavior. Portions of the pain triangle interrupted by pharmacological interventions are shown.

to tolerate the stresses imposed by continuous pain. Chronic pain often leads to anxiety and depression, which in turn exacerbate the pain. This cycle ultimately leads to adoption of a "pain lifestyle" in which polypharmacy and polysurgery become overrepresented in a patient's medical history. If secondary gain such as increased attention from family members or financial reward becomes an issue, there is less incentive to recover from a pain syndrome. Pain may also mask underlying psychological or physical abuse and can present itself as a symptom of emotional need (51).

A distinction can usually be made between the "pain patient" and the patient who is in pain. The patient who is in pain will exhibit findings that are seen more often with acute pain, such as pacing, grimacing, or alterations in heart rate and blood pressure. These individuals will likely fully recover psychologically from the painful episode once adequate pain control is achieved. Even in many such patients with chronic pain, reliance on medications is stable at a minimal level, and the patient demonstrates a high degree of self-dependence in overcoming pain-related disability. Interaction with health care providers is not extensive, and the patient exhibits self-motivation in returning to a premorbid lifestyle.

The pain patient, by contrast, is an individual who has suffered pain for long enough to exhibit notable changes in lifestyle, such as a discharge from employment and heavy reliance on family members or the health care system to offer relief. These patients may be tearful and anxious and may also exhibit symptoms of acute pain that abate when the patient is distracted during conversation. Patients with extreme pain behaviors will visit and/or call their health care providers often and may manipulate their medication regimens without the advice of a health care provider. Patients who use their medications more often than directed may be required to "contract" with their provid-

ers, a system in which the patient is given a specific quantity of medicines for a predetermined period of time. Pain patients may have difficulty establishing realistic goals for their therapy and will request a "cure" for their pain syndrome, though none may exist.

EVALUATION OF PAIN

A simple "PQRST" mnemonic can aid the practitioner in evaluating pain. P represents the *palliative* or *precipitating* factors associated with the pain, such as diet, stress, or physical exertion. Q represents the *quality* of the pain, that is, whether it is sharp, dull, constant, aching, shooting, or the like. R stands for *"region"* or *"radiation"* and is used to locate the pain. S is the patient's *subjective* description of the pain's *severity* and its effects on daily habits and lifestyle. For example, does pain cause waking or appetite loss? Finally, T represents the *temporal*, or *time-related*, nature of the pain. It is useful to ask the patient whether the pain is worse in the evening or the morning, whether it is related to any habitual daily activity, and other questions that are designed to detect diurnal, weekly, or monthly patterns. Women may experience differences in pain at various points in their menstrual cycles, as estrogen induces hyperalgesia (52).

In addition to knowing how, where, and when the pain began and what leads to its continuation, other pertinent facts about a patient's lifestyle are germane to accurate pain assessment. A pain questionnaire will aid in the evaluation and treatment of the chronic pain patient in the ambulatory care setting (53).

Detailed information about the pain should be gathered to supplement the more general "PQRST" scale. It is necessary to determine what help the patient requests and whether his or her goals are consistent with the treatment that is offered. Chronic pain patients cannot expect to be pain-free, as underlying degenerative pathophysiology is

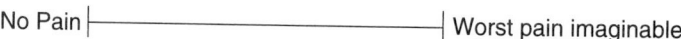

No Pain ├────────────────────────────┤ Worst pain imaginable

Figure 52.4. VAS pain scale. The subject is asked to draw a hash mark at a point on the line corresponding to his or her pain. A ruler is used to measure the placement of the mark, and a number value (in centimeters) is assigned to the measurement.

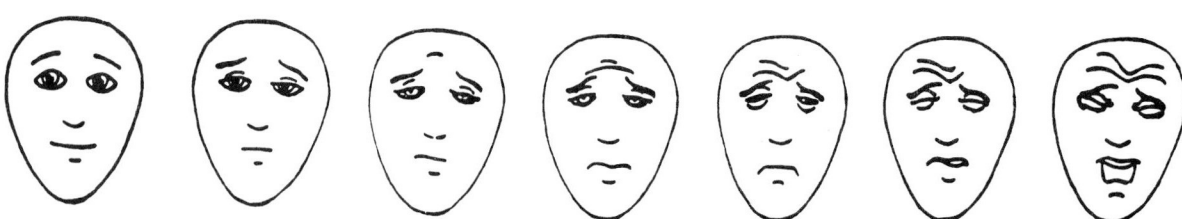

Figure 52.5. The faces pain scale for assessment of pain in pediatric patients. Children are asked to point to the face that best describes their pain. (Source: From Bieri D, Reeve RA, Champion GD, Addicoat L, Ziegler JB. The faces pain scale for the self-assessment of the severity of pain experienced by children: development, initial validation, and preliminary investigation for ratio scale properties. Pain 41:139–150, 1990.)

often permanent. Changes in aspects of lifestyle such as exercise and exertion, employment, and emotional approaches to living with chronic pain may reduce its dominance in one's life, however.

Location of the pain is ascertained with anatomical drawings on which the patient marks areas where the pain is worse. For pain intensity, a visual analog scale (VAS) is a reproducible method to objectively measure and quantify pain. The VAS is a 10-cm line without subdivision marks. The left extreme of the line is labeled "no pain." The rightmost extreme of the line is labeled "worst pain imaginable" (Figure 52.4). The patient is asked to draw a hash mark on the line at the point that best corresponds to his or her pain. Successive VAS scales are compared over time to evaluate response to therapy.

An important portion of any questionnaire is concerned with past medication history as well as current pain medication and other treatments. From this portion of the evaluation, proper selection of analgesics, analgesic adjuncts, and patient compliance can be assessed. Patients who are compulsive in their consumption of pain medications or patients who are on subtherapeutic doses of appropriate medication can be identified.

Finally, a checklist of problems related to major organ systems should be included. Patients who complain of multiple somatic symptoms along with pain may be experiencing depression or another affective disorder. Correction of the underlying depression may lead to remission of pain and somatic complaints.

Assessing pediatric pain is particularly difficult, as young children are often unable to adequately verbalize descriptors of pain intensity and quality. For children a modified visual scale, the Faces Pain Scale (Figure 52.5), can be used (54).

CLINICAL PAIN SYNDROMES

An algorithm for medication selection in various pain syndromes is illustrated in Figure 52.6. Cancer pain arises at the primary site as a result of tumor expansion, nerve compression or infiltration by the tumor, malignant obstruction, or infections in a malignant ulcer. It may also occur at distant metastatic sites. Furthermore, treatment for tumors such as radiation therapy may lead to mucositis and subsequent pain. Some of the more commonly encountered symptoms of cancer pain occur in the musculoskeletal tissue and in the nervous system. Although

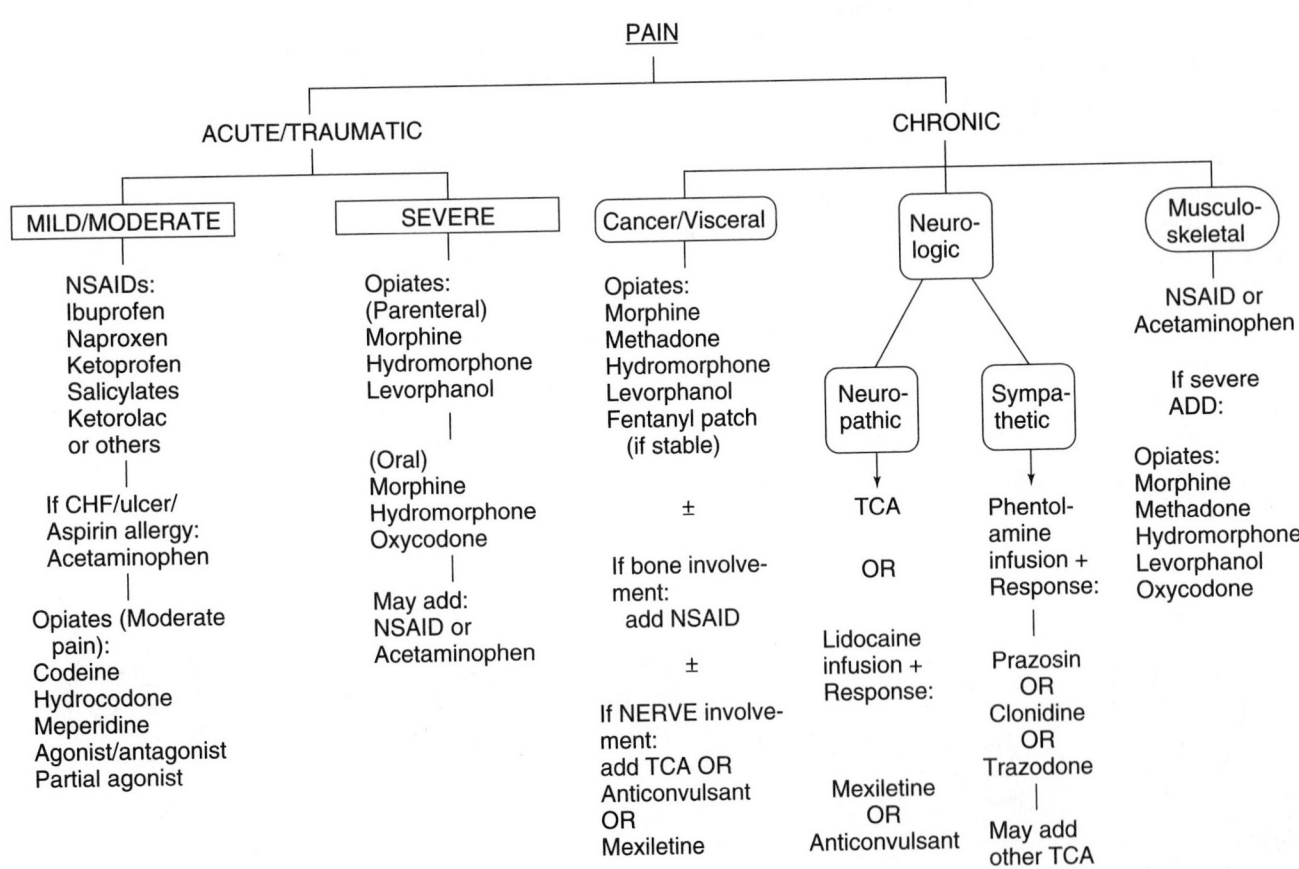

Figure 52.6. Medication selection in the treatment of pain.

Table 52.3.
Principles of Analgesia for Cancer Pain

1. Choose appropriate analgesic(s).
2. Determine the dose by individual requirement.
3. Time doses to a regular schedule (not prn).
4. Anticipate pain; do not "chase" it.
5. Minimize sedation or untoward effects.
6. Use the oral route whenever feasible.
7. Treat nausea and constipation early.
8. Use adjuvant medications whenever necessary.
9. Tolerance and dependence are not problems.

the majority of bony metastases do not produce pain, infiltration of bone is the most common cause of cancer pain. A constant, unpleasant, burning sensation often indicates compression of somatic nerves by tumor. This pain can also be accompanied by an intermittent lancinating pain (55).

For cancer pain, analgesics should be given at regular intervals and in adequate doses (refer to Table 52.3). Medication should never be prescribed on a "prn" basis, as the objective is to maintain maximum possible patient comfort at all times through maintenance of therapeutic levels. Oral medication is preferred, especially long-acting drugs, unless factors prohibit such administration. Such factors include malignant bowel obstruction or severe nausea from emetogenic chemotherapeutic agents. Sublingual narcotic administration has also been studied; the more lipophilic agents provide better analgesia than the less lipophilic morphine, presumably because of improved absorption. An alkaline pH also enhances the sublingual absorption of most opioids. Rectal administration of suppositories may suffice, although this method is less reliable because of variable absorption of drugs from the rectal mucosa. Parenteral infusion is a dependable method of analgesic delivery and can be used in the home as well as the hospital environment with portable, programmable infusion pumps. Many such pumps are now available with syringe drivers that require infrequent changes of the syringe. Medication can thus be prepared by a home health care agency and supplied to the patient on a regular basis (56, 57).

Treatment of mild to moderate cancer pain should begin with nonnarcotic analgesics. When these drugs alone are ineffective, they are combined with intermediate-potency opioid agonists such as codeine or its derivatives. NSAIDs are effective in relieving many symptoms of bone-associated cancer pain, as are corticosteroids. However, the extensive adverse effect profile of the corticosteroids makes the nonsteroidal agents preferable. Bony metastases release prostaglandin E_2, which sensitizes peripheral nociceptors. NSAIDs act by inhibiting elaboration of PGE_2. In addition to relieving pain, the nonsteroidals reduce stiffness, swelling, and tenderness (58). Finally,

potent opioid agonists such as morphine or methadone should be used in the pain management regimen (59). A common agent for treating advanced cancer pain is morphine because of its potency and dosing flexibility. It is generally well tolerated by patients with a terminal illness. Alternatives include hydromorphone, methadone, and levorphanol. Diacetylmorphine (heroin) is not available in the United States and does not possess any advantages in treating pain, since it is hepatically metabolized in vivo to morphine, its active analgesic component. Heroin has a slightly faster onset of action than morphine but a shorter duration of analgesia. It is more soluble, allowing intramuscular administration; however, methadone is as appropriate an alternative to morphine (60).

Analgesic adjuvants such as tricyclic antidepressants may be added to the drug regimen for cancer pain, particularly if there is neural involvement. The benefits of analgesia may be enhanced by the psychotropic effects of the drugs on depression. Other adjuncts include antihistamines, phenothiazines, anticonvulsants, and amphetamines (58, 61).

Neuropathic pain can arise from either discrete or generalized sites of nerve injury or may be idiopathic. Two common neuropathic pain syndromes are postherpetic neuralgia ("shingles") and peripheral neuropathies arising from various causes such as diabetes mellitus or acquired immune deficiency syndrome (AIDS). Less common are neuropathies induced by agents such as dideoxycytidine, an antiretroviral drug. Neuropathic pains are most often sharp, lancinating, burning, hot, electrical, shocking, or searing. They can be intermittent or constant and may involve paresthesias manifested by tingling or numbness of a limb. Neuropathic pain is relatively unresponsive to opioids, but this may be a function of inadequate dosing and underlying patient variables rather than due to the pharmacology of the opioids (62).

Postherpetic neuralgia (PHN) is a persistent, often lifelong pain syndrome resulting from infection with varicella-zoster virus (herpes zoster). The infection is initially manifested by fever, headache, lymphadenopathy, and malaise. These symptoms are followed by increasing pain or itching over a local area known as a dermatome, which is innervated by a specific nerve branch. Treatments for acute herpes zoster infection include systemic corticosteroids, antiviral agents, interferon, adenine arabinoside, and cimetidine. More invasive procedures, including somatic and sympathetic nerve blocks with local anesthetics and/or corticosteroids, have proven to be efficacious (63). Rarely, herpes zoster can leave an elderly or immunocompromised patient with permanent nerve damage resulting in persistent pain that is characterized as lancinating, burning, or itching. Areas that are commonly affected by postherpetic neuralgia are the cervical, cranial/trigeminal, thoracic, and lumbar regions. Herpes zoster is a reactivation of a latent virus that was originally acquired through acute varicella ("chicken pox") infection. The afferent nerve pathways undergo degeneration and interruption, causing deafferentation followed by nerve reorganization (64). The cornerstone of treatment of PHN is the use of tricyclic antidepressants. In addition to their pain-remitting effects, tricyclic antidepressants can also treat the vegetative signs of depression such as sleep disturbance or anorexia (65). Anticonvulsants are also used; carbamazepine and valproic acid have been employed in doses of 600 to 1200 mg/day and 500 to 1500 mg/day, respectively. These drugs reduce complaints of lancinating pain. They are gradually adjusted upward from low starting doses, particularly for elderly patients (66). Topical local anesthetics also help to reduce pain of the affected dermatome. A cream containing capsaicin, a purified derivative of red chili peppers, can be applied directly to the area of itching and inflammation. Studies comparing this agent to placebo have shown a favorable response; however, the use of capsaicin is accompanied by 1 or more days of intense burning, since it acts as a nerve ending counterirritant by stimulating and then desensitizing afferent C fibers (67). Intravenous administration of lidocaine (5 mg/kg) has also been beneficial in treating PHN, as has its oral congener, mexiletine. Sympatholytic agents such as clonidine may prove to be beneficial as well. Baclofen is also useful for refractory PHN pain of the trigeminal distribution (68, 69).

Diabetic neuropathy is usually reported as distal sensorimotor loss and is a long-term complication of diabetes mellitus. Like PHN, diabetic neuropathies respond well to the tricyclic antidepressants. Intravenous lidocaine has been administered with encouraging results, and mexiletine may also prove to be useful in treating this condition. Aldose reductase inhibitors that counteract hyperglycemia-induced metabolic changes at peripheral nerve sites show future promise for reversing early changes associated with functional nerve loss (70, 71).

Phantom limb pain has been described variously as burning, tingling, throbbing, shooting, and stabbing. Neurosurgical procedures are not permanently successful in reducing this type of pain. Biofeedback has a role in increasing temperature and blood perfusion and in reducing discomfort at the amputation site. Anticonvulsants are helpful in reducing paroxysms of pain, as are tricyclic antidepressants (72). Calcitonin may also play a role in the treatment of phantom limb pain (73).

A syndrome known as sympathetically maintained pain, reflex sympathetic dystrophy (RSD), causalgia, or posttraumatic spreading neuralgia predominates in areas of the extremities that are innervated by thoracolumbar branches of the nervous system. It may coexist with other forms of neuropathic pain. Causalgia is marked by burning pain, allodynia, and hyperpathia and occurs in a hand or foot

following nerve injury. RSD is continuous pain in a portion of an extremity following injury and is associated with sympathetic hyperactivity (49). Causes include multiple fractures or surgery to a localized area without involvement of a major nerve. Manifestations of RSD, in addition to burning pain stimulated by activity of the extremity, include vascular phenomena of coldness, numbness, or pain with changes in skin color. Trophic changes such as shiny, hairless skin or loss of bone mass may occur later. Reflex Sympathetic dystrophy may be life-long. Treatment involves vasoactive agents such as prazosin as well as analgetic medications. Initial episodes usually respond to local glucocorticoid injections; more refractory cases respond to regional sympathetic blockade with local anesthetics or instillation of a sympatholytic agent such as guanethidine. Topical application of clonidine or capsaicin to the affected area is promising (74, 75).

Myofascial pain arises from the muscles (myalgias), bones, joints (arthralgias), or connective tissue. Like a neuropathy, it can be idiopathic, iatrogenic, or injurious in origin. Muscle pain arising from exertion or strain is easily treated with the NSAIDs, as is bone pain following dental or orthopedic procedures. Idiopathic musculoskeletal pain includes myositis and fasciitis, which are treated with local injections of anesthetics. Inflammatory diseases of muscle include polymyositis, dermatomyositis, and polymyalgia rheumatica. Flares may respond to low-dose intermittent steroids, for example, prednisone 10 to 60 mg/day tapered over a 2-week period (76).

Examples of iatrogenic, or drug-induced, musculoskeletal pains include those arising from the use of zidovudine (AZT), an agent that is used in treating AIDS, and amphetamine or phencyclidine overdose leading to rhabdomyolysis and myoglobinuria (77). In 1989 an illness associated with consumption of L-tryptophan for insomnia was reported that included myalgia, weakness, fever, arthralgia, dyspnea, rash, extremity edema, and pneumonia. A striking component in all cases was marked eosinophilia. Within 8 months, approximately 1500 cases of eosinophilia-myalgia syndrome were recorded, and many patients died from the illness. The acute phase was notable for severe myalgia followed by proximal muscular weakness. Sensory and motor neuropathy were late complications and mimicked rheumatic diseases such as systemic sclerosis, polymyalgia rheumatica, and fibrositis. A contaminant of L-tryptophan that caused a dramatic increase of eosinophils and subsequent release of toxic granule-related proteins was suspected. Patients did not respond adequately to NSAIDs, hydroxychloroquine sulfate, or penicillamine. High-dose corticosteroids had a modicum of success, though these drugs were often discontinued because of severe muscle cramping. Intramuscular injections of local anesthetic and steroid combinations (e.g., lidocaine/triamcinolone or bupivacaine/hydrocortisone) produced short-term reduction of myalgic pain. In extreme cases the pain was opioid-responsive (78).

Sickle cell disease results in acute infarctions and necrosis of organs secondary to vasoocclusive episodes or "crises." Painful episodes are attributed to tissue injury from obstruction of blood flow by the deformed erythrocytes; however, a small population of people who are affected with sickle cell disease report constant pain that persists between such episodes. Similarly, hemophilia may cause spontaneous bleeding into joints (hemarthroses) during flares of the disorder. NSAIDs and acetaminophen are the mainstay of therapy for mild to moderate pain. Opiate analgesics such as meperidine, morphine, or hydromorphone are reserved for severe acute episodes and are dosed according to duration of action and relative potency. Consideration of hepatic or renal dysfunction due to venoocclusion of these organs is required. When a crisis begins to abate, narcotic tapering is instituted, pharmacologic emphasis being placed on the nonopioid drugs (79).

PRINCIPLES OF PAIN MANAGEMENT

Pain therapy is begun with nonnarcotic analgesics when possible, followed by the stepwise addition of opioids and analgesic adjuncts (see Figure 52.7).

Opioid Analgesics

Opioids include natural and synthetic agents. They reduce moderate to severe pain and are unique in their ability to do this without producing loss of consciousness. All opioids have the potential for tolerance, habituation, and addiction. There are three classes of opioids: the phenanthrene derivatives, which include morphine, codeine, hydromorphone, levorphanol, oxymorphone, oxycodone, hydrocodone, dihydrocodeine, and opium; the phenylpiperidine

derivatives, which include meperidine (pethidine), fentanyl, sufentanil, and alfentanil; and the diphenylheptane derivatives, which include methadone and propoxyphene (see Table 52.4). Several agonist/antagonist combinations and partial opioid agonists are also available that are weaker than their pure agonist counterparts and are thus purported to be less habituating.

Potent Opioids

Morphine and other potent opioids are used to treat severe acute, chronic, or terminal malignant pain. They can be given orally, rectally, as continuous subcutaneous or intravenous infusions, intramuscularly, or directly into the CNS via epidural or intrathecal administration. The CNS route allows minute doses without sensory, motor, or sympathetic dysfunction. Newer methods of administration include the transdermal, intranasal, and buccal routes.

Required doses of opioids vary according to a patient's prior exposure, severity of pain, hepatic or renal function, and route of administration. The oral:parenteral morphine ratio is approximately 5:1, owing to a large first-pass effect. Oral preparations include short-acting tablets and elixirs as well as extended-release tablets. Conversion from short-acting to longer-duration formulations requires consideration of active drug and metabolite accumulation. One approach is to reduce the total daily dose by 25%, divide this amount by three or four, and then administer the resulting amount every 8 or 6 hours, respectively. In increasing the dose, an extra tablet is initially added at night to eliminate daytime somnolence, followed by the addition of subsequent tablets until effective analgesia is noted.

Morphine and hydromorphone exert major pharmacodynamic effects on μ and κ receptors. Large doses of morphine can reduce systemic vascular resistance, produc-

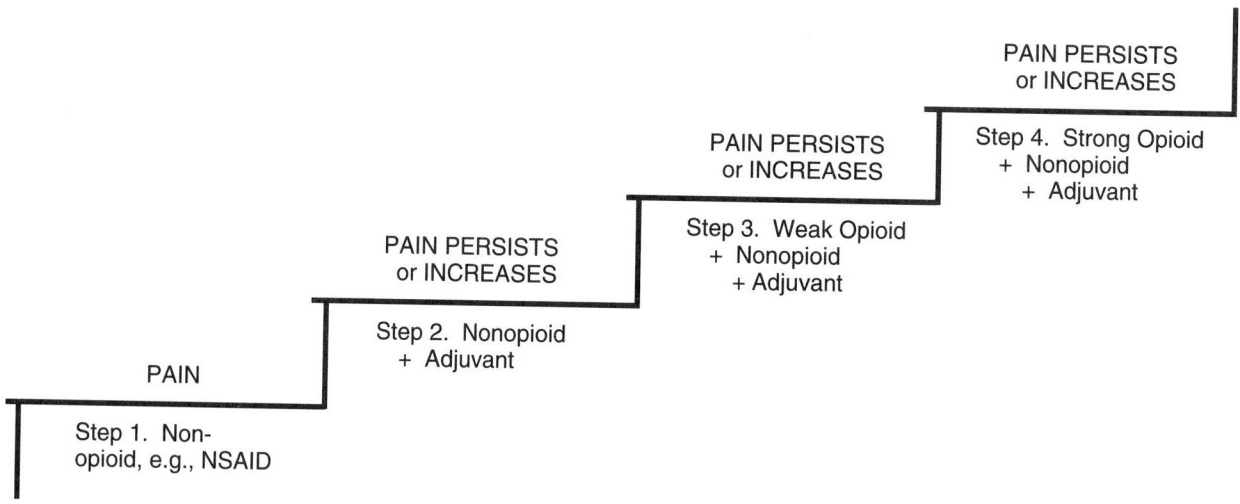

Figure 52.7. Analgesic stepladder for chronic pain management. (Source: Adapted from World Health Organization. Cancer Pain Relief. Geneva: World Health Organization, 1986.)

Table 52.4.
Centrally Acting Analgesic Characteristics

	IM Dose (mg)[a]	Oral Equiv.[a]	Routes	Onset (min)	Duration (hr)	$t_{1/2}$ (hr)	Notes
Opioid agonists for severe pain							
Phenanthrenes:							
Morphine (various)	10	60[b]	PO, SC, IV, IM, PR	IV: 5, PO: 60	3–6	2–3	
Hydromorphone (Dilaudid)	1.5	7.5	PO, SC, IV, IM, PR	See morphine	3–6	2–4	
Levorphanol (Levo-Dromoran)	2	4	PO, SC, IM	30–90	4–6	4–12	Accumulates
Oxymorphone (Numorphan)	1.5	6	PO, SC, IV, IM 10–90	3–6	3–4		
Phenylpiperdines:							
Fentanyl (Sublimaze)	0.1	N/A	IV, spinal, buccal, patch	10	1–2	3–4	Duration dose-related?
Sufentanil (Sufenta)	10 µg	N/A	IV, IM, SC, intraspinal	10	2–4		
Diphenylheptanes:							
Methadone (Dolophine)	10	10	PO, SC, IM	SC, IM = 60	6–8	21–25	Accumulates
Opioids for mild to moderate pain							
Phenanthrenes:							
Codeine	120	200	PO, SC, IV, IM	See morphine	3–6		
Hydrocodone (various)	N/A	30	PO	30–60	3–4		
Oxycodone (Percocet)	N/A	20	PO	30–60	4–6		
Dihydrocodeine (various)	N/A	30	PO	30–60	4–6		
Phenylpiperidines:							
Meperidine (Demerol)	100	400	PO, SC, IV, IM	15–60	1–3	3–4	Can provoke seizures
Pentazocine (Talwin)	30–60	150	PO, SC, IV, IM	10	3–4	2–4	Dysphoric
Diphenylheptanes:							
Propoxyphene (Darvon)	N/A	65–130	PO	60–90	4–6	6–12	Hepatotoxic
Partial agonists/antagonists							
Buprenorphine (Buprenex)	0.3	N/A	SC, IV, IM	15	4–6	2–3	Not naloxone reversible
Butorphanol (Stadol)	2	N/A	SC, IV, IM, intranasal	15–45	3–4	2–3	Dysphoric
Nalbuphine (Nubain)	10	N/A	SC, IV, IM	15	4–6	4–6	Respiratory ceiling
Dezocine (Dalgan)	10–15	N/A	SC, IV, IM	15	3–6		
Opioid antagonists							
Naloxone (Narcan)	0.4–0.8	N/A	IV	10	2–3	1–1.5	
Naltrexone (Trexan)	N/A	50	PO	30–60	24–72	9–17	Duration dose-dependent

[a]Based on single doses.
[b]Multiple dose conversion = 30 mg oral morphine = 10 mg IM morphine.

ing a transient fall in blood pressure. Hydromorphone has less potential to produce nausea, vomiting, constipation, sedation, or euphoria than morphine does and can be used as a substitute when these adverse effects warrant a therapeutic alternative. Concentrated parenteral preparations are useful for opioid-tolerant cancer patients for whom high narcotic requirements have posed a problem because of the volume of drug that must be administered. Though high-dose infusions of morphine or hydromorphone are associated with muscle rigidity and spasm, all narcotics can cause muscular rigidity, presumably by accumulation in the sensitive regions of the brain (80).

Oral morphine is variably absorbed, with a bioavailability of approximately 20 to 30%. It is also absorbed rectally. Peak analgesia occurs about 20 to 60 min after a dose and lasts longer in opioid-naive individuals. The major metabolite of morphine is morphine-3-glucuronide, which is inactive. Minor active metabolites include morphine-6-glucuronide and normorphine, with a small amount biotransformed to codeine. Approximately 90% of morphine is excreted unchanged by the kidneys, most of the remaining 10% being excreted via biliary elimination (81).

Parenteral hydromorphone and levorphanol are about five times as potent as morphine, with oral to parenteral ratios of 5:1 and 2:1, respectively. Both are available as tablets and as parenteral formulations for intravenous, intramuscular, or subcutaneous use. Hydromorphone can also be administered intraspinally or rectally (82). Hydromorphone, a semisynthetic opioid, has a more rapid onset and shorter duration of action than morphine does. Hydromorphone is converted mainly to a glucuronide metabolite, with urinary excretion (83). Levorphanol is a potent, semisynthetic opioid agonist for moderate to severe pain, including intractable pain in terminally ill patients. It produces more sedation and smooth muscle stimulation than does morphine in equianalgesic doses and has the same potential for habituation or addiction as naturally occurring opioids. Like methadone, it has a long half-life and a longer duration of action than morphine, meperidine, or hydromorphone. Levorphanol is well absorbed and, like hydromorphone, undergoes hepatic metabolism to a glucuronide conjugate excreted by the kidneys. Peak analgesia occurs approximately 20 to 90 min after intravenous or subcutaneous injection, respectively. Duration of analgesia may be shorter in opioid-tolerant individuals (84). Levorphanol is often used as a substitute when large requirements lead to frequent morphine dosing.

Meperidine is used in treating moderate traumatic or postoperative pain and, like morphine, is given for pain from myocardial infarction or for sedation for patients with pulmonary edema. However, caution is advised when there is atrial flutter or supraventricular tachycardia, as meperidine can increase systemic vascular resistance and the heart rate. Parenteral meperidine reduces rigors associated

with amphotericin-B administration and is used as a premedication for patients who are receiving this antifungal agent. Some preparations contain metabisulfite preservatives that produce anaphylaxis or hypersensitivity reactions, especially in asthmatic patients. Parenteral meperidine has one-tenth the potency of morphine. Because it is poorly absorbed, oral doses are 25% as effective as parenteral doses. Meperidine is available as tablets, an oral solution, and an injectable preparation. It is metabolized to meperidinic acid, which is excreted by the kidneys as a glucuronide metabolite. Of greater importance is normeperidine, which can accumulate with renal impairment to induce CNS stimulation and tonic-clonic seizures. Approximately one-third of meperidine is converted to this N-demethyl metabolite, which has twice the convulsant activity and a fraction of the analgesic potency of meperidine and has a half-life of 12 to 16 hr. Meperidine is shorter-acting than morphine and produces the same degree, but a shorter duration, of respiratory depression. It is often administered during labor because of less extensive placental penetration that reduces respiratory and CNS depression in the newborn infant (85). Oral combinations with promethazine or acetaminophen and parenteral combinations with promethazine or atropine also exist, though there is little rationale for using such fixed-dose combinations because patient-specific dosing is preferred. Combination products are more expensive than individual constituents and can produce additive side effects without providing additional benefit.

Methadone was initially approved only for narcotic detoxification until the 1980s, when labeled use was extended to analgesia. It is useful in the treatment of terminal painful conditions, as the longer duration of action allows for less frequent dosing. Methadone has unique pharmacokinetic properties: Oral absorption is nearly complete, and the half-life is 13 to 47 hr, with an average of 25 hr. Analgesic duration increases from 4 to 6 hr for a single dose to 6 to 8 hr after repeated administration. However, CNS depression persists up to 36 hr after overdose, an important factor in reversing the effects with the opioid antagonist naloxone. The half-life of naloxone is about 60 to 90 min. A patient will require naloxone by continuous infusion until the critical period has ended (82).

Methadone is equivalent to morphine on a single dose basis; however, with repeated administration, accumulation in CNS and lipid tissues occurs. The total dose can be decreased 10%/day until a stable analgesic regimen is obtained. In detoxifying opioid-dependent patients with chronic pain, a "blind taper" can be used in which an oral solution of methadone is mixed with acetaminophen elixir or cherry syrup. The methadone dose is thus decreased gradually while the same total volume administered to the patient is maintained. Methadone, like meperidine, was synthesized in Germany during the 1940s to treat war casualties when morphine supplies were exhausted. Methadone is available as tablets, oral solution, and parenterally for intramuscular use.

Narcotic Analgesics for Mild to Moderate Pain

Codeine (methylmorphine) is a natural opioid derivative that is produced in the liver on metabolism of morphine. It is a less potent analgesic than morphine, as are its derivatives hydrocodone and dihydrocodeine. Oxycodone, a third codeine derivative, exhibits intermediate potency. Propoxyphene is also less potent than its structural analog methadone. All of these drugs are effective for mild to moderate pain.

Tramadol is a new agent that possesses activity at both opioid and monoaminergic pathways in the CNS. It demonstrates weak opioid receptor affinity, particularly at the μ receptors. It has been used in place of more potent opioid analgesics for treatment of acute pain and may also be useful in treating chronic pain syndromes. Advantages of tramadol include lower abuse liability and reduced potential for respiratory depression. Disadvantages include adverse effects such as dizziness, dry mouth, sedation, and constipation (86).

Agonist/Antagonists

Agonists and antagonists have varying effects at different opioid receptors, and their affinity for any particular receptor is dose-related. A characteristic of agonist/antagonist combinations is a "ceiling" effect with regard to analgesia and respiratory depression (28). This means that doses above the threshold or ceiling do not increase the degree of analgesia or the potential for respiratory failure. Butorphanol, a synthetic opiate agonist/antagonist, is available parenterally and as an intranasal spray. Pentazocine, a benzomorphan derivative, does not decrease the propulsive activity of the intestines in therapeutic doses (39). It is contraindicated for patients with myocardial infarction because it may increase blood pressure and systemic vascular resistance. It has been combined with naloxone in oral preparations to discourage its abuse. Nalbuphine may have less psychotomimetic effects than does either butorphanol or pentazocine (87).

Partial Agonists

Buprenorphine and dezocine have less reported abuse liability than morphine does but can precipitate withdrawal in narcotic-addicted patients. Dezocine is a nonscheduled opioid analgesic that is approved for parenteral administration. Both agents are indicated for postoperative or posttraumatic acute pain. Like other opioids, they are metabolized by glucuronidation. In addition, dezocine appears to have a sulfate metabolite. Side effects of these agents include constipation or diarrhea, hypertension or hypotension, nausea, vomiting, anxiety, and sedation.

Dezocine reportedly has high μ receptor affinity, moderate δ and κ receptor affinity, and low ς receptor affinity. The threshold dose of dezocine for respiratory depression is 30 mg (88).

Narcotic Antagonists

Naloxone is a short-acting, specific opioid receptor antagonist that is used to reverse the untoward side effects of narcotics, such as pruritus and respiratory depression. It is a competitive saturable inhibitor of the opioid receptor and is usually administered in doses of 0.1 to 0.2 mg as needed. Care should be taken not to administer an excessive amount, as large doses will also reverse opioid analgesia and may precipitate symptoms of withdrawal (81). Naltrexone is an oral opioid antagonist and, because of its extended duration of action, may be dosed as infrequently as twice weekly.

NONOPIOID ANALGESICS

Nonsteroidal Antiinflammatory Drugs

Aspirin and other NSAIDs are useful for the treatment of pain from injury, surgery, trauma, arthritis, or cancer. The NSAIDs are especially effective in the management of bone pain secondary to tumor metastases (89). Though acetaminophen does not possess antiinflammatory properties, it is the most commonly used nonprescription pain reliever. NSAIDs differ from opioid analgesics in several ways: An analgesic ceiling exists for these agents, they are antipyretics, and they do not induce tolerance or physical or psychological dependence. In addition, their actions—with the exception of that of acetaminophen—occur through inhibition of cyclooxygenase. Cyclooxygenase acts as a catalyst in the formation of prostaglandins, which sensitize nociceptors to the effects of pain-eliciting substances such as bradykinin. Because of predominant action in the peripheral nervous system, NSAIDs and acetaminophen work synergistically with the centrally acting opioids. NSAIDs also have central effects that contribute to their analgesic activity, as they are thought to reduce C-fiber activity in the thalamus (90, 91).

The NSAIDs are approximately equipotent, and no structure-activity relationship exists for these agents. Only ibuprofen and ketoprofen are believed to be superior analgesics at equivalent doses. Patient response varies considerably, so a patient who does not obtain therapeutic efficacy with one drug at a maximum dose should be given an alternative agent (49).

Absorption of the NSAIDs occurs in the stomach and duodenum. The rate of absorption increases with slower gastric emptying and decreases when food or antacids are present in the stomach, although the total amount of drug absorbed is unchanged. Extent of absorption can be affected by the salt formulation. Currently, two products are available in the salt form: naproxen sodium and diclofenac potassium. Both agents are rapidly absorbed and thus are believed to reduce dyspepsia associated with gastric residence time. In addition, they possess a more rapid onset of action, making them useful for treatment of migraine headache and other acute pain syndromes in the ambulatory setting. NSAIDs are eliminated primarily through biotransformation in the liver, the metabolites being excreted by the kidney. Some NSAIDs may undergo enterohepatic recirculation (92).

The propionic acid class of agents includes ibuprofen, naproxen, fenoprofen, flurbiprofen, ketoprofen, and oxaprozin. ketoprofen is unique in that it also inhibits the lipooxygenase enzyme, the result being decreased leukotriene production. Whether this has clinical relevance is unknown. In single-dose comparisons, ketoprofen proved to be as effective in treating cancer pain as an acetaminophen and codeine combination (93).

Ketorolac is a pyrrolacetic acid that is structurally related to zomepirac, tolmetin, and indomethacin and possesses potent analgesic with moderate antiinflammatory activity. For postoperative pain, ketorolac is as effective as morphine, meperidine, or pentazocine, although the onset of action occurs slightly later. Like other NSAIDs, it inhibits platelet aggregation and can prolong bleeding time, induce gastric ulceration, or impair renal function. The most common side effects are somnolence and other central effects such as nausea and dizziness. Available for intramuscular and intravenous administration, it is well absorbed, with a time to maximum effect of approximately 45 min. The major metabolite is a glucuronide, and elimination is mostly renal, approximately 90% being excreted in the urine. The usual dose is 30 to 60 mg as a single dose or 30 mg every 6 hr as needed. The maximum daily dose should not exceed 120 mg/day. Doses should be reduced by half for elderly patients, patients with decreased creatinine clearance, or patients who weigh less than 110 lb (50 kg). The major role of ketorolac is acute postoperative analgesia when opioids are undesirable, as it is nonhabituating and does not appear to decrease respiratory drive (94). There is little rationale to support the use of ketorolac for a patient who is tolerating oral medications or one for whom intramuscular narcotics are appropriate, and conversion to an oral NSAID such as ibuprofen or naproxen is indicated. Oral ketorolac is also available for the treatment of acute pain, with a recommended maximum therapeutic duration of 5 days.

Anthranilic acids are also called fenamates, and although mefenamic acid is reported to have greater prostaglandin inhibition at the myometrium, it does not provide greater analgesia than do other NSAIDs. Frequently reported adverse effects, such as diarrhea and CNS impairment, have limited its use.

Piroxicam has an extended plasma half-life and is given once daily (95). Other once-daily NSAIDs include oxaprozin, nabumetone (a nonacidic prodrug that is metabolized to an acetic acid), and sustained-release ketoprofen. However, these drugs are unsuitable for treatment of acute or chronic pain, as plasma levels drop below analgesic threshold before the end of the dosing interval. They are useful for treatment of rheumatologic conditions, since antiinflammatory action persists beyond the duration of analgesia, and once-daily dosing enhances patient compliance.

ANALGESIC ADJUNCTS

Antidepressants

The human response to pain includes the "fight or flight" reaction to physical or emotional stresses. Two simultaneous phenomena occur: corticoadrenal and sympathetic responses. The first results in production of endogenous glucocorticoid steroids to mobilize energy sources and inhibit prostaglandins. The sympathetic response induces an outpouring of norepinephrine (a catecholamine) and serotonin (an indoleamine) within neuronal synaptic junctions. Tricyclic antidepressants that inhibit the reuptake and storage of these neurogenic amines have analgesic properties that are related to their ability to increase pain tolerance (see Table 52.5) (96, 97). This effect occurs in the absence of depression, and the onset of analgesia is often more rapid than the antidepressant effect (98). In addition, vegetative symptoms that are associated with chronic pain, such as sleep disturbance and depression, are reduced by central serotonin enhancement. Serotonergic processes are an integral part of endogenous pain inhibitory mechanisms, so tricyclic antidepressants have proven useful as adjuncts in chronic pain management (99). Patients should be instructed that 1 to 3 weeks or more of treatment are typically required before such antinociception occurs (100).

The antidepressants include several classes of agents, which can be organized into three categories: the tricyclic antidepressants (TCAs), the monoamine oxidase inhibitors (MAOIs), and newer heterocyclic compounds. Clinical effects include improvement in mood and sleep, anxiolysis, and a decreased perception of pain. The tricyclic agents are commonly used in the management of neurogenic pain conditions. The MAOIs have been used infrequently for treatment of painful conditions and are reserved for patients who are refractory to the TCAs. Some clinicians prefer them for migraine headache management, however. MAOIs are more difficult to use because of food and drug interactions, and their benefits in treating pain have not been well documented. Newer nontricyclic agents include serotonin-specific reuptake inhibitors (SSRIs), venlafaxine, and buproprion, an aminoketone that, like MAOIs, is

Table 52.5.
Antidepressants That Are Used as Analgesic Adjuvants

Medication	Daily Dose	Conc. (ng/mL)	Receptor Blockade		Adrenergic	
			Cholinergic	Histaminergic	α₁	α₂
Tertiary amines						
Amitriptyline	75–300 mg	110–250ᵃ	Very high	Very high	High–very high	Moderate
Doxepin	30–300 mg	30–150ᵇ	Moderate	Very high	High–very high	Moderate
Imipramine	75–300 mg	100–350ᵃ	Moderate–high	Moderate	High	Insignificant
Secondary amines						
Amoxapine	100–300 mg	Not established	None–slight	Slight	Slight–moderate	Slight
Desipramine	75–300 mg	125–250	Slight	Slight	Moderate	None–slight
Nortriptyline	50–150 mg	50–150	Moderate	Moderate	Slight–moderate	Insignificant
Protriptyline	15–60 mg	100–200	Moderate–high	Slight	Moderate	Insignificant
Bicyclic						
Fluoxetine	20–60 mg	160–700ᵃ	None–slight	None–slight	None–slight	None–slight
Triazolopyridine						
Trazodone	150–600 mg	800–2100	None–slight	Moderate	Very high	Moderate

ᵃParent compound + active metabolite.
ᵇParent compound alone.

reserved for people with refractory depression. None of these have been thoroughly studied for their effects on chronic pain.

The most commonly used antidepressant for painful conditions is amitriptyline in doses of 50 to 300 mg/day. Individuals who have chronic pain usually have poor sleep habits, and this drug is useful in overcoming insomnia or nighttime waking. An agent with fewer anticholinergic effects, such as nortriptyline, may be substituted for amitriptyline. Desipramine, an active metabolite of imipramine, is also less sedating and has fewer anticholinergic effects than does its parent compound.

Analogs of fluoxetine with shorter half-lives accumulate more slowly in slow metabolizers such as the elderly. Paroxetine is an SSRI that is modeled after the prototype agent zimelidine, and it significantly decreases symptoms of painful diabetic neuropathy without withdrawal effects or changes in nerve function measurements. Paroxetine at 40 mg/day also does not have the autonomic side effects that frequently limit the use of TCAs (101).

Neuroleptics

Of the neuroleptics, fluphenazine will potentiate the effects of amitriptyline in patients with diabetic neuropathies and central (poststroke) pain. It also aids sleep onset and is typically given in small doses of 1 mg at bedtime, up to a maximum of 3 mg/day in divided doses or all at bedtime (102). Methotrimeprazine is available as a treatment for mild to moderate pain. Its duration of action is equal to that of morphine, and it possesses analgesic equivalence to morphine or meperidine without similar habituating/addictive potential or likelihood of respiratory depression. It has been underused in chronic pain management because of sedative and anticholinergic effects that de-

crease patient tolerance. The use of other neuroleptics is controversial, and phenothiazine analgesia is unproven with the exception of these agents (103).

Anticonvulsants

The mechanism of action of carbamazepine and valproate is suppression of spontaneous neuronal firing. Lancinating, burning pains are best treated by these drugs, which are typically long-acting but can induce their own metabolism. Carbamazepine and valproate are prescribed for tic douloureux (trigeminal neuropathy), cranial nerve disorders, neural invasion by cancerous tumor, radiation fibrosis, surgical scarring, deafferention, and other neuralgic syndromes. Doses of carbamazepine and valproate are the same as those used for treatment of convulsive disorders. Plasma levels should be monitored, as side effects may include bone marrow suppression, ataxia, diplopia, nausea, lymphadenopathy, and hepatic dysfunction. Periodic liver function tests, blood counts, and serum drug levels should be obtained for patients who are on chronic therapy (104). Recently released agents such as lamotrigine and gabapentin may be of some use in the treatment of chronic neurogenic pain states in patients for whom treatment with antidepressants or other anticonvulsants has been unsuccessful.

Other Agents

Lidocaine is also given for neuropathic syndromes and, like all local anesthetics, enters the CNS after intravenous administration. Mexiletine has been used for lidocaine-responsive patients who require a longer-acting substitute, as the effects of lidocaine are short-lived. Both agents reduce neuronal firing through stabilization of sodium-conducting channels in nerve cell membranes. When administered systemically, they diffuse into the peripheral nerves. Analgesic doses of mexiletine are the same as those needed for antiarrhythmic effects, that is, approximately 10 mg/kg/day to produce plasma levels of 0.75 to 2.0 μg/mL. The use of tocainide, an oral lidocaine analog, is not advised because of a higher incidence of serious adverse effects such as aplastic anemia. Side effects of both lidocaine and mexiletine include dizziness, lightheadedness, ataxia, nausea, and vomiting. High doses of these agents can lead to tremor and convulsions. Gastrointestinal effects of mexiletine can be reduced by taking the medication with food or antacids (105).

Two centrally acting α_2 agonists, clonidine and guanethidine, are also used for pain management. They reduce sympathetic outflow from the CNS by presynaptic inhibition of norepinephrine release. Clonidine may interact with opioid receptors by inducing the release of the endogenous peptide dynorphin and has been used with some success in suppressing the symptoms of opioid withdrawal that are attributed to a hyperadrenergic state, including agitation, diarrhea, and sweating. This drug may also be used during surgery to reduce inhalation and opioid anesthetic requirements, as it potentiates morphine analgesia. Unlike morphine, however, clonidine is not reversed by naloxone, though its actions can be blocked by κ-specific antagonists. Clonidine may also prove useful for patients with spinal cord injury and neuropathic and sympathetically mediated pain syndromes. It is available as an oral tablet or as a patch that provides constant blood levels of the drug for 5 to 7 days, thus increasing compliance. Clonidine may produce orthostatic hypotension, so a candidate for therapy should first receive a baseline evaluation of blood pressure (106, 107). Guanethidine, with a mechanism of action similar to that of clonidine, is also used for patients with sympathetic pain. Guanethidine produces significant vasodilation, counteracting the vasoconstriction due to sympathetic hyperactivity, with resultant warming of an affected extremity and a reduction in pain. Guanethidine holds promise in the treatment of pain associated with rheumatoid arthritis, as patient response to regional guanethidine blockade has been favorable (108).

Prazosin is an agent that is used for the relief of sympathetically mediated pains such as reflex sympathetic dystrophy. It has high specificity and affinity for the α_1-adrenergic receptor. Like clonidine, it produces vasodilation with significant orthostasis. Prazosin should be dosed initially at bedtime to reduce the risk of syncope due to a precipitous drop in blood pressure. Doses can be gradually increased according to patient response and tolerance of side effects. Other agents that are used to relieve sympathetically mediated pain include intravenous phentolamine and oral phenoxybenzamine. However, these agents are nonselective for the α_1 receptor and also produce α_2-adrenergic effects. A test infusion of phentolamine can be used to predict guanethidine or prazosin response (109).

Benzodiazepines such as diazepam are used for skeletal muscle relaxation and anxiolysis in the treatment of acute pain, while clonazepam has been used in the management of neuropathic and atypical facial pain. Side effects include sedation, cognitive impairment, and sometimes profound depression, all of which decrease the pain patient's activity. Some researchers believe that benzodiazepines may even exacerbate pain. In addition, they produce habituation and serious withdrawal reactions, including seizures. The elderly are more susceptible to these effects. Therefore tricyclic antidepressants are more rational choices for relieving the insomnia and anxiety that accompany chronic pain (110).

Antihistamines such as hydroxyzine and promethazine have been used to augment the sedative effects of opioids. They may have some analgesic activity, although their use is controversial.

Dextroamphetamine 5 to 10 mg/day can be used for patients with cancer pain to overcome the sedation of opioids. It also relieves some of the vegetative effects of depression that often accompany a terminal diagnosis (111). Methylphenidate 5 to 10 mg/day has also been used for these purposes.

ADVANCES IN PAIN THERAPY: INNOVATIVE METHODS OF DRUG DELIVERY
Patient-Controlled Analgesia (PCA)

Patient-controlled devices take advantage of intravenous bolus injections to produce rapid analgesia along with slower infusion to produce steady-state opioid concentrations for sustained pain control. Since opioid kinetics vary greatly between patients, the rates of infusion must be tailored. Many computerized PCA devices are available that rely on the principle of a baseline infusion plus optional bolus and "rescue" doses. Boluses are self-administered and can be controlled by a predetermined lockout period. PCA is useful for patients with chronic malignant pain, allowing a greater degree of ambulation and independence. Many PCA devices are compact enough to be worn on a belt or carried in a pocket (112).

Intraspinal

Opiates that are administered into the spinal fluid provide important information about nociceptive pharmacology, in addition to being clinically useful tools for pain relief. They are justified for patients with malignant pain, those for whom neurolytic techniques have failed, those with acquired tolerance to systemic opioids, and those whose pain undergoes a sudden exacerbation, such as postsurgical amputees. Morphine was the first opioid to be used in this manner. Unfortunately, spinal opioids may produce a greater degree of urinary retention, biphasic respiratory depression, urticaria, pruritus, nausea, and vomiting than do opioids that are administered parenterally or orally. Agents that undergo significant migration up the spinal column toward the brain are most often associated with these side effects, as drug polarity influences such cephalad migration. Morphine is more polar than meperidine and undergoes a greater degree of migration, leading to delayed respiratory depression. This agent reaches the respiratory center approximately 3 hr after administration. Because of this, efforts have been made to reduce the severe side effects through combinations of opioids and local anesthetics such as bupivacaine. By taking advantage of analgesic synergism via different mechanisms of action, smaller doses of each drug may be administered.

Several other analgesic opioid and nonopioid drugs have been studied since the introduction of intraspinal morphine. Spinally infused opioids have the potential for precipitating abstinence syndrome when they are withdrawn, but it is not clear whether intraspinal opioids produce differences in the development of narcotic tolerance when compared to oral administration. Changes in opioid receptor number and/or drug-receptor affinity due to chronic occupation of the opioid receptors are believed to account for the tolerance phenomenon, but removal of the opioid for a period of 7 to 14 days can result in recovery of drug efficacy. Long-term spinal infusion of opioids does not cause permanent sensory or motor functional loss or histophysiologic changes, though it may lead to mild dorsal column degeneration. Disadvantages include the risk of infection or puncture of the dura mater and catheter displacement (113, 114).

The entire volume of CSF turns over approximately every 5 hr. Any drug that is placed into the CSF is rapidly distributed and eliminated into systemic circulation. Bulk flow of CSF toward the brain will cause a lumbar injection of an opioid to reach the brainstem, leading to effects such as drowsiness and vomiting within 2 to 4 hr. A bolus will cause concentrated drug to reach the brainstem, whereas a continuous infusion pump will allow a steady state to be reached after five drug half-lives. Distribution across the dura from epidural administration occurs within 10 to 40 min. More lipid-soluble agents, such as methadone, will distribute along the spinal cord in a very limited manner because of rapid crossing of the dura and consequent migration out of the CSF (115).

The action of morphine in the spinal cord makes it ideal for powerful and relatively selective inhibition of pain information processing. Repeated bolus administration and continuous infusion of narcotics into the epidural space for terminal cancer pain have both demonstrated utility and efficacy. An implantable pump allows continuous infusion of opioids or other agents into the spinal space without requiring an external port. In addition, the lack of repeated bolus injections theoretically limits the development of narcotic tolerance. Spinal morphine has the advantage of providing adequate pain relief for patients who are unable to tolerate other forms of the drug. Cancer patients who are receiving highly emetogenic antineoplastic drugs, for example, may lose significant amounts of oral drug by vomiting. A third advantage of this method of drug delivery is facilitation of ambulation, allowing a patient to leave the hospital. Epidural administration of narcotics or other analgesic agents has also found use in the postoperative and obstetrical settings for short-term pain relief (2 to 5 days) following surgical procedures (116, 117).

Intrathecal opioid administration has received widespread attention. In vitro and in vivo data suggests a strong inverse relationship between intrathecal potency and lipophilicity for morphine, normorphine, methadone, meperidine, fentanyl, and buprenorphine. This can be explained by the rapid migration of highly lipophilic agents out of the CSF. Generalizations about relative intravenous or intramuscular narcotic efficacy do not correlate with intrathecal or epidural potency, and specific δ receptor agonists may prove useful for spinal infusion with minimal μ receptor cross-tolerance. Similarly, clonidine via intrathecal administration shows promise for producing analgesia without morphine cross-tolerance. Hormones as diverse as somatostatin and calcitonin have been administered intraspinally for analgesia. Intrathecal baclofen is employed for treatment of intractable pain and spasm due to spinal injury. Like clonidine, baclofen can potentiate morphine analgesia or produce analgesic effects alone. Intrathecal methadone 5, 10, and 20 mg has been used for patients following orthopedic surgery; however, because of its higher side effect profile and lower efficacy when compared with morphine, it is not widely used via the intraspinal routes (118–122).

Fentanyl is a synthetic opioid derivative of the 4-anilinophenyl-piperidine class and is approximately 100 times more potent than morphine. It is used clinically as an analgesic that is administered either intraspinally or intravenously and as a preoperative anesthetic agent because of its potency, rapid onset, and short duration of action. Recently, a buccal preparation of fentanyl was made available for preoperative sedation when the parenteral route is undesirable. Fentanyl is a highly lipophilic agent, so it has rapid uptake and elimination, and orally the drug undergoes extensive first-pass metabolism. Parenteral administration has therefore been the typical route, but large initial doses, which are required to sustain analgesia, lead to a risk of overdose. Stable levels can be achieved through continuous intravenous administration when the infusion rate matches the plasma elimination rate. Transdermal administration has widened the clinical use of this agent because it also supplies the drug at a stable rate. Transdermal fentanyl is available in four strengths, with patches releasing 25,

50, 75, or 100 μg/hr. These patches are most applicable in the treatment of stable terminal cancer pain. Each patch lasts approximately 72 hr, but several days are required to reach steady-state concentrations. Supplemental doses of a short-acting analgesic should be used as needed during the initial 24 hr of application for breakthrough pain. Similarly, the drug is not rapidly eliminated if the patch must be removed because of untoward effects. Transdermal patches are noninvasive and offer an advantage in facilitating patient mobility. Conversion to an oral opioid can be done easily if such conversion becomes feasible. Sufentanil, another synthetic phenylpiperidine derivative that is approximately 10 times more potent than fentanyl and more lipophilic, may also find use with this novel route of administration in the future (39). Unlike previous permeability studies with other drugs, percutaneous penetration of these weak bases depends on pH but not on the anatomical location of the patch (123).

Morphine can be administered directly into the brain's cerebral ventricles for the treatment of cancer pain. Morphine that is administered in this way is effective and naloxone-reversible. The disadvantages of this technique are the risks of meningitis, nausea, vomiting, and pruritis (124).

Intrapleural administration of bupivacaine has been performed for patients with rib fractures and patients with abdominal and thoracic pain following surgery. It exemplifies the many newer modalities that are available to the practitioner (125).

Agents Under Investigation

N-methyl-d-aspartate (NMDA) is an excitatory amino acid in the CNS that has been discovered to produce hyperalgesia of CNS origin. Glutamate may play a similar role in activating pain systems. Research into NMDA receptor antagonists has offered an exciting hint at the future of pharmacologic agents for pain management. Ketamine, a commercially available anesthetic, is one such NMDA antagonist. Unfortunately, it is available only parenterally and produces occasional adverse reactions, such as dysphoria and hallucination. Dextrorphan, the demethylated metabolite of dextromethorphan, though not yet commercially available, is another agent that is undergoing investigation (126, 127).

Cholecystokinin antagonists have gained attention for their role in analgesia based on observations that morphine-induced analgesia can be antagonized in vivo by cholecystokinin. Administration of proglumide, an investigational agent, potentiates morphine-induced analgesia in both animals and humans. Calcium-channel blockers may also potentiate morphine analgesia by modulation of calcium availability to the cell. These drugs, like proglumide, are devoid of any analgesic activity when they are given alone. Endogenous opioid peptides (endorphins,

dynorphins, and enkephalins) have not proven to be superior to exogenous opioids in the management of pain. Their analgesic effects are of short duration, and they produce the same side effects as drugs like morphine do. Other nonopioid endogenous peptides have been suggested for their roles in pain modulation. Specific δ receptor agonists have risen to the forefront of opioid research. Recent evidence suggests that they may produce analgesia without inducing habituation. Opioid peptides also show promise as therapeutic agents, since they differ from opioids in several ways. Peptide analogs of enkephalins undergo degradation by placental enzymes, thus inhibiting or preventing their transfer across placental membranes. This would make them ideal agents in obstetrics. Moreover, no δ receptors have yet been demonstrated in fetal brain tissue; therefore the safety margin of future δ-specific peptides is increased. A third advantage the peptides may have over opioids is degradation to constituent amino acids instead of active and possibly toxic metabolites. There is less potential for renal or hepatic damage with such peptides. Fourth, peptide δ agonists, as was mentioned, are likely to have less dependence and abuse liability than μ or κ agonists. Patients who have become tolerant to μ agonists such as morphine may benefit from little or no analgesic cross-tolerance with the δ opioid peptides (128).

NONPHARMACOLOGIC MODALITIES
Surgical

Cordotomy is a method of severing the sympathetic chains that emanate from the spinal cord. Indications for such intervention are short life expectancy and specific unilateral or focal pain. In percutaneous cordotomy a lesion is produced in the spinothalamic tract, most often at the level of the first or second cervical vertebra. This method has virtually replaced open cordotomy, in which a quadrant of the spinal cord is almost completely severed at the cervical or thoracic level. Pain relief by either technique is transient, rarely lasting more than 2 years. The advantage of cordotomy includes analgesia without significant loss of motor function or touch sensation (129).

Neuroablative Blocks/Chemoneurolysis

Chemical destruction of nerves (neurolysis) is used at spinal nerve roots and is a relatively simple and painless procedure that can be done with minimal equipment. It is shorter-acting than cordotomy but, unlike cordotomy, can be done in elderly patients and those in poor general health. Agents that are used include absolute alcohol and phenol.

Nervous System Stimulators

Various types of central and peripheral nervous system stimulators are used for neurogenic, neuropathic, and ischemic pain syndromes. Dorsal column stimulators (DCS) operate on a principle similar to that of transcutaneous electrical nerve stimulators; both produce analgesia by inducing partial depolarization of neurons. DCS consists of an electrode that is placed in the epidural space and attached to a programmable continuous-pulse pacemaker implanted into a subcutaneous pocket in the abdomen. A sensory thalamic stimulator (STS) consists of an electrode that is placed into the thalamus of the brain. DCS and STS are used in cases of intractable neurogenic pain that is unresponsive to medications or other therapies. Peripheral nerve stimulators are implantable devices that are most successful in pain syndromes caused by injury to a peripheral nerve. Newer stimulators are taking the form of thermal, vibrotactile, and magnetic stimulators, though these methods have not evolved sufficiently for widespread use in pain management (130).

SPECIAL CONSIDERATIONS IN ANALGESIC PHARMACOTHERAPY

Narcotics exert anticholinergic effects that can be compounded by the concomitant use of anticholinergic agents such as diphenhydramine, hydroxyzine, tertiary tricyclic antidepressants, or atropine. The most serious consequence of combined use of these drugs is precipitation of an anticholinergic crisis, which is manifested by psychosis; tachycardia; cardiac conduction abnormalities with possible first-, second-, or third-degree heart block; coma; and death by cardiorespiratory failure.

Patients with chronic pain often use alcohol to decrease their suffering. They may drink themselves into a stupor to achieve pain relief through decreased consciousness. Combining analgesics and ethanol produces additive CNS depression with mood changes, depression of respiratory drive, and the danger of lethal overdose. Alcohol in combination with NSAIDs can lead to increased CNS side effects of the NSAIDs, such as disorientation and dizziness, as well as increased gastric irritation and ulceration.

Like alcohol and antihistamines, narcotics can potentiate effects of barbiturates, meprobamate, or benzodiazepines, including transient delirium and respiratory failure. Of particular concern is the interaction between fentanyl and midazolam, an ultra-short-acting benzodiazepine that is used in preoperative anesthetic "cocktails." This combination produced a few deaths from cardiorespiratory failure until lower doses of midazolam with more judicious perioperative monitoring of the patient were instituted (131).

Patients with obstructive respiratory diseases such as asthma and emphysema or structural abnormalities such as kyphoscoliosis are at greater risk of respiratory-drive depression due to opioids. Half of the usual starting dose should be prescribed, and the medication should then be titrating upward with careful attention to respiratory rate and oxygen saturation. Narcotic suppression of the cerebellar chemoreceptor response to carbon dioxide can have catastrophic consequences for patients whose response to carbon dioxide is already blunted from chronic respiratory disease.

Patients with hepatic failure are at potential risk for drug-induced sequelae when they are given opioids or NSAIDs because of the inability of the liver to glucuronidate these agents for renal excretion. In addition, the NSAIDs have been shown to induce hepatocellular necrosis. Acetaminophen is an agent that is commonly combined with centrally acting opioids. In patients with hepatic dysfunction secondary to alcoholic cirrhosis or hepatitis, chronic doses can precipitate hepatic failure. Cirrhosis also affects the disposition of opioids, as meperidine, pentazocine, and propoxyphene all exhibit increased bioavailability and decreased clearance (132, 133).

Most of the opioids are conjugated and demethylated in the liver to form normetabolites as well as glucuronide metabolites, both of which are excreted by the kidneys. In patients with renal impairment these metabolites accumulate and produce side effects that last longer than the biological half-lives of the parent compounds. This is particularly true of morphine, dihydrocodeine, propoxyphene, and meperidine. Methadone appears to be safe to use for patients with renal dysfunction when it is administered at 12- or 24-hr intervals (134, 135).

INTERDISCIPLINARY PAIN MANAGEMENT

Multidisciplinary methods of pain management are the focus of effective treatment for complex chronic pain syndromes. The goal of centers that use these methods is not to "cure" pain, as this is often unachievable, but to ease the suffering of chronic pain patients and to reduce their reliance on opioids and other analgesics. These centers strive to improve pain control and improve both psychological and physical functioning and conditioning by involving specialists in the fields of anesthesia, neurology/neurosurgery, physical therapy, pharmacy, physiatry, psychology, and nursing.

CONCLUSION

Pain management has progressed a great deal scientifically throughout the last century, due in large part to the introduction of more effective pharmacologic agents and the development of a better understanding of their use. Though ancient civilizations did not understand the reason behind applying electric fish to an area that was affected by neuropathic pain, or of using acupuncture to induce analgesia, they did learn through trial and error the methods available to them which produced a therapeutic response. Likewise, there is still a great deal for practitioners to learn about the mechanisms and treatments for pain.

The pharmacist has a unique role in developing useful medicinal tools to ease suffering brought on by acute or chronic pain. Through rational drug prescribing habits and education of both patients and caregivers, effective regimens can be designed to increase pain control while decreasing untoward drug side effects. The pharmacist can assist in implementing such regimens to reduce drug dependence and overall drug use while increasing patient activity. A movement toward pharmacist involvement with pain management teams is gaining momentum, as government and third-party insurers seek ways to reduce the financial burden of chronic pain in terms of dollars spent and work days lost due to disability.

The pharmacist's role in researching non-traditional medicines for pain relief is also integral. In studies involving the use of lidocaine and antidepressants for relief of chronic pain, pharmacists have served as co-investigators. Even in the areas of traditional pain management, they can monitor medication compliance and efficacy. In the multidisciplinary setting, the pharmacist can provide counseling and guidance to patients who are adjusting their intake of antidepressants, anticonvulsants, or other non-opioid medications while providing direction in decreasing opioid use. A lucid understanding of pharmacology and pharmacokinetics is invaluable in this setting, since opioid habituation and symptoms of withdrawal are highly undesirable and counterproductive. Many clinic settings allow the pharmacist to see patients on a regular basis, documenting pain relief scores, monitoring side effects, determining when and by how much medication doses should be increased or decreased, selecting alternatives to non-tolerated medications, and obtaining pharmacokinetic data or other laboratory parameters. Using the pharmacist's knowledge of real or potential drug interactions can assist in designing regimens which will be most useful in treating patients with acute or chronic debilitating pain syndromes.

Through rational drug-prescribing habits and education of both patients and caregivers, effective regimens can be designed to increase pain control while decreasing untoward side effects. A lucid understanding of pharmacology and pharmacokinetics is invaluable, since opioid habituation and symptoms of withdrawal are highly undesirable and counterproductive.

REFERENCES

1. Melzack R, Wall PD. On the nature of cutaneous sensory mechanisms. Brain 85:331–356, 1962.
2. Hardy JD, Wolff HG, Goodell H. Pain Sensations and Reactions. Baltimore: Williams and Wilkins, 1952.
3. Bonica JJ. The Management of Pain, Second Edition. Philadelphia: Lea & Febiger, 1990, Chap. 1.
4. Melzack R, Wall PD. Pain mechanisms: a new theory. Science 150:971–979, 1965.
5. Bonica JJ. The Management of Pain. Philadelphia: Lea & Febiger, 1953.
6. Livingston WK. Pain Mechanisms. New York: Macmillan, 1943.
7. Ganong WF. Review of Medical Physiology. Los Altos, CA: Lange Medical Publications, 1985, p. 105.
8. Wall PD. Presynaptic control of impulses at the first central synapse in the cutaneous pathway. In: Physiology of Spinal Neurons: Progress in Brain Research 12. Amsterdam: Elsevier, 1964, pp. 92–118.
9. Peters ML, Schmidt AJM. Human pain responsivity. Pain 41:117–121, 1990.
10. Fields HL. Pain. New York: McGraw-Hill, 1987, pp. 13–28.
11. Adriaensen H, Gybels J, Handwerker HO, Van Hees J. Response properties of thin myelinated (A-δ) fibers in human skin nerves. J Neurophysiol 49:111–122, 1983.
12. Price DD, Hu JW, Dubner R, Gracely RH. Peripheral suppression of first pain and central stimulation of second pain evoked by noxious heat pulses. Pain 3:57–68, 1977.
13. Torebjork HE. Afferent C units responding to mechanical, thermal and chemical stimuli in human non-glabrous skin. Acta Physiol Scand 92:374–390, 1974.
14. Torebjork HE, Hallin RG. Perceptual changes accompanying controlled preferential blocking of A and C fibre responses in intact human skin nerves. Exp Brain Res 16:321–332, 1973.
15. Wall PD, McMahon SB. Microneuronography and its relation to perceived sensation: a critical review. Pain 21:209–229, 1985.
16. Willis WD. The origin and destination of pathways involved in pain transmission. In: Wall PD, Melzack R (eds.). Textbook of Pain, Second Edition. New York: Churchill Livingstone, 1989, pp. 112–123.
17. Vierck CJ, Luck MM. Loss and recovery of reactivity to noxious stimuli in monkeys with primary spinothalamic cordotomies, followed by secondary and tertiary lesions of other cord sectors. Brain 102:233–238, 1979.
18. Wall PD, Sweet WH. Temporary abolition of pain in man. Science 155:108–109, 1967.
19. Yaksh TL, Aimone LD. The central pharmacology of pain transmission. In: Wall PD, Melzack R (eds.). Textbook of Pain, Second Edition. New York: Churchill Livingstone, 1989, p. 190.
20. Perl ER. Sensitization of nociceptors and its relation to sensation. In: Bonica JJ, Albe-Fessard D (eds.). Advances in Pain Research and Therapy, Vol. I. New York: Raven Press, 1976, pp. 17–28.
21. Beck PW, Handwerker HO. Bradykinin and serotonin effects on various types of cutaneous nerve fibres. Pfluegers Arch 347:209–222, 1974.
22. Taiwo YO, Bjerknes LK, Goetzl EJ, Levine JD. Mediation of primary afferent peripheral hyperalgesia by the cAMP second messenger system. Neuroscience 32:577–580, 1989.
23. Ferreira SH. Prostaglandins, aspirin-like drugs, and analgesia. Nature 240:200–203, 1972.
24. Taiwo YO, Levine JD. Characterization of the arachidonic acid metabolites mediating bradykinin and noradrenaline hyperalgesia. Brain Res 458:402–406, 1988.
25. Levine JD, Lau W, Kwiat G, Goetzl EJ. Leukotriene B$_4$ produces hyperalgesia that is dependent on polymorphonuclear leukocytes. Science 225:743–745, 1984.
26. Levine JD, Moskowitz MA, Basbaum AI. The effect of gold, an anti-rheumatic therapy, on substance P levels in rat peripheral nerve. Neurosci Lett 87:200–202, 1988.
27. Yaksh TL. Multiple opioid receptor systems in brain and spinal cord: parts 1 and 2. Eur J Anaesth 1:171–243, 1984.
28. DiFazio CA. Pharmacology of narcotic analgesics. Clin J Pain 5(suppl 1):S5–S7, 1989.

29. Millan MJ. Kappa-Opioid receptors and analgesia. Trends Pharmacol Sci 11:70–76, 1990.

30. Carmody JJ. Opiate receptors: an introduction. Anaesth Intensive Care 15:27–37, 1987.

31. Goldstein A, James IF. Multiple opiate receptors: criteria for identification and classification. Trends Pharmacol Sci 5:503–505, 1984.

32. Ferreira SH, Nakamura M. II. Prostaglandin hyperalgesia: the peripheral analgesic activity of morphine, enkephalins, and opioid antagonists. Prostaglandins 18:191–200, 1979.

33. Levine JD, Taiwo YO. Involvement of the mu-opiate receptor in peripheral analgesia. Neuroscience 32:571–575, 1989.

34. DeLander GE, Hopkins CJ. Spinal adenosine modulates descending antinociceptive pathways stimulated by morphine. J Pharmacol Exp Ther 239:88–93, 1986.

35. Duggan AW, North RA. Electrophysiology of opioids. Pharmacol Rev 35:219–282, 1983.

36. Martin WR. A homeostatic and redundancy theory of tolerance to and dependence on narcotic analgesics. Res Publ Ass Res Nerv Ment Dis 46:206–225, 1968.

37. Foley KM. Treatment of cancer pain. N Engl J Med 313:84–95, 1985.

38. Bozarth MA, Wise RA. Anatomically distinct opiate receptor fields mediate reward and physical dependence. Science 224:516–517, 1984.

39. Jaffe JH, Martin WR. Opioid analgesics and antagonists. In: Gilman AG, Goodman LS, Rall TW, Murad F (eds.). The Pharmacological Basis of Therapeutics, Seventh Edition. New York: Macmillan, 1985, pp. 491–531.

40. Chisholm RJ, et al. Narcotics and spasm of the sphincter of Oddi: a retrospective study of operative cholangiograms. Anaesthesia 38:689–691, 1983.

41. Romagnoli A, Keats AS. Ceiling effect for respiratory depression by nalbuphine. Clin Pharmacol Ther 27:478–485, 1980.

42. Tamsen A, Gordh T. Epidural clonidine produces analgesia. Lancet i:231–232, 1984.

43. Howe JR, Wang JY, Yaksh TL. Selective antagonism of the antinociceptive effect of intrathecally applied alpha-adrenergic agonists by intrathecal prazosin and intrathecal yohimbine. J Pharmacol Exp Ther 224:552–558, 1983.

44. Schmauss C, Hammond DL, Ochi JW, Yaksh TL. Pharmacological antagonism of the antinociceptive effects of serotonin in the rat spinal cord. Eur J Pharmacol 90:349–357, 1983.

45. Max MB, et al. Effects of desipramine, amitriptyline, and fluoxetine on pain in diabetic neuropathy. N Engl J Med 326:1250–1256, 1992.

46. Post C, Gordh T Jr, Jansson I, Hartvig P, Gillberg PG. Interactions between spinal noradrenergic and cholinergic mechanism of anti-nociception abstract. Pain 13 (suppl 4):13:408, 1987.

47. Panerai AE, Sacerdote P, Bianchi M, Ripamonte C, Manfredi L, Tiengo M, Mantegazza P. Neuropharmacological approach to nociception. In: Lipton S, Tunks E, Zoppi M eds. Advances in Pain Research and Therapy, Vol. 13: The Pain Clinic. New York: Raven Press, 1990, pp. 41–44.

48. Dickenson AH, Brewer CM, Hayes NA. Effects of topical baclofen on C-fibre evoked neuronal activity in the rat dorsal horn. Neuroscience 14:557–562, 1985.

49. Merskey H (ed.). IASP Committee on Taxonomy, Classification of chronic pain: descriptions of chronic pain syndromes and definitions of pain terms. Pain 12 (suppl 3): 12:S28–S217, 1986.

50. American Pain Society. Principles of analgesic use in the treatment of acute pain and chronic cancer pain, Second Edition. Clin Pharm 9:601–611, 1990.

51. Sternbach RA. Clinical aspects of pain. In: Sternbach RA (ed.). The Psychology of Pain, Second Edition. New York: Raven Press, 1986, pp. 223–239.

52. Levine JD, Taiwo, YO. β-Estradiol induced catecholamine-sensitive hyperalgesia: a contribution to pain in Raynaud's phenomenon. Brain Res 487:143–147, 1989.

53. Fields HL. The Medical Center at the University of California, San Francisco Pain Questionnaire, copyright 1988.

54. Bieri D, Reeve RA, Champion GD, Addicoat L, Ziegler JB. The faces pain scale for the self-assessment of the severity of pain experienced by children: development, initial validation, and preliminary investigation for ratio scale properties. Pain 41:139–150, 1990.

55. Foley KM. Cancer pain syndromes. J Pain Symp Manag 2:T3-T7, 1987.

56. Ferrer-Brechner T. Rational management of cancer pain. In: Raj PP (ed.). Practical Management of Pain. Chicago: Year Book Medical Publishers, 1986, pp. 312–328.

57. Inturrisi CE. Newer methods of opioid drug delivery. In: IASP Refresher Course on Pain Management: Book of Abstracts, Vol. 1. Hamburg, West Germany: International Association for the Study of Pain, 1987, pp. 27–39.

58. Bennett A. The role of biochemical mediators in peripheral nociception and bone pain. Cancer Surv 7:55–67, 1988.

59. World Health Organization. Cancer Pain Relief. Geneva: World Health Organization, 1986.

60. Halpern LM. Psychotropics and ataractics and related drugs. Adv Pain Res Ther 2:275–283, 1979.

61. Inturrisi CE, Max MB, Foley KM, et al. The pharmacokinetics of heroin in patients with chronic pain. N Engl J Med 210:1213–1217, 1984.

62. Portenoy RK, Foley KM, Inturrisi CE. The nature of opioid responsiveness and its implications for neuropathic pain: new hypotheses derived from studies of opioid infusions. Pain 43:273–286, 1990.

63. Satterthwaite JR. Acute herpes zoster: diagnosis and treatment. Pain Management 3:17–28, 1990.

64. Portenoy RK, Duma C, Foley KM. Acute herpetic and postherpetic neuralgia: clinical review and current management. Ann Neurol 20:651–664, 1986.

65. Loeser JD. Postherpetic neuralgia: a review of pathophysiology and treatment. Presented at the Annual Meeting of the American Pain Society, Washington, DC, Nov. 8, 1986.

66. Davis EH. Clinical trials of tegretol in trigeminal neuralgia. Headache 9:77–82, 1969.

67. Bernstein JE, Korman NJ, Bickers, DR, Dahl MV, Lawrence LE. Topical capsaicin treatment of chronic postherpetic neuralgia. J Am Acad Dermatol 21:265–270, 1989.

68. Chabal C, Russell LC, Burchiel KJ. The effect of intravenous lidocaine, tocainide and mexiletine on spontaneously active fibers originating in rat sciatic neuromas. Pain 38:333–338, 1989.

69. Max MB, Schafer SC, Culnane M, Dubner R, Gracely RH. Association of pain relief with drug side effects in postherpetic neuralgia: a single-dose study of clonidine, codeine, ibuprofen, and placebo. Clin Pharmacol Ther 43:363–371, 1988.

70. Bach FW, Jensen TS, Kastrup J, Stigsby B, Dejgard A. The effect of intravenous lidocaine on nociceptive processing in diabetic neuropathy. Pain 40:29–34, 1990.

71. Masson EA, Boulton AJM. Aldose reductase inhibitors in the treatment of diabetic neuropathy: a review of the rationale and clinical evidence. Drugs 39:190–202, 1990.

72. Sherman R, Sherman C, Gall N. A survey of current phantom-limb pain treatment in the United States. Pain 8:85–99, 1980.

73. Jaeger H, Meier C. Calcitonin in phantom limb pain: a double-blind study. Pain 48:21–27, 1992.

74. Fine PG. The pharmacologic management of sympathetically maintained pain. Hosp Form 23:796–808, 1988.

75. Davis KD, Campbell JN, Raja SN, et al. Topical application of an α-2 agonist relieves hyperalgesia in sympathetically-maintained pain [Abstract]. Pain 16 (suppl) 16:S421, 1990.

76. Currie S. Inflammatory myopathies: polymyositis and related disorders. In: Walton JN (ed.). Disorders of Voluntary Muscle, Fourth Edition. Edinburgh: Churchill Livingstone, 1981, pp. 525–568.

77. Lane RJM, Mastaglia FL. Drug-induced myopathies in man. Lancet ii:562–566, 1978.

78. Criswell LA, Sack KE. Tryptophan-induced eosinophilia myalgia syndrome. West J Med 153:269–274, 1990.

79. Shapiro BS. The management of pain in sickle cell disease. Pediatr Clin North Am 36:1029–1055, 1989.

80. Melzacka M, Nebelhut T, Havemann U, Vetulani J, Kuschinsky K. Pharmacokinetics of morphine in striatum and nucleus accumbens: relationship to pharmacological actions. Pharmacol Biochem Behav 23:295–301, 1985.

81. Hoskin PJ, Hanks GW, Aherne GW, et al. The bioavailability and pharmacokinetics of morphine after intravenous, oral and buccal administration in healthy volunteers. Br J Clin Pharmacol 27:499–505, 1989.

82. AHFS Drug Information. Bethesda, MD: American Society of Hospital Pharmacists, 1994, pp. 1286–1326.

83. Reidenberg MM, Goodman H, Erle H, et al. Hydromorphone levels and pain control in patients with severe chronic pain. Clin Pharmacol Ther 44:376–382, 1988.

84. Foley KM. Controversies in cancer pain: Medical perspectives. Cancer 63:2257–2265, 1989.

85. Kaiko RF, Foley KM, Grabinsky PY, et al. Central nervous system excitatory effects of meperidine in cancer patients. Ann Neurol 13:180–185, 1983.

86. Lee RC, McTavish D, Sorkin EM. Tramadol: a preliminary review of its pharmacodynamic and pharmacokinetic properties, and therapeutic potential in acute and chronic pain states. Drugs 46:313–340, 1993.

87. Meyers FJ, Meyers FH. Management of chronic pain. Am Fam Physician 36:139–146, 1987.

88. O'Brien JJ, Benfield P. Dezocine: a preliminary review of its pharmacokinetic properties, and therapeutic efficacy. Drugs 38:226–248, 1989.

89. Stambaugh JE. The use of nonsteroidal anti-inflammatory drugs in chronic bone pain. Orthop Rev 18:54–60, 1989.

90. McCormack K. The spinal actions of nonsteroidal anti-inflammatory drugs and the dissociation between their anti-inflammatory and analgesic effects. Drugs 47(Suppl 5):28–45, 1994.

91. Jurna I, Brune K. Central effect of the non-steroid anti-inflammatory agents, indomethacin, ibuprofen, and diclofenac, determined in C fibre-evoked activity in single neurones of the rat thalamus. Pain 41:71–80, 1990.

92. Harris RH, Vavra I, Ketoprofen. In: Rainsford KD (ed.). Anti-inflammatory and Anti-rheumatic Drugs, Vol. II: Newer Anti-inflammatory Drugs. Boca Raton, FL: CRC Press, 1985, pp. 151–170.

93. Sunshine A, Olson NZ. Analgesic efficacy of ketoprofen in postpartum, general surgery, and chronic cancer pain. J Clin Pharmacol 28:S47–S54, 1988.

94. Buckley MMT, Brogden RN. Ketorolac: a review of its pharmaco-dynamic and pharmacokinetic properties, and therapeutic potential. Drugs 39:86–109, 1990.

95. Wiseman EH. Pharmcologic studies with a new class of nonsteroidal anti-inflammatory agents–the oxicams–with special reference to piroxicam (Feldene). Am J Med 72:2–8, 1982.

96. Krishnan KRR, France RD. Antidepressants in chronic pain syndromes. Am Fam Physician 4:233–237, 1989.

97. Lee R, Spencer PS. Antidepressants and pain: a review of the pharmacological data supporting the use of certain tricyclics in chronic pain. J Int Med Res 5(1 suppl):146–156, 1977.

98. Feinmann C. Pain relief by antidepressants: Possible modes of action. Pain 23:1–8, 1985.

99. Messing RB, Lytle LD. Serotonin-containing neurons: their possible role in pain and analgesia. Pain 4:1–21, 1977.

100. Magi G. The use of antidepressants in the treatment of chronic pain. Drugs 42:730–748, 1991.

101. Sindrup SH, Gram LF, Brøsen K, Eshøj O, Mogenson EF. The selective serotonin reuptake inhibitor paroxetine is effective in the treatment of diabetic neuropathy syndromes. Pain 42:135–145, 1990.

102. Davis JL, Lewis SB, Gerich JE, et al. Peripheral diabetic neuropathy treated with amitriptyline and fluphenazine. JAMA 238:2291–2292, 1977.

103. McGee JL, Alexander MR. Phenothiazine analgesia: fact or fantasy. Am J Hosp Pharm 36:633–650, 1979.

104. Hatangdi VS, Boas RA, Edwards EG. Postherpetic neuralgia: management with antiepileptic and tricyclic drugs. Adv Pain Res Ther 1:583–587, 1976.

105. Chabal C, Russell LC, Burchiel KJ. The effects of intravenous lidocaine, tocainide and mexiletine on spontaneously active fibers originating in rat sciatic neuromas. Pain 38:333–338, 1989.

106. Crawley JN, Laverty R, Roth RH. Clonidine reversal of increased norepinephrine metabolite levels during morphine withdrawal. Eur J Pharmacol 57:247–250, 1979.

107. Maze M, Segal IS, Bloor BC. Clonidine and other alpha₂ adrenergic agonists: strategies for the rational use of these novel anesthetic agents. J Clin Anesth 1:146–157, 1988.

108. Levine JD, Fye K, Heller P, Basbaum AI, Whiting-O'Keefe Q. Clinical response to regional intravenous guanethidine in patients with rheumatoid arthritis. J Rheumatol 13:1040–1043, 1986.

109. Exton JH. Mechanisms involved in α-adrenergic phenomena. Am J Physiol 248 (Endocrinol Metab 211):E633–E647, 1985.

110. King SA, Strain JJ. Benzodiazepines and chronic pain. Pain 40:3–4, 1990.

111. Forrest WH, Brown BW, Brown CR et al. Dextroamphetamine with morphine for the treatment of postoperative pain. New Engl J Med 296:712–715, 1977.

112. Barkas G, Duafala ME. Advances in cancer pain management: a review. Patient-controlled analgesia. J Pain Symp Manag 3:150–160, 1988.

113. Magora F. The spinal route. In: Lipton S, Tunks E, Zoppi M (eds.). Advances in Pain Research and Therapy, Vol. 13: The Pain Clinic. New York: Raven Press, 1990, pp. 309–314.

114. Max MB, Inturrisi CE, Kaiko RF, et al. Epidural and intra-thecal opiates: cerebrospinal fluid and plasma profiles in patients with chronic cancer pain. Clin Pharmacol Ther 38:631–641, 1985.

115. Gourlay GK, Cherry DA, Plummer JL, Armstrong PJ, Cousins MJ. The influence of drug polarity on the absorption of opioid drugs into CSF and subsequent cephalad migration following lumbar epidural administration: application to morphine and pethidine. Pain 31:297–305, 1987.

116. Rawal N, Arner S, Gustaffson LL, Alvin R. Present state of extradural and intradural opioid analgesia in Sweden: A nation wide follow-up survey. Br J Anaesth 59:791–799, 1987.

117. Onofrio BM, Yaksh TL. Long-term pain relief produced by intrathecal morphine infusion in 53 patients. J Neurosurg 72:200–209, 1990.

118. Dickinson AH, Sullivan AF, McQuay HJ. Intrathecal etorphine, fentanyl and buprenorphine on spinal nociceptive neurones in the rat. Pain 42:227–234, 1990.

119. Coombs DW, Saunders RL, Fratkin JD, et al. Continuous intrathecal hydromorphone and clonidine for intractable cancer pain. J Neurosurg 64:890–894, 1986.

120. Mollenholt P, Post C, Paulsson I, Rawal N. Intrathecal and epidural somatostatin in rats: can antinociception, motor effects and neurotoxicity be separated? Pain 43:363–370, 1990.

121. Yaksh TL, Reddy SVR. Studies in the primate on the analgetic effects associated with intrathecal actions of opiate, α-adrenergic agonists and baclofen. Anesthesiology 54:451–467, 1981.

122. Jacobson L, Chabal C, Brody MC, Ward RJ, Wasse L. Intrathecal methadone: a dose-response study and comparison with intrathecal morphine 0.5 mg. Pain 43:141–148, 1990.

123. Roy SD, Flynn GL. Transdermal delivery of narcotic analgesics: pH, anatomical, and subject influences on cutaneous permeability of fentanyl and sufentanil. Pharmaceut Res 7: 842–847, 1990.

124. Yaksh TL, Stevens CW. Properties of the modulation of spinal nociceptive transmission by receptor-selective agents. In: Dubner R, Gebhart GF, Bond MR (eds.). Proceedings of the Fifth World Congress on Pain. Amsterdam: Elsevier, 1988, pp. 417–435.

125. Rocco A, Reiestad F, Gudman J, McKay W. Intrapleural administration of local anesthetics for pain relief in patients with multiple rib fractures. Reg Anaesth 12:10–14, 1987.

126. Kolkehar R, Meller ST, Gebhart GF. Characterization of the role of spinal N-methyl-D-aspartate receptors in the nociceptor in the rat. Neuroscience 57:385–395, 1993.

127. Øye I, Paulsen O, Mauset A. Effects of ketamine on sensory perception: evidence of a role of N-methyl-D-aspartate receptors. J Pharmacol Exp Ther 260:1209–1213, 1992.

128. Rapaka RS, Porreca F. Development of delta opioid peptides as nonaddicting analgesics. Pharmaceut Res 8:1–8, 1991.

129. Siegfried J. Neurosurgical treatment of neurogenic pain. In: Lipton S, Tunks E, Zoppi M (eds.). Advances in Pain Research and Therapy. Vol. 13: The Pain Clinic. New York: Raven Press, 1990, pp. 207–215.

130. McGlone FP, Marsh D. Stimulators for treatment of pain. In: Lipton S, Tunks E, Zoppi M (eds.). Advances in Pain Research and Therapy, Vol. 13: The Pain Clinic. New York: Raven Press, 1990, pp. 79–82.

131. Forster A, Morel D, Bachmann M, Gemperle M. Respiratory depressant effects of different doses of midazolam and lack of reversal with naloxone: a double-blind randomized study. Anesth Analg 62:920–924, 1983.

132. Seeff LB, Cuccherini BA, Zimmerman HJ, et al. Acetaminophen hepatotoxicity in alcoholics. Ann Intern Med 104:399–404, 1986.

133. Neal EA, Meffin PJ, Gregory PB, Blaschke TF. Enhanced bioavailability and decreased clearance of analgesics in patients with cirrhosis. Gastroenterology 77:96–102, 1979.

134. Wolfert AI, Sica DA. Narcotic usage in renal failure [Editorial]. Int J Artif Organs 11:411–415, 1988.

135. Kreek MJ, Schecter AJ, Gutjahr CL, Heath M. Methadone use in patients with chronic renal disease. Drug Alcohol Depend 5:197–205, 1980.

CHAPTER 53

ANXIETY DISORDERS

MARSHALL CATES, BARBARA G. WELLS, and G. WILLIAM THATCHER

Anxiety is an unpleasant feeling of apprehension or fearful concern. It can be a normal, reasonable, and expected response to a stressful situation or perceived danger, or it can be an excessive, irrational feeling state that signifies a mental disorder. The distinction between the two may be difficult to make. Generally, in the former, anxiety serves adaptive purposes, whereas in the latter, it is clearly maladaptive.

ETIOLOGY AND PATHOPHYSIOLOGY

Various psychodynamic, psychoanalytic, behavioral, cognitive, genetic, and biologic theories have been proposed to explain the etiology and pathophysiology of anxiety disorders. The anxiety disorders discussed in this chapter are a heterogeneous group of disorders and probably have no single unifying etiology. Several of the anxiety disorders have a familial pattern suggestive of a genetic component (1).

Neurotransmitter systems involved in the generation of anxiety include the serotonergic, noradrenergic, dopaminergic, adenosinergic, and the benzodiazepine-GABA system. The biologic theories best understood are the noradrenergic and benzodiazepine-GABA receptor models.

According to the noradrenergic model, the autonomic nervous system of patients with anxiety disorders becomes overactive to various stimuli. This model may have particular relevance for panic disorder. It is clear that patients with anxiety disorders exhibit symptoms of peripheral autonomic hyperactivity, including tremulousness, palpitations, and hyperventilation (2). The locus ceruleus (LC) is a brain stem nucleus that contains 70% of the noradrenergic neurons in the brain. It has extensive projections to the limbic system, cerebral cortex, and cerebellar cortex. Uncontrollable and threatening stimuli activate the LC. In general, drugs with anxiolytic or antipanic efficacy (e.g., tricyclic antidepressants and benzodiazepines) decrease neuronal firing in the LC (3). Alprazolam decreases corticotropin releasing factor (CRF) concentrations in the LC (4). Drugs that stimulate LC activity (e.g., caffeine and yohimbine) are usually anxiogenic, and patients with anxiety disorders are often more susceptible to the anxiogenic effects of these drugs (5).

Gamma-Aminobutyric acid (GABA) is the major inhibitory neurotransmitter. Two types of GABA receptors have been described, $GABA_A$ receptors that are coupled to chloride channels, and $GABA_B$ receptors that are coupled to calcium and possibly cAMP. When GABA interacts with the $GABA_A$ receptor, this facilitates opening of the chloride channel linked to the receptor. The result is augmentation of chloride ion influx intraneuronally (hyperpolarization), making depolarization less likely (6). Benzodiazepines facilitate the actions of GABA by binding to $GABA_A$ receptors and inducing a conformational change that increases the affinity of the receptor for GABA (7).

The clinical response to pharmacologic challenges and interventions has led to various hypotheses concerning etiology. The selective serotonin reuptake inhibitors (SSRIs), such as fluoxetine, are now widely used in the treatment of anxiety disorders, thus focusing interest on the serotonergic neurotransmitter system (8). Treatment with SSRI medications has reversed the abnormalities found in positron emission tomography (PET) studies in some anxiety disorders (9). The only medications that are effective in obsessive–compulsive disorder (OCD) are highly selective serotonin reuptake inhibitors (9). Serotonin reuptake inhibition seems to be the necessary property for the antipanic effect of antidepressant medications (10). Buspirone has a partial agonist effect on the $5-HT_{1A}$ serotonin receptor and is used in treating various anxiety disorders (7). Unfortunately, serotonergic systems have a relatively large number of known receptor subtypes, making serotonin systems difficult to study. Various pathophysiologic studies have yet to firmly substantiate the role of serotonin in the etiology of these diverse disorders (9).

The hypothalamic–pituitary–adrenal axis (HPA) also plays a role in anxiety disorders. Perceived threat or stress activates the HPA axis and one of its components, CRF. CRF plays an important role in the generation of anxiety by activating the LC. CRF released by hypothalamic neurons eventually leads to the release of cortisol from the adrenal gland and the cortisol interacts with the HPA axis to inhibit CRF production. Evidence suggests that CRF is responsible for integrating the endocrine, autonomic, and behavioral responses of an organism to stress. Cortisol levels are low in one type of anxiety disorder (posttraumatic stress disorder), and it is postulated that these patients are more sensitive to the feedback inhibition of the HPA axis by cortisol (4, 11).

EPIDEMIOLOGY

The National Comorbidity Survey (NCS), supported by the United States Alcohol, Drug Abuse, and Mental Health Administration, provides the most recent information on the epidemiology of anxiety disorders (12). The lifetime prevalence rate for anxiety disorders overall is 24.9%. In the 12 months prior to the NCS survey, 17.2% of the population experienced an anxiety disorder. This data suggests anxiety disorders are more chronic than affective or substance abuse disorders.

Panic disorder, with or without agoraphobia (phobic avoidance behaviors), has a lifetime prevalence rate in women of 5%, and in men of 2% (12). The lifetime prevalence of generalized anxiety disorder is 5.1%, and the diagnosis of this disorder is somewhat more frequent in females (12). Obsessive–compulsive disorder has a lifetime prevalence rate of 2.3% (13). Although the lifetime prevalence rate of posttraumatic stress disorder for the general population is about 1%, traumatized populations such as combat veterans and refugees can have a lifetime prevalence rate of 30–50% and a current rate of 10 to 38% (14). Social phobia is the most common of the anxiety disorders with a lifetime prevalence rate of 13.3%, and it is somewhat more common in women than men (12).

Comorbidity is a major factor in determining adequate treatment and outcome. One study reported 28% of patients with panic disorder and 21% of those with social phobia had a history of major depression in their lifetimes (15). The NCS study states comorbidity is generally associated with a more serious course and that one-sixth of the population has a lifetime history of three or more mental disorders. Uncomplicated panic disorder has a lifetime rate of suicide attempts of 7% (the rate for the population without a mental disorder is 1%), and comorbid panic disorder has a rate of 26.3% (16).

DIAGNOSIS AND CLINICAL FINDINGS

Evaluation of the anxious patient requires a thorough physical examination, psychiatric examination (including the mental status examination), appropriate laboratory workup, and an understanding of the patient's history, including a drug history. It is important to determine whether the symptoms of anxiety represent situational anxiety or an anxiety disorder. Situational anxiety is a normal response to a stressful situation and usually lasts only two to three weeks. Short-term treatment with an antianxiety agent may be helpful, but more prolonged therapy is unnecessary.

A variety of medical conditions may cause anxiety symptoms (Table 53.1). If prominent symptoms of anxiety are judged to be a direct physiologic consequence of a medical condition, and if certain criteria are met, these symptoms are labeled in the Diagnostic and Statistical Manual of Mental Disorders, Fourth Edition (DSM-IV) as Anxiety Disorder Due to a General Medical Condition (2). Furthermore, knowledge that one has a chronic and perhaps disabling medical illness can precipitate anxiety that may in turn complicate treatment and rehabilitation (17).

Anxiety may also be a symptom of an underlying primary psychiatric disorder. Almost all major psychiatric illnesses may be associated with symptoms of anxiety. These include schizophrenia, major depression, dysthymia, mania, delirium, dementia, and substance-use disorders (18). Anxiety related to substance abuse is categorized in the DSM-IV as Substance-Induced Anxiety Disorder.

When symptoms of anxiety are secondary to an underlying medical or psychiatric illness, treatment of the primary illness is the treatment of choice. Use of an antianxiety agent may also be necessary, preferably short term.

Several pharmacologic agents are known to produce anxious symptoms, most notably central nervous system (CNS) stimulants and depressants. CNS stimulants most commonly incriminated include albuterol, amphetamines, cocaine, fenfluramine, isoproterenol, and methylphenidate. Nonprescription drugs well known to cause anxiety include caffeine, nicotine, and decongestants (e.g., ephedrine, pseudoephedrine, oxymetazoline, phenylephrine, phenylpropanolamine, and naphazoline) (19). The elderly and patients with panic disorder may be especially sensitive to the anxiety-producing effects of these agents. CNS depressants (e.g., alcohol, narcotic analgesics, barbiturates, meprobamate, benzodiazepines) may cause anxiety and agitation as a paradoxical reaction, but far more commonly,

Table 53.1.
Medical Disorders Associated with Anxiety

Cardiovascular:	
Arrhythmias	Hypertension
Angina	Mitral valve prolapse
Myocardial infarction	Congestive heart failure
Respiratory:	
Chronic obstructive pulmonary disease	Pneumonia
Pulmonary embolism	Hyperventilation
Endocrine:	
Hyperthyroidism	Hypoglycemia
Hypothyroidism	Pheochromocytoma
Gastrointestinal:	
Ulcerative colitis	Irritable bowel syndrome
Peptic ulcer disease	
Metabolic:	
Vitamin B_{12} deficiency	Porphyria
Inflammatory:	
Rheumatoid arthritis	Lupus erythematosus
Neurological:	
Neoplasms	Encephalitis
Miscellaneous:	
Chronic infections	Malignancies

Table 53.2.
DSM-IV Classification of Anxiety Disorders

Panic disorder
   with agoraphobia
   without agoraphobia
Agoraphobia without history of panic disorder
Specific phobia
Social phobia
Obsessive–compulsive disorder
Posttraumatic stress disorder
Acute stress disorder
Generalized anxiety disorder
Anxiety disorder due to a general medical condition
Substance-induced anxiety disorder
Anxiety disorder not otherwise specified

anxiety associated with the use of these agents is part of the physiologic withdrawal phenomenon following abrupt discontinuation of chronic administration of these agents (18).

The official classification of anxiety disorders, according to the American Psychiatric Association, is detailed in the DSM-IV (Table 53.2) (2). This manual also specifies the diagnostic criteria and differential diagnosis for each disorder.

The DSM-IV specifies criteria for panic attack separate from the disorders because panic attacks occur in the context of several different anxiety disorders. A panic attack is a discrete period of intense fear or discomfort that is accompanied by at least four somatic or cognitive symptoms (Table 53.3). Panic attacks have a sudden onset, quickly intensify, and usually reach their apex in 10 minutes or less. They are often accompanied by a sense of impending doom, and an intense sense of fear is usually present where people often feel they are about to die, are having a heart attack, or are "going crazy" (2).

Generalized Anxiety Disorder (GAD)

The essential feature of GAD is excessive and unrealistic worry that is difficult to control about several life circumstances for 6 months or longer. The anxiety must be accompanied by at least three of the following six symptoms: restlessness, being easily fatigued, difficulty concentrating, irritability, muscle tension, and disturbed sleep. Many individuals with GAD also experience somatic symptoms and depressive symptoms. This disorder very frequently is a comorbid condition with mood disorders, with other anxiety disorders, and with substance abuse disorders. Physical symptoms that might be associated with stress (e.g., headache, irritable bowel syndrome) often occur with GAD. The course of GAD is chronic but fluctuating (2).

Panic Disorder (PD)

The essential criterion of this disorder is the occurrence of recurrent, unexpected panic attacks followed by at least 1 month of persistent concern of experiencing further attacks; worry about the possible implications or consequences of the episodes; or a significant change in the individual's behavior secondary to the attacks. Unexpected panic attacks are those that are not set off by specific circumstances. The individual needs at least two unexpected attacks for the diagnosis, but most patients have more than two and will have other attacks that are related to anticipating an attack or being in a situation that generates fear (2,20). The frequency of the attacks is quite variable from daily attacks for a week followed by weeks or months of no attacks to once a week for months (2).

Most patients who seek treatment have also developed some symptoms of agoraphobia, a fear of being in places or situations where help may be unavailable or where escape might be difficult or embarrassing. As a result of this, patients often come to avoid these situations, placing travel restrictions on themselves or venturing out only in the presence of a companion. Common agoraphobic situations include being alone away from home; being in a crowd; standing in line; being on a bridge; and traveling in a bus, train, or car. Although PD without agoraphobia may cause limited or no social or occupational impairment, PD with agoraphobia is associated with constriction in lifestyle. In severe cases, patients may be unable to leave the house alone (2).

PD is often a chronic relapsing illness that may require lifetime treatment. Fifty to 65% of individuals with PD will have a comorbid diagnosis of major depressive disorder with the depression preceding the panic disorder in one-third of the cases (2). Between 8 and 30% of individuals with PD will have another comorbid anxiety disorder (2).

Obsessive–Compulsive Disorder (OCD)

The essential feature of OCD is recurrent obsessions or compulsions that cause marked distress; are time consum-

Table 53.3.
Symptoms Associated with a Panic Attack[a]

Palpitations or tachycardia
Sweating
Trembling or shaking
Sensations of shortness of breath or smothering
Feeling of choking
Chest pain
Nausea or abdominal distress
Feeling dizzy, lightheaded, or faint
Feelings of unreality or feelings of being detached from oneself
Fear of losing control or going crazy
Fear of dying
Numbness or tingling sensations
Chills or hot flashes

[a]Adapted from reference 2.

ing; or interfere significantly with normal occupational functioning, social activities, or relationships (2).

Obsessions are persistent ideas, thoughts, impulses, or images that are experienced as intrusive and senseless. Examples include recurrent thoughts of harming a loved one, recurrent blasphemous thoughts, or recurrent thoughts of contamination. The obsessions are not simply excessive worries about real-life problems. The person recognizes that the obsessions are the product of his or her own mind. Compulsions are repetitive, intentional, purposeful behaviors performed in response to an obsession in a certain stereotyped fashion. However, the activity is not realistically connected with the obsession it is designed to neutralize, or it is clearly excessive. Usually the person recognizes the behavior is excessive or unreasonable. Although the behavior provides some decrease in anxiety, these persons do not derive pleasure from carrying out the activity. Examples of common compulsions are repetitive handwashing, counting, checking, and touching. When these patients resist a compulsion or are prevented from performing the compulsive behavior, there is a sense of mounting anxiety (2).

Patients with OCD are often moderately to severely impaired. Avoidance behavior due to obsessions is common, and in some cases acting on compulsions may become the major life activity. Complications of OCD include abuse of alcohol or antianxiety agents (2).

Posttraumatic Stress Disorder (PTSD)

PTSD may occur when a person reacts with intense fear, helplessness, or horror on exposure to a traumatic event. The person must experience, witness, or be confronted with an event that involves actual or threatened death or serious injury, or a threat to the physical integrity of self or others (2).

Directly experienced traumatic events include military combat, violent personal assault, being kidnapped or taken hostage, being a prisoner of war, incarceration in a concentration camp, natural or man-made disasters, and severe automobile accidents. Witnessing the serious injury or death of another or learning about such events that occur to a family member or close friend may also induce PTSD (2).

The individual with PTSD persistently reexperiences the traumatic event through recurrent, intrusive thoughts or images, recurring nightmares, or flashbacks where the actual event seems to be recurring. Individuals tend to avoid any situations where they are reminded of the traumatic event. People with PTSD have a numbing of general responsiveness, which includes such things as markedly diminished interest in activities previously enjoyed, feelings of detachment or estrangement from others, and the inability to develop closeness or loving feelings toward others. They often have a sense they will not live

long, or have a career, or get married and have children (sense of foreshortened future). Individuals with PTSD are often unable to recall an important aspect of the traumatic event (2). Symptoms of dissociation are quite common and may include a sense of loss of time, the person finding himself or herself somewhere but not knowing how he or she got there, the person being outside his or her body, and the person being confused about who or where he or she is (21).

Another distinguishing aspect of PTSD is extensive and persistent symptoms of increased arousal, including such things as difficulty sleeping, irritability or outbursts of anger, difficulty concentrating, hypervigilance, and exaggerated startle response (2).

Extensive comorbidity is associated with this disorder, and the vast majority of individuals with PTSD will also experience at sometime such comorbidities as various other anxiety disorders, major depressive disorder or dysthymia, or substance-use disorder (most commonly, alcohol abuse) (14).

The more severe and violent the trauma, the more likely an individual will develop PTSD, and the more likely it will be persistent with significant comorbidity. Some patients with PTSD will improve and have little to very mild symptoms and do quite well overtime; however, others will have a more persistent symptomatic course or have a waxing and waning of symptoms (14).

Social Phobia (SP)

SP is characterized by a marked and persistent fear of social or performance situations in which embarrassment may occur. The anxiety may be associated with a variety of situations (generalized SP), or it may be more specific (discrete SP). When exposed to the social or performance situation, an immediate anxiety response (e.g., palpitations, tremors, sweating, gastrointestinal discomfort, diarrhea, muscle tension, blushing, confusion) is invariably provoked and may take the form of a situationally bound or situationally predisposed panic attack. The social situation or performance is usually avoided or endured with dread. Adults usually perceive their fears as unreasonable (2).

To avoid embarrassment, individuals with SP may avoid eating, drinking, or writing in public for fear that others will see them tremble. They may avoid using public lavatories and fear speaking in public. The main cognitive characteristic is fear of negative evaluation. They often are hypersensitive to criticism or rejection, have difficulty being assertive, have low self-esteem, and have poor social skills (2).

Comorbidity with other anxiety disorders, substance abuse, and depression is very common (22). Diagnosis of SP is made only if there is significant impairment of the person's daily routine, occupational functioning, or social life (2).

NONPHARMACOLOGIC APPROACHES

Just as the last decade has brought psychopharmacologic advances in the treatment of anxiety disorders, there have been significant gains in the effectiveness of nonpharmacologic interventions. Cognitive therapy and behavior therapy have been well researched and have often been combined to treat the various disorders.

The effectiveness of cognitive-behavioral therapy in PD has been reported to be as high as 80% with the effect lasting up to 2 years (23, 24). It appears in the long-term treatment of PD that cognitive-behavioral treatment may be very helpful (25). This type of treatment focuses on the fear of symptoms of anxiety. Patients often make catastrophic interpretations of the meaning of panic symptoms (e.g., "I am having a stroke" or "I am about to go insane"), and these cognitions are thought to maintain a high level of anticipatory anxiety and to cue the next panic attack. The therapy is aimed at the elimination of this fear of symptoms and its associated anxiety and avoidance. Further, stepwise exposure to feared bodily sensations combined with cognitive restructuring helps patients decrease catastrophic misinterpretations of somatic symptoms of panic (25). Therapist-guided or -instructed exposure to phobic situations is an important aspect of this therapy (20). Alprazolam may interfere with cognitive-behavioral therapy because it may prevent the controlled elicitation of anxiety during therapy sessions (26). According to Taylor, the thoughtful integration of cognitive-behavioral therapy and pharmacotherapy produces an optimal outcome. He suggests that many patients require some medication before they are able to undertake intensive exposure therapy and that psychological interventions can facilitate withdrawal of medication and prepare patients for long-term treatment (27).

SP is felt to be amenable to the combination of cognitive-behavioral therapy and pharmacotherapy (28). Cognitive-behavioral therapy, applied relaxation therapy, and traditional psychodynamic psychotherapy have been found to be helpful in patients with GAD (27, 29, 30). OCD is a particularly difficult problem to treat, but combining pharmacotherapy with other interventions is probably the most efficacious approach. Combining either clomipramine or fluoxetine with the behavioral treatments of exposure with response prevention (not allowing the compulsion to occur) was associated with a 75% rate of significant improvement in one study (31). PTSD usually requires both pharmacotherapy and nonpharmacologic interventions, which may include individual, group, and family psychotherapies (32, 33).

ANTIANXIETY MEDICATIONS

Commonly used antianxiety medications include benzodiazepines (BZDs), buspirone, beta-blockers, tricyclic antidepressants (TCAs), monoamine oxidase inhibitors (MAOIs), and selective serotonin reuptake inhibitors (SSRIs).

Benzodiazepines (BZDs)

INDICATIONS

Currently available BZD antianxiety agents are alprazolam (Xanax), chlordiazepoxide (Librium), clonazepam (Klonopin), clorazepate (Tranxene), diazepam (Valium), halazepam (Paxipam), lorazepam (Ativan), oxazepam (Serax), and prazepam (Centrax). All these agents are FDA-approved for the treatment of anxiety except clonazepam, which is technically an anticonvulsant. As a class, BZDs are very widely prescribed, accounting for approximately 5% of prescriptions written in the United States (6). The most common indication for BZD therapy is GAD. Double-blind, randomized clinical trials have shown that BZDs clearly reduce the symptoms of GAD more effectively than placebo (34).

Numerous controlled trials have established the efficacy of alprazolam as an antipanic agent (35), and it is currently the only FDA-approved drug to treat PD. There is growing evidence that clonazepam, diazepam, and lorazepam also have antipanic efficacy (36).

Clonazepam was reported to significantly improve 85% of SP patients with long-term treatment despite gradual dosage reduction during the study period (37). Alprazolam is another BZD considered effective for SP (8).

BZDs have not been well studied in the treatment of PTSD. Alprazolam failed to improve PTSD-specific symptoms in a double-blind, placebo-controlled crossover study (38).

MECHANISM OF ACTION

BZDs may exert antianxiety effects through the potentiation of the inhibitory neurotransmitter, GABA. BZD-binding sites have been identified in cortical and limbic forebrain areas in the CNS. These receptors are linked to GABA receptors. When BZDs interact at the BZD receptor, the affinity of the GABA receptor for GABA is increased. This causes an amplification of the GABA-mediated chloride ion influx intracellularly, with resultant hyperpolarization (6). BZDs inhibit firing in the LC (18).

PHARMACOKINETICS

The pharmacokinetics of the BZD antianxiety agents are summarized in Table 53.4. Subtle differences in the pharmacokinetic profiles may aid clinicians in selecting the most appropriate agent. When immediate effects are desired, as in treatment of acute anxiety or in as-needed treatment of anxiety, it is important to select an agent with rapid onset. In treating anxiety of a more chronic nature with more prolonged dosing, this becomes less important. Similarly, if panic attacks occur between doses of alprazolam, it may be helpful to switch the patient

Table 53.4.
Pharmacokinetic Profile of the Benzodiazepine Antianxiety Agents[a]

Generic Name	Time to Peak Plasma Concentration (hrs)	Elimination Half-Life[b] (hrs)	Protein Binding (%)	Metabolic Pathway	Clinically Important Metabolites
Alprazolam	1–2	12–15	80	Oxidation	None
Chlordiazepoxide	1–4	5–30	96	Oxidation	Desmethchlordiazepoxide Demoxepam N-DMDZ[c] Oxazepam
Clonazepam	1–4	20–50	85	Nitroreduction	None
Clorazepate	1–2	Prodrug	97	Oxidation	N-DMDZ Oxazepam
Diazepam	0.5–2	20–80	98	Oxidation	N-DMDZ Oxazepam
Halazepam	1–3	7–14	97	Oxidation	3-Hydroxyhalazepam N-DMDZ Oxazepam
Lorazepam	2–4	10–20	85	Conjugation	None
Oxazepam	2–4	5–20	97	Conjugation	None
Prazepam	6	Prodrug	97	Oxidation	3-Hydroxyprazepam N-DMDZ Oxazepam

[a]Modified from reference 40.
[b]Parent compound.
[c]N-Desmethyldiazepam; half-life = 36–200 hours.

to clonazepam since the longer half-life of elimination seems to be associated with a more sustained duration of action (35).

The highly lipophilic BZDs, diazepam and clorazepate, are rapidly absorbed and distributed into the CNS. As a result, an anxiolytic effect can be anticipated within 1 hour of dosing with these agents. This rapid entry into the CNS may be associated with a "rush" in some patients that may contribute to the likelihood of abuse. Similarly, the highly lipophilic agents are rapidly distributed peripherally to inactive storage sites (adipose tissue). This accounts for the short duration of action seen with single dosing of clorazepate and diazepam (39). Lorazepam and oxazepam are less lipophilic. This results in a slower onset of antianxiety effect but a more prolonged effect than might be expected based on half-life because extensive tissue distribution does not occur (40).

Clorazepate and prazepam are prodrugs and do not have antianxiety activity until they are converted to the metabolite, N-desmethyldiazepam (N-DMDZ). Clorazepate is converted rapidly in the acidic gastric environment to N-DMDZ by a pH-dependent process. Administration of antacids may elevate the pH of the stomach and decrease the rate of N-DMDZ formation. Conversion of prazepam to N-DMDZ is a much slower process since transformation occurs in the liver. Consequently, several hours are required to achieve peak plasma concentrations of

N-DMDZ after administration of prazepam. Prazepam would not be an appropriate drug to choose when acute (rapid) antianxiety effects are desired.

In the unusual circumstance that an intramuscular preparation is to be used, lorazepam provides the most predictable absorption. Diazepam and chlordiazepoxide intramuscular injections can be painful and are absorbed erratically (39).

With chronic dosing, the rate and extent of accumulation depend on clearance and half-life of elimination of parent compound and active metabolites. The BZDs are biotransformed by two primary metabolic processes, hepatic microsomal oxidation (N-dealkylation and aliphatic hydroxylation) and glucuronide conjugation. Oxidation may be impaired by aging, liver disease, and concurrent administration of drugs that inhibit oxidative processes. In this situation, greater plasma concentrations and total body stores at steady state would be expected (39). Conjugation is not affected by these factors.

As shown in Table 53.4, several BZDs are converted to N-DMDZ, which is an active metabolite with a half-life of 36 to 200 hours. Further oxidation converts N-DMDZ to oxazepam, which is then conjugated and excreted. Extensive accumulation of N-DMDZ at steady state provides a long duration of antianxiety effects, allowing once or twice daily dosing if desired. In the presence of impaired oxidation, prolonged half-life and increased accumulation may be associated with excessive sedation and ataxia in some patients (39).

Alprazolam, oxazepam, and lorazepam have short-to-intermediate half-lives of elimination, so a shorter time is required to achieve steady-state accumulation and plasma concentrations. Alprazolam is oxidized to alpha-hydroxyalprazolam, which is present in small amounts and probably does not contribute substantially to clinical efficacy. Oxazepam and lorazepam do not undergo oxidation; they are simply glucuronidated and excreted (39). For this reason, oxazepam and lorazepam are considered good choices for the patient suspected of having impaired oxidative processes.

Patients with hypoalbuminemia may have a significantly greater free (pharmacologically active) fraction of BZDs that are highly protein bound. For these patients, lorazepam or alprazolam would be a rational choice because of its lower percentage of protein binding.

DOSING

BZDs with long half-lives of elimination may be dosed once daily at bedtime, thereby providing hypnotic effects as well as daytime antianxiety effects (see Table 53.5). Agents with

shorter half-lives (oxazepam, lorazepam, alprazolam) are usually administered in divided daily doses. Patients should be started on low doses and titrated upward to the lowest effective dose. Treatment duration should be as brief as possible.

All the BZDs have similar efficacy in the treatment of GAD if appropriate doses are employed. Approximate equivalent doses, relative to diazepam 5 mg, are alprazolam 0.25 mg, clonazepam 0.25 mg, lorazepam 1 mg, clorazepate 7.5 mg, chlordiazepoxide 10 mg, prazepam 10 mg, oxazepam 15 mg, and halazepam 20 mg.

The total daily dose for BZDs in PD tends to be approximately twice that required for GAD (41). Some PD patients need up to 10 mg/d or more of alprazolam, 6 mg/d of clonazepam, 60 mg/d of diazepam, or 16 mg/d of lorazepam for optimal therapeutic effectiveness.

ADVERSE EFFECTS

Overall, BZDs are very well tolerated by most patients. By far the most common adverse effects of BZDs involve depression of the CNS. Side effects such as sedation, ataxia, and incoordination tend to be more common during the initial phase of therapy and diminish with continued

Table 53.5.
Dosing of Antianxiety Medications[a]

Antianxiety Agent	Initial Dose[b]	Titration[b]	Maximum Dose[c]
BZDs:			
Alprazolam	0.25 mg tid	0.25–0.5 mg/d q 2–4 d	1 mg qid
Chlordiazepoxide	5 mg tid	5–10 mg/d q 2–4 d[d]	100 mg qhs
Clonazepam	0.5 mg bid	0.5–1.0 mg/d q 2–4 d[d]	3 mg bid
Clorazepate	7.5 mg bid	3.75–7.5 mg/d q 2–4 d[d]	60 mg qhs
Diazepam	5 mg bid	2–5 mg/d q 2–4 d[d]	40 mg qhs
Lorazepam	1 mg tid	0.5–1.0 mg/d q 2–4 d	5 mg bid
Oxazepam	10 mb tid	10–15 mg/d q 2–4 d	30 mg tid
Buspirone	5 mg tid	5 mg/d q 2–3 d	20 mg tid
Beta-blockers:			
Atenolol	25 mg qam	25 mg/d q 3–4 d	100 mg qam
Propranolol	10 mg tid	20–40 mg/d q 2–3 d	120 mg tid
TCAs:			
Clomipramine	25 mg qhs	25 mg/d q 2–4 d	250 mg qhs
Imipramine[e]	25–50 mg qhs	25 mg/d q 2–4 d	300 mg qhs
Nortriptyline	25 mg qhs	25 mg/d q 2–4 d	150 mg qhs
MAOIs:			
Phenelzine	15 mg qam	15 mg/d q 3–4 d[f]	45 mg bid
Tranylcypromine	10 mg qam		30 mg bid
SSRIs:			
Fluoxetine	20 mg qam	20 mg/d q 2–4 wk	80 mg qam
Fluvoxamine	50 mg qhs	50 mg/d q wk	150 mg bid
Paroxetine	20 mg qam	10 mg/d q wk	50 mg qam
Sertraline	50 mg qam	50 mg/d q wk	200 mg qam

[a]These are intended as general guidelines only. Elderly patients usually require approximately one-half the doses required for younger adults.
[b]SSRI- and TCA-treated PD patients require lower initial doses and slower titrations (see text).
[c]BZD-treated PD patients may require higher doses (see text).
[d]After initial response, titrate q 1–2 weeks because of long half-life.
[e]Similar dosing strategies for amitriptyline, desipramine, and doxepin.
[f]Until 60 mg/d, then increase further only if there is no improvement after 8–12 weeks.

Table 53.6.
Common or Serious Adverse Effects of Antianxiety Medications

BZD
Drowsiness, weakness/fatigue, ataxia, slurred speech, confusion/ disorientation, incoordination, impaired memory, paradoxical agitation/excitement, dizziness, nausea

Buspirone
Nausea, dizziness, headache, insomnia, agitation, drowsiness, dysphoria

Beta-blocker
Depression, nightmares, insomnia, weakness/fatigue, lethargy, hypotension, bradycardia, dizziness, heart failure, bronchospasm, exacerbation of peripheral vascular disease or Raynaud's Disease, masks hypoglycemic symptoms in diabetics

TCA
Sedation, orthostatic hypotension, dry mouth, blurred vision, constipation, urinary retention, weight gain, slowed atrioventricular conduction, tremor, seizures, sexual dysfunction

MAOI
Orthostatic hypotension, dry mouth, constipation, drowsiness, insomnia, overstimulation, agitation, sexual dysfunction, edema, weight gain, dizziness, hypertensive crisis

SSRI
Nausea, anxiety, insomnia, nervousness, diarrhea, anorexia, dizziness, weight loss, dry mouth, headache, tremor, sweating, sexual dysfunction

treatment. Elderly patients, debilitated patients, and patients with hepatic or renal disease are more likely to experience CNS adverse effects (42). Impaired memory reported with BZD use is termed anterograde amnesia because loss of memory is for events occurring after drug ingestion. In addition, a paradoxical reaction involving excitement, aggressiveness, and confusion may occur, especially in the elderly (see Table 53.6) (40).

DRUG INTERACTIONS

Drug interactions involving BZDs are shown in Table 53.7. Caution is recommended when combining alcohol, opioid analgesics, or other CNS depressants with BZDs because of additive/synergistic CNS depression. Many drug interactions involve the induction or inhibition of the oxidative metabolism of BZDs; these interactions are of little concern when BZDs such as lorazepam or oxazepam are employed.

DEPENDENCE, WITHDRAWAL, ABUSE, AND TOLERANCE

Physiologic dependence is defined by the emergence of withdrawal symptoms on discontinuation of therapy. BZD dependence is well documented, and a mild withdrawal syndrome occurs in up to 44% of patients receiving therapeutic doses of BZDs for 4 to 6 weeks (43). Mild withdrawal symptoms include anxiety, insomnia, irritability, anorexia, diaphoresis, and sensitivity to light and sound. In more severe cases, withdrawal may include confusion,

depersonalization, myoclonus, nausea, delirium, and psychosis. The onset of withdrawal usually occurs 1 to 2 days after discontinuing (or reducing the dose of) short-to-intermediate half-life BZDs and 5 to 10 days after discontinuing (or reducing the dose of) the long half-life entities. Although prominent withdrawal symptoms generally subside within 1 to 3 weeks, mild symptoms may persist for several months (6). Withdrawal is more likely to occur and to be severe if the duration of therapy has been long and if high doses have been used. Withdrawal may also

Table 53.7.
Drug-Drug Interactions with the Benzodiazepine Antianxiety Agents[a,b]

Drug	Effect
Antacids	Decreased rate of diazepam and chlordiazepoxide absorption; decreased rate and extent of DMDZ conversion from clorazepate
Beta-blockers	Propranolol and metoprolol cause a small reduction in oxidative metabolism of diazepam and DMDZ
Cimetidine	Decreased oxidative metabolism of most BZDs
Digoxin	Elevated digoxin serum concentrations with signs/symptoms of toxicity reported with addition of alprazolam or diazepam
Disulfiram	Decreased oxidative metabolism of BZDs
Ethanol	Inhibition of BZD metabolism; additive or synergistic CNS depression
Erythromycin	Inhibition of oxidative metabolism of triazolam, and possibly other BZDs
Hydantoins	Increased and decreased phenytoin serum concentrations reported with addition of diazepam or chlordiazepoxide; increased oxazepam elimination
Isoniazid	Decreased oxidative metabolism of diazepam and triazolam
Levodopa	Worsening of parkinsonian symptoms
Nefazodone	Inhibition of metabolism of alprazolam and triazolam
Oral contraceptives	Decreased clearance of diazepam, chlordiazepoxide, triazolam, and perhaps alprazolam; metabolism of oxazepam, lorazepam, and temazepam may be increased
Probenecid	May increase lorazepam levels by decreasing clearance
Rifampin	Increased oxidative metabolism of diazepam and N-DMDZ
Theophyllines	Antagonism of CNS depressant effects of BZDs
Valproic acid	Decreased oxidative metabolism of diazepam; protein binding of diazepam may also be altered

[a]Based on information from reference 42.
[b]This is not intended to be an all-inclusive list.

be more severe following the use of the shorter half-life drugs lorazepam, oxazepam, and alprazolam (40).

Two other discontinuation syndromes are described that may be confused with withdrawal. Relapse is simply the return of the original symptoms of anxiety, which may occur weeks to months after drug discontinuation. Rebound refers to a return of the original symptoms, but with greater intensity. This may occur hours to days after drug discontinuation, and it is followed by recovery to pretreatment status (6).

BZDs should be discontinued gradually, by one-eighth to one-fourth of the total dose every few weeks to allow careful monitoring and to reduce the risk of withdrawal or rebound. Substituting a long half-life BZD for a short-to-intermediate half-life drug before downward tapering may reduce the severity of withdrawal symptoms (6). It has been suggested that alprazolam may not be cross-tolerant with other BZDs, but substitution of clonazepam for alprazolam has been used successfully (44).

It is crucial to recognize that abuse is a separate issue from dependence. Abuse is persistent or sporadic excessive drug use inconsistent with or unrelated to acceptable medical practice. Individuals with a history of alcohol or other drug abuse are at greatest risk of becoming BZD abusers. In individuals without this history, BZD abuse is unusual (45). Diazepam, followed by alprazolam and lorazepam, has been judged to have the greatest liability for abuse among the BZDs (6).

Although tolerance develops to the sedative, muscle relaxant, and anticonvulsant properties of the BZDs, tolerance does not appear to develop to the antianxiety or antipanic effects in most patients (46). Consequently, most patients are unlikely to attempt to escalate the dose.

PATIENT EDUCATION

Patients should be told about the expected benefits, expected length of therapy, common side effects, and precautions to be observed with any medications they are taking. Detailed patient education information can be found in the USP-DI published by the United States Pharmacopeial Convention, Inc. (47). Patients should be told that although they will likely experience some antianxiety and/or antipanic effects during the first weeks, they should maintain regular contact with the prescriber as long as they are taking this medication. The prescriber should regularly assess side effects and make a decision on the need to continue drug therapy. If depression emerges or becomes more pronounced, the prescriber should be notified (47).

Patients should be told that BZDs can cause drowsiness and decrease coordination. Patients should be warned against driving a car or operating dangerous machinery until they know how the drug affects them.

Patients should understand that with continued dosing, their medication can cause a physical dependence and that stopping the medication abruptly may result in withdrawal side effects. They should, therefore, not discontinue medication abruptly without first checking with the prescriber, who may elect to gradually taper the dose downward before discontinuing it (47).

Female patients of child-bearing potential should understand that taking BZDs during pregnancy may be associated with risks, including birth defects (if taken during the first trimester), physiologic dependence in the baby, and other selected problems in the newborn, such as drowsiness, slow heart beat, and difficulty breathing (47).

Buspirone

INDICATIONS

Buspirone is a member of a unique chemical class called the azapirones. It is structurally dissimilar to previously marketed agents and exhibits no cross-tolerance with the BZDs. It is approved for the management of anxiety and for the short-term relief of symptoms of anxiety. Buspirone lacks anticonvulsant, muscle relaxant, and hypnotic properties. Several double-blind studies in GAD have demonstrated that buspirone has antianxiety activity superior to placebo and equal to that of benzodiazepines (48, 49).

Buspirone was found to be as effective as clomipramine in treating obsessive-compulsive and depressive symptoms in OCD patients in a 6-week, double-blind, controlled study (50). However, studies examining buspirone as monotherapy or adjunct therapy for OCD have yielded mixed results.

Nine of 11 SP patients completing an 8-week open trial of buspirone showed moderate to marked improvement (51). Buspirone has not been well studied in the treatment of PTSD, and it is commonly considered to be ineffective in the treatment of PD.

MECHANISM OF ACTION

The mechanism of action of buspirone in exerting antianxiety effects is poorly understood, but it clearly does not interact with benzodiazepine receptors and may increase rather than decrease brain noradrenergic and dopaminergic activity. Buspirone is a $5HT_{1A}$ partial agonist and reportedly inhibits spontaneous firing in the dorsal raphe. 5HT has a complex role in anxiety and interacts in multiple ways with other neurotransmitters. The effect of buspirone in treating anxiety may involve multiple neurotransmitter systems in the midbrain; hence the term "midbrain modulator" (6).

PHARMACOKINETICS

Buspirone is absorbed rapidly and undergoes extensive first-pass metabolism. After oral administration, plasma concentrations of unchanged buspirone are low. Peak plasma concentrations of 1 to 6 ng/ml occur 40 to 90 minutes after a single oral dose of 20 mg. Food may decrease the presystemic clearance of buspirone, resulting in an increased area under the plasma-concentration-time curve and an increased peak-plasma concentration. Buspirone demonstrates nonlinear pharmacokinetics. Therefore, a dosage increase may result in a greater increase in steady-state plasma concentrations than would have been predicted. Buspirone is approximately 95% protein bound. It is metabolized primarily by oxidative mechanisms producing several hydroxylated metabolites, one of which is active, 1-pyrimidinylpiperazine (1-PP). 1-PP probably contributes little or nothing to antianxiety effects. The mean half-life of elimination of unchanged buspirone after single doses of 10 to 40 mg is 2 to 3 hours. Although not studied extensively, clearance appears to be unaffected by age, but it decreases markedly in patients with cirrhosis and to a lesser extent in patients with renal impairment (52).

DOSING AND ONSET OF ACTION

Because of its short half-life, buspirone is generally given in three divided doses per day. The most common maintenance range is 20 to 30 mg/d (53), but many clinicians now advocate the use of 30 to 60 mg/d in order to achieve optimal response (see Table 53.5) (8).

Unlike BZDs, at least 1 to 2 weeks are required before onset of antianxiety activity, and maximal effects may require up to 6 weeks.

ADVERSE EFFECTS

In general, buspirone causes less sedation and fewer psychomotor difficulties than BZDs. Dizziness, nausea, and headache occur with a frequency greater than 5% (53). Drowsiness can be seen with doses greater than 20 mg/d, and dysphoria has been reported with doses exceeding 30 to 40 mg/d (see Table 53.6).

DRUG INTERACTIONS

Concurrent use of buspirone and MAOIs is not recommended because an elevation in blood pressure may occur. The concurrent administration of trazodone and buspirone has been reported to cause a three- to sixfold elevation in ALT levels; however, the combination is frequently used clinically with little difficulty. Buspirone may displace digoxin from plasma proteins. Serum haloperidol concentrations may be increased by buspirone. Levels of buspirone metabolites may be increased by cimetidine (6). Unlike the benzodiazepines, buspirone lacks a pharmacokinetic interaction with alcohol and does not potentiate the impairment in psychomotor performance caused by alcohol (40).

DEPENDENCE, WITHDRAWAL, AND ABUSE

Unlike BZDs, buspirone does not produce physical dependence, withdrawal symptoms, or abuse (6).

PATIENT EDUCATION

As with most medications, patients taking buspirone should inform the clinician if they are pregnant, plan to become pregnant, or are breast-feeding. Patients are well advised to not drive or engage in other potentially hazardous activities until they know how the medication affects them.

Patients should be well educated on the relatively low sedative profile (relative to BZDs) and on the delayed onset of therapeutic effects. If patients are educated on the lack of potential for causing physiologic dependence, they are more likely to willingly sacrifice immediate sedative and antianxiety effects and comply with treatment.

Beta-Blockers

INDICATIONS

Propranolol is considered to be a less effective antianxiety agent than BZDs. Propranolol may be considered useful in selected GAD patients with prominent cardiovascular symptoms of anxiety, such as tachycardia, palpitations, and tremor (6).

Single-dose beta-blocker treatment is likely to be effective for performance anxiety (54). Atenolol appeared to be more helpful in discrete SP than in generalized SP in a placebo-controlled study; however, the sample size of the subtype was too small to draw definitive conclusions (55).

Propranolol-treated PTSD patients were reported to have fewer intrusive thoughts and nightmares and to experience less explosiveness and autonomic instability (56).

Beta-blocker therapy for PD is considered controversial. Thus far, two controlled trials evaluating propranolol in PD offered conflicting results (36).

PHARMACOKINETICS

Propranolol is almost completely absorbed after oral administration but undergoes extensive first-pass metabolism. Propranolol exhibits high lipid solubility and is highly bound to plasma proteins. The elimination half-life is approximately 3 to 5 hours (57).

Atenolol is about 50% absorbed after oral administration and exhibits minimal hepatic metabolism. Lipid solubility and protein binding are considered to be very low. Atenolol is eliminated primarily unchanged in the urine, and the half-life is about 6 to 7 hours (57).

DOSING

Propranolol is usually dosed every 8 hours, whereas atenolol can be dosed once daily. Propranolol doses used in treatment of most anxiety symptoms are 40 to 360 mg/d although standard doses have not been firmly established (42). For treating SP, 40 to 120 mg/d of propranolol is recommended, and for performance anxiety, 10 to 20 mg as a single dose, taken 1 hour before the performance, may be effective (see Table 53.5) (42).

Several problems exist with respect to dosing of beta-blockers. First, the dosage must be titrated against common side effects as well as efficacy. Many patients cannot be titrated upward to sufficient anxiolytic doses because of bradycardia and/or hypotension. Second, beta-blockers should not be abruptly discontinued, but rather gradually tapered to avoid adverse cardiovascular effects and rebound anxiety (58).

ADVERSE EFFECTS

Beta-blocker therapy is generally well tolerated if patients are well selected. Beta-blockers are contraindicated in patients with sinus bradycardia, greater than first-degree atrioventricular block, congestive heart failure, and bronchial asthma. They can worsen Raynaud's syndrome and other peripheral vascular diseases. In addition, beta-blockers can mask symptoms of hypoglycemia in diabetics. CNS side effects, such as depression and nightmares, are more likely to be seen with propranolol than atenolol because of differences in lipid solubility and CNS penetration. Common side effects such as bradycardia and hypotension necessitate careful monitoring of the patient's vital signs (see Table 53.6).

DRUG INTERACTIONS

When given along with oral hypoglycemics or insulin, beta-blockers may impair glycemic control and may mask symptoms of hypoglycemia. When taken with sympathomimetics having both alpha- and beta-adrenergic effects, beta-blockade results in unopposed alpha-adrenergic activity, which can lead to significant elevations in blood pressure and excessive bradycardia. Beta-blockers can potentiate the antihypertensive effects of other hypotension-producing drugs. Beta-blockers can inhibit the hepatic metabolism of theophylline, and mutual inhibition of therapeutic effects is possible with this drug combination (57).

Tricyclic Antidepressants (TCAs)

INDICATIONS

TCAs are not traditionally considered to be treatments for GAD; however, results from several placebo-controlled studies have confirmed their efficacy. One such study revealed comparable efficacy of imipramine, trazodone, and diazepam in treating GAD patients who did not have comorbid major depression or PD. Although diazepam-treated patients showed the most improvement during the first 2 weeks of treatment, imipramine exhibited somewhat better anxiolytic efficacy when compared to diazepam during the last 6 weeks of treatment (59).

Imipramine is the most widely studied TCA in treating PD, and its efficacy is now well established. More recently, clomipramine has been reported by some investigators to be superior to imipramine in the treatment of PD, and one study reported the efficacy of doses as low as 25 mg/d (8).

Clomipramine is well-documented in several double-blind trials to be effective in treatment of OCD, and it is currently one of only three drugs with FDA-approval for this indication.

The TCAs have the most solidly established efficacy in treatment of core-intrusive PTSD symptoms. Imipramine and amitriptyline have produced positive results in placebo-controlled studies involving veterans with PTSD (60).

PHARMACOKINETICS

TCAs are rapidly and completely absorbed following oral administration, but bioavailability is limited because of first-pass metabolism. Plasma levels vary widely between individuals because of genetic differences in hepatic metabolism, lipid solubility, and/or extent of protein binding (57).

TCAs are very lipid soluble, and protein binding is greater than 90%. TCAs are metabolized primarily by the liver to active metabolites. Amitriptyline and imipramine are demethylated to nortriptyline and desipramine, respectively. Doxepin and clomipramine also have demethylated active metabolites. Many TCAs also have hydroxylated metabolites (57).

The elimination half-life varies widely between various TCAs and among individuals but is considered approximately 24 hours for most agents (57).

DOSING

In low to moderate doses, the entire dose of a TCA can usually be administered once daily at bedtime to take advantage of its sedative effect. Ordinarily, TCA therapy for PD is initiated at a relatively low dose (imipramine 10 to 25 mg/d) and increased gradually to maximize compliance and minimize side effects, especially a hyperstimulatory reaction. Patients treated with TCAs for PTSD, GAD, and PD respond to a wide range of doses although typically the antidepressant dosing range of the TCA (50 to 300 mg/d) is required. Patients treated with clomipramine for OCD usually require 150 to 250 mg/d (see Table 53.5).

ADVERSE EFFECTS

The most common side effects seen with TCAs include sedation, orthostatic hypotension, and anticholinergic effects. Twenty percent of PD patients taking TCAs experience a hyperstimulatory reaction characterized by intensification of anxiety symptoms, agitation, tachycardia, and insomnia. Medication compliance suffers in many patients who manifest this side effect (61). Patients who experience this side effect require low initial doses and very gradual upward titration (see Table 53.6).

DRUG INTERACTIONS

Concurrent use of MAOIs with TCAs has resulted in hypertensive crisis, hyperpyretic episodes, convulsions, and death. The combination has been used safely when both drugs are cautiously initiated simultaneously or when the MAOI is gradually added to the TCA; however, a TCA should never be added to an existing MAOI regimen. It is recommended that TCA–MAOI combination therapy be undertaken only under the supervision of a clinician experienced in prescribing this combination. TCAs can antagonize the antihypertensive action of clonidine and guanethidine. Concurrent use of sympathomimetics with TCAs may potentiate cardiovascular effects, possibly resulting in arrhythmias, tachycardia, or severe hypertension. Medications that can increase plasma TCA levels, possibly resulting in toxicity, include cimetidine, phenothiazines, fluoxetine, sertraline, and paroxetine (57).

Monoamine Oxidase Inhibitors (MAOIs)

INDICATIONS

Phenelzine blocked panic attacks in 100% of PD patients and 95% of agoraphobic patients in an open trial (62). In addition, many placebo-controlled trials have shown the MAOIs, particularly phenelzine, to be effective antipanic agents. Unfortunately, the side effect profile and dietary restrictions preclude the routine use of MAOIs in most PD patients despite good efficacy.

Seventy-four patients with SP completed an 8-week double-blind, randomized, placebo-controlled study comparing phenelzine and atenolol. The overall response rates were 64% for phenelzine, 30% for atenolol, and 23% for placebo. Patients with generalized SP were preferentially responsive to phenelzine (55).

Several open studies suggested possible effectiveness of phenelzine in treating PTSD. The efficacy of phenelzine was confirmed in an 8-week, double-blind, randomized trial in 34 veterans comparing imipramine, phenelzine, and placebo. Patients in both active treatment groups improved. Treatment-responsive symptoms included nightmares, flashbacks, and intrusive recollections, but not avoidance (63).

PHARMACOKINETICS

MAOIs are rapidly and completely absorbed from the gastrointestinal tract, undergo rapid oxidative metabolism in the liver, and are renally eliminated (57).

DOSING

MAOIs are usually administered on a twice-daily schedule. The usual therapeutic dosage range for phenelzine in treatment of anxiety disorders is 45 to 90 mg/d (see Table 53.5).

ADVERSE EFFECTS

Common adverse effects of MAOIs include weight gain, orthostatic hypotension, edema, and sexual dysfunction (acronym: WOES). Drowsiness is more common with phenelzine, whereas tranylcypromine tends to cause overstimulation. Insomnia can be problematic with both phenelzine and tranylcypromine. MAOIs cause fewer anticholinergic effects than TCAs but more problematic orthostatic hypotension (64). Because of this side effect profile as well as dietary and drug restrictions (see "Drug Interactions"), patients generally prefer other antianxiety medications to MAOI therapy (see Table 53.6).

DRUG INTERACTIONS

The serotonin syndrome and hypertensive crisis are potentially lethal reactions attributed to drug interactions with MAOIs. The serotonin syndrome is a hyperserotonergic state manifested by confusion, restlessness, myoclonus, hyperreflexia, diaphoresis, shivering, tremor, diarrhea, and/or fever. Drugs such as clomipramine (and other TCAs), meperidine, SSRIs, tryptophan, dextromethorphan, and trazodone can cause the serotonin syndrome when taken concurrently with MAOIs. Hypertensive crisis, manifested by hypertension, severe headache, stiff or sore neck, nausea, and vomiting, can be caused by using MAOIs with sympathomimetics (ephedrine, pseudoephedrine, amphetamines, phenylephrine, phenylpropanolamine, levodopa, and so on), tyramine-containing foods, and TCAs (65).

Selective Serotonin Reuptake Inhibitors (SSRIs)

INDICATIONS

Currently available SSRIs include fluoxetine, sertraline, paroxetine, and fluvoxamine.

Drugs with clearly established efficacy in the treatment of OCD have serotonin-reuptake-inhibiting properties. Controlled studies have revealed positive effects of fluoxetine, sertraline, and fluvoxamine on obsessive–compulsive symptoms; fluoxetine and fluvoxamine are approved by the FDA for treatment of OCD. Fluoxetine was found to be as effective as clomipramine in treating OCD, but with fewer side effects (66).

Although not extensively evaluated, the SSRIs have been used successfully in the treatment of PD. In one study, 19 of 25 patients showed a moderate-to-marked improvement on fluoxetine (67).

A significant reduction in symptoms occurred when PTSD patients took fluoxetine in a double-blind, placebo-controlled study. Of particular interest is the apparent ability of the SSRIs to treat the avoidance and numbing symptoms of PTSD in trials thus far (60).

Three open trials have examined fluoxetine's efficacy in SP, and all yielded moderately effective results (68).

PHARMACOKINETICS

The SSRIs are generally well absorbed orally although the rate of absorption is slow (t_{max} = 5-8 hr). Food may decrease the rate, but not the extent, of the absorption of fluoxetine, whereas it may increase the C_{max} and bioavailability of sertraline. All the SSRIs are highly protein bound (more than 95%) except fluvoxamine, which is only 77% protein bound (69).

The SSRIs undergo extensive hepatic metabolism. Fluoxetine and sertraline are metabolized to active metabolites norfluoxetine and desmethylsertraline, respectively. It should be noted, however, that desmethylsertraline retains only a small fraction of the pharmacologic activity of the parent drug. Paroxetine and fluvoxamine have no active metabolites. The half-lives of fluoxetine and norfluoxetine are 2 to 3 days and 7 to 9 days, respectively. The half-lives of sertraline and desmethylsertraline are 26 hours and 62 to 104 hours, respectively. The half-life of paroxetine is approximately 10 to 16 hours, and that of fluvoxamine is 15 hours. Following multiple administration of fluoxetine or paroxetine, $t_{1/2}$ and AUC values are greatly increased, possibly due to these drugs inhibiting their own metabolism. Sertraline exhibits linear pharmacokinetics over its clinically relevant dosage range (69).

DOSING

SSRIs are generally dosed once daily in the morning to avoid insomnia; however, fluvoxamine is initiated as a single daily dose at bedtime, with daily doses exceeding 100 mg given in two divided doses. One must bear in mind that changes in the dose of fluoxetine are not fully reflected in the plasma for several weeks because of the long elimination half-life of both parent drug and active metabolite (42). Sertraline, paroxetine, and fluvoxamine, however, can have doses adjusted at weekly intervals.

In treating most patients with anxiety disorders, typical antidepressant doses of the various SSRIs are required. Starting doses are lower (fluoxetine 5 mg/d; sertraline 25 mg/d), and titration is more gradual when treating PD because of possible hyperstimulatory reactions (see Table 53.5).

ADVERSE EFFECTS

SSRIs are relatively free of anticholinergic, orthostatic, and sedative effects. Sexual dysfunction is a common side effect of SSRIs. Common reasons for the discontinuation of SSRIs include nervousness, nausea, insomnia, and anxiety (42). A hyperstimulatory reaction can occur in SSRI-treated PD patients as previously described for TCAs (see Table 53.6).

DRUG INTERACTIONS

SSRIs should not be used concurrently with MAOIs because of the risk of precipitating the serotonin syndrome. A sufficient washout phase should be observed after discontinuation of either medication before therapy is initiated with the other. A full 5 weeks should lapse after discontinuing fluoxetine before a MAOI is initiated. Concurrent use with tryptophan can result in agitation, restlessness, and gastrointestinal distress (57). All SSRIs, especially fluoxetine, can increase TCA levels to possible toxicity (69). Fluvoxamine inhibits the metabolism of propranolol, warfarin, theophylline, and carbamazepine. Fluoxetine inhibits the metabolism of carbamazepine and diazepam. Paroxetine reduces digoxin clearance, and prolongs bleeding time in patients receiving warfarin. Sertraline inhibits the metabolism of diazepam and warfarin (69).

PHARMACOTHERAPY OF ANXIETY

Anxiety disorders that have been shown to respond to psychopharmacologic agents include GAD, PD, OCD, PTSD, and SP.

Generalized Anxiety Disorder (GAD)

Pharmacotherapy of GAD should be used as part of a comprehensive treatment plan that includes nondrug approaches, such as psychologic and behavioral therapies (6). The BZDs, buspirone, TCAs, and to a lesser extent, the beta-blockers are the most appropriate pharmacologic alternatives (see Table 53.8 and Fig. 53.1).

All BZDs are considered to be equally effective as antianxiety agents, and selection of one agent over another

Table 53.8.
Efficacy of Various Drug Classes in Treatment of Anxiety Disorders

	GAD	OCD	PD	PTSD	SP
BZD	X		X[a]		X[a]
Buspirone	X				
B-blocker					X
TCA	X	X[b]	X	X	
MAOI			X	X	X
SSRI		X	X	X	X

[a]High potency (i.e., alprazolam, clonazepam)
[b]Clomipramine

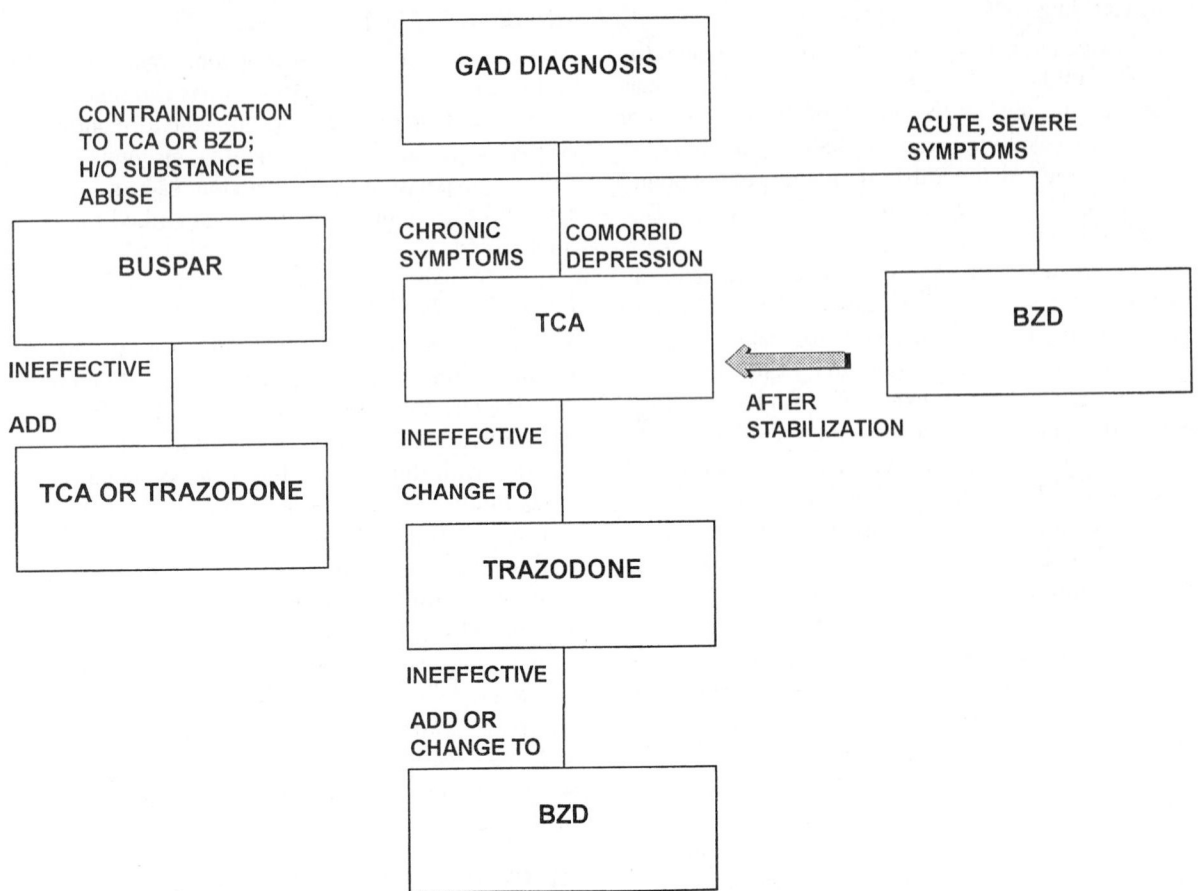

Figure 53.1. Algorithm for treatment of generalized anxiety disorder (adapted from Workman EA, Tellian FF. Practical Handbook of Psychopharmacology. Ann Arbor: CRC Press, 1994, ch 7).

is usually based on pharmacokinetic properties and the patient's clinical situation, medical status, and history of response and tolerability. Approximately three-fourths of GAD patients treated with BZDs demonstrate at least moderate improvement (6). Predictors of response include acuteness of symptoms, presence of a precipitating stress, high level of psychic and somatic anxiety, low level of depression and interpersonal problems, lack of previous treatment or good response to previous treatment, expectation of recovery, desire for medications, awareness that symptoms are psychologic, and improvement during the first week of treatment (6).

In treating GAD, the lowest effective BZD dose for the shortest possible period should be used. Periodic attempts at drug discontinuation should be made after assessments of patient needs. Many clinicians attempt to gradually discontinue BZDs after several months of therapy. For patients who relapse, intermittent treatment (lasting weeks to months) coinciding with the fluctuating nature of the illness is often effective. Some patients may need to continue the medication long term because of frequent relapses, persistent stresses, inability to resolve conflict, or

risk of suffering physical harm from chronic anxiety (6). Major risks associated with long-term use (e.g., dependence and impaired psychomotor function) must be weighed against the benefits of BZD therapy (6).

Buspirone therapy offers several advantages over BZD therapy. Because buspirone carries no obvious risk for abuse, dependence, or withdrawal, it is an appropriate choice for GAD patients with a prior history of drug abuse and patients likely to need long-term treatment. Buspirone causes fewer CNS side effects such as sedation and psychomotor and cognitive impairment, and does not enhance the sedation or psychomotor impairment of alcohol or other CNS depressants. The major disadvantage of buspirone is that it takes several weeks before a significant effect occurs, whereas BZDs exert their effects quickly. Thus, buspirone is not an appropriate choice for patients requiring immediate relief of anxiety. Moreover, buspirone must be taken on a continuous basis to exert anxiolysis, so it cannot serve as an as-needed medication. The dosing of buspirone is more cumbersome because it generally requires a three-times-daily schedule (8).

Response rates achieved with buspirone are comparable to those seen with BZDs (41). However, evidence suggests that the psychological symptoms of anxiety respond to buspirone better than the physical symptoms of anxiety (70). Furthermore, it is a common belief that former users of BZDs may respond less well to buspirone (41). A potential reason for this peculiarity is that the subjective effect of buspirone compares unfavorably with the sedative-euphoric effects of BZDs (70). Another explanation is that patients recently withdrawn from BZDs and placed on buspirone experience BZD withdrawal, which goes unblocked by the noncross-tolerant azapirone (70). Lastly, patients who have previously experienced rapid anxiety relief with a BZD may be dissatisfied with the delayed onset of antianxiety effects associated with buspirone. When switching a patient from a BZD to buspirone, it is appropriate that buspirone be added to BZD treatment for 2 to 4 weeks before the BZD taper begins (6).

Results from several well-controlled studies suggest that TCAs may have a significant role in the treatment of GAD (8). Antidepressants are useful for chronic subpanic anxiety and anxiety associated with depression (6). The inherent concerns associated with chronic BZD use make TCA therapy a particularly attractive alternative for long-term management of GAD. In terms of cost, generic preparations of the TCAs are considerably less expensive than buspirone (41). A disadvantage of TCA therapy is a greater incidence of side effects that may be problematic for anxious patients (41). Patients nonresponsive to TCA therapy may benefit from trazodone. Trazodone is a nontricylic antidepressant that may improve anxiety as well as depressive symptoms. Trazodone can cause sedation as well as orthostatic hypotension. TCA therapy should be initiated with small doses and titrated upward gradually in order to minimize these effects (8). The onset of the anxiolytic action is gradual, and the effectiveness of the TCA tends to increase over subsequent weeks (8).

Combination strategies have been used in cases of treatment-resistant anxiety. Although not systematically examined, selected individuals may benefit from various combinations involving BZDs, buspirone, TCAs, and beta-blockers (41).

Panic Disorder (PD)

Psychopharmacologic agents with proven efficacy in the treatment of patients with PD are shown in Table 53.8. The efficacy of BZDs and antidepressants is not solely restricted to panic attacks, but includes other components of the disorder such as anticipatory anxiety, depression, and phobic avoidance (36).

Alprazolam is the BZD traditionally used for treating PD, but other high-potency agents considered effective include clonazepam, lorazepam, and diazepam (8). A daily dose of between 2 and 6 mg is usually sufficient for most PD patients taking alprazolam, but higher doses are sometimes required (41). In general, total daily doses for BZDs in PD tend to be much higher than those in GAD (41). A switch from alprazolam to clonazepam has been deemed beneficial for patients experiencing interdose symptom breakthrough presumably due to clonazepam's longer half-life (36). Patients failing to respond to one BZD may respond to another one (41).

One advantage of BZD therapy in PD is the rapid onset of effect, which typically occurs within 1 to 2 weeks (41). Further, the BZDs have an overall favorable side effect profile (8) and are better tolerated than antidepressants (36). However, sedation is a troublesome side effect that affects a substantial number of PD patients taking BZDs, especially early in treatment (36). Another disadvantage of BZD therapy is the difficulty discontinuing treatment because of withdrawal and reemergence of panic (41). Whereas dependence and withdrawal are realistic concerns, patients with PD rarely abuse BZDs, and abuse is more likely to occur among patients with a personal or family history of drug or alcohol abuse (71). It should be noted that comorbidity of PD and alcoholism is not uncommon (36). There is no evidence of tolerance to BZDs, and hence increasing dosage requirements with long-term treatment of PD (8).

Advantages of antidepressants relative to BZDs include lack of concern over dependence, withdrawal, or abuse and antidepressant efficacy as well as antipanic efficacy (8). Disadvantages of antidepressants include a delayed onset of effects (4 to 6 weeks) and hyperstimulatory reactions that complicate therapy and affect compliance (8). Antidepressants should be chosen for those PD patients with a history of substance abuse, those with prominent depression, or those who do not tolerate BZDs (see Fig. 53.2) (71).

Imipramine and clomipramine are the two TCAs most studied for PD, but other TCAs, such as desipramine and nortriptyline, are probably effective as well (8). TCAs have the advantage of once-daily dosing, but have the disadvantage of causing side effects that prevent dose increases to optimal levels in a substantial portion of PD patients (8). Recent research conducted to examine therapeutic plasma levels of TCAs in PD and agoraphobia has revealed that imipramine levels of approximately 125 to 150 ng/ml and desipramine levels above 125 ng/ml may be optimal (8).

Some clinicians believe that MAOIs may have superior efficacy, particularly in treatment-resistant patients (41). However, the potential dangerous side effects and drug interactions of MAOIs restrict their use in PD (36). MAOIs should be reserved for the most severely ill or treatment-refractory patients (see Fig. 53.2) (71).

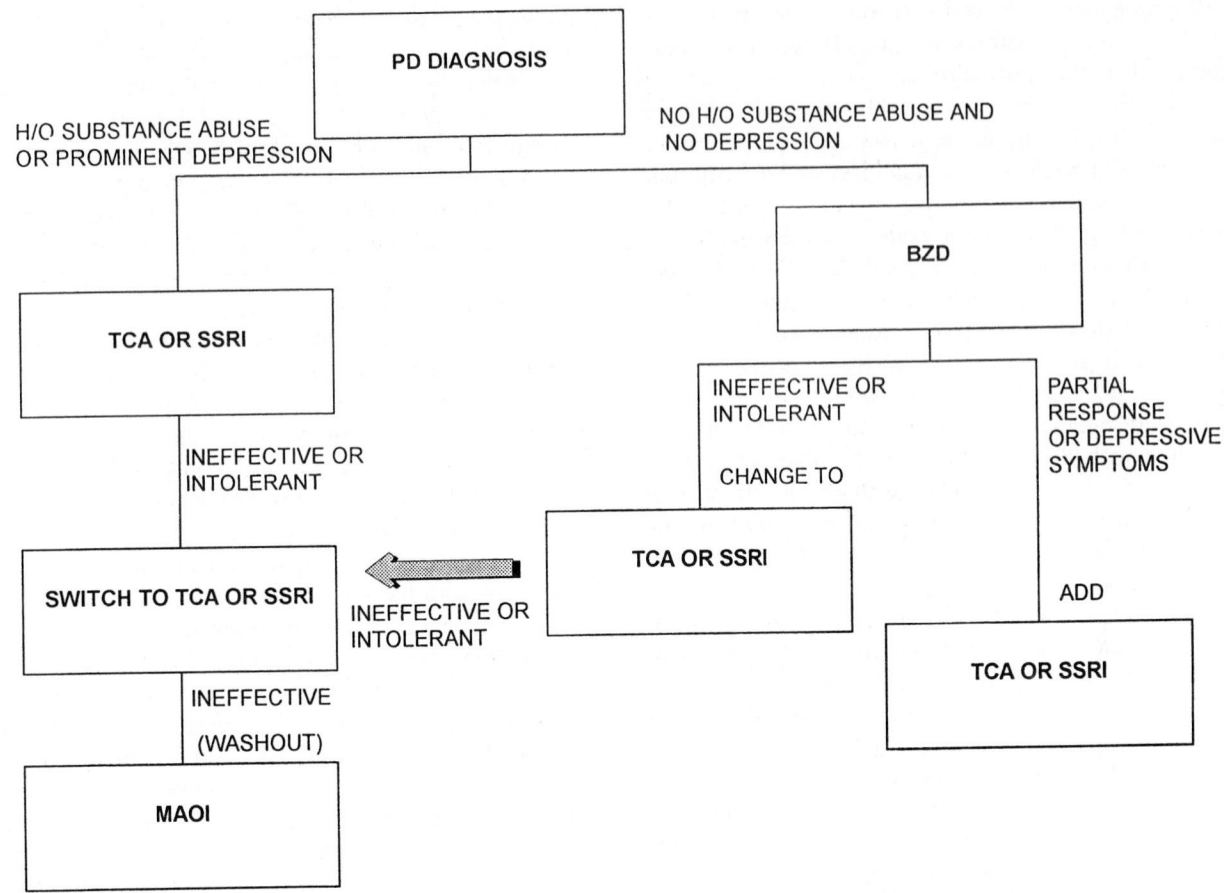

Figure 53.2. Algorithm for treatment of panic disorder.

SSRIs share the aforementioned advantages of antidepressants over BZDs, and they have a favorable side effect profile compared to TCAs and MAOIs. Thus, many clinicians now consider SSRIs to be first-line treatment for PD (8,41). Hyperstimulatory reactions occur in some patients, but fluoxetine is well tolerated by most patients when treatment is initiated at 5 mg/d and titrated cautiously (8).

Various clinical scenarios have dictated combined BZD and antidepressant use in PD. Antidepressants can be added when depressive symptoms emerge during BZD monotherapy (8). Combination therapy may also be used in cases of treatment-resistant PD (41). Finally, combination therapy early in treatment followed by a taper of the BZD has been used as a strategy to avoid the long-term use of BZDs and to circumvent the slow onset of action of antidepressants (36).

PD is a chronic illness (41), but some patients enjoy periods without panic attacks (36). A treatment period of 6 to 12 months followed by a gradual discontinuation phase has been suggested for BZDs (36). One-year maintenance treatment with imipramine can protect against relapse, even with a much lower dose than required during acute

treatment (8). However, many PD patients may require several years of drug therapy; indefinite therapy may be the plight of some patients (71).

Behavioral treatment is also effective for PD. The combination of behavioral treatment and drug treatment may be optimal for many PD patients. Unfortunately, nearly one-half of PD patients continue to experience some degree of symptoms during the course of their illness despite treatment (8).

Obsessive–Compulsive Disorder

Drugs that inhibit serotonin reuptake, such as clomipramine and the SSRIs, are clearly beneficial in the treatment of OCD (Table 53.8). These drugs can decrease the devastating symptoms and improve the patient's quality of life (72). However, there are caveats concerning pharmacotherapy of OCD. First, these drugs may be more effective for obsessions than for compulsions (72). Second, only approximately a 40 to 60% reduction in symptomatology is seen with pharmacotherapy alone, so many patients will continue to be symptomatic even after adequate trials of medications (8). Superior response may be seen with the combination of pharmacotherapy and behavior therapy, such that 80% of patients experience at least moderate improvement with the combined modalities (73). Further, behavior therapy may quicken the response to medications and reduce the likelihood of relapse after medication discontinuation (8).

Concerning comparative efficacy, clomipramine may be slightly more effective than the SSRIs, but clomipramine therapy is more problematic than SSRI therapy because of its typical TCA side-effect profile, seizure risk, and toxicity on overdose (73). Patients may respond differentially to the various SSRIs, so sequential trials may be worthwhile in light of nonresponse to a particular agent (8).

In order to minimize side effects, starting doses of these agents should be low, and dose escalation should be gradual (73). The SSRIs are more likely than clomipramine to cause an initial hyperstimulatory effect (73). Up to 250 mg/d of clomipramine may be required for maximum effect, and the dosage ranges for the SSRIs are comparable to those used in treating depression. Although individual patients may preferentially respond to higher doses of the SSRIs, comparable efficacy can generally be achieved with relatively lower doses (8). Doses may be reduced in the maintenance phase once a response has been achieved (73).

Response of OCD symptoms to pharmacotherapy occurs slowly, such that improvement may be noted after about 3 to 4 weeks, and a graded improvement continues

up to 10 to 12 weeks (73). Duration of treatment is debated; however, most practitioners agree that drug treatment should be continued for at least 1 year before gradual discontinuation is considered (73). Relapse may be a likely consequence of medication discontinuation (72).

Treatment-resistant patients may respond to augmentation with agents such as lithium, buspirone, or fenfluramine (Fig. 53.3). These agents may act by enhancement of serotonin function (74). Although touted as effective in case reports and open trials, the augmentation potential of these agents has been disappointing in controlled studies (8). Nevertheless, in refractory patients, augmentation strategies are justified since individual patients may experience beneficial results (8).

Posttraumatic Stress Disorder (PTSD)

Pharmacotherapeutic studies have demonstrated that the symptoms of PTSD respond to medication (Table 53.8), but it is also clear that most patients receiving pharmacotherapy experience limited gains and continue to meet the diagnostic criteria for PTSD even after successful treatment. The treatment plan should be a broadly based one, including various combinations of psychopharmacologic, psychodynamic, and behavioral treatments (60). Furthermore, pharmacotherapy may enhance the efficacy of the other forms of treatment (60).

The goals of pharmacotherapy in PTSD include reduction of intrusive symptoms, improvement of avoid-

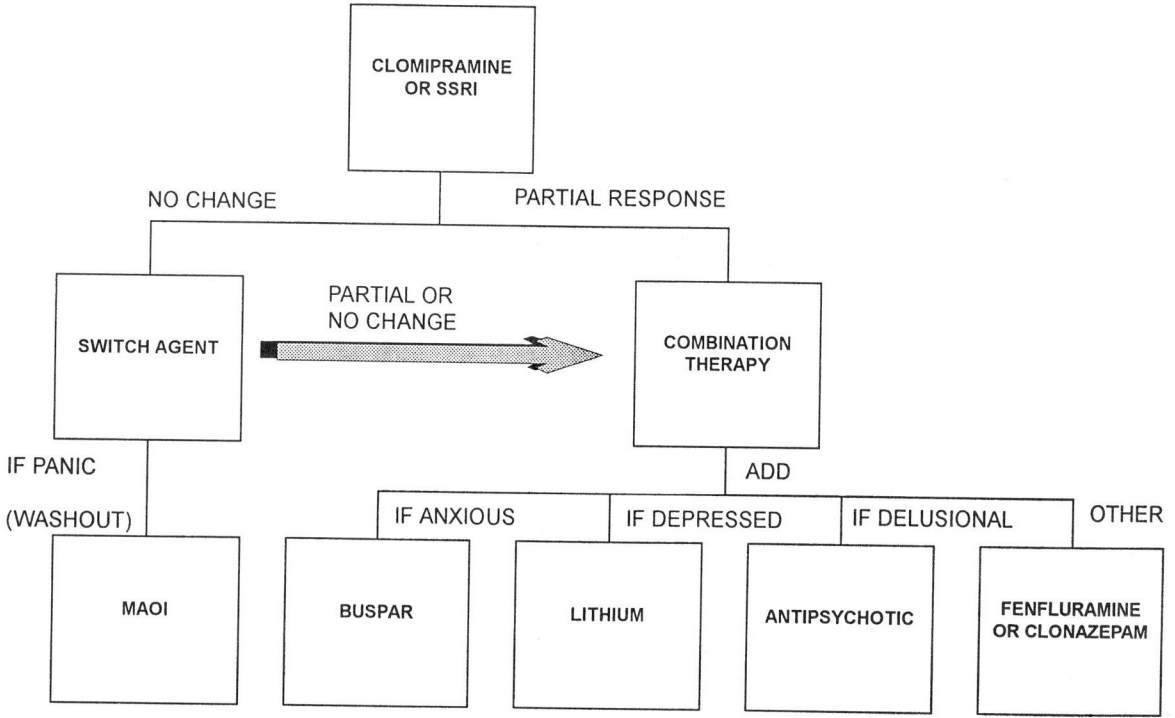

Figure 53.3. Algorithm for treatment of obsessive–compulsive disorder (adapted from reference 74).

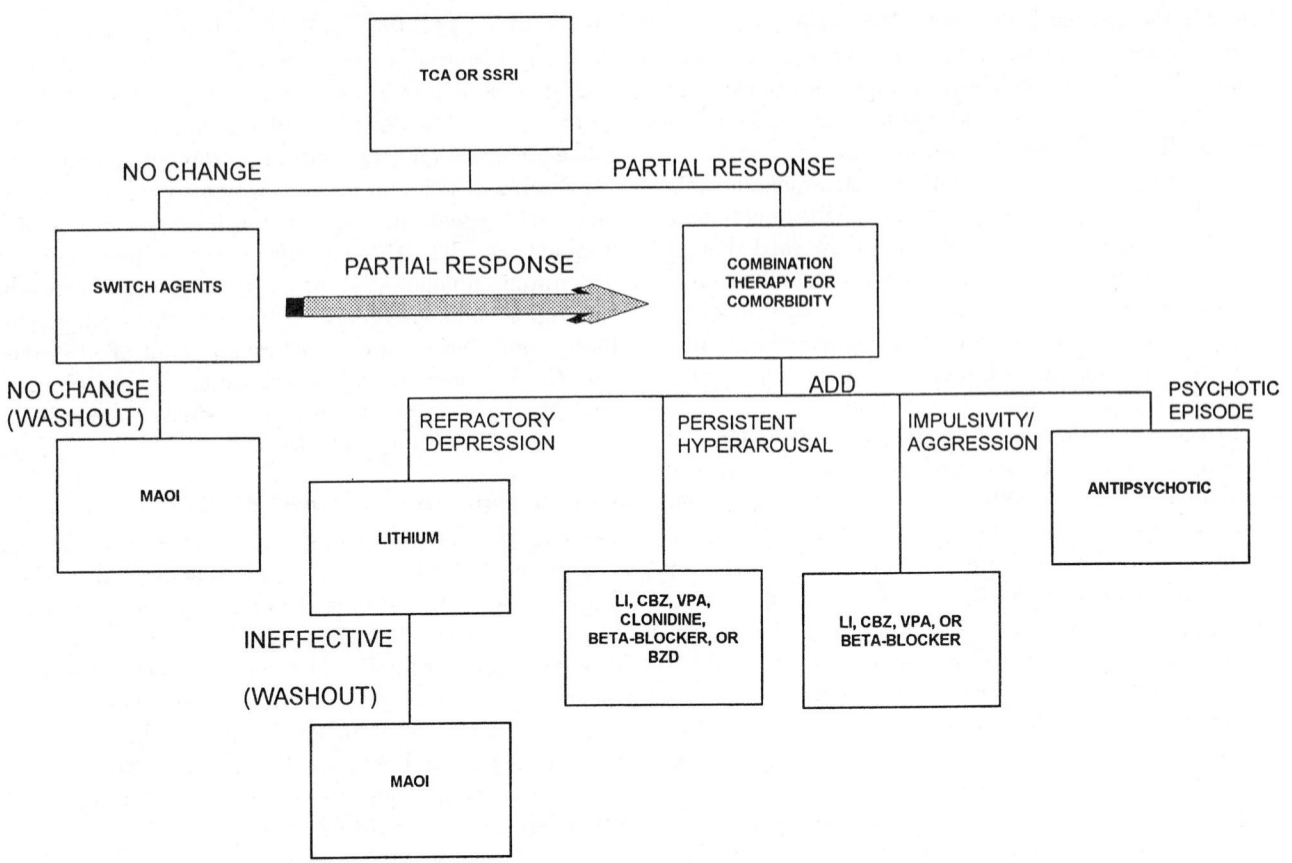

Figure 53.4.   Algorithm for treatment of posttraumatic stress disorder (adapted from references 60 and 77).

ance symptoms, reduction of hyperarousal, relief of depression, control of impulsivity, control of psychotic features, and facilitation of psychotherapy (75). Interestingly, the symptom picture of PTSD can fluctuate over the course of the illness; thus, treatment goals may differ from time to time in the same patient (76).

Placebo-controlled studies have disclosed both positive and negative outcomes with respect to efficacy of pharmacotherapy for core PTSD symptoms. Although these studies are limited in quantity, several conclusions have been drawn about factors that differentiate positive from negative trials. First, positive trials have involved drugs with prominent serotonergic effects, such as amitriptyline, imipramine, phenelzine, and fluoxetine. Two of the 3 negative trials involved the nonserotonergic agents alprazolam and desipramine. Next, positive trials have tended to use high drug doses, whereas negative trials have employed lower doses. Finally, positive trials have had a treatment duration of up to 8 weeks, whereas negative trials have had a treatment duration of only 4 to 5 weeks (75).

Patients with PTSD often do not respond to a single medication because of persistent core symptoms as well as comorbid symptoms (see Fig. 53.4). Silver and his colleagues proposed the popular therapeutic strategy of using an antidepressant for initial pharmacologic treatment, assessing response after an adequate trial, then addressing comorbid symptoms with combination drug therapy (77). The TCAs appear to be effective for intrusive symptoms and for anxiety and depressive symptoms, but not as effective for avoidance symptoms (60). The SSRIs may differ from other medications by improving avoidance and numbing symptoms in addition to intrusive symptoms (60). The MAOIs have largely been relegated to a treatment-resistant role for reasons previously discussed. Hyperarousal symptoms, often persistent despite antidepressant therapy, and impulsive symptoms are best treated with propranolol or the mood-stabilizing drugs lithium, carbamazepine, or valproic acid. BZD therapy should be used cautiously because of the prevalence of substance abuse in this patient population, as well as the ability of BZDs to induce depression and cause behavioral disinhibition.

It may take 8 weeks or longer before beneficial effects of pharmacotherapy are evident in PTSD symptoms (60), and maximum effects may take several months. Pharmacotherapy may need to be continued for years in patients with chronic PTSD (76).

Many pharmacotherapeutic questions remain unanswered at this time. These include whether medication response varies with the type of trauma, determination of the mechanisms of action of various drugs, rates of relapse after drug discontinuation, and efficacy of drug therapy relative to psychotherapy (60).

Social Phobia (SP)

Cognitive-behavioral techniques are recognized as being quite effective for SP (41), and recently pharmacologic therapy has shown utility as a valid primary treatment option (78). The goal of drug treatment is to decrease both the fear and avoidance associated with SP. Drugs of choice in treating SP are listed in Table 53.8.

High-potency BZDs are effective for SP, with response onset occurring within 2 weeks. Typical effective doses are 1.5 to 2 mg/d of clonazepam or 3 mg/d of alprazolam (41). The long-term benefits of BZD therapy appear to be maintained over time with no obvious tolerance and minimal adverse effects (8). However, high relapse rates following BZD discontinuation (68) and potential BZD abuse in a population with a high comorbidity of alcoholism are concerning (41).

Beta-blockers are clearly effective for performance anxiety (discrete type of SP) when given about 1 hour prior to the feared event (41). Beta-blockers are probably of little benefit in the treatment of generalized SP, but a trial for acute and maintenance therapy of discrete SP is worthwhile (8).

Phenelzine has the best demonstrated efficacy in the treatment of SP, and MAOIs are especially effective for patients with generalized SP (8). Eight weeks of treatment may be required for full therapeutic effects, but approximately two-thirds of patients eventually respond to MAOI therapy (41). Of significance is the fact that a large proportion of patients maintain clinical improvement after discontinuation of MAOI therapy (78). MAOI therapy is complicated, unfortunately, by troublesome side effects and dietary restrictions.

Fluoxetine has been touted as a particularly effective treatment of SP in open trials; however, double-blind, placebo-controlled trials are sorely needed to assess the utility of the SSRIs in this disorder. It has been suggested that patients with either generalized or discrete SP are likely to respond to fluoxetine treatment (78). Interestingly, investigators have not noted hyperstimulatory effects in the

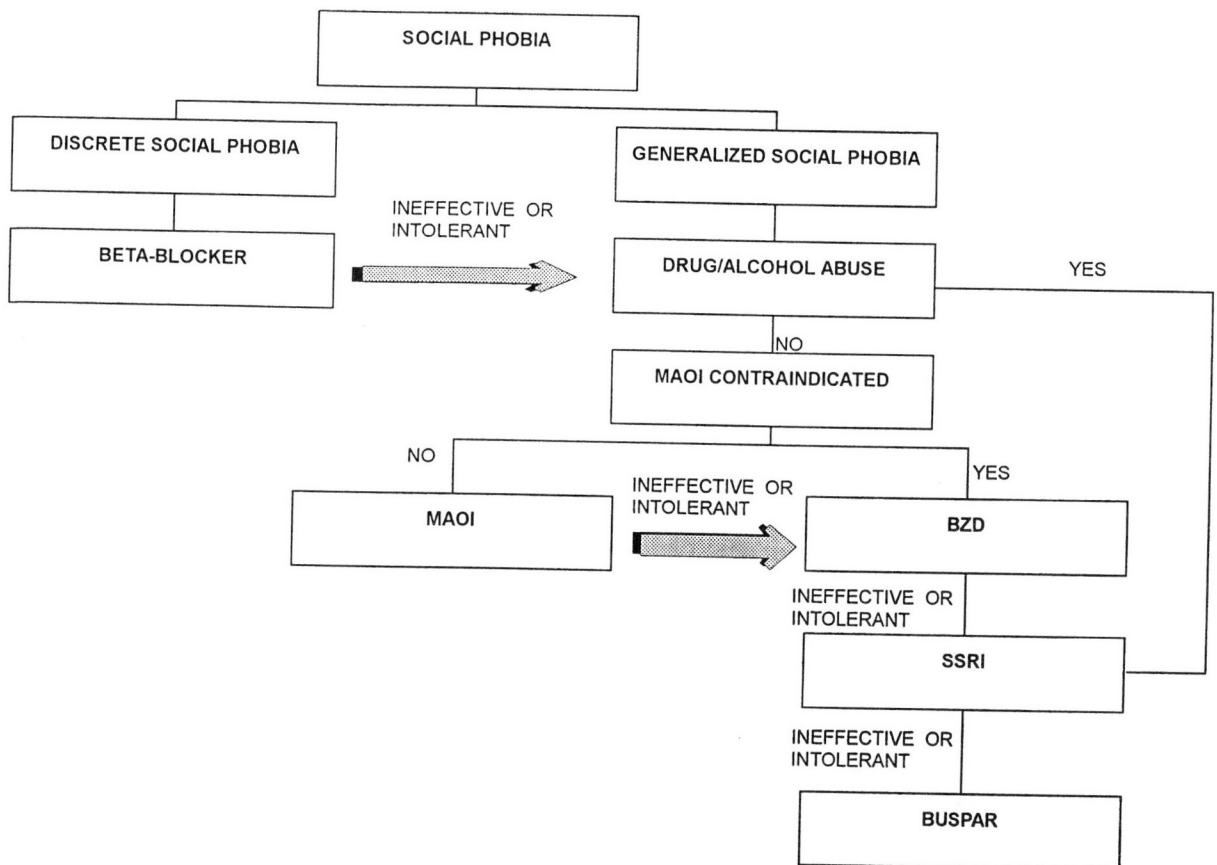

Figure 53.5. Algorithm for treatment of social phobia.

early stages of SSRI treatment of SP in contrast to what is seen frequently in PD (68).

A pharmacologic treatment algorithm is depicted in Figure 53.5. This algorithm is based on the following clinical guidelines:

1. MAOIs and BZDs are clearly effective short-term treatments for SP (8).
2. BZDs are considered first-choice medications only if MAOIs are contraindicated (8).
3. It may be useful to determine the effectiveness of beta-blocker therapy in discrete SP before committing the patient to longer-term continuous treatment with a MAOI or BZD (8).
4. The efficacy of SSRIs in treating SP is less well established, but they would be especially desirable treatment alternatives for SP patients who are poor candidates for other medications because of alcohol or drug abuse.

Additional study is required to further delineate the efficacy of different drug treatments, to determine the optimal duration of drug therapy, and to examine the potential role of combined psychotherapeutic interventions (78).

CONCLUSION

Our understanding of the anxiety disorders, their pathophysiology, epidemiology, and treatment, continues to advance. Not all patients with anxiety disorders should receive pharmacotherapy, and many of those who are appropriate candidates for antianxiety medications should also have the benefit of nonpharmacologic interventions. Accurate diagnosis is crucial to the selection of the most rational pharmacotherapy. It is now recognized that many patients with anxiety disorders have marked morbidity and that some patients are, in fact, profoundly disabled by their illness. These patients deserve the same meticulous assessment and concern as that afforded patients with chest pain. It is the responsibility of health care providers to take an active role in educating patients about their therapy, monitoring for therapeutic benefit and real and potential drug-related problems, and intervening whenever possible to maximize positive clinical outcomes.

REFERENCES

1. Weissman MM. Family genetic studies of panic disorder. J Psychiatr Res 27(Suppl 1):69–78, 1993.
2. American Psychiatric Association. Diagnostic and Statistical Manual of Mental Disorders, DSM-IV. Washington, D.C.: American Psychiatric Association, 1994, pp 393–444.
3. Charney DS, Heninger GR. Noradrenergic function and the mechanism of action of antianxiety treatment. I. The effect of long-term alprazolam treatment. Arch Gen Psychiatry 42: 458–467, 1985.
4. Owens MJ, Vargas MA, Nemeroff CB. The effects of alprazolam on corticotropin-releasing factor neurons in the rat brain: implications for a role for crf in the pathogenesis of anxiety disorders. J Psychiatr Res 27(Suppl1):209–220, 1993.
5. Charney DS, Heninger GR, Breier A. Noradrenergic function in panic anxiety. Arch Gen Psychiatry 41:751–763, 1984.

6. Dubovsky SL. Generalized anxiety disorder: new concepts and pharmacologic therapies. J Clin Psychiatry 51(Suppl):3–10, 1990.
7. Hyman SE, Nestler EJ. The Molecular Foundations of Psychiatry. Washington, D.C.: American Psychiatric Press, Inc., 1993, pp 150–157.
8. Brawman-Mintzer O, Lydiard RB. Psychopharmacology of anxiety disorders. Psychiatr Clin North Am, Annual of Drug Therapy 1:51–79, 1994.
9. Insel TR, Winslow JT. Neurobiology of obsessive compulsive disorder. Psychiatr Clin North Am 15:813–824, 1992.
10. Humble M, Wistedt B. Serotonin, panic disorder and agoraphobia: short-term and long-term efficacy of citalopram in panic disorders. Int Clin Psychopharmacol 6(Suppl 5):21–39, 1992.
11. Southwick SM, Bremner D, Krystal JH, Charney DS. Psychobiologic research in post-traumatic stress disorder. Psychiatr Clin North Am 17:251–264, 1994.
12. Kessler RC, McGonagle KA, Zhao S, et al. Lifetime and 12-month prevalence of DSM-III-R psychiatric disorders in the United States. Arch Gen Psychiatry 51:8–19, 1994.
13. Weissman MM, Bland RC, Canino GJ, et al. The cross national epidemiology of obsessive compulsive disorder: the cross national collaborative group. J Clin Psychiatry 55(Suppl 3):5–10, 1994.
14. Tomb DA. The phenomenology of post-traumatic stress disorder. Psychiatr Clin North Am 17:237–250, 1994.
15. Swinson RP, Cox BJ, Woszczyna BA. Use of medical services and treatment for panic disorder with agoraphobia and for social phobia. Can Med Assoc J 147:878–883, 1992.
16. Johnson J, Weissman MM, Klerman GL. Panic disorder, comorbidity, and suicide attempts. Arch Gen Psychiatry 47:805–808, 1990.
17. Schuckit MA. Anxiety related to medical disease. J Clin Psychiatry 44:31–36, 1983.
18. Hayes PE, Dommisse CS. Current concepts in clinical therapeutics: anxiety disorders, part I. Clin Pharm 6:140–147, 1987.
19. Cameron OG. The differential diagnosis of anxiety: psychiatric and medical disorders. Psychiatr Clin North Am 8:3–23, 1985.
20. Agras WS. The diagnosis and treatment of panic disorder. Annu Rev Med 44:39–51, 1993.
21. Bremner JD, Steinberg M, Southwick SM, et al. Use of the structured clinical interview for DSM-IV dissociative disorders for systematic assessment of dissociative symptoms in posttraumatic stress disorder. Am J Psychiatry 150:1011–1014, 1993.
22. Rosenbaum JF, Pollock RA. The psychopharmacology of social phobia and comorbid disorders. Bull Menninger Clin 58(Suppl A):A67–A83, 1994.
23. Margraf J, Barlow DH, Clark DM, et al. Psychological treatment of panic: work in progress on outcome, active ingredients, and follow-up. Behav Res Ther 31:1–8, 1993.
24. Beck AT, Sokol L, Clark DA, et al. A crossover study of focused cognitive therapy for panic disorder. Am J Psychiatry 149:778–783, 1992.
25. Otto MW, Gould RA, Pollack MH. Cognitive-behavioral treatment of panic disorder: considerations for the treatment of patients over the long term. Psychiatric Annals 24:307–315, 1994.
26. Sanderson WC, Wetzler S. Observations on the cognitive behavioral treatment of panic disorder: impact of benzodiazepines. Psychotherapy 30:125–132, 1993.
27. Taylor CB. Psychopharmacologic treatment of anxiety disorders. In The American Psychiatric Press Textbook of Psychopharmacology. Washington, D.C., American Psychiatric Press, in press, ch 32.
28. Barlow DH. Comorbidity in social phobia: implications for cognitive-behavioral treatment. Bull Menninger Clinic 58(Suppl A):A43–A57, 1994.
29. Borkovec TD, Costello E. Efficacy of applied relaxation and cognitive-behavioral therapy in the treatment of generalized anxiety disorder. J of Consulting Clinical Psychology 61:611–619, 1993.

30. Durham RC, Allan T. Psychological treatment of generalized anxiety disorder: a review of the clinical significance of results in outcome studies since 1980. Br J Psychiatry 163:19–26, 1993.

31. Munford PR, Hand I, Liberman RP. Psychosocial treatment for obsessive-compulsive disorder. Psychiatry 57:142–152, 1994.

32. McFarlane AC. Individual psychotherapy for post-traumatic stress disorder. Psychiatr Clin North Am 17:393–408, 1994.

33. Allen SN, Bloom SL. Group and family treatment of posttraumatic stress disorder. Psychiatr Clin North Am 17:425–437, 1994.

34. Bradwejn J. Benzodiazepines for the treatment of panic disorder and generalized anxiety disorder: clinical issues and future directions. Can J Psychiatry 38(Suppl 4):S109–S113, 1993.

35. Tesar GE. High-potency benzodiazepines for short-term management of panic disorder: the U.S. experience. J Clin Psychiatry 51(Suppl 9):4S–10S, 1990.

36. Rosenberg R. Drug treatment of panic disorder. Pharmacol and Toxicol 72:344–353, 1993.

37. Davidson JRT, Ford SM, Smith RD, et al. Long-term treatment of social phobia with clonazepam. J Clin Psychiatry 52(Suppl 11):16–20, 1991.

38. Braun P, Greenberg D, Dasberg H, et al. Core symptoms of posttraumatic stress disorder unimproved by alprazolam treatment. J Clin Psychiatry 51:236–238, 1990.

39. Greenblatt DJ, Shader RI, Abernethy DR. Current status of benzodiazepines, part I. New Engl J Med 309:354–358, 1983.

40. Dommisse CS, Hayes PE. Current concepts in clinical therapeutics: anxiety disorders, part II. Clin Pharm 6:196–215, 1987.

41. Roy-Byrne P, Wingerson D, Cowley D, et al. Psychopharmacologic treatment of panic, generalized anxiety disorder, and social phobia. Psychiatr Clin North Am 16:719–735, 1993.

42. Guze B, Richeimer S, Szuba M. The Psychiatric Drug Handbook. St. Louis: Mosby-Year Book, Inc., 1992, ch 2,4,7.

43. Power KG, Jerrom DWA, Simpson RJ, et al. Controlled study of withdrawal and rebound anxiety after six week course of diazepam for generalized anxiety. Br Med J 290:1246–1248, 1985.

44. Perry PJ, Alexander B, Liskow BI. Psychotropic Drug Handbook, ed. 6. Cincinnati: Harvey Whitney Books Company, 1991, p 289.

45. Busto U, Seller EM, Naranjo CA, et al. Patterns of benzodiazepine abuse and dependence. Br J Addict 81:87–94, 1986.

46. Pollack MH. Long-term management of panic disorder. J Clin Psychiatry 51(Suppl 5):11S–13S, 1990.

47. United States Pharmacopeial Convention. USP-DI, ed 14. Rockville, MD, United States Pharmacopeial Convention, 1994.

48. Rickels K. Buspirone in clinical practice. J Clin Psychiatry 51(Suppl 9):51S–54S, 1990.

49. Strand M, Hetta J, Rosen A, et al. A double-blind controlled trial in primary care patients with generalized anxiety: a comparison between buspirone and oxazepam. J Clin Psychiatry 51(Suppl 9):40–45, 1990.

50. Pato MT, Pigott TA, Hill JL, et al. Controlled comparison of buspirone and clomipramine in obsessive-compulsive disorder. Am J Psychiatry 148:127–129, 1991.

51. Munjack DJ, Bruns J, Baltazar PL, et al. A pilot study of buspirone in the treatment of social phobia. J Anx Dis 5:87–98, 1991.

52. Gammans RE, Mayol RF, Labudde JA. Metabolism and disposition of buspirone. Am J Med 80:41S–51S, 1986.

53. Mead Johnson Pharmaceutical Division/Bristol Myers. Buspar package insert. Evansville, IN, 1990.

54. Agras WS. Treatment of social phobias. J Clin Psychiatry 51(Suppl 10):52S–55S, 1990.

55. Liebowitz MR, Schneier F, Campeas R, et al. Phenelzine vs atenolol in social phobia. Arch Gen Psychiatry 49:290–300, 1992.

56. Kolb LC, Burris BC, Griffiths S. Propranolol and clonidine in the treatment of post traumatic stress disorder of war. In van der Kolk BA (ed): Post Traumatic Stress Disorders Psychological and Biological Sequelae. Washington, D.C., American Psychiatric Press, 1984, pp 29–42.

57. United States Pharmacopeial Convention. USP-DI, ed 14. Rockville, MD, United States Pharmacopeial Convention, 1994.

58. Noyes R. Beta-adrenergic blocking drugs in anxiety and stress. Psychiatr Clin North Am 8:119–132, 1985.

59. Rickels K, Downing R, Schweizer E, et al. Antidepressants for the treatment of generalized anxiety disorder: a placebo-controlled comparison of imipramine, trazodone, and diazepam. Arch Gen Psych 50:884–895, 1993.

60. Sutherland SM, Davidson JRT. Pharmacotherapy for posttraumatic stress disorder. Psychiatr Clin North Am 17:409–423, 1994.

61. Noyes R, Garvey MJ, Cook BL, et al. Problems with tricyclic antidepressant use in patients with panic disorder or agoraphobia: results of a naturalistic follow-up study. J Clin Psychiatry 50:163–169, 1989.

62. Buigues J, Vallejo J. Therapeutic response to phenelzine in patients with panic disorder and agoraphobia with panic attacks. J Clin Psychiatry 48:55–59, 1987.

63. Frank JB, Kosten TR, Giller EL, et al. A randomized clinical trial of phenelzine and imipramine for posttraumatic stress disorder. Am J Psychiatry 145:1289–1291, 1988.

64. Rabkin J, Quitkin FM, Harrison W, et al. Adverse reactions to monoamine oxidase inhibitors. Part I. a comparative study. J Clin Psychopharmacol 4:270–278, 1984.

65. Maxmen JS. Psychotropic Drugs Fast Facts. New York: W.W. Norton & Company, 1991, p 104.

66. Pigott TA, Pato MT, Bernstein SE, et al. Controlled comparisons of clomipramine and fluoxetine in the treatment of obsessive-compulsive disorder. Arch Gen Psychiatry 47:926–932, 1990.

67. Schneier FR, Liebowitz MR, Davies SO, et al. Fluoxetine in panic disorder. J Clin Psychopharmacol 10:119–121, 1990.

68. Liebowitz MR. Pharmacotherapy of social phobia. J Clin Psychiatry 54 (Suppl 12):31–35, 1993.

69. van Harten J. Clinical pharmacokinetics of selective serotonin reuptake inhibitors. Clin Pharmacokinet 24(3):203–220, 1993.

70. Sussman N. The uses of buspirone in psychiatry. J Clin Psychiatry 12:3–19, 1994.

71. Shelton RC. Pharmacotherapy of panic disorder. Hosp and Comm Psychiatry 44:725–726, 1993.

72. Jackson CW, Morton A, Lydiard RB. Pharmacologic management of obsessive-compulsive disorder. South Med J 87:310–320, 1994.

73. Rasmussen SA, Eisen JL, Pato MT. Current issues in the pharmacologic management of obsessive compulsive disorder. J Clin Psychiatry 54(Suppl 6):4–9, 1993.

74. McDougle CJ, Goodman WK, Price LH. The pharmacotherapy of obsessive-compulsive disorder. Pharmacopsychiat 26(Suppl):24–29, 1993.

75. Vargas MA, Davidson J. Post-traumatic stress disorder. Psychiatr Clin North Am 16:737–748, 1993.

76. Davidson J. Drug therapy of post-traumatic stress disorder. Br J Psychiatry 160:309–314, 1992.

77. Silver JM, Sandberg DP, Hales RE. New approaches in the pharmacotherapy of posttraumatic stress disorder. J Clin Psychiatry 51(Suppl 10):33–38, 1990.

78. Social phobia: an overview of treatment strategies. J Clin Psychiatry 54:165–171, 1993.

CHAPTER 54

MOOD DISORDERS

GLEN L. STIMMEL

Disturbances of mood include both full and partial manic and/or depressive episodes. Mood disorders involve prolonged disturbance of the expression of emotion that go beyond brief emotional upset from negative life experiences. At least one of ten people in the United States will experience a diagnosable mood disorder in their lifetime. Such a high prevalence in the general population suggests that clinicians in all treatment settings will encounter patients with mood disorders and must be familiar with their recognition and treatment.

ETIOLOGY

Although the exact etiology of mood disorders is not known, much is known about neurotransmitter systems and their relationship to mood disorders. The most clearly established biologic fact regarding mood disorders is the existence of a genetic substrate, with genetic loading greatest in bipolar illness. Some 60 to 65% of bipolar patients have a positive family history of mood disorder. Since recurrence is fundamental to most mood disorders, hypotheses that incorporate sleep and circadian rhythm as well as kindling and sensitization are being investigated. A compelling convergence of information from CT, MRI, PET, and SPECT studies of patients with depression suggests this disorder is associated with regional brain dysfunction. The many symptoms of depression are closely associated with changes in cerebral blood flow and/or metabolism in the frontal-temporal cortex and caudate nucleus (1). Much more is known about the mechanism of action of antidepressants, which provides only indirect evidence concerning an etiology for mood disorders.

Many drugs are reported to cause depression, but establishing a direct causative relationship is very difficult. Since major depression has a lifetime prevalence of greater than 6% in the United States, no drugs have been reported to cause depression with such frequency. Of greater concern is use of these drugs in patients with a history of depressive illness. These drugs include many antihypertensives (reserpine, propranolol, methyldopa, clonidine), hormones (estrogen, progesterone), corticosteroids, and several anti-Parkinson agents (levodopa, amantadine) (2).

DIAGNOSTIC CLASSIFICATION

There are two major categories of mood disorders (Table 54.1) (2, 3). The bipolar disorders are typically characterized by distinct episodes of mania and depression separated

by intervals without mood disturbance. Most bipolar patients with one or more manic episodes will eventually have a depressive episode. At any one time, a bipolar patient may be manic, hypomanic, depressed, or euthymic (normal mood) between episodes. Hypomania is a predominately elevated, expansive, or irritable mood but much less severe than a manic episode. In 50 to 60% of instances, a manic episode will be immediately preceded or followed by a major depressive episode with no euthymic period between. *Bipolar I Disorder is the more classic picture of manic and depressive episodes, whereas Bipolar II Disorder is characterized by major depressive episodes and hypomanic episodes.* The depressive episodes of bipolar disorders are clinically indistinguishable from major depressive disorder. Bipolar patients may have mixed episodes, in which both manic and depressive symptoms are present at the same time. Bipolar patients with at least four episodes of mania or depression in one year are termed rapid cyclers (4).

Cyclothymia is a milder form of bipolar illness. It is a chronic mood disturbance of greater than two years characterized by numerous periods of depression and hypomania. In the first two years, the depressive episodes are not severe enough to meet criteria for major depression, and hypomanic symptoms never reach the severity of a manic episode. Intervals of normal mood last no more than 2 months between episodes of depression and hypomania. Cyclothymic patients do not develop psychotic symptoms, rarely require hospitalization, only occasionally require drug treatment, but may often abuse alcohol or other drugs in an attempt to self-treat their mood fluctuations. Cyclothymia is frequently found in relatives of bipolar patients and is thought to represent a mild form of bipolar disorder.

Major depression includes patients who experience only one episode of depression and those who have recurrent depressive episodes. Patients with major depression are commonly referred to as unipolar. The frequency of episodes is quite variable, with some patients having episodes separated by many years of normal functioning, whereas others have frequent clusters of episodes.

Dysthymia is a chronic mood disturbance of greater than two years in which the severity of depressed mood and associated symptoms are insufficient to meet criteria for major depression (Table 54.2). Periods of normal mood last only a few days to a few weeks, but never more than 2

Table 54.1.
Classification of Mood Disorders

Bipolar Disorders
  Bipolar I
  Bipolar II
  Cyclothymic
Depressive Disorders
  Major Depression
  Dysthymia

Table 54.2.
Dysthymic Disorder

Depressed mood most of the day, more days than not, for 2 years
Characteristic symptoms while depressed (2 or more required):
  Poor appetite or overeating
  Insomnia or hypersomnia
  Low energy or fatigue
  Low self-esteem
  Poor concentration or indecisiveness
  Feelings of hopelessness
Symptoms cause significant distress or impaired social or occupational
  functioning

Adapted from reference 3.

months at a time. Dysthymic patients do not have psychotic symptoms and rarely require hospitalization.

PREVALENCE

The lifetime prevalence of bipolar I disorder is 0.4 to 1.6%, whereas bipolar II disorder is 0.5%, and cyclothymic disorder is 0.4 to 1.0%. Bipolar I and cyclothymia is equally common in men and women, whereas bipolar II is more common in women. The lifetime risk for major depression in community samples has varied from 10 to 25% for women, and 5 to 12% for men, whereas the lifetime prevalence of dysthymic disorder is 6% (3). Women are two to three times more likely to develop dysthymia than men. The point prevalence of major depression is 5 to 9% for women and 2 to 3% for men, making major depression a more common chronic disorder than most all chronic medical disorders. The prevalence of major depression in the elderly living in the community is 3%, lower than younger adults, but 15 to 25% of those living in nursing homes (5).

Recognition and diagnosis of major depression is a serious concern. About one-third to one-half of patients with major depression are unrecognized by primary care physicians and are often given sedative-hypnotic drugs rather than antidepressants (6).

ONSET, COURSE, AND OUTCOME

Bipolar I disorder is a recurrent disorder. After experiencing one manic episode, more than 90% of patients have future manic episodes. Studies completed prior to the availability of lithium suggest, on average, bipolar patients experience four episodes every ten years. With age, the interval between episodes tends to decrease. Although most bipolar patients recover completely from their episodes, about 20 to 30% continue to have mood lability and interpersonal or occupational difficulties. About 5 to 15% of bipolar I patients are rapid cyclers (four or more mood episodes in one year). Cyclothymic disorder, which usually begins by early adult life, has a slow insidious onset and a chronic course. About 15 to 50% of cyclothymic patients will subsequently develop bipolar I or II disorder.

Major depression may begin at any age, though on average, it begins in the mid-20s. After the first major depressive episode, about 50 to 60% of patients will have a second episode. After two episodes, 70% will have a third episode, and after three episodes, 90% will have future episodes. About two-thirds of major depressive episodes fully recover and become asymptomatic, with the remainder having either partial or no remission of symptoms. The ultimate risk of completed suicide in patients with major depression is 15%, and for bipolar I and II it is 10 to 15%, which is 30 times the risk of the general population (7).

CLINICAL FEATURES

Manic Episode

The essential feature of a manic episode is a distinct period of elevated, expansive, or irritable mood accompanied by at least three of the symptoms listed in Table 54.3 that have been present at least 1 week. Common examples of excessive involvement in pleasurable activities that may cause great harm to the patient and/or family include unrestrained buying sprees, sexual indiscretions, or foolish business investments. Whereas most manic episodes have a predominance of euphoria and grandiosity, others may

Table 54.3.
Clinical Features of Mania

Distinct period of persistently elevated, expansive, or irritable mood
  lasting at least one week, characterized by at least three of:
  Inflated self-esteem or grandiosity
  Decreased need for sleep
  More talkative than usual, pressure to keep talking
  Flight of ideas, subjective experience that thoughts are racing
  Distractibility
  Increase in goal-directed activities, psychomotor agitation
  Excessive involvement in pleasurable activities that have a high po-
    tential for painful consequences (e.g., sexual, illegal, financial)
Marked impairment in occupational functioning or usual social activi-
  ties, necessity to hospitalize to prevent harm to self or others, or
  psychotic symptoms (hallucinations, delusions)
Hypomania
  Same symptoms, lasting at least 4 days, but without impaired social
    or occupational functioning and no psychotic symptoms or need
    for hospitalization

Adapted from reference 3.

show a more dysphoric and paranoid pattern. The onset of mania is usually sudden and dramatic. Frequently, manic patients do not recognize that they are ill and, therefore, resist treatment. Lability of mood, that is, rapid mood shifts, is also common. The manic patient often has considerable impairment in social and occupational functioning though many bipolar patients have a good work history between episodes. The acute course of a manic episode has been described in terms of three stages. Stage I corresponds to hypomania, in which euphoria predominates. These patients are perceived as happy, hyperactive, somewhat tangential in thinking, impulsive, distractable, and hyperverbal but not psychotic or markedly impaired in occupational or social functioning. Stage II, usually called acute mania, finds the euphoria replaced by irritability and anger. The racing thoughts of Stage I lead to definite flights of ideas, with rapid shifting from one thought to another. Grandiose or paranoid ideas become more intense and often become fixed false beliefs (delusions). With early treatment, few patients progress to Stage III, which can be indistinguishable from any florid psychosis, including schizophrenia or an organic psychosis. The rate of progress through these stages can be very rapid, but the sequence of symptom progression is usually consistent and predictable. An untreated manic episode usually lasts less than 4 months and ends as abruptly as it began (2, 8).

Major Depressive Episode

Depression is characterized by a persistent depressed mood or loss of interest or pleasure in nearly all activities. One of these symptoms must be accompanied by at least four other symptoms (Table 54.4) (3). Major depression is diagnosed when at least five of the nine symptoms are present most of the day, nearly every day, for at least 2 weeks. Most depressed patients will describe their mood as sad, hopeless, or blue. In children and adolescents, the mood may be irritable rather than sad. Some patients will deny depressed mood but will describe loss of interest and

Table 54.4.
Clinical Features of Major Depression

Five or more of the following symptoms present nearly every day for 2
  weeks, representing a change from previous functioning:
  Depressed mood most of every day[a]
  Marked decreased interest or pleasure in most all activities[a]
  Appetite or weight change (>5% body weight in 1 month)
  Insomnia or hypersomnia
  Psychomotor agitation or retardation
  Fatigue or loss of energy
  Worthlessness, excessive guilt
  Decreased ability to think or concentrate, indecisiveness
  Recurrent thoughts of death, suicidal ideation or attempt

[a]One of these symptoms must be one of the five symptoms.
Adapted from reference 3.

Table 54.5.
Subtypes of Major Depression

Double Depression
  Dysthymia with superimposed major depressive episode
Major Depression with Psychotic Features
  Most common symptom is delusions
Major Depression with Atypical Features
  Mood reactivity–mood brightens in response to positive event
  Plus two of following symptoms:
    Increased appetite, weight gain
    Hypersomnia
    Leaden paralysis (heavy leaden feeling of arms and legs)
    Interpersonal rejection sensitivity (long-standing)
Major Depression with Seasonal Pattern
  Commonly episodes begin in fall or winter, remit in spring
  Must have 2 years of regular seasonal pattern

caring, or an inability to experience pleasure in normal activities (anhedonia). Sleep and appetite are typically decreased though occasionally both may be increased. Sleep disturbance is typically middle or terminal insomnia, waking up during the night or waking up too early and not being able to return to sleep. Change in weight must exceed 5% of body weight in a month. Psychomotor agitation is often manifested as pacing; wringing of the hands; pulling or rubbing hair, skin, or clothing; and outbursts of shouting. Psychomotor retardation is manifest as slowed speech, increased pauses in speech, slowed body movements, and sometimes, muteness (2,3). Symptoms of a major depression usually develop over days to weeks. An untreated episode usually lasts 6 months or longer.

TREATMENT OF DEPRESSION

Treatment options for depression include various psychotherapies, electroconvulsive therapy (ECT), light therapy, monoamine oxidase inhibitors (MAOIs), tricyclic antidepressant drugs (TCAs), and the newer nontricyclic antidepressant drugs. Selection of a treatment option depends primarily on the type and subtype of depression (Table 54.5). Treatment of a depressive episode in a bipolar patient usually requires both lithium and an antidepressant drug. Although the remainder of this chapter will focus on treatment of major depression and bipolar disorders, depressive subtypes whose treatment is different will be considered first.

Dysthymia

Patients with dysthymia often receive inappropriate antidepressant drug therapy. Dysthymic patients have a mood of depression that is mild but persistent, and often receive long-term small-dose antidepressant drug treatment that provides no therapeutic benefit beyond the value of regular interactions with the treating clinician. Psychotherapy is the most effective treatment for dysthymia, but drug therapy can be effective if given in adequate doses and duration similar to treatment of major depression (9, 10).

Double Depression

Dysthymic patients can have a superimposed major depressive episode. Up to 20% of patients hospitalized with a major depressive episode have underlying dysthymia. Antidepressant drugs will be effective in treating the major depressive episode, but some patients will return only to their baseline, which is dysthymia. The chronic mild depression remains, and the unsuspecting clinician will incorrectly view the patient as a partial responder and continue to increase antidepressant dosage or change drugs. Thus an adequate history is necessary on all patients being treated for major depression to establish a realistic therapeutic endpoint (11).

Major Depression with Psychotic Features

Patients with major depressive disorder may have psychotic symptoms, delusions being most common. The presence of delusions means that antidepressant drug therapy alone will be much less effective. Electroconvulsive therapy (ECT) is the most effective treatment for psychotic depression. When drugs are used, higher doses and longer duration of treatment is necessary, and most patients will benefit from using an adjunctive antipsychotic drug. Antidepressant drug treatment alone for delusional depression has been shown to be effective only in 41% of patients, whereas a combination of an antidepressant and an antipsychotic drug has a response rate of 78% (12, 13). Fixed combination products (e.g., Triavil) are not recommended since use of the antipsychotic is needed for only a few weeks, whereas the antidepressant will be used for at least 6 months. During treatment, it is also usually necessary to adjust and titrate the dose of one of the two drugs, which is difficult or impossible with a fixed combination drug product.

Major Depression with Atypical Features

Major depression with atypical features is characterized by many symptoms that are opposite that typically seen in major depression. For these atypical major depressions, monoamine oxidase inhibitors (MAOIs) have been shown to be at least as effective, if not more effective, than tricyclic antidepressants (TCAs) (14, 15).

Major Depression with Seasonal Pattern

A more recently recognized subtype of mood disorder is major depression with a seasonal pattern to the episodes. These patients are predominately women (60 to 90%), whose episodes regularly begin in the fall or winter, with full remission in the spring. This syndrome is most commonly seen in northern latitudes where sunlight is limited in the winter (3). Light therapy is effective in about 60% of these patients though it seldom eliminates all depressive symptoms. The intensity and duration of light exposure are more important than the time of day that light is administered. Typical treatment involves 2 hr of bright light (2500 lux) daily either in the morning or evening, with most symptom response seen in the first week.

The mechanism is not clear but may involve suppression of melatonin secretion, and/or circadian phase-shifting (16, 17).

Treatment Options for Major Depression and Bipolar Depression

PSYCHOTHERAPY

Once-a-week interpersonal psychotherapy has been shown to be equal in efficacy to antidepressant drug therapy for ambulatory depressed patients, and the combination of both is superior to each alone. Maintenance drug therapy is effective in reducing relapse rates and preventing symptom return, whereas psychotherapy improves psychosocial function, interpersonal relationships, and day-to-day coping. Pharmacotherapy and psychotherapy should be viewed as complementary and necessary components of an effective total treatment plan (18, 19). The American Psychiatric Association's Practice Guideline states interpersonal psychotherapy is useful for depressed patients amid recent conflicts with significant others and for those having difficulty adjusting to an altered career or social role or other life transition (20).

ELECTROCONVULSIVE THERAPY (ECT)

ECT remains the most effective treatment for major depression. ECT is more effective, more rapid in onset of effect, and safer in patients with cardiovascular disease than TCAs. Disadvantages of ECT compared to TCAs include frequent relapse after treatment termination, temporary memory loss, a significant social stigma concerning its use, and in some states, legal barriers to its use. Following a successful course of ECT, there is a 50% risk of relapse during the next 12 months unless maintenance antidepressant drugs are given. Although ECT has a history of misuse and overuse, drug modification of ECT by anesthetic and neuromuscular blocking drugs, and unilateral rather than bilateral ECT, now make it a safe, effective, and humane treatment option (21, 22). In addition to a valuable treatment option for major depression, ECT is especially effective and indicated for treatment of delusional depression and treatment-resistant depression. Although a highly charged political and emotional issue, ECT should be viewed as a treatment option that can be life saving for patients who otherwise would not recover from their depressive illness.

STIMULANTS

Controversy continues among clinicians regarding the role of psychostimulants in the treatment of depression. Nine of ten placebo-controlled studies do not support stimulants as effective in outpatients with mild to moderate depression (23). Stimulants have no place in the treatment of major depression. The best evidence for efficacy is brief, low-dose therapy in apathetic institutionalized geriatric patients, with the expectation that depressed mood will only partially improve. Methylphenidate 20 to 30 mg/day for 2 to 4 weeks is usually tolerated well, with exacerbation of preexisting anxiety the only consistent adverse effect.

MONOAMINE OXIDASE INHIBITORS (MAOIs)

After nearly 20 years of being viewed as less effective and more toxic than TCAs, MAOIs have become recognized as effective agents for selected patients. Table 54.6 lists currently available antidepressants. MAOIs are most effective in atypical depression, panic disorder, and some phobic disorders and are an alternative treatment for patients with major depression who fail to respond to other antidepressants (24, 25).

Phenelzine and tranylcypromine are equal in efficacy and very similar in their adverse effects. MAOIs should be given in divided doses, with the last dose administered no later than 6 PM to prevent drug-induced insomnia. The initial dose should be low (e.g., phenelzine 15 mg twice daily) to allow assessment of adverse effects before titration up to a therapeutic dose (Table 54.7). Similar to TCAs, MAOIs have a delay in onset of clinical efficacy of several weeks. Inhibition of MAO enzyme and subsequent in-

Table 54.6.
Available Antidepressant Drugs

Monoamine Oxidase Inhibitors
  Phenelzine (Nardil)
  Tranylcypromine (Parnate)
Tricyclics
  Amitriptyline (Elavil, Endep)
  Nortriptyline (Pamelor)
  Protriptyline (Vivactil)
  Imipramine (Tofranil, Janimine)
  Trimipramine (Surmontil)
  Desipramine (Norpramin, Pertofrane)
  Doxepin (Sinequan, Adapin)
Tetracyclic
  Maprotiline (Ludiomil)
Dibenzoxazepine
  Amoxapine (Asendin)
Phenylpiperazines
  Trazodone (Desyrel)
  Nefazodone (Serzone)
Selective Serotonin Reuptake Inhibitors (SSRIs)
  Fluoxetine (Prozac)
  Sertraline (Zoloft)
  Paroxetine (Paxil)
Monocyclic Aminoketone
  Bupropion (Wellbutrin)
Serotonin/Norepinephrine Reuptake Inhibitor
  Venlafaxine (Effexor)

Table 54.7.
Effective Antidepressant Dosage Ranges

Drug	Dose mg/day
Amitriptyline	150–300
Nortriptyline	50–150
Protriptyline	30–60
Imipramine	150–300
Desipramine	150–250
Trimipramine	150–300
Doxepin	150–300
Maprotiline	150–225[a]
Amoxapine	200–600
Trazodone	200–600
Nefazodone	300–500
Fluoxetine	20–40
Sertraline	50–200
Paroxetine	20–50
Bupropion	300–450[a]
Venlafaxine	150–375
Phenelzine	45–90
Tranylcypromine	20–60

[a]Maximum daily dose due to risk of seizures.

creased synaptic neurotransmitter levels is not an immediate effect but requires 2 to 4 weeks for peak effect.

Common adverse effects with MAOIs include orthostatic hypotension, delayed ejaculation and anorgasmia, weight gain, and edema. Orthostatic hypotension may often limit the rate of dosage titration. MAOIs also lower supine blood pressure, which does not occur with TCAs. In contrast to TCAs, MAOIs do not prolong cardiac conduction and have little effect on heart rate. For these reasons, MAOIs may offer some advantages to patients with angina and conduction defects, whereas TCAs may be preferred for patients with preexisting dysrhythmias (26). Phenelzine is the MAOI most likely to cause weight gain, whereas tranylcypromine does not (27). Generalized edema is more commonly seen with phenelzine and usually subsides within a week. The anticholinergic effects are less frequent and severe compared to TCAs. Restlessness, agitation, and insomnia can occur, and MAOIs can switch bipolar patients into mania. Unlike TCAs, MAOIs do not lower seizure threshold (28).

Severe hypertensive reactions following ingestion of food containing high amounts of tyramine are rare, but the risk can and should be minimized by careful patient education. MAO inhibition prevents the metabolism of tyramine in the GI tract and liver, causing release of norepinephrine. The clinical result is a sudden onset, painful throbbing occipital headache and, if severe, may progress to severe hypertension, profuse sweating, pallor, palpitation, and occasionally death. The severity of the reaction depends on many factors. Six mg of tyramine produces mild elevation of blood pressure, 10 mg has a marked pressor effect, and 25 mg can result in severe hypertensive crisis. Only a few foods must be absolutely restricted: all aged cheeses, concentrated yeast extracts, pickled fish (herring), sauerkraut, and broad bean pods (fava beans) (25, 29). Although foods have received the most attention in regard to hypertensive reactions, several drugs are more dangerous than these foods when combined with MAOI drugs. These drugs include sympathomimetics (ephedrine, phenylpropanolamine); stimulants (amphetamine, methylphenidate); levodopa, meperidine, buspirone, and venlafaxine; and SSRIs (30).

Changing a patient from a MAOI to a TCA or from a TCA to a MAOI is safely done with a 2-week washout period between the two drug treatments. But rarely is there such luxury of time when dealing with a severely depressed patient. Fortunately, the more common clinical situation involves switching a patient from a TCA to a MAOI when the TCA has failed. This switch can be done without a washout period because there is no immediate double effect on neurotransmitters. Changing from a MAOI to a TCA, however, cannot be done quickly since there is an immediate doubling of effect of neurotransmitter levels. TCAs block presynaptic reuptake of neurotransmitters and do so immediately, whereas MAOIs slowly increase levels of neurotransmitters released into the synapse over several weeks (31).

MECHANISM OF ACTION

Although MAOIs increase synaptic catecholamines by inhibition of MAO enzyme, most antidepressants are potent inhibitors of the uptake of either norepinephrine, serotonin, or both into the presynaptic nerve ending. Many antidepressants are also potent antagonists of other neurotransmitter receptors. TCAs are histamine H_1 receptor blockers, with doxepin, trimipramine, and amitriptyline several hundred times more potent than diphenhydramine. Least potent H_1 blockers include protriptyline and desipramine. These potencies correlate well with their sedative properties. TCAs block muscarinic receptors, which leads to peripheral and central anticholinergic effects. Amitriptyline and protriptyline are most potent, whereas the nontricyclics are virtually devoid of this effect. Alpha$_1$-adrenergic blockade helps explain the occurrence of postural hypotension and reflex tachycardia seen with some antidepressants. Doxepin, trimipramine, and amitriptyline are the most potent, whereas protriptyline and desipramine are the least potent alpha$_1$-adrenergic blockers. Blockade of 5-HT reuptake also contributes to orthostatic hypotension because of effects on serotonergic neurons in the brainstem vasomotor center. Imipramine and nortriptyline, for example, have about equal activity at alpha$_1$-adrenergic receptors, yet imipramine causes significantly more orthostatic hypotension than nortriptyline. The difference between these two drugs is that imipramine is a much more potent 5-HT reuptake blocker, and nortripyline is more

potent as a 5-HT receptor blocker. TCAs are very weak antagonists of dopamine (D-2) receptors, whereas beta-adrenergic, GABA, opiate, and benzodiazepine receptors are not antagonized by TCAs (32). In contrast, SSRIs, bupropion, and venlafaxine have little effect on muscarinic, adrenergic, and histaminic receptors.

Although it has long been known that antidepressant drugs increase neurotransmitter levels by reuptake blockade, their proposed mechanism of antidepressant action has moved past this simplistic notion, and depression is no longer thought to be caused by a deficiency of these neurotransmitters. Chronic administration of antidepressants causes different effects on neurotransmitters and receptors than is seen with acute administration. With chronic administration, sensitivities of several neurotransmitter receptors are altered in response to the acute effects of increased neurotransmitter levels from reuptake blockade. These changes in receptor sensitivity develop over 2 to 4 weeks, which coincides with the time necessary to see clinical antidepressant response. The major functional consequence of chronic TCA treatment is a gradual facilitation of postsynaptic alpha$_1$-adrenergic receptor function, as well as increased physiologic sensitivity to 5-HT in the brain. There is also a downregulation (fewer receptor sites) and decreased sensitivity of alpha$_2$-adrenergic autoreceptors and beta-adrenergic receptor function (33). Much is known about the acute and chronic effects of TCA treatment on neurotransmitter systems and their relative sensitivities, but the exact mechanism of action of antidepressants is not yet precisely defined.

Tricyclic Antidepressants (TCAs)

PHARMACOKINETICS

TCAs are tertiary and secondary amines with pKa's in the range of 8 to 10 and a high degree of lipid solubility. These basic drugs are rapidly and well absorbed following oral administration, and most undergo significant first-pass metabolism. Peak plasma levels occur within 2 to 6 hr for all TCAs except protriptyline, which peaks in 6 to 12 hr. Systemic availability is markedly reduced by pronounced hepatic first-pass metabolism. TCAs are widely distributed; most are highly protein bound and have high volumes of distribution of 15–37 liters/kg. Secondary amine TCAs tend to have slightly longer elimination half-lives averaging 12 to 44 hr, whereas the tertiary amine TCAs range from 10 to 25 hr. Protriptyline is the exception with an elimination half-life of 67 to 89 hr. Tertiary amine TCAs are demethylated to their respective secondary amine compounds, which are then hydroxylated, glucuronidated, and excreted. The hydroxy metabolites were once considered to be inactive, but recently have been shown to contribute to antidepressant efficacy and cardiotoxicity. The rate of hydroxylation can vary greatly among individuals, resulting in variation of steady-state plasma levels as high as 30-fold in individuals given the same oral dose (28, 34).

PLASMA LEVELS

Four TCAs have a well-established correlation of plasma level range with antidepressant response—nortriptyline, desipramine, amitriptyline, and imipramine. Other TCAs have proposed therapeutic levels but should not be viewed as well established (Table 54.8) (28, 34). Nortriptyline's minimum effective concentration is 50 ng/ml, with an upper limit of 150 ng/ml, above which therapeutic response declines. Nortriptyline is the only TCA to consistently demonstrate this curvilinear response, or so-called therapeutic window. Imipramine response has been shown to correlate with plasma levels of imipramine plus its metabolite desipramine at concentrations greater than 200 ng/ml. No decline in response is found at higher levels, with beginning toxicity seen above 500 ng/ml and significant toxicity becoming apparent when levels reach 1000 ng/ml. Desipramine and amitriptyline are less adequately studied, but a linear relationship seems to exist between plasma level and therapeutic effect. All other antidepressants have insufficient data to allow a definitive correlation between plasma level and response. Blood samples for TCA concentration determination should be drawn after absorption and distribution is complete, typically 10 to 12 hr after the last dose. Indications for TCA plasma level determinations include lack of response at usual therapeutic doses, significant adverse effects at relatively low doses, suspected noncompliance, stopping or starting cigarette smoking or known enzyme inducers or inhibitors, and use of TCAs in the very young and elderly. Patients given nortriptyline are definite candidates for plasma level monitoring since the maximum therapeutic plasma level of 150 ng/ml can be unknowingly exceeded and full response never achieved as the dosage is increased beyond the therapeutic window. Patients given imipramine, amitriptyline, or desipramine should have one steady-state measurement assuming compliance is not a concern. Repeat levels would be indicated in situations listed previously that can alter TCA elimination or when noncompliance is suspected. For all the other antidepressants, plasma level monitoring is not

Table 54.8.
Therapeutic Antidepressant Plasma Levels

	ηg/ml
Nortriptyline	50–150
Imipramine (plus Desipramine)	>200
Desipramine	100–160
Amitriptyline (plus nortriptyline)	75–175

Adapted from reference 34.

indicated since the cost is high, and correlation with clinical response is uncertain (34).

NONTRICYCLIC ANTIDEPRESSANTS

TCAs have a slow onset of effect of several weeks, are not effective in one-third of patients with major depression, have troublesome anticholinergic effects and serious cardiovascular effects, and a 2-week supply can be fatal in overdose. Thus far, newer antidepressants do not offer a faster onset of effect, and all are equally effective, but not more effective than TCAs. The nontricyclic antidepressants do offer advantages in terms of adverse effects and safety in overdose though most also have their own unique disadvantages compared to TCAs.

Maprotiline has been shown to be an equally effective antidepressant that offers no clinically important differences from other TCAs. Seizures are about three times more likely with maprotiline than TCAs, causing the initially recommended dosage range of 150 to 300 mg daily to be changed to a maximum of 225 mg. An unanswered question is if maprotiline is equal in efficacy to TCAs with its lowered maximum daily dosage. In 13 cases of fatal overdosage with maprotiline alone, the ingested dose ranged from 1.75 to 6 g, making it equally toxic in overdose compared to TCAs. Compared to TCAs, maprotiline overdose involves more seizures, more delirium, and less cardiac arrhythmias (35, 36). Amoxapine is unique among antidepressants since it possesses some antipsychotic activity and may cause extrapyramidal effects and tardive dyskinesia because of its hydroxy metabolite's dopamine blocking activity. Although amoxapine could be considered an option for psychotic depression, it suffers from the disadvantage that the amount of antipsychotic activity is not predictable, and as a "fixed combination" product, there is not the needed flexibility of dosage titration of each drug, nor the ability to discontinue the antipsychotic and continue treatment with the antidepressant. For nonpsychotic depressions, amoxapine is not an appropriate choice since it is the only antidepressant reported to cause extrapyramidal effects, tardive dyskinesia, and neuroleptic malignant syndrome. Amoxapine is less potent than most TCAs, meaning that the daily dosage must be higher (Table 54.7). Of eight documented fatalities with amoxapine alone, the lethal dose ranged from 2.6 to 6 g, which also provides no additional safety in overdose compared to TCAs. Amoxapine toxicity has fewer cardiac effects, but carries an increased risk of renal failure, seizures, and irreversible neurologic damage (36–38).

Trazodone was the first of the newer antidepressant drugs to offer several significant advantages over TCAs. Efficacy studies completed prior to marketing showed trazodone to be equal to TCAs. Postmarketing experience has led many clinicians to question whether trazodone is as effective as the TCAs. The differences between earlier studies and clinical use is a matter of dosage. Trazodone is one-half as potent as TCAs such as amitriptyline and imipramine, meaning trazodone must be given in daily doses of 200 to 600 mg. Many clinicians often abandon trazodone at doses of 200 to 300 mg, claiming it to be ineffective (39). Some patients cannot tolerate the sedation at daily doses of 400 to 600 mg. In doses of 100 to 400 mg daily, it can be given in a single daily bedtime dose with no loss of efficacy and less daytime sedation (40). Trazodone commonly causes orthostatic hypotension, but administration of dosing after meals usually minimizes this effect. Trazodone has no anticholinergic effects, making it a useful consideration for patients who must avoid anticholinergic effects. Of 43 cases of trazodone overdose, the greatest 9.2 g, there was uneventful recovery. Trazodone has no effect on cardiac conduction in contrast to TCAs that slow cardiac conduction. Trazodone is safer in patients with angina and cardiac conduction defects. This lack of effect on cardiac conduction means trazodone has no antiarrhythmic effect, however, and there are case reports of some ventricular arrhythmias being aggravated by trazodone (36, 41).

Since 1982, 207 cases of abnormal penile erectile activity have been reported with trazodone. These cases include increased nocturnal tumescence, return of erectile activity in previously impotent males, and true priapism. Priapism is defined as sustained penile erection unaccompanied by sexual desire and often painful. Fifty-two of these cases required surgical intervention, with about half leading to permanent impotence. Priapism has been reported with many drugs, most commonly with phenothiazine antipsychotics, antihypertensives (mostly prazosin), as well as trazodone (42). Other common causes include sickle cell disease, solid tumors, leukemia, and trauma. Drug-induced priapism is caused by the inhibition of sympathetically controlled detumescence through direct alpha-blockade. The majority of cases with trazodone occur at daily doses of 150 mg or less, and most occur within the first 28 days of treatment. The incidence of priapism with trazodone is estimated to be between 1 in 1000 and 1 in 10,000. Male patients given trazodone should be advised to report prolonged erections, with emphasis given to the need for early reporting and intervention. Once priapism occurs, it should be regarded as a urologic emergency. Any erection lasting longer than 4 hr must be treated quickly before local hypoxia occurs. Untreated priapism after 72 hr may lead to fibrosis of the corpora cavernosa and gangrene. Early recognition allows pharmacologic treatment with no risk of permanent impotence. Through angiocatheters, deoxygenated blood can be removed, and irrigation with saline and an alpha agonist (e.g., phenylephrine) is often successful in promoting detumescence (43). Only one case of a priapism equivalent in females has been reported

although there are case reports of clitoral enlargement and increased libido in women receiving trazodone (42, 44).

Trazodone has become a commonly used hypnotic drug alone, as well as an adjunctive hypnotic for patients with persistent insomnia while taking fluoxetine or bupropion (45). There is little support for trazodone's use as a SSRI potentiator of efficacy despite such widespread clinical use (46).

Bupropion is a monocyclic antidepressant, unique as a mild dopamine uptake inhibitor with no direct effect on norepinephrine, serotonin, or monoamine oxidase, and essentially devoid of anticholinergic, antihistaminic, and adrenergic effects. An active metabolite is reported to block norepinephrine reuptake. Elimination $t_{1/2}$ is 10 to 20 hr, but an active hydroxy metabolite has a $t_{1/2}$ of greater than 24 hr. Bupropion produces no clinically significant effect on cardiac conduction, orthostatic hypotension, or sexual function; has minimal anticholinergic effect; and causes little or no weight gain. Frequent adverse effects include insomnia, agitation, headache, and nausea (47). Its lack of sedation and its activating effect may be advantageous for patients with decreased psychomotor activity and lethargy. Disadvantages of bupropion include seizures and the inability to dose once daily. With daily doses of 450 mg or less, seizures are observed in 0.4% of patients, with a 1-year cumulative incidence of 0.5% (48). Bupropion is contraindicated in patients with psychotic disorders since its dopamine agonist effect may increase psychotic symptoms. Although still too early to assess, bupropion seems to offer additional safety in overdose compared to TCAs. The original efficacy studies were done at daily doses of 300 to 750 mg, but seizures at the higher doses caused the maximum recommended daily dose to be decreased to 450 mg. Subsequent studies have demonstrated antidepressant efficacy when compared to placebo at lower daily doses of 300 to 450 mg (49). Bupropion must be dosed three times daily, with a maximum single dose of 150 mg to minimize the seizure risk. The initial dose is 100 mg twice daily, increasing to 100 mg three times daily no sooner than 3 days after the start of therapy. After several weeks, the dosage may be increased to a maximum of 450 mg/day in divided doses in those not responding to 300 mg/day.

Selective Serotonin Reuptake Inhibitors (SSRIs)

The SSRIs have virtually replaced TCAs as first-line agents in the treatment of depression. Although no more effective than TCAs, patient tolerance of adverse effects is better with SSRIs, and SSRIs are more convenient to use since the initial starting dose is often the effective dose, thus requiring no dosage titration (50). SSRIs are potent and specific serotonin reuptake inhibitors with negligible binding to alpha or beta adrenergic, muscarinic, serotonin, dopamine, or histamine receptors. Table 54.9 summarizes clinically important SSRI pharmacokinetic information

Table 54.9.
SSRI Pharmacokinetics

Drug	Protein Binding (%)	Elimination Half-Life (hr)	Inhibition P450 IID6
Fluoxetine	94	94–704	Significant
Sertraline	98	26	Modest
Paroxetine	95	21	Significant

(34). The unique very long half-life of fluoxetine has clinical implications in regard to frequency of dosing adjustments and persistence of effects for weeks after discontinuation of fluoxetine. Sertraline is most highly protein bound and is unique as the only SSRI whose absorption may increase by up to 40% in the presence of food. All three SSRIs are potent inhibitors of the hepatic isoenzyme IID6 though sertraline is 7 to 10 times less potent than fluoxetine (34). All three SSRIs have flat dose–response curves in terms of antidepressant response, meaning increasing doses beyond the lower effective dose range does not increase therapeutic benefit but does increase adverse effects. SSRIs show equal antidepressant efficacy, but fewer adverse effects are seen with either sertraline or paroxetine than with fluoxetine. Agitation, anxiety, and insomnia are more common with fluoxetine than with sertraline or paroxetine, whereas other adverse effects are similar in frequency (51, 52). The most common adverse effects from SSRIs include nausea, insomnia, nervousness, and sexual dysfunction. Delayed ejaculation and anorgasmia are common with all three SSRIs, and are directly dose related, meaning the most effective treatment, when clinically feasible, is to decrease the SSRI dose. SSRIs essentially lack sedative, anticholinergic, cardiovascular effects, and weight gain seen with TCAs. SSRIs are very safe in overdose compared to TCAs. Although a 2-week supply of a TCA alone can be fatal in overdose, patients have had uneventful recoveries from single overdoses of 3000 mg of fluoxetine, 4000 mg of sertraline, and 850 mg of paroxetine (53, 54).

Fluoxetine's effective antidepressant dose for most patients is 20 mg administered in the morning. Although the manufacturer recommends a daily dosage range of 20 to 80 mg, increased response is seldom seen in doses above 20 mg, and some patients will respond to daily doses of only 5 to 10 mg (55). Akathisia, or severe motor restlessness, has been reported with fluoxetine, which is clinically indistinguishable from antipsychotic-induced akathisia (56). Anorexia and weight loss can be considered to be a positive or negative effect for a depressed patient. Most fluoxetine studies for depression that mention weight change indicate weight loss of 1 to 2 kg over 5 to 6 weeks. Case reports and a few controlled studies for obesity suggest weight loss of up to 5 kg over 8 weeks. There is no information on whether the weight loss is maintained after the initial loss (57). Though many questions remain regarding weight loss

with fluoxetine, its lack of weight gain is a definite advantage over TCAs for some patients.

The emergence of intense suicidal preoccupation during fluoxetine treatment has been adequately studied and refuted (58). The initial six case reports of intense suicidal preoccupation after treatment with fluoxetine, and subsequent completed suicides during fluoxetine treatment, have raised clinical and legal concerns (59). However, emergence of suicidal ideation during treatment with antidepressants is not unique to fluoxetine, but a component of necessary clinical monitoring of any severely depressed patient (60). A primary clinical concern with SSRIs is the potential for many drug–drug interactions. Fluoxetine and paroxetine significantly impair oxidative metabolism, resulting in increased plasma levels and adverse effects of drugs that rely on the P450IID6 isoenzyme. Addition of fluoxetine or paroxetine to TCAs causes as much as a fourfold increase in TCA plasma levels, and adverse effects of antipsychotics can be aggravated by addition of fluoxetine (61, 62). Combination of SSRIs with MAOIs can lead to a serotonin syndrome, consisting of confusion, hypomania, myoclonus, hypertension, tremor, and diarrhea. One death has resulted from initiation of MAOI therapy shortly after discontinuation of fluoxetine (63). These interactions may occur up to 5 weeks after discontinuation of fluoxetine (61, 63).

Sertraline may be dosed either in the morning or evening since it is less likely than fluoxetine to cause insomnia. Most depressed patients will respond to a daily dose of either 50 or 100 mg. Although many patients successfully treated with fluoxetine continue taking it, sertraline and paroxetine have become preferred SSRIs for new patients because of their more favorable elimination half-lives and because they cause less insomnia and restlessness (64).

Paroxetine causes the least insomnia and restlessness of the three SSRIs and is more likely to cause sedation. Its effective daily dose is 20 mg, with few patients benefiting from an increased dose. As the newest SSRI antidepressant, its actual differences or possible advantages have not yet been fully determined.

Venlafaxine is a potent serotonin/norepinephrine reuptake inhibitor, modest dopamine reuptake inhibitor, with little effect on cholinergic, histaminergic, and adrenergic receptors. This difference from TCAs suggests less anticholinergic, sedation, weight gain, and cardiovascular effects. Unlike SSRIs, venlafaxine is not highly protein bound and is not a potent inhibitor of hepatic metabolizing enzymes. Venlafaxine can be dosed either twice or three times daily. The effective daily dosage range for most patients is 150 to 275 mg, whereas severely depressed patients may require up to 375 mg. Common adverse effects include nausea, insomnia or somnolence, dizziness, sweating, and sexual dysfunction. Venlafaxine may cause a dose-related increase in diastolic blood pressure, making regular blood pressure monitoring mandatory. Sustained elevation in blood pressure (more than 10 mm Hg above baseline on three consecutive visits) is found in 7% of patients receiving 200 to 300 mg/day, and 13% if the daily dose is above 300 mg (65, 66).

Nefazodone is a postsynaptic 5-HT-2A receptor antagonist with presynaptic serotonin reuptake inhibition. Like all newer antidepressants, it has been shown to be equal in efficacy to imipramine for major depression with a similar onset of effect. Although similar to trazodone in structure in pharmacology, it has less sedation and orthostatic hypotension and no reported cases of priapism. Compared to TCAs, nefazodone has much less sexual dysfunction and less insomnia and activating effects. The most common adverse effects with nefazodone include sedation, nausea, dizziness, and dry mouth. Nefazodone's effective daily dosage range is 300 to 500 mg, which must be given in a divided twice daily schedule. Whereas the SSRIs are inhibitors of the P450IID6 isoenzyme, nefazodone only weakly inhibits the IID6 but is a potent inhibitor of the IIIA4 isoenzyme. Drugs that rely on IIIA4 for their metabolism include terfenadine, astemizole, triazolam, and alprazolam, so their plasma levels and adverse effects may increase if nefazodone is added (67, 68).

INITIATION OF TREATMENT

With TCAs, drug therapy should begin with small and divided doses to assess tolerance of side effects, sedation and orthostatic hypotension in particular. For a healthy hospitalized young adult, 25 mg three times daily for imipramine would be reasonable. If that dose is tolerated well, it can be quickly titrated upward to 50 mg three times daily within the first 3 or 4 days. Dosage increments should be done more slowly in outpatients whose appointments are usually weekly. Once the lower end of the therapeutic dosage range is reached (Table 54.7), dosage can be increased weekly. The expected pattern of response is that the physical manifestations of depression will show improvement within the first week, and the psychological symptoms will show initial improvement after 2 to 4 weeks of an effective dosage (Table 54.4). If the patient given imipramine 150 mg daily for 1 week shows improvement in physical symptoms (sleep, appetite, energy), then the dosage should remain at 150 mg with the expectation that the pessimism and dysphoric mood will respond after another week or two. If no change is noted in physical symptoms after 1 week at 150 mg daily, the dose should be increased in 50-mg increments weekly until response in physical symptoms is seen. When an effective dosage level is achieved, most patients will benefit from once daily bedtime dosing. Adverse effects may slow the rate of upward dosage titration, whereas patients given a more sedating antidepressant drug may initially benefit from

most or all of the dose administered at bedtime. Initial dosing of SSRIs is far easier than most other antidepressants since there is no need to start low and titrate to the lower end of an effective dosing range. The initial dose for SSRIs is usually the effective dose. During the final trimester of pregnancy, the mean dose of TCA required is 1.6 times the mean dose when the patients were not pregnant (69).

The elderly are more sensitive to both the therapeutic and toxic effects of antidepressants due to reductions in neurotransmitters, increased receptor site sensitivity, and age-related alterations in the pharmacokinetics of antidepressants (70). Initial daily doses in geriatric patients should be 10 mg for all TCAs, whereas trazodone can begin at 25 mg daily. Dosage titration should be done more slowly in the elderly, but dose increases should be continued until clinical response or significant adverse effects are seen to prevent undertreatment (71). Fluoxetine and paroxetine have more age-related differences in clearance than sertraline. Plasma levels of fluoxetine and norfluoxetine at 20 mg/day can be twice that in the young and 70% higher with paroxetine, whereas sertraline's clearance is about 40% less in the elderly than the young (34). Thus initial doses of fluoxetine and paroxetine should be reduced by one-half, but most elderly patients can be given the same initial dose of sertraline of 50 mg.

Treatment-Resistant Depression

In controlled trials, approximately 30% of patients with major depression do not respond to the first antidepressant given, and in actual practice, many more patients fail to receive an adequate dose or duration of treatment. Up to 70% of patients given antidepressants fail to take 25 to 50% of their prescribed dose (70). Reasons for noncompliance include patients stopping the drug once depressive symptoms resolve after 1 to 2 months, disbelief in the value of medication, and adverse effects (73). The first approach to nonresponse is to reassess diagnosis and ensure the adequacy of dose, duration, and plasma levels with the first drug treatment (74). Many studies of so-called treatment-resistant depression show less than one-half these patients received at least 200 mg of imipramine or its equivalent for at least 4 weeks (75). A 6 to 8 week trial at the top end of the dosage range (Table 54.7) constitutes an adequate trial, and if symptoms remain unresponsive, an alternative drug should be considered. There are no clear guidelines for choosing an alternative antidepressant. It should have a favorable adverse effect profile for the patient and should be of a different chemical subclass. Because all TCAs primarily affect norepinephrine and have similar effects on receptor sensitivities, the serotonin-specific drugs represent commonly used alternatives for a TCA-resistant patient. Despite this common clinical practice, studies to evaluate differential efficacy suggest that serotonin and noradrenergic-selective drugs are not necessarily more effective alternatives to each other, and nonresponse to one SSRI does not predict nonresponse to another SSRI (76). The differences in adverse effects determine how quickly one can switch from an ineffective drug to an alternative drug (Table 54.10). Differences in sedation and orthostatic hypotension are of most concern, whereas switching from a drug high in anticholinergic activity to one without may cause cholinergic rebound effects. Use of two different antidepressant trials at the top end of their dosage range for at least 6 weeks each, along with plasma level monitoring, represents a logical initial approach to the treatment-resistant patient.

Two antidepressant failures suggest the use of augmentation therapy. Lithium and triiodothyronine (T_3) are the most effective antidepressant adjunctive treatment options. T_3 (25 to 50 mcg/day) has the advantage of an onset of effect usually within 1 week, whereas lithium (600 to 900 mg/day) requires 3 to 6 weeks (74, 77). The potential benefit of augmentation drugs must be weighed against increasing depressive morbidity and the likelihood of increased adverse effects of the combination therapy. The risks of combination therapy are more often greater than the potential benefit in the elderly, particularly when lithium is added to antidepressants (78).

CONTINUATION AND MAINTENANCE THERAPY

Once a depressive episode has successfully responded to drug treatment, the clinician must decide how long to continue drug therapy. Treatment is divided into continuation and maintenance therapy (Table 54.11). Continuation

Table 54.10.
Antidepressant Adverse Effect Profiles

Drug	Sedation	Anticholinergic Effect	Orthostatic Hypotension
Amitriptyline	4	4	4
Trimipramine	4	3	4
Doxepin	4	3	4
Maprotiline	3	2	3
Trazodone	3	0	3
Nefazodone	2	1	2
Amoxapine	2	2	3
Imipramine	2	2	3
Protriptyline	1	4	2
Nortriptyline	2	2	2
Desipramine	1	2	3
Fluoxetine	−1	0	0
Sertraline	0	0	0
Paroxetine	1	1	0
Bupropion	−1	1	0
Venlafaxine	0	0	0
MAOIs	−1	1	4

1 is low, 4 is high.

Table 54.11.
Ideal Pharmacological Treatment of Depression

Acute phase: 6–8 weeks at full therapeutic doses; aim is remission of symptoms

Continuation phase: 4–9 months at full dose for all patients; aim is to prevent relapse

Maintenance phase: 1–2 years at full dose for patients with three or more prior depressive episodes, or lifelong if more than two episodes in 5 years; aim is to prevent recurrence of future depressive episodes

therapy is defined as the time that the underlying pathophysiology of the depressive episode continues to run its course. Since the natural duration of an untreated major depressive episode is approximately 6 months, continuation therapy is usually defined as at least 6 months after onset of the depressive episode. All depressed patients should receive continuation antidepressant therapy. When antidepressant drugs are discontinued immediately after drug response, relapse is almost certain. The first 8 weeks following discontinuation of drug therapy is the period of highest risk of relapse. Presence of even mild symptoms in patients with a previous baseline of better functioning between episodes suggests that the depressive episode has not run its course, and drug therapy should not be discontinued. Although it is still common clinical practice to decrease the maintenance antidepressant dose by 30 to 50% of the dose necessary to treat the acute depressive episode, the risk of relapse is much higher (79). Both continuation and maintenance therapy must be at the same dose used to treat the acute episode. Maintenance therapy is the period when the patient would normally be between episodes of depression, and the drug is being used to prevent future episodes. Maintenance antidepressant therapy is recommended for 1 to 2 years after continuation therapy in patients with an established history of 3 or more major depressive episodes, and lifelong for patients who have had 3 or more in 5 years (20, 80, 81).

Antidepressant Withdrawal

When it is necessary to discontinue an antidepressant drug, it must be done by gradual tapering of the dose rather than abrupt discontinuation. A variety of withdrawal effects from TCAs can occur with abrupt discontinuation, including excessive anxiety, restlessness, insomnia, and autonomic symptoms such as diaphoresis, diarrhea, hot and cold flashes, and piloerection. The mechanism of these withdrawal symptoms are related to rebound cholinergic effects as well as noradrenergic hyperactivity (82). Estimates of the frequency of withdrawal effects with abrupt discontinuation of TCAs ranges from 20 to 55%. Patients who experience these effects often fear they are becoming depressed again. Prevention of withdrawal effects is best achieved by decreasing the antidepressant dose by no more than 25% every 1 to 2 weeks. Discontinuation of an antidepressant drug must be done with careful monitoring since early signs of relapse is a major concern in addition to possible withdrawal effects. Patients should be educated regarding the possibility of withdrawal effects and urged to not abruptly discontinue drug therapy on their own. Withdrawal effects are not a concern when switching from one antidepressant to another with a similar profile of adverse effects.

MANAGEMENT OF ADVERSE EFFECTS

Sedation and Anticholinergic Effects

Sedation can be selected or avoided based on drug choice, and excessive sedation can usually be managed by switching to a once daily bedtime dosing schedule. For patients with significant daytime psychomotor agitation, a divided schedule of a more sedating antidepressant may be most appropriate. Common anticholinergic effects include dry mouth, blurred near vision, and constipation. These effects can also be minimized by a once daily bedtime dosing schedule. There is no treatment of proven value for dry mouth and blurred near vision except changing dosing schedule or decreasing dosage. Many patients experience some decrease in severity of these effects after 2 weeks of treatment. Constipation requires more careful attention, since if untreated, it can progress to fecal impaction and ileus. Because constipation is caused by decreased GI motility, resulting in hard, dry stools, the best treatment is use of a stool softener and increased fluid intake. Docusate 100 to 500 mg daily, with increased fluid intake, is usually effective. Treatment need not be continuous but given for treatment periods of 4 to 7 days. Less common, but of more concern, are urinary retention and central anticholinergic intoxication effects. Men with prostatic hypertrophy are at risk for urinary retention, as are patients with any preexisting difficulty in initiating urination. Central anticholinergic intoxication manifests as confusion, delirium, and sometimes, psychotic symptoms. Urinary retention may require acute treatment with catheterization and bethanechol, but both urinary retention and central intoxication indicate a significant reduction in antidepressant dosage or switch to an alternative drug with very low anticholinergic effect. Bethanechol 10 mg three times daily has been shown to reduce subjective complaints of anticholinergic effects from nortriptyline in an elderly population (84).

Cardiovascular Effects

Cardiovascular effects of concern with TCAs include orthostatic hypotension, tachycardia, and decreased cardiac conduction. Orthostatic hypotension is a common effect of TCAs and trazodone (Table 54.10). About 20% of patients given imipramine will be seriously affected by orthostatic hypotension, with 10% requiring dosage reduction and/or discontinuation. Subjective complaints of dizziness and lightheadedness often decrease with time, but no tolerance develops to the objective drop in systolic blood pressure. Orthostatic hypotension is of concern in patients with impaired cardiac conduction or congestive heart failure, and in patients taking antihypertensive drugs. MAOIs cause orthostatic hypotension with more frequency than TCAs and also cause a fall in supine blood pressure (85, 86). Venlafaxine has the unique effect of increasing diastolic pressure.

Sinus tachycardia resulting from the TCAs' anticholinergic effect of vagal inhibition of the SA node is of clinical concern only in patients with ischemic heart disease and marginally compensated congestive heart failure. TCAs have properties similar to Class I antiarrhythmic drugs like quinidine and lidocaine. Clinically, imipramine has been shown to have an antiarrhythmic effect, suppressing ventricular premature contractions. TCAs have little effect on A-V nodal conduction but do prolong conduction below the A-V node. These effects are of no clinical significance in patients who show no evidence of preexisting conduction defects. Of concern, however, are patients whose pretreatment ECG show prolonged PR interval, higher degrees of A-V block, bundle-branch or fascicular block, or intraventricular conduction delay. For these patients, trazodone, SSRIs, bupropion, and MAOIs represent safer treatment options (85, 86).

Other Adverse Effects

Several types of sexual dysfunction are commonly caused by antidepressants. TCAs, SSRIs, venlafaxine, and MAOIs are more likely to impair ejaculation and cause an orgasmia than impair erection (87). Drug-induced sexual dysfunction is often difficult to identify in depressed patients who often have decreased libido as a symptom of depression. When most symptoms of depression have improved, yet sexual dysfunction continues or worsens, drug-induced dysfunction should be suspected. The delayed ejaculation and anorgasmia from SSRIs can be treated with serotonin antagonists or yohimbine. Continuous use of cyproheptadine, however, may also interfere with the antidepressant effect, so PRN dosing is recommended (88, 89). Delayed ejaculation and anorgasmia is such a common effect with serotonergic drugs that SSRIs can be used in treating premature ejaculation (90).

Weight gain is common with TCAs and MAOIs. Patients can gain 2 pounds per week for many weeks on TCAs. MAOIs can also cause edema of the legs and ankles that will contribute to weight gain. When compliance is threatened because of weight gain, SSRIs or bupropion offer an alternative that do not contribute to continued weight gain and may cause slight weight loss.

All antidepressants and ECT have been shown to switch some bipolar patients from depression to hypomania or mania. When a patient is switched to mania or hypomania, the antidepressant should be discontinued and lithium initiated. TCAs have been reported to be capable of exacerbating psychotic symptoms in schizophrenic patients though the evidence is scarce. Bupropion and venlafaxine may exacerbate preexisting psychotic symptoms because of their mild dopamine agonist activity.

Seizures are an uncommon but serious adverse effect of antidepressants. Most seizures occur in patients with an identifiable predisposition. Risk of seizures is directly dose related, and the TCAs, maprotiline, and bupropion carry the highest risk. The SSRIs, trazodone, and MAOIs have the lowest risk of seizures (91).

TCA toxicity in overdose is manifest as CNS effects (toxic psychosis, seizures, coma with respiratory depression), cardiovascular effects (sinus and supraventricular tachycardias, impaired conduction leading to A-V block, intraventricular block, ventricular arrhythmias or fibrillation, and asystole), and peripheral anticholinergic effects (urinary retention, decreased bowel sounds, ileus). Treatment consists of first preventing absorption and interfering with enterohepatic recirculation by gastric lavage and activated charcoal. Physostigmine is not an antidepressant antidote and should be reserved for treating supraventricular tachycardias causing significant problems. Fluids require careful monitoring since too vigorous hydration may lead to pulmonary edema. Intensive cardiac monitoring can be discontinued when plasma levels fall below 500 ng/ml for drugs like amitriptyline or imipramine, or when the ECG has been normal for more than 2 days (92). An ingestion of a 2-week supply of any TCA, amoxapine, and maprotiline represents a serious medical emergency and can be fatal. Clinicians must exercise care in selecting the amount of medication given to depressed patients and not routinely give 1-month supplies to all patients. For patients with a history of overdose suicide attempts or who are currently suicidal, an antidepressant safer in overdose should be used. Trazodone, bupropion, and SSRIs all have much greater safety in overdose.

Drug of Choice

Factors important in selecting an antidepressant drug for a patient include history of response, medical status of the patient, presenting symptoms, and differences in adverse effect profile among antidepressants. There are no differences among antidepressant drugs in relative overall efficacy, no differences in efficacy for certain types of symptoms except for atypical depression and delusional depression previously discussed, and no differences in onset of effect. Although it is not possible to predict which drug will be effective, individual patients do sometimes show a better response to particular drugs. It is for this reason that history of response should be a major factor in drug selection. The drug history should include a determination of which antidepressant drugs have been used in the past, which one was most effective, what type of adverse effects were experienced, and which drugs are viewed positively or negatively by the patient. For many patients, this information will be a more important drug selection factor than differences in adverse effect profile among antidepressant drugs. Patient attitude, though of no pharmacologic value, is crucial to future patient compliance with drug therapy.

All TCAs cause the same type of adverse effects, but there are significant differences in relative incidence of sedation, anticholingeric, and orthostatic hypotensive effects. The nontricyclic antidepressants have a much different adverse effect profile than TCAs (Table 54.10). Sedation is often a desirable effect since most depressed patients have insomnia, and some patients have psychomotor agitation. Use of a more sedating antidepressant with bedtime dosing also eliminates the need for a hypnotic drug. Patients with significant psychomotor retardation, even if there is significant insomnia, usually do best with a less sedating antidepressant. The relative frequency of anticholinergic effects varies greatly among antidepressant drugs. Compared with antipsychotic drugs, thioridazine is about equal to desipramine, meaning antidepressant drugs as a class are much more likely to cause anticholinergic effects. Dry mouth, blurred near vision, and constipation are usually only bothersome effects for most patients and can be minimized by once daily bedtime dosing. For some patients, however, anticholinergic effects can become intolerable. Orthostatic hypotension does not present a significant problem for most patients properly educated about its cause and how to prevent dizziness and syncope. For the elderly with decreased cerebral perfusion or for patients taking other drugs with hypotensive effects, SSRIs or bupropion may offer a significant advantage. As can be seen, there is no drug with an ideal adverse effect profile. A patient's medical history, drug history, and current symptoms must all be considered in selecting the most appropriate antidepressant drug.

PATIENT COUNSELING

A primary purpose of counseling is to enhance compliance. The major reasons for antidepressant noncompliance include recovery from the depressive episode and symptoms, disbelief in the value or need for drug treatment, and adverse effects. Thus, counseling must address these areas of concern. Five specific areas of antidepressant counseling are necessary (Table 54.12). Because alcohol may worsen or contribute to the depressive symptoms, it is always best to advise depressed patients to avoid alcohol. For antidepressants with sedative and/or orthostatic hypotension, alcohol will aggravate these two effects. Patients can be told

Table 54.12.
Antidepressant Counseling

Antidepressants treat a physical biological reason for the depression. Depression is not a personality flaw or weakness.

There is no need for concern regarding addiction or dependence on antidepressant drugs.

All antidepressants require several weeks of continuous use before symptoms improve. "Be patient and don't give up on the drug too soon."

Most patients will require 6–12 months of therapy to effectively treat a depressive episode. Stopping the drug therapy too soon greatly increases the risk of relapse. "Keep taking the medication even after the symptoms improve."

For every adverse effect mentioned, the clinician must discuss what the patient should do if one occurs.

they will "get drunk more quickly and may become very dizzy and even fall." Counseling should focus on the possible consequences of drinking while taking an antidepressant, rather than merely telling the patient he or she absolutely cannot drink. Such absolute dictates will more likely result in noncompliance since when the patient does drink, he or she will obediently avoid taking the antidepressant drug.

TREATMENT OF BIPOLAR PATIENTS
Cyclothymia

Lithium prophylaxis is the preferred treatment for cyclothymic patients who require drug therapy. Although there are no published studies comparing various treatment alternatives for cyclothymia, clinical experience suggests that lithium can decrease the frequency of cycling and/or the severity of the hypomanic or depressive episodes. There is some concern that antidepressant drugs alone may in fact increase the frequency of cycling in both bipolar and cyclothymic patients (93).

Acute Mania

Lithium is the treatment of choice for acute manic episodes. It remains a more effective and more specific treatment than antipsychotic and anticonvulsant drugs. Because lithium has a lag time in onset of effect of 7 to 10 days, an antipsychotic drug often must be given with lithium for the first 1 to 2 weeks. High-potency antipsychotics like haloperidol or fluphenazine are usually preferred over low-potency antipsychotics like chlorpromazine because of their virtual lack of sedative and cardiovascular effects unless both sedation is desirable and psychotic symptoms must be treated (94, 95). Once lithium plasma levels are within therapeutic range, the antipsychotic drug should be tapered and discontinued to allow assessment of lithium's efficacy alone. Use of high-potency benzodiazepines have more recently become preferred

over antipsychotic drugs as an adjunctive treatment to lithium. Lorazepam orally or intramuscularly, and clonazepam are equally effective in managing manic symptoms while waiting for onset of lithium effect and cause fewer adverse effects than antipsychotic drugs (96, 97). An antipsychotic drug is preferred when psychotic symptoms are significant, whereas a benzodiazepine is preferred when symptoms are primarily decreased sleep and agitation (98). A reasonable expectation of lithium efficacy for an acute manic episode is remission or remarkable improvement of manic symptomatology in 60 to 80% of patients after 2 weeks (94). There is some suggestion that lithium nonresponse may be episode specific. The 20 to 40% of patients who do not respond to lithium for an acute manic episode are not necessarily unresponsive to lithium for future episodes (99). This is contrary to the common clinical practice of labeling a patient a lithium nonresponder and seeking alternative drugs for prophylaxis and future manic episodes.

Prophylaxis

Lithium is the most effective treatment for preventing future manic and depressive episodes in bipolar patients (100). Lithium is somewhat more effective in preventing manic episodes than depressive episodes. Combination of manic and depressive episode relapse rate studies shows 34% relapse in 1 year for lithium treated patients and 79% relapse with placebo (101). Bipolar patients who receive antidepressant drugs should be given lithium to prevent the antidepressant drug from switching the patient into a hypomanic or manic state (102). Despite its efficacy, lithium prophylaxis is not indicated for every bipolar patient. The decision to initiate lithium prophylaxis depends on the history of episode frequency and the impact of another episode on the patient, and his or her job and family. Bipolar patients with good insight into their illness, who can recognize early signs of relapse, who have a good family support system, who do not have significant residual symptoms between episodes, and whose episodes are less frequent than every 2 years may not need lithium prophylaxis.

Lithium Discontinuation

There are no clear guidelines concerning which patients may be candidates for discontinuation of lithium treatment. Rapid discontinuation in patients stable on lithium for years results in 50% of patients having another mood episode within 5 months, and the monthly risk of an episode is 28 times higher than during lithium treatment (103). Because half of the patients relapsed within 3 months, suggestive of a mood rebound phenomenon, a slow gradual tapering and discontinuation of lithium is recommended. Current clinical practice reflects an attitude of only rarely considering the discontinuation of lithium therapy so that patients are not subjected to the high risk of relapse. An unresolved controversy is the suggestion from four cases that lithium discontinuation not only increases the risk of relapse, but previously lithium-responsive patients become nonresponsive when lithium is reinstituted (104).

LITHIUM PHARMACOKINETICS

Lithium carbonate is virtually totally absorbed from the gastrointestinal tract within 8 hr of oral administration, with peak blood levels achieved in 2 to 4 hr. Peak concentration from a single 600 mg dose is 0.45 to 0.85 mEq/L. Initial distribution volume corresponds to the extracellular fluid space, with a final volume of distribution of 0.8 to 1.2 liters/kg. Tissue uptake is not uniform, with levels in the brain, thyroid, and saliva exceeding plasma levels. Lithium is not bound to proteins or metabolized, but excreted unchanged in the urine. Lithium is freely filtered through the glomerulus, about 80% being reabsorbed in the proximal tubule, competing with sodium. Average plasma elimination half-life is 18 to 24 hr (105, 106). Compared to younger patients, elderly patients eliminate lithium more slowly from a smaller volume of distribution. Elimination half-life of lithium in the elderly is about 25% longer than in younger patients, typically ranging up to 36 hr. The elderly require one-third to one-half fewer lithium doses than younger patients (107).

Blood Levels

There is very good correlation of clinical response and adverse effects to lithium levels. For acute mania, levels of 0.9 to 1.2 mEq/L are often adequate, whereas levels as high as 1.5 mEq/L are occasionally necessary. Maintenance levels of 0.6 to 0.8 mEq/L are effective for many patients, but relapse rates are lower if levels are maintained at 0.6 to 1.2 mEq/L (108, 109). Levels above 1.5 mEq/L are regularly associated with signs of toxicity, and levels above 2.0 mEq/L result in serious toxicity. The narrow range between therapeutic and toxic levels makes plasma level monitoring mandatory for all patients receiving lithium. A 12-hr interval between the last dose and drawing the blood sample in a patient receiving the same divided daily dose for at least 1 week will yield a standardized lithium level that is reproducible.

Use of erythrocyte lithium concentrations have not been adopted clinically but remain only of research interest. The only clinical use of the RBC lithium to plasma lithium ratio is as an assessment of lithium compliance. The noncompliant patient who takes lithium only a few days before his or her clinic appointment will have an apparent therapeutic plasma level, but the ratio will be very low. Similarly, the patient with relatively stable plasma levels but significant swings in the ratio over repeated visits is probably not compliant (110).

LITHIUM DOSING

For acute manic episodes, a daily dose of 1500 mg to 2400 mg is usually necessary to achieve a plasma level near 1.0 mEq/L. The initial dose, however, should be small and divided to assess tolerance of initial adverse effects. A typical starting dose of 300 mg three times daily is conservative and can be increased by 300 mg increments every 2 or 3 days if necessary. More aggressive therapy may be necessary for inpatients whose manic symptoms are severe or whose history of response indicates the need for higher doses. A plasma level drawn 2 or 3 days after initiation of therapy can be used to calculate the steady-state level at that dose, with subsequent 300-mg dosage increments yielding a plasma level increase of 0.15 to 0.35 mEq/L (Table 54.13) (111). Its relatively simple pharmacokinetics allows consideration of lithium-loading doses and prediction of dosage based on a single test dose. A loading dose of 30 mg/kg of slow-release lithium administered in 3 divided doses over a 6-hr period has been shown to accurately predict a 12-hr plasma level of 1.0 mEq/liter without adverse effects (112). A number of studies have attempted to predict lithium dosage based on a single test dose and plasma level determination, as well as a priori predictive dosing methods with relatively positive results (113, 112). Once the desired lithium level is reached and reproduced on the same daily dosage, monthly plasma level determinations are sufficient. Initiation of lithium for prophylaxis should be done very conservatively since the patient is not symptomatic and no adverse effects are desired. A starting dose might be 300 mg twice daily with weekly dosage increments of 300 mg following steady-state plasma level determinations. An oral daily dose of 900 mg to 1200 mg will usually yield lithium plasma levels within the maintenance range of 0.6 to 0.8 mEq/liter.

Table 54.13.
Lithium Steady-State Prediction

Day	Lithium Received	Plasma Level (mEq/L)
1	900	—
2	900	—
3	900	0.51

Blood drawn on morning of day 3 prior to lithium administration, so 0.51 represents two days of 900 mg. Assume 24-hour half-life, 0.51 represents 75% of steady-state level at 900 mg/day:

Estimated steady-state level at 900 mg/day = $100/75 \times 0.51 = 0.68$ mEq/L.

For each 300 mg/day added, the new steady-state level will increase 0.15–0.35 mEq/L. Thus, increase dose by 300 mg to reach desired level of 1.0:

Estimated steady-state level at 1200 mg/day = $(0.68 + 0.15)$ to $(0.68 + 0.35) = 0.83$ to 1.03 mEq/L.

Before lithium is begun, a physical examination and history should focus on detection of cardiovascular, endocrine, and renal disease. Baseline tests should include serum creatinine, blood urea nitrogen, complete blood count, urinalysis, thyroid function tests, electrolytes, serum calcium, and an ECG if the patient is over 40 or has cardiovascular disease.

Concern about adverse renal effects of lithium has led to investigation of once daily or every other day dosing regimens. Most evidence suggests that trough plasma lithium concentrations are more important than peak concentrations in causing nephrotoxicity. A disadvantage of daily or every other day dosing schedules is the possibility of increased adverse effects,especially gastrointestinal and neurologic, which can be minimized by using a slow-release lithium preparation. Whether the total daily dose is divided into two, three, or four doses does not appear to alter the 12-hr steady-state serum lithium concentration. Once daily dosing at bedtime, however, will increase the 12-hr concentration by 12 to 33%. Because the kinetics of single daily dose lithium influence the standardized 12-hr serum level, patients should be stabilized on a twice daily dosing schedule, with a switch to once daily if the daily dose is 900 mg or less, or if renal dysfunction occurs (108).

LITHIUM ADVERSE EFFECTS

Adverse effects and their relationship to therapeutic or toxic lithium levels, as well as nondose-related adverse effects are listed in Table 54.14. Although the list is long, most patients with a therapeutic lithium level experience few if any significant adverse effects. The most common

1141Table 54.14.
Lithium Adverse Effects

Dose Related (Therapeutic Levels)	Nausea, diarrhea Polyuria polydipsia Cognitive impairment Fine hand tremor Muscle weakness ECG T-wave alteration
(Signs of Toxicity)	Coarse hand tremor Persistent nausea, diarrhea Slurred speech, confusion Seizures Increased deep tendon reflexes Irregular pulse, hypotension Coma
Nondose Related	Nephrogenic diabetes insipidus Goiter hypothyroidism Hypercalcemia Weight gain Macropapular or acneiform reactions Leukocytosis

adverse effects are polyuria, polydipsia, and weight gain. The most bothersome adverse effects that lead to noncompliance, however, are weight gain, confusion, and mental slowness (115).

Dose-Related Adverse Effects

Adverse effects seen with therapeutic lithium levels are worse in the first week or two of therapy and for most patients are bothersome but not severe. When plasma levels are maintained near 0.7 mEq/L, the frequency and severity of these effects are much less than previously reported frequencies in which mean levels were 0.85 mEq/L. Diarrhea occurs in 20% of patients with higher blood levels versus 6% of those with lower blood levels; polydipsia 70% versus 60%; and tremor 45% versus 15% (116).

Gastrointestinal effects are most apparent during the first week of lithium therapy, and usually result from the peak plasma level being too high. If further dividing the daily dosage does not treat the nausea, a slow-release lithium preparation will further reduce the steepness of rise of the peak plasma level and usually eliminates GI complaints. Almost 25% of patients will continue to experience polyuria and secondary polydipsia after 1 to 2 years of lithium therapy. For most patients, however, it is of little concern and does not interfere with continued treatment. Cognitive impairment is usually manifest as confusion, mental slowness, poor concentration, and memory problems. Although it is difficult to distinguish lithium-induced cognitive effects from those caused by depressed mood, patients attribute these symptoms to lithium and may become noncompliant. Muscle weakness is present in about 30% of patients initially, but disappears quickly. Fine hand tremor is noticeable in more than 50% of patients initially and may persist. Lithium tremor is an intentional hand tremor, worsening with voluntary movement; is not an extrapyramidal symptom; and is not responsive to anticholinergic drugs. Most patients are initially unaware of the tremor, which becomes noticeable only when delicate movements are attempted such as drinking coffee or eating soup. Management of the tremor includes reduction of lithium dose if clinically possible, reduction in caffeine intake, and as a last resort, addition of a beta-adrenergic blocking agent. Propranolol 40 to 80 mg daily or metroprolol 50 to 100 mg daily are effective treatments (117). About 50% of patients given lithium in the therapeutic range will demonstrate T-wave flattening, and cases of reversible sinus node abnormalities and other conduction disturbances have been reported rarely.

Lithium Toxicity

Lithium toxicity is usually seen when the plasma level exceeds 1.5 mEq/L though many cases of lithium toxicity have been reported with therapeutic levels, particularly in the elderly. Many of the effects seen at therapeutic levels worsen, and central effects of slurred speech, increased confusion, or seizures predominate in lithium toxicity. Patients and family members should be familiar with these effects and should be instructed to temporarily discontinue lithium and immediately contact their physician if these effects are seen. Lithium intoxication represents a serious medical emergency. Mild intoxication can quickly become serious intoxication when the nausea and diarrhea causes the patient to not eat. Several days of fasting and diarrhea dramatically decreases sodium intake and increases sodium loss, causing significant lithium reabsorption and higher lithium levels. Hemodialysis is indicated when the lithium plasma level exceeds 4.0 mEq/L, the patient has renal failure, or if electrolyte and fluid balance cannot be maintained. For levels between 2.0 and 4.0 mEq/liter, most patients can be treated with supportive care. Use of diuresis to hasten lithium elimination is no longer recommended, and diuretics that act distally may actually increase lithium retention. Lithium levels should be measured every 3 hr to follow the decline and aid in decision making. Fatalities are uncommon and are usually due to renal failure or cardiovascular collapse, whereas persistent neurologic and renal sequelae are more common (118, 119).

Nondose-Related Adverse Effects

A variety of nondose-related effects are possible with lithium, many of which develop only with long-term lithium therapy. The polyuria and polydipsia seen in many patients may progress in a few patients to a nephrogenic diabetes insipidus, manifest as 3 or more liters of urine output per day and a urine-specific gravity as low as 1.002 to 1.005 following a 12-hr water deprivation test. This nephrogenic diabetes insipidus is unresponsive to vasopressin and is usually fully reversible on discontinuation of lithium therapy. Lithium blocks the effect of antidiuretic hormone on adenylate cyclase, which reduces water reabsorption in the distal tubules and collecting ducts, leading to polyuria. Because many patients need to continue lithium therapy in spite of this adverse effect, attention has focused on treatment rather than discontinuation of lithium therapy. Hydrochlorthiazide has been used to reduce extracellular volume and thus decrease urine output, but increased lithium reabsorption with resultant increased lithium levels and hypokalemia are significant clinical concerns. Amiloride is equally effective and causes volume contraction similar to that seen with thiazide diuretics, but also blocks reuptake of lithium into the cells of the distal tubules and collecting ducts. Amiloride has the advantage of a very weak natriuretic effect, predisposing less to lithium toxicity, and no hypokalemia. Treatment of lithium-induced diabetes insipidus should begin with amiloride 5 to 10 mg twice daily, and if no response is seen,

a thiazide diuretic can be added (116, 120). Renal function monitoring (urine-specific gravity, serum creatinine, and BUN) should be done in all lithium patients every 6 to 12 months.

The potential for actual functional renal damage with long-term lithium therapy, and its possible relationship to the persistence of nephrogenic diabetes insipidus, is much less clear. Large prospective studies of renal function in patients receiving long-term lithium therapy have found no evidence of progressive deterioration of renal function, but only an impaired renal concentrating ability. Up to 5% of patients on long-term lithium therapy will develop serum creatinine levels above 2.0 mg/dL (116, 121).

Lithium may also cause several endocrine and metabolic adverse effects. In about 5% of patients, lithium will induce a diffuse nontender goiter, and an equal number of patients may become hypothyroid. Lithium inhibits the synthesis and release of thyroid hormone from the thyroid gland as well as inhibiting the action of thyroid stimulating hormone (TSH). The most consistent laboratory finding is an elevated TSH seen in the first several months of therapy in about 30% of patients. An elevated TSH persisting for more than 3 months implies impaired thyroid reserve and indicates replacement with L-thyroxine. An adequate dose will produce a normal TSH assay in 6 weeks. To prevent the development of these complications, thyroid function should be monitored every 6 to 12 months. Evaluation of thyroid function should include inspection of the patient's neck for signs of goiter and eyes for exophthalmos, and TSH, T_3, T_4, and free thyroxine index. Hypercalcemia is occasionally seen in lithium-treated patients although its significance is not clearly understood. Complications of hyperparathyroidism and hypercalcemia have not been reported in lithium-treated patients, but baseline and yearly serum calcium levels should be part of routine lithium monitoring.

Weight gain is a common and significant adverse effect of lithium. In the first year of therapy, patients gain an average of 4 kg, with 20% of patients gaining more than 10 kg. Intake of high-caloric fluids is commmon because of the polyuria and polydipsia, which contributes to weight gain. Weight measurement must be a routine part of lithium monitoring (115). Lithium may aggravate psoriasis and acne, and may cause maculopapular eruptions, exfoliative dermatitis, and hair loss. Aggravated acne or psoriasis is often responsive to common treatments, but discontinuation of lithium may sometimes be necessary because of these effects. Hair loss, though rare, can be significant and cause for discontinuation of therapy. Thyroid function must be evaluated in cases of hair loss to determine if hypothyroidism is the cause (122). Leukocytosis during lithium therapy is secondary to neutrophilia accompanied by lymphocytopenia. The mean increase is 3000 to 4000/cu mm, and is without the shift to the left seen in an infectious process. Although a benign effect, it is useful to obtain a baseline complete blood count before lithium therapy.

LITHIUM AND PREGNANCY

Any woman of childbearing age should be using a contraceptive method while taking lithium, lithium should be discontinued before a planned pregnancy, and lithium should be discontinued as soon as an unplanned pregnancy has been discovered. The teratogenicity of lithium is well established, with demonstrated malformations of the heart and large vessels. Because the cardiovascular system is formed during the 3rd to 9th week after conception, lithium is contraindicated in the first trimester of pregnancy. Lithium may be used if necessary in the second and third trimesters, but lithium should be discontinued or the dosage decreased by 50% several weeks prior to the delivery date. The dehydration associated with labor and fluid shifts during delivery may lead to lithium toxicity in the mother. Maternal lithium levels of 1.0 mEq/L at term have been associated with neonatal toxicity manifest by cyanosis, bradycardia, impaired respiratory function, "floppy baby syndrome," and nephrogenic diabetes insipidus. Lithium therapy should be resumed a few days after delivery with a reduced dose to counteract the increased risk of postpartum mania and depression. Lithium does pass from the mother's blood to milk. Infants breast-fed by mothers taking lithium have serum lithium concentrations 10 to 50% of the mother's serum lithium concentrations, causing most clinicians to recommend that women taking lithium abstain from nursing their children (123, 124).

DRUG INTERACTIONS WITH LITHIUM

Relatively few drug interactions are of concern with lithium, but most are of great clinical concern since they may quickly lead to lithium toxicity if not recognized and prevented. Thiazide diuretics will reduce lithium clearance within several days, causing lithium levels to rise as much as 50%. When a thiazide diuretic must be used in a patient receiving lithium, the lithium dosage must be decreased and lithium levels monitored more closely. Nonsteroidal antiinflammatory drugs, particularly indomethacin, declofenac, naproxen, and ibuprofen decrease renal clearance of lithium, thus increasing serum lithium levels by 20 to 60% after 3 to 7 days of concurrent use. Sulindac and aspirin do not significantly affect lithium levels (125). Angiotensin-converting enzyme inhibitors and calcium channel blockers may also cause substantial increases in lithium levels (100 to 200%) (125). Additive neurotoxicity is possible with anticonvulsants and antipsychotic drugs, requiring more careful monitoring. Electroconvulsive therapy (ECT) should be used cautiously in a patient receiving lithium since memory loss and confusion are increased, and lithium can

potentiate and prolong the effect of neuromuscular blocking agents (126).

ALTERNATIVES TO LITHIUM

Increasing attention has been devoted to alternative drugs to lithium for the treatment of acute manic episodes as well as for prophylaxis in bipolar patients. Such drugs are needed since both rapid cyclers and mixed bipolar patients are less responsive to lithium, and some patients discontinue lithium because of adverse effects. Carbamazepine and valproate are effective for both acute manic episodes and prophylaxis of bipolar disorder. Efficacy of these agents has been demonstrated both alone and in combination with lithium. Carbamazepine demonstrates an overall response rate of 62% in acute mania and 72% prophylactically. Valproate shows a mean response rate of 63%. Many of the patients in these studies were unresponsive to lithium (98). Most carbamazepine studies added carbamazepine to lithium, so its efficacy alone is not well established (127, 128). Valproate has shown efficacy alone for typical bipolar patients, as well as rapid-cycling patients, and possible efficacy for prophylaxis (127, 128). Previous lithium response or nonresponse appears to have no relationship to valproate effectiveness. Carbamazepine's usual dosage range is 400 to 1200 mg/day, with a lower initial dose of 200 mg once or twice daily. A serum level range for bipolar disorder has not been established, but levels should be between 6 and 12 ug/ml, which is consistent with efficacy and less adverse effects. Then initial dose of valproate is 250 mg twice daily. The usual effective dosage range for valproate is 750 to 2500 mg/day, with levels between 45 and 100 ug/ml. A loading dose of 15 mg/kg, with the goal of reaching a level of 45 ug/ml quickly results in a more rapid onset of clinical effect, usually within 5 days, if GI effects can be tolerated. Clonazepam is not a useful alternative treatment for bipolar disorder and is not considered an antimanic drug. Both clonazepam (1 to 4 mg/day) and lorazepam (2 to 6 mg/day) are useful as adjunctive medication for acute mania to ensure sleep and reduce hyperactivity (98, 128).

CONCLUSION

Mood disorders are very common, and effective treatments are available for most patients. Because of the slow onset of clinical effect and many possible adverse effects, patient education regarding antidepressant drugs is critical. Advances in antidepressant therapy include increased use of therapeutic plasma level monitoring and introduction of newer antidepressant drugs with unique differences compared to tricyclic antidepressants. Lithium remains the standard for treatment of bipolar illness, but valproate and carbamazepine are increasingly used as effective alternative antimanic drugs. Careful patient monitoring is necessary for all three antimanic drugs to minimize the likelihood of adverse effects and drug interactions. The high prevalence of mood disorders requires pharmacists in all practice settings to be familiar with their appropriate treatment.

REFERENCES

1. Cummings JL. The neuroanatomy of depression. J Clin Psychiatry 54(suppl 11):14–20, 1993.
2. Hirschfeld RMA, Goodwin FK, Mood disorders. In: Talbott JA, Hales RE, Yudofsky SC. Textbook of Psychiatry. Washington DC, American Psychiatric Press, 1988, pp 403–441.
3. American Psychiatric Association. Diagnostic and Statistical Manual of Mental Disorders, 4th edition, Washington DC: American Psychiatric Association. 1994, pp 317–391.
4. Maj M, Magliano L, Pirozzi R, et al. Validity of rapid cycling as a course specifier for bipolar disorder. Am J Psychiatry 151:1015–1019, 1994.
5. Anon. Diagnosis and treatment of depression in late life: the NIH consensus development conference statement. Psychopharmacol Bull 29:87–100, 1993.
6. Katon W, von Korff M, Lin E, et al. Adequacy and duration of antidepressant treatment in primary care. Med Care 30:67–76, 1992.
7. Blumenthal SJ. Suicide: a guide to risk factors, assessment, and treatment of suicidal patients. Med Clin N Amer 72:937–971, 1988.
8. Garvey MJ, Tuason VB. Mania misdiagnosed as schizophrenia. J Clin Psychiatry 41:75–78, 1980.
9. Markowitz JC. Psychotherapy of dysthymia. Am J Psychiatry 151:1114–1121, 1994.
10. Howland RH. Pharmacotherapy of dysthymia: a review. J Clin Psychopharmacol 11:83–92, 1991.
11. Keller MB, Lavori PW, Endicott J, et al. "Double depression": two year followup. Am J Psychiatry 140:689–694, 1983.
12. Spiker DG, Weiss JC, Dealy RS, et al. The pharmacological treatment of delusional depression: part I. Am J Psychiatry 142:430–436, 1985.
13. Spiker DG, Perel JM, Hanin I, et al. The pharmacological treatment of delusional depression: part II. J Clin Psychopharmacol 6:339–342, 1986.
14. Quitkin FM, Harrison W, Liebowitz M, et al. Defining the boundaries of atypical depression. J Clin Psychiatry 45(7, sec 2):19–21, 1984.
15. Quitkin FM, McGrath PJ, Stewart JW, et al. Atypical depression, panic attacks, and response to imipramine and phenelzine. Arch Gen Psychiatry 47:935–941, 1990.
16. Wirz-Justice A, Graw P, Krauchi K, et al. Light therapy in seasonal afffective disorder is independent of time of day or circadian phase. Arch Gen Psychiatry 50:929–937, 1993.
17. Lafer B, Sachs GS, Labbate LA, et al. Phototherapy for seasonal affective disorder. Am J Psychiatry 151:1081–1083, 1994.
18. Frank E, Kupfer KJ, Perel JM, et al. Three year outcomes for maintenance therapies in recurrent depression. Arch Gen Psychiatry 47:1100–1105, 1990.
19. Weissman MM. Psychotherpay in the treatment of depression: new technologies and efficacy. In: Treatment of Psychiatric Disorders, vol. 3, Washington DC, American Psychiatric Association, 1989, pp 1814–1823.
20. American Psychiatric Association. Practice guideline for major depressive disorder in adults. Am J Psychiatry 150(4,suppl):1–26, 1993.
21. Fink M. Myths of shock therapy. Am J Psychiatry 134:991–996, 1977.
22. Welch CA. Electroconvulsive therapy. In: Treatment of Psychiatric Disorders, vol. 3, Washington DC, American Psychiatric Association, 1989, pp 1803–1813.
23. Satel SL, Nelson JC. Stimulants in the treatment of depression: a critical overview. J Clin Psychiatry 50:241–249, 1989.
24. Nies A. Differential response patterns to MAO inhibitors and tricyclics. J Clin Psychiatry 45(7, sec. 2):70–77, 1984.
25. Brown CS, Bryant SG. Monoamine oxidase inhibitors: safety and efficacy issues. Drug Intell Clin Pharm 22:232–235, 1988.
26. Goldman LS, Alexander RC, Luchins DJ. Monoamine oxidase inhibitors and tricyclic antidepressants: comparison of their cardiovascular effects. J Clin Psychiatry 47:225–229, 1986.
27. Cantu TG, Korek JS. Monoamine oxidase inhibitors and weight gain. Drug Intell Clin Pharm 22:755–759, 1988.
28. Bryant SG, Brown CS. Major affective disorders, part I and II. Clin Pharm 5:304–318 and 385–395, 1986.
29. Shulman KI, Walker SE, MacKenzie S, et al. Dietary restriction, tyramine, and the use of monoamine oxidase inhibitors. J Clin Psychopharmacol 9:397–402, 1989.
30. Walker JI, Davidson J, Zung WWK. Patient compliance with MAO inhibitor therapy. J Clin Psychiatry 45(7, sec 2):78–80, 1984.
31. Kahn D, Silver JM, Opler LA. The safety of switching rapidly from tricyclic antidepressants to monoamine oxidase inhibitors. J Clin Psychopharmacol 9:198–202, 1989.
32. Richelson E. Pharmacology of antidepressants in use in the United States. J Clin Psychiatry 43(11, sec 2):4–11, 1982.
33. Baldessarini RJ. Current status of antidepressants: clinical pharmacology and therapy. J Clin Psychiatry 50:117–126, 1989.
34. Preskorn SH. Pharmacokinetics of antidepressants. J Clin Psychiatry 54(suppl 9):14–34, 1993.
35. Stimmel GL. Maprotiline. Drug Intell Clin Pharm 14:585–590, 1980.
36. Coccaro EF, Siever LJ. Second generation antidepressants: a comparative review. J Clin Pharmacol 25:241–260, 1985.
37. Lydiard RB, Gelenberg AJ. Amoxapine—an antidepressant with some neuroleptic properties? Pharmacotherapy 1:163–178, 1981.
38. Madakasira S. Amoxapine-induced neuroleptic malignant syndrome. DICP 23:50–51, 1989.
39. Bryant SG, Hokanson JA, Brown CS. A drug utilization review of prescribing patterns for trazodone versus amitriptyline. J Clin Psychiatry 51(9,suppl):27–29, 1990.
40. Fabre LF. Trazodone dosing regimen: experience with single daily administration. J Clin Psychiatry 51(9,suppl):23–36, 1990.
41. Georgotas A, Forsell TL, Mann JJ, et al. Trazodone hydrochloride. Pharmacotherapy 2:253–265, 1982.
42. Thompson JW, Ware MR, Blashfield RK. Psychotropic medication and priapism: a comprehensive review. J Clin Psychiatry 51:430–433, 1990.
43. Dittrich A, Albrecht K, Bar-Moshe, et al. Treatment of pharmacological priapism with phenylephrine. J Urology 146:323–324, 1991.
44. Gartrell N. Increased libido in women receiving trazodone. Amer J Psychiatry 143:781–782, 1986.
45. Nierenberg AA, Adler LA, Peselow E, et al. Trazodone for antidepressant-associated insomnia. Am J Psychiatry 151:1069–1072, 1994.
46. Nierenberg AA, Cole JO, Glass L. Possible trazodone potentiation of fluoxetine: a case series. J Clin Psychiatry 53:83–85, 1992.
47. Preskorn SH, Othmer SC. Evaluation of bupropion hydrochloride, the first of a new class of atypical antidepressants. Pharmacotherapy 4:20–34, 1984.
48. Davidson J. Seizures and bupropion: a review. J Clin Psychiatry 50:256–261, 1989.
49. Lineberry CG, Johnston JA, Raymond RN, et al. A fixed-dose (300 mg) efficacy study of bupropion and placebo in depressed outpatients. J Clin Psychiatry 51:194–199, 1990.

50. Montgomery SA, Henry J, McDonald G, et al. Selective serotonin reuptake inhibitors: meta-analysis of discontinuation rates. Int Clin Psychopharmacol 9:47–53, 1994.

51. Aguglia E, Casacchia M, Cassano GB, et al. Double-blind study of the efficacy and safety of sertraline versus fluoxetine in major depression. Int Clin Psychopharmacol 8:197–202, 1993.

52. DeWilde J, Spiers R, Mertens C, et al. A double-blind, comparative, multicentre study comparing paroxetine with fluoxetine in depressed patients. Acta Psychiatr Scand 87:141–145, 1993.

53. Stokes PE. Fluoxetine: a five-year review. Clin Therapeutics 15:216–243, 1993.

54. Caracci G. Unsuccessful suicide attempt by sertraline overdose. Am J Psychiatry 151:147, 1994.

55. Schweizer E, Rickels K, Amsterdam JD, et al. What constitutes an adequate antidepressant trial for fluoxetine? J Clin Psychiatry 51:8–11, 1990.

56. Lipinski JF, Mallya G, Zimmerman P, et al. Fluoxetine-induced akathisia: clinical and theoretical implications. J Clin Psychiatry 50:339–342, 1989.

57. Kinney-Parker JL, Smith D, Ingle SF. Fluoxetine and weight: something lost and something gained? Clin Pharm 8:727–733, 1989.

58. Fava M, Rosenbaum JF. Suicidality and fluoxetine: is there a relationship? J Clin Psychiatry 52:108–111, 1991.

59. Teicher MH, Glod C, Cole JO. Emergence of intense suicidal preoccupation during fluoxetine treatment. Am J Psychiatry 147:207–210, 1990.

60. Damluji NF, Ferguson JM. Paradoxical worsening of depressive symptomatology caused by antidepressants. J Clin Psychopharmacol 8:347–349, 1988.

61. Ciraulo DA, Shader RI. Fluoxetine drug-drug interactions: antidepressants and antipsychotics. J Clin Psychopharmacol 10:48–50, 1990.

62. Preskorn SH. Recent pharmacologic advances in antidepressant therapy for the elderly. Am J Med suppl 94:(suppl 5A):2S–12S, 1993.

63. Feighner JP, Boyer WF, Tyler DL, et al. Adverse consequences of fluoxetine-MAOI combination therapy. J Clin Psychiatry 51:222–225, 1990.

64. Grimsley SR, Jann MW. Paroxetine, sertraline, and fluvoxamine: new selective serotonin reuptake inhibitors. Clin Pharm 11:930–957, 1992.

65. Feighner JP. The role of venlafaxine in rational antidepressant therapy. J Clin Psychiatry 55(9,suppl A):62–68, 1994.

66. Montgomery SA. Venlafaxine. A new dimension in antidepressant pharmacotherapy. J Clin Psychiatry 54:119–126, 1993.

67. Dopheide JA, Stimmel GL, Yi DD. Focus on nefazodone: a serotonergic drug for major depression. Hosp Formul 30:205–212, 1995.

68. Rickels K, Schweizer E, Clary C, et al. Nefazodone and imipramine in major depression: a placebo-controlled trial. Br J Psychiatry 164:802–805, 1994.

69. Wisner KL, Perel JM, Wheeler SB. Tricyclic dose requirements across pregnancy. Am J Psychiatry 150:1541–1542, 1993.

70. Salzman C. Practical considerations in the pharmacologic treatment of depression and anxiety in the elderly. J Clin Psychiatry 51(1, suppl):40–43, 1990.

71. Stimmel GS, Gutierrez MA. Psychiatric Disorders. In Delafuentes JC, Stewart RB: Therapeutics in the Elderly, 2nd ed, Cincinnati, Harvey Whitney Books, 1995, pp 324–343.

72. Perel JM. Compliance during tricyclic antidepressant therapy: pharmacokinetic and analytic issues. Clin Chem 34:881–887,1988.

73. Blackwell B. Antidepressant drugs: side effects and compliance. J Clin Psychiatry 43(11, suppl):14–18, 1982.

74. Phillips KA, Nierenberg AA. The assessment and treatment of refractory depression. J Clin Psychiatry 55(suppl 2):20–26, 1994.

75. Post RM. Treatment of refractory mood disorders. In: Review of Psychiatry, vol.9, Washington DC, American Psychiatric Press, 1990, pp 7–202.

76. Nolen WA, vandePutte JJ, Dijken WA, et al. Treatment strategies in depression. Part I and II. Acta Psychiatr Scand 78:668–675, 676–683, 1988.

77. Joffe RT, Singer W, Levitt AJ, et al. A placebo-controlled comparison of lithium and triiodothyronine augmentation of tricyclic antidepressants in unipolar refractory depression. Arch Gen Psychiatry 50:387–393, 1993.

78. Austin LS, Arana GW, Melvin JA. Toxicity resulting from lithium augmentation of antidepressant treatment in elderly patients. J Clin Psychiatry 51:344–345, 1990.

79. Kupfer DJ, Frank E, Perel JM, et al. Five-year outcome for maintenance therapies in recurrent depression. Arch Gen Psychiatry 49:769–773, 1992.

80. Depression Guideline Panel. Depression in Primary Care: Detection, Diagnosis, and Treatment. Quick Reference Guide for Clinicians, Number 5. Rockville, MD. US Dept HHS, Agency for Health Care Policy and Research. AHCPR Publication No 93-0552. April 1993.

81. Greden JF. Antidepressant maintenance medication: when to discontinue and how to stop. J Clin Psychiatry 54(8, suppl): 39–45, 1993.

82. Charney DS, Heninger GR, Sternberg DE, et al. Abrupt discontinuation of tricyclic antidepressant drugs: evidence for noradrenergic hyperactivity. Brit J Psychiatry 141:377–386, 1982.

83. Cole JO, Bodkin JA. Antidepressant drug side effects. J Clin Psychiatry 51(1,suppl):21–26, 1990.

84. Rosen J, Pollock BG, Altieri LP, et al. Treatment of nortriptyline's side effects in elderly patients: a double-blind study of bethanechol. Am J Psychiatry 150:1249–1251, 1993.

85. Jefferson JW. Cardiovascular effects and toxicity of anxiolytics and antidepressants. J Clin Psychiatry 50:368–378, 1989.

86. Roose SP, Glassman AH. Cardiovascular effects of tricyclic antidepressants in depressed patients with and without heart disease. J Clin Psychiatry Monograph 7(2):1–18, 1989.

87. Balon R, Yeragani VK, Pohl R, et al. Sexual dysfunction during antidepressant treatment. J Clin Psychiatry 54:209–212, 1993.

88. Katz RJ, Rosenthal M. Adverse interaction of cyproheptadine with serotonergic antidepressants. J Clin Psychiatry 55:314–315, 1994.

89. Jacobsen FM. Fluoxetine-induced sexual dysfunction and an open trial of yohimbine. J Clin Psychiatry 53:119–122, 1992.

90. Waldinger MD, Hengeveld MW, Zwinderman AH. Paroxetine treatment of premature ejaculation. Am J Psychiatry 151:1377–1379, 1994.

91. Rosenstein DL, Nelson JC, Jacobs SC. Seizures associated with antidepressants: a review. J Clin Psychiatry 54:289–299, 1993.

92. Preskorn SH, Irwin HA. Toxicity of tricyclic antidepressants—kinetics, mechanism, intervention: a review. J Clin Psychiatry 43:151–156, 1982.

93. Wehr TA, Goodwin FK. Rapid cycling in manic-depressives induced by tricyclic antidepressants. Arch Gen Psychiatry 36:555–559, 1979.

94. Goodwin FK, Zis AP. Lithium in the treatment of mania. Arch Gen Psychiatry 36:840–844, 1979.

95. Shopsin B, Gershon S, Thompson H, et al. Psychoactive drugs in mania: a controlled comparison of lithium, chlorpromazine, and haloperidol. Arch Gen Psychiatry 32:34–42, 1975.

96. Busch FN, Miller FT, Weiden PJ. A comparison of two adjunctive treatment strategies in acute mania. J Clin Psychiatry 50:453–455, 1989.

97. Bodkin JA. Emerging uses for high-potency benzodiazepines in psychotic disorders. J Clin Psychiatry 51(5,suppl):41–46, 1990.

98. Gerner RH, Stanton A. Algorithm for patient management of acute manic states: lithium, valproate, or carbamazepine? J Clin Psychopharmacol 12(suppl 1):57S–63S, 1992.

99. Carroll BJ. Prediction of treatment outcome with lithium. Arch Gen Psychiatry 36:870–878, 1979.

100. Prien RF, Kupfer DJ, Mansky PA, et al. Drug therapy in the prevention of recurrences in unipolar and bipolar affective disorders. Arch Gen Psychiatry 41:1096–1104, 1984.

101. Klerman GL. Long term treatment of affective disorders. In: Lipton MA, DiMascio A, Killam KF. Psychopharmacology: A Generation of Progress. New York: Raven Press, 1978. pp 1303–1311.

102. Nasrallah HA, Lyskowski J, Schroeder D. TCA-induced mania: difference between switchers and nonswitchers. Biol Psychiatry 17:271–275, 1982.

103. Suppes T, Baldessarini RJ, Faedda GL, et al. Risk of recurrence following discontinuation of lithium treatment in bipolar disorder. Arch Gen Psychiatry 48:1082–1088, 1991.

104. Post RM, Leverich GS, Altshuler L, et al. Lithium discontinuation-induced refractoriness: preliminary observations. Am J Psychiatry 149:1727–1729, 1992.

105. Amdisen A. Serum level monitoring and clinical pharmacokinetics of lithium. Clin Pharmacokinet 2:73–92, 1977.

106. DeVane CL. Fundamentals of Monitoring Psychoactive Drug Therapy. Baltimore, MD, Williams and Wilkins, 1990, pp 82–138.

107. Hardy BG, Shulman KI, Mackenzie SE, et al. Pharmacokinetics of lithium in the elderly. J Clin Psychopharmacol 7:153–158, 1987.

108. Jefferson JW. Lithium: a therapeutic magic wand. J Clin Psychiatry 50:81–86, 1989.

109. Gelenberg AJ, Kane JM, Keller MB, et al. Comparison of standard and low serum levels of lithium for maintenance treatment of bipolar disorder. N Engl J Med 321:1489–1493, 1989.

110. Frazer A, Mendels J, Brunswick D, et al. Erythrocyte concentrations of the lithium ion: clinical correlates and mechanisms of action. Am J Psychiatry 135:1065–1069, 1978.

111. Gutierrez MA, Walker NR, Kramer BA. Evaluation of a new steady-state lithium prediction method. Lithium 2:57–59, 1991.

112. Kook KA, Stimmel GL, Wilkins JN, et al. Accuracy and safety of a priori lithium loading. J Clin Psychiatry 46:49–51, 1985.

113. Lobeck F. A review of lithium dosing methods. Pharmacotherapy 8:248–255, 1988.

114. Browne JL, Huffman CS, Golden RN. A comparison of pharmacokinetic versus empirical lithium dosing techniques. Ther Drug Monitoring 11:149–154, 1989.

115. Gitlin MJ, Cochran SD, Jamison KR. Maintenance lithium treatment: side effects and compliance. J Clin Psychiatry 50:127–131, 1989.

116. Jefferson JW. Lithium: the present and the future. J Clin Psychiatry 51(suppl,8):4–8, 1990.

117. Zubenko GS, Cohen, BM. Comparison of metoprolol and propranolol in the treatment of lithium tremor. Psychiatric Research 11:163–164, 1984.

118. Hansen HE, Amdisen A. Lithium intoxication. Quart J Med 47:123–144, 1978.

119. Rose SR, Klein-Schwartz, Oderda GM, et al. Lithium intoxication with acute renal failure and death. Drug Intell Clin Pharm 22:691–694, 1988.

120. Battle DC, von Riotte AB, Gaviria M, et al. Amelioration of polyuria by amiloride in patients receiving longterm lithium therapy. New Engl J Med 312:408–414, 1985.

121. Gitlin MJ. Lithium-induced renal insufficiency. J Clin Psychopharmacol 13:276–279, 1993.

122. Deandrea D, Walker NR, Mehlmauer M et al. Dermatological reactions to lithium: a critical review of the literature. J Clin Psychopharmacol 2:199–204, 1982.

123. Schou M. Lithium treatment during pregnancy, delivery, and lactation: an update. J Clin Psychiatry 51:410–413, 1990.

124. Cohen LS, Heller VL, Rosenbaum JF. Treatment guidelines for psychotropic drug use in pregnancy. Psychosomatics 30:25–33, 1989.

125. Ragheb M. The clinical significance of lithium-nonsteroidal anti-inflammatory drug interactions. J Clin Psychopharmacol 10:350–354, 1990.

126. Small JG, Milstein V. Lithium interactions: lithium and electroconvulsive therapy. J Clin Psychopharmacol 10:346–350, 1990.

127. Stuppaeck C, Barnas C, Miller C, et al. Carbamazepine in the prophylaxis of mood disorders. J Clin Psychopharmacol 10:39–42, 1990.

128. Post RM. Non-lithium treatment for bipolar disorder. J Clin Psychiatry 51(suppl, 8):9–16, 1990.

129. Bowden CL, Brugger AM, Swann AC, et al. Efficacy of divalproex vs lithium and placebo in the treatment of mania. JAMA 271:918–924, 1994.

130. Calabrese JR, Delucchi GA. Spectrum of efficacy of valproate in 55 patients with rapid-cycling bipolar disorder. Am J Psychiatry 147:431–434, 1990.

CHAPTER 55

SCHIZOPHRENIA

GLEN L. STIMMEL

The emphasis on community treatment, the chronic shortage of public psychiatric beds, and the closing of many state mental hospitals have ensured that virtually all health care settings now treat schizophrenic patients. Community hospitals and health maintenance organizations now provide care to many psychiatric patients, and community pharmacy practitioners increasingly serve residential care facilities and board and care facilities. Thus schizophrenia and other major psychiatric disorders, whose treatment is largely pharmacologic, is now part of all pharmacists' responsibilities and practice.

Schizophrenia is one of the more misunderstood psychiatric disorders. Schizophrenia is not a split personality. Portrayal of schizophrenia as a Dr. Jekyll-Mr. Hyde syndrome or as multiple personality is inaccurate. Multiple personality disorder exists but is classified as a personality disorder, not a psychotic disorder. While schizophrenic patients may at times be psychotic and bizarre, between psychotic episodes they often remain in total control of their behavior, feelings, and thoughts.

ETIOLOGY AND PREVALENCE

There is no clear causal explanation for schizophrenia. Schizophrenia is best viewed as a set of syndromes with a large continuum of pathophysiologic disruptions. The simple hypothesis of overactive dopaminergic pathways is not adequate to explain schizophrenia. Schizophrenics have diminished dopaminergic autoregulatory functions and disturbed homoeostatic function within the dopaminergic system and between other systems. Underactivity of the medial frontal cortex, caudate nucleus, and thalamus is a consistent finding in newly diagnosed schizophrenics, along with structural findings of bilateral enlarged ventricles and decreased brain volumes in the temporal lobes, amygdala, and hippocampus. Structural changes in the temporal areas have been correlated with positive symptoms of hallucinations and thought disorder, while frontal lobe hypoactivity has been associated with the negative symptoms of schizophrenia (1). There is increased genetic vulnerability to schizophrenia. While the risk in the general population is about 1%, the risk for a first-degree relative is 10%. In dizygotic twins the rate of concordance is 10%; in monozygotic twins it is 40 to 50%, a finding suggesting that nongenetic factors are also important even in the presence of genetic vulnerability (2).

Schizophrenia is not synonomous with psychosis. Psychosis has many causes and is merely a clinical descriptor that is defined as being out of touch with reality. Psychosis can be caused by many drugs (e.g., amphetamines, hallucinogens, anticholinergics, alcohol, phencyclidine) as well as sedative-hypnotic withdrawal, and psychotic symptoms may accompany dementias and delirium from many causes (infectious, metabolic, and endocrine). Psychotic symptoms are also very common in mood disorders, including mania and some major depressive disorders. The diagnostic criterion of a minimum 6-month duration of symptoms for schizophrenia ensures that schizophrenia can usually be distinguished from the briefer-duration drug-induced psychoses.

In the United States the total lifetime prevalence for schizophrenia ranges from 0.5 to 1.0% (3). The prevalence rates for schizophrenia appear to be very similar in different countries and cultures.

DIAGNOSIS AND CLINICAL FINDINGS

Schizophrenia is best understood as a thought disorder. The essential features of schizophrenia include the presence of characteristic psychotic symptoms during the active phase of the illness, deterioration from a previous level of social and occupational functioning, and continuous signs of the disturbance for at least 6 months (Table 55.1). If an illness otherwise meets the criteria but has a duration of between 1 and 6 months, it is termed schizophreniform disorder. Psychotic symptoms with an acute onset that last less than 1 month are termed brief psychotic disorder.

Characteristic symptoms of schizophrenia involve disturbances in perception, content, and form of thought; bizarre behavior; poverty of speech; blunting of emotional expression; avolition; and lack of interest in and impaired attention to others or the environment (Table 55.2). No single symptom is diagnostic of schizophrenia; the diagnosis requires a constellation of symptoms in addition to impaired occupational or social functioning.

Changes in Perception

Perception disturbance primarily involves hallucinations, in which there is a sensory awareness without a sensory stimulus. While perceptual disturbance is possible in any of the five senses, auditory hallucinations are the most common in schizophrenia. Voices or noises are perceived as coming from outside the head, not from within the mind

Table 55.1.
Diagnostic Criteria for Schizophrenia

Two or more of the following symptoms present at least 1 month:
  Delusions
  Hallucinations
  Disorganized speech
  Grossly disorganized or catatonic behavior
  Negative symptoms
Significant decline in social and/or occupational functioning
Some of above symptoms continuously present for 6 months

Source: Adapted from (3).

Table 55.2.
Symptoms of Schizophrenia

Positive symptoms
  Hallucinations
  Delusions
  Formal thought disorder
  Bizarre behavior
Negative symptoms
  Alogia
  Affective blunting
  Avolition
  Anhedonia
  Attentional impairment

Source: Adapted from (4).

as through imagination, and are distinct from the person's own thoughts. Most characteristic of schizophrenic auditory hallucinations are two or more voices conversing with one another or voices that maintain a running commentary on the person's thoughts or behavior. Visual and tactile hallucinations are possible in schizophrenia but are more characteristic of a drug-induced psychosis.

Content of Thought

The major disturbance in content of thought involves delusions, defined as fixed false beliefs. Delusions can vary in theme and content; they may be somatic, religious, referential, or persecutory. Common delusions in schizophrenia include persecutory or paranoid beliefs, in which the person believes that he or she is being followed, spied on, or tormented. Referential ideas or delusions are also common, in which a person believes that song lyrics, another's gestures, or television reports are specifically directed at him or her. So-called Schneiderian symptoms include a variety of bizarre delusions, such as a belief of thought insertion or withdrawal or thought broadcasting or a belief that one's body or actions are being controlled by an outside force. False beliefs or concerns that are not firmly held are termed ideation (e.g., paranoid ideation, ideas of reference).

Form of Thought

A formal thought disorder is regarded as the symptom that is unique to schizophrenia. Disorganized thinking may be manifested as "loose associations" or "derailment," in which the patient may shift from one thought to another without any awareness that the topics are unrelated. Other common descriptors include tangentiality, circumstantiality, or, in the most severe cases, derailment of thought processes. The tangential patient is one whose thinking goes off on a tangent, never to return to the original thought. The circumstantial patient talks in general terms around an idea but never addresses the topic directly. These symptoms must be severe enough to substantially impair effective communication. "Concrete thinking" is the loss of an ability to think in abstract terms.

Bizarre Behavior

Disorganized behavior may be mainfested in many ways, from problems in performing the activities of daily living to childlike silliness, catatonic motor behaviors, or unpredictable agitation. Examples include disheveled or unusual dress or grooming, poor hygiene, inappropriate sexual behavior, untriggered swearing or shouting, and bizarre or rigid posture. Stereotypical behavior (non-goal-directed repetitive movements) and odd mannerisms are common in chronic schizophrenic patients.

Alogia

Poverty of speech is manifested by very brief empty responses to questions that appear to be related to a lack of thoughts rather than any resistance to speaking.

Affect

Disturbances of affect involve blunting, flattening, or inappropriateness of the expression of the mood. This can be manifested as an unchanging facial expression, decreased spontaneous movements, poverty of gestures, poor eye contact, lack of vocal inflection, and slowed speech. These symptoms may be interpreted by others as apathy or indifference and must be differentiated from antipsychotic drug-induced pseudoparkinsonism, as well as depression.

Other Symptoms

Most schizophrenics will have some disturbance in self-initiated goal-directed activity (avolition) that interferes with work and other role functioning. Many schizophrenics do not comfortably relate to the world around them and have great difficulty in interpersonal relationships. This is manifested as social withdrawal and isolation, emotional detachment, and lack of friends. Anhedonia, a lack of interest and motivation in other people or activities, may be present in some schizophrenics.

Positive and Negative Symptoms

Schizophrenic symptoms are classified as either positive or negative symptoms, which correlate with different neural substrates and differential responsiveness to drug therapy (Table 55.2) (4). Positive symptoms reflect increased dopamine function; negative symptoms correspond to hypoactive prefrontal dopaminergic pathways. Traditional antipsychotic drugs are generally very effective in treating the positive symptoms of schizophrenia but are less effective in treating the negative symptoms. The newer atypical antipsychotic drugs, clozapine and risperidone, are effective in treating positive symptoms but are more effective in treating negative symptoms.

Onset, Course and Outcome

The first psychotic episode in schizophrenia commonly occurs in the late teens or early twenties. For many, the onset of psychosis is insidious; prodromal symptoms of social withdrawal, loss of interest in work or school, and deterioration in hygiene are common. The natural course and outcome of schizophrenia are typically very poor (5, 6). Some individuals display exacerbations and remissions of symptoms, while others remain chronically ill. For most, schizophrenia is a chronic disorder with incomplete recovery, persistent dysfunction, and a progressive deteriorating course. There is some evidence that antipsychotic drugs can alter the natural course of the illness; effectively treating an acute psychotic episode does provide for a better outcome for at least several years. Several 15- to 35-year follow-up studies of schizophrenics show that about two-thirds were economically completely incapacitated and were functioning marginally or worse at follow-up. Only 6 to 20% of patients at follow-up were completely free of psychiatric symptoms and judged to be recovered (5).

SCHIZOAFFECTIVE DISORDER

Distinguishing an acutely manic bipolar patient from an acutely psychotic schizophrenic patient is often very difficult because so many symptoms are common to the two disorders. Likewise, the patient with a major depression with psychotic features may be very difficult to distinguish from the schizophrenic with a secondary depression. The diagnostic criteria for schizoaffective disorder require the presence of a manic or major depressive disorder concurrent with symptoms that meet criteria for schizophrenia. During an episode, delusions or hallucinations must be present for at least 2 weeks without any prominent mood symptoms (3). Schizoaffective disorder is unfortunately too convenient a diagnosis and is made too often in place of adequate diagnostic assessment. Most patients who are given this diagnosis are found on follow-up to have either schizophrenia or bipolar disorder. Although primarily a diagnostic issue, the validity of a diagnosis of schizoaffec-

tive disorder is crucial, since these patients often receive unnecessary polypharmacy.

TREATMENT

Antipsychotic drug therapy is only one component of effective therapy for schizophrenic disorders. Drug treatment can eliminate or reduce symptoms of schizophrenia, but psychological, vocational, and social therapies are most effective in facilitating day-to-day coping and improving long-term outcome of schizophrenia (6).

TYPICAL ANTIPSYCHOTIC DRUGS

Pharmacology

More than a dozen antipsychotic drugs are available for use in the United States (Table 55.3), although only about six are commonly used in the treatment of schizophrenia. The aliphatic and piperidine phenothiazines are commonly referred to as low-potency drugs, while the piperazine phenothiazines, thiothixene, and haloperidol are commonly called high-potency drugs. This terminology of low and high potency refers only to the milligram doses that are used for these drugs as well as their similar adverse effect profiles; it does not suggest any difference in effectiveness.

Antipsychotic drugs have in common an ability to antagonize dopaminergic, muscarinic, histaminic, and α-adrenergic neurotransmitter receptors, although the relative affinity for each receptor varies greatly among the drugs. Both the therapeutic effffects and many of the

Table 55.3.
Available Antipsychotic Drugs

Phenothiazines
  Aliphatic
    Chlorpromazine (Thorazine)
    Trifluopromazine (Vesprin)
  Piperidine
    Thioridazine (Mellaril)
    Mesoridazine (Serentil)
  Piperazine
    Trifluoperazine (Stelazine)
    Fluphenazine (Prolixin, Permitil)
    Perphenazine (Trilafon)
    Acetophenazine (Tindal)
    Prochlorperazine (Compazine)
Thioxanthenes
  Thiothixene (Navane)
Butyrophenones
  Haloperidol (Haldol)
Dibenzoxazepines
  Loxapine (Loxitane)
Dihydroindolones
  Molindone (Moban)
Dibenzazepines
  Clozapine (Clozaril)
Benzisoxazole
  Risperidone (Risperdal)

Table 55.4.
Oral Dosage and Potency

Drug	Acute Dosage (mg/day)	Maintenance Dosage (mg/day)	Potency*
Haloperidol	10–60	3–20	2
Fluphenazine	10–60	3–20	2
Thiothixene	20–80	5–30	4
Trifluoperazine	20–80	5–30	5
Perphenazine	8–64	4–32	10
Loxapine	40–160	20–80	10
Molindone	50–200	20–100	10
Clozapine	300–600	150–400	50
Thioridazine	400–800	100–300	100
Chlorpromazine	400–1000	100–300	100
Risperidone	4–16	4–8	—

*Chlorpromazine 100 mg has equal antipsychotic activity to haloperidol 2 mg.

adverse effects of antipsychotic drugs can be explained by their antagonism of neurotransmitter receptors (7).

The antipsychotic activity of these drugs is related to antagonism of D-2 receptors in the mesolimbic area. Antagonism of the D-2 receptors in other areas of the brain explains the occurrence of extrapyramidal effects and endocrinologic effects. Antagonism of muscarinic (acetylcholine) receptors explains the occurrence of anticholinergic effects. Antipsychotic drugs antagonize histamine receptors, with a much greater affinity for H_1 receptors than for H_2 receptors. This antagonism explains the occurrence of sedation, drowsiness, and appetite stimulation and contributes to their hypotensive effects. Molindone's virtual lack of H_1 blockade explains the lack of weight gain and the reported weight loss effect of its use compared to that of other antipsychotic drugs. Finally, α_1 blockade explains the occurrence of postural hypotension and reflex tachycardia, while α_2 blockade explains the mechanism of blocking the antihypertensive effect of drugs such as clonidine and methyldopa. The most potent α_1 blockers are mesoridazine, chlorpromazine, and thioridazine; molindone has virtually no effect on α_1 receptors. Most antipsychotic drugs do not have sufficient α_2 blockade effect to be of clinical significance, but when it is advisable to avoid this effect, haloperidol is preferred.

Treatment of Acute Psychosis

Once a particular drug has been selected for a patient, the lower end of the daily dosage range is given in divided doses initially (e.g., haloperidol 5 mg twice a day or thiothixene 5 mg five times a day) (Table 55.4) (8, 9). Beginning with a divided dose allows evaluation of tolerance of adverse effects and a patient's subjective response to the medication. The initial dose can then be titrated upward by 25 to 33% increments weekly. If there is no change in target symptoms after 1 week, an increased dosage may be necessary; partial reduction of psychotic

symptomatology after 1 week suggests that the dosage be left at its current level. This titration schedule must be slowed in treating the elderly or patients who are experiencing adverse effects. The schedule can be accelerated in treating hospitalized patients whose psychotic symptoms and agitation are severe.

Full therapeutic effect from a given dosage is seen at 6 to 8 weeks, but at least some response should be seen within 1 week to justify maintaining the current dose. Psychomotor agitation and insomnia are likely to resolve first; auditory hallucinations, delusions, and thought disorder typically require several weeks of treatment for significant improvement. If no improvement is seen at the top end of the dosage range, the diagnosis should be reevaluated, drug compliance should be questioned, and an alternative drug should be considered. If partial response is seen at the top end of the dosage range, the dose can be increased further. The one exception is thioridazine, whose pigmentary retinopathy at high doses restricts its maximum daily dosage to 800 mg. Some acutely psychotic patients will require very high doses for response, such as haloperidol 60 mg or more daily. These patients should, however, constitute a minority of patients in a treatment facility. The best candidate for high-dose therapy is the patient whose psychosis is acute, who has a past history of brief episodes, and whose physical examination and medical history are unremarkable. Nonresponse to one antipsychotic drug suggests a trial of different classes of antipsychotic drugs used for at least 4 weeks in doses in excess of 500 mg/day chlorpromazine equivalents. Failure of three antipsychotic drugs justifies consideration of clozapine, risperidone, or adjunctive drugs (9).

Table 55.4 also lists the relative potency of antipsychotic drugs. Potency bears no relationship to effectiveness but refers only to the milligram equivalency of antipsychotic effect. These potency relationships are only approximations and do not take into account the significant differences in adverse effects among the drugs. Thus a patient who needs to be switched from haloperidol 25 mg to an equivalent dose of chlorpromazine would need 1250 mg. However, while this is an equivalent antipsychotic dose, it could not be given to most patients because of chlorpromazine's significant adverse effects of sedation, orthostatic hypotension, and anticholinergic effects.

Dosing Strategies

Attempts have been made to hasten the response of acute psychotic episodes by rapidly administering intramuscular doses of the high-potency drugs. Fluphenazine hydrochloride or haloperidol is given intramuscularly, 5 to 10 mg every hour until resolution of symptoms, excessive sedation, or intolerable adverse effects occur. Often patients may receive 40 to 100 mg within the first 24 hr of therapy. While this is an appealing concept, indications for such rapid titration are very few. Such rapid dosing is most effective for quick control of psychotic agitation and bizarre acting out of psychotic ideation. This technique does not shorten the time these drugs require to exert their therapeutic benefit for the core psychotic symptoms of thought disorder, delusions, and hallucinations when compared to traditional dosing regimens, and such high doses cause more adverse effects. Doses of oral haloperidol or fluphenazine 5 to 20 mg daily are equally effective and are better tolerated than high-dose therapy (9, 10). An equally effective treatment for acute psychotic agitation is use of a benzodiazepine as an adjunct to the antipsychotic drug. This treatment allows elimination of PRN antipsychotic orders, fewer adverse effects, and up to a 50% reduction of antipsychotic drug dose. Lorazepam is the preferred parenteral drug, since it is quickly and reliably absorbed; clonazepam or alprazolam orally (1 to 4 mg daily) is equally useful (11, 12).

Dosage Schedule

Once an effective dose is found, all antipsychotic drugs can be shifted to once-daily bedtime dosing. Once-daily dosing is equally effective, enhances compliance, reduces anticholinergic effects, often eliminates the need for a hypnotic drug, and decreases cost. Occasionally, a patient may require or prefer the daytime sedative effect that a divided dosing schedule provides.

Maintenance Therapy

Once an acute psychotic episode has resolved and the patient is free of overt psychotic symptoms, a decision must be made about maintenance drug therapy. A comparison of controlled studies of continuing antipsychotic drugs versus placebo treatment for 6 weeks to 2 years found an overall relapse rate of 58% in placebo-treated patients and 16% in drug-treated patients (13). For the schizophrenic patient who is stabilized on drug therapy and is virtually asymp-

tomatic for several years, low-dose maintenance therapy is preferred over an attempt to taper and discontinue drug treatment. Although 60 to 80% of patients will relapse within 1 year when they are placebo-treated, all will relapse within 3 years when they are untreated (9, 14). Comparison of a targeted, intermittent treatment approach to continuous drug treatment found that the continuous drug treatment approach was superior in preventing relapse and hospitalization (14, 15).

Very-low-dose maintenance therapy has been evaluated with the use of fluphenazine decanoate. While 25 mg intramuscularly every 2 weeks is the usual maintenance dose, low-dose studies have found that 5 to 10 mg intramuscularly every 2 weeks is an effective dose for many patients. Risk of relapse is higher with 5 mg than with 25 mg after 2 years, but raising the dose to 10 mg intramuscularly every 2 weeks is usually sufficient to treat and prevent psychotic exacerbation (16). All stable chronic schizophrenic patients should be tapered down to a very-low-maintenance dose with careful monitoring. Chronically psychotic patients with persistent symptoms relapse much more frequently with low-dose therapy; schizophrenic patients who are in remission benefit most. A reasonable goal for maintenance therapy is to reduce the antipsychotic dosage to one-half the discharge dose by the end of 1 year (17, 18). However, 10 to 15% of chronic patients will continue to require high-dose maintenance therapy of greater than 15 mg/day of haloperidol or its equivalent (19).

Depot Formulations

The use of fluphenazine decanoate or haloperidol decanoate represents a unique option for maintenance drug therapy. The advantage of these preparations is that a patient can be given an intramuscular injection every 2 to 4 weeks rather than ingesting capsules or tablets daily. Depot drugs are indicated for patients who respond well to antipsychotic drugs but are consistently noncompliant or refuse to take oral medication. Studies of relapse rates find an average difference of 15% favoring depot therapy compared to oral antipsychotic drug therapy. While depot therapy is used in 40 to 60% of treated schizophrenics in many European countries, estimates in the United States are only 10 to 20% of patients (20). Depot therapy is not an appropriate treatment for an acute psychotic episode, owing to variable onset and duration of depot drugs. Treatment of acute psychotic symptoms requires the flexibility of dosage titration that is offered by oral or nondepot intramuscular preparations. The contribution of depot drugs to maintenance drug therapy is substantial, considering the magnitude of noncompliance with antipsychotic drugs. There are several danger areas, however, that must be avoided in using these preparations. The ease and convenience of depot therapy can result in routine, nonindividualized doses and schedules. Continuous monitoring is needed to ensure that staff convenience remains secondary to actual patient needs. Drug usage evaluation in a group of patients who are receiving depot antipsychotics should reveal varying doses and different frequency of injections. Initiation of a depot preparation should not be viewed as a life sentence to depot therapy. Once a patient demonstrates the capability of assuming responsibility in other daily activities, a switch from depot to oral medication should be considered.

Fluphenazine decanoate (FD) is best initiated after oral treatment has resolved acute psychotic symptoms. The techniques of conversion from oral therapy to depot therapy are many, though most are based on clinical experience rather being than validated by clinical trial. If it is known early that the patient will be converted to FD for maintenance, it is easiest to give the patient oral fluphenazine for the acute phase of the psychosis. If the patient happens to be taking another antipsychotic orally, it is not necessary to convert to oral fluphenazine before instituting the FD. The average initial dose of FD following successful treatment of an acute psychotic episode is 12.5 to 75 mg intramuscularly every 2 weeks. A practical approach to conversion that this author has developed is to convert on the basis of the relationship between the usual oral and FD dosage ranges. The oral dose of fluphenazine for treatment of an acute episode is 10 to 60 mg daily; the usual FD dose initially is 12.5 to 75 mg every 2 weeks. To maintain this relationship, take the daily oral fluphenazine dose or its equivalent, increase it to the nearest 0.5 mL amount of FD (25 mg/mL), and give that amount every 2 weeks. For example, 10 mg orally equals 12.5 mg (0.5 mL), and 25 mg orally equals 25 mg (1.0 mL). Because of the delayed onset of effect with FD, conversion from oral fluphenazine to FD is not a simple matter of stopping one and starting the other. Although the peak plasma concentration of fluphenazine occurs within 2 days after a single FD injection, it is often necessary to reduce but continue oral treatment until the second injection is given. With continuous dosing, FD requires at least 6 weeks to reach steady state (21). For maintenance therapy, FD dosage can be gradually reduced, most patients requiring 12.5 to 25 mg every 2 to 3 weeks.

Haloperidol decanoate (HD) is now the preferred depot antipsychotic because of its less frequent administration. While HD and FD are virtually identical in efficacy and adverse effect profile, dose and frequency of administration are different. The initial dose of HD is 10 to 20 times the oral dose of haloperidol, up to a maximum initial dose of 100 mg. If the calculated monthly dose exceeds 100 mg, the balance of the first month's dose can be given in a second injection 3 to 7 days later. For geriatric or hepatically impaired patients a tenfold to fifteenfold conversion should be used initially. A loading dose

technique has been described of giving 20 times the oral dose, using 100 to 200 mg of depot every 3 to 7 days to reach the calculated amount, with a maximum of 450 mg (22). The target monthly maintenance dose should be approximately 10 to 15 times the oral daily dose. A monthly maintenance dose of 200 mg provides better prevention of relapse than do lower doses. Experience with doses over 500 mg is limited, and administration of more than 5 mL should be divided into two equal injections given in two sites. Peak haloperidol concentrations occur between 3 to 9 days, with an apparent half-life of 3 weeks, and the steady state level with multiple dosing is reached after 12 to 16 weeks. The frequency of adverse effects, notably extrapyramidal effects, is the same as or less than with oral haloperidol, although the severity of extrapyramidal effects tends to be worse with depot therapy than with oral therapy. In contrast, FD tends to cause more extrapyramidal effects than does oral fluphenazine (20, 23). HD is available as 50 and 100 mg/mL; FD is available as 25 mg/mL. While HD doses seem low in relation to their oral equivalents, efficacy at these low doses reinforces recent efforts to significantly lower the maintenance doses that are used for most schizophrenic patients.

Plasma Levels

Therapeutic plasma concentrations for antipsychotic drugs are not well established. Fixed-dose studies of haloperidol show that acutely psychotic patients respond best when plasma levels range from 3 to 40 ng/mL; a majority of the studies suggest a range of 5 to 15 ng/mL. There is some suggestion of a therapeutic window, with clinical response decreasing when levels are either above or below that range (24). Minimal evidence exists for the other antipsychotic drugs (9, 25). Plasma levels are not routinely used in the clinical management of schizophrenic patients.

DRUG INTERACTIONS

Most drug interactions with antipsychotic drugs are predictable on the basis of known pharmacologic and pharmacokinetic information. Most antipsychotic drugs are lipophilic and highly protein-bound and have large apparent volumes of distribution. Antipsychotics are extensively metabolized by the liver through microsomal oxidation and conjugation reactions, making them susceptible to enzyme inducers and inhibitors. Common drug interactions include additive sedative, hypotensive, and anticholinergic effects. Cigarette smoking has been shown to increase clearance of many antipsychotic drugs by 50 to 150% (26).

ADVERSE EFFECTS

Extrapyramidal Effects

Extrapyramidal symptoms (EPS) are the most significant adverse effect in terms of frequency and reason for patients' noncompliance with antipsychotic drug therapy.

There are three categories of EPS: dystonic reactions, pseudoparkinsonism, and akathisia. A fourth category, tardive dyskinesia, while technically an extrapyramidal effect, will be treated separately, since its cause, mechanism, and treatment in many aspects are opposite to those of the first three. EPS are described in Table 55.5 (27, 28).

Dystonic reactions involve an acute spasm of a muscle group, which is frightening and often painful for the patient. About 90% of all dystonic reactions occur in the first 72 hr of therapy and can occur after a single dose. Dystonic reactions are most frequent in younger patients and in males (29). The high-potency drugs are more likely to cause dystonic reactions than are the low-potency drugs. Haloperidol in acute psychotic patients causes dystonia in up to 65% of patients (30). Dystonic reactions are generally brief and are most responsive of all EPS to treatment. Laryngospasm is the only potentially life-threatening EPS, since it can interfere with respiration.

Pseudoparkinsonism manifests similarly to Parkinson's disease. Early signs or more mild forms consist of a

Table 55.5.
Extrapyramidal Effects

Dystonic reactions
    Oculogyric crisis: fixed upward gaze
    Torticollis: neck twisting
    Opisthotonus: arching of back
    Trismus: clenched jaw
    Others: spasm of muscle group resulting in facial grimaces; exaggerated posturing of head or jaw; difficulty in speech, swallowing, breathing (laryngospasm)
Pseudoparkinsonism
    Akinesia
        Rigidity and immobility
        Stiffness and slowness of voluntary movement
        Masklike facial expression
        Drooling (sialorrhea)
        Stooped posture
        Shuffling, festinating gait
        Slow, monotonous speech
    Tremor
        Regular rhythmic oscillations of extremities, especially hands and fingers
        Pill-rolling movement of fingers
Akathisia
    Inability to sit still, constant pacing
    Continuous agitation and restless movements
    Rocking and shifting of weight while standing
    Shifting of legs, tapping of feet while sitting
Tardive dyskinesia
    Mouth: rhythmical involuntary movements of tongue, lips, or jaw; protrusion of tongue; puckering of mouth; chewing movements (bucco-linguo-masticatory triad)
    Choreiform: irregular purposeless, involuntary quick movements of the extremities; flailing movements
    Athetoid: continuous wormlike slow movements of the extremities
    Axial hyperkinesis: to-and-fro clonic movements of spine

reduction of facial expression and arm movements. Of special concern is akinesia, which can sometimes be misdiagnosed as depression, demoralization, and/or negative symptoms of schizophrenia. Pseudoparkinson symptoms typically begin after several weeks of antipsychotic drug therapy and may occur up to 3 months after initiation of treatment. Pseudoparkinsonism is more commonly seen in the elderly and is usually very responsive to treatment. Parkinsonian tremor, rigidity, and bradykinesia do occur naturally in 20 to 30% of untreated schizophrenics and should be assumed to be drug-induced (31).

Akathisia is the most common and troublesome EPS. It is often difficult to distinguish akathisia from psychotic agitation; as a result, antipsychotic dosage may be increased, thus worsening the akathisia. Akathisia has no preference for any age group and has its onset days to weeks after drug therapy begins. Akathisia is the least likely EPS to respond to treatment and is the primary cause of antipsychotic drug noncompliance. Akathisia is caused more by the high-potency drugs (28).

The approximate frequency of EPS caused in patients treated with thioridazine is 10 to 15%, that for chlorpromazine is 20 to 25%, and that for fluphenazine and haloperidol is 40 to 50%. The severity of akathisia is often greater with depot drugs. It is not uncommon to be forced to discontinue depot drugs because of intolerable and untreatable akathisia and to switch to another drug that has less of a likelihood of causing EPS. Patients who are receiving lithium in addition to an antipsychotic drug, as well as those with organic brain syndromes, have a greater likelihood of EPS (32).

The pathophysiology of EPS is now understood to be much more complex than a simple model of cholinergic-dopaminergic balance in the striatum. Blockade or dysregulation of dopamine-2 receptors appear to be responsible for most EPS. Additionally, γ-aminobutyric acid (GABA), adrenergic, and cholinergic influences on nigrostriatal dopaminergic activity can directly affect whether EPS will be manifested, and drugs affecting each of these systems can be used as treatments for EPS. Dystonias are the result of rapid shifts in dopaminergic transmission, whereas pseudoparkinsonism results from postsynaptic dopaminergic blockade. Akathisia is thought to result from dopaminergic dysregulation in limbic or cortical pathways; this would explain why it is the EPS that is most resistant to treatment (1).

DRUG TREATMENT OF EPS

Commonly used drugs and doses to treat EPS are listed in Table 55.6. The two most commonly used anticholinergic drugs are trihexyphenidyl and benztropine. They are equal in efficacy and adverse effects, but benztropine is twice as potent as trihexyphenidyl. The duration of effect of benztropine is longer than that of trihexyphenidyl, allowing

Table 55.6.
Drugs Used to Treat Extrapyramidal Effects

Drug	Daily Oral Dose (mg)	Daily Dosing Frequency	IM/IV Dose (mg)
Benztropine (Cogentin)	2–6	1–2	2
Trihexyphenidyl (Artane, Tremin)	4–15	3–4	—
Diphenhydramine (Benadryl)	100–300	3–4	50
Amantadine (Symmetrel)	200–400	2–3	—

benztropine to be given once daily or at most twice daily. Trihexyphenidyl must be given at least three times daily. When benztropine is given once daily, it should be given in the morning. Bedtime dosing is of no value, since the extrapyramidal tracts shut down during sleep and EPS are not present during the night. Diphenhydramine is a less effective oral treatment for EPS but is an effective drug parenterally for dystonic reactions.

Acute dystonic reactions are best treated with parenteral diphenhydramine 50 mg or benztropine 2 mg. Nonresponse within 1 min for intravenous dosing or 15 to 20 min for intramuscular dosing justifies administration of a second dose. For pseudoparkinsonism, oral benztropine 1 to 2 mg twice daily or trihexyphenidyl 2 mg three or four times daily is the usual starting dose, maximum doses usually being 6 mg and 15 mg, respectively. While pseudoparkinsonism is usually responsive to anticholinergic agents, akathisia accompanied by pseudoparkinsonism responds only to anticholinergic drugs (28). The two classes of drugs that are commonly used to treat akathisia are benzodiazepines and β-adrenergic antagonists. Diazepam 15 to 30 mg daily, lorazepam 2 to 5 mg daily, and propranolol 20 to 80 mg daily are most commonly used to treat akathisia. Case reports suggest that other benzodiazepines (clonazepam) and β-blockers (nadolol, pindolol) are also effective in the treatment of akathisia. The variety of treatment approaches to akathisia suggests that there is no optimal treatment approach, and many patients will not be effectively treated. The best treatment for akathisia remains antipsychotic dosage reduction if this is clinically possible, trials of drug treatments, and, as a last choice, switching to another antipsychotic drug that is less likely to cause EPS (33).

Amantadine is considered an alternative drug for EPS when anticholinergic drugs fail or cause intolerable adverse effects. Amantadine causes no anticholinergic effects, thus offering a useful alternative for elderly patients and patients whose medical status could be worsened by these effects. Amantadine also causes no significant effect on memory or time perception, whereas anticholinergic drugs

impair storage of new information and perception of time (34). A daily dose of amantadine 200 mg equals the efficacy of 8 mg of trihexyphenidyl.

The literature in the 1970s recommended against the automatic prescribing of an anticholinergic agent when antipsychotic drugs are initiated (35). This literature fails to take into account the fact that more recent prescribing trends favor use of the high-potency antipsychotics in higher doses than were used in the 1970s, thus creating a much greater potential for EPS and, in particular, dystonic reactions. The use of benztropine 2 mg twice daily for the first week of high-potency antipsychotic therapy has been shown to significantly reduce dystonic reactions, while placebo-treated patients who were given high-potency drugs experienced a 47% incidence of dystonic reaction (36). Most studies suggest that prophylaxis reduces the rate of dystonia by twofold in all patients and by fivefold to eightfold in patients who are given high-potency antipsychotic drugs (35). Anticholinergic prophylaxis is justified when at least two risk factors for developing an EPS are present: the patient has a history of EPS, the patient is a young male, and a high-potency antipsychotic drug is being administered. In these cases, prophylaxis is a high-benefit, low-risk treatment.

The appropriate duration of anticholinergic drug treatment is not well established, but after 2 to 3 months the anticholinergic drug dose should be reduced gradually, and if no EPS recur, the drug should be discontinued. Withdrawal of unnecessary anticholinergic agents is desirable to minimize adverse effects of memory impairment and anticholinergic effects (37, 38).

Tardive Dyskinesia

Tardive dysinesia (TD) is a late-appearing effect that looks like an EPS, but its cause and treatment are very different. The clinical features of TD are the bucco-linguomasticatory triad (Table 55.5). These mouth movements are usually mild, and many patients are unaware of them until others point them out. TD often appears as if the patient is chewing gum or has ill-fitting dentures. The more severe cases may include movements of fingers, toes, arms, and legs. Although rare, severe axial movements may interfere with walking, respiratory dyskinesia may make breathing labored, and intense facial grimacing can produce marked discomfort as well as social and physical disability (39). The jerky choreiform movements are often made to look like purposeful movements, such that a patient will be constantly readjusting glasses, hair, or clothing. Observation of fingers and toes at rest may reveal constant involuntary dyskinetic movement. Not all movements are drug-induced, however. In elderly patients, dyskinesias can spontaneously develop independent of antipsychotic drug therapy. Up to 23% of schizophrenics with no exposure to antipsychotic drugs will show some movement disorder on evaluation, 15% showing specific oral-facial dyskinesias (40).

Unlike EPS, TD typically appears on antipsychotic dose reduction or discontinuation, improves when antipsychotic dosage is increased, worsens with administration of anticholinergic drugs, and may persist for months or years after antipsychotic drugs are discontinued. All antipsychotic drugs are capable of causing TD. Clozapine may be the one exception, since it has much less affinity for the D_2 receptor. Prevalence of TD cannot be precisely stated, since so many variables enter in considering a long-term adverse effect. Prospective studies in all age groups suggest a 20% risk of persistent TD after 5 years of cumulative antipsychotic drug exposure, with an incidence of about 4% per year for the first 5 to 6 years. Higher incidence rates have been consistently found in older populations (41). Increasing age remains the most consistent factor associated with increased risk of TD. Other risk factors include female sex in older populations and diagnosis of affective disorder. Patients with moderately severe TD have more drug-free periods in their drug histories than do patients with mild TD (42). Follow-up of patients for up to 10 years suggests that the severity of TD does not increase over time but either remains constant or decreases despite continued antipsychotic drug treatment (9, 43).

The pathophysiology of TD can be deduced from the clinical observation of changes various drugs induce. Improvement of symptoms is seen with an increase in dose of antipsychotic drug, and worsening of symptoms that is seen with an anticholinergic drug or a decrease in dose of antipsychotic drug suggests a relative striatal hyperdopaminergic activity. TD is thought to result from long-term blockade of striatal dopaminergic receptors with resultant hypersensitivity of those receptors. It has been suggested that TD remains reversible if only hypersensivity develops but becomes irreversible if dopaminergic receptors undergo structural changes and/or an increased number of dopaminergic receptors develop (44, 45). Early in therapy, there is up-regulation of dopamine-2 receptors, with later denervation supersensitivity that causes a further proliferation of dopamine-2 receptors in the parts of the striatum that control mouth, lip, and tongue motion. On dosage reduction or discontinuation of treatment, younger patients are more able to down-regulate their dopamine-2 receptors and have reversal of TD symptoms than are older patients (46).

Treatment approaches to TD are based on an understanding of its pathophysiology. Symptoms should improve on administration of GABA-ergic agonists, noradrenergic antagonists, dopaminergic antagonists, or cholinergic agonists (47). Studies of all treatment attempts can be summarized as being at best only moderately effective for up to several months but not effective in the long-term management of irreversible TD. Most recently, vitamin E,

in doses of 1600 IU/day, has shown efficacy in trials of up to 12 weeks (48). Although there is no consistently effective treatment of TD, there are several necessary steps in the management of the patient with TD. First, any anticholinergic drug should be discontinued, and the antipsychotic drug dose should be lowered as far as is clinically possible. Clozapine has been suggested as the antipsychotic drug that is least likely to contribute to a worsening of TD and may become the drug of choice for patients with severe TD. Because treatment of TD is so disappointing, prevention becomes most important. While TD is an acceptable risk for patients who have schizophrenia, with its possibility of severe disruptive psychotic episodes, antipsychotic drugs should not be used casually for nonpsychotic indications. Anxiety disorders, insomnia, personality disorders, gastrointestinal disorders, and long-term management of bipolar patients are more effectively treated with other drug classes. Patients who receive maintenance antipsychotic drug therapy should be assessed for presence of early signs of TD at least semiannually. Early signs include wormlike muscular movements on the surface of the tongue, facial tics such as frequent blinking, and choreoathethoid finger or toe movements. Early detection is crucial in identifying TD while it is still reversible.

Anticholinergic Effects

Peripheral anticholinergic effects may commonly accompany thioridazine and chlorpromazine therapy. Additionally, patients who are taking high-potency drugs often require anticholinergic agents for EPS, so they too are often bothered by dry mouth, blurred near vision, and constipation. These effects are directly dose-related and are additive. Usually, anticholinergic effects are bothersome but not significant unless there is preexisting prostatic hypertrophy, glaucoma, or constipation. Anticholinergic effects can often be minimized by switching to once-daily bedtime dosing or by decreasing antipsychotic or anticholinergic drug dosage. The dry mouth and blurred vision are worse in the beginning of therapy, and some tolerance develops. Patients should be instructed that these effects should decrease after the first 2 weeks of therapy. There is no treatment of proven value except alteration of dosage or dosing schedule. Constipation is the more serious concern that should be a part of routine monitoring. The reduction in gastrointestinal motility and secretions typically results in constipation characterized by hard, dry stools. Use of stool softeners represents the most appropriate treatment, such as docusate 100 to 500 mg daily accompanied by increased fluid intake. Treatment need not be continuous but may be on an interrupted basis for 4 to 7 days at a time. Patients often will also require some education regarding normal physiology and the role of exercise and diet. Untreated constipation can become a significant medical concern and emergency. Fecal impaction, ileus, the

Table 55.7.
Relative Adverse Effect Profiles°

Drug	Sedation	Extra-pyramidal	Anticholinergic	Postural Hypotension
Haloperidol	1	4	1	1
Fluphenazine	1	4	2	1
Thiothixene	2	3	2	1
Trifluoperazine	2	3	2	1
Perphenazine	2	3	2	1
Molindone	1	2	1	1
Loxapine	2	2	2	2
Chlorpromazine	4	2	3	4
Thioridazine	4	1	4	4
Clozapine	4	<1	4	4
Risperidone	1	1	1	2

°1 is low, 4 is high.

megacolon requiring surgery, and fatalities have resulted from untreated chronic constipation caused by antipsychotic drugs. Rarely, more severe anticholinergic effects can occur such as urinary retention and a central anticholinergic intoxication characterized by confusion, delirium, and psychotic symptoms. Urinary retention is a particular problem in older men with benign prostatic hypertrophy. Treatment may require catheterization and bethanechol, accompanied by significant reduction of dosage of the causative drug or change to another drug that has much less anticholinergic activity (Table 55.7). Central anticholinergic effects are of most concern in the elderly and patients with dementia. A patient's entire drug regimen must be reviewed to detect all drugs that are capable of contributing to the anticholinergic effect, including antihistamines and tricyclic antidepressants.

Cardiovascular Effects

The most frequent cardiovascular effect caused by antipsychotic drugs is orthostatic hypotension. It is much more common with the aliphatic and piperidine phenothiazines and is unusual with the high-potency drugs except when they are given parenterally (27). Orthostatic hypotension is most common in the first hours or days of treatment, and most patients develop a compensatory tolerance to the subjective effect of dizziness during the first week of therapy. This effect must be part of initial patient education, since it is easy to prevent. When an aliphatic or piperidine phenothiazine is first given or when dosage is increased, patients should be warned to rise slowly from a sitting or reclining position. Elderly patients and patients who are taking other drugs with hypotensive effects are at much greater risk of significant hypotensive effects.

Treatment of orthostatic hypotension usually requires only elevating the feet while the patient is in a prone position. Nonresponse, which is unusual, will then require administration of fluids and, in rare cases, pressor agents. Pure α-adrenergic agents are preferred over a drug like epinephrine to overcome the antipsychotic drug's α-adrenergic blockade. Thioridazine, and to a lesser extent chlorpromazine, may induce electrocardiogram changes, T-wave abnormalities in particular. Doses above 300 mg daily are necessary to see this effect in most patients. This change is thought to represent a benign disturbance of myocardial repolarization and does not represent a clinical concern.

Neuroleptic Malignant Syndrome

Neuroleptic malignant syndrome (NMS) is an uncommon but serious adverse effect that occurs in 1.4% of patients who are treated with antipsychotic drugs. NMS is characterized by (a) fever; (b) severe EPS such as lead-pipe rigidity, trismus, choreiform movements, and opisthotonus; (c) signs of autonomic instability such as tachycardia, labile hypertension, diaphoresis, and incontinence; and (d) fluctuating levels of consciousness. Some cases have been followed by permanent neurological sequelae, including dementia and signs of parkinsonism. Through 1980 there was a mortality rate of 22% in reported cases; the mortality rate has now dropped to 4% in the last 50 cases reported because of improved early recognition and treatment (49). Fatalities have been associated with rhabdomyolysis and myoglobinuria with acute renal failure, cardiovascular collapse, intravascular thrombosis with pulmonary embolism, and respiratory arrest.

NMS typically occurs after 3 to 9 days of treatment with antipsychotic drugs and is not related to dose or previous antipsychotic drug exposure. Once NMS begins, symptoms rapidly progress over 24 to 72 hr. Symptoms usually last 5 to 10 days after discontinuation of oral antipsychotic drugs and 13 to 30 days after discontinuation of depot drugs. NMS occurs more often in patients under 40 years of age, is almost twice as common in males as in females, and in 40% of cases occurred in patients with affective disorder rather than schizophrenia.

Early diagnosis of NMS is crucial to successful treatment. The antipsychotic drug should be quickly discontinued, and supportive measures should be provided, particularly hydration. Though controlled trials are not likely to be possible, dantrolene and dopaminergic agonists such as bromocriptine and levodopa have been effective in treating many cases of NMS. Because many patients who experience NMS will require resumption of an antipsychotic drug, rechallenge is usually necessary. A waiting period of 5 days before rechallenge, and preferably 2 weeks after complete resolution of the NMS, is recommended (50, 51). Depot antipsychotic drugs are usually not given to patients who have a history of NMS.

Endocrine Effects

Common endocrine effects of antipsychotic drugs include galactorrhea and menstrual irregularities in females, with a prevalence of 30% (52). Galactorrhea results from suppression of prolactin inhibitory factor in the median eminence of the hypothalamus by antipsychotic drugs, allowing secretion of prolactin from the anterior pituitary. No specific treatment is necessary, and lowering the dosage may lessen or eliminate this effect. The patient should be assured that it is a reversible effect. There is no information concerning a differential incidence of galactorrhea among antipsychotic drugs; all typical antipsychotic drugs should be capable of causing this effect, since it is caused by dopaminergic blockade in the hypothalamus. Amenorrhea and irregular menses are common in psychiatric patients. A 1942 (pre–drug era) study of schizophrenic women of childbearing age showed an 18% incidence of amenorrhea, and 31% had delayed or prolonged menstrual cycles (53). With the introduction of antipsychotic drugs, the incidence seems not to have increased. All women of childbearing age should have a menstrual history taken to use as a baseline before drug therapy is initiated. Women who experience amenorrhea should be cautioned not to view the antipsychotic drug as a reliable contraceptive.

Phenothiazines, thiothixene, and haloperidol cause weight gain; loxapine and molindone may cause slight weight loss (54). This difference for some patients can represent a useful clinical difference. The mechanism of weight change is unknown, but it may be due to a combination of effects on several neurotransmitters. A high affinity for blockade of H_1 and D_2 receptors correlates with weight gain, and serotonin agonist effects contribute to weight loss. Molindone may have a central anorexigenic effect via serotonin agonist activity, coupled with its low affinity for H_1 and D_2 receptors.

Temperature Regulation

Antipsychotic drugs interfere with normal temperature regulation. The most common effect is relative poikilothermia, in which the environmental temperature can produce either hypothermia or hyperthermia. Hyperthermia is more frequently reported by patients who are taking antipsychotic drugs in hot, humid climates. Hyperthermia not only results from central effects on temperature regulation, but is also aggravated by an increased peripheral vasodilation and diminished heat loss due to decreased sweating from anticholinergic effects.

Sexual Dysfunction

The most frequent adverse effect is a disorder of ejaculation. Most common is absence of ejaculation on masturbation or sexual intercourse. Some patients also report suprapubic pain on orgasm. In addition to their affecting α-adrenergic receptors in the pelvic plexus, thus interfering with the ejaculatory mechanism, antipsychotic drugs with high anticholinergic effects can also relax the internal sphincter muscle of the bladder, resulting in retrograde ejaculation by reflux of semen into the bladder. Patients should be reassured that these effects are reversible, and if necessary, a drug with less anticholinergic activity can be substituted. Impotence or ejaculation complaints should not be routinely assumed to be drug-induced, since sexual dysfunction is a common component of psychiatric disorders.

Pigmentary Effects

Pigmentation in the skin and eye occurs with high-dose, long-term use of low-potency phenothiazine drugs. Piperazine phenothiazines and thioxanthenes can also contribute to pigmentation, but the risk is very low, since they are given in tens of milligrams instead of hundreds of milligrams daily. Haloperidol, loxapine, and molindone do not cause pigmentation and represent alternative treatment options. Ocular pigmentation involves the cornea and lens, while skin pigmentation may range from a slate gray to a metallic purple color and is confined to skin that is exposed to sunlight. The color changes are so gradual that the patient may not notice. Any patient with skin pigmentation should be referred for ophthalmologic examination, since there is close correlation of skin and eye changes. Patients who have received a daily dose of 600 mg or 200 g of chlorpromazine in 1 year have a 30% likelihood of eye pigmentation (55). These pigmentary changes are slowly reversible over a period of months once the patient has been switched to an antipsychotic that is incapable of causing pigmentation. Thioridazine is unique in its ability to cause pigmentary retinopathy when given in doses over 1200 mg daily for several months. Because retinal pigmentation can directly interfere with visual acuity, thioridazine has an absolute dosage limit of 800 mg daily to prevent this effect.

Allergic Reactions

Skin eruptions take a variety of forms, but the most common reaction is a rash on the face, neck, upper chest, and extremities that occurs within 14 to 60 days. Often allergic skin reactions are mild and transitory and can be treated with antihistamines without discontinuing the antipsychotic drug. Allergic skin manifestations must be differentiated from photosensitivity reactions, which are characterized by erythematous lesions in sun-exposed areas of the body.

Other Adverse Effects

All antipsychotic drugs except loxapine have been associated with hepatic toxicity, though it is rare and of little concern except for patients with preexisting hepatic dysfunction. Cholestatic jaundice with chlorpromazine typically occurs within the first 4 weeks of therapy, and most cases have classic prodromal symptoms that precede the jaundice by about 1 week. Laboratory findings are consistent with those seen in other types of obstructive jaundice. Onset of prodromal symptoms is usually abrupt. Chlorpromazine-induced hepatitis is usually short-lived and self-limiting. With the exception of clozapine, hematologic effects of antipsychotic drugs are varied but extremely rare. Agranulocytosis, the most significant hematologic effect, has an abrupt onset in which the leukocyte count drops rapidly, reaching its low point in 2 to 5 days. Ninety percent of cases occur within the first 8 weeks of phenothiazine drug therapy, whereas clozapine-induced agranulocytosis often has a delayed onset of 6 to 8 weeks and will usually occur within the first 6 months of treatment. Agranulocytosis begins with symptoms of localized infection, usually in the pharynx, and includes fever, pharyngeal erythema, and adenopathy (56).

Seizures occur in approximately 1% of patients who take antipsychotic drugs. A history of seizures is not an absolute contraindication to use of an antipsychotic drug. Among typical antipsychotic drugs, thioridazine, molindone, thiothixene, fluphenazine, and haloperidol are least associated with seizure production, while seizures have been reported most with chlorpromazine and to a moderate extent with trifluoperazine and perphenazine. Clozapine is by far the most likely psychotropic drug to cause seizures, with a 1 year prevalence of approximately 10%. Of additional significant importance, however, are drug factors that increase the likelihood of seizures, including (a) rapid dosage titration, (b) abruptly switching from one antipsychotic drug to another, (c) use of two antipsychotics simultaneously, and (d) discontinuation of concurrently used benzodiazepines (57).

NEWER ANTIPSYCHOTIC DRUGS

While the clinical effect of typical antipsychotic drugs is explained by their blockade of dopamine$_2$ (D$_2$) receptors, newer antipsychotic drugs have been developed that have unique and atypical effects. Newer drugs are being developed that include selective dopamine agonists or partial agonists, serotonin agonists and antagonists, mixed dopamine and serotonin antagonists, and atypical components of these effects (58). The first two of these antipsychotic drugs to be marketed in the United States are clozapine and risperidone.

Clozapine

Clozapine was the first marketed atypical antipsychotic drug with unique pharmacological effects and indications, but unfortunately, it also has unique significant adverse effects. Clozapine has more affinity for D$_1$ and D$_4$ receptor

blockade than D$_2$ receptor blockade and also has serotonin$_2$ (5-HT$_2$) receptor blockade. It has been suggested that the combination of D$_2$ and 5-HT$_2$ blockade and/or the D$_1$ and D$_4$ effects accounts for the drug's unique effects. Both of these hypotheses are actively being investigated with nearly two dozen compounds, with various combinations of receptor effects in clinical testing (58).

Clozapine is more effective than typical antipsychotic drugs for refractory schizophrenia, is as effective for the positive symptoms of schizophrenia, and is more effective for the negative symptoms (59, 60). Clozapine is the drug of choice for patients who have failed adequate trials of several antipsychotic drugs. Up to 40% of these patients will respond favorably to clozapine (61). Thus efficacy of clozapine should be carefully evaluated, and the drug should be continued only when the benefits are significant enough to outweigh the risks of serious adverse effects. Clozapine's unique efficacy means that some patients are successfully treated for the first time in many years, while others experience tremendous disappointment when the drug fails. The clinician must be aware of and cope with patient and family expectations, cure and rescue fantasies, family conflicts from improved functioning, and adaptation acceptance if treatment fails (62). Despite the high cost of the drug and its associated intense and costly adverse-effect-monitoring requirements, clozapine has been shown to be a cost-effective treatment of resistant schizophrenia because of reduced cost of hospitalization (63). Initial dosing of clozapine must be very low (e.g., 25 to 50 mg) and must be titrated up slowly because of adverse effects. While the maximum daily dose is 900 mg, most patients will benefit from daily doses of 300 to 600 mg with fewer adverse effects (64).

Frequent adverse effects include sedation, orthostatic hypotension, anticholinergic effects, fever, and excessive salivation. Seizures are dose-related, with a frequency up to 2% with therapeutic doses but 14% when daily doses exceed 600 mg (64). Agranulocytosis is the other major adverse effect of concern, occurring in up to 26% of patients. Clozapine agranulocytosis is characterized by a white blood cell (WBC) count of less than 2000 cells/m^3, a polymorphonuclear leukocyte count of less than 500 cells/m^3, and relative lymphopenia. Weekly WBC monitoring is a mandatory component of treatment, and deaths have occurred in the United States despite weekly WBC monitoring. Substantial weight gain has been reported in a majority of patients receiving clozapine (64). Case reports of adverse effects of clozapine include neuroleptic malignant syndrome, priapism, pancreatitis, and hyponatremia. Extrapyramidal effects are rare with clozapine, a unique advantage compared to typical antipsychotic drugs (65). Overall, clozapine represents a valuable option for treatment-resistant patients and those with prominent negative symptoms. Clozapine should be reserved for patients who cannot be treated with other agents and when benefits are clear and outweigh the potential for the many serious adverse effects.

Risperidone

Risperidone combines potent 5-HT$_2$ receptor blockade with weaker D$_2$ antagonism. This combination yields additional efficacy for negative symptoms of schizophrenia and less EPS than do typical antipsychotic drugs. It has lower affinity for α_1-adrenergic and H$_1$ receptors and neglible affinity for D$_1$ and muscarinic receptors. Risperidone has a curvilinear dose-response curve, with an optimum daily dose range of 4 to 8 mg. Adverse effects are minimized by initiating risperidone at 1 mg twice daily, increasing by 2 mg weekly. Risperidone is more effective, particularly for negative symptoms, and causes fewer EPS than haloperidol does. Higher doses of risperidone (12 to 16 mg) cause EPS that are similar to those seen with haloperidol. The most common adverse effects include agitation, anxiety, insomnia, EPS, headache, and nausea. Orthostatic hypotension is possible during initial dose titration (66, 67).

Clozapine and risperidone share the similarities of greater efficacy for negative symptoms and less EPS than typical antipsychotic drugs. Clozapine has an established efficacy for treatment-resistant schizophrenia but a much greater risk of serious adverse effects of agranulocytosis and seizures. Initial comparative studies show equal efficacy, clozapine causing more sedation and weight gain, risperidone causing more EPS (68).

DRUG OF CHOICE

An examination of factors that are important in the drug selection process provides a useful way to present the clinically significant differences among antipsychotic drugs. The drug of choice for a patient should ideally be the most effective and have the least side effects for that patient, and the patient should have a positive past history of response to the drug. For compliance reasons the patient should have a positive attitude or at least a neutral attitude toward the drug selected. There is no single drug that can, before it is used, be predicted to be more effective than any other. The one exception is the greater efficacy of clozapine and risperidone for negative symptoms. However, equivalent efficacy does not suggest that all patients will respond equally well to any given antipsychotic drug. While it is not possible to predict the most effective drug, individual patients do sometimes show better response to particular drugs. It is for this reason that past history of response should be a major factor in selecting a drug. Important questions to ask in the drug history include "Which drug helped you most in the past?" and "With which side effects have you had the most difficulty?". Most schizophrenic patients have been treated with several or many different

drugs and often have definite opinions about individual drugs. If a negative attitude is elicited about a particular drug, it makes no sense to choose that drug again, since compliance will likely be very poor. Some chronic patients have very negative attitudes about almost all the antipsychotic drugs and will refuse to take them if they are prescribed. In this case, drug selection becomes a matter of reviewing the record to find a drug that the patient has not tried. Other patients are firmly committed to taking one drug and will refuse to try anything else in spite of other considerations such as side effects. These two types of patients make a strong case for the need for a very liberal formulary of antipsychotic drugs. In terms of efficacy, there is no need for more than maybe two drugs on a formulary. In terms of side effects, maybe four or five drugs could be justified. But in terms of patient attitudes and past history, virtually all antipsychotic drugs should be available for use in the treatment of schizophrenic disorders. It has also been shown that a patient's early subjective response to an antipsychotic drug can be used as a predictor of symptomatic outcome (69). Response to questions such as "How does the medication agree with you?", "Did it make you feel calmer?", "Did it affect your thinking?", and "Do you think this would be the right medicine for you?" were rated on the basis of euphoric or dysphoric responses after a test dose of chlorpromazine. During the subsequent hospital stay, patients with an early euphoric response improved more than did patients with an early dysphoric response. The early dysphoric response persists, since 88% of the dysphoric responders eventually refused to continue taking chlorpromazine because of persisting dysphoria compared to only 23% of the early euphoric responders. Thus in addition to seeking a patient's past history of response and attitude, it is worthwhile to assess a patient's early subjective response to an antipsychotic drug.

The final factor that is important in drug selection is the clinically important differences in frequency of adverse effects. The relative frequencies of four of the most common adverse effects are listed in Table 55.7. Unfortunately, there is no drug that is least likely to cause all adverse effects. Rather, drug selection requires tailoring the drug to the individual patient. Sedation may be an undesirable effect for some patients, while it may be advantageous for the patient with significant agitation or insomnia. A past history of EPS or noncompliance due to EPS might suggest the use of thioridazine rather than haloperidol or fluphenazine, or a history of severe EPS might justify use of clozapine or risperidone. For the patient with dementia, glaucoma, prostatic hypertrophy, or chronic constipation, a drug that is low in anticholinergic effects is most desirable. For the patient who is already taking another drug with orthostatic hypotensive effects or for elderly patients in whom hypotension can decrease cerebral blood flow and worsen confusion, a drug that is low in orthostatic hypotensive effects would be most desirable. Information from a patient's medical history, past drug history, and current symptoms must be used in selecting the most appropriate drug.

CONCLUSION

Schizophrenia is a chronic thought disorder that is manifested by various psychotic symptoms and usually a gradual decline in functioning. Drug treatment is most effective in treating the acute psychotic symptoms and preventing relapse with maintenance therapy. Antipsychotic drug selection must be individualized for each patient. The drug of choice should be determined by an evaluation of the patient's past history of drug response and adverse effects, the patient's attitude toward individual drugs that may affect compliance, and clinically significant differences in antipsychotic drugs' adverse effect profiles. Most schizophrenics will require lifelong drug treatment to prevent psychotic exacerbations of their illness. Although antipsychotic drugs cause many adverse effects, most of these can be ameliorated by patient education, manipulation of dosage and schedule, and sometimes adjunctive drug treatments. Thus patients who are being treated with antipsychotic drugs require careful monitoring to maximize response and minimize adverse effects. The philosophy of community mental health care means that most care givers (pharmacist, nurse practitioner, physician's assistant, etc.), regardless of practice setting, will care for schizophrenic patients and must have some expertise and experience in this area of therapeutics.

REFERENCES

1. Ereshefsky L, Tran-Johnson TK, Watanabe MD. Pathophysiologic basis for schizophrenia and the efficacy of antipsychotics. Clin Pharm 9:682–707, 1990.
2. Carpenter WT, Buchanan RW. Schizophrenia. New Engl J Med 330:681–690, 1994.
3. American Psychiatric Association. Diagnostic and statistical manual of mental disorders. 4th ed. Washington, DC: American Psychiatric Association, 1994:273–315.
4. Andreasen NC, Swayze III VW, Flaum M, et al. The neural mechanisms of mental phenomena. In: Andreasen NC, ed. Schizophrenia: from mind to molecule. Washington DC: American Psychiatric Press, 1994.
5. Black DW, Yates WR, Andreasen NC. Schizophrenia, schizophreniform disorder, and delusional disorders. In: Talbott JA, Hales RE, Yudofsky SC, eds. Textbook of psychiatry. Washington, DC: American Psychiatric Press, 1988:357–402.
6. Davis JM, Andriukaitis S. The natural course of schizophrenia and effective maintenance drug treatment. J Clin Psychopharmacol 6(suppl 1):2S–10S, 1986.
7. Richelson E. Pharmacology of neuroleptics in use in the United States. J Clin Psychiatry 46(8, sect 2):8–14, 1985.
8. Ortiz A, Gershon S. The future of neuroleptic psychopharmacology. J Clin Psychiatry 47(5, suppl):3–11, 1986.
9. Kane JM. The current status of neuroleptic therapy. J Clin Psychiatry 50:322–328, 1989.
10. Baldessarini RJ, Cohen BM, Teicher MH. Significance of neuroleptic dose and plasma level in the pharmacological treatment of psychoses. Arch Gen Psychiatry 45:79–91, 1988.
11. Bodkin JA. Emerging uses for high-potency benzodiazepines in psychotic disorders. J Clin Psychiatry 51(5, suppl):41–46, 1990.
12. Barbee JG, Mancuso DM, Freed CR, et al. Alprazolam as a neuroleptic adjunct in the emergency treatment of schizophrenia. Am J Psychiatry 149:506–510, 1992.
13. Davis JM, Andriukaitis S. The natural course of schizophrenia and effective maintenance drug treatment. J Clin Psychopharmacol 6:2S–10S, 1986.
14. Davis JM, Kane JM, Marder SR, et al. Dose response of prophylactic antipsychotics. J Clin Psychiatry 54(3, suppl):24–30, 1993.
15. Carpenter WT Jr, Hanlon TE, Heinrichs DW, et al: Continuous versus targeted medication in schizophrenic outpatients: outcome results. Am J Psychiatry 147:1138–1148, 1990.
16. Marder SR, Van Putten T, Mintz J, et al. Low and conventional dose maintenance therapy with fluphenazine decanoate. Arch Gen Psychiatry 44:518–521, 1987.
17. Johnson DAW. Antipsychotic medication: clinical guidelines for maintenance therapy. J Clin Psychiatry 46(5, sect 2):6–15, 1985.
18. Heresco-Levy U, Greenberg D, Lerer B, et al. Trial of maintenance neuroleptic dose reduction in schizophrenic outpatients: two year outcome. J Clin Psychiatry 54:59–62, 1993.
19. Brotman AW, McCormick S. A role for high-dose antipsychotics. J Clin Psychiatry 51:164–166, 1990.
20. Glazer WM, Kane JM. Depot neuroleptic therapy: an underutilized treatment option. J Clin Psychiatry 53:426–433, 1992.
21. Jann M, Ereshefsky L, Saklad SR. Clinical pharmacokinetics of the depot antipsychotics. Clin Pharmacokinetics 10:315–333, 1985.
22. Ereshefsky L, Toney G, Saklad SR, et al. A loading-dose strategy for converting from oral to depot haloperidol. Hosp Community Psychiatry 44:1155–1161, 1993.
23. Hemstrom CA, Evans RL, Lobeck FG. Haloperidol decanoate: a depot antipsychotic. Drug Intell Clin Pharm 22:290–295, 1988.
24. Khot V, DeVane CL, Korpi ER, et al. The assessment and clinical implications of haloperidol acute-dose, steady-state, and withdrawal pharmacokinetics. J Clin Psychopharmacol 13:120–127, 1993.
25. Sramek JJ, Potkin SG, Hahn R. Neuroleptic plasma concentrations and clinical response: in search of a therapeutic window. Drug Intell Clin Pharm 22:373–380, 1988.
26. Goff DC, Baldessarini RJ. Drug interactions with antipsychotic agents. J Clin Psychopharmacol 13:57–67, 1993.
27. Simpson GM, Pi EH, Sramek JJ Jr. Adverse effects of antipsychotic agents. Drugs 21:138–151, 1981.
28. Fleischhacker WW, Roth SD, Kane JM. The pharmacologic treatment of neuroleptic-induced akathisia. J Clin Psychopharmacol 10:12–21, 1990.
29. Keepers GA, Casey DE. Prediction of neuroleptic-induced dystonia. J Clin Psychopharmacol 7:342–345, 1987.
30. Remington GJ, Voineskos G, Pollock B, et al. Prevalence of neuroleptic-induced dystonia in mania and schizophrenia. Am J Psychiatry 147:1231–1233, 1990.
31. Caligiuri MP, Lohr JB, Jeste DV. Parkinsonism in neuroleptic-naive schizophrenic patients. Am J Psychiatry 150:1343–1348, 1993.
32. Addonizio G, Roth SD, Stokes PE, et al. Increased extrapyramidal symptoms with addition of lithium to neuroleptics. J Nerv Ment Dis 176:682–685, 1988.
33. Tonda ME, Guthrie SK. Treatment of acute neuroleptic-induced movement disorders. Pharmacotherapy 14:543–560, 1994.
34. Gelenberg AJ, VanPutten T, Lavori PW, et al. Anticholinergic effects on memory: benztropine versus amantadine. J Clin Psychopharmacol 9:180–185, 1989.

35. Arana GW, Goff DC, Baldessarini RJ, et al: Efficacy of anticholinergic prophylaxis for neuroleptic-induced acute dystonia. Am J Psychiatry 145:993–996, 1988.

36. Winslow RS, Stillner V, Coons DJ, et al. Prevention of acute dystonic reactions in patients beginning high-potency neuroleptics. Am J Psychiatry 143:706–710, 1986.

37. Baker LA, Cheng LY, Amara IB. The withdrawal of benztropine mesylate in chronic schizophrenic patients. Brit J Psychiatry 143: 584–590, 1983.

38. Siris SG. Adjunctive medication in the maintenance treatment of schizophrenia and its conceptual implications. Br J Psychiatry 163(suppl 22):66–78, 1993.

39. Singh H, Simpson GM, Tardive dyskinesia. In: Wolf ME, Mosnaim AD, eds. Tardive dyskinesia. Washington DC: American Psychiatric Press, 1988:69–84.

40. Fenton WS, Wyatt RJ, McGlashan TH. Risk factors for spontaneous dyskinesia in schizophrenia. Arch Gen Psychiatry 51:643–650, 1994.

41. Morgenstern H, Glazer WM. Identifying risk factors for tardive dyskinesia among longterm outpatients maintained with neuroleptic medications. Arch Gen Psychiatry 50:723–733, 1993.

42. Yassa R, Nair NPV, Iskandar H, et al. Factors in the development of severe forms of tardive dyskinesia. Am J Psychiatry 147:1156–1163, 1990.

43. Gardos G, Casey DE, Cole JO, et al. Ten year outcome of tardive dyskinesia. Am J Psychiatry 151:836–841, 1994.

44. Baldessarini RJ. Clinical and epidemiologic aspects of tardive dyskinesia. J Clin Psychiatry 46(4, sect 2):8–13, 1985.

45. Klawans HL, Carvey P, Tanner CM, et al. The pathophysiology of tardive dyskinesia. J Clin Psychiatry 46(4, sect 2):38–41, 1985.

46. Seeman P. Tardive dyskinesia, dopamine receptors, and neuroleptic damage to cell membranes. J Clin Psychopharmacol 8:3S–9S, 1988.

47. Jeste DV, Lohr JB, Clark K, et al. Pharmacologic treatments of tardive dyskinesia in the 1980s. J Clin Psychopharmacol 8:38S–48S, 1988.

48. Adler LA, Peselow E, Rotrosen J, et al. Vitamin E treatment of tardive dyskinesia. Am J Psychiatry 150:1405–1407, 1993.

49. Pearlman CA. Neuroleptic malignant syndrome: a review of the literature. J Clin Psychopharmacol 6:257–273, 1986.

50. Wells AJ, Sommi RW, Crismon ML. Neuroleptic rechallenge after neuroleptic malignant syndrome: case report and literature review. Drug Intell Clin Pharm 22: 475–480, 1988.

51. Rosebush PI, Stewart TD, Gelenberg AJ. Twenty neuroleptic rechallenges after neuroleptic malignant syndrome in 15 patients. J Clin Psychiatry 50:295–298, 1989.

52. Zito JM, Sofair JB, Jaeger J. Self-reported neuroendocrine effects of antipsychotics in women: a pilot study. DICP Ann Pharmacother 24:176–180, 1990.

53. Ripley HS, Papanicolaou GN. The menstrual cycle with vaginal smear studies in schizophrenia, depression and elation. Am J Psychiatry 98:567–573, 1942.

54. Doss FW: The effect of antipsychotic drugs on body weight: a retrospective review. J Clin Psychiatry 40:528–530, 1979.

55. Wheeler RH, Bhalerao VR, Gilkes MJ. Ocular pigmentation, extrapyramidal symptoms and phenothiazine dosage. Br J Psychiatry 115:687–690, 1969.

56. Swett C. Outpatient phenothiazine use and bone marrow depression. Arch Gen Psychiatry 32:1416–1418, 1975.

57. Cold JA, Wells BG, Froemming JH. Seizure activity associated with antipsychotic therapy. DICP Ann Pharmacother 24:601–606, 1990.

58. Lieberman JA. Understanding the mechanism of action of atypical antipsychotic drugs. Br J Psychiatry 163(suppl 22):7–18, 1993.

59. Ereshefsky L, Watanabe MD, Tran-Johnson TK. Clozapine: an atypical antipsychotic agent. Clin Pharm 8:691–709, 1989.

60. Breier A, Buchanan RW, Kirkpatrick B, et al. Effects of clozapine on positive and negative symptoms in outpatients with schizophrenia. Am J Psyhciatry 151:20–26, 1994.

61. Clozapine Study Group. The safety and efficacy of clozapine in severe treatment-resistant schizophrenic patients in the UK. Br J Psychiatry 163:150–154, 1993.

62. Kotcher M, Smith TE. Three phases of clozapine treatment and phase-specific issues for patients and families. Hosp Community Psychiatry 44:640–647, 1993.

63. Meltzer HY, Cola P, Way L, et al. Cost effectiveness of clozapine in neuroleptic-resistant schizophrenia. Am J Psychiatry 150:1630–1638, 1993.

64. Lieberman JA, Kane JM, Johns CA. Clozapine: guidelines for clinical management. J Clin Psychiatry 50:329–338, 1989.

65. Safferman A, Lieberman JA, Kane JM, et al. Update on the clinical efficacy and side effects of clozapine. Schizophr Bull 17:247–261, 1991.

66. Cohen LJ. Risperidone. Pharmacotherapy 14:253–265, 1994.

67. Marder SR, Meibach RC. Risperidone in the treatment of schizophrenia. Am J Psychiatry 151:825–835, 1994.

68. Remington GJ. Clinical considerations in the use of risperidone. Can J Psychiatry 38(suppl 3):S96–S100, 1993.

69. Van Putten T, May PRA. Subjective responses as a predictor of outcome in pharmacotherapy. Arch Gen Psychiatry 35:477–480, 1978.

CHAPTER 56

SLEEP DISORDERS

MICHAEL Z. WINCOR and MONICA CYR

On average, we spend one-third of our lives sleeping, yet many of us take this psychophysiologic phenomenon for granted. Only when it becomes disturbed do we pay some attention to it; even then, we probably heed the warnings of daytime fatigue less than we should. We do not know why, but we definitely need to sleep, and the exact sleep need varies a great deal among individuals. It has been found in various national surveys that during a year, 25 to 35% of the adult population have some complaint concerning sleep (1). Up to 17% of the population experience the problem as serious. The serious insomniacs tend to be older women with high levels of psychic distress and somatic anxiety as well as multiple health problems. Between 2 and 4% of those surveyed use hypnotics or other psychotherapeutic agents to promote sleep. The vast majority of hypnotic users take these drugs for short periods (1 day to 2 weeks); only 11% (0.3% of all adults) report using the drugs regularly for a year or more (2). An additional 3 to 4% use nonprescription sleep aids. However, a small survey of community pharmacists indicated little involvement in counseling patients about over-the-counter sleep aids (3). Although insomnia and daytime sleepiness are two of the most common human complaints, most serious insomniacs (85%) are untreated by either prescription or nonprescription hypnotics. The significant impact of sleep disturbances on the many aspects of our lives is becoming increasingly clear. The U.S. Department of Transportation estimates that up to 10% of automobile accidents are directly related to sleepiness, accounting for $29 billion in fatalities and disabling injuries (4). It is estimated that of the 25% of Americans who perform shift work, at least 60% have a chronic sleep disorder (3). Sleep disorders also are estimated to be responsible for 52% of work-related accidents at a cost of $24 billion (5). With a fundamental understanding of sleep disorders, the pharmacist can make an important contribution not only in encouraging patients to seek proper evaluation, but also in educating the patient on prescription medications and nonpharmacologic approaches, and advising patients on selection of over the counter sleep aids as well.

SLEEP PHYSIOLOGY

Sleep has been studied in various ways. Behaviorally, one can observe changes in body position, responsiveness to external stimuli, and eyelid closure. Anatomically, sleep-regulating centers in the brainstem have been identified.

Neurochemically, various neurotransmitters are involved in sleep mechanisms. Not long ago, we simply pointed to norepinephrine as being involved in wakefulness and dreaming sleep, and serotonin as being involved in nondreaming sleep. Then it became clear that there is an interaction between the cholinergic systems and the noradrenergic systems. In the future, contributions of other neurotransmitters and various endogenous peptides will likely be elucidated (6, 7).

Electrophysiology and Sleep Stages

Currently, the standard method for observing and measuring sleep is electrophysiologic (8). In the laboratory, sleep is recorded polygraphically, with electroencephalograms (EEGs), electro-oculograms (EOGs) from each of the two eyes, and electromyograms (EMGs) generally of the mentalis and submentalis muscles. Two EOGs, one EEG, and one EMG are the minimal recordings used for scoring sleep stages. A number of other physiologic variables may be needed to identify specific sleep disorders, as will be discussed. The entire recording process is often referred to as polysomnography. Today, by means of portable devices, such recordings are possible in the patient's home.

By means of these recordings, sleep can be divided into nonrapid eye movement (NREM) sleep, which is further subdivided into stages 1 through 4 and rapid eye movement (REM) sleep. Wakefulness is characterized by a low-voltage, fast EEG; high muscle tone; and various types of eye movements, including blinks. Stage 1 sleep is characterized by a low-voltage, mixed-frequency EEG; slightly decreased muscle tone; and slow, rolling eye movements. The subjective experience of this transition stage varies widely among individuals, some experiencing it as wakefulness, others as drowsiness, and yet others as sleep. Stage 2 is characterized by sleep spindles and K-complexes on EEG and is recognized as unequivocal sleep. Stages 3 and 4 are characterized by high-amplitude, slow activity in the EEG known as delta waves; hence, these two stages together are often referred to as delta sleep. Delta sleep appears to be the deep, restorative sleep that most people (especially insomniacs) think of when they visualize sleep.

REM sleep is characterized by a low-voltage, mixed-frequency EEG, in many ways quite similar to that seen in stage 1, but with very low muscle tone and bursts of bilaterally conjugate rapid eye movements. It appears as though the sleeper is watching a movie or observing some activity. Classical dreaming occurs in REM sleep; dream reports can be obtained 80 to 90% of the times that subjects are awakened during or at the end of REM periods. Brain and autonomic activity may be greater and more variable than during relaxed wakefulness.

Physiologic Changes During sleep

Physiologically, much activity occurs during sleep. While heart rate and respiratory rate are slow and regular during NREM sleep, they, along with blood pressure, become irregular with rapid changes in REM sleep. In the male, erections occur regularly during REM sleep. Body temperature descends to its lowest in the early morning, while, during REM sleep, the sleeper is poikilothermic (cold-blooded). Cortisol levels are lowest at sleep onset, while growth hormone is released during delta sleep. Melatonin secretion increasees in sleep and can be suppressed by bright light.

Function of Sleep

Although the function of sleep is not clearly understood, it is believed that NREM sleep serves to restore, rejuvenate, and revitalize the body. Slow-wave sleep seems to play an important role in thermoregulation and tissue repair. Metabolic rate decreases during sleep, with a fall not only in body temperature, but also a decrease in glucose consumption and production of catabolic hormones. On the other hand, along with the increase in growth hormone seen in delta sleep, there is an increase in skeletal muscle protein synthesis during sleep. Slow-wave sleep may have a role in maintaining immune function. It would appear, then, that adequate sleep is critical for growing children and individuals with healing wounds or infections.

REM sleep may be needed to sort through short-term memory stores, deleting unnecessary data and laying down important information in long-term memory. REM sleep may also play a role in maintaining noradrenergic receptor sensitivity. Whatever its role, REM sleep appears to be of vital physiologic importance in that REM deprivation leads to a dramatic REM rebound during recovery sleep (9).

Sleep Cycle

The architecture of sleep in the normal young adult is cyclic. The sleeper quickly passes from wakefulness through stages 1 and 2, spending a moderate block of time in delta sleep. Some 90 minutes after sleep onset, the sleeper enters the first REM period of the night, which may last only 5 to 7 minutes. The cycle is repeated four to five times each night. As the night progresses, less time is spent in delta sleep, with most delta sleep occurring in the first half of the night. REM periods become longer and more intense, both physiologically and psychologically, as the night goes on. The final REM period of the night may last as long as 30 to 60 minutes.

Most individuals who recall a dream in the morning are waking from this REM period and remembering the dream's content. In general, one spends approximately 75% of the night in NREM sleep and the remaining 25% of the night in REM sleep.

In the elderly, however, the typical sleep architecture described here may be quite different, with a considerable decrease in delta sleep, an increase in light sleep, an increase in awakenings during the night, and a generally more disrupted night of sleep. There may be a slight decrease in total sleep time during the night, compared with young adults, but how much daytime napping and specific sleep pathology (e.g., sleep apnea and periodic limb movements) contribute to this apparent decrease is unclear. Even in randomly selected, non-complaining, elderly individuals, the combined incidence of sleep apnea and periodic limb movements is as high as 58% (10–12).

The parameters that can be measured objectively in the sleep laboratory, which are of particular interest with respect to insomnia and drug effects on sleep, are listed in Table 56.1. Latency to sleep onset (or sleep latency) is defined as the length of time taken to fall asleep after getting into bed. The number of awakenings and number of stage shifts during the night indicate how disrupted sleep has been. REM intensity, or the frequency of bursts of rapid eye movements, may at times be a more subtle indicator of changes in REM sleep than simply the total number of minutes spent in REM sleep during the night. Finally, other physiologic measurements may include electrocardiogram, respiration, oxygen saturation, and activity of the anterior tibialis muscles.

DIAGNOSIS AND CLINICAL FINDINGS

In the 1970s, a group of clinically oriented sleep researchers developed an organization, the Association of Sleep Disorders Centers, as well as a scheme for classifying sleep disorders (13). Simply stated, disorders of initiating and maintaining sleep (DIMS) were equivalent to insomnia, the disorders of excessive somnolence (DOES) were equivalent to excessive daytime sleepiness, the disorders of the sleep–wake schedule involved disturbances of biologic

Table 56.1.
Sleep Parameters

Latency to sleep onset
Total sleep time
Sleep stage durations
Sleep stage percentages of total sleep time
Number of awakenings during the night
Number of stage shifts during the night
REM intensity
Other physiologic measurements

Table 56.2.
International Classification of Sleep Disorders (ICSD)ᵃ

1. Dyssomnias
   A. Intrinsic sleep disorders
   B. Extrinsic sleep disorders
   C. Circadian rhythm sleep disorders
2. Parasomnias
   A. Arousal disorders
   B. Sleep–wake transition disorders
   C. Parasomnias usually associated with REM sleep
   D. Other parasomnias
3. Medical/psychiatric sleep disorders
   A. Associated with mental disorders
   B. Associated with neurologic disorders
   C. Associated with other medical disorders
4. Proposed sleep disorders

ᵃAdapted from Diagnostic Classification Steering Committee of the American Sleep Disorders Association (Thorpy MJ, chair). International Classification of Sleep Disorders—Diagnostic and Coding Manual. Rochester, MN: American Sleep Disorders Association, 1990.

rhythms, and the parasomnias included a number of miscellaneous disorders associated with sleep, sleep stages, or partial arousals. There was a considerable amount of overlap in possible etiologies among the major categories of disorders, with the exception of the parasomnias. In fact, the determining factor in applying a label to the patient was often the nature of the subjective complaint (e.g., "Doctor, I'm not sleeping well at night" versus "Doctor, I'm always sleepy").

As sleep-disorder clinicians worked with this classification scheme over the years, an international effort for revision and modification began. The result was *The International Classification of Sleep Disorders* (ICSD) (14), a very extensive listing and description of the sleep disorders (as outlined in Table 56.2). It was published by what is now called the American Sleep Disorders Association, in cooperation with the European Sleep Research Society, the Japanese Society of Sleep Research, and the Latin American Sleep Society. A bit earlier, however, a committee of the American Psychiatric Association was revising its official *Diagnostic and Statistical Manual of Mental Disorders* (DSM-III-R). The result was a somewhat abbreviated nomenclature for the sleep disorders most likely to be encountered in a psychiatric practice (15). It is outlined in Table 56.3 for the sake of completeness; however, since the ICSD is the more exhaustive, international classification, it will serve as the basis of this discussion. Eighty-four specific sleep disorders are described in the ICSD. It is beyond the scope of this chapter to cover each of them in detail; however, each of the major categories is expanded in Tables 56.4 through 56.7 to provide the reader with an idea of the progress made in the past 15 years in identifying and classifying sleep disorders.

The entire field of sleep-disorders medicine is in its infancy, at most approaching adolescence. For many of the sleep disorders, both etiology and prevalence are as yet unclear (in instances where these are established or even postulated, such information will be mentioned). The remaining discussion is focused on the disorders that have been best studied, are seen most frequently, or are most likely to have a pharmacotherapeutic component to treatment. Particular emphasis is placed on insomnia and the use of hypnotics.

PARASOMNIAS

The parasomnias, as indicated in Table 56.5, include 23 distinct disorders. Only sleepwalking (somnambulism), sleep terrors (pavor nocturnus), and nightmares are discussed in detail here.

Somnambulism

Sleepwalking, or somnambulism, is a phenomenon occurring in delta sleep. At least one episode of sleepwalking is seen in about 15% of children, and in 2 to 5% of adults. Peak prevalence occurs between 4 and 8 years of age. Typically, the sleeper sits up, gets out of bed, walks around, and returns to bed. The individual appears to be navigating well, but critical skills and reactivity are impaired (e.g., if you were to rearrange the furniture in the house, the sleepwalker would probably stumble over it). Fortunately, the disorder is usually "outgrown." Treatment consists primarily of protecting the individual from harm. This may include locking doors and windows at night and giving the

Table 56.3.
DSM-IV Classification of Sleep Disordersᵃ

PRIMARY SLEEP DISORDERS
Dyssomnias
307.42	Primary insomnia
307.44	Primary hypersomnia
347	Narcolepsy
780.59	Breathing-related sleep disorder
307.45	Circadian rhythm sleep disorder
307.47	Dyssomnia not otherwise specified

Parasomnias
307.47	Nightmare disorder
307.46	Sleep terror disorder
307.46	Sleepwalking disorder
307.47	Parasomnia not otherwise specified

SLEEP DISORDERS RELATED TO ANOTHER MENTAL DISORDER
| 307.42 | Insomnia related to . . . |
| 307.44 | Hypersomnia related to . . . |

OTHER SLEEP DISORDERS
| 780.xx | Sleep disorder due to . . . (a medical condition) |
| ___.__ | Substance-induced sleep disorder |

ᵃAdapted from American Psychiatric Association. Diagnostic and Statistical Manual of Mental Disorders, 4th ed. Washington, DC: American Psychiatric Association, 1994.

Table 56.4.
ICSD Classification of Dyssomnias[a]

Disorders that are characterized by difficulty in initiating or maintaining sleep or by excessive sleepiness

Intrinsic sleep disorders

Developing within the body or from causes within the body

307.42-0 Psychophysiologic insomnia

Somatized tension and learned sleep-preventing associations resulting in a complaint of insomnia and associated decreased functioning during wakefulness

307.49-1 Sleep state misperception

A complaint of insomnia or excessive sleepiness without objective evidence of sleep disturbance

780.52-7 Idiopathic insomnia

A lifelong inability to obtain adequate sleep that is presumably due to an abnormality of the neurologic control of the sleep–wake system

347 Narcolepsy

Characterized by excessive sleepiness typically associated with cataplexy and other REM sleep phenomena such as sleep paralysis and hypnagogic hallucinations

780.54-2 Recurrent hypersomnia

Characterized by recurrent episodes of excessive sleepiness that typically occur weeks or months apart

780.54-7 Idiopathic hypersomnia

Characterized by a normal or prolonged major sleep episode and excessive sleepiness consisting of prolonged (1–2 hours) sleep episodes of NREM sleep, presumably due to a central nervous system abnormality

780.54-8 Posttraumatic hypersomnia

Excessive sleepiness as a result of a trauma to the central nervous system

780.53-0 Obstructive sleep apnea syndrome

Characterized by repetitive episodes of upper airway obstruction that occur during sleep, usually associated with a reduction in blood oxygen saturation

780.51-0 Central sleep apnea syndrome

Characterized by a cessation or decrease of ventilatory effort during sleep, usually with associated oxygen desaturation

780.51-1 Central alveolar hypoventilation syndrome

Characterized by ventilatory impairment, resulting in arterial oxygen desaturation that is worsened by sleep, which occurs in patients with normal mechanical properties of the lung

780.51-1 Periodic limb movement disorder

Characterized by periodic episodes of repetitive and highly stereotyped limb movements that occur during sleep

780.52-5 Restless legs syndrome

Characterized by disagreeable leg sensations, usually prior to sleep onset, that cause an almost irresistible urge to move the legs

780.52-9 Intrinsic sleep disorder NOS

An intrinsic dyssomnia not otherwise specified (i.e., none of the above)

Extrinsic sleep disorders

Developing from causes outside the body

307.41-1 Inadequate sleep hygiene

Due to the performance of daily living activities that are inconsistent with the maintenance of good quality sleep and full daytime alertness

780.52-6 Environmental sleep disorder

Due to a disturbing environmental factor that causes a complaint of either insomnia or excessive sleepiness

289.0 Altitude insomnia

An acute insomnia, usually accompanied by headaches, loss of appetite, and fatigue, that occurs following ascent to high altitudes

307.41-0 Adjustment sleep disorder

Temporally related to acute stress, conflict, or environmental change causing emotional arousal

307.49-4 Insufficient sleep syndrome

Occurs in an individual who persistently fails to obtain sufficient nocturnal sleep required to support normally alert wakefulness

307.42-4 Limit-setting sleep disorder

Primarily a childhood disorder that is characterized by the inadequate enforcement of bedtimes by a caretaker, with resultant stalling or refusal to go to bed at an appropriate time

307.42-5 Sleep-onset association disorder

Characterized by impaired sleep onset due to the absence of a certain object or set of circumstances

780.52-2 Food allergy insomnia

Disorder of initiating and maintaining sleep due to an allergic response to food allergens

780.52-8 Nocturnal eating (drinking) syndrome

Characterized by recurrent awakenings, with the inability to return to sleep without eating or drinking

780.52-0 Hypnotic-dependent sleep disorder

Characterized by insomnia or excessive sleepiness that is associated with tolerance to or withdrawal from hypnotic medications

780.52-1 Stimulant-dependent sleep disorder

Characterized by a reduction of sleepiness or suppression of sleep by central stimulants, and resultant alterations in wakefulness following drug abstinence

780.52-3 Alcohol-dependent sleep disorder

Characterized by the assisted initiation of sleep onset by the sustained ingestion of ethanol that is used for its hypnotic effect

780.54-6 Toxin-induced sleep disorder

Characterized by either insomnia or excessive sleepiness produced by poisoning with heavy metals or organic toxins

780.52-9 Extrinsic sleep disorder NOS

An extrinsic dyssomnia not otherwise specified (i.e., none of the above)

Circadian rhythm sleep disorders

Related to the timing of sleep in the 24-hour day

307.45-0 Time zone change (jet lag) syndrome

Characterized by varying degrees of difficulty in initiating or maintaining sleep, excessive sleepiness, decrements in subjective daytime alertness and performance, and somatic symptoms (largely gastrointestinal) following rapid travel across multiple time zones

307.45-1 Shift work sleep disorder

Insomnia or excessive sleepiness that occurs as transient phenomena in relation to work schedules

307.45-3 Irregular sleep–wake pattern

Temporally disorganized and variable episodes of sleep and waking behavior

780.55-0 Delayed sleep phase syndrome

Characterized by the major sleep episode being delayed relative to the desired sleep time, resulting in sleep-onset insomnia or difficulty in awakening at the desired time

780.55-1 Advanced sleep phase syndrome

Characterized by the major sleep episode being advanced relative to the desired sleep time, resulting in symptoms of compelling evening sleepiness, an early sleep onset, and an awakening that is earlier than desired

780.55-2 Non-24-hour sleep–wake disorder

Characterized by chronic steady patterns composed of 1- to 2-hour daily delays in sleep onset and wake times

780.55-9 Circadian rhythm sleep disorder NOS

A circadian rhythm dyssomnia not otherwise specified (i.e., none of the above)

[a]Adapted from Diagnostic Classification Steering Committee of the American Sleep Disorders Association (Thorpy MJ, chair). International Classification of Sleep Disorders—Diagnostic and Coding Manual. Rochester, MN: American Sleep Disorders Association, 1990.

Table 56.5.
ICSD Classification of Parasomnias[a]

Undesirable physical phenomena occurring predominantly during sleep, including disorders of arousal, partial arousal, and sleep stage transition

Arousal disorders

Disorders of impaired arousal from slow wave (delta) sleep

307.46-2 Confusional arousals
Characterized by confusion during and following arousals from sleep, most typically from deep sleep in the first part of the night

307.46-0 Sleepwalking
Characterized by a series of complex behaviors that are initiated during slow wave (delta) sleep, resulting in walking during sleep

307.46-1 Sleep terrors
Characterized by a sudden arousal from slow wave (delta) sleep with a piercing scream or cry, accompanied by autonomic and behavioral manifestations of intense fear

Sleep–wake transition disorders

Occurring in the transition from wakefulness to sleep, from sleep to wakefulness, or, more rarely, from one stage of sleep to another; regarded as altered physiology rather than pathophysiology

307.3 Rhythmic movement disorder
Characterized by stereotyped, repetitive movements involving large muscles, usually of the head and neck, which typically occur immediately prior to sleep onset and are sustained into light sleep

307.47-2 Sleep starts
Characterized by sudden, brief contractions of the legs, sometimes also involving the arms and head, which occur at sleep onset

307.47-3 Sleep talking
The utterance of speech or sounds during sleep without simultaneous subjective detailed awareness of the event

729.82 Nocturnal leg cramps
Characterized by painful sensations of muscular tightness or tension, usually in the calf, but occasionally in the foot, that occur during the sleep episode

Parasomnias usually associated with REM sleep

307.47-0 Nightmares
Frightening dreams that usually awaken the sleeper from REM sleep

780.56-2 Sleep paralysis
Characterized by an inability to perform voluntary movements either at sleep onset (hypnagogic or predormital form) or upon awakening (hypnopompic or postdormital form) either during the night or in the morning

780.56-3 Impaired sleep-related penile erections
Inability to sustain a penile erection during sleep that would be sufficiently large or rigid to engage in sexual intercourse

780.56-4 Sleep-related painful erections
Characterized by penile pain that occurs during erections, typically during REM sleep

780.56-8 REM sleep-related sinus arrest
A cardiac rhythm disorder that is characterized by sinus arrest during REM sleep in otherwise healthy individuals

780.59-0 REM sleep behavior disorder
Characterized by the intermittent loss of REM sleep electromyographic (EMG) atonia and by the appearance of elaborate motor activity associated with dream mentation

Other parasomnias

306.8 Sleep bruxism
A stereotyped movement disorder characterized by grinding or clenching of the teeth during sleep

780.56-0 Sleep enuresis
Characterized by recurrent involuntary micturition that occurs during sleep

780.56-6 Sleep-related abnormal swallowing syndrome
Characterized by inadequate swallowing of saliva, resulting in aspiration, with coughing, choking, and arousals or awakenings from sleep

780.59-1 Nocturnal paroxysmal dystonia (NPD)
Characterized by repeated, stereotyped dystonia or dyskinetic (ballistic, choreoathetoid) episodes that occur during NREM sleep

780.59-3 Sudden unexplained nocturnal death syndrome (SUND)
Characterized by sudden death during sleep in apparently healthy young adults, particularly of Southeast Asian descent

780.53-1 Primary snoring
Characterized by loud upper airway breathing sounds in sleep, without episodes of apnea or hypoventilation

770.80 Infant sleep apnea
Characterized by central or obstructive apneas that occur during sleep

770.81 Congenital central hypoventilation syndrome
Characterized by hypoventilation, which is worse during sleep than wakefulness, and unexplained by primary pulmonary disease or ventilatory muscle weakness

798.0 Sudden infant death syndrome
Unexpected sudden death in which a thorough postmortem investigation fails to demonstrate an adequate cause for death

780.59-5 Benign neonatal sleep myoclonus
Characterized by asynchronous jerking of the limbs and trunk that occurs during quiet sleep in neonates

780.59-9 Other parasomnia NOS
A parasomnia not otherwise specified (i.e., none of the above)

[a]Adapted from Diagnostic Classification Steering Committee of the American Sleep Disorders Association (Thorpy MJ, chair). International Classification of Sleep Disorders—Diagnostic and Coding Manual. Rochester, MN: American Sleep Disorders Association, 1990.

sleepwalker a first-floor bedroom. Medications that may exacerbate or induce sleepwalking (e.g., thioridazine, chloral hydrate, lithium, fluphenazine, perphenazine, and desipramine) should be discontinued if possible. Theoretically, sleepwalking could be reduced by suppressing delta sleep. Most benzodiazepines suppress delta sleep, and in an adult with frequent episodes, especially with a history of injury to self or others, a benzodiazepine may be a very appropriate and efficacious intervention. However, in the case of childhood sleepwalking, the benefit of treatment over simply protecting the individual from injury is questionable in light of the unknown risks of long-term exposure of the child's developing central nervous system to benzodiazepines (16).

Sleep Terrors

Sleep terrors (pavor nocturnus or night terrors), also a delta sleep phenomenon, is seen in approximately 3% of children

Table 56.6.
ICSD Classification of Sleep Disorders Associated with Medical/Psychiatric Disorders[a]

Associated with mental disorders
292-299   Psychoses
          Insomnia or excessive sleepiness commonly associated with psychiatric disorders characterized by the presence of delusions, hallucinations, incoherence, catatonic behavior, or inappropriate effect that causes impaired social or work functioning
296-301   Mood disorders
          Insomnia typically and, rarely, excessive sleepiness associated with psychiatric disorders characterized by either one or more episodes of depression, or partial or full manic or hypomanic episodes
300   Anxiety disorders
          A sleep-onset or maintenance insomnia due to excessive anxiety and apprehensive expectation about one or more life circumstances associated with psychiatric disorders characterized by symptoms of anxiety and avoidance behavior
300   Panic disorder
          Sudden awakenings from sleep associated with panic episodes that are characterized by discrete periods of intense fear or discomfort, with several somatic symptoms that occur unexpectedly and without organic precipitation
303   Alcoholism
          Insomnia or excessive sleepiness associated with excessive alcohol intake, both abuse and dependence
Associated with neurologic disorders
330-337   Cerebral degenerative disorders
          Insomnia, excessive sleepiness, abnormal movement activity, or circadian rhythm disturbances associated with slowly progressive conditions characterized by abnormal behavior or involuntary movements, often with evidence of other motor system degeneration
331   Dementia
          Delirium, agitation, combativeness, wandering, and vocalization without ostensible purpose occurring during the early evening or nighttime hours associated with the loss of memory and other intellectual functions due to a chronic, progressive degenerative disease of the brain
332-333   Parkinsonism
          Insomnia associated with the group of neurologic disorders characterized by hypokinesia, tremor, and muscular rigidity
337.9   Fatal familial insomnia
          A progressive disorder that begins with a difficulty in initiating sleep and leads within a few months to total lack of sleep and later to spontaneous lapses from quiet wakefulness into a sleep state with enacted dreams (oneiric stupor)

345   Sleep-related epilepsy
          Facilitatory effects of sleep on epileptic activity in disorders characterized by an intermittent, sudden discharge of cerebral neuronal activity
345.8   Electrical status epilepticus of sleep
          Characterized by continuous and diffuse spike-and-slow-wave complexes persisting through NREM sleep
346   Sleep-related headaches
          Severe, mainly unilateral headaches that often have their onset during sleep
Associated with other medical disorders
086   Sleeping sickness
          A protozoan-caused illness characterized by an acute febrile lymphadenopathy followed, after a period of latency usually of 4 to 6 months, by an excessive sleepiness associated with a chronic meningoencephalomyelitis
411-414   Nocturnal cardiac ischemia
          Characterized by myocardial ischemia that occurs during the major sleep episode
490-494   Chronic obstructive pulmonary disease
          Altered cardiorespiratory physiology during sleep or a complaint of insomnia associated with a disorder characterized by a chronic impairment of airflow through the respiratory tract between the atmosphere and gas exchange portion of the lung
493   Sleep-related asthma
          Asthma attacks that occur during sleep
530.1   Sleep-related gastroesophageal reflux
          Characterized by regurgitation of stomach contents into the esophagus during sleep
531-534   Peptic ulcer disease
          Awakenings from sleep with pain or discomfort in the abdomen, resulting in a complaint of insomnia, associated with a disorder characterized by gastric or duodenal ulceration by acid and pepsin
729.1   Fibrositis syndrome
          Unrefreshing, light sleep and chronic fatigue associated with a disorder characterized by diffuse musculoskeletal pain, and increased tenderness in specific localized anatomic regions, but without laboratory evidence of contributing articular, nonarticular, or metabolic disease

[a]Adapted from Diagnostic Classification Steering Committee of the American Sleep Disorders Association (Thorpy MJ, chair). International Classification of Sleep Disorders—Diagnostic and Coding Manual. Rochester, MN: American Sleep Disorders Association, 1990.

and less than 1% of adults. It is characterized by extreme vocalizations, motility, and autonomic variability. Recall of frightening content is minimal or absent. Hence, the phenomenon may be more disturbing to others in the house than to the child experiencing it. The parents of the child may hear a "blood-curdling" scream; run into the sleeper's bedroom; and find the child wet from perspiration, breathing forcefully, and experiencing tachycardia. Fortunately, the absence of frightening content results in nothing psychologic with which to associate the event. Generally, there is amnesia for the event. Again, treatment consists primar-

ily of waiting for the disorder to be "outgrown" since sleep terrors are typically observed in children between the ages of 4 and 12 years and resolve spontaneously during adolescence. The same reservations about use of delta sleep suppressants discussed in regard to somnambulism apply for this disorder (16).

Nightmares

Unlike sleep terrors, nightmares ("bad dreams") occur in REM sleep (in about 5% of the general population) and are associated with elaborate and frightening content. There is less motility and autonomic variability than in sleep terrors. It is estimated that 10 to 50% of children between 3 and 6 years of age suffer from enough nightmares to disturb the parents. Approximately 50% of the adult population admit to having at least an occasional nightmare, and perhaps 1% experience frequent nightmares (one or more per week). After REM suppressant drug withdrawal is ruled out as the cause, psychological intervention is the usual treatment.

Table 56.7.
ICSD Classification of Proposed Sleep Disorders[a]

	Disorders for which insufficient or inadequate information is available to substantiate their unequivocal existence
307.49-0	Short sleeper
	An individual who habitually sleeps substantially less during a 24-hour period than is expected for his or her age group
307.49-2	Long sleeper
	An individual who consistently sleeps substantially more (although with basically normal sleep architecture and physiology) in 24 hours than the conventional amount of sleep for his or her age group
307.47-1	Subwakefulness syndrome
	An inability to sustain daytime alertness without polysomnographic evidence of nocturnal sleep disruption or severe excessive sleepiness
780.59-7	Fragmentary myoclonus
	Characterized by jerks that consist of brief involuntary "twitchlike" local contractions involving various areas of both sides of the body in an asynchronous and asymmetrical manner during sleep
780.8	Sleep hyperhidrosis
	Characterized by profuse sweating that occurs during sleep
780.54-3	Menstrual-associated sleep disorder
	Characterized by a complaint of either insomnia or excessive sleepiness that is temporally related to the menses or menopause
780.59-6	Pregnancy-associated sleep disorder
	Characterized by either insomnia or excessive sleepiness that develops in the course of pregnancy
307.47-4	Terrifying hypnagogic hallucinations
	Terrifying dream experiences that occur at sleep onset that are similar to, or at times indistinguishable from, those taking place within sleep
780.53-2	Sleep-related neurogenic tachypnea
	Characterized by a sustained increase in respiratory rate during sleep, which occurs at sleep onset, is maintained throughout sleep, and reverses immediately upon return to wakefulness
780.49-4	Sleep-related laryngospasm
	Characterized by episodes of abrupt awakenings from sleep with an intense sensation of inability to breathe and stridor
307.42-1	Sleep choking syndrome
	Characterized by frequent episodes of awakening with a choking sensation

[a]Adapted from Diagnostic Classification Steering Committee of the American Sleep Disorders Association (Thorpy MJ, chair). International Classification of Sleep Disorders—Diagnostic and Coding Manual. Rochester, MN: American Sleep Disorders Association, 1990.

This may be as simple as a parent providing comfort and reassurance to a child with an occasional nightmare or as complex as intensive psychotherapy for an adult with frequent, highly disturbing nightmares (16).

SLEEP APNEA

Definition and Overview

Sleep apnea, a sleep-induced respiratory impairment, is a condition characterized by episodes of cessation of breathing (17). Each apneic episode, often lasting 20 to 30 seconds, is terminated by a brief arousal from sleep during which breathing resumes. There may be as many as several hundred of these "mini-arousals" during a single night, but the patient may not be aware of their occurrence. The patient may instead complain of morning headache, irritability, and general difficulty with daytime functioning. Often, the bed partner is the best source of information, reporting that the patient snores very loudly or has periods in which breathing stops followed by gasps for air. Often there is a recent history of weight gain associated with onset of symptoms. Sleep apnea generally has an onset in adulthood, usually over the age of 30, probably with a prevalence of 1 to 2% of the population, and, in the case of obstructive sleep apnea, is at least eight times more prevalent in men than in women. Although the incidence is high in the elderly, many are asymptomatic (i.e., they have no complaints that would have brought this condition to the attention of a physician or sleep-disorders specialist). Common complications of sleep apnea include arrhythmias, systolic or diastolic hypertension, and signs of pulmonary arterial hypertension and right-sided heart failure.

Sleep apnea is often described as obstructive, central, or mixed. Obstructive sleep apnea is caused by something obstructing the airway. The problem may be the tongue falling back across the airway, enlarged tonsils, or some other craniofacial abnormality. Respiratory effort continues as is demonstrated by strain gauge recordings around the thorax and abdomen in the absence of nasal and oral airflow (measured by a device attached to the face below the nostrils). In central sleep apnea, respiratory effort ceases, indicating a problem in the respiratory centers of the brain, with resultant absence of nasal and oral airflow. In mixed sleep apnea, there seems to be a cessation of central respiratory effort, followed by an obstructive event, and then even when respiratory effort resumes, there is no airflow. In any of these cases, as oxygen saturation falls (which can be measured with an earlobe oximeter), the brain automatically produces a mini-arousal resulting in resumption of breathing. Whether the patient complains of insomnia or excessive daytime sleepiness is subjective, but obstructive sleep apnea seems to be more highly associated with complaints of excessive daytime sleepiness, whereas central sleep apnea appears to be more closely associated with complaints of insomnia (18).

Treatment

Treatment varies with the type of sleep apnea under consideration. For obstructive sleep apnea, sometimes simple weight loss or removal of enlarged tonsils may solve the problem. Sometimes preventing the patient from sleeping on his or her back, by sewing a tennis ball to the back of the night shirt, can lead to a significant decrease in apneic episodes. When life-threatening complications of repeated episodes of hypoxemia (e.g., arrhythmias, pulmonary hypertension, right ventricular failure) are present, aggressive intervention should be considered. A rather elegant plastic surgical procedure, performed in some patients, is the uvulopalatopharyngoplasty (UPPP), which involves major reconstruction of the pharyngeal airspace. Unfortunately, in many cases, long-term follow-up has been lacking. Other, less dramatic surgical procedures—some involving laser surgery—have more recently been performed. A most useful and commonly employed approach is continuous positive airway pressure (nasal CPAP) (19). This involves the use of a small device that sits beside the bed, connected by a tube to a facial mask worn by the patient throughout the night. The device, initially calibrated during one or two nights in a sleep-disorders center, provides a continuous flow of air that keeps the airway open. For the many patients who are appropriately counseled and learn to tolerate the noise, mucosal drying, and minor discomfort of the facial mask, the technique can have a major impact on the quality of sleep and resultant daytime functioning. Finally, various dental appliances designed to pull the tongue forward and maintain an open airway are being tested.

The single most important pharmacologic intervention in the treatment of any type of sleep apnea is the careful avoidance of all drugs that have central nervous system (CNS) depressant activity. These include anxiolytics, hypnotics, narcotics, and alcohol. Any agent that can interfere with the ability of the brain to produce an apnea-terminating mini-arousal is potentially lethal. Even CNS depressants that appear to have little or no effect on respiration during wakefulness must be avoided since some evidence indicates differential effects during sleep. Preliminary data indicate that a subset of patients with central sleep apnea may be an exception to this rule of avoiding CNS depressants. In fact, triazolam improved sleep quality, increased total sleep time, and decreased apneic episodes (20). However, until these findings are confirmed in further studies, it remains safest to avoid CNS depressants in all patients with sleep apnea. Active pharmacologic intervention in treating sleep apnea has met with mixed, fairly unimpressive results. Tricyclic antidepressants, particularly protriptyline, have been used in both obstructive and central sleep apnea. Protriptyline may act by decreasing REM sleep or by increasing oropharyngeal muscle tone (21). Respiratory stimulants, such as medroxyprogesterone

(22) and acetazolamide (23), show only limited efficacy, with no studies demonstrating long-term effectiveness.

NARCOLEPSY

Definition and Overview

Narcolepsy, along with obstructive sleep apnea, is a major cause of excessive daytime sleepiness and is found in approximately 0.1% of the population. Its onset is often during adolescence. Patients suffering with narcolepsy are extremely sleepy throughout the day and find themselves falling asleep at inopportune moments. There are four classic features: excessive daytime sleepiness, cataplexy, sleep paralysis, and hypnagogic hallucinations. Cataplexy is described as brief (lasting only seconds to minutes) episodes of muscle weakness that may result in the patient collapsing. These episodes are often precipitated by emotionally charged stimuli (e.g., laughter, anger, excitement). Sleep paralysis and hypnagogic hallucinations occur during the transition between wakefulness and sleep. Sleep paralysis involves inhibition of the musculature before the individual is unconscious. This is particularly frightening because the patient is aware of the paralysis. Hypnagogic hallucinations are brief dream-like events but perhaps more fragmented and bizarre than a typical dream (18, 24).

Sleep-laboratory findings strongly suggest that narcolepsy involves a dysregulation of REM sleep. In addition to cataplexy and sleep paralysis (which represent the loss of muscle tone in REM sleep), narcoleptics have sleep-onset REM periods (i.e., instead of the normal latency of 90 minutes following sleep onset to the first REM period, they can make a transition from wakefulness immediately to REM sleep). The genetic basis of the disorder is supported by an extremely strong association between the human leucocyte antigen-DR2 phenotype (HLA-DR2) and narcolepsy (25).

Treatment

Treatment consists of both pharmacologic and nonpharmacologic interventions. The patient and family members must be educated about the disorder to dispel the misconception that the patient is simply a lazy, unmotivated, nonproductive individual. There are local and national support groups. In addition, careful scheduling of daytime naps can be particularly helpful. The patient may feel fairly refreshed for up to several hours after a 15- or 20-minute nap.

Pharmacologic treatment is directed toward the excessive daytime sleepiness on the one hand and the cataplexy on the other (26). CNS stimulants are used for the sleepiness. Hesitation in prescribing amphetamines (due to concerns over abuse, tolerance, and dependence) has led to the more common use of methylphenidate, starting at 2.5 mg twice daily. Occasionally, pemoline is started at a dose of 18.75 mg per day. For the cataplexy, imipramine (in the past) and now, more commonly, the less sedating protriptyline (at an initial dose of 5 mg titrated up to 60 mg daily) have been used.

General principles of pharmacologic management include using the lowest effective dose possible, with gradual titration and careful monitoring for therapeutic and adverse effects (particularly the anticholinergic and hypotensive effects of the tricyclic antidepressant), and temporarily withdrawing the stimulant when tolerance has developed. It is ideal if the temporary withdrawal can be scheduled at a time when a return of daytime sleepiness will have the least impact on the general functioning of the patient (e.g., during a vacation break from work or school). Cataplexy, in some patients, can be treated on an as-needed basis. A patient who recognizes specific situations with which the cataplexy is associated can use the protriptyline for a day or two before and during the time of expected occurrence.

INSOMNIA

Definition and Dimensions

Insomnia is a problem that 95% of all adults have experienced at least once in their lives. It must be defined in terms of both amount of sleep and its perceived quality. No absolute number of hours of sleep per se constitutes insomnia since sleep need among individuals is highly variable. The individual who sleeps 5 hours per night, needs only 5 hours per night, and functions in his or her daily activities at peak performance does not have insomnia. However, the individual who needs 8 hours per night, sleeps only 7 with a perception of fragmented sleep, and complains of daytime impairment may indeed be suffering from insomnia. Hence, insomnia must be seen as a perceived relative decrease in the quantity and/or quality of sleep along with some perceived consequences in waking life. These perceptions take the form of a subjective complaint by the patient. In many respects, insomniacs' sleep is not that dramatically different from that of good sleepers, but they perceive it as poor sleep. Unfortunately, at present, there is no definitive way to measure the quality of sleep in the sleep laboratory; however, it appears likely that fragmentation of sleep (as indicated by arousals, stage shifts, and perhaps subtle findings in EEG frequencies) is most closely associated with perceived quality (16, 27).

Insomnia can be viewed from various perspectives. The severity (i.e., from mild to severe) will clearly have implications with respect to treatment decisions. Whether the insomnia is transient or chronic is important in both diagnosis and treatment. Finally, the pattern of a typical night may be characterized by difficulty falling asleep, difficulty staying asleep (numerous awakenings during the night), early morning awakening (3 to 4 hours earlier than

Table 56.8.
Non-Drug Factors Associated with Long-Term Insomnia

Psychiatric Disorders	Medical/Neurologic Disorders (cont.)
• Mood disorders	• Asthma
• Anxiety disorders	• Bronchitis
• Somatoform disorders	• Chronic obstructive pulmonary
• Eating disorders	disease
• Personality disorders	• Chronic liver failure
Chronic Pain	• Chronic renal failure
Alcohol/Substance Abuse	• Congestive heart failure
Sleep Disorders	• Cystic fibrosis
• Sleep apnea	• Dementia
• Periodic limb movement	• Epilepsy
disorder	• Gastroesophageal reflux
• Restless legs syndrome	• Head injury
• Delayed sleep phase syndrome	• Hyperthyroidism
Psychophysiologic Conditioning	• Hypoglycemia
Shift Work	• Malignancy
Medical/Neurologic Disorders	• Menopause
• Angina	• Parkinson's disease
• Arthritis	• Peptic ulcer disease

expected, with an inability to return to sleep), or some combination of these problems.

Etiology

The actual neurochemical or pathophysiologic bases for the various types of insomnia are, in general, unknown. There are numerous "causes" for insomnia. Many of the drug and non–drug factors associated with insomnia are listed in Table 56.8 and 56.9. Medical causes include pain of various types (e.g., arthritis, pruritus, duodenal ulcer). Pain not only interferes with the ability to fall asleep but also may lead to increased nocturnal arousals and a generally "lighter" sleep. Nocturia may be part of a medical disorder or a result of too late a dose of a diuretic; the result in either case is fragmentation of sleep. Psychologic or psychiatric causes of insomnia can be as common as worry or excitement (e.g., over an important examination or job interview). Almost everyone is familiar with an occasional bout of insomnia associated with emotional arousal. In addition, it is almost certain that some type of sleep disturbance will accompany an acute episode of any of the major psychiatric disorders (e.g., schizophrenia, major depression, mania), and often the sleep disturbance is one of the diagnostic criteria. The ICSD has 19 specific mental, neurologic, and medical disorders with which sleep disturbances are associated. Additional causes may include disruption of circadian rhythms (e.g., jet lag or work shift change), change of environment (e.g., sleeping for the first night or two in a hotel room in a strange city), sleep apnea, periodic limb movements, stimulant drugs, drug dependence, and drug withdrawal.

Classification by Duration

Often it is useful to classify insomnia as transient, short-term, or persistent (also called long-term or chronic). This distinction is valuable for both diagnosis and treatment decisions. Transient insomnia occurs in an otherwise normal sleeper, has a duration of only several days, and is often associated with an acute stress or disruption of the biological clock (e.g., jet lag or change in work schedule). Short-term insomnia is very similar to transient insomnia except that its duration is 1 to 3 or 4 weeks. It, too, is often associated with some situational stress (e.g., loss of a loved one, family conflict, work conflict) or serious medical illness.

Persistent insomnia has a duration longer than 3 or 4 weeks and is often associated with psychiatric or medical conditions. Sleep apnea syndrome and the association of insomnia with psychiatric disorders have already been discussed. Periodic limb movement disorder (also called periodic leg movements, nocturnal myoclonus, or PMS for periodic movements during sleep) is characterized by periodic (every 20 to 40 seconds), stereotypic, myoclonic movements of the anterior tibialis or other limb muscles during sleep, resulting in arousals. Like the arousals of sleep apnea, the patient may experience several hundred per night and yet not be aware of them the following day. Often, as with sleep apnea, the bed partner will voice the complaint, in this case about the sleeper's "kicking" throughout the night. The condition is age related, showing a marked increase in incidence in individuals over 40 years of age. A related condition that can affect the ability to fall asleep is restless legs syndrome. This is characterized by uncomfortable sensations in the legs at rest, which can be relieved by movement; hence, the patient feels the need to get out of bed and move around.

A number of biological rhythm disorders can be associated with a complaint of persistent insomnia, for example, delayed sleep phase syndrome (28). The patient wants to fall asleep at 11:00 PM and awaken at 7:00 AM. He gets into bed at 11:00 PM and finds that he cannot fall asleep for 4 or 5 hours. When he wakes up (usually with the help of an alarm or two) at 7:00 AM to meet his and society's daily demands, he feels unrefreshed and tired. This pattern is repeated night after night. If he is asked how late he would sleep if he did not have to get out of bed at 7:00 AM, he would probably say 11:00 AM or noon; hence, he could indeed sleep 8 hours. The patient's ability to sleep simply does not coincide with the period set aside for sleep; his body (i.e., his internal biological clock) is not sleepy at the time that he wants to be sleeping.

Drugs and alcohol can be associated with insomnia in numerous ways. Any drug with stimulant properties can disrupt sleep, especially if taken late in the day. The use of CNS depressants, including alcohol, can lead to dependence; then, on withdrawal, it is common to see more disturbed, restless sleep. Even within a single night, alcohol can disrupt sleep. Although it may make the individual feel more relaxed and able to fall asleep, the short duration of action may allow a mild withdrawal in the middle of the night, associated with more disrupted sleep and increased dreaming due to an REM rebound (i.e., early in the night, the alcohol suppresses REM sleep, and as the effect of the alcohol wears off, there is a tendency to make up the lost REM sleep later in the night).

Psychophysiologic insomnia may be transient, short-term, or persistent. It is a conditioned or learned insomnia that the sleeper has associated with the bed, bedroom, or sleep process. The harder the patient tries, the more difficult it becomes to sleep. The patient becomes more and more focused on the inability to sleep and the resultant daytime impairment. Interestingly, such individuals sleep remarkably well in the laboratory or in a strange hotel room, away from the conditions with which insomnia is associated, or at times when they are not thinking about trying to fall asleep (e.g., while watching TV or reading).

Finally, sleep-related gastroesophageal reflux, characterized by regurgitation of gastric contents or fluid into the esophagus during sleep, can awaken the patient from sleep, with heartburn or a sour taste in the mouth.

Table 56.9.
Drugs Associated with Insomnia

• Alcohol	• Corticosteroids	• Oral contraceptives
• Amphetamines	• Decongestants	
• Antipsychotics	• Diuretics	• Phenytoin
• Appetite suppressants	• Hypnotics (chronic use)	• Quinidine
		• Reserpine
• Beta agonists/ blockers	• Levodopa	• Selective serotonin reuptake inhibitors
• Bupropion	• Methyldopa	
• Caffeine	• Methysergide	• Theophylline
• Clonidine	• MAO inhibitors	• Thyroid preparations
• Cocaine	• Nicotine	• Tricyclic antidepressants

Epidemiology

As stated earlier, 35% of all adults will be afflicted with insomnia in a given year. Other surveys estimate that this is the percentage of people who have a sleep problem at any given time (1). The results of a prevalence study of randomly selected elderly (age 65 and older) individuals indicate that sleep apnea can be found in 24%, and periodic limb movements during sleep can be found in 45%, with 10% showing both (11, 12).

The largest analysis of patients studied objectively in sleep-disorders centers found that the most prevalent diagnosis for a complaint of insomnia was insomnia associated with psychiatric disorders (35%). Approximately half had a major affective disorder, and half had personality disorders; less than 5% had major psychoses. Psychophysiologic insomnia (15%) was the second most frequent diagnosis, followed by drug and alcohol dependence (12.4%). Nearly 9% of people with complaints of insomnia had no significant sleep pathology. Sleep apnea syndromes accounted for 6.2% of insomnia. Only 2.9% of the patients were diagnosed with circadian rhythm disorders; however, this category may be underrepresented because of a lesser awareness at that time (29).

The results, unfortunately, may not be representative of the population at large since they represent findings in sleep-disorders centers. Most individuals with a sleep problem probably do not seek medical attention. No adequate, large-scale epidemiologic study has yet been done in the general population (i.e., individuals seen in a primary care practice or in a community pharmacy). The most common sleep disorders may be adjustment sleep disorder (i.e., transient situational insomnia), insomnia associated with anxiety disorders, psychophysiologic insomnia, inadequate sleep hygiene, insomnia associated with mood disorders, obstructive sleep apnea syndrome, delayed or advanced sleep phase syndromes, shift work sleep disorders, alcohol/hypnotic/stimulant-dependent sleep disorders, and periodic limb movement disorder.

Treatment

Treatment of insomnia depends highly on the type. Again, an extremely important distinction exists between persistent or chronic and transient or short-term insomnia. Hypnotics are reserved primarily for transient or short-term insomnia. The persistent insomnias often have other specific interventions of choice. For instance, delayed sleep phase syndrome is treated by chronotherapy (28, 30). Since the patient with delayed sleep phase syndrome can sleep but is sleepy at the wrong time of the 24-hour day, chronotherapy is a means of adjusting the internal clock in 2- to 3-hour blocks each day until sleep occurs at the desired time. The persistent insomnias associated with major psychiatric disorders are most appropriately treated with the specific class of agents targeted for the particular disorder. For example, the patient with a major depressive disorder should be receiving an antidepressant as the primary drug treatment. The sleep disturbance, one symptom of the depressive episode, will be one of the first target symptoms to respond to the treatment. For the psychotic patient, selection and titration of an antipsychotic would be the most appropriate treatment. If the insomnia is associated with drug dependence or drug withdrawal, gradual tapering of the offending agent or the equivalent amount of a cross-tolerant long-acting agent is the primary treatment. If the insomnia is associated with a stimulant, in many cases, the agent should simply be discontinued abruptly.

In the case of insomnia associated with medical disorders, adjunctive, short-term use of a benzodiazepine to promote sleep may be reasonable, while a specific treatment is directed to the primary problem. Further, there are times when a patient is best served by education. The elderly individual whose sleep has become more fragmented, or the "short sleeper" whose sleep need is small and who shows no daytime impairment, may simply need assurance that he or she is sleeping normally.

Periodic limb movements of sleep, a persistent insomnia, is an exception to the general rule of not using hypnotics for chronic insomnias because it is occasionally treated with these agents. Originally treated with clonazepam (Klonopin), it appears that an equivalent response can be obtained with any benzodiazepine (31). The benzodiazepines do not significantly reduce the number of movements, but patients report an improved quality of sleep and feeling more refreshed in the morning. For restless legs syndrome, codeine and related compounds (e.g., oxycodone) or carbamazepine (Tegretol), typically one Percodan tablet or 200 mg of carbamazepine given at bedtime, have helped some patients (32). More recently, considerable success has been demonstrated using levodopa/carbidopa at bedtime, for both periodic limb movements and restless legs syndrome (32).

Some general rules of sleep hygiene can be recommended for both persistent and transient insomnias (Table 56.10). In addition, other nonpharmacologic approaches are available. These include desensitization, meditation, biofeedback, stimulus control, and others (33). There are, however, times when hypnotics should be and are appropriately used.

HYPNOTICS

The Ideal Hypnotic

It is helpful to describe the ideal hypnotic. Although it does not exist, keeping the ideal characteristics in mind helps place the existing agents into perspective. Ideally, the drug should induce sleep rapidly after ingestion. It should maintain sleep for the entire duration expected, without lasting so long that it produces a "morning hangover" and impaired daytime performance. It should not induce development of tolerance or dependence when used over a number of consecutive nights, and abrupt withdrawal should not result in a drug-withdrawal or rebound insomnia. It should have a wide margin of safety, and it should make abnormal sleep normal while not making the sleep of a normal sleeper abnormal. Finally, it should have no potential for drug–drug interactions.

Classification and Pharmacology of Selected Agents

Many of the more commonly used hypnotic agents are presented in Table 56.11. Note that for the elderly, dosing

Table 56.10.
Sleep Hygiene—Suggestions for Improved Sleep

1. Set a regular time to go to bed and a regular time to wake up.
    Regularity is a key component to improving sleep. You must set these times and adhere to them as diligently as possible. At least as important as a regular bedtime is the establishment of a regular wake-up time. No matter how long it took to fall asleep, no matter how little sleep you have had, and no matter how flexible your morning schedule is, there should be no "sleeping in." This would only further confuse and disorganize the internal biological clock (i.e., the circadian pacemaker).
2. Engage in regular, moderate exercise early in the day; do not exercise vigorously in the evening.
    Heavy exercise too late in the evening can lead to a worsening of sleep in all but the best-conditioned athlete; therefore, for most of us, heavy exercise should be scheduled earlier in the day.
3. Generally avoid daytime naps.
    The idea is to consolidate sound, solid sleep through the night. Satisfying some of your sleep need during the day may prevent this. The exception is the individual who routinely takes a daytime nap (e.g., the "siesta"); such an individual generally has a somewhat shorter than average night of sleep.
4. Eat a light snack or beverage before bedtime if hungry; do not eat heavy or spicy food in the evening and do not eat late evening meals or drink large quantities of liquids in the evening.
    A heavy meal late in the evening can severely disrupt sleep in the patient with gastroesophageal reflux (e.g., "heartburn"). Too much liquid can result in multiple awakenings to go to the bathroom.
5. Make the bedroom as comfortable and secure as possible.
    You should attempt to see that the bedroom is dark and quiet, and is neither too hot nor too cold. Although minor fluctuations in room temperature and firmness of the mattress probably have little impact on sleep, extremes can be disturbing. A sense of security can also be quite important.
6. Use the bedroom only for activities associated with sleep.
    Although many of us, while in bed, use the bedroom for watching television, preparing work for the following day, eating snacks, and paying bills, the individual with a sleep problem needs to set the bedroom aside for sleep only. (Sexual activity may be an exception.) In addition, just as warm milk and cookies become a ritual for some children prior to bedtime, some adults must develop a similar relaxing ritual that can be a part of the stimulus for a sleep response.

7. If not asleep within 30 minutes, move to another room and engage in a boring or relaxing activity.
    Get out of bed, leave the bedroom, and do something nonstimulating; for some, this would be watching a late night talk show on television and for others it might be reading one's professional journals. After some 30 to 60 minutes, another attempt should be made to fall asleep. The idea is to not spend too much time in bed awake; an association between the bed and an inability to fall asleep can simply compound the problem.
8. Sleep only as much as needed to feel refreshed and alert during the day.
    Sleep need varies considerably among individuals. Discover for yourself what your sleep need is and satisfy it. Spending extra time in bed awake, thinking that you need to sleep more, may associate the bedroom with wakefulness rather than sleep.
9. Avoid or minimize caffeine (coffee, tea, soft drinks), alcohol, and tobacco.
    Each individual must discover how late such use can be tolerated. However, for the very sensitive, caffeine intake may need to be discontinued each day by noon. Although alcohol is often used as a self-treatment for relaxation and sleep induction, its rapid elimination during the first half of the night may result in some degree of withdrawal, characterized by increased dreaming and nightmares, as well as a general disruption of sleep, during the latter half. In addition, nicotine may be stimulating in some individuals.
10. Avoid routine hypnotics.
    Although hypnotics can be very effective for short-term treatment of a variety of insomnias, long-term use may result in a type of drug-dependence insomnia, characterized by sleep that is even worse than it was before use of the drug.

If your sleep difficulty persists in spite of following the preceding suggestions and perhaps even a brief trial of nonprescription hypnotics, discuss your problem with your physician or pharmacist. Consider learning relaxation techniques or hypnosis. Some people simply need to be able to relax sufficiently to allow sleep to occur. Consider psychotherapy; since at least 35% of all patients seen in sleep disorders centers for complaints of insomnia have an identifiable psychiatric or psychologic cause, some form of psychotherapy or psychiatric treatment may be helpful.

---

should begin at or below the low end of the dosage ranges shown. The old-time barbiturates lost popularity as a result of their narrow margin of safety; moderately high abuse potential; potential drug–drug interactions as a result of liver enzyme induction; suppression of delta and REM sleep, with an REM rebound following abrupt discontinuation; and loss of efficacy in inducing and maintaining sleep within 14 consecutive nights of use at a consistent dose (34).

The older nonbarbiturate nonbenzodiazepines were thought to be superior to the barbiturates because of their lack of the barbiturate structure. However, with the exception of chloral hydrate, they share many of the disadvantages of the barbiturates, and they have additional ones as

well. For instance, methaqualone, which is no longer available, was found to have an even higher abuse potential than the barbiturates. Glutethimide, in an overdose situation, presents the emergency room staff not only with a CNS depressant overdose but also with anticholinergic toxicity. In several European countries, agents such as ethchlorvynol, glutethimide, and methyprylon are not available. Although there has been controversy over their ability in the United States for the past 22 years, they remain on the market. Chloral hydrate, an exception, lacks some of these disadvantages, but it does displace other protein-bound drugs (e.g., warfarin), it causes gastrointestinal irritation in some individuals, and in the higher doses (1 to 2 g) needed for some patients, it may lose its effectiveness in inducing and maintaining sleep at least as rapidly as the barbiturates (35).

The antihistamines, primarily diphenhydramine and doxylamine, are used by taking advantage of their sedative side effects. Some would argue that this drug class is a good choice for patients with a high potential for abusing the benzodiazepines (i.e., those with a history or current problem of substance abuse). Unfortunately, little research into the hypnotic efficacy of these drugs has been done in the sleep laboratory. By subjective report, patients assess the soporific effect of diphenhydramine 50 mg to be equivalent to 60 mg of pentobarbital (36). Increasing the dose of diphenhydramine does not produce a linear increase in hypnotic effect, but it does produce greater anticholinergic side effects, which can be particularly troublesome in the elderly. Not only are they bothered by constipation, urinary retention, dry mouth, and blurred near vision, but they are also particularly sensitive to the central anticholinergic effects of confusion, disorientation, impaired short-term memory, and, at times, visual and tactile hallucinations. Hence, the patient should be monitored for and counseled about these side effects as well as drug interactions with other CNS depressants.

One amino acid, L-tryptophan, became popular as a natural hypnotic since it is a precursor to serotonin, a neurotransmitter that seems to be significantly involved in NREM sleep. L-tryptophan has never been approved by the FDA as a hypnotic; it has been sold as a food supplement. The overall efficacy of this agent is unclear.

Positive response is unpredictable since the predictors of response have not been identified (37). Some 1500 cases (including 24 fatalities) of an eosinophilia–myalgia syndrome associated with the use of L-tryptophan have been reported to the U.S. Centers for Disease Control (CDC) in Atlanta (38). The CDC defines this L-tryptophan-associated eosinophilia–myalgia syndrome as (1) an increase of eosinophils to counts above 1000/mm^3, (2) myalgia that interferes with daily activities, and (3) the absence of some other identifiable cause (e.g., parasites, leukemia). Although the nature of this association is unclear (for instance, there has been strong speculation that some contaminant was accidentally introduced through use of a new strain of bacillus in the production process into the bulk supplies shipped from overseas), as of this writing, the FDA and CDC have recommended that people stop using the agent and that physicians stop prescribing it. If it should come back into use, it should be noted that it is not a totally innocuous substance. Most commonly, people are bothered by its gastrointestinal irritation, which previously pregnant women have compared with morning sickness. In addition, chronic use has been associated with both niacin and pyridoxine deficiencies. The combination of L-tryptophan and a monoamine oxidase inhibitor (e.g., phenelzine or tranylcypromine) or fluoxetine can produce a "serotonin syndrome," characterized by disorientation, agitation, hyperthermia, hyperreflexia, diaphoresis, ocular oscillations, and myoclonic jerking. Finally, low doses have been associated with changes in liver ultrastructure in normal rats and have been lethal in rats with adrenal insufficiency.

Melatonin, endogenously synthesized from serotonin and secreted by the pineal gland, has now become a popular "natural" self-treatment for a variety of disorders. Exogenous melatonin products have not been approved by the FDA but are available in health food stores. Limited studies of doses generally ranging from 0.3 to 5 mg demonstrate efficacy in treating insomnia and jet lag (39, 40). Large controlled trials are still needed as long-term efficacy is unclear and little is known about adverse effects. In addition, the sources and purity of the products sold in health food stores are uncertain.

The benzodiazepines come closest to the ideal hypnotic. Indeed, this was one of several major conclusions of the Consensus Development Conference on Drugs and Insomnia at the National Institute of Mental Health in November 1983 (41). Three significant conclusions to this discussion were that (1) hypnotics should be used primarily in the treatment of transient or short-term insomnia (e.g., situational, jet lag, and work shift change); (2) when pharmacotherapy is indicated, a benzodiazepine is generally the drug of choice; and (3) selection of the specific agent should be based on its pharmacokinetic and pharmacodynamic characteristics in relation to the individual

Table 56.11.
Hypnotics—Classification and Dosages

Generic Name	Trade Name	Dosage Range
Barbiturates		
Pentobarbital	Nembutal	100–200 mg
Secobarbital	Seconal	100–200 mg
Amobarbital	Amytal	100–200 mg
Nonbarbiturate nonbenzodiazepines		
Ethchlorvynol	Placidyl	0.5–1.0 g
Glutethimide	Doriden	0.5–1.0 g
Chloral hydrate	Noctec	0.5–2.0 g
Antihistamines		
Diphenhydramine	Benadryl, Sominex-2	25–100 mg
Doxylamine	Unisom	25–100 mg
"Natural" Products		
L-Tryptophan	Trofan	1.0–4.0 g
Melatonin	—	0.3–5.0 mg
Benzodiazepines		
Flurazepam	Dalmane	15–30 mg
Temazepam	Restoril	15–30 mg
Triazolam	Halcion	0.125–0.5 mg
Quazepam	Doral	7.5–15 mg
Estazolam	ProSom	1.0–2.0 mg
BZD$_1$—Receptor Specific Nonbenzodiazepines		
Zolpidem	Ambien	5–10 mg

Table 56.12.
Benzodiazepine Pharmacokinetics and Doses

Generic Name	Trade Name	Peak Plasma Levels (hrs)	Half–Life (hrs)	Dosage Range (mg)
Alprazolam	Xanax	1–2	12–15	0.75–4
Chlordiazepoxide	Librium	0.5–4	5–30	15–100
Clonazepam	Klonopin	1–2	18–50	1.5–20
Clorazepate	Tranxene	1–2	30–100	15–60
Diazepam	Valium	0.5–2	20–80	4–40
Estazolam	**Prosom**	**2**	**10–24**	**1–2**
Flurazepam	**Dalmane**	**0.5–1**	**47–100**	**15–30**
Halzepam	Paxipam	1–3	14	60–160
Lorazepam	Ativan	1–6	10–20	2–4
Oxazepam	Serax	2–4	5–20	30–120
Prazepam	**Centrax**	**6**	**30–100**	**20–60**
Quazepam	**Doral**	**2**	**39**	**7.5–15**
Temazepam	**Restoril**	**2–4**	**9.5–12.4**	**15–30**
Triazolam	**Halcion**	**0.5–2**	**1.5–5.5**	**0.125–0.25**

Items in bold have indications as hypnotics.

patient and situation. Table 56.12 lists the benzodiazepines including their pharmacokinetics.

Flurazepam was the first of the benzodiazepines marketed as a hypnotic. Its favorable profile, as compared with the barbiturates and the nonbarbiturate nonbenzodiazepines, includes a wider margin of safety, lower abuse potential, and fewer drug–drug interactions. In addition, it produces little or no REM suppression at lower doses (15 mg), and even at higher doses (30 mg), REM suppression is not followed by an REM rebound on abrupt discontinuation of the drug, probably because of the slow elimination of its long-acting active metabolite, N-desalkylflurazepam. Whether it demonstrates no withdrawal phenomena has yet to be clarified; one may need to look at sleep patterns several weeks beyond discontinuation of the drug. It has the additional advantage of remaining effective at a consistent dose for at least 28 consecutive nights of use. It does suppress delta sleep, and the long-acting metabolite (with an elimination half-life of 47 to 200 hours) accumulates over time. This can cause impaired daytime functioning, especially in the elderly, leading to falls resulting in injuries (42). Peak plasma levels are achieved within 30 to 60 minutes.

Temazepam has the advantage of a short-to-intermediate elimination half-life of 9 to 15 hours. However, it can be as long as 20 to 30 hours in the elderly, so one must watch for possible accumulation and morning hangover with repeated use. It shares many of the properties of flurazepam with respect to effects on sleep. In doses of 15 to 30 mg, it increases total sleep time and decreases the frequency and duration of nocturnal awakenings in insomniac patients. It suppresses delta sleep, and, although there is a decrease in REM sleep during the first half of the night, there is a corresponding increase in the second half. However, there is an ongoing

question about its ability to shorten sleep latency significantly in the patient who has difficulty falling asleep because it can take 1 to 2 hours to work. Initial studies of the drug included two dosage forms: a hard gelatin capsule with a powder inside (available in the United States) and a soft gelatin capsule containing a solution of the drug in polyethylene glycol. With the soft gelatin capsule, the drug appears to be absorbed more quickly. This formulation issue has yet to be adequately addressed by the manufacturer.

Triazolam is unique in being ultrashort to short acting, with an elimination half-life of 2 to 3 hours (5.5 at the most). Peak plasma levels are achieved within 30 to 80 minutes. Triazolam appears to be absorbed about as quickly as flurazepam but eliminated much more rapidly. Although it suppresses REM sleep in the first half of the night, there appears to be compensation for this in the second half (probably as drug levels are decreasing). It seems to have little effect on delta sleep, which distinguishes it from flurazepam, temazepam, and other benzodiazepines. It is least likely of the benzodiazepines to produce morning hangover. Indeed, at the 0.25-mg dose, the effect is equal to that with placebo. Like flurazepam and temazepam, it increases the general quality of sleep, decreases nocturnal awakenings, and increases total sleep time (43–47).

There has been some concern among clinicians and the public that triazolam is more likely to produce psychomotor impairment, psychologic adverse effects, and anterograde amnesia than other benzodiazepines. However, rather than a unique risk of triazolam, this may be a function of the dose and pattern of use, potency, combination with other CNS depressants, and the mechanism of adverse drug reaction reporting (48). In a meeting of the FDA's Psychopharmacological Drugs Advisory Committee (September 22, 1989), the consensus was that the issue of amnesia should receive greater attention in the product labeling (i.e., the package insert) and that patient information should be developed about the use and risks of the entire class of benzodiazepine hypnotics.

In fact, the FDA requested that all manufacturers of benzodiazepine hypnotics comply with these recommendations: (a) modify the warnings section of the package insert; (b) provide a patient package insert; and (c) distribute their products in unit-of-use packs containing a maximum of 10 doses. Not all manufacturers accepted these recommendations which, of note, refer only to benzodiazepine hypnotics.

Some of the concern over triazolam has been associated with "traveler's amnesia." This is the situation in which an individual flying across a number of time zones decides to force sleep during the flight with a short-acting hypnotic, perhaps having ingested some ethanol on the plane as well. Later the traveler has little or no recall for a number of hours following ingestion of the drug (e.g., arrival at the airport and subsequent activities). Until we fully understand this form of anterograde amnesia, it may simply be safer to readjust the internal biological clock after arriving at our destination. Whatever the actual incidence (as yet still unclear) of psychomotor impairment, psychological adverse affects, and anterograde amnesia, especially at the lower doses currently being recommended and used, it is prudent to carefully monitor and counsel patients using triazolam.

Quazepam and estazolam are the two benzodiazepines most recently marketed in the United States. Where estazolam, the second triazolobenzodiazepine hypnotic, stands in our benzodiazepine hypnotic armamentarium is yet to be established. It appears to decrease sleep latency and nocturnal awakenings, while increasing total sleep time and improving depth of sleep and sleep quality (49). Peak plasma levels are achieved within 0.5 to 4 hours, although with the doses generally employed, onset of action appears to be similar to that seen with flurazepam and triazolam. The half-life of elimination is 8 to 28 hours. Based on its onset of action and elimination half-life, it appears to be a "faster-acting temazepam." This would place it in the position of being an agent that can significantly decrease sleep latency (a distinct advantage over temazepam) and provide a duration of action intermediate between flurazepam and triazolam. However, results of objective sleep laboratory studies are mixed with respect to estazolam's ability to significantly decrease latency to sleep onset.

Although quazepam has an intriguing specificity for the BZD_1 benzodiazepine receptor subtype, the clinical significance of this property is unclear. Indeed, although the parent compound has a 39–hour half-life of elimination, one of its metabolites, N-desalkyl-2-oxoquazepam, is identical to N-desalkylflurazepam, which is the long-acting active metabolite of flurazepam. Therefore, one would expect that, clinically, its properties would be very similar to those of flurazepam. Peak plasma levels are achieved in 1 to 2 hours (50). With greater use, we may discover that it offers few, if any, advantages over flurazepam.

Zolpidem is the most recently approved hypnotic in the United States; it is an imidazopyridine compound with a number of intriguing characteristics. It is not a benzodiazepine; however, the molecule is designed in such a way that it binds selectively to the BZD_1 receptor. Its specificity distinguishes it from all the other currently marketed benzodiazepine hypnotics except quazepam; and the fact that it does not have any nonspecific, benzodiazepine-receptor binding metabolites distinguishes it from quazepam.

Pharmacologically, zolpidem's BZD_1 receptor specificity seems to account for its strong hypnotic activity, with minimal anxiolytic, muscle relaxant, and anticonvulsant activity even at higher doses than recommended for insomnia (although at extremely high doses, the specificity appears to be lost). This is certainly advantageous in a hypnotic; however, theoretically, one would exercise extreme caution in attempting to switch a patient from long-term and/or high-dose use of a benzodiazepine to zolpidem. Zolpidem would not be expected to protect the patient from withdrawal symptoms of increased anxiety, muscle disturbances, or convulsions. In addition, in patients for whom a single bedtime dose of a sedative-hypnotic is desired in order to help the patient sleep at night and have a carryover anxiolytic effect throughout the day, zolpidem would not appear to be appropriate.

Zolpidem is rapidly absorbed, resulting in a rapid onset of action. It has a mean plasma elimination half-life of 2.3 hours in healthy subjects, 2.9 hours in the elderly, and close to 10 hours in patients with hepatic cirrhosis. It is metabolized to three major pharmacologically inactive metabolites.

With respect to specific effects on sleep, zolpidem decreases latency to sleep onset (sleep occurring within 20 to 30 minutes following ingestion), increases total sleep time, decreases the number of awakenings during the night, and subjectively improves the quality of sleep. Although some evidence exists for a slight suppression of REM sleep when using higher–than–recommended doses, in most studies the drug appears to have little effect on this stage of sleep. Unlike most benzodiazepines, zolpidem does not suppress delta sleep; in fact, in one study, delta sleep was increased in healthy, young adults.

Zolpidem, in lower doses (5 to 10 mg), appears to provide a full night of sleep with little or no daytime impairment or effects on memory. It appears to have a lower abuse potential than the benzodiazepines. In fact, at very high doses, it produces nausea, dizziness, anxiety, and dysphoria; such effects would discourage many recreational drug users. Rebound insomnia has been minimal or absent following abrupt discontinuation of zolpidem. In a sleep laboratory study lasting 4 weeks, no evidence of tolerance was seen polysomnographically. Subjectively, patients receiving zolpidem for 5 weeks or no longer report no significant changes in efficacy over time.

Adverse effects associated with zolpidem (in doses of 10 mg or less) have primarily been headache, drowsiness, dizziness, lethargy, nausea, myalgia, and sinusitis. The incidence of headache and drowsiness seems to be age-related. And drowsiness, nausea, and anterograde amnesia appear to be dose-related, increasing significantly at a dose of 20 mg. Falls and confusion can be seen in the elderly if treated with doses in excess of 10 mg (which is twice the recommended starting dose for this population). Except for what appears to be additive CNS depressant effects when zolpidem is used in combination with chlorpromazine or imipramine, no drug interactions have been noted with haloperidol, cimetidine, ranitidine, warfarin, or digoxin (51).

Based on currently available data, zolpidem seems likely to move into a significant position in our hypnotic armamentarium. How significant that position will be hinges, in large part, on whether or not patients respond well to the recommended lower doses (5 mg in the elderly and 10 mg in the healthy nonelderly) without needing the higher doses associated with an increased incidence of adverse effects. As we have seen all too often in past years, much excitement is generated regarding new and unique agents prior to extensive postmarketing experience in the U.S., only to be dampened by the less–than ideal realities discovered upon clinical use in large numbers of patients. As always, cautious optimism is in order.

Drug-Withdrawal Insomnia and Rebound Insomnia

When barbiturates were used more commonly for the treatment of insomnia, drug-withdrawal insomnia was described as a phenomenon associated with the abrupt discontinuation of the hypnotic after long-term use (52). After chronic REM suppression, discontinuation led to an REM rebound, accounting for as much as 40% of total sleep time. This REM rebound was accompanied by very intense and frightening dreams as well as a generally disrupted night of sleep. The patient, not understanding the nature of the phenomenon, was likely to immediately return to chronic, high-dose use. With gradual tapering of the drug or an equivalent amount of a longer-acting agent and patient education about the possibility of temporarily increased dreaming and decreased quality of sleep, patients are better able to tolerate discontinuation of their hypnotics.

More recently, rebound insomnia has been described as a phenomenon associated with the abrupt discontinuation of the shorter-acting benzodiazepines (e.g., temazepam and triazolam) (53). It involves a worsening of sleep, even

beyond what it was like before the patient was started on the drug. The exact incidence of the phenomenon is unclear, but it is prudent to warn the patient about a possible transient worsening of sleep immediately after stopping the drug. Gradual tapering of the drug, rather than abrupt discontinuation, may lessen the severity of these withdrawal symptoms (54). As an example, a patient taking 0.25 mg of triazolam every night for several weeks could reduce the dose by half (to 0.125 mg) for three nights, by half again (to one half of a 0.125-mg tablet) for the next three nights, and then finally discontinue the medication.

Problems and Controversies

Two important issues with insomnia and hypnotics are that no one drug is ideal for every insomniac and that not all insomniacs should be treated with hypnotics. As previously stated, hypnotics are to be used almost exclusively for the treatment of transient or short-term insomnia. The implication is that a thorough assessment will be made of every patient with a complaint of insomnia. Although hypnotic-induced sleep may be unnatural in some respects, an ultimate measure of efficacy must be seen as optimal daytime performance (55, 56).

Some prescribers and patients believe that all hypnotics should be avoided because of the possible development of dependence. If they are used appropriately—for brief periods and at low doses—the risk is low. Also, drug-dependence insomnia, in which sleep worsens with long-term use of hypnotics even while the patient continues to take the drug, should not be a problem. In many respects, our society has been responsible for many of the transient insomnias (e.g., jet lag, work shift change, and situational) and must take responsibility, either pharmacologically or nonpharmacologically, for dealing with the problem.

General Clinical Guidelines

A careful diagnostic assessment is necessary before treating any insomnia. The health care provider can play a major role in assessing sleep and arousal disorders. See Tables 56.13 and 56.14 for ideas on what types of questions to ask in screening a patient. Don't allow your own experiences to interfere with your assessment. Unfortunately, because most of us have had at least an occasional bout of insomnia, we may too easily assume that everyone else's problem is similar to our own. Clarify the complaint and do a drug history. Assess the possibility that the problem is drug-induced. Look for stimulating drugs such as sympathomimetic decongestants or caffeine. Look for CNS depressant withdrawal such as moderate-to-heavy ethanol intake at dinner time. Assess the contribution of street drugs. In addition, look for sedating drugs as causes of excessive daytime sleepiness. Finally, find out what, if anything, has worked for the same problem in the past. Ask if the

Table 56.13.

Important Questions to Ask in Assessing a Sleep Complaint

- How long have you had this problem?
- What is your normal bedtime/sleep pattern and has it changed recently?
- How long do you usually sleep? Do you go to sleep at about the same time each night? Do you take daytime naps?
- How long does it take you to fall asleep? How often do you wake up during the night? What time do you wake up? Are you able to fall back to sleep?
- Have you been experiencing pain, worry, stress, work or family problems recently that could be associated with your sleep problem?
- Do you suffer from any emotional or physical illness?
- Do you consume any drugs, alcohol, or caffeine-containing foods or beverages?
- Has your bed partner observed any snoring or unusual movements?
- How do you feel upon awakening and during the day—tired, depressed, sleepy, irritable?
- Do any of your relatives suffer from poor sleep?
- Does anything help your sleep—sleeping pills, exercise, or sleeping in another room?

problem is one of insomnia or excessive daytime sleepiness. Patients may be excessively sleepy secondary to obstructive sleep apnea or narcolepsy. If it's a case of self-induced sleep deprivation (e.g., studying for examinations), caffeine tablets may be appropriate short-term, but evaluate possible drug-disease interactions (e.g., hypertension) and tell the patient about sleep hygiene. If the complaint is insomnia, determine if it is transient or chronic. If transient, a nonprescription sleep aid containing doxylamine or diphenhydramine may be worth a try for a few nights; but tell the patient about anticholinergic effects and consider alternatives if the antihistamine is either ineffective or intolerable. If the insomnia is chronic, the patient deserves as meticulous an evaluation as the patient who comes in with a complaint of chronic stomach pain or unremitting, chronic headache. There are many reasons for chronic insomnia, and a number of them are treatable. Finally, be prepared for appreciation and praise. If only one patient a year is identified with a treatable and responsive chronic insomnia, the change in quality of life will make that patient forever grateful.

Until now, once a decision has been made to treat insomnia pharmacologically, benzodiazpines have been the treatment of choice; pharmacokinetic differences play a major role in selecting a benzodiazepine. Zolpidem offers one more option. Drug selection must take into account onset of action and duration with respect to single versus multiple dosing and past history of response. If possible daytime impairment associated with accumulation of long-acting active metabolites (especially in the elderly) is a concern, avoid flurazepam and quazepam; choose one of the shorter-acting benzodiazepines or zolpidem. Also,

recall that accumulation becomes a much greater concern with continuous use over several nights than with infrequent p.r.n. use (in which drug action is terminated as quickly as it can be redistributed out of brain tissue). If the possible delayed onset of action of temazepam is a concern, choose the more rapidly acting flurazepam, triazolam, zolpidem, or, perhaps, estazolam. If possible anterograde amnesia is a concern, use very low doses, caution the patient, and consider avoiding hypnotic use in situations in which the drug effect may not have worn off by the time the individual needs to be awake, alert, and fully functioning. The choices do not always have to be limited to the agents specifically marketed as hypnotics. For instance, diazepam is superior to flurazepam in onset of action and yet shares the property of accumulation of a long-acting active metabolite under multiple-dosing conditions. In general, the choice of drug depends upon pharmacokinetic profile and benefits sought.

The hypnotics should be avoided in patients with sleep apnea, patients who use alcohol or other CNS depressants heavily, pregnant patients, and individuals in whom alert nighttime performance is mandatory (e.g., firemen, pilots). Although the benzodiazpines are relatively safe, one must be cautious in giving them to patients with a high suicidal risk. Patients who overdose often use combinations of agents, frequently washing down everything with alcohol. Combination of benzodiazepines with alcohol can be fatal. Most likely, an additive or synergistic mechanism is the basis for the interaction, resulting in impaired psychomotor functioning and excess sedation. Acute ethanol ingestion appears to enhance benzodiazepine absorption, decrease the volume of distribution and impair elimination (due to hepatic enzyme inhibition). Zolpidem has additive, not synergistic, effects when combined with alcohol and it is recommended that the two not be taken in combination.

The benefit that the patient is seeking must be determined. Ideally, the patient is looking for both improved sleep and improved daytime functioning. Simply increasing the number of hours of sleep is generally not a sufficient reason for prescribing hypnotics. Once the hypnotic is chosen, the lowest effective dose to achieve a

Table 56.14.

Important Questions to Ask in Monitoring Hypnotic Therapy

- Is your sleep improved?
- Are you taking the medication as it was prescribed?
- Have you increased your dose or taken a second dose at night?
- Are you experiencing undesirable sleepiness in the morning or during the day?
- Are you awakening early?
- Have you noticed changes in your mood, behavior, or memory?
- Are you more nervous, irritable, or anxious than usual?
- Are you having problems with dizziness, unsteadiness, or lightheadedness?

clear-cut benefit is used. This requires following the patient regularly, quantifying the results, and educating the patient about the need to begin with a low dose and give it an adequate trial. For flurazepam, this is 15 mg; with triazolam in an elderly patient, the dose is 0.125 mg, or perhaps even half a 0.125-mg tablet; for zolpidem, the dose is 5 mg in the elderly and 10 mg in the healthy adult. The importance of starting with a low dose cannot be overstated. For instance, with flurazepam the optimal effect may not be experienced for 2 to 3 days; this may be due to slow accumulation of N-desalkylflurazepam. In addition, especially in the elderly, daytime sequelae must be monitored. These are important educational and monitoring roles for the health care provider. Questions that should be asked of patients when monitoring hypnotic effects and side effects are listed in Table 56.13. Drug-drug and drug-disease interactions should be identified and avoided. Examples of drug-drug interactions include additive CNS depression when the hypnotics are combined with other CNS depressants; and accumulation of flurazepam, quazepam, and their long-acting metabolite N-desalkylflurazepam in the presence of cimetidine (which interferes with oxidative metabolic processes). A primary drug-disease interaction is the use of an agent requiring oxidative metabolic transformation (e.g., flurazepam and quazepam) in the presence of liver disease or old age. If one of the older nonbenzodiazepines is being prescribed, the effect of liver enzyme induction must be kept in mind, in addition to additive effects with other CNS depressants. With zolpidem, recall that the elimination half-life is increased approximately four-fold in the presence of hepatic cirrhosis.

The issue of hypnotic use in chronic insomnia is complex. Few data are available regarding the efficacy and safety of hypnotics when taken for more than 1 to 2 months. In addition, there is no evidence to indicate that chronic hypnotic use will produce lasting, objective improvement in sleep and daytime function in the persistent insomnias. Therefore, if hypnotics are prescribed, the goal with chronic insomnia should be pulsed, intermittent treatment and periodic medical reevaluation. Indeed, for many chronic insomniacs, the underlying problem is a psychiatric condition, drug or alcohol dependence, sleep apnea, or delayed sleep phase syndrome. Treatments specific to the disorder and nonpharmacologic approaches should be tried first. If psychiatric and medical disorders have been ruled out and nonpharmacologic approaches have failed, referral to a sleep-disorders center would be appropriate. In the rare instances in which a thorough sleep evaluation has been done and a hypnotic is used in treating a chronic insomnia (e.g., periodic limb movement disorder), the patient should be evaluated frequently for improvement in both sleep and daytime functioning, as well as the persistence of the therapeutic effect at a constant dose. The reason for this, at least with the typical benzodiazepines, is that longer-term use carries an increased risk of dependence, tolerance with resulting escalation of dose, and difficult withdrawal.

Patient education should include emphasis on short-term use, discussion of possible daytime sedation and impairment with the longer-acting agents, the importance of avoiding other CNS depressants, and the risks of tolerance and dependence if used for too long and/or at excessively high doses. Where hypnotics are to be used for extended periods, it may be useful to suggest skipping a night or two once in a while. This allows the patient to see if the drug is still really needed, and perhaps it can reduce the development of tolerance. When the drug is discontinued—ideally in a gradual, tapered style—the patient must be told about possible temporary withdrawal phenomena.

PROGNOSIS

Insomnia and the other sleep disorders can be crippling for many people. As life becomes more complex, it would not be surprising to see an increase in the incidence of transient insomnia. However, with appropriate assessment and treatment, the transient insomnias can be managed, to improve both nighttime sleep and daytime performance. Although there may be no cures for many persistent insomnias such as sleep apnea, increased understanding of these disorders is leading to prevention of harm to patients by inadequate assessment or inappropriate use of hypnotics. Further, with better assessment and increased referral by pharmacists, many patients with some of the persistent insomnias (e.g., psychiatric disorders and delayed sleep phase syndrome) can be helped significantly.

CONCLUSION

Sleep is a fascinating psychophysiologic phenomenon that is cyclic and can be measured electrophysiologically. Much is now known about sleep and its disorders, but sleep-disorders medicine is still in its infancy. Millions of our patients are afflicted by a variety of sleep disorders. They are a heterogeneous group of disorders capable of producing major social or occupational disability; disturbed sleep can be crippling for many people. Sleep complaints deserve the same meticulous assessment and concern as that afforded a complaint of chest pain, flank pain, or coughing up blood. Disorders of excessive daytime sleepiness (obstructive sleep apnea and narcolepsy), insomnia (transient as well as persistent types), and unusual behaviors and mental activity during sleep (sleepwalking, sleep terrors, and nightmares) have been described. Not all sleep complaints should be treated with hypnotics; indeed, some of the sleep disorders may be worsened by hypnotics or other drugs.

Hypnotic use is generally most appropriately reserved for the treatment of transient or short-term insomnias. Although a number of hypnotics are available, the benzodiazepines and zolpidem are currently accepted as the drugs of choice; selection within the group is based primarily on differences in pharmacokinetic profiles. The health care provider has the opportunity to play an important role in assessing, recommending treatment, or recommending further evaluation for the many patients with complaints of insomnia or excessive daytime sleepiness. In addition, you can play a major role in educating the patient about therapy and monitoring for therapeutic and adverse effects. With careful diagnosis and treatment tailored to the individual and the particular problem, more people will be sleeping better and performing considerably better in their daily activities.

REFERENCES

1. Bixler EO, Kales A, Soldatos CR, et al. Prevalence of sleep disorders in the Los Angeles metropolitan area. Am J Psychiatry 136:1257–1262, 1979.
2. Mellinger GD, Balter MB, Uhlenhuth EH. Insomnia and its treatments. Arch Gen Psychiatry 42:225–232, 1985.
3. Wincor MZ, Johnson KA. Non-prescription hypnotics: purchase and pharmacist-patient interaction in the community pharmacy. Presented to the 14th European Symposium on Clinical Pharmacy. Stockholm, October, 1985.
4. The involvement of sleep in motor vehicle crashes. National Highway Traffic Safety Administration memorandum. Washington, DC: U.S. Department of Transportation, National Highway Traffic Safety Administration, U.S. Government Printing Office, November 22, 1985.
5. Leger D. The cost of sleep-related accidents: a report for the national commission on sleep disorders research. Sleep 17:84–93; 1994.
6. Hobson JA, Lydic R, Baghdoyan HA. Evolving concepts of sleep cycle generation: from brain centers to neuronal populations. Behav Brain Sci 9:371–448, 1986.
7. Siegel JM. Mechanisms of sleep control. J Clin Neurophysiol 7:49–65, 1990.
8. Rechtschaffen A, Kales A, eds. A Manual of Standardized Terminology, Techniques and Scoring System for Sleep Stages of Human Subjects. (Publication 204, Public Health Service Publications.) Washington, DC: U.S. Government Printing Office, 1968.
9. Karni A, Tanne D, Rubenstein BS, et al. Dependence on REM sleep of overnight improvement of a perceptual skill. Science 265:679–682, 1994.
10. Bliwise DL. Sleep in normal aging and dementia. Sleep 16:40–81, 1993.
11. Ancoli-Israel S, Kripke DF, Klauber MR, et al. Sleep-disordered breathing in community-dwelling elderly. Sleep 14:486–495, 1991.
12. Ancoli-Israel S, Kripke DF, Klauber MR, et al. Periodic limb movements in sleep in community-dwelling elderly. Sleep 14:496–500, 1991.
13. Sleep Disorders Classification Committee, Association of Sleep Disorders Centers. Diagnostic classification of sleep and arousal disorders. Sleep 2:1–137, 1979.
14. Diagnostic Classification Steering Committee of the American Sleep Disorders Association (Thorpy MJ, chair). International Classification of Sleep Disorders—Diagnostic and Coding Manual. Rochester, MN: American Sleep Disorders Association, 1990: 396.
15. American Psychiatric Association. Diagnostic and Statistical Manual of Mental Disorders, ed. 3, revised. Washington, DC: American Psychiatric Association, 1987:297–313.
16. Kales A, Soldatos CR, Kales JD. Sleep disorders: insomnia, sleepwalking, night terrors, nightmares, and enuresis. Ann Intern Med 106:582–592, 1987.
17. Guilleminault C. Obstructive sleep apnea syndrome: a review. Psychiatr Clin North Am 10:607–621, 1987.
18. Kales A, Vela-Bueno A, Kales JD. Sleep disorders: sleep apnea and narcolepsy. Ann Intern Med 106:434–443, 1987.
19. Handelsman H, Carter E. Continuous Positive Airway Pressure for the Treatment of Obstructive Sleep Apnea in Adults. (Health Technology Assessment Reports 1986, no 3.) Rockville, MD: National Center for Health Services Research and Health Care Technology Assessment, 1986.
20. Bonnet MH, Dexter JR, Arand DL. The effect of triazolam on arousal and respiration in central sleep apnea patients. Sleep 13:31–41, 1990.
21. Whyte KF, Gould GA, Airlie MA. Role of protriptyline and acetazolamide in the sleep apnea/hypopnea syndrome. Sleep 11:463–472, 1988.
22. Strohl KP, Hensley MJ, Saunders NA, et al. Progesterone administration and progressive sleep apneas. JAMA 245:1230–1232, 1981.
23. Tojima H, Kunitomo F, Kimura H, et al. Effects of acetazolamide in patients with the sleep apnea syndrome. Thorax 43:113–118, 1988.
24. Dement WC, Carskadon MA, Guilleminault C, et al. Narcolepsy: diagnosis and treatment. Prim Care 3:609–623, 1976.
25. Inoko H, Ando A, Tseuji K, et al. HLA-DQ chain DNA restriction fragments can differentiate between healthy and narcoleptic individuals with HLA-DR2. Immunogenetics 23:126–128, 1986.
26. Aldrich MS. Narcolepsy. N Eng J Med 323:389–394, 1990.
27. Carskadon MA, Dement WC, Mitler MM, et al. Self reports versus sleep laboratory findings in 122 drug-free subjects with complaints of chronic insomnia. Am J Psychiatry 133:1382–1388, 1976.
28. Weitzman ED, Czeisler CA, Coleman RM, et al. Delayed sleep phase syndrome. Arch Gen Psychiatry 38:737–746, 1981.
29. Coleman R, Roffwarg H, Kennedy S, et al. Sleep-wake disorders based on a polysomnographic diagnosis: a national cooperative study. JAMA 247:997–1003, 1982.
30. Czeisler CA, Kronauer RE, Allan JS, et al. Bright light induction of strong (Type O) resetting of the human circadian pacemaker. Science 244:1328–1333, 1989.
31. Mitler MM, Browman CP, Menn SJ, et al. Nocturnal myoclonus: treatment efficacy of clonazepam and temazepam. Sleep 9:385–392, 1986.
32. Krueger BR. Restless legs syndrome and periodic movements of sleep. Mayo Clin Proc 65:999–1006, 1990.
33. Morin CM, Culbert JP, Schwartz SM. Nonpharmacological interventions for insomnia: a meta-analysis of treatment efficacy. Am J Psychiatry 151:1172–1180, 1994.
34. Kales AK, Bixler EO, Kales JD, et al. Comparative effectiveness of nine hypnotic drugs: sleep laboratory studies. J Clin Pharmacol 17:207–213, 1977.
35. Kales A, Allen C, Scharf MB, et al. Hypnotic drugs and their effectiveness: all night EEG studies of insomniac subjects. Arch Gen Psychiatry 23:226–232, 1970.
36. Teutach G, Mahler DL, Brown CR, et al. Hypnotic efficacy of diphenhydramine, methapyrilene, and pentobarbital for nighttime sedation. Clin Pharmacol Ther 17:195–201, 1975.
37. Schneider-Helmert D, Spinweber CL. Evaluation of L-tryptophan for treatment of insomnia: a review. Psychopharmacology 89:1–7, 1986.
38. Raphals P. Disease puzzle nears solution. Science 249:619, 1990.
39. Zhdanova IV, Wirtman RJ, Lynch HJ, et al. Sleep-inducing effects of low doses of melatonin ingested in the evening. Clin Pharmacol Ther 57:552–558, 1995.
40. Petrie K, Dawson AG, Thompson L, et al. A double-blind trial of melatonin as a treatment for jet lag in international cabin crew. Biol Psychiatry 33:526–530, 1993.

41. National Institute of Mental Health, Consensus Development Conference. Drugs and insomnia: the use of medications to promote sleep. JAMA 251:2410–2414, 1984.

42. Ray WA, Griffin MR, Downey W. Benzodiazepines of short and long elimination half-life and the risk of hip fracture. JAMA 262:3303–3307, 1989.

43. Dement WC. Rational basis for the use of sleeping pills. Pharmacology 27(suppl 2):3–38, 1983.

44. Wincor MZ. Insomnia and the new benzodiazepines. Clin Pharm 1:425–432, 1982.

45. Kales A, Kales JD. Sleep laboratory studies of hypnotic drugs: efficacy and withdrawal effects. J Clin Psychopharmacol 3:140–150, 1983.

46. Rickels K. Clinical trials of hypnotics. J Clin Psychopharmacol 3:133, 1983.

47. Greenblatt DJ, Harmatz JS, Englehardt N, et al. Pharmacokinetic determinants of dynamic differences among three benzodiazepine hypnotics. Arch Gen Psychiatry 46:326–332, 1989.

48. Griffiths RR, Lamb RJ, Ator NA, et al. Relative abuse liability of triazolam: experimental assessment in animals and humans. Neurosci Biobehav Res 9:133–151, 1985.

49. Pierce MW, Shu VS. Efficacy of estazolam: the United States clinical experience. Am J Med 88(suppl 3A):6–11, 1990.

50. Kales A. Quazepam: hypnotic efficacy and side effects. Pharmacotherapy 10:1–12, 1990.

51. Langtry HD, Benfield P. Zolpidem: a review of its pharmacodynamic and pharmacokinetic properties and therapeutic potential. Drugs 40:291–313, 1990.

52. Kales A, Bixler E, Tan T, et al. Chronic hypnotic-drug use: ineffectiveness, drug-withdrawal insomnia, and dependence. JAMA 227:513–517, 1974.

53. Kales A, Scharf M, Kales J. Rebound insomnia: a new clinical syndrome. Science 201:1039–1041, 1978.

54. Schweizer E, Rickels K, Case G, et al. Long-term therapeutic use of benzodiazepines—II. Effects of gradual taper. Arch Gen Psychiatry 47:908–915, 1990.

55. Gillin JC, Byerley WF. The diagnosis and management of insomnia. N Engl J Med 322:239–247, 1990.

56. Everett DE, Avorn J, Baker MW. Clinical decision-making in the evaluation and treatment of insomnia. Am J Med 89:357–362, 1990.

CHAPTER 57

ATTENTION DEFICIT HYPERACTIVITY DISORDER

STEPHEN C. COOKE

Attention Deficit/Hyperactivity Disorder (ADHD) is a childhood disorder characterized by persistent patterns of inattention, hyperactivity, and impulsivity (1). Although all children are at times inattentive and restless, a child who is diagnosed with ADHD exhibits inattention and hyperactivity to a degree that is both debilitating and greater than that exhibited by other individuals at a comparable level of development. Associated features may include low frustration tolerance, temper outbursts, mood lability, poor self-esteem, academic underachievement, and oppositional behavior. Left untreated, ADHD may lead to school failure and rejection by peers, teachers, siblings, and parents. Even when ADHD is properly treated with medication, children will often continue to exhibit "learned behaviors" (low self-esteem, poor academic skills) that are secondary to behaviors originally induced by the disease. These continued behaviors often take time and nonpharmacologic interventions such as group, family, or individual therapy to resolve.

Evolving concepts of this disorder have contributed to the dynamic nature of the diagnostic criteria that have been found in the Diagnostic and Statistical Manual (DSM) over the years. The Diagnostic and Statistical Manual, Second Edition (DSM-II), characterized "hyperkinetic reaction of childhood" as a reaction disorder caused by suppression or internalization of interpersonal problems (2). A decade later, the DSM-III classified the disease as Attention Deficit Disorder (ADD), with or without hyperactivity (3). In the DSM-III-R the symptom criteria were further modified to stress the importance and core inclusion of hyperactivity (4). The new DSM-III-R classification, Attention Deficit Hyperactivity Disorder (ADHD), reflected that emphasis. In addition, the diagnosis of ADD without hyperactivity was dropped in favor of Undifferentiated Attention Deficit Disorder. The current edition, DSM-IV, combines both of the subtypes found in the DSM-III-R into one category but allows the clinician to diagnostically indicate a predominating symptom pattern (1). DSM-IV criteria also require that symptoms be present in more than one setting (e.g., home and school) to reduce the risk of false-positive diagnoses.

Careful diagnosis of any disorder is important, but special caution should be taken in considering a psychiatric diagnosis for a school-age child. The effects of social stigma at this level of development can be particularly cruel and debilitating, often having long-reaching effects on the psyche of a maturing child. In many settings, the diagnosis of ADHD has a "me-too" effect in that other children who may be doing poorly academically may be unduly diagnosed because of social pressures rather than clinical parameters. Diagnosis, therefore, should be made with strict adherence to criteria to avoid a diagnosis based on parental or teacher "dissatisfaction with performance."

ETIOLOGY

ADHD is thought to have a biological basis, but the precise cause remains unknown. Several causative factors have been suggested; they are summarized in Table 57.1. Reports in the literature on the influence of thyroid abnormalities, environmental toxins, deficits in the behavioral inhibition system, and poor prenatal care are present but are not convincing. Dietary consumption of simple sugars (which abound in the average American child's diet) have long been popularly held to be at fault in this disorder. Several studies, however, have refuted this idea (5, 6). Perhaps the most logically based, yet still unproven, hypothesis suggests that the anatomical and developmental immaturity of the catecholamine system is to blame. This hypothesis is supported by the high prevalence of ADHD in children and the frequent remission of symptoms with maturity. There also appears to be a familial link in ADHD, but a causative gene has yet to be identified.

PREVALENCE/OCCURRENCE

For school-age children in the United States, the estimated prevalence of ADHD is 3 to 5% (7). Males are 4 to 9 times more likely to be affected by ADHD (8). Reasons for this are unclear. Studies also suggest that 30 to 70% of children with ADHD will continue to be symptomatic as adults (4, 9). However, data in this area remains limited and is complicated by the changing presentation of symptoms over time.

DIAGNOSIS/CLINICAL FINDINGS

The proper diagnosis of ADHD requires the cooperation and astute observation of individuals who are in direct care

Table 57.1.
Postulated Causative Factors in Attention Deficit/ Hyperactivity Disorder

Prenatal or perinatal insult
Neurotransmitter (norepinephrine) deficiency or breakdown
Neurochemical lesions
Congenital anomalies
Low CNS arousal level
Genetic disorders
Exposure to environmental toxins

relationships with the individual in conjunction with a knowledgeable clinician. As with other disorders, a differential diagnosis must be considered in evaluating an individual for ADHD. Other related disorders that must first be considered include mental retardation, oppositional behavior, personality disorders, mood disorders, and substance abuse (1). There are no current laboratory tests that have proven to be diagnostic for ADHD. Children and adults with ADHD are usually physically healthy with no associated physical defects or anomalies being identified.

Table 57.2 outlines the diagnostic criteria found in the DSM-IV for ADHD. The essential feature for proper diagnosis of ADHD is a consistent pattern of hyperactivity/ impulsivity and/or inattention that is maladaptive and more pronounced than is seen in developmental peers. Symptom presence must also be judged to be severe enough to cause decreased productivity and interpersonal difficulty among peer and teacher/parent relationships. Usually recognized in retrospect, symptoms must also be recognized to have been present before the age of seven. New DSM-IV criteria also require that symptoms be present in at least two distinct environments. Symptom clusters are divided between predominantly inattentive and hyperactive/ impulsive subtypes. Emphasis of an individual's symptoms in either one of these clusters will lead the clinician to classify the disorder as either ADHD, Predominantly Inattentive Type or ADHD, Predominantly Hyperactive-Impulsive Type. A symptom profile that is distributed across both clusters will result in a diagnosis of ADHD, Combined type. Symptoms must be continuously present for at least 6 months for proper diagnosis.

Inattention, though usually more problematic during school, can manifest itself in many situations. Individuals often make careless mistakes, paying little attention to details or instruction. They give partial effort to many tasks instead of completing one entire assignment. They quit easily, especially as complexity or difficulty increases. Homework, if done or not lost, is often messy and incomplete and will appear to have been done in a haphazard manner. Though these individuals are present in body during a lesson, their minds seem to be elsewhere. They are literally unavailable to the learning experience.

Failure to follow through on requests is common, as are partially completed or ignored chores. Compared with other students, these individuals lack organizational ability and poorly grasp time/task management skills. They are easily distracted and will quickly abandon current tasks to investigate or focus on even the most trivial stimuli. In social settings, individuals with ADHD easily lose the focus of a conversation, often switching from one topic to the next. During conversation they quickly lose interest and often appear bored or disinterested. They have difficulty following prescribed rules of conduct as well as game rules during play time.

The hyperactive child appears to be an amazing and endless source of energy that can seldom be repressed. Though an active, curious child is looked on as healthy in our society, the child with ADHD exhibits hyperactivity to a problematic degree. Children with ADHD are often described as being constantly "on the go" or "driven by a motor." They have trouble remaining seated for any length

Table 57.2.
DSM–IV Diagnostic Criteria for ADHD[a]

A. Six (or more) symptoms of either inattention or hyperactivity for greater than 6 months

   Inattention
   (1) Often fails to give close attention to details or makes careless mistakes in schoolwork, work, or other activities
   (2) Often has difficulty sustaining attention in tasks or play activities
   (3) Often does not seem to listen when spoken to directly
   (4) Often does not follow through on instructions and fails to finish assignments
   (5) Often has difficulty organizing tasks and activities
   (6) Often avoids or dislikes tasks that requires sustained mental effort
   (7) Often loses things necessary for tasks or activities (e.g., toys, books, assignments)
   (8) Is often easily distracted by extraneous stimuli
   (9) Is often forgetful in daily activities

   Hyperactivity-impulsivity
   (1) Often fidgets with hands or feet or squirms in seat
   (2) Often leaves seat in classroom or situations in which remaining seated is expected
   (3) Often runs or climbs about excessively when inappropriate
   (4) Often has difficulty playing quietly
   (5) Is often "on the go" or acts as if "driven by a motor"
   (6) Often talks excessively
   (7) Often blurts out answers before questions have been completed
   (8) Often has difficulty awaiting turn
   (9) Often interrupts or intrudes on others

B. Symptoms present before age 7
C. Impairment from symptoms is present in two or more distinct settings (e.g., school, work, home)
D. Clear evidence of significant impairment in social, academic, or occupational functioning

[a]Adapted from (1).

of time and will squirm and fidget. Their hyperactivity is also manifested by an inability to play quietly when expected, by running or playing raucously when inappropriate, and also by excessive talking. Disciplinary action arising out of disruptive behavior during class is common, as is an inability to get through "quiet time" without incident. As a child with ADHD matures, the presentation of hyperactivity symptoms changes. Toddlers with ADHD are like wind-up race cars, into everything, climbing everywhere, and dashing here and there with no apparent purpose. Their behavior is very tiring and frustrating to those who are responsible for their care, and resentment toward a "problem child" can begin to build at any early age. School-age children with ADHD are still hyperactive but to a lesser degree than toddlers. They squirm and fidget at school, unable to remain seated for any length of time. They are often distracting to other children and the teacher, playing with a pencil, tapping their fingers, kicking the chair in front of them, focusing on anything but the task or lesson at hand. Adolescents with ADHD usually learn to suppress the hyperkinetic movements but are still plagued by feelings of restlessness and an inability to participate in solitary work such as reading.

Impulsivity in a child can often lead to the child's being tagged as disruptive or disrespectful. Impulsivity can manifest itself as impatience, immediate expression regardless of setting, or blurting out answers, comments, or emotions. Impulsive children often interrupt conversations or speak out of turn, showing great frustration when they are not allowed to talk. Impulsive individuals will grab inappropriate objects (a hot skillet, fragile items), intrude into other children's space or things, and seemingly act with no regard to impending consequence.

MEASURES OF EFFICACY

Several behavioral and performance measures have been developed to help determine the impact of therapy on the progression of this disorder. Developed primarily for research, these scales are now increasingly being used in the clinical setting. The Conners Parent Questionnaire (CPQ) is a parent-rated scale that measures conduct, learning difficulty, impulsivity, somaticism, and anxiety (10). The Conners Teacher Rating Scale (CTRS) is a teacher-rated scale that measures conduct, hyperactivity, and inattentiveness (11). The abbreviated Conners Parent-Teacher Questionnaire (CAPTQ) is a shortened hybrid of the CPQ and the CTRS that may prove useful. This scale quickly (only 11 items) allows the clinician to systematically assess the efficacy of treatment.

While the Conner scales primarily measure behavior, several other tests are used routinely in research to assess performance-based abilities. The Seat Movement (STMT) scale measures the amount of movement a child makes while performing learning-based activities (12). Other tests

such as the Matching Familiar Figures Test (MFFT) measure impulsivity (13), and the Continuous Performance Test (CPT) evaluates attention span (14).

TREATMENT OVERVIEW

Psychosocial Treatment

As was mentioned, many children who are successfully diagnosed and treated pharmacologically still exhibit maladaptive learned behaviors that are secondary to chronicity of disease. Therefore, most children (as well as their families) benefit from an approach that views medication as a component of the total therapy, not as the final solution. Results are usually better when pharmacologic treatment is paired with some form of nonpharmacologic therapy such as behavior therapy, individual therapy, or family counseling. Behavior therapy focuses on recognition and reinforcement of positive behaviors. Individual therapy allows one-on-one counseling to help the individual learn coping skills and mechanisms while providing a structured relationship that is free from prejudice and judgment. Family therapy is useful because of the profound "ripple effect" of psychiatric disorders. For the individual with ADHD, below-average performance and poor behavior often encourage judgment, disappointment, and eventual dysfunction within a family. Family therapy seeks to involve all members of a family in a supportive, nonjudgmental framework that is beneficial to all. Family avoidance of the problem is common and usually leads to further dysfunction and continued withdrawal of individuals with this disorder.

Pharmacologic Treatment

Pharmacotherapy for hyperactive children dates back to 1937, when Bradley first reported using amphetamine for behaviorally disordered children. Since that time, ADHD has had the benefit of having more research published than on any other childhood psychiatric disorder. Despite this volume of research, psychopharmacology in the pediatric field has shown little progress beyond the use of stimulants. Most pharmacologic experience outside of stimulants and tricyclic antidepressants has been anecdotal, and few guidelines exist to guide practitioners who employ these agents. Lack of experience with medication in this area has led to therapy modalities that pursue unlikely expectations and treatment goals. It is important to remember that medication use in ADHD will reduce problematic symptoms as well as improve the patient's potential for learning but should not be construed to be curative. Realistic expectations of psychopharmacology are essential to therapeutic success and should be communicated in depth and with clarity to family members and patient alike.

General treatment considerations initially focus on correct psychiatric workup according to the DSM-IV and should include a global overview of social, educational, and cognitive functioning. Information should come from as many sources as possible (parent, teacher, student) and should include enough data to rule out potential etiologies other than ADHD. Once the diagnosis of ADHD is clear and pharmacotherapy is deemed beneficial, selection of an appropriate pharmacologic agent should be made. The patient's age, weight, severity of illness, coexisting conditions, and target symptoms are all considered in choosing an appropriate agent. Effective communication is a must at this stage among caretakers, clinicians, and patient. It is important to provide medication information, which can be critical to the success of therapy. Patient and parents should be educated about potential and expected benefits as well as potential risks and should understand the role that medication plays in treatment. Pharmacologic agents should be started at the lowest possible dose, being titrated slowly to the desired effect while the patient is monitored for adverse effects. Parents should also be reminded that approximately 20 to 25% of individuals who respond poorly to one agent will respond favorably to another (15). Once the initial goals have been met in the acute phase, long-term goals of therapy should be established and regularly evaluated to ensure efficacy. Prudent therapy should also include drug-free periods or "drug holidays." After stabilization for 6 months or longer, a drug-free period that coincides with a school break is recommended. To test the continued need for these agents, medication should not be reintroduced until a few weeks after the return to school. Initial results of behavior and performance in these first weeks of school can give valuable clues to the need for continued pharmacotherapy. If the patient is removed from medication, follow-up should be made 6 months to 1 year after drug discontinuation to assess the patient's clinical status and recent performance. Parents and patient should also be educated about potential warning signs and symptoms that might signal the need for reintroduction of therapy.

STIMULANTS

Since Bradley first used racemic amphetamine in the 1930s, stimulants have remained the drug of choice for hyperactive children. Amphetamine remained in predominant use into the 1960s, when methylphenidate was introduced. Although methylphenidate was initially touted as being much safer and more effective, research shows differences in efficacy between the two agents to be relatively small (16, 17). Magnesium pemoline represents the third stimulant that is useful in treating ADHD. Studies show that approximately 70% of children who are treated with stimulants will show significant improvement in inattention, hyperactivity, and impulsivity (18). Improvements in relationships with adults and peer groups are also similarly improved (19). However, variable improvement is often seen in achievement, despite good behavioral response.

Stimulants are sympathomimetic drugs that are structurally similar to catecholamines that are found in the body. These compounds are thought to act in both the peripheral nervous system and the central nervous system, primary effects being seen in the dopaminergic and noradrenergic transmission systems (20). Several studies of neurotransmitter involvement in ADHD have shown the complexity and multineurotransmitter interplay that are necessary for the development and subsequent improvement of ADHD symptoms (21, 22). These studies suggest that the exact mechanism of action of stimulant-mediated improvement of ADHD symptoms is not yet clearly understood.

The clinical use of stimulants should begin with a low or subtherapeutic dose. This lower dosage can serve as a test dose and can alert the clinician to sensitivity or troublesome side effects. Slow titration while monitoring for improvement of agreed-on target symptoms and emergence of side effects allows for familial adjustment and greater acceptance, and therefore compliance, by the patient. In fact, some researchers have shown that while lower doses improve cognitive functioning, higher doses are more efficacious at controlling behaviors (23). There may be a therapeutic window in which both cognitive improvement and behavioral control can be achieved. Advancing beyond this point could lead to improved behavioral management at the expense of cognitive functioning.

A comparison of stimulants with placebo finds that decreased appetite, insomnia, stomachache, and headache are the most commonly reported adverse effects associated with stimulant therapy (24). These effects tend to be transient, and adequate education of the patient and family can help to allay fears and to increase the chance for accurate compliance with treatment. Methylphenidate and dextroamphetamine have been shown to stimulate the noradrenergic system somewhat more than pemoline does, resulting in a greater incidence of tachycardia, palpitations, and hypertension associated with their use. Baseline and subsequent measurement of blood pressure and heart rate are recommended and should become a regular component of each follow-up visit. However, serious complications such as myocardial hypertrophy or significant electrocardiogram (ECG) changes rarely occur (25).

Growth suppression has been reported during long-term stimulant therapy (26). Factors contributing to this phenomenon include the use of dextroamphetamine, doses greater than 40 mg/day of methylphenidate, doses greater than 20 mg/day of dextroamphetamine, treatment duration of more than 2 years, and multiple daily dosing (27). Most studies show that a growth rebound usually occurs when the stimulant is discontinued or when routine drug holidays are used. Thus, although stimulants can have a significant effect on childhood growth, a compensating growth spurt

Table 57.3.
Signs and Symptoms of Acute Stimulant Ingestion and Abuse

Restlessness	Anxiety	Severe agitation
Tremor	Paranoia	Muscular tension
Hallucinations	Amnesia	Repetitive movements
Flushing	Grimacing	Reckless behavior

leaves eventual height and size uncompromised (28).

Another area of particular concern is the reported incidence of medication-induced tic disorders with stimulant use (29). Stimulants have long been thought to worsen tic and movement disorders, especially in underlying disorders such as Tourette's syndrome. This strongly suspected risk is now being challenged by several researchers who show that some tic disorders may actually improve with long-term methylphenidate administration (30, 31). Additional results are needed to further clarify this issue. Current guidelines, therefore, still require careful monitoring and informed consent. Children with a personal or familial history of tic disorders are considered to be at a greater risk for developing a chronic tic disorder, and stimulant medication is relatively contraindicated in these patients.

Abuse and/or addiction is a concern with chronic administration of stimulants. Most adolescents are more likely to divert drugs for the sake of peers rather than for their own use (32). However, some case studies suggest that the adolescent with a substance abuse history may be at a greater risk of stimulant abuse (33). Monitoring for diversion and signs of stimulant abuse (see Table 57.3) should be routine. Pemoline doesn't share the abuse potential and street value that methylphenidate and dextroamphetamine possess and represents a viable alternative to the other stimulants. Other drug classes with lower abuse potential are available and efficacious and should also be considered when abuse or diversion is feared.

In general, methylphenidate, dextroamphetamine, and pemoline all provide rational therapeutic options for stimulant-treated ADHD. The stimulants increase attention span while decreasing impulsivity and motor activity. Stimulant efficacy is best documented when correct DSM-IV diagnostic criteria are used, target symptoms are severe and clearly delineated, and the dosages used are therapeutic and carefully adjusted to response and avoidance of toxicity.

METHYLPHENIDATE

Methylphenidate is the most commonly prescribed medication for the treatment of ADHD. Several studies have documented methylphenidate's efficacy in improving both behavior and performance measures (34, 35). Although some studies suggest that the efficacy of methylphenidate is superior to that of dextroamphetamine (36), other studies suggest just the opposite (17). In reality, methylphenidate and dextroamphetamine are usually efficacious in most clinical situations; and if a therapeutic failure occurs with one, success is probable with the other (37). Compared with dextroamphetamine, methylphenidate seems to have greater effect on the reuptake of norepinephrine and dopamine with less effect on neurotransmitter release. Conversely, dextroamphetamine inhibits reuptake to a lesser degree, inhibits the enzyme monoamine oxidase, and at high doses causes the release of norepinephrine, dopamine, and serotonin. These differing mechanisms suggest at least one reason why failure with one stimulant does not necessarily preclude efficacy with another.

The usual starting dose of methylphenidate is 0.3 mg/kg/day, adjusted to facilitate the 5-mg, 10-mg, and 20-mg tablet sizes that are available. Although best absorbed on an empty stomach, the drug is usually given with meals to minimize the anorectant effect, maximize compliance, and reduce the incidence of gastrointestinal complaints. Methylphenidate is completely and well absorbed from the gastrointestinal tract following oral administration, has a short half-life (see Table 57.4), and has a rapid onset of behavioral effect (38). Because of methylphenidate's short half-life, multiple daily dosing is usually necessary to achieve a consistent daytime response. In addition, most children begin to exhibit rebound behavioral dyscontrol approximately 4 to 5 hr after the last dose (39). Therefore, most children are dosed once at breakfast and then again at noon to provide adequate control throughout the school day. Delaying the administration of this second dose until later in the afternoon is not recommended, as insomnia and agitation usually result. This requires that a second dose usually be given at school. While this may present some logistical problems, it may also provide an opportunity for both teachers and parents

Table 57.4.
Kinetic and Dosing Parameters of CNS Stimulants in the Treatment of ADHD[a]

Parameter	Methylphenidate	Dextroamphetamine	Pemoline
Elimination half-life	2–3 hr	6–7 hr	2–12 hr (8.6 mean)
Time to peak (T_{max})	1–3 hr	3–4 hr	1–5 hr
Onset of effect	~1 hr	~1 hr	2–3 weeks
Dosing interval	4–6 hr	4–6 hr	8–12 hr
Daily dose range			
mg/kg/day	0.3–1.5	0.2–1.0	0.5–3.0
mg/day	10–60	5–40	37.5–112.5

[a]From (38).

to communicate concerning the child's progress and parent-teacher expectations. Open communication between parents and teachers also allows for the comparison of notes concerning the child's behavior, providing a more complete and therefore more accurate clinical picture. Methylphenidate is also available in a sustained-release formulation that allows once-daily dosing. However, this product is considerably more expensive, and studies have not shown superiority over the standard formulation (40).

The initial dosage may be advanced by increments of 2.5 to 5.0 mg (0.1 mg/kg) daily every 2 weeks until a response is seen. If no response is seen after 1 month at higher doses, an alternative agent should be considered. The end target dose is approximately 0.6 mg/kg/day divided, with no one dose exceeding 20 mg and no total daily dosage exceeding 60 mg. Termination of drug therapy, whether permanent or for a drug holiday, should always be done gradually. Immediate withdrawal of methylphenidate can lead to rebound hyperactivity and behavioral problems. Tapering the total methylphenidate dose over a few days can significantly reduce the possibility of this occurring.

One area of current interest is the search for an optimal therapeutic serum concentration that could be used in dosing to achieve maximum efficacy while avoiding adverse effects. The large intraindividual differences in metabolism rates and plasma concentrations at fixed doses have made clinical application of current findings difficult. Some investigators have shown a positive correlation between plasma concentrations and clinical result (41); other investigators have not (42). Currently, no guidelines exist to facilitate dosing to target levels. Plasma levels can be useful, however, when questions of compliance arise.

The most frequent adverse effects of methylphenidate appear to be dose-related and include insomnia, nervousness, and loss of appetite. These effects are compared with those of other commonly used agents in Table 57.5. Lower doses (0.6 mg/kg as compared to 1.0 mg/kg or greater) and avoidance of late afternoon dosing can reduce the incidence of agitation and difficulty falling asleep. However, if paradoxical excitation and stimulation continue to be a problem during methylphenidate therapy, the total daily dosage should be reduced or the drug should be discontinued. Methylphenidate should also be avoided in patients with an underlying or predominant anxiety disorder. Stimulant therapy has been shown to exacerbate the condition of these patients; they will better tolerate the use of nonstimulant agents such as tricyclic antidepressants. Dosing methylphenidate with meals reduces the incidence of gastrointestinal complaints as well as the incidence of appetite suppression.

Caution should be observed with the concomitant use of methylphenidate and anticoagulants, anticonvulsants, and/or tricyclic antidepressants. Case studies have shown that methylphenidate may inhibit the metabolism of these

Table 57.5.
Common Side Effects Seen with Medications used in ADHD

Drug	Adverse Effects
Stimulants	Insomnia, decreased appetite, weight loss, agitation, increase in heart rate and blood pressure, abnormal liver function tests (with pemoline), growth suppression (reversible), behavior exacerbation with sudden withdrawal
Tricyclic antidepressants	Anticholinergic (dry mouth, constipation, blurred vision), weight loss, sedation, irritability, mild cardiovascular changes (orthostasis, tachycardia); serious cardiovascular changes (arrhythmias, conduction disturbances) are less common
Monoamine oxidase inhibitors	Severe dietary restrictions (avoidance of tyramine), weight gain, drowsiness, insomnia, potential for hypertensive crisis with tyramine or stimulant/ decongestant ingestion
Bupropion	Dry mouth, GI upset, headache, non-specific rash: seizure induction generally avoided when individual doses are <150 mg and daily doses are <450 mg.
Fluoxetine	Nausea, nervousness, insomnia, anorexia
Clonidine	Sedation, hypotension, dry mouth, depression; rebound hypertension with sudden withdrawal

agents, and symptoms of toxicity may result (43). Controlled studies have yet to fully support these case reports. Clinicians should therefore monitor individuals on these combinations for evidence and signs of toxicity.

DEXTROAMPHETAMINE

Dextroamphetamine is the second most widely used medication in the treatment of ADHD. Dextroamphetamine is considered to have a more direct action on dopaminergic and noradrenergic transmitters than methylphenidate does. This differing mechanism is one reason that a trial of dextroamphetamine is justified when a therapeutic failure occurs with methylphenidate.

Like methylphenidate, dextroamphetamine has a short half-life that dictates multiple daily dosing. The initial starting dose is 5 mg once or twice daily, which can then be increased by 5 mg weekly until target symptoms are well controlled or problematic side effects emerge. Total daily dosage should not exceed 40 mg, and individual doses should not exceed 10 mg. Like methylphenidate, dextroamphetamine should be given with breakfast and again at the midday meal to reduce stomach upset and insomnia. Dextroamphetamine is currently available as 5-mg, 10-mg, and 20-mg tablets and is less expensive than methylphenidate. There is little advantage in using the sustained-release form of dextroamphetamines. Dextroamphetamine is preferred over the levoamphetamine or racemic configuration because of its established efficacy and quick onset of action (44). However, a new product under the trade name Adderal is being marketed that combines the neutral sulfate salts of dextroamphetamine and amphetamine with the dextro isomer of amphetamine saccharate and d,1 amphetamine aspartate. This "new" product is actually a reintroduced formulation of Obetrol, an anorectant agent that was used primarily in the 1970s and early 1980s. It is doubtful that this new stimulant combination will dramatically alter the current treatment of ADHD.

Side effects of dextroamphetamine tend to be transient and usually decrease to negligible levels within a few weeks of therapy initiation. Dextroamphetamine has a side effect profile that is similar to methylphenidate's, though central nervous system (CNS) stimulation and insomnia have been reported to be more severe with the former. Persistent overstimulation and insomnia can usually be reduced by dose reduction or by switching to methylphenidate. If dextroamphetamine is discontinued in favor of methylphenidate, dose reduction should take place over a few days.

Dextroamphetamine possesses the highest street value of any of the stimulants. As was mentioned earlier, most patients who are treated for ADHD do not abuse the drug themselves but divert their medication for the benefit of others. Caution should be taken with individuals who have a prior history of substance or alcohol abuse, and parents should make every effort to be aware of the drug's use and disposition.

PEMOLINE

The third stimulant that is available for the treatment of ADHD is magnesium pemoline. Pemoline has a much longer half-life than standard preparations of either methylphenidate or dextroamphetamine and can therefore be dosed once daily, usually in the morning. Pemoline is generally considered to have a slower onset of action than the other stimulants (15). Therefore, behavioral improvement may not be seen for up to 2 weeks after pemoline is started. Initial daily doses begin at 18.75 mg, with weekly increases of 18.75 mg daily until a favorable response is seen. The upper dosage range for optimal benefit is generally considered to be between 56.25 and 75.0 mg daily. Doses that are higher than this should be reserved for adolescents, as improvement in children is not usually seen

at greater doses. The maximum total daily dose for all age groups should not exceed 112.5 mg. Pemoline is also available as a 37.5-mg chewable tablet, which may aid in compliance with younger children. In contrast, methylphenidate and dextroamphetamine should never be crushed or chewed, as an increased stimulant effect can occur secondary to increased absorption brought about by altering the dosage form.

Pemoline is considered to be a second therapeutic choice following rational use of the other stimulants. Pemoline has demonstrated its efficacy in several well-controlled trials (45, 46). It has been shown to be superior to placebo and slightly less efficacious than, or equally efficacious as, methylphenidate. In addition, one pharmacodynamic study suggested that pemoline doses calculated at 1 to 2 mg/kg to achieve a plasma concentration of greater than 2 µg/mL can lead to a more rapid and measurable onset of action than was previously thought (47).

Most clinicians feel that pemoline has less abuse potential and certainly less street value than the other stimulants. Pemoline, therefore, offers another therapeutic option when abuse is feared or present.

Pemoline exhibits a side effect profile that is similar to those of the other stimulants and is therefore just as likely to cause irritability, insomnia, and loss of appetite. Long-term use of pemoline has been associated with significantly increased liver enzymes and potential hepatic failure in 1 to 2% of patients (48). These hepatic effects are thought to be due to hypersensitivity, and enzyme levels usually return to normal when pemoline is discontinued. Even though most patients with increased liver function tests will be asymptomatic, baseline and periodic liver function tests are warranted and should become part of an annual evaluation.

TRICYCLIC ANTIDEPRESSANTS

Tricyclic antidepressants such as imipramine and desipramine are the drugs of choice for children who fail to respond to stimulant therapy or who cannot tolerate their adverse effects. Numerous well-controlled studies have documented the efficacy of these agents over placebo but have not been able to demonstrate superiority over treatment with stimulants (34, 35). One interesting finding is that patients who have failed stimulant therapy have been shown to have the greatest response to tricyclic treatment, a result suggesting that perhaps these patients represent a subpopulation of ADHD (49). This group may suffer from greater anxiety and depression, hence the greater effect seen with tricyclic treatment. Future diagnostic criteria may identify these individuals, leading to improved treatment modalities for patients such as these.

The onset of action with the tricyclic antidepressants is reported to be slower than that seen with stimulants, positive effects usually being seen within 2 weeks. In addition, some researchers have reported a therapeutic tolerance that develops within 2 to 3 months of tricyclic treatment (50). The extent and significance of this remain unclear. Tricyclics have the advantage of a longer duration of action, single daily dosing, no insomnia or symptom rebound, and no risk of abuse or addiction. Tricyclics also have particular benefit for children who have comorbid affective disorders (35), nocturnal enuresis (51), or sleep disturbances and when there is abuse or a history of substance abuse.

The initial dose of imipramine or desipramine is 25 to 50 mg, divided into multiple doses to reduce the severity of potential side effects. Once the patient demonstrates that he or she can tolerate these agents, the dosing can be made once daily, usually at bedtime. Doses can be increased by 25 to 50 mg weekly until a positive response is evident. While most drug references suggest that total daily doses not exceed 2.5 mg/kg/day of imipramine or its equivalent, recent studies suggest that up to 5 mg/kg/day may be required to produce efficacy (49). Similar doses have been used with success to treat both childhood depression (52) and school phobia (53). Use of higher doses is consistent with the belief that children metabolize and eliminate tricyclics at a more efficient rate than do adults. Unlike the stimulants, tricyclics should be continued on weekends, and at no time should the dose be rapidly withdrawn. If a tricyclic is discontinued at any point in therapy, a taper of the dose over several days is warranted to prevent rebound hyperactivity and other withdrawal effects.

The adverse effect profile of the tricyclic antidepressants in children is similar to that seen in adult populations. Typical side effects include sedation, anticholinergic effects, and cardiovascular changes. Sedation associated with tricyclic use is usually transient, and doses can be given once daily at bedtime to minimize this effect. Anticholinergic effects usually include dry mouth and constipation and may also include blurry vision and urinary hesitancy. Desipramine has less anticholinergic activity than does imipramine and should be used when anticholinergic effects become bothersome but a tricyclic is still required. Common cardiovascular effects include orthostasis and tachycardia but can include more serious effects such as arrhythmias and heart block. A relationship between decreased cardiac conduction and plasma tricyclic concentrations has been observed. Imipramine and desipramine concentrations that approach 250 ng/mL have been shown to be associated with more serious cardiac effects (54). Therefore, exceeding 300 ng/mL of imipramine or desipramine in children is not currently recommended. Three sudden deaths in children receiving desipramine at normal doses have been reported (55). Details in these cases remain somewhat obscure, but doses and plasma concentrations were found to be within an acceptable range. Although tricyclic use in children with a normal ECG is acceptable, these agents are contraindicated for children who have a history of acquired or congenital cardiac disease or murmurs or have a family history of cardiomyopathy or diastolic hypertension. Tricyclic use should be preceded by a complete medical history and workup, including baseline ECG, blood pressure, and heart rate. An ECG should also be taken during tricyclic titration and again at steady state to identify vulnerable children. Nortriptyline may have some benefit, as its active metabolites might be less cardiotoxic than those of other tricyclics. Tricyclics have also been shown to cause paradoxical irritability, tearfulness, and aggression (56). Other CNS side effects may include insomnia, nightmares, and forgetfulness.

Comparatively, tricyclics are less effective than stimulants on both behavioral and performance measures; are more effective than placebo, especially on behavioral measures; and may show preferential efficacy in ADHD patients who also exhibit marked anxious or depressed features.

OTHER ANTIDEPRESSANTS

Because stimulants have been shown to weakly inhibit the enzyme monoamine oxidase, monoamine oxidase inhibitors such as clorgyline and tranylcypromine have been evaluated in the treatment of ADHD. One study that compared the efficacy of these two agents to that of dextroamphetamine showed that similar effects were seen in improving behavior while reducing hyperactivity (57). The monoamine oxidase inhibitors exhibited an onset of action that was significantly shorter than that usually seen in major depression. Study results show that both agents were well tolerated, with mild side effects that included fatigue, drowsiness, and appetite suppression. Clinical use of the monoamine oxidase inhibitors is self-limiting. The potential for developing a hypertensive crisis secondary to stimulant or tyramine ingestion is usually enough to dissuade regular use by most clinicians. Many think that it would be too difficult to monitor and control what the average school-age child consumes and are not willing to accept this potential liability.

Bupropion is an atypical antidepressant that exhibits primarily dopaminergic activity. Unlike the tricyclic compounds, bupropion does not significantly inhibit the reuptake of either serotonin or norepinephrine. Bupropion was removed from the market in the mid-1980s because of its association with a high incidence of epileptic seizures. This agent was reintroduced in 1989 with dosage guidelines and strict warnings about its effects on the seizure threshold. Bupropion's efficacy in the ADHD child has been compared to placebo in one study (58). Doses of 3 to 6 mg/kg were administered to 20 children with DSM-III diagnosed ADD-H. Improvement was seen on teacher-rated hyperactivity and also on global assessment scores, but other measures showed no significance over placebo. Bupropion was shown to be well tolerated.

Nortriptyline is a tricyclic compound that may have benefit in this population because of possible decreased cardiotoxicity of its metabolites. Studies show that moderate improvement is seen in approximately 76 to 90% of patients, with marked improvement seen in 48% (59, 60). Adverse effects seen in these studies were described as mild and included lethargy, gastrointestinal distress, weight gain, orthostasis, and insomnia. Interestingly, one study showed that children who were dosed to the therapeutic range of nortriptyline (50 to 100 ng/mL) were significantly more likely to be responders.

Fluoxetine has also been examined in this population in one study that used 0.6 mg/kg/day in 19 children with DSM-III-R diagnosed ADHD (61). Greater improvement was noted in behavior than in performance. One-third of study patients reported adverse effects that included sedation, rash, and akathisia.

Controlled studies of these agents are necessary to adequately determine their role in the management of ADHD. Studies using agents with differing mechanisms of action are also needed to further illuminate the etiology, psychopathology, and course of this disease.

OTHER AGENTS

Clonidine is a centrally acting α-2-adrenergic agonist that is most commonly used in the United States as an antihypertensive. Controlled studies have documented clonidine's efficacy over placebo on both performance and behavior measures at levels similar to those of methylphenidate (62, 63). The usual dose for school-aged children is 0.15 to 3.0 mg/day in divided doses to minimize its hypotensive effects. Sedation and mild drowsiness are the primary side effects that are seen with clonidine use, especially during the first few weeks of treatment. Mild hypotension, orthostasis, and depression have also been reported with its use but are usually present to a clinically insignificant degree. Rebound hypertension and marked deterioration in behavior have been noted after sudden withdrawal. The availability of a transdermal delivery system, the lack of apparent abuse potential, and no evidence of rebound dyscontrol during the evening hours may lead to increased usage of clonidine in the future.

Antipsychotics such as chlorpromazine, haloperidol, and thioridazine have been used in the treatment of ADHD with limited efficacy (64). These agents have been shown to reduce hyperactivity but do not improve cognitive functioning and attention span. Antipsychotics are less effective than either the stimulants or tricyclic antidepressants and should be reserved for only the most disturbed children. When used, these agents should be given in the lowest possible doses to avoid the decreased cognitive functioning and learning impairment that are often noted with higher doses. In addition, adverse reactions such as extrapyramidal effects and tardive dyskinesia severely limit the utility of this class of drugs for most patients.

Benzodiazepines and barbiturates are ineffective in the treatment of ADHD and may worsen the condition through paradoxical excitement and agitation (65, 66). Amantadine (67) and levodopa/carbidopa (68), although similar to other effective dopaminergic agents, have also been shown to have little or no efficacy. Other agents that have been shown to be ineffective include caffeine (69), fenfluramine (70), lithium (71), and anticonvulsants (72). Special diets such as the Feingold diet, which are free of salicylates and food additives, have been shown to be marginally effective (5).

SPECIAL POPULATIONS

Females

Although most ADHD patients are males, the 1980s saw a consistent increase in the proportion of females receiving treatment for this disease. In 1989 the overall prevalence of ADHD in girls was 3% (73). Early studies reported wide differences in response rates, genetic predisposition, and associated features. More recent studies have shown that both sexes exhibit similar socioeconomic and demographic backgrounds, males showing a higher incidence of familial dysthymia, alcoholism, and bipolar disorder (74). Phobias were found more often in females, and conduct disorder was found predominantly in males. Recent studies have also shown an equivocal and beneficial response rate to methylphenidate in both sexes (75). Currently, treatment guidelines are similar for both sexes.

Tourette's Syndrome

As many as 50% of patients with Tourette's syndrome will also meet criteria for ADHD (76). The antipsychotic medications such as haloperidol and pimozide that are used to treat Tourette's syndrome are not effective in managing the symptoms of ADHD. In fact, these medicines place the ADHD-diagnosed child at a greater risk of serious adverse effects such as extrapyramidal side effects, tardive dyskinesia, and cognitive impairment. The reports of stimulant-induced exacerbation of tics are also of concern to clinicians (29). Recent studies, however, have reexamined this association. One study showed that while low doses (5 mg/day) of methylphenidate worsened the severity of tics of three children with comorbid ADHD and Tourette's syndrome, higher doses (15 mg/day) showed an amelioration of tic symptoms (30). Another study retrospectively compared six pairs of monozygotic twins with Tourette's syndrome in whom only one individual of each pair had received stimulant treatment (31). No significant difference in the onset of Tourette's was noted between the two groups. All twelve individuals eventually developed the full syndrome. While cases such as these cast doubt on an association between stimulants and tic disorders, further and more conclusive evidence is needed. Until this occurs, comorbid ADHD and Tourette's syndrome can be effectively treated by using nonstimulant medications such as desipramine, nortriptyline, or clonidine. Selegiline, a MAO-B inhibitor, has recently been shown to improve ADHD symptoms in a group of 29 children with ADHD and Tourette's syndrome (77). Exacerbation of tics was noted in only two patients.

Adult Populations

Studies suggest that 30 to 70% of children with ADHD will continue to exhibit symptoms as adults (4). As with children, stimulants and tricyclic antidepressants remain the primary agents that are used in adults with residual symptomatology. Evidence exists that effective treatment of ADHD during childhood will ultimately lead to a better outcome as an adult (78). This study showed that adults who were treated with methylphenidate as children for a minimum of 3 years had less psychiatric treatment, had fewer automobile accidents, achieved a higher educational level, and reported a more positive outlook on life than did untreated adults.

TREATMENT OVERVIEW AND CONCLUSIONS

Stimulants are currently the most efficacious and least toxic of the drugs that are available for the treatment of ADHD. Common side effects such as insomnia, gastrointestinal upset, anorexia, and agitation are usually mild and transient and do not pose a significant deterrent to successful management of this disorder. Initial growth suppression that has been reported with stimulants is offset by an eventual growth spurt, and inconclusive information exists concerning tic exacerbation with or without comorbid Tourette's syndrome. Methylphenidate is the most widely used agent in ADHD. However, dextroamphetamine and pemoline are both viable options and should be evaluated when methylphenidate fails or it cannot be tolerated. Tricyclic compounds are regarded as second-line therapy because of their lower reported efficacy and potentially troublesome side effect profile. The cardiac toxicities that are seen with tricyclic antidepressants are of particular concern, and adequate monitoring for ECG abnormalities, heart rate, and blood pressure should be done routinely to avoid more serious complications. Tricyclic antidepressants may provide a useful option for ADHD patients who also exhibit comorbid anxiety, depression, enuresis, or substance abuse. Other agents such as clonidine, bupropion, and fluoxetine may prove useful in the future if further controlled studies continue to document their efficacy.

REFERENCES

1. American Psychiatric Association. Diagnostic and statistical manual of mental disorders, 4th ed. Washington, D.C.: American Psychiatric Association, 1994.
2. American Psychiatric Association. Diagnostic and statistical manual of mental disorders, 2nd ed. Washington, D.C.: American Psychiatric Association, 1968.
3. American Psychiatric Association. Diagnostic and statistical manual of mental disorders, 3rd ed. Washington, D.C.: American Psychiatric Association, 1982.
4. American Psychiatric Association: Diagnostic and statistical manual of mental disorders, 3rd ed, revised. Washington, D.C.: American Psychiatric Association, 1987.
5. Wender PH. Food additives and hyperkinesis. Am J Dis Child 131:1204–06, 1977.
6. National Advisory Committee on Hyperkinesis and Food Additives. Final report to the Nutrition Foundation, October 1980. New York: Nutrition Foundation, 1980.
7. Safer DJH, Krager JM. A survey of medication treatment for hyperactive/inactive students. JAMA 260:2256–58, 1988.
8. Cantwell D. The hyperkinetic syndrome. In: Rutter M, Hersov L, ed. Child psychiatry: modern approaches. London: Blackwell Scientific Publications, 1977.
9. Silver LB. Attention-deficit hyperactivity disorder. Washington, D.C.: American Psychiatric Press, 1992.
10. Conners CK. A teacher rating scale for use in drug studies with children. Am J Psychiatry 126:886–88, 1969.
11. Guy W, ed. ECDEU assessment manual for psychopharmacology. Department of Health Education and Welfare Publication no. ADM 76-338, revised. Washington, D.C.: U.S. Government Printing Office, 1976.
12. Sprague RL, Toppe LK. Relationship between activity level and delay of reinforcement. J Exp Psychol 3:390–97, 1966.
13. Kagin JH. Reflection-impulsivity: the generality of dynamics of conceptual temp. J Abnorm 7:17–24, 1966.
14. Rosvoid A, Mirsky A, Sarason I, et al. A continuous performance test of brain damage. J Consult Psychol 30:343–50, 1956.
15. Dulcan MK. Using psychostimulants to treat behavioral disorders of children and adolescents. J Child Adolesc Psychopharmacology 1:7–20, 1990.
16. Millicap JG. Drugs in management of hyperkinetic and preceptually handicapped children. JAMA 206:1527, 1968.
17. Winsberg BG, Yepes LE, Bialar I. Pharmacologic management of children with hyperactive/aggressive/inattentive behavior disorders. Clin Pediatr 15:471–74, 1976.
18. Gittelman-Klein R. Review of clinical psychopharmacological treatment of hyperkinesis. In: Klein F, Gittelman-Klein R, eds. Progress in psychiatric drug treatment. New York: Brunner Mazel 1975:661–74.
19. Jacobvitz D. Treatment of attentional and hyperactivity problems in children with sympathominetic drugs: a comprehensive review. J Am Acad Child Adolesc Psychiatry 29:677–88, 1990.
20. Gilman AG, Rall T. The pharmacological basis of therapeutics, 8th ed. New York: Pergamon Press, 1990.
21. Rogeness GA, Javor MA, Pliska SR. Neurochemistry and child and adolsecent psychiatry. J Am Acad Child Adolesc Psychiatry 31:765–81, 1992.
22. Lou HC, Hendriksen L, Bruhn P. Focal cerebral dysfunction in developmental learning disabilities. Lancet 335:8–11, 1990.
23. Brown R, Sleator EK. Methylphenidate in hyperkinetic children: differences in dose effects on impulsive behavior. Pediatrics 64:408–10, 1979.
24. Barkley RA, McMurray MB, Edelbrock CS, et al. Side effects of methylphenidate in children with attention deficit hyperactivity disorder: a systemic, placebo-controlled evaluation. Pediatrics 86:184–92, 1979.
25. Boileau RA, Ballard JE, Spraque RL, et al. Effect of methylphenidate on cardiorespiratory responses in hyperactive children. Res Quart 47:184–92, 1990.
26. Dickinson LE, Lee J, Ringdahl IC, et al. Impaired growth in

hyperkinetic children receiving pemoline. J Pediatr 94:538–41, 1979.

27. Safer D, Allen R, Barr E. Depression of growth in hyperactive children on stimulant drugs. N Engl J Med 287:217–18, 1972.

28. Gittelman-Klein R, Mannuzza S. Hyperactive boys almost grow up, III: methylphenidate effects on ultimate height. Arch Gen Psychiatry 45:1131–34, 1988.

29. Riddle MA, Hardin MT, Cho SC, et al. Desipramine treatment of boys with attention deficit hyperactivity disorder and tics: preliminary clinical experience. J Am Acad Adolesc Psychiatry 27:811–14, 1988.

30. Sverd J, Gadow KD, Paolicelli LM. Methylphenidate treatment of attention-deficit hyperactivity disorder in boys with Tourette's syndrome. J Am Acad Child Adolesc Psychiatry 28:574–79, 1989.

31. Price RA, Leckman JF, Pauls DL, Cohen DJ, Kidd KK. Gilles de Tourette's syndrome: tics and central nervous system stimulants in twins and non-twins. Neurology 36:232–37, 1986.

32. Clampit MK, Pirkle JB. Stimulant medication and the hyperactive adolescent: myths and facts. Adolescent 18:811–22, 1983.

33. Jaffe SL. Intranasal abuse of prescribed methylphenidate by an alcohol and drug abusing adolescent with ADHD. J Am Child Adolesc Psychiatry, 30:1773–74, 1991.

34. Rapoport J, Quinn PO, Bradbard G, et al. Imipramine and methylphenidate treatment of hyperactive boys. Arch Gen Psychiatry 30:789–93, 1974.

35. Garfinkel BD, Wender PH, Sloman L, et al. Tricyclic antidepressant and methylphenidate treatment of attention deficit disorder in children. J Am Acad Child Adolesc Psychiatry 141:906–08, 1984.

36. Gross MD. Imipramine in the treatment of minimal brain dysfunction in children. Psychosomatics 14:282–85, 1973.

37. Elia J, Borcherding BG, Rupoport JL, Keysor CS. Methylphenidate and dextroamphetamine treatment of hyperactivity: are there true non-responders? Psychiatry Res 36:141–55, 1991.

38. American Hospital Formulary Service. Drug information. Bethesda, MD: America Society of Hospital Pharmacists, 1994.

39. Safer DJ, Allen RP. Single daily dose methylphenidate in hyperactive children. Disorders of the Nervous System 34:325–28, 1973.

40. Fitzpatrick PA, Klorman R, Brumaghim JT, et al. Effects of sustained-release and standard preparations of methylphenidate on attention deficit disorder. J Am Acad Child Adolesc Psychiatry 31:226–34, 1992.

41. Kupietz SS, Winsburg BG, Sverd J. Learning ability and methylphenidate (Ritalin) plasma concentrations in hyperkinetic children. J Am Acad Child Adolesc Psychiatry 21:27–30, 1982.

42. Gualtieri CT, Wargin W, Kanoy R, et al. Clinical studies of methylphenidate serum levels in children and adults. J Am Acad Adolesc Psychiatry 21:26–9, 1982.

43. Fischer KC, Wilson WP. Methylphenidate and hyperkinetic state. Disorders of the Nervous System 32:695–98, 1971.

44. Arnold LE, Huestis RD, Smeltzer DJ, et al. Levoamphetamine vs. dextroamphetamine in minimal brain dysfunction. Arch Gen Psychiatry 33:292–301, 1976.

45. Conners CK, Taylor E. Pemoline, methylphenidate, and placebo in children with minimal brain dysfunction. Arch Gen Psychiatry 37:922–30, 1980.

46. Stephens R, Pelham WE, Skinner R. The state-dependent and main effects of pemoline and methylphenidate on paired-associated learning and spelling in hyperactive children. J Consult Clin Psychol 52:104–13, 1984.

47. Sallee FR, Stiller RL, Perel JM. Pharmacodynamics of pemoline in attention deficit disorder with hyperactivity. J Am Acad Child Adolesc Psychiatry 31:244–51, 1992.

48. Pratt DS, Dubois RS. Hepatoxicity due to pemoline: a report of two cases. J Pediatr Gastroenterol Nutr 10:239–41, 1990.

49. Biederman J, Baldessarini RJ, Wright V, et al. A double-blind controlled study of desipramine in the treatment of ADD: efficacy. J Am Acad Child Adolesc Psychiatry 28:777–84, 1989.

50. Gualtieri CT, Hicks RE. Neuropharmacology of methlyphenidate and a neural substrate for childhood hyperactivity. Psychiatr Clin North Am 8:875–92, 1985.

51. Rapoport JL, Mikkelsen FJ, Zavadil A, et al. Childhood enuresis, II: psychopathology, tricyclin concentration in plasma and antienuresis effect. Arch Gen Psychiatry 37:1146–52, 1980.

52. Preskorn SH, Puig-Antich J, Perel JM, et al. Plasma levels of imipramine (IMI) and desmethylimipramine (DMI) and clinical response in prepubertal major depressive disorder. J Am Acad Child Adolesc Psychiatry 18:616–27, 1979.

53. Gittelman-Klein RM, Klein DF. Controlled imipramine treatment of school phobia. Arch Gen Psychiatry 25:204–07, 1971.

54. Biederman J, Baldessarini RJ, Wright V, et al. A double-blind placebo controlled study of desipramine in the treatment of ADD, II: serum drug levels and cardiovascular findings. J Am Acad Child Adolesc Psychiatry 28:903–11, 1989.

55. Riddle MA, Nelson JC, Kleinman CS, et al. Sudden death in children receiving norpramin: a review of three reported cases and commentary. J Am Acad Child Adolesc Psychiatry 30:104–08, 1991.

56. Pallmeyer TP, Petti TA. Effects of imipramine on aggression and dejection in depressed children. Am J Psychiatry 136:1472–73, 1979.

57. Zametkin A, Rapoport JL, Murphy DL, et al. Treatment of hyperactive children with monoamine oxidase inhibitors, I: clinical efficacy. Arch Gen Psychiatry 42:962–66, 1985.

58. Casat CD, Pleasants DZ, Schroeder DH, et al. Bupropion in children with Attention Deficit Disorder. Psychopharmacol Bull 25:198–200, 1989.

59. Sual RC. Nortriptyline in attention deficit disorder. Clin Neuropharmacol 8:382–84, 1985.

60. Wilens TE, Biederman J, Geist D, et al. Nortriptyline in the treatment of ADHD: a chart review of 58 cases. J Am Acad Child Adolesc Psychiatry 32:343–49, 1993.

61. Barrickman L, Russell N, Kuperman S, et al. Treatment of ADHD with fluoxetine: a preliminary trial. J Am Acad Child Adolesc Psychiatry 30:762–67, 1991.

62. Hunt RD, Minderaa RB, Cohen D. Clonidine benefits children with attention deficit disorders and hyperactivity: a report of a double-blind placebo controlled trial. J Am Acad Child Adolesc Psychiatry 24:617–29, 1985.

63. Hunt RD. Treatment effects of oral and transdermal clonidine in relation to methylphenidate: an open pilot study in ADHD. Psychopharmacol Bull 23:111–14, 1987.

64. Winsberg BG, Yepes LE. Antipsychotics (major tranquilizers, neuroheptics). In: Werry JS, ed. Pediatric psychopharmacology: the use of behavior modifying drugs in children. New York: Brunner Mazel, 1978:234–74.

65. Millichap J. Drugs in the management of minimal brain dysfunction. Ann NY Acad Sci 205:321–24, 1973.

66. Conners CK, Taylor E, Meo G, Kurtz MA, Fournier M. Magnesium pemoline and dextroamphetamine: a controlled study of children with minimal brain dysfunction. Psychopharmacology 26:321–36, 1972.

67. Mattes J, Gittelman R. A pilot trial of amantadine in hyperactive children. New Clinical Drugs Evaluation Unit (NCDEU) meeting. Key Biscayne, Florida, May 1979.

68. Langer DH, Sweeney KP, Bartenbach DE, et al. Evidence of lack of abuse or dependence following pemoline treatment: results of a retrospective survey. Drug and Alcohol Dependence 17:213–27, 1986.

69. Firestone P, Davey J, Goodman JT, et al. The effects of caffeine and methylephenidate on hyperactive children. J Am Acad Child Adolesc Psychiatry 17:445–56, 1978.

70. Donnelly M, Rapoport JL, Potter WZ, et al. Fenfluramine and dextroamphetamine treatment of childhood hyperactivity: clinical and biochemical findings. Arch Gen Psichiatry 46:205–12, 1989.

71. Greenhill LL, Reider RO, Wender PH, et al. Lithium carbonite in the treatment of hyperactive children. Arch Gen Psychiatry 28:636–40, 1973.

72. Erenberg G. Drug therapy in minimal brain dysfunction: a commentary. J Pediatr 81:359–65, 1972.

73. Szatmari P, Offord DR, Boyle MH. Ontario Child Health Study: prevalence of attention deficit disorder with hyperactivity. J Child Psychol Psychiatry 30:219–30, 1989.

74. Farone SV, Biederman J, Keenan K, Tsuant MT. A family genetic study of girls with DSM-III Attention Deficit Disorder. Am J Psychiatry 148:112–17, 1991.

75. Pelham WE, Walker JL, Sturges J, Hoza J. Comparative effects of methylphenidate on ADD girls and ADD boys. J Am Acad Child Adolesc Psychiatry 28:773–76, 1989.

76. Comings DE, Comings BG. Tourette's syndrome and attention deficit disorder with hyperactivity [Letter]. Arch Gen Psychiatry 44:1023–26, 1987.

77. Jankovic J. Deprenyl in attention deficit associated with Tourette's syndrome. Arch Neurol 50: 286–88, 1993.

78. Hechtman L, Weiss G, Perlman T. Young adult outcome of hyperactive children who received long-term stimulant treatment. J Am Acad Child Adolesc Psychiatry 23:261–69, 1984.

CHAPTER 58

OBESITY AND EATING DISORDERS

MARTIN J. JINKS and MARK W. GARRISON

OBESITY

Leave gourmandizing, know that the grave doth gape for thee thrice wider than for other men.

—William Shakespeare

Despite these perceptive words, Shakespeare and his contemporaries admired an ample form. Suppleness denoted a person graced by God and was the hallmark of the opulent and idly rich. Rubens would certainly have scoffed at the idea of Twiggy as a model of beauty. It took the industrial revolution to give obesity a bad reputation. Mechanization caused voluntary or forced reduction in average activity without a decrease in caloric intake, and obesity became the single most prevalent metabolic disorder in the United States.

Obesity can be defined as a condition occurring from the sum total of environmental, emotional, and familial factors that have as the lowest common denominator an abnormal energy balance usually resulting from excessive caloric intake and inadequate caloric loss. In simplest terms, obesity exists when there is excess energy stored as body fat. More specifically, body mass index (BMI), the parameter that is frequently used to characterize body weight, is a value that normalizes an individual's weight based on height. It can be calculated by dividing the patient's weight in kilograms by the height of the individual in meters squared (kg/m^2). In general, patients with a BMI between 25 and 30 are classified as overweight, and those with one greater than 30 are considered obese and at increased risk for health complications (1). Others classify obesity based on the relationship between actual and ideal body weight. In males, moderate obesity is present when adipose comprises more than 25% of ideal weight. The upper limit in females is 30%. Massive obesity is defined by adiposity in excess of 100% of ideal weight (2).

PREVALENCE

Currently it is estimated that close to 50% of men and women in the United States have some degree of obesity. Over age 50, 34% of men and 49% of women are moderately obese, and the overall incidence of adults seriously overweight ranges 5 to 7% (2, 3). A detailed account of the prevalence of obesity in the United States has been previously published (4). On average, approximately 25% of adults in the United States at any given time are attempting to lose weight through some type of weight reduction program (1).

The incidence of obesity appears to be increasing over time. Evaluation of military records reveals a consistent pattern of weight increase in servicemen over the years 1918, 1943, and 1950 (5). The degree of body fat is influenced by age, gender, race, and extent of physical activity.

At the start of life, adipose tissue comprises approximately 12% of body weight, and it rapidly increases to an average of 25% at 6 months of age. During early adulthood, the percentage of body fat in males is 15 to 18% and in females, 20 to 25%. A gradual increase in body fat occurs with age approaching an average of 30 to 40% in adult men and women (5).

Differences in racial background and socioeconomic status appear to influence body fat, but it is often difficult to accurately distinguish the individual effect that each of the factors has. Reports demonstrate a greater prevalence of obesity in black versus white women; however, the reverse is true with males—obesity is more likely to occur in white rather than black men (6). Furthermore, individuals in lower socioeconomic classes tend to have a higher rate of obesity relative to their middle- and upper-class counterparts. This relationship holds true particularly in females and does not appear as pronounced in males (5).

As one might expect, an inverse relationship exists between level of physical activity and development of obesity. Individuals with sedentary life-styles or a physical handicap that restricts activity are prone to obesity. Increasing the degree of physical exercise is associated with a reduction in body fat as lean body mass increases; however, this relationship is rapidly reversed on discontinuation of the energy expenditure.

PATHOGENESIS

In a small percentage of patients, obesity has an identifiable organic cause (7). Weight gain in excess of 1 kg/day invariably implies fluid retention and is frequently a signal of cardiovascular, renal, or hepatic disorders (8). Medications can also produce weight gain by inducing fluid retention in susceptible individuals, through either direct (steroids and related drugs) or indirect (medicinals high in sodium) mechanisms. Only rarely is obesity a symptom of a specific endocrinopathy, such as insulinoma or Cushing's disease. These uncommon disorders are easily differentiated by their peculiar fat distribution, attendant symptoms, and history of sudden appetite changes.

Idiopathic obesity is a complex interplay of physiologic, hereditary, psychologic, and metabolic influences that have as their ultimate manifestation chronic dietary indiscretion.

Physiologic Factors

Since the discovery nearly 80 years ago that obesity can be induced surgically in animals, a great deal of interest has developed in the relationship between abnormal appetite and possible aberrations within the hypothalamus. Lesions in the ventromedial nucleus of the hypothalamus (satiety center) result in hyperphagia, whereas lesions in the lateral hypothalamic areas (feeding center) result in cessation of eating (9, 10). Factors controlling these centers are unknown but have been associated with endocrine and metabolic determinants.

Obese individuals exhibit behavior that might indicate a derangement in the satiety center. When obese and nonobese individuals are allowed to ingest freely, the nonobese regulate food intake based on internal cues, such as hunger sensations and caloric density of the food, while obese individuals regulate food intake by external cues such as time and environment, regardless of the caloric density of the food (11).

In the first year of life, the number of existing fat cells is relatively fixed. Storage of excess energy is accommodated by increasing the size of adipose cells (hypertrophic). Prior to adolescence, the number of adipose cells multiply as young children grow. In obese children, this rate of multiplication is greater than in nonobese children, resulting in a larger number of adipose cells (hypercellular) throughout life. In contrast, adult-onset obesity is primarily the result of hypertrophic obesity (12).

Weight loss is more rapid and prolonged in persons with hypertrophic obesity compared to hypercellular obesity. Attempting to reduce weight to norms in hypercellular individuals is very difficult and can result in extreme hunger symptoms similar to those seen with starvation as well as psychologic and physical disability (13).

Since evidence favors the increased likelihood of chubby infants becoming obese adults (14), preventive measures are important. These measures include avoiding overfeeding of infants, encouraging the use of unsugared foods, keeping junk foods and snacks out of the house, and encouraging activity.

Genetic Factors

The role of heredity in obesity is a matter of great speculation and research. Often environmental factors pertaining to food intake greatly confound this issue, making it difficult to determine the true impact of genetics on obesity. Studies involving adopted children and twins have been performed in an attempt to overcome these environmental influences. Results reflect little correlation in relative body weight between adopted children and their adoptive parents; however, definite trends do exist when the weights of the children are compared to their biologic parents (15). Furthermore, the body weight of twin siblings appears to correlate well, identical twins showing greater correlation than fraternal twins (16). These observations lend support to a genetic component of obesity.

Statistically, when both parents are of normal weight, the incidence of having an obese child is approximately 9%. If one or both parents are obese, there is a 50 and 80% incidence of obese offspring, respectively (15).

Psychologic Factors

Familial and cultural eating habits are implanted in individuals at an early age. As a society, we place great emphasis on food—to most, one of life's enduring pleasures is a rich, hearty meal. The obese patient carries this gratification to an extreme level.

Obese individuals often exhibit an immense appetite for psychologic reasons. Overeating may be a manifestation of anxiety or depression, where the pleasures of food serve as a substitute for the satisfactions missed from other sources. As a result, the obese characteristically dine until the food is completely gone or until they are overtly uncomfortable, while the nonobese usually stop eating when their hunger is gone.

Because obesity is often associated with neurotic traits, overeating is commonly considered to be a behavioral defect. In the pathologically obese, where no distinct underlying problem exists, psychologic factors undoubtedly play a major role. Obviously, obesity is a complicated mix of psychologic, genetic, and metabolic influences that manifest as abnormal appetite and resultant overweight.

Metabolic Factors

Insulin refractoriness is the most significant metabolic deviation in obesity, since insulin regulates the major pathways for fat accumulation and storage. Insulin-induced lipogenesis is an attractive hypothesis to explain the cause of obesity, but current evidence suggests that insulin refractoriness is more a result than a cause of obesity.

Adrenal overactivity is a common finding in massively obese patients. This is reflected by elevated urinary corticosteroids, mild hirsutism, borderline hypertension, and glucose intolerance (17). Again, these abnormalities are most likely the result of obesity rather than a cause, since they develop in nonobese subjects following gorging and disappear as weight returns to normal.

Metabolic enzyme deficiency may also result in abnormalities in thermogenic dissipation of calories in obese patients. Cellular enzyme systems account for much of thermogenic calorie loss, and there is evidence that the obese may have inefficient catalytic rates (18). Impaired hormonal control by catecholamines and insulin may be involved, but this hypothesis is controversial (19).

DIAGNOSIS

Individuals with massive obesity, peculiar fat distribution, or sudden, rapid weight gain require extensive evaluation. However, common idiopathic obesity does not usually demand elaborate evaluation techniques.

Table 58.1.
Disorders Associated with Obesity

Hypertension
Congestive heart failure
Diabetes
Cerebrovascular disease
Gall bladder disease
Hyperlipidemia
Respiratory distress syndrome (Pickwickian)
Obstetric complications
Osteoarthritis
Varicose veins
Flat feet
Hiatus hernia
Intertriginous dermatitis

Quantifying obesity is not difficult. The patient who is 136 kg (300 lb) overweight is readily recognized as obese. Moderately obese patients are easily diagnosed using standard height-weight charts. These charts have a 90% correlation with much more elaborate densitometry and radioisotope dilution techniques (2). However, height-weight charts are not without deficiencies, and the easiest and most accurate method of quantifying body fat involves measuring triceps, subscapular, or suprailiac skinfold thickness with constant pressure calipers. Skinfold thickness measurements coupled with height-weight data give a convenient and accurate evaluation of the degree of obesity.

COMPLICATIONS

Many serious disorders are associated with severe obesity (Table 58.1). Significant excess weight is clearly detrimental to longevity, and a definite statistical link exists between obesity and hypertension, diabetes, cardiovascular disease, and gastrointestinal disorders (Figs. 58.1 and 58.2). This link pertains primarily to moderate and severe obesity, since the marginally or slightly obese individual compares favorably in longevity to nonobese persons. In addition, significantly underweight persons are also at risk for digestive and pulmonary disease.

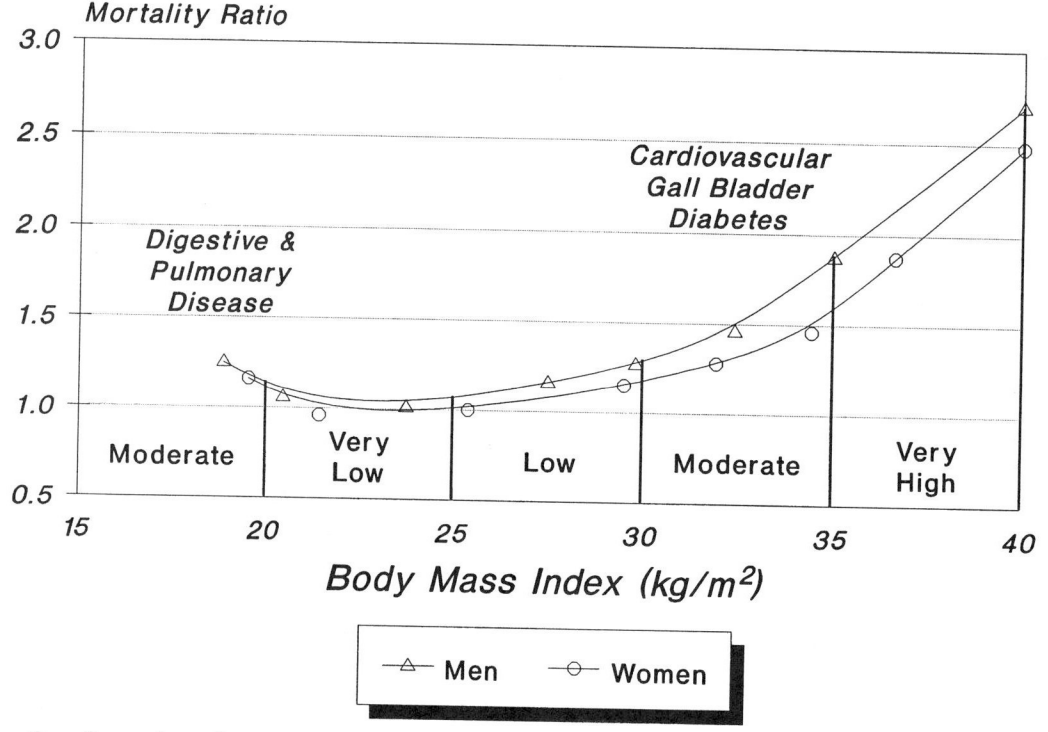

Figure 58.1. Overall mortality risk at various levels of body mass index. (Reprinted with permission from Bray GA, Gray DS. Obesity. Part I-pathogenesis. West J Med 149:429, 1988.)

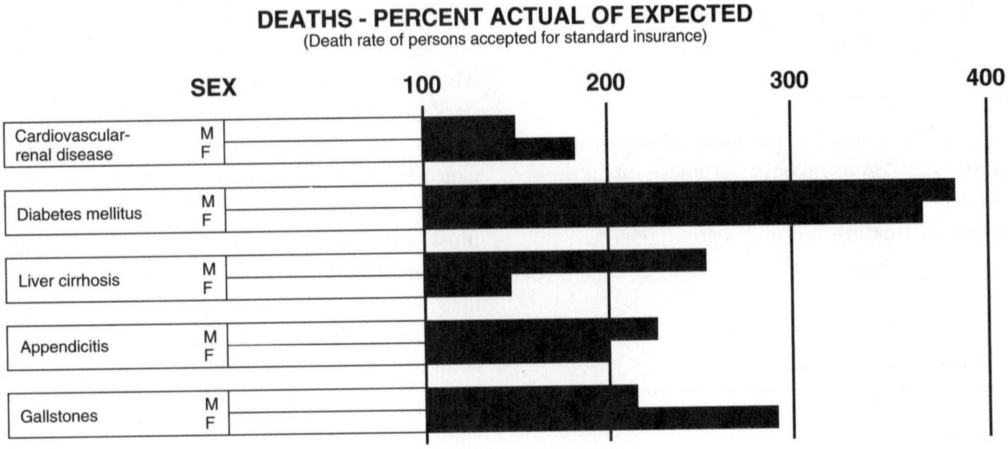

DEATHS - PERCENT ACTUAL OF EXPECTED
(Death rate of persons accepted for standard insurance)

Figure 58.2. Relationship between obesity and serious medical disorders. (Reprinted with permission from the Metropolitan Life Insurance Company).

Massive obesity during pregnancy is associated with a sevenfold increase in toxemia, a tenfold increase in diabetes, and a twofold risk of maternal mortality (20). Substantial excess weight is also associated with altered pharmacokinetics of certain drugs (21, 22). A detailed review of the morbidity and mortality associated with obesity has recently been reported (23, 24).

Despite evidence of the detrimental effects of obesity on health, the prevalent factor motivating most individuals to lose weight is not health but cosmetic ideals.

TREATMENT

Successful approaches to the management of obesity are often difficult and pose a significant challenge to individuals interested in reducing their weight. There is no "standard treatment" that is effective in most or even a large fraction of obese patients, and weight reduction programs must be designed to fit the personality, life-style, and health status of each patient. Success depends on the individual's motivation, on behavioral modification, and on the establishment of reasonable goals and expectations. Crash programs and demands for extreme alterations from established life-styles are uniformly unsuccessful in the long run and potentially dangerous.

A comprehensive weight reduction program incorporates components of caloric restriction, exercise, behavioral modification, and possibly pharmacologic and invasive approaches. The critical factor is that caloric expenditures exceed caloric demands, and that permanent change in caloric intake must be achieved to maintain desired weight.

Regulation of Caloric Intake

Modest reduction of caloric intake through dieting and setting realistic goals and expectations is the most palatable and easily available method of treatment. A good diet

prevents the patient from becoming too hungry and noncompliant. The importance of learning good eating habits and familiarity with the caloric content of various foods should be strongly emphasized.

The primary goal of any diet is to reduce the caloric intake below expenditure so that excess energy stored in the form of fat can be used. Weight loss should not exceed 1 kg (2 lb) per week unless close medical supervision is involved (25). Any program resulting in weight loss of more than 0.3 kg (0.7 lb) per day usually involves more fluid than tissue loss. Obligatory water loss accounts for the accelerated weight loss frequently observed during the initial weeks of dieting. Although use of diuretics for weight reduction exploits this phenomenon, this practice is both illusory and hazardous (26).

In obese subjects, approximately a 3500-calorie deficit is required to lose 0.5 kg (1 lb) of tissue. To achieve this deficit, a bewildering array of diets have been advocated, each differing in ratios of carbohydrate, fat, and protein, and each claiming superiority over all the others. Easy weight loss diets tend to exploit the obese individual who is not ready for a permanent level of change and discipline. Items like dietary drinks offer easy, short-term solutions, but their simplicity and convenience merely put off the essential need to learn about food and food values. Diet books appear with great regularity, and despite their guarantees and initial effectiveness, few effectively induce the permanent solutions of discipline and life-style changes.

"Crash diets" are dangerous in susceptible individuals when applied to extremes. Diets involving limited foods, such as the "Beverly Hills Diet," promote nutritional misinformation and can result in severe health problems (27, 28). "Very low calorie diets" (VLCDs) consisting of 200 to 500 kcal/day are designed to cause a calorie deficit while preserving lean body mass. One such diet, the "Last

Chance Diet," resulted in dozens of cardiovascular fatalities due to negative nitrogen balance and consequent protein tissue loss (29). The Cambridge and Optifast diets are other VLCDs that incorporate higher quality protein sources (egg albumin, casein, or soy) and adequate nutritional content; however, concern persists that such diets are inherently dangerous when used as sole nutritional sources (1, 30, 31). The use of VLCDs should be restricted to patients with moderate to severe obesity who are under close medical supervision, with special attention to cardiovascular monitoring (31).

With all VLCDs, fluid and electrolyte abnormalities, arrhythmias, dehydration, ketoacidosis, hyperuricemia, alopecia, and teratogenesis are potential complications. These diets are contraindicated in patients with diabetes, cardiovascular disorders, kidney and liver disease, and pregnancy.

Diets based on starvation represent an extreme form of caloric restriction with intake less than 200 kcal/day. Starvation diets are associated with very rapid and significant reductions in body weight; however, their use is limited due to potential side effects, the need for extremely close medical supervision, and the high percentage of weight regain that occurs following discontinuation of the diet.

Exercise

The inclusion of physical exercise in a weight reduction program can be a valuable supplement to dieting. Regular exercise increases energy expenditure, favoring adipose reduction and prolonged maintenance of weight loss. Due to reductions in caloric intake associated with dieting, individuals may experience a compensatory decrease in their basal metabolic rate (BMR) of up to 40% in 6 months (32). Regular exercise generates an increase in BMR that counteracts this adaptive response to dieting.

In order for exercise to be useful, it must be regular, of high quality, and consistent with the patient's life-style. Aggressive exercise should be avoided at the onset due to the lack of conditioning and potential for injury. A regimen of thrice weekly exercise that expends in excess of 300 kcal over at least 30 minutes is recommended (33). The selection of an activity of moderate intensity and longer duration is preferred because the longer time frame favors utilization of fat stores. In mild to moderate obesity, exercise results in a significant reduction in adipose tissue; however, in some instances overall body weight may not change significantly due to increases in lean body mass.

Unfortunately, quality exercise is not acceptable to many obese patients. They often turn to "effortless" weight reduction devices, such as mechanical vibrators, inflatable weight-reducing clothing or "spot reducers." As one author

noted, these devices are little better than doing nothing, and the primary reduction often occurs in the exerciser's wallet (33).

Behavioral Modification

Behavior therapy can also facilitate weight reduction, especially in the long-term management of massively obese patients who require assistance in accepting the seriousness of their problem. The primary goal of behavioral treatment is to modify behaviors that are associated with or promote eating (34). Therapy can be divided into three separate components. First, self-monitoring forces obese individuals to record, on a daily basis, the type of food items and when and where they were eaten. The purpose of daily record keeping is to increase the individual's awareness and identify specific eating patterns or behaviors. Once these patterns are identified, the second phase of behavioral therapy focuses on breaking the relationship between repetitive patterns or events (external cues) and actual ingestion of the meal. Often this is done through assigning specific times and places for eating meals, chewing food a specific number of times, or taking sips of water between each bite. Finally, behavioral modification incorporates a system of positive self-feedback to reinforce and maintain an optimal attitude toward weight reduction. The majority of studies evaluating the effectiveness of behavioral therapy on weight reduction indicate a greater duration or maintenance of weight loss compared to programs that lack a behavioral modification component (35).

A number of self-help programs such as Weight Watchers, NutriSystems, Overeaters Anonymous, and Take Off Pounds Sensibly (TOPS), provide several obese individuals important psychologic support and motivation to bring about permanent weight control measures. Membership in these programs is enormously large, with Weight Watchers alone claiming several million active members.

Appetite Suppressants

Obese patients who are adequately instructed on dietary management and are treated with appetite suppressants tend to lose more weight on average than patients on diet alone. In a review of over 200 studies of appetite suppressants involving 10,000 patients, pooled data demonstrate an average loss of 0.25 kg (0.56 lb) per week more versus placebo (36). However, since these drugs are typically labeled for durations of 2 to 4 weeks only, the average patient will lose only one additional kilogram when they are employed as recommended. When appetite suppressants are used, it becomes critical for the patient to realize that improved dietary compliance is the goal of therapy and diet, not the drug, is responsible for weight loss. Drug use is only temporary, and restoration of drug-free dieting through behavior change is the desired outcome.

Unfortunately, the routine use of appetite suppressants in the initial phases of a weight reduction program may detract from the importance of dietary/behavioral measures and provide a psychologic escape from the need to change lifelong eating habits. A comparison of patients treated with either pharmacotherapy or behavioral therapy indicates that, while pharmacotherapy produces more weight loss, the benefits are short-lived and weight is rapidly regained when the drug is discontinued. At the end of a 1-year follow-up, patients treated with behavioral therapy alone weighed significantly less than patients treated with drugs alone. Also, combined pharmacotherapy and behavioral therapy produced results inferior to behavioral therapy alone (37).

Appetite suppressants should be reserved for use in situations where (a) a reducing diet has been established and an unsatisfactory response observed; (b) a plateau is reached after initial success with dieting alone; or (c) a relapse is encountered after a prolonged period of progress. Unfortunately, many physicians prescribe appetite suppressants early in therapy because they cannot resist the pressures placed on them by patients, who have invariably experienced failure with do-it-yourself dieting and present to the physician expecting more. Better long-term results could be realized if physicians would lend their esteem and credibility to dietary/behavioral approaches, including vigorous monitoring for compliance, rather than undermining the importance of self-motivated dieting by prescribing appetite suppressants in the initial stages. However, some of the newer agents have shown promise in long-term management and it may be appropriate to use these agents in the initial stages of therapy.

Pharmacology

Appetite suppressants are thought to exert their effect directly on the hypothalamic satiety center, which is under adrenergic control. Most suppressants will augment brain catecholamine action, with the exception of fenfluramine, which acts specifically on serotonin. Fenfluramine and mazindol also affect peripheral energy metabolism, such as triglyceride and glucose uptake and utilization, but the relationship of these effects to appetite suppression is unclear (38). Many authorities feel the drugs act by inducing euphoria and suppressing appetite as a manifestation of a psychologic defect.

Conventional wisdom holds that tolerance develops rapidly to the anorectic effects of these agents, as evidenced by the decelerating weight loss curves with continued use. This belief has led to recommendations that appetite suppressants be limited to short-term use. However, most appetite suppressants appear to maintain weight loss for the duration of administration, and discontinuation

following long-term use results in a rapid rebound of increased appetite and weight regain (39). Therefore, tolerance to the appetite suppressant effects may not be significant at doses usually employed, and long-term treatment may be plausible for selected patients (40). In addition, it has been demonstrated that phentermine, diethylpropion, and mazindol were as effective, cheaper, and less prone to drug abuse when administered intermittently (i.e., 4 weeks every second month) for an extended period of time (41).

The antidepressant fluoxetine is a selective inhibitor of serotonin reuptake that is currently being evaluated for the management of obesity. Study results suggest similar rates of effectiveness and fewer side effects relative to currently available anorectic agents (42). Fluoxetine was approved by the FDA for the treatment of depression in 1988; however, its use in the treatment of obesity has not yet been approved. Another recently approved serotonin reuptake inhibitor antidepressant, sertraline, has also been reported to produce weight loss. The low abuse potential and their ability to effectively reduce weight make serotonergic agents a welcome addition to the potential agents used to treat obesity. Excellent reviews of the various drug therapies for the treatment of obesity have recently been published (43, 44).

Abuse Potential

Because several of these agents are reinforcing (i.e., euphorigenic) central nervous system stimulants, their misuse potential is high. However, misuse of these agents is not typically associated with anorectic use in motivated, obese patients. Misuse is more a result of indiscriminate prescribing with subsequent diversion for nonmedical, "recreational" use. Among the anorectic drugs, amphetamines account for the greatest number of abuse episodes, with estimates that over 10% of the legitimately manufactured amphetamines wind up in the hands of abusers (40). Therefore, stimulants in controlled substance class II are no longer used in the treatment of obesity (43).

In December 1978, the Advisory Review Panel on OTC Miscellaneous Internal Drug Products found the nonprescription ingredient phenylpropanolamine (PPA) safe and effective for weight control. The widespread promotion of PPA as the "ultimate diet pill" and its close association with prescription ingredients (e.g., Dexatrim, Dex-A-Diet, Acutrim, etc.) led to special problems of misuse. PPA is the most common ingredient in "lookalike" counterfeit drugs, which are packaged in tablets and capsules to look virtually identical to amphetamines and sold as "legal stimulants."

Drug Selection

No superiority has been shown for the appetite-suppressant effects of any of these agents. Aside from physician preference, product selection is primarily deter-

Table 58.2.
Appetite Suppressants Used to Treat Obesity

Drug (Common Trade Name)	Usual Doses (mg)	Frequency of Administration[a]
Schedule II[b,c]		
Amphetamine (Biphetamine)	5–10	TID (before meals)
Dextroamphetamine (Dexedrine)	5–10	TID (before meals)
	10–15	QD (before breakfast)
Methamphetamine (Desoxyn)	2½–5	BID–TID (before meals)
	10–15	QD (before breakfast)
Phenmetrazine (Preludin)	25	BID or TID (before meals)
	75	QD (midmorning)
Schedule III[b]		
Benzphetamine (Didrex)	25–50	QD (midmorning)
Phendimetrazine (Plegine, Phenazine)	35	BID–TID (before meals)
	105	QD (before breakfast)
Schedule IV[b]		
Diethylpropion (Tenuate)	25	TID (before meals)
	75	QD (midmorning)
Fenfluramine (Pondimin)	20–40	QD (before lunch)
Phentermine (Ionamin, Fastin)	8–15	TID (before meals)
	30	QD (before breakfast)
Nonscheduled		
Fluoxetine[d] (Prozac)	40–60	QD (before breakfast)
Phenylpropanolamine[e] (Dexatrim, Acutrim)	25–37.5	BID–TID (before meals)
	50–75	QD (midmorning)

[a]TID, three times daily; BID, twice daily; QD, once daily.
[b]Drug Enforcement Agency (DEA) controlled substance schedule.
[c]Agents in controlled substance schedule II should no longer be used in the management of obesity.
[d]Investigational agent not yet approved by the Food and Drug Administration (FDA).
[e]Available over-the-counter.

mined by trial and error using the entire spectrum of available agents (Table 58.2). Patients that cannot tolerate an agent from one chemical class may benefit from agents in another class. Restlessness, insomnia, tremors, tachycardia, nausea, diarrhea, constipation, dry mouth, and mydriasis are commonly reported side effects. In susceptible patients, elevated blood pressure and cardiac arrhythmias may occur. Agents acting on serotonin (fenfluramine, fluoxetine, and sertraline) are an exception, producing fewer adverse effects than other drugs, but they can cause headaches, sleep disturbances, decreased libido, and sexual dysfunction (41).

Pulmonary hypertension has been reported in two patients receiving 120 mg/day and 160 mg/day of fenfluramine continuously for 8 months (45). In addition, depression has been reported with fenfluramine when the drug was abruptly discontinued (43).

The duration of action can also help determine the best anorectic agent for a given patient. If overeating occurs in the evening, little benefit is derived from morning doses. Likewise, long-acting agents are irrational when dietary indiscretion is limited to a particular time of day. In both instances, short-acting agents are preferred. Patients who overindulge in the evening but suffer from drug-induced insomnia may benefit from fenfluramine, which exhibits

unique sedating properties (41, 46). Combinations of anorectic agents with other ingredients, such as barbiturates or phenothiazines, probably possess no greater efficacy and exhibit an expanded array of side effects.

Persons receiving appetite suppressants should be advised about stimulant side effects, dry mouth, and possible insomnia. Dry mouth is minimized by sucking on sugarless hard candy. Insomnia from long-acting agents can be minimized by taking the dose early in the day. Patients receiving serotonergic agents should be warned about possible insomnia, somnolence, and nausea. Drug interactions can occur with all of these agents, and caution should be exercised when they are used concomitantly with monoamine oxidase inhibitors, antihypertensives, tricyclic antidepressants (TCAs), and caffeine. Lithium toxicity has been reported to be precipitated by mazindol (47).

Appetite suppressants should also be dispensed with caution to pregnant patients. In studies involving amphetamines and morpholines, an increased incidence in oral clefts was noted when the drug was taken during the first 56 days of pregnancy (48).

Bulk Forming Agents

Bulk formers are indigestible hydrophilic colloids that swell when hydrated to give a sense of repletion. Clinical studies have been contradictory, and bulk can be easily obtained through dietary means with the addition of high fiber fruits and vegetables. These are less expensive and more palatable, and should become a part of the patient's lifelong diet anyway.

In addition, various inhibitors of carbohydrate and lipid absorption as well as lipid synthesis inhibitors are being evaluated as potential weight reducing agents (42). Gastrointestinal side effects appear to limit the effectiveness of these agents, and further studies are needed to characterize their potential role in the management of obesity.

Thermogenic Agents

Use of thyroid hormone has been advocated for the treatment of obesity due to its thermogenic properties. Its early use was based on the incorrect observation that obesity was accompanied by an abnormally low BMR. This observation was later shown to be an artifact due to the poor correlation between body surface area and BMR in grossly obese patients (8). Currently, advocates claim thyroid hormone may prevent the compensatory drop in BMR caused by caloric restriction. Critics argue that very substantial doses of thyroid (6 to 14 grains) are required to even slightly increase BMR, and these pharmacologic doses can have deleterious cardiovascular effects in obese patients already predisposed to heart problems. In view of the risks, use of thyroid hormone in obese individuals should be avoided unless there is clear evidence of thyroid deficiency (49).

Additional drugs that appear to enhance thermogenesis include ephedrine, caffeine, nicotine, growth hormone, and investigational β-agonists (35, 42, 50). Furthermore, a synergistic thermogenic effect has been documented when a combination of ephedrine and caffeine is administered (51). A limited number of studies have evaluated these agents, and, despite an apparent effect on increased energy expenditure, associated side effects tend to limit the usefulness of these agents.

Invasive Treatment Approaches

At the extreme end of the treatment continuum, more invasive approaches to obesity are available and include mandibular fixation, vagotomy, surgical manipulation of the gastrointestinal tract, and liposuction. These methods should be restricted to use in morbidly obese individuals refractory to the previously mentioned approaches.

Limited data suggest that fixation of the mandible (jaw wiring) can effectively reduce weight by restricting solid food intake. Although this particular procedure is associated with significant weight reduction, rapid weight regain is encountered in roughly 70% following removal of the wires (35). Truncal vagotomy is another approach and involves surgical interruption of the vagal nerve in an attempt to reduce the stimuli responsible for triggering eating. Unfortunately, the additional side effects associated with such a procedure limit its usefulness (35).

Jejunoileal and gastric surgery involve bypassing a significant portion of the small intestine and stomach, respectively. Weight loss with either proceeds more slowly than with fasting and, unfortunately, may stop quite short of ideal weight. Jejunoileal bypass works by inducing a malabsorptive state and is associated with significant digestive discomfort, nutrient malabsorption, polyarthritis, fatty liver degeneration, oxalate nephrolithiasis, and tuberculosis (3, 52, 53). Gastric bypass surgery produces a decreased gastric reservoir, which results in epigastric distress or vomiting when the capacity is exceeded. Gastric bypass may have fewer long-term complications but is technically more difficult and associated with a higher incidence of early postoperative complications. Nevertheless, despite these many complications, surgery remains the only viable solution in selected patients to avoid permanent disability or death.

Liposuction should be viewed more as a cosmetic method for body contouring than as a means of weight reduction. A frequently misconstrued notion is that significant amounts of adipose tissue can be eliminated via liposuction. If excessive tissue is extracted, serious complications such as blood loss, nerve damage, infection, and disfiguration of the skin contour may occur. Furthermore, successful operations tend to involve younger individuals in which the elasticity of the skin structure is intact (35). Therefore, the number of obese individuals potentially able to benefit from the procedure is limited. For these reasons, liposuction should not be advocated for managing obesity.

CONCLUSION

In virtually all cases, obesity can be preventable. When it occurs, the cure is uniquely simple and noninvasive. Despite this, a significant fraction of the population is suffering from what can be depicted as a "human energy crisis." This is due largely to the insensitivity of our society to the unfavorable health outcomes associated with sustained obesity and the unwillingness of obese individuals to undertake lifetime treatment (i.e., good dietary habits). Our acceptance of obesity as a benign condition leads to poor motivation and poor patient compliance.

Health care professionals play an important role in the management of obesity. As has been emphasized, the use of drugs, though temporarily beneficial, can detract from the attainment of permanent solutions. The health professional is in an important position to put the many components of treatment into perspective and, with educational and reinforcing techniques, assist the obese patient to achieve lasting results.

EATING DISORDERS

The two common eating disorders (EDs) are anorexia nervosa (AN) and bulimia. AN is a syndrome characterized by self-starvation, extreme weight loss, body image disturbance, and an intense fear of becoming obese (54). Some investigators recognize two separate subgroups of AN based on the presence of bulimic symptoms (55). Bulimia was described as a clinical entity in the 1980s and is characterized by binge eating, usually followed by some form of purging such as self-induced vomiting, laxative abuse, or associated behaviors such as diuretic use, diet pill use, or compulsive exercising (56, 57). Almost half of anorectics have bulimic symptoms, and one-third of bulimics have a history of anorexia or a major depressive disorder (58). Thus, most eating-disordered patients fall on a spectrum between the purely food restrictive anorectic and the binge-and-purge bulimic (59).

ETIOLOGY AND INCIDENCE

An intense preoccupation with food is common to both anorectics and bulimics. Bulimia is characterized by mild or marked weight fluctuations, while severe weight loss is found in AN. The bulimic's weight typically does not fluctuate to the dangerously low levels seen in AN. The most common type of ED is normal-weight bulimia, which involves patients who are within 10 percent of ideal weight despite purging (60). A normal weight, coupled with characteristic secretiveness regarding binge-and-purge behavior, makes these patients very difficult to detect.

This preoccupation with food stems in part from the cultural value Western society places on thinness, that fat is disgusting and weight gain means one is bad or out of control. Susceptible individuals have an unfettered drive to achieve society's ideal figure. AN usually begins between the ages of 12 years and the mid-30s, but most commonly first afflicts females in their early teens. Commonly, the teenager perceives a real or imagined weight problem and progresses from a modest effort to lose weight to a compulsive preoccupation with food restriction. *Anorexia* is a misnomer because most patients do not lose their appetites.

Bulimia has a similar pattern of onset. It begins later in adolescence and usually after a period of being overweight. Unsuccessful attempts at dieting, coupled with self-imposed or family pressure to lose weight, lead the individual, either accidentally or through a friend, to the discovery that self-induced vomiting or laxative use is a convenient way to reduce weight. This ultimately escalates into the binge-and-purge bulimic behavior.

Ninety percent of anorectic and bulimic patients are young females, often from middle- or upper-class backgrounds (54, 60). Five to ten percent of adolescent girls and young women are affected to some degree, and it is estimated that the incidence of AN and bulimia has doubled over the past two decades (61, 62). Up to 2 percent of teenage girls from upper socioeconomic backgrounds develop AN, and 3 to 5 percent of college women suffer from bulimia. Twenty percent of patients with EDs have a history of alcohol or other drug abuse (60).

DIAGNOSIS

EDs are classified as psychiatric illnesses. Diagnostic criteria from the fourth edition of the American Psychiatric Association's *Diagnostic and Statistical Manual* (DSM-IV) (63) are presented in Table 58.3.

COMPLICATIONS

The complications of AN are mainly those of starvation. The most consistent medical findings, aside from cachexia, are amenorrhea and estrogen deficiency (64). Thirty percent of anorexic teenage girls do not menstruate until

Table 58.3.
DSM IV Criteria for Anorexia Nervosa and Bulimia Nervosa

Anorexia Nervosa

A. Refusal to maintain body weight at or above a minimal normal weight for age and height (e.g., weight loss leading to maintenance of body weight 15% below that expected; or failure to make expected weight gain during period of growth, leading to body weight 15% below that expected).

B. Intense fear of gaining weight of becoming fat, even though underweight.

C. Disturbance in the way in which one's body weight, size, or shape is experienced, undue influence of body weight or shape on self-evaluation, or denial of the seriousness of the current low body weight.

D. In females, absence of at least three consecutive menstrual cycles when otherwise expected to occur (primary or secondary amenorrhea). *A woman is considered to have amenorrhea if her periods occur only following hormone (e.g., estrogen) administration.*

Bulimia Nervosa

A. Recurrent episodes of binge eating. An episode of binge eating is characterized by both of the following:
   (1) eating, in discrete period of time (e.g., within any 2-hour period), an amount of food that is definitely larger than most people would eat during a similar period of time and under similar circumstances
   (2) a sense of lack of control over eating during the episode (e.g., a feeling that one cannot stop eating or control what or how much one is eating)

B. Recurrent inappropriate compensatory behavior in order to prevent weight gain, such as self-induced vomiting; misuse of laxatives, diuretics, enemas, or other medications; fasting; or excessive exercise.

C. The binge eating and inappropriate compensatory behaviors both occur, on average, at least twice a week for 3 months.

D. Self-evaluation is unduly influenced by body shape and weight.

E. The disturbance does not occur exclusively during episodes of Anorexia Nervosa.

their 30s (56). Decreased fertility has also been observed in both men and women with AN. In extreme cases, every physiologic system may be disturbed, including the endocrine, cardiovascular, renal, gastrointestinal, and hematologic systems (65). Postural hypotension is observed in roughly 60% of patients (56). Bradycardia is reported in up to 87% (59), and cardiac arrhythmias, a common cause of death, may be precipitated by a diminished heart muscle mass, hypokalemia, or other severe electrolyte imbalance (54). Mortality associated with AN, excluding suicide, may be as high as 9%, and suicide may account for an additional 2 to 5% of deaths (66). In the untreated or poorly treated patients, the mortality rate approaches 20% (56).

Complications associated with bulimia tend to be less severe and involve the consequences of chronic bingeing and purging. Unlike the anorectic, whose emaciation attracts attention, the bulimic may be near ideal weight, which makes it easier for the patient to hide the problem. If weight loss is substantial, menstrual irregularities are common (54). Subtle changes in serum electrolytes may be seen in chronic vomiters, and laxative and diuretic abuse further contribute to hypokalemia with muscle weakness and fasciculations. Frequently, bulimic patients present with the characteristic "chipmunk face" secondary to parotid gland swelling. Increased susceptibility to infections and complaints of frequent sore throats, poor dentition, and scarring on the fingers and nails may also be present in chronic vomiters. Vomiting following use of central nervous system depressants, such as alcohol, predisposes patients with bulimia to aspiration pneumonia. A particularly dangerous practice is the repeated induction of vomiting with syrup of ipecac. Chronic absorption of ipecac can lead to a potentially fatal cardiotoxicity (67). A comprehensive list of complications associated with AN and bulimia are compared and reviewed in Table 58.4.

TREATMENT

The treatments of AN and bulimia are among the most unsatisfactory in clinical medicine. Despite several trials with a number of different pharmacologic agents, optimal drug therapies have not been identified. To complicate matters, anorectic patients and their families tend to deny the existence and severity of the illness and fail to obtain adequate medical and psychiatric care (54). Bulimia patients are more likely to seek treatment but have a low tolerance for extended compliance, which leads to a high relapse rate (68).

Table 58.4.
Complications of Anorexia Nervosa and Bulimia

Manifestation	Anorexia Nervosa	Bulimia
Endocrine/Metabolic	Amenorrhea	Menstrual irregularities
	Osteoporosis	
	Euthyroid sick syndrome	
	Decreased norepinephrine secretion	
	Decreased somatomedin C	
	Elevated growth hormone	
	Decreased or erratic vasopressin secretion	
	Abnormal temperature regulation	
	Hypercarotenemia	
Cardiovascular	Bradycardia	Ipecac poisoning
	Hypotension	
	Arrhythmias	
Renal	Increased blood urea nitrogen	Hypokalemia (diuretic induced)
	Decreased glomerular filtration rate	
	Renal calculi	
	Edema	
Gastrointestinal	Decreased gastric emptying	Acute gastric dilation, rupture
	Elevated hepatic enzymes	Constipation
		Parotid enlargement
		Dental-enamel erosion
		Esophagitis
		Mallory-Weiss tears, esophageal rupture
		Hypokalemia (laxative induced)
Hematologic	Anemia	
	Leukopenia	
	Thrombocytopenia	
Pulmonary		Aspiration pneumonia

Reprinted with permission from Herzog DB, Copeland PM. Eating disorders. N Engl J Med 313:295–303, 1985.

Psychotherapy is the mainstay of treatment of EDs, producing a full or partial recovery in 75% (69). Psychotherapy includes individual, group, family, and behavioral therapy, with the primary objective of helping patients to overcome denial of the problem and to reconstruct self-identity and self-confidence.

In addition to psychotherapy, the benefits of pharmacologic intervention for ED patients has been studied. Recent review articles have evaluated the various agents used in the management of ED (55, 70). Studies have suggested a possible link between EDs and major depressive illness, including a blunted dexamethasone suppression test (65) and lowered urinary metabolites of norepinephrine (71). More than 20 percent of bulimic patients satisfy *DSM-III-R* criteria for major depressive illness (72). Other evidence disputes a definitive connection between EDs and depression. One of the best studies demonstrating the effectiveness of the tricyclic antidepressant (TCA) desipramine in bulimia carefully excluded subjects with major depressive disorder (73), suggesting that the drug may have a direct antibulimic effect. In addition, AN and bulimia are associated with changes in noradrenergic, serotonergic, and opioid systems, which are thought to perpetuate pathologic eating behavior (74). Thus, drugs modifying activity of these neurotransmitters may potentially be useful in the treatment of EDs.

There is little evidence to suggest that psychotropic medications offer significant advantages to patients with AN already receiving behavioral therapy (55). In contrast, the use of various antidepressants in patients with bulimia has demonstrated beneficial results. Double-blind controlled studies with imipramine, desipramine, and phenelzine produced a striking reduction in bingeing behavior in bulimics (73, 75, 76). Antidepressants are preferred to monoamine oxidase inhibitors because they preclude dietary restriction problems in patients with diet-indiscreet illness. Also, the phenelzine study group exhibited a high dropout rate, indicating poor patient acceptability of this monoamine oxidase inhibitor. In another study, amitriptyline produced disappointing results compared to controls, but suboptimal amitriptyline doses (150 mg/day) and mixed therapy, including psychotherapy for both study and control groups, may have confounded the results (77). Based on current evidence, desipramine and imipramine are the preferred TCAs for treatment of bulimia (78). Doses for these agents are essentially the same as those used for major depressive disorders and are administered for a duration of at least 6 to 8 weeks. In successful treatment of bulimia with antidepressants alone, most patients relapsed after the drug was stopped, emphasizing that drugs are only a part of a multifocal strategy. Optimal duration of therapy is unknown. However, bulimic patients have been successfully maintained on antidepressants for 2 years or more (79).

There have been several recent clinical trials evaluating the effectiveness of a new category of antidepressants in the management of bulimia. Open labeled trials have shown fluoxetine, a serotonin reuptake inhibitor, to be associated with a significant reduction in the number of binge-and-purge bulimic episodes (80-83). This beneficial effect was observed regardless of whether depression was present in the patient. The use of fluoxetine in patients unresponsive to TCAs has also been reported (84). In addition, a large, multicentered controlled trial concluded that fluoxetine, in a dose of 60 mg/day, was more effective at decreasing the frequency of bulimic episodes when compared to placebo or standard antidepressant doses of fluoxetine (20 mg/day) (85). Other controlled trials, which also involved some form of psychotherapy, failed to demonstrate an advantage of fluoxetine over placebo (86, 87).

Relative to the TCAs and monoamine oxidase inhibitors, fluoxetine is fairly well tolerated. As discussed in the treatment of obesity, fluoxetine produces a variety of side effects but rarely do these adverse events result in the discontinuation of therapy. Other attractive attributes include once-daily dosing, and unlike the TCAs, fluoxetine has been associated with weight loss that poses less threat to the bulimic patient. The use of fluoxetine in the management of bulimia has been recommended to the FDA for approval; however, official FDA approval is still pending.

In contrast to fluoxetine, open studies of trazodone, another serotonergic antidepressant, produced mixed results and even worsening of bulimic behavior (88, 89). In 1986, a trial of bupropion in a bulimic population resulted in a relatively high incidence of seizures, which forced the temporary withdrawal of bupropion from the market (90). A number of other drug modalities have been employed in EDs. In a double-blind study of 72 patients with AN, cyproheptadine in high doses (32 mg/day) produced modest weight gain compared to amitriptyline and placebo (91). The anticonvulsants phenytoin, carbamazepine, and valproic acid have all been studied in the treatment of bulimic patients (92–94). Results have been generally disappointing, but there have been isolated cases of symptomatic improvement. There may be a subgroup of binge eaters, whose behavior is secondary to a neurologic disorder analogous to epilepsy, who may be more likely to respond to an anticonvulsant agent (95). In addition, the opiate antagonists naloxone and naltrexone, lithium, d-fenfluramine, and other agents have been studied (55). Clearly, further controlled studies in larger numbers of patients are warranted to establish the safety and specific role of these agents in the management of EDs.

As for a general recommendation for treatment of EDs, one investigator (55) recommends some form of behavioral or psychotherapy as the initial therapy for

Table 58.5.
Recognizing Patients with Eating Disorders

- Typical ED patient is a female in early to late teens who (1) exhibits weight loss or no significant weight gain during development (AN), or (2) exhibits frequent significant weight fluctuations (bulimia).
- Young women fitting ED stereotype who repeatedly purchase laxatives, enemas, appetite suppressants, syrup of ipecac, or diuretics.
- Complaints of irregular menstrual cycles or amenorrhea
- History of depression or alcohol/other drug abuse
- Other nonspecific complaints, e.g., swollen parotid glands, poor dentition, frequent sore throats from vomiting; abdominal complaints from laxative abuse, etc.

patients with bulimia. For those individuals who do not responded after a prolonged course of psychotherapy, the use of fluoxetine, or perhaps a TCA, should be considered for the treatment of bulimia. As for patients with AN, several pharmacologic agents have been studied with disappointing results. Due to these dismal results, the mainstay of acute therapy for AN should focus on restoration of normal body weight. Even if patients with AN show signs of depression, progressive weight gain tends to correct the depression without the need for antidepressants. Therefore, the use of antidepressants play a limited role in the management of AN.

RECOGNIZING EATING DISORDERS

Health care professionals can play an important role in recognizing and counseling patients with EDs. ED patients exhibit typical symptoms and behaviors, which are listed in Table 58.5. Based on these symptoms and behaviors, rapid judgments may need to be made about whether a patient is suffering from one of these serious, potentially life-threatening disorders. Since many of the drugs misused by bulimics are purchased without a prescription, the use of stimulant laxatives, enemas, appetite suppressants and syrup of ipecac by young women should be monitored. Suspicious use of diuretic agents, such as furosemide or thiazides, in apparently healthy young women should also be questioned. In one study of 275 bulimic patients, 34 percent admitted to using a prescription diuretic for weight control (96). Finally, the health care professional must be knowledgeable about community services available to help ED victims once they are identified. Appropriate referral to regional or local support groups can be extremely helpful at getting these individuals the necessary care.

CONCLUSION

Current evidence suggests that there is a relationship between depression or other neurotransmitter abnormalities and EDs, particularly bulimia. Antidepressants probably are effective in treating depression in ED patients; moreover, they appear to provide symptomatic relief in

patients who are not clinically depressed. At the present time, a trial of antidepressants is considered appropriate in patients with EDs if behavioral therapy is unsuccessful.

It must be remembered that these patients are often noncompliant and tend to misuse and overuse drugs. Relapses are heralded by excessive purchases of laxatives, syrup of ipecac, over-the-counter weight control products, and surreptitious diuretic use.

Through vigilance of patient compliance in psychotherapy and pharmacotherapy strategies, and observing for evidence of relapses, health care professionals play an important role in the interdisciplinary management of patients with EDs.

REFERENCES

1. Edwards KI. Obesity, anorexia, and bulimia. Med Clin North Am 77:899–910, 1993.
2. Gray DS. Diagnosis and prevalence of obesity. Med Clin North Am 73:1–13, 1989.
3. Van Itallie TB, Kral JG. The dilemma of morbid obesity. JAMA 246:999–1003, 1981.
4. Kuczmarski RJ. Prevalence of overweight and weight gain in the United States. Am J Clin Nutr 55(suppl 2):495S–502S, 1992.
5. Bray GA, Gray DS. Obesity. Part I-pathogenesis. West J Med 149:429–441, 1988.
6. Pi-Sunyer FX. Obesity. In: Modern nutrition in health and disease, ed 7. Philadelphia: Lea & Febiger, 1988:795.
7. Tan T, Handford HA, Soldatos CR. Current therapy of eating disorders II: obesity. Rational Drug Therapy 18:1, 1984.
8. Thorn GW, Cahill GF. Gain in weight; obesity. In: Harrison's principles of internal medicine, ed 7. New York: McGraw-Hill, 1974:232.
9. Anand BK. Nervous regulation of food intake. Physiol Rev 41:667–672, 1961.
10. Celesia GG, Archer CR, Chung HD. Hyperphagia and obesity, relationship to medial hypothalamic lesions. JAMA 246:151–153, 1981.
11. Schacter S. Obesity and eating: internal and external values differentially affect the eating behavior of obese and normal subjects. Science 161:751–756, 1968.
12. Knittle JL, Timmers K, Ginsberg-Fellner F, et al. The growth of adipose tissue in children and adolescents. J Clin Invest 63:239–246, 1979.
13. Stunkard A, Rush J. Dieting and depression reexamined–a critical review of reports of untoward responses during weight reduction for obesity. Ann Intern Med 81:526–533, 1974.
14. Charney E, Goodman HC, McBride M, et al. Childhood antecedents of adult obesity. N Engl J Med 295:6–9, 1976.
15. Price RA, Cadoret RJ, Stunkard AJ, et al. Genetic contributions to human fatness: an adoption study. Am J Psychiatry 144:1003–1008, 1987.
16. Stunkard AJ, Foch TT, Hrubec Z. A twin study of human obesity. JAMA 256:51–54, 1986.
17. Danowski TS. The management of obesity. Hosp Pract (April):11:39–46, 1976.
18. Bondy PK. Metabolic obesity? N Engl J Med 303:1057–1058, 1980.
19. Newsholme EA. A possible metabolic basis for the control of body weight. N Engl J Med 302:400–405, 1980.
20. Edwards LE, Dickes WF, Alton IR, et al. Pregnancy in the massively obese: course, outcome, and obesity prognosis of the infant. Am J Obstet Gynecol 131:479–483, 1978.
21. Sketris I, Lesar T, Zaske DE, et al. Effect of obesity on gentamicin pharmacokinetics. J Clin Pharmacol 21:288–293, 1981.

22. Cheymol G. Clinical pharmacokinetics of drugs in obesity. An update. Clin Pharmacokinet 25:103–114, 1993.

23. Sjostrom LV. Morbidity of severly obese subjects. Am J Clin Nutr 55(suppl 2):508S–515S, 1992.

24. Sjostrom LV. Mortality of severly obese subjects. Am J Clin Nutr 55(suppl 2):516S–523S, 1992.

25. Stunkard AJ, Sorensen TIA, Hanis C, et al. Adoption study of human obesity. N Engl J Med 314:193–198, 1986.

26. Van Itallie TB, Yang M. Diet and weight loss. N Engl J Med 297:1158–1161, 1977.

27. Mazel J. The Beverly Hills diet. New York: Macmillan, 1981.

28. Mirkin GB, Shore RN. The Beverly Hills diet: dangers of the newest weight loss fad. JAMA 246:2235–2237, 1981.

29. Anon. Protein diets. FDA Drug Bull 8:2, 1978.

30. Wadden TA, Stunkard AJ, Brownell KD, Van Itallie TB. The Cambridge diet—more mayhem? JAMA 250:2833–2834, 1983.

31. Felig P. Very-low-calorie diets. N Engl J Med 310:589–591, 1984.

32. Straw WE, Sonne AC. The obese patient. J Fam Pract 9:317–323, 1979.

33. Franklin BA, Rubenfire M. Losing weight through exercise. JAMA 244:377–379, 1980.

34. Brownell KD, Kramer FM. Behavioral management obesity. Med Clin North Am 73:185–201, 1989

35. Bray GA, Gray DS. Obesity. Part II-treatment. West J Med 149:555–571, 1988.

36. Scoville BA. Review of amphetamine-like drugs by the Food and Drug Administration: clinical data and value judgments. In: Bray GA, ed. Obesity in perspective. Washington, DC: U.S. Government Printing Office, 1976:441–443.

37. Craighead LW, Stunkard AJ, O'Brien RM. Behavior therapy and pharmacotherapy for obesity. Arch Gen Psychiatry 38:763–768, 1981.

38. Sullivan AC, Comai K. Pharmacologic treatment of obesity. Int J Obes 2:167–189, 1978.

39. Stunkard AJ. Anorectic agents: a theory of action and lack of tolerance in a clinical trial, In Garattini S, ed. Anorectic agents: mechanisms of action and of tolerance. New York: Raven Press, 1981.

40. Anon. The Green Sheet. Dec. 5, 1977.

41. Galloway SML, Munro JF, Farquhar DL. The current status of anti-obesity drugs. Postgrad Med J 60:19–26, 1984.

42. Wilson MA. Treatment of obesity. Am J Med Sci 299:62–68, 1990.

43. Bray GA. Use and abuse of appetite suppressant drugs in the treatment of obesity. Ann Intern Med 119(part 2):707–713, 1993.

44. Silverstone T. Appetite suppressants: a review. Drugs 43:820–836, 1992.

45. Douglas JG, Munro JF, Kitchin AH, et al. Pulmonary hypertension and fenfluramine. Br Med J 283:881–836, 1981.

46. Duhault J, Beregi L, deBoistesselin R. General and comparative pharmacology of fenfluramine. Curr Med Res Opin 6:3(suppl 1), 1979.

47. Hendy MS, Dove AF, Arblaster PG. Mazindol-induced lithium toxicity. Br Med J 280:684–685, 1980.

48. Milkovich R, van den Berg BJ. Effects of antenatal exposure to anorectic drugs. Am J Obstet Gynecol 129:637–642, 1977.

49. Bray GA. Drug treatment of obesity. Am J Clin Nutr 55(suppl 2):538S–544S, 1992.

50. Astrup A, Toubro S, Christensen NJ, Quaade F. Pharmacology of thermogenic drugs. Am J Clin Nutr 55(suppl 1):246S–248S, 1992.

51. Astrup A, Toubro S, Cannon S, Hein P, Madsen J. Thermogenic synergism between ephedrine and caffeine in healthy volunteers. A double blind placebo controlled study. Metabolism 40:323–329, 1991.

52. Bruce RM, Wise L. Tuberculosis after jejunoileal bypass for obesity. Ann Intern Med 87:574–576, 1977.

53. Kral JG. Overview of surgical techniques for treating obesity. Am J Clin Nutr 55(suppl 2):552S–555S, 1992.

54. Herzog DB, Copeland PM. Eating disorders. N Engl J Med 313:295–303, 1985.

55. Walsh BT, Devlin MJ. The pharmacologic treatment of eating disorders. Psychiatr Clin North Am 15:149–160, 1992.

56. Giannini AJ, Newman M, Gold M. Anorexia and bulimia. Am Fam Physician 41:1169–1176, 1990.

57. Mitchell JE, Hatsukami D, Pyle RL, Eckert ED. The bulimia syndrome: course of the illness and associated problems. Compr Psychiatry 27:165–170, 1986.

58. Newman MM and Halmi KA. The endocrinology of anorexia nervosa and bulimia nervosa. Neurol Clin 6:195–212, 1988.

59. Brotman AW, Rigotti N, Herzog DB. Medical complications of eating disorders: outpatient evaluation and management. Compr Psychiatry 26:258–272, 1985.

60. Mickley D. Evaluating common eating disorders—ten questions to ask your patient. Female Patient 13:33, 1988.

61. Pope HG, Hudson JI, Yurgelun-Todd D, Hudson MS. Prevalence of anorexia nervosa and bulimia in three student populations. Int J Eating Disord 3:45–49, 1984.

62. Pope HG, Hudson JI, Yurgelun-Todd D. Anorexia nervosa and bulimia among 300 women shoppers. Am J Psychiatry 141:292–294, 1984.

63. American Psychiatric Association. Diagnostic and statistical manual of mental disorders, 4th ed., revised. Washington, D.C.: American Psychiatric Association, 1994.

64. Warren MP, Vande Weile RL. Clinical and metabolic features of anorexia nervosa. Am J Obstet Gynecol 117:435–449, 1973.

65. Weiner H. The physiology of eating disorders. Int J Eating Disord 4:347–351, 1985.

66. Seidensticker JF, Tzagournis M. Anorexia nervosa—clinical features and long term follow-up. J Chronic Dis 21:361, 1968.

67. Adler AG, Walinsky P, Krall RA, Cho SY. Death resulting from ipecac syrup poisoning. JAMA 243:1927–1928, 1980.

68. Mitchell JE, Davis L, Goff G. The process of relapse in patients with bulimia. Int J Eating Disord 4:457–463, 1985.

69. Adams C, Koop L, Toce P. Current ideologies of eating disorders: an overview. Am Pharm NS28:41–46, 1988.

70. Kennedy SH, Goldbloom DS. Current perspectives on drug therapies for anorexia nervosa and bulimia nervosa. Drugs 41:367–377, 1991.

71. Biederman J, Herzog DB, Rivinus T, et al. Urinary MHPG in anorexia nervosa patients with and without a major depressive disorder. J Psychiatr Res 18:149–160, 1984.

72. Bond WS, Crabbe S, Sanders MC. Pharmacotherapy of eating disorders: a critical review. Ann Pharmacother 20:659–662, 1986.

73. Hughes PL, Wells LA, Cunningham CJ, Ilstrup DM. Treating bulimia with desipramine: a double-blind, placebo-controlled study. Arch Gen Psychiatry 43:182–186, 1986.

74. Fava M, Copeland PM, Schweiger U, Herzog DB. Neurochemical abnormalities of anorexia nervosa and bulimia nervosa. Am J Psychiatry 146:963–971, 1989.

75. Pope HG Jr, Hudson JI, Jonas JM, Yurgelun-Todd D. Bulimia treated with imipramine: a placebo-controlled, double-blind study. Am J Psychiatry 140:554–558, 1983.

76. Walsh BT, Stewart JW, Roose SP, et al. Treatment of bulimia with phenelzine; a double-blind, placebo-controlled study. Arch Gen Psychiatry 41:1105–1109, 1984.

77. Mitchell JE, Groat R. A placebo-controlled, double-blind trial of amitriptyline in bulimia. J Clin Psychopharmacol 4:186–193, 1984.

78. Kim LE, Middleton RK. Antidepressants used in bulimia. Ann Pharmacother 23:882–885, 1989.

79. Mitchell PB. The pharmacological management of bulimia nervosa: a critical review. Int J Eating Disord 7:29–35, 1988.

80. Wilcox JA. Fluoxetine and bulimia. J Psychoactive Drugs 22:81–82, 1990.

81. Trygstad O. Drugs in the treatment of bulimia nervosa. Acta Psychiatr Scand 82:34–37, 1990.

82. Freeman C, Hampson M. Fluoxetine as a treatment for bulimia nervosa. Int J Obes 11(suppl 3):171–177, 1987.

83. Solyom L, Solyom C, Ledwidge B. The fluoxetine treatment of low-weight, chronic bulimia nervosa. J Clin Psychopharmacol 10: 421–425, 1990.

84. Mitchell JE, Pyle RL, Eckert ED, et al. Response to alternate antidepressants in imipramine non-responders with bulimia nervosa. J Clin Psychopharmacol 9:291–293, 1989.

85. Fluoxetine Bulimia Nervosa Collaborative Group. Fluoxetine in the treatment of bulimia nervosa: a multicentered, placebo-controlled, double-blind trial. Arch Gen Psychiatry 48:139–147, 1992.

86. Fichter MM, Leibl K, Rief W, et al. Fluoxetine versus placebo: a double blind study with bulimia inpatients undergoing intensive psychotherapy. Pharmacopsychiatry 24:1–7, 1991.

87. Marcus MD, Wing RR, Ewing L, et al. The assessment of binge eating severity among obese persons. Addict Behav 7:47–52, 1982.

88. Wold P. Trazodone in the treatment of bulimia. J Clin Psychiatry 44:275–276, 1983.

89. Pope HG, Hudson JI, Jonas JM. Antidepressant treatment of bulimia: preliminary experience and practical recommendations. J Clin Psychopharmacol 3:274–281, 1983.

90. Carson SW. Bupropion, is it here to stay? Ann Pharmacotherapy 23:704–705, 1989.

91. Halmi KA, Eckert E, LaDu TJ, et al. Anorexia nervosa: treatment efficacy of cyproheptadine and amitriptyline. Arch Gen Psychiatry 43:177–181, 1986.

92. Wermuth BM, Davis KL, Hollister LE, et al. Phenytoin treatment of the binge-eating syndrome. Am J Psychiatry 134:1249–1253, 1977.

93. Kaplan AS, Garfinkle PE, Darby PL, et al. Carbamazepine in the treatment of bulimia. Am J Psychiatry 140:1225–1226, 1983.

94. Herridge PL, Pope HG Jr. Treatment of bulimia and rapid cycling bipolar disorder with sodium valproate: a case report. J Clin Psychopharmacol 5:229–230, 1985.

95. Moore SL, Rakes SM. Binge eating-therapeutic response to diphenylhydantoin: case report. J Clin Psychiatry 43:385–386, 1982.

96. Russell G. Bulimia: an ominous variant of anorexia nervosa. Psychol Med 9:429–448, 1979.

CHAPTER 59

ALCOHOLISM

THEODORE G. TONG and JEFFREY N. BALDWIN

Alcohol is the most misused drug in the United States today. Alcohol abuse and alcoholism are estimated to have cost the United States $136.3 billion in 1990, mostly from lost productivity and employment (1). According to knowledgeable estimates, the incidence of alcoholism in the United States ranges from 9 to 14 million, about 10% of the total number of adult Americans who use alcohol (2). This rate increases to 30 to 50% when close relatives are alcoholic (3). It is a condition far more common than generally perceived, with only 3 to 5% of the country's alcoholic population classified as the "skid row" or public inebriate type. Alcoholics come from all levels of our society; the majority will be found in the working and homemaking population.

The largest percentage of American alcoholics are between the ages of 35 and 50 years. Professionals and businesspeople have high rates of alcohol consumption and alcoholism. The proportion of alcohol use in the younger school-age population and "problem drinking" among women have increased and appear to be continuing trends (4, 5). Although the prevalence of alcohol misuse among the elderly is lower, detection of the problem is difficult, and it is frequently unrecognized. Vulnerability of the older alcoholic to the harmful effects of alcohol is much greater (2). Alcoholism is among America's major health concerns along with cancer and heart disease and problems related to alcohol abuse and alcoholism.

Alcoholism is an illness that can shorten one's life span considerably. About 25% of hospitalized individuals have an alcohol-related problem, and 20% of the total national health expenditure for hospital care is spent on alcohol-related illness (2, 6). Alcohol is involved in half of all fatalities from fire and highway traffic accidents, 67% of homicides, and 33% of suicides (2). Death rates from alcohol abuse in the major risk age groups are more than twice those for the general population. Alcoholism is a treatable illness when diagnosed in its early stages. Unfortunately, there is a serious deficit of accessible and high-quality alcoholism treatment services. Moreover, the majority of the services available are designed to deal with only the later stages of alcoholism.

Alcoholism, like other diseases such as hypertension and diabetes mellitus, can be considered a biological disease with genetic predisposition that is activated by environmental factors (6, 7). Thus, a "biopsychosocial" approach is usually used in the identification, treatment, and ongoing recovery support systems for alcoholics. Difficulty in differentiating between alcohol abuse and alcoholism (alcohol dependence) may be cited by some as a reason for questioning the disease concept. However, other diseases such as hypertension may be equally difficult to define when borderline. A recent survey found that about 89% of the surveyed population considered alcoholics to be ill, yet 47% also felt that the alcoholic was morally weak (8). This reveals a fairly strong public sentiment that alcoholism represents "willful misconduct" and represents an important societal impediment in the identification and treatment of the disease.

Alcohol abuse involves persistent patterns of heavy alcohol consumption with associated health or social consequences. Alcoholism is differentiated from abuse by the presence of craving, tolerance, and physical dependence that result in behavioral changes and loss of control over drinking. Persons who are alcoholic experience both psychologic and physical dependency and tolerance. Psychologic dependency is perhaps the single most important factor and involves the compulsive use of and craving for a drug. Physical dependency is characterized by a series of physiologic events that occur when the drug is discontinued, including the withdrawal or abstinence syndrome. Tolerance develops when the continued use of a drug is required and increasing doses are needed to produce the same effect.

Although the most important feature of addictive disorders is the psychologic dependency, it is the least understood. A person may be made physically dependent on alcohol, but abuse may not be recognized or diagnosed as such until behavioral effects secondary to psychologic dependence are present. Many persons consume alcoholic beverages, but relatively few develop physical and psychologic dependency on the drug. A commonly held belief is that if someone does not drink daily, or drinks only alcoholic beverages with relatively low alcohol content, such as wine or beer, they cannot be alcoholic. The quantity, type, and frequency of alcohol consumption are relatively unimportant; loss of control over consumption once initiated and continued use despite clear evidence of adverse consequences (social, physical, legal) are more important in the diagnosis of alcoholism.

PHARMACOLOGY

Alcohol is a psychoactive agent that can be characterized pharmacologically as a sedative-hypnotic drug. At low doses, the action of alcohol is an excitatory and stimulatory effect due to its depression of inhibitory centers in the brain. In a dose–response relationship, at sufficient doses, alcohol produces a depressant action. Although alcohol is able to provide relief of anxiety and sedation at one dose level, it produces sleep and depression of the central nervous system and respiratory system at higher levels.

Alcohol is present in a variety of popular beverages: Beer and ale are products of the fermentation of cereal grains and contain 3 to 6% alcohol; wine results from the fermentation of yeast on sugars present in fruits and contains 11 to 20% alcohol; brandy is produced from the distillation of wine products and usually contains 40% alcohol; hard liquors are the distillates of fermented products such as grain and are available as gin, rye, bourbon, scotch, and vodka and contain approximately 40 to 50% alcohol. Hard liquors are commonly labeled with a proof number that is twice the alcohol concentration by volume. Nonalcoholic (N.A.) beers and wines rarely contain no alcohol; they often contain less than 1% alcohol, but this may be enough to cause a relapse in a recovering alcoholic. Such individuals should generally be advised to avoid products containing any alcohol.

METABOLISM

Alcohol is efficiently and rapidly absorbed by the stomach and small intestine in 30 to 120 minutes after ingestion. Absorption is direct and complete by simple (passive) diffusion; alcohol distributes freely in body tissues and fluids. Its volume of distribution ranges from 0.58 to 0.70 liter/kg of body weight. The concentration of alcohol in the brain rapidly approaches that in the blood.

Factors that modify alcohol absorption are volume, dilution, rate of ingestion, and presence of food in the stomach. Protein and water both slow, whereas carbonation facilitates, the absorption of alcohol. Gastric alcohol dehydrogenase (ADH), which is involved in gastric metabolism of alcohol, is about 80% higher in nonalcoholic males than females, whereas chronic alcoholism results in a decrease of about 40% in men and 15% in women. This may help explain why alcohol blood levels in females, corrected for size, are relatively higher than males and may partially explain the greater susceptibility and early onset of liver and brain damage in female alcoholics (9). Alcohol crosses the placenta and may be found in the milk of lactating mothers.

The liver is the main site of the first step in the oxidation of ethyl alcohol. Ethanol is oxidized by alcohol dehydrogenase to acetaldehyde, which subsequently is oxidized by acetaldehyde dehydrogenase (ALDH) to acetate or acetyl coenzyme A. This enters the Kreb's cycle to form carbon dioxide and water and also participates in protein and fat synthesis. Both oxidizing enzymes are responsible for converting nicotinamide adenine dinucleotide (NAD) to its reduced form, NADH, which contributes to the many metabolic abnormalities (e.g., hyperlipidemia, ketoacidosis, hyperlactacidemia, hyperuricemia) associated with chronic alcohol ingestion. Genetic predisposition to alcoholism may be in part explained by the presence of an inactive form of ALDH2 isoenzyme in many alcoholics that impairs acetaldehyde metabolism. Acetaldehyde accumulation may lead to an increase in aldehyde condensation products, such as tetrahydropapaveroline and salsolinol, collectively known as tetrahydroisoquinolines (THIQs), and beta-carbolines; infusion of these substances in rats and monkeys causes them to drink large quantities of alcohol. They probably have a relationship to the development of tolerance and habituation. Inactive ALDH2 isoenzyme may therefore be implicated in the pathogenesis of alcohol-induced tissue toxicity and dependence (7, 10, 11). A distinct microsomal ethanol-oxidizing system (MEOS) has also been characterized; this may be involved in increasing the clearance of alcohol and other drugs from the blood (12, 13).

Although most drugs are known to be metabolized or cleared from the body in a fixed percentage ("first order") of the dose taken, alcohol is unique in that nonlinear or saturation elimination kinetics is followed and, therefore, removed from the blood in a fixed amount ("zero order") over time. Most of the ingested dose of alcohol is eliminated by liver metabolism. In a 70-kg (approximately 150-lb) person, the rate of alcohol metabolism approximates 7 g/hr. At this rate of metabolism, the blood alcohol level will decline at a rate of nearly 15 mg/100 ml/hr. An average "shot" of distilled spirit, 86 proof, contains about 15 g of ethyl alcohol; because body water approximates 65% of body weight in a 70-kg person, the blood ethyl alcohol content after one "shot" will be 15 g/50 liters, or 30 mg/dl, with 50 liters being the approximate volume of total body water calculated from the percentage of weight. If taken in one swallow, it will take approximately two hours for the blood ethyl alcohol level to return to zero. Within one hour after drinking five 12-ounce cans of beer, four 4-ounce glasses of table wine, five 1-ounce glasses of liqueur, five 1-ounce shots of distilled spirits, or three 3-ounce martinis, a 70-kg person would have a blood ethanol concentration of 100 mg/dl (the amount legally defined as intoxication in many states; some now use 50 to 80 mg/dl). There is, however, wide variability observed in individual ethanol metabolism, so blood ethanol concentrations may vary considerably among persons who consume these amounts.

Ethanol elimination by the kidneys, lungs, and through sweat is minimal with approximately 2 to 10% cleared by these routes depending on the amount of alcohol ingested.

Table 59.1.
Blood Ethanol Concentrations and Clinical Effects in the Nontolerant Adult Drinker

Blood Ethanol Level (mg/100 ml)	Clinical Effects
20–99	Slight changes in mood and feelings progressing to muscular incoordination, impaired sensory function, personality and behavioral changes (talkative, noisy, morose)
100–199	Marked mental impairment, incoordination, clumsiness and unsteadiness in standing or walking, ataxia, prolonged reaction time, gross intoxication
200–299	Nausea, vomiting, diplopia, marked ataxia
300–399	Hypothermia, severe dysarthria, amnesia, stage 1 anesthesia
400–700	Coma, respiratory failure, and death

Exercise or administration of thyroid hormone, oxygen, glucose, or multivitamins does not increase the rate of alcohol oxidation. Whether or not there are ethnic differences for developing tolerance to alcohol is still unclear (12, 14).

BLOOD ALCOHOL CONCENTRATIONS AND INTOXICATION

The relationship between blood ethyl alcohol concentration and clinical signs and symptoms of intoxication is variable and depends on the rate of ingestion, amount consumed, alterations in absorption, metabolism, excretion, and chronicity of exposure (Table 59.1). The correlation of the blood alcohol concentration to behavioral effects has obvious important medical and legal importance. As a consequence of tolerance, higher blood alcohol concentrations may be required to produce clinical effects in alcoholics than in occasional drinkers. There are drinkers who exhibit such extreme degrees of tolerance to alcohol that they will appear sober even with blood alcohol concentrations two to three times higher than the limit permitted by law for driving an automobile. The lethal blood alcohol level is variable but in the range of 400 to 700 mg/dl. The lethal level may be substantially lowered when opiates, neuroleptics, or other sedative-hypnotics are taken along with an excessive amount of alcohol.

DIAGNOSIS OF ALCOHOLISM

The diagnosis of alcoholism is difficult because of societal stigmatization of the disease, denial, and imprecise diagnostic criteria. The clinical signs and subtleties of the condition are varied, elusive, and without reliable parameters. Objective laboratory verification of the diagnosis is frequently unavailable or incomplete. Although a specific genetic marker for alcoholism has been recently suggested (15), this is not universally accepted and likely represents only one of a number of factors (e.g., multiple gene loci, environment, gender, ethnicity) that affect predisposition. Reliable biochemical or genetic markers for diagnosing alcoholism are not available. Much depends on the experience and motivation of the observer in deciding whether a patient is suffering from alcoholism or not. Unfortunately, many physicians and other health professionals are poorly educated concerning the diagnosis of alcoholism, and therefore underdiagnose and mismanage alcohol-related problems. The first recognition of alcoholism often occurs during a hospitalization when an advanced manifestation of alcoholism, such as ascites or cirrhosis, is being treated. Many patients with unrecognized alcoholism probably experience minor withdrawal symptoms, such as agitation and insomnia, during hospital stays or when admitted to nursing homes. Although not absolute, the DSM-IV criteria established by the American Psychiatric Association can serve as a convenient starting point for the diagnosis of alcohol dependence (16).

Early identification of an existing alcohol problem is important because the prognosis from treatment is much more promising when the difficulty is recognized early in its course. Clues that provide early recognition can be found in the demographic, social, familial, and cultural characteristics of alcohol consumers (17). Frequent episodes of drinking to the point of intoxication, an inability to control the intake of alcohol, alcoholic "blackout" periods (loss of memory while intoxicated, not passing out), drinking despite strong social contraindications such as job loss, legal problems such as drunk driving arrests, or family or marital discord resulting from pathologic drinking are signs of the presence of this condition. Common early physical signs and symptoms of alcoholism include hypertension, gastritis, diarrhea or irritable colon, burns, bruises, red face, puffy face and eyes, enlarged nose with prominent veins, reddened conjunctiva, obesity, insomnia, or impotence. Several identification or screening tests in common clinical use [Michigan Alcoholism Screening Test (MAST), the abbreviated MAST, and CAGE (Cutting down drinking, Annoyed by criticism of drinking, Guilty about drinking, and Eye-openers)] were recently studied; Cyr and Wartman (18) found that, in addition to one of these tests, the specific questions "Have you ever had a drinking problem?" and "When was your last drink?" were helpful in establishing a diagnosis of alcoholism.

Equally important in obtaining assistance for the alcoholic is getting them to agree to be evaluated for the problem. Denial is a common characteristic of chemical dependency, including alcoholism. Although some patients may respond to a personal expression of concern from a friend, employer, or physician, many patients require a formal intervention to get help. A formal intervention normally is a carefully planned confrontation of the individual during which those who have observed alcohol-related behaviors report these in objective terms and define an ultimatum that the individual get help or suffer consequences such as loss of job, family, friends, or other significant support. Interventions are normally coordinated by someone such as a counselor; in some specific professions, interventions may also be done by trained teams of intervenors from within the profession. Normally, the individual is encouraged to obtain the formal evaluation or enter formal treatment as soon as possible, preferably that day. This helps assure compliance and reduces the risk of suicide at a time when this is a major risk.

MAJOR ADVERSE EFFECTS FROM ALCOHOL

Alcohol affects almost every organ system in the body. The more important and known medical complications and pathologic consequences from excessive alcohol consumption are summarized in Table 59.2 (19).

Alcoholic Liver Disease

There are three distinct histologic patterns of alcohol-induced liver disease. All three may coexist simultaneously and do not represent a single progression. Cirrhosis may occur in the absence of prior hepatitis (35). The risk of developing alcoholic liver disease is related to the quantity and duration of alcohol consumption. Factors such as genetics, nutritional state, and environment also predispose to the development of alcoholic liver disease (22). Alcoholic "fatty liver" disease is the most common alcohol-induced hepatic abnormality, occurring in 90 to 100% of chronic alcoholics.

The postulated mechanism for fatty accumulation in the liver is that an increase in the NADH:NAD ratio during ethanol oxidation is responsible for accumulation of hepatic triglycerides. Uncomplicated fatty liver is usually asymptomatic or presents as nausea, vomiting, and right upper quadrant abdominal pain, rarely presenting with the usual signs of liver disease such as ascites, jaundice, or splenomegaly. Mild, usually reversible, elevation of liver enzymes is the most frequent laboratory finding. Not as relatively benign as once believed, fatty liver can progress to liver failure and death occasionally.

Alcoholic hepatitis is a much more serious disorder; 10 to 30% of alcoholics develop this complication, usually after years of excessive drinking or after an abrupt increase in alcohol intake. Liver injury results from the degenerative effects of alcohol on subcellular structures. The clinical course of alcoholic hepatitis ranges from acute or chronic asymptomatic, mild, severe, and fulminant forms. It is often an incidental diagnosis when hepatomegaly and mild elevations in liver function study results are detected during a physical examination. Some patients who develop the fulminant course will rapidly progress to liver failure. The death rate in cases of severe alcoholic hepatitis is substantial.

The pathogenesis of alcoholic cirrhosis has not been determined completely. Although approximately half of the survivors from alcoholic hepatitis subsequently will experience cirrhosis of the liver, this condition may develop in the absence of any previously documented hepatitis. The liver is characterized as being finely nodular or grossly deformed, which may be smaller or larger than normal. Laboratory findings include hyperbilirubinemia, hypoalbuminemia, and prolonged prothrombin time. Complications from cirrhosis include encephalopathy, portal hypertension with bleeding at the esophageal varices, portal vein thrombosis, and hepatorenal syndrome. As many as 30,000 deaths occur each year from alcohol-induced cirrhosis.

Alcohol and the Heart

Cardiac dysfunction may account for up to 50% of the difference between normal death rates and those in alcohol-abusing or dependent individuals. Modest to moderate consumption of alcohol (up to two drinks per day) may reduce the risk for myocardial infarction and death, possibly by increasing the level of high-density lipoprotein (HDL) cholesterol and antithrombotic activity (36–38). Although there seems little doubt that modest to moderate alcohol consumption can exert a protective effect against coronary heart disease, consumption of well beyond two drinks per day is associated with an increasing occurrence of coronary heart disease. Along with cigarette smokers, chronic excessive drinkers are at higher risk for hypertension, ischemic heart disease, and stroke.

Recognition of alcoholic cardiomyopathy has been made difficult by its similarity to two other types of alcohol-related cardiomyopathies (24, 25). Nutritional deficiency in thiamine can lead to an unusual type of cardiac disorder ("wet beriberi heart disease"), which is characterized by a state of high output failure, fluid retention, and cardiac dilatation. Another cause of cardiomyopathy has been associated with excessive consumption of beer containing cobalt, an added foaming agent. There are patients with a history of alcoholism who have heart disease that is unrelated to either of these possible causes. Evidence that alcohol is metabolized in the heart to fatty acid ethyl esters that interfere with mitochondrial function to cause cardiomyopathy have been suggested. With continued abstinence, alcohol-induced cardiomyopathy may be reversible in some patients (39, 40).

As many as 24% of cases of hypertension may have alcohol as a primary cause. Blood pressure elevation occurs with acute intoxication and often parallels the severity of alcoholism with chronic use.

Alcohol and the Hematopoietic System

The association of anemia, macrocytosis, and alcoholism was long held to be attributable to nutritional deficiencies. Studies have shown that there is a direct role of alcohol on

Table 59.2.
Complications of Alcoholism

Complication	Usual Onset	Comments
Increased morbidity and mortality	Chronic	Most common causes are cirrhosis, cancers of respiratory and gastrointestinal tracts, accidents, suicide, and ischemic heart disease (19).
Fluid and electrolyte abnormalities	Acute	Alcohol has diuretic action as blood alcohol concentration increases. Stable or decreasing blood alcohol concentrations result in antidiuresis. Hyperosmolarity, hypokalemia, hypophosphatemia, and hypomagnesemia are common. Mild lactic acidemia may contribute to asymptomatic elevation of uric acid due to interference with renal secretion of uric acid (19).
Hypoglycemia	Acute or chronic	Alcohol depletes liver glycogen stores and decreases gluconeogenesis, blood sugar may drop precipitously. Stupor and coma, apart from the direct effects of alcohol on the nervous system, are experienced. A dramatic but relatively uncommon complication (20).
Hyperglycemia	Acute	During early phases of alcohol withdrawal, blood sugar may be elevated because of increased release of catecholamines. Alcoholic pancreatitis and decreased peripheral glucose utilization are contributing factors.
Hyperketonemia	Acute	Alcoholic patients frequently develop hyperketonemia and metabolic acidosis in the absence of hyperglycemia. Often the patient is hypoglycemic and without glycosuria. This is presumably due to alcohol-induced starvation ketosis. Insulin is not administered.
Hypothermia	Acute	Occurs frequently as a result of prolonged exposure to cold (not uncommon in unconscious or stuporous state); pancreatitis and meningitis may also contribute.
Liver disease		Best known sequela of chronic alcoholism and a leading cause of morbidity. Three common liver diseases are often associated with alcoholism: acute fatty liver, alcoholic hepatitis, and alcoholic cirrhosis. Individual sensitivity is variable and the degree of liver dysfunction does not appear to be related only to the amount of alcohol ingested. Nutritional status, genetic composition, and immunologic factors appear to interact in the development of alcoholic liver disease (21).
Acute fatty liver	Acute	Develops in nearly all who ingest alcohol excessively (defined by some as an intake of at least 70 g ethyl alcohol daily) even for only a few days. Treatment: to stop drinking and give a diet with adequate vitamin and protein replacement (21).
Alcoholic hepatitis	Acute or chronic	Apparently a toxic inflammatory response of the liver in 10–30% of chronic or acute alcoholics. A high percentage who continue to drink with alcoholic hepatitis develop cirrhosis within 5–10 years. Most patients require 8–12 weeks to show improvement from the acute stage. Treatment is supportive, an adequate diet, vitamin supplements, bed rest, and stopping drinking. In severe cases, liver failure (hepatic coma), variceal bleeding, and hepatorenal syndrome often are present. Clinical features are similar to those of other forms of toxic or viral liver injury. Hepatomegaly, jaundice, splenomegaly, fever, and ascites are common. Corticosteroids may be of benefit in fulminant cases, but their exact role in treatment of this disorder is still being investigated. Some studies have failed to show any benefit from their use (21).
Alcoholic or Laennec's cirrhosis	Chronic	Symptoms are frequently nonspecific in character; e.g., fatigue, weight loss, lethargy. Other physical signs include: slight hepatomegaly, splenomegaly, ascites, gynecomastia, spider angiomas, and palmar erythema. About 10–30% of alcoholics develop alcoholic cirrhosis, usually after drinking heavily for 10–15 years. The three most common causes of death in alcoholic cirrhosis are: bleeding esophageal varices, liver failure (encephalopathy and coma), and infection. The only treatment is to stop drinking (21).
Portal hypertension	Acute or chronic	A sequela of hepatitis. Return of blood from abdominal viscera to the heart is impaired as pressure rises and collateral blood vessels enlarge. All abdominal organs become congested; splenomegaly and ascites result (21).
Ascites	Acute or chronic	Seen often in patients with portal hypertension and may be worsened by alcoholic liver disease and a low serum albumin. A low sodium diet, spironolactone, and sometimes diuretics are helpful. As liver disease improves, ascites will often resolve. Careful monitoring of electrolytes must be done when diuretics and aldosterone antagonists are used (21).
Esophageal varices	Acute	These thin-walled, collateral blood vessels of the portal system are prone to hemorrhaging. Hemorrhage usually occurs when the portal pressure rises because of expanded plasma volume, worsening liver involvement, or increased intraabdominal pressure. Thin walls and accompanying esophagitis are also contributing causes.

(continued)

Table 59.2. *(Continued)*

Complication	Usual Onset	Comments
Encephalopathy	Acute	The central nervous system is depressed by toxins; e.g., ammonia that reaches it through shunted blood that has bypassed liver. The patient is usually lethargic, has "flapping tremor," deterioration of fine movement, and unable to perform any purposeful activity before lapsing into coma. The central nervous system is more sensitive than usual to anoxia, sedative-hypnotics, opiates, or tranquilizers. Coma is frequently precipitated by gastrointestinal hemorrhage, hypokalemia, infection or large amounts of nitrogen from dietary sources such as proteins (22).
Gastrointestinal problems; e.g., pancreatitis, gastritis, peptic ulcer	Acute or chronic	Acute pancreatitis occurs more commonly in alcoholics and is most often seen in persons who have been drinking heavily for 8–10 years or more. Often no characteristic clinical picture except for abdominal pain is present. Nausea and vomiting are common. It is one of the more frequent causes for hospitalization of alcoholics following a drinking bout. Other manifestations of this condition include shock, hypocalcemia, hyperglycemia, marked fluid loss, or dehydration.
		Acute gastritis, often hemorrhagic, is common in alcoholics and is worsened by the chronic use of aspirin. The incidence of peptic ulcer is probably higher in alcoholics than nonalcoholics. Tearing of the gastroesophageal mucosa (Mallory-Weiss syndrome) with severe bleeding may occur as consequence of vomiting; this should be considered a medical and surgical emergency.
Malabsorption	Chronic	Changes in gastrointestinal morphology and decreased enzyme activity in the intestinal tract have been observed in chronic alcoholic patients, even with an adequate diet. Thiamine, vitamin B_{12}, folate, xylose, iron, and fat malabsorption occur. Alcohol consumption and poor diet are major contributors to malabsorption.
Hyperlipidemia	Acute or chronic	Alcohol ingestion induces an elevation of serum triglycerides in persons with type IV hyperlipoproteinemia. Because alcoholic liver disease begins with fatty infiltrates, hypertriglyceridemia may be an early contributory factor to the hepatic and cardiac disorders from alcohol.
Cardiomyopathies	Acute or chronic	Alcohol presumably affects the heart by depressing ventricular activity, reducing myocardial uptake of free fatty acids, enhancing uptake of triglycerides, and causing myocardial cell injury. Direct toxic effects of alcohol on the myocardium, multiple vitamin deficiencies, inadequate protein intake, and electrolyte disturbances are all contributory (23, 24).
Myopathy	Acute or chronic	Generalized and occasionally focal muscle weakness develops during or following heavy drinking bout. Muscle edema, pain, and cramps are common and may be accompanied by tenderness and edema. Elevated muscle enzymes (creatine phosphokinase and aldolase) may be present. In severe cases, myoglobulinuria can occur. Mortality is high (50%) when alcoholic myopathy occurs concomitantly with hyperkalemia and renal failure (25).
Infection	Acute or chronic	Acute and chronic alcohol ingestion decreases resistance to bacterial infection, especially in the respiratory tract. Most pulmonary infections in alcoholics are due to Pneumococcus. Susceptibility to Klebsiella and Haemophilis organisms is also greater. Because they are debilitated, alcoholics are at a higher risk of reactivated tuberculosis; it has been claimed that 20% of patients with active tuberculosis are alcoholics. Aspiration pneumonia is also a major complication. Absence of elevation of white blood cell counts or temperature should not preclude the possibility of infections in an alcoholic (26).
Hematologic disorders; e.g., anemia, leukopenia, thrombocytopenia	Chronic	Four major factors contribute to hematologic disorders: poor diet, blood loss, liver disease, and alcohol itself. Folate deficiency is probably the most important hematologic abnormality in alcoholics. Good diet alone cannot protect against the bone marrow toxicity of alcohol if a major portion of calories are ingested as ethanol. Stopping of alcohol, a nutritious diet including folic acid and multivitamins, and treatment of other medical complications nearly always reverse hematologic abnormalities (27, 28).
Neurologic disorders, polyneuropathy	Chronic	A degenerative process of nerve and brain tissues secondary to nutritional deficiency is common with a long history of alcoholism. Clinical and pathologic features of polyneuropathy are almost identical with beriberi. Subjective sensory disturbances and loss of reflexes and motor activity occur. Recovery is slow and often incomplete, even with complete alcohol abstinence (22, 29).
Wernicke's disease	Acute or chronic	The clinical presentation includes ocular disturbances (e.g., nystagus), muscle weakness or paralysis, diplopia, ataxia, disorientation, and confusion frequently accompanying signs of thiamine deficiency. It can be treated by giving thiamine (22, 29).

(continued)

Table 59.2. *(Continued)*

Complication	Usual Onset	Comments
Korsakoff's psychosis	Acute or chronic	More apparent disturbances in this disorder are cognitive defect and personality changes. Memory may be affected to exclusion of other components of mental function. Recent memory is affected the most. Other clinical features often are confusion and confabulation. Recovery is slow and usually incomplete, despite treatment with thiamine and other vitamins and cessation of drinking (22, 29).
Amblyopia	Chronic	A disorder of the optic nerve occuring alone or in conjunction with other neuropathies; manifested by blurred vision (22).
Skin disorders	Chronic	Skin disorders are common (30–50%) in alcoholic patients and can result from vitamin deficiency diseases such as scurvy or pellagra. Neglected skin disorders often result in secondary infections; seborrhea, lacerations, abrasions, acne, scabies, and pediculosis are also frequent. When common skin conditions (e.g., psoriasis, eczema are not responding to the usual treatment measures, alcoholism may play a role (30).
Teratogenesis	Chronic	Multiple congenital defects, prenatal growth retardation, and delay in development are fetal abnormalities that result from heavy alcohol abuse during pregnancy (31).
Neonatal intoxication and withdrawal)	Chronic	Ethanol crosses the placental barrier freely. The clearance rate of alcohol is reduced in premature infants. Substantial impairment of motor activity, alertness, and respiration are reported in neonates after ethanol infusion just before delivery (32).
Sexual impotence, loss of libido	Chronic	Experienced frequently by male alcoholics. Endocrine effects of alcohol, characteristics of hypogonadism (i.e., gynecomastia), loss of facial hair, spider angiomata, and testicular atrophy, and testosterone deficiency are seen.
Cancer	Chronic	Excessive use of alcohol combined with tobacco has been implicated in greater risks for cancers, particularly of the head, neck, mouth, pharynx, larynx, esophagus, and liver. Alcohol may be a cocarcinogen promoting the activity of true carcinogens (33).

suppression of folate metabolism, depletion of folate from body stores, and malabsorption of folate. The direct toxicity of alcohol on erythropoiesis is demonstrated by vacuolation of erythroid and myeloid precursors (28, 29). A sideroblastic or "iron-loading" anemia can result from the impairment by alcohol of iron incorporation and metabolism in the red blood cell. Alcohol affects iron absorption by increasing jejunal absorption of iron, as reflected in hemochromatosis and a rise in serum iron levels. Iron deficiency anemia due to gastritis and to gastrointestinal bleeding also can occur. Alcoholic thrombocytopenia occurs in 25 to 30% of acutely ill alcoholics; platelets often have shorter than normal life spans, and thrombopoiesis is ineffective because of marrow suppression and folate deficiency.

Fetal Alcohol Syndrome

The relation between heavy alcohol consumption in pregnancy and fetal abnormalities has been suspected since antiquity. In 1973, Jones and his colleagues described a unique clustering of fetal defects in offspring of mothers with chronic alcoholism as the fetal alcohol syndrome (39). Clarren and Smith (32) characterized this pattern of malformation as follows: (1) prenatal and postnatal growth deficiency; (2) central nervous system dysfunction, including physiologic depression, hypotonia, irritability and jitteriness, mental retardation, and poor coordination and hyperactivity during childhood; (3) craniofacial abnormalities, including short palpebral fissures, short upturned nose, hypoplastic philtrum, flat mid-face, and thinned upper lip; (4) other major organ system defects such as abnormalities of the eyes, ears, and mouth, heart murmurs, septal defects, genitourinary abnormalities, hemangiomas, and musculoskeletal problems such as hernias. Longitudinal studies show these children to experience immunodeficiency. No "catch-up" seems to occur in terms of either behavior or intellect in the impaired child with the fetal alcohol syndrome.

The reported incidence of fetal alcohol syndrome is rare, affecting 1:300 to 1:2000 infants. Estimates of the proportion of women who drink heavily during pregnancy range from 2 to 13%, depending on the population studied and survey methodologies.

Many factors may influence the phenotypic outcome of pregnancy in the alcoholic mother, including variable dose exposure at variable gestational periods as well as the genetic background of the individual fetus. Alcohol, like other teratogens, does not uniformly affect all those exposed to it. Rather, there seems to be a continuum of effects of alcohol on the fetus with increasingly severe outcomes generally associated with higher intakes of alcohol by the mother (40).

It should also be noted that alcohol readily enters breast milk, thereby providing alcohol to the nursing infant. There appears to be no established safe amount of alcohol or a safe time to drink it during pregnancy and lactation.

There have been numerous case reports and studies of alcohol use during pregnancy, both in humans and in animal models. The limitations of these studies include variations in population characteristics, nutritional status, techniques for reporting alcohol consumption patterns, and other outcome variables. Most of the studies lack adequate control groups, and thus it is difficult to separate direct effects of alcohol on the fetus from indirect effects by environmental, maternal, and genetic factors. Despite these limitations, these studies appear to be generally consistent in their findings that maternal alcohol abuse is related to adverse effects on fetal growth and development. Abstinence is the preferred course of action during pregnancy and breast-feeding. However, the stress of total abstinence for some pregnant women may endanger the fetus; some physicians suggest limited alcohol use (1 to 2 drinks a week), when needed, stressing the need for adequate nutrition (41).

ACUTE ALCOHOL INTOXICATION

Intoxication from alcohol, like that of other sedative-hypnotics, is characterized by depressed deep tendon reflexes, slurred speech, staggering gait, stupor, and coma through a generalized depression of the central nervous system. Nystagmus and ataxia may also be present.

The lethal dose of alcohol varies in adults: It ranges from 5 to 8 g/kg of body weight. This is lower in children, approximately 3 to 4 g/kg of body weight is considered at risk. The therapeutic index of alcohol is about 1:5, which is low in comparison with other sedative-hypnotic drugs. Diazepam and chlordiazepoxide, for example, have a therapeutic index of approximately 1:7000. Occasionally, alcohol substitutes such as methanol or isopropyl alcohol are ingested. There are differences in the clinical manifestations following ingestion of these agents that distinguish each (Table 59.3).

Diagnosis

The severity of the acute intoxication depends on the blood alcohol level and individual tolerance. Levels below 50 mg/dl, or 0.05%, rarely produce significant effects in adults. In children, signs of alcohol intoxication are often prominent at this level. The presence or absence of the odor of alcohol on a patient's breath cannot be used to establish a

Table 59.3.
Toxicities of Alcohol Substitutes

Substance	Sources	Signs and Symptoms	Management
Methanol (methyl alcohol "denatured alcohol")	Found in solvents, denaturant, antifreeze; toxic amounts attained through inhalation and ingestion	Intractable metabolic acidosis and optic nerve injury can result in 12–24 hours after ingestion. Toxic metabolites are formic acid and formaldehyde. Find both metabolites in urine.	Approximate lethal dose: 1–4 ml/kg in adult. Treat by administering intravenous ethanol to block the generation of toxic metabolites by alcohol dehydrogenase. Administer sodium bicarbonate. Peritoneal dialysis and hemodialysis can be useful.
Isopropanol (isopropyl alcohol)	Found in rubbing alcohol, solvents; toxic amounts attained through inhalation and ingestion	Severe hypoglycemia, acidosis, and coma; hypothermia and convulsions also occur. Infants and children at risk of hypoglycemia. Gastrointestinal irritant. Acetone on breath, in urine, and serum in absence of hyperglycemia or glycosuria.	Approximate lethal dose: 250 g for adult. Alkalinization to correct metabolic acidosis may be helpful. Manage primarily with support.
Ethylene glycol	Found in antifreeze	Clinical abnormalities of the central nervous and cardiopulmonary systems. Oxidation of ethylene glycol by alcohol dehydrogenase to oxalic acid and calcium oxalate, which precipitate in kidney. Oliguria and acute renal failure can occur.	Approximate lethal dose: 100 mg for adult. In children, much lower doses are associated with renal, cardiac, and central nervous system toxicity. Treatment by administration of intravenous ethanol. Alkalinization to correct metabolic acidosis and to solubilize calcium oxalate useful. Hemodialysis has been successful in removing ethylene glycol.

diagnosis of alcohol intoxication. Unique odors should still be noted since they may offer a diagnostic clue to the overall clinical condition of a toxic patient. The plasma osmolality can be a useful indicator since the relationship of osmolality with plasma alcohol is linear. A rise of approximately 25 to 30 milliosmoles/kg H_2O reflects a 100 mg/dl, or 0.1%, increase in plasma alcohol. Concomitant conditions such as trauma, blood loss, infection, multiple drug use, and hypoglycemia will often complicate the recognition and assessment of an intoxicated patient; therefore, the measurement or estimate of the blood alcohol level or comparable analysis of urine, saliva, and expired air is valuable for confirming alcohol intoxication and for establishing an appropriate treatment plan (41).

Other toxicological tests, particularly for barbiturates and other sedative drugs, as well as salicylates, may be indicated to detect suspected commonly occurring poly-drug toxicity. In addition, specific laboratory studies for liver function, renal function, serum electrolytes with particular attention to the potassium, magnesium, and phosphate levels and the anion gap, arterial blood gases, blood ketones, and glucose should be performed routinely. The urine should be examined for the appearance of any crystal-like material or myoglobin. Following a prolonged drinking binge, myoglobinuria, hyperkalemia, and increased serum creatine kinase levels secondary to alcohol myopathy may occur. An electrocardiogram should be taken, and changes characteristic of abnormal calcium, magnesium, and potassium levels or presence of hypoxia or hypothermia should be recognized. An abdominal radiographic examination (KUB) may offer useful clues to the identity of materials ingested in any possible multiple overdose involving an acutely alcohol-intoxicated patient. Some common drugs often taken in suicide attempts such as phenothiazines; tricyclic antidepressants; heavy metals, including iron, arsenic, and halides, iodides, and bromides; chloral hydrate; and enteric-coated tablets are radiopaque. Radiographs of the skull and chest are also advisable at the time of initial examination.

Management

The basic treatment for acute alcohol intoxication is to maintain and support vital functions (i.e., maintain a patent airway and adequate blood pressure, avoid aspiration) until no longer needed during the detoxification process, which takes from 7 to 10 days (33, 42). In the comatose patient, particularly if this involves accidental ingestion of alcohol by a child, acute alcoholic hypoglycemia and other possible causes of coma such as subdural hematoma should be ruled out. Central nervous system stimulants should not be used. The major problems encountered in the management of acute alcohol intoxication are (1) pneumonia, a leading cause of morbidity; (2) overhydration; and (3) complications from unnecessary therapeutic maneuvers.

The possible presence of alcohol should not be overlooked when evaluating a suspected acute case of drug intoxication. One study revealed that almost one of every five acute drug-overdosed patients in whom the presence of alcohol was unsuspected or thought to be irrelevant was found to have high blood levels of alcohol. The notion that acute alcohol intoxication is benign should be dispelled. Diagnosis of any drug intoxication should include a blood ethanol determination in addition to other laboratory tests.

Alcoholic coma is a life-threatening situation that usually responds well to supportive treatment. Establishment of a clear airway and assisted ventilation are essential in this condition. Oxygenation and volume replacement with intravenous fluids generally improves the hypotension. Patients who are experiencing protracted vomiting may have substantial fluid deficits. If alcoholic hypoglycemia is suspected or if the blood glucose is at 70 mg/dl or lower, 50 to 100 ml of 50% glucose should be given intravenously. Thiamine 100 mg given to prevent the possible exacerbation of the Wernicke-Korsakoff syndrome should be administered before or along with the glucose. In circumstances where the recent ingestion of drugs is suspected, gastric lavage can be carefully performed in the unconscious patient with appropriate guarding of the airway to avoid the risk of aspiration. Emetics, such as syrup of ipecac, given to prevent the further absorption of drugs taken in an overdose should be used with great caution in any acutely intoxicated conscious alcoholic patient since tearing of the gastroesophageal mucosa may occur as a life-threatening consequence of ipecac-induced protracted vomiting.

The use of 10% and 40% solutions of fructose given either orally or intravenously in attempts to accelerate the metabolism of ethanol is not recommended. The minimal benefits from such an effort are outweighed by the disadvantages. Adverse effects from fructose include nausea, vomiting, hyperuricemia, worsening of metabolic acidosis, and volume depletion. Increasing the rate of clearance of alcohol from the body also leads to more rapid development of the alcohol withdrawal symptoms (46). Administration of naloxone to reverse alcohol-induced coma has been reported to produce some antagonistic effects in acute alcohol intoxication. In cases described, the responses were quite variable; in some, improvement was only slight. Difficulties were encountered when trying to exclude concomitant opiate use in those patients reported to have responded, (to noloxone) and failed attempts to reproduce these findings in the laboratory have left this issue of naloxone use as an antagonist to alcohol-induced coma unresolved (44, 45).

Treatment of hepatic encephalopathy precipitated by alcohol is to reverse the precipitating factors and lower serum ammonia levels. The immediate approach to bleeding esophageal varices is blood replacement, possible administration of vasopressin, and use of a Sengstaken-Blakemore tube if necessary. Injection of sclerosant solutions can be given for bleeding varices of the esophagus. Sodium morrhuate and sodium tetradecyl sulfate are variceal sclerosing agents available. Reduction of increased blood flow in the portal collateral system and increased intrahepatic resistance with vasoconstrictors, such as vasopressin and somatostatin, or beta-adrenergic blockers, are beneficial in lowering variceal pressures. Surgery may be required to further decompress the varices by shunting the flow of the hepatic portal circulation after the patient has stabilized. This condition is further characterized by sodium retention, progressively worsening oliguria, and eventually azotemia.

A toxic psychosis associated with acute alcohol intoxication occasionally presents as an emergency situation. It is characterized by a markedly impaired sensorium with confusion, amnesia, and disorientation. There is frequently a sudden onset of aggressive and hostile behavior with associated psychotic symptoms, including hallucinations and delusions. The treatment of this agitated phase can be accomplished with sedation to produce a calm, but still arousable, condition. Benzodiazepines and haloperidol can be used judiciously in these circumstances.

A number of considerations should be kept in mind when treating and caring for the patient acutely intoxicated or overdosed with alcohol. The symptoms of acute alcohol intoxication and response to treatment both vary among patients. Factors such as age, weight, tolerance, and concomitant ingestion of other drugs must be considered. Polydrug abuse in the adult with alcohol intoxication should be suspected, and withdrawal from barbiturates or opiates may be a further complication. In children, the toxicological effects of ingredients contained in alcoholic solutions that are used for cough and colds, pain and allergic symptoms, or sleep should be considered. Medical and surgical illnesses may contribute to the toxicological problems of acute alcohol poisoning. The basis of treatment should be to maintain and support vital functions and to individualize all aspects of care and treatment (41).

CLINICAL FEATURES OF ACUTE ALCOHOL ABSTINENCE (WITHDRAWAL) SYNDROME

An acute abstinence, or withdrawal, syndrome is a common problem experienced by the alcoholic when alcohol is discontinued abruptly; delirium tremens (DTs) is the most severe form. The severity of the withdrawal syndrome cannot always be predicted on the basis of the quantity or duration of alcohol ingestion. Although most patients experience only minor and moderate symptoms, described often as a "hangover," it is difficult to rule out the possibility that progressively more severe and even life-threatening withdrawal reactions may occur. There is a wide variability in the severity and duration of this syndrome; 5 to 6% of

those undergoing this experience will progress to the most severe stage: delirium tremens.

The early physiologic and behavioral effects of acute alcohol abstinence experienced (8 to 36 hours after cessation of drinking) include anorexia; tremors ("shakes"); flushing; increased blood pressure, pulse, respiration rate, and temperature; intermittent hallucinations; seizures ("rum fits"); sleep disturbance; and sweating. Mild-to-moderate withdrawal may stimulate the alcoholic to resume drinking in order to reverse the symptoms. A common finding in the later progression of alcoholism is the use of morning drinks ("eye openers") to reduce these effects from drinking the previous night. Late effects, experienced two to six days after cessation of drinking, may include severe tremors, marked agitation, profound disorientation, excitation, persistent visual and auditory hallucinations, marked sleep disturbances, fever, tachycardia, and other life-threatening complications. Patients experiencing major alcohol withdrawal symptoms or delirium tremens, estimated to occur in 5% of hospitalized withdrawing alcoholics, are seriously ill. Patients with DTs are febrile, disoriented, agitated, and will often have an accompanying concurrent medical problem such as infection or coma. Although the mortality rate for this condition has decreased during the past 50 years, deaths from the DTs still occur (variously estimated at 5 to 20%), particularly in patients with underlying or alcohol-associated diseases such as pancreatitis, cirrhosis, gastrointestinal bleeding, pneumonia, or sepsis.

It should not be taken for granted that the intoxicated or bizarre behavior in alcoholics is an effect of alcohol; hypoxia, hyperosmolarity, hypomagnesemia, or hypoglycemia may be contributing to it (41).

The exact pathophysiologic mechanism for the acute alcohol withdrawal syndrome is uncertain. With hyperventilation and respiratory alkalosis, a corresponding rise in arterial pH and fall in serum magnesium takes place. Central nervous system excitability, altered sleep patterns, and other signs of withdrawal are experienced, probably as a result of decreased cerebral blood flow and oxygen delivery to the brain and electrolyte imbalance.

Management

The object of detoxification is to remove alcohol from the body with as few withdrawal symptoms as possible. This process involves the substitution and slow withdrawing of a long-acting sedative-hypnotic drug for the shorter-acting one, alcohol. Some patients in cases of mild withdrawal may not require drugs for relief. In the past 30 years, many different drugs and drug combinations have been described in the medical literature for the treatment of acute alcohol withdrawal (33, 46–53).

A review of studies that investigated the effectiveness of drugs in treating the withdrawal syndrome suggests that many such studies are poorly controlled and lack objective comparisons of effects. In carefully conducted studies, some drugs have not been shown to be necessarily or universally much more effective than placebos. The major benefit of the antianxiety agents may be, in many instances, for the nursing and medical staff as the patient is made more manageable.

Drug Therapy

BENZODIAZEPINES

The sedative-hypnotic drugs of this group, compared to others in this class of agents, are longer-acting, safer, do not produce gastritis, and have antiseizure activity. They are used also because of the convenient dosage forms available. Diazepam and chlordiazepoxide can be administered by oral and intravenous routes, often in gradually tapering doses. Lorazepam is available in oral and parenteral dosage forms. Clorazepate and oxazepam are available in the oral form. The usual therapeutic endpoint in the management of acute alcohol withdrawal symptoms is to produce a calmed but awake patient, using whatever doses are required to achieve this endpoint (33, 55).

The pharmacokinetics of these drugs in patients undergoing alcohol withdrawal or in patients with mild liver impairment have aroused a great deal of clinical and research interest. The elimination half-lives of oxazepam, lorazepam, chlordiazepoxide, clorazepate, and diazepam are 8, 16, 16, 24, and 32 hours, respectively, with wide individual variations existing. In patients with alcohol cirrhosis, the elimination of diazepam from the body is presumably decreased because of decreased clearance by the liver and increased tissue distribution. Because the major metabolites of benzodiazepines, with the exception of oxazepam and lorazepam, are also psychoactive, accumulation of effects during chronic administration of these drugs should be evaluated carefully in patients with cirrhosis. No evidence suggests that any one of the benzodiazepines is better than another for use in acute alcohol detoxification. Most studies on the use of benzodiazepines in this situation have been conducted with chlordiazepoxide. Oxazepam and lorazepam might be considered the drugs of choice, particularly in patients with liver disease who are likely to have impaired metabolism of these drugs.

Dose requirements of these drugs for detoxification are quite variable. The usual range for diazepam is 30 to 200 mg during the first 24 hours, but a few cases may require 1000 mg or more. Withdrawing alcoholics may require more sedative-hypnotic drug than other agitated patients, probably because of tolerance and decreased sensitivity (54). Some alcoholic patients are calmed only by doses that would be severely depressive in nonalcoholic patients. Because dose requirements are variable, no fixed dose schedule can be predicted for a given patient. In a patient

undergoing a mild-to-moderate withdrawal syndrome, an initial oral dose of 20-mg diazepam can be administered orally, followed by 10 to 20 mg every 2 to 3 hours. However, elderly patients should receive only 10 mg initially, followed by doses every 4 to 6 hours if needed. If chlordiazepoxide is the preferred drug, 25 to 100 mg can be given every 2 to 6 hours, depending on symptoms. A total dose of 400 to 600 mg may be needed by extremely tolerant individuals with severe symptoms. In the elderly patient, 50 mg two to four times a day should be sufficient for symptom relief. Treatment with benzodiazepines can even be successfully addressed for patients experiencing mild withdrawal symptoms without coexisting illnesses (49).

Every patient should be reevaluated and drug requirements reassessed every few hours until initial sedation is achieved and then at least daily during the maintenance phase. Standing orders for repetitive doses are not advisable. Predetermined, fixed-dosing regimens contribute often to unnecessary oversedation of the patient undergoing withdrawal. In cases of severe withdrawal, intravenous diazepam should be cautiously administered in a dose of 10 to 30 mg every 30 or more minutes until the patient is calm. Once calmed, a maintenance regimen of 10 to 20 mg can be given intravenously or orally as needed during the day and in the evening to enable sleep. Because of the risks of hypotension and respiratory depression, the patient should be assessed before and periodically after every intravenous dose of a sedative-hypnotic drug. Intramuscular administration of the benzodiazepines should be avoided because of its slow and erratic absorption. With the shorter-acting benzodiazepines, loading doses are not required; however, in order to maintain blood levels sufficient to sustain relief from withdrawal symptoms, doses of oxazepam and lorazepam at 15 to 30 mg and 1 to 4 mg, respectively, need to be given at 6- to 8-hour intervals. Withdrawing these drugs during the detoxification process should be accomplished by lowering their dose rather than by lengthening their administration interval beyond 8 hours.

PHENOTHIAZINES

The phenothiazines have not been shown to be any more effective than the sedative-hypnotic drugs and should not be used. They can result in increased seizures, impaired thermoregulation, extrapyramidal effects, and postural hypotension. The syncope and arrhythmias that can result from these drugs can produce serious consequences in the acutely withdrawing alcoholic. At high doses, delirium can occur as a result of their anticholinergic effects.

BUTYROPHENONES

Haloperidol in oral doses of 5 to 10 mg or 5 mg intramuscularly has been advocated for use in treating hallucinations and acute agitation associated with alcohol. Producing less sedation, hypotension, and hypothermia when contrasted to the phenothiazines, haloperidol, like other dopamine antagonists, however, may cause extrapyramidal and rarely centrally mediated anticholinergic reactions. Extreme caution should be exercised with the use of this drug since the central nervous system depression from the concomitant alcohol may be additive or potentiated.

LITHIUM

Lithium carbonate may also be an effective medication for the treatment of the acute alcohol withdrawal syndrome. Subjective symptoms of alcohol withdrawal appear to ameliorate when lithium is administered before discontinuation of the alcohol (53). The mechanism is unknown because catecholamine release, heart rate, blood pressure, and dopamine beta-hydroxylase are not affected.

CLONIDINE

Clonidine, a centrally acting inhibitor of adrenergic vasomotor centers used in the treatment of hypertension, has been compared with benzodiazepines in the management of acute alcohol withdrawal. Used successfully to treat opiate withdrawal, clonidine can also relieve the tremors, tachycardia, systolic hypertension, and diaphoresis secondary to alcohol withdrawal and appears to be as effective as chlordiazepoxide. Since the ability of clonidine to protect against withdrawal seizures is uncertain, the role of the drug should remain limited to being given only in those situations where the risks of seizures and serious medical or psychiatric complications are minimal (55).

PHENYTOIN

Phenytoin has been advocated for routine use in acute alcohol withdrawal to prevent seizures, but there is no evidence that the drug actually prevents seizures associated with alcohol abstinence. Prospective studies have examined the benefits of phenytoin in preventing additional seizures in alcohol withdrawal once the initial seizure has been experienced. Whether prophylaxis with phenytoin during alcohol withdrawal reduces the risk for seizures is unclear. The study most often referred to as showing that the risk is reduced compared chlordiazepoxide alone and in combination with phenytoin 100 mg given orally three times a day for five days. Although the combination was concluded to be more effective, the phenytoin blood levels were considerably lower than those usually required for seizure control (56).

The seizures associated with acute alcohol withdrawal ("rum fits") are usually self-limiting and frequently do not require anticonvulsant medication. The episode is brief, consisting usually of a single grand-mal-like seizure and only occasionally appears as repeated seizures. This usually occurs in patients with a history of traumatic epilepsy or seizure onset in childhood or adolescence. In the postictal period following alcohol withdrawal seizures, very few will show electro-encephalographic abnormalities. In the acute situation during status epilepticus, small doses (2 to 4 mg) of intravenous diazepam or lorazepam can be administered. Patients who present with or are suspected to have alcohol withdrawal seizures require careful observation and need thorough evaluation for traumatic, infectious, or metabolic causes. Withholding anticonvulsant medications over a 6- to 12-hour period may permit an opportunity to characterize any subsequent seizure that might occur (57).

Long-term antiepileptic drug therapy is unproven and not indicated for alcohol-withdrawal seizures. Focal seizures suggest a central nervous system lesion and are not alcohol related. Patients with status epilepticus or focal seizures may experience greater risks for seizures during alcohol withdrawal. Prophylactic use of phenytoin during the detoxification process might offer some reduction of seizure risk in these circumstances.

PROPRANOLOL

Theoretically, a beta-adrenergic blocking drug such as propranolol should be beneficial in preventing the adrenergic overactivity that occurs during alcohol withdrawal. The alcohol withdrawal syndrome is likely to be mediated in part by the autonomic system (58). Few clinical studies on the use of beta-blockers in alcohol withdrawal have been published. A trial comparing atenolol, a beta-blocker, with placebo in a large group of hospitalized alcohol-withdrawing patients showed the drug had an ameliorating effect on symptoms. Because beta-blockers lack anticonvulsant activity, both groups also received oxazepam 15 or 30 mg four times a day. The results showed a shorter duration of hospital stay, a reduced need for benzodiazepines during hospitalization, and a more rapid return of vital signs to normal in the atenolol-treated patients (59). Propranolol has been shown to be effective in reducing tremor, blood pressure, heart rate, and urinary and total catecholamine levels in alcohol-withdrawing patients.

Potential hazards include the precipitation of congestive heart failure, asthmatic attacks, and peripheral vascular insufficiency, and the masking of symptoms of hypoglycemia. Benefits from the use of beta-adrenergic blockers should, nevertheless, be weighed carefully in each case against the risks before being considered a therapeutic agent for acute alcohol withdrawal syndrome.

PARALDEHYDE

The difficulty in administering this drug, the variability in dose response, and the currently recommended use of safer drugs (e.g., benzodiazepines) have reduced the use of paraldehyde in treating alcoholic withdrawal (46). This traditional and once popular drug was used widely in the treatment of alcohol withdrawal. A major complication of this drug is the ability to produce an acidosis from its acetaldehyde and acetic acid metabolites, which further complicate an already altered acid–base status. Paraldehyde is primarily metabolized in the liver, and thus, its potential for hepatotoxicity should be recognized, particularly when administered to a patient where severe hepatic impairment may exist. Oral or rectal administration is impractical in an acutely agitated alcoholic and causes local irritation of mucous membranes.

ETHANOL

The use of alcohol in the management of acute alcohol withdrawal symptoms is hazardous because of its short duration of action and the risk of continuing the metabolic, endocrine, and neurologic disturbances and pathologies.

ANTIHISTAMINES-HYDROXYZINE

These drugs have been recommended by some and are sometimes used although clinical investigations suggest only equivocal therapeutic benefits. They are less effective in seizure control, and their antianxiety effects have not been well established. Toxic doses of antihistamines may produce anticholinergic symptoms such as delirium and tachycardia that may be confused with acute alcohol withdrawal.

THIAMINE (VITAMIN B₁)

The most serious consequences of thiamine deficiency experienced by chronic alcoholics are neuromuscular effects. Wernicke's syndrome and Korsakoff's syndrome, characterized by ophthalmoplegia, ataxia, peripheral neuropathy, and progressive confusion, are manifestations of the deficiency (23, 60). Thiamine is routinely administered intravenously (100 to 200 mg) to withdrawing alcoholics as a preventive measure. Because glucose solutions are invariably administered to such patients, deficient stores of thiamine may be further depleted as a result.

VITAMIN K

Vitamin K may be used particularly in patients with alcoholic hepatitis or cirrhosis because prothrombin production is frequently impaired.

FOLIC ACID

The moderate to severe anemia seen in alcoholics is usually of the megaloblastic type caused by folic acid deficiency. A combined megaloblastic anemia and microcytic anemia indicating iron deficiency usually results from blood loss in addition to nutritional deficits (24).

FLUIDS, GLUCOSE, AND ELECTROLYTES

It is important to correct fluid and electrolyte imbalances, particularly sodium, potassium, and magnesium, accompa-

nying acute withdrawal (61, 62). In some patients, water is retained and renal resorption of sodium, potassium, and chloride is increased contrary to the notion that all acutely withdrawing alcoholics are dehydrated from the diuresis produced by alcohol (20). An observation common in patients with severe alcohol withdrawal is hypomagnesemia with serum levels ranging from 0.7 to 1.4 mEq/L. Since symptoms of withdrawal such as tremor, hyperreflexia, and seizures are similar to those associated with this condition, the administration of magnesium is thought to aid in reducing the severity and even preventing some of these symptoms.

Summary

The following considerations should be kept in mind when treating and caring for the alcoholic patient in the acute withdrawal phase. The acute alcohol withdrawal syndrome and response to treatment will vary among alcoholic patients. Polydrug abuse occurs in the chronic alcoholic, and withdrawal from barbiturates or opiates would further complicate therapy. An opiate-dependent person who is also dependent on alcohol is generally detoxified from the alcohol while being maintained on methadone. Benzodiazepines are the drugs of choice for treating the acute alcohol withdrawal syndrome because they are distinctly safer than other medications. Patient variables may influence the pharmacokinetics of benzodiazepines, the dose, and the route of administration. The doses of the medication used to treat withdrawal symptoms should be tapered to avoid delayed withdrawal symptoms. Complete eradication of withdrawal symptoms may indicate overmedication. Medical and surgical illness may worsen the acute withdrawal syndrome. Nondrug factors such as staff attitude and ward environment can be effective in helping with the anxiety, insomnia, depression, and other problems that often occur during acute detoxification. There is no evidence that drug therapy during acute alcohol detoxification modifies the outcome of long-term treatment of alcoholism. Detoxification is the first, not the final, step in therapy for alcoholism. The most important factors in successful treatment of and recovery from alcoholism are the motivation of the patient to stop drinking and ongoing participation in recovery support programs, such as Alcoholics Anonymous (AA).

ACUTE INTOXICATION FROM ALCOHOL SUBSTITUTES

Occasionally, alcohol substitutes such as methanol, ethylene glycol, isopropyl alcohol, or paraldehyde are ingested. Often the availability and relative low cost of products containing alcohol substitutes make it convenient for persons intent on drinking alcohol to seek out these products. Many of these products are readily found around the home; they are sweet smelling and pleasant tasting, often colorless, and appear innocuous enough to young children who might be attracted to them. Many of these products are packaged in an attractive manner and not in child-resistant containers, thus contributing to risks of accidental ingestion. There are differences in the clinical manifestations following ingestion of these agents that distinguish each (see Table 59.3).

Methanol

Following ingestion, methanol is rapidly absorbed and distributed throughout the total body water, similarly to ethanol. The toxic dose is extremely variable; as little as 4 ml has been reported to cause blindness though no permanent impairment was demonstrated after an alleged 500 ml had been consumed. Methanol is metabolized by alcohol dehydrogenase enzymes in the liver to formaldehyde and formic acid. The rate of this process is independent of the dose and blood concentration and is approximately one-seventh the rate for ethanol metabolism. Formic acid accumulation is associated with the clinical symptoms experienced.

Methanol produces slight central nervous system depression; unlike ethanol, inebriation is not often observed. Optic nerve and retinal injury from the toxic metabolites develop within 12 to 24 hours following acute exposure. An asymptomatic period of up to a day may follow an acute methanol poisoning before the onset of headache, nausea, and vomiting. Severe abdominal pain, occasionally presumed mistakenly to be the result of ethanol-induced pancreatitis, is experienced. Central nervous system depression, coma, and respiratory failure take place late in the course. The breath odor of alcohol or methanol is frequently not present. In the later stages of the intoxication, the breath odor of formalin and Kussmaul respiration may be noticed. Visual disturbances will occur. They range in severity from mild diminished vision to total blindness, very often accompanied by photophobia, pain, and conjunctival changes. Eye examination will show dilated, nonreactive pupils with optic disk hyperemia and retinal edema. The early recognition of the clinical presentation of acute methanol intoxication is commonly hampered by the effects of concomitant excessive ethanol ingestion.

Laboratory findings in acute methanol intoxication usually include metabolic acidosis, with a large anion gap and moderate ketonemia. Serum amylase is often markedly elevated. A significant leukocytosis is also part of this poisoning. Urine analysis will yield albuminuria with slight to moderate acetonuria. Differential diagnostic considerations would necessarily include diabetic ketoacidosis; lactic acidosis; uremic acidosis; and acute intoxication from ethylene glycol, paraldehyde, isoniazid, or salicylates. Detection of methanol and formic acid in the urine would confirm methanol poisoning.

Early diagnosis and vigorous treatment of methanol poisoning can be sight- and life-saving. A methanol blood level can be obtained. It is estimated that for each 40 mg/dl of methanol in blood, there is an accompanying rise in plasma osmolality of 15 mOsm/kg H_2O. Sodium bicarbonate to reverse the metabolic acidosis and ethanol, either intravenously or orally, should be administered. Ethanol with its greater affinity for alcohol dehydrogenase can competitively inhibit the generation of the toxic metabolites of methanol. Blood ethanol levels of 100 mg/dl or higher are required to saturate the liver enzyme alcohol dehydrogenase. A loading dose of ethanol of 0.6 g/kg body weight, or about 40 g for a 70-kg person, is needed to achieve this desired concentration in the blood. This dose can be given conveniently by mouth with four 1-ounce "shots" of 80-proof whiskey or intravenously as 500 ml of a 10% ethanol solution. Maintenance doses of ethanol should average 7 to 10 g/hr or 109 mg/kg/hr. Hemodialysis is an effective method to treat methanol poisoning and should be initiated promptly where the blood methanol level is greater than 50 mg/dl. The rapidity of blood methanol level reduction appears to be critical for a favorable outcome. Doses of ethanol required to maintain a blood level of 100 mg/dl should be increased to 237 mg/kg/hr. Therefore, a total of 17 g of ethanol must be given hourly during dialysis for a 70-kg person to satisfactorily maintain the desired ethanol blood level. Blood levels of ethanol should be monitored frequently until the methanol has been cleared from the blood (63).

If an acute ingestion of methanol has taken place within several minutes to a few hours from the time of ingestion to initiation of treatment, further gastrointestinal absorption should be decreased with activated charcoal and removal by emesis or lavage. Respiratory and circulatory support should be established and maintained. Forced diuresis does not enhance elimination of either methanol or its metabolites.

Ethylene Glycol

The initial symptoms of acute ethylene glycol poisoning are similar to those for acute ethanol intoxication except for differences in their onset and duration. The earliest sign of ethylene glycol intoxication is inebriation. A breath odor of alcohol is conspicuously absent in persons who have ingested only ethylene glycol. Central nervous system depression and gastrointestinal distress are experienced early in the course. During the first 12 hours, hypertension and leukocytosis are frequently seen. Symptoms may progressively worsen until pulmonary edema, convulsions, respiratory failure, and coma occur (30). Ethylene glycol itself is relatively nontoxic, but its metabolic products are responsible for considerable toxicity. Severe metabolic acidosis, similar to that experienced with acute methanol poisoning, is seen. Glyoxylic acid, oxalic acid, and hippurate are the acid breakdown products of ethylene glycol that cause this profound acidosis. The overproduction and accumulation of lactate and other organic acids also contribute to the acidosis. Acute oliguric renal failure can occur. This is usually severe and believed to be irreversible although survival from this condition has occurred. There is marked renal pathology, including focal hemorrhagic necrosis, oxalate crystals in the convoluted renal tubules, and epithelial cell destruction. Calcium oxalate crystals, considered an important diagnostic marker for ethylene glycol poisoning, are frequently but not always seen on urinalysis. Urinalysis normally shows albumin, red blood cells, and casts.

Myopathy is another common feature of ethylene glycol poisoning. Searching for signs of ethylene glycol is not often helpful for establishing an early diagnosis. Blood ethylene glycol, if rapidly available, is more useful. Serum osmolality can be used to provide an estimation of the toxic ethylene glycol concentration. For every 50 mg/dl of ethylene glycol, the plasma osmolality is increased by 10 mOsm/kg H_2O. A high anion and osmolal gap with metabolic acidosis is quite characteristic of this poisoning. Treatment of acute ethylene glycol poisoning is focused on preventing the metabolism to the toxic metabolites and enhancing its elimination from the body. Ethanol inhibits the metabolism of ethylene glycol by competing for alcohol dehydrogenase. The monitoring and pharmacokinetic considerations of ethanol administration that has been described for methanol are applicable for ethylene glycol. The necessity for rapid treatment in ethylene glycol cannot be overstated. Since the half-life of ethylene glycol is approximately 3 hours, ethanol administration should be initiated promptly. Alkalinization should be attempted with consideration for risks of volume overload and exacerbation of existing electrolyte imbalance.

Hemodialysis readily eliminates ethylene glycol and its metabolites from the body. Blood ethylene glycol levels should be closely monitored since redistribution of the alcohol from tissue to the body water often occurs after dialysis. Repeated dialysis may be necessary to completely clear the ethylene glycol. Support of vital functions such as ventilation, perfusion, and volume are important as in all acute overdoses involving the alcohols.

Isopropyl Alcohol

Isopropyl alcohol is rapidly absorbed following ingestion. Peak plasma levels with distribution throughout body fluids and tissues may be reached within an hour. Inhalation of isopropyl alcohol vapors can produce considerable systemic absorption. With the exception of children, skin absorption is minimal. Coma has been experienced by children who were bathed with excessive amounts of rubbing alcohol. Isopropyl alcohol is metabolized in the liver by alcohol dehydrogenase enzymes to form acetone. Only 15% of this alcohol, when consumed, is eliminated as acetone via the saliva, lungs, and kidneys. The remainder is further converted to acetate, formate, and carbon

dioxide. The rate of isopropyl alcohol metabolism to acetone is slower than that of ethanol. Both isopropyl alcohol and acetone are central nervous system depressants. Tolerance to the toxic levels of both is experienced similarly to the ethanol tolerance seen in chronic alcoholics. Toxic symptoms can occur with an ingestion of as little as 20 ml. Deaths from ingestion of 4 to 8 ounces of 70% isopropyl alcohol have been reported. The symptoms of acute isopropyl alcohol intoxication are similar to those of acute ethanol intoxication except for the absence of any early stimulatory phase. Dizziness, headache, confusion, flushing sensation, ataxia, stupor, hypothermia, and hypotension may be felt. Nausea, vomiting, diarrhea, and severe gastritis occasionally accompanied by bleeding are frequent. Children are often hypoglycemic. Respiratory failure and death can occur within a few hours following a sufficient ingestion of isopropyl alcohol. Marked hypotension, renal dysfunction, and hepatic dysfunction are ominous predictors of outcome on such occasions.

Volume for volume, the toxicity of isopropyl alcohol is considered twice that of ethanol. Toxic symptoms are noticed when blood isopropyl alcohol levels reach 50 mg/dl. In children, symptoms are likely to occur at even lower levels. Coma is associated with levels greater than 120 mg/dl. The range of blood isopropyl alcohol between fatal and severe nonfatal intoxication is narrow. Acetonuria and acetonemia in the absence of glucosuria, hyperglycemia, or acidemia in an acutely intoxicated patient should arouse suspicion of acute isopropyl alcohol poisoning. Unlike ethanol, there is no fixed relationship between the concentration of isopropyl alcohol in the blood and urine, therefore, blood level determination in such circumstances is necessary.

There is no specific treatment for an acute isopropyl alcohol overdose. Usual methods for preventing further and continuous absorption, giving symptomatic and supportive treatment to maintain vital function, should be used. Forced diuresis is of little value. Hemodialysis has been shown to be life-saving in severe and unresponsive isopropyl alcohol poisoning. Repeated gastric lavage to prevent continued reabsorption of isopropyl alcohol has been reported to successfully reverse severe acute toxic symptoms. Use of serial activated charcoal may be effective in removing this alcohol. Many manufacturers of rubbing alcohol have begun to substitute ethanol for isopropyl alcohol, presumably because it is less toxic. Whenever dealing with a history of acute rubbing alcohol ingestion, determine which of these alcohols is in the product prior to treatment.

MANAGEMENT OF CHRONIC ALCOHOLISM

Although the period of detoxification is relatively short, it may take months for the physiologic processes to return to normal. Treatment of the chronic alcoholic is enhanced by maintaining a prolonged alcohol-free period after detoxification.

It is commonly thought that alcoholism is primarily a manifestation of underlying psychiatric problems, and most methods of treatment and dealing with those problems will not succeed while the patient continues to drink. A variety of pharmacotherapeutic approaches are available for management of chronic alcoholism, including use of medications either alone or in combination with behavior modification techniques. Although some recovering alcoholics feel that recovery requires total abstinence from any medication, successful recovery maintenance may depend on pharmacotherapy under the direction of a physician experienced in addiction medicine.

Disulfiram

This drug is considered best used in the context of a close physician–patient or therapist–patient relationship with attempts at behavioral modification (64). Even though disulfiram has been available and used for more than 40 years, a consensus of its therapeutic utility has still not been developed. This is due to methodologic problems inherent in studies in which there is a lack of accurate definitions for the stages of the disorder and an absence of a method to assess compliance.

MECHANISM OF ACTION

When administered alone, disulfiram is relatively nontoxic, but in the presence of alcohol, it alters alcohol metabolism. Disulfiram causes an increase in the blood acetaldehyde levels by interfering with acetaldehyde dehydrogenase action, producing an acetaldehyde syndrome. It also inhibits dopamine beta-hydroxylase, leading to the release and depletion of norepinephrine stores. The patient becomes flushed and develops a scarlet appearance; as the vasodilation continues, palpitations, chest pain, hyperventilation, headache, tachycardia, weakness, hypotension, and syncope occur. Respiratory difficulty, nausea, vomiting, blurred vision, and vertigo may also occur. The reaction may be produced by as little as a few milliliters of alcohol and can last from 30 minutes to several hours. The action of disulfiram may last up to ten days after the patient's last dose. At higher blood alcohol levels, more marked symptoms, including cardiac arrhythmias, heart failure, and death, are experienced.

TREATMENT OF THE DISULFIRAM–ALCOHOL REACTION

The intensity and duration of symptoms are related to the disulfiram dosage, the amount of alcohol consumed, and individual sensitivity. Blood alcohol levels as low as 5 to 10 mg/dl can cause a mild reaction. Although the disulfiram–alcohol reaction is usually short-lived and without major sequelae, death can occur. In many fatal cases, the disulfiram dose was excessive, but in others, there was no apparent explanation. In these inexplicable cases, the causes of death were intracranial hemorrhage, acute myocardial infarction, pulmonary edema, and cerebral edema (65).

There are reports of antidotal treatment of the disulfiram–alcohol reaction with ascorbic acid, iron salts, or antihistamines, but the results are not definitive. Intravenous administration of ascorbic acid (0.5 to 2.0 g) is based on experimental evidence that ascorbic acid appears to reverse the disulfiram inhibition of cellular oxidation.

Table 59.4.
Considerations in Use of Disulfiram

Assessment	Management	Evaluation
Assess for informed consent, motivation, social stability.	Adequate blood level may take up to 4 days, although effect begins within 12 hours. The effect may last up to a week after discontinuation of disulfiram.	Check for side effects (usually transient, lasting 2 weeks), drowsiness, fatigue, impotence, acneform eruption, metallic taste.
Persons with moderate to severe hypertension, psychiatric problems, suicidal ideation should not receive this drug.	Metallic taste may cause anorexia; good oral hygiene may decrease taste.	Nausea and vomiting, dizziness, hypotension, headache, syncope, and flushed face in disulfiram-alcohol reaction.
Interview patient.	Tell patient to avoid alcohol; give list of OTC drugs and foods containing alcohol. Paraldehyde may cause reaction and should not be given. Give with caution concurrently with central nervous system depressants; may potentiate their effects. Patient should carry appropriate medical alert identification with this drug.	Check for other medications being taken; i.e., phenytoin, barbiturates, isoniazid, metronidazole, or warfarin. Disulfiram can potentiate their therapeutic or toxic effects.

However, nonspecific supportive measures such as placing the patient in Trendelenburg posture, administration of oxygen, infusion of fluids and solutes, and (if needed) vasopressor agents are more beneficial than the unproven use of these questionable antidotes. Table 59.4 summarizes the special factors to be considered in the use of disulfiram.

PHARMACOKINETICS

Disulfiram is rapidly absorbed from the gastrointestinal tract; it achieves full pharmacologic action in approximately 12 hours. Disulfiram is eliminated slowly; approximately 20% still remains in the body after a week.

ADVERSE EFFECTS

Although disulfiram is relatively safe in most cases, it can cause acneform eruptions, fatigue, tremor, restlessness, impotence, and a garlicky or metallic taste in the mouth. With large doses, psychologic depression occurs, probably as a result of interference in dopamine beta-hydroxylase activity in the brain. Disulfiram has also been shown to retard the metabolism of oral anticoagulants, isoniazid, and other drugs (see Table 59.6). Any patient receiving disulfiram should be warned to avoid medications that contain alcohol, particularly over-the-counter preparations such as some cough and cold medicines, tonics, antihistamines, body and after-shave lotions, colognes, mouthwashes, and alcohol sponges (66).

DOSAGE

The usual initial dosage of disulfiram is 250 to 500 mg/day for 5 to 7 days. The dosage may then be reduced to 125 to 250 mg/day.

Sedative-Hypnotic Drugs

Anxiety, depression, and insomnia are common in chronic alcoholics. Under most circumstances, these symptoms can be treated supportively, without psychotropic medications. The indiscriminate prescribing of antianxiety agents is all too frequent, and they have a high abuse potential in the alcoholic population. There is no evidence to support outpatient use of psychotropic drugs in the long-term treatment of alcoholism. The use of placebos for relief of anxiety may be worthwhile when basic behavioral problems are dealt with concomitantly.

Antidepressants

Antidepressants for patients in need of therapy for chronic and severe depression should be considered only after careful evaluation of the patient. Antidepressant drugs are too frequently a convenient means of suicide in the depressed alcoholic patient. When antidepressants are prescribed for an alcoholic patient, the patient should be warned that the concomitant use of alcohol or other central nervous depressing agents with these drugs will produce severe impairment of motor and sensory function.

Lithium

There are studies that suggest that lithium, which is indicated for manic depressive disorders, may prevent the progress of primary alcoholism; however, results of these investigations indicate that a comprehensive evaluation of lithium for further evidence of its efficacy is needed (67). The dual diagnosis of other psychiatric illnesses accompanying alcoholism has been increasing, with manic-depressive illness a not infrequent diagnosis. In such cases, lithium therapy may support recovery and might affect the course of alcoholism.

Diet

Malnutrition is commonplace among alcoholics (31). Chronic alcohol consumption results in impaired digestion and absorption of essential nutrients. Nearly all alcoholics have diminished food intake while drinking because alcohol presumably suppresses appetite. Alcohol represents "empty calories" lacking in nutritive value. In excess, alcohol also prevents adequate gastrointestinal absorption of nutrients and contributes to debilitated and malnourished conditions. Nutritional problems that alcoholics are most susceptible to are deficiencies of protein, water-soluble vitamins, and minerals (Table 59.5).

Accumulation of fluids with resultant ascites is a frequent complication of alcoholic cirrhosis. It is secondary to nutritional, endocrine, and metabolic disorders resulting from alcoholism. The basis of management is to supply a normal or fortified diet with restricted sodium intake to replace only daily losses. "Hidden sources" of sodium such as intravenously administered fluids, including plasma and drugs, may be responsible for unexpected reaccumulation of fluids in these patients. Careful monitoring for problems that are related to nutritional balance of the hospitalized alcoholic patient is essential for successful management and care.

Nondrug Treatment Methods

Often alcoholics enter treatment under threat from family, employer, or the courts; they may not at first want the help. Treatment initially attempts to break through the denial systems and help the alcoholic realize that alcoholism is a disease that can be treated. Recovery from alcoholism is a life-long process. Relapse is only one drink away for the alcoholic; they will usually consider themselves "recovering" rather than "recovered" alcoholics.

Several techniques for behavioral modification are used with the chronic alcoholic. Individual psychotherapy is useful in those patients who are intelligent, well-motivated, and financially secure. Group psychotherapy allows for

Table 59.5.
Nutritional Problems Associated with Alcoholism

Source	Signs and Symptoms	Comments
Protein	Fatty liver and hypoalbuminemia may be result of deterioration of liver function or low protein intake. Others: hypocholesterolemia, edema, normocytic anemia.	Association of alcohol with liver disease complicates the interpretation of many clinical signs of protein deficiency. Alcoholic liver disease is not prevented by eating well or limiting alcohol consumption only to certain types of beverages. Administration of protein to patients with severe active alcoholic cirrhosis can precipitate hepatic coma. When protein is poorly tolerated or the patient becomes progressively disoriented, showing asterixis or flapping temors, administration of protein should be discontinued.
Water-soluble vitamins, vitamin B complexes, thiamine	The signs and symptoms are variable depending on severity of the deficiency: ophthalmoplegia, sixth-nerve palsy, nystagmus, weakness, ataxia, peripheral neuropathies, confusion, amnesia, coma, heart failure, Wernicke's syndrome, "beriberi" heart disease, sudden death.	Most common deficiency in alcoholics. Polyneuropathy is the mildest and most common form of thiamine deficiency. Depressed tendon reflexes, muscle cramps, weakness, paresthesias and pain develop. The lower extremities are most often affected. Prognosis grave and must be recognized early. Treatment is to give thiamine. Administration of glucose without thiamine may further deplete stores of thiamine. Thiamine deficiency-induced heart failure does not respond well to digitalis or diuretics. Animal studies suggest that thiamine deficiency reduces myocardial oxygen consumption due to deficiency of the coenzyme thiamine pyrophosphate. Average requirement is 1.5 to 2 mg thiamine for adult per day. Alcoholics often will require more; 100 to 200 mg results in dramatic reversal of signs and symptoms.
Niacin	Weakness, photosensitive dermatitis, stomatitis, gastritis, diarrhea, peripheral neuropathy, dementia, encephalopathy	Alcoholic pellagra is the result of the lack of dietary nicotinic acid or its precursor, tryptophan. Niacin contributes to formation of specific coenzyme nucleotides (NAD) which participate in intracellular metabolism and cell respiration. Replacement dose is 200 mg niacinamide three times a day.
Riboflavin	Weakness, photosensitive dermatitis, stomatitis, gastritis, diarrhea, peripheral neuropathy, dementia, encephalopathy	Riboflavin deficiency usually accompanies alcoholic pellagra. Riboflavin is an essential constituent of coenzymes responsible for oxidative and electron transport processes. Replacement dose is 10 mg per day.
Pyridoxine	Irritability, anemia, insomnia, peripheral neuropathy, ataxia, skin lesions	Pyridoxine is responsible for a variety of enzymatic activities particularly related to nitrogen metabolism.
Ascorbic acid	Anorexia, petechial ecchymoses, gingivitis and bleeding gums, dry mouth, loss of hair, perifollicular hemorrhages, purpuric lesions, ecchymoses, itchy dry skin, weakness, lethargy	Ascorbic acid is a coenzyme involved in the metabolism of amino acids. Usual amount recommended is 10 mg/day.
Folic acid	Macrocytic anemia, reticulocytosis	Deficiency of folic acid is the primary cause of macrocytic anemia in chronic alcoholics. Alcohol directly affects the hematopoietic activity and interferes with utilization of folic acid. Must discontinue alcohol. Usual amount recommended for replacement is 1.0 mg daily.
Magnesium	Lethargy, muscle weakness, coarse athetoid movements, gross tremors of hands and tongue, mental changes, convulsions, stupor, coma	Alcohol promotes the renal excretion of magnesium. Renal effect and inadequate diet cause significant depletion. Symptoms of acute alcohol withdrawal are often complicated by coexisting magnesium depletion. The total body magnesium deficits are not reflected by serum magnesium levels.
Potassium	Weakness; lethargy	Poor dietary intake of potassium and loss by diuresis, vomiting, and diarrhea contribute to hypokalemia.

interaction among alcoholics to deal with difficulties they have in common. An estimated success rate of 80 to 90% of health professionals and 70% of employed people who participate in a full-recovery program for at least 2 years can be contrasted with a 4-year sobriety rate of less than 5%

for "skid row" alcoholics. In managing the chronic alcoholic, the goal is to achieve and maintain sobriety or prolong the periods of sobriety to give the patient time to learn to identify and avoid factors that may promote drinking, or so-called slips.

The preferred full-recovery program includes (1) education about the disease of alcoholism; (2) abstinence from alcohol and other psychoactive substances (not forever, but "one day at a time," as is recommended by Alcoholics Anonymous); (3) group therapy (regular attendance at Alcoholics Anonymous meetings or the equivalent; formal, interactive group therapy, preferably for at least 2 years; and family therapy, including participation of family members in Al-Anon or similar support group meetings). Initially, treatment may involve formal participation in an inpatient (residential) treatment program, usually for several weeks, followed by intensive outpatient therapy for a number of weeks, then regular "after-care" meetings, usually through the treatment provider. Difficult cases may require more prolonged inpatient therapy, whereas relatively uncomplicated, low-risk cases may be totally managed on an outpatient basis.

Employee assistance programs are available through most major employers; these programs often require employees to sign a recovery agreement. Such agreements assure understanding of the terms of continued employment, encourage ongoing sobriety, and provide employers with assurance of compliance. Random drug screening at employee expense is often a stated condition of the agreement.

For individuals who have inadequate support systems in place at home to assure sobriety during outpatient therapy or early in the recovery process following such therapy, "half-way" houses may be used. These provide a community living environment with fairly rigid rules, ongoing group therapy, and requirements, such as maintaining employment, that encourage responsibility and social adaptation during sobriety. Half-way houses are most often used by individuals recovering from drug addictions other than alcohol and by those with multiple addictions.

The group support approach of AA takes a more structured and evangelistic attitude in dealing with alcoholics; it has returned many alcoholics to sobriety and helped maintain ongoing recovery. Basic tenants of AA's 12 steps are acceptance of the disease nature of alcoholism, acceptance of an external locus of control in life, "cleaning house" (guilt reduction through the process of confession and maintenance of ongoing honesty), and helping other alcoholics. AA is a private organization whose members offer mutual support to one another to remain free of alcohol. Meetings occur regularly. Individuals in early recovery are often encouraged to attend 90 AA meetings in 90 days; this encourages the alcoholic to maintain frequent contact with a support system and forces him or her to attend a number of different meetings. Since AA meetings vary in format and character, the recovering alcoholic can eventually identify meetings that meet his or her specific needs and schedules. Other similar groups such as the

Salvation Army and Volunteers of America also have help groups for assisting in the recovery of alcoholics. Alcoholism resources listed in the yellow pages of telephone books can identify these and other treatment and support resources in the community. Many support groups exist for specific populations, such as lawyers, physicians, pharmacists, and nurses. These exist to provide support for problems unique to recovery for each group and are not intended to replace participation in other support groups, such as AA.

ALCOHOL–DRUG INTERACTIONS

Because approximately 70 to 80% of adults consume alcoholic beverages, it is almost inevitable that medications either prescribed by a physician or bought over the counter will be taken concomitantly with alcohol or while alcohol is still in the body. Often these preparations are sources of the alcohol that interacts with prescribed medications to produce untoward effects in the unsuspecting patient (68).

Cimetidine, ranitidine, and nizatidine, but not famotidine, have been shown to decrease gastric alcohol dehydrogenase activity, resulting in increased alcohol absorption and effects (68, 69).

Alcohol administration in high concentrations results in increased metabolism by MEOS, with concurrent inhibition of metabolism of drugs that undergo microsomal degradation. The repeated administration of alcohol has been shown to cause nonspecific hepatic microsomal enzyme induction, resulting in increased clearance of both alcohol and microsomally metabolized drugs, such as barbiturates (70–72). Following withdrawal of alcohol, enhanced hepatic metabolism of drugs may persist for some time, requiring higher doses of affected drugs. Metabolic pathways such as N-desmethylation of the longer-acting benzodiazepines and oxidation and glucuronidation are inhibited by acute alcohol intake. With chronic use, however, metabolism increases. This explains partially the "tolerance" to the action of sedatives observed in some chronic alcoholics. Warfarin, phenytoin, tolbutamide, procainamide, and isoniazid are nonpsychoactive drugs subject to hepatic microsomal enzyme activity. The plasma half-lives of these drugs are markedly decreased in some chronic and heavy users of alcohol as a result of their increased rate of clearance. Clinical reports of problems from such interactions, however, are few. Variable and unpredictable response to drugs in the alcoholic should suggest the possibility of some metabolic alteration of drug kinetics. It has become increasingly evident that toxicity to certain drugs and chemicals is enhanced in chronic alcoholics as a result of this mechanism. The hepatotoxic risk with acetaminophen usage or with carbon tetrachloride ingestion is increased in chronic alcoholics because of increased formation of toxic metabolites of these chemicals caused by MEOS induction.

Table 59.6.
Summary of Selected Alcohol-Drug Interactions

Drugs Interacting with Alcohol	Mechanism	Effect	Significance
Anticoagulants (oral): warfarin	Metabolism enhanced with chronic alcohol abuse	Diminished anticoagulant effect	Moderate
	Metabolism reduced with acute alcohol intoxication	Increased anticoagulant effect	Moderate
Antihistamines	Additive	Increased central nervous system (CNS) depression	Moderate
Aspirin (and other salicylates)	Additive	Increased occult blood loss and damage to gastric mucosa	Moderate
Acetaminophen	Metabolism enhanced in chronic alcohol abuse	Increased risk for hepatotoxicity	Moderate
	Metabolism reduced in acute alcohol intoxication	Reduced risk for hepatotoxicity	Moderate
Anticonvulsants: phenytoin (Dilantin) and others	Metabolism enhanced with chronic alcohol abuse	Diminished anticonvulsant effect	Moderate
	Metabolism reduced with acute alcohol intoxication	Increased anticonvulsant effect	Moderate
Antimicrobials: isoniazid	Metabolism enhanced in chronic alcohol abuse	Diminished isoniazid effect	Moderate
		Increased incidence of isoniazid hepatitis	Not established
cefoperazone, cefamandole, metronidazole chloramphenicol, griseofulvin	Metabolism of alcohol reduced	Disulfiram-like reaction	Minor to moderate
Antidiabetic agents:	Additive	Hypoglycemia effect increased	Moderate
sulfonylureas, tolbutamide (Orinase), glipizide (Glucotrol)	Metabolism enhanced in chronic alcohol abuse	Decreased effect	Moderate in chronic alcoholic
acetohexamide (Dymelor)	Accumulation of acetaldehyde	Disulfiram-like reaction	Moderate
phenformin (DBI)	Alteration of biochemical pathway	Lactic acidosis	Major
insulin	Interferes with hepatic gluconeogenesis	Increased hypoglycemic effects	Moderate but major if liver is damaged
Antihypertensives: methyldopa (Aldomet)	Additive	Sedation	Minor to moderate
reserpine, methyldopa (Aldomet), guanethidine (Ismelin), hydralazine (Apresoline)	Additive	Postural hypotensive effect increased	Minor to moderate
Disulfiram (Antabuse)	Inhibits intermediate metabolism of alcohol	Abdominal cramps, flushing, vomiting, confusion, hypotension	Major
Monoamine oxidase inhibitors: pargyline, tranylcypromine, procarbazine	Alteration of tyramine metabolism additive	Increased CNS depression, hypertensive crisis	Moderate to major
Narcotic analgesics: meperidine (Demerol), morphine, methadone	Additive	Increased CNS depression	Major
Nonbarbiturates: (ethchlorvynol, glutethimide, meprobamate)	Tolerance with chronic alcohol use	Diminished CNS effect	Minor to moderate
chloral hydrate	Additive with acute alcohol intoxication and competition	Increased CNS depression	Moderate
Nonsteroidal antiinflammatory drugs: indomethacin	Additive	Possible additive, gastric mucosal damage	Minor
Sedative-hypnotics: barbiturates (phenobarbital, pentobarbital, secobarbital)	Additive or metabolism enhanced with acute alcohol intoxication	Increased CNS depression	Major
Tranquilizers: phenothiazines (Thorazine, etc.)	Additive	Impaired coordination and judgment, also increased CNS depression	Moderate

Alcohol is primarily a central nervous system depressant. When combined with other drugs with similar depressing action on the central nervous system, an additive or synergistic effect occurs. This is the most important type of interaction between alcohol and other drugs.

Alcoholics taking tolbutamide and other antidiabetic drugs, chloramphenicol, griseofulvin, quinacrine, or metronidazole have reported a mild "disulfiramlike" reaction (Table 59.6). Alcohol consumption during ceforanide, cefotetan, cefamandole, or cefoperazone therapy may precipitate a disulfiramlike reaction. Some alcoholic beverages such as chianti wines contain appreciable amounts of tyramine that, when taken by patients using monoamine oxidase-inhibiting (MAOIs) drugs (i.e., procarbazine, pargyline), cause an acute hypertensive episode. Interference with tyramine metabolism by the MAOIs results in the release of norepinephrine from the sympathetic nerve terminal.

Alcohol as a Therapeutic Agent

There is a prevailing notion that alcohol may have some usefulness in the treatment of a variety of disorders and conditions. Clinical evidence, however, is not encouraging

Table 59.7.
"Therapeutic" Use of Alcohol

Proposed Use	Actual Effect
Relief of anxiety	Anxiety often worsens when blood alcohol level falls, as in withdrawal.
Bedtime sedation	Sleeplessness is less common as blood alcohol level declines.
Improvement of nutrition	Blood sugar levels become more labile; although each gram of alcohol = 7.1 calories on oxidation, "empty" calories are gained. Overall nutrition not improved with alcohol because vitamins, minerals or other essential dietary materials are absent in alcoholic beverages.
Diuresis of edema	Diuretic response to alcohol occurs when blood alcohol level is on the rise; antidiuresis, hypersomality, and fluid retention occur as blood alcohol concentration falls.
Anemia	Iron metabolism and bone marrow function are affected, and folate antagonism contributes to anemia in spite of frequent presence of iron in wines.
Lowering of blood sugar in diabetics	Lowering of blood sugar is negligible. In fact, alcohol produces more labile blood sugar levels.
Heart disease	The alcohol metabolite acetaldehyde is toxic to myocardium and not effective as a coronary vasodilator. Alcohol is a myocardial depressant. Although alcohol enhances coronary blood flow, myocardial oxygen consumption simultaneously increases.
Antiinfective	Chronic alcoholism predisposes to systemic infections.

about the role of alcohol in therapy, and it may actually worsen many conditions for which its use has been suggested (Table 59.7).

Intravenous administration of 10% volume/volume alcohol has been used with some success to delay premature labor and prolong gestation. The efficacy of this method has been compared with ritodrine to delay premature labor by inhibiting uterine contractions. Ritodrine, a synthetic sympathomimetic amine, was considered more effective. Blood alcohol levels of 100 to 150 mg/dl are required to inhibit uterine contractions. Studies of placenta and cord blood alcohol levels following delivery showed they were slightly less than that of the mother. In fact, neonatal depression of respiratory and circulatory activity after administration of alcohol before delivery have been reported.

CONCLUSION

Much confusion has arisen amid a widely publicized 1976 report by the Rand Corporation on alcoholism that seems to imply that some alcoholics can return to social drinking (73). The goal of alcohol abstinence by the alcoholic has been long advocated. For instance, Alcoholics Anonymous considers abstinence the only goal for anyone with an alcohol problem. Careful evaluation of data from this report does not support the notion that alcoholics can safely return to drinking. What it did point out was that after an 18-month period, relatively few alcoholics were practicing long-term abstinence despite an impressive improvement rate (70%). Most had intermittent periods of abstinence interspersed with "controlled" drinking. Relapse to uncontrolled drinking by those who continued to drink in a "controlled" manner and those who continued abstinence was found to be no different. Major methodologic problems are suggested by the large number (more than 80%) of subjects lost to follow-up at the end of the 18-month study period. The same investigators in a 1980 follow-up report sharply modified their original claims; however, this has accomplished little to discourage the many and vocal advocates of "controlled drinking" for alcoholics (74).

Abstinence from alcohol should not be a goal for treatment but rather a means to an end. The treatment of alcoholism is best accomplished if conducted in a relationship of understanding and trust with others. This can be a concerned and interested friend or spouse, or a professional, or members of a therapeutic or rehabilitation group. Dependence on alcohol is no different in any significant way from dependency on other addictive drugs such as opiates and barbiturates. Although there are differences in social attitudes toward drinking and drug abuse, many features of alcohol and "hard drugs" are remarkably similar. The similarities and differences should be appreciated and understood by those who are involved in the treatment, care, and rehabilitation of alcohol-dependent patients.

ACKNOWLEDGMENTS

The authors acknowledge and thank Dr. Linda R. Bernstein, Clinical Associate Professor, School of Pharmacy, University of California San Francisco, coauthor (with Theodore G. Tong) of "Alcoholism and Substance Abuse in Clinical Pharmacy," Clinical Pharmacy and Therapeutics, 4th ed, Ch 40, for contributing to the discussion on "Fetal Alcohol Syndrome" that appears here.

REFERENCES

1. Harwood HJ, Kristiansen P, Rachal JV. Social and economic costs of alcohol abuse and alcoholism. Issue Report No. 2. Research Triangle Park, NC: Research Triangle Institute, 1985.
2. West LJ, Maxwell DS, Noble EP, et al. Alcoholism. Ann Intern Med 100:405–416, 1984.
3. Cotton NS. The familial incidence of alcoholism. J Stud Alcohol 40:89–116, 1979.
4. Committee on Adolescence, American Academy of Pediatrics. Alcohol use and abuse: a pediatric concern. Pediatrics 79:450–453, 1987.
5. Blume SB. Women and alcohol. JAMA 256:1467–1470, 1986.
6. Seventh Special Report to the U.S. Congress on Alcohol and Health. Rockville, MD: National Institute on Alcohol Abuse and Alcoholism, 1990:1–41.
7. Wallace J. The new disease model of alcoholism. West J Med 152:502–505, 1990.
8. Blum TC, Roman PM, Bennett N. Public images of alcoholism: data from a Georgia survey. J Stud Alcohol 50:5–14, 1989.
9. Frezza M, di Padora C, Pozzata G, et al. High blood alcohol levels in women. N Engl J Med 322:95–99, 1990.
10. Morgan MY, Sherlock S. Sex-related differences among 100 patients with alcoholic liver diseases. Br Med J 1:939–941, 1977.
11. Ehrig T, Bosron WF, Ting-Kai L. Alcohol and aldehyde dehydrogenase. Alcohol & Alcoholism 25:105–116, 1990.
12. Mendelson JH. Biologic concomitants of alcoholism: Parts I and II. N Engl J Med 283:24, 71–81, 1970.
13. Lieber CS. Metabolism and metabolic effects of alcohol. Med Clin N Amer 68:3–31, 1984.
14. Vessell ES, Page PG, Passananti GT. Genetic and environmental factors affecting ethanol metabolism in man. Clin Pharmacol Ther 12:192–201, 1971.
15. Blum K, Noble EP, Sheridan PJ, et al. Allelic association of human dopamine D_2 receptor gene in alcoholism. JAMA 263:2055–2060, 1990.
16. American Psychiatric Association. Diagnostic and Statistical Manual of Mental Disorders, 4th edition. Washington, DC: American Psychiatric Association, 1994.
17. Ewing JA. Detecting alcoholism: the CAGE questionnaire. JAMA 252:1905–1907, 1984.
18. Cyr MG, Wartman SA. The effectiveness of routine screening questions in the detection of alcoholism. JAMA 259:51–54, 1988.
19. Eckardt MJ, Harford TC, Kaelbar CT, et al. Health hazards associated with alcohol consumption. JAMA 246:648–666, 1981.
20. Kaysen G, Noth RH. The effects of alcohol on blood pressure and electrolytes. Med Clin N Amer 68:221–246, 1984.
21. Williams HE. Alcoholic hypoglycemia and ketoacidosis. Med Clin North Am 68:33–38, 1984.
22. Pimstone NR, French SW. Alcoholic liver disease. Med Clin North Am 68:39–56, 1984.
23. Nakada T, Knight RT. Alcohol and the central nervous system. Med Clin North Am 68:121–131, 1984.
24. Segel LD, Klausner SC, Harney-Gnadt JJ, et al. Alcohol and the heart. Med Clin North Am 68:147–161, 1984.
25. Demakis JG, Proskey A, Rahimtoola SH. The natural course of alcohol cardiomyopathy. Ann Intern Med 80:293, 1974.
26. Haller RG, Knochel JP. Skeletal muscle disease in alcoholism. Med Clin North Am 68:91–103, 1984.
27. Adams HG, Jordan C. Infections in the alcoholic. Med Clin North Am 68:179–201, 1984.
28. Eichner ER. The hematologic disorder of alcoholism. Am J Med 54:621, 1973.
29. Larkin EC, Watson-Williams EJ. Alcohol and blood. Med Clin North Am 68:105–120, 1984.
30. Scully RE, Galdabini JJ, McNeely BU. Case records of the Massachusetts General Hospital: Case 38-1979: ethylene glycol poisoning. N Engl J Med 301:650–657, 1979.
31. Leevy C, Baker H. Vitamins and alcoholism. Am J Clin Nutr 21:1325, 1968.
32. Clarren SK, Smith DW. The fetal alcohol syndrome. N Engl J Med 298:1063, 1978.
33. Sellers EM, Kalant H. Alcohol intoxication and withdrawal. N Engl J Med 294:757–762, 1976.
34. Breeden JH. Alcohol, alcoholism and cancer. Med Clin North Am 68:163–177, 1984.
35. Lieber CS. Alcohol and the liver: 1984 update. Hepatology 4:1243–1260, 1984.
36. Altura BM. Introduction to the symposium and overview. Alcoholism (NY) 10:557–559, 1986.
37. Klatsky AL. Epidemiology of coronary heart disease: influence of alcohol. Alcohol Clin Exp Res 18:88–96, 1994.
38. Rubin R, Rand ML. Alcohol and platelet function. Alcohol Clin Exp Res 18:105–110, 1994.
39. Lange LG, Kinnunen PM. Cardiovascular effects of alcohol. Adv Alcohol Subst Abuse 6:47–52, 1987.
40. Klatsky AL. The cardiovascular effects of alcohol. Alcohol & Alcoholism 22(suppl 1):117–124, 1987.
41. Purdie FR, Honigman B, Rosen P. Acute organic brain syndrome: a review of 100 cases. Ann Emerg Med 10:455–461, 1981.
42. Khantzian EJ, McKenna GJ. Acute toxic withdrawal reactions associated with drug use and abuse. Ann Intern Med 90:361, 1979.
43. Coarse JF, Cardoni AA. Use of fructose in the treatment of acute alcoholic intoxication. Am J Hosp Pharm 32:518, 1975.
44. Lyon LJ, Antony J. Reversal of alcoholic coma by naloxone. Am Intern Med 96:464–465, 1982.
45. Mattila MJ, Nuotto E, Seppala T. Naloxone is not an effective antagonist of ethanol. Lancet 1:775–776, 1981.
46. Thompson WL, Johnson AD, Maddrey WC. Diazepam and paraldehyde for treatment of severe delirium tremens. Ann Intern Med 82:175–180, 1975.
47. Kaim SC, Klett J. Treatment of delirium tremens. Q J Stud Alcohol 33:1065,1072, 1972.
48. Sellers EM, Naranjo CA, Harrison M, et al. Diazepam loading: simplified treatment of alcohol withdrawal. Clin Pharmacol Ther 34:822–826, 1983.
49. Hayashida M, Alterman AL, McClellan AT, et al. Comparative effectiveness and cost of inpatient and outpatient detoxification of patients with mild to moderate alcohol withdrawal syndrome. N Engl J Med 320:358–365, 1989.
50. Sellers EM, Cooper SD, Zilm DH, et al. Lithium treatment of alcohol withdrawal. Clin Pharmacol Ther 20:199, 1976.
51. Miller WC Jr, McCurdy L. A double-blind comparison of the efficacy and safety of lorazepam and diazepam in the treatment of the acute alcohol withdrawal syndrome. Clin Therap 6:364–368, 1984.

52. Greenblatt DJ, Greenblatt M. Which drug for alcohol withdrawal? J Clin Pharmacol 12:429–431, 1972.

53. Saitz R, Mayo-Smith MF, Roberts MS, et al. Individualized treatment for alcohol withdrawal: a randomized double-blind controlled trial. JAMA 272:519–523, 1994.

54. Kloz UA, Avant GR, Hoyumpia A, et al. The effects of age and liver disease on the disposition and elimination of diazepam in adult man. J Clin Invest 55:347, 1975.

55. Baumgartner GR, Rowen RC. Clonidine versus chlordiazepoxide in the management of acute alcohol withdrawal syndrome. Arch Intern Med 147:1223, 1987.

56. Sampliner R, Iber FL. Diphenylhydantoin control of alcohol withdrawal seizures. JAMA 230:1430–1432, 1974.

57. Brown CG. The alcohol-withdrawal syndrome. West J Med 138:579–581, 1983.

58. Mendelson JH. Propranolol and behavior of alcohol addicts after acute alcohol ingestion. Clin Pharmacol Ther 15:571, 1974.

59. Kraus ML, Gottlieb LD, Horwitz RI, et al. Randomized clinical trial of atenolol in patients with alcohol withdrawal. N Engl J Med 313:905–909, 1985.

60. Victor M, Adams RD. On the etiology of the alcoholic neurologic diseases with special reference in the role of nutrition. Am J Clin Nutr 9:379, 1961.

61. Vetter WR, Cohn LH, Reichgott M. Hypokalemia and electrocardiographic abnormalities during acute alcohol withdrawal. Arch Intern Med 120:536, 1967.

62. Beard JD, Knott DH. Fluid and electrolyte balance during acute withdrawal in chronic alcoholic patients. JAMA 204:135, 1968.

63. McCoy HG, Cipolle RJ, Ehlers SM, et al. Severe methanol poisoning: application of a pharmacokinetic model for ethanol therapy and hemodialysis. Am J Med 67:804–807, 1979.

64. Fuller RK, Branchey L, Brightwell DR, et al. Disulfiram treatment of alcoholism: a Veterans Administration Cooperative study. JAMA 256:1449–1455, 1986.

65. Elenbaas RM, Ryan JL, Robinson WA, et al. On the disulfiram-like activity of moxalactam. Clin Pharmacol Ther 32:347–355, 1982.

66. Tong TG, Bernstein LR. Alcoholism. In: Herfindal GT. Clinical Pharmacy and Therapeutics, 3rd ed. Baltimore, Williams & Wilkins, 1983:146–155.

67. Dorus W, Ostrow DG, Anton R, et al. Lithium treatment of depressed and nondepressed alcoholics. JAMA 262:1646–1652, 1989.

68. Caballeria J, Baraona E, Rodamilans M, et al. Effects of cimetidine on gastric alcohol dehydrogenase activity and blood ethanol levels. Gastroenterology 96:388–392, 1989.

69. Caballeria J, Baraona E, Rodamilans M, et al. Cimetidine and alcohol absorption. Gastroenterology 97:1067–1068, 1989.

70. Lane EA, Guthrie S, Linnoila M. Effects of ethanol on drug and metabolite pharmacokinetics. Clin Pharmacokin 10:228–247, 1985.

71. Hoyumpa AM, Schenker S. Ethanol-drug interaction. Annu Rev Med 33:113–149, 1982.

72. Lieber CS. Interaction of ethanol with drugs, hepatotoxic agents, carcinogens and vitamins. Alcohol & Alcoholism 25:157–176, 1990.

73. Armour DJ, Polich JM, Stambul HB. Alcoholism and Treatment. The Rand Corporation, R-1739-NIAAA, New York, John Wiley and Sons, 1978.

74. Polich JM, Armour DJ, Braiker HV. The Course of Alcoholism Four Years After Treatment. The Rand Corporation, R-2433-NIAAA, 1980.

CHAPTER 60

DRUG ABUSE

JAMES C. EOFF III and RITA G. BATES

Drug abuse in the United States reached epidemic proportions during the 1980s. Combined efforts at the local, state, and federal levels to attempt to curtail this problem have been implemented. There has been moderate success of the national "war on drugs" and state efforts like the "drug free" and "just say no" programs. However, recent statistics indicate that drug use among junior and senior high school students is once again increasing. The overall cost of drug abuse to our society continues to be great. Crime and violence continue to increase, with 65% of all crimes being drug related. Drug abuse contributes to rising medical costs both through rehabilitation and treatment programs and significantly through treatment of medical consequences such as the spread of infectious diseases (e.g., AIDS, hepatitis). Drug abuse is responsible for thousands of deaths by accidental overdosage and suicide and half of the 45,000 traffic fatalities in the United States are drug or alcohol related. Drug abuse also causes higher taxes to pay for the prevention, treatment, and rehabilitation programs, not to mention the burden to the criminal justice system, including the courts, prisons, and law enforcement agencies. Drug abuse disrupts families and schools, and it lowers productivity and causes loss of creative potential. All health professionals need to be involved in education and prevention programs to help control and eliminate this problem to society.

Drug abuse is the self-administration of a drug that deviates from the approved medical or society patterns within a given society. People misuse drugs for a number of reasons. The primary factors in young people are peer pressure and the fear of being different, the desire to "fit in." Other well-known reasons for drug abuse are curiosity, boredom, escape, pleasure seeking, insecurity, and rebellion involving a desire to prove independence. Different classifications of drug abusers range from the experimental user who tries drugs only one or two times for curiosity, to the recreational user who occasionally uses drugs, to the heavy user who administers the drug every day. Compulsive drug users (drug dependence) have a compelling desire to continue self-administration of a drug either to experience its effects or to avoid the discomfort of its absence. This terminology is used in most reports of drug abuse and has generally replaced the term *drug addiction*. Physical dependence refers to an altered physiologic state resulting from the chronic administration of a drug, which requires the continued administration of the drug to prevent a characteristic set of withdrawal symptoms for that particular drug. Psychological dependence refers to a pattern of behavior directed to the procurement and use of a drug, based on an attitude that the effects produced by this drug are essential to maintain an optimal state of well-being. Tolerance is the condition in which the body is accustomed to the drug so that the larger doses of the drug must be taken to obtain the same effects produced by the smaller dose when the drug is first taken. Some authorities hold that genetically inherited traits may result in progression of addictive diseases when individuals are exposed to certain drugs. Though we do not know as much as we would like to about the biochemical basis for the addictive process, which may be the same for all drugs, the pharmacologic and psychosocial aspects have been described and vary considerably from drug to drug. The most common substances used for alteration of consciousness are the opiates, the central nervous system sedatives, the central nervous system stimulants, the psychedelics, and a few inhalants.

OPIATES

Opiates can be divided into three groups on the basis of their origin (Table 60.1). Morphine and codeine are naturally occurring constituents of the crude plant preparation of opium. The semisynthetic agents are chemical derivatives of morphine and codeine. Lastly, the synthetic drugs produce the same pharmacologic effects as the natural agents. Opium is the dried crude exudate of the incised unripe poppy pod. Opium contains about 10% morphine, 1% codeine, and 18 other alkaloids. Heroin is a semisynthetic narcotic drug that was quickly marketed as a "cure" for morphine addiction shortly after its discovery in 1874. Several new synthetic drugs have a potency 600 times that of heroin (1).

The potential for dependence on opiates is high. The most common abusers of narcotics fall into the following categories: street addicts, drug-dependent health professionals, infants of addicted mothers, abusers of prescription opiates, and methadone maintenance patients. Heroin is converted to morphine in the body. It was once believed that the rapid onset of action and marked euphoric properties of heroin produce a greater potential for dependence than with other semisynthetic or naturally

Table 60.1.
Narcotics and Related Compounds

Naturally Occurring and Derivatives
  Opium
  Morphine
  Codeine
  Tincture of opium
  Camphorated tincture of opium (Paregoric)
Semisynthetic Derivatives
  Heroin (diacetylmorphine)
  Oxycodone (Percodan, Percocet, Tylox)
  Hydrocodone (various)
  Oxymorpyhone (Numorphan)
  Hydromorphone (Diaudid)
Synthetic Agents
  Meperidine (Demerol)
  Loperamide (Imodium)
  Diphenoxylate (Lomotil)
  Anileridine (Leritine)
  Fentanyl (Innovar, Sublimaze)
  Methadone (Dolophine)
  L-Acetylomethandol (LAAM)
  Propoxyphene (Darvon)
  Pentazocine (Talwin)
  Butorphanol (Stadol)
  Nalbuphine (Nubain)

occurring agents. However, addicts have difficulty differentiating between heroin, morphine, and synthetic narcotics given in equivalent doses. Tolerance develops rapidly to most of the effects of heroin, with the exception of pupillary constriction and constipation. Tolerance for opiates disappears after complete withdrawal and may result in unintentional overdosage following weeks or months of abstinence if the previous doses are taken.

Acute Intoxication—Overdose

A large percentage of chronic heroin users have experienced an overdose on at least one occasion. A number of factors can contribute to accidental overdoses of opiates. A major factor is considerable confusion about the precise quantity of heroin taken because of variation in the concentration of street heroin, which may range from 1 to 90%. The amount of powder that looks like a user's customary dose may contain a dose of heroin many times greater. On some occasions, an overdose occurs soon after the addict has completed a jail sentence, during which time tolerance to heroin is lost.

Some of the "designer drugs," (e.g., alpha-methyl-fentanyl, referred to as China White) are much more potent (on an equivalent weight basis) than the compounds they are derived from and are sometimes inadequately mixed with inactive powdered ingredients, causing a very high concentration of active drugs in one dose (2). "Mexican tar" is another example of a product with a particularly high concentration of heroin. It was available on the streets

in a higher concentration than had previously been available and was responsible for a number of opiate overdoses. Multiple-drug use may produce an overdose when the additive effects of agents such as CNS depressants are combined with opiates.

Patients may have been treated through one of several "street methods" for resuscitation, such as the intravenous administration of salt, vinegar, or milk solutions. Salt and vinegar intravenous injections are extremely painful and may produce sclerosing of the veins, abscesses, infections, and hypernatremia. Intravenous milk may also cause lipoidal pneumonia and microscopic pulmonary emboli. External pain such as slapping the face, ice baths, and pinching the nipples or testicles are commonly used to attempt to revive the unconscious patient. Neither stimulation nor painful injections have any positive effect on a significant opiate overdose, and they may simply produce additional trauma and complicate the medical condition further.

Another street treatment known as speed reversal is the use of CNS stimulants (e.g., cocaine or methamphetamine) intravenously. These agents do not reverse the respiratory depressant effects of opiates and may produce serious additional adverse effects (e.g., convulsions, hypertension, arrhythmias), producing further complications requiring treatment of stimulant overdosage in addition to the opiate overdosage.

To escape apprehension by authorities, bags or balloons of opiates are sometimes swallowed to hide evidence. If these rupture or are released in the intestinal tract, they can produce an overdose.

Opiate overdose produces a profound coma, depressed respiration (as low as 2 to 4 per minute), and cyanosis. The pupils are symmetric and pinpoint, characteristic of the narcotic effect. However, if hypoxia or asphyxia has occurred, mydriasis may develop at this state. As the respiratory rate becomes slower, the blood pressure drops, and bradycardia, hypothermia, and pulmonary edema are commonly seen.

Management of Opiate Intoxication

Naloxone is the opiate antagonist of choice (3). It is a specific pure opioid antagonist with no agonist properties of its own. It lacks the adverse effects associated with nalorphine and levallorphan, which have both antagonist and agonist activity and are likely to worsen the respiratory depressant effects, especially in cases of overdoses of a mixture of nonopiate depressant drugs. Nalorphine and levallorphan may also produce CNS stimulant effects leading to hallucinations and acute psychosis.

Naloxone should be administered in an initial dose of 0.4 mg intravenously followed by a second dose within 10 to 20 minutes if the first dose does not revive the patient. The peak effect of naloxone occurs within 1 to 2 minutes, but the agent is very short acting, lasting only 30 to 60 minutes. The patient must be monitored carefully since the toxic effects of the opiates may last for 6 to 8 hours requiring multidose administration of the naloxone. Propoxyphene, codeine, pentazocine, and fentanyl derivatives may require larger doses of naloxone, and their durations of action are longer than those of other opiates, so the acutely intoxicated patient must be monitored from 12 to 24 hours. In these cases, it is more convenient to infuse naloxone in a dose sufficient to produce antagonistic effects, usually 0.8 to 1.2 mg per hour. Naloxone has a very high therapeutic index, with patients tolerating 80 to 100 mg of the drug intravenously with few side effects (4). As the dose of opiate antagonist is increased, an opiate-withdrawal syndrome may be precipitated. A serious attempt should be made to determine if any street therapies have been tried. In addition to opiate antagonist therapy, there should be close monitoring as well as mechanical support of respiration and blood pressure.

Opiate-Withdrawal Syndrome

Withdrawal can be precipitated by the administration of an opiate antagonist (5). If compulsive opiate users do not receive their drugs, a predictable sequence of signs and symptoms occurs, depending on the degree of tolerance, dose of the drug, and duration of use (Table 60.2). Anxiety, hyperactivity, lacrimation, rhinorrhea, and yawning appear within hours after the last dose depending on the half-life of the particular opiate. This is followed by a restless sleep that may last only a few hours as the withdrawal progresses. Initial symptoms of opiate withdrawal are followed by marked chills, excessive sweating, and pilomotor activity producing waves of gooseflesh of the skin (i.e., resembling that of a plucked turkey). This symptom is the basis of the term cold turkey used to describe abrupt withdrawal without treatment. Abdominal cramps, anorexia, nausea, vomiting, and diarrhea follow. Musculoskeletal pains of the back along with muscle spasms and kicking movements have been referred to as kicking the habit. As the syndrome approaches peak intensity, the patient exhibits increasing irritability, insomnia, anorexia, lacrimation, and increases in

Table 60.2.
Narcotic Withdrawal and Abstinence Symptoms

Dilated pupils	Vomiting
Elevation of pulse rate	Diarrhea
Elevation of blood pressure	Dehydration
Elevation of temperature	Weakness
Elevation of respiratory rate	Chills
Muscle aches	Rhinorrhea
Irritability	Lacrimation
Twitching	Gooseflesh
Tremulousness	Yawning
Nausea	Restlessness

heart rate and blood pressure. Leukocytosis is common, and white cell counts are often above $14,000/mm^3$. Weight loss, dehydration, ketosis, and acid–base imbalance follow the vomiting, sweating, diarrhea, and failure to take foods and fluids. Although cardiovascular collapse has been reported during the peak of the withdrawal, this is a rare phenomenon. In fact, death due to narcotic withdrawal is very rare. Without treatment, the withdrawal syndrome subsides, with most of the observable signs and symptoms disappearing in 7 to 10 days. Total restoration of the physiologic equilibrium can take much longer and varies with the patient, the length of the dependence, and the total daily dose of the drug. Administration of any opiate will completely suppress the symptoms of withdrawal at any point if appropriate doses are administered (depending on the individual's tolerance) (6, 7).

All opiates produce similar withdrawal signs and symptoms. However, depending on the particular agents and their length of action, symptoms may vary in duration and severity. For example, methadone withdrawal is less intense, develops more slowly, and is more prolonged because of the longer duration of action of methadone. Symptoms are rare within the first 24 to 48 hours after the last dose. A similar picture of withdrawal as that with heroin or morphine is observed, with peak effects occurring in 5 to 6 days and subsiding within 2 or 3 weeks. Meperidine, a much shorter-acting synthetic narcotic, may produce withdrawal effects within 3 hours of the last dose, which reach their greatest intensity within 8 to 12 hours and subside rapidly within 3 to 5 days. The pupils may not be widely dilated, and there are fewer autonomic signs and symptoms with meperidine withdrawal. Nausea, vomiting, and diarrhea are not as common as the nervousness, restlessness, and muscle twitching characteristic of meperidine abstinence.

Patients who have received 2 weeks of recommended doses of morphine 3 or 4 times daily may experience minor withdrawal symptoms when therapy is abruptly discontinued or an opiate antagonist is administered. Treatment of pain with opiates should be limited when possible, and patients should be withdrawn gradually to minimize the withdrawal symptoms. Patients on narcotics less than 2 weeks seldom experience more than mild anxiety, irritability, insomnia, and restlessness.

Infant Dependence

Since opiates cross the placenta, babies born to narcotic-dependent mothers will be physically dependent. With heroin dependence, signs of withdrawal appear within 24 hours of birth and include irritability, excessive crying, tremors, hyperactivity, increased respiratory rate, frantic sucking of fists, sneezing, vomiting, and fever. These same signs will occur in 2 or 3 days in babies born to methadone-dependent mothers (8). Withdrawal symptoms in babies born to mothers maintained on methadone are generally more intense; however, infant mortality is reduced in mothers maintained on methadone because of the clinic environment resulting in greater likelihood of appropriate prenatal care (9). Teratogenic effects have not been linked to methadone. Withdrawal of the opiate can be fatal to the fetus especially in the first trimester, so dependent mothers should remain on methadone until after birth. Other agents used to treat infant opiate withdrawal, in addition to paregoric, are tincture of opium, phenobarbital, diazepam, chlorpromazine, and clonidine (10). Mild symptoms may not require replacement therapy. If symptoms persist and become more severe, paregoric (0.2 ml), orally every 3 to 4 hours and increased as needed until symptoms are controlled, provides effective relief.

Management of Detoxification with Methadone

Hospitalized patients who are opiate dependent are usually not withdrawn until their acute medical or surgical problems are treated. These patients are generally placed on methadone for short-term replacement therapy to avoid complication of their medical problems. Methadone is usually not administered until physiologic signs of the withdrawal syndrome are present. Doses of 5 to 10 mg are initiated and titrated to prevent further withdrawal signs or symptoms. Total daily doses of 10 to 20 mg may be sufficient. The dose is titrated as low as possible without allowing withdrawal symptoms to continue (11). After the medical or surgical illness is treated, the patient should choose between detoxification or enrolling in a methadone-maintenance program (12). Some patients refuse therapy and are simply discharged. Long waiting lists and program prerequisites may make methadone maintenance less attractive. The most convenient alternatives are detoxification with methadone, naltrexone–clonidine combination, or clonidine alone (13–15). Detoxification is only a small part of the treatment that must include behavior modification, support groups, and so on, with the ultimate goal to transform the opiate addict into a "recovering," psychologically and emotionally stable, responsible, and productive member of society. Unfortunately, failure/relapse rates remain high in most programs.

Methadone is a synthetic opiate with a duration of action up to 24 hours. It possesses pharmacologic effects identical to those of morphine and carries a full dependence potential. The slow onset of action of methadone produces a less intense "rush" effect. However, methadone continues to be a desired street substitute for heroin among addicts even though they consider the high it provides inferior to other opiates.

The initial phase of treatment of opiate dependence is detoxification, which is the substitution of the abused opiate with methadone to minimize withdrawal symptoms, followed by progressively decreasing doses until the patient is drug free. Detoxification can be carried out by a daily or every other day reduction of up to 20% of the total methadone dose, while keeping the withdrawal symptoms minimal (16). Most programs can complete this process within 14 to 21 days, depending on the dose and severity (length of time) of dependence. Since street products vary in percentage of heroin, it is difficult to determine an exact dosage for replacement. The conversion used is 1 mg methadone substituted for 2 mg heroin, 4 mg morphine, and 20 mg meperidine (17). If there is no evidence of how much narcotic is being ingested on a daily basis, a daily dose of 10 to 20 mg is initiated and increased until withdrawal signs are minimal. Since 20% reduction in dose is well tolerated with minimum withdrawal symptoms, the dose is reduced accordingly. Doses larger than 40 mg per day must be documented by the medical director of the program. Many clinicians question the benefits of larger doses of methadone in order to avoid possible euphoric effects that reinforce drug dependence.

During detoxification, patients most often receive their methadone dose in liquid form that must be taken at the clinic in the presence of staff. Methadone may produce sedation and drowsiness, excessive sweating, constipation, and decreased libido. Methadone should be used only after opiate addiction is clearly established because fatalities have resulted from overdoses of methadone in nontolerant persons (18).

Methadone Maintenance

The treatment of heroin addiction varies from program to program and ranges from an aggressive narcotic abstinence of the cold turkey approach with abrupt cessation and no supportive therapy to maintenance with a substitute narcotic agent (e.g., long-acting methadone). Methadone maintenance involves placing the addict on a large enough dose of methadone to prevent withdrawal symptoms without producing euphoria. Initial doses of 10 to 20 mg per day are titrated up to 60 to 80 mg per day. A single daily oral dose is given to maintain contact with the patient and prevent the patient hoarding or selling the drug on the street. Since methadone is less likely than other narcotics to produce euphoria and tolerance develops rapidly, the craving for narcotics disappears at approximately 40 mg per day. Higher doses appear to block the euphoric effects of additional use of other narcotics. Longer-acting narcotics (L-acetyl methadone) (LAAM) have been tested in clinical trials since they can be given every 3 days instead of daily (19). Other methadone analogs are D-acetylmethadol and 1-methadyl acetate.

Methadone maintenance allows addicts a chance to escape from the illegal drug scene and refocus their goals and lifestyles. Controversy continues to surround long-term methadone-maintenance programs, and many practitioners see the replacement of illegal heroin with legally sanctioned methadone as incomplete and nonsuccessful therapy. Proponents think that time away from the illegal street scene will foster the attitudes and values necessary to conquer the dependency at a later time (18).

Supportive Treatment

A nonnarcotic technique for withdrawal involves management of the symptoms with a variety of nonnarcotic medications. Anxiety, irritability, and apprehension are usually treated with long-acting minor tranquilizers such as chlordiazepoxide (Librium) since the shorter-acting agents produce euphoric effects of their own that may reinforce or substitute a dependence. Phenobarbital is also effective in the treatment of anxiety. Insomnia can be managed with short-acting benzodiazepines (triazolam) or diphenhydramine. Gastrointestinal symptoms of cramps, diarrhea, and nausea may be managed with the belladonna alkaloids or dicyclomine, and with promethazine or prochlorperazine if vomiting is present. Analgesic therapy is usually limited to nonsteroidal antiinflammatory agents (e.g., ibuprofen), which are also effective for musculoskeletal pain.

Clonidine, a centrally acting alpha$_2$-agonist, can suppress some components of the opiate-withdrawal syndrome. The use of the drug in the outpatient clinic has been very effective. Clonidine side effects such as orthostatic hypotension and sedation have been reduced by use of the sustained-release patches. After 2 days of oral clonidine therapy of 0.4 to 1.2 mg in daily divided doses, two Catapres-TTS-2 patches are applied. The patches should be replaced in 1 week, for a total therapy of 2 weeks (20, 21). Combination therapy of clonidine with nonsteroidal antiinflammatory agents for pain and sleep medications has been very successful.

The opiate antagonists have been used to produce a block of the euphoric efforts of opioids. If a drug is needed to break the conditioning of a drug-seeking behavior, opiate antagonist may be used. Naloxone and naltrexone can block the euphoria of opiates and prevent development of physical dependence. Naltrexone is an orally effective narcotic antagonist and relatively free of side effects (22–24). Doses of 50 mg daily up to 150 mg Monday, Wednesday, and Friday will block opiate effects. Unlike methadone, naltrexone is nonaddictive and without reenforcing properties. Poor compliance has limited this agent's use. However, some individuals who are motivated to abstain have found additional help and long-term success with this drug (25, 26).

Medical Complications of Opiate Dependence

Most medical complications of narcotic abuse are indirect and depend more on the method of use than on the direct effects of the drugs (e.g., toxic and withdrawal reactions; see (Table 60.3). The repeated use of unsterile needles and

Table 60.3.
Medical Complications of Intravenous Drug Use

Skin	Abscesses, cellulitis, edema, emboli, excoriation, jaundice, macules, nodules, purpura, "tracks," ulcers
Lymph nodes	"Addict's lymphadenopathy," lymphatic hyperplasia
Eyes	Emboli from talc and cornstarch, quinine amblyopia, scleral icterus
Mouth	Poor dental hygiene
Pulmonary	Infections secondary to aspiration, bronchiectasis, atelectasis, septic emboli, tuberculosis, pulmonary hypertension, decreased vital capacity, asthma, noncardiogenic pulmonary edema
Cardiovascular	Arrhythmias, endocarditis complicated by systemic and pulmonary emboli, vasculities, gangrene
Hematologic	Anemia, hemolysis, malaria, neutropenia
Neurologic	Subarachnoid hemorrhage, neuropathies, meningitis, central and peripheral emboli, nerve damage
Gastrointestinal	Hepatomegaly, hepatitis, splenic abscess, portal hypertension, constipation, bowel obstruction, hemorrhoids
Genitourinary	Heroin nephropathy, vasculitis, glomerulonephritis secondary to hepatitis or infection, myoglobinuria from muscle destruction, acute tubular necrosis, acute renal failure
Extremities	Phlebitis, edema, arthritis, rhabdomyolysis, tetanus
Immunologic	False-positive VDRL, rheumatoid factor, hypergammaglobulinemia, serologic abnormalities, increased risk for acquired immunodeficiency syndrome (AIDS)
"Cotton fever"	Pyrogenic reaction, shaking chills, headache, vomiting, gastrointestinal pain, leukocytosis shortly after intravenous administration subsiding in an hour or two

syringes has led to acute viral hepatitis, bacterial endocarditis, aseptic abscesses, embolism, thrombophlebitis, and cellulitis. *Staphylococcus aureus* is the most common infecting organism, followed by streptococci, Gramnegative bacilli (*Pseudomonas* and *Serratia*), and fungi (*Candida*). One study reported a 60% incidence of AIDS among addicts who commonly share needles and syringes (27). Some of the other infectious diseases transmitted in this fashion are tetanus, viral hepatitis, tuberculosis, and syphilis (28).

A common practice of self-administration of heroin is the use of cotton to filter out adulterants. Allergic reactions caused by the tiny cotton fibers may cause shaking, chills, fever, tachycardia, and a low-grade fever mimicking sepsis within 30 minutes of injection. These symptoms commonly subside within 2 to 4 hours. Pulmonary complications may be secondary to injection of these and other foreign body emboli (e.g., starch, talc, or cotton fibers). Many patients with significant embolic complications have been previous users of methylphenidate or pentazocine. Subcutaneous use of heroin (skin popping) frequently produces infection at the site, with *Staphylococcus aureus* being the most frequent organism. Tetanus is also a possible serious infection (29).

CENTRAL NERVOUS SYSTEM DEPRESSANTS

The most widely used and abused sedative–hypnotic drug is alcohol. Chapter 59 goes into detail on alcohol abuse, the many medical and social problems associated with alcohol abuse, and its management.

Barbiturates and other sedative–hypnotic drugs produce their effects through generalized depression of the central nervous system, and are all capable of producing dependence when used chronically even at recommended therapeutic doses. Short-acting barbiturates such as pentobarbital, secobarbital, and amobarbital were the major sedative-hypnotics used and abused prior to the 1970s. Physician awareness of their dependence, liability, and toxicities coupled with stringent DEA controls has dramatically decreased both their use and abuse. However, a host of nonbarbiturate sedative-hypnotics appeared on the market, with meprobamate introduced in the 1950s as the first of many "minor tranquilizers" to be released. Several other nonbarbiturate agents were also used (glutethimide, methyprylon, ethinamate, ethchlorvynol, and methaqualone) but have been primarily replaced by the increasing use of benzodiazepines. However, there are marked similarities of all agents that depress the central nervous system in producing the same type of dependence and withdrawal syndrome (30, 31).

Acute intoxication from combined use of alcohol with the barbiturates and benzodiazepines is a frequent problem. In addition, the number of attempted suicides with sedative-hypnotics is the largest of any class of prescription drugs. Some patients have accidentally overdosed on the barbiturates because, though there is considerable tolerance to the sedative and intoxicating effects, the lethal dose is not much greater in addicts than in normal individuals. Consequently, acute barbiturate poisoning may be accidentally superimposed on chronic intoxication at any time. Benzodiazepines appear to be safer than barbiturates and related sedatives since an acute overdosage is much less likely to produce fatal respiratory depression. However, the combination of alcohol and benzodiazepines is a serious problem that can be life threatening.

The signs and symptoms of barbiturate poisoning relate to their CNS depressant effects. Initial signs of minor intoxication resemble those of alcohol inebriation and progress in severe intoxication to slurred speech, ataxia, and coma. Lowered blood pressure and depressed respiration and tendon reflexes are common. Cerebral hypoxia

and respiratory acidosis may lead to hypotension and arrhythmias. The patient develops shock, a weak but rapid pulse, cold and sweaty skin, increased hematocrit, and renal ischemia. Pulmonary complications and renal failure are the most common causes of death from severe barbiturate poisoning (32).

The basic treatment of barbiturate intoxication is general supportive care and maintenance of vital functions, which may include mechanical respiration, dialysis, and intensive-care continuous monitoring. Initial treatment should also prevent further intestinal absorption of the drug. Gastric lavage should be considered within the first 2 to 4 hours after the overdose, followed by repeated doses of activated charcoal given orally to decrease absorption of drug remaining in the intestinal tract. However, forced diuresis, urinary alkalization, and giving repeated doses of charcoal have not been shown to be more successful than general supportive care (33, 34). Use of CNS stimulants increases mortality and has no place in the treatment of sedative–hypnotic overdose. Special attention must be given to maintenance of the patient's airway and the prevention of pneumonia. Oxygen should be administered, and mechanical ventilation used when indicated. Patients with severe hypotension or shock must be rehydrated. Hypovolemia must be corrected with caution; overhydration may contribute to pulmonary edema. Should renal failure occur, the most effective method of eliminating barbiturate is hemodialysis.

The original contact with sedative-hypnotics is most commonly through a physician's prescription. Development of dependence may be gradual, beginning with prolonged use of these agents for anxiety or insomnia, progressing through increased doses at night for insomnia, to multidoses in the daytime for sedation, until drug use becomes a major part of the user's life. In such situations, a fine line separates therapeutic need and physical dependency. Neither the prescriber nor the patient may recognize a dependence until the patient attempts to withdraw from the drug.

Withdrawal Syndrome

There are marked similarities between the withdrawal syndromes of the barbiturates and the nonbarbiturate minor tranquilizers. The term *general depressant-withdrawal syndrome* refers to the manifestation and withdrawal from any of these agents. Initial withdrawal signs and symptoms include restlessness, anxiety, sleep disturbances, tremulousness, and gastric distress. Withdrawal signs and symptoms of shorter-acting sedatives appear within 24 hours and reach a peak in 2 to 3 days, including agitation, delirium, psychoses, postural hypotension, hyperthermia, cardiovascular collapse, tonic–clonic seizures, and even death. Presence of these later symptoms should be considered signs and symptoms of major withdrawal, and they require hospitalization. Abstinence from the longer-acting sedatives does not produce withdrawal symptoms until the 2nd or 3rd day, and they reach their peak much more slowly. Seizures may not occur until the 7th to 10th day.

Major signs of physiologic dependence and withdrawal have been observed after 30 to 60 days of use of depressants at minimum or threshold doses two to three times maximum recommended therapeutic doses. Daily doses of secobarbital and pentobarbital of 600 to 800 mg per day for 30 to 60 days have been reported as the minimum dose to produce physical dependence. Thirty percent of patients taking 400 mg per day experience significant symptoms. The withdrawal or abstinence syndrome has been described for almost every sedative–hypnotic drug, but the doses and times to produce withdrawal are not as well defined as with the barbiturates. Abrupt discontinuation of doses as low as 30 mg diazepam per day for 3 months has resulted in seizures. Obviously, the longer the therapy and the higher the daily dose, the more likely that serious withdrawal symptoms will occur on discontinuing the drug. In addition, it takes 5 days or longer for the longer-acting benzodiazepines to produce significant symptoms of abstinence after discontinuing the drug, resulting in a withdrawal that might last 2 to 3 weeks (35–41). In addition to the classic withdrawal symptoms, patients who are taking lower than threshold doses required to produce physical dependency may exhibit a rebound phenomenon with the abrupt discontinuation of the drug. Patients abruptly discontinuing commonly prescribed doses of benzodiazepines have experienced insomnia, anorexia, REM rebound, irritability, and anxiety, which could be mistaken for the symptoms that the drug was originally prescribed for or reemergence of these symptoms (42, 43). All patients taking benzodiazopines longer than 1 month should gradually taper their dose over a period of several weeks to avoid this effect.

Sedative Detoxification

Because of the severity of general depressant withdrawal, successful management must involve tapering the patient off the sedative agents slowly. Most treatment centers will not detoxify the patient with the drug that is causing the dependence because of the strong association with the patient's drug of choice and the dependence. All sedatives and hypnotics can be withdrawn by benzodiazepines. The longer-acting benzodiazepines are considered the agents of choice for substitution withdrawal because of their anticonvulsant effects and wide margin of safety.

Some clinicians use phenobarbital for substitution withdrawal. The dose of phenobarbital is 30 mg for each 100 mg of pentobarbital or secobarbital or for each 5 mg of diazepam, 25 mg of chlordiazepoxide, or 50 mg of butalbital. The total daily dose may be as high as 600 or 700

mg of phenobarbital and is administered in three or four divided doses. Some clinics orally administer 120-mg doses of phenobarbital hourly until sedative effects and/or horizontal nystagmus appear, and this total dose is then given in divided daily doses (44–46). A stabilization period of 1 to 2 days for short-acting drugs and 3 to 4 days for long-acting drugs is used. The patient is monitored for slurred speech, nystagmus, or ataxia during this stabilization period. Minor signs and symptoms of withdrawal may be treated with clonidine. After the patient is stabilized, the total daily dose of phenobarbital is decreased 30 mg per day (47). If patients requiring detoxification have mixed addictions of the opiate-sedative type, they are maintained on sufficient amounts of methadone until detoxification from the sedative-hypnotic is completed (48).

Benzodiazepine Detoxification

Benzodiazepines (Table 60.4) have cross-tolerance with each other, alcohol, and other sedative–hypnotic drugs. Any benzodiazepine can be substituted for another benzodiazepine or barbiturate, so conversion for equivalent doses can be calculated. The long-acting benzodiazepines (e.g., chlordiazepoxide) are preferred to the shorter-acting benzodiazepines by some clinicians (Table 60.5) (35). Long-acting agents may be more effective than short-acting agents in suppressing withdrawal symptoms, thereby producing a gradual, smooth transition to the abstinent state, improving patient compliance, and reducing morbidity (49, 50).

Medications should be prescribed on a regular schedule. Addicts need the structure of a drug schedule; they do not do well with as-needed prescriptions because their basic problem is loss of control over drugs. Unlike alcohol withdrawal, benzodiazepine withdrawal is not usually marked by hypertension and tachycardia, so as-needed doses are not necessary. It is difficult to differentiate drug-seeking behavior from withdrawal-related anxiety or from anxiety caused by another disorder. Only anxiety secondary to benzodiazepine withdrawal should be treated with increasing doses of benzodiazepines. Alternative treatment is indicated for anxiety associated with another disorder (e.g., panic disorder) (35).

Table 60.4.
Short- and Long-Acting Benzodiazepines

Short-Acting Agents	Long-Acting Agents
Triazolam (Halcion)	Chlordiazepoxide (Librium)
Oxazepam (Serax)	Diazepam (Valium)
Temazepam (Restril)	Halazepam (Paxipam)
Lorazepam (Ativan)	Clorazepate (Tranxene)
Alprazolam (Xanax)	Prazepam (Centrax)
	Clonazepam (Klonopin)
	Flurazepam (Dalmane)

Table 60.5.
Signs and Symptoms of Benzodiazepine Withdrawal

Neuropsychiatric	Hyperexcitability
Ataxia	Agitation
Depersonalization	Anxiety
Depression	Hyperactivity
Fasciculations	Insomnia
Formications	**Gastrointestinal**
Headache	Abdominal pain
Hyperventilation	Constipation
Malaise	Diarrhea
Myalgia	Nausea
Paranoid delusions	Vomiting
Paresthesias	**Cardiovascular**
Pruritus	Chest pain
Tinnitus	Flushing
Tremors	Palpitations
Visual hallucinations	**Genitourinary**
	Incontinence
	Loss of libido
	Urinary urgency, frequency

Table 60.6.
Common Signs and Symptoms of Acute Amphetamine Intoxication

Restlessness	Paranoia
Anxiety	Delusional thoughts
Tremor	Visual hallucinations
Muscle tension	Auditory hallucinations
Repetitious body movement	Physical malnutrition
Facial grimacing	Needle tracks and abscesses
Dystonia	Hypertensive crisis
Temporary amnesia	Cardiac arrhythmias

CENTRAL NERVOUS SYSTEM STIMULANTS

Caffeine is the most universal, socially accepted stimulant in the world, in the form of coffee, tea, and soft drinks, and has a wide margin of safety and rare toxicity. Use of central nervous system stimulants was recorded in ancient Asian and African writings. Amphetamines are the prototype prescription CNS stimulant, and they were heavily prescribed for weight control until the 1970s when the DEA moved most of them to schedule II controlled substances and limited their production.

The over-the-counter diet pills contain phenylpropanolamine. Phenylpropanolamine has a limited effect on suppressing appetite, but it is not defined as habit forming because it is not self-administered by animals and does not produce the increase of energy, alertness, and euphoria of the amphetamines. Serious adverse effects of excessive use of these over-the-counter diet aids (including sudden death) have rarely been reported (51–53). "Look-alikes" are nonprescription tablets and capsules manufactured in colors, shapes, and sizes to resemble the prescription stimulants and marketed as diet aids. These agents most commonly contain phenylpropanolamine, pseudoephedrine, ephedrine, caffeine, and/or a combination of these. They are commonly advertised as appetite suppressants but sold illicitly for methamphetamine, dextroamphetamine, or cocaine.

Amphetamines were first used for treatment of depression and fatigue, increasing alertness, and as an anorexiant to suppress appetite. Because of a rapid tolerance that develops within a few weeks, these drugs have no medical place in the previously mentioned conditions. Accepted medical uses for the amphetamine agents today are limited to hyperkinesia, attention-deficit disorder, and narcolepsy.

Amphetamines are sympathomimetic agents that produce systemic stimulation of the central nervous system. In addition to increasing alertness, amphetamines produce an elevation of mood, a sense of increased energy, and decreased appetite. Amphetamines initially increase productivity slightly, alleviate fatigue, and produce a euphoric sense of well-being, which can produce a quick, psychological habituation to the drug. Coupled with a rapid development of tolerance requiring increased doses on a weekly basis, dependence is common. Tolerance to the recommended 15-mg-per-day dosage leads to use of 80 to 100 times the initial dosages. Some users have been reported to inject up to 1 g of the drug several times daily without apparent toxicity.

Chronic users have not only used intravenous injections of amphetamines, but have also started "freebasing" methamphetamine (ice) and smoking it, similar to cocaine. The method of freebasing will be explained when cocaine abuse is presented. Chronic amphetamine users, known as speed freaks, tend to be hostile, impulsive, aggressive, mentally unstable, and subject to wide swings in behavior, including violence (Table 60.6) (53). An amphetamine binge or "speed run" is the continuous round-the-clock use of amphetamines for several days without sleep. The patient is referred to as strung out and may become hostile, overactive, and impulsive. Prolonged periods of paranoia and delusions can result. The fully developed toxic syndrome is characterized by vivid visual, auditory, and sometimes tactile hallucinations. An acute psychotic episode induced by amphetamines does not generally respond to "talk-down" therapy. Mild nonviolent patients are treated with oral benzodiazepines, and more seriously agitated patients should receive parenteral haloperidol (Haldol). If the patient is combative and hostile, physical restraints are indicated until the drug therapy controls the patient. After several days of a speed run, the patient usually "crashes" from exhaustion.

In chronic users, a tolerance builds up to most of the sympathomimetic effects, and the blood pressure may be normal. It is very difficult to differentiate the toxic syndrome from a schizophrenic reaction. Chronic use of high-dose amphetamine has also been reported to produce microvascular neurologic damage and depletion of dopamine in the caudate nucleus (54). Other complications of chronic use are malnutrition due to appetite suppression and perception of "crank bugs" (i.e., imagining bugs crawling under the skin). The intravenous use of these agents carries with it all the medical complications of other agents abused in this fashion (e.g., infectious diseases, microemboli, abscesses, hepatitis, AIDS, "cotton fever"). Intravenous injections of methamphetamines may produce a systemic necrotizing angiitis and generalized spasm of the cerebral blood vessels. Cardiac arrhythmias and cerebral hemorrhages have been reported. Severe abdominal pain mimicking acute appendicitis is also seen.

Amphetamine overdosage-toxicity may result if an individual has lost tolerance and self-administers the previous dosage. Toxicity developing if the amphetamine dose has been increased too rapidly before tolerance develops is referred to as overramped, with patients characterized by consciousness without the ability to move or speak. Physiologic signs and symptoms include high blood pressure and an extremely rapid pulse, intense pain, increased temperature, severe agitation, and insomnia. Higher doses produce cardiac arrhythmias, seizures, hallucinations, cardiomyopathy, and myocardial infarction. Dehydration associated with malnutrition, vomiting, and diarrhea is also possible. Death from overdosage is usually caused by cardiovascular collapse.

Abrupt cessation following chronic or high-dose amphetamine use will produce an abstinence syndrome that may last up to 1 week. Symptoms include fatigue, muscle aches, depression, headache, gastrointestinal disturbances, and craving for the drug. Withdrawal from amphetamines is not life threatening and does not require gradual reduction of dose. Psychotic conditions, depression, and sleep disturbances may persist for months and require psychiatric management. Treatment of acute amphetamine withdrawal is supportive in nature: benzodiazepines are appropriate for mild-to-moderate symptoms, and haloperidol can be given if sedation is required. Chlorpromazine and other phenothiazines should not be given to treat mental or physiologic disturbances caused by amphetamine reactions. There is a great risk of impulsive self-destructive behavior in the chronic amphetamine abuser. Treatment of the chronic amphetamine abuser is difficult with a high frequency of relapse. The number of chronic amphetamine users has been dramatically reduced in the past 2 decades, with a corresponding increase in cocaine abuse.

Cocaine

Cocaine is a local anesthetic drug with significant CNS-stimulant effects. Widespread abuse of cocaine began in the late 1800s, shortly after its isolation from the *Erythroxylon coca* plant. The use of cocaine goes back many

centuries in Peru, Bolivia, Ecuador, and Colombia. Local natives in the upper Andes regularly chewed or sucked plugs of moistened coca leaves, smeared with a pinch of lime (ashes or limestone) to extract the cocaine from the leaves. Chewing coca leaves satisfies hunger, eliminates fatigue, and imparts a feeling of great physical strength to its users working in the high altitudes (55). Cocaine is still obtained from the natural plant source. As an alkaloid, it is extracted from the plant with organic solvents, precipitated into a paste, and then usually converted to the hydrochloride salt, producing a white powder. The purity of street cocaine varies considerably. Pure cocaine is most commonly diluted with adulterants ("cut" or "stepped on") to help dealers support their own habits and/or increase their profit margin. Cheaper local anesthetics, mannitol, lactose, glucose, corn starch, flour, and talc are some of the agents used to cut the pure form. Samples of street cocaine may vary from 25 to 75%. Because of the high demand and popularity of the drug and the large profits, suppliers have increased the availability of higher-quality product on the street. It is estimated that there are more than 5 million regular users in the United States alone, with 30 million who have experimented with the drug. The Drug Enforcement Agency estimates range as high as 200 tons of cocaine sold on the street annually, representing a multibillion-dollar business.

In addition to the crystalline powder form of cocaine found on the street, "freebase" and "crack" became increasingly popular in the 1980s. Freebase is prepared by mixing cocaine hydrochloride with an alkali solution such as sodium bicarbonate, then extracting with a solvent, usually ethyl ether. This not only separates the cocaine from the adulterants but also cleaves the hydrochloride salt, leaving the free alkaloidal cocaine base as a colorless, transparent, crystalline substance, insoluble in water. The most common form of cocaine seen today is crack, a base form of cocaine prepared by dissolving the hydrochloride salt in water and alkali (bleach or sodium bicarbonate) (56). The free alkaloidal base precipitates out, leaving a brittle, milky-colored solid that crackles when it burns, hence the nickname crack. After the product is dried, it is broken into small pieces or chips known as rocks and usually sold in small glass vials or metal tubes.

Cocaine can be administered in a number of different ways (57). The oldest known method of using cocaine is orally, chewing the moistened leaves placed between the cheek and gum like a plug of chewing tobacco. The drug is also effective when ingested orally although gastrointestinal absorption is slower and incomplete. However, these routes of administration do not produce as fast or as intense a high, or rush, and are rarely seen in the United States. The most common method of self-administration of cocaine is smoking crack, either by itself, in a pipe, or sprinkled in marijuana cigarettes called primo joints (58).

Because of its purity, crack produces the quickest and most intense cocaine high, taking effect within 8 to 10 seconds with a very short duration of 10 to 20 minutes.

Another route of administration of cocaine is inhalation through the nose, or snorting. There is a ritual of using the drug by this method that involves placing the powder on a hard surface (counter top, book, or mirror), separating and chopping the powder into a small particle size, dividing the powder into a small narrow "line" or "hit," then sniffing the powder into the nostril with a rolled-up dollar bill or a short straw. A small spoon, "coke spoon," is a device to measure out single doses of the drug sufficient for one sniff. One line of street cocaine would usually contain 5 to 10 mg of cocaine, whereas one coke spoon may contain only half this amount.

Another method of use is freebasing. Using a modified water pipe with several layers of stainless steel screens fitted in the bowl, the freebase is placed on the top screen, melted to an oil, and heated slowly to vaporize the drug for inhalation. Absorption of cocaine through the lungs is very rapid, and users experience a more intensive, euphoric (rush) effect. Many users report binges lasting up to 3 or 4 days of uncontrolled craving and repeated drug use via freebasing. Freebase smokers and the intravenous cocaine users seldom return to intranasal use (59).

Other patterns of cocaine drug use are smoking the crude paste with marijuana or tobacco and intravenous injection. Most users claim the euphoric rush of intravenous use to be of lower intensity than that with freebasing or crack smoking. Only a very small percentage of cocaine users administer the drug intravenously. A preparation called speed ball is a combination of heroin and cocaine administered together intravenously.

Pharmacologic Effects

The local anesthetic activity of cocaine is due to a direct effect on the nerve cell membrane to prevent the generation and conduction of nerve impulses. Cocaine affects the sympathetic nervous system by blocking the reuptake of catecholamines at adrenergic nerve endings, thus potentiating both inhibitory and excitatory responses of sympathetically innervated structures to endogenous and exogenous serotonin, norepinephrine, and epinephrine. Although cocaine blocks the reuptake of dopamine in the

Table 60.7.
Signs and Symptoms of Cocaine Toxicity

	CNS	*Circulatory*	*Respiratory*
Phase I (Early Stimulation)	Euphoria/elation	Initial decreased pulse rate, then increased	Increased respiratory rate
	Mydriasis	Increase blood pressure	Dyspnea
	Talkativeness	Skin pallor (vasoconstriction)	
	Excited/flighty	PVCs	
	Restless/irritable		
	Nausea, vomiting		
	Vertigo		
	Sudden headache		
	Cold sweats		
	Tremor/twitching (especially face, fingers)		
	Generalized tics		
	Preconvulsive movements		
	Pseudohallucinations		
	Verbalizaton of impending doom		
Phase II (Advanced Stimulation)	Decreased responsiveness to stimuli	Increase pulse rate	Gasping, rapid or irregular respiratory rate
	Generalized hyperflexia	Increase blood pressure initially followed by decreased blood pressure due to decreased cardiac output with ventricular arrhythmias	Cheyne-Stokes progressive hypoxia
	Increased DTRs	Rapid pulse, weak and irregular	
	Incontinence	Peripheral then central cyanosis	
	Convulsions, status epilepticus		
	Malignant encephalopathy possible		
Phase III (Depressive)	Flaccid paralysis of muscle	Ventricular fibrillation	Agonal gasps
	Coma	Circulatory failure	Respiratory faiure
	Pupils fixed and dilated	Ashen gray cyanosis	Gross pulmonary edema
	Loss of reflexes	No palpable pulse	Paralysis of medullary brain center
	Loss of vital support functions	Cardiac arrest	Death
	Paralysis of medullary brain center	Paralysis of medullary brain center	
	Death	Death	

brain initially, it appears that chronic use actually depletes dopamine stores (60). The mechanism of reinforcing action and effects associated with cocaine may be related to this increase of synaptic concentration of dopamine.

Cocaine is generally considered to have a rapid onset and short duration of action, depending somewhat on the method of administration (61). The onset is 2 to 3 minutes when the drug is snorted, less than 1 minute when it is injected, and 8 to 10 seconds when it is smoked. The elimination half-life of cocaine is 60 to 75 minutes, with peak plasma concentration occurring between 30 and 60 minutes, depending on the route of administration (intravenous versus snorting). The physiologic effect of cocaine outlasts the euphoria and tends to correlate with the blood levels of the drug. However, most users want to repeat the use of the drug within 20 to 30 minutes after the first dose. This may indicate that the rate of rise of cocaine concentration in the brain is the major factor responsible for the subjective euphoric effects and the "rush," rather than the serum concentrations (62).

Cocaine produces many classic sympathomimetic manifestations (Table 60.7). Cocaine has powerful CNS-stimulant effects producing euphoria, restlessness, talkativeness, and gregariousness. Other physiologic effects include dry mouth, sweating, mydriasis, hyperthermia, tachycardia, increased blood pressure, vasoconstriction, increased muscle activity, tics, chills, and increased respiratory rate initially, followed by Cheyne–Stokes respiration with continued drug use. The euphoric rush, often referred to by users as being "better than orgasm," reinforces and contributes to repeated self-administration. Abusers claim they cannot control their dose and may go on a "binge" or "run" of cocaine for several days.

Medical Complications of Cocaine

The cardiovascular effects of cocaine are due to the increased central sympathetic stimulation. The initial effects of tachycardia, palpitations, angina, and hypertension will return to normal within several hours, depending on the dosage and whether the drug is being used repeatedly. However, increasing numbers of patients are developing life-threatening arrhythmias and infarctions (63). Ventricular tachycardia, fibrillation, and premature ventricular contractions have been reported (64, 65). These users frequently complain of chest pain from alveolar hemorrhage (crack lung) and may experience pulmonary edema, pneumonia, or respiratory depression. Other serious cardiovascular effects seen with cocaine use are myocardial infarction, life-threatening ventricular arrhythmias, hypertensive crisis, endocarditis, thrombosis, and rupture of the ascending aorta (66–68). Many patients who have experienced the cardiovascular toxicities had no underlying heart disease previously. These effects have been reported following all routes of ad-

Table 60.8.
Medical Complications of Cocaine Use

System or Condition	Complication Examples
Cardiovascular	Myocardial infarction, premature ventricular contraction, ventricular tachycardia, ventricular fibrillation, congestive heart failure, chest pain, endocarditis, hypertension, pneumopericardium, rupture of ascending aorta, thrombosis, thrombophlebitis
CNS	Stroke, subarachnoid hemorrhage, intracranial hemorrhage, cerebral vasculitis, hyperpyrexia, dysphagia, dysarthria
Respiratory	Alveolar hemorrhage (crack lung), pneumonia, pneumomediastinum, pulmonary edema, pneumothorax, respiratory arrest
Ophthalmic	Retinopathy, central retinal artery occlusion
Pregnancy	Abrupt placenta fetal hypoxemia, fetal death in utero, spontaneous abortion, preterm labor, convulsions in breast feeding baby, feeding disorder, teratogenicity
Psychiatric	Panic disorder, psychosis and violence
Miscellaneous	Renal artery thrombosis, midline granuloma, subcutaneous emphysema, nasal problems, rhadomyolysis, sexual dysfunction, various infectious diseases and other complications with IV drug use (Table 60-3).

ministration and with both large and small doses (Table 60.8) (69–72).

Pulmonary complications have increased dramatically with freebasing and the smoking of crack. Alveolar hemorrhage (crack lung), pulmonary edema, pneumomediastinum, pneumothorax, pneumopericardium, pneumonia, and respiratory arrest are commonly seen in regular users of cocaine (73–75). Stroke and subarachnoid and intracranial hemorrhage are some of the life-threatening CNS effects reported with cocaine use (76–78). High doses of cocaine have been associated with tonic–clonic convulsions (79). Intravenous use of cocaine has been associated with a variety of infectious diseases such as hepatitis, AIDS, bacterial endocarditis, and other complications (80). Cocaine may lead to cardiac arrhythmias, severe hypotension, hypothermia, seizures, and renal and respiratory failure (81). Myocardial infarction and cardiac failure within 2 to 3 hours following cocaine use in young adults without prior heart disease have been reported (82–85). Toxic effects of acute cocaine exposure may be precipitated by physical exertion. Cases of sudden death following freebase use are probably caused by arrhythmias. Cocaine overdose has also been frequently reported in individuals smuggling cocaine. "Body packing" involves swallowing plastic bags filled with cocaine in order to pass through immigrations, with a plan to retrieve the containers from bowel movements. Occasionally, these bags will rupture in the gut, and in other cases, the plastic may be semipermeable, allowing absorption of cocaine (43, 86–88).

Treatment of Overdosage

Treatment of acute cocaine intoxication includes general supportive care, fluid and electrolyte replacement, maintenance of vital functions (blood pressure, airway), and monitoring for suspected hyperadrenergic crisis (e.g., hypertension, arrhythmias) (89). Mild-to-moderate cocaine intoxication is self-limiting and lasts no longer than 2 to 3 hours without treatment. If symptoms progress in severity or persist longer than an hour, the patient should be monitored for arrhythmias with an ECG since cardiac arrhythmias are the major cause of death due to cocaine toxicity. Respiratory arrest, seizures, myocardial infarction, or cardiovascular collapse are all possible, and preparations should be made to manage any of these conditions should they arise. Ventricular arrhythmias are treated with lidocaine or phenytoin and may require cardioversion. Supraventricular arrhythmias have been managed effectively with the nonselective beta-blocker propranolol (Inderal) in mild-to-moderate cocaine toxicity. There is a danger of unexpected hypertension because of unopposed alpha-adrenergic activity, so propranolol should be avoided in major toxicity (90–92). Several reports have indicated that labetalol may be more effective in managing cocaine toxicity (93). Intravenous nitroprusside sodium may be used to control hypertensive emergencies. Naloxone may be given to comatose patients suspected of cocaine intoxication since some addicts use narcotics with cocaine. Seizures may be treated by diazepam, phenytoin, or phenobarbital (94). Anxiety and restlessness may be treated with benzodiazepines, and acute psychotic reactions with haloperidol (95). Caution is advised because haloperidol may lower the seizure threshold and increase the risk of convulsions.

Cocaine Withdrawal

There is no doubt that cocaine produces severe dependence. Animals given cocaine will continuously self-administer the drug. Many addictionologists claim that cocaine dependence is the most difficult drug dependence to treat. Furthermore, abrupt discontinuation of cocaine following chronic use results in depression, fatigue, craving

Table 60.9.
Phases of Cocaine Abstinence[a]

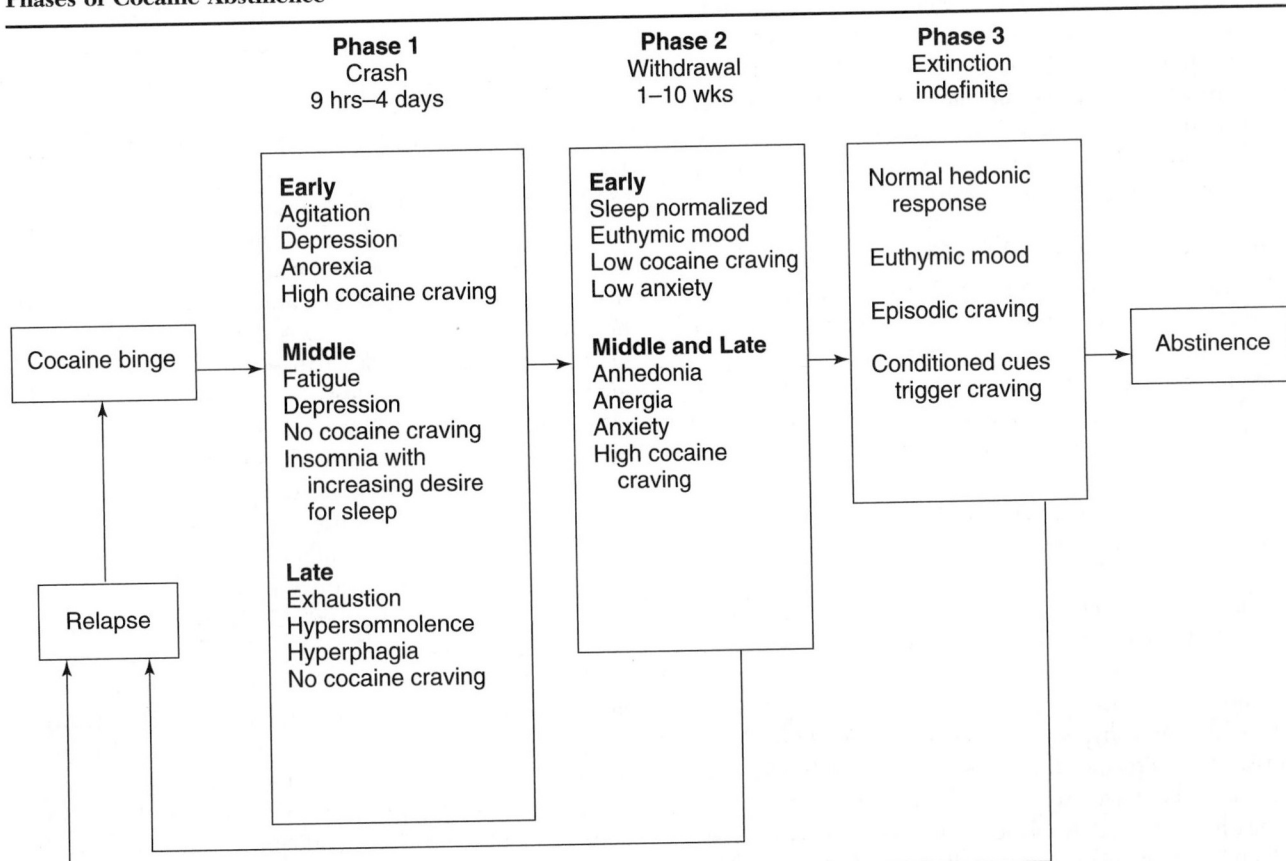

[a]Modified from Hall WC, Talbert RL, Ereshefsky L. Cocaine abuse and its treatment. Pharmacotherapy 10:47–65, 1990.

for the drug, social withdrawal, eating and sleep disturbances, REM rebound, and electroencephalographic changes. These effects generally last less than a week, with the exception of the abnormal sleep patterns, which may last several weeks (96). These signs and symptoms are significant enough to meet the criteria for withdrawal syndrome as evidence of physical dependence (97, 98). The three phases of cocaine withdrawal are outlined in Table 60.9 (99).

Abrupt discontinuation of cocaine use is not life threatening and does not cause the major physiologic withdrawal symptoms associated with narcotics and sedatives. Pharmacologic treatment of chronic cocaine dependence is limited, unless efforts are made to include support and behavioral modification modeled after the Alcoholics Anonymous treatment program. The treatment modalities that are under investigation include the use of carbamazepine, tricyclic antidepressants, which produce an alteration of dopamine receptors (100); bromocryptine (Parlodel), which restores dopamine depletion (101); lithium carbonate, which decreases the euphoria of cocaine through unknown mechanisms; and methylphenidate. The benefits of these agents are still under evaluation (102–104).

PSYCHEDELICS

A wide variety of natural alkaloids and synthetic chemicals have been taken for their mind-altering and psychedelic effects. Other names used for this class of compounds are hallucinogens, psychotomimetics, and entactogens. In addition to their psychedelic effect, each of these drugs also has a wide range of physiologic and psychological effects. A classic physical dependence has not been observed with the prototype hallucinogenic agents. Tolerance is seen with chronic use, and psychological dependence is possible but rare. The normal drug-use cycle is an occasional self-administration for curiosity and to "explore the inner self." Adverse effects vary from agent to agent and depend not only on dose and duration of use but also on the user's personality and underlying psychiatric conditions.

The classic hallucinogenic agent is lysergic acid diethylamide (LSD, acid, white lightning, cubes, window panes, dots, blotteracid), first synthesized by Albert Hoffman at Sandoz laboratories in 1938. Five years later, he accidentally discovered the intense visual hallucinations associated with this drug. Self-experimentation and illicit use of LSD peaked in the early 1970s, and it dropped steadily through that decade into the 1980s because of public attention to the serious adverse effects of this compound. However, the mid-1980s saw a resurgence in LSD use, particularly in high school students, because of its low cost and increased availability and a renewed interest in self-exploration of the inner self.

LSD is a very potent agent active at doses averaging from 50 to 150 mcg. LSD is usually taken orally, with an onset of 30 to 40 minutes. The first symptoms are mild-to-moderate sympathomimetic effects (pupillary dilation, tachycardia, sweating, blurred vision, and so on) followed by the sensory, psychological, and cognitive effects of profound visual hallucinosis and the sensation of disordered integration of sensory input (Table 60.10) (105). For example, users may visualize sounds or music, feel odors, and hear color, and inanimate objects can assume lifelike qualities. The peak intensity of effects is variable, depending on the dose, and occurs within the first 2 or 3 hours and then wears off over the next 5 to 10 hours. Most users return to a normal psychological state within 10 to 12 hours after ingestion. The user's personality and experience with LSD along with environmental factors play an important part in the sensory and psychological effects seen with the drug.

The most common adverse effect is a temporary episode of panic and fear referred to as a bad trip (106). Although this is most common with first-time users, it is also possible with repeat users with increased dosages. Some users can control themselves by relaxation techniques involving breathing exercises and removing any external stimuli that might be producing acute stress. If the patient cannot control the bad trip, treatment is generally supportive and involves talking down the anxiety and fear. This is also referred to as reality therapy and involves the reassurance that these adverse effects are drug related and will soon wear off. Placing the user in a quiet, relaxed setting and removing stress-producing stimuli are also helpful. If this method is not effective, oral benzodiazepines are useful in calming the patient and relieving the panic. However, since benzodiazepines do not reverse the LSD effects, talk-down reassurance should be continued. Even though antipsychotics antagonize the LSD effects, they are usually not needed and have produced orthostatic hypotension and anticholinergic toxicities. Sedative doses of a benzodiazepine like flurazepam 30 to 60 mg should be used if panic reactions continue after initial therapy, which will allow the patient to sleep through the remainder of the drug effects (107).

Flashbacks are an acute but transient recurrence of past or all LSD experiences following a period of normal consciousness. The duration is usually a matter of hours. These events are more common in frequent users of LSD and may occur several years after the last LSD exposure. The incidence of flashbacks has been reported to range from 10 to 80%. However, most people who experimented only a few times with the drug have never had a flashback. Treatment of flashbacks is the same as for an acute anxiety-panic attack.

A small number of cases are reported of what appears to be permanent changes in patterns of thought and behavior developing after repeated use of large doses of LSD. These individuals have been referred to as acid burnouts or acid casualties, and they exhibit a condition indistinguishable from chronic undifferentiated schizophrenia (108).

Table 60.10.
Signs and Symptoms of Hallucinogenic Reactions

Sensory	Psychological	Cognitive	Physiologic
Altered perception of color, objects, size, and shape	Anxiety	Impaired memory, recall, attention	Dilated pupils
Distortion of time, direction, and distance	Panic	Reduced mental performance	Tremor
Synethesias (e.g., "seeing sounds," "hearing colors")	Depression	Difficulty with problem solving	Piloerection ("gooseflesh")
	Mood alterations		Sweating
	Paranoid ideation		Dizziness
	Hallucinations (when sufficiently large doses are taken)		Weakness
			Paresthesias
			Ataxia
			Blurred vision
			Hyperreflexia
			Elevated blood pressure
			Hyperactivity
			Coma
			Elevated temperature
			Nausea
			Vomiting
			Hunger
			Tachycardia
			Bleeding (in massive LSD overdoses; thought to be evidence of platelet dysfunction)
			Clonic movements
			Blood pressure decline (in severe overdoses)

Whether such conditions would have resulted without the drug is unclear. It is possible that the drug simply exacerbated or unmasked an existing schizophrenia (109). Evidence linking these effects to direct neurologic toxicity (brain damage) is inconclusive at this time.

A number of mothers using LSD during pregnancy gave birth to children with birth defects. All these cases involved multidrug use during pregnancy, preventing clear evidence that LSD is teratogenic when taken by either parent before or during pregnancy. However, all drugs used in pregnancy have a potential for producing teratogenic or fetotoxic effects, and they should be avoided, especially during the first trimester.

Mescaline (3,4,5-trimethoxyphenylethylamine) is chemically similar to norepinephrine and its precursor, dopamine. Mescaline and its derivatives have been referred to as the hallucinogenic amphetamines. Mescaline occurs naturally in peyote, a plant preparation obtained from the mescal cactus. The dome-shaped head of this plant is made up of one or more discs (buttons) that have the potential for flowering and contain the principle peyote hallucinogen, mescaline. The peyote or mescal buttons are brown and hard and only rarely available in a powdered form. The buttons are usually softened by the user's saliva before being swallowed and contain, in addition to mescaline, numerous other phenylethylamines and isoquinoline alkaloids. This accounts for the common differences and effects of peyote and mescaline.

Mescaline and peyote have a slow onset, and initial effects are often unpleasant. Nausea, profuse perspiration, and static tremors are common for the first 1 to 2 hours followed by an hallucinogenic experience similar to that with LSD (110). The psychomimetic effects, lasting 8 to 12 hours, include alterations of sight, smell, touch, and hearing, but less mental reorganization than with LSD. Although some illicit users claim to prefer mescaline to LSD, most street samples of mescaline are, in fact, LSD, PCP, or combinations of LSD and PCP and contain no mescaline.

Other phenethylamine derivatives of mescaline include TMA (3,4,5-trimethoxyphenylisopropylamine) and DOM (STP) 2,5-dimethoxy-4-methyl phenylisopropanolomine. The original STP (serenity, tranquility, and peace) was, in fact, a variety of drug mixtures, and not all of them contained DOM; today, STP is a common synonym for DOM. These related conjurors produce a sense of euphoria and talkativeness; however, unlike amphetamines, they impair rather than improve concentration and rarely cause anorexia. They provide a mild psychedelic experience in lower doses and effects similar to mescaline and LSD in larger doses.

Another related chemical entity, MDA (3,4–methylenedioxyamphetamine) was synthesized in 1910, but its psychedelic effects were not discovered until the 1960s. MDA possesses both psychedelic and amphetaminelike effects. Initial effects with doses of 50 to 150 mg are described as euphoric and a sense of detachment or out-of-body experience. The drug has been used experimentally for introspection and to facilitate psychotherapy. Larger doses have produced hallucinations similar to the LSD experience (111). The N-methylation of MDA produces MDMA (methylenedioxymethamphetamine) (111). Street names for this drug are ecstasy, ice, XTC, M & M's, and Adam and Eve. This drug appears to increase talkativeness and has a reputation as an aphrodisiac. Initial sympathomimetic activity includes a mild rise in blood pressure, tachycardia, increased motor activity, and mild anxiety lasting 30 minutes to 1 hour. This state is followed by the relaxed introspection and euphoria seen with MDA. Users claim the psychedelic effects are easier to manage, increasing its popularity among college students as a "recreational drug" (113–118). This drug has a low therapeutic index, with the possibility of chronic and possibly permanent neurologic toxicity at two to four times the hallucinogenic dose. There appears to be a selective destruction of tryptaminergic nerves in the cerebral cortex and hypothalamus in animals. Long-term recovery may occur but is generally incomplete (119). Chronic users experience a withdrawal syndrome marked by severe depression (known as crash) and bruxism (120–122).

Compounds related to LSD and resembling serotonin are DMT (dimethyltryptamine), psilocybin, psilocin, harmine, and bufotenine. Psilocybin is a naturally occurring psychedelic found in mushrooms and used by the Mexican Indians. Psilocybin is commonly taken by mouth and is one of the most rapidly acting psychedelics used orally. Initial effects are seen within 15 minutes after ingestion of doses 4 to 8 mg, reaching a peak effect in 1 to 2 hours. Total duration is 5 to 6 hours unless the dosage is increased above 8 mg. Physiologic effects include increased pulse rate, respiratory rate, and body temperature; dilated pupils; and elevated systolic blood pressure; followed by an LSD-type hallucinogenic experience. As with the other exotic psychedelics (mescaline and DOM), most street sales of this compound contain LSD, PCP, amphetamines, or a combination of these or other drugs.

DMT (dimethyltryptamine) is one of the derivatives that has been isolated from the "hallucinogenic snuffs" used by the South American Indians. In its pure form, DMT is a very short-acting agent with effects lasting less than 1 hour. Because of its short-acting effects, DMT is sometimes referred as the businessman's psychedelic or businessman's trip.

Other agents that have been used recently to produce hallucinogenic effects are the anticholinergic preparations used in the treatment of extrapyramidal effects, trihexiphenidyl (Artane) and benztropine (Cogentin). These agents may produce effects ranging from mild CNS stimulation to a toxic delirium. High doses of these agents

produce euphoria, confusion, hallucinations, and paranoia and may result in a state resembling toxic psychosis.

Phencyclidine

Phencyclidine (PCP) was developed in the 1950s as a general anesthetic for veterinary and human use under the trade name of Sernyl. Although it was approved and marketed for human use for a short period, the postoperative delirium and unpleasant side effects resulted in withdrawal of the drug from the market in 1965. Phencyclidine was then marketed for veterinary use only in 1967 as Sernylan, until 1978 when it was classified as a schedule I controlled substance and removed from the market. Parke Davis continues to market a similar arylcycloalkylamine compound, ketamine, which causes similar adverse effects to PCP in a few patients and has also appeared with increasing frequency on the street scene as "monkey morphine." PCP appeared on the street scene in the late 1960s under the street names of hog, PeaCe Pill, crystal, flakes, and angel dust. Its popularity increased in the mid-1970s, frequently as a substitute for less-available drugs such as THC, peyote, mescaline, psilocybin, and LSD. Publicity about serious adverse effects led to a decline in PCP use in the late 1980s (123). PCP can be used orally, injected, or snorted, but it is most commonly smoked to allow users to monitor the dosage more carefully. PCP can be applied to tobacco, parsley, or marijuana (laced or dusted joint, or killerweed). It is also sold in combination with a variety of other drugs and many times substituted for street drugs that are difficult to obtain, such as THC, peyote, psilocybin, mescaline, or LSD.

In small doses, PCP produces intoxication, with staggering gait, ataxia, slurred speech, numbness of the extremities, and a dissociative feeling. Horizontal and/or vertical nystagmus is often present and diagnostic. Muscular rigidity, sweating, apathy, and a blank stare may develop. Users report feelings of depersonalization and disordered thoughts. The effects of PCP generally last 4 to 6 hours depending on the dosage. With doses in excess of 5 mg, a more pronounced analgesic effect is noticed. Hostile or unusual behavior is possible as doses are increased (124). The patient may show agitation, combativeness, and psychosis. Users perceive a superhuman strength, invulnerability, and body image distortions. Blood pressure is likely to be increased along with heart rate. Increased salivation, fever, repetitive movements, and muscular rigidity have also been reported. With increasing doses, analgesia is increased. Users do not perceive pain. Anesthesia, stupor, or coma and convulsions may occur though the eyes may remain open. With higher doses, prolonged coma, muscle rigidity, opisthotonic posturing, and convulsions may occur. Nystagmus may or may not be present at toxic doses. Respiratory depression, seizures, acidosis, and rhabdomyolysis are also possible (125). Hypoglycemia and increased CPK, AST, ALT, and uric acid levels are also present. Isolation of patients from external stimuli to the degree compatible with support of vital functions and control of self-destructive or violent behavior is recommended. Recovery is usually rapid although some reports of overdosage include symptoms that last for several weeks. Mental status may take several days to weeks to return to normal. A psychotic phase has been reported for several weeks in some patients after a single dose of PCP.

Treatment of bad trips or an overdose of PCP often requires emergency care because the patient is often violent and combative in behavior. Benzodiazapines are used to calm the patient. Attempts to talk down the patient are generally ineffective and may often trigger violent behavior. Hostile and combative patients may require haloperidol to protect the patient and others from violent behavior. Chlorpromazine is not recommended because of possible hypotensive effects and augmenting the anticholinergic actions of PCP (126). Treatment of overdosage is otherwise symptomatic and aimed at supporting vital functions (127). Hypersalivation may require suction, and respiratory depression may require artificial ventilation. Convulsions have been successfully treated with diazepam, and hypertension has been treated with hydralazine, sublingual nifedipine, nitroprusside, or phentolamine. Anticonvulsants should be used to prevent seizures and excessive muscle contractions since these along with hyperthermia may aggravate rhabdomyolysis.

There is considerable gastric recirculation of PCP when it reaches the alkaline environment of the duodenum. Continuous gastric suction can be of value in the treatment of an overdose. Other clinicians prefer to use repeated doses of activated charcoal to enhance elimination of the drug from the intestine. Urinary secretion of PCP is increased when urinary pH is acidic. However, since only a small percentage of the drug is excreted renally, urinary acidification may not play an important role in the elimination of the compound.

Serious neurologic and psychological disorders have been reported with chronic PCP use, ranging from personality changes, confusional states, to psychotic states that may be long lasting. Patients with schizophrenia may be especially vulnerable to the psychotogenic effects of PCP. Other disorders that have been commonly reported with chronic PCP use are anxiety, nervousness, paranoia, delusions, memory disturbances, speech problems, anxiety, and mood swings ranging from social withdrawal and isolation to highly aggressive violent behavior that may last up to 1 year after cessation of drug use. Psychotic states have been reported to last several weeks after a single dose of PCP. Flashbacks have been reported to recur over a period of up to 2 months after discontinuing PCP use.

Chronic use of PCP can lead to both psychological and physical dependence. Monkeys with implanted catheters will not administer LSD to themselves, but they do self-administer PCP (128). Chronic users have reported continuous difficulty with memory, speech, and visual disturbances lasting up to 1 year after discontinuing the drug. Severe depression, nervousness, and personality changes are often resistant to treatment. The recovery phase of users discontinuing PCP is often marked with severe depression, stimulating recurrent drug abuse.

Marijuana

Marijuana is the flowering tops and leaves of the hemp plant known as *Cannabis sativa* (grass, pot, weed, Mary Jane). The dried leaves are most commonly smoked as cigarettes (joint, reefer, doobie, number) or in a pipe. The drug may be ingested orally in a prepared food (brownies) or beverage, but onset is slow (45 to 60 minutes) and absorption incomplete. Although all parts of the male and female plant contain psychoactive substances, the highest concentrations are found in the flowering tops. The dried resinous exudate of the tops is called hashish. More than 60 cannabinoids have been isolated from marijuana. The euphoric and psychoactive effects may be due to a combination of several of them. However, delta-9-tetrahydrocannabinol (THC) is the agent believed to produce most of the characteristic effects. Hundreds of other compounds are produced by pyrolysis when marijuana is smoked and may be important in the long-term toxic effects of chronic use.

Another form of the drug, "hashoil," is extracted from the plant with organic solvents and may contain a concentration of up to 50 to 60% THC. However, much of the "pure THC" or hashoil that is found on the street is often PCP. The major effects of marijuana are seen in the central nervous system and range from a mild relaxation and sedation to euphoria. Intoxication with marijuana is known as being stoned or high. Users commonly describe a increased sense of well-being; giddiness; alteration of time and space perception; and subjective enhancement in senses of touch, taste, smell, and sound. Users experience unusual hunger and craving for food referred to as the munchies. Some users claim that the drug increases their creativity and awareness of their surroundings. Many of the subjective effects appear to depend on the expectations of the user and the circumstances under which the drug is used. Other physiologic effects are a mild increase in heart rate, dry mouth and throat, dryness of the eyelids, and conjunctival reddening. Performance of simple motor tasks and reaction times are unimpaired in small doses but are significantly affected by doses equivalent to one or two cigarettes. Driving performance is clearly impaired for 4 to 8 hours, well beyond the time that the user thinks the subjective effects of the drug have worn off. Impairment produced by marijuana is additive to that of alcohol if the two are used concurrently. The effects of smoking marijuana occur rapidly within 5 to 10 minutes, may last 2 to 3 hours, depending on the dose, and are occasionally followed by a period of drowsiness (129).

Relative to opiates, cocaine, depressants, and hallucinogens, emergency treatment of marijuana intoxication is rare (130, 131). Occasionally, a first-time user may experience a syndrome known as a panic attack, consisting of anxiety, disorientation, and paranoid feelings. Previous users of the milder forms of marijuana may also experience this reaction if exposed to more potent forms of cannabis or THC. Treatment for this reaction is primarily reassurance and talking down the fear and panic exhibited. Placing the patient in quiet surroundings and avoiding stimulants are also beneficial. Panic attacks seldom last more than 2 to 3 hours and may be relieved by small doses of benzodiazepines if talk-down therapy is not fully effective. Patients with combative or aggressive behavior may have been using a product known as super weed that has been "laced" with phencyclidine (PCP).

Tolerance to the effects of marijuana clearly exists even though chronic users have described a "reversed tolerance" and claim that smaller doses of the drug are necessary to produce the desired effects (132, 133). This effect is probably related to the manner of use and the expectations of the user. Chronic, high-dose cannabis users may experience an abstinence or withdrawal syndrome on abrupt discontinuation of use. Signs and symptoms include irritability, restlessness, nervousness, anorexia, weight loss, insomnia, and REM rebound. Onset of this syndrome is several hours after the last dose, and it lasts 4 to 5 days. Since withdrawal is not life threatening, treatment involves little more than supportive therapy with short-term, low doses of benzodiazepines.

In addition to the slowed psychomotor response while under the influence of the drug, there is a decrease in short-term memory that is reversible on discontinuing the drug (134–136). Several reported physiologic effects produce concern. The respiratory effects of long-term marijuana use produce chronic cough, laryngitis, bronchitis, and pathologic changes like those in chronic tobacco smokers (137–141). Chronic smoking of one marijuana cigarette daily will decrease vital lung capacity equal to that seen after chronic smoking of one pack of tobacco cigarettes daily (142–144). In addition, the smoke from a marijuana cigarette contains high concentrations of several key carcinogenic agents found in tobacco smoke (145). Another concern is the possibility of pulmonary fibrosis from smoking marijuana that has been sprayed with paraquat, other herbicides, or other insecticides. However, the latest reports indicate that smoking destroys paraquat by pyrolysis (146).

Other effects of marijuana are decreased testosterone concentrations and a reversible decreased spermatogenesis in males. Females experience decreased FSH and LH concentrations in the normal ovulatory cycle. Although THC crosses the placenta, there are no reports in humans of teratogenic effects directly attributable to marijuana alone (147–149). However, avoiding any unnecessary drug during pregnancy is advisable. Children born to mothers who were chronic marijuana smokers during pregnancy may be at increased risk for learning disabilities such as attention-deficit disorders (150, 151). *Salmonella* and *Aspergillus* contaminants have been reported to produce infections (152, 153).

Chronic use of marijuana has been implicated in producing psychological changes and production of what has been called an amotivational syndrome characterized by diminished drive, ambition, and motivation; loss of effectiveness; impairment of judgment, concentration, memory, and communication skills; and inability to set goals or manage stress. Cessation may lead to gradual improvement over several weeks but may require months. It is difficult to determine whether these effects were present prior to and not caused by marijuana use, but they are observed very commonly. Several studies have implicated marijuana with structural brain damage, but much controversy exists about these (154, 155). Seizures have occurred in some epileptics.

There has been much recent information on the dangers of passive tobacco smoke. Concern could also be expressed over potential problems of passive marijuana smoke although intoxication is rarely reported from passive inhalation of marijuana. However, there are numerous reports of cannabis metabolites detected in the urine of the passive inhaler (156–158). THC metabolites may be present in the urine up to 2 months after heavy chronic use.

Marijuana is considered, along with alcohol and tobacco products, as one of the major "gateway" drugs. Although this does not imply that users of marijuana will all progress to more dangerous drugs (e.g., cocaine), use of one or more of these commonly available agents is part of the history of most drug dependencies.

VOLATILE SUBSTANCES—INHALANTS

Many volatile liquids produce an intoxicated state when inhaled. Young children and adolescents most commonly experiment with this method of producing distorted consciousness. A wide variety of industrial solvents, anesthetics, and other chemicals may produce intoxication and coma (Table 60.11). They can be divided into three groups: (1) commercial solvents: toluene, xylene, benzene, naphtha, hexane, acetone, trichloroethylene, carbon tetrachloride, and many other volatile solvents found in model airplane glue, plastic cements, paint thinner, gasoline, cleaning fluids, nail polish remover, and lighter fluid; (2)

Table 60.11.
Commonly Abused Solvent Products

Glue	Toluene, xylene, acetone, benzene, n-hexane
Cleaning fluids	Trichloroethylene, toluene, carbon tetrachloride, tetrachlorethylene, 1,1,1-trichloroethane
Petrochemicals (gasoline)	Hydrocarbons, lead
Aerosols	Flurocarbons
Lighter fluid	Butane
Acrylic paint	Toluene
Paints, varnishes, thinning lacquers	Trichloroethane, methylene chloride, toluene, alcohols, ketones
Cements	Acetone, toluene, hydrocarbons, trichlorethylene, hexane
Dyes	Acetone, methylene chloride
Nail polish remover	Acetone, amyl acetate, alcohol

Table 60.12.
General Effects of Inhaled Volatile Solvents

Common Acute Effects	Rare Dangers
Euphoria	"Sudden sniffing death"
Drowsiness	Suffocation
Headache	
Nausea	
Partial amnesia	
Visual disturbance	
Hallucination	
Ataxia	
Impaired judgment	
Reduced muscle and reflex control	
Tolerance	
Metabolic acidosis	
High anion gap	
Hypokalemia	

aerosols: propellants in many household and commercial aerosols sprays, gases containing chlorinated or fluorinated hydrocarbons, including insecticides, deodorants, hairsprays, and nonstick coating substances; and (3) anesthetics: nitrous oxide (laughing gas) and, less frequently, chloroform and ether. Nitrous oxide is available commercially as a whipped-cream propellant and as a tracer gas to detect pipe leaks to reduce preignition in racing cars. Anesthetics have been abused since their discovery in the early 1800s. Glue sniffing became widespread in the late 1950s, and experimentation with many other inhalants proliferated during the 1960s. These compounds are commonly sniffed for their intoxicating effects. Solvents can be "bagged," or sprayed into a plastic bag prior to inhalation, or "huffed," sprayed into a cloth and held to the mouth.

Although there is a wide range of chemical entities, nearly all the abused volatile substances produce CNS depression. Decreased inhibition may produce an apparent stimulant effect and initial sense of euphoria preceding the classic sedative effects of ataxia, dizziness, impaired judgment, slurred speech, and somnolence. At larger doses, hallucinations and delusions, including a sense of omnipotence or unusual strength, may lead to impulsive behavior. The initial euphoric effects may last only a few minutes, with the depressant effects gradually wearing off in 1 to 2 hours. At very high doses, loss of consciousness may occur, and recovery can take several hours.

All the inhalants share the hazard of inducing an intoxicated state in which judgment and motor function are impaired (Table 60.12). Accidents have occurred, including fatalities where suffocation is the major cause of death. Most commonly, this occurs when the user becomes unconscious with the apparatus used covering the nose and mouth. High concentrations of any aromatic hydrocarbon can cause coma and death (159, 160). In addition to

asphyxiation and trauma, reports of death due to sudden cardiac ventricular arrhythmias are most commonly preceded by physical exercise (161). Other adverse effects are direct organ toxicities associated with specific compounds (161). Chronic long-term inhalation of benzene may cause bone marrow aplasia, neurosis, and fatty degeneration of the liver and heart (163). Gasoline not only contains benzene, but some types contain enough lead to produce systemic lead poisoning (164–166). Toluene may produce permanent, neurologic dysfunction of the cerebral cortical, cerebellar, auditory, pyramidal track, brain stem, and peripheral nervous system (167–171). Hepatic and renal damage (renal tubular acidosis) have also been reported with chronic use (172).

Nitrous oxide has been recreationally abused since its discovery in 1844. However, it is a safe and valuable anesthetic when used appropriately, as is seen commonly in "painless" dental practice today. Misuse can cause hypoxia and asphyxia, leading to permanent nerve damage and/or death when oxygen is not inhaled in appropriate concentrations with the gas. End-organ toxicity is rare with occasional use of nitrous oxide. However, chronic use of this gas has been reported to produce a number of transient neurotoxicities such as progressive paresthesia or neuropathy similar to vitamin B-12 deficiency (173). Contaminants of some consumer kits for production of nitrous oxide may produce respiratory distress (174). Intoxication with nitrous oxide clearly impairs muscle coordination and delays reaction time, decreasing the ability to drive.

A growing number of users of organic nitrites include abuse of amyl nitrite and its nonprescription analogs, butyl and isobutyl nitrite, which are sold as liquid incense or room deodorizers under such trade names as (Rush, Lockerroom, Sweat, Bolt, Quicksilver, Jock, Hardware, Aroma of Men, and Heart On). Commonly known as poppers, snappers, or disco drugs, these products have

Table 60.13.
Organic Nitrites Effects

Physiologic Effects	Adverse Effects
Vasodilation	Giddiness
Venous pooling	Headache
Hypotension	Nausea
Reflex tachycardia	Vomiting
Reduced cerebral blood flow	Flushing
Tissue hypoxia	Dermatitis
Sphincter relaxation	Methemoglobinemia
Tolerance	Weakness
	Dizziness
	Syncope
	Shortness of breath
	Chest pain
	Tracheobronchitis
	Increased intraocular pressure

been popularized as aphrodisiacs among male homosexuals (175). The major pharmacologic effects of the nitrites is a significant vasodilation due to their smooth muscle relaxant effect (Table 60.13). Peak effects following inhalation occur within seconds, last less than a minute, and may be followed by flushing, headaches, and dizziness. Hypotensive reflex tachycardia is common and may lead to syncope. Methemoglobinemia and death have been rarely reported following chronic use of these compounds and are more likely to occur if they are ingested (176, 177).

Nicotine

Approximately 50 million Americans regularly smoke cigarettes despite serious health consequences, declining social acceptability, and numerous educational programs and antismoking campaigns. Between 80 and 90% of smokers have tried to quit smoking, but most have been unable to maintain long-term abstinence (178, 179).

Cigarette smoking is a complex addiction, with both behavioral and pharmacologic components (180). The addictive substance in tobacco is nicotine. Nicotine is one of the most addictive, dependency-causing drugs known. Milligram for milligram, nicotine is 10 times more potent than heroin. But unlike heroin, cigarette smoking retains a certain amount of social acceptability (181).

Depending on the pH of the nicotine-delivery vehicle, nicotine can be readily absorbed from the respiratory tract, buccal mucosa, and skin. Nicotine ingested through smoke (pH 5.5) is readily absorbed in the lungs and is quickly transported to the brain. Chewing tobacco, snuff, and nicotine chewing gum are alkaline, which facilitates the absorption of nicotine across mucous membranes. Oral ingestion of nicotine results in low systemic concentrations because of extensive first-pass metabolism in the liver (182).

Nicotine acts via two major neuronal pathways in the brain: the mesolimbic–dopaminergic system and the locus

ceruleus. The mesolimbic–dopaminergic system is the motivational behavioral center of the brain. When stimulated, this center produces a calming effect and a significant sense of well-being. The locus ceruleus mediates stress reactions, vigilance, and alertness. As such, it is one of the prime physiologic enhancers of the higher mental functions. In effect, nicotine gives the smoker a "double whammy." Nicotine makes the smoker feel good while enhancing the higher cognitive functions (183).

MEDICAL CONSEQUENCES OF NICOTINE

Cigarette smoking is the most devastating preventable cause of disease and premature death in the United States. More than 5 million years of life were lost prematurely in 1990 as a result of smoking. Table 60.14 shows the distribution by disease of smoking-related deaths in 1990 (184).

Of the more than 4000 substances in cigarette smoke, 43 are known carcinogens. Smoking accounts for 30% of all cancer-related deaths. Cigarette smoking significantly increases the risk of cardiovascular disease, including coronary heart disease (CHD), stroke, sudden death, aortic aneurysm, and peripheral vascular disease. The risk is directly correlated with the number of cigarettes smoked; however, smoking even as few as one to four cigarettes per day substantially increases the risk (185, 186).

Lung cancer is the most important of the smoking-related cancers; smoking caused 85% of cases and 119,920 deaths in 1990. Cigarette smoking is the leading cause of pulmonary illness and related deaths in the United States. Chronic obstructive pulmonary disease (COPD) is the fifth leading cause of death in our country, and most deaths from COPD are attributable to smoking (184, 185, 187).

In addition to being responsible for a large percentage of lung cancers, smoking is associated with cancers of the mouth pharynx, larynx, esophagus, stomach, pancreas, uterine cervix, kidney, ureter, and bladder and accounts for about 30% of all deaths from cancer (188). Other possible health consequences of cigarette smoking include peptic ulcer disease, cataracts, and, in women, reduced fertility and osteoporosis (185). Smokeless tobacco also has serious

Table 60.14.
Smoking-Related Deaths in the United States in 1990[a]

Cause of Death	No. Deaths
Cardiovascular disease	179,820
Lung cancer	119,920[b]
Cancer other than lung cancer	31,402
Respiratory disease	84,475
Disease in infants[c]	1,711
Burns	1,362

[a]Data from Centers for Disease Control and Prevention
[b]Includes deaths associated with exposure to environmental tobacco smoke
[c]Persons less than one year of age

health consequences. The use of smokeless tobacco increases the risk of oropharyngeal cancers fourfold (189).

In summary, the economic health costs of tobacco use are enormous. The total expenditures are believed to exceed $100 billion per year (190).

SMOKING CESSATION METHODS—NONPHARMACOLOGIC INTERVENTION

Nicotine dependence may be treated successfully with unassisted or assisted cessation programs. The most frequent unassisted cessation method employed is where the patient simply decides to quit. This cold turkey method is used by more than 80% of smokers attempting to quit. Other unassisted methods include intake limitation, brand changing (reduced tar), and nonprescription aids (191). Assisted methods include support groups; programs offered by the American Cancer Society, American Lung Association, or American Heart Association; and physician-assisted cessation. Some smokers also seek assistance through hypnosis or acupuncture therapy.

SMOKING CESSATION METHODS—PHARMACOLOGIC INTERVENTION

The only pharmacologic agent with FDA-approved labeling for use in smoking-cessation therapy is nicotine. Since nicotine gum and patches were first marketed, more data have become available on their effectiveness, and new formulations of the drug have been developed. Recent data indicate that treatment with nicotine patches double or triple long-term smoking cessation rates (191). Manufacturers recommend wearing the patches for 4 to 12 weeks, but the optimal duration of patch use is unknown; 8 weeks' treatment appears to be as effective as longer therapy. Nicotine in gum (nicotine polacrilex) is available in 2 and 4 mg doses. Manufacturers recommend using nicotine gum for 4 to 6 months, but the optimal duration is unknown. Patches are generally better tolerated than nicotine gum. Skin irritation is the most frequently reported adverse effect with the nicotine patch. The gum may cause flatulence; indigestion; nausea; an unpleasant taste; hiccups; and a sore mouth, throat, and jaw. Nicotine nasal spray and nicotine inhaler are new formulations currently under investigation (192).

Other agents such as buspirone, a nonbenzodiazepine antianxiety drug, and various antidepressants have also been tried as aids to smoking cessation. Further research is needed to define the role of these agents in the treatment of nicotine dependence, either alone or in combination with nicotine replacement therapy (192).

Nicotine dependence is difficult to treat, but effective use of available options can greatly enhance a smoker's chances of quitting. All smokers should be educated about the risks of tobacco use and the benefits of quitting, and they should be advised to quit.

CONCLUSION

Drug abuse is a complex multifaceted problem. There have been no simple or universally successful solutions. Increased public awareness programs, coordinated educational programs in elementary and junior high schools, increased law enforcement efforts to decrease the availability of illicit drugs, and more severe punishment from the judicial system have been the mainstays of coordinated efforts at both the local and national levels to decrease most forms of drug abuse among young people. However, at the same time, alcohol abuse is at an all-time high in teenagers and is occurring at younger ages. Health professionals have a unique responsibility regarding drug abuse and should be proactive in drug abuse education and prevention programs.

REFERENCES

1. Ziporyn T. A growing industry and menace: makeshift laboratory's designer drugs. JAMA 256(22):3061, 1986.
2. LaBarbera M, Wolfe T. Characteristics, attitudes and implications of fentanyl use based upon reports from self-identified fentanyl users. J Psychoactive Drugs 15(4):293, 1983.
3. Moore RA, Rumack BH, Conner CS, et al. Naloxone underdosage after narcotic poisoning. Am J Dis Child 134:156, 1980.
4. Jasinski DR, Martin WR, Haertzen CA. The human pharmacology and abuse potential of N-allylnoroxymorphone (Naloxone). J Pharmacol Exp Ther 157:420, 1967.
5. Heishman SJ, Stitzer ML, Bigelow GE, Liebson IA. Acute opioid physical dependence in postaddict humans: naloxone dose effects after brief morphine exposure. J Pharmacol Exp Ther 248:127–134, 1989.
6. Freitas PM. Narcotic withdrawal in the emergency department. Am J Emerg Med 3:456–460, 1985.
7. Hodding GC, Jann M, Ackerman IP. Drug withdrawal syndromes: a literature review. West J Med 133:383–391, 1980.
8. Ostrea EM, Chavez JS, Strauss ME. A study of factors that influence the severity of neonatal narcotic withdrawal. J Pediatr 88:642, 1976.
9. Bashore RA, Ketchum JS, Staisch KJ. Heroin addiction and pregnancy. West J Med 134:506, 1981.
10. Rosen TS. Infants of addicted mothers. In Farnoff AA, Martin RJ (eds): Neonatal-Perinatal Medicine St. Louis, CV Mosby, 1114, 1987.
11. Futz JM Jr, Senay EC. Guidelines for the management of hospitalized narcotic addicts. Ann Inter Med 82:815–818, 1975.
12. Gossop M, Johns A, Green L. Opiate withdrawal: inpatient versus outpatient programmes and preferred versus random assignment to treatment. Br Med J 293:103–104, 1986.
13. Vining E, Kosten TR, Kleber HD. Clinical utility of rapid clonidine-naltrexone detoxification for opioid abusers. Br J Addiction 83:567–574, 1988.
14. Brewer C, Rezae H, Bailey C. Opioid withdrawal and naltrexone induction in 48-72 hours with minimal drop-out, using a modification of the naltrexone-clonidine technique. Br J Psychiatry 153:340–343, 1988.
15. Senft RA. Experiences with Clonidine-Naltrexone for Rapid Opiate Detoxification. J Sub Abuse Treat 8:257–259, 1991.
16. Strain EC, Stitzer ML, Liebson IA, Bigelow GE. Dose-Response Effects of Methadone in the Treatment of Opioid Dependence. Ann Int Med 119:23–27, 1993.
17. Jaffe JH. Drug addiction and drug abuse. In Gilman AG, Rall TW, Nies AS, et al. (eds): The Pharmacological Basis of Therapeutics, ed. 8. New York, Macmillan, 1990.

18. Newman RG. Methadone treatment: defining and evaluating success. N Engl J Med 317:447, 1987.

19. Judson BA, Goldstein A, Inturrisi CE. Methadylacetate (LAAM) in the treatment of heroin addicts. Arch Gen Psychiatry 40:834–840, 1983.

20. Gossop M. Clonidine and the treatment of the opiate withdrawal syndrome. Drug Alcohol Depend 21:253–259, 1988.

21. Gold MS, Pottash AC, Sweeney DR. Opiate withdrawal using clonidine. JAMA, 243:343, 1980.

22. Crabtree B. Review of naltrexane, a long-acting opiate antagonist. Clin Pharm 3:273–280, 1984.

23. Kleber HD. Naltrexone. J Subst Abuse Treat 2:117, 1985.

24. Gonzales JP, Brogden RN. Naltrexone: a review. Drugs 35:192–213, 1988.

25. Gram DH, Marmo J, Holden R. Naltrexone treatment—the problem of patient acceptance. J Subst Abuse Treat 6:119–122, 1989.

26. Preston KL, Bigelow GE. Pharmacological advances in addiction treatment. Int J Addict 20(6 & 7):185, 1985.

27. Steel PM, Haverkos HW. Epidemiologic Studies of HIV/AIDS and Drug Abuse. Am J Drug Alcohol Abuse 18:167–175, 1992.

28. Cherubin CE, Sapira JD. The Medical Complications of Drug Addiction and the medical Assessment of the Intravenous Drug User: 25 Years Later. Ann Intern Med 119:1017–1028.

29. Brittle RP. Infections and Injection Drug Use. J Infect 25:121–131, 1992.

30. Khantzian EJ, McKenna GJ. Acute toxic and withdrawal reactions associated with drug use and abuse. Ann Intern Med 90:361, 1979.

31. Woods JH, Katz JL, Winger G. Abuse liability of benzodiazepines, Pharmacol Rev 39:251–419, 1987.

32. Arieff AJ, Friedmann EA. Coma following non-narcotic drug overdose: management of 200 adult patients. Am J Med Sci 266:405, 1973.

33. Hadden J, Johnson K, Smith S. Acute barbiturate intoxication concepts of management. JAMA 209:893, 1969.

34. Pond SM, Olson KR, Osterloh JD. Randomized study of the treatment of phenobarbital overdose with repeated doses of activated charcoal. JAMA 251:3104–3108, 1984.

35. Miller NS, Gold MS. Identification and treatment of benzodiazepine abuse. Am Fam Physician 40:175–183, 1989.

36. Owen RT, Tyrer P. Benzodiazepine dependence: a review of the evidence. Drugs 25:385, 1983.

37. Rifkin A, Quitkin F, Klein DF. Withdrawal reaction to diazepam. JAMA 236:2171, 1976.

38. Smith DS, Wesson DR. Benzodiazepine dependency syndromes. J Psychoactive Drugs, 15:85, 1983.

39. Rosenberg HC, Chiu TH. Time course for development of benzodiazepine tolerance and physical dependence. Neurosci Biobehav Rev 9:123–131, 1985.

40. Busto U, Sellers EM, Naranjo CA. Withdrawal reaction after long-term therapeutic use of benzodiazepines. N Engl J Med 313:854–859, 1986.

41. Sanchez-Craig M, Cappell H, Busto U, Kay G. Cognitive-behavioural treatment for benzodiazepine dependence: a comparison of gradual versus abrupt cessation of drug intake. Br J Addict 82:1317–1327, 1987.

42. Woods JH, Katz JL, Winger G. Use and abuse of benzodiazepines: issues relevant to prescribing. JAMA 260:3476–3480, 1988.

43. Kales A, Scharf MB, Kales JD. Rebound insomnia: a potential hazard following withdrawal of certain benzodiazepines. JAMA 241:1692, 1979.

44. Robinson GM, Sellers EM, Janecek E. Barbiturate and hyposedative withdrawal by a multiple oral phenobarbital loading dose technique. Clin Pharmacol Ther 30(1):71, 1981.

45. Smith DE, Wesson DR. Phenobarbital technique for treatment of barbiturate dependence. Arch Gen Psychiatry 24:56–60, 1971.

46. Robinson GM, Sellers EM, Janecek E. Barbiturate and hyposedative withdrawal by a multiple oral phenobarbital loading dose technique. Clin Pharmacol Ther 30:71–76, 1981.

47. Martin PR, Kapur BM, Whiteside EA. Intravenous phenobarbital therapy in barbiturate and hyposedative withdrawal reactions: a kinetic approach. Clin Pharmacol Ther 26:856–864, 1979.

48. Wesson DR, Smith DE. Treatment techniques for narcotic withdrawal and special reference to mixed narcotic-sedative addiction. J Psychedelic Drugs 4:118, 1971.

49. Perry PJ, Alexander B. Sedative/hypnotic dependence: patient stabilization, tolerance testing, and withdrawal. Drug Intell Clin Pharm 20:532–537, 1986.

50. Harrison M, Busto U, Naranjo CA. Diazepan tapering in detoxication for high-dose benzodiazepine abuse. Clin Pharmacol Ther 36:527–533, 1984.

51. Mueller SM. Neurologic complications of phenylpropanolamine use. Neurology 33:650, 1983.

52. Dietz AJ. Amphetamine-like reactions to phenylpropanolamine. JAMA 245(6):601, 1981.

53. Ellinwood EH. Assault and homicide associated with amphetamine abuse. Am J Psych 127:1170, 1971.

54. Schmidt CJ, Gibb JW. Role of dopamine in the neurotoxic effects of methamphetamine. J Pharmacol Exp Ther 233:539, 1985.

55. Kleber HD. Cocaine abuse: historical, epidemiological, and psychological perspectives. J Clin Psychiatry 49:2(suppl),3–6, 1988.

56. Washton AM, Gold MS, Pottash AC. Crack: early report on a new drug epidemic. Postgrad Med, 80(5):52, 1986.

57. Gawin FH, Ellinwood EH, Jr. Cocaine and other stimulants: actions, abuse, and treatment. N Engl J Med 318:1173–1182, 1988.

58. Siegel RK. Cocaine smoking. J Psychoactive Drugs 14(4):313, 1982.

59. Perez-Reyes M, DiGuiseppi S, Ondrusek G. Free-base cocaine smoking. Clin Pharmacol Ther 32(4):459, 1982.

60. Dakis CA, Gold MS. New concepts in cocaine addiction: the dopamine depletion hypothesis. Neurosci Biobehav Rev 9:469, 1985.

61. Jeffcoat AR, Perez-Reyes M, Hill JM. Cocaine disposition in humans after intravenous injection, nasal insufflation (snorting), or smoking. Drug Metab Dispos 17:153–159, 1989.

62. Chow MJ, Ambre JJ, Ruo TI. Kinetics of cocaine distribution, elimination, and chronotropic effects. Clin Pharmacol Ther 38:318, 1985.

63. Isner JM, Estes NAM III, Thompson PD. Acute cardiac events temporally related to cocaine abuse. N Engl J Med 315:1438–1443, 1986.

64. Itkonen J, Schnoll S, Glassroth J. Pulmonary dysfunction in "freebase" cocaine users. Arch Intern Med 144:2195, 1984.

65. Warner EA. Cocaine Abuse. Ann Intern Med 119:226–235, 1993.

66. Karch SB, Billingham ME. The pathology and etiology of cocaine-induced heart disease. Arch Pathol Lab Med 112:225–230, 1988.

67. Cregler LL. Adverse consequences of cocaine abuse. J Natl Med Assoc 81:27–38, 1989.

68. Isner JM, Estes NAM III, Thompson PD. Acute cardiac events temporally related to cocaine abuse. N Engl J Med 315:1438–1443, 1986.

69. Lang RA, Cigarroa RG, Yancy CW. Cocaine-induced coronary-artery vasoconstriction. N Engl J Med 321:1557–1562, 1989.

70. Cregler LL, Mark H. Special report: medical complications of cocaine abuse. N Engl J Med 315(23):1495, 1986.

71. Baldwin WA, Rosenfeld BA, Brelos MJ, Buchman TG, Deutshman CS, Moore RD. Substance Abuse Related to Admission to Adult Intensive Care. Chest 103:21–25, 1993.

72. Nademanee K, Gonelick DA, Josephson MA. Myocardial Ischemia During Cocaine Withdrawal. Ann Int Med 111:876–879, 1989.

73. Ettinger NA, Albin RJ. A review of the respiratory effects of smoking cocaine. Am J Med 87:664–668, 1989.

74. Itkonen J, Schnoll S, Glassroth J. Pulmonary dysfunction in "freebase" cocaine users. Arch Intern Med 144:2195, 1984.

75. McCarrol KA, Roszler MH. Lung Disorders due to Drug Abuse J Thorc Imaging 6:30–35, 1991.

76. Golbe LI, Merkin MD. Cerebral infarction in a user of freebase cocaine (crack). Neurology 36:1602, 1986.

77. Kaku DA, Lowenstein DH. Emergence of Recreational Drug Use as a Major Risk Factor for Stroke in Young Adults. Ann Int Med 113:821–827, 1990.

78. Mody CK, Miller BL, McIntyre HB, Cobb SK, Goldberg MA. Neurologic complications of cocaine abuse, Neurology 38:1189–1193, 1988.

79. Lathers CM, Tyau LSY, Spino MM, Agarwal I. Cocaine-induced seizures, arrhythmias and sudden death. J Clin Pharmacol 28:584–593, 1988.

80. Cregler LL, Mark H. Medical complications of cocaine abuse. N Engl J Med 315:1495–1500, 1986.

81. Sharff JA. Renal infarction associated with intravenous cocaine use. Ann Emerg Med 13:1145, 1984.

82. Isner JM, Chorkshi SK. Cocaine and vasospasm. N Engl J Med 321:1604–1606, 1989.

83. Nademanee K, Gorelick DA, Josephson MA. Myocardial ischemia during cocaine withdrawal. Ann Intern Med 111:876–880, 1989.

84. Pasternack PF, Colvin SB, Baumann FG. Cocaine induced angina pectoris and acute infarction in patients younger than 40 years. Am J Cardiol 55:847, 1985.

85. Howard RE, Hueter DC, Davis GJ. Acute myocardial infarction following cocaine abuse in a young woman with normal coronary arteries. JAMA 245(1):95, 1985.

86. Vandette JM, Cornish LA. Medical Complications of illicit cocaine use. Clin Pharm 8:401–411, 1989.

87. Caruana DS, Weinbach B, Goery D. Cocaine packet ingestion: diagnosis, management, and natural history. Ann Intern Med 100:73, 1984.

88. Roberts JR, Price D, Goldfrank L. The bodystuffer syndrome: a clandestine form of drug overdose. Am J Emerg Med 4:24, 1986.

89. Gay GR. Clinical management of acute and chronic cocaine poisoning. Ann Emerg Med 11:562, 1982.

90. Deriet RW. Cocaine intoxication. Postgrad Med 86:245–253, 1989.

91. Lacombe S, Stanislov SW, Marken PA. Pharmacologic Treatment of Cocaine Abuse. DICP, Ann Pharmacotherapy 25: 818–823, 1991.

92. Ramoska E, Sacchetti AD. Propranolol-induced hypertension in treatment of cocaine intoxication. Ann Emerg Med 14:1112, 1985.

93. Dusenberry SJ, Hicks MJ, Mariani PJ. Labetalol treatment of cocaine toxicity. Ann Emerg Med 16(2):235, 1987.

94. Jonsson S, O'Meara M, Young JB. Acute cocaine poisoning: importance of treating seizures and acidosis. Am J Med 75:106, 1983.

95. Louie AK, Lannon RA, Keller IA. Treatment of cocaine-induced panic disorder. Am J Psychiatry 146:40–44, 1989.

96. Fischman MW. Behavioral pharmacology of cocaine. J Clin Psychiatry 318:1173–1182, 1988.

97. Kalivas PW, Duffy P, DuMars LA, Skinner C. Behavioral and neurochemical effects of acute and daily cocaine administration in rats. J Pharmacol Exp Ther 245:485–492, 1988.

98. O'Brien CP, Childress AR, Arndt IO, McLellan T, Woody GE, Maany I. Pharmacological and behavioral treatment of cocaine dependence: controlled studies. J Clin Psychiatry, 49:17–22, 1988.

99. Hall WC, Talbert RL, Ereshefsky L. Cocaine abuse and its treatment. Pharmacotherapy 10:47–65, 1990.

100. O'Brien CP, Childress AR, Arndt IO. Pharmacological and behavioral treatments of cocaine dependence: controlled studies. J Clin Psychiatry 49:2(suppl):3–6, 1988.

101. Dackis CA, Gold MS. Bromocriptine as a treatment for cocaine abuse. Lancet, 1(8438):1151, 1985.

102. Gawin R, Kleber H. Pharmacologic treatment of cocaine abuse. Psychiatr Clin North Am 9(3):573, 1986.

103. Resnick RB, Resnick EB. Cocaine abuse and its treatment. Psychiatr Clin North Am 7(4):713, 1984.

104. Gawin FH, Kleber HD, Byck R, Rounsaville BJ, Kosten TR, Jatlow PI, Morgan C. Desipramine facilitation of initial cocaine abstinence. Arch Gen Psychiatry 46:117–121, 1989.

105. Sanders-Bush E, Burris KD, Knoth K. Lysergic acid diethylamide and 2,5-dimethozy-4 methylamphetamine are partial agonists at serotonin receptors linked to phosphoinositide hydrolysis. J Pharmacol Exp Ther 246:924–928, 1988.

106. McGlothlin WH, Arnold DO. LSD revised: 10 year follow up of medical LSD users. Arch Gen Psychiatry 24:35, 1971.

107. Hollister LE. Drug-induced psychiatric disorders and their management. Med Toxicol 1:428, 1986.

108. McWilliams S, Tuttle R. Long term psychological effects of LSD. Psychol Bull 79:341, 1973.

109. Vardy MM, and Kay SR. LSD psychosis or LSK-induced schizophrenia? Arch Gen Psychiatry 40:877–883, 1983.

110. Schuckit MA. The hallucinogens and related drugs. In Woods SM (ed) Drug and Alcohol Abuse: A Clinical Guide to Diagnosis and Treatment. New York, Plenum Press, pp 137–151, 1984.

111. Glass G. Psychedelic drugs, stress, and the ego. J Nerv Ment Dis 156:232, 1973.

112. Shulgin AT. The background and chemistry of MDMA. J Psychedelic Drugs 18(4):291, 1986.

113. Hayner GN, McKinney H. MDMA—the dark side of ecstasy. J Psychedelic Drugs 18(4):341, 1986.

114. Dowling GP, McDonough ET, Bost RO. Eve and ecstasy—a report of five deaths associated with the use of MDEA and MDMA. JAMA 257(12):1615, 1987.

115. Ricaurte G, Bryan G, Strauss L. Hallucinogenic amphetamine selectively destroys brain serotonin nerve terminals. Science 229:986, 1985.

116. Schmidt CJ, Wu L, Lovenberg W. Methylenedioxymethamphetamine: a potential neurotoxic amphetamine analog. Eur J Pharmacol 124:175, 1986.

117. Gehlert DR, Schmidt CJ, Wu L. Evidence for specific methylenedioxymethamphetamine (ecstasy) binding sites in the rat brain. Eur J Pharmacol 119:135, 1985.

118. Stone DM, Stahl DC, Hanson GR. The effects of 3,4-methylenedioxyamphetamine (MDA) and 3,4-methylenedioxymethamphetamine (MDMA) on monoaminergic systems in the rat brain. Eur J Pharmacol 128:41, 1986.

119. Battaglia G, Yeh SY, O'Hearn E, Molliver ME, Kuhar MJ, De Souza EB. 3,4-Methylenedioxymethamphetamine and 3,4-methylenedioxyamphetamine destroy serotonin terminals in rat brain: quantification of neurodegeneration by measurement of [^{3}H]paroxetine-labeled serotonin uptake sites. J Pharmacol Exp Ther 242:911–916, 1987.

120. Verebey K, Alrazi J, Jaffe JH. Complications of "ecstasy" (MDMA). JAMA 259:1649–1650, 1988.

121. Lamb RJ, Griffitys RR. Self-injection of d,1-3,4-methylenedioxymethamphetamine (MDMA) in the baboon. Psychopharmacology (Berlin) 91:268–272, 1987.

122. Peroutka SJ, Newman H, Harris H. Subjective effects of 3,4-methylenedioxymethamphetamine in recreational users. Neuropsychopharmacology 1:273–278, 1988.

123. Davis BL. The PCP epidemic: a critical review. Int J Addict 17:1137, 1982.

124. McCarron MM, Schulze BW, Thompson GA. Acute phencyclidine intoxication: incidence of clinical findings in 1000 cases. Ann Emerg Med 10:237, 1981.

125. Patel R, Connor G. A review of thirty cases of rhabdomyolysis associated renal failure among phencyclidine users. Clin Toxicol 23:547, 1986.

126. Giannini AJ, Eighan MS, Loiselle RH. Comparison of haloperidol and chlorpromazine in the treatment of phencyclidine psychosis. J Clin Pharmacol 24:202, 1984.

127. Aronow R, Miceli JN, Done AK. A therapeutic approach to the acutely overdosed PCP patient. J Psychedelic Drugs 12:259, 1980.

128. Nabeshima T, Fukaya H, Yamaguchi K, Ishikawa K, Furukawa H, Kameyama T. Development of tolerance and supersensitivity to phencyclidine in rats after repeated administration of phencyclidine. Eur J Pharmacol 135:23–33, 1987.

129. Dewey WL. Cannabinoid pharmacology. Pharmacol Rev 38:151–178, 1986.

130. Weil AT. Adverse reactions to marijuana. N Engl J Med 282(18):997, 1970.

131. Weil AT, Zinberg NE, Nelson JM. Clinical and psychological effects of marijuana in man. Science 162:1243, 1968.

132. Jones RT, Benowitz N. Clinical studies of cannabis tolerance and dependence. Ann NY Acad Sci 282:221, 1976.

133. Nowlan R, Cohen S. Tolerance to marijuana: heart rate and subjective "high." Clin Pharmacol Ther 22(5):550, 1977.

134. Vachon L, Sulkowski A, Rich E. Marijuana effects of learning, attention and time estimation. Psychopharmacologia 39–41, 1974.

135. Abel E. Marijuana and memory: acquisition and retrieval. Science 128:194, 1971.

136. Dornbush RL, Fink M, Freedman AM. Marijuana, memory and perception. Am J Psychiatry 128:194, 1971.

137. Huber GL, Simmons GA, McCarthy CR. Depressant effect of marijuana smoke on antibacterial activity of pulmonary alveolar macrophages. Chest 68:769, 1975.

138. Henderson RL, Tennant FS, Guerry R. Respiratory manifestations of hashish smoking. Arch Otolaryngol 95:248, 1972.

139. Abramson HA. Respiratory disorders and marijuana use. J Asthma Res 11:97, 1974.

140. Waldman MM. Marijuana bronchitis. JAMA 211:501, 1970.

141. Wu TC, Tashkin DP, Djahed GB, Rose JE. Pulmonary hazards of smoking marijuana as compared with tobacco. N Engl J Med 318:347–351, 1988.

142. Tashkin DP, Shapiro BJ, Lee YE. Subacute effects of heavy marijuana smoking on pulmonary function in healthy men. N Engl J Med 294(3):125, 1976.

143. Tashkin DP, Calvarese BM, Simmons MS. Respiratory status of seventy-four habitual marijuana smokers. Chest 78:699, 1980.

144. Gong H Jr, Taskin DP, Simmons MS. Acute and subacute bronchial effects of oral cannabinoids. Clin Pharmacol Ther 35:26, 1984.

145. Hoffman D. On the carcinogenicity of marijuana smoke. Res Adv Phytochem 9:63, 1975.

146. Landrigan PJ, Powell KE, James LM. Paraquat and marijuana: epidemiological risk assessment. Am J Public Health 73:784, 1983.

147. Fried PA, Buckingham M, VonKulmiz P. Marijuana use during pregnancy and perinatal risk factors. Am J Obstet Gynecol 146:992, 1983.

148. Linn S, Schoenbaum SC, Monson RR. The association of marijuana use with outcome of pregnancy. Am J Public Health 73:1161, 1983.

149. Greenland S, Staisch KJ, Brown N. The effects of marijuana use during pregnancy. Am J Obstet Gynecol June:408, 1982.

150. Hollister LE. Cannabis—1988. Acta Psychiatr Scand (Suppl. 345) 78:108–118, 1988.

151. Hollister LE. Health aspects of cannabis. Pharmacol Rev 38:1–20, 1986.

152. Taylor DN, Wachsmuth IK, Shangkuan YH. Salmonellosis associated with marijuana: a multistate outbreak traced by plasmid fingerprinting. N Engl J Med 306(21):1249, 1982.

153. Kagen SL. Aspergillus: an inhalable contaminant of marijuana. N Engl J Med 304(8):483, 1981.

154. Hannerz J, Hindmarsh T. Neurological and neuroradiological examination of chronic cannabis smokers. Ann Neurol 13:207, 1983.

155. Co BT, Goodwin DW, Gado M. Absence of cerebral atrophy in chronic cannabis users. JAMA 237(12):1229, 1977.

156. Morland J, Bugge A, Skuterud B. Cannabinoids in blood and urine after passive inhalation of cannabis smoke. J Forensic Sci 30(4):997, 1985.

157. Cone EJ, Johnson RE. Contact highs and urinary cannabinoid excretion after passive exposure to marijuana smoke. Clin Pharmacol Ther 40(3):247, 1986.

158. Perez-Reyes M, DiGuiseppi S, Mason AP. Passive inhalation of marijuana smoke and urinary excretion of cannabinoids. Clin Pharmacol Ther 34(1):36, 1983.

159. Anderson HR, Macnair RS, Ramsey JD. Deaths from abuse of volatile substances: a national epidemiological study. Br Med J 290:304, 1985.

160. King GS, Smialek JE, Troutman WG. Sudden death in adolescents resulting from the inhalation of typewriter correction fluid. JAMA 253:1604, 1985.

161. Boon NA. Solvent abuse and the heart. Br Med J 21:722, 1987.

162. Engstrand DA, England DM, Huntington RW. Pathology of paint sniffer's lung. Am J Forensic Med Pathol 7(3):232, 1986.

163. Vigliani E, Forni A. Benzene and leukemia. Environ Res 11:122, 1976.

164. Coulehan JL, Hirsch W, Brillman J. Gasoline sniffing and lead toxicity in Navajo adolescents. Pediatrics 71(1):113, 1983.

165. Hansen KS, Sharp FR. Gasoline sniffing, lead poisoning, and myoclonus. JAMA 240(13):1375, 1978.

166. Robinson RO. Tetraethyl lead poisoning from gasoline sniffing. JAMA 240(13):1373, 1978.

167. Bass M. Death from sniffing gasoline. N Engl J Med 299(4):203, 1978.

168. Lazar RB, Ho SU, Melen O. Multifocal central nervous system damage caused by toluene abuse. Neurology 33:1337, 1983.

169. Streicher HZ, Gabow PA, Moss AN. Syndromes of toluene sniffing in adults. Ann Intern Med 94:758, 1981.

170. Fischman CM, Oster JR. Toxic effects of toluene: a new cause of high anion gap metabolic acidosis. JAMA 241(16):1713, 1979.

171. Rosenberg NL, Kleinschmidt-KeMasters BK, Davis KA. Toluene abuse causes diffuse central nervous system white matter changes. Ann Neurol 1988.

172. Moss AH, Gabow PA, Kaehny WD. Fanconi's syndrome and distal tubular acidosis after glue sniffing. Ann Intern Med 92(1):69, 1980.

173. Heyer EJ, Simpson DM, Bodis-Wollner J. Nitrous oxide: clinical and electrophysiologic investigation of neurologic complications. Neurology 36:1618, 1986.

174. Messina FV, Wynne JW. Homemade nitrous oxide: no laughing matter. Ann Intern Med 96(3):333, 1982.

175. Everett G. Effects of amyl nitrite ("poppers") on sexual experience. Med Aspects Human Sexuality 6:146, 1972.

176. Cohen S. The volatile nitrites. JAMA 241(19):2077, 1979.

177. Sharp CW, Stillman RC. Blush not with nitrites. Ann Intern Med 92(5):700, 1980.

178. The health benefits of smoking cessation. A report of the Surgeon General: Office on Smoking and Health, Department of Health and Human Services, Rockville, Md: publication no. (CDC) 90-8416, 1990.

179. Fagerstrom KO. Effects of nicotine chewing gum and follow-up appointments in physician-based smoking cessation. Prev Med 13:517–527, 1984.

180. Report of the Surgeon General. The Health Consequences of Smoking: Nicotine Addiction. US Department of Health and Human Services, Washington, DC: Publication no.(CDC) 88-8406, 1989.

181. Sachs DPL. Advances in smoking cessation treatment. Current Pulmonology, Simmons, ed. Chicago, Ill: Year Book Medical Publishers 12:139–198, 1991.

182. Benowitz NL. Cigarette smoking and nicotine addiction. Med Clin North Am 76:415–437, 1992.

183. Grenhoff J, Svensson R. Pharmacology of nicotine. Br J Addict 84:477–492, 1989.

184. Cigarette smoking-attributable mortality and years of potential life lost—United States, 1990. Centers for Disease Control and Prevention, MMWR 42:645–649, 1993.

185. Bartecchi CE, MacKenzie TD, Schrier RW. The human costs of tobacco use (first of two parts). N Engl J Med 330:907–912, 1994.

186. McBride PE. The health consequences of smoking: cardiovascular diseases. Med Clin North Am 76:333–353, 1992.

187. Sherman CB. The health consequences of cigarette smoking: pulmonary diseases. Med Clin North Am 76:355–375, 1992.

188. Cancer facts and figures—1993. New York: American Cancer Society, 1993.

189. Gottlieb A, Pope SK, Rickert VI. Patterns of smokeless tobacco use by young adolescents. Pediatrics 91:75–78, 1993.

190. MacKenzie TD, Bartecchi CE, Schrier RW. The human costs of tobacco use (second of two parts). N Engl J Med 330:975–980, 1994.

191. Fiore MC, Smith SS, Jorenby DE. The effectiveness of the nicotine patch for smoking cessation—A meta-analysis. JAMA 271:1940–1947, 1994.

192. Use of nicotine to stop smoking. Medical Letter 37:6–8, 1995.

CHAPTER 61

IMMUNIZATIONS

CINDY D. STOWE, STEPHANIE J. PHELPS, and EMILY B. HAK

Active and passive immunization can protect an individual from infectious diseases and even help to eliminate certain diseases. For example, in 1972 the World Health Organization declared that smallpox had been eradicated by a successful worldwide vaccination program, and in 1994, the International Commission for the Certification of Poliomyelitis Eradication in the Americas declared that wild poliovirus transmission had been interrupted in those countries (1). To further illustrate the importance of immunizations in children, the National Childhood Immunization Initiative of 1993 has a goal of achieving immunization rates of 90% by 1996 in children who are 2 years old (2). In order to achieve this goal, federally funded programs have been established to expand clinic hours, increase awareness of immunization programs, decrease immunization cost, track immunization rates, and encourage collaboration between federal and local vaccination programs.

Active immunization is the process of administering a microorganism or its products to stimulate the host's immunologic response to that antigen. Immunization with either vaccine or toxoid results in long-term but not necessarily lifelong protection against a specific disease. Vaccines are composed of live or inactivated microorganisms (e.g., bacteria, viruses) or immunogenic components of microorganisms. Vaccines comprised of immunogenic components of microorganisms such as subvirion, purified surface antigen, or acellular components have minimal risk for febrile reactions while maintaining immunogenicity. Use of recombinant DNA technology to manufacture vaccines can remove the risk for transmission of infectious diseases such as human immunodeficiency virus (HIV) or hepatitis. Live vaccines stimulate an immunologic response similar to natural infection (e.g., including S-IgA as with polio vaccination) and usually result in lifelong immunity. The response induced by killed or inactivated vaccines is sufficient to confer long-lasting immunity; however, it may not be lifelong, and revaccination may be required for continued immunity. Polysaccharide vaccines are less immunogenic and, in some cases, have been conjugated to proteins to increase the antibody response.

Unlike vaccines, toxoids are modified nontoxic exotoxins that retain the ability to stimulate an immunologic response. Revaccination at scheduled intervals ensures continued immunity. Adsorption of a toxoid to a carrier (e.g., aluminum phosphate, aluminum hydroxide, calcium phosphate) delays absorption and increases antigenicity. Unfortunately, these agents may increase tissue irritation at the injection site.

The most common routes of administration of vaccines and toxoids are subcutaneous (s.c.), intramuscular (i.m.), or intradermal (i.d.) injection. Immunizations must be given according to the manufacturer's recommended route or the desired immunologic response may not be stimulated. Vaccines or toxoids given i.m. should be given in the anterolateral aspect of the thigh in infants and the deltoid muscle in children or older individuals. The buttocks should be avoided because the large amount of fat present can interfere with absorption and because of the potential for damaging the sciatic nerve. While studies are limited, available data suggest that immunization against several diseases with killed or inactivated vaccines can be accomplished at the same time. Injections should be administered at different sites unless efficacy with a combination product has been demonstrated. The immunologic agents discussed in the text are listed in Tables 61.1 and 61.2.

The antibody response usually begins soon after immunization, but adequate antibody concentrations to protect against disease may not be achieved for weeks. Therefore, individuals should not be considered immune from disease immediately following immunization. In some cases, the response to the initial vaccine dose is insufficient to protect against disease or protection wanes with time; thus, many vaccines require more than 1 dose.

Passive immunity results from direct administration of nonspecific (e.g., immunoglobulin) or specific antibodies (e.g., antitoxin) and is a prophylactic measure. This increase in antibodies from exogenous sources provides protection for a relatively short time period. Reexposure to the disease after the metabolism and degradation of the exogenous antibodies may result in infection. In addition, the administration of specific or nonspecific immunoglobulins may prevent the desired antibody response to concurrent active immunization. In some cases concurrent vaccination and immunoglobulin administration may be warranted, as in the case of rabies and perinatal hepatitis B exposure.

Table 61.1.
Immunizations

Diseases	Immunization Type	Route°	Additives†
Diphtheria	Toxoid	IM	aluminum, thimerosal
Hepatitis A	Inactivated viral antigen	IM	aluminum, formalin, phenoxyethanol
Hepatitis B	Inactivated viral antigen (recombinant)	IM	aluminum, yeast protein, thimerosal
Haemophilus influenzae (Hib)			
PRP-D	Bacterial polysaccharide, PRP,‡ conjugated to diphtheria toxoid	IM	thimerosal
HbOC	Bacterial oligosaccharide, PRP,‡ conjugated to diphtheria CRM$_{197}$	IM	thimerosal
PRP-OMP	Bacterial polysaccharide, PRP,‡ conjugated to meningococcal outer membrane protein	IM	thimerosal, aluminum
PRP-T	Bacterial polysaccharide, PRP,‡ conjugated to tetanus toxoid	IM	sucrose, formalin
Influenza	Inactivated virus—2 type A & 1 type B (whole & split virus)	IM	egg antigen
Measles	Live attenuated virus	SC	neomycin, egg antigen
Meningococcal	Bacterial polysaccharides—4 serotypes	SC	diluent—thimerosal
Mumps	Live attenuated virus	SC	neomycin, egg antigen
Pertussis	Inactivated bacteria or acellular inactivated bacteria	IM	thimerosal
Pneumococcal	Bacterial polysaccharides—23 serotypes	IM, SC	phenol or thimerosal
Polio			
OPV	Live attenuated virus	PO	streptomycin, neomycin, sorbitol
eIPV	Enhanced inactivated virus	SC	streptomycin, neomycin, polymyxin B, phenoxyethanol
Rabies	Inactivated virus adsorbed or grown in human diploid-cell	IM, ID^a	aluminum
Rubella	Live attenuated virus	SC	neomycin
Tetanus	Toxoid	IM	aluminum, thimerosal
Tuberculosis	Bacillus Calmette-Guerin (BCG), live attenuated bacteria	ID, SC	buffered diluent
Typhoid			
Parenteral	Inactivated bacteria	SC, ID^b	phenol
	Bacterial polysaccharide	IM	phenol
Oral	Live attenuated bacteria	PO	ascorbic acid, amino acid mixture
Varicella	Live attenuated virus	SC	neomycin
Yellow fever	Live attenuated virus	SC	egg antigen

°Route abbreviations: SC, subcutaneous; ID, intradermal; IM, intramuscular; PO, oral.
†Preservatives may not be contained in single dose units of those with preservative in multidose vials.
‡PRP, polyribosyl-ribitol-phosphate.
^{a}The ID dose is different from the IM, and is used only for preexposure vaccination.
^{b}Booster may be given ID.
Adapted from reference 3.

Specific groups of individuals require special consideration prior to vaccination. Immunization of pregnant women, immunocompromised individuals, or dialysis patients may require modification of an immunization schedule or dose and consideration of the type of immunization (e.g., live vs. killed vaccine). Individuals traveling to countries where specific infectious diseases are endemic may require immunization or prophylactic therapies to prevent endemic diseases. Patients with hypersensitivity reactions to vaccine components (e.g., egg protein, stabilizers, preservatives) may require desensitization prior to immunization.

Proper storage and reconstitution of vaccines and immunoglobulin products are necessary to ensure potency and concentration. Products ready for injection usually require refrigeration and protection from freezing. Lyophilized vaccines may require storage under refrigeration and protection from heat or freezing. The package insert should be consulted for proper storage conditions and reconstitution instructions.

New or improved products to provide immunity and more effective immunization schedules are being evaluated. The American Academy of Pediatrics (AAP) Committee on Infectious Diseases publishes current recommendations in the *Red Book,* which is revised every 3 to 5 years (3). As new information becomes available, revised recommendations are published in *Pediatrics, The Journal of the American Medical Association* (JAMA), and the *Morbidity and Mortality Weekly Review* (MMWR).

ACTIVE IMMUNIZATIONS

Ontogenic Events

The immune system begins to develop early in fetal life. At 7 weeks small lymphocytes appear in the circulation, and at 9 weeks, B cells primarily involved in the humoral immune response are seen in fetal liver. At term birth, all of the components of the immune system are present and

functional, but immunoglobulin production is low. However, active transport of maternal IgG across the placenta results in IgG serum concentrations 5 to 10% greater than in the mother. While neonates can produce all classes of immunoglobulins, they cannot produce specific antibodies against all antigens. At birth, there is no immunologic memory, complement concentrations are reduced, opsonin activity is poor, and neutrophil chemotaxis and phagocytosis are reduced. By 1 year of age, the complement concentrations in both the classic and alternative pathways have reached adult values. By 2 years of age, memory response to polysaccharide antigen is present, immune complex diseases begin to appear, and IgM concentrations

Table 61.2.
Antigenic Composition of Immunizations

Immunization	Antigenic Component (amount)
DTP°	diphtheria toxoid from *Cornynebacterium diphtheria* endotoxin (12.5 Lf)
	tetanus toxoid from *Clostridium tetani* endotoxin (5 Lf)
	whole-cell pertussis from *Bordetella pertussis* endotoxin (4 protective units)
DTaP	
Acel-Imune	diphtheria toxoid from *Cornynebacterium diphtheria* endotoxin (7.5 Lf)
	tetanus toxoid from *Clostridium tetani* endotoxin (5 Lf)
	pertussis: FHA (86%), PT (8%), pertactin (4%), agglutinogen (2%)
Tripedia	diphtheria toxoid (6.7 Lf)
	tetanus toxoid (5 Lf)
	pertussis: FHA (50%), PT (50%)
DT	diphtheria toxoid from *Cornynebacterium diphtheria* endotoxin (6.6–15 Lf)
	tetanus toxoid from *Clostridium tetani* endotoxin (5–10 Lf)
Td	diphtheria toxoid from *Cornynebacterium diphtheria* endotoxin (1.5–2 Lf)
	tetanus toxoid from *Clostridium tetani* endotoxin (5–10 Lf)
OPV	polio virus: types 1,2,3 (10^5 infective titers)
eIPV	polio virus: type 1 (≥40 D antigen units), type 2 (8 D antigen units), type 3 (32 D antigen units)
MVR	measles virus: Enders' attenuated Edmonston strain (1000 $TCID_{50}$)
	mumps virus: Jeryl Lynn (B level) strain (20,000 $TCID_{50}$)
	rubella virus: Wistar RA 27/3 strain (1000 $TCID_{50}$)
Hib	
PRP-D	Hib capsular polysaccharide-PRP (25 µg) & diphtheria toxoid (18 µg)
HbOC°	Hib capsular oligosaccharide-PRP (10 µg) & CRM_{197} protein (25 µg)
PRP-OMP	Hib capsular polysaccharide-PRP (15 µg) & group B meningococcal OMP (250 µg)
PRP-T	Hib capsular polysaccharide-PRP (10 µg) & tetanus toxoid (20 µg)
HBV	HBsAg gene in a plasmid is inserted into baker's yeast (*S. cerevisiae*)
Varicella	varicella virus Oka/Merck strain (≥1350 PFU)
Hepatitis A	hepatitis A HM-175 strain (adult: 1440 ELISA viral antigen units; pediatric: 360 ELISA viral antigen units
Influenza	2 type A & 1 type B influenza viruses (amounts and specific strains may change yearly)
Meningococcal	*N. meningitidis* serotypes A, C, Y, and W-135 bacterial capsular polysaccharide (50 µg of each serotype)
Pneumococcal	*S. pneumoniae* 23 polysaccharide serotypes (25 µg of each)
BCG	tuberculosis *M. bovis* strain
	Danish substrain *M. bovis* (1–8×10^8 CFU per 2 mL)
	Tice substrain *M. bovis* (8–26 million CFU per mL)
HDCV	rabies virus (not <2.5 IU/mL)
RVA	
Typhoid	
Typhoid vaccine	inactivated *S. typhi* Ty2 strain (5×10^8 organisms/mL)
Typhim Vi	capsular polysaccharide (25 µg of purified virulence [Vi] antigen)
Vivotif Berna	live (2–6×10^9 CFU) & nonviable (5–50×10^9 CFU) *S. typhi* strain Ty21a per capsule
Yellow fever	yellow fever from the 17D strain (5.04 $\log_{10}$ PFU)

Lf, flocculating units, antitoxin content; LPF, lymphocytosis-promoting factor; PT, pertussis toxin; FHA, filamentous hemagglutinin; $TCID_{50}$, tissue culture infective dose 50%; PRP, polyribosyl-ribitol-phosphate; PFU, plaque-forming units; ELISA, enzyme-linked immunosorbent assay; CFU, colony-forming units.
°Tetramune combination of DTP & HbOC.

reach adult values. Secretory IgA reaches maximal concentration by 2 to 4 years; however, the capacity for production of specific antibodies of the IgA class matures slowly, and adult values are not reached until puberty. Adult concentrations of IgG are reached by 4 to 6 years of age.

The age at which an infant can respond appropriately to a specific immunization depends on the disappearance of transplacentally acquired antibodies and the capability of the immune system to respond to specific antigens. For example, concentrations of maternally derived antibodies to measles, mumps, or rubella may be present in sufficient concentration to prevent the desired antibody response for the first year of life; therefore, immunization for these viruses is delayed. Likewise, infants respond poorly to immunization with polysaccharide capsular antigens from organisms such as *Streptococcus pneumoniae* and *Haemophilus influenzae* type b (Hib). To stimulate the appropriate antigen-antibody response to Hib in infants, the polysaccharide has been conjugated to a variety of different proteins. For other unconjugated polysaccharide vaccines such as that of *S. pneumoniae*, vaccination is delayed until 2 years of age, when the desired response can be elicited.

Misconceptions regarding contraindications and precautions to immunization result in a significant number of missed opportunities for vaccination. Sound clinical judgment under those conditions viewed as precautions and strict adherence to absolute contraindications should minimize missed vaccination opportunities and avoidable adverse events. In general, pediatric immunizations begin when an infant is 6 to 8 weeks of age. Healthy preterm infants should begin immunizations at the same chronologic age as term infants, and to ensure an adequate response, the full dose should be used (3–5).

In 1993 the National Immunization Program of the CDC coordinated a meeting between the AAP, the American Medical Association, and the American Academy of Family Practice to develop a single pediatric immunization strategy that was acceptable to all participants (6). This schedule allows a certain degree of flexibility and can minimize the number of physician or clinic visits required to comply with the recommendations.

Diphtheria, Pertussis, and Tetanus

DIPHTHERIA

Corynebacterium diphtheriae is the causative agent for diphtheria, a highly contagious disease transmitted by aerosolized droplets. The mucous membranes of the upper respiratory tract are usually the site of local infection, but ocular and genital mucous membranes and even the skin can be infected. The toxin causes local tissue inflammation and necrosis that may form an exudate and further progress to a gray or black membrane. Local lesions may be sufficiently deep to allow hematogenous spread. Mild infection resembles the common cold, while severe disease resulting from the delayed action of the diphtheria toxin may result in cardiomyopathy, neuropathy, or liver necrosis. A single intravenous dose of diphtheria antitoxin is the specific treatment for the complications of diphtheria, but the appropriate antibiotics are required to kill the organism. Active infection does not necessarily confer immunity, and all individuals should be immunized throughout life (3, 4).

TETANUS

The spores of *Clostridium tetani* are commonly found in soil and dust and are responsible for the disease commonly referred to as "lockjaw." Once introduced into a wound, *C. tetani* can be converted to the vegetative form that elaborates a neurotoxic exotoxin responsible for the disease. Local infection results in pain, muscle rigidity, and muscle spasm in adjacent areas. The disease is generalized to involve virtually every muscle, including those necessary for respiration. The individual with tetanus can be neurologically alert but unable to respond. In addition, intense pain or airway obstruction, cyanosis, and asphyxia can be associated with muscle spasms. Treatment includes supportive care, administration of tetanus immune globulin, tetanus toxoid, and tetanus antitoxin. Occasionally, active infection does not necessarily provide permanent immunity, so patients with tetanus should be immunized during convalescence. As immunity to tetanus wanes with time, all individuals should be reimmunized throughout life (3, 4).

PERTUSSIS

Humans are the only known reservoir for pertussis or "whooping cough," an acute respiratory infection that usually results from *Bordetella pertussis*. A milder form may be caused by *Bordetella parapertussis*. For the initial 1 to 2 weeks of infection (catarrhal stage), pertussis resembles an upper respiratory tract infection. During the following 2 to 4 weeks (paroxysmal stage), the cough worsens and may be severe enough to result in asphyxia and cerebral anoxia, leading to seizures, coma, and permanent neurologic damage. Exhaustion from coughing, dehydration, and weight loss are frequent findings. During the weeks to months of recovery (convalescent stage), the number and severity of coughing episodes gradually decreases. In adults, pertussis may go unrecognized because the symptoms are often atypical, and a severe persistent cough may be the only overt symptom of infection. Treatment includes administration of antimicrobials to limit the spread of the organism and supportive care. Active infection with pertussis appears to provide lifelong immunity (3).

Table 61.3.
Pediatric Immunization Schedule

Age	Hepatitis B[A]	Oral Polio	Diphtheria, Tetanus, Pertussis[B]	H. influenza type b[B]	Measles, Mumps, Rubella
Birth	$HBV_{(1)}$				
2 months	$HBV_{(1 \text{ or } 2)}$	OPV[a]	DTP[a]	$Hib_{(3 \text{ or } 4)}^{a}$	
4 months	$HBV_{(2)}$	OPV	DTP	$Hib_{(3 \text{ or } 4)}$	
6 months	$HBV_{(1 \text{ or } 2)}$	OPV[b]	DTP	$Hib_{(3)}$	
12 months				$Hib_{(4)}$	
15 months			DTP/DTaP[c]	$Hib_{(3)}^{d}$	
4–6 years		OPV	DTP/DTaP		MMR[e]
11–12 years					
14–16 years			Td[f]		MMR[e]

[A]HBV may be given in either of 2 schedules:
  (1) Birth, 1–2 months, 6–18 months (if mother HBsAg + also receive HBIG 0.5 mL within 12 hours of birth).
  (2) 1–2 months, 4 months, 6–18 months.
[B]There are 2 schedules for Hib conjugate vaccines:
  (3) HbOC (HibTITER), PRP-T (ActHIB), or DTP/HbOC (Tetramune) and PRP-T reconstituted with DTP by Connaught: 2, 4, 6, & 15 months.
  (4) PRP-OMP (PedvaxHIB): 2, 4, & 12 months.
  Combination of DTP & Hib may be used when both are required. PRP-D should only be used as a booster in children > 12 months of age or primary immunization at ≥ 15 months of age.
[a]DTP, OPV, & Hib may be given as early as 6 weeks of age.
[b]OPV may be given with MMR & Hib at 15 months or anytime between 6 & 18 months.
[c]DTP 4 can be administered as early as 12 months of age provided that the interval since the previous dose of DTP is at least 6 months. DTaP is currently recommended only for use as the 4th and 5th doses of the DTP series among children aged 15 months to 6 years.
[d]After the primary infant Hib series is completed, any of the licensed Hib may be used as a booster dose at age 12–15 months.
[e]MMR first dose may be given at 12 to 15 months, and second dose is given at 11 to 12 years (preferred) or at 4–6 years of age (regimen consists of two doses following the first birthday).
[f]Td given to children > 7 and adults: repeat every 10 years throughout life.
Adapted from references 3 and 4.

IMMUNIZATIONS

Diphtheria and tetanus toxoids and whole-cell pertussis vaccine (DTP) are combined and given as a single immunization (Table 61.1). Because of the adverse events seen with the whole-cell pertussis vaccine, acellular pertussis vaccines that demonstrate efficacy and a decreased incidence of side effects were developed (7, 8). Two acellular pertussis vaccines in combination with diphtheria and tetanus toxoids (DTaP) have been approved for use in the United States as the fourth and fifth immunization in children over 15 months of age (7–10). Acel-Imune (Lederle, Takeda Chemical) and Tripedia (Connaught, BIKEN/Tanabe) are currently available (Table 61.2). Development of second and third generation acellular vaccines is ongoing. The second generation acellular vaccines use 1 to 5 individually purified and inactivated pertussis antigens. The third generation acellular vaccines will contain genetically derived immunogenic components (7). Currently the specific antigens needed to stimulate the appropriate immune response are unknown (7, 8).

The DTP and both of the DTaP immunizations contain similar amounts of diphtheria and tetanus toxoid but differ in their pertussis component (Table 61.2). Because of the increased incidence of adverse effects in older children and adults given the whole-cell pertussis vaccine and the larger dose of diphtheria toxoid contained in DTP, DTaP, and DT, the product used in those over 7 years old contains less diphtheria toxoid and the same amount of tetanus toxoid (Td), and does not contain a pertussis component (Table 61.2). Despite limited indications for single immunization, each is available individually (11).

SCHEDULE

Immunization with DTP begins at 6 to 8 weeks of age (3, 4, 6). Three primary immunizations are given at least 1 month apart, followed by booster doses at 15 to 18 months and prior to school enrollment at 4 to 6 years of age. The DTaP can be substituted for the fourth and fifth DTP in children over 15 months to 7 years of age (9, 10). For increased compliance and convenience, the DTP immunization is usually scheduled to coincide with polio, hepatitis B, and H. influenzae type b vaccination (Table 61.3). Immunity against diphtheria and tetanus wanes with time, and repeated vaccination every 10 years with Td is recommended.

The adverse effects seen with DTP immunization are usually mild and self-limiting but have a significantly higher incidence than is seen with the DT. Local reactions, including redness, swelling, or pain at the injection site, occur in about 50% of patients immunized with DTP but in only 8 to 10% of patients immunized with DT. Seizures and hypotonic-hyporesponsive episodes occur in 1 out of 1750 doses, fever ≥ 40.5°C in 1 of every 330 doses, and persistent crying in 1 of every 100 immunizations with

DTP (12). Use of 15 mg/kg of acetaminophen at the time of immunization and at 4 and 8 hours after immunization decreased the incidence of fever (>38°C) from 44 to 27% and decreased the incidence of local and systemic effects for the primary DTP immunization series (13). Use of a eutectic mixture of local anesthetics, EMLA cream, containing lidocaine and prilocaine decreased pain and crying associated with DTP immunization to a greater degree than placebo; however, there was no effect on fear of immunization (14). Compared to DTP, immunization with DTaP results in fewer local reactions and a decreased incidence of systemic effects such as fever, fussiness, persistent crying, drowsiness, and anorexia (15). DTP immunization was postulated as a cause of Sudden Infant Death Syndrome (SIDS); however, no controlled study has found a positive relationship between DTP immunization and SIDS.

Children who experience an immediate anaphylactic reaction should not receive further doses of DTP and the specific allergen should be identified (4, 11). Children who develop encephalopathy should not receive the pertussis vaccine, but should continue the primary immunization schedule with DT after the neurologic status has stabilized (11). Fever (≥40.5°C), collapse or shocklike state, and persistent, inconsolable crying lasting over 3 hours within 48 hours of receiving DTP, or seizures within 3 days of DTP are not absolute contraindications to further DTP dosing (11). However, under these circumstances the benefits must be weighed against the risks of continued dosing. If the vaccination series is to continue without the pertussis component, the DT should be used.

DTP immunization may result in an increased risk for a seizure in children with a preexisting neurologic disorder or provide the first pyrogenic stimulus for a febrile seizure (11). Recently a prospective trial was undertaken to elucidate the causes and risk factors for serious systemic DTP reactions (16). Seizures occurring after DTP immunization were similar to febrile seizures in control patients, and the *B. pertussis* endotoxin in the DTP vaccine was felt to be the cause (16). Similar to other febrile seizures, they are usually uncomplicated and rarely resulted in permanent neurologic injury. However, more serious neurologic side effects have been temporally associated with the DTP immunization, and retrospective studies suggested that the pertussis component was responsible. Unfortunately, the age at which congenital or other preexisting serious neurologic disease becomes obvious coincides with the time routine pediatric immunizations are being administered. This coincidental relationship coupled with the desire to establish a cause for serious neurologic disease has influenced the linkage of pertussis vaccine to serious central nervous system sequelae.

After the whole-cell pertussis vaccine was introduced, the incidence of the disease decreased from over 250,000 cases with 7500 deaths in 1934 to only 2300 reported cases per year in the 1970s (11). During the 1980s, the number of cases increased in some areas despite attainment of greater than 90% vaccination rates. This increased incidence of pertussis may have been due to vaccine failures or to a gradual decrease in immunity after vaccination. Studies have shown that immunity following pertussis immunization decreases after 3 years (17). Pertussis in adolescents and adults has a low incidence of morbidity and mortality (8, 18). However, it is becoming clear that adolescents and adults serve as the primary reservoir in the transmission of pertussis to susceptible infants and children and that immunization of those under 7 years of age is not sufficient to eradicate disease. The incidence of pertussis in adolescents is predicted to be 1.2 to 8.2% (19). In 11.2% of households with culture proven pertussis, the source of the infection was an adult (20). To evaluate immunization of adults with an acellular pertussis vaccine, healthy adults were given one of three concentrations of pertussis antigen in combination with 2 Lf units of diphtheria toxoid and 5 Lf units of tetanus toxoid or Td alone (21). Those who received the acellular pertussis vaccine experienced an antibody response, antibody concentrations declined 50% by 1 year, and adverse effects were not different among the four groups (21). There was no difference in the response to diphtheria or tetanus toxoids (21). It is foreseeable that pertussis vaccination will someday continue throughout life as does administration of diphtheria and tetanus toxoids.

Polio

Humans are the only known reservoir for the enteroviruses responsible for poliomyelitis. Infection with either type 1, type 2, or type 3 wild-type polio virus may result in disease that may be progressive. About 90% of poliovirus infections are asymptomatic. In 4 to 8% of individuals the illness is minor, consisting of fever, malaise, headache, and nausea. While most with these symptoms do not progress past the first stage or abortive poliomyelitis, about 20% progress to the nonparalytic aseptic meningitis stage with symptoms consisting of a stiff neck and spine. The nonparalytic stage may progress further to either spinal (paralytic) or bulbar (cranial) poliomyelitis. Rarely, the spinal and bulbar forms occur together.

IMMUNIZATION

The first polio vaccine, developed by Jonas Salk in 1954, was an inactivated polio vaccine (IPV) that contained antigens for types 1, 2, and 3 polio viruses. Since the IPV did not confer long-term protection against polio, an enhanced potency IPV (eIPV) that more efficiently stimulates an antibody response was developed and licensed and replaced the Salk vaccine (Tables 61.1 and 61.2) (22). Adverse effects described with eIPV include erythema and tenderness at the injection site, fever, and urticarial rash.

In 1961 Albert Sabin developed a live, attenuated oral polio vaccine (OPV) that protects against poliovirus types 1, 2, and 3, and induces gastrointestinal immunity (Tables 61.1 and 61.2). OPV results in lifelong immunity, is less expensive, and is easy to administer. Use of OPV for immunization has virtually eradicated naturally occurring polio from the United States. After OPV dosing, the virus persists in the throat for 1 to 2 weeks after vaccination. Because the OPV is a live virus vaccine, it replicates in the gastrointestinal tract and the virus is shed via stool for as long as 6 to 8 weeks after immunization. This may improve immunization rates, since during the period of viral shedding, unimmunized close contacts such as other infants in day care settings may ingest the virus and indirectly become immunized. Although the ACIP and AAP recommend OPV for primary pediatric polio immunization, the eIPV is also effective in preventing poliomyelitis (3, 11).

SCHEDULE

OPV immunization begins at 6 to 8 weeks of age and is followed by a second dose at approximately 4 months of age (Table 61.3). The third dose of OPV may be given as early as 6 months of age or delayed until 18 months of age. A fourth booster dose is given prior to school enrollment. Because of intestinal replication and carriage of the live virus, repeat immunization may not be effective if given more frequently than every 6 weeks. However, during epidemics or when traveling to an endemic area, accelerated vaccination may be warranted and the interval may be as short as 4 weeks.

The use of eIPV is indicated in those unimmunized adults who are traveling to an endemic or epidemic area of polio, immunosuppressed individuals including children with HIV infection, and close household contacts of immunosuppressed individuals who require polio vaccination. The primary immunization series with eIPV begins at 6 to 8 weeks of age, the same age as with OPV. The second dose is given at 3 or 4 months of age and the third dose at 6 to 12 months after the second. A fourth dose is given prior to school entry (3). Three doses of eIPV are required for primary immunization. Repeat booster immunizations after this series are not needed. Routine polio immunization of previously unimmunized adults is not recommended.

During the weeks following OPV immunization, immunocompromised individuals, those receiving immunosuppressants (e.g., steroids, chemotherapy) and unimmunized adults (>18 years) who come in contact with anyone shedding the live virus are at risk of contracting polio from the rarely excreted mutant wild-type virus. There is an extremely low risk of 1 case per 6.8 million doses that a wild-type mutant may emerge from the attenuated virus pool, resulting in active disease in the vaccine or a close

contact. In fact, since 1979 all cases of poliomyelitis in the United States have been associated with OPV or have been imported. Contraindications to OPV include those who are immunocompromised or in close contact with an immunocompromised individual.

While wild-type poliovirus transmission has been interrupted in the United States, outbreaks of polio continue in other countries, and polio vaccination will be required in the Americas because of the risk for imported disease. Currently research is being directed toward the eradication of wild-type poliomyelitis globally and elimination of OPV associated poliomyelitis (23). A polio vaccination regimen that includes initial immunization with eIPV followed by OPV has been proposed as a means of decreasing the incidence of vaccine associated polio (23).

Measles, Mumps, Rubella

MEASLES

Rubeola, or measles, is caused by the RNA virus *Morbillivirus*. This highly contagious disease is spread by direct contact with infectious droplets or by airborne spread. Following 10 days of incubation, a prodrome characterized by Koplik spots on the buccal and pharyngeal mucosa, fever, conjunctivitis, photophobia, cough, and coryza occurs. During this time measles may be transmitted via aerosolized droplets. Following the prodrome, a high fever develops, and a maculopapular rash starts on the neck and face and progresses down the body. Complications such as otitis media, croup, and diarrhea are common in young children. Encephalitis occurs in approximately 1 of every 1000 cases, while death has occurred in 3 of every 1000 cases reported since 1989 (3).

MUMPS

Also known as *epidemic parotitis*, mumps is caused by a paramyxovirus. It is highly contagious and is transmitted by aerosolized droplets. The 3-week incubation period is characterized by fever, neck muscle pain, headache, and malaise. This is followed in a matter of hours by unilateral or bilateral parotid gland swelling in approximately one third of all cases. Age-related complications associated with mumps are common and include encephalitis in approximately 1 in 6000 cases, orchitis or epididymitis in up to 45% of postpubertal males, and oophoritis in 7% of postpubertal females. A small number of males with orchitis may become sterile as a result of testicular infection. Mumps immunization has decreased the incidence by 98%, but mumps outbreaks continue to occur (3).

RUBELLA

German or 3-day measles is a contagious disease caused by an RNA virus whose only known host is man. Following a 2- to 3-week incubation period, rubella is characterized by mild catarrhal symptoms culminating with an erythematous maculopapular, discrete rash, slight fever, and enlarged, tender cervical lymph nodes. Symptoms last for up to 7 days. Complications are uncommon but include arthritis and neuritis, usually in adolescent and older females (3).

The most significant problem with rubella is the potential for fetal infection. Fifty to eighty percent of infants born to mothers who contracted rubella during the first trimester will have congenital rubella syndrome. The incidence decreases to 10 to 20% if the infection occurs during the second trimester and is rare if infection occurs during the third trimester. Relatively common manifestations of congenital rubella syndrome noted at birth include low birth weight, hepatomegaly, splenomegaly, congenital heart disease, or cataracts. While newborns may be asymptomatic, up to 70% are eventually diagnosed with hearing loss, congenital heart disease, mental retardation, or cataracts.

IMMUNIZATION

The measles, mumps, and rubella live, attenuated virus vaccines (MMR) contain measles and mumps viruses grown in chick embryo cell cultures and rubella virus grown in human diploid cell culture (Tables 61.1 and 61.2). Each component vaccine of the MMR is available individually as well as either measles-rubella or mumps-rubella combinations (24). The MMR vaccine has undergone several modifications in the vaccine composition, timing of vaccination, and number of doses recommended (3).

Immunization with MMR has resulted in a highly significant decrease in the incidence of measles, mumps, and rubella. The number of measles cases reported has drastically declined from 27,786 cases reported in 1990 to 281 cases in 1993 (2). This dramatic decrease in the incidence of measles followed the recommendation for a second MMR vaccination. The incidence of mumps and rubella has remained low and has continued to decline into the early 1990s (2). It is important to note that the incidence of congenital rubella syndrome parallels the incidence of rubella and is amplified when outbreaks occur in unvaccinated populations of women who are of childbearing age (25). Although individuals immunized with MMR can shed virus in the saliva and tears, there is no risk for disease transmission.

SCHEDULE

MMR is administered twice. The first immunization is given at 12 to 15 months of age and the second by the age of 11 to 12 years (Table 61.3). Ninety to ninety-five percent of individuals immunized at 15 months of age will develop long-lasting immunity. However, outbreaks of measles and mumps have occurred in highly vaccinated communities. Thus, a second immunization is required to ensure a higher degree of protection. During a measles outbreak, infants over 6 months and under 1 year of age should receive the monovalent measles vaccine or the MMR if the monovalent vaccine is not available. These infants should receive 2 additional doses of MMR according to the previously described schedule. Individuals born prior to 1957 likely had measles infection and do not require immunization. Those born after 1957 are considered susceptible unless they have had 2 doses of MMR after 12 months of age or documentation of measles immunity. In addition, most colleges and medical institutions require that incoming students or employees document that they have received two measles immunizations or provide evidence of immunity (3, 4).

Several factors related to the MMR vaccine must be considered before administration. MMR and the individual vaccines are live virus vaccines and should not be administered to severely immunosuppressed individuals with the exception of children with HIV infection. These children should receive the first dose of MMR between 12 and 15 months of age. Those who are to receive immunosuppressive doses of steroids, chemotherapy, or radiation should be immunized either 2 weeks prior to or 3 months after therapy (4, 26). Those who receive immune globulin for measles prophylaxis can be given MMR 5 months after a dose of 0.25 mL/kg in healthy individuals or 6 months after a dose of 0.5 mL/kg in immunosuppressed individuals (27). Individuals with anaphylactic egg allergies may require desensitization prior to vaccination (Table 61.4) (3, 28). Finally, women who are pregnant or who intend to become pregnant within 3 months should not be immunized with the rubella vaccine because of the theoretical risk for congenital rubella syndrome (3).

Adverse effects associated with MMR have been reported in 0.5 to 4% of vaccinees. Burning at the injection site is probably due to the low pH of the vaccine. Local

Table 61.4.
Management of Immunizations in Individuals with Egg Allergy

1. *Scratch, prick, puncture test.* 1:10 dilution (in physiologic saline) applied as a scratch, prick, or puncture on forearm. The test is read after 15–20 minutes. Positive test is denoted by a wheal ≥ 3 mm more than that produced by the control (physiologic saline applied as scratch, prick, or puncture at another site).
2. *Intradermal test.* 0.002 mL of 1:100 dilution (in physiologic saline) is injected intradermally. Wheal > 5 mm more than produced by the control (physiologic saline injected intradermally at another site).
3. *Desensitization.* The following should be administered subcutaneously at 15- to 20-minute intervals.
   0.05 mL of 1:100 dilution in physiologic saline
   0.05 mL of 1:10 dilution in physiologic saline
   0.05 mL of full strength vaccine
   0.1 mL of full strength vaccine
   0.15 mL of full strength vaccine
   0.2 mL of full strength vaccine

Adapted from references 3 and 28.

reactions following measles vaccination include induration, erythema, vesiculation, edema, and soreness at the injection site. Infants may experience irritability, fever, drowsiness, conjunctivitis, generalized rash, and a willingness to stay in bed. From 6 to 11 days after immunization, a transient rash, fever up to 39.4°C, and other symptoms consistent with subclinical measles infection such as headache, cough, sore throat, photophobia, and malaise may occur. Although rare, seizures have been reported during the febrile episode, particularly in children under 2 years of age. Systemic reactions to mumps vaccine are rare, but mild fever has been reported. While rare, systemic effects to rubella vaccination resemble those seen with rubella infection and appear to be age related. A transient arthralgia occurring 2 to 6 weeks after immunization has been reported in 1 to 3% of children and in up to 40% of adult females (3).

National Childhood Vaccine Compensation Act

All vaccines and toxoids can produce adverse effects that are predominantly mild and self-limiting. While extremely rare, certain adverse events temporally associated with immunization have resulted in severe permanent injury or death. Serious side effects temporally related to immunization must be reported to the U.S. Department of Health and Human Services through the Vaccine Adverse Event Reporting System (VAERS) (3). VAERS functions as the system for monitoring and tracking suspected serious adverse events after the administration of any vaccine. This replaces the CDC's Monitoring System for Adverse Events following immunizations and the Food and Drug Administration's (FDA) Adverse Reaction Reporting System (29).

Historically, compensation for injury related to immunization was through litigation between the injured party and vaccine manufactures or health care professionals who prescribed or administered vaccines. A few lawsuits of sufficient magnitude forced some manufacturers to suspend production of vaccines and toxoids and threatened the viability of the national immunization program. Because of the importance of this program, the federal government passed the National Childhood Vaccine Compensation Act in 1988 to provide financial assistance to children who experienced serious adverse reactions that were temporally related to vaccination. This would decrease the financial burden previously assumed by vaccine manufacturers. To finance and establish this program, the government appropriated funds for 5 years and placed a tax on each vaccine, with the amount of tax directly related to the possibility of severe adverse reaction (30). Vaccines that are covered include diphtheria toxoid, tetanus toxoid, and whole-cell pertussis; measles, mumps, and rubella; and oral and inactivated polio. Funds are available to provide treatment and rehabilitation costs not covered by private insurance, with

damages awarded for pain and suffering not exceeding $250,000. If parents of children who experienced vaccine-related severe adverse effects accept compensation via this route, they give up the right to institute legal proceedings against the manufacturer or individuals who prescribed or administered the vaccine (31).

Haemophilus Influenzae

Haemophilus influenzae can cause meningitis, epiglottitis, pneumonia, septic arthritis, osteomyelitis, cellulitis, otitis media, and pericarditis in infants and young children. Most of the invasive diseases associated with *H. influenzae* are caused by encapsulated strains, most commonly type b (Hib). Hib is carried in the nasopharynx in as many as 5% of people and may be transmitted by asymptomatic carriers via aerosolized droplets. Up to 75% of Hib infections occur in children under 18 months of age. However, children up to 5 years of age may develop serious neurologic morbidity including mental retardation and deafness (25 to 50%), and mortality occurs in 3 to 10% of patients with Hib meningitis. Risk factors for acquiring Hib disease include young age, day care attendance, anatomic or functional asplenia, malignancies, and ethnicity, with native Americans, Alaskan Eskimos, and African Americans being at increased risk. Active disease in those over 24 months of age results in lifelong immunity (3).

IMMUNIZATION

In 1985, the first Hib polyribosyl-ribitol-phosphate (PRP) capsular polysaccharide vaccine was licensed in the United States. Children 24 months of age or older achieved adequate seroconversion to confer protection against Hib disease. However, younger children who were most likely to acquire the infection failed to respond. Additionally, native Americans and Alaskan Eskimos did not have the desired immunologic responses to immunization regardless of age. This was thought to be related to socioeconomic factors, genetics, differences in infecting strains of Hib, or environmental factors due to ethnicity (3, 32).

To increase immunogenicity, the PRP capsular polysaccharide was conjugated to various protein carriers. Four conjugated vaccines are licensed in the United States: diphtheria toxoid conjugate (PRP-D), diphtheria CRM_{197} protein conjugate (HbOC), meningococcal outer-membrane protein conjugate (PRP-OMP), and tetanus toxoid conjugate (PRP-T) (Tables 61.1 and 61.2). A fifth product that combines DTP with the HbOC, Tetramune (Lederle-Praxis), has also been approved (3).

The carrier proteins in PRP-T, PRP-D, and HbOC are chemically and immunologically similar to the toxoids contained in DTP. Vaccination with diphtheria or tetanus toxoids may be required to elicit an optimal anti-PRP antibody response. Therefore, if the DTP or DT vaccine is not given, the PRP-OMP should be used for Hib immunization to ensure optimal anti-PRP antibody to the conjugate vaccine. Immunization with any of the conjugated vaccines does not provide immunity against diphtheria, tetanus, or meningococcal disease (3, 4, 6).

The incidence of systemic Hib disease has decreased by about 85% since the introduction of the conjugated vaccines (33, 34). This decreased incidence occurred with most children from 12 to 23 months of age having received only a single immunization and with 36% of those children having received 3 immunizations (34). Otitis media and upper respiratory infections are caused frequently by nontypeable *H. influenzae,* so the incidence of these diseases is not affected by Hib immunization.

SCHEDULE

Infants should be immunized starting at 2 months of age (Table 61.3). The HbOC and PRP-T require a primary series of 3 doses given at 2, 4, and 6 months of age, with the final dose, a booster, given at 15 months of age. The PRP-OMP dosing schedule consists of 2 primary immunizations at 2 and 4 months with the booster dose given at 12 months of age. Any of these conjugate vaccines may be used in infants 2 to 12 months of age. These can be given at the same time as polio vaccine, DTP, DTaP, or MMR. If it is not possible to use the same conjugate vaccine throughout, the primary series should consist of 3 immunizations. PRP-D is indicated only for use in those over 12 months of age. Recently, a novel combination of vaccines has been approved for use in an effort to decrease the number of injections associated with immunization. The DTP vaccine by Connaught can be combined in the same syringe with the PRP-T and given as a single injection. Alternatively, Tetramune, the HbOC and DTP combination vaccine can be used.

Children who are at increased risk for Hib disease, such as those with HIV infection, immunoglobulin deficiency, functional or anatomic asplenia, Hodgkin's disease, sickle-cell disease, and recipients of a bone marrow transplant or chemotherapy, may have a decreased response to Hib conjugate vaccination. Children with solid tumors have a 50% response rate to PRP-D, and leukemic children have an 80% response rate (35). Preterm infants do not appear to respond as well to PRP-OMP as term infants (36). Recent reports show that infants and children with sickle cell disease (37) and those after bone marrow transplant (38) have a good response to Hib vaccination.

If Hib disease is contracted at under 24 months of age, the patient should start the immunization process 1 month after the onset of illness, and any Hib immunization prior to the Hib infection should be ignored. Infants at increased risk for Hib and who either have received one vaccination prior to 12 months of age or who have received no Hib doses and are over 12 months and under 5 years of should receive two Hib conjugate immunizations separated by 2 months (3). Unvaccinated

children over 5 years of age with sickle cell disease or asplenia should receive a single Hib immunization. Those with HIV, immunoglobulin (IgG2) deficiency, after bone marrow transplant, or with malignancy should receive 2 doses separated by 1 to 2 months.

Hib vaccines cause few local (e.g., induration tenderness in under 5%) or systemic (e.g., fever in about 2%) reactions. For the HbOC vaccine, adverse events following the first and second doses were less frequent than after the third dose. Following the third dose, approximately 2% of patients had a fever and local redness. Adverse reactions to PRP-OMP have been rare as well, with only 4.3% of patients experiencing a fever after the second dose (39).

RIFAMPIN PROPHYLAXIS (H. INFLUENZAE)

The Hib bacteria continue to colonize the nasopharynx even after the infection has been treated with systemic antibiotics. Rifampin is used to eliminate nasopharyngeal colonization of Hib in the index case (patient with systemic disease) and in asymptomatic carriers, thereby decreasing the occurrence of secondary Hib infections. Regardless of immunization history, all patients with systemic Hib should be treated with rifampin (3, 40). Nasopharyngeal colonization with encapsulated or pathogenic Hib occurs in 2 to 5% of all children, however, the incidence of pathogenic Hib colonization increases to between 9 to 20% of parents, 20% of patients in institutions, up to 58% of children in day care centers, and 60 to 70% of the index case's siblings (40).

Recommendations for rifampin prophylaxis against secondary infection are controversial (3). Generally, all pediatric and adult household contacts (e.g., individuals living with the index case or nonresidents who spent over 4 hours a day with the index case for 5 to 7 days prior to diagnosis) in homes where at least one unvaccinated contact is under 48 months of age should receive prophylaxis. Rifampin is not needed if household members under 48 months of age have completed Hib vaccination. All members of households with infants under 12 months of age who have not received the primary immunization series and booster should receive prophylaxis. Children who are immunocompromised and their household members should receive rifampin prophylaxis regardless of immunization status.

The efficacy of large-scale prophylaxis of children in day care centers has not been well established. Because recommendations vary from state to state and even within a state, the local health department should be contacted for information concerning prophylaxis criteria. Children and personnel in day care centers that house children under 2 years of age for longer than 25 hours a week may require rifampin prophylaxis. Unvaccinated or incompletely vaccinated children should receive a dose of conjugate vaccine. If all children in the day care are older than 2 years of age, rifampin prophylaxis is not necessary regardless of vaccination status. Unvaccinated or incompletely vaccinated children should receive a dose of Hib vaccine.

Prophylaxis should be initiated as soon as possible after identification of the index case, because the majority of secondary cases occur within 1 week after hospitalization of the index case (3). Furthermore, those individuals identified as requiring prophylaxis should be treated during the same time period to prevent nasopharyngeal recolonization within a group. A single 20-mg/kg dose not to exceed 600 mg of rifampin administered once a day for 4 days is 95% effective (3, 41). The dose of rifampin for infants under 1 month of age has not been established; however, some experts recommend reducing the daily dose to 10 mg/kg (3). Rifampin is not marketed in a dosage form suitable for pediatric use; however, a rifampin suspension extemporaneously compounded from the powder in rifampin capsules and simple syrup provides an acceptable method of delivering the prescribed dose (42). Rifampin is a potent inducer of hepatic microsomal enzymes, so potential drug interactions must be considered. In addition, patients taking rifampin should be counseled about the orange discoloration of body secretions (sweat, tears, urine, etc.); in particular, patients should be advised of the permanent discoloration of soft contact lenses that may occur during therapy.

Hepatitis B

The hepatitis B virus (HBV), a 42-nm, DNA virus of the class hepadnaviridae is a major cause of acute and chronic hepatitis, cirrhosis, and hepatocellular carcinoma. Worldwide, more than 250 million chronic carriers, some of whom are asymptomatic, provide a reservoir for viral transmission (3).

The likelihood of becoming chronically infected with HBV varies inversely with the age at which infection occurs. A very small percentage of infants born to hepatitis B surface antigen (HBsAg) positive mothers become infected in utero. However, 80 to 90% will become infected during or after birth if left untreated. The carrier state can be prevented in about 90% of infants who are treated with the vaccine and hepatitis B immune globulin (HBIG). Thus, identification of HBsAg positive mothers is important. Others who are at increased risk of becoming infected with HBV include those who require frequent blood products, such as those with hemophilia or those who require hemodialysis, since there is a possibility that these products may contain the virus.

Most of those who become infected acquire the disease as adolescents or adults. Health care workers, hospital staff, clients or staff of institutions for the mentally retarded, recipients of clotting factors, household contacts of HBV carriers, hemodialysis patients, homosexually active males, persons with multiple heterosexual partners, and intravenous drug abusers are at increased risk for HBV infection

and require preexposure hepatitis B vaccine. Persons requiring postexposure hepatitis B vaccine include infants born to carrier mothers, those with accidental percutaneous or permucosal exposure to infected blood, sexual partners of persons with acute HBV infection, and household contacts of persons with acute HBV infection (3).

To decrease HBV transmission and eradicate the disease, universal immunization against HBV must be achieved (43). Several strategies have been proposed in order to begin to address this problem. HBV vaccine is recommended for all infants as part of the routine childhood immunization schedule (Table 61.3) (3, 6, 43). However, HBV immunization of infants is not routine in this country, and most states do not require evidence of HBV immunization prior to school entry (44). In order to facilitate the immunization of children and adolescents against HBV, many immunization clinics provide HBV vaccine at little to no cost as part of the Childhood Immunization Initiative.

An analysis of hepatitis B vaccination strategies evaluated the most cost-effective approach to universal hepatitis B vaccination. This study recommended that all women who give birth be screened and neonates born to HBsAg positive mothers be vaccinated and receive HBIG. Also recommended was universal vaccination at 10 years of age followed by revaccination at 20 years of age (45). Adults at high risk would also receive HBV vaccine.

IMMUNIZATION

Two HBV vaccines are licensed for use in the United States (Table 61.5). Recombivax HB (Merck, Sharp, Merck & Co.) and Engerix-B (SmithKline Beecham) are produced using recombinant DNA technology (Tables 61.1 and 61.2). Because the dose of the Recombivax HB to achieve

Table 61.5.
Dosages of HBV Vaccine

Recipient Criteria	Recombivax HB μg (mL)	Engerix-B μg (mL)
Infants of HBsAg negative mothers	2.5 (0.5[a])	10 (0.5)
Infants of HBsAg positive mothers[b]	5 (0.5[c]) or (1.0[a])	10 (0.5)
Children < 11 years	2.5 (0.5[a])	10 (0.5)
Children & adolescents (11–19 years)	5 (0.5[c])	20 (1.0)
Adults ≥ 20 years	10 (1.0[c])	20 (1.0)
Dialysis patients & other immunosuppressed adults	40 (1.0[d])	40 (2.0[e])

[a]Pediatric formulation.
[b]Should receive HBIG (0.5 mL) at a separate site along with the first dose of vaccine.
[c]Adult formulation.
[d]Dialysis formulation.
[e]Two 1.0-mL doses given at one site in a 4-dose schedule at 0, 1, 2, and 6–12 months.
Adapted from references 3 and 43.

the desired antibody response in hemodialysis patients would deliver over 1.25 mg of aluminum, which is the maximum amount allowed by the FDA, a formulation with increased antigen and decreased aluminum has been developed. The recombinant HBV vaccines have no real or theoretical potential for contamination with HIV. The plasma derived HBV vaccine is no longer produced in the United States; however, it can be obtained from Merck & Co. for individuals with yeast allergy.

SCHEDULE

The primary immunization series consists of 3 doses with the second and third doses given 1 and 6 months after the first (Table 61.3). Infants born to HBsAG positive mothers should receive their first dose of vaccine (Table 61.5) and 0.5 mL of HBIG at a separate injection site within 12 hours of birth. Ideally, the second dose will be given at 1 month of age and the third at 6 months of age.

In infants and children under 11 years of age, three doses (Table 61.5) are given with at least 1 month between the first and second doses and at least 2 months (preferably 4 months) between the second and third doses. This schedule can be started at birth or adapted to coincide with other routine pediatric immunizations (3, 6). Ideally, children will have completed HBV immunization by 18 months of age. One advantage in immunizing those under 11 years of age is that the dose is half that administered to individuals over 11 years of age, which results in significant cost savings. The same 3-dose schedule is used for individuals 11 years of age or older. Patients undergoing hemodialysis or who are immunosuppressed require larger doses to induce antibody concentrations that are considered protective.

Long-term follow-up in children and adults indicates that immune memory remains for 5 to 9 years despite the fact that antibody titers decline (43). Routine measurement of anti-HBsAg is not recommended, except in hemodialysis patients, those with HIV, and those at occupational risk. Additional doses should be given when titers fall below 10 mIU/mL (3). Currently routine booster doses of HBV are not recommended. The need for boosters will continue to be assessed as our knowledge about the duration of effect of this vaccine increases.

The most common side effect of these vaccines is soreness at the injection site and fever in 1 to 6% of vaccines. Occasionally malaise, headache, chills, and gastrointestinal symptoms occur and may persist for a few days. Immediate hypersensitivity reactions have been reported rarely (3). For a thorough discussion of hepatitis B, see Chapter 27.

Delayed or Missed Immunizations

Should a child under 7 years of age fail to receive all recommended immunizations on time, it is not necessary to repeat immunizations that have already been given. Rather, the immunizations that have not been given should be administered at the recommended intervals. Unimmunized children 15 months to 5 years of age can be given DTP, OPV, MMR, HBV, and any one of the Hib vaccines at the same time (3, 32). Those children over 5 years old should be given all the named immunizations except the Hib vaccine, which is no longer required. The second DTP, HBV, and OPV should be given 2 months after the initial immunization, and the third HBV and DTP 2 months after the second doses. Six to twelve months after the third DTP, a second dose of MMR and booster doses of DTP and OPV are given. DTaP can be substituted for DTP as the fourth and fifth dose in the series for those 15 months to 7 years of age (3).

Unimmunized children over 7 years but under 18 years of age should be immunized with Td, OPV, HBV, and MMR with these being repeated in 2 months. A third immunization with Td, OPV, and HBV is given after 6 to 12 months to complete the primary series. All individuals should receive Td every 8 to 10 years.

OTHER IMMUNIZATIONS

Varicella

Varicella-zoster virus, a herpesvirus, is responsible for both varicella (chickenpox) and herpes zoster (shingles). Varicella is spread by aerosolized droplets and is the primary varicella-zoster infection in children under 10 years old. Varicella is highly contagious, with over 90% secondary infection rates for household contacts. The incubation period ranges from 10 to 20 days after exposure. Prodromal symptoms consist of malaise, fever, and anorexia. The constantly pruritic rash has an abrupt onset about 24 hours later and consists of small red papules that progress to fluid-filled vesicles. Individuals are contagious from 1 to 2 days before onset of the rash until 5 to 6 days later, when the lesions have dried and crusted. Because the disease is highly contagious, most children between 5 and 10 years of age have chickenpox with an uncomfortable but uncomplicated course and usually no serious sequelae. Children who are immunocompromised have a more complicated course, a prolonged recovery, and potentially serious sequelae (3).

Herpes zoster results from reactivation of the latent virus and is more common in those over 10 years old. The virus is thought to gain access to sensory nerves during varicella, when the virus is present in the fluid-filled vesicles. The virus remains latent or dormant in most individuals. Reactivation of the virus results in shingles usually involving the thoracic, cervical, lumbar, or sacral nerves.

IMMUNIZATION

The live, attenuated varicella vaccine was developed by removing fluid from a vesicle in a child with chickenpox and isolating and attenuating the virus by serial passages through various cell cultures (Tables 61.1 and 61.2). In 1995 Varivax by Merck became the first varicella vaccine licensed in the United States. It is anticipated that a MMR-varicella combination vaccine will become available in the future.

SCHEDULE

Varicella vaccination has recently been recommended by the AAP and it consists of a single dose given to children 1 through 12 years of age. The need for booster doses is unknown at this time. While one immunization results in protection in 95% of healthy children, it is less effective in adolescents, adults, and immunocompromised children (46). In those 13 years of age or older, 2 doses are given from 1 to 2 months apart. Vaccination should be avoided for at least 3 months following administration of immunoglobulin. About 17% of normal, healthy individuals experience rash and fever after immunization. The rate of adverse effects is increased to 47% in immunocompromised patients.

The protective effects of this vaccine were demonstrated by a decrease in the rate of postexposure infection and a milder course in immunized children who developed disease. In addition, the occurrence of zoster infection was less in those who had breakthrough varicella than in those who had naturally occurring varicella. This may relate to the decreased number of fluid-filled lesions that occur in those who have been vaccinated and still have breakthrough varicella. A cost-effectiveness evaluation determined that routine immunization of healthy children would result in a net savings in medical costs as well as parental work loss (47). Despite the fact that this is a live virus vaccine, it is indicated in children with acute lymphocytic leukemia (ALL). While the incidence of vaccine related adverse effects is greater in these patients, the resultant breakthrough disease is significantly milder when it occurs (48).

Hepatitis A

Hepatitis A is an RNA virus classified as a picornavirus. This highly contagious disease is transmitted by the fecal-oral route and is commonly called *infectious hepatitis.* Worldwide, 1.4 million cases are reported each year, and it is believed that the actual number of cases are several times that number. Each year in the United States, 143,000 individuals contract and 80 individuals die from hepatitis A. The estimated cost is $200 million (49).

IMMUNIZATIONS

Havrix, marketed by SmithKline Beecham Biologicals, is the first hepatitis A vaccine licensed in the United States (Table 61.1). Pediatric and adult formulations are available (Table 61.2) (50). A second hepatitis A vaccine, Vaqta, has been developed and is under investigation by Merck (51).

Each 0.6-mL dose of Vaqta consists of 25 units of hepatitis A virus antigen, 0.3 mg of aluminum, and thimerosal as a preservative.

SCHEDULE

Ideally, the immunization should be given at least 2 weeks prior to expected hepatitis A exposure. In adults an initial injection is given followed by a booster in 6 to 12 months. Children from 2 to 18 years are given an initial dose, a second dose 1 month later, and a booster in 6 to 12 months.

A randomized, controlled cross-over trial in Thai children found that hepatitis A occurred in 38 of 598 control patients who received hepatitis B immunization and 2 of 583 hepatitis A immunized patients (50). The duration of protection conferred by vaccination is unknown; however, a European study reported that adults who received 720 ELISA units had increased antibody titers for 4 years. These investigators extrapolated their data and suggested that protection may last as long as 20 years (50).

In order to provide immediate protection to individuals exposed to hepatitis A, immune globulin is given concurrently with the hepatitis A vaccine. When immune globulin is given at the same time as the vaccine, antibody titers are lower than in individuals who receive the vaccine alone (52). An additional booster may be required in these individuals (52). Adverse effects include local pain, which occurs more often in those who receive hepatitis A vaccine compared to HBV (50). For a thorough discussion of hepatitis A, see Chapter 27.

Influenza

Influenza viruses are orthomyxoviruses of three antigenic types, A, B, and C. Types A and B cause disease. Influenza is spread by direct contact and is characterized by the abrupt onset of fever, headache, malaise, muscle aches, and cough. Later, respiratory symptoms become more prominent, and nausea and vomiting may occur. Influenza can present as a variety of clinical syndromes ranging from a sepsislike picture in the very young to mild symptoms in usually healthy adults (3).

Influenza type A is subclassified by hemagglutinin (H), which can be subtype H1, H2, or H3, and neuraminidase (N), which can be subtype N1 or N2. Antigenic shifts are major variations in either the H or N antigens; antigenic drifts are minor variations within the same subtype and are the primary reason that new variants of influenza occur (3, 53).

IMMUNIZATION

The changes in influenza patterns are evaluated in March and April of each year. The vaccine is formulated based on the influenza strains that are expected to be prevalent in the upcoming influenza season. At least 6 months are required for production, quality control, and distribution. The vaccine is available as an inactivated, whole virus vaccine and a split (subvirion) virus vaccine made from two type A and one type B virus strains (Tables 61.1 and 61.2).

SCHEDULE

Generally, the vaccine is given in the fall 1 month before the expected influenza season begins. From 2 weeks to 6 months after vaccination, antibody concentrations should be protective. Since immunity declines after 6 months, annual revaccination is necessary to ensure protection from disease.

Children between the ages of 6 months and 8 years should receive 2 doses of the split virus vaccine separated by a month the first time the immunization is given. Children 6 to 35 months of age should be given a 0.25-mL dose, and those 3 to 8 years of age should receive a 0.5-mL dose. For subsequent influenza immunizations, only 1 dose is required. Individuals over 9 years old are given a single 0.5-mL dose of whole or split virus each year.

In general, few adverse effects are associated with the influenza vaccine. The whole virus is a better antigen, but adverse effects are greater than those seen with split virus vaccines, which contain only the antigenic portions of the virus. The most common adverse effects include pain, induration, and erythema at the injection site. Flulike symptoms of fever, chills, myalgia, and malaise may begin within 12 hours and are more common in children given the whole virus vaccine. Febrile seizures have been reported.

A placebo controlled study in hospital employees vaccinated against influenza showed that 325 mg of acetaminophen given at the time of immunization and 4, 8, and 12 hours later decreased soreness associated with the immunization, and those who received 650 mg on the same schedule had decreased soreness and less nausea (54). Because chick embryo cultures are used to manufacture this vaccine, individuals with egg allergies may require a graded protocol for vaccine administration or desensitization prior to influenza immunization (Table 61.4) (27, 28).

Influenza and pneumococcal vaccines can be administered concurrently at different sites, thereby increasing compliance. Conversely, the influenza vaccine should not be given within 3 days of the whole-cell pertussis immunization, since both can cause fever. Individuals 15 months of age or older can receive the DTaP and the influenza vaccines at the same time (3).

Although the vaccine is recommended for the general population, the CDC has defined high-risk target groups that may receive the greatest benefit from vaccination. These include individuals with chronic cardiovascular disease, renal disease, diabetes mellitus, hemoglobinopathies (sickle cell disease), or pulmonary disorders (cystic fibrosis, bronchiectasis, obstructive pulmonary disease, asthma, and class 3 tuberculosis). From September through March, unvaccinated hospitalized patients in any high-risk group should receive influenza vaccination as part of routine discharge procedures. Individuals over 65 years of age, individuals in chronic-care facilities, and health care personnel who may spread nosocomial infections should be vaccinated (55). Likewise, patients who are pharmacologically or functionally immunosuppressed should be immunized. Children who are not in a high-risk group do not need to be immunized (3).

In spite of the recommendations that influenza immunization be given to high-risk populations, typically immunization rates are low. The federally funded influenza immunization program (through Medicare) has been successful in increasing influenza immunization rates from about 40% to 60% in those over 65 years of age. Immunization rates tend to be higher in older individuals with other risk factors such as diabetes or heart disease and in those who are more educated (55). Important factors in the failure of the elderly to receive influenza immunizations are the lack of awareness of the Medicare program and lack of transportation to obtain the immunization. Those who have had adverse effects from previous "flu shots" tend to avoid reimmunization (56).

Meningococcus

Neisseria meningitidis is a Gram-negative diplococcus that causes meningococcemia with or without meningitis. Onset of fever, chills, malaise, and the characteristic rash is abrupt. Within hours of the initial symptoms the disease can progress to disseminated intravascular coagulation, shock, coma, and death. Individuals with asymptomatic colonization of the upper respiratory tract frequently transmit the disease via infected droplets. Meningococcal infections occur more frequently in children under 5 years of age, with most disease occurring in those 6 to 12 months of age. Disease transmission requires close personal contact (e.g., family members, day care attendance, military). About 3% of households will experience more than one secondary case of meningococcal disease. While 9 serotypes have been identified, groups B, C, Y, and W-135 are the most common cause of disease in the United States.

IMMUNIZATION

The current quadrivalent polysaccharide vaccine provides protection against serotypes A, C, Y, and W-135 (Table 61.2) but does not provide protection against serotype B, the major cause of disease in children (Table 61.1). The immunologic response to types C, Y, and W-135 is poor in infants. However, this vaccine is very effective in preventing disease secondary to serotype A in children over 3 months of age (57). By 2 years of age, children have an adequate immune response to serotype C (58).

SCHEDULE

With the exception of military personnel, routine immunization with meningococcal vaccine is not recommended. However, individuals over 2 years old who have functional or anatomic asplenia or complement deficiency should receive the vaccine (0.5 mL per dose) (Table 61.1). Immunization of a child 3 to 18 months of age during an epidemic should include two 0.5 mL doses administered 3 months apart. The duration of protection in children under 4 years of age is probably under 3 years for serotype A (3). Adverse effects seen with meningococcal vaccine include mild local and systemic effects. Fever is more common in younger children but is rarely above 38.5°C (58).

RIFAMPIN PROPHYLAXIS (N. MENINGITIDIS)

As with Hib infection, *N. meningitidis* colonizes the nasopharynx and is spread through direct contact. Secondary cases may not develop symptoms for several weeks after disease exposure (3). Because of the disease severity, all household contacts and children in day care centers should receive prophylactic antibiotics within 24 hours of diagnosis of the index case (3). Also, rifampin is indicated for individuals who have come in contact with oral secretions (e.g., kissing, sharing beverages, or food) from the index case. Hospital personnel who care for a child with meningococcal disease have a very low risk for acquiring the disease; thus prophylaxis is not recommended unless biologic fluid exposure occurs prior to antibiotic administration. Neither the vaccine or chemoprophylaxis prevents 33% of cases that occur within 72 hours of the disease onset in the index case; therefore, follow-up surveillance after exposure and chemoprophylaxis is essential. Rifampin 10 mg/kg up to 600 mg per dose is given every 12 hours for 2 days. Alternatively, the same regimen recommended for Hib disease prophylaxis can be used (3). In neonates, the rifampin dose is decreased to 5 mg/kg given every 12 hours for 2 days.

Pneumococcus

Streptococcus pneumoniae, the leading pathogen in community-acquired pneumonia, is the second most common cause of meningitis in the United States and is the cause of otitis media in over a million pediatric patients each year. An estimated 40,000 individuals die each year from pneumococcal pneumonia and meningitis (59). Although there are over 80 pneumococcal capsular polysaccharide serotypes worldwide, most pneumococcal disease is caused by 10 serotypes.

IMMUNIZATION

In 1983, the first pneumococcal vaccine that contained 14 serotypes was replaced by a vaccine containing 23 capsular polysaccharides, representing 85 to 98% of disease isolates worldwide (60). Approximately 88% of serotypes causing adult bacteremia and meningitis, 85% causing acute otitis media, and nearly 100% of the serotypes causing pediatric bacteremia and meningitis are contained in the current vaccine (61). As with other polysaccharide vaccines, the pneumococcal vaccine is poorly immunogenic with efficacy ranging from 48 to 70%. The duration of immunity conferred by vaccination is unknown. Increasing immunogenicity by conjugating the polysaccharides with different protein carriers such as diphtheria or tetanus toxoids as was done with Hib protein conjugate vaccines is being investigated (62, 63).

SCHEDULE

The pneumococcal vaccine is indicated in individuals over 2 years of age who are at high risk for acquiring serious pneumococcal infection (Tables 61.1 and 61.2) (3, 60). Groups at high risk include those with sickle cell anemia, anatomic or functional asplenia, chronic renal failure, nephrotic syndrome, Hodgkin's disease, and immunosuppression, including children with HIV infection. Also, the vaccine is indicated in healthy individuals over 65 years of age (55). Ideally, patients undergoing elective splenectomy or those to be treated with immunosuppressive medications should be vaccinated at least 2 weeks before the procedure or initiation of therapy (3). If this is not possible, the vaccine can be given 3 months after the completion of therapy. Influenza and pneumococcal vaccines can be administered concurrently at different sites.

The need for repeat vaccination with the pneumococcal vaccine has been discussed and debated for years (64). Currently it is recommended that children under 10 years of age who are at high risk for severe pneumococcal disease should be revaccinated within 3 to 5 years of previous immunization. Older children and adults with severe risk for pneumococcal disease should be revaccinated 6 years after the initial vaccination (64).

Few serious adverse effects are associated with initial immunization with the pneumococcal vaccine. Discomfort, induration, and erythema at the injection site occur in 40 to 90% of patients. Systemic effects occur less frequently but include fever, weakness, muscle aches, chills, headache, nausea, and photophobia. Patients with immune thrombocytopenia have experienced exacerbations of disease following pneumococcal immunization.

Tuberculosis

Tuberculosis (TB) is a necrotizing bacterial infection caused by *Mycobacterium tuberculosis*. Occasionally, *Mycobacterium bovis* has caused human disease in the United States. After many years of decline, the incidence of TB in the United States has recently increased because patients with AIDS develop TB secondarily. In addition to the increased incidence, there has been an increase in multiple drug-resistant TB (65).

Children should receive either the multiple puncture or the Mantoux TB skin test at the time of the first MMR immunization (about 15 months of age), before school entry (about 6 years of age), and during adolescence (14 to 16 years of age). Children in high-risk groups including those who are contacts of adults with TB or those with HIV, immunosuppression, Hodgkin's disease, lymphoma, diabetes mellitus, chronic renal failure, and malnutrition should receive annual TB skin tests (3).

IMMUNIZATION

Bacillus Calmette-Guerin (BCG) vaccine is available for immunization against TB (Tables 61.1 and 61.2). Between 10 and 14 days after immunization, a lesion develops at the immunization site. Maximal effects are noted by 4 to 6 weeks, and by 6 months the lesion usually has completely healed and faded. In some patients, there may be a residual scar; however, the lack of a scar following BCG vaccination does not indicate vaccine failure.

SCHEDULE

A single immunization is given, followed by application of a tuberculin skin test 2 to 3 months after immunization. If the skin test is negative, a second dose of the vaccine should be administered. Because a positive tuberculin skin test is an end point of BCG vaccination, this test is not useful for identifying TB after BCG vaccination. Routine vaccination against TB using BCG vaccine is not recommended.

A meta-analysis of studies conducted worldwide reported that the incidence of TB was decreased by 50% in those vaccinated with BCG (65). In addition, the duration of protection is not known, but sensitivity to tuberculin skin testing has persisted for 7 to 10 years. In spite of lack of agreement on the efficacy of BCG, vaccination should be considered in those in close contact with infected patients who are untreated, ineffectively treated, or resistant to treatment; health care workers where other control measures do not prevent an annual new infection rate greater than 1%; and other groups with an excessive new infection rate in whom surveillance and treatment programs fail or are not feasible. Because of the risk for development of disease secondary to live vaccine administration, BCG is contraindicated in patients who are immunosuppressed or have burns, symptomatic HIV, or skin infections (3).

Adverse effects include skin ulceration at the injection site, regional adenitis, and occasionally, lupoid reactions. Osteitis has been reported in BCG vaccinated neonates, and the incidence appears to depend on the specific vaccine used. For a thorough discussion of tuberculosis, see Chapter 64.

Rabies

Rabies is an acute viral disease caused by a RNA virus of the rhabdovirus group that affects the central nervous system. Known natural reservoirs for rabies include skunks, foxes, raccoons, and bats, but all mammals can be affected. Transmission is primarily by infected secretions, usually saliva. The incubation period for rabies is between 20 and 60 days but may be over 6 months. Following the initial inoculation, the virus remains close to the wound; however, migration along a neuronal pathway to the central nervous system ultimately occurs. The clinical manifestations of rabies can be divided into three stages; a nonspecific prodrome, an acute encephalitis, and a profound dysfunction of brainstem centers. Recovery without intervention is rare and occurs slowly.

The most effective effort in decreasing rabies in humans is the extensive rabies vaccination program conducted in domestic animals (66). Twenty cases of rabies were reported in humans in the United States from 1980 to 1995. Of these cases, half were imported, a few were associated with an animal bite, and most were diagnosed at autopsy. Rabies has occurred secondary to corneal transplant from a donor that unknowingly had rabies. As a result of these 20 cases, over 800 individuals who were exposed to rabies required prophylaxis that cost $850,000 (66, 67).

IMMUNIZATION

The original vaccine developed by Pasteur was a suspension of fragments of rabies virus from infected spinal cords. Because of adverse effects, the vaccine was modified several times. Work in the early 1960s led to development of the human diploid-cell rabies vaccine (HDCV), which is more immunogenic and has fewer side effects than previous vaccines. Both i.m. (Imovax rabies) and i.d. (Imovax rabies I.D.) dosage forms of the HDCV are available (Table 61.1). A second rabies vaccine, rabies vaccine absorbed (RVA), has been prepared by growing virus in cell culture (Table 61.2) (68).

SCHEDULE

Preexposure Prophylaxis. Individuals who have a high risk for exposure to rabies, such as veterinarians or dog catchers, should receive preexposure prophylaxis against rabies. The preexposure immunization schedule is 1 mL of the RVA or HDCV or 0.1 mL i.d. of Imovax rabies I.D. given on days 0, 7, and 28 (3 doses). For those who will have continuing exposure, antibody concentrations should be measured every 6 months and a booster vaccination with 1 mL i.m. of the HDCV or RVA or 0.1 mL of Imovax rabies I.D. given when concentrations are below 0.5 IU/mL or a virus neutralization titer is > 15. Rabies immune globulin (RIG) should not be given to individuals who are immunized preexposure.

RVA or HDCV should be administered i.m. for preexposure rabies prophylaxis in individuals receiving chloroquine or mefloquine for malaria prophylaxis. In this situation, i.d. injection of rabies vaccine may not result in an appropriate antibody response.

Postexposure Prophylaxis. Those who have not been immunized previously and who are acutely exposed to rabies should be immunized with 1 mL of HDCV or RVA given i.m. on days 0, 3, 7, 14, and 28 (3). Additionally, RIG 20 IU/kg should be given as soon as possible but not longer than 8 days after exposure, with half the dose instilled at the site of the bite and the remainder administered i.m.

Vaccination causes local discomfort, swelling, erythema, and induration in up to 90% of individuals, which usually subsides in 1 to 3 days. Up to 10% of patients have systemic reactions that include nausea, vomiting, abdominal pain, headache, malaise, and low-grade fever. An immune complex–like reaction has been reported in up to 7% of individuals receiving booster vaccination and is characterized by urticaria with or without arthralgia, arthritis, or angioedema (69). Anaphylactic reactions have been reported rarely. Once initiated, rabies prophylaxis should not be discontinued because of local or mild systemic reactions to the vaccine.

VACCINATION FOR TRAVEL

Travel to developing countries may include exposure to diseases that are rarely encountered in the United States. Immunization or prophylactic measures will help decrease the likelihood of developing specific diseases that are endemic in certain areas of the world. Prior to travel outside the United States, the CDC should be contacted regarding information about immunizations or prophylactic medications and other measures that are advised or required for entrance into individual countries. This should be done as early as possible before anticipated travel, because immunizations for various diseases not be able to be administered at the same time, and others require a series of doses to induce adequate immunity (70, 71).

Cholera

Previously, an International Certificate of Vaccination against cholera was required to gain entrance to several countries. However, the vaccine only provides protection in 40 to 60% of vaccinees, the duration of effect is relatively short, and the vaccine is not effective against the most common serotype that is now responsible for disease. For these reasons, cholera vaccination is no longer recommended and no country requires documentation of cholera vaccination prior to entry. Experimental attenuated live oral cholera vaccines are more effective and have fewer side effects; however, none have yet been approved for use.

Typhoid

Typhoid vaccination is recommended for individuals who travel to rural areas of tropical countries or to areas where there are unsanitary conditions and an increased risk for disease exposure. Although immunization results in antibody production in 50 to 90% of individuals, the degree of immunity is not great and can be readily overcome with a large inoculum.

IMMUNIZATION

Inactivated, live (Vivotif Berna), and capsular polysaccharide vaccines are available to the general public (Tables 61.1 and 61.2). A fourth acetone-inactivated typhoid vaccine is provided by the U.S. government for military use.

SCHEDULE

The primary series of the phenol-inactivated typhoid vaccine consists of 2 doses given up to 4 weeks apart. The dose for children 6 months to 10 years old is 0.25 mL and for individuals over 10 years is 0.5 mL. A booster is required every 3 years if reexposure is expected. The booster dose is better tolerated if given by the i.d. route (dose 0.1 mL).

The primary immunization series with Vivotif Berna, the oral typhoid vaccine, consists of 1 capsule every other day for 4 doses. Capsules are stored in the refrigerator and should be taken with cool water about 1 hour before a meal. This vaccine is contraindicated in children under 6 years old, those with an acute febrile illness or an acute gastrointestinal illness, and individuals receiving sulfa drugs or antibiotics. The same dose and schedule is repeated every 5 years if reexposure to typhoid is expected.

The primary immunization with the polysaccharide vaccine is administered as a single 0.5-mL dose. A booster dose should be given every 2 years if reexposure to typhoid is expected. This vaccine is not recommended for use in children under 2 years of age (72).

The inactivated vaccine contains significant quantities of endotoxin and often results in 1 to 2 days of discomfort at the injection site, fever, malaise, and headache. Serious systemic adverse reactions are rare and may be decreased by using the i.d. route of administration. Adverse effects with the oral vaccine include nausea, vomiting, abdominal cramps, and urticarial rash. The incidence of fever and headache are not different between the live vaccine and the polysaccharide vaccine but are significantly greater with the inactivated vaccine (72). Overall, adverse effects with the attenuated, live oral vaccine are less than with the other two, and the capsular polysaccharide vaccine has fewer side effects than the inactivated vaccine.

Yellow Fever

The vaccine is recommended for persons who will be traveling to rural endemic areas or laboratory workers who may be exposed to the virus (71, 73). There is a single yellow fever vaccine available in the United States (Tables 61.1 and 61.2).

SCHEDULE

A single 0.5-mL dose induces immunity that persists for over 10 years. Infants under 4 months of age should not be vaccinated because of the increased risk of encephalitis. Immunization of infants from 4 to 9 months of age should be based on estimates of risk of exposure (70). The vaccine is available in centers of high risk designated by certain state health departments.

Reactions to the yellow fever vaccine are generally mild. Up to 10% of individuals have mild headaches, myalgia, or low-grade fever from 5 to 10 days after immunization. Immediate hypersensitivity reactions are rare. Yellow fever vaccine should not be given to those who are immunocompromised or experience anaphylactic reactions to eggs. An immunization waiver from a physician or official immunization center stating the contraindication may be sufficient to gain entrance into certain countries. Should there be a high risk for yellow fever and immunization a requirement, skin testing may be performed to determine the allergic potential of the vaccine. If necessary a desensitization protocol can be followed to achieve full immunization (Table 61.4).

Cholera and yellow fever vaccines should be given at least 3 weeks apart because of reported decreases in antibody response to both vaccines with concomitant administration. However, if time constraints do not permit, the ACIP recommends they be administered at the same time but at different sites (73).

Malaria

Since no vaccine is available currently, chemoprophylaxis remains the primary method for malaria prevention. The choice of therapy depends on the organism endemic to the area being visited. Usually therapy is with chloroquine 300 mg (base) given once per week, started 1 week prior to travel and continued for 4 to 6 weeks after exposure (70, 71, 74). The pediatric dose is 5 mg/kg up to 300 mg of the base drug. Adverse effects associated with chloroquine therapy include dizziness, headache, gastrointestinal problems, and pruritus. An alternative agent for nonpregnant females and those over 8 years old is doxycycline, which can be started 1 to 2 days prior to travel in a dose of 2 mg/kg up to 100 mg per day and continued for 4 to 6 weeks after exposure. Doxycycline causes photosensitivity and may be upsetting to the gastrointestinal tract.

For those who use chloroquine, 3 tablets of Fansidar (75 mg pyrimethamine and 1500 mg sulfadoxine) should be available for use in the event that a febrile illness occurs when professional medical care is not available. Those with a history of hypersensitivity to sulfonamides, pregnant women near term and infants under 2 months of age should not receive pyrimethamine-sulfadoxine. While rare, pyrimethamine-sulfadoxine has been associated with Stevens-Johnson syndrome, and therapy should be discontinued immediately upon appearance of a rash.

Those traveling to areas known to have chloroquine-resistant malaria should receive one 250-mg dose of mefloquine salt (228 mg base) 1 week prior to arrival in the malarious area, and prophylaxis should continue with weekly doses until 4 weeks after exposure (75). The pediatric dose is 1/4 tablet for those 15 to 19 kg, 1/2 tablet for 20 to 30 kg, 3/4 tablet for 31 to 45 kg, and one 250 mg tablet for over 45 kg. Children under 15 kg, pregnant women in the first trimester, individuals with epilepsy, and those with severe psychiatric disorders should not receive mefloquine. Individuals receiving β-blockers, calcium-channel blockers, chloroquine, quinidine or quinine, or valproic acid should not receive mefloquine because of the risk for drug interactions. With mefloquine, gastrointestinal disturbances and dizziness are reported. Occasionally, hallucinations and seizures have been reported; however, these are more frequent with higher doses than those used for malaria prophylaxis. An alternative to mefloquine is doxycycline in the previously described doses.

Travelers to areas endemic for *Plasmodium vivax* or *Plasmodium ovale* should be aware of the risk for relapse after infection with these organisms. To prevent relapse in individuals who have prolonged exposure to malaria, 15 mg primaquine (base) is taken daily for 14 days or 45 mg primaquine (base) once a week for 8 weeks beginning the last 2 weeks of chloroquine prophylaxis after the traveler has left the malarious area. The pediatric dose of primaquine (base) is 0.3 mg/kg/day up to 15 mg. The CDC may be consulted for the appropriateness of therapy and an acceptable method to deliver primaquine in small doses. Primaquine is contraindicated in pregnancy and may cause hemolysis in individuals with G6PD deficiency.

Passive Immunity

Passive immunity results from parenteral administration of immune globulin or antitoxin that contains antibodies to disease. Certain precautions should be undertaken when administering these products. Individuals with an IgA deficiency may have anti-IgA antibodies, resulting in a risk of serious adverse effects when products with IgA are infused.

Immune globulin may interfere with the desired antibody response, therefore, in most cases immune globulin should not be given for 2 weeks after immunization. Because of potential inactivation of the vaccine by immune globulin, immunization with a live virus vaccine should, in general, be delayed for at least 3 months after immune globulin administration. When concomitant administration of immune globulin and a live virus vaccine occurs, the immunization should be repeated in 3 months unless seroconversion is documented. Immune globulin does not interfere with the antibody response to the OPV or yellow fever live virus vaccines. In the case of perinatal hepatitis B exposure or rabies, the vaccine and immunoglobulin should be administered at the same time but at different sites.

IMMUNE GLOBULIN

Immune globulin is used to provide exogenous antibodies to individuals who are immunodeficient, have certain autoimmune or infectious diseases, or who are exposed to infectious diseases. Specific products are available for i.m. and i.v. use. Immune globulin provides passive immunity from disease and this immunity will wane with time.

Immune globulin for i.v. (IVIG) or i.m. (IGIM) use is prepared from over 1000 donors to ensure a broad spectrum of antibody content. Because of concern over potential transmission of viral diseases such as hepatitis and HIV, all donor units are tested prior to fractionation. Additionally, newer fractionation techniques are effective in removing or inactivating HIV in donor units spiked with the virus. The risk for transmission of HIV via immune globulin remains theoretical, and no cases of infection have been directly attributed to infusion of immune globulin. Several cases of hepatitis C were associated with the IVIG products manufactured by Baxter Healthcare Corporation, Gammagard and Polygam. These products were withdrawn from the market and the extraction process modified to include a solvent detergent treatment designed to inactivate viruses. The brand name has been changed to Gammagard S/D and Polygam S/D to indicate the change in manufacturing technique (76). Immune globulin is produced by a variety of manufacturers and varies in immune globulin concentrations, manufacturing techniques, additives, product form, and FDA-approved indications. IVIG is a purified immune globulin product, and because it can be infused intravenously, it allows administration of a larger dose of immune globulin than can be achieved with IGIM.

The protein content of IGIM is about 165 mg/mL, with a stabilizer, glycine, and a preservative, thimerosal, included. IGIM is used to provide passive immunity to individuals within 2 weeks of exposure to certain diseases. This may include hepatitis A, non-A non-B hepatitis, measles, and rubella. A dose of 0.02 mL/kg given prior to or within 2 weeks of exposure to hepatitis A is 80 to 90% successful in preventing infection (3). Within 6 days of measles exposure, an IGIM dose of 0.25 mL/kg in healthy individuals, or 0.5 mL/kg in immunosuppressed or immunodeficient individuals up to a total dose of 15 mL, can be given to decrease morbidity or prevent the disease. Measles vaccination should be deferred 5 months in those who receive 0.25 mL/kg and 6 months in those receiving 0.5 mL/kg (23). Because of the relatively large volume required, the dose may need to be divided and administered at different sites. Adverse effects associated with IGIM are primarily pain at the injection site, and less commonly, flushing, headache, chills, and nausea (3). IGIM should not be infused intravenously because of the risk for serious side effects.

Primary immunodeficiency resulting from an immune globulin deficiency or from impaired function is the major indication for IVIG. In patients with IgG subclass deficiency, IVIG is reserved for those who have recurrent infections. Treatment of idiopathic thrombocytopenic purpura and infection prophylaxis in patients with chronic lymphocytic leukemia, in bone marrow transplant patients over 17 years of age, and in children with HIV are approved indications for IVIG.

IVIG infusion is efficacious in preventing or reducing the number of infectious episodes in patients with immunodeficiency. Serum IgG concentrations below 200 mg/dL (normal is 1500 mg/dL) are associated with an increased risk for sudden, overwhelming bacterial infection. Increasing serum concentrations to over 400 mg/dL is felt to be sufficient in most cases (77). Although the lowest effective dose is 150 mg/kg, an IVIG dose of 200 to 400 mg/kg per month is used in most patients (77).

In addition to approved uses, 2 g/kg IVIG as a single dose is the standard of care in Kawasaki disease, and when given within 7 days of onset, the incidence of coronary vasculitis and subsequent development of aortic aneurysm is significantly reduced (77). IVIG has also been used to improve immunity and decrease infection in patients with burns, multiple myeloma, cytomegalovirus, and neonatal sepsis (77). For sepsis prophylaxis in high-risk neonates, IVIG doses sufficient to attain an IgG serum concentration of 700 mg/dL have been used (77).

Up to 10% of patients who receive IVIG experience adverse reactions including nausea, vomiting, chills, fever, malaise, fatigue, dizziness, headache, urticaria, tightness in the chest, flushing, dyspnea, and pain in the chest, hip, or back. These effects are usually related to the rate of infusion and are managed by stopping the infusion until the symptoms subside and restarting the infusion at a lower rate. Pretreatment with acetaminophen, diphenhydramine, and/or glucocorticoids has been used to decrease side effects. Patients with IgA deficiency are at risk for the development of anaphylaxis due to anti-IgA antibody formation and should receive immune globulin products with as low a concentration of IgA as possible.

HYPERIMMUNE GLOBULINS

Passive immunity against specific diseases can be provided by immune globulin products with high concentrations of specific antibodies. These products are made from the serum of individuals with increased concentrations of the specific antibody. All plasma used to prepare hyperimmune globulin products is negative for HBsAg. Products contain glycine as a stabilizer and most contain thimerosal as a preservative. Currently available hyperimmune globulin products include cytomegalovirus (CMVIG) (3, 78, 79); hepatitis B (HBIG) (3, 43); tetanus (TIG) (3); rabies (RIG) (3, 45); Rhesus or Rh₀ (D) (RhIG) (81); and varicella zoster (VZIG) (3, 82). These products

Table 61.6.
Hyperimmune Globulins

Product[a]	Route[b]	Use	Comments
CMVIG	IV	renal, liver, & bone marrow transplant	Doses range from 100–150 mg/kg/week. Some controversy remains as to whether or not the benefits of CMVIG outweigh the increased cost over IVIG. (78–80).
HBIG	IM	postexposure to hepatitis B infection with concurrent administration of HBV vaccine	*Neonates* born to HBsAg positive mothers should receive 0.5 mL within 12 hours of birth as well as infants who have care givers with acute hepatitis B (3, 43). *Adults* should receive 0.06 ml/kg up to 5 mL within 24 hours of percutaneous exposure & within 14 days of sexual contact (3, 43).
RIG	IM	postexposure to rabies concurrently with HDCV or RVA	A dose of 20 IU/kg should be administered within 8 days of initiation of the vaccination schedule. Not to be used in individuals previously vaccinated (3, 45).
RhIG	IM	Rh-negative mother following delivery of a Rh-positive fetus	The standard dose of 300 µg will suppress 15 mL of Rh-positive packed RBC or 30 mL of whole blood. Ideally, given within 72 hours of delivery but it may be given up to 28 days following delivery. RhIG should be given regardless of the duration of pregnancy. RhIG is effective in preventing subsequent infant deaths from erythroblastosis fetalis (3, 81).
TIG	IM	postexposure in tetanus-prone wounds & active tetanus infection	The postexposure dose is 250–500 units and treatment dose ranges from 3000 to 6000. Td should be given if minor wound and > 10 years since Td, if major wound and > 5 years since Td, and in individuals who have not completed the immunization series (3).
VZIG	IM	postexposure to high-risk individuals	The dose is 125 units/10 kg (maximum dose of 625 units or 5 vials). VZIG is primarily used to decrease the morbidity and mortality in high risk individuals (< 15 years old who have not had varicella, who are immunocompromised, and are exposed to varicella) and infants born to mothers who develop varicella 5 days before or 2 days after delivery, and premature infants < 28 weeks gestation. Administer within 48 hours for maximum benefit and no later than 96 hours following exposure (3, 82).

[a]CMVIG, cytomegalovirus immune globulin; HBIG, hepatitis B immune globulin; RIG, rabies immune globulin; RhIG, Rh (rhesus) immune globulin or Rh$_o$(D); TIG, tetanus immune globulin; VZIG, varicella-zoster immune globulin.
[b]Route abbreviations: IM, intramuscular; IV, intravenous.

are listed in Table 61.6. Concurrent administration of active immunization with hyperimmune globulin has been previously discussed. CMVIG is administered i.v., and the adverse reactions related to this product are similar to those of IVIG. All of the other products are administered i.m., and their adverse effects consist most commonly of local pain and tenderness at the site of injection. Other adverse events such as fever, rash, and rarely anaphylactic shock may occur. Other hyperimmune globulin products are being studied and may find a place in therapy for a specific disease such as *Pseudomonas aeruginosa* immune globulin in cystic fibrosis.

ANTITOXIN

Antitoxins differ from hyperimmune globulins because they are derived from equine serum. Products derived from animal sera may result in severe allergic reactions including anaphylaxis, and therefore require special precautions prior to administration. First, a careful history of past allergic responses (especially to horses or other animals) should be elicited, since these individuals may be extremely sensitive to antitoxin. Prior to administration a scratch test or "eye test" should be performed to determine an individual's sensitivity. If these tests are negative, an intradermal test using a small amount of very dilute antitoxin is performed (3). Failure to elicit a positive response to the test dose does not eliminate the risk for a systemic reaction. Indications for the use of antitoxin are very limited, and these products should be used by an appropriately trained individual with the necessary precautions taken (emergency kit available). Antitoxins are available through the CDC for the treatment of diphtheria, tetanus, and botulism.

Usually antitoxin is given i.m.; however, in some cases, i.v. infusion may be indicated. The risk for a systemic reaction with i.v. infusion is increased; thus, doses should be dilute, infused very slowly, and the patient observed for adverse effects.

IMMUNOCOMPROMISED HOST

Immunocompromised patients may respond poorly to immunization. The response to live virus vaccines may result in enhanced or prolonged viral replication and potentially result in systemic disease. The immune response to inactivated vaccines, although less than in normal individuals, is usually adequate.

Generally, patients who are immunosuppressed due to disease (e.g., malignancy, immune deficiency syndromes) or who are receiving immunosuppressants (e.g., high-dose steroids, chemotherapy, irradiation) should not be given live virus vaccines (OPV, MMR, oral typhoid, BCG, and yellow fever) because of the risk for development of active disease. The exception is infants and children with HIV infection, who should receive influenza and measles vaccines. In addition, immunocompromised individuals are at risk for the development of polio should they come in contact with an individual immunized with OPV who is shedding live virus via stool. Infants and children who are close contacts of immunosuppressed individuals can be immunized against polio using eIPV.

Individuals with asymptomatic HIV infection may be safely immunized with inactivated vaccines. Both the AAP and ACIP recommend that children with HIV receive routine pediatric immunizations with the appropriate vaccines (DPT, eIPV, MMR, Hib) regardless of symptoms (57). While MMR is a live virus vaccine, no adverse effects were reported in 42 children with HIV who received MMR either during or following measles infection, and the current recommendation is that children with HIV receive MMR. In addition, the AAP and ACIP recommend immunizing children with symptomatic HIV infection against pneumococcal and influenza infections (3, 83).

Cancer patients may be immunosuppressed due to the malignancy, nutritional status, or anticancer therapy (e.g., irradiation, chemotherapy). Patients with active malignant disease should not be given live vaccines. While killed vaccines and toxoids may be given, the immune response to the immunization depends on the chemotherapeutic agent being used and may be inadequate to confer immunity. Whenever possible, vaccination should occur before radiation or chemotherapy. Patients over 2 years old with Hodgkin's lymphoma should be immunized with pneumococcal and Hib vaccines 10 to 14 days before therapy is started. Patients who have not received chemotherapy for 3 to 4 weeks may have an adequate antibody response to influenza vaccine. Live virus vaccines can be given to patients who are in remission from leukemia when 3 months have lapsed since the last chemotherapy was administered.

After immunosuppressive therapy has been discontinued, a quantitatively normal immunologic response usually develops 3 to 12 months later. Corticosteroids given as replacement therapy (e.g., Addison's disease); short courses of high-dose steroids (<2 weeks); topical steroid therapy; long-term alternate-day therapy with low-to-moderate doses of short-acting steroids; or single-dose intraarticular, bursal, or tendon injection are not usually immunosuppressive, and live virus vaccine administration is not contraindicated in these patients (3).

Functional (e.g., sickle cell disease) or anatomic asplenia results in an increased risk of infection from encapsulated microorganisms that appears to be greater in children. Pneumococcus is the most common encapsulated pathogen in splenectomized individuals. Immunization with the pneumococcal, meningococcal, and Hib vaccines are recommended for all asplenic individuals over 2 years old. Because the response to pneumococcal vaccine is poor, prophylactic penicillin is recommended for sickle cell patients under 5 years of age. It is not clear at what age penicillin prophylaxis can be stopped.

PREGNANCY AND LACTATION

In determining the need for active immunization during pregnancy or lactation, the potential benefits and risks must be considered (4, 82). In general, passive immunization with immune globulin is considered safe for pregnant women (3, 4). The consequences of natural infection and the likelihood of exposure must be balanced against the risk of immunization for the mother and child. In most cases, the decision to immunize must be made with limited or no data available regarding the risk for congenital anomalies or other adverse outcomes. Active immunizations that are needed should be administered during the third trimester whenever possible. The ACIP and AAP publish guidelines that assist in managing complex or unusual situations.

Active immunization with toxoids is relatively safe when performed in the third trimester. In fact, it is desirable to fully immunize previously unimmunized pregnant women against diphtheria and tetanus, preferably during the third trimester of pregnancy (3, 4). Furthermore, those who have not received a Td booster within the last 10 years should receive Td prior to delivery.

Inactivated viral and bacterial vaccines present less risk than live vaccines because these organisms will not replicate. Pregnant women in high-risk groups should be immunized for influenza at the appropriate time of year (53). The risks of pneumococcal immunization to the fetus are unknown; therefore, the risk of infection in a high-risk mother must be weighed against the potential harm to the fetus (4).

Immunization with the MMR live, attenuated virus vaccine is contraindicated in pregnancy. Because of the potential risk of fetal rubella infection, women who are of child-bearing age who are vaccinated with these agents should be counseled to avoid conception for 3 months following immunization. While immunization with MMR should be avoided immediately prior to and during pregnancy, recently published findings of women who inadvertently received the rubella vaccine within 3 months of conception reported no evidence that the vaccination was responsible for congenital rubella syndrome (3, 84).

If unimmunized and pregnant, a woman anticipating travel outside the United States and exposure to wild polio virus should be immunized with OPV or eIPV (3). If travel to an area with a high risk for contracting yellow fever cannot be postponed, the yellow fever vaccine should be given (4, 52). Malaria prophylaxis with chloroquine or hydroxychloroquine is not contraindicated in pregnancy. However, travel to areas with *P. falciparum* that is resistant to chloroquine or hydroxychloroquine should be avoided, since both mefloquine and doxycycline are contraindicated in pregnancy (74).

The postpartum period is thought to be a good time to review immunization status and update any necessary immunizations. While there may be transfer of antibody to the infant who is fed with human milk, lactation is not a contraindication to immunization with any agent (3). Breast feeding is not adversely affected by immunizations in the infant or mother. Most live vaccines are not transferred to breast milk. Rubella virus has been found in breast milk; however, it is well tolerated by the infant. Infants who are breast fed should be immunized according to the usual schedule.

PHARMACEUTICAL CONSIDERATIONS

Knowing specifics about individual vaccine preparation including manufacturing techniques and added excipients is essential to minimize adverse reactions to vaccines. The package insert provides information about manufacturing procedures and provides a list of all excipients for vaccines and immunobiologics.

Should an allergic reaction occur, it is generally related to (a) viral vaccines grown in embryonic egg culture, (b) antibiotics or preservatives, (c) stabilizers, or (d) antitoxin or antisera of animal origin (Table 61.2). Individuals who experience anaphylactic reactions to eggs or egg products may experience a similar reaction to a viral vaccine grown in egg culture. MMR and influenza vaccines are grown in egg culture; however, they are highly purified and can generally be safely given to patients with a nonanaphylactic-type egg allergy. Desensitization or a graded protocol can be used successfully for vaccines grown in egg cell cultures to immunize individuals with egg allergies (Table 61.4) (28). Trace amounts of antibiotics or preservatives (e.g., neomycin, thimerosal) added to immunobiologics may be responsible for hypersensitivity reactions. However, a causal relationship between the trace amounts of antibiotics in vaccines and adverse effects has not been established. Delayed minor reactions attributed to neomycin or streptomycin have been reported between 48 and 96 hours after immunization with MMR. Anyone with a history of anaphylactic reaction to neomycin or streptomycin should not receive vaccines that contain these antibiotics. No vaccine contains penicillin. Mercury may accumulate in individuals who receive repeated courses of IGIM. Those who are sensitive to mercury may experience a reaction; however, no specific causal relationship has been reported.

Antisera or antitoxins of animal origin are the most likely agents to cause allergic reactions. Horse serum is used to produce diphtheria, tetanus, and botulism antitoxins; equine antirabies serum; and antivenins. Biologics of equine origin are inherently immunogenic; thus, all patients should undergo a scratch test or eye test using a dilution of the product to be administered prior to treatment.

Safe handling and storage of vaccines and immunobiologics is essential to ensure vaccine potency and prevent vaccine failure (85). Pharmacists should be familiar with the usual appearance of immunobiologics to help validate that product integrity was maintained during transport and to assure that product degradation did not occur during storage. The shelf life should be validated and expiration dates noted, and the appropriate storage conditions should be maintained. Care must be taken to ensure timely reconstitution prior to immunization to maintain potency and prevent vaccine failure. The package insert should be consulted for specific information about the appropriate handling and storage of each vaccine.

FUTURE

A renewed commitment to preventive medicine has focused attention on development of safer and more efficacious immunizations, simplifying schedules, increasing supplies, and producing new immunizations for diseases that currently are not preventable (86). The goal of the Childhood Immunization Initiative is to have over 90% of 2-year-old children in the United States immunized by 1996 (2). Influenza and pneumococcal immunizations are covered by Medicare, which has increased the number of elderly individuals who are immunized (55). Cytomegalovirus, herpes simplex, and HIV vaccines are currently being investigated (87). Vaccines against a number of bacteria with polysaccharide cell walls, such as *P. aeruginosa, N. meningitidis* serotype A, *Escherichia coli* K1, and *S. pneumoniae,* are being investigated. Many of these require an alteration of the bacterial antigenic component and protein conjugation in order to stimulate the appropriate immunogenic response (63). Work continues in the development of avirulent polio vaccines to eliminate the small risk for polio infection that exists with the current OPV. While immunizations of today are usually composed of attenuated or inactivated microorganisms, immunizations of the future may be derived from a component of an organism that stimulates the immunologic response, be an "empty" viral particle, or be manufactured using recombinant DNA technology. In addition, different techniques of administration are being explored, including intranasal aerosols or nose drops and time-release capsules. The further development of safer, more effective vaccines will have a positive impact on decreasing infectious diseases provided immunizations are administered to the appropriate target population.

REFERENCES

1. Anonymous. Certification of poliomyelitis eradication—the Americas, 1994. MMWR 43(39):720–722, 1994.
2. Anonymous. Reported vaccine-preventable diseases—United States, 1993, and the childhood immunization initiative. MMWR 43(4):57–60, 1994.
3. American Academy of Pediatrics. Report of the Committee on Infectious Diseases. Red Book 23, 1994.
4. General recommendations on immunization. Recommendations of the Advisory Committee on Immunization Practices (ACIP). MMWR 43(RR-1):1–38, 1994.
5. Bernbaum J, Draft A, Samuelson J, et al. Half-dose immunization for diphtheria, tetanus, pertussis: response of preterm infants. Pediatrics 83:471–476, 1989.
6. Hall CB. The recommended childhood immunization schedule of the United States (Commentary). Pediatrics 94:135–137, 1995.
7. Cherry JD. Acellular pertussis vaccines—a solution to the pertussis problem. J Infect Dis 168:21–24, 1993.
8. Edwards KM. Acellular pertussis vaccines—a solution to the pertussis problem? J Infect Dis 168:15–20, 1993.
9. Pertussis vaccination: acellular pertussis vaccine for reinforcing booster and booster use. Supplementary ACIP statement. Recommendations of the Advisory Committee on Immunization Practices (ACIP). MMWR 41(RR-1):1–10, 1992.
10. Pertussis vaccination: acellular pertussis vaccine for the fourth and fifth doses of the DTP series. Update to supplementary ACIP statement. Recommendations of the Advisory Committee on Immunization Practices (ACIP). MMWR 41(RR-15):1–5, 1992.
11. Diphtheria, tetanus, and pertussis: recommendations for vaccine use and other preventive measures. Recommendations of the Advisory Committee on Immunization Practices (ACIP). MMWR 40(RR-10):1–28, 1991.
12. Cody CL, Baraff LJ, Cherry JD, et al. Nature and rates of adverse reactions associated with DTP and DT immunizations in infants and children. Pediatrics 68:650–660, 1981.
13. Ipp MM, Gold R, Greenberg S, et al. Acetaminophen prophylaxis of adverse reactions following vaccination of infants with diphtheriapertussis-tetanus toxoids-polio vaccine. Pediatr Infect Dis J 6:721–725, 1987.
14. Uhari M. A eutectic mixture of lidocaine and prilocaine for alleviating vaccination pain in infants. Pediatrics 88:719–721, 1993.
15. Bernstein HH, Rothstein EP, et al. Comparison of a three-component acellular pertussis vaccine with a whole-cell pertussis vaccine in 15-through 20-month-old infants. Pediatrics 93:656–659, 1994.
16. Blumberg DA, Lewis K, Mink CAM, et al. Severe reactions associated with diphtheria-tetanus-pertussis vaccine: detailed study of children with seizures, hypotonic-hyporesponsive episode, high fevers, and persistent crying. Pediatrics 91:1158–1165, 1993.
17. Halperin SA, Bortolussi R, MacLean D, et al. Persistence of pertussis in an immunized population: results of the Nova Scotia enhanced pertussis surveillance program. J Pediatr 115:686–693, 1989.
18. Bass JW, Stephenson SR. The return of pertussis. Pediatr Infect Dis J 6:141–144, 1987.
19. Cromer BA, Goydos J, Hackell J, et al. Unrecognized pertussis infection in adolescents. Am J Dis Child 147:575–577, 1993.
20. Aoyama T, Takeuchi Y, Goto A, et al. Pertussis in adults. Am J Dis Child 146:163–166, 1992.
21. Edwards KM, Decker MD, Graham BS, et al. Adult immunization with acellular pertussis vaccine. JAMA 269:53–56, 1993.
22. Adenyl-Jones SC, Faden H, Ferdon MB, et al. Systemic and local immune responses to enhanced-potency inactivated poliovirus vaccine in premature and term infants. J Pediatr 120:686–689, 1992.
23. Abraham R, Minor P, Dunn G, et al. Shedding of virulent poliovirus revertants during immunization with oral poliovirus vaccine after prior immunization with inactivated polio vaccine. J Infect Dis 168:1105–1109, 1993.
24. Measles, Mumps, Rubella package inserts from Merck & Co., Inc., 1994.
25. Anonymous. Rubella and congenital rubella syndrome-United States, January 1, 1992–May 7, 1994. MMWR 43(21):391–401, 1994.
26. Use of vaccines and immune globulins in persons with altered immunocompetence. Recommendations of the Advisory Committee on Immunization Practices. MMWR 42(RR-4):1–18, 1993.
27. American Academy of Pediatrics Committee on Infectious Diseases. Recommended timing of routine measles immunization for children who have recently received immune globulin preparations. Pediatrics 93:682–685, 1994.
28. Miller JR, Orgel HA, Meltzer EO. The safety of egg-containing vaccines for egg-allergic patients. J Allergy Clin Immunol 71:568–573, 1983.
29. Anonymous. Vaccine adverse event reporting system-United States. Curr Trends MMWR 41:730–733, 1990.
30. Bartell LA, Charney SA. National vaccine injury compensation act: a viable alternative to litigation? J Pharm Pract 2:36–44, 1989.
31. Clayton EW, Hickson GB. Compensation under the National Childhood Vaccine Injury Act. J Pediatr 116:508–513, 1990.
32. Greenberg DP, Vadheim CM, Partridge S, et al. Immunogenicity of *Haemophilus influenzae* type B tetanus toxoid conjugate vaccine in young infants. J Infect Dis 170:76–81, 1994.
33. Schoendorf KC, Adams WG, Kiley JL, et al. National trends in *Haemophilus influenzae* meningitis mortality and hospitalization among children, 1980 through 1991. Pediatrics 93:663–668, 1994.
34. Anonymous. Progress toward elimination of *Haemophilus influenzae* type B disease among infants and children-United States. 1987–1993. Current Trends MMWR 43:144–148, 1994.
35. Shenep JL, Feldman S, Gigliotti F, et al. Response of immunocompromised children with solid tumors to a conjugated vaccine for *Haemophilus influenza* type b. J Pediatr 125:581–584, 1994.
36. Washburn LK, O'Shea TM, Gillis DC, et al. Response to *Haemophilus influenzae* type B conjugate vaccine in chronically ill premature infants. J Pediatr 123:791–794, 1993.
37. Newcome W, Santosham M, Bengston S, et al. Immunogenicity of *Haemophilus influenzae* type B polysaccharide and *Neisseria meningitidis* outer membrane protein complex conjugate vaccine in infants

and children with sickle cell disease. Pediatr Infect Dis J 12:1026–1027, 1993.

38. Guinan EC, Molrine DC, Antin JH, et al. Polysaccharide conjugate vaccine responses in bone marrow transplant patients. Transplantation 57:677–684, 1994.

39. *Haemophilus* B conjugate vaccines for prevention of *Haemophilus influenza* type B disease among infants and children two months of age and older. Recommendations of the Immunization Practices Advisory Committee (ACIP). MMWR 40(RR-1):1–7, 1991.

40. Phelps SJ, Hogue SL, Saluk S, et al. Rifampin prophylaxis for *Hemophilus influenzae* infections. Hosp Pharm 25:861–864, 1990.

41. Shapiro ED, Wald ER. Efficacy of rifampin in eliminating pharyngeal carriage of *Haemophilus influenzae* type b. Pediatrics 66:5–8, 1980.

42. Committee on Extemporaneous Formulations. Handbook on extemporaneous formulations. Bethesda, MD: American Society of Hospital Pharmacists Special Projects Division(ASHP), 1987:43.

43. American Academy of Pediatrics Committee on Infectious Diseases. Universal hepatitis B immunization. Pediatrics 89:795–800, 1992.

44. Freed GL, Bordley WC, Clark SJ, et al. Universal hepatitis B immunization of infants: reactions of pediatricians and family physicians over time. Pediatrics 93:747–751, 1994.

45. Bloom BS, Hillman AL, Fendrick AM. A reappraisal of hepatitis B virus vaccination strategies using cost-effective analysis. Ann Intern Med 118:298–306, 1993.

46. Drawl-Klein LA, O'Donovan CA. Varicella in pediatric patients. Ann Pharmacother 27:938–49, 1993.

47. Lieu TA, Cochi SL, Black SB, et al. Cost-effectiveness of a routine varicella vaccination program for US children. JAMA 271:375–381, 1994.

48. Gershon AA, Steinberg SP, Gelb L, et al. Live attenuated varicella vaccine use in immunocompromised children and adults. Pediatrics 78(suppl):757–762, 1986.

49. Hadler SC. Global pattern of hepatitis A virus infection changing patterns. In: Hollinger FB, Lemon SM, Margolis H, eds. Viral hepatitis and liver disease. Baltimore: Williams & Wilkins, 1991:14–20.

50. Innis BL, Snitbhan R, Kunasol P, et al. Protection against hepatitis A by an inactivated vaccine. JAMA 271:1328–1334, 1994.

51. Werzberger A, Mensch B, Kuter B, et al. A controlled trial of a formalin-inactivated hepatitis A vaccine in healthy children. N Engl J Med 327:453–457, 1992.

52. Green MS. Cohen D, Lerman Y. Depression of the immune response to an inactivated hepatitis A vaccine administered concomitantly with immune globulin. J Infect Dis 168:740–743, 1993.

53. Prevention and control of influenza: part I, vaccines. Recommendations of the ACIP. MMWR 43(RR-9):1–13, 1994.

54. Aoki FY, Yassi A, Cheang M, et al. Effects of acetaminophen on adverse effects of influenza vaccination in health care workers. Can Med Assoc J 139:1425–1430, 1993.

55. Fieback N, Beckett W. Prevention of respiratory infections in adults. Arch Intern Med 154:2545–2557, 1994.

56. Nichol KL, Lofgren RP, Gapinski J. Influenza vaccination. Knowledge, attitudes and behavior among high-risk outpatients. Arch Intern Med 152:106–110, 1992.

57. Greenwood BM, Hassan-King M, Whittle HC. Prevention of secondary cases of meningococcal disease in household contacts by vaccination. Br Med J 1:1317–1319, 1978.

58. Peltola H, Safary A, Kayhty H, et al. Evaluation of two tetravalent (ACYW$_{135}$) meningococcal vaccines in infants and small children: a clinical study comparing immunogenicity of O-acetyl-negative and O-acetyl positive group C polysaccharides. Pediatrics 76:91–96, 1985.

59. Butler JC, Breiman RF, Campbell JF, et al. Pneumococcal polysaccharide vaccine efficacy. JAMA 270:1826–1831, 1993.

60. Immunizations Practices Advisory Committee (ACIP). Pneumococcal polysaccharide vaccine. MMWR 38:64–76, 1989.

61. Klein JO. The epidemiology of pneumococcal disease in infants and children. Rev Infect Dis 3:S246–S253, 1981.

62. Musher DM, Watson DA, Domingues EQ. Pneumococcal vaccination: work to date and future prospects. Am J Med Sci 300:45–52, 1990.

63. Dintzis RZ. Rational design of conjugate vaccines. Pediatr Res 32:376–385, 1992.

64. American Academy of Pediatrics. Committee on Infectious Diseases. Recommendations for using pneumococcal vaccine in children. Pediatrics 75:1153–1158, 1985.

65. Colditz GA, Brewer TF, Berkey CS, et al. Efficacy of BCG vaccine in the prevention of tuberculosis. JAMA 271:698–702, 1994.

66. Fishbein DB, Robinson LE. Rabies. N Engl J Med 329:1632–1638, 1993.

67. Human rabies-Miami. 1994. MMWR 43(42):773–775, 1994.

68. Centers for Disease Control. Rabies vaccine, adsorbed: a new rabies vaccine for use in humans. MMWR 37:217–223, 1988.

69. Immunizations Practices Advisory Committee (ACIP). Systemic allergic reactions following immunization with human diploid cell rabies vaccine. MMWR 33:185–187, 1984.

70. Hill DR, Pearson RD. Health advice for international travel. Ann Intern Med 108:839–852, 1988.

71. Wolfe MS. Vaccines for foreign travel. Pediatr Clin North Am 37:757–769, 1990.

72. Typhoid Immunization. Recommendations of the Advisory Committee on Immunization Practices (ACIP). MMWR 43(RR-14):1–7, 1994.

73. Immunizations Practices Advisory Committee (ACIP). Yellow fever MMWR 39(RR-6):1–6, 1990.

74. Immunizations Practices Advisory Committee (ACIP). Recommendations for the prevention of malaria among travelers. MMWR 39(RR-3):1–10, 1990.

75. Centers for Disease Control. Revised dosing regimen for malaria prophylaxis with mefloquine. MMWR 39(36):630, 1990.

76. Schneider L, Geha R, Magnuson WG. Outbreak of hepatitis C associated with intravenous immunoglobulin administration-United States, October 1993–June 1994. MMWR 43(28):505–509, 1994.

77. Phelps SJ, Reynolds MA, Tami JA, et al. ASHP therapeutic guidelines for intravenous immune globulin. ASHP Commission on Therapeutics. Clin Pharm 11:117–136, 1991.

78. Snydman DR, Werner BG, Tilney NL, et al. Final analysis of primary cytomegalovirus disease prevention in renal transplant recipients with a cytomegalovirus-immune globulin: comparison of the randomized and open-label trials. Transplant Proc 23:1357–1360, 1991.

79. Snydman DR, Werner BG, Dougherty NN, et al. A further analysis of the use of cytomegalovirus immune globulin in orthotopic liver transplant patients at risk for primary infection. Transplant Proc 26(suppl 1):23–7, 1994.

80. Glowacki LS, Smaill FM. Meta-analysis of immune globulin prophylaxis in transplant recipients for the prevention of symptomatic cytomegalovirus disease. Transplant Proc 25:1408–1410, 1993.

81. Duerbeck NB, Seeds JW. Rhesus immunization in pregnancy: a review. Obstet and Gynecol 48:801–810, 1993.

82. Immunizations Practices Advisory Committee (ACIP). Recommendations on varicella-zoster immune globulin for the prevention of chickenpox. MMWR 33:84–100, 1984.

83. Onorato IM, Markowitz LE, Oxtoby MJ. Childhood immunization, vaccine-preventable diseases, and infection with human immunodeficiency virus. Pediatr Infect Dis J 7:588–595, 1988.

84. Saballus MK, Lake KD, Wager GP. Immunizing the pregnant woman. Postgrad Med 81:103–113, 1987.

85. Casto DT, Brunell PA. Safe handling of vaccines. Pediatrics 87:108–112, 1991.

86. Ellis RW, Douglas RG. New vaccine technologies. JAMA 271:929–931, 1994.

87. Gershon AA. Vital vaccines of the future. Pediatr Clin North Am 37:689–707, 1990.

CHAPTER 62

UPPER RESPIRATORY TRACT INFECTIONS

WILLIAM L. GREENE

Upper respiratory infections are those afflicting the apparatus of the upper airways. Pharyngitis, laryngitis, sinusitis, and other syndromes affecting these structures are sometimes associated with one another and may progress from one type of infection to another. Indeed, at times it is difficult to distinguish the different upper respiratory infections from one another, since similar symptoms and signs occur. The upper respiratory tract consists of the nose, paranasal sinuses, trachea, pharynx, and larynx. Airflow through the nose is turbulent, only about 10 to 15% of the flow going directly to the lower airways. While the lower airways are easily described as open channels with many branches, the nasal vault is a chamber with structures that deflect airflow. Three turbinates inside each nostril force air to flow over, under, and around each structure, creating many currents. The turbinates significantly expand the nasal surface area, increasing the efficiency of the humidifying, warming, and filtering functions of these passages (1).

Adjacent to the nasal passages are the frontal, maxillary, and ethmoid sinuses (Figure 62.1). Each of these spaces communicates with the nasal cavity through small openings referred to as the sinus ostia. Posterior to the nasopharynx are the eustachian tubes, which communicate with the middle ears. While the sinus ostia remain open unless there is an abnormality, the eustachian tubes remain closed 99% of the time. In general, these passages open only during swallowing, enabling equilibration of the pressures of the middle ear with atmospheric pressure.

THE COMMON COLD

The term "common cold" actually refers to a syndrome that is caused by any one of a number of infectious viruses. These infections share common signs and symptoms and are clinically indistinguishable from one another. Generally, one is said to "have a cold" when one experiences some combination of rhinorrhea, congestion, sneezing, sore throat, and nonproductive cough. This syndrome is self-limiting but causes significant discomfort and contributes to lost productivity through absenteeism at work. Children are more commonly afflicted than are adults; among adults, those residing with young children are at highest risk.

Pathogenesis

Investigations into the cause of the cold have determined that more than 200 viruses from five different viral families are associated with this condition. The most common etiologic agent is the rhinovirudae; over 100 distinct serotypes have been described. The virus is highly stable in the environment, and this factor doubtless contributes to its epidemiology. Adenoviruses, coronaviruses, influenza viruses, parainfluenza viruses, respiratory syncytial virus, and enteroviruses also induce colds. In as many as one-third of studied cases, pathogens have not been identified. Reinfections with the same virus may occur; these tend to exhibit milder symptoms. With the influenza virus, topical inoculation is more likely to induce the cold syndrome, while inhalation tends to induce infection of the lower airways (2).

In temperate climates, each cold-producing virus fills a distinct seasonal niche. In general, incidence of infection increases in early fall, peaks in midwinter, and drops to low levels during the summer. The incidence of most other upper respiratory infections follows a similar pattern. The role for climate and temperature changes in this seasonality is not well understood.

Transmission of influenza and rhinoviruses may occur via aerosolization and inhalation, but the most important means of spread is direct contact with respiratory secretions of infected individuals (3). An incubation period of 1 to 4 days follows inoculation. Symptoms reach their peak in approximately 5 days, and complete recovery usually requires another 3 to 5 days. Viral shedding mirrors symptoms, peaking in 3 to 4 days and becoming undetectable in approximately 7 days.

Cold symptoms result from an immune response to the infection. Viral replication takes place in the ciliated epithelium of the nasal turbinates and nasopharynx. Interferon production and mobilization of cytotoxic cells such as T lymphocytes and natural killer cells limit the infection; these defensive mechanisms also result in some destruction of epithelial cells. The most significant and consistent result of this immune reaction is the production of hyperemia and edema of the submucosa. Swelling of the mucosa and exudation of seromucinous fluid result in narrowing of the airways and production of symptoms.

Clinical Findings, Complications, and Diagnosis

Although some colds are preceded by a prodrome of chilly sensations and vague discomfort, the first symptom of a cold is usually a dry, scratchy, sore throat. Rhinorrhea, sneezing, and nasal stuffiness follow soon thereafter. Loss

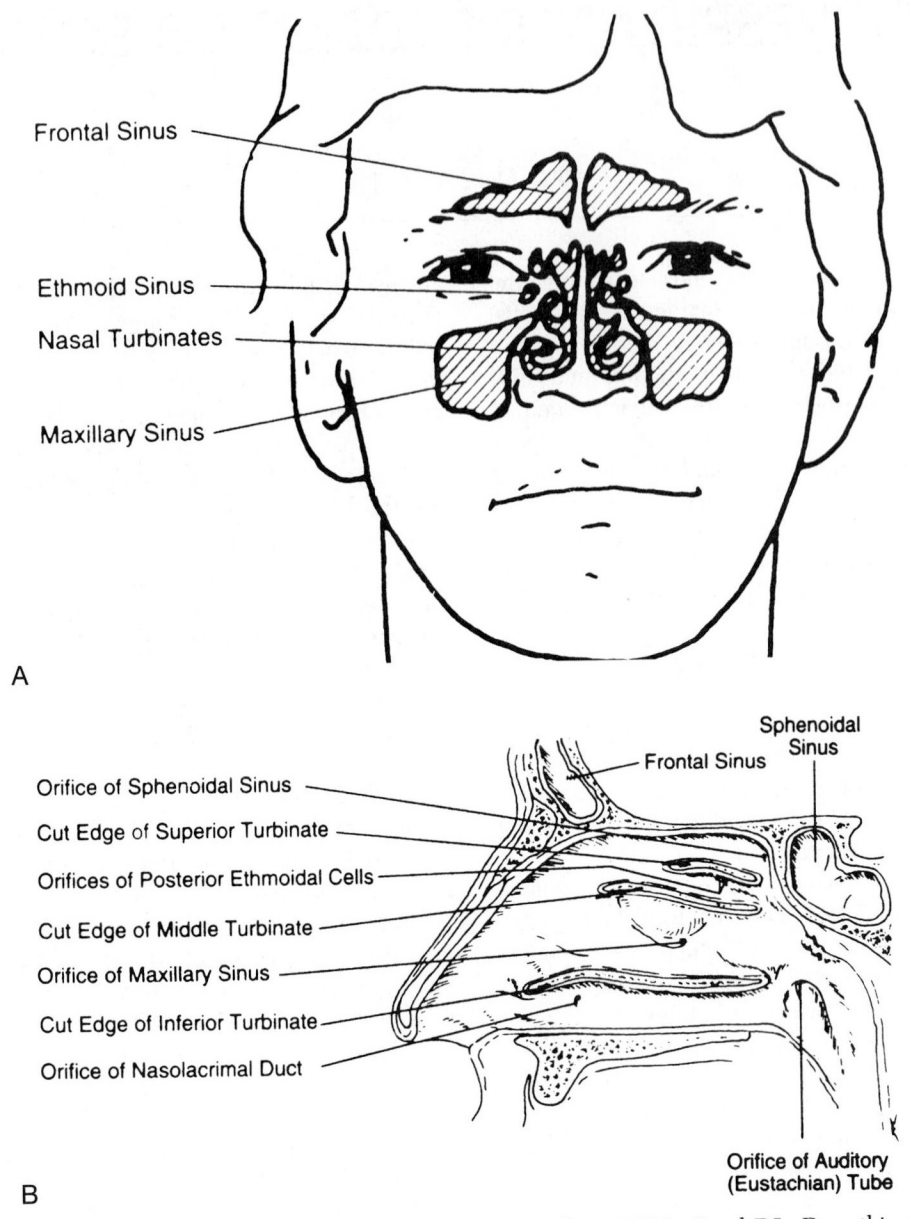

Figure 62.1. **A.** Coronal and **B.** sagittal views of the sinuses. From Williams JW Jr, Simel DL. Does this patient have sinusitis?: diagnosing acute sinusitis by history and physical examination. JAMA 270:1242, 1993, with permission.

or alteration of the sense of smell may occur, and a nasal voice quality may be imparted because of the nasal congestion. Other symptoms may include malaise, myalgias, subjective feeling of a fever, headache, hoarseness, and nonproductive cough. Temperature is rarely taken by the patient or parent. As was noted above, symptoms usually resolve after 5 to 7 days in adults; children may experience a slightly longer duration of illness.

The diagnosis of this infection is presumptive and is based on clinical presentation. No laboratory test is broadly available for determination of the cause of a cold, so knowledge of the seasonal relationship of the major virus groups forms the basis for assigning etiologic diagnosis.

The presence of group A streptococci should be ruled out by objective means, as it is the only uncomplicated upper respiratory illness that requires specific therapy. Hoarseness is a clinical finding that exhibits a negative correlation with group A streptococcal infection. Occasionally, the common cold may be confused with allergic rhinitis. Examination of a nasal smear for the presence of eosinophils will help to rule out the common cold.

Inflammation resulting from the cold may occasionally produce complications such as otitis media and acute sinusitis (4, 5) due initially to occlusion of ostia of the paranasal sinuses or dysfunction of the eustachian tube. These complications should especially be suspected in the child who develops fever 3 to 5 days after onset of a cold. The possibility of these complications emphasizes the need for performance of a complete examination of the pharynx, nasal cavity, ears, and sinuses. Other potential but less common complications of the cold include systemic bacterial infections, Guillain-Barré syndrome, and asthma attacks (6).

Treatment

A vast amount of research has focused on various prevention and treatment strategies for the common cold. No specific treatment for the common cold is currently available, and the vast array of pathogens that are involved in pathogenesis complicates efforts directed toward therapy. Thus, management of the common cold remains focused on symptoms. Goals of treatment include symptom relief, minimization of communicability, and prevention of complications. Antibiotics are not useful unless a secondary bacterial infection results. Measures such as bed rest, application of petroleum jelly to the nares, saline throat gargles, and saline nose drops often provide some degree of relief. Clearing of nasal passages by use of a bulb syringe may be helpful, especially in infants (7). Antihistamines and decongestants are often used to control symptoms; unfortunately, little scientific evidence supports the use of some of these agents. Many fixed-combination products that are available "over the counter" (OTC) contain subtherapeutic doses of one or more active ingredients. At the same time,

the effects of multiple agents may be unpredictable and even dangerous. The American Association of Poison Centers has reported that OTC cold medications are a frequent cause of unintentional ingestion in preschool children; approximately 20% of these children require treatment in a health care facility, and a few experience major morbidity (8). Significant toxicity can even arise from intended ingestions (7). Thus, reliance on supportive measures is preferred over the use of antihistamines or decongestants in young children. With few exceptions in any age group, if antihistamines or decongestants are needed, one or more single products should should be used at the appropriate dose. In an effort to communicate about the safety and efficacy of OTC remedies, the Food and Drug Administration (FDA) has developed a classification scheme (9). Category I agents are both safe and effective, category II drugs are neither safe nor effective, and Category III agents are those for which insufficient data is available to permit a final classification. Table 62.1 lists FDA Category I OTC drugs. Only in selected cases are fixed-combination products most appropriate. Table 62.2 lists drug classes that are commonly used for symptomatic relief of colds, with their common adverse effects and drug interactions.

Antihistamines

While antihistamines are frequently and effectively used for the treatment of allergic rhinitis (where histamine is

Table 62.1.
FDA Category I (Safe *and* Effective) Cough and Cold Agents

Class/Drug	Max. Dose: 2–5 yrs old	Max. Dose: 6–11 yrs old	Max. Dose: Adults
Antihistamines	No drug in this class is deemed safe and effective (Category I)		
Decongestants, topical			
Ephedrine 0.5%	None recommended	1–2 drops q4h	3 drops/sprays q4h
Naphazoline 0.05%	None recommended	Not recommended	2 drops/sprays q4h
Naphazoline 0.025%	None recommended	2 drops/sprays q6h	Same as 6–11 year old
Oxymetazoline 0.05%	Not recommended	3 drops/sprays morning & evening	Same as 6–11 year old
Oxymetazoline 0.025%	3 drops/sprays a.m. & p.m.	—	—
Phenylephrine 0.5% & 1%	Not recommended	Not recommended	2 drop/sprays q4h
Phenylephrine 0.2% & 0.25%	Not recommended	2 drops/sprays q4h	Same
Phenylephrine 0.125%	1 drop/spray q4h	—	—
Xylometazoline 0.1%	Not recommended	Not recommended	3 drops/sprays q8h
Xylometazoline 0.05%	3 drops/sprays q8h	Same as 2–5 year old	—
Decongestants, oral			
Phenylephrine	2.5 mg q4h	5 mg q4h	10 mg q4h
Phenylpropanolamine	6.25 mg q4h	12.5 mg q4h	25 mg q4h
Pseudoephedrine	15 mg q6h	30 mg q6h	60 mg q6h
Expectorants			
Guaifenesin	100 mg q4h	200 mg q4h	400 mg q4h
Antitussives			
Codeine	5 mg q4h	10 mg q4h	20 mg q4h
Dextromethorphan	5 mg q4h	10 mg q4h	20 mg q4h
Diphenhydramine	6.25 mg q4h	12.5 mg q4h	25 mg q4h
Camphor up to 11%	Apply externally to throat/chest		

Source: Taken from (9).

Table 62.2.
Adverse Effects and Drug Interactions of Drugs That Are Commonly Used to Treat the Common Cold

Drugs	Potential Adverse Effects	Potential Drug Interactions
Antihistamines	Sedation, drying of secretions, paradoxic stimulation, urinary retention, constipation, blurred vision, exacerbation of glaucoma, hypersensitivity	Alcohol & other sedating agents (additive sedation), itraconazole, ketoconazole, fluconazole, erythromycin (arrhythmias)
Sympathomimetics	Rhinitis medicamentosa, irritation, elevated blood pressure, cardiac stimulation, hyperglycemia, CNS stimulation, sleep disturbance, headache, urinary retention, exacerbation of glaucoma	MAOIs & selegeline (hypertensive crisis)
Analgesics	Vary by agent. Noteworthy: GI bleed & renal dysfunction (ASA & NSAIDs)	Antihypertensives (ablation of effect on blood pressure), alcohol (hepatotoxicity with acetaminophen), warfarin (increased bleeding risk, especially with ASA), lithium (lithium toxicity with ASA & NSAIDs), oral hypoglycemics (hypoglycemia with ASA), methotrexate (increased toxicity with ASA & NSAIDs)
Antitussives	Sedation, nausea, lightheadedness, constipation, pruritus, hypersensitivity, mucosal drying, exacerbation of glaucoma (diphenhydramine)	Alcohol, other sedatives (added sedation), MAOIs & selegeline (serotonin syndrome with dextromethorphan), quinidine (nausea, vomiting, nervousness, tremor, convulsions with quinidine)
Expectorants	Nausea, vomiting	None noted with guaiafenesin

involved in disease pathology), the role of antihistamines for management of cold-associated symptoms is questionable. Any beneficial effect of these drugs may depend on anticholinergic or sedative side effects. Anticholinergic effects may decrease nasal and pharyngeal secretions, while sedation may alter the patient's perception of cold symptoms. Modest effects of selected antihistamines have been documented in various clinical trials, but methodological problems are common in this literature (10). Most studies do not show positive effects; the few studies that demonstrate some difference reveal meager benefits of the drugs. Although the FDA has previously classified several of the antihistamines as effective OTC agents, placebo-controlled studies have clearly demonstrated that agents such as brompheniramine (11), chlorpheniramine (12), and terfenadine (13) contribute little to the relief of cold symptoms. When one considers this consistent lack of benefit of antihistamines for treatment of colds in combination with the significant risk of these products, it is difficult to recommend their use. In testimony before the U.S. House of Representatives in 1992, Hendeles argued that "antihistamines . . . provide no measurable relief for patients suffering from the common cold" (14). The final monograph for cough and cold products in the *Federal Register* does not contain a section on antihistamines.

Decongestants

Decongestants used singly or in combination products are among the most common drugs used in the treatment of cold symptoms. α-Adrenergic agonists may be administered topically or orally; they either directly or indirectly interact with the sympathetic nervous system to produce constriction of the microvasculature of the engorged nasal mucosa. Decreased blood flow and venous capacitance results, leading to diminished vascular leakage, improved sinus drainage, and clearing of the airways. The documented benefits of these agents have included decreased nasal resistance, decreased nasal mucus weights, and reduction of sneezing and congestion (15).

Topical administration of the decongestants (Table 62.1) leads to rapid, effective relief of the nasal congestion associated with a cold. However, their utility is limited by the potential for development of tolerance and rebound nasal congestion (rhinitis medicamentosa). Rhinitis medicamentosa is a severe reengorgement of the nasal mucosa that occurs on withdrawal of drug and that may be associated with local ischemia and membrane irritation. This effect is usually noted after the patient has used the drug routinely for more than 3 to 4 days. Other adverse effects are occasionally noted with topical administration (Table 62.2). The patient who uses topical sympathomimetics should be counseled about the regimen, the need to limit use of the drug to a few days, and the need to limit frequency of use.

Method of administration is important to ensure optimal benefit from the topical decongestants. In general, sprays are preferred over drops for all but small children because of better coverage of the nasal mucosa. The spray should be inhaled while the patient is upright. A few minutes after inhalation of one spray in the affected nostril, the nose should be blown to decrease mucus blockage; an additional spray can be administered if needed. Younger children (e.g., <6 years) should receive drops because of their smaller nares. The head should be tilted back during administration of drops and for a few minutes thereafter.

The oral decongestants include phenylpropanolamine (PPA), pseudoephedrine (PSE), and phenylephrine (PE). These drugs exhibit pharmacologic effects that are similar to those of the topical agents but in general have a slower onset, lower intensity, and (in some cases) longer duration of action. Because of the lower intensity of vasoconstriction, the potential for rebound congestion is much lower; no cases have been associated with use of the oral drugs. Sustained-release products delay the time to achieve peak concentrations and effectively prolong the duration of action of pseudoephedrine.

These drugs exert their stimulatory effects on other areas of the body where sympathetic stimulation is involved, and adverse effects are usually a consequence of this effect (Table 62.2). Generally, systemic vasoconstriction is insufficient to cause elevated blood pressure, but this effect is noted in predisposed individuals. Stimulation of the cardiovascular system or central nervous system is the most common presentation of adverse effects. Pseudoephedrine exhibits the lowest potential for cardiovascular or central nervous system stimulation. All these drugs should be used with caution by patients who have hypertension, hyperthyroidism, diabetes mellitus, ischemic heart disease, narrow-angle glaucoma, benign prostatic hypertrophy, and urinary retention; they are contraindicated for patients receiving monoamine oxidase inhibitors or selegiline.

Analgesics

Analgesics have long been used in the treatment of the common cold. Aspirin, acetaminophen, and the nonsteroidal antiinflammatory agents exhibit equivalent analgesic effects when given in equipotent doses. Various investigations have examined the possibility that these drugs may alter the course of symptoms or viral shedding associated with these infections. Examination of the effect of aspirin has yielded conflicting results (16, 17), while treatment with ibuprofen has been demonstrated to decrease the number of days of viral shedding (18). A recent study of naproxen did not demonstrate a similar effect on viral shedding, even though symptom scores improved (19). For children, acetaminophen 10 mg/kg every 4 hours is the preferred analgesic and antipyretic, since aspirin administration is associated with development of Reye's syndrome. Adults who are chronic alcoholics should not use more than perhaps one dose per day of acetaminophen because of increased risk of heptotoxicity (see Chapters 27 and 28). All of these agents will decrease symptoms of malaise, fever, and myalgias.

Although caffeine is a common ingredient in combination cough-and-cold preparations, it is doubtful that it contributes significantly to patient comfort. Caffeine does augment pain relief when combined with analgesics, but it also carries a significant risk of multiple side effects. The risk of disturbances such as alteration of sleep pattern, altered mood, increased blood pressure, increased gastric acid secretion, and provocation of cardiac arrhythmias militates against its routine use.

Antitussives and Expectorants

Coughing associated with a cold is generally nonproductive and may interfere with sleep. Such coughs are easily suppressed by various available antitussive agents, including codeine, hydrocodone, noscapine, dextromethorphan, diphenhydramine, and benzonatate. With the exception of benzonatate, these drugs act by depressing the medullary cough reflex. Benzonatate exerts a local anesthetic action in the airways. Dextromethorphan is the safest of these agents; the narcotics and diphenhydramine have the added benefit of causing sedation, which may aid sleep. If the cough becomes productive, therapy should aim for minimization of excessive coughing while maintaining the ability to eliminate secretions. The risks of therapy with these drugs are generally addressed in Table 62.2.

Topical anesthetics are available in a number of different preparations, including gargles, sprays, and lozenges. These agents act to anesthetize oropharyngeal tissue to decrease pain and irritation. Although these drugs are weak cough suppressants, they often prove to be soothing. Excessive use may inhibit the gag reflex, thereby increasing the risk of aspiration.

Expectorants including guaifenesin, terpin hydrate, syrup of ipecac, ammonium chloride, potassium guaiacol sulfonate, and potassium iodide have for many years been promoted for treatment of colds. These agents are purported to decrease sputum viscosity, thereby facilitating expectoration. It has also been suggested that they exert an antitussive effect. Even though these drugs are widely used, no clear evidence exists to demonstrate a beneficial effect of their use for treatment of colds (14). Nevertheless, guaifenesin has been rated by the FDA as a Category I agent.

Anticholinergic Agents

The role of the parasympathetic nervous system in the generation of nasal symptoms associated with a cold is not clear. Nevertheless, studies of systemic and topical administration of anticholinergic agents have been conducted. Orally administered atropine exerts no beneficial effect on cold symptoms or nasal secretions (20). In contrast, topical ipratropium has been found to reduce secretions, probably via competition at muscarinic receptors that control rhinorrhea. In one study, intranasal application of 84 μg per nostril 4 times daily for 4 days resulted in a statistically significant 28% mean reduction of nasal discharge (21). An earlier study using thrice-daily administration for 5 days demonstrated an average 40% reduction of mucus weights (22). Side effects were minor and included dry mouth, dry nasal passages, and nosebleed. This therapy appears promising but requires further validation and quantification of *clinical* significance. An FDA advisory panel has recommended approval of 6% ipratropium nasal spray for this indication.

Interferon and Zinc

The interferons have elicited much excitement as potential agents for treatment of the common cold. α- and β-interferons are produced by virus-infected cells and protect the cells with which they come into contact by inducing a state of infection resistance. Intranasal delivery of exogenous interferon is known to protect humans from experimental and naturally occurring colds (23). Unfortunately, studies in families have revealed consistent effects only against the rhinoviruses, and the prolonged administration of effective doses has proven to cause multiple nasal symptoms such as stuffiness and nosebleed. Thus, the treatment has proved to cause some of the same symptoms that it was intended to cure. The possibility of beneficial effects with improved tolerance of other interferons has yet to be demonstrated.

Studies in the mid-1970s demonstrated that zinc chloride inhibited the in vitro replication of rhinovirus by preventing the formation of viral capsid proteins. As a result of this finding, various clinical trials have been conducted using multiple different forms of zinc lozenges. At least seven placebo-controlled double-blind trials have been conducted, many yielding positive results. Unfortunately, a high incidence of adverse effects and patient intolerance, coupled with problems in methodology such as inadequate blinding, cast the clinical implications of these trials into doubt. In short, zinc seems to exert a positive effect on the common cold, but problems with study design and poor tolerance of treatment limit the ability to conclude that this therapy is beneficial for patient management (24).

Vitamin C

In 1970 and 1971, Linus Pauling published multiple works in which he made the case for the utility of vitamin C for treatment or prevention of the cold. Since that time, controversy has existed as to the utility of this approach to treatment or prevention. A recent review of the published literature on this topic demonstrated that all placebo-controlled studies conducted since 1971 have found a reduction in the duration of symptoms associated with the cold (25). The mean reduction in these studies is 23%; some suggestion of a dose-related effect is observed. The mechanism of the beneficial effects of vitamin C is unknown but may be related to its antioxidant properties. It is postulated that neutrophils responding to the infection release large amounts of oxidizing compounds into the local environment. Large amounts of vitamin C may protect against the harmful effects of these compounds.

The apparent beneficial effects of vitamin C must be balanced against possible risks. No long-term study has demonstrated the safety of high-dose vitamin C. Adverse effects of regularly ingested high doses of ascorbic acid may include diarrhea, oxalate or urate renal stones, mobilization of calcium from bones, hyperglycemia, and possible drug interactions, including inhibition of the effect of warfarin (26). Finally, the clinical significance of the observed benefits is difficult to determine. Thus, the real role of regular ingestion of large doses of vitamin C for treatment of the cold has not yet been resolved.

Other Approaches

The potential for enhancement of host immunity has been noted since the first successful culture of rhinoviruses. Early vaccines that were directed against specific viral serotypes have produced resistance to infection with the same virus, but the large number of existing serotypes renders development of a broadly effective vaccine seemingly impossible. Yet, as the structure of the different viruses becomes better appreciated, the potential for success in this direction increases significantly. It has already been suggested that it may be possible to develop a vaccine that would facilitate the generation of antibodies against conserved sequences of the viruses (27). In addition to these vaccines, research has examined the possibility of blocking viral attachment or replication. Studies with inhibitors of viral attachment such as monoclonal antibodies to cell receptors, competitors for the receptor, and capsid-binding agents (e.g., dichloroflavin or disoxaril) have yielded disappointing results, but work is ongoing. McKinlay and colleagues (28) have summarized much of the work examining these approaches.

An innovative approach directed at treatment of the cold has been to use inhalation of heated humidified air to increase the temperature of the nasal passages to a level at which viral replication will cease. Early results with this approach were very encouraging; dramatic benefits were sometimes noted (29). Unfortunately, a number of inconsistencies were noted in these studies, and subjects who were given the 43°C treatment often complained of local discomfort. More recent trials have failed to verify the effectiveness of this approach. Current opinion on this therapy is that any noted positive effect is either too dependent on the specifics of treatment method or too small to be reproducible and practical (30).

PHARYNGITIS

Inflammation of posterior oral cavity tissue is known as pharyngitis or pharyngotonsillitis. This disorder is a common malady, affecting humans in a seasonal pattern similar to that seen with the common cold. In temperate climates the peak prevalence of sore throat is generally during the colder months of the year.

Table 62.3.
Implicated Pathogens for Acute Pharyngitis and Tonsillitis

Viral Agents	Bacterial Agents	Other Pathogens
Rhinoviruses	Group A streptococci	*Mycoplasma pneumoniae*
Coronaviruses	Group B streptococci	*Chlamydia pneumoniae*
Adenoviruses	Group C streptococci	*Treponema pallidum*
Influenza A	Corynebacteria	
Influenza B	*Arcanobacterium haemolyticum*	
Parainfluenza viruses	*Yersinia enterocolitica*	
Herpes simplex virus	*Neisseria gonorrhoeae*	
Epstein-Barr virus	*Staphylococcus aureus*	
Human immunodeficiency virus	*Haemophilus influenzae*	
	Bacteroides fragilis	

Microbiology of Pharyngitis

A number of different pathogens have been implicated in the causation of sore throat. Table 62.3 lists potential bacterial and viral causes. The most common viral causes of this disorder are rhinovirus (perhaps 20%), coronavirus, adenovirus, influenza A and B, and parainfluenza virus. Human immunodeficiency virus infection may present with sore throat as an early manifestation. Group A β-hemolytic streptococci (GAS) are causative agents in 15 to 30% of all of these cases. The identification of this organism is important because of the sequelae that are often associated with untreated infections, including acute rheumatic fever, glomerulonephritis, and pyogenic abscesses. Other bacteria are less commonly identified. In cases of recurrent infection, the β-lactamase-producing *Staphylococcus aureus*, *Haemophilus influenza*, and *Bacteroides fragilis* should be considered as possible pathogens. *Neisseria gonorrhoeae* should be suspected in patients who practice oral sex. *Mycoplasma pneumoniae*, *Chlamydia pneumoniae*, and *Treponema pallidum* are infrequent causes of sore throat.

Pathogenesis and Complications

The pathogenesis of pharyngitis involves direct invasion of the pharyngeal mucosa by the various pathogens. Direct person-to-person spread of the pathogen is the predominant means of transmission. Hyperemia, edema, inflammatory exudate, hemorrhage of the pharyngeal walls and tonsils, and formation of a fibrinous membrane composed of leukocytes, necrotic cells, and bacteria may develop, depending on the pathogen. Mucosal cell changes that favor increased adherence may play a significant role in bacterial infections (31). These cell changes may result from viral infection.

The possible role of altered immunity in the pathogenesis of these infections has been examined in multiple trials. Increasing evidence implicates transient immaturity or minor defects of the immune system as contributory to recurrent or chronic infections of the nasopharynx. Secretion of lower amounts of IgA and IgG2 due to immune

Table 62.4.
Potential Implication of Clinical Findings Associated with Pharyngitis

Clinical Finding	Potential Implication
Mild sore throat	Rhinovirus, *Mycoplasma pneumoniae*
Severe sore throat	Adenovirus, influenza, herpes simplex, coxsackie A, streptococci
High fever (>39.4°C)	Streptococci
Conjunctivitis	Adenovirus
Cough, coryza, mild erythema	Influenza
Vesicles & ulcers of the anterior & posterior labial mucosa, with gingival stomatitis	Herpes simplex (acute)
Small vesicles in the posterior pharynx	Herpangina (coxsackie A virus)
Associated fatigue, malaise, headache, adenopathy	Mononucleosis
Associated truncal maculopapular rash, myalgia, and lethargy	HIV (primary infection)

system immaturity may predispose younger children to various bacterial infections (32). A reduced capacity to generate B cells may also play a significant role (33), particularly in recurrent tonsillitis.

Nearly all of the various causes of pharyngitis are self-limiting, with the exception of streptococcal infection. This infection may lead to development of acute rheumatic fever, glomerulonephritis, or suppurative complications such as otitis media, sinusitis, peritonsillar abscess, bacteremia, and postanginal sepsis (septic jugular thrombophlebitis). Treatment decreases the incidence of rheumatic fever and suppurative complications but not of glomerulonephritis.

Clinical Findings and Diagnosis

Pharyngitis presents with a wide range of symptoms; variable clinical findings may be helpful in differentiating among the causative agents with a modest level of confidence, as noted in Table 62.4. In addition to the severe sore throat and high fever noted in the table, streptococcal infections usually present with abrupt onset, headache, malaise, dysphagia, gray-white tonsillar exudate, and tender submandibular lymph nodes. Unfortunately for diagnostic purposes, a remarkably milder presentation may also be seen.

The definitive diagnosis of sore throat is often difficult, but the goal is to differentiate between benign viral infection and group A β-hemolytic streptococcal infection or rarer viral or bacterial causes (e.g., herpetic or bacteria other than GAS). History of exposure to others who are similarly infected is helpful, as is knowledge of the seasonality of the various pathogens. Streptococcal infection is most common during the winter and spring months and occurs most frequently in children 3 to 18 years of age. Because its presentation is variable, the diagnosis must be confirmed. The most accurate method of diagnosis is to perform culture of carefully obtained material on blood agar culture medium. Unfortunately, it is often difficult to obtain a useful specimen from an uncooperative child, and 2 days are required to determine the results of the test. The recent availability of rapid office-based tests for streptococcal antigen has helped to improve the accuracy and rapidity of diagnosis (34). These tests exhibit a relatively low degree of sensitivity, and therefore it has been recommended that negative test results be confirmed with culture (35). A recent examination of the cost-effectiveness of various approaches to this question has indicated that this is indeed the most efficient method for diagnosis (36). In this setting, it must be remembered that up to 50% of children with positive cultures for Streptococcus pyogenes may simply be carriers and not be actually infected.

Treatment

Therapy for pharyngitis is predicated on the determined or presumed etiology. Viral sore throat is generally managed symptomatically by using warm saline gargles (1 teaspoon salt per 8 ounces warm water), rest, and analgesics as necessary. If the sore throat is due to influenza A, then amantadine or rimantadine may be used effectively for therapy. If the sore throat is due to herpetic infection in the immunocompromised patient, acyclovir should be used. Aspirin is best avoided because of its potential causative role in the genesis of Reye's syndrome. Acetaminophen and ibuprofen are useful at increasing the rate of resolution of sore throat; some data suggests a greater rate of resolution when ibuprofen is used than with acetaminophen (37). The clinical significance of this is unknown. Topical agents such as the demulcents and anesthetics/antiseptics may play a role. The usefulness of nonprescription anesthetics such as benzocaine (5 to 20%), phenol or phenol-containing salts, and benzyl alcohol is controversial. These as well as hard candy may be soothing; sugarless candy is preferred to avoid cariogenesis.

Specific therapy for pharyngitis is most commonly considered when GAS is implicated. Currently accepted regimens for treatment of this infection are listed in Table 62.5. Delaying initiation of therapy pending results of culture will not diminish the beneficial effects of therapy on complications but may slow resolution of symptoms. Penicillin remains the drug of choice for *S. pyogenes* (38, 39), and various regimens are apparently equally effective. Intramuscular administration of a single injection of benzathine or benzathine plus procaine penicillin is as effective as a 10-day oral regimen of penicillin (40) but is painful. Compliance may be a factor in consideration of treatment approach. Recent data suggests that a twice-daily regimen of penicillin V is as effective as the standard 3 or 4 times daily regimen (41, 42). At least one study has also indicated that amoxicillin can be effective if given once daily (43). For patients who are allergic to penicillin, erythromycin is usually the preferred alternative. Sulfonamides, trimethoprim, tetracyclines, and chloramphenicol are not acceptable in this setting because of high rates of streptococcal resistance to these antibiotics (38). A 10-day course of oral penicillin increases the probability of eradication of this organism (44).

For cases of recurrent infection, failure to respond to penicillin, or management of the chronic carrier of GAS, no clear consensus now exists as to the optimal approach to therapy. Treatment failures and patients with relapses may be most effectively treated with a β-lactamase-resistant antibiotic such as amoxicillin/clavulanate or cephalosporin (45). Concurrent administration of rifampin during the final 4 days of a 10-day course of penicillin may also improve response in these settings (46). Eradication of the "carrier state" should particularly be considered whenever there is apparent recurrent transmission within families, in families with a history of rheumatic fever, during outbreaks of GAS in closed or semiclosed communities, or when tonsillectomy is being considered to eradicate carriage. In this setting, the combined penicillin/rifampin regimen is effective, and clindamycin appears to offer promise (47).

SINUSITIS

Sinusitis is inflammation of the mucosal lining of one or more of the paranasal sinuses, including the ethmoid, maxillary, sphenoid, and frontal sinuses (Figure 62.1). Although "inflammation" is the simple definition of the disease, sinusitis has come to refer to infectious inflammation of these structures. The epidemiology of this disorder is currently unclear, but it is estimated that approximately 0.5% of upper respiratory tract infections in children are complicated by sinusitis (48) and that 0.02% of the adult population may have chronic sinusitis (49). Slavin (50) has stated that sinusitis is present in "some 31 million Americans." This infection may be classified as acute, subacute, or chronic. Acute sinusitis exhibits nasal conges-

Table 62.5.
Antimicrobials Regimens for Treatment of Pharyngitis and Sinusitis[a]

Agent	Dose: Pharyngitis[b]	Dose: Sinusitis[b]	Comments
Benzathine Pcn G	<27.3 kg = 600,000 u i.m. ≥27.3 kg = 1.2 MU i.m.	Not recommended	Single dose Single dose
Penicillin VK	250 mg p.o. t.i.d.	Not recommended	
Erythromycin estolate	20–40 mg/kg/day p.o., 2–4× daily	Not recommended	Max. 1 g/day
EES[c]	40 mg/kg/day p.o. 2–4× daily	Not recommended	Max. 1 g/day
Amoxicillin	40 mg/kg/day (P) or 250 mg (A) 2–3× daily	40 mg/kg/day (P) or 500 mg (A) p.o. 2–3× daily	
Cephalexin	25–50 mg/kg/day (P) or 1 g (A) in 2 doses	Not recommended	
Cefadroxil	30 mg/kg/day (P) or 1 gm/day (A) in 1–2 doses	Not recommended	
Clindamycin	8–16 mg/kg/day (P) or 600 mg/day (A) in 3 doses	Not recommended	
Clarithromycin	7.5 mg/kg (P) or 250 mg (A) p.o. q12h	7.5 mg/kg (P) or 500 mg (A) p.o. q12h	
Dicloxacillin	12.5 mg/kg/day (P) or 500 mg/day (A) in 4 doses	Not recommended	
Cotrimoxazole	Not recommended	8/40 mg/kg/day (P) or 1 DS tab b.i.d.	Less activity against group A strep- tococci
Erythromycin/ sulfisoxazole	Not recommended (see erythromy- cin)	50/150 mg/kg/day t.i.d.	
Cefaclor	40 mg/kg/day (P) or 250 mg (A) t.i.d.	40 mg/kg/day (P) or 500 mg (A) t.i.d.	
Cefuroxime axetil	10 mg/kg (P) or 250 mg (A) b.i.d.	15 mg/kg (P) or 500 mg (A) b.i.d.	Tablets as small as 125 mg
Cefixime	8 mg/kg/day (P); 400 mg q.d. (A)	8 mg/kg q.d. (P); 400 mg q.d. (A)	Higher incidence of GI side effects; less effective against pneumococ- cus
Cefprozil	15 mg/kg/day (P) b.i.d. or 500 mg (A) q.d.	15 mg/kg/day (P) or 500 mg (A) b.i.d.	
Cefpodoxime proxetil	10 mg/kg/day (P) or 100 mg (A) b.i.d.	10 mg/kg/day (P) or 200 mg (A) b.i.d.	
Loracarbef	7.5 mg/kg/day (P) or 200 mg (A) b.i.d.	15 mg/kg/day (P) or 400 mg (A) b.i.d.	
Amoxicillin/clav. acid	40 mg/kg/day or 250 mg t.i.d.	40 mg/kg/day or 500 mg t.i.d.	Take with food; high rate of GI side effects

Source: Taken from FDA-approved literature and published trials.
[a]Drugs of choice for prevention of rheumatic fever include benzathine penicillin i.m. or penicillin VK p.o.; erythromycin is the preferred alternative in the penicillin-allergic patient. Duration of therapy is 10 days for pharyngitis, and 14 days for acute sinusitis.
[b](P) = dose for child; (A) = dose for adult.
[c]Erythromycin ethysuccinate.

tion, submucosal edema and epithelial cellular debris for up to 3 weeks; subacute sinusitis exhibits signs and symptoms of inflammation persisting between 3 weeks and 2 months, and chronic sinusitis persists for a period of greater than 2 months (51). The occurrence of sinusitis appears to parallel that of other acute upper respiratory infections, peaking in the fall, winter, and spring months. Sinusitis is more frequently noted in adults than in children.

Pathophysiology

The pathophysiology of sinusitis begins with compromise of the normal physiology of the sinuses. Most commonly, viral infection (the common cold) induces inflammation of the sinuses, which leads to excess secretions, compromise

in the normal action of mucociliary cells, and impaired drainage of the sinuses through the ostia (50). These alterations result in the production of an environment that is favorable for bacterial growth, and bacteria that have gained access through the ostia or by other means then proliferate. Alteration of breathing patterns (i.e., increased mouth breathing) also contributes to infection by decreasing the movement of air through the sinuses; decreased oxygen tension thereby results, further favoring growth of microbes. The reaction of inflammatory cells further contributes to this pathology by production of proteases and other enzymes that are destructive of sinus mucosa. Thus, a negative cycle is established.

In addition to upper respiratory infection such as the cold, a number of local and systemic factors predispose the patient to the development of sinusitis. These include allergic rhinitis, overuse of topical decongestants, hypertrophied adenoids, deviated nasal septum or other structural abnormalities, nasal polyps, tumors, swimming and diving, cigarette smoking, dental infection or extraction/injections, local trauma induced by nasotracheal intubation, immune deficiency, bronchiectasis, and dysfunctional cilia. Allergic and infectious rhinitis are the most commonly implicated determinants of this disorder.

Microbiology

A number of studies have closely examined the microbiology of acute sinusitis. Studies using direct aspiration and culture of sinus contents have identified organisms in acute sinusitis that are remarkably consistent with those noted in otitis media. Viral infection accounts for up to 30% of cases, usually involving rhinovirus, influenza, or parainfluenza viruses (52). In community-acquired infections, *Streptococcus pneumoniae* or nontypable *Haemophilus influenzae* is found in up to 75% of cases for adults and children. Anaerobes, streptococcal species, *Moraxella catarrhalis, Staphylococcus aureus,* and other species make up the balance of infecting pathogens for adults (53). *Moraxella catarrhalis* is noted in approximately 20% of pediatric cases. Otherwise, similar organisms are noted in children as in adults.

Little is known about the microbiology of subacute sinusitis, but in chronic sinusitis the infectious flora changes somewhat. Similar organisms as noted above are found in this setting, but the incidence of anaerobic strains and *Staphylococcus aureus* increases. Anaerobic strains include primarily *Bacteroides* species, *Peptostreptococcus,* and *Fusobacterium* species. In addition to these organisms, patients can experience acute exacerbations with the "usual" strains of bacteria.

Certain patient groups will be predisposed to involvement of "unusual" pathogens. Hospital-acquired sinusitis is more commonly due to Gram-negative enteric organisms and staphylococci, often in combination (54). Sinusitis in patients with cystic fibrosis is likely to involve *Pseudomonas aeruginosa.* Immunocompromised patients may be predisposed to infection with *Aspergillus niger, Candida,* or *P. aeruginosa. Rhizopus* species (*Mucor*) is associated with uncontrolled hyperglycemia in diabetics but is fortunately rare (55). Although *P. aeruginosa* and *Legionella pneumophila* have been noted as pathogens causing sinusitis in patients with acquired immune deficiency syndrome, infecting pathogens in general appear to be similar to those noted in HIV-negative patients.

The complications of sinusitis result from extension of the suppurative process. Infection may progress to involve the soft tissue, the orbit, bone, or the intracranial space. Abscesses, meningitis, osteomyelitis, or cellulitis may result. In this case, hospitalization and aggressive management with intravenous antibiotics or surgical therapy may be needed.

Clinical Findings and Diagnosis

The signs and symptoms of sinusitis are in many ways similar to those noted for other upper respiratory infections. Acute sinusitis exhibits rhinorrhea, which is often purulent, generally with a combination of one or more of the following: midfacial or periorbital pain or fullness, congestion, fever, cheek swelling, and conjunctival swelling. Headache, maxillary toothache, altered sense of taste or smell, and nasal quality of the voice may also be present. A history of antecedent upper respiratory infection may be helpful as an indicator of progression of disease. Unfortunately, multiple other abnormalities present with similar findings, and the diagnosis may be difficult to establish on clinical grounds. The presence of maxillary toothache, purulent secretions in the nasal meatus, poor response to decongestants, and history of colored nasal discharge have a positive correlation with the presence of sinusitis. The degree of sensitivity and specificity of any one of these findings is low, but as the number of these signs and symptoms present increases, the likelihood of infection drastically increases (57). Transillumination of the sinuses may also contribute to the diagnosis. Williams and Simel have concluded that when the four signs and symptoms noted above are present and transillumination yields an opaque sinus field, the odds of sinusitis are very high (57). In contrast, the lack of any of these signs or symptoms should virtually exclude the diagnosis. Objective data including radiography and computerized tomagraphy (CT) scan can provide confirmatory evidence of infection. In children this infection is insidious and is often found in conjunction with otitis media. The same signs and symptoms are noted as in adults, but a good history is rarely obtained; clear or purulent discharge and persistent cough are the most sensitive findings in this population but are not specific. Sinusitis should especially be considered in children when the signs and symptoms of an upper respiratory infection (URI) persist beyond the usual 7- to 10-day course (58).

Objective documentation of the microbiology of the infection is difficult. Nasal exudates are contaminated by strains colonizing the nasal passages. Direct sinus puncture avoids this contamination and will usually result in identification of organism(s) and antimicrobial sensitivity. This approach is invasive and should be reserved for the difficult case that is unusually severe, when extension is suspected or documented, in treatment failure, when severe immunosuppression is present, and in the setting of nosocomial infection.

The findings of subacute and chronic sinusitis are generally less pronounced but are more protracted than with acute sinusitis. Nonspecific signs of fatigue, general malaise, and poor health may be more pronounced than the above-noted local findings. Chronic infection may mimic asthma, allergic rhinitis, or chronic bronchitis. Many cases of chronic infection may be related to odontogenic infection (49). Chronic infection carries a greater risk of producing complications.

Treatment of Sinusitis

The medical management of sinusitis relies on a number of different interventions, usually in combination, to hasten recovery of the patient and prevent complications. Treatment options include saline nasal spray or irrigation (nasal toilet), mucolytics, decongestants, corticosteroids, and antibiotics. Goals of therapy include restoration and improvement of sinus function, eradication of causative organism(s), symptomatic relief, and prevention of complications and chronicity. Some patients (as many as 45%) will respond to therapy without the need for antimicrobials. For this reason it is reasonable in milder cases of acute presentation to initiate other measures first, followed by antibiotics only if the patient fails to improve within 48 to 72 hours. In many of these cases as well as in the moderate to severe clinical presentation, antimicrobials will be required.

Antibiotic therapy for acute sinusitis should be directed toward the infecting pathogens. Table 62.6 displays data from in vitro evaluation of recent (1992–1993) clinical isolates of common upper respiratory pathogens from around the United States. Empiric therapy directed at *Streptococcus pneumoniae*, nontypable *Haemophilus influenzae*, and *Moraxella catarrhalis* is appropriate and should be continued for a duration of 10 to 14 days. If the patient has not responded within 72 hours, an alternative

antibiotic should be considered. When slow improvement is seen, duration of therapy should in general be extended for approximately 7 days after resolution of signs and symptoms (59). Studies of sinusitis from the 1970s and early 1980s revealed a low incidence of β-lactamase-producing strains, but this enzyme is now present in as many as 50% of *H. influenzae* and the majority of *M. catarrhalis* strains (53). Barry and colleagues found this enzyme in 30% of *H. influenzae* and 92% of *M. catarrhalis* tested (54). The implication of this finding is that antibiotics that are resistant to the effects of this enzyme should be more frequently considered. In spite of this, recent trials of antibiotic therapy of acute sinusitis have not demonstrated a lower response rate for patients who are treated with amoxicillin (inactive versus β-lactamase-producing strains) (53, 59, 60). Thus, it is rational to use amoxicillin as initial therapy for management of the patient presenting with his or her first case of acute uncomplicated sinusitis (59, 61). Cotrimoxazole or erythromycin/sulfisoxazole is a suitable first-line alternative. When the patient has failed to show evidence of response within approximately 72 hours, or if β-lactamase strains are suspected, then cotrimoxazole, erythromycin/sulfisoxazole, cefaclor, cefuroxime axetil, cefixime, cefpodoxime proxetil, cefprozil, loracarbef, clarithromycin, azithromycin, or amoxicillin/clavulanate should be initiated. Consideration of prior therapy, tolerance, and cost will help to guide selection. For chronic sinusitis, selection of the agent should take into account the increased prevalence of staphylococci and anaerobes and the potential for selection of resistant strains by any previous therapy the patient has received. In addition, this infection should be treated for longer periods of time, generally about 4 weeks. Subacute sinusitis may not require

Table 62.6.
Relative Activity of Selected Oral Antibiotics Against Common Bacterial Pathogens of the Upper Respiratory System (% Susceptible at Breakpoint)[a]

Agent	Streptococcus pyogenes	Haemophilus influenzae	Moraxella catarrhalis	Streptococcus pneumoniae[b]
Amoxicillin	100	67	7	0.5 μg/mL
Cotrimoxazole	97	94	99	>4 μg/mL
Erythromycin	97	1	97	4 μg/mL
Clarithromycin	99	79	98	2 μg/mL
Azithromycin	97	>99	99	8 μg/mL
Amoxicillin/clavulanate	100	99	100	0.5 μg/mL
Cefaclor	100	91	>99	8 μg/mL
Cefuroxime	100	98	97	2 μg/mL
Cefixime	>99	>99	>99	8 μg/mL
Cefprozil	100	89	92	2 μg/mL
Loracarbef	100	92	88	32 μg/mL

Source: Taken from (54).
[a]Number of species tested: *S. pyogenes* (764), *H. influenzae* (619 β-lactamase negative and 271 β-lactamase positive), *M. catarrhalis* (53 β-lactamase negative and 645 β-lactamase positive), *S. pneumoniae* (799).
[b]622 strains were penicillin-susceptible, 119 were intermediate, and 58 were high-level penicillin-resistant; since no specific minimum inhibitory concentration (MIC) breakpoints have been set for this organism and most of the tested drugs, results for this organism are expressed as the MIC 90% for penicillin-*intermediate* strains.

antimicrobials, since at least one trial has demonstrated that an equivalent number of these patients respond to nonantimicrobial therapy as compared with antibiotics (62). If antimicrobials are used, their choice should be based on the same factors as those noted for acute sinusitis.

Adjunctive therapy for sinusitis is often helpful. "Nasal toilet" involves the use of saline nasal sprays or irrigations to facilitate clearing of secretions. Alkalinization of these solutions may facilitate mucolytic effects. Facial pain may also be relieved somewhat by use of moist heat to the face and by the inhalation of steam either in a hot shower or through hot moist towels. Mucolytics appear to offer some benefit in sinusitis. Saturated solution of potassium iodide (SSKI) has been used historically, but it has been essentially replaced by organic iodides. These agents are effective in bronchitis but have not been studied in sinusitis. Guaifenesin has been shown to thin secretions and improve nasal congestion (63), but large doses (2400 mg/day) must be used. These doses may result in gastrointestinal intolerance. Antihistamines should be avoided unless otherwise indicated, as they offer no therapeutic benefit and significantly increase the viscosity of secretions. Intranasal steroids effectively reduce edema and are most useful in the later stages of treatment of subacute or chronic sinusitis (64).

Decongestants are very important in the overall management of sinusitis, even though their efficacy has not been rigorously studied. Judicious application of topical decongestants will diminish local edema and improve access for air and for elimination of secretions. Care must be taken to limit duration of therapy with topical agents to 3 or 4 days to minimize the possibility of rebound congestion. Use of systemic decongestants is supported by reviewers (64), but these drugs have not been compared to topical agents and may induce significant adverse effects involving the sympathetic nervous system.

CROUP (ACUTE LARYNGOTRACHEOBRONCHITIS)

Croup is an infection that has been known for many years, having first been described in 1765 (65). Infection with a number of different viruses has been implicated in the causation of this disease, but the parainfluenza viruses (predominantly Type 1) are most commonly incriminated. *Mycoplasma pneumoniae* has occasionally been noted in some studies to produce this disorder. Croup most commonly occurs in young boys, usually at less than 3 years of age. As is seen with other viral URIs, there is a seasonal occurrence, peaking in late fall and early winter.

As with the common cold, the primary mode of transmission is direct contact. Incubation lasts 2 to 6 days, and children may shed the virus for as long as 2 weeks after onset. Infection induces inflammatory changes in the upper respiratory tract, which spread to involve the laryngotracheal structures and at times the lower respiratory tract. Edema of the submucosa of the subglottic area induces narrowing of this relatively fixed airway. Obstruction to airflow results, causing a compensatory increase in respiratory effort. If the child fatigues, respiratory failure can ultimately ensue.

The typical presentation of this illness is that of a young child with a 1- to 3-day history of URI symptoms associated with a barking or "brassy" nonproductive cough and hoarseness. Tachypnea and stridor are usually present, as is fever. The child may appear anxious, may be sitting forward, and often will be using accessory muscles in the breathing effort. A hallmark of this disease is its vacillating course, resulting in rapid clinical changes even within an hour. In milder infection it is common for the child to improve in the morning and to worsen at night. The course of this infection is usually 3 to 4 days; cough may persist for a number of days thereafter. Objective data such as white blood cell count is not helpful, as it is usually not elevated; hypoxemia and hypercapnea are noted in more severe cases, which usually require hospitalization. Diagnosis is confirmed either radiographically or endoscopically (66).

Management of croup may use any of several options, including inhalation of humidified air, inhalation of epinephrine, systemic corticosteroids, and intubation. Because bacteria are rarely involved, antibiotics are not indicated. Humidification is often the first treatment that is initiated for the patient with croup. This may involve simple exposure of the child to the air of a cool night or to a warm running shower or may be as extensive as the use of humidification tents. Although anecdotal reports attest to the usefulness of aggressive humidification, little objective data supports this practice. In one trial, use of high humidification in the treatment of croup produced no therapeutic benefit up to 12 hours after initiation (67). Thus, parental reassurance and support may be as beneficial as these measures (68).

Racemic epinephrine is the cornerstone of therapy for severe croup. This agent induces sympathomimetic effects that lead to vasoconstriction of the subglottic area, thereby resulting in relief of edema. β-Agonist effects on the airways may also contribute to the beneficial effects that are seen by improving airflow in the lower airways. Use of this drug will generally lead to symptomatic improvement within 10 minutes. Delivery of drug to the airways may be achieved by intermittent positive pressure breathing or by simple nebulization; the recommended dose is 0.25 mL of a 2.25% solution for children less than 6 months old and 0.5 mL of the solution for older children. Repeated treatments are usually necessary because of recurrence of symptoms; a decrease in the frequency of required treatments may signal resolution of the episode. Even though use of this drug does not alter the natural history of the disease, it may minimize the need for intubation (66).

The question of whether corticosteroids are beneficial in the treatment of croup generates much controversy. Questions and concerns about study design, definition of croup for patients evaluated, and definition of endpoints of therapy render interpretation of results difficult at best (69). Any beneficial effect of steroids is attributed to their effect on decreasing capillary endothelial permeability and stabilizing lysosomal membranes, thereby inhibiting the inflammatory reaction. The onset of effect of these agents is slow, however, requiring a minimum of 3 hours to produce any substantial change; effects may also be dose-related. The most commonly recommended steroid is dexamethasone in a single dose of at least 0.6 mg/kg. Use of this drug appears to decrease the need for repeated doses of epinephrine and to improve recovery (70, 71) and may prevent the need for intubation (72). However, hospital stay is not shortened by this therapy. Since the risk of giving a single dose of dexamethasone is very small and no trials have reported adverse effects of this therapy, it is reasonable to treat with a single intramuscular dose of 0.6 mg/kg upon admission to the hospital.

SUPRAGLOTTITIS (EPIGLOTTITIS)

Acute supraglottitis, also known as epiglottitis, is an infection of the epiglottis and adjacent structures. Although little data is available concerning the epidemiology of this infection, it has been responsible for approximately 1 in 1000 to 2000 admissions to pediatric hospitals (73) and 1 in 100,000 admissions to adult hospitals (74). This malady presents as a severe upper respiratory infection, which may progress rapidly to fatal airway obstruction. *Haemophilus influenzae* type B is the most frequent causative organism, accounting for 80 to 100% of incriminated pathogens (75). Other pathogens that are associated with production of this infection in both children and adults include *Streptococcus pneumoniae*, other streptococci, *Staphylococcus aureus*, *H. influenzae* non type B, and *H. parainfluenzae*.

The pathogenesis of this syndrome involves infection by the offending agent, which induces inflammatory changes and edema of the epiglottitis, aryepiglottic folds, arytenoids, and false vocal chords. It is presumed that the offending agent produces infection by direct invasion, but the precise cause of infection is unclear. The noted inflammatory changes rapidly progress to produce airway obstruction. Thus, management of these patients is emergent, requiring placement of an artificial airway.

The pediatric patient with epiglottitis manifests no viral prodrome. Initial signs and symptoms include sore throat, irritability, lethargy, and fever. This presentation rapidly worsens over a period of 4 to 8 hours as the child complains of severe sore throat, pain on swallowing, and dyspnea and begins to look toxic. Fever usually will exceed 101°F, and tachycardia is present out of proportion to the fever. The child will be using accessory muscles in the breathing effort

and will often be sitting upright with neck extended and hands on knees to maximize the size of the supraglottic airway. Severe inspiratory stridor is noted, and drooling and muffled voice are common (66).

Although the same findings may be present in adults, the presentation is much more variable. Prolonged prodromal illness is frequently seen in this population, and patients may already have been treated for presumed pharyngitis. In both children and adults, cervical lymphadenopathy is often present. Examination of the epiglottis and supraglottic structures is diagnostic and reveals the presence of severe inflammation and watery edema. This examination should be undertaken only in the operating suite with appropriate support personnel and equipment that would enable placement of an artificial airway. Soft tissue radiographs may be helpful in confirming the diagnosis but should not delay appropriate (emergent) therapy. It is important to note that the epiglottis will occasionally appear normal. Laboratory data generally reveals leukocytosis with "left shift"; cultures of supraglottic structures and blood should be obtained. Because of the very serious nature of this infection, the child with acute febrile dysphagia should be considered to have supraglottitis until this has been ruled out.

Management involves placement of an artifical airway (endotracheal intubation). Following this step, cultures of the epiglottic structures and blood should be obtained. Intravenous therapy with antibiotics that are active against the noted microorganisms should be initiated; pending culture results, agents that are active against β-lactamase-producing type B *H. influenzae* are appropriate. Conventional therapy has involved ampicillin 200 mg/kg/day plus chloramphenicol 75 to 100 mg/kg/day in divided doses given every 6 hr. Recent studies support the use of cefotaxime (100 to 150 mg/kg/day in 4 doses), cefuroxime (100 to 200 mg/kg/day in 3 doses), or ceftriaxone (100 mg/kg/day in 1 dose) as effective alternatives (76, 77). Therapy should be continued for 5 to 10 days; shorter courses may be possible (78). Conversion from intravenous to oral antimicrobial therapy may be indicated, depending on the rapidity of response, organisms and sensitivities identified on culture, and extubation; usually, the oral route can be used, beginning within 2 days of extubation. Intravenous hydration should be maintained while the patient is intubated, but overhydration should be avoided to decrease the risk of pulmonary edema. Nebulized bronchodilators and corticosteroids have no role in the management of this disorder. If the patient has had any significant (usually household or day-care) contact with children under 6 years of age, the patient and each contact should receive a course of rifampin 20 mg/kg/day (maximum of 600 mg/day) in 4 divided doses for 4 days. This regimen is intended to eradicate colonizing strains of the infecting organism and should be completed before discharge from the hospital. Immunization of the patient who has experienced an episode of supraglottitis due to type B *H. influenzae* does not appear to be warranted, since second episodes are rare, probably indicating effective immunity. The possibility that this infection may occur emphasizes the need for consistent immunization against type B *H. influenzae*. Evidence to date indicates significant progress toward elimination of these infections, primarily attributed to consistent use of this vaccine (79).

CONCLUSION

Optimal management of upper respiratory infections requires a complete understanding of the differing predisposing factors, microbiology, natural history, and potential for complications associated with each distinct infection. Acute, subacute, and chronic presentations may be managed in significantly different ways; intimate knowledge of recent and remote patient history and underlying diseases plays an important role in determining the best approach. The pharmacotherapist who is involved in the care of these patients must keep abreast of changes in microbiology of these diseases and should be intimately familiar with the activity, pharmacokinetics, and pharmacodynamics of antibiotics that may be used for therapy. Knowledge of data supporting or refuting the usefulness of associated therapies will aid in minimizing risk while maximizing benefit of treatment, particularly as some of these treatments are released by the FDA to become over-the-counter products. Finally, pharmacist awareness of the cost-effectiveness of various treatments fills a significant niche in the health care team.

REFERENCES

1. Fireman P. Pathophysiology and pharmacotherapy of common upper respiratory diseases. Pharmacotherapy 13(6, pt 2):101s–109s, 1993.
2. Douglas RG Jr. Influenza in man. In: Kilbourne ED, ed. The influenza viruses and influenza. New York: Academic Press, 1975: 395–447.
3. Hendley JO, Gwaltney JM Jr. Mechanisms of transmission of rhinovirus infection. Epidemiol Rev 10:242–58, 1988.
4. Arola M, Ziegler T, Ruuskanen O, et al. Rhinovirus in acute otitis media. J Pediatr 113:693–95, 1988.
5. Elkhatieb A, Hipskind G, Woerner D, Hayden FG. Middle ear abnormalities during natural rhinovirus colds in adults. J Infect Dis 168:618–21, 1993.
6. Hogg JC. Adenoviral infection and childhood asthma. Am J Respir Crit Care Med 150:2–3, 1994.
7. Gadomski A, Horton L. The need for rational therapeutics in the use of cough and cold medicine in infants. Pediatrics 89:774–76, 1992.
8. Litovitz TL, Holm KC, Clancy C, et al. 1992 annual report of the American Association of Poison Control Centers Toxic Exposure Surveillance System. Am J Emerg Med 11:494–555, 1993.
9. Bryant BG, Lombardi TP. Cold, cough, and allergy products. In: Handbook of nonprescription drugs, 10th ed. Washington, DC: American Pharmaceutical Association. 1993:89–115.
10. Luks D, Anderson M. Over-the-counter cold remedies [Letter]. JAMA 270:1812–13, 1993.
11. Crutcher JE, Kantner TR. The effectiveness of antihistamines in the common cold. J Clin Pharmacol 21:9–15, 1981.
12. Howard JC Jr, Kantner TR, Lilienfield LS, et al. Effectiveness of antihistamines in the symptomatic management of the common cold. JAMA 242:2414–17, 1979.
13. Berkowitz RB, Tinkelman DG. Evaluation of oral terfenadine for treatment of the common cold. Ann Allergy 67:593–8, 1991.
14. Hendeles L. Efficacy and safety of antihistamines and expectorants in nonprescription cough and cold preparations. Pharmacotherapy 13:154–8, 1993.
15. Johnson DA, Hricik JG. The pharmacology of alpha-adrenergic decongestants. Pharmacotherapy 13(6, pt 2):110s–115s, 1993.
16. Mogabgab WJ, Pollock B. Re: increased virus shedding with aspirin treatment of rhinovirus infection. JAMA 235:801, 1976.
17. Rubemis M, Dirda V. Increased virus shedding with aspirin treatment of rhinovirus infections. JAMA 231:1248–51, 1975.
18. Sperber SJ, Swaltney JM Jr, Sorrentino JV, Hayden FG. Pseudoephedrine alone or combined with ibuprofen as treatment for experimental rhinovirus colds. Program and Abstracts of the Twenty-Seventh Interscience Conference on Antimicrobial Agents and Chemotherapy (ICAAC) 27:184, Abstract 501, 1987.
19. Sperber SJ, Hendley O, Hayden FG, et al. Effects of naproxen on experimental rhinovirus colds: a randomized, double-blind, controlled trial. Ann Intern Med 117:37–41, 1992.
20. Doyle WJ, Riker DK, McBride TP, et al. Therapeutic effects of an anticholinergic-sympathomimetic combination in induced rhinovirus colds. Ann Otol Rhinol Laryngol 102:521–7, 1993.
21. Dockhorn R, Grossman J, Posner M, Zinny M, Tinkleman D. A double-blind, placebo-controlled study of the safety and efficacy of ipratropium bromide nasal spray versus placebo in patients with the common cold. J Allergy Clin Immunol 90(6, pt 2):1076–82, 1992.
22. Gaffey MJ, Haden FG, Boyd JC, Gwaltney JM Jr. Ipratropium bromide treatment of experimental rhinovirus infection. Antimicrob Ag Chemother 32:1644–47, 1988.
23. Tyrrell DAJ. A view from the common cold unit. Antiviral Res 18:102–25, 1992.
24. Potter YJ, Hart LJ. Zinc lozenges for treatment of common colds. Ann Pharmacother 27:589–92, 1993.
25. Hemila H. Does vitamin C alleviate the symptoms of the common cold?: a review of current evidence. Scand J Infect Dis 26:1–6, 1994.
26. Dykes MHM, Meier P. Ascorbic acid and the common cold: evaluation of its efficacy and toxicity. JAMA 231:1073–79, 1975.
27. Rossman MG. The canyon hypothesis. Viral Immunol 2:143–61, 1989.
28. McKinlay MA, Pevear DC, Rossmann MG. Treatment of the picornavirus common cold by inhibitors of viral uncoating and attachment. Ann Rev Microbiol 46:635–54, 1992.
29. Tyrrell DAJ. Hot news on the common cold. Ann Rev Microbiol 42:35–47, 1988.
30. Monto AS. The common cold: cold water on hot news. JAMA 271:1122–24, 1994.
31. Fainstein V, Musher DM, Cate TR. Bacterial adherence to pharyngeal cells during viral infection. J Infect Dis 141:172–76, 1980.
32. Rynnel-Dagöö B, Forsgren J, Freijd A, Lindberg K. Rationale for antibiotic therapy in pediatric ear, nose and throat infections: immunologic issues. Pediatr Infect Dis J 13:s15–s20, 1994.
33. Korsrud F, Brandtzaeg P. Influence of tonsillar disease on the expression of J chain by immunoglobulin-producing cells in human palatine and nasopharyngeal tonsils. Scand J Immunol 13:271–80, 1981.
34. Dobkin D, Shulman ST. Evaluation of an ELISA for group A streptococcal antigen for diagnosis of pharyngitis. J Pediatr 110:566–69, 1987.
35. Campos JM. Laboratory diagnosis of group A streptococcal pharyngitis. Infect Dis Clin Pract 2:303–07, 1994.
36. Lieu TA, Fleisher GR, Schwartz JS. Cost-effectiveness of rapid latex agglutination testing and throat culture for streptococcal pharyngitis. Pediatrics 85:246–56, 1990.

37. Bertin L, Pons G, d'Athis P, et al. Randomized, double-blind, multicenter, controlled trial of ibuprofen versus acetaminophen (paracetamol) and placebo for treatment of symptoms of tonsillitis and pharyngitis in children. J Pediatr 119:811–14, 1991.

38. Dajani AS, Bisno AL, Chung KJ, et al. Prevention of rheumatic fever: a statement for health professionals by the Committee on Rheumatic Fever, Endocarditis, and Kawasaki Disease of the Council on Cardiovascular Disease in the Young, the American Heart Association. Circulation 78:1082–86, 1988.

39. Markowitz M, Gerber MA, Kaplan EL. Treatment of streptococcal pharyngotonsillitis: reports of penicillin's demise are premature. J Pediatr 123:679–85, 1993.

40. Peter G. Streptococcal pharyngitis: current therapy and criteria for evaluation of new agents. Clin Infect Dis 14 (Suppl 2):s218–s223, 1992.

41. Gerber MA, Markowitz M. Management of streptococcal pharyngitis reconsidered. Pediatr Infect Dis J 4:518–26, 1985.

42. Krober MS, Weir MR, Themelis MJ, van Hamont JE. Optimal dosing interval for penicillin treatment of streptococcal pharyngitis. Clin Pediatr (Phila) 29:646–48, 1990.

43. Shvartzman P, Tabenkin H, Rosentzwaig A, Dolginov F. Treatment of streptococcal pharyngitis with amoxycillin once a day. Br Med J 306:1170–72, 1993.

44. Peter G, Smith AL. Group A streptococcal infections of the skin and pharynx. N Engl J Med 297:311–17, 365–70, 1977.

45. Bass JW. Antibiotic management of group A streptococcal pharyngotonsillitis. Pediatr Infect Dis J 10 (suppl 10):s43–s49, 1991.

46. Chaudhary S, Bilinsky SA, Hennessy JL, et al. Penicillin V and rifampin for the treatment of group A streptococcal pharyngitis: a randomized trial of 10 days penicillin vs. 10 days penicillin with rifampin during the final 4 days of therapy. J Pediatr 106:481–86, 1985.

47. Tanz RR, Poncher JR, Corydon KE, Kabat K, Rogev R, Shulman ST. Clindamycin treatment of chronic pharyngeal carriage of group A streptococci. J Pediatr 119:123–28, 1991.

48. Wald ER. Epidemiology, pathophysiology and etiology of sinusitis. Pediatr Infect Dis 4 (suppl 6):s51–s54, 1985.

49. Melen I, Lindahl L, Andreasson L, Rundcrantz H. Chronic maxillary sinusitis: definition, diagnosis and relation to dental infections and nasal polyposis. Acta Otolaryngol (Stockh) 101:320–27, 1986.

50. Slavin RG. Medical management of nasal polyps and sinusitis. J Allergy Clin Immunol 88:141–46, 1991.

51. Stankiewicz J, Osguthorpe JD. Medical treatment of sinusitis. Otolaryngol Head Neck Surg 110:361–62, 1994.

52. Sogg A. Long term results of ethmoid surgery. Ann Otol Rhinol Laryngol 98:699–701, 1989.

53. Gwaltney JM Jr, Scheld WM, Sande MA, Sydnor A. The microbial etiology and antimicrobial therapy of adults with acute community-acquired sinusitis: a fifteen-year experience at the University of Virginia and review of other selected studies. J Allergy Clin Immunol 90 (3, pt 2):457–62, 1992.

54. Barry AL, Pfaller MA, Fuchs PC, Packer RR. In vitro activities of 12 orally administered antimicrobial agents against four species of bacterial respiratory pathogens from U.S. medical centers in 1992 and 1993. Antimicrob Ag Chemother 38:2419–25, 1994.

55. Humphrey MA Simpson GT, Grindlinger GA. Clinical characteristics of nosocomial sinusitis. Ann Otol Rhinol Laryngol 96:687–90, 1987.

56. Parnes LS, Brown DH, Garcia B. Mycotic sinusitis: a management protocol. J Otolaryngol 18:176–80, 1989.

57. Williams JW Jr, Simel DL. Does this patient have sinusitis?: diagnosing acute sinusitis by history and physical examination. JAMA 270:1242–46, 1993.

58. Manning SC. Pediatric sinusitis. Otolaryngol Clin North Am 26:623–38, 1993.

59. Wald ER. Antimicrobial therapy of pediatric patients with sinusitis. J Allergy Clin Immunol 90(3, pt 2):469–73, 1992.

60. Felstead SJ, Daniel R. Short-course treatment of sinusitis and other upper respiratory tract infections with azithromycin: a comparison with erythromycin and amoxycillin. European Azithromycin Study Group. J Int Med Res 19:363–72, 1991.

61. Giebink GS. Criteria for evaluation of antimicrobial agents and current therapies for acute sinusitis in children. Clin Infect Dis 14 (suppl 2):s212–s215, 1992.

62. Dohlman AW, Hemstreet MPB, Odrezin GT, Bartolucci AA. Subacute sinusitis: are antimicrobials necessary? J Allergy Clin Immunol 91:1015–23, 1993.

63. Wawrose SF, Tami TA, Amoils CP. The role of guaifenesin in the treatment of sinonasal disease in patients infected with the human immunodeficiency virus (HIV). Laryngoscope 102:1225–28, 1992.

64. Mabry RL. Therapeutic agents in the medical management of sinusitis. Otolaryngol Clin North Am 26:561–70, 1993.

65. Hall CB. Acute laryngotracheobronchitis (croup). In: Mandell GL, Douglas RG Jr, Bennett JE, eds. Principles and practice of infectious diseases, 3rd ed. New York: Churchill Livingstone, 1990:499–505.

66. Cressman WR, Myer CM III. Diagnosis and management of croup and epiglottitis. Pediatr Clin North Am 41:265–76, 1994.

67. Bourchier D, Dawson KP, Fergusson DM. Humidification in viral croup: a controlled trial. Aust Paediatr J 20:289–91, 1984.

68. Henry R. Moist air in the treatment of laryngotracheitis. Arch Dis Child 58:577, 1983.

69. Tunnessen WW, Feinstein AR. The steroid-croup controversy: an analytic review of methodologic problems. J Pediatr 96:751–56, 1980.

70. Postma DS, Jones RO, Pillsbury HC. Severe hospitalized croup: treatment trends and prognosis. Laryngoscope 94:1170–75, 1984.

71. Super DM, Cartelli NA, Brooks LJ, Lembo RM, Kumar ML. A prospective randomized double-blind study to evaluate the effect of dexamethasone in acute laryngotracheitis. J Pediatr 115:323–29, 1989.

72. Kairys SW, Olmstead EA, O'Connor GT. Steroid treatment of laryngotracheitis: a meta-analysis of the evidence from randomized trials. Pediatrics 83:683–93, 1989.

73. Takala AK, Eskola J, Peitola H, Makela PH. Epidemiology of invasive *Haemophilus influenzae* type B disease among children in Finland before vaccination with *Haemophilus influenzae* type B conjugate vaccine. Pediatr Infect Dis J 8:297–302, 1989.

74. MayoSmith MF, Hirsch PJ, Wodzinski SF, Schiffman FJ. Acute epiglottitis in adults: an eight-year experience in the state of Rhode Island. New Engl J Med 314:1133–39, 1986.

75. Crysdale WS, Sendi K. Evolution in the management of acute epiglottitis: a 10-year experience with 242 children. Int Anesthesiol Clin 26:32–8, 1988.

76. Haemophilus influenzae infections. In: Report of the Committee on Infectious Diseases. Chicago: American Academy of Pediatrics, 1991:220–29.

77. Barker KF, Patel B. Adult epiglottitis: cefuroxime is effective [Letter]. Br Med J 308:919, 1994.

78. Sawyer SM, Johnson PD, Hogg GG, et al. Successful treatment of epiglottitis with two doses of ceftriaxone. Arch Dis Child 70:129–32, 1994.

79. Anonymous. Progress toward elimination of *Haemophilus influenzae* type B disease among infants and children: United States, 1987–1993. Morbid Mortal Weekly Rep 43:144–47, 1994.

CHAPTER 63

LOWER RESPIRATORY TRACT INFECTIONS

J. EDWIN UNDERWOOD, Jr

Pneumonia is defined as an inflammation of the lung caused by bacteria, viruses, or, less commonly, noninfectious agents such as drugs or chemicals. The principle site of infection is the alveolus and the surrounding interstitial tissues (1). In the early 1900s, bacterial pneumonia was referred to as "the Captain of the men of death" (2). Today, despite numerous available antibiotics, the advent of broader-spectrum antibiotics, and improved diagnostic methods, pneumonia remains an infectious disease that is responsible for significant morbidity and mortality. Pneumonia is the sixth most common cause of death and the most common cause of infectious death in the United States (3). In the United States, community-acquired pneumonia occurs in up to 4 million people each year (4), and approximately 1 million of these require hospitalization (5). Nosocomial (hospital-acquired) pneumonia is the second most common hospital-acquired infection, occurring in approximately 300,000 patients every year (6). It is estimated that the total cost of treating this illness is $23 billion ($14 billion in direct care costs and $9 billion in lost wages) (3). The biggest challenge confronting clinicians is identifying the cause and selecting the appropriate treatment. Initial therapy is usually empiric, based on clinical judgment. The clinician must have a solid understanding of the body's defenses and the etiology, pathogenesis, clinical presentation, and pharmacotherapy of pneumonia.

HOST DEFENSES AND PATHOGENESIS

The body's defense mechanisms against lower respiratory tract infections comprise a complex, integrated system. Intact defense mechanisms help to maintain a nearly sterile environment from the larynx to the terminal airways and can be divided into four groups: (a) mechanical, (b) phagocytic, (c) immunologic, and (d) secretory. A delicate balance exists between host defenses and exposure to infectious pathogens. Pneumonia occurs when this balance is disrupted. Specifically, infection occurs when there is a defect in the host defenses, exposure to a particularly virulent organism, exposure to an overwhelming number of organisms, or a combination of any of these events. Four pathological mechanisms are involved in the development of pneumonia: (a) aspiration of oropharyngeal secretions, (b) inhalation of aerosolized organisms, (c) hematogenous spread, and (d) contiguous spread by direct extension of infections from adjacent tissues.

The lung defenses originate in the upper respiratory tract (URT), which consists of the anterior nares, nasopharynx, oropharynx, and larynx. The basic aerodynamic design of the URT provides the initial and important filtration barrier against potential pathogens and foreign material. Large particles are filtered and trapped by the hair and mucus in the nares. Swirling air currents in the URT cause impaction of smaller particles that penetrate through the nares, trapping them on the mucus membranes of the nasopharynx to be expelled or swallowed.

The lungs consist of branching airways (bronchi) that end as thin-walled sacs called alveoli. The surface of the lower respiratory tract is lined with mucus-secreting cells interspersed among ciliated columnar epithelial cells; these make up the mucociliary transport system. This transport system stops short of the alveoli and consists of millions of cilia that beat approximately one thousand times per minute, creating an efficient transport system for foreign material, macrophages, and lung secretions away from the smaller airways (7). Smaller particles that escape the initial filtration defense mechanisms of the URT are removed by the mucociliary escalator into the oropharynx, where they are coughed up and swallowed or expectorated. Dysfunction of the mucociliary transport system results in the inability to effectively remove matter, including microorganisms, from the lower airways and may be caused by several factors, which are listed in Table 63.1. Chronic lung disease, aging, and smoking result in a disproportionate ratio of mucus-secreting cells to ciliated epithelial cells. The mucus-secreting cells overwhelm the mucociliary escalator with excessive secretions, hindering efficient function. This situation provides an environment for bacterial overgrowth, called colonization. Subsequently, the person becomes colonized with pathogenic organisms, making him or her more susceptible to development of pneumonia.

Particles that are smaller than 1 μm may escape the mucociliary transport system and reach the alveoli. Alveolar macrophages are the predominant resident phagocytic cells found in the alveoli, interstitial spaces, and surfaces of the airways (7). Their primary responsibility is to handle foreign material and microorganisms that have successfully surpassed the mucociliary transport system. Low numbers of microorganisms reaching this level are easily removed by alveolar macrophage ingestion (phagocytosis) in the immunocompetent host (Figure 63.1) (8). Encapsulated

Table 63.1.

Factors That Diminish Mucociliary Transport of Cellular and Bacterial Debris from the Lower Airways

Smoking	Cystic fibrosis
Chronic bronchitis	Viral infection
Immotile cilia syndrome	Aging
COPD	Inhalation of toxic substances
Asthma	Hyperoxia

Table 63.2.

Factors Associated with Diminished Alveolar Macrophage Activity and Chemotaxis

Chronic	Acute
Alcohol ingestion	Bacterial endotoxin
Advanced age	Hypoxemia
Diabetes mellitus	Metabolic acidosis
Sickle cell disease	Pulmonary edema
Malnutrition	Uremia
Immunosuppressive drugs	Hyperoxia
Corticosteroid treatment	Mechanical obstruction
Hypogammaglobulinemia	Viral infection
Chronic obstructive pulmonary disease	
Acquired immune deficiency syndrome	
Malignancies	
Cystic fibrosis	

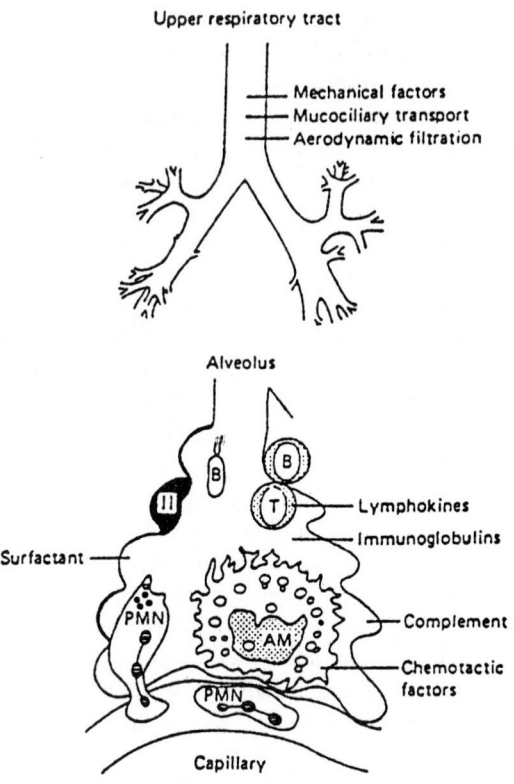

Figure 63.1. Defense mechanisms of the lung. (Source: Reprinted with permission from Reynolds HY. Host defense impairments that may lead to respiratory infections. Clin Chest Med 8(3):344, 1987.)

bacteria such as *Streptococcus pneumoniae* and certain types of *Haemophilus influenzae* require opsonization before phagocytosis can take place. Phagocytes containing bacteria remnants are removed by way of the mucociliary escalator and expectorated or swallowed. It has been estimated that 5 million macrophages leave the lung by this route every hour (9).

If the host is challenged by a virulent pathogen or a high number of organisms, alveolar macrophages and the few available resident polymorphonuclear neutrophils (PMNs) are unable to resolve the insult. When this occurs, chemotactic agents and immunoglobulins recruit extrapulmonary PMNs via the alternative and classical pathways of the complement system (Figure 63.1). Recruitment of

extrapulmonary PMNs results in a more intense inflammatory response, which causes exudation and edema, resulting in the classic pathogenic episode of pneumonia. Numerous factors may interfere with the phagocytic activity of alveolar macrophages, recruitment of PMNs, or host immunity and may predispose the patient to the development of pneumonia (Table 63.2). Pulmonary secretions in the mucosal airway and alveoli consist of surfactant, transferrin, immunoglobulins, complement, and free fatty acids that are bacteriocidal and contribute to host defenses (7).

Viruses compromise ciliary function and impair alveolar macrophage activity. In addition, interactions may occur between respiratory viruses and bacteria that increase either the severity or the likelihood of bacterial pneumonia (7). Patients who become infected with the influenza A virus are at a higher risk for the development of a secondary bacterial pneumonia, predominantly by *Staphylococcus aureus* and *Streptococcus pneumoniae*.

Cell-mediated immunity is an important host defense mechanism that enhances phagocytosis in response to cytokine production but may also result in lung injury leading to pneumonia. T cells are important in eliminating pathogens such as *Mycobacterium* spp., *Mycoplasma pneumoniae*, *Legionella* spp., and fungi that can survive inside the macrophage. In addition to being susceptible to pneumonia secondary to defects in cellular immunity, individuals with acquired immunodeficiency syndrome (AIDS) are more susceptible to pneumonia caused by encapsulated organisms such as *Streptococcus pneumoniae* and *Haemophilus influenzae* because of defects in humoral immunity. The reader should refer to Chapter 72 for an in-depth discussion of pneumonia in patients with AIDS.

The oropharynx contains a consistent variety of microbial flora, including Gram-positive, Gram-negative, and anaerobic organisms called normal flora (Table 63.3). Normal oral secretions contain approximately 10^8 aerobic organisms per milliliter and ten times as many anaerobic organisms. These present a large bacterial challenge to the lung daily (10). In the immunocompetent host, IgA, lysozyme, and glycoproteins found in saliva and mucosal surfaces inhibit bacterial adherence to oropharyngeal mucosa. Thus, in the normal host, few pathogenic Gram-negative bacteria are able to bind to the mucosa of the upper airways and oropharynx; this binding is a critical first step in colonization (9). The prevalence of Gram-negative pathogens in the oropharynx of normal subjects is very low, even when the patient is exposed to a hospital environment (9). However, patients who are chronically ill, elderly, and postsurgical show a higher incidence of colonization with pathogenic Gram-negative organisms, including *Pseudomonas aeruginosa*, because of a lack of cell-surface glycoproteins in the oropharynx (7). These pathologic mechanisms can alter the sensitive balance that exists between microorganisms residing in the oropharynx (7), predisposing the host to colonization and, ultimately, pneumonia. Table 63.4 lists some factors that may increase oropharyngeal bacterial colonization. This concept is an important prerequisite for the development of nosocomial pneumonia and also for the development of community-acquired pneumonia (CAP) in the elderly. The balance of oropharyngeal flora and the beneficial effects of colonization resistance exerted by mouth anaerobes is also disturbed by the administration of antibiotics (11).

Aspiration of oropharyngeal contents is the most common route for microbial access to the lower respiratory tract and is the most frequent mechanism for the development of both community-acquired and nosocomial

pneumonia. Microaspiration of oral secretions is a normal physiologic phenomenon that occurs in 70% of healthy subjects during sleep (12) and rarely leads to infection in the normal host with intact defense mechanisms. Normal epiglottic closure and cough reflex resulting in expulsion from the lung are important pulmonary defense mechanisms that aid in preventing aspiration. Coughing allows aspirated material, excessive secretions, and foreign material in the trachea or major bronchi to be removed quickly from the airways. Factors that compromise epiglottic closure and the ability to cough are associated with a higher incidence of pneumonia (Table 63.5).

There is strong evidence for a causal relationship between gastric colonization with Gram-negative bacilli and the development of nosocomial pneumonia due to aspiration of these organisms (13). Normal gastric pH and gastrointestinal (GI) motility serve as protective factors against overgrowth of endogenous and exogenous sources of bacteria in the stomach. Upper GI bleeding due to stress ulceration is a significant cause of morbidity and mortality among critically ill hospitalized patients (14). However, the use of antacids and H-2 antagonists in the intensive care unit (ICU) for stress ulcer prophylaxis is associated with gastric colonization with Gram-negative organisms. A direct relationship exists between the increase in gastric pH and the number of Gram-negative organisms that are isolated from the stomach (13). The significance of this association is still being studied. In a prospective randomized trial, Driks and colleagues observed a lower rate of pneumonia and a significantly lower mortality rate in mechanically ventilated ICU patients who are treated with sucralfate than in patients who are treated with H-2 antagonists combined with antacids for stress ulcer prophylaxis (15). However, the lower rate of pneumonia that was observed in this study did not reach statistical significance. Despite the established efficacy of sucralfate in preventing stress ulceration, further studies are needed that clearly establish its superiority to other agents in preventing nosocomial pneumonia in critically ill patients who are receiving stress ulcer prophylaxis.

There is additional evidence that supports the reduction or elimination of Gram-negative bacteria in the GI

Table 63.3.
Normal Flora of the Oropharynx

Streptococcus pneumoniae	*Haemophilus influenzae*
Streptococcus pyogenes	*Neisseria* spp.
Streptococcus viridans	Corynebacteria
Staphylococcus aureus	*Lactobacillaceae*
Moraxella (Branhamella) catarrhalis	Various anaerobes

Table 63.4.
Factors That Increase Gram-Negative Bacterial Colonization

Malnutrition	Prolonged hospitalization
Chronically ill	Antacids
Advanced age	H-2 blockers
Nursing home residence	Antibiotic use
Postsurgical patients	Ventilator assistance
Cigarette smoking	Intensive care unit stay

Sources: From (6), (7), (12), and (16).

Table 63.5.
Factors That Decrease the Cough Reflex and Increase the Risk of Aspiration Leading to Pneumonia

Delayed gastric emptying	General anesthesia
Supine position during enteral feeding	Drugs that impair mental status
Alcohol intoxication	Nasogastric intubation
Seizure	Endotracheal intubation
Stroke	Tracheostomy

Sources: From (9) and (11).

tract to minimize the occurrence of nosocomial pneumonia in the ICU setting (16). Selective decontamination of the digestive tract has been used as an effective means of preventing nosocomial pneumonia in mechanically ventilated ICU patients (13). However, results from these trials should be accepted with caution because of study flaws and legitimate concerns about bacterial resistance (13, 14).

Inhalation of aerosolized organisms is a less common pathogenic mechanism that is responsible for causing pneumonia. However, for organisms such as *Legionella pneumophila* and *Mycobacterium tuberculosis*, this is a primary means of access to the lower respiratory tract to cause infection. In addition, airborne transmission of viral agents such as respiratory syncytial virus (RSV) and influenza A is the most common cause of nosocomial pulmonary infections on pediatric wards and may be significant in adult hospital settings as well (9). Respiratory devices, particularly those that deliver aerosols, provide a potential source of microorganisms when used in the hospital setting. Nosocomial pneumonia may occur by this mechanism in any hospitalized patient. However, when these devices are used for patients who are receiving mechanical ventilation support, the URT defense mechanisms and cough reflex are bypassed by the endotracheal tube, allowing microorganisms direct access to the lower respiratory tract. Pneumonia resulting from the use of these devices has caused some researchers to refer to this as direct inoculation (9). Proper cleaning of respiratory equipment and good infection control procedures are essential and are associated with a reduced incidence of nosocomial pneumonia in the hospital and ICU settings.

Hematogenous seeding of the lungs and contiguous spread by direct extension of infections from adjacent tissues are rare pathogenic mechanisms that cause pneumonia. Right-sided endocarditis and septic pelvic thrombophlebitis are infections that may cause pneumonia when the infecting organism in these respective sites travels through the bloodstream and seeds the lung tissue. Hematogenous spread may also be a unique mechanism causing pneumonia due to *Escherichia coli* in the patient with urosepsis (9). Contiguous spread is very uncommon but has occurred in patients with hepatic abscess (17, 18).

CLINICAL EVALUATION AND DIAGNOSIS

The diagnosis of pneumonia is based on clinical, radiologic, laboratory, and microbiologic findings. No single test is capable of diagnosing the cause of pneumonia. An adequate history is helpful and should be obtained from all patients. Mandell and colleagues recommend that the history should attempt to define (a) the clinical setting of the pneumonia, (b) any defects in host defense mechanisms that may predispose the patient to develop pneumonia, and (c) exposure to specific pathogens (19). The age

of the patient and any underlying diseases should be noted. Diagnosis of pneumonia may be more complicated for patients who have a history of chronic obstructive pulmonary disease (COPD) or congestive heart failure (CHF) and those who present with atypical symptoms.

Physical examination is an essential component in evaluating the patient with pneumonia. Abnormal vital signs include fever, tachypnea, and tachycardia. The pulse usually increases by 10 beats per minute for every degree centigrade of temperature elevation (19). Bradycardia may suggest pneumonia caused by *Mycoplasma pneumoniae*, *Chlamydia* spp., *Legionella* spp., or infection with a viral agent (19). While tachypnea and tachycardia may be present in many patients with pneumonia, these are the most sensitive yet least specific signs of pneumonia in the elderly (20). Auscultation of the lung reveals fine crackling rales and diminished breath sounds over the affected area. Percussion dullness is evident in approximately 30% of patients and indicates the presence of consolidation (3). The patient may exhibit restricted movement on the affected side and obtain relief by lying on that side (21). Cyanosis due to hypoxia occurs secondary to poor ventilation and may suggest severe pneumonia and the need for hospitalization.

Laboratory evaluation usually reveals an elevated white blood cell count with an increased number of immature banded neutrophils (left shift). Approximately 20 to 30% of patients will have positive blood cultures, and isolation of a pathogen from this source strongly suggests the cause of the pneumonia (4, 22). Therefore, two sets of blood cultures should be obtained from all patients with pneumonia. Blood samples for arterial blood gases and routine chemistry should be obtained from the patient who presents with severe symptoms, dehydration, or cyanosis or who requires hospitalization.

Classic symptoms of bacterial pneumonia include fever, chills, pleuritic chest pain, and cough productive of purulent sputum. Ten to thirty percent of patients with bacterial pneumonia also complain of headache, nausea, vomiting, abdominal pain, diarrhea, myalgia, and arthralgia (3). In 1938, Reimann first separated pneumonia syndromes into "typical" and "atypical" on the basis of observations of the clinical presentation (23). He recognized that some patients failed to exhibit the classic symptoms of bacterial pneumonia (fever, rapid onset of infection, purulent sputum production, and an elevated white blood cell count), while others were observed to atypically have a milder fever, a more insidious onset of infection, cough without production of purulent sputum, a normal white blood cell count, and an overall milder infection. Atypical presentations may also be associated with more nonspecific extrapulmonary manifestations such as abdominal pain, diarrhea, and confusion. Pneumonia that is caused by *Mycoplasma pneumoniae*, *Chlamydia* spp., *Legionella* spp., viruses, and others account for some of these atypical presentations.

It should be noted that elderly patients and those who are chronically ill, who account for a large proportion of pneumonia cases, often fail to demonstrate the classic symptoms of pneumonia, despite being infected with a typical bacterial pathogen. Pneumonia in the elderly is more often associated with a lower incidence of fever, cough, and sputum production and a higher incidence of mental status changes, tachypnea, tachycardia, bacteremia, and death (24). A number of studies have found that distinguishing between typical and atypical presentations is not useful (23). Caution should be exercised in interpreting the presenting signs and symptoms as being "typical" or "atypical." Nevertheless, the reader should be knowledgeable about the distinctions between them because they can be helpful, and the terms are widely accepted and used in clinical settings, albeit sometimes incorrectly.

A lateral and posterior-anterior (PA) chest radiograph is one of the most important tools used to diagnose pneumonia (19, 25–27). The chest radiograph also serves to establish a baseline to gauge therapeutic response to antimicrobial therapy and to assess complications (25). Complications usually require hospitalization; they include pleural effusion, abscess, empyema, and cavitation. If a significant pleural effusion is present, a diagnostic thoracentesis for culture and sensitivity should be performed. The classic pneumonia chest radiograph usually reveals an infiltrate (area of consolidation) in one or more lobes of the lung, either unilaterally or bilaterally (8). Often, however, the radiograph displays a pattern of nonlobar or diffuse involvement termed bronchopneumonia. Underlying illnesses, especially exacerbation of CHF, malignancy, COPD, and adult respiratory distress syndrome, increase the difficulty of radiologic interpretation, thereby obscuring the diagnosis of pneumonia in these patients (28). Chest radiographs of patients who are dehydrated at initial presentation may be less likely to reveal evidence of pneumonia. Despite this purported observation, it has not consistently been demonstrated in animal and human models and is validated only from a few case reports (3, 28). Although certain radiologic patterns may be observed that suggest the presence of a specific pathogen, an etiologic diagnosis cannot be made by the appearance of the chest radiograph alone.

Despite controversy over the reliability of microscopic examination of the sputum Gram stain, it remains the primary tool in determining the cause of pneumonia and should be obtained from all patients with CAP (25). The Gram stain of an adequate sputum sample allows the clinician to make a presumptive diagnosis as to the cause of the pneumonia and promptly initiate the appropriate antibiotic. Much of the controversy surrounding the Gram stain's reliability is its reported lack of sensitivity and specificity in some clinical trials. Strict criteria have been established and should be used in microscopically examining the Gram stain. An adequate sample contains more than 25 PMNs and fewer than 10 squamous epithelial cells per low power field and a predominating pathogen (29). When these criteria are used, contamination with oropharyngeal flora is less likely, and sensitivity may be as high as 85% in determining the cause of the pneumonia (19, 26). Specimens that meet these criteria are also suitable for culture, allowing antibiotic sensitivities to be established. Unfortunately, children, the elderly, and uncooperative patients cannot always elicit a deep enough cough to produce an adequate sputum sample; this hinders the identification of a pathogen. In such cases an induced sputum collection using nebulized albuterol or saline may be helpful. Proper technique in the procurement of the sputum sample is very important as well. Improper collection will result in a Gram stain that is representative of saliva and oropharyngeal flora and may result in a false positive culture of bacteria that are not part of the inflammatory process. A Gram stain with high numbers of PMNs and low numbers of squamous epithelial cells but without bacteria is suggestive of atypical pathogens, including *Legionella* spp., *Chlamydia* spp., *Mycoplasma pneumoniae*, and viral agents (25).

When an adequate sputum sample cannot be obtained, invasive diagnostic procedures may be used to determine the cause of the pneumonia. Transtracheal aspiration (TTA) is an invasive procedure in which a 14-gauge needle is inserted through the cricothyroid membrane into the trachea below the level of the larynx but not reaching the lower peripheral airways (22, 25). At this position the tracheobronchial tree is normally sterile, and the isolation of a pathogen usually indicates the cause of the pneumonia (9). TTA is particularly helpful in diagnosing pneumonia caused by anaerobic pathogens (8, 9). However, TTA has fallen into disfavor and is used less often because of the risk of complications. Sputum Gram stains that met the criteria of > 25 PMNs and < 10 squamous epithelial cells per low power field closely reflected specimens that were obtained from similar patients in one study (29). Hence, collection of an adequate sputum sample may supersede the need for TTA for most patients. In addition, TTA is an unreliable tool in the diagnosis of nosocomial pneumonia because of the presence of colonizing organisms in the area being sampled, resulting in a higher incidence of false positive bacterial cultures.

Fiber-optic bronchoscopy is another invasive procedure that is used for diagnosing the presence and cause of pneumonia. It is a relatively safe procedure but is not without risks of complications. Therefore, it is usually reserved for critically ill or immunocompromised patients and mechanically ventilated patients with nosocomial pneumonia. Fiber-optic bronchoscopy gives the experienced pulmonologist direct access to the lower airways with the ability to visualize and sample tissues and secretions. Protected specimen brush (PSB) and broncho-alveolar lavage (BAL) are two diagnostic procedures that are used with fiber-optic bronchoscopy. If correctly used, both have high sensitivity and specificity in determining the cause of pneumonia. A potential advantage of BAL over PSB is its ability to sample a larger area of the lung and allowing the clinician to microscopically examine the specimen after the procedure (22). Samples that are obtained by using either PSB or BAL are suitable for culture using quantitative techniques.

Transthoracic needle aspiration is an invasive proce-dure that is seldom used in the diagnosis of pneumonia because of its risks of serious complications and the evolution of safer fiber-optic bronchoscopy techniques.

Open lung biopsy provides the least contaminated specimens. However, because of risks of complications and controversy over its benefits, it is usually reserved for diag-nosing complicated or unresolving pneumonia in patients with AIDS and other immunosuppressed patients (22).

Three immunoassays that are used for the identification of bacterial and viral antigens include counterimmuneelec-trophoresis (CIE), agglutination, and enzyme-linked im-munosorbent assay (ELISA) (19). CIE has been used to detect antigens in various body fluids, including urine, serum, sputum, and pleural fluid (8). Currently, because of their expense and variable sensitivity, these tests are used primarily to confirm a clinical diagnosis when necessary (19) and have yet to find their diagnostic niche in evaluating pneumonia. Other methods using DNA probes, poly-merase chain reactions, and monoclonal antibodies are being studied and may be valuable diagnostic tests in the future (4). Serologic titers using immunofluorescence may be performed but, because of their delayed response, are more helpful for epidemiologic purposes than for diag-nosis.

GENERAL TREATMENT OF PNUEMONIA

The treatment of pneumonia involves selection of the appropriate antibiotic(s) and, when required, the provision of supportive care. The patient's age, coexisting diseases, and the setting in which the pneumonia occurs may suggest the most likely infecting organism.

Many antibiotics are currently available and are effec-tive in the treatment of pneumonia. Antibiotic choice should be individualized for the patient and take into consideration the spectrum of activity, pharmacokinetics, adverse effects, clinical efficacy, and cost. The need for hospitalization and whether the patient's condition neces-sitates parenteral antibiotic therapy must also be consid-ered. Generally, drugs that are used for initial empiric therapy should have a reasonably broad spectrum of activity covering the most likely pathogens. Every effort

should be made to obtain sputum specimens, blood cultures, and other appropriate diagnostic specimens before initiation of antibiotics. However, this should not significantly delay the first dose. Once the causative organism has been reliably identified and antibiotic sensi-tivities have been established, a narrow-spectrum agent should be substituted.

If an effective antibiotic is selected, a clinical response will usually occur in the first 48 to 72 hr in the immunocompetent patient. Therapy should not be changed during the first 72 hr unless the patient exhibits significant clinical deterioration (4) or specific diagnostic information, such as culture and sensitivity data, becomes available, permitting an appropriate change.

Successful antibiotic treatment requires that the agent reach an effective concentration at the site of infection. If the patient has coexisting bacteremia, serum drug concen-trations are equally important. Most antibiotics reach the infected lung by passive diffusion across the blood-bronchoalveolar barrier. Diffusion depends on the degree of ionization, concentration gradient, and pharmacokinetic properties of the drug (size, lipid solubility, and protein binding) (30). Antibiotics that are un-ionized and lipophilic penetrate into lung tissue most readily, and inflamed lung tissue may enhance the permeability of drugs as well (30). Since albumin is too large to gain access to the lung by passive diffusion through pulmonary capillary pores, a high affinity for protein binding may decrease the drug's ability to penetrate lung tissue (1). Hence, it is important to consider all of the pharmacokinetic and pharmacodynamic properties of a drug in evaluating its efficacy for the treatment of pneumonia.

In addition, the most cost-effective agent should be chosen. This decision should include consideration of length of hospital stay. For example, the most cost-effective therapy may be a more expensive antibiotic that gets the patient out of the hospital faster than a less expensive antibiotic would permit.

Empiric treatment of CAP should always cover the most common pathogen, Streptococcus pneumoniae. If intravenous antibiotics are required initially, a switch to oral therapy can usually be made between day 3 and day 6 of therapy. However, a change to oral therapy should be made only when the patient's clinical condition has stabilized and fever has subsided (4).

The American Thoracic Society has established guide-lines for the initial management of adults with CAP (4). These guidelines have taken into consideration the severity of the pneumonia at initial presentation and the presence of either coexisting illness or advanced age. Table 63.6 is based on these recommendations and is a useful guide for empiric treatment of the patient with CAP.

Empiric antibiotic treatment for nosocomial pneumo-nia requires a recognition of the difference between the

Table 63.6.

Frequently Encountered Pathogens in Patients with Community-Acquired Pneumonia (CAP) and Reasonable Empiric Therapy; Based on Age, Coexisting Disease, and Severity at Presentation[a]

CAP Requiring Outpatient Treatment		CAP Requiring Hospitalization	
Group 1: Patients ≤ 60 Years or Older & No Coexistent Disease	Group 2: Patients > 60 Years Old AND/OR Coexistent Disease	Group 3: Patients Requiring Hospitalization	Group 4: Patients with Severe CAP
Common pathogens S. pneumoniae M. pneumoniae C. pneumoniae H. influenzae Respiratory viruses	Common pathogens S. pneumoniae H. influenzae S. aureus Aerobic Gram-negative bacilli Respiratory viruses	Common pathogens S. pneumoniae H. influenzae Legionella spp. S. aureus C. pneumoniae Polymicrobial (including anaerobes) Aerobic Gram-negative bacilli Respiratory viruses	Common pathogens S. pneumoniae Legionella spp. M. pneumoniae Aerobic Gram-negative bacilli Respiratory viruses
Less common pathogens Legionella spp. S. aureus M. tuberculosis Endemic fungi Aerobic Gram-negative bacilli	Less common pathogens M. catarrhalis Legionella spp. M. tuberculosis Endemic fungi	Less common pathogens M. pneumoniae M. catarrhalis M. tuberculosis Endemic fungi	Less common pathogens H. influenzae M. tuberculosis Endemic fungi
Empiric therapy Erythromycin OR azithromycin[b]	Empiric therapy Cefuroxime axetil or TMP/SMX[c] or amoxicillin/clavulate + or − erythromycin[d]	Empiric therapy IV cefuroxime or cefotaxime or ceftriaxone + or − erythromycin[e]	Empiric therapy Erythromycin[e] + ceftazidime + gentamicin or tobramycin

Source: From (4) and (23).
[a]Excludes patients with AIDS.
[b]Azithromycin should be used only for mild to moderate infections.
[c]TMP/SMX = trimethoprim/sulfamethoxazole.
[d]Erythromycin should be added if Legionella spp. is suspected.
[e]Rifampin can be added if Legionella spp. is documented.

pathogens and those that cause CAP. Empiric treatment may incorporate combination therapy with a β-lactam and aminoglycoside or broad-spectrum monotherapy. Aminoglycosides have been favored for empiric treatment of nosocomial pneumonia because of synergism with β-lactam antibiotics, rapid killing rate, postantibiotic effect, and activity against Gram-negative pathogens, including *Pseudomonas aeruginosa*. Because of limitations, monotherapy with aminoglycosides should be avoided in the treatment of pneumonia. The infected lung tissues and secretions are more acidic than normal, and this has a negative effect on the activity of aminoglycosides (1). In addition, aminoglycosides are water-soluble and do not readily pass into lung tissue. Both factors require that therapeutic peak serum concentrations of gentamicin or tobramycin be maintained above 6 mg/L to ensure satisfactory lung penetration and improved patient outcomes (31, 32). These shortcomings have prompted research in the area of aerosolized and endotracheal administration of aminoglycosides to overcome their phar-

macokinetic disadvantages. Both methods attempt to provide a greater concentration of drug at the site of infection while limiting systemic adverse effects. Despite these theoretical advantages, the role of these administration methods in clinical practice remains controversial but deserves continued study (33). Empiric monotherapy may be acceptable with some antimicrobial agents, and a wide array of selections are possible. It is imperative that one be familiar with the institution's microbial flora and susceptibility patterns before choosing the empiric agent. The institution's antibiogram should be used in making empiric therapeutic decisions.

COMMUNITY-ACQUIRED PNEUMONIA

The annual incidence of community-acquired pneumonia (CAP) in the United States is 2 million to 4 million; as many as 20% of patients require hospitalization (4, 23). Most patients can be treated in the ambulatory setting with oral agents; the mortality rate of these patients is less than 5%. In contrast, the mortality rate for CAP patients who require hospitalization is as high as 25%, and these patients account for a significant amount of hospital resources (4, 23). CAP can occur during any time of the year but is most often encountered during late fall through late spring. Certain pathogens may exhibit seasonal and geographic variation. A pathogen is not identified in up to 50% of pneumonia cases (23); the result is empiric therapy throughout the clinical course. Therefore, it is essential to know the most likely cause in order to initiate the appropriate antimicrobial agent (Table 63.6). Typically, patients present with a sudden onset of a chill followed by fever, pleuritic chest pain, and cough productive of purulent sputum. Factors that are predictive of a more severe course and death due to pneumonia include advanced age, absence of chest pain, tachypnea, hypotension, confusion, elevated blood urea nitrogen, leukopenia, leukocytosis, and digoxin toxicity (3).

Pneumococcal Pneumonia

Streptococcus pneumoniae is the most common cause of CAP. It accounts for 10 to 25% of all cases of CAP (25, 34) and may actually be responsible for as many as 60% of cases (28). Most patients with pneumococcal pneumonia present with an abrupt onset of fever, chills, pleuritic chest pain, and a cough productive of purulent, rust-colored sputum. However, elderly or chronically ill patients may present with only tachypnea, tachycardia, and changes in mental status. A Gram stain of the sputum reveals many PMNs, few epithelial cells, and many lancet-shaped Gram-positive diplococci. A physical exam and chest radiograph are consistent with evidence of bacterial pneumonia. Uniquely, up to 40% of patients have evidence of *Herpes simplex* (fever blisters) (19). Laboratory evaluation reveals an elevated white blood cell count of 10,000 to 35,000 cells/mm^3 with an increased number of immature banded neutrophils.

The drug of choice for pneumococcal pneumonia in most areas of the United States is still penicillin. Although penicillin-sensitive pneumococci are also sensitive to other penicillin derivatives, none of these derivatives are more active than penicillin, and some are considerably less active (8).

The Centers for Disease Control and Prevention recently reported penicillin resistance in 6.6% of pneumococcal isolates in the United States (35). Penicillin resistance was also recently reported in 29% of nasopharyngeal isolates in Memphis, Tennessee, and 61% of isolates at a day care center in Kentucky (36). Other countries such as New Guinea, Spain, Israel, Poland, and South Africa have a higher incidence of pneumococcal resistance to penicillin. Up to 62% of isolates in these countries exhibit minimum inhibitory concentrations (MICs) for penicillin ranging from intermediately sensitive (≥1.0 µg/mL) to highly resistant (≥2.0 µg/mL) (34). Researchers at Vanderbilt University Hospital recently observed intermediate- or high-level resistance to penicillin and an inverse relationship between the age of the patient and the prevalence of resistance in 32% of pneumococcal isolates (35). Currently, most pneumococcal strains in this country are highly sensitive to penicillin (MICs < 0.02 µg/mL). Nevertheless, appropriate therapy should be dictated on the basis of the geographic pattern of penicillin resistance, especially in children or others who have been exposed to many antibiotics.

Uncomplicated, mild pneumococcal pneumonia can usually be treated in the outpatient setting with 1 to 2 g of penicillin V given in four divided doses for 7 to 10 days. Some clinicians may opt to give a single intramuscular injection of 600,000 units of procaine penicillin G followed by oral therapy. Patients with complicated or severe pneumococcal pneumonia who require hospitalization can be effectively treated with aqueous penicillin G in a dose of 5 to 10 million units/day in divided doses (19). In geographic regions where penicillin resistance is prevalent or likely, an intravenous third-generation cephalosporin such as cefotaxime 1 g every 8 hr or ceftriaxone 1 g every 24 hr should be used empirically until culture and sensitivity data is available. Recent evidence suggests that ceftizoxime should be avoided in these situations because of an observed lower level of in vitro activity against *S. pneumoniae* compared to cefotaxime or ceftriaxone, particularly in areas with intermediate- or high-level resistance to penicillin (35).

When appropriate therapy is initiated, a favorable response and defervescence are usually seen within 48 to 72 hr. As a general rule, a switch from intravenous to oral therapy may be made at this time to complete the full course of therapy. Chest radiograph abnormalities may persist for up to 4 to 6 weeks, especially in the elderly or patients with underlying pulmonary disease. Those who develop complications such as pneumococcal meningitis, endocarditis, bacteremia, or arthritis should receive 20 million units of aqueous penicillin G intravenously per day in divided doses. In geographic regions with a high prevalence of penicillin resistance, high-dose vancomycin in combination with cefotaxime has been advocated for the patient with pneumococcal meningitis (35).

Erythromycin 1 to 2 g daily or most first- and second-generation cephalosporins are effective alternatives for the penicillin-allergic patient. However, up to 15% of penicillin-allergic patients are also allergic to cephalosporins, and their use should be guided by the severity of the penicillin allergy or history of previous exposure to cephalosporins. In general, cephalosporins should be avoided for patients who have experienced anaphylaxis to penicillin. The newer semisynthetic macrolide antibiotics clarithromycin and azithromycin can be recommended only for "mild" infections at this time and when oral therapy is considered appropriate. Other secondary alternatives include clindamycin, trimethoprim/sulfamethoxazole (TMP/SMX), and intravenous vancomycin. Despite widespread use, excellent lung tissue penetration, and increased Gram-positive coverage of ofloxacin compared to ciprofloxacin, currently available systemic quinolone antibiotics are not good choices because of unreliable pneumococcal sensitivities and reported treatment failures. Aminoglycosides are not effective, and tetracyclines are unreliable for treatment of *Streptococcus pneumoniae*.

Significant risk factors for the development of pneumococcal pneumonia include age greater than 50, smoking, residence in a nursing home, neutropenia, seizure disorder, and asplenia or splenic dysfunction. Other high-risk groups include patients with cardiovascular disease, COPD, diabetes mellitus, AIDS, chronic renal or hepatic failure, Hodgkin's disease, or sickle cell disease; those receiving chemotherapy or immunosuppressive therapy; and alcoholics. Patients who have these risk factors or fall into high-risk groups have an increased likelihood of pneumonia complications, higher mortality rates, and a greater need for hospitalization due to pneumococcal pneumonia (37) and should receive active immunization with the polyvalent pneumococcal vaccine. The vaccine consists of 23 types of purified, capsular polysaccharide antigens, which represent the majority of *Streptococcus pneumoniae* types that are responsible for pneumococcal infections in the United States. Its efficacy depends on the recipient's ability to produce antibodies in response to the vaccine. Despite controversy over the vaccine's reduced efficacy in immunocompromised patients and the elderly, its benefits are generally considered to outweigh the risks of not receiving the vaccination. The vaccine is clearly of benefit for high-risk patients who are otherwise immunocompetent (38, 39). The influenza vaccine is also recommended for high-risk patients to reduce complications and the potential for secondary bacterial pneumonia.

Haemophilus influenzae

Haemophilus influenzae makes up part of the normal flora of the URT in virtually all people older than 1 year of age (40). Approximately 5% of *H. influenzae* exist as the encapsulated form; 95% are nonencapsulated. *H. influenzae* type B is responsible for most childhood URT infections, and vaccination has become increasingly important. *H. influenzae* is now recognized as a significant pathogen causing lower respiratory tract (LRT) infections in adults, especially among alcoholics, people with AIDS, the elderly, and individuals who have chronic pulmonary diseases. Three-quarters of adult patients present with a worsening cough, tachypnea, and low-grade fever, which may indicate acute exacerbation of chronic bronchitis. In these patients the sputum Gram stain is unreliable because colonization with *H. influenzae* and other Gram-negative

pathogens is common. A smaller percentage of patients present with a more sudden onset of symptoms, fever, purulent sputum production, and pleuritic chest pain, which indicate pneumonia rather than bronchitis. A sputum Gram stain will show many PMNs and a predominance of Gram-negative coccobacilli, which are indicative of *H. influenzae*. A chest radiograph may reveal lobar involvement, and a high percentage of patients will have blood cultures that are positive for the organism, confirming the etiology.

Ampicillin and amoxicillin were once considered the drugs of choice for treatment of LRT infections caused by *H. influenzae* and are still considered to be alternatives for treating URT infections in some patients. Ampicillin resistance due to plasmid-mediated β-lactamase production is being encountered more frequently in the community setting. For hospitalized patients, empiric antimicrobial choice should be reasonably broad and may include a second-generation cephalosporin such as cefuroxime 750 mg intravenously every 8 hr or the third-generation cephalosporins cefotaxime 1 g intravenously every 8 hr or ceftriaxone 1 g intravenously every 24 hr. Ampicillin/sulbactam 1.5 g intravenously every 6 hr may also be considered when β-lactamase-producing *H. influenzae* is suspected. Antimicrobial therapy may later be streamlined on the basis of culture and sensitivity information.

A variety of other agents are effective against ampicillin-resistant strains, including TMP/SMX, ciprofloxacin, and ofloxacin. Empiric quinolones should not be chosen if pneumococcus cannot be ruled out. Azithromycin is a secondary alternative for mild infections and only when oral therapy is considered appropriate. The MIC for erythromycin is not sufficient to treat most infections caused by *H. influenzae*; therefore, erythromycin should not be used. Despite additive or synergistic activity of clarithromycin and its 14-hydroxy metabolite, this agent has exhibited failure to eradicate *H. influenzae* in some patients with CAP and bronchitis when given in an oral dose of 25 mg twice a day (41). More clinical trials and experience are necessary before clarithromycin can be recommended for LRT infections caused by this organism. Combination agents containing a β-lactam and β-lactamase inhibitor such as amoxicillin/clavulanic acid, ticarcillin/clavulanic acid, ampicillin/sulbactam, or piperacillin/tazobactam are also effective against β-lactamase-producing strains of *H. influenzae*. Ticarcillin/clavulanic and piperacillin/tazobactam are seldom necessary in these instances because of their broad spectrum of activity and the availability of more cost-effective agents. Amoxicillin/clavulanic acid, TMP/SMX, cefuroxime axetil, and cefixime are suitable for ambulatory patients and for switching from intravenous to oral therapy if β-lactamase producers are causing the infection. Cefixime should be avoided if *S. aureus* or pneumococcus cannot be ruled out. Newer oral third-generation cephalosporins, loracarbef and cefprozil, and the older second-generation cephalosporin, cefaclor, may be considered secondary alternatives for ambulatory patients but are usually not justified owing to lack of cost-effectiveness.

Moraxella (Branhamella) catarrhalis

M. catarrhalis is part of the normal flora of the URT and, until recently, was considered to be nonpathogenic. It is now recognized as a relatively common cause of exacerbation of bronchitis, sinusitis, otitis media, and pneumonia in patients with underlying pulmonary disease. Up to 15% of CAPs may be attributed to this pathogen (25). Smoking, COPD, chronic corticosteroid use, and viral illness may allow overgrowth of this organism, potentially leading to the development of pneumonia. Patients usually present with mild to moderate symptoms, which are sometimes indistinguishable from those of bronchitis. Chills, fever, and pleuritic chest pain are present in fewer than 33% of patients, but evidence of pneumonia on chest radiograph may be as high as 43% (42). White blood cell counts may be mildly elevated, and bacteremia is uncommon. A sputum Gram stain, if obtainable, may show a predominance of Gram-negative, kidney bean-shaped diplococci (43). There is evidence that β-lactamase production by these organisms has increased in recent years (42). This may, in part, account for the fact that *M. catarrhalis* has become a legitimate pathogen in recent years. Historically, ampicillin and amoxicillin were considered effective antibiotics against *M. catarrhalis*. Today, β-lactamase producers are resistant to both agents, regardless of the MIC (42).

Antibiotics that are used to treat infections caused by β-lactamase-producing strains of *M. catarrhalis* include TMP/SMX, amoxicillin/clavulanic acid, cefuroxime and most other second-generation cephalosporins, ciprofloxacin, ofloxacin, and third-generation cephalosporins. Ampicillin is the drug of choice for non-β-lactamase-producing strains. Erythromycin, clarithromycin, and azithromycin (for mild infections) are alternative agents. When available, culture and sensitivity information should be used to guide therapy.

ATYPICAL PNEUMONIA

Several pathogens have been identified as being "atypical" on the basis of the contrast of presenting signs and symptoms with those of pneumonia caused by "typical" bacterial pathogens. Atypical presentations may also be associated with more extrapulmonary manifestations. Pneumonia caused by *Mycoplasma pneumoniae*, *Chlamydia* spp., *Legionella* spp., and viruses account for some of these atypical presentations. Other, less common causes of community-acquired atypical pneumonia syndromes include *Chlamydia psittaci* (psittacosis), *Coxiella burnetii* (Q fever), *Francisella tularensis* (tularemia), *Mycobacte-*

rium tuberculosis (TB), fungi, and respiratory viruses (influenza A and B, adenovirus, parainfluenza, and RSV).

Legionella Pneumonia

Legionella spp. are Gram-negative bacilli that cause pneumonia in adults more commonly than in children. *Legionella* spp. are ubiquitous to aquatic environments, and outbreaks of pneumonia have been associated with excavation, construction, cooling towers, ventilation systems, and shower heads. Institutional outbreaks causing nosocomial pneumonia have been associated with contaminated water supplies. *Legionella* spp. are often grouped with other atypical pathogens but are capable of causing severe, life-threatening pneumonia. In the community, peak incidence occurs between late summer and early fall and may be as high as 30% in some geographic locations, but this type of pneumonia is encountered less often in most areas (44). Specific predispositions to infection include smoking, age greater than 60, alcoholic liver disease, and high-dose corticosteroid use in institutionalized patients. *Legionella pneumophila* is responsible for the majority of cases of Legionnaire's disease, a rapidly progressive and severe form of *Legionella* pneumonia. Patients present with an abrupt onset of high fever, chills, and cough with a small amount of nonpurulent sputum production. Many patients complain of extrapulmonary symptoms including diarrhea, nausea, vomiting, headache, and confusion. However, none of the clinical features, with the possible exception of bradycardia, reliably distinguish *Legionella* pneumonia from that caused by other typical bacteria. Laboratory evaluation reveals an elevated white blood cell count, hypophosphatemia, and elevated liver enzymes in most patients. If enough sputum is available, identification of the organisms is possible by direct immunofluorescence. Serologic indirect immunofluorescent antibody determination may be used to detect *Legionella* spp. However, most patients do not become seropositive until convalescence, during the third to sixth week, so this test is impractical for acute therapy and more useful for epidemiologic purposes. A very sensitive, specific, and rapid radioimmunoassay that detects *Legionella* spp. antigen in the urine is currently available.

Intravenous erythromycin 1 g four times a day is the treatment of choice for *Legionella* pneumonia. Intravenous therapy may be switched to oral erythromycin 500 mg four times a day to complete a 21-day course of therapy when clinical improvement occurs. In very severe cases of Legionnaire's disease the addition of oral rifampin in a dosage of 300 to 600 mg every 12 hr may be helpful (44). However, rifampin should not be used alone. If the patient is intolerant to erythromycin, alternative agents include tetracycline and doxycycline. Anecdotal reports have also described the successful use of other agents, including TMP/SMX, imipenem/cilastatin, and ciprofloxacin (8).

Legionella spp., including *Legionella pneumophila*, are not susceptible to β-lactam antibiotics.

Mycoplasma pneumoniae

Mycoplasma pneumoniae is one of the smallest known free-living organisms (45). It does not have a cell wall and has properties of both viruses and bacteria. *M. pneumoniae* is more likely to cause pharyngitis or a self-limiting URT infection than pneumonia. However, atypical CAP due to this organism is common, accounting for up to 20 to 30% of pneumonia cases in adults under 30 years of age and up to 50% of cases in people living in close quarters (45, 46). Endemic outbreaks of *Mycoplasma* pneumonia have been observed in college dormitories and military installations. *Mycoplasma* pneumonia is relatively uncommon in the elderly, occurring in fewer than 3% of patients over 60 years of age (47), although it may occur in the older person, especially if he or she is exposed to young adults or children with the infection. The incidence of pneumonia varies from year to year. It generally peaks every 4 years and is most prevalent in the fall; however, it may occur during any time of the year (46). *Mycoplasma* pneumonia may manifest as anything from a mild, self-limiting influenza-type illness to severe life-threatening pneumonia. The onset of pneumonia is gradual, and patients present with a variety of complaints, including a worsening sore throat, nonproductive cough that is worse at night, headache, low-grade fever, general malaise, myalgias, and earache. Although a rare finding, *Mycoplasma pneumoniae* should be strongly suspected in the patient with erythema multiforme and atypical pneumonia symptoms (44). As with other atypical pathogens, a relative bradycardia in relationship to the patient's temperature may be noted. A chest radiograph most commonly reveals a pattern of bronchopneumonia. Definitive diagnosis of *Mycoplasma pneumoniae* is made by isolation of the organism or demonstration of an appropriate antibody response (45). Elevated cold agglutinin titers greater than 1:64 occur in a majority of patients during the second to third week of illness. Other diagnostic techniques using indirect immunofluorescence, ELISA, or polymerase chain reaction may gain popularity in the future.

Determination of *Mycoplasma pneumoniae* as the causative pathogen is often impractical, and therapy is usually presumptive on the basis of clinical evaluation and history. Most people with *Mycoplasma* pneumonia can be treated as outpatients with oral erythromycin 500 mg every 6 hr for 14 days. Erythromycin is usually chosen as first-line therapy because of its additional activity against *Streptococcus pneumoniae* and *Legionella* spp. Tetracycline 500 mg every 6 hr and doxycycline 100 mg twice a day for 14 days are also effective treatments for *M. pneumoniae* but are not ideal choices if empiric *Streptococcus pneumoniae* coverage is also desired. Clarithromycin 250 to 500 mg

every 12 hr and azithromycin 500 mg on day 1 followed by 250 mg for 4 days are considered alternative regimens for mild infections. Azithromycin may be the most helpful for patients who are intolerant of the GI side effects of erythromycin. However, GI side effects associated with erythromycin may be avoided by using oral preparations that can be taken with food or that are enteric-coated. Estolate salts of erythromycin should be avoided because of a high incidence of liver toxicity. β-lactam antibiotics are not effective because *M. pneumoniae* does not have a cell wall.

Chlamydia pneumoniae

Chlamydia pneumoniae, also designated TWAR strain, is an obligate intracellular Gram-negative pathogen that causes atypical pneumonia. It is transmitted from human to human and accounts for up to 10% of all cases of CAP (45). Prevalence increases through adolescence up to age 40 and is uncommon in the very young and very old. Of special interest is recent evidence of a possible association of this organism with atherosclerosis and coronary artery disease in men (48). Further analysis is warranted before a true relationship can be suggested. *C. pneumoniae* most commonly causes sinusitis, pharyngitis, or bronchitis rather than pneumonia. When pneumonia does occur, approximately 50% of patients report severe pharyngitis and hoarseness in the previous 1 to 3 weeks (45). Pneumonia is usually classified as mild to moderate but may be severe in some, especially older adults or chronically ill patients. Fatal infections have been reported in patients with underlying COPD and CHF (45). Patients generally present with a low-grade fever, a nonproductive cough, and a normal white blood cell count. A chest radiograph may show a diffuse process, and consolidation is uncommon. One clue to the presence of *C. pneumoniae* as the causative pathogen is a "low-grade eosinophilia" (44).

The two most common serologic tests for *C. pneumoniae* are IgM complement fixation and microimmunofluorescence. Etiologic diagnosis is usually a presumptive one based on clinical findings and history. For this reason and because standard "atypical" antibiotic regimens usually cover *C. pneumoniae*, the true incidence of this organism may be underrecognized. Furthermore, because of its self-limiting nature, many patients do not seek treatment or progress to the development of pneumonia.

The treatment of choice for pneumonia caused by *C. pneumoniae* is tetracycline 500 mg by mouth every 6 hr or doxycycline 100 mg every 12 hr for 14 to 21 days to prevent relapse. Ciprofloxacin and ofloxacin are considered secondary agents, and clarithromycin may be used secondarily for mild infections. Tetracyclines and quinolones should be avoided for pregnant women and children. No firm guidelines exist for erythromycin dosing. If erythromycin is used, care should be taken to avoid underdosing and premature discontinuation to prevent relapse.

NOSOCOMIAL PNEUMONIA

Nosocomial pneumonia deserves special mention because of its frequency of occurrence, high incidence of morbidity and mortality, and different treatment approach. This infection also increases costs of care because of prolongation of hospitalization and expensive antibiotic and supportive therapy. The basic mechanisms involved in the pathogenesis of pneumonia that were previously discussed also apply in this setting. Colonization of the oropharyngeal cavity with Gram-negative bacilli with subsequent microaspiration of these organisms and inhalation of aerosolized organisms via respiratory equipment are the primary mechanisms resulting in nosocomial pneumonia. Table 63.4 lists factors associated with Gram-negative colonization of the oropharyngeal cavity. Hematogenous spread occurs less commonly. Patients who are cared for in the ICU and those who are receiving mechanical ventilation support are at greatest risk for the development of nosocomial pneumonia. It is estimated that 300,000 patients develop this infection each year (6). It is the second most common hospital-acquired infection, behind urinary tract infections, and carries an overall mortality rate

between 20 to 50%, making it the leading cause of death among the nosocomial infections (12, 14). The highest postoperative nosocomial pneumonia rates involve patients who have undergone thoracic or abdominal surgery, and the overall highest rates occur in patients who are receiving mechanical ventilation support in the ICU (6). Among nursing home patients, nosocomial pneumonia is one of the most common reasons for hospitalization.

Approximately 60% of nosocomial pneumonias are caused by aerobic Gram-negative bacilli; the remaining 40% are attributed to Gram-positive organisms, polymicrobial sources, or anaerobic pathogens (9, 49). A review of 15,499 isolates in the National Nosocomial Infection Study revealed that *Pseudomonas aeruginosa*, *Enterobacter* spp., *Klebsiella pneumoniae*, and *Staphylococcus aureus* were the most common pathogens associated with nosocomial pneumonia in the participating institutions (50). Pathogens arise primarily from overgrowth of the patient's endogenous flora or from exogenous sources via respiratory equipment and the hands of hospital personnel. In general, the etiology of nosocomial pneumonia is influenced by the patient's underlying illness, the type of unit in which care

Table 63.7.
Empiric Antibiotic Regimens for Nosocomial Pneumonia Based on Likely Pathogen, Severity, and Concurrent Illness

Mild to Moderate Pneumonia and No Underlying Diseases	Mild to Moderate Pneumonia with Risk Factors or Underlying Disease[a,b]	Severe Pneumonia

Common Pathogens
  S. aureus
  Klebsiella spp.
  Entrobacter spp.
  E. coli
  Proteus spp.
  H. influenzae
  Serratia marcescens
	Common Pathogen:
	PLUS:
	  Anaerobes
	  Legionella spp.
	  Pseudomonas aeruginosa[c,d]
		Common Pathogens
		PLUS:
		  Pseudomonas aeruginosa[c]

Empiric Treatment
  Cefazolin + gentamicin
  OR
Ampicillin/sulbactam
  OR
Second-generation cephalosporin:
  cefuroxime
  OR
Nonantipseudomonal third-generation
  cephalosporin:
cefotaxime or
ceftriaxone or
ceftizoxime
  OR
Fluoroquinolone:
ciprofloxacin or ofloxacin
	Empiric Treatment[b]
	  Add IV vancomycin (if MRSA is suspected)
	  Add clindamycin or
	  metronidazole + penicillin or
	  ampicillin/sulbactam (if anaerobes are suspected)
	  Add erythromycin (if Legionella spp. is suspected)
		Empiric Treatment[e]
		  Antipseudomonal penicillin (piperacillin,
		  azlocillin, mezlocillin, ticarcillin)
		  OR
		Antipseudomonal cephalosporin (ceftazidime)
		  OR
		Aztreonam
		  OR
		Imipenem/cilastatin
		  OR
		Fluoroquinolone (ciprofloxacin, ofloxacin)
		PLUS
		Aminoglycoside (gentamicin or tobramycin)

Source: From (55).
[a]Macroaspiration, thoracic or abdominal surgery, corticosteroid use, diabetes mellitus, coma, closed head injury.
[b]Includes previous regimens for common pathogens and additional coverage as listed.
[c]Risk factors for this organism include prolonged hospitalization, intensive care unit stay, prior course of antibiotics, and mechanical ventilation.
[d]Treat as severe pneumonia.
[e]Additional coverage against S. aureus, anaerobes, or Legionella spp. should be added if these pathogens are also suspected.

is being provided, unit and institutional antibiotic use, and the hospital's microbial flora and antibiotic sensitivity patterns. Reasonable empiric antibiotic treatments for nosocomial pneumonia can be found in Table 63.7.

Diagnosis of nosocomial pneumonia is usually made by the recognition of new or progressive infiltrates on chest radiograph, new onset of fever, leukocytosis, and cough or tracheal secretions containing purulent material. A sputum Gram stain and culture may be less reliable, owing to the presence of upper airway colonization. Blood, pleural fluid, and sputum for culture and Gram stain all may be used to determine the cause of infection and guide antimicrobial therapy. Diagnosis for the mechanically ventilated patient is even more challenging and may require the use of invasive procedures such as bronchoscopy using BAL or PSB or open lung biopsy for the immunosuppressed patient.

GRAM-NEGATIVE BACILLIARY PNEUMONIA

A multitude of Gram-negative organisms have been implicated as causes of nosocomial pneumonia, including the Enterobacteriaceae (*Klebsiella* spp., *Enterobacter* spp., *Escherichia coli*, *Proteus* spp., *Morganella* spp., *Serratia marcescens*, and *Providencia* spp.), *Pseudomonas aeruginosa*, *Acinetobacter* spp., and *Xanthomonas maltophillia*. *Pseudomonas aeruginosa* may be more common in patients with COPD and those receiving mechanical ventilation support (51). The clinician must often initiate empiric therapy before the pathogen has been identified.

Empiric treatment of Gram-negative bacillary pneumonia should take into account diagnostic information and the institution's antibiogram and should attempt to cover all likely pathogens. Microbial susceptibility patterns are different among institutions and may differ from unit to unit within the same institution. Therefore, one must keep in mind that no single antibiotic or combination of antibiotics is suitable for every clinical situation. If *P. aeruginosa* alone is suspected, an antipseudomonal β-lactam such as ticarcillin, piperacillin, or ceftazidime plus an aminoglycoside such as gentamicin or tobramycin is an acceptable first-choice regimen. Regimens that include an antipseudomonal β-lactam plus an aminoglycoside decrease the development of resistance and achieve a synergistic bactericidal effect. Because of a high mortality rate associated with *P. aeruginosa* pneumonia, therapy should be aggressive. Gentamicin or tobramycin may be administered as a 1 to 2 mg/kg loading dose (52) followed by a maintenance dosage to achieve peak serum concentrations of 6 mg/L and trough serum concentrations less than 2 mg/L. Aminoglycoside dosing should be based on the patient's weight, renal function, and serum concentration data. Alternatively, larger doses of aminoglycosides given over an extended interval (e.g., every 24 to 48 hr rather than every 8 hr) are appealing because they achieve

high therapeutic peak serum concentrations while allowing trough serum concentrations to fall below 2 mg/L before the next does is administered and because of the postantibiotic effect that aminoglycosides have against Gram-positive and Gram-negative bacteria. Several studies have described equal efficacy and less nephrotoxicity in once-a-day gentamicin dosing compared to an every 8 to 12 hr dosing regimen (53, 54).

Other antipseudomonal regimens include an aminoglycoside plus ofloxacin, ciprofloxacin, imipenem/cilastatin, or aztreonam. A quinolone combined with an antipseudomonal β-lactam or aminoglycoside is not a synergistic combination but may have additive effects against *P. aeruginosa*.

Double β-lactam combinations are undesirable because they do not achieve synergy and may induce β-lactamase production that easily inhibits both agents, leading to a quick development of resistance (55). The addition of the β-lactamase inhibitors clavulanic acid and tazobactam to ticarcillin and piperacillin, respectively, does not enhance their intrinsic activity against *P. aeruginosa*. Clavulanic acid and tazobactam lack affinity for the β-lactam that is responsible for the inactivation of enzymes produced by this organism. Therefore, ticarcillin/clavulanic acid and piperacillin/tazobactam are unnecessary if only infections caused by *P. aeruginosa* are being treated. However, they may be of benefit in treating resistant or polymicrobial infections caused by other β-lactamase producing Gram-negative bacilli and anaerobes.

Third-generation cephalosporins such as cefotaxime or ceftriaxone are acceptable choices for treating pneumonia caused by Gram-negative organisms unless *Enterobacter* spp., *P. aeruginosa*, or anaerobes are suspected. Pneumonia caused by *Enterobacter* spp. can usually be treated with ciprofloxacin alone or with an extended-spectrum penicillin, such as piperacillin, plus an aminoglycoside. The resistance of this organism is increasing in many hospitals, and third-generation cephalosporins, especially ceftazidime, should be avoided when *Enterobacter* spp. are suspected.

When reliable culture and sensitivity information is available, it should be used to guide antimicrobial therapy.

Staphylococcus aureus

Staphylococcus aureus is a coagulase-positive Gram-positive coccus that appears in clusters on the Gram stain. It has been implicated in up to 14% of nosocomial pneumonias (33) and usually results from either aspiration or hematogenous spread. It is most commonly seen in comatose patients and those with head trauma (55). Pneumonia caused by *Staphylococcus aureus* also occurs in the community setting after recovery from influenza. Patients typically exhibit an abrupt onset of fever, chills, dyspnea, pleuritic chest pain, cough productive of purulent sputum, and an elevated white blood cell count; approximately 20% of patients are bacteremic (26). A chest radiograph reveals multilobar infiltrates or bilateral involvement (26). Release of extracellular toxins by this organism can result in extensive lung tissue destruction, causing cavitation or a necrotizing pneumonia. Many strains of S. aureus produce penicillinase, which inactivates penicillin and so requires the use of an antistaphylococcal penicillin.

Intravenous nafcillin 1 to 2 g every 4 to 6 hr for 10 to 14 days is an effective first choice. If necrotizing pneumonia is present, therapy for up to 6 weeks may be necessary. Methicillin is not recommended because of an increased risk of interstitial nephritis. An intravenous first-generation cephalosporin such as cefazolin 1 g every 8 hr may also be an appropriate first choice when the level of staphylococcal resistance to methicillin is low or when culture and sensitivity data allows such a choice (19). If oral therapy is subsequently initiated, nafcillin should be avoided because of poor absorption. Dicloxacillin, cloxacillin, cephalexin, or cephradine may be used when oral therapy is desired. However, these agents will not effectively treat methicillin-resistant Staphyllococcus aureus (MRSA).

Intravenous vancomycin may be used for the patient who is allergic to penicillin and cephalosporin and should be the first choice when MRSA is cultured or strongly suspected. If MRSA growth has a high frequency in a particular unit or hospital, the clinician may opt to use intravenous vancomycin empirically until culture and sensitivity information indicates otherwise. Increasingly, vancomycin is the initial empiric choice for nosocomial pneumonia when S. aureus is suspected. Nevertheless, prudence is necessary in using this agent, primarily because of the emergence of vancomycin-resistant enterococci. The usual intravenous vancomycin dosage is 1 g every 12 to 24 hr, but the dose should be based on the patient's weight, renal function, and serum concentration data. Oral vancomycin is not well absorbed and is not effective for the treatment of systemic infections.

ASPIRATION PNEUMONIA AND LUNG ABSCESS

Aspiration of large amounts of oropharyngeal or gastric contents can introduce a significant number of pathogens into the lower airways, causing "aspiration" pneumonia. This event is termed macroaspiration, in contrast to microaspiration, which is the primary cause of other pneumonias. Because of the high incidence of anaerobic organisms causing these infections, the terms "aspiration pneumonia" and "anaerobic pneumonia" are often used synonymously.

Patients with seizure disorders, neurologic disorders, and lung cancer; stroke victims with dysphagia; alcoholics; drug abusers; debilitated elderly patients; and intubated patients, especially in the setting of periodontal disease, are at greatest risk for the development of aspiration pneumonia (Table 63.5). In addition, medications that cause sedation, reduce consciousness, or inhibit the cough reflex may predispose patients to macroaspiration leading to pneumonia. Aspiration pneumonia may occur in either the community or hospital setting and is usually a polymicrobial infection involving a variety of anaerobic and aerobic organisms. In the community setting a mixture of normal mouth anaerobic organisms predominates in as many as 88% of cases, while as few as 35% of anaerobic organisms are identified in nosocomial aspiration pneumonia (56). The role of anaerobes in community-acquired aspiration pneumonia may be overlooked because of the similarity of the presentation and Gram stain appearance of atypical and anaerobic pneumonia (57). In the hospital setting, several pathogens may be present, including Staphylococcal aureus, Gram-negative bacilli, and anaerobes.

Aspiration pneumonia has an insidious onset, and many patients do not seek medical attention until later in the course, after complications develop (57). Complications of aspiration pneumonia may be serious and include empyema or abscess resulting in necrosis of lung tissue. Patients usually present with a low-grade fever, a moderately increased white blood cell count, weight loss, and anemia. Cough becomes productive with putrid, foul-smelling sputum in up to 60% of patients after the development of abscess or empyema (57).

The chest radiograph appearance may reflect the patient's position at the time of the aspiration event and may also reveal abscess or cavitation. Involvement of the posterior segments of the upper lobes is usually consistent with aspiration in the recumbent position; lower lobe involvement generally indicates aspiration in the upright position (57). A sputum Gram stain reveals many PMNs and a variety of Gram-positive and Gram-negative organisms, usually mimicking the normal flora. For this reason, some investigators believe that a significant number of atypical pneumonia presentations may be unrecognized as anaerobic infections (57). Anaerobic pneumonia should be strongly suspected in the patient who presents with a slow onset of pneumonia symptoms and is at high risk for aspiration. The diagnosis of aspiration pneumonia is usually made on a presumptive basis because of the difficulty of obtaining appropriate specimens and the inability of most laboratories to perform antibiotic sensitivity testing for anaerobic organisms. In addition, aspiration pneumonia has historically responded to therapy when the appropriate empiric agent is selected. Several studies have identified Fusobacterium spp., Bacteroides melaninogenicus, and Peptostreptococcus spp. as the three most common pathogens associated with aspiration pneumonia (56, 57). Definitive diagnosis in these studies was made from uncontaminated specimens obtained by using a variety of invasive procedures. Other anaerobic organisms, microaerophilic streptococci, and aerobic streptococci also play an important role in these infections and should also be covered by empiric therapy.

Treatment of aspiration pneumonia involves the appropriate antibiotic and drainage of the abscess or empyema when present. Penicillin V covers most anaerobes that exist above the diaphragm and aerobic and microaerophilic streptococci that cause aspiration pneumonia. Early trials showed that oral penicillin V 3 g/day was as effective as aqueous penicillin G and established penicillin as the drug of choice for aspiration pneumonia (57). More recently, up to 55% of *Fusobacterium* spp. and *B. melaninogenicus* have been identified in vitro to produce β-lactamase and exhibit resistance to penicillin (57).

Clindamycin is active against most staphylococci, streptococci, and anaerobes, including β-lactamase-producing *B. fragilis* and other *Bacteroides* spp., thus making it a more attractive treatment choice for anaerobic pneumonia. Several studies have demonstrated a higher number of treatment failures and relapses with penicillin compared to clindamycin (58, 59). For these reasons, intravenous clindamycin 600 every 8 hr or 300 to 450 mg every 6 hr orally has become the regimen of first choice of most clinicians.

Metronidazole is also a very effective antibiotic against anaerobic pathogens, including β-lactamase producers. However, treatment failures have been encountered with this agent, most likely because of its inability to cover microaerophilic and aerobic streptococci. Hence, if metronidazole is used, it should be combined with penicillin to cover these additional organisms.

Lung abscess and empyema are usually treated initially with parenteral agents and surgical drainage until the patient is afebrile. A prolonged course of oral therapy with clindamycin or metronidazole plus penicillin V for 4 to 6 weeks is necessary until complete resolution or stabilization of the chest radiograph, which may take longer than 10 weeks (57). Patients should be counseled that adequate treatment duration and compliance are important to prevent relapse. For patients with nosocomial aspiration pneumonia, empiric antibiotic therapy should cover anaerobes and Gram-negative bacilli. A logical empiric treatment option would be a third-generation cephalosporin such as ceftriaxone or cefotaxime plus clindamycin. Intravenous vancomycin should be added if there is a high prevalence MRSA in the setting where the patient develops aspiration pneumonia.

CONCLUSION

Despite the availability of newer antibiotics and improved diagnostic methods, pneumonia remains an infectious disease that causes significant morbidity and mortality. In the United States, CAP occurs in approximately 4 million people and nosocomial pneumonia occurs in approximately 300,000 patients each year.

The biggest challenge confronting the clinician is identifying the causative organism and selecting the proper antibiotic. An adequate history is important in guiding empiric therapy and should describe the clinical setting of the pneumonia, any host defense defects, and any exposure to specific pathogens. The chest radiograph and sputum Gram stain along with clinical and laboratory signs and symptoms are the primary tools that are used for diagnosing pneumonia and determining the cause.

Empiric antimicrobial therapy should usually cover a broad spectrum and must take into account the setting of the pneumonia (community-acquired or nosocomial), as well as variations in institutional and geographical bacterial susceptibility patterns. Once the causative organism has ben reliably identified through culture and sensitivity testing, therapy may be streamlined to a narrow-spectrum, cost-effective agent.

REFERENCES

1. Mandell LA. Antibiotics for pneumonia therapy. Med Clin North Am 78(5):997–1014, 1994.
2. Osler W. The principles and practice of medicine. 4th ed. New York: D. Appleton, 1901:108.
3. Marrie TJ. Community acquired pneumonia. Clin Infect Dis 18:501–15, 1994.
4. American Thoracic Society. Guidelines for the initial management of adults with community acquired pneumonia: diagnosis, assessment of severity, and initial antimicrobial therapy. Am Rev Respir Dis 148:1418–26, 1993.
5. Paz HL, Wood CA. Pneumonia and chronic obstructive pulmonary disease. Postgrad Med 90(5):77–86, 1991.
6. Winter JH. The scope of lower respiratory tract infection. Infection 19(suppl 7):359–64, 1991.
7. Busse WW. Pathogenesis and sequalae of respiratory infections. Rev Infect Dis 13(suppl 6):477–85, 1991.
8. Mullenix TA, Prince RA. Lower respiratory tract infections. In: Herfindal ET, Gourley DR, Hart LL, eds. Clinical pharmacy and therapeutics. 5th ed. Baltimore: Williams & Wilkins, 1992:1080–91.
9. Stratton CW. Bacterial pneumonias: an overview with emphasis on pathogenesis, diagnosis, and treatment. Heart Lung 15(3):226–44, 1986.
10. Johanson WG. Introduction to pneumonia. In: Wyngaarden JB, Smith LH, Bennett JC, eds. Cecil textbook of medicine. 19th ed. Philadelphia: WB Saunders, 1992:409–13.
11. Thompson R. Prevention of nosocomial pneumonia. Med Clin North Am 78(5):1185–95, 1994.
12. Craven DE, Steger KA, Barat LM, et al. Nosocomial pneumonia: epidemiology and infection control. Intensive Care Med 18(suppl): 3–9, 1992.
13. Heyland D, Mandell LA. Gastric colonization by Gram-negative bacilli and nosocomial pneumonia in the intensive care unit patient: evidence for causation. Chest 101(1):187–92, 1992.
14. Scheld WM, Mandell GL. Nosocomial pneumonia: pathogenesis and recent advances in diagnosis and therapy. Rev Infect Dis 13 (suppl 9):43–51, 1991.
15. Driks MR, Craven DE, Celli BR, et al. Nosocomial pneumonia in intubated patients given sucralfate as compared with antacids or histamine type 2 blockers. N Engl J Med 317:1376–82, 1987.

16. Hamer DH, Barza M. Prevention of hospital-acquired pneumonia in critically ill patients. Antimicrob Agents Chemother 37(5):931–38, 1993.

17. LaForce FM. Bacterial pneumonia. In: Gorbach SL, Bartlett JG, Blacklow NR, eds. Infectious diseases. Philadelphia: WB Saunders, 1992.

18. Bartlett JG. Aspiration pneumonia. In: Gorbach SL, Bartlett JG, Blacklow NR, eds. Infectious diseases. Philadelphia: WB Saunders, 1992.

19. Donowitz GR, Mandell GL. Acute pneumonia. In: Mandell GL, Douglas RG, Bennett JE. Principles and practice of infectious diseases. 4th ed, vol 1. New York: Churchill Livingstone, 1995:619–32, 1769.

20. Stein D. Managing pneumonia acquired in nursing homes: special concerns. Geriatrics 45(3):39–47, 1990.

21. Cluff LE, Johnson JE. Pneumonia. In: Cluff LE, Johnson JE, eds. Clinical concepts of infectious diseases. Baltimore: Williams & Wilkins, 1972.

22. Lode H, Schaberg T, Raffenberg M, et al. Diagnostic problems in lower respiratory tract infections. J Antimicrob Chemother 32(suppl A):29–37, 1993.

23. Campbell GD. Overview of community acquired pneumonia: prognosis and clinical features. Med Clin North Am 78(5):1035–47, 1994.

24. Whitson B, Campbell GD. Community-acquired pneumonia: new outpatient guidelines based on age, severity of illness. Geriatrics 49(3):24–36, 1994.

25. Brown RB. Community-acquired pneumonia: diagnosis and therapy of older adults. Geriatrics 48(2):43–50, 1993.

26. Marrie TJ. Pneumonia. Clin Geriatr Med 8(4):721–34, 1992.

27. Levy M, Dromer F, Brion N, et al. Community-acquired pneumonia: importance of initial noninvasive bacteriologic and radiologic investigations. Chest 92(1):43–8, 1988.

28. Fein AM, Niederman MS. Severe pneumonia in the elderly. Clin Geriatr Med 10(1):121–42, 1994.

29. Murray PR, Washington JA. Microscopic and bacteriologic analysis of expectorated sputum. Mayo Clin Proc 50:339–44, 1975.

30. Aoun M, Klastersky J. Drug treatment in the hospital: what are the choices? Drugs 42(6):962–73, 1991.

31. McCormack JP, Jewesson PJ. A critical re-evaluation of the "therapeutic range" of aminoglycosides. Clin Infect Dis 14:320–39, 1992.

32. Moore RD, Smith CR, Lietman PS. Association of aminoglycoside plasma levels with therapeutic outcome in Gram-negative pneumonia. Am J Med 77:657–62, 1984.

33. Reed MD, Witte MK. Lower respiratory tract infections. In: DiPiro JT, Talbert RL, Hayes PE, et al., eds. Pharmacotherapy: a pathophysiological approach. 2nd ed. Norwalk, CT: Appleton & Lange, 1993:1543–59.

34. Marrie TJ. New aspects of old pathogens of pneumonia. Med Clin North Am 78(5):987–93, 1994.

35. Centers for Disease Control and Prevention. Resistant Streptococcus pneumoniae: Kentucky and Tennessee. MMWR 43:23–31, 1994.

36. Haas DW, Stratton CW, Griffin JP. Diminished activity of ceftizoxime in comparison to cefotaxime and ceftriaxone against Streptococcus pneumoniae. Clin Infect Dis 20:671–76, 1995.

37. Hedlund JU, Kalin ME, Ortqvist AB, et al. Antibody response to pneumococcal vaccine in middle-aged and elderly patients recently treated for pneumonia. Arch Intern Med 154:1961–65, 1994.

38. Sims RV, Steinmann WC, McConville JH, et al. The clinical effectiveness of pneumococcal vaccine in the elderly. Ann Intern Med 108:653–57, 1988.

39. Shapiro ED, Berg AT, Austrian R, et al. The protective efficacy of polyvalent pneumococcal polysaccharide vaccine. N Engl J Med 325(21):1453–60, 1991.

40. Moxon ER, Wilson R. The role of Haemophilus influenzae in the pathogenesis of pneumonia. Rev Infect Dis 13(suppl 6):518–26, 1991.

41. McEvoy GK, Litvak K, Welsh OH, et al. AHFS drug information. Bethesda, MD: American Society of Hospital Pharmacists, 1994:208.

42. Verghese A, Berk SL. Moraxella (Branhamella) catarrhalis. Infect Dis Clin North Am 5(3):523–35, 1991.

43. Hampson NB, Woolf RA, Springmeyer SC. Oral antibiotics for pneumonia. Clin Chest Med 12(2):395–407, 1991.

44. Cunha BA. Atypical pneumonias: clinical diagnosis and empirical treatment. Postgrad Med 90(5):89–101, 1991.

45. Martin RE, Bates JH. Atypical pneumonia. Infect Dis Clin North Am 5(3):585–601, 1991.

46. Clyde WA Jr. Clinical overview of typical Mycoplasma pneumoniae infections. Clin Infect Dis 17(Suppl 1):32–6, 1993.

47. Lynch JP. Community-acquired pneumonia: what new trends mean in practice. J Resp Dis 13(11):1619–43, 1992.

48. Saikku P. The epidemiology and significance of Chlamydia pneumoniae. J Infect Dis 25(suppl 1):27–34, 1992.

49. Meduri GU. Diagnosis of ventilator-associated pneumonia. Infect Dis Clin North Am 7(2):295–325, 1993.

50. Horan T, Culver D, Jarvis W, et al. Pathogens causing nosocomial infections. CDC: The antimicrobial newsletter 5:65–7, 1988.

51. Silver DR, Cohen IL, Weinberg PF. Recurrent Pseudomonas aeruginosa pneumonia in an intensive care unit. Chest 101(1):194–98, 1992.

52. Chelluri L, Warren J, Jastremski MS. Pharmacokinetics of a 3 mg/kg body weight loading dose of gentamicin in critically ill patients. Chest 95(6):1295–97, 1989.

53. Prins JM, Buller HR, Kuijper EJ, et al. Once versus thrice daily gentamicin in patients with serious infections. Lancet 341:335–39, 1993.

54. Nicolau DP, Belliveau PP, Nightingale CH, et al. Implementation of a once-daily aminoglycoside program in a large community teaching hospital. Hosp Pharm 30(8):674–76, 679–80, 1995.

55. Niedderman MS. An approach to empiric therapy of nosocomial pneumonia. Med Clin North Am 78(5):1123–39, 1994.

56. Lorber B, Swenson RM. Bacteriology of aspiration pneumonia: A prospective study of community- and hospital-acquired cases. Ann Intern Med 81:329–31, 1974.

57. Bartlett JG. Anaerobic bacterial infections of the lungs and pleural space. Clin Infect Dis 16(suppl 4):248–55, 1993.

58. Gudiol F, Manresa F, Pallares R, et al. Clindamycin versus penicillin for anaerobic lung infections: high rate of penicillin failures associated with penicillin-resistant Bacteroides melaninogenicus. Arch Intern Med 150:2525–29, 1990.

59. Levison ME, Mangura CT, Lorber B, et al. Clindamycin compared with penicillin for the treatment of anaerobic lung abscess. Ann Intern Med 98:466–71, 1983.

CHAPTER 64

TUBERCULOSIS

CAROLINE S. ZEIND, GRETA K. GOURLEY, and CATHY E. CORBETT

Tuberculosis (TB) has emerged as the single leading cause of death from any single infectious agent (1). An estimated one-third of the world's population is latently infected with *Mycobacterium tuberculosis,* the causative agent of tuberculosis (1, 2). The resurgence of tuberculosis in the United States is due to many factors, including the human immunodeficiency virus (HIV) pandemic, a degeneration in the health care infrastructure, and increases in the number of cases reported among foreign-born people (3). The progressive and ultimately profound reduction in cell-mediated immunity that HIV infection causes is considered to be the most powerful risk factor for the activation of latent *M. tuberculosis* infection (4). The rising prevalence of multidrug-resistant tuberculosis (MDR-TB) in the United States is a serious concern (2, 5, 6). The majority of outbreaks of MDR-TB have involved people who are infected with HIV (6). Patient noncompliance with drug treatment for *M. tuberculosis* is a major cause of relapse and drug resistance (7). Adherence to the recommendations for the treatment of tuberculosis among adults and children that were provided in a joint statement of the American Thoracic Society (ATS) and the Centers for Disease Control and Prevention (CDC) will help to prevent the development of more cases of MDR-TB, reduce the occurrence of treatment failure, and reduce the transmission of tuberculosis in the United States (8).

ETIOLOGY

Mycobacterium tuberculosis, or the tubercle bacillus, is a member of the genus Mycobacteriaceae, order Actinomycetales. It, along with *M. bovis* and *M. Africanum,* which are also species of this order, cause tuberculosis in humans. Currently, disease due to *M. bovis* and *M. Africanum* is rare in the United States (9, 10).

M. tuberculosis infects humans, other primates, and other mammalians that are in contact with humans. The only reservoir of the organism, however, is humans (9).

The bacilli are aerobic rods, which are slow growing (4 to 6 weeks) and acid-fast. Because of these latter characteristics, identification and susceptibility testing took several weeks in the recent past. Time for these processes has been reduced significantly with the advent of radiometric testing (9). Acute infection is generally present when *M. tuberculosis* is cultured, whereas identification of

other microorganisms may simply depict colonization or disease process (11).

INCIDENCE

The incidence of TB in the United States in 1993 was 26,287 cases (9.8 cases per 100,000 population). This represented a 5.2% decrease from 1992 (26,673; 10.5 cases per 100,000) but a 14% increase over 1985 (22,201). The 1985 rate represents the lowest number of TB cases since 1953, when national reporting was started. The 33 states that reported fewer cases in 1993 included California, New York, and Texas. Before 1993 these three states had reported the greatest increase in cases since 1985 (12, 13).

The demographics of sex and age group are similar to those in 1989. Males are reported to contract the disease at a rate that is two times higher than that of females. Risk is lowest in the 5- to 14-year-old age group. Case reports are greatest in non-Hispanic whites in the 65 or older age group. Among minorities the greatest number of cases is seen in the 26- to 44-year-old age group (13).

In 1993, foreign-born individuals represented approximately one-third (29.1%) of tuberculosis cases in the United States. This represents a 6.5% increase over 1987. Of these people, 38% were from Mexico and 45% were from Asia. These figures represent a 2% and a 9% increase over 1987 statistics, respectively. The percent of cases of tuberculosis in the 65-year-old age group in 1993 was 23%. This represents a 6.7% decrease since 1982 (11, 13).

Some of the factors contributing to the 14% increase or resurgence of tuberculosis between 1985 and 1993 were identified in the introduction. Possible reasons cited by the CDC for the decrease of 5.2% for reported TB cases in 1993 include:

1. effectiveness of prevention and control measures implemented during 1989 to 1993,
2. delayed reporting due to use of the new surveillance reporting form and change to a computerized data system, and
3. underreporting because of modification of the acquired immunodeficiency syndrome (AIDS) surveillance case definition in January 1993 (12).

TRANSMISSION IN THE 1990s

The long-held concept that only 10% of tuberculosis cases are the result of recent infection, the rest being due to reactivation of a latent infection, is being reconsidered (13). It is becoming apparent that more tuberculosis cases now are due to recent infection. Two studies, one from San Francisco and the other from New York City, have found that more than 30% of today's tuberculosis cases are the result of recent infection (15, 16). In both studies, the authors used DNA fingerprinting to distinguish recently acquired infections due to *M. tuberculosis* from remote latent infections. Recent infections were inferred in cases with the same DNA fingerprinting pattern that appeared in a particular cluster. Small and colleagues analyzed DNA fingerprints of isolates from 473 patients with tuberculosis and found that 191 appeared to have active tuberculosis due to recent infection. Forty-four clusters were identified, 20 of which consisted of only two people and the largest of which consisted of 30 people. Clearly, a single patient can cause dozens of active cases; one of the index patients apparently infected 29 other patients, accounting for 16% of tuberculosis cases. Recent infection accounted for 31% of TB cases reported to the city's public health department from 1991 to 1992 (15). Alland and colleagues analyzed DNA fingerprints of isolates from 104 patients and identified 39 patients who had recently acquired infections. These patients belonged to 12 clusters. In this inner-city community, recently transmitted tuberculosis accounted for approximately 40% of cases between 1989 and 1992 (16). As these two studies demonstrate, recent infection contributes significantly to the increase in tuberculosis in the 1990s.

Several risk factors for recent tuberculosis infection have been identified. Recent studies found that nearly two-thirds of the patients with HIV or AIDS had clustered strains (15-17).

HIV infection not only appears to dramatically increase susceptibility to acquiring tuberculosis infection but also involves a rapid accelerated progression from infection to disease (18, 19). Daley and colleagues studied an outbreak of tuberculosis using DNA fingerprinting that occurred in an HIV residential facility. In only 5 months, 12 cases of tuberculosis were diagnosed among 31 residents; one patient developed active disease within 4 weeks after exposure. Approximately 50% of those who were exposed developed either a newly positive skin test (13%) or active disease (37%). In contrast, of 28 staff members with possible exposure, 6 seroconverted but none developed active disease (19).

In addition, exogenous reinfection with *M. tuberculosis* is more likely to occur in patients with AIDS. Small and colleagues analyzed DNA fingerprinting on serial positive isolates of *M. tuberculosis* on 17 patients in New York City after the institution of drug therapy (6). In four of the patients the serial DNA fingerprint patterns showed dramatic changes, indicating exogenous reinfection. Furthermore, the reinfecting strain was identical, indicating

probable recent infection from a common source (6). Exogenous reinfection with *M. tuberculosis* can no doubt occur either during therapy for the original infection or following completion of drug therapy.

PATHOGENESIS

Tuberculosis is nearly always transmitted through the air by infectious particles called droplet nuclei. When a person with active pulmonary or laryngeal tuberculosis coughs, sneezes, speaks, or sings, these particles are emitted in droplets that can remain suspended in the air for several hours. Transmission may occur if another person inhales the droplet nuclei. Three factors determine the probability that tuberculosis will be transmitted: (a) the infectiousness of the person with tuberculosis, (b) the environment in which the exposure occurred, and (c) the duration of the exposure. The upper respiratory tract is the body's first line of defense against the transmission of tuberculosis. Therefore, most immunocompetent people who are exposed to tuberculosis do not become infected. Particles smaller than five microns in diameter may reach the alveoli, and infection may begin. The bacilli are initially ingested and multiply within the alveolar macrophages and then are spread throughout the body by the lymphatic and circulatory systems (see Figure 64.1) (11, 20). Within 2 to 10 weeks after infection, a healthy immune system intervenes, halting the multiplication of the bacterium and preventing further spread. This cell-mediated response is manifested by the delayed-type hypersensitivity reaction of the purified protein derivative (PPD) skin test. Most people who are infected with tuberculosis will have a positive reaction to the PPD skin test within 2 to 10 weeks after infection, a condition known as latent infection. Cell-mediated immunity effectively contains the infection in 90% of immunocompetent people, and no clinical disease develops. In the remaining 10%, half will develop disease within the first year or two because of ineffective immunity, and the other half will develop disease later in life (20).

HIV infection has dramatically altered the natural history of tuberculosis because of its profound effects on cell-mediated immunity. HIV infection favors the development of acute infection with *M. tuberculosis* because of poor control of initial infection. It appears that in most HIV-infected people, *M. tuberculosis* may be due to recent transmission rather than reactivation of a latent infection (21). It is also clear that HIV infection is the most potent risk factor for the development of active tuberculosis among people who were previously infected with *M. tuberculosis*. AIDS patients have a 170 times greater risk for the development of active tuberculosis than do people who have no known risk factor (22). In comparison to the 10% lifetime risk among people who have tuberculosis

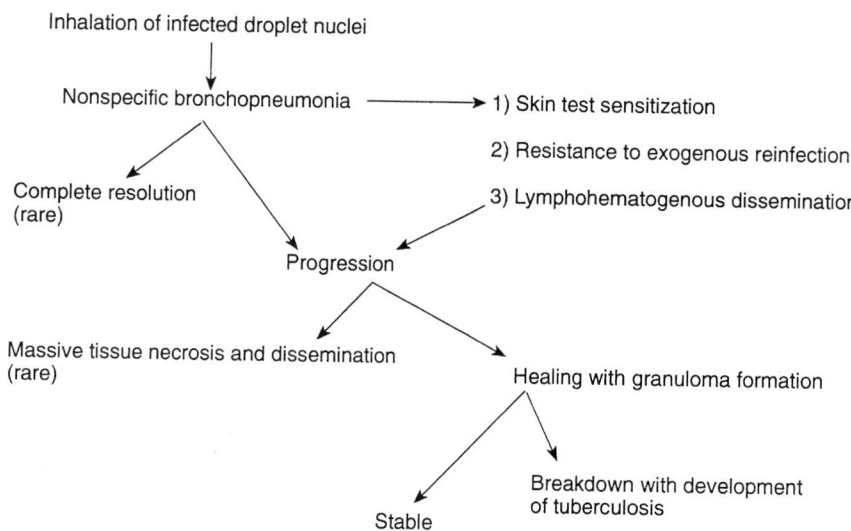

Figure 64.1. Results of infection with *M. tuberculosis*. (Source: From Hooker KD, Jost PM. Tuberculosis. Chapter 62. In: Herfindal ET, Gourley DR, Hart LL, eds. Tuberculosis in Clinical Pharmacy and Therapeutics, 5th edition. Baltimore: Williams & Wilkins, 1992, pp. 1093.)

infection without HIV infection, HIV-infected people develop reactivation disease at a rate of 8% per year (23). In light of these findings, pulmonary tuberculosis was added to the list of indicator diseases in the 1993 AIDS Surveillance case definition.

IDENTIFICATION OF INDIVIDUALS WITH TB INFECTION

The Mantoux tuberculin skin testing is the standard method of identification of individuals with *M. tuberculosis* infection. It is the intradermal injection of purified protein derivative (PPD) of killed tubercle bacilli, usually on the inner forearm. The reaction to the Mantoux test should be examined by a trained health care worker 48 to 72 hr after the injection for induration (20).

A tuberculin reaction of ≥5 mm of induration is considered positive for the highest-risk groups, which include people with HIV infection, people who have had close contact with a person with infectious tuberculosis, people who have chest radiographs that are consistent with previous tuberculosis, and injecting drug users whose HIV status is not known. A tuberculin reaction of ≥10 mm of induration is considered positive for other high-risk groups, which include people who have several medical conditions that increase the risk that tuberculosis will progress to disease. Such conditions include HIV infection, substance abuse, diabetes, silicosis, prolonged systemic corticosteriod therapy, hematologic and reticuloendothelial disease, end-stage renal disease, chronic malabsorption syndromes, intestinal bypass or gastrectomy, or low body weight (≥10% below ideal body weight). Other high-risk groups are injecting drug users who are HIV seronegative; foreign-born people who come from high-prevalence areas (such as Latin America, Asia, and Africa); residents of long-term care settings (such as nursing homes, mental institutions, and correctional facilities); medically underserved, low-income populations, including high-risk racial and ethnic groups (such as Blacks, Native Americans, Asians and Hispanics); local populations who have been identified as high-prevalence groups (such as homeless people or farm workers); and children in one of the high-risk groups noted above. A tuberculin reaction of ≥15 mm of induration is considered positive for individuals who have no known risk factors for tuberculosis (20).

Health care providers should identify individuals who are in high-risk groups, and tuberculin skin testing should be included as part of their routine evaluation. Individuals who have a positive reaction once active disease is excluded should be considered for preventive therapy (20).

ANERGY

A negative reaction to the tuberculin skin test does not rule out tuberculosis infection or disease. In the immunosuppressed person, delayed-type hypersensitivity responses may disappear. This state, known as anergy, can be seen in people with overwhelming miliary or pulmonary tuberculosis, in the administration of immunosuppressive agents or corticosteroids, or in HIV infections and other conditions. Approximately, 10 to 25% of people with tuberculosis are anergic. Furthermore, approximately one-third of people with HIV infection and more than 60% of people with AIDS may have skin test reactions <5 mm even though they are infected with *M. tuberculosis* (20).

Because of the occurrence of anergy to PPD among people with HIV infection, they should be evaluated for delayed-type hypersensitivity anergy at the time of PPD testing. Companion testing with two delayed-type hypersensitivity antigens is recommended. In general, people who mount a delayed-type hypersensitivity response have a negative PPD reaction and are considered not to be infected with *M. tuberculosis*. Individuals who show no evidence of delayed-type hypersensitivity responsiveness and are tuberculin negative should also be considered for isoniazid prevention therapy, which involves an estimated ≥10% risk of tuberculous infection (24).

MULTIDRUG-RESISTANT TUBERCULOSIS (MDR-TB)

MDR-TB is defined as a case of tuberculosis caused by a strain of M. tuberculosis that exhibits resistance to two or more antituberculosis agents (2). The emergence of drug-resistant tuberculosis in New York City was noted by Frieden and colleagues (25). The authors examined drug resistance in 466 isolates (90%) available from 518 patients with positive cultures for M. tuberculosis during April 1991. Overall, 33% had isolates that were resistant to at least one drug. Of these, 26% of isolates were resistant to isoniazid, 22% to rifampin, and 19% to both drugs. In the 239 patients who had been previously treated, 44% of isolates were resistant to at least one drug. In the 227 patients who had never been treated, 23% of isolates were resistant to at least one drug. Such resistance was only 10% in 1982 to 1984 (25). This problem with MDR-TB is occurring throughout the United States.

The CDC has noticed several factors that have contributed to several outbreaks of MDR-TB in hospitals and correctional facilities from 1990 through 1992 (26, 27). Mortality among these patients was extraordinarily high, ranging from 43% to 89%. In addition, the median interval from diagnosis to death was very short, only 4 to 16 weeks. Some of these factors include patient noncompliance with therapy, suboptimal treatment regimens, overall poor response to therapy when both INH and rifampin resistance is present, prolonged infectiousness, severe immunosuppression, inadequate infection control measures, and susceptible contacts in the same area as increased numbers of tuberculosis patients (26, 27).

The first three factors were emphasized by Goble and colleagues, who retrospectively reviewed treatment of 171 patients with pulmonary tuberculosis that was resistant to INH and rifampin (28). This largely immunocompetent group had the disease for a median of six years and received a median of six antituberculous drugs. All patients were noted to have an isolate that was resistant to a median of six drugs. Despite individually tailored regimens, an overall response rate of only 56% was seen. Rifampin resistance was associated with suboptimal or irregular dosing and/or the administration of rifampin as the single effective agent (28). The prolonged infectiousness of inadequately treated patients with MDR-TB is associated with AFB sputum smear positivity and higher numbers of tuberculin-positive contacts than susceptible tuberculosis cases (29, 30). Thus, transmissibility is higher, as has been noted in nosocomial outbreaks.

The last three factors were emphasized in a study by Edlin and colleagues that evaluated an outbreak of MDR-TB among hospitalized patients with AIDS (31). The authors compared exposure among 18 AIDS patients who had developed MDR-TB with that among 30 controls who had contracted a susceptible strain of tuberculosis. The patients with MDR-TB were more likely to have been hospitalized on the same ward and in rooms near patients with infectious drug-resistant tuberculosis. In addition, of 16 patient rooms that were tested with air flow studies, only one had the recommended negative pressure ventilation (31).

CLINICAL FEATURES AND DIAGNOSIS

The majority of cases of tuberculosis are pulmonary. The symptoms of pulmonary tuberculosis include a productive cough, chest pain, and hemoptysis. Systemic symptoms include fever, night sweats, chills, easy fatigability, anorexia, and weight loss. Approximately 15% of tuberculosis cases are extrapulmonary, and the specific symptoms depend on the site of involvement. For a person who is suspected of having tuberculosis, a medical evaluation should include a medical history, including assessing whether the patient has medical conditions, especially HIV infection, that increase the risk for tuberculosis disease; a physical examination; a tuberculin skin test; a chest radiograph; and appropriate bacteriologic or histologic examinations. When extrapulmonary tuberculosis is suspected, a variety of clinical specimens other than sputum (e.g., urine, cerebrospinal fluid, pleural fluid, pus, or biopsy specimens) may be needed for examination (20).

The clinical features of tuberculosis that occur in HIV-infected patients vary depending on the severity of underlying immunosupression (32, 33). The earlier tuberculosis develops in the HIV-infected patient, the more "typical" its clinical presentation; the later it occurs, the more "atypical" its features (34).

Theur and colleagues compared the clinical features of tuberculosis in HIV-seropositive and seronegative patients and found that the site of disease, drug toxicity, and relapse rate did not differ significantly (32). Tuberculosis was the first clinical manifestation of cellular immunodeficiency in 88% of seropositive patients, the median absolute CD4+ lymphocyte count being 327/mm^3. It is thought that tuberculosis tends to occur early in the course of HIV infection, presumably because of its relative virulence. The lungs were the most frequent site of disease in both groups. Extrapulmonary disease was noted with equal frequency in both groups; however, only seronegative patients had only extrapulmonary tuberculosis. The most frequent extrapulmonary sites of disease in the seropositive group were the lymph nodes and the genitourinary system. In the seronegative group, the pleura and meninges were the most frequent extrapulmonary sites of disease. Tuberculin skin test results at the time of diagnosis did not appear impaired, despite HIV infection; 80% of the HIV seropositive patients tested had a tuberculin reaction of 9 mm or more, as did 90% of seronegative patients. No difference was noted between the two groups in smear and culture positivity of initial sputum, and no significant differences in time to sputum conversion were noted. Radiographic findings for patients with HIV infection were not distinguishable from those patients who were seronegative. Seropositive patients responded well to standard antituberculosis chemotherapy, and the frequency of adverse reactions to drug therapy did not differ significantly. Therefore, it appears that HIV-related tuberculosis is "typical" in its clinical features when it presents in the less immunocompromised state, as was noted in this study (32).

The "atypical" clinical presentation of tuberculosis in AIDS patients versus non-AIDS patients was clearly demonstrated by Chaisson and colleagues (33). Although the lungs remained the most frequent site of involvement in both groups, 60% of the AIDS group had at least one extrapulmonary site of disease compared to 28% of the non-AIDS group. In the AIDS group, the most common sites of extrapulmonary involvement were lymphatic (31%), urogenital (14%), bone marrow or blood (both 11%), and musculoskeletal (9%), the central nervous system, skin, and soft tissue each accounting for 3% of cases. Nonsignificant tuberculosis skin tests were seen more commonly in the AIDS group. Chest radiographs showed predominantly diffuse or miliary infiltrates in the AIDS group but predominantly focal infiltrates and/or cavitation in the non-AIDS group. A generally favorable response to treatment was seen, and although adverse drug reactions were seen more frequently in the AIDS group, no treatment failures occurred due to drug intolerance. Overall survival, however, was exceedingly poor, though death was almost always due to other complications of AIDS (33).

What about the HIV-infected patient with MDR-TB? Fischl and associates compared in HIV-infected patients the clinical presentation and outcome of 62 patients with MDR-TB diagnosed from 1988 through 1990 with 55 control patients with drug-susceptible or monoresistant isolates (35). Overall, patients with MDR-TB were more likely to have an AIDS-defining illness (76%) than controls were (29%) and were more likely to have widely disseminated disease. Cases were almost three times more likely to have both pulmonary and extrapulmonary disease than controls were. The presence of more widely disseminated disease was felt to reflect acquisition of tuberculosis late in the course of HIV infection with overwhelming miliary spread without the constraints of an adequate immune response. In further support of this were that histopatho-

logic features noted during autopsies showed overwhelming miliary disease with extensive necrosis, poor or absent granuloma formation, marked inflammatory changes with a predominance of neutrophils at all stages of necrosis, microabscesses, and numerous acid-fast bacilli. Of the 62 patients with MDR-TB, 4% converted to smear negative and 84% had persistently or intermittently positive smears. Patients with MDR-TB were more likely on initial chest radiograph to have had alveolar infiltrates, interstitial infiltrates with a reticular pattern, and cavitation. For MDR-TB cases the median survival time from the time of diagnosis of tuberculosis was 2.1 months, compared with 14.6 months in the drug-susceptible controls. The highest number of fatalities was noted in those patients who had AIDS and MDR-TB, the median survival time in this group being only 1.5 months, compared to 14.8 months in those without AIDS and MDR-TB (35).

CHEMOTHERAPEUTIC STRATEGIES

The availability of antituberculous agents has revolutionized the prognosis of patients with tuberculosis and tuberculosis infection (36). Streptomycin was introduced for the management of tuberculosis during the 1940s. It soon became apparent that streptomycin monotherapy frequently resulted in treatment failure that was associated with in vitro resistance to the drug (37, 38). In the 1950s and 1960s, isoniazid and aminosalicylic acid were combined with streptomycin in a regimen that cured tuberculosis in nearly all patients. Treatment programs were very successful because they were carried out in hospitals, where compliance could be ensured. As a consequence, acquired drug resistance was uncommon. During the late 1960s, therapy was shifted to the outpatient setting. Unfortunately, reduced compliance to antituberculous regimens in the outpatient setting has led to rising rates of treatment failure, relapse, and acquired drug resistance (39-44).

Most patients with tuberculosis can be cured with adherence to chemotherapeutic regimens (36). The goal of drug therapy of active tuberculosis is twofold: (a) to cure the sick and (b) to impede the transmission of tubercle bacilli in the community. In people with tuberculosis infection, isoniazid therapy prevents disease in the treated person while sparing others the potential of becoming infected from contact with that person (8). On the basis of controlled clinical trials, three basic principles for the treatment of tuberculosis (disease) have evolved: (a) regimens for treatment of disease must contain multiple drugs to which the organisms are susceptible, (b) the drugs must be taken regularly, and (c) drug therapy must continue for a sufficient period of time (8, 45). The aim of therapy is to provide the most efficacious regimen with the least toxicity possible for the shortest period of time.

Three subpopulations of the tubercle bacilli can potentially coexist during an infection (9). Antituberculous agents are targeted toward various sites of mycobacterial growth in the body (Table 64.1) (11). The most numerous population consists of extracellular bacteria; these organisms are killed most readily by isoniazid and streptomycin and to a lesser extent by rifampin. The second population is composed of organisms that seek out the acidic environment of caseating granulomas. Rifampin exhibits the greatest activity in killing these organisms. The final population of organisms exists within the activated macrophages (intracellular). Because of the acidic environment within macrophages, the activity of most antituberculous agents is inhibited. Pyrazinamide possesses the greatest activity against this population.

Current antituberculous regimens use combinations of agents to eliminate extracellular organisms from the sputum, decrease infectivity, and destroy slowly dividing organisms within granulomas and macrophages (46-48). By combining various agents, regimens as short as 6 months' duration can be used while minimizing drug resistance.

Microbial resistance to antituberculous agents may be classified as either initial or secondary (8). Initial resistance occurs in patients who have not received previous antituberculous therapy. Various risk factors for initial resistance include coming from a country with a high prevalence of drug-resistant tuberculosis, exposure to a patient with drug-resistant tuberculosis, and greater than 4% primary resistance to isoniazid within the community. Secondary resistance occurs in patients who have been treated with antituberculous agents in the past. The quality of tuberculosis treatment programs will affect the development of both types of resistance. Inadequate treatment programs allow the emergence of resistant organisms, producing secondary resistance in patients who are inadequately treated. Once these organisms are transmitted and tuberculosis disease develops, the infected person has "primary" resistant disease. The management of patients who have drug-resistant disease will be discussed later in the chapter.

ANTITUBERCULOUS AGENTS IN CURRENT USE

Isoniazid

Since its introduction in 1952, isoniazid, or isonicotinicyl hydrazine (INH), has been the most widely used antituberculous agent (8). The drug exhibits many qualities of an ideal agent: It is bactericidal, relatively nontoxic, inexpensive, and well-absorbed orally or parenterally.

Although the mechanism of action is unknown, INH appears to inhibit the biosynthesis of mycolic acids, which are important constituents of the mycobacterial cell wall (49). The drug is actively transported into the bacterium, where it acts to kill rapidly multiplying extracellular bacteria and inhibits the growth of dormant organisms existing within macrophages and in caseating granulomas (50).

INH is generally administered as a single dose of 300 mg for adults and 10 to 20 mg/kg (maximum 300 mg) for children (3). Rapid and complete absorption occur following oral administration, achieving peak concentrations of 3 to 5 µg/mL after a 3- to 5-mg/kg dose (51). When INH is administered orally with food, a reduction in the extent of absorption and peak plasma concentration of INH may occur. Aluminum-containing antacids may decrease gastrointestinal absorption of INH (52). The drug is widely distributed throughout the body; significant quantities have been detected in the pleural, ascitic, and cerebrospinal fluids; caseous material; saliva; skin; and muscle (8, 53).

Metabolism via the hepatic p-450 mixed oxidase system accounts for 70 to 90% of the elimination of INH. Several metabolic pathways are involved, acetylation being the major pathway (54, 55). After acetylation by the liver, the drug is excreted as a metabolite by the kidneys; it appears unchanged in the urine, along with other metabolites, including hydrazones (36). The relative fractions of INH, acetylisoniazid, and hydrazones in the urine differ considerably among patients. The rate of acetylation of INH is genetically controlled (56). Individuals are categorized as either fast or slow acetylators, depending on the rate of acetylation of INH in the liver. Approximately 45 to 65% of the American and northern European populations are classified as slow acetylators. Inuit (Eskimos) and Orientals are primarily rapid acetylators. The elimination rate of INH depends on acetylator phenotype, half-lives of approximately 0.5 to 2 hr being observed in the fast acetylators and 2 to 5 hr in slow acetylators (50). Patients who are slow acetylators may be more susceptible to the side effects related to higher concentrations, such as peripheral neuropathy (36). It has been postulated that

Table 64.1.
Principal Activity and Site of Action of the Major Antituberculous Agents[a]

Agent	Activity	Site of Action
Isoniazid (NH)	Bactericidal	Intracellular bacilli, extracellular bacilli, bacilli in caseous lesions
Rifampin (RMP)	Bactericidal	Intracellular bacilli, extracellular bacilli, bacilli in caseous lesions
Pyrazinamide (PZA)	Bactericidal	Intracellular bacilli
Streptomycin (STM)	Bactericidal	Extracellular bacilli
Ethambutol (EMB)	Bacteriostatic	Intracellular bacilli, extracellular bacilli

[a]From Hooker KD, Jost PM. Tuberculosis. In: Herfindal ET, Gourley DR, Hart LL, eds. Tuberculosis in Clinical Pharmacy and Therapeutics, 5th ed. Baltimore: Williams & Wilkins, 1992, p. 1096.

hepatotoxicity is more common in rapid acetylators, owing to the production of larger amounts of the metabolite acetylhydrazine (57). The acetylhydrazine metabolite is thought to be involved in the development of INH-induced hepatotoxicity (55). More recent data suggests that rapid acetylators are not at increased risk for hepatitis from INH and that the rate of acetylation is unlikely to be of therapeutic significance (58, 59).

Only a small amount of INH is eliminated unchanged by the kidneys. Therefore, dosage adjustments in patients with renal dysfunction is necessary only for individuals who are slow acetylators with a creatinine clearance less than 10 mL/min (60, 61). A reduction of the daily dose by 50% is recommended for these individuals as well as for those with severe hepatic disease to prevent accumulation of the drug and to reduce the potential for hepatotoxicity. In patients who are undergoing dialysis, significant amounts of INH are removed from the blood by hemodialysis and peritoneal dialysis. Dosage adjustments may be necessary.

Peripheral neuropathy appears to be a dose-dependent adverse effect of INH (8, 50). It is uncommon at a dose of 5 mg/kg, occurring in 2% of patients receiving INH. At higher dosages, peripheral neuropathy may develop in 10 to 20% of the patients. Peripheral neuropathy is most likely caused by INH-induced depletion of pyridoxine stores and/or competitive inhibition with pyridoxine in its role as a cofactor in the synthesis of synaptic neurotransmitters (62). Pyridoxine (15 to 50 mg/day) should be given with INH to people who have conditions in which neuropathy is common (diabetes, uremia, alcoholism, malnutrition) (8, 50). For pregnant women and people who have a seizure disorder, it is also recommended that pyridoxine be given with INH. As was previously mentioned, patients with slow acetylation may be more susceptible to the development of peripheral neuropathy (36).

Hepatotoxicity associated with the use of INH occurs in approximately 1 to 2% of the patients (54, 55). In the majority of the cases, transaminase values return to pretreatment values despite continuation of INH; however, in rare cases, progressive liver dysfunction, jaundice, bilirubinuria, and severe and often fatal hepatitis have occurred. Although the mechanism of hepatitis is unknown, it is probably associated with hepatic metabolites (55). Age appears to be the most significant factor in determining the risk of INH-induced hepatotoxicity. A U.S. Public Health Service Surveillance Study evaluated the toxicity of INH in 13,838 patients (63). The results of this study indicated that the rate of hepatitis increased directly with increasing age to 65 years. The rate of hepatitis was 0% in patients who were less than 20 years old; 0.3% in patients 20 to 34 years old; 1.2% in patients 35 to 49 years old; and 2.3% in patients 50 to 64 years old. However, recent studies have demonstrated that hepatitis may occur in approximately 4% of patients older than 65 years of age who are receiving the drug (64). Excessive or chronic alcohol consumption has also been identified as a risk cofactor (8, 62).

Baseline measurement of liver enzymes levels should be performed for patients receiving INH and should be followed up periodically (50). Patients should be questioned monthly for signs and symptoms of liver disease and should be instructed to report to their physician any of the prodromal symptoms of hepatitis (e.g., malaise, fatigue, weakness, anorexia, or nausea). Should these symptoms appear or if the signs that are suggestive of hepatic damage occur (e.g., liver enlargement with tenderness, jaundice, or dark urine), prompt discontinuation of INH is warranted; this usually prevents progression (see Table 64.2) (8). Some clinicians recommend discontinuation of INH if transaminase values exceed five times normal in treating disease and three times normal in giving preventive therapy.

Other rare adverse effects that are reported with INH administration include various central nervous system (CNS) toxicities (i.e., hallucinations, convulsions), dermatologic (i.e., acne, allergic rashes), hematologic (i.e., aplastic anemia), and gastrointestinal effects.

Several drug interactions have been reported with the use of INH in combination with other agents (50, 65). INH is an inhibitor of several cytochrome P-450-dependent microsomal pathways (66, 67). Acetylation is the major pathway; therefore, acetylator phenotyping may be a factor to consider in the interaction on INH with various agents (67, 68). INH inhibits the metabolism of several agents, including phenytoin, disulfiram, carbamazepine, warfarin, benzodiazepines, and vitamin D; increased serum concentrations may occur with concomitant use of INH (65).

Results of studies examining the interaction between INH and phenytoin indicate that phenytoin intoxication occurs mainly in slow acetylators of INH (67-69). In patients who are receiving INH and phenytoin concomitantly, it is necessary to monitor phenytoin serum levels, especially in slow acetylators of INH. A reduction in the

Table 64.2.

Signs and Symptoms of Hepatic Damage or Other Adverse Effects[a]

- Unexplained anorexia
- Nausea
- Vomiting
- Dark urine
- Icterus
- Rash
- Persistent paresthesias of hands and feet
- Persistent fatigue
- Weakness or fever of >3 days
- Abdominal tenderness (especially right upper quadrant)

[a]From American Thoracic Society. Treatment of tuberculosis and tuberculosis infection in adults and children. Am J Respir Crit Care Med 150:1372, 1994.

dosage of phenytoin is warranted for patients who are exhibiting clinical symptoms of phenytoin intoxication and/or toxic serum phenytoin levels.

As was mentioned previously, concomitant administration of INH and food results in impaired absorption of INH; the peak concentration, the mean concentration, and the total amount of drug are reduced (70, 71). Since aluminum-containing antacids may decrease gastrointestinal absorption of INH, administration of INH at least 1 hr before taking antacids is recommended (52). More studies evaluating INH absorption with antacids and laxatives are necessary (52, 72).

INH is also an inhibitor of monoamine and diamine oxidase (73). There are reported cases of adverse reactions such as skin flushing, palpitations, headache, nausea and vomiting, and itching in patients who are receiving INH and ingesting foods with high histamine or tyramine content (73-83). These reactions were attributed to monoamine and diamine oxidase inhibition by INH. Patients should be counseled to take INH on an empty stomach and to avoid foods with high histamine or tyramine content (selected fishes, cheeses, and wines) (65).

INH may possibly exhibit enzymatic induction of certain agents (65). In patients who are receiving INH, rifampin, and ketoconazole concomitantly, decreases in ketoconazole concentrations have been reported; this interaction appears to involve an additive affect of INH and rifampin to reduce ketoconazole concentrations (84, 85).

The potential interaction between INH and theophylline has been examined in various European and U.S. studies (86-88). In studies using INH at dosages of 400 mg/day or 10 mg/kg/day, a reduction in theophylline clearance was observed (86, 87). A study in the United States that used INH at a dosage of 300 mg/day reported a mean 16% increase in theophylline clearance (88). On the basis of the results of these studies, it appears that INH at dosages of 300 mg/day does not cause clinically significant decreases in theophylline clearance (89). In patients who are receiving larger daily doses of INH (e.g., 400 mg or 600 mg) or possibly in underweight individuals who are receiving 300 mg/day this interaction may be significant. A summary of clinically significant INH interactions is provided in Table 64.3 (65). Included are INH interactions that require further study and should be considered in monitoring therapy.

Rifampin

Rifampin (RMP) is a semisynthetic derivative of rifamycin B that is an antibiotic produced by *Streptomyces mediterranei* (50). RMP exhibits a broad spectrum of activity that includes activity against *Neisseria, Staphylococcus, Haemophilus*, most streptococci, and several species of En-

Table 64.3.
Isoniazid Interactions[a]

Agent	Comments	Management
Phenytoin[b]	Mainly occurs in slow acetylators of INH. If rifampin given concurrently, phenytoin levels decrease (i.e., induction effect outweighs INH's inhibitory effect).	Monitor serum phenytoin levels. May need to decrease phenytoin dose.
Carbamazepine[b]		Monitor serum carbamazepine levels. May need to decrease carbamazepine dose.
Ketoconazole[b]	INH has an additive effect with rifampin to decrease ketoconazole concentrations.	Monitor. Adjust dose if necessary.
Food[b] Cheese, fish, wine[b]	May delay and decrease absorption of INH.	Take INH on an empty stomach. Avoid foods with high histamine or tyramine content. Monitor patients for flushing, palpitations, headache, itching, nausea, and vomiting.
Antacids (aluminum hydroxide) Anticoagulants	May delay and decrease absorption of INH. Reported only at INH dose of 9 mg/kg/day.	Give INH at least one hour before meals. Monitor INH. May need to decrease anticoagulant dose.
Benzodiazepines	Rifampin's effect if given concomitantly should be considered.	May need to decrease dose of select benzodiazepines.
Vitamin D		Monitor vitamin D levels as well as calcium phosphate levels in select patients.
Theophylline	Potential decrease in theophylline clearance appears to occur at INH doses greater than 300 mg daily. If rifampin is given concurrently, theophylline levels decrease (i.e., induction effect outweighs INH's inhibitory effect).	Monitor serum theophylline levels.

[a]Adapted from 65: Baciewicz AM, Self TH. Isoniazid interactions. South Med J 78(6):714–718, 1985.
[b]Clinical significance established.

terobacteriaceae. The drug is bactericidal for *M. tuberculosis*, most strains being inhibited in vitro by concentrations of 0.5 µg/mL. Its mechanism of action entails inhibition of DNA-dependent RNA polymerase of mycobacteria and other microorganisms, preventing chain initiation. RMP exhibits greater activity than INH against slower or intermittently growing organisms that are present in macrophages (90). RMP is unique in its ability to destroy the organisms in semisolid caseous material. When it is used in combination with INH, synergy is obtained, thus enabling the duration of treatment for tuberculosis to be shortened from 18 to 24 months to 6 to 9 months (91).

RMP is generally administered as a single dose of 600 mg daily or biweekly for adults and 10 to 20 mg/kg (maximum 600 mg) for children. The drug is well absorbed from the gastrointestinal tract, peak serum concentrations of approximately 7 µg/mL being achieved within 2 to 4 hr. However, because of considerable interpatient variation, peak plasma concentrations of the drug may range from 4 to 32 µg/mL (92-95). Although the peak plasma concentrations may be slightly reduced when RMP is administered with food, this difference is not known to be clinically significant (36). The drug is 60 to 90% protein-bound and penetrates well into the tissues, including the CNS, liver, lungs, bone, saliva, and tears (96, 97). Rifampin may impart an orange discoloration to the urine, feces, sputum, tears, and sweat. Soft contact lenses may be permanently discolored; patients should be counseled accordingly (50).

Following absorption from the gastrointestinal tract, RMP is eliminated in the bile, where it undergoes enterohepatic circulation (50). At this time, the drug is deacetylated to desacetylrifampin, a metabolite with antibacterial activity similar to that of the parent compound. Intestinal reabsorption is decreased by deacetylation; thus, metabolism promotes elimination of the drug. The serum half-life of RMP initially ranges from 1.5 to 5 hr. Because RMP is a potent inducer of hepatic microsomal enzymes, it induces its own metabolism, thus shortening its half-life to 2 to 3 hr. The half-life of RMP may be increased in the presence of hepatic dysfunction, and dosage adjustments may be necessary. In patients with renal impairment, adjustment of dosage is not necessary.

In recommended doses, RMP is generally well tolerated (98, 99). Significant adverse reactions occur in fewer than 4% of patients with tuberculosis. The most common adverse effects are gastrointestinal upset (i.e., nausea and vomiting, 1.5%), rash (0.8%), and fever (0.5%). Although uncommon in recommended doses, an influenzalike syndrome may occur with intermittent administration of doses of rifampin greater than 10 mg/kg (100). The patient may complain of fever, chills, malaise, arthralgias, and headache. The syndrome may also include interstitial nephritis, acute renal failure, eosinophilia, thrombocytopenia, hemolytic anemia, and shock.

Elevations in hepatic enzymes occur in approximately 10 to 15% of patients when RMP is administered alone (101). In combination with INH, elevations in serum transaminases may occur in 20 to 30% of patients (102). This usually occurs within the first 8 weeks of therapy. The development of hepatitis in patients with normal hepatic function is rare. Alcoholism, chronic liver disease, and old age may increase the risk of hepatotoxicity with the administration of RMP alone or in combination with INH. Whether the combination of INH and RMP increases the incidence of hepatotoxicity remains controversial.

RMP induces hepatic microsomal enzymes and may enhance the elimination of several drugs, including theophylline, warfarin, oral contraceptive agents, phenytoin, cyclosporin, glucocorticoids, methadone, ketoconazole, and/or hypoglycemic agents (103-105). These interactions may result in decreased efficacy of these agents, such as reduced efficacy of oral contraceptives, including several reports of unplanned pregnancy (106, 107). Potentially clinically significant rifampin drug interactions that have been reported more recently include interactions with haloperidol, several antiarrhythmics, diltiazem, fluconazole, and select benzodiazepines (105). On initiation of rifampin therapy the appropriate management of these interactions is essential to prevent therapeutic failures and potential toxic reactions after rifampin is discontinued. Table 64.4 provides a summary of rifampin interactions with recommendations for management (105).

Patients who are taking RMP should be monitored for signs of hepatotoxicity, renal function, and skin appearance (50). For females who use oral contraceptives, another form of contraception during therapy should be recommended. Adherence to the prescribed dosing regimen is important since, interrupted therapy may cause an increase in the incidence of toxicity.

Ethambutol

Ethambutol (EMB), or d-ethylenediimino-di-l-butanol dihydrochloride, is a synthetic antimycobacterial agent that is generally considered to be tuberculostatic in the recommended doses (50). Its precise mechanism of action is unknown, although the drug has been shown to inhibit the incorporation of mycolic acid into the mycobacterial cell wall (108). Inhibition of mycobacterial growth requires approximately 24 hr. In vivo activity of EMB appears to be targeted toward actively dividing mycobacteria. Most strains of *M. tuberculosis* are inhibited in vitro by concentrations of 1 to 5 µg/mL (8). The peak plasma concentration 2 to 4 hr after a 15 mg/kg oral dose is approximately 5 µg/mL (50).

Approximately 75 to 85% of EMB is absorbed from the gastrointestinal tract (50). Administration of the drug with food does not interfere with absorption. Either single daily doses of 15 to 25 mg/kg or a 50 mg/kg twice-weekly

Table 64.4.
Rifampin Drug Interactions[a]

Agent	Comments	Management
Anticoagulants, oral[b]		Increase anticoagulant dose based on monitoring of INH.
Beta-blockers		May need to increase propanolol or metoprolol dose.
Chloramphenicol		Monitor serum chloramphenicol concentrations; if necessary, increase dose.
Contraceptives, oral[b]	Document patient counseling in chart.	Use other forms of birth control.
Cyclosporine[b]		Monitor serum cyclosporine concentrations. Increased dose is most likely.
Digitoxin[b]		Monitor serum digitoxin concentration. Monitor for arrhythmia control and signs and symptoms of heart failure. Increase dose if necessary.
Digoxin	In patients with decreased renal function, this interaction is most likely to be significant.	Monitor serum digoxin concentrations. Monitor for arrhythmia control and signs and symptoms of heart failure.
Glucocorticoids[b]		Increase glucocorticoid dosage twofold to threefold.
Ketoconazole[b]		Avoid this combination if possible. If administered, space rifampin and ketoconazole doses by 12 h. Monitor serum ketoconazole concentrations, and increase dose if necessary.
Methadone[b]		Increase methadone dose. Control withdrawal symptoms.
Phenytoin[b]		Monitor phenytoin serum levels. Increase dose if necessary.
Quinidine[b]		Monitor serum quinidine levels. Monitor for arrhythmia control. Increase dose if necessary.
Sulfonylureas	Monitor for blood glucose on discontinuation of rifampin therapy.	Monitor blood glucose control. Increase sulfonylurea dose if necessary.
Theophylline[b]		Monitor serum theophylline levels. Increased dose is most likely.
Verapamil[b]	Alternative agent recommended because even a very large increase in oral verapamil dose may not be sufficient.	Use alternative agent if possible. If utilized, monitor serum verapamil levels. Monitor patient for clinical response.
Haloperidol	Initial study indicates that serum concentrations and half-life are reduced by about 50%.	Monitor serum haloperidol levels. Change dosing regimen if necessary.
Tocainide	Approximately a 30% decrease in tocainide serum half-life was reported in one trial in healthy subjects.	Monitor arrhythmia control. Increase dose if necessary.
Disopyramide	Initial study reported a reduction in disopyramide serum half-life by about 50%.	Monitor arrhythmia control. Increase dose if necessary.
Propafenone		Monitor arrhythmia control. Monitor plasma propafenane concentrations. Increase dose if necessary.
Diltiazem	Alternative agent recommended because even a very large increase in oral diltiazem dose may not be sufficient (similar interaction with verapamil).	Use an alternative agent if possible.
Fluconazole	A 22% decrease in fluconazole serum half-life was reported in one trial in healthy subjects.	May need to increase fluconazole dosage. Monitor signs and symptoms of infection.
Diazepam	a 300% increase in diazepam oral clearance has been reported.	Monitor clinical response. Increase diazepam dose if necessary.

[a]Adapted from Borcherding SM, Baciewicz AM, Self TH. Update on rifampin drug interactions II. Arch Intern Med 152:711–715, 1992. In addition to this reference, see (103) and (104) for further information; for each interaction, when rifampin is discontinued, enzyme induction effect is slowly reduced over 1 to 2 weeks.
[b]Major clinical significance is well established.

regimens may be chosen. Although EMB penetrates well into most tissues and fluids, cerebrospinal fluid (CSF) concentrations are low, even in the presence of meningeal inflammation. About two-thirds of an oral dose of EMB is eliminated in the urine; approximately 50% is excreted unchanged via glomerular filtration and tubular secretion. Hepatic metabolism occurs through oxidation, and two inactive metabolites, an aldehyde and a dicarboxylic acid derivative, are formed. Up to 15% of the drug is excreted in the urine in the form of these inactive metabolites (109).

About 20% is excreted as unchanged drug in the feces. The serum half-life is approximately 4 hr in patients with normal renal function and may increase to 7 hr or longer in patients with renal failure (50). Dosage adjustment is required for patients who have renal impairment; patients whose creatinine clearance is between 10 and 50 mL/min require a 50% reduction in the normal dose; for patients whose creatinine clearance is less than 10 mL/min, a 65% dose reduction is necessary (110). No dosage adjustment is required for patients with hepatic dysfunction.

EMB is a relatively safe drug and produces very few adverse effects when the recommended dosages are used (50). The most toxic effect of EMB is retrobulbar neuritis, which is characterized by decreased visual acuity, loss of red-green color vision, and central scotomata (111). This appears to be a dose-related phenomenon that is more common at doses above 50 mg/kg/day. The occurrence is reported to be 5% in patients who are receiving daily doses of 25 mg/kg and less than 1% in patients who are being treated with 15 mg/kg/day (50). In patients with renal impairment, the frequency of ocular toxicity is increased because of accumulation of the drug. Baseline examination of visual acuity should be performed before initiation of EMB therapy, followed by monthly eye examinations. Patients should be instructed to report any changes in visual acuity and seek medical attention immediately. Caution should be exercised in prescribing EMB for children who are too young for assessment of visual acuity and red-green color discrimination. The use of possible alternative agents should be considered. Other adverse effects of EMB include hypersensitivity reactions (rash, anaphylactic shock), neuritis, gastrointestinal intolerance, headache, and hyperuricemia. Increased concentration of urate in the blood is most likely due to decreased clearance of renal urate (112).

Pyrazinamide

Pyrazinamide (PZA), a synthetic pyrazine analog of nicotinamide, exhibits bactericidal activity against mycobacteria in an acid environment (50). Although its precise mechanism is unknown, the drug is slowly bactericidal against the slow-growing bacilli within the acidic pH of the macrophages (113). The unique intracellular activity of the drug has led to the encorporation of PZA into the initial phase of therapy. The drug has recently been used in short-course regimens with INH and RMP for the treatment of tuberculosis (114). The minimum inhibitory concentration (MIC) in an acid environment is 20 µg/mL against *M. tuberculosis*, although the tubercle bacilli within the monocytes are killed by concentrations of 12.5 µg/mL (50). PZA is well absorbed from the gastrointestinal tract, peak serum concentrations occurring approximately 2 hr after ingestion. Following doses of 20 to 25 mg/kg, peak serum concentrations range from 30 to 50 µg/mL. The drug is widely distributed throughout the body, including

the CSF. PZA is primarily excreted by glomerular filtration, but it is also hydrolyzed and hydroxylated. In people with normal renal function, the elimination half-life is 9 to 10 hr. When a patient has renal impairment, minor dosage adjustments may be required. The usual dosage is 15 to 30 mg/kg/day (maximum 2 g), 50 to 70 mg/kg twice weekly (maximum 4 g), or 50 to 70 mg/kg thrice weekly (maximum 3 g).

The most common and toxic effect of PZA is dose-dependent hepatotoxicity (50). In early studies using high doses of 3 g/day (40 to 50 mg/kg), a 15% incidence of hepatotoxicity was reported. Transient, asymptomatic elevations of serum transaminase levels are the earliest abnormalities produced by the drug. Initial 2-month regimens consisting of INH, RMP, and PZA, which use PZA at a dosage of 15 to 30 mg/kg, do not indicate a significant increase in hepatotoxicity (115, 116). Other adverse effects include hypersensitivity reactions, photosensitivity, gastrointestinal intolerance, dysuria, malaise, fever, and arthralgias (50). Salicylates usually provide symptomatic relief of PZA-related arthralgia (8). PZA may cause elevations in prothrombin time (by decreasing prothrombin concentration or activity) and serum bilirubin levels (50). Because PZA inhibits renal tubular secretion of uric acid, hyperuricemia occurs frequently (117). Although acute gout is uncommon, in individuals with a history of gout precipitation of an acute gouty attack may be a problem. In these cases, discontinuation of the drug may be warranted.

Streptomycin

Streptomycin (STM), an aminoglycoside antibiotic, was the first clinically effective drug to become available for the treatment of tuberculosis (50). The drug is bactericidal in an alkaline environment and acts by inhibiting protein synthesis. Because aminoglycosides are poorly absorbed from the gastrointestinal tract, STM must be administered parenterally. The drug is highly effective within the extracellular environment; however, it diffuses poorly into granulomas and macrophages and lacks activity in the intracellular environment. The majority of strains of *M. tuberculosis* are inhibited in vitro at a concentration of 8 µg/mL. Following an intramuscular dose of 15 mg/kg, peak serum concentration levels averaging approximately 40 µg/mL are achieved. Excretion is primarily renal, the majority of drug being excreted unchanged in the urine. The half-life in blood ranges from 2 to 5 hr in individuals with normal renal function. In patients with renal insufficiency, the dose should be reduced. Bennett and associates recommend extending the dosing interval in the following siutations: For patients with a glomerular filtration rate between 10 and 50 mL/min, the dosing interval should be adjusted to 24 to 72 hr; for patients with a glomerular filtration rate less than 10 mL/min, the dosing interval should be adjusted to 72 to 96 hr (61). A reduction in serum concentrations by 66% has been noted during a 12-hr dialysis (118). STM has moderate tissue penetration. It does not enter the CSF except in the presence of meningeal inflammation (50).

Ototoxicity is the major toxic effect of STM (8). This usually results in vertigo and ataxia, although hearing loss may also occur. Other adverse effects include hypersensitivity and fever. Nephrotoxicity occasionally occurs, although STM has less adverse effect on the kidneys than do kanamycin and capreomycin. The risk of nephrotoxicity may be increased for patients who are receiving other nephrotoxic drugs concomitantly or patients with preexisting renal insufficiency. It is recommended that a total cumulative dose of no more than 120 g be given unless there are no other therapeutic options. In individuals who are older than 60 years of age, both ototoxicity and nephrotoxicity are more common. All patients who are receiving STM should have baseline hearing and renal function tests, as well as periodic monitoring for changes. Several drug interactions are possible with concomitant administration of STM. As with other aminoglycosides, STM interacts with neuromuscular blocking agents (e.g., pancuronium, turocurarrine) (119). This interaction may result in prolonged respiratory depression.

Paraaminosalicylic Acid

Paraaminosalicylic acid (PAS) is a tuberculostatic agent that is rarely used in current antituberculous regimens (50). It is a structural analog of paraaminobenzoic acid (PABA); thus, its mechanism of action appears to be similar to that of sulfonamides, competitive antagonism of PABA. Most strains of M. tuberculosis in vitro are inhibited at concentrations of 1 μg/mL. The usual dose in adults and children is 150 mg/kg by mouth (maximum 10 to 12 g/d), administered in divided doses. The drug is well absorbed from the gastrointestinal tract and distributes throughout the total body water, achieving high concentrations in the pleural fluid and caseous tissue. However, concentration levels in the CSF are low, possibly because of active transport outward (120). Following a single 4-g oral dose, plasma concentrations ranging from 75 to 100 μg/mL are achieved within 1 to 2 hr. The high doses are necessary because the drug has an elimination half-life of about 1 hr (50). More than 80% of the drug is eliminated in the urine; approximately 50% is in the form of an acetylated compound. For patients with renal dysfunction, the dosage should be reduced. A significant sodium load is present in a dose when the tablet preparation is used (8). If the delayed-release granule formulation is used, the dose should be administered with acidic food or drink.

The frequency of adverse effects associated with the use of PAS ranges from 10 to 30% (50). The most frequent complaint is gastrointestinal upset (nausea, vomiting, anorexia, diarrhea, and epigastric pain), which may contribute to patient noncompliance. Other adverse effects include hypersensitivity reactions in 5 to 10% of patients, thrombocytopenia, and rarely hepatitis. Probenicid blocks the renal excretion of PAS, resulting in increased plasma concentrations of PAS. Caution should be exercised with this combination because of the possibility of PAS toxicity. Patients should be counseled about compliance with the medication. The drug should be administered in two to four equally divided doses with meals to minimize gastric irritation (50).

Ethionamide

Ethionamide is an oral agent that is structurally similar to INH but has less activity (50). It is used as a second-line agent in combination with other antituberculous agents following failure with the primary regimens. Its precise mechanism of action is unknown, although it appears to involve protein synthesis inhibition. The majority of M. tuberculosis strains are inhibited by concentrations of 0.6 to 2.5 μg/mL. The activity of this agent may be either tuberculostatic or tuberculocidal, depending on the susceptibility of the organism and on drug concentration at the site of infection. Rapid resistance occurs in vitro, and cross-resistance occurs between ethionamide and INH. The recommended daily dose is 15 to 20 mg/kg, with a maximum dosage of 1 g/day (8). Absorption is rapid from the gastrointestinal tract following oral administration (50). Peak concentrations of approximately 20 μg/mL are achieved in 3 hr following a 1-g dose. The serum half-life is approximately 3 hr. Ethionamide is evenly distributed into the blood and various organs. Metabolism is predominantly hepatic.

The most common adverse effects of ethionamide are anorexia, nausea, and vomiting. For most patients it is necessary to gradually increase the dose to the full amount. A useful approach to maintaining treatment is the administration of ethionamide at bedtime with an antiemetic drug taken 30 min before the dose and occasionally a hypnotic (8). Other adverse effects include arthralgias, impotence, photosensitivity dermatitis, gynecomastia, hypothyroidism, hepatitis, and a metallic taste in the mouth. The frequency of hepatitis associated with ethionamide does not appear to be greater than that associated with PZA. Patients should have hepatic enzymes monitored monthly. The drug should be discontinued if the hepatic enzymes reach five times normal levels, even in the absence of symptoms.

Cycloserine

Cycloserine is an antituberculous agent that is an analog of the amino acid D-alanine. Like ethionamide, the drug is limited to certain situations (8). Most strains of M. tuberculosis are inhibited by concentrations of 5 to 20 μg/mL, and the drug is considered to be bacteriostatic (50). Cycloserine inhibits the processes that incorporate D-alanine in bacterial cell wall synthesis. The drug is available in 250-mg capsules. Following the usual dose of 15 to 20 mg/kg/day, the drug is rapidly absorbed from the gastrointestinal tract. Cycloserine distributes into most body fluids and tissue, including the CSF. The most common adverse effects of the drug involve the CNS. Emotional and behavioral disturbances, including psychosis, have been reported. These reactions tend to appear within the first 2 weeks of therapy and usually disappear on discontinuation of the drug. Manifestations of the CNS effects of cycloserine are more likely to occur in patients who have a history of psychological problems or who have a chronic psychiatric condition. The mental status of these patients should be assessed regularly to monitor for these adverse effects. Other adverse effects include convulsions and peripheral neuropathy, especially when the drug is used in combination with INH. Consequently, 150 mg/day of pyridoxine should be administered with cycloserine. Cycloserine inhibits the hepatic metabolism of phenytoin, especially when it is taken with INH (8). If necessary, the dosage of phenytoin should be reduced. Cycloserine is contraindicated for people who have a history of epilepsy, depression, or severe anxiety (50). The risk of CNS effects may be increased with concurrent use with ethionamide, INH, and alcohol.

Capreomycin and Kanamycin

Capreomycin and kanamycin are injectable aminoglycoside antibiotics that may be used in combination with other effective antituberculous drugs (8). The concurrent administration of more than one aminoglycoside should be avoided. Capreomycin and kanamycin both inhibit protein synthesis and are tuberculostatic. Capreomycin is available in 1-g vials; kanamycin is available in 75-mg, 500-mg, and 1-g vials. The usual daily dosage of both agents is 15 to 30 mg/kg given intramuscularly, with a maximum daily dosage of 1 g. The frequency of renal toxicity is similar, and regular monitoring of serum creatinine is necessary. Auditory toxicity appears to be more common with kanamycin than with streptomycin and capreomycin. Monthly audiometry is recommended in patients who are receiving kanamycin. Vestibular toxicity is uncommon. Capreomycin may produce damage to the eighth cranial nerve, resulting in high-frequency loss before vestibular dysfunction occurs. Recommendations with these agents include an audiogram performed at baseline and repeated at least every other month while the patient is receiving therapy and periodic examinations for vestibular function. In older patients the maximal daily dosage of capreomycin should be limited to 750 mg.

Thiacetazone

Thiacetazone is an antituberculous agent that is biochemically related to INH (8). The drug is not available in the United States; however, it is used in many developing countries because it is very inexpensive. Its activity is

bacteriostatic, and it is more toxic than INH. Thiacetazone, at the usual adult dosage of 150 mg/day, is commonly combined in a single tablet with 300 to 400 mg of INH. Gastrointestinal complaints, including nausea and vomiting, occur in up to 10% of patients. Other adverse effects that are less frequently reported include jaundice (<1%), reversible bone marrow suppression (0.2%), and rashes (3.9%). Cutaneous reactions that are associated with the use of thiacetazone may be severe. If the drug is not discontinued, an exfoliative dermatitis or Stevens-Johnson syndrome may occur. These reactions appear to be more frequent in HIV-infected individuals. Thiacetazone is not contraindicated in this population. The vestibular toxicity that is associated with the use of streptomycin may be potentiated by the concurrent use of thiacetazone.

Potentially Effective Antituberculous Agents

New agents that have been evaluated in children or adults for antituberculous activity include amikacin, quinolones, rifamycin derivatives, clofazimine, and β-lactams (121). Although these agents have not been tested in multidrug regimens for treating tuberculosis, the increase in the number of multidrug-resistant tuberculosis cases may create more situations in which the usefulness of these agents must be considered (8). Since these agents have not yet been fully evaluated in well-designed, randomized trials for tuberculosis treatment or prophylaxis, they should not be used to replace any of the previously recommended agents until efficacy is established. The following agents discussed either are licensed or are available through an investigational new drug (IND) request in the United States. Recommendations for dosages and intervals for the use of these drugs as antituberculous agents have not been established. Consultation with tuberculosis experts for adjustments in dosages is necessary if these agents are used for infants and children.

Amikacin is tuberculocidal against *M. tuberculosis* in vitro (8). The drug is administered intramuscularly as a single daily dose of 15 mg/kg five times weekly. If the drug is administered intravenously, a single daily dose of 15 mg/kg is given over 30 min. One hour after intramuscular administration of a 7.5-mg/kg single dose, the average peak serum concentration is 21 μg/mL (121). The MIC for amikacin is about 4 to 8 μg/mL for a broad range of strains of *M. tuberculosis* (122).

Several fluoroquinolones exhibit in vitro activity against *M. tuberculosis*. Ofloxacin and ciprofloxacin are quinolones that appear to be most active against *M. tuberculosis*, with inhibitory concentrations of approximately 1 μg/mL for a variety of strains of *M. tuberculosis* (123-125). Data concerning the use of these agents for the treatment of tuberculosis is limited (126, 127).

Rifabutin is a semisynthetic derivative of rifamycin S that exhibits in vitro activity against certain rifampin-resistant strains of *M. tuberculosis* (128). The MICs of rifabutin for strains of *M. tuberculosis* that are rifampin-susceptible are low: <0.06 µg/mL. However, the MICs for rifampin-resistant strains are substantially higher than those of rifampin-susceptible strains (range: 0.27 to 16.0 µg/mL). This indicates cross-resistance between rifabutin and rifampin. The wide range of MICs for rifampin-resistant strains implies varying degrees of susceptibility to rifabutin. The potential role of rifabutin in tuberculosis is not known at this time.

Clofazimine is an oral phenazine dye that is weakly bactericidal against *M. leprae* (36). The drug exerts in vitro and in vivo activity against mycobacteria, including *M. tuberculosis*. The efficacy of clofazimine in the treatment of tuberculosis has not been established (123).

Amoxicillin is an aminopenicillin with a broad spectrum of antibacterial activity against many Gram-positive and Gram-negative microorganisms. The in vitro activity against *M. tuberculosis* is greatly enhanced by the addition of a β-lactamase inhibitor to amoxicillin (129). The β-lactamase inhibitors (e.g., clavulanic acid) lack intrinsic antimycobacterial activity; however, they inhibit the enzyme that is partially responsible for the resistance of *M. tuberculosis* to β-lactam antibiotics. To date, there are no in vivo studies using this drug combination against *M. tuberculosis*. One concern in using these agents in the treatment of tuberculosis is the poor penetration of β-lactam antibiotics into mammalian cells (130).

Other agents that are currently under investigation include sulfonamides, macrolides, and folate antagonists (44).

INITIAL TREATMENT REGIMEN

Tables 64.5 and 64.6 provide initial treatment regimens for children and adults. Over the past 45 years, many studies evaluating the use of antituberculosis regimens have provided specific information about the use of combination therapy. On the basis of the results of these studies, the CDC and ATS provide several important generalizations (8):

1. Isoniazid should be used in any treatment regimen for the entire duration of therapy unless contraindications are present or the organisms are resistant to the drug.
2. Although there are some reports of good results with 4-month regimens, in general, relapse rates are unacceptably high. An exception is the adult who is carefully evaluated and found to have sputum-culture-negative pulmonary tuberculosis. For such adults the success rate with 4-month regimens has been high.
3. Rifampin and isoniazid should be used for the entire duration of therapy when 6-month regimens are chosen.
4. In treatment regimens of less than 9 months' duration, efficacy is enhanced by the administration of pyrazinamide during the initial phase of therapy.
5. The efficacy of a regimen is decreased when ethambutol or

Table 64.5.
Drugs for the Initial Treatment of Tuberculosis in Children and Adults[a]

Drug	Daily Dose		Twice Weekly		Thrice Weekly	
	Children	Adults	Children	Adults	Children	Adults
First-line agents						
Isoniazid (mg/kg)	10–20, max. 300 mg	5, max. 300 mg	20–40, max. 900 mg	15 max., max. 900 mg	20–40, max. 900 mg	15 max., max. 900 mg
Rifampin (mg/kg)	10–20, max. 600 mg	10, max. 600 mg	10–20, max. 600 mg	10, max. 600 mg	10–20, max. 600 mg	10, max. 600 mg
Pyrazinamide (mg/kg)	15–30, max. 2 g	15–30, max. 2 g	50–70, max. 4 g	50–70, max. 4 g	50–70, max. 3 g	50–70, max. 3 g
Streptomycin (mg/kg)	20–40, max. 1.0 g	15, max. 1.0 g	25–30, max. 1.5 g	25–30, max. 1.5 g	25–30, max. 1.5 g	25–30, max. 1.5 g
Ethambutol (mg/kg)	15–25, max. 2.5 g	15–25, max. 2.5 g	50, max. 2.5 g	50, max. 2.5 g	25–30, max. 1.5 g	25–30, max. 1.5 g
Second-line agents						
p-Aminosalicylic acid (mg/kg)	150, max. 12 g	150, max. 12 g				
Ethionamide (mg/kg)	15–20, max. 1 g	15–20, max. 1 g				
Cycloserine (mg/kg)	15–20, max. 1 g	15–20, max. 1 g				
Capreomycin (mg/kg), Kanamycin (mg/kg)	15–30, max. 1 g	15–30, max. 1 g				

[a]Adapted from Centers for Disease Control. Initial therapy for tuberculosis in the era of multidrug resistance: recommendations of the Advisory Council of the Advisory Council for the Elimination of Tuberculosis. MMWR Morb Mortal Wkly Rep 42 (RR-7):1–8, 1993.

Table 64.6.

Regimen Options for the Preferred Initial Treatment of Children and Adults: Tuberculosis Without HIV Infection[a]

Option 1[b]	Option 2[b]	Option 3[b]
Administer daily INH, RMP, and PZA for 8 weeks followed by 16 weeks of INH and RMP daily or 2–3 times/week.[c] If INH resistance rate is not <4%, EMB or STM should be added to the initial regimen until susceptibility to INH and RMP is demonstrated.[d]	Administer daily INH, RMP, PZA and STM or EMB for 2 weeks followed by 2 times/week[c] administration of the same drugs for 6 weeks (by DOT) and subsequently with 2 times/week administration of INH and RMP for 16 weeks (by DOT).[d]	Treat by DOT, 3 times/week[c] with INH, RMP, PZA, and EMB or STM for 6 months.[d]

[a]Adapted from Centers for Disease Control. Initial therapy for tuberculosis in an era of multidrug resistance: recommendations of the Advisory Council for the Elimination of Tuberculosis. MMWR Morb Mortal Wkly Rep 42 (No. RR-7):1–8, 1993.
[b]For patients with tuberculosis and HIV infection, options 1, 2 or 3 can be used, but treatment regimens should continue for a total of 9 months and at least 6 months beyond culture conversion.
[c]Any regimen that is administered 2 times/week or 3 times/week should be monitored by DOT for the duration of therapy.
[d]With any of the options, consult a TB medical expert if the patient is symptomatic or smear- or culture-positive after 3 months.

streptomycin, in the recommended dosages, is substituted for pyrazinamide in the initial phase of therapy.

6. Following an initial daily phase of treatment as short as 2 weeks, the intermittent administration of appropriately adjusted doses of the antituberculosis agents provides results that are similar to those of daily administration. Four drug regimens that are administered three times weekly throughout the duration of treatment provide equally good results in adults. Data is not available concerning thrice-weekly regimens in children. Experience with other intermittent regimens suggests that equal efficacy may be achieved with thrice-weekly regimens in children.

These guidelines are applicable only when the tuberculosis is caused by organisms that are susceptible to the standard antituberculous agents. Community rates of initial resistance to INH have remained low (<4%) in some areas of the United States (8). Local data is useful in determining whether the population in general is at low risk for drug resistance or whether specific subgroups in the population can be defined that are at low risk (131). In areas in which rates of initial resistance to antituberculous drugs are low, continued surveillance of drug susceptibility patterns is necessary to ensure that low rates of drug resistance continue.

Recently, an increase in the frequency of outbreaks of disease caused by multiple-drug-resistant organisms has been reported (26, 132). The organisms that were isolated during these outbreaks were resistant to both INH and RMP and frequently to EMB, as well as to other agents. In these situations the response to treatment with standard initial regimens is poor. Since most cases of MDR-TB have occurred among HIV-infected adults, there have been transmission of infection and progression to disease among their contacts.

When initiating therapy for tuberculosis, physicians should be aware of the prevalence of drug resistance in their communities, as well as the epidemiologic features of people who are most likely to be carrying these organisms

(8). Patients with newly diagnosed tuberculosis should have drug susceptibility testing performed on the organisms that were initially isolated. The earliest identification of growth can be achieved by radiometric or colorimetric detection techniques. If performance of full drug susceptibility studies is not possible, testing for resistance to rifampin can identify strains that are likely to have multiple drug resistance.

The minimal duration of treatment for all children and adults with culture-positive tuberculosis is 6 months, which should include an initial phase of INH, RMP, and PZA for a 2-month period (132). The initial regimen should also include EMB (or STM in children who are too young to be monitored for visual acuity) until the results of drug susceptibility studies are available, unless there is a low likelihood of drug resistance (i.e., primary resistance to INH in the community is less than 4% and the patient has no known exposure to a drug-resistant case, is not from a country where the prevalence of drug resistance is high, and has not received prior therapy with antituberculous agents). Following the initial phase of a 2-month period of therapy, a second phase of treatment consisting of INH and RMP should last for 4 months. If the clinical response to therapy is slow or suboptimal, treatment should be prolonged.

Directly observed therapy (DOT) is an option to consider on initiation of antituberculous therapy (8). In DOT the patient is observed by a health care provider or other responsible person as the patient ingests the antituberculous medications. DOT may be administered to patients in a clinical setting, as well as in the patient's home, place of employment, school, or other mutually agreed-on setting. Daily, twice-weekly, or thrice-weekly antituberculous medications can be administered with DOT. DOT should be considered in all patients who are treated for tuberculosis and *is strongly recommended in patients with HIV infection; there appears to be a reduced degree of safety in treating patients with HIV infection, and patient compliance to antituberculosis therapy is crucial.* The various options that are available for administration with DOT are listed in Table 64.6 (3, 133, 134). Although these specific regimens have not been studied in children, the results achieved in adults suggest potential benefits in children.

Efficacy has also been achieved with 9-month regimens using INH and RMP (135). Initial drug regimens should also include EMB or STM (or STM in children who are too young to be monitored for visual acuity) until the results of drug-susceptibility studies are available, unless there is little possibility of drug resistance. Following an initial 1 or 2 months of daily therapy, INH and RMP may be administered twice weekly (136).

In adults with sputum-smear-negative and sputum-culture-negative active pulmonary tuberculosis, a shorter duration of therapy is possible (8). In these patients, 4-month therapy with INH and RMP, preferably with PZA for the first 2 months, provides results that are equivalent to those for patients with culture-positive disease who are treated with longer regimens (137, 138). This regimen is also recommended for adult tuberculin reactors who have silicosis and are sputum-smear-negative and sputum-culture-negative or for adult reactors with a chest radiograph that is suggestive of old, healed tuberculosis (8). An acceptable alternative therapy is a regimen of INH therapy for 12 months.

MONITORING FOR ADVERSE EFFECTS

Baseline measurements of hepatic enzymes, bilirubin, and serum creatinine; a complete blood count; and a platelet count (or estimate) are required for adults who are treated for tuberculosis (8). A serum uric acid level should be measured if PZA is used. Baseline examination of both visual acuity and red-green color perception is necessary for patients who are to be treated with EMB. Baseline tests are useful in detecting abnormalities that may complicate a regimen; adjustments in dosages may be necessary on the basis of these values. They also provide a means of comparison with measurements obtained during therapy if an adverse reaction is suspected. For children, baseline tests, except for visual acuity, are not necessary unless a complicating condition exists or is clinically suspected.

All patients, adults and children, who are receiving antituberculosis therapy should be monitored clinically for adverse drug effects and should be instructed to look for symptoms that are associated with common adverse effects of their medications (8). Medical personnel should follow patients at least monthly during therapy and ascertain whether symptoms suggesting drug toxicity are present. In general, routine laboratory monitoring for toxicity in patients with normal baseline test is not necessary. Should symptoms suggest drug toxicity, appropriate laboratory testing should be performed to confirm or exclude such toxicity.

EVALUATION OF RESPONSE TO THERAPY

Patients with Positive Pretreatment Sputum

Patients with positive bacteriology (*M. tuberculosis* identified in sputum) should be evaluated by repeated examinations of sputum following initiation of antituberculosis therapy (8). Sputum examinations should be performed at least at monthly intervals until sputum conversion is documented. More than 85% of patients with positive pretreatment cultures should convert to negative after 2 months of therapy with regimens consisting of INH and RMP.

Patients in whom sputum cultures do not convert to negative following 2 months of therapy should be reevaluated, and drug susceptibility tests should be repeated (8). If drug resistance is not demonstrated, the treatment should be continued with DOT. If resistant organisms are present, modification of the treatment regimen is necessary and must include at least two drugs to which the organisms are susceptible. Administration of the modified regimen should be provided with DOT. Bacteriologic evaluations should be performed at least at monthly intervals thereafter until cultures convert to negative.

Patients whose sputum converts to negative following 2 months of therapy require at least one further sputum smear and culture performed at the completion of therapy (8). Chest radiographs during therapy are not as useful as sputum examination; on completion of therapy a chest radiograph provides a baseline for comparison with future radiographs. Routine follow-up is not necessary for patients with susceptible organisms who exhibit a prompt and adequate bacteriologic response following therapy with regimens containing INH and RMP.

Patients with Negative Pretreatment Sputum

Extensive efforts, including induction of sputum by inhalation of hypertonic saline, should be made to establish a microbiologic diagnosis for adults with radiographic abnormalities that are consistent with tuberculosis (8). Consideration should be given to bronchoscopy and bronchoalveolar lavage for patients who are not able to produce a satisfactory sputum specimen. If another diagnosis is not established, presumptive therapy for tuberculosis may be warranted. Response to therapy in these patients can be provided by clinical evaluation and chest radiograph. A chest radiograph that shows no improvement after 3 months of antituberculosis therapy implies that the abnormality is due to another process or is the result of previous (not current) tuberculosis. If the tuberculin reaction is positive and other diagnoses have been ruled out, INH and RMP therapy can be continued for a total duration of 4 months. If tuberculosis is suspected in a child, microbiologic data can be obtained from early morning gastric aspirates or urine. In children with pneumonia that is unresponsive to standard treatments or with HIV infection, aggressive efforts should be made to establish a diagnosis. When culture and susceptibility information is not available from the adult contact, specimens for smear, culture, and susceptibility tests should be obtained from children.

Management of Patients Whose Treatment Has Failed or Who Have Relapsed

Patients whose sputum does not convert to negative are considered treatment failures. A current sputum specimen should be obtained, and susceptibility testing should be performed at this time. The currently used regimen may be continued while the results are pending, or at least three drugs that are not part of the current regimen can be added. Once the results of the susceptibility testing are available, the regimen should be adjusted accordingly, and DOT should be used.

Unlike patients who are treatment failures, patients who relapse after completion of a regimen containing INH and RMP with organisms that are susceptible to the drugs at the start of therapy usually maintain susceptibility to these agents (139). In general, the management of these patients involves reinstitution of the regimen that was previously used with DOT. If drug susceptibility testing reveals resistant organisms, the regimen must be modified and reinstituted.

Management of Patients Who Have Drug-Resistant Disease

In managing patients who have organisms that are resistant to one or more drugs, the basic principle is to administer at least two drugs for which susceptibility has been demonstrated (8). For patients who demonstrate INH resistance, the recommended 6-month, four-drug regimen is effective (140). On documentation of isolated INH resistance, INH should be discontinued, and PZA should be continued throughout the entire 6-month duration of therapy. For patients who are receiving the 9-month regimen without PZA, INH should be discontinued on documentation of isolated INH resistance. If the initial regimen included EMB, treatment consisting of RMP and EMB should be continued for a 12-month minimum (141). If EMB was not initially included in the initial regimen, drug susceptibility tests should be repeated, INH should be discontinued, and two new agents (e.g., EMB and PZA) should be added. Adjustments to this regimen can be made, if necessary, once the results of the susceptibility tests are available.

Good data is not available on the efficacy and duration of therapy of various regimens that are used for patients with organisms that are resistant to both INH and RMP. On discovery of drug resistance, it is likely that many patients will demonstrate resistance to other first-line agents. It is recommended that at least three new agents be used to which the organism is susceptible, with continuation of this regimen until sputum conversion is documented; completion of therapy with at least 12 months of two-drug therapy is necessary. Antituberculosis therapy for a total duration of 24 months is sometimes given empirically. Although the role of the new agents mentioned previously is unknown, these agents are being used in such cases. In patients in whom the majority of disease can be resected, surgery may provide substantial benefit and improvement in cure rate (142).

SPECIAL TREATMENT CIRCUMSTANCES
Children and Adolescents

Treatment principles for tuberculosis in children and adolescents are essentially the same as those for adults (11, 143). A high rate of success has been observed with 9-month regimens that include isoniazid and rifampin (144). Six-month regimens with three-drug therapy consisting of isoniazid, rifampin, and pyrazinamide have also shown success (11, 145). Dosing of these drugs should be based on body weight (11). The daily, twice-weekly, and thrice-weekly doses that are used for children are noted in Table 64.5 (3). Follow-up evaluations on successful completion of treatment are the same as those described for adults (8).

In addition to the basic pharmacotherapy, eight treatment considerations delineated in the ATS treatment recommendations include the following:

1. *Greater dissemination occurs in individuals who are younger than 4 years of age.* This heralds the need for prompt and vigorous therapy once diagnosis is suspected.
2. *Generally, treatment of primary intrathoracic tuberculosis is identical to treatment of pulmonary tuberculosis.* An exception to this recommendation is applicable in the case of drug nonresistance. When this is true, rifampin and isoniazid for 6 months supplemented with pyrazinamide in the first 2 months is sufficient.
3. *Sputum specimens are less helpful in diagnosis.* Dependence on the culture and sensitivity from the adult case source may be necessary. If drug resistance is suspected and adult isolates are unavailable, early morning gastric aspirates, bronchoalveolar lavage, or tissue diagnosis may be required.
4. *Bacteriologic examinations are less reliable in response evaluation.* Clinical and radiologic examinations are of greater importance in evaluation. Hilar adenopathy may require 2 to 3 years of complete radiographic resolution so that a normal chest radiograph is not a necessary criterion for halting therapy.
5. *Ocular toxicity is difficult to monitor.* Streptomycin and pyrazinamide are useful alternatives to ethambutol.
6. Bone and joint disease, disseminated disease, and meningitis require 12 months of treatment, compared with extrapulmonary tuberculosis (including cervical adenopathy), which can be treated the same as pulmonary tuberculosis.
7. *Directly observed therapy (DOT) is preferred except in cases in which compliance is not an issue.*
8. *Management of the newborn whose mother (or other house-*

hold contact) has tuberculosis is based on individual considerations. Separation of the mother and infant should be minimized. Recommendations are based on the unique circumstances and include:

a. Mother (or household contact) with a *positive tuberculosis skin test and no evidence of disease.* The infant should be tested with a Montoux test (5 tuberculin units PPD) at 4 to 6 weeks of age and at 3 to 4 months of age. If prompt testing of the family is not possible, prophylaxis of the infant with isoniazid (10 mg/kg/day) should be considered until skin testing of the family is found to be negative for active tuberculosis. If follow-up can be arranged, hospitalization of the infant is not required. Isoniazid prophylaxis for the mother should also be entertained.

b. Mother with *current disease* but ruled to be *noncontagious at delivery.* Rigorous study of household members and extended family is required. If chest radiograph and Montoux done at 4 to 6 weeks of age are negative, these should be repeated at 3, 4, and 6 months of age. When the mother adheres to treatment, separation from the mother is not necessary, and she may breast-feed. Even though the skin test and radiograph are negative for disease, the infant should be given isoniazid until 6 months of age. If the Montoux is negative at 6 months of age and no active disease exists in family members, isoniazid may be discontinued. The infant should be examined monthly. Bacillus Calmette-Guérin vaccine may be used for the infant if the mother has AFB-positive sputum (or smear), noncompliance is documented, and DOT is impossible. The infant's response to the vaccine may be inadequate.

c. Mother with *current disease* and thought to be *contagious* at delivery. Separation of the mother and the infant must be maintained until a noncontagious state is ensured; then recommendations for a mother who is noncontagious at time of delivery prevail.

d. Mother exhibiting *hematogenous spread* of tuberculosis. Congenital tuberculosis in the infant should be suspected, a skin test and a radiograph should be done, and treatment should be initiated promptly. If findings are negative for congenital tuberculosis, the infant and the mother should be separated until the mother is ruled to be noncontagious. Isoniazid should be given until the infant is 6 months old; if the skin test is positive at that time, isoniazid therapy should be continued until the infant is 9 months old (8, 143).

Pregnancy and Lactation

The benefits outweigh the risks that are involved in the treatment of tuberculosis in pregnant women. Also, tuberculosis during pregnancy does not warrant a therapeutic abortion. Treatment should include the use of isoniazid and rifampin and ethambutol (unless primary isoniazid resistance is unlikely). Pyridoxine is recommended when isoniazid is used. Because of inadequate teratogenic data, pyrazinamide is not recommended. Other drugs that should be avoided include streptomycin, kanamycin, and capreomycin, cycloserine, or ethionamide. Of

these, streptomycin is the only one with documented teratogenic effects (i.e., interference with ear development and congenital deafness) (8, 146, 147).

Small concentrations of antituberculosis drugs are present in breast milk. Nursing should not be abandoned, because this does not cause toxicity in the newborn; nor should it be considered an effective treatment for prevention in the nursing infant (8, 148). In cases in which both the infant and the mother are receiving antituberculosis drugs, breast-feeding should probably be discontinued (11).

Associated Disorders

Tuberculosis has been observed to occur in combination with disorders that can be grouped into two classes: (a) immune-altering disorders and (b) illnesses occurring in the same social and cultural environment as TB. Disorders that alter the immune status include HIV infection, hematologic or reticuloendothelial malignancies, immunosuppressive therapy, chronic renal failure, malnutrition, and culture-positive silicotuberculosis (8, 149). Two prominent disorders that relate to the social and cultural environment are chronic alcoholism (hepatitis and cirrhosis) and neuropsychiatric disorders. Therapy adjustments may be required, as well as steps toward correcting the existing disorder. Examples include (a) extension of therapy by 2 months with culture-positive silicotuberculosis; (b) avoidance of streptomycin, kanamycin, and capreomycin with decreased renal function; lengthening of intervals and measurement of blood concentrations for dosage adjustments in severely impaired renal function; (c) routine monitoring of liver function and complications of potentially hepatotoxic drugs in the case of hepatic dysfunction; and (d) the use of DOT in neuropsychiatric patients (8, 150-152).

TREATMENT OF TUBERCULOSIS INFECTION (PREVENTIVE THERAPY)

Treatment of tuberculosis in people who are infected is termed "preventive therapy." It does not include treatment of individuals with active disease or those who have been exposed but are not yet infected. Preventive therapy refers to the reduction or eradication of the bacterial population in "healed" or radiographically nonvisible lesions. Effectiveness of a 12-month regimen of isoniazid for preventive therapy for those with a positive skin test lasts for 20 years; in the absence of reinfection this coverage is believed to last for life. For primary prophylaxis (the person has been exposed but is not yet infected), isoniazid is effective only while the patient is receiving the drug (8, 153).

The risk of inducing isoniazid resistance is enhanced when isoniazid is used solo in a person with current disease; therefore, the recommended regimens for treatment (multidrug) are indicated until the diagnosis is clarified. If current disease is ruled out, multidrug treatment can be stopped after 4 months in adults and after 6 months in children (8, 137).

PEOPLE FOR WHOM PREVENTIVE THERAPY IS RECOMMENDED

The ATS has delineated individuals with a positive skin test and specified medical maladies, group membership, and findings on completion of specific evaluations (see the section below entitled "Screening Procedures") who should be considered for isoniazid preventive treatment. These individuals should be considered regardless of age. They include the following:

1. HIV-infected individuals, those who have diagnosed risk factors for HIV, and those who are undiagnosed but who are suspected of having AIDS (may also consider for HIV-infected individuals who are tuberculin-negative but belong to a group with a high prevalence rate.) (23, 24).
2. Close contacts of newly diagnosed tuberculosis patients.
3. Recent tuberculin skin test converters (≥10 mm increase in a 2-year period in people less than 35 years of age or ≥15 mm increase in people 35 years of age or older).
4. Patients with the following medical maladies, which are known to increase risk of tuberculosis:
   a. diabetes mellitus;
   b. long-term systemic adrenocorticosteroid therapy;
   c. immunosuppressive therapy;
   d. specific hematologic and reticuloendothelial diseases, e.g., leukemia or Hodgkin's disease;
   e. end-stage renal disease; and
   f. clinical instances yielding significant rapid weight loss or chronic malnutrition, such as intestinal bypass surgery for obesity, gastrectomy, or chronic alcoholism.
5. Injection drug users who are HIV-seronegative and have a tuberculin reaction ≥10 mm (8, 20, 154).

In the absence of the prior risk factors, individuals in the following groups who are less than 35 years of age and have a positive (≥10 mm) skin test should be considered for preventive treatment:

1. Foreign-born people from Latin America, Asia, and Africa.
2. Medically underserved low-income populations.
3. Residents of long-term care facilities (e.g., correctional institutions, nursing homes, and psychiatric institutions).
4. Staff of long-term health care facilities, schools, or child-care facilities, if they are diagnosed with tuberculosis and have a tuberculin reaction ≥10 mm (8, 154).

SCREENING PROCEDURES

Specific evaluations must be completed before institution of isoniazid preventive therapy for the individuals cited above. These evaluations include:

1. *Tuberculin skin test.*
   a. A reaction ≥ 5 mm is considered positive in people with HIV infection, close contacts of infectious individuals, and those with fibrotic lesions on chest radiograph.
   b. a reaction ≥10 mm is considered positive in other at-risk individuals, including infants and children younger than 4 years of age.
   c. A reaction ≥15 mm is considered positive in people who are not in a high-risk category or who are not exposed to a high-risk environment.
2. *Chest radiography.* Every person with a positive skin test should have a chest radiograph.
3. *Medical evaluation and bacteriologic examinations.* These should be conducted if the chest radiograph is consistent with pulmonary tuberculosis. Evaluation should also be conducted when extrapulmonary tuberculosis is suspected.
4. *Interview for exclusion of those who have a history of adequate treatment for tuberculosis (preventive/disease).*
5. *Interview for exclusion of those who have had an adequate course of isoniazid preventive therapy.*
6. *Determine whether contraindications exist for isoniazid preventive therapy.* These include:
   a. prior isoniazid-related hepatic injury;
   b. severe, adverse isoniazid reactions; and
   c. acute or unstable hepatic disease.
7. Delineate individuals who require special precautions. They include those with the following factors present:
   a. greater than 35 years of age,
   b. long-term therapy with any other medication,
   c. daily ethanol use,
   d. prior discontinuation of isoniazid therapy due to possible related side effects,
   e. current chronic liver disease,
   f. peripheral neuropathy or other conditions that might predispose to such,
   g. pregnancy (preventive therapy should generally be delayed until after delivery except when recent infection or high-risk medical condition (e.g., HIV infection) is present),
   h. injection drug use, and
   i. being a Black or Hispanic female (demonstrated increased risk of fatal hepatitis, especially during the postpartum period) (8, 154, 155).

ADMINISTRATION OF ISONIAZID PREVENTIVE THERAPY

Isoniazid is given solo for prevention in a once-daily dose of 300 mg/day for adults and 10 to 15 mg/kg body weight per day, not to exceed 300 mg/day, for children. Only a month's worth of therapy should be dispensed at any given time. Adherence to therapy for at least 6 months is strongly advised. HIV-infected individuals should receive 12 months of treatment. Children, according to the American Academy of Pediatrics, should receive 9 months of therapy. For adults and children for whom high-risk status has been determined and adherence may be questionable, directly observed therapy (DOT) is advisable. Another option, when DOT is not possible, is administration of isoniazid twice weekly in a dose of 15 mg/kg (8, 143).

MONITORING PREVENTIVE THERAPY AND INDICATIONS FOR DISCONTINUANCE OF THERAPY

Individuals who are receiving preventive therapy (or a responsible adult in the case of children) should be counseled about the signs and symptoms of isoniazid-adverse events (see Table 64.2) (8) and the need to report to their health care provider when such occur. In addition, these people should be interviewed monthly about this issue. When adverse effects occur, the patient should be evaluated, including biochemical tests for hepatitis (11, 8).

Several factors are associated with an increased risk for isoniazid-associated hepatitis. They include:

1. being older than 35 years of age (a transaminase test should be obtained before initiating therapy and then monthly during therapy),
2. daily use of ethanol,
3. chronic liver disease,
4. injection drug use, and
5. being a postpubertal Black or Hispanic woman (8).
6. Individuals with these factors should have more frequent liver function studies; however, these are not a substitute for a monthly clinical evaluation. When any of the liver tests are three to five times above the normal range, discontinuation of isoniazid should be considered (8, 11).

SITUATIONS WARRANTING THE USE OF AN ALTERNATIVE FORM OF TUBERCULOSIS PREVENTIVE THERAPY

Close Contacts of Isoniazid-Resistant Cases

Child contacts and high-risk individuals (e.g., immunocompromised hosts) should be treated with rifampin when isoniazid resistance is apparent. Some clinicians would support adding a second drug such as ethambutol. Administration of standard therapeutic doses for 6 months in adults and 9 months in children is recommended (8).

High Probability of Multidrug-Resistant Infection

If organisms are resistant to both isoniazid and rifampin, except in cases of high risk, ongoing observation without preventive therapy is recommended (156). Consideration should be given to preventive treatment using ethambutol and pyrazinamide daily for 6 months at the usual therapeutic doses in high-risk cases (e.g., HIV infection). When resistance to ethambutol is present, pyrazinamide plus a fluoroquinolone (ofloxacin or ciprofloxacin, which are FDA-approved only for patients who are older than 18 years of age) is recommended for 6 months (8).

Intolerance to Isoniazid

When isoniazid intolerance is known, rifampin in standard therapeutic doses for 6 months for adults and 9 months for children is recommended. Some clinicians may add a second drug such as ethambutol (8).

Infants and Children in Compromised Circumstances in Which Bacille Calmette-Guérin (BCG) Vaccine* Is Recommended

BCG vaccine is recommended in tuberculin-negative infants and children in the following situations:

1. Intimate and prolonged exposure to untreated or ineffectively treated individuals with infectious pulmonary tuberculosis when removal from contact is not feasible and long-term preventive therapy is not possible.
2. Ongoing contact with individuals who have tuberculosis that is resistant to isoniazid and rifampin.
3. Residence in an area where the rate of new infection is greater than 1% annually and where customary surveillance and treatment programs are not feasible. Such areas include those where there is:
   a. limited access to health care,
   b. cultural or social nonacceptance of usual health care, and
   c. an inability to effectively use existing accessible care.

Though BCG is an alternative to preventive therapy in cases discussed earlier, it should not be used in cases in which there is other active infection, depressed host immunity (e.g., HIV infection, therapy with immunosuppressive drugs), or pregnancy (8, 11, 24, 157).

CONCLUSION

Unfortunately, tuberculosis is not a conquered disease of the past. The resurgence of tuberculosis and the rising prevalence of MDR-TB in the United States indicate that the battle is being lost (158). More recently, factors have been identified that are contributing to the deteriorating situation regarding tuberculosis. These include the problems of homelessness, substance abuse, and the HIV epidemic (158).

Chemotherapy continues to be the cornerstone of effective antituberculosis therapy, enabling TB to be a curable and preventable disease (8). In the past, for various reasons, the potential benefits of chemotherapy were not seen (159). These include the long duration of drug-taking, as well as the difficulties of organizing health care services that have the ability to provide diagnostic, treatment, and prevention measures effectively and efficiently (159). Recently, various strategies have been developed to ensure effective therapy of TB. The guidelines provided by the CDC/ATS list various options for initial treatment of TB (8). Directly observed therapy (DOT) will eliminate noncompliance by patients and can be administered two or three times weekly. On initiation of therapy, monitoring the patient for adverse effects and response to therapy is necessary. The overall clinical and social management of patients with tuberculosis and their contacts is the ultimate goal. In this setting, the success of chemotherapy is achieved (8).

---

*BCG should be administered only according to package labeling.

REFERENCES

1. Snider DE Jr, La Montagne JR. Neglected global tuberculosis problem: a report of the 1992 World Congress on Tuberculosis. J Infect Dis 169:1189–96, 1994.

2. Riley LW. Drug-resistant tuberculosis. Clin Infect Dis 17(Suppl 2):S442–6, 1993.

3. Centers for Disease Control. Initial therapy for tuberculosis in the era of multidrug resistance: recommendations of the Advisory Council for the Elimination of Tuberculosis. MMWR Morb Mortal Wkly Rep 42(No. RR-7):1–8, 1993.

4. Rose DN, Schecter CB, Sacks HS. Preventive medicine for HIV infected patients: an analysis of isoniazid prophylaxis for tuberculin reactors and for anergic patients. J Gen Intern Med 7:589–94, 1992.

5. Iseman MD. A leap of faith: what can we do to curtail intrainstitutional transmission of tuberculosis. Ann Int Med 117:271–3, 1992.

6. Small PM, Shafer RW, Hopewell PC, et al. Exogenous reinfection with multidrug-resistant mycobacterium tuberculosis in patients with advanced HIV infection. N Engl J Med 328(16):1137–44, 1993.

7. Weiss SE, Slocum PC, Blais FX, et al. The effect of directly observed therapy on the rates of drug resistance and relapse in tuberculosis. N Engl J Med 330 (No. 17):1179–84, 1994.

8. American Thoracic Society. Treatment of tuberculosis and tuberculosis infection in adults and children. Am J Respir Crit Care Med 149:1359–74, 1994.

9. Des Prez RM, Heim CR. Chapter 229: *Mycobacterium tuberculosis.* In: Principles and practice of infectious diseases (3rd edition). Edited by Mandell GL, Douglas RG, and Bennett JE. New York: Churchill Livingstone, 1990:1877–1906.

10. Daniel TM. Chapter 127: Tuberculosis. In: Harrison's principles of internal medicine (12th edition). Edited by Wilson JD, et al. New York: McGraw-Hill, Inc., 1991:637–38.

11. Hooker KD, Jost PM. Chapter 62: Tuberculosis. In: Clinical pharmacy and therapeutics (5th edition). Edited by Herfindal ET, Gourley DR, and Hart LL. Baltimore: Williams & Wilkins, 1992: 1092–1108.

12. Centers for Disease Control. Expanded tuberculosis surveillance and tuberculosis morbidity: United States, 1993. MMWR Morb Mortal Wkly Rep 44(No. 20):361–66, 1994.

13. Centers for Disease Control and Prevention. Reported tuberculosis in the United States, 1993. October 1994:1–5.

14. Horwitz O, Edwards PQ, Lowell AM. National Tuberculosis Control Program in Denmark and the United States. Health Serv Rep 88:502, 1973.

15. Small PM, Hopewell PC, Singh SP, et al. The epidemiology of tuberculosis in San Francisco: a population based study using conventional and molecular methods. N Engl J Med 330:1703, 1994.

16. Alland D, Kalkut GE, Moss AR, et al. Transmission of tuberculosis in New York City: an analysis by DNA fingerprinting and conventional epidemiologic methods. N Eng J Med 330:1701, 1994.

17. Hamburg MA, Frieden TR. Tuberculosis transmission in the l990s [Editorial]. N Eng J Med 330:1750, 1994.

18. Graham NMH, Chaisson RE. Tuberculosis and HIV infection: epidemiology, pathogenesis, and clinical aspects. Ann Allergy 71:421, 1993.

19. Daley CL, Small PM, Schecter GF, et al. An outbreak of tuberculosis with accelerated progression among persons infected with the human immunodeficiency virus: an analysis using restriction-fragment-length polymorphisms. N Engl J Med 327:231, 1992.

20. Core curriculum on tuberculosis: what the clinician should know (3rd edition). Atlanta: Centers for Disease Control, 1994.

21. Centers for Disease Control. Management of persons exposed to multidrug-resistant tuberculosis. MMWR Morb Mortal Wkly Rep 41(No. RR-11):61–71, 1992.

22. Hamburg MA, Frieden TR. Tuberculosis transmission in the 1990's [Editorial]. N Eng J Med 330:1750, 1994.

23. Selwyn PA, Hartel D, Lewis VA, et al. A prospective study of the risk of tuberculosis among intravenous drug users with HIV infection. N Eng J Med 320:545, 1989.

24. Centers for Disease Control. Purified protein derivative (PPD)-tuberculin anergy and HIV infection: guidelines for anergy testing and management of anergic persons at risk of tuberculosis. MMWR Morb Mortal Wkly Rep 40(No. RR-5):27–32, 1991.

25. Frieden TR, Sterling T, Pablos-Mendez A, et al. The emergence of drug-resistant tuberculosis in New York City. N Engl J Med 328:521, 1993.

26. Centers for Disease Control. Nosocomial transmission of multidrug-resistant tuberculosis among HIV-infected persons: Florida and New York, 1988-1991. MMWR Morb Mortal Wkly Rep 40:585, 1991.

27. Doole SW, Jarvis WR, Martone WD, et al. Multidrug-resistant tuberculosis [Editorial]. Ann Intern Med 117:277, 1992.

28. Goble M, Iseman MD, Madsen LA, et al. Treatment of 171 patients with pulmonary tuberculosis resistant to isoniazid and rifampin. N Engl J Med 328:527, 1993.

29. Beck-Sague C, Dooley JW, Hutton MD, et al. Hospital outbreak of multi-drug resistant *Mycobacterium tuberculosis* infections. JAMA 278:1280, 1992.

30. Snider DE Jr., Kelly GD, Cauthen GM, et al. Infection and disease among contacts of tuberculosis cases with drug-resistant and drug-susceptible bacilli. Am Rev Respir Dis 132:127, 1985.

31. Edlin BR, Tokar JI, Grieco MN, et al. An outbreak of multi-drug resistant tuberculosis among hospitalized patients with the acquired immunodeficiency syndrome. N Engl J Med 327:1514, 1992.

32. Theuer CP, Hopewell PC, et al. Human immunodeficiency virus infection in tuberculosis patients. J Infec Dis 162:8, 1990.

33. Chaisson RE, Schecter GF, et al. Tuberculosis in patients with acquired immunodeficiency syndrome: clinical features, response to therapy and survival. Am Rev Respir Dis 136:570, 1987.

34. Hopewell PC. Impact of human immunodeficiency virus infection on the epidemiology, clinical features, management, and control of tuberculosis. Clin Infect Dis 15:540, 1992.

35. Fischl MA, Daikos GL, et al. Clinical presentation and outcome of patients with HIV infection and tuberculosis caused by multiple-drug-resistant bacilli. 177:184, 1992.

36. Van Scog RE, Wilkowske CJ. Antituberculous agents. Mayo Clin Proc 67:179–187, 1992.

37. Mitchison DA. Development of streptomycin resistant strains of tubercle bacilli in pulmonary tuberculosis: results of simultaneous sensitivity tests in liquid and on solid media. Thorax 5:144–61, 1950.

38. Canetti G. Present aspects of bacterial resistance in tuberculosis. Am Rev Respir Dis 92:687–703, 1965.

39. Hobby GL. Primary drug resistance in tuberculosis: a review. Am Rev Respir Dis 86:839–46, 1962.

40. Hobby GL. Primary drug resistance in tuberculosis: a review. Am Rev Respir Dis 87:29–36, 1963.

41. Doster B, Caras CJ, Snider DE. A continuing survey of primary drug resistance in tuberculosis, 1961 to 1968: a U.S. Public Health Service cooperative study. Am Rev Respir Dis 113:419–27, 1976.

42. Kopnoff DE, Kilburn JO, Glassroth JL, et al. A continuing survey of tuberculosis primary drug resistance in the United States: March 1975 to November 1977: a United States Public Health Service cooperative study. Am Rev Respir Dis 118:835–42, 1978.

43. Snider DE, Cauthen GM, Farer LS, et al. Drug-resistant tuberculosis. Am Rev Respir Dis 144:732, 1991.

44. Iseman MD. Treatment of multidrug-resistant tuberculosis. N Engl J Med 329(11):784–91, 1993.

45. Perez-Stable EJ, Hopewell PC. Chemotherapy of tuberculosis. Semin Respir Med 9:459, 1988.

46. Aquinas SM. Short-course therapy for tuberculosis. Drugs 24:118–32, 1982.

47. Angel JH. The case for short-course chemotherapy of pulmonary tuberculosis. Drugs 27:1–8, 1983.

48. Stratton MA, Reed MD. Short-course drug therapy for tuberculosis. Clin Pharmacy 5(12):977–87, 1986.

49. Takayama K, Schnoes HK, Armstrong EL, et al. Site of inhibitory action of isoniazid in the synthesis of mycolic acids in *Mycobacterium tuberculosis*. J Lipid Res 16:308–17, 1975.

50. Mandell GL, Sande MA. Drugs used in the chemotherapy of tuberculosis and leprosy. In: The pharmacologic basis of therapeutics (8th edition). Edited by Gilman AG, Goodman LS, and Gilman A. New York: Macmillan, 1990:1146–1159.

51. Dickinson JM, Aber VR, Mitchison DA. Bactericidal activity of streptomycin, isoniazid, rifampin, ethambutol, and pyrazinamide alone and in combination against *Mycobacterium tuberculosis*. Am Rev Respir Dis 116:627–35, 1977.

52. Hurwitz A, Schlozman DL. Effect of antacids on gastrointestinal absorption of isoniazid in rat and man. Am Rev Respir Dis 109:41–7, 1974.

53. Holdiness MR. Cerebrospinal fluid pharmacokinetics of antituberculous antibiotics. Clin Pharmacokinet 10:532–34, 1985.

54. Maddrey WC, Boitnott JK. Isoniazid hepatitis. Ann Intern Med 79:1–12, 1973.

55. Mitchell JR, Zimmerman HJ, Ishak KG. Isoniazid liver injury: clinical spectrum, pathology and probable pathogenesis. Ann Intern Med 84:181–92, 1976.

56. Evans DAP, Manley KA, McKusick VA. Genetic control of isoniazid metabolism in man. Br Med J 2:485–91, 1960.

57. Mitchell JR, Thorgeirsson UP, Black M, et al. Increased incidence of isoniazid hepatitis in rapid acetylators: possible relation in hydrazine metabolites. Clin Pharmacol Ther 18:70–79, 1975.

58. Alexander MR, Louie SG, Guernsy BG. Isoniazid-associated hepatitis. Clin Pharmacy 1:148–53, 1982.

59. Martinez-Roig A, Cami J, Llorens-Terol J, et al. Acetylation phenotype and hepatotoxicity in the treatment of tuberculosis in children. Pediatrics 77:912–15, 1986.

60. Anderson RJ, Gambertoglio JG, Schrier RW. Clinical use of drugs in renal failure. Springfield, IL: Charles C. Thomas, 1976.

61. Bennett WM, Aronoff GR, Morrison G, et al. Drug prescribing in renal failure: dosing guidelines for adults. Am J Kidney Dis 3: 155–93, 1983.

62. Girling DJ. Adverse effects of antituberculous drugs. Drugs 23:56–74, 1982.

63. Kopanoff DE, Snider DE Jr, Caras GJ. Isoniazid-related hepatitis: a U.S. Public Health Service cooperative surveillance study. Am Rev Respir Dis 117:991–1001, 1978.

64. Stead WW, To T. The significance of the tuberculin skin test in elderly persons. Ann Intern Med 107: 837–42, 1987.

65. Baciewicz AM, Self TH. Isoniazid interactions. South Med J 78 (No. 6):714–18, 1985.

66. Maukkassah SF, Bidlack WF, Yang WCT. Mechanism of the inhibitory action of isoniazid on microsomal drug metabolism. Biochem Pharmacol 30:1651–58, 1981.

67. Kutt H, Brennan R, Dehejia H, et al. Diphenylhydantoin intoxication. Am Rev Respir Dis 101:377–84, 1970.

68. Brennan RW, Dehejia H, Kutt H, et al. Diphenylhydantoin intoxication attendant to slow inactivation of isoniazid. Neurology 20:687–93, 1970.

69. Miller RR, Porter J, Greenblatt DJ. Clinical importance of the interaction of phenytoin and isoniazid. Chest 75:356–58, 1979.

70. Melander A, Danielson K, Hanson A, et al. Reduction of isoniazid bioavailability in normal men by concomitant intake of food. Acta Med Scand 200:93–7, 1976.

71. Männiströ P, Mäntylä R, Klinge R, et al. Influence of various diets on the bioavailability of isoniazid. J Antimicrob Chemother 10:427–34, 1982.

72. Mattila MJ, Takki S, Jussila J. Effects of sodium sulphate and castor oil on drug absorption from the human intestine. Ann Clin Res 6:19–24, 1974.

73. Hauser MJ, Baier H. Interactions of isoniazid with foods. Drug Intell Clin Pharm 16:617–18, 1982.

74. Smith CK, Durack DT. Isoniazid and reaction to cheese. Ann Intern Med 78:520–21, 1978.

75. Lejonc JL, Gusmini D, Brochard P. Isoniazid and reaction to cheese [Letter]. Ann Intern Med 91:793, 1979.

76. Uragoda CG, Lodha SC. Histamine intoxication in a tuberculous patient after ingestion of cheese. Tubercle 60:59–61, 1979.

77. Lejonc JL, Schaeffer A, Brochard P, et al. Hypertension artérielle paroxystique provoquée sous isoniazide par l'ingestion de gruyère: deux cas. Ann Med Interne 131:346–48, 1980.

78. Uragoda CG, Kottegoda SR. Adverse reactions to isoniazid on ingestion of fish with a high histamine content. Tubercle 58:83–9, 1977.

79. Senanayake N, Vyravanathan S, Kanagasuriyam S. Cerebrovascular accident after a "skipjack" reaction in a patient taking isoniazid. Br Med J 2:1127–28, 1978.

80. Uragoda CG. Histamine poisoning in tuberculous patients after injestion of tuna fish. Am Rev Respir Dis 121:157–59, 1980.

81. Aloysius DJ, Uragoda CG. Histamine poisoning on ingestion of tuna fish. J Trop Med Hyg 86:13–15, 1983.

82. Uragoda CG. Histamine poisoning in tuberculosis patients on ingestion of tropical fish. J Trop Med Hyg 81:243–45, 1978.

83. Uragoda CG. Histamine intoxication with isoniazid and a species of fish. Ceylon Med J 23:109–10, 1978.

84. Brass C, Galgiani JN, Blaschke TF, et al. Disposition of ketoconazole, an oral antifungal in humans. Antimicrob Agents Chemother 21:151–58, 1982.

85. Englehard D, Stutman HR, Marks MI. Interaction of ketoconazole with rifampin and isoniazid. N Engl J Med 74:18–47, 1983.

86. Hoglund P, Nillson LG, Paulsen O. Interaction between isoniazid and theophylline. Eur J Resp Dis 70:110–16, 1987.

87. Samigun M, Santoso B. Lowering of theophylline clearance by isoniazid in slow and rapid acetylators. Br J Clin Pharmac 29:570–73, 1990.

88. Thompson JR, Buckart GJ, Self TH, et al. Isoniazid-induced alterations of theophylline pharmacokinetics. Curr Ther Res 32: 921–25, 1982.

89. Thompson JR, Self TH. Theophylline and isoniazid. Br J Clin Pharmac 30:909, 1990.

90. Thornsberry C, Hill BC, Swenson JM, et al. Rifampin: spectrum of antibacterial activity. Rev Infect Dis 5(Suppl 3):S412–17, 1983.

91. Wehrli W. Rifampin: mechanisms of action and resistance. Rev Infect Dis 5(Suppl 3):S407–11, 1983.

92. Fox W. Whither short-course chemotherapy? Br J Dis Chest 75:331–57, 1981.

93. Kucer A, Bennett N. The use of antibiotics: a comprehensive review with clinical emphasis (3rd edition). Philadelphia: Lippincott, 1979.

94. Koup JR, Williams-Warren J, Viswanathan CT, et al. Pharmacokinetics of rifampin in children. II: oral bioavailability. Ther Drug Monit 8:17–22, 1986.

95. Council on Drugs, American Medical Association. Evaluation of a new antituberculous agent. JAMA 220:414–15, 1972.

96. McCracken GH, Ginsberg CM, Zweighaft TC, et al. Pharmacokinetics of rifampin in infants and children: relevance to prophylaxis against *Haemophilus influenzae* type b disease. Pediatrics 66:17–21, 1980.

97. Sippel JE, Mikhail IA, Girgis NI, et al. Rifampin concentrations in cerebrospinal fluid of patients with tuberculosis meningitis. Am Rev Respir Dis 109:579–80, 1974.

98. Furesz S. Clinical and biological properties of rifampicin. Antibiot Chemother 16:316–51, 1970.

99. Grosset J, Leventis S. Adverse effects of rifampin. Rev Infec Dis 5 (Suppl 3):S440–46, 1983.

100. Flynn CT, Rainford DJ, Hope E. Acute renal failure and rifampicin: danger of unsuspected intermittent dosage. Br Med J 2:428, 1974.

101. Girling DJ, Hitze HL. Adverse reactions to rifampicin. Bull WHO 57:45–9, 1979.

102. Gronhagen-Riska C, Hellstrom PE, Froseth B. Predisposing factors in hepatitis induced by isoniazid-rifampin treatment of tuberculosis. Am Rev Respir Dis 118:461–66, 1978.

103. Baciewicz AM, Self TH. Rifampin drug interactions. Arch Intern Med 144:1167, 1984.

104. Baciewicz AM, Self TH, Bakemeyer WB. Update on rifampin drug interactions. Arch Intern Med 147:565, 1987.

105. Borcherding SM, Baciewicz AM, Self TH. Update on rifampin drug interactions II. Arch Intern Med 152:711–15, 1992.

106. Gupta KC, Joshi JV, Anklesria PS, et al. Plasma rifampicin levels during oral contraception. J Assoc Phys India 36:365–66, 1988.

107. Skolnick, JL, Stoler BS, Katz DB, et al. Rifampin, oral contraceptives, and pregnancy. JAMA 236(No. 12):1382, 1976.

108. Takayama K, Armstrong EL, Kunugi KA. Inhibition by ethambutol of mycolic acid transfer into the cell wall of *Mycobacterium smegmatis.* Antimicrob Agents Chemother 16:240, 1979.

109. Peets EA, Sweeney WM, Place VA. The absorption, excretion and metabolic fate of ethambutol in man. Am Rev Respir Dis 91:51–8, 1965.

110. Holdiness MR. Clinical pharmacokinetics of the antituberculous drugs. Clin Pharmacokinet 9:511–44, 1984.

111. Liebold JE. The ocular toxcity of ethambutol and its relation to dose. Ann NY Acad Sci 135:904–09, 1966.

112. Postlethwaite AE, Bartel AG, Kelly WN. Hyperuricemia due to ethambutol. N Engl J Med 286:761–62, 1972.

113. Mackandess GB. The intracellular activity of pyrazinamide and nicotinamide. Am Rev Tuberc 74:718–28, 1956.

114. Zierski M, Bek E. Side effects of drug regimens used in short course chemotherapy for pulmonary tuberculosis: a controlled study. Tubercle 61:41–9, 1980.

115. Pilheu JA, De Salvo MC, Koch O, et al. Liver alterations in antituberculosis regimens containing pyrazinamide. Chest 80:720–24, 1981.

116. Steele MA, Des Prez RM. The role of pyrazinamide in tuberculosis chemotherapy. Chest 94:845, 1988.

117. Cullen JH, Early LJA, Fiore JM. The occurrence of hyperuricemia during pyrazinamide-isoniazid therapy. Am Rev Tuberc Pulm Dis 74:289–92, 1956.

118. Edwards KDG, Whyte HM. Streptomycin poisoning in renal failure. Br Med J 1:752, 1959.

119. Hansten PD, Horn JR. Drug interactions (6th edition). Philadelphia: Lea & Febiger, 1989.

120. Spector R, Lorenza WV. The active transport of para-aminosalicylic acid from the cerebrospinal fluid. J Pharmacol Exp Ther 185:642–48, 1973.

121. Peloquin CA. Antituberculous drug pharmacokinetics. In: Drug susceptibility in the chemotherapy of mycobacterial infections. Edited by Heifets, LB. Boca Raton, FL: CRC Press, 1991.

122. Heifets LB. Drug susceptibility in the management of chemotherapy of tuberculosis. In: Drug susceptibility in the chemotherapy of mycobacterial infections. Edited by Heifets LB. Boca Raton, FL: CRC Press, 1991.

123. Cynamon MH, Klemens SP. New antimycobacterial agents. Clin Chest Med 10:355–64, 1989.

124. Leysen DC, Haemers A, Pattyn SR. Mycobacteria and the new quinolones. Antimicrob Agents Chemother 33:1–5, 1989.

125. Physicians' desk reference (47th edition). Montvale, NJ: Medical Economics Company, 1993.

126. Tsukamura M, Nakamura E, Yoshii S, Amanott R. Therapeutic

127. Yew WW, Kwan SY, Wing KM, et al. *In vitro* activity of ofloxacin against *Mycobacterium tuberculosis* and its clincial efficacy in multiple resistant pulmonary tuberculosis. J Antimicrob Chemother 27:227–36, 1990.

128. Heifets LB, Lindholm-Levy PF, Iseman MD. Rifabutine: minimum inhibitory and bactericidal concentrations for *Mycobacterium tuberculosis.* Am Rev Respir Dis 137:719–21, 1988.

129. Wong CS, Palmer GS, Cynamon MH. *In vitro* susceptibility of *Mycobacterium tuberculosis, Mycobacterium bovis,* and *Mycobacterium kansasii* to amoxycillin and ticarillin in combination with clavulanic acid. J Antimicrob Chemother 22:863–6, 1988.

130. Parenti F. New experimental drugs for the treatment of tuberculosis. Rev Infect Dis 11:S479–83, 1989.

131. Centers for Disease Control. Nosocomial transmission of multidrug-resistant TB in health-care workers and HIV-infected patients in an urban hospital: Florida. MMWR Morb Mortal Wkly Rep 39:718, 1990.

132. Combs DL, O'Brien RJ, Geiter LJ. USPHS tuberculosis short-course therapy trial 21: effectiveness, toxicity, and acceptability. The report of final results. Ann Intern Med 112:397, 1990.

133. Cohn DL, Catlin BJ, Peterson KL, et al. A 62-dose, 6-mo therapy for pulmonary and extrapulmonary tuberculosis: a twice-weekly, directly observed, and cost-effective regimen. Ann Intern Med 112:407, 1990.

134. Hong Kong Chest Service/British Medical Research Council. Five-year follow-up of a controlled trial of five 6-month regimens of chemotherapy for pulmonary tuberculosis. Am Rev Respir Dis 136:1339, 1987.

135. Slutkin G, Schecter GF, Hopewell PC. The results of 9-month isoniazid-rifampin therapy for pulmonary tuberculosis under programs in San Francisco. Am Rev Respir Dis 138:1622, 1988.

136. Dutt AK, Moers D, Stead WW. Short-course chemotherapy for tuberculosis with mainly twice-weekly isoniazid and rifampin: community physicians' seven-year experience with mainly outpatients. Am J Med 77:223, 1984.

137. Hong Kong Chest Service/Tuberculosis Research Centre, Madras/British Medical Research Council. A controlled trial of 3-month, 4-month and 6-month regimens of chemotherapy for sputum-smear negative pulmonary tuberculosis: results at 5 years. Am Rev Respir Dis 139:871, 1989.

138. Dutt AK, Moers D, Stead WW. Smear- and culture-negative pulmonary tuberculosis: four-month short course chemotherapy. Am Rev Respir Dis 139:867, 1989.

139. Snider DE, Long MW, Cross FS, et al. Six-months isoniazid-rifampin therapy for pulmonary tuberculosis. Am Rev Respir Dis 129:573, 1984.

140. Singapore Tuberculosis Service/British Medical Research Council. Clinical trial of six-month and four-month regimens of chemotherapy in the treatment of pulmonary tuberculosis. Am Rev Respir Dis 119:579–85, 1979.

141. Zierski M. Prospects of retreatment of chronic resistant pulmonary tuberculosis: a critical review. Lung 154:91, 1977.

142. Iseman MD, Madsen L, Goble M. Surgical intervention in the treatment of pulmonary disease caused by drug-resistant *Mycobacterium tuberculosis.* Am Rev Respir Dis 141:623, 1990.

143. American Academy of Pediatrics. Report of the committee on infectious diseases (22nd edition). Elk Grove, IL: American Academy of Pediatrics, 1991:487–508.

144. Abernathy AS, Dutt, Stead WW, Mowers, DJ. Short-course chemotherapy for tuberculosis in children. Pediatrics 72:801, 1983.

145. Starke, JR. Multidrug chemotherapy for tuberculosis in children. Pediatr Infect Dis J 9:785–93, 1990.

146. Briggs, GG, Freeman, RK, Yaffe, JJ. Drugs in pregnancy and lactation (3rd edition). Baltimore: Williams & Wilkins, 1990: 327–28, 565, 924–36.

147. Snider DE, Layde RM, Johnson MW, Lyle, MA. Treatment of tuberculosis during pregnancy. Am Rev Respir Dis 122:65, 1980.

148. Snider, DE, Powell KE. Should women taking antituberculosis drugs breastfeed? Arch Intern Med 144:589, 1984.

149. Mangura, BT Reichman, LB. Tuberculosis: guidelines for preventive therapy. J Respir Dis 15:109–21, 1994.

150. Hong Kong Chest Service/Tuberculosis Research Center, Madras/British Medical Research Council. A controlled clinical comparison of 6 and 8 months of antituberculosis chemotherapy in the treatment of patients with silicotuberculosis in Hong Kong. Am Rev Respir Dis 144:272–7, 1991.

151. Andrew, OT, Schoenfeld, PY, Hopewell PC, Humphrey MH. Tuberculosis in patients with end-stage renal disease. Am J Med 68:59, 1980.

152. Cross, FS, Long, MW, Banner, AS, Snider, DE. Rifampin-isoniazid therapy of alcoholic and nonalcoholic tuberculosis patients in a U.S. Public Health Service Cooperative therapy trial. Am Rev Respir Dis 122:350, 1980.

153. Comstock, GW, Gaum C, Snider DF. Isoniazid prophylaxis among Alaskan Eskimos: a final report of the Bethel isoniazid studies. Am Rev Respir Dis 119:827–30, 1979.

154. Centers for Disease Control. Screening for tuberculosis and tuberculosis infection in high-risk populations and the use of preventive therapy for tuberculosis infection in the United States: recommendations of the Advisory Committee for Elimination of Tuberculosis. MMWR Morb Mortal Wkly Rep 39:1–12, 1990.

155. Snider DE, Caras GJ. Isoniazid-associated hepatitis deaths: a review of available information. Am Rev Respir Dis 145:484–97, 1992.

156. Centers for Disease Control. Management of persons exposed to multidrug-resistant tuberculosis. MMWR Morb Mortal Wkly Rep 41:59–71, 1992.

157. Immunization Practices Advisory Committee and Advisory Committee for the Elimination of Tuberculosis. Use of BCG vaccines in the control of tuberculosis. MMWR Morb Mortal Wkly Rep 37:663, 1988.

158. Iseman MD, Cohn DL, Sbarbaro JA. Directly observed treatment of tuberculosis: we can't afford not to try it. N Engl J Med 328 (No. 8):576–78, 1993.

159. Johnston RF, Wildrick KH. The impact of chemotherapy in the care of patients with tuberculosis. Am Rev Respir Dis 109:636, 1974.

CHAPTER 65

URINARY TRACT INFECTIONS

DIANE R. ROMAC

Urinary tract infections remain as one of the most common infectious diseases for which medical treatment is sought. These infections are responsible for approximately 7 million office visits in the United States annually, ranking second only to respiratory tract infections. In addition, over 1 million hospital admissions annually are complicated by an urinary tract infection. Research continues in an attempt to resolve the controversial issues that remain and to seek new and better approaches to treatment.

DEFINITIONS

The urinary tract consists of the urethra, prostate gland (in males), urinary bladder, ureters, and kidneys. The term *urinary tract infection* (UTI) describes a variety of conditions relating to the components of the tract in which the common base is the presence of microorganisms in significant quantities.

UTI may be evident solely by the presence of bacteria in the urine (bacteriuria) or signs and symptoms of bacterial invasion of one or more components of the tract. It should be recognized that, however localized the infection is initially, once any component of the tract is invaded, the entire tract is at risk for infection.

UTIs can be designated as asymptomatic or symptomatic, complicated or uncomplicated, and acute, chronic, or recurrent. The terms *asymptomatic, symptomatic, chronic,* and *acute* are self-explanatory. An uncomplicated UTI is defined as an infection in which there is no structural or neurologic abnormality of the urinary tract that interferes with the normal flow of urine in the voiding mechanism of an otherwise healthy patient. A complicated UTI is the result of the presence of a congenital abnormality or distortion of the tract; a stone, indwelling catheter, enlarged prostate gland, neurologic deficit; an infection of a normal tract in a patient with an underlying disease; or one that is hospital acquired.

The term *recurrent* refers to the recurrence of an UTI in a given patient. The recurrent infection is further categorized into relapse or reinfection. If an UTI is a relapse, it is the result of invasion by the same specific serotype of microorganism, usually within 14 days of completion of antibacterial therapy for the preceding UTI. Relapse accounts for approximately 20% of recurrent attacks. The remaining 80% of recurrent infections can be termed *reinfection,* occur weeks to months after successful treatment, and are the result of a completely different microorganism or the same microorganism but of a different serotype.

EPIDEMIOLOGY

In general, UTIs occur predominantly in females. It is only during the first year and after the fifth decade of life that the incidence of UTIs in males is high or begins to increase. These latter findings are attributable to the higher incidence of congenital abnormalities in the males in the former instance, and the development of prostatic hypertrophy and interference with urinary flow in the latter instance. One review quantified the incidence of UTIs, pooling data from 17 studies, and is presented in Table 65.1 (1).

Approximately 10 to 20% of all females will have at least one UTI in their lifetime. During the childbearing years, women appear to have a particular predisposition to UTIs. Several factors increase the risk of infection, including sexual intercourse, use of a diaphragm or spermicide, and delayed postcoital micturition (2, 3).

Bacteriuria occurs in 4 to 7% of pregnant females, an incidence similar to that in nonpregnant women. However, if left untreated, bacteriuria can develop into symptomatic pyelonephritis in an estimated 23 to 40% of pregnant women (4). Increased incidence of bacteriuria may be seen in patients with diabetes mellitus, renal transplants, advanced age, and other immunocompromising conditions. In the diabetic population, women appear to have a two-to threefold higher incidence of bacteriuria then nondiabetic women, while diabetic men and children do not appear to be further predisposed to UTI (5). Urologic manipulation is another well-known risk factor for UTI, with catheterization and cystoscopy accounting for over 500,000 UTIs annually. UTIs represent the most common site for hospital acquired infections, and account for 30 to 46% of all nosocomial infections (6). The majority of these infections, greater than 80%, are associated with the use of catheters (7, 8).

PATHOGENESIS

Microorganisms invade the urinary tract by two routes: through the urethra and by hematogenous spread. The hematogenous route is much less common and results from seeding the kidney from a primary site of infection such as a carbuncle, osteomyelitis, endocarditis, or empyema (9). The UTI thus becomes a secondary infection. The

Table 65.1.
Prevalence of Bacteriuria in Various Populations

Population	Sex (%)	
	Male	Female
Community based		
Infants	2	0.5
Young children	0.1	1.5
College students	<0.01	5
Adults (30 to 65 years old)	0.1	10
Elderly persons		
65 to 85 years old	5	15
>85 years old	15	25
Patient based		
Adults (medical clinic)	4	6
Adults (urology clinic)	8	—
Adult inpatient		
<70 years old	7.5	30
>70 years old	25	30
Institutionalized elderly persons	>30	>30
Patients after instrumentation		
Urethral catheterization	5	5
Transurethral procedures	20	40

Percentages are approximations derived from a wide range of values from many studies in diverse settings; in these studies, specimens were obtained by various methods, and different definitions of bacteriuria were used.
Adapted from Lipsky BA. Urinary tract infections in men. Ann Intern Med 110(2):138–150, 1989.

hematogenous route has been the primary pathway implicated in the development of renal candidiasis and occurs in approximately 90% of patients with another source of candidal infection (10).

The most common route of invasion of microorganisms into the urinary tract is via the urethra. The source of these organisms is the fecal reservoir of enteric bacteria, as is evident from the 75 to 80% correlation of the causative microorganisms in bacteriuria and those cultured from a rectal swab. In females, bacteria progressively colonize the perineum, vagina, urethra, and bladder. Bacteria that adhere to the bladder mucosa remain behind after voiding, colonize, and produce infection. These bacteria may further ascend into the kidneys, causing upper tract infection (9). Urologic manipulation can introduce bacteria into the bladder by contamination at the time of instrument insertion, by bacterial migration, and by breaks in the sterility of the catheter system. Normally bacteria inhabit the distal third of the urethra. Thus, the introduction of an instrument through the urethra can contaminate the bladder. With an indwelling urinary catheter, microorganisms can migrate from the periurethral area into the bladder via the fluid that separates the urethral mucosa and the catheter. Loss of sterility of the catheter system can contribute to catheter-associated UTIs. This can occur if the closed collecting system is broken or disconnected at any time, if retrograde urine flow occurs from bag to

bladder, or if cross-contamination of patients in close proximity occurs as a result of improper hand cleansing of hospital personnel caring for the patients. Other factors that increase the rate of catheter-associated UTIs include age, sex, duration of the catheterization, catheter care techniques, training of the health care personnel inserting the catheter, and clustering of catheterized patients. Elderly, debilitated men appear to be at highest risk for developing this form of infection.

A major intrinsic defense mechanism against UTI is the washing out of bacteria that occurs with each urinary void (3). This defense mechanism is compromised if urinary flow is slowed or obstructed, or if a postvoid residual urine develops. Since urine is a good culture medium, urinary stasis provides an ideal environment for bacterial growth. Obstructed or decreased urine flow can occur with urologic tumors, strictures, stones, or prostatic hypertrophy. postvoid residual urine can occur with neurologic lesions affecting the bladder or sphincter musculature, including bladder spasticity or flaccidity; with drugs, including anticholinergic and anesthetic medications; with advanced age; or with poor micturition habits.

Changes in the urinary tract also occur with advanced age and contribute to the increased incidence of UTI in the elderly. Genitourinary complications are more frequent in the elderly and include cystoceles, rectoceles, bladder diverticula, and ureteric reflux (5). The decrease in estrogen production in elderly females has also been implicated in the development of UTI. The increased frequency of concurrent diseases also cause changes in bladder function and control.

Vesicoureteral reflux (VUR) provides a mechanism for bacteria to ascend from the bladder to the kidney. This reflux occurs when the anatomic valve at the vesicoureteral junction is incompetent. This lesion may result from a congenital abnormality and is present in approximately 30 to 50% of all children with UTI (11). VUR can also occur during pregnancy due to a distortion of the bladder.

CAUSATIVE AGENTS

The enteric bacteria—*Escherichia coli, Proteus, Klebsiella, Enterobacter, Enterococcus,* and *Pseudomonas*—are responsible for the vast majority of UTIs (Table 65.2). The predominant infecting agent is *E. coli,* accounting for over 80% of initial infections and approximately 50% of recurrent infections. The majority of acute, uncomplicated UTIs are caused by enteric gram-negative organisms. Once thought to be a urinary contaminant, *Staphylococcus saprophyticus* UTIs have increased and now account for 5 to 15% of UTIs in young women (2). When a UTI is hospital acquired or if the urinary tract is complicated by obstruction, stone, catheter, or other urologic manipulation, the causative microorganism is often difficult to predict. The use of repeated courses of antiinfectives and the presence of these complicating factors tend to select out organisms other than *E. coli* and also result in an increased frequency of mixed infections. Organisms causing these infections commonly include *Proteus mirabilis, Klebsiella pneumoniae, Pseudomonas aeruginosa, Enterobacter* species, *Staphylococcus aureus, Enterococcus faecalis,* and *Candida albicans* (3). Certain urease-producing organisms such as *P. mirabilis, K. pneumoniae,* and *P. aeruginosa,* can lead to the development of complicated infections by predisposing to struvite formation (11).

CLINICAL PRESENTATION

The clinical presentation of UTI can be divided into those findings associated with lower tract and upper tract infections. Classically the signs and symptoms of lower tract infection have an abrupt onset and include dysuria, frequency, urgency, and a vague lower abdominal discomfort. Grossly, the urine is turbid, dark, and foul smelling. Urinalysis reveals pyuria (more than 5–10 white blood cells (WBCs) per high-power field), bacteriuria, and hematuria in approximately 50% of patients. Leukocytosis in a peripheral blood smear is absent unless the upper tract or prostate is involved.

The presentation of prostatitis is similar to that of a lower UTI; however, fever, perineal pain, and urethral discharge may also be present. A rectal examination reveals an enlarged, tender, firm prostate gland. In an acute prostatic infection, leukocytosis is present. In a chronic infection the patient will also typically complain of a lumbosacral backache.

The classic presentation of an upper UTI includes nonspecific complaints of headache, malaise, nausea, and vomiting. In association with these nonspecific findings, the patient may also complain of suprapubic pain, costovertebral angle (CVA) tenderness, fever (to 39°C), and chills. Urinalysis will reveal bacteria, pyuria, and WBC casts in most patients. Hematuria and proteinuria will be detected in approximately 10 to 15% of patients, especially in the first few days of infection. Examination of the blood reveals a leukocytosis with a predominance of polymorphonucleocytes and band forms on the differential count. Blood cultures are positive for the infecting organism in approximately 20% of patients. In addition to these upper tract findings, lower tract symptoms can also be present.

Unfortunately, not all UTIs present with classic findings. For example, both upper and lower tract UTIs can be asymptomatic. Asymptomatic UTIs can occur in any patient but are found most commonly in elderly patients. In addition, symptoms may not be classic, such as infants who may present with nonspecific findings of poor feeding, vomiting, and fever (11). Elderly patients may present with delirium, confusion, lethargy, abdominal pain, and loss of interest in eating, drinking, or social activities (12).

Laboratory studies may also prove to be atypical. Although pyuria can be a good predictor of an UTI, not all women with UTI will have pyuria on urinalysis. Conversely, pyuria can occur without bacteriuria. In this latter instance, vaginal contamination of the specimen, tuberculous infection, tumor, a foreign body, or medications can cause inflammation of the tract. Similarly, dysuria in the absence of UTI can be caused by irritation of the bladder or urethra by medications, including methenamine and cyclophosphamide, or by other genitourinary conditions in up to 50% of patients presenting with dysuria (13).

DIAGNOSIS

The diagnosis of UTI should be based on the demonstration of a significant quantity of bacteria in the urine. In addition, although other factors may not definitively diagnose an UTI, together they may be good predictive factors. A study involving three different groups of women (approximately 250 per group) found five common clinical

Table 65.2.
Etiologic Organisms of Urinary Tract Infections (UTIs)

Organism	% of Total UTIs	% of Inpatient UTIs	% of Outpatient UTIs
Gram-negative			
Escherichia coli	51.5	30.6	72.5
Proteus species	5.0	4.6	5.3
Klebsiella species	6.6	8.9	4.3
Pseudomonas species	4.8	9.7	0.0
Other coliforms	6.8	10.3	3.3
Gram-positive			
Enterococcus species	7.8	13.9	1.6
Staphylococcus species	9.6	6.2	13.0
Others	1.2	2.3	0.0
Yeast	6.7	13.5	0.0
	100.0	100.0	100.0

Data from Bronsema DA, Adams JR, Pallares R, et al. Secular trends in rates and etiology of nosocomial urinary tract infections at a university hospital. J Urol 150:414–416, 1993; and Gruneberg RN. Antibiotic sensitivities of urinary pathogens, 1971–1982. J Antimicrob Chemother 14:17, 1984.

findings as having high predictive value for positive urinary culture results: (a) history of UTI, (b) back pain, (c) urinalysis with more than 15 WBC per high-power field (HPF), (d) urinalysis with more than 5 red blood cells (RBCs) per HPF, and (e) urinalysis with more than a "few" bacteria. Patients without any findings had negative urine cultures, whereas 73% of women with two or more findings and 86% of women with four or five findings had positive urinary cultures (14).

Several studies have shown that pyuria accompanied by lower UTI symptoms is a good predictor of true infection (13). Gram stain examination of the urine may provide information as to whether the microorganism is gram-positive or gram-negative, but does not specifically identify the organism nor does it provide quantitative information. Gram staining can be also misleading, as is evidenced by a 20% error rate.

Consequently, the most reliable method of diagnosing the UTI is the properly performed urine culture and sensitivity.

Collection of the Specimen

Collection of urine for culture and sensitivity testing is performed by one of three different methods: the suprapubic needle aspirate, single catheterization, or the midstream void collection. Each method has a different accuracy potential and a different level of bacteriuria indicative of the presence or absence of UTI.

Suprapubic aspiration is performed by inserting a needle in the midline, 2 cm above the symphysis pubis, and aspirating the urine. The sample is then cultured. A colony count of 5×10^3/mL or greater of the same organism is diagnostic of an UTI. A single culture using this technique is 99% accurate in detecting infection. Suprapubic aspiration is most commonly employed in neonates and infants, where specimens collected by other methods are frequently contaminated and yield two or more bacterial strains (11). This method may also be necessary to obtain a specimen from patients with spinal cord injury.

The single or in-and-out catheterization method can alleviate the problem of contamination of the specimen in the debilitated patient or may be useful in the patient who cannot void or follow the instructions. However, the procedure itself can introduce bacteria into the bladder. The patient's periurethral area is cleansed and a catheter is aseptically inserted; the urine is drained, the catheter removed, and an aliquot of urine is cultured. A bacterial colony count of 1×10^5/mL or greater of the same microorganism is diagnostic of UTI. This method is 95% accurate in detecting UTIs.

The most common technique for obtaining urine for culture is the midstream void method. The patient's periurethral area is cleansed with soap. The female patient is asked to separate her labia to avoid contamination.

During the midpoint of the void, an aliquot of urine is collected and this specimen is cultured. If the patient is asymptomatic, midstream samples from two separate voids should be obtained; if symptomatic, a single specimen is sufficient. A bacterial colony count of 1×10^5/mL or greater of the same microorganism is diagnostic of UTI. This method is 95% accurate in detecting UTIs. Over recent years, the traditional colony count of 1×10^5/mL as diagnostic of UTI has been disputed. Several studies have shown that women with bacterial counts as low as 1×10^2/mL and who are symptomatic have been culture positive and have benefited from treatment. One study found that one third of all acute dysuric episodes in ambulatory women who had positive culture results were characterized by 10^2 to 10^4 organisms/mL of midstream urine (13).

Collection of the urine specimen from a patient with an indwelling catheter can be obtained with relative ease. The catheter is clamped closed a short distance from the meatus for 1 hour. After this interval, the clamp is released and a few milliliters of urine are allowed to drain before the clamp is reapplied. An alcohol swab is used to wipe clean the area on the catheter between the meatus and clamp. Finally, a needle and syringe are used to aspirate the urine from the catheter just distal to the meatus. The sample is then cultured.

Culture and Sensitivity Testing

The standard method of identifying, quantitating, and determining the sensitivity and resistance pattern to antiinfectives of the invading microorganism is the culture and sensitivity test. The most popular tests are the Kirby-Bauer method and microdilution testing. After 24 hours of incubation, the organism can be identified. Usually the antimicrobial sensitivities of the organism can be determined within 48 hours.

The concentration required to determine susceptibility varies with the agent and may reflect the concentration achievable in either the urine or the serum. The concentration used by a laboratory should be investigated by the practitioner in order to gain the proper perspective of the sensitivity and resistance pattern of the microorganism. Many antiinfectives are excreted and concentrated in their active form in the urine. Therefore, sensitivities that used the antiinfective concentration achievable in the serum will not reflect the true resistance/sensitivity pattern of the microorganism in the urine and may underestimate the drug's ability to eradicate the infection. In addition, when treating an upper tract infection, the organism must also be susceptible in serum.

Methods other than the standard culture and sensitivity test for urinary infections are available. These methods are designed primarily to circumvent the cost and time factors required by the culture and sensitivity test. These alternative methods are most useful for diagnosis of uncomplicated UTIs or for posttherapy follow-up of complicated or upper tract infections. Since these tests do not provide information on organism identification or sensitivity testing, they are not useful in patients requiring an exact diagnosis for proper treatment. These patients include those that have (a) recurrent or relapsing infection, (b) upper tract infection, (c) nosocomial infection, (d) infection associated with a catheter or instrumentation, and (e) kidney stones or other complicating factors.

Localization Studies

A positive culture and sensitivity test only confirms that bacteria are present in the bladder. It provides no information regarding the presence or absence of infection in the kidney. Various tests, including renal concentrating ability and antibody titers, have been devised in an attempt to determine if pyelonephritis is present. Since in pyelonephritis the kidney often loses its ability to concentrate urine, a test of this function has been devised. This test unfortunately requires ureteral catheterization and can be influenced by other noninfectious renal conditions (e.g., analgesic nephropathy), but it still remains the most reliable diagnostic test.

The use of serum antibody titers to the infecting microorganism is based on the fact that patients who have classic upper UTIs have higher titers than patients with classic cystitis. However, since there is considerable overlap, the test is not definitive.

Another test for differentiating upper from lower tract UTIs is the presence or absence of antibody-coated bacteria in urinary sediment. Theoretically, upper tract infections should evoke an immune response and the bacteria would be coated with antibody (ACB positive). UTIs confined to the lower tract should not produce antibody (ACB negative). Several factors, including poor standards for test results, have prevented widespread use of the test.

The intravenous pyelogram (IVP) is another study that can provide evidence of pyelonephritis. Classically, in the early stages, localized scarring and calyceal distortion are present. In advanced cases of pyelonephritis, the above findings plus cortical scarring are found.

The indications for using localization studies in males revolve around the infrequent occurrence of UTIs. The presence of an infection, especially in boys and men under 50 years of age, usually indicates a structural deformity within the tract, which can sometimes be corrected with surgical intervention. Localization studies should be done with the first infection in all children less than 5 years of age, first infections in any male child, and recurrent infections in any female child (11). Up to 50% of those with their first proven case of symptomatic UTI will have a structural abnormality. Urinary tract abnormalities, including VUR,

can cause renal scarring in 10 to 15% of children, with most of the damage to the kidney occurring before the age of 2 years (11). Studies have shown that early renal scarring predisposes to later development of hypertension and renal insufficiency. Therefore, rapid diagnosis and effective early management of UTI in infants and children is crucial.

Since the incidence of UTIs in women is quite high as a result of their anatomic predisposition, localization studies are usually not performed on a routine basis. Studies have shown that only a small percentage of women have abnormalities of their urinary tract (3). In addition, the outcome of these studies rarely influences clinical management. Therefore, these studies are usually reserved for those women with relapsing infections after long-term therapy, atypical features of infection, or fever and flank pain persisting 72 hours after treatment (2).

THERAPY

The therapeutic approaches available for the patient with urinary tract infection can be broadly classified as eradicative, prophylactic, suppressive, and preventative. The approach used depends on the extent of the current illness; the patient's past history of UTIs; the patient's urologic status (complicated or uncomplicated); and the presence or absence of other diseases that will predispose or affect the severity of current and future UTIs.

Eradicative Therapy

The goal of eradicative therapy is the sterilization of the urinary tract. The approach is used when there is bacterial colonization occurring in any part of the tract. It is indicated prior to the institution of prophylactic or suppressive therapy and prior to insertion of an indwelling catheter or other urologic manipulation should an infection be present.

The efficacy of eradicative therapy is usually more dependent on the host environment than on the choice of drug. In the patient with a complicated infection, the structural abnormality, whether it be a stone, renal disease, prostatic hypertrophy, or vesicoureteral or ureterovesical reflux, can negatively affect the outcome of therapy by preventing adequate antimicrobial-organism contact. Similarly, should the patient have a disease such as diabetes mellitus, which predisposes or otherwise modifies the patient's response to infection, the outcome of therapy can be adversely affected. Control or correction of the underlying predisposing factors is essential to effective eradicative therapy.

The ideal antimicrobial agents for the treatment of UTI should meet the following criteria: a low rate of allergic/untoward reactions, once daily dosing, complete upper gastrointestinal absorption so as not to change bowel flora, high urinary levels with glomerular filtration and secretion, minimal change in vaginal flora, excellent gram-negative coverage, low cost, and minimal development of resistance. To date, many agents are available for the treatment of UTI, but none satisfy all the requirements for the ideal agent.

The drug that is selected should reflect variables encountered in the individual patient. In this regard, the patient's immunologic status, age, sex, allergy history, renal and hepatic function, and previous urologic history can influence the choice of antimicrobial used. In women who are pregnant, the selection of an agent should be viewed also from the perspective of potential teratogenic or neonatal toxicity; for example, tetracyclines and tooth discoloration, sulfonamides, and kernicterus.

Aside from these patient variables, the sensitivity of the organism to the available agents is a factor that must be considered. Finally, the relative differences of the agents themselves, including pharmacokinetics, cost, dosage form availability, and toxicity, are practical considerations that influence the choice of agents.

The agents available for the treatment of UTIs can be divided into two groups: (a) agents available for the treatment of acute, uncomplicated UTIs in the outpatient setting (Table 65.3) and (b) agents used in the treatment of serious and/or complicated UTIs (Table 65.4). These agents will be discussed in the following sections.

Asymptomatic Bacteriuria

Asymptomatic bacteriuria (ABU) is defined as the presence of bacteria of 10^5 cfu/mL or greater, in two or more midstream urine samples, in a patient without any symptoms of UTI (11). The significance of ABU is debatable, but most studies have failed to demonstrate increased morbidity or mortality associated with untreated ABU (12).

In the U.S. Preventative Task Force guidelines for screening of asymptomatic bacteriuria by dipstick urinalysis, routine screening is not recommended for asymptomatic persons. The one clear exception is the routine screening of all pregnant women, since early detection and treatment can prevent symptomatic infections (15). The task force favored the routine use of urine culture over dipstick urinalysis in pregnant women to prevent the occurrence of false-negative testing (15). As stated previously, 2 to 10% of pregnant women will have ABU detected by these screening methods. Both maternal and perinatal morbidity have been associated with UTIs, including low birth weight, prematurity, premature labor, hypertension/preeclampsia, maternal anemia, and amnionitis (16). The treatment of ABU in pregnant women is essential with follow-up to document eradication followed by continued surveillance throughout the remainder of the pregnancy. The agents most commonly used in pregnancy include penicillins, cephalosporins, and nitrofurantoin (4). TMP/SMZ is also used, although some consider trimethoprim contraindicated in pregnancy due to folate antagonism and

sulfonamides have the potential to cause kernicterus in the newborn when used in the last trimester of pregnancy. Treatment duration is debatable, but most authors conclude that single-dose or short 3-day courses should be adequate to eradicate the bacteriuria while minimizing fetal exposure to the drug (4).

ABU is common in the elderly, occurring in 20 to 50% of females and in 5 to 20% of males over 80 years of age (12). These patients may be chronically or intermittently colonized with bacteria, but in most cases a positive culture represents ABU and not a true infection. Many episodes of ABU will clear spontaneously, but greater than 50% will recur frequently. Pyuria will be present in approximately 90% of these infections. None of the studies to date have proven that treatment of ABU in the elderly is beneficial or impacts long-term morbidity or mortality. A recently published study conducted over a 9-year period in elderly, ambulatory women failed to identify bacteriuria as a risk factor for mortality, and its treatment did not lower the mortality rate (17). In fact, treatment may do more harm than good by causing adverse drug reactions and predisposing patients to the development of resistant organisms (5, 12, 17). Due to the lack of benefit of treating elderly patients with ABU, routine screening is not recommended (17).

ABU also occurs frequently in patients with neurogenic bladder dysfunction secondary to spinal cord injury. Treatment has not been shown to be very effective, with 1-week posttreatment eradication rates of only 47% in patients treated with 7 to 14 days of antibiotics and 41% in those patients treated for at least 28 days (18). In addition, of the patients whose urine was cleared, 93% in the 7- to 14-day treatment and 85% in the 28-day treatment had relapsed or were reinfected within 30 days posttreatment. Development of antimicrobial resistance after 28 days of treatment was also demonstrated with trimethoprim/sulfamethoxazole, ampicillin, gentamicin, and ciprofloxacin, with a statistically significant increase in MICs in the ciprofloxacin group. In these patients with ABU, treatment should be withheld due to the threat of emerging resistant organisms, risk of adverse drug reactions, and unnecessary expense.

ABU in children occurs at a rate of 1 to 3% in infants, 1% in preschool children, 1.2 to 1.8% of schoolgirls, and 0.03% of schoolboys (11). Screening for ABU in children is not indicated except for those at increased risk for bacteriuria and subsequent renal damage, including children with systemic or immunologic diseases, known abnormalities of the urinary tract, stones, neurogenic bladder or voiding dysfunction, or family history of urinary tract abnormalities, and girls less than 5 years of age with recurrent UTIs. Single-dose or short-course treatment should be adequate therapy for ABU detected in these high-risk children.

Table 65.3.
Eradicative Agents for Acute, Uncomplicated UTI

Class	Medication	Adult Dose	Half-Life (hr) Normal	Half-Life (hr) Anuric	Common Toxicity	Comments
Cephalosporins	Cefaclor	250–500 mg p.o. q 8 h	0.5–1	3	Gastrointestinal, hypersensitivity; blood dyscrasias; neurotoxicity; moniliasis	Approximately 5–16% cross-sensitivity with penicillins; although categorized as second generation, may not offer greater Gram-negative coverage
	Cefadroxil	500–1000 mg p.o. q 12 h	1.1	20–25	As above	As above
	Cephalexin	250–500 mg p.o. q 6 h	0.5–1.2	10–20	As above	As above
	Cephradine	250–500 mg p.o. q 6 h	0.7–2	8–15	As above	As above
Penicillins	Amoxicillin	250–500 mg p.o. q 8 h	0.7–1.4	7.4–21	Hypersensitivity; rash; gastrointestinal; blood dyscrasias	Better gastrointestinal absorption than ampicillin; lower frequency of diarrhea, rash
	Amoxicillin-clavulanate	250–500 mg p.o. q 8 h; each tablet contains 125 clavulanic acid	As above	As above	As above	As above + clavulanic acid helps prevent inactivation of amoxicillin through β-lactamase inhibition; for resistant organisms
	Ampicillin	250–500 mg p.o. q 6 h	As above	As above	As above	Lower absorption with food; higher rate of diarrhea, rash; usual DOC in pregnancy
	Bacampicillin	400 mg p.o. q 12 h	As above	As above	As above	Prodrug of ampicillin; good gastrointestinal absorption; lower rate of diarrhea, rash
Sulfonamides	Sulfacytine	250 mg p.o. q 6 h	4–8	10	Hypersensitivity; gastrointestinal blood dyscrasias; crystalluria	Caution in patients with liver dysfunction or asthma; maintain adequate fluid intake; contraindicated in term pregnancy
	Sulfamethizole	500–1000 mg p.o. q 6–8 h	4–8	10	As above	As above
	Sulfamethoxazole	1 gm p.o. q 8–12 h	7–17	30	As above	Greater risk of crystalluria over sulfisoxazole because of slower absorption and excretion; alkalinization of urine usually unnecessary
	Sulfisoxazole	1 gm p.o. q 6 h	4–8	10	As above	Relatively high solubility even in acid urine; risk of crystalluria low; alkalinization of urine usually unnecessary

(continued)

Table 65.3. *(Continued)*

Class	Medication	Adult Dose	Half-Life (hr) Normal	Half-Life (hr) Anuric	Common Toxicity	Comments
Tetracyclines	Tetracycline	250–500 mg p.o. q 6 h	6–12	57–120	Gastrointestinal, rash; superinfection; dental staining	Contraindicated in last half of pregnancy and in children <8 years; avoid antacids, dairy products
	Doxycycline	50–100 mg p.o. q 12 h	14–25	20–30	As above	As above + administration with food or milk OK; high lipid solubility affords good prostatic penetration
	Minocycline	100 mg p.o. q 12 h	11–26	12–30	As above + vestibular disturbances	As above
Miscellaneous	Cinoxacin	500 mg p.o. q 12 h	1–1.5	16	Gastrointestinal headache; dizziness; hypersensitivity	Chemically related to nalidixic acid—cross-resistance may occur
	Nalidixic acid	1 g p.o. q 6 h	1–2.5	21	Gastrointestinal, headache; visual disturbances; drowsiness; glucose 6-phosphate dehydrogenase hemolysis	Development of resistance may occur within 48 hr; low use since introduction of fluoroquinolones
	Nitrofurantoin	50–100 mg p.o. q 6 h	0.5	?	Gastrointestinal; eosinophilic pulmonary infiltrate; glucose 6-phosphate dehydrogenase hemolysis; peripheral neuropathy; hepatotoxicity	Contraindicated with creatinine clearance of < 40 mL/min; no development of resistance
	Trimethoprim	100 mg p.o. q 12 h	8–11	26	Rash; gastrointestinal; blood dyscrasias	Contraindicated in pregnancy; use with caution in patients with folate deficiency because of megaloblastic anemia; penetrates prostatic tissue and fluid
	Trimethoprim/ Sulfamethoxazole	160 mg/800 mg (double-strength tablet) p.o. q 12 h	As above	As above	As above + see Sulfonamides	As above + see Sulfonamides. Usual DOC for most types of UTIs

Acute, Uncomplicated UTI

The vast majority of women with urinary tract symptomatology have simple, uncomplicated UTIs. Although debate still exists concerning optimal therapy, especially related to treatment duration, most clinicians now agree that short-course treatment is adequate for the majority of these infections (2, 19). In the past, traditional treatment regimens consisted of 7- to 10-day antibiotic courses. Numerous studies have been undertaken to demonstrate therapeutic efficacy of short-term antibiotic therapy, including single-dose, 3-day, and 5-day regimens (20). Three-day regimens are the most widely accepted duration for short-course treatment (20, 21). The efficacy is equivalent to longer treatment periods, and many of the advantages of single-dose treatment are retained. In addition, typical symptoms last approximately 3 days, so patients will not be as apt to assume that their treatment has failed (2, 21).

Although many of the studies have shown single-dose therapy to be as effective as 7- to 10-day treatment, they have often involved small numbers of highly selected patients. Opponents point out that these studies do not parallel true patient populations, so the results cannot be extrapolated to the general population (20). Due to these factors, many practitioners hesitate to adopt single-dose therapy as routine clinical practice, especially until definitive data is collected from large-scale double-blind trials.

Single-dose therapy does offer several advantages, including a lower rate of adverse drug reactions, cost-effectiveness, better patient compliance, minimal change of bacterial flora, and a lower frequency of developing bacterial antibiotic resistance. Studies have shown that a majority of women with lower tract infections will be cured by single-dose treatment when the organisms are sensitive, whereas less than half of the women with upper tract involvement will respond. Patient selection is very important in determining appropriate candidates for single-dose therapy. Indications for optimal patient inclusion are female, acute uncomplicated UTI, lack of systemic symptoms, duration of local symptoms less than 48 hours, infrequent recurrence, and good follow-up available.

Single-dose studies have been carried out using several drugs including trimethoprim-sulfamethoxazole (TMP/SMZ), amoxicillin, cefaclor, kanamycin, fluoroquinolones, tetracycline, and others (20, 22). The two most important factors in predicting efficacy of single-dose treatment are the organism's susceptibility to the antibiotic and the duration of effective antimicrobial levels in the urine. Agents with a long plasma half-life and urinary concentrations above the MIC 90 for at least 24 to 48 hours are the most effective (20). Highest cure rates with single-dose therapy have been reported with TMP/SMZ 320/1600 mg, trimethoprim 600 mg, ofloxacin 400 mg, and ciprofloxacin 500 mg (19, 20). β-Lactam drugs, such as amoxicillin and cephalosporins, have had lower cure rates, primarily due to resistance (especially in the case of amoxicillin) and faster excretion rates (20). TMP/SMZ is the drug of choice for single-dose treatment of uncomplicated UTIs when single-dose therapy is to be employed (19, 20). Trimethoprim alone can also be used in patients with sulfa allergies. Fluoroquinolones should be reserved for patients with multiple drug allergies or intolerance, or suspected or proven resistant organisms.

Although short-course therapy, including single-dose treatment, is not routinely advocated in children due to the increased incidences of urinary tract abnormalities or upper tract involvement, more trials are examining this population for efficacy of shortened treatment (23–25). Often it is difficult to administer antibiotics to young children, so single-dose treatment may be especially advantageous. Several comparative trials and small studies have yielded results with single-dose treatment comparable to 7- to 10-day treatment regimens (23). Critics point out that inadequate sample sizes, poor study designs, inadequate follow-up, and differing methodology make the analysis of these studies inconclusive (26). In a recent analysis of 12 clinical trials evaluating single-dose treatment in 320 infants and children, overall cure rates were 89% (23). Single-dose therapy was most effective in children with a lower UTI and in those with a normal urinary tract. Highest cure rates were achieved with an IM

aminoglycoside (96%) and TMP/SMZ (90%), which proved to be far superior to amoxicillin (75%). Therefore, single-dose treatment is probably most effective in children with no known abnormalities of the urinary tract, including young girls with acute or recurrent cystitis or children with ABU (11, 19, 25). Recommended doses for TMP/SMZ are 30 to 40 mg/kg or trimethoprim 6 to 9 mg/kg (25). Further study is required to determine the optimal duration of treatment in children.

Single-dose therapy has not been shown to be effective in the treatment of upper urinary tract infections and is inappropriate for use in the patient with known renal involvement. In addition, short-term therapy is not indicated in the treatment of UTIs in pregnant women, elderly women, and diabetics, so standard treatment of 7 to 10 days is routinely recommended (12). Uncomplicated infections are rare in males but have been associated with a lack of circumcision and HIV infection (27). Males under 65 years with acute, uncomplicated UTIs should be treated for 7 days. Elderly males presenting with an initial symptomatic UTI should be treated for 14 days, and those with recurrent symptomatic infections often require treatment for 6 to 12 weeks (5). Elderly females with UTIs have significantly poorer outcomes when treated with short course therapy than younger women. Single-dose treatment may be effective in only one third of elderly patients (12). Most females over 65 years will be cured within 3 days if there is no involvement of the upper tract (5). Therefore, minimum treatment duration should be 3 days, although most clinicians still advocate 7-day treatment.

Treatment of uncomplicated UTI is often done empirically without culture and sensitivity testing. Infections in pregnant, elderly, diabetic, or male patients should be guided by culture and sensitivity data. These patients may not have typical infecting organisms or sensitivities to antimicrobials, so success of eradicative therapy will depend on appropriate selection of an antimicrobial agent. Many agents have been shown to be effective in the treatment of UTI with standard 7- to 10-day courses. The preferred agents include TMP/SMZ and nitrofurantoin (28).

The majority of community-acquired pathogens remain sensitive to commonly prescribed antimicrobials. The in vitro susceptibilities of 295 isolates from adult female outpatients are presented in Table 65.5 (29). The breakpoint criteria for sensitivity were based on serum levels for all drugs except nitrofurantoin and nalidixic acid, and therefore underestimate the ability of these agents to eradicate the UTI. This is because most antibiotics concentrate in the urine and achieve much higher levels than in the serum.

Comparative clinical trials with newer agents such as the quinolones have not shown superiority over established regimens for the treatment of uncomplicated infections. In

Table 65.4.
Commonly Used Eradicative Agents in Complicated UTI

Drug Class/ Medications	Spectrum	Dose	Adjust Dose in Renal Impairment	Toxicity	Comments
Aminoglycosides Gentamicin Tobramycin Amikacin	Gram-negatives, including *Pseudomonas aeruginosa*	(3–5 mg/kg/day i.v. q 8–12 h) (15 mg/kg/day i.v. q 8–12 h)	Yes	Nephrotoxicity; ototoxicity; neuromuscular blockade	Monitor serum levels: G, T A Peak 4–8 15–30 Trough <2 5–10 Gentamicin least expensive; reserve amikacin for resistant organisms; empiric drugs of choice
Antifungals Amphotericin B	*Candida*	50 mg/L sterile H₂O continuous irrigation	No	Minimal because of local effect—minimal systemic absorption	Continual irrigation for 5 days; efficacy is controversial and may be dependent on host factors
Flucytosine	*Candida*, *Cryptococcus* spp.	50–150 mg/kg/day p.o. q 6 h	Yes	Gastrointestinal; hematologic disorders; rash; elevation of hepatic enzymes	Nausea/vomiting may be reduced by spacing capsules over 15 min
Fluconazole	*Candida*, *Cryptococcus* spp.	50–100 mg p.o. qd	Yes	Minimal toxicity	High urinary concentrations
Cephalosporins	Gram-negatives (3rd gen. > 2nd gen. > 1st gen.)			Hypersensitivity; gastrointestinal; blood dyscrasias, phlebitis; superinfection; positive Coombs' anemia test	3rd generation most active vs. gram-negatives; good empiric coverage for nosocomial UTIs
Cefazolin	As above	1 g i.v. q 8 h	Yes	See class	1st generation; organisms may be resistant
Cefixime	As above	200 mg p.o. q 12 h	Yes	See class	3rd generation; oral form
Cefotaxime	As above	1–2 g i.v. q 6–8 h	Yes	See class	Enhanced gram-negative coverage; 3rd generation
Ceftazidime	As above + *Pseudomonas*	0.5–1 g i.v. q 8–12 h	Yes	See class	3rd generation; most active vs. *Pseudomonas*
Ceftizoxime	As above	0.5–1 g i.v. q 8–12 h	Yes	See class	As above with slightly lower activity vs. *Pseudomonas*
Penicillins				Hypersensitivity; gastrointestinal; blood dyscrasias; neurotoxicity; thrombophlebitis; superinfection	Extended-spectrum PCNs offer good gram-negative coverage as well as enterococcus; well tolerated
Ampicillin	*E. coli, Proteus* spp., *Enterococcus* spp.	0.5–1 g i.v. q 6 h	Yes	See class	Organisms may be resistant
Carbenicillin-indanyl sodium	Gram-negative, *Pseudomonas*	382–764 mg p.o. q 6 h	Yes	See class	Good prostatic penetration
Mezlocillin	As above	2–3 g i.v. q 6 h	Yes	See class, possibly lower	

Agent	Spectrum	Dose	Toxicity		Comments
Piperacillin	As above	2–3 g i.v. q 6 h	See class + bleeding abnormalities; electrolyte imbalances	Yes	Greatest in vitro activity vs. *Pseudomonas*; prostatic penetration
Ticarcillin–clavulanate potassium	As above	3.1 g i.v. q 6 h	See class	Yes	As above + greater activity vs. gram-negative organisms because of addition of clavulanate to prevent inactivation of ticarcillin through β-lactamase inhibition
Miscellaneous					
Aztreonam	Gram-negative including *Pseudomonas*	500 mg–1 gm i.v. q 8–12 h	Gastrointestinal; phlebitis; rash; hypersensitivity; superinfection	Yes	Monobactam; reserve for resistant organisms; alternate when AGLY contraindicated
Imipenem–Cilastatin	Gram-negative, *Pseudomonas* gram-positive	250–500 mg i.v. q 6 h	Gastrointestinal; blood dyscrasias; hypersensitivity; neurotoxicity; superinfection	Yes	Reserve for serious infections resistant to other available agents; use with AGLY in pseudomonal infection
Quinolones			Gastrointestinal; neurotoxicity; hypersensitivity; superinfection		Newer oral agents with good gram-negative coverage; reserve for use against multiply resistant strains; contraindicated in pregnant women and children; avoid concurrent antacid administration
Ciprofloxacin	Gram-negative, *Pseudomonas*, Gram-positive	250–750 mg p.o. q 12 h or 200–400 mg i.v. q 12 h	See class	Yes	Greatest in vitro antimicrobial activity of the quinolones; good prostatic penetration; higher serum levels
Enoxacin	As above	200–400 mg p.o. q 12 h	See class	Yes	Empty stomach
Lomefloxacin	As above	400 mg p.o. qd	See class + photosensitivity	Yes	
Norfloxacin	As above	400 mg p.o. q 12 h	See class	Yes	Effective concentrations only in urine, for lower UTI only; empty stomach
Ofloxacin	As above	200 mg p.o./i.v. q 12 h	See class	Yes	Equivalent levels when given by PO or IV route; empty stomach

Table 65.5.
In Vitro Antimicrobial Susceptibilities of Isolates from Ambulatory Bacteriuric Women as Determined by Kirby-Bauer Assay: Experience in One Clinic

Organism	Number of Isolates	AMP	CEPH	NA	NITRO	SULFA	TCN	TMP-SMX	One or More	All
Escherichia coli	223	69	96	98	98	73	76	96	100	48
Proteus species	22	91	95	95	32	68	5	91	100	0
Klebsiella species	17	6	88	100	82	75	76	88	100	6
Pseudomonas species	10	0	0	0	0	0	0	0	0	0
Enterococcus	10	90	40	20	90	20	30	50	100	0
Other	13	15	31	100	54	77	69	92	100	8

AMP, ampicillin; CEPH, cephalothin; NA, nalidixic acid; NITRO, nitrofurantoin; SULFA, sulfonamides; TCN, tetracycline; TMP/SMX, trimethoprim-sulfamethoxazole.
Adapted from Fowler JE. Urinary Tract Infection and Inflammation. Chicago: Year Book Medical Publishers, 1989.

those patients with UTIs due to organisms resistant to the preferred agents, alternate 10-day drug regimens include cephalosporins, amoxicillin-clavulanate, and fluoroquinolones.

Pyelonephritis

In the treatment of mild pyelonephritis, where the patient is not acutely ill and able to tolerate oral antibiotic therapy, most patients can be treated as an outpatient. Again, there is some controversy regarding treatment duration, but most studies advocate treatment for 10 to 14 days (2). In keeping with the trend toward shorter treatment durations, one group is advocating 5-day treatment for acute uncomplicated pyelonephritis (30). They have performed four prospective studies in hospitalized patients with severe UTIs, treating them for 5 days, with cure rates above 90% in patients receiving an aminoglycoside and above 80% in patients treated with a β-lactam or quinolone. Response to parenteral antibiotics usually occurs within 24 to 48 hours, at which time oral treatment can commence and the patient be discharged to home to complete the 5-day course. Longer treatment durations are associated with decreased patient compliance and have not been shown to offer improved patient outcomes. More study is required before shorter treatment durations for pyelonephritis can be advocated.

Culture and sensitivity testing in upper tract infections is important to ensure appropriate antibiotic coverage. The empiric regimen of choice for acute, uncomplicated pyelonephritis in the outpatient is TMP/SMZ. Since approximately 20 to 30% of organisms causing pyelonephritis are resistant to amoxicillin and first-generation cephalosporins, they are rarely used for empiric treatment (2). Culture and sensitivity data may warrant the use of newer, more expensive agents including quinolones, amoxicillin plus clavulanate, or oral third-generation cephalosporins such as cefixime. The availability of these oral antibiotics has been a significant advantage in the treatment of mild cases of pyelonephritis. Prior to their

development, many patients required hospitalization to receive parenteral antibiotic therapy to ensure adequate coverage of the infecting organisms. Due to their extended spectrum and enhanced susceptibilities, these agents can effectively eradicate these infections and substantially reduce costs when compared to hospitalization and parenteral antibiotic therapy. Adequate follow-up and post-therapy cultures are essential to document bacterial eradication.

The acutely ill patient with pyelonephritis is hospitalized and immediately started on empiric parenteral antimicrobial therapy until results of urine culture and sensitivity tests are known. Empiric therapy usually consists of an aminoglycoside, TMP/SMZ, an extended-spectrum penicillin, a third-generation cephalosporin, or a quinolone. Although ampicillin was traditionally added to an aminoglycoside in the past, there is little, if any, evidence that the combination offers any advantage over monotherapy. The likely organisms should be susceptible to monotherapy, and enterococcus is rare in this population (30). When susceptibility is known, appropriate therapy is continued with the least expensive agent providing adequate coverage of the infecting organism. Therapy is converted to an oral regimen when the patient has been afebrile for 48 hours, and is continued for a minimum of 2 weeks (2).

Complicated Infections

Complicated infections usually present more of a therapeutic challenge because they are often (a) caused by multiply resistant organisms, (b) difficult to eradicate, and (c) precursors to chronic conditions and renal damage. It is important to attempt to correct the underlying problem (catheter, stone, enlarged prostate, etc.) if possible, as eradicative therapy is not usually successful or long term if the condition remains. Approximately 50% of complicated infections will recur within 4 to 6 weeks, even with appropriate antimicrobial therapy. Most complicated infections are treated for a minimum of 14 days, and antibiotic selection must be guided by results of culture and sensitivity data. Complicated infections can lead to bacteremia with a resultant mortality of 10 to 20% (28). In a group of 247 patients with moderate to severe UTI, 32% of the patients had bacteremia. Of these patients, 17.5% died during hospitalization, compared with a 5% mortality rate in 167 nonbacteremic patients with UTI. There was a 47% incidence of resistant organisms in this population. Three predictive factors were associated with resistant pathogens: male gender, antibiotic therapy in the previous month, and increased age (28).

One study evaluated 416 male and 387 female outpatients with complicated infections treated with either an oral cepham or a quinolone (31). Bacterial eradication (82% vs. 91.7%) and clinical response (75.7% vs. 87.1%) were both significantly lower in the male patients than in the female patients. Interestingly, there were also significant differences in the pathogens isolated from male and female patients. In male patients, the incidence of *Staphylococcus*, the subtotal of gram-positive bacteria, *Enterobacter* species, *Serratia* species, and *Pseudomonas* species were significantly higher than those in female patients. The incidences of *E. coli*, *Klebsiella* species, and the subtotal of gram-negative bacteria were significantly higher in the female patients. Although bacterial eradications was similar in both sexes of patients when infected with the same organism, male patients were predominantly infected with the organisms that were more difficult to eradicate.

In males, the majority of UTIs are considered to be complicated due to an anatomic or urologic abnormality, recent catheterization, or urologic surgery (27). These infections are difficult to eradicate, have a high rate of recurrence, and often require prolonged treatment courses to achieve adequate antimicrobial levels in both the kidney and prostate. Bacterial prostatitis is the most common cause of acute complicated or chronic recurrent UTI in men (27). In bacterial prostatitis, the efficacy of eradicative therapy depends on the ability of the medication to penetrate into the prostate gland and activity against the usual urinary tract pathogens. In acute bacterial prostatitis, penetration of the drug into the prostatic tissue and fluid is higher as a result of inflammation (32). The patient is usually hospitalized and treated with parenteral antibiotics. After the patient has been afebrile for 48 hours, the medication is changed to an oral agent. Trimethoprim, doxycycline, carbenicillin, quinolones, and azithromycin achieve high prostatic concentrations (32). Doxycycline and azithromycin may not always offer good gram-negative coverage, and both carbenicillin and ciprofloxacin are usually reserved for resistant organisms. Therefore, trimethoprim, with good gram-negative coverage, is the drug of choice in prostatic infections. It is usually given in combination with sulfamethoxazole, which does not penetrate the prostate gland well, in a dose of one double-strength tablet twice daily. These patients require long-term treatment of 4 to 6 weeks, followed by long-term suppression, treatment of relapses, or surgical correction (27).

Nosocomial infections contribute significantly to morbidity and mortality, cost of treatment, and length of stay in the hospitalized patient. An estimated 5 to 10% of all hospitalized patients will develop a nosocomial infection (6). Treatment duration ranges from 14 to 21 days. Nosocomial UTI is frequently associated with catheter use, and in a national surveillance study of 42,509 surgical patients, 96% of those patients who acquired UTI had a catheter in place (8). In the patient who develops asymptomatic bacteriuria while catheterized, antibiotic therapy is not indicated and may in fact lead to the development of resistant organisms. In many cases, the urine will clear spontaneously after catheter removal. In the symptomatic patient, every attempt should be made to remove the catheter before initiating therapy.

When selecting empiric therapy in patients with suspected nosocomial or complicated UTIs, the likely pathogens must be considered. *E. coli* accounts for only 30% of nosocomial UTIs with *Pseudomonas, Proteus, Klebsiella, Enterobacter, Serratia, Enterococcus, Staphylococcus, Citrobacter*, coagulase-negative *Staphylococcus* and *Candida* being other likely pathogens (6). Many of these hospital-acquired strains are often resistant to the more frequently used antibiotics. Empiric therapy is initiated after urine and blood cultures have been obtained. The usual drugs of choice for nosocomial UTI are a combination regimen of an aminoglycoside (gentamicin) and ampicillin. Alternate regimens include third-generation cephalosporins, extended-spectrum penicillins, quinolones, imipenem, or aztreonam (2). If the gram stain reveals a gram-negative organism, monotherapy with gentamicin is usually adequate treatment. Antibiotic therapy can be adjusted once culture and sensitivity data are obtained. New antimicrobials are constantly introduced and add to the armamentarium of agents available for the treatment of serious UTIs. These drugs such as aztreonam, imipenem, and quinolones, should be reserved for use in patients with infections due to multiply resistant organisms, or if a patient cannot tolerate first-line agents due to allergy or toxicity. The restriction of these antibiotics is important for cost-containment measures and to help prevent widespread bacterial resistance.

The importance of restricting the use of newer, broad-spectrum antibiotics was recently emphasized in a study comparing resistance rates to ciprofloxacin. MIC data from two hospitals were compared, one with no antibiotic restrictions (uncontrolled) and the other with an antibiotic restriction policy in place (controlled) (33). Ciprofloxacin resistance occurred more frequently at the institution without restrictions in prescribing. Significantly increased resistance rates were noted in the following isolates for the uncontrolled versus the controlled institutions, respectively: *Serratia* species 79% vs. 12%, *Providencia* species 59% vs. 38%, *P. mirabilis* 48% vs. 0%, *Pseudomonas* species 32% vs. 10%, and *Morganella morganii* 10% vs. 0%. Therefore, indiscriminate use of these agents must be eliminated to preserve their usefulness where required. Fluoroquinolone use should be limited to (a) infections caused by multiply resistant organisms sensitive to quinolones, (b) infections where parenteral antibiotics would be required either in an outpatient or in a hospitalized patient who would otherwise be ready for discharge, and (c) infections where other oral agents have failed or are not tolerated.

When used appropriately, the advantages of the oral quinolones can be preserved. One of the most important benefits may be in cost reduction in the treatment of patients who would otherwise require parenteral antibiotics. Eliminating or decreasing hospital stay is a goal most clinicians have in the care of their patients with complicated or nosocomial UTI.

Another pathogen to consider in nosocomial UTIs is fungus. Fungi, especially *C. albicans,* are becoming more prevalent pathogens in nosocomial infections, including UTIs. Risk factors associated with fungal UTIs include previous antimicrobial therapy, urinary tract abnormality, history of diabetes, Foley catheterization, and an immunosuppressed state (10). The significance of candiduria is debatable, and many infections clear spontaneously without treatment. More study is needed to determine which type of fungal infections require treatment. Fungi can cause both lower and upper UTIs, and may be a cause of fungemia in certain patients. Although amphotericin B bladder irrigations have been the standard therapy for many years, the efficacy has never been proven through randomized clinical trials and definitive guidelines for treatment do not exist (10, 34). Traditionally, 50 mg/L amphotericin B has been the recommended concentration for a continuous bladder irrigation for 5 days (10, 35). Recently, concentrations of 5 to 10 mg/L amphotericin B instilled intermittently for a period of 2 days have been advocated to be as effective with a lower theoretical risk for bladder uroepithelial damage (36). Amphotericin B topical bladder irrigations are not effective in the treatment of upper tract candidal infections. Although intravenous amphotericin B has minimal urinary excretion, it has been effective in the treatment of fungal UTI. However, due to the toxicities associated with amphotericin B, other agents have been explored.

Fluconazole is available both intravenously and orally, and 70 to 80% of the drug is excreted unchanged in the urine (35). The drug has been shown to be well tolerated and effective in the treatment of both upper and lower UTIs. In the currently available data, clinical response rates achieved with fluconazole have ranged from 71 to 100% (35). Lower eradication rates were seen in patients with indwelling catheters. An additional benefit of fluconazole therapy may be in the prevention of dissemination of the disease in critically ill patients with a resultant reduction in septic morbidity and mortality (37). More trials are needed to determine optimal dosage and duration of treatment, but fluconazole appears to be a promising agent in the treatment of fungal UTI.

Whatever the source of nosocomial or complicated infections, follow-up cultures 7 to 10 days after eradicative therapy are necessary to detect and treat persistence of the pathogen or suprainfection if it occurs.

Prophylactic Therapy

Prophylactic therapy is used to prevent infection in patients who have uncomplicated urinary tracts and a history of closely spaced, recurrent UTIs. Since recurrent, uncomplicated UTIs are primarily a problem of women and are usually reinfections, a prophylactic agent should continue to be effective in low doses to minimize side effects (Table 65.6). Primary prophylaxis is aimed at preventing acquisition of infection from a small number of microbes from a source outside the urinary tract (e.g., periurethral flora, instrumentation). Secondary prophylaxis prevents the emergence of infection from a site within the urinary tract (e.g., latent infection in the prostate, kidney, stone) (38).

Women who have three or more UTIs per year generally benefit from prophylaxis. At this rate, it is also cost-effective to use prophylaxis when compared to treatment costs-office visits, urinalysis, medication, and time. In addition, prophylaxis is indicated in children with greater than 3 UTIs per year or in those children less than 5 years of age with VUR or other abnormalities of the urinary tract (11). Prophylactic therapy should not be instituted until an existing infection is cleared using eradicative therapy.

Table 65.6.
Prophylactic and Suppressive Agents for UTIs

Drug	Dose	Comments
Methenamine mandelate	1.0 g qid	Requires urine pH of <5.5; contraindicated in renal insufficiency, dehydration; can cause dysuria, gastrointestinal irritation; avoid concurrent use with sulfonamides
Methenamine hippurate	1.0 g bid	As above
Nitrofurantoin	50–100 mg q hs	See Table 65.3
Trimethoprim-sulfamethoxazole	½–1 tab q hs	See Table 65.3

Several antiinfectives appear to be effective as prophylactic agents: TMP/SMZ, nitrofurantoin, methenamine, and others. Since uncomplicated reinfections are the result of periurethral contamination by colonic flora, the prophylactic agent should not alter the sensitivity-resistance pattern of these bacteria. Both methenamine and nitrofurantoin do not affect the sensitivity of these organisms and thus remain effective with continued use (19, 38). The effectiveness of trimethoprim is based on the ability to achieve bactericidal concentrations in vaginal fluid and thus inhibit periurethral colonization of enteric flora (19, 38).

Three options are available for prophylactic therapy: long-term prophylaxis, postcoital prophylaxis, and self-treatment. Long-term prophylaxis is indicated in the patient with very frequent, closely spaced reinfections and requires daily or alternate day treatment. The doses are much lower than those required for eradicative therapy. Nitrofurantoin 50 mg, trimethoprim 100 mg, ½ tablet of trimethoprim-sulfamethoxazole (80–400 mg/tablet), and norfloxacin 200 mg, all at bedtime, have been demonstrated to be effective prophylactic measures (5, 19). Recent reports have shown doses of trimethoprim-sulfamethoxazole as low as ½ tablet 3 times weekly to be as effective as daily dosing with infection rates of < 0.2/ patient year. A long-term prophylaxis study of 11 women demonstrated excellent results with this dosage regimen (39). Although the study was small, infection rates dropped from an average of 3 to 5 UTIs per year to 0.14 per patient year. In addition, these women were predisposed to UTI due to underlying conditions: diabetes, 3 patients; renal transplant, 1; cancer patient on chemotherapy, 1; and one patient with systemic lupus erythematosus. Five of the seven UTIs were caused by resistant organisms (*E. coli, Staphylococcus epidermidis, S. faecalis*) that were sensitive to nitrofurantoin and ampicillin. In the 5-year study, no significant adverse reactions occurred. TMP/SMZ appeared to be a safe and effective agent for long-term prophylaxis in the patient predisposed to UTI. The development of resistant organisms in the infections that do occur appears to be the only potential problem and needs to be further assessed with larger research trials.

Nitrofurantoin has also been shown to be effective in the prophylaxis of recurrent UTI (38, 40). A recent double-blind, placebo-controlled, 3-month crossover study was performed to assess the efficacy of nitrofurantoin prophylaxis in 56 pediatric patients with recurrent UTIs due to neurogenic bladder (41). During the daily treatment arm of the study, the infection rate decreased significantly from 39% in the placebo group to 19% in the nitrofurantoin group. No adverse reactions occurred. The drug is well absorbed in the gastrointestinal tract and only achieves therapeutic concentrations in the urinary tract. Therefore, the drug does not alter normal bacterial flora. Another advantage of the drug is the lack of development of

Table 65.7.
Urinary Acidifying Agents

Agent	Dose	Comments
Ascorbic acid	6 g/day in divided doses	Titrate dose and urine pH; caution with patients who are receiving other medications, whose clearance will be affected by acidic pH
Ammonium chloride	2–3 g p.o. q 6 h	As above; caution in patients with decreased hepatic or renal function; effectiveness limited by renal compensation; can cause systemic acidosis

resistance among sensitive organisms despite use of the drug for almost 40 years. The disadvantage of the drug is the potential for serious adverse drug reactions, including pulmonary fibrosis and liver toxicity, with long-term use. Although the incidence of these side effects is low, patients receiving nitrofurantoin therapy should receive careful monitoring for adverse effects.

Methenamine mandelate has been studied in a single bedtime dose of 1.0 gram; however, this is less effective than the other agents. Consequently, full doses of 0.5 to 1.0 gram of methenamine 4 times a day in addition to urinary acidification to a pH of 5.5 or lower are required if this agent is used for prophylaxis (Table 65.7) (29).

Methenamine hippurate, a different salt form of the drug, was evaluated in a double-blind crossover study in a dose of 1 gram twice daily (42). Patients received 6 months of drug or placebo and then were crossed over to the other agent. Prophylaxis continued for 2 years. A significant difference was noted between the two groups, with an infection rate of 2.1 per patient year in the placebo group versus 0.8 per patient year in the methenamine group. The drug provided effective prophylaxis and was well tolerated. This salt form may be more efficacious because patient compliance is better with the simplified regimen. Methenamine does not alter normal flora and resistance does not develop, since the agent is only an antiseptic. In comparison with the other prophylactic regimens, methenamine does have a higher infection rate and may not be as effective in patients with high recurrence rates.

Currently, the majority of patients are placed on prophylactic therapy for 6 months and then the agent is discontinued. If the infection recurs, the patient again goes through the eradication treatment and is placed back on prophylactic therapy. Prophylaxis has not been shown to alter the natural course of UTIs, as demonstrated by rapid reinfection after the agent is discontinued in most studies, and therefore may need to be continued indefinitely in the patient who suffers from unrelenting recurrences (29).

Although not an antimicrobial, vaginal estrogen cream has recently been studied as prophylactic treatment for recurrent UTIs in postmenopausal women. Estrogen deficiency is thought to play a major role in the pathogenesis of recurrent UTIs in older women. Estrogens promote colonization of the vagina with lactobacilli, which in turn maintain a low vaginal pH, thus inhibiting bacterial growth. A randomized, double-blind placebo controlled trial of intravaginal estriol cream was conducted in 93 postmenopausal women (43). The study demonstrated a significant reduction in UTIs from 5.9 episodes per patient-year to 0.5 episodes per patient-year.

UTIs are a common occurrence in renal transplant recipients, occurring in 35 to 50% of patients not receiving antimicrobial prophylaxis (44, 45). The highest incidence of bacteriuria occurs in the first 6 months following transplantation. TMP/SMZ 160/800 mg daily has been shown to be effective in reducing the incidence of UTI to 5% compared with 38% in a similar group receiving placebo (45). Ciprofloxacin 250 mg daily has also been shown to be an effective prophylactic agent in renal transplant patients unable to tolerate TMP/SMZ; however, *Pneumocystis carinii* pneumonia developed in 14% of the ciprofloxacin treated patients versus 0% in the TMP/SMZ group. Therefore, a follow-up study is being conducted to evaluate ciprofloxacin prophylaxis combined with aerosolized pentamidine to prevent both UTI and pneumocystis pneumonia in renal transplant recipients unable to tolerate TMP/SMZ.

Due to the association of sexual intercourse with UTI and concern over long-term continuous prophylaxis, more studies are now being done to assess the effectiveness of postcoital prophylaxis. Postcoital prophylaxis is indicated in women with less frequent reinfections, who clearly associate sexual intercourse with the development of UTI. Excellent results have been achieved with several agents including TMP/SMZ, nitrofurantoin, cephalexin, nalidixic acid, and cinoxacin (46). In a study of 33 pregnant women (39 pregnancies) with a history of recurrent UTIs, postcoital prophylaxis with either cephalexin 250 mg or nitrofurantoin 50 mg significantly reduced the frequency of UTI (46). The incidence dropped from 130 UTIs in the 7 months before prophylaxis to only 1 UTI in 8.6 months after prophylaxis was initiated. This regimen is advocated for any woman with a history of recurrent UTIs who intends to become pregnant and for any woman who develops a UTI early in pregnancy. Potential benefits of this type of prophylaxis include lower cost, better tolerance, and increased patient compliance. The possible disadvantages of this prophylactic regimen, as well as continuous prophylaxis, are adverse drug reactions and the possible emergence of resistant organisms. Therefore, all patients

on any prophylactic regimen who acquire an acute UTI would require a urine culture with sensitivity testing to ensure effective eradicative therapy.

Self-treatment is the final option available for women with infrequent recurrences, although it is not truly prophylactic. The patient is instructed to initiate single-dose or short-course therapy with the selected antimicrobial at the first sign of an impending UTI. Self-treatment is less costly than continuous prophylaxis or standard treatment procedures, and it also has a decreased rate of adverse drug reactions. In order for this regimen to be effective, patient selection is crucial.

Suppressive Therapy

Long-term suppressive therapy is used primarily to reduce the frequency of recurrence and acute exacerbations of chronic infections. In contrast to prophylactic therapy, suppressive treatment decreases the population of microbes already present in the urinary tract (38). This form of therapy is indicated in patients who have a persistent focus of infection from which the microorganism cannot be eradicated. Examples of this type of infection include men with chronic bacterial prostatitis, patients with urinary calculi or other structural defects in the urinary tract, and patients with neurogenic bladder requiring chronic intermittent catheterization. Prior to instituting suppressive therapy, an attempt to clear the urine of active infection should be made. Suppressive treatment usually requires larger doses of antimicrobials than prophylactic therapy. If effective, suppressive treatment is continued as long as the focus of infection persists.

In these patients, the goals of suppressive therapy are to decrease the episodes of recurrent infection and maintain sterile urine. The antimicrobials used for suppressive therapy are similar to those used for prophylactic regimens. TMP/SMZ 80/400 mg, fluoroquinolones, nitrofurantoin 50 to 100 mg, and trimethoprim, all dosed once daily, have been shown to be effective agents (27). Methenamine may also be useful for long-term use due to lack of resistance or toxicity. In a recent study, the lowest rates of bacteriuria and clinical UTI among 302 patients requiring chronic intermittent catheterization was in the group of patients taking methenamine (47). The hippurate salt can be dosed 1 gram twice daily, with urinary acidification to maintain pH at 5.5 or less.

Preventive Therapy

Preventive measures are those that attempt to minimize the chance of developing an UTI. These measures are directed toward patient populations that are at particular risk of infection. Included in this group are patients who are or are about to be catheterized or have some other form of urologic manipulation, diabetics, and debilitated or otherwise compromised patients.

Since urologic manipulation is such a well-known risk factor for UTIs, the need for performing the procedure should be weighed against the potential risks. Should the necessity be compelling, proper preparation of both the patient and the practitioner in order to minimize the risk of infection should be made and the procedure should be performed using aseptic techniques.

The urinary catheter poses a special predisposing problem and has been studied extensively. The frequency of catheter-associated UTIs is related to a variety of factors, including the method and duration of catheterization, the health care personnel inserting the catheter, the catheter system, and catheter care. The Centers for Disease Control (CDC) have developed recommendations for the use of the indwelling catheter. Although the complete recommendations are too extensive for discussion in this text, a summary is presented (48):

1. Indwelling catheters should be used only when indicated and for as short a time as is possible.
2. Insertion should be done by adequately trained personnel using aseptic technique.
3. A sterile closed drainage system should always be used.
4. At no time should the collecting bag be above the level of the patient's bladder. The urine flow should be "downhill" and unobstructed, but should be suspended off the floor to prevent bacterial contamination.
5. Any closed collecting system that is contaminated by inappropriate technique, accidental disconnection, or the like should be replaced.
6. If a patient is catheterized for 2 weeks or less, a routine catheter change is not required except when obstruction, contamination, or other malfunction of the system occurs.
7. In patients who are chronically catheterized, replacement is not necessary until a malfunction or obstruction occurs.
8. Patients who are catheterized should be in separate rooms, and not in adjacent beds, to avoid cross-contamination.
9. Bacteriologic monitoring of the urine of catheterized patients may be useful; however, the cost-effectiveness requires evaluation.
10. Urine samples should be obtained from the aspiration port using aseptic technique.
11. The urethral meatus should be cleansed daily, with water used to reduce encrustations.
12. The use of systemic antibiotics may delay the development of bacteriuria but does not prevent it. In light of cost, adverse reactions, and development of resistance, prophylactic antimicrobial therapy is not recommended as routine practice. However, its use may be warranted in patients who require short-term catheterization and are at high risk of complications from UTI.

The routine use of antibiotic irrigations, antiseptic instillation into the drainage bag, or meatal care with antimicrobial ointments have not been shown to be effective in preventing or reducing the incidence of UTI (3).

Maintenance of the patient in a well-hydrated state is a simple and worthwhile preventive measure that inhibits or minimizes the risk of developing pyelonephritis. The value of maintaining hydration is based on its effect on the activity of phagocytes in the renal medulla. Dehydration and resultant hypertonicity of the urine in the renal medulla inhibit leukocyte mobilization and phagocytic activity (49).

Follow-up

One of the most important yet most frequently omitted components in the total treatment of UTIs is adequate follow-up. While many clinicians do not insist on follow-up cultures after treatment for acute, uncomplicated UTIs, they should be performed routinely after therapy for complicated infections, those involving the upper tract, and in pregnant women. Cultures should be obtained 7 to 10 days after treatment ends to ensure clearance of even long-acting antimicrobials. After achievement of sterile urine, cultures are only repeated for symptomatic episodes of bacteriuria.

PROGNOSIS

The prognosis for UTIs is highly variable, even with adequate therapy. Urologic structural abnormalities, presence of an indwelling catheter, and prostatitis favor the potential for recurrent infections. Concurrent predisposing conditions such as immunosuppression, pregnancy, diabetes, sex, age, debility, and urologic manipulation favor the spread of infection beyond the urinary tract.

There is a high recurrence rate with children: 26% in neonates, 30 to 40% in girls and 10 to 18% in boys. The prognosis is poor if these infections are not diagnosed early and treated adequately. In fact, 5 to 25% of these cases will progress to end-stage renal disease (11). Following an episode of bacteriuria during pregnancy, the possibility of recurrence is markedly enhanced when compared to patients who did not have bacteriuria during pregnancy (30 versus 5%). Of note is the increased incidence, approximately 20%, of urologic abnormalities on radiographs on follow-up examination in the patients who had bacteriuria during pregnancy. Elderly men, especially those with prostatitis, also are prone to recurrent infections. Eradication rates average 50%, even with long-term therapy.

Metastatic infections secondary to UTIs can occur. Men appear to be more prone to developing metastases from lower UTIs and women more prone to developing metastases from upper tract infections. In general, predisposing factors to developing these ectopic infections include an abnormal urinary tract, urologic manipulation, and impaired host defenses as seen in diabetes, malignancy, cirrhosis, uremia, malnutrition, anemia, and collagen vascular diseases. The sites of metastases reported include skeletal (59%), endocarditis (29%), chest (4%), eye (2%), and miscellaneous (3%). Of note is that within the skeletal metastatic lesions, 83% were to the vertebrae (50).

The uncomplicated UTI has the most favorable prognosis. In women with this type of infection up to 94% of uncomplicated infections can be eradicated.

CONCLUSION

UTIs are one of the most common infectious diseases and therefore are encountered in virtually all types of practices. A thorough knowledge of the pathogenesis, clinical course, and therapeutic choices are essential to the rational management of this disease state. To be an effective member of the health care team one must understand the controversies, therapeutic options, and the rationale for drug selection in the management of UTI. Based on this knowledge, appropriate therapy of these infections can ensure optimal patient outcomes.

REFERENCES

1. Lipsky BA. Urinary tract infections in men. Ann Intern Med 110(2):138–150, 1989.
2. Stamm WE, Hooton TM. Management of urinary tract infections in adults. N Engl J Med 329(18):1328–1334, 1993.
3. Forland M. Urinary tract infection. How has its management changed? Postgrad Med 93(5)71–86, 1993.
4. Tan JS, File TM. Treatment of bacteriuria in pregnancy. Drugs 44(6):972–980, 1992.
5. Nicolle LE. Urinary tract infection in the elderly. J Antimicrob Chemother 33(suppl A):99–109, 1994.
6. Bergogne-Berezin E, Decre D, Jolly-Guillou ML. Opportunistic nosocomial multiply resistant bacterial infections-their treatment and prevention. J Antimicrob Chemother 32(suppl A):39–47, 1993.
7. Bronsema DA, Adams JR, Pallares R, et al. Secular trends in rates and etiology of nosocomial urinary tract infections at a university hospital. J Urol 150:414–416, 1993.
8. Horan TC, Culver DH, Gaynes RP, et al. Nosocomial infections in surgical patients in the United States, January 1986–June 1992. Infect Control Hosp Epidemiol 14(2):73–80, 1993.
9. Sobel JD. Pathogenesis of urinary tract infections. Inf Dis Clin North Am 1(4):751–772, 1987.
10. Gubbins PO, Piscitelli SC, Danziger LH. Candidal urinary tract infections: a comprehensive review of their diagnosis and management. Pharmacotherapy 13(2):110–127, 1993.
11. Zelikovic I, Adelman RD, Nancarrow PA. Urinary tract infections in children–an update. West J Med 157:554–561, 1992.
12. McCue JD. Urinary tract infections in the elderly. Pharmacotherapy 13(2Pt2):51S–53S, 1993.
13. Stamm WE. Protocol for diagnosis of urinary tract infection: reconsidering the criterion for significant bacteriuria. Urol Suppl 32:6–12, 1988.
14. Wigton RS, Hoellerich VL, Ornato JP, et al. Use of clinical findings in the diagnosis of urinary tract infection in women. Arch Intern Med 145:2222, 1985.
15. Pels RJ, Bor DH, Woolhandler S, et al. Dipstick urinalysis screening of asymptomatic adults for urinary tract disorders. JAMA 262(9):1220–1224, 1989.
16. Schieve LA, Handler A, Hershow R, et al. Urinary tract infection during pregnancy: its association with maternal morbidity and perinatal outcome. Am J Public Health 84(3):405–410, 1994.

17. Abrutyn E, Mossey J, Berlin JA, et al. Does asymptomatic bacteriuria predict mortality and does antimicrobial treatment reduce mortality in elderly ambulatory women? Ann Intern Med 120(10):827–833, 1994.
18. Waites KB, Canupp KC, DeVivo MJ. Eradication of urinary tract infection following spinal cord injury. Paraplegia 31:645–652, 1993.
19. Bailey RR. Management of lower urinary tract infections. Drugs 45(suppl 3)139–144, 1993.
20. Stamm WE. Controversies in single dose therapy of acute uncomplicated urinary tract infections in women. Infection 20(suppl 4):S272–S275, 1992.
21. Brumfitt W, Hamilton-Miller JMT. Consensus viewpoint on management of urinary infections. Antimicrob Chemother 33(suppl A):147–153, 1994.
22. Pfau A, Sacks TG. Single dose quinolone treatment in acute uncomplicated urinary tract infection in women. J Urol 149:532–534, 1993.
23. Khan AJ. Efficacy of single-dose therapy of urinary tract infection in infants and children: a review. J Natl Med Assoc 86(9):690–696, 1994.
24. Lidefelt KJ, Bollgren I, Wiman A. Single dose treatment of cystitis in children. Acta Paediatr Scand 80:648–653, 1991.
25. Bailey RR. What evidence is there for the use of single-dose therapy for urinary tract infections in children? Infection 22(suppl 1):S14–S15, 1994.
26. Moffatt M, Embree J, Grimm P, et al. Short-course antibiotic therapy for urinary tract infections in children. Am J Dis Child 142:57–61, 1988.
27. Schaffer AJ. Urinary tract infection in men-state of the art. Infection 22(suppl 1):S19–S21, 1994.
28. Leibovici L, Greenshtain S, Cohen O, et al. Toward improved empiric management of moderate to severe urinary tract infections. Arch Intern Med 152:2481–2486, 1992.
29. Fowler JE. Urinary tract infection and inflammation. Chicago: Year Book, 1989.
30. Bailey RR. Duration of antimicrobial treatment and the use of drug combinations for the treatment of uncomplicated acute pyelonephritis. Infection 22(suppl 1):50–52, 1994.
31. Kawada Y. Comparison of complicated urinary tract infections in men and women. Infection 22(suppl 1):55–57, 1994.
32. Leigh DA. Prostatitis–an increasing clinical problem for diagnosis and management. J Antimicrob Chemother 32 (suppl A):1–9, 1993.
33. Thomson KS, Sanders WE, Sanders CC. USA resistance patterns among UTI pathogens. J Antimicrob Chemother 33(suppl A):9–15, 1994.
34. Jacobs LG, Skidmore EA, Cardoso LA, et al. Bladder irrigation with amphotericin B for treatment of fungal urinary tract infections. Clin Infect Dis 18:313–318, 1994.
35. Voss A, Meis JF, Hoogkamp-Korstanje JA. Fluconazole in the management of fungal urinary tract infections. Infection 22(4):247–251, 1994.
36. Sanford JP. The enigma of candiduria: evolution of bladder irrigation with amphotericin B for management–from anecdote to dogma and a lesson from Machiavelli. Clin Infect Dis 16:145–147, 1993.
37. Nassoura Z, Ivatury RR, Simon RJ, et al. Candiduria as an early marker of disseminated infection in critically ill surgical patients: the role of fluconazole therapy. J Trauma 32(2):290–295, 1993.
38. Kunin CM. Chemoprophylaxis and suppressive therapy in the management of urinary tract infections. J Antimicrob Chemother 33:51–62, 1994.
39. Nicolle LE, Harding GK, Thomson M, et al. Efficacy of five years of continuous, low-dose trimethoprim-sulfamethoxazole prophylaxis for urinary tract infection. J Infect Dis 157(6):1239–1242, 1988.

40. Vahlensieck W, Westenfelder M. Nitrofurantoin versus trimethoprim for low-dose long-term prophylaxis in patients with recurrent urinary tract infections. Int Urol Nephrol 24(1):3–10, 1992.

41. Johnson HW, Anderson JD, Chambers GK, et al. A short-term study of nitrofurantoin prophylaxis in children managed with clean intermittent catheterization. Pediatrics 93(5):752–755, 1994.

42. Cronberg S, Welin CO, et al. Prevention of recurrent acute cystitis by methenamine hippurate: double blind controlled crossover long term study. Br Med J 294:1507–1508, 1987.

43. Raz R, Stamm WE. A controlled trial of intravaginal estriol in postmenopausal women with recurrent urinary tract infections. N Engl J Med 329(11):753–756, 1993.

44. Fox BC, Sollinger HW, Belzer FO, et al. A prospective, randomized, double-blind study of trimethoprim-sulfamethoxazole for prophylaxis of infection in renal transplantation: clinical efficacy, absorption of trimethoprim-sulfamethoxazole, effects on the microflora, and the cost-benefit of prophylaxis. Am J Med 89:255–274, 1990.

45. Hibberd PL, Tolkoff-Rubin NE, Doran M, et al. Trimethoprim-sulfamethoxazole compared with ciprofloxacin for the prevention of urinary tract infection in renal transplant recipients: a double-blind, randomized controlled trial. Online J Curr Clin Trials, Doc. No. 15, 1992.

46. Pfau A, Sacks TG. Effective prophylaxis for recurrent urinary tract infections during pregnancy. Clin Infect Dis 14:810–814, 1992.

47. Bakke A, Vollset SE. Risk factors for bacteriuria and clinical urinary tract infection in patients treated with clean intermittent catheterization. J Urol 149:527–531, 1993.

48. Stamm WE. Guidelines for prevention of catheter-associated urinary tract infections. Ann Intern Med 82:386–390, 1975.

49. Seiler WO, Stahelin HB. Practical management of catheter-associated UTIs. Geriatrics 43(8):43–45, 1988.

50. Siroky MB, Moylan RA, Austin G, et al. Metastatic infection secondary to genitourinary tract sepsis. Am J Med 61:351, 1976.

CHAPTER 66

INTRAABDOMINAL INFECTIONS

JOAN E. KAPUSNIK-UNER

Intraabdominal infections present serious clinical problems because they are difficult to diagnose and successfully treat. Such infections generally occur after leakage of bacteria from the gastrointestinal (GI) tract into the sterile environment of the peritoneal cavity. The resulting infections may be a diffuse peritonitis or localized abscesses. Primary peritonitis may seemingly occur spontaneously, so it is sometimes referred to as spontaneous bacterial peritonitis (SBP) and is usually found in adult patients with a history of alcoholic cirrhosis and ascites (1). Secondary peritonitis is usually associated with one or a combination of processes such as abdominal trauma, surgery, or intrinsic obstructive, neoplastic, or inflammatory GI disease.

The concept of mixed bacterial infection is especially relevant to these intraabdominal processes (2). As many as 400 anaerobic and aerobic species of microorganisms have been found to be present as part of the normal intestinal flora. Thus, when infection occurs after GI content spillage, multiple organisms may be responsible. However, the mere presence of an organism (i.e., on culture) does not guarantee its pathogenicity. Enterobacteriaceae are able to produce endotoxins and thus can trigger septic shock. *Bacteroides* spp. have a virulence factor, the polysaccharide capsule, which explains in part their pathogenicity. The presence of other organisms such as *Enterococcus* spp. has not reproducibly caused morbidity or mortality.

Even after identification of the pathogens, clinical outcome may be influenced by other factors, including the bacterial load at the site of infection (i.e., the inoculum size) and immunologic variables relating to local host defenses, as well as the general systemic immune response, the progression or severity of the underlying intrinsic GI disease, the success of surgical interventions performed, and whether the antimicrobial agents administered penetrate to the site of infection and are pharmacologically active in that environment. These factors should be considered prior to selection of therapy, as well as when assessing clinical response.

Patients who receive dialysis via continuous ambulatory peritoneal dialysis (CAPD) are a particular challenge with regard to treatment of peritonitis (3). These patients are reported to have a high incidence of infection arising from bacterial contamination caused during the technical aspects of CAPD. The advantages of CAPD compared to hemodialysis have been tempered by this constant risk of peritonitis. Therefore, successful treatment of intraabdominal infections in these patients holds a separate significance.

ETIOLOGY-INTESTINAL MICROFLORA

The great majority of intraabdominal infections are caused by Enterobacteriaceae and anaerobes from the GI tract. In general though, the normal GI tract bacterial flora is of low virulence. The number of bacterial species and the colony counts increase as one moves from the mouth down along the GI tract. This flora is stable early in childhood and for the most part does not differ with geographic location, race, diet, or increasing age. In a human stomach there usually exist fewer than 10^4 colony forming units/mL (cfu/mL) of aerobic and anaerobic microflora. Acidity and normal GI motility are factors that inhibit bacterial growth in this region (4). Trauma or diseases of the stomach and duodenal region may compromise these protective factors. Thus, medical conditions such as a gastric ulceration, achlorhydria, obstructing duodenal ulcer, carcinoma, an upper GI bleed, or certain drug therapies may result in the abnormal proliferation of the local flora (e.g., anaerobic streptococci, *Streptococci viridans*, lactobacilli, and yeast).

The microflora of the proximal small bowel is similar to that which is observed in the stomach, though increased numbers of Enterobacteriaceae and *Bacteroides* spp. may be found. Peristalsis is most rapid in the jejunum and upper ileum, which explains in part the low bacterial counts relative to the distal ileum. Injury or disease of this upper portion of the GI tract results in relatively low bacterial inocula into the peritoneal cavity. Thus, the number and severity of clinical infections related to such injuries would be fewer compared to injuries of the large bowel. Between the proximal and terminal ileum is a bacterial transition zone where the composition of organisms changes toward greater numbers of aerobic and anaerobic gram-negative bacilli, and counts are up to 10^8 cfu/mL.

The highest concentration of microorganisms in the GI tract is in the colon. As many as 10^{11} cfu/g of organisms are present and account for roughly one third of the total weight of the GI contents. Anaerobes outnumber aerobes by a factor of 1 to 100–1,000, with *Bacteroides* spp. being the predominant bacteria (5). Under the usual conditions within the lumen of the GI tract, anaerobic organisms behave as harmless commensals, but when introduced into surrounding host tissues and the peritoneal cavity they express their pathogenic potential. Certain underlying clinical conditions, such as compromised vascular supply or tissue necrosis may predispose a patient to anaerobic infections. Such clinical situations are associated with confined tissue spaces with a low oxidation-reduction potential and hypoxia, and thus provide an environment for uncontrolled anaerobic proliferation. Although more than 400 species of anaerobes reside in the colon and 200 in the oral cavity, only few produce the majority of clinical anaerobic infections. *Bacteroides fragilis* accounts for only about 5% of the colonic microflora, yet causes many times the incidence of clinical infection, compared to any other *Bacteroides* spp.

Primary peritonitis infections (e.g., SBP) are usually caused by a single pathogen, and in 80 to 85% of cases three organisms have been responsible, *Escherichia coli,* streptococci, and *Klebsiella* spp. In contrast, secondary peritonitis infections usually involve mixed microflora, both aerobic and anaerobic bacteria. Within this setting of mixed bacteria, there appears to be the potential for synergism. Enterobacteriaceae have been demonstrated to lower oxygen tension or redox potential within the peritoneal cavity, thus promoting growth of obligate anaerobes. Conversely, there is some evidence that the presence of low virulence anaerobic organisms enhances the pathogenicity of aerobic gram-negative bacilli, such as *E. coli, Klebsiella* spp., and *Proteus mirabilis.* A variety of obligate anaerobes have been observed to interfere with intracellular bacterial killing by polymorphonuclear leukocytes (PMNs), as well as PMN chemotaxis and phagocytosis (6).

Results from observations in humans and in the animal model of intraabdominal sepsis reveal a biphasic disease process. After intraabdominal inoculation of intestinal flora, animals initially developed acute peritonitis, predominantly from aerobic gram-negative bacilli and less frequently from enterococci (7). This phase was associated with a 40% mortality rate. Surviving animals later developed intraabdominal abscesses, which were culture positive most often for obligate anaerobes. However, in this model when a large inoculum of a single strain of bacteria was used (5×10^7 cfu/mL), no strain alone, aerobic or anaerobic, was able to induce abscesses. This evidence reaffirms the significance of synergism for abscess formation.

The microbiology of peritonitis in CAPD patients reveals that most cases are due to the aerobic organisms commonly residing on skin. Most episodes, 70%, are caused by gram-positive cocci (*S. aureus, S. epidermidis,* and streptococci). Less frequently, 25%, Enterobacteriaceae cause infection, and infrequently, 5%, anaerobes, mycobacteria, and fungi are the cause. It is thought that anaerobic organisms rarely cause infection in this group of patients because of the high oxygen tension present in the dialysate.

PATHOGENESIS OF PERITONITIS

The pathogenesis of primary peritonitis is not well understood and may result from bacterial spread from hematogenous or lymphatic sources, or from microperforation (e.g., transmural migration) of an otherwise intact GI tract. Secondary peritonitis from traumatic injury or GI disease results in the following situations when the first-line host defense mechanisms become overwhelmed: (a) when the infecting inoculum is very large; (b) when the bacterial contamination is due to mixed flora that acts synergistically to evade the first-line defenses; and (c) in the presence of a foreign body (e.g., CAPD catheter) when host defenses are not efficient and intraleukocytic sequestration of organisms occurs (8).

A general understanding of anatomic relationships within the peritoneal cavity is important for determining the possible sources of intraabdominal infection, as well as anticipating the extent and routes of spread of infection. The peritoneal cavity in males is a completely closed space, whereas in females it is perforated by the free ends of the fallopian tubes. This distinction is important because pelvic peritonitis often accompanies pelvic inflammatory disease (PID), especially if infection of the fallopian tubes is severe. Organs found within the peritoneal cavity include the stomach, jejunum, ileum, transverse and sigmoid colon, cecum, liver, gallbladder, pancreas, spleen, and appendix. The peritoneal cavity has various pouches and recesses into which bacteria or infected exudate may potential collect and become loculated. The peritoneal cavity is lined by a serous membrane. This membrane consists of a mesothelial cell monolayer beneath which are lymphatics, blood vessels, and nerve endings. The peritoneal space usually contains sufficient fluid to maintain surface moistness, which facilitates movement of the viscera. This moist peritoneal membrane is also highly permeable so that solutes and water are quickly transported in a bidirectional manner.

Host defense mechanisms generally combat bacterial invasion of the peritoneal cavity. Humoral and cellular immune defense mechanisms form the initial response to bacterial contamination, and the regional lymphatic circulation clears the bacterial debris. Intraabdominal infection results when these first-line host defenses are overwhelmed because (a) the infecting inoculum is very large, (b) the bacterial contamination is caused by mixed bacterial flora (anaerobic and aerobic), which act synergistically to evade host defenses, or (c) a foreign body renders host defenses inefficient. The peritoneal membrane is next to respond by exuding a fluid containing opsonins, antibodies, complement, PMNs, and macrophages into the peritoneal cavity. This inflammatory response is presumably facilitated by means of local vasodilation and increased vascular permeability. Inflammation increases the membrane's permeability so that the transport of large molecules and protein is enhanced. This may additionally improve an antimicrobial agent's ability to penetrate into the peritoneal cavity during peritonitis.

INCIDENCE, PROGNOSTIC FACTORS, AND OUTCOMES

Primary peritonitis (SBP) in adults with cirrhosis and ascites is reported to occur in as many as 8 to 27% of patients and has a resulting mortality rate of approximately 50%. The overall mortality rate in these patients may be as high as 95% because SBP is often accompanied by severe hepatic failure.

Most patients with secondary peritonitis can be placed in one of three categories: penetrating abdominal trauma, appendicitis, or other (9). Generally patients are young males and have a very low rate of morbidity and mortality, although the prognosis of secondary peritonitis is closely associated with early diagnosis and prompt surgical intervention. A mathematical equation has been derived to predict the risk of posttrauma infection in patients with penetrating abdominal trauma. Factors entering the equation were age, ostomy formation (performed for all left colonic injuries), shock, number of organs injured, and amount of blood or blood products administered prior to the time of surgery (10). Postoperative complication rates have also been associated with extent of organ failure or numbers of organs affected, duration/stage of illness, the adequacy of surgical procedures, and the presence of other chronic underlying illnesses including immunosuppression. An important outcome indicator is length of hospital stay, which has been measured to be 7 to 14 days for most intraabdominal infections, though in patients with complications it can be a great deal longer.

CLINICAL FEATURES AND DIAGNOSIS

Systemic Symptoms

General malaise, prostration, nausea, vomiting, diarrhea, fever, dehydration, leukocytosis with a left shift, and electrolyte imbalance are systemic symptoms that may be observed in patients with intraabdominal infections. Intraabdominal abscesses may often "smolder" for long periods of time with no or inconsistent symptoms.

Aerobic and anaerobic gram-negative bacteria may release endotoxin, a lipopolysaccharide from the bacterial cell wall into the blood stream, which is responsible for some of the serious clinical symptoms observed. These are septic shock, adult respiratory distress syndrome (ARDS), and disseminated intravascular coagulation (DIC). None of these clinical findings is specific to intraabdominal infections though, and they may occur to a varying degree in patients or may not be observed at all. Hypotension may also be exacerbated by reduced intravascular volume secondary to the massive influx of fluid from the vascular space into the peritoneum during peritonitis.

Abdominal Signs and Symptoms

Abdominal pain and tenderness may be localized or general (11). Specific abdominal pain on respiration or coughing and rebound tenderness or tenderness on gentle percussion are signs of acute peritonitis. The musculature that is overlying the area of inflamed peritoneum may become spastic. Involuntary muscle rigidity of the entire abdominal wall ("guarding") may develop with diffuse peritonitis. This muscle rigidity, though, is frequently absent or difficult to elicit in the latter stages of peritonitis, in obese patients, or in patients with significant third-spacing of fluid (e.g. ascites).

Specific Objective Findings

The serous fluid in the peritoneal cavity is normally clear yellow with a low specific gravity (less than 1.016) and has low protein concentration (usually less than 3 g/mL), with albumin being the predominant protein. Fibrinogen is not normally present. Solute concentrations are similar to those observed in plasma. A few leukocytes (<300/mL) and desquamated serosal cells may also be found.

Infected peritoneal fluid is visibly cloudy. Measurements used for immediate diagnosis include pH below 7.34 and PMN count above 500/mL. Other predictive measures include a fluid lactate concentration above 25 mg/dL and a fluid glucose concentration below 60 mg/dL. Diagnostic sensitivity improves when multiple parameters are used to establish the diagnosis (12).

Specimens from the infected tissue or fluid should be obtained during surgery or by needle aspirate and directly cultured for both anaerobic and aerobic bacteria. Gram stain of specimens may also more quickly help to identify pathogens, so that empiric antimicrobial therapy can be tailored to the patient. The Gram staining procedure is especially important in situations where the patient has been on antibiotics prior to obtaining the specimen, when cultures may never turn positive.

The diagnosis of intraabdominal abscesses has been improved, particularly with use of computed tomography scans (CT scans) (13). Isotope scans and ultrasonography are much less useful because of nonspecific and false-positive results. Also, CT-guided needle aspiration procedures or placement of percutaneous drains is established as one of the most significant surgical adjuncts in the management of intraperitoneal infection developed in the last decade.

TREATMENT

Surgical Management

Management of intraabdominal infections is initially based on any necessary operative procedures to repair GI perforations or injury. As important are debridement procedures for removal of any necrotic material and infectious foci. This includes drainage of abscesses and debridement of infected, necrotic tissue or bowel. The goal of surgical procedures is to debulk the infection and devitalized tissue, which would then allow antibiotics and host defenses to have an impact. Deaths do occur from undrained intraabdominal abscesses (14).

The indication for Tenckhoff catheter removal in CAPD patients with peritonitis has not been established. It is felt by some that continuing regular CAPD in patients with peritonitis improves outcome because infectious exudate can be physically removed by each dialysis. Others feel that it is important to remove the catheter (thus losing dialysis access) because curing an infection that involves a foreign body (i.e., the catheter) is extremely difficult. A conservative recommendation would be, if a patient has not responded to therapy alone within 5 days, removal of the Tenckhoff catheter should be considered. Experience with fungal and *Pseudomonas* peritonitis in CAPD suggests that early catheter removal is indicated (3).

General Measures

Support of intravascular volume with fluid therapy is essential to maintain adequate blood pressure and renal perfusion. The use of so-called volume expanders, such as albumin and hetastarch, has not been shown to be essential in this setting, and they are expensive. Electrolyte imbalances and metabolic acidosis should be corrected with intravenous therapy.

Oral intake of foods should be temporarily discontinued and nasogastric (NG) suction started as soon as peritonitis is suspected to prevent gastrointestinal disten-sion. Suction is continued until peristaltic activity returns and the patient begins to pass flatus. NG suction may contribute to the patient's overall fluid loss and dehydration, as well as acid-base and electrolyte problems.

Administration of oral medications should be discontinued in patients receiving NG suctioning. The gastrointestinal absorption of oral medications under such circumstances may be erratic due to changes in pH and motility. The drug may also be inadvertently removed from the GI tract by the suctioning procedure.

Antimicrobial Therapy

The choice of empiric antimicrobial therapy for intraabdominal infections is often controversial and has been reviewed (15, 16). Primary peritonitis infections (e.g., SBP) are usually caused by a single pathogen, and in 80 to 85% of cases three organisms have been responsible, *E. coli*, streptococci, and *Klebsiella* spp. Thus therapy for SBP is often more narrow than that instituted for secondary peritonitis. In fact SBP has been prevented by antimicrobial prophylaxis in high-risk cirrhosis patients (17).

Treatment of secondary peritonitis will be the focus of the remainder of this chapter. Antibiotics directed against only aerobic organisms were used prior to the technical improvements made in anaerobic culturing and sensitivity methods (18), which revealed the true incidence of anaerobic abscess infections. Now, parenteral therapy for both anaerobic and aerobic organisms of the GI flora is recommended based on observations in animal models of intraabdominal sepsis and from clinical experience. Data

Table 66.1.
Summary of Culture Results from Intraabdominal Infection Studies

Aerobic Organism	Study 1 (n = 161)	Study 2 (n = 144)	Study 3 (n = 48)	Study 4 (n = 162)
Enterococcus spp.	19	17	6	23
Streptococci	14	33	6	36
Staphylococci	7	24	8	10
E. coli	99	67	40	57
Proteus spp.	9	10	8	6
Enterobacter spp.	5	0	2	14
Klebsiella spp.	30	13	0	15
Pseudomonas spp.	15	10	2	15
Miscellaneous Aerobes	22	14	2	9
Candida spp.	0	4	4	9
Streptococci	0	1	13	4
Peptococci	0	4	19	4
Peptostreptococci	8	6	17	n/a
Fusobacterium	35	3	4	6
Clostridium spp.	29	36	31	18
Bacteroids fragilis	100	66	52	23
Other *Bacteroides* spp.	19	36	58	21
Miscellaneous anaerobes	0	25	8	22

Note: Percentages in each study do not add up to 100% because each culture may have been positive for more than one organism.
Percentage (%) of positive cultures by organism.
Data is from blood and peritoneal cultures; reported in Lau WY et al. (19), Harding et al. (20), Jones et al. (21), and Solomkin et al. (22).

Table 66.2.

Antimicrobials for Empiric Therapy of Intraabdominal Infections: Description of Spectrum of Activity

Generic Name (Trade Name)	Usual Adult Daily Dosage	Activity Against *Bacteroides fragilis*	Activity Against Enterobacteriaceae	Activity Against *Enterococcus* spp.
Metronidazole (Flagyl)	500 mg q8h	yes	no	no
Clindamycin (Cleocin)	600–900 mg q8h	yes	no	no
Chloramphenicol (Chloromycetin)	50 mg/kg/day, divide q6h	yes	yes	no
Cefuroxime (Zinacef, Kefurox)	750 mg or 1.5 g q8h	no	yes	no
Cefotetan (Cefotan)	1–2 g q12h	yes	yes	no
Cefoxitin (Mefoxin)	1–2 g q6–8h	yes	yes	no
Cefmetazole (Zefazone)	1–2 g q6–8h	yes	yes	no
Cefotaxime (Claforan)	1–2 g q6–8h	some	yes	no
Ceftizoxime (Ceftizox)	1–2 g q6–8h	yes	yes	no
Ceftazidime (Fortaz, Tazidime, Tazicef)	1–2 g q8h	no	yes	no
Ceftriaxone (Rocephin)	1–2 g q24h	no	yes	no
Cefepime (Maxipime)	1–2 g q12h	no	yes	no
Ampicillin and Sulbactam (Unasyn)	1.5–3 g q6h	yes	yes	yes
Ticarcillin and Clavulanic Acid (Timentin)	3.1 g q4h	yes	yes	some
Piperacillin and Tazobactam (Zosyn)	4.5 g q6h	yes	yes	yes
Imipenem (Primaxin)	500 mg q6–8h	yes	yes	no
Gentamicin or Tobramycin	5–10 µg/mL peak < 2 trough	no	yes	no
Vancomycin (Vancocin)	1 g q12h (trough 5–10 µg/mL)	no	no	yes
Penicillin G	1–2 mg q4–6h	no	no	yes
Ampicillin	1–2 g q4–6h	no	some	yes
Mezlocillin (Mezlin)	4 g q6h	some	yes	yes
Piperacillin (Pipracil)	4 g q6h	some	yes	yes
Ticarcillin (Ticar)	3 g q4h	some	yes	some
Aztreonam (Aztactam)	1 g q6–8h	no	yes	no
Ofloxacin (Floxin)	400 mg q12h	no	yes	no
Ciprofloxacin (Cipro)	400 mg q12h	no	yes	no

from four clinical studies spanning the last 15 years have been compiled (see Table 66.1) to give a snapshot of how often and what types of mixed infection pathogens are recovered from patients with varying intraabdominal infections.

There are an extensive number of acceptable antibiotic monotherapy regimens or combination regimens for the treatment of intraabdominal infections (23). All regimens must include coverage for Enterobacteriaceae and *B. fragilis* (24). Each reasonable regimen has subtle advantages or disadvantages in a specific patient. The following descriptions of antibiotic therapies will not give exact recommendations for therapy, but will provide a necessary framework and some important details for the formulation of patient-specific therapy (see Table 66.2). Controversy still arises regarding the need for empiric coverage of *Enterococcus* spp. organisms, with most experts still feeling that this coverage is not necessary. Exceptions to this recommendation would be for patients exhibiting signs of septic shock or if the blood or peritoneal fluid Gram stain reveals a predominance of gram-positive cocci. Empiric therapy that includes antistaphylococcal and antipseudomonal activity is not routinely necessary unless there are known predisposing factors.

Selection of empiric antimicrobial therapy should follow a careful thought process that considers first the suspected site(s) and source of infection, along with the most likely pathogens. Empiric therapy should be chosen to include, as narrowly as possible, only those suspected organisms. It is helpful to classify the infection as either community acquired or nosocomial and appropriate susceptibility data should then be applied to the antibiotic selection process. Using the antibiotic(s) with the narrowest spectrum possible will additionally reduce the incidence of secondary drug-resistance, superinfections, and confusion when assessing clinical response.

The unique pharmacologic properties of each potential antimicrobial must next be considered with regard to (a) ability to penetrate to the site of infection, (b) inoculum effect (stability toward β-lactamases produced by a large gram-negative bacterial inocula), and (c) activity in an infection environment, one of low metabolic activity (as in abscesses), and one of lower pH, and in more anaerobic conditions. Last are the considerations of potential adverse reactions, dosing, and costs, which enter the schema for final antimicrobial selection. Table 66.2 includes antimicrobial agents that have been used either as monotherapy or in combination with one another to treat intraabdominal infection. The drug dosage in adults is provided as well as a description of the spectrum of activity.

Penicillin or ampicillin can be used to provide antibacterial coverage for aerobic/anaerobic gram-positive cocci from the oropharyngeal or upper GI regions. Cephalosporins also are active against these organisms as well as Enterobacteriaceae. Additionally, some of the second- and third-generation cephalosporins have broader antibacterial activity including many anaerobic gram-negative bacilli.

Aminoglycosides are often used to provide specific antimicrobial activity against aerobic gram-negative bacilli that are found in the GI tract. However, as currently dosed, these agents have a narrow therapeutic-toxic serum concentration range that makes dosage adjustments and monitoring more complicated. Single-daily dosing may make these drugs more useful. Aminoglycosides are highly active in vitro against most strains of facultative aerobes, which are important in producing bacteremia and early mortality in intraabdominal infections. This efficacy was illustrated in an animal model of intraabdominal sepsis (25) and has since been a component of the standard of therapy. Aztreonam and quinolones have a similar narrow spectrum of activity.

Various extended spectrum penicillin and second- and third-generation cephalosporins have been more recently used instead of aminoglycosides, as their activity against most aerobic gram-negative bacilli is comparable. The combination of a penicillin plus an aminoglycoside compares to cefoxitin, with regard to susceptibility of aerobic gram-negative bacilli and anaerobic/aerobic gram positive streptococci, and it includes enterococci. The toxicity issue for aminoglycosides remains their limiting factor. The incidence of aminoglycoside-induced nephrotoxicity in patients being treated for intraabdominal infections has been reviewed (26). There is growing interest in the use of aminoglycosides as once-daily large doses (27). This dosage scheme is thought to have less potential for ototoxicity and nephrotoxicity, since this regimen does not allow drug accumulation in patients with normal renal function (28).

No cephalosporin has antimicrobial activity against enterococci. Penicillins (penicillin, ampicillin, mezlocillin, piperacillin) and vancomycin, when given alone, are bacteriostatic for this organism. The combination of one of these latter agents plus an aminoglycoside is bactericidal against enterococci, which is another reason such combinations are used when treating intraabdominal sepsis with septic shock.

Antimicrobial agents, such as B. fragilis, with good activity against obligate anaerobes reduce the incidence of abscesses, a later complication of intraabdominal infections. This coverage is needed in addition to, not instead of, therapy for aerobes. Chloramphenicol has a broad spectrum of activity against anaerobes, but few studies have evaluated its efficacy (20). In addition, the potential for serious toxicity (e.g., aplastic anemia and bone marrow suppression) has minimized its usefulness as a first-line drug.

Clindamycin has been used successfully for treatment of abdominal abscesses. The value of clindamycin has been reduced, though, by the problems of drug-induced diarrhea, pseudomembranous colitis, and emerging clindamycin-resistant B. fragilis, which has been reported to be higher than 20% in some regions (29). Metronidazole has been directly compared to clindamycin for the treatment of serious intraabdominal infections due to anaerobic organisms and demonstrated equal efficacy and probably better safety. Metronidazole is bactericidal with a narrow spectrum of antianaerobic bacterial activity. During pregnancy and lactation metronidazole should be avoided if possible because of concerns of teratogenicity.

Cefoxitin was the first of the β-lactams to show in vitro activity against B. fragilis and is still very useful (30). It has been shown to be safe and effective for the treatment of community-acquired mixed flora intraabdominal infections, whether given alone or with an aminoglycoside. Caution must be taken, though, because not all of the second- and third-generation cephalosporins are appropriate for single-drug therapy. Each has its own problems: cefuroxime, ceftazidime, ceftriaxone, and cefipime are only active against Enterobacteriaceae; cefmetazole lacks widespread acceptance (the methyl-tetrazole ring infers potential toxicity); and cefotetan, cefotaxime, and ceftizoxime have only moderate B. fragilis activity. Imipenem is very potent, is stable against many types of β-lactamases, and has excellent activity against all suspected gram-negative organisms (aerobic and anaerobic). However, it is expensive and potentially neurotoxic, and therefore is often reserved for short-term empiric therapy in seriously ill patients thought to have multiply resistant pathogens.

Special considerations must be taken into account when considering intraperitoneal drug administration in CAPD patients with peritonitis. Studies have shown a loss of activity of some antibiotics in dialysis fluid due to the low pH and high osmolarity of the dialysate solution. Aminoglycosides specifically have shown reduced bactericidal activity when the test media pH is lowered to pH 5.5, which simulates the pH of infected dialysate solution. Also, combining β-lactams and aminoglycosides in the same peritoneal dialysis bag should not be routinely done, as there may be significant inactivation of the aminoglycoside depending on the β-lactam employed. These are important considerations when CAPD patients treated with aminoglycosides are not clinically responding as expected.

COMPLICATIONS
Paralytic Ileus

Adynamic or paralytic ileus occurs to some extent with any peritoneal injury or surgery, including peritoneal inflammation. Early in the course of peritoneal irritation, the intestine may have a transient period of hyperperistalsis, but soon after motility decreases or is even absent to the point of obstruction. Severity and duration depend on the type of insult, but usually will last from 2 to 3 days, even in an uncomplicated surgical case. Studies indicate that the pathogenesis of this condition involves neurogenic, hormonal, and local factors. The adrenergic response to intraabdominal inflammation stimulates the sympathetic pathways of the intestine, resulting in the slowing of peristalsis. The accumulation of gas and fluids within the bowel lumen distends the intestinal wall to the point at which intraluminal pressure exceeds capillary perfusion pressure causing bowel ischemia.

Symptoms of paralytic ileus include progressive abdominal distension and vomiting of pooled gastric contents and biliary secretions. Localized pain and profuse vomiting only occur if there is complete bowel obstruction and strangulation. Therapy consists of GI tract rest, NG suction and treatment of the underlying GI disease.

Abdominal Adhesions

As a normal host defense the body attempts to isolate infections of the abdomen into localized pockets. The peritoneum exudes large quantities of fibrin into the peritoneal fluid while fibrinolytic activity is reduced. The result is the formation of a network of fibrinous strands between the loops of bowel and the adjacent visceral surfaces. If the fibrin is not reabsorbed, the strands are invaded by fibroblasts and develop a blood supply. Fibrin strands transform into firm adhesive bands. The absence of peristalsis allows these adhesions to more easily form. Surgical treatment may be necessary to free these attachments.

CONCLUSIONS

In the patient with intraabdominal sepsis, the crucial therapy modality is prompt, adequate surgical intervention. Parenteral antibiotics are also used to decrease the incidence of bacteremia and abscess formation. By necessity the empiric antimicrobial regimen is selected based on clinical considerations. Thus, every clinician must be aware of the differences of the microflora at various levels of the GI tract, along with their usual antimicrobial susceptibility. This data are then used to formulate empiric therapies. Therapy usually includes antimicrobial coverage for the aerobic gram-negative bacilli, Enterobacteriaceae, that cause early infection morbidity, as well as coverage for *B. fragilis,* which causes late infection morbidity.

REFERENCES

1. Bhuva M, Ganger D, Jensen D. Spontaneous bacterial peritonitis: an update on evaluation, management, and prevention. Am J Med 97:169–175, 1994.
2. Gorbach SL. Intraabdominal infections. Clin Infect Dis 17:961–967, 1993.
3. Horton MW, Deeter RG, Sherman RA. Treatment of peritonitis in patients undergoing continuous ambulatory peritoneal dialysis. Clin Pharm 9:102–118, 1990.
4. Nichols RL. Intraabdominal sepsis: characterization and treatment. J Infect Dis 135:S54–S57, 1977.
5. Hentges DJ. The anaerobic microflora of the human body. Clin Infect Dis 16(suppl 4):S175–S180, 1993.
6. Ingham HR, Tharagonnet D, Sisson PR, Selkon JB, Codd AA. Inhibition of phagocytosis in vitro by obligate anaerobes. Lancet 2:1252–1254, 1977.
7. Onderdonk AB, Shapiro ME, Finberg RW, Zaleznik DF, Kasper DL. Use of a model of intraabdominal sepsis for studies of the pathogenicity of *Bacteroides fragilis.* Rev Infect Dis 6:S91–S95, 1984.
8. Buggy BP, Schaberg DR, Swartz RD. Intraleukocytic sequestration as a cause of persistent *Staphylococcus aureus* peritonitis in continuous ambulatory dialysis. Am J Med 76:1035–1039, 1984.
9. DiPiro JT. Considerations for therapy of mixed infections: focus on intraabdominal infection. Pharmacotherapy 15:15S–21S, 1995.
10. Nichols RL, Smith JW. Risk of infection, infecting flora and treatment considerations in penetrating abdominal trauma. Surg Gynecol Obstet 177(suppl):50–54, 1993.
11. Levison ME Bush LM. Peritonitis and other intra-abdominal infections. In: Mandell GL, Bennett JE, Dolin R, eds. Mandell, Douglas and Bennett's principles and practice of infectious diseases, 4th ed. New York: Churchill Livingstone, 1995:705–740.
12. Garcia-Tsao G, Conn HO, Lerner E. The diagnosis of bacterial peritonitis: comparison of pH, lactate concentration and leukocyte count. Hepatology 5:91–96, 1985.
13. Wilson SE. A critical analysis of recent innovations in the treatment of intra-abdominal infection. Surg Gynecol Obstet 177(suppl):11–17, 1993.
14. Fry DE, Garrison RN, Heitsch RC, Calhoun K, Polk HC. Determinants of death in patients with intraabdominal abscess. Surgery 88:517–522, 1980.
15. McClean KL, Sheehan GJ Harding GKM. Intraabdominal infection: a review. Clin Infect Dis 19:100–116, 1994.
16. Shands JW Jr. Empiric antibiotic therapy of abdominal sepsis and serious perioperative infections. Surg Clin North Am 73:291–306, 1993.
17. Singh N, Gayowski T, Yu VL, Wagener MM. Trimethoprim-sulfamethoxazole for the prevention of spontaneous bacterial peritonitis in cirrhosis: a randomized trial. Ann Intern Med 122:595–598, 1995.
18. Wexler HM. Susceptibility testing of anaerobic bacteria-the state of the art. Clin Infect Dis 16(suppl 4):S328–S333, 1993.
19. Lau WY, Teoh-Chan CH, Fan ST, Yam WC, Lau KF, Wong SH. The bacteriology and septic complication of patients with appendicitis. Ann Surg 200:576–581, 1984.
20. Harding GKM, Buckwold FJ, Ronald AR, Marrie TJ, Brunton S, Koss JC, Gurwith MJ, Albritton WL. Prospective, randomized, comparative study of clindamycin, chloramphenicol, and ticarcillin, each in combination with gentamicin in therapy for intraabdominal and female genital tract sepsis. J Infect Dis 142:384–393, 1980.
21. Jones RC, Thal ER, Johnson NA, Golihar LN. Evaluation of antibiotic therapy following penetrating abdominal trauma. Ann Surg 201:576–585, 1985.
22. Solomkin JS, Dellinger EP, Christou NV, Busuttil RW. Results of a multicenter trial comparing imipenem/cilastatin to tobramycin/clindamycin for intra-abdominal infections. Ann Surg 212:581–591, 1990.
23. DiPiro JT, Cue JI. Single-agent versus combination antibiotic therapy in the management of intraabdominal infections. Pharmacother 14:266–272, 1994.
24. Bohnen JMA, Solomkin JS, Dellinger EP, Bjornson HS, Page CP.

Guidelines for clinical care: anti-infective agents for intra-abdominal infection–a surgical infection society policy statement. Arch Surg 127:83–88, 1992.

25. Nichols RL, Smith JW, Fossedal EN, Condon RE. Efficacy of parenteral antibiotics in the treatment of experimentally induced intraabdominal sepsis. Rev Infec Dis 1:302–312, 1979.

26. Ho JL, Barza M. Role of aminoglycoside antibiotics in the treatment of intra-abdominal infection. Antimicrob Agents Chemother 31:485–491, 1987.

27. Kapusnik JE, Hackbarth CJ, Chambers HF, Carpenter T, Sande MA.

Single-large daily dose versus conventional intermittent dosing of tobramycin for the treatment of guinea pigs with *Pseudomonas aeruginosa* pneumonia. J Infect Dis 158:7–12, 1988.

28. Gilbert DN. Once daily aminoglycoside therapy. Antimicrob Agents Chemother 35:339–345, 1991.

29. Rasmussen BA, Bush K, Tally FP. Antimicrobial resistance in Bacteroides. Clin Infect Dis 16(suppl 4):S390–S400, 1993.

30. Johnson CC. Susceptibility of anaerobic bacteria to beta-lactam antibiotics in the United States. Clin Infect Dis 16(suppl 4):S371–S376, 1993.

CHAPTER 67

GASTROINTESTINAL INFECTIONS

SHAWN R. AKKERMAN and VICTOR LAMPASONA

Gastroenteritis (GE) remains a major cause of morbidity and mortality worldwide, particularly among children, in whom 1.5 billion episodes of diarrhea and 4 million associated deaths occur each year (1). In the United States, children under 5 years of age experience 20 to 35 million episodes of diarrhea, 10% of which result in doctor visits, over 200,000 hospitalizations, and 400 deaths annually (2). Recent studies also suggest that GE is becoming an important and rising cause of mortality in elderly adults in developed countries (3, 4). The most common symptom of acute infectious GE is diarrhea, which is often mild, self-limiting, and responsive to appropriate oral fluid and electrolyte therapy and nutritional management. The need for intravenous fluids, antibiotics, and antidiarrheal agents should be determined based on the likely pathogen, the patient's clinical status, and accepted indications, as these interventions are infrequently necessary or helpful.

ETIOLOGY AND EPIDEMIOLOGY

Viruses are the leading cause of GE around the world; the most common are rotavirus and Norwalk virus. Bacterial GE is less frequent and is caused by *Salmonella*, *Shigella*, *Campylobacter*, *Yersinia*, *Vibrio*, and *Escherichia coli*. Parasites, such as *Giardia lamblia*, *Entamoeba histolytica*, and *Cryptosporidium*, may also be associated with diarrheal diseases; these are discussed with other intestinal parasites in Chapter 73.

This discussion is limited to organisms that are common, are of increasing epidemiologic importance, or primarily affect immunocompetent patients. Information about GE in the immunocompromised setting, other viral infections, overgrowth of normal flora, antibiotic-induced *Clostridium difficile* colitis, and agents that cause diarrhea through food poisoning may be found in other references (5–8).

Viruses

Five major categories of human GE viruses have been defined: rotavirus, enteric adenovirus, Norwalk virus, calicivirus, and astrovirus (9). These viruses may be predominantly associated with an endemic type of disease pattern (rotavirus, enteric adenovirus) or with an epidemic or outbreak disease pattern (Norwalk, calicivirus, astrovirus).

Rotavirus is the single most important cause of dehydrating diarrhea in both developed and developing countries (10). Rotavirus GE is felt to be seasonal, first appearing in the fall in the western United States, moving eastward, and reaching the Northeast by late winter and spring (11, 12). It primarily affects infants and children between 3 and 24 months of age, but adults may become infected after close contact with an infected child (13). Although usually considered an endemic disease, outbreaks of rotavirus GE can occur and are common, especially in day-care centers (13, 14). The virus is transmitted by the fecal-oral route and is excreted in the feces throughout the illness. The incubation period is approximately 2 days. Diarrhea may be severe and is often accompanied by vomiting and fever. The duration of illness may range from 3 to 8 days (9, 13, 14).

Enteric adenoviruses are specific strains (serotypes 40 and 41) that, unlike other adenoviruses, do not cause conjunctivitis or respiratory tract symptoms. Endemic adenoviral GE is not seasonal, primarily affects children under the age of 2, and is the second most common cause of severe viral diarrhea in children (13). It is transmitted via the fecal-oral route and has an 8- to 10-day incubation period. The presentation is one of watery diarrhea followed by 2 or 3 days of low-grade fever and vomiting. The illness often lasts for 5 to 12 days, longer than other forms of viral GE (9, 13).

Norwalk virus is one of a class of small, round structured viruses that are often associated with epidemics or outbreaks of GE. Such outbreaks occur in families, camps, schools, nursing homes, hospitals, cafeterias, and sports teams, and on cruise ships. The virus may be acquired by the fecal-oral route or airborne transmission, or may result from consuming contaminated drinking or swimming water or inadequately cooked shellfish. Although also known as "winter vomiting disease," infection can occur year-round, affecting adults and older children but not infants or younger children (9). The incubation period is 12 to 48 hours, followed by the abrupt onset of nausea and vomiting with or without diarrhea (13). The duration of illness is brief (1 or 2 days) and, in contrast to rotavirus, usually does not result in significant dehydration (14).

Astroviral and caliciviral GE occur most commonly in infants and young children but with less frequency than other viral GE pathogens. Both have been associated with outbreaks in day-care centers and nursing homes or with the ingestion of contaminated water or shellfish (13). One

Table 67.1.
Clinical and Epidemiologic Characteristics of Viral Gastroenteritis

Virus	Epidemiology	Transmission	Incubation	Symptoms	Duration
Rotavirus	Winter peak; endemic/ epidemic	Fecal-oral, food, water	2 days	Water diarrhea, fever, vomiting	3–8 days
Adenovirus	Year-round; endemic	Fecal-oral	8–10 days	Diarrhea, fever, vomiting, respiratory symptoms	5–12 days
Norwalk virus	Year-round with winter peak; epidemic	Fecal-oral, shellfish, water	12–48 hours	Nausea, vomiting, with/ without diarrhea	1–2 days
Astrovirus	Winter peak; epidemic	Fecal-oral, shellfish, water	1–2 days	Mild diarrhea, fever, vomiting	2–3 days
Calicivirus	Year-round; epidemic	Fecal-oral, shellfish, water	1–4 days	Mild diarrhea, fever, vomiting	4–5 days

study also suggests that astrovirus is an important causative agent of diarrhea in HIV-infected patients and may be more common than bacterial or parasitic pathogens in this setting (15). The important clinical and epidemiologic characteristics of viral gastroenteritis pathogens are summarized in Table 67.1.

Bacteria

Salmonella spp. are Gram-negative bacilli of the Enterobacteriaceae family and can basically be divided into nontyphoidal and typhoidal (*S. typhi,* the causative agent of typhoid fever) species. *S. enteritidis* is the predominant nontyphoidal species, has many serotypes, and is responsible for the majority of cases of *Salmonella*-induced GE. Infection is usually the result of ingestion of contaminated water or food, particularly meat, poultry, or dairy products (10, 16). A recent review of 380 outbreaks of *S. enteritidis* in the United States from 1985 to 1991 implicates eggs and egg-containing products as the most important source of these infections. Previously thought to be more confined to the Northeast, such outbreaks have now spread throughout the United States (17). Transmission of *Salmonella* occurs via the fecal-oral route. Certain domestic animals may be a vector for this organism as well. One example is turtles, whose commercial sale in the United States has been prohibited due to their common carriage of this organism (16). The incubation period is approximately 6 to 48 hours after ingestion. *Salmonella* GE presents as watery diarrhea, which often contains blood and mucus, and usually abates within 3 to 7 days. Infants less than 6 months of age, HIV-infected persons, and patients with sickle cell disease are particularly susceptible to disseminated disease following GE. Sequelae include meningitis, osteomyelitis, myocarditis, and pneumonia (10, 16, 18). Chronic carriage of the organism is common, especially in children (19).

Shigella spp. are Gram-negative rods that are known to cause a type of GE in humans that is also referred to as bacillary dysentery. Four types of *Shigella* have been implicated: *S. sonnei* (most prevalent in industrialized countries), *S. flexneri* (most important between the 1920s and 1930s), *S. boydii* (rare), and *S. dysenteriae* (the most virulent and not commonly seen in developed countries since early this century). Because *Shigella* is relatively acid resistant and requires a very small inoculum to cause disease, it is easily transmitted from person to person via the fecal-oral route (10). *Shigella* infections occur more often in the summer and fall, and are the primary cause of bacterial GE in day-care centers (16, 18). While shigellosis is more common in children from 6 months to 10 years of age, a recent report suggests that changing levels of immunity to *S. sonnei* may support periodic hyperendemic rates of shigellosis in older patient populations (20). Following transmission, the incubation period is 24 to 48 hours. The patient with shigellosis initially presents with high fever, abdominal cramping, and profuse, watery diarrhea, which lasts about 24 hours. After this period, the diarrhea becomes less frequent and may contain blood and mucus. Illness duration is approximately 4 or 5 days. The most common complication is neurotoxicity with seizures, which occurs in 10 to 40% of infected children (16).

Campylobacter spp. are spiral-shaped Gram-negative bacilli known to cause systemic as well as gastrointestinal illnesses. *C. jejuni* is the most common species associated with acute GE in humans and is one of the organisms implicated as a cause of traveler's diarrhea (16). Animal reservoirs of this organism include cattle, sheep, swine, fowl, cats, and dogs. *Campylobacter* GE is more common in the summer and has a bimodal infection frequency, occurring mostly in children less than 1 year old and in young adults (10, 16). Outbreaks have been associated with contaminated water, raw meat, poultry, clams, and unpasteurized dairy products or contact with young dogs or cats (21). Transmission is by the fecal-oral route followed by an incubation period of 1 to 7 days. Initial clinical symptoms are fever, headache and myalgias that last for 12 to 24 hours. Acute GE symptoms ensue with abdominal cramping, fever, and a secretory diarrhea that may contain mucus and blood (10, 18). Symptoms often resolve within 5 to 7 days, but in severe cases may persist for several weeks.

Escherichia coli is a Gram-negative rod that is a common inhabitant of the human gastrointestinal tract. GE can be caused by five different types of the organism. There are different virulence properties among the types, some of which may overlap. The primary types are enterotoxigenic *E. coli* (ETEC) and enterohemorrhagic *E. coli* (EHEC). Less frequent, but equally important, are enteropathogenic *E. coli* (EPEC), enteroaggregative *E. coli* (EAggEC), and enteroinvasive *E. coli* (EIEC) (22).

ETEC is the predominant cause of traveler's diarrhea in adults and infantile diarrhea in developing countries. It has also been associated with outbreaks due to ingestion of contaminated food or water. Both ETEC and *Shigella* were responsible for the majority of GE cases experienced by U.S. troops during Operation Desert Shield (23). ETEC symptoms such as low-grade fever, abdominal cramping, and watery diarrhea follow a 1- to 3-day incubation period (24). Illness usually remits in about 3 to 5 days.

EHEC may cause diarrhea, hemorrhagic colitis, hemolytic uremic syndrome (HUS), and postdiarrheal thrombotic thrombocytopenic purpura. *E. coli* O157:H7 is the best-described strain in this class to date. Since its discovery in 1983, it has received much public and scientific attention as a result of several deaths in outbreaks linked to ingestion of contaminated hamburger meat (25). One report of an outbreak connected with contaminated swimming water confirmed that a small inoculum of organism, similar to *Shigella*, is sufficient to cause disease (26). The incubation period is 3 to 4 days, at which time patients experience some abdominal pain

and fever. Within 1 or 2 days, nonbloody diarrhea follows and may be accompanied by vomiting. The diarrhea becomes bloody within 1 or 2 more days and usually lasts about 4 to 10 days. Approximately 10% of *E. coli* O157:H7 infections in children less than 10 years old progress to HUS. If it occurs, HUS will develop within 1 week after the onset of diarrhea. Complications of HUS may include seizures, stroke, renal failure, hypertension, glucose intolerance, and death (22).

Yersinia enterocolitica is another Gram-negative coccobacillus that causes GE in both children and adults. It is a major cause of bacterial GE in Europe and Canada with a preference for colder climates. It is felt to be an important but underrecognized pathogen in the United States as well (27). Modes of transmission include ingestion of contaminated foods, water, or unpasteurized milk. Swine and pork products have been associated with several outbreaks of *Yersinia* GE tied to the consumption of contaminated chitterlings (pig intestines) (28). Symptoms of *Yersinia* GE are abdominal pain, vomiting, fever, and blood-streaked diarrhea. The illness may last 7 to 21 days, with continued excretion of the organism for weeks after symptoms subside (18, 27).

Other miscellaneous Gram-negative organisms have been reported to cause clinical GE in certain patient groups. *Vibrio* spp. are a cause of GE in the United States and around the world. The primary pathogenic species are *V. cholerae* (the causative agent of cholera) and *V. parahaemolyticus*. Of recent interest is the significant emergence of cholera on the North and particularly the South American and Indian continents (29). Noncholera *Vibrio*, *Aeromonas*, and *Plesiomonas* spp. share an association with water. Infection due to these organisms is usually linked with the ingestion of raw or undercooked

Table 67.2.

Clinical and Epidemiologic Characteristics of Bacterial Gastroenteritis

Bacteria	Transmission	Incubation	Symptoms	Duration	Complications
Salmonella spp.	Fecal-oral; eggs, milk, meat, turtles	6–48 hours	Water, mucoid, bloody diarrhea	3–7 days	Osteomyelitis, meningitis, pneumonia, myocarditis
Shigella spp.	Fecal-oral; food, water	24–48 hours	Fever, diarrhea cramping	4–5 days	Seizures, HUS
Campylobacter spp.	Fecal-oral; water, dairy, meat, pets	1–7 days	Fever, cramping, secretory diarrhea	5–7 days	None (with *C. jejuni*)
ETEC[a]	Fecal-oral; food, water	1–3 days	Watery diarrhea, cramping	3–5 days	None
EHEC[b]	Fecal-oral; hamburger, water	3–4 days	Fever, vomiting, bloody diarrhea	4–10 days	HUS, TTP, seizures, renal failure, stroke
Yersinia spp.	Fecal-oral; water, milk, pork	2–11 days	Fever, diarrhea, abdominal pain	1–3 weeks	Bacteremia, ileitis, arthritis
V. cholerae	Fecal-oral; water, shellfish	6–48 hours	Profuse, watery diarrhea	5–7 days	Renal failure, acidosis, hypoglycemia

[a]Enterotoxigenic *Escherichia coli*
[b]Enterohemorrhagic *Escherichia coli*

seafood, often shellfish, or contaminated water (18, 27, 30). The important clinical and epidemiologic characteristics of bacterial GE pathogens are summarized in Table 67.2.

Pathogens on the Horizon

Several organisms, some newly identified (*Cyclospora, picobirnavirus*) and others not previously associated with diarrheal diseases (*Bacteroides fragilis*), have been shown to be associated with GE illness (15, 27, 31). Their roles as potential pathogens require further investigation before their relationship to GE can be substantiated.

PATHOGENESIS

Host Defenses

Among the host factors that act against pathogenic organisms, four have been well established as defense mechanisms: (a) gastric acidity, (b) peristalsis, (c) resident microflora, and (d) immune response. Most enteric pathogens do not reach the intestine due to the highly acidic environment of the stomach. They may survive if they are relatively acid resistant (e.g., *Shigella*) or if a large inoculum of organism is ingested (10). Additionally, food, achlorhydria, gastric resection, or iatrogenic factors, such as antacids, H2 antagonists, or H+/K+ ATPase inhibitors, may reduce gastric pH and increase the risk of GE in certain patients. Slowed intestinal motility may allow colonization and increased contact time of enteropathogens with the intestinal mucosa. Impaired motility may be caused by antiperistaltic compounds such as diphenoxylate or loperamide or by underlying diseases such as stroke (32). Antibiotics (especially broad-spectrum compounds) decrease normal flora of the gastrointestinal tract and allow inappropriate overgrowth of pathogenic or colonizing nosocomial organisms known to cause GE.

A recent report of an investigation into an outbreak of nosocomial *S. enteritidis* infections affecting 28% of the patients in a 1045-bed hospital indicated that diabetics requiring insulin or oral hypoglycemics were at an increased risk of infection. The increased risk may be due to decreased gastric acid and/or impaired motility, both well-recognized complications of diabetes mellitus (33). This report underscores the need to consider underlying diseases when evaluating a patient's risk for GE.

Finally, immature or compromised immune status predisposes patients to enteric infections. Conversely, active or passive immunity (e.g. breast-milk antibody) aids in the prevention of GE (34, 35). Immune responses to GE organisms have been and continue to be the focus of intense research efforts to develop effective and inexpensive methods of prophylaxis against GE illnesses. The reader is referred to several excellent articles on the subject of vaccine development for bacterial and viral enteric pathogens (36, 37).

Diarrheal Pathophysiology and Virulence Mechanisms

One of the main functions of the small intestine and colon is the absorption and secretion of fluids, ions, and nutrients. These processes take place in the villus-crypt units that line the small intestinal mucosa. GE pathogens impair absorption and/or increase secretion. The result is too much water in the stool or diarrhea (38).

Water absorption occurs passively and is linked to two pathways of active sodium transport in the villi. In the first pathway, water is pulled from the intestine into the vasculature along an osmotic gradient created by the transport of sodium from the intestine into the mucosal cell. This occurs via a sodium/chloride cotransport mechanism that is inhibited by cyclic AMP and GMP. Some GE pathogens produce toxins that activate adenyl cyclase, leading to increased cAMP levels. Increased amounts of cAMP cause (a) reduced active sodium and water absorption and (b) increased active secretion of chloride. These effects result in more water and electrolyte volume in the stool and diarrhea (38, 39).

The second pathway involves the cotransport of sodium with nutrients, such as glucose and amino acids, across the intestine into the mucosal cell. This mechanism is not nearly as important in the production of diarrhea as in the treatment of it. Administration of a glucose-containing solution promotes sodium and water absorption via this pathway and aids in rehydration of the patient with diarrhea (38).

The secretion of fluid and electrolytes into the intestine is the function of the crypt cells. GE organisms may invade and destroy the surface villi. This leads to greater proliferation of crypt epithelium and increased secretion of water and electrolytes into the stool (38, 39). Secondary lactose intolerance may occur due to destruction of mucosal brush border enzymes (13).

Other means by which GE pathogens are able to cause diarrhea include (a) production of enterotoxins and secretogogues (e.g., prostaglandins, interleukins), which stimulate secretion; (b) damage and ulceration of the intestinal epithelium with leakage of serous fluid, blood, and cells into the lumen; and (c) altered intestinal myoelectric activity and transit secondary to enterotoxins, cytotoxins, or organism invasion (38, 39). A summary of the organisms with their associated pathogenic mechanisms is provided in Table 67.3.

Electrolyte Depletion

In addition to increased fluid losses resulting from the pathogenic mechanisms described above, these infectious processes result in a disregulation of sodium and bicarbonate homeostasis and electrolyte losses. In the parietal cell, H_2CO_3 dissociates into hydrogen and bicarbonate. The bicarbonate is secreted into the intestine along with

Table 67.3.
Pathogenic Mechanisms of Enteric Organisms

	Rotavirus	Norwalk	Salmonella spp.	Shigella spp.	E. coli	Vibrio spp.	Yersinia spp.	Campylobacter spp.
Increased Secretion								
Enterotoxins			+		+	+		
Prostaglandins			+					
Crypt proliferation	+	+				+		
Decreased Absorption								
Villi destruction	+	+			+			
Cytotoxins							+	
Epithelial invasion				+	+	+		+
Altered Transit		+?	+	+	+	+	+	+

Adapted from references 34, 38, 39.

sodium, and the hydrogen is reabsorbed into the blood. In the diarrheal process, the sodium loss increases, causing a concomitant increase in bicarbonate loss into the intestine. This allows more hydrogen to be reabsorbed into the blood, resulting in systemic metabolic acidosis. Potassium loss increases secondary to interference with reabsorption or to activation of the aldosterone system as a result of hyponatremia or hypovolemia.

CLINICAL PRESENTATION

GE syndromes can be classified as either inflammatory or noninflammatory. Inflammatory GE is characterized by fever and abdominal cramping with small-volume, bloody, mucoid diarrhea. Microscopic stool examination often reveals the presence of numerous fecal leukocytes. This is indicative of cytotoxin-induced damage and organism invasion of the colonic mucosa that causes blood, serous fluid, and white blood cells to leak into the lumen (10, 38). Inflammatory diarrheal illnesses often are more severe and may cause systemic symptoms such as vasculitic rashes, arthritis, and bacteremia (34, 38).

Noninflammatory GE is characterized by low-grade fever, nausea and vomiting, and large-volume, watery, diarrhea. In contrast to inflammatory GE, diarrhea is the result of nondestructive pathogenic mechanisms (e.g., enterotoxin, altered transit) that primarily affect absorptive and secretory processes. Therefore, no cellular components, such as red or white blood cells, should be present on microscopic stool examination due to the lack of intestinal epithelial damage (10, 38).

A careful history, including recent travel, antibiotic use, family or other contact illnesses, weight loss, recent food or water ingestion, and underlying diseases should be obtained. Evaluation of the appearance, quantity, and duration of diarrhea is also important. Actual examination of a stool specimen for blood, mucus, and leukocytes is preferable to a description of the stool by the patient. With these data and knowledge of the epidemiology setting and likely GE organisms, a presumptive causative

agent can usually be identified. Stool cultures may be useful in diagnosis but should be reserved for unresponsive diarrheal illness or patients with signs of inflammatory or systemic disease. Such testing is costly and should be appropriately requested in order to isolate suspected pathogens that require special media and procedures (10). As fluid and nutritional therapies are the cornerstone of GE management, physical assessment of signs of dehydration and electrolyte abnormalities is crucial. The health-care provider should know when other diagnostic procedures, such as radiologic or endoscopic evaluations, are necessary and refer patients quickly to the appropriate medical source. Information on the differential diagnosis of infectious and noninfectious diarrhea can be found elsewhere (5).

TREATMENT
Fluid and Electrolyte Therapy

The cornerstone of treatment for all types of infectious GE is fluid and electrolyte replacement. Therapy consists of two phases: (a) the rehydration phase, in which water and electrolytes are given to replace existing losses, and (b) the maintenance phase, which includes both replacement of ongoing fluid and electrolyte losses and adequate dietary intake (40). Fluid may be given by the oral or intravenous (IV) route. The degree of dehydration and the patient's ability to maintain oral intake determine the method of fluid repletion to be used. Evaluation of the degree of dehydration includes assessment of objective (skin turgor, mucous membranes, sunken eyes or fontanelle, pulse, blood pressure) and subjective signs (mental status, thirst, lethargy, extremities).

Oral rehydration therapy (ORT) is preferred in all cases of mild to moderate dehydration and for the prevention of subsequent dehydration (10). ORT is as effective in achieving rehydration and provides several advantages compared to IV therapy (41). ORT is less invasive, less costly, and less likely to result in overhydration, and allows for rapid institution of therapy in the home setting (13, 42). It has revolutionized the management of infectious GE in endemic areas but, for reasons that are unclear, remains greatly underused in developed countries such as the United States (10, 43, 44).

Indications for the use of IV hydration are severe dehydration (≥10% fluid deficit), hypovolemic shock, or inability to take oral therapy (e.g., coma, uncontrolled vomiting, ileus). Less than 2% of community cases and less than 10% of patients requiring medical attention will meet the criteria for IV therapy (10). Two populations are at greatest risk from dehydration and may require IV hydration more frequently: infants, who have a higher surface area to fluid volume ratio, and elderly adults, who may experience more serious sequelae as a result of concomitant atherosclerotic disease (18, 32). When indicated, IV therapy should consist of an isotonic solution (such as Ringer's lactate) and be infused within 4 to 6 hours (10). Sodium, potassium, and bicarbonate should be carefully monitored and replaced appropriately based on measured losses and serum concentrations. Table 67.4 indicates the clinical signs and appropriate treatments associated with different degrees of dehydration for patients with GE.

The choice of which oral rehydration solution (ORS) to use in the management of GE-induced diarrhea is an important one. The optimal ORS should be isotonic and contain adequate amounts of water, sodium, potassium, and bicarbonate (18). Glucose is also a necessary component to enhance sodium and water absorption via mucosal glucose/sodium cotransport mechanisms. Other carbohydrates, such as fructose and sucrose, can also be used but may be less effective (45). In 1975, the World Health Organization (WHO) and the United Nations International Children's Emergency Fund (UNICEF) developed a single ORS formula for use in the treatment of diarrhea (40). This ORS contains (in mmol/L): sodium, 90; potassium, 20; chloride, 80; citrate 30; and glucose 111 (2%). It is available in packets for easy mixture, it has been shown to be effective in the management of diarrhea, and it has dramatically reduced the number of dehydration-related deaths in developing countries since its institution. Several premixed oral rehydration solutions are commercially available and are listed in Table 67.5. The American Academy of Pediatrics (AAP) recommends that solutions used for rehydration contain 75 to 90 meq/L of sodium and those for hydration maintenance or prevention of dehydration contain 40 to 60 meq/L of sodium, in order to prevent hypernatremia (46). An ORS with 75 to 90 meq/L should always be used in the setting of highly purging diarrhea (e.g., >10 mL/kg/hr) and, when used for maintenance, should be administered with other low-sodium fluids (e.g., breast milk, formula, water) (40). It should be noted that "clear liquids" often found in the home, such as cola, ginger ale, fruit juice, and Gatorade, are not recommended for treatment. These solutions often contain excess sugar and inadequate bicarbonate and electrolytes, and can cause osmotic diarrhea (34, 40, 44). However, they can be used for prevention of dehydration and in milder cases of diarrhea. Free water alone should always be avoided, since this may result in hyponatremia.

Recently, other substrates have been investigated for use in ORS formulas. Cereal-based oral rehydration solutions deliver larger amounts of carbohydrate to the lumen than glucose-based solutions and are able to further increase fluid absorption without an increase in osmotic load. Rice-based solutions have been found to be equally

Table 67.4.
Clinical Assessment and Management of Diarrhea

Degree of Dehydration	Signs[a]	Rehydration Therapy (within 4 hours)	Replacement of stool fluid losses	Dietary Therapy[b]
Mild (3–5%)	Slightly dry buccal membranes, increased thirst	ORS[c] 50 mL/kg	10 mL/kg or ½–1 cup of ORS for each diarrheal stool	Breast milk, or half- or full-strength lactose-containing milk or undiluted lactose-free formula
Moderate (6–9%)	Sunken eyes and/or fontanelle, poor skin turgor, dry buccal membranes	ORS 100 mL/kg	Same as above	Same as above
Severe (≥10%)	Signs of moderate dehydration with one of the following: rapid thready pulse, cyanosis, cold extremities, rapid breathing, lethargy, coma	IV fluids (Ringer's lactate), 20 mL/kg/hr until pulse, perfusion, and mental status return to normal; then 50–100 mL/kg of ORS	Same as above	Same as above

[a]If patient exhibits no signs of dehydration, rehydration therapy is not indicated. Begin maintenance therapy and replacement of stool losses.
[b]Children who tolerate solid food can continue their usual diet, but foods high in simple sugars and fats should be avoided.
[c]Oral rehydration solution.
Adapted from reference 40.

Table 67.5.
Comparison of Oral Rehydration Solutions

ORS	Carbohydrate		Sodium (meq/L)	Potassium (meq/L)	Chloride (meq/L)	Base (meq/L)
	Concentration (g/L)	Source				
WHO-ORS	20	Glucose	90	20	80	30
Rehydralyte	25	Glucose	75	20	65	30
Pedialyte	25	Glucose	45	20	35	30
Infalyte	30	Rice syrup	50	25	45	34
Elderlyte	25	Glucose	45	20	35	30
Resol	20	Glucose	50	20	50	34
Rice-based	50	Starch (rice)	60–90	20	80	30

Adapted from references 10, 18, 32.

effective, with reduced duration and volume of diarrhea (10, 47). They can be easily prepared at home and in developing countries, and offer a "bridge" between the transition from fluid to food (48). Health-care providers should be familiar with the different available ORS products and their appropriate uses and should encourage parents of young children to have a supply of ORS at home at all times for early use when diarrhea occurs (40).

Although the past standard of practice has been to withhold food until diarrhea is resolved, recommendations now are to institute feeding within the first 24 hours of the onset of diarrhea (46). There are data to suggest that early feeding reduces the severity and duration of diarrhea, aids in intestinal mucosa repair, and may prevent malnutrition (34, 49). For infants, breast-feeding or full-strength, lactose-free formula should be reinstated after rehydration. For older children, a regular diet should be resumed consisting of frequent but small amounts of starches, cereals, soup, yogurt, vegetables and fresh fruits (40). In general, lactose- or sorbitol-containing foods, caffeine, and foods high in simple sugars or fat should be avoided.

Other Supportive Therapy

The benefits and risks of antidiarrheal therapy in the treatment of infectious GE depend on the particular product, the infectious agent, and the age of the patient. Indeed, it could be argued that diarrhea is itself a host defense mechanism, designed to expel the pathogen, and should not be suppressed (39). Use of antidiarrheal agents, when indicated, should in no way interfere with or shift the focus from appropriate fluid, electrolyte, and nutritional therapy (40).

Antimotility agents such as tincture of opium, diphenoxylate-atropine, and loperamide may reduce the frequency of stool in milder cases of GE seen in adults and older children in developed countries. However, risks associated with these agents include side effects (atropinism, sedation), ileus, toxic megacolon, and increased bowel wall invasion and organism excretion (38, 50). Antimotility

agents should not be given to infants, elderly adults, or any patient with an inflammatory, bloody diarrhea, usually indicating infection with an invasive pathogen (32, 50, 51). In cases of mild to moderate diarrhea, particularly traveler's diarrhea, loperamide may be useful in reducing the duration of symptoms. When indicated, the regimen to be used is loperamide 4 mg as a single dose, then 2 mg after each loose stool, not to exceed 16 mg/day.

Kaolin-pectin suspension adds bulk and produces firmer stools, but does not reduce stool volume (38). Bismuth subsalicylate (BSS) demonstrates antimicrobial activity against enteropathogens such as E. coli, Salmonella, Shigella, and Campylobacter, and is effective in the treatment of traveler's diarrhea (52). Other potential mechanisms for its efficacy include antisecretory activity, enterotoxin inactivation, and prevention of bacterial attachment to intestinal mucosa (50). The regimen for BSS is 60 mL every 2 hours for each stool up to 4 doses, then 30 mL every 6 hours as needed (32). An alternative regimen is 2 tablets 4 times daily. The primary side effect of BSS is blackened stools. Tinnitus, encephalopathy, and salicylate toxicity have been reported with chronic use. Patients with hypersensitivity to aspirin or who are taking oral anticoagulants should not be treated with BSS (50, 53).

Other antidiarrheal agents that are under investigation include α_2-adrenergic agonists, berberine, somatostatin, phenothiazines, chloride channel blockers and antiinflammatory drugs, such as indomethacin and glucocorticoids (50). The future role of these agents in the management of infectious GE remains to be determined.

Antimicrobial Therapy

There are no effective antimicrobial agents for viral GE. The use of antibiotics to treat bacterial GE depends on the infecting organism, the severity and chronicity of the infectious process, and the effectiveness of the antibiotic in reducing the severity or carrier state of the illness. Since many of the GE infections experienced by ambulatory patients are self-limiting, antibiotic therapy is not routinely recommended unless the infection is severe or disseminated, or the patient is chronically symptomatic or debilitated.

Antimicrobial Resistance

A major factor in the prevalence of multiresistant strains of pathogenic organisms is the indiscriminate use of antibiotics in humans and animals. The use of antibiotics is clearly related to the development of plasmid-mediated resistance in microorganisms, particularly in the presence of suboptimal concentrations. Multiresistant *Salmonella*, *Shigella*, and ETEC have been associated with epidemics in developing countries (54). A recent example was the identification of ETEC and *Shigella* isolates in U.S. troops with GE during Operation Desert Shield that exhibited high levels of resistance to trimethoprim/sulfamethoxazole, tetracycline, and ampicillin (23). Resistance to selected antimicrobial agents varies widely, changes with time, and depends on the agent, organism strain, and the year or specific geographic location (55). To minimize the development of resistant strains of bacteria, antibiotics must be carefully chosen, based on susceptibility testing and the severity of the condition.

Antibiotics of Choice

The primary goals of antibiotic therapy in the management of infectious GE are to decrease the duration of symptomatic illness, prevent complications, and reduce the excretion of pathogenic organisms and further spread of disease (56). The utility of such therapy depends on the specific organism involved and the timely institution of therapy. Antibiotics appear to be of most value in *Shigella*, ETEC, cholera, and *Campylobacter* infections, and the least value in *Salmonella* or *Yersinia* GE. They may be of some value in noncholera *Vibrio*, *Aeromonas*, or *Plesiomonas* infections in certain patients. Table 67.6 lists the drug(s) of choice by causative agent and the conditions under which antibiotic therapy is considered

most appropriate. Table 67.7 lists the usual drug, dose, side effect, and monitoring parameters by drug entity for agents used in the management of infectious GE.

Ampicillin has been evaluated for use in *Shigella* and *Salmonella* GE. It is very effective in GE caused by *Shigella* ampicillin-sensitive strains only. In fact, prior to the mid 1970s, oral ampicillin was considered the drug of choice for GE caused by *Shigella*. However, more than half of the *Shigella* strains currently encountered are resistant to ampicillin. Ampicillin has not been shown to affect the duration or severity of diarrhea due to *Salmonella* GE but may be useful in systemic or disseminated infections due to this organism (57, 58). These infections appear to be more common in infants less than 3 months of age.

Tetracycline has been successfully used to treat GE caused by *Shigella* and ETEC. Resistance of both organisms to tetracycline has been increasing, relegating it to use as an alternative drug or when susceptibility data are available (23). Tetracycline is the drug of choice for *V. cholerae* due to its efficacy and low cost (56). Tetracycline should not be given to pregnant women or children under the age of 12 years because of the potential for unwanted permanent staining of the teeth. It is also associated with photosensitivity reactions, probably secondary to accumulation in the skin. Patients taking tetracycline should be advised to take appropriate precautions (e.g., sunscreen) when exposed to sunlight.

Chloramphenicol has been used to treat systemic *Salmonella* and *Campylobacter* infections caused by susceptible strains. This compound is associated with bone marrow suppression, both dose related and idiosyncratic. If chloramphenicol is used, judicious monitoring of all hematopoietic cell lines is necessary to limit toxicity. Serum chloramphenicol drug concentrations should be less than 25 mg/L in order to reduce the probability of dose-related bone marrow suppression.

Table 67.6.
Antibiotics of Choice for Bacterial Gastroenteritis

Organism	Indication	Drug(s) of Choice[a]	Alternative Drugs[a]
Salmonella spp.	Disseminated disease or high-risk patient	TMP/SMX, FQ	Amox, Amp, Chloro, TG Ceph
Shigella spp.	GE (dysentery)	TMP/SMX	Amp, Tetra; FQ, Norflox (if resistance likely)
Campylobacter spp.	GE, Bacteremia	Erythro	FQ, Chloro, Doxy, Gent
ETEC	Moderate-severe traveler's diarrhea	TMP/SMX	FQ, Norflox, Doxy
V. cholerae	GE	Tetra	FQ, TMP/SMX, Chloro
Yersinia spp.	Bacteremia	Chloro, Gent	Doxy, TMP/SMX, FQ, TG ceph
Aeromonas spp.[b]	Persistent diarrhea	TMP/SMX	FQ, Norflox, Chloro, Tetra, Gent, TG Ceph
Plesiomonas spp[b]	GE	TMP/SMX	FQ, Chloro, Doxy

[a]TMP, SMX, timethoprim/sulfamethoxazole; FQ, fluoroquinolone (e.g., ciprofloxacin, ofloxacin, etc., except norfloxacin); Amox, amoxicillin; Amp, ampicillin; Chloro, chloramphenicol; TG Ceph, third generation cephalosporin; Tetra, tetracycline hydrochloride; Norflox, norfloxacin; Erythro, erythromycin; Doxy, doxycycline; Gent, gentamicin; Clinda, clindamycin.
[b]Strain-specific susceptibility testing should be used to guide treatment.
Adapted from references 74, 75.

Table 67.7.
Antibiotic Dosing and Monitoring Data

Drug	Dose	Adverse Effects	Monitoring Parameters
Ampicillin	Adult: 500 mg q6h, or 50–100 mg/ kg/day Children: 50–200 mg/kg/day	Rash (3%), diarrhea, nausea (10%) Hypersensitivity, hematologic—less common	Skin changes: (rash onset 4–5 days) GI: assess changes in symptoms despite cure of infection
Trimethoprim/ sulfamethoxazole (TMP/SMX), Cotrimoxazole	Adult: TMP/SMX, 160/800 mg q12h Children > 6 weeks: TMP/SMX, 5/25 mg/kg q12h	Rash (5%), Stevens-Johnson syndrome (rare), bone marrow suppression (anemia, neutropenia), nephrotoxicity; increased incidence of adverse effects in AIDS patients	Skin changes: progressive rash with periorbital or oral blisters may indicate SJS—discontinue drug Hematologic: CBC with differential, platelet count Nephrotoxicity: serum creatinine, urine output
Tetracycline HCl	Adult: 250–500 mg q.i.d. Children > 12 years: 25–30 mg/kg/ day divided q.i.d. (do not give orally with agents or food containing di- or trivalent cations—Fe, Ca, Mg, Al)	Nausea, vomiting, epigastric pain (common): photosensitivity; antianabolic effect aggravates uremia	GI: assess changes in symptoms despite cure of infection Photosensitivity: apply sunscreen
Doxycycline	Adult: 100 mg qd or b.i.d. Children > 12 years: 4–5 mg/kg/day in 2 doses for 1st day, followed by 2–2.5 mg/kg in 2 doses	Dental and bone effects (permanent staining of teeth least likely with doxycycline), hematologic reactions, hepatotoxicity (rare, results in fatty infiltration of the liver)	Hematologic: CBC, platelet count
Erythromycin	Adult: 250–500 mg q.i.d. Children: 30–50 mg/kg/day divided q.i.d.	Nausea, vomiting, abdominal cramping (15–60%), hepatotoxicity (cholestatic jaundice; estolate most, ethyl succinate least), reversible ototoxicity with high IV doses; Inhibitor of cP450 hepatic metabolism of theophylline, cyclosporine, warfarin; increases bioavailability of digoxin	GI: assess changes in symptoms despite cure of infection Hepatic: monitor liver transaminases, total bilirubin Drug interactions: monitor theophylline, cyclosporine, and digoxin levels; monitor INR (or PT) to assess warfarin pharmacodynamics
Chloramphenicol	Adult: 500 mg q.i.d. Children: 25–100 mg/kg/day divided q.i.d.	Nausea, vomiting, diarrhea; aplastic anemia (1 in 500–100,000 patients treated, irreversible), gray syndrome (infants and children), bone marrow suppression (dose related); inhibits metabolism of tolbutamide, phenytoin, dicumarol	GI: assess changes in symptoms despite cure of infection Hematologic: CBC with differential, reticulocyte count Monitor serum levels with dosage adjustment Drug interactions: monitor phenytoin levels
Ciprofloxacin Norfloxacin Ofloxacin	Adult: 500–750 mb b.i.d. 400 mg b.i.d. 200–400 mg b.i.d. Children: not recommended (do not give orally with agents or food containing di- or trivalent cations—Fe, Ca, Mg, Al—may result in inadequate absorption)	Nausea, vomiting, diarrhea (5%), CNS (headache, dizziness, tremors, restlessness—more common with eldery and renally impaired); Drug interactions: may cause elevations in theophylline concentrations	GI: assess changes in symptoms despite cure of infection CNS: evaluate changes in mental status, consider reduced dosage in elderly and renally impaired Drug interactions: monitor theophylline levels

Trimethoprim/sulfamethoxazole (TMP/SMX) remains an important drug in the armamentarium used to treat bacterial GE. It is considered the drug of choice for GE caused by ETEC, *Aeromonas,* and *Plesiomonas* (27, 59). TMP/SMX is also effective in the treatment of *Shigella* and ampicillin-resistant *Salmonella* infections (58). TMP/SMX may cause rash, vomiting, fever, Stevens-Johnson syndrome, hemolytic anemia, and bone marrow suppression. It is less likely than tetracycline to cause photosensitivity

reactions when used in the management of ETEC (traveler's diarrhea). Because the majority of this compound is excreted unchanged by tubular secretion in the kidney, the dose should be reduced in patients with severe renal dysfunction.

Erythromycin is considered the drug of choice for treating infectious GE caused by *C. jejuni,* due to its ability to shorten the duration of organism excretion in stool (60). There are conflicting data with regard to the ability of early antibiotic therapy to shorten the duration of diarrhea (60, 61). The drug is usually given orally, but may need to be given intravenously in cases of disseminated disease. One of the major adverse effects of erythromycin is gastrointestinal intolerance, typically manifested by nausea and abdominal cramping, which can be seen with both the oral and IV routes of administration. Reversible cholestatic jaundice has been seen with erythromycin, primarily with the estolate salt of the drug. Liver transaminases should be monitored in patients receiving all salt forms of this compound if therapy is to be used long-term. Reversible hearing loss and phlebitis may be seen with the IV form of erythromycin as well.

The aminoglycoside compounds can be used in the treatment of systemic *Campylobacter* and *Yersinia* infections or GE caused by EPEC, *Aeromonas*, or *Pseudomonas*. When used in the management of GE, these compounds are administered orally. Although they are not appreciably absorbed from the gastrointestinal tract due to their highly polar nature, caution should be used in patients in whom the integrity of the gastrointestinal lining is known to be compromised. In this setting, absorption may occur, resulting in measurable systemic drug concentrations. The aminoglycosides are known to be nephro- and ototoxic. When used for systemic disease, these agents are given intravenously and dose adjustments based on renal function must be made. Serum drug concentrations and renal function parameters must also be monitored.

Quinolone compounds have become widely accepted as useful agents to eradicate many common organisms causing GE. Nalidixic acid, in a dose of 55 mg/kg/day in 4 divided doses, was the first quinolone used to treat multiply resistant *Shigella*, *Salmonella*, ETEC, and *Campylobacter* infections (62, 63). Other, newer fluoroquinolones, such as ciprofloxacin, norfloxacin, and ofloxacin, have been successfully used in the management of *Shigella*, *Campylobacter*, and systemic *Salmonella* infections (62–66). Fluoroquinolone compounds have also become primary agents in the treatment and prophylaxis of ETEC infections (59, 67, 68). Although fluoroquinolones have been shown to shorten the course of illness with *Salmonella* GE, their use in this setting is not currently recommended due to reports of persistent disease and development of resistance (69, 70). The broad-spectrum activity of the fluoroquinolones against several of the most common pathogens has led some to study their use as empiric agents in the treatment of bacterial GE (69). Although seemingly good candidates for empiric use, fluoroquinolones should not be used in this setting due to serious concern over further spread and development of resistance (63, 69). The common dosages of ciprofloxacin, norfloxacin, and ofloxacin appear to be 500 to 750 mg, 400 mg, and 200 mg, twice daily, respectively. These agents are not approved for use in children because of arthropathy in immature animals. Based on experience

with these compounds in children with cystic fibrosis, these concerns may be overrated and have little clinical significance (71). Further studies are clearly needed to confirm or disprove their safety in children, who could greatly benefit from the use of these agents in the management of infectious GE.

Other agents having activity against enteropathogens, such as *Salmonella*, *Shigella*, *Yersinia*, and *Aeromonas*, include newer oral and IV cephalosporins, amoxicillin-clavulanic acid, aztreonam, and imipenem (16, 27, 72–74).

CONCLUSION

Infectious GE remains a significant cause of morbidity and mortality worldwide. Most cases of GE are viral, are self-limiting in nature, and may be endemic or cause outbreaks related to contaminated water or food. The primary treatment for all types of infectious GE is administration of appropriate oral fluids and electrolytes, and nutritional therapy. For bacterial GE, antibiotic therapy is not often useful or indicated for several reasons-lack of data showing improved outcome, turnaround time of microbiologic procedures (organism identification and susceptibility testing), and concerns over developing organism resistance. Adjunctive therapies, such as antidiarrheal agents, may have benefit in mild cases of viral GE but should be used with caution in bacterial GE. Future interventions will be predominantly prophylactic and include better food and water processing techniques, improved sanitation, and the development of effective vaccines.

REFERENCES

1. Bern C, Martines J, de Zoysa I, et al. The magnitude of the global problem of diarrhoeal diseases: a ten year update. Bull World Health Organ 70:705–714, 1992.
2. Glass RI, Lew JF, Gangarosa RE, et al. Estimates of morbidity and mortality for diarrheal diseases in American children. J Pediatr 118:S27–S33, 1991.
3. Gangarosa RE, Glass RI, Lew JF, et al. Hospitalizations involving gastroenteritis in the United States, 1985: the special burden of the disease among the elderly. Am J Epidemiol 135:281–290, 1992.
4. Lew JF, Glass RI, Gangarosa RE, et al. Diarrheal deaths in the United States 1979 through 1987. JAMA 265:3280–3284, 1991.
5. Mandell GL, Bennett JE, Dolin R. Principles and practice of infectious diseases. New York: John Wiley & Sons, 1995, vol 1, ch 76, 77, 79–81.
6. Kelly CP, Pothoulakis C, LaMont JT. *Clostridium difficile* colitis. N Engl J Med 330:257–262, 1994.
7. Bartlett JG. Antibiotic-associated diarrhea. Clin Infect Dis 15:573–581, 1992.
8. Smith PD, Quinn TC, Strober W, et al. Gastrointestinal infections in AIDS. Ann Intern Med 116:63–77, 1992.
9. Blacklow NR, Greenberg HB. Viral gastroenteritis. N Engl J Med 325:252–264, 1991.
10. Northrup RS, Flanigan TP. Gastroenteritis. Pediatr Rev 15:461–471, 1994.
11. Ho MS, Glass RI, Pinsky PF, et al. Diarrheal deaths in American children; are they preventable? JAMA 260:3281–3285, 1988.

12. Ansari SA, Springthorpe VS, Sattar SA. Survival and vehicular spread of human rotaviruses: possible relation to seasonality of outbreaks. Rev Infect Dis 13:448–461, 1991.

13. Lieberman JM. Rotavirus and other viral causes of gastroenteritis. Pediatr Ann 23:529–535, 1994.

14. Taterke JA, Cuff CJ, Rubi DH. Viral gastrointestinal infections. Gastroenterol Clin North Am 21:303–330, 1992.

15. Grohmann GS, Glass RI, Pereira HG, et al. Enteric viruses and diarrhea in HIV-infected patients. N Engl J Med 329:14–20, 1993.

16. Stutman HR. *Salmonella, Shigella,* and *Campylobacter:* common bacterial causes of infectious diarrhea. Pediatr Ann 23:538–543, 1994.

17. Mishu B, Koehler J, Lee LA, et al. Outbreaks of *S. enteritidis* infections in the United States, 1985–1991. J Infect Dis 169:547–552, 1994.

18. Laney DW, Cohen MB. Approach to the pediatric patient with diarrhea. Gastroenterol Clin North Am 22:499–516, 1993.

19. Buchwald DS, Blaser MJ. A review of human salmonellosis II. duration of excretion following infection with nontyphi *Salmonella.* Rev Infect Dis 6:345–356, 1984.

20. Lee LA, Shapiro CN, Hargrett-Bean N, et al. Hyperendemic shigellosis in the United States: a review of surveillance data for 1967–1988. J Infect Dis 164:894–900, 1991.

21. Altekruse SF, Hunt JM, Tollefson LK, et al. Food and animal sources of human *Campylobacter* infections. JAVMA 1:57–61, 1994.

22. Tarr PI. *Escherichia coli* O157:H7: clinical, diagnostic and epidemiologic aspects of human infection. Clin Infect Dis 20:1–10, 1995.

23. Hyams KC, Bourgeois AL, Merrel BR, et al. Diarrheal disease during Operation Desert Shield. N Engl J Med 325:1423–1428, 1991.

24. Afghani B, Stutman HR. Toxin-related diarrheas. Pediatr Ann 23:549–555, 1994.

25. Bell BP, Goldoft M, Griffin PM, et al. A multistate outbreak of *Escherichia coli* O157:H7-associated bloody diarrhea and hemolytic uremic syndrome from hamburgers: the Washington experience. JAMA 272:1349–1353, 1994.

26. Keene WE, McAnulty JM, Hoebly FC, et al. A swimming-associated outbreak of hemorrhagic colitis caused by *Escherichia coli* O157:H7 and *Shigella sonnei.* N Engl J Med 331:579–584, 1994.

27. San Joaquin VH. *Aeromonas, Yersinia,* and miscellaneous bacterial enteropathogens. Pediatr Ann 23:544–548, 1994.

28. Lee LL, Taylor J, Carter GP, et al. *Yersinia enterocolitica* O:3: an emerging cause of pediatric gastroenteritis in the United States. J Infect Dis 163:660–663, 1991.

29. Lacey SW. Cholera: calamitous past, ominous future. Clin Infect Dis 20:1409–1419, 1995.

30. Holmberg SD. Vibrios and *Aeromonas.* Infect Dis Clin North Am 2:655–676, 1988.

31. Wurtz R. Cyclospora: a newly identified intestinal pathogen of humans. Clin Infect Dis 18:620–623, 1994.

32. Bennet RG, Greenough WB. Approach to acute diarrhea in the elderly. Gastroenterol Clin North Am 22:517–533, 1993.

33. Telzak EE, Greenberg MS, Budnick LD, et al. Diabetes mellitus–a newly diagnosed risk focator for infection from *Salmonella enteritidis.* J Infect Dis 164:538–541, 1991.

34. Guerrant RL, Bobak DA. Bacterial and protozoal gastroenteritis. N Engl J Med 325:327–340, 1991.

35. Guarino A, Canani RB, Russo S, et al. Oral immunoglobulins for treatment of acute rotaviral gastroenteritis. Pediatr 93:12–16, 1994.

36. Dellert SF, Cohen MB. Diarrheal disease: established pathogens, new pathogens, and progress in vaccine development. Gastroenterol Clin North Am 23:637–654, 1994.

37. Levine MM, Noriega F. Vaccines to prevent bacterial enteric infections in children. Pediatr Ann 22:719–725, 1993.

38. Park SI, Giannella RA. Approach to the adult patient with acute diarrhea. Gastroenterol Clin North Am 22:483–497, 1993.

39. O'Loughlin EV, Scott RB, Gall DG. Pathophysiology of infectious diarrhea: changes in intestinal structure and function. J Pediatr Gastroenterol Nutr 12:5–20, 1991.

40. Center for Disease Control and Prevention. The management of acute diarrhea in children: oral rehydration, maintenance and nutritional therapy. MMWR 41:1–20, 1992.

41. Santosham M, Burns B, Nadkarni V, et al. Oral rehydration therapy for acute diarrhea in ambulatory children in the United States: a double blind comparison of four different solutions. Pediatr 76:159–166, 1985.

42. Listernick R, Zieserl E, Davis AT. Outpatient oral rehydration in the United States. Am J Dis Child 140:211–215, 1986.

43. Santosham M, Greenough WB. Oral rehydration therapy: a global perspective. J Pediatr 118:544–551, 1991.

44. Snyder JD. Use and misuse of oral therapy for diarrhea: comparison of U.S. practices with the American Academy of Pediatrics recommendations. Pediatr 87:28–33, 1991.

45. Farthing MJ. History and rationale of oral rehydration and recent developments in formulating an optimal solution. Drugs 36:80–90, 1988.

46. American Academy of Pediatrics Committee on Nutrition. Use of oral fluid therapy and post-treatment feeding following enteritis in children in a developed country. Pediatr 75:358–361, 1985.

47. Khiri-Maung U, Greenough WB. Cereal-based oral rehydration therapy I. clinical studies. J Pediatr 118:572–579, 1991.

48. Anon. Cereal-based oral rehydration solutions–bridging the gap between fluid and food. Lancet 339:219–220, 1992.

49. Brown KH, Gastanaduy AS, Saavedra JM, et al. Effect of continued oral feeding on clinical and nutritional outcomes of acute diarrhea in children. J Pediatr 112:191–200, 1988.

50. Powell DW, Szauter KE. Nonantibiotic therapy and pharmacotherapy of acute infectious diarrhea. Gastroenterol Clin North Am 22:683–707, 1993.

51. Motala C, Hill ID, Mann MD, et al. Effect of loperamide on stool output and duration of acute infectious diarrhea in infants. J Pediatr 117:467–471, 1990.

52. Gorbach SL. Bismuth therapy in gastrointestinal diseases. Gastroenterology 99:863–875, 1990.

53. Okhuysen PC, Ericsson CD. Traveler's diarrhea: prevention and treatment. Med Clin North Am 76:1357–1373, 1992.

54. Murray BE. Resistance of *Shigella, Salmonella,* and other selected enteric pathogens to antimicrobial agents. Rev Infect Dis 8:S172–S181, 1986.

55. Murray BE. Problems and mechanisms of antimicrobial resistance. Infect Dis Clin North Am 3:423–439, 1990.

56. Ashkenazi S, Cleary TG. Antibiotic treatment of bacterial gastroenteritis. Pediatr Infect Dis J 10:140–148, 1991.

57. Nelson JD, Kusmiesz H, Jackson LH, et al. Treatment of *Salmonella gastroenteritis* with ampicillin, amoxicillin or placebo. Pediatr 65:1125–1130, 1980.

58. Grisant KA, Jaffe DM. Dehydration syndromes: oral rehydration and fluid replacement. Emerg Med Clin North Am 9:565–588, 1991.

59. Ericsson CD, Johnson PC, Dupont HL, et al. Ciprofloxacin or trimethoprim/sulfamethoxazole as initial therapy for traveler's diarrhea. Ann Intern Med 106:216–220, 1987.

60. Williams D, Schorling J, Barrett LJ, et al. Early treatment of *Campylobacter jejuni* enteritis. Antimicrob Agents Chemother 37:248–250, 1989.

61. Salazar-Lindo E, Sack B, Chea-Woo E et al. Early treatment with erythromycin of *Campylobacter jejuni*-associated dysentery in children. J Pediatr 109:355–360, 1986.

62. Akalin HE. Quinolones in treatment of acute bacterial diarrhoeal diseases. Drugs 45(suppl 3):114–118, 1993.

63. Dupont HL. Use of quinolones in the treatment of gastrointestinal infections. Eur J Clin Microbiol Infect Dis 10:325–329, 1991.

64. Akalin HE, Firat M, Unal S, et al. Clinical efficacy of single dose or one day treatment with ofloxacin in shigellosis. Rev Infect Dis 11:S1152–1153, 1989.

65. Mandal BK. *Salmonella typhi* and other salmonellas. Gut 35:726–728, 1994.

66. Bennish ML, Salam MA, Khan WA, et al. Treatment of shigellosis II. Comparison of one or two dose ciprofloxacin with standard 5-day therapy. Ann Intern Med 117:727–734, 1992.

67. Wistrom J, Norrby SR. Antibiotic prophylaxis of traveler's diarrhea. Scand J Infect Dis 70: S111–S129, 1990.

68. Ericsson CD, Dupont HL. Traveler's diarrhea: approaches to prevention and treatment. Clin Infect Dis 16:616–626, 1993.

69. Wistrom J, Jertborn M, Ekwall E, et al. Empiric treatment of acute diarrheal disease with norfloxacin. Ann Intern Med 117:202–208, 1992.

70. Howard AJ, Joseph TD, Bloodworth LLD, et al. The emergence of ciprofloxacin resistance in *Salmonella typhimurium*. J Antimicrob Chemother 26:296–298, 1990.

71. Kubin R. Safety and efficacy of ciprofloxacin in pediatric patients. Infection 21:65–73, 1993.

72. Ashkenazi S, Amir J, Waisman Y, et al. A randomized double-blind study comparing cefixime and trimethoprim/sulfamethoxazole in the treatment of childhood shigellosis. J Pediatr 123:817–821, 1993.

73. Cherubin CE, Eng RHK, Smith SM, et al. Cephalosporin therapy for salmonellosis. Questions of efficacy and cross resistance with ampicillin. Arch Intern Med 146:2149–2152, 1986.

74. Mandell GL, Bennett JE, Dolin R. Principles and practice of infectious diseases. New York: John Wiley & Sons, 1995, vol II, ch 192, 194, 201, 205, 208, 214.

75. Gorbach SL, Bartlett JG, Blacklow NR. Infectious diseases. Philadelphia: WB Saunders, 1992, ch 86.

CHAPTER 68

INFECTIVE ENDOCARDITIS

STEVEN L. BARRIERE

Endocarditis is an infection of the inner lining of the heart and the mucosa that underlies it. However, the term refers most commonly to an infection of a heart valve. The heart wall, papillary muscles, and chordae tendineae can be involved in the infection, but the complications and clinical manifestations arise from the involvement of the tricuspid, mitral, or aortic valves (1, 2).

Subacute disease is an indolent infection that may produce signs and symptoms over periods as long as several months before a diagnosis is made. Acute infection is of rapid onset, with fulminant symptoms. Classically, patients with subacute disease have all of the "typical" manifestations of the disease (see below). However, the diagnosis is now suspected in any febrile illness of unclear cause, so progression to chronicity is becoming less common (2, 3).

ANATOMY

As mentioned above the tissues involved in endocarditis are primarily the tricuspid, mitral, and aortic valves; the valve of the pulmonary artery is rarely infected. The tricuspid valve is a common site of infection in intravenous drug users. The mitral and aortic valves are also involved in this group of patients, as well as in patients with underlying valve pathology. Damage to the mitral and aortic valves leads to more severe hemodynamic alterations than tricuspid disease (1, 2).

The sites of the lesions are the atrial surfaces of the mitral and tricuspid valves and the ventricular surface of the aortic valve. Lesions of the chordae, the atrial or ventricular walls, and the pulmonary artery or aorta are considered satellite infections to the primary valvular involvement (1).

There has been a significant trend in recent years toward an increase in the age of patients with endocarditis (2, 3). This is at least partly due to marked decreases in the prevalence of rheumatic heart disease, the longevity of persons in modern society, and increasing numbers of older patients with prosthetic cardiac valves (3). This has also led to a recognition of additional forms of heart disease that predispose to the development of endocarditis (2).

PATHOPHYSIOLOGY

Four factors are necessary in the pathogenesis of the infection: (a) a previously damaged cardiac valve, (b) a platelet-fibrin thrombus, (c) bacteremia, and (d) bacterial adherence (1). In published series of patients with en-

docarditis, the mitral valve is involved in 66 to 86%, the aortic valve in 45 to 55%, the tricuspid valve in 5 to 20%, and the pulmonic valve in only 1% (2, 3). Correlating the pressure gradient across these valves with the relative frequency of infection makes a strong argument for mechanical stress as an important factor in the pathogenesis of endocarditis. Similarly, the hemodynamic alterations that occur across an incompetent valve result in abnormal "jets" of blood that may damage the endocardium and provide a locus for infection. This change in hemodynamics also creates a low-pressure "sink," which sets up an additional site for infection. A bacterial aerosol (bacteremia) flows from the high-pressure source (left ventricle) through the narrowed orifice (incompetent mitral valve) into the low-pressure area (left atrium). The development of vegetations just distal to the orifice has been demonstrated with this model. Vegetations in endocarditis are most commonly found on the low-pressure side of the valve (1, 2).

Once the endothelial surface of the valve is traumatized by the jet effects, collagen is exposed, and a sterile platelet-fibrin thrombus is formed. This is referred to as nonbacterial thrombotic endocarditis (NBTE) (1, 2).

The next critical factor in the pathogenesis of the infection is bacteremia. The microorganism is delivered to the valve surface by the bloodstream. The ability of the organisms to adhere to the valve surface correlates directly with their ability to produce endocarditis (2, 4). This process is complex, but is associated with bacterial dextran and the production and local deposition of other exopolysaccharides, among other factors (2).

ETIOLOGY

Infection due to viridans streptococci has declined over the last 3 decades. Half or more of all cases of endocarditis were due to these organisms 30 years ago. Now approximately one-fourth to one-third are caused by these streptococci (2, 3). Enterococci are the causative pathogens in approximately 10 to 15% of cases, and other streptococci account for an additional 10 to 15% of cases. Staphylococci account for 25 to 35% of all cases and account for the majority of isolates among intravenous drug users (2, 5). Gram-negative bacteria such as *Serratia marcescens* and *Pseudomonas aeruginosa* have been reported to be responsible for as many as 11% of cases (6), again, frequently occurring in habitual intravenous drug users. Nearly 20%

1347

of cases of endocarditis involving prosthetic valves are due to gram-negative bacilli (6). Fungi, particularly *Candida albicans,* are seen in 5% of cases or less (1, 2).

Intravenous drug users develop endocarditis more frequently than the general population, probably because of frequent nonsterile intravenous injections. The bacteriology of endocarditis in this population is composed of staphylococci (50 to 60%), streptococci (15%), and Gram-negative bacilli and fungi (25 to 35%) (6). Anaerobes and other organisms produce only a few cases of disease in this population.

The other group of patients who are at special risk for developing endocarditis are those who have prosthetic cardiac valves. Prosthetic valve endocarditis (PVE) occurring within the first 2 months after surgery (early PVE) is caused by organisms introduced during surgery. The most frequently cultured organisms are staphylococci, especially coagulase-negative staphylococci. Infections occurring beyond 2 months (late PVE) are caused by the same organisms that produce diseases on native valves (i.e., primarily streptococci). Fungi are a major concern in these patients. Endocarditis is especially devastating in patients with prosthetic valves, since fatal complications can occur quickly (7, 8).

BACTEREMIA

Infecting organisms must reach the cardiac tissues by means of the general circulation. Bacteremia and fungemia are the initiating events in the genesis of the actual infection (as noted above).

Viridans streptococci, nonenterococcal group D streptococci, and other facultative organisms are normal flora of the nasopharynx. Enterococci and Gram-negative bacilli usually arise from the urinary or gastrointestinal tracts. Staphylococci are found on the skin and may colonize the nasopharynx. Fungi may arise from the bowel, as can certain Gram-negative and anaerobic organisms. Fungi may also colonize certain areas of skin and thus gain entrance to the circulation via intravenous catheters (1, 2).

Distinguishing the presence of endocarditis in a bacteremic patient may be very difficult. For example, numerous investigations have been carried out attempting to differentiate uncomplicated *S. aureus* bacteremia from endocarditis. In 1976, Nolan and Beaty defined bedside-predictive criteria in 105 retrospectively-analyzed cases of *S. aureus* bacteremia (9). The criteria were (a) nosocomial or community acquisition; (b) presence or absence of an obvious primary focus of infection; and (c) presence or absence of metastatic sequelae of the bacteremia (e.g., kidney or CNS infection or infarct). Community-acquired bacteremia from an inapparent primary focus and with metastatic sequelae characterized patients with *S. aureus* endocarditis (10). It must be noted that this study and others that have confirmed its results had a preponderance of intravenous drug abusers in the patient population. Studies in nonad-

Table 68.1.
Incidence and Types of Bacteremia

Procedure	Incidence of Bacteremia	Organisms
dental extraction	30–80%	streptococci diphtheroids coagulase-negative staphylococci
periodontal surgery	30–90%	as above plus anaerobes
tooth brushing, flossing	0–50%	streptococci, staphylococci
tonsillectomy	30–40%	streptococci
upper GI endoscopy	10%	as for dental procedures
lower GI endoscopy	5–10%	enterococci enteric Gram-negative bacilli
liver biopsy	5–10%	streptococci, staphylococci enteric Gram-negative bacilli
cystoscopy, urethral dilation	20–80%	enteric Gram-negative bacilli enterococci

dict populations have shown disparate results. In contrast, patients with enterococcal or viridans streptococcal bacteremia and other risk factors or compatible clinical findings are highly likely to have endocarditis (2, 4).

Endocarditis has been described following bacteremias arising from such disparate sources as genitourinary infection and the use of an oral irrigation device. In addition, transient bacteremias with the potential for producing endocarditis have been described following tooth extraction, periodontal surgery, liver biopsy, endoscopy or sigmoidoscopy, and manipulations of the genitourinary tract (Table 68.1).

DIAGNOSIS AND CLINICAL FEATURES

The classical signs and symptoms of endocarditis such as Osler's nodes, Janeway lesions, clubbing of the fingers, splinter hemorrhages, and retinal lesions are all seen infrequently in modern clinical medicine (2, 4). The primary reason for this is the high index of suspicion for the disease in a patient with fever of unknown cause, leading to early diagnosis prior to the development of the more chronic findings. The most common signs and symptoms are a heart murmur or a change in a previously noted murmur, fever, embolic episodes, splenomegaly, skin manifestations (primarily petechiae), weakness, dyspnea, sweats, anorexia, weight loss, malaise, and cough (2, 4). These are not present in all cases, but the most crucial criterion for the diagnosis of the disease is positive blood cultures.

The bacteremia of endocarditis is qualitatively continuous, but quantitatively variable. Negative blood cultures may be due to uremia, poor bacteriologic technique, fastidious organisms (e.g., the HACEK group [*Haemophilus* spp., *Actinobacillus actinomycetemcomitans*, *Cardiobacterium hominis*, *Eikenella corrodens*, *Kingella kingii*]), nonbacterial disease (e.g., Q fever, fungi, viruses), or prior antibiotic therapy (11). The number of blood cultures necessary to establish or exclude the diagnosis has been determined to be at least three and perhaps as many as five. In practice, three cultures taken over a 24-hour period in a patient who is not critically ill should produce a very high yield. In acutely ill patients, 2 to 3 samples of blood should be taken rapidly from different sites before starting antibiotic therapy.

Most of the classic signs and symptoms are due to either emboli from the infected endocardium or local vasculitis. Subacute disease is characterized by one or more of the classic signs or symptoms, but acute disease present with hemorrhage, embolus, or metastatic infection (meninges, eye, kidneys) (2).

Echocardiography has become an important tool for the diagnosis of endocarditis (2, 4). Three recent developments have greatly enhanced its value: two-dimensional (2D) echocardiography, the introduction of color-flow doppler technology, and the development of transesophageal imaging. The latter has facilitated higher resolution imaging, by moving the transducer from outside of the chest wall to immediately adjacent to the heart. In contrast to transthoracic echocardiography (TTE), transesophageal echocardiography (TEE) is much more sensitive (>95% detection of vegetations vs. only ca. 75% for TTE) (4). Additionally, smaller vegetations (≤ 10 mm) are readily detected by TEE whereas only 25 to 70% of vegetations this size are found with TTE.

Table 68.2.
Proposed New Criteria for Diagnosis of Infective Endocarditis

Definite infective endocarditis
  Pathologic criteria
    Microorganisms: demonstrated by culture or histology in a vegetation, *or* in a vegetation that has embolized, *or* in an intracardiac abscess, *or*
    Pathologic lesions: vegetation or intracardiac abscess present, confirmed by histology showing active endocarditis.
  Clinical criteria (using specific definitions listed in Table 68.3)
    Two major criteria, *or*
    One major criterion plus three minor criteria, *or*
    Five minor criteria
Possible infective endocarditis: findings consistent with infective endocarditis, that fall short of *Definitive* but not *Rejected.*
Rejected
  Firm alternate diagnosis explaining evidence of infective endocarditis, *or*
  Resolution of endocarditis syndrome wth antibiotic therapy for 4 days or less, *or*
  No pathologic evidence of infective endocarditis at surgery or autopsy, after antibiotic therapy for 4 days or less.

Adapted from reference 12 with permission.

Table 68.3.
Definitions Used in the New Criteria for Infective Endocarditis

Major Criteria
  Positive blood culture for infective endocarditis
    Typical microorganism for infective endocarditis from two separate blood cultures: viridans streptococci, *S. bovis*, HACEK group, *or* community-acquired *S. aureus* or enterococci in the absence of a primary focus; *or*
    Persistently positive blood culture, defined as microorganism consistent with infective endocarditis from:
      Blood cultures drawn more than 12 hours apart, *or*
      All of 3, or a majority of 4 or more separate blood cultures, with first and last drawn at least 1 hour apart.
  Evidence of endocardial involvement
    Positive echocardiogram for infective endocarditis
    Oscillating intracardiac mass on valve or supporting structures or in the path or regurgitant jets, or on iatrogenic devices, in the absence of an alternative anatomic explanation, *or*
    Abscess, *or*
    New partial dehiscence of prosthetic valve, *or*
    New valvular regurgitation (increase or change in preexisting murmur not sufficient)
Minor Criteria
  Predisposition: predisposing heart condition or intravenous drug use
  Fever: ≥ 38.0°C (100.4°F)
  Vascular phenomena: arterial embolism, septic pulmonary infarcts, mycotic aneurysm, intracranial hemorrhage, Janeway lesions
  Immunologic phenomena: glomerulonephritis, Osler's nodes, Roth spots, rheumatoid factor
  Echocardiogram: consistent with infective endocarditis, but not meeting major criterion above
  Microbiologic evidence: positive blood culture, but not meeting major criterion above, or serologic evidence of active infection with organism consistent with infective endocarditis.

Adapted from reference 12 with permission.

The laboratory parameters (other than cultures) used to establish the diagnosis of endocarditis include elevated titers of rheumatoid factor; increased erythrocyte sedimentation rate; normochromic, normocytic anemia; and a decline in renal function with hematuria (2).

Endocarditis in intravenous drug users is frequently heralded by neurologic dysfunction or pulmonary emboli (2, 4, 6). This may misdirect the efforts toward a diagnosis, which again points to the importance of obtaining sufficient blood cultures in the febrile patient with a history of symptoms compatible with endocarditis.

All of the above and a history consistent with risk factors compatible with endocarditis put the disease at the top of the list of possible diagnoses. Risk factors associated with the development of endocarditis include intravenous drug abuse, underlying heart disease, or the presence of an indwelling prosthetic device.

Durack et al. have recently proposed new criteria for the diagnosis of infective endocarditis (Tables 68.2 and 68.3) (12). The new criteria combine the definitions put forth by von Reyn et al. (13) but also acknowledge the important role for newer techniques in echocardiography.

TREATMENT

The cure of infective endocarditis requires the sustained application of antimicrobial agents that are capable of killing the organisms causing the infection (2, 4). Sequestration of the infecting organisms within valvular vegetation protects them from antibodies and macrophages, and in addition, results in slowed microbial metabolism. This slowed replication leads to relative insusceptibility to many antibiotics and requires that the organisms be killed by the antibiotics used (4). This has been proven clinically by the failure of bacteriostatic antibiotics such as the tetracyclines, erythromycin, and chloramphenicol to cure endocarditis. This relative impermeability of antibiotics and slowed microbial replication also require the use of prolonged, high-dose antimicrobial therapy.

The bactericidal or fungicidal activity of the patient's serum during therapy may be assessed in infections caused by more resistant organisms (enterococci, Gram-negative bacilli, fungi, and in some cases, staphylococci) or if treatment with oral antibiotics is to be used after a shortened course of parenteral therapy. Bactericidal activity should be present after no less than 1:8 dilutions of serum (Fig. 68.1) (2). This has been found to correlate with good outcome in the therapy of endocarditis and other infectious diseases. However, it has been demonstrated that peak titers of 1:64 or above and trough titers of 1:32 or more are associated with 100% bacteriologic cure rates (14). Titers of 1:8 were predictive of success 93 and 97.5% of the time, for peak and trough, respectively. However, this study also revealed that the serum bactericidal titer test could not predict either bacteriologic failure or clinical outcome.

Empiric therapy is often instituted before the results of culture and sensitivity tests are known, especially in patients who are acutely ill. The choice of empiric therapy is based on the history, the physical examination, and the course of the disease. For example, an elderly man with evidence of chronic disease and a history of enterococcal urinary tract infections should be treated for enterococcal endocarditis. Likewise, an IV drug user with acute disease should be treated for staphylococcal, enterococcal, and Gram-negative endocarditis until culture results are ob-

tained. Table 68.4 lists drugs of first choice and alternative drugs for the treatment of the most common causes of endocarditis.

Streptococcal Infection

Most streptococci (except enterococci) are usually highly susceptible to penicillin G or ampicillin, and therapy with either of these drugs alone is adequate in nearly all cases (2, 4, 15). Abundant glycocalyx production by viridans streptococci has been associated with delayed antimicrobial sterilization in the rabbit model of endocarditis. Dextranase and other enzymes have also been found to augment the effect of antimicrobials (especially β-lactams) in vitro by decreasing glycocalyx production, but its clinical utility is unknown (2).

Therapy for 2 weeks, rather than the usual 4 weeks, has been evaluated and found to be effective as long as a combination of penicillin and an aminoglycoside is used (15). This shorter regimen is cost-beneficial, but it may be more toxic because of the aminoglycoside. This regimen should not be used in the elderly, patients in shock, those with PVE or extracardiac foci of infection, or those infected with less susceptible streptococci (15). Some nonenterococcal streptococci may also be relatively resistant to penicillin G (minimal inhibitory concentration (MIC) above 0.1 mg/L) and should be treated with penicillin G or ampicillin plus an aminoglycoside (streptomycin or gentamicin) (15) (Table 68.4).

Enterococcal Infection

Group D streptococci include *Enterococcus* spp. and *Streptococcus bovis*. The latter organism is susceptible to penicillin G. Enterococci, however, are only moderately susceptible (MIC = 1 to 2 mg/L), and therapy with a penicillin alone has resulted in a high failure rate. Addition of an aminoglycoside results in synergistic killing of the organism in vitro and produces improved cure rates (15). Penicillinase-resistant penicillins or cephalosporins plus an aminoglycoside, although sometimes shown to provide in vitro killing of enterococci, have not demonstrated this effect in vivo.

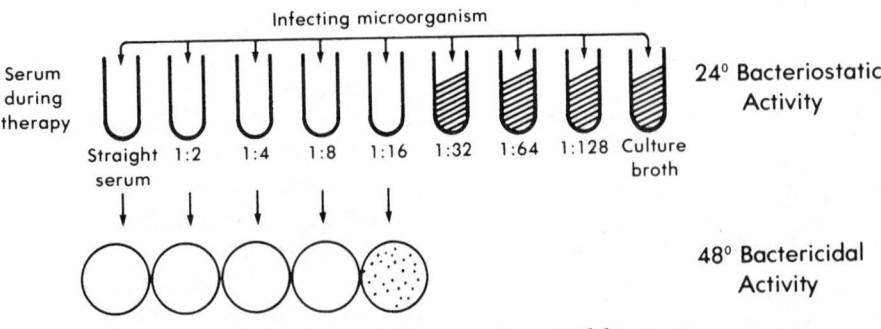

Figure 68.1.   The serum bactericidal test.

Table 68.4.
Antimicrobial Therapy for Endocarditis

Organisms	Regimen(s) of Choice	Daily Dosage	Alternatives	Daily Dosage	Comments
Streptococci (viridans & others) (penicillin MIC < 0.1 mg/L)	Penicillin G *or* Ampicillin	200,000–300,000 U/kg IV 150 mg/kg IV	Cefazolin Vancomycin	75–100 mg/kg IV 20–30 mg/kg IV	Total duration of treatment is 4 weeks. Addition of gentamicin (1 mg/kg Q 8–12 hr) or streptomycin (7.5 mg/kg [up to 500 mg] Q 12 hr) may be used to reduce duration of treatment to 2 weeks in uncomplicated cases. Some clinicians may opt to give an aminoglycoside for the first 2 weeks in all patients with "susceptible" isolates. Caution should be taken in patients who are susceptible to aminoglycoside toxicity.
Streptococci (viridans & others) (penicillin MIC > 0.1 & < 0.5 mg/L)	Penicillin G or Ampicillin *plus* Gentamicin or Streptomycin	Higher doses above As above	As above	As above	Total duration of treatment is 4 weeks. The aminoglycoside should be given for the first 2 weeks.
Enterococci & streptococci with penicillin MIC > 0.5 mg/L	Penicillin G *or* Ampicillin *plus* Gentamicin *or* Streptomycin	400,000 U/kg IV 200 mg/kg IV 2–3 mg/kg IV 15 mg/kg IV (Max: 1 gm)	Vancomycin *plus* Gentamicin *or* Streptomycin	30 mg/kg IV Same Same	Total duration of treatment is 4–6 weeks. Combination therapy is given for the entire duration. Cephalosporins are *not* suitable alternatives to penicillin. Consideration should be given to desensitization of penicillin-allergic patients. Choice of the aminoglycoside depends upon susceptibility testing. Penicillinase-producing enterococci should be treated with ampicillin/sulbactam. Multiply resistant (including vancomycin) enterococci are isolated infrequently but therapy choices are suboptimal (see text).
Staphylococci Methicillin-susceptible	Penicillinase-resistant penicillin *with or without* Gentamicin	150–200 mg/kg IV As above	Cefazolin *with or without* Gentamicin *or* Vancomycin + Rifampin	As above Same 30 mg/kg IV/ 600 mg/d	Duration of treatment is 4 to 6 weeks. The aminoglycoside is sometimes given for the first 3 to 5 days to accelerate clearance of the organism from blood cultures, but caution should be taken in patients at risk for toxicity. Patients with prosthetic valve infection should be treated with gentamicin plus rifampin (900 mg/day) in addition to the primary antimicrobial for the entire duration of treatment.
Methicillin-resistant	Vancomycin	30 mg/kg IV	TMP/ SMX ± Rifampin Ciprofloxacin + Rifampin	10/50 mg/kg/ 600 mg 1500 mg/ 600 mg	
Pseudomonas aeruginosa	Aminoglycoside *plus* Antipseudomonal penicillin *or* Ceftazidime	High dose 300 mg/kg IV 100 mg/kg IV	Imipenem Aztreonam Ciprofloxacin	60 mg/kg IV 100 mg/kg IV 1200 mg IV	Surgery is often necessary. Choice of regimen is dependent upon susceptibility testing and patient tolerance (see text).
Fungi (Candida & others)	Amphotericin B	0.5–1.0 mg/kg IV	Fluconazole Itraconazole	? ?	Little to no experience has been gained with imidazoles in this setting. Surgery is nearly always needed for cure. Addition of flucytosine may be synergistic against some isolates of *Candida*. Rifampin has also been used in combination.

In vitro, over 50% of enterococci are highly resistant to streptomycin (MIC ≥ 2000 mg/L). These organisms are not killed *in vitro* by the penicillin/streptomycin combination (2). Gentamicin is recommended over streptomycin in combination with a penicillin when high-level resistance is found. High-level gentamicin resistance is common now in some isolates of enterococci, and rarely, in viridans streptococci (2, 15, 16). These organisms are not killed by the penicillin/gentamicin combination. In some centers, as many as 60% of *E. faecium* isolates are resistant to high levels of gentamicin (2, 4, 16). Approximately 30 to 50% of these gentamicin-resistant strains are, however, susceptible to streptomycin, and the penicillin/streptomycin combination will be bactericidal (16).

Increasing numbers of enterococci are being found that are resistant to multiple antimicrobials, including all aminoglycosides, penicillins, and glycopeptides (e.g., vancomycin). Treatment options for these situations are limited. In patients with ampicillin-sensitive, multiply aminoglycoside-resistant strains, the traditional penicillin/aminoglycoside combination is unlikely to be effective (16). Therapy with high-dose penicillin G or ampicillin alone for 6 to 8 weeks may be effective, but the supporting data, especially long-term follow-up, are limited (2, 16). Other treatments, reported to be effective in anecdotal cases, include addition of a fluoroquinolone (e.g., ciprofloxacin) to the penicillin or penicillin/aminoglycoside regimen. Experimental models of endocarditis suggest that continuous intravenous infusion of the daily dose of the penicillin is more effective than intermittent bolus administration of the same dose. However, human data are lacking.

Isolates of enterococcus (especially *E. faecium*) are increasingly found to be resistant to penicillins by virtue of the production of β-lactamase or by alteration of penicillin-binding proteins (PBPs). The β-lactamase producing strains are effectively treated with a β-lactam/β-lactamase inhibitor combination (e.g., ampicillin/sulbactam) plus an aminoglycoside (if the isolate is aminoglycoside susceptible). The presence of penicillin resistance mediated by PBP alteration necessitates the use of vancomycin (or teicoplanin where available) in combination with an aminoglycoside. This is suboptimal therapy because the glycopeptides are less rapidly bactericidal than β-lactams (2, 4). However, there are no other proven treatment options available at the present.

Finally, glycopeptide-resistant enterococci, though still uncommon, have also emerged. These organisms are often resistant to all cell wall-active agents and may also be resistant to aminoglycosides. Hence, therapy selection is difficult. In vitro data suggest that exposure of these isolates to low concentrations of vancomycin (10 mg/L) renders the organism hypersusceptible to β-lactams (16). However, experimental studies utilizing such regimens have rendered conflicting data. Anecdotal clinical reports of the effectiveness of minocycline and chloramphenicol have been communicated, but these data are also limited. Trimethoprim-sulfamethoxazole should not be used for enterococcal infection because these organisms are capable of bypassing the folate reductase blockade by utilizing preformed folates (2). Rifampin, in combination with other antimicrobials, produces indifferent or antagonistic effects against enterococci and also should probably be avoided (2). The most reliable management for endocarditis caused by multiply resistant strains of enterococci appears to be surgical replacement of the valve accompanied by the best available medical therapy for prolonged periods (2, 15). Investigational agents with good in-vitro activity against vancomycin-resistant enterococci (e.g., RP59500, a pristinamycin derivative) are currently being tested.

In penicillin-allergic patients with streptococcal endocarditis, vancomycin or a cephalosporin (except in enterococcal infection) are acceptable alternatives (2). However, a cephalosporin should probably not be given to a patient with a history of an IgE-mediated, immediate reaction to penicillin (e.g., anaphylaxis, laryngeal edema).

Staphylococcal Infection

Staphylococcus aureus is nearly always resistant to penicillin G, necessitating the use of a β-lactamase-resistant antibiotic (e.g., isoxazolyl penicillins or cephalosporins).

Staphylococcal endocarditis is best treated with a penicillinase-resistant penicillin (10, 15). Oxacillin and nafcillin appear to be significantly less toxic than methicillin. Ampicillin combined with sulbactam is active in vitro against *S. aureus* and has been used with success in staphylococcal infections other than endocarditis. However, data from experimental endocarditis studies in the animal model have been equivocal.

First-generation cephalosporins such as cefazolin should be as effective as penicillinase-resistant penicillins. Failures reported when cefazolin was used to treat *S. aureus* endocarditis may be due to the relative instability of cefazolin to certain types of staphylococcal β-lactamases (17, 18). Therefore, it must be used with caution in this patient population. Cephalothin is more β-lactamase stable and may be a more suitable alternative. Newer second- and third-generation cephalosporins are less active in vitro against staphylococci, and although they are very β-lactamase stable, should not be used.

Patients with immediate hypersensitivity reactions to β-lactams or who are infected with methicillin-resistant staphylococci should receive vancomycin (10, 15). As noted above, vancomycin is less rapidly bactericidal than β-lactams. Small and co-workers treated four IV drug abusers with vancomycin for *S. aureus* endocarditis (19). Two patients had recurrence of positive blood cultures 2 days after completing a 4-week course of vancomycin. Two other patients were cured only after modification of their regimens because of persisting bacteremia after 7 to 16 days of therapy. Time-kill studies performed with nafcillin and vancomycin for 10 isolates of *S. aureus* showed that vancomycin was less rapidly bactericidal than nafcillin. Several other investigators have documented the suboptimal efficacy of vancomycin in this situation. Based on such data, vancomycin should only be used when absolutely indicated (4, 10, 15).

Another therapeutic attempt to improve in vivo effectiveness of the therapy of *S. aureus* endocarditis has been the addition of gentamicin to a penicillinase-resistant penicillin. This has been effective in an animal model and in scattered case reports. A large multicenter study was performed to assess the benefit of adding gentamicin to nafcillin, compared with nafcillin alone. The results indicated that although the duration of bacteremia was shorter with the combination therapy, the overall cure rate was no different between the two groups (20). However, these patients were predominantly young IV drug users, in whom endocarditis (almost always a tricuspid valve infection) appears to be easier to treat. Shorter course therapy (2 weeks) is also possible in these patients with uncomplicated tricuspid valve infection (21). The mortality rate of this infection in patients over 50 years of age is very high, and these patients should be treated aggressively (10, 21). The addition of an aminoglycoside should be weighed against the potential toxicity in an older patient. Rifampin also has excellent in vitro activity against staphylococci and may also be considered for addition to β-lactam or vancomycin regimens to enhance bactericidal activity (10). There have been studies assessing the efficacy of ciprofloxacin for treating *S. aureus* (particularly methicillin-resistant *S. aureus* [MRSA]) endocarditis. Results have been promising, but rapid emergence of resistance does occur, and the addition of another agent such as rifampin is required (10). Infection due to MRSA, particularly common in IV drug-user populations necessitates the use of vancomycin. Gentamicin may be added for the first 3 to 5 days to hasten clearing of bacteremia. An additional treatment alternative is trimethoprim/sulfamethoxazole with or without rifampin (10). This has also been shown to be effective in the treatment of right-sided endocarditis due to MRSA.

Staphylococcus epidermidis is often resistant to the semisynthetic penicillins. Endocarditis due to these organisms, often found on prosthetic valves, should be treated with a 2- or 3-drug regimen: vancomycin plus an aminoglycoside and, possibly, rifampin (22).

Several studies have evaluated the use of teicoplanin (not commercially available in the United States) for the treatment of Gram-positive endocarditis. Early studies using relatively low doses were disappointing, since several failures occurred (23, 24). It was found that the high serum protein binding of the drug limited the in vivo bactericidal activity (25). Studies with higher doses have been conducted, and in general, have been effective. The drug was reasonably well tolerated.

Other Infections

The treatment of other forms of endocarditis is less well established. Infections due to Gram-negative bacilli, fungi, and anaerobes are extremely difficult to cure with antimicrobial therapy alone and often require surgical intervention to repair the valve or replace the infected valve with a prosthesis. The prime indications for surgery are the development of emboli, impending heart failure, persistent bacteremia, fungal infection, pericarditis, or relapse following "adequate" therapy (26).

Gram-negative bacillary endocarditis should be treated with bactericidal antibiotics to which the infecting organisms are sensitive. Unfortunately, the most common organisms found in this category are not relatively antibiotic-susceptible *E. coli* or *Proteus mirabilis*, but rather *Serratia marcescens* and *Pseudomonas aeruginosa*. Both of these organisms are relatively resistant to most antibiotics, and many isolates are resistant to all available agents except amikacin, the fluoroquinolones, and imipenem.

The empiric treatment of Gram-negative endocarditis should include an aminoglycoside at maximal doses in combination with a β-lactam compound (2, 4). Extended-spectrum cephalosporins (cefotaxime, ceftizoxime, ceftriaxone, etc) and penicillins (piperacillin, mezlocillin), fluoroquinolones, and imipenem may provide bactericidal therapy for endocarditis caused by aerobic Gram-negative bacilli. TMP/SMX is a valuable antimicrobial for the treatment of many extraurinary infections including endocarditis. Bactericidal activity of the patient's serum must be assured, however. Ciprofloxacin has been used to treat Gram-negative endocarditis (27). The major disadvantage is the emergence of resistance, as seen with Gram-positive infections. One solution may be to combine ciprofloxacin with another agent such as a broad-spectrum penicillin or cephalosporin to prevent the emergence of resistance, but these regimens are largely untested in the clinical setting.

Anaerobic Gram-negative organisms such as *Bacteroides fragilis* and related genera present a special problem due to drug resistance (2, 4). Many other anaerobic organisms are highly susceptible to penicillin G. Metronidazole has also been shown to be highly bactericidal in vitro against *B. fragilis*, and isolated reports have shown it to be effective in treating anaerobic infections other than endocarditis. Clindamycin and chloramphenicol are bacteriostatic and should be avoided. Cephamycins (cefoxitin, cefotetan, cefmetazole), imipenem, and β-lactam/β-lactamase inhibitor combinations (e.g., ampicillin/sulbactam, piperacillin/tazobactam, ticarcillin/clavulanate) are also active in vitro against *B. fragilis* and may be considered (2).

Fungal endocarditis is virtually impossible to cure without surgery, and even with optimal therapy, the mortality rate is very high. This is probably due to the invasiveness of the organisms, the large vegetations produced on the valve, the lack of fungicidal activity with available antifungal agents, and the negligible penetration of the antifungal agent into the vegetation (2). The mainstay of therapy is amphotericin B given for a prolonged period. Dosage should be tailored to the patient's tolerance. The addition of 5-flucytosine (5-FC) for the treatment of *Candida* infections should be based on in vitro susceptibility and, perhaps, synergy studies. 5-Flucytosine is hematotoxic, however, which is manifested primarily in the presence of renal failure as a consequence of drug accumulation. The toxicities include agranulocytosis and hepatic necrosis. Fluconazole produces in vitro activity against many fungi, including *Candida albicans, Cryptococcus* spp., and *Histoplasma* spp. (2). There is potential for it to be used in fungal endocarditis but there are no data to support this use.

Coxiella burnetii, the agent of Q fever, can produce endocarditis. The treatment is long-term medical therapy with doxycycline plus either rifampin or a fluoroquinolone (2).

Prosthetic Valve Infection

Prosthetic valve replacement is becoming more widespread because of advances in surgical and life-support techniques. Along with this has come an increase in infections involving these valves (PVE). The mortality rate from this infection has been reported to be as high as 90%, depending on the onset and types of organisms, with an overall mortality figure approaching 70%.

The greatest mortality in PVE is associated with an onset within the first few months after surgery, with Gram-negative bacillary, fungal, or *S. aureus* infections, aortic valve involvement, and the presence of CHF (2, 4). The most common infecting organisms are staphylococci (40 to 60%) and streptococci (30 to 40%). Early PVE (occurring within 2 to 3 months of surgery) is generally caused by organisms implanted at surgery (e.g., staphylococci, fungi, Gram-negative bacilli). Late PVE (>3 months postsurgery) is associated with organisms producing infection on native valves (*S. aureus*, viridans streptococci, and enterococci).

Therapy with antibiotics alone has resulted in a cure rate of approximately 40%, but many patients have required replacement of the infected prosthesis to achieve cures (26). Parenteral antibiotics should be used for a minimum of 6 weeks in endocarditis occurring on natural valves. Early replacement of infected prostheses should be considered in all patients except those with uncomplicated streptococcal or mitral valve PVE (26).

Anticoagulant therapy for the treatment of endocarditis (other than that necessary for the management of a prosthetic valve) is contraindicated due to the risk of hemorrhage. The theoretical benefit of decreasing vegetation size is unfounded in the clinical setting.

COMPLICATIONS

Complications in infective endocarditis are due to the disease, the antibiotics used, or both. The overall mortality for all forms of infective endocarditis is approximately 25 to 30%. However, the mortality ranges from 10 to 15% in penicillin-sensitive streptococcal endocarditis to 90% or more in fungal infection. A poor prognosis is associated with advanced age, serious underlying cardiac or other disease, aortic or mitral valve involvement, infection of a prosthetic valve, presence of emboli, and infection with Gram-negative bacilli or fungi (2).

Patients with subacute disease may develop renal insufficiency. This may be due to one or more of several factors: nephrotoxicity of antimicrobials, metastatic abscess within the kidney from infected emboli (predominantly staphylococcal infection), infarction of the kidney from compromised blood flow caused by aseptic emboli, or immune-complex nephritis caused by deposition of immunoglobulins and complement on the glomerular basement membrane (2).

Involvement of the central nervous system occurs in nearly one-third of all patients with endocarditis. The predominant manifestations are stroke and hemorrhage. Less common are meningitis, toxic encephalopathy, mononeuritis, convulsions, and visual impairment. The visual impairment is usually due to emboli or infarction but may be caused by secondary endophthalmitis, which may rapidly progress to loss of the eye. The most common

Table 68.5.
Cardiac Conditions*

Endocarditis Prophylaxis Recommended
  Prosthetic cardiac valves, including bioprosthetic and homograft valves
  Previous bacterial endocarditis, even in the absence of heart disease
  Most congenital cardiac malformations
  Rheumatic and other acquired valvular dysfunction, even after valvular surgery
  Hypertrophic cardiomyopathy
  Mitral valve prolapse with mitral regurgitation
Endocarditis Prophylaxis Not Recommended
  Isolated secundum atrial septal defect
  Surgical repair without residua beyond 6 months of secundum atrial septal defect, ventricular septal defect, or patent ductus arteriosus
  Previous coronary artery bypass graft surgery
  Mitral valve prolapse without mitral regurgitation†
  Physiologic, functional, or innocent heart murmurs
  Previous Kawasaki disease without valvular dysfunction
  Previous rheumatic fever without valvular dysfunction
  Cardiac pacemakers and implanted defibrillators

*This table is not meant to be all-inclusive.
†Individuals who have a mitral valve prolapse associated with thickening and/or redundancy of the valve leaflets may be at increased risk for bacterial endocarditis, particularly men who are 45 years of age or older.
From JAMA 264:2919–2922, 1990. Copyright 1990, American Medical Association.

Table 68.6.
Dental or Surgical Procedures*

Endocarditis Prophylaxis Recommended

Dental procedures known to induce gingival or mucosal bleeding, including professional cleaning

Tonsillectomy and/or adenoidectomy

Surgical operations that involve intestinal or respiratory mucosa

Bronchoscopy with a rigid bronchoscope

Sclerotherapy for esophageal varices

Esophageal dilation

Gallbladder surgery

Cystoscopy

Urethral dilation

Urethral catheterization if urinary tract infection is present†

Urinary tract surgery if urinary tract infection is present†

Prostatic surgery

Incision and drainage of infected tissue†

Vaginal hysterectomy

Vaginal delivery in the presence of infection†

Endocarditis Prophylaxis Not Recommended‡

Dental procedures not likely to induce gingival bleeding, such as simple adjustment of orthodontic appliances or fillings above the gum line

Injection of local intraoral anesthetic (except intraligamentary injections)

Shedding of primary teeth

Tympanostomy tube insertion

Endotracheal intubation

Bronchoscopy with a flexible bronchoscope, with or without biopsy

Cardiac catheterization

Endoscopy with or without gastrointestinal biopsy

Cesarean section

In the absence of infection: urethral catheterization, dilation and curettage, uncomplicated vaginal delivery, therapeutic abortion, sterilization procedures, or insertion or removal of intrauterine devices

---

*These procedures listed in this table are not meant to be all-inclusive.

†In addition to prophylactic regimen for genitourinary procedures, antibiotic therapy should be directed against the most likely bacterial pathogen.

‡In patients who have prosthetic heart valves, a previous history of endocarditis, or surgically constructed systemic-pulmonary shunts or conduits, physicians may choose to administer prophylactic antibiotics even for low-risk procedures that involve the lower respiratory, genitourinary, or gastrointestinal tracts.

From JAMA 264:2919–2922, 1990. Copyright 1990, American Medical Association.

complications of endocarditis involve the lung (pulmonary emboli) and congestive heart failure from valvular insufficiency (2, 4).

Valve replacement is indicated for many intractable complications of endocarditis. These include severe heart failure, an infecting organism that is resistant to available antimicrobials, and instability of an infected prosthetic valve (26).

PREVENTION OF ENDOCARDITIS

Bacteremia from most sources is usually transient and nearly always inconsequential in the normal individual. However, in the patient with congenital or acquired heart disease or a prosthetic valve, any bacteremia may lead to

endocarditis (28). In assessing the risk of a bacteremia to an individual patient, important considerations include the incidence of bacteremia with a given procedure (Table 68.1), as well as the most likely organisms, the type of cardiac abnormality, and perhaps, the concentration of the bacteria in the bloodstream. In general, Gram-positive cocci infect congenital defects or acquired valvular diseases, while Gram-negative aerobic bacilli and fungi are common pathogens in prosthetic valve infection. It has been estimated that as many as 15% of all cases of endocarditis are related to dental surgical procedures (2). In a recent survey of failures of endocarditis prophylaxis, over 90% of the cases occurred after a dental procedure and 75% were caused by viridans streptococci (28).

General measures to reduce the risk of bacteremia are to avoid manipulation or instrumentation of infected areas, procedures that may traumatize mucous membranes usually colonized with a normal flora (e.g., mouth), and intravenous catheterization with plastic devices. Topical antiseptic agents do not decrease the incidence of bacteremia during dental procedures.

Only indirect evidence from animal studies demonstrates the effect of prophylactic systemic antibiotics in bacteremia-producing procedures. No controlled trials of endocarditis prophylaxis are available, and the recommended regimens are derived from experiments in the rabbit model. In the aforementioned survey, only 12% of patients received prophylactic regimens consistent with the American Heart Association (AHA) recommendations (29). More recent surveys also document low compliance with AHA guidelines. However, the AHA recommends the use of prophylactic antimicrobials prior to, during, and

Table 68.7.
Recommended Standard Prophylactic Regimen for Dental, Oral, or Upper Respiratory Tract Procedures in Patients Who Are at Risk*

Drug	Dosing Regimen
	Standard Regimen†
Amoxicillin	3.0 g orally, 1 hr before procedure, then 1.5 g 6 hr after initial dose.
	Amoxicillin/Penicillin-Allergic Patients
Erythromycin *or*	Erythromycin ethylsuccinate 800 mg, or erythromycin stearate 1.0 g orally 2 hr before procedure; then half the dose 6 hr after the initial dose
Clindamycin	300 mg orally 1 hr before procedure and 150 mg 6 hr after the initial dose

---

*Includes those with prosthetic heart valves and other high-risk patients

†Initial pediatric doses are as follows: amoxicillin 50 mg/kg; erythromycin ethylsuccinate or erythromycin stearate 20 mg/kg; and clindamycin 10 mg/kg. Follow-up doses should be half the initial dose. **Total pediatric dose should not exceed total adult dose.** The following weight ranges may be used for the initial pediatric dose of amoxicillin: < 15 kg: 750 mg; 15 to 30 kg: 1500 mg; and > 30 kg: 3000mg (full adult dose).

From JAMA 264:2919–2922, 1990. Copyright 1990, American Medical Association.

Table 68.8.
Alternate Prophylactic Regimens for Dental, Oral, or Upper Respiratory Tract Procedures in Patients Who Are at Risk

Drug	Dosing Regimen*
Patients Unable to Take Oral Medications	
Ampicillin	Intravenous (IV) or intramuscular administration (IM) of ampicillin 2.0 g, 30 min before procedure; then IV or IM administration for ampicillin 1.0 g or oral administration of amoxicillin 1.5 g 6 hr after the initial dose
Ampicillin/Amoxicillin/Penicillin-Allergic Patients Unable to Take Oral Medication	
Clindamycin	IV administration of 300 mg 30 min before procedure and IV or oral administration of 150 mg 6 hr after the initial dose
Patients Considered High Risk and Not Candidates for Standard Regimen	
Ampicillin, gentamicin and amoxicillin	IV or IM administration of ampicillin 2.0 g plus gentamicin 1.5 mg/kg (not to exceed 80 mg), 30 min before procedure; followed by amoxicillin 1.5 g orally 6 hr after the initial dose; alternatively, the parenteral regimen may be repeated 8 hr after the initial dose
Penicillin-Allergic Patients Considered High Risk	
Vancomycin	IV administration of 1.0 gm over 1 hour, starting 1 hr before procedure; no repeated dose necessary

*Initial pediatric doses: ampicillin 50 mg/kg; clindamycin 10 mg/kg; gentamicin 2.0 mg/kg; and vancomycin 20 mg/kg. Follow-up dose should be half the initial dose. **Total pediatric dose should not exceed total adult dose.**
From JAMA 264:2919–2922, 1990. Copyright 1990, American Medical Association.

Table 68.9.
Regimens for Genitourinary/Gastrointestinal Procedures

Drug	Dosing Regimen*
Standard Regimen	
Ampicillin, gentamicin and amoxicillin	IV or IM administration of ampicillin 2.0 gm plus gentamicin 1.5 mg/kg (not to exceed 80 mg), 30 min before procedure; followed by amoxicillin 1.5 gm orally 6 hr after the initial dose; alternatively, the parenteral regimen may be repeated 8 hr after the initial dose
Ampicillin/Amoxicillin/Penicillin-Allergic Patients	
Vancomycin and gentamicin	IV administration of vancomycin 1.0 gm over 1 hour plus IV or IM administration of gentamicin 1.5 mg/kg (not to exceed 80 mg) 1 hr before the procedure; may be repeated once 8 hr after the initial dose
Alternate Low-Risk Patient Regimen	
Amoxicillin	3.0 gm orally 1 hr before the procedure; then 1.5 gm 6 hr after the initial dose

*Initial pediatric doses: ampicillin 50 mg/kg; amoxicillin 50 mg/kg; gentamicin 2.0 mg/kg; and vancomycin 20 mg/kg. Follow-up dose should be one-half the initial dose. **Total pediatric dose should not exceed total adult dose.**
From JAMA 264:2919–2922, 1990. Copyright 1990, American Medical Association.

after a procedure likely to produce a bacteremia (29). These include all dental procedures likely to induce gingival bleeding, tonsillectomy/adenoidectomy, surgical procedures or biopsy involving respiratory mucosa, bronchoscopy, incision and drainage of infected tissue, and various genitourinary and gastrointestinal procedures. Table 68.5 lists cardiac conditions for which prophylaxis is recommended and those where it is not felt to be necessary (29). Table 68.6 lists dental or surgical procedures where

prophylaxis is or is not recommended. The AHA guidelines for prophylaxis are summarized in Tables 68.7 through 68.9 (29).

CONCLUSION

Endocarditis is a potentially life-threatening infection that requires early recognition and aggressive treatment for successful management. Organisms causing the disease have become progressively more difficult to treat, and combinations of antibiotics are frequently used to achieve synergistic bactericidal effects. Infections due to multiply resistant pathogens such as the enterococcus and coagulase-negative staphylococci are increasing in prevalence. Surgical removal of the infected valve is often necessary to achieve cure in cases of Gram-negative bacillary and fungal infection. Newer antimicrobials such as extended-spectrum cephalosporins, imipenem, and the fluoroquinolones may have a role in replacing aminoglycosides for the treatment of Gram-negative infections. Prevention of infection is best achieved by recognition of patients at risk, identification of clinical situations likely to produce bacteremia, and use of the recommended prophylactic regimens.

REFERENCES

1. Sullam PM, Drake TA. Sande MA. Pathogenesis of endocarditis. Am J Med 78(6B):110–115, 1985.
2. Scheld WM, Sande MA. Endocarditis and intravascular infections. In: Mandell GL, Bennett JE, Dolin R, eds. Principles and practice of infectious diseases, 4th ed. New York: Churchill Livingstone, 1995:740–783.
3. Harris SL. Definitions and demographic characteristics. In: Kaye D, ed. Infective endocarditis. New York: Raven Press, 1992:1.
4. Molavi A. Endocarditis: recognition, management, and prophylaxis. Cardiovasc Clin 23:139–174, 1993.

5. Chambers HF, Korzeniowski OM, Sande MA, et al. *Staphyloccoccus aureus* endocarditis: clinical manifestations in addicts and non-addicts. Medicine 62:170–177, 1983.

6. Levine DP, Crane LR, Zervos MJ. Bacteremia in narcotic addicts at the Detroit Medical Center. II. Infectious endocarditis: a prospective comparative study. Rev Infect Dis 8:374–396, 1986.

7. Karchmer AW, Archer CL, Dismukes WE. *Staphylococcus epidermidis* causing prosthetic valve endocarditis: microbiologic and clinical observations as guides to therapy. Ann Intern Med 98:447–455, 1983.

8. Wilson WR, Danielson GK, Giuliani ER, Ceraci JE. Prosthetic valve endocarditis. Mayo Clin Proc 57:155–160, 1982.

9. Nolan CM, Beaty HM. *Staphylococcus aureus* bacteremia–current clinical patterns. Am J Med 60:495–501, 1976.

10. Mortara LA, Bayer AS. *Staphylococcus aureus* bacteremia and endocarditis–new diagnostic and therapeutic concepts. Infect Dis Clin North Am 7:53–67, 1993.

11. Pazin CJ, Saul S, Thompson SE. Blood culture positivity: suppression by outpatient antibiotic therapy in patients with bacterial endocarditis. Arch Intern Med 142:263, 1982.

12. Durack DT, Lukes AS, Bright DK, et al. New criteria for diagnosis of infective endocarditis. Am J Med 96:200–209, 1994.

13. Von Reyn CF, Levy BS, Arbeit RD, Friedland G, Crumpacker CS. Infective endocarditis: analysis based on strict case definitions. Ann Intern Med 94:505–511, 1981.

14. Weinstein MP, Stratton CW, Ackley A, et al. Multicenter collaborative evaluation of a standardized serum bactericidal test as a prognostic indicator in infective endocarditis. Am J Med 78:262–269, 1985.

15. Bisno AL, Dismukes WE, Durack DT, et al. Antimicrobial treatment of infective endocarditis due to viridans streptococci, enterococci, and staphylococci. JAMA 261:1471–1477, 1989.

16. Eliopoulos GM. Aminoglycoside-resistant enterococcal endocarditis. Infect Dis Clin North Am 7:117–133, 1993.

17. Sabath LD. Reappraisal of the antistaphylococcal activities of first generation (narrow-spectrum) and second-generation (expanded spectrum) cephalosporins. Antimicrob Agents Chemother 33:407–411, 1989.

18. Kernodle DS, Classen DC, Burke JP, Kaiser AB. Failure of cephalosporins to prevent *Staphylococcus aureus* surgical wound infections. JAMA 263:961–966, 1990.

19. Small PM, Chambers HF. Vancomycin for *Staphylococcus aureus* endocarditis in intravenous drug abusers. Antimicrob Agents Chemother 34:1227–1231, 1990.

20. Karchmer AW. Staphyloccocal endocarditis. Laboratory and clinical basis for antibiotic therapy. Am J Med 78(6B):116–127, 1985.

21. Chambers HF. Short-course combination and oral therapies of *Staphylococcus aureus* endocarditis. Infect Dis Clin North Am 7:69–79, 1993.

22. Whitener C, Caputo G, Weitekamp MR, Karchmer AW. Endocarditis due to coagulase-negative staphylococci. Infect Dis Clin North Am 7:81–95, 1993.

23. Hirschel B. Early termination of a prospective, randomized trial comparing teicoplanin and flucloxacillin for treating severe staphylococcal infections. J Infect Dis 155:187–190, 1987.

24. Glucpczynski Y, Lagast H, Van der Auwera P et al. Clinical evaluation of teicoplanin for therapy of severe infections caused by Gram-positive bacteria. Antimicrob Agents Chemother 29:52–71, 1986.

25. Stratton CW, Weeks LS. Effect of human serum on the bactericidal activity of daptomycin and vancomycin against staphylococcal and enterococcal isolates as detemmined by time-kill kinetic studies. Diagn Microbiol Infect Dis 13:245–252, 1990.

26. Alsip SG, Blackstone EH, Kirklin JW, Cobbs CG. Indications for cardiac surgery in patients with active infective endocarditis. Am J Med 78(6B):138–148, 1985.

27. Gudiol F, Cabellos C, Pallares R, Linares J, Ariza J. Intravenous ciprofloxacin therapy in severe infections. Am J Med 87(5A):221–224, 1989.

28. Durack DT. Current issues in prevention of infective endocarditis. Am J Med 78(6B):149–156, 1985.

29. Dajani AS, Bisno AL, Chyung KJ, et al. Prevention of bacterial endocarditis—recommendations by the American Heart Association. JAMA 264:2919–2922, 1990.

CHAPTER 69

CENTRAL NERVOUS SYSTEM INFECTIONS

LISA M. AVERY and CONSTANCE M. PFEIFFER

Central nervous system (CNS) infections are caused by a variety of pathogens, including bacteria, viruses, fungi, and parasites. These infections can occur in the meninges (meningitis) or the brain itself (encephalitis and brain abscesses) or may be associated with indwelling CNS devices (shunt infections). Prompt diagnosis and aggressive treatment are of the utmost importance in managing CNS infections because of the significant morbidity and mortality that can result.

ANATOMY

The central nervous system consists of the brain and the spinal cord. The brain is protected by the skull. Between the skull and the brain are three membranes called the meninges. The outermost membrane, which lines the skull, is the dura mater. The innermost membrane, which is in direct contact with the brain, is the pia mater. The arachnoid lies between the outermost and innermost membranes and is separated from the pia mater by the subarachnoid space.

Cerebrospinal fluid (CSF) flows through the subarachnoid space into the spinal column. CSF is produced at a rate of 0.5 mL/min by the choroid plexus and flows unidirectionally from the lateral ventricles to the third and fourth ventricles and then to the subarachnoid space. This unidirectional flow is important in administering drugs directly into the CSF; therapeutic levels of antibiotic will be achieved below the site of injection but not above it. Drugs can be introduced directly into the CSF by a variety of routes (Figure 69.1). Intraventricular injection is the most invasive, consisting of a subcutaneous reservoir with a catheter that is placed directly into one of the lateral ventricles. In intrathecal administration a needle is inserted into the subarachnoid space. Intracisternal administration is the injection of drug at the base of the skull.

ETIOLOGY

Various factors influence the suspected etiology of meningitis. Age (Table 69.1), underlying risk factors (e.g., a compromised immune system), and seasonal variations can be useful in directing empiric therapy. In adults, three organisms—*Neisseria meningitidis*, *Streptococcus pneumoniae*, and *Haemophilus influenzae*—are most commonly responsible for meningitis. Gram-negative meningitis is extremely rare in adults; however, meningitis due to enteric organisms, most frequently *Escherichia coli*, is common in

neonates. The elderly (usually defined as those older than 50 years of age) are more likely than other adults to develop meningitis due to *Listeria monocytogenes*, although *S. pneumoniae* and *N. meningitidis* are the most common pathogens in this group as well as in adults aged 18 to 50.

Age should not be the only criterion that is used in empiric antibiotic therapy selection. Several other factors should influence the decision-making process. Nosocomial meninigitis or open head trauma increases the index of suspicion for Gram-negative and staphylococcal infections. Patients with indwelling shunts may develop *Staphylococcus epidermidis* meningitis (which is frequently methicillin-resistant). Predisposing factors for the development of certain types of meningitis include alcoholism, asplenia, bacterial pneumonia, sinusitis, head trauma, and immunosuppression. Sickle cell disease increases the likelihood of *S. pneumoniae* meningitis.

Physical examination of the patient can also yield important information as to the likely pathogen. Particular signs and symptoms can implicate one organism over another. Petechial rash is commonly a presenting sign with *N. meningitidis* infection (a macular rash may also occur with *S. pneumoniae* meningitis). Changes in mental status and neurologic abnormalities are more common in *S. pneumoniae* infections. The clinical presentation of meningitis associated with the different pathogens will be discussed in more detail later.

Use of laboratory data, physical signs, age, and past medical history allows swift and effective implementation of appropriate empiric therapy.

PATHOGENESIS

Pathogens infect the meninges through three pathways: hematogenous seeding, direct inoculation (trauma, neurosurgery), or contiguous spread from a parameningeal focus (e.g., sinusitis, dental surgery). Organisms such as *S. pneumoniae* and *H. influenzae* type b are able to cross the mucosal barrier into the CNS because of encapsulation, which makes them resistant to phagocytosis in the bloodstream, and virulence factors that promote mucosal attachment. *N. meningitidis* use pili on their cell surface to attach to and breach the mucosal barrier.

Once pathogens have entered the CNS, a cascade of events occurs. The presence of bacterial cell wall products triggers the production of cytokines, including interleukin-1, tumor necrosis factor, and prostaglandin E2, which

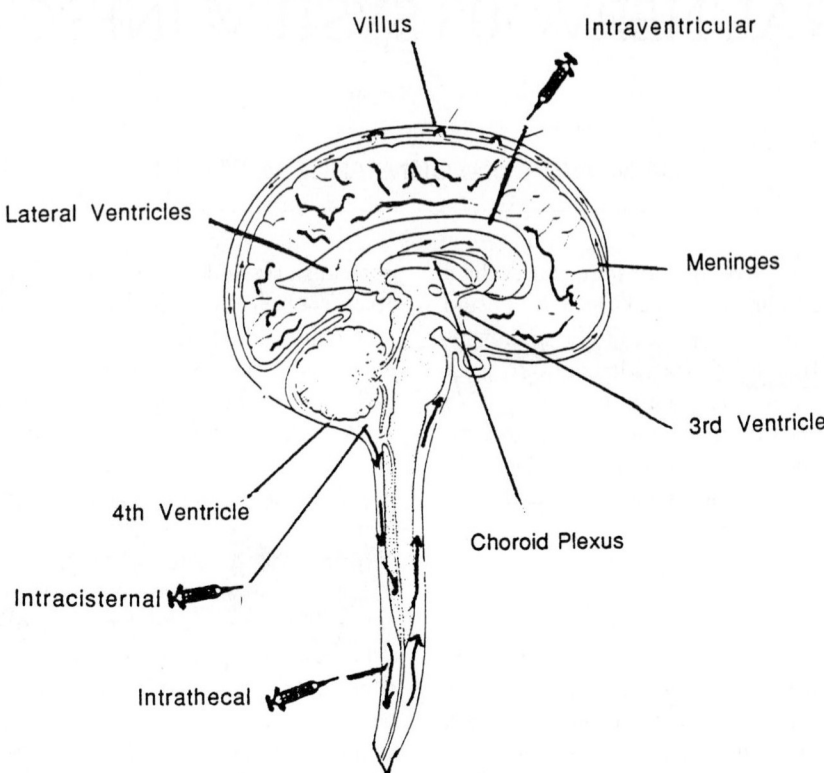

Figure 69.1. Sites of CSF administration.

Table 69.1.
Common Meningitis Pathogens by Age Group

Age Group	Common Pathogens	Empiric Treatment
Neonates	Group B streptococcus	Ampicillin + aminoglycoside
	Listeria monocytogenes	
	Gram-negative bacilli	
Infants (1–3 months)	Group B streptococcus	Ampicillin + cefotaxime or ceftriaxone
	Listeria monocytogenes	
	Gram-negative bacteria	
	Haemophilus influenzae	
3 months to 18 years	*Haemophilus influenzae*	Cefotaxime or ceftriaxone
	Neisseria mengitidis	
	Streptococcus pneumoniae	
18–50 years	*Streptococcus pneumoniae*	Ampicillin or penicillin G
	Neisseria mengitidis	
Elderly (>50 years)	*Streptococcus pneumoniae*	Ampicillin + cefotaxime or ceftriaxone
	Neisseria mengitidis	
	Listeria monocytogenes	
	Gram-negative bacilli	

initially lead to increased blood flow to the brain. These cytokines also increase the permeability of the blood-brain barrier by interfering with the integrity of capillary tight junctions, thus allowing cerebral edema to occur. Cytotoxins released from neutrophils and possibly the bacteria itself also contribute to the development of cerebral edema.

Intracranial pressure rises secondary to increased blood flow and edema, resulting in decreased cerebral perfusion. The inflammatory process can result in vasculitis and thrombotic events that contribute to the overall cerebral ischemia, which may ultimately result in significant neurologic sequelae.

MENINGITIS

Diagnosis

Before instituting antimicrobial therapy for suspected meningitis, it is imperative that a rapid diagnosis be made to ensure prompt, appropriate therapy. A lumbar puncture is used to confirm the diagnosis and identify the pathogen. Before this procedure is performed, a patient is evaluated for papilledema and focal neurologic signs such as hemiparesis, aphasia, ataxia, and visual field defects, which may suggest an extreme increase in intracranial pressure. A computerized tomographic scan or magnetic resonance imaging may be performed to rule out a mass lesion, brain abscess, or subdural empyema. If any of these tests are positive, a lumbar puncture is contraindicated because of the risk of brain herniation. A lumbar puncture will provide important information through measurement of the CSF pressure and the collection of CSF. The opening pressure is increased in meningitis, >200 mm H$_2$O, (normal is <150 mm H$_2$O). Pressures greater than 600 mm H$_2$O may be consistent with intracranial masses. A repeat tap may be performed to confirm the diagnosis or to monitor therapy at a later date.

The CSF is evaluated for turbidity, cytology, glucose, and protein. A normal CSF sample should be colorless and clear. In bacterial meningitis the CSF may be cloudy, but in fungal and viral meningitis the fluid is generally clear. A pleocytosis (increased number of white blood cells) with a predominance of neutrophils is consistent with bacterial meningitis (Table 69.2). A lymphocytic pleocytosis is consistent with fungal, mycobacterial, and viral infections, although viral meningitis may have a neutrophilic predominance on initial presentation. The glucose concentration in normal CSF fluid is 50 to 60% of the serum glucose, 3 to 6.1 mmol/L (70 to 110 mg/dL). For an accurate assessment of CSF glucose a plasma glucose sample should be obtained before the lumbar puncture. This is especially important for diabetic patients whose plasma glucose may be elevated, making the amount of glucose in the CSF appear normal. In bacterial, fungal, and mycobacterial infections the CSF:blood glucose ratio is generally less than 0.5, while in viral

meningitis this ratio is normal. An elevated protein concentration is a sign of disruption of the blood-brain barrier. Normal protein concentrations range between 20 and 40 mg/dL. Although protein elevation is a nonspecific finding, in meningitis it is generally elevated (100 to 500 mg/dL); however, in viral meningitis the concentrations are somewhat lower (50 to 100 mg/dL).

A Gram stain of the CSF provides a tool for rapid diagnosis in bacterial meningitis. A causative organism will be detected in 60 to 80% of untreated patients and 40 to 60% in patients who received prior antibiotic therapy (1). For example, a Gram stain showing Gram-positive diplococci would be consistent with pneumococcus. The diagnostic accuracy of the Gram stain is related to the concentration of the bacteria and the particular microorganism involved. Concentrations greater than 10^5 colony-forming units are associated with a positive Gram stain (1). Acid-fast stain or india ink stain is used if tuberculous or cryptococcal meningitis, respectively, is suspected. CSF cultures are positive in 70 to 80% of cases of bacterial meningitis and can help to direct antibiotic therapy. Blood cultures are positive in 40 to 60% of patients with *Haemophilus influenzae*, meningococcus, and pneumococcal meningitis. Respiratory and urinary tract cultures may also provide useful information. As in other types of infection, the patient may have a peripheral leukocytosis (white blood cell count > 10,000 m^3). Rapid diagnostic tests play a role in identifying the causative organism, especially in patients who were previously on antibiotics, when the Gram stain is negative. In the past, counterimmunoelectrophoresis (CIE) was used to detect bacterial antigens in the CSF. CIE has been replaced with the more sensitive and rapid latex particle agglutination test. These tests detect the polysaccharide antigen of *H. influenzae* type b, *S. pneumoniae*, *N. meningitidis*, *E. coli* K1, and group B *Streptococci* from either CSF, serum, or urine. These specimens are combined with specific antibodies and coated onto latex particles. If the antigen for the given organism is present, the particles will clump together; the results are available in minutes. The Limulus amoebocyte lysate test, prepared from the amebocytes of the horseshoe

Table 69.2.
Cerebral Spinal Fluid Characteristics in Meningitis

Pathogen	Number of Cells (cells/mm^3)	Differential	Glucose (CSF:blood)	Protein (mg/dL)
Normal	<5	Lymphocytes Monocytes	0.5–0.6	20–40
Bacterial	1000–100,000	Neutrophils (PMN)	<0.5	100–500
Fungal	10–1000	Lymphocytic	<0.5	100–500
Mycobacterial	100–400	Lymphocytic	<0.5	100–500
Viral	10–1000	Lymphocytic (PMN early)	0.5–0.6	50–100

crab, detects endotoxin-producing Gram-negative organisms. This test is also not widely used. Polymerase chain reaction techniques are currently being investigated for use in rapid diagnosis of CNS infections.

Clinical Symptoms

Symptoms of meningitis may occur acutely, within 24 hr, or insidiously, over 1 to 7 days. Acute meningitis is associated with a higher fatality rate (50%) and is most commonly caused by bacteria. Subacute meningitis is caused by either viral, mycobacterial, fungal, or bacteria infection and is generally associated with a lower mortality rate (<25%) (2). A patient with either acute or subacute meningitis may present with symptoms of meningeal inflammation such as vomiting, headache, lethargy, confusion, or neck stiffness (nuchal rigidity). Fever, rigors, myalgias, and photophobia are seen as well. Less commonly, patients experience focal symptoms such as seizures, cranial nerve palsies, or hemiparesis. The clinical presentation in neonates and the elderly is more insidious. Neonates and young infants lack the meningeal signs and symptoms but may display hypothermia or hyperthermia, listlessness, lethargy, high-pitched crying, nausea, vomiting, anorexia, poor eating habits, irritability, and seizures. Late clinical manifestations in infants include neck stiffness and full fontanelles. The elderly may present with confusion or possibly a concurrent upper respiratory infection.

On physical examination, patients may have nuchal rigidity, positive Kernig's or Brudzinski's sign, and papilledema. Kernig's sign occurs when the patient is lying in the supine position and the thigh is flexed perpendicular to the abdomen with the knee also in the flexed position. In a patient with meningitis, as the leg is extended, the patient resists leg extension. Brudzinski's sign is evident when neck flexion results in flexion of the hips and knees. A petechial or purpuric rash that occurs predominantly on the extremities is consistent with *N. meningitidis*, although it may also occur with streptococci or *H. influenzae* infections.

Treatment Principles

Several factors relating both to the structure and chemical properties of antimicrobials must be considered in determining the drug of choice. The agent should have a low molecular weight and be less complex in structure to passively diffuse across the blood-brain barrier (BBB). Since only free drug is capable of transversing the BBB, agents that are highly protein-bound are also at a disadvantage. Another property that is associated with the diffusion across the membrane is the lipid solubility of the drug. Since the BBB is a continuous lipid bilayer, the more lipophilic an agent is, the higher is the degree of penetration. The degree of ionization of an antibiotic also plays a

role. Nonionized agents are less polar and therefore more lipid-soluble.

The chemical properties of antibiotics are not the only factors to be considered. The BBB is an integral component of this equation, acting as a regulator of drug concentrations both entering and exiting the CSF. Meningeal inflammation enhances the penetration of antibiotics into the brain tissue (Table 69.3). Although the exact mechanism is unknown, it may be related to the impairment of active transport pumps and the disruption of the tight junctions of the capillaries. The penicillins achieve low concentrations when the meninges are normal; but with inflammation, therapeutic concentrations are achievable. Since the percentage of antibiotic penetration is associated with the degree of inflammation, when inflammation decreases, as occurs with the healing process, the percentage falls. It is important clinically not to decrease the dose of antimicrobial therapy on the basis of a patient's improvement. Steroids have also been related to a decrease in inflammation, a decrease in BBB permeability, and a decrease in CSF concentration. To control the exiting of substances, the CSF has a series of active transport pumps. These stereospecific carriers remove weak organic acids such as penicillin, ampicillin, nafcillin, and cefazolin from the CSF through the choroid plexus, thus removing the antibiotic from the site of action, the subarachnoid space. These "exit pumps" are saturable and may be inhibited by weak organic acids such as probenecid and salicylates.

The pharmacodynamic properties of the antimicrobial must also be considered in selecting an appropriate agent to treat meningitis. Similar to endocarditis and osteomyelitis, the antibiotic that is chosen for treatment of meningitis must be bactericidal. This is an important factor because, compared to the serum, the CSF has

Table 69.3.
Cerebral Spinal Fluid Penetration

Achieve Adequate Concentration in CSF without Inflammation	Achieve Adequate Concentration in CSF with Inflammation	Do Not Achieve Adequate Concentrations
Sulfonamides	Penicillins	Aminoglycosides
Trimethoprim	Imipenem/cilastatin	Clindamycin
Chloramphenicol	Aztreonam	Vancomycin
Isoniazid	Cephalosporins	Polymyxin
Metronidazole	Quinolones	Macrolides
	Ciprofloxacin	
	Ofloxacin	
Quinolones	Rifampin	Tetracycline
Enoxazcin		
Pefloxacin		
Fluconazole		Amphotericin B
Flucytosine		Ketoconazole
Pyrazinamide		Itraconazole

Table 69.4.
Antibiotics Used in Treating CNS Infections

Drug	Dose	Side Effects	Monitor
Penicillins		Leukopenia	CBC[c], Scr[d], BUN[e], LFTs[f]
		Anemia	
Penicillin G	500,000 U/kg/day (3–4 MU q4h)	GI upset	
PCN-ase resistant	>12 g/day	Hepatotoxicity[a]	
		Interstitial nephritis	
Cephalosporins		GI upset	CBC, Scr, BUN
Ceftriaxone	2–4 g/day	Biliary sludging[b]	
Ceftazidime	2–3 g q8h		
Cefotaxime	2 g q4h		
Aminoglycosides	Gentamycin/tobramycin:	Nephrotoxicity	WBC[g], Scr, BUN, audiogram
Gentamicin	IT: 8–10 mg/day	Ototoxicity	
Tobramycin	IV: 2 mg/kg load		
Amikacin	Amikacin:		
	IT: 20–30 mg/day		
	IV: 15 mg/kg load		
Vancomycin	IV: 1 g q12h	Red Man's syndrome	Scr, BUN, audiogram
	Intraventricular: 10 mg/day	Nephrotoxicity	
		Ototoxicity	
		Leukopenia	
Chloramphenicol	IT: 25 mg/kg q6h	Aplastic anemia	CBC with reticulocyte count
	IV: 75–100 mg/kg/day or 4–6 g divided q6h	Thrombocytopenia	
		Leukopenia	
		Gray baby syndrome	
TMP-SMX	10 mg/kg/day divided q8h	GI upset	WBC[h], PLT, K+, BUN, Scr
		Rash	
		Leukopenia	
		Thrombocytopenia	
		Nephrotoxicity	
		Hyperkalemia	
Amphotericin B	IT: 25–300 μg q48–72h (max. 500 μg–1 mg)	Fever	Mg^{++}, K+, BUN, Scr, LFTs, CBC
	IV: 0.5–0.8 mg/kg/day	Chills	
		Nephrotoxicity	
		Hypokalemia	
		Hypomagnesemia	
Fluconazole	400 mg on day 1, then 200 mg/day	GI upset	LFTs, Scr, BUN
		Elevated liver Enzymes	
Flucytosine	150 mg/kg/day divided q6h	Myelosuppression	Scr, BUN, CBC, LFTs
		Anemia	
		Hepatitis	

[a]Oxacillin. [b]Ceftriaxone. [c]CBC complete blood count. [d]Scr serum creatinine. [e]BUN blood urea nitrogen. [f]LPT's liver function tests. [g]WBC white blood cell count. [h]PLT platelets.

decreased complement, phagocytic activity, and immunoglobulins, features that impair the killing of encapsulated bacteria. Agents such as erythromycin, clindamycin, and tetracycline are bacteriostatic and should not be used for treatment of meningitis. They also should not be used together with a bactericidal agent, since this combination may cause antagonism. Concentrations of bactericidal agents must exceed the minimum bactericidal concentration (MBC) of the organism by at least eightfold to tenfold to achieve the maximum rate of bacteria kill (3).

Table 69.4 lists the antibiotics that are used in treating CNS infections.

Streptococcus Pneumoniae

S. pneumoniae, commonly called pneumococcus, is a Gram-positive coccus that is seen on Gram stain in pairs or short chains. It is an encapsulated organism with 85 different serotypes. Most patients with this infection have an acute onset of symptoms and are more likely to experience an alteration in their level of consciousness and/or focal neurologic defects.

Empiric therapy for *S. pneumoniae* in the past included penicillin or ampicillin. Patients who are allergic to penicillin may respond to chloramphenicol or vancomycin. Although penicillin has been the first-line agent, there has been an increase in the rates of pneumococcal resistance to penicillin therapy. The first reports of resistant pneumococci occurred in the late 1970s. Now resistance rates in the United States are as high as 12 to 15% in some areas (4). Risk factors for the development of resistance include frequent antibiotic use and the use of prophylactic antibiotics to prevent chronic infections, such as otitis media (5). This resistance is caused by an alteration in affinity for penicillin-binding proteins and could be manifested as either intermediate resistance (minimum inhibitory concentration (MIC) between 0.1 and 1.0 µg/mL) or high-level resistance (MIC > 1.0). High-dose penicillin therapy results in a CSF concentration from 0.1 to 1.0 µg/mL, which is below the MIC for all organisms with high-level resistance and is not recommended as first-line therapy (6, 7). Empiric therapy for a patient with proven or suspected pneumococcal meningitis in an area with high rates of penicillin-resistant organisms should be vancomycin until sensitivity results are available. Organisms that are resistant to penicillin are also resistant to chloramphenicol and tetracycline in 83% of cases (8). Imipenem/cilastin has been reported to be effective in treating both intermediate and resistant strains but may increase the risk of seizures (9). Treatment of intermediate strains includes either high-dose penicillin (500,000 units/kg/day) or the third-generation cephalosporins. Ceftriaxone or cefotaxime achieves high CSF concentrations; however, there have been increasing numbers of case reports of cephalosporin-resistant isolates. If the MIC is greater than 1.0 µg/mL for ceftriaxone or cefotaxime, these agents may not be adequate therapy (10). Vancomycin, the drug of choice for high-level penicillin resistance, is sometimes used in combination with either rifampin or chloramphenicol (4, 11). The duration of therapy is 10 days.

To prevent pneumococcal infection, a 23-valent polysaccharide vaccine (Pneumovax R) has been available since 1983. Because 90% of all pneumococcal isolates are covered, the vaccine should be highly recommended to patients who meet the criteria for immunization. Proper vaccination will decrease the incidence of infections from this pathogen, including resistance strains. This vaccine is recommended for immunocompetent adults who are more than 65 years old and individuals with chronic illnesses such as cardiovascular or pulmonary disease, diabetes mellitus, alcoholism, cirrhosis, or CSF leaks. Immunocompromised adults or children with asplenia, splenic dysfunction, Hodgkin's disease, lymphoma, multiple myeloma, chronic renal failure, or nephrotic syndrome should also be vaccinated, as should adults caring for children with HIV infection (12). The vaccine is not recommended for children younger than 2 years of age, since they mount a poor immunologic response to the vaccine. The usual dose of the current vaccine is given as a one-time dose of 0.5 mL (25 µg of each polysaccharide antigen) either subcutaneously or intramuscularly. Side effects consist of local reactions at the injection site, low-grade fever, weakness, myalgia, and rash, although the incidence is low. Chemoprophylaxis is recommended for children with functional or anatomic asplenia. Prophylaxis with penicillin G or V may be given at a dose of 125 mg orally twice a day for children less than 5 years of age and 250 mg orally twice a day for children aged 5 or older (12).

Neisseria Meningitidis

N. meningitidis is a Gram-negative organism and the second most common cause of bacterial meningitis in the United States, with a fatality rate of approximately 10% despite antibiotic therapy (12). The incidence of endemic meningococcal disease increases in the late winter and early spring. Children 6 to 12 months of age, military recruits, asplenic patients, and patients with C3 and C5–9 complement deficiencies have increased incidence of meningococcal disease. Asymptomatic colonization of the upper respiratory tract is common, and transmission from person to person occurs through inhalation of droplets of respiratory secretions. Close contacts of *N. meningitidis*–infected patients are at increased risk for development of disease.

Neisseria meningitidis has multiple serogroups that are known to cause invasive disease. Serogroup B accounts for the majority (>50%) of *N. meningitidis* meningitis cases, followed by serogroup C (approximately 25%) and serogroup W-135 (15%). Serogroups A and Y account for most of the remaining cases in the United States (14). Although serogroup A is an infrequent cause of endemic disease in the United States, it is the most common cause of epidemic disease elsewhere in the world (12).

Clinical features of *N. meningitidis* infection include rapid onset of meningococcemia with fever, chills, malaise, and a rash. The rash may be maculopapular, petechial, or urticarial. In fulminant disease the rash may become purpural and is associated with a syndrome of disseminated intravascular coagulation, shock, coma, and death (Waterhouse-Friderichsen syndrome). This may occur within a few hours of presentation despite adequate antibiotic therapy. Other signs of meningococcal meningitis are common to infection with other pathogens.

The drug of choice for the treatment of meningococcal meningitis is intravenous penicillin G 3 to 4 million units every 4 hr for 7 days (13, 15–17). Cefotaxime or ceftriaxone is used as a second-line agent for patients who are allergic to penicillin. Chloramphenicol may be used for patients with allergy to both penicillin and cephalosporins. Penicillin does not eradicate *N. meningitidis* from the nasopharynx. Patients must be treated with rifampin 10 mg/kg (maximum 600 mg) orally every 12 hr for 2 days to avoid a carrier state (16). Respiratory isolation should be instituted for 24 hr after therapy initiation to avoid airborne transmission.

Household, child care center, and nursery school contacts should be given antibiotic prophylaxis as soon as possible after discovery of exposure to the primary case. Prophylaxis of medical care workers is not recommended unless exposure to respiratory secretions (through mouth-to-mouth resuscitation, intubation, or suctioning) occurs before antibiotics have been administered. The drug of choice for prophylaxis is rifampin, administered in the same dosing regimen as is used for nasopharynx eradication (12, 13). A 4-day regimen of 20 mg/kg/day (maximum 600 mg) is also effective (13). Ceftriaxone (250 mg for adults, 125 mg for children under 12 years of age) given as a single intramuscular dose has been proven to be more effective than rifampin in eradicating serogroup A *N. meningitidis*; however, efficacy has not been confirmed for other strains (18). Sulfisoxazole and ciprofloxacin have also been used with some success (13).

A quadrivalent meningococcal vaccine is commercially available. The vaccine is active against serogroups A, C, Y, and W-135. Unfortunately, no vaccine is available with activity against serogroup B, the most frequent cause of meningococcal infection. The vaccine is given as a single 0.5-mL dose and consists of 50 μg of each of the purified bacterial capsular polysaccharides. Routine vaccination of children is not recommended, since infants are the highest risk group and generally exhibit a poor response to all but the serogroup A component (13, 19). Vaccination should be considered for children more than 2 years of age in high-risk groups, including functional or anatomically asplenic patients and those with terminal complement component deficiency. The vaccine may be considered an adjunct to antibiotic prophylaxis and may be useful in containing outbreaks of meningococcal disease due to the represented serogroups. Military recruits are routinely vaccinated, owing to the frequency of serogroup C infection in this population (13).

Haemophilus Influenzae **Type b**

H. influenzae type b is an encapsulated Gram-negative pleomorphic coccobacillus. Approximately 30 to 50% of children carry *Haemophilus* spp. asymptomatically in the nasopharynx, generally as the nonvirulent, nonencapsulated species. These nonencapsulated strains are the common cause of otitis media, sinusitis, or bronchitis. Up to 80% of adults are carriers (3). Colonization by the type b conjugate is infrequent, ranging from 2% to 5%. Children younger than 2 years of age are at the highest risk of developing infection from this organism, along with adults who have predisposing factors such as sickle cell disease, asplenia, immunodeficiency status, malignancy, head trauma, neurosurgery, sinusitis, otitis media, or CSF leak. Alaskan Eskimos and Apache and Navajo Indians are also at increased risk because of genetic factors. Commonly, patients present after an upper respiratory infection or

otitis media. Complications of *H. influenzae* meningitis include deafness, blindness, seizure disorders, behavior disorders, and a deterioration in school performance.

The previous empiric therapy for this pathogen was ampicillin. Because of the increase in frequency of plasmid-mediated β-lactamase production up to 12 to 40%, chloramphenicol was added to ampicillin therapy. Since the development of broad-spectrum cephalosporins such as ceftriaxone and cefotaxime, these agents have become first-line empiric therapy. They also have excellent in vitro activity against the most commonly encountered meningeal pathogens, they have few serious adverse reactions, and they have been shown to rapidly sterilize CSF cultures. Unlike chloramphenicol, the third-generation cephalosporins do not require monitoring of serum drug concentrations; do not affect the metabolism of other agents via cytochrome p450 such as phenytoin, rifampin, carbamazepine, and phenobarbital; and do not cause bone marrow suppression. Ceftazidime was also used in the treatment of bacterial meningitis, but clinical studies showed an increase in hearing loss of children who were treated with ceftazidime, possibly because of a delayed sterilization of CSF fluid (20). Duration of therapy is 7 to 10 days in uncomplicated cases.

Chemoprophylaxis is recommended to stop contact spread, as with meningococcus. Rifampin is used because it eradicates nasopharyngeal carriage of *H. influenzae* type b (21). Minocycline is an alternative, although its CNS side effects discourage its use. Rifampin prophylaxis is recommended for all household contacts, children and adults, if there is one unvaccinated contact younger than 4 years of age. In households with a fully vaccinated, immunocompromised child, all members should receive rifampin prophylaxis because of the possibility of inadequate immune response to the vaccine. Since most secondary cases occur within the first week after the patient has been hospitalized, prophylactic therapy should be administered promptly. Some benefit may be gained from therapy instituted up to 7 days after the index case. If the family does require prophylaxis for one of the above reasons, the index patient should also receive rifampin prophylaxis before being discharged from the hospital (21).

The recommendations are not fully defined for patients from a day care center or nursery school. Rifampin is indicated if one case of *H. influenzae* meningitis occurs at a day care facility that is attended by unvaccinated children younger than 2 years of age whose contact time is greater 25 hr/week. Unvaccinated children should receive a dose of conjugate vaccine and then complete the vaccination series. If the children are older than 2 years of age, there is no need for rifampin. If two or more cases of invasive disease occur within 60 days, then all children and supervisory personnel should promptly receive rifampin therapy. Rifampin 20 mg/kg (maximum 600 mg) should be given orally for 4 days. Formal dosing guidelines are not available for children younger than 1 month of age, but some experts recommend 10 mg/kg (maximum 600 mg) daily for 4 days (21). If the child cannot swallow the capsules, rifampin powder may be mixed in applesauce before administration, or a 1% suspension in simple syrup can be compounded. Side effects include GI disturbances, headache, drowsiness, dizziness, and elevated liver enzymes. The use of rifampin is contraindicated for pregnant women.

Since the development of the vaccine, the incidence of *H. influenzae* type b meningitis has declined by more than 90% (22). *Haemophilus influenzae* type b (Hib) conjugate vaccine contains antigenic capsular polysaccharide ribosyl-ribitol phosphate (PRP). It is coupled to carrier proteins such as diphtheria toxoid (PRP-D), *Neisseria meningitidis* protein (PRP-OMP), tetanus toxoid (PRP-T), or diphtheria CRM197 (mutant) protein (HbOC). Current recommendations are three doses of either HbOC or PRP-T given at 2, 4, and 6 months or two doses of PRP-OMP given at 2 and 4 months. PRP-D is not recommended for children younger than 12 months of age. Booster doses of any of the four conjugate vaccines are given at 12 to 15 months of age. The vaccine does not affect nasopharyngeal carriage.

Listeria Monocytogenes

L. monocytogenes is a Gram-positive aerobic bacillus that may be mistaken for diphtheroids that are part of the normal skin flora. Pregnant women, newborns, elderly people, and immunocompromised individuals are predisposed to listeria infections. The incidence of listeria is greatest in the summer and early fall. Contaminated cole slaw, milk, and cheeses have been the source of outbreaks; patients present with food poisoning (2). Antibiotics with activity against listeria include penicillin G, ampicillin, erythromycin, sulfamethoxazole/trimethoprim, chloramphenicol, rifampin, tetracyclines, and aminoglycosides; but only sulfamethoxazole/trimethoprim and aminoglycosides are bactericidal.

In bacterial meningitis, when listeria is a suspected pathogen, empiric therapy should consist of a third-generation cephalosporin combined with ampicillin. The addition of ampicillin is necessary because cephalosporins have no activity against this organism. The treatment of choice for documented listeria includes ampicillin in combination with an aminoglycoside administered either intravenously and or intrathecally. The aminoglycoside is added because of its documented in vitro synergy (23, 24). Trimethoprim/sulfamethoxazole is an alternative therapy for patients with penicillin allergy.

Gram-Negative Bacterial Meningitis

Gram-negative organisms are a relatively infrequent cause of meningitis. Patients who are more likely to develop Gram-negative meningitis include the elderly, neonates, the immunocompromised, and patients with a history of recent trauma or neurosurgery. Enterobacteriaceae (especially *Escherichia coli* and *Klebsiella* spp.) and *Pseudomonas* spp. are the most frequently implicated Gram-negative pathogens. Gram-negative meningitis in the elderly patient generally has a poor prognosis and involves a protracted clinical course.

Before the introduction of drugs such as ceftazidime and cefotaxime, aminoglycoside therapy with or without chloramphenicol resulted in mortality rates of 40 to 90% (25). While aminoglycosides cover a wide range of Gram-negative pathogens, they do not penetrate into the CSF in adequate amounts. Therefore, when these antibiotics are used, they must be delivered directly into the CSF by intrathecal administration. Preservative-free formulations of gentamicin or amikacin are used in doses of 8 mg/day and 20 to 30 mg/day, respectively (16). However, even with intrathecal administration, therapeutic aminoglycoside levels are not obtained in the ventricles. Ventriculitis is frequently associated with Gram-negative meningitis and may require intraventricular aminoglycoside administration through a reservoir.

Treatment of Gram-negative bacterial meningitis was revolutionized by the advent of third-generation cephalosporins, which result in cure rates of 78 to 94% (15, 26). The greatest experience in Gram-negative infections is with cefotaxime; this is currently the empiric drug of choice for the treatment of Gram-negative bacterial meningitis (17, 27, 28). The usual dosage of cefotaxime is 2 g every 4 hr. Trimethoprim/sulfamethoxazole is occasionally used when β-lactam antibiotics cannot be tolerated; however, recurrences with this regimen are common.

If *Pseudomonas* is implicated, ceftazidime 2 to 3 g every 8 hr plus intrathecal and systemic aminoglycoside therapy may be used empirically (17). Once sensitivity to ceftazidime has been established, the aminoglycoside can be discontinued. Imipenem/cilastatin should be reserved for treatment of nosocomial meningitis due to multiple-resistant Gram-negative organisms only, owing to its propensity to induce seizures (29). Treatment of Gram-negative bacterial meningitis should be guided by in vitro susceptibility patterns once a final identification of the organism is made, and therapy should be continued for 14 days after cultures become negative.

Use of Corticosteroids in Meningitis

The use of corticosteroids as adjunctive therapy in meningitis is controversial. The pathogenesis of meningitis, as reviewed earlier, consists of the release of cytokines that cause brain edema, increased intracranial pressure, and enhanced BBB permeability. Steroids inhibit the synthesis of these cytokines, thus blocking the cascade of events. CSF inflammation has been shown to normalize more rapidly with steroid therapy. More important, the addition of dexamethasone to cephalosporin therapy has resulted in a reduction of neurologic sequelae, especially hearing loss, in children. The results of a metaanalysis of three studies using ceftriaxone and dexamethasone showed a relative risk of developing persistent neurologic and/or audiologic sequelae for children who are treated with ceftriaxone and placebo to be 2.29 (95% CI : 1.20–4.39) (30). The majority of cases in these clinical trials were due to *H. influenzae*. Currently, the Infectious Diseases Committee of the American Academy of Pediatrics advocates the use of dexamethasone for the adjunctive treatment of meningitis caused by *H. influenzae* (21).

There are also arguments against the use of steroids. The data does not currently provide firm evidence on the use of these agents in treating *S. pneumoniae* and *N. meningitidis* infections. Steroids may reduce the penetration of antibiotics into the CSF. A rabbit model of meningitis showed a decrease in CSF concentrations and a delay in CSF sterilization when either ceftriaxone or vancomycin was combined with dexamethasone. This may be detrimental when the MIC of the pathogen is increased and the achievable concentration at the site of infection is decreased. Side effects of steroids are also a concern. There has been an increase in reports of secondary fevers and an increased risk of gastrointestinal bleeding with the short-term steroid regimen.

The exact timing of the steroid dose has also been investigated. Since antimicrobial therapy can cause an increase in the release of endotoxin, which stimulates cytokine production, the administration of the steroid prior to the initial antibiotic dose is recommended. The usual dose is 0.15 mg/kg intravenously every 6 hr for 4 days (31). In an effort to decrease potential side effects, a 2-day regimen of 0.4 mg/kg intravenously every 12 hr has shown equal efficacy (32).

Fungal Meningitis

The two most common causes of fungal meningitis are *Cryptococcus neoformans* and *Coccidioides immitis*. Bird droppings, rotten fruits and vegetables, wood rot, and soil contain *C. neoformans*. Infection occurs through inhalation of the aerosolized spores, which results in primary pulmonary disease that disseminates to the CNS. The onset of disease is gradual, over days to weeks, and is most prevalent in immunosuppressed individuals. Patients most commonly experience headache along with alteration in mental status, nuchal rigidity, fever, and papilledema. Diagnosis is made by india ink stain, culture, and latex agglutination test, which identifies the circulating capsular antigen, in serum of CSF. With these three methods the diagnosis can be made in 98 to 99% of cases (33).

The preferred treatment regimen in non-HIV-infected individuals is the combination of intravenous amphotericin

B 0.5 to 0.8 mg/kg/day and oral flucytosine 100 to 150 mg/kg/day for 6 weeks. A total of 1 to 2 g of amphotericin B should be administered. Amphotericin B is not a benign agent. It may cause nephrotoxicity, electrolyte abnormalities, infusion-related toxicities, anemia, thrombocytopenia, and phlebitis. Not only is amphotericin B fairly toxic, it also achieves low CSF concentrations. Flucytosine (5-FC) is associated with bone marrow suppression, nausea and vomiting, and liver abnormalities. Fluconazole is a synthetic triazole-derivative antifungal agent that achieves good CSF concentration, is available as an oral agent, and is better tolerated than amphotericin B is. Studies have shown efficacy with fluconazole as primary therapy for HIV-infected patients who present with good prognostic signs (34, 35). The usual dose is 400 mg on day 1, then 200 to 400 mg/day thereafter for 10 to 12 weeks. There is a high rate of relapse, so chronic suppressive therapy is often given. Maintenance therapy may consist of either amphotericin B 1.0 mg/kg/week or oral fluconazole 200 mg daily.

Coccidioidomycosis is caused by *C. immitis*. This fungus is present in the soil of the southwestern United States, Mexico, and Central America. Hyphal segment fragments release arthroconidia, the infectious particles, which are aerosolized and inhaled. Once the fungus has been inhaled, it disseminates within 3 to 6 months to the skin, musculoskeletal system, and meninges. In tissues the spherules develop and form endospores. People who are at increased risk of CNS infection include immunocompromised individuals, infants, the elderly, noncaucasians (incidence is highest in Blacks, Filipinos, and Asians), males, and pregnant women. Headache is the most common symptom of fungal meningitis. Symptoms of meningeal irritation are usually absent. Approximately 90% of patients die within 12 months without active treatment (36). Amphotericin B either intrathecally, intracisternally, and/or intravenously is used. The azoles also have activity against coccidioidomycosis. Comparative trials with the azoles and amphotericin B are not available, but because of the advantages of azoles, fluconazole, itraconazole, and ketoconazole may be used. As in treating cryptococcal meningitis, maintenance therapy is required, since the relapse rate is high.

Viral Meningitis

In aseptic meningitis, meningeal signs and symptoms are present, as are CSF abnormalities consistent with meningitis, but Gram stain and cultures are negative for bacteria or fungi. The most common causes of aseptic meningitis are viruses, particularly enterovirus, herpes, lymphocytic choriomeningitis, and mumps. Drugs have also been implemented in aseptic meningitis; these are listed in Table 69.5.

Enteroviruses are members of the picornavirus family and consist of poliovirus, coxsackie A and B virus, and

Table 69.5.
Drug-Related Causes of Aseptic Meningitis Syndrome

Ibuprofen
Trimethoprim/sulfamethoxazole
Sulindac
Naproxen
Tolmentin
Diclofenac
OKT3 (muromonab)
Carbamazepine
Immune globulin
Phenazopyridine
Vaccines: mumps and rubella

echovirus. These agents are the most common cause of aseptic meningitis. Transmission of these viruses occurs via fecal-oral and respiratory routes. Infants, children, and adults younger than 40 years of age are at risk for development of enteroviral infections. Symptoms are either gradual or abrupt and are similar to those of bacterial meningitis. Focal neurologic symptoms are uncommon. An increased incidence of infections is usually seen in the late summer and early fall in temperate climates. Enteroviral infections are self-limited. Patients are given supportive care, including hydration and pain control.

ENCEPHALITIS

Etiolgy

Encephalitis is a direct infection of the brain parenchyma. Viruses are by far the most common pathogen associated with encephalitis, although fungi, rickettsiae, and protozoans have also been implicated. Because of the relative frequency of viral encephalitis, it will be the main focus of the discussion here. Viruses that are associated with encephalitis include arboviruses, varicella zoster, herpes simplex, measles, mumps, cytomegalovirus, HIV, and rabies (37).

Pathogenesis

The virus enters the CNS by hematogenous spread. The organism may enter the bloodstream through the respiratory or GI tract or may be introduced through an insect or animal bite. Viral replication occurs at the site of entry, followed by spilling into the systemic circulation and, finally, infection of distant sites, including the CNS. In the CNS, cell dysfunction due to viral invasion and inflammatory changes are similar to those seen in meningitis.

Clinical Symptoms

Clinical manifestations include a prodrome for several days that may consist of myalgia, fever, malaise, rash, or mild upper respiratory symptoms. Following the prodromal period, headache, drowsiness, change in mental status, and meningismus signify the development of encephalitis. As the infection progresses, drowsiness and confusion increase and may eventually lead to coma. Seizures are common, and focal signs associated with the area of the brain where the infection is concentrated may appear. Intracranial pressure may also be elevated.

Diagnosis

The symptoms of viral encephalitis mimic those of a large range of other disease states, including bacterial meningitis, fungal or protozoan encephalitis, brain abscess, neoplasm, and drug overdose. These etiologies should be ruled out quickly. A peripheral blood smear should be examined for parasites, and blood cultures should be obtained promptly. Increased intracranial pressure should be ruled out before lumbar puncture is performed. Computed tomography, electroencephalogram, or magnetic resonance imaging should be performed to identify any focal lesions, masses, or cerebral edema. Focal infarctions in the temporal lobes may be indicative of herpes simplex infection. The CSF exhibits leukocytosis, usually predominately lymphocytes, although PMNs may be present in early stages. Red cells may be present if a necrotizing component is present, as is seen in herpes simplex encephalitis. In addition, glucose concentration is normal, the protein level is elevated, and organisms are often not found on Gram stain.

Symptoms are also generally nonspecific for the different viruses; however, several organisms (e.g., herpes simplex, rabies) demonstrate tropism for certain areas of the brain. The resulting focal signs can increase the index of suspicion for a particular pathogen. Because of the commonality of symptoms of encephalitis, patient history can be an important consideration in determining the probable causative pathogen. Signs of infection outside the CNS may be helpful in diagnosing cases of encephalitis secondary to varicella, measles, mumps, and herpes simplex. Cytomegalovirus encephalitis is generally seen in infants and immunocompromised individuals, including organ transplant patients and patients with AIDS. Travel history, season, or evidence or a history of an insect or animal bite may also provide clues to pathogen identity. Japanese encephalitis is the most common arbovirus infection worldwide and is endemic in Japan, southeast Asia, China, India, and the Philippines. Eastern equine encephalitis occurs along the Atlantic and Gulf coasts of the United States and occurs mainly in summer and autumn. Evidence of a dog, cat, or raccoon bite increases suspicion for rabies infection, especially in endemic areas. Brain biopsy has been used when herpes simplex virus is suspected; however, there is no guarantee that the area biopsied contains virus, so the yield can be quite low. Despite efforts to determine the causative organism, no identification is made in approximately one-third of cases.

Treatment Principles

Treatment of viral encephalitis is, with the exception of herpes simplex virus, primarily symptomatic. Anticonvulsants are used to control seizure activity; adequate nutrition, hydration, and oxygen are provided as needed; and cerebral edema is treated with intubation and hyperventilation, diuretics, or corticosteroids. The use of dexamethasone in these patients is controversial because of the theoretical inhibition of interferon synthesis, which may impair host defense mechanisms against the virus (37).

Herpes simplex virus should be treated with intravenous acyclovir 10 mg/kg over 1 hr every 8 hr for 10 days. Rapid institution of acyclovir treatment has been shown to decrease mortality to 30% (38).

BRAIN ABSCESS

Pathogenesis

Approximately 1 in 10,000 hospital admissions are due to brain abscesses. A brain abscess is a potentially life-threatening infection that is precipitated by a focal suppurative process within the brain parenchyma. Contiguous infection, hematogenous dissemination, or direct trauma may be the cause. Paranasal sinus, middle ear, mastoid, and dental infections result in contiguous spread either by direct extension or through vascular channels. The result is generally a single abscess. Multiple metastatic abscesses are caused by hematogenous spread from pulmonary infections, osteomyelitis, dental abscess, endocarditis, and skin pustules. Children with cyanotic congenital cardiac anomalies, such as tetralogy of Fallot, are also at increased risk for development of brain lesions by hematogenous spread. Bone fragments and debris caused by neurosurgery and cranial trauma may serve as a nidus of infection. Approximately 25% of cases do not have an identifiable focus.

Brain abscesses are the result of either bacteria, fungi, or parasitic infections that seed an area of necrosis in the brain. The pathology of brain abscess formation can be divided into four stages (39). Stage 1 is an early cerebritis that occurs on days 1 to 3. Days 4 to 9 mark the beginning of stage 2 or the late cerebritis phase. Fibroblasts produce the reticulin network that is the framework for the collagen capsule. At this stage there is maximal edema. On days 10 through 13 the capsule becomes more developed around the necrotic center. This stage is termed the early encapsulation stage. The capsule serves as a protective structure, since it controls the spread of infection and limits the destruction of brain parenchyma. Encapsulation is completed in stage 4, the late capsule stage.

Etiology

The identification of the causative organism can be aided by considering the cause of the infection (Table 69.6). *Staphylococcus aureus* is present in 10 to 15% of cases,

Table 69.6.
Brain Abscess: Common Pathogens by Risk Factor

Cause	Pathogens	Recommended Therapy
Sinusitis	*Streptococci, Staphylococci,* Anaerobes, *H. influenzae*	Third generation cephalosporin and metronidazole
Otitis media/ mastoiditis	*Streptococci, Bacteroides,* Gram-negatives	Third-generation cephalosporin and metronidazole
Dental infections	*Fusobacterium, Bacteroides, Streptococci*	Penicillin and metronidazole
Cranial trauma and neurosurgery	*S. aureus, Streptococci*	Nafcillin or vancomycin (MRSA)

most commonly after trauma or surgery. Frontal lobe abscesses are caused by concurrent sinusitis with *S. aureus*, aerobic and anaerobic streptococci, and *Haemophilus influenzae*. Temporal lobe or cerebellar abscesses are the result of otitis media. Causative organisms include *Streptococci, Bacteroides fragilis*, and Gram-negative bacilli. Dental infections may result in frontal lobe abscess caused by mouth flora, such as *Fusobacteria* spp., *Bacteroides* spp., and streptococci. Children with right-to-left shunts are more prone to develop anaerobic, streptococcal (including *S. viridans*), and *Haemophilus* infections. Infants and neonates develop brain abscess caused by the Gram-negative organisms *Proteus* spp. and *Citrobacter* spp. Immunocompromised patients are at an increased risk of fungal abscesses caused by *Candida, Aspergillus, Cryptococcus neoformans, Blastomyces* spp., *Histoplasma* spp., *Mucor*, and *Rhizopus*. *Listeria monocytogenes* and *Nocardia asteroides* also cause infections in immunocompromised individuals. *Toxoplasma gondii* causes brain abscess in patients with AIDS.

Clinical Symptoms

Brain abscess occurs more commonly in males (2:1) within the first two decades of life. The clinical symptoms of patients with brain abscesses are nonspecific and depend on the size, location, and number of lesions; the virulence of the organism; the host response; and the severity of the cerebral edema that accompanies the abscess. Patients may have either abrupt symptoms or insidious onset over weeks. Most patients develop a constant progressive headache that is not relieved by analgesics. Nausea and vomiting occur as a sign of increasing intracranial pressures. Patients may have a low-grade fever, (<101.5°F), focal neurologic deficits, and change in mentation. The spectrum of consciousness can range from mild confusion to a coma. There is a worse prognosis associated with an obtunded or comatose individual. In a study of 45 consecutive cases the most common symptoms were headache (72%), fever (42%), seizure (35%), nausea, vomiting (35%), and confusion (26%) (40). Symptoms may also provide clues to the area of the brain that is infected. Parietal lobe abscesses are associated with the development of hemiparesis; ataxia and nystagmus may be caused by a cerebellar lesion. Symptoms in infants include vomiting, irritability, seizures, poor feeding, enlarging head circumference, and a bulging fontanelle.

Diagnosis

Unlike meningitis, diagnosis of brain abscesses does not depend on CSF findings. Lumbar punctures are contraindicated, since the diagnostic usefulness is poor and the risks are high. Blood and urine cultures are also rarely helpful. The peripheral white blood cell count may be mildly elevated (>15,000/mm^3), as may the erythrocyte sedimentation rate (45 to 50 mm/hr). Computed tomography (CT) scans and magnetic resonance imaging aid in making the early diagnosis and monitoring therapy. The sensitivity of these procedures exceeds 95%, and they are useful to confirm the exact location of the lesion. To identify the causative organism, aspiration of the abscess should be performed. This sample is then stained and cultured for potential pathogens, including both aerobic and anaerobic organisms.

Treatment Principles

Once the diagnosis has been confirmed, antibiotic therapy alone or combined with surgery is the cornerstone of treatment. Surgical procedures include excision or aspiration of the purulent material. These procedures not only remove the purulent material, but also decrease the mass effect and intracranial pressure. Controversy exists as to whether antibiotics alone can cure an abscess.

Antibiotics that are used for the treatment of brain abscesses must be bactericidal and able to achieve high tissue concentrations in the brain. This does not always correlate with CSF concentrations. Antibiotics such as chloramphenicol, metronidazole, penicillin, nafcillin, vancomycin, trimethoprim/sulfamethoxazole, and third-generation cephalosporins achieve therapeutic concentrations. Another consideration in choosing appropriate therapy is that the agents should not be inactivated by either the acid environment or purulent material present in the abscess. Agents such as aminoglycosides are inactivated by acid and penicillin G, whereas chloramphenicol may be inactivated by the purulent milieu. Appropriate empiric therapy is included in Table 69.4. The duration of therapy ranges from 4 to 8 weeks but depends on the patient's response. Corticosteroids have been used as adjuvant therapy, although no significant benefit has been observed in survival. Steroids reduce cerebral edema and mass effect but also reduce the host defense mechanism along with decreasing antibiotic concentrations. This may cause a delay in killing of the organism. Generally, steroids are recommended only for patients who have a significant mass effect that is responsible for the observed neurologic deficit.

Long-term neurologic sequelae may result from brain abscesses. These include seizures, cognitive dysfunction, and focal neurologic deficits. Mortality associated with brain abscesses ranged from 40 to 60% in the preantibiotic era (41, 42). Now with availability of the CT scan, diagnosis is made earlier, and mortality rates range from 0 to 24% (43). Recurrence ranges from 5 to 10% and occurs within 6 weeks of treatment. This may be due to inadequate antibiotic therapy, an incorrect antibiotic regimen, failure to aspirate a large abscess, presence of a foreign body, or failure to eradicate the underlying source of infection.

SHUNT INFECTIONS

Pathogenesis

Hydrocephalus is an abnormal increase in the amount of cerebrospinal fluid that results in enlargement of the ventricles, which can result in brain atrophy. To relieve this pressure, ventriculoperitoneal (VP) and ventricular atrial (VA) shunts are placed. A VP shunt relieves pressure by draining CSF into the peritoneal cavity; VA shunts drain into the right atrium. The shunts are composed of a proximal ventricular catheter, a one-way valve or subcutaneous reservoir, and a distal catheter inserted into the peritoneum or right atrium (44). Since the CSF shunts interfere with the normal host defenses, they are associated with infections (45). Infection rates are between 2 and 40% (46). Bacteria are introduced either retrograde from the distal end of the shunt, through wound or skin infections, by hematogenous spread, or most commonly by colonization at the time of surgery.

Organisms that make up the skin flora are the most common pathogens in shunt-related infections. *Staphylococcus epidermidis* produces a "slime layer" that is composed of an exopolysaccharide substance that not only increases its adherence to the foreign body, but also decreases the activity of various antibiotics. Second to *S. epidermidis*, *S. aureus* is also isolated in the majority of cases. Gram-negative organisms, such as *E. coli*, *Klebsiella* spp., *Proteus* spp., and *Pseudomonas* spp. may cause infections. *H. influenza*, *S. pneumoniae*, *N. meningitidis*, and fungal infections occur less frequently.

Clinical Symptoms and Diagnosis

The symptoms of shunt infections are nonspecific. The most common problems are symptoms related to the malfunctioning of the shunt, such as headache, nausea, lethargy, and changes in mental status. Patients may have fever higher than 100°F. If a VP shunt is in place, abdominal symptoms may be present, but if a VA device is inserted, it may result in chronic bacteremia and septic pulmonary emboli. Diagnosis is made on the basis of blood cultures, CSF Gram stain, and cultures taken directly from the reservoir. The CSF sample will have increased protein and neutrophils, but the glucose concentration may be normal.

Treatment

Effective treatment consists of antibiotics, removal of the shunt either by externalization of the distal ends of the catheter or by complete removal. Antibiotics can be given intraventricularly through the reservoir and/or intravenously. Treatment of *S. epidermidis* and methicillin-resistant *Staphylococcus aureus* includes vancomycin 2 g/day with the addition of rifampin 10 to 20 mg/kg/day. Vancomycin can also be given intraventricularly at a dose of 10 mg/day for adults. The goal is to maintain both serum and CSF vancomycin trough concentrations between 10 and 20 µg/mL. Elevated vancomycin concentrations may cause neurotoxicity; therefore CSF levels are helpful to maintain therapy within the therapeutic range (45). An alternative therapy would be trimethoprim/sulfamethoxazole 10 to 20 mg/kg/day with or without rifampin (44). Methicillin-sensitive *S. aureus* is treated with penicillinase-resistant penicillins such as nafcillin and oxacillin at doses greater than 12 g/day. Gram-negative organisms other than *Pseudomonas* sp. respond to treatment with either ceftriaxone or cefotaxime. Intravenous ceftazidime 2 g every 8 hr, with the addition of an aminoglycoside in some cases, is used for treatment of *Pseudomonas aeruginosa*.

CONCLUSION

Central nervous system infections are serious, potentially life-threatening events that require aggressive and rapid antibiotic therapy. Prompt administration of antibiotics may not only improve survival, but also decrease long-term neurologic sequelae. The choice of appropriate antibiotic therapy is guided not only by the spectrum of activity, but also by the ability to penetrate the CNS. Adjunctive steroid administration is of proven benefit in *H. influenzae* meningitis; however, its usefulness in other types of meningitis is unclear.

REFERENCES

1. Greenlee JE. Approach to diagnosis of meningitis, cerebrospinal fluid evaluation. Infect Dis Clin North Am 4(4):583–99, 1990.
2. Wispelwey B, Tunkel AR, Scheld WM. Bacterial meningitis in adults. Infect Dis Clin North Am 4(4): 645–59, 1990.
3. Mandell GL, Bennett J, Dolin R. Principles and practice of infectious diseases. 4th ed. New York: Churchill Livingstone, 1995:Chap. 64.
4. John CC. Treatment failure with use of third generation cephalosporin for penicillin-resistant pneumococcal meningitis: case report and review. Clin Infect Dis 18:188–93, 1994.
5. Breiman RF, Butler JC, Tenover FC, Elliott JA, Facklam RR. Emergence of drug-resistant pneumococcal infections in the United States. JAMA 271:1831–35, 1994.
6. Hieber JP, Nelson JD. A pharmacological evaluation of penicillin in children with purulent meningitis. N Engl J Med 297:410–13, 1977.
7. Ramirez JA, Raff MJ. Penicillin-resistant *Streptococcus pneumoniae*: clinical implications for therapy. Infect Med 10:9, 1993.
8. Pallares R, Gudiol F, Linares J, Ariza J, Rufi G, Murgui L, Dorca J, Viladrich PF. Risk factors and response to antibiotic therapy in adults with bacteremic pneumonia caused by penicillin-resistant pneumonococci. N Engl J Med 317:18–22, 1987.
9. Aseni F, Otero MC, Perez-Tamarit D, Rodriguez-Escribano I, Cabedo JL, Gresa S, Canton E. Risk/benefit in the treatment of children with imipenem-cilastin for meningitis caused by penicillin-resistant pneumococcus. J Chemotherapy 5(2):133–34, 1933.
10. Friedland IR, Shelton S, Paris, M, Rinderknecht S., Ehrett S., Krisher K, McCracken GH. Dilemmas in diagnosis and management of cephalosporin-resistant *Streptococcus pneumoniae* meningitis. Pediatr Infect Dis J 12:196–200, 1993.
11. Sloas MM, Barrett FF, Chesney PJ, English BK, Hill BC, Tenover FC, Leggiadro RJ. Cephalosporin treatment failure in penicillin- and cephalosporin-resistant *Streptococcus pneumoniae* meningitis. Pediatr Infect Dis J 11:662–66, 1992.
12. Lieberman JM, Greenberg DP, Ward JI. Prevention of bacterial meningitis, vaccines and chemoprophylaxis. Infect Dis Clin North Am 4(4):703–729, 1990.
13. Committee on Infectious Diseases, American Academy of Pediatrics, Meningoccal Infections. In: Peter G, ed. 1994 Redbook: report of the Committee on Infectious Diseases. 23rd ed. Evanston, IL: American Academy of Pediatrics, 1994:323–27.
14. Band JD, Chamberland ME, Platt T, et al. Trends in meningococcal disease in the United States, 1975–1980. J Infect Dis 148:754–58, 1983.
15. Tunkel AR, Wispelwey B, Scheld WM. Bacterial meningitis: recent advances in pathophysiology and treatment. Ann Intern Med 112:610–23, 1990.
16. Luby JP. Southwestern Internal Medicine Conference: Infections in the central nervous system. Am J Med Sci 304:379–91, 1992.
17. Kaplan SL. New aspects of prevention and therapy of meningitis. Infect Dis Clin North Am 6:197–213, 1992.
18. Schwartz B, Al-Ruwais A, A'Ashi J, et al. Comparative efficacy of ceftriaxone and rifampin in eradicating pharyngeal carriage of group A *Neisseria meningitidis*. Lancet i:1239–42, 1988.
19. Goldschneider I, Lepow ML, Gotschlich EG, et al. Immunogenicity of group a and group c meningococcal polysaccharides in human infants. J Infect Dis 128:769–72, 1973.
20. Schaad UB, Suter S., Gianella-Borradori A., Pfenninger J, Auckenthaler R., Bernath O, Chelseaux JJ, Wedgwood J. A comparison of ceftriaxone and cefuroxime for the treatment of bacterial meningitis in children. N Engl J Med 322(3):141–47, 1990.
21. Committee on Infectious Diseases, American Academy of Pediatrics, Haemophilus influenza infections. In: Peter G, ed. 1994 Redbook: report of the Committee on Infectious Diseases. 23rd ed. Evanston, IL: American Academy of Pediatrics, 1994:203–216.
22. Adams WG, Deaver KA, Cochi Sl et al. Decline of childhood *Haemophilus influenzae* type b (Hib) disease in the Hib vaccine era. JAMA 269:221–26, 1993.
23. Trautmann M, Wagner J, Chahin M, Weinke T. *Listeria meningitis*: report of ten recent cases and review of current therapeutic recommendations. J Infect 10:107–14, 1985.
24. Hansen PB, Jensen TH, Lykkegaard S, Kristensen HS. *Listeria monocytogenes* meningitis in adults: sixteen consecutive cases, 1973–1982. Scand J Infect Dis 19:55–60, 1987.
25. Cherubin CE, Marr JS, Sierra MF, Becker S. Listeria and gram negative bacillary meningitis in New York City, 1972–1979. Am J Med 71:199–209, 1981.

26. Cherubin CE, Corrado ML, Nair SR, Gombert ME, Landesman SH, Humbert G. Treatment of gram negative bacillary meningitis: role of new cephalosporin antibiotics. Rev Infect Dis 4(Suppl):S453–64, 1982.

27. Jacobs RF. Cefotaxime treatment of gram negative enteric meningitis in infants and children. Drugs 35(Suppl 2):185–89, 1988.

28. Kaplan SL, Patrick CC. Cefotaxime and aminoglycoside treatment of meningitis caused by gram-negative enteric organisms. Pediatr Infect Dis J 9:810–14, 1990.

29. Calandra GB, Brown KR, Grad LC, et al. The efficacy results and safety profile of imipenem/cilastatin from the clinical research trials. J Clin Pharmacol 28:120–27, 1988.

30. Schaad UB, Kaplan SL, McCracken GH. Steroid therapy for bacterial meningitis. Clin Infect Dis 20:685–90, 1995.

31. Lebel MH, Frey BJ, Syrogrannopoulos GA. Dexamethasone therapy for bacterial meningitis: results of two double-blind, placebo controlled trials. N Engl J Med 319:964–71, 1988.

32. Syrogiannopoulos GA, Lorida AN, Theodoridou MC, Pappas IG, Babilis GC, Economidis JJ, Zoumboulakis DJ, Berotis NG, Matsoniotis NS. Dexamethosone Therapy for Bacterial Meningitis in Children 2 verses 4 day regimen. J Infect Dis 169:853–8, 1994.

33. Medoff G., Kobayashi GS. Systemic fungal infections: an overview. Hosp Pract 2:41–52, 1991.

34. Saag MS, Powderly WG, Cloud GA, et al. Comparison of amphotericin B with fluconazole in the treatment of acute AIDS-associated cryptococcal meningitis. N Engl J Med 326:83–9, 1992.

35. Nightingale SD. Initial therapy for acquired immunodeficiency syndrome–associated cryptococcosis with fluconazole. Arch Intern Med 155:538–40, 1995.

36. Stevens DA. Coccidioidomycosis. N Engl J Med 332(16):1077–82, 1995.

37. Anderson M. Management of cerebral infection. J Neurol Neurosurg Psychiatry 56:1243–58, 1993.

38. Whitley RJ, Alford CA, Hirsch MS, et al. Vidarabine versus acyclovir therapy of herpes simplex encephalitis. N Engl J Med 314:144–49, 1986.

39. Britt RH, Enzmann DR. Clinical stages of human brain abscesses on serial CT scans after contrast infusion: computerized tomographic, neuropathological and clinical correlations. J Neurosurg 59:972–89, 1983.

40. Chun CH, Johnson JD, Hofstetter M, Raff MJ. Brain abscess: a study of 45 consecutive cases. Medicine 65(6):415–31, 1986.

41. Garfield J. Management of supratentorial intracranial abscess: a review of 200 cases. Br Med J 2:7, 1969.

42. Bellar AJ, Sahar A, Praiss I. Brain abscess: review of 89 cases over 30 years. J Neurol Neurosurg Psychiatry 36:757, 1973.

43. Small M. Dale BAB. Intracranial suppuration, 1969–1982: a 15 year review. Clin Otolaryngol 9:315, 1984.

44. Gorbach Sl, Bartlett JG, Blacklow NR. Infectious diseases. 9th ed. Philadelphia: WB Saunders, 1992:Chap. 169, 172, 174.

45. Luer MS, Halton J. Vancomycin administration into the cerebrospinal fluid: a review. Ann Pharmacother 27:912–21, 1993.

46. Kaufmann BA, Tunkel AR, Pryor JC, Dacey RG. Meningitis in the neurosurgical patient. Infect Dis Clin North Am 4:677–701, 1990.

CHAPTER 70

BONE AND JOINT INFECTIONS

MARTIN L. JOB and HEWITT W. MATTHEWS

Osteomyelitis and septic arthritis are the principal infections of the bones and joints. They involve separate infectious entities with specific etiologies, pathogenesis, and treatment. Both of these infections require prompt and accurate diagnosis to prevent serious tissue destruction and permanent bone damage and deformity. In contrast to other arthritic diseases, proper diagnosis and treatment can usually result in a cure. The discussion in this chapter is limited to infections of bacterial origin.

OSTEOMYELITIS

The term "osteomyelitis" is most commonly associated with bacterial infections of the bone, although other causative organisms such as viruses and fungi have also been isolated. Despite the advent of modern antimicrobial therapy, enhanced imaging methods, and newer orthopedic techniques, osteomyelitis continues to pose a diagnostic and therapeutic challenge. Furthermore, more aggressive procedures such as hip replacement, bone grafting, other reconstructive surgeries, and radiation therapy, as well as intravenous drug abuse, have contributed to the complexity of this disease. Controversy still remains regarding the appropriate antibiotic treatment and its duration.

Classification and Epidemiology

The classification of osteomyelitis depends on the source of bacterial spread to the bone. Other variables such as precipitating factors and the patient's age usually dictate which bones are involved. Osteomyelitis is usually divided into three principal categories: hematogenous, contiguous, and contiguous with vascular insufficiency (Table 70.1). These can be acute or chronic, depending on the onset of symptoms and the duration of the clinical manifestations.

Hematogenous osteomyelitis refers to infections whose source of contamination is the bloodstream. The disease is commonly seen in children and young adults below the age of 20 but has been reported with increasing frequency in adults over 50 years of age. Hematogenous osteomyelitis accounts for approximately 20% of the cases of all bone infections (1, 2). Hematogenous spread of infection of the bone frequently involves a bacterial embolus from a distant focus (3).

Contiguous osteomyelitis refers to infections in which contamination of the bone arises with contact from nearby infected tissue or from direct inoculation from an exogenous source. Unlike hematogenous osteomyelitis, con-tiguous osteomyelitis is most predominant in adults, particularly those who are older than 50 years of age, and accounts for the majority of all cases of osteomyelitis (1).

Osteomyelitis resulting from contiguous spread may also occur in patients who suffer from vascular insufficiency. These patients are generally older (between 50 and 70 years of age) and have underlying diseases that contribute to their vascular insufficiency. Similarly, these infections also develop as an extension of an existing localized infection. Because this type of osteomyelitis often involves various bones and different bacterial etiologies, its therapy generally differs from that of other types of osteomyelitis (4).

The term "chronic osteomyelitis" remains somewhat confusing and, in some cases, without a satisfactory definition. It is often described as an extension of both acute hematogenous and contiguous osteomyelitis. It frequently occurs in adults as a result of surgery or trauma. It often involves osteomyelitis of the lower extremities and the development of local ischemia. This may result in lower success rates of treatment with either antibiotics, debridement, or both. Although the causative organism in this situation may be similar to those in the acute process, the medical management is more difficult and challenging (5).

Etiology

The most common etiologic agents in bacterial osteomyelitis are shown in Table 70.2. *Staphylococcus aureus* represents the most common pathogen that is implicated in hematogenous osteomyelitis (6). It is isolated in 60 to 90% of the cases in children. *Haemophilus influenzae* type b accounts for about 20% of cases in children younger than 2 years of age. Group B streptococci and *Escherichia coli* are common pathogens associated with osteomyelitis during the neonatal period (7). In children older than 5 years of age, the most commonly isolated pathogens are *S. aureus*, Group A streptococci, and *Streptococcus pneumoniae* (8).

In adults, *Staphylococcus aureus* is also the most common causative organism and is isolated in 50 to 75% of cases. *S. epidermidis* has been isolated in approximately 30% of cases. In addition, Gram-negative bacilli may be isolated in up to 30% of cases, streptococci having been isolated in fewer than 10% of cases. Other organisms such as fungi, *Pseudomonas aeruginosa*, and *Mycobacterium* spp. have also been isolated (9, 10).

1373

Table 70.1.
Major Types of Osteomyelitis

	Hematogenous	Contiguous	Contiguous with Vascular Insufficiency
Age distribution	1–20 years, >50 years	>50 years	>50 years
Bones involved	Long bones, vertebrae	Femur, tibia, skull, mandible	Feet, toes
Major clinical findings	Initial episode	Initial episode	Initial and recurrent
	Fever	Fever	Pain
	Local tenderness	Erythema	Swelling
	Local swelling	Swelling	Erythema
	Limitation of motion	Sinus	Drainage
	Recurrent	Recurrent	Ulceration
	Drainage	Drainage	
		Sinus	

Source: Modified from (44).

Table 70.2.
Common Etiologic Agents in Bacterial Osteomyelitis

Neonate (<1 month)	Infants and Children (1 month to 5 years)	Children and Adolescents (5–16 years)	Adults (>16 years)
S. aureus	S. aureus	S. aureus	S. aureus
Group B streptococcus	H. influenzae	Group A streptococcus	Streptococci (including enterococci)
E. coli	Group A streptococcus		Gram-negative bacilli
			Anaerobes

Polymicrobial infections are common in adult osteo-myelitis and may include three or more pathogens. Anaerobes such as *Bacteroides fragilis*, *Bacteroides* spp., *Fusobacterium*, *Clostridium*, and microaerophilic cocci can also be significant pathogens in osteomyelitis (11, 12).

Risk Factors

Risk factors that favor the development of osteomyelitis are outlined in Table 70.3. Identification and knowledge of these factors can aid in early diagnosis and perhaps prevention of these infections.

Bacteremia is one of the most important risk factors for the development of acute hematogenous osteomyelitis. Although this by itself may not be sufficient to cause infections, it may be more significant when associated with trauma (10). Since most blood-borne infections originate from a source, identification of risk factors that are associated with the promotion of bacteremia must be considered. For example, septic foci associated with acute pharyngitis, minor lacerations, cellulitis, and cutaneous abscesses have been implicated as sources of bacteremia in children with acute osteomyelitis (3). Nonpenetrating trauma is common in children with acute hematogenous osteomyelitis (11). As many as 30% of children with this infection have experienced minor injury within 2 weeks before the onset of the disease. Invasive procedures, such as umbilical catheters and frequent heel sticks, and complicated delivery are associated with bacteremia in

neonates (13, 14). Certain underlying diseases such as sickle cell anemia and related hemoglobinopathies have been associated with osteomyelitis due to *Salmonella* species. Respiratory infections are a focus of infection in 12 to 26% of cases (12).

Hematogenous osteomyelitis is less common in adults and is found predominantly in patients who require long-term use of intravenous catheters, patients undergoing hemodialysis, and intravenous drug abusers.

Certain underlying diseases such as infections of the urinary tract, respiratory tract, and soft tissue are associated with vertebral osteomyelitis, which is usually found in the elderly (10, 11).

Infection of the bone by nonhematogenous spread may evolve from either direct inoculation or contiguous spread from an adjacent focus. Direct inoculation can occur from a variety of sources, such as penetrating trauma from open injuries to bone, reduction of fractures, orthopedic and diagnostic procedures, gunshot wounds, and animal bites (10). Contiguous spread from an adjacent soft tissue infection is the most important risk for osteomyelitis in adults. Foci for bone infections in this situation include soft tissue infections close to the bone, as in the case of osteomyelitis of the mastoid bone, which can originate from malignant otitis media or other paranasal sinus infections. Osteomyelitis of the mandible has also been observed in patients with poor oral hygiene or chronic infections of the teeth. Postoperative wound infections

Table 70.3.
Common Risk Factors Associated with the Development of Osteomyelitis

Hematogenous	Contiguous	Contiguous with Vascular Insufficiency
Bacteremic foci	Direct inoculation	Diabetes mellitus
Noninvasive	Penetrating trauma	Peripheral vascular disease
Acute pharyngitis	Open reduction of fracture	Pressure sores
Minor laceration	Gunshot wounds	
Cellulitis	Orthopedic procedures	
Cutaneous abscesses	Diagnostic procedures	
Sickle cell anemia	Animal bites	
Respiratory infections	Puncture wounds	
Invasive	Adjacent foci	
Intravenous catheters	Surgery	
Intravenous drug abusers	Postoperative wound infections	
Hemodialysis	Soft tissue infections	
Heel sticks		
Nonpenetrating trauma		

following orthopedic correction of the skeleton, neurosurgery, median sternotomy, and oral surgery are major contiguous sources of osteomyelitis. Osteomyelitis of the foot following puncture wounds, often referred to as "tennis shoe cellulitis," has also been identified as a major cause of infections. These risk factors differ from penetrating trauma in the sequence in which the skeletal infection develops (11, 13).

Diabetes mellitus and severe atherosclerosis are the most common risk factors for patients with vascular insufficiency. These conditions often predispose patients to chronic draining ulcers and cellulitis of the feet and toes and promote the development of osteomyelitis (11). Pressure sores in chronically debilitated bedridden patients are also a major risk factor (15).

Osteomyelitis should be suspected when decubiti fail to respond to standard antibiotic therapy and debridement.

Any situation such as osteomyelitis of the lower extremity following severe local trauma, misdiagnosis, inadequate surgical drainage, or inappropriate treatment would be considered a risk factor for chronic osteomyelitis.

Pathophysiology and Clinical Manifestations

Several unanswered questions remain in describing the pathogenesis of osteomyelitis. For example, what is the significance of prior injury, acute injury, or trauma to the actual development of osteomyelitis? In addition, it is unclear why certain pathogens, such as *S. aureus*, appear to have a greater affinity for bone as well as other factors that enhance its ability to invade osseous tissue.

In acute hematogenous osteomyelitis in children the long, tubular, rapidly growing bones such as the femur, tibia, and humerus are predominantly affected. The infectious process usually begins in the sinusoidal veins in the metaphyseal region of the bone. The anatomic features and vascular structure favor the growth of

microorganisms in this site, since these capillaries lack phagocytic lining cells (Fig. 70.1). Also, capillary blood flow in this region is slower and more turbulent. Following invasion of the pathogen, a typical inflammatory response ensues. Bacterial and neutrophilic enzymes are released that contribute to the breakdown of the bone, removal of calcium, and eventual necrosis. In addition, the cortical section of the bone and the metaphyses are much thinner in children than in adults. There is also less adherence of the periosteum to the underlying cortex of the bone. This situation favors the extension of the suppurative process from the metaphysis through the cortex and into the periosteum, resulting in the accumulation of pus in the subperiosteal space. Pressure can build up, causing ischemia to nutrient arteries and eventual necrosis of the bone (16).

This has generally been considered the traditional explanation for the pathogenesis of acute hematogenous osteomyelitis in children. Research using an avian model, which closely resembles human disease, suggests this explanation may not be accurate. In the avian model, bacteria attach to the exposed growth plate cartilaginous matrix adjoining the extending tips of the metaphyseal vessels. Bacteria proliferate, resulting in vascular occlusion and abscess formation. The bacteria can become enclosed in a slimelike substance composed of extracellular complex sugars referred to as glycocalyx, which can act as a barrier and prevent natural host defenses or antibiotics from reaching the bacteria. These changes would somewhat refute the concept of sluggish blood flow as the principle explanation for bacterial deposition (17, 18).

Since bacteremia is the major source of infection in acute hematogenous osteomyelitis, patients occasionally present with signs and symptoms of acute sepsis, fever being the most common. The fever may be accompanied

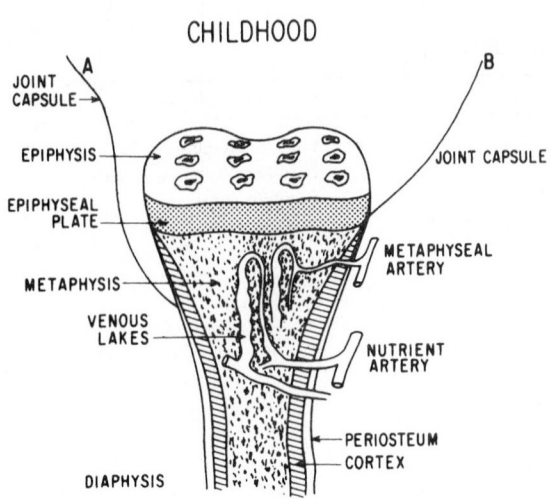

Figure 70.1 Major structures of the bones of a child. (From: Gutman LT. Acute, subacute, and chronic ostecmyelitis and pyogenic arthritis in children. Curr Probl Pediatr 15(12):1–72, 1985. Copyright 1985. Chicago: Year Book Medical Publishers; reproduced with permision.)

by chills, muscle ache, headache, nausea, and vomiting. In staphylococcal osteomyelitis the incidence of sepsis is quite high, occurring in 56 to 73% of the cases. Moderate fever, often the only presenting symptom, may occur along with pain, swelling, tenderness, decreased range of motion in an adjacent joint, or suppuration at the involved site (3, 6). In about one-third of cases of hematogenous osteomyelitis a subacute form of the infection occurs, in which case the child may present only with mild muscular pain and no systemic findings (19).

In adults the vertebrae appear to be the most common site of involvement for acute hematogenous osteomyelitis. This is partly due to the well-vascularized flat bone that is adjacent to the cartilage as well as the persistent marrow cavity. Patients often present with fever, malaise, chills, back pain, and stiffness. Although symptoms may be more than those in children and may consist only of pain, local suppuration is uncommon (7). Paralysis can occur if the diagnosis is not made promptly (11).

In osteomyelitis resulting from contiguous spread, almost any bone in the body may be involved. Infections in this situation are most predominant in the bones that are more prone to fracture or open reduction, such as the femur or tibia. Other bones that are frequently involved include the skull and mandible, the osteomyelitis resulting from dental or sinus infections. Infections of the bones of the feet have occurred secondary to puncture wounds (11). Osteomyelitis of the sternum has been associated with medial sternotomy incisions. Major symptoms are generally confined to the infected adjacent tissues and usually present as pain, tenderness, swelling, and redness. Fever may be present during the initial episode. During recurrent

infections, systemic symptoms may be absent, pain and drainage from a sinus tract or ulcer being the predominant clinical findings (11).

Chronic osteomyelitis involves advanced bone destruction and necrosis secondary to the continued inflammatory process. The common characteristics for all types of chronic osteomyelitis are the presence of vascular thrombosis and/or necrotic bone commonly referred to as a sequestra. It provides a bacterial milieu for persistence of the infection and perpetuation of the inflammatory process. This results in eventual vascular thrombosis and further development of necrotic bone (16). In addition, glycocalyx formation acts as a barrier to hormonal and cellular host defenses while enhancing the attachment of microorganisms to the bone or foreign bodies (18). Several conditions have been proposed as criteria for defining chronic osteomyelitis. These include findings such as (a) abnormal or radiologic evidence of infection for 6 weeks or longer, (b) radiologic evidence of sequestrum formation, (c) bone infections associated with vascular insufficiency or foreign bodies, and (d) persistence of infection or relapse following treatment. The presence of any one of these findings constitutes chronic osteomyelitis (20).

Diagnosis and Laboratory Findings

Several laboratory findings may be useful in the diagnosis of osteomyelitis. Positive identification of the infecting pathogen is one of the most important diagnostic aides and is useful in selecting appropriate antibiotic therapy. Positive blood cultures occur in approximately 60 to 75% of cases (16) of untreated acute hematogenous osteomyelitis. However, isolation of organisms from other tissues or fluids may also aid in the diagnosis.

Culture diagnosis of osteomyelitis due to contiguous spread or vascular insufficiency may be more complex. Since infection occurs from a contiguous abscess, cellulitis, or penetration of the overlying skin, specimens obtained from subcutaneous or other surrounding tissues need to be evaluated. These may be obtained either by direct needle biopsy or at the time of surgical debridement. Caution should be exercised in evaluating culture specimens obtained from superficially draining sinus tracts. The results in this case may be misleading and not indicative of the actual pathogen at the site of infection (11).

In chronic osteomyelitis, blood cultures are rarely studied. When tissue and blood cultures are negative, direct subperiosteal or metaphyseal needle aspiration is required to make a definitive diagnosis. Subsequent evaluation of a Gram stain is useful for initiating therapy (6).

Roentgenographic changes may not be evident until at least 10 to 14 days after the onset of clinical illness. However, radiographic signs indicating changes in the deep tissues, as evident from a loss of normally defined planes between the muscles, may be present during early stages of the disease. Therefore, early radiographs show only changes of the adjacent tissue and not of the bone (6).

Radionuclide imaging or bone scan using technetium pyrophosphate-labeled compounds may reveal indirect evidence of osteomyelitis and is a useful test with a high degree of sensitivity. A fixed quantity of an intravenous radioactive compound is administered. The patient's skeletal system is imaged or scanned approximately 2 to 4 hr later. The scan is repeated in 24 hr. The ratio of uptake is determined between the two scanning intervals. Often referred to as the "four-phase" bone scan, this method enables the clinician to distinguish osteomyelitis from cellulitis, since technetium will disappear more rapidly from the soft tissue than from bone (21). Abnormal findings are related to the enhanced ability of the inflamed tissues to take up the labeled compound due to increased blood flow of the infected areas. Technetium scanning, however, is not specific for infections and may be positive in the presence of other inflammatory processes such as trauma, tumor, or arthritis. It is less accurate in the diagnosis of acute hematogenous osteomyelitis (10).

Gallium-67 citrate is a more selective imaging radionuclide. The outcome of gallium scanning is directly related to the ability of the polymorphonuclear leukocytes to take up the radioactive compound. Since leukocytes concentrate at the site of bacterial infection, an abnormal finding or "hot spot" would be detected in the area of the infected bone. Gallium scans are quite useful in detecting acute osteomyelitis in the very early stages of the disease, when conventional radiographs are of limited value, or if the technetium scan yields negative results (22). Gallium scanning is associated with higher levels of radiation and should be reserved for cases in which the diagnosis cannot be established by conventional methods. It is an excellent test to distinguish early acute osteomyelitis from septic arthritis or when the technetium studies are normal (16).

Magnetic resonant imaging has recently emerged as the preferred imaging technique for the diagnosis of osteomyelitis and soft tissue infections and is superior to computer-assisted tomography (CT scan) in establishing the level of involvement of the infection. A CT scan is preferred for establishing cortical bone destruction, sequestra, or as a guide for drainage or biopsy (23).

Other clinical laboratory observations that are of diagnostic importance include leukocytosis and elevated erythrocyte sedimentation rate (ESR). The white blood cell count may be normal in 40 to 75% of the patients during initial examination for acute osteomyelitis (6). The ESR is generally normal within the first 36 hr of the disease but will progressively rise in some cases to values greater than 100 mm/hr. The ESR is not a reliable laboratory test for

patients on corticosteroids, patients with sickle cell disease, or neonates (10).

Serologic tests designed to detect the presence of teichoic acid antibodies (TAA) have been used in the diagnosis of acute osteomyelitis due to *S. aureus*. The cell wall structure of *S. aureus* is comprised of three major components: peptidoglycan, techoic acid, and protein A. Teichoic acid is the largest component and accounts for as much as 40% by weight of the total cell wall. During severe *S. aureus* infections, antibodies that are directed against the teichoic acid antigenic portions of the wall are formed. In osteomyelitis, TAA may not be detectable in the acute phase of the infection but may be useful in the diagnosis of chronic osteomyelitis. These antibodies can be detected by using counterimmunoelectrophoresis (CIE) and gel diffusion techniques and may be useful in the diagnosis of bone infections caused by this organism (24, 25).

Medical Management

Since the treatment of osteomyelitis involves a protracted commitment to antibiotic therapy, careful evaluation and diagnosis are of paramount importance. Early diagnosis precludes serious damage to the tissue and avoids complications associated with recurrent or chronic bone infections.

The diagnosis and subsequent choice of therapy may be difficult, particularly in the early stages of the disease. Many of the clinical manifestations, such as white blood cell count, radiographs, and radionuclide scans, may be within normal limits. Furthermore, blood cultures may be positive in only 50% of the cases, and superficial sinus drainage cultures may be unreliable. Therefore, antibiotic therapy, particularly during the initial phase of treatment, is largely empiric and is based predominantly on patient factors such as age, history before the onset of symptoms, site of infection, and other underlying risk factors. The clinician must evaluate all these parameters and come to some reasonable conclusion regarding the most likely causative organism.

Antibiotic Therapy

Staphylococcus aureus is the predominant organism in most cases of hematogenous osteomyelitis; therefore, it is prudent to include in the initial empiric therapy an antibiotic that is capable of eradicating this organism. The penicillinase-resistant penicillins such as nafcillin and oxacillin are useful antistaphylococcal agents (10, 11). These antibiotics are bactericidal and relatively inexpensive. They have the disadvantage that neither agent is effective against *E. coli*, a common cause of neonatal osteomyelitis. Therefore, the use of a first- or second-generation cephalosporin such as cefazolin or cefuroxime may be an appropriate choice for the newborn (7). Other disadvantages of penicillins include frequent administration and their association with severe anaphylaxis and allergic reactions such as fevers, rash, and neutropenia (6).

First-generation cephalosporins such as cephalothin or cefazolin have relatively few adverse effects and are effective alternatives in most penicillin-allergic patients. These agents have the advantage of retaining excellent activity against *S. aureus* while providing adequate coverage against *E. coli*. Cefazolin has an added advantage in that it may be administered every 8 hr (12).

A second-generation cephalosporin such as cefuroxime has antistaphylococcal activity similar to that of first-generation cephalosporins. It also possesses extended Gram-negative coverage against *H. influenzae* and, therefore, may be useful as empiric therapy in children with hematogenous osteomyelitis when this organism is suspected (9).

Third-generation cephalosporins such as cefotaxime and ceftizoxime retain good activity against *S. aureus* and are effective in osteomyelitis caused by this organism. Traditionally, these agents are more costly and less active against *S. aureus* than are first-generation cephalosporins (26). Cefotaxime is among the third-generation cephalosporins that are most active against *S. aureus*, with minimum inhibitory concentrations approaching those of the first-generation cephalosporins. This activity has been related to the synergistic effect of its active metabolite, desacetylcefotaxime (27). Since this antibiotic possesses excellent activity against common Gram-negative organisms, such as Enterobacteriaceae and *H. influenzae*, it may be useful for empiric therapy when these pathogens are suspected (10).

Ceftriaxone has emerged as a potential safe and effective agent in the treatment of osteomyelitis. It is active against most common pathogens. Its long half-life and once-a-day dosing make it particularly attractive for home care therapy (28).

For patients who are allergic to β-lactam antibiotics, clindamycin is an effective alternative in the treatment of staphylococcal osteomyelitis (10, 29, 30).

Strains of methicillin-resistant *S. aureus* (MRSA) have emerged as potential pathogens in osteomyelitis. Although cephalosporins may appear to be active when disk diffusion methods are used, the organism is generally resistant when it is tested by using microdilution techniques. Therefore, vancomycin remains the only antibiotic that is effective in vivo for the treatment of osteomyelitis due to MRSA (31).

Teicoplanin is a new glycopeptide antibiotic that is being investigated for the treatment of serious staphylococcal infections, including osteomyelitis. In a recent trial involving patients with bone and joint infections due to sensitive and resistant staphylococci, teicoplanin was shown to be effective and generally well tolerated for most patients. Teicoplanin has advantages in that it has a long half-life and can be administered on a once-daily schedule.

The drug may be given intramuscularly; this makes it very suitable for outpatient use. Teicoplanin also does not require routine serum concentration measurements (32).

Osteomyelitis arising from a contiguous spread is similar to that of hematogenous osteomyelitis in that *S. aureus* remains the predominant organism. However, it is not unusual that bone infections in this category involve mixed etiologies. Organisms such as *P. aeruginosa*, and *Proteus* spp. are also frequently isolated. Under these circumstances an aminoglycoside should be empirically added in combination with the traditional antistaphylococcal agent until culture reports can be obtained. Once the organism has been identified, the antibiotic regimen can be adjusted according to the sensitivities (10, 12).

The prolonged use of aminoglycoside therapy may cause nephrotoxicity, particularly in elderly or diabetic patients. Broad-spectrum β-lactam antibiotics such as cefotaxime, ceftizoxime, ceftazidime, and ceftriaxone have been suggested as agents for monotherapy in the treatment of mixed-etiology bone infections (26, 28). Cefotaxime and ceftizoxime are considered the most active third-generation cephalosporins against *S. aureus*, ceftriaxone being less active. Additionally, all three agents are quite active against common Enterobacteriaceae. They have the disadvantage of not being effective against *P. aeruginosa*. Ceftazidime is less active against *S. aureus* but is the most active cephalosporin against *P. aeruginosa*. Cefotaxime, ceftizoxime, ceftriaxone, and ceftazidime are associated with a low incidence of side effects (26, 28).

Anaerobic bacteria have been isolated in some cases of both acute hematogenous and contiguous spread osteomyelitis. Acute hematogenous osteomyelitis as a result of anaerobic bacteremia is relatively uncommon and is responsible for about one-third of cases of all anaerobic osteomyelitis. Intraabdominal infections are often a source of anaerobic bacteremia. Chronic osteomyelitis related to prior trauma is considered one of the most common forms of osteomyelitis of the long bones. These infections may be of mixed anaerobic and aerobic etiologies. Chronic anaerobic osteomyelitis has also been associated with implantation and infection of prosthetic devices (33). The most common form of chronic osteomyelitis due to anaerobes is that related to underlying peripheral vascular disease. This syndrome is almost always associated with long-standing diabetes and, in nondiabetics, with severe peripheral vascular disease. The small bones of the feet are most commonly involved. There is generally a small ulcer surrounding the affected area. Anaerobic osteomyelitis of the mandibles or the cranial or facial bones have also been reported. The relatively high concentration of anaerobic bacteria from the oral cavity are responsible for these infections (34). Pressure ulcers may also predispose elderly patients to bone infections. Osteomyelitis may occur in up to one-third of patients with nonhealing pressure ulcers.

The infectious process may be polymicrobic, including anaerobic bacteria (35).

The clinical presentation of anaerobic osteomyelitis is similar to those of aerobic disease. Certain signs such as foul-smelling sinus tract drainage, bone biopsy, or purulence as well as the presence of gas on radiograph, multiple pleomorphic organisms on Gram-stain, or negative aerobic cultures may be clues. Penicillin G remains the most active agent against anaerobic bacteria other than *B. fragilis*. For infections due to *B. fragilis*, clindamycin and metronidazole remain highly effective agents. Clindamycin is also very active against *S. aureus* and has good penetration into the osseous tissue. Other agents, such as cefoxitin, cefotetan, mezlocillin, and piperacillin, although less active against *B. fragilis* than are the former compounds, have been used in the treatment of anaerobic infections (33, 34). β-Lactamase inhibitor combinations such as ampicillin/sulbactam, ticarcillin/clavulanic acid, and piperacillin/tazobactam are uniquely suited for treating these infections, since these combinations cover not only anaerobes but also many of the other more common Gram-positive and Gram-negative pathogens that are isolated in osteomyelitis. Clinical trials supporting the use of these agents in osteomyelitis have been limited.

Antibiotic therapy for bacterial osteomyelitis is summarized in Table 70.4.

Oral Antibiotic Therapy

In an attempt to reduce hospital stay and costs, there have been numerous clinical trials involving oral antibiotic therapy in the treatment of osteomyelitis. In most instances, therapy was initiated with a parenteral antibiotic and completed with an appropriate oral agent. A variety of oral agents were used, including penicillins, cephalexin, clindamycin, and fluoroquinolones (36, 37). Aggressive monitoring of the patient included measurements of the ESR, roentgenologic evaluation, and complete blood counts. In some cases, patients underwent surgical drainage when the initial bone aspirate contained purulent material. Antibiotic serum bactericidal titers remain one of the best predictors of successful outcomes in the treatment of acute hematogenous osteomyelitis. Twofold serial dilutions of the patient's own antibiotic-containing serum is tested against a known inoculum of the infecting organism. Favorable outcomes were seen when peak bactericidal levels were achieved at titers greater than 1:8. If the patient's bactericidal concentration was less, the antibiotic dose was increased to provide the appropriate titer. Serum bactericidal titers have been studied most often in patients receiving oral antibiotic therapy following a brief initial course of parenteral therapy (38).

Overall, these studies indicated that the treatment of acute osteomyelitis with an initial brief period of parenteral therapy followed by appropriate oral therapy and aggressive patient monitoring is effective. Although these results are encouraging, there are several limitations that need to be considered before embarking on oral therapy. For example, in almost all cases the patients involved were children with acute staphylococcal osteomyelitis of recent onset. The pathogen was positively identified, and there was aggressive patient monitoring. Surgical intervention was performed when needed. Compliance was enforced to ensure proper antibiotic consumption and to avoid relapse or failure. This is critical to prevent

Table 70.4.
Empiric Antibiotic Therapy for the Treatment of Bacterial Osteomyelitis

Age Group	Likely Organisms	Antibiotics of Choice (Dose, Route, and Frequency of Administration)
Neonates (<4 weeks)	S. aureus Group B streptococcus E. coli	Nafcillin or oxacillin 50 mg/kg/day i.v. q12h plus gentamicin 5 mg/kg/day i.v. q12h or cefazolin 40 mg/kg/day i.v. q12h
Infants and children (1 month to 5 years)	S. aureus Group A streptococcus H. influenzae	Cefuroxime 75–150 mg/kg/day i.v. q8h or cefotaxime or ceftizoxime 100–200 mg/kg/day i.v. q8h
Children and adolescents (6–16 years)	S. aureus Group A streptococcus	Nafcillin or oxacillin 100–200 mg/kg/day i.v. q6h or cefazolin 50–100 mg/kg/day i.v. q8h
Adults (>16 years)	S. aureus Nonenterococcal streptococcus Enterobacteriaceae Enterococcal streptococci[a] P. aeruginosa[b] Anaerobes[c]	Nafcillin or oxacillin 150 mg/kg/day i.v. q6h or cefazolin 50–150 mg/kg/day i.v. plus aminoglycoside (e.g., gentamicin or tobramycin 5 mg/kg/day i.v. or amikacin 15 mg/kg/day i.v.) or monotherapy with cefotaxime or ceftizoxime 100–150 mg/kg/day q8h

[a]If enterococci are cultured, use ampicillin 2 g i.v. q6h plus an aminoglycoside; for penicillin-allergic patients, use vancomycin 0.5–1 g i.v. q12h plus an aminoglycoside.

[b]Piperacillin 3 g i.v. q4h or ceftazidime 2–3 g i.v. q8h plus tobramycin 5 mg/kg i.v. q day.

[c]For anaerobes other than *B. fragilis*, penicillin G 2 million units i.v. q4h. For *B. fragilis*, clindamycin 900 mg i.v. q8h or metronidazole 500 mg i.v. q6h or cefoxitin 2 g i.v. q6h.

exacerbation, progression of a chronic infection, or permanent bone destruction.

In many cases of osteomyelitis the infecting organism is not identifiable, nor is the onset of symptoms recent. In the past the availability of an appropriate oral agent against a variety of Gram-negative organisms was limited. Fluoroquinolone antibiotics such as ciprofloxacin and ofloxacin have been demonstrated to be effective for oral therapy in the treatment of Gram-negative osteomyelitis, including that due to *P. aeruginosa*. Ciprofloxacin given at a dose of 750 mg twice a day achieved clinical success rates that were similar to those of conventional intravenous therapy (39). The efficacy of fluoroquinolones in the treatment of staphylococcal osteomyelitis has not been established. In addition, the rising development of resistance to staphylococci and *P. aeruginosa* may limit the use of these agents in the treatment of bone infections. Careful assessment of in vitro microbiological data is warranted to ensure adequate bactericidal activity (11, 40).

The optimal time for switching from parenteral to oral therapy has not been well established. Oral therapy should be applied only to certain types of osteomyelitis and is influenced by factors such as recent onset of illness, positive identification of the organism, aggressive monitoring, availability of a suitable oral agent, and good patient compliance. Serum bactericidal levels should be used for all patients receiving oral therapy. Peak titers should be maintained at 1:8 (7). Other authors recommend monitoring trough levels to achieve titers of 1:2 or greater (10).

Combination Therapy

Although combination antibiotic therapy has been used with success in selected infections, this approach has not been adequately evaluated in the treatment of osteomyelitis for acute hematogenous osteomyelitis. Single-agent therapy is effective in the treatment of most common pathogens. For contiguous spread osteomyelitis, traditional empiric therapy has been the combination of a β-lactam antibiotic and an aminoglycoside (10).

Broad-spectrum β-lactam antibiotics have been used as monotherapy in the treatment of osteomyelitis. Reviews of patient cases suggest that ceftazidime is effective as monotherapy for the treatment of serious Gram-negative bacillary osteomyelitis. (41). Furthermore, evaluations of large numbers of clinical trials suggest that β-lactam antibiotics, particularly third-generation cephalosporins, are effective as monotherapy for osteomyelitis due to susceptible organisms when there is appropriate surgical debridement (42). However, strains of *P. aeruginosa* have emerged that are resistant to ceftazidime and imipenem. This creates reason for concern and suggests that combination with an aminoglycoside be used for this pathogen (26).

Preliminary data suggests the use of oral rifampin in combination with a parenteral penicillinase-resistant penicillin for the treatment of chronic staphylococcal osteomyelitis. Rifampin appears to act synergistically with antistaphylococcal agents when used in combination. The combination of rifampin and β-lactam antibiotics or fluoroquinolones has been used as heroic treatment in nonremovable prosthetic osteomyelitis (11).

Duration of Therapy

The optimal length of therapy for the treatment of osteomyelitis has not been adequately defined. One controlled study reported a significantly higher percentage of failures for patients who received parenteral antibiotics for 3 weeks or less than for patients whose therapy continued for greater than 3 weeks. The addition of oral antibiotics did not appear to influence the outcome of therapy (43). The current standard is to treat the infection for a minimum of 4 weeks with high-dose parenteral therapy. However, this can vary depending on the etiology of the infection. For example, *H. influenzae, Neisseria meningitidis,* and *Streptococcus pneumoniae* can be treated with shorter courses in a minimum of 14 days. *Staphylococcus aureus* and enteric Gram-negative organisms usually require a minimum of 4 weeks (7). Most clinicians prefer to use the amelioration of clinical signs and the normalization of laboratory parameters such as white blood cell count and ESR in determining the precise length of therapy (6).

The length of treatment for chronic osteomyelitis is even less well defined, since infections in this situation may involve significant necrosis of the bone and formation of sequestra. Traditional recommendations include at least 4 to 6 weeks parenteral therapy followed by 2 months of oral therapy. These guidelines were developed from patients with chronic staphylococcal osteomyelitis and may not be appropriate for infections of Gram-negative origin (44). Other studies suggest better cure rates following 3 months of appropriate intravenous antibiotic therapy (45). Patients with chronic osteomyelitis often require extensive debridement, bone reconstruction, and muscle flaps. The duration of therapy for these patients has ranged from 14 days to 6 weeks. Some researchers suggest that longer courses of therapy provide no additional benefit and may even increase morbidity and that postoperative antibiotic courses of 10 to 14 days are adequate (5).

Home Antibiotic Therapy

Administration of antibiotics on an outpatient basis has emerged as a viable alternative to hospitalization in the long-term treatment of selected infectious diseases such as endocarditis and osteomyelitis. Numerous studies have demonstrated the safety and cost-effectiveness of outpatient intravenous therapy compared to in-hospital administration.

In most cases, patients receive a brief in-hospital course of antibiotic therapy. During the hospital stay, patients are observed for untoward effects and overall tolerability of the regimen. Once they are clinically stable, patients may be sent home, depending on the reliability of their home environment for safe and adequate care. Patients should also have other family or home members who are willing to learn and assume the responsibilities of home drug administration (46). Drugs are administered through a peripheral venous access such as intermittent needle therapy (INT), a central catheter such as a peripheral intravenous central catheter, or directly through a Hickman-Broviac catheter. The INT administration has a disadvantage in that the needle must be replaced every 3 days. Also, patients often complain of local pain and inflammation. Central catheters generally remain in place for the duration of therapy. Hickman-Broviac catheters have the disadvantage of usually requiring minor surgery and general anesthesia for insertion. Home patients generally receive several doses of prepackaged antibiotics. Ambulatory patients return to the hospital or physician's office on a weekly or twice-weekly basis for their drug supply. Drugs are delivered to debilitated patients by the home health care team. The intravenous catheter care is provided by contracted health nursing services. A pharmacist has both dispensing and drug-monitoring responsibilities (47). Some hospitals have developed their own home health care programs. It has been shown that hospital-based distribution of home antibiotics is an efficacious, safe, and cost-effective alternative to prolonged hospitalization in the treatment of osteomyelitis (48).

Antibiotic Bone Concentrations

Numerous studies have been devoted to the issue of antibiotic penetration into normal and infected bone. Antibiotic bone concentrations have been determined by assaying aliquot of solutions containing bone fragments that have been agitated in an appropriate buffer at an optimal pH. Unfortunately, data extracted from these studies varies considerably and has produced conflicting recommendations with regard to which agents are appropriate. Factors such as time of sample collection, extraction techniques, methods of assay, and source of specimen (whether normal or osteomyelitic bone) all have contributed to the confusion. These studies indicate that most antibiotics that have been tested are able to permeate capillary membranes of normal and osteomyelitic bones. It is proposed that these agents cross capillary membranes by simple passive diffusion as well as other processes.

Concomitant serum concentrations measured at steady state appear to be similar to those of the interstitial fluid space in the osseous tissue. Therefore, serum concentrations appear to be an adequate reflection of bone fluid concentrations (49). Serum and bone levels of β-lactam antibiotics have been evaluated in patients with chronic osteomyelitis following debridement. Despite adequate serum concentrations there was only minimal penetration into the necrotic bone (50).

In summary, it appears that most antibiotics are capable of penetrating and distributing into both normal and osteomyelytic bone, although high-dose therapy is often used. Serum concentrations appear to be an adequate indicator of interstitial bone concentrations. Antibiotic penetration into necrotic bone appears to be minimal.

OTHER TREATMENT MODALITIES

Local Antibiotic Therapy

Although systemic antibiotic therapy seems to be the mainstay in the treatment of osteomyelitis, it has several disadvantages, particularly in the chronic form of this disease. These include potential side effects following prolonged therapy, questionable penetration of antibiotics into necrotic or ischemic tissue, and protracted hospitalization. As a result, a number of techniques have been developed that provide direct local application of antibiotics.

Antibiotic-impregnated polymethylmethacrylate bone cement beads have been used extensively in the United Kingdom but only on a limited basis in the United States. Several antibiotics, including aminoglycosides, penicillins, clindamycin, cephalosporins, lincomycin, streptomycin, and vancomycin, have been incorporated into bone cement. In this system the polymethylmethacrylate (PMMA) bone cement bead serves as a carrier for the antibiotic. The release of antibiotic from the bead follows a bimodal pattern. The beads are designed to release approximately 5% of the antibiotic within the first 24 hr and the remainder over several weeks or months. The beads may be used individually for packing empty voids following surgery or strung on a multifilament stainless steel wire in the form of chains for direct attachment to the bones. The chains consist of either 10, 30, or 60 beads. Impregnated PMMA beads have the advantage of providing high local antibiotic tissue levels with minimal serum concentrations. The incidence of toxicity and allergic reactions are significantly lower than occur in the use of systemic antibiotics. Antibiotic-impregnated beads have been useful as therapy in the treatment of soft tissue infections and osteomyelitis. The addition of systemic antibiotics is generally not required, reducing the need for extensive nursing care and decreasing the duration of hospital stay. Unfortunately, the use of PMMA beads is not without limitations and disadvantages. These include strict mandatory patient immobilization and bed rest. Also, the introduction of another foreign body may lead to local inflammation and the possibility of reinfection. Finally, an additional surgical procedure is required to remove the beads and chains (51, 52). Documented well-controlled studies supporting the use of antibiotic impregnated beads are still lacking.

Antibacterial solutions, usually iodophor, may also be directly instilled through a closed continuous suction irrigation system. This is often done in cases of chronic osteomyelitis or in large areas of avascular tissue. This system requires a considerable amount of monitoring by the nursing staff and involves the risk of secondary infection through the drains (44). Disappointing results have been reported with the use of suction irrigation, and it may be limited only to short periods of use (10).

Hyperbaric Oxygen Therapy

Hyperbaric oxygen (HBO) therapy has been used in the treatment of osteomyelitis. In this method, the patient is placed in a monoplace hyperbaric chamber and is subjected to oxygen pressures greater than sea level, usually 2 atmospheres. The duration of therapy ranges from 90 min to 2 hr, depending on the level of refractoriness of the infection and subsequent results of each treatment. As many as 60 treatments may be given to a single patient. Beneficial effects have been observed in patients with chronic or refractory osteomyelitis.

Limited clinical studies have documented that intermittent short-term, high-dose oxygen inhalation has been associated with increased vascularity as well as enhancing both bone and soft tissue healing in ischemic tissue. HBO has been shown to be effective in controlling infections that are caused by anaerobic and microaerophilic bacteria. Common organisms such as *S. aureus* and *P. aeruginosa*, however, are susceptible only at pressures that are unsafe for human exposure. Effectiveness of HBO for these organisms is postulated to be related to the enhancement of leukocyte bactericidal activity by elevating intermedullary oxygen tension. Several studies have demonstrated beneficial effects of HBO when it is used in the treatment of chronic refractory osteomyelitis. However, flaws in the designs of these studies make the interpretation of the results difficult. Unfortunately, there have been no randomized well-controlled perspective studies to support the routine use of HBO therapy. In addition, HBO is expensive; this has created difficulty in terms of third-party reimbursement (53).

Currently, HBO is recommended only in advanced stages of osteomyelitis in which adequate surgical debridement or reconstruction in well-vascularized areas cannot be performed. HBO may be useful as suppressive therapy when surgical outcomes are poor and definitive therapy is less than optimal. It may also be useful to improve outcome when surgical grafts are performed or in cases of difficult reconstruction or compromised muscle flaps. No harmful effects of HBO have been reported. HBO is adjunctive therapy and should always be used in conjunction with surgery and antibiotics. The cost-effective use of HBO as a standard regimen in the treatment of osteomyelitis is controversial (54).

Surgical Intervention

In the majority of cases of acute hematogenous osteomyelitis, surgical intervention is not required other than as a necessary diagnostic procedure such as bone aspiration. However, some cases do not respond to pharmacologic management, and surgical intervention is required either for exploration or for drainage of an abscess (16). On the other hand, in adult osteomyelitis, surgical intervention is usually required to drain abscesses and close fistula tracts. With chronic infection, surgery is almost certainly required to excise necrotic bone and remove sequestra. Patients will often require skin or muscle flaps to close overlying skin or fill empty cavities (5). The timing and approach of surgery as adjunctive treatment in osteomyelitis have not been well studied.

The decision to remove external fixation devices in an area of infected bone depends on whether union of the bone has been accomplished. If bone union occurs, infection can be treated with the presence of the device. However, most authorities agree that if the union fails, the removal of the fixation device is warranted (55).

Prognosis

Favorable prognosis depends largely on the type of osteomyelitis and whether the appropriate medical interventions are implemented as soon as possible after the onset of symptoms. Under these circumstances it appears that acute osteomyelitis is associated with the best overall prognosis, having an approximately 80% cure rate when parenteral antibiotics are maintained for more than 4 weeks and appropriate surgical intervention is used. Similar results are also seen in children who receive initial parenteral antibiotics followed by an appropriate oral agent if peak bactericidal levels greater than 1:8 are maintained (38).

In the case of chronic osteomyelitis the prognosis is substantially less favorable. Success rates vary from study to study depending on the criteria, such as healing of drained sinuses or changes in laboratory parameters. Original observations in the management of chronic osteomyelitis have defined success rates as high as 90% and as low as 20%. Later studies have shown that proper surgical debridement of dead bone and sequestra along with appropriate antibiotic treatment may increase the follow-up success rate to 50%. Patients for whom surgery was contraindicated or was unsuccessful may require long-term suppressive antibiotics to control their infections (44).

Conclusion

Osteomyelitis is a serious infection of the bone and, when left untreated, can result in significant bone loss and deformity. Infection can be transmitted directly via the bloodstream or can spread from adjacent tissue. The majority of cases are caused by *S. aureus*, although other pathogens such as Enterobacteriaceae, *P. aeruginosa*, and anaerobes have also been isolated. The medical management of osteomyelitis involves a comprehensive clinical assessment of patient factors, culture material, roentgenographic studies, complete blood counts, and appropriate antimicrobial therapy. Most β-lactam and aminoglycoside antibiotics penetrate normal and osteomyelitic bone adequately but do not penetrate necrotic bone. The majority of cases of the acute form can be treated with monotherapy for a minimum of 4 weeks and are associated with a favorable prognosis. Selected patients can be treated successfully with oral antibiotics when there is aggressive monitoring and forced compliance. Chronic osteomyelitis may require several months of treatment with intravenous and oral antibiotics and is associated with a less favorable prognosis. Patients may require surgical intervention to remove necrotic bone fragments as well as undergo extensive bone reconstruction and muscle flaps. Hyperbaric oxygen may be useful as adjunctive therapy for chronic refractory patients. The administration of antibiotics at home has been shown to be a safe and cost-effective alternative to prolonged hospitalization.

INFECTIOUS ARTHRITIS

"Infectious arthritis" and "septic arthritis" are interchangeable terms that are used to describe inflammatory reactions of the joint space, synovium, synovial fluid, and articular cartilage following invasion by a variety of microorganisms. Infectious arthritis constitutes a medical emergency requiring immediate treatment to prevent permanent damage to the joint. Bacteria are the most common cause of joint infections, but fungi, viruses, and chlamydia have also been isolated. This discussion deals exclusively with bacterial arthritis.

Etiology

The bacteria that cause infectious arthritis are primarily age-dependent. The most common bacteria that have been isolated for varying ages of children and adults are outlined in Table 70.5. *S. aureus* is the most common organism

isolated in newborns. Group B streptococci and Enterobacteriaceae, especially *E. coli*, have also been isolated and may be important pathogens. *H. influenzae* is the predominant pathogen in infants and children below 2 years of age, followed by *S. aureus* and streptococci, but is virtually absent in late childhood and adolescence. *S. aureus* and Group A streptococci are the most common pathogens in the latter two age groups. Occasionally, Gram-negative bacteria have also been isolated in this age group (7, 56). *Neisseria gonorrhoeae* is the most predominant organism in sexually active young adults. *S. aureus* is the most common pathogen in the overall adult population. Gram-negative bacilli have also been isolated in adults. Anaerobic bacteria have been isolated as a complication of traumatic injuries (57). *S. epidermidis* is the most common pathogen isolated in prosthetic joint infections (58). *S. aureus* and *P. aeruginosa* are the most common pathogens in intravenous drug abusers (57).

Risk Factors

Bacteremia is generally considered the most important predisposing factor, since hematogenous spread from a distant foci represents the most common mechanism for joint infections (55). There are, however, a number of additional risk factors that may also predispose a patient to infectious arthritis (Table 70.6). Identification of these risk factors can also assist in the diagnosis. For example, patients with chronic illness such as diabetes mellitus and serious underlying diseases such as malignancy are more vulnerable to septic arthritis. Adults with previous joint damage, such as that from rheumatoid arthritis, osteoarthritis, gout, and recent joint trauma, also appear to be at high risk for infectious arthritis (59). Patients with impaired host defense systems either through direct immunosuppressive therapy, such as from systemic or intraarticular corticosteroid, or from primary malignancy, such as lymphoma, are at risk (60). Infections in these patients are usually associated with Gram-negative bacilli. Intravenous drug abusers have a high rate of infections caused by *P. aeruginosa* or *S. aureus* species (57). There is a rising incidence of septic arthritis in hemophiliacs. This increase is observed primarily in patients who are infected with the human immunodeficiency virus (HIV) (60).

Table 70.5.
Common Etiologic Agents in Bacterial Arthritis

Neonates (<1 month)	Infants and Children (1 month to 5 years)	Children and Adolescents (5–16 years)	Sexually Active Adults	Adults with Underlying Illness
S. aureus Group B streptococcus Enterobacteriaceae	*H. influenzae* *S. aureus* *Streptococcus* spp.[a]	*S. aureus* Group A streptococcus Occasionally gram-negative bacteria	*N. gonorrhoeae* Occasionally *S. aureus*	*S. aureus* Enterobacteriaceae *P. aeruginosa* *Streptococcus* spp[a].

[a]Includes *Streptococcus pneumoniae*, Group A and B streptococci

Extraarticular foci of infections can also predispose patients to joint infections. For example, cutaneous infections can result in bacteremic spread of *S. aureus* or *Streptococcus pyogenes*. Similarly, patients with pulmonary infections may be at risk for bacteremia spread of *S. pneumoniae* to the joint. Genitourinary and gastrointestinal tract infections have also been associated with Gram-negative septic arthritis (57). Infectious arthritis resulting from direct inoculation is rare and occurs mostly in patients who have prosthetic joints or are receiving steroid injections (55).

In infants and children the underdeveloped immune system and lack of antibody response probably contribute to the predominance of *H. influenzae* joint infections. Bacteremic spread from extraarticular sites can also predispose children to joint infections. Meningitis, phar-yngitis, and cutaneous infections are among the most common sources of septic foci in children (56).

Pathophysiology

Microorganisms generally make their way to the joint via bacteremic spread from a distant focus. Infectious arthritis rarely begins from a contiguous focus as is the case in osteomyelitis. Acute septic arthritis is relatively uncommon in children. The majority of the cases involve only a single joint. In older children the knee is the most commonly involved joint; in infants the hip is more commonly affected. Other joints that are involved include the sterno-clavicular, shoulder, and sacroiliac (7, 9).

Infectious arthritis rarely develops from direct inoculation, such as from injury or surgical procedures. Once the organism reaches the joint, factors that favor the penetration of the organism into the synovium are not completely understood but may include the state of the patient's immune defense system, previous joint injury, or the presence of other forms of arthritis. Special properties and virulence of the microorganism may also play a role, as in the case of Gram-positive cocci and *N. gonorrhoeae*, which have a particular affinity for bone and joint tissue and are frequent causes of infectious arthritis (59).

Once the organism invades the joint, the initial lesion usually develops in the microvasculature of the synovial membrane (Fig. 70.2). At this site the bacteria proliferate and release their toxic factors. A typical inflammatory response develops from subsequent formation of antigen-

Table 70.6.
Risk Factors Associated with the Development of Infectious Arthritis

Corticosteroid therapy
Diabetes mellitus
Rheumatoid arthritis
Gout
Osteoarthritis
Intravenous drug abuse
Hematologic malignancies
Hemophilia
Extraarticular foci of infection

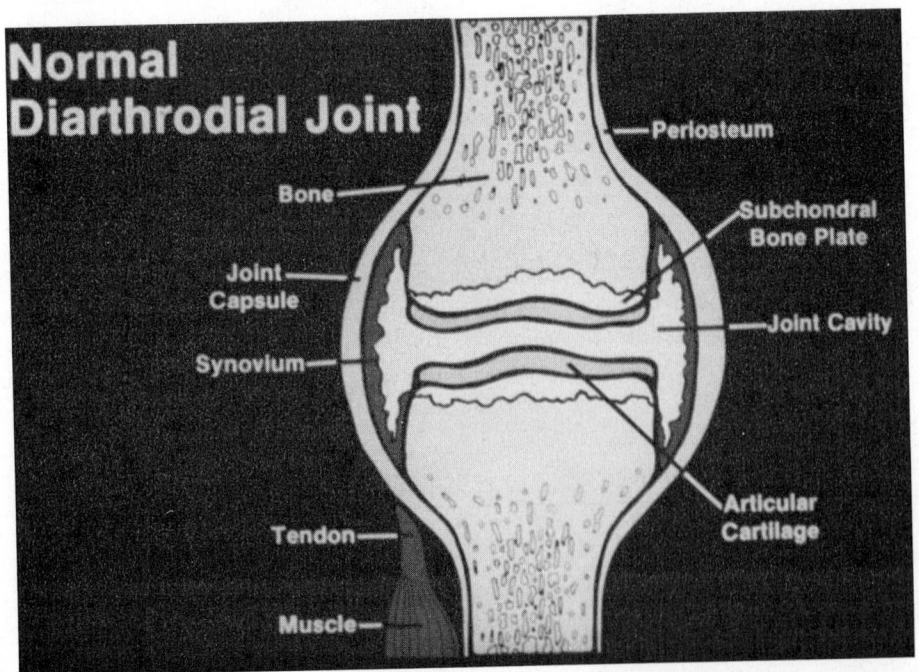

Figure 70.2 Major structures of the joint. (From the Arthritis Teaching Slide Collection, copyright 1980. Used by permission of the Arthritis Foundation.)

antibody complexes, complement activation, and phagocytic cell stimulation. During the latter process, lysosomal enzymes are released, resulting in the formation of microabscesses that eventually extend into the synovial tissue and joint space. Intraarticular pressure increases, enhancing synovial and capsular erosion. The continued inflammatory process may lead to destruction of the cartilage and invasion of the adjacent bone, causing osteomyelitis (59).

Clinical Manifestations and Diagnosis

Septic arthritis generally presents as monoarticular pain, swelling, and redness that is sometimes associated with fever and chills. The patient has substantial limitation in the range of motion of the joint as a result of the swelling and tenderness (Table 70.7). There is a diffuse periarticular tenderness, and effusion is invariably present in the majority of the cases (61). Children with infectious arthritis of the hip can present with fever, apprehension, and irritability. The child assumes a position that enhances comfort to the affected joint. There is usually limited spontaneous motion in the affected extremity, referred to as "pseudo-paralysis" (56). In the case of gonococcal arthritis, patients present with systemic symptoms such as fever and skin lesions. Gonococcal arthritis is usually disseminated and polyarticular. The majority of patients with gonococcal arthritis usually present with symptoms of tenosynovitis, an inflammation of the tendon sheath (62).

Rapid microbiologic assessment of the synovial fluid is the most useful diagnostic procedure in the evaluation of septic arthritis. Any patient who presents with a tender, swollen joint, a limited range of motion, and signs of infection should undergo immediate joint aspiration and drainage. A delay in this procedure can result in permanent destruction of the joint and bone, particularly in children. A Gram stain of the aspirated fluid can assist in differentiating between Gram-positive and Gram-negative infection, although differentiation between streptococci and staphylococci may be difficult, owing to the inability of the latter organism to cluster. Chemical evaluation of the joint leukocyte count can be useful in distinguishing septic arthritis from other causes of in-

Table 70.7.
Clinical Symptoms of Infectious Arthritis

Monoarticular pain
Swelling and redness in the joint
Fever
Chills
Limitation in joint range of motion
Gonococcal syndrome
   Fever
   Skin lesions
   Tenosynovitis

flammatory joint reaction such as gout, pseudogout, and rheumatoid arthritis. Synovial leukocyte counts in infectious arthritis are usually similar to the peripheral blood count. In patients with bacterial infection the ratio of polymorphonuclear neutrophil leukocytes in synovial fluid is generally higher (59, 61).

Evaluation of blood cultures may yield positive results in up to 35 to 40% of patients (61). Positive blood cultures for gonococci are not as reliable, occurring in only 3% of the cases. N. gonorrhoeae, however, may be recovered from other infectious sites, such as the genitourinary tract, in 50 to 80% of cases of gonococcal arthritis (62). The ESR is elevated in the majority of patients and can reach levels greater than 100 mm/hr (61).

Early roentgenographic evaluation of the joint is generally nonspecific, showing only joint effusion or soft tissue swelling. Radionuclide imaging, such as technetium-99 and gallium-67 citrate scanning, is also used in the diagnosis of infectious arthritis. As in osteomyelitis, the technetium-99 scan may be positive for inflammatory reactions as a result of noninfectious etiologies. In this situation the gallium scan may be more useful (16).

Medical Management

Appropriate medical management of septic arthritis involves a comprehensive microbiologic assessment, antibiotic therapy, and aspiration and immobilization of the joint. Prompt initiation of these measures will avoid destruction of the cartilage and permanent disabling damage to the joint.

Initial microbiologic evaluations should include a Gram stain to determine the morphology of the organism until definitive culture results can be obtained. If the Gram stain and cultures cannot be performed, empiric therapy should be started. Factors such as age, clinical manifestations, and underlying disease states should be considered in choosing an appropriate regimen.

Antibiotic Therapy

Initial therapy for infectious arthritis should always include an agent to cover S. aureus. For newborns who are less than 1 month of age, empiric therapy should begin with a penicillinase-resistant penicillin (Table 70.8). A third-generation cephalosporin such as cefotaxime should be added to cover Gram-negative bacilli such as E. coli (57). For infants and young children a second-generation cephalosporin such as cefuroxime is a good choice for empiric therapy, since this agent is active against the two most predominant pathogens, S. aureus and H. influenzae, including β-lactamase-producing strains (7). Third-generation cephalosporins such as cefotaxime, ceftizoxime, or ceftriaxone are also very active against H. influenzae and would be useful in the treatment of bacterial arthritis when this organism is suspected (57).

Table 70.8.
Empiric Antibiotic Therapy for the Treatment of Bacterial Arthritis

Age Group	Likely Organisms	Antibiotics of Choice (Dose, Route, and Frequency of Administration)
Neonates (<4 weeks)	S. aureus Group B streptococcus Enterobacteriaceae	Nafcillin or oxacillin 50 mg/kg/day i.v. q12h plus cefotaxime 100–150 mg/kg/day i.v. q12h
Infants and children (1 month to 5 years)	H. influenzae S. aureus Streptococcus species[a]	Cefuroxime 75–150 mg/kg/day i.v. q8h or nafcillin or oxacillin 150 mg/kg/day or cefazolin 40 mg/kg/day q8h plus cefotaxime[b] 100–200 mg/kg/day i.v. q8h
Children and adolescents (5–16 years)	S. aureus Group A streptococcus Occasionally Gram-negative bacteria	Nafcillin or oxacillin 100–200 mg/kg/day i.v. q6h or cefazolin 50–100 mg/kg/day i.v. q8h
Sexually active adults Adults with underlying illness, immunosuppressed	N. gonorrhoeae S. aureus Enterobacteriaceae P. aeruginosa Streptococcus spp.	Ceftriaxone 1 g i.v. qd Nafcillin or oxacillin 150 mg/kg day i.v. q6h or cefazolin 150 mg/kg/day i.v. q8h plus piperacillin 200–300 mg/kg/day i.v. q4h or ceftazidime 80–100 mg/kg i.v. q8h or monotherapy ticarcillin/clavulanic acid 175 mg/kg/day i.v. q6h

[a]Includes *S. pneumoniae,* Group A and B streptococci.
[b]May substitute ceftizoxime, ceftazidime or ceftriaxone.

For older children and adolescents, *S. aureus* and Group A streptococci have been the most commonly isolated organisms. *H. influenzae,* Enterobacteriaceae, and *N. gonorrhoeae* have occasionally been isolated but are rare. Initial therapy with a penicillinase-resistant penicillin or a first-generation cephalosporin is adequate (7).

When gonococci are suspected in sexually active healthy adults, the Centers for Disease Control and Prevention currently recommends the use of ceftriaxone for treatment (63).

In the adult population, both Gram-positive and Gram-negative organisms, including *P. aeruginosa,* have been isolated. A reliable Gram stain is the most valuable diagnostic tool for empiric therapy. If Gram-positive cocci are identified, a penicillinase-resistant penicillin or a first-generation cephalosporin is appropriate. When Gram-negative bacilli are suspected or identified, therapy should include an antipseudomonal penicillin such as piperacillin or a third-generation cephalosporin such as ceftazidime. This is particularly true for patients who have known urinary tract infections or sepsis. Ticarcillin/clavulanate may also be useful, since this combination is active against *S. aureus* and most Gram-negative organisms, including *P. aeruginosa.* For hospitalized patients, in whom there is a high prevalence of MRSA, therapy should be initiated with vancomycin (57, 61). Antibiotics can be adjusted pending culture and sensitivity results.

Successful treatment of infectious arthritis is contingent on the antibiotic's ability to adequately penetrate the joint space and achieve sufficient synovial antibacterial levels. In general, penicillins and cephalosporins easily penetrate into joint fluid and achieve synovial concentrations similar to those measured in the serum. This is in contrast to aminoglycosides, the activity of which is decreased in joint fluid, despite achieving adequate

concentrations. This poor activity is related to low pH and to the presence of purulent material in the synovium, both of which reduce the antibacterial activity in this group of agents. Therefore, aminoglycosides should generally be avoided in the treatment of infectious arthritis. For these reasons, β-lactam antibiotics are considered the first-line agents for treating infections of the joint (61).

To ensure adequate treatment, high-dose parenteral antibiotics should be administered for a minimum of 14 days, although the precise length of therapy usually depends on the organism being treated. For example, streptococci and haemophilus spp. generally require no more than 2 weeks of therapy, whereas staphylococci and Gram-negative organisms should be treated for at least 4 weeks. *P. aeruginosa* may require as much as 6 to 8 weeks of therapy for adults. Gonococcal arthritis responds quite well to ceftriaxone therapy and can be treated in as little as 1 week. Direct installation of antibiotics into the joint space is not recommended, since this can result in chemical synovitis (59).

Oral antibiotics have been used successfully without recurrence in the treatment of infectious arthritis. As in osteomyelitis, oral antibiotic therapy provides less costly treatment and is more convenient for the patient than parenteral antibiotics. Only oral antibiotics that have adequate absorption to provide sufficient bactericidal concentrations should be considered. Similarly, patient compliance and follow-up are of paramount importance. It is recommended that bactericidal titers of 1:8 should be achieved to ensure adequate killing (38, 61).

Adjunctive Therapy

In addition to antibiotic therapy, closed-needle arthrocentesis is indicated as adjunctive therapy. The removal of purulent material containing harmful enzymes and bacterial toxins not only reduces the risk of further damage to cartilage but also improves the antibiotic activity. Aspiration of the joint may be performed repeatedly if needed. Closed-needle aspiration is generally preferred over surgical drainage. Exceptions are in the cases of septic arthritis of the hip, in which needle aspiration is often anatomically difficult to perform, or when the purulent material is too thick to pass through the standard aspiration needle (55).

Immobilization of the joint also plays a key factor in successful treatment by helping to decrease inflammation, relieve pain, and reduce the risk of further damage. Larger weight-bearing joints may require splints or traction for initial immobilization. When the inflammation subsides, the patient may begin slow passive range of movements to prevent permanent disability or contracture. Use of weight-bearing joints is recommended only when all signs of the inflammatory process have ceased and no effusion is observed (7, 61).

Prognosis

The overall prognosis for septic arthritis is generally favorable. Nongonococcal septic arthritis has been associated with a mortality rate of 10%. The majority of deaths occur in patients with underlying risk factors such as sepsis, rheumatoid arthritis, and malignancy. Functional impairment or continuation of infection has been reported in as many as 25 to 33% of children and adults.

The successful outcome of the infection is usually contingent on several factors. For example, the prognosis for children is correlated with several parameters, such as the particular joint involved, type of organism, adequate drainage, appropriate antibiotic coverage, and time of initiation of treatment relative to the onset of symptoms. Infections of the hip are associated with the highest rate of sequelae, and the morbidity in these cases may not be evident until months or years later. The patient may display such signs as limitation in motion, joint fusion, deformity, and limb shortening. S. aureus is the organism that has the greatest propensity for causing chronic problems (55, 59).

The delay in seeking appropriate medical care has often been cited as a major predictor for long-term morbidity, although this prognostic indicator has been challenged in regard to children (55). In adults the outcome of treatment is considerably poorer if the offending organism is not eradicated from the synovial fluid within 6 days of initiating therapy or if the patient is over 60 years old (61).

Conclusion

Infectious arthritis is a serious infection of the joint and surrounding tissue that requires immediate treatment to prevent permanent damage. Most infections are transmitted through the blood from distant foci. Patients who have previous joint damage, as from rheumatoid arthritis, osteoarthritis, gout, and trauma, also appear to be at risk. The most common causative organism is S. aureus,

although other pathogens such as Enterobacteriaceae, P. aeruginosa, and N. gonorrhoeae have also been isolated. Treatment of infectious arthritis involves prompt aspiration of the joint fluid, rapid identification of the organism, and appropriate antibiotic therapy. Most β-lactam antimicrobial agents achieve therapeutic concentrations in joint spaces. The duration of therapy can range from 7 to 21 days, depending on the offending pathogen. Further needle aspiration may be required during therapy. Immobilization of the joint is recommended to prevent the risk of further damage to the joint and surrounding cartilage. Infectious arthritis retains an overall favorable prognosis when the appropriate medical management is provided.

REFERENCES

1. Waldvogel FA, Medoff C, Swartz M. Osteomyelitis: a review of clinical features, therapeutic considerations, and unusual aspects. N Engl J Med 282:198–206, 1970.
2. Nelson JD. Acute osteomyelitis in children. Infect Dis Clin North Am 4:513, 1990.
3. Anderson JR, Scobie WG, Watt B. The treatment of acute osteomyelitis in children: a 10-year experience. J Antimicrob Chemother 7(suppl A):43–50, 1981.
4. Kerstein MD. Osteomyelitis associated with vascular insufficiency. Curr Ther Res Clin Exp 16:306–310, 1974.
5. Anthony JP, Mathes SJ. Update on chronic osteomyelitis. Clin Plast Surg 18(3):515–522, 1991.
6. Waldvogel FA, Vasey H. Osteomyelitis: the past decade. N Engl J Med 303:360–370, 1980.
7. Dagan R. Management of acute hematogenous osteomyelitis and septic arthritis in the pediatric patient. Pediatr Infect Dis J 12:88–93, 1993.
8. Jackson MA, Nelson JD. Etiology and medical management of acute suppurative bone and joint infections in pediatric patients. J Pediatr Orthop 2:313–323, 1982.
9. Hughes LO, Aronson J. Skeletal infections in children. Curr Opin Pediatr 6:90–93, 1994.
10. Dirschl DR, Almekinders LC. Osteomyelitis: common causes and treatment recommendations. Drugs 45(1):29–43, 1993.
11. Bamburger DM. Osteomyelitis: a common sense approach to antibiotic and surgical treatment. Postgrad Med 94(5):177–184, 1993.
12. Cierny G. Classification and treatment of adult osteomyelitis. In: Evarts CMC, ed. Surgery of musculoskeletal system. 2nd ed., vol. 5. London: Churchill Livingston, 1990:4337–4380.
13. Wald ER. Risk factors for osteomyelitis. Am J Med 78(suppl 6B):206–212, 1985.
14. Puczynski MS, Dvonch VM, Menendez CE. Osteomyelitis of the great toe secondary to phlebotomy. Clin Orthop 190:239–240, 1985.
15. Sugarman B, Hawes S. Musher DM, et al. Osteomyelitis beneath pressure sores. Ann Intern Med 143:683–688, 1983.
16. Gutman L. Acute, subacute and chronic osteomyelitis and pyogenic arthritis in children. Curr Probl Pediatr 15(12):1–72, 1985.
17. Norden CW. Lessons learned from animal models of osteomyelitis. Rev Infect Dis 10:103–110, 1988.
18. Marrie TJ, Costerton JW. Mode of growth of bacterial pathogens in chronic polymicrobial human osteomyelitis. J Clin Microbiol 22:924–933, 1985.
19. Roberts JM, Drummond JS, Breed AL, et al. Subacute hematogenous osteomyelitis in children: a retrospective study. J Pediatr Orthop 2:249–254, 1982.
20. Braun TL, Lorber B. Chronic osteomyelitis. In: Schlossberg D, ed. Orthopedic infections. New York: Springer-Verlag, 1988:9–20.

21. Israel O, Gips S, Jerushalmi J, et al. Osteomyelitis and soft tissue infection: differential diagnosis with 24 hr/ratio of Tc-m MDP uptake. Radiology 163:725, 1987.

22. Schuwauker DS, Park HM, Mock BH, et al. Evaluation of complicating osteomyelitis with Tc-99m MDP, IN-111 granulocytes and GA-67 citrate. J Nucl Med 25:849–853, 1984.

23. Magid D. Computed tomographic imaging of the musculoskeletal system. Radiol Clin North Am 32:255–273, 1994.

24. Tuazon CU. Teichoic acid antibodies in osteomyelitis and septic arthritis caused by *Staphylococcus aureus*. J Bone Surg 64(A):762–765, 1982.

25. Wise FA, Tosolin FA. Detection of teichoic acid antibodies in *Staphylococcus aureus* infections. Pathology 24(2):102–108, 1992.

26. Gentry LD. Role for newer beta-lactam antibiotics in the treatment of osteomyelitis. Am J Med 78(suppl 6A):134–139, 1985.

27. Stratton CW, Kernodle DS, Eades SO, et al. Evaluation of cefotaxime alone and in combination with desacetyl cefotaxime against strains of *Staphylococcus aureus* that produce variants of staphylococcal beta-lactamase. Diagn Microbiol Infect Dis 12:57–65, 1989.

28. Tice AD. Osteomyelitis. Hosp Prac 28(suppl)2:36–39, 1993.

29. Glover SC, Padfield C, McKendrick MW, et al. Acute osteomyelitis in a district general hospital. Lancet 1:609–611, 1982.

30. Kaplan SL, Mason EO, Feigin RD. Clindamycin versus nafcillin or methicillin in the treatment of *Staphylococcus aureus* osteomyelitis in children. South Med J 75:138–143, 1982.

31. Sheftel, TG, Mader JT, Pennick JJ. Methicillin-resistant *Staphylococcus aureus,* osteomyelitis. Clin Orthop 198:231–239, 1985.

32. Weinberg WG. Safety and efficacy of teicoplanin for bone and joint infections: results of a community-based trial. South Med J 86(8):891–897, 1993.

33. Mathisen GE. Bone and joint infections. In: Finegold SM, George WL, eds. Anaerobic infections in humans. San Diego: Academic Press, 1989:507–527.

34. Templeton WC, Wawrukiewicz A, Melo JC. Anaerobic osteomyelitis of long bone. Rev Infect Dis 5:692–712, 1983.

35. Alvarez OM, Childs EJ. Pressure ulcers: physical, supportive, and local aspects of management. Clin Podiatr Med Surg 8(4):869–890, 1991.

36. Black J, Hunt HL, Godley PJ, et al. Oral antimicrobial therapy for adults with osteomyelitis or septic arthritis. J Infect Dis 155:968–972, 1987.

37. Gentry LO. Prescribing considerations in fluoroquinolone therapy. Pharmacother 12:398–488, 1993.

38. Prober CG, Yeager AS. Use of the serum bactericidal titer to assess the adequacy of oral antibiotic therapy in the treatment of acute hematogenous osteomyelitis. J Pediatr 95:131–135, 1979.

39. Gentry LD, Rodriquez GG. Oral ciprofloxacin compared with parenteral antibiotics in the treatment of osteomyelitis. Antimicrob Agents Chemother 34:40–43, 1990.

40. Sable CA, Scheld WM. Fluoroquinolones: how to use (but not overuse) these antibiotics. Geriatrics 48:41–51, 1993.

41. Bach MC, Cocchetto DM. Ceftazidime as single-agent therapy for gram-negative aerobic bacillary osteomyelitis. Antimicrob Agents Chemother 31:1605–1608, 1987.

42. Gentry LO. Antibiotic therapy for osteomyelitis. In: Norden CW, ed. Infectious disease clinics of North America. Philadelphia: WB Saunders, 1990:3–499.

43. Dich VQ, Nelson JD, Holtelin KC. Osteomyelitis in infants and children. Am J Dis Child 129:1273–1278, 1975.

44. Norden CW. Osteomyelitis. In: Mandell GL, Douglas RG, Bennett JE, eds. Principles and practice of infectious diseases. 3rd ed. New York: John Wiley, 1990:903–922.

45. Wagner VQ, Collier BD, Rytel MW. Long term intravenous antibiotic therapy in chronic osteomyelitis. Arch Intern Med 145:1073–1078, 1985.

46. Brown RB. Selection and training of patients for outpatient intravenous antibiotic therapy. Rev Infect Dis 13(suppl 2):S147–S151, 1991.

47. Tice AD. An office model of outpatient parenteral antibiotic therapy. Rev Infect Dis 12(suppl 2):S184–S188, 1991.

48. Smego RA, Grainer BR. Home intravenous antimicrobial therapy provided by community hospital and a university hospital. Am J Hosp Pharm 42:2185–2189, 1985.

49. Fitzgerald RH. Antibiotic distribution in normal and osteomyelitic bone. Orthop Clin North Am 15:537–545, 1984.

50. Perry HP, Ritterbusch JK, Burdge RE, et al. Cefamandole levels in serum and necrotic bone. Clin North Am 15:537–545, 1984.

51. Henry SL, Seligson D, Mangino P, Popham GJ. Antibiotic-impregnated beads. I: bead inplantation versus systemic therapy. Orthop Rev 20(3):242–7, 1991.

52. Popham GJ, Mangino P, Seligson D, Henry SL. Antibiotic-impregnated beads. II: factors in antibiotic selection. Orthop Rev 20(4):331–337, 1991.

53. Kindwall ER. Uses of hyperbaric oxygen therapy in the 1990s. Cleve Clin J Med 59:517–528, 1992.

54. Calhoun JH, Cobos JA, Mader JT. Does hyperbaric oxygen have a place in the treatment of osteomyelitis? Orthop Clin North Am 22:467–471, 1991.

55. Waldvogel FA. Treatment of osteomyelitis and septic arthritis. Bull NY Acad Med 58:733–749, 1982.

56. Shaw BA, Kasser JR. Acute septic arthritis in infancy and childhood. Clin Orthop 257:212–225, 1990.

57. Brooks GF, Pons VG. Septic arthritis. In: Hoeprich PD, Jordan MC, Ronald AR, eds. Infectious diseases, 5th ed. Philadelphia: JB Lippincott, 1994:1382–1389.

58. Inman RD, Gallegos KV, Brause BD, et al. Clinical and microbiological features of prosthetic joint infections. Am J Med 77:47–53, 1994.

59. Freeland AE, Senter BC. Septic arthritis and osteomyelitis. Hand Clin 5:533–552, 1989.

60. Goldenberg DL. Septic arthritis and other infections of rheumatologic significance. Rheum Dis Clin North Am 17(1):49–56, 1991.

61. Smith JW. Infectious arthritis. Inf Dis Clin North Am 4(3):523–538, 1990.

62. Keat AK. Sexually transmitted arthritis syndromes. Med Clin North Am 74(6):1617–1631, 1990.

63. Anonymous. 1993 sexually transmitted diseases treatment guidelines. Morbid Mortal Week Rep 42(RR-14), September 24, 1993.

CHAPTER 71

SEXUALLY TRANSMITTED DISEASES

THOMAS C. HARDIN

Sexually transmitted diseases (STDs), which are occasionally referred to as venereal diseases, are infections that are caused by a variety of pathogenic microorganisms, as summarized in Table 71.1. These diseases are generally grouped together because they are spread through sexual contact, although sexual contact is not the only means of disease transmission. It is generally accepted that patients with one sexually transmitted disease are at greater risk for the development of other sexually transmitted diseases, either concurrently or at some later point in time. Additionally, sexual partners of patients with diagnosed STDs are at high risk for the development of STDs. Over the past decade, primarily because of concern about transmission of the human immunodeficiency virus (HIV), much effort has been directed toward changes in sexual practices to reduce the potential for transmission of disease by sexual contact (1). Nevertheless, sexually transmitted diseases continue to be an important public health concern, with annual costs for treatment of non-AIDS STDs in the United States of over 5 billion dollars (2).

This chapter has been organized into three general sections: a review of common urethritis syndromes, discussion of infections associated with genital ulceration, and limited comments on some other less common sexually transmitted diseases. Several diseases that are transmitted by sexual contact, such as hepatitis, HIV infection, and AIDS, and parasitic infections are discussed in other chapters of this text.

Several general treatment goals are applicable to the clinical management of all patients with sexually transmitted diseases. Important treatment objectives include eradication of the infectious pathogen, elimination or reduction of symptoms, prevention of associated long-term sequelae, and interuption of disease transmission. The recommended therapeutic options discussed are aimed at these goals. It is important to remember also that for every patient with an STD requiring therapy, there is at least one and often several infected sexual partners who should be identified and treated.

URETHRITIS SYNDROMES

The sexually transmitted disease that is most commonly seen in STD clinics, student health care facilities, and private practice offices is urethritis, or inflammation of the urethra, which usually presents clinically as a urethral discharge that may be accompanied by dysuria or burning on urination. Clinically, urethritis is usually divided into either gonococcal or nongonococcal syndromes on the basis of the infecting pathogen. Nationwide, nongonococcal urethritis is much more common than gonococcal urethritis (gonorrhea) (3). However, gonorrhea tends to be seen more frequently in STD clinics, possibly because of differences in socioeconomic factors.

While the usual clinical features of gonococcal and nongonococcal urethritis differ to some degree, as shown in Table 71.2, there is sufficient overlap in presentation to make distinguishing between the two syndromes difficult (4). The incubation period for gonococcal urethritis can be as short as a few days; the majority of cases develop symptoms within a week of the initial infection. By contrast, the clinical symptoms of nongonococcal urethritis usually develop gradually over the course of several weeks. While the presence of a urethral discharge is characteristic of both gonococcal and nongonococcal urethritis, the nature of the discharge may be useful in distinguishing between the two syndromes. With gonococcal urethritis the discharge is obviously purulent and often associated with painful, burning urination. The discharge seen in nongonococcal urethritis is typically mucoid or mucopurulent, and dysuria is present in fewer than 50% of cases. A clear urethral discharge suggests nongonococcal urethritis.

Gonorrhea

Gonorrhea is the most common communicable disease in the United States, particularly in young adults between the ages of 16 and 30 (5). The actual incidence of gonorrhea is unclear because of the large number of asymptomatic carriers and unreported cases. The infection, which primarily affects the epithelium and mucous membranes of the lower genital tract, may also involve the oropharynx and anus. It is caused by *Neisseria gonorrhoeae*, a Gram-negative aerobic coccus that usually grows in pairs (diplococci). Humans appear to be the only natural host for this intracellular pathogen. Transmission of gonorrhea is almost always by sexual intercourse, though perinatal transmission of the disease may occur. The incidence of gonorrhea is reported to be 10 times greater in nonwhites than in whites. Other risk factors for gonorrhea include low socioeconomic status, urban residence, single marital status, and a previous history of gonococcal infections. The rate of male to female transmission of gonorrhea during

Table 71.1.
Sexually Transmitted Pathogens and Associated Disease

Pathogen	Clinical Syndrome/Disease
Bacteria	
Neisseria gonorrhoeae	Gonorrhea
Treponema pallidum	Syphilis
Haemophilus ducreyi	Chancroid
Calymmatobacterium granulomatis	Granuloma inguinale
Gardnerella vaginalis	Nonspecific vaginitis
Mycoplasma	
Ureaplasma urealyticum	Nongonococcal urethritis
Chlamydia	
Chlamydia trachomatis	Nongonococcal urethritis
	Lymphogranuloma venereum
Virus	
Herpes simplex	Herpes genitalis
Human immunodeficiency virus	AIDS
Hepatitis A, B, and C	Hepatitis
Human papillomavirus	Condylomata acuminata
Poxvirus	Molluscum contagiosum
Parasites	
Trichomonas vaginalis	Trichomoniasis
	Nonspecific vaginitis
Giardia lamblia	Giardiasis
Entamoeba histolytica	Amebiasis
Phthirus pubis	Pediculosis
Sarcoptes scabiei	Scabies

sexual intercourse is reported to be higher than transmission from female to male. The risk of transmission from an infected female to her male partner approaches 20% per episode of unprotected vaginal intercourse; transmission risk from an infected male to his female partner has been reported to be closer to 50% per episode (6).

CLINICAL PRESENTATION AND DIAGNOSIS

As was mentioned above, the clinical presentation of gonorrhea, or gonococcal urethritis, is usually characterized by profuse, purulent urethral discharge that is associated with dysuria. Many cases of gonorrhea in men are asymptomatic and resolve spontaneously over the course of several weeks without specific treatment. However, up to 10% of untreated cases may be further complicated by the development of acute epididymitis, periurethral abscess, acute prostatitis, seminal vesiculitis, or urethral strictures. In women, gonorrhea primarily involves the endocervix as well as the urethra. Most women will develop acute symptoms within 10 days of infection, consisting of increased vaginal discharge and dysuria. Progression to salpingitis may occur in up to 15% of untreated women and usually is characterized by the development of acute abdominal or pelvic pain. In addition, over 40% of women with gonorrhea are also coinfected with *Chlamydia trachomatis* and/or *Trichomonas vaginalis* (5). Approximately 15% of women with untreated gonorrhea will progress to develop pelvic inflammatory disease, which may be associated with

infertility and ectopic pregnancies if inadequately managed.

Infectious involvement of other body sites by *N. gonorrhoeae* can also be seen. Pharyngeal gonococcal infection, developed following orogenital sexual activity with an infected partner, is more common in females and homosexual males. The presentation is often asymptomatic, but symptoms resembling acute streptococcal pharyngitis may occur. Anorectal gonorrhea is reported to accompany gonococcal urethritis in up to 40% of women and homosexual men. Anal transmission of *N. gonorrhoeae* in women is generally by perianal contamination with vaginal discharge, while in men it is through receptive anal intercourse with an infected partner. Most cases of anorectal gonorrhea are asymptomatic, but anal pruritus, constipation, tenesmus, and rectal bleeding have been observed in association with this condition (6). Ocular gonococcal infection most frequently involves the conjunctiva and is often considered secondary to autoinoculation from fingers contaminated through sexual contact with an individual with urogenital gonorrhea. Gonococcal conjunctivitis may be serious and requires timely initiation of aggressive antibiotic therapy to prevent corneal ulceration. Disseminated gonococcal infection secondary to hematogenous spread is uncommon but is often considered the cause of septic arthritis in otherwise healthy young adults. Most patients with disseminated gonococcal infection do not have signficant fevers or elevated white blood cell counts but do frequently present with monoarticular arthritic complaints in the wrist, knee, or ankle (any joint can be involved). In addition, a striking pustular, erythematous rash, located primarily on the extremities, is also common in patients with bacteremia secondary to *N. gonorrhoeae* (5, 6).

Newborns who are exposed to gonococci in utero or during delivery are at risk for the development of gonococcal ophthalmia neonatorum, a sight-threatening infection of the conjunctiva. Fortunately, this condition is rare today in the United States because of the use of aggressive ophthalmia prophylaxis following delivery.

Table 71.2.
Comparison of Usual Clinical Presentation of Urethritis Syndromes

Characteristic	Gonococcal Urethritis	Nongonococcal Urethritis
Incubation	Frequently short (days)	More prolonged (weeks)
Onset of symptoms	Rapid	Gradual
Discharge	Purulent	Mucoid
Gram stain of discharge	Gram-negative intracellular cocci	Many neutrophils, no bacteria
Presence of dysuria	More common	Less common

The diagnosis of gonorrhea is best made by identification of *N. gonorrhoeae* from a specimen taken from an involved site. In women, cultures taken from the cervix produce the highest yield, but urethral cultures are also acceptable. Men should have both urethral and anal cultures performed. Cultures can become positive within 24 to 48 hr, yielding the diagnosis. Culturing of the organism is not only important for diagnosis; in areas where drug-resistant *N. gonorrhoeae* is a concern, susceptibility testing may be important in determining therapeutic options (5, 7). An alternative diagnostic technique that is frequently used in clinics to evaluate the collected specimen is Gram staining. If intracellular Gram-negative diplococci are observed, a presumptive diagnosis of gonorrhea is made, pending confirmation by subsequent culture. In males, Gram-stain evaluation of the urethral discharge is both highly sensitive and highly specific; therefore, culture confirmation is not considered necessary. However, the Gram-stain is not considered acceptable as the sole method to diagnose gonococcal infection of the pharynx or rectum or in women with endocervical infection

(6). Rapid diagnostic tests based on detection of gonococcal antigens or cellular components do not have better sensitivity or specificity than Gram stain and culture and are therefore rarely used.

TREATMENT

A number of treatment options for the management of gonococcal disease are available to the practicing clinician. Most cephalosporins, fluoroquinolones, and macrolides have potent in vitro and in vivo activity against *N. gonorrhoeae*. Historically, penicillins, tetracyclines, and sulfonamides were used widely as therapy for gonococcal infections, but widespread resistance now prevents their clinical use. Table 71.3 summarizes the current Centers for Disease Control (CDC) treatment recommendations for gonococcal infections (8). Since there are several choices, selection of a specific therapeutic regimen must be based on careful consideration of efficacy and safety, patient preference, and costs.

Many clinicians consider intramuscular ceftriaxone to be the treatment of choice for noncomplicated gonorrhea;

Table 71.3.
Current Treatment Recommendations for Gonococcal Infections

Diagnosis	Drug Regimen	Cost[a]	Alternatives/Comments
Uncomplicated gonorrhea	Ceftriaxone 125 mg IM as single dose Or	$5.30	Spectinomycin 2 g IM as single dose in patients who cannot tolerate first line medications, but it should not be used alone for pharyngeal infection; other quinolones may also be used, as can other oral and parenteral second- and third-generation cephalosporins; quinolone antibiotics contraindicated in pregnancy and children.
	Cefixime 400 mg PO as single dose Or	$6.00	
	Ciprofloxacin 500 mg PO as single dose Or	$3.00	
	Ofloxacin 400 mg PO as single dose PLUS	$3.50	
	Doxycycline 100 mg PO bid × 7 days Or	$4.00[b]	
	Azithromycin 1000 mg PO as single dose	$32.50	
Disseminated gonococcal infection (adults)	Ceftriaxone 1 gm IM/IV q 24 hr Or	$30.70	Spectinomycin 2 mg IM q 12 hr can be used for persons with β-lactam allergy.
	Cefotaxime 1 mg IV q 8 hr Or	$34.35	
	Ceftizoxime 1 gm IV q 8 hr	$34.20	
Continue for 24–48 hr after clinical improvement, then continue therapy for 7 more days with either:			
	Cefixime 400 mg PO bid Or	$12.00	
	Ciprofloxacin 500 mg PO bid	$6.00	
Disseminated gonococcal infection (infants)	Ceftriaxon 25–50 mg/kg IV/IM in single daily dose for 7 days Or	$ variable	Treatment should be continued for 10–14 days if meningitis is present.
	Cefotaxime 25 mg/kg IV/IM q 12 hr for 7 days	$ variable	
Gonococcal ophthalmia neonatorum	Ceftriaxone 25–50 mg/kg IV/IM as a single dose (up to 125 mg)	$ variable	Topical therapy alone is inadequate and is not necessary with systemic antibiotic therapy.
Gonococcal conjunctivitis (adult)	Ceftriaxone 1 gm IM as single dose	$30.70	Infected eye should also be flushed with saline.

Source: From (7, 8).
[a]Based on 1994 Red Book AWP for daily drug costs or total drug costs for single dose regimens.
[b]Variable based on generic availability of doxycycline.

this choice is based on extensive clinical evaluations demonstrating effective clearing of gonococcal infections from all sites (5, 7). Also, resistance to ceftriaxone has not been reported to date, so concern about potential treatment failure due to inactivity of the selected therapeutic agent is reduced. Previous treatment guidelines recommended an intramuscular ceftriaxone dose of 250 mg, but single doses as low as 62.5 mg have been reported to produce 100% cure rates in noncomplicated gonorrhea (7). The currently recommended ceftraixone regimen of 125 mg allows for a smaller volume for intramuscular injection and a lower drug cost. There is also limited data suggesting that intramuscular ceftriaxone provides adequate coverage for incubating syphilis as well, a characteristic that other treatment options do not have (9).

Cefixime is the only oral cephalosporin that is recommended for the treatment of gonococcal infections. An oral cefixime dose of 400 mg is effective for urethral disease but has not been well studied for pharyngeal infection and does not provide activity against incubating syphilis (10).

The fluoroquinolones, ciprofloxacin and ofloxacin, are also effective and inexpensive oral alternatives for the treatment of uncomplicated gonorrhea but are contraindicated for use during pregnancy and for children under the age of 18. Ofloxacin, unlike ciprofloxacin, is active against *C. trachomatis* but requires prolonged dosing for successful treatment of chlamydial infections. The fluoroquinolones provide no activity against *T. pallidum*. Gonococcal resistance to the fluoroquinolones has been widely reported in Asia, Australia, and the United Kingdom, and there have been reports of decreasing susceptibility to fluoroquinolones in several regions of the United States (11).

Recently, a 95% cure rate for uncomplicated gonorrhea with a single 2000-mg oral dose of azithromycin was reported (12). Unfortunately, azithromycin is expensive and causes too much gastrointestinal intolerance to be considered an option for routine treatment of gonorrhea. However, it may prove useful for patients who are unable to tolerate standard therapies. One benefit of a single dose of azithromycin for gonorrhea is that it also provides coverage for any chlamydial infection that may be present.

Spectinomycin was once a commonly used alternative to β-lactam treatment of gonorrhea. Today it is useful only for patients with urogenital or anal infections who are unable to tolerate therapy with either a cephalosporin or fluoroquinolone (5, 7).

Disseminated gonococcal infections are best treated with a prolonged course of intravenous ceftriaxone, cefotaxime, or ceftizoxime. Therapy should be continued for 24 to 48 hr after significant clinical improvement, then followed with a suitable oral agent for another 7 days. Gonococcal endocarditis and meningitis require several weeks of intravenous antibiotic therapy (6). Topical therapy with either 1% silver nitrate, 1% tetracycline, or 0.5% erythromycin, as recommended by the American Academy of Pediatrics for immediate postpartum administration to all newborns, is insufficient to treat gonococcal ophthalmia neonatorum in a baby born to a mother with active gonorrhea. A single intramuscular or intravenous dose of ceftriaxone appears to be adequate treatment for both gonococcal ophthalmia neonatorum and gonococcal conjunctivitis in adults (5).

Routine follow-up is not necessary for patients who are treated with a regimen recommended in the CDC guidelines because of the very low treatment failure rates that have been reported. Patients who are treated with alternative regimens should be evaluated within 3 to 7 days to ensure resolution of symptoms. In most cases, persistence of clinical signs and symptoms indicates reinfection rather than treatment failure or may indicate coinfection with another infectious pathogen, such as *C. trachomatis*. In either case the patient needs another diagnostic workup along with aggressive identification and treatment of all recent sexual partners.

Nongonococcal Urethritis

Sexually transmitted urethritis can also be caused by organisms other than *N. gonorrhoeae*. When these organisms are considered as a group, nongonococcal urethritis is more frequent in the United States today than is gonorrhea. The most common cause of nongonococcal urethritis, responsible for up to 55% of cases, is *Chlamydia trachomatis*, an obligate intracellular parasite that has features of both bacteria and viruses (13, 14). *Chlamydia* spp., like viruses, requires host cellular material for replication, yet maintain their cellular identity like bacteria. It is estimated that almost 50% of individuals with gonorrhea are coinfected with *C. trachomatis*. The most common cause of postgonococcal urethritis in heterosexuals is chlamydia (15). Other pathogens that can also produce a urethritis syndrome include the bacteria *Ureaplasma urealyticum*, identified in approximately 20 to 40% of cases, and the parasite *Trichomonas vaginalis*, seen in fewer than 10% of patients (13, 14). However, approximately 20 to 30% of men with urethretis will fail to demonstrate either gonococcal or common nongonococcal pathogens on evaluation. These cases of urethritis may be due to yeasts, viruses, and other bacteria that are difficult to culture or identify (13).

CLINICAL PRESENTATION AND DIAGNOSIS

As was stated above, the clinical presentation of nongonococcal urethritis cannot be distinguished easily from the clinical features of gonococcal urethritis. Common symptoms of nongonococcal urethritis in men include dysuria, polyuria, and the presence of a mucoid urethral discharge that occur within several weeks after exposure (13). The majority of women with chlamydial urethral infections are clinically asymptomatic, making the identification of these individuals almost impossible (15).

The identification of the infecting organism for most cases of nongonococcal urethritis is hampered because the two most common pathogens associated with nongonococcal urethritis, *C. trachomatis* and *U. urealyticum*, cannot be cultured by routine laboratory procedures. Therefore, the diagnosis of nongonococcal urethritis has generally depended on the presence of a characteristic urethral discharge (microscopically greater than 4 polymorphonuclear leukocytes per oil immersion field on a smear of an intraurethral swab specimen), the exclusion of gonorrhea, and a clinical response to therapy. Serologic tests that are specific for chlamydia and tissue-culturing techniques appear to be unnecessary for the management of STDs in general clinical practice (13). Rapid office tests using an enzyme immunoassay for the diagnosis of chlamydia infections are now available and are reported to offer excellent sensitivity and specificity (16).

TREATMENT

A number of antibiotic regimens have been evaluated for the clinical managment of nongonococcal urethritis. According to these studies and generaly clinical experience, the optimal drug, dosage, and duration of therapy remain uncertain. The recent CDC treatment guidelines for sexually transmitted diseases recommend a regimen of doxycycline 100 mg orally twice a day for 7 days (8). Azithromycin orally as a single 1000-mg dose is equivalent to doxycycline in the treatment of nongonococcal urethritis (17, 18). Both doxycycline and azithromycin have cure rates greater than 95% in cases of nongonococcal urethritis (19). With doxycycline the clinician has a very inexpensive 7-day regimen but one that requires patient compliance because of multiple daily dosing. The toxicities of doxycycline are mild, nausea and vomiting being the most commonly reported and phototoxicity a potential concern. Azithromycin represents an expensive alternative. A single 1000-mg oral dose can be administered under direct patient observation to ensure compliance. It has a very acceptable side effect profile, diarrhea, nausea, dizziness, and headache being reported in fewer than 3% of treated patients.

Alternative regimens that have been indicated by the CDC include erythromycin base 500 mg and erythromycin ethylsuccinate 800 mg orally four times a day for 7 days (8). Many patients cannot tolerate these high doses of erythromycin because of gastrointestinal side effects. If necessary, lower dosages of 250 mg for the base or 400 mg for the ethylsuccinate salt can be used, but the duration of treatment should be extended to 14 days (13). If a pregnant woman needs treatment of nongonococcal urethritis, erythromycin base should be used.

Ofloxacin has been studied clinically in the treatment of nongonococcal urethritis. On the basis of the limited data available, ofloxacin appears to be similar to doxycycline in efficacy, with treatment success rates of nearly 100% (19, 20). The dose of ofloxacin that has been used most often is 100 mg orally twice daily for 7 days. Larger doses (up to 400 mg/day) administered for shorter periods of time (5 days) have also been used for a limited number of patients. Ofloxacin currently represents a more expensive alternative to doxycycline that does not provide the opportunity for improved patient compliance; therefore its clinical usefulness is limited. Ciprofloxacin has limited activity against *C. trachomatis* and should not be considered a therapeutic option for the treatment of nongonococcal urethritis (21).

As with the treatment of gonorrhea, no specific patient follow-up is required unless symptoms persists after completion of therapy or recur shortly afterward. Patients should be informed to refer recent sexual partners for evaluation and treatment, regardless of the presence of clinical signs and symptoms of infection. Additionally, patients should be instructed to abstain from sexual intercourse until treatment has been completed and there is evidence that the infection has been cured. An alternative to abstinence would be careful use of a condom and a contraceptive foam.

Chlamydia trachomatis can be the cause of sexually transmitted diseases other than nongonococcal urethritis. The CDC recommendations for treatment of any chlamydial STD are summarized in Table 71.4.

Table 71.4. Treatment Recommendations for STDs Caused by *Chlamydia trachomatis*

Diagnosis	Drug Regimen	Alternatives/Comments
Nongonococcal urethritis	Doxycycline 100 mg PO bid for 7 days	Azithromycin 1000 mg PO as a single dose is an expensive alternative; erythromycin base 500 mg or erythromycin ethyl-succinate 400 mg PO qid for 7 days is also effective and is recommended during pregnancy.
Uncomplicated endocervical or rectal infection	Doxycycline (as above) OR Azithromycin 1000 mg PO as a single dose	Ofloxacin 300 mg PO twice daily for 7 days or erythromycin as shown above, especially in pregnancy.
Ophthalmia neonatorum	Erythromycin 50 mg/kg/day PO in 4 divided doses for 10–14 days	
Lymphogranuloma venereum	Doxycycline 100 mg PO every 12 hr for 21 days	Erythromycin base 500 mg PO 4 times a day for 21 days or sulfisoxazole 500 mg PO 4 times a day for 21 days. Surgery may be required for full healing.

ULCEROGENIC GENITAL INFECTIONS

The development of genital ulcerations is associated with several sexually transmitted diseases, particularly syphilis, genital herpes simplex infections, and chancroid. Each of these diseases will be discussed separately.

Syphilis

Syphilis is an important contagious disease that can present clinically with many different manifestations. Therefore it is worthy of the title "the great imposter" (22, 23). Syphilis, or "lues" as it has been called, has played a major role in the development of the New World from the days of Christopher Columbus to modern times. The incidence of syphilis in the United States reached a peak during World War II, then declined following the introduction of penicillin in the late 1940s. In the 1960s the number of reported cases of syphilis rose slightly, then plateaued until the mid-1980s, when the incidence again began to rise. In 1990 over 50,000 cases were reported in the United States, up nearly 10% from 1989 (24). The reported incidence of 20 cases per 100,000 individuals represents a 75% increase from 1985. These recent changes are thought to reflect a reduction in syphilis in homosexual males, while the incidence among heterosexuals is increasing rapidly, particularly in women and newborns. This increase is probably related to a pattern of trading sex for drugs. The majority of new cases occur in 15- to 30-year-old individuals, and many cases present with concurrent infection with the human immunodeficiency virus (HIV). Although syphilis is most commonly transmitted through sexual intercourse, it can also be passed through the placenta (congenital syphilis), by the administration of fresh human blood, by kissing or touching active lesions, or by accidental inoculation (25).

PATHOGENESIS AND CLINICAL PRESENTATION

The spirochete, *Treponema pallidum* subspecies *pallidum*, is the causal agent of syphilis. This unicellular organism is elongated and tightly coiled and divides approximately every 30 hr. The human is the only natural host. Unfortunately, the organism cannot be grown in vitro. The disease is usually transmitted by direct contact with an active infectious lesion, which teems with approximately 10^7 organisms per gram of tissue (23). The organisms can penetrate intact skin or mucous membranes and, within hours, invade regional lymphatics and blood vessels. Dissemination throughout the body is rapid. Any organ system can be infected, including the central nervous system.

Syphilis can be divided clinically into five stages: incubating, primary, secondary, latent, and tertiary (late) syphilis (23, 24, 26). The *incubation* period usually lasts about 3 weeks, appears to be directly related to the size of the inoculum, and may range from 3 days to 3 months.

During this period the individual is asymptomatic and noninfectious, and serologic tests are usually negative.

The hallmark of *primary syphilis* is the development of a painless chancre at the site of initial inoculation, consisting of spirochetes, histiocytes, and plasma cells. Multiple chancres may occur; this feature is usually observed in HIV-infected individuals. Spirochetes can be easily identified by using darkfield microscopy, silver staining, or specific immunofluorescent or immunoperoxidase stains of transudate or tissue from the lesion. Not all patients develop a chancre, and some chancres are atypical in appearance or so small and inconspicuous that they are not noticed. Painless regional lymphadenopathy (bubo) can be present. Chancres quickly erode and ulcerate, developing a smooth base with raised borders that usually heals spontaneously within several weeks, accompanied by resolution of lymphadenopathy.

Secondary syphilis, or disseminated syphilis, is a generalized illness that develops approximately 2 to 8 weeks after contact and may begin before complete resolution of the chancre. The presentation is most often characterized by classic lesions of the skin and mucous membranes (26). The rash most often starts as reddish or copper-colored macular lesions appearing on the truncal extremities but may also appear maculopapular, papular, or pustular. The soles of the feet and palms of the hands are frequently involved. It is not uncommon to also detect similar nonpainful lesions on mucous membranes. These lesions usually persist for up to a week. Generalized lymphadenopathy is also often present. Constitutional symptoms are common and include headache, fever, sore throat, malaise, myalgias, arthralgias, anorexia, and weight loss. Condylomata lata are flat, hypertrophic lesions resembling warts that develop in moist areas and contain spirochetes. Involvement of other organ systems is possible and may include the development of immune-complex glomerulonephritis, syphilitic hepatitis, and synovitis. The central nervous system (CNS) is asymptomatically involved in nearly 30% of cases of secondary syphilis. Unless there is clinical evidence of CNS infection, evaluation of the cerebrospinal fluid (CSF) is not indicated. Serologic tests will be positive in 65 to 85% of cases of secondary syphilis.

Latent syphilis refers to a period of time during which there are no clinical manifestations of disease but the serological tests for syphilis are positive. *Early latent syphilis*, generally considered to be the first 4 years, is the time when relapses of secondary syphilis may occur, and the patient is considered to be infectious. Over 90% of relapses, most often mucocutaneous in nature, will occur in the first year, and it is widely believed that each relapse is clinically less florid than the previous episode. *Late latent syphilis* may continue for the balance of the patient's life or may progress to tertiary syphilis. During late latent syphilis, relapses are rare, and the patient is not considered to be infectious. Nevertheless, in utero transmission of disease is possible during latent syphilis.

If untreated, approximately 30% of patients will progress to late (tertiary) syphilis, a slowly progressive disease that can affect any system in the body years after initial infection. Clinically, late syphilis is often classified as either neurosyphilis, cardiovascular syphilis, or gummatous syphilis (late benign syphilis), a condition that is characterized by the development of hyperimmune granulomas, known as *gummas*, that often involve the skin and the bones.

About 10% of untreated patients will progress to the development of neurosyphilis. As was mentioned above, CNS involvement is initially asymptomatic and can be detected only by evaluation of the CSF. Under ideal situations, all patients should have evaluation of the CSF at 1 year after diagnosis and treatment of syphilis to detect evidence of residual CNS disease, such as pleocytosis, increased protein, decreased glucose, or positive nontreponemal antigen test. Examination of the CSF is also indicated for all HIV-positive patients with syphilis. The clinical manifestations of symptomatic neurosyphilis may include focal or generalized seizures, visual disturbances, paresthesias, altered reflexes, speech disturbances, pupillary abnormalities, dementia, and stroke. *Tabes dorsalis*, resulting from degeneration of the dorsal columns of the spinal cord, is characterized by ataxia with a wide-based gait, impotence, urinary incontinence or retention, paroxysms of intense shooting pain (usually in the legs), and loss of reflexes.

Congenital syphilis results from transplacental transmission of spirochetes to the fetus in utero. Babies who are born to mothers who acquire syphilis during pregnancy are at a higher risk of developing congenital syphilis than are those whose mothers acquired syphilis before pregnancy. While nearly 75% of cases of congenital syphilis are diagnosed after the age of 10, some cases manifest very early after birth. Early cases often present with rhinitis and a diffuse maculopapular rash that may result in significant epithelial sloughing. Additionally, there may be generalized osteochondritis and perichondritis, eventually leading to bone destruction. Neonatal death from congenital syphilis is usually due to pneumonia, pulmonary hemorrhage, or hepatic failure. Patients with late congenital syphilis may present with Hutchinson's triad, which includes Hutchinson's teeth (short, narrow, barrel-shaped incisors with a central notch), interstitial keratitis (photophobia, eye pain, tearing), and nerve deafness.

DIAGNOSIS

The most direct method for establishing the diagnosis of syphilis is demonstration of *T. pallidum* on darkfield microscopic examination of fluid or tissue taken from a suspicious cutaneous lesion or lymph node (22, 23, 27).

Because *T. pallidum* is susceptible to environmental changes, it is recommended that any clinical specimen taken from a patient with suspected syphilis be examined immediately. Because of their highly characteristic spiral shape and motility, viable treponemes are easy to distinguish under microscopic examination. Since nonpathogenic spirochetes can be members of the normal oral flora, darkfield microscopic examination of material from the oral cavity may not be useful in diagnosing syphilis. An alternative to darkfield microscopy that has been implemented in many clinical laboratories is the use of a direct fluorescent antibody test (DFA-TP), which has greater specificity for *T. pallidum* and does not require immediate examination (28).

In the absence of suitable pathological specimens to examine, the diagnosis of syphilis can be based on serologic testing (23, 29). The serologic tests that are used in the diagnosis of syphilis are classified as either nontreponemal or treponemal. Two commonly used nontreponemal antibody tests, VDRL (which stands for Venereal Disease Research Laboratory) and rapid plasma reagin (RPR), are quantitative measurements of antibodies against cardiolipin and are reported as serum titers that correlate with disease activity. These tests are inexpensive and easy to perform and are therefore often used for routine screening of patients. However, the test may remain reactive at low titers after treatment (sero-fast state) or become negative after 5 to 10 years, even without treatment (serorevert) (29). In some patients with secondary syphilis a prozone phenomenon may occur, leading to a false negative VDRL test. This is due to an excess of antibody relative to antigen and may be corrected by dilution of the patient's serum before testing (28). These tests can be used for patient monitoring and evaluation of therapy. Titers should fall and become nonreactive within 1 year after successful treatment of primary syphilis and within 2 years after effective treatment of secondary syphilis. Patients who are treated for late syphilis usually become nonreactive after a period of up to 5 years (30). Other nontreponemal tests that have been used include the reagin screen test (RST), the automated reagin test (ART), and the unheated serum reagin test (USR) (27).

Specific treponemal antibody tests, such as the fluorescent treponemal antibody-absorbed test (FTA-abs), are very sensitive and specific. The positive predictive value of the FTA-abs test is 100% for the initial or any subsequent symptomatic case of syphilis. Unfortunately, since this specific treponemal test usually remains positive for life, despite treatment, it is much less reliable in the evaluation of asymptomatic patients with a previous history of treated syphilis (31). Two additional treponemal antibody tests that are useful in the diagnosis of syphilis are the microhemagglutination assay for antibodies to *T. pallidum* (MHATP) and the hemagglutination treponemal test for syphilis

(HATTS). These tests are less expensive and easier to perform than the FTS-abs test but are also somewhat less sensitive in diagnosing early syphilis (31).

TREATMENT

Four basic principles guide the current treatment strategy for syphilis: (a) the requirement of a minimum treponemicidal antibiotic concentration, (b) maintenance of continuous antibiotic concentration above this minimal concentration, (c) adequate duration of therapy, and (d) the fact that the response to treatment is inversely related to the duration of the infection (32). The specific CDC recommendations for the preparation, dosage, and duration of therapy are based on the stage and clinical manifestations of the disease at the time of treatment and are summarized in Table 71.5 (33).

On the basis of over 40 years of experience, the drug of choice for the treatment of all stages of syphilis is parenteral penicillin G (33, 34). *T. pallidum* is highly sensitive to the effects of penicillin, with reported minimal treponemicidal concentrations of 0.018 μg/mL in infected tissues. Unfortunately, there have been no adequately controlled clinical trials to clearly define the optimal penicillin regimen for the treatment of various stages of syphilis. In addition, the data addressing non-penicillin therapy is extremely limited. The current treatment guidelines for syphilis use benzathine penicillin G as first-line therapy for primary, secondary, and latent syphilis. Alternative therapeutic options for patients with significant penicillin allergy are limited. The use of doxycycline, 100 mg orally every 12 hr, or tetracycline, 500 mg orally every 6 hr, is considered an acceptable

Table 71.5.
Recommended Treatment Regimens for All Stages of Syphilis in Non-HIV-Infected Patients

Stage of Disease	Adult Regimen	Child Regimen	Adult Penicillin Allergy
Sexual contact to infectious case of syphilis	Benzathine PCN G, 2.4 million units IM as single-dose therapy		Doxycycline, 100 mg PO BID for 14 days OR Tetracycline, 500 mg PO QID for 14 days
Primary or secondary syphilis	Benzathine PCN G, 2.4 million units IM as single-dose therapy	Benzathine PCN G, 50,000 units/kg IM as single-dose therapy (max. 2.4 MU)	Doxycycline, 100 mg PO BID for 14 days OR Tetracycline, 500 mg PO QID for 14 days
Early latent syphilis (<1 yr duration)	Treat as primary or secondary syphilis		
Late latent syphilis (>1 yr duration)	Benzathine PCN G, 2.4 million units IM weekly for 3 doses	Benzathine PCN G, 50,000 units/kg IM weekly for 3 doses (max. 2.4 MU/dose)	Doxycycline, 100 mg PO BID for 28 days OR Tetracycline, 500 mg PO QID for 28 days
Late syphilis (not neurosyphilis)	Treat as late latent syphilis		
Neurosyphilis	Aqueous PCN G, 12–24 million units IV daily (2–4 MU q 4 h) for 10 to 14 days OR Procaine PCN G, 2.4 million units IM daily plus probenecid 500 mg PO 4 times a day, both for 10 to 14 days (acceptable regimen only if compliance can be assured)		Desensitize; IV aqueous PCN G
Pregnancy	Treat as appropriate with parenteral penicillin.		Desensitize; Parenteral penicillin
Congenital syphilis		Aqueous PCN G, 100,000–150,000 units/kg/day, administered as 50,000 units/kg IV q 12 h during the first 7 days of life, and q 8 h thereafter, for 10 to 14 days OR Procaine PCN G, 50,000 units/kg IM daily as single dose for 10 to 14 days	

Source: From (33).

Table 71.6.
Oral Penicillin Desensitization Protocol[a]

Penicillin V Suspension Dose[b]	Amount (units/mL)	mL	Units	Cumulative Dose (units)
1	1,000	0.1	100	100
2	1,000	0.2	200	300
3	1,000	0.4	400	700
4	1,000	0.8	800	1,500
5	1,000	1.6	1,600	3,100
6	1,000	3.2	3,200	6,300
7	1,000	6.4	6,400	12,700
8	10,000	1.2	12,000	24,700
9	10,000	2.4	24,000	48,700
10	10,000	4.8	48,000	96,700
11	80,000	1.0	80,000	176,700
12	80,000	2.0	160,000	336,700
13	80,000	4.0	320,000	656,700
14	80,000	8.0	640,000	1,296,700

Source: From (35).

[a]The penicillin dose should be diluted in 30–45 mL of water and administered orally.

[b]Interval between individual doses is 15 minutes.

Table 71.7.
Recommended Treatment Regimens for Syphilis in HIV-Infected Patients

Stage of Disease	Adult Regimen	Alternative Regimen
Primary and secondary	Benzathine PCN G, 2.4 million units IM as single-dose therapy (Some experts suggest multiple doses.)	None; desensitize and treat with penicillin
Latent	Benzathine PCN G, 2.4 million units IM weekly for 3 doses	None; desensitize and treat with penicillin

alternative treatment. Erythromycin, 500 mg orally every 6 hr, has undergone limited evaluation but appears to be associated with high treatment failure rates (22, 33, 34). The use of first-generation cephalosporins has shown limited efficacy but unacceptably high treatment failure rates. More recently, ceftriaxone has undergone clinical studies in small numbers of patients with syphilis, and the results are promising (9, 29). The usual daily dose of ceftriaxone is 250 mg intramuscularly for 10 to 14 days in treating primary and secondary syphilis and 1 g intravenously for 14 days in treating neurosyphilis. Unfortunately, adequate clinical trial data does not exist at this time to clearly define the appropriate use of ceftriaxone in the treatment of syphilis (22, 23, 29).

Parenteral penicillin G is the only therapy that is documented to be effective in the management of syphilis during pregnancy and neurosyphilis; therefore, patients who are allergic to penicillin should be treated with penicillin following desensitization. Patients who have

positive skin tests to either the major or minor determinants of penicillin allergy can usually be safely desensitized over a 4- to 6-hr period using oral penicillin V suspension as outlined in Table 71.6 (35). Once desensitized, patients should be maintained on penicillin continuously until completion of the treatment course.

Many clinicians treat primary and secondary syphilis in HIV-infected patients more aggressively than in non-HIV-infected patients, using three intramuscular doses of benzathine penicillin G administered at weekly intervals, as suggested in Table 71.7.

Often within the first 24 hr of treatment for early syphilis, the patient will experience a Jarisch-Herxheimer reaction, an acute, benign, febrile episode that is commonly accompanied by myalgias, transient adenopathy, and headache lasting for several hours. This reaction is thought to be caused by release of treponemal antigens due to destruction of the organism by antibiotics. It is important that the clinician recognize this reaction as being independent of the drug regimen and not consider it to be an allergic reaction to the therapeutic agent used. If necessary for patient comfort, acetaminophen or aspirin can be used for symptomatic relief.

The CDC recommends serologic follow-up of patients who are treated for syphilis in order to evaluate the therapeutic outcome. Quantitative nontreponemal tests should be performed at 3 and 6 months after completion of therapy for primary and secondary syphilis and at 6 and 12 months for latent disease (33). For patients with neurosyphilis, examination of the CSF every 6 months until the cell count is normal is recommended. If the cell count remains abnormal at 24 months, retreatment is suggested. A quantitative nontreponemal test every 2 to 3 months until it is nonreactive is recommended as a follow-up for congenital syphilis. The adequacy of treatment for syphilis during pregnancy should be evaluated with nontreponemal serologic testing on a monthly basis. Women who fail to demonstrate a fourfold reduction in titer over a 3-month period or who show a fourfold increase in titer between tests should be retreated.

Herpes Genitalis

Genital herpes, or herpes genitalis, is an acute inflammatory infection caused by the double-stranded DNA herpes simplex virus (HSV) (36). Genital herpes is the most commonly encountered cause of genital ulceration in the United States and can involve male and female genital tracts with equal prevalence. It is estimated that over 30 million Americans are currently infected with genital herpes (37).

HSV type-2 (HSV-2) is the predominant viral type associated with herpes genitalis, but HSV type-1 (HSV-1) can also produce indistinguishable genital disease. Primary genital herpes develops after transmission of the virus by direct contact of the recipient's mucous membranes or skin with infected secretions or mucocutaneous surface of an infected sexual partner. There appears to be no risk of HSV transmission from inanimate objects or by aerosolization (38). After inoculation there is an incubation period ranging from 2 to 20 days when the HSV replicates locally in epithelial cells, eventually causing a localized inflammatory response and ulceration. The virus also migrates via peripheral neurons to the sacral ganglia, where it remains for life. Periodic reactivation of symptomatic disease or asymptomatic viral shedding occurs, but the physiologic, immunologic, and emotional factors that contribute to this reactivation are poorly understood at present (39).

CLINICAL PRESENTATION AND DIAGNOSIS

The clinical manifestations and recurrence rates of genital herpes are influenced by the viral type and numerous host-related factors, such as gender, immunocompetence, site of infection, and previous infection with HSV (36). Individuals with HSV-1 or HSV-2 infections in the absence of serum HSV antibody to either HSV-1 or HSV-2 (first episode, primary) tend to have severe presentations of the disease. Individuals who have serum antibodies to HSV-1 (first episode, nonprimary) have less severe manifestations of primary disease with HSV-2; patients with serum antibodies to HSV-2 seldom develop genital HSV-1 infection (36).

A significant percentage of patients with primary HSV infection experience a prodromal flulike syndrome with fever, headache, malaise, and diffuse myalgias. After a brief incubation period of 2 to 20 days (average of 4 to 7 days), local symptoms develop, consisting of genital itching, tenderness, and dysuria. Typically, the lesions start as painful papules or vesicles that spread rapidly over the genital region, often clustering together to form large areas of shallow ulceration. The pain and irritation gradually increase over the first week, reaching maximum intensity between days 7 and 11 of infection, then slowly recede over the next week. Over the course of several weeks, the cutaneous ulcers will crust over and eventually reepithelialize. Crusting does not occur with lesions on mucous membranes (36). Viral shedding occurs during the period from development of the initial lesion until approximately the eleventh or twelfth day of illness.

The symptoms of recurrent HSV infection are similar to those seen with primary episodes. The symptoms often appear to be more severe in women than men, possibly because of the extent of involved mucosal surface. In general, recurrent symptoms are milder than those seen with primary infection, and the recurrences usually last from 5 to 7 days.

Complications of genital herpes infection occur most frequently after primary episodes and usually result from the spread of genital disease or by autoinoculation of the virus. HSV infection of the rectum, pharynx, and eye are not unusual. Central nervous system involvement can include aseptic meningitis, transverse myelitis, or sacral radiculopathy. Blood-borne dissemination of HSV infection may accompany primary mucocutaneous infection in immunocompromised patients or during pregnancy. HSV infection of neonates who were exposed during pregnancy or delivery is associated with extremely high morbidity and mortality, with a case-fatality rate approaching 50% (40).

Since a number of other diseases are associated with genital ulceration, the diagnosis of herpes genitalis often requires laboratory testing. The easiest, but least sensitive and specific, technique is examination of cells scraped from the base of a typical lesion or ulcer (Tzanck smear) and stained by Giemsa or Papanicolaou stain (36). Evidence of multinucleated giant cells with intranuclear inclusions is characteristic of HSV infection. Identification of HSV in tissue culture processed from a specimen taken from a symptomatic patient is the most sensitive and specific method for confirmation of primary HSV infection but is expensive and time-consuming to perform. Serologic demonstration of HSV infection is useful for confirming the diagnosis of primary HSV infection, for determining the HSV serotype (if a serotype-specific assay is used), and for distinguishing between primary and reactivated infections, since recurrent genital herpes rarely induces a significant increase in anti-HSV antibodies (39, 41).

TREATMENT

The goals in treating herpes genitalis are to decrease the duration and severity of active infection, prevent associated complications, decrease the frequency of recurrence, and reduce the period of viral shedding and infectivity (36). To date, only acyclovir has been shown to be effective in the clinical management of genital herpes. Acyclovir, a guanosine analog, is selectively taken up by HSV-infected cells and undergoes serial phosphorylation to the active form, acyclovir triphosphate. This triphosphorylated moiety acts to inhibit HSV DNA polymerase and viral replication. Both HSV-1 and HSV-2 are inhibited by concentrations of acyclovir that are achieved in serum and body tissues at the currently recommended dosages (41).

Commercially, acyclovir is available for intravenous, oral, and topical administration. Only oral and intravenous use of acyclovir is associated with reductions in viral shedding, decreases in the severity and duration of symptoms, and the speeding of healing of first-episode HSV genital infections. The use of 5% acyclovir topical ointment in cases of genital herpes should be discouraged because of lack of demonstrated efficacy (41). The recommended acyclovir regimens for herpes genitalis are summarized in Table 71.8. In first-episode cases, prompt initiation of acyclovir is associated with reduction in symptoms within 48 hr (36, 39). Acyclovir dosages should be reduced for patients with significant renal dysfunction. There is no advantage to using parenteral acyclovir instead of oral acyclovir except for patients with severe disease or complications who require hospitalization and cannot take acyclovir orally.

Since recurrent episodes of genital herpes in immunocompetent patients are self-limited, acyclovir therapy has little benefit unless it is started at the beginning of the prodrome or when lesions are first noted (36). Daily dosing of acyclovir for chronic suppressive therapy to prevent recurrences in patients with more than six episodes per year has been reported to reduce the frequency of

recurrences by nearly 75%. If suppressive therapy is started, the current recommendation is to discontinue therapy after 12 months of continuous treatment in order to reassess the patient's rate of recurrence (37). While the potential for adverse effects from long-term acyclovir administration and the possibility of developing acyclovir-resistant strains of HSV are concerns, no clinical data exists to confirm cumulative acyclovir toxicities or changes in HSV susceptibility patterns to acyclovir following prolonged acyclovir use for up to 3 years (36, 42). However, there have been limited reports of apparent acyclovir-resistant strains of HSV in patients with genital herpes. Foscarnet, 40 mg/kg intravenously every 8 hr until clinical resolution, is the recommended treatment alternative in such cases (37).

The safety of systemic acyclovir therapy during pregnancy has not been clearly established, although there is currently no evidence to suggest that acyclovir is teratogenic in humans (37, 40, 41). Current recommendations are to avoid acyclovir therapy for HSV infections during pregnancy unless there is life-threating infection as evidenced by encephalitis, hepatitis, or pneumonitis (37). Women who do receive acyclovir during pregnancy should be reported to the cooperative CDC–Burroughs Wellcome Co. registry (1-800-722-9292, ext. 58465).

Patients with genital herpes should be advised to refrain from sexual activity while genital lesions are present. In addition, sexual partners of infected individuals should be evaluated and counseled about the lifelong nature of the disease.

Chancroid

Chancroid is a sexually transmitted disease caused by *Haemophilus ducreyi*, a small, Gram-negative, facultative anaerobic bacillus that is particularly hard to grow in culture. While most experts agree that genital herpes and primary syphilis are responsible for the majority of ulcerative genital lesions in developed countries, chancroid accounts for most of the genital ulcers in Third World and developing societies (43, 44). Nevertheless, since the early 1980s, there have been several significant outbreaks of chancroid in the United States and Canada. Men, especially uncircumcised men (43), have a higher incidence of infection than women.

For several years, the epidemiologic relationship between the presence of genital ulcers, such as chancroid, and heterosexual transmission of the human immunodeficiency virus has been recognized, particularly in Africa. It is believed that contact between the infectious ulcer of one sexual partner and mucus membranes of the other partner leads to this viral transmission. Therefore, identification and treatment of patients with chancroid, as well as other infections that lead to the formation of genital ulcers, are important in limiting the spread of HIV.

Table 71.8.
Recommended Acyclovir (ACV) Regimens for Treatment of Herpes Genitalis

Type of Infection	Recommended Regimen	Alternative IV Regimen
First-episode of genital herpes	ACV 200 mg PO 5 times daily for 7–10 days or until clinical resolution	ACV 5–10 mg/kg IV every 8 hr for 5–7 days or until clinical resolution
First-episode of herpes proctitis	ACV 400 mg PO 5 times daily for 10 days or until clinical resolution	As above
Recurrent infection	ACV 200 mg PO 5 times daily, or 400 mg PO 3 times daily, or 800 mg PO 2 times daily for 5 days, initiated within 48 hr of onset of lesions	
Chronic suppression	ACV 400 mg PO 2 times daily or 200 mg PO 3 times daily	

Source: From (37).

CLINICAL MANIFESTATIONS AND DIAGNOSIS

The incubation period for chancroid ranges from 3 to 10 days. The chancre starts as a tender, papulelike lesion with surrounding erythema and progresses over several days to an eroded, pustular ulcer that is frequently quite painful, particularly in men (43). Many women with chancroid are asymptomatic. With time, several of these small lesions can merge to form giant ulcers. The presence of painful inguinal lymphadenitis is seen concurrently in approximately 50% of cases and is often unilateral. Inflammed lymph nodes can progress to the development of formed buboes, which may rupture spontaneously in severe cases. Superinfection of the ulcerative lesions by enteric aerobic and anaerobic pathogens may further complicate the condition (43).

The definitive diagnosis of chancroid is dependent on the identification of *H. ducreyi* from culture on special media of samples collected from the ulcer or bubo. Since the proper techniques and media for culture are not widely available, the diagnosis is generally made by the exclusion of other diseases that produce inguinal ulceration, such as herpes genitalis, lymphogranuloma venereum, and syphilis, in a patient with suppurative inguinal adenopathy and a clinical response to empiric therapy (43, 44).

TREATMENT

The CDC recommends systemic antibiotic therapy with any one of the following regimens: azithromycin 1000 mg orally as a single dose, ceftriaxone 250 mg intramuscularly as a single dose, or erythromycin base 500 mg orally every 6 hr for 7 days (44). Each of these regimens has proven to be highly effective in non-HIV-infected patients with chancroid. Most clinicians will not consider single-dose therapy for HIV-infected patients because of reported higher treatment failure rates seen in these patients with single-dose regimens (45).

Alternative regimens that have not been evaluated as well include amoxicillin 500 mg plus clavulanic acid 125 mg orally 3 times daily for 7 days and ciprofloxacin 500 mg orally twice daily for 3 days (43, 45). Cefotaxime is also an effective treatment option for chancroid, but multiple doses are required for optimal cure rates. Three successive daily intramuscular doses of 1 g cefotaxime produced a 95% cure rate; a single 1-g intramuscular dose cured only 53% of patients (45). Other cephalosporins have not been studied as therapy for chancroid. Trimethoprim plus sulfamethoxazole (cotrimoxazole) is no longer a recommended treatment option for chancroid because of reports of developing resistance of *H. ducreyi* to this combination (45).

Patients should be reexamined several days after starting therapy to ensure that symptomatic improvement is observed. The time for complete healing may be several weeks, and significant scarring of tissues is common.

Relapse after apparent healing has been reported in up to 5% of cases (43). All known recent sexual contacts of the patient with chancroid should be evaluated and treated if necessary.

SELECTED OTHER SEXUALLY TRANSMITTED DISEASES

Trichomoniasis

Trichomoniasis is a common condition caused by the flagellated, motile protozoan *Trichomonas vaginalis* (46). In the United States, approximately 3 million females are treated for trichomoniasis annually; the incidence among males is unknown (47). Individuals who have multiple sexual partners or are concurrently infected with another STD appear to be at increased risk for trichomoniasis. This supports the belief that trichomoniasis is an STD. Transmission between sexual partners is further confirmed by reports of recovery of *T. vaginalis* from 66 to 100% of female sexual partners of infected men and 30 to 40% of male partners of infected women (48). For unclear reasons, trichomoniasis appears to be less common in women who use barrier contraception or oral contraceptives. Nonvenereal transmission can also occur from contact with colonized materials, such as towels and clothing. Neonates can acquire the organism during normal vaginal delivery (49).

CLINICAL PRESENTATION AND DIAGNOSIS

Trichomoniasis appears to be an asymptomatic and self-limited disease in most men and neonates, often requiring no specific therapy (50, 51). Up to 50% of women with vaginal trichomoniasis are asymptomatic. However, symptoms may develop following an incubation period ranging from 1 to 4 weeks. Frequent complaints include malodorous grayish or yellow-green vaginal discharge, dysuria, pruritis in the genital area, and vulvovaginal tenderness. Signs and symptoms appear to be exacerbated during menstruation, possibly because of increased vaginal pH facilitating an increase in organism growth (51). Laboratory findings include an elevated vaginal pH (>4.5) and large numbers of neutrophils seen on microscopic evaluation on the wet mount prep of the discharge. Evaluation of a wet mount prep from a vaginal swab remains the easiest, cheapest, and most widely used diagnositic technique employed (46). Traditional stains, such as the Gram, Giemsa, and acridine orange stains, are not helpful in the diagnosis of trichomoniasis but should be done on all samples because of the high likelihood of concurrent disease in infected patients (46). Culture of *T. vaginalis* from collected specimens is the most sensitive diagnostic technique available but requires up to 48 hr for necessary growth, reducing the clinical usefulness of culture for clinical diagnosis (51).

TREATMENT

The treatment of choice for trichomoniasis in both men and women is oral metronidazole (46, 52). With the recent availability of metronidazole gel as a treatment for bacterial vaginosis, topical metronidazole for trichomoniasis has been considered. Systemic therapy is superior to topical intravaginal treatment for women because organisms in the urinary tract are treated as well, reducing the chance of relapse (51). A single 2-g oral dose of metronidazole has been shown in several clinical trials to be equivalent to regimens of 250 mg orally 3 times daily or 500 mg orally twice daily for 7 days for women, providing cure rates of between 82% to 88% (46, 51, 52). This probably holds true for men as well, although data is lacking to confirm this belief. A metronidazole regimen of 375 mg orally twice daily for 7 days has recently been recommended for approval as an alternative regimen by the Food and Drug Administration (FDA) Anti-Infective Advisory Committee (52). As with any STD, it is important to treat all sexual partners as well to prevent reinfection. When sexual partners are treated simultaneously with metronidazole, the cure rate increases to greater than 95% (46). Infants with symptomatic trichomoniasis or with prolonged (>4 weeks) colonization following birth can be treated with parenteral metronidazole, 10 to 30 mg/kg/day for 7 days (51). No specific follow-up is required unless signs and symptoms of infection continue.

Metronidazole therapy is associated with some well-recognized side effects, particularly mild nausea and dysgeusia, which appear to be worse with large single doses. Peripheral neuropathy, presenting as numbness and paresthesias, is also associated with metronidazole therapy, especially in patients who take large doses for prolonged periods of time. Metronidazole can interfere with alcohol metabolism by blocking alcohol dehydrogenase, producing an "Antabuse-like" reaction consisting of severe nausea, vomiting, and flushing when the two are taken concomitantly. The use of metronidazole during pregnancy is relatively contraindicated, particularly during the first trimester. Recent data suggests that metronidazole use during the second and third trimesters of pregnancy is safe; however, most clinicians do not consider specific therapy for trichomoniasis to be necessary during pregnancy unless the symptoms are severe (51).

When the clinician is faced with an apparent failure of metronidazole to resolve a case of trichomoniasis, consideration must be given to the possibility of failure due to poor compliance to the prescribed regimen, reinfection of the patient by an infected sexual partner, or the potential of infection by a metronidazole-resistant organisms. Although *T. vaginalis* resistance to metronidazole appears to be increasing, alternative therapies are limited (49). Current therapeutic options for infections caused by suspected or known metronidazole-resistant organisms include treatment for 7 to 10 days with daily oral doses of 2 g of metronidazole, with or without concurrent use of metronidazole 0.5% gel intravaginally (51).

Lymphogranuloma Venereum (LGV)

Lymphogranuloma venereum (LGV) is caused by the invasive L_1, L_2, and L_3 serotypes of *Chlamydia trachomatis*, the same pathogen that is associated with the development of nongonococcal urethritis in many patients (53). LGV is a relatively rare disease in the United States and must be differentiated clinically from such other conditions as lymphoma, syphilis, chancroid, plague, tularemia, and genital herpes. Like other STDs, LGV is more common among individuals with multiple sexual contacts, in urban rather than rural areas, and in lower socioeconomic populations (54).

CLINICAL PRESENTATION AND DIAGNOSIS

The most common clinical manifestation of LGV is tender inguinal lymphadenopathy, which is most commonly unilateral in presentation. This inguinal adenopathy appears 2 to 6 weeks after the development of an unremarkable herpetiform vesicle at the site of inoculation. The initial vesicle often goes unnoticed, particularly in women. Within 2 weeks, the inflamed inguinal node (bubo) may progress to fluctuance and rupture through the skin, forming sinus tracts that are slow to heal. This occurs in fewer than 30% of cases (54). The remaining cases slowly form firm inguinal masses without suppuration. In females and homosexual males, LGV can alternatively present as perianal or perirectal inflammation that can progress to the formation of colonic fistulas or strictures. These patients can present with rectal bleeding or rectal discharge of pus. In severe cases, patients may appear systemically ill. Laboratory findings are usually nonspecific and may consist of slightly elevated white blood cell counts, elevated erythrocyte sedimentation rate, and mild increases in hepatic transaminases.

The diagnosis of LGV is based largely on the clinical presentation of significant inguinal adenopathy in the absence of another etiology. Isolation of *C. trachomatis* from an aspirated swollen bubo is possible in up to one-third of cases but requires special culture techniques that are not available in most laboratories. Serological documentation of antichlamydial antibodies by microimmunofluorescence (MIA) or enzyme-linked immunosorbent assay (ELISA) appears to be sensitive and more specific than complement fixation (CF) but can lead to false positives because of the widespead prevalence of other chlamydial infections in the population that is at risk.

TREATMENT AND PROGNOSIS

The recommended treatment of choice for LGV is doxyclycline, 100 mg orally twice daily for 21 days, as shown in Table 71.4 (54, 55). Alternative antibiotic regimens include erythromycin, 500 mg orally four times daily for 21 days, or sulfisoxazole, 500 mg orally four times daily for 21 days. Erythromycin is the treatment of choice for pregnant females. While it is expected that the macrolide clarithromycin and the azalide azithromycin should offer similar efficacy to that of erythromcyin as alternative therapy to doxycycline, insufficient clinical data is available to support their widespread use at this time. Swollen, inflamed lymph nodes may require surgical aspiration or incision and drainage for optimal care.

In general, appropriate antibiotic therapy and surgical intervention, if necessary, cure LGV and prevent further tissue damage and scarring. However, patients should be followed clinically until resolution of presenting signs and symptoms of the disease. Sexual partners should be evaluated and treated appropriately if urethral or cervical chlamydial infection is detected.

Condylomata Acuminata

Condylomata acuminata, or genital warts, are venereal infections caused by human papilloma virus (HPV) (56). Genital HPV infection is the second most common venereal disease seen in STD clinics in the United States; it is responsible for over 1 million office visits annually. Papilloma viruses are double-stranded DNA viruses that often produce squamous epithelial tumors. The virus has been shown to penetrate and infect the basal cell layer, the only site of actively dividing cells in the epithelium. Over 70 types of HPV have been identified; they contribute to a wide range of lesions, including plantar warts, laryngeal carcinoma, and cervical dysplasia. The HPV virus types that are considered to be primarily responsible for genital warts are HPV-6 and HPV-11 (57). These HPV are easily transmitted during sexual intercourse. Genital warts are almost always the result of anal intercourse, particularly in homosexual men.

The natural history of untreated genital warts is variable. Some may grow larger, some regress, and many stay the same over time. Several years ago, it was commonly believed that, if left untreated, large genital warts would progress to malignancy. As techniques to identify particular types of HPV became available, it became more clear that the risk of genital warts progressing to cancerous lesions was very small (58). The HPV types that are most strongly associated with the development of cervical cancer are not the same types that are associated with genital warts. Additionally, the rates of noncervical genital cancers are extremely low in the United States, while the prevalence of genital HPV infections are very high.

CLINICAL PRESENTATION AND DIAGNOSIS

Condylomata acuminata can frequently be rather asymptomatic, with only occasional anogenital pruritis and burning (56). These lesions are usually known as flat condylomas and are identified as shiny white plaques following the application of dilute (3 to 5%) acetic acid solution to the site. The common locations for these flat warts are the penis, anus, vagina, vulva, and cervix. Large, hyperplastic, exophytic warts with raised, pinkish-colored papules represent the classic condylomata acuminata (59). These larger lesions may be associated with increased pain, bleeding, burning, and soiling of undergarments.

Condylomata acuminata should be differentiated from other anogenital growths, such as molluscum contagiosum, moles, and skin tags. HPV cannot be grown in tissue culture; therefore, diagnosis is based on gross clinical appearance and confirmed by biopsy (59). Histological evidence of koilocytosis, the characteristic finding of HPV infection, can be observed with appropriate staining techniques, such as the Papanicolaou smear. Recently, newer techniques, such as DNA hybridization and polymerase chain reaction, have expanded the ability to identify specific HPV types, but these procedures are not currently useful for clinical screening (58).

TREATMENT

The treatment options for genital warts are frequently associated with significant pain and expense and with frustrating results because of poor responses or recurrences (56, 60). Many experts believe that recurrences of genital warts are much more commonly due to reactivation of subclinical infection than to reinfection by a sexual partner (61). Eradication of genital HPV infection is not accomplished by any therapeutic option that is currently available. While aggressive techniques for removal of the warts do produce cosmetic benefits, the surrounding tissues usually remain subclinically infected with HPV.

The plant resin podophyllin, applied as a 10 to 25% solution in compound tincture of benzoin, has traditionally been the most common initial treatment. Podophyllin has been shown to inhibit mitosis, leading to cell death. Topical applications of limited amounts (<0.5 mL per application) are made to the lesions and followed by thorough washing in 1 to 4 hr (61). Applications can be repeated weekly as needed. In several clinical trials, podophyllin treatment was associated with initial clearance of warts in 32 to 79% of patients, with recurrence within 9 months seen in 27 to 65% of patients (58). Systemic absorption of topically applied podophyllin can occur. The use of podophyllin is contraindicated during pregnancy.

Podofilox (podophyllotoxin), the most biologically active component of podophyllin, was approved by the FDA for the self-treatment of external genital warts and is now available by prescription as a 0.5% solution (62). Limited topical application of podofilox (<0.25 mL per application) is made to warts twice daily for 3 days, followed by a 4-day period of no treatment. Treatment cycles can be repeated as needed for up to four cycles. Complete clearance of warts has been described in 45 to 88% of patients, with recurrence within 3 months observed in 33 to 60% of these patients (58). Local irritation associated with the use of podofilox is usually mild but does appear to be more frequent than that reported with podophyllin use. Podofilox has not been approved for the treatment of perianal, rectal, vaginal, or urethral warts. Like podophyllin, podofilox is contraindicated during pregnancy.

An alternative treatment option is trichloroacetic acid (85%) applied to the genital warts followed by powdering of the area with talc or baking soda to remove excess unreacted acid. Application can be made at weekly intervals as required (56). Cryotherapy using liquid nitrogen or a cryoprobe produces results similar to those reported with podofilox and podophyllin (58). In limited uncontrolled studies, topical 5% 5-fluorouracil has been reported to produce complete clearance of vulvovaginal warts in up to 68% of women, with 6- to 12-month recurrence rates of less than 10%. Intralesional injection of interferon-α 2b for external genital warts produced complete clearing in 44 to 60% of patients, and no recurrences were seen in these patients with limited short-term follow-up (58). When intralesional interferon injection was combined with topical podophyllin, the response observed was superior to that seen with podophyllin alone, particularly in non-HIV-infected patients who had warts for less than 1 year. Systemic interferon administration in combination with other treatment options has not been associated with any improvement in response rates. The use of CO_2 laser therapy has produced disappointing results in limited clinical evaluations (58).

Currently, the primary goal of therapy for condylomata acuminata is removal of wart tissue for cosmetic reasons. The choice of treatment should be based on patient preferences, convenience, costs, and clinician experience (56).

SUMMARY

All health care professionals have a responsibility to contribute to the efforts to reduce the ever-expanding prevalence of sexually transmitted diseases. Infected patients and their sexual partners must be identified, treated appropriately, consistent with recently published guidelines, and counseled about the nature of their disease and methods that can be used to reduce the transmission of all STDs.

Advances in drug therapy have led to safe and effective treatment regimens for most STDs that are also relatively inexpensive and easy to follow. Compliance has been enhanced for several diseases through the development of regimens requiring only a single dose of medication. Additional newer therapies are currently undergoing evaluation.

This chapter reviews the major sexually transmitted diseases seen in the United States and provides an expanded discussion of the recently published treatment guidelines for sexually transmitted diseases released by the Centers for Disease Control and Prevention. For more in-depth discussions of epidemiology, pathogenesis, and pathophysiology of specific diseases, texts and published reviews addressing individual STDs are recommended.

REFERENCES

1. Piot P, Islam MQ. Sexually transmitted diseases in the 1990s: global epidemiology and challenges for control. Sex Transm Dis 21(Suppl 2):S7–S13, 1994.
2. Centers for Disease Control and Prevention. Addressing emerging infectious disease threats: a prevention strategy for the United States. Atlanta, GA: U.S. Department of Health and Human Services, Public Health Service, 1994.
3. Centers for Disease Control and Prevention. Summary of notifiable diseases, United States, 1993. MMWR Morb Mortal Wkly Rep 42(53):1–73, 1994.
4. Rothenberg R, Judson FN. The clinical diagnosis of urethral discharge. Sex Transm Dis 10:24–8, 1983.
5. Adimora AA, Hamilton H, Holmes KK, Sparling PF. Sexually transmitted diseases: companion handbook. 2nd ed. New York: McGraw-Hill, 1994:25–40.
6. Handsfield HH, Sparling PF. Neisseria gonorrhoeae. In: Mandell GL, Bennet JE, Dolin R, eds. Principles and practice of infectious diseases. 4th ed. New York: Churchill Livingstone, 1995:1909–26.
7. Moran JS, Levine WC. Drugs of choice for the treatment of uncomplicated gonococcal infections. Clin Infect Dis 20(Suppl 1):S47–S65, 1995.
8. Centers for Disease Control and Prevention. 1993 sexually transmitted diseases treatment guidelines. MMWR Morb Mortal Wkly Rep 42(RR-14):47–83, 1993.
9. Hook EW, Roddy RE, Handsfield HH. Ceftriaxone therapy for incubating and early syphilis. J Infect Dis 158:881–84, 1988.
10. Handsfield HH, McCormack WM, Hook EW, et al. A comparison of single dose cefixime with ceftriaxone as treatment for uncomplicated gonorrhea. N Engl J Med 325:1337–1341, 1991.
11. Centers for Disease Control and Prevention. Decreased susceptibility of Neisseria gonorrhoeae to fluoroquinolones: Ohio and Hawaii, 1992–1994. MMWR Morb Mortal Wkly Rep 43(18):325–27, 1994.
12. Handsfield HH, Dalu ZA, Martin DH, et al. Multicenter trial of single-dose azithromycin vs. ceftriaxone in the treatment of uncomplicated gonorrhea. Sex Transm Dis 21:107–11, 1994.
13. Adimora AA, Hamilton H, Holmes KK, Sparling PF. Sexually transmitted diseases: companion handbook. 2nd ed. New York: McGraw-Hill, 1994:271–80.
14. Bowie WR, Wang SP, Alexander ER, et al. Etiology of non-gonococcal urethritis: evidence for Chlamydia trachomatis and Ureaplasma urealyticum. J Clin Invest 59:735–42, 1977.
15. Martin DT. Chlamydial infections. Med Clin North Am 74:1367–88, 1990.
16. Coleman P, Varitek V, Muchahwar IK, et al. Testpack chlamydia: a new rapid assay for the detection of Chlamydia trachomatis. J Clin Microbiol 27:2811–14, 1989.
17. Martin DH, Mroczkowski TF, Dalu ZA, et al. A controlled trial of a single dose of azithromycin for the treatment of chlamydial urethritis and cervicitis. N Engl J Med 327:921–25, 1992.
18. Whatley JD, Thin RN, Mumtaz G, et al. Azithromycin vs doxycycline in the treatment of non-gonococcal urethritis. Int J STD AIDS 2:248–51, 1991.

19. Weber JT, Johnson RE. New treatments for *Chlamydia trachomatis* genital infection. Clin Infect Dis 2(Suppl):S66–S71, 1995.

20. Augenbraun MH, Cummings M, McCormack WM. Management of chronic urethral symptoms in men. Clin Infect Dis 15:714–15, 1992.

21. Hooton TM, Rogers MR, Medina TG, et al. Ciprofloxacin compared with doxycycline for nongonococcal urethritis: ineffectiveness against *Chlamydia trachomatis* due to relapsing infection. JAMA 264:1418–21, 1990.

22. Adimora AA, Hamilton H, Holmes KK, Sparling PF. Sexually transmitted diseases: companion handbook. 2nd ed. New York: McGraw-Hill, 1994:63–86.

23. Tramont EC. *Treponema pallidum* (syphilis). In: Mandell GL, Bennet JE, Dolin R, eds. Principles and practice of infectious diseases. 4th ed. New York: Churchill Livingstone, 1995:2117–33.

24. Centers for Disease Control. Primary and secondary syphilis: United States, 1981–1990. MMWR Morb Mortal Wkly Rep 40(19):314–23, 1991.

25. Hook EW, Marra CM. Acquired syphilis in adults. N Engl J Med 326:1060–69, 1992.

26. Chapel TA. The signs and symptoms of secondary syphilis. Sex Transm Dis 7:161–65, 1980.

27. Fitzgerald TJ. Treponema. In: Balow A. Hausler WJ, Herrmann KL, Isenberg HD, Shadomy HJ, eds. Manual of clinical microbiology, 5th ed. Washington, DC: American Society for Microbiology, 1991:567–571.

28. Larsen SA. Syphilis. Clin Lab Med 9:545–557, 1989.

29. Quinn TC, Zenilman J, Rompalo A. Sexually transmitted diseases: advances in diagnosis and treatment. Adv Intern Med 39:149–96, 1994.

30. Romanowski B, Sutherland R, Fick GH, et al. Serologic response to treatment of infectious syphilis. Ann Intern Med 114:1005–09, 1991.

31. Zenker PN, Rolfs RT. Treatment of syphilis, 1989. Rev Infect Dis 12(Suppl 6):S590–S609, 1990.

32. Wolters EC. Treatment of neurosyphilis. Clin Neuropharmacol 10:143–54, 1987.

33. Centers for Disease Control. 1993 sexually transmitted diseases treatment guidelines. MMWR Morb Mortal Wkly Rep 42(RR-14):1–102, 1993.

34. Rolfs RT. Treatment of syphilis, 1993. Clin Infect Dis 20(Suppl 1):S23–S38, 1995.

35. Wendel GD, Stark BJ, Jamison RB, Molina RD, Sullivan TJ. Penicillin allergy and desensitization in serious infections during pregnancy. N Engl J Med 312:1229–32, 1985.

36. Adimora AA, Hamilton H, Holmes KK, Sparling PF. Sexually transmitted diseases: companion handbook. 2nd ed. New York: McGraw-Hill, 1994:135–154.

37. Centers for Disease Control and Prevention. 1993 sexually transmitted diseases treatment guidelines. MMWR Morb Mortal Wkly Rep 42(RR-14):22–6, 1993.

38. Guinan ME, Wolinsky SN, Reichman RC. Epidemiology of genital herpes simplex virus infection. Epidemiol Rev 7:127–32, 1985.

39. Kinghorn GR. Genital herpes: natural history and treatment of acute episodes. J Med Virol Suppl 1:33–8, 1993.

40. Blanchier H, Huraux JM, Hurauz-Rendu C, Sainte-Croix BA. Genital herpes and pregnancy: preventive measures. Eur J Obstet Gynecol Reprod Biol 53:33–8, 1994.

41. de Ruiter A, Thin RN. Genital herpes: a guide to pharmacologic therapy. Drugs 47:297–304, 1994.

42. Fife KH, Crumpacker CS, Mertz GJ, et al. Recurrence and resistance patterns of herpes simplex virus following cessation of ≤ 6 years of chronic suppression with acyclovir. J Infect Dis 169:1338–41, 1994.

43. Adimora AA, Hamilton H, Holmes KK, Sparling PF. Sexually transmitted diseases: companion handbook. 2nd ed. New York: McGraw-Hill, 1994:87–92.

44. Centers for Disease Control and Prevention. 1993 sexually transmitted diseases treatment guidelines. MMWR Morb Mortal Wkly Rep 42(RR-14):20–2, 1993.

45. Schulte JM, Schmid GP. Recommendations for treatment of chancroid, 1993. Clin Infect Dis 20(Suppl 1):S39–S46, 1995.

46. Adimora AA, Hamilton H, Holmes KK, Sparling PF. Sexually transmitted diseases: companion handbook. 2nd ed. New York: McGraw Hill, 1994:212–22.

47. Kent HL. Epidemiology of vaginitis. Am J Obstet Gynecol 165:1168–76, 1991.

48. Muller M, Rein ME. Trichomonas vaginalis. In: Holmes KK, Mardh PA, Sparking PF, et al., eds. Sexually transmitted diseases. 2nd ed. New York: McGraw-Hill, 1990:481–92.

49. Grossman JH, Galash RP. Persistent vaginitis caused by metronidazole-resistant trichomoniasis. Obstet Gynecol 76:521–22, 1990.

50. Kriega JN, Jenny C, Verdon M, et al. Clinical manifestations of trichomoniasis in men. Ann Intern Med 118:844–949, 1993.

51. Rein MF. Trichomoniasis vaginalis. In: Mandell GL, Bennet JE, Dolin R, eds. Principles and practice of infectious diseases. 4th ed. New York: Churchill Livingstone, 1995:2493–97.

52. Centers for Disease Control and Prevention. 1993 sexually transmitted diseases treatment guidelines. MMWR Morb Mortal Wkly Rep 42(RR-14):70–2, 1993.

53. Perine PL, Osoba AO. Lymphogranuloma venereum. In: Holmes KK, Mardh PA, Sparling PF, et al., eds. Sexually transmitted diseases. 2nd ed. New York: McGraw-Hill, 1990:195–204.

54. Adimora AA, Hamilton H, Holmes KK, Sparling PF. Sexually transmitted diseases: companion handbook. 2nd ed. New York: McGraw Hill, 1994:56–62.

55. Centers for Disease Control. 1993 sexually transmitted diseases treatment guidelines. MMWR Morb Mortal Wkly Rep 42(RR-14):26–7, 1993.

56. Adimora AA, Hamilton H, Holmes KK, Sparling PF. Sexually transmitted diseases: companion handbook. 2nd ed. New York: McGraw Hill, 1994:162–74.

57. Reid R, Greenberg M, Jenson AB, et al. Sexually transmitted papilloma viral infections. I: the anatomic distribution and pathologic grade of neoplastic lesions associated with different viral types. Am J Obstet 156:212–18, 1987.

58. Stone KM. Human papillomavirus infection and genital warts: update on epidemiology and treatment. Clin Infect Dis 20(Suppl 1):S91–S97, 1995.

59. Howley PM, Schlegel R. The human papillomaviruses: an overview. Am J Med 85:155–172, 1988.

60. Kraus ST, Stone KM. Management of genital infection caused by human papillomavirus. Rev Infect Dis 12(Suppl 6):S620–S632, 1990.

61. Centers for Disease Control and Prevention. 1993 sexually transmitted diseases treatment guidelines. MMWR Morb Mortal Wkly Rep 42(RR-14):83–8, 1993.

62. Anonymous. Podofilox for genital warts. Med Lett Drugs Ther 33:117–18, 1991.

CHAPTER 72

HUMAN IMMUNODEFICIENCY VIRUS (HIV) INFECTION AND ACQUIRED IMMUNODEFICIENCY SYNDROME (AIDS)

JOAN E. KAPUSNIK-UNER

Acquired immunodeficiency syndrome (AIDS) was first recognized and described before the discovery of the causative retrovirus in mid-1981, when an unusual cluster of patients was reported as having *Pneumocystis carinii* pneumonia (PCP). AIDS is a clinical syndrome that is the result of infection and disease with the human immunodeficiency virus (HIV), which causes profound immunosuppression (1). The effects of HIV on the body's host defense mechanisms are gradual and eventually render the patient susceptible to cancers and opportunistic infections. In the late stage of the illness, patients may have a constellation of symptoms and diseases. A more specific AIDS case definition that is used for patient surveillance will be described below. Therapeutic advances against HIV have been unprecedented since the syndrome was recognized in 1981; the first antiretroviral agent was approved by the Food and Drug Administration (FDA) by 1987. Goals to be achieved in the next decade of this epidemic, our modern-day plague, include control of viral transmission, vaccine development, and the widespread availability of effective therapy for suppressing HIV.

ETIOLOGY AND PATHOGENESIS

HIV is an RNA retrovirus that can be divided further into subgroups, HIV-1 and HIV-2. The more common viral strain is HIV-1, which has been extensively studied. HIV is known to be transmitted by direct inoculation with infected blood, body fluids, or secretions. Therefore, transmission may occur during intimate sexual contact, by direct exposure to contaminated blood or blood-products, and by direct in utero transmission. It is clearly established that infection with HIV results in selective defects in immune function. The most prominent feature in the immunopathogenesis of HIV infection is the depletion of the CD4 (helper, inducer) subset of T lymphocytes. B-cell dysfunction is also present in patients with HIV infection.

The outer envelope of HIV includes a critical structure known as gp120, which interacts with CD4 cell receptor molecules. These receptors, which are found on T cells, are also found on other cells throughout the body; thus widespread HIV binding and infection occurs. HIV-1

viral replication preferentially and continuously occurs in lymphoreticular tissues (i.e., lymph nodes, spleen, gastrointestinal-associated lymphoid cells and macrophages). Viral kinetics, organism replication, and clearance have recently been described to be extremely dynamic. Continuous de novo viral infection, replication, and rapid cell turnover occur; the viral half-life is reported to be as short as 2 days. Thirty percent or more of the body's total viral load is replenished daily (2).

Mechanisms and factors that are associated with disease pathogenesis have been proposed, including increased expression of specific cytokines (e.g., interleukin-6, tumor necrosis factors α and β) causing immune system activation, which plays a major role in persistent viral replication. Also, a reduction in the expression of other cytokines (e.g., interleukin-2 and interleukin-4) has been observed. A clear picture of disease pathogenesis remains to be elucidated but involves the following steps: rapid, early dissemination of virus; seeding of virus in lymphoid tissue; partial host immune responses that down-regulate viral expression; persistent viral replication; sequestration of extracellular virus into the germinal centers of lymph nodes; chronic activation of T lymphocytes and secretion of immune system-activating cytokines; accelerated viral replication; destruction of lymphoid tissue; escape of virus into peripheral blood cells; and direct killing of CD4 cells.

Disease progression has been noted to occur at various rates for individual patients. Rates of progression are likely due to a combination of factors, including unique viral strain characteristics and host factors. Patients have been classified by some into groups that describe the time course of disease progression: "fast progressors," who move from initial viral infection to AIDS within 4 years; "normal progressors," who develop AIDS within 10 to 12 years after initial infection; "slow progressors," who have long-term HIV infection and have stable but low CD4 cell counts; and "long-term nonprogressors," who continue to be HIV-antibody positive, to have high CD4 cell counts (>500/ mm^3) and to be asymptomatic for 10 to 16 years. The latter two groups of patients are being closely studied to identify their more efficient immune system responses.

INCIDENCE/OCCURRENCE

AIDS/HIV statistics worldwide are very difficult to determine because of low reporting, even in areas of endemic infection such as Africa, and because of the different AIDS definitions that are used. The World Health Organization estimates that by the year 2000, approximately 40 million people will be infected with HIV, and there will be approximately 10 million AIDS cases worldwide. Since 1981, more than 440,000 people in the United States have been reported to have AIDS, and there have been 270,000 reported deaths. The greatest impact has been on males age 25 to 44, for whom AIDS has become the leading cause of death (3). The AIDS epidemic in women continues to worsen in the United States, where women currently comprise 18% of AIDS cases compared to only 7% in 1985. AIDS in women disproportionally affects racial and ethnic minorities (4).

The population groups that are at greatest risk for HIV transmission in the United States include men who have sex with men, intravenous drug users, people who received blood or blood products before the institution of routine HIV screening and testing and infants (5) born to HIV-infected mothers. Outside of the United States, heterosexual transmission of HIV through intercourse is the major risk factor. Many experts believe that widespread education about "safe sex" and selective education for intravenous drug users about avoiding needle sharing and about needle-cleansing techniques have made a major impact on HIV transmission. This educational effort must be continuous and must reach all age, gender, cultural, and ethnic groups to truly influence the future incidence of HIV infection.

DIAGNOSIS

Patients who are infected with HIV have several manifestations of illness, including the acute symptoms of viral infection (e.g., flulike syndrome); unexplained thrombocytopenia with bleeding; an asymptomatic phase; and AIDS with symptoms, including those from opportunistic infections and cancers, wasting, and HIV-related dementia. The Centers for Disease Control (CDC) has published criteria for the case definition of AIDS (see Table 72.1) (6). The criteria have been revised several times over the last decade to better describe and include patients with severe immune suppression from HIV. The most recent revision was expanded to include HIV-infected patients with one of the following conditions: (a) invasive cervical cancer, (b) pulmonary tuberculosis, (c) recurrent bacterial pneumonias, and (d) any individual with a CD4 T-lymphocyte cell count less than 200/mm^3, irrespective of concurrent symptoms. The CD4 T lymphocyte is the most commonly used "surrogate marker" of HIV infection. The CD4 defect in HIV-infected adults may be assessed and monitored by

Table 72.1.

Summary of the CDC's 1993 Surveillance Case Definition for AIDS among Adolescents and Adults

Bacterial pneumonia, recurrent (more than one episode in one year)
Candidiasis of esophagus, bronchi, trachea, or lungs
Cervical cancer, invasive
Coccidioides immitis infection, extrapulmonary
Cryptococcus neoformans infection, extrapulmonary
Cryptosporidiosis, chronic intestinal infection > 1 month duration
Cytomegalovirus infection, other than liver, lymph nodes, or spleen, and including retinitis
Herpes simplex virus infection, chronic ulcerative disease > 1 month duration, or bronchitis, pneumonitis, or esophagitis
HIV-related encephalopathy
HIV-related wasting syndrome (>10% of baseline body weight *plus* chronic diarrhea or chronic weakness and fever for > 30 days)
Histoplasma capsulatum infection, extrapulmonary
Isosporiasis, chronic intestinal infection > 1 month duration
Kaposi's sarcoma
Lymphoma: Burkitt's, immunoblastic, or primary of the brain
Mycobacterium avium complex, *M. kansasii* or other *Mycobacterium* species infection, extrapulmonary
Mycobacterium tuberculosis, any site including lungs
Pneumocystis carinii pneumonia
Progressive multifocal leukoencephalopathy
Salmonella septicemia, recurrent
Toxoplasma gondii encephalitis

Source: From (6).

using the absolute CD4 count; a normal count is in the range 500 to 1100/mm^3. The CD4 percentage (normal is >29%) or CD4/CD8 ratio (helper/suppressor cell ratio; normal is 2 to 1) is also used for monitoring disease progression. In HIV infection this ratio inverts, with CD8 cells predominating.

Antibodies against HIV are detectable by using various serological testing methods. Antibody-testing of blood is the most widespread method of determining HIV infection, though false-positive and false-negative results can occur. HIV-antibody testing is usually done with the sensitive enzyme-linked immunosorbent assay (ELISA) method, and positive results are confirmed with a second procedure, the Western blot method. Confirmation of all positive results is necessary, since false-positive ELISA results have been reported in patients with collagen vascular disease, chronic hepatitis, and other conditions. The diagnosis of HIV infection from antibody testing in neonates is difficult because of the possible presence of passive maternal HIV antibodies, which persist for many months.

An important issue with regard to antibody testing is that false-negative results occur when a patient is newly HIV-infected. At this stage, patients can transmit the virus (i.e., "are infectious"), but sufficient time has not elapsed for adequate antibody production for detection with the HIV-antibody assay. The FDA has recently approved an

HIV test system that detects antibodies in oral fluid specimens (7). This test is even less sensitive than blood testing methods but is a less invasive test for the patient and potentially is a safer test for health care workers, since infected blood is not obtained nor processed. More sensitive test methods for earlier detection of infection are needed. HIV culture techniques are used in many research studies but are not available for routine clinical diagnoses. Financial considerations, as well as high false-negative rates, make currently used culture methods impractical. The HIV p24 antigen, HIV p24 antibody, and β-2-microglobulin tests have also been used. However, β-2-microglobulin increases are not specific for HIV disease progression, and HIV p24 tests are less well standardized, less sensitive, and not routinely available, and results have not been as helpful in the clinical decision-making process.

Excitement has grown in anticipation of FDA approval and the availability of tests that measure "viral burden." The branched-chain HIV DNA test (Chiron Corporation) and the polymerase chain reaction HIV RNA test (Roche Molecular Systems) are sensitive and fast techniques for quantifying HIV in plasma or tissue. It is predicted that these tests will be used as tools for making an earlier diagnosis, including infection in children. They will be useful for monitoring disease progression in all patient groups and will be used as a monitoring tool (i.e., serial measurements to be performed) for assessing the efficacy of antiretroviral drug therapies.

CLINICAL FINDINGS

Individuals with HIV infection who are asymptomatic may remain so for many years. The reasons for disease progression and for observing unpredictable rates of progression are not well understood. An array of mild-to-moderate nonspecific symptoms can be observed early in HIV infection (previously termed AIDS-related complex, ARC). Symptoms include persistent fevers, night sweats, weight loss, headaches, lymphadenopathy, skin rashes, diarrhea, thrush, recurrence of varicella zoster virus infection (i.e., shingles), and hematological abnormalities, including severe thrombocytopenia. All of these symptoms are nonspecific for HIV infection, and patients need to be routinely assessed for other potential disease processes. With further progression of HIV disease and immunosuppression, patients are observed to have opportunistic infections and neoplasms. The diagnosis of AIDS is made during this late stage of HIV infection. The current CDC case definition of AIDS, published in 1993, includes several categories of potential AIDS diagnoses. AIDS is diagnosed when specific infectious diseases/neoplasms are present that are otherwise rare illnesses (e.g., Kaposi's sarcoma, *Pneumocystis carinii* pneumonia, cryptococcal meningitis, *Candida* esophagitis, *Toxoplasma* encephalitis, and disseminated atypical mycobacterial infection). Patients with

HIV infection are also known to have frequent, severe, and recurrent problems with bacterial infections. These will not be discussed here but have been recently reviewed in the literature (8, 9). Wasting syndrome and malnutrition are common in patients with HIV infection as a result of many factors, including decreased food intake because of malaise and anorexia; gastrointestinal (GI) disorders such as vomiting, diarrhea, and malabsorption; and factors related to hypermetabolism from infection and endocrine disorders.

Pediatric AIDS patients differ in their clinical presentation and rate of disease progression compared to adolescents and adults. They may have rapid progression of HIV infection in the first year of life, which manifests as failure to thrive or as neurodevelopmental delay. Since HIV infection in children may be masked by the presence of passive maternal antibodies and disease progression differs from that in adults, the CDC has separately classified HIV infection in children under the age of 13 years (10).

MEDICAL TREATMENT WITH ANTIRETROVIRAL THERAPY

It has been challenging to select and evaluate therapies for patients with the various stages of HIV infection. Definitions for therapy "cure" and "failure" have been especially difficult to establish. Success is not defined by the usual infectious diseases criteria of microbiologic cure and resolution of clinical symptoms. Rather, treatment success is measured by parameters such as improved survival, delay in disease progression, improved functional status (Karnofsky's performance status), restoration of neurologic function, and a lower attack rate or prolonged time until occurrence of first or new opportunistic infections (OIs). These successful outcomes have been observed in several subpopulations of patients who have received antiretroviral therapy early in their disease course. Appropriate antimicrobial prophylaxis for *Pneumocystis carinii* pneumonia (PCP) has also been a factor for these positive outcomes.

Zidovudine (AZT)

Zidovudine (Retrovir) was the first FDA-approved antiretroviral agent that has been shown in controlled studies to be "effective." However, progression of disease and death do still occur while patients are taking AZT therapy. AZT is a thymidine analog that is triphosphorylated by cellular kinase enzymes to become the active drug moiety. Because of the structural similarity to thymidine triphosphate, zidovudine triphosphate is used as a substrate by the viral RNA-dependent DNA polymerase enzyme, reverse transcriptase. Zidovudine triphosphate is integrated into the DNA where the drug's 3'-azido groups prevent the formation of the normal 5'-3'phosphodiester linkages. AZT thus acts as a chain terminator of viral DNA synthesis. Data from AZT trials is summarized in Table 72.2.

Table 72.2.
Summary of Zidovudine (AZT) Trials

Study Description	Endpoints	Results
BW 002 Placebo vs. AZT 1500 mg/day AIDS/ARC patients (7, 8, 9)	Survival	Improved with AZT
ACTG 016 Placebo vs. AZT 1200 mg/day Milder HIV infection (not AIDS or ARC) (10)	Disease progression	Delay if CD4 200–500 No effect CD4 >500
Veterans Affairs Cooperative Study AZT in mild HIV infection (11) CD4 200–500 AZT 1500 mg/day Deferred vs. immediate therapy	Survival Progression to AIDS	No survival differences Delay in progression
ACTG 019 Placebo vs. AZT (12, 13) CD4 above vs. below 500 AZT 500 or 1500 mg/day	Time to disease progression CD4 cell count Survival time	Delay in progression if CD4 <500 Efficacy of 500 mg = 1500 mg/day AZT increased CD4 in all patients No differences in survival No delay in progression if CD4 >500
Concorde Placebo vs. AZT 1000 mg/day (14) Asymptomatic; matched CD4 Deferred vs immediate therapy	Disease progression	No long-term (3 year) delay in progression Early (55 week) delay in progression
EACG 020 Placebo vs. AZT 1000 mg/day (15) CD4 >400 Asymptomatic	Progression AIDS/ARC Drop in CD4	Delay in progression at any CD4 count AZT less decline in CD4
ACTG 002 AZT in AIDS patients (20) 1500 mg vs. 600 mg/day	Survival Onset of OIs	Increase time of survival both dosages Delay OIs both dosages Higher dosage has more side effects

In early 1987 the 6-month follow-up data from a placebo-controlled study (BW 002) reported AZT to be effective in the management of two adult HIV-infection subpopulations (11). These groups were (a) patients with AIDS with confirmed PCP and (b) advanced ARC patients with an absolute CD4 count less than 200/mm^3. In this initial study, the probability of survival was improved for post-PCP and ARC patients in the AZT group compared to the placebo group. There was also a significantly decreased probability of developing other opportunistic infections. The results of this study were reviewed, and FDA approval for AZT was given in March 1987. The initial dosage recommendation was "high-dose" therapy of 200 mg (two 100-mg capsules) every 4 hr around the clock (1200 mg/day). Further follow-up of these patients to 21 months revealed continued improved survival in the AZT-treated patients (12, 13). Another placebo-controlled trial from the AIDS Clinical Trials Group (ACTG 016) enrolled patients with milder HIV disease (i.e., no AIDS or ARC diagnoses) and monitored disease progression. AZT-treated patients with baseline CD4 counts between 200 and 500 had a delay in disease progression, defined as a new diagnosis of ARC or AIDS (14). Patients with a baseline CD4 count greater than 500 did not progress over the study period, and

therefore no difference was observed between placebo- and AZT-treated patients. The Veterans Affairs Cooperative Study Group study of patients with mild HIV-related symptoms found no differences in survival after 28 months but found that early treatment slowed progression to AIDS (15).

In 1990 a large collaborative study (ACTG 019) reported the efficacy of AZT for patients with asymptomatic HIV infection (16). Analysis of the data has shown that patients with a CD4 count less than 500/mm^3 benefit from AZT therapy. Of the 1338 participants who were followed for two years, 33 cases of AIDS were diagnosed in the placebo control group, compared to 11 and 14 cases in the 500-mg/day and 1500-mg/day AZT groups, respectively. Success was assessed to be a significant reduction in the rate of disease progression in both the low-dose (500 mg/day) and high-dose (1500 mg/day) groups. For ACTG 019 patients who started with a CD4 count greater than 500 (n = 1637), the data revealed differences in immediate versus delayed therapy (17). Patients showed an earlier decline in CD4 count (to 400/mm^3) if therapy was delayed. However, survival time and the onset of first opportunistic infection were equivalent in delayed and immediate therapy groups. The discordant results of clinical disease progression and CD4 count again call into question the value of surrogate markers, such as the CD4 count, as a study endpoint.

The Concorde trial also studied the timing of initiating AZT therapy (immediate versus delayed therapy) and found no benefits for most patients (18). By contrast, the European-Australian Collaborative Group protocol 020 studied asymptomatic patients with CD4 counts greater than 400 mm^3 at enrollment (19). This study showed that there was a delay in time to an AIDS or ARC diagnosis for all patients, including patients with initial CD4 counts greater than 500 mm^3. Thus, the controversy surrounding early antiretroviral therapy (i.e., when the CD4 is greater than 500/mm^3) in HIV continues (20).

Adverse reactions were common in the initial placebo-controlled study (BW 002), with 84% and 72% of patients in AZT and placebo groups, respectively, reporting at least one adverse event (21). Weakness, headache, diarrhea, abdominal pain, and fever were symptoms that occurred commonly in both study groups. Nausea, myalgia, and insomnia were the only adverse experiences that were reported with significantly greater frequency in the AZT group. Headaches occurred at the same frequency but were more severe in the AZT-treated patients. Macrocytosis developed within weeks in most patients on AZT. By week six, anemia with hemoglobin levels less than 7.5 g/dL developed in 24.5% and 4.4% of AZT and placebo patients, respectively (p < 0.001). Neutropenia (<500 cells/mm^3) occurred in 16.1% and 2.2% of AZT and placebo patients, respectively (p <0.001). Leukopenia and neutropenia were most marked in the patients who had low CD4 counts and AIDS at study entry. Thirty-one percent of AZT patients and 11% of placebo patients received transfusions during the study period (p ≤ 0.05). Additionally, multiple transfusions were required in 21% of AZT patients compared to only 4% in placebo groups. Overall, platelet counts were observed to increase to a greater extent in patients receiving AZT compared to placebo. A quality-of-life analysis was done as part of the ACTG 019 study of asymptomatic HIV-infected patients (22). The authors of this study suggested that the delay in disease progression from AZT was equal to the time of decreased quality-of-life due to drug side effects.

Administration of exogenous recombinant erythropoietin (EPO), a glycoprotein growth factor, has been reported to improve outcome in AZT-induced anemia (23). In the bone marrow, erythropoietin stimulates erythrocyte maturation, thus increasing the oxygen-carrying capacity of blood, resulting also in improvement of the patient's symptoms from their anemic state. In a randomized, double-blind, placebo-controlled trial of 63 AIDS patients receiving concomitant AZT, 29 patients in the EPO group received 100 units/kg three times per week. Both the number of patients needing transfusions and the actual

number of transfusions per patient decreased for EPO recipients compared to placebo recipients. EPO response was characterized to be most effective in patients with a ≤ 500 IU/L baseline endogenous erythropoietin concentration. These patients were observed to have a greater rise in hematocrit values when they were given EPO. Recommendations for widespread use of EPO in patients on AZT are not appropriate. However, EPO is a useful therapeutic modality to be initiated on a case-by-case basis when symptomatic anemia persists despite AZT dosage reduction.

Since 1987 there have been other important advances in our knowledge about the rational use of AZT. A dose-comparison study (ACTG 002) was done involving 524 post-PCP AIDS patients who were randomized to receive one of two AZT treatment regimens (24). One group received "standard therapy" (1500 mg/day); the other group was given an initial dosage of 1200 mg/day for 1 month followed by a lower dosage of 100 mg every 4 hr (600 mg/day). Results revealed that the two groups had comparable survival rates and frequencies of opportunistic infections. However, the low-dose (600 mg/day), regimen was associated with a significantly lower incidence of hematologic toxicity. Lower dosages of AZT (300 mg/day), might be less toxic and equally efficacious (25), but this regimen needs to be more thoroughly evaluated. The currently recommended AZT dose for adults is 600 mg/day. It is not known, however, whether this regimen is as effective as higher dosages for the treatment of HIV encephalopathy (dementia) or thrombocytopenia. Patients with these conditions may need the higher dosages.

Initial results from a study of 88 children (ages 4 months to 11 years) who were given oral AZT 180 mg/m^2 every 6 hr were optimistic and reported clinical, immunologic, and virologic improvements (26). Subsequently, many studies of children have used AZT monotherapy at various dosages or as combination therapy. The more frequent occurrences of central nervous system (CNS)-related HIV disease in children has led to the recommendation of higher AZT dosages than those given to adults (e.g., 180 mg/m^2/dose) (27). The pharmacokinetics of AZT in children are similar to those in adults, except that children younger than 2 months of age have reduced drug clearance. The future holds promise when there is data on the pharmacokinetics of the active intracellular AZT-triphosphate compound; this data will help us to optimize drug dosing for adults and children.

The rate of HIV transmission from an infected mother to her infant has been estimated to between 15% and 40%; approximately half of these children are infected in utero and 14% are infected from breastfeeding. Most of the in utero transmission has been reported to occur late in pregnancy. Some of the most significant effects of AZT have been recently described in this patient population. In a placebo-controlled trial, AZT was reported to reduce maternal-infant HIV transmission (28). HIV-infected women who had not been receiving antiretroviral therapy were randomized to placebo versus AZT antepartum 500 mg/day and intrapartum 2 mg/kg loading dose intravenously over 1 hr followed by a maintenance infusion of 1 mg/kg/hr until delivery. Neonates who were born to mothers in the treatment arm of the study were also given AZT 2 mg/kg orally four times a day for 6 weeks. Transmission rates measured at 1 year and older were found to be 8.4% in the AZT group compared to 22.5% for placebo.

The emergence of AZT-resistant isolates of HIV is not surprising, considering that nucleoside analogs reduce viral replication only by approximately 90%. The high rates of viral replication along with the presence of chronic active infection and limited antiviral effectiveness present ideal conditions for the emergence of resistance. More rapid clinical progression may result from resistance to AZT; therefore a change in therapy should be instituted when a clinical decline is apparent (29). In vivo and in vitro studies have demonstrated that mutant isolates can be selected for that are resistant to any or all of the nucleoside analogs. Exact mechanisms of resistance are yet to be determined.

General therapy recommendations for adults who are infected with HIV are that individuals who have not been diagnosed with AIDS should be offered AZT when their CD4 count is approximately 500/mm^3. Optimally, there should be two consecutive counts below 500/mm^3 that were obtained a few weeks apart before therapy is initiated. In the near future, viral burden tests may help to guide this decision. All pregnant women with HIV infection should receive AZT per the study protocol described above or be enrolled in a new drug regimen study. The optimal time to initiate antiretroviral therapy in children is not known, and the CD4 count is not a good surrogate marker in this patient group. The Working Group on Antiretroviral

Table 72.3.
Prescribing Guidelines for Antiretroviral Agents
Initiation of Therapy

Clinical Status	CD4 Count/mm^3	Recommendation
Adults		
Asymptomatic	>500	No treatment
Asymptomatic	200–500	Offer treatment
Symptomatic	200–500	Treat
Asymptomatic	<200	Treat
Symptomatic	<200	Treat
Pregnant	Any	Treat mother and neonate
Children	Evidence of significant immunosuppression or HIV-associated symptoms/diseases	
<1 year	<1750 (<30%)	
1–2 years	<1000 (25%)	
2–6 years	<750 (20%)	
>6 years	<500 (20%)	

Therapy of the National Pediatric HIV Resource Center has made some recommendations based on the age of the child and symptoms (23). Guidelines for initiating antiretroviral therapy are listed in Table 72.3. A summary of AZT dosage recommendations for various ages and stages of HIV infection are given in Table 72.4. These recommendations have taken into consideration recently published guidelines (30).

Didanoside (DDI)

Didanosine (Videx) was approved by the FDA in 1991 as monotherapy for both children and adults who were intolerant to, or had failed on, AZT. This antiretroviral agent is a nucleoside analog with several pharmacokinetic/pharmacodynamic features that differ from those of AZT (31). DDI has poorer bioavailability because it is acid labile. It does not penetrate the blood-brain barrier (21% of plasma concentration) as well as AZT does and so may be less useful in the treatment of HIV-related CNS disease. The active metabolite of DDI, DDATP, was found to have a long intracellular half-life (12 to 24 hr), which compares favorably to the short 3-hr half-life of AZT's active metabolite. Possible pharmacodynamic advantages include DDI's improved activity in monocyte/macrophages, a reservoir for HIV.

DDI studies have been designed to answer various questions relative to AZT use:

1. Is a switch from AZT to DDI beneficial?
2. Which monotherapy is more effective?
3. Is combination therapy more efficacious than monotherapy?

Two Phase I studies of DDI in adults with AIDS/ARC have been published. One study reported significant decreases in p24 antigen levels and increases in CD4 cell counts in 37 patients receiving the drug twice a day (over a dose range of 0.4 to 66 mg/kg/day) (32). Fifty percent of patients reported an increase in energy or an improved sense of well-being, and 50% had significant weight gain; approximately 25% had both weight gain and subjective improvement. In a second Phase I study using once-daily dosing of oral DDI 1.6 to 30.4 mg/kg/day, efficacy was also reported (33). Data for children was available and contributed to the original FDA approval (34, 35).

With respect to answering question 1 above, results from controlled trials ACTG 116B/117 were positive (36). In these studies, patients who were on AZT for at least 4 months were randomized to receive either AZT or DDI. Overall, patients (with any CD4 count) appeared to benefit from the switch to DDI on the basis of two clinic endpoints: delay of OI or delay of death. Another study from the Community Program for Clinical Reseach on AIDS corroborates that switching therapy to DDI after "some" treatment with AZT delays death or the onset of new OIs (37). The answer to question 2 was resolved in ACTG 116A

OI = opportunistic infection

Table 72.4.
Dosage Recommendations for Antiretroviral Agents

Drug	Patient	Recommendation
ZIDOVUDINE 100 mg capsule 50 mg/5 mL oral solution 10 mg/mL intravenous	**ADULT**	**200 mg po TID (lower dose if not tolerated)** May need increased dosage for HIV-related dementia and HIV-related thrombocytopenia
	PREGNANT	Antepartum 100 mg 5 times/day Intrapartum 2 mg/kg IV loading dose over 1 hr then 1 mg/kg/hr IV until delivery (cord clamped)
	CHILD	180 mg/m^2 q6h (not to exceed 200 mg q6h)
DIDANOSINE	NEONATE–3 MONTHS	2–3 mg/kg q6h
	ADULT	200 mg po BID if ≥60 kg (2 tablets/dose for maximum buffer)
Tablets: 25, 50, 100, and 150 mg Chewable or dispersible tablets with aspartame **and buffer**		125 mg po BID if <60 kg (2 tablets/dose for maximum buffer)
Buffered powder sachets: 100, 167, 25, 375 mg	ADULT	250 mg po BID if ≥60 kg 167 mg po BID if <60 kg FORMULATIONS
Pediatric powder to be admixed with antacid (final concentration 10 mg/mL)	CHILD 1.1–1.4 m^2 0.8–1.0 m^2 0.5–0.7 m^2 ≤0.4 m^2	100 mg po BID tabs or 125 mg po BID powder 75 mg po BID tabs or 94 mg po BID powder 50 mg po BID tabs or 62 mg po BID powder 25 mg po BID tabs or 31 mg po BID powder (2 tablets/dose for maximum buffer if >1 year old)
ZALCITABINE 0.375 and 0.75 mg tablets	**ADULT**	**0.75 mg po TID (lower dose if not tolerated)**
	CHILD <13 years	No current recommendations
STUVUDINE 15, 20, 30, & 40 mg capsules	**ADULT**	**40 mg po BID if ≥60 kg** 30 mg po BID if <60 kg
	CHILD 5 mo.–15 years	0.125–4 mg/kg/day

(AZT-naive or less than 16 weeks of AZT). Patients with AIDS/ARC and a CD4 less than 300 or asymptomatic patients with a CD4 less than 200 were enrolled. AZT 600 mg/day was preferable to either DDI dosage, with fewer AIDS-defining illnesses or deaths occurring. A small study has been published that answers question 3. Patients received either combination AZT and DDI or alternating monotherapies (38). Patients who received the combination therapy had greater increases in their CD4 count at 1 year, as well as significant weight gain. Lower daily doses of both DDI (250 mg/day) and AZT (300 mg/day) were used in this study.

Evaluation of safety revealed DDI to be tolerated by most patients, with an estimated maximum dosage of 12 mg/kg/day. The major dose-limiting side effects are painful peripheral neuropathy and life-threatening pancreatitis. Also, asymptomatic elevations of levels of liver enzymes, amylase, and uric acid were frequently observed. Impressive was the lack of hematologic toxicity, compared to those reported for AZT. Studies of children report side effects that are similar to those found in adults, though retinal depigmentation and vision changes have been reported in

a few children. Data from the expanded access study of DDI that enrolled over 21,000 patients identified a low CD4 count (≤ 100/mm^3) and an AIDS diagnosis as risk factors for experiencing DDI intolerance (39).

The rapid rate of DDI decomposition at the low pH and temperatures that are found in the GI tract has resulted in three unique drug formulations: as buffered (antacid), chewable-dispersible tablets; in single-dose sachets of a powder mixture that includes DDI and a citrate-phosphate buffer; and as a pediatric powder to be admixed with antacid. Adult patients should always take two tablets per dose of DDI for adequate amounts of the buffering agent. Patients should also be instructed to take DDI on an empty stomach and not to drink beverages that contain alcohol because of the potential increased risk of pancreatitis. Patients should also be warned to avoid medications that have drug-drug interactions with antacids (e.g., ketoconazole).

Zalcitabine (DDC)

Zalcitabine (Hivid) is the most potent dideoxynucleoside analog and was approved by the FDA in 1992 for combination therapy with AZT. It has since been proven to be useful as a monotherapy agent. Development of this drug somewhat lagged behind that of DDI because in early studies, DDC caused severe peripheral neuropathy. Like DDI, DDC has poor CNS penetration compared to AZT, but the oral bioavailability is better for DDC, and the drug is formulated as a small, easy-to-swallow tablet. Experience with children is limited at this time. However, since CNS penetration is low, outcomes will probably not be as favorable in children.

As with DDI, DDC monotherapy has been shown to be effective for patients who are experiencing disease progression while they are on AZT alone (33). In drug-naive patients the combination of AZT and DDC produced a significant effect on surrogate marker endpoints. A sustained increase in CD4 count and a decrease in p24 antigenemia were observed in patients compared to those who continued to receive AZT (40). In a recently published study of advanced HIV patients who had tolerated AZT for 6 months or longer, combination therapy with AZT and DDC was compared to AZT and DDC monotherapies. This meant that patients on AZT were either switching to DDC or adding DDC to their AZT regimen. The intent of this study was to assess clinical endpoints, time to disease progression or death, while also monitoring surrogate markers (41). Approximately 1000 patients were enrolled in this study and were monitored for disease progression for 18 months. No difference in survival or time to disease progression was noted for any of the treatment groups nor with subgroup analysis. However, DDC-containing regimens did produce a greater increase in CD4 counts. Thus, patients who have been on AZT do benefit from either a switch to DDC monotherapy or the addition of DDC or combination therapy.

The toxicity that is reported for DDC is similar in spectrum to that for DDI, except that apthous oral ulcers and rash are more frequently reported. Like DDI, DDC is not generally thought to cause serious hematologic toxicity, but dose-limiting side effects include peripheral neuropathy and rarely symptomatic pancreatitis.

Stavudine (D4T)

Stavudine (Zerit) is a nucleoside analog with good oral bioavailability and good CNS penetration. Limited data is available on this drug, since it received fast-track FDA approval in 1994. D4T was approved for adults with advanced HIV infection who had failed on, or were intolerant to, AZT and DDI. Approval was based on data from studies involving over 11,000 patients, 264 patients in phase I/II studies and the remainder from the expanded access program. D4T was studied in ARC/AIDS patients with positive results (42). An analysis of the parallel track data that was presented to the FDA revealed that D4T 20 mg orally twice a day and 40 mg orally twice a day were equally efficacious at 40 weeks and that 40 mg twice a day

was significantly more toxic (i.e., involved peripheral neuropathy). Later data analyses revealed a better response with higher doses.

The major toxicity from D4T has been peripheral neuropathy, which is clearly dose-related, occurring at a rate of 15% at a dose of 0.5 mg/kg/day and 30% at a dose of 2 mg/kg/day. Elevation in serum liver enzyme levels has also been reported. The safety and effectiveness of D4T for children and as part of a combination regimen are yet to be determined.

Lamivudine (3TC)

Lamivudine (Epivie®) was recently approved by the FDA. It was previously made available through an expanded access program for patients with CD4 counts less than 300/mm^3 who have been intolerant or have failed on all other available antiretroviral agents. The combination of 3TC and AZT is reported to be very potent, increasing CD4 count and decreasing viral burden, effects that are reported to be more sustained than for other agents. No clinical outcome data on the 3TC/AZT combination has been published to date.

Other Investigational Antiretroviral Agents

Nevarapine is a nonnucleoside dipyridodiazepinone that inhibits the reverse transcriptase enzyme. As monotherapy, nevarapine is not projected to be useful because resistance develops rapidly. Initial reports of a triple drug regimen that included nevarapine were positive; viral replication was almost completely suppressed, and resistant mutants could not evolve. ACTG 241 results are pending that studied AZT plus DDI with and without 3TC. A high incidence of rash has been reported in patients receiving 3TC >400 mg/day. Data from other trials is also pending. The drug L-697,661, with a similar mechanism of action, has also been studied, but resistance with monotherapy quickly evolved (43).

A series of proteinase inhibitor drugs, also known as protease inhibitors (e.g., saquinavir, Invirase; ABT-538; and indinavir, Crixivan), are being studied by many pharmaceutical companies. Many have revealed encouraging preliminary data when the drugs are used in combination therapies utilizing surrogate marker endpoints (44, 45).

Trichosanthin (compound Q) is an exciting anti-HIV compound because of its unique ability to treat acutely infected T cells and also chronically infected macrophages/ monocytes. In humans this drug has been reported to improve surrogate markers. Adverse reactions have been the limiting factor for this agent's development. Side effects included mild and reversible myalgias, hypoalbuminemia, and delayed fevers. Most significantly, 6 of 51 patients developed dementia at 36 to 60 hr after infusion. Two patients progressed to coma, which reversed within 12 hr with dexamethasone therapy.

PREVENTION MEASURES

Educational programs in the community and schools are critical for teaching the facts about the risk of transmission and the consequences of exposure to HIV. Opinions differ as to the age at which children should receive counseling about "safe sex," but few would dispute that safe sex is critical. Health care practitioners play an important role in this educational effort. Condom use is advocated as the major protective measure for stopping transmission of HIV. The additional use of nonoxynol-9 spermicidal preparations during intercourse increases anti-HIV efficacy and is therefore highly recommended. Many women in the United States are unaware that they are at risk for HIV infection and often remain undiagnosed until the onset of AIDS. Recurrent, refractory candida infections (vaginal and other) may be in the first sign of immunosuppression from HIV. Medical referral for such patients is encouraged and may lead to earlier detection of HIV. Health care practitioners should also actively distribute prepared materials (available from the CDC, the U.S. Public Health Service, and other agencies) concerning high-risk activities, safe sex, condom use, early signs of HIV, and how and where to get HIV testing and counseling. Health care practitioners need to be informed about the current issues and controversies surrounding HIV infection and treatments.

OCCUPATIONAL EXPOSURE TO HIV

The AIDS epidemic has led to a concern about potential occupational exposure to HIV. One study estimated the rate of infection after accidental exposure from needle stick injuries to be 0.4% (46). The implementation of universal infection control precautions may reduce the incidence of occupational exposures but will not entirely eliminate the risk of infection with HIV from accidental inoculation. Health care institutions and employee health services are faced with the difficult decision of whether or not to empirically give postexposure AZT prophylaxis. Two programs that described institution-specific policies and procedures on this matter have been reported in detail (47). A dosage regimen of 200 mg orally five times a day for 1 month has been suggested, but many individuals cannot tolerate this regimen and dose-adjust accordingly. A 3TC/AZT combination is also being tested for postexposure prophylaxis in health care workers.

COMPLICATIONS: KAPOSI'S SARCOMA AND HUMAN PAPILLOMAVIRUS

In addition to opportunistic infections, HIV-infected individuals are also at high risk for developing certain cancers. Kaposi's sarcoma (KS) is an endothelial neoplasm of either capillary of lymphatic origin and is the most commonly observed neoplasm in patients with HIV infection (48). A diagnosis of KS actually classifies a patient as having AIDS on the basis CDC criteria. The KS lesion may appear as a nontender red to purple nodule with associated edema. KS can also be an invasive systemic disease. Recently, a herpesvirus has been isolated in KS tissue (49), which may be a major breakthrough in the understanding of KS epidemiology and pathogenesis and may lead to new therapies for this complication. Some experts believe that because of this new information it is reasonable to begin acyclovir therapy when KS is initially diagnosed. The duration of therapy is not known. Local treatments of KS skin lesions include liquid nitrogen or intralesion vinblastine, as well as systemic therapy with antineoplastic drugs (e.g., vincristine, adriamycin, or bleomycin). The addition of AZT to the regimen of KS patients has been shown to improve outcomes. The use of immunomodulating compounds, such as α-interferon, in the treatment of Kaposi's sarcoma has also been somewhat effective. Clinical trials of recombinant interleukin-4, which down-regulates interleukin-6, are underway.

AZT and α-interferon have been given in combination and have shown an antitumor effect as well (50). A dose-escalation study of α-interferon plus AZT was conducted as an open, nonrandomized trial in patients with KS. The ability of patients to tolerate the interferon was directly related to their dose of AZT. The three oral AZT regimens that were studied were 250 mg every 4 hr, 100 mg every 4 hr, and 50 mg every 4 hr. At a minimum of 6 weeks after starting AZT, patients were begun on daily subcutaneous dosages of interferon, which was initiated at 5 million units (MU) per day, increasing every 2 weeks to a maximum tolerated dose or to 35 MU/day. Only patients who received the 50 mg every 4 hr regimen of AZT were able to tolerate more than 15 MU/day of interferon. At the two higher AZT dosages, neutropenia, thrombocytopenia, and hepatic dysfunction were the primary toxicities. Of the 22 patients who received a stable dose of both drugs for 12 weeks, 11 patients had a complete or partial antitumor response and 9 showed an anti-HIV effect as measured by converting to either HIV culture-negative (n = 6) or p24 antigen-negative (n = 3). Further studies are underway with new agents and unique formulations of adriamycin that may improve therapy outcomes for patients with KS.

Three types of human papillomavirus (HPV) are widespread throughout the population. At present, HPV infection is the most common sexually transmitted disease in the United States. Condylomata acuminatum is the sexually transmitted HPV that causes recurrent and persistent anogenital warts. HPV infection of the cervix can cause premalignant tumor as well as squamous cell carcinoma. The most recent CDC AIDS definitions include women with cervical squamous cell carcinoma. Annual PAP smears are recommended for all HIV-positive women for early detection of atypical squamous cells or cervical cancer. These women appear to be at greater risk for this disease, treatment failures, and recurrence (51). The treatment of this viral-induced disease usually consists of physically removing the affected tissue. This may be done by several methods using either surgical or chemical debridement.

COMPLICATIONS: OPPORTUNISTIC INFECTIONS ASSOCIATED WITH HIV DISEASE

Principles of Treatment

HIV attacks various cellular components of the immune system that are necessary host defenses in the fight against pathogen invasion and clinical infectious diseases. The resultant immunodeficiency state predisposes the HIV-infected patient to a wide variety of so-called opportunistic infections (OIs). The treatment of OIs in AIDS patients may consist of multiple-drug therapy, including antibacterial, antifungal, antiparasitic, antiviral, and antimycobacterial agents. Table 72.5 lists commonly observed opportunistic pathogens in HIV-infected patients; this is by no means a complete listing.

Patients with HIV infection should be evaluated and monitored in a continuous fashion for degree of immuno-suppression. A complete blood count with differential, CD4 count, and anergy skin testing may be used to assess the immune status. The severity of HIV infection, in addition to the severity of the OI, may dictate the type and duration of treatment. A comprehensive treatment regimen for a given OI may be divided into three distinct stages: primary prophylaxis, acute treatment, and secondary prophylaxis. The first stage of therapy, primary prophylaxis, is therapy that is initiated before the development of a clinical infection. This may or may not be instituted before the patient's actual exposure to the pathogen. Thus two distinct situations are possible for primary prophylaxis: Antibiotics are started before contact with the potential pathogen, or antibiotics are given after exposure to the potential pathogen but before development of clinical disease. Of these two primary prophylaxis scenarios, the latter applies in most cases for AIDS patients. The U.S. Public Health Service has guidelines for the prevention of OIs in people who are infected with HIV (52). For example, primary prophylaxis is instituted for prevention of tuberculosis or PCP when an individual patient's risk of developing an acute infection is perceived to be imminent on the basis of an assessment of the

Table 72.5.
Opportunistic Infections (OIs)[a] Commonly Observed in Individuals with HIV Infection

	SITE OF INFECTION
FUNGAL PATHOGENS	
Pneumocystis carinii	Pneumonia
Cryptococcus neoformans	Meningitis
Candida albicans (other *Candida* species)	Oral/pharyngeal, esophageal, vaginal
Endemic mycoses	
Coccidioides immitis	Disseminated
Histoplasma capsulatum	Disseminated
Blastomyces dermatitidis	Disseminated
PARASITIC PATHOGEN	**SITE OF INFECTION**
Toxoplasma gondii	Encephalitis
Cryptosporidium	Diarrhea
Strongyloides stercoralis	Disseminated infection, "hyperinfection"
Microsporidium	Diarrhea
VIRAL PATHOGEN	**SITE OF INFECTION**
Cytomegalovirus	Retinitis, gastrointestinal
Herpes simplex virus I & II	Chronic, ulcerative oral/genital lesions
Varicella zoster virus	Shingles or recurrent herpes zoster infection
Kaposi's sarcoma–associated herpes viruses	Kaposi's sarcoma
Human papillomavirus	Anogenital warts, cervical squamous cell carcinoma
Hepatitis B and C	Chronic active hepatitis
MYCOBACTERIAL PATHOGENS	**SITE OF INFECTION**
Mycobacterium tuberculosis	Pulmonary and/or extrapulmonary
Mycobacterium avium complex	Disseminated
Other atypical *Mycobacterium* species	Various
BACTERIAL PATHOGENS	**SITE OF INFECTION**
Streptococcus pneumoniae	Upper/lower respiratory tract, sepsis
Listeria monocytogenes	Meningitis, disseminated
Staphylococcus aureus	Impetigo, sinusitis, IV-line infection, skin infection
Salmonella species	Gastroenteritis, sepsis, disseminated, with recurrences
Pseudomonas aeruginosa	Upper/lower respiratory tract, skin, with recurrences
Treponema pallidum	Primary, secondary, tertiary with CNS involvement

[a]OIs that are seen with increased severity and frequency in HIV-positive patients.

patient's immune status. Specific criteria exist for initiating PCP prophylaxis when the CD4 count is less than 200/mm^3 or the percentage of CD4 is less than 20% (53). Guidelines also exist specifically for children (see the description below).

The next stage of therapy is the acute treatment of an OI. A review of recent advances in the management of AIDS-related OIs has been published (54). When it is available, such therapy should consist of bactericidal antimicrobial agents, much as one would give "cidal" antimicrobial therapy to an immunocompromised cancer patient. Unfortunately, this is neither possible nor practical for some of the OIs that are encountered in AIDS patients, such as toxoplasmosis, for which oral sulfadiazine and pyrimethamine are "static" and are currently the therapy of choice. Combination regimens are often used because of their theoretical additive or synergistic effects. Also, adequate drug penetration to the multiple sites of infection (e.g., the CNS) may be improved when more than one antimicrobial agent is used. Unfortunately, patients with HIV infection have in general been observed to be much less tolerant to drugs and experience adverse effects with greater frequency and intensity. Thus, combination regimens are not routinely recommended (e.g., flucytosine and amphotericin B for cryptococcal meningitis).

The duration of acute treatment of opportunistic infections in patients with AIDS may be guided by experience from other patient groups as well as individual patient response. In general, therapy will be more prolonged than for other patients. The goal of acute treatment is to reverse most signs and symptoms of infection and to improve the quality of life.

The last stage of antimicrobial therapy is the secondary prophylaxis regimen, which is instituted after the completion of acute treatment. The goal of secondary prophylaxis is to prevent relapses or recurrences of clinical infection. Secondary prophylaxis may also be termed maintenance or suppressive therapy. Secondary prophylaxis may be very prolonged; it may be necessary for a patient's entire lifetime, as in the case of cryptococcal meningitis, which has a high recurrence rate. The drug doses that are employed for suppressive regimens are usually lower than those used for acute treatment but are highly variable and may need to be titrated on the basis of the patient's response or intolerance.

Pneumocystis Carinii Pneumonia (PCP)

Pneumocystis carinii is an organism, newly reclassified as a fungus on the basis of RNA sequencing data, that is commonly observed to be part of human respiratory tract normal flora. Clinical infection with *P. carinii* has been reported to occur in situations of host immune suppression, such as in patients with specific cancers or after organ transplantation. Infection involving the lung is the most common clinical presentation and is well described. In the 1980s, AIDS became the most common underlying immune disorder predisposing individuals to PCP. In the United States, PCP occurs in the majority of AIDS patients and is the AIDS case-defining diagnosis for many.

PCP is, however, distinctive in the AIDS patient population compared to other immunosuppressed patient groups. The infection is more insidious, the patients are symptomatic for a longer period of time before acute respiratory decompensation, and therapy is quite often complicated by the occurrence of adverse drug reactions. Because PCP ultimately develops in up to 80 to 90% of AIDS patients, institution of primary prophylaxis is recommended for HIV-infected individuals who have profound immunosuppression. Such treatment is recommended for patients with a CD4 count of approximately 200 cell/mm^3. This preventive measure may in part be responsible for improvements that have recently been observed in the long-term survival of AIDS patients.

The most frequent presenting symptoms of acute PCP are shortness of breath, dyspnea, fever, and cough. An elevated serum lactate dehydrogenase level and a chest radiograph with diffuse interstitial markings may be clues to the presence of this pneumonia. Although patients with PCP often complain of cough, they rarely produce sputum. Currently, *P. carinii* culture techniques are not reliable except in the research setting. The diagnosis in many cases is presumptive, but a definitive diagnosis can be made by Giemsa and silver stain procedures that are performed on induced sputum specimens for microscopic examination and identification of the organism.

After diagnosis or just before (24 to 48 hr) an induced sputum is performed, patients may be started on acute treatment (see Table 72.6). Patients with PCP who have been on AZT for at least 6 weeks before diagnosis appear to have a better prognosis. Trimethoprim/sulfamethoxazole (TMP/SMX) is considered to be the drug of choice for PCP unless the patient has a significant history of drug intolerance or allergy. TMP/SMX drug desensitization protocols have been used, but their role has not been clearly established. When an allergy history reveals mild intolerance or allergy, a T/S rechallenge may be indicated. This should not be done if there is any indication of previous Stevens-Johnson syndrome or anaphylaxis.

For acute PCP treatment, either the oral or parenteral route of administration may be used, as the bioavailablity of TMP/SMX is close to 100%. Parenteral therapy is recommended only if the patient has evidence of GI intolerance or suspected malabsorption or when the patient is too ill for oral medications. Parenteral TMP/SMX is usually selected as empiric therapy for the hospitalized patient, therapy being switched to oral when improvement and stabilization occur. Therapy is given for a total of 14 to

Table 72.6.
Drug Therapy for Acute Treatment and Prophylaxis of *Pneumocystis Carinii* Pneumonia in Adults

Therapy	Dosage	Route
Trimethoprim/sulfamethoxazole (TMP/SMX)	T: 15–20 mg/kg/day (divided q6–8h; 400 mg maximum/IV dose)	IV or PO
Pentamidine	3–4 mg/kg QD	IV
Trimethoprim/dapsone (TMP/D)	T: 15–20 mg/kg/day (divided q6–8hr)	PO
	D: 100 mg QD	PO
Clindamycin/primaquine (C/P)	C: 900 mg q6–8hr	IV/PO
	P: 15–30 mg base QD	PO
Atovaquone	750 mg po BID (for suspension)	PO
Trimetrexate/leucovorin (T/L)	T: 45 mg/m^2	IV
	L: 20 mg/m^2 q6hr *for 24 days*	PO/IV
PROPHYLAXIS		
Trimethoprim/sulfamethoxazole (TMP/SMX)	One double-strength tablet QD (160 mg/800 mg) or QOD, or 3×/week	PO
	One single-strength tablet QD (80 mg/400 mg)	PO
Dapsone	100 mg QD	PO
	50 mg BID	PO
Dapsone plus pyrimethamine plus leucovorin	D: 50 mg QD & P: 50 mg qweek & L: 25 mg qweek	PO
	D: 200 mg qweek & P: 75 mg qweek & L: 25 mg qweek	PO
Pentamidine aerosol	300 mg qmonth	Via Respirgard II Nebulizer

Atovaquone, clindamycin plus primaquine, and IV/IM pentamidine are not routinely recommended for prophylaxis.

21 days. Adverse reactions to TMP/SMX occur in most patients but require drug discontinuation in fewer than 50% of patients. Nausea and vomiting are often a problem but may be minimized by dividing the total daily dosage into smaller doses given at more frequent intervals (e.g., every 6 hr). Hyponatremia and fluid overload may also be managed by administering more concentrated TMP/SMX solutions and by using diluents other than in D5W (55). Other adverse reactions from T/S include hematologic toxicities (anemia, neutropenia, and thrombocytopenia), skin rashes, hyperkalemia, and liver transaminase enzyme elevation. TMP/SMX-induced adverse reactions, for the most part, are not serious and are reversible. It is generally felt that the lower dose based on the trimethoprim component (15 mg/kg/day) may result in less toxicity (e.g., bone marrow, electrolyte abnormalities, liver, kidneys).

In a prospective, randomized study of AIDS patients with PCP, there was no statistical difference in efficacy or the frequency of adverse reactions from TMP/SMX or intravenous pentamidine (56). Adverse reactions associated with pentamidine administration are potentially serious and can be irreversible (e.g., pancreatic dysfunction). Adverse reactions from pentamidine include nephrotoxicity, elevation of liver transaminase enzymes, hypocalcemia, hypoglycemia, pancreatitis followed by hyperglycemia and insulin-dependent diabetes mellitus, infusion-related hypotension, and thrombocytopenia.

Therapeutic alternatives to TMP/SMX and pentamidine include the oral regimen of dapsone plus trimethoprim, which has been shown in mild-to-moderately ill

patients to be as effective as TMP/SMX and less toxic (57). In another study, dapsone alone was not as effective as TMP/SMX. Atovaquone has been shown to be less efficacious in mild-to-moderate PCP but better tolerated than TMP/SMX (58). If a patient fails to improve on initial intravenous therapy, a switch is often made to parenteral clindamycin plus primaquine (59), or steroids can be added to the regimen. "Salvage therapy" for PCP may be tried with drugs such as trimetrexate. The efficacy and toxicity data for trimetrexate alone is pending, but this is a potentially toxic regimen to be given along with an expensive leucovorin "rescue" and requires prolonged intravenous therapy.

The administration of corticosteroids along with antimicrobial therapy has improved outcome in certain patients with PCP (60). Adults or children (older than 13 years of age) with documented or suspected PCP complicating HIV infection should be given corticosteroids if they have moderate or severe pulmonary dysfunction. This dysfunction is defined as a partial arterial oxygen pressure of ≤ 70 mm Hg or an arterial-alveolar gradient of >35 mm Hg. Early treatment with corticosteroids reduces the risk of respiratory failure and death from PCP. In studies revealing these beneficial effects of adjunctive corticosteroids, steroid therapy was begun early, within 24 to 72 hr of initiating antipneumocystis therapy. The corticosteroid regimen that is currently recommended is as follows: On days 1 through 5, prednisone 40 mg orally every 12 hr; on days 6 through 10, prednisone 40 mg orally once a day; on days 11 through 21, prednisone 20 mg orally once a day.

PCP Prophylaxis

All patients who have had an episode of PCP should receive secondary prophylaxis. Without prophylaxis there is a 60% chance of developing PCP in the next year. The same regimens that are recommended for primary prophylaxis of PCP can be considered for secondary prophylaxis (see Table 72.6). Many studies have evaluated various drug regimens (61). Recommendations for infants and children differ from those for adults. Since the CD4 count is used as an indicator for initiating PCP prophylaxis, it must be recognized that the normal CD4 count changes with age. Thus, separate PCP prophylaxis recommendations are necessary for children of various age groups, as well as for infants who were exposed perinatally to HIV (62). For HIV-infected adults and children, any prophylaxis regimen, once begun, should be continued indefinitely. Several doses of TMP/SMX are being recommended for adults (e.g., one single-strength tablet per day or one double-strength tablet every day, every other day or three times a week); lower dosages are thought to be as effective and better tolerated. Individuals who are receiving sulfadiazine plus pyrimethamine for toxoplasmosis encephalitis therapy or prophylaxis do not need to take additional drugs for PCP prophylaxis; the same cannot be said for patients who are receiving clindamycin plus pyrimethamine.

An early AIDS/PCP prophylaxis study was done involving adult patients with KS receiving TMP/SMX as primary prophylaxis (63). The twice-daily 160 mg/800 mg regimen administered for 2 years was compared to placebo. TMP/SMX was observed to prevent or delay an initial episode of PCP. No patient (0 of 30) developed PCP while receiving TMP/SMX compared to an incidence of 53% in the placebo group (16 of 30). Significantly, no patient in the TMP/SMX group died of PCP. Adverse reactions were observed in 50% of patients receiving TMP/SMX, only 5 (17%) of whom had to discontinue therapy because of severe erythroderma or neutropenia and fever. Of these 5 patients, PCP developed in 80% (4 of 5) within 5 months of discontinuing prophylaxis.

Aerosolized pentamidine 300 mg/month and dapsone 100 mg/day are slightly less effective than T/S but are reasonable alternatives for TMP/SMX-intolerant or -allergic patients (64). In the same study, dapsone 50 mg/day was less efficacious. The most common adverse effects that are reported during aerosol treatments are cough and, less frequently, wheezing. Systemic side effects have been reported but are rare after aerosol pentamidine administration. Other potential limitations of aerosol pentamidine include lack of protection against extrapulmonary disease and direct pulmonary toxicity, such as bronchospasm or pneumothorax.

Cryptococcal Meningitis

Disseminated cryptococcal infection and meningitis can occur in individuals who do not have HIV-induced immunodeficiency but is rare. Meningitis is the most common manifestation of cryptococcosis in AIDS patients, with an incidence of 7 to 10%. The cerebrospinal fluid (CSF) glucose concentration, protein concentration, and cell count are frequently normal, although the glucose has also been observed to be less than 2.8 mmol/L (50 mg/dL). Analysis of the CSF usually reveals positive results with India ink staining, culture, and antigen titer testing. The most common presenting symptoms in AIDS patients with cryptococcal meningitis has been headache and fever. Other symptoms of meningitis include nausea and vomiting, photophobia, malaise, stiff neck, focal neurologic abnormalities, mental status changes, seizures, and papilledema. Flame hemorrhages of the retina occur less commonly. Before the use of amphotericin B, cryptococcal meningitis was a uniformly fatal disease.

The therapy of choice is somewhat debated, depending on the initial patient presentation. The two available parenteral antifungal agents are amphotericin B, the "gold standard," and fluconazole. Patients with altered mental status should receive amphotericin B (0.3 to 0.6 mg/kg/day as tolerated) (65). A high CSF cryptococcal antigen titer (>1:1024) and a low CSF white blood cell count (≤ 20) are also associated with increased mortality and thus are parameters that indicate that amphotericin should be selected. The addition of flucytosine 100 to 75 mg/kg/day divided every 6 hr (Ancobon; 5-fluorocytosine, 5-FC) is recommended if the patient does not respond quickly and only if the hematologic parameters, especially the neutrophil count, are stable.

There has been some success with fluconazole as an initial treatment of cryptococcal meningitis compared to amphotericin plus 5FC (66), but this therapy is not routinely recommended for severely ill patients. New data on the combination regimen of fluconazole plus flucytosine is very encouraging (67). Response rates at 10 weeks were better than seen in historical data on amphotericin B or fluconazole monotherapy studies. Treatment with other "azoles" (ketoconazole and itraconazole) has been disappointing.

Intrathecal administration of amphotericin B for the treatment of cryptococcal meningitis is usually reserved for seriously ill patients who have relapsed on maximal systemic amphotericin B or for patients who are unable to receive adequate doses of intravenous amphotericin because of progressive amphotericin-induced nephrotoxicity. The complications that are associated with the insertion and use of an Omaya reservoir include fever, pain, tinnitus, headache, chemical ventriculitis, and infection.

5-FC is well absorbed after oral administration (76 to 79%) and distributes well into most body fluid and tissues, including the CSF. Unlike amphotericin B, 5-FC is almost exclusively eliminated by the kidneys, and patients with renal dysfunction (e.g., from amphotericin B) do require dosage adjustment. 5FC toxicities include leukopenia (20%) and thrombocytopenia (10%); diarrhea and rash have been reported to occur in 8% of patients. Toxicities related to amphotericin B therapy include infusion-related side effects, as well as the acute and chronic adverse reactions that are related to organ system toxicities. Infusion-related toxicities can usually be managed, and therapy can be continued. These may include fever, hypotension, chills, myalgias, nausea, and vomiting. Therefore, vital signs should be monitored closely during therapy. Premedication or symptomatic relief with intravenous fluids, diphenhydramine, aspirin, antiemetics, or acetaminophen may be required. Infusion-related thrombophlebitis may be ameliorated by the addition of heparin (500 to 1000 units) and hydrocortisone (15 to 25 mg) to the intravenous infusion. The infusion rate may also be slowed, but this measure is not always effective. Infusion-related shaking chills or rigors may improve with the administration of meperidine.

The more chronic toxicities from amphotericin, such as hematologic effects, include normochromic, normocytic anemia, and thrombocytopenia. Nephrotoxicity from amphotericin B is not preventable, nor is it predictable. Reported nephrotoxic effects include renal arteriolar vasoconstriction, which is associated with decreased glomerular filtration rate, tubular degeneration, nephrocalcinosis, decreased tubular concentrating ability, and renal tubular acidosis with potassium wasting. Sodium loading is a technique that has diminished amphotericin-induced nephrotoxicity in animal models; administration of normal saline >2 L/day is recommended for humans. Dosage adjustment may also help to minimize impending renal toxicity. Various liposomal amphotericin B preparations are being studied in the hope that these preparations will be as effective and less nephrotoxic.

Although the overall treatment response rate for AIDS patients with cryptococcal meningitis is similar to that observed for other populations, infection does not appear to be eradicated. In AIDS patients a marked relapse rate of at least 40% has been noted, which suggests that secondary prophylaxis or suppressive therapy is necessary (68). Suppressive therapy with fluconazole 200 mg/day orally is recommended for all AIDS patients (69). Primary prophylaxis for cryptococcal meningitis is not routinely recommended. Fluconazole prophylaxis has been shown to be somewhat effective (70), but the patients who are at highest risk are not easily identifiable. Administering fluconazole broadly may have significant negative consequences for *Candida* species resistance as well as great fiscal impact. Some experts have recommended routine primary prophylaxis with fluconazole for all patients with a CD4 count less than 50/mm³, but the outcomes (clinical and fiscal) of this recommendation are yet to be described.

Oral/Pharyngeal Candidiasis and Candida Esophagitis

Oropharyngeal candidiasis (thrush) is the most common fungal infection that is reported in AIDS patients. Infection usually causes mild inflammation and local discomfort but does not become invasive with symptomatic fungemia. Fungal throat swab cultures have been studied as a screening test but do not appear to be useful, since *Candida* species organisms are common commensal oropharyngeal and pulmonary flora.

Good oral hygiene is tantamount to a therapeutic success for preventing recurrent, resistant disease. Topical treatment, even for the more symptomatic cases of thrush, is usually adequate. Initial treatment with nonabsorbable antifungal agents including nystatin or clotrimazole is recommended. There is no proven benefit in the use of combined topical regimens. Initial treatment should not be on an as-needed schedule. For thrush, it is recommended that one clotrimazole 10-mg troche be given four to five times daily until clinical resolution of signs and symptoms. The dose of nystatin suspension is 100,000 to 1,500,000 units, "swish and swallow," every 4 to 6 hr. Nystatin may also be administered topically by instructing the patient to suck on a vaginal tablet (100,000 units per tablet) three to four times daily. The vaginal tablet or pastille preparations may actually provide more oral mucosal contact time for the drug to exert its effect. Compliance may be a problem with nystatin suspension because it has a bitter taste; clotrimazole troches and nystatin pastilles are more palatable. Troches or lozenges should be dissolved slowly in the mouth, not swallowed whole. Systemic antifungal therapy with ketoconazole or fluconazole is generally not warranted for thrush. However, intermittent short courses of fluconazole 100 mg/day orally may be useful for patients who have more resistant infection. Ketoconazole is less desirable because of potential drug-drug interactions and its poor bioavailability. Itraconazole is being used in cases of suspected fluconazole-resistant disease with some success, though cross-resistance among "azole" agents does occur. Topical amphotericin B 0.1% solution may be useful in the most resistant cases, but this therapy has not been established.

Esophageal candidiasis can occur without preceding symptoms of thrush and usually presents with difficulty or pain on swallowing. Other symptoms may include anorexia, nausea, fevers, and GI upset. The diagnosis of esophageal candidiasis is usually made by endoscopic examination. Systemic therapy is indicated for this invasive fungal infection; most patients respond to fluconazole 100 to 200 mg/day orally. Duration of therapy may be prolonged (e.g., 2 to 3 weeks), as clinical response is variable. Continuous, suppressive therapy is necessary only for specific patients who have frequent, painful recurrences. Good oral hygiene is imperative in controlling these difficult cases. Routine secondary prophylaxis is not recommended, since fluconazole-resistant strains of *Candida albicans* (71) or intrinsically resistant strains (e.g., *Candida kruzeii, Torluopsus glabrata*) (72) may result and recurrent infections would then require parenteral amphotericin B.

Toxoplasmosis

Toxoplasmic encephalitis in AIDS patients may represent a newly acquired infection or reactivation of a latent infection (73). Serologic findings in one study suggested that most disease results from recrudescence rather than new, primary infection. Most patients have had one or more OIs before developing focal necrotizing encephalitis due to *Toxoplasma gondii*, and the CD4 count is usually below 75 to 100/mm^3. Focal neurologic findings and a decreased level of consciousness, seizures, or fever are common presenting symptoms. The CSF in patients with toxoplasmic encephalitis will usually reveal a mononuclear pleocytosis with an elevated protein and a normal or low glucose concentration. In general, serial lumbar punctures should not be done for monitoring *Toxoplasma* antibody titers because of the potential for herniation in these patients with CNS mass lesions and increased intracranial pressures. Computed tomography or magnetic resonance imaging scans are recommended for diagnosis and monitoring and also to guide brain biopsy or excision. Currently, many centers are treating patients who have clinical and radiographic findings that are suggestive of CNS toxoplasmosis without biopsy confirmation. Demonstration of tachyzoite forms, but not cysts, in tissue sections or smears of body fluid (e.g., brain biopsy tissue or CSF) establishes the diagnosis of acute toxoplasma infection.

The most effective drug therapy for AIDS patients has been pyrimethamine plus sulfadiazine. Optimal dosages of these agents have not been established; however, it is recommended that adult AIDS patients receive a loading dose of pyrimethamine 100 to 200 mg twice a day for one day, followed by 50 to 100 mg/day. The dose of sulfadiazine is 1.5 to 2 g four times a day (74). Despite the fact that the serum elimination half-life of pyrimethamine is approximately 100 hr, most practitioners continue to administer this drug once daily because of concerns about interpatient pharmacokinetic variability, patient compliance, and GI intolerance. Patients who are receiving sulfadiazine/pyrimethamine for acute toxoplasmosis are also getting adequate PCP prophylaxis.

Toxicity that is attributable to pyrimethamine or sulfadiazine therapy has been reported in as many as 60% of individuals. Neutropenia, thrombocytopenia, and rash were most common during therapy. Crystalluria occurs in patients whose fluid intake is inadequate because this sulfonamide is not very water-soluble (compared to sulfamethoxazole and sulfisoxazole). The concomitant use of leucovorin (i.e., folinic acid) with pyrimethamine/sulfadiazine is routinely recommended to prevent their

dose-related bone marrow-suppressive effects. Leucovorin may be given orally or parenterally, 5 to 25 mg/day, as "rescue treatment." Leucovorin does not antagonize the antiparasitic activity of pyrimethamine, whereas folic acid may; therefore the latter should not be administered concurrently.

Alternatively, patients who are allergic to sulfa drugs may be given clindamycin plus pyrimethamine with somewhat comparable efficacy (75). The oral or intravenous dose of clindamycin 600 to 1200 mg four times a day that are used to treat acute CNS toxoplasmosis are much higher than those that are used to treat bacterial infections but have generally been well tolerated. A small study evaluating therapy with pyrimethamine and azithromycin also looks promising (76). Other therapies that are being studied include atovaquone, trimetrexate, tetracyclines, and investigational agents.

AIDS patients with toxoplasmosis should receive secondary prophylaxis or maintenance suppressive therapy (77). Although there is not a consensus about the "appropriate" dosage for such maintenance regimens, pyrimethamine plus sulfadiazine should be given indefinitely: 25 to 50 mg pyrimethamine with sulfadiazine 500 mg to 1.0 g four times a day or clindamycin 300 to 600 mg three times a day. Twice-weekly sulfadiazine plus pyrimethamine regimen has also been effective for maintenance therapy (78). For efficacy and tolerance reasons, sulfadiazine is preferred over clindamycin for long-term maintenance therapy. An added benefit of sulfadiazine (plus pyrimethamine) maintenance therapy is that it is also effective prophylaxis for PCP.

The role of these drugs or others for primary prophylaxis of toxoplasmosis is less well established. Individuals who are at highest risk for toxoplasmic encephalitis are IgG antibody-positive (i.e., have had previous exposure) and have a CD4 count ≤ 75 to 100 mm^3. This subset of HIV patients would already be taking trimethoprim/sulfamethoxazole for PCP prophylaxis. It is felt that TMP/SMX, given in adequate doses for PCP prophylaxis, is also effective for primary toxoplasmosis prophylaxis. When dapsone 100 mg/day is used for PCP prophylaxis, pyrimethamine 50 to 75 mg/week plus leucovorin 25 mg should be added for toxoplasmosis prophylaxis.

Cryptosporidial Diarrhea

Cryptosporidiosis is a protozoal parasitic infection of the GI tract that is a cause of severe diarrhea in humans and animals. Transmission is by ingestion of oocysts that have been excreted in the feces of infected humans or animals. Thus, person-to-person transmission occurs, as well as transmission by eating contaminated foods or drinking from a contaminated water supply. Prevention measures include proper hand-washing and food-preparation techniques. The risk of acquiring cryptosporidium from municipal water supplies varies from city to city (79). Oocysts can be eliminated from water that is intended for drinking by boiling it for 1 min. Common symptoms of cryptosporidiosis include epigastric cramping pain, nausea, fever, malaise, vomiting, anorexia, weight loss, and watery diarrhea. The diarrhea can be severe and debilitating and can progress to malabsorption and malnutrition. The patient must be carefully supported with fluids and electrolytes. The diarrhea should be controlled with bulk agents and antidiarrheals. No antimicrobial therapy has been shown to consistently improve symptoms or eradicate *Cryptosporidium* from the stool in AIDS patients, though prolonged treatment with azithromycin or paromomycin has been used by some (80). Research efforts, including antimicrobial susceptibility testing, have been impeded by the inability to grow the organism in vitro. Reports have been published that describe the lack of efficacy of various agents, including the oral antibiotics spiramycin, clindamycin, atovaquone, furazolidone, quinine, and the antisecretory agent octreotide. Immunomodulation studies using oral formulations of bovine anti-*Cryptosporidium* immunoglobulin are ongoing.

Cytomegalovirus (CMV) Infection

CMV infection is common in normal hosts, as many as 50% of people being seropositive by adulthood. However, for most the initial infection does not result in clinical disease. CMV is responsible for most congenital and perinatal infections that cause morbidity in neonates. Organ transplant recipients who are taking immunosuppressive drugs are at risk for morbidity and mortality resulting from recurrences of latent CMV infection. Treatment of CMV infections with antiviral agents had been unsuccessful until the mid-1980s, when ganciclovir (Cytovene, DHPG) became available (81). In 1991 the FDA approved foscarnet (Foscavir), which has shown in vitro activity against CMV and other herpesviruses as well as in vivo efficacy (82).

CMV is a herpesvirus and, like herpes simplex virus, can cause acute, latent, and chronic persistent infection. Subclinical CMV infection is reported to occur in the majority of HIV-infected individuals, as is evidenced by serologic testing. CMV is commonly found to coexist in the lung with other pathogens. Thus, its role in clinical infection (pneumonia) is not always clear, and therefore it is not routinely treated. Gastrointestinal disease, including esophageal ulceration, is now being more frequently observed as AIDS patients live longer. Retinitis is the most common CMV infection manifestation in HIV patients. It is usually an end-stage opportunistic infection when the CD4 count is less than 50 mm^3. CMV retinitis may result in unilateral or bilateral blindness. The diagnosis of CMV retinitis is usually based on ophthalmologic examination. Subjective findings are unilateral peripheral vision loss, and objective ophthalmic findings include white, fluffy patches of retinal opacifications and retinal hemorrhage. The histologic verification of this diagnosis is difficult and is rarely pursued. Isolation of virus from the blood or urine constitutes an important piece of confirmatory data in patients with ophthalmic findings.

Ganciclovir and foscarnet are currently the two available parenteral agents for the management of CMV infection. They have been compared in a prospective, randomized study and were shown to be equally effective (83). However, the survival data analysis favored patients in the foscarnet group. This may have resulted from this agent's additional activity against HIV, as well as the fact that patients who were randomized to ganciclovir more frequently had to stop their AZT because of potentiated bone marrow-suppressive effects. Foscarnet is potentially more desirable for patients who have low platelet counts ($\leq 20,000/mm^3$), as thrombocytopenia is a notable side effect of ganciclovir. Foscarnet should be avoided, if possible, for patients with significant renal insufficiency, as nephrotoxicity is a frequent adverse effect. After a discussion of the risks and benefits, patients should be offered a choice of either agent. Because of logistical and adverse reaction considerations, ganciclovir is most often given as empiric treatment of acute CMV retinitis (84). Therapy begins with 5 mg/kg intravenously every 12 hr for 14 days. During this so-called induction phase of therapy, the patient is monitored closely for disease progression. The intraocular penetration of ganciclovir is generally adequate for disease control. Intravitreous ganciclovir administration has been useful in rare cases. Concomitant administration of granulocyte colony-stimulating factor (G-CSF) may be necessary if severe neutropenia cannot be controlled with ganciclovir dosage adjustments.

Foscarnet is an antiviral drug with broad-spectrum activity, including activity against HIV and herpesviruses. Like ganciclovir, foscarnet is not capable of eradicating infection but acts only to control disease by suppressing viral replication. Consequently, relapses of the CMV infection are common after discontinuation of either ganciclovir or foscarnet therapy. Initial induction therapy with foscarnet is to be administered intravenously by intermittent infusion (60 mg/kg every 8 hr or 90 mg/kg every 12 hr) until disease stabilization or improvement, which is usually recommended to be 2 weeks. Combination therapy with ganciclovir and foscarnet has been used for refractory patients, but this combination may also prove to be a strategy of giving lower doses of both agents in an effort to minimize neutropenia and nephrotoxicity. Studies with an investigational agent, cidofovir (HPMPC, Vistide) are ongoing and look promising, though this agent is known to cause nephrotoxicity.

Adverse effects from ganciclovir include bone marrow toxicity, specifically neutropenia (13% dose-limiting) and thrombocytopenia (5% dose-limiting), which are usually reversible but may be more problematic in patients who are receiving other bone marrow-suppressing drugs (zidovudine, pyrimethamine, or trimethoprim/sulfamethoxazole). Toxicity appears to be somewhat dose- and/or duration-dependent; therefore, regimens may be altered to minimize neutropenia before therapy has to be discontinued. G-CSF may need to be coadministered to patients who are unable to tolerate adequate doses of ganciclovir. Ganciclovir is eliminated by the kidneys, so dosage alterations are necessary for patients with renal insufficiency. Toxicities from foscarnet are mostly related to abnormalities in calcium, magnesium, and phosphorus concentrations. Nephrotoxicity from intermittent infusion regimens has been reported (10 to 23% dose-limiting) but is less serious than earlier reports from continuous infusions. It is recommended to discontinue foscarnet therapy when the serum creatinine approaches 3.0 mg/dL. Other adverse reaction that have been reported include neurotoxicity, diabetes insipidus, hypertension, and genital ulcers. Foscarnet is eliminated by the kidneys, so dosage adjustments must be made for renal insufficiency.

Secondary prophylaxis or chronic suppression/maintenance therapy is imperative for CMV retinitis and is not necessary for other CMV disease. Ganciclovir 5 to 6 mg/kg/day has been given intravenously five to seven times a week. This regimen has been selected because of the long elimination half-life of ganciclovir's intracellular active metabolite. Maintenance therapy with foscarnet 60 mg/kg/day for seven days of the week is recommended, as this agent has a shorter elimination half-life. In December 1994 the FDA reviewed data from three studies comparing intravenous to oral ganciclovir and approved oral ganciclovir for secondary prophylaxis (maintenance therapy) of CMV retinitis. Because of this drug's poor bioavailability, patients are required to take 3 g/day (1 g orally three times a day).

Primary prophylaxis of CMV retinitis with oral ganciclovir is not routinely recommended. The highest-risk patients groups are yet to be identified. When data becomes available, careful consideration should be made in interpreting it. Reasons to oppose the widespread use of CMV prophylaxis include the fact that ganciclovir treatment is efficacious and prophylaxis may promote CMV resistance. Also neutropenia is common with oral ganciclovir, making other therapies (pyrimethamine, trimethoprim/sulfamethoxazole, and AZT) more toxic, and the cost of primary prophylaxis should be directly assessed with respect to a particular patient's risk of disease (e.g., depending on the CD4 count). Ganciclovir prophylaxis can never take the place of careful, routine ophthmalogic examinations.

Herpes Simplex and Varicella Zoster Virus Infections

Many patients with HIV have severe, recurrent outbreaks of herpes simplex virus (HSV) type I and type II infection.

Chronic, progressive infection with HSV is included in the CDC's definition of AIDS. In HIV-positive patients an episode of shingles or herpes zoster infection, which is a recrudescent infection with varicella zoster virus (VZV), can also be very severe and refractory to therapy. It is felt that herpes zoster infection is a predictor of AIDS in people who are at risk for acquiring HIV.

Acyclovir remains first-line therapy for HSV-1, HSV-2, and VZV infections. However, dosing may require titration in patients with HIV based on clinical response (85, 86). Dosing for acute treatment of HSV is 200 mg orally five times a day or 400 mg orally three times a day for 7 to 10 days, or longer if needed. VZV infection requires higher doses, 800 mg orally five times a day. Parenteral acyclovir is sometimes necessary because of the severity of disease. Treatment should continue until all vesicular lesions crust or epithelialize, and symptoms resolve.

Routine prevention of mild recurrent HSV disease with chemoprophylaxis is not warranted. When severe recurrences occur, suppressive therapy should be considered with acyclovir (200 mg three times a day or 400 mg twice a day). Primary drug resistance to acyclovir has been documented but is rarely problematic. The emergence of acyclovir-resistant HSV after several courses of acyclovir has occurred, and treatment with foscarnet will usually be successful. Foscarnet has also been useful in the treatment of acyclovir-resistant VZV infection (87). The role of famciclovir (Famvir) and valaciclovir (the valyl-ester of acyclovir; Vattrex) remains to be elucidated. These agents have improved bioavailability and are reported to have improved outcomes with regards to VZV-induced postherpetic neuralgia (88).

A controversy exists about the use of acyclovir along with AZT to improve long-term survival of HIV patients. Several retrospective and prospective studies have confirmed or refuted the reported beneficial effects of this combination. Patients and health care providers appear to be divided on this issue. Because acyclovir is very well tolerated and is widely taken for HSV suppression, this drug continues to be used liberally with or without AZT. This is a therapeutic dilemma that will need to be resolved in the future.

Atypical Mycobacterial Infection

Mycobacterium avium-intracellulare complex (MAC) is a commonly encountered group of environmental organisms. *M. avium* is present in dust, dirt, and the public water supply. Human disease with MAC was described before AIDS but was infrequent. Most cases were pulmonary infections in patients with preexisting pulmonary disease and was rarely known to cause disseminated illness. The epidemic of disseminated MAC is concurrent with the AIDS epidemic (89). A major risk factor for this infection appears to be the level of HIV-induced immunosuppression and correlates with CD4 cell count; this infection is rare in patients with counts greater than 50 to 75/mm^3. The pathogenesis of this disease is not well understood. Colonization occurs and can be longstanding; therefore, positive cultures from nonsterile sites (e.g., sputum and stool) are not routinely helpful in distinguishing patients with normal colonization from those with disseminated MAC disease. Antimicrobial sensitivity testing is not routinely performed, since these tests are difficult to perform and there are no current standardized methods. Symptoms of dissemination disease include fevers, night sweats, weight loss, abdominal pain, diarrhea, pancytopenia, and hepatosplenomegaly with liver enzyme elevation. Blood cultures and bone marrow aspirate cultures are often positive.

Most atypical mycobacteria, including MAC, are known to be more intrinsically drug-resistant than *Mycobacterium tuberculosis*. Serotype strains of MAC that cause infection in AIDS patients also are also known to be more virulent. Thus the limited response to therapies is not surprising. Therefore, when treatment is indicated, multidrug therapy for MAC disease is recommended to prevent the emergence of resistance and improve efficacy.

No therapy to date has been shown to prolong survival of AIDS patients with disseminated MAC infection, but improvement of symptoms may occur. Further study on disease pathogenesis, in vitro culture-susceptibility techniques, and drug therapy is needed. There is lack of consensus about which drugs should empirically be used. Therapy recommendations include ethambutol 15 mg/kg plus a macrolide-clarithromycin 500 to 1000 mg twice a day or azithromycin 500 mg/day. Depending on the severity of illness, one to three of the following agents may be added to this regimen: a quinolone-ciprofloxacin 750 mg twice a day or ofloxacin 400 mg twice a day; clofazamine 100 mg/day; a rifamycin-rifampin 600 mg/day or rifabutin 300 mg/day; and intravenous amikacin 7.5 mg/kg/day.

Primary prophylaxis for MAC infection is also an area in which there is much debate. Rifabutin was approved by the FDA on the basis of prophylaxis data published from two studies (90). Rifabutin was shown to reduce the frequency of MAC bacteremia and symptoms associated with MAC disease. The long-term benefits of such prophylaxis have not been established, and the potential of such therapy to induce MAC or *M. tuberculosis* (MTB) resistance needs to be considered. A comprehensive cost versus benefit analysis of rifabutin or clarithromycin prophylaxis for patients who are at highest risk (i.e., CD4 count less than 50 to 75/mm^3) remains to be performed. There have been several reports of uveitis as a possible adverse reaction to rifabutin after a mean of 2 months of high-dose therapy. Potential drug-drug interaction because of liver cytochrome P-450 induction are felt to be less for rifabutin than for rifampin.

Mycobacterium Tuberculosis Infection

The most common mycobacterial infections in HIV-positive individuals are with MAC, but infections caused by MTB are much more likely to be cured. Because the CD4 cells and macrophages play a central role in host antimycobacterial defenses, dysfunction or depletion of these cells by HIV disease places people at risk for disease reactivation or at higher risk of acquiring primary infection. The incidence of tuberculosis in AIDS patients is disproportionately higher at almost 500 times the incidence than that observed in the general population. Also, extrapulmonary forms of the infection are more likely to occur, including lymphatic and disseminated-miliary disease. Patients with tuberculosis may have pulmonary symptoms and radiographic lung infiltrates in any lung zone, often associated with mediastinal or hilar lymphadenopathy. Specimens (e.g., sputum, blood, urine, or bone marrow) should be obtained for acid-fast staining and culture before therapy is instituted. Tuberculin skin testing (PPD) can also be helpful in making the diagnosis, especially if a previous negative test result is known. False-negative results often occur even when skin tests are placed properly because of profound immunosuppression. This anergic response may be confirmed by also placing skin test controls (e.g., candida, mumps) with the PPD skin test, although these controls are not routinely recommended.

Infection control measures with respiratory precautions should be instituted when a patient is hospitalized and is suspected of having pulmonary tuberculosis. Multiple-drug chemotherapy should be started after adequate specimens are obtained for acid-fast staining and culture (91). Most patients respond well to standard oral therapy with isoniazid 300 mg/day, rifampin 600 mg/day, and ethambutol 15 to 25 mg/kg/day and/or pyrazinamide 20 to 30 mg/kg/day. Vitamin B6 should be given with this regimen, as INH-induced neuropathy may be a problem in AIDS patients. Both ethambutol and pyrazinamide are recommended to be given if INH resistance is suspected. They need to be administered only for the first 2 months of therapy when cultures are pending to assess isoniazid susceptibility. The appropriate duration of therapy for the HIV-infected person is unknown; however, at least 6 months of a recommended regimen, preferably with directly observed therapy, is optimal. The prevalence of multiple-drug-resistant (MDR) tuberculosis has steadily increased in the United States over the past few years from 2% to 9% (92). As many as six drugs may be indicated as empiric therapy of suspected MDR tuberculosis. The choice of these agents should be based on local patterns of resistance.

Drug monitoring for adverse reactions to antimycobacterial agents can be difficult because of multiorgan system toxicities. Patients with HIV infection are commonly taking various other agents that cause similar toxicities, such as those that cause liver toxicity or bone marrow suppression. Rarely does therapy for *M. tuberculosis* have to be interrupted if treatment is carefully monitored. (See Chapter 64, "Tuberculosis.")

CONCLUSION

In summary, HIV disease is a continuum of clinical conditions, ranging from an asymptomatic state to AIDS with OIs and cancers. The early institution of antiretroviral therapy has delayed disease progression; therefore it is recommended for adult patients with a CD4 cell count of less than $500/mm^3$. Optimal therapy has yet to be described, though monotherapy does not produce a prolonged effect. Combination and alternating antiretroviral regimens are being studied. The pharmacodynamics of antiretroviral agents and their active intracellular metabolites needs to be better studied and correlated with efficacy data using the new "viral load" tests. Regimens that contain immunomodulators may also improve the efficacy for HIV infection and OIs. Vaccine development will help to fight this battle. The successful treatment of opportunistic infections in AIDS patients remains a challenge as therapies are routinely disrupted because of adverse drug reactions. Thus, more intensive therapy monitoring is required for HIV patients. An appropriate health care maintenance program is essential for improving and prolonging quality of life (see Table 72.7). Primary and secondary prophylaxis regimens have been recommended for various OIs in an attempt to decrease the incidence of acute and recurrent disease. Signs of malnutrition and wasting need to be recognized so that pharmacologic interventions and nutritional supplementation may be undertaken to decrease early morbidity and mortality.

Table 72.7.
Health Care Maintenance Program for HIV-Positive Patients Monitoring Parameters and Interventions

LABORATORY STUDIES
Screening for sexually transmitted diseases
   Hepatitis B serologies
   Syphilis: RPR or VDRL test
Toxoplasmosis IgG antibodies
Cryptococcal serum antigen
CD4 T-lymphocyte count
Complete blood count with differential,
Platelet count, blood chemistry profile
VACCINATIONS
Hepatitis B series (if negative serology and engaging in high-risk activities)
Pneumococcal
Influenza virus, annually
Tetanus booster
GENERAL PREVENTATIVE CARE
History and physical exam
Medication and allergy history
Chest radiograph
Tuberculosis skin testing (PPD): Do annually only if previous result *is not known* to be positive.
Pelvis and breast examination
PAP smear, annual
Safe sex counseling
Dental examination
Ophthalmologic examination
Nutritional assessment: weight and diet
General well-being: Karnofsky's performance scale
Education
   Safe sex
   Oral hygiene
   Environmental/occupationl
   Pets
   Food
   Water
   Travel
PREVENTATIVE THERAPY
Do not recommend routine herpes simplex virus, cytomegalovirus, or antifungal primary prophylaxis.
Antiretroviral therapy (CD4 count < 500 mm³). The addition of acyclovir is not recommended.
Pneumocystis carinii pneumonia (PCP) prophylaxis (CD4 count < 200/mm³ or <20%)
Mycobacterium avium complex dissemination (CD4 count < 50–75/mm³)
Toxoplasmosis encephalitis (only if positive IgG antibodies and CD4 count < 75–100)
Mycobacterium tuberculosis: if skin test results positive and no signs of active disease
Recurrent bacterial infections in children: IV immune globulin (not necessary if already taking TMP/SMX)

REFERENCES

1. Nowak MA, McMichael AJ. How HIV defeats the immune system. Scientific American 271:58–65, 1995.
2. Wei X, Ghosh SK, Taylor ME, et al. Viral dynamics in human immunodeficiency virus type 1 infection. Nature 373:117–22, 1995.
3. Centers for Disease Control. Update: acquired immunodeficiency syndrome: United States, 1994. MMWR 44:64–7, 1995.
4. Centers for Disease Control. Update: AIDS among women: United States, 1994. MMWR 44:81–4, 1995.
5. Peckham C, Gibb D. Mother-to-child transmission of human immunodeficiency virus. N Engl J Med 333:298–302, 1995.
6. Centers for Disease Control. 1993 revised classification system for HIV infection and expanded surveillance case definition for AIDS among adolescents and adults. MMWR 41:1–19, 1992.
7. Department of Health and Human Services. Statement on FDA approval of AIDS virus test system based on oral fluid samples. Public Health Service Memo, December 23, 1994.
8. Keller DW, Breiman RF. Preventing bacterial respiratory tract infections among persons infected with human immunodeficiency virus. Clin Infect Dis 21(Suppl 1):S77–S83, 1995.
9. Angulo FJ, Swerdlow DL. Bacterial enteric infections in persons infected with human immunodeficiency virus. Clin Infect Dis 21(Suppl 1):S84–S93, 1995.
10. Centers for Disease Control. Classification system for human immunodeficiency virus (HIV) infection in children under 13 years of age. MMWR 36:225–36, 1987.

11. Fischl MA, Richman DD, Grieco MH, et al. The efficacy of azidothymidine (AZT) in the treatment of patients with AIDS and AIDS-related complex. N Engl J Med 317:185–91, 1987.

12. Richman DD, Andrews J. Results of continued monitoring of participants in the placebo-controlled trial of zidovudine for serious human immunodeficiency virus infection. Am J Med 85:208–13, 1988.

13. Fischl M, Richman DD, Causey DM, et al. Prolonged zidovudine therapy in patients with AIDS and advanced AIDS-related complex: AZT Collaborative Working Group. JAMA 262:2405–10, 1989.

14. Fischl M, Richman DD, Hansen N, et al. The safety and efficacy of zidovudine (AZT) in the treatment of persons with mildly symptomatic human immunodeficiency virus type (HIV) infection: a double-blind, placebo-controlled trial: The AIDS Clinical Trials Group. Ann Intern Med 112:727–37, 1990.

15. Hamilton JD, Hartigan PH, Simberkoff MS, et al. A controlled trial of early versus late treatment with zidovudine in symptomatic human immunodeficiency virus infection. N Engl J Med 326:437–43, 1993.

16. Volberding PA, Lagakos SW, Koch MA, et al. Zidovudine in asymptomatic human immunodeficiency virus infection: a controlled trial in persons with fewer than 500 CD4-positive cells per cubic millimeter. N Engl J Med 322:941–49, 1990.

17. Volberding PA, Lagakos SW, Grimes JM, et al. The duration of zidovudine benefit in persons with asymptomatic HIV infection. JAMA 272:437–42, 1994.

18. Concorde Coordinating Committee. Concorde: MRC/ANRS randomised double-blind controlled trial of immediate and deferred zidovudine in symptom-free HIV infection. Lancet 343:871–81, 1994.

19. Cooper DA, Gatell JM, Kroon S, et al. Zidovudine in persons with asymptomatic HIV infection and CD4 cell counts greater than 400 per cubic millimeter. N Engl J Med 329:297–303, 1993.

20. Collier AC. Early intervention in HIV infection: where are we? AIDS Res Hum Retroviruses 10:893–99, 1994.

21. Richman DD, Fischl MA, Grieco MH, et al. The toxicity of azidothymidine (AZT) in the treatment of patients with AIDS and AIDS-related complex. N Engl J Med 317:192–97, 1987.

22. Lenderking WR, Gelber RD, Cotton DJ, et al. Evaluation of the quality of life associated with zidovudine treatment in asymptomatic human immunodeficiency virus infection. N Engl J Med 330:738–43, 1994.

23. Fischl M, Galpin JE, Levine JD, et al. Recombinant human erythropoietin for patients with AIDS treated with zidovudine. N Engl J Med 322:1488–93, 1990.

24. Fischl MA, Parker CB, Pettinelli C, et al. A randomized controlled trial of a reduced daily dose of zidovudine in patients with the acquired immunodeficiency syndrome. N Engl J Med 323:1009–14, 1990.

25. Collier AC, Bozzette S, Coombs RW, et al. A pilot study of low-dose zidovudine in human immunodeficiency virus infection. N Engl J Med 323:1015–21, 1990.

26. McKinney RE, Maha MA, Connor EM, et al. A multicenter trial of oral zidovudine in children with advanced human immunodeficiency virus disease. N Engl J Med 324:1018–25, 1991.

27. Pizzo PA, Wilfert C. Antiretroviral therapy for infection due to human immunodeficiency virus in children. Clin Infect Dis 19:177–96, 1994.

28. Connor EM, Sperling RS, Gelber RG, et al. Reduction of maternal-infant transmission of human immunodeficiency virus type I with zidovudine treatment. N Engl J Med 331:1173–80, 1994.

29. D'Aquila RT, Johnson VA, Welles SL, et al. Zidovudine resistance and HIV-1 disease progression during antiretroviral therapy. Ann Intern Med 122:401–08, 1995.

30. Sande MA, Carpenter JC, Cobbs CG, et al. Recommendations from a state-of-the art panel. JAMA 270:2583–89, 1993.

31. Hartman NR, Yarchoan R, Pluda JM, Thomas RV, Marczyk KS, Broder S, and Joghns DG. Pharmacokinetics of 2′,3′-dideoxyadenosine and 2′,3′-dideoxyinosine in patients with severe human immuno-

deficiency virus infection. Clin Pharmacol Ther 47:647–54, 1990.

32. Lambert JS, Seidlin M, Reichman RC, et al. 2′,3′-dideoxyinosine (DDI) in patients with the acquired immunodeficiency syndrome or AIDS-related complex. N Engl J Med 322:1333–40, 1990.

33. Cooley TP, Kunches LM, Saunders CA, et al. Once-daily administration of 2′,3′-dideoxyinosine (DDI) in patients with the acquired immunodeficiency syndrome or AIDS-related complex. N Engl J Med 322:1340–45, 1990.

34. Butler KM, Husson RN, Balis FM, et al. Dideoxyinosine in children with symptomatic human immunodeficiency virus infection. N Engl J Med 324:137–44, 1991.

35. Mueller BU, Butler KM, Stocker VL, et al. Clinical and pharmacokinetic evaluation of long-term therapy with didanosine in children with HIV infection. Pediatrics 94:724–31, 1994.

36. Kahn JO, Lagakos SW, Richman DD, et al. A controlled trial comparing continued zidovudine with didanosine in human immunodeficiency virus infection. N Engl J Med 327:581–87, 1992.

37. Abrams DI, Goldman AI, Launer C, et al. A comparative trial of didanosine or zalcitabine after treatment with zidovudine in patients with human immunodeficiency virus infection. N Engl J Med 330:657–62, 1994.

38. Yarchoan R. A randomized pilot study of alternating or simultaneous zidovudine and didanosine therapy in patients with symptomatic human immunodeficiency virus infection. J Infect Dis 169:9–17, 1994.

39. Schindzielorz A, Pike I, Daniels M, et al. Rates and risk factors for adverse events associated with didanosine in the expanded access program. Clin Infect Dis 19:1076–83, 1994.

40. Meng TC, Fischl MA, Boota AM, et al. Combination therapy with zidovudine and dideoxycytidine in patients with advanced human immunodeficiency virus infection: a phase I/II study. Ann Intern Med 116:13–20, 1992.

41. Fischl MA, Stanley K, Collier AC, et al. Combination and monotherapy with zidovudine and zalcitabine in patients with advanced HIV disease. Ann Intern Med 122:24–32, 1995.

42. Browne MJ, Mayer KH, Chafee SB, et al. 2′,3′-didehydro-2′3′-dideoxythymidine (d4T) in patients with AIDS or AIDS-related complex: a phase I trial. J Infect Dis 167:21–9, 1993.

43. Pollard RB. Use of proteinase inhibitors in clinical practice. Pharmacotherapy 14(6PT2):21S–9, 1994.

44. Kitchen VS, Skinner C, Ariyoshi K, et al. Safety and activity of saquinavir in HIV infection. Lancet 345:952–55, 1995.

45. Saag MS, Emini EA, Laskin OL, et al. A short-term clinical evaluation of L-697,661, a non-nucleoside inhibitor of HIV-1 reverse transcriptase. N Engl J Med 329:1065–72, 1993.

46. Becker CE, Cone JE, Gerberding JL. Occupational infection with human immunodeficiency virus (HIV). Ann Intern Med 110:653–56, 1989.

47. Henderson DK, Gerberding JL. Prophylactic zidovudine after occupational exposure to the human immunodeficiency virus: an interim analysis. J Infect Dis 160:321–27, 1989.

48. Safai B, Johnson KG, Myskowski PL, et al. The natural history of Kaposi's sarcoma in the acquired immunodeficiency syndrome. Ann Intern Med 103:744–50, 1985.

49. Chang Y, Cesarman E, Pessin MS, et al. Identification of herpesvirus-like DNA sequences in AIDS-associated Kaposi's sarcoma. Science 266:1865–69, 1994.

50. Kovacs JA, Deyton L, Davey R, et al. Combined zidovudine and interferon-alpha therapy in patients with Kaposi's sarcoma and the acquired immunodeficiency syndrome. Ann Intern Med 111:280–87, 1989.

51. Vernon SD, Holmes KK, Reeves WC. Human papillomavirus infection and associated disease in persons with human immunodeficiency virus. Clin Infect Dis 21(Suppl 1):S21–S24, 1995.

52. Kaplan JE, Masur H, Holmes KK, et al. USPHS/IDSA guidelines for the prevention of opportunistic infections in persons infected with

human immunodeficiency virus: an overview. Clin Infect Dis 21(Suppl 1):S12–S31, 1995.

53. Centers for Disease Control. Recommendations for prophylaxis of *Pneumocystis carinii* pneumonia for adults and adolescents infected with human immunodeficiency virus. MMWR 41(RR–4):1–11, 1992.

54. Lane HC, Laughton BE, Falloon J. et al. Recent advances in the management of AIDS-related opportunistic infections (NIH conference). Ann Intern Med 120:945–55, 1994.

55. Jarosinski PF, Kennedy PE, Gallelli JF. Stability of concentrated trimethoprim-sulfamethoxazole admixtures. Am J Hosp Pharm 46:732–37, 1989.

56. Wharton M, Coleman DL, Wofsy CB, et al. Trimethoprim-sulfamethoxazole for *Pneumocystis carinii* pneumonia in the acquired immunodeficiency syndrome. Ann Intern Med 105:37–44, 1986.

57. Medina I, Mills J, Leoung G, et al. Oral therapy for *Pneumocystis carinii* pneumonia in the acquired immunodeficiency syndrome. N Engl J Med 323:776–82, 1990.

58. Hughes W, Leoung G, Kramer F, et al. Comparison of atovaquone (BW566C80) with trimethoprim-sulfamethoxazole to treat *Pneumocystis carinii* pneumonia in patients with AIDS. N Engl J Med 328:1521–27, 1993.

59. Black JR, Feinberg J, Murphy RL, et al. Clindamycin and primaquine therapy for mild-to-moderate episodes of *Pneumocystis carinii* pneumonia in patients with AIDS: AIDS Clinical Trials Group 044. Clin Infect Dis 18:905–13, 1994.

60. The National Institutes of Health–University of California Expert Panel for Corticosteroids as Adjuvant Therapy for Pneumocystis Pneumonia. Special Report: consensus statement on the use of corticosteroids as adjuvant therapy for *Pneumocystis carinii* pneumonia in the acquired immunodeficiency syndrome. N Engl J Med 323:1500–04, 1990.

61. Simonds RJ, Hughes WT, Feinberg J, and Navin TR. Preventing *Pneumocystis carinii* pneumonia in persons infected with human immunodeficiency virus. Clin Infect Dis 21(Suppl 1):S44–S48, 1995.

62. Centers for Disease Control. 1995 revised guidelines for prophylaxis against *Pneumocystis carinii* pneumonia for children infected with or perinatally exposed to human immunodeficiency virus. MMWR 44(RR–4):1–11, 1995.

63. Fischl MA, Dickinson GM, La Voie L. Safety and efficacy of sulfamethoxazole and trimethoprim chemoprophylaxis for *Pneumocystis carinii* pneumonia in AIDS. JAMA 259:1185–89, 1988.

64. Bozzette SA, Finkelstein DM, Spector SA, et al. A randomized trial of three antipneumocystis agents in patients with advanced human immunodeficiency virus infection. N Engl J Med 332:693–99, 1995.

65. Saag MS, Powderly WG, Cloud GA, et al. Comparison of amphotericin B with fluconazole in the treatment of acute AIDS-associated cryptococcal meningitis. N Engl J Med 326:83–9, 1992.

66. Larsen RA, Leal MAE, Chan LS. Fluconazole compared with amphotericin B plus flucytosine for cryptococcal meningitis in AIDS. Ann Intern Med 113:183–87, 1990.

67. Larsen RA, Bozzette SA, Jones BE, et al. Fluconazole combined with flucytosine for treatment of cryptococcal meningitis in patients with AIDS. Clin Infect Dis 19:741–45, 1994.

68. Chuck SL, Sande MA. Infections with *Cryptococcus neoformans* in the acquired immunodeficiency syndrome. N Engl J Med 321:794–99, 1989.

69. Bozzettee SA, Larsen RA, Chiu J, et al. A placebo-controlled trial of maintenance therapy with fluconazole after treatment of cryptococcal meningitis in the acquired immunodeficiency syndrome. N Engl J Med 324:580–84, 1991.

70. Powderly WG, Finkelstein DM, Feinberg J, et al. A randomized trial comparing fluconazole with clotrimazole troches for the prevention of

fungal infections in patients with advanced human immunodeficiency virus infection. N Engl J Med 332:700–05, 1995.

71. White A, Goetz MB. Azole-resistant *Candida albicans*: report of two cases of resistance to fluconazole and review. Clin Infect Dis 19:687–92, 1994.

72. Newman SL, Flanigan TP, Fisher A, et al. Clinically significant mucosal candidiasis resistant to fluconazole treatment in patients with AIDS. Clin Infect Dis 19:684–86, 1994.

73. Luft BJ, Remington JS. Toxoplasmosic encephalitis in AIDS. Clin Infect Dis 15:211–22, 1992.

74. St Georgiev V. Management of toxoplasmosis. Drugs 48:179–88, 1994.

75. Dannemann B, McCutchan JA, Israelski D, et al. Treatment of toxoplasmic encephalitis in patients with AIDS: a randomized trial comparing pyrimethamine plus clindamycin to pyrimethamine and sulfadiazine. Ann Intern Med 116:33–43, 1992.

76. Saba J, Morlat P, Raffi F, et al. Pyrimethamine plus azithromycin for treatment of acute toxoplasmic encephalitis in patients with AIDS. Eur J Clin Microbiol Infect Dis 12:853–56, 1993.

77. Richards FO, Kovacs JA, Luft BJ. Preventing toxoplasmic encephalitis in persons with human immunodeficiency virus. Clin Infect Dis 21(Suppl 1):S49–S56, 1995.

78. Podzamczer D, Miro JM, Bolao F, et al. Twice-weekly therapy with sulfadiazine-pyrimethamine to prevent recurrent toxoplasmic encephalitis in patients with AIDS. Ann Intern Med 123:175–80, 1995.

79. Centers for Disease Control. Assessing the public health threat associated with waterborne cryptosporidiosis: report of a workshop. MMWR 44:RR–6:1–19, 1995.

80. Petersen C. Cryptosporidiosis in patients infected with the human immunodeficiency virus. Clin Infect Dis 15:903–09, 1992.

81. Markham A, Faulds D. Ganciclovir. Drugs 48:455–84, 1994.

82. Wagstaff AJ, Bryson HM. Foscarnet. Drugs 48:199–226, 1994.

83. Studies of Ocular Complications of AIDS Research Group and AIDS Clinical Trials Group. Mortality of patients with acquired immunodeficiency syndrome treated with either foscarnet or ganciclovir for cytomegalovirus retinitis. N Engl J Med 326:213–20, 1992.

84. Jacobson MA. Current management of cytomegalovirus disease in patients with AIDS. AIDS Research Hum Retroviruses 10:917–23, 1994.

85. McGrath BJ, Newman CL. Genital herpes simplex infections in patients with the acquired immunodeficiency syndrome. Pharmacotherapy 14:529–42, 1994.

86. Stewart JA, Reef SE, Pellett PE, et al. Herpesvirus infection in persons infected with human immunodeficiency virus. Clin Infect Dis 21(Suppl 1):S114–S20, 1995.

87. Safrin S, Berger TG, Gilson I, et al. Foscarnet therapy in five patients with AIDS and acyclovir-resistant varicella-zoster virus infection. Ann Intern Med 115:19–21, 1991.

88. Tyring S, Barbarash RA, Nahlik JE, et al. Famciclovir for the treatment of acute herpes zoster: effects on acute disease and postherpetic neuralgia. Ann Intern Med 123:89–96, 1995.

89. Hawkins CC, Gold JWM, Whimbey E, et al. *Mycobacterium avium* complex infections in patients with the acquired immunodeficiency syndrome. Ann Intern Med 105:184–88, 1986.

90. Nightingale SD, Cameron DW, Gordin FM, et al. Two controlled trials of rifabutin prophylaxis against *Mycobacterium avium* complex infection in AIDS. N Engl J Med 329:828–33, 1993.

91. Castro KG. Tuberculosis as an opportunistic disease in persons with human immunodeficiency virus. Clin Infect Dis 21(Suppl 1):S66–S71, 1995.

92. Jacobs RF. Multiple-drug-resistant tuberculosis. Clin Infect Dis 19:1–10, 1994.

CHAPTER 73

MYCOTIC AND PARASITIC INFECTIONS

DONNA CARR, CATHY E. CORBETT, and PETER J. S. KOO

MYCOTIC INFECTIONS

Mycotic infections can be classified into superficial and systemic. These fungi usually cause infection in humans as a result of accident or opportunism. Except for a few dermatophytes these fungi do not require the human for the propagation of the species. Dermatophytes do not invade living tissue, but they survive on the dead tissue structures of the stratum corneum of the skin, the hair, and the nails, and they depend on person-to-person or object-to-person transmission. These dermatophytes exist as saprophytes and can be found anywhere in the world.

Fungi causing systemic infections are almost always soil saprophytes with the ability to adapt to a host and therefore cause disease. These fungi are usually dimorphic; they can either grow in the soil as mycelial forms that are responsible for spore production or as budding yeast while in a host. Infection is usually acquired by inhalation of the airborne spores. These dimorphic fungi are generally restricted to distinctive geographic environments. Subclinical infections of the population in these endemic areas are common.

Another important category of fungal infection is caused by the opportunistic fungi. These organisms are generally not infective to the normal healthy host. However, they produce disease in the host who is compromised due to acquired immunodeficiency syndrome (AIDS), diabetes, neoplastic disease, or immunosuppression from drugs. Tissue response varies greatly from no response to pyogenic or granulomatous reactions. These fungi are committed mycelial forms and are not restricted to a particular geographic area.

Subcutaneous mycoses usually occur through trauma to the host. They have some ability to adapt to dimorphism. Clinically, they cause diseases known as chromomycosis and mycetoma. They are diverse varieties of soil organisms. In the tissue these organism form grains, granules, and sclerotic bodies. Infections develop slowly and so is recovery. Most of these subcutaneous mycotic organisms are confined to limited geographic areas.

SYSTEMIC MYCOSES

Aspergillosis

"Aspergillosis" has been used to describe the disease responsible for allergy, colonization, or tissue invasion by the *Aspergillus* spp. *Aspergillus* usually infects the pulmo-nary system of the human host, but extrapulmonary systemic infections involving the major organs and central nervous system can also occur (1). There are many *Aspergillus* species, however, the two most important pathogens are *A. fumigatus* and *A. flavus* (1–4). The prognosis of invasive aspergillosis depends on the immune status of the host. In patients who are immunosuppressed, mortality rates of greater than 90% have been reported. However, prompt diagnosis, early therapy and resolution of neutropenia may decrease mortality rates to less than 15% (5).

EPIDEMIOLOGY

Aspergillus spp. is an ubiquitous fungus found in the air, dust, soil, decaying vegetation, and in hay or grain storehouses (1, 2, 4, 5). This fungus grows well in most compost piles, and in temperatures greater than 45°. *A. fumigatus*, the most common species, is usually seen as the cause of aspergillosis infections. *A. flavus* is the second most common species, and is usually seen as an invasive disease in immunosuppressed patients (1–3). Less virulent and/or less common species such as. *A. niger*, *A. nigulans* and *A. terreus* have been pathogenic in organ transplant populations (5). Other *Aspergillus* species have been reported to be invasive pathogens in humans, especially the immunocompromised patient (2).

CLINICAL MANIFESTATIONS

The most common manifestation of aspergillosis is pulmo-nary invasion. Symptoms include persistent or recurrent fevers not responsive to antibiotic therapy. Respiratory symptoms include cough, pleuritic pain, hemoptysis and shortness of breath. Symptoms of sinusitis include nasal discharge, epistaxis, sinus tenderness and nasal eschar (1, 3, 4, 6). Extrinsic asthma, allergic alveolitis, and broncho-pulmonary aspergillosis (BPA) are hypersensitivity reac-tions usually seen in normal hosts (1–4). Invasive aspergil-losis is seen among patients receiving immunosuppressive therapy, bone marrow transplant patients, and HIV-infected patients (1, 2, 4–7). The airborne conidia (spores) are approximately 2.5–3.0 μm in diameter. They can invade the lungs by inhalation, and migrate into the alveoli (1, 2, 4, 5). *Aspergillus* can also invade the nose, paranasal sinuses, external ear, and traumatized skin. Once into the tissue, the fungus can invade the submucosa, cartilage and disseminate into the adjacent blood vessels. The hyphae multiply and grow into 'fungus balls' after colonizing into damaged bronchi and preexisting pulmonary cavities. Inflammatory and vascular changes occur, leading to hemoptysis, a common and sometimes fatal complication (1). Symptomatic pulmonary aspergillosis has rarely been reported in AIDS patients (6). However, when it is reported the patient is usually in the advanced stages of AIDS with CD4 counts <50 cells/mm^3 (8). Neutropenia has been identified as the most important risk factor for invasive aspergillosis in AIDS patients (6–8). Other possible risk factors include corticosteriod use, prolonged courses of antibiotics, diabetes, hepatic disease, underlying lung disease, such as tuberculosis, and alcohol, marijuana or intravenous drug use (6–8). Granulocytes are the host's major defense against aspergillosis infection. They act on the mycelial form of the fungus while macrophages kill the conidia (1, 8).

DIAGNOSIS

A definitive diagnosis of aspergillosis is usually demonstrated by histologic examination of tissue microscopically and by cultures. Aspergillus may be colonizing and not invading tissue, however an isolated culture or the appearance of hyphae from sputum, urine, stool, cornea, or wound are strongly suggestive of the diagnoses. This is particularly true in the immunocompromised host and should not be ignored (1, 3, 4, 9, 10). On radiographic examination, a localized consolidation as a wedge-shaped peripheral infiltrate may be present, however, a majority of patients have negative findings in early disease. Computed tomography (CT) scans may be of benefit in early detection and in showing the extent of infection. Nodular and cavitary infiltrates with a halo surrounding the area may be seen on films (3, 4). In advanced disease, CT scans of the brain, liver, spleen and other organs have shown necrotic lesions diagnostic of disseminating infection (3). Invasive procedures for diagnosing have been used, such as needle aspiration or open lung biopsy (3).

TREATMENT

Alleviation of the symptoms is the mainstay of therapy in BPA. Steriods are the treatment of choice, since BPA is a hypersensitive response and not an infectious process. Prednisone (1mg/kg/day) is given until the chest roentgenogram has cleared, then the same dose is continued every other day for 3 to 6 months, then gradually tapered. Bronchodilators, along with physiotherapy may also be used to help alleviate symptoms (2, 4).

Surgical excision has been successful in treating invasive aspergillosis of the brain, paranasal sinuses, and in non-invasive colonization of the sinuses. In patients with massive hemoptysis, surgical excision of the aspergilloma may be indicated, however, most aspergillomas are managed by conservative measures (1, 3, 7). Transthoracic

intracavitary instillation of amphotericin B has been used to treat inoperable cases of aspergillomas. The number of cases have been small and long-term benefits have not been established (1). Surgical removal of an infective prosthetic heart valve may aid in the effectiveness of antifungal therapy, but the mortality in endocarditis remains high (1, 3).

Neutropenia. Intravenous amphotericin B remains the treatment of choice for aspergillosis infection, however response to therapy is still poor in the immunocompromised patient (1–4). Invasive pulmonary aspergillosis was detected in patients receiving amphotericin B at doses of 0.5mg/kg/day empirically. This leads to doses being increased to 1.0–1.5 mg/kg/day in the severely neutropenic patient, until marrow recovery is evident (1, 3–6).

The use of itraconazole, a newer azole antifungal agent, has shown to be effective in aspergillosis infections (1, 3, 5, 8, 11, 12). Noncomparative trials suggest that the efficacy of itraconazole may be similar to that of amphotericin B (14–16). In a recent open-label trial conducted by the National Institute of Allergy and Infectious Diseases (NIAID), Mycoses Study Group, itraconazole (200mg twice a day with meals) was significantly effective in the treatment of invasive aspergillosis in immunocompromised patients. Efficacy varied depending on the site of disease and underlying immunosuppression. For example, failure rates were 14% with pulmonary and tracheobronchial disease, 7% with solid organ transplantation, 14% in neutropenia, contrasting with failure rates of 63% and 44% with CNS involvement and extrapulmonary infections respectively (5, 11). In life-threatening situations a loading dose of 200mg three times a day for the first 3 days, followed by 200mg twice daily, has been suggested by the manufacturer (13). A comparative trial of itraconazole and amphotericin B in patients with invasive aspergillosis is currently ongoing (14–16).

Combination Therapy. Combination therapy of rifampin and flucytosine (5-FC) with amphotericin B have also been advocated. However treatment failure rates with either amphotericin B alone or in combination with rifampin or flucytosine have ranged from 13 to 100% (3–5, 8, 12). Outcomes improved in patients whom the infection was identified early and amphotericin B therapy was initiated soon thereafter. Flucytosine penetrates well into the CNS, eye and, bone compared to amphotericin B. Flucytosine has been reported to cause bone marrow toxicity, especially in patients with renal dysfunction or when receiving concomitant amphotericin B therapy. Therefore, patients with existing myelosuppression should not be given 5-FC (12). Doses ranging from 50mg/kg up to 200mg/kg daily in 4 divided doses have been advocated (13). Rifampin has no antifungal activity itself, however, in combination with amphotericin B, it has been shown to be synergistic, and occasionally additive or indifferent in in vitro studies.

Itraconazole with amphotericin B demonstrated the same results (5, 12).

Empiric Treatment and Prophylaxis. Because of the difficulty in diagnosing invasive aspergillosis, empiric therapy has been suggested in treating high-risk patients. Studies have shown that in neutropenic patients with persistent fever, amphotericin B begun 4 to 7 days after initiation of broad-spectrum antibiotic therapy, had a favorable result (3, 17–21). Because low dose amphotericin may not be effective, higher doses of > 1.0mg/kg/day have been advocated by some as empiric treatment (3, 20).

Amphotericin B has been used in certain immunocompromised populations as prophylactic treatment. Doses have ranged from 0.1mg/kg/day to 0.25mg/kg/day with varying success against invasive infection (3, 22–25). Some data suggest that itraconazole given prophylactically may prevent invasive aspergillosis, however, experience is limited and further investigation is needed (3, 26). Instillation of amphotericin B nasally has been used to prevent invasive aspergillosis in neutropenic patients, however efficacy has not been shown (1, 27, 28). Itraconazole, with or without intranasal amphotericin, has been suggested also, but no studies to date have been conducted (1, 29).

Cryptococcosis

Cryptococcosis is a systemic infection caused by the fungus *Cryptococcus neoformans*. Older names for the disease are torulosis, European blastomycosis and Busse-Buischke's disease. There are reports of other *Cryptococcus* species causing disease, but documentation of these cases has been questioned (30, 31). *Cryptococcal* infection is an important pathogen particularly in AIDS patients, because of its high incidence of occurrence and mortality in this population. It affects the central nervous system, primarily, however, nonmeningeal cases have been reported. Relapse of the disease is extremely high ≥ 50%. Lifelong antifungal treatment given prophylactically has been effective in preventing reoccurrence (30, 32).

EPIDEMIOLOGY

Cryptococcus is a yeast-like encapsulated fungus (4–6 μm in diameter). Four serotypes, A,B,C,D, of *C. neoformans* have been identified based on their antigenic specificity of the polysaccharide capsule (30, 33). Serotypes A and D have been found in pigeon feces, soil, and farm produce. Serotypes B and C are more restricted to tropical and subtropical areas, particularly in areas surrounding Eucalyptus trees (30, 32, 34, 35). It is believed the disease occurs after the fungus is aerosolized and inhaled, but cases of cryptococcosis rarely occur in clusters. There is no occupational predisposition and histories of exposure to pigeons, dust, or Eucalyptus trees are unfounded (30). It is thought that exposure to *C. neoformans* is common, due to

the fact that normal subjects react to skin testing, but they manifest no evidence of infection or develop a self-limited pneumonitis. Therefore the host must have a natural defense mechanism that keeps non-immunocompromised patients disease free (32). In immunocompromised patients, such as those with defects of cell-mediated immunity (transplant recipients, patients with lymphomas, and patients infected with HIV), *Cryptococcus* is an opportunistic fungus. It occurs in animals, however, animal to human transmission has not been documented (30, 34). Only in transplant tissue has transmission from person to person been seen (30, 36). It is not clear what factors predispose humans to cryptococcosis, however its prevalence in AIDS patients is 5–10% in the United States, and higher in central Africa (8, 30, 34).

CLINICAL MANIFESTATIONS

The central nervous system is the most common site of *Cryptococcus* infections. More often its presentation is seen acutely in immunocompromised patients, especially in AIDS patients (30, 37). However, it may present insidiously, delaying diagnosis for weeks (30, 32, 38). Fever is the most common finding, seen in approximately 62 to 88% of cases (32, 37, 39). Complaints of headache, nausea, dizziness, irritability, clumsiness, confusion or obtundation have been noted. The patient may develop symptoms of decreased visual acuity, diplopia, and facial numbness or weakness, as a result of cranial nerve involvement, and may progress on to total visual loss. Seizures, choreoatheoid movements, myoconic jerks, and dementia, may present late in the course of the disease (30). The most common nonmeningeal site of *Cryptococcus* infections is found in the lungs. The patient may be asymptomatic, or may produce scant, blood-tinged sputum. In HIV patients who present with pulmonary involvement, common findings are cough and dyspnea, seen in 5–28% of patients. Focal and interstitial infiltrates, lymphadenopathy, and pleural effusion are findings upon chest radiography (32). Mortality has been reported as high as 42% in AIDS patients who have cryptococcosis pneumonia (8, 32, 40). Meningitis is diagnosed in the majority of HIV patients presenting with respiratory involvement, therefore, it is essential the central nervous system be evaluated if cryptococcosis is diagnosed from any site (32, 41, 42). Other less common areas of involvement include skin, bone, joint, and organs, such as heart, kidney, adrenal, intestine, eye, and liver (30, 32, 39).

DIAGNOSIS

Routine laboratory is of no diagnostic value, because findings are usually normal in patients with widespread *Cryptococcus* infections (30). In nonimmunosuppressed patients, CSF is usually abnormal, exhibiting depressed glucose, elevated protein concentrations, and leukocyte counts of 20/mm³ or higher. In contrast, AIDS patients have minimal or no abnormalities of CSF, but *Cryptococci* may grow in cultures (30, 32, 37, 39, 43). Specific tests for *Cryptococcal* infection with visualization of the organism on Gram or India ink stain may give a more definite diagnosis in these patients (8, 30, 32). Serologic testing has been described for detecting the fungus early. The screening method of latex agglutination detects antigen in the CSF or serum with 90% or more of patients with *Cryptococcal* meningitis. The antigen may be detected in any tissue or body fluid (30, 32). Radiological techniques such as CT scans and MRIs have not been found to be useful in the diagnosis of *Cryptococcus* (8, 30, 32). In diagnosing pulmonary infections in the AIDS patients, bronchoalveolar lavage and pleural fluid cultures are useful tests (32, 41). In nonpulmonary sites, biopsy of the lesion is required to determine infection (32).

TREATMENT

Non-AIDS. Amphotericin B in combination with 5-FC have been the treatment of choice in non-AIDS *Cryptococcal* meningitis. Doses of 0.3mg/kg/day of amphotericin B IV plus 150mg of 5-FC in four divided doses have been used for 6 weeks treatment regimens (30, 44). The combined therapy reduces the incidence of resistance to 5-FC. Serum levels of 5-FC should be monitored, especially when high doses of amphotericin B are used, since amphotericin-induced azotemia may increase the risk of 5-FC accumulation. Flucytosine doses should be decreased to 75–100mg/kg/day and monitoring serum levels with the range of 25 and 60 µg/ml when renal dysfunction is evident (30, 45, 46). In nonimmunocompromised patients, the length of therapy is generally 4 weeks, however this shorter therapy is limited to those who have negative cultures and India ink smears in large CSF samples after 2 weeks or less of therapy. In immunocompromised patients the therapy should be extended beyond 6 weeks, because of higher relapses (30, 44). Therapy may be discontinued when weekly cultures are negative for 4 weeks (30, 47). Intrathecal amphotericin B, delivered intracisternally by an implanted subcutaneous reservoir, has been used rarely in some patients (30, 48, 49).

In most non-AIDS patients, *Cryptococcal* infections of the skin, bone, or other organs should be treated with amphotericin B/5-FC combination therapy. Total doses of 2 to 3gms of amphotericin B are most often the end-point of therapy (30). It has been found in patients who have pulmonary cryptococcosis, without any identifiable predisposing immunologic defects, that the infection may resolve without the use of antifungal therapy. As long as CSF and urine cultures are negative, the lesion remains small, and the patient has no predisposing factors (such as corticosteroid therapy, immunosuppressing chemotherapy), antifungal may be delayed (30, 50). Fluconazole therapy may

prove to be of value in this group of patients, however, the dose, duration and efficacy are not known (30, 50).

AIDS. *Cryptococcal* infections is the most common life-threatening fungal infection in AIDS patients, with mortality rates being as high as 60%, even with treatment (8). Pulmonary infections have similar outcomes to meningeal involvement. The primary objective of therapy is to control the infection, decrease early mortality, prevent relapse, and maintain quality of life. *Cryptococcal* infection can occur at any time during the course of HIV infection, especially when CD4 counts are < 200cell/mm³ (32).

The increased risk of toxicity in AIDS patients when amphotericin B/5-FC combined therapy was given, prompted the search for alternative treatments (30, 32). Fluconazole has been investigated because of its lower toxicity profile, dosage forms, and excellent penetration into cerebrospinal fluid for treatment of *Cryptococcal* meningitis (14). In initial studies, fluconazole demonstrated efficacy in some patients who were not responding to amphotericin B. (32, 51, 52). Also, studies of fluconazole in the initial treatment of *Cryptococcal* meningitis in AIDS showed a 67 to 75% response rate (32, 52). Laren et al., compared fluconazole with amphotericin B plus 5-FC for treatment of AIDS related *Cryptococcal* meningitis in a small, randomized trial. Fluconazole 400mg was compared with amphotericin B 0.7mg/kg/day and 5-FC 150mg/kg/day. Of 14 patients randomly assigned to receive fluconazole, 8 failed; compared to none of the 6 patients who received the combination therapy. Also, the conversion to negative CSF cultures were longer in the fluconazole group (32, 53). In a larger study, Saag et al. compared 200mg/day fluconazole with 0.3mg/kg/day amphotericin B in the initial treatment of *Cryptococcal* meningitis in 194 AIDS patients (54). Treatment was considered successful if the patient had two consecutive negative CSF cultures by the end of a 10 week treatment period. Treatment was successful in 40% of patients who received amphotericin B, and 34% of patients who received fluconazole (P = 0.40). There was no significant difference between the overall mortality in the two groups, 14% in the amphotericin versus 18% in the fluconazole (P = 0.48); however, mortality was significantly higher in the fluconazole group during the first two weeks of therapy. It has been suggested that the treatment doses may have been too low (30, 32, 54). Berry et al. reported higher doses of fluconazole (800mg/day) have been tolerated in patients who have failed to improve with other antifungals (55). Berry et al. and Haubrich et al. have demonstrated safe and responsive therapy with high dose fluconazole (800mg/day) given as initial or salvage treatment in *Cryptococcal* infections (55, 56). Combination therapy of fluconazole and 5-FC may be more effective than fluconazole alone in *Cryptococcal* meningitis. A phase II trial of high dose fluconazole in combination with

5-FC is currently in progress to determine efficacy and safety (57). Itraconazole has been used to treat presumptive *Cryptococcal* meningitis in a small study, however, more research is needed to determine its efficacy (32, 58). The experimental use of liposomal amphotericin B and amphotericin B lipid complex (ABLC) have shown reduced toxicity and efficacy in *Cryptococcal* meningitis, however these dosage forms are not currently available in the United States.

Maintenance Therapy. All AIDS patients who have survived *Cryptococcal* meningitis after successful primary treatment must receive lifelong maintenance therapy to prevent relapse. Two regimens have been given as maintenance doses; amphotericin B IV at a dose of 1mg/kg/week, and oral fluconazole 200mg/day. In a recent multicenter study comparing these two regimens, fluconazole was superior to amphotericin B by demonstrating fewer relapses and fewer adverse events (32, 59). Also, a double-blinded, placebo controlled trial further showed its effectiveness as first line treatment (32, 60). A large, prospective trial is underway to determine intraconazole's usefulness in preventing relapses (30).

Prophylaxis. Fluconazole, given 100mg daily, in patients with CD4 counts of < 50/mm^3, has shown to be effective in protecting AIDS patients against *Cryptococcal* meningitis. This regimen is not completely protective; therefore, fluconazole may be considered useful in some patients (32, 61).

Candidiasis

Candida organisms are yeasts that have been described as thrush dating as far back to the time of Hippocrates and Galen. The first well-documented case of *Candida* was described by Zenker in 1861, and the first case of *Candida* endocarditis was found in 1940 (62). In the United States *Candida* species are now the fourth most common organism cultured from blood in hospitalized patients. Candida is now considered an emerging pathogen which have been responsible for infections such as arthritis, endocarditis, osteomyelitis meningitis, peritonitis and others. With the increasing use of broad spectrum antibiotics, incidence of HIV infection, surical procedures, organ transplantation, and implantable prosthetic devices, the increase of *Candida* infections has risen significantly. *Candida* infections are the most frequently diagnosed fungal infection in HIV patients (62, 63).

EPIDEMIOLOGY

Candida organisms are small (4–6 µm), thin-walled, ovoid yeast cells. They form smooth, creamy white, colonies resembling staphylococcal colonies (62, 64). There are more than 150 species of *Candida*, but only 10 are thought of as being important pathogens in humans. These are *C. albican, C. guilliermondi, C. krusei, C. parapsilosis, C. stellatoidea* (now considered *C. albicans*), *C. tropicalis, C. pseudotropicalis, C. lusitaniae, C. rugosa,* and *C. glabrata.* Because certain *Candida* species are more pathogenic, species identification is important (62). *Candida albicans* has been found in soil, food, hospital environments, inanimate objects, and animal sources. It is a normal commensal of man, and are found on diseased skin, throughout the gastrointestinal tract, sputum, the female genital tract, and in the urine of patients with indwelling Foley catheters (62, 64, 65). *Candida* can colonize indwelling central venous catheters from the skin, which serves as a portal entry for organisms to seed the blood. Human to human transmission is possible, for example; thrush in a newborn infant being acquired from the mother's vagina with a preexisting *Candida* infection (62).

CLINICAL MANIFESTATIONS

Candida infection can be divided into two types of clinical manifestations, either mucocutaneous or deep organ involvement. The mucocutaneous layers where the infection is exhibited is the esophageal, vagina, gastrointestinal tract, oral and pharyngeal areas, and the cutaneous layers of the skin (62). Thrush is one specific form of candida, appearing as white, creamy patches on the tongue and mucus membranes of the oral cavity. The use of inhaled steroids have increased the incidence of this infection (62, 66). Thrush is commonly seen, also, in the immunocompromised host, such as cancer and AIDS patients (62, 65). Herpes simplex virus and cytomegalovirus may occur concomitantly with *Candida* esophagitis (62). *Candida* vaginitis is the most common infection seen in diabetes, patients on antibiotics, and pregnancy. It is thought that birth control pills may be a predisposing factor for vaginal candidiasis (62). *Candida* may present as confluent eruptions that spread over the trunk, thorax and extremties, however, it may be found around the fingers, toes, hair follicles, genitalia, paronychia, and perianal area. Diaper rash is a common manifestation of cutaneous *Candida* (62).

Chronic mucocutaneous candidiasis (CMC) is a persistent condition that effects the skin, mucus membranes, and nails as a result of a T-cell immune defect. The lesions may be so severe that disfiguration may occur. Addison's disease and hypoparathyroidism has been associated with this disorder (62, 64).

Candida can infect major organ systems, such as the parenchymal and meningeal layers of brain tissue, usually a complication of disseminated candidiasis. *Candida albicans* has been the species most identified in 90% of all CNS *Candida* infections (62).

Other organ involvement is seen in the respiratory tract, and myocardium. Endocarditis caused by *Candida* has been associated with underlying factors, such as defective valves, heart disease, heroin addicts, cancer chemotherapy, implantable prosthetic valves, prolonged intravenous catheters, and bacterial endocarditis (62, 64, 65).

Colonization of the urine by *Candida* can frequently be seen in patients on antibiotics and indwelling Foley catheters and may not indicate an infectious process. Urinary tract infections may be classified as primary; from the ascending route, or secondary; from the hematogenous route, the later being the most common form of candidiasis infection (62).

Once, rarely seen, but now more frequently reported are *Candida* arthritis, osteomyelitis, costochondritis, myositis, peritonitis, vasculitis, and *Candida* infections of the gallbladder, spleen, and pancreas. *Candida* may infect the eye as a result of eye surgery, or hematogenous spread (62).

Disseminated candidiasis may infect multiple organ systems, most commonly the kidneys, myocardium, brain and the eye. Only 15 to 40% of patients are diagnosed early, because of the absence of positive blood cultures (62). In the immunosuppressed patient, those with neoplastic disease, burn patients, and those with complicated post operative courses, candidemia almost always means the patient has disseminated disease (62, 64, 65).

DIAGNOSIS

The diagnosis for *Candida* in the mucous membranes or cutaneous areas is made by the clinical appearance of the lesion, and by scraping the tissue for a specimen. The use of gram staining and the use of a 10% potassium hydroxide solution identifies the hyphae, pseudohyphae and yeast forms. The fungus grows well in blood cultures and agar plates. A rapid identification test is by placing the organism in serum and observing small projections from the cell surface within 90 minutes (8, 62, 67). Endoscopy with biopsy of the tissue is the procedure most often used to diagnose *Candida* esophagitis and gastritis (62, 68). In CNS candidiasis, CT scan may show abcess secondary to parenchymal involvement. Spinal fluid pleocytosis is a common finding with *Candida* meningitis (62). In the respiratory tract, biopsy of the pulmonary tissue is usually necessary to make a definitive diagnoses (62, 69). Blood cultures are general positive in patients who have *Candida* endocarditis (62, 70). Echocardiography and transesophageal echocardiography are frequently used to detect vegetative growth (62). Serological testing has been used to diagnose *Candida* arthritis, however, the incidence of false positives is high, especially in the immunosuppressed and post operative patient. Percutaneous needle aspiration is used to determine osteomyelitis caused by this organism, because blood cultures are usually negative. CT scan, Ultrasonography (US), Magnetic Resonance Imagining (MRI), radiologically guided needle aspiration, and laparoscopic techniques have been used to diagnose deep organ involvement (62).

TREATMENT

Oral Candida Infections. In the immunocompetent patient treatment of oral *Candida* infection has been successful with nystatin suspension, 100,000 units 3 to 6 times a day. Nystatin vaginal tablets and clotrimazole troches dissolved orally four times a day have also been effective treatment for oral thrush. Topical nystatin or amphotericin B cream have been used for angular chelitis. Diaper rash caused by *Candida* can be managed with nystatin powder or cream in combination with a corticosteroid. *Candida* vaginitis has been successfully treated with clotrimazole or nystatin suppositories, or miconazole or clotrimazole cream. Ketoconazole and fluconazole have been used, also, to treat vaginitis in refractory infections (62, 64).

Chronic Mucocutaneous Candidiasis (CMC). In early stages of chronic mucocutaneous candidiasis (CMC), nystastin and clotrimazole may be useful, however in advanced disease ketoconazole or short courses of IV amphotericin B followed by ketoconazole as maintenance therapy should be initiated (64, 71). Relapse rates are significantly high when treatment is discontinued, therefore life-long therapy is required. Immunostimulating factors have been investigated such as transfer factor, a cell-free leukocycte extract that transfers delayed hypersensitivity reaction to anergic patients. Other experimental agents have been with levamisole, thymosin fraction 5, lymphocyte transfusion, thymus transplant, and cimetidine (62, 72, 73).

Ocular Candidiasis. Ocular candidiasis must be treated with parenteral amphotericin B or in refractory cases, combined therapy with amphotericin B and 5-FC should be used (62, 64).

Candidemia. In a randomized study comparing fluconazole (400mg qd) with amphotericin B (0.5 to 0.6mg/kg/day) for the treatment of candidemia in patients without neutropenia conducted by Rex et al., the efficacies of the two drugs were not significantly different (65, 74). A study in neutropenic patients comparing these two agents has not been completed, therefore, the efficacy of fluconazole compared to amphotericin has not been determined in this group of patients (65). Some authorities suggest that fluconazole may be used only in neutropenic patients who meet the following criteria: 1) are clinically stable, 2) no evidence of hematogenous dissemination, 3) the candidemia has occurred in association with an intravascular catheter, 4) not receiving an azole as a prophylactic, and 5) *Aspergillus* infections are not common at the institution. Intravenous amphotericin B should be used in neutropenic patients if this criteria is not met until further data is available (65).

Fluconazole should be avoided in *Candida krusei* and *C. torulopsis glavrate* because these species are resistant to this drug. Amphotericin B should be used whether the patient is neutropenic or not (65).

Itraconazole has been studied in one small trial comparing it to amphotericin B with or without 5-FC. Efficacy was comparable in both groups, however, subtherapeutic blood levels were seen in some patients who failed itraconazole (65, 75).

Intravascular catheters. Patients should be classified into two groups, either ICU patients or cancer patients, to address whether intravascular catheters should be changed or removed. In a study involving ICU patients comparing amphotericin B with fluconazole, data showed that in patients whom all intravascular catheters were changed when the patients were found to have *Candida*, the duration of the infection was shortened (65, 74). However, in cancer patients with Hickman or Broviac catheters amphotericin B has been used successfully without the removal of the catheter (65, 76). Some authorities suggest these catheters should be changed when feasible, and amphotericin B should be administered when catheter change is not an option (62, 65).

Patients who have developed *Candida* peritonitis and who are on chronic ambulatory peritoneal dialysis (CAPD) may be treated with the addition of amphotericin B to the dialysis fluid to achieve a concentration of 2 to 4 µg/ml (62). Others have recommended fluconazole as a loading dose of 200mg to 400mg followed by 50 to 200mg qd. The peritoneal catheter should be removed whenever possible, to eliminate the source of infection (62, 65).

Chronic Hematogenous Disseminate Candidiasis. Though rare, chronic hematogenously disseminated candidiasis is most often treated with longterm amphotericin B (total dose of 5gms), and 5-FC (65, 77, 79). No randomized studies have been conducted, however, in retrospective studies, initial treatment with amphotericin B followed by a fluconazole resulted in a 91% response rate (65, 79, 80). In another study using this regimen, a superinfection with *Aspergillus* was documented in 3 out of 20 patients, therefore, it is recommended that amphotericin B be used in combination with 5-FC (65, 79).

Candiduria. Currently a large study, conducted by the NIAID Mycoces Study Group, is underway to determine the optimal treatment of candiduria, however, preanalysis data is not available (65). Patients who present with candiduria should be investigated further for evidence of urinary tract obstruction, because of the risk of dissemination. The presence of white blood cell casts in the urine and pyuria are often indicative of an infection. Candiduria should be treated in all immunocompromised patients irrespective of their symptoms, and, if possible, the Foley catheter and antibiotics should be discontinued (65). Once systemic candidiasis is ruled out, the immunocompromised

patient should be treated with fluconazole 50 to 100mg qd for 2 to 3 days (65). An alternative therapy is with amphotericin B bladder irrigation as a continuous infusion via three-way Foley catheter (50mg/L sterile water for injection) (65, 81). A reduced dose of amphotericin B (10mg/L) infused into the bladder intermittently to reduce local irritation has been used with success by Sanford. Two hundred to 300mls is instilled into the bladder and the catheter is cross clamped for 60 to 90 minutes (65, 82). If the candiduria persists, then an upper urinary tract infection or 'fungus balls' should be suspected and systemic treatment should be initiated, or the fungus balls surgically removed (65).

Central Nervous System Infections. Central nervous system candidiasis is treated with combined amphotericin B and 5-FC. Intrathecal instillation is not recommended, except in severe cases. If a shunt is present, it should be removed if possible (62, 65, 83).

Endocarditis. Medical and surgical treatment is necessary to reduce the mortality rate of *Candida* endocarditis. Once the diagnosis is made, treatment with amphotericin B should be initiated and removal of the valve surgically should be performed as soon as possible. Once the valve is removed, 6 to 10 weeks of amphotericin B is given to reduce the incidence of relapse. Patients should be followed for 2 years after this therapy (65).

Oral Candidiasis in AIDS. Oral candidiasis is a significant problem in AIDS patients and those with defects in cell-mediated immunity. In a large randomized study Pons et al. found oral fluconazole (100mg qd) and oral clotrimazole (10mg 5 times a day) have shown to be equally efficacious in the treatment of oral candidiasis. Relapses occurred more frequently in the clotrimazole group compared to the fluconazole group (65, 84). A randomized, double-blind study comparing fluconazole (50mg qd) and ketoconazole (200mg qd) for 28 days was conducted by DeWit et al. Clinical remission was achieved at the end of therapy in 100% of patients who received fluconazole, versus 75% in those treated with ketoconazole (85). De Wit et al. also have studied single-dose fluconazole (150mg) compared to fluconazole (50mg qd for 7 days). Clinical cure was demonstrated on day 7 in 85% of patients treated with the single-dose fluconazole versus 96% in the daily regimen (not clinically significant) (86).

Oral nystatin may be useful in the treatment of esophageal candidiasis, however, in severe disease ketoconazole or fluconazole may be the better choice. In AIDS patients, fluconazole showed an advantage over ketoconazole in patients treated for esophageal candidiasis in a study conducted by Laine et al. (87). Itraconazole has been compared to ketoconazole in a double-blinded study by Smith et al. in HIV positive patients. Clinical responses were equal at 4 weeks of therapy in both treatment groups, however, 80% of patients had relapse infections within 3 months in both groups (88). A study comparing itraconazole (200mg qd) with fluconazole (50mg qd) in patients with oral and esophageal candidiasis is currently underway. Preliminary results suggest that both drugs are equally effective (89). Also, de Repentigny et al. compared itraconazole (200mg qd) and ketoconazole (200mg qd) in oral, pharyngeal or esophageal candidiasis. There were no significant differences in efficacy in either group, however, time to relapse was greater with itraconazole compared to ketoconazole (90).

Blastomycosis

Blastomycosis is a rare but nevertheless important mycotic disease that causes a systemic granulomatous infection characterized pathologically by a combination of supparative and granulomata (91, 92). Unlike many fungal infections that are opportunistic, Blastomycosis usually occurs in healthy hosts, however, recent data suggest that it may occur more commonly in the immunocompromised host than previously appreciated (91, 93).

EPIDEMIOLOGY

Blastomyces dermatitis, a dimorphic fungus, occurs primarily in the Southcentral and Midwestern United States, the Central Provinces of Canada, and wide portions of Africa (93, 94). Cases of endemic or sporadic Blastomycosis account for the majority of cases and usually occur in young to middle-aged adults and are reported more often in men than women (91, 92). Epidemics of blastomycosis that are related to a point-source exposure also occur in which patients of all ages and both sexes are involved (91, 92). The ecologic niche of the organism in 2 outbreaks involving a point source was identified by Klein and co-workers (95, 96). The organism was isolated from soil containing vegetation or from decomposed wood (95, 96).

CLINICAL MANIFESTATIONS

The usual portal of entry in humans is the lungs with disease at other body sites the result of dissemination from a primary pulmonary infection, even if not clinically apparent (92). Clinical disease from dissemination most commonly involves the skin, bone, and genitourinary tract (92). In the immunocompromised host, those with solid organ transplants, on glucocorticoids or receiving cytotoxic chemotherapy for hematologic malignancies or solid tumors, Pappas et al. noted the disease to be more aggressive with multiple organ and central nervous system involvement relatively common (93). Overall, mortality was much higher in the immunocompromised hosts than immunocompetent hosts (29% vs. 3.2%) (93). Blastomycosis, in a few patients with AIDS, occurs late and is frequently fatal with overwhelming disseminated disease that commonly includes involvement of the CNS with a high early mortality (97).

DIAGNOSIS

The diagnosis is made by the identification of the organisms characteristic size, refractile cell wall, and single broad-based buds from clinical specimens followed by cultures (91, 92).

TREATMENT

The majority of immunocompetent hosts have a self-limited illness from acute pulmonary blastomycosis (98). Those patients with progressive acute or chronic pulmonary disease, and disseminated disease require therapy (98). The NIAID, Mycoses Study Group, compared low dose ketoconazole (400mg/day) with high dose ketoconazole (800mg/day) in the immunocompetent patient treated for at least 6 months (99). The study showed a 79% cure rate in the low dose group compared to a 100% cure rate in the high dose group which was associated with a greater toxicity (99). In the treatment of nonmeningeal, non life-threatening blastomycosis, it was recommended that ketoconazole be initiated at a dose of 400mg/day which may be increased to 600–800mg/day if needed (99).

Dismuke et al, noted itraconazole to be a highly effective therapy for nonmeningeal, non life-threatening blastomycosis with a 95% success rate for patients treated for more than 2 months (100). It was recommended for those patients who have progression or persistence of disease on 200mg/day that the dose be increased to 400mg/qd (100). Because of its greater efficacy and tolerability in comparison to ketoconazole, itraconazole is considered by most to be the agent of choice for the majority of immunocompetent patients with nonmeningeal, non life-threatening blastomycosis (14, 100). In patients with severe or acute life-threatening forms of blastomycosis, such as the appearance of Acute Respiratory Distress Syndrome (ARDS), or the person with CNS involvement with blastomycosis, amphotericin B remains the initial treatment of choice (91).

Immunocompromised Hosts. Amphotericin B should be used as initial therapy in most immunocompromised hosts with blastomycosis with a cumulative total dose of a least 1 gram (93). Controversy exits whether to continue amphotericin B until a patient is disease free or to switch to an oral azole after initial therapy with amphotericin B (93). In those patients converted to azole therapy following amphotericin B, it should be administered for at least 6 months and until disease free (93). Azole therapy may also play a role in those patients who have responded to a primary course of amphotericin B but require long-term suppressive therapy (93). Clinicians should be cautious in using the newer azoles as primary therapy in the immunocompromised host with blastomycosis until more data is available, and consider their use only in patients with limited disease and a stable underlying condition (93).

Coccidiodomycosis

Coccidiodomycosis is a disease known by many names such as valley fever, San Joaquin Valley Fever or 'desert fever' or 'cocci.' There has been renewed interest in the disease because endemic areas are experiencing population growth and along with increased travel and tourism the number of infected people may increase (101, 102). In addition, coccidioidomycosis is a significant opportunistic infection among HIV-infected person living in a coccidioidal area and was added to the CDC's surveillance case definition for AIDS in 1987 (103, 104).

EPIDEMIOLOGY

Coccidioidomycosis is caused by *Coccidioides immitis*, a dimorphic fungus, that is endemic to certain areas of the Western Hemisphere, including the low deserts of the Southwestern United States (102, 105). Its natural habitat is the soil, and the infection is caused by inhalation of airborne infectious arthrospores (101, 102). Localized epidemics have been reported in areas where soil disturbances have occurred, such as following the 1978 dust storms in California and after the 1993 earthquake in Los Angeles (101, 102). However, increasingly, cases are being recognized outside the endemic areas such as acquired infection from tomatoes, fruit or cotton bales from endemic areas; travelers to an endemic area; or as reactivation of a previously latent infection in former residents of an endemic area (101, 102, 106).

CLINICAL FEATURES

Infections can be divided into 3 broad groups and include pulmonary infection, pulmonary complications or disseminated (extrapulmonary) disease (105). Primary pulmonary infection usually remains asymptomatic in 60% of infected persons (101, 102, 105). About 40% have symptomatic infection one to three weeks after exposure and range from a 'flu-like' illness to overt pneumonia (101, 102). After initial infection, a small percentage of patients (5%) develop pulmonary residua such as nodules or cavities (101, 102, 105). Nodules are remnants and represent residual granulomatous organization of a former pneumonia (102, 105). Coccidioidal cavities are usually peripheral and thin walled and can carry a risk of complications such as hemoptysis, persistent enlargement of pyopneumothorax (102, 105). Less frequently, the initial pneumonia does not resolve, and a progressive pneumonia or chronic lung infection develop (101, 102, 105). Diabetics or those with a compromised immune system are especially susceptible to chronic pulmonary disease which can be fibrocavitory with bronchiectasis, empyema or bronchopleural fistulas as sequela (101, 102, 105). Approximately 0.5% of patients develop disseminated (extrapulmonary) disease, and common sites of involvement are the meninges, bone and joints, skin, and soft tissue (101, 102, 105). Dissemination is far more common in dark-skinned races, men, pregnant women and the immunocompromised, host (101, 102). Results of a prospective study of HIV-infected person in an endemic area noted that CD4 lymphocytic counts less than $250/mm^3$ and a diagnosis of AIDS were risk factors associated with the development of active disease. A diffuse reticulonodular pattern on a chest radiograph is common in these patients (104).

DIAGNOSIS

The organism can be demonstrated by visualization of its distinctive spherule and culture from clinical specimens (101, 102, 105). In the absence of histopathologic findings or positive cultures two serologic tests may provide a presumptive diagnosis (101, 102, 105). The precipitin antibody (IgM) can be detected in 75% of patients with primary infection and generally occur 1 to 3 weeks after onset of symptoms (101, 102, 105). Complement-fixing antibody (IgG) can be detected in 50 to 90% of patients with primary symptomatic infection and generally occur 3 months after onset of symptoms (101, 102, 105). An elevated IgG antibody titer is a marker of disseminated disease with 61% of patients with titers of at least 1:32 and 41% have titers of at least 1:64 (101–103). In meningitis, which is the most serious complication of disseminated disease, serum antibody titers as well as CSF cultures may be negative (101, 102, 105). However, IgG antibody titer is present in CSF in 70% of patients on initial examination, and as the disease progresses, in almost all (101, 102).

TREATMENT

Patients with severe primary infection and those with high complement-fixing antibody titers, because of the concern for dissemination, should be treated (101, 102, 105). Other factors that should be assessed to determine the need for therapy in primary infection include a high inoculum exposure; increased susceptibility; persistent symptoms for over 6 weeks; extensive, enlarging, or persistent pulmonary involvement; and concurrent noncoccidioidal disease (101, 102). Ketoconazole at 400mg/day has been recommended as initial therapy for progressive nonmeningeal forms of coccidioidomycosis, however, relapses can be seen (102, 107). Itraconazole at 400mg/day has been noted to be less toxic than ketoconazole, may be more effective than ketoconazole, and was associated with fewer relapses for treatment for nonmeningeal coccidioidomycosis (108). Fluconazole has favorable response rates in the treatment of nonmeningeal coccidioidomycosis at 400 to 600mg/day (109, 110). The optimal duration of azole therapy remains to be defined, but based on relapse rates, a prolonged course after disease activity is apparent and is probably needed (101, 102).

In disseminated (extrathoracic) disease, therapy is always indicated (101, 102). An approach that has been suggested is to treat with amphotericin B until the disease becomes inactive, or for a total of 2 to 3 months (101). With coccidioidal meningitis, traditional treatment is usually intrathecal therapy with amphotericin B which is commonly given along with systemic amphotericin B (0.5–1.0gm) as well (102). Fluconazole and itraconazole offer an alternative treatment of meningeal disease at the same doses as recommended for nonmeningeal disease with associated high rates of response (101, 102, 111, 112). However, after azole therapy is stopped very high rates of relapse have been suggested (101, 102, 113).

HIV. In the HIV-infected adult and adolescent primary prophylaxis for *Coccidioides immitis* may be considered in those with CD4 counts of 50/mm^3 and in the endemic geographic region with fluconazole 200mg po qd or itraconazole 200mg qd as an alternative (61).

Histoplasmosis

Histoplasmosis is a dimorphic fungus of nearly worldwide distribution. It is the most common systemic mycosis in the United States (114). It is an important opportunistic pathogen in patients with impaired T-cell mediated immunity, particularly those with AIDS, lending to its inclusion in the CDC's 1987 revised surveillance definition for AIDS (103, 114).

EPIDEMIOLOGY

Histoplasma capsulatum, a soil saprophyte, is endemic to the Central and Southeastern United States and areas of Latin America (115, 116). Humid environmental conditions with moderate temperatures and shady environment favor its growth (114). Bird droppings and bat excrement accelerate its sporalution in the soil (114). These unique growth factors help explain the localization of the organism into so-called microfoci (114). Rural exposure to these microfoci occur with such activities as spelunking, cleaning chicken coops or bird roosts (114). Spores can be found 10 years after birds have abandoned their roosts. Urban exposure occurs when these microfoci are disturbed during such activities as excavation, demolition, and construction for urbanization (114). During such activities, highly infectious spores can be spread by the wind over large areas.

CLINICAL MANIFESTATIONS

A variety of clinical manifestations may follow infection with *H. capsulatum*, depending not only on the immunity of the host but on the degree of exposure (114, 117, 118). Although it is an inhalationally acquired mycoses occasionally reactivation may account for some cases of disseminated disease in areas of low endemicity, in those immunocompromised hosts who had resided in endemic

areas prior (114, 119–121). Analysis by Dr. Wheat and colleagues of 2 major urban outbreaks have made important contributions to the clinical, diagnostic, and therapeutic aspects of *H. capsulatum* infection (118). Several acute self-limited syndromes were noted during the outbreak and constituted the majority of symptomatic cases (114, 118). Acute pulmonary histoplasmosis, a flu-like illness, was the most common presenting manifestation, occurring in 56% of patients (118). Other acute self-limited manifestations that occurred in about 10% of symptomatic cases, included rheumatologic syndromes and pericarditis (114, 118). Cavitary histoplasmosis with clinical findings similar to tuberculosis occurred in approximately 10% of clinically recognized cases (118). Disseminated disease developed in 9% of clinically recognized cases and age greater than 54 years old and immunosuppression were the only risk factors noted (118).

During continued study by Wheat et al, of a third outbreak in Indianapolis, 26% of 239 patients with AIDS were diagnosed with histoplasmosis (122). Only 22% of these patients had just disseminated histoplasmosis with approximately 40% having another concurrent opportunistic infection (122). Unusual clinical manifestation noted in the AIDS patients compared to literature reports were a syndrome resembling septicemia, coagulopathy, hemolysis, an oral lesion of the mandible with a draining fistula, rhabdomyolysis with renal failure and unexplained renal failure with thrombocytopenia (122).

DIAGNOSIS

Currently a variety of tests can be utilized for the diagnosis of histoplasmosis and include fungal cultures, fungal stains, serologic test for antibodies, and antigen detection (123). Dr. Wheat has suggested an approach to the diagnosis of histoplasmosis based on the sensitivity, specificity, and the turn-around-time of the test for the different clinical manifestations of the disease (123) (See Table 73.1).

TREATMENT

The NIAID Mycoces Study Group compared low dose (400mg/day) ketoconazole with high dose (800mg/day) ketoconazole in the immunocompetent patient treated for

Table 73.1.

Summary of Suggested Work-Up for Histoplasmosis

	Self Limited	Severe Acute Pulmonary	Chronic Pulmonary	Disseminated
Serology	+++	+	+++	++
Antigen	+	+++	+	+++
Histology		+++	+	++
Culture		+	+++	+++

With permission from Indiana University-Purdue University Indianapolis, and Histoplasmosis Reference Laboratory, Dec. 21, 1995.

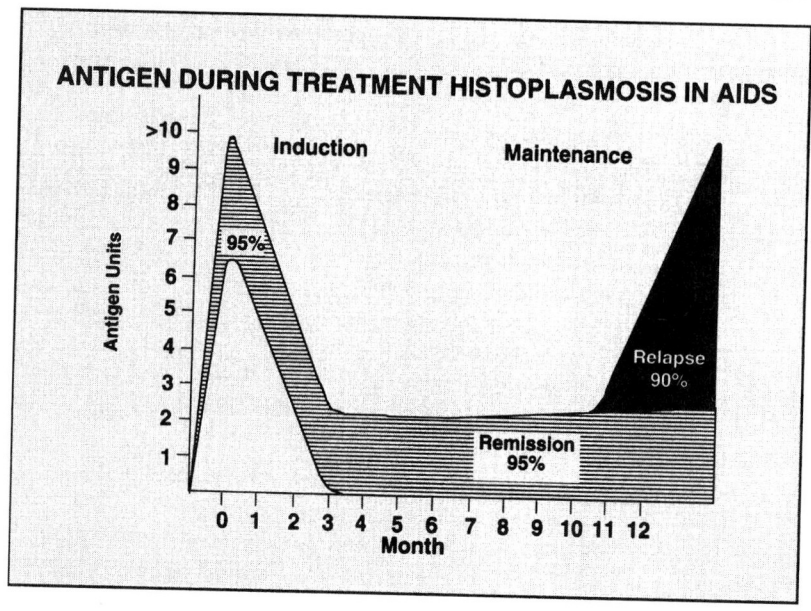

Figure 73.1 With permission from Indiana University-Purdue University Indianapolis, and Histoplasmosis Reference Laboratory, Dec. 21, 1995.

at least 6 months. The overall success rate was 85%, however, toxicity was greater in the high dose group. The study concluded that ketoconazole is effective for immunocompetent patients with non life-threatening, nonmeningeal forms of histoplasmosis. It recommended an initial dose of ketoconazole at 400mg/day, and increased to 600–800mg/day if needed (124). In a large multicenter study itraconazole was found to be highly effective therapy for nonmeningeal, non life-threatening histoplasmosis (125). Itraconazole at 400mg/day over six months appears to be better tolerated than ketoconazole, but at greater expense (14, 125).

Amphotericin B would still be recommended as the initial treatment in those patients with severe or acute life-threatening disease (122, 124).

AIDS/Induction. In patients with AIDS the goal of treatment is suppression since disseminated disease cannot be cured (122). Treatment for disseminated histoplasmosis is usually divided into two phases, an initial period of induction therapy followed by maintenance therapy to prevent relapse (122). One recommended approach would be a gram of amphotericin B initially followed by weekly doses of 50 to 80mg until a cumulative dose of 2 grams, then biweekly doses of 50–80mg continued indefinitely (126). Ketoconazole is not effective as either induction or maintenance therapy as relapse rates of 50 to 60% have been noted (122). Itraconazole has been shown to be a safe and effective agent for induction therapy in patients with AIDS who have mild disseminated histoplasmosis (127). In those patients with moderately severe or severe disease, amphotericin B should be used, and, after achieving clinical improvement, be changed to itraconazole (127).

Maintenance. Itraconazole has been found to be a safe and effective alternative to amphotericin B for maintenance therapy at 200mg twice daily (128). In addition, fluconazole at 200mg/day is another reasonable choice for chronic suppressive therapy in AIDS patients who are unable to tolerate itraconazole secondary to drug interaction, malabsorption, or side effects (129). In patients with AIDS, antigen detection can be used for monitoring therapy and to identify relapses. A suggested approach would be to obtain an antigen level at the initiation and completion of therapy and then every 4 months during suppressive therapy. Antigen concentrations should fall and usually become undetectable within 3 months after initiation of therapy. Guidelines have been proposed for interpretation of antigen increase during therapy with recommendation to aid the clinician (14, 123). (See Fig. 73.1) (See Table 73.2).

Prophylaxis. Primary prophylaxis may be considered for histoplasmosis in HIV infected adults and adolescents with itraconazole (200mg/day), and fluconazole (200mg qd) as an alternate when with CD4 counts are less than 50/mm^3, and in an endemic geographic area (61).

CONCLUSION

Superficial mycotic infections rarely cause serious systemic disease, and a successful treatment often includes the prevention of reinfection, even after the initial infection is successfully treated. Systemic mycotic infections often result from accidental exposure, and they frequently have only limited clinical symptoms or disease in a healthy individual. However, when a host's immune system is suppressed because of disease (e.g., AIDS) or immunosuppressant drugs, these fungi, such as *Aspergillus, Histo-*

Table 73.2.
Interpretation Antigen Increases During Treatment

Increase	Interpretation	Implication	Recommendation
0 to 1.9	Stable	None	None
2.0 to 4.0	Mild increase	Possible failure	Culture
			Repeat antigen
			Review therapy
>4.1	Moderate-marked increase	Probable failure	Culture
			Intensify therapy

With permission from Indiana University-Purdue University Indianapolis, and Histoplasmosis Reference Laboratory, Dec. 21, 1995.

plasma, *Blastomyces, Coccidioides, Cryptococci* and *Candida*, can become opportunistic infective organisms. Opportunistic mycotic infections in immunocompromised individuals require more aggressive therapy. Even with appropriate treatment these individuals can often have relapses and require prolonged drug therapy.

PARASITIC INFECTIONS

Parasites infect humans in all regions of the world, but there is a particularly high prevalence in areas with mild climates and poor sanitation. In those underdeveloped regions, there is an abundance of species and infected-host reservoirs. Many of these parasites require special environment conditions for both reproduction and survival. Other parasites may require an intermediary host for transmission and completion of their life cycle. These intermediary hosts gain access to humans, because of inadequate preventive measures or hard-to-change cultural habits in these endemic areas. In contrast to the more developed countries in the temperate zones where degenerative, cardiovascular, and malignant diseases are the major causes of disability and death, the underdeveloped countries have to deal with diseases that afflict their young. Infections and malnutrition are sometimes so severe that 40 to 50% of the population may die before reaching the age of 50. Eating habits can also determine the incidence of parasitic infection. The practice of eating raw or partially cooked foods increases the risk of getting a parasitic infection.

Parasitic infections are not always limited to the endemic areas. Infections are frequently observed in the migrant population or in travelers, who acquire their infection in endemic areas. Thus, healthcare practitioners outside the tropics and subtropics must also have adequate knowledge of the diagnosis and treatment of parasitic diseases.

Enterobiasis

Enterobiasis (pinworm, threadworm, or seatworm) infection is an infection of the human gastrointestinal tract by *Enterobius vermicularis* (130–132). It is one of the most common parasitic infections in temperate and well-sanitized areas today. In the United States, 5 to 15% of the general population is estimated to harbor this helminth. The highest prevalence is in school-age children, followed by children of preschool age and mothers of infected children. The infection rate is lowest among adults. Infection can be transmitted directly by oral-fecal contact or indirectly through clothing, bedding, food, or dust contaminated with viable eggs. Since this parasitic infection is readily transmitted from individual to individual, it is entirely possible that every member of the household is infected (133).

CLINICAL MANIFESTATIONS

Pinworm infection may be asymptomatic, but the most frequent symptom is intense pruritus ani produced by the migrating female helminth and the presence of eggs (134–138). This intense pruritus ani may cause secondary dermatitis, eczema, and bacterial infection from the host's constant scratching. Parasitic vulvovaginitis and urinary tract infection due to enterobiasis may occur in young girls (139, 140). Rare infections of the peritoneal cavity and the female genital tract may also occur (141–146). Behavioral changes, including inattention, irritability, and lack of cooperation, can occur in children infected with pinworm.

DIAGNOSIS

Stool examination for pinworm infection is of little value, since adult worms are only occasionally found in heavy infections, but the *Enterobius* eggs are almost always present in the perianal areas. The most satisfactory method of diagnosing pinworm infection is by the use of a perianal swab made of a wooden tongue blade and clear transparent tape. The tape is then placed on a glass slide and examined under a microscope for *Enterobius* ova. The swabs should be used in the morning before bathing and defecation. The eosinophil count is usually normal in enterobiasis. Other household members should also be screened for enterobial infection.

TREATMENT

Numerous anthelmintics are available for the treatment of *Enterobius* infection, among them are mebendazole, albendazole, piperazine citrate, pyrantel pamoate, pyrvinium pamoate, and thiabendazole (137–152). See Table 73.3. Besides medical management of pinworm infection with pharmacological agents, treatment should also include prevention of reinfection and screening of the other household members. Personal hygiene and adequate sanitary facilities are important in the prevention of pinworm infection. The therapeutic agent of choice for the management of enterobiasis is mebendazole, because it is easy to give and has minimal side effects. Usually a

Table 73.3.
Treatment of Helminthic Infections

Enterobiasis
Mebendazole (Vermox) (257–259)
Dose: adult and child over 2 years of age
  A single dose of 100 mg and repeat in 2 weeks
Side effects
  Occasional abdominal cramps and diarrhea have been reported. Rarely it can cause leukopenia.
Piperazine citrate (Antepar) (260)
Dose: adult and child
  65 mg/kg not to exceed 2.5 g daily for 7 days and repeat in 2 weeks
Side effects (261, 262)
  Occasionally can cause nausea, vomiting, diarrhea, abdominal cramps, and headaches. On rare occasions it can cause transient vertigo, incoordination, muscle weakness, lethargy, erythema multiforme, urticaria, and visual disturbances. It can also exacerbate underlying seizure disorders and cause other CNS toxicity, especially in patients with renal dysfunction.
Pyrantel pamoate (Antiminth) (263, 264)
Dose: adult and child
  A single dose of 11 mg/kg not to exceed 1 g and repeat in 2 weeks
Side effects
  Occasionally causes abdominal cramps, diarrhea, dizziness, headaches, rash, and fever. A transient rise in AST has been reported.
Pyrvinium pamoate (Povan) (see text)
Dose: adult and child
  A single dose of 5 mg/kg not to exceed 250 mg and repeat in 2 weeks
Side effects
  Pyrvinium pamoate turns the stool red and can stain clothing. Occasionally it can cause nausea, vomiting, and diarrhea. Pyrvinium pamoate can also cause photosensitivity on rare instances.
Thiabendazole (Mintezol) (see text)
Dose: adult and child
  25 mg/kg twice daily not to exceed 3.0 g per day for 1 day only and repeat in 2 weeks
Side effects
  Side effects include anorexia, headache, nausea, vomiting, and dizziness. On rare occasions it can also cause fever, chills, urticaria, and pruritis.

Ascariasis
Mebendazole (Vermox) (265, 266)
Dose: adult and child
  100 mg orally twice daily for 3 days
Side effects (267)
  Abdominal cramps and diarrhea have been reported and occasionally it can cause leukopenia.
Piperazine citrate (Antepar) (see text)
Dose: adult and child
  75 mg/kg orally once daily not to exceed 3.5 g per day for 2 consecutive days
Side effects
  Adverse reactions can include nausea, vomiting, diarrhea, abdominal cramps, and headaches. Muscle weakness, vertigo, incoordination, lethargy, urticaria, erythema multiforme, and visual disturbance also rarely occur. In patients with renal dysfunction, CNS toxicities can occur as well.
Pyrantel pamoate (Antiminth) (see text)
Dose: adult and child
  A single dose of 11 mg/kg not to exceed 1 g
Side effects
  Abdominal cramps, diarrhea, headache, dizziness, rash, and fever can occasionally occur. Transient increases in AST have been reported.
Thiabendazole (Mintezol) (see text)
Dose: adult and child
  25 mg/kg orally twice daily not to exceed 3.0 g per day for 1 day and repeat in 2 weeks
Side effects
  Occasional side effects include anorexia, headache, nausea, vomiting, and dizziness. In rare instances pruritis, fever, chills, and urticaria can occur.
Trichuriasis (268–270)
Mebendazole (Vermox) (271–273)
Dose: adult and child over 2 years of age
  100 mg twice daily for 3 days is the treatment of choice
Side effects
  Generally well tolerated, but occasional abdominal cramps and diarrhea can ocur. On rare instances leukopenia can also occur.

---

single-dose treatment is adequate, but it should be repeated in 2 weeks to prevent reinfection.

Ascariasis

Ascariasis (153–158) (roundworm) infection is an infection of the human gastrointestinal tract by *Ascaris lumbricoides*. *Ascaris* infection occurs worldwide, with the highest incidence in the tropics. In the United States this disease is most prevalent in the southern states among preschool and early school-aged children. Approximately 4 million people in the United States and one fourth of all the world population are believed to be infected by this parasite (159, 160). Ascariasis is transmitted via ingestion of food or soil contaminated with feces containing viable *Ascaris* eggs (161). Direct person-to-person transmission does not occur because the eggs require a minimum soil incubation of 2 weeks.

CLINICAL MANIFESTATIONS

Symptoms caused by ascariasis are often vague and variable or absent. However, children with a heavy parasitic burden may have symptoms of abdominal pain, vomiting, sleep disturbance, intestinal obstruction, and malnutrition (172–174). Individuals who ingest large numbers of *Ascaris* eggs may develop fever, cough, ascaris pneumonitis, and prominent eosinophilia secondary to the large number of migrating larvae. Other rare but more serious complications include appendicitis, intestinal perforation, obstruction of hepatic, pancreatic, or common bile ducts and aspiration of the worm (165–170).

DIAGNOSIS

The diagnosis is made based upon demonstration of *Ascaris* ova in the stool or the recovery of a passed adult worm. On occasion the diagnosis is made upon visualizing the adult worm in the intestine by x-ray with or without contrasting material. Administrating barium can increase the x-ray visualization of the adult worm after the barium is passed, because the barium is adsorbed onto the surface of the *Ascaris* and sometimes stored in their alimentary canal (171).

TREATMENT (See Table 73.3)

Treatment of ascariasis involves treatment of the disease and prophylaxis. Several drugs are available for the treatment of ascariasis, among them are mebendazole, albendazole, piperazine citrate, and pyrantel pamoate. These agents have replaced some of the older and more toxic agents. Pyrantel pamoate is the treatment of choice, but mebendazole, albendazole, and piperazine citrate are also extremely effective in eradicating this intestinal parasite. Mebendazole and piperazine citrate should be used with some caution in children under 2 years old or in patients with seizure disorders. Prophylaxis against ascariasis should include good hygiene, especially with respect to proper disposal of human feces, and prevention of ingestion of contaminated soil. The time-honored method of fasting before treatment and purging after treatment has proved to be unnecessary. Unless the patient has total intestinal *Ascaris* obstruction, these pharmacological agents are effective in eradicating the worm and symptoms. It is quite common to see an increase in abdominal symptoms prior to the expulsion of the *Ascaris*.

Trichuriasis

Trichuriasis (172, 173) (whipworm or trichocephaliasis) is an infection of the large intestinal tract of the human by the parasite *Trichuris trichiura*. Trichuriasis has a geographic distribution like that of ascariasis. It is quite common for a patient to have ascariasis and trichuriasis simultaneously. The prevalence of trichuriasis is highest among young children in the tropics. In the United States approximately 2.2 million individuals are estimated to have trichuriasis. Among them, more than 40% are children. Trichuriasis is transmitted via ingestion of soil contaminated with feces containing viable eggs. Direct person-to-person transmission usually does not occur because the eggs require a minimum of 10 days in the soil to mature.

CLINICAL MANIFESTATIONS

Trichuris (174–177) infections usually produce no clinical symptoms unless a large worm burden is present. Severe infestation of *Trichuris* can produce symptoms including dysentary, mucoid stools, abdominal cramps, weight loss, prolapsed rectum, and malnutrition. Moderate eosinophilia and stool Charcot-Leyden crystals may also be found.

DIAGNOSIS

The diagnosis (178) depends upon recovery of *Trichuris* eggs from the stool or visualizing the adult worms through sigmoidoscopy or colonoscopy. Three stool samples should be collected on alternate days and preserved in P.V.A. (polyvinyl alcohol fixative) for shipment or laboratory analysis. This method of stool sampling allows screening for other concurrent parasitic infection as well.

TREATMENT (See Table 73.3)

Mebendazole is the drug of choice for the treatment of trichuriasis, although other agents such as albendazole and thiabendazole may also work (179–180). Thiabendazole is not recommended for use during pregnancy. Mebendazole should be used with caution in children under 2 years old and during pregnancy. Mild trichuriasis is usually self-limiting and requires no treatment, but it may be a source of infection for other family members and contacts.

Treatment of trichuriasis should also include screening of all household members and playmates (when children are involved). Follow-up stool-screening of the patient and other household members will ensure eradication of the parasite. However, the most important treatment is improved hygiene and fecal disposal.

Amebiasis

Amebiasis (181–190) (amebic dysentery, amebic colitis, or amebic enteritis) refers specifically to an infection of the human host by the protozoan *Entamoeba histolytica*. Amebiasis occurs in temperate areas worldwide. The *E. histolytica* cysts passed in the stool are immediately infective, and person-to-person transmission can occur. Unlike the cysts, the motile trophozoites are not infective because they are easily destroyed by stomach acid after ingestion. The most common mode of transmission of amebiasis is from person to person. The asymptomatic cyst-passer is an important source of infection, especially if the individual is involved in food preparation. Other modes of transmission may involve a contaminated water source, houseflies, cockroaches, and sexual contact. The exact incidence of amebiasis is not known, but the prevalence is highest in areas of poor water quality or poor sanitation. Amebiasis also has a relatively high incidence among the homosexual population.

CLINICAL MANIFESTATIONS

The clinical manifestations (191–198) of amebiasis vary greatly, depending upon the site infected. The most common site of amebic infection is the intestine. Infected individuals may have mild diarrhea, bloody dysentery, or no symptoms at all. Thus, amebiasis is known as the great imitator. Amebiasis can also disseminate to other organs such as the liver, lungs, and brain. The most frequent extraintestinal organ involved is the liver. Liver abscesses may occur many years after the primary intestinal infestation; therefore, liver involvement should be treated at the time of treating the intestinal amebiasis. The factors that determine the virulence of amebiasis are poorly understood, but some evidence indicates that the pathogenesis of the disease requires the presence of symbiotic bacteria.

DIAGNOSIS

The stools from a patient with suspected amebiasis should be examined over a period of 7 to 10 days. If direct on-location examination of the stool is not possible, the stool specimens should be preserved in P.V.A. fixative for transport and future examination. The stool should be passed into the container directly or onto paper and then transferred to the container with wooden sticks. The specimens collected during sigmoidoscopy examination may also be examined. The most difficult part of making a correct diagnosis is laboratory interpretation errors. A positive stool finding is the only indisputable evidence for diagnosing intraluminal amebiasis. However, the indirect hemagglutination (I.H.A.) test for amebiasis is valuable for diagnosis of extraluminal amebiasis. The usefulness of this test is limited by its inability to differentiate currently active extraluminal amebiasis from old dormant extraluminal amebic infection. An I.H.A. titer above 1:512 is a reasonably good indicator of recent extraluminal infection. Less than 50% of patients with hepatic amebiasis have a positive stool examination result, while 95 to 100% of them will have a positive I.H.A. titer above 1:128. Liver function tests are generally not very helpful in detecting hepatic amebiasis because 75% of these patients have normal liver function test results. However, a radioisotope scan is of value if an amebic abscess is present. When stool examinations are performed correctly, 90% of the intestinal amebiasis cases can be accurately diagnosed by three formed and one purged sample, and a 95% accuracy level can be achieved from six samples taken from patients with diarrhea. Diarrhea can be induced by giving the patient magnesium sulfate (170–177).

TREATMENT (See Table 73.4)

The treatment of amebiasis (207–208) is not as clearly defined as that of the other parasitic infections. The currently available drug treatment of amebiasis remains less than optimal, and opinions among the experts are divergent. This confusion is compounded by the toxicities of some of the most active drugs. Because there are increasing numbers of reports of treatment failures after using a single agent for amebic dysentery, the therapeutic regimen is now comprised of two active agents, one for the intestinal amebiasis and the other for the possible extralu-

minal infection. It is necessary to repeat the stool examination 6 months after treatment to confirm total eradication of the organism.

Since no single drug is adequate in curing both types of amebiasis, a luminal and extraluminal amebicide must be employed for patients with only intestinal or hepatic amebic infection. The combination of metronidazole followed by diloxanide furoate or paromomycin is generally well tolerated and adequate for this purpose, but other drug combinations can also be used. These regimens are generally not recommended during pregnancy because of the possible teratogenicity and fetal toxicity. Other agents used for treating amebiasis include chloroquine phosphate and iodoquinol. Although emetine and emetine hydrochloride have been used very effectively for treatment of extraluminal amebic infections in the past, Cardiotoxicity limits their current use. Sterilization of contaminated water by boiling or treating with iodine or household bleach kills the amebic cysts.

Scabies

Scabies (219–225) (itch mite, or seven-year itch) belong to the family of *Sarcoptidae* itch mites. Scabies infections occur most frequently when overcrowding and poor sanitation exist. It also appears to be cyclic. Scabies mites are most readily spread through close bodily contact for prolonged periods of time. Only the female mite is implicated in transmission, and she can survive apart from the host for 2 to 3 days. She is activated by warmth and perspiration of the skin and burrows into the stratum corneum. The mite will live for approximately 2 months in the host and lay a total of several hundred eggs during her lifespan. The incubation period is 3 to 4 days for the eggs, and 10 to 12 days for the larval stage. Fortunately for the human host only 1% of eggs hatch successfully.

CLINICAL MANIFESTATIONS

Most clinical symptoms (226–227) are caused by the female mite moving through the burrows. She leaves secretions and excreta that elicit erythema, edema, and severe itching. The most common parts of the body infested by scabies mite include the arms, hands, feet, and especially in the skin folds, but other areas such as the belt line, scrotum, penis, and the skin around the nipples in women can also be infected. The most severe form of scabies is often seen in immunocompromised patients, where crusty scabs may cover the entire body. This type of severe scabies infestation has been called *crusted scabies* or *Norwegian scabies*.

DIAGNOSIS

The diagnosis (228–231) of scabies is made based on clinical presentation of intestine pruritus with associated

Table 73.4.
Treatment of Protozoal Infections

Amebiasis (274–278)
Intestinal amebiasis:
Diiodohydroxyquin (various)
Dose
  Adult: 650 mg orally 3 times daily for 20 days
  Child: 40 mg/kg orally in 3 divided doses daily, not to exceed 2 g
    per day, for 20 days
Side effects
  Occasional abdominal cramps, diarrhea, weakness, rash, acne,
    pruritis ani, optic atrophy, and blindness in children with pro-
    longed exposure. Diiodohydroxyquin may cause deafness in
    children from prenatal exposure, and it should be avoided
    during pregnancy.
Diloxanide furoate (Furamide)
Dose
  Adult: 500 mg taken orally 3 times daily for 10 days
  Child: 20 mg/kg/day given in 3 divided doses daily, not to exceed 1.5
    per day, for 10 days
Side effects
  Frequently causes flatulence and other gastrointestinal symptoms
    such as cramps, diarrhea, vomiting, and nausea. Occasional urti-
    caria has also been reported.
Metronidazole (Flagyl) (see text)
Dose
  Adult: 750 mg taken orally 3 times daily for 10 days
  Child: 50 mg/kg/day given in 3 divided doses daily, not to exceed
    2250 mg per day, for 10 days
Side effects (see text)
  Metronidazole at amebicidal doses may exhibit disulfiram-like
    side effects when alcohol is taken. Other side effects may in-
    clude occasional anorexia, nausea, vomiting, diarrhea, flatu-
    lence, blurred vision, headaches, confusion, disorientation, de-
    pression, and a metallic taste in the mouth. Leukopenia may
    occur. Recently, metronidazole has been reported to be carci-
    nogenic in rodents and mutagenic in bacteria; therefore this
    drug is relatively contraindicated for at least the first trimester
    of pregnancy.

Paromomycin (Humatin)
Dose: adult and child
  25–30 mg/kg/day orally in 3 divided doses, not to exceed 2.0 g per
    day, for 10 days
Side effects
  Gastrointestinal disturbances including nausea, vomiting, diarrhea,
    and abdominal cramps are most common. These side effects are
    frequently associated with doses in excess of 2.0 g as a total daily
    dose. On rare occasions, eighth-nerve damage and nephrotoxicity
    can also occur, since paromomycin is an aminoglycoside.
Extraintestinal amebiasis
Chloroquine (Aralen) (see text)
Dose
  Adult: 600 mg of base (1 g of chloroquine phosphate) taken orally
    once daily, for 2 to 3 weeks.
  Child: 10 mg base (16.67 mg of chloroquine phosphate) per kilo-
    gram per day, not to exceed 300 mg base (500 mg of chloroquine
    phosphate) given orally once daily, for 2 to 3 weeks.
Side effects
  Nausea, vomiting, rashes, corneal opacity, alopecia, muscle weak-
    ness, and exfoliative dermatitus have been occasonally observed.
    Rare blood dyscrasias and deafness can also occur.
Metronidazole (Flagyl) (see text)
Dose
  Adult: 750 mg orally 3 times daily for 10 days, or 2.0 g taken
    orally once daily for 3 days. These two regimens are equally effec-
    tive.
  Child: 50 mg/kg/day given in 3 divided doses, not to exceed 2250
    mg per day, for 10 days.
Side effects
  Metronidazole may have effects similar to disulfiram when taken
    with alcohol. Other side effects include nausea, vomiting, diarrhea,
    anorexia, flatulence, blurred vision, headaches, confusion, disorien-
    tation, and depression. Leukopenia has also been observed in some
    patients. Metronidazole is relatively contraindicated during the first
    trimester of pregnancy because of recent reports of mutagenicity
    and carcinogenicity in bacteria and rodents, respectively.

burrow lesions measuring 1 to 10 mm in length. The distribution of excoriation marks can help with the diagnosis, but are not conclusive. Skin scrapings of suspicious areas may contain mites or eggs when examined under the microscope, and a positive finding is diagnostic of scabies.

TREATMENT (See Table 73.5)

Good personal hygiene is the foremost treatment for scabies infections, and reinfection is common when infested clothing or bedding is used. Treatment should include laundering of all clothing, especially bedclothes, treating all household contacts, and application of scabicides after a thorough bath. The scabicides used include (γ)-benzene hexachloride, crotamiton, benzyl benzoate, sulfur ointment, and 5% permethrin. Permethrin is considered by some experts as the drug of choice. Even after adequate treatment, the itching may persist for days, which should not be construed as a sign of reinfection,

superinfection, or treatment failure. Overtreatment is common and can lead to toxicity with (γ)-benzene hexachloride. A second course of treatment is necessary at 7 to 10 days after the initial course in only less than 5% of the cases. (γ)-Benzene hexachloride use should be discouraged in infants, young children, and pregnant women. Sulfur ointment can be the alternative agent for these patients. Sulfur ointment has an unpleasant odor, and it will stain clothing. Permethrin 5% is often used in the treatment of (γ)-benzene-hexachloride-resistant scabies, and it has been used successfully in place of crotamiton in children (231–239).

Pediculosis

Pediculus (241–244) (human lice) belongs to the family of Pediculidae, and three species that infest humans. These species are (a) *Pediculus humanus corporis/humanus*, body lice; (b) *Pediculus humanus capitis*, head lice; and (c) *Phthirus pubis*, crab or pubic lice.

Table 73.5.
Treatment of Human Lice and Scabies

SCABIES
% γ-Benzene hexachloride (see text)
Cream or lotion
Directions
  Warm bath at night
  Apply lotion or cream with soft brush from neck down
  Allow application to dry
  Repeat application of lotion or cream in the morning
  Second warm bath in the evening
  This 24-hr procedure may be repeated in 4–7 days
Cautions
  Avoid overtreatment
  Symptoms may persist for 1 month after adequate treatment
  Avoid use of GBH on face or urethral meatus
Crotamiton 10% (see text)
Cream or lotion
Directions
  Warm bath at night
  Apply lotion or cream from neck down thoroughly in a massage motion
  Reapply lotion or cream in 24 hr
  Second warm bath 48 hr after the second application
Cautions
  Avoid the head, grossly inflamed areas, or excoriated areas
Permethrin 5% (see text)
Cream
No reported adverse effects on animal reproductive systems or teratogenicity, effects on humans are not known
Directions
  Warm bath at night
  Apply cream from the head to the bottoms of feet, and leaving it on for 8 hr
  Thoroughly wash entire body
Cautions
  Itching and erythema may increase transiently after initial application of permethrin in some patients
  May produce burning or tingling sensation after application
Sulfur ointment (see text)
2.5%, 5%, 10% in petrolatum
This is the preferred treatment in infants, young children, and pregnant women
Directions
  Warm bath at night
  Apply ointment over entire body from neck down nightly for 3 consecutive nights
  Final bath 24 hr after final application
Cautions
  Avoid the head
  The ointment will stain clothing
  The ointment has an unpleasant sulfur odor
Benzyl benzoate 25% (see text)
Solution
Directions
  Warm bath at night
  Apply solution by hand or spray over body from neck down for 3 consecutive nights
  Final bath 24 hr after last application
Cautions
  Avoid the head
BODY LICE
1% γ-Benzene hexachloride (see text)
Shampoo
Directions
  Sterilize clothing, bedding by laundering and hot drying, dry cleaning, or ironing
  Use 1 ounce of shampoo for adult (less for children) and lather trunk and extremities for at least 4 min, then rinse thoroughly

Repeat procedure in 7 days
Cautions
  Same as in the treatment for scabies
1% Malathion or 0.2% pyrethrins or 0.3% allethrin with 1:10 piperonyl butoxide in an inert dusting powder
Directions
  (This procedure is used in cases of heavy infestation or where cleaning facility is not available)
  Dust body and clothing with duster or a sifter can
  Pay special attention to seams and insides of the clothing
Cautions
  Avoid excessive use of the dust
  Avoid inhalation of dust or contamination of foods
HEAD AND CRAB LICE (see text)
0.5% Malathion
Solution in 78% alcohol
Directions
  Clean and wash affected area
  Apply solution to hair until the underlying skin is moist
  Leave solution on for 8 hr
  Rinse off solution and comb out nits and dead lice with a fine-tooth comb
Cautions
  This solution contains 78% alcohol and is a flammable hazard; avoid open flames or dryers before rinsing off solution
  Malathion has an unpleasant sulfur odor
1% Permethrin
Cream
Directions
  Clean and wash affected area
  Massage liberal quantities of solution into hair for at least 1 min
  Rinse area thoroughly and comb out nits and dead lice with a fine-tooth comb 10 min after application (although not necessary)
  May repeat procedure in 5 days if condition persists
Caution
  May case local pruritis or irritation upon application of the cream.
  Local irritation and erythema occur in 1.2% of patients
1% γ-Benzene hexachloride
Shampoo
Directions
  Clean and wash affected areas well
  Apply 1 ounce of shampoo for adult (proportionally less for children) and work into hair for at least 4 min
  Thoroughly rinse out shampoo and remove nits with a fine-tooth comb
  Procedure may be repeated in 7–10 days
  Sterilize bedding and clothing used within the past 7 days
Cautions
  Same as in the treatment of scabies
Pyrethrins 0.16%, piperonyl butoxide 2.0%, and deodorized kerosene 5.0%
Liquid or gel
Directions
  Clean and wash affected area
  Massage liberal quantities of solution into hair for at least 1 min
  Rinse area thoroughly and comb out nits and dead lice with a fine-tooth comb within 10 min after application
  May repeat procedure in 24 hr
Cautions
  Avoid face and excessive contact with solution
Physostigmine 2.0% or ammoniated mercury 2.0% or ophthalmic petrolatum
Ointment
Used primarily for treatment of eye-lash infestations
Directions
  For infestation involving eye-lashes one of these ointments may be applied twice daily for 7–10 days
Cautions
  Avoid excessive use

Pediculus humanis corporis/humanus (Body Lice)

Like the other ectoparasites, body lice are cosmopolitan in distribution. This species has been implicated in the transmission of diseases such as relapsing fever, trench fever, and epidemic typhus (245, 246). Body lice are most commonly found in the seams of clothing where tight contact with the body occurs, especially in areas of the axilla, perineum, belt line, neck, and shoulders. The female louse has a life-span of 3 to 4 weeks and can lay up to 300 eggs during this time. The eggs hatch in 11 to 13 days, depending on conditions, and mature to adults in 10 to 20 days. The adult parasite feeds 2 to 3 times daily. The adult and the eggs can survive without the host for up to a month. Body lice are transmitted through direct contact with a louse-infested individual, bedding, or clothing.

CLINICAL MANIFESTATIONS OF BODY LICE

Most of the clinical symptoms are caused by the adult louse feeding on the host daily by digging through the skin with its claws and sucking the blood. The saliva and excreta produce the intense itching and irritation. Together, they produce the classic clinical presentation.

DIAGNOSIS OF BODY LICE

The diagnosis is based on the intense itching, excoriation, and infection from the scratching and finding the adult louse or the eggs in the seams of the clothing from the suspected infested individual.

TREATMENT OF BODY LICE (See Table 73.5)

Since communal infections are common, treatment must include all members of the household or group and sterilization of all possible vehicles of transmission such as clothing, bedding, and cosmetic objects. The most effective method of sterilization in endemic areas is the application of insecticide-containing dusting powders. The agents used to treat body lice include (γ)-benzene hexachloride, permethrin, malathion, carbaryl, and mobam. Malathion and (γ)-benzene hexachloride can be used as a 1% dusting powder in treating outbreaks of infestations, but now there are reports of strains of pediculi that are resistant to them. Treatment with (γ)-benzene hexachloride must be repeated in 7 to 10 days, because it is not ovicidal. (γ)-Benzene hexachloride should be used with caution on infants, children, and pregnant women. Bedding and clothing should be washed in hot water or dry-cleaned. Secondary bacterial infections often accompany body lice infestation as a result of poor hygiene and excoriation, and these secondary infections may require appropriate antibiotic therapy (247–248).

Pediculus Humanus Capitis (Head Lice)

Head lice are similar to body lice in geographic distribution. These organisms are typically found on the hair located around the back of the head and ears. The adult female has a life-span of 33 to 40 days, and can lay 50 to 100 eggs, which she attaches individually to a hair shaft with a cement substance. The eggs hatch in 1 to 3 weeks, reach maturity in 10 to 20 days. As with body lice, the adult head louse can survive without a host for up to 10 days. The infestation is communicated by shared hats, combs, brushes, and towels and by direct contact.

CLINICAL MANIFESTATIONS OF HEAD LICE

Pruritis is a cardinal clinical symptom, and excoriation frequently leads to impetigo and pyoderma.

DIAGNOSIS OF HEAD LICE

The itching and the sequelae of scratching usually cause the patient to seek medical help. The diagnosis of head lice is made when adult lice or nits are found.

TREATMENT OF HEAD LICE (See Table 73.5)

Treatment of head lice involves cleaning and washing affected areas of the scalp and applying the pediculocide such as (γ)-benzene hexachloride, malathion, permethrin, or pyrethrins. Permethrin 1% cream is 95 to 98% effective with just a single application (249–255). Systemic absorption of such a short-term permethrin application is not known, but it is detectable in hair for several days after a single 10–min application. The nits must be physically removed with a fine-tooth comb (256), because they are attached to the hair shaft by a cement-like substance. Resistance to (γ)-benzene hexachloride has been reported, but there are no reported cases of resistance to malathion or carbaryl. Both malathion and carbaryl will kill not only the adult lice, but the nymphs and eggs as well. A second application is a must when (γ)-benzene hexachloride is used, and it may be necessary with the other agents if the infestation is severe.

Secondary impetigo and pyoderma will require appropriate antibiotic therapy.

Phthirus pubis (Pubic Lice or Crabs)

The pubic louse is also distributed worldwide. These organisms infest primarily the pubic hairs, but not to the exclusion of other areas. Infestation of the eye-lashes and other hairy areas can also occur. The life-span of the female louse is about 20 to 30 days, and she can produce approximately 50 eggs during this period. The eggs hatch in approximately 1 week, and develop into mature adults in 15 to 17 days. The adult crab louse can live for a maximum of 42 hr without feeding, and the eggs can stay viable for up to a month under ideal conditions. The route of transmission is almost always sexual contact, but in rare circumstances, transmission can occur by sharing bedding, underwear, or other objects.

CLINICAL MANIFESTATIONS OF PUBIC LICE OR CRABS

Pruritis and the host's inflammatory response to the crab louse saliva and excreta at the site of feeding accounts for most of the clinical symptoms. Secondary infection can occur as a result of scratching and excoriation. The crab lice are usually confined to the pubic regions, but occasional infestation of other hairy areas such as the axilla, eye-lashes, beards, and chest also occurs, resulting in irritation and inflammation.

DIAGNOSIS OF PUBIC LICE OR CRABS

The diagnosis of crab louse infestation is based on the clinical symptoms, distribution of the feeding sites of the pubic lice, and the isolation of either the adult louse or the eggs that are cemented to the hair shaft.

TREATMENT OF PUBIC LICE OR CRABS
(See Table 73.5)

Treatment of crab louse infestation is very similar to the treatment of head lice. It requires cleaning and washing the affected areas and application of a delousing agent. Since crab lice is a sexually transmitted infestation, the treatment must also include sexual partners. The delousing agents used include (γ)-benzene hexachloride, pyrethrin, and physostigmine or ammoniated mercury for eye-lash involvement. No resistance to the treatment has been reported.

CONCLUSION

Parasitic diseases constitute the major cause of death in less developed areas of the world, where sanitation is inadequate or poor. The clinical presentation of these parasitic infections may vary, depending upon the host's immune system and the parasitic burden. When treating parasitic infections, one must also treat the cause of the parasitic infection by improving the sanitation of the endemic areas. Preventive measures such as purifying the drinking water and eating only cooked vegetables will reduce the risk of getting parasitic infections.

REFERENCES

1. Bennett JE. *Aspergillus species*. In Mandell, Douglas and Bennetts' Principles and Practice of Infectious Diseases, ed. 4. New York: Churchill Livingstone Inc., 1995, pp 2306–2311.
2. Cunha BA. Invasive Aspergillosis. Internal Medicine, Special Report. New Jersey: Medical Economics, 1995, p. 2.
3. Wingard JR, et al. Aspergillus infections in immuno-compromised cancer patients. Internal Medicine, Special Report. New Jersey: Medical Economics, 1995, pp 4–10.
4. Levitz SM, et al. Aspergillosis. Inf Dis Clin of North America 3:1–18, 1989.
5. Patterson TF. Invasive aspergillosis in organ transplantation. Internal Medicine, Special Report. New Jersey: Medical Economics, 1995, pp 11–14.
6. Denning DW, Follansbee SE, Scolaro M et al. Pulmonary aspergillosis in the acquired immunodeficiency syndrome. N Engl J Med 324:(10)654–661, 1991.
7. Minamoto GY, Barlam TF, Vander Els NJ. Invasive Aspergillosis in patients with AIDS. Clin Inf Dis 14:16–74, 1992.
8. Koll BS, Pawleck BJ. Fungal Infection in the AIDS patient. Internal Medicine, Special Report. New Jersey: Medical Economics, 1995, pp 15–24.
9. Kusne S, Torre-Cisnero J, Manez R, et al. Factors associated with invasive lung aspergillosis and the significance of positive *aspergillosis* cultures after liver transplantation. J Infect Dis 166:1379–83, 1992.
10. Yu VL, Muder RR, Poorsattar A. Significance of isolation of *Aspergillus* in the respiratory tract in the diagnosis of invasive pulmonary aspergillosis. N Engl J Med 81:249–54, 1986.
11. Denning DW, Lee JY, Hostetler JS et al. NIAID Mycoses Study Group Multicenter Trial of Oral Itraconazole Therapy for Invasive Aspergillosis. AM J Med 97;135–144, 1994.
12. Lutz JE, Stevens DS. Treatment of invasive aspergillosis. Internal Medicine, Special Report. New Jersey: Medical Economics, 1995, pp 25–31.
13. AHFS Drug Information. American Society of Health Systems Pharmacist, Inc. 1995, p 85.
14. Como JA, Dismukes WE, et al. Oral azole drugs as systemic antifungal therapy. N Engl J Med 330:2663–2722, 1994.
15. Denning DW, Tucker Rm, Hanson LH, Stevens DA. Treatment of invasive aspergillosis with itraconazole. Am J Med 86:791–800, 1989.
16. Dupont B. Itraconazole therapy in aspergillosis, study in 49 patients. J Am Acad Dermatol 23:607–614, 1990.
17. Pizzo PA, Robichaud KH, Gill FA et al. Emperic antibiotic and antifungal therapy for cancer patients with prolonged fever and granulocytopenia. AM J Med 72:101, 1982.
18. EORTC International Antimicrobial Therapy Cooperative Group: Empiric antifungal therapy in febrile granulocytopenic patients. AM J Med 86:668, 1989.
19. Suger AM. Empiric treatment in fungal infections in the neutropenic host: Review of the literature and guidelines for use. Arch Intern Med 150:2258, 1990.
20. Walsh TJ, Lecciones J, et al. Empiric therapy with amphotericin B in febrile granulocytopenic patients. Rev Inf Dis 13:496, 1991.
21. Karp JE, Merz WG, Charache P. Response to empiric amphotericin B during antileukemic therapy-induced granulocytopenia. Rev Inf Dis 13:592, 1991.
22. O'Donnell MR, Schmidt GM, Tegtmeier BR, et al. Prediction of systemic fungal infection in allogenic marrow recipients: Impact of amphotericin B prophylaxis in high risk patients. J Clin Oncol 12:827, 1994.
23. Rousey SR, Russler S, Gottlieb M, et al. Low-dose amphotericin B prophylaxis against invasive *aspergillus* infection in allogenic marrow transplantation. Am J Med 91:484, 1991.
24. Riley OK, Pavia AT, Beatty PG, et al. The prophylactic use of low-dose amphotericin B in bone marrow transplant patients. Am J Med 97:509, 1994.
25. Perfect JT, Klotman ME, Gilbert CC, et al. Prophylactic intravenous amphotericin B in neutropenia autologous bone marrow transplant recipients. J Infect Dis 165:891, 1992.
26. Tricot G, Joosten E, Boogaerts MA, et al. Ketoconazole vs. itraconazole for antifungal prophylaxis in patients with severe granulocytopenia; Preliminary results of two nonrandomized studies. Rev Inf Dis 9 (supp 1):594, 1987.
27. Beyer J, Barzen G, Risse G, et al. Aerosol amphotericin B for prevention of invasive pulmonary aspergillosis. Antimicrob Agents Chemother 37:1367–1369, 1993.

28. Jeffery GM, Beard ME, Ikram RB, et al. Intranasal amphotericin B reduces the frequency of invasive aspergillosis in neutropenic patients. AM J Med 90:685–92, 1991.

29. Todeschini G, Muraru C, Bonesi R, et al. Oral intraconazole plus nasal amphotericin B for prophylaxis of invasive aspergillosis in patients with hematological malignancies. Eur J Microbiol Infect Dis 12:614–18, 1993.

30. Diamond, RD. *Cryptococcus Neoformans*, In Mandell, Douglas and Bennetts' Principles and Practice of Infectious Diseases, ed. 4. New York: Churchill Livingstone Inc., 1995, pp 2331–2340.

31. Krajdens, Summerbell RC, Kane J, et al. Normally saprobic *cryptococcus* isolated from *Cryptococcus neoformans* infections. J Clin Micro 29:1883–1887, 1991.

32. White MH, Armstrong D, et al. Cryptococcosis. Inf Dis North Am 8:383–397, 1994.

33. Wilson DE, Bennett JE, Bailey JW. Serologic grouping of Cryptococcus neoformans. Proc Soc Exp Biol Med 127:820–823, 1968.

34. Levitz, SM. The ecology of *Cryptococcus neoformans* and the epidemiology of cryptococcosis. J Infect Dis 13:1163–9, 1991.

35. Ellis DH, Pfeifta TJ. Natural habitat of *Cryptococcus neoformans var. gattii*. J clin Microbiol 28:1642–4, 1990.

36. Gottesdiener KM. Transplanted infections: Donor to host transmission with the allograft. Ann Intern Med 110:1001–6, 1989.

37. Chuck SL, Sande MA. Infections with *Cryptococcus neoformans* in the acquired immunodeficiency syndrome. N Engl J Med 321:794–9, 1989.

38. Dismukes WE. Cryptococcal meningitis in patients with AIDS. J Infect Dis 157:624, 1988.

39. Clark RA, Greer D, Atkinson W, et al. Spectrum of *Cryptococcus neoformans* infection in 68 patients infected with human immunodeficiency virus. Rev Infect Dis 12:768, 1990.

40. Cameron ML, Bartlett JA, Gallis HA, et al. Manifestation of pulmonary *cryptococcus* in patients with acquired immunodeficiency syndrome. Rev Infect Dis 13:64, 1991.

41. Checkani V, Kamholz SL. Pulmonary manifestation of disseminated cryptococcosis in patients with AIDS. Chest 98:1060, 1990.

42. Clark, RA, Greer D, Valainis GT, et al. *Cryptococcus neoformans* infection in HIV-1–infected patients. J Acquir Immun Defic Syndr 3:480, 1990.

43. Powderly WG, Saag MS, Cloud GA, et al. A controlled trial of fluconazole or amphotericin B to prevent relapse of *cryptococcal* meningitis in patients with the acquired immunodeficiency syndrome. N Engl J Med 326:793–8, 1992.

44. Bennett JE, Dismukes WE, Duma RJ, et al. A comparison of amphotericin B alone and combined with flucytosine in the treatment of *cryptococcal* meningitis. N Engl J Med 301:126–31, 1979.

45. Francis P, Walsh TJ. Evolving role of flucytosine in immunocompromised patients: New insights into safety, pharmacokinetics, and antifungal therapy. Clin Infect Dis 15:1003–8, 1992.

46. Armstrong D. Treatment of opportunistic fungal infections. Clin Infect Dis 16:1–9, 1993.

47. Dismukes EW, Cloud G, Gallis HA, et al. Treatment of *cryptococcal* meningitis with combination amphotericin B and flucytosine for four as compared with six weeks. N Engl J Med 317:334–41, 1987.

48. Diamond RD, Bennett JE. A subcutaneous reservoir for intrathecal therapy of fungal meningitis. N Engl J Med 288:186–8, 1973.

49. Polsky B, Depman MR, Gold JWM, et al. Intraventricular therapy of *cryptococcal* meningitis via a subcutaneous reservoir 94:24–8, 1986.

50. Kerkering TM, Duma RJ, Shadomy S. The evolution of pulmonary cryptococcosis: Clinical implications from a study of 41 patients with and without compromising host factors. Ann Int Med 94:611–16, 1981.

51. Byrne WF, Wajszczuk CP. *Cryptococcal* meningitis in AIDS: Successful treatment with fluconazole after failure of amphotericin B. Ann Int Med 108:384, 1988.

52. Jones PD, Marriott D, Speed BR. Efficacy of fluconazole in *cryptococcal* meningitis. Diagn Microbiol Infect Dis 12:235s, 1989.

53. Larsen RA, Leal MAE, Chan LS. Fluconazole compared with amphotericin B plus flucytosine for *cryptococcal* meningitis in AIDS, A randomized trial. Ann Int Med 113:183, 1990.

54. Saag MS, Powderly WG, Cloud GA et al. Comparison of amphotericin B with fluconazole in the treatment of acute AIDS-associated *cryptococcal* meningitis. N Engl J Med 326:83–89, 1992.

55. Berry AJ et al. Use of high-dose fluconazole as salvage therapy for *cryptococcal* meningitis in patients with AIDS. Antimicrob Agents Chemo 36(3):690–692, 1992.

56. Haubrich R et al. High-dose fluconazole for treatment of *cryptococcal* disease in patients with human immunodeficiency virus infection. J Infect Dis 170:238–242, 1994.

57. Howe M. Opportunistic Infections (Part XII) Cryptococcosis. AIDS Information Newsletter, VA Med Center, San Francisco: In Opportunistic Infections and Related Disorders: From AM FAR's AIDS/HIV Treatment Directory. Vol. & No. 4: Jan 1995.

58. Denning DW, Tucker RM, Hanson LH, et al. Itraconazole therapy for *cryptococcal* meningitis and cryptococcosis. Arch Intern Med 149:2301, 1989.

59. Powderly WG, Keath EJ, Little JR, et al. Resistant *Cryptococcus Neoformans* in a patient with AIDS [abstract 1164]. Thirtieth Interscience Conference on Antimicrobial Agents and Chemotherapy, Ammerican Society for Microbiology, Atlanta, Georgia, Oct 21–24, 1990.

60. Bozzett SA, Larsen RA, Chiu J, et al. A placebo-controlled trial of maintenance therapy with fluconazole after treatment of *cryptococcal* meningitis in the acquired immunodeficiency syndrome. N Engl J Med 324:580, 1991.

61. CDC.USDHS/IDSA Guidelines for the Prevention of Opportunistic Infections in persons Infected with Human Immunodeficiency Virus: A Summary MMWF 44 (No RR-8):1–34, 1995.

62. Edwards JE et al. *Candida Species*, In Mandell, Douglas and Bennetts' Principles and Practice of Infectious Diseases, ed. 4. New York: Churchill Livingstone Inc., 1995, pp 2289–2306.

63. Wenzel RP, Pfaller MA. *Candida Species*: Emerging hospital bloodstream pathogens. Infect Control Hosp Epidemiol 12:523–4, 1991.

64. Crislip MA, Edwards JE. Candidiasis. Infect Dis North Am 3:103–133, 1989.

65. Filler SG, Edwards JE. When and How to Treat Serious Candidal Infections: Concepts and Controversies. In Current Clinical Topics in Infectious Diseases, Chapter 15, 1–18, 1995.

66. Douglass JA, Bowes G. Inhaled corticosteriods in asthma. Med J 152:475–6, 479, 1990.

67. Reynolds R, Braude AI. The filament-inducing property of blood for *Candida albicans*: Its nature and significance. Clin Res Prac 7:417–20, 1956.

68. Wheeler RR, Peacock JE Jr, Cruz JM, et al. Esophagitis in the immunocompromised host: Role of esophagoscopy in diagnosis. Rev Infect Dis 9:88–96, 1987.

69. Buff SJ, McLeiland R, Gallis HA, et al. *Candida albicans* pneumonia, Radiographic appearance. AJR 128:645–8, 1982.

70. Seelig MS, Speth CP, Kozinn PJ, et al. Patterns of *Candida* endocarditis following cardiac surgery. Importance of early diagnosis and therapy (an analysis of 91 cases) Prog Cardiovasc Dis 27:125–60, 1974.

71. Rosenblatt HM, Steihmer. Therapy for chronic mucocutaneous candidiasis. Am J Med, 1983.

72. Kirkpatrick CH. Chronic mucocutaneious candidiasis. In Bodey's Candidiasis: Pathogenesis. Diagnosis and Treatment, 2nd ed. New York; Raven Press: 167–84, 1993.

73. Filler SG, Edwards JE Jr. Chronic mucocutaneous candidiasis. In Murphy, Friedman, Bendinellis' Fungal Infections and Immune Response, New York: Plenum Press 117–33, 1993.

74. Rex JH. A randomized trial comparing fluconazole with amphotericin B for the treatment of candidemia in patients without neutropenia. N Engl J Med 331:1325–1330, 1994.

75. Heykants, J et al. The clinical pharmacokinetics of itraconazole: an overview. Mycoses 32(suppl 1);67–87, 1989.

76. Kulak K, Maki DG. Treatment of Hickman catheter-related candidemia without removing the catheter. In Programs and Abstracts of the 32nd Interscience Conference on Antimicrobial Agents and Chemotherapy, Atlanta. Washington, DC: American Society for Microbiology 249. Abstract 831, 1992.

77. Pizzo PA, Walsh TJ. Fungal infection in the pediatric cancer patient. Semin Oncol 17:6–9, 1990.

78. Blade J, Lopez-Guillermo A, Rozman C, et al. Chronic systemic candidiasis in acute leukemia. Ann Hematol 64:240–244, 1992.

79. Anaissie E, Boey GP, Kantayian H, et al. Fluconazole therapy for chronic disseminated candidiasis in patients with leukemia and prior amphotericin B therapy. Am J Med 91:142–150, 1991.

80. Kauffman CA, Bradley SF, Ross SC. Hepatosplenic candidiasis; successful treatment with fluconazole. Am J Med 91:137–141, 1991.

81. Jacobs LG, Skidmore EA, Cardoso LA, Ziv F. et al. Bladder irrigation with amphotericin B for treatment of fungal urinary tract infections. Clin Infec Dis 18:313–318, 1994.

82. Sanford JP. The enigma of candiduria: evolution of bladder irrigation with amphotericin B for management—from anecdote to dogma and a lesson from Machiavelli. Clin Infect Dis 16:145–147, 1993.

83. Smego RA, Perfect JR, Durack DT. Combined therapy with amphotericin B and 5–Flurocytosine for Candida meningitis. Rev Infect Dis 6:791–801, 1984.

84. Pon V, Greenspan D, DeBruin M. The Multicenter Study Group: Therapy for oropharyngeal candidiasis in HIV-infected patients: a randomized, prospective multicenter study of oral fluconazole vs. clotrimazole troches. JAIDS 6:1311–6, 1993.

85. DeWit S, et al. Comparison of fluconazole and ketoconazole for oropharyngeal candidiasis in AIDS. Lancet 8641:746–8., 1989.

86. DeWit S, et al. Single-dose vs. 7 days of fluconazole treatment for oral candidiasis in HIV-infected patients: a prospective, randomized pilot study. JID 168:1332–3, 1993.

87. Laine L, et al. Fluconazole compared to ketoconazole for the treatment of candida esophagitis in AIDS. Ann Int Med 117:655–660, 1992.

88. Smith DE. Itraconazole vs. ketoconazole in the treatment of oral and oesophageal candidiasis in patients infected with HIV. AIDS 5:1367–1371, 1991.

89. Soubry R. Comparison of itraconazole oral solution and fluconazole capsules in the treatment of oral esophageal candidiasis in HIV-infected patients. Preliminary results VII Intl Conf AIDS, Florence. Vol 1:108(WA 1064), 1991.

90. deRep L, et al. Itraconazole vs. ketoconazole in HIV-positive patients with oropharyngeal and/or esophageal candidiasis. 32nd ICAAC, abstract 1117, 1992.

91. Bradsher RW: Blastomycosis. Clin Infect Dis 14(suppl 1):S82–90, 1992.

92. Chapmman SW. Blastomycosis, In Mandell, Douglas and Bennetts' Principles and Practice of Infectious Diseases, ed. 4. New York: Churchill Livingstone Inc., 1995, pp 2353–2365.

93. Pappas PG, Threlkeld MG, Bedsole GD, Cleveland KO, et al. Blastomycosis in immunocompromised patients. Medicine 72:311–325, 1993.

94. Sarosi GA, Davis SF. Blastomycosis. Am Rev Respir Dis 120:911–938, 1979.

95. Klein BS, Vergeront JM, Weeks RJ, et al. Isolation of Blastomyces dermatitidis in soil associated with a large outbreak of blastomycosis in Wisconsin. N Engl J Med 314:529–534, 1986.

96. Klein BS, Vergerpont JM, DiSalvo AF, et al. Two outbreaks of blastomycosis along rivers in Wisconsin: isolation of Blastomyces dermatitidis from riverbank soil and evidence of its transmission along waterways. Am Rev Respir Dis 136:1333–1338, 1987.

97. Pappas PG, Pottage JC, Powderly WG, et al. Blastomycosis in patients with the acquired immunodeficiency syndrome. Ann Intern Med 116:847–853, 1992.

98. Saag MS, Dismukes WE. Treatment of histoplasmosis and blastomycosis. Chest 93:848–851, 1988.

99. National Institute of Allergy and Infectious Diseases, Mycoses Study Group. Treatment of blastomycosis and histoplasmosis with ketoconazole. Ann Intern Med 103:861–872, 1985.

100. Dismukes WE, Bradsher RW, Cloud GC, et al. Itraconazle therapy for blastomycosis and histoplasmosis. AMJ Med 93:489–497, 1992.

101. Stevens DA. Coccidioidomycosis. N Engl J Med 332:1077–1082, 1995.

102. Stevens DA. Coccidioides immitis. In Mandell, Douglas and Bennetts' Principles and Practice of Infectious Diseases, ed. 4. New York: Churchill Livingstone Inc., 1995, pp 2365–2375.

103. CDC Revision of the CDC Surveillance Case Definition for Acquired Immunodeficiency Syndrome. MMWR 36:15–145, 1987.

104. Ampel NM, Dols CL, Galgiani JN. Coccidioidomycosis during human immuno-deficiency virus infection: Results of a prospective study in a coccidioidal endemic area. Am J Med 94:235–240, 1993.

105. Knoper SR, Galgiani JN. Coccicioidomycosis. Infec Dis Clinics of North America 2(4):861–875, 1988.

106. Rothman PE, Harris JC. Coccidioidomycosis, possible fomite transmission: A review and report of a case. Am J Dis Chold 118–792, 1969.

107. Galgiani JN, Steven DA, Graybill JT, et al. Ketoconazole therapy of progressive Coccidioido-mycosis: Comparison of 400 and 800–mg doses and observations at higher doses. AM J Med 84:603–610, 1988.

108. Graybill Jr, Stevens DA, Galgiani JN, et al. Itraconazole treatment of Coccidioidomycosis. Am J Med 89:282–290, 1990.

109. Cantanzaro A, Fiever T, Friedman P. Fluconazole in the treatment of persistent coccidioidomycosis. Chest 97:666–669, 1990.

110. Diaz M, Negroni R, Montero-gei F, et al. A Pan-American's-Year Study of fluconazole therapy for deep mycoses in the immunocompetent host. Infect Dis 14(suppl 1):S68–S76, 1992.

111. Tucker RM, Denning DW, Dupont B, Stevens DA. Itraconazole therapy for chronic coccidioidal meningitis. Ann Intern Med 112:108–112, 1990.

112. Galgiani JN, Catanzavo A, Cloud GA, et al. Fluconazole therapy for coccidioidal meningitis. Ann Intern Med 119:28–35, 1993.

113. Dewsnup DH, Galgiani JN, Graybill JR, et al. Is it safe to stop azole therapy of Coccidioides immitis meningitis? (abstract No. 9) In Galgini, JN, ed. Proceedings of the 36th Annual Meeting of the Coccidioidomycosis Study Group, 1992.

114. Wheat LJ. Histoplasmosis. Infect Dis Clin North Am 2(4):841–857, 1988.

115. McKinsey DS, Driks MR, et al. Histoplasmosis in HIV disease. The AIDS Reader 203–209, 1993.

116. Wheat LJ, Connolly-Stringfield P, Blair R, et al. Histoplasmosmosis relapse in patients with AIDS: Detection using Histoplasma capsulatum variety capsulatum antigen levels. Ann Inter Med 115:936–941, 1991.

117. Zarabi CM, Thomas R, Adesokan A. Diagnoses of systemic histoplasmosis in patients with AIDS. Southern Medical Journal 85:1171–1175, 1992.

118. Wheat LJ. Histoplasmosis: Epidemiology, Clinical Manifestations, Diagnosis, and Therapy. Medical Grand Rounds 2(4):364–374, 1983.

119. Davies SF, Khan M, Savosi GA. Disseminated histoplasmosis in immunologically suppressed patients. Am J Med 64:94–100, 1978.

120. Kauffman CA, Isreal KS, Smith JW, et al. Histoplasmosis in immunosuppressed patients. AM J Med 64:923–932, 1978.

121. Mandell W, Goldberg DM, Nev HC. Histoplasmosis in patients with the acquired immune deficiency syndrome. Am J Med 81:974–978, 1986.

122. Wheat LJ, Connolly-Stringfield PA, Baker RL, et al. Disseminated histoplasmosis in the acquired immune deficiency syndrome: Clinical findings, diagnosis and treatment, and review of the literature. Medicine 69:361–374, 1990.

123. Wheat LJ. Diagnosis of Histoplasmosis. Indiana University-Purdue University, Indianapolis and Histoplasmosis Reference Laboratory, 1994.

124. National Institute of Allergy and Infectious Disease Mycoses Study Group. Treatment for blastomycosis and histoplasmosis with keto-conazole. Ann Intern Med 103:861–872, 1985.

125. Dismukes WE, Bradsher RW, Cloud GC, et al. Itraconazole therapy for blastomycosis and histoplasmosis. Am J Med 93:489–497, 1992.

126. McKinsey DS, Gupta MR, Riddler SA, et al. Long term amphotericin B therapy for disseminated histoplasmosis in patients with the acquired immunodeficiency syndrome. Ann Intern Med 111(8): 655–659, 1989.

127. Wheat LJ, Hafner R, Korzun AH, Limjoco MT, et al. Itraconazole treatment of disseminated histoplasmosis in patients with the acquired immunodeficiency syndrome. Am J Med 98:336–342, 1995.

128. Wheat LJ, Hafner R, Wultsohn M, et al. Prevention of relapse of histoplasmosis with itraconazole in patients with the acquired immunodeficiency syndrome. Ann Intern Med 118:610–616, 1993.

129. Norris S, Wheat J, McKinsey DS, et al. Prevention of relapse of histoplasmosis with fluconazole in patients with acquired immunodeficiency syndrome 96:504–508, 1994.

130. Benenson AS. Control of Communicable Diseases in Man, Ed. 12. An official Report of the American Public Health Association, 1975.

131. Chan CT. Enterobiasis among schoolchildren in Macao. Southeast Asian J Trop Med Public Health 16(4):549–553, 1985.

132. Libbus MK. Enterobiasis. Nurse Pract 8(8):17–18, 1983.

133. Saxena KK, et al. Family infection in enterobiasis. Indian Journal of Pediatrics, 1988 55(4):627–630, 1988.

134. Cram EB. Studies on oxyuriasis XXVII. Summary and conclusion. Am J Dis Child 65:46–59, 1943.

135. Johnston TS. Diagnosis and treatment of five parasites. Drug Intell Clin Pharm 15:103–110, 1981.

136. Royer A, et al. Pinworm infestation in children; the problem and its treatment. Can Med Assoc J 86:60–65, 1962.

137. Blumenthal DS. Current Concept. Intestinal Nematodes in the United States. N Engl J Med 297:1437–1439, 1978.

138. Markell EK. Intestinal nematode infections. Pediatr Clin North Am 32(4):971–986, 1985.

139. Simon RD. Pinworm infestation and urinary tract infection in young girls. Am J Dis Child 128:21–22, 1974.

140. Sachdev YV, et al. Enterobius vermicularis infestation and secondary enuresis. J Urol 113:143–144, 1975.

141. Beckman EN, Holland JB. Ovarian enterobiasis—a proposed pathogenesis. Am J Trop Med Hyg 30(1):74–76, 1981.

142. Snow P, Cartwrit G. Enterobius in an unusual location [letter] JAMA 240:2046, 1978.

143. Bak M, Bodo M. Vaginal enterobiasis [letter]. Acta Cytol (Baltimore) 26(2):264–265, 1982.

144. McDonald GSA, et al. Ectopic Enterobius vermicularis. Gut 13:621–626, 1972.

145. Brook STJ Jr, et al. Pelvic granuloma due to Enterobius vermicularis. JAMA 179:492–494, 1962.

146. Knuth KR, et al. Pinworm infestation of the genital tract. Am Fam Physician, 38(5):127–130, 1988.

147. Bambalo TS, et al. Treatment of enterobiasis with pyrantel pamoate. Am J Trop Med Hyg 18:50–52, 1969.

148. Miller MJ, et al. Mebendazole, an effective anthelmitic for trichuriasis and enterobiasis. JAMA, 230:1412–1414, 1974.

149. Beck JN. Treatment of pinworm infections with reduced single dose of pyrvinium pamoate. JAMA 189:511, 1964.

150. Brown HW, et al. Treatment of enterobiasis and ascariasis with piperazine. JAMA 161:515, 1956.

151. Jagota SC. Albendazole, a broad-spectrum anthelminthic, in the treatment of nematode and cestode infection: a multicenter study in 480 patients. Clin Ther 8(2):226–231, 1986.

152. Anthelmintic Study Group on Enterobiasis: A comparative evaluation of mebendazole, piperazine and pyrantel in threadworm infection. Indian Pediatr 21(8):623–628, 1984.

153. Most H. Office management of common intestinal parasites. Drug Ther 3:39–45, 1973.

154. Arfaa F. Selective primary health care: strategies for control of disease in the developing world. XII. Ascariasis and trichuriasis. Rev Infect Dis 6(3):364–373, 1984.

155. Marsden PD. The treatment and control of parasitic diseases. Rev Infect Dis 4(4):885–890, 1982.

156. Nwanyanwu OC, Moore JS, Adams ED. Parasitic infections in Asian refugess in Fort Worth. Tex Med 85(12):42–45, 1989.

157. Bonar S, Burrell M, West B, et al. Recurrent cholangitis secondary to oriental cholangiohepatitis. J Clin Gastroenterol 11(4):464–468, 1989.

158. Tankhiwale SR, et al. Single dose therapy of ascariasis—a randomized comparison of mebendazole and pyrantel. J Commun Dis 21(1):71–74, 1989.

159. Warren KS. Helminthic disease endemic in the United States. Am J Trop Med Hyg 23:723–730, 1974.

160. Schultz MG. The surveillance of parasitic diseases in the United States. Am J Trop Med Hyg 23:744–751, 1974.

161. Raisanen S, et al. Epidemic ascariasis—evidence of transmission by imported vegetables. Scand J Prim Health Care 3(3):189–191, 1985.

162. Tripathy K, et al. Effects of Ascaris infection on human nutrition. Am J Trop Med Hyg 20:212–218, 1971.

163. Gupta MC. Intestinal parasitoses and malnutrition. Trop Gastroenterol. 6(4):175–187, 1985.

164. Blumenthal DS, et al. Effects of Ascaris infection on nutritional status in children. Am J Trop Med Hyg 25:682–690, 1976.

165. Hamadto HA, et al. Relation between intestinal parasitosis and appendicitis. J Egypt Soc Parasitol 16(1):111–116, 1986.

166. Radin DR, Vachon LA. CT findings in biliary and pancreatic ascariasis. J Comput Assist Tomogr, 10(3):508–509, 1986.

167. Baird JK, et al. Fatal human ascariasis following secondary massive infection. Am J Trop Med Hyg 35(2):314–318, 1986.

168. Bambirra EA, et al. Tumoral form of ascariasis: report of a case. J Trop Med Hyg 88(4):273–276, 1985.

169. Jenkins MO, et al. Intestinal obstruction due to ascariasis: report of thirty-one cases. Pediatrics 13:419–425, 1954.

170. Katz Y, et al. Intestinal obstruction due to Ascaris lumbricoides mimicking intussusception. Dis Colon Rectum 28(4):267–269, 1985.

171. Arene FO, Akabogu OA: Intestinal parasitic infections in pre-school children in the Niger Delta. J Hyg Epidemiol Microbiol Immunol 30(1):99–102, 1986.

172. Croll NA, Ghadirian E. Wormy persons: contributions to the nature and patterns of overdispersion with Ascaris lumbricoides, Ancylostoma duodenale, Necator americanus and Trichuris trichiura. Trop Geogr Med 33(3):241–248, 1981.

173. Annan A, et al. An investigation of the prevalence of intestinal parasites in pre-school children in Ghana. Parasitology, 92(Pt 1): 209–217, 1986.

174. Jung RC, et al. Clinical observations on Trichocephalus trichiuras (whipworm) infestation in Children. Pediatrics 8:548–557, 1952.

175. Layrisse M, et al. Blood loss due to infections with *Trichuris trichiura*. Am J Trop Med Hyg 16:613–619, 1967.

176. Lotero H, et al. Gastrointestinal blood loss in *Trichuris* infection. Am J Trop Med Hyg 23:1203–1204, 1974.

177. Cooper ES, Bundy DA, MacDonald TT, et al. Growth suppression in the Trichuris Dysentery Syndrome. Eur J Clin Nutr 44(4):285–291, 1990.

178. Melvin DM, et al. Laboratory Procedures for the Diagnosis of Intestinal Parasites. (DHEW Publication no. [CDC] 75–8282), Atlanta: Centers for Disease Control, 1974.

179. Bundy DA, et al. Population dynamics and chemotherapeutic control of *Trichuris trichiura* infection of children in Jamaica and St. Lucia. Trans R Soc Trop Med Hyg, 79(6):759–764, 1985.

180. Bundy DA, et al. Rate of expulsion of *Trichuris trichiura* with multiple and single dose regimens of albendazole. Trans R Soc Trop Med Hyg 79(5):641–644, 1985.

181. Brooks JL, Kozarek RM. Amebic colitis. Preventing morbidity and mortality from fulminant disease. Postgrad Med 78(1):267–274, 1985.

182. Martinez-Palomo A, Martinez-Baez M. Selective primary health care: strategies for control of disease in the developing world. X. Amebiasis. Rev Infect Dis 5(6):1093–1102, 1983.

183. Judson FN. Sexually transmitted viral hepatitis and enteric pathogens. Urol Clin North Am 11(1):177–185, 1984.

184. Kean BH. Venereal amebiasis. NY State J Med 76:930–931, 1976.

185. Mildvan D, et al. Venereal transmission of enteric pathogens in male homosexuals. JAMA, 238:1387, 1977.

186. Schmerin MJ, et al. Amebiasis. An increasing problem among homosexuals in New York City. JAMA 238:1387, 1977.

187. Irani D, McGavran MH. Amebiasis: still present and lethal in Texas. Tex Med 82(5):34–36, 1986.

188. Steffen R. Epidemiologic studies of travelers' diarrhea, severe gastrointestinal infections, and cholera. Rev Infect Dis 8(suppl 2):S122–130, 1986.

189. Krogstad DJ, et al. Amebiasis: epidemiologic studies in the United States, 1971–1974. Ann Int Med 88:89–97, 1978.

190. Ma P, Visvesvara GS, Martinez AJ, et al. *Naegleria* and *Acanthamoeba* infections: review. Reviews of Infectious Diseases 12(3):490–513, 1990.

191. Jones RW. Amoebic liver abscess presenting thirty-two years after acute amoebic dysentary. Proc Soc Med 68:593–595, 1975.

192. Seidel J. Primary amebic meningoencephalitis. Pediatr Clin North Am 32(4):881–892, 1985.

193. Greenstein AJ, et al. Amebic liver abscess: a study of 11 cases compared with a series of 38 patients with pyogenic liver abscess. Am J Gastroenterol 80(6):472–478, 1985.

194. Del-Campo C, Del-Campo M. Thoracic complications of amebiasis. Can J Surg 25(2):119–121, 1982.

195. Bia FJ, Barry M. Parasitic infections of the central nervous system. Neurol Clin 4(1):171–206, 1986.

196. Mirelman D, et al. *Entamoeba histolytica*: effect of growth conditions and bacterial associates on isoenzyme patterns and virulence. Exp Parasitol 62(1):142–148, 1986.

197. Salata RA, Ravdin JI. Review of the human immune mechanisms directed against *Entamoeba histolytica*. Rev Infect Dis 8(2):261–271, 1986.

198. Guerrant RL. Amebiasis: introduction, current status, and research questions. Rev Infect Dis 8(2):218–227, 1986.

199. Juniper K Jr, et al. Serologic diagnosis of amebiasis. Am J Trop Med Hyg 21:157–168, 1972.

200. Khan AH, Das SR. Rapid micro-IHA test with FACL-SRBCs in serodiagnosis of amoebiasis. Indian J Med Res 83:377–379, 1986.

201. Healy GR. Immunologic tools in the diagnosis of amebiasis: epidemiology in the United States. Rev Infect Dis 8(2):239–246, 1986.

202. Walsh JA. Problems in recognition and diagnosis of amebiasis. estimation of the global magnitude of morbidity and mortality. Rev Infect Dis 9–2):228–238, 1986.

203. Salata RA, et al. Patients treated for amebic liver abscess develop cell-mediated immune responses effective in vitro against *Entamoeba histolytica*. J Immunol 136(7):2633–2639, 1986.

204. Ravdin JI. Pathogenesis of disease caused by *Entamoeba histolytica*: studies of adherence, secreted toxins, and contact-dependent cytolysis. Rev Infect Dis 8(2):247–260, 1986.

205. Kim CW. The diagnosis of parasitic diseases. Prog Clin Pathol 6:267–288, 1975.

206. Korelitz BI. When should we look for amebae in patients with inflammatory bowel disease? J Clin Gastroenterol 11(4):373–375, 1989.

207. Campbell WC. The chemotherapy of parasitic infections. J Parasitol 72(1):45–61, 1986.

208. Ferrante A. Amphotericin B doses for primary amoebic meningoencephalitis [letter]. Lancet 2(8497):35–36, 1986.

209. Abuabara SF, et al. Amebic liver abscess. Arch Surg 117(2):239–244, 1982.

210. Culbertson CG. Amebic meningoencephalitis. Antibiot Chemother, 30:28–53, 1981.

211. Ellis CJ. Antiparasitic agents in pregnancy. Clin Obstet Gynaecol 13(2):269–275, 1986.

212. Powell SJ. Therapy of Amebiasis. Bull NY Acad Med Ser 2, 47:469–477, 1971.

213. Oakley GP. The neurotoxicity of the halogenated hydroxyquinolines, JAMA 225:395–397, 1973.

214. Behrens MM. Optic atrophy in children after diiodohydroxyquin therapy, JAMA 228:693, 1974.

215. Coher HG, et al. Comparison of metronidazole and chloroquin for the treatment of amebic liver abscess. Gastroenterology 69:35–41, 1975.

216. Anon. Is Flagyl dangerous? Med Lett Drug Ther 17:53–54, 1975.

217. Tsar SH. Experience in the therapy of amebic liver abscesses on Taiwan. Am J Trop Med Hyg 22:24–29, 1973.

218. Thoren K, Hakansson C, Beagstrom T, et al. Treatment of asymptomatic amebiasis in homosexual men. Clinical trials with metronidazole, tinidazole, and diloxanide furoate. Sex Transm Dis 17(2):72–74, 1990.

219. Orkin M. Resurgence of Scabies. JAMA 217:593, 1971.

220. Parlette HL. Scabietic infestations of man. Cutis 16:47, 1975.

221. Currier RW. Lice and scabies control. Iowa Med 76(2):80, 82, 1986.

222. Crissey JT. Scabies and pediculosis pubis. Urol Clin North Am 11(1):171–176, 1984.

223. Gurevitch AW. Scabies and lice. Pediatr Clin North Am 32(4):987–1018, 1985.

224. Wolf R, et al. Norwegian-type scabies mimicking contact dermatitis in an immunosuppressed patient. Postgrad Med 78(1):228–230, 1985.

225. Honig PJ. Arthropod bites, stings, and infestations: their prevention and treatment. Pediatr Dermatol 3(3):189–197, 1986.

226. Richey HK, et al. Scabies: diagnosis and management. Hosp Pract [Off] 21(2):124A–124C,124H,124K–124L passim, 1986.

227. Mellanby K. The development of symptoms. Parasitic infection and immunity in human scabies. Parasitology 35:197, 1944.

228. Oakes RC, et al. Atopic dermatitis. A review of diagnosis, pathogenesis, and management. Clin Pediatr (Phila), 22(7):467–475, 1983.

229. Minster J. Nursing management of patients with scabies and lice. Nurs Clin North Am 15(4):747–756, 1980.

230. Buntin DM. Cutaneous features of sexually transmitted diseases. Recognition and treatment. Postgrad Med 78(7):121–128, 1985.

231. Fragola LA Jr, Watson PE. Common groin eruptions: diagnosis and treatment. Postgrad Med, 69(5):159–163, 166–169, 172, 1981.

232. Taplin D, et al. A comparative trial of three treatment schedules for the eradication of scabies. J Am Acad Dermatol 9(4):550–554, 1983.

233. Taplin D, et al. Eradication of scabies with a single treatment schedule. J Am Acad Dermatol 9(4):546–550, 1983.

234. Burgess I, et al. Aqueous malathion 0.5% as a scabicide: clinical trial. Br Med J [Clin Res], 292(6529):1172, 1986.

235. Moberg SA, et al. An epidemic of scabies with unusual features and treatment resistance in a nursing home. J Am Acad Dermatol 11(2 Pt 1):242–244, 1984.

236. Shacter B. Treatment of scabies and pediculosis with lindane preparations: an evaluation. J Am Acad Dermatol 5(5):517–527, 1981.

237. Amer M, et al. Treatment of scabies: preliminary report. Int J Dermatol 20(4):289–290, 1981.

238. Permethrin for scabies. Med Lett Drugs Ther 32(813):21–22, 1990.

239. Taplin D, Meinking TL, Chen JA, et al. Comparison of crotamiton 10% cream (Eurax) and permethrin 5% cream (Elimite) for the treatment of scabies in children. Pediatr Dermatol 7(1):67–73, 1990.

240. Bourgeois M, et al. Mercury intoxication after topical application of a metallic mercury ointment. Dermatologica, 172(1):48–51, 1986.

241. NuHall G. The Biology of *Pediculus humanus*. Parasitology 10:80, 1917.

242. Orkin M. Treatment of today's scabies and pediculosis. JAMA 236:1136, 1976.

243. Couch JM, et al. Diagnosing and treating *Phthirus pubis palperbrarum*. Surv Ophthalmol, 26(4):219–225, 1982.

244. Monheit BM, Norris MM. Is combing the answer to headlice? J Sch Health 56(4):158–159, 1986.

245. Geigy R. Relapsing fevers. In Wienman D, Ristie M (eds): Infectious Blood Diseases of Man and Animals, vol 2. New York, Academic Press, 1968, pp 175–216.

246. Zolrodovskii PF, Golinevich EH. Wolhynian on five-day fever. In The Rickettsial Diseases. 2nd Edition, Pergammon Press, London, 1960;630.

247. Maibach HI. Therapeutic Agents for Human Skin Infections. JAMA 230:759, 1974.

248. Meinking TL, et al. Comparative efficacy of treatments for pediculosis capitis infestations. Arch Dermatol 122(3):267–271, 1986.

249. Bowerman JG, Gomez MP, Austin RD, et al. Comparative study of permethrin 1% cream rinse and lindane shampoo for the treatment of head lice. Pediatr Infect Dis J 6(3):252–255, 1987.

250. Taplin D, et al. Permethrin 1% creme rinse for the treatment of *Pediculus humanus* var *capitis* infestation. Pediatr Dermatol 3(4):344–348, 1986.

251. Permethrin for head lice. Med Lett Drugs Ther 28(722):89–90, 1986.

252. Brandenburg K, et al. 1% permethrin cream rinse vs 1% lindane shampoo in treating pediculosis capitis. Am J Dis Child 140(9):894–896, 1986.

253. Edling C, et al. New methods for applying synthetic pyrethroids when planting conifer seedlings: symptoms and exposure relationships. Ann Occup Hyg 29(3):421–427, 1985.

254. Ares-Mazas E, et al. The efficacy of permethrin lotion in pediculosis capitis. Int J Dermatol 24(9):603–605, 1985.

255. Flannigan SA, Tucker SB. Variation in cutaneous sensation between synthetic pyrethroid insecticides. Contact Dermatitis 13(3):140–147, 1985.

256. Monheit BM, Norris MM. Is combing the answer to headlice? J Sch Health 56(4):158–159, 1986.

257. Keystone JS, Murdoch JK. Mebendazole. Ann Intern Med 91:582–586, 1979.

258. Pena C, et al. Mebendazole, an effective broad-spectrum anthelmintic. Am J Trop Hyg 22:592–595, 1973.

259. el Kalla S, Menon NS. Mebendazole poisoning in infancy. Ann Trop Paediatr 10(3):313–314, 1990.

260. Swartzwelder JC, et al. The use of piperazine for the treatment of human helminthiases. Gastroenterology 33:87–96, 1957.

261. Belloni C, et al. Neurotoxic side-effects of piperazine. Lancet 2:369, 1967.

262. Miller CG, et al. Neurotoxic side-effects of piperazine. Lancet 1:895, 1971.

263. Desowitz RS, et al. Anthelmintic activity of pyrantel pamoate. Am J Trop Med Hyg 19:775–778, 1970.

264. Vallarejos VM, et al. Experience with the anthelmintic pyrantel pamoate. Am J Trop Med Hyg 20:842–845, 1971.

265. Feldmeier H, et al. Flubendazole versus mebendazole in intestinal helminthic infections. Acta Trop (Basel) 39(2):185–189, 1982.

266. Abadi K. Single dose mebendazole therapy for soil-transmitted nematodes. Am J Trop Med Hyg 34(1):129–133, 1985.

267. Katz M. Adverse metabolic effects of antiparasitic drugs. Rev Infect Dis 4(4):768–770.

268. Varma TK, Shinghal TN, Saxena M, et al. Studies on the comparative efficacy of mebendazole, flubendazole and niclosamide against human tapeworm infection. Indian J Public Health 34(3):163–168, 1990.

269. Walden J. Parasitic diseases. Other roundworms. *Trichuris*, hookworm, and *Strongyloides*. Prim Care 18(1):53–74, 1991.

270. Upatham ES, Viyanant V, Brockelman WY, et al. Prevalence, incidence, intensity and associated morbidity of intestinal helminths in south Thailand. Int J Pharasitol Apr; 19(2):217–228, 1989.

271. Sargent RG, et al. A clinical evaluation of mebendazole in the treatment of trichuriasis. Am J Trop Med Hyg 23:375–377, 1974.

272. Wagner ED, et al. Morphologically altered eggs of *Trichuris trichiura* following treatment with mebendazole. Am J Med Hyg 23:154–157, 1974.

273. Wagner ED, et al. In vivo effects of a new anthelmintic mebendazole (R-17, 635) on the eggs of *Trichuris trichiura* and hookworm. Am J Trop Med Hyg 23:151–153, 1974.

274. Krogstad, DJ, et al. Amebiasis. N Engl J Med 298:262–265, 1978.

275. Rees PH. Amoebiasis--*Entamoeba histolytica* infections: a review. East Afr Med J 63(1):81–84, 1986.

276. Viswanathan R, et al. An ameboma--lest we forget. J Indian Med Assoc 84(1):18–20, 1986.

277. Most H. Treatment of common parasitic infections of man encountered in the United States. N Engl J Med 287:698–702, 1972.

278. Levine GI. Sexually transmitted parasite diseases. Clin Off Pract 18(1):101–108, 1991.

CHAPTER 74

SURGICAL ANTIBIOTIC PROPHYLAXIS

RONALD L. BRADEN

Administration of prophylactic antibiotics in certain surgical procedures can decrease postoperative infections, decrease the length of hospital stay, and reduce the overall cost of care. Haley and colleagues demonstrated that surgical wound infections can be responsible for an additional week of hospitalization and an increase of approximately 20% in the overall cost of care (1). This cost is estimated to exceed $1.5 billion per year in the United States.

Inappropriate or indiscriminate use of prophylactic antibiotics can increase cost of care by increasing drug cost, increasing drug toxicity, increasing microorganism resistance, and increasing laboratory costs. Prophylactic antibiotics can account for up to 30% of total antibiotic use in some hospitals, and inappropriate usage remains a problem (2).

PRINCIPLES OF ANTIBIOTIC PROPHYLAXIS

Prophylactic antibiotics are indicated when the risk of postoperative infection is high or the consequence of infection is excessive morbidity or mortality (3). Antibiotic selection should be based on spectrum of antimicrobial activity, pharmacokinetic profile, drug toxicity, and positive results from well-controlled clinical trials. The benefit of the prophylactic antibiotic must always clearly outweigh its risks.

Classification of Surgical Wounds

The Ad Hoc Committee of the Committee on Trauma of the National Research Council developed a standard classification of surgical wounds in 1964 (4). This classification identified four basic categories of wound contamination and the resultant postoperative infection rate that is expected within each category (Table 74.1).

Risk Factors for Infection

The risk of postoperative infection depends on patient factors, intraoperative factors, and perioperative management. Factors that have been identified as increasing the risk of postoperative infection are listed in Table 74.2. Regardless of the procedure classification, emergency operations have a higher postoperative infection rate than does the same elective procedure. Institutions that do a high volume of an operative procedure have a lower postoperative infection rate than do institutions where the procedure is performed less frequently (5). Also operative

procedures of longer duration have a higher postoperative infection rate, regardless of wound classification.

CHOICE OF ANTIBIOTIC REGIMEN

Antimicrobial Spectrum

The antimicrobial agent chosen should have activity against the most common pathogens that cause surgical wound infections (Table 74.3). The agent does not need to have antibacterial activity against all pathogens that are endogenous to the surgical site; agents with an excessively broad spectrum of activity increase the risk of microbial resistance without an increase in effectiveness. Third-generation cephalosporins demonstrate this point; despite increased antimicrobial activity, these agents have not proven to be superior to first-generation cephalosporins in any operative procedure (6).

Pharmacokinetics

The pharmacokinetic profile of the prophylactic agent is also an extremely important factor. Burke demonstrated

Table 74.1.
National Research Council Wound Classification Criteria

Classification[a]	Criteria
Clean (<2%)	Elective (not urgent or emergency), primarily closed; no acute inflammation or transection of gastrointestinal, oropharyngeal, genitourinary, biliary, or tracheobronchial tracts; no technique break (e.g., elective inguinal herniorrhaphy)
Clean-contaminated (<10%)	Urgent or emergency case that is otherwise clean; elective, controlled opening of gastrointestinal, oropharyngeal, biliary, or tracheobronchial tracts; minimal spillage and/or minor technique break; reoperation via clean incision within 7 days; blunt trauma, intact skin, negative exploration (e.g., vagotomy and pyloroplasty)
Contaminated (20%)	Acute, nonpurulent inflammation; major technique break or major spill from hollow organ; penetrating trauma <4 hr old; chronic open wounds to be grafted or covered (e.g., acute, nonperforated, nongangrenous appendicitis)
Dirty (40%)	Purulence or abscess; preoperative perforation of gastrointestinal, oropharyngeal, biliary, or tracheobronchial tracts; penetrating trauma >4 hr old (e.g., perforated appendicitis with abscess)

Source: Adapted from (3).
[a]Wound infection rates appear in parentheses.

the importance of adequate serum concentrations of the prophylactic antibiotic at the time of incision in experimental animals (7). Since most antibiotics distribute rapidly into tissue compartments after intravenous administration, elimination half-life and volume of distribution become the most important pharmacokinetic variables. Intraoperative

factors such as blood loss, fluid replacement, and alteration of blood flow to the liver and kidneys may cause significant alterations in the elimination half-life and volume of distribution of prophylactic antibiotics. Guglielmo and colleagues demonstrated a significant increase in volume of distribution and elimination half-life of cefamandole in patients undergoing elective vascular surgery (8). These authors also report low serum concentrations of the antibiotic at the time of prosthetic graft placement, which would theoretically place the patient at increased risk of postoperative infection. Additional information is needed to recommend dosage adjustment for these patients, but continued close observation of surgical wound infection rates is warranted at this time.

Timing of Antibiotic Administration

The most common error that is encountered in surgical prophylaxis is in the timing of antibiotic doses. As was previously stated, Burke demonstrated the importance of adequate serum concentrations of the prophylactic antibiotic at the time of incision in experimental animals (7). This finding was confirmed by Polk and colleagues in a prospective clinical trial in which inappropriate time of drug administration was an independent risk factor for postoperative infection (9). Classen and colleagues prospectively monitored the timing of antibiotic prophylaxis and studied the occurrence of surgical wound infections in patients

Table 74.2.
Factors Associated with Increased Risk of Postoperative Infection

Patient Factors	Perioperative Factors	Intraoperative Factors
Extremes of age	Long preoperative	Intraoperative con-
Undernutrition	hospitalization	tamination
Obesity	No preoperative	Lengthy operation
Associated problems	shower	Excessive electro-
Diabetes	Early shaving of site	cautery
Hypoxemia	Hair removal	Foreign material
Remote infection	Prior antibiotic	Wound drainage
Corticosteroid	therapy	High hematocrit
therapy		wound fluid
Recent operation		Epinephrine wound
Chronic		injection
inflammation		Intraoperative
Prior site		hypotension
irradiation		Massive transfusion
		Alcohol/hexachloro-
		phene skin prepa-
		ration

Source: Adapted from (3).

Table 74.3.
Recommendations for Prophylactic Antibiotic Agents by Site

Operations	Bacteria	Antibiotic Agent	Dose
Cardiac: all with cardiopulmonary bypass	*Staphylococcus aureus* *Staphylococcus epidermidis*, diptheroids, Gram-negative enterics	Cefazolin (Vancomycin)	1–2 g preinduction, 1–2 g every 8 h for 48 hr
Noncardiac vascular: aortic resection and prosthetic bypass	*S. aureus, S. epidermidis*, diphtheroids, Gram-negative enterics	Cefazolin (Vancomycin)	1 g preinduction, 2 postoperative doses
Orthopedic: insertion of prosthetic joints open operations	*S. aureus, S. epidermidis*	Cefazolin	1 g preinduction
Neurosurgery	*S. aureus, S. epidermis*	Cefazolin (Vancomycin)	1 g preinduction
Head and neck: operations involving the mucous membranes and deep tissue	Oral aerobes and anaerobes, *S. aureus*, streptococci	Cefazolin	2 g preinduction
Gastroduodenal: ulcer patients treated with H$_2$ blockers, bleeding duodenal ulcer, gastric cancer	Oropharyngeal flora and Gram-negative enterics, *S. aureus*	Cefazolin	1–2 g preinduction
Biliary: all open and laproscopic procedures	Gram-negative enterics, *S. aureus, Enterococcus fecalis*, clostridia	Cefazolin	1–2 g preinduction
Colorectal: operations that open the colon and/or rectum	Enteric aerobes and anaerobes	Oral neomycin/ erythromycin Cefoxitin	Operating room day 1: 1 g at 1:00, 2:00, and 11:00 P.M. 1 g preinduction
Appendenctomy: simple appendicitis	Enteric aerobes and anaerobes	Cefoxitin, cefotetan, or cefmetazole	1 g preinduction
Cesarean section	Enteric aerobes and anaerobes, *E. fecalis*, group B streptococci	Cefazolin	1 g after umbilical cord is clamped
Hysterectomy	Enteric aerobes and anaerobes, *E. fecalis*, group B streptococci	Cefazolin	1 g preinduction

Source: Adapted from (3).

undergoing elective clean or clean-contaminated surgical procedures (10). Patients receiving prophylactic antibiotics during the 2 hours prior to incision had the lowest overall surgical wound infection rate. "On call" dosing of prophylactic antibiotics may result in early administration and inadequate tissue concentrations at the time of incision. Therefore, this practice should be strongly discouraged.

Duration of Prophylaxis

Antibiotics that are continued longer than 24 to 48 hr do not decrease the risk of surgical wound infection but may increase toxicity, increase cost, and alter the microflora of the institution (11). Single-dose prophylaxis of most operative procedures provides the optimal balance of reducing surgical wound infections while decreasing adverse drug effects (12).

SURGICAL PROCEDURES AND SUGGESTED ANTIBIOTIC REGIMENS

Cardiac Operations

Cardiac operations are classified as clean surgical procedures and pose a low risk of surgical wound infection. However, in cardiac operations that involve placement of prosthetic material, such as prosthetic valve replacement, the excessive morbidity and mortality of endocarditis and mediastinitis mandate the use of prophylactic antibiotics. The pathogens that are most commonly responsible for postoperative infection include *Staphylococcus aureus*, *Staphylococcus epidermidis*, and diptheroid species. In most institutions, first-generation cephalosporins have good activity against these pathogens and have remained the standard against which other antibiotics are compared. Cefazolin, a first-generation cephalosporin with a relatively long elimination half-life, has remained the most commonly prescribed prophylactic agent. Several investigations have compared newer cephalosporins, with varying results. Slama and colleagues compared cefamandole, cefazolin, and cefuroxime (13). Their results indicate that cefamandole and cefuroxime are both superior to cefazolin in overall wound infection rates. However, other investigators have been unable to reproduce these results, and the choice of agent remains an area of controversy (14, 15). The choice of agent in this setting should be based on individual institution sensitivities, but the literature supports cefazolin as the prophylactic agent of choice in cardiothoracic operations.

Noncardiac Vascular Operations

Like cardiac operations, noncardiac vascular procedures are classifies as clean, and the most common pathogens are *S. aureus* and *S. epidermidis*. The incidence of postoperative infection is increased with insertion of vascular prosthesis or in procedures involving the groin (16–18). Several authors have demonstrated the efficacy of three-dose cefazolin prophylaxis, and cefazolin remains the prophylactic agent of choice in these procedures (19, 20). Prophylactic antibiotics have not been shown to improve outcome in carotid endarterectomy or brachial artery repair without insertion of prosthetic material and therefore are not indicated (3). In institutions that have a significant incidence of methicillin-resistant *S. aureus*, vancomycin is an acceptable alternative agent.

Orthopedic Operations

Like the previously described operations, orthopedic procedures are clean and pose a low risk of infection. However, the associated morbidity and mortality of prosthetic joint infections are extremely high and warrant the use of prophylactic antibiotics. The most common pathogens are *S. aureus* and *S. epidermidis*. Cefazolin is the prophylactic agent of choice and has shown a significant reduction in postoperative infections and demonstrated adequate tissue and bone concentration, and it has a low risk of toxicity (21). Duration of therapy is somewhat more controversial, but courses longer than 48 hr offer no added benefit, and strictly intraoperative doses appear promising (21, 22).

Neurosurgical Operations

The benefit of prophylactic antibiotics has not been well documented in clean neurosurgical operations without shunt placement, although this practice is common. *S. aureus* and *S. epidermidis* are the predominate pathogens, with Gram-negative aerobes being somewhat more common in cerebrospinal fluid (CSF) shunt infections. A review of the literature published by Haines supports the use of prophylactic antibiotics, but recommendations about specific agents remains difficult (23). Prophylactic agents that are used include cefazolin, cloxacillin, penicillin, piperacillin, and vancomycin as monotherapy and cefazolin plus gentamicin and gentamicin plus vancomycin as combination therapy. All agents have been shown to reduce postoperative infection rates, but the data is not overwhelming (24–27). Limited data is available regarding CSF shunt procedures, but applying knowledge from other areas involving prosthetic material would mandate the use of prophylactic antibiotics because of the extreme morbidity and mortality associated with these procedures. From the available literature, cefazolin monotherapy appears effective in reducing the surgical wound infection rate in neurosurgical operations and should be considered the preferred prophylactic agent.

Head and Neck Operations

Head and neck operations should be divided into two categories: clean procedures, in which no transection of the oropharyngeal tract occurs, and clean-contaminated procedures, in which transection of the oropharyngeal tract does occur. Clean procedures include parotidectomy, hyroidectomy, and submandibular-gland excision. The infection rate for these procedures is low, and routine prophylactic antibiotics are not recommended (28). Clean-contaminated procedures that were performed without prophylactic antibiotics have produced surgical wound infection rates of 24 to 87%, and appropriate perioperative antibiotics have been shown to reduce the postoperative infection rate by approximately 50% (29). The predominant pathogens in clean-contaminated head and neck procedures are the normal flora of the mouth and oropharynx. Multiple prophylactic antibiotic regimens have been proven effective in reducing surgical wound infection rates. However, the preferred regimens are cefazolin 2 g or clindamycin plus gentamicin. Duration of therapy should not exceed 24 hr.

Gastroduodenal Operations

Surgical wound infection rates of the gastroduodenal tract have been documented to be a function of stomach pH. Disease states or drugs that increase pH are well known to increase the incidence of postoperative infection (30). The predominant pathogens in gastroduodenal operations are normal mouth flora, skin flora, and, to a lesser extent, bowel flora. Several cephalosporins have been proven to be effective in reducing postoperative infection rates. Cefazolin has been studied in a single-dose regimen and appears to have equal efficacy to that of multidose regimens. The preferred regimen is cefazolin 1 to 2 g as a single dose at the induction of anesthesia (31, 32).

Biliary Tract Operations

The postoperative infection rate of biliary tract operations is directly related to the presence or absence of microorganisms in the bile. The infection rate of patients with positive bile cultures is reported to be approximately 36%; the infection rate of patients with sterile bile is <5% (33, 34). Risk factors for positive bile cultures include acute cholecystitis, biliary tract obstruction, and age greater than 70 (35). The most common organisms found in biliary tract surgery are *Escherichia coli*, *Klebsiella*, enterococci, streptococci, and staphylococci. Cephalosporins have shown good activity in biliary tract surgery, and a metaanalysis by Meijer and colleagues concluded that perioperative antibiotics should be used for all patients who are undergoing biliary tract surgery. Although patients with sterile biliary tracts appear to gain little or no benefit, preoperative identification of these patients is not possible (36). Cefazolin is the preferred agent and should be given as a single preinduction dose.

Appendectomy

The incidence of surgical wound infections following appendectomy is highly variable and depends on the status of the appendix at the time of surgery. In uncomplicated appendicitis the infection rate is reported to be 4 to 9% without perioperative antibiotics and 1 to 5% with antibiotics (37). The most common pathogens that are isolated after appendectomy are anaerobic organisms such as *Bacteroides fragilis* and aerobic Gram-negative organisms such as *Escherichia coli*. Streptococci, staphylococci, and enterococci are identified less frequently but may be associated with antibiotic treatment failure. Antibiotic regimens that have been found to be effective in significantly reducing postoperative complications have included cefoxitin, cefotaxime, mezlocillin, and clindamycin (37, 38). The first-generation cephalosporins, cefazolin and cephalothin, have not been proven to be effective in reducing postoperative infections and do not appear to be appropriate prophylactic agents (39, 40). The preferred regimen in uncomplicated appendicitis seems to be cefoxitin, cefotetan, or cefmetazole given as a single-dose preinduction regimen (38). Antibiotic use in complicated appendicitis is classified as treatment, not prophylaxis, and is therefore not included in the discussion.

Colorectal Operations

Surgical wound infections are responsible for excessive morbidity and mortality following elective colorectal surgery and mandate use of effective prophylactic antibiotics. Risk factors for postoperative infections include impaired host defenses, age greater than 60 years, hypoalbuminemia, inadequate bowel preparation, and bacterial contamination of the surgical wound (41). The goal of surgical prophylaxis in colorectal surgery is to reduce the risk of wound contamination by bacteria spilled from the colon and rectum during the surgical procedure. This is accomplished most effectively by use of mechanical bowel preparation, preoperative oral antibiotics, and parenteral perioperative antibiotics (3). Mechanical bowel preparation reduces fecal bulk but does not significantly alter the concentration of microorganisms in the stool and does not decrease surgical wound infection rates (42). Addition of oral antibiotics such as erythromycin and neomycin to mechanical bowel preparation further decreases postoperative infections, and the addition of a perioperative parenteral cephalosporin such as cefoxitin, cefotetan, or cefmetazole can further decrease postoperative infection rate to <10% for elective colorectal procedures (43). The preferred prophylactic regimen would include the following: (a) 4 L of a polyethylene glycol-electrolyte lavage solution given the day before surgery plus (b) oral neomycin sulfate 1 g and erythromycin base 1 g given after the bowel preparation is completed at 1:00, 2:00, and 11:00 P.M. the day before surgery plus (c) cefoxitin or a similar agent at induction of anesthesia.

Cesarean Section

The risk of postoperative infection in cesarean section appears to be related to host factors and can be divided into high- and low-risk populations. High-risk patients are women who have not received prenatal care, are under-nourished, have undergone multiple vaginal exams, have prolonged labor, and/or have undergone frequent invasive monitoring. The risk of postpartum endometritis is reported to be as high as 85% for high-risk patients and 5 to 10% for low-risk patients (44). Appropriate prophylactic antibiotics can reduce the incidence of postoperative infection by 50 to 70%, as has been documented by controlled clinical trials (45). The preferred prophylactic regimen is cefazolin 1 g given after umbilical cord clamping. Administration of the drug after cord clamping is intended to minimize toxicity to the infant.

Hysterectomy

The incidence of postoperative infection following vaginal hysterectomy without prophylactic antibiotics is reported to be as high as 40%. Appropriate prophylactic antibiotics can reduce this incidence to <10% (46). Risk factors for postoperative infection include low socioeconomic status, extremes of age, obesity, diabetes, and prior instrumentation. Postoperative infections are caused by a variety of aerobic and anaerobic organisms, *Bacteroides* species being the predominant anaerobe. Single-dose cefazolin has proven to be as effective as extended- spectrum cephalosporins and is the preferred prophylactic agent (46).

CONCLUSION

In summary, prophylactic antibiotics play a significant role in the perioperative management of surgical patients. The resultant decrease in postoperative infections serves to decrease morbidity and mortality, which in turn can limit the length of the hospital stay and cut health care delivery costs in general. In using antibiotic prophylaxis, however, several criteria should be emphasized to extend its safety and efficacy. First, the antibiotic's benefit should outweigh the risks of treatment, and consideration should be given to appropriate spectrum of antimicrobial activity. In addition, antibiotic dosing should be scheduled such that adequate tissue concentrations are achieved during the critical period while postoperative duration of prophylaxis is limited to the shortest effective length. Being aware of these considerations will allow successful antibiotic prophylaxis and help to ensure a successful surgical result.

REFERENCES

1. Haley RW, Schaberg DR, Crossley KB, et al. Extra charges and prolongation of stay attributable to nosocomial infections: a prospective interhospital comparison. Am J Med 70:51–8, 1981.
2. Wenzel RP. Preoperative antibiotic prophylaxis. N Engl J Med 326:337–39, 1992.
3. Page CP, Bohnen JMA, Fletcher JR, et al. Antimicrobial prophylaxis for surgical wounds: guidelines for clinical use. Arch Surg 128:79–88, 1993.
4. Ad Hoc Committee of the Committee on Trauma, Division of Medical Sciences, National Academy of Sciences–National Research Council. Postoperative wound infections: the influence of ultraviolet irradiation of the operating room and various other factors. Ann Surg 160(Suppl 2):23, 1964.
5. Farber BF, Kaiser DL, Wenzel RP. Relation between surgical volume and incidence of postoperative wound infection. N Engl J Med 305:200, 1981.
6. DiPiro JT, Bowden TA, Hooks VH. Prophylactic parenteral cephalosporins in surgery: are the newer agents better? JAMA 252:3277, 1984.
7. Burke JF. Effective period of preventive antibiotic action in experimental incisions and dermal lesions. Surgery 50:161, 1961.
8. Guglielmo BJ, Salazar TA, Rodondi LC, et al. Altered pharmacokinetics of antibiotics during vascular surgery. Am J Surg 157:410–12, 1989.
9. Polk HC, Lopez-Mayor JF. Postoperative wound infection: a prospective study of determinant factors and prevention. Surgery 66:97–103, 1969.
10. Classen DC, Evans RS, Pestonik SL, et al. The timing of prophylactic administration of antibiotics and the risk of surgical wound infection. N Engl J Med 326:281–86, 1992.
11. Guglielmo BJ, Hohn DC, Koo PJ, et al. Antibiotic prophylaxis in surgical procedures: a critical analysis of the literature. Arch Surg 118:943, 1983.
12. DiPiro JT, Cheung RPF, Bowden TA, et al. Single dose systemic antibiotic prophylaxis of surgical wound infections. Am J Surg 152:552–59, 1986.
13. Slama TG, et al. Randomized comparison of cefamandole, cefazolin, and cefuroxime prophylaxis in open-heart surgery. Antimicrob Agents Chemother 29:744–51, 1986.
14. Conklin CM, et al. Determinants of wound infection incidence after isolated coronary artery bypass surgery in patients randomized to receive prophylactic cefuroxime or cefazolin. Ann Thorac Surg 46:172, 1988.
15. Gentry LO, et al. Antibiotic prophylaxis in open-heart surgery: a comparison of cefamandole, cefuroxime, and cefazolin. Ann Thorac Surg 46:167–72, 1988.
16. Szilagi DE, Smith RF, Elliott JP, Vrandecic MP. Infection in arterial reconstruction with synthetic grafts. Ann Surg 186:321–33, 1972.
17. Goldstone J, Moore WS. Infection in vascular prostheses: clinical manifestations and surgical management. Am J Surg 128:225–33, 1974.
18. Landreneau MD, Raju S. Infections after elective bypass surgery for lower limb ischemia: the influence of preoperative transcutaneous arteriography. Surgery 90:956–61, 1981.
19. Kaiser AB, Clayson KR, Mulherin JL Jr, et al. Antibiotic prophylaxis in vascular surgery. Ann Surg 188:283–89, 1978.
20. Pitt HA, Postier RG, MacGowan WAL, Frank LW. Prophylactic antibiotics in vascular surgery: topical, systemic, or both? Ann Surg 192:356–64, 1980.
21. Van Meirhaeghe J, Verdonk R, Verschraegen G, Myny P, Paeme G, Classen H. Flucloxacillin compared with cefazolin in short-term prophylaxis for clean orthopedic surgery. Arch Orthop Trauma Surg 108:308–13, 1989.
22. Nelson CL. Prevention of sepsis. Clin Orthop 222:66–72, 1987.
23. Haines SJ. Efficacy of antibiotic prophylaxis in clean neurosurgical operations. Neurosurgery 24:401–05, 1989.
24. Geraghty J, Feely M. Antibiotic prophylaxis in neurosurgery. J Neurosurg 60:724–26, 1984.

25. Bullock R, van Dellen JR, Ketelbey W, Reinach SG. A double-blind placebo-controlled trial of perioperative prophylactic antibiotics for elective neurosurgery. J Neurosurg 69:687–91, 1988.

26. van Ek B, Dijkmans BA, van Dulken H, Mouton RP, Hermans J, van Furth R. Effect of cloxacillin prophylaxis on the bacterial flora of craniotomy wounds. Scand J Infect Dis 22:345–52, 1990.

27. Cartmill TD, al Zahawi MF, Sisson PR, et al. Five days versus one day of penicillin as prophylaxis in elective neurosurgical operations. J Hosp Infect 14:63–8, 1989.

28. Johnson JT, Wagner RL. Infection following uncontaminated head and neck surgery. Arch Otolaryngol Head Neck Surg 113:368–69, 1987.

29. Friberg D, Lundberg C. Antibiotic prophylaxis in major head and neck surgery when clean-contaminated wounds are established. Scand J Infect Dis Suppl 70:87–90, 1990.

30. Gatehouse D, Dimock F, Burdon DW, et al. Prediction of wound sepsis following gastric operations. Br J Surg 65:551, 1978.

31. Pories WJ, Van Rij AM, Burlingham BT, Fulghum RS, Meelheim D. Prophylactic cefazolin in gastric bypass surgery. Surgery 90:426–32, 1981.

32. Lewis RT, Goodall RG, Marien B, Park M, Lloyd-Smith W, Wiegand FM. Efficacy and distribution of single dose preoperative antibiotic prophylaxis in high-risk gastroduodenal surgery. Can J Surg 34:117–22, 1991.

33. Cainzos M, Potel J, Puente JL. Prospective randomized controlled study of prophylaxis with cefamandole in high risk patients undergoing operations upon the biliary tract. Surg Gynecol Obstet 160:27–32, 1985.

34. Stone HH, Hooper CA, Kolb LD, et al. Antibiotic prophylaxis in gastric, biliary and colonic surgery. Ann Surg 184:443–52, 1976.

35. Chetlin SH, Elliot DW. Preoperative antibiotics in biliary surgery. Arch Surg 107:319–23, 1973.

36. Meijer WS, Schmitz PIM, Jeeke J. Meta-analysis of randomized, controlled clinical trials of antibiotic prophylaxis in biliary tract surgery. Br J Surg 77:282–90, 1990.

37. Bauer T, Vennits B, Holm B, et al. Antibiotic prophylaxis in acute nonperforated appendicitis: The Danish Multicenter Study Group III. Ann Surg 209:307–11, 1989.

38. Winslow RE, Dean RE, Harley JW. Acute nonperforating appendicitis: efficacy of brief antibiotic prophylaxis. Arch Surg 113:651–55, 1983.

39. Donovan IA, Ellis D, Gatehouse D, et al. One-dose antibiotic prophylaxis against wound infection after appendectomy: a randomized trial of clindamycin, cefazolin sodium and a placebo. Br J Surg 66:193–96, 1979.

40. Panichi G, Pantosti AL, Marsiglio F. Cephalothin or cefoxitin in appendectomy? J Antimicrob Chemother 6:801–04, 1980.

41. Nichols RL. Prophylaxis for elective bowel surgery. In: Wilson, SE, Williams RA, Finegold S, eds. Intra-abdominal infections. New York: McGraw Hill, 1982:267–85.

42. Bartlett J, Condon R, Gorbach S, et al. Veterans Administration Cooperative Study on bowel preparation for elective colorectal operations: impact of oral antibiotic regimen on colonic flora, wound irrigation cultures and bacteriology of septic complications. Ann Surg 188:249–54, 1978.

43. Stellato TA, Danziger LH, Gordon N, et al. Antibiotics in elective colon surgery: a randomized trial of oral, systemic, and oral/systemic antibiotics for prophylaxis. Am Surg 56:251–54, 1990.

44. Amstey MT, Sheldon GW, Blyth JF. Infectious morbidity after primary cesarean section in a private institution. Am J Obstet Gynecol 136:205–10, 1980.

45. Mugford M, Kingston J, Chalmers I. Reducing the incidence of infection after cesarean section: implications of prophylaxis with antibiotics for hospital resources. Br Med J 299:1003–06, 1989.

46. Soper D, Yarwood R. Single-dose antibiotic prophylaxis in women undergoing vaginal hysterectomy. Obstet Gynecol 53:879–82, 1987.

CHAPTER 75

INFECTIONS IN THE IMMUNOSUPPRESSED PATIENT

WILLIAM J. McINTYRE and MICHAEL D. PARR

The human immune system serves many functions, including homeostasis, surveillance, and defense. Defects in host defense can lead to a variety of infectious complications. This chapter will review specific defects in the immune system and the infectious complications associated with those defects. It will primarily discuss the treatment of infection in neutropenic patients. However, many of the principles and treatments discussed in the section on neutropenia can also be applied to other immunocompromised patients. Discussion of Acquired Immune Deficiency Syndrome (AIDS) and the associated opportunistic infections will be covered in another chapter of this text.

DEFECTS IN THE IMMUNE SYSTEM

An immunocompromised state is created by defects in the immune system. Immunodeficiency or immunosuppression occurs in patients as a result of either inherited or acquired disorders of the immune system. Inherited disorders are usually diagnosed shortly after birth and include diseases such as Severe Combined Immune Deficiency Syndrome (SCIDS) and agamma-globulinemia. Acquired disorders can occur at any point in a patient's life and can be induced by chemotherapy, immunosuppressive agents (e.g., azathioprine, cyclosporine, and corticosteroids), radiation, or viruses (e.g., HIV). The severity of the immunodeficiency varies in both inherited and acquired disorders. The types of infections seen in these patients are related to their specific defect and the severity of that defect. Defects can be seen in any component of the immune system. Most often, these defects can be generally classified into disorders of the mucocutaneous barriers, granulocytes, cellular immunity, complement synthesis, and antibody formation (1, 2).

The mucocutaneous barriers of the skin, respiratory, gastrointestinal, and genitourinary tracts provide the body's initial primary defense against pathogens. The loss of mucocutaneous barriers offers a way for pathogens to gain access to the host's internal organs. Breaches in mucocutaneous barriers are produced by a number of medical devices (central venous catheters, Foley catheters, endotracheal tubes), procedures (surgery), and treatments (chemotherapy and radiation). Mechanical

malfunctions may also occur, such as loss of the mucociliary mechanism of the lungs and decreased saliva production by salivary glands, resulting in a decreased ability to clear organisms from the bronchopulmonary tree and gastrointestinal tract (1).

Effects on granulocytes can be quantitative or functional. A number of investigators have correlated the incidence of infection to the total granulocyte count, also called the absolute neutrophil count (ANC). A patient's ANC is determined by multiplying the total white blood cell count (WBC) by the percentage of circulating granulocytes (mature granulocytes plus band-immature white cell forms) obtained from a white blood cell (WBC) differential. In general, patients are said to be neutropenic or granulocytopenic if their total granulocyte count falls below 1000 cells per cubic millimeter (mm^3). However, some institutions use the more strict criteria of ANC of 500 cells/mm^3 to define neutropenia. As the total granulocyte count falls below 1000 cells per mm^3, the rate of infection increases. When the total number of granulocytes falls below 100 cells per mm^3, the incidence of infection approaches 100% (3).

Granulocytopenic patients are particularly susceptible to infections by bacteria. The duration of granulocytopenia also has a profound effect on the rate of infectious mortality. The longer the patient is granulocytopenic, the greater the risk of infection by organisms. Granulocytes can also have functional abnormalities, which can be inherited or iatrogenic. Certain chemotherapeutic drugs, such as asparaginase and the vinca alkaloids, cause functional abnormalities that alter the granulocyte's ability to migrate and phagocytose bacteria, thus increasing the patient's susceptibility to infection.

The cellular immune system consists primarily of macrophages and T lymphocytes. These cells protect against certain types of infection. Cellular immunity provides protection against specific fungi, viruses, and protozoans. Impairment of cellular immunity is seen in patients who receive immunosuppressive agents (e.g., the corticosteroids, cyclosporine) and in patients with certain types of cancer (e.g., Hodgkin's lymphoma).

Defects in complement synthesis, antibody production, and in monocyte–macrophage systems can lead to recurrent pneumonia and sepsis by encapsulated organisms, such as *Streptococcus pneumoniae*. This increase in infection is due to a loss of ability to opsonize bacteria. Opsonization describes the ability of antibodies and/or complement to attach to a pathogen, thereby enhancing its phagocytosis by monocytes and macrophages. Defects in opsonization and in the macrophage–monocyte system are seen in patients with complement deficiencies (angioedema), impaired antibody function (chronic lymphocytic leukemia), and decreased macrophage function (splenectomy).

Knowing the specific immune deficiency that a patient is experiencing will help predict likely pathogens and aid in choosing the appropriate initial therapies. However, rarely will patients have just one specific deficiency. In immunocompromised hosts, most often a number of the components of the immune system are usually affected. This point is well illustrated in patients undergoing cancer treatment. In many patients with cancer, the disease itself will predispose the patient to infection. Tumors can invade normal tissues leading to tissue destruction, necrosis, and loss of normal barriers. The loss of barriers provides a place for bacteria to invade and grow. Tumor invasion of the bone marrow can lead to "crowding out" of normal hematopoietic cells, thus resulting in leukopenia. In addition, hematologic tumors, such as lymphoma, leukemia, and myeloma, may directly impair cell-mediated and antibody-mediated immunity.

Each cancer treatment modality affects host defenses. For the delivery of chemotherapy and supportive care, patients will often require central venous catheters and Foley catheters. Again, these devices provide a site for pathogenic invasion particularly by gram-positive bacteria and fungi. Mucocutaneous barriers may be further compromised by radiation and chemotherapy-induced mucositis. Patients with mucositis have a predilection for developing infections by gram-negative bacteria and *candida* spp. In addition to producing bone marrow suppression and neutropenia, individual antineoplastic agents may affect specific functions of the immune system as illustrated in Table 75.1 (4). Prolonged treatment with antineoplastic drugs not only affects granulocytes, but will impact cellular immunity as well. Compromised cellular immunity increases the risk of developing an opportunistic fungal or viral infection.

Among the most immuncompromised patients who have the condition because of an inherited disorder are children with SCID. SCID is an autosomal disorder characterized by a lack of cellular and humoral immunity. Patients with SCID fail to produce antibodies on exposure to an antigen and fail to respond to cutaneous skin testing (anergy). During the first year of life, patients frequently present with opportunistic infections caused by *candida*, *pneumocystis carnii*, and viruses.

Table 75.1.
Examples of Chemotherapy Agents Effect on Immune System

Effect	Sample Agent
Myelosuppression	Alkylating agents
	Antimetabolites
Impaired cellular immunity	Cyclophosphamide
	Corticosteroids
Impaired antibody dysfunction	Cyclophosphamide
	Corticosteroids
	Alkylating agents
	Antimetabolites
Impaired chemotaxis	Vincristine
Phagocyte dysfunction	Corticosteroids

In the past, SCIDS was fatal unless the patient received a bone marrow transplant or was maintained in a protective environment—"bubble children." Recently, new approaches have been attempted. Forty percent of the patients with SCID have a deficiency in adenosine deaminase (ADA) (5). ADA is responsible for preventing the toxic accumulation of deoxyadenosine in lymphocytes. Replacement therapy using pegademase bovine (polyethylene-glycol modified ADA bovine, Adagen®) at 15 IU/kg intramuscularly once a week has been demonstrated to be of benefit in some patients. Gene therapy is currently being evaluated as a possible means to incorporate the ADA gene into the patient's lymphocytes (6).

Among the most severe of the iatrogenic immunocompromised states is found in patients undergoing bone marrow transplantation (BMT). The myelotoxic BMT conditioning regimens consists of high-dose chemotherapy and/or radiation that produce severe and prolonged neutropenia. To prevent graft-versus-host disease in patients receiving donor bone marrow (allogenic BMT), T cell function must be suppressed. This is achieved either through purging the donor marrow of T cells or through the use of immunosuppressive agents, such as cyclosporine, methotrexate, and corticosteroids. Deficiencies in both antibody function and cellular immunity have been found to exist for up to two years following bone marrow transplantation.

By far, the largest group of immunosuppressed patients are those receiving antineoplastic agents. Once neutropenia develops, these patients are highly susceptible to infection. Fever in a neutropenic patient is treated as a medical emergency; death due to sepsis may occur within 48 to 72 hours if the appropriate antibiotics are not initiated immediately. The rest of this chapter will focus on the treatment of the neutropenic patient.

THE NEUTROPENIC PATIENT

Over the past 20 years, great strides have been made in the treatment of infections in the neutropenic patient. Even

Table 75.2.
Causes of Death in Neutropenic Patients

Complication	Percentage of Patients with Findings
Infection	35%
Hemorrhage	27%
Progression of cancer	18%
Miscellaneous	20%
Renal insufficiency	
Myocardial infarction	
Carcinoma meningitis	
Acute pulmonary edema	

though the initial morbidity and mortality from infection has diminished substantially, infection is still the leading cause of death in cancer patients (see Table 75.2) (7). The reasons for this are not completely clear despite improvements in antibiotic therapy. The treatment of cancer, however, has been refined, and chemotherapeutic regimens are becoming much more aggressive. Therefore, more patients are developing neutropenia for a longer period and, consequently, the greater are their chances of developing a life-threatening infection. Investigators have also shown that the more advanced the cancer, the greater the chance the patient will die of an infection (7). Fungal organisms are becoming increasingly implicated as the cause of infections and death in the neutropenic patient. In one study, up to 58% of the cancer patients at autopsy had pathologic signs of an invasive fungal infection (8). Infection due to fungi are often more difficult to eradicate than bacterial infections.

BACTERIAL INFECTIONS

Diagnosing an infection in a granulocytopenic patient can be difficult. The classic signs of infection (e.g., redness, swelling, tenderness, heat) are absent because of the lack of granulocytes. Often, the only sign of infection is fever, and fever is not always due to infection. Fever can be induced by the administration of blood products and medications, further complicating the diagnosis. In actuality, infection is documented in only approximately 60% of the neutropenic patients presenting with fever (see Table 75.3) (1). Therefore, most often antibiotics are initiated without any documented evidence of the infective organism (empiric).

Because the treatment must be initiated empirically, the clinician must know what organism to suspect. In 80% of the culture documented infections in neutropenic patients, the infecting organism will be either a gram-negative or a gram-positive bacteria. The most common organisms are *Pseudomonas aeruginosa, Escherichia coli, Klebsiella pneumoniae, Staphylococcus aureus,* and *Staphylococcus epidermidis.* The other 20% of the documented

infections are due to fungi, viruses, or protozoans. Prior to the release of methicillin, the majority of the infections were due to gram-positive bacteria. Subsequently, gram-negative bacteria became the primary cause of infection in neutropenic patients. In general, the pattern appears to be changing again, and infections due to *Pseudomonas aeruginosa* are dropping, with infections due to gram-positive organisms increasing. *Staphylococcus epidermidis* has become a major pathogen because of central venous catheter (e.g., Hickman Catheters) use in cancer patients (9,10). The increased incidence of infection by *S. epidermidis* is important because this organism is often methicillin resistant. The point that needs to be emphasized is that the primary group of organisms causing infections in this patient population is always changing. Therefore, it is important for the clinician to know the primary pathogens cultured from neutropenic patients at their institution (11).

The sources for infection in neutropenic patients are primarily from the gastrointestinal tract (i.e., normal flora from the mouth and alimentary canal) and the respiratory tract (see Table 75.4). Pizzo and colleagues (12) demonstrated that 80% of infections arise from organisms that colonize the patient. However, 50% of these organisms were acquired by the patient in the hospital and may be resistant to standard antibiotics. It would appear from these data that surveillance cultures (cultures employed to monitor colonization) would supply beneficial information. However, investigation has shown that routine surveillance cultures are not cost effective (13). The reasons surveillance cultures are of limited value are as follows: (1) no one site of colonization was consistently predictive for the offending pathogen; (2) other potential pathogens were usually cultured at the same time; (3) if a useful culture was obtained, it was usually after initiation of antibiotics; and (4) the current practice of employing broad-spectrum antibiotics will cover the vast majority of potential pathogens in the neutropenic host (13). Therefore, surveillance cultures should not be used to routinely monitor colonization of patients.

Table 75.3.
Outcome of Infection in the Febrile Neutropenic Patient

Evidence of Infection	Percentage of Patients with Findings
Documented infection	60%
Microbiologically documented infection with bacteremia	20%
Microbiologically documented infection without bacteremia	20%
Clinically documented infection	20%
Fever of undetermined origin	20%
Fever of noninfectious origin (e.g., blood product, medication)	20%

Table 75.4.
Source of Infection in a Neutropenic Patient

Oral cavity
Trachea, bronchi, or lungs
Intestine and esophagus
Nose and sinuses
Intravenous catheter sites

Antibacterial Therapy

When granulocytopenic patients develop a fever, a careful physical examination should be performed to locate any possible source of infection. The patient's medication and transfusion records should be checked to ensure that the fever is not related to either of these potential causes. Prior to initiating antibiotic therapy, the patient must be cultured extensively. Culture specimens should be obtained from the following fluids or sites: sputum, urine, throat, and blood. A duplicate set of blood cultures should be obtained if a patient has a central venous catheter (i.e., one set from the central venous catheter and one set from a peripheral venipuncture). Duplicate cultures may help determine if the central venous catheter is infected. In the case of an infected catheter, blood cultures from the catheter may be positive, whereas peripheral blood cultures are negative. Any area that appears infected, such as a venipuncture site or bone marrow aspiration site, should also be cultured. After the appropriate cultures have been collected, empiric antibiotic therapy should be initiated immediately to prevent early mortality.

Antibiotic therapy will be empiric and designed to cover the most common pathogens seen at the institution. Antibiotic therapy in the febrile neutropenic patient has traditionally employed combination therapy with either two or three drug regimens. However, with the introduction of the new broad-spectrum third-generation cephalosporins (e.g., cefoperazone and ceftazidime) and the carbapenems (imipenem/cilastatin), single-agent therapy is a consideration. In selecting empiric therapy, three principles should always be followed. First, antibiotics must be administered at the maximum prescribed dose. Next, broad-spectrum therapy should be selected whether the clinician decides to administer single or combination therapy. Finally, the antibiotic(s) chosen must take into account the resistance patterns of the institution (9).

Many antibiotic combinations have been investigated in the treatment of infections in the neutropenic patient. Antibiotic combinations fall into four categories:

1. Antipseudomonal β-lactam plus an aminoglycoside
2. Semisynthetic penicillin plus a third-generation cephalosporin (double β-lactam)
3. Third-generation antipseudomonal cephalosporin or carbapenem (monotherapy)
4. Vancomycin added to any of the preceding regimens

Other factors also important in the selection of antibiotics include rapidity of bactericidal activity, efficacy in the neutropenic patient, pharmacokinetics of the antibiotics, potential for synergy between the antibiotics, and toxic effects (9). Table 75.5 lists a number of studies investigating the treatment of infections in the granulocytopenic patient. In general, early morbidity and mortality is seen from gram-negative organisms. Therefore, the majority of regimens initially cover gram-negative bacteria (8). Recently however, *Group A streptococcus* has been associated with fulminant infections. When reviewing the literature, it becomes obvious that the majority of antibiotic studies demonstrate a 65 to 97% overall response rate when appropriate antibiotic combinations are used. Therefore, Table 75.5 is not a list of the "ideal" combinations, but provides a reference point when comparing antibiotic combinations.

When combination antibiotic regimens are employed, the antibiotics included in the combination should be synergistic. The organism should be susceptible to at least two of the antibiotics for the patient to receive the maximum benefit from the combination regimen. In neutropenic patients, Klastersky and colleagues (23) demonstrated that if two synergistic antibiotics (against the cultured organism) were employed, the cure rate of infection was 80%. If the antibiotics used were not synergistic, the cure rate was only 49%. Even if the combination of antibiotics employed does not demonstrate true synergy, studies have shown as long as the agents are active against the cultured organism, the response rate is improved when compared to regimens in which only one of the antibiotics shows activity (24, 25). In addition, the bactericidal activity of the antibiotics is important to consider. Bactericidal activity can be measured by drawing

Table 75.5.
Antibiotic Combinations Studied in the Neutropenic Patient

Drugs	Overall Percentage of Responses	References
Semisynthetic Penicillins and Aminoglycosides		
Carbenicillin-Gentamicin	83%	14
Ticarcillin-Amikacin	80%	15
Ticarcillin-Gentamicin	97%	16
Third-Generation Cephalosporin-Aminoglycoside		
Moxalactam-Amikacin	83%	15
Ceftazidime-Tobramycin	71%	17
Cefoperazone-Amikacin	88%	18
Semisynthetic Penicillins and Third-Generation Cephalosporins		
Piperacillin-Moxalactam	77%	19
Ticarcillin-Moxalactam	65%	20
Miscellaneous Combinations		
Piperacillin-Vancomycin	72%	21
Co-trimoxazole-Ticarcillin	7%	2

peak serum samples of the antibiotics administered and performing serial dilutions of the serum, which is then cultured with the infecting organism from the patient. A peak bactericidal serum titer of 1:16 or greater correlated with a favorable clinical response in 87% of infected neutropenic patients (25). Trough bacterial serum titers provided no additional information.

Some investigators have challenged the need for an aminoglycoside in empiric regimens. It is important to note that aminoglycosides have been found to be less effective in neutropenia patients (26). In one study, the addition of an aminoglycoside to an antipseudomonal penicillin had no advantage over the antipseudomonal penicillin alone (27). If aminoglycosides are employed in an antibacterial regimen, peak and trough level of the aminoglycoside should be monitored regularly. Concentrations of gentamicin or tobramycin that should be attained in this patient population are between 6 and 8 mcg/ml for the peak level and between 1 and 2 mcg/ml for the trough level (28).

With the introduction of the third-generation cephalosporins, there has been renewed interest in monotherapy (single-agent therapy) in the treatment of infections in neutropenic patients. Good results have been obtained in trials with monotherapy. The benefits of single-agent therapy in the neutropenic patient include (1) avoidance of nephrotoxicity can be avoided because aminoglycosides are not being employed, and (2) patients receive less intravenous fluid, and less expensive therapy, compared to traditional combination therapy. However, single-agent therapy does have some drawbacks. With single-agent therapy, the infecting organism must be covered by the antibiotic being employed. If not, the patient basically has no antibiotic coverage. The third-generation cephalosporins have gaps in their coverage (i.e., gram-positive organisms). Further, the demonstrated beneficial effects of synergism cannot be used. The third-generation cephalosporins have theoretical advantages because they provide broad coverage against gram-negative bacteria, they attain high bactericidal concentrations in the serum, and many have long plasma half-lives. Imipenem/cilastatin has also been shown to be effective as a single agent. Ceftazidine and imipenem/cilastin have been compared in a randomized trial. Both regimens were equally efficacious in the management of neutropenic fever (32). However, the addition of anaerobic coverage (metrodiazole and clindamycin) was more frequent in patients treated with ceftazidine, whereas patients treated with imipenem/cilastatin experienced more episodes of nausea. More than half the patients in the trial required modification of their initial monotherapy. Table 75.6 lists some of the studies that have investigated single-agent therapy. In all these studies, the investigators recommended either close monitoring of the patient for treatment failures or the addition of a second agent initially to cover for gram-positive organisms. Therefore, at the

Table 75.6.

Single-Agent Antibiotic Therapy Studies in Neutropenic Patients

Drug	Average Dose	Overall Percentage of Response	Reference
Ceftazidime	2 g q 8 h	95%	28
Ceftazidime	2 g q 8 h	60%	17
Cefoperazone	6 g q 12 h	77%	18
Moxalactam	1.5 g q 8 h	80%	29
Imipenem/ Cilastatin	500 mg q 6 h	74%	30

present time, single-agent therapy is not recommended without close observation of the patient. These regimens may require early modification. It is recommended that monotherapy be limited to patients with an ANC of 500 to 1000 experiencing short periods of neutropenia (31).

Fungal Infections

If febrile neutropenic patients do not respond to antibacterial agents within 4 to 7 days and no evidence of bacterial infection is documented, antifungal therapy should be initiated (33). After bacteria, fungi are the next most likely cause of infection in the neutropenic patient. The incidence of fungal infection increases dramatically in patients with prolonged granulocytopenia (1, 3, 7, 8). A major obstacle in the treatment of fungal infections is making the diagnosis. Fungal cultures can be negative in the presence of a true fungal infection (8). In addition, no good serologic tests for the diagnosis of fungal infections currently exist (33). On the other hand, fungal organisms can be cultured from a number of different sites and fluids, including nares, throat, sputum, and stool in patients. Often, fungal organisms cultured from these sites represent only colonization; yet, in the febrile neutropenic, the risk is too great, and treatment should be initiated. A true diagnosis of fungal infection can be made only when the culture is obtained from a sterile site or by histology (3).

The majority of these in infections are due to *Candida albicans*. However, other *candida* species like *C. glabrata*, *C. krusei* , and *C. tropicalis* must be considered. *Candida* species tend to infect the mucus membranes of the gastrointestinal and urinary tracts but can also cause cutaneous or disseminated infections. Other common fungal pathogens include *Aspergillus, Fusarium,* and *Trichosporon* species.

Aspergillus rarely causes infection in immunocompetent patients. In an immunosuppressed patient, the organism is pathogenic and often fatal. In most cases, patients acquire the organism by inhalation of *Aspergillus* spores dispersed in the air. Because *Aspergillus* is normally present in the soil, fungal spores may seed the air in areas near excavation or construction. Outbreaks of *Aspergillus* during periods of construction support this. *Aspergillus* infection occurs primarily in two sites of the body: the sinuses and the lungs. The risk factors for the infection include prolonged granulocytopenia (for more than 30 days), severe neutropenia (ANC less than 100 for more than 7 days), and graft-versus-host disease. Although prolonged granulocytopenia is the major risk factor for the development of fungal infection, broad-spectrum antibiotic and corticosteroid therapy can influence the development of fungal infection (35).

Aspergillosis actually is a rare disease, but it is extremely difficult to treat (36). Treatment of the infection must be extremely aggressive with resection of the infected area if possible followed by amphotericin B. The *Aspergillus* organism is only moderately sensitive to amphotericin B. Rifampin or flucytosine have been used in combination with amphotericin B to increase the efficacy (37). There have been, however, no *in vivo* studies demonstrating a benefit from the addition of these medications (37).

Amphotericin B remains the "gold standard" for fungal infections. However, the possibility of severe side effects makes many clinicians somewhat reluctant to initiate amphotericin B as empiric therapy. Fluconazole has gained increased acceptance as empiric therapy.

Amphotericin B has activity against *Candida albicans* but limited efficacy against *Aspergillus* and *Cryptococcus*. The dose of amphotericin B is 0.5 to 1.0 mg per kilogram of body weight per day. The manufacturer of amphotericin B recommends that a test dose of 1 mg be administered and followed by slow titration up to the calculated maintenance dose to limit adverse reactions. However, in neutropenic patients with a documented fungal infection, the dose should be escalated rapidly to the maintenance dose. Early initiation of amphotericin B may decrease the risk of invasive fungal disease (11). The duration of amphotericin B therapy depends on whether a positive diagnosis of a fungal infection has been made. The patient with a verified fungal infection should receive a total of 500 to 3000 mg of amphotericin B. If no positive diagnosis of a fungal infection has been made, the drug may be stopped when the total neutrophil count is above 500 cells per mm (3, 33).

Amphotericin B side effects can fall into two categories: immediate and dose related. Immediate side effects include fever, chills, and rigor. Patients receiving amphotericin B can be pretreated with acetaminophen, diphenhydramine, and hydrocortisone in an attempt to eliminate the immediate symptoms. Often, pretreatment is not effective, and the patient must endure the side effects. Long-term adverse effects from amphotericin B include renal toxicity and, rarely, bone marrow suppression. If patients develop renal toxicity due to amphotericin B, they will lose large amounts of potassium and magnesium. If renal failure does develop, it is usually reversible once the drug has been discontinued.

Ketoconazole is an oral antifungal agent with good activity against *Candida albicans* (36). An imidazole derivative, ketoconazole is effective only against fungal organisms in a growth phase. This medication is indicated only for superficial *candida* infection and should never be prescribed when an invasive process is suspected or diagnosed. Side effects include adrenal suppression and hepatotoxicity. The usual dose of ketoconazole is 200 to 400 mg every day. Ketoconazole requires an acidic environment for absorption from the gastrointestinal tract.

Fluconazole is the first of a new class of broad-spectrum bis-triazole antifungal agents. The fungaistatic activity of fluconazole is related to the inhibition of fungal P-450 sterol C-14 alpha-demethylation, resulting in an accumulation of 14 alpha-methyl sterols in the fungus. Fluconazole is currently approved for use in oropharyngeal candidiasis, systemic candidal infections, and cryptococcal meningitis. Its role in treatment of neutropenic patients remains to be defined (37). It is promising because of its lack of toxicity compared to amphotericin B. The usual oral dose for systemic candidiasis is 400 mg the first day, followed by 200 mg every day for 4 weeks. For esophageal candidiasis, the dose is 200 mg the first day followed by 100 mg every day for 2 weeks. Because fluconazole is eliminated by the kidneys, the dose must be adjusted in renal insufficiency. The use of fluconazole in cryptococcal meningitis will be discussed in the chapter on AIDS. Itraconazole, an oral triazole, has an increased spectrum against *Aspergillus*. Its role in the treatment of granulocytopenic has yet to be clearly defined (38).

Antiviral Therapy

Viral infections can be seen in patients with acute leukemia who are neutropenic because of aggressive chemotherapy, but the infections occur more frequently in organ transplant patients (i.e., kidney, heart, liver, and bone marrow) (39). Patients receiving organ transplants may be severely immunosuppressed in order to prevent rejection of their transplanted organ. Viruses are responsible for up to 33% of deaths in the transplant population (40). The mortality from viral infection [particularly from cytomegalovirus infection (CMV)] is extremely high in bone marrow transplant patients (41, 42). Viral infection can be either a primary infection in which the host was infected for the first time or a reactivated infection where the virus has been harbored in a nerve (e.g., Herpes) or in a WBC (e.g., CMV). The main goal in the treatment of viral infections is to prevent the spread of the virus systemically (i.e., to the brain, lungs, gastrointestinal tract, and so on). At no time during a patient's immunosuppression should he or she receive live or attenuated viral vaccines since these vaccines may result in viral infection.

Herpes virus infections can be caused by either type I or type II viruses. In the immunocompromised host, approximately 85% of the infections affect the oral cavity with the other 15% involving genital area (43). An oral herpes infection is usually diffuse and can be extremely painful, preventing the patient from taking in adequate oral nutrition. The herpetic lesion can serve as a focus for bacterial infections (43). Herpes infections frequently occur within the first 17 days after the initiation of chemotherapy in bone marrow transplant patients (42).

The treatment of choice for herpes virus infections is acyclovir (44, 45). Acyclovir has significantly reduced herpes infections as a cause of death in bone marrow transplant patients (42). Acyclovir is a prodrug that is metabolized by viral thymidine kinase. The metabolized drug is a potent inhibitor of herpes simplex and varicella zoster DNA polymerases. Acyclovir has been shown to be highly effective in the treatment of herpes in a number of different studies (43, 45). The intravenous dose employed in the treatment of herpes simplex is 5 mg per kilogram of body weight every 8 hours (or 250 mg per m^2 every 8 hours). There are a few side effects from acyclovir. Patients can develop a thrombophlebitis in peripheral veins due to the alkaline nature of the drug. Good urine output should be maintained to prevent crystallization of the drug in the renal tubules. The dose of acyclovir should be adjusted in renal failure. Topical acyclovir alone should not be prescribed in widespread disease because of an increased risk of disseminated viral disease (40).

Varicella-zoster, a communicable virus, causes chickenpox in childhood on initial exposure (primary disease). In immunosuppressed patients, the virus may reactivate, usually occurring along a dermatomal pattern. Disseminated varicella can cause pneumonia, encephalitis, hepatitis, and pancreatitis. In an investigation of children receiving chemotherapy for malignancies who subsequently developed a varicella infection, 32% progressed to disseminated disease, and 7% died of the infection (46). The greatest risk of developing disseminated varicella occurred in patients whose total granulocyte count was below 500 cells/mm^3. Children with malignancies, immunosuppressed patients, and bone marrow transplantation patients who are exposed to a child with chickenpox should receive passive immunization with varicella-zoster immune globulin (VZIG). The dose of VZIG is based on the patient's body weight and the titer to varicella in the serum. Varicella-zoster can be treated with either vidarabine or acyclovir. Vidarabine has been shown to be effective in the treatment of zoster if it is initiated within 72 hours from the onset of the symptoms (46). The intravenous dose of vidarabine is 10 mg per kilogram of body weight per day given as an infusion over 12 hours. However, the side effects of vidarabine such as gastrointestinal distress, megaloblastic anemia, hallucinations, and seizures have limited its clinical usefulness. The treatment of choice for varicella-zoster is acyclovir; it has demonstrated efficacy in the treatment of zoster (48). The best results are seen when the drug is administered early in the course of the disease (46). The intravenous dose of acyclovir in the treatment of a varicella infection is higher than in a herpetic infection (10 mg per kilogram of body weight every 8 hours or 500 mg/m^2 every 8 hours).

Cytomegalovirus is an opportunistic virus that causes few symptoms in an immunocompetent patient (48) but becomes a serious pathogen in immunosuppressed patients. CMV in the bone marrow transplant population is responsible for 15 to 20% of all deaths. Infection from CMV can cause pneumonia, retinitis, hepatitis, and bone marrow suppression (41). The disease can be primary in origin or can be caused by reactivation of the virus. The infection also can be transmitted by a blood transfusion that has CMV harbored in WBCs (41, 47). Infection in the lungs is usually the most severe form. Patients with CMV pneumonia present with fever, dyspnea, and a nonproductive cough. On chest radiograph, the infection appears as an interstitial pneumonia with bilateral infiltrates. Respiratory function deteriorates rapidly, with patients often dying of respiratory failure.

Current options for the treatment of CMV disease are limited. A number of antiviral medications have been tried to treat the disease, including vidarabine, acyclovir, and interferon, but none of these drugs have demonstrated efficacy in controlling the infection (47, 49). Only ganciclovir, foscarnet, and intravenous immunoglobulin (IVIG) have demonstrated activity against CMV. Studies with ganciclovir have been conducted in bone marrow transplant patients with documented CMV pneumonia (49). Despite good *in vitro* activity against CMV, ganciclovir alone did not change the outcome of the disease. Similarly, in limited trials, foscarnet was of limited value. The combination of ganciclovir and IVIG has been the most effective treatment of CMV. Combination therapy of IVIG and ganciclovir has been reported to increase survival although mortality was still high (50). Single agent ganciclovir and foscarnet may be useful in the treatment of pneumonia in less immunocompromised patients (e.g., AIDS and renal transplant patients) (51) and in patients who have CMV infections in organs other than the lung (e.g., liver, gastrointestinal tract).

The Epstein-Barr virus has been associated with pneumonia and leukopenia in the immunosuppressed patient population. Epstein-Barr-virus–associated lymphoma development has also been described in bone marrow transplant patients receiving bone marrow that has been T-cell depleted (52). High-dose acyclovir and alpha-interferon have been employed to treat the infection (53).

Decontamination Therapy

Prophylactic antibiotics and protective environment procedures have been beneficial in certain neutropenic patient populations. Theoretically, the number of infections in all neutropenic patients could be reduced because 80% of the documented infections arise from endogenous bacterial and fungal flora (12). Therefore, if the number of organisms colonizing a patient are decreased or completely eliminated, the infection rate in these patients could be reduced. If a prophylactic regimen employed to decrease colonization were effective, morbidity and mortality would also be reduced. In addition, complications from systemic antibiotics would be decreased because patients would not require antibiotics as often. Techniques that can be used to decrease the rate of infection include (1) bolstering the host defense mechanisms, (2) reducing damage to natural body barriers, (3) reducing the acquisition of new organisms from the environment, and (4) suppressing the potential pathogenic organisms currently colonizing the patient (12). The benefits of these techniques, however, have been shown only in patients with prolonged neutropenia.

The first three techniques are measures employed in the general care of the patient. Procedures to enhance host defenses include proper nutrition, use of immunostimulants, and resolution of neutropenia as rapidly as possible. The most important aspect of bolstering the host defense is proper nutrition. If the patient has good nutritional intake, his or her response to stress and infection will be improved.

Protection of natural barriers helps limit access of potential pathogens to the systemic circulation. Limiting the number of venipuncture and bone marrow aspirations will decrease the number of breaks in the skin. Rectal administration of drugs should be avoided to avert the induction of enteric bacteria into the blood. Invasive procedures such as urinary catheterization should be avoided to prevent colonization. Health care personnel and visitors should wash their hands thoroughly each time they enter a patient's room to help prevent the transfer of organisms from patient to patient. Attention to these general aspects of infection control can help reduce infectious complications in the neutropenic patient.

A technique that can decrease the rate of infection by more than 50% is protected environment isolation (54). Protective isolation involves the use of laminar air flow rooms and total microbial suppression. Laminar air flow rooms use high-efficiency particulate air filters (e.g., HEPA filters) to remove bacteria, fungi, and spores from the air. It is combined with good housekeeping methods and food and beverages with low-microbial content (cooked meats and no fresh fruits or vegetable) to decrease exposure to pathogens. Patients in protective isolation also receive total microbial suppression that includes both antibacterial and antifungal prophylaxis. Topical antiinfective cleaners are applied to decontaminate the skin, and oral nonabsorbable antibiotics are given to clean the gastrointestinal tract. Examples of nonabsorbable antibiotics employed include

vancomycin (500 mg) and gentamicin (160 mg) given orally 3 to 4 times a day (55). Fungal prophylaxis will be discussed later in the chapter.

The preceding regimen of protective environment isolation does decrease the rate of infection in neutropenic patients; however, it also has some major drawbacks. The first concerns patient compliance; patients in this protected environment are not allowed to leave their room during the period of neutropenia (which can last, in some cases, 2 months or longer). These isolation techniques thus place a great deal of psychological stress on the patient and decrease compliance. The nonabsorbable antibiotic regimens that are used are not very palatable, and compliance after several weeks is poor. In addition, if a patient stops taking the oral antibiotic, he or she can be colonized with organisms that are resistant to many antibiotics, and ultimately they become infected with these resistant organisms (12). Finally, facilities for protective isolation are expensive, and many hospitals cannot afford these techniques.

An alternative method of microbial prophylaxis is called selective decontamination, which involves the use of antimicrobial agents to selectively suppresses gram-negative organisms. Selective decontamination involves a concept of colonization resistance. The concept of colonization resistance states that anaerobic bacteria provide protection in the gastrointestinal tract from colonization with pathogenic bacteria, and if the anaerobic bacteria are killed off, colonization with pathogenic organisms will occur. Therefore, if antibacterial agents are given orally that suppress gram-negative organisms, but leave anaerobic flora intact, colonization with more virulent organisms should not be seen. The two antimicrobial agents that have been administered as selective decontaminants are co-trimoxazole (trimethopriml/sulfamethoxazole) and nalidixic acid. The drug that has been studied the most for this effect is co-trimoxazole. Results from the various studies have been somewhat contradictory. The dose of co-trimoxazole in studies investigating selective decontamination ranges from one single-strength tablet to one double-strength tablet orally 2 to 3 times a day. From the studies, co-trimoxazole appears to decrease the rate of infection in patients who are neutropenic for a prolong period (more than 7 days) (56–60). Patients with short-term neutropenia, however, do not realize any benefits from co-trimoxazole prophylaxis (60). Co-trimoxazole has been compared to nalidixic acid in antibacterial prophylaxis (61). Both of the therapies were efficacious, but the investigator stated that both regimens had disadvantages. Both the co-trimoxazole and nalidixic acid group produced resistant organisms that colonized the gastrointestinal tract and could have lead to superinfection. The primary disadvantage of co-trimoxazole is the possible inhibition of WBC production, which in turn, could prolong the neutropenia. In several studies, the period of neutropenia was longer when compared to the control group (61). Ciprofloxacin has been shown to be an effective alternative to co-trimoxazole (62). However, a question of increased fungal overgrowth is a concern (62). In summary, it appears that both total microbial decontamination and selective decontamination are effective in decreasing the incidence of infections when used appropriately, but should be administered only to patients who are expected to have an extremely prolonged neutropenic episode (12, 61, 63).

Antifungal Prophylaxis

Antifungal agents are administered prophylactically to decrease the incidence of superficial fungal infections and fungal colonization caused by *Candida albicans*. The agents that are used include nystatin suspension (15 ml orally 4 times a day), clotrimazole troches (10 mg orally 5 times a day), ketoconazole (200 to 400 mg orally once a day), and fluconazole (200 to 400 mg daily). One of these medications is usually combined with an antibacterial prophylactic regimen to give broad-spectrum coverage for both fungal and bacterial organisms. All these drugs are efficacious in the treatment of superficial fungal infection and suppression of *candida* in the gastrointestinal tract, but both nystatin suspension and clotrimazole troches can cause nausea and vomiting. Ketoconazole may be more effective than nystatin, but in a comparison study, there was an increase in colonization of torulopsis (64). Therefore, the selection of an antifungal prophylactic agent should be made according to the patient's preference.

Antiviral Prophylaxis

Antiviral prophylaxis is aimed primarily at the herpes simplex virus and CMV. In both cases, antiviral prophylaxis should be administered only to patients who are going to be severely immunosuppressed (i.e., acute leukemic patients undergoing induction therapy and bone marrow transplant patients). The prophylactic antiviral of choice for Herpes simplex virus is acyclovir (6, 66). Acyclovir is given at the same dose used for treatment, 5 mg/kg every 8 hours. The use of prophylactic medication in the prevention of CMV infection appears to be effective. In several studies, intravenous immunoglobulins have been administered to bone marrow transplant patients to prevent CMV pneumonitis (67, 68). These include CMV-selected immunoglobulins (CMV-IVIG) and IVIG. CMV-IVIG are primarily prepared by pooling CMV-positive plasma with extremely high titers to CMV (67). The result showed a decreased incidence of CMV pneumonia. Cost must be a consideration since IVIG therapy is expensive. Therefore, the administration of IVIG for viral prophylaxis is limited to high-risk populations (e.g., bone marrow transplant patients).

Prophylaxis Against *Pneumocystis Carinii*

Pneumocystis carinii is a protozoal organism that can cause opportunistic infections in immunosuppressed patients. Patients who are infected with this develop pneumonia and respiratory failure. Studies have demonstrated that one double-strength co-trimoxazole tablet twice a day or three times per week can prevent development of this infection in severely suppressed patients (70–72).

The Role of Colony Stimulating Factors in Neutropenia

The hematopoietic growth factors, granulocyte-macrophage colony stimulating factor (GM-CSF) and granulocyte colony stimulating factor (G-CSF), have both been used in the treatment and prophylaxis for neutropenia. GM-CSF produces an increase in granulocytes, monocytes, and eosinophils. G-CSF effects the precursors of the neutrophil lineage. In addition, the administration of these agents may cause the release of other stimulating factors that may directly or indirectly affect other cell lines, such as erythrocytes and platelets. Through stimulating monocyte and myeloid precursors, these agents have been shown to decrease the duration of neutropenia and thereby decrease the risk of infection (73, 74). The American Society of Clinical Oncology has recommended the following guidelines for use of hematopoietic growth factors as shown in Table 75.7.

At standard doses, both GM-CSF and G-CSF are well tolerated; side effects are usually limited to fever, chills, rash, fluid retention, and bone pain. Higher dose have been identified with more serious adverse effects, such as pulmonary edema and effusions. The frequency of bone pain increases in proportion to the dose. Nonsteroidal antiinflammatory agents have been reported to relieve this pain.

The efficacy and safety of administering granulocyte transfusions therapeutically and prophylactically in neutropenic patients has been investigated. Therapeutic granulocyte transfusions have demonstrated some benefit in neutropenic patients with documented infection (75). Studies looking at the potential benefits of administering granulocytes prophylactically have shown no advantage in the groups receiving transfusions (76, 77), and in one study, the granulocyte group did slightly worse (77). Adverse reactions seen from the transfusions, such as pulmonary infiltrates, increased incidence of cytomegalovirus infections, and cross-matching problems, also limit the utility of this therapy. Therefore, at the present time, granulocyte transfusion should be administered only to patients with a documented infection that is not responding to appropriate antibiotic therapy (75).

Table 75.7.
ASCO Guidelines for CSF Use

Generally Recommended

Myelosuppressive regimens with an incidence of neutropenia > 40%

In patients experiencing febrile neutropenia in prior episodes of chemotherapy, where chemotherapy dose reduction is not indicated

Following autologous bone marrow transplantation

Mobilization for collection of peripheral blood progenitor cells

Special Uses

In patients with prolonged neutropenia or at high risk of spesis

In neutropenic patients with myelodysplasia

With caution, in patients with acute myeloid leukemia after initial
therapy

Not Generally Recommended

In afebrile neutropenic patients

After allogeneic bone marrow transplantation

Not Reemmended

Concurrent with chemotherapy

To support dose intensity outside a clinical trial

For acute myeloid leukemia priming outside a clinical trial

Recommended Dosages

Neutropenia

G-CSF 5 μg/kg/d SC started 24–72 hr postchemotherapy until
ANC ≥ 10,000/μL

GM-CSF 250 μg/kg/d IV over 2 hr or SC started 24–72 hr postchemotherapy until ANC ≥ 10,000/μ/L

BMT

G-CSF 10–20 μg/kg/d SC started 24–72 hr postchemotherapy until
ANC ≥ 10,000/μL

GM-CSF 250 μg/kg/d IV over 2 hr or SC started 24–72 hr postchemotherapy until ANC ≥ 10,000/μL

DURATION OF THERAPY

The duration of antibiotic therapy in a neutropenic patient
is a topic of debate in the literature. If a patient's neutropenia and fever resolves during treatment with antibiotic(s),
the antibiotic(s) can be discontinued 7 days after the febrile
episode. The controversy involves patients who are still
neutropenic 7 days after defervescing. A study performed
by Pizzo and colleagues (78), investigated the duration of
antibiotic therapy in this patient population. Neutropenic
patients in this study were randomized either to continue
antibiotics after being afebrile for 7 days or to have their
antibiotics discontinued. The patients in the group who
continued to receive antibiotic therapy developed no further infectious complications. However, in the group in
which the antibiotics were discontinued, 41% of the patients were restarted on antibiotics within 2 days because of
recurrence of fever and/or clinical signs of infection. No
superinfection occurred in the group that continued to
receive antibiotics. Some clinicians still feel that antibiotics
should be discontinued after the patient has been afebrile
for several days to reduce the possibility of superinfection
(9). Factors that must be considered in the decision to stop
antibiotics in a patient that is still neutropenic include the
degree of neutropenia, existing sources of infection (muco-
cytsis), and the stability of the patient (31).

Patients whose fever is persistent for more than 3 days
should be reevaluated (31). Possible considerations include
resistance to current regimens, inadequate doses of antibiotics, and nonbacterial causes (31). Evidence of progressive
disease suggests the need to reassess the current antibiotic
regimen; if vancomycin was not a part of the initial regimen, it should be added. Persistent fever after 1 week of
therapy usually dictates the addition of antifungal therapy.
Fungal therapy should be continued for 2 weeks; if no locus
for a fungal infection is found, antifungal therapy may be
stopped. Empiric use of antiviral therapy is usually recommend only if evidence of viral disease exists (31). Should
fever persist despite the addition of amphotericin B,
anaerobic coverage should be considered.

In patients with persistent fever and pulmonary infiltrates while on broad-spectrum antibiotics, other opportunistic infections must be considered (79, 80). In addition
to *Aspergillus*, pulmonary infiltrates may be caused by
other fungal organisms, such as *Zygomycetes, Cryptococcus,* and *Histoplasma* (78). Other potential pathogens
include mycobacteria, *Chlamydia, Nocardia, Legionella,*
and Pneumocystitis. Bronchoalveolar lavage may be helpful in delineating the causative organism although open
lung biopsy maybe necessary. Table 75.8 contains a listing
of pathogens in the immune-compromised patient and
appropriate antibiotic therapy.

In culture-positive patients, antibiotic therapy may be
targeted toward the cultured organism. However, broad-
spectrum coverage should be maintained because of the
possibility of a mixed infection. Culture-positive patients
should receive a 10-to 14-day course of appropriate
antibiotic therapy.

MONITORING THERAPY

In monitoring a neutropenic patient, the clinician should
focus on two areas. Foremost is the status of the patient's
neutropenia and establishing the identity of the infecting
organism. The second task is to monitor the patient for
drug side effects and toxicities, and to make the appropriate
adjustments in therapy accordingly.

Once the initial work-up is complete and empiric
therapy is started, the clinician should focus on delineating
the causative organism and monitoring the status of the
patient for signs of a worsening condition, sepsis, and drug
toxicity. As stated earlier, granulocytopenic patients may
not present with typical symptoms of infection. The patient
must be carefully watched for subtle changes. Complaints
of fatigue, changes in mood, or changes in mentation may
be the only signals of a deteriorating condition. Vital signs
must be carefully monitored for signs of sepsis, such as
increases in heart rate, increases in respiratory rate, and
decreases in blood pressure. The state of the neutropenia
should be accessed daily by obtaining complete blood
counts with differential. Attempts to identify the causative

Table 75.8.
Medications to Treat Infections in Immunosuppressed Patients[a]

Organism	Drug	Dosing Regimens
Mycobacterial infection		
Mycobacterium avium-intracellulare	Isoniazid	300 mg orally daily
	Rifampin	600 mg orally daily
	Pyridoxine hydrochloride	10–100 mg orally daily given with isoniazid
	Ethambutol hydrochloride	25 mg/kg/day orally for six weeks then 15 mg/kg/day
	Streptomycin	0.75–1.0 g daily IM for two months then 2–3 times a week
	Capreomycin	15 mg/kg/day IM
	Ethionamide	500–1000 mg orally daily in 1–3 divided doses
	Cycloserine	750–1000 mg orally daily in 2–4 divided doses
	Pyrazinamide	25 mg/kg/day orally
Resistant *M. avium-intracellulare*	Rifabutin	150–300 mg orally daily
	Clofazimine	300 mg orally daily in three divided doses
	Co-trimoxazole (TMP-SMZ)	Oral: 20 mg/kg day TMP + 100 mg/kg/day SMZ in four divided doses
		Intravenous: 15 mg/kg/day TMP + 75 mg/kg day SMZ in four divided doses
Toxoplasma gondii	Pentamidine isoethionate	4 mg/kg/day IM or intravenously
	Sulfadiazine	1 g orally four times daily
	plus	
	Pyrimethamine	25 mg orally daily
	plus	
	Folinic acid	10 mg orally daily
Giardia lamblia	Quinacrine hydrochloride	100 mg orally three times daily
	Metronidazole	250–500 mg orally three times daily
Isospora belli	Co-trimoxazole	Trimethoprim 160 mg/sulfamethoxazole 800 mg orally, four times daily
Fungal Infections		
Candida albicans		
Oral thrush	Nystatin	500,000 units swish in mouth 4–6 times daily
	Clotrimazole	10 mg orally five times daily
Esophagitis	Ketoconazole	400 mg orally daily
	Fluconazole	200 mg, 100 mg daily
Transient fungemia	Amphotericin B	0.3 mg/kg/day i.v.
Disseminated disease with or without pneumonia	Amphotericin B	0.6 mg/kg/day i.v.
Cryptococcus neoformans		
Meningeal	Amphotericin B	0.3 mg/kg/day i.v.
	plus	
	Flucytosine	150 mg/kg/day orally in four divided doses
Nonmeningeal	Fluconazole	400 mg, then 200 mg daily
	Ketoconazole	400 mg orally daily
Histoplasma capsulatum	Amphotericin B	0.6 mg/kg/day i.v.
Pseuda ilescheria	Miconazole	600 mg intravenously every 8 hours
Aspergillus	Amphotericin B	0.6 mg/kg/day i.v.
	Amphotericin B	0.3 mg/kg/day i.v.
	Flucytosine	150 mg/kg/day orally in four divided doses
Coccidiodes immitis	Amphotericin B	0.6 mg/kg/day i.v.
	Ketoconazole	400 mg orally daily (for the treatment failures)
Chlamydia pneumoniae	Tetracycline	500 mg qid for 10–14 days
Nocardia asteroides	Sulfonamides	1 g every 4 hours

[a]Adapted from a table that appeared in an article by Furio and Wordell, reference 64.

organism must be rigorously pursued. Obtaining of daily blood cultures has been advocated.

The side effects from antibiotic therapy are going to depend on the antibiotic(s) chosen. Close monitoring is indicated in this population because many of the patients are on multiple agents. Concurrent or prior exposure to one agent may predispose the patient to the toxicities of other agents. Certain side effects are very common to the neutropenic patient. Nephrotoxicity can be seen as a result of aminoglycosides. Studies investigating the incidence of nephrotoxicity from aminoglycosides show a range between 0 to 15% (28, 29, 30). The incidence of nephrotoxicity may be higher when the aminoglycosides are combined with other nephrotoxic drugs such as cephalothin (30), amphotericin B, or vancomycin. Ototoxicity may also occur with aminoglycosides, with an incidence ranging from 6.2 to 17% (28, 31).

Fluid and electrolyte problems may also occur secondary to antibiotics. Patients receiving semisynthetic penicillins often lose large amounts of potassium in their urine during therapy because of the potassium-wasting effect of the penicillin. Additional amounts of potassium and magnesium can also be lost if the patient is receiving amphotericin B. Thus, serum potassium and magnesium levels should be monitored closely in patients prone to potassium wasting. The use of co-trimoxazole (generic for sulfamethoxazole-trimethoprim combinations) in neutropenic patients to treat infection may inhibit granulopoiesis and increase the duration of granulocytopenia (33). Finally, combination antibiotic therapy along with the administration of amphotericin B and acyclovir can substantially increase the amount of fluid a patient is receiving. This increase in fluid is due to the additional diluent that is required to administer the drug intravenously. The result may be volume overload and edema.

Prognosis

The prognosis for immunosuppressed patients without correction of their underlying disease or removal of the causative agent is poor. In the majority of cases, the patient will remain immunocompromised and have recurrent bouts of infection.

CONCLUSION

The treatment of infections in the immunocompromised host is difficult and requires close monitoring for any signs or symptoms of infection. Patients must be treated aggressively and promptly to prevent morbidity and mortality. Gram-negative infections are still the most frequently encountered. However, the incidence of gram-positive infections is on the rise once again. The importance of knowing the trends at the individual institution cannot be overemphasized. Initial treatment remains empiric. Monotherapy is increasing in popularity, but combination therapy still remains the standard of practice. In patients who remain febrile, the use of antifungal therapy is indicated. Colony stimulating factors are indicated in specific situations. The guidelines expressed in this chapter represent a generalized approach to the treatment of the immunosuppressed patient. Nonetheless, each patient must be treated on an individual basis.

REFERENCES

1. Schimpff SC. Overview of empiric antibiotic therapy for the febrile neutropenic patient. Rev Infect Dis, 7:5734–5740, 1985.

2. Cone LA, Woodard D, Heim NA. Clinical experience in the diagnosis and treatment of infection in the compromised host. Clin Therapeut, 4(Suppl):45–53, 1981.

3. Pizzo PA. Granulocytopenia and cancer therapy. Cancer, 5 4:2649–2661, 1984.

4. Haskell CM. Ed Cancer Treatment Philadelphia, W.B. Sanders Co. 1990.

5. Hirschlorn R. Overveiw of biochemical abnormalities and molecular genetics of adenosine deaminase deficiency. Pediatric Reseach, 33(1 Suppl):S35–S41, 1993.

6. Blaese R. Development of gene therapy for immunodeficiency: adenosine deaminase deficiency. Pediatric Research, 33(1 Suppl); S49–S53, 1993.

7. Schlier JP, Weerts D, Klastersky J. Causes of death in febrile granulocytopenic cancer patients receiving empiric antibiotic therapy. Eur J Cancer Clin Oncol, 20:55–60, 1984.

8. Armstrong D, Young LS, Meyer JD, et al. Infectious complications of neoplastic disease. Med Clin North Am 55:729–745, 1971.

9. Bodey GP. Antibiotics in patients with neutropenic. Arch Intern Med, 144:1845–1851, 1984.

10. Wade JC, Schimpff SC, Newman KA, et al. Staphylococcus epidermidis: An increasing cause of infection in patients with granulocytopenia. Ann Intern Med, 97:503–508, 1982.

11. Klastersky J,. Management of infection in granulocytopenic patients. J Antimicro Chem Ther, 12:102–104, 1983.

12. Pizzo PA, Schimpff SC. Strategies for the prevention of infection in the myelosuppressed or immunosuppressed cancer patients. Cancer Treat Rep, 67:223–233, 1983.

13. Kramer BS, Pizzo PA, Robichaud KJ. Role of serial microbiologic surveillance and clinical evaluation in the management of cancer patients with fever and granulocytopenia. Am J Med, 72:561–568, 1982.

14. Lau WK, Young LS, Black RE, et al. Comparative efficacy and toxicity of amikacin/carbenicillin versus gentamicin/carbenicillin in leukopenic patients: A randomized prospective trial. Am J Med, 62:959–966, 1977.

15. DeJongh CA, Wade JC, Schimpff SC, et al. Empiric antibiotic therapy for suspected infection in granulocytopenic cancer patients. A comparison between the combination of moxalactam plus amikacin and ticarcillin plus amikacin. Am J Med, 73:89–96, 1982.

16. Love LJ, Schimpff SC, Hahan DM, et al. Randomized trial of empiric antibiotic therapy with ticarcillin in combination with gentamicin, amikacin or netilmicin in febrile patients with granulocytopenia and cancer. Am J Med, 66:603–610, 1979.

17. Fainstein V, Bodey GP, Bolivar ER, et al. A randomized study of ceftazidime compared to ceftazidime and tobramycin for the treatment of infection in cancer patients. J Antimicro Chemother, 12(Suppl A):101–110, 1983.

18. Piccart M, Klastersky J, Lagast MH, et al. Single-drug versus combination empirical therapy for gram-negative bacillary infections in febrile cancer patients with and without granulocytopenia. Antimicro Agents and Chemo, 26:870–875, 1984.

19. Wintson DJ, Baines RC, Ho WC, et al. Moxalactam plus piperacillin versus moxalactam plus amkacin in febrile granulocytopenic patients. Am J Med, 77:442–450, 1984.

20. Fainstein V, Bodey GP, Bolivar R, et al. Moxalactam plus ticarcillin or tobramycin for treatment of febrile episodes in neutropenic cancer patients. Arch Intern Med, 144:1766–1770, 1984.

21. Jade AL, Bolivar R, Fainstein V, et al. Piperacillin plus vancomycin in the therapy of febrile episodes in cancer patients. Antimicro Agent Chemo, 26:295–299, 1984.

22. Keating MJ, Lawson R, Grose W, et al. Combination therapy with ticarcillin and sulfamethoxazole-trimethoprim for infection in patients with cancer. Arch Intern Med, 141:926–930, 1981.

23. Klastersky J. Treatment of severe infections in patients with cancer.

The role of new acyl-penicillins. Arch Intern Med, 142:1984–1987, 1982.

24. Young LS. Use of aminoglycoside in immunocompromised patients. Am J Med, 79(Suppl A):21–27, 1985.

25. Sculier JP, Klastersky J. Significance of serum bactericidal activity in gram negative bacillary bacteremia in patients with and without granulocytopenia. Am J Med, 76:429–435, 1984.

26. Bodey GP. Aminoglycoside use in the compromised host. In: Whelton A Neu HC, eds. The Aminoglycosides. New York: Marcel Dekker, 1982:557–583.

27. Bodey GP, Fainstein V, Rolston K, Elting L. Empiric therapy for the granulocytopenic patient.

28. Pizzo PA, Hathorn JW, Hiemenz J, et al. A randomized trial comparing ceftazidime alone combination antibiotic therapy in cancer patients with fever and neutropenic. N Engl J Med, 315:552–558, 1986.

29. Stambaugh JE, McAdams J. The efficacy and safety of moxalactam in the treatment of acute bacterial infections in immunosuppressed patient with cancer. Curr Ther Research, 31:864–871, 1982.

30. Mortimer J, Miller S, Black D, Kwok K, Kirby WM. Comparison of cefoperazone and mezlocillin with imipenem as empiric therapy in febrile neutropenic cancer patients. Am J Med, 85(suppl.):21–30, 1988.

31. Hughes WT, Armstrong D, Bodey GB, Feld R, et al. Guidelines for the use of antimicrobial agents in neutropenic patients with unexplained fever. J Infect Dis, 161:381–396, 1990.

32. Freifeld AG, Walsh T, Marshall D, Gress J, et al. Monotherapy for fever and neutropenia in cancer patients; a randomized comparison of ceftazidine versus imipenem. J Clin Oncol, 13:165–176, 1995.

33. Cohen J. Empirical antifungal therapy in neutropenic patients. J Anti-micro Chemo Ther, 13:409–411, 1984.

34. Schubert MM, Peterson DE, Meyers JD, et al. Head and neck aspergillosis in patients undergoing bone marrow transplantation. Cancer 57:1092–1096, 1986.

35. Gerson SL, Talbot GH, Hurwitz S, et al. Prolonged granulocytopenia: The major risk factor for invasive pulmonary aspergillosis in patient with acute leukemia. Ann Intern Med, 100:345–351, 1984.

36. Meunier-Carpentier F. Treatment of mycoses in cancer patients. Am J Med, 74(Suppl):74–78, 1983.

37. Preston Sl, Briceland LL. Fluconazole for antifungal prophylaxis in chemotherapy-induced neutropenia. AM J Heatlh-Syst Pharm, 52:164–173, 1995.

38. Jennings TS, Hardin TC. Treatment of apergilosis with itraconazole. Annals of Pharmacotherapy, 27(10):1206–1211, 1993.

39. Prentice HG, Hann IM. Antiviral therapy in the immunocompromised patient. Brit Med Bull, 41:367–373, 1985.

40. Burns WH, Saral R. Opportunistic viral infections. Brit Med Bull, 41:46–49, 1985.

41. Wong KK, Hirsch MS. Herpes virus infections in patients with neoplastic disease, diagnosis and therapy. Am J Med, 76:464–478, 1984.

42. Straus SE, Smith HA, Brickman C, et al. Acyclovir for chronic mucocutaneous herpes simplex virus infection in immunosuppressed patients. Ann Intern Med, 96:270–277, 1982.

43. Wade JC, Newton B, McLaren C, et al. Intravenous acyclovir to treat mucocutaneous herpes simplex virus infection after bone marrow transplantation. Ann Intern Med 96:265–269, 1982.

44. Whitley RJ, Soong SJ, Dolin R, et al. Early vidarabine therapy to control the complications of herpes zoster in immunosuppressed patients. N Engl J Med, 307:971–975, 1982.

45. Balfour HH, Bean B, Laskin OL, et al. Acyclovir halts progression of herpes zoster in immunocompromised patients. N Engl J Med, 308:1448–1453, 1983.

46. Balfour HH, McMonigal KA Bean B. Acyclovir therapy of varicella-zoster virus infections in immunocompromised patients. J Antimicro Chemother, 12(Suppl. B):169–179, 1983.

47. Skinhj P, Anderson HK, Moller J, et al. Cytomegalovirus infection after bone marrow transplantation: Relation of pneumonia to postgrafting immunosuppressive treatment. J Med Virol, 14:91–99, 1984.

48. Meyer JD, Wade JC, McGuffin RW, et al. The use of acyclovir for cytomegalovirus infections in the immunocompromised host. J Antimicro Chemother, 12:Suppl. B, 181–193, 1983.

49. Shepp DH, Dandliker PS, Miranda P, et al. Activity of 9-[2-Hydroxy-1-(hydroxymethyl) ethoxymethyl]guanine in the treatment of cytomegalovirus pneumonia. Ann Intern Med, 103:368–373, 1985.

50. Emamuel D, Cunningham I, Jules-Elysee K, et al. Cytomegalovirus pneumonia after bone marrow transplantation successfully treated with the combination of ganciclovir and high dose intravenous immune globulin. Ann Intern Med, 09:777–782, 1988.

51. Bach MC, Bagwell SP, Knapp NP, et al. 9 (1,3-dihydroxy-2-propoxymethyl) guanine for cytomegalovirus infection in patients with the acquired immunodeficiency syndrome. Ann Intern Med, 103: 381–382, 1985.

52. Papadopoulos EB, Ladanyi M, Emanuel D, Mackinnon S, et al. Infusions of donor leukocytes to treat Epstein-Barr virus-associated lymphoproliferative disorders after allogeneic bone marrow transplantation. N Engl J Med, 330(17):1231–1233, 1994.

53. Taguchi Y. Purtilo DT. Okano M. The effect of intravenous immunoglobulin and interferon-alpha on Epstein-Barr virus-induced lymphoproliferative disorder in aliver transplant recipient. 57(12): 1813–1815, 1994.

54. Schimpff SC. Infection prevention during profound granulocytopenia. New approaches to alimentary canal microbial suppression. Ann Intern Med, 93:358–361, 1980.

55. Malarme M, Meunier-Carpentier F, Klastersky J. Vancomycin plus gentamicin and co trimoxazole for prevention of infections in neutropenic cancer patients (a comparative, placebo-controlled pilot study). Eur J Cancer Clin Oncol, 17:1315–1322, 1981.

56. Kauffman CA, Liepman MK, Bergman AG. Trimethoprim/ sulfamethoxazole prophylaxis in neutropenic patients. Am J Med, 74:599–607, 1983.

57. Riben PD, Louie TJ, Lank BA, et al. Reduction in mortality from gram negative sepsis in neutropenic patients receiving trimethoprim/ sulfamethoxazole therapy. Cancer, 51:1587–1592, 1983.

58. Wade JC, Schimpff SC, Hargadon MT, et al. A comparison of trimethoprim/sulfamethoxazole plus nystatin with gentamicin plus nystatin in the prevention of infections in acute leukemia. N Engl J Med, 304:1057–1062, 1981.

59. Martino P, Venditti M, Concetta M, et al. Co-trimoxazole prophylaxis in patients with leukemia and prolonged granulocytopenia. Am J Med Sci, 287:7–9, 1984.

60. Weiser B, Lange M, Fialk MA, et al. Prophylactic Trimethoprim-sulfamethoxazole during consolidation chemotherapy for acute leukemia: A controlled trial. Ann Intern Med, 95:436–438, 1981.

61. Wade JC, deJongh CA, Newman KA, et al. Selective Antimicrobial modulation as prophylaxis against infection during granulocytopenia: trimethoprim-sulfamethoxazole vs. nalidixic acid. J Infect Dis, 147:624–633, 1983.

62. Dekker A. Rozenberg-Arska M, Verhoef J. Infection prophylaxis in acute leukemia: a comparison of ciprofloxacin with trimethoprim-sulfamethoxaozole and colistin. Ann Intern Med, 06:7–12, 1987.

63. Denning D, Flulle HH. Hellriegel KP. Chemoprophylaxis of bacterial infection in granulocytopenic patients. Okologie 19:57–58, 1987.

64. Shepp DH, Klosterman A, Siegel MS, et al. Comparative trial of ketoconazole and nystatin for prevention of fungal infection in neutropenic patients treated in a protective environment. J Infect Dis, 152:1257–1263, 1985.

65. Hann IM, Prentice HG, Blacklock HA, et al. Acyclovir prophylaxis against herpes virus infections in severely immunocompromised patients: randomized double blind trial. Brit Med J, 287:384–388, 1983.

66. Prentice HG. Use of acyclovir for prophylaxis of herpes infections in severely immunocompromised patients. J Antimicro Chemother, 12(Suppl B):153–159, 1983.

67. Condie RM, O'Reilly RJ. Prevention of cytomegalovirus pneumonia with high-dose intravenous, hyperimmune; native, unmodified cytomegalovirus globulin. Am J Med, 76(Suppl):134–141, 1984.

68. Winton DJ, Ho WG, Lin CH, et al. Intravenous immunoglobulin for modification of cytomegalovirus infection associated with bone marrow transplantation. Am J Med, 76(Suppl):128–133, 1984.

69. Purdy BD, Plaisance KI. Infection with the human immunodeficiency virus: Epidemiology, pathogenesis, transmission, diagnosis, and manifestations. Am J Hosp Pharm., 6:1185–1209, 1989.

70. Gualtieri RJ, Donowitz GR, Kaiser DL, et al. Double-blind randomized study of prophylactic trimethoprim/sulfumethoxazole in granulo- cytopenic patients with hematologic malignancies. Am J Med, 74:934–940, 1983.

71. Gordin FM, Simon GL, Wafsy CB, et al. Adverse reactions to t rimethoprim-sulfamethoxazole in patients with the acquired immunodeficiency syndrome. Ann Intern Med, 100:495–499, 1984.

72. Small CB, Harris CA, Friedland GH, et al. The treatment of pneumocystis carinii pneumonia in acquired immunodeficiency syn drome. Arch Intern Med, 145:837–840, 1985.

73. Nemunaitis J, Singer JW, Buckner D, Durnam D. Use of recombinant human granulocyte-macrophage colony-stimulating factor in graft failure after bone marrow transplantation. Blood, 76(1):245–253, 1990.

74. Glaspy JA, Golde DW. Granulocyte colonyy-stimulating factor: Preclinical and clinical studies. Semin Oncology, 19:386–394, 1992.

75. American Society of Clinical Oncology. American Scoiety of Clinical Oncology recommendations for the use of hematopoietic colony-stimulating factors:evidence=based, clinical practice guidelines. J Clin Oncol 1994;12:2471–2508.

76. Young LS. Prophylactic granulocytes in the neutropenic host. Ann Intern Med, 96:240–241, 1982.

77. Winston DJ, Ho WG, Gale RP. Therapeutic granulocyte transfusion for documented infections. Ann Intern Med, 97:509–519, 1982.

78. Strauss RG, Connett JE, Gale RP, et al. A controlled trial of prophylactic granulocyte transfusions during initial induction chemotherapy for acute myelogenous leukemia. N Engl J Med 305:597–603.

79. Pizzo PA. Evaluation of fever in the patient with cancer. Eur J Cancer Clin Oncol, 25(supp):9–16, 1989.

80. Pizzo PA, Robichaud KJ, Gill FA, et al. Duration of empiric antibiotic therapy in granulocytopenic patients with cancer. Am J Med, 67:194–200, 1979.

CHAPTER 76

BACTEREMIA AND SEPSIS

ALAN H. MUTNICK, STEPHEN C. BERGQUIST, and ELIZABETH A. BELTZ

Bacteremia refers to the presence of viable bacteria in the bloodstream. The presence of fungi, parasites, viruses, and other pathogens in the blood should be described in a similar fashion (fungemia, parasitemia, viremia, and so on) (1). Sepsis is a term that has been used to describe the physiologic events that take place in the body in response to an infection (2, 3). These events are triggered by either bacteria themselves or their toxic byproducts that are released into the circulation.

Bacteremia is defined as bacteria in the blood confirmed by blood cultures. Bacteremia may be low grade and transient (i.e., dental cleaning or manipulations) or high grade and constant (i.e., bacterial endocarditis). It may be associated with primary or secondary infectious processes. Nosocomial bacteremia may be associated with peripheral and central intravenous devices, intravascular hemodynamic monitoring devices, hemodialysis catheters, and total parenteral nutrition solutions.

Appropriately drawn blood cultures are crucial to the appropriate diagnosis and/or confirmation of bacteremia (as discussed later in this chapter). Choice of antimicrobial agents should be based on the clinical presentation, gram stain results, and suspected infectious source. Antimicrobial therapy may then be modified based on confirmatory blood culture results. Removal of foreign bodies such as intravascular catheters may be appropriate and should always be considered in addition to appropriate antimicrobial therapy. Duration of antibiotic therapy is determined by primary site of infection; causative organism(s), and the removability status of infected foreign bodies.

OVERVIEW

The American College of Chest Physicians/Society of Critical Care has attempted to more accurately define the term *sepsis* in order to standardize terminology used and to eliminate confusion among clinicians and researchers (4). Because of the consensus feeling that other noninfectious events can trigger a clinical response within the body, a recommendation was made to use the phrase, "Systemic Inflammatory Response Syndrome" (SIRS) as a general description for an inflammatory process, independent of its cause (4). Consequently, "sepsis" becomes a subset of SIRS and would involve those "SIRS" cases that are the result of an infectious process (Fig. 76.1).

As can be seen from Figure 76.1, patients within circle A develop an infection. The etiology of the infection could include bacteria, fungi, parasites, viruses, and so on. Many of these infections are able to exist within the bloodstream and result in bacteremias, fungemias, parasitemias, viremias, and so on. Each of these bloodstream pathogens is able to induce physiologic changes such as (1) body temperature greater than 38°C or less than 36°C; (2) heart rate greater than 90 beats per minute; (3) respiratory rate greater than 20 breaths per minute or $PaCO_2$ less than 32 torr; and (4) alterations in white blood cell count such as a white blood cell count greater than 12,000/cu mm, a count less than 4000/cu mm, or the presence of more than 10% immature white blood cells (bands) and resulting in sepsis as shown in area B. However, those infectious processes resulting in sepsis as well as those noninfectious processes (for example, burns, pancreatitis, and trauma) are able to induce physiologic changes such as (1) body temperature greater than 38°C or less than 38°C; (2) heart rate greater than 90 beats per minute; (3) respiratory rate greater than 20 breaths per minute or $PaCO_2$ less than 32 torr; and (4) alterations in white blood cell count such as a white blood cell count greater than 12,000/cu mm, a count less than 4000/cu mm, or the presence of more than 10% immature white blood cells (bands) are considered to make up circle C (1).

According to this newly proposed classification, all patients with sepsis suffer from SIRS, but the converse is not always true because other etiologic events besides sepsis contribute to the development of SIRS. As will become evident later in this chapter, confusion and inability to have consistent definitions for the various clinical entities that encompass sepsis have made it difficult to compare therapeutic modalities, develop consistency among clinical trials, and identify the incidence of this clinical entity among patient populations.

PATHOPHYSIOLOGY

The initial event believed responsible for activating the *sepsis cascade* involves the release of a toxin into the circulation (5). The form of toxin released into the circulation depends on the invading pathogen. Endotoxins are released into the circulation from select Gram-negative bacteria, whereas Gram-positive or yeast cell-wall products and viral or fungal antigens are believed to be capable of activating the sepsis cascade as well (6, 7).

After the toxin gains access to the circulation, it is able to stimulate the release of numerous mediators that

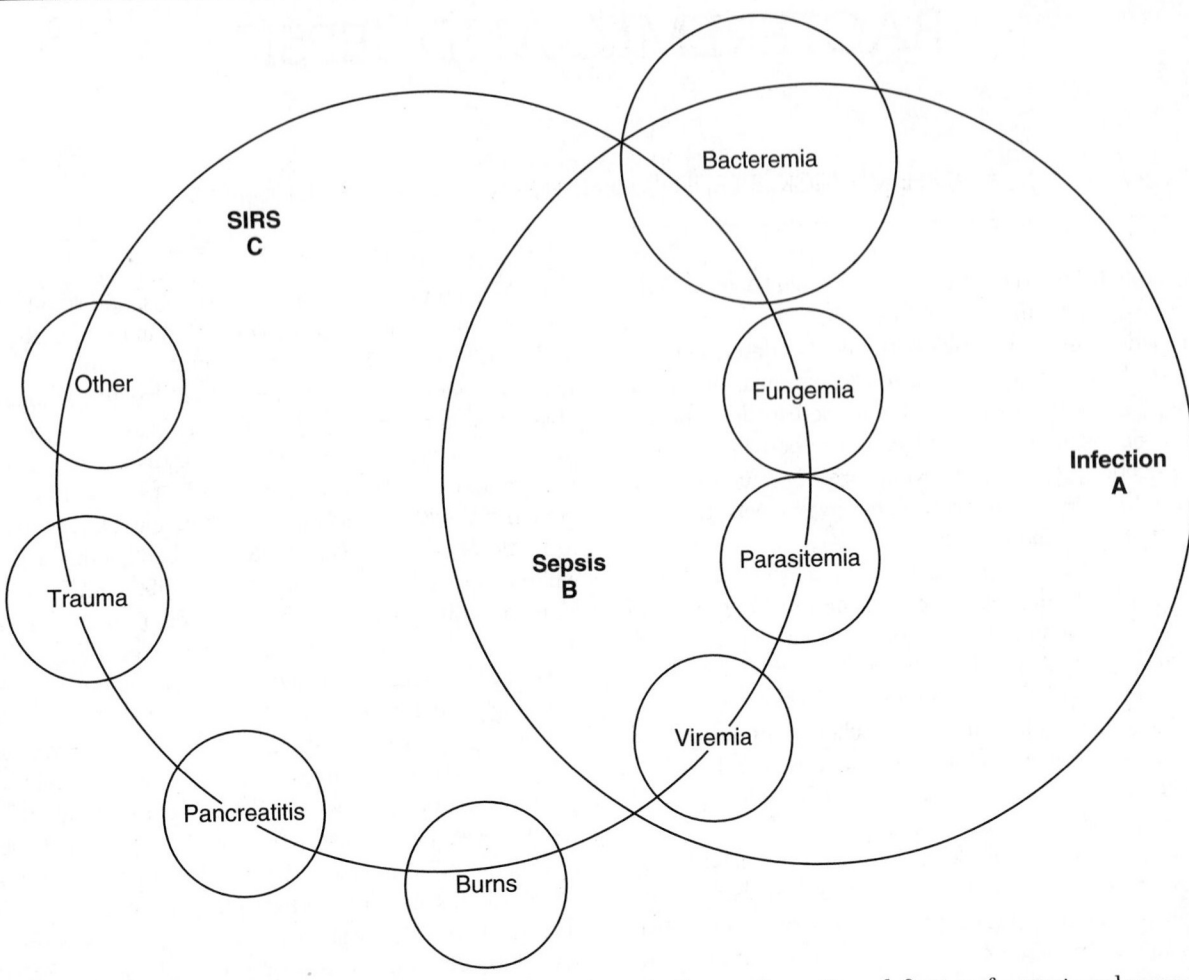

Figure 76.1. The relationship between SIRS sepsis, infection, and bacteremia. Adapted from Bone RC, Balk RA, Cerra FB, Dellinger RP, Fein AM, et al. The ACCP/SCCM Consensus Conference Committee: definitions for sepsis and organ failure and guidelines for the use of innovative therapies in sepsis. Chest 101:1644–1655, 1992.

result in endothelial damage and activation of the coagulation cascade and complement system (Fig. 76.2). As depicted in Table 76.1, each mediator released is capable of inducing various physiologic changes that depend on the specific mediator. If the body becomes unable to restore normal physiologic function, the generalized inflammatory response produces the clinical signs of sepsis. As endothelial damage continues in a specific site, sepsis evolves into **severe sepsis** (previously referred to as septic syndrome), which, if associated with systolic blood pressure less than 90 mm Hg, becomes *sepsis-induced hypotension*, which, if allowed to persist despite fluid resuscitation along with the presence of hypoperfusion abnormalities or organ dysfunction, results in *septic shock* (4).

We have attempted to oversimplify the important triggering events so that the reader can gain an appreciation for the changes occurring during the sepsis cascade. However, it would be inappropriate to assume that the process is as straightforward as our description may lead one to believe. In fact, the chemical mediators may have different effects on various organ systems and may stimulate as well as inhibit various events within the sepsis cascade. Additionally, different chemical mediators may or may not be present in significant concentrations under different septic events. Many questions still exist about the exact pathophysiologic events that take place during the sepsis process.

EPIDEMIOLOGY

As mentioned earlier, the lack of consistency in defining the clinical entities of sepsis has made it difficult to determine the true incidence of this potentially life-threatening condition. The purpose of the recently completed "Consensus Conference" was to develop a working definition for the various clinical entities and provide a framework for future clinical research, epidemiologic evaluation, and therapeutic modalities (1).

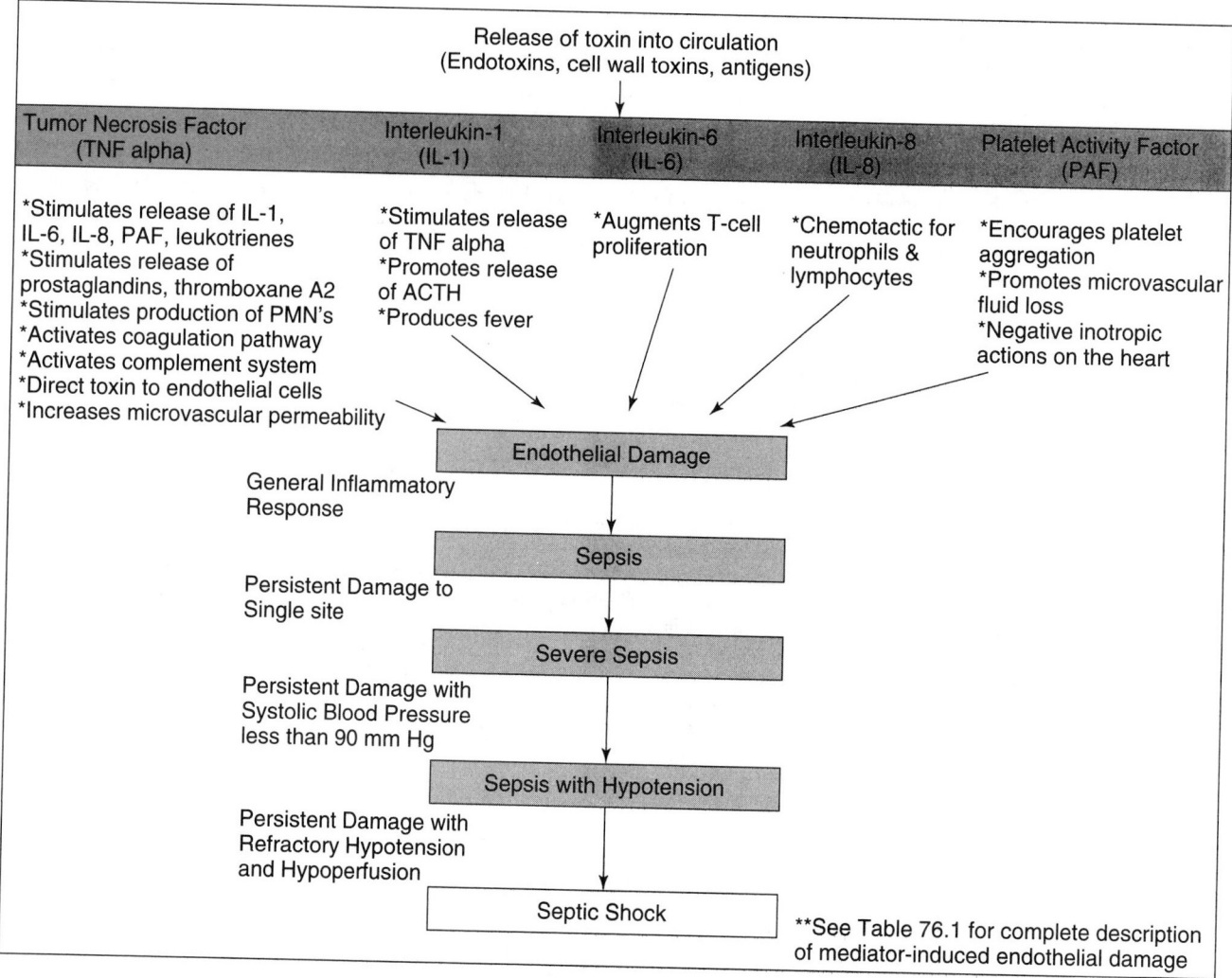

Figure 76.2. Sepsis—cascade pathway.

Recent reports from national publications reveal a significant increase of 139% in the incidence of septicemia during the years 1979 through 1987, from 73.6 to 175.9 cases per 100,000 persons (8). In this report, septicemia was considered a disease associated with the presence and persistence of pathogenic microorganisms or their toxins in the blood. Though the aforementioned incidence uses a working definition that is in close agreement to that developed by the Consensus Conference, incidences of septic shock developing in patients with septicemia have a rather large variability. Reports in the literature have suggested the development of septic shock in 17% of patients presenting initially with coagulase-negative staphylococcal infections (9), in 47% of patients with bacteremia (10), and in 30% in patients with nonbacteremias (10).

What has become clear in the literature is that the development of septic shock offers a poor prognosis, with mortality rates reported to be as high as 90% and as low as 10% (10–16). Once again, disparity in the incidents

reported may be a reflection of differences in defining the various clinical entities as sepsis.

CLINICAL MANIFESTATIONS OF SEPSIS

The clinical presentation of sepsis is not easily defined because of the numerous biologic mediators that are released in response to sepsis and their respective impact on the patient. Additionally, the duration of illness, degree of endotoxin release, and underlying comorbidities may present with differing degrees of organ dysfunction.

The recent recommendations from the American College of Chest Physicians/Society of Critical Care Medicine Consensus Conference (4) require that two or more of the following conditions must exist as a result of infection in order for a patient to be considered septic:

1. Temperature greater than 38°C or less than 36°C
2. Heart rate greater than 90 beats per minute

Table 76.1.
Select Mediators of Endothelial Damage in Sepsis and their Selected Actions[a]

Mediator	Major Effects
Tumor necrosis factor alpha (TNF alpha)	• Stimulates release of interleukin-1, interleukin-6, interleukin-8, platelet-activating factor, leukotrienes, thromboxane A_2, prostaglandins; may be able to stimulate macrophages directly to promote its own release • Has only a weak effect on T cells • Stimulates production of polymorphonuclear (PMN) cells by bone marrow; enhances phagocytic activity of PMN cells • Promotes adhesion of endothelial cells, PMN cells, eosinophils, basophils, monocytes, and occasionally, lymphocytes • Activates common pathway of coagulation and complement system • Direct toxin to vascular endothelial cells; increases microvascular permeability • Acts directly on hypothalamus to cause fever
Interleukin-1 (IL-1)	• Stimulates release of TNF alpha, interleukin-6, interleukin-8, platelet-activating factor, leukotrienes, thromboxane A_2, prostaglandins; may also be capable of stimulating its own production • Activates resting T cells to produce lymphocytes and other products; supports B-cell proliferation and antibody production; is cytotoxic for insulin-producing B cells • Promotes adhesion of endothelial cells, PMN cells, eosinophils, basophils, monocytes, and occasionally lymphocytes • Promotes PMN cell activation and accumulation • Increases endothelial precoagulant activity and endothelial release of plasminogen activator inhibitor • Acts synergistically with TNF alpha; enhances tissue cell sensitivity to TNF alpha • Promotes release of adrenocorticotropic hormone • Acts directly on hypothalamus to produce fever
Interleukin-6 (IL-6)	• Acts as a helper cell for T- and B-cell activation; interacts synergistically with IL-1 to affect thymocyte proliferation; in combination with TNF alpha, augments T-cell proliferation • Promotes PMN cell activation and accumulation
Interleukin-8 (IL-8)	• Is chemotactic for both neutrophils and lymphocytes; induces tissue infiltration of both • Inhibits endothelial–leukocyte adhesion and decreases the hyperadhesion induced by them
Platelet-activating factor (PAF)	• Stimulates release of TNF alpha, leukotrienes, thromboxane A_2 • Promotes leukocyte activation and subsequent free-radical formation • Encourages platelet aggregation leading to thrombosis • Markedly alters microvascular permeability, thereby promoting microvascular fluid loss • Stimulates calcium influx-efflux in endothelial cells; causes cells to retract and lose reciprocal contact and promotes albumin diffusion in endothelial cells • Exerts a negative inotropic effect on the heart; lowers arterial blood pressure • May attenuate effects of endotoxin on hyperglycemia and hyperlactacidemia • May cause gastrointestinal ulceration, specifically in the duodenum and jejunum • Induces blood–brain damage and vasoconstriction; may be neurotoxic
Thromboxane A_2	• Promotes release of endothelium-derived relaxing factor; may stimulate prostacyclin production • Causes platelet aggregation and neutrophil accumulation • Increases vascular permeability • Produces vasoconstricton of vascular beds and pulmonary bronchoconstriction
Leukotreine B_4	• Promotes neutrophil chemotaxis and adhesion of neutrophils to endothelium • Is weakly chemotactic for eosinophils • Increases vascular permeability
Leukotriene C_4, D_4, E_4	• Stimulate release of prostacyclin • Decrease coronary blood flow and myocardial contractility; increase pulmonary vascular resistance • Have mild vasoconstrictive effects and enhance vasoconstrictive effects of epinephrine and norepinephrine
Prostacyclin	• Inhibits platelet aggregation and adhesion • Inhibits thrombus formation; may have fibrinolytic activity • Acts synergistically with prostaglandin E_2 to increase the effects of serotonin and bradykinin on vascular permeability • Causes vasodilation and increased blood flow • Exerts beneficial effects on tissue perfusion during the early stages of sepsis • Produces smooth muscle relaxation

[a]For a more comprehensive listing of all mediators, the reader is referred to Bone RC. The pathogenesis of sepsis. Ann Int Med 115:457–469, 1991.

3. Respiratory rate greater than 20 breaths per minute or $PaCO_2$ less than 32 torr
4. White blood cell count greater than 12,000/cu mm, less than 4000/cu mm, or greater than 10% immature (band) forms

Additionally, the conference provided the following guidelines in order to differentiate the varying dynamic changes that may be associated with sepsis and its comparison to severe sepsis, septic shock, and multiple organ dysfunction syndrome:

Severe Sepsis

1. Sepsis associated with organ dysfunction, hypoperfusion, or hypotension
2. Clinical manifestations, including lactic acidosis, oliguria, or an alteration in mental status

Septic Shock

1. Sepsis with hypotension, despite adequate fluid resuscitation, along with abnormalities of inadequate perfusion, lactic acidosis, oliguria, and acute alteration in mental status

Multiple Organ Dysfunction Syndrome

1. Presence of altered organ status in an acutely ill patient so that normal homeostasis cannot be maintained

Because of the dynamic changes that occur in the patient with sepsis, the patient may present with routine findings such as fever, tachycardia, tachypnea, leukocytosis, and a "shift to the left"; there are similar findings for many other infectious as well as noninfectious processes. However, under the right conditions—poor nutritional status, debilitated or compromised host state, virulent organisms, and release of significant toxins—the patient may quickly progress to other findings suggestive of the various sequelae associated with sepsis.

In the remaining sections of this chapter, the reader will be introduced to the various clinical strategies used to reduce the morbidity and mortality associated with sepsis. However, as will become apparent during the discussion, the release of multiple chemical mediators, along with their varying effects on different organ systems, requires multiple treatment modalities in order to combat the aggressive nature of the various clinical entities associated with sepsis.

CLINICAL SYMPTOMS AND DIAGNOSIS

The clinical presentation of the sepsis syndrome can be quite variable because of the patient's underlying condition(s), particularly the presence of leukopenia. The sepsis syndrome is a dynamic process with symptoms that may progress rapidly in a given patient. The primary physical symptoms associated with bacterial etiologies of sepsis syndrome as described by Young include fever, chills, hyperventilation, hypothermia, skin lesions, and/or changes in mental status (14). Hyperventilation may precede the onset of fever and chills in many patients. The presence of skin lesions may be useful in identifying the etiology of a potential pathogen. Ecthyma gangrenosum lesions have been commonly associated with Pseudomonas aeruginosa bacteremia. Erythroderma is often seen with staphylococcal or streptococcal infections. Mental status changes could be seen in central nervous system infection or might be complicated by concomitant drug therapy.

Complications observed in the sepsis syndrome secondary to bacterial etiologies include hypotension, bleeding (disseminated intravascular coagulation (DIC)), leukopenia, thrombocytopenia, and organ failure, for example, lung (acidosis, cyanosis), kidney (oliguria, anuria, acidosis), liver (jaundice), and heart (congestive heart failure). The appearance and progression of these complications and symptoms are variable and may be influenced by under-

lying disease processes (14). The appropriate management of these complications is critical to a positive clinical outcome and will be discussed in a subsequent section of this chapter.

The presence of predisposing factors such as surgery, organ transplantation, chemotherapy, or recent trauma may assist in the diagnosis and provide clues to potential pathogens. Data on previous or current antimicrobial therapy as well as gram stain and culture results are important in defining the possible etiologic agent. Two sets of blood cultures should be drawn from different peripheral sites at the time of first clinical suspicion of bacteremia or sepsis (17). Ideally, these cultures should be performed prior to the initiation of antimicrobial therapy. Cultures of urine, sputum, and other obvious sources of infection should also be performed and sent expeditiously to the microbiology laboratory. Gram stain results for collected specimens should be available within hours of specimen collection and will be valuable in the selection of initial antimicrobial therapy. It must be noted, however, that bacteremia is present in only about 45% of patients with sepsis. Therefore, negative blood culture results should not militate against the proper clinical diagnosis and initiation of appropriate supportive therapies.

COMPLICATIONS OF SEPSIS

Adult Respiratory Syndrome (ARDS)

Adult respiratory distress syndrome (ARDS), also referred to as acute respiratory distress syndrome, is defined as acute respiratory failure characterized by increased microvascular and epithelial permeability pulmonary edema, with a major oxygenation defect and relatively normal cardiac function (18). ARDS was first described during World War I as a syndrome associated with thoracic trauma, but the first description involving nontraumatic etiologies occurred in 1967 (18).

ETIOLOGY

ARDS always occurs in the face of recognized clinical predispositions and usually occurs within the first 72 hours of insult (18, 19). These predisposing conditions may be direct insults to the lungs such as pneumonia, aspiration of gastric contents, or toxic inhalations, or they may be indirect insults, including sepsis, trauma, and pancreatitis (18–20). Sepsis is a leading cause of ARDS, and it is estimated that 30 to 40% of patients with bacterial sepsis will develop ARDS (18, 20, 21). The mortality from ARDS is reported to be 40 to 60% (19, 21, 22).

DIAGNOSIS

The diagnostic workup for ARDS includes a chest radiograph that shows a progression to diffuse, alveolar infiltrates (23). Arterial blood gas results show a hypoxemia with a ratio of PaO_2 to percentage oxygen inspired of ≤200 (18).

Invasive hemodynamic monitoring is usually necessary to distinguish ARDS from congestive heart failure (cardiogenic pulmonary edema) since the chest radiograph is similar in appearance in both circumstances (23). Because ARDS is from a noncardiogenic origin pulmonary edema, readings from a pulmonary artery catheter would be expected to show a relatively normal cardiac output with a relatively normal pulmonary capillary wedge pressure (estimating left ventricular end-diastolic pressures) (19, 24).

Pathology, usually seen only on autopsy, shows virtually airless lungs, heavy with fluid on gross examination (21). Microscopic findings vary depending on the phase of ARDS (21). Initially, alveolar spaces are filled with proteinaceous fluid and inflammatory cells (acute phase) progressing through a subacute or organizing phase with a final fibrotic phase (21).

THERAPY

Therapy of ARDS is primarily supportive aimed at maintaining homeostasis (gas exchange, organ perfusion, and aerobic metabolism) while the acute lung injury resolves. The mainstay of supportive therapy is mechanical ventilation, which is closely monitored and customized to the individual patient (19, 25). The goal is to maximize oxygenation with minimal compromise of cardiac output and minimal lung injury secondary to barotrauma and/or delivery of toxic percentages of oxygen (greater than 50%) (25).

Although ARDS is due to an increased permeability of pulmonary vasculature rather than volume overload, most physicians prefer to minimize patients' pulmonary capillary wedge pressures as much as possible while still maintaining an adequate cardiac output and blood pressure with adequate perfusion of end-organs (19, 26). Diuretics are useful, but volume status must be carefully monitored (26).

Few pharmacologic interventions have been shown to clearly offer benefit in ARDS. Large studies are lacking in the literature, but agents that have been studied and found to offer no benefit include exogenous surfactant, acetylcysteine (an antioxidant), ibuprofen, and alprostadil (19). Clinical trials involving ketoconazole and pentoxifylline require larger study groups to evaluate their role in sepsis; however, neither treatment looks promising (19). The use of corticosteroids has been a subject of great controversy in ARDS. Although studies have not found corticosteroids to be useful in the early or later phases of ARDS (27–29), and in fact, may predispose the patient to infections, these agents may be useful during the fibroproliferative stage (30, 31). Some authors recommend initiating a 1- to 2-week trial of corticosteroids 1 to 2 weeks after the onset of ARDS in patients with severe disease with no sign of improvement (19).

A promising agent is inhaled nitric oxide. Nitric oxide acts as a selective pulmonary vasodilator. Its use in neonatal pulmonary hypertension is well described. Although its use in ARDS is still under investigation, it may prove useful for patients in whom conventional maneuvers have not optimized the patient's oxygenation (19).

Antibiotics should be targeted to known infections as much as possible although empiric broad spectrum coverage is appropriate in sepsis when the etiologic agent(s) have not yet been identified. Prophylactic antibiotics have not been shown to be useful. Additionally, their use may promote antibiotic resistance (19).

RECOVERY

Recovery from ARDS may take several weeks. Supportive care and measures to prevent complications such as nosocomial pneumonia, stress ulcers, and deep vein thromboses continue to be the mainstay of therapy for patients with ARDS (19).

Disseminated Intravascular Coagulation (DIC)

Disseminated intravascular coagulation (DIC) is a common complication of sepsis and occurs when the normal balance between fibrin formation and the fibrinolytic system is disrupted. This results in the stimulation of the coagulation process and fibrin formation (32). DIC is associated with many clinical entities, including infections, trauma, and malignancy (32).

DIAGNOSIS

DIC is best diagnosed with a combination of coagulation tests (32). Because fibrinogen is converted to fibrin in DIC, fibrinogen levels are usually low, and fibrinogen degradation products are elevated (32). Plasmin generation and subsequent lysis of factors V and IX cause an increase in prothrombin time and thrombin time (32). Partial thromboplastin time is prolonged because of consumption and degradation of factors V, VIII, IX, and XI. Platelet counts are also typically low (32).

Clinically, the patient with DIC typically presents with bleeding (often profuse) accompanied by thrombotic disorders. For example, the patient may have necrosis of the skin secondary to thromboses at the same time they are bleeding profusely from puncture sites and into organs. Microvascular thrombi may lead to organ damage (32).

THERAPY

The primary treatment of DIC is to treat the underlying cause and to support the patient while healing occurs (32). Fresh frozen plasma is commonly given as necessary (32).

Although controversial, heparin (which inhibits thrombin formation) may be used in patients for whom supportive measures are inadequate. When used for DIC, heparin is given as a continuous infusion at a low dose (300 to 500 units per hour) (32). Other anticoagulants, such as warfarin, have been used unsuccessfully (32).

INITIAL APPROACH TO ANTIBIOTIC THERAPY

The initial choice of antibiotic therapy in a patient with presumed sepsis will be empiric in most instances. Selection of therapy should be based on:

1. Suspected site of infection and likely bacterial pathogen
2. Community- or hospital-acquired organism
3. Bacterial susceptibility or resistance patterns in a given hospital or community
4. Patient factors such as allergy history or presence of organ dysfunction

Antibiograms based on hospital or patient care unit-specific antibiotic susceptibilities are very useful in the initial selection of antibiotic(s). In a prospective surveillance study of 1,754 patients in 80 U.S. hospitals with sepsis syndrome, 389 Gram-negative blood isolates were identified (33). Table 76.2 summarizes the identities of these isolates. Based on this information and other published data, it would seem that the initial empiric antibiotic therapy of patients with suspected sepsis syndrome should include a combination of antibiotics to cover a wide spectrum of Gram-negative as well as Gram-positive organisms, including streptococci and staphylococci (MRSA and coagulase-negative species). Combination antibiotic therapy further affords (1) coverage for "polymicrobial" bacteremia, (2) prevention of the development of bacterial resistance by eradicating subpopulations of bacteria resistant to one of the drugs of the combination, (3) additive or synergistic bactericidal effects over that achieved with single-drug therapy.

Given the environmental and patient factors described previously, the initial empiric antibiotic therapy combination might include:

1. An extended spectrum penicillin (piperacillin, mezlocillin) or third-generation cephalosporin combined with an aminoglycoside.
2. If anaerobes are suspected (GU, trauma, or GI source), metronidazole can be added to the first combination, or a

Table 76.2.
Frequency of Gram-Negative Isolates of 1754 Patients with Sepsis Syndrome in 80 U.S. Hospitals[a]

Organism	Number of Isolates (%) (N = 389)
E. coli	155 (39.85)
Klebsiella sp	49 (12.6)
Enterobacter sp.	29 (7.46)
Pseudomonas sp.	46 (11.83)
Bacteroides sp.	11 (2.83)
Proteus sp.	15 (3.86)
Mixed	30 (7.71)
Miscellaneous	54 (13.88)

[a]Adapted from Conboy K, et al. Sepsis syndrome and associated sequelae in patients at high risk for gram-negative sepsis. Pharmacotherapy 15:66–77, 1995.

penicillinase-inhibitor beta lactam combination such as piperacillin-tazobactam or ticarcillin-clavulanate can be substituted and combined with an aminoglycoside. Imipenem can also be combined with an aminoglycoside.

3. If an indwelling intravascular catheter is a possible source, add vancomycin to the antibiotics chosen in either 1 or 2 above. (14, 34).

Antibiotics administered to treat the sepsis syndrome must always be given by intravenous routes. It is still unresolved whether intermittent or continuous intravenous administration of antibiotics is optimal. Doses of antibiotics must be modified based on the degree of hepatic and/or renal function. Initial regimens may require frequent modification because of the dynamic nature of the sepsis process. Individualization of drug therapy using pharmacokinetic models is particularly important with the aminoglycoside antibiotics. Peak aminoglycoside serum concentrations of 8 to 12 times the minimum inhibitory concentration of the bacteria have been associated with a positive clinical outcome (35). Extended interval aminoglycoside therapy may offer promise in the therapy of serious Gram-negative infections (36, 37). Its role in the therapy of the sepsis syndrome has not been clearly defined at this time. Modification of the initial antibiotic regimen may be required after culture and susceptibility data from initial blood, urine, sputum, and/or wound specimens become available.

The clinical condition of the patient may deteriorate somewhat after initial antibiotic therapy is initiated. It is thought that this may be due to release of bacterial endotoxin secondary to bactericidal effects of the antimicrobials.

The optimal duration of antibiotic therapy in the sepsis syndrome is difficult to define. It depends on a number of factors such as site of infection, bacterial organism(s), concomitant medical problems, and degree of immunocompetence. Typically, the duration of therapy should be 10 to 14 days or longer if infection persists at the primary site (14).

ADJUNCTIVE AND SUPPORTIVE THERAPIES

Aside from antibiotics, a patient with sepsis or septic shock requires prompt stabilization of respiratory and hemodynamic parameters. Stabilization of respiratory function is achieved with supplemental oxygen, close monitoring of arterial blood gases, and, if necessary, mechanical ventilation (38).

Hypotension is commonly present and should be initially treated with rapid fluid administration to raise the blood pressure and achieve adequate tissue perfusion (38). It should be noted that the institution of positive pressure mechanical ventilation will, transiently, decrease the patient's blood pressure. This transient hypotension usually responds to fluids. If fluid administration does not achieve the desired effects or if the patient develops signs of fluid

Table 76.3.
Vasoactive Drugs Used in Sepsis

Drug	Dose[a]	Receptor Activity
Dopamine	2–20 mcg/kg/min	Dopaminergic, Alpha, Beta
Norepinephrine	2 mcg/min and titrate	Alpha, Beta
Epinephrine	0.05–0.2 mcg/kg/min	Alpha, Beta
Phenylephrine	20–200 mcg/min	Alpha-1
Dobutamine	2–15 mcg/kg/min	Beta-1

[a]Dosage guidelines only. Must be titrated to desired effect.

overload, a sympathomimetic agent should be used (38). Dopamine is the agent initially used in most cases. At low doses (2 to 5 mcg/kg/min), dopamine acts on the dopaminergic receptors, increasing renal blood flow (39). At higher doses (5 to 10 mcg/kg/min), beta receptors are stimulated to a greater degree than alpha receptors, whereas at doses greater than 10 mcg/kg/min, the effect is primarily on alpha receptors, causing an increased systemic vascular resistance (39). At this point, dopamine has essentially the same effects as norepinephrine. When either agent is used, it should be titrated to achieve an adequate blood pressure to maintain tissue perfusion. Other agents (Table 76.3) may also be used to increase blood pressure.

Keep in mind that as the vasoconstrictor effects increase, blood flow is decreased to many organs, including the kidneys, liver, and gastrointestinal tract. Therefore, the minimal dose necessary to maintain an adequate blood pressure should be employed. In some cases, dobutamine may be employed to increase myocardial contractility and cardiac output.

Hemodynamic parameters are usually monitored by invasive means in the critically ill septic patient. This may involve the placement of an arterial line to provide continuous blood pressure monitoring and placement of a pulmonary artery catheter to monitor fluid status and cardiac output (38).

The use of corticosteroids as adjunctive therapy in sepsis has been well studied. Two recent placebo-controlled trials demonstrated no reduction in mortality (13, 29). In fact, a higher mortality rate was seen in the corticosteroid group that was attributed to secondary infections. Therefore, the use of corticosteroids is not recommended as adjunctive therapy for sepsis.

IMMUNOTHERAPY OF SEPSIS

Even with appropriate antibiotic therapy and other adjunctive therapies, sepsis may progress to shock, cellular damage, and the death of the patient. The core endotoxin components of the cell wall of Gram-negative bacteria act as messengers or signals for macrophages to release biologically active "triggers" such as tumor necrosis factor (TNF) and other cytokines as detailed earlier in this chapter. These cytokines produce many of the manifestations of sepsis syndrome, including hypothermia, tachypnea, tachycardia, and organ dysfunction. Blocking or modification of the actions of endotoxin and/or these cytokines may provide the ability to augment or blunt the physiologic and pathologic manifestations of sepsis and its sequelae. It is thought that early clinical interventions with these treatment modalities might save lives in septic patients.

Ziegler and colleagues conducted a study using human antiserum to endotoxin produced by E. coli J5 (J5 antiserum) in bacteremic patients. Deaths due to sepsis were reduced 22% compared to the control group (39%). In patients with profound shock, mortality was reduced 44% compared to controls (77%) (40). This study provided the first clinical evidence that augmentation of endotoxin effect might improve patient outcome in Gram-negative bacteremia and shock. Prophylactic administration of J5 antiserum in high-risk surgical patients improved outcome in infected patients in a later study (41). Although these early results were promising, widespread use of antiendotoxin antiserum is not feasible because of the large number of volunteers needed in order to generate the antiserum. Additionally, the risk of disease transmission as well as lack of predictable interlot consistency in potency militate against common clinical application. The application of monoclonal antibody technology avoids some of these problems and has led to the development of monoclonal antibodies directed against endotoxin and tumor necrosis factor (TNF-alpha) (42–46).

Two large randomized controlled trials were conducted to evaluate the use of human monoclonal antiendotoxin antibody (HA1A) and murine monoclonal antiendotoxin antibody (E5) in the treatment of Gram-negative sepsis and shock. Ziegler and colleagues conducted a randomized double-blind trial involving 543 patients with sepsis. Patients were randomized to be treated with HA1A or placebo. Two hundred (37%) patients had Gram-negative bacteremia proven by blood cultures. Forty-nine percent of patients with Gram-negative bacteremia receiving placebo died. Thirty percent of patients receiving HA1A died. In the 196 patients with Gram-negative bacteremia who were followed to hospital discharge or death, 45 of 93 (48%) given placebo were discharged alive compared to 65 of 103 (63%) of patients treated with HA1A (47).

Greenman and colleagues conducted a prospective, randomized, double-blind, placebo-controlled trial of E5 in 486 patients with Gram-negative sepsis. A total of 316 patients had confirmed Gram-negative sepsis. Administration of E5 resulted in significantly greater survival in patients with Gram-negative sepsis without shock. Resolution of organ failure was more frequent in these patients, with 19 of 35 (54%) receiving E5 compared to 8 of 27 (30%) in the placebo group (48).

Critical review and analysis of these studies by the scientific community produced much controversy and debate (49). The widespread use of these agents in patients with Gram-negative bacteremia was associated with certain dilemmas (50):

1. Which patients should be treated?
2. Which products should be used?
3. Must these agents be used in suspected Gram-negative bacteremia?
4. Can a patient be retreated if necessary?

The projected high cost of these agents ($4000 per treatment course of HA1A and annual costs of $1.3 to $2.3 billion) mandated further evaluation and scrutiny of the routine use of these agents in all patients with suspected Gram-negative bacteremias (51).

Development of hospital-specific as well as general guidelines for patient selection and use occurred prior to the anticipated FDA approval in 1992 in an attempt to assure rational cost-effective use (52). Recent trials of HA1A and E5 have shown that these agents have no effect on patient mortality (53, 54). Because of questions of study design and other factors, the FDA approval has not occurred at the time of this writing. Continuing clinical trials with these agents are in progress.

Tumor necrosis factor-alpha (TNF-alpha) appears to have a central role in the release of cytokines that cause the pathophysiologic changes associated with the sepsis syndrome and other inflammatory conditions (55, 56). Its nomenclature is based on its early use in oncologic studies. Injection of endotoxin induces a rise in TNF concentrations, which is associated with onset of chills, headache, fever, and tachycardia. Elevated TNF levels have been associated with adverse outcomes in sepsis (57). Antibodies to TNF-alpha might, therefore, provide an effective treatment modality for the sepsis syndrome (58).

A large multicenter prospective trial of monoclonal antibody to human tumor necrosis factor-alpha (TNF-alpha MAb) versus placebo in 994 patients was performed. Septic patients with shock (N = 478) demonstrated a trend toward a reduction in all-cause mortality at 3 days after infusion. There was no significant difference in all-cause mortality between patients who received TNF-alpha MAb and those who received placebo. Serious adverse effects were reported in 4.6% of treated patients (59). Further studies will likely focus on the subset of patients with sepsis syndrome and shock.

Further clinical studies will need to be performed to evaluate the role of specific monoclonal antibodies in the treatment of sepsis. Recently, soluble interleukin-1 (IL-1) receptor and IL-1 receptor antagonists have shown promise in animals and in human phase II trials. These products of technology show much promise, but they must be used in a focused, cost-effective manner if they are to become available in the future.

CONCLUSION

The successful management of sepsis with its attendant high mortality relies on early clinical suspicion and rapid diagnosis. Use of traditional treatment modalities such as prompt fluid resuscitation and early institution of broad spectrum antibiotic therapy, including ventilatory and blood pressure support, are fundamental to the clinical management of this syndrome. Because of the rapid decline in organ function, prompt modifications of drug dosing and application of therapeutic drug monitoring to patient management are required. The optimal cost-effective application of newer technology such as the use of monoclonal antibodies is awaiting further results of ongoing clinical trials. Only through continued research and the proper application of the results to the management of the septic patient can the overall outcome of this syndrome be improved.

REFERENCES

1. Bone RC, Balk RA, Cerra FB, Dellinger RP, Fein AM, et al. The ACCP/SCCM Consensus Conference Committee: definitions for sepsis and organ failure and guidelines for the use of innovative therapies in sepsis. Chest 101:1644–1655, 1992.
2. Balk RA, Bone RC. The septic syndrome: definition and clinical implications. Crit Care Clin 5:1–8, 1989.
3. Ayres SM. SCCM's new horizons conference on sepsis and septic shock. Crit Care Med 13:864–866, 1985.
4. Members of the American College of Chest Physicians/Society of Critical Care Medicine Consensus Conference Committee. Definitions for sepsis and organ failure and guidelines for the use of innovative therapies in sepsis. Crit Care Med 20:864–874, 1992.
5. Bone RC. The pathogenesis of sepsis. Ann Int Med 115:457–469, 1991.
6. Tracey KJ, Lowry SF, Cerami A. Cachectin/TNF-alpha in septic shock and septic adult respiratory distress syndrome (editorial). Am Rev Resp Dis 138:1377–1379, 1988.
7. Fong Y, Lowry SF, Cerami A. Cachectin/TNF: a macrophage protein that induces cachexia and shock. J Parenter Enterol Nutr 12:72S–77S, 1988.
8. Increase in national Hospital Discharge Survey rates for septicemia— United States. 1979-1987. MMWR 39:31–34.
9. Martin MA, Pfaller MA, Wenzel RP. Coagulase-negative staphylococcal bacteremia. Ann Intern Med 110:9–16, 1989.
10. Bone RC, Fisher CJ Jr, Clemmer TP, Slotman GH, Metz CA, et al. Sepsis syndrome: a valid clinical entity. Crit Care Med 17:389–393, 1989.
11. Tran DD, Groeneveld AB, van der Meulen J, Nauta JJ, Strack van Schijndel RJ, et al. Age, chronic disease, sepsis, organ system failure, and mortality in a medical intensive care unit Crit Care Med 18:474–479, 1990.
12. Dunn DL. Immunotherapeutic advances in the treatment of gram negative bacterial sepsis. World J Surg 11:233–240, 1987.
13. The Veteran's Administration Systemic Sepsis Comparative Study Group. Effect of high-dose glucocorticoid therapy on mortality in patients with clinical signs of systemic sepsis. N Engl J Med 317:659–665, 1987.

14. Young LS. Gram-negative sepsis. In: Mandell GL, Douglas RG, Bennett JE, eds. Principles and Practice of Infectious Diseases, 3rd ed. New York: Churchill Livingstone, 1990:611–636.

15. Sprung CL, Caralis PV, Marcial EH, Pierce M, Gelbard MA, et al. The effects of high-dose corticosteroids in patients with septic shock. A prospective, controlled study. N Engl J Med 311:1137–1143, 1984.

16. Parker MM, Parillo JE. Septic shock: hemodynamics and pathogenesis. JAMA 250:3324–3327, 1983.

17. Chandrasekar PH, Brown WJ. Clinical issues of blood cultures. Arch Int Med 154:841–849, 1994.

18. Hyers TM. Prediction of survival and mortality in patients with adult respiratory distress syndrome. New Horizon 1:466–470, 1993.

19. Kollef MH, Shuster DP. The acute respiratory distress syndrome. N Eng J Med 332:27–37, 1995.

20. Fowler AA, Hamman RF, Good JT Jr, et al. Adult respiratory distress syndrome: risk with common predispositions. Ann Int Med 98:593–597, 1983.

21. Goldsberry DT, Hurst JM. Adult respiratory distress syndrome and sepsis. New Horizon 1:342–347, 1993.

22. Suchyta MR, Clemmer TP, Elliott CO, et al. The adult respiratory distress syndrome: a report of survival and modifying factors. Chest 101:1074–1079, 1992.

23. Wheeler AP, Carroll FE, Bernard GR. Radiographic issues in adult respiratory distress syndrome. New Horizon 1:471–477, 1993.

24. Parrillo JE, Parker NM, Natanson C, et al. Septic shock in humans: advances in the understanding of pathogenesis, cardiovascular dysfunction, and therapy. Ann Int Med 113:227–242, 1990.

25. Marini JJ. New options for the ventilatory management of acute lung injury. New Horizon 1:489–503, 1993.

26. Shuster DP. The case for and against fluid restriction and occlusion pressure reduction in adult respiratory distress syndrome. New Horizon 1993;1:478–488.

27. Bernard GR, Luce JM, Sprung CL, et al. High-dose corticosteroids in patients with the adult respiratory distress syndrome. N Engl J Med 317:1565–1570, 1987.

28. Luce JM, Montgomery AM, Marks JD, et al. Ineffectiveness of high-dose methylprednisolone in preventing parenchymal lung injury and improving mortality in patients with septic shock. Am Rev Resp Dis 138:62–68, 1988.

29. Bone RC, Fisher CJ Jr, Clanner TP, et al. Early methylprednisolone treatment for septic syndrome and the adult respiratory distress syndrome. Chest 92:1032–1036, 1987.

30. Hooper RG, Kearl RA. Established ARDS treated with a sustained course of adrenocorticosteroids. Chest 97:138–143, 1990.

31. Meduri GU, Belenchia JM, Estes RJ, et al. Fibroproliferative phase of ARDS: clinical findings and effects of corticosteroids. Chest 100:943–952, 1991.

32. ten Cate H, Brandjes DPM, Wolters HJ, et al. Disseminated intravascular coagulation: pathophysiology, diagnosis, and treatment. New Horizon 1:312–323, 1993.

33. Conboy K, Welage LS, Walawander CA, et al. Sepsis syndrome and associated sequelae in patients at high risk for gram-negative sepsis. Pharmacotherapy 15:66–77, 1995.

34. Conte JE Jr. Empiric antibiotic therapy. In: Manual of Antibiotics and Infectious Diseases, 8th ed. Baltimore: Williams and Wilkins, 1995: 54–61.

35. Moore RD, Lietman PS, Smith CR. Clinical response to aminoglycoside therapy: importance of the ratio of peak concentration to minimal inhibitory concentration. J Infect Dis 155:98–99, 1987.

36. Marik PE, Lipman J, Kobillski S, et al. A prospective randomized study comparing once versus twice-daily amikacin dosing in critically ill adult and pediatric patients. J Antimicrob Chemother 28:753–764, 1991.

37. Nicolau DP, Freeman CD, Belliveau PP, et al. Experience with a once-daily aminoglycoside program administered to 2,184 adult patients. Antimicrob Agents Chemother 39:650–655, 1995.

38. Light RB. Septic shock. In: Principles of Critical Care. New York: McGraw-Hill, 1992:1172–1185.

39. Complete prescribing information, Intropin® (dopamine HCl injection). August 1992.

40. Ziegler EJ, McCutchan JA, Fierer J, et al. Treatment of gram-negative bacteremia and shock with human antiserum to a mutant escherichia coli. N Engl J Med 307:1225–1230, 1982.

41. Baumgartner J-D, Glauser MP, McCutchan JA, et al. Prevention of gram-negative shock and death in surgical patients by antibody to endotoxin core glycolipid. Lancet 2:59–63, 1985.

42. Chmel H. Role of monoclonal antibody therapy in the treatment of infectious disease. Am J Hosp Pharm 47(suppl 3):S11–S15, 1990.

43. Wenzel RP. Anti-endotoxin monoclonal antibodies—a second look. N Engl J Med 326:1151–1152, 1992.

44. Zarowtiz BJ. Human monoclonal antibody against endotoxin. Ann Pharmacother 25:778–783, 1991.

45. Olsen KM, Campbell GD. E5 monoclonal immunoglobulin M antibody for the treatment of gram-negative sepsis. Ann Pharmacother 25:784–790, 1991.

46. Pennington JE. Therapy with antibody to tumor necrosis factor in sepsis. Clin Infect Dis 17(suppl 2):S515–S519, 1993.

47. Ziegler EJ, Fisher CJ, Sprung CL, et al. Treatment of gram-negative bacteremia and septic shock with HA-1A human monoclonal antibody against endotoxin. N Engl J Med 324:428–436, 1991.

48. Greenman RL, Schein RMH, Martin MA, et al. A controlled clinical trial of E5 murine monoclonal IgM antibody to endotoxin in the treatment of gram-negative sepsis. JAMA 266(8):1097–1102, 1991.

49. Warren HS, Danner RL, Munford RS. Antiendotoxin monoclonal antibodies. N Engl J Med 326:1153–1156, 1992.

50. Bone RC. Monoclonal antibodies to endotoxin: new allies against sepsis? JAMA 266(8):1125–1126, 1991.

51. Schulman KA, Glick HA, Rubin H, et al. Cost-effectiveness of HA-1A monoclonal antibody for gram-negative sepsis. JAMA 266(24):3466–3471, 1991.

52. Wenzel RP, Andriole VT, Bartlett JG, et al. Antiendotoxin monoclonal antibodies for gram-negative sepsis: guidelines from the IDSA. Clin Infect Dis 14:973–976, 1992.

53. Bone RC, Balk RA, Fein AM, et al. A second large controlled clinical study of E5, a monoclonal antibody to endotoxin: results of a prospective, multicenter, randomize, controlled trial. Crit Care Med 23:994–1009, 1995.

54. McCloskey RV, Straube RC, Sanders C, et al. Treatment of septic shock with human monoclonal antibody HA1A. Ann Intern Med 121:1–5, 1994.

55. Beutler B, Cerami A. Cachectin: more than a tumor necrosis factor. N Engl J Med 316:379–384, 1987.

56. Michie HR, Spriggs DR, Manoque KR, et al. Tumor necrosis factor and endotoxin induce similar metabolic responses in human beings. Surgery 104:280–286, 1988.

57. Casey LC, Balk RA, Bone RC. Plasma cytokine and endotoxin levels correlate with survival in patients with the sepsis syndrome. Ann Int Med 119:771–788, 1993.

58. Dinarello CA, Gelfand JA, Wolff SM. Anticytokine strategies in the treatment of the systemic inflammatory response syndrome. JAMA 269(14):1829–1835, 1993.

59. Abraham E, Wunderink R, Silverman H, et al. Efficacy and safety of monoclonal antibody to human tumor necrosis factor alpha in patients with sepsis syndrome. JAMA 273(12):934–941, 1995.

CHAPTER 77

SKIN AND SOFT TISSUE INFECTIONS

JEANNE HAWKINS VAN TYLE and NEETA BAHAL O'MARA

SKIN AND SOFT TISSUE INFECTIONS

Bacteria normally colonize the skin without causing infection. Normal skin flora include a variety of aerobic and anaerobic bacteria and fungi (Table 77.1). The body's best defense against bacterial infection is an intact skin barrier. A variety of bacterial infections of the skin may occur (Table 77.2). Infections may be primary or secondary. The common etiologic agents and empiric treatment options will vary depending on the infection, as summarized in Table 77.2. This chapter will discuss a number of the more common skin infections, including cellulitis, impetigo, erysipelas, periorbital cellulitis, decubitus ulcers, and diabetic foot ulcers.

Cellulitis is defined as an acute, spreading infection of the skin and subcutaneous tissues (1). It may occur when the barrier is broken, as in a cut, bite, or abrasion. Other etiologies of cellulitis include a focus such as osteomyelitis causing contiguous spread or through the blood (hematogenous spread). While cellulitis may affect patients of all ages, more than one-half of patients who develop cellulitis have an underlying condition such as drug or alcohol abuse, obesity, diabetes mellitus, peripheral vascular disease or preexisting edema (2).

Although any organism may cause cellulitis, the most common bacterial causes are group A streptococci and *Staphylococcus* species (1). In addition, in certain populations, other organisms are prevalent (Table 77.3). For example, patients with diabetes may develop cellulitis caused by multiple organisms including Gram-negative organisms and anaerobic organisms (see the section entitled "Diabetic Foot Infections"). *Haemophilus influenzae* was considered a common pathogen in children before the introduction of the *Haemophilus influenzae* vaccine.

Cellulitis most commonly affects the head, neck, and upper and lower extremities. The most common signs and symptoms associated with cellulitis include pain, tenderness, erythema, swelling, and warmth at the site of infection (2). Less frequently, patients will have lymphangitis (streaks of erythema spreading from the area of cellulitis) and enlarged and tender lymph nodes. Some patients may experience a prodrome, which may include chills, malaise, anorexia, nausea, and vomiting (2). Fever and elevation in white blood cell count may occur in some patients but are not present in all.

Diagnosis of the pathogenic organism by needle aspiration of the infected area may provide identification in up to 60% of the cases (3), but other investigators report lower yields (4, 5). In general, needle aspiration and cultures of the infected area are unnecessary in uncomplicated cases, since empiric therapy is effective in the majority of cases (6). Cultures should be considered (a) if the infection is considered complex; (b) if there is an increased risk of complications, such as in very young or elderly patients, in patients with diabetes or peripheral vascular disease, or in immunosuppressed patients; and (c) for those who have failed a standard course of antibiotics (7, 8).

TREATMENT

Nonpharmacologic therapy of cellulitis consists of rest and elevation of the affected area, analgesics, and the application of moist heat. Moist heat is preferred to minimize edema around the infected site (8) and to promote suppuration and drainage (9). Surgery may be necessary if an abscess is present. Depending on the severity, extent, and location of the infection, the patient may be treated with oral antibiotics as an outpatient or as an inpatient using intravenous antibiotics. Patients with deep infections of the hand, orbital or facial cellulitis, or deep human or animal bites and patients who are seriously ill are often hospitalized and treated initially with parenteral antibiotics. Following improvement, patients may complete therapy with oral antibiotics.

Choosing the best antibiotic for the treatment of cellulitis is based on a number of factors, including the most likely causative organism, penetration of the antibiotic to the site of infection, current medications, medication allergies, patient compliance, and cost. The most likely organism may vary depending on the age of the patient and concomitant diseases such as diabetes mellitus or human immunodeficiency virus (HIV) infection (Table 77.3). Commonly used outpatient antibiotic regimens in the treatment of uncomplicated cellulitis are provided in Table 77.4.

Empiric therapy of uncomplicated cellulitis should be effective against *Streptococcus* and *Staphylococcus* species. Table 77.4 summarizes commonly used outpatient antibiotic regimens in the treatment of uncomplicated cellulitis. While penicillin or erythromycin therapy is effective against streptococci, they do not reliably treat β-lactamase-producing staphylococci. Therefore, oral therapy with a β-lactamase-stable penicillin such as dicloxacillin or a cephalosporin such as cephalexin is preferred until the causative agent is identified. If intravenous therapy is indicated, empiric therapy with a β-lactamase-stable penicillin such as nafcillin or oxacillin or a first-generation cephalosporin such as cefazolin may be used. For patients who reside in a nursing home or who have been hospitalized for a prolonged period of time, methicillin-resistant *Staphylococcus aureus* (MRSA) should be considered, and vancomycin therapy may be necessary until culture and sensitivity results are known.

Once the causative organism is known, therapy may be tailored to provide the most appropriate antibiotic for the organism that is identified. If streptococci are identified as the causative organism, oral penicillin VK (250 to 500 mg four times a day) or intravenous penicillin G (1,000,000 to 2,000,000 units every 4 to 6 hr) may be used. Oral erythromycin (250 to 500 mg four times a day) and intravenous erythromycin (500 mg every 6 hr) are suitable alternatives for a patient who is allergic to penicillins and cephalosporins. If MRSA is identified, intravenous vancomycin should be used.

A variety of the newer intravenous antibiotics have been evaluated in the treatment of cellulitis. A number of investigators have evaluated the use of ceftriaxone (Rocephin) for pediatric and adult patients with cellulitis (10). Advantages cited include activity against the most common pathogens associated with cellulitis and the ability to administer once daily while maintaining sustained tissue concentrations above the mean inhibitory concentration for the common pathogens. Ampicillin-sulbactam (11) (Unasyn) and ticarcillin-clavulanate (12) (Timentin),

Table 77.1.
Microorganisms Commonly Found on the Human Skin (Normal Flora)

Bacteria
  Staphylococcus epidermidis[a]
  Diphtheroids
    Corynebacterium spp.[a]
    Propionibacterium acnes[a]
  Staphylococcus aureus
  Streptococcus species
    Streptococcus pyogenes
  Peptococci
  Mycobacterium spp.
  Bacillus spp.
Fungi
  Malassezia furfur[a]
  Candida spp.

[a]Most frequent organisms.

Table 77.2.
Common Bacterial Infections of the Skin

Lesion	Common Etiologic Agents	Treatment Options
Primary infections		
Cellulitis	Group A streptococcus, *Staphylococcus aureus*	Oral 1st-generation cephalosporin, azithromycin,[a] clarithromycin[b]
Impetigo	Group A streptococcus, *Staphylococcus aureus*	Oral 1st- or 2nd-generation cephalosporin, AM/CL, azithromycin,[a] clarithromycin, mupirocin
Erysipelas	Group A streptococcus	PRSP or cefazolin
Periorbital cellulitis	Group A streptococcus, *Staphylococcus aureus*, Enterobacteriaceae	Parenteral 1st-generation cephalosporin; PRSP; TC/CL; AM/SB; 2nd/3rd-generation parenteral cephalosporin
Secondary infections		
Chronic ulcers (decubitus)	Polymicrobic, may include: Coliform bacteria, Peptostreptococci, Enterococci, *Bacteroides* spp, *Proteus* spp., *Clostridium perfringens*, *Pseudomonas aeruginosa*	Cefoxitin + APAG Imipenem + cilastatin TC/CL PIP/TZ CIP + clindamycin
Diabetic foot ulcers	Polymicrobic, may include: *Staphylococcus aureus*, *Bacteroides fragilis*, *Clostridium perfringens*, *Pseudomonas aeruginosa*, Peptostreptococci, Enterococci, *Proteus* spp.	Cefoxitin + APAG Imipenem + cilastatin TC/CL PIP/TZ CIP + clindamycin

[a]FDA-approved indication.
[b]Unlabeled use.
AM/CL = amoxicillin + clavulanate.
PRSP = penicillinase-resistant synthetic penicillin.
APAG = antipseudomonal aminoglycoside.
CIP = ciprofloxacin.
AM/SM = ampicillin + sulbactam.
TC/CL = ticarcillin + clavulanate.
PIP/TZ = piperacillin + tazobactam.

β-lactamase-stable penicillins, have also been used successfully in the treatment of cellulitis infections. While many of the newer agents have demonstrated efficacy equivalent to that of traditional therapies of cellulitis, cost is generally higher and should be considered in selecting these newer agents. In addition, the antibiotic that is most active against the causative agent and has the narrowest spectrum should be chosen, so as not to promote the development of antimicrobial resistance.

Fluoroquinolones such as ciprofloxacin (Cipro) should be used cautiously in the treatment of cellulitis. While the fluoroquinolones possess excellent activity against Gram-negative bacteria, the efficacy against streptococci and staphylococci is equivocal. The emergence of ciprofloxacin-resistant *S. aureus* has been noted, especially in areas where fluoroquinolones are widely used (13, 14). To reduce the spread of resistance, the overuse of the fluoroquinolones should be avoided.

In patients who may have Gram-negative organisms (diabetic patients, patients experiencing prolonged hospitalization, and immunocompromised patients), empiric therapy should be broadened to include the likely pathogens. Typically, an aminoglycoside such as gentamicin or tobramycin may be added to a penicillin or cephalosporin. If anaerobic organisms are suspected, the antibiotic regimen should include clindamycin or metronidazole. Another alternative is the use of a penicillin (ampicillin-sulbactam, ticarcillin-clavulanate) or a cephalosporin (cefoxitin, cefotetan) that has activity against anaerobic organisms (12).

IMPETIGO

Impetigo is one of the most common, contagious, superficial bacterial skin infections and occurs predominantly in children. Initially, impetigo presents as vesicles that become pustules that rupture to form honey-crusted lesions. The most common causative organism is group A streptococci, although *S. aureus* may be present. It is unclear whether *S. aureus* is a primary cause or represents a secondary invader of the infected site.

Treatment

The most effective therapy of impetigo is controversial (15). Although some investigators claim that systemic therapy is necessary, others argue that topical therapy is sufficient. Penicillin therapy has long been considered the drug of choice (1). This, however, is being questioned. In one study, only 53% of patients responded to oral penicillin V therapy, while cloxacillin therapy was effective in 100% (16). Consequently, therapy with a β-lactamase-resistant antibiotic (cloxacillin, dicloxacillin, cephalexin, cefuroxime axetil, cefadroxil, amoxicillin-clavulanic acid, or erythromycin) may be preferred (17–19). Erythromycin therapy should be avoided in geographical areas where there is a high rate of erythromycin-resistant *S. aureus*.

Table 77.3.
Common Microorganism Causing Cellulitis in Specific Populations

Normal healthy population	Group A streptococci, *Staphylococcus aureus*
Children	Group A streptococci, *Staphylococcus* spp., *Hemophilus influenza*
Diabetic patients	*Staphylococcus* spp., *Streptococcus* spp., Gram-negative organisms, anaerobic organisms
Hospitalized patients (10)	*Staphylococcus* spp. (including coagulase negative staphylococci), *Streptococcus* spp., Gram-negative organisms (*Haemophilus* spp., *E. coli*, Klebsiella)

Table 77.4.
Commonly Used Outpatient Antibiotic Regimens in the Treatment of Uncomplicated Cellulitis

Generic Name	Brand Name	Adult Dose	Pediatric Dose
Penicillin antibiotics			
Penicillin V	Pen-Vee K, V-Cillin K, others	250–500 mg q6–8	15–62.5 mg/kg/day divided q6–8
Dicloxacillin	Dynapen, Pathocil, others	125–250 mg q6	12–25 mg/kg/day divided q6*
Amoxicillin-clavulanate	Augmentin	250–500 mg (of amoxicillin) q8	20–40 mg/kg/day (of amoxicillin) divided q8h
1st-generation cephalosporin antibiotics			
Cephalexin	Keflex, Keftabs, others	250–500 mg q6–12	25–50 mg/kg/day divided q6–12
Cefadroxil	Duricef, Ultracef	1 g as single dose or divided q12	30 mg/kg/day divided q12
Cephradine	Velosef	250–500 mg q6–12	25–50 mg/kg/day divided q6–12
Macrolide antibiotics			
Erythromycin	ERYC, Ery-Tab, EES, others	250–500 mg q6	30–50 mg/kg/day divided q6
Clarithromycin	Biaxin	250 mg q12	15 mg/kg/day divided q12
Azithromycin	Zithromax	500 mg then 250 mg q.d.	N/A
Others			
Clindamycin	Cleocin, others	150–450 mg q6	20–30 mg/kg/day divided q6

*Dosing of dicloxacillin. According to AHFS, the pediatric dose for skin and skin structure infections is 12.5 mg/kg (25 mg/kg is the dose for mild to moderate and systemic infections).

Mupirocin ointment (Bactroban), a topical antibiotic, has activity against Gram-positive organisms including group A streptococci and *S. aureus*. It is applied as a 2% ointment to the affected area two or three times daily. A number of studies (17, 20–23) comparing oral erythromycin to topical mupirocin have supported the efficacy of topical mupirocin. Consequently, topical mupirocin may be the treatment of choice for patients whose lesions are not widespread (17). Regardless of the agent used, impetigo should respond to treatment within 7 days. If no improvement is seen, antimicrobial resistance or noncompliance with the prescribed regimen should be considered.

ERYSIPELAS

Erysipelas is a skin infection that presents with the acute onset of a fiery red rash, hence the nickname "St Anthony's fire." The rash typically occurs in the lower extremities but may also occur on the face or ears (24). It affects people of all ages but appears to be more prevalent in neonates, infants, and the elderly. The most common etiology is group A streptococci, but other streptococcus species, *Haemophilus influenzae*, and staphylococci have been implicated. Bacteria enter through a break in the skin such as a scratch, cut, or lesion such as that from chickenpox (9). Patients often develop blisters and malaise, myalgia, chills, fever, nausea, and vomiting. Diagnosis is made by inspection of the rash and on clinical appearance.

Treatment

While nonpharmacologic therapy (bed rest, elevation of the affected area, and cool, moist dressings) is helpful, antibiotic therapy is the mainstay of therapy. Without antibiotics the mortality rate may be as high as 80% in neonates (25). Penicillin is the drug of choice. It may be administered orally or intravenously, depending on the severity of the infection. Other agents that may be used include ampicillin, amoxicillin, erythromycin, clindamycin, and cephalosporins such as cefazolin, cephalexin, cephadroxil, cefuroxime axetil, or cefaclor (9, 26). In nonimmunized children, empiric therapy with a second-generation cephalosporin such as cefaclor, cefuroxime axetil, or cephradine may be necessary to ensure adequate treatment for *H. influenzae* in addition to streptococci (9).

PERIORBITAL CELLULITIS

Periorbital cellulitis is an infection that most commonly affects infants and children. Periorbital cellulitis involves the superficial area around the eye and may represent a medical emergency. The eyelid is edematous, erythematous, warm, and tender. In addition, fever and leukocytosis are present (27).

Periorbital cellulitis is often preceded by an upper respiratory tract infection, sinusitis, or conjunctivitis. At other times, it may follow trauma such as a scratch, abrasion, or insect bite (28). The most common causative organisms include staphylococcus species, streptococcus species, and *Haemophilus influenzae*. The incidence of *H. influenzae* periorbital cellulitis has declined dramatically in recent years following the routine administration of *H. influenzae* type b vaccine to children 2 months of age and older.

Treatment

Empiric antibiotic therapy with parenteral antibiotics should be effective against the most likely pathogens. Streptococcus and staphylococcus should be suspected in all infants and children, while *H. influenzae* may be an important pathogen in nonimmunized infants and children. Intravenous penicillins such as nafcillin or oxacillin or a first-generation cephalosporin such as cefazolin is effective against streptococci and most staphylococcus species. Second-generation cephalosporins such as cefuroxime are effective against *H. influenzae* in addition to streptococci and staphylococci. A clinical response such as reduction in fever and resolution of symptoms typically occurs within 24 to 72 hr. Following such a response, oral antibiotic therapy with amoxicillin/clavulanic acid, trimethoprim-sulfamethoxazole, or cefadroxil or other broad-spectrum cephalosporin should be continued for 7 to 10 days (27, 28). Cefixime, a third-generation agent, may not be active against *S. aureus*.

PRESSURE SORES (DECUBITUS ULCERS, BED SORES)

Pressure ulcers are a serious problem that affects approximately 9% of all hospitalized patients and 23% of all nursing home patients, according to the Agency for Health Care Policy and Research (AHCPR) (29). Pressure sores (29–37) result from ischemic necrosis and ulceration of tissues overlying a bony prominence that has been subjected to prolonged pressure against an external object such as a bed, wheelchair, cast, or splint. This pressure may be sufficient to occlude small vessels and result in irreversible ischemic

Table 77.5.
Classification of Pressure Sores[a]

Grade	Description	Treatment
I	Lesion involves only the epidermis; nonblanchable erythema of the intact skin.	Relief of pressure and local wound care
II	Partial thickness loss; ulcer extends into the dermis.	Relief of pressure and local wound care
III	Full thickness loss; deep ulcer extends into the subcutaneous tissue and fascia.	Relief of pressure and surgery and systemic antibiotics if needed
IV	Ulcer extends into muscle, bone, or joint.	Radical surgery and systemic antibiotics to treat osteomyelitis if present

[a]This classification for pressure ulcers has been recommended by The National Pressure Ulcer Advisory Panel (30).

changes. These lesions often develop into infected ulcers. Immobility is the most important risk factor.

Four factors that are critical to formation of pressure sores are pressure, shearing forces, friction, and moisture. Shearing forces relate to the sliding of parallel surfaces of tissue in unequal fashion, as when the head of the bed is raised and the patient slides toward the foot of the bed. Friction generated by pulling a patient across a bed sheet may result in tissue trauma and development of an ulcer. Moisture from perspiration or incontinence may lead to maceration and skin irritation, which weaken the epidermal barrier. These lesions are most often seen in patients who have diminished or absent sensation, as patients with spinal cord injury (38) or degenerative neurologic disease or those who are debilitated, demented, emaciated, or paralyzed (39). Other risk factors for the development of pressure sores include advanced age, poor nutrition, and low arteriolar pressure.

Pressure sores most commonly occur in tissues over the sacrum and the heels and may involve skin, muscle, and bone. More than 95% of pressure sores are located on the lower body. Clinical staging (29, 30) or grading helps to guide management (Table 77.5). Stage I lesions involve only the epidermis, Stage II ulcers extend into the dermis, Stage III ulcers are deep lesions that extend into the subcutaneous tissues, and Stage IV lesions extend into muscle and bone. Deep lesions frequently require months to heal and extensive surgical treatments. Figure 77.1 illustrates the classification of lesions based on depth of lesion and tissue involvement.

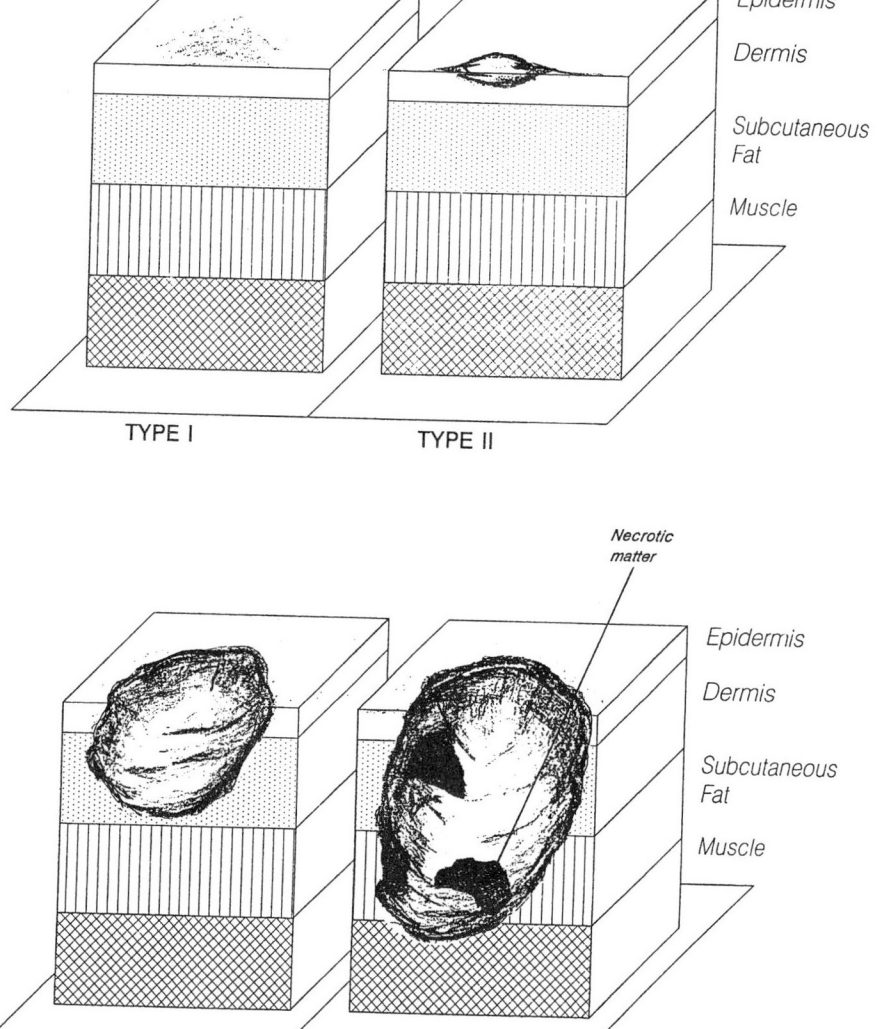

Figure 77.1. Classification of lesions based on depth of lesion and tissue involvement.

Accurate identification of patients who are increased risk is essential to the prevention of pressure sores. Several authors have proposed risk assessment scales (40–43). One such scale, The Braden Scale (41–43), is composed of six subscales that reflect sensory perception, skin moisture, activity level, mobility, nutritional status, and friction and shear. A score of 16 or less out of a possible 23 points predicts development of an ulcer. The Braden Scale has shown high reliability with different assessors, including nurse's aides, licensed practical nurses, and registered nurses. The size, number, and location of pressure ulcers need to be documented to allow evaluation of the effectiveness of the treatments. The key to prevention is early recognition of predisposing factors and measures to prevent pressure on sensitive areas, frequent position changes, frequent visual skin inspection, and keeping the predisposed skin areas clean and dry. Durable medical goods and special supplies are useful in these patients. The use of "sheepskin" or "egg-crate" mattresses has been suggested, but objective data suggests that they do not lower pressures sufficiently to prevent pressure sores. Many institutions have nursing policies that combine air mattresses with frequent repositioning.

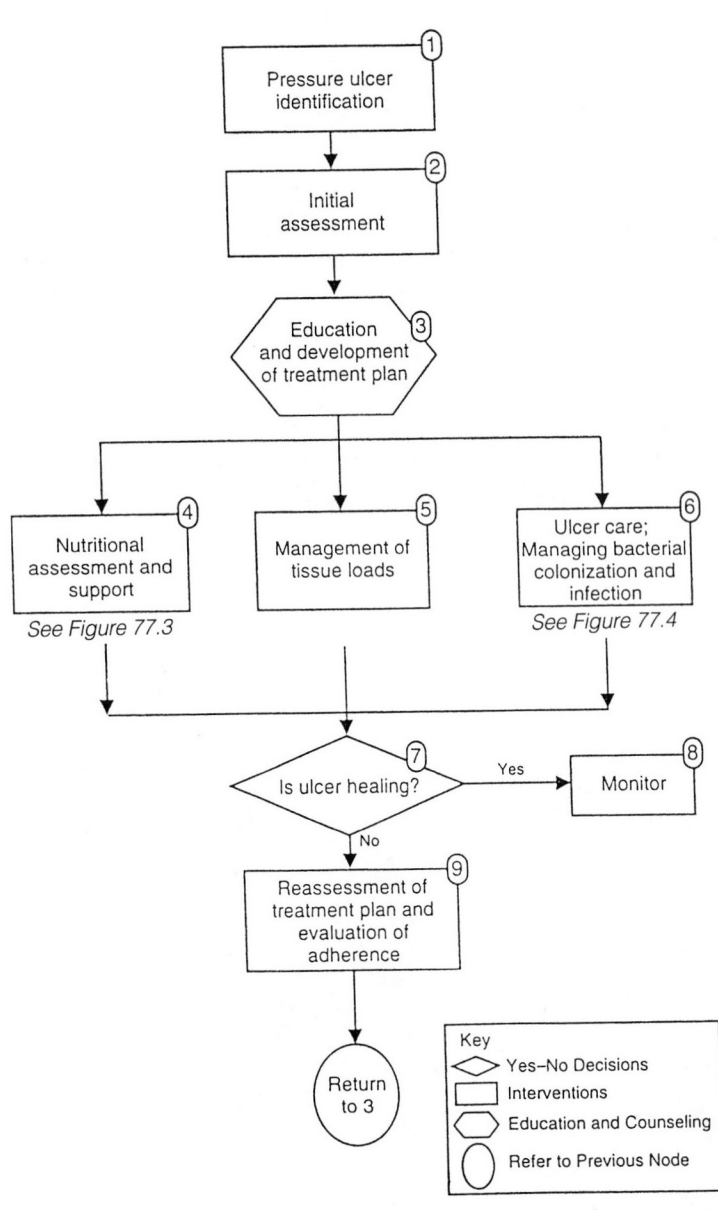

Figure 77.2.   Overview of activities related to pressure ulcer treatment.

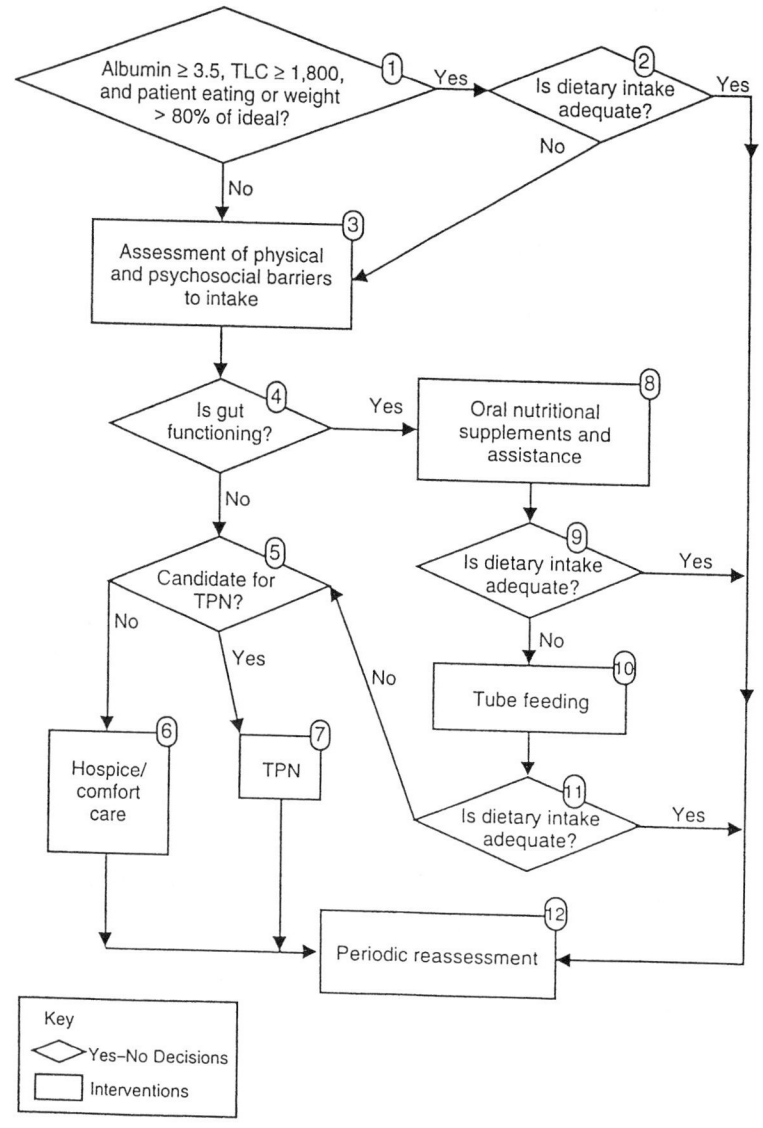

Note: TLC = total lymphocyte count; TPN = total parenteral nutrition.

Figure 77.3. Algorithm to help clinicians ensure the diet of an individual with a pressure ulcer contains nutrients.

Treatment

In the treatment of an ulcer, one must consider that it is much like an iceberg with only a small visible surface but an extensive unknown base. Many treatments for pressure ulcers have been recommended without adequate evidence to support their use. The treatment of Stage I and Stage II lesions is primarily local. If the patient cannot adequately oxygenate the tissue, systemic antibiotics are unlikely to have high penetration into the area. Figure 77.2 is an algorithm that provides an overview of the activities related to pressure ulcer treatment (29).

Attention to nutritional status is essential in the management of pressure ulcers at all stages (44). Figure 77.3 provides an algorithm to help clinicians ensure that the diet of the individual with a pressure ulcer contains nutrients that are adequate to support healing (29). Hypoalbuminemic patients have been shown to be at higher risk for the development of pressure sores and to exhibit slower rates of healing. Nutritional monitoring with attention to dietary protein is essential. In addition, ascorbic acid supplementation (500 mg twice daily) and zinc sulfate have been suggested, but study flaws make interpretation of this treatment difficult.

The mainstay of therapy is local care (45). Management of an established ulcer involves treatment of underlying medical conditions, proper nutrition and hydration, and the use of dressings or procedures that facilitate repair of tissue. The goal of therapy is to produce a local wound environment that enhances wound healing. Table 77.6 summarizes local wound therapies for pressure ulcers. The environment to promote wound healing is one that is warm, moist, and clean and that has an adequate blood supply. This promotes wound healing by permitting the formation of healthy granulation tissue. Polyurethane films such as Tegaderm or OpSite may help to reduce friction between skin and bedsheets and may prevent further skin maceration. OpSite is a semipermeable, transparent, polyurethane film that permits evaporation of perspiration but is impermeable to bacterial entry. DuoDerm is an impermeable, opaque, hydrocolloid dressing that forms a gellike wound covering on absorption of wound exudate. This is helpful to prevent and treat Grade I lesions.

Debridement is the process of cleaning an open wound by removal of foreign material and dead tissue so that healing may occur. Removal of dead tissue is necessary to remove devitalized tissue, to prevent the dead tissue from promoting infection, and to start reepithelialization of the area. Figure 77.4 outlines initial care of the pressure ulcer, including debridement and wound care (29). Extensive necrotic material can be removed rapidly and effectively by surgical debridement. Most clinicians prefer irrigation that follows surgical debridement. The role of pharmaceutical debriding agents is less well defined. Many products that

are used as debriding agents are applied to the wound on gauze. Mechanical debridement through the use of gauze dressings may allow earlier development of granulation tissue. Mechanical debridement with wet-to-dry dressings is painful and may also traumatize the wound (46). Wet-to-moist or wet-to-wet debridement may accomplish the same result while causing less discomfort to the patient. Gauze interacts physically with the wound surface and can cause debridement by dry-to-dry debridement, wet-to-dry debridement, or wet-to-wet debridement.

Absorbent materials such as dextranomer (Debrisan) microbeads have been used on moist ulcers. Dextranomer is a sterile, chemically inert, hydrophilic substance that removes exudate from the wound surface via a capillary action mechanism. It is available as a paste or bead preparation. When sprinkled onto open wounds, these products are thought to act through the formation of a gel that removes fluids, microbes, and debris from the wound through capillary forces.

Enzymatic debridement has been used to clean pressure sores that are covered with eschar. Eschar is a descriptive term for the scab or slough produced by the wound. Travase (casein in mineral oil and polyethylene glycol) is a sutilain that acts to selectively digest necrotic soft tissue by proteolytic actions. A moist environment is necessary for optimal enzymatic activity. The wound is cleaned and irrigated with normal saline. A thin layer of Travase ointment is applied to the site and covered with a moist dressing. The site should be cleansed and redressed 3 to 4 times a day for best results. The action of the casein is impaired by certain agents such as benzalkonium chloride, hexachlorophene, nitrofurazone, and thimerosal that may be used as preservatives in other products. Antibiotics such as penicillin, neomycin, and streptomycin do not affect the enzyme activity. Santyl is collagenase in white petrolatum. Collagenase is able to dissolve undenatured collagen fibers that retard healing. Collagenase is effective within a narrow pH range of 6 to 8. Collagenase ointment is applied directly to deep wounds with a tongue depressor or onto a sterile gauze. In the presence of an infection the topical antibiotic should be applied first. It is used once daily and is compatible with neomycin-polymyxin B-bacitracin ointment. Elase is fibrinolysin and deoxyribonuclease in petrolatum. The enzyme activity is probably exhausted at the end of 24 hr. Desoxyribonuclease is isolated from bovine pancreas. It acts to depolymerize deoxyribonucleic acids and DNA in necrotic tissue. The wound should be cleaned with saline, then gently dried before use of the ointment. The dressing is changed two to three times a day with warm saline flushes during dressing changes.

It is doubtful whether antiseptics (see Table 77.7) have any beneficial effects on open ulcers. The contact time between antiseptic and microbe is too brief for bactericidal

Table 77.6.
Local Wound Therapy for Pressure Ulcers

Therapy	Examples	Notes
Cleanse with normal saline or lactated ringers		Avoid antiseptic solutions.
MED (moist environment dressings)	Cutinova hydro	
Enzymatic debridement	Elase, Travase	May also damage healing tissue.
Skin barrier products (used primarily with stages I and II)	Polyurethane: OpSite Tegaderm Bioclusive, EnsureIt	
	Hydrogel: Vigilon Geliperm IntraSite	Dressings interact with wound exudate producing a soft moist gel that enables removal of the dressings with little damage to the newly formed tissue. Dressings stay in place for 1 to 7 days.
	Hydrocolloid: Duoderm, Comfeel, Restore	Opaque and impermeable to oxygen and water.

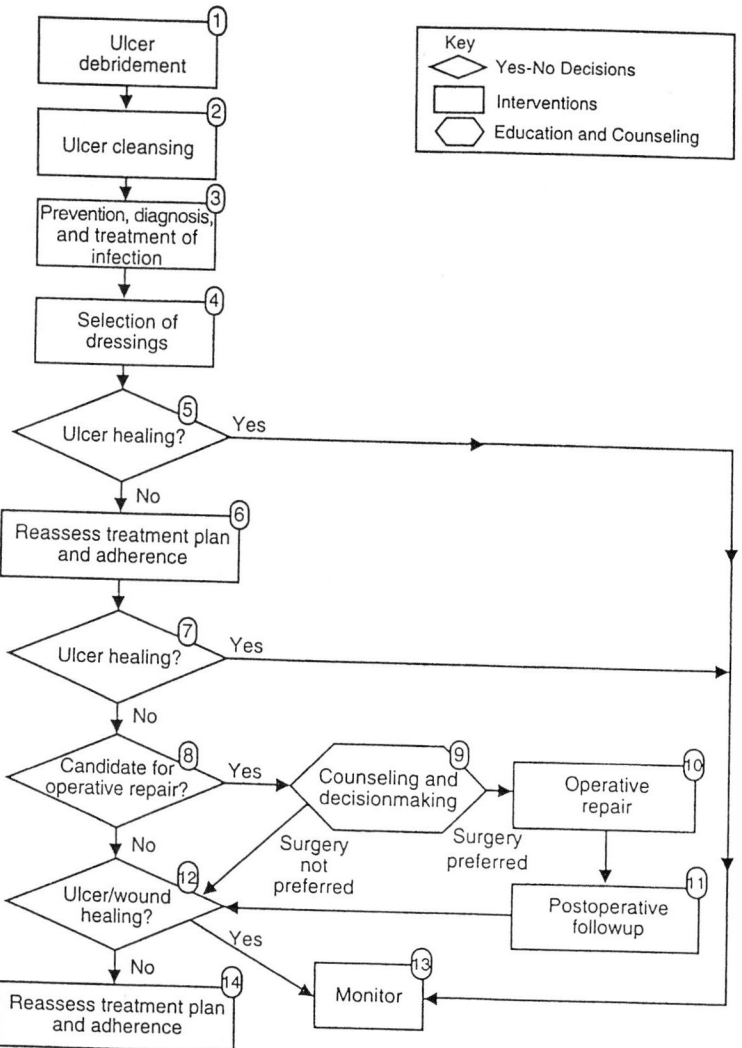

Figure 77.4. Initial care of the pressure ulcer.

effects, and antiseptics may inhibit wound healing locally. The clinical practice guidelines published by AHCPR specifically state that antiseptics should not be used in the treatment of pressure sores. Normal saline is the recommended cleansing solution for most pressure ulcers.

The topical antibiotics (Table 77.8) do not penetrate deeper tissues. Antibiotic dressings may not enhance healing and may induce microbial resistance. Neomycin-based products may produce allergic reactions. Infected pressure sores require culture and sensitivity testing with appropriate parenteral antibiotics if bacterial infection is documented (47). Figure 77.5 from AHCPR guides the clinician through a preferred pathway for managing bacterial colonization and local and systemic infection. A 2-week trial of topical antibiotics (e.g., an agent such as silver sulfadiazine) for clean pressure ulcers that are not

Table 77.7.
Topical Antiseptic Agents

Generic	Trade	Note or Caution
Chlorhexidine	Hibiclens	Associated with corneal opacification.
Povidone-iodine	Betadine	Associated with hypothyroidism.
Hydrogen peroxide	Various	Cytotoxic; may impair healing; no longer recommended.
Acetic acid	Various	Cytotoxic; may impair healing; no longer recommended.
Sodium hypochlorite	Dakin's solution	Cytotoxic; may impair healing; no longer recommended.

Note: chemicals used as antiseptics may kill the microflora in a wound but may also damage delicate, newly forming skin. The AHCPR Clinical Practice guidelines do not recommend any topical antiseptic (29).

Table 77.8.
Topical Antibiotic Agents

Suggested role in pressure ulcers with purulent drainage and/or foul
    odor
Silver sulfadiazine
Gentamicin
Bacitracin
Mupirocin (Bactroban)
Metronidazole gel (MetroGel) *(not currently FDA-approved)*

healing should be considered. Silver sulfadiazine is a broad-spectrum agent with activity against Gram-positive and Gram-negative bacteria. It has been used in treating pressure ulcers and infected leg ulcers (48). Topical metronidazole may be effective in treating infected ulcers that produce a characteristic foul odor. A number of studies (49–51) have employed once- or twice-daily application of topical metronidazole with promising results. This is not currently an FDA-approved indication. In a study by Pierleoni (51), 1% topical metronidazole was applied to a

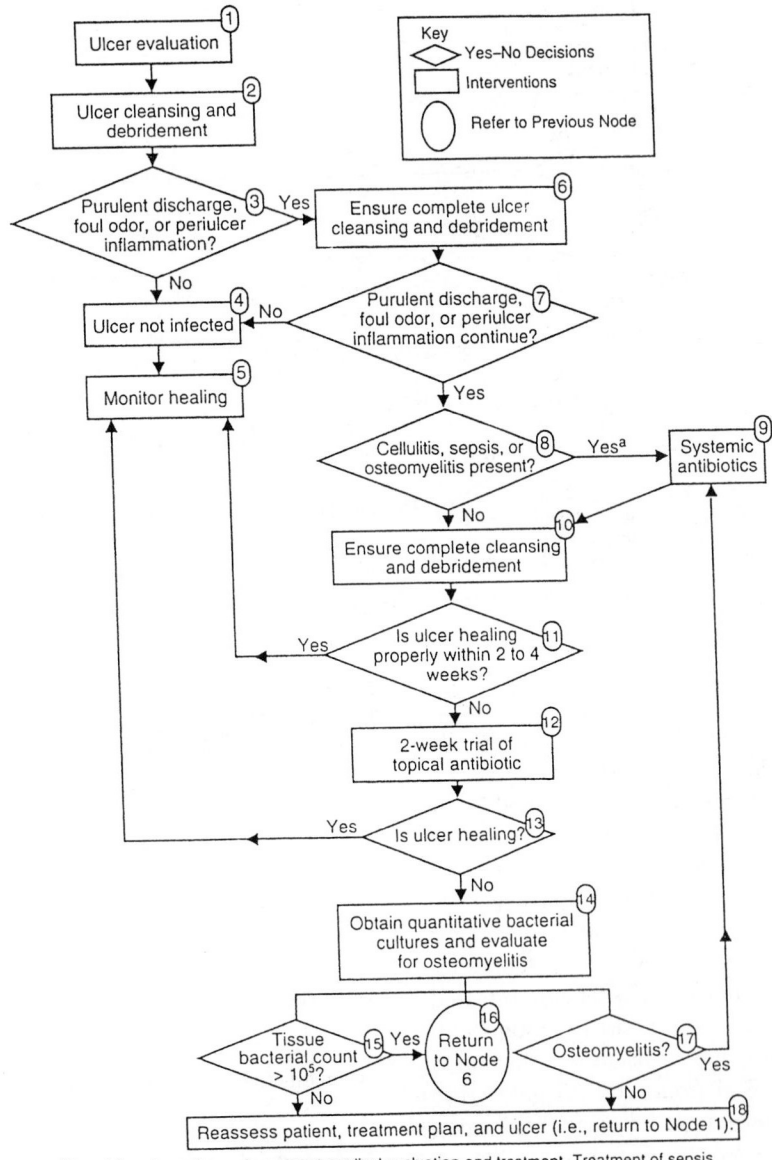

ᵃSuspicion of sepsis requires urgent medical evaluation and treatment. Treatment of sepsis
is not discussed in this guideline.

Figure 77.5.   Preferred pathway for managing bacterial colonization and local and systemic infection.

sterile gauze in infected decubitus ulcers every 8 hr. Microbiologic efficacy was documented. It may be combined with oral therapy in suspected or documented susceptible anaerobic infections. A commercially available gel contains metronidazole 0.75% in a water-soluble gel (MetroGel).

Systemic antibiotics (52) are indicated only when there is evidence of advancing cellulitis, sepsis, bacteremia, or osteomyelitis. Since debridement of ulcers may result in transient bacteremia in about 50% of patients, prophylaxis for bacterial endocarditis seems prudent in patients with artificial valves or other risk factors who require debridement.

BACTERIAL DIABETIC FOOT INFECTIONS

The foot of the diabetic is susceptible to all forms of trauma (53–55). Common results from trauma are infection and gangrene. Foot infections are the most common complication of diabetes requiring hospitalization. This complication accounts for more than 20% of all hospitalizations and is the most common cause of foot amputation in diabetic patients (56).

Many factors are involved in the development of diabetic foot ulcers (57); three major factors are neuropathy, vascular insufficiency, and immunologic defects. Neuropathy, which includes sensory disturbances and autonomic neuropathy with anhidrosis, vasodilation, edema, and erythema, causes structural and functional changes in the foot that alter weight bearing, muscle function, and support and normal pain sensations. Classic neuropathic ulcers occur most frequently on the plantar surfaces of the foot. Vascular insufficiency and angiopathy are risk factors for foot infections. Finally, diabetics are impaired hosts. Granulocytes from poorly controlled diabetics exhibit defects in phagocytosis. Because of these and other factors, the diabetic foot ulcer and infection present unique management problems. These ulcers may involve only superficial tissues or may involve deeper tissues and structures. A grading system using a six-point scale (0 to 5) has been proposed by Wagner (58).

Typical signs and symptoms of infection may not be present, since the neuropathy renders infection and gangrene relatively painless in the diabetic patient. For this reason, prophylactic foot care is essential. If an ulcer is detected, all weight bearing should be eliminated. Early incision, drainage, and identification of the organisms may prevent the need for further surgery.

Deep tissue cultures provide the most reliable microbiologic information. Bacteriologic investigations reveal a polymicrobic spectrum (average of three to six organisms) in most diabetic infections. Both aerobes and anaerobes are common. *Staphylococcus aureus*, *S. epidermidis*, *Corynebacterium*, Group D streptococci, and anaerobic Grampositive cocci are reported most frequently (59–62).

Treatment

Objective data concerning the efficacy of various antibiotic treatments is lacking. The selection of antibiotic treatment depends on assumptions made from available studies (59, 60), many of which are inappropriately designed. Systemic antibiotic treatment is clearly indicated when there is evidence of cellulitis, septicemia, or osteomyelitis (63, 64). However, some general therapeutic concepts can be suggested. Since diabetics are impaired hosts and have granulocyte defects, bactericidal antibiotics are preferred, and prolonged courses of treatment may be necessary. The prevalence of vascular insufficiency suggests the need for higher doses to obtain adequate tissue penetration. These infections are presumed to be polymicrobic with aerobes and anaerobes. Empiric therapy should provide broad coverage until culture results are available. The higher incidence of renal insufficiency in diabetic patients requires cautious use and careful monitoring of nephrotoxic agents such as the aminoglycosides. Table 77.9 lists agents

Table 77.9.
Antibiotic Regimens for Infected Diabetic Foot Ulcers

Appearance	Microbiologic	Possible Treatment Regimen
Limited in extent	Aerobic Gram (+) cocci	p.o. Clindamycin 300 Q.I.D. × 14 d p.o. (1st-generation Cephalosporin) cephalexin 500 mg Q.I.D. × 14 d p.o. amoxicillin + clavulanate I.V. cefazolin
Chronic, recurrent, limb-threatening	Polymicrobic (both aerobes and anaerobes)	Cefoxitin 1–2 g I.V. q6–8h *or* Oral ciprofloxacin 750–100 mg p.o. B.I.D. + clindamycin 300 mg p.o. Q.I.D.
	If septic	Imipenem + cilastatin or ticarcillin + clavulanate or piperacillin + tazobactam or PRSP + APAG + clindamycin or vancomycin + metronidazole + azetreonam

PRSP = penicillinase-resistant synthetic penicillin.
APAG = antipseudomonal aminoglycoside.

that may be useful in the treatment of diabetic foot infections. Even with careful treatment and monitoring, amputation may be necessary under certain conditions.

Supportive Care

Other considerations in the care of the diabetic foot ulcer should recognize that healing of an ulcer may take a long time because of the underlying poor circulation and tissue oxygenation. Nutritional monitoring and support are essential. Anemia should be corrected to enhance tissue oxygenation. While it is usually more difficult to control blood glucose in diabetic patients with active infections, adequate glucose control is essential to enhance treatment success. During the acute infection, diabetic patients may require higher doses of oral sulfonylurea agents or insulin. Major complications include sepsis syndrome, development of contiguous osteomyelitis, and transient bacteremia during ulcer manipulation. Since debridement of ulcers may result in transient bacteremia, prophylaxis for bacterial endocarditis would seem prudent in patients with artificial valves or other indications who require debridement.

CONCLUSION

The treatment of skin and soft tissue infections is common. It demands a knowledge of the anticipated flora and the host's normal defense mechanisms. The infections result in morbidity and extended health care needs. Decubitus ulcers and diabetic foot ulcers result from an interplay of the host factors and tissue invasion and result in chronic care dilemmas. The health care practitioner should be informed and knowledgeable about the therapeutic management issues of skin and soft tissue infections.

REFERENCES

1. Swartz MN. Cellulitis and superficial infections. In: Mandell GL, Douglas RG Jr, Bennett JE, eds. Principles and practices of infectious diseases, 3rd ed. New York: Churchill Livingstone, 1990:796–807.
2. Ginsberg MB. Cellulitis: analysis of 101 cases and review of the literature. South Med J 74:530–533, 1981.
3. Fleisher G, Ludwig S, Campos J. Cellulitis: bacterial etiology, clinical features and laboratory findings. J Pediatr 97:591–593, 1980.
4. Hook EW III, Hooton TM, Horton CA, et al. Microbiologic evaluation of cutaneous cellulitis in adults. Arch Intern Med 146:295–297, 1986.
5. Sigurdsson AF, Gudmundsson S. The etiology of bacterial cellulitis as determined by fine-needle aspiration. Scand J Infect Dis 21:537–542, 1989.
6. Powers RD. Soft tissue infections in the emergency department: the case for the use of "simple" antibiotics. South Med J 84:1313–1315, 1991.
7. Sachs MK. The optimum use of needle aspiration in the bacteriologic diagnosis of cellulitis in adults. Arch Intern Med 150:1907–1912, 1990.
8. Lindbeck G, Powers R. Cellulitis. Hosp Pract (Off Ed) 28 (suppl 2):10–14, 1993.
9. Ben-Amitai D, Ashkenazi S. Common bacterial skin infections in childhood. Pediatr Ann 22:225–233, 1993.
10. Gainer RB. Ceftriaxone in the treatment of serious infections: skin and soft tissue infections. Hosp Pract (Off Ed) 26 (suppl 5):24–30, 1991.
11. Campoli-Richards DM, Brogden RN. Sulbactam/ampicillin: a review of its antibacterial activity, pharmacokinetic properties, and therapeutic uses. Drugs 33:577–609, 1987.
12. File TM Jr, Tan JS. Ticarcillin-clavulanate therapy for bacterial skin and soft tissue infections. Rev Infect Dis 13 (suppl 9):S733–S736, 1991.
13. Walker RC, Wright AJ. The fluoroquinolones. Mayo Clin Proc 66:1249–1259, 1991.
14. Ball P. Emergent resistance to ciprofloxacin amongst *Pseudomonas aeruginosa* and *Staphylococcus aureus*: clinical significance and therapeutic approaches. J Antimicrob Chemother 26(suppl F):165–179, 1990.
15. Dagan R. Impetigo in childhood: changing epidemiology and new treatments. Pediatr Ann 22:235–240, 1993.
16. Schachner L, Talpin D, Scott GB, Morrison MA. A therapeutic update of superficial skin infection. Pediatr Clin North Am 30:397–403, 1983.
17. Dagan R, Bar-David Y. A double blind study comparing erythromycin and mupirocin for treatment of impetigo in children: implication of a high prevalence of erythromycin-resistant *Staphylococcus aureus* strain. Antimicrob Agents Chemother 36:287–290, 1992.
18. Jacob RF, Brown WD, Chartrand S, et al. Evaluation of cefuroxime axetil and cefadroxil suspension for the treatment of pediatric skin infections. Antimicrob Agents Chemother 36:1614–1618, 1992.
19. Blumer JL, Lemon E, O'Horo J, Snodgross DJ. Changing therapy for skin and soft tissue infections in children: have we come full circle? Pediatr Infect Dis J 6:117–122, 1987.
20. Goldfarb J, Crenshaw D, O'Hord J, Lemon E, Blomer JL. Randomized clinical trial of topical mupirocin versus oral erythromycin for impetigo. Antimicrob Agents Chemother 32:1780–1783, 1988.
21. Britton JW, Fajardo JE, Krafte-Jacos B. Comparison of mupirocin and erythromycin in the treatment of impetigo. J Pediatr 117:827–829, 1990.
22. McLinn S. Topical mupirocin vs systemic erythromycin treatment for pyoderma. Pediatr Infect Dis J 7:785–790, 1988.
23. Barton LL, Friedman AD, Sharky AM, Schneller DJ, Sweirkosz EM. Impetigo contagiosa. III: comparative efficacy of oral erythromycin and topical mupirocin. Pediatr Dermatol 6:134–138, 1989.
24. Canoso JJ, Barza M. Soft tissue infections. Rheum Dis Clin North Am 19:293–307, 1993.
25. Fekety FR Jr. Erysipelas. In: Demis DJ, ed. Clinical dermatology, vol 3, sect 16. Philadelphia: JB Lippincott, 1992:1–4.
26. Kahn RM, Goldstein EJC. Common bacterial skin infections. Postgrad Med 93:175–182, 1993.
27. Malinow I, Powell KR. Periorbital cellulitis. Pediatr Ann 22:241–246, 1993.
28. Siddens JD, Gladstone GJ. Periorbital and orbital infections in children. J Am Osteopath Assoc 92:226–230, 1992.
29. Bergstrom N, Bennett MA, Carlson CE, et al. *Pressure ulcer treatment:* clinical practice guideline. Quick Reference Guide for Clinicians, No. 15. Rockville, MD: U.S. Department of Health and Human Services, Public Health Service, Agency for Health Care Policy and Research. AHCPR Pub. No. 95–0653, Dec. 1994.
30. National Pressure Ulcer Advisory Panel. Pressure ulcer prevalence, cost and risk assessment: consensus development conference statement. Decubitus 2:24–28, 1989.
31. Allman RM. Pressure ulcers among the elderly. N Engl J Med 320:850–853, 1989.
32. Brandeis GH, Morris JN, Nash DJ, et al. The epidemiology and natural history of pressure ulcers in elderly nursing home residents. JAMA 264:2905–2909, 1990.

33. Young JB, Dobrzanski S. Pressure sores: epidemiology and current management concepts. Drugs Aging 2:42–57, 1992.

34. Goode PS, Allman RM. The prevention and management of pressure ulcers. Med Clin North Am 73:1511–1524, 1989.

35. Leigh IH, Bennett G. Pressure ulcers: prevalence, etiology, and treatment modalities. Am J Sur 167(1A Suppl):25S–30S, 1994.

36. Longe RL. Current concepts in clinical therapeutics: pressure sores. Clin Pharm 5:669–681, 1986.

37. Spoelhof GD, Ide K. Pressure ulcers in nursing home patients. Am Fam Phys 47:1207–1215, 1993.

38. Ditunno JF Jr, Formal CS. Chronic spinal cord injury. N Engl J Med 330:550–556, 1994.

39. Hunter SM, Cathcart-Silberberg T, Langemo DK, et al. Pressure ulcer prevalence and incidence in a rehabilitation hospital. Rehab Nurs 17:239–242, 1992.

40. Gosnell DJ. Assessment and evaluation of pressure sores. Nurs Clin North Am 22:339–415, 1987.

41. Bergstrom N, Braden BJ, Laguzza A, et al. The Braden Scale for predicting pressure sore risk. Nurs Res 36:205–210, 1987.

42. Bergstrom N, Demuth PJ, Braden BJ. A clinical trial of the Braden Scale for predicting pressure sore risk. Nurs Clin North Am 22:417–428, 1987.

43. Bergstrom N, Braden B. A prospective study of pressure sore risk among institutionalized elderly. J Am Geriatr Soc 40:747–758, 1992.

44. Telfer NR, Moy RL. Drug and nutrient aspects of wound healing. Dermatol Clin 11:729–737, 1993.

45. Howell JM. Current and future trends in wound healing. Emerg Med Clin North Am 10:655–663, 1992.

46. Stuzin J, Engrav L, Buehler P. Care of open wounds. Compr Ther 8:32–34, 1982.

47. Rogers KG. The rational use of antimicrobial agents in simple wounds. Emerg Med Clin North Am 10:753–766, 1992.

48. Payne CM, Bladin C, Colchester AC, et al. Argyria from excessive use of topical silver sulphadiazine [Letter]. Lancet 340:126, 1992.

49. Jones PH, Willis AT, Ferguson IR. Treatment of anaerobically in-fected pressure sores with topical metronidazole. Lancet 1, 214, 1978.

50. Baker PG, Haig G. Metronidazole in the treatment of chronic pressure sores and ulcers. Practitioner 225:569–573, 1981.

51. Pierleoni EE. Topical metronidazole therapy for infected decubitus ulcers. J Amer Geriatr Soc 32:775–781, 1984.

52. Leaper DJ. Prophylactic and therapeutic role of antibiotics in wound care. Am J Surg 167(suppl 1A):15S–19S, 1994.

53. Burton CS III. Management of chronic and problem lower extremity wounds. Dermatol Clin 11:767–773, 1993.

54. Kertesz D, Chow AW. Infected pressure and diabetic ulcers. Clin Geriatr Med 8:835–852, 1992.

55. Laing P. Diabetic foot ulcers. Am J Surg 167(suppl 1A):31S–36S, 1994.

56. Newman LG, Waller J, Palestro CJ, et al. Unsuspected osteomyelitis in diabetic foot ulcers. JAMA 266:1246–1251, 1991.

57. Caputo GM, Cavanagh PR, Ulbrecht, et al. Assessment and management of foot disease in patients with diabetes. N Engl J Med 331:854–860, 1994.

58. Wagner FW. The dysvascular foot: a system for diagnosis and treatment. Foot Ankle 2:64–122, 1981.

59. Peterson LR, Lissack LM, Canter K, et al. Therapy of lower extremity infections with Ciprofloxacin in patients with diabetes mellitus, peripheral vascular disease, or both. Am J Surg 86:801–808, 1989.

60. Lipsky BA, Pecoraro RE, Larson SA, et al. Outpatient management of uncomplicated lower-extremity infections in diabetic patients. Arch Intern Med 150:790–797, 1990.

61. Wheat LJ, Allen SD, Henry M, et al. Diabetic foot infections. Arch Intern Med 146:1935–1940, 1986.

62. Mertz PM, Ovington LG. Wound healing microbiology. Dermatol Clin 11:739–747, 1993.

63. Gentry LO. Therapy with newer oral β-lactam and quinolone agents for infections of the skin and skin structures: a review. Clin Infect Dis 14:285–297, 1992.

64. Leichter SB, Schaefer JC, O'Brian JT. New concepts in managing diabetic foot infections. Geriatrics 46:24–30, 1991.

CHAPTER 78

ACUTE LEUKEMIAS

MICHELLE H. SANDERS and WILLIAM R. CROM

The leukemias are a group of neoplastic diseases of the blood-forming cells of the bone marrow, which result in the proliferation and accumulation of immature and generally defective blood cells in both the bloodstream and the bone marrow (1). The involved cells are usually leukocytes, but several different forms of the disease may be manifested, according to which leukocyte cell line is involved (Fig. 78.1). The leukemias are universally fatal if untreated, usually due to complications resulting from the leukemic infiltration of the bone marrow and replacement of normal hematopoietic precursor cells. These fatal complications are usually hemorrhage and infection (1). The natural history of untreated leukemia has led to the classifications of "acute" and "chronic" leukemia, referring to the rapidity of death, with average survival for untreated acute leukemia of about 3 months. Patients with chronic leukemia generally have more differentiated types of malignant cells and survive without treatment somewhat longer. However, with modern therapy, many patients with acute leukemia may survive for several years even if they eventually succumb to the disease, and indeed, for these patients, leukemia is a chronic disease.

Acute leukemia is classified according to the predominant cell type involved. Because of significant differences in age distribution, responses to treatment, and prognosis, the acute leukemias are commonly divided into acute lymphocytic leukemia (ALL) and acute nonlymphocytic leukemia (ANLL). ANLL can be further divided into additional subtypes, depending on the cell line involved (Figs. 78.1 and 78.2): myelocytic, myelomonocytic, monocytic, promyelocytic, erythrocytic, and several other very rare types. However, because response to treatment is similar for all these relatively uncommon types of leukemia, they are generally treated in the same fashion and referred to collectively as ANLL. In this chapter, ALL and ANLL will be discussed separately with regard to pathophysiology, treatment, and prognosis.

EPIDEMIOLOGY AND ETIOLOGY

Approximately 25,700 new cases of acute leukemia are identified each year in the United States, according to the National Cancer Institute's Surveillance, Epidemiology,

and End Results (SEER) program (2). About 20,400 Americans die each year from leukemia. Overall, leukemias and lymphomas account for about 6% of all new cancer cases and about 8% of cancer deaths (2).

The causes of acute leukemias are generally not known. Viruses have been shown to produce some types of leukemia in animals (e.g., feline leukemia), and the Epstein-Barr virus has been implicated as the causative agent of African Burkitt's lymphoma, as well as some types of nasopharyngeal carcinoma (3). Currently, attention is being focused on the isolation of the human T-cell leukemia virus (HTLV) from a human lymphoma. Individuals who have previously been exposed to radiation, with or without antineoplastic drugs, are also at greater risk to develop leukemia. In addition, numerous genetic derangements (particularly Down's syndrome) have been associated with a higher incidence of acute leukemia. However, in the majority of cases in both children and adults, the cause of leukemia cannot be identified, and probably numerous factors interact to result in the malignant condition.

Despite differences in appearance and clinical behavior, all hematologic neoplasms have in common the fact that they are clonal; that is, all cells composing the malignant population in a given patient are derived from a single mutant precursor cell (4). The neoplastic clones have two important features compared to normal cells. First, they appear to possess an advantage over normal hematopoietic clones that results in growth of the malignant population at the expense of normal cells. Second, there is an imbalance between proliferation and differentiation. Most malignant populations are made up of poorly differentiated cell types that ordinarily would not proliferate or be found in the bloodstream in large numbers. However, the malignant transformation of these cells results in immature cell types that proliferate but do not further differentiate.

It is useful to review the process of normal production of cellular blood elements. As shown in Figure 78.1, all lymphoid and hemopoietic blood cells are derived from a small population of pluripotent stem cells. These stem cells have virtually unlimited potential for self-renewal and are capable of responding to physiologic needs by inducing production of progenitor cells committed to mature separately into lymphoid cells, erythroid cells,

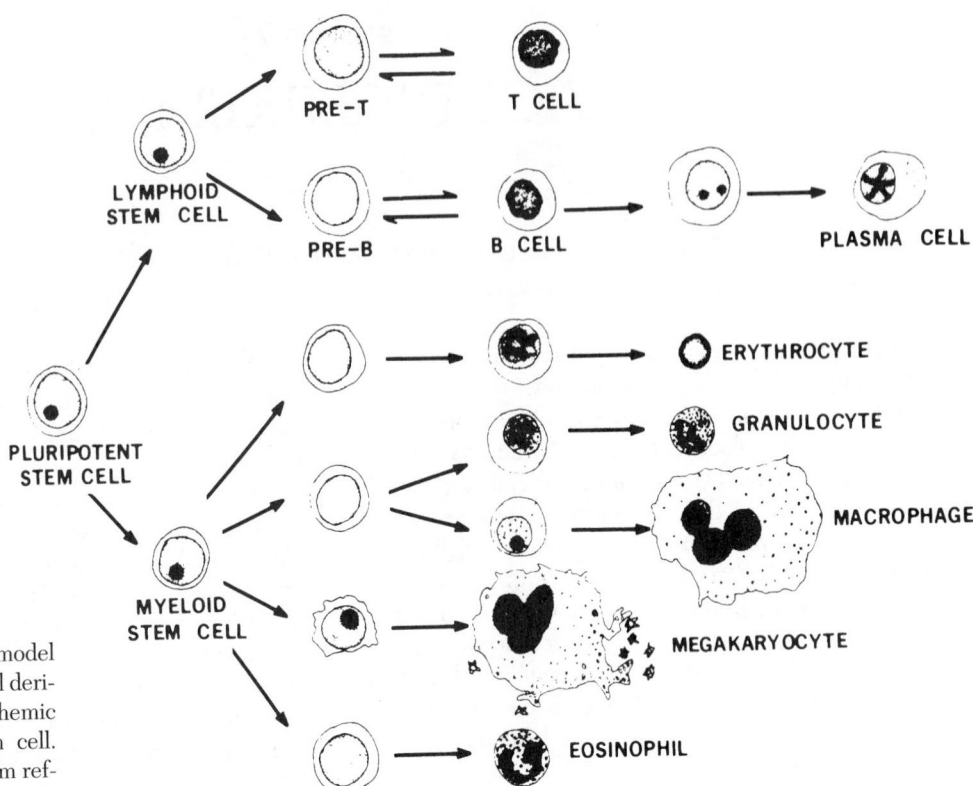

Figure 78.1. A schematic model of hematopoiesis showing clonal derivation of mature lymphoid and hemic cells from a pluripotent stem cell. (Reprinted with permission from reference 4.)

megakaryocytes, granulocytes, and monocytes. As maturation proceeds in the various cellular lineages, proliferative capacity becomes progressively restricted until eventually it is lost completely. Therefore, mature cells must be continually replaced as they complete their life cycle. Various stimulatory factors, such as erythropoietin, thrombopoietin, and colony-stimulating factors, regulate the proliferation and differentiation of committed precursor cells, derived from the pluripotent stem cells. Leukemia cells do not undergo terminal differentiation and thus do not lose their proliferative potential. The leukemic cell population continues to expand, and normal bone marrow elements may be "crowded out," resulting in the characteristic signs of bone marrow failure, which generally bring patients to medical attention.

CLASSIFICATIONS OF ACUTE LEUKEMIA

Acute leukemia is classified depending on the cell of origin. However, additional classifications of leukemia have been developed to further identify differences in the clinical course, response to treatment, and prognosis of various types of acute leukemia. An important development introduced in the 1970s is the French–American–British (FAB) system of nomenclature that is now widely used to classify the morphologic subgroups of acute leukemias (5). The FAB system is summarized in Table 78.1.

In addition to the FAB system, both immunologic and biochemical markers are used to classify and identify subtypes of leukemia cells. Immunologic "markers" refer to the surface immunoglobulin (SIg) found on the cell membrane of malignant leukocytes or to their cytoplasmic immunoglobulins (CIg). As normal cells undergo differentiation, these markers change and may be used to determine the degree of differentiation achieved by the malignant cell line. This permits identification of the type of cell involved and leads to further classification.

The development of hybridoma techniques and unlimited quantities of specific monoclonal antibodies has led to more precise identification of specific immunologic markers in the classification of ALL and to a revised immunologic classification system (Table 78.2). The classification of ALL is now made on the basis of the pattern of reactivity to a panel of lineage-associated monoclonal antibodies (6, 7). ALL is broadly classified as having a T-lineage (based on positive reactions with monoclonal antibodies CD3, CD7 plus CD5 or CD2, or both) or a B-lineage (based on positive reactions with antibodies CD19 and CD22). B-lineage classification includes three major subtypes: B-cell (expression of surface immunoglobulin heavy chains and either κ or λ light chains), pre-B (presence of cytoplasmic immunoglobulin), and early pre-B (no surface and cytoplasmic immunoglobulins). Transitional B-cells, which express cytoplasmic and surface immunoglobulin chains and surrogate light-chain proteins, appear to define a clinically distinct form of ALL. T cells may also be classified according to the degree of differentiation (early,

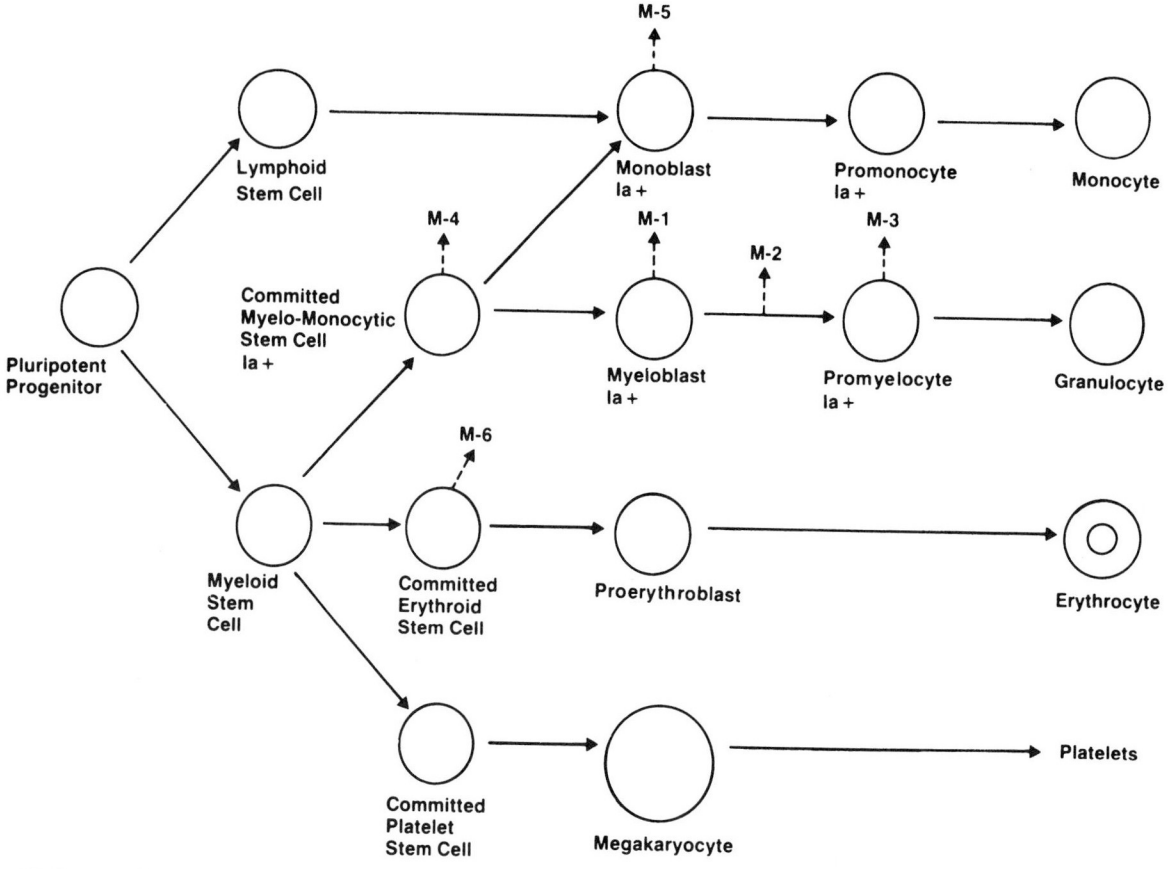

Figure 78.2. Myeloid differentiation and relationship to FAB classification of AML. M1, undifferentiated myeloid; M2, early (?) differentiated myeloid; M3, promyelocytic; M4, myelomonocytic; M5, monocytic; M6, erythroleukemia. (Reprinted with permission from reference 8.)

Table 78.1.
The French–American–British (FAB) Cooperative Group Classification of Acute Leukemias

FAB Designation	Common Terms (Abbreviations) for Leukemic Subgroups	Predominating Cell Type
L1	Acute lymphocytic leukemia, childhood (ALL)	Microlymphoblasts
L2	Acute lymphocytic leukemia, adult (ALL)	Mixed lymphoblasts, prolymphoblasts
L3	Burkitt's-type leukemia	Lymphocytes
M0	Minimal myeloid differentiation	Undifferentiated
M1	Acute myelocytic leukemia, undifferentiated; acute myelogenous, acute granulocytic	Myeloblasts
M2	Acute myelocytic leukemia, differentiated	Mixed myeloblasts, promyelocytes
M3	Acute progranulocytic leukemia	Hypergranular promyelocytes
M4	Acute myelomonocytic leukemia (AMML)	Mixed myelocytes, monocytes
M5	Acute monocytic leukemia (AMOL)	Monocytes
M6	Erythroleukemia	Mixed erythroblasts, erythrocytes, myelocytes
M7	Megakaryoblastic leukemia	Megakaryoblasts

intermediate, or late), but this classification of T-cell ALL has limited clinical significance (7). The prognosis of these various subgroups of ALL will be discussed later.

Biochemical markers refer to altered concentrations of intracellular enzymes, which may be found in various forms of leukemia. Terminal deoxynucleotidyl transferase (TdT) is an intracellular enzyme that is generally not detected in mature lymphocytes but is found in most patients with ALL, excluding those with the B-cell subtype. It may also be found in up to 5% of ANLL cases. Myeloperoxidase and Sudan black stain, on the other hand, are positive predominantly in cases of nonlymphocytic leukemia. The

Table 78.2.
Classification of ALL by Morphologic Characteristics, Immunophenotype, and Chromosome Number[a]

Category	Frequency %
FAB morphological classification system	
L1	80
L2	17
L3	3
Immunophenotype	
Early pre-B	57
Pre-B	25
Transitional pre-B	1
B-cell	2
T-cell	15
Ploidy	
Hypodiploid (<45 chromosomes)	7
Diploid (normal 46 chromosomes)	8
Pseudodiploid (46 chromosomes, with abnormalities)	42
Hyperdiploid (47 to 50 chromosomes)	15
Hyperdiploid (>50 chromosomes)	27
Triploid/tetraplid (>65 chromosomes)	1

[a]On the basis of 500 consecutive newly diagnosed cases (ages ≤ 18 years) treated at St. Jude Children's Research Hospital (from references 6 and 7).

Table 78.3.
Frequency of the More Common Presenting Complaints Among Children with ALL

Finding	Percent
Fever	61
Pallor	55
Hemorrhage	52
Anorexia	33
Fatigue	30
Bone pain	23
Abdominal pain	19
Joint pain	15
Lymphadenopathy	15
Weight loss	13

periodic acid-Schiff (PAS) reaction is positive in ALL and is useful in differentiating it from ANLL (6).

In actual practice, the classification of a particular case of acute leukemia is based on the combination of morphology and immunologic and biochemical studies. These studies generally correlate with one another, and are used to confirm the suspected classification of any particular case. Figure 78.2 shows the correlation between FAB classification, immunologic markers, and biochemical markers for subgroups of ALL and ANLL, respectively.

CLINICAL PRESENTATION AND DIAGNOSIS

The initial presenting symptoms of acute leukemia differ very little for ALL and ANLL. The complaints that most often bring patients to medical attention are fever, pallor, purpura, and pain (8). These symptoms result from bone marrow failure. Anemia occurs because of inadequate erythrocyte production, infections are due to inadequate neutrophil production, and bleeding is due to inadequate platelet production. In addition, infiltration of leukemia cells into the liver, spleen, or lymph nodes may result in hepatosplenomegaly, lymphadenopathy, and bone and joint pain. Table 78.3 lists the frequency of presenting complaints among patients with ALL. These complaints may be present for a few days or even a few weeks; rarely, there may be a history of these symptoms for several months prior to diagnosis. The most common symptom at diagnosis is the presence of fever, occurring in about 60% of patients. Although patients may be neutropenic at diagnosis, fever appears to be due to the leukemia itself since 70% of these patients become afebrile within 72

hours of beginning induction therapy without antibiotics (9). Nevertheless, empiric antibiotic therapy is usually instituted in febrile, neutropenic leukemia patients at diagnosis since the risk of serious systemic infections in such patients cannot be ignored.

Newly diagnosed patients with leukemia may have a total white blood cell (WBC) count that is markedly elevated, normal, or markedly depressed. A very high circulating WBC count is associated with a poorer prognosis, but even in these patients, most of the white cells in the circulation are immature blast forms that are incapable of mounting a response to bacterial infections. Therefore, most patients with leukemia are at an increased risk of opportunistic infections at diagnosis.

The diagnosis of acute leukemia is not usually difficult to establish. A bone marrow aspirate is performed to allow examination of the cellular elements of the bone marrow. It is often hypercellular, with 60 to 100% blast cells. A minimum of 25% blast cells is considered adequate to establish the diagnosis of acute leukemia, but most commonly this is an all-or-none diagnosis, and the pattern is obvious. Abnormal cells found in the peripheral blood, may be suspicious for acute leukemia but usually are not considered diagnostic, because bizarre mononuclear cells may be seen in the blood of patients with viral illnesses. If blasts or other unidentified cells are seen in the peripheral blood, the diagnosis must be confirmed by a bone marrow examination.

PRINCIPLES OF THERAPY

The modern cure-oriented approach to the treatment of any malignant condition usually involves some combination of surgery, radiation, and chemotherapy. Although surgery is important in the treatment of solid tumors, it is impossible to surgically remove tumor tissue in leukemia, and therefore surgery has a minor supportive role.

Radiation therapy has a more important role in leukemia, but it is not used alone as a curative modality. It is important in the treatment of either occult or overt central nervous system (CNS) leukemia. High-dose radiotherapy is also used to obliterate functional bone marrow as part of the preparation for bone marrow transplants. It may also be used in individual cases to reduce the size of an infiltrative leukemic mass, particularly where functional impairment of an organ or joint is involved.

Drug Therapy

Drug therapy remains the primary modality for the treatment of acute leukemias. Beginning with the use of aminopterin in childhood ALL in 1948 (10), additional effective agents have been identified and introduced into routine clinical use. The mechanisms of action and common toxicities of the drugs routinely used to treat acute leukemia today are summarized in Table 78.4. This table includes investigational agents effective in the treatment of acute leukemia.

For all phases of leukemia, it has been clearly demonstrated that drugs used in combination are superior to single agents. The rationale for combination therapy is that several effective agents with different mechanisms of action are more likely to destroy different subpopulations of leukemia cells and reduce the potential for development of drug resistance. The practical problem in the design of clinical treatment programs is to use the optimal number of agents in the most effective dosages and sequence. Several principles guide the use of combination chemotherapy for malignant diseases: (1) each of the drugs used should have demonstrated single-agent activity against the tumor; (2) the drugs should have different mechanisms of action; (3) the drugs used should have minimally overlapping toxicities; and (4) the maximal optimal doses should be used, scheduled with respect to specific tumor cell kinetics.

The optimal use of anticancer drugs is limited by our incomplete understanding of their mechanisms of action, mechanisms of resistance to them, and their interactions. In addition, our understanding of the biology of tumors and the factors that control their growth is incomplete. Current research directed at elucidating the cellular mechanisms that govern both the reproduction of malignant cells and their response to anticancer drugs is expected to improve our use of the drugs currently available, as well as lead to the development of new agents.

Bone Marrow Transplantation

Bone marrow transplantation is a treatment modality that has an important role in the treatment of ANLL, particularly during first remission. Transplantation has also been useful in producing cures in patients with ALL who have relapsed and receive a transplant during their second remission, or during first remission in ALL patients with a poor prognosis, such as those who are Philadelphia chromosome positive. This procedure requires that the patient receive total body irradiation, with or without high-dose drug therapy (cyclophosphamide, busulfan, and etoposide have all been used), to kill residual leukemia cells and produce irreversible bone marrow suppression. Bone marrow is obtained from either an HLA-matched donor (allogeneic), an identical twin (syngeneic), or from the patient in remission (autologous). Bone marrow is harvested from the iliac crest of the donor and then intravenously infused into the patient. Engraftment usually occurs in about 2 to 3 weeks.

Bone marrow transplants have a number of potential hazards. First, there is the complication of graft-versus-host disease (GVHD), which results from T lymphocytes in the donor marrow reacting against host tissue. GVHD is either an acute or a chronic disease. Acute and chronic GVHD differ by the cellular mechanism and time to occur posttransplant. Acute GVHD usually occurs 7 to 100 days posttransplant and is believed to be mediated by the cell line. Histologically, acute GVHD appears as an infiltrate of mononuclear lymphocytes. Chronic GVHD resembles an autoimmune response and occurs more than 100 days posttransplant. Both forms of GVHD affect the skin, liver, and gastrointestinal tract. The patients present with abdominal cramping; severe diarrhea; guaiac-positive ("guaiac-positive") stools; itching rash on soles, palms, and trunk; and elevated bilirubin, transaminases, and alkaline phosphatase. The incidence of GVHD ranges from 20 to 70% and increases with HLA disparity, increased age of recipient, conditioning regimens with irradiation, and type of disease treated (less in patients with aplastic anemia). GVHD accounts directly or indirectly for 15 to 40% of the deaths in transplant patients. GVHD is treated or prevented with high-dose corticosteroids, or with cyclosporine, methotrexate, or a combination, to inhibit proliferation of T lymphocytes. GVHD treatment has also included monoclonal antibodies and antithymocyte globulin (11–15).

Second, there is the risk of infection as a result of immunosuppression. Viral and fungal infections are especially common and difficult to treat. Patients on high-dose corticosteroids or those with a prolonged engraftment phase are at increased risk for infection. Viral and fungal infections may occur, particularly interstitial pneumonitis (caused by *Pneumocystis carinii* or cytomegalovirus and other viruses), which may occur in 25 to 60% of patients. The incidence of these infections has been significantly decreased with the prophylactic use of sulfamethoxazole and trimethoprim for *Pneumocystis carinii* and ganciclovir and immune globulin for cytomegalovirus (16–18). Infection is the second leading cause of death in allogeneic transplants and the first leading cause in autologous transplants.

A third complication is veno-occlusive disease (VOD) of the liver. It is a fibrous obliteration (either partial or complete) of small hepatic venules leading to thrombosis,

Table 78.4.
Principal Toxicities and Clinical Indications for Drugs Used to Treat Leukemia

Drug	Acute	Delayed	Indications
Plant Alkaloids			
Etoposide	Nausea and vomiting; hypotension with rapid administration; hypersensitivity reactions (2 to 20%); irritant with extravasation	Bone marrow depression; alopecia, oral ulceration	ANLL (induction-200 mg/m² CI for 3 days) ALL (150–300 mg/m² weekly pairs)
Vincristine	Vesicant reaction with extravasation; mild emetogenicity	Neurotoxicity: peripheral neuropathy, jaw pain, paralytic ileus, foot drop, decreased reflexes, constipation; alopecia; bone marrow depression	ALL (remission induction and continuation: 1–1.5 mg/m² weekly pairs)
Antimetabolites			
Cladribine (2-CDA)	Mild nausea and vomiting; rash	Bone marrow depression; immunosuppression	8.9 mg/m²/day × 5 days CI
Cytarabine	Nausea, vomiting, diarrhea	Bone marrow depression; central nervous system toxicity; interstitial pneumonitis	ALL (200–300 mg/m² weekly or alternating pairs) If intrathecally: 28–36 mg ANLL (100 mg/m² CI days 1–7 or 250 mg/m² CI days 1–5)
Fludarabine	Nausea and vomiting	Bone marrow depression; megaloblastosis; oral ulceration; fever and arthralgias; diarrhea; alopecia; rash on soles and palms	50–150 mg/m²/day × 5 days over 30 minutes IV
Mercaptopurine	Occasional nausea and vomiting	Bone marrow depression; liver damage	ALL (continuation therapy: 75–100 mg/m²/day)
Methotrexate	Dose-related nausea and vomiting; diarrhea (usually mild); rash	Bone marrow depression; oral and gastrointestinal ulceration; nephrotoxicity (high doses); hepatic cirrhosis (low-dose) and elevated liver transaminases; pulmonary infiltration (fibrosis/pneumonitis); CNS toxicity (high-dose and intrathecal therapy)	ALL (intrathecal 6–12 mg, low doses orally or IV 40 mg/m² dose, high doses IV 1500–5000 mg/m² over 2 to 24 hours)
Thioguanine	Occasional nausea and vomiting 1 or 2 days after administration	Bone marrow depression	ANLL (100 mg/m² daily to twice daily days 1–7)
Antibiotics			
Daunorubicin	Nausea and vomiting; diarrhea; vesicant—local reactions at infiltration site; red urine, 1 or 2 days after administration	Bone marrow depression; cardiotoxicity; stomatitis; alopecia; potentiation of radiation	ANLL (30–60 mg/m² CI over 3 days) ALL (25 mg/m² IV once a week for 2 to 3 weeks) ANLL (30 mg/m² CI over 3 days)
Doxorubicin	Nausea and vomiting; diarrhea; local reactions at infiltration site; red urine, 1 or 2 days after administration	Bone marrow depression; cardiotoxicity; stomatitis; alopecia; potentiation of radiation	
Alkylating Agents			
Cyclophosphamide	Nausea and vomiting (sometimes delayed)	Bone marrow depression; immunosuppression; alopecia; hemorrhagic cystitis; sterility; secondary malignancies; SIADH	ALL (150–300 mg/m² IV alternating weekly pairs)
Miscellaneous			
Asparaginase	Nausea and vomiting; fever; anaphylaxis; local reaction	Hepatotoxicity; hyperglycemia; pancreatitis; abdominal pain; coagulation defects; CNS depression	ALL induction (10,000 U/m²/day IM QOD to weekly for 6–9 doses)

endophlebitis, fibrosis, and portal hypertension with ascites. The incidence of VOD approaches 20% and usually occurs within the first 3 to 4 weeks of transplant. Factors that influence incidence are age, history of liver disease, high doses of alkylating agents, radiation, elevated liver enzymes (i.e., SGOT) prior to transplant, and diagnosis other than ALL. Treatment for the disease is primarily supportive, fluid and sodium restriction, and diuretics. Disease mortality in patients with VOD range from 7 to 50% (19–23).

Finally, there is the risk of leukemic relapse even following the intensive therapy administered prior to bone marrow transplantation. With autologous transplants, there is the additional risk that leukemic cells may remain in the patient's bone marrow that is reinfused following systemic treatment. Brenner and colleagues (24) recently used gene marking techniques to demonstrate that, in some acute nonlymphocytic leukemia patients who relapsed following bone marrow transplant, the source of the relapse was from leukemia cells that had been marked ex vivo prior to reinfusion into the patient. This study demonstrates the need for improved bone marrow purging techniques when using autologous marrow transplants to treat leukemias.

ACUTE LYMPHOCYTIC LEUKEMIA

ALL is the most common malignancy of childhood but is quite rare in persons over 15 years of age. The incidence in children is about 2.5 per 100,000, and it is slightly higher in boys than girls (2). There is also a higher incidence of leukemia in children with various genetic abnormalities, particularly Down's syndrome.

Childhood ALL represents one of the success stories of recent years in cancer treatment. Long-term survival in children receiving modern therapy is now about 73%. Several distinct phases of therapy, each with a specific rationale, have been developed, and current efforts to improve the cure rate of ALL have focused on refining and optimizing therapy for each of these phases.

Induction Therapy

Complete remission, defined as the complete eradication of all detectable disease, may be produced in at least 95% of patients with ALL. Patients in complete remission have no evidence of leukemia and may lead relatively normal lives while in remission. However, patients in remission may have as many as 10^8 leukemia cells in their bodies, but this mass of cells remains clinically undetectable. Remission induction therapy is capable of eradicating up to 99.9% of the total body burden of malignant cells, but since patients may have 10^{10} to 10^{12} leukemia cells at diagnosis, a substantial number of cells remains to be eliminated after patients achieve a clinical complete remission.

The objectives of initial remission induction are to (1) eradicate as many leukemia cells as possible, within the limits of biologic tolerance, and (2) reestablish normal hematopoiesis and general good health. "Standard" remission induction therapy generally consists of two or more drugs. Prednisone and vincristine are almost always used, and this combination produces a complete remission in more than 90% of patients. However, the intensity of the initial treatment influences the duration of remission, and addition of a third agent, either asparaginase or an anthracycline (daunorubicin or doxorubicin), appears to increase the fraction of patients who remain in continuous complete remission (CCR) and are eventually cured (25–27). Therefore, induction regimens generally include at least three drugs: prednisone, vincristine, and either asparaginase or an anthracycline.

Consolidation Therapy

Consolidation therapy refers to a period of intensive therapy administered after achievement of complete remission. The purpose of consolidation therapy is to secure the complete remission by eradicating as many of the remaining leukemic cells as possible, within the limits of biologic tolerance. Consolidation therapy may consist of different combinations of agents or may consist of repeated courses of the regimen used to achieve the initial clinical remission.

Central Nervous System Therapy

An important site of initial relapse in patients who achieve a complete remission is the CNS. Following conventional induction therapy alone, up to 60% of patients may have their initial reappearance of malignant blast cells in the CNS (28), probably because of poor penetration across the blood–brain barrier by the drugs used to induce remission. The precise definition of CNS disease has been somewhat controversial. The two most commonly accepted definitions of CNS disease are as follows: (1) the total cerebrospinal fluid (CSF) white blood cell count (greater than 5 cells/μL) and the presence of blast cells in the CSF or with cranial nerve palsy and (2) the presence of any number of blasts regardless of cell counts in the CSF.

Presence of the CNS as a "pharmacologic sanctuary" for ALL led to the recognition that specific CNS therapy is an essential component of treatment for this disease. Proposed by George and Pinkel in the 1960s (29), CNS therapy has reduced the CNS relapse rate to less than 10% (28). The mainstay of CNS therapy has been cranial irradiation, either with spinal irradiation or intrathecal methotrexate. The dose originally used was 2400 cGy delivered over 2 to 3 weeks, but more recently, it has been shown that 1800 cGy provides adequate treatment, with less toxicity and morbidity (30). Intrathecal methotrexate has been used with success in place of spinal irradiation, resulting in less myelosuppression and growth abnormalities (31). The usual dose for patients more than 3 years of age is 12 mg/m² (32). Cytarabine or hydrocortisone, or both, may be added to methotrexate to further improve the effectiveness of CNS therapy. Recent data have suggested that the treatment for CNS disease should be intensified based on prognostic factors as well as on the CNS disease at diagnosis reserving cranial irradiation and multiple intrathecal doses for those at greater risk for relapse. Therefore, the non-T-cell, non-B-cell ALL patients with less than 5 cells/μL in the CSF, regardless of blasts, would receive less CNS prophylaxis and no irradiation in the context of highly effective chemotherapy (33, 34).

Another approach to CNS treatment is the use of high-dose methotrexate intravenously, without irradiation (35). This therapy consists of methotrexate in dosages of 500 mg/m^2 or more, infused over 24 hours. The long infusion time is intended to improve penetration of methotrexate across the blood–brain barrier. Although cerebrospinal fluid (CSF) methotrexate concentrations are typically only 1% or less of the concurrent plasma concentrations (36), use of high-dose methotrexate allows prolonged high plasma concentrations to achieve cytocidal methotrexate concentrations in the CSF. Leucovorin "rescue" is then administered to prevent excessive and intolerable toxicity to normal tissues. High-dose intravenous methotrexate may be combined with intrathecal methotrexate to further boost CSF concentrations. Doses as high as 33.6 gm/m^2 have been used (37) to achieve CSF concentrations of 10 μM from intravenous methotrexate alone. However, no improvement in overall survival has been shown as a result of using this approach. In general, high-dose methotrexate may result in a slightly higher CNS relapse rate than cranial irradiation with intrathecal methotrexate (38), but overall disease-free survival does not appear to be different. This suggests that high-dose methotrexate may improve control of disease in the bone marrow as well. In addition, cranial irradiation results in more significant CNS toxicities than does high-dose methotrexate.

The optimal dosage of high-dose methotrexate in the treatment of ALL has not been defined. One study (39) has identified a relationship between plasma methotrexate concentration and the probability of relapse. Patients received 15 courses of methotrexate, 1000 mg/m^2, given as a 200 mg/m^2 loading dose, followed by 800 mg/m^2 over 24 hours. This therapy was delivered as CNS therapy and during the first 75 weeks of continuation therapy. Patients who achieved steady-state plasma concentrations greater than 16 μM for at least half their courses were more likely to remain in complete continuous remission than patients whose plasma concentrations were lower. The variability in plasma concentrations was due solely to interpatient differences in drug elimination since all patients were treated with identical methotrexate dosages. This study provides insight into how best to use methotrexate in ALL and offers guidance in selecting a dosage of methotrexate that will yield optimal cytotoxic exposure and the most efficacious

results. A potential role for prospective pharmacokinetic monitoring of high-dose methotrexate to improve its therapeutic benefit in ALL patients is also discussed.

The preceding data for the use of CNS prophylaxis and HDMTX for control or prevention of CNS disease and/or relapse is in the context of intense systemic therapy. Recent data suggest that the addition of epipodophyllotoxins to the systemic therapy may result in better CNS cytotoxicity because of documented CNS penetration (40). Other approaches to improve control of CNS disease include the use of dexamethasone instead of prednisone during continuation therapy (41).

Continued (Maintenance) Therapy

In patients who have a achieved a complete remission, only a small proportion (perhaps 15%) will be long-term survivors if no additional therapy is administered (42). Continuation, or maintenance, therapy appears to be necessary to eradicate the remaining leukemia cells that are undetectable during remission. The growth fraction of leukemia cells is relatively small, and the cell–cycle time is fairly long. Therefore, only a small fraction of the total number of leukemia cells is susceptible at any given time to the effects of most anticancer drugs that are cell–cycle phase-specific agents. Hence, a prolonged period of exposure to anticancer drugs is necessary to further reduce the malignant population. Most commonly, continuation therapy has consisted of a two-drug combination of mercaptopurine and methotrexate (42). Mercaptopurine is given orally in dosages of 50 to 90 mg/m^2/day, and methotrexate is given either orally, intravenously, or intramuscularly at dosages of 15 to 30 mg/m^2/week.

The optimal duration of continuation therapy is not known, and current guidelines are based on empiric trial-and-error approaches. Most treatment programs use a duration of 2 to 6 years for continuation therapy. In determining the length of continuation therapy, the risk of off-therapy relapses must be considered in comparison to the risks of undesirable toxic effects of the therapy. Therapy may be stopped after 30 months of continuous complete remission or at least 12 months of continuous remission after an isolated nonmedullary relapse (CNS or testes). Results of several large long-term studies indicate that 70% of patients who have therapy electively stopped in this fashion will remain disease-free and be long-term survivors (42).

Although continuation therapy is well tolerated, a significant problem is relapse while on therapy. A substantial fraction (perhaps 40%) of patients relapse during the continuation phase of therapy, presumably as a result of the development of resistant disease. In addition, continuation therapy is immunosuppressive and associated with the risk of opportunistic infections. Therefore, alternative strategies have been employed to overcome both the development of resistance and to reduce the risk of infections and other complications.

Approaches to prevent bone marrow relapse during remission have included increasing the number of drugs administered during remission, periodic repetition of the agents used to induce the initial remission (referred to as "reinforcement" pulses), and intermittent rather than continuous chemotherapy. Use of more than two agents simultaneously does not appear to improve the rate of disease-free survival but does increase the toxicity of the therapy (43). A recent approach to improving event-free survival includes a delayed reintensification phase, or reinduction (33).

One approach to the continuation therapy of ALL is rotational use of non-cross-resistant anticancer drugs early in therapy. This concept is based on the somatic mutation theory of Luria and Delbrück (44) and its further development by Goldie and Coldman (45, 46). This hypothesis states that intense early therapy and sequential or rotational use of multiple non-cross-resistant agents during continuation therapy will reduce the likelihood of the emergence of a drug-resistant subpopulation of leukemia cells. Bone marrow relapses while on continuation therapy account for the largest fraction of patients who succumb to ALL, and this is undoubtedly due to the development of resistance, either by mutation or by selection, to the methotrexate–mercaptopurine combination usually administered during this phase of therapy. The rationale for administering additional non-cross-resistant agents during continuation therapy is to reduce the opportunity for resistance to be manifested to the primary combination. Therefore, other effective agents such as etoposide, cyclophosphamide, cytarabine, teniposide, or additional anthracyclines may be administered during continuation therapy in addition to the more customary methotrexate and mercaptopurine. However, the negative aspect is the increase in toxicity that may be encountered with some of these other agents. Since up to 50% of patients may be cured with the relatively well-tolerated methotrexate–mercaptopurine combination, additional more toxic drugs during continuation therapy may result only in more morbidity for patients who may be cured with less aggressive therapy. This dilemma points out the need to develop a better understanding of the various subtypes of ALL and significant prognostic factors in order to more readily identify those patients who would be expected to do well with less intense therapy.

Prognostic Factors

Numerous variables have been identified that are associated with the likely prognosis for ALL. These factors are used in much the same way that staging is used for solid tumors: to provide patients and families some indication of the likely outcome of treatment and to develop treatment

plans appropriate for the type of disease. Table 78.5 lists some of the most widely recognized factors. Age at diagnosis is important, with children under 2 years of age and those over 10 years of age having a higher mortality rate with current standard therapy. Several studies have shown that boys have a slightly greater risk of relapse than girls, even after accounting for nonmedullary relapses in the testes, which apparently act as a pharmacologic sanctuary from systemic anticancer drugs. WBC count at diagnosis is universally recognized as an important prognostic factor since higher WBC counts represent a greater tumor burden and are associated with a poorer outcome. T-cell and B-cell leukemias, identified by the reaction of their SIgs with specific monoclonal antibodies, have a poorer prognosis than leukemia expressing other SIgs. Many series have shown that nonwhite patients may have a poorer prognosis though there has been speculation that this may be due at least partly to socioeconomic factors that may cause delays in diagnosis and treatment. A thymic or mediastinal mass on chest roentgenograms is a high-risk feature although this is often associated with T-cell disease. Patients with lymphoblasts detectable in the CSF at diagnosis have a poorer prognosis.

Genetic characteristics, in addition to clinical factors, also have prognostic significance. Ploidy, defined as the number of chromosomes present in leukemic clones, is an established prognostic factor. The types and frequency of various ploidies are summarized in Table 78.2. Patients who have leukemic cell clones with more than 53

Table 78.5.
Adverse Prognostic Factors at Diagnosis of ALL

Age	
	<2 years
	>10 years
Sex	
	Male
Race	
	Nonewhite
Physical findings	
	Hepatosplenomegaly
	Lymphadenopathy
	Mediastinal mass (on chest roentgenogram)
	Lymphoblasts in CNS
Hematologic findings	
	Elevated WBC count
	Elevated hemoglobin
	Decreased platelets
FAB morphology	
	L2, L3
Immunologic markers	
	T-cell or B-cell leukemia
Cytogenetics	
	DNA index < 1.16
	Translocations
	Philadelphia chromosome

chromosomes, or a ratio of DNA content greater than 1.15 times normal (sometimes referred to as the "DNA index"), are more responsive to treatment, and patients with this type of disease have a better prognosis (47). Cytogenetic studies have shown that leukemia clones that exhibit various types of translocations result in a poorer prognosis.

These risk factors often cosegregate; patients with T-cell leukemia often have a high WBC count, for example. Therefore, none of these factors should be regarded as having completely independent prognostic value, and any treatment plan that uses these factors to individualize therapy should consider how these factors interact and correlate with one another. It appears highly likely that as our understanding of the molecular biology of leukemia improves, the genetically oriented prognostic factors will gradually replace the more traditional clinical factors in assigning risk categories and designing treatment regimens. On the other hand, any prognostic factor is important relative only to the treatment currently used. If a major new treatment advance is developed, all currently used prognostic factors could lose their predictive value.

ACUTE NONLYMPHOCYTIC LEUKEMIA

ANLL differs in many respects from ALL, particularly with regard to its age distribution and prognosis. Whereas ALL is primarily a childhood disease, ANLL is primarily a disease of adults. In addition, in both children and adults, it has proved much more resistant to treatment, and in order to achieve a cure, most patients require much more intense, toxic, and myelosuppressive therapy than that required for ALL. The most successful treatment programs available today result in cure rates of no more than about one-third of all patients with ANLL. In addition, the more intense therapy results in greater morbidity and mortality, particularly in older patients, and may limit the amount of effective therapy that can be administered. Bone marrow transplants have a more well-established role in the treatment of ANLL for those patients who have an acceptably matched donor.

Although early attempts to treat ANLL used the same drugs that had been found to be successful in ALL, the two groups of diseases are quite different in their biologic characteristics and their responses to therapy. The two most effective agents in the treatment of ANLL are cytarabine and daunorubicin. Almost all current treatment protocols administer 5 to 10 days of cytarabine by continuous infusion. Daunorubicin is administered daily for 2 or 3 days, either prior to cytarabine or simultaneously at the beginning of the cytarabine continuous infusion. This combination will result in complete remissions in up to 75% of patients (48–50). However, the challenge in the treatment of ANLL is to maintain remission. Relapses are usually due to resistant disease in the bone marrow; isolated extramedullary relapses are uncommon. In addi-

tion, relapses generally occur earlier than with ALL, during the first year following diagnosis. Therefore, most current treatment regimens have emphasized early intense therapy, but use a shorter duration of therapy, relative to ALL. Other drugs that may be used in the treatment of ANLL are etoposide, thioguanine, and the investigational agents 5-azacytidine and amsacrine. Recently, a new antimetabolite, cladribine or 2-chlorodeoxyadenosine, has been shown to produce a high complete response rate as a single agent in both relapsed (51) and newly diagnosed (52) pediatric patients with ANLL. Fludarabine, a fluorinated purine that is resistant to deactivation by deaminase enzymes, has also shown activity when combined with cytarabine in adult ANLL (53). Further studies of both these agents in combination with established agents used to treat ANLL are needed to establish their role in the therapy of this disease. Current treatment approaches for both adults (54) and children (55) with ANLL have recently been reviewed.

Treatment of the CNS is of lesser importance in ANLL since the primary reason for treatment failure is bone marrow relapse. Although lymphoblasts are found in the CSF more frequently in ANLL than in ALL, treatment of the CNS is often limited to intrathecal drugs, with irradiation administered at the end of therapy to patients with CNS disease at diagnosis. CNS treatment delivered earlier has no effect on disease-free survival because of the inadequacy of systemic therapy and bone marrow relapses. Intrathecal therapy usually consists of methotrexate, cytarabine, and hydrocortisone.

Splenectomy has been evaluated as a treatment for ANLL and has shown no substantial therapeutic benefit and had little impact on the clinical course of the disease (56).

With the limitations of current therapy, the most promising new treatment modality available to ANLL patients is bone marrow transplants. The optimal time for a transplant is as soon as possible after achieving a clinical remission. This procedure is complicated by the occurrence of both acute and chronic GVHD, and only a limited number of ANLL patients (25 to 40%) have compatible bone marrow donors. Therefore, bone marrow transplants do not offer a universal cure for this disease. Use of autologous transplants also shows promise. However, the established risk of relapse due to residual leukemia cells in the marrow, as discussed, limits this approach until better purging techniques are developed.

Prognostic Factors

Prognostic factors for ANLL are less well defined than for ALL primarily because the overall survival is much poorer. Nevertheless, a number of variables have been identified that are associated either with a poor likelihood of achieving a clinical remission or with a short duration of

Table 78.6.
Adverse Prognostic Factors at Diagnosis of ANLL

Age
>60 years
<2 years
Gender
Male
Symptomatic preleukemic interval
Treatment-induced leukemia
Following treatment for Hodgkin's disease or other malignancy
Physical findings
Hepatosplenomegaly
Significant infection or hemorrhage
Leukemia cells in the CNS
Hematologic findings
Elevated WBC count (>100,000/ul)
Decreased hemoglobin
Severe thrombocytopenia
Marrow infiltration >75%
FAB morphology
M5
Cytogenetics
All abnormal karyotypes
Philadelphia chromosome
Monosomy 7

remission. These factors are summarized in Table 78.6. Variables associated with a poor prognosis are advancing age, the presence of a hemorrhage or significant infection (particularly in adults), hepatosplenomegaly, and a prolonged symptomatic interval preceding diagnosis. Like ALL, patients with a high WBC count have a poorer prognosis. In addition, the degree of bone marrow involvement, the presence of Auer rods, and elevated serum lysozyme concentrations carry a poor prognosis. Cytogenetic studies have not identified specific abnormalities that are associated with prognosis, but all abnormal karyotypes are unfavorable, including the presence of the Philadelphia chromosome (a classic marker for chronic myelocytic leukemia).

SUPPORTIVE THERAPY

The improving prognosis of acute leukemias is due in large part to the advancements in supportive care that have occurred over the past 10 years. Deaths during induction therapy due to hemorrhage, infections, and metabolic derangements have been reduced as a consequence of the improved ability to manage these complications. In addition, deaths during remission due to opportunistic infections are less frequent today, and certain types of lethal infections, notably *Pneumocystis carinii* pneumonia, have been virtually eradicated from the leukemia patient population. Use of central venous catheters has also simplified the delivery of complicated chemotherapy regimens although these devices are associated with significant complications of their own. The use of enteral and parenteral

nutritional support has also been important in the management of these patients. All these factors have permitted the routine use of more intense therapies in an attempt to develop effective, curative therapy for acute leukemia.

Infection in the immunosuppressed granulocytopenic cancer patients remains a significant cause of morbidity and mortality. The risk of life-threatening septicemia or pneumonia increases dramatically as the patient's granulocyte count decreases and the duration of the granulocytopenia increases (57). Since immunosuppressed patients are unable to mount a response to infectious organisms, common clinical signs of infection (leukocytosis, purulence) may be absent. Therefore, fever is of supreme importance in diagnosing infections in the granulocytopenic patient, and the presence of fever in such patients should be regarded as a medical emergency. Infections that are not promptly treated progress rapidly, and death from septicemia or pneumonia may occur in a few hours. Prompt institution of empiric broad-spectrum antibiotic coverage will prevent mortality in most cases.

A potentially lethal opportunistic infection for immunosuppressed patients is *Pneumocystis carinii* pneumonia. This organism is ordinarily innocuous and is found virtually everywhere in the environment. However, in immunosuppressed cancer patients, who are not necessarily granulocytopenic, this organism can produce a potentially fatal infection, and in the past has been a major cause of death during remission for ALL patients. Low daily doses of trimethoprim/sulfamethoxazole (TMP/SMX) administered prophylactically during remission prevented this infection in virtually all immunosuppressed ALL patients (58). Equally efficacious protection can be achieved by administering this combination for only 3 consecutive days each week (59). This reduced exposure has the advantage of fewer adverse effects, primarily, the occurrence of systemic mycoses. Although neutropenia has been reported as an unwanted consequence of prophylaxis with TMP/SMX in some studies, no difference in neutropenia was detected in this study. For those few cases that are intolerant to TMP/SMX, dapsone is a viable alternative and has been found to be safe and effective (60).

Tumor lysis syndrome (TLS) is a complication of the initial antileukemic therapy in some patients, particularly those with a very high initial WBC count. TLS refers to the metabolic disturbances found with a very brisk response to induction therapy that results in significant cell death and the release of intracellular nucleoproteins into the circulation. The purine byproducts of these nucleoproteins are metabolized by xanthine oxidase to uric acid, which in high concentrations can produce obstructive urate nephropathy. The metabolic disturbances include hyperuricemia, hyperphosphatemia, hyperkalemia, and hypocalcemia. Patients may also experience acute renal failure. There is a clear association with hyperuricemia and acute renal failure

(61, 62). Other factors that influence the risk of acute renal failure in those with TLS include hyperphosphatemia, glomerular filtration rate prior to therapy, xanthinuria, intravascular volume depletion, and infiltration of renal parenchyma by malignant cells (61–63). Therefore, the goals of treatment of TLS is to prevent renal failure and worsening of metabolic disturbances. This is primarily done through increasing the excretion of the aforementioned metabolic contents. Vigorous hydration and urinary alkalinization (to increase the solubility of uric acid in the urine) should be instituted in patients with an initial high WBC count. Overzealous alkalinization of the urine may lead to massive phosphate crystalluria because phosphate precipitates at alkaline pH. The goal of alkalinization should be to maintain urine pH between 6.5 and 7.0 (64).

Administration of allopurinol, a xanthine oxidase inhibitor, prevents the production of uric acid and the development of nephropathy. However, the concern for xanthine nephropathy must be considered during allopurinol therapy, especially if impaired renal function decreases the elimination of allopurinol. This would require a dosage decrease in allopurinol. Currently, there is an investigational agent, the enzyme urate oxidase, which converts uric acid to the water soluble metabolite allantoin, thereby lowering plasma uric acid concentrations as well as urinary uric acid excretion (65).

Because of the bone marrow suppressive effects of both the disease and its therapy, most patients need extensive support with blood products, including platelet, erythrocyte, and occasionally, granulocyte transfusions. Hemorrhages, particularly, are a cause of significant morbidity and mortality in leukemia patients, and the ability to collect platelets either from whole blood or by plasmapheresis is essential in the modern therapy of leukemia. The hematocrit may be decreased as a result of decreased erythrocyte production, and packed red blood cells may be required to maintain the hematocrit at adequate levels. Granulocyte transfusions have no apparent role in the prevention of infection but, along with antibiotic therapy, may be effective in treating documented sepsis. However, because of the cost of preparing granulocyte transfusions, the very short life span of transfused granulocytes in the patient, and the serious side effects of granulocyte transfusions, this procedure is usually reserved for only the most gravely ill patients.

Cytokines (granulocyte colony stimulating factor [G-CSF] and granulocyte-macrophage colony stimulating factor [GM-CSF])have been widely used in the treatment of patients with solid tumors and lymphomas to shorten the length and severity of neutropenia following treatment with antineoplastic drugs. The use of cytokines in acute leukemias has been less widespread. Although occasional patients may benefit from cytokine support during treatment for acute lymphocytic leukemia, in general, the treatment does not produce prolonged neutropenia, and

the benefit of cytokine use has not been established. Our institution is currently completing a double-blind placebo-controlled trial of G-CSF therapy during induction therapy, but the results have not been unblinded at this time. In acute nonlymphocytic leukemia, cytokine use initially was avoided because of concern that cytokines which stimulate the growth and release of cells from the myelocytic lineage could potentially stimulate growth of leukemia cells as well. However, two recent double-blind, placebo-controlled studies (66, 67) have evaluated the use of GM-CSF to reduce the length and severity of neutropenia in elderly patients being treated for primary acute myelocytic leukemia. The results of these studies were somewhat different. In the larger study (66), 388 patients greater than 60 years of age were evaluated, and no significant benefit of cytokine treatment was identified. The authors conclude that GM-CSF use cannot be recommended in such patients. However, in the smaller study, 124 patients between 55 and 70 years of age were evaluated, and GM-CSF treatment was associated with shorter time to neutrophil recovery, reduction in overall treatment-related toxicity, reduction in infectious toxicity, and longer survival time. This paper concluded that GM-CSF treatment was safe and efficacious in this group of patients. Further evaluation of cytokine support in elderly patients with acute myelocytic leukemia is needed to clearly define the role of such therapy.

Disseminated intravascular coagulation (DIC) is an occasional but life-threatening complication of ANLL, particularly for patients with progranulocytic leukemia, and results in severe hemorrhages. It is characterized by thrombocytopenia, hypofibrinogenemia, decreased factor V levels, and increased levels of fibrin split products. It is treated with low-dose heparin.

CONCLUSION

Tremendous advances have been made in the treatment of the acute leukemias over the past 10 years, and the successes that have been achieved in the treatment of childhood ALL serve as a model for treatment of other human malignancies. Today, acute leukemias are potentially curable diseases in many patients, and considerable prolongation of a useful and productive life can be achieved for many others. Current research efforts in immunology and molecular biology are likely to lead to powerful new treatments.

REFERENCES

1. Clarkson B. The acute leukemias. In: Thorn GW, Adams RD, Braunwald E, Isselbacher KJ, Petersdorf RG. Harrison's Principles of Internal Medicine, 8th ed. New York: McGraw-Hill, 1977:1767–1777.
2. Wingo PA, Tong T, Bolden S. Cancer statistics. CA Cancer J Clin 45:8–30, 1995.
3. Gallo RD, Wong-Staal F. Retroviruses as etiologic agents of some animal and human leukemias and lymphomas and as tools for

elucidating the molecular mechanism of leukemogenesis. Blood 60:545–556, 1982.

4. Altman AJ, Schwartz AD. Malignant Diseases of Infancy, Childhood and Adolescence. Philadelphia: W. B. Saunders Company, 1983: 187–238.

5. Bennett JM, Catovsky D, Daniel M-T, et al. Proposals for the classifications of the acute leukemias; French-American-British (FAB) co-operative group. Br J Haematol 33:451–458, 1976.

6. Pui C-H, Behm FG, Crist WM. Clinical and biologic relevance of immunologic marker studies in childhood acute lymphoblastic leukemia. Blood 82:343–362, 1993.

7. Pui C-H. Childhood leukemias (medical progress). N Engl J Med 332:1618–1630, 1995.

8. Fernbach DJ. Natural history of acute leukemia. In: Sutow WW: Fernbach DJ, Vietti TJ. Clinical Pediatric Oncology, 3rd ed. St. Louis: The C. V. Mosby Company, 1984:332–377.

9. Freeman AI, Pantazopoulos N, DeCastro L, et al. Infections in children with acute leukemia. Med Pediatr Oncol 1:67–73, 1975.

10. Farber S, Diamond LK, Mercer RD, et al. Temporary remissions in acute leukemia in children produced by folic antagonist 4-amethopteroylglutamic acid (aminopterin). N Engl J Med 238:787–793, 1948.

11. Storb R, Deeg HJ, Pepe M, et al. Methotrexate and cyclosporine versus cyclosporine alone for prophylaxis of graft-versus-host disease in patients given HLA-identical marrow grafts for leukemia: long-term follow-up of a controlled trial. Blood 73:1729–1734, 1989.

12. Shepherd JD, Shore TB, Reece DE, et al. Cyclosporine and methylprednisolone for prophylaxis of acute graft-versus-host disease. Bone Marrow Transplant 3:553–558, 1988.

13. Kennedy MS, Deeg HJ, Storb R, et al. Treatment of acute graft-versus-host disease after allogeneic transplantation: Randomized study comparing corticosteroids and cyclosporine. Am J Med 78:978–983, 1985.

14. Ramsay NK, Kersey JH, Robison LL, et al. A randomized study of the prevention of acute graft-versus-host disease. N Engl J Med 306:392–397, 1982.

15. Martin PJ, Remlinger K, Hansen JA, et al. Murine monoclonal anti-T cell antibodies for treatment of refractory acute graft-versus-host disease. Transplant Proc 16:1494–1495, 1984.

16. Winston DJ, Ho WG, Bartoni K, et al. Ganciclovir prophylaxis of cytomegalovirus infection and disease in allogeneic bone marrow transplant recipients. Results of a placebo-controlled, double-blind trial. Ann Intern Med 118:179–184, 1993.

17. Goodrich JM, Bowden RA, Fisher L, et al. Ganciclovir prophylaxis to prevent cytomegalovirus disease after allogeneic transplant. Ann Intern Med 118:173–178, 1993.

18. Schmidt GM, Horak DA, Niland JC, et al. A randomized, controlled trial of prophylactic ganciclovir for cytomegalovirus pulmonary infection in recipients of allogeneic bone marrow transplants; The City of Hope-Stanford-Syntex CMV Study Group. N Engl J Med 324:1005–1011, 1991.

19. Rollins JB. Hepatic veno-occlusive disease. Am J Med 81:297–306, 1986.

20. Jones RJ, Lee KS, Beschorner WE, et al. Venoocclusive disease of the liver following bone marrow transplantation. Transplantation 44:778–783, 1987.

21. Dulley FL, Kanfer EJ, Appelbaum FR, et al. Venoocclusive disease of the liver after chemoradiotherapy and autologous bone marrow transplantation. Transplantation 43:870–873, 1987.

22. Ozkaynak MF, Weinberg K, Kohn D, et al. Hepatic venoocclusive disease post-bone marrow transplantation in children conditioned with busulfan and cyclophosphamide: incidence, risk factors, and clinical outcome. Bone Marrow Transplant 7:467–474, 1991.

23. Heslop HE, Benaim E, Brenner MK, et al. Response of steroid-resistant graft versus host disease to lymphoblast antibody CBL1. Lancet 346:805–806, 1995.

24. Brenner MK, Rill DR, Moen RC, et al. Gene-marking to trace origin of relapse after autologous bone-marrow transplantation. Lancet 341:85–86, 1993.

25. Jacquillat C, Weil M, Gemon MF, et al. Combination therapy in 130 patients with acute lymphoblastic leukemia (protocol 06 LA 66-Paris). Cancer Res 33:3278, 1973.

26. Ortega JA, Nesbit ME Jr, Donaldson MH, et al. L-asparaginase, vincristine and prednisone for induction of first remission in acute lymphocytic leukemia. Cancer Res 37:535, 1977.

27. Sackman JF, Pavlovsky S, Penalver JA, et al. Evaluation of induction of remission, intensification and central nervous system prophylactic treatment in acute lymphoblastic leukemia. Cancer 34:418, 1974.

28. Aur RJA, Simone JV, Hustu HO, et al. A comparative study of central nervous system irradiation and intensive chemotherapy early in remission of childhood acute lymphocytic leukemia. Cancer 29:381, 1972.

29. George P, Pinkel D. CNS radiation in children with acute lymphocytic leukemia in remission (abstract). Proc Amer Assoc Cancer Res 6:22, 1965.

30. Nesbit ME, Robison LL, Littman PS, et al. Presymptomatic central nervous system therapy in previously untreated childhood acute lymphoblastic leukaemia: comparison of 1800 rad and 2400 rad. A report for Children's Cancer Study Group. Lancet 1:461, 1981.

31. Aur RJA, Hustu HO, Verzosa MS, et al. Comparison of two methods of preventing central nervous system leukemia. Blood 42:349, 1973.

32. Bleyer WA. Clinical pharmacology of intrathecal methotrexate. II. An improved dosage regimen derived from age-related pharmacokinetics. Cancer Treat Rep 61:1419–1425, 1977.

33. Tubergen DG, Gilchrist GS, O'Brien RT, et al. Improved outcome with delayed intensification for children with acute lymphoblastic leukemia and intermediate presenting features: a Children's Cancer Group phase III trial. J Clin Oncol 11:527–537, 1993.

34. Gilchrist GS, Tubergen DG, Sather HN, et al. Low numbers of CSF blasts at diagnosis do not predict for the development of CNS leukemia in children with intermediate-risk acute lymphoblastic leukemia: a Childrens Cancer Group report. J Clin Oncol 12:2594–2600, 1994.

35. Freeman AI, Weinberg V, Brecher ML, et al. Comparison of intermediate-dose methotrexate with cranial irradiation for the post-induction treatment of acute lymphocytic leukemia in children. N Engl J Med 308:477–484, 1983.

36. Evans WE, Crom WR, Yalowich JC. Methotrexate. In: Evans WE, Schentag JJ, Jusko WJ. Applied Pharmacokinetics; Principles of Therapeutic Drug Monitoring, 2nd ed. Spokane: Applied Therapeutics, Inc., 1986:1009–1056.

37. Balis FM, Savitch JL, Bleyer WA, et al. Remission induction of meningeal leukemia with high-dose intravenous methotrexate. J Clin Oncol 3:485–489, 1985.

38. Freeman AI, Weinberg VE, Brecher ML, et al. Comparison of intermediate-dose methotrexate with cranial irradiation for the post-induction treatment of acute lymphocytic leukemia in children. N Engl J Med 308:477–484, 1983.

39. Evans WE, Crom WR, Abromowitch M, et al. Clinical pharmacodynamics of high-dose methotrexate in acute lymphocytic leukemia; identification of a relation between concentration and effect. N Engl J Med 314:471–477, 1986.

40. Relling MV, Mahmoud H, Pui C-H, et al. Intravenous etoposide therapy achieves potentially cytotoxic concentrations in cerebrospinal fluid of children with acute lymphoblastic leukemia (meeting abstract). Proc Annu Meet Am Assoc Cancer Res 35:A1438, 1994.

41. Jones B, Freeman AI, Shuster JJ, et al. Lower incidence of meningeal leukemia when prednisone is replaced by dexamethasone in the treatment of acute lymphocytic leukemia. Med Pediatr Oncol 19:269–275, 1991.

42. Simone JV, Rivera G. Management of acute leukemia. In: Sutow WW,

Fernbach DJ, Vietti TJ. Clinical Pediatric Oncology, 3rd ed. St. Louis: The C. V. Mosby Company, 1984:378–402.

43. Aur RJA, Simone JV, Verzosa JS, et al. Childhood acute lymphocytic leukemia: study VIII. Cancer 42:2123, 1978.

44. Luria SE, Delbrück M. Genetics 28:491–511, 1943.

45. Goldie JH, Coldman AJ. A mathematical model for relating the drug sensitivity of tumors to their spontaneous mutation rate. Cancer Treat Rep 63:1727–1733, 1979.

46. Goldie JH, Coldman AJ, Gudauskas GA. Rationale for the use of alternating non-cross-resistant chemotherapy. Cancer Treat Rep 66:439–449, 1982.

47. Williams DL, Tsiatis A, Brodeur GM, et al. Prognostic importance of chromosome number in 136 untreated children with acute lymphoblastic leukemia. Blood 60:864–871, 1982.

48. Lister TA, Rohatiner AZS. The treatment of acute myelogenous leukemia in adults. Semin Hematol 19:172–192, 1982.

49. Gale RP. Advances in the treatment of acute myelogenous leukemia. N Engl J Med 300:1189–1199, 1979.

50. Gale RP, Foon KA, Cline M, et al. Intensive chemotherapy for acute myelogenous leukemia. Ann Intern Med 94:753–757, 1981.

51. Santana VM, Mirro J Jr, Kearns C, et al. 2-Chlorodeoxyadenosine produces a high rate of complete hematologic remission in relapsed acute myeloid leukemia. J Clin Oncol 10:364–370, 1992.

52. Santana VM, Hurwitz CA, Blakley RL, et al. Complete hematologic remissions induced by 2-chlorodeoxyadenosine in children with newly diagnosed acute myeloid leukemia. Blood 84:1237–1242, 1994.

53. Gandhi V. Fludarabine for treatment of adult acute myelogenous leukemia. Leuk Lymphoma 11(suppl 2):7–13, 1993.

54. Stone RM, Mayer RJ. Treatment of the newly diagnosed adult with de novo acute myeloid leukemia. Hematol Oncol Clin North Am 7:47–64, 1993.

55. Hurwitz CA, Mounce KG, Grier HE. Treatment of patients with acute myelogenous leukemia: review of clinical trials of the past decade. J Pediatr Hematol Oncol 17:185–197, 1995.

56. Dahl G, Kalwinsky D, Kumar M, et al. A randomized trial of splenectomy in childhood acute nonlymphocytic leukemia (ANLL) (abstract). Proc Amer Assoc Cancer Res and Amer Soc Clin Oncol 22:480, 1981.

57. Schimpff SC. Therapy of infection in patients with granulocytopenia. Med Clin North Am 61:1101–1118, 1977.

58. Hughes WT, Kuhn S, Chaudhary S, et al. Successful chemoprophylaxis for *Pneumocystis carinii* pneumonitis. N Engl J Med 297:1419–1426, 1977.

59. Hughes WT, Rivera GK, Schell MJ, et al. Successful intermittent chemoprophylaxis for *Pneumocystis carinii* pneumonitis. N Engl J Med 316:1627–1632, 1987.

60. Slavin MA, Hoy JF, Stewart K, et al. Oral dapsone versus nebulized pentamidine for Pneumocystic carinii pneumonia prophylaxis: an open randomized prospective trial to assess efficacy and haematological toxicity. AIDS 6:1169–1174, 1992.

61. Kjellstrand CM, Cambell DC II, von Hartitzsch B, et al. Hyperuricemic acute renal failure. Arch Intern Med 133:349–359, 1974.

62. Jones DP, Stapleton FB, Kalwinsky D, et al. Renal dysfunction and hyperuricemia at presentation and relapse of acute lymphoblastic leukemia. Med Pediatr Oncol 18:283–286, 1990.

63. Band PR, Silverberg DS, Henderson JE, et al. Xanthine nephropathy in a patient with lymphosarcoma treated with allopurinol. N Engl J Med 283:354–357, 1970.

64. Jones DP, Mahmoud H, Chesney RW. Tumor lysis syndrome: pathogenesis and management. Pediatr Nephrol 9:206–212, 1995.

65. Masera G, Jankovic M, Zurlo MG, et al. Urate-oxidase prophylaxis of uric acid-induced renal damage in childhood leukemia. J Pediatr 100:152–155, 1982.

66. Stone RM, Berg DT, George SL, et al. Granulocyte-macrophage colony-stimulating factor after initial chemotherapy for elderly patients with acute myelogenous leukemia. N Engl J Med 332:1671–1677, 1995.

67. Rowe JM, Anderson JW, Mazza JJ, et al. A randomized placebo-controlled phase III study of granulocyte-macrophage colony-stimulating factor in adult patients (>55 to 70 years of age) with acute myelogenous leukemia: a study of the Eastern Cooperative Oncology Group (E1490). Blood 86:457–462, 1995.

CHAPTER 79

MALIGNANT LYMPHOMAS

REBECCA S. FINLEY and CLARENCE L. FORTNER

The lymphoreticular system constitutes the anatomic basis of both cellular and humoral immunity. Lymphocytes are the principal cellular component of the lymphoreticular system and are widely distributed in the body both singly and in aggregated centers (most commonly the lymph nodes). Reticulum cells and cells of the monocyte–macrophage series are also included in this system. Lymphoid cells originate in the bone marrow, undergo differentiation, and migrate by way of the blood and lymphatic vessels to populate the other lymphoreticular tissues (Fig. 79.1). T lymphocytes are processed through the thymus gland and are responsible for cell-mediated immunity. T lymphocytes are the predominant lymphocytes in peripheral blood and occupy the deep cortex of the lymph nodes. B lymphocytes are derived from the bone marrow and confer humoral immunity. B lymphocytes constitute only 10 to 15% of circulating lymphocytes and predominate in the follicles of the lymph nodes.

Lymphoreticular malignancies may manifest in either the bone marrow and peripheral blood or in one of the centers of aggregation (Fig. 79.2). When they present as extramedullary tumors arising primarily in the lymph nodes or other sites, these tumors are referred to as malignant lymphomas; when the bone marrow is the major site of the disease, they are classified as leukemias. Malignant lymphomas are generally separated into Hodgkin's disease and non-Hodgkin's lymphomas (NHLs). The term *non-Hodgkin's lymphomas* represents multiple diseases with diverse morphologic and clinical features.

Most lymphomas can be classified by their cellular origin. The precise cellular origin of Hodgkin's disease has not yet been firmly established. It has been suggested that it is derived from an immature lymphoid stage of development that undergoes malignant transformation prior to B or T cell differentiation and that the different subtypes of Hodgkin's disease arise from different lymphoid progenitor cell lines (1, 2). In adults, most NHLs are derived from B lymphocytes, with only about 15% of T cell origin in developed countries such as the United States (3).

For unexplained reasons, the incidence of lymphomas in the United States appears to be rising. The American Cancer Society estimated that during 1995 there will be 7800 new cases of Hodgkin's disease and 50,900 new cases of NHL diagnosed, with 1450 and 22,700 deaths attributed to each disease (4). The incidence of NHL increases steadily from childhood to age 80, and it is more common

in males than females (5). Hodgkin's disease exhibits a bimodal incidence curve, with the first peak occurring in the late 20s, after which there is a decline in incidence until about age 45. After age 45, the incidence increases steadily with age. Hodgkin's disease is also more common in males than females (6).

The etiology of malignant lymphomas is largely unknown. A potential infectious etiology of Hodgkin's disease has been suggested. The Epstein-Barr virus (EBV) has been indirectly associated with the disease in several ways. First, there has been a small, but consistent increased risk of Hodgkin's disease among persons who have had infectious mononucleosis (7–9). Further, the proportion of Hodgkin's disease patients with elevated titers of antibody against the EBV is larger than expected, and enhanced activation of EBV may precede the development of Hodgkin's disease (10–12). EBV has also been detected in Hodgkin's disease biopsy specimens (13, 14). It is not clear whether EBV has a direct role in the development of Hodgkin's disease or whether EBV infection is a result of a decreased immune competency that is linked to the pathogenesis of Hodgkin's disease (12). Epidemiologic studies have also reported clustering of patients with Hodgkin's disease in a high school (15, 16). Familial studies suggested an increased risk in first-degree relatives, especially siblings of young adult patients (17). There is also an association of Hodgkin's disease with certain leukocyte antigens (18). Overall, there is insufficient evidence to support the hypothesis that Hodgkin's disease is transmitted by person-to-person contact.

Patients with primary immunodeficiency diseases (e.g., Wiscott-Aldrich syndrome, ataxia-telangiectasia), and those receiving chronic immunosuppressive therapy (e.g., renal and cardiac transplant, chronic renal disease, inflammatory bowel disease, systemic lupus erythematosus) appear to have an increased risk of NHL (3, 19, 20). Other diseases that may predispose to the development of lymphomas include Klinefelter's syndrome, sarcoidosis, and Sjogren syndrome (3). Lymphomas now account for many of the cancers in patients with the acquired immunodeficiency syndrome (AIDS)(21). Ionizing radiation may also induce lymphomas, as evidenced by the increased incidence in survivors of Hiroshima and patients irradiated for ankylosing spondylitis (3, 22). Other environmental and occupational exposures that have been associated with an increased risk of NHL include other

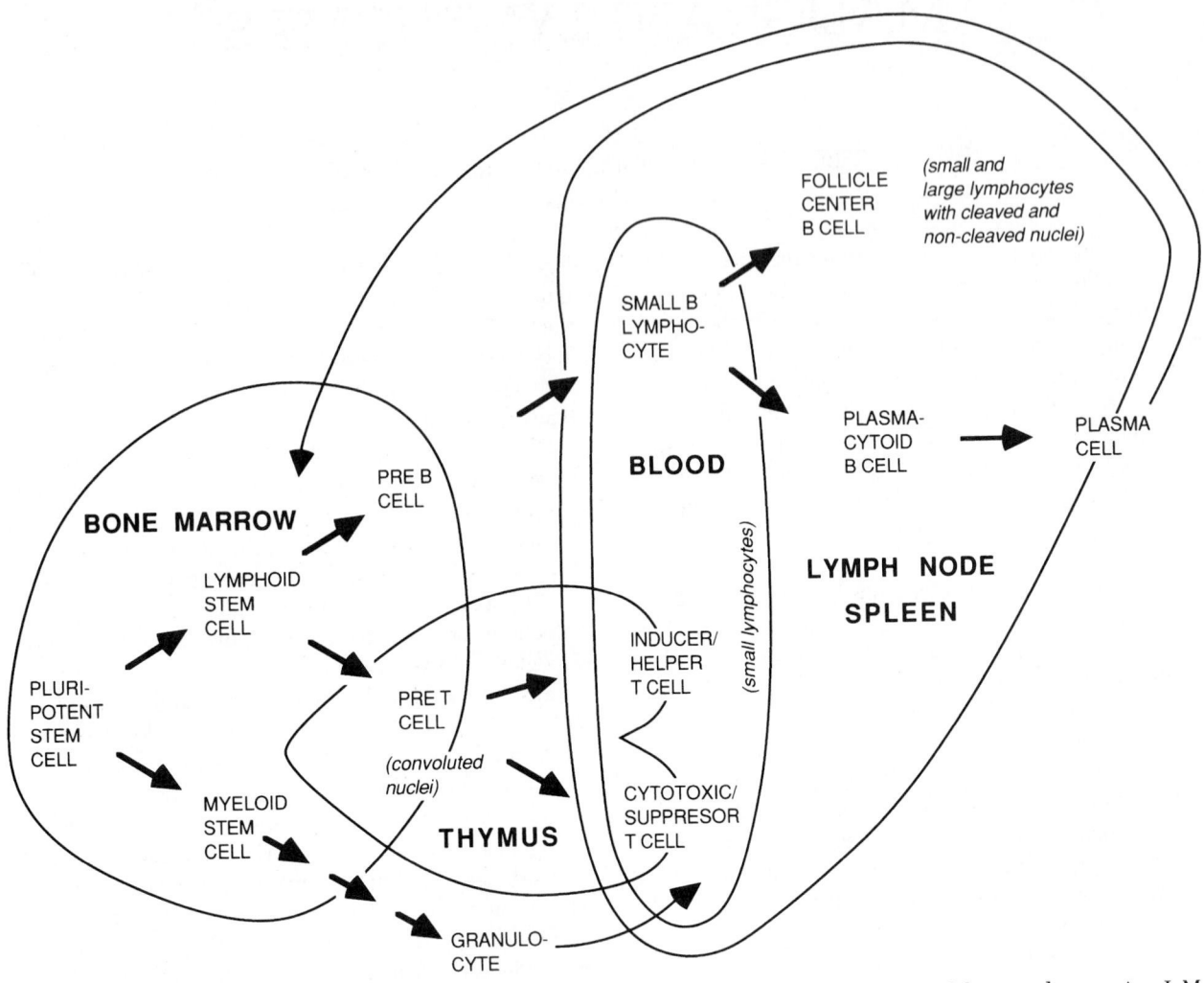

Figure 79-1. Tissue distribution of lymphocytes. From Aisenberg AC. Cell lineage in lymphoproliferative disease. Am J Med 74:680, 1983.

toxins, pesticides, solvents, hair dye, woodworking, and some cancer chemotherapy drugs (23).

The only documented viral associations of lymphomas have been that of Burkitt's lymphoma in Africans with the EBV and the human T cell leukemia virus (HTLV-I) in adult T cell leukemia and lymphoma (24, 25).

PATHOLOGY

The diagnosis and classification of malignant lymphoma can be made only by biopsy and histopathologic examination under a light microscope.

A biopsy specimen of Hodgkin's disease reveals a heterogeneous cellular population of normal-appearing lymphocytes (predominantly helper T cells), eosinophils, plasma cells, and Reed-Sternberg cells. These Reed-Sternberg (R-S) cells, the characteristic malignant cells of Hodgkin's disease, are multinucleated giant cells that are usually necessary to make a pathologic diagnosis. The

normal-appearing host inflammatory cells that surround the R-S cells are like the body's response to the tumor. Although 35 to 40% of cases have cytogenic abnormalities, no specific chromosomal marker has been identified. A mononuclear variant of the R-S cell, sometimes called the Hodgkin's disease cell, is also seen in some biopsy specimens (2). The histopathology of Hodgkin's disease is divided according to the Rye classification into four major subgroups (Table 79.1)(26). This classification has been widely accepted because of its simplicity, and in the past, it provided a crude correlation with prognosis, but the availability of highly curative treatments has diminished this importance (27). The lymphocyte-predominant, mixed-cellularity, and lymphocyte-depleted histologies can be differentiated from one another based on the increased frequency of R-S cells (28). The nodular sclerosis histology is characterized by bands of collagen that partly or completely divide the lymphoid tissue into nodules.

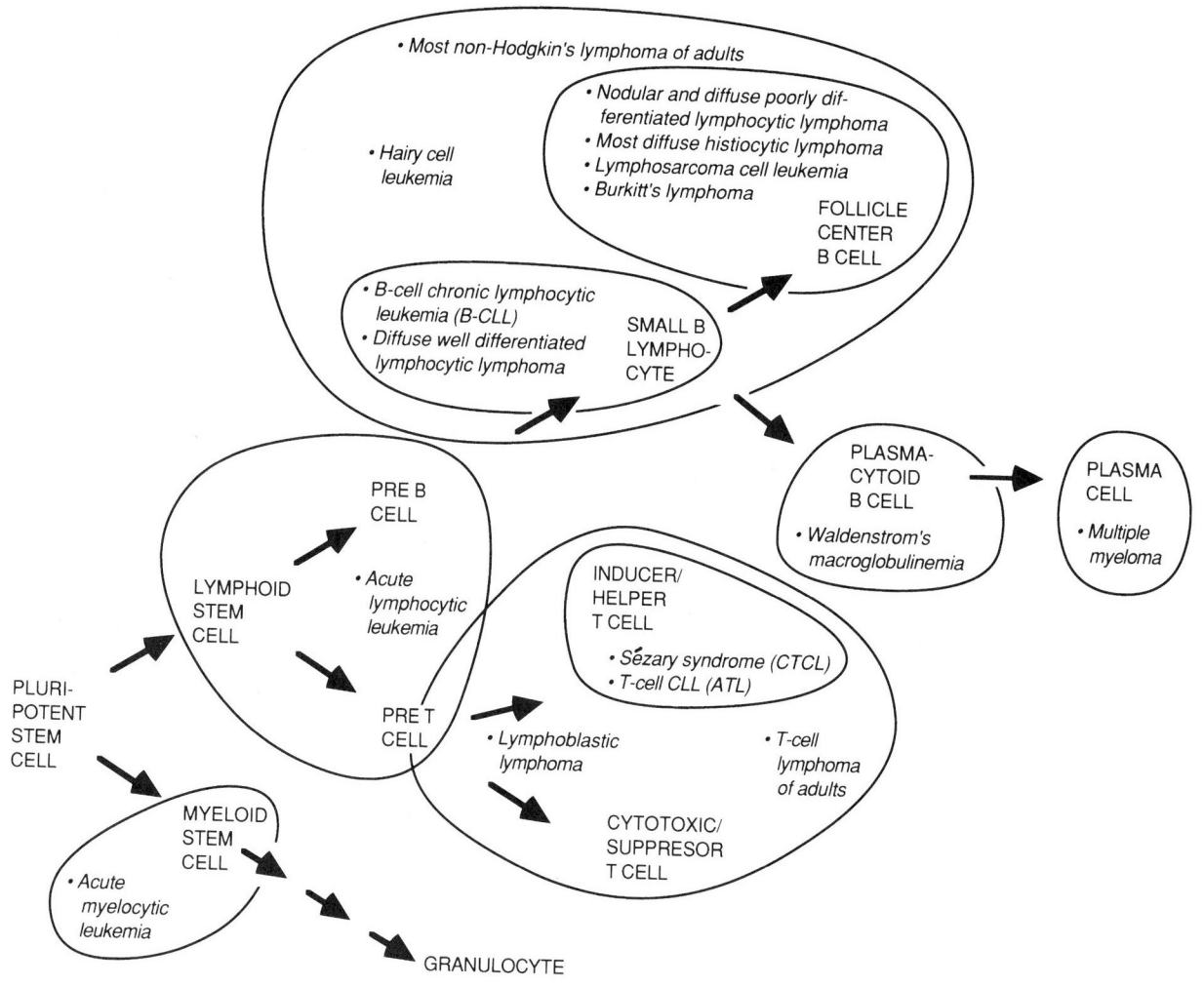

Figure 79-2. Cell lineage in lymphoproliferative disease. From Aisenberg AC. Cell lineage in lymphoproliferative disease. Am J Med 74:682, 1983.

The lymphocyte-predominant histology is characterized by a cellular proliferation of benign-appearing lymphocytes, and at least three important subtypes exist (29). It is more common in men and most often occurs in patients under 35 years. Most patients have clinically localized disease at diagnosis and are asymptomatic. The prognosis is usually favorable.

The mixed-cellularity subtype contains a proportion of neoplastic cells intermediate between the lymphocyte-predominant and lymphocyte-depleted histologies. This type is also more common in older patients and in men. Patients may present in any clinical stage and often experience systemic symptoms. This histology carries an intermediate prognosis.

Lymphocyte-depleted Hodgkin's disease is characterized by a predominance of abnormal and R-S cells, with a relative paucity of lymphocytes. This subtype is most commonly seen in older patients, who have sympto-matic and disseminated disease. This is also the most common type of Hodgkin's disease seen in patients with AIDS.

Nodular-sclerosing Hodgkin's disease is more commonly found in women and most frequently occurs in adolescents and young adults. It is associated with a good prognosis, especially in localized disease.

Hodgkin's disease cells release various cytokines that produce local and systemic reactions. These cytokines include interleukin-1, interleukin-2, interleukin-5, interleukin-6, tumor necrosis factor, interferon gamma, granulocyte-macrophage colony-stimulating factor, granulocyte colony-stimulating factor, macrophage colony-stimulating factor, and tumor growth factor-beta. It is believed that release of these cytokines contributes to the "B" symptoms (i.e., fever, night sweats, weight loss), and tumor growth factor-beta may play a role in the fibrosis of nodular sclerosing Hodgkin's disease (30).

Table 79.1.
Rye Classification of Histologic Subtypes Found in Hodgkin's Disease

1. **Lymphocyte predominance**
   A. Lymphocytic and/or histiocytic diffuse: sinusoids of lymph nodes become filled with lymphocytic cells and general normal architecture of the lymph node becomes obscured; this picture does not occur uniformly throughout the node and normal foci may be found; the lymph node capsule is not invaded by lymphocytes in early stages of the disease.
   B. Nodular proliferative type: this form differs little from the diffuse form except for the tendency of the lymphocytic cells to be placed into poorly defined large and closely arranged nodules.
2. **Nodular sclerosis**
   This tissue type is characterized by formation of bands of connective tissue that intercommunicate and separate the cellular and necrotic areas into islands.
3. **Mixed cellularity**
   Presents a picture between lymphocyte predominance and lymphocyte depleted and characterized by having a variable number of lymphocytes and the presence of neutrophils, eosinophils, and plasma cells.
4. **Lymphocyte depleted**
   A. Diffuse fibrosis: characterized by widespread disorderly fibrosis with depletion of lymphoid cells and eventually of all other cellular elements.
   B. Reticular type: lesions in this category have no significant characteristics other than a predominance of Reed-Sternberg cells to distinguish them from other diffuse, fibrotic, mixed or even nodular sclerotic lesions.

Unlike Hodgkin's disease, the cellular origin of the various NHLs is well established. The classification of NHLs is based on their cellular origin, morphologic and immunologic characteristics of the malignant cells. Six different histologic classification systems have been used over the years. In the past, the Rapport system, based solely on morphology, has been most commonly used (31).

Many attempts have been made to develop a classification system that will integrate morphologic and prognostic information with the evolving knowledge of the functional classification of lymphocytes. From 1976 until 1980, the National Cancer Institute sponsored a multiinstitutional study in which 12 pathologists evaluated the reproducibility and comparability of the 6 major classification systems. It was concluded that although each of the systems had particular merits, none was clearly superior to the others. These pathologists reached a consensus (Working Formulation of Non-Hodgkin's Lymphomas) to group lymphomas according to biologic aggressiveness, or grade (Table 79.2) (32). The groups of NHLs in this classification represent points on a spectrum rather than distinct types of disease.

The major groups (low-, intermediate-, and high-grade) of the Working Formulation are based primarily on differences in survival. The presence of a follicular or nodular pattern is an important prognostic indicator. These tumors are usually not rapidly proliferating, and their course is often indolent. However, they can disseminate throughout the lymphoid system and present with stage III

Table 79.2.
Comparison of the Rappaport and "Working Formulation" Classifications for Non-Hodgkin's Lymphomas

Rappaport (31)	"Working Formulation" (32)
	Low-Grade Malignancy
Lymphocytic, well differentiated	A. Malignant lymphoma: small lymphocytic consistent with chronic leukemia; plasmacytoid
Nodular (follicular) lymphocytic, poorly differentiated	B. Malignant lymphoma: follicular, predominantly small cleaved by diffuse areas; sclerosis
Nodular (follicular) mixed lymphocytic and histiocytic	C. Malignant lymphoma: follicular mixed, small cleaved, and large cell sclerosis
	Intermediate-Grade Malignancy
Nodular (follicular) histiocytic	D. Malignant lymphoma: follicular, predominantly large-cell diffuse areas sclerosis
	E. Malignant lymphoma: diffuse small cleaved cell sclerosis
Diffuse lymphocytic, poorly differentiated	F. Malignant lymphoma: diffuse mixed, small, and large cell sclerosis,
Diffuse mixed, lymphocytic and histiocytic	epithelioid cell component
	G. Malignant lymphoma: diffuse large cell cleaved cell, noncleaved cell
Diffuse histiocytic (with or without sclerosis)	sclerosis
	High-Grade Malignancy
	H. Malignant lymphoma: large cell, immunoblastic plasma cytoid clear
Diffuse histiocytic (with or without sclerosis)	cell polymorphous epithelioid cell component
	I. Malignant lymphoma: lymphoblastic convoluted cell, nonconvoluted cell
Lymphoblastic (with or without convoluted cells)	J. Malignant lymphoma: small cleaved, Burkitt's tumor; follicular areas
Diffuse, undifferentiated (Burkitt's and non-Burkitt's type)	K. Miscellaneous: composite mycosis fungoides, histiocytic, extramedullary plasmacytoma

or IV disease. Slightly less than half of the NHLs are composed of follicular histologies. The natural history of some follicular lymphomas is progression to a diffuse pattern (where the lymphoma diffusely replaces the normal follicular architecture of the lymph node) as well as a shift from the small, relatively slowly proliferating cells to large, more rapidly proliferating cells. The proliferation rate of NHLs can be measured by estimating the proportion of cells in the S phase of the cell cycle using flow cytometry. Within any given subcategory of NHL, tumors with a higher proliferative rate have been associated with a poorer treatment outcome (33). This may be due to a rapid emergence of resistance. Immunologic characteristics may also affect the natural history, response to treatment, and overall prognosis of NHL. Although controversial, the prognosis of patients with T cell-derived NHL is probably worse than that of patients with B cell tumors (33).

The large-cell lymphomas comprise both B and T cell neoplasms, and although they are aggressive (they spread rapidly), they are potentially curable with intensive chemotherapy. Although the natural history of small-cell lymphomas is less aggressive than that of large-cell lymphomas (patients with low-grade lymphomas may survive for long periods without therapy), they are seldom completely cured with chemotherapy.

Although the large-cell lymphomas usually progress rapidly if not treated and the small-cell lymphomas generally have a more indolent course, Burkitt's lymphoma, which comprises noncleaved small cells, is an exception to this principle and carries a poor prognosis. Burkitt's lymphoma is of B lymphocyte origin and has been recognized as a clinicopathologic entity for many years. In the United States, Burkitt's lymphoma accounts for less than 5% of NHL. Although a definite association of Burkitt's lymphoma in African children with EBV has been established, EBV-positive tumors are rare in Americans.

T cell NHL are far less common than B cell lymphomas, especially in adults. Tumors of differentiated T cells frequently arise in the lymph nodes and skin (e.g., mycosis fungoides and Sezary syndrome) or may be widespread (i.e., T cell leukemia). The cellular appearance of T cell malignancies varies and may include cytologic types ranging from small, atypical lymphoid cells to large and often convoluted lymphoid cells. Mycosis fungoides, a cutaneous T cell lymphoma, is characterized by proliferation of mature T cells (helper or inducer cells). Its prognosis is related to the stage of the disease, with most patients having a chronic course. The Sezary syndrome is closely related to mycosis fungoides and generally represents a leukemic phase.

Lymphoblastic lymphoma represents less than 10% of NHLs and is closely related to T cell acute lymphoblastic leukemia. It is more common in adolescents and young adults and, without very aggressive treatment, has a poor prognosis. About one-half of lymphoblastic lymphomas are characterized morphologically by convoluted nuclear configurations.

It has become evident in the past few years that not all NHLs fit well into the Working Group Classification (e.g., anaplastic large cell, monocytoid B cell), and several groups have already proposed new classification schemes (34).

PRESENTATION AND NATURAL HISTORY

Most patients with malignant lymphomas have superficial lymphadenopathy. Although superficial lymphadenopathy in adults is most frequently related to an acute infectious process, discrete hard lymph nodes, particularly if they are fixed or matted, should be biopsied. The cervical nodes are the most common site of presentation in Hodgkin's disease (65 to 80%), but this presentation is less common in NHL (30 to 40%). Supraclavicular and mediastinal lymphadenopathy are also common in Hodgkin's disease. Twenty to 35% of patients with NHL have disease only outside the lymph nodes. The majority of these lymphomas exhibit a diffuse histologic pattern. The most commonly involved extranodal site is the head and neck area, followed by the gastrointestinal tract. Other primary extranodal sites include the skin, central nervous system, liver, lung, testes, and bone marrow. When bone marrow involvement occurs, half the patients show variable degrees of blood invasion (35).

Hodgkin's disease is believed to be unifocal in origin, probably beginning with a single cervical or retroperitoneal lymph node. Spread occurs to adjacent nodes via lymph channels and either by direct extension into adjacent organs or by blood vessel invasion with dissemination to the spleen, bone marrow, liver, bone, and other organs. Lymph node involvement begins with a few malignant cells surrounded by normal lymphocytes. As the disease progresses, there is a tendency toward a worsening of the histology, with depletion of normal lymphocytes, an increased number of malignant cells, destruction of the lymph node architecture, and onset of symptoms. Effective therapy may interrupt this progression.

In NHL, with disease initially confined to the lymph nodes, there is a tendency to spread to contiguous lymphatic sites or occasionally, to adjacent extranodal sites. In contrast to Hodgkin's disease, NHL spreads more rapidly to distant nodal and extranodal sites via the blood stream, similar to the metastatic dissemination of many other tumors. Presentation of NHL depends on the histology of the disease. Low-grade NHL may initially present with slowly progressive, nontender peripheral lymphadenopathy that may wax and wane spontaneously, whereas intermediate- and high-grade NHL generally progress steadily.

In rare cases, Hodgkin's disease may present with massive mediastinal adenopathy causing superior vena cava obstruction with headache; congestion of the face; subcutaneous edema involving face, neck, and thorax; and cough and dyspnea (see "Complications"). Lymphoblastic lymphoma may also present with mediastinal adenopathy, which may also produce vena cava obstruction. NHL, and less commonly Hodgkin's disease, may present with massive retroperitoneal adenopathy that may obstruct the ureters or the inferior vena cava, giving rise to ascites and edema in the lower extremities.

At initial presentation, 20% of patients with NHL and 30 to 40% percent of patients with Hodgkin's disease experience systemic or constitutional symptoms (fever, night sweats, weight loss, and pruritus). These symptoms may develop about the same time as the lymph node enlargement or may occasionally precede the detection of adenopathy. These symptoms generally subside rapidly with treatment, and their appearance at any time in the course of the disease represents an unfavorable prognostic sign. In patients with Hodgkin's disease, the frequency of systemic symptoms increases with the stage of disease, age of the patient, and unfavorable histology.

Lymphomas Associated with the Acquired Immunodeficiency Syndrome

Since the AIDS epidemic began in 1981, the number of reports of lymphoma in patients with AIDS and the AIDS-Related Complex (ARC) has steadily increased. In 1985, the Centers for Disease Control (CDC) amended its case definition of AIDS to include patients with high-grade, B cell non-Hodgkin's lymphoma and documented HIV infection (36). In 1993, Pluta and colleagues reported that HIV-infected patients with profound immunodeficiency were at greatest risk of developing non-Hodgkin's lymphoma and particularly primary CNS lymphoma (37). This was especially seen in those patients with less than 50 CD4 cell/ul. These results suggest NHL as a late complication for patients with HIV infection. Further, in a combined cohort of 116 patients with AIDS and ARC receiving antiretroviral therapy, the estimated probability of NHL developing after 36 months was 19%.

The incidence of lymphoma associated with HIV infection is not unexpected because various other immunodeficiency disorders have also been associated with an increased incidence of lymphomas (3, 19, 20). Non-Hodgkin's lymphomas of several histologic types, including Burkitt's lymphoma (38), immunoblastic lymphoma (39), and lymphoblastic lymphoma (40) as well as Hodgkin's disease (41), have been reported in patients with AIDS (21); however, most patients have had high-grade, B cell lymphomas. Early reports indicated that many of these lymphomas presented at advanced stages, with unusual clinical features, including prodromal manifestations, a high frequency of extranodal and central nervous system involvement, and an usually poor prognosis with respect to the histologic subtypes (21).

In a series of NHLs in 90 homosexual men, 62% of the lymphomas were high grade, 29% were immediate grade, and 7% were low grade (21). In 46% of these patients, the diagnosis of AIDS preceded the recognition of the lymphoma, and an additional 15% of patients developed AIDS following the diagnosis of the lymphoma. All but two of these patients had extranodal involvement. Thirty-eight patients (42%) had involvement of the central nervous system, and 30 patients (33%) had bone marrow involvement. These frequencies are far in excess of that expected in de novo NHL. The response to treatment and survival in this series was poor in comparison to treatment results in other patients with similar types of lymphoma. Many other reports have now confirmed that the lymphomas in AIDS are highly aggressive and frequently involve extranodal sites, including the CNS, gastrointestinal tract, bone marrow, liver, lung, rectum, heart, bile duct, and pleura (41). It has been estimated that up to 25% of HIV-associated NHL are confined to only the CNS.

DIAGNOSIS AND STAGING

Decisions regarding appropriate therapy for a patient with a lymphoma depend on the correct morphologic diagnosis and accurate assessment of the extent of disease. Diagnosis of malignant lymphoma requires histopathologic confirmation of lymph node biopsy. When lymphadenopathy is present, one or more complete nodes must be excised. Needle biopsies are generally not adequate. When primary extranodal lymphoma presents with regional or distant adenopathy, both sites should be examined histologically to ensure a correct diagnosis. When the primary disease is only extranodal in certain sites (e.g., stomach, breast, testicle), a diagnosis of carcinoma is often made on clinical grounds, and NHL is discovered from the surgical pathology.

Staging systems have been developed to facilitate therapeutic planning and communication of data concerning the natural history of the disease and treatment outcomes. The Ann Arbor staging system (Table 79.3) was developed in 1971 for use in Hodgkin's disease and was revised in 1989 (42). It has also been used for staging NHL. In Hodgkin's disease, this system has been reproducible and predictive of response to therapy. The Ann Arbor Classification is divided into four stages, and each stage is further subdivided into A (asymptomatic) and B (symptomatic) groups. As the disease progresses from stage I to stage IV, the prognosis becomes worse. The presence of symptoms (designated B) confers a worse prognosis. The clinical symptoms associated with Hodgkin's disease are general rather than specific; they are unexplained weight loss of more than 10% of the body weight, unexplained

Table 79.3.

Ann Arbor Classification for the Staging of Hodgkin's Disease[a]

Stage I:	Disease involvement of a single contiguous lymph node region (I) or of a single localized extralymphatic organ or site (I_E) on the same side of the diaphragm.
Stage II:	Disease involvement of two or more contiguous lymph node regions on the same side of the diaphragm (II) or localized involvement of an extralymphatic organ or site and of one or more lymph node regions on the same side of the diaphragm (II_E). An optional recommendation is that the number of node regions involved be indicated by a subscript (e.g., II_3).
Stage III:	Disease involvement of lymph node regions on both sides of the diaphragm (III). III_1 indicates with or without involvement of splenic, hilar, celiac, or portal nodes. III_2 indicates involvement of para-aortic, iliac, or mesenteric nodes. May also be accompanied by localized involvement of an extralymphatic organ or site (III_E) or by involvement of the spleen (III_S), or both (III_{SE}).
Stage IV:	Diffuse or disseminated disease involvement of one or more extralymphatic organs or tissues with or without associated lymph node enlargement. The extralymphatic sites of involvement should be identified by symbols.

[a]Each stage subdivided into A (asymptomatic) and B (symptomatic). Symptoms are (a) weight loss greater than 10% of body weight, (b) unexplained fever with temperature above 38°C (100.4°F), and (c) night sweats.
Suffix "X" to designate bulky disease as > ⅓ widening of the mediastinum or > 10 cm maximum dimension of nodal mass.
The number of anatomical regions involved should be indicated by a subscript.
Staging should be identified as clinical stage (CS) or pathologic stage (PS).

Table 79.4.

Staging Procedures for Hodgkin's Disease and Non-Hodgkin's Lymphomas

Required Procedures

1. Detailed history with special attention to the presence (and duration) or absence of systemic symptoms (i.e., fever, unexplained sweating, unexplained weight loss)
2. Careful physical examination with special attention to all lymph node areas
3. Adequate surgical biopsy reviewed by an experienced hemopathologist
4. Routine laboratory tests, including complete blood count, erythrosedimentation rate, liver and renal function tests, serum uric acid
5. Radiologic examination of the chest, gastrointestinal tract, and skeletal system of any areas of bone tenderness
6. Bilateral bone marrow biopsy
7. Computed tomography (CT) scan of chest
8. Abdominal computed tomography scan

Procedures Necessary Under Certain Circumstances

1. Biolateral lower extremity lymphography
2. Exploratory laparotomy and splenectomy

fever with temperature above 38°C (100.4°F), and night sweats. A patient may experience additional symptoms such as pruritus or alcohol-induced pain, but they generally do not correlate with the severity of disease and are not considered in the staging evaluation.

In patients in whom localized extranodal disease is contiguous to involved lymph nodes (often in the lungs or vertebrae adjacent to involved lymph nodes), staging is based on the appropriate lymph node involvement followed by the subscript E, which denotes direct extension. These patients have a more favorable prognosis than those with clearly disseminated (stage IV) disease. In general, the E designation is used in patients with extranodal disease so limited in extent and location that it can be easily irradiated.

The diaphragm has key significance in the staging of Hodgkin's disease. It is the reference point from which the extent (or stage) of Hodgkin's disease is measured. If the disease is confined to lymph nodes on only one side (above or below) of the diaphragm, the disease is considered to be localized, and the prognosis is generally better than if the disease were more disseminated and present on both sides of the diaphragm.

Procedures necessary for accurate clinical staging of Hodgkin's disease are listed in Table 79.4. A detailed patient history is obtained, making note of the presence or absence of symptoms, and a thorough physical examination must be performed, giving particular attention to areas of bone tenderness and the size of the liver and spleen. Laboratory tests and procedures that are conducted are designed to detect any clinical abnormality that may implicate a specific organ or organ system invaded by Hodgkin's disease. Further pathologic staging is then necessary to definitively diagnose Hodgkin's disease in tissues that have been implicated by the clinical staging procedures. Pathologic staging involves biopsy and microscopic examination of the suspicious tissue. More aggressive staging techniques have included exploratory laparotomy and splenectomy. In the past, these procedures have made tremendous contributions in staging accuracy and knowledge of the natural history of Hodgkin's disease; however, the role of staging laparotomy is under reevaluation, and computerized tomography (CT) or magnetic resonance imaging (MRI) are now the most commonly used procedures for evaluation of the abdomen. Current recommendations specify that laparotomy should be performed only if management decisions depend on the identification of abdominal disease, and in some of these situations, laparoscopy combined with needle marrow biopsies may substitute for this procedure. Laparotomy is of most value in identifying those patients eligible for treatment with radiation therapy alone (i.e., patients with negative laparotomy results). If systemic chemotherapy is already considered essential to the patient's management, based on noninvasive studies, then staging laparotomy becomes superfluous. Although the overall morbidity is low, laparotomy plus splenectomy increases the risk of sepsis from encapsulated organisms (i.e., *Streptococcus pneumoniae, Hemophilus influenzae*), varicella zoster infection, and bowel obstruction resulting from adhesions among the intestinal loops. Therefore, the decision to perform such a staging procedure must be carefully weighed, especially because a CT or MRI scan is easy to administer and noninvasive.

The distribution of Hodgkin's disease (at initial diagnosis) according to stage is stage I, 13%; stage II, 38%; stage III, 35%; and stage IV, 14% (43). Data collected over the years have revealed some interesting statistics regarding the correlation of the clinical stage of Hodgkin's disease with histologic tissue type. Patients presenting with the lymphocyte-predominant variety have a strong association with clinical stages I and II, whereas the lymphocyte-depleted variety is seen mainly in patients with clinical stages III and IV. The mixed-cellularity variety occurs in all clinical stages of the disease, without any strong correlations. The nodular sclerosis variety is seen primarily in patients with clinical stage II disease and is the one histologic subtype that presents with a distinctive anatomic pattern of distribution, namely, a predilection to involve the lower cervical lymph nodes and mediastinum (44). The lymphocyte-predominant, lymphocyte-depleted, and mixed-cellularity types exhibit a variable propensity for anatomical involvement when compared within the same clinical stage.

Non-Hodgkin's Lymphoma

Non-Hodgkin's lymphomas are not as predictable in their patterns of involvement, nor do they reflect discrete changes in their prognosis with changes in stages, as seen with Hodgkin's disease. Despite these limitations, to date, the Ann Arbor staging system has been most widely used in defining patient groups in clinical trials. More recently, other factors that have prognostic significance such as the maximal diameter of the largest tumor, the specific sites of extranodal involvement, the patient's performance status, and LDH concentrations are being incorporated into new staging systems (45). In contrast to those with Hodgkin's disease, patients with NHL are more likely to have disseminated disease, so local therapeutic options such as surgery and radiation therapy are less commonly used. Therapeutic options in NHL are also more likely to be limited because of the advanced age or concomitant illnesses of the patient. Because of the divergent clinical features of patients with NHL, no rigid or routine staging plan is appropriate for all patients. Many of the staging procedures used in Hodgkin's disease (Table 79.4) are used for the NHLs although they are less applicable because of the high prevalence of extranodal disease. These staging procedures should be carefully considered with regard to the histologic subtype, the individual patient, and the anticipated and available therapy. Extensive staging procedures should be reserved for clinical trials or for patients

in whom a specific therapeutic alternative, such as radiation therapy, is available.

As in Hodgkin's disease, a thorough physical examination and routine laboratory tests are aimed at the detection of potential sites of involvement. Although the bone marrow is frequently involved in NHL, peripheral blood abnormalities are uncommon. Bilateral bone marrow aspirations and biopsies are generally indicated in follicular lymphomas or clinically advanced diffuse histologies. The frequency of bone marrow involvement ranges from 5 to 15% in patients with diffuse "histiocytic" lymphoma (DHL) to 55 to 85% of patients with nodular, poorly differentiated lymphoma (NPDL). Although relatively uncommon in DHL, bone marrow involvement may predict central nervous system involvement, and patients with this finding should receive a lumbar puncture with examination of the cerebrospinal fluid.

Gastrointestinal studies are indicated in patients with abdominal symptoms or masses and in patients with nasopharyngeal lymphomas, to obtain prognostic information, to plan therapy, and to establish involvement or impending obstruction of the gastrointestinal or genitourinary tract. Although lymphangiography has been widely used for assessment of retroperitoneal and intraabdominal disease, computed tomography scanning has largely replaced this procedure. As in Hodgkin's disease, there is no justification for routine staging laparotomy, and this procedure should be used only when it will influence management decisions.

TREATMENT

The treatment of malignant lymphomas centers mainly on radiation therapy and chemotherapy. Surgery, although useful in the management of many other malignancies, does not play a major role in the therapy of lymphomas. Today, the only roles for surgery in lymphomas are (1) initial staging and diagnostic procedures; (2) relief of obstruction related to a localized lymph node enlargement not responding to therapy; (3) management of a gastrointestinal lymphoma to reduce the rate of perforation or hemorrhage; and (4) management of complications of lymphomas such as hypersplenism.

Lymphomas were recognized early on as being very responsive to radiation therapy, and until the end of the 1960s, radiation therapy was the only successful modality that could, under appropriate circumstances, achieve cure in some malignant lymphomas. Although radiation therapy has been used since the early 1900s, it was not until the 1950s, the era of megavolt radiation (using ^{60}Co and linear accelerators), that the use of large fields, exposing entire lymph node chains to radiation in the range of 3500 to 4000 rads ("rad" stands for radiation-absorbed dose and equals 100 ergs/g tissue) was possible. With these advances in technique, the therapeutic results of patients with all types of lymphomas have improved progressively.

Radiation therapy essentially has the same effect on cellular biochemistry as do the alkylating agents employed in chemotherapy. Deoxyribonucleic acid (DNA) replication is prevented by interfering with cross-links necessary to maintain the double-helix DNA molecule. Proliferating tissue, characteristic of malignancies, is especially radiosensitive because of its constant DNA production necessary for cell division. The epithelial lining of the gastrointestinal tract is also rapidly dividing tissue, and frequently encountered side effects with radiation therapy are radiation-induced pharyngitis, esophagitis, and gastroenteritis. The rapid production of cells in the bone marrow makes this site very susceptible to radiation-induced bone marrow suppression. It is therefore important that vital, uninvolved organs and viscera be shielded during radiation therapy to minimize radiation-induced toxicities.

Possible radiation fields used for the treatment of lymphomas are described in Table 79.5 and Figure 79.3.

The use of drugs in the management of neoplastic diseases was developed after the end of World War II, and lymphomas and leukemias were among the first tumors to respond to such chemotherapy. In general, with single-agent chemotherapy, the complete response rate has rarely exceeded 20 to 30%, so the treatment of lymphomas relies on the use of drug combinations. Combination chemotherapy uses drugs with different mechanisms of action that attack proliferating cells at different stages of cell replication.

Table 79.5.
Radiation Therapy Fields Used in the Management of Lymphomas

Mantle: Encompasses mediastinal, hilar, and bilateral supraclavicular, infraclavicular, cervical, and axillary node chains, with lead shields shaped to lungs, heart, and spinal cord

Inverted-Y: Encompasses splenic or splenic pedicle, para-aortic, iliac, inguinal, and femoral node chains, with lead shields for rectum and bladder, iliac and upper femoral bone marrow, and "gap" at junction with mantle fields

Para-aortic/hepatic: Encompasses splenic hilar and para-aortic node chains and entire right lobe of liver, usually joined across another "gap" by a separate pelvic field

Waldeyer: Encompasses preauricular nodes and lymphatic tissues of Waldeyer's ring when clinically involved or when adenopathy is present in high cervical nodes

Total nodal: Encompasses all lymph nodes regions above the diaphragm (cervical, supra- and infraclavicular, axillary, mediastinal) and all lymph node regions below the diaphragm (periaortic, retroperitoneal, inguinal, and splenic regions)

Subtotal nodal: Encompasses the mantle plus para-aortic, spleen and pedicle fields

Involved field: Encompasses only the known involved sites

Extended field: Encompasses known involved sites plus contiguous uninvolved regions

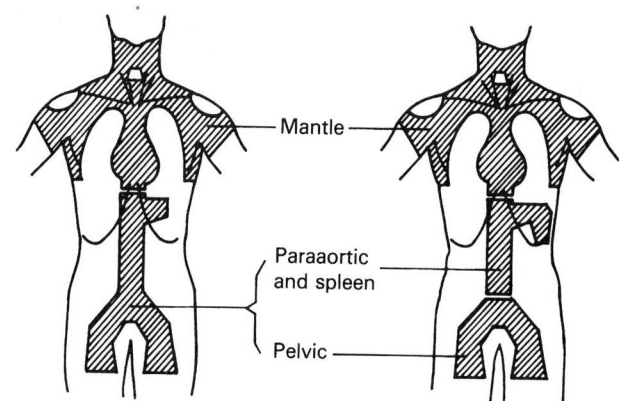

Figure 79-3. "Mantle" and "Inverted Y" radiation fields used in the management of lymphomas. From Rosenberg S and Kaplan HS. Hodgkin's disease and other malignant lymphomas. Calif Med 113(4):23–38, 1970.

Although the great majority of cytotoxic drugs can produce objective response in lymphomas, it was only in 1970 with the four-drug regimen known as MOPP (mechlorethamine, vincristine, procarbazine, and prednisone) that DeVita and colleagues showed that chemotherapy could induce a high rate of complete remission in advanced Hodgkin's disease (46). Later, the ability of chemotherapy to produce long-term remissions (compatible with cure) in Hodgkin's disease and certain NHL histologies was confirmed.

After radiation therapy or chemotherapy has been administered to a patient with lymphoma, the patient's response to treatment must be assessed. Standard criteria are generally used for the objective evaluation of treatment response (Table 79.6) so that various therapies may be compared in a consistent manner. Objective reduction of the disease manifestations usually begins within the first month after the start of treatment. However, this depends on the histologic type of lymphoma and is usually more rapid in Hodgkin's disease than in NHL.

Selection of the appropriate type of therapy depends on confirmation of the histologic subtype and the extent of the disease, as well as any patient-specific factors (e.g., age,

Table 79.6.
Criteria for Treatment Response

Complete remission (CR): Disappearance of all signs and symptoms of the disease. This includes the return to normal of all previously abnormal parameters and a negative second biopsy of known involved extranodal sites.

Partial remission (PR): A reduction of greater than 50% in the product of the longest perpendicular diameters of all measurable lesions.

Minimal response (MR) or no change: A reduction of less than 50% in the product of the longest perpendicular diameters of all measurable lesions.

Treatment failure (TF): Increase in size of any lesion and/or appearance of new lesion(s).

concomitant illness) that may influence the patient's ability to withstand treatment. With few exceptions, the initial approach to management of malignant lymphomas must have curative intent, regardless of disease extent and histologic type.

Hodgkin's Disease

EARLY STAGE (I, II, III$_A$)

Stage I and II are very amenable to radical external beam radiation therapy (i.e., high doses of radiation with curative intent) because in these stages the disease is present in a few well-defined, focal areas (47). Treatment may be limited to the known involved sites (i.e., involved field, IF), given to only the known involved sites plus contiguous uninvolved regions (i.e., extended field, EF), or delivered to all major lymphoid regions (i.e., total nodal irradiation, TNI). It is generally recommended that local tumor masses receive "boost therapy" to a minimum dose of 4,000 to 4,400 rads, whereas apparently uninvolved areas treated for subclinical disease appear to be controlled adequately with doses of 3,000 to 3,500 rads. One hundred fifty to 220 rads per day are usually administered 5 days each week, so the total duration of treatment is 4 to 6 weeks.

Using either TNI or subtotal nodal irradiation (sTNI), the 10-year relapse-free survival rate (which is often equated to cure) in patients with pathologic stage I and II is 75 to 80% (48–50). If only the IF is irradiated, the response rate has been poorer (38%) than with TNI although overall survival was comparable at 5 years (90%) because most patients who relapse after radiation will respond to chemotherapy (51). The use of combined chemotherapy and radiation appears to reduce the relapse rate, but it does not improve the overall survival (52). sTNI is not associated with significantly more toxicity than experienced with IF although it dramatically improves relapse-free survival; therefore, this technique is generally considered the standard approach for stages I and II disease. Systemic symptoms, age, histologic subtype, and limited extranodal extension do not appear to affect the prognosis of stages I and II patients treated with radiation (53). About 50% of patients with a large (more than one-third the largest transverse chest diameter) mediastinal mass relapse when treated with radiation therapy alone (54). Therefore, most investigators advocate the use of chemotherapy plus irradiation, whereas others believe that chemotherapy should be reserved for those patients who do relapse following radiation (43).

Some evidence indicates that treatment of early-stage disease with chemotherapy alone is at least as effective as radiation therapy. When patients with stages I$_B$, II$_A$, or III$_A$ disease were randomized to receive either radiation or MOPP chemotherapy, Longo and colleagues reported a CR rate of 96% in each arm of the study. At a median follow-up of 7.5 years, 35% of patients in the radiation group and 13% of patients who received MOPP therapy had relapsed. The projected 10-year disease-free survival for radiation therapy patients is 60 versus 86% for MOPP-treated patients (p=.009) although overall survival was not significantly different (55). Chemotherapy has certain advantages. Systemic chemotherapy eliminates the need for the patient to undergo a laparotomy or splenectomy and the associated morbidity. However, the acute toxicities associated with chemotherapy may be worse than those associated with radiation. Further follow-up of this and other similar trials is necessary to assess late and chronic treatment-related side effects.

For patients with stage III$_A$ disease, the 5-year relapse-free survival when treated with radiation alone is only 35 to 66% although overall survival ranges from 80 to 92% at 5 years, emphasizing the effectiveness of salvage treatment (43). Currently, it is believed that radiation therapy alone is inadequate in stage III$_A$ and that combination chemotherapy is the treatment of choice (56). Several clinical studies have reported improved relapse-free survival with the use of chemotherapy plus radiation (57–59). Other studies suggest that combined modality therapy does not increase the long-term disease-free survival rate when compared to chemotherapy alone (60, 61). In addition, combined modality therapy is associated with more toxicity (62).

STAGES III$_B$ AND IV

Chemotherapy with or without radiation therapy is the treatment of choice for patients with stage III$_B$ or IV Hodgkin's disease. Stage IV disease is not well suited for radiation therapy since sites of the disease in this stage may be so numerous and diffuse that localized radiation cannot be effectively administered. Parenchymal organs cannot tolerate curative doses of radiation, and the presence of Hodgkin's disease in these areas precludes the use of radical radiation. Stage IV disease is therefore treated primarily with systemic chemotherapy, which has access to all sites of disease. "Spot" radiation is also used in stage IV disease for palliative treatment to anatomic areas of disease involvement not responding to chemotherapy and causing pain, tenderness, or obstruction.

A drug combination that has been very successful in obtaining the induction of remissions in Hodgkin's disease is MOPP (mechlorethamine or Mustargen®, vincristine or Oncovin®, prednisone, and procarbazine). Pioneered by DeVita and colleagues (46), MOPP therapy has endured and is still considered by many to be a valuable front-line chemotherapy for Hodgkin's disease (Table 79.7) (63, 64). After 20 years of experience with this regimen at the NCI, 159 of 198 patients (80%) achieved a complete remission, with 54% of these patients remaining disease free at 20 years. MOPP therapy is given in cycles that repeat every 28 days. More than 1,000 patients have been treated with the MOPP regimen in reported clinical trials. The average CR rate has been 67% (44 to 87%) with a long-term disease-free survival of at least 50% in all studies (33, 65). Patients should receive a minimum of six complete cycles of therapy

Table 79.7.
MOPP Regimen with Dosing Adjustments

Mechlorethamine	6 mg/m^2 IV days 1 and 8
Vincristine (Oncovin^R)	1.4 mg/m^2 IV days 1 and 8
Procarbazine	100 mg/m^2 PO days 1 through 14
Prednisone[a]	40 mg/m^2 PO days 1 through 14, cycles 1 and 4 only

Repeat cycle every 4 weeks
  Six cycles minimum

WBC Count	Platelet Count	Dose Adjustment
≥4000/mm^3	100,000/mm^3	100% all drugs
3000–4000/mm^3	100,000/mm^3	100% vincristine, 50% procarbazine and mechlorethamine
2000–3000/mm^3	50,000–100,000/mm^3	100% vincristine, 25% procarbazine and mechlorethamine
1000–2000/mm^3	50,000/mm^3	50% vincristine, 25% procarbazine and mechlorethamine
<1000/mm^3	50,000/mm^3	No therapy

[a]No dosage adjustment required.

at maximally tolerated doses. When doses have been attenuated, lower remission and survival rates have been reported (65, 66). Although it appears that full-dose chemotherapy predicts the best response, it is possible that patients with worse prognosis disease are unable to tolerate full-dose treatment. When patients are considered to be in complete remission, which must be determined by appropriate restaging, two more cycles of chemotherapy should be given. Once complete remission has been achieved, there is no real advantage in prolonging treatment or administering any type of maintenance therapy. Similar chemotherapy regimens have yielded comparative results and toxicities (Table 79.8). In addition to MOPP and MOPP derivatives, other novel combination chemotherapy regimens have shown excellent results when used as first-line therapy. Bonadonna and colleagues first described the ABVD regimen (doxorubicin or Adriamycin^R, bleomycin, vinblastine, and dacarbazine) (Table 79.8) in patients who had relapsed following MOPP (67). Following their very positive results, they undertook a prospective study to evaluate MOPP versus MOPP alternating with ABVD.

Goldie and Coldman proposed that during treatment malignant cells may mutate and become resistant to therapy (72). The use of alternating, non-cross-resistant chemotherapy regimens has been suggested as a possible means of improving the complete response rate and lengthening the median duration of disease-free survival by exposing tumor cells to an increased number of cytotoxic

Table 79.8.
Other Combination Chemotherapy Regimens Used in Hodgkin's Disease

Acronym	Agents	Dose (mg/m^2)	Treatment Days	Frequency of Cycles	Reference
ABVD	Doxorubicin	25	1, 15	Every 28 days	(67)
	Bleomycin	10	1, 15		
	Vinblastine	6	1, 15		
	Dacarbazine	375	1, 15		
MVPP	Mechlorethamine	6	1, 8	Every 28 days	(68)
	Vinblastine	10	1, 8, 15		
	Procarbazine	100	1–15		
	Prednisolone	40	1–15		
MVVPP	Mechlorethamine	0.4 mg/kg	1	Every 57 days	(69)
	Vincristine	1.4 (max 2 mg)	1, 8, 15		
	Vinblastine	6	22, 29, 36		
	Prednisone	40	1–22, then taper		
	Procarbazine	100	22–43		
MOPP/APB	Mechlorethamine	6	1	Every 28 days	(70)
	Vincristine	1.4 (max 2 mg)	1		
	Prednisone	40	1–14		
	Procarbazine	100	1–7		
	Doxorubicin	35	8		
	Bleomycin	10	8		
	Vinblastine	6	8		
EVA	Etoposide	100	1–3	Every 28 days	(71)
	Vinblastine	6	1		
	Doxorubicin	50	1		

drugs. This strategy offers the possibility of reducing treatment failures caused by overgrowth of singly, doubly or even multidrug-resistant phenotypes. The ABVD regimen consists of drugs that are individually non-cross-resistant with the agents in the MOPP regimen. This combination has demonstrated a complete response rate as high as the MOPP regimen and has been proved to be effective in patients resistant to MOPP therapy. In a randomized study of patients with advanced Hodgkin's disease, alternating monthly cycles of MOPP and ABVD (MOPP/ABVD) were compared to MOPP therapy alone. The rates of complete response (89 versus 74%) and 8-year relapse-free survival (73 versus 45%) were superior for the MOPP/ABVD regimen, with a similar incidence of serious toxicities (73, 74).

Klimo and Connors reported the results of a similar hybrid regimen (MOPP/ABV) (Table 79.8), which administered seven drugs in single monthly cycles. This regimen omitted the dacarbazine and increased the dose of doxorubicin from 25 mg/m^2 to 35 mg/m^2, and 13% of the patients also received some local radiation therapy. The complete response rate was 97.5%, and at a median follow-up of 3.5 years, the overall survival rate was 93.5% and the relapse-free survival was 90.5% (70). Recently, Glick and colleagues reported a complete response rate of 81% and a 22-month relapse-free survival of 80% using this hybrid regimen (75).

Over the past 25 years, it has become apparent that several factors influence the overall long-term response to Hodgkin's disease therapies. Factors that have a negative impact on potential cure include age (over 40 years), stage of disease, number of extranodal sites, and constitutional symptoms(76–78). After chemotherapy is initiated, the rate of tumor regression and the dose intensity (i.e., amount of drug administered per unit of time) also appear to influence the duration of response and survival (64, 79). Review of outcome data has shown that the best overall results are seen in patient subsets who received chemotherapy at closest to the intended dose and schedule (without dosage attenuation or delay between cycles) (28). The dose intensities of the mechlorethamine, procarbazine, and vincristine have each been suggested to correlate with outcome in MOPP or MOPP-derivative regimens (64, 74, 79–83). For example, although the original MOPP regimen includes 1.4 mg/m^2 of vincristine, many clinicians have limited each dose to a maximum of 2 mg. Using full doses is associated with significant neurotoxicity, but no patient was permanently disabled if a sliding-scale dose, taking into account the patient's symptoms, was used to adjust the dose. Conversely, no study using the 2-mg dose maximum has shown results as good as the original regimen, and retrospective analyses have shown that the dose of vincristine does make an impact on treatment results (56).

The most common dose-limiting toxicity of many of the other drugs used in Hodgkin's disease regimens is myelosuppression. Therefore, the use of colony-stimulating factors in combination with chemotherapy regimens may allow for a higher dosage intensity to be tolerated.

Despite the success of first-line therapies (both radiation and chemotherapy) for Hodgkin's disease, 20 to 50% of patients will either be initially refractory to or relapse following primary treatment (84). Chemotherapy such as the MOPP or ABVD regimens is also appropriate therapy for patients whose Hodgkin's disease relapses following radiation therapy (63, 85). DeVita and colleagues reported that 94% of patients whose disease recurred following local irradiation achieved a complete remission with MOPP therapy (63).

The optimal management for patients who relapse following primary chemotherapy (e.g., MOPP) or for those failing initial chemotherapy is not clearly established. At the NCI, 59% of 32 patients who relapsed after MOPP achieved a complete remission when retreated with MOPP therapy. Patients whose first complete remission was longer than 1 year were more likely to achieve a second complete remission. The duration of the second remission was also longer in patients whose initial remission was longer than a year (86). Overall, about 35% of patients who relapse after initial chemotherapy-induced complete remission have a long-term disease-free survival (28).

A number of other antineoplastic agents, including doxorubicin, carmustine, lomustine, vinblastine, dacarbazine, and bleomycin, have demonstrated important activity in Hodgkin's disease. These agents have been assembled in various combinations (Table 79.8). Patients resistant to MOPP should receive one of the established non-cross-resistant regimens. The most widely used regimen in this situation has been the ABVD regimen, which produced complete remissions in 60% of 54 MOPP-resistant patients with a 17-month median disease-free survival (63). In relapsed patients who initially received ABVD, retreatment with ABVD may be difficult because of the risks of cumulative doxorubicin cardiotoxicity and bleomycin pulmonary toxicity. One promising regimen includes etoposide, vinblastine or vincristine, and doxorubicin (EVA). In patients who have previously relapsed following MOPP or are MOPP resistant, a 41% complete response rate and a 2-year failure-free survival rate of 38% has been reported (71). This regimen incorporated yet another active agent, etoposide (87), into the treatment of Hodgkin's disease. This regimen has the potential advantage of less emetogenic complications and pulmonary toxicity than many of the other second-line regimens.

Patients who fail first-line therapy are much less likely to respond to other conventional therapies (67). Even if such patients do achieve a complete remission with second-line therapy, it is likely to be of only brief duration.

Prognosis is influenced by the stage of the disease at initial diagnosis and at relapse, the status of "B" symptoms at relapse, the patient's performance status, whether it is a first or later relapse, the number of failed chemotherapy regimens, whether it is relapsed or refractory disease, and the duration of the prior remission. (88)

The use of high-dose chemotherapy with allogeneic or autologous bone marrow transplant may offer better chances of long-term survival (89–91). With this treatment approach, the complete response rates have ranged from 40 to 70%, and 20 to 49% of patients appear to have a long remission (more than 2 years) (92–100). Best treatment results are seen in patients with low tumor volumes, good performance status, and chemotherapy-sensitive disease (i.e., showing some indication of tumor response prior to BMT). Rapport and colleagues reported a projected 3-year event (relapse)-free survival for patients with minimal disease (all areas ≤ 2 cm) of 70 versus 15% for patients with bulky disease (101). In one series, HLA-identical allogeneic marrow recipients had a statistically lower relapse rate compared to recipients of autologous marrow although survival, event-free survival, and nonrelapse mortality were not different (91). Clinical trials have reported 8 to 20% treatment-related deaths. Many of these deaths and other treatment morbidities are associated with the profound myelosuppression prior to bone marrow engraftment. Numerous trials using colony-stimulating factors have now reported accelerated myeloid recovery, fewer febrile days, and shorter hospitalizations (102, 103).

Non-Hodgkin's Lymphoma

The management for non-Hodgkin's lymphomas depends on many factors, including the age of the patient, presence of concomitant disease, and the stage and histologic subgroup of the primary disease.

LOW-GRADE NHL

Less than 10% of patients with favorable prognosis (low-grade) histologies (Table 79.2) have localized disease (i.e., stage I or II) at the time of diagnosis. Local or regional radiation therapy is generally very effective in achieving disease control in the irradiated areas (104). If patients relapse following radiation therapy, it is usually in unirradiated nodal or extranodal sites. However, because of the indolent nature of this disease, asymptomatic patients may not require immediate therapy.

More than 50 to 75% of patients with low-grade lymphomas have stage III or IV disease at initial diagnosis (105, 106). Few of these patients can be cured. Treatment options for patients with favorable histologies and advanced disease include total nodal irradiation, total body irradiation, single-agent chemotherapy, and combination chemotherapy. Radiation therapy alone (TLI) appears to be most effective in patients with less than five sites of disease involvement, no systemic symptoms, and small tumor masses (less than 10 cm); however, patients may continue to relapse for up to 10 years following therapy (107).

A number of agents, including mechlorethamine, melphalan, chlorambucil, cyclophosphamide, vincristine, vinblastine, doxorubicin, carmustine, fludarabine, and etoposide have activity against the follicular lymphomas. Although complete response rates as high as 65% have been reported with several of these agents, and the duration of relapse-free survival may be up to 50 months, this type of therapy is not considered to be curative (108, 109). Using new molecular biologic techniques, it appears that many patients with follicular NHL in apparent complete remission still have cells containing cytogenetic evidence of the disease (110). In an attempt to improve on the results observed with single-agent therapy, a number of combination chemotherapy regimens have been developed. Initially, one of the most widely used regimens was the CVP (cyclophosphamide, vincristine, and prednisone) regimen (Table 79.9). Although studies with this regimen suggested higher complete response rates than with single-agent therapy, the overall disease-free survival and survival were not significantly altered. In response to this information, a number of more aggressive regimens (with and without radiation therapy) have been investigated. Trials using regimens such as CHOP-bleo, CMOPP, M-BACOD, COPP, and carmustine, cyclophosphamide, vincristine, and dexamethasone have now reported higher long-term disease-free survival rates (114, 120–122). Overall survival has not been improved, but this is probably due to the long survival (median more than 8 years) observed even in patients who do not achieve a CR.

The follicular low-grade NHL has shown responsiveness to alpha interferon. In an NCI-sponsored trial, 13 (4 complete responses, 9 partial responses) of 24 patients responded to a regimen of 50 million units/m^2 given three times weekly. The responses included both lymph node and extranodal disease. The median duration of response was 8 months (123). Other dosages and schedules as well as combination therapy with cytotoxic drugs or other biologic agents (e.g., monoclonal antibodies) are under investigation. A more recent report showed that patients who received interferon alfa combined with CHOP (cyclophosphamide, doxorubicin, vincristine, prednisone) chemotherapy had longer remission and a higher rate of survival than those treated with CHOP alone (124). Patients who do not achieve CR often receive various palliative therapies for many years. A longer duration of disease-free survival is almost certainly associated with a better quality of life for the patient and fewer treatment-related side effects. Unfortunately, many patients with low-grade lymphomas still cannot be cured with currently available treatment.

Table 79.9.
Combination Chemotherapy Regimens Used in Non-Hodgkin's Lymphoma

Acronym	Agents	Dose (mg/m²)	Treatment Days	Frequency of Cycles	Reference
C-MOPP or COPP	Cyclophosphamide	650	1, 8	Every 28 days	(111)
	Vincristine	1.4 (max 2 mg)	1, 8		
	Procarbazine	100	1–14		
	Prednisone	100	1–14		
CVP	Cyclophosphamide	400	1–5	Every 21 days	(112)
	Vincristine	1.4 (max 2 mg)	1		
	Prednisone	100	1–5		
CHOP	Cyclophosphamide	750	1	Every 21 days	(113)
	Doxorubicin	50	1		
	Vincristine	1.4 (max 2 mg)	1		
	Prednisone	100	1–5		
CHOP-bleo	Same as above plus bleomycin	15	1, 5		(114)
M-BACOD	Methotrexate	3000	14	Every 28 days	(115)
	Bleomycin	4	1		
	Doxorubicin	45	1		
	Cyclophosphamide	600	1		
	Vincristine	1	1		
	Dexamethasone	6	1–5		
	Leucovorin				
MACOP-B	Methotrexate	400	8, 36, 64	Only one cycle is given	(116)
	Doxorubicin	50	1, 15, 29, 43, 57, 71		
	Cyclophosphamide	350	1, 15, 29, 43, 57, 71		
	Vincristine	1.4	8, 22, 36, 50, 64, 78		
	Bleomycin	10	22, 50, 78		
	Prednisone	75 (total)	1–63, taper, 64–78		
ProMACE	Prednisone	60	1–14		(117)
	Methotrexate	500	15		
	Doxorubicin	25	1, 8		
	Cyclophosphamide	650	1, 8		
	Etoposide	120	1, 8		
ProMACE CytaBOM	Cyclosphosphamide	650	1	Every 21 days	(117)
	Doxorubicin	25	1		
	Etoposide	120	1		
	Prednisone	60	1–15		
	Cytarabine	300	8		
	Bleomycin	5	8		
	Vincristine	1.4	8		
	Methotrexate	120	8		
	Leucovorin	25q 6	9		

Another approach to managing asymptomatic patients with advanced disease is to delay therapy until the disease progresses. This approach is appealing, especially in older patients who are less likely to tolerate the side effects of chemotherapy. However, recent data support therapy at initial diagnosis. Young and colleagues reported similar survival durations, but higher complete response rates and disease-free survival rates in patients receiving therapy at diagnosis (125).

Patients with these indolent lymphomas respond repeatedly and usually undergo multiple treatment regimens with inevitable relapse after varying durations of response. Such patients eventually die of unrelated causes, toxicity of the therapy, progressive disease, or transition to a more aggressive type of lymphoma. High-dose chemotherapy with autologous bone marrow or peripheral stem cell transplantation often results in complete response with several groups reporting event-free survivals of greater than 3 to 4 years (126, 127). However, it is uncertain if the cure rate is increased (128).

INTERMEDIATE-GRADE AND HIGH-GRADE NHL

Patients with pathologic stage I and contiguous stage II intermediate-grade or high-grade histologies may often be managed with radiation therapy. Combination chemotherapy using regimens, including doxorubicin, yield high cure rates (greater than 75%) in patients with clinical stage I and nonbulky stage II diffuse NHL. Often three cycles of a regimen such as CHOP followed by irradiation of the involved area are recommended. In some patients, combined radiation and chemotherapy may improve overall survival (129).

For the majority of patients with stage II disease and for all patients with stages III and IV of intermediate- and high-grade histologies, systemic chemotherapy is required. Although a number of single agents are active in these diseases, few patients achieve complete remission, and the duration of response is usually short (130). Unlike the indolent nature of the follicular histologies, patients with these more aggressive histologies may succumb to their disease rapidly unless they respond to therapy. However, the prognosis of many of these histologies has improved with the use of intensive combination chemotherapy. For greater than 20 years, it has been recognized that many patients with aggressive histology lymphomas can be cured with various regimens although no single regimen has emerged as superior.

CHOP is a first-generation regimen that has been widely used over the past 2 decades. It has consistently produced complete remissions in 45 to 55% of patients and cure in approximately 30 to 35%. With the intent of increasing the percentage of long-term, disease-free survivors, many other regimens have been used in clinical trials (Table 79.9). These regimens have used other active agents such as doxorubicin, bleomycin, etoposide, cytarabine, etoposide, and methotrexate. With currently used regimens, complete remission rates have ranged from 60 to 85%, depending on the regimen, histologic subtype, and other prognostic factors. Many of these patients remain disease-free for more than 5 years after initial treatment.

In addition to combining active drugs, many regimens have used innovative approaches to scheduling in an attempt to maximize response while maintaining acceptable degrees of toxicity. Examples of such regimens include the M-BACOD and the ProMACE combinations, in which the relatively nonmyelosuppressive high-dose methotrexate with leucovorin rescue is given between the myelosuppressive agents to prevent regrowth of the lymphoma between cycles of the treatment. A 75% CR rate was reported for M-BACOD, and initial projections predicted that 55 to 60% of patients would be cured (115). The MACOP-B regimen includes weekly administration of active agents for 12 weeks, with myelosuppressive and nonmyelosuppressive intravenous agents given on alternating weeks. The reported complete response rate with this regimen is 84%, with a predicted median duration of response of greater than 2 years. This initial evidence suggests that this regimen is as effective as other regimens although it can be administered in one-half the time or less (116). Other regimens have also reported CR rates exceeding 80%, and it has been estimated that approximately 70% of patients who achieve a CR are cured of the disease (117). Despite

the reported success of these (and similar regimens) at single institutions, a large, multiinstitutional, randomized trial reported that remission rates and overall survival at 3 years did not differ significantly whether CHOP, MACOP-B, m-BACOD, or ProMACE-CytaBOM was used. Because fewer severe toxicities and fatalities were in the CHOP group, these investigators concluded that it remains the best available treatment (131).

In these aggressive lymphomas, only patients who achieve a complete response will have a long, disease-free survival. Factors that appear to adversely affect the ability to attain a complete response include advanced stage of the disease, the presence of systemic symptoms, bone marrow or liver involvement, gastrointestinal masses greater than 10 cm in diameter, a hemoglobin of less than 12 g/dl, and a lactate dehydrogenase greater than 250 units (132). Other factors that may also adversely affect the prognosis include more than three sites of disease involvement, advanced age, or a slow rate of response to initial therapy (133). Variability in response rates to similar regimens in different clinical trials may be due to a different mix of prognostic factors in the patient population. If patients with poor prognostic factors do attain a complete remission, then overall survival does not appear to be compromised.

Patients with NHLs who respond to chemotherapy should receive a minimum of six courses of therapy. If they appear to be in clinical complete remission after pathologic restaging, two more cycles of chemotherapy should be given. Although the aggressive treatment regimens are effective, they also produce serious side effects. In patients experiencing toxicity, it is often tempting to prolong the interval between courses of therapy to allow more recovery time. However, the specified schedule must be adhered to, whenever possible, to produce the best results. In many cases, prolongation by even 1 week may be associated with rapid tumor regrowth. Few clinical trials have directly addressed the significance of a dose intensity in the aggressive lymphomas. The National Cancer Institute of Canada clinical trials group compared standard BACOP with BACOP that included escalated doses of doxorubicin in patients with previously untreated, advanced intermediate- and high-grade non-Hodgkin's lymphoma. The standard dose doxorubicin group received 25 mg/m^2 on days 1 and 8 of each cycle, and the escalated dose group received 40 mg/m^2. There were no differences in response rate, disease-free survival, and survival during a median 65 months follow-up; however, because of granulocytopenia (no colony-stimulating factor was given), only 47% of patients were able to tolerate the escalated dose of doxorubicin beyond the first cycle (134). A meta analysis of 22 studies, however, suggested that dose-intensity may correlate with remission rate in advanced-stage intermediate-grade lymphoma (135). The availability of colony-stimulating factors has reduced morbidity related to neutropenia somewhat when using the high-dose regimens.

Maintenance chemotherapy following achievement of a complete response does not appear to prolong survival in most types of NHL, but it is indicated in patients with lymphoblastic lymphoma and Burkitt's lymphoma. Patients with bone marrow involvement (leukemia-like), lymphoblastic lymphoma, and Burkitt's lymphoma may benefit from prophylactic intrathecal methotrexate if they did not receive high-dose methotrexate as part of their systemic therapy.

Patients who are not responsive to initial chemotherapy or who relapse in less than 1 year should be given non-cross-resistant regimens. However, the results of salvage treatments for NHLs are far less encouraging than those described for Hodgkin's disease. Patients whose initial remission exceeds 1 year may benefit from retreatment with the original regimen, but only 5 to 10% of patients who relapse after chemotherapy-induced CR have a long-term disease-free survival (i.e., cure) with conventional chemotherapy regimens (136).

The use of high-dose chemotherapy with or without total body irradiation combined with autologous or allogeneic bone marrow transplant may offer an improved prognosis for some subsets of NHL patients (91, 101, 137, 138). The patients who are most likely to derive benefit from early intervention using this type of therapy are those who achieve a CR following salvage chemotherapy, those who achieve only a PR following initial chemotherapy, and those with poor prognostic features who achieve a CR following initial chemotherapy (139). When used as salvage therapy in patients who have relapsed or had refractory disease to first-line therapy, CR rates of 40 to 60% have been reported, with 15 to 20% long-term survivors (140–143). Higher cure rates (35 to 40%) have been reported for subgroups of patients who underwent this treatment approach when their tumors remained sensitive (i.e., after first relapse).

OTHER NHL

Lymphoblastic lymphomas (T cell type) generally occur in adolescent and young adult males. These patients are more likely to have bone marrow, mediastinal, and central nervous system involvement than those with other lymphomas. Regimens similar to those used to treat acute lymphoblastic leukemia with central nervous system prophylaxis and maintenance chemotherapy have reported encouraging results.

Three other relatively rare intermediate histologies (Rappaport) are nodular "histiocytic" lymphoma (NH), diffuse mixed lymphoma (DML), and diffuse poorly differentiated lymphoma (DPDL). Aggressive chemotherapy regimens in these diseases have produced complete response rates in the range of 40 to 60% with median

durations of response of 20 to 40 months. However, of this group, only NH is known to be cured with chemotherapy.

Systemic chemotherapy is the treatment of choice for Burkitt's lymphoma. Surgical reduction of the tumor prior to chemotherapy may improve the outcome because the overall prognosis of the disease is directly proportional to the volume of the tumor (144). Although aggressive chemotherapy regimens have achieved durable systemic remissions, many patients have relapses in the central nervous system. Therefore, such regimens should be augmented with intermittent intrathecal methotrexate or cytarabine prophylaxis. Initial chemotherapy must contain high doses of cyclophosphamide, and commonly used regimens also use vincristine, doxorubicin, prednisone, and high-dose methotrexate. Regimens such as these are producing 2-year disease-free survival rates in the range of 50 to 70% (145).

There are five well-established treatment modalities for mycosis fungoides and Sezary syndrome: (1) topical therapy with mechlorethamine, (2) photochemotherapy with psoralen and ultraviolet light, (3) electron beam therapy to the whole body, (4) systemic chemotherapy, and (5) alpha interferon. Patients with disease limited to plaque lesions (without erythroderma or other tissue involvement) generally respond well to topical mechlorethamine or photochemotherapy, but most patients experience relapse within a few years. Electron-beam irradiation also produces complete responses in most patients with only plaque lesions and in some patients with more extensive disease although relapse generally occurs within 3 years. Systemic chemotherapy is reserved for patients with disease that has spread to other organs. Combination chemotherapy regimens used in mycosis fungoides are similar to those used in other NHLs. Although these regimens produce complete responses in about 25% of patients, the duration of response is usually brief (3).

Treatment of HIV-Associated Lymphomas

Patients with AIDS-related lymphomas have a much poorer prognosis than individuals with similar histologies who are not infected with the HIV. Within the AIDS-associated lymphoma group, patients with poor Karnofsky performance status, a history of AIDS prior to the diagnosis of lymphoma, bone marrow involvement, other extranodal involvement, or a CD4 cell count of less than 100/dl have all been reported to have a shorter survival (146, 147).

Because of the aggressiveness and extent of these lymphomas, intensive chemotherapy regimens similar to those used in intermediate and high-grade non-HIV lymphoma have been used. Complete response rates have been somewhat less than those reported for those regimens in the non-HIV population, but several investigators have reported significant complete response rates (greater than

50%) (148–151). Complete response rates have been highest in patients without the poor prognostic factors mentioned earlier. Despite these encouraging responses, many investigators have reported median survivals of less than 1 year (147, 148, 150, 151) with patients either dying from AIDS-related complications (e.g., opportunistic infections), treatment toxicity, or recurrent disease.

The high incidence of treatment-related complications and mortality has led to the use of less intensive regimens. The AIDS Clinical Trials Groups reported the results of a low-dose m-BACOD regimen with CNS and *Pneumocystis carinii* prophylaxis followed by zidovudine. Forty six percent of 42 patients achieved a complete response, and at the time of publication, the median duration of complete response exceeded 14 months (152). A subsequent follow-up study demonstrated that higher dosages of chemotherapy could be administered in combination with granulocyte-macrophage colony stimulating factor (153).

Evidence suggests that patients without poor prognostic signs and who are able to tolerate combination chemotherapy and achieve a complete response may experience a 1- to 2-year disease-free survival. Unfortunately, with currently available therapeutic options, few patients attain a long-term disease-free survival. Therefore, less intensive (lower-dose) regimens that are associated with fewer complications and comparable response and survival outcomes are reasonable at this time.

Another new regimen involving a 96-hour infusion of cyclophosphamide, doxorubicin, and etoposide in 21 patients demonstrated a CR rate of 62% and a median survival of 21 months (55). Two cycles of this regimen resulted in significantly decreased CD4 count and lymphocyte count. Most patients required dose reduction for hematologic toxicity and the mean dose intensity achieved with approximately 75% of the intended dose intensity. Currently, no standard therapy is available for patients considered to be refractory or relapsed after initial therapy has failed. These patients may find investigational therapies helpful.

Methyl-glyoxal-bis guanylhydrazone (MGBG), an investigational agent, may be considered in relapsed or refractory patients with AIDS lymphoma (55). MGBG provides another mechanism of action in that it interferes with polyamine biosynthesis. It also crosses the blood–brain barrier and has no significant myelotoxicity. Response rates of 50% have been reported. Further use of another investigational agent, a monoclonal antibody (anti-B4) conjugated with ricin, has been used in relapsed or refractory patients with AIDS lymphoma (56). This agent was administered at low dosage over 28 days and may be associated with tumor responses with acceptable toxicity. Results from ongoing clinical trials such as these and additional new therapies are in great demand.

COMPLICATIONS

Patients with malignant lymphomas may experience a wide variety of complications, which may be secondary to either the disease or the therapy (Table 79.10). Although many of the disease-related complications have been reduced or eliminated through the use of more effective therapies, the use of more aggressive treatment regimens has resulted in more treatment-related complications. Additionally, the increased cure rate for Hodgkin's disease and many of the NHLs has stimulated concern for late and long-term treatment-associated toxicities.

Many disease-related complications result from infiltration or obstruction of organs, tissues, or blood vessels by the lymphoma. Rapidly growing lymphomas (e.g., nodular sclerosing Hodgkin's disease, lymphoblastic lymphoma) may produce obstruction of the superior vena cava. Patients with this complication frequently present with shortness of breath; swelling of the face, neck, and upper extremities; headache; and sensations of choking. The occurrence of superior vena cava syndrome should be considered an oncologic emergency. Therapy must often be initiated before a tissue diagnosis is made (if this is the initial presentation of the lymphoma) and includes immediate radiation therapy to the mass, diuretics, and combination chemotherapy.

Lymphoma masses may occasionally cause compression of the spinal cord. Initially, this is generally more common in Hodgkin's disease than in NHL; however, it is more common overall in relapsed or refractory NHL and HIV-associated lymphomas. The most common presenting symptom is central back pain. As the degree of compres-

Table 79.10.

Serious Complications Associated with Malignant Lymphomas

Disease related
  Superior vena cava obstruction
  Spinal cord compression
  Central nervous system infiltration
  Renal failure
  Immunologic abnormalities
  Pleural effusion
  Hemolytic anemia
Treatment related
  Chemotherapy related
    Granulocytopenia and infection
    Tumor lysis syndrome
    Gonadal injury/sterility
    Secondary leukemia
    Organ damage secondary to specific agents
  Radiation therapy related
    Tumor lysis syndrome
    Pneumonitis
    Pericarditis
    Hypothyroidism

sion progresses, other neurologic symptoms develop (e.g., motor dysfunction, paresthesias, incontinence), and paraplegia may result if not treated. Appropriate therapy depends on the extent of compression. If detected early enough, chemotherapy and/or radiation therapy may elicit a rapid improvement. In some more advanced spinal cord compressions, emergency surgery (laminectomy) followed by radiation therapy may be required. Corticosteroids are also used to prevent edema or promote its resolution. These agents may also have a direct oncolytic effect as well (157).

Some lymphomas (mostly diffuse NHL where there is bone marrow involvement) may infiltrate the central nervous system and develop meningeal seeding (leptomeningeal involvement). Signs of this complication include headache, nausea and vomiting, and lethargy. Confirmation of meningeal involvement is made by examination of the cerebrospinal fluid, and treatment includes corticosteroids and intrathecal chemotherapy agents (e.g., methotrexate, cytarabine) and radiation therapy. Intracerebral lymphomas may also occur, but these are generally primary tumors (now most commonly seen in patients with HIV) and not complications of other systemic disease.

Renal failure in patients with lymphoma may be due to infiltration of the kidneys or obstruction of the ureters by the lymphoma. Infiltration of the kidneys is usually treated with systemic therapy (although low-dose, local radiation therapy may occasionally be used), and ureteral obstruction may be treated with local radiation therapy combined with systemic chemotherapy.

As would be anticipated from the nature of the disease, immunologic abnormalities commonly occur in patients with malignant lymphomas. Abnormalities in delayed hypersensitivity, particularly cutaneous anergy, develop with extensive involvement of lymphatic tissues or severe lymphocytopenia. Depressed cell-mediated immunity (T lymphocyte) is associated with a high risk of opportunistic infections, including tuberculosis, salmonellosis, toxoplasmosis, and herpes zoster. This is particularly true in patients with Hodgkin's disease. In some cases, infection may precede diagnosis of the disease (158). Furthermore, patients may continue to have an underlying T cell function deficit that persists after they are in remission (159). Radiation and chemotherapy also contribute to the decreased immunologic functions and subsequent infectious complication.

Granulocytopenia secondary to myelosuppressive chemotherapy also predisposes patients to serious infections. Gram-negative bacilli (i.e., *Escherichia coli*, *Klebsiella pneumoniae*, and *Pseudomonas aeruginosa*) and Gram-positive cocci (*Staphylococcus aureus* and *Staphylococcus epidermidis*) are the most common pathogens responsible for infections during granulocytopenia. As chemotherapy regimens have become more aggressive, especially those used in NHL, the degree and duration of granulocytopenia have increased, placing more patients at risk of infectious complications. Fortunately, the availability of colony-stimulating factors (filgrastim and sargramostim) has ameliorated this risk substantially.

Acute and chronic toxicities associated with the administration of combination chemotherapy are determined by the individual agents included in the treatment regimen. In addition to myelosuppression, these toxicities may include nausea and vomiting, mucositis, neurotoxicity, cardiotoxicity, skin changes, and pulmonary toxicity. Many of these toxicities are avoidable or reversible if the clinician(s) managing the patient are familiar with the agents being used and their associated risks. The major long-term complications of chemotherapy of lymphomas are sterility and the risk of secondary malignancies.

Testicular function in adult men is particularly susceptible to injury by many chemotherapeutic agents. The MOPP regimen has been reported to cause azoospermia and germinal aplasia in more than 80% of men receiving this regimen (160). Although chemotherapy-associated azoospermia is generally persistent, recovery may be observed in a small portion of patients several years following the cessation of therapy. A comparison of the MOPP and ABVD regimens revealed that azoospermia occurred in 100% of MOPP-treated men but in only 15 to 35% of those receiving ABVD therapy. In addition, spermatogenesis almost always recovered in the ABVD-treated men (161, 162). This information may be important in planning treatment for young men with Hodgkin's disease who are concerned about preservation of fertility following treatment.

Gonadal injury also occurs in women following combination chemotherapy. Ovarian failure is associated with arrest of follicular maturation or frank destruction of ova and follicles. Unlike the profound effects of the MOPP regimen on testicular function, it appears to produce ovarian dysfunction and amenorrhea in only 40 to 50% of women (86, 163). Ovarian injury from MOPP therapy is correlated with age at treatment, with older patients (over age 35) much more likely to experience persistent amenorrhea (164). Persistent amenorrhea also appears to be less common following ABVD therapy than following MOPP therapy (161).

The potential of myelodysplasia and secondary malignancies, particularly acute nonlymphocytic leukemia, is a well-documented complication associated with Hodgkin's disease or its therapy. Several studies have provided convincing evidence that the risk of leukemia varies markedly with the form of therapy for Hodgkin's disease. Secondary leukemias occur in 2 to 3% of patients who have received MOPP with or without radiotherapy, and the 10-year cumulative risk of such patients is between 5 and 10% (165–168). Leukemia has usually developed between

3 and 10 years after initiation of treatment for Hodgkin's disease, and most patients have been in complete remission of the Hodgkin's disease when the leukemia develops (165). The risk of acute leukemia following ABVD therapy appears to be negligible. Patients with Hodgkin's disease are also at increased risk of developing NHL. Non-Hodgkin's lymphomas apparently occur more frequently after combined radiation and chemotherapy (169). Patients with Hodgkin's disease may also have a slight increased risk of developing solid tumors (165, 168). In particular, excess lung cancer risk has been observed in patients who received radiation therapy (in the irradiated field) (168). Patients treated for NHL also have an increased risk of developing acute nonlymphocytic leukemia, and the intensity of therapy appears to be correlated with the likelihood of developing a secondary leukemia (165).

Complications following radiation therapy are largely related to the field that has been irradiated although fatigue generally occurs in most patients. Nausea, vomiting, mucositis/esophagitis, diarrhea, and anorexia commonly occur following abdominal radiation, whereas dryness of the mouth and throat, dysphagia, alteration in taste, and increased dental caries may occur following irradiation of the head and neck regions. Bone marrow depression may occur during the abdominal–pelvic irradiation and may require interruption of treatment. In addition to these acute side effects, long-term complications may pose more serious problems. Long-term effects are usually related to the volume of normal tissue that has been irradiated, the total dose given, and the size of the daily dose administered. They include radiation pneumonitis, pericarditis, nephritis, hepatitis, growth retardation (in children), and hypothyroidism.

CONCLUSION

The lymphomas are malignant disorders that originate from lymphoreticular cells. These disorders may disseminate via contiguous lymphatics or the bloodstream to other lymph nodes and other organ systems. Malignant lymphomas are generally separated into Hodgkin's disease and non-Hodgkin's lymphomas, but the term *non-Hodgkin's lymphomas* represents multiple diseases with diverse morphologic and clinical features. The prognosis and treatment of each lymphoma are related to the histopathology and the anatomic extent of disease determined by staging procedures. Most lymphomas are sensitive to radiation therapy as well as many chemotherapeutic agents. Combination chemotherapy regimens are now successful in curing many patients with Hodgkin's disease and high-grade non-Hodgkin's lymphomas. In addition, many other patients experience a significant prolongation of disease-free survival following chemotherapy. It is likely that high-dose chemotherapy with bone marrow transplantation and biologic response modifiers (e.g., interferon) will

assume a much more prominent role in the management of lymphomas.

Management of patients with lymphomas requires not only an understanding of the disease process and its appropriate therapy but also an understanding of the variety of complications that may arise secondary to the disease or its therapy. These complications include opportunistic infections, obstruction by the tumor, secondary malignancies, and chemotherapy- and radiation-associated toxicities. Anticipation and appropriate management of these complications can greatly reduce the overall morbidity experienced by the patient.

REFERENCES

1. Diehl V, vonKalle C, Fonatsch C, et al. The cell origin in Hodgkin's disease. Semin Oncol 17:660–672, 1990.
2. Slivnick DJ, Nawrocki JF, Fisher RI. Immunology and cellular biology of Hodgkin's disease. Hematol Oncol Clin N Am 3:205–220, 1989.
3. DeVita VT, Jaffe ES, Mauch, Longo DL. Lymphocytic lymphomas. In DeVita VT, Hellman S, Rosenberg SA, eds. Cancer. Principles and practice of oncology, ed 3. Philadelphia, J.B. Lippincott and Co., p. 1741.
4. American Cancer Society, Facts and Figures, 1991. New York, American Cancer Society, 1991.
5. Cantor KP, Fraumeni JF. Distribution of non-Hodgkin's lymphoma in the United States between 1950 and 1975. Cancer Res 40:2645–2652, 1980.
6. MacMahon B. Epidemiological evidence of the nature of Hodgkin's disease. Cancer 10:1045–1054, 1957.
7. Miller RW, Beebe GW. Infectious mononucleosis and the empirical risk of cancer. J NCI 50:315–321, 1973.
8. Connolly RR, Chistene BW. A cohort study of cancer following infectious mononucleosis. Cancer Res 34:1172–1178, 1974.
9. Rosdahl N, Larsen SO, Clemmensen J. Hodgkin's disease in patients with previous mononucleosis, 30 years experience. Br Med J 2:253–256, 1974.
10. Gottlieb-Stematsky T, Vonsover A, Ramot B, et al. Antibodies to Epstein-Barr virus in patients with Hodgkin's disease and leukemia. Cancer 36:1640–1645, 1975.
11. Evans AS, Gutensohn NM. A population-based case-control study of EBV and other viral antibodies among persons with Hodgkin's disease and their siblings. Int J Cancer 34:149–157, 1984.
12. Mueller N, Evans A, Harris NL, et al. Hodgkin's disease and Epstein-Barr virus. Altered antibody pattern before diagnosis. N Engl J Med 320:689–695, 1989.
13. Staal SP, Ambinder R, Beschorner WE, et al. A survey of Epstein-Barr Virus DNA in lymphoid tissue. Frequent detection in Hodgkin's disease. Am J Clin Pathol 91:1–5, 1989.
14. Weiss L, Movahed LA, Warnke RA, et al. Detection of Epstein-Barr viral genomes in Reed-Sternberg cells of Hodgkin's disease. N Engl J Med 320:502–506, 1989.
15. Vianna NJ, Greenwald P, Davies JNP. Extended epidemic of Hodgkin's disease in patients with previous mononucleosis, 30 years experience. Br Med J 2:253–256, 1974.
16. Vianna JH, Dolan AK. Epidemiological evidence for transmission of Hodgkin's disease. NEJM 289:499–502, 1973.
17. Grufferman S, Cole P, Smith PG, Lukes RJ. Hodgkin's disease in siblings. NEJM 296:248–250, 1977.
18. Prazak J, Hermanska Z. Study of HLA antigens in patients with Hodgkin's disease. Eur J Haematol 43:50–53, 1989.

19. Penn I. The incidence of malignancies in transplant recipients. Transplant Proc 7:323,1975.

20. Matas AJ, Hertel BF, Rosai J, et al. Post-transplant malignant lymphoma. Distinctive morphologic features related to its pathogenesis. Am J Med 61:716, 1976.

21. Ziegler JL, Beckstead JA, Volberding PA, et al. Non-Hodgkins lymphoma in 90 homosexual men. Relation to generalized lymphadenopathy and the acquired immunodeficiency syndrome. N Engl J Med 311:565–570, 1984.

22. Anderson RE, Nishiyama H, Yohei I, Kenzo T, Nobukazo O. Pathogenesis of radiation related leukemia and lymphoma. Speculations based primarily on experience of Hiroshima and Nagasaki. Lancet 1:1060–1062, 1972.

23. Rabkin CS, Devesa SS, Zahm SH, Gail MH. Increasing incidence of non-Hodgkin's lymphoma. Semin Hematol 30:286–296, 1993.

24. Reedman BM, Klein G. Cellular localization of an Epstein-Barr virus (EBV)-associated complement fixing antigen in producer and nonproducer lymphoblastoid cell lines. Int J Cancer 11:499–520, 1973.

25. Blattner WA, Gibbs WN, Saxinger C, et al. Human T-cell leukaemia/lymphoma virus-lymphomareticular neoplasia in Jamaica. Lancet 2:61–64, 1983.

26. Lukes RJ, Butler JJ, Hicks ED. Natural history of Hodgkin's disease as related to its pathologic picture. Cancer 42:1039–1045, 1978.

27. Parker BA, Green MR. Hodgkin's disease. In: Moosa AR, Schimpff SC, Robson MC, eds: Comprehensive textbook of oncology, ed 2. Baltimore, Williams and Wilkens, 1991, p. 1257.

28. Hellman S, Jaffe ES, DeVita VT. Hodgkin's disease. In: Devita VT, Hellman S, Rosenberg SA, eds. Cancer. Principles and practice of oncology, ed 3. Philadelphia, J.B. Lippincott and Co., p. 1696–1741.

29. Poppema S, Kaiserling E, Lennert K. Nodular paragranuloma and progressively transformed germinal centers: ultrastructural and immunohistologic findings. Virchows Arch (Cell Pathol) 31:211–225, 1979.

30. Kradin ME, Agnarsson BA, Ellingsworth LR, Newcom SR. Immunohistochemical evidence of a role for transforming growth factor beta in the pathogenesis of nodular sclerosing Hodgkin's disease. Am H Pathol 136:1209–1214, 1990.

31. Rappaport H. Tumors of the hematopoietic system. In Atlas of Tumor Pathology, Sec III, Fasc 8. Washington DC, Armed Forces Institute of Pathology, 1966.

32. National Cancer Institute sponsored study of classification of non-Hodgkin's lymphomas. Summary and description of a working formulation for clinical usage. Cancer 49:2112–2135, 1982.

33. Armitage JO. Treatment of Non-Hodgkin's lymphoma. NEJM 328:1023–1030, 1993.

34. Harris NL, Jaffe ES, Stein H, et al. A revised European-American classification of lymphoid neoplasms: a proposal from the International Lymphoma Study Group. Blood 84:1361–1392, 1994.

35. Foucar K. Incidence and patterns of bone marrow and blood involvement by lymphoma in relationship to the Lukes-Collins classification. Blood 54:1417–1422, 1979.

36. Centers for Disease Control. Revision of the case definition of acquired immunodeficiency syndrome for national reporting - United States. MMWR 34:373–375, 1985.

37. Pluta JM, Venzon DJ, Tosato JL et al. Parameters Affecting the Development of Non-Hodgkin's Lymphoma in Patients with Severe Human Immunodeficiency Virus Infection Receiving Antiretroviral Therapy. J Clin Onco Vol 11 No 6(June):1099, 1993.

38. Ziegler JL, Drew WL, Miner RC, et al. Outbreak of Burkitt's-like lymphoma in homosexual men. Lancet 2:631–633, 1982.

39. Snider WD, Simpson DM, Aronyk KE, Nielson SL. Primary lymphoma of the nervous system associated with acquired immunodeficiency syndrome (letter). N Eng J Med 308:45, 1983.

40. Ciobanu N, Adreeff M, Safai B, Koziner B, Mertelsmann R. Lymphoblastic neoplasia in a homosexual patient with Kaposi's sarcoma. Ann Intern Med 98:151–155, 1983.

41. Ioachim HL, Cooper MC, Hellman GC. Lymphomas in men at high risk for acquired immune deficiency syndrome. Cancer 56:2831–2842, 1985.

42. Lister TA, Crowther D, Sutcliffe SB, et al. Report of a committee convened to discuss the evaluation and staging of patients with Hodgkin's disease: Cotswolds Meeting. J Clin Oncol 7:1630–1636, 1989.

43. Portlock CS. Hodgkin's disease. Med Clin N Am 68:629–740, 1984.

44. Berard C, Thomas LB, Axtell LM. The relationship of histopathological subtype to clinical stage of Hodgkin's disease of diagnosis. Cancer Res 31:1776, 1971.

45. Coiffer B, Gisselbrecht C, Vose JM et al. Prognostic factors in aggressive malignant lymphomas: description and validation of a prognostic index that could identify patients requiring a more intensive therapy: The Groupe d'Etudes des Lymphomes Agressifs. J Clin Oncol 9:211–219,1991.

46. DeVita VT, Serpick A, Carbone P. Combination chemotherapy in the treatment of advanced Hodgkin's disease. Ann Intern Med 73:881, 1970.

47. Hoppe RT. Radiation therapy in the management of Hodgkin's disease. Semin Oncol 17:704–715, 1990.

48. Leslie NT, Mauch PM, Hellman S. Stage IA to IIB supradiaphragmatic Hodgkin's disease: Long-term survival and relapse frequency. Cancer 55:2072–2078, 1985.

49. Lee CK, Appli DM, Bloomfield CD, Levitt SH. Curative radiotherapy for laparotomy-staged IA, IIA, IIA Hodgkin's disease: An evaluation of the gains achieved with radical radiotherapy. Int J Radiat Oncol Biol Phys 19:547–549, 1990.

50. Farah R, Ultmann J, Griem M, et al. Extended mantle radiation therapy for pathologic stage I and II Hodgkin's disease. J Clin Oncol 6:1047–1058, 1988.

51. Gladstein E. Radiation in Hodgkin's disease: Past achievements and future progress. Cancer 39:837–842, 1977.

52. Koziner B, Myers J, Cirrincione C, et al. Treatment of stages I and II Hodgkin's disease with three different therapeutic modalities. Am J Med 80:1067–1078, 1986.

53. Hoppe RT, Coleman CN, Cox RS, et al. The management of stage I-II Hodgkin's disease with irradiation alone or combined modality therapy: The Stanford experience. Blood 59:455–465, 1982.

54. Mauch P, Goodman R, Hellman S. The significance of mediastinal involvement in early stage Hodgkin's disease. Cancer 42:1039–1045, 1978.

55. Longo DL, Glatstein E, Duffy PL, et al. Radiation therapy versus combination chemotherapy in the treatment of early-stage Hodgkin's disease: seven year results of a prospective randomized trial. J Clin Oncol 9:906–917, 1991.

56. Longo DL. The use of chemotherapy in the treatment of Hodgkin's disease. Semin Oncol 17:716–735, 1990.

57. Stein RS, Golomb HS, Wiernik PH, et al. Anatomic substages of stage IIIA Hodgkin's disease: Followup of a collaborative study. Cancer Treat Rep 66:733–741, 1982.

58. Hoppe RT, Cox RS, Rosenberg SA, et al. Prognostic factors in pathologic stage III Hodgkin's disease. Cancer Treat Rep 66:743–749, 1982.

59. Mouch PM, Rosenthal DS, Canellos GP, et al. Improved survival for stage IIIA and IIIB Hodgkin's disease patients treated with combined radiation therapy (RT) and chemotherapy. Proc Am Soc Clin Oncol 2:213, 1983.

60. Lister TA, Dorreen MS, Faux M, et al. Treatment of stage III$_A$ Hodgkin's disease. J Clin Oncol 1:745–749, 1983.

61. Crowther D, Wagstaff J, Deaken D, et al. A randomized study comparing chemotherapy alone and chemotherapy followed by

radiotherapy in patients with pathologically staged III$_A$ Hodgkin's disease. J Clin Oncol 2:892–897, 1984.

62. Brookman MA, Longo DL. Concomitant illness in patients treated for Hodgkin's disease. Cancer Treat Rev 13:77–111, 1986.

63. DeVita VT, Simon RM, Hubbard SM, et al. Curability of advanced Hodgkin's disease with chemotherapy: long-term follow up of MOPP treated patients at NCI. Ann Intern Med 92:587, 1980.

64. Longo DL, Young RC, Wesley M, et al. Twenty years of MOPP therapy for Hodgkin's disease. J Clin Oncol. 4:1295–1306, 1986.

65. Wiernik PH. Chemotherapy of Hodgkin's disease. Prin Pract Oncol 2:1–12, 1988.

66. van Rijswijk RE, Haanen C, Dekker AW, et al. Dose intensity of MOPP chemotherapy and survival in Hodgkin's disease. J Clin Oncol 7:1776–1782, 1989.

67. Harker WG, Kushlan P, Rosenberg SA. Combination chemotherapy for advanced Hodgkin's disease after failure of MOPP: ABVD and B-CAVe. Ann Intern Med 101:440–446, 1984.

68. Nicholson WM, Beard MEJ, Crowther D, et al. Combination chemotherapy in generalized Hodgkin's disease. Br Med J 3:7–10, 1976.

69. Farber LR, Prosnitz LR, Cadman EC, et al. Curative potential of combined modality therapy for advanced Hodgkin's disease. Cancer 46:1590–1517, 1980.

70. Klimo P, Connors JM. An update on the Vancouver experience in the management of advanced Hodgkin's disease treated with the MOPP/ABV hydrid program. Semin Hematol 25:34–40, 1988.

71. Canellos GP, Anderson BA, Peterson BA, Gottlieb AJ. EVA: etoposide, vinblastine, doxorubicin (adriamycin)—an effective regimen for the treatment of Hodgkin's disease in relapse following MOPP. A study of the Cancer and Leukemia Group B. Proc Am Soc Clin Oncol 10:273, 1991.

72. Goldie JH, Coldman AJ. A mathematical model for relating the drug sensitivity of tumors to their spontaneous mutation rate. Cancer Treat Rep 63:1727–1733, 1979.

73. Santoro A, Bonadonna G, Bonfante V, et al. Alternating drug combinations in the treatment of advanced Hodgkin's disease. N Engl J Med 306:770–775, 1982.

74. Bonadonna G, Valgussa P, Santoro A. Alternating non-cross-resistant combination chemotherapy or MOPP in stage IV Hodgkin's disease. Ann Intern Med 104:739–746, 1986.

75. Glick J, Tsiatis A, Schilsky R, et al. A randomized phase III trial of MOPP/ABV hydrid vs. sequential MOPP-ABVD in advanced Hodgkin's disease: preliminary results of the intergroup trial. Proc Am Soc Clin Oncol 10:271, 1991.

76. Oliver IN, Wolf MM, Cruickshank D, et al. Nitrogen mustard, vincristine, procarbazine, and prednisolone for relapse after radiation in Hodgkin's disease. Cancer 62:233–239, 1988.

77. Pillai GN, Hagemeister RB, Valasquez WS, et al. Prognostic factors for stage IV Hodgkin's disease treated with MOPP, with or without bleomycin. Cancer 55:691–697, 1985.

78. Wagstaff J, Gregory WM, Swindell R, et al. Prognostic factors for survival in stage III$_B$ and IV Hodgkin's disease: a multivariate analysis comparing two specialist treatment centres. Br J Cancer 58:487–492, 1988.

79. Carde P, MacKintosh FR, Rosenberg SA. A dose and time response analysis of the treatment of Hodgkin's disease with MOPP chemotherapy. J Clin Oncol 1:146–153, 1983.

80. Canellos GP. Can MOPP be replaced in the treatment of advanced Hodgkin's disease? Semin Oncol 17(suppl 2):2–6, 1990.

81. Levis A, Vitolo U, CioccaVasina MA, et al. Predictive value of the early response to chemotherapy in high-risk stages II and II Hodgkin's disease. Cancer 60:1713–1719, 1987.

82. Green JA, Dawson AA, Fell LF, et al. Measurement of drug dosage intensity in MVPP therapy in Hodgkin's disease. Br J Clin Pharmacol 9:511–514, 1980.

83. Van Rijswijk, RE, Haanen C, Dekker AW, et al. Dose intensity of MOPP chemotherapy and survival in Hodgkin's disease. J Clin Oncol 7:1776–1782, 1989.

84. Gibbs GE, Peterson BA, Kennedy BJ, et al. Long-term survival of patients with Hodgkin's disease: treatment with cyclophosphamide, vinblastine, procarbazine, and prednisone. Arch Intern Med 141:897–900, 1981.

85. Santoro A, Viviana S, Villarreal CJ, et al. Salvage chemotherapy in Hodgkin's disease irradiation failures: superiority of doxorubicin-containing regimens over MOPP. Cancer Treat Rep 70:343–348, 1986.

86. Fisher RI, DeVita VT, Hubbard SM, et al. Prolonged disease-free survival in Hodgkin's disease with MOPP reinduction after first relapse. Ann Intern Med 90:761–763, 1979.

87. Taylor RE, McElwin TJ, Barrett A, et al. Etoposide as a single agent in relapsed advanced lymphomas-a phase II study. Cancer Chemother Pharmacol 7:175–177, 1982.

88. Canellos GP. Is there an effective salvage therapy for advanced Hodgkin's disease? Ann Oncol 2(suppl 1):1–7,1991.

89. Vose JM, Bierman PJ, Armitage JO. Hodgkin's disease: the role of bone marrow transplantation. Semin Oncol 17:749–757, 1990.

90. Williams SF, Bitran JD. The role of high-dose therapy and autologous bone marrow reinfusion in the treatment of Hodgkin's disease. Hematol Oncol Clin N Am 3:319–329, 1989.

91. Anderson JE, Litzow MR, Appelbaum FR, et al. J Clin Oncol 11:2342–2350, 1993.

92. Jagannath S, Armitage JO, Dicke KA, et al. Prognostic factors for response and survival after high-dose cyclophosphamide, carmustine, and etoposide with autologous bone marrow transplantation. J Clin Oncol 7:179–185, 1989.

93. Carella AM, Congiu AM, Gaozza E, et al. High-dose chemotherapy with autologous bone marrow transplantation in 50 advanced resistant Hodgkin's disease patients: an Italian Study Group report. J Clin Oncol 6:1411–1416, 1988.

94. Gribben JG, Linch DC, Singer CRJ, et al. Successful treatment of refractory Hodgkin's disease by high-dose combination chemotherapy and autologous bone marrow transplantation. Blood 73:340–344, 1989.

95. Goldstone AH. EBMT experience of autologous BMT (ABMT) in non-Hodgkin's lymphoma and Hodgkin's disease. Bone Marrow Transplant 1(suppl):289–292, 1986.

96. Phillips GL, Solff SN, Herzig RH, et al. Treatment of progressive Hodgkin's disease with intensive chemoradiotherapy and autologous bone marrow transplantation. Blood 73:2086–2092, 1989.

97. Vose JM, Bierman PJ, Armitage JO. Hodgkin's disease: the role of bone marrow transplantation. Semin Oncol 17:749–757, 1990.

98. Jones RJ, Piantadosi S, Mann RB, et al. High-dose cytotoxic therapy and bone marrow transplantation for relapsed Hodgkin's disease. J Clin Oncol 8:527–537, 1990.

99. Reese DE, Barnett MJ, Conners JM et al. Intensive chemotherapy with cyclophosphamide, carmustine, and etoposide followed by autologous bone marrow transplantation for relapsed Hodgkin's disease. J Clin Oncol 1991;9:1871–1879.

100. Desch CE, Lasala MR, Smith TJ, Hillner BE. The optimal timing of autologous bone marrow transplantation in Hodgkin's disease patients after a chemotherapy relapse. J Clin Oncol 10:200–209, 1992.

101. Rapoport AP, Rowe JM, Kouides PA, et al. One hundred autotransplants for relapsed or refractory Hodgkin's Disease and lymphoma: value of pretransplant disease status for predicting outcome. J Clin Oncol 11:2351–2361, 1993.

102. Taylor K Mc, Jagannath S, Spinolo JA, et al. Recombinant human granulocyte colony-stimulating factor hastens recovery after high-dose chemotherapy and autologous bone marrow transplantation in Hodgkin's disease. J Clin Oncol 7:791–799, 1989.

103. Nemunaitis J, Singer JW, Buchner CD, et al. Use of recombinant human granulocyte-macrophage colony-stimulating factor in autologous marrow transplantation for lymphoid malignancies. Blood 72:834–836, 1988.

104. Portlock CS. Management of the low-grade non-Hodgkin's lymphomas. Semin Oncol 17:51–59, 1990.

105. Chabner BA, Johnson RE, Young R, et al. Sequential non-surgical and surgical staging of non-Hodgkin's lymphomas. Ann Intern Med 85:149–154, 1976.

106. Rosenberg SA. Validity of Ann Arbor staging of the non-Hodgkin's lymphomas. Cancer Treat Rep 61:1023–1027, 1977.

107. Paryani SB, Hoppe RT, Cox RS, et al: The role of radiation therapy in the management of stage III follicular lymphomas. J Clin Oncol 2:841–848, 1984.

108. Portlock CS: Management of the indolent non-Hodgkin's lymphomas. Semin Oncol 7:292–301, 1980.

109. Hoppe RT, Kushlan P, Kaplan HS, et al: The treatment of advanced stage favorable histology non-Hodgkin's lymphoma: a preliminary report of a randomized trial comparing single agent chemotherapy, combination chemotherapy, and whole body irradiation. Blood 58:592–598, 1981.

110. Gribben JG, Freedman AS, Woo SD, et al. All advanced stage non-Hodgkin's lymphomas with polymerase chain reaction amplifiable breakpoint of bcl-2 have residual cells containing the bcl-2 re-arrangement at evaluation and after treatment. Blood 78:3275–3280, 1991.

111. DeVita VT, Canellos GP, Chabner BA, et al. Advanced diffuse histiocytic lymphoma, a potentially curable disease. Results with combination chemotherapy. Lancet 1:248–250, 1975.

112. Portlock CS, Rosenberg SA. Chemotherapy of the non-Hodgkin's lymphomas: The Stanford experience. Cancer Treat Rep 61:1049–1055, 1977.

113. Armitage JO, Dick FR, Corder MP, et al. Predicting therapeutic outcome in patients with diffuse histiocytic lymphoma treated with cyclophosphamide, adriamycin, vincristine, and prednisone (CHOP). Cancer 50:1695–1702. 1982.

114. Merchant N, McLaughlin P, Fuller L, et al. Follicular (nodular) mixed lymphoma: a review of 65 cases. Proc Am Soc Clin Oncol 3:249, 1984.

115. Skarin AT, Canellos GP, Rosenthal DS, et al. Improved prognosis of diffuse histiocytic and undifferentiated lymphoma by use of high dose methotrexate alternating with standard agents. (M-BACOD). J Clin Oncol 1:91–98, 1983.

116. Klimo P, Connors JM. MACOP-B chemotherapy for the treatment of diffuse large-cell lymphoma. Ann Intern Med 102:596–602, 1985.

117. Urba WJ, Duffy PL, Longo DL. Treatment of patients with aggressive lymphomas: an overview. J NCI Monographs 10:29–37, 1990.

118. Fisher RI, DeVita VT, Hubbard SM. Diffuse aggressive lymphomas: Increased survival after alternating flexible sequences of ProMACE and MOPP chemotherapy. Ann Intern Med 98:304–309, 1983.

119. Longo DL, DeVita VT, Duffy PL, et al. Superiority of ProMACE-CytaBOM over ProMACE-MOPP in the treatment of advanced diffuse aggressive lymphoma: results of a prospective randomized trial. J Clin Oncol 9:25–38, 1991.

120. Anderson KC, Skarin AT, Rosenthal DS, et al. Combination chemotherapy for advanced non-Hodgkin's lymphomas other than diffuse histiocytic or undifferentiated histologies. Cancer Treat Rep 68:1343, 1984.

121. Case DC Comparison of M-2 protocol with COP in patients with nodular lymphoma. Oncology 41:159, 1984.

122. Ezdinli EZ, Anderson JR, Melvin F., et al. Moderate versus aggressive chemotherapy of nodular lymphocytic poorly differentiated lymphoma. J Clin Oncol 3:769, 1985.

123. Foon KA, Sherwin SA, Abrams PG. Treatment of advanced non-Hodgkin's lymphoma with recombinant leukocyte A interferon. N Engl J Med 311:1148–1152, 1984.

124. Smalley RV, Andersen JW, Hawkins MJ, et al. Interferon alfa combined with cytotoxic chemotherapy for patients with non-Hodgkin's lymphoma. NEJM 327:1336–1341, 1992.

125. Young RC, Longo DL, Gladstein E, et al. The treatment of indolent lymphomas: watchful waiting versus aggressive combined modality treatment. Semin Hematol 25:11–16, 1988.

126. Colombat P, Binot C, Linassier C, et al. High dose chemotherapy with autologous marrow transplantation in follicular lymphomas. Leuk Lymphoma 7(suppl):3–6, 1992.

127. Bierman P, Vose J, Armitage J, et al. High dose therapy followed by autologous hematopoietic rescue for follicular low grade non-Hodgkin's lymphoma (NHL). Proc Am Soc Clin Oncol 11:317, 1992.

128. Rohatiner AZS, Lister TA. Myeloablative therapy for follicular lymphoma. Hematol Oncol Clin North Am. 5:1003–1012, 1991.

129. Longo DL, Glatstein E, Duffey P, et al. Treatment of Localized aggressive lymphomas with combination chemotherapy followed by involved-field radiation therapy. J Clin Oncol 7:1295–1302, 1989.

130. Jones SE, Rosenberg SA, Kaplan ES, et al. Non-Hodgkin's lymphomas: Single agent chemotherapy. Cancer 43:417–425, 1972.

131. Fisher RI, Gaynor ER, Dahlberg S, et al. Comparison of a standard regimen (CHOP) with three intensive chemotherapy regimens for advanced non-Hodgkin's lymphoma. NEJM 328:1002–1006, 1993.

132. Fisher RI, Hubbard SM, DeVita VT, et al. Factors predicting long-term survival in diffuse mixed, histiocytic, or undifferentiated lymphoma. Blood 58:45–50, 1981.

133. Vose JM, Armitage JO, Weisenburger DD, et al. The importance of age in survival of patients treated with chemotherapy for diffuse large-cell lymphoma-rapidly responding patients have more durable remissions. J Clin Oncol 4:160–164, 1986.

134. Meyer RM, Quirt IC, Skillings JR, et al. Escalated as compared with standard doses doxorubicin in BACOP therapy for patients with non-Hodgkin's lymphoma. NEJM 329:1770–1776, 1993.

135. Meyer RM, Hryniuk WM, Goodyear MDE. The role of dose intensity in determining outcome in intermediate-grade non-Hodgkin's lymphoma. J Clin Oncol 9:339–347, 1991.

136. Cabanillas F. Experience with salvage regimens at M.D. Anderson Hospital. Ann Oncol 2(suppl 1):31–32, 1991.

137. Kessinger A, Nademanee A, Forman SJ, Armitage JO. Autologous bone marrow transplantation for Hodgkin's and Non-Hodgkin's lymphoma. Hematol Oncol Clin N Am 4:577–587, 1990.

138. Williams SF. The role of bone marrow transplantation in the non-Hodgkin's lymphomas. Semin Oncol 17:88–95, 1990.

139. Haq R, Sawka CA, Franssen E, Berinstein NL. Significance of a partial or slow response to front-line chemotherapy in the management of intermediate-grade or high-grade non-Hodgkin's lymphoma: a literature review. J Clin Oncol 12:1074–1084, 1994.

140. Phillips GL, Herzig RH, Lazarus HM, et al. Treatment of resistant malignant lymphoma with cyclophosphamide, total body irradiation, and transplantation of cryopreserved autologous marrow. N Engl J Med 310:1557–1561, 1984.

141. Armitage JO, Gingrich RD, Klassen LW, et al. Trial of high-dose cytarabine, cyclophosphamide, total-body irradiation, and autologous marrow transplantation for refractory lymphoma. Cancer Treat Rep 70:871–875, 1986.

142. Takvoran T, Canellos GP, Ritz J, et al. Prolonged disease free survival after autologous bone marrow transplantation in patients with non-Hodgkin's lymphoma with a poor prognosis. N Engl J Med 316;1499–1505.

143. Armitage JO. Treatment of non-Hodgkin's lymphoma. NEJM 328:1023–1030, 1993.

144. Magrath I, Lee YJ, Anderson T, et al. Prognostic factors in Burkitt's lymphoma: importance of total tumor burden. Cancer 45:1507–1515, 1980.

145. Ziegler JL. Burkitt's lymphoma. N Engl J Med 305:735–745, 1981.

146. Levine AM, Loureiro C, Sullivan-Halley J, et al. HIV-related lymphoma: prognostic factors predictive of survival. Blood 1988;72: 247a, 1988.

147. Kaplan LD, Abrams DI, Feigal E, et al. AIDS-associated non-Hodgkin's lymphoma in San Francisco. JAMA 261:719–724, 1989.

148. Gill PS, Levine AM, Krailo M, et al. AIDS-related malignant lymphoma: results of prospective treatment trials. J Clin Oncol 5:1322–1328, 1987.

149. Bermudez MA, Grant KM, Rodvien R, Mendes F. Non-Hodgkin's lymphoma in a population with or at risk for acquired immunodeficiency syndrome: indications for intensive chemotherapy. Am J Med 86:71–76, 1989.

150. Knowles DM, Chamulak GA, Subar M, et al. Lymphoid neoplasia associated with the acquired immunodeficiency syndrome (AIDS). Ann Intern Med 108:744–753, 1988.

151. Lowenthal DA, Straus DJ, Campbell SW, et al. AIDS-related lymphoid neoplasia. Cancer 61:2325–2337, 1988.

152. Levine AM, Wernz JC, Kaplan L, et al. Low dose chemotherapy with central nervous system prophylaxis and zidovudine maintenance in AIDS-related lymphoma: a multi-institutional trial. Blood 74:897a, 1989.

153. Walsh C, Wernz J, Laubenstein L, et al. Phase I study of M-BACOD and GM-CSF in AIDS-associated non-Hodgkin's lymphoma: preliminary results. Blood 74:466a, 1989.

154. Sparano JA, Wiernik PH, Dutcher JP, et al. Infusional Cyclophosphamide (C), Doxorubicin (D), and Etoposide (E) in HIV-Related Non-Hodgkin's Lymphoma (NHL): A followup report of a Highly Active Regimen. Blood 82:1530, 1993.

155. Levine AM, Weiss G, Tulpule A, et al. MGBG: A highly active drug in relapsed or refractory AIDS Lymphoma. Proc ASCO 13:11, 1994.

156. Tulpule A, Anderson LJ, Levine AM, et al. Anti-B4 (CD 19) monoclonal antibody, conjugated with ricin (B4 blocked ricin:B4BR) in refractory AIDS-Lymphoma. Proc ASCO 13:10, 1994.

157. Posner JB, Howieson J, Cvitkovic E. "Disappearing" spinal cord compression: Oncolytic effect of glucocorticoids (and other chemotherapeutic agents) on epidural metastases. Ann Neurol 2:409–413, 1977.

158. Hohl RJ, Schilsky RL. Nonmalignant complications of therapy for Hodgkin's disease. Hematol Oncol Clin N Am 3:331–343, 1989.

159. Vanhaelan CPJ, Fisher RI. Increased sensitivity of T cells to regulation by normal suppressor cells persists in long-term survivors with Hodgkin's disease. Am J Med 72:385–390, 1982.

160. Schilsky RL, Sherins RJ. Adverse effects of treatment: Gonadal dysfunction. In DeVita VT, Hellman S, Rosenberg SM: Cancer Principles and Practice of Oncology, ed 2. Philadelphia, J.B. Lippincott and Co., 1985, p. 2032.

161. Santoro A, Viviani S, Zucali R, et al. Comparative results and toxicity of MOPP vs ABVD combined with radiotherapy in PS IIB, III Hodgkin's disease. Proc Am Soc Clin Oncol 2:223, 1983.

162. Bonadonna G, Santoro A. ABVD chemotherapy in the treatment of Hodgkin's disease. Cancer Treat Rev 9:21–35, 1982.

163. Chapman RM, Sutcliffe SB, Malpas JS. Cytotoxic-induced ovarian failure in women with Hodgkin's disease. I. Hormone function. JAMA 242:1877–1881, 1979.

164. Schilsky RL, Serins RJ, Hubbard SM, et al. Long term follow up of ovarian function in women treated with MOPP chemotherapy for Hodgkin's disease. Am J Med 71:552–556, 1981.

165. Li FP. Adverse effects of treatment: Second cancers. In DeVita VT, Hellman S, Rosenberg SA: Cancer Principles and Practice of Oncology, ed. 2. Philadelphia, J. B. Lippincott and Co., 1985, p. 2040.

166. Pedersen-Bjergaard J, Larsen SO. Incidence of acute nonlymphocytic leukemia, preleukemia, and acute myeloproliferative syndrome up to 10 years after treatment of Hodgkin's disease. N Engl J Med 307:965–971, 1982.

167. Coltman CA, Dixon DO. Second malignancies complicating Hodgkin's disease: A Southwest Oncology Group 10-year follow-up. Cancer Treat Rep 66:1023–1033, 1982.

168. VanLeeuwen FE, Somers R, Taal BG, et al. Increased risk of lung cancer, non-Hodgkin's lymphoma and leukemia following Hodgkin's disease. J Clin Oncol 7:1046–1058, 1989.

169. Krikorian JG, Burke JS, Rosenberg SA, et al. Occurrence of non-Hodgkin's lymphoma after therapy for Hodgkin's disease. N Engl J Med 300:452–458, 1979.

CHAPTER 80

BREAST CANCER

SUZANNE M. FIELDS JONES and HOWARD A. BURRIS III

Approximately 182,000 new cases of breast cancer will be diagnosed in the United States during 1995, with an American woman having approximately an 11% chance of developing breast cancer during her lifetime (1). Women under the age of 30 are rarely diagnosed with breast cancer, but the incidence rate increases dramatically after the age of 30 and plateaus around the age of 50. Less than 1% (approximately 1400 cases) of the cases diagnosed annually occur in men, but the prognosis is generally poorer for male patients. Although public awareness and early detection of breast cancer have significantly increased over the past 40 years, the mortality rate from the disease has changed very little. An estimated 46,240 people will die with breast cancer in 1995. Breast cancer is the second most common cause of cancer death in women, surpassed only recently by lung cancer. A great deal of controversy exists regarding the appropriate clinical management of particular patient subsets, such as women with node-negative disease or postmenopausal women with node-positive disease, and the appropriate use of mammography as a screening tool. Resolution of these controversies will require the willingness of both physicians and patients to participate in randomized, controlled clinical trials and analysis of long-term outcomes of clinical trials.

ETIOLOGY

The etiology of breast cancer is unknown, but several predisposing risk factors for the disease have been determined. These factors can be divided into three major categories: genetic, endocrine, and environmental factors (Table 80.1).

Women who have a first-degree relative (e.g., mother and/or sister) with breast cancer have a twofold to threefold increased risk of developing breast cancer (2, 3). This risk may be increased further if more than one first-degree relative is diagnosed with the disease, the relative is a young age at the time of diagnosis, or the relative presents with bilaterial breast cancer (4). Women with endometrial, ovarian, or colon cancer may also have an increased risk of developing breast cancer because of the transmission of an autosomal dominant trait for the disease (2). Patients who have breast cancer as part of cancer family syndromes are frequently diagnosed at an earlier age, and the disease is often bilateral. Recent research has revealed a gene on the long arm of chromosome 17 known as BRCA1, which is responsible for an inherited predis-

position to breast and ovarian cancer (5). This discovery could be beneficial for screening, counseling, and treating the subset of patients with a genetic predisposition for the disease. Finally, women who have a personal history of breast cancer have a higher probability than the average woman of developing primary breast cancer in the contralateral breast (3).

Patients with benign breast disease have an increased risk of developing breast cancer if they have proliferative lesions with atypical hyperplasia (2, 3). Their risk is increased further if there is also a positive family history for breast cancer. Patients in these higher risk groups may warrant close monitoring for breast cancer development, but other patients with benign breast disease (e.g., fibrocystic or "lumpy breast") should be treated like the general population. Both endogenous and exogenous hormones have also been associated with an increased risk for breast cancer. The incidence of breast cancer appears to correlate with prolonged high levels of estrogen in the bloodstream, which would occur in women with long menstrual histories. As a result, women with early menarche (under 12 years of age) or late menopause (over 55 years of age) are at higher risk for the development of breast cancer (6, 7). Nulliparous women are also at a greater risk for breast cancer than parous women. However, the age at which a woman experiences her first full-term pregnancy also influences her risk of developing breast cancer. A first full-term pregnancy after the age of 35 increases the risk for breast cancer because of hormonal changes and latent breast tissue differentiation that occur during pregnancy, particularly the first pregnancy (3, 6). Theoretically, increasing the number of menstrual cycles with either oral contraceptive use or postmenopausal hormone-replacement therapy could be associated with an increased risk of breast cancer. However, the studies that have been published in this area to date still show some conflicting results. Most studies have been conducted retrospectively with numerous hormone preparations and have shown no relation between oral contraceptives and breast cancer. Furthermore, the protection from the morbidity and mortality of cardiovascular disease and osteoporosis experienced with postmenopausal estrogen replacement must be considered when weighing the risks and benefits of therapy.

In a metaanalysis of the case-control studies available in the literature through 1989, a positive trend in the risk

Table 80.1.
Risk Factors for Breast Cancer Development

Personal history of breast cancer
Family history of breast cancer in first-degree relatives
Proliferative benign breast disease
Early menarche, late menopause
Nulliparity
First pregnancy after age 35
Exogenous estrogens (postmenopausal, oral contraceptives)
Obesity (menopausal weight gain, fat distribution)
Dietary factors: alcohol, high-fat diet
Radiation
Endometrial, ovarian, or colon cancer

of breast cancer was noted among premenopausal women who used oral contraceptives for an extended period prior to their first term pregnancy (8). Several studies have also suggested an increased risk of breast cancer in women taking oral contraceptives during the perimenopausal period (6). Prolonged duration of postmenopausal hormone-replacement therapy has also been associated with an increased risk of breast cancer in studies conducted in both Europe and the United States (9). Additional large prospective studies will be required to determine the true association between exogenous estrogen administration and the risk of breast cancer. However, decreased exposure of breast cells to estrogens and progestogens could be obtained by using the combination of a gonadtropin-releasing hormone agonist and very low-dose hormone replacement for contraception (10). This type of contraception could possibly be beneficial in reducing the lifetime risk of breast cancer and should be explored further because of the large number of women using combination-type oral contraceptives.

Based on the incidence rates of breast cancer in various countries, it would appear that environmental factors contribute to the development of breast cancer in women. Western countries, such as the United States, have high breast cancer rates, whereas Eastern countries like Japan have a low incidence of the disease. Furthermore, when people migrate from Japan to the United States they acquire the higher incidence rates of their new environment (11). The difference in breast cancer rates is thought to be partially due to dietary differences between the two populations, specifically, the amount of fat that is consumed in the diet. Data obtained from several large studies have failed to show a direct correlation between high-fat diets and the risk of breast cancer, but a diet consisting of less than 30% fat is recommended (12, 13). Obesity has also been associated with increased estrogen levels, but has only been directly associated with an increased risk of breast cancer in postmenopausal women (2, 11). More recent research indicates that the weight gain and increases in central body fat that occur during menopause are associ-

ated with an increased risk of postmenopausal breast cancer, possibly due to the concomitant alterations in ovarian hormones, glucose metabolism, and breast cancer growth factors that occur (14). Women who are physically active during adolescence and young adulthood may also have a decreased risk of developing breast cancer possibly due to infrequent or irregular menstrual cycles and maintaining a lean body weight (15). Although several logical explanations support the protective effect of exercise in protecting against breast cancer development, no studies have conclusively demonstrated this relationship (16). The combination of all or several of these factors probably contributes to the development of breast cancer in many women.

Several prospective and case-control studies have consistently demonstrated a positive correlation between alcohol consumption and the risk of breast cancer. These studies are somewhat difficult to compare because the amount and type of alcohol consumed has varied with each study (17). However, a metaanalysis of 16 studies did uncover a dose–response relationship between alcohol consumption and breast cancer risk (18). The combined data indicates that women who consume two drinks per day have a 40 to 70% increased risk for breast cancer compared to women who did not drink at all.

Survivors of the atomic bomb blast during World War II have experienced an increased incidence of breast cancer because of radiation exposure (3, 19). Similar breast cancer incidence rates have also been reported in women treated with radiation for mastitis and women receiving multiple fluoroscopies for the treatment of tuberculosis. There is a 10- to 15-year latency period between radiation exposure and tumor development, and women over 40 years of age at the time of exposure appear to experience little or no increased risk for breast cancer. Some physicians have expressed concern about the use of repeated screening mammographies in women because of the link between radiation exposure and breast cancer. However, the amount of radiation a woman is exposed to during a mammogram is extremely low, and there have been no case reports to date of breast cancer development secondary to mammography screening.

BREAST ANATOMY AND TUMOR DEVELOPMENT

Human breast tissue is composed primarily of connective tissue and fat. There is also an elaborate duct system within the breasts that is used during lactation. Breast tissue has an abundant blood supply and an extensive lymphatic network. Lymphatic drainage of the mammary tissues flows into the axillary, interpectoral, and internal mammary lymph nodes. This is important because breast cancer commonly spreads via the lymphatic system, and metastatic disease is frequently discovered in the regional lymph nodes at the time of diagnosis (Fig. 80.1).

A woman's breast tissue and glands begin to develop around the time of puberty because of the influence and interaction of sex hormones. However, the amount of breast development occurring at puberty is limited, and the majority occurs during the first pregnancy. The large amounts of estrogen and progesterone produced by the ovaries during pregnancy stimulate rapid growth and terminal differentiation of immature breast tissue. A delay in the terminal differentiation of breast tissue until a later age may help explain why women who become pregnant for the first time after the age of 35 have an increased risk for breast cancer development since immature cells are more susceptible to cycling estrogen effects and estrogens are known to initiate tumor growth (20).

The development of breast cancer occurs when breast cells lose their normal differentiation and proliferation controls. The proliferation of these abnormal, or tumor cells, is influenced by various hormones, oncogenes, and growth factors (Fig. 80.2) (21, 22). There is now strong evidence to suggest that estrogen directly and indirectly stimulates the growth of tumor cells (23). Furthermore, there are numerous growth factors that also play a role in tumor development that are secreted by the breast cancer cells themselves. These factors can be classified as either autocrine (if they stimulate their own growth) or paracrine (if they have an effect on other cells). Examples of the autocrine growth factors include transforming growth factor-alpha (TGF-α) and insulinlike growth factors I and II (IGF-I and IGF-II). Transforming growth factor-beta (TGF-β), platelet-derived growth factor (PDGF), and pro-cathepsin D (52K protein) are all paracrine growth factors. The exact mechanism of tumor development is not completely understood presently, but tremendous progress has been made in this area in the past few years with the discovery of the autocrine and paracrine growth factors.

Furthermore, the mechanism of action of several of the hormonal agents used for the treatment of breast cancer involves the alteration of the growth factors involved in tumor development.

DETECTION AND DIAGNOSIS

Early detection of breast cancer is critical because patients with limited stage disease have a better prognosis. Three complementary screening techniques have been shown to be effective for breast cancer detection: breast self-examination (BSE), physical examination by a physician, and mammography.

A large majority of breast cancers are discovered by patients themselves during regular breast self-examinations. Breast self-examination is a simple procedure that should be performed by all women over the age of 20 on a monthly basis. In a prospective study involving more than 200 women diagnosed with breast cancer, Huguley and colleagues demonstrated that women who performed breast self-examinations had a better prognosis than women who did not do self-examinations (24). Women conducting self-examinations were generally diagnosed with earlier stage disease and had a higher 5-year survival rate than women not performing self-examinations (76.7 versus 60.9%). Currently, the American Cancer Society recommends that all women should perform monthly breast self-examinations, and numerous educational brochures and breast models are available to aid women in this procedure. However, in order for breast self-examination to be an effective screening tool, women must conduct thorough monthly examinations.

A physical examination conducted by a trained physician is also an important screening technique for breast cancer detection. The American Cancer Society recommends that women over the age of 40 have a yearly physical

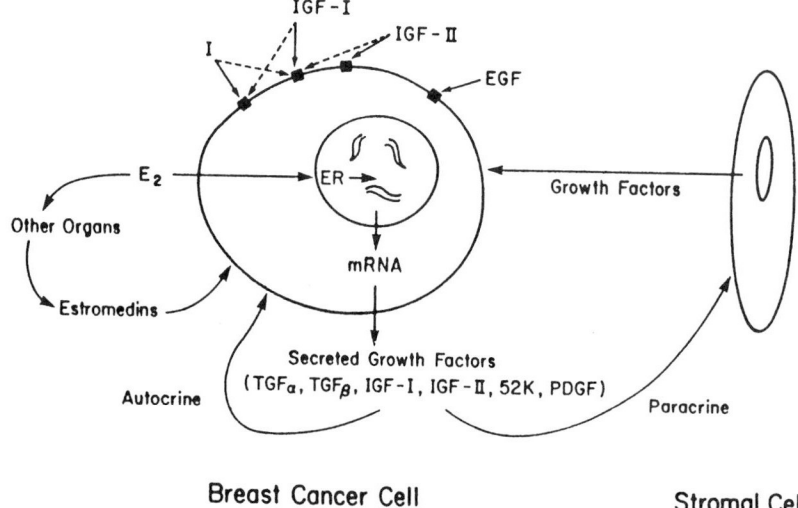

Figure 80.1. Breast tissue drainage and its relationship to tumor metastases. From Copeland EM III, Bland KI. The breast. In: Sabiston DC, Jr, ed. Essentials of Surgery. WB Saunders, Philadelphia, 1987, with permission.

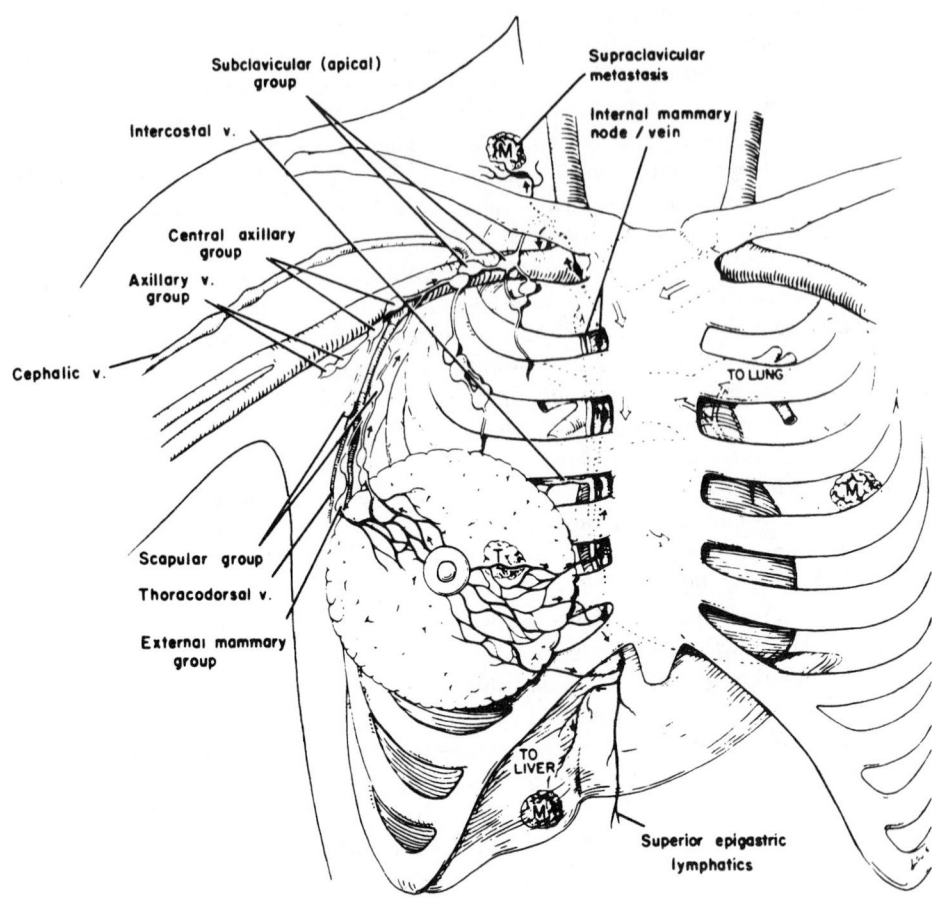

Subclavicular (apical)
group

Supraclavicular
metastasis

Intercostal v.

Internal mammary
node / vein

Central axillary
group

Axillary v.
group

Cephalic v.

TO LUNG

Scapular group

Thoracodorsal v.

External mammary
group

TO
LIVER

Superior epigastric
lymphatics

Figure 80.2. Proposed schema for breast cancer cell development. From Osborne CK, Arteaga CL. Autocrine and paracrine growth regulation of breast cancer: Clinical implications. Breast Cancer Res Treat. 15:3–11, 1990, with permission.

examination by their physician. Women between the ages of 20 and 40 should have a physical examination by their physician every 3 years. Although mammography is more sensitive for detecting small breast tumors than physical examination, approximately 10% of palpable masses are missed by mammography (25). Therefore, it is critical that both physical examinations and screening mammography be performed. When the two procedures are used together, it is estimated that greater than 90% of diagnosed breast cancers are detected (26).

The importance of physical examination and mammography as a screening tool to detect breast cancer has been confirmed with two large, randomized prospective clinical trials: The Health Insurance Plan of Greater New York (HIP) and the Breast Cancer Detection Demonstration Project (BCDDP). The HIP study randomized 31,000 women between the ages of 40 and 64 to receive an initial screening examination plus mammography with three annual follow-up screenings (27). The matched control group for the study consisted of 31,000 additional women who received only routine medical care. At the 5-year analysis, a 38% reduction in breast cancer mortality was noted in the patients receiving annual physical examinations and mammography compared with the control group.

Furthermore, the reduction in mortality has persisted throughout 18 years of follow-up and remains at 23% (28). The BCDDP enrolled 280,000 women between the ages of 35 and 72 at centers throughout the United States who were screened with physical examination and mammography (29). The women were also instructed about breast self-examination and were encouraged to perform monthly examinations. During the study period, 4443 breast cancers were diagnosed, and approximately one-third of these were less than 1 cm in size at the time of diagnosis. Furthermore, more than 80% of the cancers detected had no axillary nodal involvement at the time of detection. The BCDDP further supported the use of screening mammography since approximately 42% of the tumors were detected by mammography alone. When the data were initially analyzed at the 5-year follow-up point, there was some question about whether women younger than 50 benefited from screening mammograms. However, the final analysis conducted after 10 years of follow-up demonstrated that screening for breast cancer with mammography is effective in younger women as well as older women (30). This finding is not surprising given the natural course of breast cancer development and progression. As a result of this study, the American Cancer Society recommended that all women receive a baseline mammography between the ages of 35 and 40, followed by repeat mammograms every 1 to 2 years between the ages of 40 and 49, and annual mammograms after the age of 50.

A great deal of controversy regarding the benefit of mammography screening in women between the ages of 40 and 49 has surfaced in the recent oncology literature. The reason for this controversy is that the clinical trial data from the individual trials were subsequently analyzed in subsets determined by patient age although the original design of the trials did not allow for this stratification (31). When analyzed by subgroup, the studies lose their statistical power because sufficient numbers of women ages 40 to 49 were not enrolled in the trials. However, when all the randomized controlled trials are analyzed in a metaanalysis, a mortality reduction of 25 to 30% is achieved in women who begin mammography screening by the age of 40. As a result of this controversy, The National Cancer Institute amended its guidelines for breast cancer screening in women under the age of 40 by eliminating the recommendation for mammography and breast physical examination. On the other hand, the American Cancer Society and the American College of Radiology feel that the data still support the screening recommendations for this age group. The current American Cancer Society guidelines for breast cancer detection are listed in Table 80.2.

The benefits of early detection by mammography have only recently begun to be realized. Since 1980, the number of women over 40 years of age who have ever had a mammogram has increased by more than 200% (33). At the same time, the incidence of breast cancer detection has increased by approximately 32%, with the majority of the tumors being diagnosed at an early stage. It is hoped that this increase in early detection and treatment will subsequently result in a decrease in breast cancer mortality.

Approximately 90% of breast masses are detected by the patients themselves through either breast self-examination or accidental contact (2). Breast cancer masses tend to be painless, solitary, unilateral, hard, irregular, and nonmobile. Patients may also present with skin changes, nipple discharge, or axillary lymphadenopathy. On presentation, any woman with suspected benign or malignant breast disease should have a mammography. Furthermore, any breast mass that suggests malignancy by mammography or on physical examination should be biopsied by either fine needle aspiration, core needle biopsy, incisional biopsy, or excisional biopsy. Although needle aspirations and core biopsies do provide enough evidence for a histologic diagnosis of breast cancer, they do not delineate the size of the tumor or allow for estrogen receptor determination of the tumor (26).

STAGING

The TNM classification system is the most commonly accepted staging system for breast cancer. Tumor size (T) is described on a scale of 0 to 4 based on characteristics of the primary tumor. Extent of lymph node involvement (N) based on location and palpability and the presence or absence of distant metastases (M) are also included in the system. In the management of breast cancer, the ipsilateral axillary, internal mammary, and pectoral nodes are all considered regional spread of the disease. Involvement of any other lymph nodes, however, is considered distant metastases. Table 80.3 summarizes the TNM staging system used for breast cancer.

PROGNOSTIC FACTORS

The natural history of breast cancer varies greatly between patients. Some patients present with extremely aggressive disease that progresses rapidly, whereas others are diagnosed with disease that follows a more indolent course. Because of these variations, the ability to predict which

Table 80.2.
American Cancer Society Guidelines for Breast Cancer Detection

Age Group	Screening Recommendation
20–39	Monthly breast self-examination
	Breast physical examination every 3 years
	Baseline mammogram at age 35–39
40–49	Monthly breast self-examination
	Yearly breast physical examination
	Mammogram every 1–2 years
>50	Monthly breast self-examination
	Yearly breast physical examination and mammogram

Table 80.3.
TNM Staging System for Breast Cancer

Stage	Tumor Size (T)	Nodal Involvement (N)	Metastases (M)
0	T_{is}[a]	Negative axillary nodes	None
I	≤2 cm	Negative axillary nodes	None
II	>2 cm ≤ 5 cm	Positive axillary nodes	None
III	>5 cm or any size with skin or chest wall fixation	Positive axillary nodes	None
IV	Any size	Any involvement	Present

[a]T_{is} = Carcinoma in situ

Table 80.4.
Prognostic Factors in Breast Cancer

Tumor size
Extent of nodal involvement
Estrogen and progesterone receptor status
Patient age
Menopausal status
Histologic grade
Cell proliferation indices
Oncogene and growth factor receptor expression
Estrogen-regulated proteins

Table 80.5.
Ten-Year Survival (%) Related to Primary Tumor Size (cm) and Level of Axillary Involvement

Axillary Status	Size of Primary Lesion (cm)		
	<2	2–5	>5
Negative	82	65	44
Positive	68	51	37

Adapted from: Harris JR, Morrow M, Bonnadonna G. Cancer of the breast. In: DeVita VT, Hellman S, Rosenberg SA, eds. Cancer, Principles & Practice of Oncology, Fourth Edition. Philadelphia, PA: J.B Lippincott Company, 1993: 1275.

patients will experience a better disease prognosis is extremely important. Table 80.4 lists the prognostic factors that have been determined in breast cancer patients to date.

The most important prognostic factor at the time of diagnosis is the extent of axillary lymph node involvement. Numerous studies have confirmed the significance of nodal involvement for predicting disease recurrence and survival. The number of affected nodes is inversely related to disease recurrence (34). Only 25 to 30% of patients with negative lymph nodes will have disease recurrence at 10 years (35). This recurrence rate increases to 55 to 65% when one to three nodes are involved, and 80 to 90% in patients with four or more positive nodes. Tumor size at the time of diagnosis is also an important prognostic factor for breast cancer (35, 36). Although large tumors have a greater tendency to metastasize to axillary lymph nodes, tumor size is also an independent predictor for breast cancer recurrence (Table 80.5). A third important prognostic factor is estrogen and progesterone receptor status. Laboratory assays for the determination of estrogen receptor content in tumors were originally developed in an attempt to predict tumor response to hormonal therapy. However, in 1977, Knight and his colleagues recognized the prognostic importance of estrogen receptor (ER) status by demonstrating a higher rate of disease recurrence in patients with ER-negative tumors (35, 37). Furthermore, in patients with node-positive disease, the presence of

progesterone receptors in tumor tissue indicates an improved disease-free survival compared to patients without progesterone receptors.

The rate of tumor cell proliferation has also demonstrated prognostic significance in breast cancer recurrence. Rate of cell proliferation can be determined using either the tritiated thymidine labeling index (TLI) or DNA flow cytometry, which determines the percentage of tumor cells actively dividing in the S-phase of the cell cycle. Both techniques indicate that patients with rapidly proliferating tumors have a decreased disease-free survival compared to patients with slowly proliferating tumors (38, 39). Additionally, flow cytometry can detect the presence of abnormal DNA content, or aneuploidy, in breast cancer cells. Patients with aneuploid tumors also appear to have a decreased disease-free survival (39). Increased levels of the HER-2/neu oncogene, a protein that promotes tumor cell development, have also been correlated with decreased disease-free and overall survival in patients with node-positive disease (40). Another important prognostic factor is the level of cathepsin D in breast cancer cells. Cathepsin D is a protease that promotes tumor cell growth and possibly disease metastasis. In women with node-negative disease, high levels of cathepsin D have been associated with a decreased disease-free and overall survival (41). A final prognostic factor for breast cancer is the vascular growth factors, such as vascular endothelial growth factor, platelet-derived endothelial cell growth factor, and fibroblast growth factors (42, 43). Early laboratory studies suggest that tumor angiogenesis is an independent and highly significant prognostic factor for lymph node involvement and that it predicts survival.

Predicting disease recurrence in patients with breast cancer is a difficult task, especially in patients with negative nodal involvement at the time of diagnosis. The ability to determine prognostic factors for disease recurrence would be extremely useful clinically since patients with a poor prognosis could be treated more aggressively initially in an attempt to prolong survival.

TREATMENT OF BREAST CANCER
Early Stage Breast Cancer

Approximately 75 to 80% of women diagnosed with breast cancer will have Stage I or II disease at the time of diagnosis. In the past, the primary treatment for breast cancer was a radical mastectomy. The goal of this treatment was to remove the breast, underlying tissues, and regional lymph nodes. However, more recent data suggest that a modified radical mastectomy, which spares the pectoralis muscles and some high axillary lymph nodes, was as effective in the treatment of primary disease as a radical mastectomy (44). Furthermore, at the NIH Consensus Conference in June 1990, it was determined that breast conservation treatment is acceptable therapy for most women with Stage I or II disease based on survival rates obtained from several randomized clinical trials (45). Ten-year follow-up of these data has recently been reported, and breast conservation treatment yields results equivalent to mastectomy (77 and 75% 10-year overall survival, respectively) (46). Breast conservation treatment is defined as lumpectomy or partial mastectomy accompanied by axillary node dissection and followed by radiation therapy. Although the local recurrence rate in women receiving breast conservation treatment is low (10 to 30%), the use of adjuvant chemotherapy or hormonal therapy may help further reduce this recurrence rate. These data have also been confirmed in subsequent clinical trials (47).

Adjuvant therapy is chemotherapy or hormonal therapy that is administered in an attempt to treat the residual micrometastatic disease that remains following surgery. In May 1988, the National Cancer Institute issued a clinical alert to physicians concerning the use of adjuvant hormonal or cytotoxic chemotherapy in the treatment of women with node-negative breast cancer (Stage I) (48). This alert was issued because of the results of four randomized clinical trials using adjuvant therapy in node-negative breast cancer patients (49–52). Although the treatment regimens used in the four trials were different, all demonstrated a statistically significant increase in disease-free survival in patients with node-negative disease (Table 80.6). However, overall survival was not prolonged significantly in any of these studies. Because the differences in disease-free survival between treated and untreated patients was relatively small and the disease-free survival in patients receiving no adjuvant therapy is 70 to 90%, many physicians question whether all patients with node-negative disease should receive adjuvant therapy (53). Furthermore, the acute and delayed toxicities as well as the cost-effectiveness of the therapy must be considered. The direct cost of treating all patients with node-negative disease may considerably outweigh the benefits achieved in disease-free survival ($338,174,200 per year to achieve a disease-free survival advantage in approximately 5000 patients) (54). Furthermore, indirect costs in the form of drug toxicities and

decreased quality of life during therapy are difficult to quantitate, but they should be included when weighing the risks and benefits of adjuvant therapy. Acute toxicities, such as nausea, vomiting, mucositis, and myelosuppression, did result in patient death in a small percentage of patients in the randomized clinical trials. Long-term toxicities in the form of secondary malignancies (i.e., leukemia following alkylating agents and endometrial cancers following tamoxifen therapy), venous and arterial thrombosis, and congestive heart failure secondary to anthracycline administration were not addressed because of the relatively short follow-up period. These delayed toxicities, however, are increasingly important when the survival benefits associated with adjuvant therapy are minimal or nonexistent (55). Until the data from these four and other clinical trials mature, the recommended treatment for Stage I breast cancer will remain controversial. Because of the discrepancies in the data collected to date, physicians are encouraged to enroll their newly diagnosed patients in large, prospectively randomized clinical trials. Outside the clinical trial setting, the decision to treat node-negative breast cancer with chemotherapy or hormonal therapy must be made on an individual basis. The presence or absence of prognostic factors and the patient's desire to receive treatment should influence the physician's final judgment concerning adjuvant therapy. For example, a woman with a small primary tumor (less than 2 cm) that possesses estrogen receptors and is diploid with a low S-phase fraction may be encouraged not to receive adjuvant therapy but to undergo close medical observation. Continued research in the area of adjuvant therapy for node-negative breast cancer is clearly warranted.

The management of Stage II breast cancer (tumor less than 5 cm with positive nodal involvement) is more straightforward based on the results of more than 100 randomized trials using systemic adjuvant therapy. Although the results of the individual trials are often contradictory, a metaanalysis indicates that systemic adjuvant therapy can prolong disease-free and overall survival in Stage II breast cancer (56). This analysis involved 133

Table 80.6.
Clinical Trials and Adjuvant Therapy for Node-Negative Breast Cancer

Trial	No. Patients	Treatment Regimen	Disease-Free Survival Treated vs. Control		P Value
Ludwig V[36]	1275	CMF × 1 month[a]	77%	73%	0.04
Intergroup[34]	406	CMFP × 6 months[b]	84%	69%	0.0001
NSABP B13[35]	679	MF × 12 months[c]	80%	71%	0.003
NSABP B14[36]	2644	TAM × 5 years[d]	83%	77%	<0.00001

[a]Cyclophosphamide 400 mg/m² IV D 1 and 8; Methotrexate 40 mg/m² IV D 1 and 8; Fluorouracil 600 mg/m² D 1 and 8 (Leucovorin 15 mg IV/PO D 1 and 8 was also given to 69% of patients).
[b]Cyclophosphamide 100 mg/m² PO D 1–14; Methotrexate 40 mg/m² IV D 1 and 8; Fluorouracil 600 mg/m² IV D 1 and 8; Prednisone 40 mg/m² PO D 1–14.
[c]Methotrexate 100 mg/m² IV D 1 and 8; Fluorouracil 600 mg/m² IV D 1 and 8 (Leucovorin 10 mg/m² PO Q6H × 6 doses).
[d]Tamoxifen 10 mg PO BID.

randomized trials in which 75,000 women were enrolled. Several conclusions concerning various patient subsets can be drawn from the pooled data.

There were 44 trials in which systemic adjuvant chemotherapy (both single agent and combination regimens) were compared with no-adjuvant therapy (56). An overall reduction in the odds of recurrence as a result of treatment in patients receiving adjuvant chemotherapy was 21%, regardless of patient age and treatment regimen. When analyzed by patient age, the reduction in the annual odds of recurrence was significantly greater in women under the age of 50 (28%) compared with older patients (17%). A concomitant decrease in the odds of death with treatment was 11% for all patients (17% for patients less than 50 years of age, 9% for patients greater than or equal to 50 years of age). Furthermore, the use of combination chemotherapy regimens appeared to be more effective than single-agent regimens, and prolonged treatment with chemotherapy (more than 6 months) had no survival advantage over short-term therapy.

Although combination chemotherapy regimens have proved to be more effective than single-agent therapy, the optimal combination regimen has not been determined. Numerous drug combinations were used in the various clinical trials, but the combination of cyclophosphamide, methotrexate, and fluorouracil (CMF) has been studied most extensively. However, doxorubicin has demonstrated the most activity of all drugs as single-agent therapy in phase II clinical trials in breast cancer and has produced increased response rates when used in combination chemotherapy regimens (57, 58). To determine whether doxorubicin should be included in standard combination chemotherapy regimens used for breast cancer, a direct comparison between CMF and a similar regimen containing doxorubicin must be conducted. Furthermore, the effect of the addition of tamoxifen to standard combination chemotherapy regimens in the treatment of premenopausal women also remains to be determined.

The metaanalysis also contained 40 trials involving adjuvant therapy with oral tamoxifen (56). The primary benefit of adjuvant tamoxifen therapy was seen in postmenopausal patients over the age of 50 years. This patient population experienced a 20% decrease in mortality and a 29% decrease in the annual odds of recurrence with adjuvant tamoxifen therapy. Premenopausal patients also experienced a decrease in mortality although not as great as in the postmenopausal patients. However, the number of young women in the trial receiving single-agent tamoxifen therapy was small, so these results are difficult to interpret. The data also suggest that various doses of tamoxifen (20, 30, or 40 mg) are equally effective and that prolonged drug administration may be more effective (i.e., 2 to 5 years versus 1 year). Further trials must be conducted to determine the optimal use of tamoxifen as systemic adjuvant therapy for breast cancer. Other questions concerning the long-term benefits and side effects of tamoxifen therapy must also be addressed and may be answered in the large, multicenter tamoxifen chemoprevention trial that is currently underway in the United States.

Tamoxifen is a weak estrogen that has both estrogenic and antiestrogenic effects. The primary mechanism of action in breast cancer involves binding of the estrogen receptor followed by inhibition of tumor cell growth (59). However, enzyme inhibition and growth factor modulation may also play a role in the mechanism of action of tamoxifen (60). Because the antitumor activity of tamoxifen is cytostatic rather than cytotoxic, the potential use of tamoxifen as chemosuppressive therapy against the development of breast cancer is being evaluated. If the drug is to be used in this setting or as long-term adjuvant therapy in early stage disease, the benefits of therapy must outweigh the risks. Fortunately, the acute toxicities associated with tamoxifen therapy are minimal and include nausea, hot flashes, mild edema, and vaginitis. Tamoxifen also has several favorable long-term effects due to its estrogenic activity on tissues other than breast. For example, tamoxifen significantly decreased total cholesterol and low-density lipoprotein cholesterol levels in postmenopausal women receiving 2 years of adjuvant therapy for node-negative breast cancer (61). Plasma high-density lipoprotein levels were also increased, resulting in lipoprotein profiles that are favorable for the prevention of coronary heart disease and artherosclerosis. Laboratory data have also suggested that tamoxifen may retard bone resorption secondary to its estrogenic activity (59, 62). Although several small studies have supported this finding, large controlled trials evaluating the effect of tamoxifen on bone mineral density must be conducted (63).

Long-term tamoxifen administration may also be associated with minimal side effects. Because of its effects on coagulation factors, tamoxifen has been reported to cause thrombophlebitis in some patients (59, 62). The development of thrombophlebitis in women participating in clinical trials has been minimal to date. Retinal changes have also been reported with long-term tamoxifen therapy. Presently, the most concerning side effect reported with long-term tamoxifen therapy is the occurrence of endometrial cancer. Scattered reports have appeared in the literature over the years of the development of endometrial cancer following tamoxifen administration (64, 65). Furthermore, in a large randomized study conducted in Scandinavia, women receiving tamoxifen had a relative risk for the development of uterine cancer that was 6.4 times greater than the patients in the control group (66). More randomized, prospective clinical trials need to be conducted in order to determine the safety of long-term tamoxifen therapy. However, these trials will require large numbers of patients and extensive follow-up. As a result, these trials may not be feasible.

In summary, the management of Stage II breast cancer depends primarily on patient age and estrogen receptor status. All premenopausal women should be treated with 6 months of adjuvant systemic chemotherapy, regardless of their estrogen-receptor status. The most commonly used adjuvant regimen is CMF. The effectiveness of hormonal therapy combined with chemotherapy remains to be established in this patient population. In postmenopausal estrogen-receptor positive patients, adjuvant endocrine therapy in the form of oral tamoxifen is the treatment of choice. Current recommendations are to administer tamoxifen in a dose of 20 mg daily for a minimum of 2 years. Postmenopausal estrogen-receptor negative patients form the only patient subset in which treatment remains undetermined. Adjuvant systemic chemotherapy has proved beneficial in this patient subset, but it remains investigational at this time. The combination of adjuvant chemotherapy and endocrine therapy may also prove to be beneficial, but it is considered investigational. However, optimal therapy has not been determined for any patient subset, and all patients should be encouraged to participate in clinical trials.

Locally Advanced Disease

Patients diagnosed with locally advanced breast cancer (Stage III disease) have tumors larger than 5 cm or direct tumor involvement of the skin or underlying chest wall. These patients also have extensive lymph node involvement. Because of the bulk of disease at the time of diagnosis, surgical management is generally not feasible. Furthermore, standard treatment modalities are minimally effective resulting in very poor survival in these patients. In an attempt to improve the overall survival rates in women with locally advanced disease, researchers began to use combined modality therapy (67). Radiation therapy, systemic chemotherapy, and surgery have all been used in various regimens in randomized clinical trials. Neoadjuvant therapy involves the use of chemotherapy prior to surgery in order to decrease the size of the tumor and improve resectability (68). Other advantages of neoadjuvant chemotherapy include earlier treatment of micrometastatic disease, intact tumor vasculature resulting in improved drug delivery, the ability to determine tumor responsiveness to chemotherapy in vivo, and the ability to customize postsurgical systemic therapy based on this response. Following neoadjuvant chemotherapy, patients may receive radiation therapy, surgery alone, or a combination of the two modalities. However, the local control rates achieved in studies using the combination of surgery and radiation therapy following chemotherapy are greater than the control rates obtained with either modality alone (68).

When all three modalities are combined, more than 90% of patients with locally advanced breast cancer are disease free following treatment, and many will remain disease free for up to 3 to 5 years. Many questions remain to be answered about the use of combined modality therapy in patients with Stage III disease at diagnosis. Some of these questions include (1) Which combined treatment regimen is the most effective? (2) How many courses of neoadjuvant therapy should be administered prior to surgery? (3) Which drugs should be used for neoadjuvant therapy? and (4) Should patients also receive systemic adjuvant therapy (either chemotherapy or endocrine therapy) postoperatively? Randomized clinical trials designed to answer some of these questions are currently being conducted, and results remain to be determined.

Metastatic Breast Cancer

Radiation therapy, hormonal therapy, and chemotherapy have all been used in the treatment of metastatic breast cancer in order to palliate the patient and possibly prolong survival. Because "cure" is not the primary goal of therapy at this point, the easiest, least toxic treatment that can provide the best possible response is generally preferred. Breast cancer can metastasize to virtually any site, but the most common sites include bone, lung, pleura, liver, soft tissue, and the central nervous system. The choice of therapy for metastatic disease is based on the site of disease involvement and the presence or absence of certain patient characteristics (2, 69). For example, patients who experience a longer disease-free survival (≥2 years) have disease that is primarily located in bone or soft tissue, have responded to primary endocrine therapy, and are late premenopausal or postmenopausal will most likely respond to endocrine therapy. The most important factor predicting response to hormonal therapy, however, is the presence of estrogen and progesterone receptors on tumor tissues. Fifty to 60% of ER-positive patients and 75 to 85% of ER- and PR-positive patients have a chance of responding to hormonal therapy, whereas those with no hormone receptors have a 90% chance of failure with hormone therapy (2). Chemotherapeutic drugs are most commonly used as palliative therapy in patients who would not be expected to respond to hormonal therapy (i.e., patients with rapidly progressive lung, liver, or bone marrow disease) or patients who have failed to respond to initial treatment with endocrine therapy (69). Radiation therapy is primarily used to control symptomatic disease such as bone metastases, metastatic brain lesions, and spinal cord compressions. Both brain and spinal cord metastases seldom respond to chemotherapy and hormonal manipulations, but they do respond somewhat to irradiation.

The most common endocrine therapies used in the management of metastatic breast cancer are listed in Table 80.7. Basically, the response rates to all types of endocrine

Table 80.7.
Endocrine Therapies used for Metastatic Breast Cancer

Class	Drug	Dose	Side Effects
Antiestrogen	Tamoxifen	10–20 mg PO BID	Disease flare, hot flashes, nausea, vomiting, edema
LHRH analogues	Leuprolide	7.5 mg SQ Q28d	Amenorrhea, hot flashes, occasional nausea
	Goserelin	3.6 mg SQ Q28d	
Progestins	Medroxyprogesterone acetate	400–1000 mg IM QWK	Weight gain, hot flashes, vaginal bleeding
	Megestrol acetate	400 mg PO QID	
Aromatase inhibitors	Aminoglutethimide	250 mg PO BID × 2 weeks then QID with Hydro-cortisone 40 mg/d	Lethargy, skin rash, postural dizziness, ataxia nystagmus
Estrogens	Diethylstilbestrol	5 mg PO TID	Nausea or vomiting, fluid retention, hot flashes, anorexia, thromboembolism, hepatic dysfunction
	Ethinylestradiol	1 mg PO TID	
	Conjugated estrogens	2.5 mg PO TID	
Androgens	Fluoxymesterone	10 mg PO BID	Deepening voice, alopeica, hirsutism, facial or truncal acne, fluid retention, menstrual irregularities, cholestatic jaundice

therapy are equivalent, so it would be prudent to begin therapy with the least toxic agent. If a patient fails to respond to initial hormonal therapy or progresses during therapy following an initial response, an alternative hormonal manipulation should be attempted since multiple responses may occur. The median duration of response to the first attempt at hormonal manipulation is usually in the range of 9 to 12 months, and the duration of any subsequent responses is generally shorter (70). Figure 80.3 contains the schema for the hormonal management of both premenopausal and postmenopausal women with metastatic breast cancer.

Ovarian ablation (oophorectomy) via surgery or radiation has been used primarily in the treatment of premenopausal women with metastatic breast cancer, and it produced response rates of 30 to 45% (71, 72). Surgery that has a mortality rate of less than 5% is generally preferred over radiation because of the possible latent side effects of radiation therapy. Although oophorectomy was used as first-line therapy for metastatic disease in premenopausal women in the past, the development of pharmacologic agents that block estrogen binding or produce medical castration has resulted in drug therapy as first-line treatment. Administration or oral tamoxifen therapy or lutenizing hormone-releasing hormone (LHRH) analogues suppresses ovarian estrogen production in premenopausal women (73). However, tamoxifen does not completely antagonize estrogen production, and menses will continue to occur. Furthermore, women who fail initial tamoxifen therapy may respond to an oophorectomy, indicating that ovarian ablation with tamoxifen may not be complete (2, 73). Following an initial stimulation of ovarian hormone production, the LHRH analogues down regulate the lutenizing hormone-releasing factor (LHRH) receptors, resulting in ablation of ovarian hormone production that is reversible on drug discontinuation. Unfortunately, the rate

at which sex hormones decline following LHRH administration is much slower than the rate of decline following surgery (1 month versus 2 to 7 days) (74). Several studies have been conducted that support the use of LHRH analogues in premenopausal women with metastatic breast cancer. The largest study, conducted by Kaufmann and colleagues, used depot goserelin administered subcutaneously every 28 days. An overall response rate of 45% was obtained, with estrogen receptor positive patients responding more frequently (75). Currently, the LHRH analogues commercially available include leuprolide (Lupron®) and goserelin (Zoladex®). Both of these agents are administered subcutaneously as depot injections every 4 weeks and are associated with minimal side effects, including amenorrhea, hot flushes, and occasional nausea. Further studies using oophorectomy, tamoxifen, or LHRH analogues as first-line therapy in premenopausal patients with metastatic breast cancer are necessary to determine the definitive choice for initial therapy. Combination endocrine therapy with tamoxifen plus an LHRH analogue is also under investigation (74). The rationale behind this combination is that tamoxifen interferes with peripheral estradiol production, whereas the LHRH analogue interferes with ovarian estradiol production. In postmenopausal women, tamoxifen therapy appears to be the first-line treatment of choice due to ease of administration and lack of serious side effects. Comparative trials between tamoxifen and other forms of endocrine therapy (i.e., estrogen, progestins, aromatase inhibitors, and androgens) have not demonstrated superiority of tamoxifen based on clinical response, but the toxicity profiles do support the use of tamoxifen initially over other therapies. Approximately 35 to 50% of patients who respond initially to tamoxifen therapy will experience a response to second-line hormonal therapy (73). Progestins, aromatase inhibitors, androgens, and pure antiestrogens are all second-line hormonal choices (76–81). The choice of second- and third-line endocrine therapy is currently based on toxicity, cost, and ease of administration rather than response due to the comparable response rates between agents. The recommended doses, routes of administration, and side effects reported with the endocrine therapies used for metastatic breast cancer are listed in Table 80.7.

Manipulation of hormone levels via oophorectomy, adrenalectomy, and hypophysectomy have fallen somewhat out of favor as therapy for metastatic breast cancer because of the morbidity and mortality associated with the procedures. Furthermore, the ability to manipulate hormones pharmacologically with decreased costs and toxicities has resulted in increased usage of endocrine therapy for the treatment of metastatic disease. Because the various endocrine therapies produce similar response rates, the choice of therapy should be based on convenience, toxicity, and cost. First-line hormonal therapy should be administered for at least 6 to 8 weeks before disease response is assessed. Following initiation of therapy, some patients may experience a flare (or worsening) of their disease that may or may not be accompanied by hypercalcemia. Therapy may need to be withheld or decreased during this initial period, but treatment can usually continue. Furthermore, 5 to 10% of patients may actually experience regression of their tumor when therapy is withdrawn (70). Clinical trials using combination endocrine therapy or the

combination of hormonal therapy and cytotoxic chemotherapy are required before their usefulness in the management of metastatic disease can be determined.

Patients with rapidly progressive disease or who do not fulfill the criteria for treatment with endocrine therapy should receive chemotherapy initially. Patients who fail to respond to endocrine therapy should also be treated with chemotherapy. The chemotherapeutic agents that have demonstrated activity in the treatment of breast cancer include doxorubicin, cyclophosphamide, 5-fluorouracil, methotrexate, mitoxantrone, vinblastine, mitomycin C, thiotepa, melphalan, and paclitaxel. The objective response rates reported with these drugs as single-agent therapy range from 20 to 50% (69, 82–84). However, higher response rates (50 to 80%) have been obtained with combination chemotherapy regimens versus single-agent therapy in the treatment of metastatic breast cancer. The chemotherapy regimens most frequently used and the common toxicities associated with the drugs in these regimens are listed in Tables 80.8 and 80.9. The choice of an initial combination chemotherapy regimen may be a difficult one. Although regimens containing doxorubicin produce slightly higher response rates than regimens without, doxorubicin-containing regimens may not be the treatment of choice. The reason for this is that patients with disease refractory to doxorubicin therapy are extremely difficult to treat. If women receive the combination of

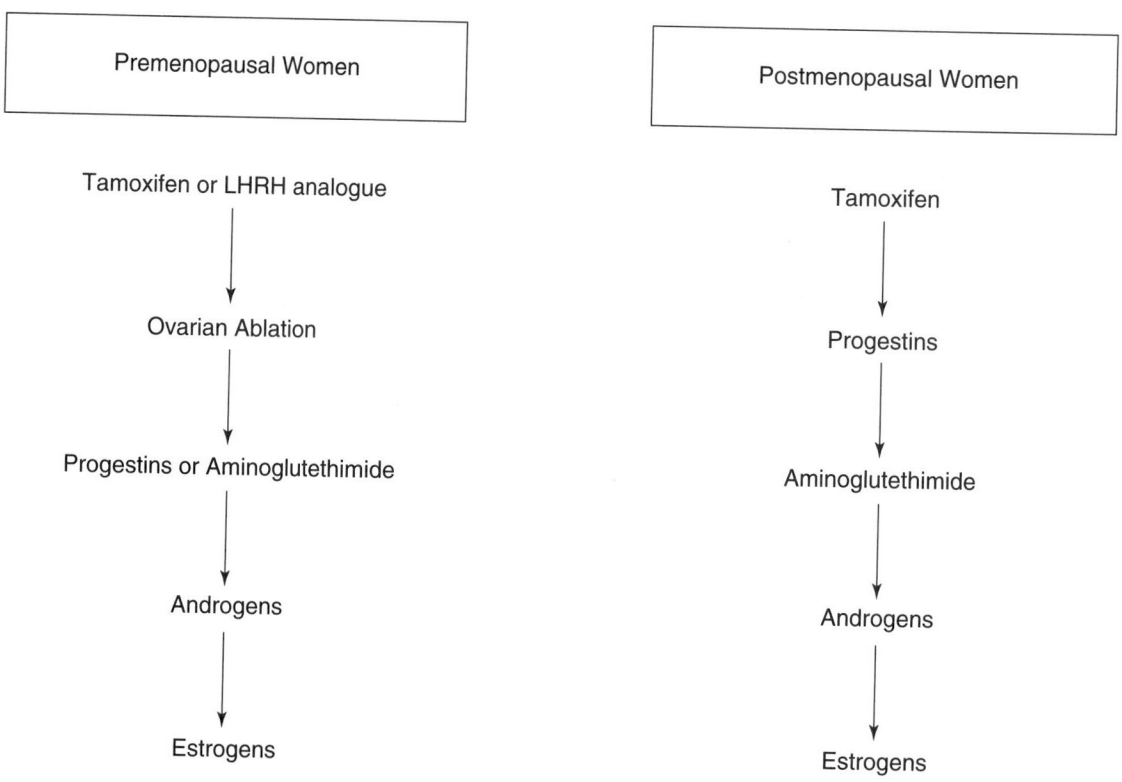

Figure 80.3. Hormonal management of metastatic breast cancer.

Table 80.8.
Combination Chemotherapy Regimens Used in the Treatment of Breast Cancer

Regimen	Drug	Dose
CMFVP "Cooper Regimen"	Cyclophosphamide	2 mg/kg/d PO
	Methotrexate	0.7 mg/kg/wk IV × 8 wk
	5-Fluorouracil	12 mg/kg/wk IV × 8 wk then qo wk
	Vincristine	35 mcg/kg/wk IV × 4–5 wk
	Prednisone	0.75 mg/kg/d reduced by 50% q10d to 5 mg/d × 3 wk
CMF ± P	Cyclophosphamide	100 mg/m²/d PO days 1–14
	Methotrexate	40 mg/m² IV days 1 and 8
	5-Fluorouracil	600 mg/m² IV days 1 and 8
	Prednisone	40 mg/m² PO days 1–14
CMF[a]	Cyclophosphamide	600 mg/m² days 1 and 8
	Methotrexate	40–50 mg/m² days 1 and 8
	5-Fluorouracil	600 mg/m² days 1 and 8
CAF[b]	Cyclophosphamide	400–500 mg/m² IV day 1
	Doxorubicin	40–50 mg/m² IV day 1
	5-Flourouracil	400–500 mg/m² IV days 1 and 8
CA	Cyclophosphamide	200 mg/m² PO days 3–6
	Doxorubicin	40 mg/m² IV day 1

[a] If dosed every 21 days, omit day 8 doses.
[b] Mitoxantrone 10 mg/m² IV day 1 may be substituted for doxorubicin in this regimen.

Table 80.9.
Toxicities of Commonly Used Antineoplastic Agents

Drug	Toxicity
Cyclophosphamide	Myelosuppression, nausea or vomiting, alopecia, hemorrhagic cystitis, stomatitis
Methotrexate	Myelosuppression, mucositis, diarrhea, nausea or vomiting, hepatic dysfunction, nephrotoxicity
5-Fluorouracil	Myelosuppression, mucositis, alopecia, nausea or vomiting, skin hyperpigmentation, chest pain, cerebellar ataxia
Vincristine	Neurotoxicity, constipation, alopecia
Doxorubicin	Myelosuppression, nausea or vomiting, alopecia, stomatitis, radiation recall, skin necrosis following extravasation cardiotoxicity (occurs more frequently with cumulative doses ≥ 550 mg/m²)
Mitoxantrone	Myelosuppression, nausea or vomiting, alopecia, mucositis, urine discoloration

cyclophosphamide, methotrexate, and fluorouracil (CMF) as adjuvant therapy or as first-line therapy for metastatic disease, they may respond to a doxorubicin-containing regimen on disease progression. The development of chemotherapeutic agents that are noncross-resistant with doxorubicin would be beneficial in this treatment setting. Because palliation is the goal of systemic chemotherapy for metastatic disease and quality of life is important, the toxicities and ease of administration of the various regimens should be considered when choosing a treatment regimen. For example, although mitoxantrone is slightly less active than doxorubicin in the management of breast cancer, its use should be considered for patients in whom drug toxicity is a problem because of the decreased toxicity profile of mitoxantrone (85). Single-agent paclitaxel at maximal doses is an attractive treatment alternative for patients who have failed prior therapy with doxorubicin since a response rate of almost 30% has been obtained with the drug in this difficult patient population. However, paclitaxel therapy is associated with a significant number of toxicities to include neutropenia, mucositis, neurotoxicity, hypersensitivity reactions, and alopecia. Single-agent mitomycin has also been used effectively in this treatment setting (86). Although not approved in the United States for the treatment of breast cancer, vinorelbine has also demonstrated significant activity in the treatment of women with metastatic disease, including women who have previously failed paclitaxel treatment (87).

Other issues that remain to be determined in the management of metastatic disease with systemic chemotherapy include the optimal duration of treatment and the standard combination regimen of choice. The use of combination chemotherapy and hormonal therapy is also being investigated for the treatment of metastatic disease.

FUTURE DIRECTIONS

Although progress has been made in the treatment of breast cancer, further improvements in therapy are essential. Current avenues of research include new methods of administration for commercially available drugs and the development of new drugs. Continuous infusion therapy and the use of liposome-encapsulated doxorubicin are two ways in which researchers are attempting to decrease the toxicities and increase the efficacy of doxorubicin administration (88, 89). The search for synergistic drug combinations using conventional agents in an attempt to increase response rates and overall survival is also being conducted. Furthermore, new therapeutic agents such as losoxantrone (an anthrapyrazole), vinorelbine (a vinca alkaloid), docetaxel (a taxane), toremifine (a hormonal agent), and vorozole (an aromatase inhibitor) are currently being used in clinical trials and have demonstrated significant activity in the treatment of breast cancer (90–92). The epidermal growth factor (EGF) receptor has an established role as an oncogene in the development and progression of breast cancer. The development of monoclonal antibodies directed against the EGF receptor is also being investigated as therapy for breast cancer (43, 93). Several novel agents that inhibit angiogenesis are also entering clinical trials to determine their activity in the treatment of breast cancer since angiogenesis plays such an important role in tumor progression (42, 43).

For many antineoplastic agents, there is a linear relationship between dose and tumor response, but the toxic effects of the drug on the marrow limit the dose that can be administered. High-dose chemotherapy intensification with or without autologous bone marrow support or peripheral blood stem cell transplantation is being investigated for the treatment of relapsed breast cancer (94, 95). In the original studies, investigators were able to administer 5 to 30 times conventional drug doses, which resulted in high response rates that were maintained for a short duration. As a result, patients are now usually treated with intensive induction chemotherapy for their disease prior to intensification therapy with autologous bone marrow support. Various treatment regimens have been used as induction therapy, and patients who exhibit stable or responsive disease will undergo a transplant as intensification therapy. Presently, 15 to 30% of transplanted women will remain disease free beyond 24 months. In an attempt to overcome drug resistance with the possibility of less toxicity, some investigators are also using double high-dose therapy (tandem transplants) with noncross-resistant preparative regimens. The use of collected peripheral blood progenitor cells to sustain hematologic parameters during tandem transplants is currently being investigated and appears to allow for the administration of dose-intensive therapy in a timely manner (96, 97). Peripheral blood progenitor cell support may also allow the administration of multiple dose-intensive cycles of therapy in the nontransplant setting. The availability of the recombinant human colony stimulating factors (i.e., granulocyte colony stimulating factor [GCSF] and granulocyte-macrophage colony stimulating factor [GM-CSF]) may help reduce the morbidity and mortality associated with both high-dose chemotherapy alone and high-dose chemotherapy with autologous bone marrow transplantation or peripheral blood progenitor cell support (98). Large cooperative group prospective randomized studies are currently underway to establish the precise role of bone marrow transplantation in the treatment of breast cancer.

CONCLUSION

The incidence of breast cancer continues to rise by approximately 1% every year. Public awareness and early detection of breast cancer have increased significantly over the past 40 years. Furthermore, the recent determination of important prognostic factors for breast cancer recurrence is helpful clinically in the determination of disease management. Appropriate clinical management of particular patient subsets has been established with the help of numerous clinical trials, but the standard treatment of some patient subsets remains to be determined. This will require willingness of both physicians and patients to participate in randomized, controlled clinical trials. Additionally, the development of new antineoplastic agents with activity in breast cancer and continued research in the areas of angiogenesis, gene therapy, and dose intensification will ideally help decrease the mortality rate of breast cancer.

REFERENCES

1. Cancer Facts & Figures—1995. American Cancer Society, Atlanta, Georgia.
2. Hutchins L, Broadwater Jr. R., Lang N, Maners A, Bowie M, Westbrook KC. Breast Cancer. DM 35:63–125, 1990.
3. Henderson IC, Harris JR, Kinne DW, Hellman S. Cancer of the Breast. In DeVita Jr VT, Hellman S, Rosenberg SA (eds): Cancer Principles and Practice of Oncology. Philadelphia, J.B. Lippincott, 1989, pp. 1197–1268.
4. Anderson DE. A genetic study of human breast cancer. J Natl Cancer Inst 48:1029–1034, 1972.
5. Lemoine NR. Molecular biology of breast cancer. Ann Oncol 5 (Suppl 4):31–37, 1994.
6. Henderson DE. Endogenous and exogenous endocrine factors. Hematol/Oncol Clin N Amer 3:577–598, 1989.
7. Jawed Iqbal M, Taylor W. Hormonal and reproductive factors—new evidence. In Stoll BA (ed): Women at high risk to breast cancer. Dordvecht, Kluwer Academic Publishers, 1989, pp. 41–46.
8. Romieu I, Berlin JA, Colditz G. Oral Contraceptives and breast cancer. Review and meta-analysis. Cancer 66:2253–2263, 1990.
9. Hulka BS. Hormone-replacement therapy and the risk of breast cancer. CA 40:289–296, 1990.
10. Spicer DV, Pike MC. Sex steroids and breast cancer prevention. Monogr Natl Cancer Inst 16:139–147, 1994.
11. London S, Willett W. Diet and the risk of breast cancer. Hematol/Oncol Clin N Amer 3:559–576, 1989.
12. Byers T. Nutritional risk factors for breast cancer. Cancer 74 (Suppl 1):288–295, 1994.
13. Willett WC, Hunter DJ. Prospective studies of diet and breast cancer. Cancer 74 (Suppl 3):1085–1089, 1994.
14. Ballard-Barbash R. Anthropometry and breast cancer. Body size—a moving target. Cancer 74 (Suppl 3):1090–1100, 1994.
15. Frisch RE, Wyshak G, Albright NL, et al. Lower prevalence of breast cancer and other cancers of the reproductive system among former college athletes compared to nonathletes. Br J Med 1985; 52:885–891.
16. Hoffman-Goetz L, Husted J. Exercise and breast cancer: review and critical analysis of the literature. Can J Appl Physiol 19:237–252, 1994.
17. Scgatzkin A, Longnecker MP. Alcohol and breast cancer. Where are we now and where do we go from here? Cancer 74 (Suppl 3):1101–1110, 1994.
18. Longnecker MP, Berlin JA, Orza MJ, et al. A meta-analysis of alcohol consumption in relation to risk of breast cancer. JAMA 260:652–656, 1988.
19. Kelsey JL, Berkowitz GS. Breast cancer epidemiology. Cancer Res 48: 5615–5623, 1988.
20. Pike MC, Krailo MD, Henderson DE, et al. Hormonal risk factors, breast tissue age and age-incidence of breast cancer. Nature 303:676–770, 1983.
21. Dawkins HJ, Robbins PD, Smith KL, Sarna M, Harvey JM, Sterrett GF. What's new in breast cancer? Molecular perspectives of cancer development and the role of the oncogene c-erbB-2 in prognosis and disease. Pathol Res Pract 189:1233–1252, 1993.
22. Morrison BW. The genetics of breast cancer. Hematol Oncol Clin North Am 8:15–27, 1994.
23. Osborne CK, Arteaga CL. Autocrine and paracrine growth regulation of breast cancer: clinical implications. Breast Cancer Res and Treat 15:3–11, 1990.
24. Huguley CM, Brown RL, Greenberg RS, Clark WS. Breast self-examination and survival from breast cancer. Cancer 62:1389–1396, 1988.
25. Kopans DB. Breast Cancer detection, diagnosis, and radiation therapy. In Rich MA, Hager JC, Keydar I (eds): Breast cancer:

progress in biology, clinical management, and prevention. Boston, Kluwer Academic Publishers, 1989, pp. 71–84.

26. Stockdale FE. Breast Cancer. In Rubenstein E, Federman DD (eds): Scientific American Medicine. New York, Scientific American Inc., 1990, pp. 1–16.

27. Shapiro S, Strax P, Venet L. Periodic breast cancer screening in reducing mortality from breast cancer. JAMA 215:1777–1785, 1971.

28. Shapiro S, Venet W, Strax P, et al. Current results of the breast cancer screening randomized trial: The Health Insurance Plan of Greater New York study. In Day NE, Miller AB (eds): Screening for Breast Cancer. Toronto, Hans Huber Publishers, 1988, pp. 3–15.

29. Baker LH. Breast Cancer Detection Demonstration Project: Five-Year summary report. CA 32:194–225, 1982.

30. Seidman H, Gelb SK, Silverberg E, LaVerda N, Lubera JA. Survival experience in The Breast Cancer Detection Demonstration Project. CA 37:258–290, 1987.

31. Kopans DB. Breast cancer screening: women 40–49 years of age. Principles and Practice of Oncology Updates 8:1–11, 1994.

32. Fletcher SW, Black W, Harris R, et al. Report of the International Workshop on Screening for Breast Cancer. J Natl Cancer Inst 85:1644, 1993.

33. Newcomb PA, Lantz PM. Recent trends in breast cancer incidence, mortality, and mammography. Breast Cancer Res Treat 28:97–106, 1993.

34. McGuire WL, Clark GM. Prognosis in breast cancer. Recent Results in Cancer Research 115:170–174, 1989.

35. Osborne CK. Prognostic factors in breast cancer. Principles and Practice of Oncology Updates 4:1–11, 1990.

36. Merkel DE, Osborne CK. Prognostic factors in breast cancer. Hematol Oncol Clin N Amer 3:641–652, 1989.

37. Clark GM, McGuire WL. Steroid receptors and other prognostic factors in primary breast cancer. Semin Oncol 15(Suppl 1):20–25, 1988.

38. Silvestrini R, Daidone MG, Valagussa P, et al. ^{3}H-Thymidine labeling index as a prognositic indicator in node-positive breast cancer. J Clin Oncol 8:1321–1326, 1990.

39. Clark GM, Dressler LG, Owens MA. Prediction of relapse or survival in patients with node-negative breast cancer by DNA flow cytometry. N Engl J Med 320:627–633, 1989.

40. Tandon AK, Clark GM, Chamness GC, Ullrich A, McGuire WL. HER-2/neu oncogene protein and prognosis in breast cancer. J Clin Oncol 7:1120–1128, 1989.

41. Tandon AK, Clark GM, Chamness GC, Chirgwin JM, McGuire WL. Cathepsin D and prognosis in beast cancer. N Engl J Med 322:297–302, 1990.

42. Harris AL, Fox S, Bicknell R, Leek R, Relf M, LeJeune S, et al. Gene therapy through signal transduction pathways and angiogenic growth factors as therapeutic targets in breast cancer. Cancer 74 (Suppl 3):1021–1025, 1994.

43. Gasparini G, Harris AL. Clinical importance of the determination of tumor angiogenesis in breast carcinoma: much more than a new prognostic tool. J Clin Oncol 13:765–782, 1995.

44. Crile G, Jr. Results of conservative treatment of breast cancer at ten and 15 years. Ann Surg 181:26–30, 1975.

45. Treatment of early-stage breast cancer. NIH Consens Dev Conf Consens Statement 1990 June 18–31; 8(6).

46. Jacobson JA, Danforth DN, Cowan KH, et al. Ten-year results of a comparison of conservation with mastectomy in the treatment of stage I and II breast cancer. N Engl J Med 332:907–911, 1995.

47. Anonymous. Report of the Council on Scientific Affairs. Management of patients with node-negative breast cancer. Arch Intern Med 153:58–67, 1993.

48. Clinical Alert from the National Cancer Institute. Br Cancer Research and Treatment 12:3–5, 1988.

49. Mansour EG, Gray R, Shatila AH, et al. Efficacy of adjuvant chemotherapy in high-risk node-negative breast cancer. An intergroup study. N Engl J Med 320:485–490, 1989.

50. Fisher B, Redmond C, Dimitrov NV, et al. A randomized clinical trial evaluating sequential methotrexate and fluovouracil in the treatment of patients with node-negative breast cancer who have estrogen-receptor-negative tumors. N Engl J Med 320:473–478, 1989.

51. Fisher B, Costantino J, Redmond C, et al. A randomized clinical trial evaluating tamoxifen in the treatment of patients with node-negative breast cancer who have estrogen-receptor-positive tumors. E Engl J Med 320:479–484, 1989.

52. Ludwig Breast Cancer Study Group. Prolonged disease-free survival after one course of perioperative adjuvant chemotherapy for node-negative breast cancer. N Engl J Med 320:491–496, 1989.

53. Hayes DF, Henderson IC. Adjuvant therapy for node-negative breast cancer patients. Advances in Oncology 6:8–18, 1990.

54. McGuire WL. Adjuvant treatment of node-negative breast cancer. (editorial) N Engl J Med 320:525–527, 1989.

55. Henderson IC, Hayes DF, Parker LM, et al. Adjuvant systemic therapy for patients with node-negative tumors. Cancer 65:2132–2147, 1990.

56. Anonymous. Systemic treatment of early breast cancer by hormonal, cytotoxic, or immune therapy. 133 randomized trials involving 31,000 recurrences and 24,000 deaths among 75,000 women. Early Breast Cancer Trialists' Collaborative Group. Lancet 339:1–15,71–85, 1992 (2 parts).

57. Namer M. Anthracyclines in the adjuvant treatment of breast cancer. Drugs 45 (Suppl 2) 4–9, 1993.

58. Hortobagyi GN, Buzdar AU. Present status of anthracyclines in the adjuvant treatment of breast cancer. Drugs 45 (Suppl 2):10–19, 1993.

59. Love RR. Tamoxifen therapy in primary breast cancer: biology, efficacy, and side effects. J Clin Oncol 7:803–815, 1989.

60. Love RR, Newcomb PA, Wiebe DA, et al. Effects of tamoxifen therapy on lipid and lipoprotein levels in post-menopausal patients with node-negative breast cancer. J Natl Cancer Inst 82:1327–1332, 1990.

61. Colleta AA, Benson JR, Baum M. Alternative mechanisms of action of anti-oestrogens. Breast Cancer Res Treat 31:5–9, 1994.

62. Love RR. Prospects for antiestrogen chemoprevention of breast cancer. J Natl Cancer Inst 82:18–21, 1990.

63. Fornander T, Rutgrist LE, Siöberg HE, Blomqvist L, Mattsson A, Glas U. Long-term adjuvant tamoxifen in early breast cancer: Effect on bone mineral density in post-menopausal women. J Clin Oncol 8:1019–1034, 1990.

64. Seoud MA, Johnson J, Weed JC Jr. Gynecologic tumors in tamoxifen-treated women with breast cancer. Obstet Gynecol 82:165–169, 1993.

65. Wolf DM, Jordan VC. Gynecological complications associated with long-term adjuvant tamoxifen therapy for breast cancer. Gynecol Oncol 45:118–128, 1992.

66. Fornander T, Cedermark B, Mattsson A, et al. Adjuvant tamoxifen in early breast cancer: occurrence of new primary cancers. Lancet 1:117–120, 1989.

67. Hortobagyi GN. Multidisciplinary management of advanced primary and metastatic breast cancer. Cancer 74 (Suppl 1):416–423, 1994.

68. Hortobagyi GN. Comprehensive management of locally advanced breast cancer. Cancer 66:1387–1391, 1990.

69. Wong K, Henderson IC. Management of metastatic breast cancer. World J Surg 18:98–111, 1994.

70. Buzdar AU. Current status of endocrine treatment of carcinoma of the breast. Semin Surg Oncol 6:77–82, 1990.

71. Schacter LP, Rozencweig M, Canetta R, Kelley S, Nicaise C, Smaldone L. Overview of hormonal therapy in advanced breast cancer. Semin Oncol 17(Suppl 9):38–46, 1990.

72. Davidson NE. Ovarian ablation as treatment for young women with breast cancer. Monogr Natl Cancer Inst 16:95–99, 1994.

73. Santen RJ, Manni I, Harvey H, Redmond C. Endocrine treatment of breast cancer in women. Endocrine Reviews 11:221–265, 1990.

74. Nicholson RI, Walker KJ, Walker RF et al. Review of the endocrine actions of lutenising hormone-releasing hormone analogues in pre-menopausal women with breast cancer. Horm Res 32(Suppl 1);198–201, 1989.

75. Kaufmann M, Jonat W, Kleeberg U, et al. Goserelin, a depot gonadotrophin-releasing hormone agonist in the treatment of pre-menopausal patients with metastatic breast cancer. J Clin Oncol 7:1113–1119, 1989.

76. Lundgren S. Progestins in breast cancer treatment. A review. Acta Oncol 31:709–722, 1992.

77. Wakeling AE. The future of new pure antiestrogens in clinical breast cancer. Breast Cancer Res Treat 25:1–9, 1993.

78. Pasqualini JR. Role of androgens in breast cancer. J Steroid Biochem Mol Biol 45:167–172, 1993.

79. Muso HB, Cruz JM. High-dose progestin therapy for metastatic breast cancer. Ann Oncol 3 (Suppl 3) 15–20, 1992.

80. Brodie AM, Santen RJ. Aromatase and its inhibitors in breast cancer treatment-overview and prospective. Breast Cancer Res Treat 30:1–6, 1994.

81. Goss PE, Gwyn KM. Current perspectives on aromatase inhibitors in breast cancer. J Clin Oncol 12:2460–2470, 1994.

82. Garber JE, Henderson IC. The use of chemotherapy in metastatic breast cancer. Hematol/Oncol Clin N Amer 3:807–821, 1989.

83. Norton L. Salvage chemotherapy of breast cancer. Semin Oncol 21 (4 Suppl 7):19–24, 1994.

84. Arbuck SG, Dorr A, Friedman MA. Paclitaxel (taxol) in breast cancer. Hematol Oncol Clin North Am 8:121–140, 1994.

85. Henderson IC, Allegra JC, Woodcock T, et al. Randomized clinical trial comparing mitoxantrone with doxorubicin in previously treated patients with metastatic breast cancer. J Clin Oncol 7:560–571, 1989.

86. Hortobagyi GN. Mitomycin: its evolving role in the treatment of breast cancer. Oncology 50 (Suppl 1):1–8, 1993.

87. Livingston RB, Ellis GK, Williams MA. Weekly vinorelbine (Navelbine®, NVB) and GCSF in taxol-refractory metastatic breast cancer (MBC): A phase I–II study. Proc Am Soc Clin Oncol 14:110, 1995.

88. Valagussa P, Brambilla C, Bonnadonna G. Chemotherapy of advanced disease. In Hoogstraten B, Burn I, Bloom JHG (eds): UICC Current Treatment of Cancer: Breast Cancer. Berlin, Springer-Verlag, 1989, pp. 233–256.

89. Treat J, Greenspan A, Forst D, et al. Antitumor activity of liposome-encapsulated doxorubicin in advanced breast cancer: Phase II study. J Natl Cancer Inst 82:1706–1710, 1990.

90. Wouters W, Snoeck E, DeCoster R. Vorozole, a specific non-steroidal aromatase inhibitor. Breast Cancer Res Treat 30:89–94, 1994.

91. Vandenberg TA. New developments in chemotherapy for metastatic breast cancer. Anticancer Drugs 5:251–259, 1994.

92. Jones al, Smith IE. Navelbine and the anthrapyrazoles. Hematol Oncol Clin N Am 8:141–152, 1994.

93. Baselga J, Mendelsohn J. The epidermal growth factor receptor as a target for therapy in breast carcinoma. Breast Cancer Res Treat 29:127–138, 1994.

94. Ayash LJ. High dose chemotherapy with autologous stem cell support for the treatment of metastatic breast cancer. Cancer 74 (Suppl 1):532–535, 1994.

95. Myers SE, Williams SF. Role of high-dose chemotherapy and autologous stem cell suppport in treatment of breast cancer. Hematol Oncol Clin N Am 7:631–645, 1993.

96. Fennelly D, Vahdat L, Schneider J, Reich L, Hamilton N, Hakes T, et al. High-intensity chemotherapy with peripheral blood progenitor cell support. Semin Oncol 221 (2 Suppl 2):21–25, 1994.

97. Williams SF. Application of peripheral blood progenitors to dose-intensive therapy of breast cancer. Breast Cancer Res Treat 26 (Suppl): S25–S229, 1993.

98. Demetri GD. The use of hematopoietic growth factors to support cytotoxic chemotherapy for patients with breast cancer. Hematol Oncol Clin N Am 8:233–249, 1994.

CHAPTER 81

LIVER TUMORS

ROBERT J. STAGG

Liver tumors are classified as primary tumors, those arising from the hepatobiliary system, or secondary tumors, those metastasizing to the liver from a primary tumor of extrahepatic origin, and as being either benign or malignant. Liver tumors, as a group, represent one of the most common malignancies in the world. In Europe and North America, metastatic adenocarcinomas are the most common liver tumors, and in Africa and Southeast Asia, primary hepatocellular carcinoma is the most prevalent hepatic malignancy. Liver tumors, both primary and metastatic, account for about 20% of cancer-related deaths in the United States. Because of the liver's vital physiologic role, tumor in the liver often governs patient survival, even in the presence of extrahepatic tumor. Primary and metastatic liver tumors will be discussed separately since they have distinct biological and clinical features.

LIVER ANATOMY AND PHYSIOLOGY

The liver is a wedge-shaped organ that is suspended from the diaphragm and lies in the right upper quadrant of the abdomen (Figure 81.1). The liver comprises three lobes: the right lobe, which is the largest; the left lobe; and the caudate lobe, which is the smallest and is located on the dorsal aspect of the liver. The right lobe is further subdivided into the anterior and posterior segments, whereas the left lobe is subdivided into the medial and lateral segments.

The liver has a dual blood supply, coming from both the portal vein and the hepatic artery. Normal hepatic parenchyma receives the majority of its blood supply from the portal vein, whereas hepatic tumors receive the majority of their blood supply from the hepatic artery (1). Several of the modalities employed in the treatment of hepatic tumors take advantage of this unique finding. The blood from both the portal vein and the hepatic artery is drained from the liver by the hepatic vein, which returns it to the inferior vena cava, immediately below the right atrium. The vena cava lies in a grove on the dorsal aspect of the liver. Each segment of the liver has its own biliary system, which join intrahepatically to form the right and left hepatic ducts and then unite as they exit the liver to form the common bile duct. The hepatic artery enters and the portal vein and bile duct exit the liver at the hilum in a region known as the porta hepatis.

The liver has a number of critical physiologic functions, including producing and excreting bile (including biliru-

bin), synthesizing proteins (including albumin, gamma globulins, and several clotting factors), and metabolizing foodstuffs, drugs, and toxins. Hepatic tumors may interfere with these physiologic functions.

Following damage by surgical resection, disease, or toxic-insult, an otherwise healthy liver is capable of regenerating to its original size. However, an impaired liver, such as a cirrhotic liver, may not be able to regenerate following such an insult. Liver regeneration occurs through hypertrophy of the remaining liver parenchyma. The liver's ability to regenerate enables it to tolerate treatment modalities, such as surgical resection, cryosurgery, and chemoembolization, which are employed in the treatment of liver tumors. Patients with cirrhotic livers may not tolerate these therapies as well. The regeneration of the liver appears to be regulated by a variety of growth factors, including epidermal growth factor (EGF), hepatocyte growth factor (HGF), transforming growth factor alpha and beta (TGF-alpha and TGF-beta), fibroblast growth factor (FGF), interleukin 1-alpha (IL-1), and hepatopoietin-B. The precise interactive role of each of these growth factors in initiating and subsequently terminating liver regeneration has not been fully elucidated. Liver regeneration is essentially complete within a few months of initiation.

PRIMARY LIVER TUMORS

Table 81.1 lists the various types of benign and malignant primary liver tumors.

Benign Primary Liver Tumors

Infantile hemangioendothelioma is a benign tumor of vasculo-endothelial origin that occurs in the first 6 months of life. Because of the vascular nature of this tumor, a bruit can sometimes be heard over the liver. Approximately one-half of the patients present with a cutaneous hemangioma. Patients may also present with hepatomegaly, congestive heart failure secondary to arteriovenous shunting, thrombocytopenia, and/or microangiopathic hemolytic anemia, and up to one-third of patients present with hemolytic jaundice (2). Asymptomatic patients can be followed without treatment since spontaneous regression of the tumor may occur within 1 year. However, patients with symptomatic congestive heart failure should be managed medically with diuretics and inotropic agents. If medical management is unsuccessful, symptoms may be controlled with steroids, radiotherapy, or hepatic arterial

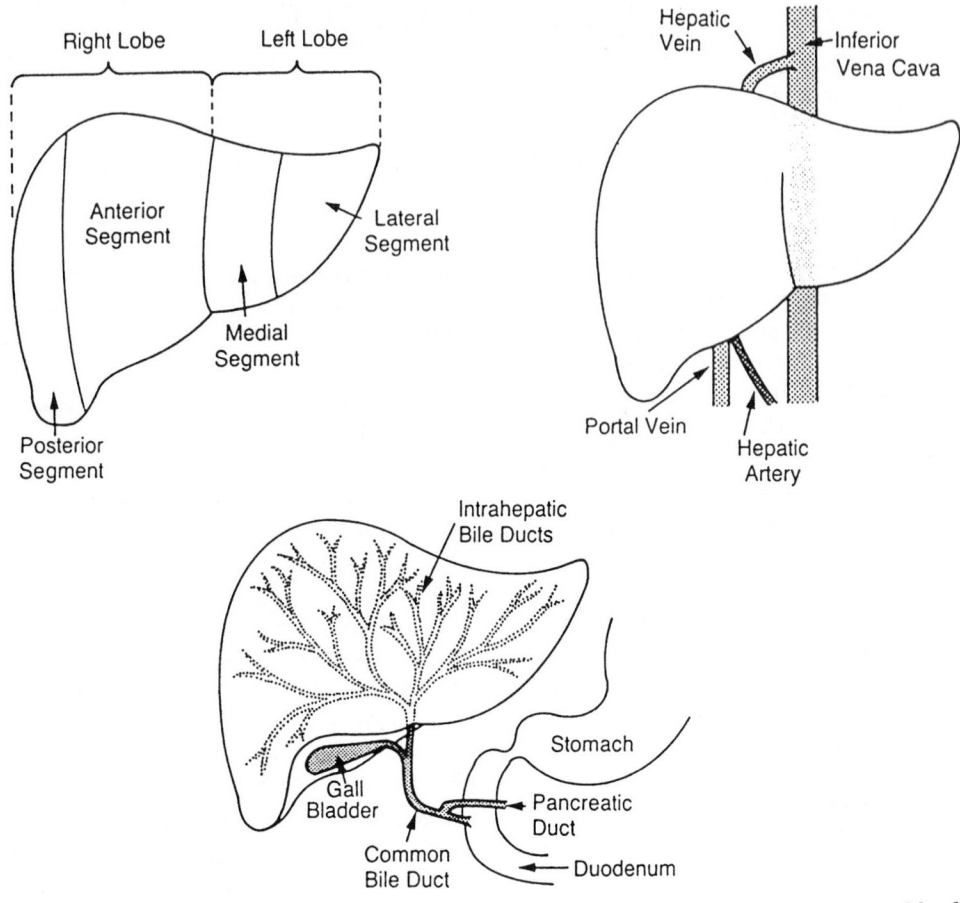

Figure 81.1. Left: Right and left hepatic lobes. Center: Hepatobiliary system. Right: Hepatic blood supply.

Table 81.1.
Primary Liver Cancers

Benign	Malignant
Infantile hemangioendothelioma	Hepatocellular carcinoma
Cavernous hemangioma	Hepatoblastoma
Hepatic cell adenoma	Intrahepatic cholangiocarcinoma
Focal nodular hyperplasia	Angiosarcoma
	Epithelioid hemangioendo-
	thelioma
	Undifferentiated sarcoma

ligation (3). Surgical resection is usually not feasible because of the large size of the tumor.

Cavernous hemangioma is the most common benign tumor of the liver, occurring in up to 7% of the population. It is a hypervascular tumor that most commonly occurs in women in the fourth, fifth, and sixth decades of life. It increases in size during pregnancy and with estrogen administration. Hemangiomas are usually asymptomatic and are most often found incidentally at autopsy. Occasionally, patients develop symptoms, including right upper quadrant pain, fever, early satiety, and/or vomiting. Only severely symptomatic patients and those having lesions

larger than 10 centimeters who are at risk for intraperitoneal hemorrhage should be treated. For such patients, surgical resection is the treatment of choice (4). Additional therapeutic modalities that have been employed include steroids, radiation, hepatic arterial ligation, and embolization (5). The prognosis of this tumor is excellent.

Hepatic adenoma occurs primarily in young women of childbearing age and usually presents as a large solitary mass in the liver. Oral contraceptives, anabolic steroids, and type 1 glycogen storage disease have been implicated in the etiology of hepatic adenoma (6). It is not known whether the development of hepatic adenoma in women taking oral contraceptives is due to the estrogen or progesterone component and whether the recent reduction in the estrogen content of many oral contraceptives will decrease the incidence of this tumor. Complete spontaneous regression, as well as progression, has been noted in women following discontinuation of an oral contraceptive. Rare cases of malignant transformation of hepatic adenoma to hepatocellular carcinoma have been reported (7). Surgical resection of a persistent hepatic adenoma is the preferred treatment because of its propensity to rupture and the possibility of malignant transformation. There is no role for radiation or chemotherapy in the management of this disease. Oral contraceptives and anabolic steroids should be strictly avoided in all patients with a history of resected or unresected hepatic adenoma.

Focal nodular hyperplasia is a hypervascular tumor that occurs most often in females and presents as an asymptomatic hepatic mass. It can occur at any age, including childhood, and is usually asymptomatic. The etiology of focal nodular hyperplasia is largely unknown, but oral contraceptives have been reported to be a possible cause (6). Patients with focal nodular hyperplasia often have coexisting congenital heart disease or other tumors, including cavernous hemangiomas, glioblastomas, astrocytomas, pheochromocytomas, and/or multiple endocrine neoplasias (8). Treatment is generally not indicated since this tumor is rarely symptomatic and is not premalignant, but surgical resection has been successfully employed in symptomatic patients (9). The long-term prognosis of this tumor is excellent.

Malignant Primary Liver Tumors

Hepatocellular carcinoma is the most prevalent malignant tumor of the liver and will be the major focus of this section. Other primary malignant tumors rarely occur, but warrant mention. Hepatoblastoma, the most common primary malignant liver tumor in young children, affects about 1 child per 100,000. It is usually diagnosed before the age of 5 but has been rarely reported in adults. It may be familial and occurs twice as frequently in males as in females. It may occur in conjunction with congenital anomalies such as tetralogy of Fallot, persistent ductus arteriosis, or extrahepatic biliary atresia. Hepatoblastoma usually presents as a solitary mass that may be encapsulated. The most common presenting symptom is abdominal swelling. Serum alphafetoprotein is elevated in the majority of cases. If untreated, hepatoblastoma is uniformly fatal. Approximately 30 to 50% of patients with hepatoblastoma are cured by surgical resection, which is the treatment of choice whenever feasible. Preoperative chemotherapy, chemoembolization, or radiation may reduce tumor bulk, allowing removal of an originally unresectable lesion (10). A small study of postoperative adjuvant chemotherapy has been conducted, but its utility remains unclear (11). Encouraging results have been obtained in a small series of patients with unresectable hepatoblastoma confined to the liver who have undergone liver transplantation although further study is needed to determine its role (9). Systemic chemotherapy for patients having unresectable primary tumors and those having metastatic disease induces responses in 30 to 40% of patients but does not significantly affect survival (12). The regimen that is most widely employed consists of cisplatin, vincristine, and 5-fluorouracil (13).

Intrahepatic cholangiocarcinoma is a tumor arising from the intrahepatic bile ducts and is the second most frequently occurring malignant primary tumor of the liver. Occasionally, tumors are found on pathologic examination to be mixtures of cholangiocarcinoma and hepatocellular carcinoma. Intrahepatic cholangiocarcinoma may arise from a peripheral bile duct or a major intrahepatic duct and has a low tendency to metastasize. Patients with Crohn's disease, sclerosing cholangitis, biliary atresia, ulcerative colitis, and hepatolithiasis are at increased risk for developing cholangiocarcinoma. The median survival of untreated patients is approximately 6.5 months although patients having small peripheral tumors may survive much longer. Surgical resection is occasionally curative and should be performed whenever possible. Adjuvant intraoperative radiotherapy is currently being investigated. Liver transplant may also have a role in the management of locally confined cholangiocarcinoma. Penn and colleagues reported the results in 109 patients with intrahepatic or hilar cholangiocarcinoma, from liver transplant centers throughout the world, who underwent orthotopic liver transplantation. The 2- and 5-year actuarial survival rates were 30 and 17%, respectively (14). Systemic chemotherapy is employed for patients with unresectable or metastatic tumor. A partial response rate of 31% was reported with intravenous chemotherapy using 5-fluorouracil, mitomycin, and doxorubicin (15). Responses have also been observed with intraarterial chemotherapy (16).

Angiosarcoma, though uncommon, is the most frequent sarcoma of the liver. It is a rapidly growing tumor that is often accompanied by thrombocytopenia. Approximately 40% of cases are associated with exposure to a carcinogen, specifically, thorium oxide (Thorotrast), vinyl chloride, arsenic, or radium (17). There can be a latency period of up to 40 years from the exposure to the carcinogen to the development of the angiosarcoma (18). It is a rapidly progressive tumor, metastasizing to the lungs, porta hepatis. lymph nodes, or spleen. Angiosarcomas occasionally rupture, leading to hemoperitoneum. Resection offers the only potential for cure and is the treatment of choice whenever feasible. Radiation and/or chemotherapy may produce partial responses in unresectable lesions although the experience with these modalities is limited (17). Patients with unresectable angiosarcoma usually survive less than 1 year.

Epithelioid hemangioendothelioma is a rare vascular tumor of the liver (19). It occurs primarily in middle age and more frequently in women than in men. In some patients, the development of epithelioid hemangioendothelioma appears to be causally related to the use of oral contraceptives. Epithelioid hemangioendothelioma causes hepatic fibrosis and frequently infiltrates the hepatic and portal veins. Clinically, it often presents similar to Budd–Chiari syndrome. Various treatments have been employed, including liver transplantation, partial hepatectomy, chemotherapy, and radiation. It can be very slow growing with 25% of patients with an unresectable tumor surviving greater than 5 years from diagnosis.

Undifferentiated (embryonal) sarcoma of the liver is a term used to describe a group of very rare pediatric sarcomas of the liver that defy categorization since they lack cellular differentiation (20). The tumor rarely metastasizes but spreads by direct invasion into adjacent organs. It is usually rapidly fatal although cures have been reported with surgical resection. Radiation and chemotherapy have been used in the treatment of unresectable lesions and metastatic disease although their utility is unclear.

Hepatocellular Carcinoma

Hepatocellular carcinoma (HCC), also known as hepatoma, accounts for 40% of childhood and 90% of adult malignant primary tumors of the liver. It is more common in males than in females. HCC rarely occurs in adults before the age of 40 and increases in frequency thereafter, with the peak incidence occurring in the sixth decade of life. HCC is uncommon in the United States, with approximately 3,000 to 4,000 cases diagnosed annually (21). However, it is one the most prevalent cancers in Asia, sub-Sahara Africa, and the South Pacific Islands and is estimated to cause 1.25 million deaths throughout the world each year.

ETIOLOGY

HCC is frequently associated with preexisting liver disease. In the United States, approximately 50% of patients with HCC have underlying cirrhosis secondary to alcohol, postnecrotic cirrhosis, or hemochromatosis (22). Primary biliary cirrhosis and the cirrhosis associated with Wilson's disease do not appear to significantly predispose patients to developing HCC. It is estimated that about 5% of all patients with cirrhosis will eventually develop HCC.

Chronic active hepatitis B infection is the most important predisposing factor worldwide (23). Epidemiologic studies reveal a high incidence of HCC in patients residing in those regions where hepatitis B is endemic. Patients chronically infected with hepatitis B have a 10- to 390-fold increased risk of developing HCC. The method by which chronic hepatitis B infection causes hepatic oncogenesis is not completely understood, but three possible mechanisms have been proposed. The first postulates that viral infection results in chronic inflammation and hepatocyte regeneration, leading to random mutations in the host genome and malignant transformation. The second theory postulates that there is targeted integration of hepatitis B regulatory genes adjacent to specific sites in the host genome, resulting in activation of host protooncogenes and/or inactivation of tumor suppressor genes and subsequent malignant transformation. The final theory postulates that random integration of the hepatitis B genome

into the host genome occurs and that malignant transformation is a direct result of the oncogenic action of the integrated viral genes or viral gene products. Whatever the exact mechanism, about 80% of the HCC worldwide is thought to be the result of prior host infection with the hepatitis B virus. Thus, the hepatitis B virus appears to rank in importance with tobacco as a human carcinogen in liver and lung cancers, respectively.

Epidemiologic data suggest that hepatitis C infection also predisposes patients to developing HCC (24). Hepatitis C infection is present in about 15% of HCC patients in the United States and 76% of patients in Japan (25, 26). Little is known about the exact mechanism by which hepatitis C produces hepatic oncogenesis.

Aflatoxin B1, a toxin produced by *Aspergillus flavus*, has also been implicated as a possible cause of HCC (27). It appears to cause HCC by producing distinct point mutations in the p53 tumor suppressor gene. Aflatoxins are present on several foodstuffs consumed in large quantities in those parts of the world having a high incidence of HCC. These include rice, peanuts, soybeans, corn, wheat, bread, milk, and cheese, especially when they are stored in unrefrigerated conditions. Aflatoxin exposure produces HCC in 100% of some susceptible animal species, whereas other species are completely unaffected.

Case reports in the literature suggest an association between sex hormone exposure and the development of HCC. Women and men have developed HCC following exposure to oral contraceptives and androgens, respectively (28, 29). However, it remains to be determined whether the ingestion of sex hormones is causally related to the development of HCC.

Finally, certain inherited metabolic disorders, including hemochromatosis, glycogen storage disease, alpha-1-antitrypsin deficiency, and tyrosinemia predispose patients to develop HCC.

PATHOLOGY

HCC is a grayish white to bright yellow tumor that is usually not encapsulated. Occasionally, however, encapsulated HCC is found in older patients and is a slower-growing and less invasive tumor than typical HCC (30). Three major categories of HCC have been described based on its macroscopic appearance. The most common type is the nodular form in which the liver is studded with tumor. The second is the massive type, which presents as a large mass and is sometimes associated with small satellite lesions. The last type is the diffuse form, which is the rarest and presents as scattered tumor throughout the liver. The diffuse form always occurs in association with cirrhosis.

Eight different histologic subtypes of HCC have been identified based on the microscopic appearance of the tumor (Table 81.2). The hepatic variant, also known as the trabecular variant, is the most common. The fibrolamellar

Table 81.2.
Histologic Variants of Hepatocellular Carcinoma

Hepatic or trabecular
Plemorphic
Adenoid or acinar
Sclerosing
Giant cell
Clear cell
Fibrolamellar
Mixed

variant is noteworthy because it is usually solitary and has a better prognosis than the other types of HCC (31). It occurs primarily in women between the ages of 15 and 30 and is not associated with cirrhosis. The clear cell variant may also be associated with a better prognosis.

HCC often infiltrates the diaphragm and invades the intrahepatic portal veins. Less often the tumor invades the hepatic vein or bile duct. Frequently, regional lymph nodes are involved with tumor, but unless this occurs in the porta hepatis, such involvement usually does not alter the patient's clinical course. At autopsy, 40 to 50% of patients with HCC are found to have distant metastases. The lung is the most common site of metastases although almost any organ can be involved. The presence of metastatic disease rarely alters the patient's outcome since the tumor burden in the liver usually determines the duration of survival.

CLINICAL PRESENTATION

Unfortunately, HCC is not usually symptomatic until there is advanced disease. The most common symptoms are abdominal pain, abdominal distension, fatigue, anorexia, weight loss, and fevers. On examination, most patients have hepatomegaly. Less often, patients present with ascites, edema, and/or jaundice. Rarely, patients present with hemorrhage secondary to esophageal varices. Although uncommon in North American patients, patients in Asia and Africa frequently (10 to 20%) present with spontaneous rupture of their HCC with intraperitoneal hemorrhage.

Many laboratory abnormalities may be present in a patient with HCC. The hepatic transaminases and alkaline phosphatase are usually elevated, and the bilirubin is elevated in up to 50% of patients. Because of the decreased synthetic ability of the liver and the cachectic state of patients, the albumin level is often decreased, and the prothrombin time (PT) and partial thromboplastin time (PTT) may be elevated. A mild anemia and a reactive leukocytosis frequently occur. Rarely, erythrocytosis is present in patients having HCC with underlying cirrhosis. Hypoglycemia occurs in two distinct subpopulations of patients with HCC. The first group are patients with good performance status who have an acquired form of glycogen storage disease, secondary to their tumor, with reduced

hepatocellular levels of glucose 6-phosphatase and a phosphorylase required for the breakdown of glycogen. The second group are terminal patients in whom hepatic gluconeogenesis is impaired. Approximately one-third of patients have high serum cholesterol levels. Finally, some patients have hypercalcemia due to either bone metastases or a parathormonelike substance produced by the tumor.

DIAGNOSIS

The diagnostic workup of a patient suspected of having HCC generally proceeds from the physician's clinical suspicion based on the patient's presenting signs and symptoms, to laboratory tests, to noninvasive radiologic studies, and then to tissue biopsy. The clinician usually first suspects the possibility of a hepatic malignancy when the patient complains of right upper quadrant pain or an enlarged liver is detected on physical examination. When these signs and symptoms occur in a patient with a prior history of hepatitis B or cirrhosis, a diagnosis of HCC must be considered.

Laboratory tests may be helpful in the diagnosis, but most are nonspecific. The most useful laboratory test is the alpha-fetoprotein (AFP). AFP is a glycoprotein synthesized by fetal liver, fetal intestine, and yolk sac cells. Levels are very high prior to birth and fall to adult levels of less than 10 ng/ml after delivery. AFP is elevated ($\geq$100 ng/ml) in about 75 to 90% of patients having HCC (32). Although levels are elevated in a few other malignant conditions, the frequency of elevated levels in patients with HCC makes this a useful initial test. When elevated, the AFP level can also be used to follow a patient's clinical course since it usually falls with response to therapy and rises with progressive disease. Ferritin levels are elevated in patients with HCC. However, it is also elevated in most patients with uncomplicated cirrhosis and thus lacks specificity (33). In addition, ferritin levels do not correlate with therapeutic response, as does AFP.

Several radiologic tests may be used to confirm the presence of a hepatic mass and to subsequently follow the course of the disease. Arteriography may be used to assist in the diagnosis of HCC when other radiographic techniques fail. On arteriographic exam, HCC typically has a dilated feeding artery with a hypervascular tumor bed. Radionuclide liver–spleen scanning with technetium sulfur colloid is simple to perform, inexpensive, and not associated with morbidity, but it is rarely used because of its inability to image the rest of the abdomen. Ultrasound is similarly inexpensive and is not associated with morbidity, but it is incapable of detecting hepatic lesions less than 1 cm in size and has limited utility in determining the presence of extrahepatic tumor. Although more expensive, computerized tomography (CT scan) and magnetic resonance imaging (MRI) are the most frequently employed methods for imaging a hepatic malignancy. Both of these techniques are more sensitive than ultrasound and allow visualization of the entire abdomen. However, the most sensitive radiographic technique for detecting a hepatic lesion is intraoperative ultrasound. This procedure should be performed whenever hepatic resection is contemplated since it is more sensitive for detecting lesions than even the surgeon's visual and tactile inspection of the liver (34).

These radiographic techniques are useful for documenting the presence of a hepatic mass and following the course of disease once the diagnosis has been confirmed and therapy has been instituted, but by themselves, they do not provide a definitive diagnosis of HCC. This requires pathologic examination of a tissue specimen. Tissue specimens may be obtained by percutaneous biopsy, peritoneoscopy with directed needle biopsy, or open biopsy at laparotomy.

PROGNOSIS

HCC is an aggressive malignancy that usually carries a grave prognosis. The reported median survival in untreated patients from the time of diagnosis varies from 1 to 6 months. Several factors are of prognostic importance (Table 81.3) (35). The most important of these is the resectability of the tumor. Surgical removal offers the only potential cure for HCC.

The performance status of the patient is of prognostic significance, with ambulatory patients surviving longer than those who are bedridden. The percentage of liver involved with tumor at the time of presentation is inversely related to the duration of survival. Additionally, the location of tumors within the liver can alter outcome. Patients with a tumor near the porta hepatis may deteriorate rapidly since a small increase in tumor volume may cause compression of

the inferior vena cava, portal vein, hepatic artery, and bile duct leading to subsequent ascites, edema, and jaundice.

The patient's baseline liver function is also important, with those patients having normal liver function tests, bilirubin, albumin, and PT and PTT having the best prognosis. Patients with ascites, edema, or esophageal varices have a poorer prognosis. Patients having the fibrolamellar or clear cell variants of HCC and those with encapsulated tumors generally survive longer. Although metastatic disease itself rarely determines outcome, its presence suggests a more aggressive tumor and is associated with a shorter survival.

Other important prognostic factors include the patient's age, sex, country of origin, and the presence or absence of cirrhosis. Patients under 45 years of age have a better prognosis than those over 45, and female patients survive longer than their male counterparts. Lastly, patients with otherwise normal livers survive longer and respond better to chemotherapy than those with cirrhosis.

PREVENTION

Since very few patients with HCC are cured, prevention of HCC is the most appealing approach to decrease the number of HCC-associated deaths. As previously discussed, hepatitis B appears to be a major etiologic factor leading to the development of HCC. Vertical transmission from mother to infant is the most common method of hepatitis B transmission in endemic areas. Vaccination of newborns with a hepatitis B vaccine can prevent vertical transmission, and thus eliminate the predisposition for subsequently developing HCC (36). Pilot data from Shanghai and Gambia have demonstrated that such a strategy is effective in preventing transmission of hepatitis B in endemic areas (37, 38). A cost–benefit analysis of newborn vaccination has shown that it is justifiable even in areas of immediate endemicity (39). However, the effect of vaccination on the incidence of HCC will not be observed for several decades because of prolonged latency between hepatitis B infection and the development of HCC.

SCREENING

Theoretically, screening high risk patients for HCC should result in the detection of the malignancy earlier, thus making potentially curative surgery feasible in a larger number of patients. However, although some early HCCs are detected by screening high-risk patients with AFP levels and ultrasound, no definitive outcome advantage has been observed (40–45).

TREATMENT

Surgical removal via resection or orthotopic liver transplantation of HCC is potentially curative and should be employed whenever feasible. Cryosurgery and intratumoral alcohol injections are two investigational modalities

Table 81.3.
Prognostic Variables in Patients with Hepatocellular Carcinoma

Factor	Favorable	Unfavorable
Resectability	Yes	No
Liver function	Normal LFTs	Abnormal LFTs
	Bilirubin <36 μmol/liter	Bilirubin >36 μmol/liter
	Normal albumin	Hypoalbuminemia
	Normal PT, PTT	Abnormal PT, PTT
	No ascites	Ascites
	No portal hypertension	Portal hypertension
Metastases	No	Yes
Performance status	Ambulatory	Bedridden
Age	<45 years	>45 years
Sex	Female	Male
Country	North America	African, Asian
Histology	Fibrolamellar variant	Nodular
	Clear cell variant (?)	Massive
	Encapsulated tumor	Diffuse
Cirrhosis	No	Yes

that may be useful in patients with potentially resectable HCCs who are not candidates for surgical resection because of underlying liver disease or other comorbid illnesses. Patients with unresectable but liver-predominant disease are most frequently treated with systemic chemotherapy, intraarterial chemotherapy (with or without Lipiodol; see the section "Intraarterial Lipiodol-Chemotherapy Injection"), or chemoembolization. Other alternatives for these patients include hepatic artery ligation, embolization, or radiation (external beam, radioimmunotherapy, or regional-administered radiotherapy). Systemic chemotherapy is the only alternative for patients who have significant extrahepatic tumor.

Surgical Resection. Surgical resection of HCC is the most widely employed modality that offers a potential for cure. Partial hepatectomy may be associated with significant morbidity and mortality (3 to 27%), especially in patients with underlying liver disease, and therefore should be attempted only with curative intent (35, 46–58). Unfortunately, the majority of patients are not candidates for surgical resection since their intrahepatic tumor is too extensive, their underlying liver disease limits their ability to withstand the surgical procedure, or they have extrahepatic disease. Approximately one-third of patients are considered candidates for resection following preoperative staging of their tumor, and of those, about two-thirds are found to be unresectable at surgery because of the presence of extrahepatic tumor or previously undiagnosed intrahepatic tumor. Thus, only about 10 to 15% of patients with HCC present with resectable disease. Occasionally, unresectable HCC may be rendered resectable with chemotherapy and/or radiation (59).

Table 81.4 summarizes the results with surgical resection for HCC. The 5-year survival rates for patients having

Table 81.4.
Results of Surgical Resection for Hepatocellular Carcinoma

Author/Year	Number of Patients	Perioperative Mortality (%)	5-Year Survival (%)	Reference
Okuda/1980	222	27	12	(35)
Adson/1981	230	—	30	(46)
Huguet/1985	42	24	15	(47)
Nagao/1986	94	20	25	(48)
Lin/1987	225	8	18	(49)
Chen/1989	120	4	32[a]	(50)
Toshihara/1990	119	15	33	(51)
Choi/1990	174	13	15	(52)
Yamanaka/1990	128	—	54	(53)
Kobayashi/1990	180	3	49	(54)
Tsuzuki/1990	119	15	39	(55)
Iwatsuki/1991	76	—	33	(56)
Gozzetti/1993	168	8	36	(57)
Kawarada/1994	149	4	39	(58)

[a]Four-year survival

undergone a potentially curative resection range from 12 to 54%. Approximately 20% of the 5-year survivors ultimately die of recurrent disease; thus, about 25% of the resected patients are cured of HCC. Although adjuvant chemotherapy is not routinely employed, a small study conducted in Asia suggests that adjuvant intraarterial chemotherapy may improve the disease-free and overall survival of patients with HCC (60).

Cryosurgery. Cryosurgery uses a probe circulating liquid nitrogen through its tip, which is inserted into a tumor intraoperatively to induce freezing temperatures within a tumor, resulting in necrosis. Intraoperative ultrasound is used to guide the freezing procedure. The use of multiple freeze–thaw cycles increases the percentage of tumor cells killed (61). Cryosurgery is relatively well tolerated. However, in the largest published experience to date, only 12 of 60 (20%) patients were alive 3 years after cryosurgery (62). Therefore, cryosurgery offers no clear advantage over standard surgical resection and should be confined to the research setting. It may ultimately be most useful in patients with resectable disease who are not candidates for partial hepatectomy due to underlying liver disease, such as cirrhosis.

Orthotopic Liver Transplantation. Orthotopic liver transplantation (OLT) has been performed in patients having locally confined but unresectable HCC. Unfortunately, the results with OLT have been disappointing with 3-year survival rates of about 50% and long-term survival rates of only 20% (56, 63–71). A retrospective review of OLT in HCC conducted at the University of Pittsburgh reported no difference in 3-year survival rates between HCC patients who underwent hepatectomy and those who underwent OLT (54). However, patients who had underlying cirrhosis had a 3-year survival rate of only 5.9% with hepatectomy compared with a 42.9% survival rate with OLT. These results, which have been confirmed in a retrospective review reported by Bismuth and colleagues, may be explained by the elimination of the cirrhotic liver (72). A prospective randomized trial of cirrhotic patients with HCC comparing surgical resection to OLT has not been conducted and thus a definitive benefit of OLT in cirrhotic patients has not been proved.

Two small subpopulations of HCC patients appear to benefit significantly from OLT. Patients with fibrolamellar HCC have a 50% disease-free survival following OLT (57, 73, 74), and patients with a small HCC discovered incidentally at the time of OLT for end-stage liver disease have an 80% likelihood of long-term survival (66).

In an attempt to improve on the results with OLT for HCC, recent studies have combined OLT with perioperative chemotherapy. In one study, doxorubicin was administered to 20 OLT patients and resulted in an estimated 3-year survival of 59% (75). In another trial, 10 patients were treated with perioperative cisplatin and alpha-interferon followed by OLT, and 9 of 10 patients were alive 1 year following OLT (76). Finally, in another study, 11 patients received preoperative chemoembolization, and 10 were alive without recurrence at a median follow-up of 33 months (77). These pilot studies suggest that perioperative chemotherapy may increase the cure rate of OLT, but a prospective randomized trial must be performed before definitive conclusions can be drawn.

Percutaneous Alcohol Injection. Percutaneous injection of absolute ethyl alcohol directly into a tumor under ultrasound guidance is capable of producing histologically confirmed complete responses in small HCCs by causing dehydration and intracellular coagulation, leading to necrosis, vascular occlusion, and fibrosis. The volume of ethyl alcohol injected depends on the size of the tumor and its vascularity, but it is generally 2 to 8 milliliters. The distribution of alcohol within the tumor during the injection is evaluated by ultrasound. Histologic evaluation of 21 HCCs treated with percutaneous alcohol injection demonstrated complete necrosis in 15 of the tumors (78). A 3-year survival of approximately 60% has been observed with percutaneous alcohol injection (78, 79). As with cryosurgery, percutaneous alcohol injection may be most useful in the rare patient who has a small solitary HCC but is unable to tolerate surgical resection because of underlying liver disease.

Radiotherapy. Standard external beam radiation is of limited benefit in the management of HCC because of the inherent intolerance of normal liver parenchyma to radiation. Doses to the liver in excess of 3,000 rads produce radiation hepatitis in a significant number of patients (80). Patients with underlying liver disease develop radiation hepatitis at even lower doses. Some partial responses to external beam radiation at doses of 2,000 to 3,000 rads fractionated over 7 days have been reported although survival does not appear to be extended (81). With new methods using three-dimensional radiation treatment, radiation ports can be designed that minimize the radiation dose to liver and allow a higher dose of radiation to be delivered to the HCC (82, 83). Whether this approach will significantly improve on the results obtained with standard external beam radiation remains to be determined.

Other approaches of delivering radiotherapy to the tumor while minimizing exposure to the normal liver tissue are under investigation. One such approach has been the administration of radioimmunoglobulin targeted to a tumor antigen. Initial studies of Iodine[131] polyclonal antiferritin antibodies plus chemotherapy and external beam radiation produced encouraging results, but a subsequent randomized trial comparing this approach to chemotherapy alone failed to produce a survival advantage (84). In addition, significant myelosuppression was observed. Attempts to decrease the bone marrow suppression by substituting the gamma-emitting Iodine[131] with the beta-emitting yttrium[90] altered the antibody-binding sites, resulting in a loss of specificity for HCC. Presently, alternative approaches to the regional delivery of radiotherapy, including intraarterial administration of Iodine[131] radiolabeled lipiodol and neutron-activated yttrium[89] containing glass microspheres, are being investigated (85, 86).

Hormonal Therapy. Some HCCs are estrogen-receptor-positive, much like some breast cancers (87). Based on this finding, patients with HCC have been treated with megesterol acetate or tamoxifen citrate (87–89). Although limited responses have been observed, hormonal therapy is felt to have limited activity and is rarely employed in the management of HCC.

Intravenous Chemotherapy. Intravenous chemotherapy is of limited benefit in altering the natural history of HCC. However, it is the only therapeutic option for patients with widely metastatic disease. The experience with single-agent chemotherapy is summarized in Table 81.5. Doxorubicin is the agent with the most reproducible activity, producing responses in about 20% of patients. It is usually administered intravenously in doses of 20 to 75 mg/m^2 every 21 days (90–98). Two similar agents, mitoxantrone and 4'epidoxorubicin, appear to have activity comparable to that of doxorubicin (99–103).

5-Fluorouracil has been administered both orally (92, 104, 105) and intravenously (105–107) to patients with HCC. By both routes, the response rates have been low. Amsacrine, dichloromethotrexate, etoposide, mitoxantrone, cisplatin, and alpha-interferon have all produced occasional responses, but the overall response rates with these agents have been low (94, 108–118). Various combination regimens have been studied, but none have improved on the results obtained with single-agent therapy.

Intraarterial Chemotherapy. Because of the discouraging results obtained with intravenous chemotherapy, administration directly into the hepatic artery has been used to increase the total drug exposure (concentration versus time) at the tumor, and thus, enhance efficacy (119, 120). The drug exposure is most dramatically increased when the agent being administered has a rapid total body clearance since intraarterial infusion enables the drug to be delivered in a high concentration to the tumor prior to its elimination from the body. An additional benefit is derived from intraarterial administration when the agent has a high first-pass hepatic extraction. The high first-pass hepatic extraction of the drug leads to a lower systemic drug exposure than with intravenous administration and thus fewer adverse effects. Table 81.6 lists the total body clearance rates and hepatic extraction ratios of chemotherapeutic agents commonly used to treat hepatic malignancies (121–126). Floxuridine, 5-fluorouracil, and doxorubicin have rapid total body clearance and high hepatic extraction ratios. Therefore, the intraarterial administration of these agents results in a substantial increase in drug

Table 81.5.

Results of Single-Agent Intravenous Chemotherapy for Hepatocellular Carcinoma

Drug	Number of Patients	Partial Responses	Response Rate (%)	Reference
Doxorubicin	41	6/41	15	(90)
	44	14/44	32	(91)
	57	9/57	16	(92)
	74	22/74	30	(93)
	28	8/28	29	(94)
	35	3/35	9	(95)
	52	6/52	11	(96)
	45	11/45	24	(97)
	109	11/109	10	(98)
	485	90/485	19	
Mitoxantrone	22	6/22	27	(99)
	20	0/20	0	(100)
	42	6/42	14	
4'-Epidoxorubincin	18	3/18	17	(101)
	13	3/13	23	(102)
	33	3/33	9	(103)
	64	9/64	14	
5-Fluorouracil	12	6/12	50	(104)
	48	0/48	0	(92)
	21	0/21	0	(105)
	10	1/10	10	(106)
	8	0/8	0	(107)
	99	7/99	7	
Amsacrine	23	3/23	13	(108)
	16	0/16	0	(109)
	20	1/20	5	(110)
	35	1/35	3	(111)
	94	5/95	5	
Dichloromethotrexate	14	0/14	0	(112)
	7	3/7	43	(113)
	21	3/21	14	
Etoposide	24	3/24	13	(114)
	38	7/38	18	(94)
	62	10/62	16	
Cisplatin	13	1/13	8	(115)
	26	4/26	15	(116)
	39	5/39	13	
Interferon	28	2/28	7	(117)
	25	2/25	8	(118)
	53	4/53	8	

Table 81.6.

Total Body Clearance and Hepatic Extraction Ratio of Drugs Administered by Hepatic Intraarterial Infusion

Drug	Total Body Clearance (ml/min)	Hepatic Extraction Ratio (%)	Reference
Floxuridine	4800	95	(121)
Doxorubicin	2000	50	(122)
5-Fluorouracil	1000	80	(123, 124)
Cisplatin	600	24	(125)
Mitomycin C	575	10	(126)

exposure at the tumor site and a decrease in systemic exposure. In contrast, cisplatin and mitomycin C have relatively slow total body clearance and low hepatic extraction ratios. Thus, intraarterial administration of these agents produces fewer changes in the tumor and less systemic drug exposure.

In the past, hepatic intraarterial chemotherapy was most commonly administered via a radiographically placed transcutaneous catheter inserted into the hepatic artery via the femoral or brachial artery. This can be successfully accomplished in about 80% of patients but is associated with several complications, including catheter migration, drug misperfusion, infection, catheter thrombosis, hepatic arterial thrombosis, and arterial emboli. To avoid catheter migration, transcutaneous catheters may be surgically placed and secured in the hepatic artery. Although this approach prevents catheter migration, the other difficulties of a transcutaneous catheter remain.

The advent of totally implantable ports and pumps in the early 1980s made the administration of long-term hepatic intraarterial chemotherapy feasible. Implanted ports are surgically placed into a subcutaneous pocket, and the catheter is inserted in a ligated gastroduodenal artery, with the tip at the hepatic artery. Implanted ports are most useful for the administration of bolus chemotherapy. Continuous-infusion chemotherapy via implanted ports requires the use of an external infusion device and is therefore technically cumbersome. Totally implantable pumps have made it feasible to administer infusional hepatic intraarterial chemotherapy in the outpatient setting (Figure 81.2). Table 81.7 lists the characteristics of the various constant flow and programmable implantable pumps. The pumps, like the ports, are placed into a subcutaneous pocket, and the catheter is inserted in a ligated gastroduodenal artery with the tip at the hepatic artery. All the devices have a drug chamber that is filled by percutaneously passing a needle into the inlet septum and injecting the next course of therapy. In addition, the pumps have a side port that may be used for bolus administration of chemotherapy.

Table 81.8 summarizes the clinical results with single-agent hepatic arterial chemotherapy in the treatment of HCC. Although the clinical trials are few and have small patient populations, the response rates are higher than those reported with intravenous chemotherapy. Single-agent intraarterial floxuridine produces responses in about 55% of patients (107, 127). Because of the high first-pass hepatic extraction of floxuridine, intraarterial infusions do not produce systemic toxicity. However, hepatobiliary toxicity may occur, including biliary sclerosis and cholecystitis. Biliary sclerosis is a potentially serious toxicity that results from floxuridine-induced inflammation and subsequent thrombosis of the peribiliary vascular plexus, which causes ischemic damage to the bile duct (128). Serious

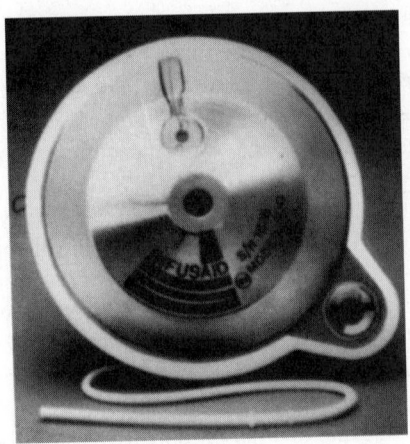
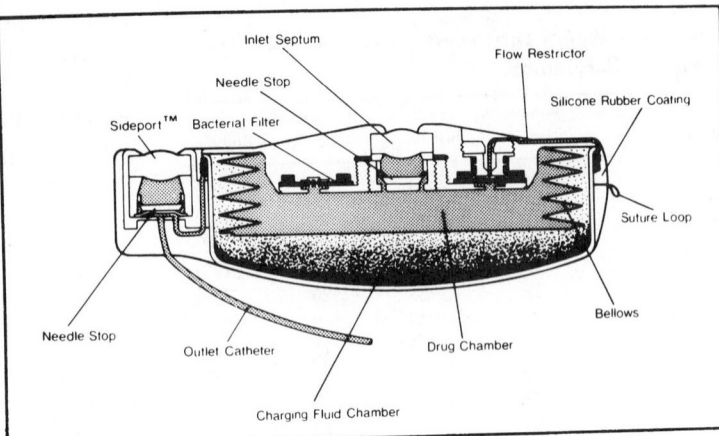

Figure 81.2. Left: Shiley-Infusoid (Norwood, Mass.) implantable pump. Right: Cross-section of implantable pump.

Table 81.7.
Implantable Pumps

Device	Diameter	Weight	Volume	Flow Rate	Side Port	Battery	Alarms	Cost
Constant flow								
Infusaid (Model 400) Single catheter	87 mm	208 g	50 ml	1–10 ml/day	Yes	No	No	$4795
Infusaid (Model 400) Double catheter	87 mm	229 g	50 ml	1–10 ml/day	Two	No	No	$5495
Infusaid (Model 600)	63 mm	100 g	23 ml	0.7 or 1.4 ml/day	Yes	No	No	$4795
Therex	77 mm	136 g	30 ml	0.5–2 ml/day	Yes	No	No	$3000
Programmable								
Infusaid (Model 1000)	9.0 cm	226 g	25 ml	0–12 ml/day	Yes	Yes	No	Unknown
Medtronics	7.0 cm	185 g	18 ml	0.1–21 ml/day	Optional	Yes	Occlusion Low battery	$6900

Table 81.8.
Results of Single-Agent Intraarterial Chemotherapy for Hepatocellular Carcinoma

Drug	Number of Patients	Partial Responses	Response Rate (%)	Reference
Floxuridine	16	9	56	(107)
	28	15	54	(127)
	44	24	55	
Fluorouracil	9	2	22	(129)
Doxorubicin	10	4	40	(93)
	4	2	50	(129)
	13	6	46	(130)
	2	1	50	(131)
	6	3	50	(132)
	19	8	42	(133)
	44	20	45	
Cisplatin	16	3	19	(134)
Mitoxantrone	22	6	27	(135)

biliary toxicity can usually be prevented with appropriate dose adjustments and careful monitoring. Prophylactic cholecystectomy is recommended if repeated courses of hepatic intraarterial floxuridine are to be administered. Additionally, gastritis and gastroduodenal ulceration have occurred as a result of misperfusion of floxuridine into the stomach and duodenum. This can be prevented by surgically ligating the arterial feeders to the stomach arising from the hepatic artery. Although 5-fluorouracil has not been tested as a single agent in the United States, results from Japan indicate that it may have activity similar to floxuridine when administered intraarterially for HCC (129). Doxorubicin also appears to have enhanced activity when infused intraarterially, with response rates of 40 to 50% (93, 129–133). Mitomycin C has been reported to have significant efficacy when administered intraarterially (33). However, detailed response data are unavailable. Finally, hepatic intraarterial cisplatin and mitoxantrone have produced some responses in patients with HCC (134, 135).

High response rates have also been reported with combination intraarterial chemotherapy. Responses were observed in 8 of 15 (53%) patients receiving an intraarterial combination of mitomycin C, 5-fluorouracil, vinblastine, vincristine, and doxorubicin (136); 8 of 12 (67%) patients receiving floxuridine, doxorubicin, and mitomycin C (137); and 8 of 13 (61%) patients receiving floxuridine, leucovorin, doxorubicin, and cisplatin (138). It remains unclear whether combination intraarterial chemotherapy is superior to single-agent treatment.

Intraarterial Lipiodol-Chemotherapy Injection. Lipiodol is an ethyl ester of the fatty acid of poppyseed oil, containing 38% iodine by weight; it is used as lymphangiogram dye. Following intraarterial injection, lipiodol concentrates in HCC. As a result of this finding, lipophilic chemotherapeutic agents have been administered intraarterially in conjunction with Lipiodol in an attempt to facilitate the delivery of the chemotherapeutic agent into the tumor cell. The drugs most commonly combined with Lipiodol have been doxorubicin and styrene-maleic acid-neocarzinostatin (SMANCS). SMANCS is a conjugation of neocarzionstatin, a proteinaceous antitumor antibiotic, and copoly styrene-maleic acid, a drug used to treat hepatic malignancies in Asia. Studies with intraarterial Lipiodol and doxorubicin or SMANCS have reported responses in 30 to 40% of patients (139). Recently, a randomized study of hepatic intraarterial cisplatin and doxorubicin versus hepatic intraarterial cisplatin, doxorubicin, and Lipiodol was conducted, and no significant response difference was observed with the addition of Lipiodol (140). Thus, the addition of Lipiodol to lipophilic chemotherapeutic agents may not be advantageous.

Hepatic Artery Ligation. Surgical ligation of the hepatic artery has been performed in patients having HCC without significant extrahepatic involvement in an attempt to produce tumor necrosis secondary to ischemia. This approach has been used as a single modality as well as in combination with chemotherapy (141, 142). Responses with hepatic arterial ligation are often transient because extrahepatic collateral arteries develop rapidly, reperfusing the tumor (143). The procedure is generally well tolerated, with hepatic pain, fever, and elevated hepatic enzymes being the most prevalent adverse events. Rarely, hepatic artery ligation causes hepatic necrosis, resulting in death. Patients with severely compromised hepatic function or portal vein thrombosis should not undergo this procedure. Although frequently employed in the past, hepatic artery ligation is rarely used today because occlusion of the hepatic artery can be accomplished radiographically (i.e., embolization), and permanent loss of the hepatic artery precludes its use for other liver-directed treatments, such as intraarterial chemotherapy or chemoembolization. Ligation of the hepatic artery has also been used to stop intraabdominal bleeding from a ruptured HCC (144), but this can also be accomplished angiographically with coiling or embolization (145); thus, it is rarely employed for this purpose.

Embolization and Chemoembolization. Two related modalities, embolization and chemoembolization, are frequently used to treat unresectable but liver-predominant HCC. Embolization of HCC involves radiographic placement of a percutaneous catheter into the hepatic artery and injection of an embolizing substance that occludes the arterial blood flow at the tumor capillary level, thus producing tumor ischemia. Embolizing substances that have been administered include Angiostat (5 × 75 U) (Target Therapeutics, Los Angeles, CA); Ethibloc (Ethicon, Hamburg, West Germany); Gelfoam cubes (1 to 3 mm) (Upjohn, Kalamazoo, MI); Ivalon particles (150 to 500 U) (Unipoint Lab, High Point, NC); and autologous blood clot. Gelfoam powder (40 to 60 U) (Upjohn, Kalamazoo, MI) has also been used, but this substance is no longer commercially available in the United States. The various embolizing substances achieve different levels and durations of arterial blockade; the optimal embolizing substance is yet to be determined. Embolization is preferred over hepatic artery ligation since it is nonsurgical and associated with fewer collateral arteries. In one study of HCC patients who had failed hepatic arterial chemotherapy, 6 of 9 patients responded to embolization (146). In Japan, 120 patients with HCC were treated with Gelfoam embolization, and 90% responded with 1-, 2-, and 3-year survival rates of 44%, 29%, and 15%, respectively (147).

Chemoembolization combines the tumor ischemia produced by embolization with prolonged high intratumoral concentrations of chemotherapy. This is accomplished by infusing embolizing microspheres that contain chemotherapeutic agents or a mixture of concentrated chemotherapy with an embolizing substance into the hepatic artery. In two studies, biodegradable albumin microspheres containing mitomycin C were used to embolize patients with HCC, and responses were observed in 7 of 7 patients and 15 of 20 patients (148, 149). In another study, chemoembolization with Gelfoam and doxorubicin, mitomycin C, and cisplatin produced responses in 12 of 50 (24%) patients and liquefaction necrosis in 70% of patients (150). Both embolization and chemoembolization are generally well tolerated, with liver pain, fever, and elevated liver function enzymes being the most prevalent adverse events. Rare cases of acute renal failure, necrosis of the bile ducts and/or gallbladder, and hemoperitoneum have been reported. Additionally, if the embolizing substance is inadvertently injected into an area other than the tumor capillary bed, necrosis of that region may result.

SECONDARY LIVER TUMORS

Metastases to the liver may occur from virtually any malignancy. Of all organs in the body, the liver is the most common site of blood-borne metastases. In an autopsy series of 9497 cancer patients, 8055 (84.8%) had metastatic disease, and 4444 (46.8%) had liver metastases (151). Liver metastases may be the only site of metastatic disease or part of a more widely metastatic process. Hepatic metastases occur most frequently in patients with primary tumors originating in organs drained by the portal vein, including tumors of the stomach, small intestine, colon, pancreas, gallbladder, and extrahepatic biliary tract. However, some malignancies such as breast cancer, lymphomas, testicular cancer, and ocular melanoma, which arise in organs having nonportal sources of venous drainage, are also associated with a high incidence of liver metastases.

The factors contributing to the high incidence of liver metastases in cancer patients are complex and not fully understood. On an ultrastructural level, the sinusoidal fenestrations of the liver may be more permeable to metastatic cells than the capillary endothelium of other organs. Further, the liver has relatively little connective tissue, which in other organs may act as a physical barrier to metastatic cells. From a physiologic standpoint, the liver, as the organ that filters the blood, may inherently be more efficient than other organs at removing metastatic cells from the blood. Lastly, in patients with tumors originating in organs drained by the portal circulation, the liver is the first organ encountered by the metastatic cells after their release into the bloodstream, and thus, is the organ presented with the highest burden of metastatic cells. The remainder of the discussion on liver metastases will focus on colorectal cancer since it is the most common tumor that metastasizes to the liver.

Colorectal Cancer Metastatic to the Liver

CLINICAL PRESENTATION

At the time of diagnosis, approximately 30 to 40% of patients with colorectal cancer have distant metastases. The liver is the most common site of metastatic involvement, followed by the lung. Often liver metastases are diagnosed incidentally during surgery in patients without antecedent signs or symptoms suggestive of hepatic involvement or during routine follow-up. The most frequent complaints in patients with symptomatic liver metastases include abdominal pain, abdominal distension, anorexia, weight loss, fatigue, jaundice, and/or unexplained fever.

DIAGNOSIS

The diagnosis of a patient suspected of having liver metastases generally proceeds from the physical exam, to laboratory tests, to radiographic imaging, and then to tissue biopsy. The most common finding on physical exam is hepatomegaly. In patients with advanced hepatic metastases, the tumor may occlude the bile duct, portal vein,

and/or inferior vena cava, resulting in jaundice, portal hypertension (ascites, esophogeal varices), and/or lower extremity edema, respectively.

Approximately 60% of patients with hepatic metastases have elevated levels of serum glutamic-pyruvate transaminase (SGPT), serum glutamic-oxaloacetic transaminase (SGOT), lactic dehydrogenase (LDH), and/or alkaline phosphatase (AP) (152). Additionally, serum bilirubin levels are often elevated in patients with advanced hepatic metastases. The greater the extent of liver involvement, the more likely these tests will be elevated. No single liver enzyme is superior to the others for detecting liver metastases. Although hepatic enzyme elevations are somewhat useful in identifying patients who may have liver metastases, elevations can occur in patients without liver metastases, and thus these tests lack specificity.

Another laboratory test that is helpful in diagnosing colorectal cancer is the carcinoembryonic antigen (CEA) level. CEA is a glycoprotein that is produced in small amounts by normal columnar epithelial cells (normal value less than 4 ng/ml). CEA is elevated in 60 to 80% of patients with colorectal cancer. Although colorectal cancer at any site may produce CEA, levels greater than 20 ng/ml are most frequently associated with liver metastases (153, 154). Approximately 70% of patients with colorectal cancer metastatic to the liver have elevated CEA levels (108). However, since CEA is elevated in a variety of other malignant and nonmalignant conditions, it lacks diagnostic specificity. Thus, its major role lies in screening patients for recurrent disease and monitoring patients known to have metastases who are receiving treatment: The CEA level tends to fall with tumor regression and to rise with disease progression.

Several radiographic techniques are helpful in diagnosing liver metastases (155, 156). Ultrasound is inexpensive and does not expose the patient to radiation. However, intestinal gas, excessive fat, and overlying ribs can interfere with imaging; thus, small lesions may be undetected. Radionuclide liver–spleen scanning using technetium sulfur colloid is easy to perform but is associated with high false-positive and false-negative results, is unable to image extrahepatic tumor, and often does not detect lesions smaller than 2 centimeters. Computerized tomography and magnetic resonance imaging are the two preferred radiographic techniques for detecting liver metastases. Although these methods are more expensive than ultrasound and radionuclide liver–spleen scanning, they more accurately detect small lesions, are more reproducible, and allow for the simultaneous imaging of the remainder of the abdomen.

Tissue biopsy to confirm the presence of liver metastases is usually unnecessary in colorectal cancer patients since data from the patient history, physical exam, laboratory tests, and radiographic studies are usually sufficient to make the diagnosis. If a tissue specimen is required to confirm the diagnosis, it may be obtained by percutaneous biopsy, peritoneoscopy with needle-directed biopsy, or open biopsy at laparotomy.

PROGNOSIS

In general, colorectal cancer metastatic to the liver carries a poor prognosis. By far, the most important prognostic factor is the resectability of the hepatic metastases. Surgical resection is the only potentially curative modality for liver metastases and should be performed whenever possible. The most important prognostic factor in patients with unresectable tumor is the extent of hepatic involvement (157). The survival in untreated patients ranges from 2 to 22 months (median of 8 to 10 months); those patients having the smallest amount of tumor survive the longest. Another important factor is the degree of histologic differentiation. Patients with well-differentiated tumors survive longer than those with poorly differentiated tumors (158). In addition, patients with a poor performance status, significant weight loss, low albumin level, ascites, elevated hepatic enzymes, and/or bilirubin level have a shortened survival.

TREATMENT

Several modalities have been employed either as single therapies or in combination in the treatment of colorectal cancer metastatic to the liver, including surgical resection, radiotherapy, hepatic arterial ligation, intravenous chemotherapy, and hepatic intraarterial chemotherapy. The following is a discussion of the results obtained with these treatments.

Surgical Resection. Surgical resection offers a potential cure for patients with colorectal cancer metastatic to the liver, and thus should be performed whenever removal of all the apparent metastatic disease can be safely accomplished. Unfortunately, this is feasible in only about 20% of

patients. The results with surgical resection of liver metastases from colorectal cancer are summarized in Table 81.9 (159–169). The operative mortality in these series ranges from 0 to 12%. The percentage of patients surviving 1 year, 3 years, and 5 years after resection is approximately 90, 45, and 30%, respectively. Patients with solitary metastases (162), those without extrahepatic disease (162), those who are female (162), those with synchronous metastases (compared with those who develop metachronous metastases) (164, 165), those with clear margins of resection (166), and those whose primary originated in the colon (compared to the rectum) (167) survive longer following resection. Recently, intraoperative ultrasound and radioimmunoguided surgery have been employed in an attempt to identify and resect inapparent hepatic tumor. The impact of these techniques is yet to be determined. Adjuvant chemotherapy is not routinely employed following the surgical removal of hepatic metastases from colorectal cancer, but results from a pilot study suggest that it may be beneficial (170).

Radiotherapy. External beam radiation plays a limited role in the management of liver metastases from colorectal cancer because of the liver's inherent radiosensitivity. As mentioned earlier, lifetime doses of greater than 3,000 rads are associated with a high incidence of radiation hepatitis (80). Fractionated doses of 1,800 to 2,400 rads can provide pain relief for patients with symptomatic metastases. However, external beam radiotherapy does not prolong survival (171). Additionally, radiotherapy has been used in combination with chemotherapy although it is unclear whether the outcome is superior to that obtained with chemotherapy alone (172).

Hepatic Arterial Ligation. As with HCC, ligation of the hepatic artery has been performed in patients with liver metastases from colorectal cancer in an attempt to produce tumor necrosis secondary to ischemia (173). Symptomatic improvement is observed in some patients following

Table 81.9.
Results of Surgical Resection for Colorectal Cancer Metastatic to the Liver

Author	Number of Patients	Operative Mortality (%)	Survival (%)			Reference
			1 year	3 year	5 year	
Marrow/1982	29	—	—	—	27	(159)
Rajpal/1982	34	11.8	84	42	—	(160)
Iwatsuki/1983	24	0	—	—	52	(161)
Adson/1984	141	4	—	—	25	(162)
Steele/1984	30	6.6	90	—	30	(163)
Fortner/1984	65	7	89	57	—	(164)
Nordlinger/1987	80	5	—	41	25	(165)
Hughes/1989	800	—	—	—	32	(166)
Adloff/1990	55	2	—	—	20	(167)
Petrelli/1991	62	8	—	—	28	(168)
van Ooijen/1992	118	7.6	—	—	21	(169)

hepatic arterial ligation, but it is usually transient. In addition, ligation of the hepatic artery prevents its future use for other liver-directed therapies, such as intraarterial chemotherapy.

Intravenous Chemotherapy. Systemic chemotherapy is of limited benefit in the treatment of patients with colorectal cancer metastatic to the liver (174). The agents possessing activity include 5-fluorouracil, mitomycin C, the nitrosoureas, methyl-CCNU and CCNU, and irenotecan (CPT-11). Intravenous 5-fluorouracil is the most commonly used agent, producing partial responses in approximately 15 to 20% of patients. Several dosage schedules have been employed, but none is significantly superior to the others (175). The most common side effects of intravenous 5-fluorouracil are nausea, vomiting, stomatitis, and myelosuppression. The cytotoxicity of 5-fluorouracil may be biochemically enhanced by the administration of leucovorin. Seven prospective randomized studies comparing 5-fluorouracil to 5-fluorouracil plus leucovorin have been conducted (176–182). Six of the studies have demonstrated a higher response rate, and two of the studies have shown a survival advantage for 5-fluorouracil plus leucovorin. As a result, 5-fluorouracil plus leucovorin has become the standard first-line systemic chemotherapy regimen. Other agents, such as phosphonacetyl-L-aspartic acid (PALA) and alpha-interferon, have also been given with 5-fluorouracil in an attempt to enhance its activity, but none has improved on the results achieved with 5-fluorouracil and leucovorin. Mitomycin C administered in doses of 10 to 15 mg/m^2 every 6 to 8 weeks also produces partial responses in about 15 to 20% of patients. However, cumulative myelosuppression and fatigue makes continued administration difficult (174); thus, mitomycin C is usually reserved for patients who have failed 5-fluorouracil. Although methyl-CCNU has activity similar to 5-fluorouracil and mitomycin C, it has been removed from the market in the United States because of its excessive toxicity (183). The experience with CCNU in the management of metastatic colorectal cancer is limited, but these agents probably have similar activity to that of methyl-CCNU. Irenotecan (CPT-11), an investigational campthothecan derivative, also appears to have activity against colorectal cancer (184). Unfortunately, combination chemotherapy has not improved on the limited activity seen with single agents.

Hepatic Intraarterial Chemotherapy. Hepatic intraarterial chemotherapy has been widely used in the treatment of colorectal cancer metastatic to the liver. (For a complete discussion of the rationale of intraarterial chemotherapy, see the section "Intraarterial Chemotherapy".) Table 81.10 summarizes the phase II results with single-agent hepatic intraarterial chemotherapy. The most commonly administered agent has been floxuridine, in part because it is available in a convenient formulation for usage in the implantable pump. It has produced partial responses ranging from

Table 81.10.

Results of Single-Agent Intraarterial Chemotherapy for Colorectal Cancer Metastatic to the Liver

Drug	Number of Patients	Response Rate (%)	Median Survival (months)	Reference
Floxuridine	81	88	26	(185)
	93	80	20	(186)
	77	83	13	(187)
	17	29	13	(188)
	24	73	22	(189)
	41	37	—	(190)
	14	36	—	(191)
5-Fluorouracil	52	67	—	(193)
	369	55	—	(194)
	24	50	9	(195)
	30	34	10	(196)
	30	57	11.9	(197)

Table 81.11.

Results of Combination Intraarterial Chemotherapy for Colorectal Cancer Metastatic to the Liver

Drugs	Number of Patients	Response Rate	Median Survival (months)	Reference
Floxuridine & 5-fluorouracil	52	81	—	(162)
	48	54	—	(198)
	64	50	22	(199)
Floxuridine & mitomycin C	12	83	15	(200)
	40	20	14	(201)
Floxuridine & dichloromethotrexate	13	69	20	(201)
5-Fluorouracil & mitomycin C	20	55	8	(202)
	30	50	11	(203)
Floxuridine & cisplatin & mitomycin	29	52	12	(204)
Floxuridine & mitomycin C & BCNU	36	70	12	(205)
5-Fluorouracil & adriamycin & mitomycin	23	35	22	(206)
Floxuridine & mitomycin & carmustine	46	47	19	(207)

29 to 88% of patients and median survival ranging from 13 to 26 months (185–191). In an attempt to further augment the activity of intraarterial floxuridine, the addition of intraarterial leucovorin was studied, but the regimen produced prohibitive hepatobiliary toxicity (192). A phase II study is currently being conducted that evaluates intraarterial floxuridine, leucovorin, and dexamethasone, with the dexamethasone being added in an attempt to diminish the hepatobiliary toxicity. 5-Fluorouracil has also been administered by hepatic intraarterial infusion with response rates

Table 81.12.

Results of Randomized Trials Comparing Intravenous to Hepatic Intraarterial Chemotherapy for Colorectal Cancer Metastatic to the Liver

Author	Number of Patients	Response Rate (%)		Survival (months)		Reference
		IV	IA	IV	IA	
Kemeny/1987	99	20	50	12	17	(208)
Hohn/1989	143	10	42	16	16.5	(209)
Chang/1987	64	17	62	11	16	(210)
Martin/1990	69	21	48	10.5	12.6	(211)
Rougier/1992	166	9	43	11	15	(212)
Mersh/1994	100	—	—	6.6	13.5	(213)

ranging from 34 to 67% and median survival of 9 to 12 months (193–198). The lower solubility of 5-fluorouracil (relative to floxuridine) prevents its use in the implantable pump, thus an external pump and a radiographically placed percutaneous catheter are required to administer the drug by continuous infusion.

To improve on the results obtained with single-agent intraarterial chemotherapy, various combination regimens have been investigated (Table 81.11). Unfortunately, the results have been similar to those obtained with single-agent intraarterial therapy, with the response rates ranging from 20 to 83%, and the median survival times from 8 to 22 months (162, 198–207). However, one combination regimen using alternating floxuridine and 5-fluorouracil may offer an advantage over other regimens since it appears to be associated with fewer side effects (199).

Six randomized trials have been conducted comparing hepatic intraarterial floxuridine with systemic chemotherapy or no treatment (Table 81.12) (208–213). All studies reported a statistically significant higher response rate in the patients treated with intraarterial therapy, and two of the studies reported a survival benefit (212, 213). The two largest studies (208, 209), both of which did not demonstrate a survival advantage for intraarterial therapy, allowed patients on the intravenous arm to receive intraarterial therapy at the time of hepatic tumor progression, thus confounding the survival analyses.

CONCLUSION

Liver tumors are a diverse group of benign and malignant tumors comprising primary tumors, which arise from the hepatobiliary system, and secondary tumors, which metastasize to the liver from neoplasms elsewhere in the body. The most prevalent primary malignancy of the liver is hepatocellular carcinoma, also referred to as hepatoma, and the most common cause of hepatic metastases is colorectal cancer. Complete surgical removal by resection or, for primary malignant tumors, liver transplantation offers a potential for cure of malignant liver tumors. Unfortunately, surgical removal is feasible in only about 10 to 15% of

patients, and of those patients, only about 30% are cured. Cryosurgery and percutaneous alcohol injection are two investigational modalities that may be useful in patients with resectable disease who are not candidates for surgical removal because of underlying liver disease, such as cirrhosis. Several therapies have been used to treat unresectable malignant liver tumors. Radiotherapy has been used, but it is of limited benefit because of the inherent intolerance of the normal hepatic parenchyma to radiation. Systemic chemotherapy has been used, but it produces responses in only 15 to 35% of patients. In patients having liver-predominant disease, more encouraging results have been obtained with liver-directed therapies such as hepatic intraarterial chemotherapy with or without Lipiodol and chemoembolization. Further research is required to develop more efficacious therapies for liver tumors.

REFERENCES

1. Bierman HR, Byron RL Jr, Kelly LH, Grady A. Studies on the blood supply of tumors in man: III. Vascular patterns of the liver by hepatic arteriography in vivo. JNCL 12:107–227, 1951.
2. Yohannan MD, Abdulla AM, Patel PJ. Neonatal hepatic hemangioendothelioma: presentation with jaundice and microangiopathic hemolytic anemia. European Journal of Pediatrics. 149:804–805, 1990.
3. Nguyen L, Shandling B, Ein S, Stephens C. Hepatic hemangiomas in childhood: Medical management or surgical management? J Pediatr Surg 17:576–579, 1982.
4. Hobbs KE. Hepatic hemangiomas: World J Surg 14:468–471, 1990.
5. Lise M, Feltrin G, Da Pian PP, Miotto D, Pilati PL, Rubaltelli L, Zane D. Giant cavernous hemangiomas: diagnosis and surgical strategies. World J Surg 16(3):516–520, 1992.
6. Nichols FC, van Heerden JA, Weiland LH. Benign liver tumors. Surg Clin North Am 69:297–314, 1989.
7. Gordon SC, Reddy KR, Livingstone AS, et al. Resolution of a contraceptive-steriod-induced hepatic adenoma with subsequent evolution into hepatocellular carcinoma. Ann Intern Med 105:547–549, 1986.
8. Wanless JR, Mawdsley C, Adams R. On the pathogenesis of focal nodular hyperplasia of the liver. Hepatology, 5:1194–1200, 1985.
9. Landen S, Siriser F, Bardoxoglou E, Maddern GJ, Careton B, Campion JP, Launois B. Focal nodular hyperplasia of the liver. A retrospective review of 20 patients managed surgically. Acta Chir Belg 93(3):94–97, 1993.

10. Takayama T, Makuuchi M, Takayasu K, et al. Resection after intra-arterial chemotherapy of a hepatoblastoma originating in the caudate lobe. Surgery 107:231–235, 1990.

11. Evans AE, Land VJ, Newton WA, et al. Combination chemotherapy (vincristine, Adriamycin, cyclophosphamide, 5-fluorouracil) in the treatment of children with hepatoblastoma. Cancer 50:821–826, 1982.

12. Tan Am, Tan CL, Phua KB, et al. Chemotherapy for hepatoblastoma in children. Ann Acad Med Singapore 19:286–289, 1990.

13. Ortega JA, Douglass E, Feusner J, et al. A randomized trial of cisplatin/vincristine/5-fluorouracil vs cisplatin/doxorubicin IV continuous infusion for the treatment of hepatoblastoma. Results from the pediatric intergroup Hepatoma Study. Proc Am Soc Clin Oncol 13:416, 1994.

14. Penn I. Hepatic transplantation for primary and metastatic cancer of the liver. Surgery 110:726–735, 1991.

15. Harvey JH, Smith FP, Schein PS. 5-Fluorouracil, mitomycin, and doxorubicin (FAM) in carcinoma of the biliary tract. J Clin Oncol 2:1245–1248, 1984.

16. Smith GW, Bukowski RM, Hewlett JS, Groppe CW. Hepatic artery infusion of 5-fluorouracil and mitomycin C in cholangio-carcinoma and gallbladder carcinoma. Cancer 54:1513–1516, 1984.

17. Locker GY, Doroshow JG, Zwelling LA, et al. The clinical features of hepatic angiosarcoma—A report of four cases and a review of the English literature. Medicine 58:48–64, 1979.

18. Azodo MV, Gutierrez OH, Greer T. Thorotrast-induced ruptured hepatic angiosarcoma. Abdom Imaging 18:78–81, 1993.

19. Dean PJ, Haggett RC, O'Hara CJ. Malignant epithelioid hemangioendothelioma of the liver in young women. Relationship to oral contraceptive use. Am J Surg Path 9:695–704, 1985.

20. Walker NI, Horn MJ, Strong RW, Lynch SV, Cohen J, Ong TH, Harris OD. Undifferentiated (embryonal) sarcoma of the liver. Pathologic findings and long-term survival after complete surgical resection. Cancer 69:52–59, 1992.

21. Boring C, Squeres T, Tong T. Cancer Statistics—1992. CA:A J for Clinicians 42:19–38, 1992.

22. Moertel CG. The liver. In Holland JF, Frei E III (eds): Cancer Medicine, pp 1541–1547. Philadelphia, Lea & Febiger, 1973.

23. Popper G, Gerber MA, Thung SN. The relation of hepatocellular carcinoma to infection with hepatitis B and related viruses in man and animals. Hepatology 2:1S–9S, 1982.

24. Zala G, Havelka J, Altorfer J, Joller-Jemelka HJ, Risti B, Meier B, Schmid M, Buhler H. Hepatitis C and hepatoma. Schweiz Me Wochenschr 122:194–197, 1992.

25. Hassan F, Jeffers LJ, De Medina M, et al. Hepatitis C-associated hepatocellular carcinoma: Hepatology 12:589–591, 1990.

26. Kiyosawa K, Sodeyama T, Tanaka E, et al. Interrelationship of blood transfusion, non-A non-B hepatitis and hepatocellular carcinoma: analysis by detection of antibody to hepatitis C virus. Hepatology 12:671–675, 1990.

27. Gerbes AL, Caselmann WH. Point mutations of the p53 gene, human hepatocellular carcinoma and aflatoxins. J Hepatol 19:312–315, 1993.

28. Palmer JR, Rosenberg L, Kaufmann DW, et al. Oral contraceptive use and liver cancer. Am J Epidemiol 130:878–882, 1989.

29. Farrell GC, Uren RF, Perkins RW, Joshua DE, Baird PJ, Kronenberg H. Androgen induced hepatoma. Lancet 1:430–431, 1975.

30. Okuda K, Musha H, Nakajima Y, et al. Clinicopathologic features of encapsulated hepatocellular carcinoma: a study of 26 cases. Cancer 40:1240–1245, 1977.

31. Ruffin MT. Fibrolamellar hepatoma. Am J Gastroenterol 85:577–581, 1990.

32. Waldmann TA, McIntire KR. The use of radioimmunoassay for alpha-fetoprotein in the diagnosis of malignancy. Cancer 34:1510–1515, 1974.

33. Okuda K, Ohtsuki T, Obata H. Natural history of hepatocellular carcinoma and prognosis in relation to treatment. Study of 850 patients. Cancer 56:918–928, 1985.

34. Salminen PM, Hockerstedt K, Edgren J, et al. Intraoperative ultrasound as an aid to surgical strategy in liver tumors. Acta Chir Scand 156:329–332, 1990.

35. Okuda K and The Liver Tumor Study Group of Japan. Primary liver cancers in Japan. Cancer 45:2663–2669, 1980.

36. Xu ZY, Liu CB, Francis DP, et al. Prevention of perinatal acquistion of hepatitis B virus carriage using vaccine: Preliminary report of a randomized, double-blind placebo-controlled and comparative trial. Pediatrics 76:713–718, 1985.

37. Sun ZT, Zhu Y, Stjernsward, et al. Design and compliance of HBV vaccination trial on newborns to prevent hepatocellular carcinoma and 5-year results of its pilot study. Cancer Detect Prev 15:313–318, 1991.

38. Fortuin M, Chotard J, Jack AD, et al. Efficacy of hepatitis B vaccine in the Gambian expanded programme on immunization. Lancet 341:1129–1131, 1993.

39. Ginsburg GM, Shouval D. Cost benefit analysis of a nation-wide neonatal inoculation programme against hepatitis B in an area of intermediate endemicity. J Epidemiol Commun Health 46:587–594, 1992.

40. Lok ASF, Lai CL. Alpha-fetoprotein monitoring in Chinese patients with chronic hepatitis B virus infection: Role in the early detection of hepatocellular carcinoma. Hepatology 9:110–115, 1989.

41. Tremolda F, Benevegnu L, Drago C, et al. Early detection of hepatocellular carcinoma in patients with cirrhosis by alpha-fetoprotein, ultrasound, and fine-needle biopsy. Hepatogastroenterology 36:519–521, 1989.

42. Colombo M, De Franchis R, Del Ninno E, et al. Hepatocellular carcinoma in Italian patients with cirrhosis. N Engl J Med 325:675–680, 1991.

43. Regan LS. Screening for hepatocellular carcinoma in high risk individuals. Arch Intern Med 149:1741–1744, 1989.

44. McMahon BJ, London T. Workshop on screening for hepatocellularcarcinoma. J Natl Cancer Inst 83:916–919, 1991.

45. Dodd GD, Miller WJ, Baron RL, et al. Detection of malignant tumors in end-stage cirrhotic livers: Efficacy of sonography as a screening technique. Am J Roentgenol 159:727–733, 1992.

46. Adson MA, Weiland LH. Resection of primary solid hepatic tumors. Am J Surg 141:18–21, 1981.

47. Huguet C, Nordlinger B, Vacher B, Parc R, Halami F, Loygue J. Surgical resection of hepatocellular carcinoma. Retrospective study of 42 cases. Gastroenterol Clin Biol 9:244–249, 1985.

48. Nagao T, Inque S, Gato S, et al. Hepatic resection for hepatocellular carcinoma. Ann Surg 205:33–40, 1987.

49. Lin TY, Lee CS, Chen KM, et al. Role of surgery in the treatment of primary carcinoma of the liver: a 31 year experience. Br J Surg 74:839–842, 1987.

50. Chen MF, Hwang TL, Jeng CB, et al. Hepatic resection in 120 patients with hepatocellular carcinoma. Arch Surg 124:1025–1028, 1989.

51. Toshihara T, Sugioka A, Veda M, et al. Hepatic resection for hepatocellular carcinoma. Surgery 107:551–560, 1990.

52. Choi TK, Edward CS, Fan ST, et al. Results of surgical resection for hepatocellular carcinoma. Hepatogastroenterology 37:172–173, 1990.

53. Yamanaka N, Okamoto, E, Toyosaka A, et al. Prognostic factors after hepatectomy for hepatocellular carcinoma. Hepatogastroenterology 37:172–173, 1990.

54. Kobayashi N, Kumada K, Yamaoka Y, et al. The outcomes of the operated hepatocellular carcinoma patients. Nippon Geka Hokan 59:369–376, 1990.

55. Tsuzuki T, Sugioka A, Ueda M, et al. Hepatic resection for hepatocellular carcinoma. Surgery 107:511–520, 1990.

56. Iwatsuki S, Starzl TW, Sheahan DG, et al. Hepatic resection versus transplantation for hepatocellular carcinoma. Ann Surg 214:221–229, 1991.

57. Gozzetti G, Mazziotti A, Grazi GL, et al. Surgical experience with 168 primary liver cell carcinomas treated with hepatic resection. J Surg Oncol 3:59–61, 1993 (Suppl).

58. Kawarada Y, Ito F, Sakurai H, et al. Surgical treatment of hepatocellular carcinoma. Cancer Chemother Pharmacol 33:S7–12, 1994.

59. Sitzmann JV, Abrams R. Improved survival for hepatocellular cancer with combination surgery and multimodality treatment. Ann Surg 217:149–154, 1993.

60. Nakashima K, Kim Y, Okada K, Iwao Y, Aramaki M, Kobyashi M, Aikawa H, Suzuki K. Prophylactic chemotherapy by regional arterial infusion in resected hepatoma patients. Gan To Kagaku Ryoho 19:1489–1492, 1992 (Suppl).

61. Ravikumar TS, Steele GS. Hepatic cryosurgery. Surg Clin North Am 69:433–440, 1989.

62. Zhou XD, Tnag ZY, Yu YQ, et al. Clinical evaluation of cryosurgery in the treatment of primary liver cancer. Cancer 61:1889–1892, 1988.

63. Hang CE, Jenkins RL, Rohrer RJ, et al. Liver transplantation for hepatic primary hepatic cancer. Transplantation 53:376–382, 1992.

64. Venook AP. Liver transplantation for primary hepatobiliary malignancy. Semin Gastrointestinal Dis 4:178–183, 1993.

65. Bismuth H, Ericzon BG, Rolles K, et al. Hepatic transplantation in Europe. Lancet 2:674–676, 1987.

66. Iwatsuki S, Gorden RD, Shaw BW, et al. Role of liver transplantation in cancer therapy. Ann Surg 202:401–407, 1985.

67. Jenkins RL, Pinson CW, Stone MD. Experience with transplantation in the treatment of liver cancer. Cancer Chemother Pharmacol 23:S104–S109, 1989 (Suppl).

68. O'Grady JG, Polson RJ, Rolles K, et al. Liver transplantation for malignant disease. Ann Surg 207:373–379, 1988.

69. Ringe B, Wittekind C, Bechstein WO, et al. The role of liver transplantation in hepatobiliary malignancy. Ann Surg 209:88–98.

70. Olthoff KM, Millis JM, Rosove MH, et al. Is liver transplantation justified for the treatment of hepatic malignancies? Arch Surg 125:1261–1268, 1990.

71. Pichlmayr R. Can liver transplantation be applied for the treatment of liver cancer? Jpn J Surg 22:187–190, 1992.

72. Bismuth H, Chiche L, Adam R, et al. Liver resection versus transplantation for hepatocellular carcinoma in cirrhotic patients. Ann Surg 218:145–151, 1993.

73. Starzl TE, Iwatsuki S, Shaw BW, et al. Treatment of fibrolamellar hepatoma with partial or total hepatectomy and transplantation of the liver. Surg Gynecol Obstet 162:145–148, 1986.

74. Ringe B, Wittekind C, Weimann A. et al. Results of hepatic resection and transplantation for fibrolamellar carcinoma. Surg Gynecol Obstet 17 5:299–305, 1992.

75. Stone MJ, Klintmalm GBG, Polter D, et al. Neoadjuvant chemotherapy and liver transplantation for hepatocellular carcinoma: A pilot study in 20 patients. Gastroenterology 104:196–202, 1993.

76. Carr BI, Selby R, Madariaga J, et al. Prolonged survival after liver transplantation and cancer chemotherapy for advanced stage hepatocellular carcinoma. Transplant Proc 25:1128–1129, 1993.

77. Venook AP, Lake JR, Robert JP, et al. Orthrotopic liver transplantation (OLT) in patients with hepatocellular carcinoma (HCC): Results using preoperative chemoembolization. Hepatology 16:45A, 1992 (abstr 4).

78. Shiina S, Hamada E, Yoshirura K, et al. Percutaneous ethanol injection therapy for hepatocellular carcinoma: Analysis of 146 patients. ProcAm Soc Clin Oncol 11:352, 1992.

79. Livraghi T, Bolondi L, Lazzaroni S, et al. Percutaneous ethanol injection in the treatment of hepatocellular carcinoma in cirrhosis. Cancer 69:925–929, 1992.

80. Ingold JA, Reed GB, Kaplan HS, Bagshw MA. Radiation hepatitis. Am J Roentgenol 93:200–208, 1965.

81. Phillips R, Murikama K. Primary neoplasms of the liver. Results of radiation therapy. Cancer 4:714–720, 1960.

82. Lawrence TS, Tesser RJ, Ten Haken RK. An application of dose volume histograms to the treatment of intrahepatic malignancies with radiation therapy. Int J Radiat Oncol Biol Phys 20:555–561, 1991.

83. Robertson JM, Lawrence TS, Dworzanin LM, et al. Treatment of primary hepatobiliary cancers with conformal radiation therapy and regional chemotherapy. J Clin Oncol 11:1286–1293, 1993.

84. Order S, Pajak T, Leibel S, et al. A randomized prospective trial comparing full dose chemotherapy to 131 I antiferitin: An RTOG study. Int J Radiat Oncol Biol Phys 20:953–963, 1991.

85. Wollner I, Knutsen C, Smith P, et al. Effects of hepatic arterial yttrium 90 glass microspheres in dogs. Cancer 61:1336–1344, 1988.

86. Leung WT, Lau WY, HO S, et al. Selective internal radiation therapy with intra-arterial 131-Iodine-Lipiodol in inoperable hepatocellular carcinoma. Proc Am Soc Clin Oncol 13:202, 1994.

87. Friedman MA, Demanes DJ, Hoffman PG. Hepatomas: Hormone receptors and therapy. Am J Med 73:362–366, 1982.

88. Paliard P, Clement G, Saez S, Chabel J, Partensky C. Treatment of hepatocellular carcinoma with tamoxifen(letter). Gastroenterol Clin Biol 8:680–681, 1984.

89. Chao Y, Wu M, Liu Y, et al. Treatment of hepatocellular carcinoma with Megace. Proc Am Soc Clin Oncol 12:205, 1993.

90. Vogel CL, Bayley AC, Brockes RJ. A phase II study of adriamycin in patients with hepatocellular carcinoma from Zambia and the United States. Cancer 39:1923–1929, 1977.

91. Johnson PJ, Williams R, Thomas H, Sherlock S, Murray-Lyon IM. Induction of remission in hepatocellular carcinoma with doxorubicin. Lancet 1:1006–1009, 1978.

92. Falkson G, Lavin P, Moertel CG, Pretorious FJ, Carbone PP. Chemotherapy studies in primary liver cancer: A prospective randomized clinical trial. Cancer 42:2149–2156, 1978.

93. Olweny CLM, Katongole-Mbidde E, Bahendeka S, Otim D, Mugerwa J, Kyalwazi SK. Further experience in treating patients with hepatocellular carcinoma in Uganda. Cancer 46:2717–2722, 1980.

94. Melia WM, Johnson PJ, Williams R. Induction remission in hepatocellular carcinoma: a comparison of VP-16 with adriamycin. Cancer 51:206–210, 1983.

95. Yang P, Sheu J, Chen D, et al. Systemic chemotherapy of hepatocellular carcinoma with adriamycin alone and FAM regimen. In Chemotherapy of Hepatic Tumors. Tokyo, Excerpta Medica, 1984, 41–47.

96. Chlebowski RT, Brezechwa-Asjukiewicz A, Cowdon A, et al. Doxorubicin for hepatocellular carcinoma: clinical and pharmacokinetic results. Cancer Treat Rep 68:487–491, 1984.

97. Choi TK, Lee NW, Wong J, et al. Chemotherapy for advanced hepatocellular carcinoma: clinical and pharmacokinetic results. Cancer Treat Rep 68:487–491, 1984.

98. Sciarrino E, Simonetti RG, Moli SL, et al. Adriamycin treatment for hepatocellular carcinoma: experience with 109 patients. Cancer 56:2751–2755, 1985.

99. Dunk AA, Scott SC, Johnson PJ, et al. Mitoxantrone as single agent therapy in hepatocellular carcinoma: a phase II study. J Hepatol 1:395–404, 1985.

100. Lai KH, Tsai YT, Lee SD, et al. Phase II study of mitoxantrone in unresectable primary hepatocellular carcinoma following hepatitis B infection. Cancer Chermother Pharmacol 23:54–56, 1989.

101. Hochester HS, Green MD, Speyer J, et al. 4'Epidoxorubicin (epirubicin) activity in hepatocellular carcinoma. J Clin Oncol 3:1525–1540, 1985.

102. Tan YO, Lim F. 4'-Epidoxorubicin as a single agent in advanced primary hepatocellular carcinoma—a preliminary experience. Ann Acad Med Singapore 15:169–171, 1986.

103. Shiu W, Leung N, Li M, et al. The efficacy of high dose 4'-epidoxorubicin in hepatocellular carcinoma. Jpn J Clin Oncol 18:235–237, 1988.

104. Kennedy PS, Lehane DE, Smith FE, Lane M. Oral fluorouracil therapy of hepatoma. Cancer 39:1930–1935, 1977.

105. Link JS, Bateman JR, Paroly WS, Durkin WJ, Peters RL. 5-Fluorouracil in hepatocellular carcinoma: Report of 21 cases. Cancer 39:1936–1939, 1977.

106. Davis HL, Ramirez H, Ansfield FJ. Adenocarcinomas of the stomach, pancreas, liver, and biliary tracts: Survival of 328 patients treated with fluoropyrimidine therapy. Cancer 33:193–197, 1974.

107. Al-Sarraf M, Go TS, Kithier K, Vaitkevicius VK. Primary liver cancer: A review of the clinical features, blood groups, serum enzymes, therapy and survival of 65 cases. Cancer 33:574–582, 1974.

108. Bukowski RM, Legna S, Saidi J, Eyre HJ, O'Bryan R. Phase II trial of M-AMSA in hepatocellular carcinoma: A Southwest Oncology Group Study. Cancer Treat Rep 66:1651–1652, 1982.

109. Cheng E, Lightdale C, Young C, Yagoda A, Fortner J, Golbey R. Phase II trial of (m-AMSA) 4'-9 (acridinylamino)-methane-sulfon-m-aniside in primary liver cancer. Am Clin Oncol 6:211–213, 1983.

110. Amrein PC, Richards F, Coleman M, et al. Phase II trial of Amsacrine in patients with hepatoma: a Cancer and Leukemia Group B study. Can Treat Rep 68:923–924, 1984.

111. Falkson G, Coetzer B, Klaasen DJ. A phase II study of m-AMSA in patients with primary liver cancer. Cancer Chemother Pharmacol 8:305–310, 1982.

112. Vogel CL, Adamson RH, DeVita VT, Johns DG, Kyalwazi SK. Preliminary clinical trials of dichloromethotrexate (NSC-29630) in hepatocellular carcinoma. Cancer Chemother Rep 56:249–258, 1972.

113. Tester WJ, Donehower RS, Eddy JL, Myers CE, Ihde DC. Evaluation of weekly escalating doses of dichloromethotrexate in patients with hepatocellular carcinoma and other solid tumors. Cancer Chemother Pharmacol 8:305–310, 1982.

114. Cavalli F, Rosencweig M, Renard J, Goldhirsch A, Hansen HH. A phase II study of oral VP-16-213 in patients with hepatocellular carcinoma. Proc Am Soc Clin Oncol 22:457, 1981.

115. Melia WM, Westaby D, Williams R. Diaminodichloride platinum(cis-platinum) in treatment of hepatocellular carcinoma. Clin Oncol 7:275–280, 1981.

116. Okada S, Okazaki N, Nose H, et al. A phase 2 study of cisplatin in patients with hepatocellular carcinoma. Oncology 50:22–26, 1993.

117. Anon. A prospective trial of recombinant human interferon 2B in previously untreated patients with hepatocellular carcinoma—The Gastrointestinal Tumor Study Group. Cancer 66:135–139, 1990.

118. Lai LL, Wu PL, Lok AS, et al. Recombinant alpha-2-interferon is superior to doxorubicin for inoperable hepatocellular carcinoma: a prospective randomized trial. J Pharmacokinet Biopharm 2:257–285, 1974.

119. Eckman WW, Patlak CS, Fenstermacher JD. A critical evaluation of the principles governing the advantages of intra-arterial infusions. J Pharmaco Biopharm 2:257–285, 1974.

120. Chen HG, Gross JF. Intra-arterial infusion of anticancer drugs: Theoretical aspects of drug delivery and review of responses. Cancer Treat Rep 64:31–40, 1980.

121. Ensminger WS, Rosowsky A, Raso V, et al. A clinical pharmacologic evaluation of hepatic arterial infusions of 5-fluoro-2'-deoxyuridine and 5-fluorouracil. Cancer Res 38:3784–3792, 1978.

122. Garnick MB, Ensminger WD, Israel M. A clinical pharmacologic evaluation of hepatic arterial infusion of adriamycin. Cancer Res 39:4105–4110, 1979.

123. Fraile RJ, Baker LH, Buroker TR, Horwitz J Vaitkevicius VK. Pharmacokinetics of 5-fluorouracil administered orally, by rapid intravenous and by slow infusion. Cancer Res 40:2223–2228, 1980.

124. Ensminger W, Stetson P, Gyves J, et al. Dependence of hepatic arterial fluorouracil pharmacokinetics on dose, route and duration of infusion. Proc Am Soc Clin Oncol 2:25, 1983.

125. Campbell TN, Howell SB, Pfeifle CE, Wung WE, Bookstein J. Clinical pharmacokinetics of intraarterial cisplatin in humans. J Clin Oncol 12:755–762, 1983.

126. Gyves JL, Ensminger W, Stetson P, et al. Clinical pharmacology of mitomycin C by hepatic arterial infusion. Proc Am Soc Clin Oncol 2:25, 1983.

127. Wellwood JM, Cady B, Oberfield RA. Treatment of primary liver cancer: Response on regional chemotherapy. Clin Oncol 5:25–31, 1979.

128. Ludwig J, Kim CH, Wiesner RH, Krom RA. Floxuridine-Induced Sclerosing Cholangitis: An ischemic cholangiopathy. Hepatology 9(2):215–219, 1989.

129. Doci A, Bignami P, Bozzetti F, et al. Intrahepatic chemotherapy for unresectable hepatocellular carcinoma. Cancer 61:1983–1987, 1979.

130. Bern MM, McDermott W, Cady B. Intraarterial hepatic infusion and intravenous adriamycin for treatment of hepatocellular carcinoma: A clinical and pharmacology report. Cancer 42:399–406, 1978.

131. Urist MM, Balch CM. Intra-arterial chemotherapy for hepatoma using adriamycin administered via an implantable infusion pump. Proc Am Soc Clin Oncol 3:146, 1983.

132. Shepherd FA, Evans WK, Fine S, Blackstein ME, Mullis B. Hepatic arterial infusion of mitoxantrone and adriamycin in the treatment of primary hepatocellular carcinoma. Proc Am Soc Clin Oncol 4:95, 1985.

133. Ukeda H, Kuroda S, Ohnoshi T, et al. Intra-arterial adriamycin for patients with hepatocellular carcinoma and metastatic carcinoma. Gan To Kagaka Ryoho 11:2579–2584, 1984.

134. Cheng E, Watson RC, Fortner J, Kemeny N, Golbey R. Regional intraarterial infusion of cisplatin in primary liver cancer. Proc Am Soc Clin Oncol 1:179, 1982.

135. Shepherd FA, Evan WK, Blackstein ME, et al. Hepatic artery infusion of mitoxantrone in the treatment of primary hepatocellular carcinoma. J Clin Oncol 5:635–640, 1987.

136. Douglas CC. Prolongation of survial with periodic percutaneous multidrug arterial infusions in patients with primary and metastatic gastrointestinal carcinoma to the liver. Proc Am Soc Clin Oncol 21:416, 1980.

137. Patt YZ, Chuang VP, Wallace S, Benjamin RS, Fuqua R, Mavligit GM. Hepatic artery chemotherapy and occlusion for palliation of primary hepatocellular and unknown primary neoplasms in the liver. Cancer 51:1359–1363, 1983.

138. Patt YZ, Charnsangavej C, Lawrence D, et al. Hepatic arterial infusion for FUDR, leucovorin, adriamycin, and platinol: Effective palliation for nonresectable hepatocellular carcinoma. Proc Am Soc Clin Oncol 11:165, 1992.

139. Kanematsu T, Matsumata T, Furuta T, et al. Lipiodol drug targeting in the treatment of primary hepatocellular carcinoma. Hepatogastroenterology 37:442–444, 1990.

140. Carr B, Iwatsuki S, Baron R. Intrahepatic arterial cisplatinum and doxorubicin with or without Lipiodol for advanced hepatocellular carcinoma (HCC): A prospective randomized study. Proc Am Soc Clin Oncol 12:219, 1993.

141. Lee YT, Irwin L. Hepatic artery ligation and adriamycin infusion chemotherapy for hepatoma. Cancer 41:12459–12555, 1978.

142. Nagasue N, Inokuchi K, Kobayashi M, Saku M. Serum alpha-fetoprotein levels after hepatic artery ligation and post-operative chemotherapy: Correlation with clinical status in patients with hepatocellular carcinoma. Cancer 40:615–618, 1977.

143. Charnsangavej C, Chuang VP, Wallace S, Soo CS, Bowers T. Angiographic classification of hepatic arterial collaterals. Radiol 144:485–494, 1982.

144. Chearanai O, Plengvanit U, Asavanich C, Damrongsak D, Sindhvananda K, Boonyapisit S. Spontaneous rupture of primary hepatoma: report of 63 cases with particular reference to the pathogenesis and rationale treatment by hepatic artery ligation. Cancer 51:1532–1536, 1983.

145. Soyer P, Levesque M, Zeittoun G, Hassen CS. Hemoperitoneum caused spontaneous rupture of hepatocellular carcinoma. Role of hepatic artery embolization in the therapeutic procedure. J Radiol 72:287–290, 1991.

146. Wallace S, Charnsangavej C, Carrasco H, Bechtel W. Infusion-Embolization. Cancer 54:2751–2765, 1984.

147. Yamada R, Sato M, Kawabata M, et al. Hepatic artery embolization in 120 patients with unresectable hepatoma. Radiology 148:397–401, 1983.

148. Fujimoto S, Miyazaki M, Endoh F, Takahashi O, Okui K, Morimoto Y. Biodegradable mitomycin C microspheres given intra-arterially for operable hepatic cancer. Cancer 56:2404–2410, 1985.

149. Ohnishi K, Tsuchiya S, Nakayama T, et al. Arterial chemoembolization of hepatocellular carcinoma with mitomycin C microcapsules. Radiology 152:51–55, 1984.

150. Venook A, Stagg R, Lewis B, et al. Chemoembolization for hepatocellular carcinoma. J Clin Oncol 8:1108–1114, 1990.

151. Weiss L, Gilbert HA (eds). Liver Metastases. Boston MA: GK Hall Medical Publishing, 1982.

152. Beck PR, Belfield A, Spooner RJ, Blumgart LH, Wood CB. Serum enzyme elevations in colorectal cancer. Cancer 43:1772–1776, 1979.

153. Kemeny MM, Sugarbaker PH, Smith TJ, et al. A prospective analysis of laboratory tests and imaging studies to detect hepatic lesions. Ann Surg 195:163–167, 1982.

154. Szymendera JJ, Nowacki MP, Szawlowski AW, Kaminska JA. Predictive value of plasma CEA levels: Preoperative and postoperative monitoring of patients with colorectal carcinoma. Dis Col Rect 25:46–52, 1982.

155. Funven P, Makuuchi M, Takayasu K, Moriyama N, Yamasaki S, Hasegawa H. Preoperative imaging of liver metastases. Comparison of angiography, CT scan, and ultrasound. Ann Surg 202:573–579, 1985.

156. Schreve RH, Terpstra OT, Ausema L, Lameris JS, van Seijen AJ, Jeekel J. Detection liver metastases. A prospective study comparing liver enzymes, scintigraphy, ultrasonography, and computed tomography. Br J Surg 71: 947–949, 1984.

157. Pettavel J, Morgenthaler F. Protracted arterial chemotherapy of liver tumors: an experience of 107 cases over a 12-year period. Prog Clin Cancer 7:217–233, 1978.

158. Goslin R, Steele G, Zamcheck N, Mayer R, Macintrye J. Factors influencing survival in patients with hepatic metastases from adenocarcinoma of the colon or rectum. Dis Col Rect 25:749–754, 1982.

159. Morrow CE, Grage TB, Sutherland DE, Najarian JS. Hepatic resection for secondary neoplasms. Surgery 92:610–614, 1982.

160. Rajpal S, Dasmahapatra, Ledesma EJ, Mittelman A. Extensive resections of isolated metastases from carcinoma of the colon and rectum. Surg Gyn Obstet 155:813–816, 1982.

161. Iwatsuki S, Shaw BW, Starzl TE. Experience with 150 liver resections. Ann Surg 197:247–259, 1983.

162. Adson MA, van Heerden JA, Adson MH, Wagner JS, Ilstrap DM. Resection of hepatic metastases from colorectal cancer. Arch Surg 119:647–651, 1984.

163. Steele G, Osteen RT, Wilson RE, Brooks DC, Mayer RJ, Zamcheck N, Ravikumar TS. Patterns of failure after surgical resection of large liver tumors. Am J Surg 147:554–559, 1984.

164. Fortner JG, Silva JS, Golbey RB, Cox EB, Maclean BJ. Multivariate analysis of a personal series of 247 consecutive patients with liver metastases from colorectal cancer. Ann Surg 199:306–316, 1984.

165. Nordlinger BN, Quilichinis M, Pac R, et al. Hepatic resection for colorectal liver metastases. Ann Surg 205:256–263, 1987.

166. Hughes K, Schilel J, Sugerbaker P, et al. Surgery for colorectal cancer metastatic to the liver. Surg Clin North Am 69:339–359, 1989.

167. Adloff M, Arnaud JP, Thebault Y, Schloegel M. Hepatic metastases of colorectal cancer. Should it be treated surgically? Report of 55 cases. Chirurgie 116:144–149, 1990.

168. Pettrelli N, Gupta B, Piedmonte M, Herrera L. Morbidity and survival of liver resection for colorectal adenocarcinoma. Dis Colon Rectum 34:899–904, 1992.

169. van Ooijen B, Wiggers T, Meijer S, et al. Hepatic resections for colorectal metastases in The Netherlands. A multiinstitutional 10-year study. Cancer 70:28–34, 1992.

170. Curley SA, Roh MS, Chase JL, Hohn DC. Adjuvant hepatic arterial infusion chemotherapy after curative resection of colorectal liver metastases. Am J Surg 166:743–746, 1993.

171. Borgelt BB, Gelber R, Brady LW, et al. The palliation of hepatic metastases: Results of Radiation Therapy Oncology Group pilot study. Int J Radiat Oncol Biol Phys 7:587–591,1981.

172. Barone RM, Byfield JE, Goldfarb PB, Frankel S, Ginn C, Greer S. Intra-arterial chemotherapy using an implantable infusion pump and liver irradiation for the treatment of hepatic metastases. Cancer 50:850–862, 1982.

173. Evans JT. Hepatic artery ligation in hepatic metastases from colon and rectal malignancies. Dis Colon Rectum 22:370, 1979.

174. Moertel CG. Chemotherapy of gastrointestinal cancer. N Engl J Med 299:1049–1052, 1978.

175. Ansfield R, Klotz J, Nealson T, et al. A phase II study comparing the utility of four regimens of 5-fluorouracil. Cancer 39:34–40, 1977.

176. Dorosow JH, Multhauf P, Leung L, et al. Prospective randomized comparison of fluorouracil versus fluorouracil and high-dose continuous infusion leucovorin calcium for the treatment of advanced measurable colorectal cancer in patients previously unexposed to chemotherapy. J Clin Oncol; 8:491–501, 1990.

177. Erlichman C, Fine S, Wong A, et al. A randomized trial of fluorouracil and folinic acid in patients with metastatic colorectal carcinoma. J Clin Oncol 6:469–475, 1988.

178. Petrelli N, Douglas HO, Herra L, et al. The modulation of fluorouracil with leucovorin in metastatic colorectal carcinoma: A prospective randomized phase III trial. J Clin Oncol 7:1419–1426, 1989.

179. Poon MA, O'Connell MJ, Moertel CG, et al. Biochemical modulation fluorouracil: Evidence of significant improvement of survival and quality of life in patients with advanced colorectal carcinoma. J Clin Oncol 7:1407–1418, 1989.

180. Valone FH, Friedman MA, Wittlinger PS, et al. Treatment of patients with advanced colorectal carcinomas with fluorouracil alone, high-dose leucovorin plus flourouracil, or sequential methotrexate, flourouracil, and leucovorin. A randomized trial of the Northern California Oncology Group. J Clin Oncol 7:1427–1436, 1989.

181. Petrelli N, Herrera L, Rustum Y, et al. A prospective randomized trial of 5-fluorouracil verus 5-fluorouracil and high dose leucovorin versus 5-fluorouracil and methotrexate in previously untreated patients with advanced colorectal carcinoma. J Clin Oncol 5:1559–1565, 1987.

182. Labianca R, Pancera G, Aitini E, et al. Folinic acid plus 5-fluorouracil versus equidose 5FU in advanced colorectal cancer. Phase III study of "GISCAD" (Italian Group for the Study of Digestive Tract Cancer). Ann Oncol 2:673–679, 1991.

183. Boice JD, Greene MH, Killen JY, et al. Leukemia and preleukemia after adjuvant treatment of gastrointestinal cancer with semustine (methyl-CCNU). N Engl J Med 309: 1079–1084, 1983.

184. Shimada Y, Yoshino M, Wakii A, et al. Phase II study of CPT-11, a new camptothecin derivative in metastatic colorectal cancer. J Clin Oncol 11:909–913, 1993.

185. Balch CM, Urist MM, Soong SJ, McGregor M. A prospective phase II clinical trial of continuous FUDR regional chemotherapy for colorectal metastases to the liver using a totally implantable pump. Ann Surg 198:567–573, 1983.

186. Niederhuber JE, Ensminger W, Gyves J, Thrall J, Walker S, Cozzi E. Regional chemotherapy of colorectal cancer metastatic to the liver. Cancer 53:1336–1343, 1984.

187. Reed ML, Vaitkevicius VK, Al-Sarraf M, et al. The practicality of chronic hepatic artery infusion therapy of primary and metastatic hepatic malignancies: ten-year results in 124 patients in a prospective protocol. Cancer 47:402–409, 1981.

188. Weiss GR, Garnick MB, Osteen RT, et al. Long-term hepatic arterial infusion of 5-fluorodeoxyuridine for liver metastases using an implanted infusion pump. J Clin Oncol 1:337–344, 1983.

189. Kemeny MM, Goldberg DA, Browning S, Metter GE, Miner PJ, Terz JJ. Experience with continuous regional chemotherapy and hepatic resection as treatment of hepatic metastases from colorectal primaries. A prospective randomized study. Cancer 55:1265–1270, 1985.

190. Kemeny N, Daly J, Oderman P, Shike M, Chun H, Petroni G, Geller N. Hepatic artery pump infusion: toxicity and results in patients with metastatic colorectal carcinoma. J Clin Oncol 2:595–600, 1984.

191. Riether RD, Khubchandani IT, Sheets JA, Stasik JJ, Rosen L. A prospective study of continuous hepatic perfusion with implantable pump. Dis Colon Rectum 28:24–26, 1985.

192. Hohn DC, Roh M, Chase J, et al. Prohibitive toxicity with hepatic arterial infusion of low-dose floxuridine and folinic acid for colorectal liver metastases. Proc Am Soc Clin Oncol 10:459, 1991.

193. Tandon RN, Bunnell IL, Cooper RG. The treatment of metastatic carcinoma of the liver by the percutaneous selective hepatic artery infusion of 5-fluorouracil. Surgery 73:118–121, 1973.

194. Ansfield FJ, Ramirez G. The clinical results of 5-fluorouracil intra-hepatic arterial infusion in 528 patients with metastatic cancer to the liver. Prog Clin Cancer 7:201–206, 1978.

195. Petrek JA, Minton JP. Treatment of hepatic metastases by percutaneous hepatic arterial infusion. Cancer 43:2182–2188, 1979.

196. Grage TB, Vassilopoulos PP, Shingleton WW, et al. Results of a prospective randomized study of hepatic arterial infusion with 5-fluorouracil versus intravenous 5-fluorouracil in patients with hepatic metastases from colorectal origin. Surgery 86:550–555, 1979.

197. Berger M. Hepatic infusion for metastatic colorectal cancer in a community hospital setting (Abstract). Proc Am Soc Clin Oncol 22:456, 1981.

198. Oberfield RA, McCafferey JA, Polio J, Clouse ME, Hamilton T. Prolonged and continuous percutaneous intra-arterial hepatic infusion chemotherapy in advanced metastatic liver adenocarcinoma from colorectal primary. Cancer 44:414–423, 1979.

199. Stagg RJ, Venook AP, Chase JL, et al. Alternating hepatic intra-arterial floxuridine and fluorouracil: A less toxic regimen for treatment of liver metastases from colorectal cancer. J Natl Cancer Inst 83:423–428, 1991.

200. Patt Y, Mavligit GM, Chaung VP, et al. Percutaneous hepatic arterial infusion (HAI) of mitomycin C and floxuridine (FUDR): an effective treatment for metastatic colorectal cancer to the liver. Cancer 46:261–265, 1980.

201. Shepard KV, Levin B, Karl RC, et al. Therapy for metastatic colorectal cancer with hepatic artery infusion chemotherapy using a subcutaneous implanted pump. J Clin Oncol 3:161–169, 1985.

202. Hatfield AK, Kammer BA, Danley RA, Miller AG, Houston JG, Harder L. Intermittent hepatic artery perfusions for symptomatic metastatic colon carcinoma. (Abstract) Proc Am Soc Clin Oncol 1:102, 1982.

203. Theodors A, Bukowski RM, Lavery I, Hewlett JS, Livingston RB, Buonocore E. Hepatic artery infusion with 5-fluorouracil and mitomycin-C in metastatic colorectal carcinoma phase II study. Med Pediatr Oncol 10:463–470, 1982.

204. Patt YZ, Boddie AW Jr, Charnsangavej C, Ajani JA, Wallace S, Soski M, Claghorn L, Mavligit GM. Hepatic arterial infusion with floxuridine and cisplatin: overriding importance of antitumor effect versus degree of tumor burden as determinants of survival among patients with colorectal cancer. J Clin Oncol 4:1356–1364, 1986.

205. Cohen AM, Schaeffer N, Higgins J. Treatment of metastatic colorectal cancer with hepatic arterial combination chemotherapy. Cancer 57:1115–1117, 1986.

206. Wils J, Schlangen J, Naus A. Phase II study of hepatic artery infusion with 5-fluorouracil, adriamycin, and mitomycin C (FAM) in liver metastases from colorectal carcinoma. Cancer Chemother Pharmacol 13:215–217, 1984.

207. Kemeny N, Cohen A, Seiter K, Conti J, Sigurdson E, Tao Y, Niedzwiecki D, Botet J, Budd A. Randomized trial of hepatic arterial floxuridine, mitomycin, and carmustine versus floxuridine alone in previously treated patients with liver metastases from colorectal cancer. J Clin Oncol 11:330–335, 1993.

208. Kemeny N, Reichman B, Oderman P, Daly J, Geller N. Update of randomized study of intrahepatic (H) vs systemic (s) infusion of fluorodeoxyuridine (FUDR) in patients with liver metastases from colorectal carcinoma (CRC). Proc Am Soc Clin Oncol 5:89, 1986.

209. Hohn DC, Stagg RJ, Fridman MA, Hannigan JF, Rayner A, Ignoffo RJ, et al. A randomized trial of continuous intravenous versus hepatic intra-arterial fluorodeoxyuridine in patients with colorectal cancer metastatic to the liver: The Northern California Oncology Group Trial. J Clin Oncol 7:1646–1654, 1989.

210. Chang AE, Schneider PD, Sugarbaker PH, Simpson C, Culnane M, Steinberg SM. A prospective randomized trial of regional versus systemic continuous 5-fluorodexyridine chemotherapy in the treatment of colorectal liver metastases. Ann Surg 206:685–693, 1987.

211. Martin JK, O'Connell MJ, Wieand HS, et al. Intra-arterial floxuridine vs systemic fluorouracil for hepatic metastases from colorectal cancer. Arch Surg 125:1022–1027, 1990.

212. Rougier P, LaPlanche A, Huguier M, et al. Hepatic arterial infusion of floxuridine in patients with liver metastases from colorectal carcinoma: Long-term results of a prospective randomized trial. J Clin Oncol 10:1112–1118, 1992.

213. Allen-Mersh TG, Earlam S, Fordy C, Abrams K. Continuous hepatic artery floxuridine infusion prolongs overall and normal-quality survival in colorectal liver metastases patients. Proc Am Soc Clin Oncol 13:202, 1994.

CHAPTER 82

GASTROINTESTINAL CANCERS

JUDY L. CHASE and BETH BRUMBAUGH BREADY

The gastrointestinal system is one of the most common sites of cancer in man. In general, surgery is the primary treatment and usually the only curative modality currently available. Advanced, surgically unresectable disease is treated with palliative chemotherapy and/or radiation. Response rates and survival of patients with advanced disease remains poor. This chapter will focus on colorectal, pancreatic, and gastric cancer. Hepatocellular (primary liver cancer) is discussed in detail in Chapter 81, "Liver Tumors." Other gastrointestinal cancers that occur less frequently and will not be covered in this chapter include esophageal, biliary, small intestine, gall bladder, and appendiceal neoplasms.

COLORECTAL CANCER

Epidemiology

In the United States, more than 150,000 new cases of colorectal cancer are diagnosed yearly, representing approximately 15% of all cancer diagnoses (1). Overall, in the United States it is estimated that approximately 1 in 17 people will develop colorectal cancer in their lifetime. North America, Australia, New Zealand, and portions of Europe have the highest incidence of the disease. Africa and other underdeveloped countries tend to have a low incidence of colorectal cancer. In the United States, the median age at diagnosis is 70 for men and 73 for women, with the age-specific incidence rising steadily from the second to the ninth decade. Approximately 50,000 deaths per year are attributed to colorectal cancer in the United States (1). The incidence appears to be relatively equally distributed between the sexes, with a slight male predominance. Colorectal cancer rates, unlike those for cancers of the lung, cervix, and prostate, show little socioeconomic correlation in the United States and other developed countries.

In the United States, the Seventh Day Adventists and Mormon religious groups have a diminished risk for colorectal cancer. The 20 to 50% reduction in risk is probably attributed to religious practices prohibiting alcohol and tobacco use and promoting some form of dietary moderation (2–3).

Etiology

A specific cause of colon cancer has not been identified. Clinical risk factors for colorectal cancer include dietary practices, genetic factors, familial syndromes, other pre-existing diseases, and advancing age (Table 82.1). Epidemiology and animal studies have determined a clear association between diets rich in animal fats and meat and poor in fiber and an increase in the risk of the disease (4). Dietary fat may enhance colorectal carcinogenesis by a number of mechanisms. Dietary fat increases the production of secondary bile acids, which promote tumorigenesis and increase the proliferative activity of intestinal crypt cells (5). Dietary fat may also enhance the damaging activity of intraluminal free fatty acids to the intestinal epithelium (6).

Another correlate of dietary fat intake and the risk of colorectal cancer is meat consumption. In industrialized countries, including the United States, meat is the major source of dietary fat, and high-fat diets tend to be high in meat intake. It is still unclear whether the association of meat with colorectal cancer reflects the effect of fat, meat in general, or certain types of meat.

A number of animal, case control human, and epidemiologic studies have assessed the influence of dietary fiber on risk of colorectal cancer. The majority have found dietary fiber to be protective. The most widely accepted mechanism reflects the stool-bulking characteristics of dietary fiber. By increasing stool bulk, the concentration of potentially carcinogenic or epithelium damaging agents are diluted out in the bowel lumen (7). A second explanation involves dietary fiber enhancing fermentation by gut bacteria. This fermentation produces short-chain fatty acids that decrease the intraluminal pH, which may decrease the solubility and ionization of both free bile acids and free fatty acids, thus reducing the risk of colorectal cancer (8). Third, some dietary fiber metabolites, such as butyrate, may have antineoplastic properties of their own (9). Other dietary factors, such as alcohol intake, have been studied and have produced conflicting data. Several epidemiologic studies have reported a direct association between alcohol ingestion and colorectal cancer, whereas other studies have found minimal or no association. A recent metaanalysis concluded that alcohol consumption and the increased risk of colorectal cancer was at best small and no clear causative role could be established (10).

Multiple genetic factors have been implicated in the development of colorectal cancer. First-degree relatives of persons with colorectal cancer have a threefold increased

Table 82.1.
Risk Factors for Colorectal Cancer

Dietary
  High animal fats and meat
  Low fiber
Genetic
  Familial adenomatous polysis syndrome
  Gardner's, Oldfield's, or Turcot's syndrome
Familial
  Familial colorectal cancer syndrome
  Hereditary adenocarcinomatosis syndrome
  Family history of colorectal cancer
Preexisting disease
  Inflammatory bowel disease
  Colorectal cancer
  Pelvic irradiation for cancer
  Neoplastic colorectal polyps
General
  All men and women over age 40
  Previous cholecystectomy
  Previous ureterosigmoidostomy

risk of developing the disease, thereby conferring a genetic etiology. Familial adenomatous polyposis is a rare inherited condition characterized by hundreds of large intestinal polyps. The majority of patients with this disease will develop colorectal cancer by age 30. The extent to which other genetic factors, either in isolation or combined with environmental factors, contributes to the development of colorectal cancer requires continued research.

Pathophysiology

Approximately 70% of all colorectal cancers occur in the sigmoid colon and rectum. The remainder occur in decreasing frequency in the ascending colon (16%), the transverse colon and splenic flexure (8%), and the descending colon (6%). Histologically, adenocarcinoma accounts for 90 to 95% of colorectal tumors. The remaining 5 to 10% of large bowel tumors are squamous cell carcinomas, undifferentiated carcinomas, rectal carcinoid, or, very rarely, sarcomas. The adenocarcinomas are further classified by grade. The grade is based on the degree of tumor differentiation, reflected by structural and cytologic features of the specimen. Grade 1 is the most differentiated, with well-formed tubules and the least nuclear polymorphism and mitoses. Grade 3 is the least differentiated, with only occasional glandular structures, and Grade 2 is intermediate between Grades 1 and 3. Poorly differentiated tumors are associated with a poor prognosis. Two histologic subtypes of colorectal adenocarcinoma, colloid or mucinous adenocarcinoma and signet ring cell carcinoma, are both associated with a more aggressive clinical course. They tend to occur more frequently in individuals less than 40 years of age. They also tend to be poorly differentiated and associated with a poor prognosis.

Colorectal adenocarcinomas tend to remain superficial for a long period of time, growing first into the lumen of the bowel, then slowly invading the deeper layers of the intestinal wall. The extent of tumor invasion into the bowel wall correlates both with the presence of lymph node metastases and, ultimately, patient survival. Colorectal cancer may spread by direct invasion of adjacent tissues and metastasize via lymphatic and hematogenous routes. The liver is the most common site of hematogenous metastases, followed by the lung. Involvement of other sites in the absence of liver or lung metastases is rare.

Clinical Presentation

The signs and symptoms of colorectal cancer are often subtle and nonspecific. Many patients may be completely asymptomatic and have colorectal cancer detected via routine screening procedures. The symptoms that are most commonly associated with colorectal cancer are the passage of blood around the stool or on the toilet paper; abdominal pain, which is frequently crampy and intermittent; and a change in bowel habits. The passage of bright red blood is most often seen with cancers of the rectum or sigmoid colon. Melena may result from right-sided colon tumors or obstructing tumors that retard the passage of fecal contents. Unexplained iron deficiency anemia may be the first sign in otherwise asymptomatic patients, especially in tumors located in the proximal colon. Any persistent change in bowel habits should be considered suspicious and deserves further evaluation. Such a change may be newly developed diarrhea, constipation, rectal pressure, or a change in stool caliber. These symptoms may mimic those of other bowel disorders such as diverticular disease, irritable bowel disease, or inflammatory bowel disease. More advanced colorectal cancer may produce unexplained weight loss. When compared to proximal colon cancers, left-sided tumors typically cause obstructive symptoms earlier in the disease course because stool in the distal colon is more solid and therefore less likely to pass easily through a narrowed lumen. Conversely, right-sided tumors can grow larger and into advanced disease and remain virtually asymptomatic.

Physical examination is usually unrevealing in early colorectal cancer. In advanced disease, a palpable abdominal mass, signs of bowel obstruction or perforation, hepatomegaly, or ascites may be present.

SCREENING

The natural history of colorectal cancer often involves a prolonged period of growth whereby many patients remain asymptomatic until advanced disease is present. Since colorectal cancer presents a major health risk to the population, routine screening of asymptomatic patients with the hope of early detection is recommended. The routine screening procedures are listed in Table 82.2. Stool

Table 81.2.
Recommendations for Screening
for the General Population

Procedure	Frequency
Digital rectal exam	Annual
Fecal occult blood tests	Annual
Flexible sigmoidoscopy/colonoscopy	Every 3–5 years

guaiac for occult blood may be useful as a means of early detection. Stool guaiac testing is not without problems. A negative test does not assure the absence of large bowel cancer and therefore should not be relied upon as the sole screening test. The primary care physician should develop a colorectal screening strategy for adult patients as part of an annual physical exam. The screening program should include stool guaiac testing, digital rectal exam, and a flexible sigmoidoscopy. Colonoscopy should be used for screening purposes in high-risk patients. Routine screening of individuals at average risk should begin at age 50. Individuals with high risk factors (personal past history of colorectal cancer or adenomas, a family history of colorectal cancer or adenomas, inflammatory bowel disease) should begin screening at an earlier age. Patients with signs or symptoms of colorectal cancer are not candidates for screening but should be referred for a definitive examination/evaluation of their entire large bowel.

DIAGNOSIS

Patients with any symptoms suggestive of colorectal cancer or a history of polyps should proceed with specific studies to establish a definitive diagnosis. The most widely used diagnostic tests are double-contrast barium enema and colonoscopy (11). Colonoscopy is somewhat more sensitive than barium enema and offers the advantages of direct visualization of the tumor and the ability to biopsy lesions for immediate tissue diagnosis. However, colonoscopy tends be more expensive than barium enema. The double-contrast barium enema involves the rectal administration of barium combined with distension of the bowel lumen with air. The barium outlines the colonic wall and may reveal lesions as small as 1 to 2 cm. However, barium enema often cannot differentiate an early colon cancer from a benign polyp. Barium enema may be helpful in assessing the remainder of the bowel in patients in which the colonoscope cannot be passed beyond the tumor because of a narrowed bowel lumen. Therefore, barium enema and colonoscopy are often used to complement each other.

There are no blood tests that are effective in identifying colorectal cancer. Carcinoembryonic antigen (CEA) is a tumor marker that can be measured in the blood and may be elevated in colorectal cancer. It is not specific to colorectal cancer, as it may be elevated in other gastrointestinal and nongastrointestinal malignancies. A marked elevation in CEA may indicate metastatic disease, especially to the liver, and may warrant further workup (12). A normal or low preoperative level does not guarantee a small or localized primary lesion. CEA may be useful in screening after curative resection and in monitoring response to treatment; however, it should not be used as the sole screening or monitoring method. Other laboratory tests that should be included in the diagnostic workup are not specific to colorectal cancer and include the usual preoperative evaluations such as complete blood count, differential, platelets, serum chemistry, liver panel, electrolytes, and coagulation profile. Chest x-ray is often requested as a part of the standard preoperative work-up but is not required for diagnosis. It may be used to rule out metastatic disease to the lung in patients with an already confirmed diagnosis of colorectal cancer. Patients with a recently diagnosed advanced colorectal cancer may also undergo CT scan or ultrasound of the abdomen to assess the presence/absence of liver metastases. However, this is not required as part of the standard diagnostic workup and is used in selected patients with symptoms or laboratory test suggestive of liver metastases. CT scan of the pelvis is recommended for large, palpable abdominal masses or rectal tumors that may be associated with genitourinary involvement. Endorectal ultrasound is a relatively new procedure that may provide more accurate assessment of the depth of invasion into the bowel wall as well as the nodal status of patients with rectal tumors. Thus, endorectal ultrasound may be able to determine the stage of rectal tumors prior to surgery.

STAGING AND PROGNOSIS

The staging of colorectal cancer has been complicated by the development of multiple staging systems, many of which use the same descriptors to represent different stages. The Dukes' and the TNM staging systems are the most widely used and are presented in Table 82.3 and 82.4. Most investigators agree that the single most important prognostic factor for survival or recurrence after curative surgical resection is stage of the cancer. The 5-year survival rate for Dukes' stage A is 80 to 90%, stage B 70 to 80%, stage C 30 to 50%, and for stage D is less than 10% (13). Stage is determined by the depth of penetration through the bowel wall, the presence and number of positive lymph nodes, and the presence of distant metastatic disease. Other factors that have a negative influence on prognosis include lymphatic vessel invasion, blood vessel invasion, mucinous or signet cell tumor type, colonic obstruction or perforation, lack of rectal bleeding, age under 40, male sex, symptomatic at diagnosis, high-grade tumors, tumors located in the rectosigmoid, and elevated preoperative CEA (14).

Table 82.3.
TMN Staging Classification for Colorectal Cancer

Primary Tumor (T)

TX	Primary tumor cannot be assessed
T0	No evidence of tumor in resected specimen
Tis	Carcinoma in situ
T1	Invades submucosa
T2	Invades muscularis propria
T3	Invades through muscularis propria into subserosa or into nonperitonealized pericolic or perirectal tissues
T4	Invades into the free peritoneal cavity or directly invades other organs (vagina, prostate, ureter, kidney)

Regional Lymph Nodes (N)

NX	Nodes cannot be assessed
N0	No regional lymph node metastases
N1	1–3 positive nodes
N2	4 or more positive nodes
N3	Central nodes positive

Distant Metastases (M)

MX	Presence of distant metastases cannot be assessed
M0	No distant metastases
M1	Distant metastases present
Stage I	T1–2, N0, M0
Stage II	T3–4, N0, M0
Stage III	T(any), N1–3, M0
Stage IV	T(any), N(any), M1

Table 82.4.
Dukes' System for Staging of Colorectal Cancer (Astler-Coler Modification)

A	Lesions limited to the mucosa, nodes negative
B1	Extension through the mucosa but within the bowel wall, nodes negative
B2	Extension through the bowel wall, nodes negative
B3	Tumors adhere to or invade adjacent structures, nodes negative
C1	B1 with positive nodes
C2	B2 with positive nodes
C3	B3 with positive nodes
D	distant metastatic disease

Treatment

SURGERY

Surgery with curative intent is the primary treatment modality for stage I, II, or III (Dukes' A, B, or C) colorectal cancers. Cancers of the colon are removed by a wide resection of the primary lesion together with all surrounding tissue that contains lymph nodes to which the tumor is likely to spread (15). The specific surgical procedure used depends upon the location of the primary tumor and its corresponding lymphatic drainage. A standard procedure for tumors of the right colon (cecum, ascending colon) is a right hemicolectomy, for left-sided tumors (transverse and descending colon) a left hemicolectomy, and for sigmoid tumors a sigmoid colectomy. Tumors in the upper portion of the rectum are usually treated with a low anterior resection with reanastomosis. Low rectal tumors often require an anteroposterior resection and colostomy. If the tumor involves adjacent organs such as the small bowel, bladder, uterus, or ovaries, then an en bloc resection of the entire area is indicated.

Resection of the primary tumor is often still warranted in patients with incurative metastatic disease found operatively or postoperatively. Resection of the primary tumor is intended to avoid local complications of cancer growth such as bleeding/hemorrhage, obstruction/perforation, and pain. Resection of the primary tumor in this setting has no impact on survival but may be associated with an improved quality of life. Patients with rectal cancer and distant metastatic disease at the time of diagnosis may receive palliative radiotherapy to the primary lesion instead of surgical resection.

RATIONALE FOR ADJUVANT THERAPY

The administration of treatments aimed at occult microscopic disease that may remain after complete surgical resection of all gross disease is termed adjuvant therapy. The goal of treatment when no disease is present is to decrease the risk of recurrences and ultimately prolong survival. Adjuvant therapy may involve systemic therapy with chemotherapy, local-regional therapy with radiation, or both, depending on the natural history of the primary neoplastic disease being treated. It is indicated when there is a high likelihood of recurrence and the potential benefit outweighs the risk of morbidity and costs. To obtain maximal benefit, the adjuvant therapy should be administered when the potential tumor burden is minimal (i.e., as soon as feasible following the primary surgical treatment), and it must be administered in maximally tolerated doses (16). For adjuvant chemotherapy, the availability of agents with proven efficacy against measurable disease is required, since there is no way to evaluate efficacy in the adjuvant setting (no measurable disease) until failure occurs.

The goal of adjuvant therapy is to decrease recurrence rates and improve overall survival of patients who have undergone potentially curative surgical resection of the primary tumor. As discussed, surgical excision is the primary treatment of colorectal cancer, with approximately 80% of patients diagnosed at a stage when all gross tumor can be surgically removed. However, nearly 50% of patients will develop recurrent disease and die from metastatic disease. Therefore, treatment directed at occult disease after complete surgical resection of the primary disease is warranted in an attempt to decrease recurrence. The risk of recurrence and ultimately survival is highly dependent on stage. The range of recurrence rates for a Dukes' stage A lesion is 0 to 13%; the range of rates for Dukes' stage B lesions is 11 to 61%; and for Dukes' stage C lesions 32 to 88% (17). Approximately 60 to 84% of recurrences become apparent within 2 years, and treatment depends on location, size, patient performance status, and prior therapy. Because the risk of recurrence after resection of a stage A colorectal tumor is low, the cost-benefit ratio does not warrant adjuvant therapy for these patients. Adjuvant therapy for stage B and C lesions will be discussed below. Because there are anatomic, natural history, and therapeutic differences between colon and rectal tumors, adjuvant therapy for each should be addressed separately.

ADJUVANT THERAPY FOR COLON CANCER

Initially, adjuvant therapy after potentially curative surgical resection for large bowel cancer was attempted using alkylating agents, nitrogen mustard and thiotepa. These drugs have not been shown to have activity in advanced colorectal cancer, and it is therefore not surprising that they were ineffective in the adjuvant treatment of colorectal cancer. Subsequent trials focused on the use of 5-fluorouracil (5-FU) and fluorodeoxyuridine (FUDR) because these drugs had produced some responses in patients with metastatic disease. These drugs were first used alone and then in combinations with other agents including semustine, vincristine, and bacillus Calmette-Guerin (BCG). None of the single-agent or combination trials resulted in decreased recurrence rates or improved survival compared to untreated controls (18).

Levamisole, an anthelmintic agent, attracted interest for cancer therapy because of its presumed immunomodulatory activity. In the early 1980s a small nonrandomized trial reported levamisole to have activity in the adjuvant setting for colon cancer (19). Subsequent trials investigated levamisole alone and in combination with 5-FU in the hope of achieving additive activity. Levamisole combined with 5-FU has been found to significantly reduce the recurrence rate. In stage C (TNM stage III) disease levamisole plus 5-FU reduced the recurrence rate by 40% and death rate by 33% compared to no adjuvant therapy (20). On the basis of these results, a Consensus Panel convened by the National Institutes of Health recommended levamisole plus 5-FU as standard adjuvant treatment for patients with stage C (TNM stage III) colon cancer (21). The dosing regimen is presented in Table 82.5. Any trials investigating the adjuvant treatment of stage C (TNM stage III) patients should incorporate levamisole plus 5-FU as the control

Table 82.5.
Adjuvant Therapy for Duke's Stage C (TMN State III) Colon Cancer

Levamisole	50 mg orally three times daily × 3 days repeated every 2 weeks × 1 year
5-FU	450 mg/m² intravenously daily × 5 days, then beginning on day 28
	450 mg/m² intravenously once a week × 48 weeks

arm. In stage B2 (TNM stage II) disease, no clear benefit of adjuvant therapy has been clearly established. Levamisole plus 5-FU produced some reduction in recurrence rates and slight improvement in survival; however, these results are not statistically significant. It is suggested that patients with stage B2 (TNM stage II) colon cancer and high risk of recurrence factors such as tumor perforation, adherence to or invasion of adjacent organs, or unfavorable cellular kinetic pattern (ploidy), be offered adjuvant treatment with levamisole plus 5-FU (18).

The toxicity associated with levamisole includes nausea, vomiting, diarrhea, and dermatitis. These side effects are infrequent and usually mild. The toxicity associated with the levamisole/5-FU combination are those anticipated with 5-FU alone and include nausea, vomiting, diarrhea, stomatitis, dermatitis, and leukopenia. Again, the toxicity is usually mild and of short duration. Overall, the levamisole/5-FU combination is generally well tolerated.

5-Fluorouracil and leucovorin have been extensively studied in the treatment of metastatic colorectal cancer. As will be discussed later, the addition of leucovorin to 5-FU increases the response rates seen in metastatic disease compared to 5-FU alone. This has prompted the extensive investigation into the role of leucovorin/5-FU, and the combination of leucovorin/levamisole/5-FU to standard levamisole/5-FU in colon cancer adjuvant trials. Most of these studies have been recently completed but await appropriate follow-up to determine the extent of benefit, optimal dose and schedule of drugs, and ultimately recurrence and survival rates (22).

ADJUVANT THERAPY FOR RECTAL CANCER

Rectal cancer, which should be distinguished from colon cancer, is characterized by an increased risk of local recurrence and a comparable risk for distant metastases compared with colon cancer. The risk of local recurrence after surgical resection of a rectal tumor depends upon disease extension beyond the rectal wall and the presence of lymph node involvement. Patients with tumor confined to the rectal wall nodal involvement have a local recurrence rate of 20 to 40%. In patients with tumor extending beyond the rectal wall and negative lymph nodes, the recurrence rate is approximately the same, 20 to 35%. Patients with both tumor extending beyond the rectal wall and positive lymph nodes have a recurrence rate that is almost double, 40 to 70% (23). Because of an increased risk of local recurrence with rectal cancer compared to colon cancer, adjuvant therapy has been approached with an increased emphasis on local-regional treatment with radiation therapy.

Postoperative radiation without chemotherapy has been shown to improve local control but has no effect on systemic recurrence or survival (24–26). Adjuvant chemotherapy without radiation has been shown to decrease the incidence of systemic failure but has had no impact on local recurrence rates or survival. Adjuvant therapy using the combined modality approach of postoperative irradiation and chemotherapy has been shown to improve both local control and survival of resected high-risk rectal cancers (26–28). The National Institutes of Health (NIH) Consensus Conference (1990) on adjuvant treatment of colon and rectal cancers recommends postoperative radiation and chemotherapy as standard adjuvant therapy for Dukes' stage B2 and C (TNM stage II and III) rectal tumors (21). The external beam pelvic radiation is usually delivered in doses of 50 to 55 Gy, combined with a 5-FU based chemotherapy regimen. In the initial combined modality adjuvant trials, the chemotherapy consisted of either 5-FU plus/minus methyl-CCNU. Current data suggest that in the adjuvant rectal setting, 5-FU alone affords equal efficacy and less toxicity than 5-FU plus methyl-CCNU when combined with radiation (27, 28). The best chemotherapy regimen is yet to be determined. Due to the positive results observed in colon cancer with continuous 5-FU, 5-FU plus levamisole, and 5-FU plus leucovorin, these chemotherapy regimens have recently been combined with radiation for the adjuvant treatment of rectal cancer, and data from these trials are awaiting appropriate follow-up. Outside of a clinical trial, patients with Dukes' stage B2 or C (TNM stage II or III) rectal cancer should receive adjuvant chemoradiation treatment with 50 to 55 Gy pelvic irradiation plus 5-FU or a 5-FU-based chemotherapy regimen.

There is some controversy regarding the sequencing of surgery and chemoradiation, as preoperative treatment appears to be equally beneficial and may be less toxic (29). A theoretic advantage of preoperative irradiation is the potential damage to cells that may be spread locally or distantly at the time of resection. The major advantage of postoperative irradiation is the ability to avoid treatment of patients at low risk for local recurrence and those who have metastatic disease that was not diagnosed prior to surgery. Currently, it is suggested that any patient with rectal cancer in which the tumor penetrates through the bowel wall or has positive lymph nodes should receive adjuvant chemo-radiation. Whether this therapy is administered pre- or postoperatively requires further clinical trials. Increased availability and expertise with endorectal ultrasound is required to determine the extent of bowel penetration and preoperative staging.

TREATMENT OF ADVANCED COLORECTAL CANCER

Single Agent Chemotherapy. Chemotherapy is usually the only feasible approach to controlling advanced (Dukes' stage D, TNM stage IV) colorectal cancer. The liver and lung are the most common sites of metastatic disease. Median survival of patients with advanced disease is usually only 6 to 10 months. For the most part, the treatment of advanced colorectal cancer is considered palliative. A few patients with small isolated liver metastases may undergo surgical resection, but this results in cure or long-term disease-free survival in only a small percentage of patients. The majority of patients with advanced or metastatic colorectal cancer may receive systemic chemotherapy that has no curative potential in an attempt to decrease symptoms and ultimately prolong survival. A number of single agents have been investigated, but the fluoropyrimidines are considered the mainstay of therapy for colorectal cancer. Until recently, bolus intravenous 5-FU administration was considered standard. A variety of bolus 5-FU schedules exist and produce response rates of 10 to 20% at best (30). 5-FU is an antimetabolite that inhibits the formation of the DNA-specific nucleoside base thymidine. The main mechanism of action is believed to be inhibition of thymidylate synthase by FdUMP, the active metabolite of 5-FU. 5-FU exerts its major cytotoxicity during the S phase of the cell cycle. The plasma half-life of 5-FU is only 10 to 20 minutes, and the inhibition of thymidylate synthase following a bolus dose is also short (31, 32). Thus, only a small fraction of cancer cells are susceptible to the toxic effects of 5-FU after bolus administration. This may theoretically limit the efficacy of 5-FU when administered by intravenous bolus. Infusional schedules have been investigated as a mechanism to overcome this limitation. 5-FU infusion durations ranging from 24 hours to greater than 10 weeks have been explored in clinical trials. Response rates for infusional 5-FU are generally 30 to 40%; however, no statistically significant survival advantage has been documented (30). The commonly used dosage schedules for infusional 5-FU are presented in Table 82.6 (33–35). The dose-limiting toxicity of infusional 5-FU is usually mucositis, but may also include diarrhea or dermatitis, whereas the dose-limiting toxicity of bolus 5-FU is usually myelosuppression, but may include mucositis and diarrhea. A distinct type of dermal toxicity, termed palmar-plantar erythrodysesthesia or hand-foot syndrome, may be seen in up to 30% of patients treated with prolonged infusions of 5-FU. This syndrome presents as painful swelling and erythema of the hands and feet and may progress to painful desquamation. It is managed by prompt discontinuation of the 5-FU infusion at the onset

Table 82.6.
Infusional 5-FU Schedules for Advanced Colorectal Cancer

Infusion Duration	5-FU Dose	Frequency	Major Toxicity
24 hours	2.6 g/m²/d	Weekly	Myelosuppression Ataxia Mucositis
4–5 days	1.0 g/m²/d	Every 3–4 wks	Mucositis
3–10 weeks	300 mg/m²/d	Continuous	Mucositis

of symptoms and reinstitution of treatment at reduced dosage after complete recovery from toxicity.

Combination Chemotherapy. Numerous combinations of chemotherapeutic agents have been explored in colorectal cancer. Most of these have combined one or more agents with 5-FU in an attempt to improve response rates. Drugs used in the combination regimens include 5-FU, cisplatin, semustine, mitomycin-C, cyclophosphamide, DTIC, hydroxyurea, methotrexate, vincristine, and doxorubicin (30). Thus far, no combination chemotherapy regimen has been shown to be superior to 5-FU alone and therefore cannot be recommended for use in colorectal cancer. No agents other than the fluoropyrimidines have adequate activity in colorectal cancer to have a significant impact.

Biochemical Modulation of 5-FU. With the exception of the fluoropyrimidines, the virtual lack of available agents with activity against colorectal cancer has stimulated the search for methods to improve response rates with 5-FU. One method of overcoming the schedule dependence of 5-FU is to prolong the inhibition of thymidylate synthase by the coadministration of a reduced folate. Leucovorin (folinic acid, LCV) has been successfully used for this purpose. Leucovorin stabilizes the covalent bond between thymidylate synthase and FdUMP and thus increases the cytotoxicity of 5-FU (36). Numerous studies have been completed using a variety of doses of leucovorin in combination with 5-FU. The response rates to 5-FU/leucovorin are 30 to 44%, a statistically significant improvement compared to 5-FU alone (37–42). There also appears to be a trend toward improved survival with 5-FU/leucovorin, but this has reached statistical significance in only two studies thus far. Despite the lack of a clear-cut survival advantage, 5-FU/leucovorin is considered standard therapy for advanced colorectal cancer by most oncologists at the present time. Doses for leucovorin have ranged from 15 to 500 mg/m^2/day, but there is now data to demonstrate that leucovorin doses of 20 mg/m^2/day effectively enhance 5-FU efficacy and are associated with less toxicity compared to high-dose leucovorin regimens (39). Currently, the most commonly accepted dosage schedule of 5-FU/leucovorin incorporates the lower dosages of leucovorin. Some of the commonly used dosage schedules for the 5-FU plus leucovorin combination are presented in Table 82.7. It should be noted that, because of its mechanism of modulation, leucovorin should always be administered prior to or concomitantly with the 5-FU. The toxicity of the 5-FU and leucovorin combinations is qualitatively different from either the bolus or infusional 5-FU alone. In general, myelosuppression is not increased over what would be expected with 5-FU alone. However, lower doses of 5-FU are usually used when combined with leucovorin. Gastrointestinal toxicity in the form of diarrhea and mucositis is significantly increased with the addition of leucovorin,

Table 82.7.

Selected Dosage Schedules for 5-FU + Leucovorin in the Treatment of Advanced Colorectal Cancer

Drug	Dose, Route and Administration	Frequency
Leucovorin	20 mg/m^2 IV push, followed by	times 5 days, repeated
5-FU	425 mg/m^2 IV push	every 4–5 weeks
Leucovorin	500 mg/m^2 IV over 2–3 hours	weekly
5-FU	600 mg/m^2 IV bolus during leucovorin	
Leucovorin	20 mg/m^2 IV push once weekly	repeat every 5 weeks
5-FU	200 mg/m^2 IV continuous infusion × 28 days	
Leucovorin	200 mg/m^2 IV push	× 5 days, repeated every 4–5 weeks
5-FU	370 mg/m^2 IV push	

and can produce life-threatening dehydration if not treated promptly. Hand-foot syndrome, which is rarely seen with bolus 5-FU, has been reported to occur frequently with the leucovorin/5-FU combination even with bolus dosing (42). A variety of other agents have been used to modulate the activity of 5-FU, including, but not limited to, methotrexate, interferon-α, dipyridamole, N-phosphonoacetyl-L-aspartate (PALA), and uridine (43–46). However, more clinical research is required to determine the exact role of modulating agents in the treatment of colorectal cancer with 5-FU.

REGIONAL CHEMOTHERAPY IN COLORECTAL CANCER

Regional chemotherapy for the treatment of colorectal cancer usually refers to hepatic arterial infusion of chemotherapy for the treatment of liver metastases. This approach offers the advantage of substantially increasing the intensity of drug delivery to the liver while minimizing the systemic side effects. It is indicated in patients who have liver-only metastases and a good performance status. The specific of hepatic arterial infusion for colorectal liver metastases is discussed in more detail in Chapter 81, "Liver Tumors".

Promising Investigational Agents. Irinotecan (CPT-11), a semisynthetic derivative of camptothecin is a potent inhibitor of topoisomerase I, thereby causing DNA strand breaks and cell death. In clinical trials approximately a 20% response rate has been seen in patients with advanced colorectal cancer who had failed a 5-FU-based chemotherapy (47). The ability to induce response in 5-FU-resistant patients makes it an attractive second-line chemotherapy option in colorectal cancer. The main toxicities associated with irinotecan are diarrhea, myelosuppression, and nausea (48).

Tomudex is a potent and specific thymidylate synthase inhibitor with activity in colorectal cancer. A 26% objective response rate has recently been reported in patients with advanced colorectal cancer (49). What makes tomudex an important agent in colorectal cancer is its lack of myelosuppresion. The major toxicity associated with tomudex is asthenia, diarrhea, nausea, and vomiting. Tomudex is usually administered intravenously once every 21 days. Tegafur (ftorafur) is a 5-FU product that has been combined with uracil to form a compound called UFT. UFT (uracil + tegafur) is administered orally and recently has been combined with oral leucovorin for the treatment of colorectal cancer. A 42% response rate has been reported in patients with advanced colorectal cancer (50). The dose-limiting toxicity of this regimen is diarrhea. The oral dosing, initial response rates, and favorable toxicity profile make UFT plus leucovorin an attractive alternative for the treatment of advanced colorectal cancer. Use of tegafur in the adjuvant setting also deserves further investigation.

Irinotecan, tomudex, and UFT plus leucovorin are all important advances in the treatment of advanced colorectal cancer. The most efficacious dose and dosing schedule, reproducible response rates, and toxicity profiles, as well as the exact role of each of these agents in the treatment of colorectal cancer, require further investigation. In addition, continued research evaluating new agents, modulating agents, combination chemotherapy, and combined modality therapies is needed.

Conclusions

Colorectal cancer is one of the most common malignancies and presents a major health problem in the United States. Prevention and early detection programs have received attention in recent years as the incidence continues to rise with a large proportion of patients diagnosed with already advanced disease. Prognosis has been directly associated with the depth of tumor invasion into or through the bowel wall. The initial treatment for colorectal cancer is surgery to remove the primary lesion and surrounding tissue. Adjuvant therapy for patients with localized disease has been shown to decrease recurrence rates and prolong survival. Treatment of advanced disease with chemotherapy remains palliative, and the results are limited by the availability of active agents. The fluoropyrimidines continue to be the most active and most commonly used agents in the treatment of colorectal cancer. Ongoing research evaluating biochemical modulation of 5-FU and identification of new agents will hopefully yield increased response rates and improved survival in the future.

PANCREATIC CANCER

Epidemiology

Pancreatic cancer is a relatively rare malignancy, with an estimated 24,000 new cases diagnosed in the United States in 1995 (1). The incidence has increased over the last several decades, probably as a result of an increased awareness of the disease and advances in diagnostic technology. In the United States pancreatic cancer is the fourth most common cause of cancer death in people over 55 years of age. Less than 5% of patients survive 5 years (1). However, the incidence and mortality have been relatively stable since 1970 except for black women, whose rates have increased slightly. It is mainly a disease of the elderly, with the median age at the time of diagnosis being 69 years; however, it may occur in young adults. There is a slight male preponderance in the incidence, which appears to vary, depending on the age of the patient at the time of diagnosis. In patients under 40 years of age, the male to female ratio is 3:1. This ratio gradually equalizes as the age of the patient increases, so that the ratio becomes 1:1 by age of diagnosis of 80 years (52). In the United States the incidence has increased in female native American Indians, black men, and both sexes of Spanish descent. The incidence is higher in urban than in rural areas and higher in industrialized nations, implying that environmental factors play a role in the etiology. Countries with a high incidence include New Zealand, Australia, Poland, Scotland, Sweden, and certain areas of Canada. Japan and China have a low incidence compared with the United States; however, the incidence rises rapidly in groups who immigrate to countries of high incidence.

Approximately 25,000 deaths/year in the United states are attributed to pancreatic cancer, making it the fourth most common cause of cancer death, behind lung, breast, and colorectal cancers (1). The median survival from the time of diagnosis for all patients with pancreatic cancer is 6 months, making it one of the most aggressive solid tumors (52). Most patients die of the disease and its complications, such as malnutrition, gastrointestinal obstruction, and liver failure.

Etiology

Many dietary and environmental factors have been implicated as possible etiologic factors in the development of pancreatic cancer, but definite causal relationships have not been established in all cases. Employees of petroleum and chemical industries appear to be at especially high risk. Workers exposed to industrial solvents or petroleum products for more than 10 years have up to a fivefold increase in incidence of pancreatic cancer. Cigarette smoking appears to be associated with a two- to threefold increase in incidence of the disease (53, 54). Some studies have suggested an association between chronic pancreatitis, alcohol, or coffee consumption and the development of pancreatic cancer, but these findings have not been confirmed.

Approximately 15% of patients diagnosed with pancreatic cancer have a history of diabetes mellitus, implying a causal relationship between diabetes mellitus and the development of pancreatic cancer (55). However, in more than half of these patients the onset of clinical diabetes preceded the diagnosis of pancreatic cancer by only a few months. This suggests that the cancer may cause the pancreatic endocrine (insulin) insufficiency. Diabetes presenting many months to years before the diagnosis of pancreatic cancer would be better evidence for a etiologic correlation.

Pathophysiology

The pancreas lies transversely in the posterior part of the upper abdomen. The head of the pancreas is on the right side of the abdomen and rests against the curve of the duodenum. The body of the pancreas lies beneath the stomach, and the tail of the pancreas extends across the abdomen to the left side. The pancreas is virtually surrounded by other organs in the upper abdomen. However, unlike other organs, it cannot be palpated because of its posterior position. Because of its position and large functional reserve, symptoms of pancreatic disease, including cancer, often do not appear until the disorder is far advanced.

The pancreas is both an endocrine and an exocrine organ. Most tumors (95%) occur in the exocrine portion. Tumors of the endocrine portion are usually benign, whereas only 2% of tumors arising in the exocrine portion of the pancreas are benign. Malignant tumors may arise from pancreatic ductal epithelial cells, acinar cells, connective tissue, or lymphatic tissue. Histologically, ductal adenocarcinoma accounts for more than 80% of all pancreatic malignancies. The head of the pancreas is the site for approximately 70% of all pancreatic tumors, with 20% occurring in the body and 10% in the tail (52).

On gross examination, tumors of the pancreas usually appear hard, gritty, and whitish. The surrounding tissue often displays evidence of chronic pancreatitis. Tumors in the head of the pancreas are usually less than 5 cm in diameter and are often associated with pancreatic and common bile duct obstruction, invasion, ulceration, and obstruction of the adjacent duodenum, and portal vein or superior mesentery artery obstruction. Tumors occurring in the tail of the pancreas are usually larger (5 to 10 cm) at the time of diagnosis and associated with splenic vein obstruction. Early subclinical metastases are characteristic of pancreatic cancer. Less than 20% of patients have disease confined to the pancreas at the time of diagnosis. Forty percent of patients have locally advanced (regional lymph nodes, adjacent organs) disease, and more than 40% have distant metastases at diagnosis. The most commonly involved distant organ is the liver, followed by lung and (less frequently) bone and brain.

Clinical Presentation

The early symptoms of pancreatic cancer tend to be very nonspecific and insidious in onset, thus making early

diagnosis of the disease difficult. Approximately 80 to 90% of patients have advanced disease at the time of diagnosis. Pain in the upper abdomen is the single most common presenting symptom and is usually the reason patients seek medical attention. The pain often mimics the pain associated with peptic ulcer disease and thus is often misdiagnosed. Other common presenting symptoms include nausea, anorexia, weight loss, and weakness. Gastrointestinal bleeding is commonly associated with tumors in the head of the pancreas, but it is rare in tumors of the body or tail. As most tumors arise in the ductal system, biliary obstruction is common. Obstructive jaundice occurs in approximately 50% of all patients with pancreatic cancer and in up to 90% of patients with tumors in the head of the pancreas. Splanchnic nerve invasion may lead to gastrointestinal motility problems, mechanical obstruction, and severe pain. Gastrointestinal obstruction is a common problem and may occur secondary to local tumor invasion, poor gastrointestinal motility, or mechanical obstruction. Anorexia and weight loss are also common symptoms. Subclinical malabsorption secondary to pancreatic insufficiency may be a cause for the weight loss, and some patients may respond to oral pancreatic enzyme supplementation.

Pancreatic cancer may spread by direct invasion of surrounding tissues or by metastasizing to distant sites. Direct invasion into the abdominal lymph nodes, liver, and gastroduodenum is often present at diagnosis. The liver and peritoneum are the most common sites of distant metastases and may be present in up to 40% of patients at the time of diagnosis. Other, less common sites of metastases include the lung, bone, and brain (52). The natural history of pancreatic cancer is highlighted by the development of widespread metastatic disease, and death is often secondary to liver failure and malnutrition.

Diagnosis

Since the symptoms of pancreatic cancer tend to be nonspecific and are often attributed to other medical conditions, a high index of suspicion is necessary to make an accurate and timely diagnosis. Pancreatic cancer should be included in the differential diagnosis of any patient presenting with unexplained jaundice, pancreatitis, weight loss, and/or nonspecific upper abdominal or back pain. The goal of the evaluation in a patient with suspected pancreatic cancer is to establish the presence/absence of a primary tumor, and if one is present to determine the extent of local and metastatic disease. The diagnostic evaluation usually begins with a physical examination to establish clinical correlations such as jaundice, weight loss, palpable mass, ascites, or metastatic disease. Blood tests are obtained to help evaluate jaundice, liver function tests, and pancreatic serum enzyme levels. Serum enzyme levels such as amylase, lipase, alkaline phosphatase, leucine aminopeptidase, and pancreatic ribonuclease may be elevated in patients with pancreatic cancer. If the tumor involves the liver, levels of lactic dehydrogenase and the transaminases may be also be elevated.

The diagnostic workup continues with noninvasive radiologic studies, then proceeds to more invasive radiologic and endoscopic procedures, and eventually to tissue biopsy. Ultrasonography of the upper abdomen is commonly used as an initial screening examination in patients suspected of having pancreatic cancer. It has the advantages of being noninvasive and relatively inexpensive, but the diagnostic yield is often limited. Computed tomography (CT) continues to be the mainstay for diagnosis, as it provides evaluation of the extent of disease (local and metastatic) and determination of resectability in patients with presumed pancreatic cancer. The most common findings on CT scan include an enlarged pancreas, a pancreatic mass, dilation of the biliary and pancreatic ducts, hepatic metastases, and retroperitoneal lymphadenopathy. Although more expensive than ultrasonography, the CT scan offers the advantages of producing superior images and allowing visualization of the entire abdomen. More invasive procedures to aid in the diagnosis of pancreatic cancer include endoscopic retrograde cholangiopancreatography (ERCP), transhepatic cholangiography, and arteriography of the pancreas, biliary tree, and vasculature.

Once a suspected pancreatic mass is identified, additional radiologic and endoscopic tests may be required to determine the extent of disease (local versus metastatic) and the surgical resectability of the tumor, if localized. If the tumor is considered unresectable or if metastatic disease is present, then histologic diagnosis should be obtained by direct fine-needle biopsy of the pancreas or percutaneous biopsy of a liver metastasis. If the tumor is considered to be possibly resectable and the patient is a surgical candidate, then the patient should be scheduled for an exploratory laparotomy. At surgery, biopsies of the pancreas, lymph nodes, and liver are obtained to confirm the diagnosis and extent of disease.

A variety of biologic substances identified in the serum of patients with pancreatic cancer may be considered tumor markers. Tumor markers are important because, depending on their sensitivity and specificity, they may aid in the differential diagnosis, identify unfavorable prognostic groups, and assist in the clinical follow-up of tumor response in patients with poorly measurable disease. At the current time, a number of potential markers have been identified, including carcinoembryonic antigen (CEA), tumor-associated carbohydrate antigen (CA 19-9), CA 125 antigen, and monoclonal antibody products (DUPAN-2, SPAN-1). CEA is elevated in approximately 50% of patients with pancreatic cancer, but it is also elevated in many other benign and malignant gastrointestinal diseases. CA 19-9 is elevated in approximately 80% of patients with

pancreatic cancer and appears to be more sensitive than CEA (56). Currently the CA 19-9 test is not routinely available and therefore not used clinically. CA 125 is elevated in less than 50% of patients with pancreatic cancer and will probably not be very clinically useful. DUPAN-2 appears to be quite specific for identifying and following patients with pancreatic cancer, but it may also be elevated in patients with other gastrointestinal malignancies or diseases (57). Further investigation into the development of more specific and sensitive tumor markers in pancreatic cancer is required before they will be considered to be consistently clinically useful.

Staging/Prognosis

The staging system used for pancreatic cancer is based on the extent of the primary tumor, regional lymph nodes, and metastatic disease (58). The TNM staging system is presented in Table 82.8. The tumor status (T) is defined by the degree of tumor extension through the pancreatic capsule; nodal status (N) by the presence of regional lymph node involvement; and metastatic status (M) by the presence of distant nodal, peritoneal, or visceral disease. The surgical staging classification based on the TNM system is defined as follows: stage I disease is localized to the pancreas and is surgically resectable; stage II disease is locally advanced and not surgically resectable; stage III disease involves the regional lymph nodes; and stage IV disease has metastatic spread. Obviously, patients with stage I disease have the best prognosis and are the only patients in which the disease is curable. Unfortunately, less than 15% of patients have stage I disease at the time of presentation. Most patients present with advanced disease (stages II, III, IV)

Table 82.8.
TNM Staging System for Pancreatic Cancer

T1	No direct extension of the primary tumor beyond the pancreas
T2	Limited direct extension to duodenum, bile ducts, or stomach
T3	Advanced direct extension (not surgically resectable)
TX	Direct extension of tumor not assessed
N0	Regional lymph nodes not involved
N1	Regional lymph nodes involved
NX	Regional lymph nodes not assessed
M0	No known distant metastases
M1	Distant metastases present
MX	Distant metastases not assessed
Stage 1	T1–2, N0, M0: No direct extension or limited extension of tumor with no regional nodal involvement
Stage 2	T3, N0, M0: Direct extension of tumor into adjacent tissue with no lymph node involvement
Stage 3	T1–3, N1, M0: Regional lymph node involvement with or without direct tumor extension, but without distant metastases
Stage 4	T1–3, N0–1, M1: Distant metastases present

and are considered unresectable and incurable. These patients have a very poor prognosis, with less than 10% of them surviving 1 year after diagnosis.

Treatment

Surgery, radiation therapy, and chemotherapy are treatment options for patients with pancreatic cancer. Since most patients present with advanced-stage disease and only those with localized (resectable) disease may be potentially cured by surgical resection, the great majority of patients require palliative treatment. Unfortunately, the treatment options for this large percentage of patients have not significantly changed the outcome in recent years.

LOCALIZED, RESECTABLE DISEASE (STAGE I)

Cancer of the pancreas usually presents in advanced stages with local invasion into vital structures, making curative surgery an option for only a small number of patients. In addition, laparotomy often reveals that the pancreatic malignancy is more advanced than was apparent on preoperative studies. Therefore, many patients thought to have potential of being cured by surgical resection may receive only palliative operations at the time of surgery. For patients who are deemed resectable at the time of surgery, a Whipple procedure is usually performed. This operation involves the en bloc removal of the distal stomach and duodenum, the first portion of the jejunum, and the head and part of the body of the pancreas. A surgical alternative is a total pancreatectomy, which may have the advantage of preventing local recurrence. However, there are disadvantages, such as pancreatic exocrine insufficiency and permanent diabetes mellitus requiring lifelong replacement therapy. Regardless of the surgical procedure performed, it is currently recommended that patients receive postoperative (adjuvant) treatment with radiation plus chemotherapy (5-fluorouracil). Radiation therapy involves 180 to 200 cGy given daily for 5 days, followed by 1-week rest, and then repeated for another 5-day course. The 5-fluorouracil (5-FU) is given as an intravenous bolus dose of 500 mg/m^2 on the first 3 days of each radiation course and then continued on a weekly schedule starting 1 month after the completion of the radiation treatments. This postoperative adjuvant therapy appears to increase the disease-free survival, compared with patients who receive no adjuvant therapy (59–62). Alternatives to postoperative adjuvant chemoradiation include the use of intraoperative radiation therapy (IORT) or neoadjuvant therapy with external beam radiation plus chemotherapy. However, the routine use of IORT and neoadjuvant therapy requires further study.

LOCALIZED, UNRESECTABLE DISEASE (STAGES II AND III)

Patients who fall into this category may be treated with a palliative surgical bypass procedure, depending on physi-

cian judgment. These palliative procedures (choledochojejunostomy or cholecystojejunostomy) are performed to treat obstructive jaundice and real or impending gastric outlet obstruction.

These operations do not prolong survival, but they usually improve the quality of life for these patients. In addition to palliative bypass surgery, these patients should be offered combined modality therapy (radiation and chemotherapy). Based on the results of a Gastrointestinal Tumor Study Group trial completed in 1988, patients with locally unresectable pancreatic cancer who receive combined modality therapy (radiation and chemotherapy) have a prolonged survival compared with patients who receive radiation therapy alone (63). The optimal combined modality treatment is yet to be determined. No multidrug plus radiation combination has been proved to be superior to 5-FU alone plus radiation, and therefore none can be recommended. Many types of investigational radiation therapy techniques are currently being tested, including intraoperative electron-beam irradiation, high-energy particle-beam irradiation, and interstitial implantation of I-125 (64–67). Currently, a major research focus is the use of preoperative radiation plus chemotherapy (neoadjuvant) to maximize tumor shrinkage and increase the resectability rates. These newer radiation therapies may improve local control, but further investigation is needed. Currently there is no standard of practice; therefore, as an alternative to external-beam irradiation plus 5-FU, these patients may be entered into investigative clinical trials.

METASTATIC DISEASE (STAGE IV)

For patients with metastatic pancreatic cancer, systemic chemotherapy is the only treatment option. Radiation therapy may be used to help provide some symptomatic palliation, but the mainstay of treatment is chemotherapy. Unfortunately, only a small number of patients benefit from chemotherapy. The most active single agents include 5-FU, doxorubicin, mitomycin C, streptozocin, ifosfamide, and methyl-CCNU. Only 10 to 30% of patients respond to these agents, and the responses rarely last more than 2 to 3 months (52). Many investigational agents are currently being studied, but only a few have shown response rates above 10% (epirubicin, neocarzinostatin) (68). To improve on the dismal results obtained with single-agent chemotherapy, combination chemotherapy has been used. Regimens such as FAM (5-FU, doxorubicin, mitomycin C) and SMF (streptozocin, mitomycin C, 5-FU) are outlined in Table 82.9. These regimens produced initial response rates of approximately 40%; however, subsequent trials have not confirmed the initial response rates. Response rates with these combination regimens have ranged from 2 to 40%, with a median of 20% (69). This is not substantially different from the results seen with single-agent 5-FU. Currently, no combination-chemotherapy regimen appears

Table 82.9.
Combination Chemotherapy Regimens for
Pancreatic Cancer

FAM	5-Fluorouracil 600 mg/m² IV bolus days 1, 8, 29, and 36
	Doxorubicin 30 mg/m² IV bolus days 1 and 29
	Mitomycin C 10 mg/m² IV bolus day 1
	Repeat cycle every 6–8 weeks
SMF	Streptozocin 1 g/m² IV over 1–2 hr days 1, 8, 29, and 36
	Mitomycin C 10 mg/m² IV bolus day 1
	5-Fluorouracil 600 mg/m² IV bolus days 1,8, 29, and 36
	Repeat cycle every 6–8 weeks

Table 82.10.
5-Fluorouracil Plus Leucovorin Administration Schedules

Daily bolus schedule
Leucovorin 20 mg/m²/day × 5 days, IV over 2 hr
5-FU 375–425 mg/m²/day × 5 days, IV over 15 min, give 1 hr after
  the start of the leucovorin infusion
Repeat every 28 days
Weekly bolus schedule
Leucovorin 20–500 mg/m² IV over 10–15 min
5-FU 600 mg/m² IV over 10–15 min following leucovorin
Repeat weekly
Bolus Schedule
Leucovorin 50–100 mg/m² IV over 10–15 min
5-FU 30 mg/kg IV over 10–15 min 1 hr after leucovorin
Repeat every 2–4 weeks as tolerated
Continuous-infusion schedule
Leucovorin 20 mg/m²/day IV over 24 hr
5-FU 500–600 mg/m²/day IV over 24 hr
Repeat daily for 4–7 days every 28 days

to be consistently superior to 5-FU alone. Biochemical modulation of 5-FU with leucovorin has proven to improve response rates in other gastrointestinal malignancies (colon, gastric), compared to 5-FU alone. A variety of treatment schedules exist for administration of 5-FU and leucovorin, ranging from bolus administration to continuous infusion (Table 82.10). The most efficacious schedule is yet to be determined. Although initial studies reported an increased response rate in patients treated with 5-FU plus LCV, subsequent studies have failed to confirm this (70–72). In addition, enhanced toxicity is often seen with the 5-FU/LCV combination, so routine use is not advocated. No standard therapy for patients with metastatic pancreatic cancer exists. Therefore, it is recommended that patients receive chemotherapy as part of a clinical trial whenever possible. Alternatively, for patients ineligible for or those who refuse clinical trials, 5-FU alone or in combination with leucovorin appear to be reasonable choices.

INVESTIGATIONAL AGENTS

Gemcitabine (Difluorodeoxycytidine) is a pyrimidine antimetabolite that appears to have activity in advanced pancreatic cancer. In a phase II trial, patients with pancreatic cancer were noted to experience a reduction in cancer related symptoms and improvement in performance status (73). Since the majority of advanced pancreatic cancer patients have multiple symptoms, recent trials have attempted to evaluate gemcitabine efficacy in terms of clinical benefit, as opposed to the more traditional objective tumor reduction. Evaluation in terms of clinical benefit has three components: pain, performance status, and lean body mass increase. Quantitative definitions of clinical benefit have been developed. In previously untreated patients, objective clinical benefit was seen in approximately 25% of patients compared to 5% in 5-FU treated controls (74). There appeared to be a slight survival advantage for patients receiving gemcitibine compared to 5-FU as well. In a phase II trial with clinical benefit being the primary end point, 27% of patients demonstrated an objective clinical benefit (75). These preliminary studies are encouraging, but additional studies are required to determine the exact role of gemcitabine in the treatment of pancreatic cancer.

Supportive Care

The presenting symptoms of pancreatic cancer almost always include nausea, vomiting, anorexia, weight loss, weakness, and pain. The clinical course is characterized by clinical wasting and pain, with survival usually measured in weeks to months. Given this scenario, supportive care of the patient with pancreatic cancer often becomes more important than treatment of the primary disease. Supportive care for this patient population includes, but is not limited to, pain control, nutritional support, and control of gastrointestinal symptoms (nausea, vomiting, constipation, gastrointestinal obstruction, etc.).

Conclusions

Pancreatic cancer is a relatively rare but highly lethal disease, resulting in the death of over 95% of patients within 5 years of diagnosis. The symptoms of this disease are vague and often attributed to more benign conditions, allowing the disease to progress to advanced stages prior to diagnosis. Only patients with very early disease are potentially curable, and the treatment of choice is surgical resection plus adjuvant radiation and chemotherapy. Effective treatments for advanced disease are still being sought. As there is no consistently effective treatment for advanced disease, these patients should be entered into clinical trials whenever possible. Since most patients experience progressive deterioration, supportive care often becomes the mainstay of therapy. Patients often require supportive care that includes control of gastrointestinal symptoms (nausea, vomiting, diarrhea, constipation, obstruction), pain control, and nutritional support.

GASTRIC CANCER

Epidemiology

In the early 1900s, the leading cause of cancer death in American males was gastric cancer; it was the third leading cause of cancer death in females at this time. Since then, the incidence of gastric cancer in the United States has decreased. The estimated cancer deaths in 1995 from gastric cancer is only 3% of all cancer deaths in males in the United States. The estimated total number of new cases of gastric cancer in the United States for 1995 is 22,800 (14,000 new cases in men; 8,800 new cases in women). Gastric cancer worldwide is most prevalent in Asia, particularly in Japan, Korea, China, Taiwan, and Singapore. Other countries with a high rate of gastric cancer include the former Soviet Union, Costa Rica, and South America (1, 76).

Etiology

The risk factors for the development of gastric cancer are believed to be associated with the environment. Diet is probably the most commonly postulated environmental factor studied in relation to gastric cancer. Diets including high concentrations of nitrates/nitrites, high salt intakes, inappropriate food storage, food spoilage/fermentation, and other factors fostering nitrosamine formation have been related to increasing the risk of developing gastric cancer (77). One proposed chemopreventive agent is ascorbic acid or Vitamin C. The mechanism of action of ascorbic acid is thought to be through this vitamin's ability to prevent the reduction of nitrous acid to N-nitroso compounds. These N-nitroso compounds are carcinogenic in the stomach (78, 79).

Another factor that may increase the risk of gastric cancer is chronic infection with Helicobacter pylori. H. pylori is commonly present in patients with severe gastritis and chronic atrophic gastritis. It is a common infection, with approximately 50% of adults over the age of 50 in North America and virtually 100% of adults in some developing or newly industrialized countries infected (77). It is estimated that the incidence of gastric cancer is 6 times higher in a 100% infected population when compared with a noninfected population (80). Still, only a small percentage of the total number of patients infected with H. pylori will actually develop gastric cancer (81). Infection with H. pylori indirectly causes gastric cancer. The chronic gastritis secondary to H. pylori leads to an increase in cell turnover and intestinal metaplasia development (82). Other risk factors increasing the occurrence of gastric cancer include family history, individuals from blood group A, and individuals with pernicious anemia, atrophic gastritis, prior gastric surgery, gastric polyps, or achlorhydria (83). Individuals from lower socioeconomic classes tend to be at increased risk for the development of gastric cancer. This increased risk is thought to be secondary to dietary and environmental factors common in this population. Smoking has also been associated with increased risk of gastric cancer. However, alcohol consumption has not been shown to increase the risk of gastric cancer.

Pathophysiology

The majority of malignant gastric cancers are adenocarcinomas, accounting for approximately 84% of all gastric neoplasms. The incidence of other, less common histologic classifications include signet ring cell tumors (8%), mucinous adenocarcinomas (3%) and diffuse type adenocarcinoma, intestinal type adenocarcinoma, papillary adenocarcinoma, undifferentiated carcinoma, adenosquamous carcinoma, and tubular adenocarcinoma, each identified in less that 2% of patients (84).

Approximately 30% of primary gastric cancers occur in the upper third of the stomach, 14% in the middle third, and 26% in the lower third. The entire stomach may be involved in up to 10% of patients (84). Gastric cancer has four major patterns of spread: direct extension into the surrounding tissues and organs such as the liver, diaphragm, pancreas, spleen, biliary tract, and transverse colon; nodal metastases, both local (perigastric, celiac axis, porta hepatis, retroperitoneal) and distant (Virchow's node, left axillary nodes); hematogenous spread to liver, lung, bone, and brain; and intraperitoneal dissemination in the pelvis (83). Intraperitoneal spread may be evidenced by the presence of peritoneal implants or ascites.

Overall the prognosis for patients diagnosed with gastric cancer is poor, mainly because only a few patients are diagnosed with early stage disease. The overall survival is strongly correlated with stage at diagnosis. The 5-year survival rate for stage I gastric cancer is 90%; stage II, 70%; stage III, 45%; and stage IV, less than 10%.

Clinical Presentation

Patients with early gastric cancer are typically men (male:female ratio 1.5:1 to 2:1) who are 44 to 70 years of age. By the time gastric cancer is diagnosed in the United States, it is usually advanced. This is primarily because the signs and symptoms of early gastric cancer are similar to those of peptic ulcer disease. The first signs and symptoms that patients may have are mild epigastric pain and dyspepsia. About 40% of patients experience nausea and vomiting. When gastric cancer is still in the early stages, weight loss is minimal, in spite of anorexia. Only one fourth of patients with early gastric cancer demonstrate signs and symptoms of upper gastrointestinal bleeding, with associated anemia. Once the disease has advanced, patients will complain of significant weight loss (>10 pounds), abdominal pain, anorexia, hematemesis, guaiac positive stools and anemia. Other physical changes that might suggest advanced gastric cancer when ob-

Table 82.11.
Common Presenting Signs/Symptoms of Gastric Cancer

Weight loss	Dysphagia
Abdominal pain	Melena
Nausea	Early satiety
Anorexia	Ulcer-type pain

served in conjunction with the previous signs include palpable lymph nodes, palpable ovarian mass, hepatomegaly, palpable abdominal mass, ascites, jaundice, and cachexia (85).

Many patients report experiencing the symptoms of mild epigastric pain for 21 to 36 months. Patients who present with advanced gastric cancer often relate having experienced symptoms for at least the previous 6 to 8 months. In general, the abdominal pain and discomfort experienced with either early or advanced gastric cancer is not relieved by food or antacids (85).

A study to better understand gastric cancer was undertaken in the late 1980s by the American College of Surgeons and involved 18,365 patients (84). Men outnumbered women in this study (63% and 37%, respectively). The median age of males was 68.4 years, and for females 71.9 years. The presenting features of these patients were evaluated and are listed in Table 82.11. The most common symptoms observed in over 50% of the patients were weight loss and abdominal pain. Other frequently encountered symptoms included nausea, anorexia, dysphagia, and melena.

Diagnosis

The differential diagnosis between peptic ulcer disease and gastric cancer must be made in these patients, since the presenting signs and symptoms are so similar. Currently, no blood test that can be used in the definitive diagnosis of gastric cancer is available. Blood tests that may be useful in determining the extent of disease include complete blood count, liver function tests (bilirubin, alkaline phosphatase, LDH, ALT, AST), and carcinoembryonic antigen (CEA). CEA is not used as a diagnostic tool, since it is elevated in only 15 to 30% of patients with advanced disease (86). CEA may be useful in assessment of response to treatment or evaluating recurrence after potentially curative surgical resection.

Historically, the diagnostic procedure performed on patients with upper gastrointestinal complaints has been the upper GI roentgenogram. However, over the last 10 to 15 years there has been a decrease in the use of upper GI roentgenogram and an increased use of upper GI endoscopy for the diagnosis of gastric symptomatology. The increase in the use of endoscopy demonstrates the usefulness of direct visualization of the stomach with an additional advantage of obtaining biopsy specimens. Thus,

esophagogastroduodenoscopy has become the diagnostic procedure of choice (84).

Endoscopic ultrasonography (EUS) can also be performed to diagnose gastric cancer and the extent of disease. The main utility of EUS is in preoperative staging by enabling evaluation of the depth of cancer invasion into the gastric wall. EUS has a 91% accuracy rate in evaluating depth of invasion and may also be useful in diagnosing perigastric metastatic lymph nodes (87).

Screening for early gastric cancer is currently being conducted in areas associated with a high risk of gastric cancer, primarily Japan, South America, and Eastern Europe. Again, esophagogastroduodenoscopy is the diagnostic procedure used in these areas (85). Another diagnostic test often ordered for patients with suspected advanced gastric cancer is a computed tomography scan of the abdomen. This test is performed to evaluate the presence/absence of distant metastases (83).

Staging and Prognosis

The staging of gastric cancer depends on the extent of the disease. This information is obtained during the diagnostic period for the patient (endoscopic procedures, radiology examinations). The TNM classification is used to describe the stage of gastric cancer as recommended by the

Table 82.12.
TNM Staging Classification for Gastric Cancer

Primary Tumor (+)	
T_{is}	Limited to mucosa; does not penetrate the basement membrane
T1	Mucosa or submucosa
T2	To or into but not through serosa
T3	Through serosa without invasion of adjacent tissue
T4a	Involves immediately adjacent structures or extends into esophagus or duodenum
T4b	Direct extension to liver, diaphragm, pancreas, abdominal wall, adrenals, kidney, retroperitoneum, or small bowel, or extraluminal extension to esophagus or duodenum
Regional Lymph Nodes (N)	
N0	No nodal involvement
N1	Perigastric nodes along lesser or greater curvature, within 3 cm of tumor
N2	Other regional lymph nodes—resectable
N3	Other intraabdominal nodes
Distant Metastases (N)	
N0	No distant metastases
N1	Distant metastases present
Stage 0	T_{is} N0 M0
Stage I	T1 N0 M0
Stage II	T2–3 N0 M0
Stage III	T1–3 N1–2 N0
	T4a N02
Stage IV	T1–4a N3 M0
	T4b Nany M0
	Tany Nany M1

American Joint Committee on Cancer (Table 82.12) (83). The percentage of patients presenting at the various stages are stage I (1–5%), stage II (10–15%), stage III (17–20%), and stage IV (72%) (102).

The prognostic factors found to be most significant in predicting poor prognosis are depth of invasion and presence of lymph node metastasis (88, 89). The 5-year survival of patients presenting with tumors invading only the mucosa is 91%; in comparison, the 5-year survival of patients presenting with tumors invading adjacent organs is 6.6%. In patients presenting with greater than 3 lymph nodes positive, 5-year survival is approximately 20%. Other factors that may have some role in predicting outcome include favorable histology (mucinous adenocarcinoma 5-year survival 38.6%) and location of the tumor (whole stomach 5-year survival 20%, upper third of stomach 5-year survival 29.1%). Five-year survival rates based on stage are as follows: stage I (90.7%), stage II (64.5%), stage III (33.4%), and stage IV (4.9%) (88).

Treatment

SURGICAL THERAPY

Surgery is the only therapeutic option that offers a potential cure for the gastric cancer patient. The amount of stomach removed should be enough to allow ample tumor-free margins, with the regional lymph nodes also being removed. Extension of the surgical margins into the adjacent organs should be done only if necessary, and a controversy surrounds the removal of other lymph nodes (i.e., those not directly involved regionally) being dissected as prophylaxis (90–95). In order to ensure tumor-free margins, either a subtotal or total gastrectomy will be performed, based on the location of the tumor in the stomach and on the pattern of spread of the tumor within the stomach. In general, tumors in the distal portion of the stomach can be best treated with a radical subtotal gastrectomy. Tumors in the middle third of the stomach often require a total gastrectomy. Tumors located in the proximal portion of the stomach and the cardia require a total gastrectomy, with the margins often extending into the distal esophagus (96, 97).

If a patient presents with locally advanced (invading other organs) or metastatic gastric cancer, surgery would only be considered with a palliative intent. Again, this could be either a subtotal or total gastrectomy, depending on the location of the obstruction. Currently, palliation from symptom-producing gastric obstruction may be achieved with endoscopic laser surgery. This often provides recanalization with minimal morbidity and mortality (97).

RADIATION THERAPY

Radiation therapy has a limited role in the treatment of gastric cancer. This is primarily due to the difficulty in delivering the required dose in the stomach area. There are many normal tissues in this area that are highly radiosensitive: the spinal cord, kidneys, liver, and small intestines. The use of intraoperative radiation therapy (IORT) is one appealing route of radiation delivery in this patient population. This method allows delivery of the required doses of radiation directly to the tumor and does not exceed the tolerance level of the normal tissues. IORT has been used in combination with external beam radiation and with chemotherapy in the adjuvant setting. Rarely, radiation therapy may be used in advanced gastric cancer for palliation of pain (98–101).

CHEMOTHERAPY

Neoadjuvant Chemotherapy. The goal of neoadjuvant chemotherapy is to improve resectability of tumors in patients with locally advanced disease by decreasing the tumor burden and, therefore, increase the survival time. Gastric cancer patients who are candidates for neoadjuvant chemotherapy are those patients who have locoregional extension of disease (stage II and III) and are considered unresectable at diagnosis or those patients who are potentially resectable, but have bulky disease or other poor prognostic factors (cardial location or enlarged lymph nodes). The advantages of giving chemotherapy to these groups of patients prior to surgery are to (a) promote tumor regression, (b) increase local control rate, (c) allow for more conservative surgical procedures, and (d) define postoperative chemotherapy regimens for patients who have responded to chemotherapy preoperatively. Problems with neoadjuvant chemotherapy include (a) development of resistant clones to chemotherapy, (b) delay of local control measures (i.e., surgery), and (c) increased risk of metastatic spread (103).

Many of the combinations of drugs used in the treatment of advanced disease have been used in the neoadjuvant setting in both patient types. Comparative trials between pre- and postoperative chemotherapy need to be completed to determine the true value of this therapy (102–105).

Adjuvant Chemotherapy. Many trials with adjuvant chemotherapy regimens have been made in an effort to improve survival rates in resected gastric cancer patients. These adjuvant regimens have been compared to surgery alone. Single agents that have been used as adjuvant chemotherapy in separate trials are thiotepa, floxuridine, and high-dose mitomycin C (106). Only mitomycin C demonstrated an increase in survival when compared to surgery alone (107).

With the advent of combination chemotherapy regimens for the treatment of unresectable gastric cancer, combination regimens in the adjuvant chemotherapy setting has increased in use. The Gastrointestinal Tumor Study Group (GITSG) reported a survival benefit in the group of patients receiving adjuvant chemotherapy with 5-fluorouracil and methyl-CCNU (108). These results, however, were not able to be duplicated in two separate confirmatory trials (109–110). 5-Fluorouracil, doxorubicin, and mitomycin C (FAM) is a regimen that has been tested extensively in the treatment of advanced disease. Two separate trials have evaluated FAM in the adjuvant setting, compared to surgery alone. Neither study demonstrated a survival advantage for adjuvant therapy over surgery alone. Other variations of the FAM regimen have been studied in the adjuvant setting, again, without affecting survival (111).

In Japan, adjuvant chemotherapy is administered earlier in the patient's course of treatment. Often, at the time of surgery, intraperitoneal mitomycin C is administered, followed by intravenous mitomycin C administration the following day. A survival benefit was noted in patients treated in this fashion. Further studies added intravenous 5-fluorouracil, which again demonstrated an improved survival advantage. The addition of immunotherapy to an adjuvant chemotherapy regimen is also common in Japanese adjuvant trials. Early administration of adjuvant chemotherapy, plus screening programs leading to early detection of gastric cancer may both be responsible for the improved survival of gastric cancer patients in Japan (106, 111–113). Additional trials need to be conducted to further define the role of adjuvant chemotherapy in gastric cancer. Due to the lack of consistent clinical data, neoadjuvant and adjuvant therapies are not currently considered standard of practice in the United States and should be practiced within the confines of clinical trials.

Chemotherapy of Advanced Disease. Numerous single agents have been tested in the treatment of advanced gastric cancer (114). Of these agents tested, 5-fluorouracil, doxorubicin, mitomycin C, and cisplatin have demonstrate activity as single agents. Because of this single-agent activity, investigators have combined these agents in a number of varying regimens (115). One of the first combinations used in advanced gastric cancer was 5-fluorouracil, doxorubicin, and mitomycin, also known as the FAM regimen (Table 82.13). In the initial study of the FAM regimen, a 42% partial response (PR) rate was reported with no complete responses (CR) observed. The median survival of responding patients was 12.5 months, compared to 5.5 months for all patients (116). Experience with the combination has since increased, and approximately 650 patients in various studies have received treatment with a FAM regimen. The overall response rate in these studies is approximately 30% (2% CR) and the median survival time is 6.9 months (114).

Numerous other combination regimens have been compared to FAM. All regimens produced a response rate that was comparable to FAM with no difference in survival. The North Central Cancer Treatment Group (NCCTG) concluded after studying FAM vs. single-agent

Table 82.13.
Combination Chemotherapy Regimens for the Treatment of Advanced Gastric Cancer

FAM[116]	5-FU	600 mg/m^2 days 1, 8, 29, 36
	Doxorubicin	30 mg/m^2 days 1, 29
	Mitomycin-C	10 mg/m^2 day 1
FAMTX[121]	Methotrexate°	1500 mg/m^2 day 1
	5-FU	1500 mg/m^2 1 hour after MTX on day 1
	Doxorubicin	30 mg/m^2 day 15
	°Leucovorin rescue started 24 hrs after MTX	
ELF[129]	Etoposide	120 mg/m^2 days 1, 2, 3
	Leucovorin	300 mg/m^2 days 1, 2, 3
	5-FU	500 mg/m^2 days 1, 2, 3
EAP[133]	Etoposide	120 mg/m^2 days 4, 5, 6
	Doxorubicin	20 mg/m^2 days 1, 7
	Cisplatin	40 mg/m^2 days 2, 8

5-fluorouracil that 5-FU should be considered the standard treatment for advanced gastric cancer, since less expense and toxicities were observed with comparable response rates (117). Other studies could not document statistically a survival advantage of one treatment over another (118, 119).

A recent four-arm study by the NCCTG compared 5-fluorouracil, doxorubicin, and methyl CCNU (FAMe); 5-fluorouracil, doxorubicin, and cisplatin (FAP); and FAMe alternating with triazinate to single agent 5-FU. Once again, single-agent 5-FU was less toxic than any of the combination regimens and the combination regimens did not demonstrate a survival advantage over the single agent (120).

The combination of high-dose methotrexate, 5-FU and doxorubicin (FAMTX, Table 82.13) produced a promising initial response rate of 63%. Other trials have resulted in lower response rates of 33 to 59%, with some severe toxicities (grade 4 neutropenia, grade 3 mucositis). FAMTX has been compared to FAM in an attempt to better define the toxicity of FAMTX in comparison to FAM, then considered standard treatment. The response rate for FAMTX in this trial was 41%; for FAM the response rate was lower than expected at 9%. Mucositis was more often observed in the FAMTX arm; thrombocytopenia was a cumulative toxicity of FAM. Overall, the toxicities of the two arms were comparable (121). Multiple modifications of the FAMTX regimen have been reported; some of these modifications have included altering drug doses, substituting drugs or adjusting the dosing schedule. None of these modification has provided survival or response advantages over other combination chemotherapy regimens (122–124).

Since single-agent 5-FU is active in the treatment of advanced gastric cancer, biochemical modulation of 5-FU has been studied in this population. Studies have reported activity in 5-FU combinations with leucovorin, interferon-α, and methotrexate. Overall response rates of these biochemically modulated regimens are in the range of 8 to 50% A higher complete and overall response rate has been observed with 5-fluorouracil and leucovorin when compared with single-agent 5-fluorouracil (125–128).

ELF chemotherapy is a combination of leucovorin, 5-FU and etoposide (Table 82.13). The original ELF regimen produced a 48% overall response rate (12% CR) (129). Modifications (l-leucovorin for d,l leucovorin; oral etoposide for intravenous etoposide) of the ELF regimen have not affected the overall response rate (130, 131). PELF chemotherapy (cisplatin, epirubicin, leucovorin, 5-FU) has been compared to a FAM regimen. Patients receiving PELF demonstrated a higher overall response rate (43%) compared to the patients in the FAM arm. However, more grade 3 and 4 toxicities were reported in the PELF arm and there was no survival advantage with PELF (132).

The final combination chemotherapy regimen studied extensively in advanced gastric cancer has been etoposide, doxorubicin, and cisplatin (EAP) (Table 82.13). Response rates using this combination of agents have ranged from 20 to 72% (133–136). Toxicities observed with EAP chemotherapy were leukopenia, thrombocytopenia, and mucositis (134). In a comparison trial of EAP versus FAMTX, both regimens produced similar response rates and toxicities; however, the toxicities associated with EAP therapy were more severe and required longer hospitalizations (135).

Another route of drug administration that has been used in advanced gastric cancer patients is intraperitoneal. This procedure is used primarily for patients with peritoneal seeding. Hyperthermic perfusion with mitomycin C (137) and intraperitoneal cisplatin (138, 139) have been reported as a safe method of direct chemotherapy administration for patients with peritoneal seeding only. Overall, the use of combination chemotherapy has improved the response rate in advanced gastric cancer patients; however, patient survival has demonstrated little improvement. Thus, new agents are continuously being screened for the treatment of advanced gastric cancer. Outside of a clinical trial the least expensive and least toxic chemotherapy regimens should be used in the treatment of advanced gastric cancer.

Conclusions

Since the signs and symptoms of early gastric cancer are so similar to those of peptic ulcer disease, gastric cancer is usually diagnosed in advanced stages. The treatment of gastric cancer depends on the stage of disease. As with other cancers of the gastrointestinal tract, surgery is the only means to achieve a cure. Patients who are able to undergo surgery for curative purposes are those with early stage disease (stage I and II). In patients with locally advanced or metastatic disease, surgery is only performed

as a palliative therapy. The role of neoadjuvant or adjuvant chemotherapy with or without radiation therapy needs to be explored further, as conflicting reports currently exist. Multiple combination chemotherapy regimens have been used in the treatment of unresectable gastric cancer, each providing the patient with varying response rates and toxicities. Unfortunately, none of the regimens provides the patient with an improved survival. Because of this, new agents continue to be studied in the treatment of gastric cancer.

REFERENCES

1. Wingo PA, Tong T, Bolden S. Cancer statistics, 1995. Calif Cancer J Clin 45:8–30, 1995.
2. Phillips RL, Kuzma JW, Lotz TM. Cancer mortality among comparable members vs non-members of the Seventh Day Adventist Church. In: Cairns J, Lyon JL, Skolnick M, eds. Cancer incidence in defined populations. Cold Spring Harbor, NY: Cold Spring Laboratory, 1980:83–102.
3. Enstrom JE. Health and dietary practices and cancer mortality among California Mormons. In: Cairns J, Lyon JL, Skolnick M, eds. Cancer incidence in defined populations. Cold Spring Harbor, NY: Cold Spring Laboratory, 1980:69–90.
4. Ziegler RG, Devesa SS, Fraumeni JF, et al. Epidemiology pattern of colorectal cancer. In: DeVita VT, Hellman S, Rosenberg SA, eds. Important advances in oncology. Philadelphia: JB Lippincott, 1986:209–232.
5. Deschner EE, Cohen BI, Raicht RF. Acute and chronic effect of dietary cholic acid on colonic epithelial cell proliferation. Digestion 21:290–296, 1981.
6. Newmark HL, Wargovich MJ, Bruce WR. Colon cancer and dietary fat, phosphate, and calcium: a hypothesis. J Natl Cancer Inst 72:1323–1325, 1984.
7. Kritchevsky D. Dietary fiber and cancer. Nutr Cancer 6:213–219, 1985.
8. Yang CS, Newmark HL. The role of micronutrient deficiency in carcinogenesis. CRC Crit Rev Oncol Hematol 7:267–287, 1987.
9. Eastwoood M. Dietary fiber and risk of cancer. Nutr Rev 45:193–198, 1977.
10. Longnecker MP, Orza MJ, Adams ME, et al. A metaanalysis of alcoholic beverage consumption in relation to risk of colorectal cancer. Cancer Causes Control 1:59–68,1990.
11. Margulis AR, Thoeni RF. The present status of the radiologic examination of the colon. Radiology 167:1–5, 1988.
12. O'Dwyer PT, Mojzcsi C, McCabe DP. Reoperation directed by carcinoembryonic antigen level: the importance of a thorough preoperative evaluation. Am J Surg 155:227–231, 1988.
13. Cohen AM, Mindky BD, Schilsky RL. Colon cancer. In: DeVita VT, Hellman S, Rosenberg SA, eds. Cancer: principles and practice of oncology, 4th ed. Philadelphia: JB Lippincott, 1993:929–977.
14. Bond JH. Screening and early detection. In: Wanebo HJ, ed. Colorectal cancer. St. Louis: Mosby, 1993:149–157.
15. Enker WE, Loffer UT, Block GE. Enhanced survival of patients with colon and rectal cancer is based upon wide anatomic resection. Ann Surg 190:350–360, 1979.
16. Steele G, Posner MR. Adjuvant treatment of colorectal adenocarcinoma. Curr Probl Cancer 17:223–269, 1993.
17. Devasa JM, Morales V, Enriques JM. Colorectal cancer: the basis for a comprehensive follow-up. Dis Colon Rectum 31:636–652, 1988.
18. Moertel CG. Accomplishment in surgical adjuvant therapy for large bowel cancer. Cancer 70:1364–1371, 1992.

19. Verhaegen H, DeCree J, DeCock W, et al. Levamisole therapy in patients with colorectal cancer. In: Terry WD, Rosenberg SA, eds. Immunotherapy of human cancer. New York: Excerpta Medica, 1982: 225–229.

20. Moertel CG, Fleming TR, Macdonald JS, et al. Fluorouracil plus levamisole as effective adjuvant therapy after resection of stage III colon carcinoma: a final report. Ann Intern Med 122:321–326, 1995.

21. NIH Consensus Conference. Adjuvant therapy for patients with colon and rectal cancer. JAMA 264:1444–1450, 1990.

22. Hamilton JM. Adjuvant therapy for gastrointestinal cancer. Curr Opin Oncol 6:435–440, 1994.

23. Gunderson LL, Martenson JA. Colorectal cancer: radiotherapy. In: Brain MC, Carbone PC, eds. Current therapy in hematology-oncology, 5th ed. St. Louis: Mosby, 1995:371–384.

24. Gastrointestinal Study Group. Prolongation of the disease-free interval in surgically treated rectal cancer. N Engl J Med 312:1465–1472, 1985.

25. Douglass HO, Mayer RJ, Thomas PRM, et al. Survival after postoperative combination treatment of rectal cancer [Letter]. N Engl J Med 315:1294, 1986.

26. Krook J, Moertel C, Gunderson LL, et al. Effective surgical adjuvant therapy for high-risk rectal carcinoma. N Engl J Med 324:709–714, 1991.

27. Weaver D, Lindblad AS. Gastrointesinal Tumor Study Group: radiation therapy and 5-fluorouracil (5-FU) with or without MeCCNU for the treatment of patients with surgically adjuvant adenocarcinoma of the rectum. Proc ASCO 9:106, 1990.

28. O'Connell M, Wieand HS, Krook J, et al. Lack of value for methyl-CCNU (MeCCNU) as a component of effective rectal cancer surgical adjuvant therapy: interim analysis of intergroup protocol 86-47-51. Proc ASCO 10:134, 1991.

29. Rougier P, Nordlinger B. Larger scale trial for adjuvant treatment in high risk resected colorectal cancers. Rationale to test the combination of loco-regional and systemic chemotherapy and to compare l-leucovorin + 5-FU to levamisole + 5-FU. Ann Oncol 2:21–28, 1993.

30. Ahlgren JD. Colorectal cancer: chemotherapy. In: Algren JD, Macdonald JS, eds. Gastrointestinal oncology. Philadelphia: JB Lippincott, 1992:339–357.

31. Macmillan WE, Wolberg WH, Welling PG. Pharmacokinetics of fluorouracil in humans. Cancer Res 38:3479–3482, 1978.

32. Washtien WL, Santi DV. Intracellular free and macromolecular-bound metabolites of 5-fluorodeoxyuridine and 5-fluorouracil. Cancer Res 39:3397–3404, 1979.

33. Seifert P, Baker LH, Reed MD, et al. Comparison of continuously infused 5-fluorouracil with bolus injection in patients with colorectal adenocarcinoma. Cancer 36:123–128, 1975.

34. Lokich JJ, Bothe A, Fine A, et al. Phase I study of protracted venous infusion of 5-fluorouracil. Cancer 48:2565–2568, 1981.

35. Ardalan B, Singh G, Silberman H. A randomized phase I and II study of short-term infusion of high-dose fluorouracil with and without N-(phosphonacetyl)-L-aspartic acid in patients with advanced pancreatic and colorectal cancers. J Clin Oncol 6:1053–1058, 1988.

36. Evans RM, Laskin JD, Hakala MT. Effect of excess folates and deoxyinosine on the activity and site of action of 5-fluorouracil. Cancer Res 41:3283–3295, 1981.

37. Petrelli N, Herrera L, Rustum Y, et al. A prospective randomized trial of 5-fluorouracil and high dose leucovorin versus 5-FU and methotrexate in previously untreated patients with advanced colorectal carcinoma. J Clin Oncol 5:1559–1565, 1987.

38. Petrelli N, Douglass HO, Herrera L, et al. The modulation of fluorouracil with leucovorin in metastatic colorectal carcinoma: a prospective phase III trial. J Clin Oncol 7:1419–1426, 1989.

39. Poon MA, O'Connell MJ, Moertel CG, et al. Biochemical modulation of fluorouracil: evidence of significant improvement of survival and quality of life in patients with advanced colorectal carcinoma. J Clin Oncol 7:1407–1408, 1989.

40. Doroshaw JH, Multhauf P, Leong L, et al. Prospective randomized comparison of fluorouracil versus fluorouracil and high dose continuous infusion leucovorin calcium for the treatment of advanced measurable colorectal cancer in patients previously unexposed to chemotherapy. J Clin Oncol 8:491–501, 1990.

41. Erlichman C, Fine S, Wong A, et al. A randomized trial of fluorouracil and folinic acid in patients with metastatic colorectal carcinoma. J Clin Oncol 6:469–475, 1988.

42. Poon MA, O'Connell MJ, Wieland HS, et al. Biochemical modulation of fluorouracil with leucovorin: confirmatory evidence of improved therapeutic efficacy in advanced colorectal cancer. J Clin Oncol 9:1967–1972, 1991.

43. Wadler SW, Schwartz EL, Goldman M, et al. Fluorouracil and recombinant alfa-2a-interferon: an active regimen against advanced colorectal carcinoma. J Clin Oncol 7:1769–1775, 1989.

44. Ardalan B, Singh G, Silberman H. A randomized phase I and II study of short-term infusion of high-dose fluorouracil with or without N-(phosphonacetyl)-L-aspartic acid in patients with advanced pancreatic and colorectal. J Clin Oncol 7:1053–1058, 1988.

45. Grem JL, Fischer PH. Enhancement of 5-fluorouracil's anticancer activity by dipyridamole. Pharmacol Ther 40:349–371, 1989.

46. Klubes P, Leyland-Jones B. Enhancement of the antitumor activity of 5-fluorouracil by uridine rescue. Pharmacol Ther 41:289–302, 1989.

47. Bugat R, Rougier P, Douillard JY, et al. Efficacy of irinotecan HCl (CPT 11) in patients with metastatic colorectal cancer after progression while receiving a 5-FU based chemotherapy. Proc ASCO 14:567, 1995.

48. Abigerges D, Chabot GG, Armand JP, et al. Phase I and pharmacologic studies of the camptothecin analog irinotecan administered every 3 weeks in cancer patients. J Clin Oncol 13:210–221, 1995.

49. Zalcberg J, Cunningham D, Green M, et al. The final results of a large scale phase II study of the potent thymidylate synthase (TS) inhibitor tomudex (ZD1694) in advanced colorectal cancer. Proc ASCO 14:494, 1995.

50. Pazdur R, Rhodes V, Lassere Y, et al. UFT plus leucovorin: a potentially effective oral regimen in colorectal carcinoma. Proc ASCO 13:590, 1994.

51. Fontham ET, Correa P. Epidemiology of pancreatic cancer. Surg Clin North Am 69:551–567, 1989.

52. Brennan MF, Kinsella T, Casper ES. Cancer of the pancreas. In: De Vita VT, ed. Cancer principles and practice of oncology. Philadelphia: JB Lippincott, 1993:849–882.

53. Mack TM, Yu M, Hanisch R, et al. Pancreas cancer and smoking, beverage consumption, and past medical history. J Natl Cancer Inst 76:49–60, 1986.

54. Olsen GW, Mandel JS, Gibson RW, et al. A case-control study of pancreatic cancer and cigarettes, alcohol, coffee and diet, Am J Public Health 79:1016–1019, 1989.

55. Karmody A, Kyle J. The association between carcinoma of the pancreas and diabetes mellitus. Br J Surg 56:362–364, 1969.

56. Steinberg W. The clinical utility of the CA '19-9 tumor associated antigen. Am J Gastroenterol 85:350–355, 1990.

57. Kiriyama E, Hayakawa T, Kondo T, et al. Usefulness of a new tumor marker, Span-1, for the diagnosis of pancreatic cancer. Cancer 65:1557–1561, 1990.

58. Beahrs OH, ed. American joint committee on cancer, manual for staging of cancer, 3rd ed. Philadelphia: JB Lippincott, 1988:109.

59. Wiley AL. Pancreatic cancer. New York: Masson Publishing, 1980:107.

60. Tepper J, Nardi G, Suit H. Carcinoma of the pancreas: review of MGH experience from 1963–1973. Cancer 37:1519–1524, 1976.

61. Gastrointestinal Tumor Study Group. Pancreatic cancer adjuvant combined radiation and chemotherapy following curative resection. Arch Surg 120:899–903, 1985.

62. Gastrointestinal Tumor Study Group. Further experience of effective adjuvant combined radiation and chemotherapy following curative resection of pancreatic cancer. Cancer 59:2006–2010, 1987.

63. Gastrointestinal Tumor Study Group. Treatment of locally unrespectable carcinoma of the pancreas: comparison of combined modality therapy (chemotherapy plus radiotherapy) to chemotherapy alone. J Natl Cancer Inst 80:751–755, 1988.

64. Whittington R, Solin L, Mohiuddin M, et al. Multimodality therapy of localized unrespectable pancreatic adenocarcinoma. Cancer 54:1991–1998, 1984.

65. Dobelbower RR, Merrick H, Ahuja R, et al. 125I interstitial implant, precision high-dose external beam therapy and 5-FU for unrespectable adenocarcinoma of pancreas and extrahepatic biliary tree. Cancer 58:2185–2195, 1986.

66. Roldan GE, Gunderson L, Nagorney D, et al. External beam versus intraoperative and external beam irradiation for locally advanced pancreatic cancer. Cancer 61:1110–1116, 1988.

67. Bagne FR, Dobelbower RR, Milligan AJ, et al. Treatment of cancer of the pancreas by intraoperative electron beam therapy: physical and biological aspects. Int J Radiat Oncol Biol Phys 16:231–242, 1989.

68. Cersosimo RJ, Hong WK. Epirubicin: a review of the pharmacology, clinical activity, and adverse effects of an adriamycin analogue. J Clin Oncol 4:425–439, 1986.

69. Haskell CM, Selch MT, Ramming KP, Exocrine Pancreas. In: Haskell CM, ed. Cancer treatment, 3rd ed. Philadelphia: WB Saunders, 1991:259.

70. Bruckner HW, Crown J, McKenna A, et al. Leucovorin and 5-fluorouracil as a treatment for disseminated cancer of the pancreas and unknown primary tumors. Cancer Res 48:5570–5572, 1988.

71. DeCaprio JA, Arbuck SG, Mayer RJ. Phase II study of weekly 5-fluorouracil (5-FU) with folinic acid (FA) in previously untreated patients with unresectable measurable pancreatic adenocarcinoma [Abstract]. Proc Am Soc Clin Oncol 8:388, 1989.

72. Crown J, Casper ES, Botet J, et al. Lack of efficacy of high dose leucovorin and fluorouracil in patients with advanced pancreatic adenocarcinoma. J Clin Oncol 9:1682–1686, 1991.

73. Casper ES, Green MR, Kelson DP, et al. Phase II trial of gemcitabine (2,2'-difluorodeoxy-cytidine) in patients with adreno-carcinoma of the pancreas. Invest New Drugs 12:29–34,1994.

74. Moore M, Andersen J, Burris H, et al. A randomized trial of gemcitabine (GEM) versus 5FU as first-line therapy in advanced pancreatic cancer [Abstract]. Proc Am Soc Clin Oncol 14:473, 1995.

75. Rothenberg ML, Burris HA, Andersen JS, et al. Gemcitabine: effective palliative therapy for pancreas cancer patients failing 5-FU [Abstract]. Proc Am Soc Clin Oncol 14:470, 1995.

76. Liu MC, Hai A, Huang AT. Cancer epidemiology in the Far East-contrast with the United States. Oncology 7:99–114, 1993.

77. Hwang H, Swyer J, Russell RM. Diet, Helicobacter pylori infection, food preservation and gastric cancer risk: are these new roles for preventive factors. Nutrition Reviews 52:75–83, 1994.

78. Tannenbaum SR, Wishnok JS, Leaf CD. Inhibition of nitrosamine formation by ascorbic acid. Am J Clin Nutr 53(suppl):247S–250S, 1991.

79. Schorah CJ, Sobala GM, Sanderson M, et al. Gastric juice ascorbic acid: effects of disease and implications for gastric carcinogenesis. Am J Clin Nutr 53:287S–293S, 1991.

80. Eurogast. An international association between Helicobacter pylori infection and the gastric cancer. Lancet 341:1359–1362, 1993.

81. Parsonnett J, Friedman GD, Vandersteen DP, et al. Helicobacter pylori infection and the risk of gastric carcinoma. N Engl J Med 325:1127–1131, 1991.

82. Graham DY. Benefits from elimination of Helicobacter pylori infection include major reduction in the incidence of peptic ulcer disease, gastric cancer, and primary gastric lymphoma. Preventive Med 23:712–716, 1994.

83. Macdonald JS, Hill MC, Roberts IM. Gastric cancer: epidemiology, pathology, detection, and staging. In: Ahlgren J, Macdonald J, eds. Gastrointestinal oncology. Philadelphia: JB Lippincott, 1992: 151–158.

84. Wanebo HJ, Kennedy BJ, Chmiel J, et al. Cancer of the stomach: a patient care study by the American College of Surgeons. Ann Surg 218:583–592, 1993.

85. Farley DR, Donohue JH. Early gastric cancer. Surg Clin North Am 72:401–421, 1992.

86. Ellis DJ, Spevis C, Kingston RD, et al. Carcinoembryonic antigen levels in advanced gastric carcinoma. Cancer 42:623–625, 1978.

87. Caletti G, Ferrari A, Brocchi E, Barbara L. Accuracy of endoscopic ultrasonography in the diagnosis and staging of gastric cancer and lymphoma. Surgery 113:14–27, 1993.

88. Kim JP, Kim YW, Yang HK, Noh DY. Significant prognostic factors by multivariate analysis of 3926 gastric cancer patients. World J Surg 18:872–878, 1994.

89. Lee WJ, Lee PH, Yue SC, et al. Lymph node metastases in gastric cancer: significance of positive number. Oncology 52:45–50, 1995.

90. Boddie AW Jr. The role of lymphadenectomy in cancer, with particular reference to gastric cancer. Int Surg 79:6–10, 1994.

91. Behrns KE, Dalton RR, van Heerden JA, Sarr MG. Extended lymph node dissection for gastric cancer: is it of value? Surg Clin North Am 72:433–443, 1992.

92. Bonenkamp JJ, van de Velde CJH, Sasako M, et al. R2 compared with R1 resection for gastric cancer: morbidity and mortality in a prospective, randomized trial. Eur J Surg 158:413–418, 1992.

93. Robertson CS, Chung SCS, Woods SDS, et al. A prospective randomized trial comparing R1 subtotal gastrectomy with R3 total gastrectomy for antral cancer. Ann Surg 220:176–182, 1994.

94. Bunt AMG, Hermans J, Boon MC, et al. Evaluation of the extent of lymphadenectomy in a randomized trial of Western- versus Japanese-type surgery in gastric cancer. J Clin Oncol 12:417–422, 1994.

95. Pacelli F, Doglietto GB, Ballantone R, et al. Extensive versus limited lymph node dissection for gastric cancer: a comparative study of 320 patients. Br J Surg 80:1153–1156, 1993.

96. Smith JW, Brennan MF. Surgical treatment of gastric cancer: proximal, mid and distal stomach. Surg Clin North Am 72:381–399, 1992.

97. Vezeridis MP, Wanebo HJ. Gastric cancer: surgical approach. In: Ahlgren J, Macdonald J, eds. Gastrointestinal oncology. Philadelphia: JB Lippincott, 1992:159–170.

98. Budach VGF. The role of radiation therapy in the management of gastric cancer. Ann Oncol 5(suppl 3):S37–S48, 1994.

99. Tepper JE. Combined radiotherapy and chemotherapy in the treatment of gastrointestinal malignancies. Semin Oncol 19(suppl 11):96–101, 1992.

100. Hallissey MT, Dunn JA, Ward LC, et al. The second British Stomach Cancer Group trial of adjuvant radiotherapy or chemotherapy in resectable gastric cancer: five-year follow-up. Lancet 343:1309–1312, 1994.

101. Calvo FA, Aristu JJ, Azinovic I, et al. Intraoperative and external radiotherapy in resected gastric cancer: updated report of a phase II trial. Int J Radiation Oncol Biol Phys 24:729–736, 1992.

102. Alexander HR, Grem JL, Pass HI, et al. Neoadjuvant chemotherapy of locally advanced gastric cancer. Oncology 7:37–41, 1993.

103. Rougier P, Lasser P, Ducreux M, et al. Preoperative chemotherapy of locally advanced gastric cancer. Ann Oncol 5(suppl 3):S59–S68, 1994.

104. Kelsen D. Neoadjuvant therapy for gastrointestinal cancers. Oncology 7:25–31, 1993.
105. Leichman L, Silberman H, Leichman CG, et al. Preoperative systemic chemotherapy followed by adjuvant postoperative intraperitoneal therapy for gastric cancer: a University of Southern California pilot program. J Clin Oncol 10:1933–1942, 1992.
106. Agboola O. Adjuvant treatment in gastric cancer. Cancer Treat Rev 20:217–240, 1994.
107. Grau JJ, Estape J, Alcobendas F, et al. Positive results of adjuvant mitomycin C in resected gastric cancer: a randomized trial on 134 patients. Eur J Cancer 29A:340–342, 1993.
108. Gastrointestinal Tumor Study Group. Controlled trial of adjuvant chemotherapy following curative resection for gastric cancer. Cancer 49:1116–1122, 1982.
109. Engstrom PF, Lavin PT, Douglass HO Jr, et al. Postoperative adjuvant 5-fluorouracil plus methyl-CCNU for gastric cancer patients: Eastern Cooperative Oncology Group Study (EST 3275). Cancer 55:1868–1873, 1985.
110. Higgins GA, Amadeo JH, Smith DE, et al. Efficacy of prolonged intermittent therapy with combined 5-FU and methyl-CCNU following resection for gastric carcinoma. A Veterans Administration Surgical Oncology Group report. Cancer 52:1105–1112, 1983.
111. Douglass HO Jr. Gastric cancer: current status of adjuvant therapy. Oncology 3:61–66, 1989.
112. Bleiberg H, Gerard B, Deguiral P. Adjuvant therapy in resectable gastric cancer. Br J Cancer 66:987–991, 1992.
113. Lise M, Nitti D, Marchet A, et al. Adjuvant treatment for gastric cancer. Anticancer Drugs 2:433–445, 1991.
114. Kelsen D. The use of chemotherapy in the treatment of advanced gastric and pancreas cancer. Semin Oncol 21(suppl 7):58–66, 1994.
115. Macdonald JS. Gastric cancer: chemotherapy of advanced disease. Hematol Oncol 10:37–42, 1992.
116. Macdonald JS, Schein PS, Woolley PV, et al. 5-fluorouracil, doxorubicin, and mitomycin (FAM) combination chemotherapy for advanced gastric cancer. Ann Intern Med 93:533–536, 1980.
117. Cullinan SA, Moertel CG, Fleming TR, et al. A comparison of three chemotherapeutic regimens in the treatment of advanced pancreatic and gastric carcinoma. Fluorouracil vs. fluorouracil and doxorubicin vs. fluorouracil, doxorubicin and mitomycin. JAMA 253:2061–2067, 1985.
118. Figoli F, Galligioni E, Crivellari D, et al. Evaluation of two consecutive regimens in advanced gastric cancer. Cancer Invest 93:257–262, 1991.
119. Kim NY, Park YS, Heo DS, et al. A phase III randomized study of 5-fluorouracil, doxorubicin, and mitomycin C versus 5-fluorouracil alone in the treatment of advanced gastric cancer. Cancer 71:3813–3818, 1993.
120. Cullinan SA, Moertel CG, Wieand HS, et al. Controlled evaluation of three drug combination regimens versus fluorouracil alone for the therapy of advanced gastric cancer. J Clin Oncol 12:412–416, 1994.
121. Wils JA, Klein HO, Wagener DJT, et al. Sequential high-dose methotrexate and fluorouracil combined with doxorubicin-a step ahead in the treatment of advanced gastric cancer: a trial of the European Organization for Research and Treatment of Cancer Gastrointestinal Tract Cooperative Group. J Clin Oncol 9:827–831, 1991.
122. Murad AM, Santiago FF, Petroianu A, et al. Modified therapy with 5-fluorouracil, doxorubicin, and methotrexate in advanced gastric cancer. Cancer 72:37–41, 1993.
123. Pyrhonen S, Kuitunen T, Nyandoto P, Kouri M. Randomized comparison of fluorouracil, epidoxorubicin and methotrexate (FEMTX) plus supportive care with supportive care alone in patients with non-resectable gastric cancer. Br J Cancer 71:587–591, 1995.
124. Roelofs EJM, Wagener DJT, Conroy T, et al. Phase II study of sequential high-dose methotrexate (MTX) and 5-fluorouracil (F) alternated with epirubicin (E) and cisplatin (P) [FEMTX-P] in advanced gastric cancer. Ann Oncol 4:426–428, 1993.
125. Wilke H, Stahl M, Schmoll HJ, et al. Biochemical modulation of 5-fluorouracil by folinic acid or alpha-interferon with and without other cytostatic drugs in gastric, esophageal, and pancreatic cancer. Semin Oncol 19(suppl 3):215–219, 1992.
126. Konishi T, Hiraishi M, Mafune K, et al. Therapeutic efficacy and toxicity of sequential methotrexate and 5-fluorouracil in gastric cancer. Anticancer Res 14:1277–1280, 1994.
127. Louvet C, deGramont A, Demuynck B, et al. High-dose folinic acid, 5-fluorouracil bolus and continuous infusion in poor-prognosis patients with advanced measurable gastric cancer. Ann Oncol 2:229–230, 1991.
128. Vanhoefer U, Wilke H, Weh HJ, et al. Weekly high-dose 5-fluorouracil and folinic acid as salvage treatment in advanced gastric cancer. Ann Oncol 5:850–851, 1994.
129. Wilke H, Preusser P, Fink U, et al. High dose folinic acid, etoposide and 5-fluorouracil in advanced gastric cancer. A phase II study in elderly patients or patients with cardiac risk. Invest New Drugs 8:65–70, 1990.
130. diBartolomeo M, Bajetta E, deBraud F, et al. Phase II study of the etoposide, leucovorin and fluorouracil combination for patients with advanced gastric cancer unsuitable for aggressive chemotherapy. Oncology 52:41–44, 1995.
131. Taal BG, Teller FGM, ten Bokkel Huinink WW, et al. Etoposide, leucovorin, 5-fluorouracil (ELF) combination chemotherapy for advanced gastric cancer: experience with two treatment schedules incorporating intravenous or oral etoposide. Ann Oncol 5:90–92, 1994.
132. Cocconi G, Bella M, Zironi S, et al. Fluorouracil, doxorubicin, and mitomycin combination versus PELF chemotherapy in advanced gastric cancer: a prospective randomized trial of the Italian Oncology Group for Clinical Research. J Clin Oncol 12:2687–2693, 1994.
133. Preusser P, Wilke H, Achterrath W, et al. Phase II study with the combination of etoposide, doxorubicin, and cisplatin in advanced measurable gastric cancer. J Clin Oncol 7:1310–1317, 1989.
134. Bajetta E, diBartolomeo M, deBraud F, et al. Etoposide, doxorubicin, and cisplatin (EAP) treatment in advanced gastric: a multicentre study of the Italian Trials in Medical Oncology (ITMO) Group. Eur J Cancer 30A:596–600, 1994.
135. Kelsen D, Atiq OT, Saltz L, et al. FAMTX versus etoposide, doxorubicin and cisplatin: a random assignment trial in gastric cancer. J Clin Oncol 10:541–548, 1992.
136. Haim M, Tsalik M, Robinson E. Treatment of gastric adenocarcinoma with the combination of etoposide, adriamycin and cisplatin (EAP): comparison between two schedules. Oncology 51:102–107, 1994.
137. Fujimoto S, Takahashi M, Kobayashi K, et al. Relation between clinical and histologic outcome of intraperitoneal hyperthermic perfusion for patients with gastric cancer and peritoneal metastasis. Oncology 50:338–343, 1993.
138. Tsujitani S, Okuyama T, Watanabe A, et al. Intraperitoneal cisplatin during surgery for gastric cancer and peritoneal seeding. Anticancer Res 13:1831–1834, 1993.
139. Jones Al, Trott P, Cunningham D, et al. A pilot study of intraperitoneal cisplatin in the management of gastric cancer. Ann Oncol 5:123–126, 1994.

CHAPTER 83

LUNG CANCER

KIMBERLY A. BERGSTROM

Lung cancer has become the leading cause of cancer death among both men and women in the United States. By the year 2000, the World Health Organization predicts that there will be 2 million cases of lung cancer annually, placing a tremendous burden on our global health care systems. Even though epidemiologic studies have convincingly linked smoking, particularly cigarette smoking, to lung cancer, both the incidence and prevalence continue to rise. This chapter will explain the classification, epidemiology, and etiology of lung cancer types; explore the pathogenesis and pathology of the disease; and review the treatment approaches to lung cancer.

CLASSIFICATION

Lung cancer types are broadly categorized into small cell lung cancer (15 to 25% of cases) and non–small cell lung cancer (75 to 85% of cases) (Fig. 83.1). Small cell lung cancers grow rapidly, are early to metastasize, and generally arise in the central regions of the lung. Non–small cell cancers comprise several cell types, including adenocarcinoma, squamous cell carcinoma, and large cell carcinoma, and often occur as a mixture of several cell types together. Non–small cell lung cancers have less of a propensity to grow rapidly or metastasize than do small cell carcinomas. Of the three non–small cell types, adenocarcinoma is the most common and tends to develop in the periphery of the lung as a small, coinlike lesion (less than 4 cm). It has an intermediate propensity for growth and metastasis. Squamous cell carcinoma represents 30 to 40% of all non–small cell lung cancers and tends to develop in the central or hilar regions of the lung. Its growth in comparison to adenocarcinoma is slow, and it tends to metastasize late. Large cell carcinomas account for approximately 10% of non–small cell lung cancers. These large cell types are characterized as having rapid growth and early metastases and the presence of carcinoembryonic antigen in the blood (1).

EPIDEMIOLOGY AND ETIOLOGY

What are the risk factors for lung cancer? Who is likely to get lung cancer and why? The worldwide incidence (new cases per year) and prevalence (number of individuals living with cancer) of lung cancer varies greatly, due mainly to smoking patterns, environmental causes, and genetic factors (2). Smoking is the largest modifiable risk factor for lung cancer. As early as the 1940s, researcher's investigating possible associations between lung cancer incidence

with urban pollutants, arsenicals, tobacco smoking, and occupation, found a strong correlation between lung cancer and cigarette smoking but found no significant association with the other risk factors. Since then, numerous studies have confirmed these initial findings. From these studies, we have learned that smokers are ten times more likely to develop lung cancer than those who have never smoked, that the risk of lung cancer increases with the number of years of smoking and greater frequency of smoking, and that smoking cessation reduces the risk of cancer, though slowly, over time (1). There is also strong evidence now linking secondhand smoke to lung cancer.

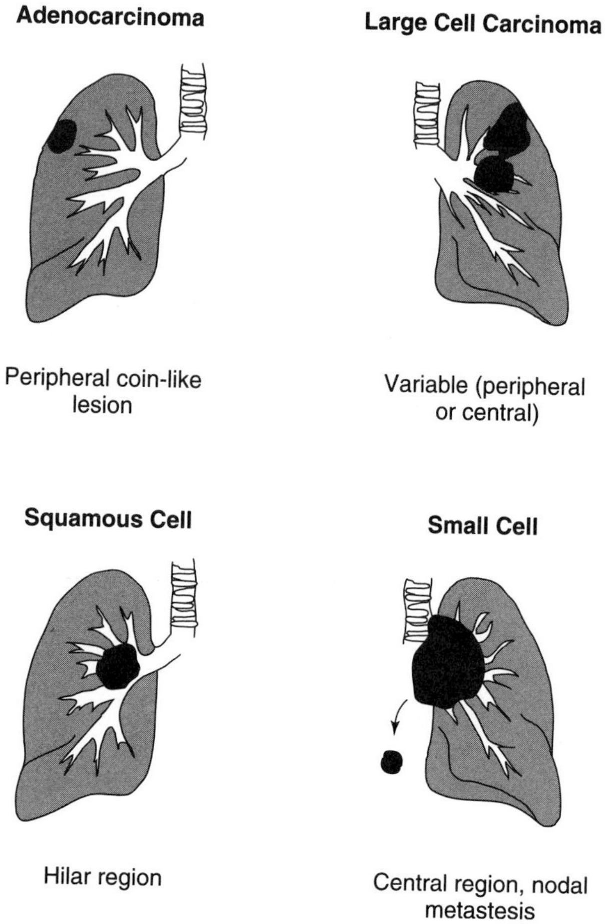

Figure 83.1 Size and location of each cellular type of lung cancer. Adapted from Harvey JC, Beattie EJ. Lung cancer. Clinical Symposia 45:2–34.

The National Research Council in 1986 performed a metaanalysis of 13 studies that showed the relative risk of lung cancer for wives of husbands who smoke to be 30% higher than for wives with nonsmoking husbands (1).

Smoking

Smoking was one of the first of several risk factors to be causatively linked with lung cancer. Occupational exposure to asbestos, radon decay products, arsenic, chromium and certain chromium compounds, ionizing radiation and gamma radiation, mustard gas, nickel, soots, tars, and vinyl chloride have also been identified as causative agents to the development of lung cancer. Of these, asbestos is the most frequent occupational cause of lung cancer, responsible for approximately 5% of lung cancers in 1981 (2). Radon decay products found in small amounts in the ground can leak into home foundations or groundwater used in the home and may contribute up to 5% of newly diagnosed lung cancers annually.

Diet

High intake of vegetables has been shown to modestly reduce the risk of lung cancer in epidemiologic studies (1). Research suggests that this effect may be due to the antioxidant effects of beta-carotene (found in green, yellow, and orange fruits and vegetables). Several ongoing chemoprevention trials are looking at whether greater intake of vitamin supplements can reduce the incidence of lung cancer in high-risk patients.

Nonmodifiable Risk Factors

Gender, race and ethnicity all play a role in either enhancing or reducing one's risk for developing lung cancer. After making adjustments for smoking, men are more likely to develop lung cancer than women. Even among nonsmokers, males have higher lung cancer mortality rates than females. Evidence also shows that after adjusting for differences in smoking behavior, black males and females have higher lung cancer rates than whites (2). And there is evidence to suggest through studies done in families, that nonsmokers who have relatives with lung cancer are two to three times more likely to develop lung cancer than nonsmokers without relatives with lung cancer (2), suggesting that there may be an inherited predisposition in some families for the development of lung cancer.

DIAGNOSIS

All patients with suspected lung cancer should undergo a physical examination, medical history, and chest radiograph (1). Blood chemistries and a complete blood count are usually taken to screen for unsuspected abnormalities, including renal and hepatic dysfunction, coagulopathies, or electrolyte imbalance. Once an abnormal finding shows up on chest radiograph, histologic examination of the tumor is necessary to confirm the diagnosis of lung cancer. Tissue for histologic examination can be obtained by one of four methods: sputum collection, percutaneous needle biopsy, fiberoptic bronchoscopy, and excision of the lesion (1).

STAGING

Staging is a quantitative assessment of the extent of disease present for the purpose of grouping like patients together to determine their prognosis, treatment strategy, and therapeutic success. It is extremely important that staging of any cancer be accurate and consistent worldwide. The American Joint Committee on Cancer (AJCC) recently revised the staging for lung cancer to better reflect modern treatment approaches to lung cancer and to resolve differences between the previous AJCC system and systems used frequently in Europe and Japan (3). The staging system is a composite of both the TNM classification, which describes the anatomic extent of disease, and the cellular classification or cell type present.

Non–small Cell Lung Cancer

The TNM staging system is described by the primary tumor size and extent (T), regional lymph node metastases (N), and distant metastases (M). Table 83.1 describes the TNM characteristics for non–small cell lung cancer. Occult stage disease is defined as bronchopulmonary secretions that contain malignant cells but where there is no other evidence of a primary tumor, regional or distant metastasis. Stage 0 describes carcinoma in situ, an encapsulated small tumor with no regional or distant metastases. Five-year survival data with treatment is not yet available for this stage. Stage I describes tumors up to or exceeding 3 cm in diameter that may or may not have invaded the main bronchus and visceral pleura. This tumor may be associated with atelectasis or obstructive pneumonitis that extends to

Table 83.1.
Staging of Non–small Cell Lung Cancer

Stage	TNM Classification	5-Year Survival Rate
Occult Stage	T_x, N_0, M_0	70–80%
Stage 0	Tis, N_0, M_0	Not available
Stage I	T_1, N_0, M_0	50% (with treatment)
	T_2, N_0, M_0	
Stage II	T_1, N_1, M_0	30% (with treatment)
	T_2, N_1, M_0	
Stage IIIa	T_1, N_2, M_0	10–15% (with treatment)
	T_2, N_2, M_0	
	T_3, N_0, M_0	
	T_3, N_1, M_0	
	T_3, N_2, M_0	
Stage IIIb	Any T, N_3, M_0	<5% (with treatment)
	T_4, Any N, M_0	
Stage IV	Any T, any N, M_2	<2% (with treatment)

Adapted from references (1, 3, 4).

the hilar regions of the lung. Stage II is described by the same primary tumor involvement as stage I with regional metastasis to the ipsilateral peribronchial and/or hilar lymph nodes, including direct extension. Stage III disease is defined by two subgroups: stage IIIa and stage IIIb. Stage IIIa describes a tumor of any size with direct extension into the bronchus, pleura, chest wall, diaphragm, parietal pericardium, and nodal metastasis in the ipsilateral peribronchial, mediastinal, subcarinal, and/or hilar lymph nodes. Stage IIIb is defined as any size tumor, including T4 with maximum nodal extension but without distant metastasis. Stage IV disease is defined as any size tumor with any amount of nodal involvement and distant metastases (1). The most common sites for distant metastasis include the central nervous system, liver, bone, bone marrow, and adrenal glands. This stage of disease carries the worst prognosis with a 5-year survival of less than 2%.

Small Cell Lung Cancer

Although it has been recommended that small cell lung cancer be staged similarly to non–small cell lung cancer, the usual extent of disease at the time of diagnosis makes that impractical. Small cell lung cancer is generally defined as limited or extensive and generally does not undergo surgical staging. Limited stage disease signifies that all known tumor can be treated within a single tolerable radiotherapy field. At the time of diagnosis, only one-third of patients will have limited stage disease confined to the hemithorax of origin, the mediastinum or the supraclavicular nodes. With treatment, the median survival for limited stage disease is 10 to 16 months. Extensive disease refers to any tumor burden greater than limited disease (3), usually defined by tumor spread beyond the supraclavicular areas. Median survival for extensive disease with current treatment options is between 6 and 12 months.

Staging Techniques

Imaging techniques are most often used for the clinical staging of lung cancer. Chest radiographs can help determine the size and extent of the tumor. Computed tomography (CT) and magnetic resonance imaging (MRI) scans are also useful in helping distinguish underlying masses from surrounding inflammation; helping evaluate chest wall invasion; and aiding the evaluation of esophageal, phrenic nerve, and pulmonary vessel invasion. Thoracentesis, the removal of pleural fluid from the pleural cavity, is often performed to determine whether malignant cells are present in the visceral or parietal pleura. Mediastinoscopy is often used routinely as a staging procedure for patients undergoing surgery because of its superiority in evaluating mediastinal masses. Thoracoscopy is used to evaluate mediastinal nodal involvement in the subaortic region.

TREATMENT

Once the tumor type is known and the cancer is staged, it is appropriate to begin treatment immediately. Because of the differences in tumor progression, and extent of disease at the time of diagnosis, the treatment of small cell lung cancer is very different from that of non–small cell lung cancer. Small cell lung cancer is most often treated with chemotherapy, whereas non–small cell lung cancer is most often treated with surgery and radiation therapy with or without chemotherapy. To better understand how each lung cancer type is treated, this chapter will review the specific treatment for each cancer type by stage of disease. Treatment guidelines for small cell and non–small cell lung cancers are represented in Figures 83.2 and 83.3 and provide a visual representation of lung cancer treatment by stage.

Non–small Cell Lung Cancer

STAGE I

Surgical resection is the treatment of choice for stage I patients and can result in cure rates of between 60 and 70% (5). Differing surgical options exist for patients with good pulmonary reserve (lobectomy) versus patients with poor pulmonary reserve (segmentectomy or wedge resection). Other surgical considerations include the size and location of the primary tumor. For patients who are not surgical candidates, radiation therapy is the treatment of choice. In this group, if the tumor is small (less than 4 cm), cure rates of 20 to 30% can be achieved.

In clinical trials looking at the adjuvant use of chemotherapy or radiation therapy after surgical resection, no benefit has been seen over surgical excision alone (4). Any use of adjuvant chemotherapy or radiation therapy for stage I patients should be done in the setting of a clinical trial.

STAGE II

As in stage I disease, many patients with stage II disease can still be cured with surgery. A number of surgical options are available, from complete lobectomy or pneumonectomy to more limited resections, including wedge excision or segmentectomy. The Lung Cancer Study Group (1), in a randomized trial comparing lobectomy to limited resection, showed higher local recurrence with limited resection but equivalent overall survival. Similar results have also been reported for segmentectomy versus lobectomy.

Radiation Therapy. Radiation therapy with curative intent is the treatment of choice for patients who are not good surgical candidates. Primary radiotherapy consists of 5500 to 6000 cGy (pronounced "gray") delivered via linear accelerator or cobalt-60 to the mid-plane of the known tumor volume using conventional fractionation

Diagnosis	Staging	Initial Work-Up	Initial Treatment	Chemotherapy Regimens	Subsequent Monitoring

Occult Stage
Tx, N0, M0
5 year survival: 70–80%
(bronchopulmonary secretions contain malignant cells on multiple samples but no other evidence of primary tumor, regional or distant metastases found)

Lab:
CBC
PT, PTT, Plts
Electrolytes, SCr, BUN
SMAC
Urinalysis

Radiology:
PA and lateral chest x-ray

Diagnostics:
Chest CT including liver and adrenals
PFT's
Xenon Scan if PFT's abnormal or pneumonectomy anticipated
Bone Scan: If alk phos elevated or bone/joint complaints
Brain CT: if neurological symptoms

Other Diagnostics:
Fine needle aspirate: for pre-op histology, cytology
Bronchoscopy: pre-thoractomy for diagnosis, staging and operative planning
Mediastinoscopy: pre-thoractomy if mediastinal nodal enlargement is present, for diagnosis, staging and operative planning

---

Stage 0
Tis, N0, M0
5 year survival rate with treatment—not available

Lab:
CBC
PT, PTT, Plts
Electrolytes, SCr, BUN
SMAC
Urinalysis

Radiology:
PA and lateral chest x-ray

Diagnostics:
Chest CT including liver and adrenals
PFT's
Xenon Scan if PFT's abnormal or pneumonectomy anticipated
Bone Scan: If alk phos elevated or bone/joint complaints
Brain CT: if neurological symptoms

Other Diagnostics:
Fine needle aspirate: for pre-op histology, cytology
Bronchoscopy: pre-thoractomy for diagnosis, staging and operative planning
Mediastinoscopy: pre-thoractomy if mediastinal nodal enlargement is present, for diagnosis, staging and operative planning

Stage 0
Surgical Resection (using least invasive procedure)
Segmentectomy
or
Wedge Resection

Investigational: Endoscopic photodynamic therapy in highly selected patients with early central tumors that extend less than 1 cm from the bronchus. (Efficacy remains to be proven)

Stage I
T1, N0, M0
T2, N0, M0
5 year survival rate with treatment: 50%

Lab:
CBC
PT, PTT, Plts
Electrolytes, SCr, BUN
SMAC
Urinalysis

Radiology:
PA and lateral chest x-ray

Diagnostics:
Chest CT including liver and adrenals
PFT's
Xenon Scan if PFT's abnormal or pneumonectomy anticipated
Bone Scan: If alk phos elevated or bone/joint complaints
Brain CT: if neurological symptoms

Other Diagnostics:
Fine needle aspirate: for pre-op histology, cytology
Bronchoscopy: pre-thoractomy for diagnosis, staging and operative planning
Mediastinoscopy: pre-thoractomy if mediastinal nodal enlargement is present, for diagnosis, staging and operative planning

Stage I
1. Surgical Resection: (curative in 60–70% of patients)
   Wedge excision — For patients with limited pulmonary reserve
   Segmentectomy
   Lobectomy: 3–5% mortality
   Pneumonectomy: 5–8% mortality
   Sleeve resection

(Lung Cancer Study group in a randomized trial comparing lobectomy to limited resection showed higher local recurrence with limited resection but equivalent overall survival. Similar results have been reported for segmentectomy vs. lobectomy)

2. Inoperable patients may be considered for radiotherapy with curative intent. Primary radiotherapy consists of 5,500–6,000 cGy delivered via linear accelerator or cobalt -60 to the mid-plane of the known tumor volume using conventional fractionation. May give boosts to the cone-down field of the primary tumor. Hyperfractionation radiotherapy (120cGy, BID) in doses of 6,960 cGy was also shown to be well tolerated with improved survival. Cure rates in this group can reach 20–30% if the tumor is small

3. No benefit has been shown to using adjuvant radiation or adjuvant chemotherapy after surgical excision of Stage I patients.

Complete history, physical exam, review of chest films, CBC, Blood chemistries.
Every 2–3 months for the first 2 years then every 4–6 months subsequently. Other diagnostics as appropriate

Complete history, physical exam, review of chest films, CBC, Blood chemistries.
Every 2–3 months for the first 2 years then every 4–6 months subsequently. Other diagnostics as appropriate

Stage II T1, N1, M0 T2, N1, M0 5 year survival rate with treatment: 30%	<u>Lab:</u> CBC PT, PTT, Plts Electrolytes, SCr, BUN SMAC Urinalysis <u>Radiology:</u> PA and lateral chest x-ray <u>Diagnostics:</u> Chest CT including liver and adrenals PFT's Xenon Scan if PFT's abnormal or pneumonectomy anticipated Bone Scan: If alk phos elevated or bone/joint complaints Brain CT: if neurological symptoms <u>Other Diagnostics:</u> Fine needle aspirate: for pre-op histology, cytology Bronchoscopy: pre-thoractomy for diagnosis, staging and operative planning Mediastinoscopy: pre-thoractomy if mediastinal nodal enlargement is present, for diagnosis, staging and operative planning	<u>Stage II</u> 1. Surgical Resection: (curative in 60–70% of patients) Wedge excision, Segmentectomy — For patients with limited pulmonary reserve Lobectomy: 3–5% mortality Pneumonectomy: 5–8% mortality Sleeve resection (Lung Cancer Study group in a randomized trial comparing lobectomy to limited resection showed higher local recurrence with limited resection but equivalent overall survival. Similar results have been reported for segmentectomy vs. lobectomy) 2. Inoperable patients may be considered for radiotherapy with curative intent. Primary radiotherapy consists of 5,500–6,000 cGy delivered via linear accelerator or cobalt -60 to the mid-plane of the known tumor volume using conventional fractionation. May give boosts to the cone-down field of the primary tumor. Hyperfractionation radiotherapy (120cGy, BID) in doses of 6,960 cGy was also shown to be well tolerated with improved survival. 3. Surgical resection plus adjuvant chemotherapy (investigational). Two randomized trials involving the use of adjuvant chemotherapy plus or minus radiation have shown increased disease free survival and one showed better overall survival.	EP (Cisplatin, Etoposide) Cisplatin 80–100 mg/M2 × 1 Etoposide 80–100 mg/M2 × 3 Repeat cycle every 21–28 days × 4–6 cycles PV (Cisplatin, Vinblastine) Cisplatin 120 mg/M2 × 1 Vinblastine 6 mg/M2 × 2 Repeat cycle every 21–28 days × 4–5 cycles CAP (Cyclophosphamide, Doxorubicin, Cisplatin) Cyclophosphamide 500 mg/M2 × 1 Doxorubicin 50 mg/M2 × 1 Cisplatin 50 mg/M2 × 1 Repeat every 28 days × 4–6 cycles	Complete history, physical exam, review of chest films, CBC, Blood chemistries. Every 2–3 months for the first 2 years then every 4–6 months subsequently. Other diagnostics as appropriate
Stage IIIa T1, N2, M0 T2, N2, M0 T3, N0, M0 T3, N1, M0 T3, N2, M0 5 year survival rate with treatment: 10–15% or >	<u>Lab:</u> CBC PT, PTT, Plts Electrolytes, SCr, BUN SMAC Urinalysis <u>Radiology:</u> PA and lateral chest x-ray <u>Diagnostics:</u> Chest CT including liver and adrenals PFT's Xenon Scan if PFT's abnormal or pneumonectomy anticipated Bone Scan: If alk phos elevated or bone/joint complaints Brain CT: if neurological symptoms <u>Other Diagnostics:</u> Fine needle aspirate: for pre-op histology, cytology Bronchoscopy: pre-thoractomy for diagnosis, staging and operative planning Mediastinoscopy: pre-thoractomy if mediastinal nodal enlargement is present, for diagnosis, staging and operative planning	<u>Stage IIIa</u> 1. Surgical Resection alone (highly selected cases) 2. Radiation Therapy alone a) Standard fractionation of 6,000 cGy b) Hyperfractionation 120 cGy twice daily in total doses up to 6,960 cGy c) Clinical trials studying fractionation schedules, radiosensitization, radiolabeled antibodies, endobronchial laser therapy, brachytherapy. 3. Neo-adjuvant chemotherapy and surgery (T1–T3, N2 patients) (experimental) × 2–3 cycles followed by surgical resection Fosella FV, et.al: Interim report of a prospective, randomized, trial of neo-adjuvant chemotherapy plus surgery vs. surgery alone for stage IIIa NSCLC (abstr. 817) Proc Am Soc Clin Onc 10:240, 1991 4. Surgical resection with adjuvant chemotherapy (experimental) 5. Surgical resection with adjuvant radiation therapy Treatment Goal: improve long term survival	MVP (Mitomycin C, Vinblastine, Cisplatin) Mitomycin 8–10 mg/M2 D1, 29 Vinblastine 3 mg/M2 D1, 8, 29, 36 Cisplatin 80 mg/M2 D1, 29 Repeat every 6 weeks × 3–6 cycles CE (Carboplatin, Etoposide) Carboplatin 300–375 mg/M2 × 1 Etoposide 100–120 mg/M2 × 3 Repeat every 21 days × 4–6 cycles	Complete history, physical exam, review of chest films, CBC, Blood chemistries. Every 2–3 months for the first 2 years then every 4–6 months subsequently. Other diagnostics as appropriate
Stage IIIb Any T, N3, M0 T4, any N, M0 5 year survival rate: <5%	<u>Lab:</u> CBC PT, PTT, Plts Electrolytes, SCr, BUN SMAC Urinalysis <u>Radiology:</u> PA and lateral chest x-ray <u>Diagnostics:</u> Chest CT including liver and adrenals PFT's Xenon Scan if PFT's abnormal or pneumonectomy anticipated Bone Scan: If alk phos elevated or bone/joint complaints Brain CT: if neurological symptoms <u>Other Diagnostics:</u> Fine needle aspirate: for pre-op histology, cytology Bronchoscopy: pre-thoractomy for diagnosis, staging and operative planning Mediastinoscopy: pre-thoractomy if mediastinal nodal enlargement is present, for diagnosis, staging and operative planning	<u>Stage IIIb</u> 1. Radiotherapy alone a) Standard Fractionation of 6,000 cGy b) Hyperfractionation 120 cGy twice daily in total doses of up to 6,960 cGy c) Clinical trials studying fractionation schedules, radiosensitization, radiolabeled antibodies. 2. Radiotherapy as above with adjuvant chemotherapy 3. Chemotherapy and concurrent radiotherapy followed by resection. (experimental) 4. Chemotherapy alone Treatment Goal: improve long term survival	CAP I (Cyclophosphamide 400, Doxorubicin 40, Cisplatin 50) Cyclophosphamide 400 mg/M2 IVB D1 Doxorubicin 40 mg/M2 IVB D1 Cisplatin 50 mg/M2 IV/1 hr D1 Repeat every 28 days × 4–6 cycles ICE (Ifosfamide, Cisplatin, Etoposide) Ifosfamide 2.5 gm/M2 D1, 2 Cisplatin 40 mg/M2 D1, 2 Etoposide 150 mg/M2 D1, 2 Repeat every 28 days × 4–6 cycles Vinorelbine (Navelbine) Vinorelbine 30 mg/M2 IV push weekly Repeat while positive response × 3 months	Complete history, physical exam, review of chest films, CBC, Blood chemistries. Every 2–3 months for the first 2 years then every 4–6 months subsequently. Other diagnostics as appropriate

Figure 83.2 Non–small cell lung cancer. *(Continued)*

Diagnosis

Staging

Stage IV
Any T, any N, M1
5 year survival rate with treatments: <2%

Recurrent Non-Small Cell Lung Cancer

Initial Work-Up

Lab:
CBC
PT, PTT, Plts
Electrolytes, SCr, BUN
SMAC
Urinalysis

Radiology:
PA and lateral chest x-ray

Diagnostics:
Chest CT including liver and adrenals
PFT's
Xenon Scan if PFT's abnormal or pneumonectomy anticipated
Bone Scan: If alk phos elevated or bone/joint complaints
Brain CT: if neurological symptoms

Other Diagnostics:
Fine needle aspirate: for pre-op histology, cytology
Bronchoscopy: pre-thoractomy for diagnosis, staging and operative planning
Mediastinoscopy: pre-thoractomy if mediastinal nodal enlargement is present, for diagnosis, staging and operative planning

Lab:
CBC
PT, PTT, Plts
Electrolytes, SCr, BUN
SMAC
Urinalysis

Radiology:
PA and lateral chest x-ray

Diagnostics:
Chest CT including liver and adrenals
PFT's
Xenon Scan if PFT's abnormal or pneumonectomy anticipated
Bone Scan: If alk phos elevated or bone/joint complaints
Brain CT: if neurological symptoms

Other Diagnostics:
Fine needle aspirate: for pre-op histology, cytology
Bronchoscopy: pre-thoractomy for diagnosis, staging and operative planning
Mediastinoscopy: pre-thoractomy if mediastinal nodal enlargement is present, for diagnosis, staging and operative planning

Initial Treatment

Stage IV
1. Chemotherapy alone (in patients with good performance status—ECOG 0, 1), give 2 courses—evaluate, continue only if response. Max 4-6 cycles.
2. External beam radiotherapy for palliative relief of local symptomatic tumor growth
3. Chemotherapy + radiotherapy (no benefit shown over chemotherapy alone, experimental)
4. Endobronchial laser therapy and/or brachytherapy for obstructing lesions.
5. Best supportive care without chemotherapy.

Treatment goal: prolong short term survival, palliate symptoms, improved quality of life.

Recurrent Disease
1. Palliative Radiotherapy
2. Chemotherapy
3. Chemotherapy and radiation
4. Surgical resection of isolated cerebral mets
5. Laser therapy or interstitial radiotherapy for endobronchial lesions

Chemotherapy Regimens

EP (Cisplatin, Etoposide)
Cisplatin   80–100 mg/M2 × 1
Etoposide   80–100 mg/M2 × 3
Repeat cycle every 21–28 days × 4–6 cycles

PV (Cisplatin, Vinblastine)
Cisplatin   120 mg/M2 × 1
Vinblastine   6 mg/M2 × 2
Repeat cycle every 21–28 days × 4–5 cycles

CAP (Cyclophosphamide, Doxorubicin, Cisplatin)
Cyclophosphamide   500 mg/M2 × 1
Doxorubicin   50 mg/M2 × 1
Cisplatin   50 mg/M2 × 1
Repeat every 28 days × 4–6 cycles

MVP (Mitomycin C, Vinblastine, Cis-platin)
Mitomycin   8–10 mg/M2 D1, 29
Vinblastine   3 mg/M2 D1, 8, 29, 36
Cisplatin   80 mg/M2 D1, 29
Repeat every 6 weeks × 3–6 cycles

CE (Carboplatin, Etoposide)
Carboplatin   300–375 mg/M2 × 1
Etoposide   100–120 mg/M2 × 3
Repeat every 21 days × 4–6 cycles

CAP I (Cyclophosphamide 400, Doxorubicin 40, Cisplatin 50)
Cyclophosphamide   400 mg/M2 IVB D1
Doxorubicin   40 mg/M2 IVB D1
Cisplatin   50 mg/M2 IV/1 hr D1
Repeat every 28 days × 4–6 cycles

ICE (Ifosfamide, Cisplatin, Etoposide)
Ifosfamide   2.5 gm/M2 D1, 2
Cisplatin   40 mg/M2 D1, 2
Etoposide   150 mg/M2 D1, 2
Repeat every 28 days × 4–6 cycles

Vinorelbine (Navelbine)
Vinorelbine   30 mg/M2 IV push weekly
Repeat while positive response × 3 months

Subsequent Monitoring

Complete history, physical exam, review of chest films, CBC, Blood chemistries.
Every 2–3 months for the first 2 years then every 4–6 months subsequently. Other diagnostics as appropriate

Drug Cost/Tx Regimen

EP $3,590.64
unsure of how many
cycles in regimen

PV Total $3,287.75

CAP Total $1,859.52

MVP Total $9,537.66

CE Total $6,216.00

CAP I Total $1,821.28

ICE Total $14,532.30

Vinorelbine
Total $3,024.00
unsure of how many
cycles in regimen

Drug Cost/Tx Cycle
*assumes 1.7m2 person

EP
Cisplatin $498.44
Etoposide $100.00
Total $598.44

PV
Cisplatin $623.05
Vinblastine $34.50
Total $657.55

CAP
Cyclophosphamide $32.70
Doxorubicin $28.00
Cisplatin $249.22
Total $309.92

MVP
Mitomycin $682.84
Vinblastine $34.50
Cisplatin $872.27
Total $1,589.61

CE
Carboplatin $936.00
Etoposide $100.00
Total $1,036.00

CAP I
Cyclophosphamide $26.16
Doxorubicin $28.00
Cisplatin $249.22
Total $303.38

ICE
Ifosfamide $2,197.44
Cisplatin $ 124.61
Etoposide $ 100.00
Total $2,422.05

Vinorelbine
Vinorelbine $252.00
Total $252.00

Drug Side Effects

Complete treatment guidelines include information pertaining to drug side effects as well as drug cost. The following provides examples of side effects and cost associated with treatment of nonsmall cell lung cancer.

Etoposide:
Major Dose-Limiting Effect:
Myelosuppression: (60–91%) nadir 7–14 days
Granulocytopenia thrombocytopenia (22–41%) nadir 9–16 days
Anemia—occasionally (up to 33%)
Common Adverse Effects:
GI: Nausea, vomiting (30–40%); alopecia (8–66%)
Rarely:
Stomatitis, transient hypotension (1–2%)
Anaphylactoid reaction, peripheral neuropathy (1–2%)
Fatigue and somnolence (up to 3%), fever, muscle cramps

Cisplatin
Major Dose Limiting:
Nephrotoxicity, occasionally nausea and vomiting

Common Adverse Effects:
Nausea and vomiting (sometimes dose limiting)
Tinnitus (9%), audiogram abnormality (24%); myelosuppression: leukopenia, thrombocytopenia (nadir 18–23 days), and anemia (25–30%); mild alopecia

Rarely:
Nephrotoxicity, electrolyte disturbances: mainly hypomagnesemia, hypocalcemia, and hypokalemia, peripheral neuropathy, anaphylactoid reactions after at least 5 doses of the drug; ocular effects: optic neuritis, bradycardia, LBBB, ST-T wave changes with CHF; elevated AST, ALT

Cyclophosphamide:
Most Common: Leukopenia, nadir occurs @ 7–14 days, recovery after 10 days, mild anemia, thrombocytopenia, hemorrhagic cystitis: 5–10% of patients; alopecia, anorexia, nausea, vomiting

Less Common: Amenorrhea, urticaria, transverse ridging of nails, skin hyperpigmentation, SIADH, hepatotoxicity

Rarely: Anaphylaxis, cardiotoxicity, pulmonary toxicity, increased incidence of transitional cell CA of the bladder.

Doxorubicin:
Most Common: Myelosuppression: mild to moderate, nausea, vomiting, diarrhea, alopecia

Less Common: Radiation cell recall reaction, radiosensitization, skin hyperpigmentation, dermal creases, fever, chills, allergic reaction, conjunctivitis

Cumulative Dose Toxicity: Cardiac—CHF cardiomyopathy

Figure 83.2 *(Continued)*

Drug Cost/Tx Regimen

EP	$3,590.64

unsure of how many cycles in regimen

PV	
Total	$3,287.75

CAP	
Total	$1,859.52

MVP	
Total	$9,537.66

CE	
Total	$6,216.00

Drug Cost/Tx Cycle
*assumes 1.7m2 person

EP	
Cisplatin	$498.44
Etoposide	$100.00
Total	$598.44

PV	
Cisplatin	$623.05
Vinblastine	$34.50
Total	$657.55

CAP	
Cyclophosphamide	$32.70
Doxorubicin	$28.00
Cisplatin	$249.22
Total	$309.92

MVP	
Mitomycin	$682.84
Vinblastine	$34.50
Cisplatin	$872.27
Total	$1,589.61

CE	
Carboplatin	$936.00
Etoposide	$100.00
Total	$1,036.00

Drug Side Effects

Ifosfamide

Common Adverse Effects:
CNS effects or encephalopathy; mild to moderate leukopenia (nadir 7–10 days), thrombocytopenia (nadir 7–14 days), hemorrhagic cystitis, dysuria, N & V, alopecia

Less Common:
Hepatotoxicity (asymptomatic), nephrotoxicity, phlebitis

Rarely:
Cardiotoxicity, polyneuropathy, pulmonary toxicity, stomatitis

Carboplatin

Major Dose Limiting: myelosuppression including thrombocytopenia

Mitomycin C

Dose Limiting myelosuppression including thrombocytopenia and leukopenia (cumulative effect)

Acute Effect: prolonged nausea and vomiting, fever, anorexia; prolonged malaise

Mucocutaneous effects: mouth ulcers, alopecia, pain on injection, thrombophlebitis, paresthesia, extravasation

Renal effects: rise in serum creatinine, BUN

Pulmonary effects: hemoptysis, dyspnea, coughing, acute bronchospasm (after administration of a vinka), occurs rarely but can be life-threatening) Hemolytic Uremic Syndrome

Vinblastine

Major Dose Limiting: Leukopenia, thrombocytopenia

GI Effects: nausea, vomiting, anorexia, diarrhea, constipation, epigastric and abdominal pain, pharyngitis, stomatitis, rectal bleeding

Nervous System Effects: numbness, paresthesias, peripheral neuropathy and neuritis, mental depression, loss of deep tendon reflexes, headache, malaise, weakness, dizziness, seizures, psychoses, dysfunction of the autonomic nervous system including urinary retention, sinus tachycardia, orthostatic hypotension

Local Effects: phlebitis and necrosis, extravasation.

Vinorelbine

Major Dose Limiting: Granulocytopenia, leukopenia

Hematologic: as above and anemia (mild)

GI Effects: nausea, vomiting, constipation, diarrhea, rise in total bilirubin, rise in SCOT

Nervous System Effects: peripheral neuropathy, asthenia

Other: injection site reactions, pain, phlebitis, alopecia, dyspnea

Carboplatin

Dose Limiting: myelosuppression, thrombocytopenia, leukopenia, anemia

GI Effects: nausea or vomiting (mild), stomatitis mucositis

GU Effects: occasional elevations in serum creatinine, BUN

Other: alopecia, neurotoxicity, skin rashes, hypersensitivity, ototoxicity, flu-like syndrome

CAP I	
Cyclophosphamide	$26.16
Doxorubicin	$28.00
Cisplatin	$249.22
Total	$303.38

CAP I	
Total	$1,821.28

ICE	
Ifosfamide	$2,197.44
Cisplatin	$ 124.61
Etoposide	$ 100.00
Total	$2,422.05

ICE	
Total	$14,532.30

Vinorelbine	
Vinorelbine	$252.00
Total	$252.00

Vinorelbine	
Total	$3,024.00
unsure of how many cycles in regimen	

Figure 83.2 (*Continued*)

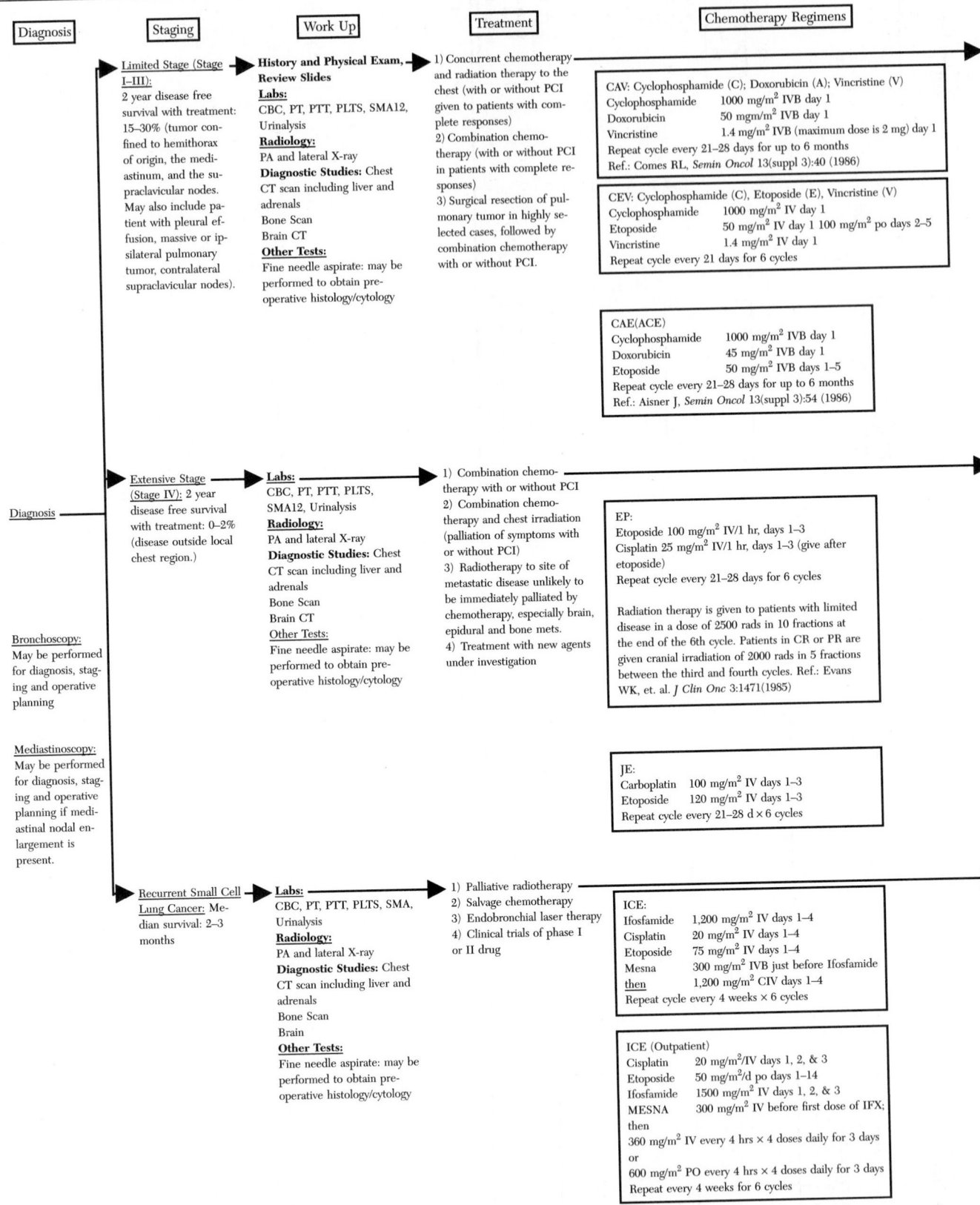

| Diagnosis | Staging | Work Up | Treatment | Chemotherapy Regimens |

Limited Stage (Stage I–III): 2 year disease free survival with treatment: 15–30% (tumor confined to hemithorax of origin, the mediastinum, and the supraclavicular nodes. May also include patient with pleural effusion, massive or ipsilateral pulmonary tumor, contralateral supraclavicular nodes).

History and Physical Exam, Review Slides
Labs: CBC, PT, PTT, PLTS, SMA12, Urinalysis
Radiology: PA and lateral X-ray
Diagnostic Studies: Chest CT scan including liver and adrenals
Bone Scan
Brain CT
Other Tests: Fine needle aspirate: may be performed to obtain preoperative histology/cytology

1) Concurrent chemotherapy and radiation therapy to the chest (with or without PCI given to patients with complete responses)
2) Combination chemotherapy (with or without PCI in patients with complete responses)
3) Surgical resection of pulmonary tumor in highly selected cases, followed by combination chemotherapy with or without PCI.

CAV: Cyclophosphamide (C); Doxorubicin (A); Vincristine (V)
Cyclophosphamide   1000 mg/m² IVB day 1
Doxorubicin   50 mgm/m² IVB day 1
Vincristine   1.4 mg/m² IVB (maximum dose is 2 mg) day 1
Repeat cycle every 21–28 days for up to 6 months
Ref.: Comes RL, *Semin Oncol* 13(suppl 3):40 (1986)

CEV: Cyclophosphamide (C), Etoposide (E), Vincristine (V)
Cyclophosphamide   1000 mg/m² IV day 1
Etoposide   50 mg/m² IV day 1 100 mg/m² po days 2–5
Vincristine   1.4 mg/m² IV day 1
Repeat cycle every 21 days for 6 cycles

CAE(ACE)
Cyclophosphamide   1000 mg/m² IVB day 1
Doxorubicin   45 mg/m² IVB day 1
Etoposide   50 mg/m² IVB days 1–5
Repeat cycle every 21–28 days for up to 6 months
Ref.: Aisner J, *Semin Oncol* 13(suppl 3):54 (1986)

Diagnosis

Bronchoscopy: May be performed for diagnosis, staging and operative planning

Mediastinoscopy: May be performed for diagnosis, staging and operative planning if mediastinal nodal enlargement is present.

Extensive Stage (Stage IV): 2 year disease free survival with treatment: 0–2% (disease outside local chest region.)

Labs: CBC, PT, PTT, PLTS, SMA12, Urinalysis
Radiology: PA and lateral X-ray
Diagnostic Studies: Chest CT scan including liver and adrenals
Bone Scan
Brain CT
Other Tests: Fine needle aspirate: may be performed to obtain preoperative histology/cytology

1) Combination chemotherapy with or without PCI
2) Combination chemotherapy and chest irradiation (palliation of symptoms with or without PCI)
3) Radiotherapy to site of metastatic disease unlikely to be immediately palliated by chemotherapy, especially brain, epidural and bone mets.
4) Treatment with new agents under investigation

EP:
Etoposide 100 mg/m² IV/1 hr, days 1–3
Cisplatin 25 mg/m² IV/1 hr, days 1–3 (give after etoposide)
Repeat cycle every 21–28 days for 6 cycles

Radiation therapy is given to patients with limited disease in a dose of 2500 rads in 10 fractions at the end of the 6th cycle. Patients in CR or PR are given cranial irradiation of 2000 rads in 5 fractions between the third and fourth cycles. Ref.: Evans WK, et. al. *J Clin Onc* 3:1471(1985)

JE:
Carboplatin   100 mg/m² IV days 1–3
Etoposide   120 mg/m² IV days 1–3
Repeat cycle every 21–28 d × 6 cycles

Recurrent Small Cell Lung Cancer: Median survival: 2–3 months

Labs: CBC, PT, PTT, PLTS, SMA, Urinalysis
Radiology: PA and lateral X-ray
Diagnostic Studies: Chest CT scan including liver and adrenals
Bone Scan
Brain
Other Tests: Fine needle aspirate: may be performed to obtain preoperative histology/cytology

1) Palliative radiotherapy
2) Salvage chemotherapy
3) Endobronchial laser therapy
4) Clinical trials of phase I or II drug

ICE:
Ifosfamide   1,200 mg/m² IV days 1–4
Cisplatin   20 mg/m² IV days 1–4
Etoposide   75 mg/m² IV days 1–4
Mesna   300 mg/m² IVB just before Ifosfamide
then   1,200 mg/m² CIV days 1–4
Repeat cycle every 4 weeks × 6 cycles

ICE (Outpatient)
Cisplatin   20 mg/m²/IV days 1, 2, & 3
Etoposide   50 mg/m²/d po days 1–14
Ifosfamide   1500 mg/m² IV days 1, 2, & 3
MESNA   300 mg/m² IV before first dose of IFX;
then   360 mg/m² IV every 4 hrs × 4 doses daily for 3 days
or   600 mg/m² PO every 4 hrs × 4 doses daily for 3 days
Repeat every 4 weeks for 6 cycles

Figure 83.3   Small cell lung cancer.

Monitoring

Chest X-Ray each Cycle
(3–4 weeks)
CBC, PLTS, SMA every
3–4 weeks, neurologic functions every 3–4 weeks
CT Chest, CT Abdomen
&
CT Brain after 4–6 cycles to
confirm PR or CR after remission
1) Chest X-Ray every 2–3
mos. year 1 then
2) Chest X-Ray every 3–4
mos. year 2
3) Chest X-Ray every 4–6
mos. thereafter

Chest X-Ray each Cycle
(3–4 weeks)
CBC, PLTS, SMA every
3–4 weeks, neurologic functions every 3–4 weeks
CT Chest, CT Abdomen &
CT Brain every 2–3 cycles
(6–12 weeks) to confirm PR
or CR after remission:
1) Chest X-Ray every 2–3
mos. year 1 then
2) Chest X-Ray every 3–4
mos. year 2
3) Chest X-Ray every 4–6
mos. thereafter

CBC, SMA
every 2–3
cycles
Chest X-Rays
every 2–3 mos.

CT Chest, CT
Abdomen, CT
Brain every 2–3
cycles

Drug Side Effects

Etoposide:
Major Dose-Limiting Effect:
Myelosuppression: (60–91%) nadir 7–14 days
Granulocytopenia thrombocytopenia (22–41%) nadir 9–16 days
Anemia—occasionally (up to 33%)
Common Adverse Effects:
GI: Nausea, vomiting (30–40%; alopecia (8–66%)
Rarely:
Stomatitis, transient hypotension (1–2%)
Anaphylactoid reaction, peripheral neuropathy (1–2%)
Fatigue and somnolence (up to 3%), fever, muscle cramps

Cisplatin
Major Dose Limiting:
Nephrotoxicity, occasionally nausea and vomiting
Common Adverse Effects:
Nausea and vomiting (sometimes dose limiting)
Tinnitus (9%), audiogram abnormality (24%); myelosuppression:
leukopenia, thrombocytopenia (nadir 18–23 days), and anemia (25–30%);
mild alopecia
Rarely:
Nephrotoxicity, electrolyte disturbances: mainly hypomagnesemia, hy-
pocalcemia, and hypokalemia, peripheral neuropathy, anaphylactoid re-
actions after at least 5 doses of the drug; ocular effects: optic neuritis,
bradycardia, LBBB, ST-T wave changes with CHF; elevated AST, ALT

Cyclophosphamide:
Most Common: Leukopenia, nadir occurs @ 7–14 days, recovery after
10 days, mild anemia, thrombocytopenia, hemorrhagic cystitis: 5–10%
of patients; alopecia, anorexia, nausea, vomiting
Less Common: Amenorrhea, urticaria, transverse ridging of nails, skin
hyperpigmentation, SIADH, hepatotoxicity
Rarely: Anaphylaxis, cardiotoxicity, pulmonary toxicity, increased incidence of transitional cell CA of the bladder.

Doxorubicin:
Most Common: Myelosuppression: mild to moderate, nausea, vomiting, diarrhea, alopecia
Less Common: Radiation cell recall reaction, radiosensitization, skin
hyperpigmentation, dermal creases, fever, chills, allergic reaction, conjunctivitis.
Cumulative Dose Toxicity: Cardiac—CHF cardiomyopathy

Vincristine:
Major Dose Limiting:
Neurotoxicity: peripheral neuropathy, peripheral paresthesias, loss of
deep tendon reflexes, other CNS manifestations, autonomic toxicities
Common Adverse Effects:
Alopecia (20–70%)
Less Common:
Cardiovascular effects: hypertension, hypotension, mild leukopenia,
mild anemia, thrombocytopenia; allergic reactions
Vincristine is a vessicant. Need to monitor for phlebitis and necrosis.

Ifosfamide
Common Adverse Effects:
CNS effects or encephalopathy; mild to moderate leukopenia (nadir
7–10 days), thrombocytopenia (7–14 days), Hemorrhagic cystitis, dys-
uria, N & V, alopecia
Less Common:
Hepatotoxicity (asymptomatic), Nephrotoxicity, phlebitis
Rarely:
Cardiotoxicity, polyneuropathy, pulmonary toxicity, stomatitis

Carboplatin
Major Dose Limiting:
myelosuppression including thrombocytopenia

Drug Cost/Tx Cycle
*assumes 1.7m2 person

CAV	
Cyclophosphamide	$ 33.50
Doxorubicin	$ 131.00
Vincristine	$ 11.00
Total	**$175.50**

CEV	
Cyclophosphamide	$ 33.50
Etoposide	$ 248.00
Vincristine	$ 11.00
Total	**$292.50**

CAE	
Cyclophosphamide	$ 7.00
Doxorubicin	$ 115.00
Etoposide	$ 66.00
Total	**$188.50**

EP	
Etoposide	$ 398.00
Cisplatin	$ 355.00
Total	**$753.00**

JE	
Carboplatin	$ 239.96
Etoposide	$ 477.36
Total	**$717.32**

ICE	
Ifosfamide	$ 1,643.76
Cisplatin	$ 368.48
Etoposide	$ 397.80
MESNA	
Total	**$2,410.04**

ICE (outpatient)	
Cisplatin	$ 250.37
Etoposide	$ 544.74
Ifosfamide	$ 959.64
MESNA	
Total	**$1,754.75**

Drug Cost/ Tx Regimen

CAV
$1,053

CEV
$1,755

CAE
$1,128

EP
$4,518

JE
$4,303.92

ICE
$14,460.24

ICE (Outpatient)
$10,528.50

(intervals of radiation therapy). A "boost" of radiation may also be given to the central portion of the primary tumor. Hyperfractionation radiotherapy, meaning smaller doses given more frequently, has also been shown to be effective. In several studies, hyperfractionated doses of 120 cGy given twice daily up to a total of 6960 cGy showed improved survival and tolerable side effects (4).

Radiation therapy has been studied in the neoadjuvant (prior to surgery) and adjuvant (postsurgery) settings in several randomized trials in patients with stage II and resectable stage IIIa disease. The results of two large randomized studies evaluating preoperative radiation therapy found that it neither increased the resection rate nor prolonged local or distant recurrence (5). Five randomized trials have also evaluated the role of radiation therapy in the adjuvant setting. None of these trials showed a survival benefit for the patients receiving adjuvant radiation therapy (5). At this time, the role of a neoadjuvant and adjuvant radiation therapy in stage II disease cannot be recommended routinely for patients with complete surgical resection.

Chemotherapy. Chemotherapy has been studied in the adjuvant setting for patients with stage II non–small cell lung cancer. Two large randomized trials have evaluated the role of adjuvant chemotherapy with or without radiation therapy. The first study, completed by the Lung Cancer Study Group (LCSG), compared adjuvant chemotherapy consisting of cyclophosphamide, doxorubicin, and cisplatin (CAP) with immunotherapy consisting of intrapleural bCG and oral levamisole. Both disease-free survival and overall median survival were extended approximately 7 months in the chemotherapy group. Whereas disease-free survival reached statistical significance, overall survival did not (6).

A second LCSG trial compared adjuvant radiation therapy (20 Gy given in 400 cGy fractions for 5 consecutive days with a 3-week rest between courses) with radiation plus CAP chemotherapy in doses similar to the first trial. In the radiation plus CAP arm, the chemotherapy was given in split courses: two cycles given on the first day of each course of radiation, and then every 4 weeks for a total of six cycles. The disease-free survival for the chemotherapy plus radiation group was significantly longer than the radiation only group (14 versus 8 months; p = 0.004), but there was no difference in overall survival (7). Additional randomized trials evaluating the use of chemotherapy in the adjuvant setting for the treatment of stage II disease should be completed before its routine use can be recommended.

STAGE III

Radiation Therapy. Although some stage IIIa patients can still be cured with surgical resection, the treatment of choice for the majority of stage III patients is radiation

therapy. The radiation regimen most commonly used today with curative intent is a total of 50 to 60 Gy of megavoltage radiation in 200 cGy fractions, 5 days per week for a total of 5 to 6 weeks (RTOG-7301) (8). The median survival is 37 to 47 weeks, and the 5-year survival rate is less than 10%. Split course dosing schedules have been compared to standard dosing methods with comparable survival rates and toxicities. However, because of the 3-week time interval between courses, many investigators feel that this method is less effective when treating patients with curative intent, due to the ability of the tumor to reseed in the period between courses. Because of the poor survival rate overall (less than 10%) with radiation therapy alone in stage III patients, investigators have looked to enhance survival with the addition of chemotherapy.

Chemotherapy. Four randomized prospective trials have evaluated whether there is a benefit to sequential administration of chemotherapy and radiation therapy over radiation therapy alone in stage IIIa and IIIb patients (9–12). Radiation therapy was given in total doses of between 55 and 65 Gy, and each study used a different chemotherapy regimen. Two of the studies showed equivalent overall 3- and 5-year survival between the chemotherapy followed by radiation therapy arm versus radiation therapy alone. The two more recent studies have continued to show a survival advantage for the chemotherapy plus radiation therapy arm at the 3-year point. A three-arm study is currently being jointly conducted by the Eastern Cooperative Oncology Group (ECOG) and the Radiation Therapy Oncology Group (RTOG). Three treatment arms include (1) standard radiation therapy alone, (2) twice daily radiation to 69.6 Gy, and (3) radiation with high-dose cisplatin and vinblastine. Preliminary results of the study show slightly better 2-year survival rates [32 versus 19% (combined)] for the chemotherapy plus radiation arm over the radiation only arms. The long-term survival benefits are yet to be determined.

Four randomized trials have also compared the effect of radiation therapy alone to radiation therapy and concurrent chemotherapy. The premise of using radiation and chemotherapy together is that the chemotherapy acts synergistically with the radiation to provide both immediate systemic and local control. All the trials compared different doses of radiation with either weekly or daily cisplatin plus radiation. In two of the trials, median survival did not differ between the two arms (13, 14). In the trial by Soresi and colleagues, the median survival for the weekly cisplatin plus radiation was 16 versus 11 months for radiation therapy alone, whereas 2-year survival differences were 40 versus 25%, respectively (15). In the trial by Schaake-Koning and colleagues, a three-arm study comparing radiation to radiation plus weekly cisplatin to radiation plus daily cisplatin, the 3-year survival rates were 2, 13, and 16%, respectively (16). Several trials of multiagent chemotherapy plus radiation versus radiation alone are being currently studied. The use of concurrent radiation and chemotherapy for the treatment of stage III non–small cell lung cancer looks promising, but until more definitive trials are completed, their combined use should be considered experimental.

Neoadjuvant Chemotherapy and Surgery. The role of combined modality therapy involving induction chemotherapy (chemotherapy given before definitive locoregional treatment) followed by surgical resection has been reported in several feasibility studies and in two small randomized trials. Rosell and colleagues reported on 44 stage IIIa patients randomized to surgery alone (22 patients) or chemotherapy (mitomycin, ifosfamide, and cisplatin) given for three courses followed by surgical resection. The overall response rate was 63% for the chemotherapy arm. Complete resection rates were 77% for the combined modality arm versus 84% for the surgery alone arm. The median disease-free survival was 6 months for the surgery alone arm and 18 months (p less than 0.001) for the neoadjuvant chemotherapy arm. Median overall survival was also significantly better for the combined modality arm (16).

Fossella and colleagues from M. D. Anderson has also reported on 30 stage IIIa patients in a study that compared surgery alone (18 patients) to three cycles of neoadjuvant chemotherapy (cyclophosphamide, cisplatin, etoposide) followed by surgical resection (12 patients). Three additional cycles of chemotherapy were given to patients who obtained a complete surgical resection and who responded to the neoadjuvant chemotherapy. The 1-year survival rate was 76% in the neoadjuvant arm compared to 34% in the surgery alone arm (17).

A follow-up report to Fossella's original study was recently published in the Proceedings of the American Society of Clinical Oncology. In the follow-up study, 60 patients had been assigned to surgery only or three cycles of neoadjuvant chemotherapy followed by surgical resection. Patients who received perioperative chemotherapy had an estimated median survival of 64 months compared to 11 months for the surgery only group, which was statistically significant by both the Wilcoxon test and log rank test. The estimated 2- and 3-year survival rates were

Table 83.2.

Patient Selection Criteria for Chemotherapy Administration in Metastatic NSCLC

- Good performance status (ECOG 0,1)
- Minimal to no weight loss
- No liver metastasis
- No bone metastasis
- Must be eligible and willing to participate in clinical trials
- Has weighed the potential benefit vs. the potential toxicity

Adapted from references (8, 28).

Table 83.3.

Single Agent Drugs Active in Non–small Cell Lung Cancer

Drugs	Response Rate
Carboplatin	11%
Cisplatin	21%
Cyclophosphamide	<15%
Doxorubicin	<15%
Etoposide	9%
Ifosfamide	>20%
Mitomycin C	15–20%
Navelbine	14–33%
Vinblastine	27%

Adapted from references (8, 20).

60 and 56% for the chemotherapy arm and 25 and 15% for the surgery only arm (18). Many more studies are underway to determine more definitively the role of neoadjuvant chemotherapy and surgery in patients with stage III disease. Until these results are available, the role of neoadjuvant chemotherapy should be considered experimental.

STAGE IV

Thirty-five percent of patients diagnosed with non–small cell lung cancer will have metastatic disease on initial presentation (19). Patients with stage IV disease are not considered curable. Therefore, the goal of treatment is to palliate symptoms, improve quality of life, and prolong life. Several studies have been performed to determine the impact of selected prognostic factors on long-term survival for patients with metastatic non–small cell lung cancer. An Eastern Cooperative Oncology Group study in 1986 reported that patients with good performance status (ECOG 0 or 1), minimal to no prior weight loss, and no subcutaneous, bone or liver metastases had a greater probability of surviving more than 1 year than patients without those prognostic factors (20). Therefore, many physicians feel that only patients who are willing to risk the toxicity of therapy for the hope of prolonged survival, and who have favorable prognostic factors, should be treated (Table 83.2).

Chemotherapy. Chemotherapy alone or combined with radiation is the treatment of choice for stage IV disease. Several single agents have been determined to be active against non–small cell lung cancer. Chemotherapeutic agents are considered active if the combined complete plus partial overall response exceeds 15%. Other drugs considered active are those whose initial response rate does not exceed 15%; however, overall survival is significantly prolonged by their use. Table 83.3 lists the single agent drugs that are active against non–small cell lung cancer.

In several randomized trials, single-drug therapy has been compared to two-drug therapy. Better response rates

Table 83.4.
Commonly Used Drug Regimens for the Treatment of Non–small Cell Lung Cancer, Their Relative Response Rates and Median Survival in Advanced Disease

Drug Regimen		Response Rate	Median Survival
PE (cisplatin, etoposide)		20–30%	25 weeks
Cisplatin	80–100 mg/m^2 × 1		
Etoposide	80–100 mg/m^2 × 3		
PV (cisplatin, vinblastine)		15–30%	33 weeks
Cisplatin	120 mg/m^2 × 1		
Vinblastine	6 mg/m^2 × 2		
CAP (cyclophosphamide, doxorubicin, cisplatin)		15–25%	25 weeks
Cyclophosphamide	500 mg/m^2 × 1		
Doxorubicin	50 mg/m^2 × 1		
Cisplatin	50 mg/m^2 × 1		
MVP (mitomycin C, vinblastine, cisplatin)		30–60%	22–37 weeks
Mitomycin C	8–10 mg/m^2 d1, 29		
Vinblastine	3 mg/m^2 d1, 8, 29, 36		
Cisplatin	80 mg/m^2 d1, 29		
Repeated every 6 weeks		14–33%	30 weeks
Vinorelbine			
Vinorelbine	30 mg/m^2 weekly		
ICE (ifosfamide, cisplatin, etoposide)		25–40%	46 weeks
Ifosfamide	2.5 gm/m^2 d1, 2		
Cisplatin	40 mg/m^2 d1, 2		
Etoposide	150 mg/m^2 d1, 2		
CE (carboplatin, etoposide)		10–30%	22 weeks
Carboplatin	300–375 mg/m^2 × 1		
Etoposide	100–120 mg/m^2 × 3		

Adapted from references (8, 20, 29).

and better overall survival were seen with the two-drug combination when compared to single-agent therapy with the exception of two trials, one in which carboplatin alone had a better median survival than etoposide plus cisplatin (32 versus 25 weeks) and one in which cisplatin alone had a median survival equivalent to mitomycin plus cisplatin (29 versus 31 weeks).

Six randomized controlled trials have also compared three-drug therapy to two-drug therapy. CAP (cyclophosphamide, doxorubicin, cisplatin) and MVP (mitomycin C, vinblastine, cisplatin) have been the most studied of the three-drug regimens. The results of those trials show no advantage in terms of either improved response or improved survival for the three-drug regimens. The three-drug regimens were, however, associated with greater toxicity. Table 83.4 lists the commonly used drug regimens for non–small cell lung cancer and their relative response rates and median survival.

Although response to chemotherapy is associated with prolonged survival, the survival benefit is minimal. Eight prospective, randomized trials have compared chemotherapy to best supportive care (BSC) in terms of survival benefit. Only three of the studies demonstrated a statistically significant difference in median survival favoring chemotherapy. The other five studies showed a survival benefit with chemotherapy, but the difference was not statistically significant (8). Since chemotherapy confers minimal benefit to overall survival, other factors such as quality of life, cost, and toxicity of therapy become important outcome indicators when making treatment decisions. None of the aforementioned studies looked at quality of life as part of their overall assessment. Although chemotherapy is our best choice for treatment of stage IV non–small cell lung cancer, less than 50% of patients will respond to the chemotherapeutic agents currently on the market. More effective chemotherapy needs to be identified. This has led to the research and development of new drugs for the treatment of non–small cell lung cancer.

New Drugs

Vinorelbine. Vinorelbine (Navelbine) is the newest drug in 15 years to be added to our drug armamentarium against non–small cell lung cancer. Vinorelbine was approved by the FDA in December 1994 for the treatment of advanced non–small cell lung cancer. It is a semisynthetic vinka alkaloid that binds to tubulin and interferes with microtubular assembly, which results in inhibition of cellular replication. It is administered weekly in doses of 30 mg/m^2 intravenous push or intravenous infusion. Because it is an extravasant, the injection site needs to be flushed with saline after administration. In studies analyzing its response rate and median survival, vinorelbine-treated patients showed median survival of 30 weeks and objective response rates in 14 to 33% of patients with advanced stage non–small cell lung cancer. In combination with intravenous cisplatin, median survival exceeded 40 weeks, and objective response rates reached 28 to 46% (21). The dose-limiting toxicity of vinorelbine is granulocytopenia. In addition, mild-to-moderate anemia is common, but thrombocytopenia is rare. Mild-to-moderate peripheral neuropathy, nausea and vomiting, constipation, and alopecia are also common. Transient elevations in liver enzymes have been observed.

Topotecan. Topotecan is an analog of camptothecan and exerts its antitumor activity through the inhibition of topoisomerase I. Topoisomerases are essential nuclear enzymes that fix problems during DNA replication such as overwinding and underwinding. Etoposide and other anthracyclines inhibit topoisomerase II, but this is the first camptothecan developed to inhibit topoisomerase I, which cleaves single-stranded DNA. Topotecan has been studied in more than 20 phase I trials and is currently being studied in phase II trials as an intravenous bolus of 1.5 to 2 mg/m^2 daily for 5 days. In an initial study by Perez-Soler and colleagues, topotecan administered at a dose of 1.5 mg/m^2 for 5 consecutive days, was able to produce a partial response in five patients (13.5%) and a minor response in three patients (22). The results of this initial trial show that topotecan has moderate activity against non–small cell lung cancer. Reported toxicities include neutropenia (dose limiting), severe to life-threatening elevations in LFTs, mild-to-moderate thrombocytopenia, alopecia, nausea, vomiting, anorexia, and fatigue (21).

CPT-11. CPT-11 (irinotecan) is another camptothecan analog that also inhibits topoisomerase I. CPT-11 is being evaluated as a single intravenous bolus every 3 weeks and a weekly intravenous bolus for 4 weeks. In a phase II trial that is ongoing, it is being used in combination with cisplatin at a dose of 60 mg/m^2 on days 1, 8, and 15, and with cisplatin on day 1 at a dose of 80 mg/m^2. Initial toxicities of the drug show that leukopenia and diarrhea are both dose limiting.

Paclitaxel. Paclitaxel (Taxol), a microtubule stabilizer, is currently FDA approved for the treatment of both advanced breast cancer and ovarian cancer. Paclitaxel has also been studied extensively in the treatment of non–small cell lung cancer. Several small studies in stage IV non–small cell lung cancer patients showed that paclitaxel as a single agent at a dose of 200 to 250 mg/m^2 over 24 hours every 3 weeks yielded overall response rates of 21 and 24% (21). In a phase II trial by Langer and colleagues, paclitaxel was given at a dose of 135 mg/m^2 over 24 hours followed by carboplatin with a dose based on a targeted AUC of 7.5, at 3-week intervals for six cycles. To date, of 16 patients evaluable for response, 2 patients have obtained a complete response, 7 patients obtained a partial response, and

1 patient obtained a minor response. The overall objective response rate was 56% (23). Survival data should be forthcoming. Paclitaxel is now currently in Phase III trials comparing low- and high-dose paclitaxel plus cisplatin to a combination of cisplatin and etoposide.

Edetrexate. An analog of methotrexate, edetrexate is a water soluble folate antagonist that blocks the synthesis of neucleotides needed for DNA synthesis by competing for the folate-binding site of the enzyme dihydrofolate reductase. Edetrexate has been studied in phase I, II, and III trials for the treatment of non–small cell lung cancer. An ongoing phase II trial at Memorial Sloan Kettering Cancer Center, is evaluating edetrexate at a dose of 80 mg/m^2 weekly for 5 weeks. Thirty-two percent of patients have partially responded to therapy. Several other phase II trials combining edetrexate with cyclophosphamide and cisplatin show overall responses in the range of 37 to 43%. Toxicities reported with edetrexate include mucositis (dose limiting), hematologic toxicities, fatigue, nausea, and vomiting (21).

Docetaxel. Docetaxel (taxotere) has been preliminarily studied in the phase II setting in stage IIIb or stage IV non–small cell lung cancer patients. Doses of 100 mg/m^2 are given intravenously over 1 hour every 3 weeks. Preliminary data show that 33 percent of patients obtained a partial response, 15 patients had no change, and 11 patients experienced progressive disease. The median duration of partial response was 14 weeks, and the projected median survival in all patients was 47 weeks. Ninety-seven percent of patients developed grade 3 or 4 neutropenia, and neutropenic infection occurred in 17% of patients. Other toxicities included alopecia, arthralgias, myalgias, hypersensitivity reactions, dermatitis, and a cumulative fluid retention syndrome of peripheral edema or pleural effusions (24). Other phase II studies are ongoing.

Gemcitabine. Gemcitabine, a pyrimidine antimetabolite with activity against many tumor types, has been studied in phase II trials. Infusions of 800 mg/m^2 to 1250 mg/m^2 over 30 minutes weekly for 3 weeks have shown response rates of approximately 20% in patients with adenocarcinoma and squamous cell carcinoma of the lung (21).

Small Cell Lung Cancer

LIMITED STAGE DISEASE

Chemotherapy is the mainstay of treatment for both limited and extensive stage small cell lung cancer. Single chemotherapeutic agents with activity against small cell lung cancer are listed in Table 83.5. Etoposide is the most useful agent alone for the treatment of small cell lung cancer. A trial of oral etoposide in an older population resulted in a 71% response rate and a median survival of 16 months for patients with limited disease, and 9 months for patients with extensive disease (1).

Combination chemotherapy is required for treating limited disease with curative intent. Most combination regimens produce partial or complete responses in greater than 80% of patients. Table 83.6 lists the most commonly used regimens to treat small cell lung cancer. The duration of treatment with any of these regimens is usually from 3 to 6 months. Maintenance therapy (treatment beyond 6 months) has not been shown to increase the duration of remission or improve survival.

The regimens most widely in use providing consistent median survival times and relatively modest toxicity are etoposide/cisplatin (EP) and cyclophosphamide/doxorubicin/vincristine (CAV). EP and CAV have been compared directly in two randomized trials of approximately 300 total patients and produced similar survival rates (25). In limited stage disease, these regimens will produce a complete response rate of greater than 50%, a median survival of greater than 14 months, and a 2-year cancer-free survival rate of between 20 and 25% (25). Subsequent studies have compared CAV alone to EP alone to CAV alternating with EP. In limited stage disease patients, the alternating combination regimens showed a survival advantage (16.8 months) over CAV alone (12.4 months) and EP alone (11.7 months), with a p value of 0.014 and 0.023, respectively (25).

CEV (cyclophosphamide/etoposide/vincristine) has been compared to CAV. There were no significant survival differences in patients with limited stage disease; however, patients with extensive disease lived longer with CEV than with CAV (p = 0.01) (25). It appears that the use of etoposide in existing regimens improves survival in extensive stage disease (25).

HIGH-DOSE CHEMOTHERAPY

Two different randomized trials have compared standard-dose CAV (cyclophosphamide/doxorubicin/vincristine) to CAV with 20 to 50% more cyclophosphamide and 20 to 75% more doxorubicin. Neither study showed differences in survival between these two dosing schedules (25). Similar clinical results have been shown when comparing high-dose EP (etoposide/cisplatin) to standard-dose EP.

RADIATION THERAPY WITH OR WITHOUT CHEMOTHERAPY

When used alone in limited stage disease, radiation therapy can cure a small fraction of patients. Up to 75% of patients with limited disease will respond to radiation. Many trials have studied combined modality treatment with radiation and chemotherapy given concurrently, interspersed between multiple cycles of chemotherapy, or at the completion of chemotherapy. Two recent metaanalyses of 11 prospective randomized trials comparing chemotherapy alone to chemotherapy plus radiation therapy showed that more patients (5%) were alive at 2 to 3 years in the combination groups compared to those who received chemotherapy alone. The studies did show a greater death rate from toxicities in the combined modality therapy, however (25). Because of these studies, the standard approach to therapy for small cell lung cancer patients with limited disease is to concurrently administer chemotherapy and radiation therapy (25, 26).

PROPHYLACTIC CRANIAL IRRADIATION

Controversy exists over whether patients should be given prophylactic cranial irradiation (PCI) in addition to treatment for their primary tumor. Prospective studies have shown that PCI reduces the likelihood of metastasis to the brain, particularly in patients with a complete response to

Table 83.5.
Single Agents with Activity Against Small Cell Lung Cancer

Drugs	Response Rate
Cisplatin	20%
Cyclophosphamide	40%
Doxorubicin	30%
Etoposide	45%
Ifosfamide	50%
Methotrexate	35%
Vincristine	40%

Adapted from references (26, 32).

Table 83.6.
Drug Therapy for the Treatment of Small Cell Lung Cancer, Response Rates, and Median Survival in Limited and Extensive Stage Disease

Drug Therapy	Response Rate	Median Survival Limited	Median Survival Extensive
CE (cisplatin, etoposide)	81%	12 months	9 months
CAV (cyclophosphamide, doxorubicin, vincristine)	63%	15 months	8 months
CAE (cyclophosphamide, doxorubicin, etoposide)	80%	14 months	10 months
CEV (cyclophosphamide, etoposide, vincristine)	61%	11 months	8 months
ICE (ifosfamide, cisplatin, etoposide)	94%	19 months	9.5 months

Adapted from references (30, 31).

therapy, but they have not shown a contribution to overall survival (25). Additionally, long-term follow-up of small cell lung cancer survivors showed CNS dysfunction in approximately 45% of patients. When given prophylactically, radiation is typically given in doses of 20 to 30 Gy in 10 to 15 fractions over 2 to 3 weeks. Studies show that PCI can effectively reduce the risk of brain metastasis from approximately 23 to 6%. Because of the controversy over PCI, it is recommended that only patients in complete remission be offered prophylactic cranial irradiation (27).

EXTENSIVE STAGE DISEASE

Sixty to seventy percent of patients initially present with extensive stage disease. The most common sites of metastasis are to the bone (35%), liver (25%), bone marrow (20%), brain (10%), extrathoracic lymph nodes (5%), and subcutaneous masses (5%).

CHEMOTHERAPY

With extensive stage disease, chemotherapy again becomes the mainstay of treatment. The same chemotherapy regimens used in limited stage disease are used in extensive stage disease. Combination chemotherapy will result in a greater than 20% overall response rate and a median survival of greater than 7 months. Very few patients will achieve a 2-year cancer-free survival. Since many of these patients have very poor performance status, aggressive chemotherapy may be difficult to tolerate. Single chemotherapy agents such as etoposide may be the best option for these patients since its use still provides a survival benefit over supportive care alone.

RADIATION THERAPY

Combination chemotherapy plus radiation therapy does not improve survival over chemotherapy alone in extensive stage patients. However, radiation therapy is still important in terms of palliating symptoms of both the primary tumor and other metastatic locations. Patients with metastasis to the brain should undergo radiation with 30 to 40 Gy administered over 2 to 4 weeks. Patients with impending bone fractures or spinal cord compression are appropriate candidates for palliative courses of radiation, usually given in doses of 30 Gy over 2 weeks.

CONCLUSION

Lung cancer continues to be a major health problem. Most patients are diagnosed in the latter stages of the disease, making treatment more difficult. The classification of lung cancer type is crucial to determining not only treatment strategy but also prognosis. Non–small cell lung cancers can be treated aggressively with surgery and radiation therapy for early stage tumors, but we continue to rely on chemotherapy and radiation therapy in combination for later stage tumors. Although vinorelbine, the first drug approved by the FDA in 15 years, has become available, its therapeutic benefit is marginal. Clearly, new agents with much greater activity against non–small cell lung cancer need to be developed. Small cell lung cancer, the solid tumor that behaves most like the leukemias, is rapidly metastatic and aggressive. Although the majority of limited stage disease patients will obtain a response to chemotherapy, the response is generally limited, and most patients go on to develop metastatic disease. Newer drugs with better overall and sustained response rates need to be developed in order for the survival outlook to change significantly. Multimodality therapy for both cancer types will continue to be explored and may contribute survival benefit for these patients. Until we have a therapeutic breakthrough, however, our best hope for significantly diminishing lung cancer is to prevent it from occurring in the first place through lung cancer awareness programs and stop-smoking campaigns.

REFERENCES

1. Harvey JC and Beattie EJ. Lung Cancer, Clinical Symposia, Vol. 45 No. 3, pp. 2–34.
2. Beckett WS. Epidemiology and Etiology of Lung Cancer. Clinics in Chest Medicine, Vol. 14, No. 1, arch 1993. pp. 1–15.
3. Stitik FP. The New Staging of Lung Cancer. Radiologic Clinics of North America. Vol. 32, No. 4, July 1994, pp. 635–643.
4. National Cancer Institute. PDQ Information for Health Care Professionals: Non–small Cell Lung Cancer. CancerFax 1-800-422-6237. October 1994, pp. 1–15.
5. Murren JR, Buzaid AC. Chemotherapy and radiation for the treatment of non–small cell lung cancer. Lung Cancer Vol. 14, No. 1, March 1993, pp. 161–169.
6. Holmes EC, Gail M. Lung Cancer Study Group. Surgical adjuvant therapy for stage II and stage III adenocarcinoma and large-cell undifferentiated carcinoma. J Clin Oncol 4:710, 1986.
7. Lung Cancer Study Group. The benefit of adjuvant treatment for resected locally advanced non–small cell lung cancer. J Clin Oncol 6:9, 1988.
8. Shepherd FA. Treatment of advanced non–small cell lung cancer. Seminars in Oncology 21:4, 1994. pp. 7–18 (suppl 7).
9. Mattson K, Holsti LR, Holsti P, et al. Inoperable non–small cell lung cancer: radiation with or without chemotherapy. Eur J Cancer Clin Oncol 24:477–482, 1988.
10. Morton RF, Jett JR, McGinnis WL, et al. Thoracic radiation therapy alone compared with combined chemo-radiotherapy for locally unresectable non–small cell lung cancer. Ann Intern Med 115:681–686, 1991.
11. Dillman RO, Seagren SL, Propert KJ, et al. A randomized trial of induction chemotherapy plus high dose radiation versus radiation alone in stage III non–small cell lung cancer. N Engl J Med 323:940–945, 1990.
12. LeChevalier T, Arriagada R, Tarayre M, et al. Significant effect of adjuvant chemotherapy on survival in locally advanced non–small cell lung cancer. J Natl Cancer Inst 84:58, 1992.
13. Trovo MG, Minatel E, Franchin G, et al. Radiotherapy (RT) versus RT enhanced by cisplatin (DDP) in stage III non–small cell lung cancer (NSCLC): A randomized cooperative study. Lung Cancer 7:158, 1991 (abstr 590).

14. Ansari R, Tokars R, Fisher W, et al. A phase III study of thoracic irradiation with or without concomitant cisplatin in locoregional unresectable non–small cell lung cancer (NSCLC): A Hossier Oncology Group (H.O.G.) Protocol. Proc Am Soc Clin Oncol 10:241, 1991 (abstr 823).

15. Soresi E, Clerici M, Grilli R, et al. A randomized clinical trial comparing radiation therapy versus radiation therapy plus cis-dichlorodiamine-platin (II) in the treatment of locally advanced non–small cell lung cancer. Semin Oncol 15:20–25, 1988 (suppl 7).

16. Rosell R, Gomez-Codina J, Camps C, et al. Randomized trial comparing preoperative chemotherapy plus surgery with surgery alone in patients with non–small-cell lung cancer. N Engl J Med 330:153–158, 1994.

17. Fossella FV, Ryan B, Dhingra H, et al. Interim report of a prospective randomized trial of neoadjuvant chemotherapy plus surgery versus surgery alone for IIIa non–small cell lung cancer (abstr 817). Proc Am Soc Clin Oncol 10:240, 1991.

18. Roth J, Fossella F, Komaki R, Ryan M, et al. A randomized trial comparing perioperative chemotherapy and surgery with surgery alone in resectable stage III non–small cell lung cancer. Proc Am Soc Clin Onc 13:334, 1994 (abstr 1106).

19. Holmes EC. Adjuvant therapy of non–small cell lung cancer. Hematological Oncology 10:21–24, 1992.

20. Finkelstein DM, Ettinger DS, Rickdeschel JC. Long term survivors in metastatic non–small cell lung cancer: an Eastern Cooperative Oncology Group Study. J Clin Oncol 4:702–709, 1986.

21. Feigal EG, Christian M, Cheson B, Grever M, Friedman M. New chemotherapeutic agents in non–small cell lung cancer. Sem Oncol 20:185–201, 1993.

22. Perez-Soler R, Glisson BS, Kane J, Lee J, et al. Phase II study of topotecan in patients with non–small cell lung cancer pre-viously untreated. Proc Amer Soc Clin Onc 13:363, 1994 (abstr 1223).

23. Langer CJ, Leighton J, Comis R, et al. Taxol and carboplatin (CBDCA) in combination in Stage IV and IIIB non–small cell lung cancer: A phase II trial. Proc Am Soc Clin Onc Vol. 13, 1994 (abstr 1122).

24. Fossella FV, Raber M, Lee JS, et al. Taxotere (Docetaxel), an active agent for recurrent/metastatic non–small cell lung cancer: preliminary report of a phase II study. Proc Amer Soc Clin Onc Vol. 13, 1994 (abstr 1114).

25. Johnson BE. Management of small cell lung cancer. Clinics in Chest Medicine Vol. 14, No. 1, 1993, pp. 173–184.

26. Idhe DC. Chemotherapy of lung cancer. N Engl J Med Vol. 327, No. 20, 1992. pp. 1434–1439.

27. Zandwijk NV. Treatment of small cell lung cancer. Recent experience of the EORTC lung cancer cooperative group. AntiCancer Research 14:313–316, 1994.

28. Ruckdeschel JC. Chemotherapy of metastatic non–small cell carci-noma of the lung. Hematological Oncology 10:25–30, 1992.

29. Ali MF, Mundia AG, Munib M, Berger S. Combination of carbo-platinum and VP-16 in advanced non–small cell lung cancer; a community hospital experience. Proc Amer Soc Clin Onc 13:363, 1994 (abstr 1225).

30. Comis RL. Clinical trials of cyclophosphamide, etoposide and vincristine in the treatment of small-cell lung cancer, Sem Onc 13:40–44, 1986 (suppl 3).

31. Bunn PA, Greco FA, Einhorn L. Cyclophosphamide, doxorubicin, and etoposide as first-line therapy in the treatment of small-cell lung cancer. Sem Onc 13:45–53, 1986 (suppl 3).

32. Aisner J. Current approaches to small cell lung cancer. Hematological Oncology 10:7–20, 1992.

CHAPTER 84

PROSTATE CANCER

CAROL BALMER

Prostate cancer is the most common cancer in the United States. More than a quarter million males are diagnosed with prostate cancer each year. Most of them are elderly; the average age at diagnosis is 70 years. Prostate cancer is highly curable when it is diagnosed while the cancer is still localized to the prostate gland. Like most cancers, prostate cancer remains curable in its advanced forms, is slow growing, and can usually be controlled for 2 years or more with a variety of hormonal and/or chemotherapy treatments.

Because it usually occurs late in life and does not grow quickly, many controversies surround its diagnosis and treatment. It remains more common to die *with* prostate cancer than *of* prostate cancer, and some clinicians question whether it should be treated at all. Treatment decisions in prostate cancer, more than any other cancer, depend on the age and medical condition of the patient.

INCIDENCE

It is estimated that 244,000 patients in the United States will be diagnosed with prostate cancer in 1995. This exceeds the number of patients diagnosed with either breast or lung cancer, the next most common cancers, by more than 30%. Prostate cancer accounts for 36% of all cancers in males and for 14% of their cancer deaths. This represents approximately 40,000 deaths annually. Only lung cancer is responsible for more cancer deaths in males (1). The incidence of prostate cancer is increasing rapidly and has more than doubled in the past 10 years. Since prostate cancer is a cancer of older men, some of the statistical increase results from a corresponding increase in the age of the U.S. population, the so-called graying of America. Improved methods of detection have also resulted in the diagnosis of prostate cancer in many patients without clinical evidence of disease, who might otherwise have remained undiagnosed.

ETIOLOGY AND EPIDEMIOLOGY

Recent studies have contributed dramatically to the understanding of prostate cancer etiology although the cause of this common cancer remains unknown. It is known that prostate cancer is a disease of elderly males. The mean age at presentation is about 70 years. In the period from 1989 to 1991, the probability of developing prostate cancer was about 1 in 10,000 for males under 39 years of age, 1 in 100 for males age 40 to 59, and 1 in 8 for those age 60 to 79. The lifetime risk was 1 in 6 (1).

It is also known that androgens are required for the development of prostate cancer. Prostate cancer does not occur in eunuchs. Differences in incidence occur in various racial or ethnic groups. Most notably, African-American men have the highest prostate cancer prevalence in the world. Their risk is 30- to 50-fold higher than the risk for Asian males in their native countries. Within the United States, African-American males are twice as likely than whites to develop prostate cancer. Japanese- and Chinese-American males have half or less than half the likelihood of developing prostate cancer than whites. It is possible that differences in androgen levels or androgen regulation may account for some of these racial differences (2). Testosterone is the primary circulating androgen. It is converted to dihydrotestosterone (DHT), which controls cell division in the prostate, by the enzyme 5-alpha reductase. Testosterone levels in young African-American males are about 15% higher than in age-matched whites, a difference that may account for the much higher risks of prostate cancer in this population. Testosterone levels are not correspondingly lower in Japanese males, but 5-alpha reductase activity is markedly lower, which could result in lower levels of DHT. This improved understanding of factors affecting prostate cancer growth has important implications for hormonal prevention strategies. Currently, a large chemo prevention trial is underway in males at high risk of prostate cancer, in which 18,000 men are randomized to long-term administration of the 5-alpha reductase inhibitor finasteride or to placebo. It is proposed that reduction of androgens by finasteride will prevent the development of prostate cancer (2).

Genetic factors are important in prostate cancer etiology. A positive family history is strongly associated with developing prostate cancer. The magnitude of risk is increased when the affected relative is diagnosed with prostate cancer at an early age and when more than one first-degree relative is affected. The exact DNA alterations responsible for this inherited predisposition are still unclear (3). Other chromosomal alterations may be important in prostate carcinogenesis, particularly loss or inactivation of tumor suppressor genes, which normally function to prevent cancerous growth (4).

Dietary factors are also associated with prostate cancer etiology. The strongest dietary association is with increased animal fat intake. A reduced consumption of red meat and dairy products is recommended to reduce the risk of

1607

prostate cancer. Retinoid and carotenoid intake may also be protective, but the data are conflicting. Prostate cancer is not associated with tobacco smoking. No occupational exposures have been convincingly linked with prostate cancer although there is some evidence that workers with cadmium exposure (alkaline battery industry), farmers, and rubber workers may have modestly increased risk (2). Benign prostatic hypertrophy (BPH), the normal overgrowth of the prostate that occurs with age, does not increase prostate cancer risk.

Recently, an association with vasectomy has been proposed. Epidemiologic evidence suggests that men who have had a vasectomy are at slightly increased risk for prostate cancer, beginning about 20 years after the vasectomy. A biologic mechanism to explain the association has not been established, and it is not yet certain that the association is causal (2, 5).

PATHOPHYSIOLOGY

The prostate is a small, walnut-shaped gland in males, about an inch and a half long. It is located at the base of the urinary bladder. It completely surrounds the first inch of the urethra and lies slightly above the rectum. This location allows palpation of part of the gland through the rectal wall (Fig. 84.1). The prostate gland is surrounded by a fibrous capsule and comprises primarily acinar or glandular tissue. The prostate's normal function is the production of a milky secretion called prostatic fluid, which adds to the volume of the semen. Its growth, and the growth of malignant prostate tissue, are controlled by androgens, particularly dihydrotestosterone (DHT).

About 98% of prostate cancers arise from glandular tissues and are adenocarcinomas. Most also arise in the periphery of the prostate, in its posterior lobe, closest to the rectum. Prostate cancers are graded pathologically by their degree of differentiation, that is, by how much (well differentiated) or how little (poorly differentiated) they resemble normal prostate tissue. This grading has prognostic value since well-differentiated tumors tend to grow more slowly and behave less aggressively than poorly differentiated tumors. The most widely used system is the Gleason grading system, in which cancers are assigned a total score from two (very well differentiated) to ten (very poorly differentiated). The DNA ploidy status of tumors is also assessed for prognostic purposes. Tumors that are primarily diploid, demonstrating 46 chromosomes like normal human somatic cells, tend to behave less aggressively than those with a high proportion of aneuploid cells, which have an irregular number of chromosomes (6).

An important tumor marker for prostate tissue is prostatic specific antigen (PSA). PSA is a glycoprotein that is a serine protease. It is produced exclusively by prostatic tissue and circulates in the blood. PSA is produced by normal and benignly hypertrophied prostate tissue as well as malignant tissue, and, therefore, is not a specific marker of prostate cancer. It is somewhat quantitative, however, with both the absolute level and the rate of increase (PSA

Table 84.1.
Clinical Uses of Prostatic Specific Antigen (PSA) Measurements

Screening asymptomatic populations in combination with digital rectal examination
Assessing clinical importance of biopsy-detected cancers
Indicating prognosis of disease
Staging prostate cancer as a guideline to appropriate initial treatment
Assessing efficacy of radical prostatectomy or radiation therapy
Monitoring patients for recurrence of disease after surgery or radiation
Evaluating objective response to hormone or chemotherapy interventions
Evaluating efficacy of new agents in prostate cancer management

Table 84.2.
Guide to Interpretation of Prostate Specific Antigen (PSA) Values

Value (ng/ml)[a]	Interpretation
0–4	"Normal range," age nonspecific
0–2.5	Age-specific normal range, ages 40–49
0–3.5	Age-specific normal range, ages 50–59
0–4.5	Age-specific normal range, ages 60–69
0–6.5	Age-specific normal range, ages 70–79
4–10	Overlap area of BPH and prostate cancer
>10	High likelihood of prostate cancer
<0.2	Expected level after radical prostatectomy

[a]Hybritech tandem assay.
Adapted from references 6, 7, and 8.

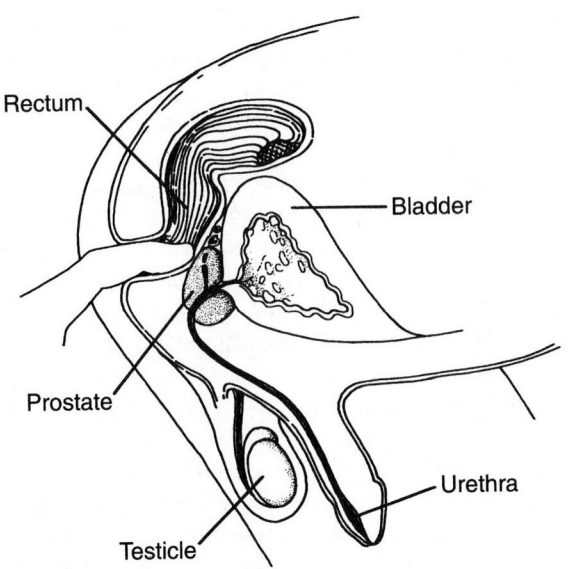

Figure 84.1 Male anatomy and digital rectal exam.

velocity) reflecting the activity of the prostate tissue growth process. PSA has many roles in the screening, diagnosis, monitoring, and management of prostate cancer (Table 84.1). New refinements of this measure, such as the PSA velocity, PSA density (which compensates for the size of the prostate gland), age-specific values (Table 84.2), and measurement of free and total forms of PSA continue to add to the specificity and clinical utility of PSA testing (7, 8). In the past 10 years, PSA has replaced prostatic acid phosphatase (PAP) as a tumor marker for prostate cancer since it is more specific. PAP remains useful primarily as an indicator of metastatic spread.

SIGNS AND SYMPTOMS

Prostate cancer follows a fairly typical natural history. It is usually a slow-growing cancer, with a long doubling time that may exceed 2 years. Although prostate cancer grows slowly, if it does become clinically detectable, it will progress relentlessly in the absence of treatment and eventually may threaten the patient's life.

Prostate cancer always begins in the prostate gland, and then spreads in one or more of three ways. It may spread locally by direct extension, penetrating the prostate capsule to invade adjacent structures such as the seminal vesicles and bladder wall. One of the most serious sequelae of local spread is urinary obstruction from compression of the urethra or bladder neck. It may also spread through the lymph system or through the blood. It is blood-borne metastatic spread that takes prostate cancer cells to the bones, which are overwhelmingly the most common site of metastases. The bones that are physically near the prostate—that is, those of the lower spine, pelvis, and proximal femurs—are the most common early sites of bony spread although prostate cancer typically affects many bones in its advanced forms. Bone metastases are typically either osteoblastic (tumor building onto bone) or a combination of osteoblastic and osteolytic (bone-dissolving) lesions. Osteoblastic tumor masses growing on the spine may cause compression of the spinal cord, with resulting paralysis. This is one of the most serious complications of prostate cancer. Other metastatic sites of spread are lungs, liver, and soft tissue, especially lymph nodes (6).

The anatomy and natural history of prostate cancer account for its presenting signs and symptoms. Prostate cancer is usually asymptomatic in its early stages since the growth in the prostate is small at first and is usually near the periphery of the gland. More advanced local prostate growth may produce urinary obstructive symptoms. The prostate physically surrounds the urethra, so its overgrowth can compress the urethra and result in these symptoms. Because most prostate cancers grow in the outer areas of the prostate, these urinary symptoms are much less commonly caused by prostate cancer than by noncancerous overgrowth of prostate tissue where the tissue overgrowth is typically in the central area of the prostate gland.

However the obstructive symptoms of prostate cancer are indistinguishable from those produced by BPH. They include difficulty in initiating the urine stream, urgency, frequency, nocturia, dribbling, and incomplete bladder emptying.

Too often, prostate cancer spreads before it produces any local symptoms that cause patients to seek medical care. The presenting symptoms are then usually attributable to metastatic spread to the bones, particularly low back pain. The evaluation of unexplained low back pain in males older than 50 should include screening tests for prostate cancer, such as a PSA. In patients with advanced disease at the time of diagnosis, the presenting symptoms may be those of spinal cord compression: lower extremity weakness or paralysis, or loss of bowel or bladder control. These cases must be treated as medical emergencies. Anemia, weakness, or weight loss may also be presenting signs of advanced disease.

SCREENING

Since prostate cancer is usually asymptomatic in its early and most curable stages, increasing public health efforts have been devoted to widespread screening of populations at risk. The American Cancer Society recommends yearly screening with a PSA and digital rectal exam for males over 50 years of age (9). Annual screening should start at 40 years for those at high risk, such as African Americans and patients with a strong family history. Some institutions offer low-cost screening tests during highly publicized events such as Prostate Cancer Awareness Weeks (10). Public figures who have been diagnosed with this disease speak in television and radio health programs to urge men to have routine prostate check-ups. Despite the potentially life-saving benefits of these screening programs, they are currently extremely controversial. The basis of this controversy can be explained by the natural history of prostate cancer.

One of the most unusual features of prostate cancer, and one that still confounds understanding, is that the histologic prevalence of prostate cancer is much greater than its clinical incidence. Autopsy series evaluating prostates from men who died from unrelated causes have demonstrated cancer in about 30% of males over 50 and in 67% of men in their 80s. These figures represent more than 10 million men in the United States who have cancer foci physically present within their prostate glands. In contrast, the 244,000 new patients diagnosed in 1995 represent only about 2.5% of these men. Most of those histologically proven cancers do not progress within the lifetime of the host and are termed latent, or clinically unimportant, cancers. Those that threaten the life or well-being of the host are called clinically important. One of the most important challenges in effective prostate cancer control and screening is to find objective criteria to distinguish between these two forms of prostate cancer (6).

The argument against widespread screening programs of asymptomatic men is that most of the prostate cancers that were detected were destined to remain asymptomatic and would never cause clinical symptoms during that person's lifetime. Because of the advanced age of prostate cancer patients, even those in whom the disease becomes clinically evident are likely to die of causes other than prostate cancer. The argument continues that diagnosis of a patient with prostate cancer may lead to unnecessary treatments, which are costly and have associated morbidity. Opponents say that this violates the medical dogma to "do no harm." Finally, prostate cancer screening has not yet been proved to directly decrease the overall mortality from prostate cancer (11).

Supporters of screening programs argue that the screening tests used (PSA and digital rectal exam) are not able to detect latent cancers. The majority of cancers that are detected by these programs have proved to be clinically important in follow-up and would have progressed locally and eventually metastasized to regional lymph nodes and distant sites. In this context, widespread screening, particularly of younger patients with greater than 10-year life expectancy, is seen as an ethical and economical public health initiative since treatment of early stage disease is less costly than treatment of advanced disease. Available data suggest that cancer screening may decrease the morbidity and mortality of prostate cancer by detecting it in its early, more curable stages (12).

DIAGNOSIS AND STAGING

The tests most widely used in screening, the PSA and digital rectal exam (DRE), are cornerstones of prostate cancer diagnosis. The PSA is the most accurate test for the detection of prostate cancer. Patients with PSA levels greater than 4 ng/ml, or greater than age-specific values listed in Table 84.2, should be evaluated next with digital rectal exam. Because most prostate cancers arise in the posterior lobe of the prostate, which can be palpated through the rectal wall (Fig. 84.1), DRE has long been a clinically useful diagnostic tool. Prostate cancers are felt as hard nodules in the otherwise rubbery glandular tissue. DRE may also detect extension of cancerous growth into tissues adjacent to the prostate. Suspicious or equivocal prostates after PSA and DRE are evaluated with transrectal ultrasound (TRUS), which can visualize prostate size, nodules, and invasion of peri-prostatic tissues. TRUS is also used to guide prostate biopsy, which is the definitive diagnostic test. The current standard of practice for prostate biopsy uses a high-speed spring-loaded gunlike biopsy device, which takes needle biopsy samples of the prostate through the rectal wall. At least six needle cores of tissue, distributed throughout the gland, are usually taken. The gunlike device has made this an outpatient procedure of little discomfort and very low morbidity, and has increased the reliability of sampling.

Once prostate cancer has been detected, the histologic grade or degree of cell differentiation (Gleason stage) and DNA ploidy status are assessed, as indicators of prognosis (see "Pathophysiology"). Limited metastatic workup, including a bone scan, chest radiograph, liver function tests, and serum phosphatases, is also performed to assess the extent and stage of the disease. Pelvic imaging studies to evaluate lymph node involvement may be performed but do not reliably detect small lymph nodes (6, 9).

Two staging systems for prostate cancer are in widespread use and have important prognostic significance.

Table 84.3.
Staging Classification Systems for Prostate Cancer

AUA[a]	Description	Tumor, Node, Metastases (TNM)	Description
A	Incidental carcinoma	T0	No evidence of primary tumor
A1	Focal	T1a	3 or fewer microscopic foci
A2	Diffuse	T1b	More than 3 microscopic foci
B	Confined to prostate	T2	Tumor present; clinically or grossly limited to gland
B1	Small, discrete nodule	T2a	Tumor 1.5 cm or less in greatest dimension, normal tissues on at least 3 sides
B2	Large or multiple nodules	T2b	Tumor >1.5 cm in greatest dimension or in more than one lobe
C	Localized to periprostatic area	T3	Tumor invades prostatic apex, into or beyond capsule, bladder neck, or seminal vesicle; not fixed
C1	No involvement of seminal vesicles	T4	Tumor fixed or invades adjacent structures other than those listed in T3
C2	Involvement of seminal vesicles		
D	Metastatic disease	N1	Metastatis in a single lymph node, 2 cm or less in greatest dimension
D1	Pelvic lymph node metastases	N2	Metastasis in single lymph node, >3 cm but <5 cm in greatest dimension
		N3	Metastasis in lymph node >5 cm in greatest dimension
D2	Bone or distant lymph node or organ or soft tissue metastases	M1	Distant metastases

[a]American Urologic Association Staging System.
Adapted from reference 13.

Table 84.4.
Risk of Death and Cure Rates by Stage of Prostate Cancer

Stage of Disease[a]	Percentage of Patients	10-Yr Survival (%)[b]	Estimated Cure Rate (%)	Prognosis
All stages	100	51	32	
Stage A	10	95	85	Treatment may be unnecessary
Stage B	30	80	65	Often curable
Stage C	10	60	25	Occasionally curable
Stage D_1	20	40	<5	Rarely curable
Stage D_2	30	10	<1	Incurable

[a]Stage is based on clinical stage, plus pelvic lymph node dissection, bone scan, and acid phosphatase.
[b]Cancer-specific survival rates.
Adapted from reference 14.

They are outlined in Table 84.3 (13). The American Urologic Association staging system, which uses an A,B,C,D format remains the most commonly used. Although most solid tumors are staged in a four-stage system (A, B, C, D or I, II, III, IV), there are some important differences in the classification pattern for prostate cancers. Stage A represents microscopic disease, which is not a stage category for other solid tumors. Stage A disease is usually found incidentally, most often at surgery for treatment of BPH. Stage B indicates one or more palpable nodules (similar to Stage A or I in most solid tumor classifications). Stage C is bulky local disease with extension outside the prostate capsule but does not include lymph node involvement. Prostate cancer is the only solid tumor in which Stage D is used to indicate pelvic lymph node involvement. This is classified as D_1 disease. Traditional metastatic spread to distant metastases, usually of bone sites, is D_2 prostate cancer.

The other staging system uses a TNM classification, which stages prostate cancer based on the primary tumor (T), lymph node involvement (N), and presence or absence of distant metastases (M).

Survival of patients with prostate cancer is closely tied to stage of disease (Table 84.4).

TREATMENT OF CLINICALLY LOCALIZED DISEASE

There are three primary treatment options for cancer that is clinically localized to the prostate gland (Stages A and B): surgery, radiation therapy, or close observation without treatment. The standard of treatment for many years has been radical prostatectomy, or surgical removal of the prostate gland, combined with pelvic lymph node dissection. This procedure offers the best chance of eradicating the disease in men whose cancer is confined to the prostate. PSA levels decline to female levels (less than 0.2 ng/ml) after successful removal of all prostatic tissue with this surgery. The survival rate at 15 years is approximately 90%. Radical prostatectomy has been technically improved in recent years but still entails significant risks of morbidity and related mortality up to 2%. The most common complications are impotence, with an incidence of 30 to 60%, and urinary incontinence (5 to 15%) (15). Impotence was nearly universal with earlier radical prostatectomy techniques since the cavernous neurovascular bundles that carry the enervation for erectile control run in channels along each side of the prostate gland. These bundles were traditionally removed with the prostate. Newer nerve-sparing surgical techniques preserve either one or both neurovascular bundles in men with localized cancer that does not involve these structures. Return of erections that are sufficient for penetration and intercourse depends on the patient's age, extent of tumor, and erectile capacity before surgery. The best success is achieved in younger males with good erectile function before surgery, in whom localized disease permits preservation of both neurovascular bundles. In most patients, the quality of erections postoperatively is not as good as that before surgery (16). Potency lost from the effects of surgery may be restored artificially with vacuum erection devices, penile injections of vasodilators, or penile prostheses (15).

Urinary incontinence is a less common but also very troublesome aftereffect of radical prostatectomy. Eighty to 95% of men recover normal urinary continence or report only stress-induced spotting within 18 months after surgery. The remainder require pads to keep their outer garments dry or are totally incontinent (16, 17). Urinary incontinence can be treated with pelvic-floor muscle exercises, anticholinergic agents or α-adrenergic agonists, anticontinence clamps, or implantation of inflatable urinary sphincters. Other complications include blood loss, urethral stricture, rectal injury, thromboembolism, and wound infection. Death occurs in 0.1 to 2% of patients (15).

Destruction of the prostate with radiation therapy is a satisfactory alternative to radical prostatectomy for men with localized prostate cancer who are not good surgical candidates because of advanced age or concomitant health problems. External beam radiation is the most commonly used method of radiation therapy. This generally requires brief radiation therapy sessions, 5 days a week, for 7 to 8 weeks. PSA levels are less likely to become undetectable after external beam radiation therapy than after surgery and also rise within 5 years after radiation therapy in most patients. These data suggest that eradication of cancerous tissue is not complete and that external beam radiation therapy does not cure prostate cancer in most patients. It is most likely to produce satisfactory results in patients with pretreatment PSA levels less than 15 ng/ml. Although long-term survival rates are lower than with surgery, the differences may not be clinically important in an elderly population (9, 18).

Rectal or bladder irritation and bleeding are the most common acute complication. These problems may be treated with anticholinergic drugs or with corticosteroid enemas. Proctitis or cystitis persists for many years in 3 to 8% of patients. Newer radiation techniques use three-dimensional conformational methods to direct the radiation dose to the prostate and produce less damage to nearby organs such as the bladder and rectum. The risk of impotence from external beam radiation is approximately the same as with nerve-sparing surgical techniques, but chronic urinary incontinence is substantially less frequent than with radical prostatectomy (15).

Brachytherapy, or interstitial radiation therapy, is a radiation therapy approach in which radioactive sources are implanted directly into the prostate, usually as seeds of radioisotopes contained in needlelike tubes. This technique delivers a high dose of radiation to the prostate with relative sparing of nearby normal tissue and may eventually prove to be a cost-effective, less toxic radiation therapy option for treatment of localized disease (19).

The third modality for treatment of localized disease is observation or so-called watchful waiting. This is currently a much-debated issue in prostate cancer management. The controversy is based on the natural history of this disease and consideration of the costs and complications of conventional surgical or radiation treatments. Since prostate cancer is a slow-growing disease, and the average age at diagnosis is about 70 years, it is statistically more common to die *with* prostate cancer than *of* prostate cancer. Forty thousand men still die of this painful, debilitating disease each year, so the difficulty of treatment planning lies in patient selection. Observation with careful follow-up is an appropriate decision choice for men with a life-expectancy of less than 10 years, who have low-grade, low-stage prostate cancers. It is most appropriate for patients with Stage A cancers that have been found incidentally. Observation may also be appropriate for patients with more advanced, but still localized, cancers although clinically evident cancers will continue to progress and may result in death. Again, those with short life-expectancy are the best candidates for watchful waiting. Younger men with a longer projected period of risk should be offered potentially curative treatment. A large randomized trial is currently underway to compare mortality and cost-effectiveness of radical prostatectomy and observation in patients with localized prostate cancer, which may ultimately resolve this controversy (15, 20, 21).

TREATMENT OF LOCALLY ADVANCED DISEASE

It is unlikely that patients with prostate cancer that has penetrated the prostate capsule and spread locally (Stage C) will be cured by either radical prostatectomy or radiation therapy. Most of these patients have clinically undetectable micrometastases at the time of diagnosis, which eventually cause recurrence of disease. Radiation therapy is the most commonly used treatment for Stage C disease. It produces 15-year survival rates, which are about half the normal survival rate. Radical prostatectomy may be used with small tumors but is rarely curative. Hormonal therapy, discussed later, may be administered investigationally before surgery to shrink the tumor mass and make it more amenable to surgical excision. This strategy is called "down staging" since the intent is to convert the tumor from Stage C to Stage B. Its value has not been proved clinically. Hormonal therapy is also employed as the primary treatment intervention in locally advanced disease. Watchful waiting may also be offered to patients with pathologically low-grade tumors. It is much less well supported in this setting since the disease-free survival is much lower in this population than in patients with low-stage localized tumors (9, 15, 20).

TREATMENT OF METASTATIC DISEASE

Hormonal therapy is the cornerstone of metastatic prostate cancer treatment. Prostate tissue growth is stimulated by androgens. This applies to normal prostate tissue, BPH, and prostate cancer although the sensitivity of individual cells or clones within the tumor mass may vary. Prostate cancer masses are heterogeneous; that is, all the cells are not identical. Some are called hormone dependent. These cells die when androgenic hormones are withdrawn. Hormone-sensitive cells stop growing until resupplied with androgen. Some prostate cancer cells are believed to be hormone independent and are unaffected by the presence or absence of androgen.

The goal of all hormonal interventions for prostate cancer management is hormonal ablation, that is, removing the stimulatory effects of male hormones from the prostate cancer cells. There are many ways to accomplish this goal. In order to put the different hormonal interventions in context, it is necessary to review the normal regulation of male hormone secretion (Fig. 84.2) (22).

Testosterone is the primary androgen or male hormone. About 90% of circulating androgens are produced in the testes; the balance (approximately 10%) is produced by the adrenal glands. This proportion varies from patient to patient, and in some patients, the adrenal gland is a very important source of androgens (6). The production of androgens is regulated by a negative feedback system that includes the hypothalamus and the pituitary in addition to the testes and adrenal glands.

Secretion of testosterone by the testes is actually controlled in the brain. The hypothalamus acts as a sensor and is sensitive to changes in the circulating levels of hormones. When it detects low levels of testosterone, the hypothalamus secretes luteinizing hormone-releasing hormone (LHRH). This is also gonadotropin-releasing hormone (GnRH). Under the stimulation of LHRH, the pituitary gland secretes luteinizing hormone (LH), a

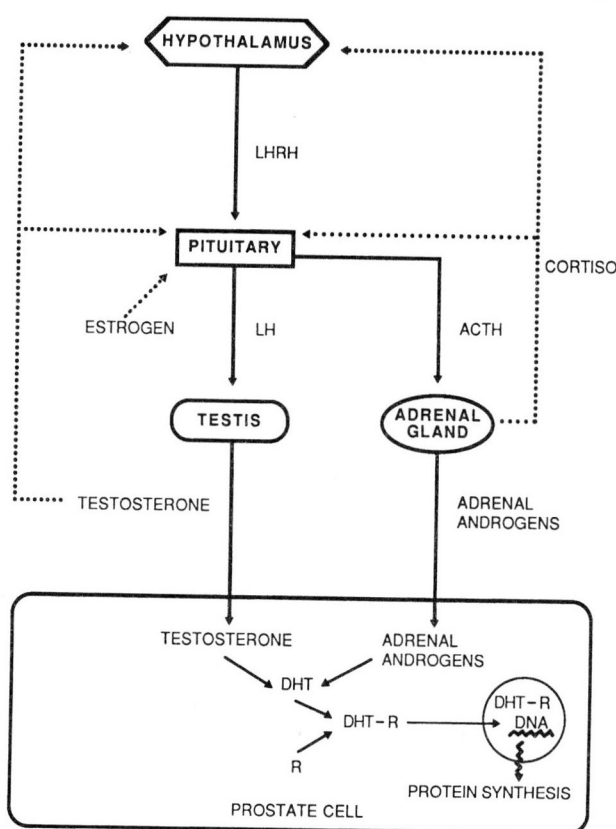

Figure 84.2 Influences of endocrine system on prostate cell growth (→), negative feedback; *LHRH*, luteinizing hormone-releasing hormone; *ACTH*, adrenocorticotropic hormone; *LH*, leuteinizing hormone; *DHT*, dihydrotestosterone; *R*, receptor.

gonadotropin. LH stimulates the Leydig cells of the testes to secrete testosterone (23). A similar feedback loop controls steroid hormone production in the adrenal glands. The adrenals cannot produce testosterone directly but produce androgenic precursors that can be enzymatically converted to testosterone in many peripheral tissues (6).

Testosterone is the main circulating androgen, but within the prostate, testosterone is transformed into dihydrotestosterone (DHT). The enzyme responsible for this conversion is 5-alpha reductase. Although both testosterone and DHT can stimulate the same androgen receptors in the prostate, DHT has greater than twice the affinity of testosterone for these receptors. DHT's actions within prostate cells are believed to be similar to other steroid hormones: DHT binds to specific receptors within the cytoplasm and is transferred to the nucleus, where the hormone-induced effects on gene transcription ultimately result in the synthesis of proteins that produce the hormone's biologic effects.

Guidelines for Hormonal Therapy

Hormonal interventions for prostate cancer control are possible at every site in the hypothalamic-pituitary-gonad–adrenal axes, at the point of conversion of testosterone to

DHT, and at the hormone receptor level. The possible hormonal interventions differ in their mechanisms, advantages, and disadvantages, but some general guidelines apply broadly to their application in the management of prostate cancer patients (15, 24, 25):

- The goal of all hormone therapy for prostate cancer is androgen ablation.
- About 85% of patients with prostate cancer will have an objective or subjective response (relief of symptoms) to first-line hormonal therapy.
- With few exceptions, all these hormonal interventions are effective and have comparable response rates. Choice of treatment depends on patient and physician preference, cost considerations, concomitant medical conditions, and rapidity of response required.
- Hormone therapy is palliative. It does not cure prostate cancer and, in general, does not prolong overall survival although disease-free survival may be lengthened.
- The average duration of response to first-line hormone therapy is 1 to 2 years.
- Second-line hormone interventions have a much lower likelihood and shorter duration of response.
- Most hormone ablative therapies produce impotence and loss of libido (sexual desire). Hot flashes and feminizing effects, such as gynecomastia (breast enlargement) and loss of male-distributed body hair, are common.

Surgical Castration

Huggins and Hodges were the first investigators to recognize the hormonal dependence of prostate cancer, and to treat it with a hormone therapy, in the early 1940s. They noted dramatic improvement in their patients with prostate cancer following treatment with surgical castration (26). Nearly 5 decades later, surgical removal of the testes (orchiectomy) remains the standard against which other hormone therapies are evaluated. It is still a widely used first-line treatment for metastatic prostate cancer. The external location of the testes makes this a minor outpatient surgical procedure with very low physical morbidity. The effects of castration on prostate cancer symptoms are very rapid. Patients may report relief of pain from bone metastases within hours of the procedure. This makes it the hormone intervention of choice in emergent situations, such as impending paralysis from spinal cord metastases. Other advantages are its relative cost-effectiveness and avoidance of noncompliance. Disadvantages include lack of acceptance by many patients, negative psychologic associations, and lack of reversibility. Impotence and loss of libido occur in nearly 100% of patients treated with orchiectomy. Hot flashes are common and troublesome.

Medical Castration—Estrogens

The availability of medical alternatives to surgical castration made hormone therapy more acceptable to many patients. Estrogens were the first form of medical castration and were widely used in prostate cancer patients in the

1960s and 1970s. Estrogens interfere with the release of LH from the pituitary, which eliminates the hormonal signal for testosterone production by the testes. Circulating testosterone levels decrease to castration levels (less than 50 nmols per liter) within 2 weeks after estrogen therapy is initiated. Estrogens also increase the synthesis of testosterone-binding proteins, which decreases the availability of free testosterone; inhibit the conversion of testosterone to DHT; and interfere with DHT binding to its receptor (24).

The most widely used estrogen has been diethylstilbestrol (DES). Its use and dosing was studied in a series of Veterans Administration Urological Research Group (VACURG) trials (27). The first VACURG trial proved that 5 mg of DES per day was as effective as, but more toxic than, orchiectomy in treating metastatic prostate cancer. Patients who received DES demonstrated a shorter overall survival than the orchiectomy patients secondary to an excess of cardiovascular deaths. The next VACURG trial compared DES at doses of 0.2, 1, and 5 mg daily. The 0.2-mg dose was not effective. The 1-mg dose produced fewer cardiovascular complications and similar response rates to 5 mg although castration levels of testosterone were not consistently achieved. Without strong objective data, an empiric 3-mg dose became the standard of practice. At these doses, the incidence of edema (15 to 20%), thrombophlebitis or embolus (5 to 10%), and myocardial infarction, angina, or congestive heart failure (about 5%) are still significant. Gynecomastia and breast tenderness, nausea, loss of libido, and impotence are common, but hot flashes do not occur. Although the use of DES fell out of favor in the 1980s with the availability of less toxic means of medical castration, there is currently a renewed interest in use of DES in 1- to 3-mg doses because of its very low cost (Table 84.5). DES costs only pennies a day if the cost of cardiovascular complications is not considered. DES is often combined with daily aspirin to reduce thromboembolic complications although there are no data to substantiate this approach (28). DES therapy should not be used in patients at high risk for thromboembolic disorders such as patients with a history of stroke. It is important that patients be counseled about the cardiovascular risks and other side effects before they make a decision to begin DES treatment.

Medical Castration—LHRH Analogs

The pharmacologic alternatives to estrogens for medical castration are the LHRH (or GnRH) analogs, leuprolide, and goserelin. Their use seems counter to the logic of androgen ablation since it is LHRH that begins the cascade of signals that results in testosterone production. Theoretically, an LHRH analog should *increase* testosterone secretion and *stimulate* the growth of prostate cancer. This is exactly what happens during the first several days of leuprolide or goserelin administration and is called the flare phenomenon. Long-term administration, however, disrupts the normal pulsatile release of LHRH and inhibits its receptors in the pituitary. This suppresses LH production and, ultimately, testosterone production. Castrate levels of testosterone are achieved within 4 weeks (24).

The LHRH analogs are as effective as DES in producing medical castration while avoiding the cardiovascular complications of estrogens and much of the gynecomastia. Disadvantages are high cost (Table 84.5), the lack of oral formulations, the need for monthly injections, a high incidence of hot flashes, and the risk of tumor flare. Flare symptoms occur in up to 10% of patients and are usually seen as a manageable increase in bone pain. Flare can be very serious in patients with tumor masses near the spinal cord or those obstructing urine flow. Special caution is required during initiation of leuprolide or goserelin therapy in these patients. Tumor flare can be prevented by concomitant administration of flutamide, discussed later.

Antiandrogens

Antiandrogens, or androgen-receptor antagonists, are compounds that block the uptake of androgens in the target organs. Antiandrogens may be steroidal or nonsteroidal. Cyproterone acetate (not available in the United States) and megestrol acetate are the most widely used steroidal antiandrogens. They are called mixed antiandrogens because, in addition to competing with testosterone and DHT for androgen receptors in the prostate, they have progestational activity, which results in suppression of LH production. Megestrol acetate is not widely used as a single agent because some of its therapeutic effects seem to be lost after 4 to 6 months of treatment. Combining it with very low doses of DES (0.1 mg daily) may improve and prolong its efficacy (24, 29).

Flutamide was the first nonsteroidal, or pure, antiandrogen available in the United States. It inhibits the uptake and binding of testosterone and DHT to nuclear receptors. Serum testosterone levels are not affected when

Table 84.5.
Dosing and Comparative Monthly Costs of Hormone Interventions

Drug	Dose	Acquisition Cost (AWP)[a]
Diethylstilbestrol	1–3 mg daily	$3.00–$9.00
Leuprolide depot	7.5 mg IM monthly	$478.00
Goserelin	3.6 mg IM monthly	$359.00
Flutamide	250 mg t.i.d.	$269.00
Casodex biglutamide	50 mg q.i.d.	$308.00
Megestrol acetate	40 mg q.i.d.	$90–$150
Ketoconazole	400 mg t.i.d.	$488.00
Aminoglutethimide	250 mg q.i.d.	$125.00

[a]Average Wholesale Price, 1995 RedBook.

flutamide is used alone, so a major advantage is that fluta-mide does not cause impotence. The high serum testoster-one levels, however, may override the competitive andro-gen blockade, and for that reason, flutamide is not ap-proved as single-agent therapy. Its use in combination regimens is discussed later. Flutamide is very expensive (Table 84.5) and causes gynecomastia, diarrhea, flushing, and liver function abnormalities. It also has a short half-life, requiring administration three times daily. Casodex bi-glutamide was approved for marketing in 1995. It is a longer–acting nonsteroidal antiandrogen which can be ad-ministered once daily (15, 24, 29).

Total Androgen Blockade

Total androgen blockade, also called combined androgen blockade (CAB), refers to combined therapy with medical castration and an antiandrogen. The rationale is to elimi-nate the effects of both testicular and adrenal androgens. Castration eliminates the testicular production, and antian-drogens prevent any physiologic effects from adrenally pro-duced androgens. Small, nonrandomized studies in the early 1980s suggested improved survival compared with historical controls treated with monotherapy. A landmark controlled trial that randomized patients to leuprolide plus either flutamide or placebo was published in 1989 (31). It demonstrated a 7-month survival advantage for patients on the combination arm. Progression-free survival was also increased. Patients with minimal metastatic disease and good performance status benefited most. At 5 years of follow-up, patients with minimal disease had a 20-month survival advantage. This was the first time that hormone therapy had been conclusively demonstrated to prolong survival. This was accomplished with a modest increase in overall toxicity although the cost of total androgen blockade was much higher than monotherapy. Combination regi-mens quickly came into widespread use. Subsequent stud-ies have confirmed the survival advantage of combined androgen blockade, particularly for patients with minimal metastatic disease. The high costs, however, may be pro-hibitive (Table 84.5). A large trial that replaces the LHRH analog injections with less costly surgical castration is un-derway (24, 25, 28).

Miscellaneous Hormonal Agents

Suppression of adrenal androgens can be achieved with aminoglutethimide or ketoconazole. Both agents block ad-renal and testicular steroid production by blocking cyto-chrome P-450. Since production of all steroid hormones is inhibited, glucocorticoid replacement is necessary. Amino-glutethimide is used primarily as a second-line treatment in patients who have progressed after treatment with other agents. Ketoconazole, an antifungal agent, lowers serum testosterone levels very rapidly. It is used short-term in patients with impending spinal cord compression when

orchiectomy is not possible. High doses are required, which may produce severe hepatitis (15, 24).

Finasteride is a 5-alpha-reductase inhibitor that inhibits the conversion of testosterone to DHT in target cells. It has minimal side effects and rarely interferes with sexual function. It has not been effective as a single agent in the treatment of metastatic prostate cancer, but is being studied as a chemopreventive agent in patients at high risk of developing cancer of the prostate (30).

Treatment of Hormone-Resistant and Hormone-Refractory Disease

Treatment options for patients who fail to respond to hormone therapy (hormone resistant, about 15% of pa-tients) or who eventually become refractory to treatment (all other patients) are very limited. Second-line hormone interventions have much lower response rates, shorter durations of effect, and greater toxicity than the first-line therapies of medical or surgical castration or combination regimens with antiandrogens. Some patients whose disease progresses on combination therapy with LHRH analogs and flutamide may benefit from stopping the flutamide (the flutamide withdrawal syndrome) (31). The mechanism of this effect is unknown, but evidence suggests that flutamide may begin to act as an androgen rather than an antiandro-gen during prolonged therapy.

Cytotoxic chemotherapy has traditionally had little benefit in these patients, either in prolonging survival or in palliating symptoms. Combination regimens have been no more successful than single-agent trials (32). Chemo-therapy has its greatest effects against rapidly dividing cells, so the very slow doubling time of prostate cancer cells may account for this general lack of activity.

Recently, some encouraging progress has been made in cytotoxic treatment of prostate cancer (33). Four commer-cially available agents have been shown to produce objec-tive response rates (complete plus partial responses) greater than 10%. These are doxorubicin, cisplatin, estra-mustine, and vinblastine. Combining these agents may in-crease the response rates. The best results at present have been obtained with combination regimens that contain estramustine. This is an unusual oral agent that combines an alkylator with an estrogen. Recent studies indicate that its mechanism of action is distinct from either of those components. It is now recognized to work as an antimitotic agent with antimicrotubule effects. In combination with vinblastine, another microtubule inhibitor, it has produced objective responses in about 30% of patients with hormone-refractory prostate cancer. This is an outpatient regimen with manageable toxicity (34). More recently, similar encouraging results have been achieved with a com-bination of estramustine and oral etoposide, a topoisomer-ase II inhibitor that has minimal activity alone in prostate cancer (35).

SUPPORTIVE CARE

Management of symptoms is an important part of the care of patients with advanced prostate cancer to manage the side effects of hormone or cytotoxic therapies and to improve quality of life when the progress of the disease cannot be controlled. Hot flashes are a common and troublesome side effect of surgical castration and LHRH analogs. These vasoactive flushes are centrally mediated and produce sensations of heat and sweating that may persist for a minute to an hour. They can occur as often as thirty or forty times in 24 hours and often awaken patients from sleep. Hot flashes can be controlled in about 75% of patients with low doses of megestrol acetate 20 mg twice daily (36). Low doses of DES and the antihypertensive clonidine have also been reported to decrease the number and severity of hot flashes. Gynecomastia secondary to DES or other hormonal agents is difficult to treat but can be prevented by prophylactic radiation therapy to each breast (37). The treatment of erectile dysfunction was discussed under radical prostatectomy.

Pain is one of the most common and troublesome side effects of prostate cancer. It is one of the most painful cancers, overall, because of the high incidence of bone metastases. Nonsteroidal antiinflammatory agents with or without opiate analgesics are effective in prostate cancer pain management. Strontium-89 is a bone-seeking radionucleotide that can give prolonged pain relief from prostate bone metastases.

FUTURE DIRECTIONS

Cryosurgery, in which the prostate gland is destroyed by freezing, is being studied as an alternative to radical prostatectomy for treatment of localized prostate cancers. The freezing causes necrosis of the prostate tissue. The procedure has lower morbidity than traditional prostatectomy but, at present, is considered less reliable and remains investigational (38).

Suramin is an investigational polysulfonated naphthylurea that has been used for many years for the treatment of sleeping sickness in Africa. Its antitumor activity appears to depend on inhibition of the effects of tumor growth factors. Suramin has significant activity in patients with hormone-refractory prostate cancer but also has a wide range of toxicities such as malaise, nephrotoxicity, neurotoxicity, chemical hepatitis, rash, edema, and adrenal insufficiency. The therapeutic-to-toxic ratio has been effectively modified by use of pharmacokinetically based dosing regimens that control plasma drug concentrations (33, 39).

One of the most exciting potential areas of research for prostate cancer is gene therapy. Recently, two genes have been linked to metastatic prostate cancer. One gene mutation of the androgen receptor may be responsible for loss of hormonal control of the disease (40). Another gene suppresses prostate metastases. These gene mutations could be targeted by new, better directed, therapies. Human studies are also underway in the first human trials using genetically modified prostate cancer cells as a vaccine to prevent recurrence.

CONCLUSION

Prostate cancer is a very common cancer that is highly curable in its localized forms but incurable once it has metastasized. Early diagnosis offers the best opportunity for cure, but widespread screening of asymptomatic patients is controversial. Many prostate cancers are biologically latent and would not produce symptoms within the life of the patient. More discriminating screening tests are needed to help distinguish between latent and clinically important cancers.

Radical prostatectomy is the recommended treatment for clinically localized cancers. It offers the best chance of cure. New surgical techniques result in fewer long-term complications. Radiation therapy is a good alternative treatment for patients who are not good surgical candidates. Watchful waiting may be appropriate in patients with low-grade tumors and a life expectancy of less than 10 years.

Hormonal therapy is the mainstay of treatment for metastatic prostate cancer. First-line treatments include medical or surgical castration, or total androgen blockade, which combines castration with antiandrogens. The choice of hormonal therapy depends on patient preference, costs, and other medical conditions. Cytotoxic chemotherapy has little role in the management of prostate cancer, but newer combination regimens of antimicrotubule agents may show some promise. Symptom management and supportive care are essential in the total care of patients with prostate cancer.

REFERENCES

1. Wingo PA, Tong T, Bolden S. Cancer statistics, 1995. CA Cancer J Clin 45:8–30, 1995.
2. Ross RK, Coetzee GA, Reichardt J, et al. Does the racial-ethnic variation in prostate cancer risk have a hormonal basis? Cancer 75:1778–1782, 1995.
3. Giovannucci E. Epidemiologic characteristics of prostate cancer. Cancer 75:1766–1777, 1995.
4. Isaacs WB, Bova GS, Morton RA, et al. Molecular genetics and chromosomal alterations in prostate cancer. Cancer 75:2004–2012, 1995.
5. John EM, Whittemore AS, Wu AH, et al. Vasectomy and prostate cancer: results from a multiethnic case-control study. J Natl Cancer Inst 87:662–669, 1995.
6. Hanks GE, Myers CE, Scardino PT. Cancer of the prostate. In: DeVita VT Jr, Hellman S, Rosenberg SA. Cancer: Principles and Practice of Oncology, 4th ed. Philadelphia: JB Lippincott Co, 1993:1073–1113.
7. Brawer MK. How to use prostate-specific antigen in the early detection or screening for prostatic carcinoma. CA Cancer J Clin 45:148–164, 1995.

8. Partin AW, Oesterling JE. The clinical usefulness of prostate specific antigen: update 1994. J Urology 152:1358–1368, 1994.

9. Ellis WJ, Lange PH. Prostate cancer. Endocrinol Metab Clin North Am 23:809–824, 1994.

10. DeAntoni EP, Crawford ED. Prostate cancer awareness week: education, service, and research in a community setting. Cancer 75:1874–1879, 1995.

11. Krahn MD, Mahoney JE, Eckman MH. Screening for prostate cancer. JAMA 272:773–780, 1994

12. Slawin KM, Ohori M, Dillioglugil O, Scardino PT. Screening for prostate cancer: an analysis of the early experience. Cancer J Clin 45:134–147, 1995.

13. Anon. Genitourinary sites. In: American Joint Committee on Cancer: Manual for Staging of Cancer, 3rd ed. Philadelphia: JB Lippincott, 1988: 177–179.

14. Scardino PT, Weaver R, Hudson MA. Early detection of prostate cancer. Hum Pathol 23:211–222, 1992.

15. Catalona WJ. Management of cancer of the prostate. N Engl J Med 331:996–1004, 1994.

16. Catalona WJ. Surgical management of prostate cancer. Cancer 75:1903–1908, 1994.

17. Zincke H, Bergstralh EJ, Blute ML, et al. Radical prostatectomy for clinically localized prostate cancer: long-term results of 1,143 patients from a single institution. J Clin Oncol 12:2254–2263, 1994.

18. Lee WR, Hanks GE, Schultheiss TE, Corn BW, Hunt MA. Localized prostate cancer treated by external-beam radiotherapy alone: sertum prostae-specific antigen-driven outcome analysis. J Clin Oncol 13:464–469, 1995.

19. Porter AT, Blasko JC, Grimm PD, Reddy SM, Ragde H. Brachytherapy for prostate cancer. CA Cancer J Clin 45:165–178, 1995.

20. Chodak GW, Thisted RA, Gerger GS, et al. Results of conservative management of clinically localized prostate cancer. N Engl J Med 330:242–248, 1994.

21. Chodak GW. The role of watchful waiting in the management of localized prostate cancer. J Urol 152:1766–1768, 1994.

22. Hirsch JD, Schwartz RN. Prostate cancer. In: Herfindal ET, Gourley DR, Hart LL. Clinical Pharmacy and Therapeutics, 5th ed. Baltimore: Williams & Wilkins, 1992:1370.

23. Rhoades R, Pflanzer R. Human Physiology, 2nd ed. Fort Worth: Saunders College Publishing, 1992:984–986.

24. Gudziak MR, Smith AY. Hormonal therapy for stage D cancer of the prostate. West J Med 160:351–359, 1994.

25. Griffiths K, Eaton CL, Harper ME, Turkes A, Peeling WB. Hormonal treatment of advanced disease: some newer aspects. Semin Oncol 21:672–687, 1994.

26. Huggins C, Stevens R, Hodges C. The effect of castration on advanced carcinoma of the prostate gland. Arch Surg 43:209–223, 1941.

27. Blackard CE. The Veterans' Administration cooperative urological research group studies of carcinoma of the prostate: a review. Cancer Chemother Rep 59:225–227, 1975.

28. McLeod DG. Hormonal therapy in the treatment of carcinoma of the prostate. Cancer 75:1914–1919, 1995.

29. The Leuprolide Study Group. Leuprolide versus diethylstilbestrol for metastatic prostate cancer. N Engl J Med 311:1281–1286, 1984.

30. Brawley OW, Thompson IM. Chemoprevention of prostate cancer. Urology 43:594–599, 1994.

31. Scher HI, Kelly WK. Flutamide withdrawal syndrome: its impact on clinical trials in hormone-refractory prostate cancer. J Clin Oncol 11:1566–1572, 1993.

32. Tannock IF. Is there evidence that chemotherapy is of benefit to patients with carcinoma of the prostate? J Clin Oncol 3:1013–1021, 1985.

33. Kreis W. Current chemotherapy and future directions in research for the treatment of advanced hormone-refractory prostate cancer. Cancer Investigation 13:296–312, 1995.

34. Hudes GR, Greenberg R, Krigel RL, et al. Phase II study of estramustine and vinblastine, two microtubule inhibitors, in hormone-refractory prostate cancer. J Clin Oncol 10(11):1754–1761, 1992.

35. Pienta KJ, Redman B, Hussain M, et al. Phase II evaluation of oral estramustine and oral etoposide in hormone-refractory adenocarcinoma of the prostate. J Clin Oncol 12:2005–2012, 1994.

36. Loprinzi CL, Michalak JC, Quella SK, et al. Megestrol acetate for the prevention of hot flashes. N Engl J Med 331:347–352, 1994.

37. Kirschenbaum A. Management of hormonal treatment effects. Cancer 75:1983–1986, 1995.

38. Onik GM, Cohen JK, Reyes GD, et al. Transrectal ultrasound guided percutaneous radical cryosurgical ablation of the prostate. Cancer 72:1291–1296, 1993.

39. Jodrell DI, Reyno LM, Sridhara R, et al. Suramin: development of a population pharmacokinetic model and its use with intermittent short infusions to control plasma drug concentration in patients with prostate cancer. J Clin Oncol 12:166–175, 1994.

40. Taplin ME, Bubley GJ, Shuster TD, et al. Mutation of the androgen-receptor gene in metastatic androgen-independent prostate cancer. N Engl J Med 332:1393–1398, 1995.

CHAPTER 85

PEDIATRIC SOLID TUMORS OF CHILDHOOD

MARTHA L. GARDNER and EDITH C. MARTINGANO

Cancer afflicts approximately 130 children per million annually. Although a rare entity in children, it is an illness that leads to significant morbidity and is second only to accidents as a cause of death in children ages 1 to 14 years (1). Approximately 50% of pediatric tumors occur in the age range of 0 to 4 years, suggesting genetic and differentiation factors contributing to disease (2). Treatment goals are complete eradication of tumor while minimizing toxicities. Unlike hematologic malignancies that use chemotherapy as a single treatment modality, therapy of solid tumors usually requires a multimodal approach. In the past 20 years, treatment of pediatric solid neoplasms has improved with less radical surgeries, better radiotherapy techniques, and the addition of aggressive combination chemotherapy. An enhanced understanding of tumor biology will undoubtedly lead to further improvements.

More than 50% of children with cancer can now achieve long-term survival, but research must continue to improve survival outcomes and tolerability of therapy (3). This is best accomplished with multicenter trials. The largest cooperative study groups in the United States are the Children's Cancer Group (CCG) and the Pediatric Oncology Group (POG). Much epidemiologic data continue to be gathered by the Surveillance, Epidemiology, and End Results program (SEER), a tumor registry of the National Cancer Institute (NCI) (see Table 85.1 and Figure 85.1) (3). This chapter will expose the reader to general principles of therapy, the more common pediatric solid tumors, clinical presentation, prognosis, multimodal treatment, and supportive care issues that arise. Oncologic terms and acronyms that are frequently referenced in the literature will also be introduced.

GENERAL PRINCIPLES OF THERAPY

The successful management of the pediatric cancer patient uses a multidisciplinary approach to treatment from the pediatric oncologist, surgeon, radiotherapist, radiologist, pathologist, and other health care professionals such as nurses, pharmacists, psychiatrists, social workers, and child life specialists. Treatment of solid malignancies can be divided into four major modalities: surgery, radiation therapy, chemotherapy, and biological therapy and immunotherapy. Surgery is the oldest treatment for solid tumors and until recently the only treatment that offered cure for the pediatric patient with cancer. The role of surgery in

pediatric cancers is threefold: (1) prevention (e.g., in patients with multiple polyposis of the colon, 50% will develop colon cancer if prophylactic colectomy is not performed); (2) diagnosis and staging (e.g., needle aspirations or biopsies for pathologic evaluation; visual inspection); and (3) treatment (e.g., primary curative total resection, debulking, adjuvant to chemotherapy or radiotherapy with delayed "second-look" resection, metastatic resection, palliation, reconstruction) (4). The present goal of surgery is to minimize disability and deformity while maximizing the extent of resection. For example, major strides in surgical limb sparing techniques that reduce functional and psychological morbidity continue to be achieved in osteosarcoma patients in contrast to the traditional surgical approach of radical extremity amputation (5).

The use of ionizing radiation to treat cancer was first reported within a year of Roentgen's discovery of radiographs in 1895 (6). The goal of radiotherapy in pediatric malignancies is to maximize local control of the primary tumor. The effective radiation dose for local control is balanced by the need to spare adjacent normal tissue from radiation damage and, ultimately, minimize growth retardation and secondary malignancies. To decrease radiation toxicity, modern techniques include fractionation of doses and dose reduction in combination with chemotherapy. Another important consideration for the use of radiation in pediatric oncology is that children must be sedated for these procedures. The health care professional must be aware of the potential side effects of the sedative agents. Long-term toxicities from radiation therapy include cardiac toxicity; learning disabilities; and the failure of soft tissues, teeth, and visual structures to develop normally, resulting in cosmetic deformities or decreased muscle mass (7).

The role of chemotherapy in solid tumors may be adjuvant to surgery (or radiation) to "debulk" prior to resection or to prevent recurrence secondary to visible or microscopic residual tumor. Chemotherapy is also used to treat unresectable metastatic disease. Fortunately, the majority of pediatric malignancies are chemotherapy sensitive. Combination chemotherapy with agents that differ mechanistically is generally employed to minimize drug resistance and allow for additive or synergistic therapeutic effects (8). Higher doses at shorter intervals, termed dose-intensive therapy, is being compared to traditional regimens for many tumor types. Intensifying drug doses can improve response rates but also augments the occurrence of serious acute side effects such as myelosuppression and mucositis, leading to more frequent emergency hospitalizations for febrile neutropenic episodes and dehydration, which often delays therapy. Many acute toxicities of chemotherapy can be prevented or minimized with individualized prospective monitoring. The use of growth factors that stimulate white blood cell production such as granulocyte colony stimulating factor (G-CSF) or granulocyte-monocyte colony stimulating factor (GM-CSF) may shorten the period and degree of neutropenia in some patients. Many patients require extensive supportive care in the form of intravenous broad spectrum antibiotics, antiemetics, blood and platelet trans-

fusions, pain management, hyperalimentation, preventive measures for mucositis, and meticulous attention to fluid and electrolyte disturbances. Pediatric patients have clearly benefited from the new, nonsedating serotonin (5-HT$_3$) receptor antagonist antiemetics (ondansetron, granisetron), which have eliminated undesired effects traditionally associated with older antiemetics (chlorpromazine, prochlorperazine, high-dose metoclopramide) (9,10). Delayed cardiomyopathies secondary to anthracycline administration may be prevented or minimized by using slower infusions and by close monitoring of cumulative doses received, generally less than 500 mg/m^2(11). The most commonly used chemotherapy agents in the treatment of pediatric solid tumors are summarized in Table 85.2.

Autologous bone marrow reinfusion after the administration of very high doses of chemotherapy or irradiation (which cause dose-limiting bone marrow suppression) is being studied in children with high-risk solid tumors in which long-term survival is thought to be less than 30%. This dose-intensive therapy has been investigated in stage III–IV neuroblastoma, disseminated Ewing's sarcoma, disseminated medulloblastoma, high-grade ependymoma, high-grade supratentorial astrocytomas, stage IV alveolar rhabdomyosarcoma, disseminated osteosarcoma, and stage IV anaplastic Wilms' tumor with mixed responses (12). Future studies are needed to define the role of high-dose chemotherapy with autologous bone marrow rescue in the treatment of pediatric solid tumors.

Biological therapy and immunotherapy are terms that are very broad in scope, incorporating the use of physiologic agents to transfer immunity or assist the patient's own immune or biological system to defend itself against cancer. Biological therapy is sometimes considered the fourth modality of cancer treatment although clinical utility

Table 85.1.
Survival Statistics of Malignant Tumors in U.S. Children, SEER Data 1983–1987

	New Cases Reported to SEER	5-Year Relative Survival (%)
Hematologic tumors		
Acute lymphocytic leukemia	814	69
Acute myelogenous leukemia	117	26
Hodgkin's disease	148	87
Non-Hodgkin's lymphomas	268	68
Solid tumors		
Brain & other nervous system	510	56
Wilms' tumor	210	85
Neuroblastoma	224	49
Retinoblastoma	100	98
Rhabdomyosarcoma	122	68
Osteosarcoma	84	53
Ewing's sarcoma	70	54

ᵃAdapted from (3).

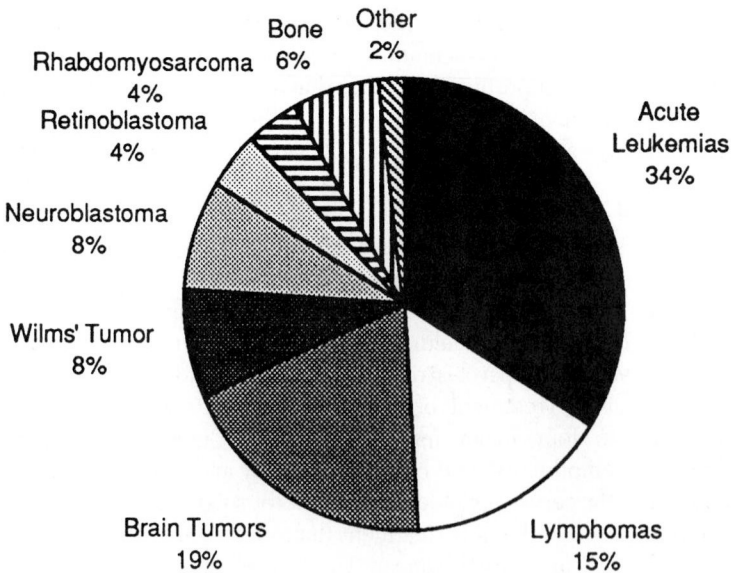

Figure 85.1. Relative incidence of pediatric malignancies (3).

Table 85.2.
Chemotherapeutic Agents Commonly Used in Pediatric Solid Tumors

Drug Synonyms and Abbreviations (in caps)	Class	Route	Toxicities	Solid Tumor Spectrum of Activity
Methotrexate MTX	Antifolate Antimetabolite	IV PO	Mild myelosuppression, mucositis, rash, hepatotoxicity, renal (high dose), neurotoxicity (high dose)	Osteosarcoma
Oxazaphosphorines Cyclophosphamide Cytoxan® CTX	Alkylators	IV PO	Myelosuppression, n/v, hemorrhagic cystitis, alopecia, water retention, SIADH, cardiac (high dose)	Rhabdomyosarcoma, Ewing's sarcoma, neuroblastoma, bone marrow transplantation (cyclophosphamide only)
Ifosfamide Ifex®, IFOS		IV	Myelosuppression, n/v, hemorrhagic cystitis, neurotoxicity, renal and electrolyte disturbances	
Platinum Analogs Cisplatin Platinol®, CDDP	Alkylators	IV	Myelosupp (WBCs), severe n/v, renal damages, electrolyte disturbances, neurotoxicity, ototoxicity, allergic reactions	Brain tumors, neuroblastoma, germ cell tumors, osteosarcoma
Carboplatin Paraplatin®, CBDCA		IV	Myelosuppression (platelets), n/v, hepatic, moderate renal toxicity	Similar spectrum to cisplatin
Doxorubicin Adriamycin®, ADR	Anthracycline Antibiotic	IV	Myelosuppression, mucositis, n/v, alopecia, vesicant, cardiac (acute and chronic)	Most solid tumors
Dactinomycin Actinomycin-D, Cosmegen®, ACT-D	Antibiotic	IV	Myelosuppression, mucositis, n/v, alopecia, hepatoxicity, vesicant	Wilms', Ewing's sarcoma, rhabdomyosarcoma
Vincristine Oncovin®, VCR	Plant alkaloid	IV	Neurotoxicity, alopecia, SIADH, hypotension, constipation, vesicant	Most solid tumors
Epipodophyllotoxins Etoposide VePesid®, VP-16	Plant alkaloids	IV PO	Myelosuppression, alopecia, n/v, mucositis, hypotension (IV formulation), allergic reactions, secondary malignancy	Brain tumors, neuroblastoma, Ewing's sarcoma, rhabdomyosarcoma
Teniposide Vumon®, VM-26		IV	Similar spectrum to etoposide	
Lomustine CeeNU®, CCNU	Nitrosourea Alkylator	PO	Delayed myelosuppression, n/v, mucositis, neurotoxicity	Brain tumors

Key: n/v (nausea/vomiting), WBCs (white blood cells)

is still in infancy stages. This modality represents the future of cancer treatment research as we gain insight into the physiology of the host–tumor relationship, host defense, and tumor biology. Interferons, interleukins, monoclonal antibodies, growth-differentiating agents such as retinoids, antisense oligonucleotides, and gene therapy are just a few examples of the types of agents being investigated.

The long-term toxicities of therapy are a result of the combination of cytotoxic agents and radiotherapy. Every attempt must be made to ensure that the child survives as a functional member of his or her family as well as society. A comprehensive support matrix must offer the child every opportunity to grow and mature as normally as possible. Treatment at a comprehensive cancer center can help reduce the problems many children experience when receiving chemotherapy. The treatment program for the child with cancer cannot focus only on tumor reduction and the physical side effects of therapy, but also must incorporate much psychosocial support. Long-term survivors of childhood cancer often have chronic complications that affect patient functioning and may include neurologic problems, cardiac and renal toxicities, infection, growth and developmental delays, diminished fertility, and secondary malignancies (12, 13). Newer, potentially less toxic anthracycline and platinum analogs, idarubicin and carboplatin, respectively, are being studied as replacements for doxorubicin and cisplatin in the hope that they can minimize late sequelae of therapy. Long-term follow-up clinics for children who survive cancer are helping us better understand these consequences and alter future therapy.

BRAIN TUMORS

Classification

Neoplasms of the brain are second only to leukemia in their frequency during childhood and are the most common solid tumors in children under 15 years. A multidisciplinary approach has allowed for improvements in diagnostic, surgical, and radiation techniques and in chemotherapeutic regimens, influencing a change in overall 5-year survival from 35% in the early 1960s to better than 60% in the late 1980s (1). The health professional's role in the care of children with brain tumors involves monitoring not only chemotherapeutic regimens and antiemetic therapy, but also assistance in special drug-related supportive care issues for cerebral edema, seizure control, endocrine therapy, antibiotic selection, pain management, and choice of medications for conscious sedation.

Classification of primary brain tumors remains a topic of controversy, and there is no universally accepted nomenclature. Tumors are frequently classified by location and are broadly divided into two categories: supratentorial neoplasms, including cerebral hemispheric and midline tumors, and infratentorial neoplasms, including brainstem and cerebellar tumors (Table 85.3) (14). Unlike adults, in which most brain tumors are located supratentorially near the cerebral hemispheres, 50 to 60% of central nervous system (CNS) tumors in children older than 1 year arise infratentorially in the posterior fossa. The most prevalent histology is glial in origin and includes a broad variety of tumor types, most commonly low-grade astrocytomas. The medulloblastoma, of primitive neuroectodermal origin, is a malignant cerebellar tumor that has a marked propensity to invade the meninges and parenchymal tissue, and is the most common distinct tumor type of childhood brain neoplasms. Midline tumors, such as craniopharyngiomas and pineal tumors, occur near the optic chiasm and often cause visual field defects, hydrocephalus, and extraocular muscle palsies (15).

Clinical Presentation and Diagnosis

Clinical manifestations of brain neoplasms depend on tumor location, age, and developmental level of the child and are often vague. Generalized symptoms include nausea, vomiting, and diffuse, frequent headaches habitually occurring in the morning on awakening. These symptoms, frequently mistaken as evidence of an infectious illness, migraine, or tension headache, may indicate the presence of increased intracranial pressure (ICP) and hydrocephalus, which is often associated with infratentorial tumors that obstruct flow of cerebrospinal fluid through the cerebral ventricles. Localizing symptoms may include gait disturbances and ataxia, seizures, visual field defects,

Table 85.3.
Distribution of Common Brain Tumors in Children, According to Location and Histologic Appearance[a]

Location and Type of Tumor	Percentage of All Brain Tumors
Infratentorial	
Primitive neuroectodermal tumor (medulloblastoma)	20–25
Low-grade astrocytoma, cerebellar	12–18
Ependymoma	4–8
Malignant glioma, brainstem	3–9
Low-grade astrocytoma, brainstem	3–6
Other	2–5
Total	45–60
Supratentorial hemispheric	
Low-grade astrocytoma	8–20
Malignant glioma	6–12
Ependymoma	2–5
Mixed glioma	1–5
Ganglioglioma	1–5
Oligodendroglioma	1–2
Choroid-plexus tumor	1–2
Primitive neuroectodermal tumor	1–2
Meningioma	0.5–2
Other	1–3
Total	25–40
Supratentorial midline	
Suprasellar	
Craniopharyngioma	6–9
Low-grade glioma, chiasmatic-hypothalamic	4–8
Germ-cell tumor	1–2
Pituitary adenoma	.05–2.5
Pineal region	
Low-grade glioma	1–2
Germ-cell tumor	.05–2
Pineal parenchymal tumor	.05–2
Total	15–20

[a]Adapted from: Pollack IF. Brain tumors in children. N Engl J Med 331:1500–1510, 1994, with permission.

neuroendocrine abnormalities, facial and extraocular muscle palsies, and hemiparesis. Diagnosis may be difficult in children less than 2 years of age because of very nonspecific, nonlocalizing signs and symptoms such as irritability, listlessness, failure to thrive, vomiting, developmental delay, and progressive macrocephaly (14).

Magnetic resonance imaging (MRI) or computed tomography (CT) are currently used to diagnose and determine size, location, and tumor density of CNS neoplasms and are also performed postoperatively to assess volume of residual tumor. For tumors with a high propensity for metastasis into the cerebrospinal fluid (CSF), such as medulloblastoma, posterior-fossa ependymoma, and germ-cell tumors, spinal MRI and a cytologic examination of CSF are performed for staging purposes. To achieve sharp images, movement during MRI and CT scans must be kept to a minimum; thus, children are often immobilized and heavily sedated prior to the exam. Pediatric patients who are lethargic or have other signs of elevated intracranial pressure need special evaluation when receiving sedation prior to diagnostic procedures. Sedative agents that decrease respiratory drive or increase ICP, such as narcotics or ketamine, should be avoided in these patients. Drug-induced hypoventilation may result in carbon dioxide retention, vasodilation, expanded intracranial vascular volume, and thus increased ICP (16). Sedative doses of agents with less effects on respiration or ICP such as benzodiazepines, pentobarbital, or chloral hydrate may be better choices for sedation in these patients.

Prognosis

Five-year survival is best in children with cerebellar astrocytomas (91%) and worst for those with brainstem gliomas (18%) (17). Less than one-third of patients in poor risk categories (high-grade astrocytomas, including glioblastoma multiforme, unresectable medulloblastomas, anaplastic ependymomas, unresectable brainstem tumors, and children less than 4 years of age) become long-term survivors.

Treatment

SURGERY

Specific management depends on tumor type and location. To determine a histologic diagnosis and reduce tumor burden, surgery is often the first task of a series of interventions. Surgical cure, however, is not frequently an obtainable goal since anatomic location of many tumors does not allow for total resection. Maximal tumor removal is balanced against the risk of inducing severe neurologic damage to the patient. Short-term external ventricular drains or long-term internal ventriculoperitoneal shunts are often placed to drain cerebrospinal fluid in patients with obstructive hydrocephalus. Table 85.4 summarizes the perioperative supportive care issues (14).

RADIOTHERAPY

Brain tumors have customarily been treated with maximum tolerated doses of 5000 to 6000 cGy administered in once-daily fractions of 180 to 200 cGy over 5 to 6 weeks. Radiation hyperfractionation, the administration of larger numbers (twice-daily doses) of smaller fractions of radiotherapy over an equivalent period, may allow for higher total doses with less morbidity and intensified tumor kill (18). Results of studies in brainstem gliomas have been mixed (19). Other advances include sophisticated approaches that allow more restricted administration of radiation to the tumor while minimizing exposure of surrounding tissue. Brainstem tumors are often surgically inaccessible; thus, primary treatment is radiotherapy with or without combination chemotherapy (14).

For neoplasms that have a propensity to metastasize throughout the neuraxis, craniospinal irradiation may be indicated (15).

Acute adverse effects of brain irradiation include transient exacerbation of local neurologic signs; radiation sickness with symptoms of nausea, vomiting, loss of appetite, drowsiness, and irritability; xerostomia and sialadenitis; hair loss; bone marrow suppression in those receiving craniospinal irradiation; skin erythema, breakdown, and hyperpigmentation; and the somnolence syndrome, a period of extreme drowsiness that may occur 4 to 8 weeks after the completion of a course of treatment with recovery in 1 to 2 weeks (20). Late side effects include significant learning disabilities, personality changes, bone and soft tissue malformations, cerebral necrosis, and retardation of linear growth due to decreased release of hormones from the hypothalamic-pituitary axis such as growth hormone and thyroid-stimulating hormone (20).

CHEMOTHERAPY

Achieving therapeutic antineoplastic drug concentrations in the brain is problematic because of poor penetration of the blood–brain barrier (BBB) by most agents. Determinants of BBB penetration embody physicochemical and pharmacokinetic drug properties and pathophysiology of the tumor itself. Chemotherapeutic agents of low molecular weight, high lipid solubility, and unionized at physiologic pH have the highest chance of crossing the BBB. Pharmacokinetic properties such as low serum protein binding and long elimination half-life may also improve drug entrance. The pathophysiology of large CNS masses creates a paradoxical situation in which permeability of the BBB is enhanced at the necrotic center, but reduced around the viable periphery of the tumor where antineoplastic effects are desired. However, clinical trials have demonstrated that some water-soluble agents (platinum analogs and classical alkylators) have significant activity in certain brain tumors that may be a result of increased BBB permeability induced by the malignancy. Efficacy of chemotherapy agents also depends on tumor growth kinetics.

Chemotherapy has been studied mostly in poor risk patients in the following situations: primary therapy for recurrent brain tumors in older studies; as adjuvant therapy after surgery and/or radiation therapy in newly diagnosed patients; and as postoperative neoadjuvant (preirradiation) therapy. Early studies demonstrated that chemotherapy could produce regression of recurrent tumors, but rarely cures. As adjuvant therapy to radiotherapy and surgery, chemotherapy regimens have significantly increased 5-year survival in children with at least partially resected supratentorial or cerebellar malignant astrocytomas (21) and in children with high-risk medulloblastomas (22, 23). Preirradiation chemotherapy regimens were conceptualized to

Table 85.4.
Common Perioperative Problems of Childhood Brain Tumors with Pharmacologic or Surgical Solutions

Perioperative Problem	Type of Tumors Involved	Preoperative and Intraoperative Management	Postoperative Management
Peritumoral edema	Large tumors; smaller tumors in critical areas such as the brainstem	Corticosteroids (e.g, dexamethasone [Decadron] at a dose of 0.05–0.1 mg/kg of body weight 4 times daily) are administered.	Corticosteroids are tapered within several days of surgery, particularly if tumor resection is extensive.
Obstructive hydrocephalus	Intraventricular or periventricular tumors	An external ventricular drain is placed before tumor resection is begun.	If the tumor resection opens the cerebrospinal fluid pathways, drainage established by ventriculostomy can often be discontinued within several days of surgery. Patients in whom progressive ventriculomegaly develops or who have an enlarging pseudomeningocele require definitive diversion of cerebrospinal fluid. Although a shunt poses a theoretical risk of peritoneal seeding of the tumor, this has not been confirmed in recent studies.[a]
Seizures	Tumors of the cerebral hemispheres; tumors that will require cerebral retraction during their removal	An anticonvulsant agent, such as phenytoin (Dilantin), is started preoperatively and continued during surgery.	In children without prior seizures, anticonvulsant drugs can generally be stopped within several months of surgery. In patients with a history of preoperative seizures who undergo complete tumor removal and are rendered seizure free, anticonvulsant agents can often be discontinued within several months of surgery.
Hypothalamic-pituitary hormonal insufficiency	Tumors arising in and around the hypothalamus	An evaluation of endocrine function is useful if the child is clinically stable. "Stress" doses (doses several times the normal maintenance dose) of a corticosteroid, such as hydrocortisone, are administered before and during surgery. Because diabetes insipidus may develop during surgery, fluid balance must be monitored closely.	Doses of corticosteroids can be decreased to maintenance levels during the first postoperative week. Fluid balance and electrolyte levels are monitored closely and controlled by administration of appropriate fluids and, if indicated, vasopressin. Detailed postoperative and, often, follow-up endocrine testing is required to determine long-term needs for hormonal replacement.

[a]See reference (14).
Adapted from: Pollack IF. Brain tumors in children. N Eng J Med 331:1500–1510, 1994, with permission.

assess drug-induced tumor responses prior to radiotherapy and to improve survival results over conventional postirradiation therapy. Further, this schedule may help avoid additive toxicity, such as prolonged myelosuppression and enhanced cisplatin ototoxicity, that may result when radiation is followed by chemotherapy; it may improve drug entry into the tumor before radiotherapy-induced vascular changes occur; and certain agents may act as radiation sensitizers (14). Children less than 3 years are at an increased risk of developing severe long-term neurologic deficits from brain irradiation because myelinization of the brain is usually not complete prior to this age. For this reason, in these children, preirradiation chemotherapy

is often preferred as initial postoperative treatment over radiation, allowing radiotherapy to be deferred for a few years until the brain is more mature (24).

The nitrosourea, CCNU, and vincristine are the prototypic agents used in malignant gliomas. CCNU is a low molecular weight, lipid-soluble, oral agent that easily crosses the BBB. Vincristine, though it penetrates the BBB poorly, has been shown to be active in the treatment of brain tumors since the late 1960s. In the latter 1970s and early 1980s, methotrexate, cyclophosphamide, and cisplatin were found to have significant activity in recurrent tumors, especially medulloblastomas. Unfortunately, the use of methotrexate and cisplatin in previously irradiated patients is constrained by a high occurrence rate of severe leukoencephalopathy and ototoxicity, respectively (25, 26). The more recent use of the analog, carboplatin, may reduce the neurotoxic, nephrotoxic, and ototoxic effects of cisplatin, but may increase the incidence of myelosuppression. Corticosteroids are often added to the chemotherapy regimen to minimize cerebral edema secondary to drug therapy. Table 85.5 summarizes common chemotherapy combinations (and their acronyms) that have been used in brain tumors (27).

Brainstem gliomas are usually unresectable, relatively unresponsive to current chemotherapeutic regimens, and generally have a median survival of less than 1 year after radiotherapy (14). Recurrent tumors are also associated with a poor prognosis. Preliminary studies of dose-intensified, marrow-ablative chemotherapy regimens, along with autologous transplantation or peripheral stem cell rescue for recurrent malignant gliomas and medulloblastoma, have shown promise. Newer studies will evaluate this strategy for newly diagnosed aggressive brain tumors, including brainstem gliomas (28).

NEUROBLASTOMA

Neuroblastoma is the most common extracranial solid tumor in children and the fourth most common pediatric malignancy. Neuroblastoma has a prevalence of 1 case per 8,000 live births. In the United States, it compromises 8 to 10% of all cancers diagnosed in children less than 15 years old or approximately 525 new cases annually. It is the most common malignant neoplasm in the newborn as well as in children between 1 and 12 months of age (9). Fifty percent of all malignancies diagnosed in the first month of life and one-third during the first year of life are neuroblastoma (9, 29). The median age at diagnosis is approximately 2 years old. Neuroblastoma is thought to be derived from the embryonic neural crest that forms the adrenal medulla and sympathetic nervous system. As a small blue round cell tumor, neuroblastoma consists of dense nests of cells separated by fibrovascular bundles. It is important for the pathologist to differentiate between neuroblastoma and the other small, round-cell tumors such as Ewing's sarcoma, lymphoma, rhabdomyosarcoma, and Askin's tumor.

Table 85.5.
Chemotherapy Combinations for Pediatric Brain Tumors[a]

Regimen	Dosage/Route	Comments
"PCV"		
CCNU	100 mg/m^2 PO, day 1 or day 2	Every 6 weeks × 8 cycles (1 year)
Vincristine[b]	1.5 mg/m^2 IV (max 2 mg), days 1, 8, ± 15	
Prednisone	40 mg/m^2 PO, days 1–14	
OR		
Procarbazine	100 mg/m^2 PO days 1–14	
"MOPP"		
Nitrogen Mustard	6 mg/m^2 IV, days 1, 8	Every 4 weeks × 12 cycles (1 year)
Vincristine[b]	14–1.5 mg/m^2 IV (max. 2 mg), days 1, 8	
Procarbazine	100 mg/m^2 PO, days 1–14	
Prednisone	40 mg/m^2 PO, days 1–14	
"8-in-1"		
Vincristine[b]	1.5 mg/m^2 IV, hour 0	Every 4–6 weeks × 10–24 cycles
CCNU	100 mg/m^2 PO, hour 0	
Procarbazine	75 mg/m^2 PO, hour 1	
Hydroyurea	1,500–3,000 mg/m^2 PO, hour 2	
Cisplatin	60–90 mg/m^2 IV, hours 3–9	
Ara-C	300 mg/m^2 IV, hour 9	
Cyclophosphamide	300 mg/m^2 IV, hour 12	
OR		
Dacarbazine	150 mg/m^2 IV, hour 12	
Methylprednisolone	300 mg/m^2 IV, hours 0, 6, 12	
Cisplatin Combinations		
Cisplatin +	90–100 mg/m^2 IV, day 1	Every 3–4 weeks
Vincristine[b]	1.5 mg/m^2 IV, day 1	Various combinations with cisplatin, which is a very active agent in medulloblastoma and ependymoma
OR		
Etoposide	150 mg/m^2 IV, day 3 and 4	
OR		
Cyclophosphamide	1000 mg/m^2 IV, day 1	

[a]Adapted from: Lanzkowsky P. Manual of Pediatric Hematology and Oncology, 2nd ed. New York: Churchill Livingstone, 1995: ch 17.
[b]Maximum dose 2.0 mg.

Table 85.6.
International Neuroblastoma Staging System and Treatment Summary[a]

Stage	Staging Criteria	Incidence	Treatment	Survival at 5 Years
1	Localized tumor confined to the area of origin, complete gross excision with or without microscopic residual disease; identifiable ipsilateral and contralateral lymph nodes negative microscopically	5%	Surgery alone, chemotherapy with recurrence	90% or greater
2a	Unilateral tumor with incomplete, gross excision; identifiable ipsilateral and contralateral lymph nodes negative microscopically	10%	Surgery plus postoperative chemotherapy with 5 courses of cyclophosphamide plus doxorubicin	70–80%
2b	Unilateral tumor with complete or incomplete gross excision; with positive ipsilateral regional lymph nodes; identifiable contralateral lymph nodes negative microscopically	10%	Surgery plus postoperative chemotherapy with 5 courses of cyclophosphamide plus doxorubicin	70–80%
3	Tumor infiltrating across the midline with or without regional lymph node involvement; or, midline tumor with bilateral regional lymph node involvement	25%	Surgery plus postoperative chemotherapy wth 5 courses of cyclophosphamide plus doxorubicin	40–70% (depending on completeness of surgical resection)
4	Dissemination of the tumor to distant lymph nodes, bone, bone marrow, liver and/or other organs (except as defined in stages 4s)	60%	Aggressive chemotherapy with cyclophosphamide plus doxorubicin then cisplatin plus teniposide plus radiotherapy; consider dose intensification with ABMT for older children	More than 60% if age at diagnosis is younger than 1 year; 20% if age at diagnosis is older than 1 year and under 2 years; 10% if age at diagnosis is over 2 years
4s	Localized primary tumor as defined for stage 1 or 2 with dissemination limited to liver, skin, and/or bone marrow.	5%	Individualized therapy, not standardized	More than 80%

[a]Adapted from: Philip T. Overview of current treatment of neuroblastoma. Am J Pediatr Hematol Oncol 14:97–102, 1992.

Mass screening for neuroblastoma using urinary excretion of catecholamine metabolites, vanillylmandelic acid (VMA), and homovanillic acid (HVA) has been performed in Japan since 1972. The evidence suggests that 65% of all childhood neuroblastomas can be detected clinically or by screening at or before 12 months of age (29). It further suggests that many of the cases detected by screening are not in the poor prognostic category. The application of mass screening is currently being evaluated to determine whether it is beneficial or harmful and at what individual and societal costs.

Clinical Presentation and Diagnosis

Neuroblastoma can occur anywhere along the sympathetic nervous system. The most common site of the primary tumor is in the abdomen [adrenal gland (40%) or a retroperitoneal paraspinal ganglion (25%)], thoracic cavity (15%), or pelvis (5%). Thoracic primaries are more common in children less than 1 year of age. Metastatic disease is identified in 50% of infants and two-thirds of older children at diagnosis. The most common sites of

metastasis are lymph node, bone marrow, bone, liver, and subcutaneous tissue. Spontaneous regression of neuroblastoma is occasionally observed in young infants; it occurs extremely rarely in older children. Further, the tumor may undergo differentiation to a more mature and benign tumor type classified as a ganglioneuroma (9, 30).

Signs and symptoms at presentation depend on the location of the primary and metastatic sites. The most common presentation is that of an abdominal or flank mass that is firm, irregular, and crosses the midline. Thoracic neuroblastoma presents as a posterior mediastinal mass and is usually found coincidentally on a routine chest radiograph. High thoracic and cervical masses can be associated with Horner's syndrome, which consists of unilateral ptosis, myosis, and anhydrosis. Paraspinal tumors may extend into the neuronal foramina of the vertebral bodies and result in symptoms related to compression of nerve roots and spinal cord. The range of symptoms include radicular pain, subacute paraplegia, and bowel and bladder dysfunction.

Physical exam should include a check for spinal cord compression and hypertension. Laboratory work-up should include a complete blood count, liver and renal function tests, and urine analysis for urinary catecholamines. Chest radiograph, CT scan or MRI, skeletal survey, abdominal ultrasound, and bone marrow aspirate and biopsy should be done to determine location, size, extent, and possible metastatic disease.

Staging and Prognosis

The most important clinical variables for neuroblastoma are the stage at diagnosis, the age of the patient at diagnosis, and the site of the primary tumor (9, 30, 31). In 1987, the International Neuroblastoma Staging System (INSS) was proposed that would lead to uniformity in staging of patients with neuroblastoma for clinical trials and biological studies worldwide (32). Table 85.6 (33) summarizes the INSS along with treatment and prognosis for each stage of patient. The INSS is based on clinical, radiographic, and surgical evaluation of the child with neuroblastoma. Patients with primary tumors of the adrenal gland appear to do worse than patients with tumors originating at other sites, particularly the thorax. Survival of patients with localized tumor surgically resected without distant metastasis is 75 to 90%; however, patients greater than 1 year old with distant metastasis at presentation have only a 10 to 30% 2-year disease-free survival (9, 31). Infants tend to have a better prognosis than older children. The presence of the *n-myc* oncogene is found predominantly in patients with advanced disease. *N-myc* amplification is associated with rapid tumor progression and a poor prognosis (34).

Treatment

The treatment of neuroblastoma is a combination of surgery, radiotherapy, and chemotherapy. The role of each is determined by stage of the tumor, age of the patient, and biological features of the tumor. Infants less than 1 year of age frequently present with a small primary tumor and metastases to skin, liver, or bone marrow (Stage IVS). Their disease often regresses spontaneously, and only supportive care is necessary. Chemotherapy remains the backbone of the multimodality treatment plan (33).

SURGERY

The goal of primary surgical procedures is to establish the diagnosis, provide tissue for biological studies, stage the tumor, and attempt to excise the tumor. Patients with localized (Stage I and II) disease require no further treatment after surgery. Delayed surgery after primary chemotherapy may convert a partial response to a complete one. Surgical complications range from 5 to 25%, with the incidence highest in abdominal tumors (30).

RADIOTHERAPY

Neuroblastoma is considered a radiosensitive tumor. Tumoricidal doses of 15 to 30 Gy are generally used to treat residual tumor after surgery or chemotherapy (9). Radiotherapy is also used in palliation of symptoms for end-stage disease. Radioactive-labeled meta-iodobenzylguanidine (MIBG) is an agent that has been used in Europe for diagnostic and therapeutic purposes. MIBG is known to be taken up by catecholamine-secreting tumors, such as pheochromocytomas and immature neuroblastoma cells. Using this specificity, MIBG radiolabeled with ^{125}I and ^{131}I has been used for both detection of neuroblastoma and evaluated for antitumor activity in small phase I and II studies, but it is currently not widely available in the United States. MIBG may be ultimately useful for the treatment of residual tumor following surgery in stage III patients or for palliation of bone pain. Use of this therapy may advantageously decrease the patient's overall exposure to radiation but increase the total dose of radiation delivered to the tumor. Myelosuppressive effects on tumor-infiltrated bone marrow have been problematic. Future studies will better define its role in the diagnosis and therapy of neuroblastoma (33).

CHEMOTHERAPY

Chemotherapy is the primary modality of treatment. Single-agent phase II trials have identified a number of effective drugs such as cyclophosphamide, cisplatin, doxorubicin, vincristine, and the epipodophyllotoxins (etoposide and teniposide), which yield a response rate of 34 to 45%. Combination chemotherapy has been shown to be more effective than single-agent therapy (33). The use of dose-intensified chemotherapy combinations has produced better immediate disease control; however, this has not translated into durable remissions (33, 35). Future treatment strategies will address the identification of new drugs and drug combinations, the role of autologous bone marrow transplantation (ABMT), and biologically based therapy such as monoclonal antibodies or interleukin-2. The differentiating effects in neuroblastoma cell lines of the retinoids (13-cis retinoic acid) has spurred ongoing investigation of clinical efficacy (36).

BIOLOGICAL THERAPY

Since neuroblastoma cells are known at times to undergo spontaneous regression or maturation to benign tumors, indicating these cells may be regulated by natural defense mechanisms, newer research strategies are focusing on biological manipulation of minimal residual disease. These strategies include exploitation of the body's own defense system with interleukin-2-stimulated natural killer cells and attempts to achieve tumor maturation with the use of vitamin B12 and retinoic acid (33). Another avenue of exploration is eradication of disease via monoclonal antibodies against the cell surface diganglioside antigen, G_{D2}, specifically located on neuroblastoma cells. Radioactive ^{131}I-coupled G_{D2} antibodies have been administered as therapy for neuroblastoma (37). Responses have been seen in patients with disseminated disease, but those with large tumor masses were resistant to this therapy. Monoclonal antibodies may also be useful in purging tumor cells from bone marrow ex vivo prior to reinfusion of autologous marrow after dose-intensive therapy.

WILMS' TUMOR

Wilms' tumor, also known as nephroblastoma, is the fifth most common pediatric malignancy. It was first described approximately 100 years ago by Max Wilms and has since been the subject of intense clinical, pathologic, therapeutic, and genetic analysis. Wilms' tumor affects approximately 1 child per 10,000 worldwide before the age of 15. The incidence is approximately three times higher for blacks in the United States and Africa than for East Asians. The median age of onset is 38 months, with cases in girls occurring, on average, 6 months later than in boys (38). The etiology of Wilms' tumor is unclear. Wilms' tumor shows a strong association with certain congenital anomalies: notably aniridia, hemihypertrophy, and malformations of the genitalia (cryptorchidism, hypospadias, pseudohermaphrodism, and gonadal dysgenesis) (38). Those with congenital abnormalities frequently have deletion of the short arm of chromosome 11. Bilateral Wilms' occurs in approximately 4 to 8% of reported cases.

Clinical Presentation and Diagnosis

Most children are found to have an asymptomatic palpable mass. Signs and symptoms appreciated on physical exam in approximately 20 to 30% of patients include malaise, pain, fever, and either microscopic or gross hematuria. Hypertension is present in about 25% of cases as a result of increased renin activity. It is important when diagnosing to distinguish Wilms' tumor from neuroblastoma. Wilms' tumor is generally intrarenal, showing intrinsic distortion of the calyceal region of the kidney, whereas neuroblastoma tends to create extrinsic displacement. Imaging studies should be done, including renal ultrasound and CT scanning of chest and abdomen. Laboratory workup should include a complete blood count, platelets, liver function tests, renal function tests, and a urinalysis (39). Metastatic disease is evident in approximately 15% of patients. The most common sites of metastases include lung (85%) and liver (15%) (39).

Staging and Prognosis

Three National Wilms' Tumor Studies (NWTS) were conducted by three cooperative groups between 1969 and 1985. More than 3000 cases were studied, and the characteristics of patients who responded poorly to treat-

ment were identified. The staging system is described in Table 85.7 (40). The most significant predictor of a poor treatment outcome was found to be histology. Wilms' tumor with anaplasia or sarcomatous features was associated with a high rate of relapse and death. The data of NWTS-2 demonstrated 54% survival for patients with unfavorable histology (UH) compared to 90% survival for patients with favorable histology (FH). The most recent NWTS demonstrated a 4-year survival for patients with favorable histology: stage I (96.5%), stage II (92.2%), stage III (73%), stage IV (78%). These studies demonstrated that patients must be stratified into two broad groups according to cytohistologic features: favorable histology and unfavorable histology (41,42).

Treatment

The treatment of Wilms' tumor requires a combination of complete surgical excision, chemotherapy, and radiotherapy. The primary focus of treatment is complete excision of the tumor, which in the prechemotherapy and radiation era resulted in a survival rate of 32%. With the addition of radiotherapy, the survival rate increased to 47%, and disease-free survival increased to 80 to 90% with adjuvant chemotherapy (38). Treatment is individualized and based on the stage and histology of the tumor. More

Table 85.7.
Staging of Wilms' Tumor (NWTS -4)[a]

I. Tumor limited to the kidney and completely excised. The surface of the renal capsule is intact. The tumor was not ruptured before or during removal. There is no residual tumor apparent beyond the margins of excision.

II. Tumor extends beyond the kidney, but is completely excised. There is regional extension of the tumor (i.e., penetration through the outer surface of the renal capsule into the perirenal soft tissues). Vessels outside the kidney substance are infiltrated or contain tumor thrombus. The tumor may have been biopsied or there has been local spillage of tumor confined to the flank. There is no residual tumor apparent at or beyond the margins of excision.

III. Residual nonhematogenous tumor confined to the abdomen. Any of the following may occur:
  a. Lymph nodes on biopsy are found to be involved in the hilus, the periaortic chains, or beyond.
  b. There has been diffuse peritoneal contamination by the tumor, such as by spillage of tumor beyond the flank before or during surgery, or by tumor growth that has penetrated through the peritoneal surface.
  c. Implants are found on the peritoneal surface.
  d. The tumor is not completely resectable because of local infiltration into vital structures.

IV. Hematogenous metastases. Deposits beyond stage III (e.g., lung, liver, bone, and brain).

V. Bilateral renal involvement at diagnosis. An attempt should be made to stage each side according to the above criteria on the basis of extent of disease prior to therapy.

[a]Adapted from: Mehta MP, Bastin KT, Wiersna SR. Treatment of Wilms' tumor. Current recommendations. Drugs 42:766–80, 1991.

than 85% of patients can be cured with current therapy, but some questions remain unanswered, including the role of whole lung radiation therapy, the efficacy of other chemotherapeutic agents with the vincristine–actinomycin-D combination, and the role of renal sparing surgery.

The results of NWTS-1, NWTS-2, and NWTS-3, showed the following: (1) Routine postoperative radiation therapy of the flank is not necessary for children with stage I FH or stage I anaplastic or stage II FH; (2) prognosis for patients with stage III FH is best when treatment programs include either actinomycin-D plus vincristine plus doxorubicin plus 1000 cGy radiation therapy or actinomycin-D plus vincristine plus 2000 cGy of flank radiation for intraabdominal rupture; (3) addition of cyclophosphamide to vincristine, actinomycin-D, and doxorubicin did not improve the prognosis for stage IV FH patients, but stage II–IV anaplastic histology may benefit from four drug therapy regimens; and (4) in general, stage II FH and stage III FH patients can be successfully treated with less intensive regimens, but better treatment is needed for stage IV disease or unfavorable histology. NWTS-4 is currently attempting to simplify, shorten, and redefine the treatment for all Wilms' patients along with comparing conventional to pulse chemotherapy (39, 41, 42).

SURGERY

Surgical excision is an essential part of treatment. Care is taken to prevent rupture of the tumor by gentle handling during resection. Inspection of the opposite kidney and the liver is performed, and local lymph nodes are biopsied if enlarged. Following surgery, histopathologic examination and staging can be completed and postoperative chemotherapy administered.

RADIATION

Not all patients require radiation therapy. NWTS-1 determined that children with completely resected tumor (FH or UH) do not benefit from radiation therapy. Controversy over the exact dose of radiation and field size is still ongoing for stage III and stage IV patients or patients with unfavorable history. In the current NWTS-4 study, external beam radiotherapy is being evaluated for stage II unfavorable histology and all stage III and stage IV patients.

CHEMOTHERAPY

Wilms' tumor was the first pediatric malignant solid tumor found to be responsive to systemic chemotherapy, specifically actinomycin-D (41, 42). Other active agents found include vincristine, doxorubicin, and cyclophosphamide. Results of the NWTS-1 demonstrated that combination chemotherapy with actinomycin-D and vincristine was significantly better than single-agent therapy for stage I FH, stage I anaplasia and stage II FH, and doxorubicin plus vincristine–actinomycin-D for stage III and IV FH.

Preoperative chemotherapy or radiation therapy is indicated for large, inoperable tumor at diagnosis. Postoperative chemotherapy is initiated as soon as possible. The current NWTS protocol is designed to evaluate the potential advantage of single-dose actinomycin D and doxorubicin versus divided doses, along with evaluation of duration of therapy, 6 months versus 15 months for stages II–IV.

THE SARCOMAS

A sarcoma is a malignant neoplasm formed by proliferation of embryonic mesenchymal cells, which normally give rise to connective tissues, including blood, bone, cartilage, and muscle tissue. Sarcomas in children can be divided into two principal categories, bone sarcomas and soft tissue sarcomas, which are further subdivided into various tumor types. Bone sarcomas occur with a peak incidence in adolescents, most commonly include osteosarcoma and Ewing's sarcoma, and constitute about 6% of all childhood tumor types. Soft tissue sarcomas are the sixth most common group of childhood cancers and are made up of a multitude of histologic types, of which the subtype rhabdomyosarcoma comprises at least one-half of all cases. A comparison chart of the most common childhood sarcomas is depicted in Table 85.8 (43).

RHABDOMYOSARCOMA

Rhabdomyosarcoma (RMS), a very aggressive tumor, is thought to arise from primitive mesenchymal tissue that mimics immature striated muscle. It occurs most frequently in children 2 to 5 years of age, has a second peak in adolescence, and has a slight male predominance. RMS has been associated with an increased incidence of maternal breast cancer as well as a surplus of cancers in siblings (44). This familial manifestation is sometimes referred to as the Li-Fraumeni Cancer Family Syndrome and may be associated with alterations in the p53 tumor suppressor gene (45). There are two major histologic subtypes of RMS, embryonal and alveolar, which may or may not have prognostic significance (46).

Clinical Presentation and Diagnosis

The RMS tumor can arise anywhere in the body, but the most common sites are the head and neck region, genitourinary tract, and extremities. Younger children tend to have embryonal histology, whereas older children have alveolar histology. Multiinstitutional trials for the treatment of RMS have been organized in both the United States and Europe, and treatment strategies for this more common entity have become the therapeutic model for other pediatric soft tissue sarcomas. Presenting signs and symptoms are widely variable, depend on the anatomic site of origin, and range from an asymptomatic mass to disturbance of a normal body function by an enlarging tumor. Tumors of the head and neck tend to occur in younger

Table 85.8.
Sites of Presentation of Sarcomas of Childhood[a]

Sarcoma Type	Primary Sites		Distant Metastatic Sites
Rhabdomyosarcoma	Head and neck	40%	Metastatic site dependent on primary
	Orbit	10%	lung (most common)
	Parameningeal (nasopharynx, sinuses, larynx, middle ear)	20%	marrow
			bone
	Other	10%	brain
	Genitourinary tract	20%	lymph nodes (infrequent)
	Bladder/prostate	12%	liver (rare)
	Vagina/uterus	2%	
	Paratesticular	6%	
	Extremities	20%	
	Trunk	10%	
	Other	10%	
Bone sarcomas			
Osteosarcoma	Distal femur	53%	Lung (most common), bone, pleura, pericardium,
	Proximal tibia	26%	kidney, adrenal gland, brain
	Proximal humerus	12%	
	Other	9%	
Ewing's sarcoma	Femur	23%	Lung, bone, bone marrow, pleura
	Ilium	13%	
	Fibula	11%	
	Rib	8%	
	Tibula	8%	
	Other	37%	

[a]Adapted from (43).

patients, are most commonly of the embryonal subtype, and may cause neurologic dysfunction secondary to extension of parameningeal lesions into the CNS. Pelvic lesions are often revealed by urinary retention, frequency, or constipation. Most children have localized or regional disease at diagnosis, but RMS may disseminate via lymphatic and hematogenous routes in about 20% of young afflicted patients. The lungs, lymph nodes, marrow, and bone are the most common sites of distant metastatic disease in newly diagnosed patients (47). Ascertaining the location and extent of disease by clinical exam, radiologic studies, and bone marrow assessment is necessary before planning therapy, and biopsy is essential for histologic diagnosis.

Staging and Prognosis

Nationally, since 1972, patients have been entered into the Intergroup Rhabdomyosarcoma Studies (IRS), which are multiinstitutional research protocols designed to investigate prognostic variables and rational therapeutic regimens for the treatment of rhabdomyosarcoma. Two major staging systems include the conventional Clinical Grouping System, a surgicopathologic staging system that is based on postsurgical categorization and was used in the IRS-I, II, and III studies, and a site-based TNM (tumor-node-metastasis) staging scheme that is being prospectively evaluated and compared in the IRS-IV study. The rationale for pretreatment staging is that (1) it will not be predetermined by extent of surgery, (2) it allows the possibility of

researching surgical questions, (3) it will facilitate comparison of IRS results with European study results, and (4) it offers a classification system that may better predict outcome (48).

Primary sites with the best prognosis are the orbit, nonparameningeal head and neck tumors, and paratesticular masses, with 5-year survival rates of greater than 80%. Currently, stage I disease is associated with about an 80% survival rate in contrast to only 20% in stage IV (metastatic) disease. Other factors that have been associated with a worse prognosis include larger tumor size; local invasiveness of the primary tumor; parameningeal head and neck primaries; retroperitoneal, trunk, and extremity disease; alveolar histology; the presence of regional lymph nodes associated with localized disease; incomplete resection; and age greater than 10 years (48–51). Response to treatment is also an important variable, but once a patient has relapsed after achieving a complete remission, survival is extremely poor.

Treatment

Rhabdomyosarcoma has a propensity to invade surrounding structures. Historically, radical surgical excisions in anatomic sites difficult to totally excise (i.e., base of skull, orbit, bladder and prostate regions) were performed that left the patient with serious cosmetic and functional deformities. Multimodal therapy with the addition of chemotherapy and radiotherapy plus innovations in supportive care have resulted in a dramatic improvement in the cure rate of nonmetastatic RMS (stages I–III), from less than 20% in older studies to 50 to 60% overall progression-free survival at 5 years in more recent series (43). Those with metastatic disease do poorly regardless of the intensity of therapy, and despite initial antitumor responses in greater than 75% of patients (47).

SURGERY

The tumor should be primarily excised with wide margins if the surgical attempt will likely result in a nonmutilating total resection; otherwise, biopsy alone may be indicated when wide excision is not possible, as in lesions of the head, neck, or pelvis. Secondary excision may become possible after debulking with chemotherapy with or without radiotherapy. Surgical exploration after chemotherapy alone is sometimes performed with the aim of avoiding radiotherapy if no residual tumor is evident.

RADIOTHERAPY

Radiation therapy in doses of 4000 to 5000 cGy is indicated when there is either local or metastatic macroscopic or microscopic residual disease that is unresectable. It may also be indicated for tumors with unfavorable histology or primary lesions of the extremity in any stage. Chemotherapy in patients with bulky disease may allow tumor reduction, permitting the use of better defined radiation fields. Patients with parameningeal lesions with extension into the brain parenchyma, meninges, or CSF, receive intrathecal chemotherapy (methotrexate, cytarabine, and hydrocortisone) plus craniospinal irradiation (47). Hyperfractionated irradiation to the primary site is being studied to determine if this method can decrease toxicity, especially the retardation of growing bone. Brachytherapy, the delivery of radiation to a carefully restricted volume via an implanted radioactive device, may be indicated for critically located, incompletely resected tumors. This internal radiation strategy may lower the radiation fibrosis in adjacent normal structures associated with external radiotherapy that inherently allows more radiation scatter (43).

CHEMOTHERAPY

Currently, all patients receive chemotherapy regardless of stage because of risk of dissemination and so as to decrease the need for radiation therapy. Treatment duration typically lasts 1 year for stage I and 2 years for stages II–IV since most relapses are seen within the first 2 years of therapy. Prototypic regimens include vincristine, actinomycin D, and cyclophosphamide (VAC), with or without doxorubicin (VACA) depending on stage of disease. The major toxicity of these combinations is severe neutropenia. Hematopoietic growth factors such as granulocyte-colony stimulating factor (G-CSF) may help shorten the duration of this side effect; its effects are being studied in IRS-IV.

Since the addition of doxorubicin in the IRS-I and II studies did not improve survival over VAC alone, and since doxorubicin is associated with serious delayed cardiotoxicity in about 2% of patients, it was not included in the current IRS-IV regimens (52, 53).

More recent studies, IRS-III and IV, are comparing VAC to newer combinations, which include agents such as ifosfamide, etoposide, cisplatin, and melphalan, and focus on more dose-intensive chemotherapy as initial therapy with the aim of improving survival and reducing the need for aggressive local control with surgery or radiotherapy. Cumulative doses of ifosfamide in excess of 72 gm/m^2 (9 gm/m^2/course for eight courses) in an IRS-IV pilot led to renal toxicity, namely, Fanconi's Syndrome (renal tubular acidosis), and decreased glomerular filtration, especially in children less than 3 years of age (54). Renal function and electrolyte status must be monitored carefully in those receiving ifosfamide, and patients frequently require chronic supplementation of potassium, phosphorous, calcium, and bicarbonate after multiple courses.

OSTEOSARCOMA

Osteosarcoma (OS) is a primary malignant sarcoma of bone and distinctly produces osteoid (extracellular matrix protein produced by bone cells). It is the most prevalent bone tumor in the first 2 decades of life and is rapidly fatal if not treated. The peak incidence occurs during the pubescent growth spurt (13 to 15 years of age) and occurs in boys more frequently than girls. Children with hereditary retinoblastoma have a significantly greater chance of later developing OS, suggesting a genetic predisposition in some patients (55, 56).

Clinical Presentation and Diagnosis

Typical symptoms that may occur over a period of a few months prior to presentation are progressive pain that becomes unremitting and severe, with or without eventual swelling near the involved bone. The presence of a limp may indicate destruction of the bone cortex, and pathologic fractures sometimes occur. Lung metastases, even if massive, are usually symptomless. A plain film of the affected area is the first diagnostic step, followed by a confirmatory biopsy. Tumor extent of the primary site is better defined by bone scanning and MRI or CT. Serum levels of alkaline phosphatase may be elevated in more than 40% of patients and may serve as a tumor marker for follow-up. The most common sites affected are the rapidly growing metaphysis of long bones—the distal femur, proximal tibia, and proximal humerus—although any bone can be affected. Swift invasion of bone cortex with contiguous spread into adjacent tissue is common. The diagnostic workup should always include conventional radiographs and CT scanning of the lungs, the major site of metastasis. Only 20% of patients initially present with visible metastatic disease; however, it is thought that the majority of patients have undetectable, micrometastatic disease at diagnosis.

Staging and Prognosis

There is no universal staging system for OS, except to differentiate local from metastatic disease. Virtually all OS lesions are high grade and tend to break through the bone cortex into extramedullary tissues early in the course of the disease. Tumor necrosis of greater than 90% after preoperative chemotherapy has been shown to be the most important positive prognostic variable in patients with OS of the extremity (57, 58). Unfavorable pretreatment prognostic variables, including large tumor burden, osteoblastic pathologic subtype, axial site of primary, age less than 10 years, male sex, and high alkaline phosphatase and LDH serum levels, have been proposed but not confirmed in all series (55, 58).

Treatment

To minimize the risk of local recurrence, surgical excision is the definitive approach to treatment of OS. With surgical resection alone, however, about 80% of patients eventually develop metastatic disease, suggesting the presence of microscopic disease at diagnosis. For this reason, treatment also consists of adjuvant systemic chemotherapy in all patients. Unlike most other solid tumors of childhood, osteosarcoma is considered to be highly radioresistant, and therefore radiotherapy is rarely used.

SURGERY

In past years, limb amputation was the primary surgical procedure, leaving the patient with serious functional deformities. With the adoption of neoadjuvant chemotherapeutic regimens and improvements in radiographic tumor definition with CT, MRI, and bone scans, orthopedic surgeons are increasingly able to perform less drastic excisional operations, known as limb-sparing procedures, in an attempt to salvage extremity function (59). Resection of limited pulmonary metastatic nodules after chemotherapy may provide long-term survival results for some patients (60).

CHEMOTHERAPY

Five-year disease-free survival in greater than 50% of patients with nonmetastatic, resectable OS can be attained with the addition of postsurgical combination chemotherapy, compared to only 20% survival with surgery alone (61, 62). Osteosarcoma is a relatively drug-resistant sarcoma, requiring intensive doses of active agents such as methotrexate with leucovorin rescue, doxorubicin, cisplatin (intravenously or intraarterially), and ifosfamide for effectiveness (63–65). Commonly used high-dose methotrexate of 12 gm/m^2 over 4 to 6 hours can cause serious myelosuppression, stomatitis, and acute renal toxicity if

proper supportive care measures are not undertaken. These side effects can be almost completely avoided by institution of adequate hydration of 2 to 3 $L/m^2/day$, alkalinization of urine with sodium bicarbonate or acetate to avoid precipitation of a methotrexate metabolite in the renal tubules, and administration of scheduled leucovorin (folinic acid) beginning 24 hours after the start of the methotrexate infusion, until the methotrexate serum concentration falls below 0.1 micromolar.

Neoadjuvant chemotherapy prior to definitive surgery has become commonplace in the therapy of OS and has several potential advantages: allows study of the in vivo effect of chemotherapy on the tumor and may help predict outcome; helps debulk the tumor bed and permits limb salvage surgery in a larger percentage of patients; and treats potential micrometastatic disease earlier on diagnosis. Postsurgical chemotherapy is administered for several months after resection, with overall treatment generally taking 6 to 9 months to complete in patients with nonmetastatic disease.

EWING'S SARCOMA OF BONE

Ewing's sarcoma of bone (ES) is a small round-cell neoplasm belonging to a family of tumors of neural histogenesis, including peripheral primitive neuroectodermal tumors, and is the second most common bone tumor of childhood. It may sometimes arise extraosseously in soft tissues. It has a male preponderance and is distinctly rare in the black population. About 65% of ES occur in the second decade of life, with only a very rare incidence in ages less than 5 years or greater than 30 (66). Treatment of ES is much different from that of osteosarcoma and more similar to the management of rhabdomyosarcoma.

Clinical Presentation

More than 90% of children present with intermittent local pain and swelling that becomes progressively persistent and severe. A syndrome of unexplained fever and leukocytosis in 20% of patients have also been reported, which occasionally leads to the incorrect diagnosis of osteomyelitis. The long tubular bones of the lower extremity are the most common sites of presentation, especially the femur, with the pelvis being the most common axial site. There is often a periosteal component that radiographically has an "onion peel" appearance. In comparison to osteosarcoma, ES produces changes more centrally in the bone somewhere between the diaphysis and metaphysis. Less than 20% of patients have clinically evident metastatic disease at diagnosis although micrometastases are thought to be present in the majority. The lung is the primary site of metastases, followed by the bone and bone marrow (66).

Staging and Prognosis

Currently, there is no accepted staging system for ES other than localized and metastatic disease. Favorable prognostic factors include small tumor size, nonmetastatic disease, a distal primary, and a normal serum lactic dehydrogenase (LDH) (66). Central axis tumors may become extremely large before symptoms and diagnostic evaluation transpire, which may be the explanation for the poorer prognosis noted in these patients.

Treatment

In contrast to osteosarcoma, ES is highly radiosensitive; therefore, surgery or radiotherapy are used for local control, and chemotherapy is always administered adjuvantly, both prior to and after local therapy, to destroy clinical or subclinical metastatic disease. Until the introduction of systemic chemotherapy in the 1960s, long-term survival for ES after surgical resection was less than 10% because of the inability to control distant spread. With current multimodal therapy, 60 to 70% of patients with localized tumors can be cured, but a less favorable prognosis is associated in those with initial metastatic disease.

LOCAL CONTROL

Radiation as a principal modality can incur local control rates of 55 to 90%. Larger tumors and central axis lesions manifest higher rates of local failure after radiation. Therefore, surgery is favored over radiotherapy for large primaries, tumors of central, expendable skeleton (i.e., small rib lesions, clavicle, body of scapula), lesions in weight-bearing bones of young children where radiation would adversely affect a major growth site, or at the site of an unmanageable pathologic fracture. Local therapy should be planned carefully so that it does not delay necessary systemic treatment. Routine use of neoadjuvant chemotherapy facilitates complete excision of previously unresectable lesions by significantly reducing the tumor's soft tissue component (67).

CHEMOTHERAPY

As single agents in the early 1960s, vincristine (V), actinomycin-D (A), and cyclophosphamide (C) were shown to be active in ES, which prompted their use in combination regimens (VAC). Doxorubicin (Adr) was also found to be an active agent in the 1970s and was added to the regimen at various institutions (VACAdr). The results of a U.S. study, the Intergroup Ewing's Sarcoma Study I (IESS-I) initiated in 1973, demonstrated that VACAdr was more effective than VAC and that delivering chemotherapy at 3-week intervals compared to 6-week intervals decreased the incidence of relapse, indicating the importance of dose intensity (68). More specifically, the dose intensity of doxorubicin compared to other agents appears to be an important determinant of a favorable outcome in both osteosarcoma and Ewing's sarcoma (64). The IESS-II study confirmed that high-dose intermittent cyclophosphamide given in VACAdr is more effective than moderate-

dose continuous cyclophosphamide similar to that used in IESS-I (69).

Two European studies have substituted ifosfamide for cyclophosphamide in VAdrCA regimens, with one study reporting superiority of ifosfamide and the other study demonstrating no benefit over conventional therapy (70, 71). Much interest has been shown for the use of an ifosfamide–etoposide (IE) combination in ES (72, 73). A recent large Childrens Cancer Group (CCG) and Pediatric Oncology Group (POG) study randomized patients with nonmetastatic ES to VAdrCA alone or VAdrCA courses alternating with IE every 3 weeks for 1 year. Primary tumor control was performed after three courses of chemotherapy by surgery, radiation, or both. Three-year event-free survival was significantly better for the VAdrCA + IE group (69%) than for the VAdrCA group (50%). However, 5% of patients in the VAdrCA + IE group suffered chemotherapy-related deaths versus 0% in the VAdrCA group (72). Although IE appears very active, the combination leads to severe myelosuppression in about 50% of patients, and this toxicity may cause treatment delays and, therefore, decrease dose intensity (66). Modern treatment with multimodal therapy can cure about 50 to 70% of patients, but for the rest, the development of more effective therapy, including high-dose chemoradiotherapy and autologous stem cell transplantation, will continue to be evaluated.

RETINOBLASTOMA

Retinoblastoma (RB) is the most common intraocular tumor of childhood and serves as the prototype and model for understanding the heredity and genetics of childhood cancer although it accounts for only a small percentage of pediatric tumors. It is a malignant tumor of the embryonic neural retina and has an incidence of 1 in 18,000 live births. An estimated 200 children per year will develop the disease (74). The tumor consists of closely packed, round, undifferentiated small cells with darkly stained nuclei and scant cytoplasm. It is congenital, though usually not recognized at birth, and affects predominantly young children (75). There is no racial or gender predilection. It may have a variable growth rate originating from single or multiple foci in one or both eyes and may be manifest in one eye many months before the other. The frequency of bilaterality ranges from 20 to 30% (74).

Clinical Presentation and Diagnosis

About 80% of all retinoblastomas are diagnosed before age 3 to 4 years, with a median age of diagnosis at 2 years (74). The hereditary form of the tumor may be transmitted by a parent or may arise from a new mutation in germ cells. The nonhereditary form arises by spontaneous mutation in somatic cells such as retinoblasts. The hereditary form accounts for approximately 60% of the cases diagnosed

(76). Approximately 40% of all retinoblastomas are inherited via an autosomal dominant gene, the Retinoblastoma gene. All the bilateral and approximately 20% of the unilateral cases are considered hereditary. Genetic counseling is recommended if the family history is positive because an affected parent has a 50% chance of transmitting the gene to the offspring.

In the United States, most cases of RB are diagnosed while the tumor remains intraocularly. Signs and symptoms depend on size and position of tumor. The most common sign is leukokoria ("white eye"), which is caused by tumor within the vitreous or retinal detachment of one or both eyes. The next most common sign is strabismus, which causes a loss of central vision. Other occasional signs are orbital inflammation, hyphema, fixed pupil, and heterochromia iridis. Metastases is generally by direct extension via the optic nerve into the meninges and by the lymphatic system or hematogenous route to bone and bone marrow. Pupillary dilation and examination under anesthesia are essential to evaluate the retina fully. Metastatic workup includes a CT of the brain, a lumbar puncture for examination of the CSF, and a bone marrow aspirate and biopsy (77).

Staging and Prognosis

The management of RB depends on the size of the tumor and extent of disease. The classification of Reese and Ellsworth is the standard scale introduced in 1963 (Table 85.9). Survival is excellent with greater than 90% for centers specializing in the treatment. Those with metastatic disease have a poorer prognosis (78). Patients generally die secondary to intracranial or distant spread.

Table 85.9.
Reese-Ellsworth Staging Classification of Retinoblastoma

Group 1 (very favorable)
A. Solitary tumor, smaller than 4 disk diameters[a] at or behind the equator.
B. Multiple tumors, none larger than 4 disk diameters, all at or behind the equator.
Group 2 (favorable)
A. Solitary tumor, 4–10 disk diameters in size, at or behind the equator.
B. Multiple tumors, 4–10 disk diameters in size, behind the equator.
Group 3 (doubtful)
A. Any lesion anterior to the equator.
B. Solitary tumors larger than 10 disk diameters behind the equator.
Group 4 (unfavorable)
A. Multiple tumors, some larger than 10 disk diameters.
B. Any lesion extending anteriorly to the ora serrata.
Group 5 (very unfavorable)
A. Tumors involving more than half the retina.
B. Vitreous seeding.

[a]1 disk diameter = 1.5 mm.

Treatment

The treatment goals of RB are to preserve life and maintain vision. The major factors determining treatment include involvement (unilateral or bilateral), size, number, and location of tumor and evidence of distant spread (79). Localized disease is controlled with surgery or irradiation, whereas advanced disease may use combined modalities. It is important that treatment be individualized.

SURGERY

Enucleation is indicated if there is no chance for useful vision even if the tumor is destroyed or if there is failure to control tumor with conservative therapy. Cryotherapy is used for small primary or recurrent tumors in the anterior part of the retina. Cryotherapy is applied by a small probe placed directly on the conjunctiva or sclera, and a whitening of the tumor occurs as it freezes. Laser photocoagulation is used when there are small primary or recurrent tumors in the posterior section of the retina. An ischemic tumor necrosis results from the application of photocoagulation. Complications from enucleation include underdevelopment of the bony orbit, which cosmetically leads to a very small eye (80).

RADIOTHERAPY

Retinoblastoma is a radiosensitive tumor (80). The purpose of radiotherapy is to control local disease while preserving vision. For optimal radiotherapy, some children must be sedated and immobilized. Total doses of 4500 to 5400 cGy over 4.5 to 6 weeks are generally used. Full cranial or craniospinal irradiation is indicated for patients with brain or dural extension. Modern techniques to minimize long-term toxicities seen previously with external beam irradiation include localized irradiation and the application of radioactive plaques to the retina (4). Complications of cataracts, retinal vascular injury, including retinopathy, vitreous hemorrhage, blindness, and bone growth abnormalities are possible.

CHEMOTHERAPY

Chemotherapy plays a small role in the treatment of RB. The prognosis for the majority of patients who receive surgery and radiotherapy alone is good. Only patients with extraocular RB or recurrent disease need to receive chemotherapy. Single-agent therapy has been studied in these children with a 47% response rate to cyclophosphamide, 33% with doxorubicin, and 16% with vincristine (79). Response rates with combination chemotherapy using vincristine, cyclophosphamide, and dactinomycin; cyclophosphamide and doxorubicin; or cisplatin and teniposide are mixed, with responses ranging from 1 to 5 months (79). Metastatic extension of RB to the cerebrospinal fluid has been treated with intrathecal methotrexate with minimal response (79).

CONCLUSION

Although childhood cancer is rare, mortality from this disease is second only to accidents as a cause of death in children. Survival outcomes for children with solid tumors have been greatly improved over the last 3 decades by a multimodal approach and intensive combination chemotherapy, and for many, there is now hope for long-term survival. Intense treatment regimens to invoke cure, however, are more toxic than past therapies, and management of patients requires extensive supportive care by a team of dedicated health care professionals. With children often surviving into adulthood, long-term follow-up of these patients is crucial to assess and ultimately prevent chronic toxicities of therapy.

REFERENCES

1. Boring CC, Squires TS, Tong T, Montgomery S. Cancer Statistics, 1994. CA Cancer J Clin 44:7–26, 1994.
2. Young JL, Ries LG, Silverberg E, Horm JW, Miller RW. Cancer incidence, survival, and mortality for children younger than age 15 years. Cancer 58:598–602, 1986.
3. Novakovic B. U.S. Childhood cancer survival, 1973–1987. Med Pediatr Oncol 23:480–486, 1994.
4. Berg SL, Grisell DL, DeLaney TF, Balis FM. Priniciples of treatment of pediatric solid tumors. Pediatr Clin North Amer 38:249–267, 1991.
5. Cohen IJ. Significant recent advances in the treatment of osteogenic sarcoma. Isr J Med Sci 29: 748–753, 1993.
6. del Regato JA, Spjut JJ, Cox JD. Cancer. Diagnosis, Treatment and Prognosis. St.Louis, CV Mosby, 1985:59–92.
7. Trott KR. Chronic damage after radiation treatment: challenge to radiation biology. Int J Radiat Oncol Biol Phy 10:907–913, 1984.
8. Goldie JH, Coldman AJ. The genetic origin of drug resistance in neoplasms: implications for systemic therapy. Cancer Res 44:3643–3653, 1984.
9. Carlsen NLT. Neuroblastoma: epidemiology and pattern of regression. Am J Pediatr Hematol Oncol 14:103–110, 1992.
10. Jacobson SJ, Shore RW, Greenberg M, Spielberg SP. The efficacy and safety of granisetron in pediatric cancer patients who had failed standard antiemetic therapy during anticancer chemotherapy. Amer J Pediatr Hematol Oncol 16:231–235, 1994.
11. Gasparini M. Anthracycline cardiotoxicity. Pediatr Hematol Oncol 11: 237–240, 1994.
12. Smith MB, Xue H, Stong L, Takahashi J, Jaffe N, et al. Forty year experience with second malignancies after treatment of childhood cancer: analysis of outcome following the development of the second malignancy. J Pedi Surg 28:1342–1349, 1993.
13. Nicholson HS, Fears TR, Byrne J. Death during adulthood in survivors of childhood and adolescent cancer. Cancer 73:3094–3102, 1994.
14. Pollack IF. Brain tumors in children. N Eng J Med 331:1500–1510, 1994.
15. Albright AL. Pediatric brain tumors. CA Cancer J Clin 43:272–288, 1993.
16. Steven JM. Anesthesia and cardiopulmonary resuscitation. In: D'Angio GJ, Sinniah D, Meadows AT, Evans AE, Pritchard J, eds. Practical Pediatric Oncology. New York: Wiley-Liss, 1992:182–191.
17. Duffner PK, Cohen ME, Myers MH, Heise HW. Survival of children with brain tumors: SEER Program, 1973–1980. Neurol 36:597–601, 1986.
18. Lassoff SJ, Allen J, Epstein F, Wisoff J. Advances in surgery: brain stem and spinal cord tumors in children. In: Bleyer A, Packer R, eds. Pediatric Neurooncology: New Trends in Clinical Research. New York: Harwood Academic Publishers, 1992:278–297.
19. Packer RJ, Boyett JM, Zimmerman RA, et al. Hyperfractionated radiation therapy (72 Gy) for children with brain stem gliomas. A Childrens Cancer Group phase I/II trial. Cancer 72:1414–1421, 1993.
20. Kun LE, Moulder JE. General principles of radiation therapy. In: Pizzo PA, Poplack DG, eds. Principles and Practices of Pediatric Oncology, 2nd ed. Philadelphia: J.B. Lippincott Company, 1993: 273–302.
21. Sposto R, Ertel IJ, Jenkin RD, et al. The effectiveness of chemotherapy for treatment of high grade astrocytoma in children: results of a randomized trial. A report from the Childrens Cancer Study Group. J Neurooncol 7:165–177, 1989.
22. Evans AE, Jenkin DT, Sposto R, et al. The treatment of medulloblastoma. Results of a prospective randomized trial of radiation therapy with and without CCNU, vincristine, and prednisone. J Neurosurg 72:572–582, 1990.
23. Packer RJ, Sutton LN, Goldwein JW, et al. Improved survival with the use of adjuvant chemotherapy in the treatment of medulloblastoma. J Neurosurg 74:433–440, 1991.
24. Duffner PK, Horowitz ME, Krischer JP, et al. Postoperative chemotherapy and delayed radiation in children less than three years of age with malignant brain tumors. N Engl J Med 328:1725–1731, 1993.
25. Friedman HS, Oakes JW. The chemotherapy of posterior fossa tumors in childhood. J Neuro-Oncol 5:217–229, 1987.
26. Schell MJ, McHaney VA, Green AA, Kun LE, Hayes FA. Hearing loss in children and young adults receiving cisplatin with or without prior cranial irradiation. J Clin Oncol 7:754–760, 1989.
27. Lanzkowsky P. Manual of Pediatric Hematology and Oncology, 2nd ed. New York: Churchill Livingstone, 1995: ch 17.
28. Finlay JL. High-dose chemotherapy followed by bone marrow "rescue" for recurrent brain tumors. In: Bleyer A, Packer R, eds. Pediatric Neuro-oncology: New Trends in Clinical Research. New York: Academic Publishers, 1992:278–297.
29. Goodman SN. Neuroblastoma screening data. AJDC 145:1415–1422, 1991.
30. Caty MG, Shamberger RC. Abdominal tumors in infancy and childhood. Pediatr Clin North Amer 40:1253–1271, 1993.
31. Evans AE, D'Angio GJ, Propert K, Anderson J, Hann H-WL. Prognostic factors in neuroblastoma. Cancer 59:1853, 1987.
32. American Joint Committee on Cancer. Neuroblastoma. In: Manual for Staging of Cancer, 2nd ed. Philadelphia: J.B. Lippincott, 1983:237.
33. Philip T. Overview of current treatment of neuroblastoma. Am J Pediatr Hematol Oncol 14:97–102, 1992.
34. Look AT, Hayes FA, Shuster JJ, et al. Clinical relevance of tumor cell ploidy and n-myc amplification in childhood neuroblastoma, a pediatric oncology group study. J Clin Oncol 9:581, 1991.
35. Johnson FL, Goldman S. Role of autotransplantation in neuroblastoma. Hem Onc Clin North Amer 7:647–662, 1993.
36. Israel MA. Disordered differentiation as a target for novel approaches to the treatment of neuroblastoma. Cancer 71:3310–3313, 1993.
37. Cheung N-KV, Burch L, Kushner BH, Munn DH. Monoclonal antibody 3F8 can effect durable remissions in neuroblastoma patients refractory to chemotherapy: a phase II trial. In: Evans AE, D'Angio GJ, Knudson AGJ, Seeger RC, eds. Advances in Neuroblastoma Research, 3rd ed. New York: Wiley-Liss, 1991:395.
38. Breslow N, Olshan A, Beckwith JB, Green DM. Epidemiology of Wilms' tumor. Med Pediatr Oncol 21:172–181, 1993.
39. Green DM, D'Angio GJ, Beckwith JB, et al. Wilms' tumor. In: Pizzo PA, Poplack DG, eds. Principles and Practices of Pediatric Oncology, 2nd ed. Philadelphia: J.B. Lippincott Company, 1993:713–737.

40. Mehta MP, Bastin KT, Wiersna SR. Treatment of Wilms' tumor. Current recommendations. Drugs 42:766–780, 1991.

41. D'Angio GJ, Evans AE, Breslow N, et al. The treatment of Wilms' tumor: the results of the national Wilms' tumor study. Cancer 38: 633–646, 1976.

42. D'Angio GJ, Evans AE, Breslow N, et al. The treatment of Wilms' tumor: The results of the second national Wilms' tumor study. Cancer 47: 2302–2311, 1981.

43. Raney RB, Hays DM, Tefft M, Triche TJ. Rhabdomyosarcoma and the undifferentiated sarcomas. In: Pizzo PA, Poplack DG, eds. Principles and Practices of Pediatric Oncology, 2nd ed. Philadelphia: J.B. Lippincott Company, 1993:769–794.

44. Hartley AL, Birch JM, Blair V, et al. Patterns of cancer in the families of children with soft tissue sarcoma. Cancer 72:923–930, 1993.

45. Malkin D, Li FP, Strong LC, Fraumeni JF, et al. Germ line p53 mutations in a familial syndrome of breast cancer, sarcomas, and other neoplasms. Science 250:1233–1238, 1990.

46. Tsokos M, Webber BL, Parham DM, et al. Rhabdomyosarcoma: a new classification scheme related to prognosis. Arch Pathol Lab Med 116:847–855, 1992.

47. Wexler LH, Helman LJ. Pediatric soft tissue sarcomas. CA Cancer J Clin 44:211–247, 1994.

48. Crist WM, Garnsey L, Beltangady MS, et al. Prognosis in children with rhabdomyosarcoma: A report of the Intergroup Rhabdomyosarcoma Studies I and II. J Clin Oncol 8:443–452, 1990.

49. Lawrence W, Geham EA, Hays DM, Beltangady M, Maurer HM. Prognostic significance of staging factors of the UICC staging system in childhood rhabdomyosarcoma: a report from the intergroup rhabdomyosarcoma study (IRS-II). J Clin Oncol 5:46–54, 1987.

50. Lawrence W, Daniel MH, Heyn R, et al. Lymphatic metastases with childhood rhabdomyosarcoma. A report from the Intergroup Rhabdomyosarcoma Study. Cancer 60:910–915, 1987.

51. Rodary C, Gehan EA, Flamant F. Prognostic factors in 951 nonmetastatic rhabdomyosarcoma in children: a report from the international rhabdomyosarcoma workshop. Med Ped Oncol 19:89–95, 1991.

52. Maurer HM, Beltangady M, Gehan EA, et al. The Intergroup Rhabdomyosarcoma Study-I. A final report. Cancer 61:209–220, 1988.

53. Maurer HM, Gehan EA, Beltangady M, et al. The Intergroup Rhabdomyosarcoma Study-II. Cancer 71:1904–1922, 1993.

54. Raney B, Ensign L, Foreman J, et al. Renal toxicity of ifosfamide in pilot regimens of the Intergroup Rhabdomyosarcoma Study for patients with gross residual tumor. Am J Pediatr Hematol Oncol 16:286–295, 1994.

55. Link MP, Eilber F. Osteosarcoma. In: Pizzo PA, Poplack DG, eds. Principles and Practices of Pediatric Oncology, 2nd ed. Philadelphia: J.B. Lippincott Company, 1993:841–866.

56. Huvos AG. Osteogenic sarcoma. In: Bone Tumors: Diagnosis, Treatment, and Prognosis. Philadelphia: W.B. Saunders Company, 1991:85–155.

57. Davis AM, Bell RS, Goodwin PJ. Prognostic factors in osteosarcoma: a critical review. J Clin Oncol 12:423–431, 1994.

58. Hudson M, Jaffe MR, Jaffe N, et al. Pediatric osteosarcoma: therapeutic strategies, results, and prognostic factors derived from a 10-year experience. J Clin Oncol 12:1988–1997, 1990.

59. Meyer WH, Malawer MM. Osteosarcoma: clinical features and evolving surgical and chemotherapeutic strategies. Pediatr Clin North Amer 38:317–348, 1991.

60. Pastorino U, Gasparini M, Tavecchio L, et al. The contribution of salvage surgery to the management of childhood osteosarcoma. J Clin Oncol 9:1357–1362, 1991.

61. Link MP, Goorin AM, Horowitz M, et al. Adjuvant chemotherapy of high grade osteosarcoma of the extremity: updated results of the Multi-Institutional Osteosarcoma Study. Clin Orthop 270:8–14, 1991.

62. Eilber F, Giuliano A, Eckardt J, et al. Adjuvant chemotherapy for osteosarcoma: A randomized prospective trial. J Clin Oncol 5:21–26, 1987.

63. Rosen G. An opinion supporting the role of high-dose methotrexate in the treatment of osteosarcoma. In: Humphrey GB, Koops HS, Molenaar WM, Postma A, eds. Osteosarcoma in Adolescents and Young Adults: New Developments and Controversies. Boston: Kluwer Academic Publishers, 1993:49–54.

64. Smith MA, Ungerleider RS, Horowitz ME, Simon R. Influence of doxorubicin dose intensity on response and outcome for patients with osteogenic sarcoma and Ewing's sarcoma. J Natl Cancer Inst 83:1460–1470, 1991.

65. Jaffe N. Pediatric osteosarcoma: treatment of the primary tumor with intraarterial cis-diamminedichloroplatinum-II (CDP)—advantages, disadvantages, and controversial issues. In: Humphrey GB, Koops HS, Molenaar WM, Postma A, eds. Osteosarcoma in Adolescents and Young Adults: New Developments and Controversies. Boston: Kluwer Academic Publishers, 1993:75–84.

66. Horowitz ME, Tsokos MG, DeLaney TF. Ewing's sarcoma. CA Cancer J Clin 42:301–320, 1992.

67. Horowitz ME, Neff JR, Kun LE. Ewing's sarcoma. Radiotherapy versus surgery for local control. Pediatr Clin North Am 38:360–380, 1991.

68. Nesbit ME, Gehan EA, Burgert O, et al. Multimodal therapy for the management of primary, nonmetastatic Ewing's sarcoma of bone: a long-term follow-up of the First Intergroup Study. J Clin Oncol 8:1664–1674, 1990.

69. Burgert O, Nesbit ME, Garnsey LA, et al. Multimodal therapy for the management of nonpelvic, localized Ewing's sarcoma of bone: Intergroup Study IESS-II. J Clin Oncol 8:1514–1524, 1990.

70. Jurgens H, Gadner H, Gobel U, et al. Update of the Cooperative Ewing's Sarcoma Studies (CESS) of the German Society of Pediatric Oncology. Med Pediatr Oncol 17:284, 1989.

71. Zucker JM, Oberlin O, Demecocq F, et al. Ifosfamide in Ewing's sarcoma. No benefit compared to cyclophosphamide but more cardiac toxicity: a report from the French Society of Pediatric Oncology. Med Pediatr Oncol 17:284, 1989.

72. Grier H, Krailo M, Link M, et al. Improved outcome in non-metastatic Ewing's sarcoma and PNET of bone with the addition of ifosfamide and etoposide to vincristine, adriamycin, cyclophosphamide, and actinomycin: a Childrens Cancer Group and Pediatric Oncology Group report. Proc Am Soc Clin Oncol 13:421, 1994.

73. Meyer WH, Kun L, Marina N, et al. Ifosfamide plus etoposide in newly diagnosed Ewing's sarcoma of bone. J Clin Oncol 10:1737–1742, 1992.

74. Devesa SS. The incidence of retinoblastoma. Am J Ophthalmol 80: 263–265, 1975.

75. Francois J, Matton M, deBie S, et al. Genesis and genetics of retinoblastoma. Ophthalmolgica 170:405–425, 1975.

76. Jensen RD, Meler RW. Retinoblastoma: Epidemiologic characteristics. N Engl J Med 285:307–311, 1971.

77. Arigg PG, Heages TR, Char DH. Computed tomography in the diagnosis of retinoblastoma. Br J Ophthalmol 67:588–591, 1983.

78. Reese AB, Ellsworth RM. The evaluation and current concept of retinoblastoma treatment. Trans Am Acad Ophthalmol Otolaryngol 65: 169–172, 1963.

79. White L. Chemotherapy for retinoblastoma: where do we go from here? Ophthalmic Paediatr Genet 12:115–130, 1991.

80. Howarth C, Meyer D, Husty O, et al. Stage-related combined modality treatment of retinoblastoma. Cancer 45:851–858, 1980.

CHAPTER 86

GYNECOLOGIC CANCER

JANET A. LYLE and KEVIN M. RODONDI

It was estimated that in 1994 there were approximately 75,300 new cases of gynecologic cancers and 25,200 deaths associated with gynecologic cancer in the United States. Together, they are the fourth most common cause of cancer death in women, preceded by lung, breast, and colorectal cancers (1). This chapter will focus on the three most common gynecologic cancers: ovarian, endometrial, and cervical. The other gynecologic cancers—vulvar, vaginal, and gestational trophoblastic neoplasia—occur less frequently.

OVARIAN CANCER

Ovarian cancer is the leading cause of gynecologic cancer death in the United States. In 1994 there were an estimated 24,000 new cases of ovarian cancer, with 13,600 deaths attributed to the disease (1).

Etiology

Although the etiology of ovarian cancer is unknown, several risk factors have been identified. The highest incidence of ovarian cancer occurs in industrialized countries, particularly northern and western Europe and North America. The exception is Japan, which has one of the lowest rates of ovarian cancer in the world. Environmental factors appear to play a role, since Japanese women who have migrated to the United States have an increased risk of ovarian cancer that by the second generation approaches the rate of white women in the United States. Asbestos and talc are the two main industrial chemicals that are associated with an increased risk of ovarian cancer. Until recently, most talc powders contained asbestos. When applied on the perineum, talc can be absorbed through the vagina or cervix, reaching the ovaries by retrograde flow. A diet that is high in meat and animal fat has also been implicated as a causative factor in several studies (2, 3).

A small subset of ovarian cancer cases have a genetic link and appear to be inherited as an autosomal dominant trait. Although familial ovarian cancer constitutes only 5 to 10% of the total ovarian cancer cases, women with two or more first-degree relatives who have ovarian cancer may have as high as a 50% chance of developing the disease. Certain reproductive and endocrine factors have also been associated with an increased risk. The two most identifiable risk factors are nulliparity or low parity and unsuppressed ovulation. The use of oral contraceptives protects against the development of ovarian cancer and may reduce the risk

by up to 40% (2, 3). Recently, prolonged use of the infertility drug clomiphene has been associated with an increased risk of borderline and invasive ovarian tumors (4).

Histology

The most common malignant ovarian tumor is epithelial ovarian cancer, representing approximately 85 to 90% of cases; the remainder are stromal tumors (<10%) and germ-cell tumors (<5%). Epithelial ovarian cancer occurs most frequently in adult white women and is more common after menarche, with a peak incidence in the 50- to 70-year age range. Stromal tumors tend to be detected at earlier stages and to have a more benign course. They are usually treated with surgery, since the response to radiation or chemotherapy is poor. Although germ-cell tumors are relatively uncommon, they are important because they occur in children and young women, usually in the nonwhite population, and display an unusual natural history. Many tend to be highly aggressive but responsive to treatment with chemotherapy (2).

Pathogenesis

Tumor dissemination occurs primarily by contiguous growth, surface shedding, and lymphatic spread. Hematogenous spread of ovarian cancer is rare. The tumor originates and grows in the ovary and invades the ovarian capsule. Pelvic structures become involved by direct contact with the tumor. The tumor is able to shed cells into the peritoneal cavity, whether or not the capsule is disrupted. These cells are carried by the peritoneal fluid to sites on the peritoneal surfaces, where they form micrometastases. Free-floating tumor cells are removed from the peritoneal cavity by lymphatic channels in the diaphragm. Common sites of tumor spread, therefore, include the peritoneum, diaphragm, omentum, bowel surfaces, and retroperitoneal lymph nodes. Distant organs are also at risk and include the liver, lungs, pleura, kidneys, bone, adrenal glands, bladder, and spleen in decreasing order of frequency (2, 5). Impairment of pleural lymphatic drainage may result in malignant pleural effusions, which can often be the first extraperitoneal sign of ovarian cancer (6).

Diagnosis and Screening

Ovarian cancer is usually asymptomatic in its early stages, and only 15 to 25% of cases are confined to the ovaries at the time of diagnosis. Because the ovaries are in a spacious pelvic cavity, the tumor can grow considerably before producing symptoms. When symptoms do develop, they are usually a sign of advanced disease and may include nausea, dyspepsia, abdominal distention, or lower abdominal pain, which is usually nonspecific and intermittent (2). Unfortunately, these symptoms are often ignored or treated symptomatically. It is therefore essential that women with abdominal symptoms have a thorough physical and pelvic exam, especially perimenopausal or post-menopausal women who have other risk factors for ovarian cancer.

If an ovarian mass is detected on pelvic exam, the diagnostic workup usually includes an ultrasound to rule out ovarian enlargement. Transvaginal ultrasound is a useful, noninvasive procedure that can define disease in the pelvis and differentiate ascites from an ovarian cyst. A computed tomography (CT) scan may be helpful in obtaining additional diagnosis and staging information, but it is costly and cannot detect tumors that are smaller than 2 cm in diameter. Although efforts at developing a screening test for ovarian cancer have focused on imaging methods, mass screening with transvaginal ultrasound has not proven to be an effective method for early diagnosis (2, 6).

Tumor markers that can detect the presence of disease are a helpful monitoring tool. CA-125 is currently the most useful marker for ovarian cancer. This antigen, identified by a monoclonal antibody to human ovarian cancer, is common to most epithelial ovarian cancers. It is elevated (>35 u/mL) in more than 80% of patients with this type of ovarian cancer but in only 1% of the normal population. Unfortunately, it is a nonspecific indicator, and elevated levels may be seen in patients with other gynecologic cancers as well as in patients with benign conditions such as pregnancy, endometriosis, pelvic inflammatory disease, hepatitis, and cirrhosis (6). It is also associated with a significant amount of false negatives in early disease. For this reason it is not a useful screening tool alone for the diagnosis of ovarian cancer. CA-125 does correlate with the stage and extent of disease and is useful in monitoring the response to therapy in patients who have elevated levels at the time of diagnosis (2). Patients with CA-125 levels that remain elevated after a course of chemotherapy are likely to have a residual tumor. Conversely, a fall in CA-125 after chemotherapy has been associated with increased patient survival (7). Other useful tumor markers in ovarian cancer are listed in Table 86.1. At this time there is no known marker that can be reliably detected in patients with small volumes of tumor.

Prognosis

The most significant prognostic indicators for ovarian cancer are the stage of the disease at the time of surgery, the amount of residual disease following initial surgical resection, and the histologic type and grade of the tumor

Table 86.1.
Clinically Useful Tumor Markers in Ovarian Cancer[a]

Marker	Types of Tumor Identified
CA-125	Nonmucinous epithelial ovarian carcinoma
CA 19-9	Mucinous epithelial ovarian carcinoma
NB/70K	Mucinous epithelial ovarian carcinoma
Alpha-fetoprotein (AFP)	Endodermal sinus tumor, embryonal cell carcinoma
Human chorionic gonadotropin (HCG)	Ovarian choriocarcinoma, embryonal cell carcinoma, mixed germ-cell tumors
Lactate dehydrogenase (LDH)	Dysgerminoma
Carcinoembryonic antigen (CEA)	Mucinous epithelial ovarian carcinoma
Lipid-associated sialic acid	Nonspecific tumor marker for high-grade cancers
Inhibin	Granulosa-cell tumor of the ovary

[a]Reprinted with permission from Deppe G. Ovarian cancer: advances in management. Surg Clin N Am 71:1285–1302, 1991.

(8). Ovarian cancer requires careful surgical exploration for proper staging of the disease. The staging classification that is most commonly used is the International Federation of Gynecology and Obstetrics (FIGO) system, which is outlined in Table 86.2. Patients undergo a thorough exploratory laparotomy, which determines the location and extent of macroscopic disease. If macroscopic disease is not found, a careful search for microscopic disease is undertaken, which includes abdominal washings and multiple biopsies. Because ovarian cancer is often asymptomatic in its early stages, up to 85% of patients have widespread abdominal disease at the time of diagnosis (FIGO stages III-IV). If surgical exploration reveals bulky abdominal disease, then cytoreductive surgery becomes the goal rather than a staging procedure (5). Accurate staging is critical for the proper management of ovarian cancer, but unfortunately, inadequate staging or understaging is common. The 5-year survival rate is 80 to 90% in patients with stage I disease and 40 to 60% in patients with stage II disease. This is significantly decreased in patients with stage III disease (10 to 15%) and stage IV disease (<5%) (8).

The histological subtype may also play a role in determining patient prognosis. Clear-cell and mucinous-cell types appear to be associated with a poorer prognosis. Approximately 10 to 20% of ovarian tumors have a histological appearance between benign cysts and malignant carcinomas and are referred to as borderline tumors. These are associated with an 80 to 90% 5-year survival rate, regardless of the stage of the disease. The value of histologic grade as an independent prognostic variable is not clearly established. Tumor grade may be the most important prognostic factor in stage I disease, but its value seems to decrease in patients with advanced disease. Patients with a well-differentiated tumor (grade 1) or a

Table 86.2.
FIGO Staging for Carcinoma of the Ovary

Stage I	Tumor limited to ovaries.
Stage IA	Tumor limited to one ovary; capsule intact, no tumor on ovarian surface, no malignant cells in ascites or peritoneal washings.
Stage IB	Tumor limited to both ovaries; capsules intact, no tumor on ovarian surface, no malignant cells in ascites or peritoneal washings.
Stage IC	Tumor limited to one or both ovaries with any of the following: capsule ruptured, tumor on ovarian surface, malignant cells in ascites or peritoneal washings.
Stage II	Tumor involving one or both ovaries with pelvic extension.
Stage IIA	Extension and/or metastases on the uterus and/or tube(s); no malignant cells in ascites or peritoneal washings.
Stage IIB	Extension to other pelvic tissues; no malignant cells in ascites or peritoneal washings.
Stage IIC	Tumor either Stage IIA or IIB with malignant cells in ascites or peritoneal washings.
Stage III	Tumor involving one or both ovaries with microscopically confirmed peritoneal metastasis outside the pelvis and/or regional lymph nodes. Liver capsule metastasis is stage III.
Stage IIIA	Microscopic peritoneal metastasis beyond the pelvis.
Stage IIIB	Macroscopic peritoneal metastasis beyond the pelvis 2 cm or less in the greatest dimension.
Stage IIIC	Peritoneal metastasis beyond the pelvis more than 2 cm in the greatest dimension and/or regional lymph node metastasis.
Stage IV	Tumor involving one or both ovaries with distant metastasis. If pleural effusion is present, there must also be positive cytology. Liver parenchymal metastasis is Stage IV.

Table 86.3.
Treatment Modalities for Ovarian Cancer After Staging/ Debulking Surgery

Stage	Treatment
IA or IB, grade 1	No further treatment
IA or IB, grade 2, 3	Intraperitoneal ^{32}P radiation therapy or combination chemotherapy
IC	Intraperitoneal ^{32}P radiation therapy, or total abdominal and pelvic radiation therapy, or combination chemotherapy
Stage II with postsurgical residual disease < 2 cm	Combination chemotherapy, or total abdominal and pelvic radiation therapy, or intraperitoneal ^{32}P radiation therapy
Stage II with postsurgical residual disease > 2 cm	Combination chemotherapy
Stage III with postsurgical residual disease < 2 cm	Combination chemotherapy or total abdominal and pelvic radiation
Stage III with postsurgical residual disease > 2 cm	Combination chemotherapy
Stage IV	Combination chemotherapy, intraperitoneal chemotherapy under investigation
Recurrent or refractory	Palliative surgery, single-agent salvage chemotherapy, or clinical trials

moderately well-differentiated tumor (grade 2) have significantly higher 5-year survival rates than do patients with poorly differentiated tumors (grade 3) (8). For patients with advanced disease (suboptimal stage III and IV) at diagnosis, younger age, good performance status, absence of ascites, and initial treatment with cisplatin-based chemotherapy have been associated with an improved overall survival (9).

Treatment

SURGERY

Early Disease. Surgery to remove the primary tumor is sufficient for the treatment of stage IA and IB ovarian tumors. After a thorough staging laparotomy, patients undergo a total abdominal hysterectomy, bilateral salpingo-oophorectomy, omentectomy, and any tumor debulking that can be accomplished. The uterus and contralateral ovary can be preserved in selected patients with early disease who desire to preserve fertility. These tumors are associated with an excellent patient survival after surgery alone, and additional therapy is not required. Patients with

poorly differentiated tumors (grade 3) and patients who have stage IC or II disease will require additional therapy with either systemic chemotherapy or intraabdominal radiation therapy. Recommended treatment modalities after surgical staging and tumor debulking are listed in Table 86.3.

Advanced Disease. Patients with advanced disease at the time of the staging laparotomy should undergo surgery to remove as much of the primary tumor and metastases as possible (cytoreductive surgery). Since complete removal of all disease is usually not possible, the goal is to reduce the tumor size to less than 1.5 to 2 cm in diameter, which can improve patient comfort and reduce the adverse metabolic effects of the tumor. Cytoreduction also leaves fewer cells that require eradication and improves blood supply to the tumor, increasing sensitivity to subsequent chemotherapy or radiation therapy. These factors can have a significant impact on overall patient survival (5, 6). A decision tree for the treatment of advanced disease after initial surgery is outlined in Figure 86.1.

A second-look operation may be helpful in evaluating the peritoneal cavity for evidence of disease. This procedure is a surgical laparotomy in a patient with no clinical evidence of disease after primary surgery and subsequent chemotherapy and is intended to determine the response to therapy. Less invasive assessments of patient response (e.g., CT scan, magnetic resonance imaging [MRI]) are not reliable in detecting residual tumor. Patients with residual disease at the time of surgery may benefit from further cytoreductive surgery, which can improve disease status

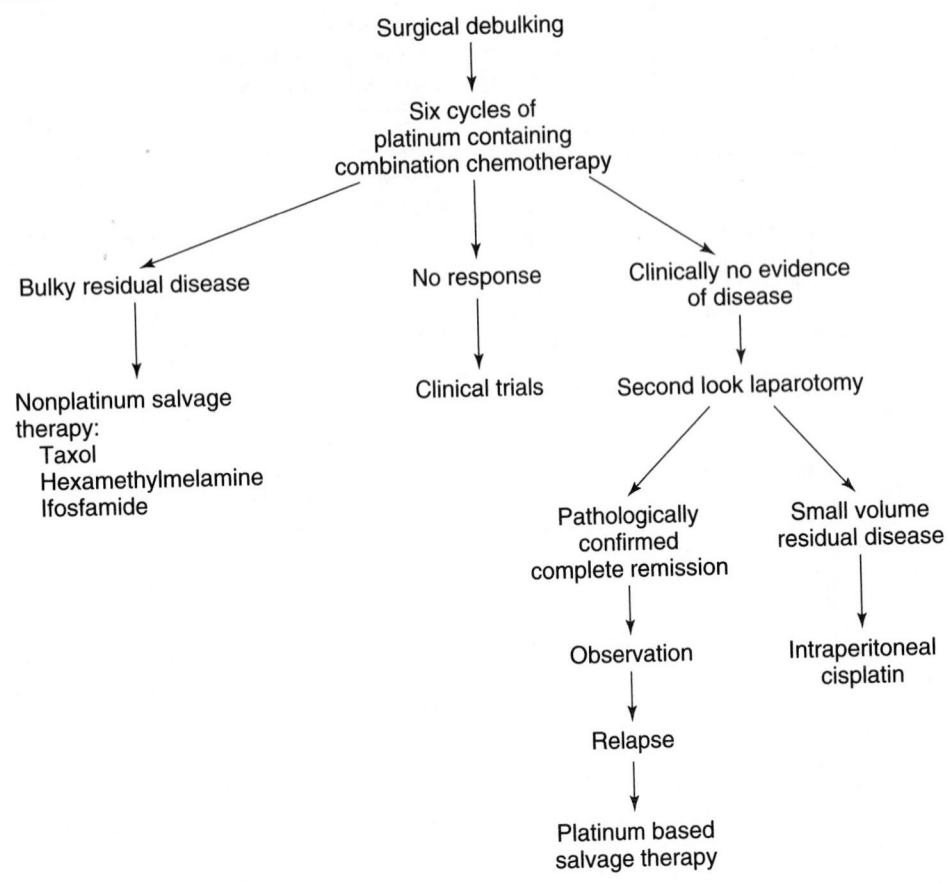

Figure 86.1. Management of advanced stage ovarian cancer. Modified with permission from Ozols RF. New approaches to management of ovarian cancer. Adv Oncol 6:9–17, 1990.

before salvage chemotherapy. A negative second look can also identify patients with chemotherapy-sensitive tumors who may be candidates for further consolidation therapy (10). However, the direct benefit of second-look operations remains controversial. Ovarian cancer will recur in 30 to 50% of patients regardless of achieving a pathologic complete response on second look. The operation is a major surgical procedure with inherent complications, and traditional second-line therapies have not demonstrated a significant effect on overall survival (11, 12). The recent development of more effective second-line and salvage therapies may add to the potential value of second-look operations in the management of ovarian cancer.

RADIATION THERAPY

Radiation may be used as primary adjuvant therapy (additional therapy administered after the primary tumor mass has been eliminated by the initial treatment modality) after surgery in patients with stage I and II ovarian cancer and in stage III patients with no evidence of macroscopic disease. Radiation must be directed to both the pelvis and the upper abdomen to avoid relapses throughout the peritoneal cavity. Many normal tissues such as the kidney

and the liver are also radiosensitive, a situation that limits the dose of radiation that can safely be administered. The dose of radiation depends on the size of the tumor and is fractionated into multiple doses delivered over several weeks. For tumors <2 cm the required dose is approximately 5000 cGy, although the dose can be increased for larger tumors or decreased in patients with microscopic disease. In advanced disease, radiation is usually reserved for inoperable tumors that are unresponsive to chemotherapy or as salvage therapy for persistent disease. Radiation can also be useful as palliation for incurable patients with symptomatic metastatic disease (2, 13). The overall toxicity of total abdominal radiation has limited its usefulness, however, and its role has declined in recent years.

The most common side effect of radiation therapy in the treatment of ovarian carcinoma is radiation enteritis. This syndrome is dose-related and may include diarrhea, nausea, vomiting, and weight loss. Gastrointestinal symptoms usually subside a few weeks after completion of therapy; however, diarrhea can persist for months in some cases. Radiation-induced hepatitis and nephritis can occur with doses exceeding 2500 cGy, especially if precautions have not been taken to minimize organ exposure during treatment. The most serious complication is small bowel damage, resulting in obstruction and requiring surgical correction. Radiation may also cause bone marrow suppression with a subsequent reduction in peripheral blood counts, which return to normal after cessation of therapy. However, irradiated bone marrow can remain impaired for extended periods, and this should be considered for patients who may subsequently receive myelosuppressive chemotherapy (2, 13).

Radioactive phosphorus (^{32}P) or chromic phosphate is a radioisotope that emits β particles with a tissue penetration range of 3 to 5 mm. It has a half-life of 14.2 days. The intraperitoneal instillation of ^{32}P may sterilize microscopic peritoneal tumor, but it cannot effectively treat larger tumors. Unfortunately, distribution may be quite variable within the peritoneal cavity because of adhesions or loculations that are secondary to surgery. The usual dose of ^{32}P is 15 to 20 mCi diluted in 1 to 1.5 L of saline, which is instilled into the peritoneal cavity. This delivers approximately 6000 cGy of radiation to the peritoneum and approximately 7000 cGy to the omentum. Because of its low toxicity, it can be useful as adjuvant therapy of unfavorable early-stage disease or as consolidation therapy in patients with negative second-look operations. The most common complication of therapy is small-bowel obstruction and stenosis, which occur in <10% of treated patients (2, 14).

CHEMOTHERAPY

Initial Therapy. Chemotherapy has become the most common form of therapy in patients with advanced ovarian cancer. Classic alkylating agents such as cyclophosphamide, melphalan, and chlorambucil have been studied the most extensively and have produced objective response rates ranging from 35 to 65% when used as single agents. Five-year survival is poor (<10%) in patients with advanced disease (15).

Cisplatin is one of the most active agents in the treatment of this disease, with overall response rates of 25 to 40% when used as a single agent. Significant side effects include nausea and vomiting, nephrotoxicity, ototoxicity, peripheral neuropathy, and bone marrow suppression. When cisplatin is incorporated into combination chemotherapy regimens, both response rates and disease-free interval are improved, and some studies have also documented an impact on overall survival. A standard chemotherapeutic regimen for advanced disease consists of six cycles of the two-drug combination of cisplatin and cyclophosphamide. Response rates range from 60 to 80%, with complete remission rates of 20 to 25% (11, 15).

Many studies have now concluded that carboplatin can be substituted for cisplatin as front-line therapy with no difference in response rates, disease-free progression, or

survival rates (10, 11). Carboplatin is a second-generation platinum compound that is less nephrotoxic, ototoxic, neurotoxic, and emetogenic than cisplatin and is therefore easier to administer. Because of carboplatin's improved therapeutic index and equal efficacy in ovarian cancer, the combination of carboplatin and cyclophosphamide is now considered an alternative therapy for patients with advanced disease. However, carboplatin is also more myelosuppressive than cisplatin and can cause significant thrombocytopenia. Pretreatment renal function correlates with the severity of hematologic toxicity. A carboplatin dose of 400 mg/m^2 is therapeutically equivalent to 100 mg/m^2 of cisplatin. Many investigators now use the Calvert formula (16) to calculate a carboplatin dose based on a target area under the curve (AUC) as follows:

$$\text{Dose (mg)} = \text{Target AUC} \times (\text{GFR} + 25)$$

Approximately 70% of the carboplatin dose is excreted in the urine, primarily as unchanged drug, and the renal clearance is closely correlated with the glomerular filtration rate (GFR). GFR can be measured directly or can be estimated by using creatinine clearance. AUC may be a better measure of drug exposure and allows for precise endpoints of therapy. A target AUC of 5 to 7 is used to maximize the dose of carboplatin and thereby increase its therapeutic efficacy without causing excessive toxicity.

Doxorubicin has a response rate of approximately 30% as a first-line single agent and has also been extensively studied in combination chemotherapy regimens. Several randomized trials have compared cisplatin plus cyclophosphamide with or without doxorubicin in advanced ovarian cancer. A metaanalysis of these trials has documented a 7% survival advantage for patients receiving the doxorubicin-containing regimens (17). It is unclear whether this was due to the addition of doxorubicin or because the doses of cisplatin and cyclophosphamide in the three-drug regimen were greater than those in the two-drug regimen in three of the trials. Because there is only a modest survival benefit and doxorubicin greatly increases the toxicity of the regimen (e.g., myelosuppression, cardiac toxicity), the combination of a platinum compound and cyclophosphamide remains first-line therapy for advanced ovarian cancer. Combination chemotherapy regimens that are used in the treatment of ovarian cancer are described in Table 86.4.

A significant-dose response relationship exists for cisplatin in the treatment of ovarian cancer. This has been seen over a dose range from 25 to 100 mg/m^2 when used as a single agent or in combination chemotherapy regimens (19). Dose-limiting side effects, especially peripheral neuropathy, limit doses of cisplatin beyond 100 mg/m^2. Consequently, most clinical trials of high-dose chemotherapy focus on carboplatin, the dose-limiting toxicity of which is bone marrow suppression, primarily thrombocy-

Table 86.4.
Selected Regimens for Ovarian Cancer

Epithelial Cell	
CP	**Cyclophosphamide** 1000 mg/m^2 i.v. day 1
	Cisplatin 50–100 mg/m^2 IV day 1
	Repeat cycle every 28 days
CC	**Cyclophosphamide** 500–750 mg/m^2 i.v. day 1
	Carboplatin 300–400 mg/m^2 i.v. day 1
	Repeat cycle every 28 days
CAP	**Cyclophosphamide** 500 mg/m^2 i.v. day 1
(PAC)	**Doxorubicin** 50 mg/m^2 i.v. day 1
	Cisplatin 50 mg/m^2 i.v. day 1
	Repeat cycle every 21 days
CAC	**Cyclophosphamide** 500 mg/m^2 i.v. day 1
(CDC)	**Doxorubicin** 40 mg/m^2 i.v. day 1
	Carboplatin 300 mg/m^2 i.v. day 1
	Repeat cycle every 28 days
CHAP	**Cyclophosphamide** 300–500 mg/m^2 i.v. day 1
(H-CAP)	**Hexamethylmelamine** 150 mg/m^2 p.o. day 1–7
	Doxorubicin 30–50 mg/m^2 i.v. day 1
	Cisplatin 50–60 mg/m^2 i.v. day 1
	Repeat cycle every 28 days
Germ Cell	
VAC	**Vincristine** 1.2–1.5 mg (maximum 2 mg) i.v. weekly for 10–12 weeks or every 2 weeks for 12 doses
	Dactinomycin 0.3–0.4 mg/m^2 i.v. days 1–5
	Cyclophosphamide 150 mg/m^2 i.v. days 1–5
	Repeat cycle every 28 days

topenia. Carboplatin is an ideal candidate for high-intensity chemotherapy regimens with hematopoietic growth factors (G-CSF, GM-CSF) and peripheral stem-cell support or autologous bone marrow transplantation. These trials are currently underway (10, 19).

Salvage Therapy. Patients who relapse after initial platinum-containing chemotherapy regimens or who have bulky residual disease following therapy are candidates for salvage chemotherapy. Retreatment with cisplatin has an established role in patients who initially respond to cisplatin- or carboplatin-based therapy and have a significant disease-free interval. The longer the interval, the more likely the response (20). Patients who do not respond to cisplatin-based chemotherapy or who have a short disease-free interval are treated with nonplatinum salvage regimens.

Paclitaxel is now recommended as second-line therapy in patients with cisplatin-resistant ovarian cancer. It is a recently approved cytotoxic agent that is very active in the treatment of ovarian cancer. Its unique mechanism of action involves binding to and stabilizing cellular microtubules, thereby inhibiting mitosis. Overall response rates of 30 to 50% have been documented in heavily pretreated patients, and up to 30% has been documented in patients who are resistant to cisplatin (21, 22). Significant side effects include bone marrow suppression, alopecia, myalgias, and peripheral neuropathy. Pretreatment with dexa-

methasone 10 to 20 mg, diphenhydramine 25 to 50 mg, and cimetidine 300 mg can reduce the incidence of hypersensitivity reactions, which are probably secondary to the cremophor vehicle (21). Doses up to 175 mg/m^2 or higher can be safely administered as a single 24-hr infusion in previously treated patients. The drug can also be administered as a 3-hr infusion with equal safety and less myelosuppression; however efficacy results are still pending (23). Current studies are evaluating the combination of paclitaxel and cisplatin as first-line therapy in the treatment of advanced ovarian cancer. The sequence of paclitaxel followed by cisplatin seems to result in less neutropenia (21). Early results are promising, but there may be an increased risk of peripheral neuropathy with this combination, and questions remain regarding proper infusion rate and timing of the two drugs. Other agents that have documented activity as second-line or salvage therapy include altretamine (hexamethylmelamine), ifosfamide, and tamoxifen. The response rates for these agents are generally less than 25% when they are used as salvage therapy (15, 20).

Intraperitoneal Chemotherapy. Intraperitoneal chemotherapy was selected as a potential treatment for ovarian cancer because the disease spreads primarily within the peritoneal cavity and direct intraperitoneal instillation of chemotherapy achieves extremely high concentrations at the site of the tumor while minimizing systemic toxicity of the drug. Optimal agents for intraperitoneal therapy have a high molecular weight and low lipid solubility, are slowly cleared from the peritoneal cavity, and are minimally toxic to the peritoneum. Cisplatin appears to be the drug of choice for intraperitoneal administration, although carboplatin, mitoxantrone, fluorouracil, methotrexate, and etoposide also demonstrate activity (24). Early results with paclitaxel show promising activity when it is administered by the peritoneal route, as levels in the peritoneal cavity are approximately 1000-fold greater than those in the plasma (25).

Intraperitoneal therapy involves the instillation of chemotherapeutic agents directly into the peritoneal cavity through a specialized catheter or a surgically placed subcutaneous port. The chemotherapeutic agent is usually diluted into 1.5 to 2 L of normal saline to ensure adequate distribution throughout the cavity. It is then instilled over 30 to 60 min, and the remainder is removed after a dwell time of approximately 6 hr. The most common complications are catheter failure and peritonitis. Peritonitis can result from the drug itself or infection, usually with *Staphylococcus epidermidis* or *S. aureus*. Intraperitoneal chemotherapy should probably be reserved for salvage therapy for patients with very small volume residual disease following systemic chemotherapy. In this setting, overall response rates of approximately 30% can be achieved with cisplatin-based therapy, most responses being seen in patients who have had high response rates to intravenous cisplatin. A survival benefit for patients treated with intraperitoneal therapy has not been documented, however, and it remains an investigational procedure. There is no evidence of substantial activity in patients with bulky residual disease (2, 24).

CERVICAL CANCER

Cancer of the cervix is the third most common female genital cancer in the United States, with an estimated 15,000 new cases in 1994 and 4,600 deaths attributed to the disease (1). It is one of the few types of cancers that can be prevented by an inexpensive mass screening program for detection of preinvasive lesions. Most deaths from this disease could be prevented by routine screening and early intervention. The peak incidence of cervical cancer is between 48 and 55 years of age, the majority of invasive cancers occurring after age 35 (26).

Etiology

Cervical cancer is more common in underdeveloped and low-socioeconomic-level populations. It is associated with sexual intercourse at a younger age, multiple sexual partners, pregnancy at a younger age, multiple pregnancies, and cigarette smoking (26). Because cervical cancer has many characteristics of a sexually transmitted disease, many infectious agents have been implicated. The strongest association is with the human papillomavirus (HPV), which is now considered the biggest risk factor for cervical cancer. Of the 22 different types of HPV identified in the human genital tract, types 16 and 18 are considered high-risk viral types leading to invasive cancer in approximately 75% of cases (26, 27). The use of diethylstilbesterol (DES) in pregnant women has been associated with an increased incidence of adenocarcinoma of the cervix and vagina in their daughters (26).

Histology

Most cervical cancers are squamous-cell carcinoma (85 to 90%), the remainder being adenocarcinoma (10 to 15%) or adenosquamous-cell carcinoma (2 to 5%). Gross cervical lesions are usually defined as either endophytic or exophytic. Endophytic lesions are located within the endocervical canal of a normal-appearing cervix and can be more extensive than they appear. These lesions may become large enough to distend the cervix, creating "barrel-shaped lesions." Exophytic lesions are cauliflowerlike and friable and bleed easily. They may be less extensive than they appear on first examination (26, 28).

Pathogenesis

Cervical carcinoma begins at the squamous-columnar junction between the endocervical canal and the cervix. The precursor lesion is referred to as dysplasia or carcinoma in situ (cervical intraepithelial neoplasia [CIN]), which precedes the development of invasive cervical cancer. Progression from dysplasia or CIN to invasive disease can be quite long, 30 to 70% of untreated patients developing invasive carcinoma over a 10-year period. The tumor becomes invasive when it breaks through the basement membrane into the underlying tissue. Cervical cancer usually progresses in a predictable manner, and tumor dissemination is generally a function of the extent of local tumor invasion. The disease can spread by direct extension into the vagina or endometrium, then to the walls of the pelvis, the bladder, and the rectum. In addition to local invasion, tumor spread can occur through the rich lymphatic network of the cervix. The risk of hematogenous spread increases with advanced stages and can result in distant metastasis (26).

Diagnosis and Screening

Patients with preinvasive cervical cancer are usually asymptomatic, and the disease is detected by a Papanicolaou (Pap) smear performed during a routine pelvic examination. Current recommendations are that every woman who is or has been sexually active or is at least 18 years of age should have an annual Pap smear and pelvic examination. If three or more consecutive exams are normal, the Pap smear may be performed less frequently at the discretion of the physician. Although Pap smears are quite accurate in detecting high-grade preinvasive lesions, false negative rates can run from 10 to 50%, emphasizing the importance of a yearly test.

Patients with early invasive disease can have symptoms of a vaginal discharge or intermittent vaginal bleeding, which commonly appear as postcoital spotting. As the lesion progresses, the vaginal discharge becomes more pronounced. In advanced disease, symptoms may include flank or leg pain, urinary frequency, hematuria, and rectal bleeding, which are indicative of pelvic invasion (26).

If dysplastic or malignant cells are discovered during screening, colposcopy should be performed to visualize abnormal areas and allow for properly directed biopsies. All visible lesions should be biopsied. Cervical conization (removal of a cone-shaped portion of tissue from the cervix) is indicated when colposcopy is inadequate or when no gross lesions are visible. Further evaluation may include a chest radiograph, cystoscopy, proctosigmoidoscopy, and a CT scan. MRI is very helpful in assessing both local and nodal disease (26).

Prognosis

The major factors influencing prognosis are stage, size of the tumor, histologic type, lymphatic node involvement, and vascular invasion. The staging of cervical cancer is based on clinical assessment of the patient and is illustrated in Table 86.5. Prognosis is worse with advancing stage,

Table 86.5.
FIGO Staging for Carcinoma of the Cervix

Stage 0	Carcinoma in situ, intraepithelial carcinoma.
Stage I	Carcinoma confined to the cervix (extension to the corpus should be disregarded).
Stage IA	Preclinical invasive carcinoma, diagnosed by microscopy only.
Stage IA1	Minimal microscopic stromal invasion.
Stage IA2	Tumors with an invasive component 5 mm or less in depth taken from the base of the epithelium and 7 mm or less in horizontal spread.
Stage IB	Tumors larger than Stage IA2.
Stage II	Invasion beyond the uterus but not to the pelvic wall or to the lower third of the vagina.
Stage IIA	Tumor without parametrial invasion.
Stage IIB	Tumor with parametrial invasion.
Stage III	Tumor extension to the pelvic wall and/or involves the lower third of the vagina and/or causes hydronephrosis or nonfunctioning kidney.
Stage IIIA	Involvement of the lower third of the vagina, with no extension to the pelvic wall.
Stage IIIB	Extension to the pelvic wall and/or causes hydronephrosis or a nonfunctioning kidney.
Stage IV	Extension beyond the true pelvis.
Stage IVA	Invasion of the mucosa of the bladder or rectum.
Stage IVB	Distant metastasis.

Table 86.6.
Treatment Modalities for Cervical Cancer

Stage	Treatment
1A	Surgery; RT if not a surgical candidate
IB, IIA	<3 cm: surgery or RT; >3 cm: RT
IIB	RT
IIIA, IIIB	RT
IVA	RT
IVB	Combination of RT and chemotherapy

RT = radiation therapy.

indicating an increase in tumor size and greater extent of spread. Patients with adenocarcinomas and adenosquamous carcinoma tend to have a less favorable prognosis than do patients with squamous-cell carcinoma of the same stage. The 5-year survival rate is 65 to 90% for stage I squamous-cell cancer (70 to 75% for adenocarcinoma) and 45 to 80% for stage II disease (30 to 40% for adenocarcinoma). Stage III disease has a 5-year survival rate of up to 61% (20 to 30% for adenocarcinoma); the 5-year survival rate of stage IV disease drops to <15% for both cell types. The size of the tumor can be useful in predicting behavior, larger tumors generally being associated with greater spread and a worse prognosis even in stage I disease. Positive lymph nodes usually indicate a larger tumor, deep invasion of the tumor, and lymphovascular spread (28, 29). Women who are infected with HIV represent a unique subset of patients who are at risk for cervical carcinoma. These patients present with more advanced disease, have a poorer response to treatment, and overall have a poorer prognosis (30).

Treatment

Surgery and radiation are the primary treatment modalities for cervical cancer and are equally effective in early disease. The use of adjuvant chemotherapy in advanced disease has not been clearly established, and most chemotherapeutic agents have limited activity in cervical cancer. Treatment modalities for cervical cancer are outlined in Table 86.6.

SURGERY

Surgery is appropriate in the treatment of early disease. Patients with carcinoma in situ (stage 0 disease) can be effectively managed by conization of the cervix, cryotherapy, or laser therapy. The latter two are quickly being replaced by a procedure called the loop electrosurgical excision, which is an outpatient procedure performed under local anesthesia. For patients with stage IA disease (<3-mm depth of invasion), a total abdominal hysterectomy is recommended. A 5-year survival rate of 85 to 90% can be achieved with a radical hysterectomy alone. In these cases there is a low risk of lymph node metastases or recurrent disease, and no adjuvant therapy is required. A total abdominal hysterectomy with bilateral pelvic lymphadenectomy is indicated for stage IB or IIA disease. Primary surgery may be preferable to radiation for a relatively young and medically fit patient. Reproductive function can be preserved and vaginal atrophy and stenosis can be avoided with a surgical approach. Postsurgical outcomes are worse for patients with large primary lesions and/or pelvic lymph node metastases (31, 32).

RADIATION

Radiation therapy is appropriate in all stages of the disease. It may be preferable to surgery for older patients, for medically inoperable patients, or for tumors that are larger than 3 to 4 cm. It is the treatment of choice for more advanced stages. As the volume of disease increases, there is a higher fraction of cells in the resting phase, and these are less sensitive to radiation therapy. There is a clear dose-response relationship with radiation for cervical cancer, and higher doses are necessary to effectively treat larger tumors.

Intracavitary radiation or brachytherapy may be used to treat stage IA disease if the depth of invasion is less than 3 mm and surgery is not an option. Brachytherapy is delivered by using applicators that are inserted in the uterus and arranged next to the cervix. These are then loaded with radioactive cesium or iridium, which delivers higher doses of radiation to the primary tumor and paracervical tissues while minimizing radiation effects to the healthy surrounding tissue. External beam irradiation combined with brachytherapy is the treatment of choice for most patients with cervical carcinoma that is more advanced than stage IIA. In this approach, high-energy photon beams deliver 4000 to 5000 cGy to the pelvis at approximately 150 to 200 cGy/day. The brachytherapy boost delivers additional radiation to the cervix and parametrium for a total tumor dose of 8000 to 10,000 cGy (26, 33).

The most common side effects during radiation therapy are acute reactions such as burning or frequency on urination, diarrhea, and bloody stools. Late tissue reactions occur in fewer than 10% of treated patients and can include vaginal stenosis, vaginal adhesions, small bowel obstruction, visceral perforation, hemorrhagic proctitis, hemorrhagic cystitis, and bladder contraction. These late reactions, which may appear months or years after therapy, are dose-related and may require surgery (33). They are more frequent in patients who have had prior abdominal or pelvic surgery or chemotherapy and in patients with underlying chronic illness such as diabetes. The tissues in which they occur are slowly proliferating tissues and normally have an excellent repair capacity. Since they tend to lose this capacity when large doses per fraction of radiation are used, hyperfractionated regimens have been developed. Hyperfractionation uses doses of 110 to 160 Gy per fraction 2 or 3 times a day and allows delivery of higher total doses with equivalent toxicity or equal total doses with less toxicity than standard once-daily fractionation (34).

CHEMOTHERAPY

Most women who have cervical cancer will be cured with surgery, radiation therapy, or a combination of the two. Patients with advanced disease or recurrent disease after surgery and radiation are good candidates for chemotherapy because of the low chance of survival with standard therapies. Unfortunately, response rates have remained low, partly because delivery is impaired by an altered blood supply and poor bone marrow reserve from previous pelvic radiation. Patients who have not received prior radiation demonstrate much higher response rates to chemotherapy, and extrapelvic disease tends to be more responsive (35). Single agents that have activity in the treatment of cervical cancer are listed in Table 86.7. Cisplatin has been the most extensively studied in the treatment of cervical cancer. Complete responses have occurred in up to 10% of treated patients, but most responses are partial and of short duration. It must be given with caution in patients with advanced disease, who often have obstruction of one or more ureters, resulting in impaired renal function. Doxorubicin and ifosfamide have also demonstrated consistent activity. Ifosfamide may be one of the most active drugs, with

Table 86.7.
Single-Agent Chemotherapy in Cervical Cancer[a]

Drug	Overall Response (%)
Alkylating agents	
Cyclophosphamide	15
Chlorambucil	25
Ifosfamide	22
Antimetabolites	
5-fluorouracil	20
Methotrexate	18
Plant alkaloids	
Vincristine	18
Antitumor antibiotics	
Doxorubicin	17
Bleomycin	10
Platinum compounds	
Cisplatin	23
Carboplatin	15

[a]Modified from (30).

response rates of approximately 30% in patients with no previous chemotherapy. Duration of response for single-agent therapy is relatively short, as is the overall survival rate. Some studies have shown higher response rates with cisplatin-based combination chemotherapy, but results are not reproducible, toxicity is greater, and an improvement in survival has not been documented (31, 35).

Intraarterial chemotherapy has also been studied because of the isolated blood supply to the tumor. Responses are limited, because it does not treat possible micrometastases outside the pelvic circulation. Hydroxyurea is an effective radiosensitizer that acts to increase the cytotoxic effect of radiation. It has improved disease-free survival in some reports, but this agent and other radiosensitizing agents (e.g., cisplatin, fluorouracil) have little effect on overall survival (25). Several small studies have addressed the role of chemotherapy delivered before radiation therapy (neoadjuvant) to try to improve local control of the disease. Results have been mixed, and there has been no effect on patient survival (36). The combination of chemotherapy and surgery may prove to be more promising.

ENDOMETRIAL CANCER

Endometrial cancer is the most common gynecologic malignancy in the United States, representing more than half of all new cases diagnosed annually. Although approximately 31,000 cases were diagnosed in 1994, only 5,900 deaths have been attributed to the disease (fewer than 2% of all cancer deaths in women) (1). This low mortality is primarily the result of early diagnosis. Endometrial cancer generally occurs in white postmenopausal women between 55 and 60 years of age. The incidence is lower in Black and Asian women (26).

Etiology

The endometrium is a complex tissue that is responsive to endogenous and exogenous fluctuations in hormonal balance. Conjugated estrogen therapy used to control symptoms in postmenopausal women without concomitant progesterone therapy (unopposed estrogen use) has been associated with an increased risk of endometrial cancer (37). Other risk factors include excessive endogenous estrogen, nulliparity, polycystic ovarian disease, late menopause, and obesity. Medical disorders such as hypertension and diabetes mellitus are also associated with the disease (26). Evidence indicates that the antiestrogen agent tamoxifen, which is used in the treatment of breast cancer, can increase the risk of endometrial cancer (38). This disease is uncommon in women who have normal menstrual cycles, presumably because of the cyclic exposure of the endometrium to progesterone. The use of a combination oral contraceptive may be protective.

Diagnosis and Screening

Abnormal vaginal bleeding is reported by almost all women with endometrial cancer, and this allows for early detection. It is usually recognizable because approximately 75% of women with the disease are postmenopausal. Pain can also be reported, but this usually signifies advanced disease. A significant percentage of patients can be asymptomatic. Endometrial cancer is diagnosed by dilatation and curettage or by endometrial biopsy. Although malignant cells can sometimes be detected in a Pap smear, this test does not reliably detect endometrial cancer. Once the diagnosis is made, the patient must undergo a thorough physical examination, pelvic examination, chest radiograph, CT scan, and possibly MRI. Cystoscopy and proctosigmoidoscopy may be helpful in some situations (26). There are no specific tumor markers for endometrial cancer, but serum CA-125 may be elevated in more than one-half of patients with the disease. A baseline level can be beneficial because if it is elevated, the level can be followed during and after treatment to evaluate the response to therapy and help to predict recurrence of the disease (39). At this time there are no adequate screening tests for endometrial cancer.

Histology and Pathogenesis

The most common cell type is adenocarcinoma, which accounts for approximately 75% of all cases. The second most common is adenosquamous carcinoma (18%), which contain both adenocarcinoma and squamous cell carcinoma cell types. Approximately 5% of endometrial cancers consist of clear-cell carcinoma, secretory carcinoma, squamous-cell carcinoma, and papillary carcinoma (40).

Endometrial cancer arises in the fundus of the uterus and can be small and focal or diffusely involve the uterine cavity. Diffuse lesions often show focal areas of ulceration or hemorrhage. Local extension accounts for disease in the

Table 86.8.
FIGO Staging for Endometrial Carcinoma

Stage 0	Atypical hyperplasia or carcinoma in situ.
Stage I	Tumor confined to the corpus uteri.
Stage IA	Tumor limited to the endometrium.
Stage IB	Invasion to up to one-half of the myometrium.
Stage IC	Invasion to more than one-half of the myometrium.
Stage II	Invasion of the cervix but not extending beyond the uterus.
Stage IIA	Endocervical glandular involvement only.
Stage IIB	Cervical stromal invasion.
Stage III	Local and/or regional spread.
Stage IIIA	Tumor invasion of the serosa and/or adnexa and/or malignant cells in ascites or peritoneal washings.
Stage IIIB	Vaginal involvement.
Stage IIIC	Metastases to the pelvic and/or paraaortic lymph nodes.
Stage IV	
Stage IVA	Tumor invasion of the bladder mucosa or the rectum and/or the bowel mucosa.
Stage IVB	Distant metastasis, including metastasis to intraabdominal lymph nodes other than paraaortic and/or inguinal lymph nodes.

ovary, vagina, or other pelvic organs and occurs in 5 to 10% of patients. The disease can also spread along the uterine cavity to the cervix, invade the uterine wall, or spread through the fallopian tubes. Cells are usually disseminated by way of the endometrial lymphatics to the pelvic and paraaortic lymph nodes and less frequently through the bloodstream. Distant metastases can occur in the lungs, inguinal and supraclavicular lymph nodes, liver, bone, and brain (26).

Prognosis

Endometrial cancer is highly curable when it is diagnosed early, and the stage of the disease at diagnosis has a direct influence on survival. The FIGO staging classification is based on a surgical staging system and is illustrated in Table 86.8. Patients with stage 0 disease have a 5-year survival rate of 100%, and patients with stage I disease have a 75 to 100% 5-year survival rate. Survival decreases as the cancer spreads outside the endometrium. The 5-year survival rate is up to 60% for stage II disease, up to 30% for stage III disease, and up to 5% for stage IV disease. Other factors that influence prognosis include histologic type and grade, depth of myometrial invasion, lymph node metastases, advanced age, and positive peritoneal cytology. Papillary, clear-cell, and squamous-cell carcinomas are associated with a less favorable prognosis. Patients with well-differentiated tumors (grade 1) tend to have disease that remains in the endometrium only or is limited to the uterine corpus. Less-differentiated tumors (grade 2 and 3) are more likely to have extrauterine spread and lymph node metastases. The greater the depth of myometrial invasion, the greater the probability of lymph node metastases and decreased survival regardless of histologic grade. Cervical involvement also increases the probability of lymph node metastases. More recent studies have found progesterone receptor levels, DNA ploidy, and proliferative activity (S-phase fraction) to be useful in identifying patients who are at high risk for extrauterine metastases (41, 42).

Treatment

SURGERY

Surgery is the treatment of choice for patients with early-stage endometrial cancer. Patients with stage I disease undergo a total abdominal hysterectomy and bilateral salpingo-oophorectomy with peritoneal cytology. Sampling of pelvic and paraaortic lymph nodes is indicated if the tumor is deeply invasive or for grade 2 and 3 tumors. It should be performed in all patients with stage II carcinoma. Patients with localized disease and well-differentiated tumors are usually curable, and no post-operative treatment is indicated if lymph nodes are negative (43).

RADIATION

Patients with stage I disease who are medically inoperable or who refuse surgery can be treated with radiation alone. Radiation is also indicated after surgery for stage I patients who have deeply invasive or high-grade tumors and in patients with stage II disease because of the high risk of extrauterine spread. These patients receive external radiation to the pelvic at a dose of about 4,000 to 5,000 cGy over a period of 5 to 7 weeks. The paraaortic lymph nodes are also irradiated if they are positive. This course of radiation may be supplemented with intracavitary radiation (brachytherapy) to increase the total dose of radiation to the primary tumor, depending on the status of the cervix. There appears to be no difference in results between preoperative and postoperative radiation. Advantages of preoperative radiation include irradiating while the uterus has an intact blood supply and reducing the tumor mass that will be surgically removed. However, postoperative radiation allows prior staging to identify patients with risk factors for recurrent disease and to determine prognosis (42). Most patients with stage II disease are not candidates for initial surgery and are treated with external pelvic irradiation and intracavitary radiation with subsequent hysterectomy for persistent disease. Patients who have more advanced disease are usually managed with whole abdominal radiation alone and paraaortic radiation if these nodes are positive.

SYSTEMIC THERAPY

Hormonal Therapy. The normal endometrium contains receptors to both estrogen and progesterone and is very sensitive to both. Progesterone exerts a maturational effect, and progestins have been used to treat advanced or

Table 86.9.
Single-Agent Chemotherapy in Endometrial Cancer[a]

Drug	Overall Response (%)
Alkylating agents	
Cyclophosphamide	11
Ifosfamide	10
Hexamethylmelamine	17
Antimetabolites	
5-Fluorouracil	21
Methotrexate	6
Plant alkaloids	
Vincristine	16
Antitumor antibiotics	
Doxorubicin	26
Epirubicin	26
Platinum compounds	
Cisplatin	25
Carboplatin	29

[a]Modified from (45).

recurrent endometrial cancer because of their systemic activity and low-grade toxicity. Responses to these agents are correlated with the presence and level of progesterone receptors. They are best suited for patients with a low tumor burden and for low-grade tumors. Agents that have been studied include medroxyprogesterone acetate, megesterol, and hydroxyprogesterone with no appreciable difference in response. Response rates of 15 to 30% have been documented, but almost all patients will eventually experience disease progression. Tamoxifen has also been studied as a single agent or in combination with progestins, with an overall response rate of approximately 20%. Like progestin therapy, responses are higher in patients with low-grade tumors and positive hormone receptors. Its use may be questioned now because of the association of endometrial cancer with chronic tamoxifen therapy in patients taking the drug for breast cancer. Hormonal therapy has not substantially altered long-term survival in patients with advanced or recurrent disease (44, 45).

Chemotherapy. Chemotherapy is most commonly used as salvage therapy in patients with advanced or recurrent disease. The single agents that have the best-documented activity in endometrial cancer include doxorubicin, cisplatin, and carboplatin. Other single agents with significant activity are listed in Table 86.9. Most responses are partial, and duration of response averages only 3 to 6 months (46). Paclitaxel has also produced some activity in early clinical trials and may show promise in this disease. Various combination chemotherapy regimens have been evaluated, most of them containing doxorubicin. These combination regimens have produced response rates of up to 60% in patients with advanced or recurrent disease, but again the duration of response has been short. There is some data indicating that disease-free survival may be extended with

Table 86.10.
Commonly Used Chemotherapeutic Agents in Gynecological Cancers

Drug	Dose	Dose Adjustment	Toxicity	Comments
Cisplatin	50–100 mg/m² i.v.	Reduce or avoid if CrCl < 50 mL/min	Nephrotoxicity, peripheral neuropathy, ototoxicity, severe nausea/vomiting	May potentiate other nephrotoxic drugs; vigorous hydration decreases risk of nephrotoxicity.
Carboplatin	300–400 mg/m² i.v.	Reduce if CrCl < 60 mL/min; avoid if CrCl < 16 mL/min	Myelosuppression	Does not require vigorous hydration like cisplatin, so can be given easily in an outpatient setting.
Cyclophosphamide	500–1000 mg/m² i.v.	Reduce if CrCl < 50 mL/min	Hemorrhagic cystitis, myelosuppression	Hydration will decrease risk of hemorrhagic cystitis.
Ifosfamide	1000–1500 mg/m²/day for 5 days with MESNA		Hemorrhagic cystitis, myelosuppresion, CNS toxicity	Hemorrhagic cystitis common at doses > 1 g if not administered with MESNA and hydration
Doxorubicin	40–50 mg/m² i.v.	Reduce if bilirubin > 1.5; avoid if bilirubin > 5	Myelosuppression, stomatitis, cardiotoxicity	Vesicant; cardiac toxicity is cumulative and more common at doses > 550 mg/m² or less with chest radiation, other cardiotoxic drugs, or older patients.
Altretamine (hexamethylmelamine)	150–260 mg/m²/day p.o. for 14 or 21 days in a 28-day cycle		Nausea and vomiting, peripheral neuropathy	GI toxicity can be reduced by giving the dose after meals.
Paclitaxel	135–175 mg/m² i.v.		Neutropenia, peripheral neuropathy, alopecia	Hypersensitivity reactions may be due to cremophor vehicle and reduced with appropriate premedications (see text).
Tamoxifen	20 mg p.o. b.i.d.		Hot flashes, fluid retention, vaginal discharge, irregular menses	Associated with an increased risk of endometrial cancer.

°MESNA is sodium 2-mercaptoethanesulfonate but is not referred to as such.

the combination of cisplatin and doxorubicin, but survival is similar to that of doxorubicin alone (44, 46). Hormones in combination with chemotherapy have not enhanced response rates, but the combination of radiosensitizing chemotherapy (e.g., fluorouracil, cisplatin) and radiation therapy has shown some beneficial results in preliminary studies (42). As there is a high incidence of significant additive toxicity with these regimens and unclear superiority over single-agent therapy, these patients should probably be considered for clinical trials.

SUMMARY

Endometrial, cervical, and ovarian cancers are the most commonly occurring gynecologic cancers. Although endometrial cancer is the most common, it is also the most curable because of early detection of the disease. Conversely, ovarian cancer has the lowest incidence of the three, yet it is the leading cause of gynecologic cancer deaths, since it is usually not detected until the disease has advanced. Improvements in the management of gynecologic cancers have centered on early diagnosis rather than innovative treatment. Surgery still represents the treatment of choice in early disease. However, new uses of chemotherapeutic agents and combined modality treatment have improved the outcome in patients with advanced disease.

REFERENCES

1. Boring CC, Squires TS, Tong T, et al. Cancer statistics 1994. CA 44:9–26, 1994.
2. Young RC, Perez C, Hoskins WJ. Cancer of the ovary. In: Devita VT, Hellman S, Rosenberg SA. Cancer Principles and practice of oncology. 4th ed. Philadelphia: JB Lippincott, 1993:1126–1263.
3. Piver MS, Baker TR, Piedmonte M, et al. Epidemiology and etiology of Ovarian Cancer. Sem Oncol 18:177–185, 1991.
4. Rossing MA, Daling JR, Weiss NS, et al. Ovarian tumors in a cohort of infertile women. N Eng J Med 331:771–776, 1994.
5. Hoskins WJ. Surgical staging and cytoreductive surgery of epithelial ovarian cancer. Cancer 71:1534–1540, 1993.

6. Deppe G and Malviya VK. Ovarian cancer: advances in management. Surg Clin North Am 71:1285–1302, 1991.

7. Mogensen O. Prognostic value of CA 125 in advanced ovarian cancer Gynecol Oncol 44:207–212, 1992.

8. Friedlander ML and Dembo AJ. Prognostic factors in ovarian cancer. Sem Oncol 18:205–212, 1991.

9. Omura GA, Brady MF, Homesley HD, et al. Long-term follow-up and prognostic factor analysis in advanced ovarian carcinoma: the gynecologic oncology group experience. J Clin Oncol 9:1138–1150, 1991.

10. McQuire WP. Primary treatment of epithelial ovarian malignancies. Cancer 71:1541–1550, 1993.

11. Ozols RF. Treatment of ovarian cancer: current status. Sem Oncol 21(suppl 2):1–9, 1994.

12. Podratz KC and Kinney WK. Second-look operations in ovarian cancer. Cancer 71:1551–1558, 1993.

13. Dembo AJ. Epithelial ovarian cancer: the role of radiotherapy. Int J Radiation Oncol Biol Phys 22:835–845, 1992.

14. Vergote IB, Winderen M, De Vos, LN, et al. Intraperitoneal radioactive phosphorus therapy in ovarian carcinoma. Cancer 71:2250–2260, 1993.

15. Sutton G. Chemotherapy of epithelial ovarian cancer: An overview. Clin Obstet Gynecol 37:461–474, 1994.

16. Calvert AH, Newell DR, Gumbrell LA, et al. Carboplatin dosage: prospective evaluation of a simple formula based on renal function. J Clin Oncol 7:1748–1756, 1989.

17. Ovarian Cancer Meta-analysis Project. Cyclophosphamide plus cisplatin versus cyclophosphamide, doxorubicin, and cisplatin chemotherapy of ovarian carcinoma: a meta-analysis. J Clin Oncol 9:1668–1674, 1991.

18. Levin L, Simon R, and Hryniuk W. Importance of multiagent chemotherapy regimens in ovarian carcinoma: dose intensity analysis. J Natl Cancer Inst 85:1732–1742, 1993.

19. Fennelly D, Vahdat L, Schneider J, et al. High-intensity chemotherapy with peripheral blood progenitor support. Sem Oncol 21(suppl 2):21–25, 1994.

20. Thigpen JT, Vance RB and Khansur T. Second-line chemotherapy for recurrent carcinoma of the ovary. Cancer 71:1559–1564, 1993.

21. Runowicz CD, Wiernik PH, Einzig AL, et al. Taxol in ovarian cancer. Cancer 71:1591–1596, 1993.

22. Trimble EL, Adams JD, Vena D, et al. Paclitaxel for platinum-refractory ovarian cancer: results from the first 1,000 patients registered to national cancer institute treatment referral center 9103. J Clin Oncol 11:2405–2410, 1993.

23. Schiller JH, Storer B, Tutsch K, et al. Phase I trial of 3-hour infusion of paclitaxel with or without granulocyte colony-stimulating factor in patients with advanced cancer. J Clin Oncol 12:241–248, 1994.

24. Markman M, Reichman B, Hakes T, et al. Intraperitoneal chemotherapy in the management of ovarian cancer. Cancer 71:1565–1570, 1993.

25. Markman M, Rowinsky E, Hakes T, et al. Phase I trial of intraperitoneal taxol: a Gynecologic Oncology Group Study. J Clin Oncol 10:1485–1491, 1992.

26. Hoskins WJ, Perez CA, Young RC, Gynecological tumors. In: Devita VT, Hellman S, Rosenberg S. Cancer principles and practice of oncology, 4th ed. Philadelphia: JP Lippincott, 1993:1152–1225.

27. Schiffman MH, Bauer HM, Hoover RN, et al. Epidemiologic evidence showing that human papillomavirus infection causes most cervical intraepithelial neoplasia. J Natl Cancer Inst 85:958–964, 1993.

28. Benda JA. Pathology of cervical carcinoma and its prognostic implications. Sem Oncol 21:3–11, 1994.

29. Perez CA, Grigsby PW, Nene SM. Effect of tumor size on the prognosis of carcinoma of the uterine cervix treated with irradiation alone. Cancer 69:2796–2806, 1992.

30. Maiman M, Fruchter RG, Guy L, et al. Human immunodeficiency virus infection and invasive cervical carcinoma. Cancer 71:402–406, 1993.

31. Thigpen T, Vance RB, and Khansur T. Carcinoma of the uterine cervix: current status and future directions. Sem Oncol 21(suppl 2):43–54, 1994.

32. Thomas GM, Stehman FB. Early invasive disease: risk assessment and management. Sem Oncol 21:17–24, 1994.

33. Marcial VA, Marcial LV. Radiation therapy of cervical cancer. Cancer 71:1438–1445, 1993.

34. Calkins A, Stitt JA, Fowler JF. New approaches to radiation therapy in locally advanced carcinoma of the cervix. Sem Oncol 21:42–46, 1994.

35. Park RC, Thigpen JT. Chemotherapy in advanced and recurrent cervical cancer: a review. Cancer 71:1446–1450, 1993.

36. Rose PG. Locally advanced cervical carcinoma: the role of chemo-radiation. Sem Oncol 21:47–53, 1994.

37. Gurpide E. Endometrial cancer: biochemical and clinical correlates. J Natl Cancer Inst 83:405–416, 1991.

38. Malfetano JH. Tamoxifen-associated endometrial carcinoma in postmenopausal breast cancer patients. Gynecol Oncol 39:82–84, 1990.

39. Fanning J, Piver MS. Serial CA 125 levels during chemotherapy for metastatic or recurrent endometrial cancer. Obstet Gynecol 77:278–280, 1991.

40. Gordon MD, Ireland K. Pathology of hyperplasia and carcinoma of the endometrium. Sem Oncol 21:64–70, 1994.

41. Homesley HD, Zaino R. Endometrial cancer: prognostic factors. Sem Oncol 21:71–78, 1994.

42. Rotman M, Aziz H, Halpern J, et al. Endometrial carcinoma: influence of prognostic factors on radiation management. Cancer 71:1471–1479, 1993.

43. Creasman WT. Limited Disease: role of surgery. Sem Oncol 21:79–83, 1994.

44. Moore TD, Phillips PH, Nerenstone SR, et al. Systemic treatment of advanced and recurrent endometrial carcinoma: current status and future directions. J Clin Oncol 9:1071–1088, 1991.

45. Lentz SS. Advanced and recurrent endometrial carcinoma: hormonal therapy. Sem Oncol 21:100–106, 1994.

46. Muss HB. Chemotherapy of metastatic endometrial cancer. Sem Oncol 21:107–113, 1994.

CHAPTER 87

SKIN CANCERS AND MELANOMAS

LAURA BOEHNKE-MICHAUD

The skin is the largest organ in the human body. It is comprised of the epidermis, dermis, and subcutaneous tissues. It performs many functions, including protection from the environment, synthesis of vitamin D, thermoregulation, and transmission of sensations of touch and temperature. Several different cell and tissue types make up the skin and its appendages (hair follicles and apocrine, eccrine, and sebaceous glands). These components can transform to produce many different benign and malignant tumors (see Table 87.1) (1). This chapter focuses on the most common and most life-threatening skin cancers: basal cell carcinoma (BCC), squamous cell carcinoma (SCC), and cutaneous malignant melanoma (CMM).

NONMELANOMA SKIN CANCERS

Epidemiology

Nonmelanoma skin cancer (NMSC) is the most common cancer in the United States and many other countries (e.g., Australia, New Zealand, United Kingdom). Basal cell carcinomas (BCC) and squamous cell carcinomas (SCC) in the United States are estimated to account for more than 800,000 new cases annually (2). The annual mortality rate from these cancers in the United States approaches 2100 deaths (2). These numbers are believed to be grossly underestimated because most cases of skin cancer are managed in a private clinic setting and are subsequently not recorded with tumor registries. Studies designed to investigate underreporting have been done in Australia and the United Kingdom and show that the incidence of NMSC is significantly underestimated in these countries (3, 4). Tumor registries divide skin cancers into two broad categories: NMSC and melanoma. This is inadequate; there is data to support that NMSCs behave differently from one another.

Etiology

UV RADIATION AND SKIN TYPE

Several factors have been determined to influence the incidence of skin cancer (see Table 87.2). Two major factors are ultraviolet (UV) radiation exposure and skin type. UV light is subdivided by wavelength into UV-A, UV-B, and UV-C. These divisions and the wavelengths involved are shown in Figure 87.1. This figure also shows the penetration of the skin by each different type of UV light and how the ozone layer protects the earth. UV-A and UV-B are considered harmful to humans, but their effects on biologic systems are still being characterized. UV-B consists of shorter wavelengths, is absorbed by the skin, and is responsible for sun-induced erythema, photoaging, and photocarcinogenesis. UV-A light is not absorbed by the ozone layer, penetrates deep into the dermal layer of the skin, and can produce erythema, immediate pigment darkening and delayed melanogenesis, and elastosis and other dermal connective tissue damage.

The amount of UV light reaching the earth's surface at any given place depends on several factors (see Table 87.3). The ozone layer determines the amount of UV-B light that penetrates the atmosphere. Many theories attribute the rise in skin cancer incidence over the past two decades to the "hole" in the ozone layer and changes in life-style (i.e., increased recreational sun exposure and decreased clothing requirements) (3). However, these assumptions have not been proven in any study to date.

Latitude is another factor that determines the amount of UV radiation that reaches the earth's surface. The incidence of skin cancer is greater in Australia than in Scandinavia; although the populations' skin colors are similar, the latitude and UV light exposure are different (1). UV light is most intense at midday and at the equator because the light has a shorter path through the earth's atmosphere (see Figure 87.2). Seasonal differences in UV radiation exist; UV radiation is most intense during the summer months when the sun is closest to the earth. Altitude also plays a role in UV radiation exposure. For every 1000 feet increase in elevation, there is a 4% increase in direct UV radiation exposure (5). Different reflective surfaces influence the amount of UV radiation exposure; sand and snow have the greatest reflective properties.

Skin type is a key factor influencing the effects of UV radiation on humans. Skin types are divided into six types based on sunburning and tanning history (see Table 87.4) (1). Types I and II have the highest risk for skin cancers. In contrast to whites, skin cancers are rare in blacks, and SCCs are more prevalent than BCCs (6). It is known that older age, freckling, and blue eyes also increase the risk for both BCC and SCC (3). SCC and BCC are most common on sun-exposed areas of the body (e.g., head, neck, and dorsum of the hands). As chronic sun exposure has changed from occupational to recreational, younger patients are being diagnosed with skin cancers. For SCC, total cumulative exposure to UV light is the primary risk factor. For

Table 87.1.
Selected Types of Skin Tumors[a]

Tumors Arising in the Epidermis	Tumors Arising in the Dermis or Subcutis
Kerotinocytic tumors	Fibrous or connective tissue tumors
Benign	Benign
Seborrheic keratosis	Dermatofibroma
Epidermal nevi	Keloid (hypertrophic scars)
Clear cell acanthoma	Malignant
Premalignant	Dermatofibrosarcoma protuberans
Actinic keratoses	berans
Large cell acanthoma	Atypical fibroxanthoma
Chondrodermatitis nodularis	Neural sheath tumors
helicis	Neurofibroma
Malignant	Neurofibromatosis
Basal cell carcinoma	Malignant neurofibroma
Squamous cell carcinoma	Vascular tumors
Tumors of Merkel's cells	
Tumors of Langerhans cells	
Tumors of melanocytic origin	
Benign	
Melanocytic nevi	
Premalignant	
Dysplastic nevi	
Malignant	
Malignant melanoma	
Tumors of epidermal appendages	
Tumors of hair follicles	
Tumors of sebaceous glands	
Tumors of apocrine glands	
Tumors of eccrine glands	

[a]For a complete list of skin tumors, see Safai (1).
Source: Adapted from (1).

Table 87.2.
Causal Factors For NMSC

UV radiation
Chemicals[a]
Chronic inflammation
Immunosuppression
Viruses[a]
Genetic factors

[a]Questionable etiologic relationship with NMSCs (see text).

BCC, risk is better correlated with the tendency to sunburn (i.e., skin type). Increases in recreational UV radiation exposure are believed to contribute to the rising incidence of skin cancer in the United States. The increased incidence is also believed to be related to decreased clothing requirements, stemming from a changing society that values tanning.

CHEMICAL CARCINOGENESIS

There are three stages of progression for chemical carcinogenesis: initiation, promotion, and carcinogenesis. Basic changes in DNA configuration take place in cells during initiation (i.e., purine and pyrimidine substitutions, dimers, deletions). Cells may progress to malignancy (if promoted effectively) or remain unchanged for life. The cells must be completely initiated for promotion to occur. Promoters cause reversible inflammation and hyperplasia. Chemical carcinogenesis was first reported in chimney sweeps of the 1700s who acquired scrotal SCC secondary to arsenic that was present in the soot of chimneys (1). Most chemical carcinogenesis data have been established from studies involving laboratory animals and are not always applicable to humans. There are several chemicals that act as initiators and promoters and may influence the risk of cancer. Tar, a compound that contains polycyclic aromatic hydrocarbons and is used to treat psoriasis, acts as an initiator. Benzoyl peroxide, used to treat acne, is a known promoter. Many other agents that are used to treat skin disorders are initiators and promoters, but long-term use of these agents has never been associated with increased incidence of malignancy (1). The two-hit theory (initiation and promotion) is accepted by scientists worldwide and seems to explain why these products are not associated with increased incidence of cancer.

CHRONIC INFLAMMATION AND IRRITATION

Chronic inflammation and irritation can predispose a patient to skin cancer in the affected area. For example, cancers can develop in an area of chronic ulcers and scars of burns. Betel nuts and chewing tobacco cause chronic irritation of the mucosal surface of the mouth and can cause SCC of the oral cavity and lip (1).

IMMUNOSUPPRESSION

Chronic UV-B exposure produces changes in the host immunity by producing generalized defects in antigen-presenting cells and by inducing the formation of suppressor T cells. UV radiation produces changes in both the number and type of Langerhans cells present in human skin (1). This may alter the immune system, allowing development and progression of skin cancers. The most common cancers in renal transplant recipients are NMSC. The incidence of SCC has been shown to be significantly higher in these individuals than in the general population, lesions developing about 3 to 5 years after transplantation. The ratio of SCC to BCC in the general population was 0.2:1 and 2.3:1 in a Toronto study of 523 renal transplant recipients (7). These factors lead us to believe that immunosuppression plays a role in the development of skin cancers, but the exact relation between UV radiation and the immune system is not well understood.

VIRAL ONCOGENESIS

There is some evidence that the presence of human papillomavirus (HVP) may be associated with an increased risk of cutaneous malignancies. HPV 5, 8, 14, 16, 17, and 33 have been associated with various epidermal carcinomas

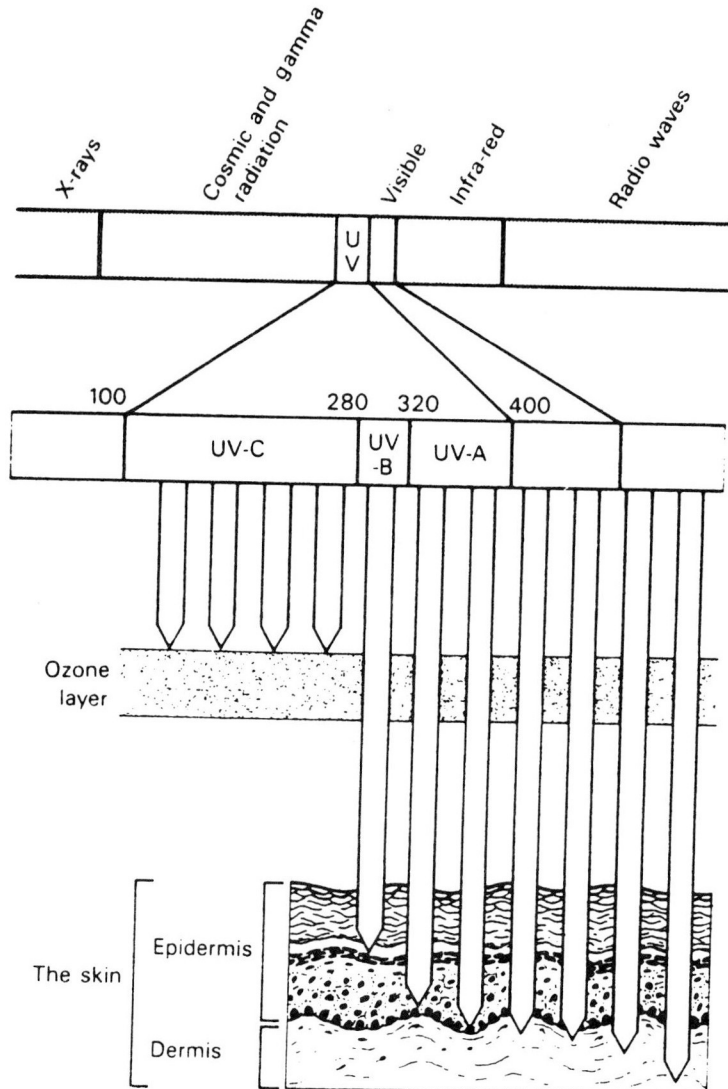

Figure 87.1. Solar electromagnetic spectrum showing depth of penetration of radiation into the skin. (Source: Reprinted with permission from Emmett AJJ, O'Rourke MGE, eds. Malignant skin tumours. New York: Churchill Livingstone, 1991:24.)

Table 87.3.
Factors Influencing UV Radiation Exposure

Amount of ozone
Latitude
Altitude
Reflective surfaces
Time of day
Season of the year
Occupation
Recreational activities
Clothing requirements (styles)

and carcinoma of the cervix (1). These appear to be oncogenic, but conclusive evidence of causality is not available.

GENETIC FACTORS

Many genetic syndromes have been associated with increased incidence of skin neoplasms. These genoderma-

toses are listed in Table 87.5. Laboratory data with human epidermal cell lines indicate that prolonged UV radiation can cause accumulation of DNA injuries and can ultimately be both mutagenic and carcinogenic to affected cells (8). Patients with xeroderma pigmentosum are known to be extremely susceptible to UV radiation-induced cancers secondary to a defect in the DNA excision repair mechanism, supporting the theory that photodamage to DNA plays a major role in UV radiation-induced carcinogenesis (1).

BASAL CELL CARCINOMA

Basal cell carcinoma represents 75 to 80% of all reported cases of nonmelanoma skin cancer (1). BCC is less invasive than SCC and rarely metastasizes, with a mortality rate of 0.12 per 100,000. The morbidity from BCC may profoundly affect the lives of these individuals with disfiguring lesions and scars from treatment. It is most commonly

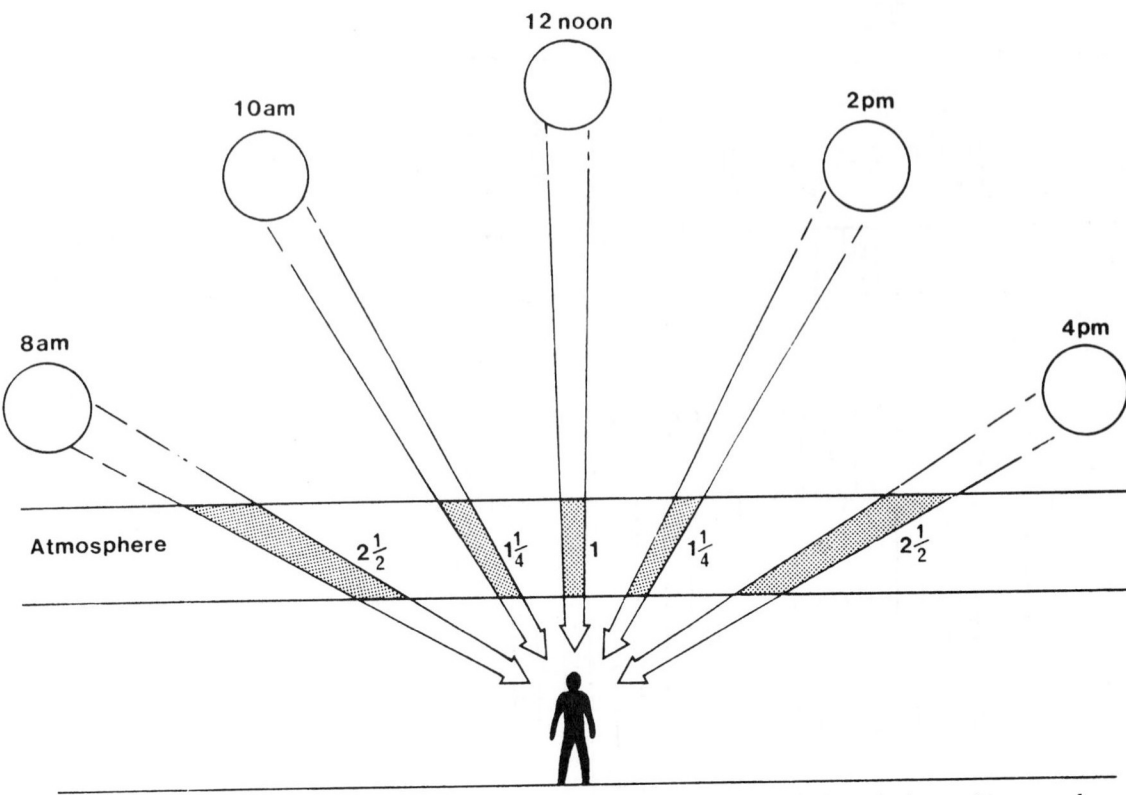

Figure 87.2. The stronger sun at midday and at the equator is related to a shorter path through the earth's atmosphere. (Source: Reprinted with permission from Emmett AJJ, O'Rourke MGE, eds. Malignant skin tumours. New York: Churchill Livingstone, 1991:7.)

Table 87.4.
Skin Types

Skin Type	Sunburning and Tanning History	Skin Color
I	Always burns, never tans	White
II	Always burns, minimal tanning	White
III	Burns often, tans gradually	Light brown
IV	Burns minimally, tans well	Moderate brown
V	Burns rarely, tans profusely	Dark brown
VI	Never burns, deeply pigmented	Black

Source: Adapted from (1).

associated with chronic sun (UV light) exposure in fair-skinned, elderly people. BCC rarely occurs under the age of 40 (although it is becoming more common). The incidence among younger people is similar, but older males have twice the incidence that females have (9). The most common sites for BCC are the face and the head and neck area (6).

Clinical Presentation

BCC arises from the basal layer of cells in the epidermis and its appendages. Malignant basal cells are not able to mature into keratinocytes and retain their ability to divide beyond the basal layer, becoming a bulky neoplasm. BCC

Table 87.5.
Genodermatoses Associated with Cancers of the Skin

Genodermatoses	Associated Skin Cancers
Xeroderma pigmentosum	Basal cell and squamous cell carcinomas
	Malignant melanomas
Basal cell nevus syndrome	Basal cell carcinomas
Familial dysplastic nevus syndrome	Malignant melanomas
Multiple self-healing epithelioma of Ferguson-Smith	Squamous cell carcinomas
Torre's syndrome	Sebaceous adenomas
	Sebaceous carcinomas
	Basal cell carcinomas
Cowden's syndrome	Hair follicle tumors
Gardner's syndrome	Cutaneous cysts (may progress to carcinoma)
Carney's syndrome	Myxomas (benign connective tissue tumor)

begins as a slow-growing, shiny, skin-colored to pink, firm, well-circumscribed, raised, dome-shaped papule (see Table 87.6). As the nodule increases in size, its center may become ulcerated, surrounded by a pearly, rolled border. Telangiectasia (a localized collection of distended blood capillaries) is often seen on the surface of the lesion. There

Table 87.6.
Characteristics of BCC and SCC

Type of NMSC	Clinical Characteristics	Site[a]	Treatment Choices[b]
BCC			
Noduloulcerative	Most common BCC (45%) Usually asymptomatic Center may become ulcerated with pearly, rolled border Multiple lesions may appear simultaneously	Nose Head and neck Trunk	C&E, Cryo, Surg, Moh's (high-risk anatomic site, aggressive clinical or histologic pattern, or > 2–3 cm)
Superficial	Dry, erythematous, scaly patches Surrounded by a fine, threadlike pearly border Associated with arsenic ingestion or exposure	Trunk Head and neck	C&E, Cryo, Surg, TC, XRT, Moh's (for multicentric or > 2–3 cm)
Pigmented	Similar presentation to noduloulcerative Dark brown pigment More common in people with dark complexion Associated with arsenic ingestion or exposure	Nose Head and neck Trunk	C&E, Cryo, Surg, Moh's (high risk anatomic site, aggressive clinical or histologic pattern, or > 2–3 cm)
Morpheaform	Flat to slightly depressed, sclerotic yellow plaques Ill-defined borders Telangiectasia most common with these lesions Ulceration not common Resistant to radiotherapy and electrodesiccation	Nose Head and neck Trunk	Surg, Moh's
Keratotic (basosquamous)	Features of both BCC and SCC Tumor keratinizes More aggressive than other types of BCC Most likely to metastasize	Ear (pre- & post-auricular sulcus)	Surg, Moh's
SCC			
Invasive	More invasive than BCC Associated with AK Firm, erythematous nodule may contain ulceration and/or telangiectasias Can arise in mucous membranes also	Upper extremities Trunk	Surg, XRT, Moh's

[a]Listed in descending order of frequency.
[b]C&E = curettage and electrodesiccation; Cryo = cryotherapy; Surg = surgical excision; Moh's = Moh's micrographic surgery; XRT = radiotherapy; TC = topical chemotherapy; Chemo = systemic chemotherapy.

are five major classifications of BCC: noduloulcerative, superficial, pigmented, morpheaform, and keratotic (basosquamous). Figure 87.3 is an illustration of the most common type of BCC: noduloulcerative.

The most common type of BCC is noduloulcerative, representing approximately 45% (10). The most common site of noduloulcerative BCC is the face, especially the nose. The head and neck area and the upper trunk are also common sites. Multiple lesions may appear simultaneously on any part of the body (1, 6).

Superficial BCC is the second most common type and manifests as dry, erythematous, scaly patches surrounded by a fine, threadlike pearly border. In contrast to noduloulcerative, pigmented, and morpheaform BCC, superficial BCC appears predominantly on the trunk. Superficial BCC, like pigmented BCC, may be associated with arsenic ingestion or exposure (6).

Pigmented BCC is similar in presentation to noduloulcerative BCC, except for the presence of a pigment (brown, black, or blue) within the lesion. This type of BCC is most often seen in people with dark complexions. This type of lesion may be associated with arsenic in-

gestion or exposure (6) and is most common on the head, neck, and face areas.

Morpheaform BCC manifests as solitary, flat or slightly depressed, sclerotic yellow plaques with ill-defined borders and are the rarest form of BCC. Telangiectasia is most common with these lesions, and ulceration is uncommon. This type of BCC is resistant to radiotherapy and electrosurgery and should be treated with surgical excision or Moh's micrographic surgery (see the section on melanoma).

Basosquamous cell carcinomas have biologic behavior and pathologic features that represent both BCC and SCC (1). This type of tumor keratinizes, is more aggressive in its growth, and is the most likely of all the BCCs to metastasize (10).

Staging

Staging of these lesions is based on the TNM staging system adopted by the American Joint Committee on Cancer (AJCC). Since BCC so rarely metastasizes even to local lymph nodes, size has been the most important factor for prognosis and treatment (see Table 87.7) (11). Most

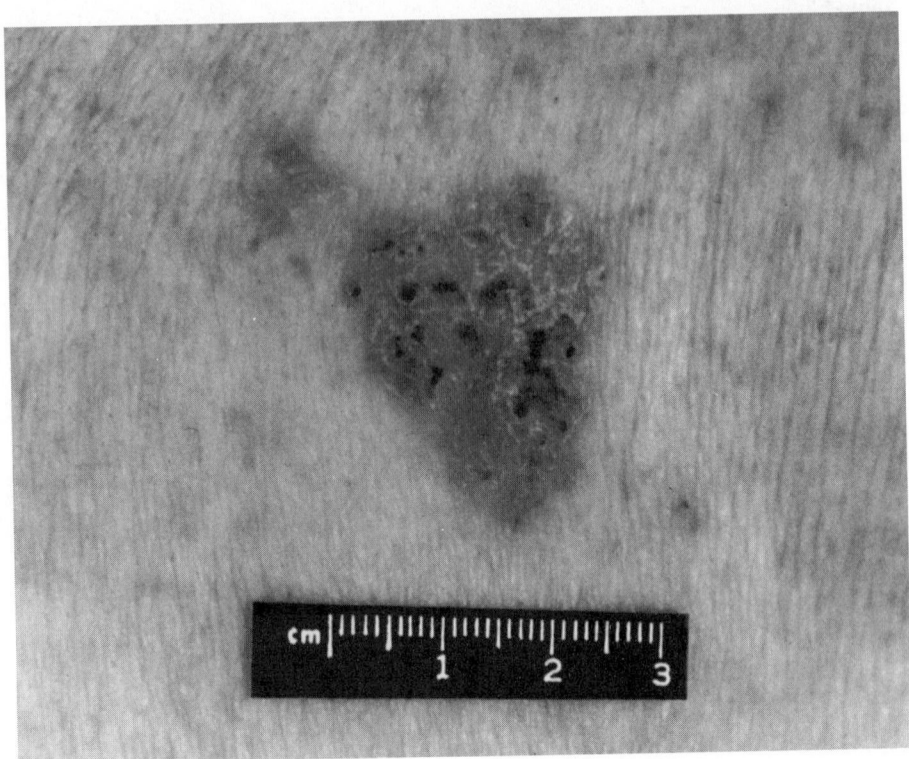

Figure 87.3. Noduloulcerative basal cell carcinoma.

Table 87.7.
AJCC Staging for BCC and SCC

Stage	Tumor (T)[a]	Nodes (N)[b]	Metastases (M)[c]
0	Tis	N0	M0
I	T1	N0	M0
II	T2	N0	M0
	T3	N0	M0
III	T4	N0	M0
	Any T	N1	M0
IV	Any T	Any N	M1

[a]Tis = Carcinoma in situ; T1 = <2 cm; T2 = 2–5 cm; T3 = >5 cm; T4 = invades extradermal structures.
[b]N0 = no regional lymph node metastases; N1 = regional lymph node metastases.
[c]M0 = no distant metastases; M1 = distant metastases.

BCCs present as T1 lesions (<2 cm). Secondary to neglect, many lesions will grow to be very large (T3, >5 cm) and may invade underlying structures. On entering the bone or blood circulation, BCC will metastasize. There have been approximately 300 reported cases of metastatic BCC in the world literature to date (1).

Prognosis

The incidence of recurrent lesions depends on the size of the lesion and the length of follow-up. Large BCC (≥2 cm) have a higher recurrence rate than do smaller tumors. Rowe and colleagues reported that 33% of BCC recurrences occurred within 1 year after treatment, 66% within

3 years, and 82% within 5 years (12). Of these recurrences, 18% did not become apparent until 5 to 10 years later; this emphasizes the need for long-term patient follow-up. Up to 70% of metastases occur in regional lymph nodes and can be surgically removed. Distant metastases occur in lungs, bones, liver, and other viscera. The average survival of patients with distant metastases is approximately 10 months. Primary tumor size and resistance of the primary tumor to surgery and radiation increase the propensity for metastases.

SQUAMOUS CELL CARCINOMA

Squamous cell is the second most common skin cancer and represents approximately 20% of all reported cases (1). SCC is more invasive and has a greater propensity for metastasis than does BCC. In 1991, Weinstock and colleagues reported age-adjusted mortality rates in Rhode Island to be 0.26 of 100,000 per year for SCC (13). SCC is most common in whites, and the incidence higher in males than in females. UV radiation is a predisposing factor for SCC. Cumulative sun exposure leads to increased incidence with increasing age. UV-A may play a role in the development of SCC, as may PUVA (psoralen plus UV-A for the treatment of psoriasis) (1). This issue is controversial, with studies also showing no increased risk of SCC with PUVA treatments. More data is needed to determine the true risks.

The presence of actinic keratoses (AK) is a risk factor for SCC. AK are the most common premalignant skin lesions and have histologic similarities to SCC in situ (see the discussion below of pathophysiology). Untreated AK can spontaneously remit, remain stable, or progress to SCC. Studies have estimated that 12 to 25% of patients with AK will eventually develop SCC (1, 9, 14). Studies were completed, controlling for as many risk factors as possible; however, the number of risk factors makes trial design very complex.

SCCs on mucous membranes are most common in individuals who have a history of heavy smoking and alcohol use. Use of chewing tobacco and use of betel nuts are also associated with development of SCC in mucous membranes.

Pathophysiology

SCC is a tumor of the keratinizing cells, arises from stratified squamous epithelium, and grows to invade the dermis. Confined to the epidermal layer, these tumors are defined as SCC in situ. Once they have invaded the dermis, they can track along tissue planes, perichondrium, or periosteum. SCC grows more rapidly than BCC but has similar invasive characteristics, causing tissue destruction. In contrast to BCC, SCC has a much greater potential for regional and distant metastases (1).

Clinical Presentation

SCC appears as a flesh-colored or erythematous raised, firm papule. It may be crusted with keratin products and may ulcerate and bleed in later stages. SCC in an area of AK has somewhat different characteristics from SCC that appears on normal skin (de novo SCC). With an SCC that

arises from an AK, the lesion appears as a plaque or a nodule with a warty scale covering (see Table 87.6). These lesions bleed easily with minor trauma and may have telangiectasias on their surface. De novo SCC may have a slightly raised, indurated border (see Figure 87.4). Invasion can occur and presents as a firm, erythematous nodule with a center core that may be ulcerated. The surface may be smooth or warty and papillomatous and may contain telangiectasias. Infiltrative lesions will often be attached to underlying tissues and cartilage. This is a sign of aggressive tumor growth. SCC occurs most commonly on the face, head, and neck, followed by the upper extremities and trunk. SCC may also present on mucous membranes with squamous epithelium. Lesions often appear in the oral cavity and lip, can invade other structures of the face, and are more likely to metastasize. These present in a similar fashion to SCC on the skin but are often diagnosed at a later stage because they are hidden within the mouth (10).

Staging

The AJCC has identified the TNM staging system as the system to be used for all skin cancers (see Table 87.7) (11). However, for SCC this is inadequate. This formal system takes into account the diameter and depth of invasion, as well as the involvement of cartilage, muscle or bone, but fails to consider other prognostic variables (see below).

Prognosis

The frequency of metastases depends on the anatomic site, histologic features, etiology, host immunosuppression, diameter, and prior treatment. Some factors have more

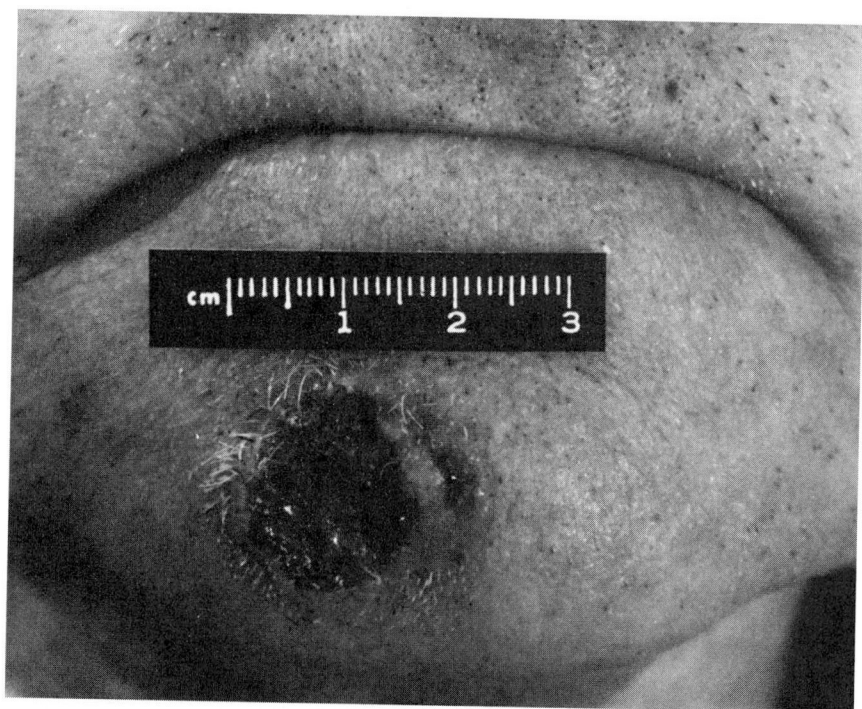

Figure 87.4. De novo squamous cell carcinoma (arising from normal tissue).

Table 87.8.
Management of NMSC

Method	Indications	5-Year DFS[a]	Comments
Curettage and Electrodessication	Superficial and noduloulcerative BCC Anatomic areas with low recurrence rates	77–97% (BCC)	Skilled, experienced practitioners' cure rates 95–97%
Cryotherapy	Best for noculoulcerative and superficial BCC and very superficial SCC Best anatomic locations are eyelid, nose, ear, chest, back, or tip of the nose	95–99% (BCC) 90% (AK)	Lack specimen for pathologic review to check margins Best results with very small tumors (<0.5 cm)
Surgical excision	Best for aggressive or large lesions Wider margins are required for SCC, morpheaform and recurrent BCC	96% (all NMSC)	Skin grafts may be required for wound closure
Moh's micrographic surgery	Lesions in which the border is not well defined Recurrent or morpheaform tumors Large tumors (>2 cm) Incompletely excised tumors Tumors within radiation dermatitis Anatomic areas with high recurrence rates	98% (BCC) 96.50% (recurrent BCC) 93% (SCC)	Very complex, time-consuming procedure Done at only a few institutions Highest DFS
Radiation	Reserved for treatment of lesions not amenable to other treatment modalities Lesions along the embryonal fusion plane Good for lesions on eyelids, periorbital region, medial triangle of cheek, earlobe, and nose	96.4% (BCC) 91.9% (SCC)	Areas of radiation are at higher risk of developing other cutaneous malignancies
Photodynamic therapy (PDT)	Not a treatment of choice yet Investigational treatment	CR[b] 88–100% (Photophrin)	Persistent photosensitivity for 8–10 weeks
Chemotherapy Topical	5-FU only approved agent Treatment of choice for multiple AK Very small superficial BCC (not amenable to other treatment modalities) Elderly patients not eligible for other treatments	79% (superficial BCC)	If used after curettage, recurrence rate is decreased
Systemic	Neoadjuvant combination chemotherapy has been investigated	CR[b] 26% PR[b] 54% (SCC skin or lip)	Not commonly used for NMSC Used in conjunction with other treatments

[a]DFS = disease-free survival.
[b]CR = complete response; PR = partial response.

prognostic significance than others. Mucosal SCC is more aggressive than cutaneous SCC and metastasizes more frequently (1, 14). SCC of the lip has a worse prognosis than cutaneous SCC but a better prognosis than SCC of the penis, scrotum, or anus (14). Histologic features that determine grading of tumor cells have been shown to be of prognostic significance. Tumors with a greater percentage of well-differentiated cells have a better prognosis than do those with a greater percentage of poorly differentiated cells (14). The cause of SCC also determines prognosis. Lesions that occur secondary to immunosuppressive disorders are more likely to metastasize than are lesions appearing secondary to UV light exposure. SCC that arises from chronic lesions, such as scars or ulcers, are associated with higher rates of metastasis than are lesions found on normal skin. Larger primary lesions (diameter > 2 cm) make up the majority of metastatic cases, and lesions that are larger than 1 cm in diameter make up the majority of recurring SCC (14). Depth of invasion of skin cancers can be classified by skin level of deepest invasion. Clark's levels

(I through V), which were initially developed for cutaneous melanomas (see the section on melanoma), have been used to study SCC (14). Depth of invasion can also be measured in millimeters. Not enough data is available to determine whether level of invasion and depth of invasion are independent prognostic variables. Perineural invasion correlates with a poor prognosis (14). The 5-year DFS rates are listed in Table 87.8.

MANAGEMENT OF NMSC

Once the diagnosis has been confirmed with biopsy, the treatment planning begins. Planning requires consideration of the type of skin cancer, anatomic location, size, the patient's general health and age, and whether the lesion is primary, recurrent, or metastatic. Because of its aggressive nature, SCC requires that a wide margin be removed or treated. Basosquamous and morpheaform BCCs have a higher rate of recurrence than do the other types of BCC and are treated more aggressively. The size of a BCC lesion determines the chance of recurrence. Tumors larger than 2 to 3 cm have a worse prognosis than do lesions smaller than 1 cm. The anatomic location of the lesion influences the rate of recurrence. Lesions that are located along the embryonal fusion planes (the midface under the eyes, periauricular and postauricular areas, the paranasal, nasolabial, and inner canthal areas) have the potential for deep invasion and higher recurrence rates (1). Cosmetic results of treatment are considered during planning. A lesion that is located on the eyelids or the tip of the nose will need to have a tissue-sparing treatment (radiation therapy or Moh's micrographic surgery). Regardless of location, the most efficacious treatment should be given (1).

The patient's general health is considered in treatment planning. Patients with coagulopathies will need a less invasive procedure to decrease the risk of bleeding, unless the problem can be corrected before surgery. If travel is a problem (e.g., the patient is elderly or debilitated or has no vehicle), procedures that require one or two office visits are better than those that require 10 to 15 office visits. The chance of infection is higher for immunosuppressed patients and should be considered in treating patients for whom compliance and cleanliness are of concern (1).

Treatment choices include curettage and electrodesiccation, cryotherapy, surgical excision (including Moh's micrographic surgery), radiation therapy, and chemotherapy (topical and systemic). These are listed in Table 87.8.

Curettage and Electrodesiccation

Curettage is performed with a curette, a pencillike instrument with a round or oval tip, sharpened on one side. The tumor is debulked down to the normal tissue; the curette and sound and texture differences are used to distinguish between normal tissue and tumor. The tumor is removed with a 2- to 3-mm margin of normal tissue. Electrodesiccation follows curettage, destroying any tumor cells remaining at the base and periphery of the excision site and producing hemostasis. This procedure uses an electrical current to produce sufficient heat, causing tissue damage at the point of contact. Increasing the amperage (current) causes more heat, deeper penetration, and more tissue damage and scarring (1).

The overall disease-free survival (DFS) rate with this procedure is 77 to 97%. The rate depends on patient selection and practitioner skill in performing the procedure. This procedure should not be used as primary treatment of lesions with more aggressive histology, larger size, longer history, or locations in high-risk anatomic areas. Skilled, experienced practitioners have DFS rates as high as 95 to 97%; less experienced dermatology residents perform less adequately, with higher recurrence rates (1).

Cryotherapy

Cryotherapy uses liquid nitrogen (−195.5°C) to freeze viable tissues. Freezing causes formation of extracellular

and intracellular ice, abnormal concentration and crystallization of electrolytes, and denaturation of lipoprotein complexes that are lethal to the cells (1). A 3- to 5-mm margin is required to maximize the cure rate. The temperature of the tissue is measured with a thermocoupler inserted underneath the tumor. A temperature that is sufficient for cell death is at least −50°C. The tissue is allowed to thaw; then the procedure is repeated for best results (1, 10).

This technique is best suited for patients who have pacemakers or are poor surgical risks. Cryotherapy is most effective in treating lesions that are less than 2 cm and are located on the eyelid, nose, ear, chest, back, or tip of the nose. This is the recommended procedure for recurrent tumors and tumors with well-defined margins. Cryotherapy is not to be used to treat morpheaform BCC, patients with cold intolerance (e.g., cryoglobulinemia, Raynaud's disease), lesions in certain anatomical locations (free margin of the eyelid, vermilion border of the lip, ala nasi, anterior and posterior ear, or scalp), or tumors larger than 3 cm. The adverse reactions that are related to cryotherapy include edema, oozing, erosions, hemorrhaging, and secondary infections. Reepithelialization may take as long as 10 weeks (10). The cosmetic results with cryotherapy are very good with the exception of hypopigmentation and hyperpigmentation. Hyperpigmentation usually fades within a few months after the procedure (1).

The DFS rate with cryotherapy is very high. One study reported a 99% 5-year DFS rate for cryotherapy to treat very small BCCs (most tumors were 0.5 cm or less) (15). Most studies report a recurrence rate of less than 5% when skilled, experienced practitioners perform the procedure (6). One disadvantage is the lack of pathologic evidence of tumor-free margins. The margins are determined by sight only. Tumor cells could be left behind, predisposing the patient to recurrence; therefore, only very superficial lesions should be treated with this technique (1, 6, 14). Use of cryotherapy for actinic keratoses is effective with a few, individual lesions and has a very low recurrence rate (10%) but is not recommended for patients with multiple AK (16).

Surgical Excision

In surgical excisions a scalpel is used to make an elliptical incision, and the entire tumor is removed with a 3- to 5-mm margin for BCC and a margin of several centimeters for SCC. The exact amount of margin required for SCC has not been determined, but it is accepted that wider margins are required for these lesions. For recurrent BCC or morpheaform BCC, a wider margin is used (e.g., 1 cm). Large tumors with deep invasion should also have wider margins removed. Regional lymph node dissection is required only when lymph nodes are clinically palpable. Skin grafts are occasionally required for closure of the wound. These grafts take 5 to 7 days to accept and 2 to 3 months to become mature and cosmetically acceptable. A skin flap, a piece of tissue that is attached on one side to the donor area and carries its own blood supply, is another option for wound closure. The decision to do surgical excision is made after all other available treatment options have been evaluated (1). The DFS rate with surgery alone for NMSC has been reported to be 96% (6, 14). Surgical excision is contraindicated for patients with coagulation disorders unless these disorders are corrected before surgery.

Moh's Micrographic Surgery

Frederick Moh first described this technique in 1930 (1, 10). The procedure is depicted in Figure 87.5. A scalpel is used to make a saucer-shaped excision with a 45° angle to provide a specimen with a beveled edge. A map is drawn to correspond to the specimen removed. The specimen is then divided, numbered, and color-coded on the edges. Corresponding numbers and color codes are marked on the map. Serial frozen sections are performed. The saucer shape and the angled edge allow for viewing of all surfaces. Any remaining tumor is marked on the map, and excision is repeated until the tumor is completely excised. With this procedure, minimal normal skin is sacrificed, and cosmetic results are usually good, depending on the size of the area excised and the anatomic location of the tumor. Occasionally, skin grafts or flaps are required for coverage of very large lesions, but these are not needed as frequently as with surgical excisions (1, 10).

Moh's micrographic surgery is indicated in cases in which the tumor recurrence rate is high (embryonal fusion planes of the midface, nasal area, or periauricular areas), the tumor border is not well defined, or there are recurrent tumors, morpheaform tumors, incompletely excised tumors, large tumors (>2 cm), or tumors within radiation dermatitis. The DFS rate with Moh's micrographic surgery is higher than that with any other treatment modality. The DFS rate has been reported to be 98% for primary BCC,

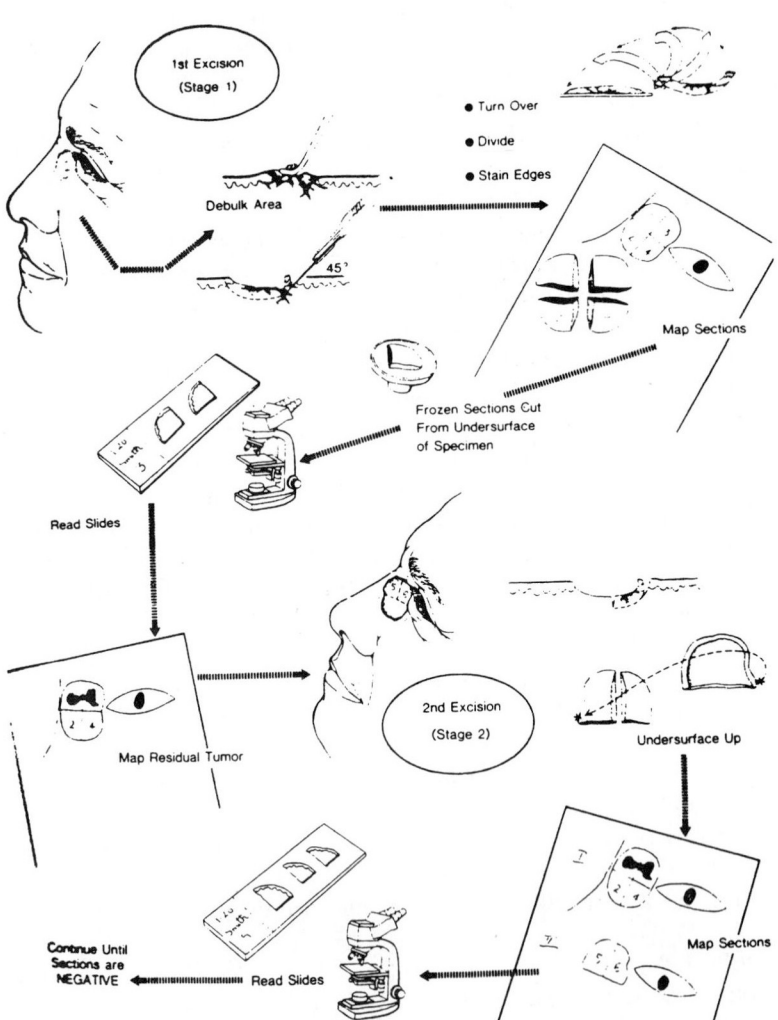

Figure 87.5. Schematic representation of the techniques of Moh's micrographic surgery. (Source: Reprinted with permission from Safai B. Cancers of the skin. In: DeVita VT, Hellman S, Rosenberg SA, eds. Cancer: principles and practice of oncology, 4th ed. Philiadelphia: JB Lippincott, 1993:1602.)

96.5% for recurrent BCC, and 93% for SCC at 5 years (17, 18).

Radiation Therapy

BCC and SCC are radiosensitive tumors. Because of the lack of pathological confirmation of clear margins and radiation-related morbidity, this method is reserved for lesions that are not amenable to other treatment modalities. Patients with tumors located on the eyelids, periorbital region and medial triangle of the cheek, earlobe, and nose are good candidates for radiotherapy. Skin cancers along the embryonal fusion plane can be successfully treated with radiation. This method of treatment is not recommended for treating tumors located on the trunk, extremities, dorsum of the hands, or scalp or those arising in sweat and sebaceous glands. It is also not recommended for tumors that are greater than 8 cm in diameter, morpheaform BCCs, intraoral lesions, or those that occur on the upper lip growing into a nostril. Radiation is a good choice for patients who are poor surgical risks and for palliation of very large tumors in elderly patients (18). DFS with this treatment modality is 96.4% for BCC and 91.9% for SCC. Immediate sequelae are erythema, loss of eyelashes when treating the eyelids, and mucositis when treating the nose. Long-term sequelae include radiation dermatitis that may manifest as atrophy, telangiectasias, hyperpigmentation or hypopigmentation, and precancerous lesions (1). Radiated areas have a higher risk for the development of other skin neoplasms (1, 10). These reasons contribute to the decision to reserve radiation for lesions that are not amenable to other treatment modalities.

Photodynamic Therapy

Photodynamic therapy (PDT) is a new technique for treatment of superficial BCC. This technique uses tumor-sensitizing drugs to selectively target tumor cells in the skin. A light is required to activate the drugs to produce free radical formation and tissue damage. Many agents are under investigation, including porphyrin-, chlorine-, and phthalocyanine-containing substances that produce free radicals when subjected to certain wavelengths of light. The first compound to reach clinical trials, a hematoporphyrin derivative (HPD, Photophrin), is given intravenously and is preferentially taken up by tumor cells. When exposed to light, the Photophrin is activated, and the tumor is killed. Complete response rates with this agent are 88 to 100% in treating BCC (19). Complete response rates with skin metastases have been reported to be 74% with lesions from a variety of primary sites (19). Generalized photosensitivity for 8 to 10 weeks after administration of this agent is a major problem. Newer agents have been developed to circumvent these problems. One agent, 5-aminolevulinic acid, has been applied topically to skin cancer lesions and illuminated with different types of light

sources (19, 20). PDT is not yet the treatment of choice for any cancer, and high recurrence rates make it inferior to other proven modalities of treatment. However, future investigations may prove to target difficult-to-treat or recurrent lesions. Further clinical studies must be done to identify the role of PDT in the treatment of primary and secondary skin cancers.

Chemotherapy

Topical chemotherapy is useful for treatment of precancers and cancers of the skin. The efficacy of topical agents depends on their ability to penetrate the lesion and be absorbed by the target cells. Fluorouracil (5-FU) is the only topical chemotherapy agent to date that has shown efficacy against NMSC and precancerous lesions (e.g., actinic keratoses). This agent is believed to preferentially penetrate sun-damaged skin, in which the protective layer is deficient. Because of its selectivity for rapidly dividing cells, 5-FU has a greater effect on premalignant and malignant cells than on normal cells. 5-FU is an antimetabolite that inhibits the action of thymidylate synthetase. Thymidylate synthetase is the enzyme that is responsible for the methylation of 2-deoxyuridylic acid to thymidylic acid, which is a key step in the synthesis of DNA and cellular reproduction.

Topical 5-FU is the treatment of choice for multiple AK. It must be applied to an entire area of skin and should not be used to "spot-treat" small areas of AK (21). A patient with AK on the face needs to have the entire face treated, not just the visible lesions. This ensures treatment of occult lesions in the affected area. Under special circumstances, superficial BCC can be treated with topical 5-FU. This is not the treatment of choice for these lesions but can be useful for patients who refuse surgery or who are not good surgical candidates. Elderly patients with multiple medical problems are excellent candidates for topical 5-FU. One disadvantage of this treatment choice is the lack of penetration into deep tissues of the dermis. The reported 5-year cumulative recurrence rate for superficial BCC that is treated with 5-FU topical therapy alone is 21% (22). This can be improved if curettage is used as primary treatment to debulk the tumor, resulting in a 6% 5-year cumulative recurrence rate (22). Topical 5-FU is contraindicated for nodular BCC and for all SCC because these lesions are more invasive. Use of 5-FU for treatment of these lesions should be reserved for patients who are not candidates for other therapies. Optimal areas for use of 5-FU are the facial areas, the dorsum of the hand, and the lower extremities. Biopsy should be performed after treatment is complete to ensure that there are no hidden cells that will put the patient at risk for recurrence. Long-term close follow-up is required for all patients with precancers and cancers of the skin but is most important for patients with more aggressive lesions.

Fluorouracil is available topically in a cream or solution (Effudex) in 1%, 2%, and 5% concentrations. Inflammation is a clinical indicator of efficacy and is expected to occur in the cancerous or precancerous area (not in normal skin). Mild to moderate inflammation is sufficient to obtain results. An increase in potency of the agent is required if there is insufficient inflammation at the treatment site. There is no clinical data demonstrating a difference between concentrations if adequate erythema is achieved. 5-FU should be administered once or twice a day for several weeks (2 to 10 weeks). Duration of therapy is determined by the location and type of lesion being treated. Lesions on the dorsum of the hands and the forearms tend to be thicker, requiring longer treatment periods. Certain types of precancerous skin disorders are more aggressive, having a higher rate of recurrence.

5-FU solution is applied with a soft brush; the cream is applied with the fingertip. Using a plastic occlusive dressing can increase the time of contact of 5-FU with the lesion, theoretically increasing the response. This method is useful in treating more aggressive lesions. Concomitant use of topical 13-all-trans-retinoic acid (tretinoin, Retin-A) enhances the effect of 5-FU (21). Steroid cream can be used to alleviate inflammation after treatment is complete without affecting overall response of the tumor (1, 21). Patients will experience photosensitivity while using 5-FU; this reaction is more severe when 5-FU is combined with tretinoin cream. Patients should be instructed to use a sunscreen and to cover with clothing when exposed to sun to prevent severe sunburns. Contact hypersensitivity to the vehicle and to the 5-FU has been reported. This reaction differs from the expected inflammation in that vesicles are seen in the area of contact and itching is reported. The therapeutic manifestations that are experienced with 5-FU are described as burning or stinging, not itching. Extemporaneous compounding of 5-FU with a different vehicle may prevent recurrence of this problem. 5-FU can cause severe irritation of the conjunctiva and nares if it is allowed to enter the eyes or nose (23). Therefore, contact with these areas should be avoided. Patients should wash their hands carefully after applying 5-FU, with instructions not to touch the eyes or nasal membranes while the fingers are still contaminated with 5-FU.

Systemic administration of 5-FU alone or with cisplatin has not been effective in the treatment of BCC. Neoadjuvant therapy is defined as any treatment that is used before definitive local therapy, in hopes of (a) determining sensitivity of the lesion, (b) decreasing the size of the lesion (limiting the amount of tissue that needs to be removed), and (c) decreasing blood flow to the lesion, making surgery less complicated. Large SCC (>5 cm) have been treated neoadjuvantly with combination chemotherapy. Sadek and colleagues, using cisplatin 100 mg/m^2 on day 1, 5-FU 650 mg/m^2/day continuous infusion over 5 days, and bleomycin

15 mg intravenous bolus on day 1 followed by continuous infusion bleomycin (16 mg/m^2/day) over 5 days, showed complete response rates of 26% and partial response rates of 54% in patients with SCC of the skin or lip greater than 5 cm in diameter (24). This strategy may be useful in improving the cosmetic results of therapy and limiting the need for extensive surgery with reconstruction. Systemic chemotherapy has also been used to treat SCC of the mucous membranes. Topical nitrogen mustard and BCNU have been used to successfully treat cutaneous T-cell lymphoma (mycoses fungoides) but are not effective against BCC or SCC.

Immune therapy with intralesional interferon-α (IFN-α) or interleukin-2 (IL-2) has been reported to be effective in treating BCC, SCC, AK, and metastatic lesions of the skin from a variety of cancers (14, 25). The administration of these drugs is required for several weeks to see a response, and the doses that are required have yet to be determined. This therapy is not without side effects. Many of the patients who receive interferon-α experience a flu-like syndrome that is associated with systemic absorption of the drug. These agents may offer an alternative to surgery, but further data is needed to determine the role of these agents in treatment of NMSCs and precancers.

Retinoids are still under clinical investigation both topically and systemically for prevention and treatment of skin cancer. In some malignant cell lines, retinoids induce cell differentiation, inhibit tumor promotion and induction, and may interfere with tumor initiation (26). Retinoids are being studied in both treatment and prevention of a number of human cancers and, being vitamin A analogs, are ideal for study in disorders of the skin. Treatment of AK and BCC with retinoids alone appears to be less effective than standard treatment modalities (26). Robinson and Kligman evaluated topical 5-FU in conjunction with topical tretinoin for treatment of AK. Response rates on the forearms were 25% for 5-FU alone and 100% for combination treatment; response rates on the hands were 0% for 5-FU alone and 90% for combination treatment (26A). Differences in side effects and relapse rates were not commented on in this report, and it has not been substantiated, but it does provide promising results. Chemoprophylaxis has been studied with both systemic and topical retinoids. Prevention of new skin cancer lesions has been reported with oral isotretinoin, oral etretinate, and topical tretinoin administered to patients with genetic dermatoses such as xeroderma pigmentosum and nevoid basal cell carcinoma syndrome (26). The doses that are required to maintain prevention are high, and withdrawal of therapy leads to regression and loss of preventive activity, requiring high-dose, chronic maintenance therapy. These agents may prove to be useful in the future but are currently investigational.

CUTANEOUS MALIGNANT MELANOMA (CMM)

Epidemiology and Risk Factors

Malignant melanoma was estimated to be the seventh most frequently diagnosed cancer in 1995, with an estimated 34,100 new cases (3% of all cancers in the United States). The mortality from melanoma was estimated to be 7200 cases in 1995, accounting for 1.3% of all cancer deaths in the United States (2). Melanoma has increased at a rate faster than that of any other cancer over the past 30 years. In 1935 the estimated lifetime risk of developing melanoma was 1 in 1500. In 1980 this incidence was 1 in 250; in 1985 it was 1 in 135. It is estimated that by the year 2000 the lifetime risk will be 1 in 90 (see Figure 87.6) (27). This increase in incidence is exponential, while the increase in mortality has been linear (see Figure 87.7) (28). This is thought to be due to early detection, secondary to screening programs, which has led to an overall increase in survival. In a study done in Alabama evaluating incidence and mortality of melanoma between 1955 and 1982, an increase in thinner, more curable lesions in the latter years was reported (29).

Whites are more commonly affected by melanomas than are nonwhites. Blacks who are diagnosed with melanoma most commonly have the acral lentiginous form. Skin, hair, and eye color have long been recognized as determinates of risk for melanoma. In a review of the literature, Armstrong and English found a relative risk ranging from 1 to 3 for people with "light" skin color (30). In this same review, they found that red hair, compared to dark brown or black hair, indicates a twofold to fourfold increase in risk and fair hair indicates less than a twofold

increase in risk. The skin's reaction to sunlight is also important in determining risk. People who burn easily rather than tanning, after relatively short exposures to UV light, are at increased risk. Interestingly, people with outdoor occupations do not have an increased risk of melanoma. The only form of melanoma that is associated with cumulative sun exposure has been lentigo maligna melanoma. All other forms of melanoma have been better associated with intermittent sun exposure, especially during childhood. Blistering sunburns during childhood or adolescence have been associated with an increased risk of developing melanoma (31). Excessive intermittent (recreational) UV radiation exposure, in conjunction with light coloring and easy burning from sunlight, seems to be the most important risk factor for developing melanoma.

Freckling, whether in adulthood or childhood, is a risk factor for developing melanoma. Benign melanocytic nevi (moles) are no longer believed to be premalignant lesions. However, people with a higher than average number of moles (more than 20) may be at increased risk for developing melanoma (27). The data in the literature is contradictory as to the number of benign melanocytic nevi that are associated with increased incidence of melanoma (30). Dysplastic nevi are characteristically different from benign melanocytic nevi at the cellular level and, in great number, are associated with a much higher incidence of melanoma than are nondysplastic nevi (see the section on etiology).

People who have had a previous melanoma are at increased risk of developing a second primary melanoma (27). Patients with the familial form of melanoma are at greater risk of developing multiple primary melanomas.

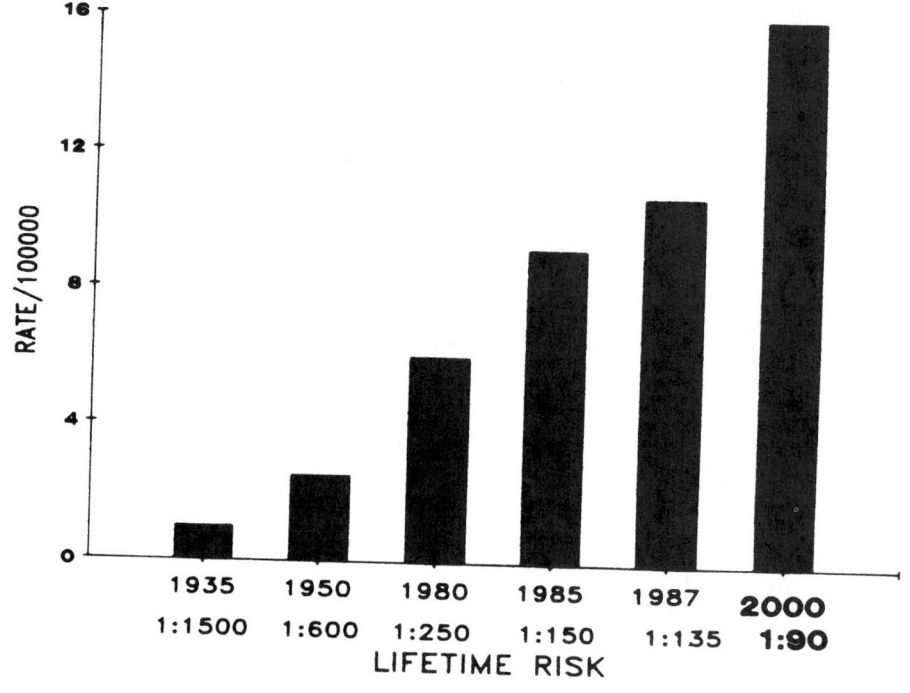

Figure 87.6. Past, current, and projected lifetime risk of a person in the United States developing malignant melanoma. (Source: Reprinted with permission from Rigel DS, Kopf AW, Friedman RJ. The rate of malignant melanoma in the US: are we making an impact? J Am Acad Dermatol 17:1050, 1987.)

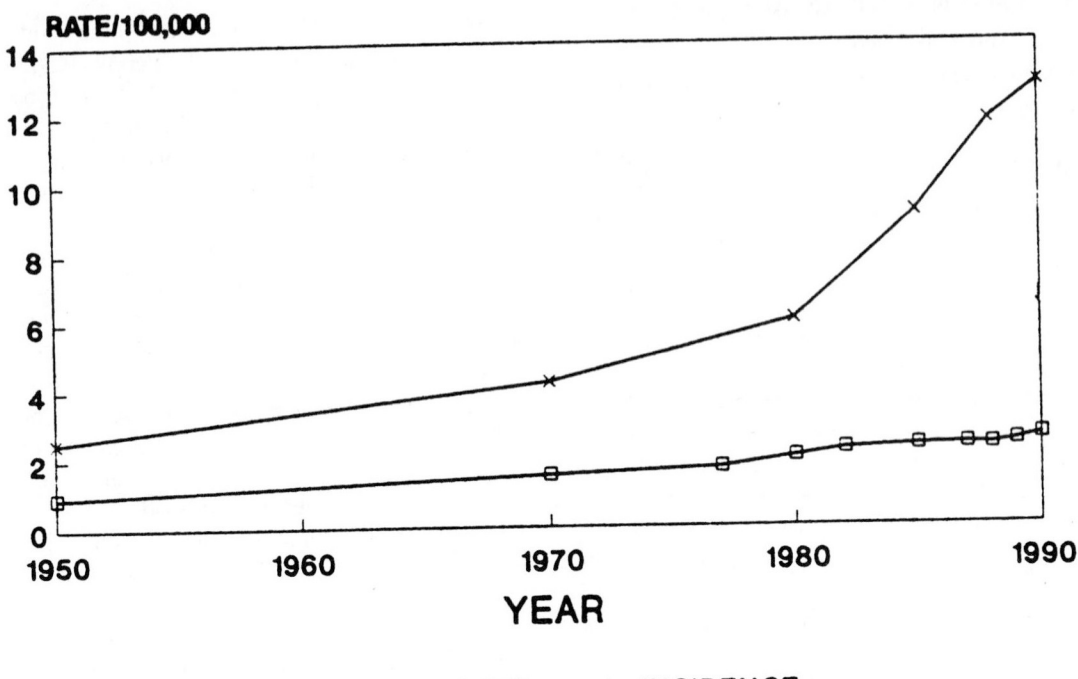

── DEATH RATE   ── INCIDENCE

Figure 87.7. Comparison of melanoma incidence and mortality rates in the United States (1990 figures estimated). (Source: Reprinted with permission from Grin-Jorgensen CM, Rigel DS and Friedman RJ. The worldwide incidence of malignant melanoma. In: Balch CM, Houghton AN, Milton GW, et al. Cutaneous melanoma, 2nd ed. Philadelphia: JB Lippincott, 1992:29.)

However, only 4 to 10% of melanoma patients describe a history of melanoma in a first-degree relative, demonstrating that familial melanoma is uncommon (27, 30). Dysplastic nevus syndrome-familial type is an autosomal dominant hereditary occurrence of melanoma in which patients typically have 10 to 100 pigmented lesions on the trunk, buttocks, and lower extremities and are at increased risk of developing melanoma (27). Xeroderma pigmentosum, a rare autosomal recessive disorder that is characterized by deficient repair of DNA damage caused by UV-B light, is associated with more than a 1000-fold increase in incidence of skin cancer, including melanoma (31). These observations lead us to believe that a relationship exists between the immune system and genetics that determines reactions to melanoma antigens (see the section on etiology).

The median age at diagnosis of melanoma is approximately 45 years of age, much younger than that of most other cancers (27). Melanoma is rare in childhood (< 15 years of age). The peak incidence for most forms of melanoma occurs at approximately 50 years of age and then declines. This distributive pattern of incidence may be related to recreational sun exposure in early adult life, which corresponds to an increased incidence of melanoma in early middle age. This pattern holds true for superficial spreading and nodular melanomas but not for lentigo

Table 87.9.
Risk Factors for CMM

Fair skin/hair coloring
Freckling
Sunburns easily/tans poorly
Blistering sunburns in childhood or adolescence
Indoor occupation/intermittent sun exposure
Personal/family history of melanoma
Benign melanocytic nevi (>20)
Dysplastic nevus

maligna melanomas (LMM). LMM is related to cumulative sun exposure, causing the incidence to increase with age and to become most common in the latter years of life (30). Melanoma incidence does not differ substantially between the sexes. Males have a greater incidence of melanoma on the trunk, and females have a greater incidence on the lower extremities, but the overall incidence is similar (30, 31). Table 87.9 lists the risk factors that are associated with cutaneous malignant melanoma.

Etiology
ULTRAVIOLET RADIATION

The precise cause of melanoma is unknown, but host factors and environmental exposures have been most extensively studied. Ultraviolet radiation is proposed to be the most important agent responsible for the development of cutaneous melanoma. People with light coloring (skin, hair, eyes) are at increased risk of developing melanoma. Also, there is a correlation between childhood exposure to UV radiation and increasing incidence of melanoma. Blistering sunburns in children and adolescents have been associated with increased risk of developing melanoma. In contrast to this data, the lack of predisposition in those with outdoor occupations tends to weaken this association. Many studies that have attempted to induce melanomas in animals with UV radiation have failed (31). Aside from lentigo maligna melanoma, melanomas do not occur most frequently on the face, the most sun-exposed area of the body (31). These facts further complicate the association between sun exposure and melanoma. Many investigators now believe that the intermittent, recreational UV radiation exposure that has become more frequent in the 1980s and 1990s has substantially contributed to the rise in incidence of this cancer and is the most important environmental risk factor for development of melanoma.

As was mentioned in the section on NMSC, UV-B radiation has been most commonly linked to skin cancers and is responsible for the erythematous reaction of the skin after excessive sun exposure. UV-A radiation is believed to have effects on the immune system that may play a role in the development of skin cancers (32). The extent of involvement of UV-A radiation in the development of melanomas has not been fully elucidated. There has been speculation about the risk posed by fluorescent lights, sun lamps, and tanning beds in the development of melanomas. The data is controversial, with studies showing an increased relative risk (33–35) and no difference in relative risk (36–38) in those who have been exposed to these types of light sources compared to the general population.

Factors that determine the extent of UV radiation exposure were discussed earlier and are listed in Table 87.3. The closer to the equator one lives, the greater the risk of developing melanoma. This is a generally well-accepted rule; however, there are exceptions. For example, Norway and Sweden (northern Europe) have higher incidences of melanoma than do Italy and France (southern Europe) (30). These anomalies may be due to the fact that ethnic skin coloring darkens with increasing proximity to the equator. Also, there are other environmental factors that determine the amount of UV radiation exposure that are not accounted for by latitude alone (e.g., altitude, reflective surfaces, time of day of exposure, season of the year).

GENETICS

Genetics plays a major role in certain types of melanoma, especially the familial form mentioned earlier. Dysplastic nevus (DN) syndrome patients characteristically have large numbers of dysplastic nevi, which are believed to increase the risk of developing melanoma and to be precursors to melanoma. Kraemer and Greene divided DN patients into five categories of risk. These categories are listed in Table 87.10 (39). Type A is associated with a risk for melanoma that is relatively low yet is slightly higher than the normal population's risk. Type D2, also referred to as dysplastic nevus syndrome-familial type, is associated with a cumulative lifetime risk that approaches 100% by age 75 (39).

OTHER ETIOLOGIC FACTORS

The effects of hormonal manipulations on the incidence of melanoma have been studied. These studies stem from the observation that nevi often undergo changes in appearance during pregnancy and puberty. This observation was attributed to changes in hormone levels in the body, especially increases in circulating estrogen. Oral contraceptives have been associated with increased incidence of melanoma in only a few studies; in all of these the increase could be attributable to chance because of the small number of cases and the lack of control for other, well-documented risk factors (e.g., sun exposure) (40, 41). The same situation exists for exogenous estrogen replacement therapy (42–44).

Table 87.10.
Categories of Risk for Dysplastic Nevus Syndrome

Category	Description	Melanoma Family History[a]	Dysplastic Nevus Family History[b]	Melanoma Risk
A	Sporadic dysplastic nevi	No	No	Low
B	Familial dysplastic nevi	No	Yes	
C	Sporadic dysplastic nevi with melanoma	Yes	No	
D1	Familial dysplastic nevi with melanoma	Yes	Yes	
D2		Yes[c]	Yes	High

[a]Blood relatives with melanoma.
[b]Two or more blood relatives with dysplastic nevi.
[c]Category D2 requires a family history of at least two blood relatives with melanoma.
Source: Adapted from Kraemer KH, Greene MH. Dysplastic nevus syndrome: familial and sporadic precursors of cutaneous melanoma. Dermatol Clin 3:225–37, 1985.

Other factors have been studied, including the effects of alcohol, tobacco, coffee, tea, dietary fat, parity, age at first pregnancy, hair dyes, surgery, prior skin problems, and viruses. None of these factors have been proven to have a consistent relationship with the risk of developing melanoma (30).

Pathophysiology

Melanomas arise from melanocytes that are located in the epidermal-dermal junction of the skin and the choroid of the eye. Melanocytes can also be found in the meninges, mucosa of the alimentary and respiratory tracts, and lymph node capsules. Melanocytes are dendritic pigmented cells that produce melanin. These cells arise from the neural crest early in fetal development. It usually takes 4 to 6 weeks for the melanocytes to migrate to their final destinations.

Melanin is synthesized from tyrosine melanosomes, organelles that are located in the cytoplasm of melanocytes. Many of the compounds that are produced along this pathway are cytotoxic and have been targets for potential therapeutic interventions. There are several types of melanin, ranging from black (eumelanin) to red-yellow (pheomelanin). Skin color depends on the type of melanin and melanosomes produced and their interactions with neighboring keratinocytes, not on the density of melanocytes in the skin (45). The differences in genetics that determine skin color, and therefore the type of melanosomes and melanin produced, have not been entirely identified to date. However, it is generally accepted that many different genes collaborate to determine skin color, texture, and anomalies.

The most important proteins that are used to identify melanomas are S-100 and HMB-45. S-100 is expressed by nearly all melanomas but is also expressed by sarcomas, nerve sheath tumors, and a subset of carcinomas. HMB-45 is more specific for melanoma cells but is not always present in metastatic melanomas (27). These proteins are used most effectively when they are applied together with a panel of markers that are specialized to identify and differentiate melanomas.

There are several types of pigmented lesions that need to be differentiated from melanoma lesions. These lesions are listed in Table 87.11. Common acquired nevi are benign in nature and, in small numbers, do not impose an increased risk of melanoma. These lesions mature through characteristic phases of growth and development, beginning as flat, focal proliferations of melanocytes within the epidermis and potentially progressing to include the dermis. Dysplastic nevi do not go through these predictable developmental stages. They manifest as asymmetrical, irregularly shaped, hazy bordered, irregularly pigmented lesions and may range in diameter from 2 mm to more than 6 mm (46). Histopathologic confirmation

Table 87.11.
Differential Diagnosis of Pigmented Cutaneous Lesions

Very Common Lesions	Uncommon Lesions
Seborrheic keratosis	Hemangioma
Subungual hematoma	Pigmented basal cell carcinoma
Compound nevus	Blue nevus
Junctional nevus	Pigmented dermatofibroma
Lentigo	Kaposi's sarcoma
	Cutaneous T-cell lymphoma
	Tattoo

must be obtained for any lesion that has these characteristics.

Melanoma cells differ from normal epidermal melanocytes in their ability to grow independently of exogenous growth factors, invade into tissues, and acquire the ability to metastasize. Melanoma cells usually have marked chromosomal anomalies with two general phases of growth. The radial growth phase is the early phase of horizontal growth with little invasion into surrounding tissue. This phase of growth is characteristically slow but is most notable to the examiner's eye. In contrast, the vertical growth phase is not recognized by examination, because of changes taking place beneath the epidermal layer of skin. Vertical growth is expressed in later phases of melanoma progression, being required for extension into the dermal or subcutaneous layers of the skin or metastases to other organs. Clark and colleagues proposed a model for tumor progression from normal melanocyte to melanoma (see Figure 87.8). (47) This theory begins with a benign nevus undergoing dysplastic changes (changes in the architecture of the cell). Most of these atypical lesions spontaneously regress over time, as is typical for most precancerous lesions, but occasionally will undergo transformation into a melanoma in situ, confined solely to the epidermal layer of the skin. During the radial growth phase, primary melanomas may develop the characteristics to invade the basement membrane of the epidermis but usually do not have the capacity to survive in the new dermal environment. These thin lesions, when removed surgically, have a very high cure rate. If they are not removed, these lesions may develop the capacity to survive in the dermal layer and potentially metastasize and survive in other tissues. Nodular melanomas do not exhibit a radial growth phase and have a greater potential for metastases from their onset. These lesions are the only exceptions to the progression theory (48).

Normal melanocytes require growth factors from other cells (paracrine growth factors) for proliferation. Some of these substances have been identified and include basic fibroblast growth factor (bFGF), insulin, insulinlike growth factor (IGF-1), hepatocyte growth factor (HGF), and c-*kit* ligand (27, 48). Melanoma cells can proliferate without the

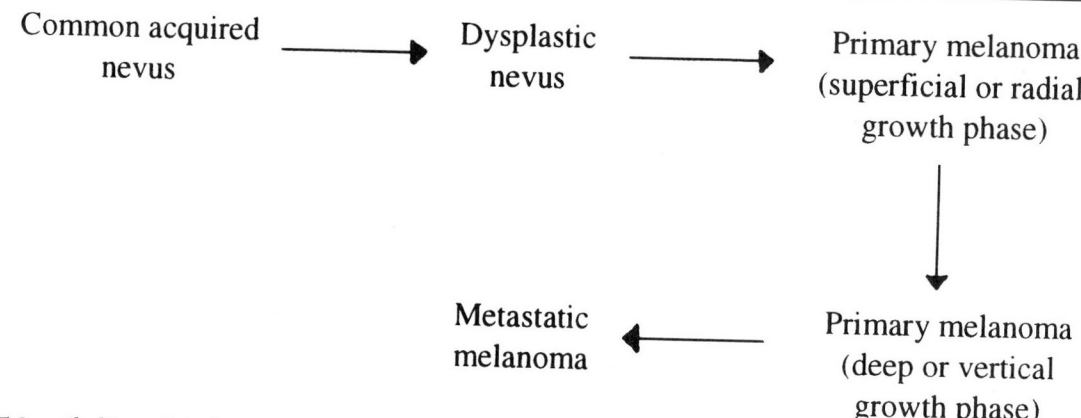

Figure 87.8. Clark's model of tumor progression from normal melanocyte to melanoma. (Source: Adapted from Balch CM, Houghton AN, Peters LJ. Cutaneous melanoma. In: DeVita VT, Hellman S, Rosenberg SA. Cancer: principles and practice of oncology, 4th ed. Philadelphia: JB Lippincott, 1993:1615.)

need for exogenous growth factors. This led to the discovery that melanomas can produce autocrine growth factors that would otherwise be supplied by the cellular environment. Several autocrine growth factors have been identified in cell culture systems of melanoma cells. The production of bFGF by melanoma cell lines in vitro has been well characterized and seems to be an early event in the progression of melanoma cells (27, 45). Melanocyte growth-stimulating activity (MGSA), platelet-derived growth factor (PDGF), transforming growth factor-α (TGF-α), interleukin-6 (IL-6), and interleukin-8 (IL-8) are also thought to be autocrine growth factors produced by melanoma cells but are less well characterized (27, 45, 48). Expression of only one of these factors is not sufficient to cause malignant transformation to melanoma. Transforming growth factor-α (TGF-α) and possibly interleukin-1 (IL-1) are believed to prevent the growth of melanoma cell lines in vitro (27, 45, 48). The relatively quiescent nature of normal melanocytes leads to the assumption that numerous negative control mechanisms work in concert to control growth. These mechanisms would need to be turned off for transformation into a highly invasive melanoma (48). Paracrine factors seem to play a role in melanoma growth and differentiation, including insulinlike growth factor and epidermal growth factor, which have been shown to stimulate growth of melanoma cells (45, 48). Adhesion molecules and angiogenesis factors are being investigated to define their role in the evolution of melanoma cells, enabling them to exist in foreign environments (e.g., other tissue sites) and metastasize (48). It is rapidly becoming evident that complex cellular systems are involved in the growth and progression of melanoma. These interactions are being investigated for development of prognostic indicators, therapeutic interventions, and predictors of response.

Many suppressor genes and oncogenes have been investigated in relation to growth stimulation and inhi-

bition. Chromosomes 1, 6, and 9 are most often found to contain abnormalities in melanomas (48). Melanoma cells have been found to abnormally express common tumor suppressor genes identified for other cancers, including p53, NF1 (neurofibromatosis-1 tumor suppressor gene), nm 23 (metastasis suppressor gene), and c-kit (oncogene expression is diminished in melanomas). Familial melanoma (dysplastic nevus syndrome) has been studied extensively to reveal the genetic link that increases these patients' susceptibility to melanoma, implicating both chromosomes 1 and 9 as possible loci for genes that are involved in susceptibility to familial melanoma (48, 49).

Clinical Presentation

Melanomas can occur anywhere on the body but are most commonly found on the lower extremities in women and on the back in men. Typical features of cutaneous melanoma are variegation, irregular raised surface, irregular border with indentations, and ulceration of the surface. The American Cancer Society has developed the ABCD rule for identification of suspected lesions (50). This rule incorporates the above features into an easily remembered acronym: A = Asymmetry, B = Border irregularity, C = Color variegations, D = Diameter greater than 6 mm (the size of a pencil tip eraser). The key for diagnosis of melanomas is recognizing that any change in a pigmented lesion is significant. Any pigmented lesion that undergoes a change in size, shape, color, texture, or sensation should be biopsied to rule out melanoma. This also includes lesions that lose color and become amelanotic. Itching, burning, or pain in a pigmented lesion should always arouse suspicion of melanoma. However, most patients present without any of these symptoms (27, 51).

Four major classifications exist for melanomas: superficial spreading, nodular, lentigo maligna, and acral lentiginous (see Table 87.12 and Figure 87.9) (27).

Table 87.12.
Classification of CMM

Subtype	% of All Melanomas	Characteristics
Superficial spreading	70	1) Initial phase of horizontal, radial growth 2) Progresses to predominantly perpendicular, vertical growth
Nodular	15–30	1) Rapid growth (over weeks to months) 2) Uniformly blue-black, dome-shaped nodule (amelanotic variants exist) 3) No discernible phase of radial growth
Lentigo maligna	4–10	1) Primarily on sun-exposed skin of elderly, most often on face 2) Closely linked to cumulative sun exposure 3) Arise from lentigo ("age spots") 4) After decades of radial growth develop nodular areas
Acral lentiginous	2–8 (in whites)	1) Most often found on palms, soles, nail beds, and mucous membranes 2) Sunlight is not involved 3) More frequent in blacks, Asians, and Hispanics

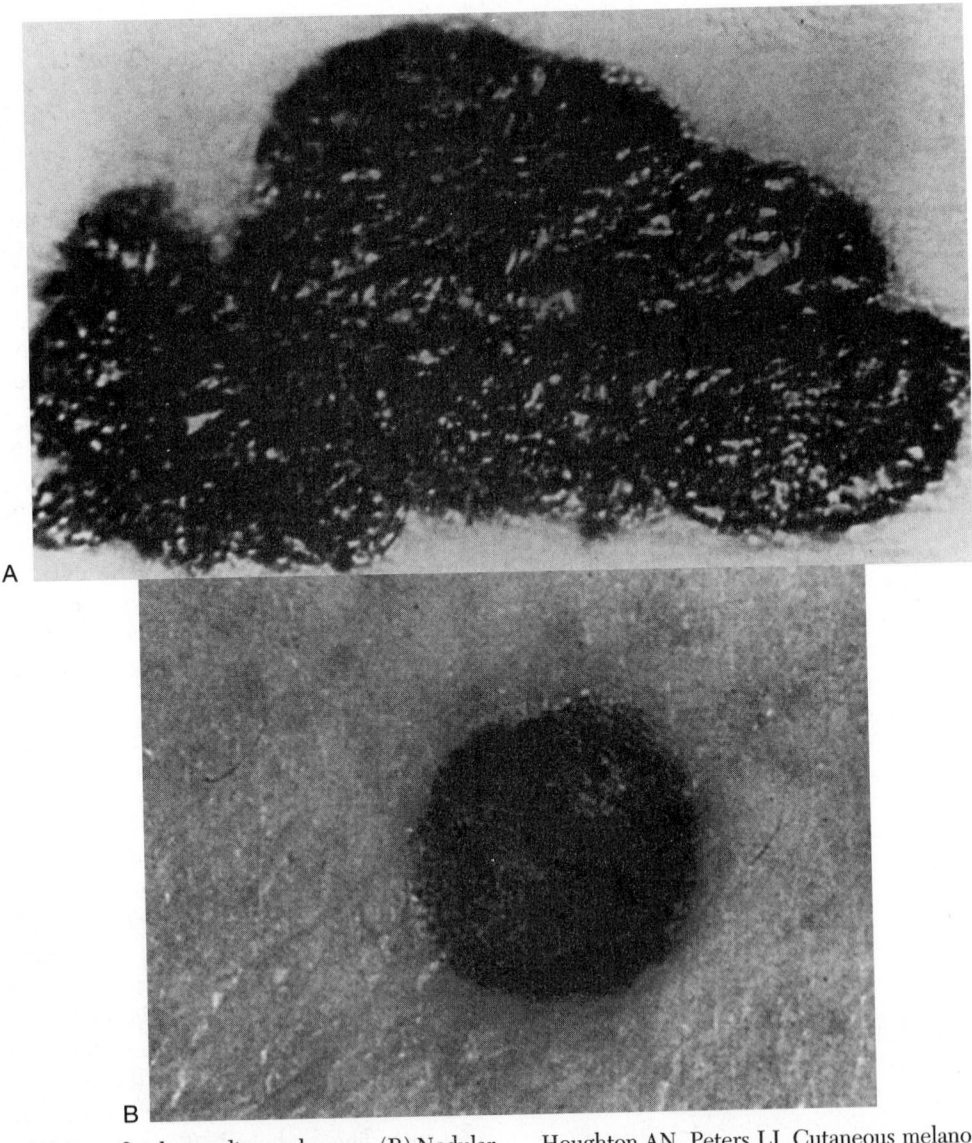

A

B

Figure 87.9. (A) Superficial spreading melanoma. (B) Nodular melanoma. (C) Lentigo maligna melanoma. (D) Acral lentiginous melanoma. (Source: Reprinted with permission from Balch CM, Houghton AN, Peters LJ. Cutaneous melanoma. In: DeVita VT, Hellman S, Rosenberg SA. Cancer: principles and practice of oncology, 4th ed. Philadelphia: JB Lippincott, 1993:1614.)

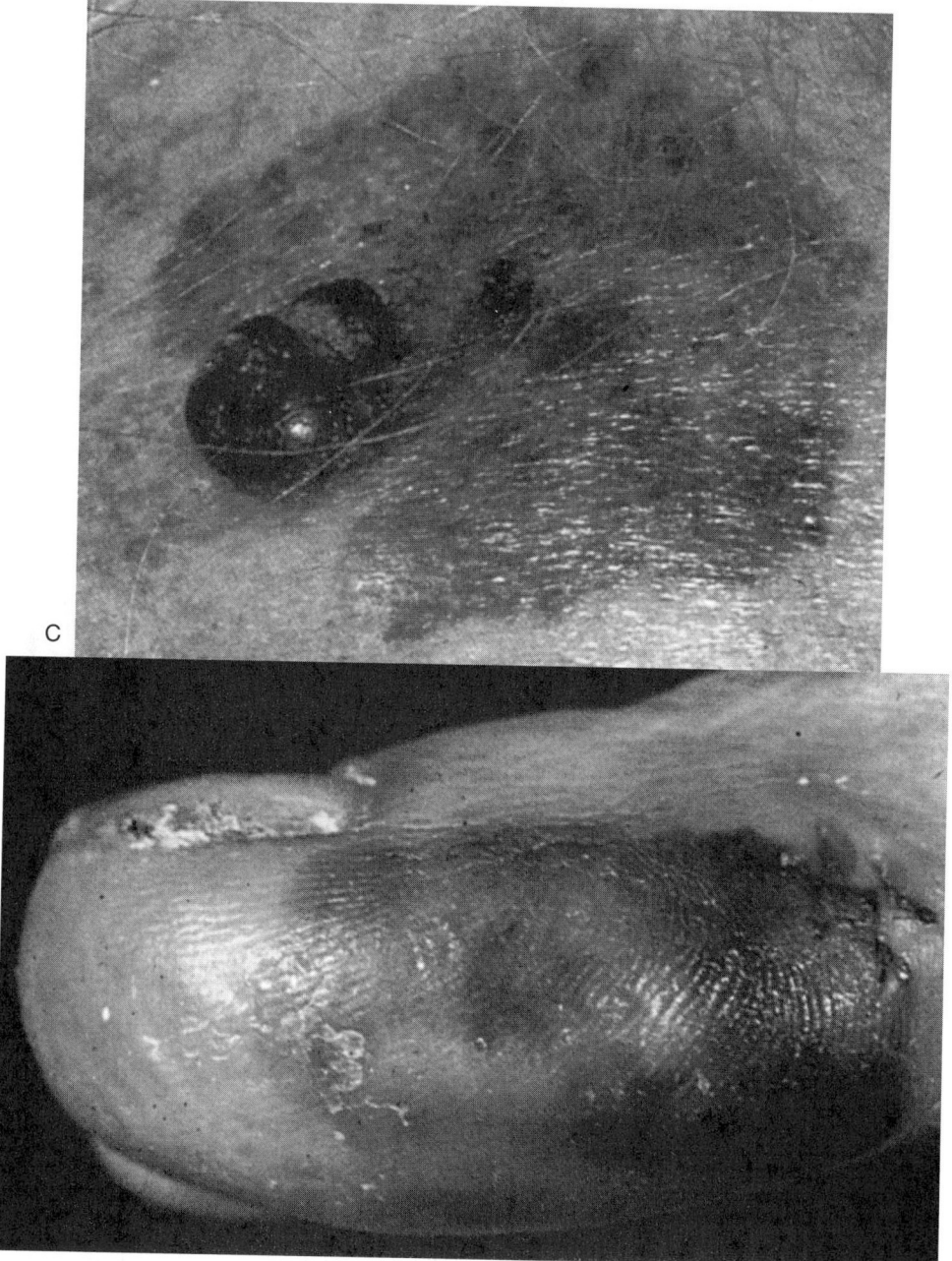

Figure 87.9. (continued)

Superficial spreading melanomas (SSM) are the most common variety, making up 70% of all melanomas. These lesions usually arise from a preexisting nevus and evolve slowly over 1 to 5 years but can also present after only a few months. The majority of existence is spent in the radial growth phase, eventually progressing to the vertical phase of growth, invading the dermis and other underlying tissues and acquiring the capacity to metastasize. Some lesions may never progress to the vertical growth phase; however, we do not have a way to determine which lesions will progress and which will not. These lesions occur at any age

after puberty and are more common in women than men. The ABCD rule applies only to superficial spreading melanomas (27).

Nodular melanoma (NM) is the second most common subset of melanomas, comprising 15 to 30% of all melanomas. These lesions are more aggressive, lacking a radial growth phase and growing undetected, vertically into the underlying structures. The undetected growth of these lesions predisposes them to late diagnosis with regional spread more likely evident at presentation. Nodular melanomas are usually present a few weeks to months before diagnosis is made. These lesions tend to arise from normal skin rather than preexisting nevi and can occur anywhere on the body. The most common areas are the trunk, head, and neck. NMs are true to their name, having a dome shape with sharply demarcated borders. Nodular melanomas are typically diagnosed between 40 and 50 years of age but can occur at any age, being more common in men than women. NMs are usually 1 to 2 cm in diameter but can be much larger. They are characteristically dark brown to black, can have blue shades, but are amelanotic (lacking pigment) in approximately 5% of cases. The ABCD rule does not apply to these characteristic lesions (27).

Lentigo maligna melanomas (LMMs) arise from lentigo malignas, certain types of "age spots," that are light brown, flat, with markedly irregular borders, usually appearing on sun-exposed areas of skin in the elderly. Approximately 5% of these lesions develop nodular areas of growth and are termed LMMs. These lesions are closely related to cumulative lifetime ultraviolet radiation exposure. The radial growth phase can last as long as 5 to 15 years or more, converting to the vertical growth phase that manifests as a nodule or papule within the lentigo maligna lesion. This form of melanoma is less common than SSM or NM and has less propensity to metastasize. LMM represents only 4 to 10% of all cutaneous melanomas. These lesions are usually located on the face, the nose and cheeks being most commonly affected. The average age at diagnosis is 70 years; LMM is very uncommon in people younger than 50 years of age. These lesions tend to be very large (>3 cm), and changes within the lesion are often overlooked because of their slow-growing nature. If neglected, LMMs have the potential to spread and become aggressive. The diagnosis requires that sun-related changes be evident in the dermis and epidermis (27).

Acral lentiginous melanomas (ALMs) are the most common melanomas in dark-skinned people such as blacks, Asians, and Hispanics, representing 35 to 60% of melanomas diagnosed but only 2 to 8% of melanomas in whites. These lesions arise on the palms, on the soles, beneath the nail plate, or in the mucous membranes and are large, the average diameter at diagnosis being 3 cm. These lesions appear to have little correlation with exposure to ultraviolet radiation. They occur most commonly in older people (the average age is in the sixties). ALM is present an average of 2.5 months before diagnosis, demonstrating its more aggressive nature. These lesions often are confused with LMM because of their light brown, flat appearance. The growth can be deceptive; the lesions can grow undetected vertically with little evidence of change from the surface. These lesions are more aggressive than SMM or LMM and therefore have a poorer prognosis. Subungual melanoma is one particular type of ALM. The median age at diagnosis is 55 to 65 years of age, and it is equally common in males and females (27).

Melanoma can metastasize anywhere in the body, presenting with characteristic dark brown to black pigmented lesions wherever it metastasizes. The most common sites of metastases at first relapse are skin, subcutaneous tissue, and distant lymph nodes. Lung, liver, bone, and the gastrointestinal tract are the next most common sites. In-transit metastases are defined as lesions that are located between the primary site of the lesion and the first major regional lymph node basin. These lesions are thought to originate from cells trapped in the lymphatics. They are usually observed in the subcutaneous or intracutaneous layer of the skin (i.e., satellitosis). Local recurrences are defined as any tumor that occurs within 5 cm of the scar of a previously excised melanoma. These lesions have a better prognosis than do in-transit metastases but are generally a sign that metastases will develop and are associated with a poor long-term survival rate (20% at 10 years) (27).

Patients with stage I, II, or III melanoma will rarely have changes in radiographic evaluations if micrometastases are present but instead will present with symptoms. Particular attention should be paid to signs or symptoms of central nervous system involvement. Also, blood in the stool and gastrointestinal symptoms can be possible indicators of metastatic disease. While some patients will remain stable for months, others will have rapid progression of disease with clinical deterioration within weeks. The clinical course of any individual patient is very difficult to predict and should be followed carefully by close monitoring of symptoms and signs relevant to the most common sites of metastases, as well as any other change in symptoms that is experienced.

Staging and Prognosis

If melanoma is suspected, biopsy is required for diagnosis. Several characteristics must be considered in determining biopsy technique. Microstaging, to determine the full thickness of the lesion, is essential and needs to be done with the initial biopsy. Therefore, excisional biopsy (removing the entire lesion) is the optimal biopsy procedure for lesions that are suspected of melanoma (31). Other characteristics that need to be considered are the location of the lesion (amount of tissue coverage) and the size of the lesion. A large lesion on the face may not be fully excisable with acceptable cosmetic results. In these cases a punch biopsy can be done in the most raised, deeply pigmented portion of the lesion, reaching its full depth. Another alternative is an incisional biopsy. Shave, needle, curettage, and saucerization biopsies are contraindicated for any primary pigmented lesion that is suspected of melanoma. These procedures may compromise the integrity of the histologic confirmation. The needle biopsy technique may be useful to document nodal metastases of melanoma (31).

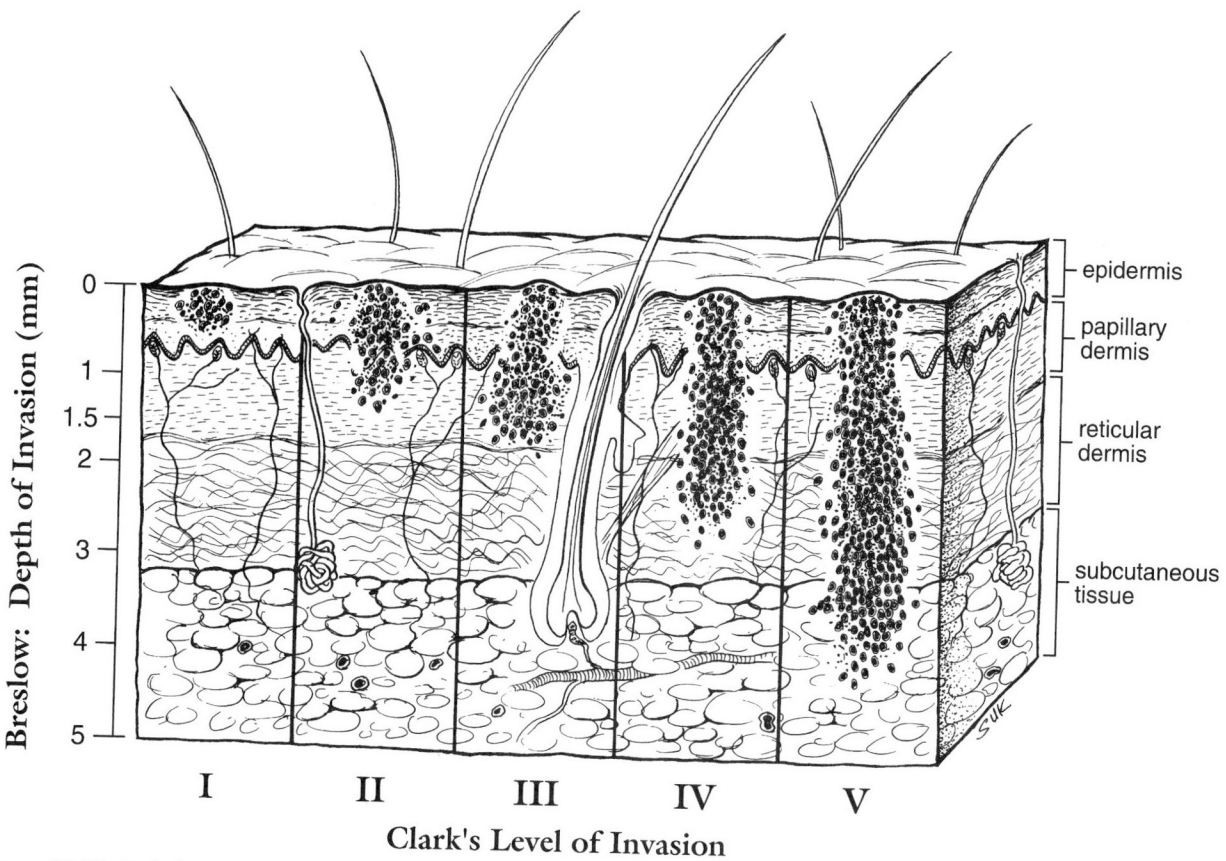

Figure 87.10. Pathologic microstaging of melanoma. Breslow's levels measure tumor thickness in millimeters and are shown on the left-hand side of the figure. Clark's levels measure the depth of invasion by tissue level of deepest penetration and are depicted across the bottom of the figure.

Microstaging, an integral part of staging and management of melanoma (see Figure 87.10), is currently accomplished by using two methods. Breslow's method uses an ocular micrometer to measure the total height (not just depth) of the lesion from the granular layer to the area of deepest penetration (52). If the lesion is ulcerated, measurements are made from the surface of the ulcer to the deepest portion of the lesion, and if the lesion is raised above the normal surface of the skin, the measurements are taken from the highest point to the deepest point of the lesion. Breslow's levels are listed in Table 87.13. Clark developed microstaging levels based on the depth of invasion into the skin rather than thickness of the lesion (see Table 87.13) (53). In several studies that looked at the prognostic significance of these two methods of microstaging, Breslow's measures of tumor thickness has demonstrated a more accurate and reproducible ability to predict the risk for metastases (52, 54).

The original three-stage system for melanoma incorporated local, regional, and distant spread of the disease into three simple stages. This staging system categorized approximately 85% of patients in stage I, preventing

Table 87.13.
Pathologic Microstaging for CMM

Breslow's Levels[a]		Clark's Levels
≤0.75 mm	I	Confined to the epidermis
0.76–1.49 mm	II	Extends into the papillary dermis
1.50–2.49 mm	III	Up to but not extending into the reticular dermis
2.50–3.99 mm	IV	Extending into the reticular dermis
≥4.00 mm	V	Extending into the subcutaneous tissue

[a]Uses an ocular micrometer to measure the total height of the lesion from the granular layer to the area of deepest penetration.

detection of discernible differences in risk for metastases and death (see Table 87.14) (29). With the observations of the prognostic significance of tumor thickness and level of invasion, the AJCC developed a new staging system incorporating these prognostic factors into the classic TNM staging system that is used for most solid tumors. The most current acceptable staging system is presented in Table 87.15 (11). Figure 87.11 illustrates the overall survival rates of patients using the new staging system, demonstrating that stage is now a better predictor of survival.

Many prognostic factors have been identified to assist in treatment planning and determination of risk with melanoma (55). Tumor thickness, as measured in millimeters, is the single most important prognostic factor for patients with stage I and II melanomas. There do not seem to be any natural breakpoints for categories of thickness; rather, a continuous correlation of survival to tumor thickness exists (55). Breslow's categories were arbitrary cut points but have been accepted for staging purposes and seem to impart some separation in terms of risk of recurrence and overall survival. Clark's levels of invasion are also of prognostic significance, with an inverse correlation between increasing level of invasion and survival. Ulceration of the primary lesion is a strong indicator of poor prognosis for stage I, II, and III melanoma. Ulceration and tumor thickness seem to be closely correlated, ulcerated lesions presenting as thicker lesions than those without ulceration. For stage I and II lesions, patients with lesions on the extremities have a better survival rate than do patients with lesions on the trunk or head and neck. Patients with lesions on the upper extremities have a slightly better survival rate than do those with lesions on the lower extremities. Gender was of prognostic significance for stage I and II lesions, women having a better survival rate than men. A primary reason for this survival advantage is that lesions in women tend to occur more commonly on the extremities and are less often ulcerated. Older patients tend to have thicker lesions and tend to have a worse prognosis than do younger patients, 50 years of age being an arbitrary cut point. When matched thickness for thickness, all of the different types of melanoma have similar prognosis except for LMM. LMM has the best prognosis, regardless of the thickness of the lesion or the patient's age.

For patients with stage III melanoma, involving regional lymph nodes, the number of metastatic lymph nodes involved was the best predictor of survival. Patients with only one lymph node involved had significantly better 10-year survival rates than did patients with two to four nodes involved and those with five or more nodes involved (40%, 18%, and 9%, respectively) (55).

The single most important prognostic variable for patients with metastatic disease is the number of metastatic sites involved. Patients with one site of metastases have a median survival of 7 months, compared to 4 months for patients with two sites and 2 months for those with three or more sites. Patients with metastases to skin, subcutaneous tissues, and distant lymph nodes, the most common sites of first relapse, have a median survival of 7 months, and 25% remain alive at one year. The next most common site of first relapse is the lung, having the best median survival of 11 months if isolated. Metastases to brain, liver, and bone impart a median duration of survival of 2 to 6 months, with a 1-year survival rate of only 8 to 10% (55). The dismal prognosis that is evident with metastatic disease, compared to local disease (stage I and II), is powerful information to advocate screening programs worldwide. These efforts will be discussed later.

Management

For melanoma, surgical excision is generally the recommended treatment of choice. Even in selected cases of metastatic disease the optimal palliative treatment includes surgical resection of the lesions. Melanomas outside of the area of the skin are generally not responsive to many treatment modalities and should be considered relatively radiotherapy-resistant and chemotherapy-resistant. While this is true, much of the research with melanoma lies in the arena of systemic therapy for metastatic melanoma and treatment of involved lymph nodes by several different modalities. Often, patients with advanced disease have a poor prognosis, and any treatment is worth trying, with the emphasis on the importance of an acceptable quality of life. Fortunately, in the

Table 87.14.
Traditional Three-Stage System for CMM

Stage	Criteria	5 Year Survival Rate (%)
I (thickness in mm)	Skin only	79
≤0.75		96
0.76–1.49		87
1.50–2.49		75
2.50–3.99		66
≥4.00		47
II Any thickness	Nodal metastases	36
III Any thickness	Distant metastases	5

Table 87.15.
AJC Staging System for CMM

T	Breslow's (mm)	Clark's	N	Stage	Criteria
1	≤0.75	II	1 Nodal mets ≤ 3 cm	I	T1 or T2, N0, M0
2	0.76–150	III	2 Nodal mets > 3 cm	II	T3 or T4, N0, M0
3	1.51–4.00	IV	M	III	Any T, N1 or N2, M0
4	>4.00	V	1 Distant mets	IV	Any T, any N, M1

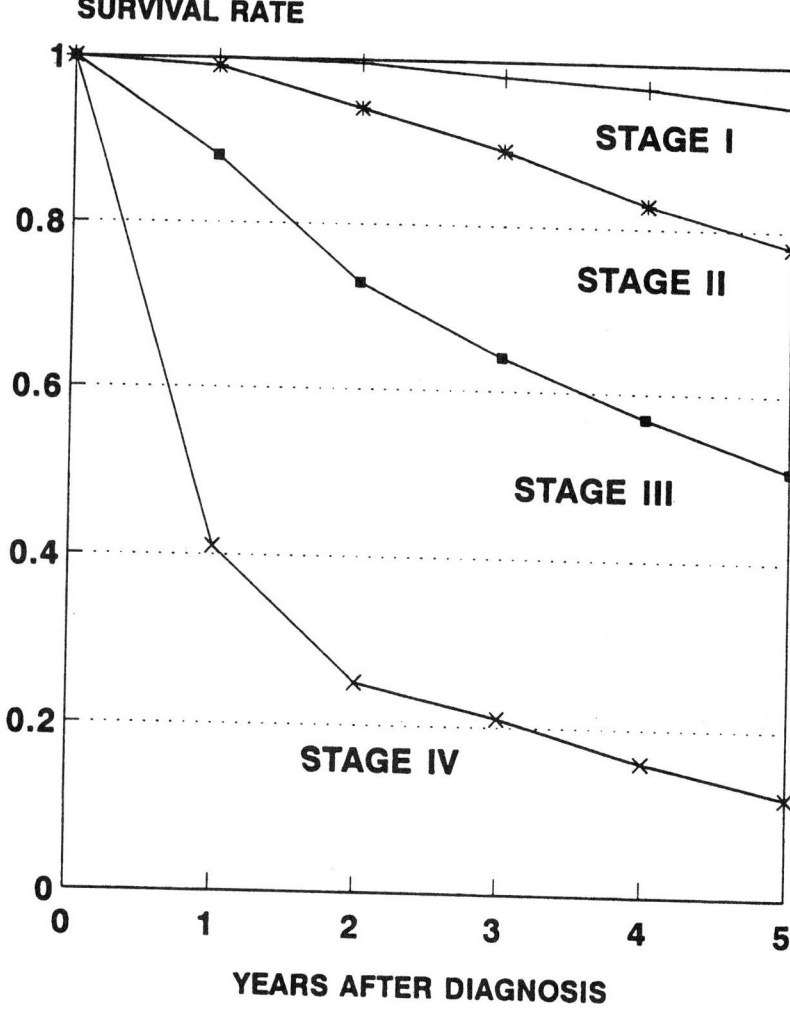

SURVIVAL RATE

STAGE I

STAGE II

STAGE III

STAGE IV

YEARS AFTER DIAGNOSIS

Figure 87.11. Relative survival rates according to the stage of disease. Data taken from 8479 patients who were diagnosed between 1977 and 1982. Patients are listed in the Surveillance, Epidemiology, and End Results Program of the National Cancer Institute. Stage I represents 4286 patients; Stage II represents 3328 patients; Stage III represents 649 patients; and Stage IV represents 216 patients. (Source: Reprinted with permission from American Joint Committee on Cancer. Manual for staging of cancer, 4th ed. Philadelphia: JB Lippincott, 1995:144.)

arena of systemic therapy (especially immunotherapy), the positive impact on survival brings hope for a future of novel immunotherapies, vaccines, and gene-targeting therapies. Table 87.16 outlines treatment strategies for CMM by stage of disease.

SURGERY

Excision of Primary Melanoma. For stage I and II melanomas the treatment of choice is surgical excision of the primary lesion, down into the subcutaneous tissue, plus a radius of normal-appearing tissue (Figure 87.12) (56). This can be done in the office with local anesthetic. With excision alone, the overall risk of local recurrence is about 3% for stages I and II (56). The prognostic significance of tumor thickness obtained from microstaging enticed investigators to challenge the standard use of radical excisions (at least 5 cm of tumor-free margin) for all melanoma lesions. Many investigators set out to prove that thinner margins are appropriate for thinner lesions without compromising these patients' overall survival, rate of metastases, or incidence of local recurrence. On the basis

of data from the World Health Organization Melanoma Programme (57) and the Intergroup Melanoma Study (58), the recommended margin of excision for lesions between 1 and 2 mm should be based on the anatomic location of the lesion and the need for a skin graft for closure versus primary closure. Those 1- to 2-mm lesions that would require a skin graft with a 2-cm excision should employ the 1-cm margin. This would lessen the risk for complications from skin grafting while maintaining a very low risk of local recurrence. Lesions between 2 and 4 mm thick should use the 2-cm margin for optimal responses. Excisional requirements for thicker lesions (>4 mm) have not been studied in a randomized, controlled manner, but the current recommendations are to excise these lesions with a 3-cm margin (59). Melanoma in situ lesions (contained in the epidermis) have a minimal risk of recurring locally and do not have the capability to metastasize. The recommended tumor-free margin for these lesions is at least 0.5 cm (60). LMM lesions are usually associated with a low risk of recurrence and can be safely excised with a 1-cm margin (27).

Table 87.16.
Treatment Strategies for CMM by Stage of Disease

Stage	Treatment of Choice	5-Year DFS (%)[a]	Comments
I and II[b]	**Surgical excision**	47–97	LMM have the best prognosis and can often be treated with thinner margins or XRT.[b]
<1.00 mm	1-cm margin		CMM on fingers or toes require digital amputation.
1.00–2.00 mm	1–2 cm margin[c]		ERLND and lymph node mapping are controversial.[c]
2.00–4.00 mm	2-cm margin		Adjuvant therapy has not been proven to prolong survival.
>4.00 mm	3-cm margin		
III	**Surgical excision of primary and involved regional lymph nodes**	20–40	Removal of the entire nodal basin is usually performed.
			Isolated limb perfusion has response rates of up to 100%.[d]
			Intralesional bCG may be used to treat satellite lesions.[a,c]
IV	**Chemoimmunotherapy**[d] **and/or surgical excision**	<5	Selected lesions in the lung, brain, and subcutaneous tissues can be resected for palliation of symptoms.
			Chemoimmunotherapy has been shown to prolong survival in patients with stage IV disease.
			Resection of isolated lung or subcutaneous metastases may prolong survival in 15–30% of patients.[c]

[a]DFS = disease-free survival; XRT = radiotherapy; ERLND = elective regional lymph node dissection; bCG = bacillus Calmette-Guerin.
[b]Information on stage I and II CMM is divided into these categories in the studies available to date. These are not the same divisions seen in the staging criteria shown in Table 87.15.
[c]See text for further information
[d]Chemoimmunotherapy = chemotherapy + IFN-α + IL-2 (see text).

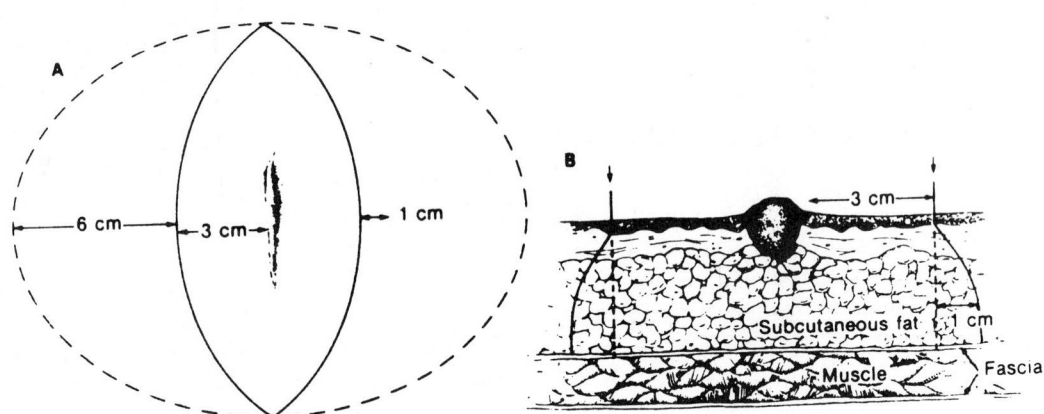

Figure 87.12. Technique of surgical excision of a primary melanoma with an elliptical excision and primary skin closure. (A) The surgical margin is 3 cm from the biopsy site. It is often necessary to mobilize the skin flaps for a distance twice that of the excised skin margin. (B) Cross-section of the excision site. The skin margin is 3 cm from the tumor. Flaps of gradually increasing thickness are raised for an additional 1 to 2 cm to remove any surrounding subdermal lymphatics. Excision of the fascia is optional. (Source: Reprinted with permission from Singletary SE, Balch CM, Urist MM, et al. Surgical treatment of primary melanoma. In: Balch CM, Houghton AN, Milton GW, et al. Cutaneous melanoma, 2nd ed. Philadelphia: JB Lippincott, 1992:271.)

For primary cutaneous melanomas on the fingers or toes, digital amputation is required. It is important to preserve enough of the digit to ensure adequate functioning. These procedures require that at least a 1-cm margin of skin be removed at the time of amputation. The ear can usually be partially amputated or wedge-resected, reserv-ing complete amputation for recurrent lesions or wide-spread disease. Ear prostheses are available for patients who require this type of surgery (56).

Elective Regional Lymph Node Dissection. Removal of normal-appearing regional lymph nodes in hopes of decreasing the incidence of local recurrence is termed an elective regional lymph node dissection (ERLND). ERLND is a controversial procedure and may or may not be associated with increasing disease-free survival or decreasing local recurrences. This procedure is based on the belief that melanoma metastasizes sequentially, going first to the regional lymph nodes then to distant sites. This hypothesis has been challenged, as has the practice of ERLND, and relies on the ability to map the lymph drainage in the area of the primary lesion. If the lymph drainage pattern is unknown (as with some lesions on the trunk), it is impossible to know which lymph nodes should be removed. Proponents of ERLND state that for patients with microscopic nodal metastases, early diagnosis can bring good survival odds, potentially preventing further distant metastases from occurring (61). Opponents of the procedure note the success with surgery alone for stage I and II melanomas as a reason not to inflict this type of morbidity on patients who may not have microscopic disease in the lymph nodes (62). Randomized studies are currently underway.

One resolution to this controversy lies in a new procedure that can stage the suspected lymph node basin without requiring full dissection. This procedure is termed intraoperative lymphatic mapping and sentinel node biopsy (63). A vital blue dye is injected into the dermis just adjacent to the primary melanoma lesion. The first node to collect the dye, the "sentinel node," is biopsied. If this node is positive for microscopic disease, then lymphadenectomy can be done. If this node is negative, the procedure can be halted, and the patient is spared an unnecessary surgery. Identification of the sentinel node is much easier in the inguinal area than in the axilla. Lymphoscintigraphy has been used to better identify the sentinel node in the axillary region. In this procedure, ^{99m}Tc-labeled colloid combined with vital blue dye is injected, and a γ-counter is used in the operating room to locate the sentinel node. This technique of lymphatic mapping with biopsy may be useful for staging purposes and to more effectively choose the patients who would benefit from adjuvant therapy.

The issue of ERLND remains one of the most controversial topics concerning patients with melanoma. Ongoing studies investigating lymph node mapping with sentinel node biopsy and subsequent ERLND (if indicated) may prove to be the treatment of choice for regional lymph node basins. Results of these studies are anxiously awaited.

Therapeutic Lymph Node Dissection. Lymphadenectomy performed on clinically apparent nodes is termed a therapeutic dissection, compared to the ERLND previously described. Clinically evident regional lymph node involvement (stage III) is managed primarily with surgical resection. The long-term disease-free survival rate after lymphadenectomy is predicted to be 20 to 40% for stage III melanoma patients. The adverse effects of lymphadenec-

tomy depend on the site of resection. The ilioinguinal lymph node basins drain the lower extremities. After resection of these basins, there is noticeable edema in approximately 26% of patients at long-term follow-up, but only 5% and 3% of patients reported pain or functional deficit, respectively (27). Leg exercises, elastic stockings, diuretics, and perioperative antibiotics have been shown to prevent edema in these patients. Complications with axillary node dissection are infections (7%), seroma (27%), hemorrhage (1%), and arm edema (1%) (27). Cervical and parotid lymph nodes can also be removed with similar complications. Complications (nerve damage) in relation to the location of these lymph nodes (close in proximity to the cranial nerves) is rarely seen but is always a possibility (27).

Surgical Management of Metastases. Patients with distant metastases have a poor prognosis, with a median survival of 5 to 8 months and a 5-year survival of less than 5%. Resections of metastatic lesions can offer palliation of symptoms but rarely affect survival rates. Resection of isolated pulmonary or subcutaneous metastases is associated with prolonged survival in up to 15 to 30% of patients (27). At this point in the disease process, emphasis is placed on quality of life rather than length of life.

RADIATION

Radiotherapy for Primary Melanomas. The use of radiation for treatment of melanoma is controversial. Initial reports of complete radioresistance among all melanomas have been challenged. With early stages of melanoma, surgery alone is the standard of care, with very high rates of cure (>95%). Treatment of primary melanomas with conventional radiation is limited to LMM lesions. Many of these lesions occur on the face in the elderly and may require extensive reconstruction if surgery is performed. Radiotherapy can be useful for these patients, with little morbidity and very good results. In one series, using fractionated doses of radiation to treat 28 patients with LMM, only two patients had recurrences, but some lesions took as long as 24 months to fully regress after radiation (64). The long-term adverse effects with radiation are skin pallor, telangiectasias, and atrophy in the area of treatment (approximately 10%) (64).

Adjuvant Radiotherapy. The use of radiotherapy after surgery has been studied in cases in which optimal resection would be disfiguring and in which the risk of local relapse is high. Ang and colleagues, in an investigation of 174 patients with cutaneous melanoma of the head and neck who were at high risk for local recurrence, concluded that adjuvant radiation can decrease local recurrence rates but has little effect on survival (65). Survival is at least equal to that seen with conventional approaches. The role for adjuvant radiation is small, but it can be instrumental if a disfiguring surgical procedure can be avoided. Radiation, in place of dissection, of the lymph node basins is possible and may be associated with less morbidity than occurs with dissection. Randomized, controlled studies need to be done to better identify the role of adjuvant radiotherapy, either to the primary sites or to the nodal basins.

Radiotherapy for Distant Metastases. Distant sites of metastases can be treated with radiation. The most common indications for radiotherapy are treatment of subcutaneous, dermal, lymph node, brain, or bone metastases. Palliation of symptoms can often be accomplished with radiotherapy that is directed toward the specific site of involvement. Spinal cord compression or other lesions that are not amenable to surgery can also be radiated for palliation. If a patient is not a surgical candidate, on the basis of other medical criteria, radiotherapy is a reasonable option for treatment of metastatic melanoma (27).

HYPERTHERMIA AND ISOLATED LIMB PERFUSION

Hyperthermia. Hyperthermia, or warming the body, has been studied in conjunction with radiotherapy and chemotherapy. Warming is accomplished with the use of a water-circulating mattress that has adjustable heating components. One rationale behind the combination of hyperthermia and radiotherapy (thermoradiotherapy) is that hyperthermia will potentially bring radio-resistant cells out of their dormant state, thereby making them more susceptible to the effects of radiotherapy. Thermoradiotherapy seems to be active, but comparative trials have not been done, and the role of this treatment modality remains controversial.

Isolated Limb Perfusion. Isolated limb perfusion with and without hyperthermia has been studied, particularly in patients with isolated lesions on the extremities (see Figure 87.13). The goal of limb perfusion is to maximize the concentration of drug in the affected limb while minimizing the systemic side effects of chemotherapy. This procedure has been used adjuvantly for subclinical micrometastases and therapeutically for in-transit metastases. Many agents have been used either alone or in combination; these include melphalan, actinomycin D, mechlorethamine, dacarbazine, cisplatin, carboplatin, tumor necrosis factor (TNF), and interferon-β (IFN-β) and interferon-γ (IFN-γ). The drug that has been most studied and most effective is melphalan, with response rates often exceeding 80% in the presence of hyperthermia (39 to 40°C) (66, 67). Survival data has not yet determined whether adjuvant isolated limb perfusion is superior to surgery alone for melanomas that are thicker than 1.5 mm. Two studies are currently underway to investigate this question. For treatment of bulky, in-transit metastases, this technique is very encouraging and should be considered standard, especially as an alternative to amputation. A combination of melphalan, TNF, and interferon-α has shown very promising results in the treatment of bulky, in-transit metastases. This combination has reported overall response rates of 100%, complete responses of 90%, and

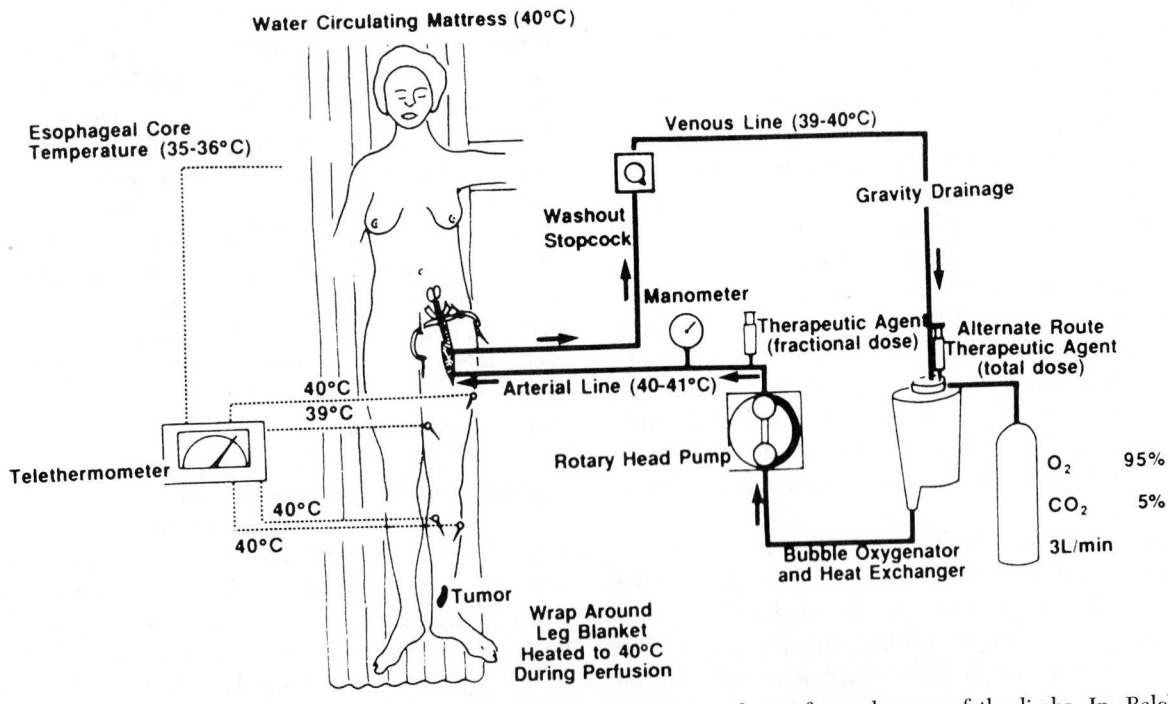

Figure 87.13. Isolated limb perfusion with hyperthermia for lower limb melanoma. (Source: Reprinted with permission from Krementz ET, Ryan RF, Muchmore JH, et al. Hyperthermic regional perfusion for melanoma of the limbs. In: Balch CM, Houghton AN, Milton GW, et al. Cutaneous melanoma, 2nd ed. Philadelphia: JB Lippincott, 1992:405.)

acceptable regional and systemic toxicity (68). The National Cancer Institutes (NCI) is currently conducting a study randomizing patients to receive isolated limb perfusion with melphalan alone or in combination with TNF, to substantiate the response rates previously described and to determine their durability.

INTRALESIONAL THERAPY

Metastatic skin lesions have been treated with a number of different agents given by intralesional injection. The most common agent used is bacillus Calmette-Guerin (bCG). This treatment has been associated with regression of lesions, sometimes with durable remissions of several months to years (69). Occasionally, satellite lesions that are adjacent to the lesion injected will also respond, demonstrating a local immune response. This type of treatment is useful only if the lesions are confined to a very small area and is not superior to surgical excision (the treatment of choice).

SYSTEMIC THERAPY

Chemotherapy. The only role for systemic chemotherapy in melanoma is for treatment of metastatic disease. Adjuvant therapy for stage I, II, and III melanoma, to date, has shown no survival advantage over surgery alone. However, adjuvant therapy for melanoma is still a major area of research because of improved response rates with newer agents and combination regimens and the overall poor prognosis of patients with local or distant spread of disease. Conventional chemotherapy has little activity against melanoma. Many agents show minimal activity, with response rates of 10 to 20% (see Table 87.17). Dacarbazine (DTIC) is the most active single-agent chemotherapy for melanoma, with responses seen in up to 25% of patients. The median duration of response is 5 to 6 months. In a review of phase III trials for DTIC in metastatic melanoma, only 5% of 580 patients achieved a complete response (70). Only 31% of these responders survived and remained disease-free at 6 years. While prolongation of survival is questionable with chemotherapy, palliation of symptoms can be accomplished for some patients, improving their quality of life, as long as the chemotherapy has minimal toxicity.

Table 87.17.
Chemotherapy Agents Having Significant Activity Against CMM

Carboplatin	Lomustine (CCNU)
Carmustine (BCNU)	Paclitaxel
Cisplatin (CDDP)	Semustine (MeCCNU)
Dacarbazine (DTIC)	Vinblastine (VBL)
Docetaxel	Vincristine
Fotemustine	Vindesine

DTIC is severely emetogenic, and up to 90% of patients vomit if they are not premedicated with strong antiemetics before treatment. Serotonin antagonists have reduced this toxicity, and the addition of dexamethasone to the antiemetic regimen further decreases nausea and emesis. A flu-like syndrome can occur with large single doses of dacarbazine, manifesting as fever, myalgia, and malaise. The onset is within 7 days and can last as long as 3 weeks (71). Another acute reaction with high-dose therapy is a severe photoreaction with exposure to sunlight; hypotension has been observed during the infusion. Myelosuppression is mild to moderate, is dose related, and predominantly affects the granulocytes and platelets. Alopecia, facial flushing, facial parasthesias, and hepatic toxicity are rarely reported (71). With the introduction of new antiemetics to control the nausea and vomiting, dacarbazine is tolerated fairly well when it is given as a single agent.

DTIC may be given in a number of different schedules and dosages. Daily schedules lasting 10, 5, and 2 days have been described, as has a single bolus injection. The most common regimens are (a) 800 to 1000 mg/m^2 as a bolus injection given once, (b) 250 mg/m^2/day for 5 days as daily bolus injections, and (c) 4.5 mg/kg/day for 10 days as daily bolus injections. These treatment regimens are repeated every 3 to 4 weeks. There is no difference in response rates with these schedules, but less nausea and vomiting occur with the lower daily doses. Doses up to 2000 mg/m^2 as single injections are associated with dose-limiting flu-like toxic reactions and hypotension. Doses up to 2500 mg/m^2 given as a continuous infusion over 24 hr have been investigated with hemibody radiation in patients with metastatic melanoma with no better responses than standard doses and much greater toxicity (71). Patients with liver metastases from melanoma have been treated with intraarterial DTIC at doses similar to those described for intravenous administration, with overall responses of 41% and less intense systemic toxicity (72). There have been a few case studies of intrathecal or intraventricular DTIC administration for leptomeningeal melanoma with questionable safety and efficacy (73, 74). A derivative of dacarbazine, temozolamide, has recently shown activity against metastatic melanoma and is being investigated in phase I and II clinical trials (75).

Nitrosoureas are less active than DTIC but are widely used in combination regimens. Carmustine (BCNU), lomustine (CCNU), semustine (methyl-CCNU), and fotemustine are most extensively studied in melanoma. These agents are lipid-soluble and cross the blood-brain barrier, but they usually lack activity against melanoma brain metastases. In contrast, fotemustine has induced some measurable responses in melanoma brain lesions (up to 25%) (76, 77). Fotemustine has also been used intraarterially for isolated hepatic metastases. In a small study of 13 patients receiving intraarterial fotemustine, response rates reached 60%, but quick relapses were seen in other visceral organs (78). Vinca alkaloids have been shown to have some activity against melanoma and are often used in combination regimens. Vindesine is used largely in Europe, where it is commercially available; vinblastine is more commonly used in the United States.

Cisplatin, in standard doses (50 to 100 mg/m^2), has demonstrated only minimal responses; but with higher doses (60 to 150 mg/m^2) with ethiofos (WR2721), response rates of 53% were seen (79). Median duration of response was 4 months, and no complete responses were demonstrated. Ethiofos is a renal protectant that is being studied in combination with cisplatin and seemed to potentiate the antitumor effects of cisplatin in this particular study. The dose-limiting toxicity in this trial was peripheral neuropathy. Unfortunately, neuroprotectants have yet to be of proven benefit, but they are being vigorously investigated. Intrahepatic chemoembolization with cisplatin and polyvinyl sponge has been investigated for liver metastases from melanoma. Responses of 25 to 50% have been reported, with durations of 2 to 19 months (80). Carboplatin, a derivative of cisplatin, has shown minimal activity (11% response rate) against melanoma as a single agent (81) but is being investigated in high-dose regimens and other combination regimens in both the adjuvant and metastatic setting.

Paclitaxel is a rather new chemotherapeutic agent with fairly promising activity against melanoma. In a review of clinical phase II studies of paclitaxel in metastatic melanoma, 73 patients were evaluable with overall response rates of 16% and stable disease in 14% (82). Median duration of response was approximately 5 months (range 1 to 17 months), again no different from historic controls. This data warrants further investigation of paclitaxel in combination regimens. Docetaxel (Taxotere), a derivative of paclitaxel, has shown more potent activity against the B16 melanoma model, a transplantable tumor model that is used in mice (83). Phase II clinical trials with taxotere in metastatic melanoma are ongoing.

Combination Chemotherapy. In response to the less than optimal results with single-agent chemotherapy, investigators began studying combination regimens. Since DTIC has minimal toxicity, adding another agent must show a clear survival advantage to warrant the added toxicity. Many two-drug regimens have been investigated but have failed to show such a survival advantage. Three-drug regimens are being investigated, but little data that compare them to single-agent DTIC is available. Some common regimens that show activity are listed in Table 87.18. The BOLD regimen has come under some scrutiny because of the inclusion of bleomycin, an agent without activity against melanoma and a pulmonary toxic agent after lifetime cumulative doses of 300 to 400 mg/m^2. The combinations that are used most frequently are combina-

Table 87.18.
Common Combination Chemotherapy Regimens Used to Treat Metastatic Malignant Melanoma

Regimen Name	Chemotherapy Agents	Dose & Schedule of Administration
BOLD	Bleomycin	15 U D1, 4 Q3–4 weeks
	Oncovin (vincristine)	1 mg/m^2 D1, 4 Q3–4 weeks
	Lomustine (CCNU)	80 mg/m^2 D1 Q3–4 weeks
	DTIC (dacarbazine)	200 mg/m^2 D1–5 Q3–4 weeks
DTIC/CDDP/ Vindesine	DTIC	250 mg/m^2 D1–5 Q3–4 weeks
	CDDP (cisplatin)	100 mg/m^2 D1 Q3–4 weeks
	Vindesine	3 mg/m^2 D1 Q3–4 weeks
CVD	Cisplatin (CDDP)	20 mg/m^2 D2–5 Q3–4 weeks
	Vinblastine (VBL)	1.6 mg/m^2 D1–5 Q3–4 weeks
	DTIC (dacarbazine)	800 mg/m^2 D1 Q3–4 weeks
Dartmouth	Cisplatin (CDDP)	25 mg/m^2 D1–3 Q3 weeks
	BCNU (carmustine)	150 mg/m^2 D1 Q6 weeks
	DTIC (dacarbazine)	220 mg/m^2 D1–3 Q3 weeks
	Tamoxifen	10 mg PO BID

tions of DTIC, cisplatin, carmustine (BCNU), vinblastine, or vindesine. In Europe the combination of DTIC, cisplatin, and vindesine has had response rates in 30 to 40% of patients treated (84). A similar regimen in which vinblastine is substituted for vindesine (CVD regimen) has been used in the United States at the MD Anderson Cancer Center. This regimen has produced response rates of up to 40% (85).

The four-drug regimen of DTIC, cisplatin, carmustine, and tamoxifen has shown response rates of up to 53% of patients treated. This regimen, developed by Del Prete and colleagues (86), is often referred to as the Dartmouth regimen and has been studied extensively by McClay and colleagues (87). The crucial component seems to be the addition of tamoxifen to the regimen. When tamoxifen was not given, the response rates fell to 10%; they rose again to 52% when tamoxifen was added back to the regimen. Tamoxifen does, however, impart more significant toxicity to the regimen with increased incidence of thromboembolic disorders and hot flashes. To date, the overall survival of patients receiving the Dartmouth regimen has not been better than that with DTIC alone, but a randomized study comparing these two regimens is underway.

The mechanism of tamoxifen in this regimen is not clear, and as a single agent, tamoxifen has no activity against melanoma. The presence of estrogen receptors in melanoma cells has not been confirmed since the advent of more accurate methods of detection for these receptors. Estrogen may play a role in melanoma cell growth that has yet to be elucidated, but it may not be related to the effects that are seen with tamoxifen. Synergy with tamoxifen has been demonstrated with cisplatin, carboplatin, nitrogen mustard, doxorubicin, and vinblastine in vitro (75). Carmustine has also been suggested to have a synergistic interaction with tamoxifen. Tamoxifen is known to bind to the p170 glycoprotein that is responsible for multidrug resistance, potentially preventing efflux of the cytotoxic drug from the cytoplasm and overcoming drug resistance. Data from McClay and colleagues did not show this to be the mechanism of synergy with cisplatin or carboplatin (88), but these agents are not generally associated with this mechanism of resistance. Other proposed mechanisms of action have included tamoxifen acting directly on melanoma cells, interacting with the cellular autocrine and/or paracrine factors involved in melanoma growth and proliferation.

High doses of chemotherapy with autologous bone marrow support have been investigated for metastatic melanoma. Overall response rates have ranged from 40 to 65%, with complete response rates as high as 15% (69). Unfortunately, to date, there has been no survival advantage with these treatments. The toxicity of these regimens makes the risk-to-benefit ratio unacceptable at this time, preventing the endorsement of such treatment outside the context of a clinical trial.

Immunotherapy. Melanomas are the single most frequent tumor type to undergo spontaneous regression (up to 3 to 4% of lesions) (75), leading to the belief that the body has an antitumor defense mechanism that is operable against some melanomas. This has directed researchers to investigate the immune system as a potential target for therapy and modulation of the natural history of melanoma.

Interferon-α (IFN-α) was one of the first immunotherapies developed to augment the body's immune system. IFN-α augments tumor cell expression of histocompatibility antigens that are necessary for immune recognition and destruction of tumor cells. Initial results with natural purified IFN-α showed infrequent responses, but responses with recombinant human IFN-α have been much better (average 20%) (75). The activity of this agent seems to be schedule-dependent, with increased responses when it is given daily or three times a week, compared to intermittent schedules. Results are dose related, the optimal dose being 12 million U/m². Unfortunately, the toxicity is also dose related. The most common adverse effects are a flu-like syndrome, consisting of myalgias, fever, headache, chills, and anorexia. With continued treatment, patients generally experience a decrease in these symptoms. Premedication with acetaminophen has proven to be helpful in tolerating these symptoms with standard doses (3 to 6 million U/m²). With high doses (>6 million U/m²), these effects are intensified and prolonged, and acetaminophen premedication is less helpful. Neutro-

penia and increases in serum transaminases occur infrequently but may require discontinuation of therapy. Responses may be delayed with IFN-α, progressing initially and subsequently responding with continued therapy. The different types of IFN-α (2a, 2b, 2c) seem to have similar activity against melanoma.

Interferon-β (IFN-β) binds to the same cell-surface receptor as IFN-α, but it is unclear whether the subsequent actions on melanoma cells are similar. The side effects of IFN-β are similar to those of IFN-α. Interferon-γ (IFN-γ) binds to a specific receptor on the cell surface and has biologic properties that are very different from those of IFN-α. Systemic administration of single-agent IFN-γ has little activity against melanoma (27).

Interleukin-2 (IL-2), initially referred to as T-cell growth factor, is produced by lymphocytes and is responsible for many immunoregulatory functions. IL-2 can amplify immune responses by promoting growth of activated T cells, resulting in enhancement of both specific and nonspecific antitumor cytotoxicity. Specific antitumor cytotoxicity is T-cell mediated, whereas nonspecific antitumor cytotoxicity is mediated by natural killer cells. Also related to the amplification of the immune response is the induction of other cytokines, including tumor necrosis factor-α (TNF-α) and IFN-γ.

IL-2 as a single agent generates response rates up to 24% in treating metastatic melanoma. When incubated with lymphatic cells in vitro, IL-2 activates the lymphoid cells to become cytotoxic to tumor cells. These lymphocytes, called lymphokine-activated killer (LAK) cells, can be administered systemically to patients in conjunction with IL-2 administration. In vitro studies of metastatic melanoma cells incubated with IL-2 have shown an increase in tumor-infiltrating lymphocytes (TIL cells). TIL cells can also be administered to patients in conjunction with IL-2. However, studies of these combinations (LAK and TIL cells with IL-2) have shown results similar to those of IL-2 alone. Responses with IL-2 may be delayed, with initial increases in tumor volume secondary to inflammation. Of these responses, a greater proportion are complete than in conventional chemotherapy. Durations of response may be prolonged in individual cases but are usually no longer than historical controls (4 to 6 months) (69).

Different doses and schedules of IL-2 have been investigated to try to maximize the antitumor response while minimizing the toxicity. Initial studies involving metastatic melanoma used high-dose IL-2 given as an intravenous bolus (6×10^5 IU/kg every 8 hours for 5 days, with a 1-week rest period between cycles), adopted from the NCI regimen for renal cell carcinoma (89). The same high doses were investigated in continuous-infusion regimens given over several days. The activity of these regimens seems to be similar against melanoma with similar toxicities. Subcutaneous administration has been most recently investigated to take advantage of the prolonged half-life that is seen with this method. Toxicity with subcutaneous administration is decreased substantially, with response data forthcoming.

Common toxicities occurring with high-dose intravenous IL-2 are listed in Table 87.19. Patients receiving the NCI regimen require intensive monitoring, since 70% of patients experience profound hypotension, requiring vasopressor support and judicious fluid administration. This phenomenon may be related to decreased peripheral vascular resistance occurring 2 to 4 hours after each injection. Capillary leak syndrome occurs quite frequently, manifesting as fluid retention with significant weight gain and pulmonary edema that leads to adult respiratory distress syndrome in some patients (69). In initial studies, 5% of patients required intubation secondary to pulmonary edema. Arrhythmias that are seen with this therapy may be related to the pressor agents that are used to treat hypotension. A pure α-sympathomimetic agent is recommended for patients who require blood pressure support. Decreased myocardial contractility occurs with this regimen, potentiating the effects associated with the capillary leak syndrome. Angina and myocardial infarction are reported in 3 to 4% of patients receiving high-dose IL-2 (90).

Table 87.19.
Toxicities Related to High-Dose Intravenous Administration of Interleukin-2ª

Capillary Leak Syndrome	Renal
Fluid retention	Oliguria
Weight gain	Azotemia
Pulmonary edema	Hepatic
Hypotension	Increased liver function
Cardiac	tests
Arrhythmias	Gastrointestinal
Decreased myocardial contractility	Nausea
Angina	Vomiting
Myocardial infarction	Diarrhea
Neurological	Stomatitis
Parasthesias	Hematologic
Constipation	Anemia
Confusion	Thrombocytopenia
Agitation	Leukopenia/leukocytosis
Hallucinations	Other
Lethargy	Rash
Somnolence	Hypothyroidism
Seizures	
Coma	
Constitutional Symptoms	
Fever	
Chills	
Myalgias	
Arthralgias	
Fatigue	

ªSee text for more information.

Renal dysfunction manifesting as oliguria and azotemia develops in nearly all patients, requiring renal-dose dopamine to enhance renal blood flow. Neuropsychiatric symptoms are common and manifest as confusion, agitation, hallucinations, lethargy, and somnolence, progressing in a few patients to seizures and coma. Severe parasthesias and constipation are also reported with this high-dose regimen of IL-2, relating to the neurotoxicity of the regimen. These effects take a few days to reverse after cessation of therapy but are fully reversible.

Gastrointestinal side effects are common with this therapy. Nausea and vomiting are reported in 87% of patients receiving high-dose therapy. Diarrhea occurs in 76% of patients and occasionally results in electrolyte abnormalities. Stomatitis occurs in up to 32% of patients and can lead to gastrointestinal ulceration and bleeding. Treatment with diphenoxylate and atropine (for diarrhea), antiemetics (for nausea and vomiting), and histamine H_2 blockers is helpful in preventing complications from these effects (90). Transient elevations in aminotransferase, alkaline phosphatase, and bilirubin are reported quite frequently, levels returning to normal several days after cessation of therapy.

Hematologic effects are common and often lead to increased incidence of sepsis, especially associated with central venous catheters. Anemia is the most common hematologic toxicity, affecting more than 50% of patients receiving high-dose IL-2 (90). Leukopenia is experienced during the first few days of therapy, secondary to demargination, followed by rebound leukocytosis. Thrombocytopenia is also common.

Constitutional symptoms consisting of fever, chills, myalgias, arthralgias, and fatigue are seen at all dose levels of IL-2. These effects are usually not severe, and the severity can be diminished by premedication with acetaminophen or indomethacin. The use of indomethacin could potentially compromise renal function; in conjunction with the effects of IL-2 on renal blood flow, this combination may be detrimental to the patient.

Toxicities related to IL-2 that is given subcutaneously are mild in comparison to those discussed above. Inflammation and induration at the injection site are commonly reported. Fever, chills, mild to moderate nausea and vomiting, and diarrhea are also reported by patients receiving IL-2 subcutaneously. The capillary leak syndrome described above is not seen with this method of administration. Response data is not available with single-agent IL-2 given subcutaneously.

Monoclonal antibodies (MoAbs) targeting specific antigens that are present on the melanoma cell surface may become the agents of the future. Several different cell surface antigens have been targeted for this type of therapy. Monoclonal antibodies act directly or indirectly to cause cell death. Antibody-dependent cellular cytotoxicity involves the MoAb binding to the cell surface target antigen, resulting in a cascade of cytotoxic events. This action is mediated by natural killer cells and monocytes (91). The indirect action of MoAbs is related to their ability to stimulate other antibodies to be released and act directly on the cells. MoAbs targeted for growth factors or their receptors are another area of research (91). As was discussed previously, the growth of melanoma cells depends on many autocrine and paracrine growth factors working together. Interference with only one of these functions may not be adequate for cell death, but investigations are underway to determine the exact role of these factors in melanoma cell growth and proliferation. This will lead to a better understanding of melanoma cellular biology and to better targeted therapy in the future. The use of MoAbs conjugated with toxins is being investigated to deliver a toxic agent directly to the melanoma cell, killing only cancer cells and sparing normal cells (91). Agents such as ricin-A-chain, vindesine, and daunorubicin are potential agents for conjugation in this manner. Radionuclides conjugated with MoAbs are also being investigated for diagnostic purposes (91). This would aid in identifying micrometastatic disease and allow for targeted therapy and better treatment choices. These approaches are investigational and are underway in the clinical setting.

The principles involved in melanoma MoAbs have also been used to develop melanoma vaccines. The goal of a vaccine is to stimulate the host immunity to reject the targeted disease cell, in this case melanoma cells. The number and type of potential antigen targets that are present on the melanoma cell surface vary among patients and between cells within the same tumor nodule. (92) This makes the development of a specific vaccine that would be generally applicable a very difficult task. The easiest technique that is used to make a vaccine is to take cells from the patient's own tumor. These cells would not produce the immune response needed because the patient's immune system would not recognize them as foreign. If these cells could be altered or combined with another agent to elicit a greater immune response, this would potentially be an effective vaccine (92). Another avenue that researchers have taken to develop a vaccine has been to use cell surface antigens that have been shed from several different cell lines and combine these into one vaccine, potentially increasing the chances of eliciting an immune response in the patient (92). Recently, several of these cell surface antigens have been cloned, opening up a new arena for development of active specific immunotherapy. Viruses can also be used to elicit tumoricidal immune responses. In ongoing studies, the vaccinia virus is being used to target melanoma cells (92).

Vaccines, and immunotherapy in general, work best against minimal tumor burden (92). Therefore, employing these agents as adjuvant therapy in early stages of melanoma has been the eventual goal of investigation. Once activity can be established in the metastatic setting, then comparative trials in earlier stages of disease will begin. Prevention of melanoma in high-risk patients by using these compounds is also of interest.

One promising new approach to cancer treatment has been the discovery of gene transfer. The process of sequencing and cloning a gene is now possible by using the polymerase chain reaction. This allows a normal gene sequence to be copied and transfected into a cancer cell to replace the defective or cancerous gene (69). Most cancers have many different genetic abnormalities, which work together to cause cells to become malignant. Therefore, this method of treating cancer is not feasible with the technology we possess today. Gene transfer can be used to introduce genes into cancer cells that encode for toxic substances, subsequently killing the cell. For example, the tumor necrosis factor gene has been transfected into TIL cells and is capable of killing melanoma cells in animal models (69). This process can be done with the gene for IL-2 as well. This causes melanoma cells to produce IL-2, leading to the melanoma's own demise (69). These theories are being tested in early clinical trials involving humans.

Combination Immuno-Chemotherapy. Single-agent chemotherapy is minimally effective against metastatic melanoma, and combination chemotherapy regimens have not proven to be better than single-agent dacarbazine. The hope for combining chemotherapy with immunotherapy is that different mechanisms of action will enhance the rate and duration of responses. Cyclophosphamide, a potent immunosuppressive agent, selectively depletes or impairs suppressor T cells. Pretreatment with cyclophosphamide causes an augmented delayed-type hypersensitivity reaction upon antigen administration. Cyclophosphamide (350 mg/m^2 intravenously) given 3 days before IL-2 ($21.6 \times 10^6 \text{ IU/m}^2$ intravenous bolus 5 days/week for 2 weeks) will augment the cytotoxicity of IL-2 (90). Objective response rates with this regimen were 26%, and the median survival for responding patients was 18 months. Of note is that four of the ten responding patients had regression of large hepatic metastases, which are usually refractory to therapy (90).

Interferon-α– causes cell surface antigen up-regulation on melanoma cells, thereby increasing susceptibility to the effects of IL-2. In one study, the combination of these two immunotherapies resulted in objective response rates of 36% with a duration of 3 to 10+ months. Three of these responses were complete. (90) This response rate was slightly higher than that with either agent alone, but this was not a direct comparison. The addition of IL-2 to dacarbazine showed no difference in response rates compared to either agent alone. The response rates ranged from 22 to 24%, and their duration was 4 to 16+ months.

Toxicity from this regimen was associated primarily with IL-2 (90).

Combination chemotherapy with the CVD regimen described above has been investigated with the addition of IL-2 and IFN-α (93). This combination appears to be sequence dependent. Alternating CVD with IL-2/IFN-α (biotherapy) every 6 weeks has shown responses similar to those obtained with CVD alone. Biotherapy administered after CVD followed by a sandwich of biotherapy/chemotherapy/biotherapy appears to be superior to CVD alone (response rates 73% and 40%, respectively). Table 87.20 outlines this regimen of CVD/BIO sequential chemoimmunotherapy. Simultaneous administration of biotherapy and CVD also appears to be superior to CVD alone (response rates 63% and 40%, respectively). However, only the sequential therapy with CVD/BIO has shown a significant increase in progression-free survival (8 months versus 4 months, $P = 0.005$) and overall survival (12 versus 9 months, $P = 0.006$) compared to CVD alone (94). A randomized trial comparing CVD alone with CVD/BIO as described in Table 87.20 is underway at the MD Anderson Cancer Center. It is important to mention that this regimen is extremely toxic, requiring hospitalization for both the chemotherapy and biotherapy portions of the regimen. Renal-dose dopamine is given as a standard for all patients during the biotherapy portion of the regimen to maintain renal perfusion during the interleukin-2 infusion. This regimen has been important for developing the sequencing aspects of chemoimmunotherapy and confirming that combining chemotherapy and biotherapy does increase survival, but more feasible outpatient regimens need to be developed to improve the quality of life of these patients.

Richards used a different chemotherapy regimen in conjunction with IL-2, IFN-α, and tamoxifen. (95) Carmustine (150 mg/m^2), dacarbazine (220 mg/m^2), and cisplatin (25 mg/m^2) were combined on days 1 through 3 and days 22 through 24. IL-2 (1.5×10^6 IU/m^2 intravenously every 8 hr) and IFN-α (6×10^6 IU/m^2 subcutaneously once daily) were given on days 4 through 8 and days 17 through 21. Tamoxifen (10 mg) was given twice daily for 6 weeks. Of the 34 patients who were evaluable, 20 (59%) had objective responses, and 8 (24%) of those were complete. This is quite impressive in comparison to other combination trials. The sites of metastases in this trial were not reported, but one patient with hepatic metastases had a complete response. This is a small, noncomparative trial that warrants further investigation.

Many different combinations of chemotherapy and immunotherapy are being investigated around the world. Many of these show greater responses than that of conventional therapy with either modality alone. These regimens have not been compared to each other, nor have they been compared to standard therapy with either chemotherapy or immunotherapy alone. Acceptance of any of these combination regimens as standards of therapy will have to wait until further evidence of a survival benefit or an increase in palliative efficacy is shown.

NO TREATMENT

Dismal responses to conventional treatment regimens and short survival spans bring to light the question of risks versus benefits. A considerable amount of toxicity is associated with the treatment regimens that are currently being investigated, especially regimens that include high-dose IL-2. If the benefits of these regimens do not include increased overall survival with good quality of life, than the benefits hardly seem worth the risks. In fact, many clinicians would consider no treatment a reasonable option

Table 87.20.
MD Anderson Chemomimmunotherapy Sequential Regimen[a]

	CVD		BIOTHERAPY	
	Cisplatin	20 mg/m^2 IV × 4 days	IFN-α	5 MU/m^2 SQ × 5 days
	Vinblastine	1.6 mg/m^2 IV × 5 days	IL-2	3 MU/m^2 IV CI over 24 hr × 4 days
	Dacarbazine	800 mg/m^2 IV × 1 day		

Day:	1–5	6–11	12–16	17–22	22–26	27–32	33–42	43–48
	CVD	BIO	BREAK	BIO	CVD	BIO	BREAK	CVD

COURSE 1   COURSE 2

Only sequential therapy (CVD ⟶ BIO), shown here, has been superior to CVD alone.[b]

[a]IFN-α = interferon-α; IL-2 = interleukin-2; BIO = biotherapy.
[b]See text for further information.

for patients with metastatic melanoma. A phase I treatment program would be an exception if the patient requests treatment. Treatment with an investigational regimen in a controlled clinical trial is the only way to ensure that these patients' options continue to expand.

OCULAR MELANOMA

Intraocular melanomas arise from uveal melanocytes residing in the uveal stroma. The majority of lesions arise within the globe (mainly from the choroid); a small percentage arise in the conjunctiva. In people older than 20 years of age, melanoma accounts for approximately 80% of all primary eye malignancies. Its incidence is approximately one-eighth that of cutaneous melanoma, with a median age of 55 and rates decreasing after the age of 70. The recent increase in incidence of cutaneous melanoma has not been seen with ocular melanoma. White people have an eightfold increased risk for ocular melanoma compared to black people and a threefold greater risk than Asian populations.

The size of the lesion is the most important prognostic indicator in ocular melanoma. Small lesions (2 to 2.5 mm in height and ≤16 mm in base diameter), which historically were treated with enucleation (removal of the eye), can be treated locally with radiation, photocoagulation, cryotherapy, ultrasonic hyperthermia, or local resection. These lesions can be safely observed if they appear dormant, the patient is elderly or not in good health, or the affected eye is the only functioning eye. Monthly exams can be done to watch the tumor, and action can be taken when necessary. Large tumors (>10 mm in height and >16 mm in base diameter or at least 2 mm in height and >16 mm in base diameter) must be treated with enucleation. Treatment of medium-sized lesions (≥2.5 mm to ≤10 mm in height and ≤16 mm in base diameter) is controversial. A trial comparing radiation with enucleation is being conducted under the auspices of the National Eye Institute. Both methods are effective, and personal choice is often the deciding factor. Immunotherapy and chemotherapy have failed to show any benefit in the primary or adjuvant treatment of medium-sized lesions. If more effective agents become available, the usefulness of treating these lesions would be to eradicate subclinical metastases that are present at the time of diagnosis (adjuvant therapy).

Metastases are present in approximately 2% of patients at diagnosis (96). The most common site of metastases is the liver. Resection of solitary hepatic lesions has been shown to be effective palliative treatment and may prolong survival. Chemoembolization of the hepatic artery has been associated with prolonged periods of remission. Systemic treatment of metastases from ocular melanoma are usually treated similarly to cutaneous metastatic melanoma, with similar results.

SCREENING AND PREVENTION

A key factor in increasing overall survival with all types of skin cancer is early diagnosis, which improves the odds of the patient evading subclinical metastases at the time of diagnosis. This is particularly true for melanoma, which is curable if detected early in its radial phase but is deadly in its later stages. Key issues that make screening for a disease successful are (a) a sensitive and specific screening tool, (b) disease prevalence that is high enough to warrant screening, (c) potential outcomes that are serious enough to warrant the expense and effort of screening, (d) a disease that is relatively slow-growing and not immediately life-threatening, (e) a screening tool that is simple, inexpensive, and acceptable to the population being screened, (f) early diagnoses that result in better overall survival rates and improved prognoses, and (g) screening leading to more effective treatment at an earlier stage (97). Skin cancer meets these criteria.

Screening for skin cancer consists of visual inspection of the skin and subsequent referral for biopsy and histologic evaluation of any suspicious lesion. This is a simple and inexpensive process but involves some challenges. Visual inspection is defined differently by different investigators. Several studies have demonstrated the impact of a trained practitioner in recognizing significant cutaneous diseases. Successful skin cancer screening programs must include the participation of such practitioners. After attending a screening program, most people are able to learn the procedure for visual self-inspection. For average-risk patients the use of self-examinations is adequate, with self-referral to a physician if any suspicious lesion is found. For high-risk patients a professional examination with mapping, documenting, and monitoring of all skin lesions is important for early detection and a positive impact on mortality. This method is both sensitive and specific as well as economically sound. For example, the National Melanoma/Skin Cancer Prevention Program in the United States relies on volunteers to provide the screenings and facilities. The prevalence of skin cancer is obviously high enough to warrant mass screening. The serious potential outcome of melanoma is also apparent, as is evidenced by the extremely high mortality rate in metastatic melanoma. However, in its radial growth phase, melanoma is slow-growing, highly curable, and not immediately life-threatening. With new treatment options such as monoclonal antibodies, vaccines, and other new agents, earlier treatment will be more effective and will lead to better overall survival rates with improved prognoses.

The most reliable method for determining the success of a screening program is a reduction in mortality from the cancer. The efficacy of screening or early detection programs has not been tested in randomized trials. Many countries around the world have shown increases in the numbers of melanomas detected and decreases in the thickness of the melanomas found. These statistical trends theoretically equate to reduced mortality, but this has not been proven.

In conjunction with disease screening, public education efforts lead not only to more effective screening programs, but also to more effective prevention. UV radiation exposure has been associated with skin cancer of all kinds. Limiting exposure to UV radiation through the use of sunscreens and protective clothing has never been shown to decrease the incidence of skin cancer in humans. However, animal studies showed that sunscreens effectively decrease the amount of UV radiation penetrating the dermis. Theoretically, this action will decrease the physiologic effects of UV radiation. Unfortunately, until the complex mechanism of action of UV radiation is outlined, these actions of prevention must be coupled with decreased time spent outdoors during periods of intense sunlight and avoidance of artificial UV sources such as tanning beds. These actions are most critical for prevention of NMSC. The association of melanoma with UV radiation is less well defined, but cutaneous melanoma may be somewhat preventable with these same measures.

Vaccines and retinoids are being investigated for prevention in high-risk populations such as patients with dysplastic nevus syndrome. These trials are in their infancy but will provide vital information concerning the pathophysiology of these diseases.

CONCLUSION

Skin cancer is often a forgotten cancer because of its generally benign nature. However, as has been demonstrated here, the incidence and importance of this set of diseases are profound. NMSC is not extremely threatening in terms of mortality but is quite detrimental in terms of morbidity and number of patients affected. Melanoma is extremely life-threatening, especially in its later stages, and poses a great threat to the general population due to its rapidly increasing incidence. Fortunately, treatment with surgery generally provides excellent results with minimal complications. The detrimental outcome that is seen with lesions that are not amenable to surgery provides the impetus for development of many new treatment modalities. These include new immunotherapies, chemotherapies, monoclonal antibodies, and vaccines. The use of new and currently available therapeutic agents in different combinations with each other and with different modalities of treatment is leading the search for better therapeutic outcomes. With the development of gene therapy on the horizon, new hopes for better survival rates are strengthened. In conjunction with all of these treatment hopes, the emphasis on prevention and screening is imperative. These tools may someday obviate the need for more effective

therapeutic modalities. Only through diligent research and education can we reach these goals.

REFERENCES

1. Safai B, Cancers of the skin. In: DeVita VT, Hellman S, Rosenberg SA. Cancer: principles and practice of oncology, 4th ed. Philadelphia: JB Lippincott, 1993:1567-1611.
2. Wingo PA, Tong T, Bolden S. Cancer statistics, 1995. CA Cancer J Clin 45:8–30, 1995.
3. Osterlind A. Etiology and epidemiology of melanoma and skin neoplasms. Curr Opin Oncol 3:355–59, 1991.
4. Roberts DL. Incidence of nonmelanoma skin cancer in West Giamorgan, South Wales. Br J Dermatol 122:399–404, 1990.
5. Diffey BL, Larko O. Clinical climatology. Photodermatology 1:30–7, 1984.
6. Hacker SM, Browder JF, Ramos-Caro FA. Basal cell carcinoma: choosing the best method of treatment for a particular lesion. Postgrad Med 93(8):101–104, 106, 108, 111, 1993.
7. Gupta AK, Cardella CJ, Haberman HF. Cutaneous malignant neoplasms in patients with renal transplants. Arch Dermatol 122: 1288–93, 1986.
8. Hart RW, Setlow RB, Woodhead AD. Evidence that pyrimidine dimers in DNA can give rise to tumors. Proc Natl Acad Sci USA 74(12):5574–78, 1977.
9. Fraser MC, Hartge P, Tucker MA. Melanoma and nonmelanoma skin cancer: epidemiology and risk factors. Semin Oncol Nurs 7 (1):2–12, 1991.
10. Vargo NL. Basal and squamous cell carcinomas: an overview. Semin Oncol Nurs 7(1):13–25, 1991.
11. American Joint Committee on Cancer. Manual for staging of cancer, 4th ed. Philiadelphia: JB Lippincott, Co, 1995:23–4.
12. Rowe DE, Carroll RJ, Day CL. Long-term recurrence rates in previously untreated (primary) basal cell carcinoma: implications for patient follow-up. J Dermatol Surg Oncol 15:315–28, 1989.
13. Weinstock MA, Bogaars HA, Ashley M, et al. Nonmelanoma skin cancer mortality. Arch Dermatol 127:1194–97, 1991.
14. Kwa RE, Campana K, Moy RL. Biology of cutaneous squamous cell carcinoma. J Am Acad Dermatol 26:1–26, 1992.
15. Kuflik EG, Gage AA. The five-year cure rate achieved by cryosurgery for skin cancer. J Am Acad Dermatol 24:1002–04, 1991.
16. Hacker SM, Flowers FP. Squamous cell carcinoma of the skin: will heightened awareness of risk factors slow its increase? Postgrad Med 93(8):115–118, 120–121, 125–126, 1993.
17. Lawrence CM. Moh's surgery of basal cell carcinoma: a critical review. Br J Plast Surg 46:599–606, 1993.
18. Albright SD. Treatment of skin cancer using multiple modalities. J Am Acad Dermatol 7:143–71, 1982.
19. Cairnduff F, Stringer MR, Hudson EJ, et al. Superficial photodynamic therapy with topical 5-aminolevulinic acid for superficial primary and secondary skin cancer. Br J Cancer 69(3):605–08, 1994.
20. Svanberg K, Andersson T, Killander D, et al. Photodynamic therapy of non-melanoma malignant tumours of the skin using topical amino levulinic acid sensitization and laser irradiation. Br J Dermatol 130:743–51, 1994.
21. Cullen SI. Topical fluorouracil therapy for precancers and cancers of the skin. J Am Geriat Soc 12:529–35, 1979.
22. Epstein E. Fluorouracil paste treatment of thin basal cell carcinomas. Arch Dermatol 121:207–13, 1985.
23. Dillaha CJ, Jansen GT, Honeycutt WM, et al. Selective cytotoxic effect of topical 5-fluorouracil. Arch Dermatol 88:247–56, 1963.
24. Sadek H, Azli N, Wendling JL, et al. Treatment of advanced squamous cell carcinoma of the skin with cisplatin, 5-fluorouracil, and bleomycin. Cancer 66:1692–96, 1990.

25. Tahery DP, Moy RL. Immunotherapy and skin cancer. J Dermatol Surg Oncol 18:584–86, 1992.

26. Peck GL. Topical tretinoin in actinic keratosis and basal cell carcinoma. J Am Acad Dermatol 15:829–35, 1986.

26A. Robinson TA, Kligman AM. Treatment of solar kenatoses with retinoic acid and 5-fluorouracil. Br J Dermatol 92:703–706, 1975.

27. Balch CM, Houghton AN, Peters LJ. Cutaneous melanoma. In: DeVita VT, Hellman S, Rosenberg SA. Cancer: principles and practice of oncology, 4th ed. Philadelphia: JB Lippincott, 1993:1612–60.

28. Grin-Jorgensen CM, Rigel DS, Friedman RJ. The worldwide incidence of malignant melanoma. In: Balch CM, Houghton AN, Milton GW, et al. Cutaneous melanoma, 2nd ed. Philadelphia: JB Lippincott, 1992:27–39.

29. Balch CM, Soong S-J, Milton GW, et al. Changing trends in cutaneous melanoma over a quarter century in Alabama, USA, and New South Wales, Australia. Cancer 52:1748–53, 1983.

30. Armstrong BK, English DR. Epidemiologic studies. In: Balch CM, Houghton AN, Milton GW, et al. Cutaneous melanoma, 2nd ed. Philadelphia: JB Lippincott, 1992:12–26.

31. Koh HK. Cutaneous melanoma. N Engl J Med 325(3):171–82, 1991.

32. Drolet BA, Connor MJ. Sunscreens and the prevention of ultraviolet radiation-induced skin cancer. J Dermatol Surg Oncol 18:571–76, 1992.

33. Swerdlow AJ, English JSC, MacKie RM, et al. Fluorescent lights, ultraviolet lamps, and risk of cutaneous melanoma. Br Med J 297:647–50, 1988.

34. Walter SD, Marrett LD, From L, et al. The association of cutaneous melanoma with the use of sunbeds and sunlamps. Am J Epidemiol 131:232–43, 1990.

35. MacKie RM, Freudenberger R, Aitchison TC. Personal risk-factor chart for cutaneous melanoma. Lancet ii:487–90, 1989.

36. Elwood JM, Williamson C, Stapleton PJ. Malignant melanoma in relation to moles, pigmentation, and exposure to fluorescent and other lighting sources. Br J Cancer 52:65–74, 1986.

37. Gallagher RP, Elwood JM, Hill GP. Risk factors for cutaneous malignant melanoma: the Western Canada Melanoma Study. Recent Results Cancer Res 102:38–55, 1986.

38. Osterlind A, Tucker MA, Stone BJ, et al. The Danish case-control study of cutaneous malignant melanoma. II: importance of UV-light exposure. Int J Cancer 42:319–24, 1988.

39. Kraemer KH, Greene MH. Dysplastic nevi and malignant melanoma. Dermatol Clin 3:225–37, 1985.

40. Ramcharan S, Pellegrin FA, Ray R, et al. The Walnut Creek contraceptive drug study. Vol III: An interim report. NIH Publication No 81-564. Washington, DC: US Government Printing Office, 1981.

41. Holly EA, Weiss NS, Liff JM. Cutaneous melanoma in relation to exogenous hormones and reproductive factors. J Natl Cancer Inst 70:827–31, 1983.

42. Holman CDJ, Armstrong BK, Heenan PJ. Cutaneous malignant melanoma in women: exogenous sex hormones and reproductive factors. Br J Cancer 50:673–80, 1984.

43. Beral V, Evans S, Shaw H. Oral contraceptive use and malignant melanoma in Australia. Br J Cancer 50:681–85, 1984.

44. Beral V, Ramcharan S, Faris R. Malignant melanoma and oral contraceptive use among women in California. Br J Cancer 36:804–09, 1977.

45. Herlyn M, Houghton AN. Biology of melanocytes and melanoma. In: Balch CM, Houghton AN, Milton GW, et al. Cutaneous melanoma, 2nd ed. Philadelphia: JB Lippincott, 1992:82–92.

46. Crutcher WA, Cohen PJ. Dysplastic nevi and malignant melanoma. Am Fam Physician 42(2):372–85, 1990.

47. Clark WH Jr, Elder ED, Guerry D IV, et al. The precursor lesions of superficial spreading and nodular melanoma. Hum Pathol 15:1147–65, 1984.

48. Lu C, Kerbel RS. Cytokines, growth factors and the loss of negative growth controls in the progression of human cutaneous malignant melanoma. Curr Opin Oncol 6:212–20, 1994.

49. Gruis NA, Bergnam W, Frants RR. Locus for susceptibility to melanoma on chromosome 1p. N Engl J Med 322(12):853–54, 1990.

50. Friedman RJ, Rigel DS, Kopf AW. Early detection of malignant melanoma: the role of physician examination and self-examination of the skin. CA Cancer J Clin 35:130–51, 1985.

51. Fitzpatrick TB, Milton GW, Balch CM, et al. Clinical Characteristics. In: Balch CM, Houghton AN, Milton GW, et al. Cutaneous melanoma, 2nd ed. Philadelphia: JB Lippincott, 1992:223–33.

52. Breslow A. Thickness, cross-sectional areas and depth of invasion in the prognosis of cutaneous melanoma. Ann Surg 172:902–08, 1970.

53. Clark WH Jr, Ainsworth AM, Bernardino EA, et al. The developmental biology of primary human malignant melanomas. Semin Oncol 2:83–103, 1975.

54. Balch CM, Murad TM, Soong S-J, et al. A multifactorial analysis of melanoma: prognostic histopathological features comparing Clark's and Breslow's staging methods. Ann Surg 188:732–42, 1978.

55. Balch CM, Soong S-J, Shaw HM, et al. An analysis of prognostic factors in 8500 patients with cutaneous melanoma. In: Balch CM, Houghton AN, Milton GW, et al. Cutaneous melanoma, 2nd ed. Philadelphia: JB Lippincott, 1992:165–87.

56. Singletary SE, Balch CM, Urist MM, et al. Surgical treatment of primary melanoma. In: Balch CM, Houghton AN, Milton GW, et al. Cutaneous melanoma, 2nd ed. Philadelphia: JB Lippincott, 1992: 269–274.

57. Veronesi U, Cascinelli N. Narrow excision (1 cm margin), a safe procedure for thin cutaneous melanoma. Arch Surg 126:438–41, 1991.

58. Balch CM, Urist MM, Karkousis CP, et al. Efficacy of 2 cm surgical margins for intermediate-thickness melanomas (1 to 4 mm): results of a multi-institutional randomized surgical trial. Ann Surg 218:262–69, 1993.

59. Timmons MJ. Malignant melanoma excision margins: marking a choice. Lancet 340:1393–95, 1992.

60. Goldsmith LA, Askin FB, Chang AE, et al. Diagnosis and treatment of early melanoma. JAMA 268:1314–19, 1992.

61. Ross MI. The case for elective lymphadenectomy. Surg Oncol Clin North Am 1:205–22, 1992.

62. Crowley NJ. The case against elective lymphadenectomy. Surg Oncol Clin North Am 1:223–43, 1992.

63. Morton DL, Wen DR, Wong JM. Technical details of intraoperative lymphatic mapping for early stage melanoma. Arch Surg 127:392–99, 1992.

64. Harwood AR. Conventional fractionated radiotherapy for 51 patients with lentigo maligna and lentigo maligna melanoma. Int J Radiat Oncol Biol Phys 9:1019–21, 1983.

65. Ang KK, Byers RM, Peters LJ, et al. Regional radiotherapy as adjuvant treatment for head and neck malignancy melanoma. Arch Otolaryngol Head Neck Surg 116:169–72, 1990.

66. Bowers GJ, Copeland EM. Surgical limb perfusion for extemity melanoma. Surg Oncol 3(2):91–102, 1994.

67. Coit DG. Isolation limb perfusion for melanoma: current trends and future directions. Melanoma Res 4(suppl 1):57–60, 1994.

68. LeJeune FJ, Liereard D, Leyvraz A, et al. Regional therapy of melanoma. Eur J Cancer 29A:606–12, 1993.

69. Ho RCS. Medical management of stage IV malignant melanoma. Cancer 75(2):735–41, 1995.

70. Houghton AN, Legha S, Bajorin DF. Chemotherapy for metastatic melanoma. In: Balch CM, Houghton AN, Milton GW, et al. Cutaneous melanoma, 2nd ed. Philadelphia: JB Lippincott, 1992: 498–508.

71. Dorr RT, Von Hoff DD. Cancer chemotherapy handbook, 2nd ed. East Norwalk, CT: Appleton-Lange, 1994:343–49.

72. Einhorn LH, McBride CM, Luce JK, et al. Intraarterial infusion therapy with 5-(3,3-dimethyl-1-triazeno)imidazole-4-carboxamide (NSC-45388) for malignant melanoma. Cancer 32(4):749–55, 1973.

73. Yamasaki T, Kikuchi H, Yamashita J, et al. Primary spinal intramedullary malignant melanoma: case report. Neurosurgery 25:117–21, 1989.

74. Champagne MA, Silver HKB. Intrathecal dacarbazine treatment of leptomeningeal malignant melanoma. J Natl Cancer Inst 84:1203–04, 1992.

75. Kirkwood JM. Systemic therapy of melanoma. Curr Opin Oncol 6:204–11, 1994.

76. Khayat D, Bizzari J-P, Frenay M, et al. Interim report of phase II study of new nitrosourea S 10036 in disseminated malignant melanoma. J Natl Cancer Inst 80:1407–08, 1988.

77. Khayat D, Lokiec F, Bizzari J-P, et al. Phase I clinical study of the new amino acid-linked nitrosourea, S 10036, administered on a weekly schedule. Cancer Res 47:6782–85, 1987.

78. Khayat D, Cour V, Bizzari JP, et al. Fotemustine (S 10036) in the intra-arterial treatment of liver metastasis from malignant melanoma: a phase II study. Am J Clin Oncol 14(5):400–04, 1991.

79. Glover D, Glick JH, Weiler C, et al. WR 2721 and high-dose cis-platin: an active combination in the treatment of metastatic melanoma. J Clin Oncol 5:574–78, 1987.

80. Mavligit G, Charnsangavej C, Carrasco CH, et al. Regression of ocular melanoma metastatic to the liver after hepatic arterial chemoembolization with cisplatin and polyvinyl sponge. JAMA 260:974–76, 1988.

81. Chang A, Hunt M, Parkinson DR, et al. Phase II trial of carboplatin in patients with metastatic malignant melanoma: a report from the Eastern Cooperative Oncology Group. Am J Clin Oncol 16(2):152–55, 1993.

82. Wiernik PH, Einzig AI. Taxol in malignant melanoma. Monographs Natl Cancer Inst 15:185–87, 1993.

83. Pazdur R, Newman RA, Newman BM, et al. Phase I trial of Taxotere: five-day schedule. J Natl Cancer Inst 84(23):1781–1788, 1992.

84. Gundersen S. Dacarbazin, vindesine, and cisplatin combination chemotherapy in advanced malignant melanoma: a phase II study. Cancer Treat Rep 71:997–99, 1987.

85. Legha SS, Ring S, Papadopoulos N, et al. A prospective evaluation of a triple-drug regimen containing cisplatin, vinblastine, and dacarbazine (CVD) for metastatic melanoma. Cancer 64:2024–29, 1989.

86. Del Prete SA, Maurer LH, O'Donnell J. Combination chemotherapy with cisplatin, carmustine, dacarbazine, and tamoxifen in metastatic melanoma. Cancer Treat Rep 68:1403–05, 1984.

87. McClay EF, Mastrangelo MJ, Berd D, et al. Effective combination chemo/hormonal therapy for malignant melanoma: experience with three consecutive trials. Int J Cancer 50:553–56, 1992.

88. McClay EF, Albright KD, Jones JA, et al. Tamoxifen modulation of cisplatin sensitivity in human malignant melanoma cells. Cancer Res 53(7):1571–6, 1993.

89. Rosenberg SA, Lotze MT, Yant JC, et al. Experience with the use of high-dose interleukin-2 in the treatment of 652 cancer patients. Ann Surg 210:474–85, 1989.

90. Brutin JK, Koeller JM. Recombinant interleukin-2. Pharmacotherapy 14(6):635–56, 1994.

91. Parkinson DR, Houghton AN, Hersey P, et al. Biologic therapy for melanoma. In: Balch CM, Houghton AN, Milton GW, et al. Cutaneous melanoma. 2nd ed. Philadelphia: JB Lippincott, 1992:522–41.

92. Hellstrom KE, Hellstrom I, Morton DL, et al. Melanoma vaccines. In: Balch CM, Houghton AN, Milton GW, et al. Cutaneous melanoma. 2nd ed. Philadelphia: JB Lippincott, 1992:542–59.

93. Buzaid AC, Legha SS. Combination of chemotherapy with interleukin-2 and interferon-alpha for the treatment of advanced melanoma. Semin Oncol 21(6):23–8, 1994.

94. Legha S, Buzaid AC, Ring S, et al. Improved results of treatment of metastatic melanoma with combined use of biotherapy and chemotherapy (biochemo) [Abstract]. Proc Annu Meet Am Soc Clin Oncol 13:394, 1994.

95. Richards JM. Sequential chemoimmunotherapy for metastatic melanoma. Semin Oncol 18(5):91–5, 1991.

96. Sahel JA, Earle JD, Albert DM. Intraocular melanomas. In: DeVita VT, Hellman S, Rosenberg SA. Cancer: principles and practice of oncology, 4th ed. Philadelphia: JB Lippincott, 1993:1662–78.

97. Cole P, Morrison AS. Issues in population screening for cancer. J Natl Cancer Inst 64:1263–72, 1980.

CHAPTER 88

PEDIATRIC AND NEONATAL THERAPY

ROBERT H. LEVIN

Pediatrics is a branch of medicine that deals with the care and treatment of the diseases of humans from birth through adolescence, with specific terminology defined for different age groups (Table 88.1). Within pediatrics, which became a specialty in the twentieth century, there are as many medical specialties as there are in adult internal medicine.

Neonates, infants, and children require unique considerations, since age-related differences in physiology alter the pharmacokinetics and pharmacodynamics of many drugs. For infants, particularly neonates, differences in drug absorption, distribution, excretion, metabolism, and sensitivity affect the use and dosing of drugs. Pediatric dosing also involves various methods of calculating doses and consideration of appropriate drug formulations. The child's family or caretakers must be included in any discussion of medical treatment that involves the administration of drugs to the child. The issue of compliance with therapeutic regimens rests on the willingness of others to assist in the child's medical care.

Healthy growth and development of children are the major focuses for "well baby" clinics. During visits to the clinics, the parents are informed about proper nutrition, breast feeding, maternal diet, and drugs to be avoided (see Chapter 92). The feeding of synthetic infant formulas, baby foods, and table foods is also discussed (see Chapter 89). Diseases are prevented by proper nutrition and the use of prophylactic agents such as immunizations (see Chapter 61). The advantages and possible adverse effects of each immunization are thoroughly discussed with the parents before the immunizations are given to the child.

DEVELOPMENTAL PHARMACOLOGY

Drug Absorption

Drugs are most frequently given to children orally. Neonates have the potential for altered drug absorption as a result of decreased production of gastric acid and reduced gastric emptying time. Neonates have a relative achlorhydria. Drugs that are absorbed in the stomach, by remaining in the stomach for an additional 6 to 8 hr, may have enhanced effects as a result of increased absorption. Although gastric acid production increases and the pH decreases rapidly over the first 24 hr of life, levels of gastric acid equivalent to those of an adult are not reached until the child is about 1 year old. This causes a decreased absorption of acidic drugs such as aspirin. As the neonate matures into infancy, the gastrointestinal transit time increases, so sustained-release drug products pass through the intestine very quickly. For example, only about 50% of a dose of Theodur Sprinkles is absorbed in children who are younger than 5 years old. The hydrolytic enzyme system of the newborn or infant may not be sufficient for absorption of certain drugs. Infants who are less than 6 months old lack the hydrolytic enzyme to split palmitic acid from chloramphenicol palmitate, which prevents its absorption. Oral phenytoin may also be inadequately absorbed in infants under 6 months old, necessitating doses greater than usual (15 to 20 mg/kg/day) to produce therapeutic serum levels (1). Finally, conditions such as diarrhea markedly decrease the absorption of orally administered drugs.

The rectal route is used more frequently for young children than for adults, since children often have difficulty swallowing medications. No specific physiologic differences influence rectal absorption of medication in children; however, problems have been documented with certain suppository dosage forms. Outdated suppositories or those that have been exposed to air may have erratic melting characteristics that cause decreased and unpredictable drug absorption, which has been reported with suppositories that contain aminophylline. Appropriate therapeutic responses occur with suppositories of aspirin, acetaminophen, prochlorperazine, promethazine, glycerin, and others.

Ointments, lotions, and creams are commonly used for topical treatment of localized skin lesions that usually occur in the diaper area of infants and on the trunk, limbs, and

Table 88.1.
Pediatric Definitions

Category	Age
Premature	<38 weeks gestation
Newborn, neonate	Birth to 1 month old
Infant, baby	1–24 months
Young child	1–5 years
Older child	6–12 years
Adolescent	13–18 years

face of children. A number of factors should be considered before selecting a topical agent. Infants, in contrast to older children, have a proportionally larger skin surface area that is capable of absorbing more topical drugs, especially if the drugs are applied to the groin or face. Inflammation increases the amount of drug that is absorbed, as does the occlusion that occurs with plastic-coated diapers. An infant's skin is very sensitive, so a number of chemicals frequently cause local irritation (e.g., parabens, methyl salicylate).

The parenteral route, which is frequently used for hospitalized children, is seldom needed for ambulatory children except for immunizations or insulin administration to diabetics. Infants have a small muscle mass, and intramuscular injections must be given in the lateral thigh rather than the arm or buttock. Absorption from intramuscular sites in neonates is slower and more erratic because of the smaller muscle mass and blood supply. Therefore the intravenous route is preferred for neonates. In treating neonates, infants, and young children, the accurate and timely administration of doses is particularly important. This requires precise dose calculation, measurement, and delivery. Microinfusion devices must deliver small volumes of fluids and medications accurately and safely. Neonatal microinfusion devices deliver intravenous fluid or medication in increments of tenths of a milliliter and have safeguards against uncontrolled free flow of fluid (2, 3).

Drug Distribution

Most drugs are distributed primarily into the aqueous portion of the body. The body weight of neonates is about 75% water; therefore the volume of distribution of many drugs is increased. For example, the volume of distribution of theophylline in a neonate is approximately 1 L/kg, compared to 0.48 L/kg in a 6-year-old. In addition, the total body water of neonates is 56% extracellular fluid, and many drugs are distributed primarily in total body water. Body water composition gradually falls to 40% extracellular and 60% intracellular water and 60% total body water by 1 year of age (Table 88.2) (4). In neonates, plasma protein concentrations are lower, and many drugs are less avidly bound to plasma proteins. This produces a higher unbound fraction of drugs such as phenytoin and sulfasoxizole, leading to an increased clearance and decreased half-life. A higher unbound fraction can also lead to increased toxicity. Thus phenytoin, which is normally 90% protein-bound, may be only 70% bound in neonates or premature infants. Serum levels of phenytoin are reported as total phenytoin levels, so a level of 10 mg/L (90% protein bound) really means that the unbound active level of the drug is 1 mg/L, while with 70% binding, the unbound level is 3 mg/L and there is the possibility of toxic effects.

Drug Metabolism

Liver metabolism is the predominant method for drug transformation. Liver enzymes are present at birth and are stimulated to proliferate by the buildup of endogenous substrate. Each of the enzyme systems matures at a different rate, but a full-term infant has sufficient enzymes at 3 days after birth to adequately metabolize endogenous substrates. Bilirubin requires metabolism through the glucuronyl transferase pathway. This pathway matures slowly, so by 1 to 2 weeks of neonatal age, it is capable of glucuronidating exogenous substances. It is at this time that drugs that depend on this pathway can be safely used. If chloramphenicol were to be given to an infant younger than 1 week old at the usual dose for children of 100 mg/kg/day, the drug would accumulate and cause cardiovascular collapse and cyanosis, which is known as "gray baby syndrome" (5). If required, chloramphenicol in a dose of 25 mg/kg/day can be used in the first week of neonatal life (6–8).

Bilirubin itself can be toxic to the newborn. The unconjugated, unbound fraction of bilirubin crosses into the brain very readily. When serum bilirubin levels reach 12 to 20 mg/dL, bilirubin will cross the blood-brain barrier and cause a yellow staining of the brain, called kernicterus. Kernicterus may progress to irreversible brain damage and death when bilirubin levels are greater than 21 mg/dL. Irreversible brain damage can also occur at lower bilirubin serum levels of 12 to 20 mg/dL if drugs such as sulfasoxizole, aspirin, or caffeine are given to the neonate. These drugs displace bilirubin from albumin and allow it to pass into the brain. Bilirubin levels over 12 mg/dL are usually treated by placing the infant under fluorescent lights. The light metabolizes the bilirubin in the skin to harmless metabolites, which are then excreted by the kidney. Other forms of treatment are phenobarbital, which induces liver enzymes, and exchange blood transfusions.

Drug Excretion

Both metabolized and unmetabolized drugs are excreted by the kidneys. Drugs are also excreted through the gastrointestinal tract, lungs, and sweat glands. With most drugs these latter pathways are of only limited importance. Neonatal kidney function matures rapidly. At birth, a full-

Table 88.2.
Percentages of Body Water[a]

Age (Weight)	Extracellular Water (%)	Intracellular Water (%)	Total Body Water (%)
Premature baby (1.5 kg)	60	40	83
Full-term baby (3.5 kg)	56	44	74
5-month-old (7.0 kg)	50	50	60
1-year-old (10.0 kg)	40	60	59
Adult male	40	60	60

[a]Developmental changes from birth to adulthood. The extracellular and intracellular water are expressed as a percentage of total body weight. Total body water is expressed as a percentage of body weight.
Source: Data from (4).

Table 88.3.
Age-Dependent Half-Life of Antibiotics in Serum

Age Group (days old)	Carbenicillin[a]		Penicillin[b]	
	Number of Patients	Average Half-Life (hr)	Number of Patients (average age in days)	Average Half-Life (hr)
1–3	13	5.7	—	—
4–7	23	4.2	7 (3.7)	3.21
8–14	13	3.4	13 (9.5)	1.74
15–21	2	2.2	6 (18.5)	1.4
22–45	4	1.5	—	—

[a]Data from (6).
[b]Data from (7).

term newborn has approximately 33% of the glomerular filtration rate and renal tubular excretion capacity of an adult. This capacity is about 15% or less in premature infants. The capacity to excrete a solute load quickly increases in the first few weeks of life to about 50% of adult levels at 1 month of age. This change is reflected in the decreasing half-lives of penicillin and carbenicillin in neonates (Table 88.3). Doses of drugs that depend to a large degree on renal excretion (e.g., aminoglycosides and penicillins) must therefore be adjusted for the neonate. For example, gentamicin is given every 12 hr for the 1-week-old neonate and every 8 hr for the 2- to 4-week-old neonate. Because of the rapidly changing characteristics of the newborn, drug level monitoring should be used in treatment with aminoglycosides. Doses should be based on the neonate's age and weight. Drugs for normal infants and older children are administered in the usual therapeutic doses with no adjustment needed for renal function. At about 9 to 12 months of age, the infant kidney is functioning at adult levels.

Drug Sensitivity

Neonates and infants are more sensitive to the effects of many drugs because of the immaturity of their organs. The central nervous system matures slowly and reaches adult levels at about 8 years of age. Because of this and the increased permeability of the blood-brain barrier, the neonate appears to be especially sensitive to the depressant effects of drugs such as phenobarbital, morphine sulfate, chloral hydrate, meprobamate, and chlorpromazine. Codeine and meperidine, however, do not produce this exaggerated effect in neonates.

The cardiovascular system usually functions adequately in the neonate and infant except in times of stress, when exaggerated responses may occur. General anesthetics may cause cardiovascular depression. Diuretics or antihypertensives in normal doses may induce severe hypotension.

The temperature-regulating system is unstable and immature in the neonate and infant. Many drugs cause wide fluctuations in temperature and have exaggerated responses in neonates and infants. Drugs in therapeutic doses that normally lower temperature, such as aspirin and acetaminophen, can also raise the temperature when taken in toxic doses (Tables 88.4 and 88.5). The skin, in addition to its immature thermal regulatory ability, increased permeability, and large surface area, is also more sensitive to drugs. This drug sensitivity may be either allergic or toxic and may occur throughout infancy and childhood. Allergic reactions are the most common and may be the immediate-onset type, such as urticaria, angioneurotic edema, and anaphylaxis, or the delayed-onset types, such as erythema multiforme or a fixed drug eruption. These drug-induced reactions mimic skin eruption caused by other processes. The most common drugs that lead to skin reactions in pediatrics are sulfonamides, tetracyclines, penicillins, isoniazid, cephalosporins, barbiturates, phenytoin, chloral hydrate, phenothiazines, narcotics, aspirin, indomethacin, iodides, griseofulvin, and topical antihistamines. A number of other adverse drug effects occur in children: (a) growth suppression with tetracycline and corticosteroids; (b) sexual precocity with androgens; (c) neurotoxicity with hexachlorophene; (d) prepubertal effects with levodopa; (e) intracranial hypertension with corticosteroids, naldixic acid, vitamins A and D, and nitrofurantoin; (f) jaundice with novobiocin, sulfonamides, and vitamin K; and (g) a bulging fontanel and tooth staining with tetracycline (9).

Drug Administration

Since the 1938 Food, Drug, and Cosmetic Act, as amended in 1962, the Food and Drug Administration (FDA) has had the responsibility of approving drugs for infants, children, and adults. The FDA requires that all drugs be tested for efficacy and safety only in adults before their approval for licensing in the United States. Information about drug use for infants, children, and adolescents is included in the package insert only if the newly licensed drug is specifically tested and indicated for treatment of children. Since 1979, the FDA has required that all drugs that are to be used for children have adequate, well-controlled clinical studies involving children before any pediatric use information can be included in the package insert or label. Therefore most

Table 88.4.
Drugs That Cause Hyperthermia

Drug	Comment

Salicylates[a]
  Aspirin
  Sodium salicylate
  Methyl salicylate (oil of
    wintergreen)
  Diflunisal
	Increase temperature with toxicity and cause sweating and dehydration.

Nonsteroidal antiinflammatory agents[a]
  Ibuprofen, naproxen
  Indomethacin
  Mefenamic acid
  Piroxicam
	Increase temperature with toxic doses.

Dinitrophenols
  Herbicides, fungicides
  Nitrophenols
  Miscellaneous pesticides
  Insecticides
	Increase temperature up to 2 days after heavy exposure, whether inhaled, ingested, or by skin contact.

Anticholinergics
  Atropine
  Scopolamine
  Belladonna
  Benztropine
  Propantheline, etc.
	High temperature can result from large doses or repeated therapeutic doses.

Sympathomimetics
  Amphetamine and congeners
  Ephedrine
  Epinephrine
  Propylhexedrine inhalers, etc.
  Cocaine
	Large doses cause chills and fever.

Para-aminophenols[a] Acetaminophen	Large doses cause sweating and chills and probably fever.

Antihistamines
  Diphenhydramine
  Hydroxyzine, etc.
	Large doses cause fever.

Boric acid	Large doses cause fever.
Thyroid preparations Levothyroxine	Large doses cause fever.
Alcohol[a]	Large doses cause fever.

Antipsychotics[a]
  Phenothiazines
    Chlorpromazine[a]
  Tricyclic antidepressants
    Amitryptyline
  Others
    MAO inhibitors
    Haloperidol
	Overdoses cause fever.

Phencyclidine (PCP)	Overdoses cause fever.

[a]Also causes hypothermia (see Table 88.5).
Source: Adapted from (8).

Table 88.5.
Drugs That Cause Hypothermia

Drug	Comment

Salicylates[a]
  Aspirin
  Sodium salicylate
  Methyl salicylate (oil of
    wintergreen)
  Diflunisal
	Lower fever in therapeutic doses.

Nonsteroidal antiinflammatory agents[a]
  Ibuprofen, naproxen
  Indomethacin
  Mefenamic acid
  Piroxicam
	Decrease temperature with therapeutic doses.

Para-aminophenol[a] Acetaminophen	Therapeutic doses will lower fever.

Phenylbutazone
  Indomethacin
  Colchicine
	Usually used for arthritis and gout but can be used to lower temperature.

Chlorpromazine[a] Other phenothiazine also	Lower fever.

Cholinergic agents
  Physostigmine
  Pilocarpine
  Neostigmine
	Large dose or repeated small doses cause profuse sweating and cold extremities.

Topical agents
  Water
  Alcohol[a]
  Volatile oils
  Menthol, etc.
	Local cooling causes lower temperature.

Sedative hypnotics
  Barbiturates
  Alcohol
  Benzodiazepines
  Diazepam
	Overdoses decrease fever, causes sympatholytic syndrome.

Opiates	Overdoses decrease fever by causing sympatholytic syndrome.
Clonidine	Overdoses decrease fever by causing symnpatholytic syndrome.
Hypoglycemic agents Tolbutamide	Overdoses decrease fever.

[a]Also causes hyperthermia (see Table 88.4).
Source: Adapted from (8).

that the necessary extensive research would cost. This leaves the pediatric health care provider with no realistic guidance from the FDA or manufacturer as to the drug's use and leaves the child a "therapeutic orphan." Alternative publications and textbooks are the only source of information on the use of these drugs in treating children. However, the FDA has finally changed its regulations and is now accepting and actively soliciting labeling supplement applications to increase the information included on labels and package inserts about drug use in treating children.

Manufacturers have until December 13, 1996, to submit these labeling supplement applications for a marketed drug if available information such as clinical trials or experience, Literature reports, or other information supports

new drugs that are approved in the United States have no pediatric information in the product insert, even if they have been successfully used in treating children.

About 80% of prescription drugs that are licensed in the United States never receive formal approval from the FDA for use in treating children because pharmaceutical companies do not want to spend the large sums of money pediatric-use labeling. This new regulation allows manufacturers to extrapolate adult clinical trial efficacy data to children if the course of the disease and effects of the drug are similar in the two populations. The included data must be accompanied by pediatric-specific information on dosing, safety, indications, pharmacokinetics, and pharmacologic considerations. In addition, the FDA is requiring manufacturers to submit pediatric-use information as part of their first application for a new drug. For the first time, children will not be "therapeutic orphans" and will be considered a special population in the drug development process. A number of professional organizations are also in the process of elaborating pediatric categories of use.

The American Society of Health-System Pharmacists, the American Academy of Pediatrics, and the FDA are discussing a system of categorizing the use of drugs in pediatrics that would be analogous to the FDA pregnancy categories A, B, C, D, and X. The proposed categories, as discussed in an article by K. Zenk (10), are as follows:

Category A: Adequate studies have not demonstrated any risk specific to pediatric patients.
Category B: Adequate studies have not been done, but no data indicating risk specific to pediatric patients have been reported.
Category C: Risks specific to pediatric patients exist with agents in the same or related therapeutic classes.
Category D: Adequate studies have not been done and no data indicating risk specific to pediatric patients have been reported; however, because of the toxicity of the drug, less toxic alternatives should be considered.
Category X: Adequate studies have demonstrated risk specific to pediatric patients.

Additional information will accompany these designations, for example, specific age of children if applicable, specific problems occurring in children, and specific therapeutic indications.

Physicians and other health care providers can also minimize costly prescription errors by being more careful when writing or filling prescriptions, according to a medication error study done by Physician Insurers of America (11). Four types of medication errors accounted for 37.4% of total liability claims in this study. These four types of errors were (a) incorrect or inappropriate dosage, (b) inappropriate medication for the medical condition being treated, (c) failure to monitor for drug side effects, and (d) communication failure between physician and patient. The other medication errors that occurred in this study were caused by illegible handwriting and related mistakes in writing prescriptions (inappropriate length of treatment, method, site, route of administration of drugs); failure to take an adequate medical history; failure to monitor drug levels, side effects, drug effects, or drug allergies; prescribing inappropriate or contraindicated medications; or pharmacist errors while filling the prescription. Antibiotics, glucocorticoids, and analgesics (narcotic, nonnarcotic, narcotic antagonists) accounted for 34.9% of the patients' liability claims to insurance companies. Errors in treating pediatric patients were most likely to be caused by drugs used for respiratory problems and from intravenous fluid use.

This study recommended a number of risk management steps, slightly modified and quoted below, that physicians might use to reduce medication errors. (These recommendations are also appropriate for other health care professionals.)

- Charting all prescriptions and refills on a medication flow sheet
- Posting medication allergies on the chart in a consistent and conspicuous manner
- Obtaining and documenting medication histories from patients and update as necessary
- Reading the medical record for contraindications to medications, allergies, and excessive number of refills
- Reviewing authoritative references before prescribing unfamiliar medications for the correct dosage, contraindications, and side effects
- Educating patients about their medications, using such resources as the AMA's *Patient Medication Instructions* or *United States Pharmacopeia* leaflet program
- Obtaining and documenting informed consent for the prescription of medications with potentially significant drug complications and side effects
- Closely monitoring patients for drug side effects
- Closely monitoring drug usage, particulary with controlled substances
- Periodically reevaluating patients who are on chronic analgesic or psychotropic therapy for the indications for, and efficacy of, continued therapy
- Obtaining specific drug allergy information for antibiotics (penicillin and sulfa), nonsteroidal antiinflammatory drugs, anticonvulsants, and diuretics.

Dosing

Children are not small adults. Doses for neonates must be tailored for their age, weight, and decreased liver and kidney function. Doses that are given on a milligram-per-kilogram basis that have established efficacy in neonates, infants, and children can be found in a number of sources (12, 13). Drugs that are very toxic, such as cancer chemotherapeutic agents, should be, for better accuracy, dosed on a milligram-per-square-meter basis. Body surface area takes into account the child's height and weight and is especially useful for children who are not normal for their age in either height or weight. If necessary, the body surface area can be calculated from a child's height and weight, or a suitable nomogram can be used (Fig. 88.1). If a dose for a drug cannot be found in appropriate texts or current publications, the drug may not be suitable for pediatric use. This should be evaluated carefully before any dose is calculated. There are many formulas to calculate doses by the child's weight, age,

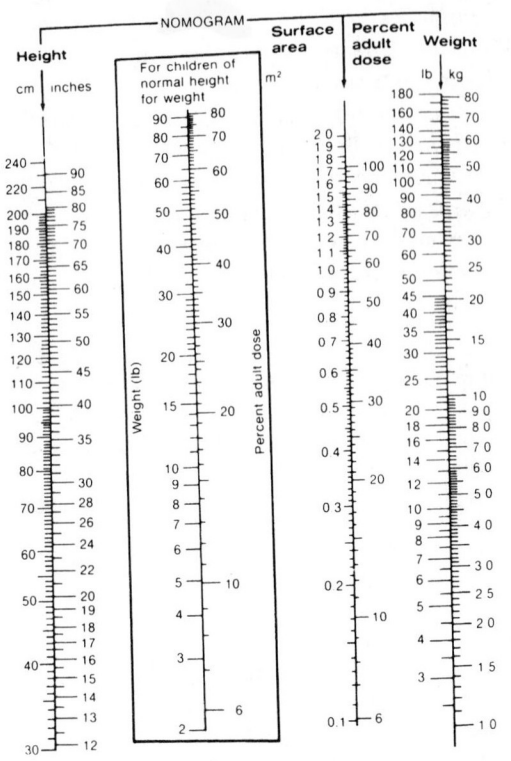

Figure 88.1. Pediatric drug therapy nomogram. (Source: From Kegel SM, Singer MI. Critical care of infants and children after the neonatal period. In: Zschoche DA, ed. Mosley's Comprehensive Review of Critical Care. St Louis: CV Mosby, 1976. Modified from Nelson WE. Textbook of Pediatrics, 8th ed. Philadelphia: WB Saunders, 1964.)

body surface area, or height; however, all are inaccurate and should not be used.

Compliance

Most compliance studies of adult ambulatory patients reveal that 50 to 70% of patients fail to complete a course of therapy. In addition, 90% of patients make at least some error in taking their medication, such as a missed dose or a dose taken at the incorrect time. In pediatrics, similar compliance problems occur. Very ill children are often unwilling to take medications. Becker et al. (14) studied mothers whose children had otitis media and were treated with oral penicillin. Mothers who were the most diligent in completing drug therapy had the following traits: (a) They were concerned about the child's health and current illness, (b) they felt that the illness was a major threat to the child's health and welfare, (c) they had confidence in the child's physician and the prescribed medication, (d) they had a more satisfactory experience with their pediatric clinic, (e) they actively endeavored to keep the child healthy and prevent future illness, and (f) they were better able to manage the problems of everyday life. In contrast, the mothers who complied less well with the medication

regiment had opposite attitudes. Additionally, these latter mothers thought that their own health was bad and were more concerned with their own health problems than with the health problems of the child. To achieve maximum success with medication regimens, therefore, health care personnel should emphasize and reinforce the traits that lead to increased compliance. Mattar and colleagues (15) reported that by emphasizing verbal and written patient instructions and providing calibrated measuring devices and calendars, pharmacists were able to achieve compliance levels of 51% in a cohort of 33 patients being treated with antibiotics for otitis media. In comparison, only 8.5% of 200 control patients were compliant.

Use of drugs that are taken only once or twice a day; are easy to swallow and palatable; and are easy to use, carry, and store should increase compliance. The person who gives medications should approach the child firmly but gently. A provocative, angry, or punishing attitude will increase the child's hostility and defensive medication-avoidance behavior. This adversary behavior affects compliance and interferes with good relationships, even in adolescents. The adolescent has all the compliance considerations of the child plus those of the adult. Therefore adolescents need to be knowledgeable about and in control of their medications.

INFANT NUTRITION

Human breast milk is the healthiest and most complete food for the full-term infant. It should be the only source of nutrition for infants up to 6 months of age (16, 17). Breast-feeding is usually supplemented with food in the child over 6 months old. In the United States, of those infants who are breast-fed, over 50% are breast-fed until at least 3 months of age. This decreases to 25% of 6-month-old infants, and fewer than 5% of 9- to 12-month-old infants are still being breast-fed. In some cultures, however, children at 4 to 6 years of age are still being breast-fed to gain needed protein. There are advantages to breast-feeding: It is less expensive than infant formula, the breast is an antiseptic environment, and breast milk has proteins that are of better biologic value than those found in infant formulas, curds that are easier to digest, and more easily absorbed fat, immunoglobulins, lysozymes, antistreptococcal enzymes, complement, lactoferrin, and macrophages that decrease infections.

Infants in the United States who are breast-fed have a lower incidence of gastrointestinal disease, respiratory disease, otitis media, and allergies than do non-breast-fed infants (18). There is also mounting evidence that breast-feeding is somewhat protective against developing obesity, allergy, arteriosclerosis, cystic fibrosis, celiac disease, early onset diabetes, and other metabolic disorders in adulthood (19). There are also advantages for the mother: Breast-feeding enhances postpartum recovery, returns women to their prepartum weight more quickly, and enhances maternal-infant bonding (16).

There are disadvantages to breast-feeding. The mother must want to nurse for it to be satisfactory and rewarding for her and the infant. The breasts must be prepared for nursing during the last trimester of pregnancy. Sometimes pain, inconvenience, engorgement, minor infections, and inflammation are associated with breast-feeding. The mother should have an adequate diet and must be careful about taking drugs that are excreted into breast milk. The mother should not breast-feed if she has active, untreated tuberculosis, breast cancer, or a serious infection. In many cases, active support and encouragement by health care personnel overcome most, if not all, of the maternal apprehension about breast-feeding. The maternal use of medications can be carefully planned to least affect the breast-feeding infant.

Normal Breast Physiology

The human breast is composed of glandular, fibrous, and adipose tissue and rests on a bed of connective tissue. The glandular tissue is composed of 15 to 20 lobes arranged radially around the nipple. Strands of fibrous tissue connect the lobes, and adipose tissue occupies the space between and around the lobes. Each lobe is divided into several lobules that are connected by alveolar tissue, blood vessels, and ducts (Fig. 88.2a) (20). Each lobule contains a small lactiferous duct. Eventually, these lactiferous ducts unite and form a single main canal for each lobe. Each of these

15 to 20 main canals becomes dilated and forms a reservoir (sinus lactiferous) for milk storage, which finally merge and pass through the nipple.

The functioning part of the breast is the alveoli or acini (sacs) in the lobule (Fig. 88.2b). Milk is produced in the acini and secreted into the lactiferous ducts. Drugs cross from the blood in the capillary beds through the acini epithelium and into the lactiferous ducts.

Normal Composition of Milk

The composition of milk is determined by the mammary gland with little or no external control (21, 22). The milk occurs in three forms: colostrum, transitional milk, and mature milk. Colostrum, which serves as a precursor of milk, may be expressed from the breasts as early as the fourth month of pregnancy, but it usually appears after parturition. It is scanty for the first few days after birth, becomes well established on the third or fourth day, and usually continues for no more than 5 days. It has, however, been know to continue for as long as 10 days. Colostrum is a transudate consisting primarily of serum albumin (3 to 5%) and cast-off epithelium (colostrum corpuscles) that has undergone fatty degeneration. It has a higher specific gravity than does mature milk (1.030 to 1.060 compared with 1.026 to 1.036) and also a higher average pH (7.7 compared with 6.8) It is richer in vitamin A, sodium, potassium, and other minerals but lower in sugar and fat. The mammary gland quickly modifies colostrum into transitional milk.

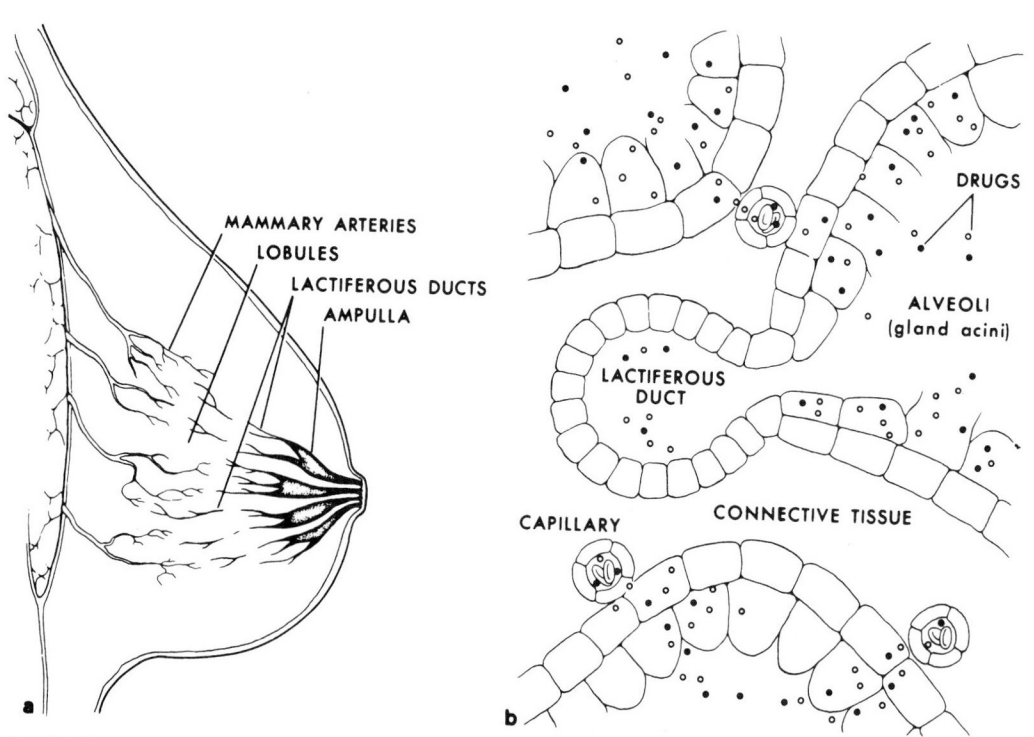

Figure 88.2. (a) Cross-section of the breast. (b) Magnified cross-section of lobule capillaries. (Source: Adapted from [18].)

Production of transitional milk usually begins within the first week of breast-feeding. It usually lasts for a few weeks, during which time a moderate increase in fat and sugar and a gradual decrease in proteins and minerals occur. Milk finally matures near the end of the first month of lactation.

Mature milk has between 0.9 and 1.6% protein, 2 to 6% fat, and 6.5 to 8% lactose. The composition of milk at the beginning of a feeding is highest in protein and lowest in fat. This is reversed toward the end of the feeding. The effect of this on the excretion of drugs is unknown.

Once established, mature milk varies little in composition (21, 22). If the mother has adequate nutritional intake, her diet can be quite varied without affecting milk composition or volume. A deficiency in maternal diet will first cause a decrease in the quantity of milk but will not affect milk composition unless the mother's tissue stores are depleted. A decreased water intake will cause maternal thirst before it affects milk production.

Control of Milk Production

The initiation and maintenance of milk production have not been adequately studied. However, the evidence regarding physiologic and endocrine factors in lactation is better understood now (18). Lactation usually begins at birth or shortly thereafter. The inhibition of lactation during pregnancy is assumed to be the result of the high estrogen or progesterone levels. The effects of estrogen on milk secretion are dose-dependent. At low endogenous levels occurring after birth, milk secretion occurs, whereas lactation is inhibited by high doses of estrogens (diethylstilbestrol or parental estrogens given postpartum). In most women, low-dose oral contraceptives do not decrease lactation even when they are taken immediately postpartum (23). Estrogens may work partly by affecting prolactin (lactogenic factor), which is secreted from the anterior pituitary.

Prolactin is currently under extensive investigation in an effort to delineate its true role during pregnancy and lactation (18). During pregnancy, prolactin, estrogen, progesterone, and human growth hormone stimulate breast development. There are high concentrations of prolactin during pregnancy and breast-feeding but low concentrations after birth in the absence of breast-feeding. If breast-feeding is successful and unrestricted, the high levels of prolactin have been reported to be contraceptive (24). This contraceptive effect is seen only in certain societies and has not been observed in the United States, where formula supplements are frequently given.

The posterior pituitary, as well as the anterior pituitary, is involved in and stimulated by breast-feeding. The release of oxytocin by the posterior pituitary initiates the letdown reflex, the expression or ejection of milk from the breast. Oxytocin stimulates the letdown reflex; prolactin stimulates milk production. The letdown reflex is responsive to other internal and external factors. The actions and sounds that are associated with nursing can initiate this reflex. In contrast, distractions such as fright, pain, and emotional distress can inhibit milk expression. It is hypothesized that the high levels of the catecholamines, adrenaline, and norepinephrine that are produced in such circumstances cause a vasoconstriction in the mammary circulation that prevents oxytocin from reaching the contractile cells (18). Excessive doses of medications that also release endogenous catecholamines (e.g., amphetamines and most decongestants) may interfere with milk secretion.

Quantity of Milk Produced

The quantity of milk that is produced depends on the infant's demand. If the infant's demand is increasing, the milk supply will adjust accordingly within 2 days and similarly if the infant's demand is decreasing. The actual secretion of milk is a discontinuous process. During feeding, there is increased milk secretion as a result of the depletion of milk stores. In all probability, drugs are excreted into milk in larger amounts when the milk is being actively secreted. To derive the total quantity of drug ingested (measured as milligrams per deciliter), it is necessary to know the quantity of milk ingested by the infant. This depends on the infant's age and weight (Table 88.6). See Chapter 92, "Drugs in Pregnancy and Lactation," for a discussion of drugs that are excreted in breast milk. If a woman cannot breast-feed, prepared infant formulas are the best substitute. These formulas are covered in Chapter 89, "Pediatric and Neonatal Nutrition."

Infants who are over 6 months old usually do not require the standard formulas with 20 cal/oz, so a reduced 16-cal/oz formula such as Advance was developed. Cow's milk plus baby food also provides adequate nutrition for this age group. If cow's milk is used, the daily intake should be kept to one quart or less. More than 1 quart/day can lead to milk intolerance, diarrhea, and iron-deficiency anemia secondary to the large intake of protein, which may cause an enteropathy. Reducing the intake of milk to less than a

Table 88.6.
Quantities of Milk Ingested

Amount at each feeding[a] (mL)	Age (weeks)
20–45	1
30–90	2
40–140	4
60–150	6
75–165	12
90–175	16
120–225	24

[a]Feedings are usually every 3–4 hr. Quantity consumed depends on the infant's weight.

quart per day and supplementing it with iron-rich infant food resolve the enteropathy and its sequelae. The infant foods that are used should have the least possible added salt, sugar, and monosodium glutamate (MSG). These substances are added to improve the taste for increased adult acceptability. The added sodium and MSG have been casually implicated in predisposing susceptible infants to developing hypertension as adults (25). The inclusion of MSG in infant food seems unwarranted. The added sugar may predispose infants to obesity by increasing the total number of fat cells.

The daily intake of infant foods for the 6-month-old should consist of two or more servings of meat, four or more servings of vegetables, one or more servings of citrus fruits, and four or more servings of bread or cereal. The size of each serving should increase as the child grows. The use of infant foods may start as early as 2 to 3 months of age with cereals and then the addition of vegetables, fruits, and meats as tolerated. Junior foods, which contain small chunks of solid food, are usually begun at 8 to 12 months of age. Adult table food is usually begun at 1 year of age. If the child receives a normal, varied diet that contains the required nutrients, no added supplements are needed. Giving a normal child additional vitamins and minerals adds nothing to health and is an unneeded monetary expense. Vitamins and minerals should be used only if nutritional deficiencies have been documented.

FEVERS IN CHILDREN

Cause

One of the most common symptoms of illness is fever, which is a mechanism for fighting off infection. It is one of the most common childhood complaints. It is important to separate mild febrile disease from a serious infection. The causes of mild fevers in children are usually upper respiratory infections and lower respiratory infections caused by assorted viruses, including influenza. Bacterial infections that cause otitis media, sore throat, urinary tract infections, or respiratory infections also quite commonly cause fever.

Complications

Children who are at the greatest risk for complications from a febrile illness, and who must be watched carefully if they develop a sudden fever, are (a) those who are less than 2 months of age with a temperature over 38°C, (b) those who are 6 to 24 months old with a temperature over 40°C, or (c) any child with a temperature over 41°C. Children younger than 2 months old do not manifest the usual signs and symptoms of systemic disease, such as fever or inflammation; it is therefore very difficult to diagnose serious disease in these infants before it becomes life-threatening. Children between the ages 6 and 24 months with a fever

Table 88.7.
Causes of Fever of Unknown Origins (FUOs)

Causes	Age <6 Yr (%)	Age 6–14 Yr (%)	Age >14 Yr (%)
Infections	65	38	36
Neoplastic diseases	8	4	19
Autoimmune diseases	8	23	13
Miscellaneous	13	17	25
Undiagnosed (FUOs)	6	18	7

have a high risk of having been infected with either *Streptococcus pneumoniae* or *H. influenzae*. Children at any age with high fevers (more than 41°C) are at great risk of having severe systemic bacterial sepsis or meningitis.

Children who have prolonged undiagnosed fevers (>38°C) for more than 2 weeks are classified as having a fever of unknown origin (FUO). There are a number of causes of FUOs, as listed in Table 88.7. These unexplained fevers require a much more extensive workup than other fevers and are generally much more serious. Most fevers are caused by infections; neoplastic disease is the least common cause of fever in 6- to 14-year-olds.

Treatment

Fever does not have to be pharmacologically treated unless it is causing morbidity or is debilitating for the patient. Fevers should be treated if the patient is irritable, very sick, or delirious or has shaking chills or seizures. In bacterial infections the fever decreases as the child recovers and provides a convenient monitoring parameter for the efficacy of antibiotics.

The two most commonly used antipyretic analgesics for treating fevers in children are aspirin and acetaminophen. The analgesic/antipyretic dose is the same on a milligram-for-milligram basis for both agents. The usual oral or rectal dose is 5 to 10 mg/kg/dose (about 65 mg/kg/day) given every 4 to 6 hr. If one agent at the maximum dose is not effective for lowering temperature, both agents can be used, either alternating doses every 2 hr or giving both at the same time every 6-8 hours. This avoids doubling the dose of either agents and causing toxicity; the toxicities of these agent are different. Aspirin causes more toxicity in children younger than 2 years old; in overdoses, aspirin leads to fluid, electrolyte, and acid-base imbalances. Acetaminophen, generally thought to be less toxic, may in high doses cause hepatic toxicity (26, 27).

Caution is needed in using analgesics to treat fevers or pain in children or adolescents younger than 19 years old with flu or varicella infections. Acetaminophen is the analgesic of choice because of the risk of developing Reye's syndrome. The syndrome usually starts in a patient who is recovering from the illness who suddenly starts to vomit and deteriorates rapidly. Some patients may slowly get better, but many go on to develop symptoms that consist of metabolic encephalopathy associated with hepatic failure. Although it is a rare disease, 204 cases were reported in 1984 and none in 1989 in the United States (28). The majority of cases of Reye's syndrome occur in children between 6 and 18 years old. Reye's syndrome may occur in children whether or not they have taken aspirin during their antecedent illness, but aspirin seems to increase the chances of developing this syndrome, possibly by altering the immune system of susceptible children and therefore increasing the virulence of the infection. It may also predispose the child to metabolic complications by acting as an additional insult (29–33).

The treatment consists of fluid and electrolyte therapy for the patient's metabolic requirements and mannitol and other agents to reduce cerebral edema. Vitamin K, barbiturates, hypothermia, or corticosteroids may also be employed. The mortality rate is between 20 and 40%, and permanent brain damage may occur in those who survive (34).

The FDA now requires a warning on all aspirin-containing products: "Children and teenagers should not use this medicine (aspirin) for chickenpox or flu symptoms before a doctor is consulted about Reye's syndrome, a rare but serious illness." Patients and parents should be alerted to this warning.

CONCLUSION

Health maintenance and disease prevention, including proper nutrition and an immunization program, are important aspects of the practice of pediatrics. Certain illnesses such as upper respiratory viral infections, otitis media, infantile diarrhea, and other febrile diseases are so common that every child can be expected to suffer several episodes before the age of 6.

Proper therapy instituted quickly can prevent these minor diseases from becoming more serious. Although many of these pediatric diseases are treated in the same way in children as they are in adults, neonates, infants, and children have unique characteristics that call for additional knowledge of drug therapy. Considerations in drug therapy in pediatrics include the influence of normal growth and development on drug absorption, distribution, and elimination as well as dosage formulation to facilitate compliance.

REFERENCES

1. Watson PD, Powell JR, Mimaki T. Anticonvulsant usage. In: Jaffe ST, ed. Pediatric pharmacology and therapeutics: principles in practice. New York: Grune & Stratton, 1980:195–212.
2. Zenk KE. Drug use in neonates. United States Pharmacist Journal 11:H2–H20, 1986.
3. Zenk KE. Special delivery: delivering IV antibiotics to children. Nursing 86 16:50–52, 1986.
4. Friis-Hansen B. Body composition during growth. Pediatrics 47:264, 1971.
5. Nelson JD. Antimicrobial drugs. In: Jaffe SJ, ed. Pediatric pharma-cology and therapeutics: principles in practice. New York: Grune & Stratton, 1980:187–198.
6. Nelson JD, McCracken GM. Clinical pharmacology of carbencillin and gentamicin in the neonate and comparative efficacy with ampicillin and gentamicin. Pediatrics 52:801, 1973.
7. McCracken GH, Ginsberg C, et al. Clinical pharmacology of penicillin in newborn infants. J Pediatr 82:692, 1973.
8. Levin RH, Maltz HE. Fluid balance in drug therapy. In: Waechter EH, Blake JB, eds. Nursing care of children. 9th ed. Philadelphia: JB Lippincott, 1976:102.
9. Tatro DA. Adverse drug reactions in children. In: Pagliaro LA, Levin RH, eds. Problems in pediatric drug therapy. Hamilton, IL: Drug Intelligence Publications, 1979.
10. Zenk KE. Challenges in providing pharmaceutical care to pediatric patients. Am J Hosp Pharm 51:688, 1994.
11. Reinso D. Pediatricians and the law: physicians can minimize costly prescription errors. News of the American Academy of Pediatrics, 10:17, 1994.
12. Zenk KE. Neonatal and pediatric dosing. In: Pagliaro LA, Levin RH, eds. Problems in pediatric drug therapy. Hamilton, IL: Drug Intelligence Publications, 1979.
13. Levin RH, Zenk KE. Medication table. In: Rudolph AM, ed. Pediatrics. 18th ed. Norwalk, CT: Appleton-Century-Crofts, 1987.
14. Becker MH, Drachman RH, Kirscht JP. Predicting mothers' com-pliance with pediatric medical regimens. J. Pediatr 81:843, 1972.
15. Mattar ME, Markello J, Jaffe SJ. Pharmaceutical factors affecting pediatric compliance. Pediatrics 55:101, 1975.
16. Lawrence RA. Breastfeeding: a guide for the medical profession. 3rd ed. St. Louis: CV Mosby, 1989:12.
17. Barness LA. Bases of weaning recommendations: supplement on dietary patterns and nutrient intake of U.S. infants. J Pediatr 117:S84–85, 1990.
18. Chen Y, Yu S, Li W. Artifical feeding and hospitalization in the first 18 months of life. Pediatrics 81:52, 1988.
19. Lawrence RA. Breastfeeding and medical disease. Med Clin North Am 73:583–603, 1989.
20. Arena J. Contamination of the ideal food. Nutrition Today 5:2, 1970.
21. Holt LE. Feeding techniques and diets. In: Barnett HL, ed. Pediatrics. 15th ed. New York: Meredith, 1972:148.
22. Jelliffe DB, Jelliffe EFP. The volume and composition of human milk in poorly nourished communities: a review. Am J Clin Nutr 31:492, 1978.
23. Gambrell R. Immediate postpartum oral contraception. Obstet Gynecol 36:101, 1970.
24. Jelliffe DB, Jelliffe EFP. Lactation, conception and the nutrition of the nursing mother and child. J Pediatr 81:829, 1972.
25. Committee on Nutrition. Sodium intake by infants in the United States. Evanston, IL: American Academy of Pediatrics, 1979.
26. APHA Project Staff. Handbook of non-prescription drugs. 7th ed. Washington, DC: American Pharmaceutical Association, 1982:123.
27. Anonymous. Aspirin or paracetamol. Lancet 2:287, 1981.
28. Centers for Disease Control. Summary of notifiable diseases, United States 1989. Morbidity and Mortality Weekly Report 38:54, 1990.
29. Anonymous. Salicylate labeling may change because of Reye's syndrome. FDA Drug Bull 12:9, 1982.
30. Waldman RJ, et al. Aspirin as a risk factor in Reye's syndrome. JAMA 247:3089, 1982.
31. Halpin TJ, Holtzhauer FJ, Campbell RJ, et al. Reye's syndrome and medication use. JAMA 248:687, 1982.
32. Starko KM, Ray CGJ, Dominguez LB, et al. Reye's syndrome and salicylate use. Pediatrics 66:859, 1980.
33. Hurwitz ES, Barrett MJ, Bregman D, et al. Public Health Service Study on Reye's syndrome and medications. N Engl J Med 313:849, 1985.
34. Rudolph AM. Pediatrics. 18th ed. Norwalk, CT: Appleton-Century-Crofts, 1987.

CHAPTER 89

PEDIATRIC AND NEONATAL NUTRITION

EMILY B. HAK and RICHARD A. HELMS

Adequate nutrition is necessary throughout life to maintain body structure and integrity. Pediatric patients require additional nutrients to meet the demands of growth and development. Failure to provide essential nutrients can result in serious sequelae, including growth retardation, impairment of the immune system, and neurologic deficits. The premature neonate presents a unique nutritional challenge to the clinician since transition to the extrauterine environment is made before the fetus is fully developed. With increasing prematurity, there are corresponding decreases in organ system maturity, lean body mass, fat stores, and micronutrient and mineral stores that affect the approach to nutrition support in the premature infant and mandate early nutrition intervention.

During the past 20 years, important advances have been made in our understanding of nutrient requirements in children. Enteral formulas to meet the specialized nutrient needs of preterm and term infants who are unable to tolerate breast milk have been developed. Likewise, commercially available enteral formulas have been designed to meet the nutritional requirements of older children who cannot or should not eat.

The most significant advancement in the nutritional care of the high-risk neonate has been the development of parenteral nutrition. Although the first report of the successful use of total parenteral nutrition in an infant occurred almost 50 years ago, only in the last 20 years has parenteral nutrition been routinely used in hospitalized and ambulatory children with a variety of surgical or medical conditions. During this time, our understanding of macronutrient and micronutrient metabolism and substrate requirements has rapidly grown. Practitioners are now able to individualize various nutrients with the parenteral nutrition solution based on age, weight, nutritional status, and disease.

NUTRITIONAL ASSESSMENT AND MONITORING

Although similar nutritional assessment techniques (1–5) are used in both children and adults (see Chapter 12, "Parenteral and Enteral Nutrition"), children require special consideration for almost all parameters assessed.

Weight

Weight is the most important assessment tool used to evaluate nutritional outcome in children. The younger the infant, the greater gain per unit of body weight. All infants receiving parenteral nutrition should have their weight measured daily unless medically prohibited. The addition or deletion of clothing, diapers, wound dressings, or arm boards used to stabilize an intravenous line can alter the apparent weight, making interpretation of daily fluctuations difficult. Furthermore, significant variation in weight can be seen when different scales are used or different care givers perform the measurement. To more reliably evaluate weight gains, an average should be made over several days since daily changes may relate to factors other than lean body mass accretion. Older children and adolescents may require less frequent weights since growth is slower and detectable changes are lower.

Intake and Output

Intake and output should be carefully assessed and summarized daily. A patient's intake consists of those delivered enterally and parenterally, including maintenance fluids, blood products, and fluid used in the delivery of medications and flushes. Output includes urine, stool, nasogastric or gastrostomy tube drainage, chest tube outputs, emesis, blood loss, ostomy drainage, and wound drainage. In an uncatheterized infant, urine and stool losses can be approximated by weighing diapers before and after elimination. If possible, urine and stool volumes should be recorded separately. Evaluation of daily weight in conjunction with daily assessment of total intake and output will aid in the evaluation of fluid balance and source of weight gain.

Growth Charts

Growth charts derived from large populations of pediatric patients in the United States allow graphical comparison of an individual child to an age-related population for length or height, weight, and head circumference (6). Preterm neonates should have their postnatal age adjusted for prematurity when using the standard growth curves or be plotted on an intrauterine growth curve or a curve developed for use in preterm neonates. Information determined from growth charts can be used as an assessment of current nutritional status and may help identify nutritional deficits and differentiate between acute and chronic malnutrition (7). For example, weight below the population standard may indicate acute malnutrition, whereas both weight and height below the population standard suggests a chronic problem (7). Periodic plotting of weight and height allow the chart to be used to assess interindividual progress and response to nutritional support (8).

Anthropometric Measurements

Anthropometric measurements can be an effective means to monitor response to nutritional support in children (8). Age-related nomograms have been developed for arm circumference and triceps skinfold (9). Using this nomogram, Frisancho, calculated age-related percentiles for arm muscle area, arm muscle diameter, and arm muscle circumference (10). Subscapular skinfold standards have also been developed (11). To minimize variability between measurements, the same trained individual and same caliper type should be used to assess a given patient.

Visceral Proteins

Serum albumin, transferrin, transthyretin (prealbumin), and retinol-binding protein are the primary visceral protein markers used in nutritional assessment (12–16). Although the half-lives of visceral proteins in children are similar to adult values, age-related normal serum concentrations usually are lower for younger patients. Transthyretin and retinol-binding protein concentrations increase following nutritional support in otherwise healthy, appropriate for gestational-age infants (17) and premature infants (18). Likewise, these markers increase in critically ill, malnourished infants receiving nutrition support (19). The availability of a micronized, inexpensive nephelometric prealbumin assay (PAB, Beckman Instruments, Inc., Brea, CA) that has been simplified may increase the clinical use of transthyretin measurements in pediatric patients.

Urine Studies

A nitrogen balance is the difference between the measurement of total nitrogen output and estimates of nitrogen intake (enteral and parenteral protein) during the same 24-hour period. Nitrogen balance is used routinely in adults because it is relatively easy, noninvasive, and a reliable assessment of adequacy of intake; however, problems exist with conducting these studies in neonates and infants (20). To collect urine in an uncatheterized pediatric patient, a urine collection bag must be placed around the genital area with an adhesive and remain affixed securely for the collection period. Collection bags that do not fit adequately, adhesives that do not stick properly, skin breakdown under the adhesive, and stool contamination of the collected urine are problematic. When a 24-hour urine collection is impractical, a 6-hour urine collection has been proposed as an alternative means of estimating nitrogen losses for nitrogen balance calculation (21). In addition to difficulties with urine collections in children, the total urine nitrogen (TUN) concentration relationship with urinary urea nitrogen is less predictable in neonates and critically ill children (22). TUN is measured using pyrochemiluminescence, a method that is not available in many hospital clinical laboratories. Despite the difficulties encountered with urine collections in neonates and infants, skilled nursing care and accurate recording of intake and output enable the clinician to make a reasonable estimate of urinary nitrogen excretion. Other measures of protein catabolism that have been used in pediatric patients include urinary 3-methylhistidine concentration to creatinine ratio (23, 24).

Immune Function

Assessments of immune function may not be helpful in assessing the nutritional status of infants and young children. The lack of an immunologic response to a specific challenge may not indicate malnutrition but may be secondary to immaturity or a lack of antigenic experience (25, 26). Only 12% of healthy infants under 7 months of age exhibited a delayed hypersensitivity response to an intradermal Candida skin test, whereas 80% of infants above 7 months of age had a positive response (26). On the other hand, Helms and colleagues noted improved lymphocyte function and enhanced expression of T-cell populations in malnourished infants receiving short-term parenteral nutrition (8, 27).

FLUID REQUIREMENTS

Fluid needs are based on water losses from skin and respiration, urine and stool output, water accumulation in newly formed tissues, and water produced from carbohydrate oxidation (28, 29). The body surface area per unit weight is greater in children than adults, resulting in increased evaporative losses and greater fluid requirements per unit weight in children. Fluid requirements are 90 to 100 ml per 100 kilocalories in children (30, 31), and decrease to 45 ml per 100 calories in adults. Maintenance fluid requirements for term infants and children can be calculated from the equations described by Holliday and Segar (Table 89.1) (31).

Fluid requirements may be altered by immaturity, activity, environment, or pathology (28, 32, 33). Soon after birth, the extracellular fluid volume contracts, and a diuresis occurs that results in weight loss (28, 34, 35). Because the percentage of extracellular fluid increases with increasing prematurity, the percentage of total body weight loss after birth is increased in premature neonates (32). Furthermore, organ immaturity (primarily kidney and skin) and greater body surface area per unit weight in the preterm neonate result in increased sensible and insensible water losses. The skin and subcutaneous tissue are thinner and more permeable in the preterm infant resulting in increased evaporative losses (36). In addition infants may be under radiant warmers to maintain normal body

Table 89.1.
Daily Maintenance Fluid Requirement for Term Infants and Children[a]

Weight	Fluid
Up to 10 kg	100 ml/kg[b]
>10 to 20 kg	1000 ml + 50 ml/kg for every kg >10 kg
>20 kg	1500 ml + 20 ml/kg for every kg >20 kg

[a]Adapted from Holliday MA, Segar WE. The maintenance need for water in parenteral fluid therapy. Pediatrics 19:823–832, 1957.
[b]Preterm infants may require 120–150 ml/kg.

temperature or require ultraviolet light therapy to treat neonatal jaundice, increasing evaporative water losses further (37, 38). Renal immaturity may result in an inability to excrete a concentrated urine, which will increase the fluid volume that preterm neonates require (39, 40). Renal function matures with increasing postconceptional age; thus, the ability of neonates to regulate water and electrolyte metabolism should improve with increasing age (41). Certain diseases common in preterm neonates have been associated with excessive fluid intake, including bronchopulmonary dysplasia (42), necrotizing enterocolitis (43), intraventricular hemorrhage (44), and patent ductus arteriosus (45).

Like adults, children with congenital cardiac or renal anomalies, increased intracranial pressure, syndrome of inappropriate secretion of antidiuretic hormone (SIADH), or pulmonary edema may require varying degrees of fluid restriction. Conversely, patients with excessive fluid losses (gastric drainage; diarrhea or increased stool or ostomy output; vomiting; chest tube drainage; burn or wound exudate; fistula drainage; or patients under radiant warmers, ultraviolet lights, or with fever) may require additional fluids to compensate for these losses. These outputs should be replaced with fluids that are equivalent in volume and electrolyte composition (Table 89.2).

PARENTERAL NUTRITION

Administration

Peripheral infusion of parenteral nutrition solutions is a reasonable alternative for patients who require short-term therapy. In small infants and children, peripheral access sites are limited and, unlike adults, veins in the dorsum of the foot or hand or scalp veins often are used to establish venous access. With peripheral access, the parenteral nutrition solution composition is limited because as osmolality increases, the risk for complications such as phlebitis and infiltration increases (see "Complications") (46).

In practice, the final osmolality for peripherally infused solutions (about 850 mOsm/liter) is similar to that used in adults. However, the dextrose concentration is usually higher (10 to 12.5%) and amino acid concentration lower (2 to 3%). Compared to plasma (295 mOsm/liter), these solutions are very hypertonic and may result in tissue irritation if infiltration occurs. Concentrations of calcium and potassium, two known tissue irritants, should be limited to 10 mEq/liter and 40 to 60 mEq/liter, respectively, in solutions infused peripherally.

Peripheral parenteral nutrition can be used successfully in pediatric patients who are relatively well-nourished and require parenteral nutrition for less than 14 days. From 50 to 75 kcal/kg/day and 2 to 3 g/kg/day of protein can be provided by this route if fluids are not restricted and fat is well tolerated.

Recently, percutaneous central venous catheters have been used in very small neonates, infants, and children who require parenteral nutrition but who have poor peripheral venous access. These catheters can be inserted into a peripheral vein and advanced into the central circulation by trained nurses at the bedside. These catheters have remained in place for an average of 24 days, which compares favorably with peripheral teflon or steel catheter life of 2 to 3 days. Not only is catheter life longer, but solutions that contain more concentrated nutrients and, therefore, are more hypertonic can be infused and the risks associated with surgical central venous catheter placement avoided (47).

Children that require extended periods of parenteral nutrition should have a central venous catheter placed surgically. The most frequently used central venous catheters for long-term access are the Broviac or Hickman catheters. If patients can accommodate a larger internal diameter catheter and there is a need for greater access, a double or triple lumen catheter can be used. Although femoral insertion of catheters is used often, the most common and convenient site for placement is the superior vena cava, with the catheter tip lying at the superior vena cava—right atrial junction (Fig. 89.1). The Dacron cuff is positioned subcutaneously near the exit site and stimulates the formation of a fibrous adhesion that anchors the catheter and prevents migration of pathogenic organisms from the skin surface to the catheter tip. The location of the exit site should be made with cosmetic considerations since scars may remain after the catheter is removed. If place-

Table 89.2.
Range of Electrolyte Composition (mEq/liter) of Gastrointestinal Secretions

Secretion	Na^+	K^+	Cl^-	HCO_3^-
Saliva	35–60	10–20	15–35	50
Gastric	10–115	5–35	10–150	0
Pancreatic	115–155	5–10	55–110	70–90
Bile	130–165	5–15	80–120	35–50
Midjejunum	70–125	5–30	70–135	10–20
Ileum	90–140	5–30	60–135	15–50
Diarrhea	25–50	35–60	20–40	35–45

ment is not done using fluoroscopy, a chest radiograph should be obtained immediately after insertion to verify catheter placement.

Totally implantable vascular-access devices can be used in larger pediatric patients who require long-term central venous access. Compared with external catheters, these catheters require less maintenance, are less noticeable, impose fewer restrictions on patient activity, and have a

lower infection rate (48, 49). In most cases, a Huber needle that is bent at a 90°% right angle is required for insertion through the skin into the port; thus, there is a needle stick each time the catheter is used. According to product literature, the central silicone port can be punctured 1000 to 2000 times depending on the brand. Careful care of the skin over the site is essential if infectious complications related to needle insertion are to be avoided.

Composition of Parenteral Nutrition Solutions

Typically, parenteral nutrition solutions for infants contain 2.5% amino acids; 10 to 25% dextrose; and electrolytes, vitamins, and minerals in amounts sufficient to meet the patient's daily requirements (Table 89.3). Older children and adolescents may require more concentrated amino acids (up to 5%) and lower concentrations of dextrose depending on the fluid volume available for infusion. Intravenous fat emulsions (10 or 20%) offer a concentrated source of calories and are used as a source of essential fatty acids. The proportion of calories from each of the major nutrients should approach the percentages in the average enteral diet: 50 to 60% carbohydrate, 30 to 40% fat (higher percentage fat in neonatal and infant diet), and 10 to 15% protein. Providing a balanced formula reduces the risk of toxicities or complications associated with excessive or inadequate administration of any single nutrient. In some institutions, the fat emulsion is added directly to the parenteral nutrition solution, referred to as a total nutrient admixture (TNA) or three-in-one (50). The use of TNAs in pediatrics is subject to several compositional limitations, including pH changes that alter calcium and phosphorous

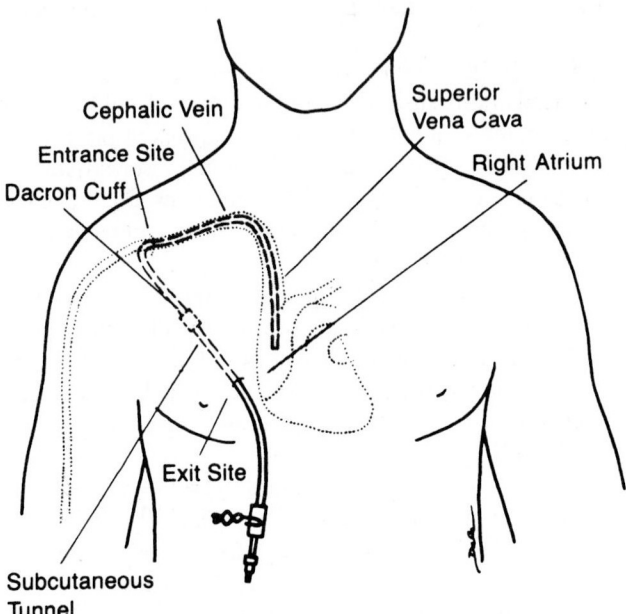

Figure 89.1. Placement of central venous catheter. The subclavian route as shown here is more commonly used in older children.

Table 89.3.
Typical Peripheral and Central Line Solutions Used in Infants and Children (per liter)

	Dextrose 10% Solutions for Peripheral Use		Dextrose 25% Solutions for Central Use	
Solution name[a]	CPF 3%	IPF 2.4%	CCF 3%	ICF 2.4%
Amino acid (g)	30[b]	24[c]	30[b]	24[c]
Dextrose (g)	100	100	250	250
Electrolytes				
Sodium	51 mEq	38.5 mEq	51 mEq	38.5 mEq
Potassium	20 mEq	20 mEq	20 mEq	20 mEq
Chloride	51 mEq	38.5 mEq	51 mEq	38.5 mEq
Acetate	12 mEq	8.2 mEq	12 mEq	8.2 mEq
Phosphate	5.5 mmol	8 mmol	5.5 mmol	8 mmol
Calcium	6 mEq	10 mEq	8 mEq	25 mEq
Magnesium	3 mEq	4 mEq	3 mEq	4 mEq
PTE[d]	NR[e]	3 ml	2 ml	3 ml
Selenium	NR	30 mcg	20 mcg	30 mcg
Multivitamin[f]				

[a]CPF, child (> 12 kg) peripheral formula; IPF, infant (< 12 kg) peripheral formula; CCF, child central formula; ICF, infant central formula.
[b]Standard crystalline amino acid formulation.
[c]Pediatric crystalline amino acid formulation (L-cysteine HCl at 40 mg/g protein (admixed at dispensing).
[d]Pediatric trace element solution, per ml: 1 mg Zn, 100 mcg Cu, 25 mcg Mn, 1 mcg Cr.
[e]NR, none required for short-term administration.
[f]Pediatric multivitamin (see dosing recommendations with vitamin section).

Table 89.4.
Electrolyte Content and pH of Commercially Available Amino Acid Products (mEq/liter)

	g/100 ml	Ac	Cl	Na	Phos[a]	pH
TrophAmine	6	56	<3	5		
	10	97	<3	5		5–6
Aminosyn-PF	7	32.5		3.4		5–6
	10	46		3.4		5–6.5
Aminosyn	7	105		5.4		5–6.5
	10	148		5.4		4.5–6
Aminosyn II	7	50.3		31.3		4.5–6
	10	71.8		45.3		5–6.5
Novamine	15	151				5–6.5
FreAmine III	8.5	72	<3	10	10	5.2–6
	10	89	<3	10	10	6–7
Travasol	8.5	73	34			6–7
	10	87	40			6–8
Cysteine HCl	5		5.7			6–8
						1.5–2

[a]Units are mmol/liter.

solubility and lipid particle instability resulting from a high divalent cation, primarily calcium, concentration. In addition, a 0.22-micron filter cannot be used with TNAs.

Protein Requirements

About 20 years ago, the protein source for parenteral nutrition solutions was protein hydrolysates; however, these products were associated with hyperammonemia, compositional variability, occasional allergic reactions, and poor nitrogen utilization (51). Early crystalline amino acid products were associated with metabolic acidosis that occurred secondary to the use of hydrochloride salt forms of several amino acids and hyperammonemia that resulted from inadequate arginine in at least one formulation. Today, the free base form of crystalline amino acids is used when possible, and those unstable as a free base, such as lysine, are usually added as the acetate salt. Since the amino acid source does vary according to manufacturer, the electrolyte content of amino acid solutions varies (Table 89.4). The distribution of amino acids present in a particular product is important since the quantity and quality of the protein infused directly affect plasma amino acids that are in active equilibrium with metabolically active cells (51, 52) (Table 89.5).

Because of the increased tissue anabolism, parenteral protein requirements in infants and children are more on a per kilogram basis than those in adults. Guidelines for protein doses can be found in Table 89.6. The preterm infant and neonate require not only quantitatively greater protein intake but also qualitatively different amino acids for optimal growth and development (53–56).

Cysteine, taurine, tyrosine, and histidine have all been described as conditionally essential amino acids for preterm neonates and infants. Enzyme immaturity in the

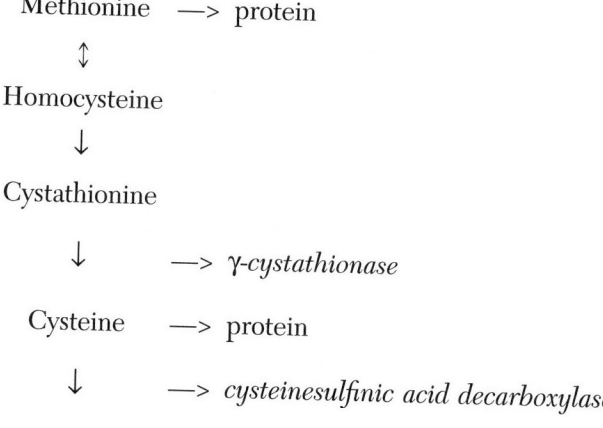

Figure 89.2. Metabolic pathway for the conversion of methionine to cysteine and taurine.

transsulfuration pathway, whereby methionine is converted to cysteine and cysteine to taurine, renders the latter two amino acids essential (Fig. 89.2). Similarly, phenylalanine hydroxylase insufficiency may limit the synthesis of tyrosine from phenylalanine. Plasma amino acid patterns in neonates and infants infused with standard amino acid products differ from those obtained in infants 2 to 3 hours after a human milk feeding, which is presumed to be ideal. Studies have shown that this concentration range is a better plasma amino acid target range than concentrations found in cord or fetal blood (57).

The differences in amino acid metabolism and the aberrant plasma amino acid concentrations described here led to the development of two pediatric-specific formulations: Aminosyn-PF (Abbott Laboratories, Chicago, IL) and TrophAmine (McGaw, Inc., Irvine, CA) (Table 89.5).

Table 89.5.
Comparison of Amino Acid Products

Amino Acid	Composition (mole %)			
	Aminosyn-PF	TrophAmine	Aminosyn	FreAmine III
L-Isoleucine	7.4	8.2	6.4	6.3
L-Leucine	11.6	14.1	8.4	8.4
L-Lysine	5.9	7.3	5.7	6.0
L-Methionine	1.5	2.9	3.1	4.3
L-Phenylalanine	3.3	3.9	3.1	4.1
L-Tryptophan	1.1	1.3	0.9	0.9
L-Threonine	5.5	4.6	5.1	4.0
L-Valine	7.1	8.8	8.0	6.8
L-Arginine	9.1	9.2	6.6	6.6
L-Histidine	2.6	4.1	2.3	2.2
L-Alanine	10.1	7.9	16.8	9.6
L-Proline	9.1	7.8	8.7	11.7
Glycine	6.6	6.4	19.9	22.5
L-Serine	6.1	4.8	4.7	6.8
L-Tyrosine	0.4	0.5	0.3	0
N-Acetyl-L-tyrosine[a]	0	1.2	0	0
L-Glutamic acid	7.2	4.5	0	0
L-Aspartic acid	5.1	3.1	0	0
L-Cysteine[b]	0	0.4	0	0
Taurine	0.7	0.3	0	0
Total	100.4	101.3	100.0	100.2

[a]As tyrosine equivalents.
[b]Admixed to Aminosyn-PF, TrophAmine.

These products vary from standard amino acid formulations in that they contain less methionine and glycine and have added the dicarboxylic amino acids (aspartate, glutamate) and taurine. Tyrosine is added in the form of N-acetyl L-tyrosine to TrophAmine. Both products require the addition of L-cysteine hydrochloride prior to infusion. They vary from each other primarily in their contents of methionine and tyrosine (lower in Aminosyn-PF) and taurine (lower in TrophAmine).

The use of the pediatric-specific amino acid formulations in preterm postsurgical infants resulted in nitrogen balance and weight gain similar to that occurring during intrauterine growth (53–55). Use of TrophAmine in term neonates and older infants resulted in appropriate-for-age weight gain and nitrogen retention (56). Pediatric-specific amino acid formulations may provide adequate growth, even when infants receive protein and, more notably, calorie intakes that are below previously described norms (58, 59). This is likely the result of optimal plasma availability of amino acids for anabolism. Beck and colleagues reported a lower incidence of cholestasis in very low-birth-weight neonates who received a pediatric amino acid formulation that is perhaps due to enhanced amino acid utilization (60). In addition, the lower solution pH allows more optimal dosing of calcium and phosphorous, and anecdotally, the incidence of metabolic bone diseases

appears to be decreased when calcium needs are more appropriately addressed (see "Complications").

Parenteral protein requirements of the older child can be met using a standard crystalline amino acid formulation. Some incremental increases in protein intake, over those found in Table 89.6, may be required for the severely catabolic patient. Adequate concurrent monitoring is essential for patient- or disease-specific adjustments in protein intake.

Caloric Requirements

Unlike adults who require nonprotein calories for basal metabolic demands, activity, and maintenance of body temperature, children require additional calories for growth and development. The most elegant work describing global and compartmental energy needs in preterm infants used indirect calorimetry (61). Enterally fed low-birth-weight infants had global energy requirements of 150 kcal/kg/day. Approximately 18 kcal/kg/day were lost in stool; thus, 132 kcal/kg/day were available for metabolizable energy. Of these 132 kcal/kg/day, basal metabolism required 63 kcal/kg/day, activity required 4 kcal/kg/day, and the remaining 65 kcal/kg/day were required for growth.

Parenteral caloric requirements for optimal growth of the preterm infant and neonate range from 85 to 135 kcal/kg/day (62, 63). However, short-term provision of lower calorie (60 to 70 kcal/kg) and pediatric amino acid intakes of 2.2 g/kg/day have been associated with a positive nitrogen balance and modest weight gain (59). Caloric requirements (per kilogram body weight) decrease during the first year of life and continue to decrease until adult needs are approached (Table 89.7). As with protein, recommendations for caloric intake are merely guidelines for the practitioner. Assessment of clinical outcome, including weight gain, height or length, nitrogen balance, visceral and somatic protein measurements, and achieve-

Table 89.6.
Parenteral Protein Requirements (g/kg/day)

Preterm	2.5–3.0
Infant/neonate	2.0–2.5
Infant	1.5–2.0
Preschool/school-age	1.0–1.5
Adolescent	0.8–1.5

Table 89.7.
Parenteral Calorie Requirements (kcal/kg/day)

Preterm infant/neonate	85–130
Infant	90–120
1–6 years	75–90
7–12 years	50–75
13–18 years	30–50

ment of developmental milestones, should be used to determine adequacy of substrate delivered.

CARBOHYDRATE

Dextrose is used almost exclusively as the carbohydrate calorie source. Neonates, particularly premature neonates, are less glucose tolerant and are at risk for developing hyperglycemic-induced hyperosomolar coma and intraventricular hemorrhage (64). Thus, initial parenteral nutrition solutions should be limited to 5 g/kg/day of dextrose and be advanced slowly by about 3 g/kg/day with close monitoring of serum glucose. Usually, older infants and children can be started with 10 g/kg/day (7 mg/kg/min) of dextrose and doses increased by 5 g/kg every 12 to 24 hours to a maximum of 30 to 35 g/kg/day if the patient has a central venous catheter and is glucose tolerant. Usually, doses of 25 g/kg/day (17 mg/kg/min) when used with concomitant fat emulsion infusion are sufficient to achieve adequate weight gain in infants. Although higher doses may not result in hyperglycemia, the maximum glucose oxidation rate may be exceeded and fat may accumulate, which is desirable in an infant, particularly if undernourished. However, the expense is inefficiency in producing fat from carbohydrate and increased CO_2 production. With increasing age, maximum exogenous glucose oxidation rates decrease from about 12.5 mg/kg/min in infants to about 5 mg/kg/min in adults. Dextrose concentrations should be advanced slowly in individuals under severe stress or those who are receiving corticosteroids since hyperglycemia may develop even when dextrose intake is modest.

For patients who are carbohydrate intolerant, insulin may be used to facilitate glucose cellular uptake. Very low-birth-weight infants are started on 0.05 unit/kg/hour, whereas older infants and children usually are started on doses of 0.1 unit/kg/hour of insulin with the dose titrated to serum glucose concentration (65). This can be accomplished best by using a concomitant insulin infusion rather than adding insulin to the parenteral nutrition solution. The insulin dose should be titrated to frequent (every 2 hours) assessments of blood glucose.

FAT

As in adults, infusion of fat emulsion prevents or reverses essential fatty acid deficiency (EFAD); provides a concentrated, isotonic source of calories; provides a more physiologic "diet"; and prolongs survival time of peripheral intravenous lines in patients receiving parenteral nutrition. Fat emulsion products are compared in Table 89.8. Unlike adults, biochemical evidence of EFAD (a triene [5, 8, 11 eicosatrienoic acid with three double bonds] to tetraene [arachidonic acid with four double bonds] ratio above 0.4) (66–69) may be evident after a few days of no fat intake in preterm neonates (Fig. 89.3). Although linolenic acid does not reverse EFAD as linoleic acid does, current evi-

Table 89.8.
Composition of 20% Fat Emulsions[a]

Ingredient or Characteristic	Liposyn III Abbott Laboratories	Intralipid Clintec Nutrition
Source		
Soybean oil (%)	20	20
Safflower oil (%)	—	—
Fatty acid distribution		
Linoleic acid (%)	54.5	50
Oleic acid (%)	22.4	26
Palmitic acid (%)	10.5	10
Linolenic acid (%)	8.3	9
Stearic acid (%)	4.2	9
Egg yolk phospholipids (%)	1.2	3.5
Glycerin (%)	2.5	1.2
Calories (per ml)	2	2.25
		2

[a]In 10% fat emulsions, the oil sources are the same for each product but the amounts are halved, resulting in a higher phospholipid-to-triglyceride ratio and a 1.1 kcal/ml concentration.

dence suggests that linolenic acid may also be essential in humans (68).

The transport of free fatty acids across the mitochondria for beta oxidation and energy production depends on carnitine acyltransferase. Neonates and infants may have a relative insufficiency of the hydroxylase required in the final step of the in vivo synthesis of carnitine. Consistent with this finding, plasma carnitine concentrations are low in preterm neonates (70) and older infants receiving carnitine-free nutrition since birth (71), resulting in a limited capacity for fat oxidation. Supplementation of 10 mg/kg/day of carnitine for 7 days in older infants resulted in increased fat utilization and plasma carnitine concentrations (71).

Fat emulsion should be initiated at 0.5 g/kg/day in premature neonates. Term infants and infants older than 1 month can usually be started at 1 g/kg/day. If serum triglyceride or free fatty acid concentrations are within acceptable limits, the fat emulsion dose can be increased by 0.25 g/kg/day to 3 g/kg/day in preterm neonates and by 0.5 to 1 g/kg/day to 4 g/kg/day in term and older infants (69). Ideally, fat emulsion is given continuously over 24 hours to promote clearance from the circulation.

Neonates, particularly premature neonates, frequently develop physiologic jaundice or unconjugated (indirect) hyperbilirubinemia because of their inability to conjugate bilirubin. Because the blood–brain barrier is immature in neonates, indirect bilirubin can cross into the brain and cause a yellow staining known as kernicterus that is associated with neurologic injury. Fatty acids and unconjugated bilirubin bind competitively to albumin; thus, unconjugated bilirubin can be displaced from high-affinity albumin binding sites by free fatty acids. Andrew and colleagues found that the molar ratio of serum-free fatty acids to albumin must exceed 6 for bilirubin to be displaced from high-affinity binding sites on albumin (72). Conversely, an in vitro study found that both Intralipid and Liposyn enhanced the reserve capacity for the binding of bilirubin to albumin (73). Therefore, hyperbilirubinemia alone should not be an absolute contraindication to the use of intravenous fat emulsion, and provision of 2 to 4% of the total daily caloric requirements as fat emulsion to prevent EFAD should not present a problem.

The effects of fat emulsion on immune function are controversial and inconsistent. Both in vitro incubation of white blood cells with fat emulsion and in vivo infusion of fat emulsion inhibit leukocyte chemotaxis, phagocytosis, bacteriocidal capacity, and lymphoproliferation (74–77). On the other hand, others report that fat either has no effect (25, 78, 79) or it restores and augments immune function (25, 80). These conflicting findings are probably secondary to the complexities (duration of exposure, lipid concentration and composition, responding cell type, and so on) of fatty acid and fatty acid metabolite interactions with immunoreactive cells. In practice, parenteral lipids are used conservatively in patients who are immunocompromised or who have sepsis, and serum triglycerides are monitored to assess tolerance.

The use of fat emulsion in neonates with pulmonary compromise is also controversial. Because fat emboli were found in pulmonary capillaries during postmortem examinations of neonates who received Intralipid, the infusion of fat emulsion in neonates with respiratory compromise was postulated to alter pulmonary function. These findings were subsequently attributed to artifact, which occurred secondary to a delay in the fixation of the lung after death (81). Neonates under 1 week of age with respiratory

distress syndrome who received 1 g/kg of Intralipid over 4 hours had lower PO_2 values than age-related neonates who received no Intralipid (82). However, in these infants, the decreased PO_2 did not correlate with elevations in serum triglyceride. Oxygen diffusion in the lungs of premature neonates was not affected by infusion of Intralipid up to 4 g/kg/day over 24 hours (83). Therefore, to avoid excessive fat concentrations in the circulation and potential changes in pulmonary microcirculation that may result in a lowering of PO_2, the total daily dose of fat emulsion should be infused over 24 hours whenever possible.

The 10 and 20% concentrations of fat emulsion contain the same amount of phospholipid that results in a higher phospholipid to triglyceride ratio in the 10% (0.12) products compared to the 20% (0.06). Infants who were randomized to 7 days of continuous infusion 10% had higher plasma concentrations of phospholipid and cholesterol than those who received 20% fat emulsion (84). In addition, the LDL cholesterol had greater total cholesterol and phospholipid concentrations in those who received 10% fat. Two-thirds of the phospholipid in 10% fat is in the form of liposomes, which may accumulate cholesterol and apoproteins and potentially alter cholesterol regulation and triglyceride metabolism. Thus, the 20% product should be used whenever possible.

ELECTROLYTE AND MINERAL REQUIREMENTS

The reader is referred to Section 2 (Chapters 9, 11, and 12) for a discussion of electrolytes and minerals. As with adults, factors such as hydration, cardiovascular status, renal function, and concurrent medications should be considered when determining electrolyte require-

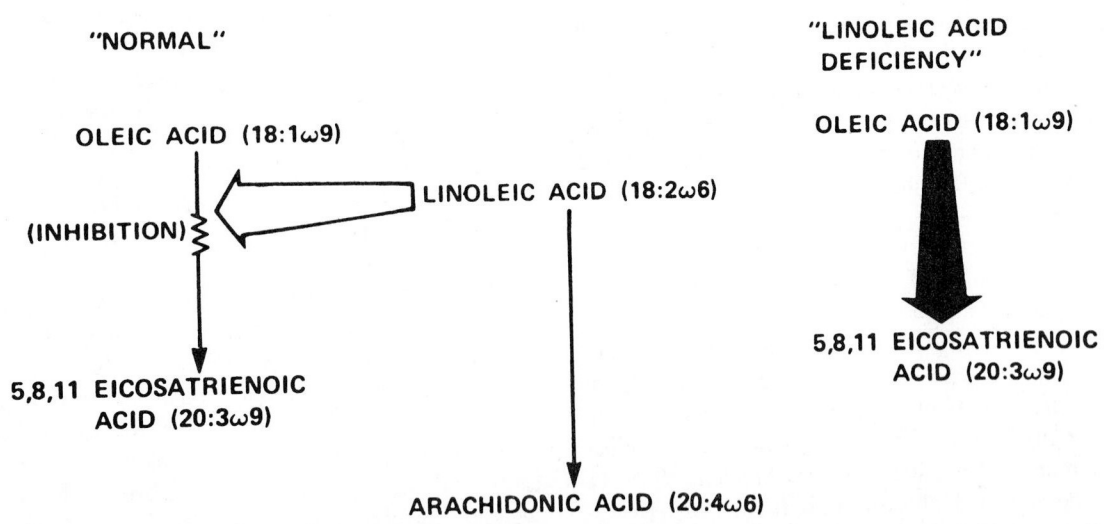

Figure 89.3. Essential fatty acid deficiency. Under "normal" conditions, the large blank arrow indicates linoleic acid's inhibition of the oleic acid conversion to 5,8,11 eicosatrienoic acid. During linoleic acid deficiency, the dark arrow depicts enzymatic elongation and desaturation of oleic acid to form abnormal 5,8,11 eicosatrienoic acid, resulting in a greater triene-to-tetraene ratio. Reprinted from Pelham LD. Rational use of intravenous fat emulsions. Am J Hosp Pharm 1981;38:202, with permission.

Table 89.9.
Daily Electrolyte Doses (mEq/kg/day)

	Preterm and Term Infants	Children
Sodium	2–8	2–5
Potassium[a]	1.4–10	2–3
Chloride	1.1–5	2–3
Magnesium	0.25–0.6	0.25–0.5
Calcium	2.5–3.5	1–2
Phosphate[b]	1–2	0.5–1

[a]Reflects patients receiving diuretics.
[b]Units are mmol/kg/day.

ments in children. In addition, age and organ maturity, particularly the kidney, should be considered in premature infants.

The daily maintenance electrolyte requirements for neonates, infants, and children are listed in Table 89.9 (85–88). As with adults, children with excessive fluid losses should receive replacement with a solution composed of comparable electrolytes (Table 89.2). Replacement fluids are delivered most efficiently using a separate intravenous infusion.

Amino acid solutions also contain various amounts of anions (usually acetate) and cations, which should be considered when determining anion distribution (Table 89.4).

Sodium

Premature infants have functionally immature kidneys that may promote excessive urinary sodium losses (89). Sodium requirements in these infants may be as high as 8 mEq/kg/day. When determining an individual's sodium needs, other sources of sodium, such as flushes, continuous infusion of normal saline through arterial lines, or medications containing sodium should be considered.

Frequent causes of abnormal serum sodium concentrations in the pediatric population are vomiting and diarrhea. Patients receiving diuretics or those with certain renal disorders (e.g., renal tubular acidosis) have increased urinary sodium losses and often require additional sodium. Parenteral nutrition solutions high in sodium may be desirable in closed head injury patients to increase serum osmolality and ultimately decrease intracranial pressure. Specific types of malignancies, pulmonary diseases, central nervous system disorders, and drugs (e.g., vincristine, carbamazepine, cyclophosphamide, barbiturates) may result in hyponatremia secondary to the syndrome of inappropriate antidiuretic hormone (SIADH).

Potassium

Several factors affect potassium homeostasis, including acid–base status, insulin, glucocorticoids, aldosterone, catecholamines, and renal potassium excretion. Vomiting, diarrhea, and draining fistulas are the primary causes of extrarenal potassium loss. In addition, metabolic alkalosis secondary to gastrointestinal losses of hydrogen ion may also result in hypokalemia. Diuretic therapy, amphotericin, and cisplatin are frequent causes of drug-associated hypokalemia. Other drugs such as the aminoglycosides and penicillins (90) promote renal potassium excretion. Hypokalemia refractory to potassium supplementation may indicate a concurrent hypomagnesemia, which must be addressed before serum potassium concentrations can be maintained. Since potassium is the principal intracellular cation, it is difficult to estimate the extent of potassium depletion by extracellular serum concentrations; therefore, frequent serum monitoring is necessary.

Usual potassium doses range from 2 to 4 mEq/kg/day; however, depending on organ maturity, presence of disease, and medications, quantities approaching 10 mEq/kg/day may be needed. Preterm infants may have increased potassium requirements secondary to increased urinary losses resulting from immature renal function.

Peripheral infusion of potassium is irritating to vessels, may be painful to the patient, and should be limited to about 40 mEq/liter for solutions infused peripherally. Patients with central venous access can receive more concentrated solutions, but the maximum rate of potassium delivery should not exceed 0.5 to 1 mEq/kg/hour considering all sources. Patients receiving more than 0.5 mEq/kg/hour should be monitored by electrocardiogram since cardiac dysrhythmias may develop when potassium is infused rapidly (91). Potassium is most efficiently replaced using continuous infusions since the transient increase in potassium serum concentration with a 1 mEq/kg dose infused over 2 hours may stimulate aldosterone and promote potassium renal elimination.

Infant serum samples are often hemolyzed because they are obtained by heel puncture, which may require considerable squeezing to obtain an adequate blood volume. Hemolysis releases intracellular potassium, causing an apparent elevation in serum potassium concentration. When hyperkalemia is noted in an asymptomatic patient, the phlebotomy method should be determined and the serum evaluated for visual evidence of hemolysis. It may be desirable to validate the serum concentration by venipuncture before aggressive treatment is undertaken.

Calcium

Calcium, the most abundant mineral in the body, is important in maintaining the functional integrity of cellular membranes, neuromuscular activity, regulation of various endocrine and exocrine secretory activities, blood coagulation, and bone metabolism. In newborns, 98% of total body calcium is present in bone. Approximately 40% of total serum calcium is bound to serum proteins, and 80 to

90% of this calcium is bound to albumin. Variations in the serum protein concentration and serum pH proportionately alter protein-bound and total serum calcium concentrations.

Calcium homeostasis is regulated by parathyroid hormone (PTH), calcitonin, and vitamin D. PTH and calcitonin respond inversely to acute changes in calcium and magnesium serum concentrations. Acute increases in these cations decrease PTH and increase calcitonin production. Likewise, an acute decrease in calcium concentration causes an increase in PTH concentration and a decrease in calcitonin, resulting in the mobilization of calcium from bone. Therefore, serum calcium concentration is neither a sensitive nor a specific measure of the adequacy of intake.

Calcium and phosphorous dose requirements are inversely related to postconceptional age. In utero calcium accretion rates at 36 weeks gestation are 5 to 7.5 mEq/kg/day of elemental calcium. It is impossible to provide this much calcium and an appropriate phosphate dose either enterally or parenterally. Interestingly, adequate bone mineralization occurs with significantly less calcium than is accreted in utero as long as the appropriate amount of phosphate is also provided. A physiologic ratio of calcium and phosphate (1.7:1 [mg:mg]) promotes retention of these minerals in premature infants and minimizes parenteral-nutrition-related bone disease (92, 93). In addition to the inherently increased calcium requirements for normal bone mineralization, premature infants often have concurrent diseases that require aggressive diuretic therapy or fluid restriction. Use of high-dose diuretics promotes calcium elimination (94) and fluid restriction limits the amount of calcium and phosphorous that can be provided because of solubility factors. Thus, these infants are at increased risk for metabolic bone disease. The pediatric amino acid products have a lower pH, and with the addition of L-cysteine, the pH is decreased further, which increases calcium and phosphate solubility. Therefore, calcium and phosphate doses can be increased to more adequately address needs.

Calcium and phosphate solubility is affected by pH, temperature, and the final calcium and phosphate concentrations. Calcium may react with phosphate to form monobasic or dibasic calcium phosphate, depending on pH. At low pH, the predominant form of calcium phosphate is monobasic, which is quite soluble. As the pH increases, more dibasic phosphate becomes available to bind with calcium, and precipitation occurs more easily (95). Solutions compounded from amino acid products with a relatively high pH, such as FreAmine III (McGaw), have a relatively low calcium phosphate solubility. On the other hand, Aminosyn-PF and TrophAmine have a low pH and, therefore, enhanced calcium and phosphate solubility (96). The addition of L-cysteine HCl further decreases the pH, allowing increased calcium and phosphate supplementation. In certain circumstances, L-cysteine HCl has been added to standard amino acid products to decrease solution pH and enhance calcium phosphate solubility (97). Increased temperatures increase calcium ionization and thereby increase the likelihood of calcium phosphate precipitation. It is common for temperatures in the nursery or near the infant to be increased. For example, infants in isolettes or those receiving ultraviolet light therapy have warmer environments that may cause solutions that are near the limit of calcium and phosphate solubility to precipitate near the infant, perhaps in the intravenous line. In some cases, precipitation has occurred within the catheter since the infusing solution was warmed by the patient's body temperature.

Because the calcium gluconate is less ionized in solution than the chloride salt, less precipitation occurs with the gluconate than with the chloride salt; thus, calcium supplementation in parenteral nutrition solutions is generally done with calcium gluconate (98). About 100 mg of calcium gluconate equals 0.46 meq or 9.2 mg of elemental calcium, and 100 mg of calcium chloride equals 1.36 meq or 27.2 mg of elemental calcium.

When compounding the solution, phosphate is added early in the process because it is concentrated (3 mmol/ml) and consumes a small volume compared to calcium; therefore, it is more likely to remain in the injection port. The addition of other additives helps clear the injection port of phosphate. Calcium is more dilute (0.456 meq/ml) than phosphate salts and is added last (99).

Phosphorus

Phosphate functions as a cofactor in multiple enzyme systems necessary for the metabolism of protein, carbohydrate, and fat, and is required for production of the high-energy bonds of adenosine triphosphate (ATP). Therapeutic refeeding of a severely malnourished patient has been associated with severe hypophosphatemia caused by total body phosphate depletion and increased intracellular shifting of phosphate during refeeding (100). Hypophosphatemia may also occur secondary to hyperparathyroidism (increased urinary phosphate excretion) or respiratory alkalosis (intracellular phosphate shifting). In addition to calcium, phosphorous is particularly important in bone growth, an important concern in pediatric patients. Phosphorus content, as the phosphate ion, in parenteral nutrition solutions is limited by solubility factors (see "Calcium").

Phosphate doses provided to neonates and infants range from 1 to 2 mmol per kg. This amount can be provided in most patients who are not fluid restricted. Dose requirements decrease to about 1 mmol per kg in older children and to 0.5 to 0.75 mmol per kg in adolescents and young adults. Since phosphate exists in two valence states that fluctuate with changing pH, phosphate requirements are usually described in millimoles or milligrams, not milliequivalents. The use of milliequivalents does not reflect the concentration of phosphorus in solution and may lead to dosing errors; 1 mmol of phosphate equals 31 mg of elemental phosphorus, and 3 mmol of phosphate is contained in either 4 meq of sodium phosphate or 4.4 meq of potassium phosphate.

Magnesium

Magnesium, the second most common intracellular cation, is necessary for numerous enzymatic reactions involving energy storage and use. Extracellular magnesium is used during neuromuscular transmission and is required for cardiovascular tone. Approximately 2% of the body's total magnesium is present in the extracellular compartment, whereas 98% is found intracellularly, primarily in bone.

Magnesium balance and serum magnesium concentration are largely determined by renal magnesium excretion, which is primarily regulated by the glomerular filtration rate, tubular reabsorption, and PTH. When necessary, the kidney can conserve or increase urinary magnesium excretion depending on the body's magnesium stores (101).

As with hypocalcemia, hypomagnesemia is often present in infants with DiGeorge syndrome and those born to diabetic mothers. Neonatal hepatitis and congenital biliary atresia are commonly associated with hypomagnesemia (102). Since magnesium is absorbed in the proximal jejunum, patients that undergo intestinal resection are at risk for developing hypomagnesemia. Similarly, patients with extensive diarrheal or ileostomy fluid losses may have increased magnesium losses. Diuretics, amphotericin, cyclosporine, and cisplatin increase urinary magnesium losses and may contribute to hypomagnesemia. Magnesium depletion may precipitate refractory hypokalemia or hypocalcemia (103). Magnesium is an intracellular cation that equilibrates rather slowly; thus, increases in magnesium content in parenteral nutrition solutions may not result in restoration of intracellular magnesium concentrations for several days. Infusion of bolus doses of magnesium results in increased amounts of magnesium urinary concentrations, and as with potassium, infusion of estimated deficits should be done with continuous infusion.

VITAMINS

The guidelines for the Recommended Dietary Allowances (RDAs) of vitamins are based on oral vitamin delivery in healthy infants and children. A pediatric parenteral multivitamin product formulated according to recommendations of the Nutrition Advisory Group (NAG) of the American Medical Association (AMA) was formulated in the early 1980s and results of studies evaluated in the mid-1980s.

Table 89.10.
Vitamin Content of MVI-Pediatric and MVI-12

Vitamin	MVI-Pediatric (5 ml)[a]	MVI-12 (10 ml)[b]
A (retinol equivalents)	2300 IU	3300 IU
D (ergocalciferol)	400 IU	200 IU
E (d,1 g tocopherol acetate)	7 IU	10 IU
K (phytonadione)	200 mcg	0
C (ascorbic acid)	80 mg	100 mg
B-1 (thiamine)	1.2 mg	3 mg
B-2 (riboflavin)	1.4 mg	3.6 mg
B-6 (pyridoxine)	1 mg	4 mg
Niacinamide	17 mg	40 mg
Dexpanthenol	5 mg	15 mg
Biotin	20 mcg	60 mcg
Folic acid	140 mcg	400 mcg
B-12 (cyanocobalamin)	1 mcg	5 mcg

[a]Contains 375 mg of mannitol, sodium hydroxide, 50 mg of polysorbate 80, 0.8 mcg of polysorbate 20, 58 mg of butylated hydroxytoluene, and 14 mcg of butylated hydroxyanisole.
[b]Contains prophylene glycol (30%), sodium citrate, citric acid, sodium hydroxide, polysorbate 20 (4.8%), butylated hydroxyanisole (0.0004%), butylated hydroxytoluene (0.0018%), and ethanolamide (2%).

Parenteral multivitamin preparations are sensitive to pH, light, and temperature. Additionally, vitamins may interact with each other or adsorb to the plastic matrix of administration sets, decreasing bioavailability (87, 99). MVI pediatric also contains vitamin K, which is not in adult parenteral vitamins, and it contains twice the amount of vitamin D as is in adult products. The pediatric and adult multivitamin products are compared in Table 89.10.

The Food and Drug Administration currently recommends that infants weighing less than 1 kg receive daily 30% (1.5 ml) of a single full dose (5 ml), and infants weighing 1 to 3 kg receive daily 65% (3.25 ml) of a single full dose. Infants and children weighing 3 kg or more up to 11 years of age should receive the full single-dose vial (5 ml) daily. The pediatric multivitamin product has been tested primarily in medically stable infants and children receiving parenteral nutrition and is effective in maintaining acceptable vitamin serum concentrations (87).

However, using the manufacturer's recommended dose in preterm infants results in increased plasma concentrations of most water soluble vitamins and low concentrations of vitamin A. Greene and colleagues suggested dosing the pediatric multivitamin product in preterm infants at 2 ml/kg/day, with the maximum of 5 ml/day to address the problem with the water soluble vitamins (87); however, this decrease in dose would also decrease the amount of vitamin A that is delivered. Of further concern in premature neonates is the possible decreased metabolism of the polysorbate emulsifiers. Because of these altered vitamin requirements and potential toxicity of the emulsifier, it has been proposed that a separate intravenous multivitamin product be developed specifically for preterm infants (87).

Children over 11 years old should receive the adult multivitamin product. This preparation contains half the vitamin D of the pediatric product, and there is no vitamin K. The remaining vitamins are present in greater amounts to address the RDA for adults (see Chapter 11).

TRACE ELEMENTS

The trace elements constitute less than 0.01% of human body weight. Despite their low body content, trace elements have essential roles in biochemical processes, including growth and development. Pediatric trace element requirements have not been well defined; hence, recommended dietary allowances (RDAs) and reports of deficiency currently guide the intravenous dosage recommendations.

Current recommendations for trace element dosing is shown in Table 89.11. Recent evidence has shown that children on long-term parenteral nutrition who receive recommended doses of chromium have plasma chromium concentrations from 5 to 10 times normal. This is likely due to significant amounts of chromium present as a contaminant in amino acid and electrolyte products that are not accounted for in chromium dosing (104, 105). It is likely that as research in this area progresses, trace element dosing in pediatric patients will change.

Since trace elements are stored during the last trimester of pregnancy, premature neonates have low body stores, which puts them at increased risk of developing deficiencies. Patients with persistent diarrhea or excessive ostomy outputs have increased zinc losses in these body fluids and thus may require additional supplementation. Copper and manganese are excreted through the biliary system, and patients with severe liver disease, including cholestasis, should not receive these trace elements (87). Conversely, patients with exterior biliary drainage or jejunostomies may have increased copper losses, resulting in increased requirements. Selenium

deficiency may result in cardiomyopathy and skeletal muscle myopathy (87). Selenium, chromium, and molybdenum are excreted primarily by the kidneys; thus, doses should be adjusted in patients with renal insufficiency. Each trace element is available as a single-entity product for patients requiring an individualized approach to supplementation.

PARENTERAL NUTRITION COMPLICATIONS

Parenteral nutrition delivers the most basic form of nutrients directly into the bloodstream, bypassing normal digestive and absorptive processes. Frequently, solutions are infused into the superior vena cava through a surgically placed catheter (Fig. 89.1). Because of the nature of the solutions and catheters and the direct link to the bloodstream, a variety of technical, metabolic, and infectious complications are associated with parenteral nutrition.

Technical

Patients who require parenteral nutrition for relatively long periods generally have central venous catheters placed specifically for this purpose. In small infants and children with limited or difficult peripheral vascular access, a central venous catheter may be required, even if parenteral nutrition is necessary for a relatively short time (106). Complications that occur at the time of catheter placement include pneumothorax, vein or cardiac perforation, chylothorax (107), and hemorrhage. Following catheter placement, the catheter hub or line may crack or break. Cracks in the hub or on the proximal (exposed) portion of the catheter can be repaired in most cases, but catheter removal may be necessary.

The infusate may extravasate into the thoracic or pericardial cavity. Solutions that are inadvertently infused through extravasated or infiltrated catheters will be resorbed, in time, after the infusion is discontinued, but significant tissue injury may result. An extravasation that occurs suddenly may result in hypoglycemia caused by the abrupt discontinuation of the infusion of concentrated

Table 89.11.
Trace Element Daily Reqirements

Trace Element	Preterm[a] Neonates	Term[a] Neonates	<5 Years Old	Older[a] Children	Adults[b]
Zinc	400 mcg/kg	300 mcg/kg	100 mcg/kg	5 mg	2.5–4 mg
Copper	20 mcg/kg	20 mcg/kg	20 mcg/kg	200 mcg	300–500 mcg
Manganese	1 mcg/kg	1 mcg/kg	2–10 mcg/kg	50 mcg	150–800 mcg
Chromium	0.2 mcg/kg	0.2 mcg/kg	0.14–0.2 mcg/kg	5 mcg	10–20 mcg
Selenium	2–3 mcg/kg	2–3 mcg/kg	2–3 mcg/kg	40 mcg	40–80 mcg
Iodide	1 mcg/kg	1 mcg/kg	1 mcg/kg		

[a]See reference (87).
[b]See reference (36).

dextrose solution into the central circulation. In addition, extravasated or infiltrated solutions may accumulate in the pleural or pericardial region, resulting in effusions that cause respiratory or cardiac decompensation.

Catheters may be accidentally removed or migrate out of position (108). This type of problem is more common with percutaneously placed catheters than with the Broviac or Hickman-type silastic catheters that are tunneled and anchored by a Dacron cuff (Fig. 89.1) (109).

Catheters located in the right atrium may stimulate dysrhythmias by coming in contact with nodal tissue. The dysrhythmias may be resolved by pulling the catheter back away from sensitive tissue.

Catheters may become occluded because of fibrin deposition (110), precipitates (111), or saponified material that accumulates within the lumen. In many instances, the catheter that is not completely occluded can be recannulated pharmacologically (112–114). Fibrinolytic agents such as urokinase, streptokinase, or tissue plasminogen activator are useful in dissolving fibrin that partially occludes a catheter. Precipitates, such as calcium phosphate, may be dissolved by decreasing the pH inside the catheter with the instillation of 0.1 N HCl in the catheter (112). Other agents such as ethanol may be used to dissolve saponified material (113).

Patients receiving peripherally infused parenteral nutrition may experience phlebitis. Infiltration of the fluid into the interstitial tissue is an expected event that is usually benign. However, infants and small children who have limited extravascular tissue space and who may not be able to communicate pain adequately are at risk for the development of complications, including localized swelling and edema, which may progress to necrosis (115). The infiltrated site can be treated with hyaluronidase injections to increase the rate of solution absorption and decrease potential tissue damage. The addition of 1 to 2 units of heparin per milliliter of dextrose amino acid solution (116) and the concomitant infusion of fat emulsion with the dextrose and amino acid solution (117) increases the length of time to infiltration in infants receiving peripherally infused parenteral nutrition.

Metabolic

Metabolic complications include electrolyte and mineral abnormalities, aberrant plasma amino acid patterns (see "Protein"), metabolic bone disease, micronutrient deficiencies, cholestasis, hypersensitivity reactions, acid–base abnormalities, and alterations in pulmonary and immunologic function (118).

Most electrolyte and mineral abnormalities and acid–base complications can be avoided with adequate monitoring and appropriate forethought when prescribing solutions. Cholestasis and metabolic bone disease are two problems that are especially worrisome in pediatric patients, and these will be discussed in more detail.

CHOLESTASIS

The etiology of cholestasis is multifactorial and complex, and it occurs most commonly in premature infants who are enterally fasted and receive long-term parenteral nutrition (119). These infants are also at risk for infection, including hepatitis, and frequently receive medications, such as furosemide, that are associated with cholestasis; thus, it remains a diagnosis of exclusion. In parenteral-nutrition-associated cholestasis, proposed mechanisms include amino acid competition with bile salts for hepatocyte uptake, enhanced production of secondary bile salts (120), and the provision of excessive calories and protein (121). Increases in glutamyl transferase (GT) and direct bilirubin (122) are early indicators but are not seen until after at least 10 days of parenteral nutrition. Initiation of small-volume enteral (trophic) feeding for gut stimulation is probably the most important intervention. Offering the patient a protein- and calorie-free period by cycling the parenteral nutrition solution off for a period during the day may be beneficial. Phenobarbital, a choleretic agent, is not effective treatment for parenteral-nutrition-associated cholestasis (123). Cholecystokinin has been proposed as a useful agent to promote bile flow and potentially treat cholestasis, but there is insufficient experience to recommend its use for this purpose (124). Finally, the use of a pediatric-specific amino acid formulation should be considered. A solution that normalizes plasma amino acid patterns should result in optimal substrate metabolism and minimize potential toxicity associated with amino acids. Cholestasis generally resolves when parenteral nutrition is discontinued.

BONE DISEASE

As with cholestasis, the etiology of metabolic bone disease is multifactorial and related to inadequate intake of calcium and phosphorous, possible end organ resistance to vitamin D, increased calcium losses in the urine due to medications (in particular loop diuretics), and aluminum intake. Because the pediatric amino acid products inherently have a lower pH, more appropriate amounts of calcium and phosphorous can be given. Adequate calcium and phosphorous dosing significantly decreases the occurrence of metabolic bone disease in infants. Aluminum is a significant contaminant in many parenteral fluids; therefore, those who receive large-volume parenteral fluids may be at risk for aluminum accumulation in bone and soft tissues, including the brain (125, 126). Amino acid manufacturers set tolerance limits for aluminum content in the individual amino acids included in their products; therefore, contaminant aluminum in these products is minimum. Patients suspected of having osteopenia and rachitic changes should be evaluated by roentgenograms or radiographic densitometry (127).

OTHER COMPLICATIONS

Hypersensitivity reactions have been reported in patients receiving parenteral nutrition. Anaphylaxis has been attributed to the amino acid solutions (128), vitamin preparations (128, 129), magnesium sulfate (128), fat emulsion (130), iron, and soybean oil (131). In addition, bradycardia (132) and diarrhea (133) have been associated with fat emulsion infusions.

A variety of hematologic abnormalities have been reported in patients receiving parenteral nutrition. Thrombocytopenia has been related to fat emulsion infusions and appears to be dose related (134). In contrast, an increased peripheral platelet count has also been described in preterm neonates on parenteral nutrition (135). Parenteral-nutrition-associated eosinophilia (135) occurs with greater frequency in premature neonates and appears to be self-limiting. Hemolysis due to lipid peroxidation of red blood cell membrane may be associated with failure to provide sufficient antioxidant (vitamin E) or antioxidant cofactors such as selenium (136). Intravascular hemolysis has been reported with rapid infusion of Intralipid in adults (137, 138).

Impairment of immune function has been described with deficiency or insufficiency of a variety of micronutrients, including zinc (139); selenium, pyridoxine, and pantothenic acid (140, 141); vitamin E (142,143); vitamins A and D (142); arginine (144); and glutamine (145).

Infectious

Infection is a serious complication associated with central venous catheters and may be a blood-borne, exit-site, or tunnel-tract infection. Organisms that commonly result in infection in pediatric patients on long-term parenteral nutrition are listed in Table 89.12 (146). In some cases, infections are polymicrobial. The incidence of central

venous line infections is inversely related to age and in pediatric patients ranges from 42 to 57% (147). Mechanisms for the development of infection include introduction of organisms into the bloodstream through the catheter, hematogenous spread, and potentially, bacterial translocation, a process in which normal bacteria present in the bowel crosses the intestinal lumen and enters the bloodstream. Because of problems with venous access in small children, central venous catheters are used for multiple purposes, increasing the risk for infection. Young children often play with their catheters or infusion sets and may chew on infusion lines or disconnect their infusion, which increases the risk for contamination. Infants who require parenteral nutrition often have bowel disease that results in frequent, loose stools that are difficult to contain. It is not uncommon for fecal material to come in contact with tubing, increasing the risk for accidental contamination of catheters or solutions. Furthermore, premature neonates have a greater risk for infection because of immune system immaturity.

In many cases, solution contamination is suspected to be the source of the infection. Dextrose amino acid solutions are very hypertonic and poorly support bacterial growth; however, yeast will grow in these solutions. On the other hand, lipid products will facilitate bacterial growth, thus, repackaging of lipid products is discouraged. *Malassezia furfur* is a fungal infection that is predominantly found in children, and it is almost exclusively associated with lipid infusion. Routine fungal cultures will not detect this organism.

Removal of infected catheters and placement of a new catheter in a different site after the infection is cleared may not be feasible in pediatric patients. Once a vein has been cannulated, collateral veins develop around the site so that blood flow to that area is not compromised. In addition, cannulated veins may become thrombosed or scarred rendering them unsuitable for subsequent catheterization. Collateral vessels are tortuous and narrow and unable to be cannulated. Therefore, the decision to remove a central line in a child who depends on this route for hydration and nutrition must be made judiciously. Placement of a catheter directly into the right atrium has been done in children without an alternative catheterization site. In patients with catheter-related sepsis who continued to require central venous access, 55 to 89% of catheter-related infections were successfully treated in situ with the administration of appropriate antibiotics (148, 149). The appropriate dosage of the antimicrobial agent(s) should be infused through the infected catheter. In addition, antibiotics or antifungals can be instilled and allowed to reside in the catheter for varying lengths of time. Daily blood cultures are obtained through the catheter lumen(s) and from a peripheral site to ensure that the microorganism is being eradicated (148, 149).

Table 89.12.
Microorganisms Cultured from Central Venous Catheters in Children Receiving Home Parenteral Nutrition[a]

Staphylococcus epidermidis	25%
Klebsiella	12%
Staphylococcus aureus	10%
E coli	6%
C parapsilosis	5%
Gram-positive organisms	43%
Gram-negative organisms	36%
Fungi	13%
Polymicrobial	11%

[a]Adapted from reference (146).

The body recognizes indwelling central venous catheters as foreign, and fibrin can accumulate inside the lumen of the catheter, particularly if the line is used for blood withdrawal (110). Microorganisms may be harbored within the fibrin, providing a nidus for infection. Even appropriate microbial therapy may not penetrate through the fibrin web and eradicate microorganisms residing inside. Although urokinase, streptokinase, TPA, and possibly HCl can dissolve the fibrin within the catheter lumen, it is less likely that fibrin around the outside of the catheter will be affected. It has been suggested that monthly treatment of central lines with a fibrinolytic decreases the number of central line infections. However, dissolution of a fibrin sheath that is harboring a large number of microorganisms will release these microorganisms into the bloodstream. The resultant bacteremia may result in an acute septic event or seed distant sites. Therefore, aseptic maintenance of central venous catheters is of paramount importance.

The catheter exit site or tunnel tract may also become infected. Local antibiotic therapy may be used to treat certain exit-site infections; however, both exit-site and tunnel-tract infections may require systemic antimicrobial therapy. In addition, more frequent central line dressing changes may be required.

ENTERAL NUTRITION

Infant Formulas

The American Academy of Pediatrics recommends that infants be breast fed whenever possible (see Chapter 88). However, many mothers elect to totally or partially bottle feed for a variety of reasons. For infants who are not breast fed exclusively, special feeding nipples for bottles are available to avoid nipple confusion. Infants who cannot be orally fed because of illness or disease may refuse the breast or bottle as they recover. Speech therapists or occupational therapists can work with infants and care givers to facilitate the transition back to oral feedings. Although this process may require a commitment of time from the primary care giver, most infants learn or relearn this skill quickly. Mothers who want to breast feed but whose infant cannot be enterally fed, initially may pump their breasts and freeze their milk until the infant is able to receive enteral feedings.

The RDA is defined as the level of intake of essential nutrients that is judged by the Food and Nutrition Board, on the basis of scientific knowledge, to be adequate to meet known nutrient needs of healthy persons (150). The RDA estimates generally exceed the nutrient requirements of most healthy infants and children, but they provide guidelines for development of enteral formulas. They do not provide guidelines for premature infants and may not provide adequate allowances for infants and children with disease or during drug therapy. The RDA requirements of energy and protein for healthy infants and children are listed in Table 89.13. Energy required for growth is greatest

Table 89.13.

Recommended Dietary Allowances (RDA) for Energy and Protein Intake[a]

	Kilocalories/kg	Grams Protein/kg[b]
Infants		
Birth–6 months	108	2.2
>6–12 months	98	1.6
>1–3 years	102	1.2
4–6 years	90	1.1
7–10 years	70	1
Males		
11–14 years	55	1
Females		
11–14 years	47	1

[a]Adapted from Recommended Dietary Allowances, ed. 10. Washington, DC, National Academy of Sciences, 1989.
[b]Standard protein: human milk.

during the newborn period. As infants grow, the total caloric requirement increases, but because of the increasing body size, the amount of kilocalories per kilogram decreases. From infancy to childhood, protein requirements decrease more rapidly than energy requirements. This reflects an increase in energy requiring activity and a decrease in growth rates (requiring protein).

The RDAs for vitamin and minerals in infants and children are listed in Table 89.14. Although infant formulas contain vitamins and minerals, it is important to determine whether their total daily intake delivers the recommended amounts. Most, but not all, infant formulas contain adequate amounts of iron. Premature infants may require additional vitamin supplementation (151).

Concentrated premature infant formulas are available to meet the needs of infants with immature gastrointestinal tracts (Table 89.15). The kilocalorie content of these formulas has been increased to 24 per ounce. Protein, carbohydrate, and fat components of these products require less complex digestive processes. The protein content in these formulas is primarily whey, which forms smaller curds that are more easily digested. In addition, whey protein has an amino acid composition high in cysteine and low in tyrosine, making it more desirable for the premature infant with immature enzymatic pathways. Lactose is the carbohydrate found in human milk; however, low lactase activity is found in the intestinal mucosa of premature infants. Thus, the lactose content of preterm formulas has been limited to 40 to 50% of the available carbohydrate. The remaining carbohydrate is provided in the form of maltodextrins or "corn syrup," which is a mixture of mono-, oligo-, and polysaccharides that relies on multiple digestive and absorptive pathways and results in enhanced utilization.

Premature infants are frequently unable to digest long chain triglycerides (LCT) because of reduced bile acid pool

Table 89.14.
Recommended Dietary Allowances (RDA) for Vitamins and Minerals[a]

	0–6 Months	>6–12 Months	>1–3 Years	4–6 Years	7–10 Years	Males 11–14 Years	Females 11–14 Years
Vitamins							
Fat soluble							
A (mcg)	375	375	400	500	700	1000	800
D (mcg)	7.5	10	10	10	10	10	10
E (mg)	3	4	6	7	7	10	8
K (mcg)	5	10	15	20	30	45	45
Water soluble							
C (mg)	30	35	40	45	45	50	50
Thiamine (mg)	0.3	0.4	0.7	0.9	1	1.3	1.1
Riboflavin (mg)	0.4	0.5	0.8	1.1	1.2	1.5	1.3
Niacin (mg)	5	6	9	12	13	17	15
B6 (mg)	0.3	0.6	1	1.1	1.4	1.7	1.4
Folate (mcg)	25	35	50	75	100	150	150
B12 (mcg)	0.3	0.5	0.7	1	1.4	2	2
Minerals							
Calcium (mg)	400	600	800	800	800	1200	1200
Phosphorus (mg)	300	500	800	800	800	1200	1200
Magnesium (mg)	40	60	80	120	170	270	280
Iron (mg)	6	10	10	10	10	12	15
Zinc (mg)	5	5	10	10	10	15	12
Selenium (mcg)	10	15	20	20	30	40	45

[a]Adapted from Recommended Dietary Allowances, ed. 10. Washington, DC, National Academy of Sciences, 1989.

size and decreased pancreatic lipase activity. Thus, 13 to 50% of fat in these formulas is provided as medium chain triglycerides (MCTs). Compared to LCTs, MCTs are easily absorbed since they do not require bile acids for solubilization, and they do not require carnitine for transport into the mitochondria where beta oxidation occurs. However, MCTs do not provide essential fatty acids, thus a portion of fat must be supplied as LCT.

The nutrient distribution in standard infant formulas available for infants under 1 year of age reflects their distribution in human milk. The composition of these products is similar (Table 89.15), and when reconstituted according to the standard formula, they contain 20 kilocalories per ounce. Infant formulas should have an osmotic load similar to that of human milk (277 to 303 mosm/kg) to avoid diarrhea induced by a high osmotic load.

The protein in the specialized infant formulas Nutramigen, Pregestimil, and Alimentum is in the form of free amino acids and peptides that result from partial acid hydrolysis of cow's milk (Table 89.16). The protein in these formulas is easily digestible; thus, they may be appropriate for infants with intestinal resection, cow's milk allergy, or other protein-allergic sensitivities. The fat content differs among these three products, with Pregestimil and Alimentum containing MCTs, whereas Nutramigen contains 100% of its fat as LCTs. Portagen, a formula with 86% of its fat as MCTs and no lactose, is available for infants with significant steatorrhea, which may occur with cystic fibrosis, pancreatic insufficiency, or intestinal resection.

Since MCTs are not transported through the lymphatic system chyle production is minimized with portagen, which makes this formula desirable for use in patients with chylothorax.

Lactose- and sucrose-free formulas (i.e., Isomil, Isomil SF, Nursoy, Prosobee; see Table 89.16) are also available for infants with disaccharidase deficiency or specific types of carbohydrate intolerance. Because all these formulas contain hypoallergenic soy protein, they may be indicated if cow's milk allergy is suspected. Low renal solute formulas (e.g., Similac PM 60/40, SMA) contain less sodium than other specialized formulas and are indicated when low sodium intake is desirable (Table 89.16). Although these formulas have a whey-to-casein protein concentration of approximately 60 to 40% (more like human milk), the carbohydrate content is solely lactose.

Formulas have been developed and marketed for children between 1 and 10 years of age (Table 89.17). The protein concentration in these products is equal to or greater than that found in infant formulas, and the percent of carbohydrate is usually greater and fat is usually less than that found in infant formulas. Calcium and phosphorous are approximately equimolar in children's formulas, whereas in infant formulas, there is a greater amount of calcium than phosphorous. In children's formulas, the renal solute load is greater than that found in infant formulas. Pediasure and Kindercal are standard children's formulas, whereas Vivonex Pediatric is designed for children who require a more elemental feeding solution.

Table 89.15.
Infant Formulas[a]

	kcal/oz	Carbohydrate Source	Protein Source	Fat Source	CHO (g)	PRO (g)	Fat (g)	Na meq	K meq	mg Ca/mg P	Fe mg	mOsm/kg H₂O
Standard infant												
Enfamil with iron	20	Lactose	Nonfat milk solids	Coconut and soybean oils	6.9	1.5	3.8	0.9	1.9	52/35	1.3	300
Similac with iron	20	Lactose	Nonfat milk	Soybean and coconut oils	7.1	1.4	3.6	0.8	1.8	49/37	1.3	290
Concentrated, premature												
Similac Special Care with iron	24	Lactose, hydrolyzed corn starch	Nonfat milk, whey protein concentrate	Coconut, soybean and coconut oils	8.5	2.2	4.3	1.5	2.6	144/72	1.2	300
Enfamil PM 24 with iron	24	Corn syrup solids, lactose	Whey, nonfat milk solids	40% MCT; coconut and soybean oils	8.9	2.4	4.1	1.3	2.1	132/67	1.2	310
Preemie SMA	24	Maltodextrins	Nonfat milk, whey	Coconut, safflower and soybean oils	8.4	1.9	4.3	1.3	1.9	72/40	0.3	280

[a]Formula content changes are possible. The authors suggest referring to the most recent publication of product literature or consulting clinical dietetics for product information.

Table 89.16.
Specialized Infant Formulas[a]

	kcal/oz	Carbohydrate Source	Protein Source	Fat Source	CHO (g)	PRO (g)	Fat (g)	Na meq	K meq	mg Ca/mg P	Fe mg	mOsm/kg H₂O
Nutramigen	20	Corn syrup solids, modified corn starch	Casein hydrolysates	Corn and soybean oils	8.9	1.9	2.6	1.4	1.9	63/42	1.3	320
Pregestimil	20	Corn syrup solids, modified corn starch	Casein hydrolysate	55% MCT; coconut, safflower and corn oils	6.9	1.9	3.7	1.4	1.9	63/42	1.3	320
Alimentum	20	Sucrose and modified tapioca starch	Casein hydrolysate	50% MCT; coconut, safflower and soybean oils	6.8	1.8	3.7	1.3	2	70/50	1.2	370
Portagen	20	Corn syrup solids, sucrose, 0.75 mg/qt lactose	Sodium caseinate	83% MCT; coconut, corn and soybean oils	7.7	2.3	3.2	1.6	2.1	63/47	1.3	236
Isomil	20	Corn syrup and sucrose	Soy protein isolate	Coconut and soybean oils	6.7	1.8	3.6	1.3	1.8	70/50	1.2	250
Nursoy	20	Sucrose	Soy protein isolate	Coconut, oleo, safflower, and soybean oils	6.9	2.1	3.6	0.8	1.9	63/44	1.3	296
ProSobee	20	Corn syrup solids, glucose polymers	Soy protein isolate	Coconut, soybean, and corn oils	6.7	2.0	3.5	1	2.1	63/49	1.3	200
SMA with iron	20	Lactose	Nonfat milk	Coconut and soybean oils	7.1	1.5	3.6	0.6	2	42/28	1.2	300
Similac PM 60/40	20	Lactose	Whey protein, sodium caseinate	Coconut and soybean oils	6.8	1.6	3.7	0.7	1.5	37/19	0.15	260

[a]Formula content changes are possible. The authors suggest referring to the most recent publication of product literature or consulting clinical dietetics for product information.

Table 89.17.
Pediatric Formulas for Use in Children from 1–10 Years[a]

	kcal/ oz	Carbohydrate Source	Protein Source	Fat Source	CHO (g)	PRO (g)	Fat (g)	Na meq	K meq	mg Ca/ mg P	Fe mg	mOsm/ kg H$_2$O
Pediasure	30	Cornstarch, sucrose	Sodium casein-ate, whey	20% MCT; coco-nut, safflower and soybean	11	3	5	1.7	3.4	97/80	1.4	310
Kindercal	30	Maltodextrin, sucrose	Calcium casein-ate, sodium caseinate, milk protein con-centrate	20% MCT; coco-nut, corn, canola, and sunflower oils	13.5	3.4	4.4	1.6	3.4	85/85	1.1	310
Peptamin Jr	30	Maltodextrin	Whey protein	60% MCT; coconut, soybean and canola oils	13.7	3	3.8	2	3.4	100/80	1.4	260
Vivonex Pediatric	24	Maltodextrin, modified starch	Free amino acids	68% MCT; coconut and soybean oils	13	2.4	2.4	1.7	3.1	97/80	1	360

[a]Formula content changes are possible. The authors suggest referring to the most recent publication of product literature or consulting clinical dietetics for product information.

Formulas are available as ready-to-feed, unit-of-use, or multiple-use containers, concentrated liquids, or dry powders. Prior to feeding, formula should be stored in a cool, dry place since temperature extremes can cause irreversible physical and chemical changes. The ready-to-feed solutions should not be diluted before feeding unless the physician prescribes a dilute formula. The concentrated liquid and dry powder formulas require dilution or reconstitution prior to feeding. Instructions for the amount of water to be added are provided on each container. Failure to dilute concentrated formulas can result in hyperosmolality and dehydration. Regular tap water that meets federal drinking water standards is acceptable for reconstituting infant formula. However, in certain situations, the physician may suggest sterilization of tap water before reconstitution, such as in the case of well water. Because salts are added to chemically softened water, it should not be used to reconstitute infant formula. Commercially prepared sterile water is not necessary for formula preparation at home. Most city water supplies are fluoridated; however, sterile water and well water are not, and supplementation may be required in infants who have formulas prepared from these sources.

Formula preparation should take place in a clean area, using clean utensils. The individual preparing the formula should have clean hands and use good technique to avoid contaminating the formula during reconstitution. Immediately after reconstitution of concentrated formula or opening a ready-to-feed multiple-use container, the portion required for an individual feeding should be put in an appropriate bottle for feeding and the remainder stored in a clean container in the refrigerator. After the infant has begun feeding, any formula left in the bottle after 2 hours should be discarded. Reconstituted formula can be stored in the refrigerator for up to 24 hours.

Smaller infants should be fed formula that is not cooler than room temperature, and they may prefer warmed formula. Older infants do not require warmed formula but may prefer it. The bottle with the required amount of formula for a single feeding can be warmed with warm, running tap water. If a bottle warmer is used, electric warmers are preferred over water-containing warmers because of the potential for bacterial contamination of the water contained in the warmer. Microwaves should never be used to warm infant formula because hot spots can develop throughout the formula and may burn the infant. In addition, the excessive heat can physically alter the formula and degrade nutrients.

Concentrated liquids and dry powder formulas can be reconstituted to provide increased amounts of all substrates included in the formula. Standard reconstitution provides 20 kcal per ounce; however, some infants require more concentrated formula because of fluid considerations. These products are often mixed with less water so that they contain 24, 27, or 30 kcal per ounce. When formulas are concentrated in this manner, the protein, electrolyte, and mineral concentrations are also increased and should be considered. Instead of concentrating formulas, other additives such as carbohydrate (e.g., polycose) or fat (e.g., MCTs) can be admixed to enhance calorie content. The manufacturers recommend that medications not be added to infant formula because of potential drug–nutrient interactions.

After the initial opening, formula powder can be covered and stored in a cool, dry place for up to 4 weeks in the original container. Refrigeration is not necessary.

However, opened liquid formula (ready-to-feed or concentrate) should be stored in the original container in the refrigerator and may be used for up to 48 hours after opening. Reconstituted formula no longer in the original container should be discarded if not used within 24 hours.

Oral electrolyte solutions, Pedialyte, Resol, and Ricelyte, are available for maintenance of fluid and electrolyte balance during mild-to-moderate diarrhea (Table 89.18). Rehydralyte contains more sodium and is better suited for use in infants with moderate-to-severe diarrhea than products containing less sodium. The World Health Organization (WHO) developed a rehydration solution formula that contains 3.5 g sodium chloride, 2.5 g sodium bicarbonate, 1.5 g potassium chloride, and 20 g glucose with distilled water added to make one liter of solution. The sodium concentration in the WHO solution is about 90 meq/L. Other liquids such as Gatorade contain less sodium and are less suitable for fluid replacement in diarrhea.

Administration

The significance of the gastrointestinal tract in immune function has been recognized, and early enteral feedings are encouraged whenever possible, even in critically ill patients. Feeding tubes are placed soon after injury in patients with burns or after trauma, and as with premature infants, low volume continuous enteral feedings are started and advanced as tolerated. In many of these patients, parenteral nutrition can be avoided entirely. In those who cannot tolerate formula advancement, low-volume continuous trophic feeds should be continued if possible.

Maturation of the gastrointestinal tract is directly related to postconceptional age, and premature neonates may not be able to be fed enterally immediately after birth. In addition, the suck-and-swallow reflex is developed at 34 to 36 weeks gestation; therefore, even with functional maturity of the gastrointestinal tract, these neonates may not be able to be orally fed. In these cases, a combination of parenteral and enteral feeding is used during the transition to full enteral, ideally oral, feedings. To begin the transition to enteral feedings, a low volume of premature formula (or human milk that is provided in most cases by the infant's mother) is infused continuously through an orogastric or nasogastric tube. Volumes are advanced very gradually if the infant tolerates the formula. Regularly during this process, gastric residuals are aspirated through the tube and the volumes measured to be sure the formula is progressing through the gastrointestinal tract. Abdominal distension and vomiting are indicative of too rapid an advancement in feedings or either outlet or intestinal obstruction. Stool consistency, volume, and frequency are monitored. During this rather slow process, parenteral nutrition is used as the primary source of substrate, but the infant is encouraged to suck a pacifier. As feedings progress, the parenteral nutrition solution is decreased, and the infant may be offered a small volume of formula (or human milk) by bottle. Infants should be weighed daily, and adequate calorie intake, considering both parenteral and enteral calories, should be maintained. Preterm neonates who develop abdominal distension and, on abdominal radiograph, have evidence of intraluminal gas (pneumotosis intestinalis) should have enteral feedings discontinued until they are evaluated for necrotizing enterocolitis. Initial therapy for this disease includes maintaining the patient NPO, parenteral nutrition, and antibiotic therapy. Surgery is required for perforation.

Feeding routes in sick neonates, infants, and children are similar to those for adults and include orogastric, nasogastric, gastrostomy, and transpyloric jejunal feeding routes. The type of illness and length of time the patient has remained NPO should be considered when reinstituting enteral feedings. Continuous low-volume feedings are often used initially; however, patients who are being fed into the stomach can be bolused with an appropriate formula and volume for age. When choosing the formula to be delivered, the feeding route should be considered.

Potential problems associated with enteral feedings include aspiration, formula intolerance, and malposition of the tube. Aspiration is a greater risk in patients with gastroesophageal reflux or intractable vomiting. Reflux precautions, including elevating the head of the bed and using low volume, more frequent or continuous feedings, are helpful. Medications that promote gastrointestinal motility, including prokinetic agents, metoclopramide, bethanechol, and cisapride, may be beneficial. The primary

Table 89.18.
Infant Electrolyte Solutions (per liter)

	kcal	Na$^+$ meq	K$^+$ meq	Cl$^-$ meq	Citrate meq	mosm
Rehydralyte	100	75	20	65	30	305
Pedialyte	100	45	20	35	30	250
Resola[a]	80	50	20	50	34	269
Ricelyte	126	50	25	45	34	
Infalyte	77	50	20	40	30	251
WHO solution	80	90	30	80	30	330

[a]Each liter contains Ca^{2+} 4 mEq, phosphate 5 mM, and Mg^{2+} 4 mEq.

manifestation of formula intolerance is diarrhea. Changing to a more elemental formula, fiber-containing formula (e.g., Pediasure with fiber), or short-term therapy with an antiperistaltic agent such as loperamide may be indicated. Patients who develop abdominal distention may have an ileus, and enteral feedings may be contraindicated. Intestinal perforation may occur with long-term therapy or by malposition of the feeding tube.

Gastrostomy-tube placement is indicated in patients with upper gastrointestinal tract anomalies (cleft palate, esophageal atresia), esophageal injury, or tracheoesophageal fistula. These tubes can be placed percutaneously in older infants and children. Button-type gastrostomy tubes are available and are aesthetically more pleasing than the standard gastrostomy feeding tubes. Infants and children requiring prolonged tube feeding, such as patients with long-term coma or severe cardiac, neurologic, or respiratory disease, should be considered for gastrostomy-tube placement. This route of administration facilitates intermittent bolus feeding.

Transpyloric jejunal feeding tubes may be used in infants and children with gastrointestinal anomalies or delayed gastric motility or after upper gastrointestinal surgery. The use of jejunostomy feeding tubes is increasing in children with the improved pediatric jejunal feeding tubes and refinement of surgical placement techniques. With jejunal feedings, continuous feedings are preferred since the small bowel cannot accommodate large volumes of fluid. Complications with jejunal feeding include malabsorption and bowel perforation (151). In addition, the formula used in patients fed via jejunostomy may need to consist of less complex substrate depending on the location of the feeding tube.

CONCLUSION

In this chapter, the reader has been apprised of the uniqueness of pediatric nutritional needs and the limitations of assessment techniques used in children. Children are not small adults, and therefore, should not be treated as such. Children (particularly neonates and infants) require quantitatively and qualitatively different nutrients than adults. Failure to address these unique substrate requirements can result in abnormal physical and neurologic growth and development. However, with an understanding of the unique needs of children, the appropriate nutrients can be provided, and normal growth can be achieved and developmental milestones can be met.

REFERENCES

1. Costa G. Determination of nutritional needs. Cancer Res 37:2419–2424, 1977.
2. Merritt RJ, Blackburn GL. Nutritional assessment and metabolic response to illness of the hospitalized child. In Susking RM (ed): Textbook of pediatric nutrition. New York, Raven Press, 1981, p 285.
3. Grant JP, Custer PG, Thurlow J. Current techniques of nutritional assessment. Surg Clin North Am 61:437–463, 1981.
4. Morriss FH. Trace minerals. Semin Perinatol 3:369–379, 1979.
5. Kerner JA, Sunshine P. Parenteral alimentation. Semin Perinatol 3:417–434, 1979.
6. Hamill PVV, Drizd TA, Johnson CL, et al. Physical growth: National Center for Health Statistics percentiles. Am J Clin Nutr 32:607–629, 1979.
7. Waterlow JC. Some aspects of childhood malnutrition as a public health problem. Br Med J 4:88–90, 1974.
8. Helms RA, Miller JL, Burckart FJ, et al. Clinical outcome as assessed by anthropometric parameters, albumin and cellular immune function in high-risk infants receiving total parenteral nutrition. J Pediatr Surg 18:564–569, 1983.
9. Gurney JM, Jelliffe DB. Arm anthropometry in nutritional assessment: nomogram for rapid calculation of muscle circumference and cross-sectional muscle and fat areas. Am J Clin Nutr 26:912–915, 1973.
10. Frisancho AR. Triceps skin fold and upper arm muscle size norms for assessment of nutritional status. Am J Clin Nutr 27:1052–1058, 1974.
11. Tanner JM, Whitehouse RH. Revised standards for triceps and subscapular skinfolds in British children. Arch Dis Child 50:142–145, 1975.
12. Ingenbleek Y, van den Schrieck H, de Nayer P, et al. Albumin, transferrin, and the thyroxine-binding prealbumin/retinol binding protein (TBPA-RBP) complex in assessment of malnutrition. Clin Chim Acta 63:61–67, 1975.
13. Rothschild MA, Oratz M, Schreiber SS. Albumin synthesis. N Engl J Med 286:748–757, 1972.
14. Awai M, Brown EB. Studies of the metabolism of I^{131}-labeled human transferrin. J Lab Clin Med 61:363–396, 1963.
15. Oppenheimer JH, Surks MI, Bernstein G, et al. Metabolism of I-131 labeled thyroxine binding prealbumin in man. Science 149:748–751, 1965.
16. Peterson PA. Demonstration in serum of two physiological forms of the human retinol-binding protein. Eur J Clin Invest 1:437–444, 1971.
17. Giacoia GP, Watson S, West K. Rapid turnover transport proteins, plasma albumin, and growth in low birth weight infants. JPEN J Parenter Enteral Nutr 8:367–370, 1984.
18. Moskowitz SR, Pereira G, Spitzer A. et al. Prealbumin as a biochemical marker of nutritional adequacy in premature infants. Pediatr 102:749–753, 1983.
19. Helms RA, Dickerson RN, Ebbert ML, et al. Retinol-binding protein and prealbumin: useful measures of protein repletion in critically ill, malnourished infants. J Pediatr Gastroenterol Nutr 5:586–592, 1986.
20. Heird WC, Winters RW. Total parenteral nutrition. J Pediatr 86:2–16, 1975.
21. Lopez AM, Wolfsdorf J, Razynski A, et al. Estimation of nitrogen balance based on a six-hour urine collection in infants. JPEN J Parenter Enteral Nutr 10:517–518, 1986.
22. Boehm KA, Helms RA, Storm MC. Assessing the validity of adjusted urinary urea nitrogen as an estimate of total urinary nitrogen in three pediatric populations. JPEN J Parenter Enteral Nutr 18:172–176, 1994.
23. Seashore JH, Huszar GB, Davis EM. Urinary 3-methylhistidine excretion and nitrogen balance in healthy and stressed premature infants. J Pediatr Surg 15:400–404, 1980.
24. Forbes GB, Bruining GJ. Urinary creatinine excretion and lean body mass. Am J Clin Nutr 29:1359–1366, 1976.
25. Lawton AR, Cooper MD. Ontogeny of immunity. In Stiehm ER, Bulginiti VA (eds): Immunologic Disorders in Infants and Children. Philadelphia, WB Sauders, 1980, p 36.

26. Shannon DC, Johnson G, Rosen FS, et al. Cellular reactivity to Candida albicans antigen. N Engl J Med 275:690–693, 1966.

27. Helms RA, Herrod HG, Burckart GJ, et al. E-Rosette formation, total T-cells and lymphocyte transformation in infants receiving intravenous safflower oil emulsion. JPEN J Parenter Enteral Nutr 7:541–545, 1983.

28. Costarino A, Baumgart S. Modern fluid and electrolyte management of the critically ill premature infant. Pediatr Clin North Am 33:153–178, 1986.

29. Heely AM, Talbot NB. Insensible water losses per day by hospitalized infants and children. Am J Dis Child 90:251–256, 1955.

30. Levine SZ, Wheatlye MA. Respiratory metabolism in infancy and in childhood: daily heat production in infants, predictions based on insensible loss of weight compared with direct measurements. Am J Dis Child 51:1300–1323, 1936.

31. Holliday MA, Segar WE. The maintenance need for water in parenteral fluid therapy. Pediatrics 19:823–832, 1957.

32. Bell EF, Oh W. Fluid and electrolyte balance in very low birth weight infants. Clin Perinatol 6:139–150, 1979.

33. Perkin RM, Levin DL. Common fluid and electrolyte problems in the pediatric intensive care unit. Pediatr Clin North Am 27:567–586, 1980.

34. Friis-Hansen B. Body water compartments in children: changes during growth and related changes in body composition. Pediatrics 28:169–181, 1961.

35. Kagan BM, Staninvoca V, Felix NS, et al. Body composition of premature infants: relation to nutrition. Am J Clin Nutr 25:1153–1164, 1972.

36. Stuart HC, Sobel EH. The thickness of the skin and subcutaneous tissue by age and sex in childhood. J Pediatr 28:637–647, 1946.

37. Williams PR, Oh W. Effects of radiant warmer on insensible water loss in newborn infants. Am J Dis Child 128:511–514, 1974.

38. Jones RWA, Rochefort MJ, Baum JD. Increased insensible water loss in newborn infants nursed under radiant heaters. Br Med J 2:1347–1350, 1976.

39. McCance RA, Maylor NJB, Widdowson EM. The response of infants to a large dose of water. Arch Dis Child 29:104–109, 1954.

40. Leake RD, Zakuddin S, Trygstad CW, et al. The effects of large volume intravenous fluid infusion on neonatal renal function. J Pediatr 89:968–972, 1976.

41. Arant BS Jr. Developmental patterns of renal functional maturation compared in the human neonate. J Pediatr 92:705–712, 1978.

42. Van Marter LJ, Leviton A, Allred EN, et al. Hydration during the first days of life and the risk of bronchopulmonary dysplasia in low birth weight infants. J Pediatr 116:942–949, 1990.

43. Goldman HI. Feeding and necrotizing enterocolitis. Am J Dis Child 134:553–555, 1980.

44. Goldberg RN, Chung D, Goldman SL, et al. The association of rapid volume expansion and intraventricular hemorrhage in the preterm infant. J Pediatr 96:1060–1063, 1980.

45. Bell EF, Warburton D, Stonestreet BS, et al. Effect of fluid administration on the development of symptomatic patent ductus arteriosus and congestive heart failure in premature infants. N Engl J Med 302:598–604, 1980.

46. Phelps SJ, Helms RA. Risk factors affecting infiltration of peripheral venous lines in infants. J Pediatr 111:384–389, 1987.

47. Oellrich RG, Murphy MR, Goldberg LA, et al. The percutaneous central venous catheter for small or ill infants. Maternal Child Nursing 16:92–96, 1991.

48. Wurzel CL, Halom K, Feldman JG, et al. Infection rates of Brovac-Hickman Catheters and implantable venous devices. Am J Dis Child 142:536–540, 1988.

49. Mirro J, Rao B, Kuman M, et al. A comparison of placement techniques and complications of externalized catheters and implantable port use in children with cancer. J Pediatr Surg 25:120–124, 1990.

50. Rollins CJ, Elsberry VA, Pollack KA, et al. Three-in-one parenteral nutrition: a safe and economical method of nutritional support for infants. JPEN J Parenter Enteral Nutr 14:290–294, 1990.

51. Stegink LD, Baker GL. Infusion of protein hydrolysates in the newborn infant: plasma amino acid concentrations. J Pediatr 78:595–602, 1971.

52. Anderson TL, Muttart CR, Bilber MA, et al. A controlled trial of glucose versus glucose and amino acids in premature infants. J Pediatr 94:947–951, 1979.

53. Helms RA, Christensen ML, Mauer EC, Storm MC. Comparison of pediatric versus standard amino acid formulation in preterm neonates requiring parenteral nutriton. J Pediatr 110:466–470, 1987.

54. Adamkin DH, McClead RE, Desai NS, et al. Comparison of two neonatal intravenous amino acid formulation in preterm infants: a multicenter study. J Perinatol 11:375–382, 1991.

55. Heird WC, May W, Helms RA, et al. Pediatric parenteral amino acid mixture in low birth weight infants. Pediatrics 81:41–50, 1988.

56. Heird WC, Dell RB, Helms RA, et al. Amino acid mixture designed to maintain normal plasma amino acid patterns in infants and children requiring parenteral nutrition. Pediatrics 80:401–408, 1987.

57. Polberger SKT, Axelsson IE, Raiha NCR. Amino acid concentrations in plasma and urine in very low birth weight infants fed protein-unenriched or human milk protein-enriched human milk. Pediatrics 86:909–915, 1990.

58. Duffy B, Gunn T, Collinge J, et al. The effect of varying protein quality and energy intake on the nitrogen metabolism of parenterally fed very low birthweight (<1600 g) infants. Pediatr Res 15:1040–1044, 1981.

59. Chessman K, Johnson M, Fernandes E, Helms R. Changing parenteral substrate requirements in neonates receiving a pediatric amino acid formulation. JPEN J Parenter Enteral Nutr 12:105, 1988. (abstract)

60. Beck R. Use of a pediatric parenteral amino acid mixture in a population of extremely low birth weight neonates: Frequency and spectrum of direct bilirubinemia. Am J Perinatol 7:84–86, 1990.

61. Reichman BL, Chessex P, Putet G, et al. Partition of energy metabolism and energy cost of growth in the very low-birth-weight infant. Pediatrics 69:446–451, 1982.

62. Kerner JA Jr. Caloric requirement. In Kerner JA Jr (ed): Manual of Pediatric Parenteral Nutrition. New York, John Wiley & Sons, 1983, p 63.

63. Zlotkin SH, Bryan MH, Anderson GH. Intravenous nitrogen and energy intakes required to duplicate in utero nitrogen accretion in prematurely born human infants. J Pediatr 99:115–120, 1981.

64. Thomas DB. Hyperosmolality and intraventricular haemorrhage in premature babies. Acta Paediatr Scand 65:429–432, 1976.

65. Collins JW Jr, Hoppe M, Brown K, et al. A controlled trial of insulin infusion and parenteral nutrition in extremely low birth weight infants with glucose intolerance. J Pediatr 118:921–927, 1991.

66. Press M, Kikuchi H, Shimoyana J, et al. Diagnosis and treatment of essential fatty acid deficiency in man. Br Med J 2:247–250, 1974.

67. Pelham LD. Rational use of intravenous fat emulsions. Am J Hosp Pharm 38:198–208, 1981.

68. Bivins BA, Bell RM, Rapp RP, et al. Linoleic acid versus linolenic acid: what is essential. JPEN J Parenter Enteral Nutr 7:473–478, 1983.

69. Committee on Nutrition, American Academy of Pediatrics. Commentary on parenteral nutrition. Pediatrics 71:547–552, 1983.

70. Schiff D, Chan G, Seccombe D, et al. Plasma carnitine levels during intravenous feeding of the neonate. J Pediatr 95:1043–1046, 1979.

71. Helms RA, Whitington PF, Mauer EC, et al. Enhanced lipid utilization in infants receiving oral L-carnitine during long-term parenteral nutrition. J Pediatr 109:984–988, 1986.

72. Andrew G, Chan G, Schiff D. Lipid metabolism in the neonate: II. The effect of Intralipid on bilirubin binding in vitro and in vivo. J Pediatr 88:279–284, 1976.

73. Burckart GJ, Whitington RF, Helms RA. The effect of two intravenous fat emulsions and their components on bilirubin to albumin. Am J Clin Nutr 36:521–526, 1982.

74. Nordenstrom J, Jarstrand C, Wienick A. Decreased chemotactic and random migration of leukocytes during Intralipid infusion. Am J Clin Nutr 32:2416–2422, 1979.

75. Tovan JA, Mahour GH, Miller SW, et al. Endotoxin clearances after Intralipid infusion. J Pediatr Surg 11:23, 1976.

76. Jarstrand C, Berghem L, Lahnborg G. Human granulocyte and reticuloendothelial system function during Intralipid infusion. JPEN J Parenter Enteral Nutr 2:663–670, 1978.

77. Ladisch S, Poplark DG, Blaese RM. Inhibition of human lympho-proliferation by intravenous lipid emulsion. Clin Immunol Immuno-pathol 25:196–202, 1982.

78. Palmbald J, Brostrom O, Lahnborg G, et al. Neutrophil functions during total parenteral nutrition and Intralipid infusion. Am J Clin Nutr 35:1430–1436, 1982.

79. Strunk RC, Murrow BW, Thilo E, et al. Normal macrophage function in infants receiving Intralipid by low-dose intermittent administration. J Pediatr 106:640–645, 1985.

80. Escudier EF, Escudier BJ, Henry-Amar MC, et al. Effects of infused Intralipids on neutrophil chemotaxis during total parenteral nutri-tion. JPEN J Parenter Enteral Nutr 10:596–598, 1986.

81. Schroder H, Paust H, Schmidt R. Pulmonary fat embolism after Intralipid therapy-a postmortem artefact? Acta Paediatr Scand 73:461–464, 1984.

82. Pereira GR, Fox WW, Stanley CA, et al. Decreased oxygenation and hyperlipemia during intravenous fat infusions in premature infants. Pediatrics 66:26–30, 1980.

83. Brans YW, Dutton EB, Andrew DS, et al. Fat emulsion tolerance in very low birth weight neonates: effect on diffusion of oxygen in the lungs and on blood pH. Pediatrics 78:79–84, 1986.

84. Haumont D, Deckelbaum RJ, Richelle M, et al. Plasma lipid concentrations in low birth weight infants given parenteral nutrition with twenty or ten percent lipid emulsion. J Pediatr 115:787–793, 1989.

85. Arnold WC. Parenteral nutrition, and fluid and electrolyte therapy. Pediatr Clin North Am 37:449–461, 1990.

86. Lorch V, Lay SA. Parenteral alimentation in the neonate. Pediatr Clin North Am 24:547–556, 1977.

87. Greene HL, Hambidge KM, Schanler R, et al. Guidelines for the use of vitamins, trace elements, calcium, magnesium, and phos-phorus in infants and children receiving total parenteral nutrition: report of the Subcommittee on Pediatr Parenteral Nutrient Requirements from the Committee on Clinical Practice Issues of The American Society for Clinical Nutrition. Am J Clin Nutr 48:1324–1342, 1988.

88. Fleming CR. Trace element metabolism in adult patients requiring total parenteral nutrition. Am J Clin Nutr 49:573–579, 1989.

89. Sulyok E, Varga F, Gyory E, et al. Postnatal development of renal sodium handling in premature infants. J Pediatr 95:787–792, 1979.

90. Stapleton FB, Nelson B, Vats TS, et al. Hypokalemia associated with antibiotic treatment. Am J Dis Child 130:1104–1108, 1976.

91. Schaber DE, Uden DL, Stone FM, et al. Intravenous KCl supplementation in pediatric cardiac surgical patients. Pediatr Cardiol 6:25–28, 1985.

92. Pelegano JF, Rowe JC, Carey DE, et al. Simultaneous infusion of calcium and phosphorus in parenteral nutrition for premature infants: use of physiologic calcium/phosphorus ratio: J Pediatr 114:115–119, 1989.

93. Koo WWK. Parenteral nutrition related bone disease. JPEN J Parenter Enteral Nutr 16:386–394, 1992.

94. Vileisis RA. Furosemide effect on mineral status of parenterally nourished premature neonates with chronic lung disease. Pediatrics 85:316–322, 1990.

95. Eggert LD, Rusho WJ, MacKay MW, et al. Calcium and phophorus compatibility in parenteral nutrition solutions for neonates. Am J Hosp Pharm 39:49–53, 1982.

96. Lenz GT, Mikrut BA. Calcium and phosphate solubility in neonatal parenteral nutrient solutions containing Aminosyn-PF or TrophA-mine. Am J Hosp Pharm 45:2367–2371, 1988.

97. Schmidt GL, Baumgartner TG, Fischlschweiger W, et al. Cost containment using cysteine HCl acidification to increase calcium/phosphate solubility in hyperalimentation solutions. JPEN J Parenter Enteral Nutr 10:203–207, 1986.

98. Henry RS, Jurgens RW Jr, Sturgeon R, et al. Compatibility of calcium chloride and calcium gluconate with sodium phosphate in a mixed TPN solution. Am J Hosp Pharm 37:673–674, 1980.

99. Niemiec PW Jr, Vanderveen TW. Compatiblity considerations in parenteral nutrient solutions. Am J Hosp Pharm 41:893–911, 1984.

100. Solomon SM, Kirby DF. The refeeding syndrome: a review. JPEN J Parenter Enteral Nutr 14:90–97, 1990.

101. Schrier RQ. Renal and Electrolyte Disorders. Boston: Little, Brown & Co, 1992, ch 6.

102. Tsang RC. Neonatal magnesium disturbances. Am J Dis Child 124:282–293, 1972.

103. Whang R, Aikawa JK. Magnesium deficiency and refractoriness to potassium repletion. J Chron Dis 30:65–68, 1977.

104. Moukarzel AA, Song MK, Buchman AL, Vargas J, Guss W, McDiarmid S, et al. Excessive chromium intake in children receiving total parenteral nutrition. Lancet 339:385–388, 1992.

105. Mouser J, Cochran EB, Helms RA, et al. Chromium concentrations in children on home TPN and the relationship to intake. JPEN J Parenter Enteral Nutr 18(suppl):33S, 1994.

106. Eichelberger MR, Rous PG, Hoelzer D, et al. Percutaneous subclavian venous catheters in neonates and children. J Pediatr Surg 16:547–552, 1981.

107. Ruggiero RP, Caruso G. Chylothorax—a complication of subclavian vein catheterization. JPEN J Parenter Enteral Nutr 9:750–753, 1985.

108. Gutcher G, Cutz E. Complications of parenteral nutrition. Semin Perinatol 10:196–207, 1986.

109. Welch GW, McKell DW, Silverstein P, et al. The role of catheter composition in the development of thrombophlebitis. Surg Gynecol Obstet 138:421–424, 1974.

110. Hoshal VL, Ause RG, Hoskins PA. Fibrin sleeve formation on indwelling subclavian central venous catheters. Arch Surg 102:353–358, 1971.

111. Breaux CW Jr, Duke D, Georgeson KE, et al. Calcium phosphate crystal occlusion of central venous catheters used for total parenteral nutrition in infants and children: prevention and treatment. J Pediatr Surg 22:829–832, 1987.

112. Duffy LF, Kerzner B, Gebus V, et al. Treatment of central venous catheter occlusions with hydrochloric acid. J Pediatr 114:102–104, 1989.

113. Pennington CR, Pithie AD. Ethanol lock in the management of catheter occlusion. JPEN J Parenteral Enteral Nutr 11:507–508, 1987.

114. Holcombe BJ, Forloines-Lynn S, Garmhausen LW. Restoring patency of long-term central venous access devices. J Intravenous Nursing 15:36–41, 1992.

115. Brown AS, Hoelzer DJ, Piercy SA. Skin necrosis from extravasation of intravenous fluids in children. Plastic Reconstruct Surg 64:145–150, 1979.

116. Alpan G, Eyal F, Springer C, et al. Heparinization of alimentation solutions administered through peripheral veins in premature infants: a controlled study. Pediatrics 74:375–378, 1984.

117. Phelps SJ, Cochran EB. Effect of the continuous administration of fat emulsion on the infiltration of intravenous lines in infants receiving peripheral parenteral nutrition solutions. JPEN J Parenter Enteral Nutr 13:628–632, 1989.

118. Baker SS, Dwyer E, Queen P. Metabolic derangements in children requiring parenteral nutrition. JPEN J Parenter Enteral Nutr 10:279–281, 1986.

119. Black DD, Suttle EA, Whitington PF, et al. The effect of short-term total parenteral nutrition on hepatic function in the human neonate: a prospective randomized study demonstrating alteration of the hepatic canalicular function. J Pediatr 99:445–449, 1981.

120. Farrell MK, Balistren WF, Sucky FY. Serum-sulfated lithocholate as an indicator of cholestasis during parenteral nutrition in infants and children. JPEN J Parenter Enteral Nutr 6:30–33, 1982.

121. Whitington PF. Cholestasis associated with total parenteral nutrition in infants. Hepatology 5:693–696, 1985.

122. Beale EF, Nelson RM, Bucciarelli RL, et al. Intrahepatic cholestasis associated with parenteral nutrition in premature infants. Pediatrics 64:342–347, 1979.

123. Gleghorn EE, Merritt RJ, Subramanian N, et al. Phenobarbital does not prevent total parenteral-associated cholestasis in noninfected infants. JPEN J Parenter Enteral Nutr 10:282–283, 1986.

124. Doty JE, Pitt HA, Porter-Fink V, et al. Cholecystokinin prophylaxis of parenteral nutrition-induced gallbladder disease. Ann Surg 201:76–80, 1985.

125. Koo WWK, Kaplan LA, Horn J, et al. Aluminum in parenteral nutrition solution—sources and possible alternatives. JPEN J Parenter Enteral Nutr 10:591–595, 1986.

126. Klein GL, Alfey AC, Shike N, et al. Parenteral drug products containing aluminum as an ingredient or a contaminment; response to FDA notice of intent. Am J Clin Nutr 53:399–402, 1991.

127. Lyon AJ, Hawkes DJ, Doran M, et al. Bone mineralization in preterm infants measured by dual energy radiographic densitometry. Arch Dis Child 64:919–923, 1989.

128. Pomeranz S, Gimmon Z, Zvi AB, et al. Parenteral-nutrition-induced anaphylaxis. JPEN J Parenter Enteral Nutr 11:314–315, 1987.

129. Bullock L, Etchason E, Fitzgerald JF, et al. Case report of an allergic reaction to parenteral nutrition in a pediatric patient. JPEN J Parenter Enteral Nutr 14:98–100, 1990.

130. Kamath KR, Berry A, Commins G. Acute hypersensitivity reaction to Intralipid. N Engl J Med 304:360, 1981.

131. Hiyama DT, Griggs B, Mittman RF, et al. Hypersensitivity following lipid emulsion infusion in an adult patient. JPEN J Parenter Enteral Nutr 13:318–320, 1989.

132. Sternberg A, Gruenevald T, Duetsch AA, et al. Intralipid-induced transient sinus bradycardia. N Engl J Med 304:422–423, 1981.

133. Connon JJ. Diarrhea possibly caused by total parenteral nutrition. N Engl J Med 301:273–274, 1979.

134. Campbell AN, Freedman MH, Pendarz PI, et al. Bleeding disorder from the "fat overload" syndrome. JPEN J Parenter Enteral Nutr 8:447–449, 1984.

135. Bhat AM Scanlon JW. The pattern of eosinophilia in premature infants. J Pediatr 98:612–616, 1981.

136. Rotruck JT, Pope AL, Banther HE, et al. Selenium: biochemical role as a component of gluthathione perioxdase. Science 179:588–590, 1973.

137. Marks LM, Patel N, Kurtides ES. Hematologic abnormalities associated with intravenous lipid therapy. Am J Gastroenterol 73:490–495, 1980.

138. McGrath KM, Zalcberg JR, Slonim J. Intralipid induced haemolysis. Br J Haematol 50:376–378, 1982.

139. Golden MHN, Harland PAEG, Golden BE, et al. Zinc and immunocompetence in protein-energy malnutrition. Lancet 1:1226–1227, 1978.

140. Hodges RE, Bean WB, Ohlson MA, et al. Factors affecting human antibody response V. Combined deficiencies of pantothenic acid and pyridoxine. Am J Clin Nutr 11:187–199, 1962.

141. Axelrod AE. Immune process in vitamin deficiency states. Am J Clin Nutr 24:265–271, 1971.

142. Kinsella JE, Lokesh B, Broughton S, et al. Dietary polyunsaturated fatty acids and eicosanoids: potential effects on the modulation of inflammatory and immune cells: an overview. Nutrition 6:24–44, 1990.

143. Meydani SN, Yogeeswaran G, Liu S, et al. Fish oil and tocopherol-induced changes in natural killer cell-mediated cytotoxicity and PGE_2 synthesis in young and old mice. J Nutr 118:1245–1252, 1988.

144. Barbul A, Sisto DA, Waserkurg HL, et al. Arginine stimulates lymphocyte immune response in healthy human beings. Surgery 90:244–251, 1981.

145. Burke DJ, Alverdy JC, Aoys E, et al. Glutamine-supplemented total parenteral nutrition improves gut immune function. Arch Surg 124:1396–1399, 1989.

146. Buchman AL, Moukarzel A, Goodson B, et al. Catheter-related infections associated with home parenteral nutrition and predictive factors for the need for catheter removal in their treatment. JPEN J Parenter Enteral Nutr 18:297–302, 1994.

147. Vargas JH, Ament ME, Berquist WE. Long-term home parenteral nutrition in pediatrics. Ten years of experience in 102 patients. J Pediatr Gastroenterol Nutr 6:24–37, 1987.

148. Flynn PM, Shenep JL, Stokes DC, et al. In situ management of confirmed central venous catheter-related bacteremia. Pediatr Infect Dis J 6:729–734, 1987.

149. Hartman GE, Shochat SJ. Management of septic complications associated with Silastic catheters in malignancy. Pediatr Infect Dis J 6:1042–1047, 1987.

150. National Research Council. Recommended Dietary Allowances, et. 10. Washington DC: National Academy Press, 1989, ch 3–9.

151. Rombeau JL, Caldwell MD. Clinical Nutrition—Enteral and Tube Feeding, Philadelphia: WB Saunders, 1990, ch 18.

152. American Academy of Pediatrics, Committee on Nutrition. Nutritional needs of low-birth-weight infants. Pediatrics 75:976–986, 1985.

CHAPTER 90

GYNECOLOGIC DISORDERS

RONALD J. RUGGIERO

Disorders of the female reproductive tract result in many gynecologic complaints and problems. In addition to the need for contraceptive measures, discussed in Chapter 91, dysmenorrhea, the premenstrual syndrome, endometriosis, vaginitis, venereal warts, and estrogen replacement therapy for hot flushes, atrophic vaginitis, and the prevention of estrogen deficiency-induced osteoporosis require rational drug management.

Teratogenicity should be considered when treating a woman with childbearing potential, and women who are taking potentially teratogenic drugs must use an effective method of contraception.

DYSMENORRHEA

It is estimated that 30 to 50% of the 35 million women of childbearing age in the United States are affected by painful menstrual periods or dysmenorrhea, and 10 to 15% of those women are incapacitated for 1 to 3 days each month. Dysmenorrhea is the greatest single cause of absenteeism from school and work among young women (1). The cost for the estimated 600 million work hours lost annually in the United States is approximately $2 billion (2).

Primary dysmenorrhea occurs during ovulatory cycles and, unlike secondary dysmenorrhea, has no detectable pelvic pathology, such as adhesions on the reproductive organs.

The chief symptom that most women experience is spasmodic pain of the lower abdomen that may radiate to the back and along the thighs. The pain is accompanied by one or more of the following systemic symptoms in more than 50% of the patients: nausea and vomiting (89%), fatigue (85%), diarrhea (60%), lower backache (60%), and headache (45%). The duration is usually 48 to 72 hours, with the pain starting a few hours prior to or just after the onset of menstrual flow (3).

The etiology of these symptoms has been determined to be related to the pharmacologic actions of prostaglandin E2 (PGE2) and prostaglandin F2alpha (PGF2alpha), which are formed from the phospholipids of dead cell membranes in the menstruating uterus. PGE2 causes disaggregation of platelets and is a vasodilator, whereas PGF2alpha mediates or potentiates pain sensations and stimulates smooth muscle contraction (1). Additionally,

estrogens can stimulate synthesis and/or release of PGF2-alpha and vasopressin (VP) that cause uterine hyperactivity, and for this reason, progestin-dominant combination oral contraceptives are often used to alleviate dysmenorrhea (4).

The goal of therapy for primary dysmenorrhea is to avoid the lower abdominal spasmodic pains and other prostaglandin-induced effects. Monitoring of the efficacy of such therapy depends solely by the subjective responses of the patient.

Table 90.1 lists drug therapy regimens currently used for primary dysmenorrhea, including nonsteroidal antiinflammatory drugs (NSAIDs) and combination oral contraceptives (COCs).

Clinically, there is no way to predict whether a certain NSAID will give maximal benefit to any given patient based on current data in the literature. Few direct comparisons of one NSAID to another have been done. Even though most studies show superiority of the active drug over placebo, no single NSAID has been found to be superior though some studies give mefenamic acid a slight edge. The initial selection should be tried for at least two to four cycles. If therapy is unsuccessful, some patients may still respond to another NSAID class, and NSAIDs are successful in 77 to 80% of dysmenorrhea patients. Ibuprofen, naproxen, or naproxen sodium are the usual initial choices, with flurbiprofen and mefenamic acid being reserved for more difficult cases.

Patients should be told that NSAIDs need not be taken until the onset of symptoms since the half-life of prostaglandins is only minutes. With the short-term use of NSAIDs for dysmenorrhea, side effects are infrequent and usually mild. Gastrointestinal irritation is best avoided by taking the NSAIDs with food or milk. Other NSAIDs such as aspirin should be avoided with the use of NSAIDs listed in Table 90.1 since they may greatly enhance their effect and toxicities such as peptic ulceration, liver damage, and renal damage. Patients with allergies to aspirin, especially anaphylactic reactions, should be cautioned never to take NSAIDs in prescription or over-the-counter preparations.

COCs relieve dysmenorrhea in 90% of patients, probably by a reduction in the amount of endometrium formed and consequently the amount of prostaglandins

Table 90.1.
Drug Therapy of Primary Dysmenorrhea

Drug	Usual Dose
NSAIDs	
Acetic acids	
Indomethacin	25 mg PO TID
Tolmetin	400 mg PO TID
Sulindac	200 mg PO q 4–6 h
Fenamates	
Mefenamic acid[a] (CDOC)[b]	500 mg PO stat, then 250 mg q 6 h
Meclofenamate	100 mg PO stat, then 50–100 mg q 6 h
Oxicams	
Piroxicam	20 mg PO daily
Proprionic acids	
Flurbiprofen	50 mg PO QID
Ibuprofen[a] (CDOC)	400 mg PO q 4 h
Naproxen[a] (CDOC)	500 mg PO stat, then 250 mg q 6–8 h
Naproxen sodium[a] (CDOC)	550 mg PO stat, then 275 mg q 6–8 h
Ketoprofen[a] (CDOC)	50 mg PO TID
Salicylic acids	
Diflunisal	1000 mg PO stat, then 500 mg q 12 h
Combination oral contraceptives (28-day cycle pack, progestin dominant)	1 daily
Alpha-adrenergic agonists[c]	
Clonidine	0.1 mg PO TID

[a]FDA approved for primary dysmenorrhea.
[b]Clinical drug of choice: (a) No single NSAID has proven superiority-proprionic acids often used initially; (b) NSAIDs may be ineffective in 20–30% of patients; (c) COCs may be ineffective in 10% of patients.
[c]Only preliminary data available, therefore last therapeutic choice.

formed. Compliance with the COC is essential for maintenance of anovulatory cycles.

Since NSAIDs do not relieve pain in 20 to 30% of patients with dysmenorrhea and COCs do not relieve pain in 10% of patients, another cause of dysmenorrhea has been proposed that includes excessive stimulation of the uterus by the adrenergic nervous system. In a recent report of four patients who failed on either NSAIDs or COCs, the alpha-adrenergic agonist clonidine in a dose of 0.1 mg three times daily worked very well (5). Clonidine may therefore be useful as the last-alternative therapy although large, well-controlled studies are needed to confirm its efficacy in primary dysmenorrhea.

PREMENSTRUAL SYNDROME

It is estimated that 30 to 50% of menstruating women experience symptoms of the premenstrual syndrome (PMS), with 20 to 30% reporting moderate to severe symptoms. Absenteeism due to PMS is costly since 60% of women are in the workforce today.

Unlike primary dysmenorrhea, there is no consensus on the definition of PMS. The most widely accepted definition

Table 90.2.
Symptoms of PMS[a]

Psychological[b]	Somatic[b]
Anxiety	Abdominal bloating
Depression	Edema
Irritability	Weight gain
Wide mood swings	Constipation
Increased appetite	Hot flashes
Aggression	Breast pain
Lethargy or fatigue	Headache
Forgetfullness and reduced concentration	Acne
Sleep disorders	Rhinitis
Phobias	Palpitations

[a]Adapted from Chihal HJ. Premenstrual syndrome: an update for the clinician. Obstet Gynecol North Am 17(2):457–479, 1990.
[b]In approximate order of frequency of occurrence.

states that the following criteria be met to document PMS (6):

1. The signs and/or symptoms must occur cyclically and recur to some degree in the luteal phase (i.e., after ovulation) of the menstrual cycle, and they are usually present to some degree each cycle.
2. During the follicular phase (i.e., prior to ovulation), the patient should be free of symptoms. There must be at least 7 symptom-free days in each cycle. Most patients do not have symptoms for several days after the onset of menses until near ovulation.
3. The combination of distressing physical, psychologic, or behavioral changes are sufficiently severe to result in deterioration of interpersonal relationships and/or interfere with normal activities.

Table 90.2 lists many of the commonly reported chief symptoms of PMS. The etiology of PMS remains as elusive as the definition and the myriad of symptoms attributed to this disorder.

The goal of drug therapy is to alleviate the symptoms of PMS. Monitoring of the efficacy of such therapy depends largely on the subjective responses of the patient and on the observations of persons close to her and the patient's health care providers.

Table 90.3 lists the drug therapy regimens of PMS. The lack of consistent definition and the paucity of carefully designed drug studies of PMS have led to less than satisfactory treatment (7). Complicating the study results is the fact that placebo responses have been as high as 60 to 80% in many studies. No one drug has been shown to be superior or satisfactory for the long-term treatment of PMS. Many early studies available were not very helpful in choosing appropriate therapy. Many case reports and uncontrolled clinical trials describe beneficial effects for the agent being studied. However, the same agent's therapeutic benefit is frequently lacking when a placebo-controlled clinical trial is performed, as is the case with

Table 90.3.
Effectiveness of the Current Drug Therapy of PMS[a,g]

Drug	Average Dose/Regimen	Average Patient Improvement[b] (%)
Spironolactone (CDOC)[c]	25 mg PO QID days 14–28	0–80
Various COCs (28's) (CDOC)	one PO daily days 1–28	0–29
Pyridoxine (CDOC)	50–500 mg PO days 1–28	0–76
Lithium	200 mg PO QID days 1–28	0–60
Mefenamic acid	500 mg PO TID days 14–28	0–92
Oil of evening primrose	3 g PO day 15 to menses	0–60
Progesterone suppositories (8) (CDOC)	200–400 mg PV days 14–28	0–60
Bromocriptine	1.25–2.5 mg PO BID day 14 to menses	0–80
Alprazolam (9)[d]	0.25–5.0 mg PO BID	37–75
Fluoxetine (60)	20 mg PO QID	0–100
Clonidine	17 ug/kg/day PO	100
GnRH agonist Leuprolide acetate (10)[e]	3.75 mg IM q 30 days	0–100[f]

[a]Data from True BL, Goodner SM, Burns EA. Review of the etiology and treatment of premenstrual syndrome. Drug Intell Clin Pharm 19:714–722, 1985; Harrison W, Sharpe L, Edicott J. Treatment of premenstrual symptoms. Gen Hosp Psychiatry 7:54–65, 1985; and Smith S, Shiff I. The premenstrual syndrome—diagnosis and management. Fertil Steril 52(4):527–543, 1989.

[b]Study results vary greatly.

[c]CDOC, clinical drug of choice. In the treatment of PMS, the CDOCs are most often tried although none are satisfactory for long-term improvement of symptoms, and the studies available are not helpful in choosing therapy.

[d]Addictive quality of alprazolam is a main drawback, and many PMS patients have a history of substance dependence, depression, and other psychiatric disorders (9).

[e]Effective for short term. Whether prolonged therapy would be safe and effective, or even necessary, remains to be determined. The only worrisome side effect is a substantial decrease in estradiol that could, with long-term use, lead to osteoporosis. The cost of GnRH agonists such as leuprolide and nafarelin is prohibitive unless they are used as a last resort.

[f]Less effective in moderately depressed and ineffective in severely depressed. Caution—More than 75% get worsening of depression.

[g]Three classes of agents have proven efficacy: benzodiazepines (especially Alprazolam), gonadotropine releasing hormone agonists (especially Leuprolide), and selective serotonin uptake inhibitors (especially fluoxetine) (60).

various forms of progesterone (13). Because of this, most clinicians use stress reduction classes, counseling, and exercise programs with drug therapy.

Patients must understand the empirical nature of the various therapies and realize that some patients have responded very well to any given drug, ancillary treatment, or combination of treatments.

In a recent double-blind, placebo-controlled, 6-month crossover study using the gonadotropin-releasing hormone agonist (GnRHa) leuprolide acetate, 3.75 mg intramuscularly monthly, or saline, both behavioral and physical symptoms of PMS were reduced and the GnRHa was well tolerated. However, those patients with moderate premenstrual depression improved but remained clinically symptomatic, and those with severe premenstrual depression showed no improvement on any efficacy measure. The differential response to leuprolide suggests that it may be of value in diagnosing distinct subtypes of PMS (10). This lends support to the theory that cyclic fluctuations in ovarian steroids are involved in the regulation of neuropeptides, which in turn modulate mood and behavior (11).

Some authors believe that 80% of patients with PMS can be treated with education, stress reduction, and dietary modifications without drugs (12, 13). Some are also studying alprazolam because of its anxiolytic and antidepressant effects during the symptomatic premenstrual days but must worry about its addiction liability. A recent study

employed 300 mg of micronized oral progesterone and 0.25 mg of alprazolam or placebo four times daily from day 18 of the menstrual cycle through day 2 of the next cycle. Oral micronized progesterone therapy was no better than placebo. In contrast, 37% of the alprazolam group experienced a 50% reduction in mental function, pain, and mood (9).

Progesterone, in various forms, has been the most commonly prescribed therapy for PMS for several decades and yet is the most controversial. For example, uncontrolled clinical trials have consistently demonstrated that progesterone suppositories are an effective treatment for PMS, and they are the basis for the widespread use of progesterone therapy in the United States. Unfortunately, progesterone deficiency has never been proved to be a cause for PMS, and most controlled clinical trials have failed to demonstrate the superiority of progesterone therapy to placebo (14). Advocates of progesterone therapy were unwilling to accept unfavorable clinical trial data because of their dilemma of having had very little in the way of alternative agents to offer their PMS patients.

The most recently studied and, often times, most effective class of agents to treat the generalized symptoms of PMS are the selective serotonin reuptake inhibitors (SSRIs). Fluoxetine 20 mg daily has shown remarkable results (15). A recent thorough risk-benefit appraisal of drugs used in the management of PMS indicates that fluox-

Table 90.4.
Danazol Therapy for Endometriosis[a,b]

Dose[c] Mild Symptoms		400 mg PO BID 100–200 mg PO BID Moderate-to-Severe Symptoms	
Side Effect	Percent	Side Effect	Percent
Weight gain	85	Decreased libido	20
Muscle cramps	52	Nausea	17
Decreased breast size	48	Headache	17
Flushing	42	Dizziness	10
Mood changes	38	Insomnia	10
Seborrhea	37	Rash	8
Depression	32	Increased libido	8
Sweating	32	Deepening voice	7
Edema	28	Increased LDL	<5
Change in appetite	28	Decreased HDL	<5
Acne	27	Increased hepatic enzymes	<5
Fatigue	25	Fetal masculinization	<5
Hirsutism	21		

[a]Data from Metzger DA, Luciano AA. Hormonal therapy of endometriosis. Obstet Gynecol Clin North Am 16(1):105–121, 1989.
[b]Clinical drug of choice (CDOC). Although approved for the treatment of endometriosis, the considerable side-effect profile and availability of newer, less troublesome therapies may have displaced danazol in this disorder.
[c]It is essential that therapy continue uninterrupted for 3 to 6 months but may be extended to 9 months if necessary. The dose may be adjusted to patient response.
Note: Cost to patient: 200 mg/day = $94 per month.
      400 mg/day = $178 per month.
      800 mg/day = $352 per month.

etine, alprazolam, and leuprolide in that order (or other members of their pharmacological classes) currently provide the best relief of generalized PMS symptoms. Despite the success of these treatments, knowledge of the potential adverse effects of these agents and their management is essential and modulates their use in some patients (15).

ENDOMETRIOSIS

Possibly 5 to 15% of all premenopausal women have endometriosis to some degree. This disorder is a common abnormal pelvic finding in women over 25 years of age and may be found in 40 to 50% of women who undergo surgery for the diagnosis and treatment of infertility. The average age at diagnosis is 28 years, and 75% of women with endometriosis are between 24 and 50 years old (16).

Endometriosis is a disorder in which there is a presence of islands of endometrium in extrauterine locations that exhibit the histologic and hormonal responsiveness of native endometrium. Cyclic change in these islands of endometrium is associated with menstrual-like bleeding and resultant localized inflammation (16).

Endometriosis most commonly occurs within the pelvis, on or within the ovaries, on the peritoneum, or beneath the serosa of pelvic viscera. Extrapelvic endometriosis, which occurs less frequently, involves locations outside the genital tract such as the bowel, rectum, appendix, umbilicus, scars, pleura, lung, kidney, ureter, bladder, and nerves (17).

The most frequent symptoms of genital tract endometriosis are secondary dysmenorrhea and pelvic pain, dyspareunia, menstrual irregularities, and infertility. Depending on the location of the extrapelvic endometriosis, the symptoms and signs vary. Interestingly, the severity of the disease does not directly correlate with the severity of the symptoms (18).

The etiology of endometriosis most widely accepted involves retrograde menstruation. This has been recently supported by findings that (1) retrograde menstruation is a common (90%) event in menstruating women with patent fallopian tubes, and (2) the anatomic distribution of endometriosis found at laparoscopy is consistent with retrograde menstruation. It has also been suggested that endometrial cells may successfully implant only in women with alterations in cell-mediated immunity and that such translocated cells may receive a stimulus for ectopic implantation and growth from activated macrophages (19). There are at least four other possible etiologies of endometriosis: (1) ectopic functioning endometrium may develop as a result of atypical development of germinal epithelium since various parts of the pelvic peritoneum are embryologically derived from totipotential coelomic epithelial cell elements; (2) metastases of normal endometrium may spread via uterine lymphatic vessels; (3) hematogenous spread via blood vessels to distant sites; or (4) cell rests of Muellerian epithelium may develop into functioning ectopic endometrial implants.

Table 90.5.
Medroxyprogesterone Acetate Therapy for Endometriosis[a]

Dose: 30–50 mg PO daily[b]	
Side Effect	Percent
Amenorrhea	70
Weight gain	60
Edema, bloating	60
Dysfunctional bleeding	20
Anxiety, irritability	20
Cyclic bleeding	10
Depression	5

[a]Data from Metzger DA, Luciano AA. Hormonal therapy for endometriosis. Obstet Gynecol Clin North Am 16(1):105–121, 1989.
[b]Cost to patient: 30 mg daily = $36 per month.
50 mg daily = $54 per month.

The goals of drug therapy of endometriosis are to ameliorate pain and to correct menstrual irregularities and infertility by the suppression of ectopic endometrial implants.

Danazol (Table 90.4) was the first hormonal agent approved by the Food and Drug Administration for the treatment of endometriosis. Although called an "antigonadotropin," its mechanism of action is much more complex in that it inhibits gonadotropin surge, inhibits the action of steroidogenic enzymes, and interacts with androgen and progesterone receptors (20).

Amenorrhea occurs with doses of 200 to 800 mg per day without significantly decreasing circulating levels of gonadotropins or estrogens. The manufacturer recommends use of a nonhormonal method of contraception since ovulation may occur and further warns that use of danazol during pregnancy could result in androgenic effects on the fetus that to date has been limited to clitoral hypertrophy and labial fusion of the external genitalia in the female fetus. The manufacturer further recommends that therapy should begin during menstruation or after a reliable pregnancy test.

Continuous progestational therapy with medroxyprogesterone acetate (MPA) by mouth is becoming popular because of its low cost and generally well-tolerated side effects compared to danazol. Although depot-medroxyprogesterone acetate (DMPA) is available, oral administration may be preferable in the patient desiring to get pregnant because of the well-documented prolonged anovulatory effect of DMPA. At a daily oral dose of 50 mg for 4 months, MPA did not adversely alter serum concentrations of lipids or lipoproteins (20). Table 90.5 lists average dose, duration, and side effects of MPA.

The inability of danazol to achieve complete ovarian suppression and its high frequency of side effects led to efforts to develop agents more effective than steroido-

genesis. Long-acting gonadotropin-releasing hormone agonists (GnRH-a) create a temporary and readily reversible "medical oophorectomy" and are currently the best therapy next to actual oophorectomy in the treatment of endometriosis. Endogenous GnRH is normally released in a circadian pattern every 60 to 90 minutes in the follicular phase. "Down-regulation" of the pituitary occurs if the peptide is given continuously or as a long-acting synthetic agonist analog. Although GnRH-a can be administered intravenously, intramuscularly, subcutaneously, intranasally, intravaginally, or rectally, only subcutaneous 28-day implants or once-daily doses, intramuscular monthly doses of depot forms, or twice-daily nasal sprays are currently used in the United States. Goserelin acetate subcutaneous implants, depot-leuprolide acetate, and intranasal nafarelin acetate have been approved for the treatment of endometriosis by the Food and Drug Administration at this time. Table 90.6 lists average dosages, routes, duration and side effects for GnRH-a preparations.

After 6 months of therapy, it has been shown that nafarelin decreased total vertebral bone mass by a mean of 5.9% at the end of treatment. Six months after completion of treatment, the total vertebral mass was still 1.4% below pretreatment levels. For this reason and since safety data for retreatment are not available, the manufacturer suggests getting bone density studies before retreating.

It is not clear which of these hormonal therapies is the most efficacious therapy for symptomatic endometriosis (20). Depot leuprolide and the goserelin implant have the advantage of avoiding compliance problems with daily injections or twice-daily nasal spraying.

Although these hormonal therapies have proved effective in relieving pain and combating the histologic manifestations of endometriosis, currently no clear evidence validates the efficacy of any medical approach in treating infertility (20).

Finally, the role of low-dose combination oral contraceptives (LDCOCs) in preventing endometriosis, in limiting progression of established disease, or in minimizing the risk of recurrence following hormonal and/or surgical therapy has not been clarified (21). Surgery is not necessarily a "last approach" in the treatment of endometriosis. Surgical techniques such as thermal ablation and cryoablation are often employed during the diagnostic laparoscopic evaluation of symptomatic patients. Only the lowest possible dose of estrogen should be used (20). The cost to the patient is $20.00 per month.

VAGINITIS (VULVOVAGINITIS)

At least one-third of all the women of childbearing age currently have one or more vulvovaginal infections. The chief symptoms are varying degrees of vaginal discharge, itching, and burning. The fear, shame, physical discomfort,

Table 90.6.
Gonadotropin-Releasing Hormone Agonists (GnRH-a) Therapy for Endometriosis[a]

GnRH-a	Dosage Regimen/Route	Duration
Nafarelin (CDOC)[b]	200 mcg in one nostril in the morning, 200 mcg in the other nostril in the evening[c]	6 months
Buserlin	300 mcg intranasally 3 times daily	6 months
Goserelin (CDOC)[d]	3.6 mg subcutaneous biodegradable implant	6 months
Leuprolide	0.5 mg subcutaneously daily	6 months
Leuprolide (CDOC)[d]	3.75 mg (depot) monthly	6 months

GnRH-a Side Effects	
Hot flashes	Decreases libido
Vaginal dryness	Decreased bone mineral content

[a]Data from Metzger DA, Luciano AA. Hormonal therapy of endometriosis. Obstet Gynecol Clin North Am 16(1):105–121, 1989; and Erickson LD, Ory SJ. GnRH analogues in the treatment of endometriosis. Obstet Gynecol Clin North Am 16(1):123–145, 1989.

[b]Clinical drug of choice.

[c]If amenorrhea does not occur after 2 months of treatment, use 1 spray (200 mcg) into both nostrils in the morning and evening (total = 800 mcg daily). Treatment should begin between days 2 and 4 of menses and not last for more than 6 months since safety data for retreatment are not available. Do not use topical nasal decongestants until 30 minutes after dosing. The manufacturer suggests use of a nonhormonal (barrier) method of contraception since the drug is Pregnancy Category X having induced major malformations in 4/80 rat fetuses at 7 times the maximum human dose.
Note: Cost to patient: 400 mcg/day = $330 per month.
                        800 mcg/day = $654 per month.

[d]Clinical drug of choice. Depot leuprolide and the goserelin implant have the advantage of avoidance of compliance with daily injections or twice daily nasal sprays. With the goserelin implant, use of the required 16-gauge needle often requires a local anesthetic before insertion.
Note: Cost to patient:
        Goserelin implant 3.6 mg/mo = $352 per month.
        SC Leuprolide 0.5 mg/day = $264 per month.
        Depot Leuprolide 3.75 mg = $378 per month.

esthetic revulsion, psychosexual problems, and embarrassment experienced as a result of vulvovaginal infections cause more unhappiness than any other gynecologic disorder, and the cost of treatment is substantial (22).

Basic Physiology and Flora

Normally, women of childbearing age have a thick, protective epithelium that is maintained by estrogen. A pH of 4.5 to 5.5 is maintained by the normal flora, consisting of a mixture of aerobic and anaerobic bacteria that break down epithelial cell carbohydrates, particularly glycogen, to lactic acid. The flora often includes clostridia, anaerobic streptococci (peptostreptococcus), aerobic group D and B-hemolytic streptococci, coliforms, and sometimes Listeria, in addition to the normally present Doderlein's bacilli (Lactobacillus species). If lactobacilli are suppressed by the administration of antibiotic drugs, yeasts or various bacteria normally present may become pathogenic by increasing in numbers and causing irritation and inflammation. After menopause, lactobacilli diminish, and a mixed flora predominates; the pH changes from acid to neutral or alkaline, which along with a thinning of the vaginal epithelium and a reduction of cervical mucus, leads to increased vaginal infections and atrophic vaginitis. Normally, cervical mucus has antibacterial activity and contains lysozyme. In some women, the vaginal introitus contains a heavy flora similar to that of the perineum and perianal area, which may predispose them to recurrent urinary tract infections. Table

Table 90.7.
Prevalence of Various Vulvovaginitides in 1000 Consecutive Patients with Lower Genital Tract Infections (Gonorrhea and Syphilis Excluded)[a]

Disorder	Incidence Number	Percentage	Percentage with One or More Other Pathogens[b]
Nonspecific vaginosis	425	42.5	23.3
Vaginal candidosis	373	37.3	17.7
Trichomoniasis	142	14.2	37.7
Herpes genitalis	94	9.4	16.4
Condylomata acuminata	72	7.2	55.6

[a]Adapted from Gardner HL. Infectious vulvovaginitis. In: Monif GR, ed. Infectious diseases in obstetrics and gynecology, 2nd ed. Philadelphia: Harper and Row, 1982:515.

[b]One patient had five infections simultaneously, 2 had four, and 126 had two. Incidences and numbers of simultaneous infections depend on the patient population studied.

90.7 includes the vulvovaginitides. Herpes genitalis is discussed in Chapter 71.

Nonspecific Vaginosis

A taxonomic controversy is responsible for the many etiologies and names proposed for nonspecific vaginosis. The former names given the disease, "Haemophilus vaginitis," "Corynebacterium vaginitis," and "Gardnerella vaginitis," reflected the suspected bacterial cause. Now, however, nonspecific vaginosis is the preferred name, pointing to the vagina as one of the body sites in which normally colonizing bacteria may become pathogenic.

Normally, lactobacilli, the predominant vaginal organism, control the growth of anaerobes and other bacteria by the production of hydrogen peroxide. If hydrogen peroxide is produced in very low levels, the mixed anaerobic and aerobic vaginal flora become free to proliferate 10- to 10,000-fold and grow Gardnerella vaginalis, which is normally present in 40 to 60% of women. Gardnerella vaginalis produces amino acids. Anaerobes produce enzymes that cleave these amino acids and form amines that increase vaginal pH, causing epithelial shedding that produces a discharge. Thus a vicious cycle starts in which an elevated pH decrease lactobacilli, anaerobes predominate, and extremely high quantities of G. vaginalis are present (23).

The chief symptom of bacterial vaginosis is vaginal discharge that has a characteristic foul "fish" odor that worsens after intercourse because of a shift to a alkaline pH in the vagina. This discharge is gray and homogeneous and frequently coats the labia. Minimal vulvovaginal itching and burning may occur.

There are four criteria to diagnose nonspecific vaginosis:

1. Homogeneous vaginal discharge
2. pH greater than 4.5
3. Presence of "clue cells" (a squamous epithelial cell whose border contains adherent G. vaginalis)
4. Positive "sniff" test (10% potassium hydroxide added to discharge releases the rotten fish odor of amines)

The goal of drug treatment of nonspecific vaginosis is to restore the normal vaginal flora and alleviate the minimal vulvar itching and burning, the gray homogeneous discharge, and the fishy odor. Monitoring the efficacy of the drug therapy does not necessitate reexamination of the patient unless symptoms persist.

Clearly, metronidazole is the CDOC and therefore is the initial choice for nonspecific vaginosis in nonpregnant women. Metronidazole, though given an approximate Pregnancy Category of B by the manufacturer, should not be used in pregnancy because of its observed mutagenicity in bacteria and carcinogenicity in animal models. In pregnancy, recent studies suggest that nonspecific vaginosis may be a factor in premature rupture of membranes and premature delivery, but they need substantiation. Until such studies have been conducted, routine treatment appears to be unnecessary or optional. Since metronidazole is contraindicated in the first trimester, and its safety in the rest of pregnancy is still in question, treatment with clindamycin 300 mg orally twice or clindamycin vaginal cream 2%, 1 applicatorful at bedtime daily for 7 days is recommended (24). Ampicillin, amoxicillin, or cephradine

Table 90.8.
Drug Treatment of Nonspecific Vaginosis[a]

Drug	Dose/Regimen
Recommended Regimen	
Metronidazole (CDOC)[b]	500 mg PO BID for 7 days (95% overall cure rate) (24)
Alternative Regimens	
Metronidazole (CDOC)[b]	2 g PO in a single dose (84% overall cure rate) (24)
Clindamycin vag cream	2%[c,d] app 1 p.v. h.s. for 7 days (24)
Metronidazole vag gel	0.75%[e] app 1 p.v. h.s. BID for 5 days (24)
Clindamycin (CDOC)[c]	300 mg PO BID for 7 days (24)
Ampicillin	500 mg PO QID for 7 days (22)
Amoxicillin	500 mg PO TID for 7 days (22)
Cephradine	250 mg PO QID for 7 days (22)
Tetracycline	500 mg PO QID for 7 days (22)

[a]The principal goal of therapy is to relieve vaginal symptoms and signs. Many authorities do not recommend treatment of asymptomatic infection. Treatment of the male sex partner, who is always asymptomatic, has not been shown to be beneficial for the patient or the male partner.
[b]Clinical drug of choice; oral metronidazole is clearly the best treatment.
[c]Clinical drug of choice; recommended in pregnancy and as an alternative to metronidazole.
[d]Clinical drug of choice; mean bioavailability is about 4%; contains mineral oil and may weaken latex condoms and diaphragms.
[e]Clinical drug of choice; preferred by some health care providers because of lack of certain systemic side effects such as mild-to-moderate gastrointestinal upset and unpleasant taste, and mean peak serum concentration is <2% that of the standard 500 mg PO dose. Data showing some efficacy with once daily dosage currently before the FDA as unpublished data, 1995.

are acceptable alternatives and can be used in pregnant patients.

No clinical counterpart of nonspecific vaginosis is recognized in the male, and treatment of the male sex partner has not been shown to be beneficial for the patient or the male partner (24).

Patients should be instructed to abstain from intercourse while taking the drug or to use condoms. It is absolutely essential to complete the full course of drug therapy because symptoms may disappear before there is bacteriologic cure.

The current drug therapies for nonspecific vaginosis are summarized in Table 90.8.

Vaginal Candidosis

Candida albicans in 90 to 95% of the cases and candida glabrata in 5 to 10% of the cases are colonized in the female genital tract and bowel and do not produce symptoms. Because of this, the terms *candidiasis* or *moniliasis* have been replaced with the term *vaginal candidosis*.

Predisposing factors to vaginal candidosis include (22):

1. Pregnancy and "pseudopregnancy" from oral contraceptives by:
   a. increased vaginal glycogen from estrogens

b. vaginal thinning from progestins
c. altered sugar metabolism
d. altered sexual habits (i.e., anal, followed by vaginal intercourse)
e. oral contraceptives may increase Candida colonization (but not infection)
2. Antibiotic therapy by:
a. increased candidal colonization by suppressing bacterial competition of the genital tract and bowel
b. reducing phagocytosis of Candida
c. direct growth stimulation of Candida
3. Diabetes mellitus, if poorly controlled, by increased glucose secretions, or alterations in the immune system

The chief symptoms of vaginal candidosis are severe itching of the vulva, vagina, or both and meatal dysuria.

The vulvitis symptoms are normally aggravated by tight clothing.

There are three criteria for the diagnosis of vaginal candidiasis:

1. Thick, white, curdlike secretions
2. pH 3.8 to 5.0
3. Long threadlike fibers of mycelia with tiny buds of conidia attached when one or two drops of 10% potassium hydroxide are added to a vaginal exudate slide (KOH preparation)

Nickerson's media is infrequently used to confirm the diagnosis before the treatments summarized in Table 90.9 are instituted.

The goal of drug treatment of vaginal candidosis is to restore normal vaginal flora and thereby alleviate the vulvar

Table 90.9.
Drug Treatment of Vaginal Candidosis

Drug/Dose	Regimen
Seven-Day Therapy	
Clotrimazole 1% Vag Cr (CDOC)[a,j]	App 1 p.v. h.s. × 7
Clotrimazole 100 mg Vag Tabs[j]	Tab 1 p.v. h.s. × 7
Miconazole Nitrate 2% Vag Cr[i,j]	App 1 p.v. h.s. × 7
Miconazole Nitrate 100 mg Vag Supp	Supp[i,j] 1 p.v. h.s. × 7
Terconazole 0.4% Vag Cr	App 1 p.v. h.s. × 7
Tioconazole 80 mg Supp[i]	Supp 1 p.v. h.s. × 7
Three-Day Therapy[b]	
Butoconazole Nitrate 2% Vag Cr[i]	App 1 p.v. h.s. × 3
Clotrimazole 1% Vag Cr[j]	App 1 p.v. BID × 3
Clotrimazole 100 mg Vag Tabs[j]	Tab 2 p.v. h.s. × 3
Econazole 150 mg Vag Tabs	Tab 1 p.v. h.s. × 3
Miconazole Nitrate 2% Vag Cr[j]	App 1 p.v. BID × 3
Miconazole Nitrate 200 mg Vag Supp	Supp[i] 1 p.v. h.s. × 3
Terconazole 80 mg Vag Supp[i]	Supp 1 p.v. h.s. × 3
One-Day Therapy[c]	
Clotrimazole 500 mg Vag Tab[d]	Tab 1 p.v. h.s. × 1
Fluconazole 150 mg PO tablet[e]	Tab 1 PO × 1
Tioconazole 6.5% Vag Oint[i]	App 1 p.v. h.s. × 1
Miscellaneous Therapies	
Ketoconazole 200 mg Oral Tab[f]	Tab 1 PO BID × 3 d
Gentian Violet Tampons 5 mg[g]	Tampon 1 p.v. one to two times daily for 3–4 hours for 12 days.
Miconazole Tampons 100 mg[h]	Tampon 1 p.v. h.s. × 5 d

[a]Clinical drug of choice would be any of the seven-day therapies.
[b]Three-day therapies are equally efficacious to seven-day therapies except for pregnant, diabetic, or corticosteroid-using women. For these conditions, use only seven-day therapy.
[c]One-day therapy, with the exception of oral fluconazole, is only good for mild or early cases. Three- and seven-day therapies are superior. In general, one-day therapy, other than with oral fluconazole, is not recommended because of poor efficacy (24).
[d]Single dose serves as a vaginal depot for at least 3 days (25).
[e]Superior to 3 days of vaginal 200 mg clotrimazole, and symptoms were relieved more rapidly (26).
[f]Should be the last treatment of choice for recurrent or persistent cases since the drug is hepatotoxic and is contraindicated in pregnancy because of its known teratogenic effects in rats manifested as limb deformities; clinically significant drug interactions may occur with terfenadine, rifampin, astemizol, phenytoin, cyclosporin A, coumarinlike agents, and oral hypoglycemics.
[g]Best treatment for Candida glabrata. Caution: purple staining.
[h]Data on file on 123 patients, Advanced Care Products, claims 5 days to be as effective as 7 days of miconazole nitrate cream with similar side effects; the manufacturer claims that the therapeutic effect is not affected by menstruation; the use of nonmedicated tampons has been associated with an increased risk of Toxic Shock Syndrome (TSS); this product is available only in California at the time of writing.
[i]Note: These creams and suppositories are oil based and may weaken latex condoms and diaphragms.
[j]Over-the-counter (OTC) preparations. If symptoms persist after use or if there is a recurrence of symptoms within 2 months, medical care should be sought (24).
Note: If any first course fails, reconfirm diagnosis with microscopic examination and treat with an alternative drug.
Note: Treatment of pregnant patients can employ any of the above medications (24) except ketoconazole.
Note: Nystatin Vag Tabs 100,000 units are intentionally left off this table because they are only fungistatic, whereas all the other therapies are fungicidal (24).

erythema; the fungal patches; the severe itching and burning of the vagina, vulva, or both; and the white, dry, curdlike vaginal discharge. Alleviation of symptoms is evidence of efficacy, and reexamination of the patient is unnecessary unless symptoms persist.

Of all the drug therapies of vaginal candidosis, only nystatin is fungistatic and is therefore no longer recommended (24). Candida glabrata is best treated with gentian violet.

Patient compliance improves as the duration of therapy decreases. Fortunately, the 3-day therapies listed in Table 90.9 are approximately as effective as the 7-day therapies (25,26). Single-day therapies, other than oral fluconazole, should be used only in uncomplicated mild or early cases, and recently many experts have recommended that 1-day therapy, other than oral fluconazole, not be used at all (24).

Patients should understand that strict regimen compliance is necessary, that creams are usually preferable to tablets or suppositories since some cream can be applied to the perineum, and that treatment should always be continued through menses, if it occurs, and when vaginal contraceptives are used. The patient should also be instructed to report any new vaginal irritation since vaginal irritation in 0 to 6.6% of users has been reported with miconazole > tioconazole > butoconazole > econazole > clotrimazole > nystatin. Irritation may necessitate changing the drug therapy. Terconazole use has been reported to cause headaches in 26% of the patients. When gentian violet is used, the patient should be advised of its permanent purple-staining characteristics. If a patient uses miconazole tampons, she must be warned of the possible increased risk of toxic shock syndrome (TSS) and should be told that TSS is a rare illness that can be fatal and is characterized by high fever (102°F or greater), hypotension, sunburnlike rash with desquamation 1 to 2 weeks after onset, vomiting, or diarrhea. If TSS symptoms occur, the patient should discontinue the tampons and contact a physician immediately.

Recurrent Vaginal Candidosis

Recurrent vaginal candidosis is usually defined as three or more episodes of symptomatic vaginal candidosis annually and effects less than 5% of women. It may be due to:

1. Intestinal reservoir: Up to 100% correlation has been found between simultaneous infestations of C. albicans in the vaginal and fecal material. A persistent intestinal reservoir may recolonize the perianal area and lead to recurrent infection (27).
2. Sexual transmission: Unequivocal proof that a colonized penis may transmit C. albicans is lacking even though circumstantial evidence shows that 5 to 25% of male partners of infected females may asymptomatically carry yeast, usually in the coronal sulcus. Some clinicians advocate treatment of the male for 7 days with a cream (see Table 90.9) (27).

3. Therapy failure: Candida blastospores invade intact epithelial cells in the superficial layers of the vaginal mucosa to a depth of several layers and may reemerge weeks or months later when the epithelial cells are normally shed. Approximately 20 to 50% of women clinically responding by culture to standard antifungal therapy are culture positive within 30 days (27).

Therefore, for recurrent vaginal candidosis, the following regimens may be employed:

1. For nonpregnant women:
   a. Ketoconazole 200 mg oral tablets one orally twice daily for 3 days (28) or fluconazole 150 mg oral tablet once
   b. Only treat male partners who experience symptomatic balanitis or penile dermatitis with a topical cream (see Table 90.9) for 7 days
2. For pregnant women:
   a. Nystatin, 500,000-unit oral tablets, one orally three times daily for 14 days, plus
   b. Clotrimazole 1% vaginal cream applied once vaginally at bedtime for 14 days
   c. Only treat males who experience symptomatic balanitis or penile dermatitis with topical antifungal creams (see Table 90.9) for 14 days

The 1993 STD Treatment Guidelines, however, state that the optimal treatment has not been established and that after confirmation by culture, maintenance therapy with ketoconazole 100 mg orally once daily can be used for up to 6 months. As part of the evaluation for predisposing conditions, HIV testing should be done in women with predisposing factors for HIV infection (24).

Trichomonas Vaginitis

Trichomoniasis is a disease of the vagina and also the lower urinary tract of men and women. Sexual transmission is well recognized although transmission by communal fomites, toilet splash, gloves, and instruments may rarely occur. Transmission to newborns of untreated mothers also occurs, and the child will require treatment. Male partners should be treated simultaneously since 80% may be culture positive (22).

The chief symptoms of Trichomonas vaginitis are variable, ranging from a mild yellow-green or gray vaginal discharge, to a moderate malodorous discharge, to itching, burning discharge with odor, to intermenstrual or postcoital bleeding. Dysuria is present in at least 10% of patients.

There are four diagnostic parameters:

1. Thick or thin white, yellow, green, or gray malodorous discharge
2. pH 5.0 to 7.5
3. Highly motile, pear-shaped, unicellular Trichomonas vaginalis seen on saline mount microscopy (a flagellated protozoan about twice the size of a white blood cell)
4. "Strawberry" vagina or cervix, seen only in about 10% of patients, due to swollen papillae projecting through vaginal secretions

The goal of drug treatment of Trichomonas vaginitis is to restore the normal vaginal flora and thereby alleviate the vaginal itching, burning, and the malodorous yellow-green or gray discharge. Reexamination is necessary only when symptoms persist.

Table 90.10 summarizes current treatment of Trichomonas vaginitis in primary and recurrent cases. Unfortunately, only metronidazole is adequately effective in the treatment and is therefore CDOC. Since 80% of male partners may be culture positive, they must be treated simultaneously.

Patient education should include discussion of the necessity of strict compliance with the simultaneous treatment for both partners and the use of condoms until the regimens are completed. A metallic taste in the mouth and brown urine may occur, and patients taking metronidazole should avoid the consumption of alcohol because of the possibility of a disulfiram-type reaction.

GENITAL AND ANAL WARTS (CONDYLOMATA ACUMINATA)

Approximately 60% of sexual partners of individuals infected with condylomata acuminata develop genital or anal warts, with an average incubation period of 2 to 3 months. The typical lesions in women are most often found in the fourchette and on the labia, and less commonly found on other parts of the vulva, perineum, and anus. In addition, cervical warts are common. During pregnancy, genital warts tend to enlarge and grow more rapidly, taking on a cauliflower appearance. They may involve both the labia and vagina rather than the perianal area and may render vaginal delivery difficult. The causative agent is the human papillomavirus (HPV). A decade ago, genital and anal warts were thought to be trivial lesions of little importance; however, today, they are recognized as one of the most important of the sexually transmitted diseases as a result of a 460% increase in 15 years in the United States. There is an estimated 2% incidence of flat condyloma of the cervix of all women of childbearing age. These data suggest that genital and anal warts are being encountered as often as herpes genitalis and gonorrhea (29).

Recently, many investigators have found that under certain circumstances certain types of HPV (most commonly types 16, 18, 31, 33, 35, 45, and 56) have been found to be strongly associated with genital dysplasia and carcinoma (30). Fortunately, most exophytic genital warts are most frequently caused by types 6 and 11 of HPV. However, a biopsy is needed in all instances of atypical, pigmented, or persistent warts. All women with anogenital warts should have a yearly pap smear (24).

The chief symptom reported by patients is an occasional itching of the lesions. The diagnosis is made by the presence of verrucose growths, usually on the vulva or genital area, and a positive sexual history.

The goal of drug treatment of genital and anal warts is to destroy the HPV-infected tissue, prevent recurrence and sexual transmission, and possibly prevent the sequellae of squamous cell genital cancer. Unfortunately, no therapy has been shown to eradicate HPV. HPV has been demonstrated in adjacent tissue after laser treatment of HPV-associated cervical intraepithelial neoplasia and after attempts to eliminate subclinical HPV by extensive laser vaporization of the anogenital area. Therefore, the goal of treatment is not the eradication of HPV (24). Sex partners should be examined for evidence of warts and treated as needed.

The CDOC at this time for vaginal and cervical warts is 5-fluorouracil (Table 90.11), along with the treatment and patient instructions for other genital and anal warts.

Treatments include cytotoxic, destructive, immunologic, and surgical methods. The cytotoxic treatment regimens with podophyllin or 5-fluorouracil and the destructive treatment with trichloroacetic acid are covered in Table 90.11.

Cryotherapy with liquid nitrogen or dry ice, electrosurgery, and carbon dioxide lasers (31) are other useful

---

Table 90.10.
Drug Treatment of Trichomonas Vaginitis[a]

A. Metronidazole CDOC 500 mg tabs: 4 PO in a single dose[a]
B. Metronidazole 500 mg BID for 7 days
  1. Male sex partners of infected women should be treated with regimen A or B.
  2. Asymptomatic women should be treated with regimen A or B.
  3. If failure occurs with either regimen, the patient should be treated with metronidazole 500 mg twice daily for 7 days.
  4. If repeated failure occurs, the patient should be treated with a single 2-gram dose of metronidazole daily for 3 to 5 days.
  5. Cases in which there are additional culture-documented treatment failure in which reinfection has been excluded should be managed in consultation with an expert who can determine the susceptibility of Trichomonas vaginalis to metronidazole.
  6. Metronidazole is contraindicated in the first trimester of pregnancy, and its safety in the rest of pregnancy is not established. However, no other adequate therapy exists. For patients with severe symptoms after the first trimester, treatment with 2 grams of metronidazole in a single dose is suggested.
  7. For lactating women, use regimen A, interrupting breast feeding for at least 24 hours after therapy.

[a]Adapted from Anon. Sexually transmitted diseases treatment guidelines. MMWR 42(RR-14):1–102, 1993.

Table 90.11.
Drug Treatment of Genital or Anal Warts (Condylomata Accuminata)[a,b]

Trichloroacetic acids 80–90% (CDOC)[c]
1. Apply skin protectant[d] to surrounding tissues.
2. Treatment is adequate if a white color develops 30–60 seconds later.
3. Patient will experience a sharp, burning pain for 15–30 minutes.

Podophyllin 10–25% in compound tincture of benzoin
1. Apply skin protectant[d] to surrounding tissues.
2. Apply < 0.5 ml per treatment; treat < 10 cm^2
3. Wash off thoroughly in 1–4 hours.
4. If four applications fail, other treatments are indicated.
5. Not for extensive lesions or pregnancy since podophyllin is absorbed and is toxic.

Podofilox 0.5% topical solution
1. Apply skin protectant[d] to surrounding tissues.
2. Apply with a cotton-tipped applicator twice daily morning and evening (every 12 hours), for 3 consecutive days, then withhold use for 4 consecutive days. This 1-week cycle of treatment may be repeated up to four times until there is no visible wart tissue. If there is incomplete response after 4 treatment weeks, alternative treatment should be considered since the safety and effectiveness of more than 4 treatment weeks have not been established.
3. Treatment should be limited to less than 10 cm^2 of wart tissue and to no more than 0.5 ml of the solution per day.
4. Systemic absorption studies did not result in detectable serum levels. However, it should be used in pregnancy only if trichloroacetic acid therapy fails.

5-Fluorouracil cream 5% (31) (CDOC)
1. Only for vaginal/cervical/penile warts.
2. Female: Insert ½ vaginal applicator (2.5 g) p.v. h.s. for 5 days.
   Male: Apply 1–2 nights weekly to entire penis; avoid the urethra; therapy is for 3 months; apply a tissue between underside of penis and scrotum, and wear a jockstrap to keep penis in place.
3. Female to apply a skin protectant[d] to vulva and urethra h.s. and a.m. after washing external genitalia.
4. Avoid during pregnancy since it may be teratogenic.

[a]Adapted from Anon. Sexually transmitted diseases treatment guidelines. MMWR 42(RR-14):1–102, 1993; and Lynch PJ. Condylomata acuminata (anogenital warts). Clin Obstet Gynecol 28:142–151, 1985 (except podofilox).
[b]Condoms should be used until warts disappear.
[c]Clinical drug of choice.
[d]Zinc oxide ointment 20%, silicone cream, or silver sulfadiazine 1% cream.

destructive treatments. Shave and scissor excision of larger lesions are acceptable surgical methods. Interferon immunotherapy is currently under study (32).

ESTROGEN REPLACEMENT THERAPY

The female climacteric is a clinical epoch secondary to the physiologic depletion of ovarian follicles. Menopause refers to the cessation of menses. A patient is postmenopausal after 1 year of amenorrhea. Statistics indicate that by age 51.1, the average age of menopause, a woman can expect to live another 28 years. Therefore, more than 32 million women in the United States 51.1 years of age and older can expect to live 40% of their lives in a state of estrogen deficiency. The consequences of this estrogen deficiency include vasomotor instability, atrophic vaginitis, and osteoporosis.

Vasomotor Symptoms

Approximately 80% of women within the first year of ovarian failure or castration experience hot flushes that are caused by a decrease in the tone of arterioles, resulting in an increased blood flow to the skin and resultant rise in skin temperature. Hot flushes appear to be synchronous with increased hypothalamic release of GnRH. Since GnRH

neurons are close to the centers that regulate temperature in the intact hypothalamus, it is likely that alpha-adrenergic stimulation of GnRH release concomitantly stimulates these centers. Although the symptoms may last for at least 5 years for 70% of this group, homeostatic adjustments eventually occur. The most likely explanation of why all women do not experience hot flushes seems to be varying amounts of endogenous estradiol (5 to 20 mcg per day versus 50 to 300 mcg per day before menopause) produced in the liver and adipose tissue. Obese women may produce twice as much estradiol as slender women.

The chief vasomotor symptoms reported by patients are described as hot flushes or hot flashes occurring over the anterior part of the body, especially the chest, neck, and face. An episode lasts usually only a few minutes and is commonly precipitated by anxiety or excitement. The vasomotor symptoms vary considerably in duration, frequency, and severity. One variation, night sweats, is experienced by some patients who usually describe awakening at night, covered in perspiration, and throwing off the bed covers.

It is estimated that following physiologic menopause, 15% of patients seek treatment for vasomotor symptoms; 50% of reproductive-age women undergoing castration

request treatment. The vasomotor symptoms themselves are not thought to be harmful, but they indicate an estrogen-deficiency state and are usually treated on request. The lowest dosage of estrogen to reduce the vasomotor symptoms to a tolerable level should be employed and reevaluated every 6 months. Reduced symptoms during the drug-free evaluation period are found within 2 to 5 years of menopause. Clinically, there is no reasonable means to follow the response to treatment other than subjective symptomatic improvement.

All potential patients for estrogen therapy should undergo a baseline evaluation, including pelvic examination, cytology, breast examination, blood pressure, and a thorough history, to rule out the following absolute and relative contraindications:

Absolute

1. Undiagnosed vaginal bleeding
2. Suspected breast cancer
3. Suspected endometrial cancer
4. Active venous thrombosis

Possibly Absolute (under debate)

1. History of breast cancer
2. History of endometrial cancer
3. Malignant melanoma

Relative

1. Uterine fibroids
2. Endometriosis
3. History of cholelithiasis
4. History of migraine
5. Hypertriglyceridemia
6. Liver disease

Patient education should include the major adverse effects of estrogen as well as instructions about the importance of yearly physical examinations repeating the baseline parameters. Patients should also be warned of the cardiovascular and neoplastic liabilities of smoking that along with estrogens may contribute to these disorders although this has not been established in the literature.

Recommended therapies for vasomotor symptoms and equivalent estrogen replacement therapy (ERT) doses and regimens (32–34) appear in Table 90.12.

Vaginal Atrophy, Atrophic Vaginitis, and Dysuria

Postmenopausal estrogen deficiency leads to a thinning of the vaginal epithelium, a decreased blood supply, dryness, and a change to a neutral or alkaline pH that predisposes to infection.

The chief symptoms are vaginal discharge secondary to infection, complaints of painful intercourse (dyspareunia) due to dryness, and dysuria. Estrogens increase the vascularity and epithelial proliferation of the vagina, allowing greater lubrication, increased protection from vaginitis, and reduced vaginal trauma from coitus. The increased vascularity resulting from estrogen therapy is associated with increased blood flow through the periurethral venous plexus, leading to small increases in periurethral pressure occasionally sufficient to correct urinary stress incontinence.

The goals of therapy are to eliminate the atrophy, dysuria, and predisposition to vaginal infections caused by estrogen deficiency.

The atrophy and dysuria can be treated with equal effectiveness by either systemic or vaginally applied estrogen. However, the response to conjugated estrogen

Table 90.12.
Treatment of Hot Flushes and Equivalent ERT Regimens[a]

Generic Name	Equivalent Regimen
Conjugated estrogens (CDOC)[b]	0.625 mg PO × 25 d/mo[c]
Esterified estrogens	0.625 mg PO × 25 d/mo[c]
Esterified estrogens with methyltestosterone 1.25 mg	0.625 mg one PO × 25 d/mo[c,g]
Estropipate	0.625 mg PO × 25 d/mo[c]
Ethinyl estradiol	0.2 mg PO × 25 d/mo[c]
17-beta estradiol	0.5 mg × 25 d/mo[c]
17-beta estradiol (transdermal)	0.05 mg patch to skin BIW[d]
Medroxyprogesterone acetate	20 mg PO daily[e]
Clonidine	0.2 mg PO BID[f]

[a]With all ERT regimens, add medroxyprogesterone acetate 2.5–10 mg 10–13 days/month to prevent endometrial hyperplasia and possible malignancy in all women who have not had their uterus removed.
[b]Clinical drug of choice; conjugated estrogens are the initial choice because of the extensive literature on their use.
[c]Over 80% of ERT patients in the United States are given conjugated estrogens. Little in the literature supports the advantage of one preparation over another if equivalent doses are used.
[d]75% effective, similar to oral ERT; up to 20% minor skin irritation (32). Least skin irritation if applied to buttocks. Recently also available as a once-weekly patch.
[e]Mechanism unknown; > 70% effective; not an approved use; may be used when estrogens are contraindicated; about one-third of women with intact uteri may have vaginal bleeding. Progestins will not prevent vaginal atrophy and may not prevent osteoporosis (33).
[f]Alpha-adrenergic agonist; < 50% effective; dry mouth and sedation limit usefulness; not an approved use; more studies needed; last choice (34).
[g]Only indicated for the treatment of moderate-to-severe vasomotor symptoms not improved by estrogens alone.

Table 90.13.
Currently Recommended Treatments for Vaginal Atrophy and Dysuria[a,b]

Generic Name	Regimen
Conjugated estrogen cream 0.625 mg/g (CDOC)[c]	0.2–1 g p.v. daily × 10, then BIW–TIW
Estropipate cream 1.25 mg/g	0.2–1 g p.v. daily × 10, then BIW–TIW
17 Beta-estradiol cream 0.1 mg/g	0.2–1 g p.v. daily × 10, then BIW–TIW
Dienestrol cream 0.01%	0.2–1 applicatorful daily × 10, then BIW–TIW

[a]Most experts recommend cyclic addition of 10–13 days of progestin monthly if the uterus is present to prevent endometrial hyperplasia and possible malignancy.

[b]These regimens are extrapolated from Dyer and Townsend (35) and differ from the manufacturer's recommendations.

[c]Clinical drug of choice.

cream may be lost after 14 days because of tissue cornification or downregulation of the estrogen receptors. This can be overcome by stopping treatment for 7 to 14 days and restarting using 0.1 mg daily rather than the 1.25- to 2.5-mg dose recommended by the manufacturer (35). For this reason, the systemic effects and topical response may be erratic. Conjugated estrogens, estropipate, and estradiol vaginal creams contain 0.625 mg/g, 1.25 mg/g, and 0.1 mg/g, respectively, and include applicators graduated from 1 to 4 g. One gram is roughly equivalent to a full applicatorful of dienestrol cream 0.01%.

The CDOC is conjugated estrogen vaginal cream since the majority of clinical data concerns its use. Patient instructions and warnings are basically the same as with oral estrogens since systemic estrogen levels may be reached. Most experts recommend the addition of 10 to 13 days of medroxyprogesterone acetate 2.5 to 10 mg daily in women with intact uteri to prevent endometrial hyperplasia and possible malignancy. Current recommended treatments for vaginal atrophy and dysuria are listed in Table 90.13.

Osteoporosis Secondary to Estrogen Deficiency

Conservatively, osteoporosis secondary to estrogen deficiency may be responsible for 100,000 wrist fractures and 250,000 hip fractures annually in the United States. The acute care cost may total $3 billion following hip fractures, and the mortality may be as high as 15 to 30%, or 27,000 to 60,000 deaths per year, for the year following a hip fracture, usually due to complications such as pneumonia, pulmonary embolism, or congestive heart failure. An additional 40,000 patients will require prolonged institutionalization (36), and this helps bring the annual total of direct and indirect costs to $7 billion (37).

In women, maximal mineral content in cortical bone of the radius occurs in the mid-30s and declines 3% per decade until menopause, at which time it declines 9% per decade until age 75, and thereafter returns to a 3% decline per decade, with as much as 66% skeletal loss by age 80. Of women over 60, 25% have spinal compression fractures, causing much pain and debilitation; by age 75, this figure reaches as high as 50% (36).

Since patients prone to osteoporosis cannot be predicted, all women who are postmenopausal or lack ovarian function or ovaries should receive ERT, when not contraindicated, soon after the diagnosis of estrogen deficiency. An exception to this may be black women, who have a greater bone mass and higher calcitonin levels than nonblack women, leading to a low risk for osteoporosis. Pure black women may need ERT only for premature surgical menopause, hot flushes, atrophic vaginitis, or estrogen-deficiency dysuria.

A decline in circulating estrogens enhances calcium efflux from bone mineral stores and increases the serum concentration of ionized calcium. This suppresses secretion of parathyroid hormone (PTH), which, in turn, reduces the synthesis of 1,25-dihydroxyvitamin D3 by the renal tubular cells. The lowered concentration of 1,25-dihydroxyvitamin D3 causes a decrease in the intestinal absorption of calcium. Studies of PTH and vitamin D have not demonstrated a consistent relationship between their levels and osteoporosis. However, calcitonin secretion progressively declines with age and estrogen deficiency. Calcitonin inhibits bone resorption and is known to be increased with ERT. Therefore, there may be beneficial effects on bone due to estrogens at nonestrogen or estrogen receptor sites.

PREVENTION OF OSTEOPOROSIS

The risks associated with hormonal therapy and the need for lifelong ERT to prevent osteoporosis have made both patients and practitioners hesitant to use ERT.

The association of endometrial cancer with ERT exists because it is well known that estrogens stimulate the growth of the endometrium and that the resultant proliferation can potentially progress to atypical hyperplasia and adenocarcinoma. However, the highest incidence of cancer is usually in users of estrogens not opposed by progestins, the lowest incidence in users of estrogen and progestin combination therapy, and intermediate incidence is in women not taking estrogens or progestins. Progestins decrease estrogen receptors in endometrial cells and induce estradiol dehydrogenase and isocitrate activity, which are the mechanisms whereby these cells metabolize estrogens (35).

Since the likelihood of developing breast cancer is higher than that of endometrial cancer in all women, and breast cancer has a less desirable outcome, it is comforting at this time to find that there is no evidence that estrogens increase the risk of breast cancer and that progestin added to ERT significantly reduced the risk of mammary malignancy in at least one study (38). Because breast cells are not cyclically shed by the action of progesterone, the protective mechanism most likely operates at the intracellular level through changes in receptors. Therefore, according to this study, progestins should be given even to those women who have had a hysterectomy, for 10 to 13 days each month, whenever they are prescribed estrogen therapy (38). Many experts disagree with this practice.

In general, epidemiologic data from case-control and cohort studies have suggested that postmenopausal estrogen confers a moderate degree of protection from coronary artery disease, with reductions in overall mortality rates for acute myocardial infarction in comparison with nonestrogen users (39).

The Postmenopausal Estrogen/Progestin Interventions (PEPI) Trial has recently shown that estrogen alone, or in combination with a progestin, improves lipoproteins and lowers fibrinogen levels without detectable effects on postchallenge insulin or blood pressure. It further showed that conjugated equine estrogens 0.625 mg daily plus 200 mg of micronized oral progesterone for 12 days of the month had the most favorable effect on HDL-C with no excess risk of endometrial hyperplasia (40).

ROLE OF CALCIUM INTAKE

Healthy postmenopausal women whose usual daily elemental calcium dietary intake is less than 400 mg lose mineral from the spine at a greater rate than those women whose intake is higher. In a recent study, in women who had undergone menopause 5 or fewer years earlier, bone loss from the spine was rapid and was not effected by supplementation with 500 mg of elemental calcium daily in addition to their normal lower-than-400-mg or 400- to 650-mg daily dietary intake. In women who had been postmenopausal for 6 years or more given placebo, bone loss was less rapid in those normally taking 400 to 650 mg. None of the women had used estrogen, glucocorticoids, or other medications known to affect calcium or bone metabolism within the past year in this double-blind, placebo-controlled, randomized trial to determine the effect of calcium on bone loss from the spine, femoral neck, and radius. During the 2-year study, those with the lower calcium intake maintained bone density at the femoral neck and radius but not the spine when treated with calcium carbonate. Although it has not been a consistent finding, increased rates of bone loss have been reported to occur for 2 to 5 years after menopause. Therefore, the authors conclude, since the median daily intake of calcium in women over 44 years of age in the United States is known to be 475 mg, healthy postmenopausal women whose usual dietary calcium intake is low should be urged to increase their calcium intake to 800 mg per day, the current recommended daily allowance (41), in order to limit bone loss (42).

Although calcium citrate malate was more bioavailable and shown to be more effective than calcium carbonate in

Table 90.14.
Oral Calcium Supplementation[a]

Generic Preparation	%Ca++	Tablet Size (mg Ca++/Tab)	#/Day to Supply 1 g	Cost/Day[b] ($)
Calcium carbonate (CDOC)[c]	40	650 (260)	4	0.36
Dibasic calcium PO4	23	500 (115)	9	0.90
Calcium lactate	13	650 (84.5)	12	0.60
Calcium gluconate	9	650 (58.5)	17	0.85

[a]Adapted from Bauwens et al (43).
[b]Based on average wholesale price, 1994 Redbook.
[c]Clinical drug of choice.

the study cited, it is not available commercially at this time (42). For those requiring calcium supplementation, calcium carbonate is usually the easiest to take calcium source since it contains the most elemental calcium per tablet. It should be taken with meals to assure adequate stomach acid secretion to facilitate absorption (43).

The main adverse effects of calcium supplementation are constipation in the elderly and possible kidney stone formation in those predisposed individuals who take at least 2000 mg of elemental calcium daily.

Dairy products are the best food source of calcium, with 8 oz of skim or whole milk containing roughly 300 mg of elemental calcium, 8 oz of yogurt having roughly 345 mg, 1 oz of cheese having 211 mg, and 8 oz of ice cream having 200 mg (43). Dietary sources may be supplemented with oral calcium salts (Table 90.14).

Current Drug Therapies to Prevent Estrogen-Deficiency Osteoporosis

The minimum effective dose of estrogen to prevent bone loss is conjugated estrogens 0.625 mg or the equivalent (44). Combining 1500-mg elemental calcium per day and 0.3-mg conjugated estrogen produced an actual increase in vertebral trabecular mass over 2 years in one study (45). For those unable to tolerate estrogens, progestins alone may be used since there is some evidence that they decrease bone turnover. Giving 150 mg of depo-medroxyprogesterone acetate intramuscularly monthly has been suggested although this has not been clearly established (46). (Note: The original article incorrectly states that 150 mg was given days 1 through 25 monthly). The 21 patients given 150 mg of depo-medroxyprogesterone acetate intramuscularly once monthly had significantly lowered urinary calcium/creatinine and hydroxyproline/creatinine ratios which were similar to the 22 patients who received oral conjugated estrogens 0.625 mg days 1 through 25 of each month. Unfortunately, the number of study patients was small and the study duration was only 3 months; therefore, the study needs to be verified with larger numbers of patients participating for a much longer duration.

In a 3-year prospective study of 200 perimenopausal women suffering from various menopausal symptoms, the 100 women who were given a triphasic oral contraceptive containing levonorgestrel and ethinyl estradiol were cleared of their various menopausal symptoms within 6 months, with no adverse effects on liver function tests, blood glucose, blood pressure, or coagulation factors, and with marked improvement in plasma lipids. At 3 years, the controls showed a loss of about 6% of bone mass compared to pretreatment levels, whereas the drug group did not lose bone mass, even though both groups averaged 1000-mg daily elemental calcium intake (47). However, with the triphasic contraceptive, the average daily intake of ethinyl estradiol is 32 mcg compared to the 20-mcg normal ERT dose.

The results of a recent study show that intermittent cyclic therapy with oral etidronate is effective in reversing the progressive loss of vertebral bone that occurs in postmenopausal osteoporosis (48). Continuous, high doses of etidronate may lead to the impairment of bone mineralization and the cessation of bone remodeling.

Therefore, to reduce bone resorption through the inhibition of osteoclastic activity, 400 mg of oral etidronate per day was given, after a 4-hour fast in the afternoon, with water for 2 weeks, since the average oral absorption is only 3% of the dose when fasting, followed by a 13-week period in which no drugs were taken. While on etidronate, 500 mg of elemental calcium and 400 units of vitamin D supplements were taken in the morning. The 15-week cycles were repeated 10 times for a total of 150 weeks, resulting in small but significant increases in the bone mineral content of vertebrae and, after approximately 1 year of treatment, a stabilization in the progression of spinal deformity and a significant decrease in the rate of new vertebral fractures. Because of the long remodeling cycle in osteoporosis, the effects of antiresorptive agents such as etidronate are not likely to be fully appreciated during the first year of therapy. Oral etidronate is well tolerated, and no significant side effects were noted during the study. A recent 4-year, prospective, randomized study in early postmenopausal women showed an additive effect of intermittent cyclical etidronate and percutaneous 17-β estradiol given daily equivalent to an oral dose of 1.5 mg daily and 200 mg of oral micronized progesterone for 12 days (HRT) each month on the bone mineral density of both the vertebrae and the hip. Furthermore, the osteomalacia associated with etidronate alone was avoided (49).

The FDA recently approved alendronate as the first drug in the bisphosphonate class to be approved for the treatment of osteoporosis in postmenopausal women. One 2-year, randomized, double-blind, placebo-controlled study showed alendronate is well tolerated at oral therapeutic doses of 5 or 10 mg daily and significantly increases

bone mineral density at the lumbar spine, hip, and total body (50).

Recently, nasal salmon calcitonin 100 IU in the morning and 100 IU in the evening has been studied for the treatment of established osteoporosis in a 1-year double-blind, placebo-controlled study (51). Further bone loss was prevented with no side effects. The patients also received 500 mg of elemental calcium daily. The FDA has approved this product for the treatment of osteoporosis after the manufacturer agreed to conduct additional studies of long-term effectiveness in preventing fractures since two clinical randomized trials demonstrated that daily use increased bone mass in the spine but not in the forearm or hip.

A 2-year prospective study of 20 women using an estradiol transdermal system releasing 0.05 mg of estradiol per day for 3 weeks with the addition of a variety of progestins for the last 10 days of the hormonal cycle validated transdermal estradiol (i.e., the prevention of osteoporosis). The study was conducted for 24 months with 24 patients as controls. The vertebral mass of the control patients, measured by dual photon absorptiometry, decreased significantly (-4.3%) (P less than .001), whereas treated women had a net gain of 5.4% (P less than .001) (52).

Long-term studies evaluating the effect of transdermal 17-beta estradiol on serum lipids are yet to be completed. One 24-week study found a significant increase in HDL cholesterol and reductions in both total serum cholesterol and LDL levels in 10 patients using a patch that released 0.1 mg of estradiol per day every day of the month (53). A more recent, small study showed that both conjugated estrogens 0.625 mg and transdermal estradiol 0.05 mg used without a progestin did not produce significant changes in lipoproteins over the course of 12 months (54). Larger numbers of patients using this therapy for a much longer duration are needed to verify this study and also the utilization of much more sophisticated lipoprotein determinations.

The onset of symptoms of osteoporosis are insidious, and the condition leads to wrist fractures and painful spinal vertebral fractures in patients in their 60s, and hip fractures in patients in their 70s.

The goals of therapy with ERT are to prevent menopausal symptoms, vaginal atrophy, dysuria secondary to estrogen deficiency, osteoporosis and cardiovascular disease. All patients should be instructed to do monthly self-breast examinations and report any lumps or retractions discovered. Additionally, patients should report any signs of jaundice such as yellowing of the skin or sclera. Finally, any irregular noncyclic bleeding should be reported since it may indicate neoplastic changes in the genital tract. It should be noted that postmenopausal patients may have withdrawl bleeding when on cyclic

Table 90.15.
Current Hormonal Replacement Therapy Regimen

Drug	Regimen	Reference
A. *Cyclic Sequential (Estrogen days 1–25 + Progestin days 13–16 through 25)*		
1. Conjugated estrogens or equivalent[a] (CDOC)[b]	0.625 mg daily days 1–25 per month	44 (see Table 90.12)
PLUS		
Medroxyprogesterone acetate or equivalent[c] (CDOC)	2.5–10 mg days 13–16 through 25 each month	59, 60
2. Conjugated estrogens or equivalent[a]	0.3 mg days 1 through 25 each month	45
PLUS		
Medroxyprogesterone acetate or equivalent[c]	2.5–10 mg days 13–16 through 25 each month	59, 60
AND		
daily elemental calcium intake	1500 mg daily	45
B. *Cyclic Combined (Estrogen days 1–25 + Progestin days 1–25)*		
C. *Continuous Sequential (Estrogen taken daily + Progestin taken days 1–12)*		
D. *Continuous Combined (Estrogen daily + Progestin daily)*		
3. Conjugated estrogens or equivalent[a,d]	0.625 mg daily	55
PLUS		
Medroxyprogesterone acetate or equivalent[c,d]	2.5–5.0 mg daily	55
4. Depomedroxy-progesterone acetate[e]	150 mg intramuscularly monthly	46
5. Levonorgestrel plus ethinyl estradiol triphasic oral contraceptive[f]	daily days 1 through 21 each month	47

[a] 97% of women with intact uteri will experience withdrawal bleeding with this regimen until age 60, and 60% of those age 60–65 will experience withdrawal bleeding (55).

[b] CDOC, clinical drug of choice.

[c] Norethindrone or norethindrone acetate 0.7–1 mg; *dl*-norgestrel 150 μg; micronized oral progesterone 150 mg twice daily (55). Further studies are ongoing to find optimal doses of all progestins (59, 60).

[d] There is no convincing proof that continuous/combined therapy reduces progestin-induced problems as compared with sequential regimens (55).

[e] Depo-medroxyprogesterone acetate usually may be used where estrogens are contraindicated. Etidronate (48), nasal salmon calcitonin (51), and calcium carbonate alone (42) may also be of benefit for patients who cannot use estrogens.

[f] Needs further study and should be last choice.

regimens of estrogen and progestin (see Table 90.15), as long as they have intact uteri.

The Role of Progestins in Hormonal Replacement Therapy

There are three reasons for adding progestin to HRT therapy: (1) to reduce the risk of estrogen-induced irregular bleeding, endometrial hyperplasia, and carcinoma; (2) to protect against breast carcinoma; and (3) to enhance the effect on bone conservation. Unequivocal data showing that progestins favorably modify the response of the breast and the skeleton to estrogens are lacking, and endometrial protection remains the only well-substantiated reason for adding progestin to estrogen regimens (55).

When used sequentially for 10 to 13 days per month, endometrial protection should occur for most patients with medroxyprogesterone acetate 10 mg, or norethindrone or norethindrone acetate 0.7 to 1.0 mg, or dl-norgestrel 150 mcg, or micronized progesterone 300 mg (55).

Many patients will experience some unwanted progestational effects: breast tenderness, bloating, edema, abdominal cramping, anxiety, irritability, and depression. The C-19-nortestosterone derivatives such as norgestrel, norethindrone, or norethindrone acetate possess some androgenic activity and thus tend to be associated with acne and greasy skin and hair. The C-21 derivatives such as medroxyprogesterone acetate are less androgenic and are more likely to be associated with depression and anxiety (55).

Oral micronized progesterone, although an attractive alternative, has a significant first-pass hepatic metabolism and therefore requires large doses and twice-daily administration. Progesterone 200 to 300 mg per day causes drowsiness in approximately 30% of patients (55). A recent study used 21 days of percutaneous 17 β-estradiol gel in a dose of 1.5 mg (low dose) for the first 6 months and 3.0 mg (high dose) for 25 days if needed to control menopausal symptoms with various doses of natural micronized progesterone. Maximal reduction of mitoses was noted on biopsies taken after 11 days of progestin. No hyperplasia was observed after 5 to 7 years of either 11 days of 200 mg or 300 mg of natural micronized progesterone (56).

In an effort to reduce patient's exposure to medroxyprogesterone side effects, cyclic hormone replacement using quarterly progestin was tried in 199 women given conjugated estrogen 0.625 mg daily and quarterly medroxyprogesterone 10 mg daily for 14 days over 1 year after having been on conjugated estrogens 0.625 mg per day with monthly cyclic medroxyprogesterone 5 or 10 mg for 1 to 5.4 years (mean 5.4 +/– 4.5 years). Endometrial hyperplasia at baseline was 0.9% and after 1 year was 1.5%. Quarterly medroxyprogesterone resulted in longer menses (7.7 +/– 2.9 versus 5.4 +/– 2.0 days) and more reports of heavier menses (31.1 versus 8.0%). Of interest, despite these problems, women preferred the quarterly regimen by nearly four to one (57).

Unfortunately, when the same researchers tried biannual medroxyprogesterone, the incidence of endometrial hyperplasia was not acceptable (Unpublished data, 1994).

Probably the greatest benefit of HRT is reduction of the risk of death from cardiovascular disease even in women normally considered to be at high risk from obesity, previous angina, or hypertension (58). It is feared that the addition of a progestin may negate the beneficial estrogen effects and possibly increase the risk of cardiovascular disease. Therefore, the minimum dose of progestin for endometrial protection should be prescribed (59).

There is also no proof that continuous, combined therapy of estrogen with progestin on a daily basis reduces the progestin-induced problems compared with sequential regimens. Additionally, there is a high incidence of vaginal bleeding in 18 to 58% of patients in 12 studies reported so far. With unopposed estrogen regimens, approximately 25% of patients experience regular withdrawl bleeding

Table 90.16.

Bleeding Patterns with Continuous Combined or Sequential Regimens of Conjugated Estrogens with Medroxyprogesterone Acetate[a]

Regimen (Estrogen/Progestin)	% Amenorrhea	% Spot-BTB
1. Continuous combined 0.625 mg/ 2.5 mg	61.4	22.3
2. Continuous combined 0.625 mg/ 5.0 mg	72.8	12.7
3. Continuous sequential 0.625 mg daily/5.0 mg days 15–28	16.1	8.1
4. Continuous sequential 0.625 mg daily/10.0 mg days 15–28	18.8	8.3
5. Continuous 0.625 mg and placebo	75.5	14.6

[a]Archer DF, Pickar JH, Bottiglioni F. Bleeding patterns in postmenopausal women taking continuous combined or sequential regimens of conjugated estrogens with medroxyprogesterone acetate. Obstet Gynecol 83:686–692, 1994.

Table 90.17.

Incidence of Endometrial Hyperplasia in Continuous Combined, Continuous Sequential Conjugated Estrogens with Medroxyprogesterone Acetate and Conjugated Estrogen Alone Regimens[a]

Regimen (Estrogen/Progestin)	Percent at 6 Months	12 Months
1. Continuous combined 0.625 mg/2.5 mg	<1	<1
2. Continuous combined 0.625 mg/5.0 mg	<1	<1
3. Continuous sequential 0.625 mg daily 5.0 mg days 15–28	<1	<1
4. Continuous sequential 0.625 mg daily 10.0 mg days 15–28	<1	<1
5. Continuous 0.625 mg and placebo	7	20

[a]Data from Woodruff JD, Pickar JH. Incidence of endometrial hyperplasia in postmenopausal women taking conjugated estrogens (Premarin) with medroxyprogesterone acetate or conjugated estrogens alone. Am J Obstet Gynecol 170:1213–1223, 1994.

during each cycle of HRT. With sequential therapies, regular bleeding occurs in about 85% of patients, appearing as a light, predictable bleeding lasting 4 to 5 days. Over time, the bleeding often becomes lighter and shorter, and in some patients amenorrhea develops (60). Table 90.16 summarizes the bleeding patterns from a 1-year, double-blind, randomized study done with 1724 postmenopausal women over 1 year (61).

Table 90.17 summarizes the incidences of endometrial hyperplasia from various HRT regimens versus continuous ERT at 6 and 12 months of treatment (62). Table 90.15 summarizes current HRT regimens to prevent osteoporosis.

CONCLUSION

The pharmacotherapies of gynecologic disorders afford varying degrees of clinical efficacy. For example, prostaglandin inhibitors are very successful in the treatment of primary dysmenorrhea. At the other end of the spectrum is the marginal success of pharmacotherapy of the premenstrual syndrome. Somewhere in between lies the success of the pharmacotherapies of endometriosis, the vulvovaginitides, and the disorders resulting from estrogen deficiency.

Three major clinical dilemmas result from these pharmacotherapies. First, the adequate treatment of the premenstrual syndrome remains elusive. Second, the validity and safety of long-term estrogen replacement with or without progestin opposition for the prevention of osteoporosis and cardiovascular disease needs further study. Finally, although not unique to gynecology, the dilemma of the teratogenic potential of all pharmacotherapies must be continually evaluated and reevaluated in women in their reproductive years.

REFERENCES

1. Smith RP. Drug therapy for dysmenorrhea. IMJ 169:22–25, 1986.

2. Dawood MY. Dysmenorrhea. Clin Obstet Gynecol 33(1):168–178, 1990.

3. Anon. Dysmenorrhea. ACOG Tech Bull 68:1–5, 1983.

4. Ekstrom P, Juchnicka E, Laudanski T, et al. Effect of an oral contraceptive in primary dysmenorrhea—changes in uterine activity and reactivity to agonists. Contraception 40(1):39–47, 1989.

5. Kleber HD, Kosten TR. Use of clonidine for dysmenorrhea in four patients. Psychosomatics 26:539–546, 1985.

6. Chihal HJ. Premenstrual syndrome: an update for the clinician. Obstet Gynecol Clin North Am 17(2):457–479, 1990.

7. Smith MA, Youngkin EQ. Managing the premenstrual syndrome. Clin Pharm 5:788–797, 1986.

8. Maddocks S, Hahn P, Moller F, et al. A double-blind placebo controlled trial of progesterone vaginal suppositories in the treatment of premenstrual syndrome. Am J Obstet Gynecol 154:573–581, 1986.

9. Freeman EW, Rickels K, Sondheimer SJ, Polansky M. A double-blind trial of oral progesterone, alprazolam and placebo in treatment of severe premenstrual syndrome. JAMA 274(1):51–57, 1995.

10. Brown CS, Ling FW, Andersen RN, et al. Efficacy of depot leuprolide in premenstrual syndrome: effect of symptom severity and type in a controlled trial. Obstet Gynecol 84(5):779–786, 1994.

11. True BL, Goodner SM, Burns EA. Review of the etiology and treatment of premenstrual syndrome. Drug Intell Clin Pharm 19:714–722, 1985.

12. Harrison W, Sharpe L, Endicott J. Treatment of premenstrual symptoms. Gen Hosp Psychiatry 7:54–65, 1985.

13. Pariser SF, Stern SL, Shank ML, et al. Premenstrual Syndrome: concerns, controversies and treatment. Am J Obstet Gynecol 153:599–604, 1985.

14. Smith S, Schiff I. The premenstrual syndrome-diagnosis and management. Fertil Steril 52(4):527–543, 1989.

15. Mortola JF. A risk-benefit appraisal of drugs used in the management of premenstrual syndrome. Drug Safety 10(2):160–169, 1994.

16. Anon. Endometriosis. ACOG Tech Bull 184:1–6, 1993.

17. Markham SM, Carpenter SE, Rock JA. Extrapelvic endometriosis. Obstet Gynecol Clin North Am 16(1):193–219, 1989.

18. Galle PC. Clinical presentation and diagnosis of endometriosis. Obstet Gynecol Clin North Am 16(1):29–41, 1989.

19. Guzick DS. Clinical epidemiology of endometriosis and infertility. Obstet Gynecol Clin North Am 16(1):43–59, 1989.

20. Metzger DA and Luciano AA. Hormonal therapy of endometriosis. Obstet Gynecol Clin North Am 16(1):105–121, 1989.

21. Erickson LD, Ory SJ. GnRH analogues in the treatment of endometriosis. Obstet Gynecol Clin North Am 16(1):123–145, 1989.

22. Gardner HL. Infectious vulvovaginitis. In: Monif GR, ed. Infectious Diseases in Obstetrics and Gynecology, 2nd ed. Philadelphia: Harper and Row, 1982:515.

23. Sweet RL. Importance of differential diagnosis in acute vaginitis. Am J Obstet Gynecol 152:945–947, 1985.

24. Anon. Sexually transmitted diseases treatment guidelines. MMWR 42 (RR-14):1–102, 1993.

25. Ritter W. Pharmacokinetic fundamentals of vaginal treatment with clotrimazole. Am J Obstet Gynecol 152:945–947, 1985.

26. Anderson GM, Barrat J, Bergan T, et al. A comparison of single-dose oral fluconazole with 3-day intravaginal clotrimazole in the treatment of vaginal candidiasis. Report of an international multicentre trial. Br J Obstet Gynecol 96:226–232, 1989.

27. Sobel JD. Epidemiology and pathogenesis of recurrent vulvovaginal candidiasis. Am J Obstet Gynecol 152:924–934, 1985.

28. Fregoso-Duenas F. Ketoconazole in vulvovaginal candidosis. Rev Infect Dis 2:620–624, 1980.

29. Lynch PJ. Condylomata acuminata (anogenital warts). Clin Obstet Gynecol 28:142–151, 1985.

30. Anon. Genital human papillomavirus infections. ACOG Tech Bull 193:1–7, 1994.

31. Ferenczy A. Comparison of 5-fluorouracil and CO2 laser for treatment of vaginal condylomata. Obstet Gynecol 64:773–778, 1984.

32. Place VA, Powers M, Darley PE, et al. A double-blind comparative study of Estraderm and Premarin in the amelioration of postmenopausal symptoms. Am J Obstet Gynecol 152:1092–1099, 1985.

33. Schiff I, Tulchinsky D, Cramer D, et al. Oral medroxyprogesterone in the treatment of postmenopausal symptoms. JAMA 244:1443–1445, 1980.

34. Laufer LR, Erlik Y, Meldrum DR, et al. Effect of clonidine on hot flashes in postmenopausal women. Obstet Gynecol 60:583–586, 1982.

35. Dyer GI, Townsend PT. Dose related changes in vaginal cytology after topical conjugated equine oestrogens. Br Med J 284:789, 1982.

36. DeFazio J, Speroff L. Estrogen replacement therapy: current thinking and practice. Geriatrics 40:32–48, 1985.

37. Anon. Hormone replacement therapy. ACOG Tech Bull 166:1–8, 1992.

38. Gambrell RD. Cancer and the use of estrogens. Int J Fertil 31:112–122, 1986.

39. Henderson BE, Ross RK, Paganini-Hill A, et al. Estrogen use and cardiovascular disease. Am J Obstet Gynecol 154:1181–1186, 1986.

40. The Writing Group for the PEPI Trial. Effects of estrogen or estrogen/progestin regimens on heart disease risk factors in postmenopausal women. JAMA 273:199-208, 1995.

41. Anon. Recommended Dietary Allowances, 10th ed. Washington, D.C.: National Academy Press, 1989:180.

42. Dawson-Hughes B, Dallal GE, Krall EA, et al. A controlled trial of the effect of calcium supplementation on bone density in postmenopausal women. N Engl J Med 323:878–883, 1990.

43. Bauwens SF, Drinka PJ, Boh L. Pathogenesis and management of primary osteoporosis. Clin Pharm 5:639–659, 1986.

44. Lindsay R, Hart M, Clark DM. The minimum effective dose of estrogen for the prevention of postmenopausal bone loss. Obstet Gynecol 63:759–763, 1984.

45. Gordan GS, Gennant, HK. The aging skeleton. Clin Geriatr Med 1:95–118, 1985.

46. Lobo RA, McCormick W, Singer F, et al. Depo-medroxyprogesterone acetate compared with conjugated estrogens for the treatment of postmenopausal women. Obstet Gynecol 63:1–5, 1984.

47. Shargil AA. Hormone replacement therapy in perimenopausal women on a triphasic contraceptive compound: a three year prospective study. Int J Fertil 30:15–28, 1985.

48. Harris ST, Watts NB, Jackson RD, et al. Four-year study of intermittent cyclic etidronate treatment of postmenopausal osteoporosis: Three years of blinded therapy followed by one year of open therapy. Am J Med 95:557–567, 1993.

49. Wimalawansa SJ. Combined therapy with estrogen and etidronate has an additive effect on bone mineral density in the hip and vertebrae: Four-year randomized study. Am J Med 99:36–42, 1995.

50. Chestnut CH III, McClung MR, Ensrud KE, et al. Alendronate treatment of the postmenopausal osteoporotic woman: Effect of multiple dosages on bone mass and bone remodeling. Am J Med 99:144–152, 1995.

51. Overgaard K, Riis BJ, Christiansen C, et al. Nasal calcitonin for the treatment of established osteoporosis. Clin Endocrin 30:435–442, 1989.

52. Ribot C, Tremollieres JM, Louvet JP, et al. Preventive effects of transdermal administration of 17-beta-estradiol on postmenopausal bone loss: A 2-year prospective study. Obstet Gynecol 75(suppl):42-55, 1990.

53. Stanczyk FZ, Shoupe D, Nunez V, et al. A randomized comparison of nonoral estradiol delivery in postmenopausal women. Am J Obstet Gynecol 159:1540–1546, 1988.

54. Erenus M, Kutlay K, Kutlay L, Pekin S. Comparison of the impact of oral versus transdermal estrogen on serum lipoproteins. Fertil Steril 61(2):300–302, 1994.

55. Whitehead MI, Hillard TC, Crook D. The role and use of progestogens. Obstet Gynecol 75(suppl):59–76, 1990.

56. Moyer DL, de Lignieres B, Driguez P, Pez JP. Prevention of endometrial hyperplasia by progesterone during long-term estradiol replacement: influence of bleeding pattern and secretory changes. Fertil Steril 59:992–997, 1993.

57. Ettinger B, Seby J, Citron JT, et al. Cyclic hormone replacement therapy using quarterly progestin. Obstet Gynecol 83:693–700, 1994.

58. Henderson BE, Ross RK, Paganini-Hill A. Estrogen use and cardiovascular disease. J Reprod Med 30(suppl):814–820, 1985.

59. Gambrell RD. Clinical use of progestins in the menopausal patient. J Reprod Med 27:531–538, 1982.

60. Lane G, Siddle NC, Ryder TA, et al. Is Provera the ideal progestogen for addition to postmenopausal estrogen therapy? Fertil Steril 45:345–352, 1986.

61. Archer DF, Pickar JH, Bottiglioni F. Bleeding patterns in postmenopausal women taking continuous combined or sequential regimens of conjugated estrogens with medroxyprogesterine acetate. Obstet Gynecol 83:686–692, 1994.

62. Woodruff JD, Pickar JH. Incidence of endometrial hyperplasia in postmenopausal women taking conjugated estrogens (Premarin) with medroxyprogesterone acetate or conjugated estrogens alone. Am J Obstet Gynecol 170:1213–1223, 1994.

CHAPTER 91

CONTRACEPTION AND INFERTILITY

JANNET M. CARMICHAEL and KARI A. WIELAND

HORMONAL BIRTH CONTROL

The use of female sex hormones to prevent the development of the female egg was suggested as early as 1940, but it was not until 1956, after the discovery of norethynodrel, that field trials were begun on what we now know as birth control pills ("the pill"). In 1960, the U.S. Food and Drug Administration (FDA) first approved the use of the combination pill. Over 50 million women in the United States have used oral contraceptives since their introduction in 1960. Today about 70 million women worldwide (13 million in the United States) use oral contraceptive products. Almost one fourth of American women 15 to 44 years of age take oral contraceptives. The pill remains a safe and acceptable contraceptive method for many women. The popularity of the pill undoubtedly relates to both its theoretical and use effectiveness (Table 91.1). In order to understand the many aspects of hormonal birth control, it is necessary to review the physiology of the menstrual cycle and the development of estrogens and progestins used in contraceptive products.

The Menstrual Cycle

The average menstrual cycle (Fig. 91.1) lasts 28 days. Several organ systems are involved in this cycle. The changes that occur at the ovaries during this 28-day cycle can be divided into three phases: the follicular phase, ovulation, and the luteal phase.

The follicular phase occupies about the first 14 days of the cycle. At the beginning of this phase, several follicles, each containing an oocyte, begin to enlarge, first independently and then in response to pituitary follicle-stimulating hormone (FSH). After 5 or 6 days one of the follicles begins to develop more rapidly. The granulosa cells of this follicle multiply, and under the influence of FSH and pituitary luteinizing hormone (LH), synthesize and release estrogens from the ovary at an increasing rate. Peripheral levels of estradiol begin to rise significantly by cycle day 7. The estrogens appear to inhibit FSH before midcycle (a negative feedback inhibition system); however, the high level and rate of increase of estrogen stimulates a surge of FSH and LH at the end of this phase, which in turn causes final-stage growth and rupture of the ovum (ovulation).

Ovulation ordinarily occurs at midcycle, on day 14 or 15. The onset of the LH surge appears to be the most reliable indicator of impending ovulation, occurring 34 to 36 hours prior to follicle rupture. Ovulation is triggered by the rapid peripheral rise in estradiol. At the time of ovulation, the granulosa cells of the follicle begin to secrete progesterone.

The luteal phase follows. Under the influence of LH, the ruptured follicle fills with blood and the surrounding theca and granulosa cells proliferate and replace the blood to form the corpus luteum. The cells of this structure produce estrogens and progesterone for the remainder of the cycle unless pregnancy occurs. If pregnancy does not occur during this cycle, the corpus luteum begins to degenerate and ceases hormone production. This drop in serum level of estrogens and progesterone results in endometrial shedding (menstruation) and the beginning of a new cycle. If pregnancy does occur, the corpus luteum remains active because it is stimulated by human chorionic gonadotropin (hCG) derived from the developing placenta, thus maintaining the high levels of progesterone and estrogen necessary for pregnancy.

The changes that occur in the uterus over the 28-day cycle can also be divided into three phases:

1. The menstrual phase starts on day 1 of the menstrual cycle with the sloughing of the old endometrium and the onset of vaginal bleeding. This phase lasts 3 to 6 days.
2. The proliferative phase is a period of growth of the endometrial lining lasting from day 6 to day 14. Estrogens from the developing follicles are responsible for this growth as well as for the growth of uterine glands and the proliferation of uterine vessels.
3. The secretory phase is primarily under the influence of progesterone. During this phase, the endometrium becomes thicker and is held in place, the uterine glands branch, and the secretory function of these glands begins. The endometrium would be prepared for implantation if pregnancy occurred.

The Estrogens

The major natural estrogens produced by women are estradiol, estrone, and estriol. Estradiol is the major secretory product of the ovary. Some estrone is also produced in the ovary, although most of it (and estriol) is formed in the liver from estradiol or converted in the peripheral tissues.

Several synthetic estrogens have been manufactured. Compared to natural estrogens, synthetic estrogens have increased biopotency when administered orally. Ethinyl estradiol administered orally is at least 200 times more

Table 91.1.
Contraceptive Effectiveness

Method	% of Women Experiencing an Accidental Pregnancy within the First Year of Use		% of Women Continuing Use at One Year
	Typical Use[a]	Perfect Use[b]	
Chance	85	85	
Spermicides	21	6	43
Periodic abstinence	20		67
Calendar		9	
Ovulation method		3	
Symptothermal		2	
Postovulation		1	
Withdrawal	19	4	
Cap			
Parous	36	26	45
Nulliparous	18	9	58
Sponge[d]			
Parous	36	20	45
Nulliparous	18	9	58
Diaphragm	18	6	58
Condom			
Female (Reality)	21	5	56
Male	12	3	63
Pill	3		72
Progestin only		0.5	
Combined		0.1	
IUD			
Progesterone T	2.0	1.5	81
Copper T 380A	0.8	0.6	78
LNg[d]	0.1	0.1	81
Depo-Provera	0.3	0.3	70
Norplant (6 capsules)	0.09	0.09	85
Female sterilization	0.4	0.4	100
Male sterilization	0.15	0.10	100

[a]Among *typical* couples who initiate use of a method (not necessarily for the first time), the percentage who experience an accidental pregnancy during the first year if they do not stop use for any other reason.

[b]Among couples who initiate use of a method (not necessarily for the first time) and who use it *perfectly* (both consistently and correctly), the percentage who experience an accidental pregnancy during the first year if they do not stop use for any other reason.

[c]Among couples attempting to avoid pregnancy, the percentage who continue to use a method for one year.

[d]Not marketed in the U.S.

Adapted with permission from Hatcher RA (2).

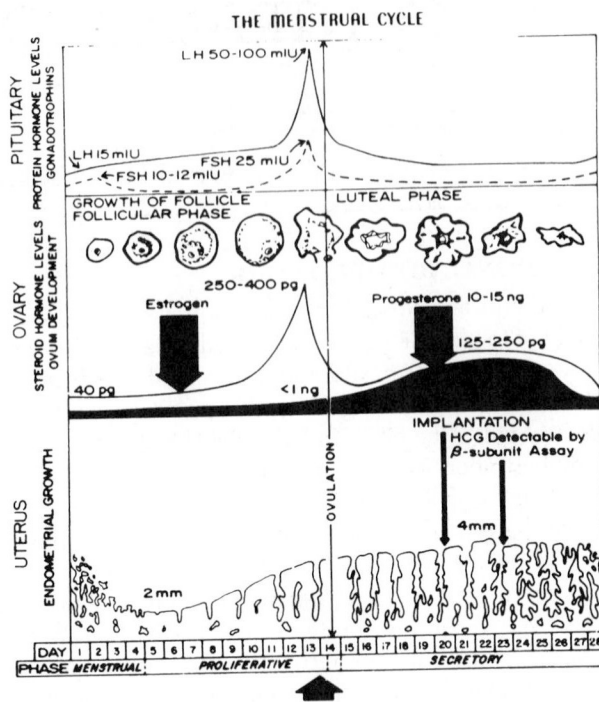

Figure 91.1. The menstrual cycle. (From Hatcher RA, Stewart GK, Guest F, Finkelstein R, Godwin C. Contraceptive technology 1976–1977. New York: Irvington Publishers, 1976; reproduced with permission.)

was once used extensively in early contraceptives, it is now seldom used due to reduced efficacy at doses below 50 μg.

Ethinyl estradiol undergoes extensive first-pass hepatic metabolism, which can result in considerable patient-to-patient variation in plasma and urine steroid concentrations. Circulating ethinyl estradiol is highly bound to albumin. It is metabolized by hepatic cytochrome P-450 oxidation. Ethinyl estradiol undergoes enterohepatic circulation and is excreted into the bile, deconjugated in the gastrointestinal system, and reabsorbed into the bloodstream. This may result in a rebound in blood levels of estrogen 10 to 14 hours after administration. The most commonly used doses of ethinyl estradiol in combined oral contraceptives are 30 to 40 μg/day.

The Progestins

Progesterone is the most important natural progestin and also serves as a precursor to the estrogens, androgens, and adrenocortical steroids. Progesterone is rapidly absorbed following parenteral administration but is poorly absorbed when given orally. Its half-life in plasma is from 3 to 90 minutes. As is the case with estrogens, it is partially stored in body fat and is almost completely metabolized in one passage through the liver. To overcome these problems, synthetic progestins were developed for use in oral contraceptives. The synthetic progestins available in oral

potent than estradiol. Only two synthetic estrogens are used in all of the various oral contraceptives on the U.S. market-ethinyl estradiol and mestranol. Ethinyl estradiol is estradiol with an ethinyl group at the 17α position. Mestranol, in addition, has a methyl group at the 3α position (Fig. 91.2).

Mestranol is metabolized in the liver to ethinyl estradiol. The amount and extent of this metabolism may vary from patient to patient. Strictly speaking, mestranol is slightly less potent than the same microgram weight of ethinyl estradiol. For practical purposes these two estrogens can be considered nearly equally potent. While mestranol

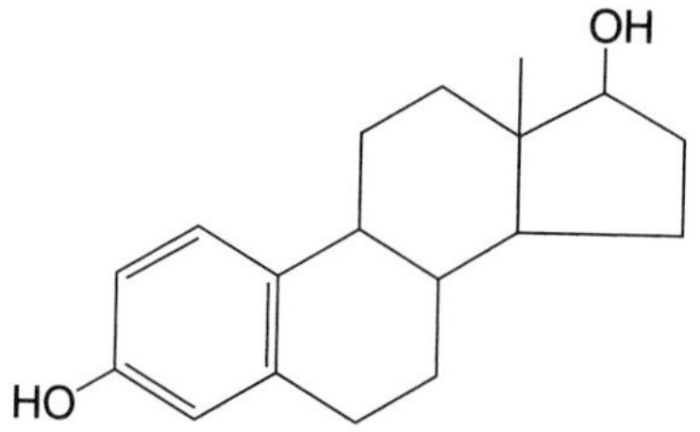

Figure 91.2. Configuration of major estrogens.

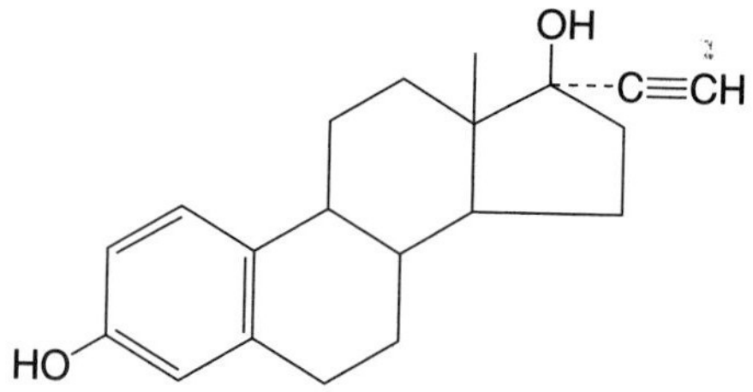

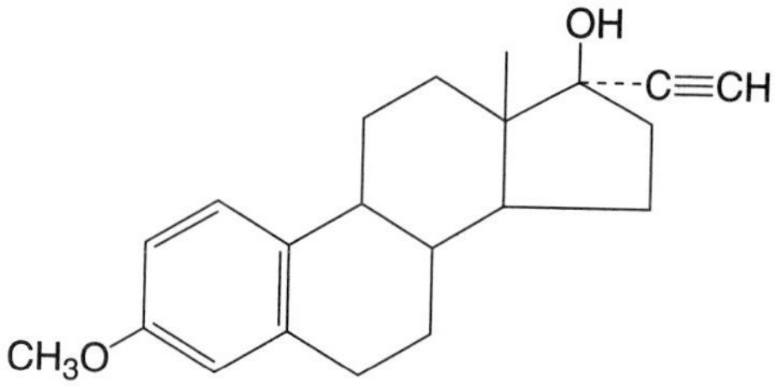

contraceptives are 19-norandrogens derived from testosterone (Fig. 91.3). There are fundamentally two types of progestins: (a) those structurally related norethindrone, and (b) derivatives of levonorgestrel.

Progestins structurally related to norethindrone include norethynodrel, norethindrone acetate, and ethynodiol diacetate. Considering the wide use of oral contraceptives, relatively little is known about the metabolism of these related compounds. Most of these structurally related products are thought to be converted to the parent compound, norethindrone, in the liver. Norethindrone is then converted and excreted as sulfates and glucuronide. Based on the ability to inhibit ovulation in clinical practice, any of the norethindrone group are considered microgram for microgram, equipotent. The minimum antiovulatory dose of norethindrone is approximately 500 μg. Wide ranges of oral bioavailability have been reported for norethindrone due to intersubject variability of first pass metabolism.

As first introduced, norgestrel was a mixture of d- and l-isomers. It has since been recognized that activity rests entirely with the levo form. Original products still contain the racemetric norgestrel, but newer products contain half the amount of levonorgestrel. There is enhanced potency of levonorgestrel and its derivatives of about fivefold to tenfold compared with norethindrone. Also, there is convincing evidence that levonorgestrel is considerably more androgenic than is norethindrone. However, there is no clear-cut evidence to show that norethindrone has an estrogenic effect. Approximately 150 μg of levonorgestrel is required to inhibit ovulation. Consistent and complete absorption may be important to reduce the level of breakthrough bleeding and drug interactions in products containing levonorgestrel (Table 91.2).

Three derivatives of levonorgestrel represent the newest generation of orally active progestins: desogestrel, norgestimate and gestodene. It appears that neither desogestrel nor gestodene is converted to levonorgestrel, but norgestimate may undergo this transformation. However, one metabolite of norgestimate, 17-deacetyl norgestimate, is likely to contribute to its pharmacologic response. Gestodene is present in high concentrations in serum after its oral administration and does not appear to be a prodrug. Desogestrel is rapidly converted to 3-keto-desogestrel and is present in high circulating concentrations.

The bioavailability, half-life, and mean binding of sex hormone–binding globulin (SHBG) can be seen for these metabolically active steroids in Table 91.2. SHBG normally binds free testosterone. Agents with high SHBG binding affinity may compete for free testosterone and lead to a increase of free (active) testosterone levels and its side affects. Levonorgestrel and in particular gestodene have markedly high binding affinity for SHBG. It is important to realize that relatively few metabolites have been identified for any steroid to date and that such work is painstakingly difficult and time-consuming. For example, while it seems likely that 17-deacetyl norgestimate, together with the parent compound, contributes significantly to the response of norgestimate, neither of these compounds has a high affinity for SHBG. However, some other metabolites of norgestimate bind strongly to SHBG, and at present it is unknown what effect these metabolites have on the androgenicity of combination oral contraceptive products containing this progestin.

Steroids may also have a direct effect on the SHBG serum levels. SHBG levels in women during combination oral contraceptive (COC) use are considered a measurement of the relative estrogen and androgen activities of the combined product, since estrogens elevate and androgens lower SHBG levels. Limited data are available on the effects of progestins alone on serum SHBG. Elevations in serum SHBG would generally be expected to cause an increase in bound testosterone and a decrease in free

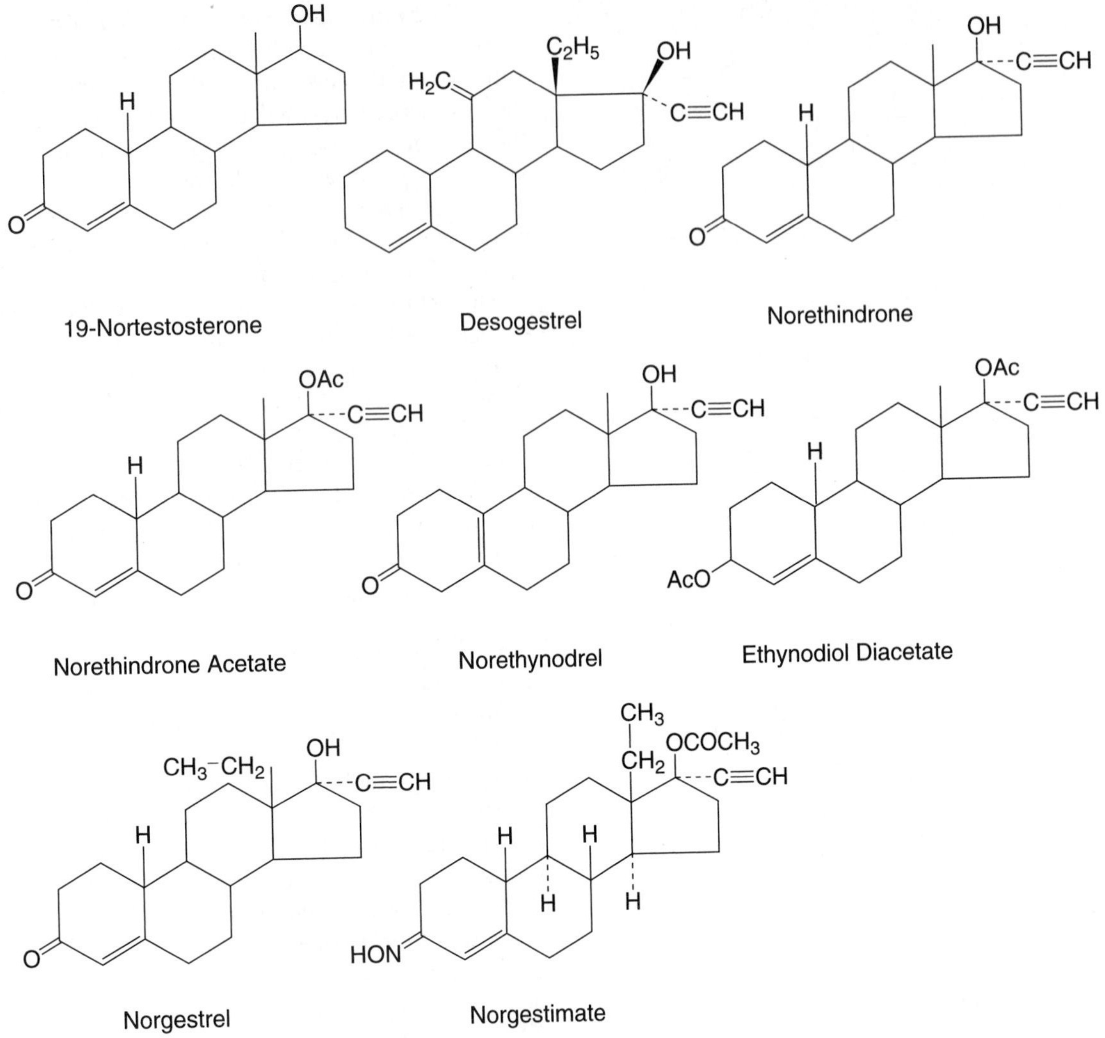

19-Nortestosterone   Desogestrel   Norethindrone

Norethindrone Acetate   Norethynodrel   Ethynodiol Diacetate

Norgestrel   Norgestimate

Figure 91.3.   Configuration of synthetic progestin.

Table 91.2.
Pharmacokinetics of Oral Contraceptive Steroids

Steroid	Bioavailability[a] (%)	$t_{1/2}$ (h)[a]	Relative Potency (μg)[a]	SHBG Relative Binding Affinity[b]
Ethinyl Estradiol	40–50	10		1
Norethindrone°	65	7.5	500	5
Levonorgestrel	100	11.4	150	7.5
Gestodene†	100	10–13	40	N/A
Desogestrel	75	N/A	60	1.75
3-Keto desogestrel‡	N/A	10–13	N/A	—
Norgestimate	90–100	45–71	250	—
17-deacetyl norgestimate‡	N/A	16–17	N/A	—

[a]Adapted from Lobo RA, Stanczyk FZ. Am J Obstet Gynecol 170:1499–1507, 1994.
[b]Adapted from McClamrock HD, Adashi EY. Am J Obstet Gynecol 168:1021–1028, 1993.
°Large intersubject and intrasubject variability exists
†Available only in Europe
‡Metabolite studied because of rapid hepatic metabolism to this compound

Table 91.3.
Biologic Activity of Oral Contraceptive Components

Class Compound	Progestational Activity[a]	Estrogenic Activity[b]	Androgenic Activity[c]
Progestins[d]			
19-Nor-testosterone progestins			
Estrane			
Norethindrone	1.0	1.0	1.0
Norethindrone acetate	1.2	1.5	1.6
Ethynodiol diacetate	1.4	3.4	0.6
5(10) Estrane			
Norethynodrel	0.3	8.3	0
Gonane			
Levonorgestrel	5.3	0	8.3
dl-Norgestrel	2.6	0	4.2
Norgestimate	1.3	0	1.9
Desogestrel	9.0	0	3.4
Gestodene	12.6	0	8.6
Pregnane progestins			
Chlormadinone acetate	1.0	0	0
Megestrol acetate	0.4	0	0
Medroxyprogesterone acetate	0.3	0	0
Estrogens[e]			
Ethinyl estradiol	0	100	0
Mestranol	0	67	0

[a]Based on amount required to induce vacuoles in human endometrium. Desogestrel, gestodene, levonorgestrel, and norgestimate based on oral stimulation of endometrium in immature estrogen-primed rabbits relative to levonorgestrel.
[b]Comparative potency based on oral rat vaginal epithelium assay.
[c]Comparative potency (oral) based on rat ventral prostate assay.
[d]Calculated on the basis of norethindrone = 1.0 in activity.
[e]Calculated on the basis of ethinyl estradiol = 100 in activity.
Adapted from Dickey (1).

testosterone, thereby causing a decrease in androgenicity profile. Estrogens in COCs induce elevation in circulating levels of SHBG, whereas progestins may significantly reduce these levels. In general, COC doses of ethinyl estradiol cause a three-to fourfold increase in the circulating levels of SHBG. Therefore, the net effect on SHBG levels in women taking COCs depends on the dose of estrogen, the type and amount of progestin, and the progestin's binding affinity to SHBG. In contrast, a comparable increase in corticosteroid-binding globulin (CSBG) is observed for all low-dose estrogen COCs, confirming that CSBG levels are estrogen dependent regardless of the progestin component.

Lower doses of the new progestins can be used to inhibit ovulation compared to levonorgestrel and especially norethindrone. Low doses of progestins produce an antifertility effect but not an antiovulatory effect. A much larger progestin dose is required for an antiovulatory effect. Comparative biologic activity has been assessed by a variety of assay methods (Table 91.3). Note that some progestins have estrogenic activity in addition to progestin effects. When these progestins are combined with an estrogen in combination pills, the resulting product is more estrogenic than a similar product with a different progestin.

The "Pill"

Two basic types of preparations are available for use as oral contraceptives: (a) the combination pill, and (b) the mini-pill. Combination oral contraceptives (COCs) are subdivided into fixed combination (monophasic), biphasic, and triphasic products. Monophasic contraceptive pills contain a fixed ratio of estrogen and progestin given daily for 21 days.

Biphasic products contain a fixed dose of estrogen (days 1–21) with a lower progestin dose on days 1 to 10 than on days 11 to 21. Only two such products are available on the U.S. market. Four triphasic products are currently available in the United States. In the triphasic pills, progestin is given throughout the cycle, the dose being increased only at midcycle in one and in the last 7 to 10 days in the other three products. Note that the dose of estrogen is fixed in three products and increased at midcycle in a fourth product (Table 91.4).

The triphasic pills are a response to the evidence that the safest combined oral contraceptive would use the lowest possible dose of both synthetic steroids. In Triphasil, for example, the progestin intake is 39% less than that in the lowest COC containing levonorgestrel. However, several fixed-dose monophasic formulations currently marketed have a lower total dose of norethindrone than the

Table 91.4.
Oral Contraceptives Available in the United States

Trade Name	Manufacturer	Estrogen	µg	Progestin	mg
Fixed Combination Contraceptives					
>50 µg of Estrogen					
Enovid 10 mg°	Searle	mestranol	150	norethynodrel	9.85
Enovid 5 mg°	Searle	mestranol	75	norethynodrel	5
50 µg of Estrogen					
Ovral	Wyeth	ethinyl estradiol	50	norgestrel	0.5
Demulen 1/50	Searle	ethinyl estradiol	50	ethynodiol diacetate	1
Ovcon-50	Mead Johnson	ethinyl estradiol	50	norethindrone	1
Genora 1/50	Rugby	mestranol	50	norethindrone	1
Nelova 1/50 M	Warner Chilcott	mestranol	50	norethindrone	1
Norethin 1/50 M	Searle	mestranol	50	norethindrone	1
Norinyl 1+50	Syntex	mestranol	50	norethindrone	1
Ortho-Novum 1/50	Ortho	mestranol	50	norethindrone	1
<50 µg of Estrogen					
Demulen 1/35	Searle	ethinyl estradiol	35	ethynodiol diacetate	1
Genora 1/35	Rugby	ethinyl estradiol	35	norethindrone	1
N.E.E. 1/35	MetroMed	ethinyl estradiol	35	norethindrone	1
Nelova 1/35E	Warner Chilcott	ethinyl estradiol	35	norethindrone	1
Norethin 1/35E	Searle	ethinyl estradiol	35	norethindrone	1
Norinyl 1/35	Syntex	ethinyl estradiol	35	norethindrone	1
Ortho-Novum 1/35	Ortho	ethinyl estradiol	35	norethindrone	1
Brevicon	Syntex	ethinyl estradiol	35	norethindrone	0.5
Genora 0.5/35	Rugby	ethinyl estradiol	35	norethindrone	0.5
Modicon	Ortho	ethinyl estradiol	35	norethindrone	0.5
Nelova 0.5/35E	Warner Chilcott	ethinyl estradiol	35	norethindrone	0.5
Ovcon-35	Mead Johnson	ethinyl estradiol	35	norethindrone	0.4
Ortho Cyclen	Ortho		35	norgestimate	0.25
Lo-Ovral	Wyeth	ethinyl estradiol	30	norgestrel	0.4
Levlen	Berlex	ethinyl estradiol	30	levonorgestrel	0.15
Levora	Hamilton	ethinyl estradiol	30	levonorgestrel	0.15
Nordette	Wyeth	ethinyl estradiol	30	levonorgestrel	0.15
Loestrin 1.5/30	Parke-Davis	ethinyl estradiol	30	norethindrone acetate	1.5
Loestrin 1/20	Parke-Davis	ethinyl estradiol	30	norethindrone acetate	1
Desogen	Organon	ethinyl estradiol	30	desogestrel	0.15
Ortho-Cept	Ortho	ethinyl estradiol	30	desogestrel	0.15
Biphasic Combination Contraceptives					
Nelova 10/11 and	Warner Chilcott				
Ortho-Novum 10/11	Ortho				
(day 1–10)		ethinyl estradiol	35	norethindrone	0.5
(day 11–21)		ethinyl estradiol	35	norethindrone	1
Jenest-28	Organon				
(day 1–7)		ethinyl estradiol	35	norethindrone	0.5
(day 8–21)		ethinyl estradiol	35	norethindrone	1
Triphasic Combination Contraceptives					
Ortho-Novum 7/7/7	Ortho				
(day 1–7)		ethinyl estradiol	35	norethindrone	0.5
(day 8–14)		ethinyl estradiol	35	norethindrone	0.75
(day 15–21)		ethinyl estradiol	35	norethindrone	1
Tri-Norinyl	Syntex				
(day 1–7)		ethinyl estradiol	35	norethindrone	0.5
(day 8–16)		ethinyl estradiol	35	norethindrone	1
(day 17–21)		ethinyl estradiol	35	norethindrone	0.5
Tri-Levlen and	Berlex				

°Not for contraceptive use.   *(continued)*

triphasic formulation containing norethindrone. Since the triphasic products have relative estrogen dominance and progestin deficiency, estrogen-related side effects can be expected to predominate. However, women with cardio-vascular or metabolic abnormalities would be excellent candidates for these products.

Three manufacturers of high-dose (greater than 50 µg estrogen) COC have discontinued production and dis-

Table 91.4. *(Continued)*

Trade Name	Manufacturer	Estrogen	μg	Progestin	mg
Triphasil	Wyeth				
(day 1–6)		ethinyl estradiol	30	norethindrone	0.05
(day 7–11)		ethinyl estradiol	40	norethindrone	0.075
(day 12–21)		ethinyl estradiol	30	norethindrone	0.125
Ortho Tri-Cyclen	Ortho				
(day 1–7)		ethinyl estradiol	35	norgestimate	0.18
(day 8–14)		ethinyl estradiol	35	norgestimate	0.215
(day 15–21)		ethinyl estradiol	35	norgestimate	0.25
Progestin-Only Contraceptives					
Micronor	Ortho			norethindrone	0.35
Nor-Q.D.	Syntex			norethindrone	0.35
Ovrette	Wyeth			norgestrel	0.075

tribution of these products as contraceptives. The use of COC with less than 50 μg of estrogen is associated with very low pregnancy rates, similar to the discontinued products, and a significantly lower incidence of serious adverse effects.

Menstrual bleeding usually begins 1 to 4 days after cessation of a 21-day cycle of COCs or during the placebo tablets of 28-day packs. The patient then resumes the same dosage exactly 7 days after the last "pill" with the 21-day dose packs. Twenty-eight-day pills have placebo or iron tablets to mark these 7 days for the patient.

The combination pill is effective for several reasons. First, ovulation is inhibited by the negative feedback inhibition that estrogens have on the hypothalamus, with the subsequent suppression of FSH and LH production. Progestogens in sufficient short-term doses (or as little as 1 mg norethindrone long-term) inhibit ovulation through suppression of the preovulatory LH surge; FSH is about half normal levels. Without FSH and LH, the ovarian follicle fails to grow and ovulation does not occur. The doses of estrogen commonly used in COC (30–40 μg) are insufficient to consistently produce an antiovulatory effect. In addition, a 0.4-mg dose of norethindrone has only about a 70% effect in inhibiting ovulation. The combination, however, inhibits ovulation by a synergistic action of estrogen and progestogen at the level of the hypothalamus. Nevertheless, in combination products containing 50 μg or less of estrogen, ovulation is probably suppressed only 95 to 98% of the time (2). The 99+% efficacy of these agents then must be attributed to synergy with the progestin. Progestins alone may inhibit ovulation via a subtle alteration in hypothalamic-pituitary-ovarian function and mid-cycle changes of FSH and LH. Additional nonovulatory mechanisms may also add to the effectiveness of the pill. Second, progestins cause thick, tenacious cervical mucus that is very resistant to sperm migration and reduces sperm survival. Third, progestins alter fallopian tube secretions, thereby indirectly affecting the motility of the ovum and sperm. Fourth, an atrophic endometrium often results from this dose of progestins by suppressing the estradiol-

induced cycle maturation of the endometrial lining. Implantation of the blastocyst is not satisfactory in an atrophic endometrium. All these effects combine to make the combination pill the most popular and effective oral contraceptive on the market.

The second type of oral contraceptive is the "mini-pill." Progestin only is given for 28 days continuously. These pills contain a smaller amount of progestin than most combination pills and no estrogen (Table 91.4). Although ovulation may be inhibited in some women on progestin-only contraception, approximately 40% of women will ovulate consistently with low-dose progestin, 40% will have anovulatory cycles, and the other 20% will sporadically ovulate (2). The aforementioned progestin effects contribute to the effectiveness of the mini-pill and other progestin-only contraceptive methods. The mini-pill is less effective than combination oral contraceptive products, especially if one or more tablets are missed. However, the mini-pill may be a good choice in lactating women or patients who are unable to take estrogens. Estrogen related side effects that may indicate a need to switch to mini-pills, subdermal implants, or medroxyprogesterone acetate, include hypertension, vascular thrombosis, chloasma, cycle weight gain, nausea, and headache.

Side Effects

ORAL CONTRACEPTIVES AND CARDIOVASCULAR DISEASE

The first serious side effects that were attributed to oral contraceptive agents related to the cardiovascular system. A critique of the epidemiologic studies on oral contraceptives and the occurrence of venous thromboembolism, stroke, myocardial infarction, and cardiovascular death has been completed elsewhere. It is generally accepted in the medical community that COC use has been shown to cause certain thromboembolic phenomena. Based on scientific weakness and bias in this literature, the debate on the link of COCs to CVD will no doubt continue. The use of low-dose COC and improved patient selection are clearly seen as a positive influence on the decline of these cardiovascular complications.

On the venous side of the circulation, very good evidence exists that increasing doses of estrogen increase the risk of venous thromboembolism. Most recent epidemiologic data would support thrombosis, not atherosclerosis, as the cause of increased cardiovascular disease in COC users. However, hypertension, impaired glucose tolerance, and hyperlipidemia are three of the major atherogenic risk factors believed to influence the occurrence of cardiovascular disease. Oral contraceptives worsen these risk factors to some degree in almost all women and become important in women with underlying disease or those who have specific susceptibility. Although laboratory values may remain within normal limits, the whole distribution of these risk factors is shifted upward. It remains to be seen whether these changes will have an effect on cardiovascular mortality.

HYPERTENSION

There seems to be no doubt that a small rise in blood pressure occurs in most patients taking oral contraceptives containing at least 50 µg of estrogen and 1 to 4 mg of progestin (4, 5). This rise in blood pressure is noted to occur in previously normotensive women and to aggravate existing hypertension. The average increase noted varies with age, becoming substantial in women about 35 or older. The time of onset and extent of increase varies between individuals. The hypertensive effect may increase with duration of oral contraceptive use (6). It has been estimated that 5% of oral contraceptive users develop frank hypertension within 5 years. This is an incidence three to six times greater than in nonusers (7, 8). In addition to producing overt hypertension in some women, oral contraceptives elevate pressure to some extent in almost all women (on the average 1 mm Hg diastolic, 5 mm Hg systolic) (9). These effects may take 6 to 12 months to manifest.

The risk of hypertension seems to be much lower when the low-dose formulations are used. One study showed no effect of oral contraceptive agents on pretreatment blood pressures in women with or without preexisting hypertension (10). However, another study (11) showed small but significant increases in both systolic and diastolic blood pressures in women who were taking a combination of 30 µg of ethinyl estradiol with either 150 µg of levonorgestrel or 2 mg of ethynodiol diacetate. This study also showed no effect on blood pressure from progestogen-only contraceptive agents.

This information has several important implications for patient follow-up. Emphasis should be placed on women 35 or older, smokers, those with a history of hypertension, the obese, and patients on COCs with higher doses of estrogen. The mechanism of COC-associated hypertension appears complex. Whereas an estrogen or a progestin alone had no effect on the occurrence of hypertension, if an estrogen is given with a progestin, there is an increased risk of hypertension. In addition, ethinyl estradiol increases the hepatic production of angiotensinogen in a dose-dependent fashion, thus increasing peripheral resistance. Although these are primarily estrogen effects, progestins may have a synergistic effect because a direct relationship between the amount of norethindrone acetate in COC and hypertension has been reported (14). One of the new progestins (gestodene) may have an antimineralocorticoid effect and thus be associated with a reduced risk of hypertension. However, this progestin is currently not available in U.S. products.

Hypertension associated with birth control pills is reversible. After discontinuing oral contraceptives, the return to normal blood pressure may take from 3 to 4 months. The patient's blood pressure should be monitored at the initiation of oral contraceptive therapy and periodically thereafter. If a large rise in blood pressure is detected, oral contraceptives should be discontinued.

LIPID METABOLISM

Estrogens appear to stimulate a significant increase in fasting serum triglyceride levels, leading to increased levels of very low-density lipoproteins (VLDL)(15). Very rarely, hyperlipidemic crisis with pancreatitis has been reported and must be attributed to the estrogen in these products (16). Certain progestins in COCs oppose this action of estrogen and lower triglyceride levels (17). Ethynodiol diacetate, however, does not have this antiestrogenic action but instead may be synergistic to increase triglycerides (18).

Much more interest has been focused on low-density lipoprotein (LDL) cholesterol because of the positive correlation between it and the risk of coronary heart disease. The inverse relationship between high-density lipoprotein (HDL) cholesterol and coronary heart disease risk has received even more attention. Thus, COCs that simultaneously elevate LDL and decrease HDL cause the most concern. Although lipid levels generally remain within normal limits, it is likely that all COCs elevate plasma triglyceride and LDL cholesterol to some extent in all users and that certain formulations do so to a marked degree. While estrogens raise HDL cholesterol levels, particularly the HDL_2 subspecies, progestins lower HDL cholesterol levels. Combination oral contraceptive products containing the more potent progestins (e.g., levonorgestrel) cause the most adverse changes (18, 19). The potency of estrogen and the potency and type (androgenicity) of progestin in COCs have important effects on lipoprotein lipids in women and may be responsible for an increased risk of arteriosclerotic disease. For these reasons, progestin-dominant COCs should be prescribed with caution in women with known risk factors for cardiovascular disease. Many of the newer products have been formulated to minimize these changes in LDL and HDL cholesterol by the use of less potent progestins, norethindrone being the most popular.

The new progestins (desogestrel and norgestimate) are reported to be less androgenic then their parent compound, levonorgestrel. As a result, these new progestins may have a more positive impact on lipid metabolism, although with some differential effects on triglycerides (20). The clinical relevance of these changes is not known at this time, especially as compared to norethindrone containing COCs.

CARBOHYDRATE METABOLISM

Women taking most older combination oral contraceptives showed a mild worsening of glucose tolerance curves (an average serum glucose increase of 11 mg/dL in 1 hr). Many normal women have shown elevations in plasma insulin response to glucose and worsening of prediabetic-type responses. Patients with established diabetes on older, high-dose COCs showed a worsening of carbohydrate intolerance. It would appear that these changes are due to the progestin components of oral contraceptives because estrogens do not effect carbohydrate metabolism (21). The impairment depends on both the type and dose of progestin. Effects are less pronounced with lower-dose preparations. Literature on the new progestins (desogestrel, gestodene, and norgestimate) concludes that carbohydrate metabolism is affected less by COCs containing these agents than by other COCs (22). Studies also show that other low-dose COCs do not change glucose tolerance and have only small effects on carbohydrate metabolism (23). Given adequate supervision, low-dose COCs may be used safely in young patients with insulin-dependent diabetes and those with a history of gestational diabetes. When COCs cause oral glucose tolerance to deteriorate and insulin levels to increase, they do so during the first 3 to 6 months and then levels stabilize (24).

MYOCARDIAL INFARCTION AND STROKE

Although the above effects of oral contraceptives on blood pressure, carbohydrates, and lipid metabolism may appear minor from a clinical standpoint, from an epidemiologic viewpoint this combination of atherogenic factors may have serious implications. A direct link between altered metabolism and increased mortality and morbidity are largely hypothetical. Much debate continues on the exact relationship of COC and the risk of myocardial infarction (MI) and stroke. Early data showed that risks while on therapy seem to increase substantially with age and the presence of such risk factors as smoking greater than 15 cigarettes daily, preexisting hypercholesterolemia, diabetes mellitus, or hypertension (25, 26). Overall, oral contraceptives were found to multiply the effects of age and other risk factors for MI and stroke, rather than just add to them (26). Because cigarette smoking is far more prevalent among women of reproductive age than any of these other risk factors, it becomes by far the most important factor.

Whereas early epidemiologic studies of high-dose oral contraceptives found significantly increased risks of developing cardiovascular disease among users of COCs, several trends have led to a reassessment of that risk. First, studies have become more sophisticated and now take into account the potentially confounding effects of cigarette smoking. Second, in recent years women have been evaluated more carefully before they begin to take oral contraceptives, and those women who have serious underlying medical problems and older women who smoke have been less likely to use oral contraceptives. Third, the formulations of oral contraceptives have changed dramatically; current formulations have a three- to fourfold decrease in estrogen dose and a onefold decrease in progestin dose compared with the formulations initially prescribed. Hence the findings of early epidemiologic studies are likely irrelevant to today's preparations (27).

Use of oral contraceptives by healthy women who do not smoke does not appear to be associated with an increased risk of either myocardial infarction or stroke (28). Data from the United States (29, 30) and the United Kingdom have documented no increase in the risk of death from cardiovascular disease among contemporary users of oral contraceptives. Data from the Oxford Family Planning association study (31) also support the hypothesis that oral contraceptives that contain less than 50 µg of estrogen are safer than higher-dose formulations.

Some evidence suggests that the pathophysiology of myocardial infarction among women who used oral contraceptives in earlier studies was thrombosis. First, most studies, including the large Nurses' Health Study (32, 33) from the United States, have found no increased risk of myocardial infarction among former users of oral contraceptives. If atherosclerosis were the cause, then the risk should remain elevated after discontinuing COCs. Corroborating evidence comes from autopsy studies of women who have died of myocardial infarction. Second, there does not appear to be a duration-related effect between length of oral contraceptive use and risk of infarction. This also argues against deposition of plaque as the pathophysiology.

COCs AND WOMEN OVER 35 YEARS OF AGE

Historically, COCs have not been prescribed for women over the age of 35. Recent data, however, indicate that the use of COCs containing less than 50 µg of estrogen is safe in healthy, nonsmoking women up to the age of 50, and is not associated with an increased risk of serious cardiovascular disease. However, COCs should not be used by women with preexisting systemic disease that may effect the cardiovascular system (e.g., hypertension, diabetes, hyperlipidemia) or by women over 35 years of age who smoke.

Women over 35 are often eager to discontinue taking daily COCs and to stop using barrier contraceptives. Tubal ligation and vasectomy are the contraceptives most often chosen in this age group. However, if a woman wants to use COCs until she is 50, has no risk factors other than age for COCs, and is not now a smoker, this option should remain open to her.

Because the average age of menopause is 51 years of age, it is possible for a women to remain on COCs her entire reproductive life. In fact, in recent years, very low-dose COCs have been recommended during the perimenopausal period in this population. These low-dose COCs decrease early vasomotor symptoms (hot flashes), maintain menstrual cycle control, and prevent pregnancy until ovarian support ceases. The lowest estrogen dose available today in COCs is 20 μg of ethinyl estradiol. This is roughly bioequivalent to four or five 0.625-mg tablets of conjugated equine estrogen. While low-dose COCs do not appear to pose any appreciably increased risk for healthy nonsmoking women in the perimenopausal years, shifting from COCs to a typical hormone replacement regimen at some point is advisable. This is an important issue, as the patient taking COCs will not be able to use spontaneous cessation of menses to identify when she reaches menopause. There is little practical value in trying to determine precisely the onset of menopause to make the transition, and simply picking the average age of menopause (between 51 and 52) should be satisfactory for evaluating whether follicular activity is still present.

If menses do not resume 3 months after stopping birth control pills or if vasomotor symptoms begin, menopausal hormone replacement therapy can be instituted safely. A small number of women will continue to cycle after this age, and it is appropriate to either await spontaneous menopause or continue COCs for another year and reevaluate their status at that time.

VENOUS THROMBOEMBOLIC DISEASE

Combination oral contraceptives have been found to increase the risks of venous thromboembolic disease (deep vein thrombosis and/or pulmonary embolism) during the first month of oral contraceptive use (30). This effect remains constant regardless of the duration of use, past use, presence of obesity, or cigarette smoking. After discontinuation of therapy, this risk seems to decline within 1 month to the level found among women who have never used the drug (34).

The most reliable source of information regarding the magnitude of risks for overt venous thromboembolic disease comes from two British cohort studies that began in 1968 (35, 36). The relative risk of thromboembolic disease in current users compared to nonusers was found to be approximately 3 times for idiopathic superficial venous thrombosis, in the range of 4 to 11 times for deep vein thrombosis or pulmonary embolism, and in the range of 1.5 to 6 times for venous thrombosis or pulmonary embolism in women with conditions that predispose to the development of thromboembolic disease. It must be kept in mind that COCs during this time contained greater than 50 μg of estrogen. The actual risk of deep vein thrombosis resulting from the use of current COC preparations, albeit low, is unknown.

Although oral contraceptives have been shown to increase the risk of death from thromboembolic disease, this effect is very rare. During over 450,000 women-years of follow-up, these studies observed only 5 fatalities from venous thromboembolic disease.

It is the estrogen component that increases the risk of thromboembolic disease. Furthermore, this effect appears to be dose related, as evidenced by a drop of one half to two thirds in the incidence of fatal or nonfatal pulmonary embolism when the dose of mestranol or ethinyl estradiol was reduced from 100–150 μg to 50–80 μg tablets (31). Because most COCs prescribed today contain less than 50 μg of estrogen, it is not surprising that this problem is seen less frequently now.

Oral contraceptives appear to cause structural and histochemical vascular changes in veins and arteries (37). A large number of changes in the process of blood coagulation have been noted, including an increase in platelet stickiness, a possible elevation of platelet count, a rise in prothrombin, and an increase in factors VII, VIII, IX, and X (38, 39).

Antithrombin III, an enzyme that inactivates thrombin, is nearly normal in women using oral contraceptives. However, antithrombin III activity is substantially decreased (40). In addition, oral contraceptives containing 75 to 150 μg of mestranol or ethinyl estradiol decrease antithrombin III activity to a greater extent than do oral contraceptives containing only 50 μg (41).

Progestins, in the low-dose pills, play some role in this effect because antithrombin III activity is reduced significantly in patients who are taking COCs that contain 30 μg of ethinyl estradiol and a member of the norethindrone family, but there is no significant change in activity in women taking 30 μg ethinyl estradiol and levonorgestrel, whether in a fixed dose or as a triphasic preparation (42).

Antithrombin III levels are lower in nonuser women of blood types A, B, and AB (especially type A) than in women of blood type O. This may account for the increase in risk of idiopathic deep venous thromboembolic disease among users and nonoral contraceptive users of blood types A, B, or AB. These changes are most important in women who smoke, since smoking also increases the risk of thromboembolic events.

TUMORIGENIC ASPECTS

Because the normal breast is hormone dependent, women who use oral contraceptive tablets may develop some mammary abnormalities. The relationship between the consumption of oral contraceptives and the development of breast disease is by no means a simple one. Oral contraceptives reduce two common benign forms of breast disease, fibroadenoma and fibrocystic disease.

To date most studies have found no overall increase in the risk of breast cancer in oral contraceptive users. Authoritative reviews of these studies have provided a reassuring picture (43–45). The aggregate relative risk of developing breast cancer is close to 1.0, with a very narrow 95% confidence interval. However, subgroup analysis have identified increased risks in certain populations, such as young women under 45 years of age, or after prolonged use. In general, these findings have been inconsistent. However, certain existing breast cancers may be worsened by the estrogen in oral contraceptive preparations. In spite of widespread oral contraceptive use and extensive observation, no increased incidence of cancer has been observed. A summary of COC risk factors for cancer of the ovary, endometrium, breast, and uterine cervix is reviewed in Table 91.5 (46).

Hepatomas may occur in women taking oral contraceptives. A wide array of different types of benign liver tumors have been reported, the most common of which are focal nodular hyperplasia and liver cell adenomas. If we compare cases of focal nodular hyperplasia before and after COC became available, it is revealed that there is little or no change with respect to incidence, age, range, location, or microscopic features of this lesion. One important difference is noted, however. Before oral contraceptives, no serious hemorrhages had been reported. Since the introduction of oral contraceptives, this tumor is sometimes fatal, with death usually due to sudden hepatic rupture and hemorrhage.

There has been an increase in the incidence of a formerly rare liver cell adenoma. Numerous cases of this adenoma, which was rarely reported before 1960, have now been reported. Risk is increased by age, duration of use, and dose of steroid.

BREAKTHROUGH BLEEDING

Bleeding between the expected episodes of menses is a common occurrence among hormonal contraceptive users and can lead to discontinuation of therapy. The term *breakthrough bleeding* (BTB) refers to bleeding that occurs other than at the time of expected menstruation and sufficient to require the use of pads or tampons. *Spotting* is defined as bleeding insufficient to require use of pads or tampons. Patients may expect some degree of breakthrough bleeding the first several months of any new contraceptive use until the body becomes accustomed to the synthetic hormones. Progestin-only mini-pills affect cycles more than COC. In addition, the dose and potency of estrogen and progestin as well as the ratio of the two may impact bleeding. If spotting continues after 3 months of use, the dose of estrogen or progestogen can be adjusted. Speroff (47) has proposed that patients receiving oral contraceptives with persistent breakthrough bleeding be treated with 7-day courses of estrogen, either ethinyl estradiol 20 μg or conjugated equine estrogens, 2.5 mg/day added to the first 7 days of the COC cycle in the patient's regular COC Packet (i.e. day 1–7 she takes regular "pill" and an estrogen tablet). Many practitioners believe this treatment works, although randomized trials are lacking. Similar treatment has been used for BTB caused by hormone implants and depot medroxyprogesterone acetate.

GALLBLADDER DISEASE

Use of oral contraceptives was originally thought to increase the incidence of gallstones and cholecystitis by at least twofold. Estrogens alter the composition of the bile.

Table 91.5.
Cancer Risks and Oral Contraceptive Use: Summary of Recent Evidence for Cancer of the Ovary, Endometrium, Breast, and Uterine Cervix

Disease	Estimated Relative Risk[a]	Risk with Duration of Use	Comments
Ovarian cancer	0.4–0.8	Decreased	Overall protective effect, especially epithelial type; most notable in nulliparous; effect after 6 months of use.
Endometrial cancer	0.4–0.6	Decreased (especially with decreased progestogen content)	Protective; most notable in nulliparous; effect after 1 year of use.
Breast cancer	0.9–1.3	No trend	Possibly no increased risk; effect less certain.
Cervical cancer	1.1–1.3	? Increased (data conflicting)	Possible slight increase but influence of sexual activity, cigarettes, cytologic screening yet to be defined.

[a]Relative risk estimate: ratio of number of observations in cases and that in control subjects.

It has been suggested that a rise in cholesterol saturation of gallbladder bile and lower bile acid levels may account for the increase in gallbladder disease. With a decrease in estrogen content, these effects may be less common. One large prospective study showed the relative risk for symptomatic gallstones in ever-users of COCs to be 1.2, in long-term users 1.5, and in current users 1.6 (48).

DEPRESSION

The incidence of depression among oral contraceptive users is approximately 5 to 6%. The symptoms noted include lethargy, loss of libido, irritability, and crying. Because of the lack of well-controlled trials and underlying prevalence of depression in this patient population, much controversy exists as to the cause. Proponents of a biochemical theory offer evidence that brain amine metabolism is altered as a result of any abnormal tryptophan metabolism. An increased requirement for vitamin B6 by pyridoxine-deficient oral contraceptive users was found. Supplementation relieved the symptoms of depression (49).

BREAST FEEDING

The World Health Organization (WHO) studied the effects of hormonal contraception on milk in women who breast-feed their children (46). Since estrogen inhibits the action of prolactin in breast tissue receptors, milk production is thought to be related to the amount of estrogen in the COC. Women who took COCs had a 42% reduction in milk volume at 18 weeks of treatment. There was a decline in volume starting at 6 weeks. No effect was seen at 6 weeks in mini-pill users, but at 18 weeks a 12% reduction in volume occurred. Those women using nonhormonal techniques had a 6% reduction in milk volume at 18 weeks.

Although specific nutrients, mainly protein, fat, and calcium, were decreased in some women using COCs, no differences in the growth of the infants in any treatment group were noted. The WHO concluded that although COCs containing 30 μg of estrogen do cause some reduction in milk volume, there are no adverse effects on infant growth. Some constituents of COCs are transferred to the infant. Although these are metabolized rapidly by the infant and, currently, there is no reason to believe that they cause harm, long-term studies have not been reported.

DRUG INTERACTIONS

Evidence indicates that certain drugs may impair the efficacy of COCs. The converse is also true; COCs may modify the action of other drugs. Mechanisms thought to be responsible for these interactions include:

1. interference with the amount of steroids absorbed or reabsorbed through enterohepatic circulation of steroid metabolites.

2. stimulating or depressing hepatic metabolism.
3. displacement of contraceptive steroids from their biologic receptor site.
4. opposing steroid action by some physiologic effect.

Gastroenteritis has long been associated with decreased gastrointestinal (GI) transit time and steroid absorption. Because ethinyl estradiol conjugates are excreted in the bile and may be broken down by gut bacteria in the colon to liberate active hormone, which can then be reabsorbed, anything that increases GI motility (e.g., diarrhea, laxatives) could reduce circulating concentrations of oral contraceptives. Likewise, ampicillin or other antibiotics, such as tetracycline or cotrimoxazole, may eliminate the gut microflora that is necessary for this enterohepatic circulation. Although this is not substantiated by detailed study in humans, numerous well-documented clinical reports have appeared of pregnancies in women who have missed no COCs but took an antibiotic agent. From a practical point of view, not many women are at risk of this interaction, but if antibiotics are prescribed for oral contraceptive users, especially during days 1 to 14, barrier concentration should be added for the remainder of the cycle.

The most clinically significant drug interactions occur with other drugs that are metabolized by the same hepatic microsomal pathway as estrogen. Case reports of failure of COCs have appeared in women taking phenytoin, primidone, barbiturates, carbamazepine, ethosuximide, rifampin, and griseofulvin (51). Conversely, estrogens are inhibitors of hepatic microsomal enzymes and may slow the metabolism of other drugs (Table 91.6). In addition, sex hormone–binding globulin (SHBG) binds common progestins with high affinity. It has been shown that SHBG's capacity to bind is significantly increased in women taking anticonvulsants. This would decrease free levels of progestins and decrease the efficacy of oral contraceptives. It has been suggested that if a young woman wishes to use a COC and is receiving treatment for a seizure disorder, she should take one of the preparations with 30 μg of estrogen. If breakthrough bleeding occurs, then an additional dose of a 20-μg estrogen should be added.(52) Valproic acid has not been associated with apparent oral contraceptive failure. If clinically appropriate for seizure control, use of valproic acid may be considered in women needing maximal assurance of contraception.

OTHER SIDE EFFECTS

Previously, tests that monitored thyroid function were affected by oral contraceptives. Thyroid function was not changed, only the laboratory tests used to measure it. Estrogens increase the thyroid-binding globulin, so tests that are used to measure thyroid function, such as protein-bound iodine thyroxine (T-4) by column and T-4 by Murphy Pattee (total T-4), will be elevated and triiodo-

Table 91.6.
Combination Oral Contraceptive (COC)
Drug Interactions

Increase COC concentrations	*Decrease COC concentrations*
Ascorbic acid	Antibiotic agents
Acetaminophen	Barbiturates
	Phenytoin
	Primidone
	Carbamazepine
	Griseofulvin
	Rifampin
Have their concentrations	*Have their concentrations*
increased by COCs	*decreased by COCs*
Alprazolam	Acetaminophen
Antipyrine	Clofibrate
Caffeine	Lorazepam
Chlordiazepoxide	Morphine
Corticosteroids	Oxazepam
Diazepam	Temazepam
Imipramine	
Metoprolol	
Nitrazepam	
Theophylline	
Triazolam	
Vitamin A	
Vitamin D	

Adapted from Shenfield GM. Drug interactions with oral contraceptive preparations. Med J Aust 114:205–211, 1986.

thyronine (T-3) resin uptake will be decreased. These tests are not used as frequently now. In order to accurately assess thyroid function in COC users, a free T-4 should be done. Abnormal thyroid values will return to normal 2 to 4 weeks after the discontinuation of oral contraceptives. Table 91.7 shows changes in this and other laboratory tests in women taking COCs.

Nausea and vomiting appear to be related to the estrogen dose of oral contraceptives. It is a common side effect and may decrease with continued use. Pharmacokinetic data suggest that the majority of estrogen is absorbed within 2 hours after oral administration. It would be wise to repeat the dose if vomiting occurs during the absorption period. Management of pill-associated nausea includes (a) use of low-dose estrogen-containing oral contraceptives, (b) reassurance if temporary nausea can be tolerated, and (c) taking the pill at bedtime so the patient will be asleep during peak serum concentrations.

Weight gain with oral contraceptives has been divided into two categories: persistent and cyclic. Persistent acyclic weight gain is thought to be secondary to the anabolic testosterone-like progestogen increase in appetite or decrease in activity. Cyclic weight gain, on the other hand, is thought to be an estrogen-related side effect, secondary to water retention.

An increase in the frequency of headache (both tension and migraine) has been noted to occur as a side effect of oral contraceptive use. Approximately half of the women who develop vascular headaches with COCs report preexisting migraine attacks. There is evidence that falling estrogen levels may incite the cerebrovascular system to respond by producing migraine headaches. Patients who develop migraine (vascular headaches) while taking oral contraceptives should discontinue the pill.

Increased corneal sensitivity, particularly contact lens discomfort, has been noted in about 1 in 5 women who take oral contraceptives (53). Changes in corneal curvature and decreased tear secretion have been blamed for this side effect in oral contraceptive users and pregnant patients. A variety of ocular changes have been attributed to the pill, ranging from retinal vascular accidents to decreases in visual acuity and color changes (54). Repeated prospective and retrospective studies failed to find a correlation between the use of birth control pills and many of these abnormalities, which are found normally in a population of women of reproductive age. However, caution should be exercised in prescribing oral contraceptives to women with known ophthalmologic disorders.

Erythema nodosum, erythema multiforme, and urticaria are hypersensitivity reactions that are occasionally seen with oral contraceptive therapy. They are rare events, occurring in at most 1 in 1000 users. Oral contraceptives should be discontinued at once. This reaction usually is attributed to the progestin component of the pill and seems to regress when patients are taken off the pill (6).

Oral contraceptives have been rarely associated with flareups of systemic lupus erythematosus (SLE)(55). However, it is more common to see SLE and antinuclear antibody (ANA) tests turn positive in patients using oral contraceptive drugs and revert to negative on discontinuation. The importance of this is unknown.

Megaloblastic anemia has been reported in oral contraceptive users for two reasons: (a) a relative folic acid deficiency, which may exist because of increased binding of folic acid, and (b) rarely a decrease in serum vitamin B_{12}. It is likely that oral contraceptives contribute to, but do not produce, this anemia in otherwise healthy women, and it responds to appropriate replacement therapy. Other vitamin deficiencies have been reported. The most marked are in the water-soluble vitamins: thiamin (B_1), riboflavin (B_2), pyridoxine (B_6), cobalamin (B_{12}), and ascorbic acid (C).

Fewer women on oral contraceptives have iron deficiency anemia. This probably reflects a decrease in menstrual flow secondary to the use of oral contraceptives, with subsequent increases in serum iron and iron-binding capacity.

Other side effects that have been attributed to the pill include acne, chloasma (skin hyperpigmentation that may be exacerbated by sun exposure when serum concentrations of estrogens are high), abnormal hair growth, changes

Table 91.7.
Potential Effects of Oral Contraceptives on the Results of a Selected Group of Laboratory Tests

Group	Specific Tests and Potential Alteration of Lab Value	
	Increased	Decreased
Carbohydrate metabolism	FBS and 2 hr postprandial Insulin level	Glucose Tolerance
Hematologic/coagulation	Coagulation factor II, VII, VIII, IX, X, XII	Antithrombin III
	Erythrocyte sedimentation rate	Erythrocyte count (total)
	Euglobulin lysis	Hematocrit
	Fibrinogen	Prothrombin time
	Leukocyte count	
	Partial thromboplastin time	
	Plasma volume, plasmin, and plasminogen	
	Platelet count, platelet aggregation, and platelet adhesiveness	
	Prothrombin time	
Lipid metabolism°	Cholesterol	
	Lipoproteins (prebata, β and α)	
	Phospholipids, total	
	Total lipids	
	Triglycerides	
Liver function/GI tests	Alkaline phosphatase	Alkaline phosphatase
	Bilirubin, SGOT, SGPT	Etiocholanolone excretion (urine)
	Cephalin flocculation	Haptoglobin (serum)
	Formiminoglutamic acid excretion after histidine (urine)	Urobilinogen excretion (urine)
	γ-Glutamyl transpeptidase	
	Leucine aminopeptidase	
	Protoporphyrin, coproporphyrin excretion (urine), uroporphyrin excretion (urine)	
	Sulfobromophthalein retention	
Metals	Copper and ceruloplasmin	Magnesium
	Iron, iron binding capacity, and transferrin	Zinc
Thyroid function	Butanole extractable iodine	Triiodothyronine resin (serum)
	Protein-bound iodine	Free thyroxin
	Thyroid-binding globulin	
	Triiodothyronine (serum)	
Vitamins	Vitamin A (blood and plasma)	Folate (serum)
		Vitamin B_2 (RBC and urine excretion)
		Vitamin B_6
		Vitamin B_{12}
		Vitamin C
Other hormones/enzyme measurements	Aldosterone (blood and urine)	Estradiol and Estriol
	Angiotensinogen	FSH (urine), LH (blood and urine)
	Angiotensin I and II	Gonadotropin excretion (urine)
	Cortisol (blood and urine)	17-Hydroxycorticosteroid excretion (urine)
	Growth hormone	17-Ketosteroid excretion (urine)
	Prolactin	Pregnanediol excretion (urine)
	Testosterone (serum)	Renin (serum)
	Total estrogens	Tetrahydrocortisone
Miscellaneous laboratory	α-1 Antitrypsin	Albumin
	Antinuclear antibody	α-amino nitrogen
	Bilirubin	Calcium (serum) and calcium excretion (urine)
	Complement-reactive protein	Complement-reactive protein
	Globulins a-1, a-2	Immunoglobulin A, G, and M
	Lactate	
	Lupus erythematosus cell preparation	
	Pyruvate	
	Sodium	

°HDL cholesterol is increased with estrogens and decreased with progestins.
Adapted with permission from Hatcher RA (2).

Table 91.8.
Side Effects That May Require Adjustment of the Estrogen/Progestogen Balance

Estrogen excess	*Progestogen excess*
Nausea, bloating	Increased appetite
Cervical mucorrhea, polyposis	Persistent weight gain
Hypermenorrhea	Tiredness, fatigue
Hyperpigmentation	Hypomenorrhea
Uterine or leg cramps	Acne, oily scalp
Hypertension	Hair loss
Migraine headache	Depression
Breast tenderness	Hirsutism
Dizziness, vertigo	Breast regression
Cyclic weight gain	Changes in libido
Fibroid growth	
Cervical eversion	
Estrogen deficiency	*Progestogen deficiency*
Irritability, nervousness	Late breakthrough bleeding
Early and/or midcycle break-	Amenorrhea
through bleeding	Hypermenorrhea
Increased spotting	Weight loss
Hot flashes	
Hypomenorrhea	
Amenorrhea	
Dyspareunia	

in libido, breast tenderness, galactorrhea, postpill amenorrhea, photosensitivity, exacerbation of acute intermittent porphyria, exacerbation of Wilson's disease, and ischemic colitis. Some of these side effects have been attributed to a particular component of birth control pills, or lack thereof, and are listed in Table 91.8.

Associated Benefits of Oral Contraceptive Use

Noncontraceptive benefits associated with COCs also are of note. In addition to the decrease in endometrial and ovarian cancer previously noted, there is a decline in the risk of rheumatoid arthritis, pelvic inflammatory disease, ectopic pregnancy, functional ovarian cysts, benign breast disease, acne, dysmenorrhea, and morbidity and mortality associated with pregnancy and childbirth. It has been estimated that the use of COCs will prevent 1 to 7 million requests for abortions annually (56).

Contraindications to Oral Contraceptive Use

The absolute and relative contraindications for the use of oral contraceptives are listed in Table 91.9.

Selection of an Oral Contraceptive Product

When selecting a combination oral contraceptive product for a patient, there are several very important considerations:

1. The product should contain the lowest effective dose of estrogen and progestin. Nearly all patients do well on products containing 35 μg or less of estrogen.

2. The product should have the minimum side effects acceptable to the patient.
3. Any problems or concomitant diseases that the patient has should be considered and minimized if possible.
4. Women with preexisting systemic disease that may affect the cardiovascular system or who smoke should discontinue use at 35 years of age.

In addition to these criteria, it is important to have an understanding of the relative estrogen and progestogen potencies of oral contraceptive products. These potencies reflect the total amount of estrogen and progestogen as well as the effects they have on each other.

Table 91.10 lists the common products on the U.S. market and their relative estrogenic, progestogenic, and androgenic potencies. Because of the large number of products available, it is important to be able to recommend a more or less potent product when an estrogen or progestogen-related side effect occurs.

The ovarian and uterine cycles are superimposed for 28 days to form the menstrual cycle. When estrogens and progestins in the form of oral contraceptive pills are added to this cycle, an attempt is made to alter the ovarian cycle without affecting the uterine cycle. However, since these synthetic agents are not identical to the naturally produced hormones, some changes from the "normal" are likely to occur (e.g., a decrease in menstrual flow, occasional spotting, or a missed period). A woman relies on her normal menstrual bleeding as a sign to indicate that she is not pregnant. If pregnancy has been ruled out, the patient should be reassured if concern is expressed over the above changes.

Risk-Benefit Ratio

For the first time in history, normal, healthy people are taking a potent medication over a long period of time. It is increasingly important to discuss the risk of this therapy with the patient, especially when the lay press, which is read most by women, tends to emphasize these risks. Perhaps some perspective can be gained if the risks of taking oral contraceptives are compared to other common risks of mortality (Fig. 91.4).

Starting COCs

COCs are usually initiated in one of two ways: (a) the first tablet of the pack is taken on the first day of menses ("day one start") or (b) the first tablet of the pack is taken on the first Sunday after the onset of menses ("Sunday start"). Many clinicians and patients prefer the Sunday start to avoid menstrual bleeding on weekends. However, the day one start has been shown to be more effective, and back-up contraceptive methods are not generally recommended once COCs are begun. In contrast, alternative methods of contraception are recommended for the first 7 days of pill use for the Sunday

Table 91.9.
Possible Contraindications to Use of Combined Oral Contraceptive Pills

Absolute contraindications:
1. Thrombophlebitis or thromboembolic disorder (or history thereof)[a]
2. Cerebrovascular accident (or history thereof)
3. Coronary artery or ischemic heart disease (or history thereof)
4. Known or suspected breast carcinoma (or history thereof)
5. Known or suspected estrogen-dependent neoplasia (or history thereof)
6. Pregnancy
7. Benign or malignant liver tumor (or history thereof)
8. Known impaired liver function at present time[b]
9. Previous cholestasis during pregnancy

Strong relative contraindications:
1. Severe headaches, particularly vascular or migraine headaches that start after initiation of oral contraceptives
2. Hypertension with resting diastolic BP or 90 mm Hg or greater, or a resting systolic BP of 140 mm Hg or greater on three or more separate visits, or an accurate measurement of 110 mm Hg diastolic or more in a single visit[c]
3. Mononucleosis, acute phase
4. Elective major surgery or major surgery requiring immobilization planned in next 4 weeks
5. Long-leg cast or major injury to lower leg
6. Over 40 years old, accompanied by a second risk factor for the development of cardiovascular disease (such as diabetes or hypertension)[o]
7. Over 35 years old and currently a heavy smoker (15 or more cigarettes a day)[o]
8. Abnormal bleeding[d]

Other considerations that may suggest that pills are not the ideal contraception:
♦ Diabetes, prediabetes or a strong family history of diabetes[e]
♦ Sickle cell disease (SS) or sickle C disease (SC)
♦ Active gallbladder disease
♦ Congenital hyperbilirubinemia (Gilbert's disease)
♦ Undiagnosed, abnormal genital bleeding[d]
♦ Over 50 years old
♦ Completion of term pregnancy within past 10 to 14 days[o]
♦ Weight gain of 10 pounds or more while on the pill
♦ Patient receiving high blood pressure treatment
♦ Cardiac or renal disease (or history thereof)[o]
♦ Conditions likely to make patient unreliable at following pill instructions (mental retardation, major psychiatric illness, alcoholism or other chemical abuse, history of repeatedly taking oral contraceptives or other medication incorrectly)
♦ Lactation[o]
♦ Family history of death of a parent or sibling due to myocardial infarction before age 50. *Myocardial infarction in a mother or sister is especially significant and indicates a need for lipid evaluation.*
♦ Family history of hyperlipedemia

[o]Refers to a contraindication to combined birth control pills, which *may not* be a contraindication to progestin-only pills or may be *less* of a contraindication to progestin-only pills than to combined pills.
[a]Some clinicians do not consider thromboembolic events related to known trauma or an intravenous needle a contraindication to pills.
[b]In areas of the world where endemic infections alter liver function tests for a high percentage of the population, few women would be started on pills if this finding were used as an absolute contraindication.
[c]The three authors who are clinicians (RAH, FHS, GKS) consider three diastolic pressures greater than 90 mm Hg a very strong contraindication to combined pills.
[d]Several reviewers of this book strongly feel that abnormal genital bleeding should be listed as an absolute contraindication to pill use. We consider it a potential rather than absolute contraindication because "abnormal" cannot be easily defined. If you, the clinician, feel that the specific patient's bleeding pattern is "abnormal" and cannot identify the cause, do not provide her with pills.
[e]Some clinicians do not consider diabetes, prediabetes, or a family history of diabetes a contraindication to combined pills and are willing to initiate pills and observe carefully. Other clinicians require that the patient's primary care physician, the endocrinologist, or the person who cares for her diabetes participate in the decision to provide OCs. The decison to provide OCs is a shared responsibility, and the primary care physician must renew approval annually.
Adapted with permission from Hatcher RA, Trussell J, Stewart FS, et al. Contraceptive technology, 1990–92, 15th ed. New York: Irvington Publishers, 1990.

start method. Some clinicians recommend an alternative method of contraception for the entire first cycle, and some feel alternative methods of birth control are unnecessary if COCs are started by the sixth menstrual day or earlier.

Patients beginning the mini-pill should be instructed to (a) begin the mini-pill on the first day of menstrual bleeding and take one tablet every day, and (b) use a backup method of birth control for the first 2 months of pill use.

Missed Pills

As a practical matter, it is important to know what to tell patients when birth control pills are missed. Certain information should be obtained before any advice is given:

Table 91.10.
Contraceptive Pill Activity

Drug	Endometrial Activity: % (Spotting, and bleeding, in third cycle of use[a,b])	Estrogenic Activity: μg (Ethinyl estradiol equivalents per day[c])	Progestational Activity: mg (Norethindrone equivalents per day[d])	Androgenic Activity: mg (Methyltestosterone per 28 days[e])
50 μg Estrogen				
Ovral	4.5	42	1.3	0.80
Genora/Norethin/Norinyl Ortho-Novum 1/50	10.6	32	1.0	0.34
Ovcon 50	11.9	50	1.0	0.34
Norlestrin 1/50	13.6	39	1.2	0.53
Demulen 50	13.9	26	1.4	0.21
Sub-50 μg Estrogen				
Monophasic				
Lo-Ovral	9.6	25	0.8	0.46
Ovcon 35	11.0	40	0.4	0.15
Desogen/Ortho-Cept	13.1	30	1.5	0.17
Levlen/Nordette	14.0	25	0.8	0.46
Ortho-Cyclen	14.3	35	0.3	0.18
Genora/Nelova/Norethin/Norinyl/ Ortho-Novum 1/35	14.7	38	1.0	0.34
Brrevicon/Modicon/Nelova 0.5/35	24.6	42	0.5	0.17
Leostrin 1.5/30	25.2	14	1.7	0.80
Loestrin 1/20	29.7	13	1.2	0.53
Demulen 1/35	37.4	19	1.4	0.21
Multiphasic				
Ortho-Novum 7/7/7	14.5	48	0.8	0.25
Tri-Levlen/Triphasil	15.1	28	0.5	0.29
Jeneset	17.3	39	0.8	0.28
Ortho-Novum 10/11	17.6	40	0.8	0.25
Ortho Tri-Cyclen	17.7	35	0.3	0.15
Tri-Norinyl	25.5	40	0.7	0.23
Progestin-Only				
Ovrette	34.9	0	0.08	0.13
Micronor/Nor-QD	42.3	1	0.12	0.13

[a]Information submitted to the United States Food and Drug Administration by the manufacturer. These rates are derived from separate studies conducted by different investigators in several population groups, and therefore, a precise comparison cannot be made, except when randomized comparative studies are used. Randomized comparative studies used are: NDA 18-985 (Ortho 7/7/7 and Jenest vs. Ortho 1 + 35); NDA 19-653 (Ortho-Cyclen vs. Lo-Ovral); Syntex laboratories study 17-6288 (Tri-Norinyl and Ortho 10/11 vs. Norinyl 1 + 35).
[b]Includes early withdrawal flow.
[c]Estrogenic activity of entire tablet—mouse uterine assay.
[d]Induction of glycogen vacuoles in human endometrium.
[e]Rat ventral prostate assay.
Adapted with permission from Dickey (1).

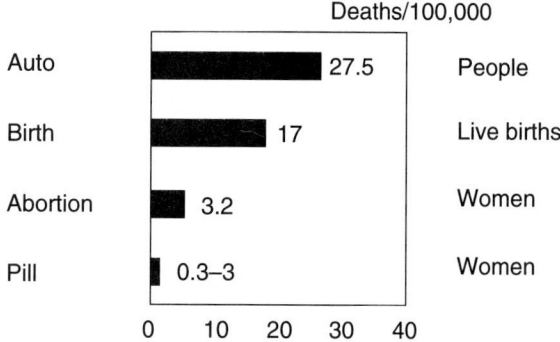

Figure 91.4. Common risks of mortality

1. What oral contraceptive product is the patient taking?
2. How long has the patient been taking oral contraceptives?
3. On which days of the menstrual cycle were pills missed?
4. How many pills were missed?

Ovulation is not always suppressed in products containing low-dose estrogen. The more estrogen and progestin in a product, the more reliable it will be at the expense of having more side effects. One missed pill would be of less consequence for a patient taking a high-dose product than for a patient taking a low-dose pill. In addition, the progestin content of the low-dose pill contributes to the contraceptive effect and must be present daily.

Modest fluctuations in the levels of FSH and LH among pill users have been observed. This might indicate that follicular development may proceed to a greater extent in some women, resulting in more breakthrough ovulation. Because women who have taken oral contraceptives for a long period of time have ovaries in a semidormant state, they are less likely to experience breakthrough ovulation as a result of a missed pill. On the other hand, women who are short-term oral contraceptive users are more likely to have mature follicles ready for ovulation; they may be more affected by a missed pill or by missing the usual dosing time by several hours. Oral contraceptives should be taken at the same time each day.

Contrary to popular belief, missing pills at midcycle is not the greatest risk. A high level of hormones early in the cycle is necessary at the level of the hypothalamus for suppression of FSH and LH. Therefore, missing pill number 2, for example, would be more likely to result in a pregnancy than missing pill number 20.

Many clinicians believe that if a patient misses one pill, that missed pill should be taken as soon as it is remembered: the next day's pill should be taken at the regular time (two pills may be taken at the same time). If two consecutive pills are missed, the medication should be doubled for the following 2 consecutive days. Barrier methods of contraception should be started immediately and used for the rest of the cycle.

This information should be evaluated with care. For example, if a patient has been taking a product that contains 50 μg of estrogen for 3 years and missed pill 18, she probably would not get pregnant. On the other hand, if a patient misses pills 2 and 3 of her second pack of 20 μg pills, she is likely to ovulate.

The triphasic oral contraceptives or mini-pills introduce an even smaller margin of error. Basal concentrations of FSH and LH are only partially depressed during the last 3 days of therapy, producing less inhibition than standard COCs. Ovulation is effectively inhibited, but after missed doses, FSH and LH concentrations recover more quickly. Excellent reviews on managing contraceptive pill patients have appeared elsewhere (1, 2, 57).

"Morning-After" Pills

The implantation of the blastocyte is inhibited by high doses of estrogen. Synthetic, natural, and conjugated estrogens have been administered as "morning-after" pills. Therapy is not recommended for routine use, but rather for cases of rape, incest, or mechanical contraceptive failure near midcycle. The interval between conception and implantation is approximately 6 days. When high-risk unprotected intercourse has occurred, it is important to begin therapy within 72 hours.

In the 1960s and early 1970s, high doses of diethylstilbestrol (DES), 25 to 50 mg/day, or ethinyl estradiol, 5 mg/day for 5 days, were used as "morning-after" therapy. Conjugated equine estrogen (Premarin), 30 mg/day orally for 5 days or 50 mg/day IV for 2 days, has been used for this purpose. Nausea and vomiting are complications of this high-dose estrogen therapy.

Although DES is an effective postcoital contraceptive agent, failures can occur. Cases of vaginal adenosis, vaginal adenocarcinoma, and cervical adenocarcinoma in young female offspring of women who took DES during pregnancy have been reported. This teratogenic effect of DES appears to occur at the ninth week of pregnancy (58). Thus, no evidence of teratogenicity has been demonstrated in association with the failure of postcoital estrogens. However, abortion should be a first consideration if these agents fail.

Today, the most popular regimen is 100 μg ethinyl estradiol and 1 mg norgestrel (i.e., two Ovral tablets) initially, repeated after 12 hours (4 tablets total). The patient should experience withdrawal bleeding within 10 days of administration. Again, treatment must be initiated within 72 hours of exposure. Experience with 1300 treatment cycles with this regimen indicates a failure rate of 1.6% (59).

Subdermal Hormonal Implants

Another method of delivering contraceptive progestogen is by subdermal implants. Norplant contains levonorgestrel (216 mg) in six silicone rods about 3.4 cm long. A small incision under local anesthesia is required to insert, in a fanlike arrangement, the device in the upper arm. The steroid is released at a relatively constant rate and provides effective contraception for 5 years.

The relatively low circulating levels of progestin are not sufficient to suppress the LH and FSH secretion completely, but levels are usually sufficient to inhibit the positive feedback of LH release and inhibit most ovulations. The annual pregnancy rate is less than 1% in women who weigh less than 150 pounds. Body weight above 70 kg results in lower serum concentrations of levonorgestrel in later years of implantation and has been associated with increased failure rates. In addition, women who rapidly metabolize steroids (those using phenytoin, carbamazepine, phenobarbital, or rifampin) may have higher pregnancy rates with Norplant or any other low-dose hormonal contraceptive. The removal of the capsules also requires an incision and local anesthesia, but fertility returns to normal promptly after removal. As with other contraceptives containing progestin only, the main side effect is irregular bleeding. About 15% of patients have the Norplant removed because of bleeding.

Two-rod systems (Norplant 2 and others) are faster, easier, and less painful, and have been studied since the early 1980s. However, production of the silastic elastomer in early products ceased before FDA approval of these products. Norplant 2 was then reformulated and is now in clinical trials. After 3 years of use, the reformulated Norplant 2 shows drug release rates, pregnancy rates and side effects similar to the 6-capsule system. Norplant 2 is less conspicuous, more rigid, and easier to remove than the original product.

Vaginal Rings

Another device that has received extensive testing is a silicone rubber vaginal ring that can be initiated and terminated by the user. The rings contain progestin, either alone or in combination with an estrogen. Sustained release of steroids is absorbed through the vaginal epithelium for contraceptive action. The rings are typically kept in the vagina for 14 to 21 days and removed to allow menstrual flow. Levonorgestrel rings were developed by the WHO and have been tested since 1972. Rings containing other combinations of progestins and estrogens are being evaluated. Estrogen was added to reduce the frequency of bleeding problems. Pregnancy rates are 3.6 per 100 women-years. The principal reasons for discontinuation are menstrual disturbances, interference with coitus, and repeated expulsion of the ring.

The "Shot"

Depot medroxyprogesterone acetate (DMPA) has been used in other countries around the world as an injectable contraceptive agent and was approved for use in the United States in 1992, 29 years after the start of clinical trials (60). The drug suppresses the preovulatory surge of LH and plasma levels of FSH decline, thus inhibiting ovulation; it also produces the progestin mucus changes and endometrial growth changes discussed earlier. Failure rates range from 0 to 1.2 pregnancies per 100 women-years.

The dose of DMPA is 150 mg intramuscularly every 90 days. Contraceptive plasma levels are reached within 24 hours, with peak concentrations within 20 days. The optimal time to initiate DMPA is within 5 days after the onset of menses. This ensures that the patient is not pregnant and prevents ovulation during the first month of use.

Women using this form of contraceptive experience very irregular menstrual bleeding patterns. After one injection 30% of users have irregular bleeding and spotting that occurs more than 11 days each month. Amenorrhea is to be expected 2 to 12 months after beginning use of the medication, with approximately 50% of women developing amenorrhea after 1 year of use. The average length of time for return of fertility after discontinuation of this drug is about 8 to 10 months. DMPA is not recommended for short-term contraception.

The same contraindications exist for DMPA as for the "pill," although it is not presently known if thromboembolic disorders increase as a result of DMPA use. Reduced bone density and unfavorable plasma lipid profiles associated with long-term use of DMPA have been reported.

Mifepristone (RU 486)/Methotrexate and Misoprostol

Mifepristone is a 19-norsteroid, an antiprogestin, used in France and China to induce an abortion. Treatment with this drug early in pregnancy leads to detachment and expulsion of the products of conception. Mifepristone has also been successfully compared with high-dose estrogen and progestogen for emergency postcoital contraception (61).

The drug has a high affinity for progesterone and glucocorticoid receptors and, to a lesser extent, for androgen receptors. It also stimulates the synthesis of prostaglandins. Both prostaglandins and withdrawal of progesterone stimulate uterine contractility.

The drug is administered orally alone or followed by a small dose of prostaglandin analog administered by vaginal suppository or intramuscularly 36 to 48 hours later. Clinical studies have shown that a single 600-mg oral dose of mifepristone can terminate early pregnancy (before 6 weeks after the onset of the last menses) in approximately 85% of cases. The incidence of complete abortion increases to about 95% when combined with a dose of prostaglandin. Bleeding begins 1 or 2 days after treatment and lasts 1 to 2 weeks. Crampy abdominal pain occurs in most patients for a few hours after administration.

Interest has been expressed recently in the use of methotrexate and misoprostol to induce early abortions. Though both drugs are approved by the FDA for other indications when given alone, safety and effectiveness concerns, including optimal dosing levels and route of administration, necessitate further research. Currently, insufficient information has been published to accurately characterize the efficacy and safety of various regimens.

MECHANICAL BIRTH CONTROL

A variety of mechanical birth control devices are available, including intrauterine devices, diaphragms, cervical caps, condoms, and spermicidal agents. The efficacy of these products in theory and in use can be seen in Table 91.1.

Intrauterine Device

The idea of inserting a foreign body into the uterus to prevent pregnancy is not new. Many years ago natural fibers such as silkworm gut as well as stones and wires containing silver and copper were used as intrauterine contraceptive devices. After World War II, artificial fibers and various types of polythene were available and were molded in many ways as intrauterine devices (IUDs). The copper-containing IUD regained popularity in the 1960s, and an IUD that slowly releases progesterone was an innovative development of the 1970s. All but two IUDs have been voluntarily withdrawn by the manufacturers from the U.S. market. Makers cite increased litigation costs as reasons for discontinuing their products. *Progesterone T* (Progestasert system by Alza), is a T-shaped unit containing a reservoir of 38 mg progesterone with barium sulfate dispersed in silicone oil. This device is associated with less blood loss and a lower frequency of primary dysmenorrhea as a result of the progesterone. The Progestasert system must be replaced annually. The *Copper-T 380A* (ParaGard-GynoPharma) is a copper-containing IUD that may be left in place for up to 8 years. The *Copper-T 380A* is believed to be the most effective IUD in current use, particularly for women over age 25. A third IUD may be approved soon-the *Levonorgestrel-IUD* (LNg-IUD by Leiras), which would contain levonorgestrel that would release at a constant rate. The newly proposed IUD would stay in place for up to 5 years.

The mechanism of action of an IUD may be from one of two mechanisms: (a) It prevents fertilization by interfering with the sperm's ability to get to the fallopian tubes from the vagina, or (b) the ovum is normally fertilized in the fallopian tube, and an IUD helps to speed the transport time of the ovum through the fallopian tube. A variety of other enzymatic and biochemical processes have been postulated.

Theoretically, the IUD is about 98 to 99% effective. Its use effectiveness is approximately the same, since very little compliance is required on the part of the patient.

The only absolute contraindications for the insertion of an IUD in a normal healthy woman are active pelvic infection and pregnancy. Because of the increased risk of pelvic inflammatory disease (PID), some clinicians do not consider the IUD for use in nulliparous women who wish to bear children in the future. Nulliparous women may also have more problems with postinsertion pain and vasovagal symptoms, which may lead to removal. However, a number of complications may follow insertion. For instance, there may be an increase in the amount of menstrual flow or spotting, as well as pain associated with the IUD, particularly for the first several months following IUD insertion. This increased blood loss may cause anemia in some patients and leads to a 10 to 15% discontinuation rate. If the woman is on anticoagulation therapy, this increase in bleeding risk must be taken into account. Moreover, all types of IUD may be expelled through the cervix. Obviously, the device can be of no value when it is absent. Patients should be taught to check for the IUD string in the vagina to make sure the device is in place. Uterine perforation is most likely to occur at the time of insertion; however, IUDs may gradually work their way through the uterine wall and may need to be removed from the abdominal cavity by laparoscopic procedures.

Women should be informed about IUD warning signs when an IUD is implanted (2). Those warning signs requiring medical attention are reflected in this mnemonic:

P: Period late (pregnancy); abnormal spotting or bleeding
A: Abdominal pain or pain with intercourse
I: Infection exposure (any STD) or abnormal discharge
N: Not feeling well, fever, chills
S: String missing, shorter, or longer

The most serious complications from IUDs are related to infections, including sepsis and in some cases death. IUD use is associated with about a threefold increased incidence of developing acute salpingitis (PID) in comparison with users of oral contraceptives and diaphragms. The Dalkon Shield was withdrawn from the market after several deaths from septic spontaneous abortions. If pregnancy occurs with an IUD in place, there is an approximate 25% increased risk of spontaneous abortion and about 5% of women will experience an ectopic pregnancy.

The Diaphragm

The diaphragm is a dome-shaped rubber cup that is available in several styles and diameters (55 to 95 mm). It is inserted into the vagina and blocks the opening to the uterus by covering the cervix with the dome of the diaphragm. The diaphragm must be fitted by a clinician and should be refitted at each annual exam or if the woman delivers a baby, aborts, or gains or loses 10 pounds or more.

It was thought that the mechanical barrier of the diaphragm would prevent sperm migration into the uterus; however, it has been shown that a diaphragm moves about during coitus (2). Therefore, its primary mechanism is to hold the spermicidal agent near the cervical os. The diaphragm should not be used without spermicidal jelly or cream. These agents also aid insertion because of their lubrication properties. The diaphragm may be used during menses.

At least a teaspoonful of spermicidal jelly or cream should be placed into the dome and spread around the inside of the rim before insertion. It takes 6 to 8 hours for the spermicidal agent to work; therefore, the diaphragm must remain in place at least 8 hours. Oil-based products (e.g., petroleum jellies and lotions) may cause deterioration. If additional lubrication is needed, use a contraceptive jelly or a water-soluble lubricant. Another applicatorful of spermicide should be inserted in the vagina, leaving the diaphragm in place, before each subsequent coitus, or if more than 6 hours has elapsed since the first insertion. There may be a possible risk of toxic shock syndrome if the diaphragm is left in place for more than 24 hours, so this is not recommended. After it has been used, the diaphragm needs to washed and stored.

The key to successful diaphragm use is motivation. Many clinicians fail to recognize the diaphragm as a viable contraceptive alternative. However, because of its mechanical action, it represents a method of contraception practically devoid of side effects. The diaphragm is not advised for use in patients who have recurrent urinary tract infections, if there is a lack of trained personal to fit the device, or if clinical time does not allow for proper user instructions.

The Cervical Cap

There has been a resurgence of interest in a barrier method smaller than a diaphragm that fits over the cervix, called a cervical cap. Two caps are available in the United States, the Prentif® and the Fem Cap®. The Prentif® cap is made of natural rubber (latex) and is thimble shaped, whereas the Fem Cap® is made of silicon rubber and shaped like a sailor's hat. It also comes with an applicator. Spermicide should fill the dome one-third full prior to insertion. The cervical cap can be left in place for a maximum of 48 hours without adding more spermicide, even if intercourse is repeated. The cervical cap should not be left in for more than 48 hours due to a increased risk of toxic shock syndrome. The Prentif is manufactured in four sizes; the Fem Cap® is available in three. Before removal the Prentif® cervical cap must be left in place for 6 hours after intercourse, while the Fem Cap® must be left in place for 8 hours after intercourse. If additional lubrication is needed, use a water-soluble lubricant or contraceptive jelly, since oil-based products may cause cervical cap deterioration. As with the diaphragm, the cervical cap needs to be washed after use, and before storage. Pregnancy rates are similar to other barrier methods; however, in parous women the cap is less effective than in nulliparous women. Because of concern about possible adverse effects on cervical tissue, caps should be used only by women with normal Pap smears. Smears should be checked after the first three months of use and annually thereafter. The cervical cap must be discontinued if the Pap smear is abnormal at the three month visit. The cervical cap is not advised (2):

1. if there is a lack of clinical time to provide appropriate instructions for the use or if education personnel lack training.
2. if the patient has had a recent full-term delivery or an abortion.
3. if the patient has vaginal bleeding (including menses).
4. if the patient has a known or suspected cervical or uterine malignancy, an abnormal Pap smear, or a current vaginal or cervical infection.

The Condom

Due to their ability to prevent sexually transmitted diseases (STDs) and pregnancy, when used consistently and properly, condoms are one of the most popular contraceptives. They are also accessible, inexpensive, and readily usable. During the 1980s, there was a dramatic increase in condom sales in the United States. Currently, condoms are made to be worn not only by men, but by women as well. Condoms that are to be worn by men are latex rubber sheaths that are worn over an erect penis during coitus. This mechanical barrier prevents transmission of the male semen into the

vagina. Although pregnancy rates are higher than in users of COCs, barrier methods are effective in preventing the transmission of venereal disease, including HIV, from either partner. Several in vitro studies have demonstrated that latex condoms prevent the transmission of viruses, specifically the herpes virus and human immunodeficiency virus (HIV) when used for vaginal, orogenital, and anogenital intercourse. In addition, *Chlamydia trachomatis* and gonorrheal infections, both frequent causes of salpingitis, can be prevented. There are also "skin" or "natural membrane" condoms, which are made of processed collagenous tissue from the intestinal caecum of lambs. This type of condom prevents pregnancy by blocking male semen into the vagina; however, they are *not* recommended for preventing the transmission of sexually transmitted diseases. People who have a latex sensitivity are able to use the natural membrane condoms. Currently, numerous synthetic products are in development that would provide protection from STDs, including HIV, as well as unintended pregnancy, for people that have a latex sensitivity.

More than 100 brands of condoms are available that are manufactured to be worn by men. They are available in different shapes, sizes, colors, and thickness. Some condoms have a small amount of spermicide (usually nonoxynol-9) applied to the inside and/or outside of the condom. Condoms are marketed rolled or unrolled, lubricated or unlubricated, and ribbed, and may have reservoir ends to collect the semen. When the condom is put on, half an inch of empty space should be left at the tip if the condom does not have a reservoir end. To prevent spillage during withdrawal, the rim of the condom should be held against the base of the penis during withdrawal, promptly after ejaculation. A condom should be used only once.

Oil-based products (e.g., petroleum jelly, hand lotion, vegetable oil) should never be used to lubricate a condom (this causes the latex to deteriorate). K-Y jelly, contraceptive foam, and saliva are good lubricants. Trying to test a condom for holes by filling it up with air or water, as well as unrolling it and then sliding it over the penis, increases the probability of breakage.

The female condom (Reality) is a polyurethane sheath (pouch) that is closed at one end and has two flexible polyurethane rings, one at each end. Polyurethane is stronger than latex and less likely to break or tear. The condom is approximately 17 cm in length and 7.8 cm in diameter. As with the latex male condoms, the female condom will help to prevent unintended pregnancy and transmission of STDs. The pouch is prelubricated on the inside with a silicone-based lubricant, with an additional bottle of lubricant provided with the condom.

The open end, with the outer ring, remains outside the vagina to cover the perineum. The inner ring is needed for insertion and to hold the pouch in place. When inserting the pouch, hold the inner ring between the thumb and middle finger while placing the index finger on the pouch between the other two fingers. While squeezing the inner ring, insert the pouch as far as possible into the vagina, to cover the cervix. The pouch should not be twisted. Removal of the pouch should occur before standing up by squeezing and twisting the outer ring and gently pulling. If the penis does not move freely in and out, if the outer ring is pushed inside, or if there is a noise during intercourse, apply more lubricant to the inside of the pouch or to the penis.

There have been some problems with the acceptability of the female condom. The visibility of the outer ring, unpleasant noises during intercourse, and problems with the initial insertion are some of the complaints voiced by users. However, many users consider the female condom an acceptable method of contraception.

Spermicidal Agents

Spermicidal products are available as film, foam, jellies, creams, suppositories and tablets. These agents may be used alone or in combination with other vaginal barrier methods. When spermicidal agents are used, they must be used prior to each ejaculation. Nonoxynol-9 is the spermicidal agent used in most of these over-the-counter (OTC) preparations. Contraceptive foam is marketed in an aerosol can or bottle with an applicator or as a tablet. The foam is the medium that holds the spermicidal agent against the cervical os. Two full applicators of foam should be inserted high in the vagina no earlier than 30 minutes before each ejaculation. Spermicides also reduce the frequency of clinical infections from sexually transmitted diseases such as chlamydia and gonorrhea. Whether spermicides reduce the risk of HIV transmission is uncertain.

Although contraceptive foam is fairly effective alone, it can be used in conjunction with a diaphragm or condom to produce a very effective method of birth control. Vaginal spermicides marketed to be used with a diaphragm are usually less potent, having a different consistency but the same active ingredient.

If a particular brand of foam is irritating to either partner, the couple should try another brand. Foam is often confused with "feminine hygiene" products. There are tablets that are supposed to foam, creams and jellies that are supposed to spread, and suppositories that are supposed to melt; sometimes they do not. The film may be used alone or with a diaphragm or condom. It is a 2″ by 2″ sheet that contains nonoxynol-9 and must be inserted on or near the cervix or in the diaphragm before intercourse to allow the sheet to melt and the spermicide to disperse. Fifteen minutes after insertion, contraception protection begins. However, it is not effective after 1 hour. It is not recommended to place the sheet on the tip of the penis, because it will not have adequate time to dissolve and the

film may not cover the cervical os. Spermicidal foams, jellies, and creams have immediate contraceptive protection, which remains effective for 1 hour. The jellies or creams used with diaphragms or caps remain effective for 6 to 8 hours. Jellies and creams need to be used by filling the applicator and inserting it properly into the vagina. Like the film, contraceptive tablets and suppositories begin their activity 10 to 15 minutes after insertion because the spermicide needs to disperse. These also provide activity for approximately 1 hour.

Douching may force sperm in the uterus and is not recommended for at least 8 hours after intercourse when using a diaphragm or foam for contraception. These products should not be used during pregnancy. The literature is not conclusive, although there have been case reports of birth defects following the use of spermicides during pregnancy. These studies were probably flawed by recall bias. Several well-designed recent studies have shown no increased risk of congenital malformations in newborns (62) or spontaneous abortuses (63) of women who conceived while using spermicides.

The Contraceptive Sponge

Until recently there was another form of vaginal contraception, a disposable, polyurethane foam sponge, slightly thicker and smaller than a diaphragm with a ribbon loop for removal. The sponge was impregnated with nonoxynol-9 and could be left in place about 24 hours. The spermicide had to be activated before insertion by adding 1 ounce of water to the sponge. It has been shown that parous women have a higher failure rate with this method than nulliparous women. At the end of 1994, the manufacturer of the Today sponge voluntarily halted production due to its inability to comply with more stringent government-directed mandates at its manufacturing facility. A few cases of toxic shock syndrome (TSS) have been reported in users of the sponge; the role of this contraceptive device as a causative agent is not clearly defined.

TOXIC SHOCK SYNDROME

Billions of tampons have been produced and used by millions of women throughout the world over the past several decades. In the last several years, a circumstantial relationship has existed between the use of tampons and several disease entities.

The first cases of TSS were described in 1978 (64). Since then a wide variety of clinical symptoms have been described. TSS generally affects previously healthy young women of childbearing age during an otherwise normal menstrual period. It usually begins with a sudden high fever (greater than 102°F) and may be accompanied by severe headache, sore throat, dizziness, vomiting, and diarrhea. Progressive hypotension may proceed to shock, coma, and death. Palmar erythema is frequent, and a diffuse sunburnlike rash has been described, which is often followed by a superficial desquamation of skin on the palms and soles within 2 or 3 weeks from the onset of the disease. A nonpurulent conjunctivitis is usually present at the disease onset.

TSS is associated with the use of highly absorbent tampons. In many cases it is possible to isolate coagulase-positive *Staphylococcus aureus* from the vagina or from focal infections of infected patients. There is concern that an increased risk of TSS with vaginal barrier forms of contraception exists. In fact, the TSS rate of women who use vaginal barrier methods is two to three per year for every 100,000 women (65). The presence of an exotoxin of *S. aureus* could certainly account for the clinical symptoms identified with this disease. Clinicians should be aware of the possibility of TSS in any menstruating woman with sudden onset of febrile illness. Prompt removal of tampons and symptomatic treatment, including support of blood pressure, may be critical. Use of β-lactamase-resistant penicillins has been shown to lower risk of the recurrence (65). In addition, patients with TSS should be instructed to permanently discontinue the use of tampons. Tampon manufacturers have decreased absorbency by removal of chemical components, such as polyester foam, carboxymethylcellulose, and polyacrylate rayon. As a result, the incidence of TSS has fallen in the last several years.

INFERTILITY

Incidence of Infertility

Infertility has been labeled "epidemic" in the United States, with 10 to 15% of couples experiencing some degree of infertility (67). Infertility is generally defined as 1 year of unprotected coitus without conception. Fifty-seven percent of couples desiring pregnancy will conceive without medical intervention in 3 months. By 6 months, this will rise to 72%. By the end of a year, 85% of couples desiring a pregnancy will have conceived. Of the remaining 15% who present with infertility, approximately half (8 in 15) will conceive spontaneously during the next year.

While there are many popular explanations for a decline in U.S. fertility, there have been no dramatic changes in the proportion of infertile couples since 1965, except among women 20 to 24 years old, for whom infertility went from 3.6% in 1965 to 10.6% in 1982. This is probably a reflection, at least in part, of increases in sexually transmitted diseases. However, there has been a dramatic increase in the demand for infertility services since 1981. From approximately 600,000 visits in 1968, the total increased to nearly 1 million in the early 1970s, and in the early 1980s the total went over 2 million visits.

Etiology

Infertility is a symptom that can be caused by numerous causative factors. In general, 37% of infertility is a problem solely of the female; another 35% is a cause found in both members of the couple. In about 8% of cases a problem is found in only the male, and no cause is found in 5% of couples. The remaining couples (15%) became pregnant during investigation (68).

There are many known causes for infertility in the male and female that can, in many cases, be successfully treated with medical or surgical techniques. It has been shown that 30–50% of all infertile women have some anatomic abnormality as the root cause. Adhesions from previous surgery, tubal obstructions from prior pelvic infections, tumors, polyps, or fibroids are just a few common example. Advances in microsurgery and laser technology have made it possible to correct many of these anatomic causes. Another 30–40% of infertile females do not ovulate (are anovulatory) or ovulate inconsistently (oligo-ovulation). Progress in understanding normal and abnormal menstrual physiology has led to the development of effective modalities for the induction of ovulation. Improvement in the treatment of ovulatory dysfunction has been one of the most successful therapeutic advances in gynecologic endocrinology. Finally 20–30% of infertile women show no demonstrable cause for their infertility, and 10% or less have a cervical barrier to fertility.

The cause of male infertility can often be determined by interpretation of the semen analysis. Up to 37% of infertile males have a varicocele, or abnormal tortuosity and dilation of the veins within the spermatic cord. In all likelihood, varicoceles exert their effects by raising testicular temperature. Testicular failure accounts for 9% of male infertility. Spermatogenesis may be deficient (oligospermia) or lacking (azoospermia) in an otherwise normal male. Virility and libido are regulated by androgens produced by Leydig cells and are unrelated to sperm production. Hypothalamic-pituitary insufficiency in males is rare but in many cases is treated with similar pharmacologic agents as the anovulatory female. Anatomic abnormalities such as obstruction (6%) or absence of the vas deferens (6%) and failure of descent of a testis can each account for another 6% of male infertility. The incidence of other semen abnormalities involving viscosity, semen volume, and agglutination account for approximately 10% of male infertility disorders. Finally, 25% of male disorders are classified as idiopathic or unknown.

Diagnosis and Clinical Findings

Because the reasons for infertility are so varied, it is very important to do a good medical history of the infertile couple. An obvious history of endometriosis, amenorrhea, frequent spontaneous abortions or anatomic abnormalities provides clues for the clinician to focus the infertility workup. However, in addition to these clues, initial workup of the infertile couple usually consists of

1. Semen analysis
2. Evaluation of pelvic anatomy: tubal patency via laparoscopy, fluoroscopically controlled hysterosalpingography (HSG), and/or hysteroscopy

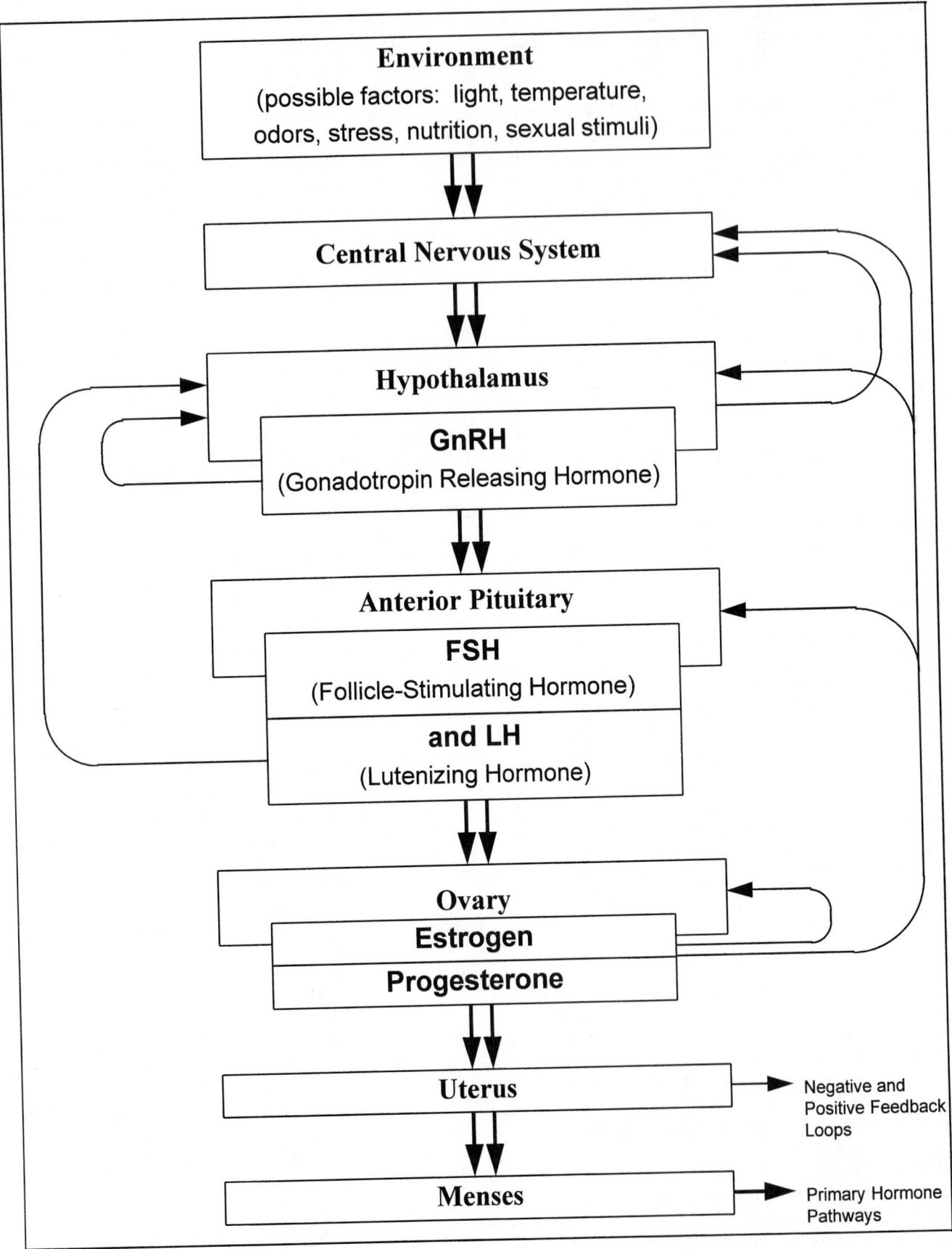

Figure 91.5. Feedback system of the hypothalamic-pituitary-ovarian axis.

3. Postcoital testing (PCT)
4. Evaluation of ovulation

The delicate balance in the hypothalamic-pituitary-ovarian axis and its feedback controls on normal follicular maturation are important to understanding the use of fertility agents. During menses the hypothalamus responds to low levels of circulating estrogen with the production and release of gonadotropin-releasing hormone (GnRH). GnRH affects the anterior pituitary to release FSH and LH. Throughout the cycle, FSH levels fluctuate via a negative feedback system involving estrogen (estradiol e-2); LH levels fluctuate by both positive and negative feedback systems involving estrogen and by the negative feedback of progesterone during the luteal phase (Fig. 91.5). This complex mechanism is exquisitely sensitive to alterations in any or all components.

CENTRAL HYPOTHALAMIC-PITUITARY AXIS FAILURE AND BROMOCRIPTINE

At least one clinical syndrome of central anovulatory dysfunction has been recognized, hyperprolactinemia. A search for galactorrhea and measurement of serum prolactin are important screening procedures for all women who are not ovulating normally (Fig. 91.6). Hyperprolactinemia (prolactin > 20) can be found in approximately 15% of women with anovulation and interferes with normal function of the menstrual cycle by suppressing the pulsatile secretion of GnRH. Suppression of prolactin restores CNS-pituitary gonadotropin function and ovarian responsiveness very quickly, and many patients will conceive within 3 or 4 months of treatment. A variety of therapeutic drugs have been associated with increased serum prolactin levels, including phenothiazines, tricyclic antidepressants, meprobamate, haloperidol, methyldopa, and isoniazid. Patients with hypothyroidism or pituitary tumor may also have hyperprolactinemia and must be ruled out as a cause. When these secondary conditions have been excluded, idiopathic hyperprolactinemia is treated with bromocriptine at a target dose of 2.5 mg BID.

Bromocriptine mesylate is a semisynthetic ergot alkaloid derivative that inhibits prolactin secretion with little effect on other pituitary hormones. It is a dopamine receptor agonist that activates postsynaptic dopamine receptors. Initial doses of 1.25 to 2.5 mg taken at bedtime or with meals to decrease GI intolerance are followed with adding a second dose after a week. The incidence of side effects is high (69%), but they are generally mild to

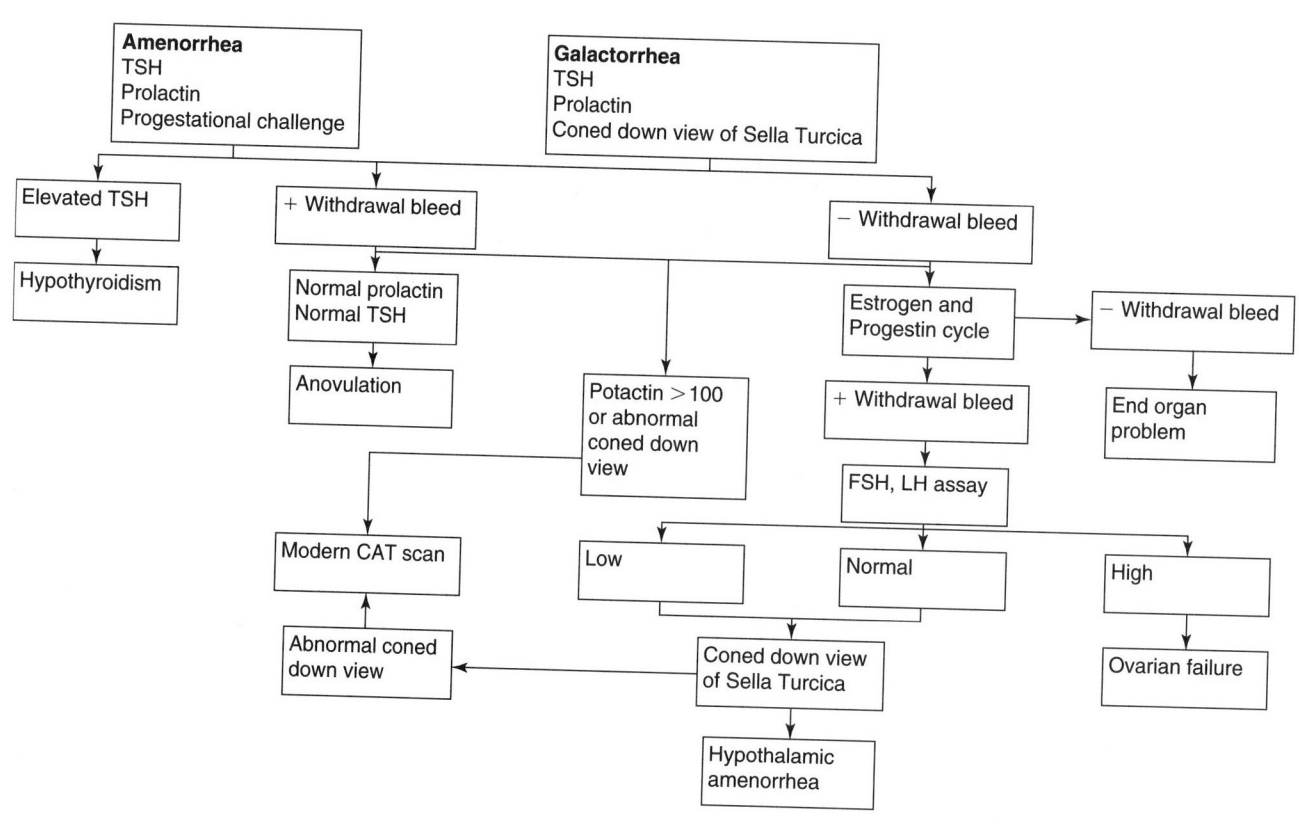

Figure 91.6. Workup of amenorrheic patients with or without galacturrhea.

moderate. The most common side effect is nausea, which occurs in 49% of women. Other side effects include dizziness, headache, or fatigue.

While the total incidence of malformations and spontaneous abortions among children conceived during bromocriptine therapy does not exceed that of the population at large, caution should be used. It may be advisable to use mechanical contraception in conjunction with therapy until normal ovulatory menstrual cycles have been restored. Once the effective dose is achieved, normal prolactin concentrations should be obtained within 1 week and menses should follow in 5 to 6 weeks. Mechanical contraception is then stopped, and bromocriptine treatment is then taken only during the follicular phase and stopped when ovulation occurs (see "Ovulation Detection"). If pregnancy does not ensue, the drug is resumed when menses begins. The drug should be discontinued as soon as a positive pregnancy test is obtained.

Ovulatory menses and pregnancy are achieved in 80% of patients with galactorrhea and hyperprolactinemia. Response is usually rapid, and if there is no evidence of ovulation (see "Ovulation Detection") within 2 months, clomiphene is added to the regimen.

OTHER ANOVULATORY DYSFUNCTIONS

FSH stimulation occurs from a nadir in blood sex steroid levels. The necessary decline in blood estrogen requires reduction of secretion, appropriate clearance and metabolism, and the absence of significant estrogen by extragonadal sources. The most common clinical example of anovulation associated with continued secretion of estrogen is pregnancy but anovulation can also be a result of an ovarian or adrenal tumor.

The clearance and metabolism of estrogen can be impaired by other pathologic conditions, such as thyroid or hepatic disease. Both hyperthyroidism and hypothyroidism can cause persistent anovulation by altering not only metabolic clearance but also the peripheral conversion rates among the various steroids. The subtle presence of hypothyroidism, which may be associated with elevated prolactin levels, demands screening with a thyroid-stimulating hormone (TSH) level and appropriate treatment with thyroid hormone.

Polycystic ovary (PCO) disease is a clinical syndrome present in women who have a history of oligomenorrhea, hirsutism, and obesity, together with a demonstration of enlarged, polycystic ovaries. The characteristic polycystic ovary emerges when a state of anovulation persists for any length of time. Because there are many causes of anovulation, there are many causes of polycystic ovaries. With persistent anovulation, the average daily production of estrogen and androgens is both increased and dependent upon increased LH stimulation. Inappropriately high LH:FSH ratios (often greater than 2 or 3:1) is

classically associated with this disease. The symptoms of this disease are a consequence of the loss of ovulation: dysfunctional bleeding, amenorrhea, hirsutism, and infertility. Each requires a specific diagnostic and therapeutic approach.

Luteal Deficiency

An inadequate luteal phase occurs when there is deficient progesterone secretion by the corpus luteum and may be a factor in women with a history of recurrent abortion. The term applies to both a short interval (less than 11 days) between ovulation and menstruation with normal peak progesterone levels and, more commonly, to a luteal phase of normal length with lower than normal progesterone levels. An inadequate luteal phase can be found in up to 30% of isolated cycles in normal women and is significant in infertility only if found in 2 cycles.

Although an inadequate luteal phase is a direct result of decreased hormone production by the corpus luteum, the underlying causes of this dysfunction can be multiple and are therefore treated differently. Regardless of the cause there is a deficiency of progesterone in the inadequate luteal phase, and replacement by exogenous progesterone has been used with success in the ovulating female. A vaginal suppository containing 25 mg of progesterone is inserted twice daily starting approximately 3 days after ovulation. Treatment is maintained until menstruation occurs or until a pregnancy is diagnosed. If the latter, a switch may be made to injections of progesterone through the 10th week of pregnancy to decrease the chance of spontaneous abortion.

Ovulation Detection

Methods to detect ovulation include charting basal body temperature (BBT), home kits for detection of increased urinary LH, endometrial biopsy showing histologic findings characteristic of the luteal phase, a single measurement of serum progesterone or urinary pregnanediol at mid-luteal phase, or ultrasound monitoring.

Once ovulation is suspected, fertilization can occur within 12 to 24 hours. The problem with most methods of detecting ovulation is that they occur after ovulation. The easiest and most inexpensive method to detect whether, and perhaps when, ovulation occurs is to chart basal body temperature (BBT). To use this method, only a special BBT thermometer and temperature charts (Fig. 91.7) are needed. A woman should take her temperature immediately upon waking and before any activity, even before leaving the bed. The BBT usually shows a distinct, biphasic pattern with an elevation during the postovulatory phase of the cycle. This elevated temperature has been attributed to the thermogenic effect of progesterone.

There appears to be no difference if the thermometer is placed orally, rectally, or vaginally, as long as it is inserted

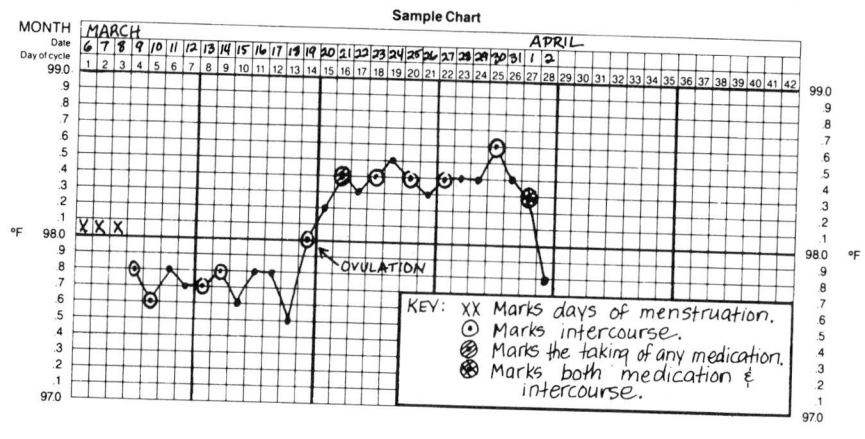

Figure 91.7. Sample basal body temperature chart. (From Carmichael JM. Pharmacologic treatment of infertility. Randolph, MA: Serono Laboratories, 1986.)

at least 5 cm and the location is consistent (69). In addition, the hour of waking should be recorded, because variation in time may affect results (70).

Luteinizing hormone (LH) urine tests are OTC products available to aid in documenting ovulation. These tests take advantage of the LH surge just prior to the ovulatory phase. Diluted urine is processed such that monoclonal antibodies selectively bind to LH in the urine. An enzyme-linked immunoassay indicates the amount of LH bound to the monoclonal antibodies via a change in color intensity. A darker color on the test, as compared to a color chart that is provided, indicates the surge in LH. Ovulation would be expected in the next 36 hours if such a color change occurs.

A variety of ovulation test kits are available and contain a series of 5 to 9 urine tests that take 4 minutes to 1 hour each morning to perform, depending on the test. During the testing period, urine is tested daily. If there is a color change or if the color change is darker than the surge guide, then the LH surge has occurred.

Conditions such as endometriosis, ovarian cysts, hyperthyroidism, and the onset of menopause can cause high LH levels that are not due to ovulation. Drugs such as the menatropins, danazol, and steroids, and initial treatment with GnRH analogs can produce a false-positive result. During clomiphene administration large amounts of LH are released; therefore urinary LH testing during or immediately after stopping clomiphene could yield false positive results. At least 2 days should elapse between the last clomiphene treatment day and LH testing. If LH testing is required in these circumstances, serum radioimmune assay techniques can be used.

A simple functional test of follicular activity involves the induction of withdrawal bleeding by progesterone administration. Upon successful induction of withdrawal bleeding, indicating unopposed estrogen stimulation, ovulation induction with clomiphene citrate is indicated.

Clomiphene Citrate

It has been approximately 40 years since the synthesis of clomiphene citrate (Serophene and Clomid). Clomiphene citrate is an orally active nonsteroidal agent distantly related to diethylstilbestrol. Despite a cumulative bibliography approaching 8,000 publications, the mechanism(s) and site(s) of action of clomiphene are still unclear (71). This knowledge gap is particularly striking in view of the widespread and highly successful use of clomiphene worldwide.

The most common indication for clomiphene has been to induce ovulation in women with absence of infrequent ovulation. It has also been used to regulate the timing of ovulation in women undergoing donor insemination. In males, it has been used to diagnose hypothalamic-pituitary axis function or as treatment of male infertility from oligospermia.

Clomiphene citrate (CC) is a weak estrogen that is capable of blocking the effects of more potent estrogens (such as estradiol) (72), thus producing a mixed agonist/antagonistic effect. Clomiphene is capable of interacting with a variety of estrogen-dependent tissues, including the hypothalamic-pituitary unit, ovary, endometrium, cervical mucus-producing glands, and vaginal mucosa.

Current concepts favor the notion that the ability of clomiphene to initiate an ovulatory sequence is due primarily, and perhaps exclusively, to its ability to interact with estrogen receptors at the level of the hypothalamus. In effect it "fools" the hypothalamus that circulating levels of estrogen are low, causing increased release of GnRH followed by increases in FSH, and LH and subsequent ovulation. Adashi (71) suggests that the overall effects of clomiphene may reflect not only the action on the hypothalamus, but the sum of its direct effects on the estrogen-dependent tissue at the hypothalamic, pituitary, and ovarian levels.

The net result at the hypothalamic level is that, in the presence of clomiphene, estradiol is incapable of exerting its negative feedback on GnRH. Thus, clomiphene will enhance FSH and LH release. This mechanism is also applicable in the male hypothalamus, since the negative feedback inhibitory effect of testosterone on GnRH secretion is produced after metabolism of testosterone to an estrogen in hypothalamic cells. In women, the drug is of no value in patients with primary pituitary or ovarian failure and is useful only in patients with hypothalamic dysfunction.

Clomiphene is readily absorbed from the gastrointestinal tract. The drug is hepatically metabolized and eliminated by the biliary tree with detectable levels in the feces for up to 6 weeks. The β elimination half-life is 5 to 7 days. Ovulation usually occurs in 4 to 10 days (average 7) after the last day of treatment during each cycle. Seventy-five percent of pregnancies occur during the first three treatment cycles.

Treatment with clomiphene in women is begun with a dose of 50 mg daily for 5 days beginning on the fifth day following spontaneous or induced bleeding. Administration of a progestin, usually oral MPA (Provera) to induce bleeding in an amenorrheic woman, although not essential, offers a convenient starting point for the cycle and confirms hypothalamic-pituitary-ovarian axis function. If ovulation, as measured by BBT or urine tests for LH, occurs without pregnancy, the same dose of clomiphene is repeated in the next treatment course. In the absence of ovulation, the daily dose should be increased to 100 mg during the next cycle, given as a single daily dose for 5 days. If there is no ovulation again, clomiphene may be increased by 50-mg increments to a maximum of 200 to 250 mg daily for 5 days. This maximum dose may be given for 3 or 4 months with no ovulation before the patient is considered a failure to clomiphene. Once an ovulatory dose has been identified, there is no need to increase the dose further. There is a significant correlation between body weight and the dose of clomiphene required for ovulation. Patients are advised to have intercourse every other day for 1 week beginning 5 days after the last dose in each cycle.

Most patients who respond do so during the first course of therapy. Six ovulatory cycles without conception constitute an adequate therapeutic trial for achievement of a pregnancy. The failure to achieve a pregnancy may be due to anovulation or, on occasion, the antiestrogenic effect of clomiphene on cervical mucus. At the time of ovulation, cervical mucus becomes thin and watery under the influence of estrogen. The thinner the mucus, the more elastic. This elastic quality is known as spinnbarkeit, and the micelles of the mucus arrange in such a fashion that sperm migration is optimal. Clomiphene behaves as an antiestrogen on cervical mucus. Therefore, if clomiphene has been administered over a long period of time without pregnancy occurring, the end-organ effect of clomiphene may be seen as inadequate cervical mucus, inadequate function of the corpus luteum, or inadequate response of the lining of the uterus. After 6 to 8 months of ovulatory clomiphene treatment, reevaluation should be undertaken. In addition, infertility of the male partner should again be considered.

In order to obtain optimal results, evaluation of clomiphene therapy should include

1. demonstration of ovulation by urine tests for LH or BBT.
2. pelvic examination to rule out ovarian enlargement and pregnancy after the first treatment cycle.
3. assessment of any side effects.

Ovulation and Pregnancy Rates Following Clomiphene Therapy

Ovulation rates range between 62 and 83%. Pregnancy rates range from 25 to 56%. It is important to counsel patients regarding side effects of clomiphene. The most common symptoms, antiestrogenic effects and menopauselike vasomotor hot flushes, occur in 11% of patients. Abdominal distension, bloating, and pain or soreness can be noted in 5.5% of women after one treatment cycle. Other minor and reversible side effects include nausea/vomiting, breast discomfort, visual symptoms, headache, heavy menses, mental depression, nervousness, insomnia, and weight gain. Many women complain that their cycles lengthen on clomiphene. Clomiphene administration mimics the normal cycle from day 1. If one counts the first day of clomiphene administration as day 1, then ovulation is expected about day 13 to 15 and menses day 28. However, because clomiphene was begun day 5, the normal cycle of CC is actually 33 days long. Beginning clomiphene earlier than day 5 of the cycle may stimulate multiple follicular maturation and may be prescribed as part of in vitro fertilization program protocols to increase egg harvest.

The frequency of multiple births with adequate patient selection and monitoring is 10% or less and is almost entirely twins (72). The abortion and congenital malformation rate in clomiphene users is not increased.

Clomiphene and Human Chorionic Gonadotropin (HCG)

When clomiphene alone is unsuccessful in inducing ovulation, it is often administered in combination with other agents. If a luteal phase defect (corpus luteum deficiency) is present, as noted by a basal body temperature elevation of less than 11 days' duration, human chorionic gonadotropin (hCG) (Profasi-HPR [Serono], A.P.L. [Ayerst], Antuitrin-S [Parke-Davis], and others) may be added to an anovulatory cycle in addition to clomiphene. The rational for hCG (which has LH-like activity) is to improve the midcycle LH surge in patients with adequate follicular development and thus improve the chance of ovulation. Accurate timing of the hCG dose may require blood estradiol levels (>400 pg/mL) or estimation of follicular size (<22 mm) by ultrasound. HCG 10,000 USP units is given as a single IM dose on the seventh day after clomiphene, when follicular maturation is at its peak (usually cycle day 12 to 16). Intercourse is advised the night of hCG administration and for the next 2 days.

Hypothalamic-Pituitary Failure

When clomiphene alone is unsuccessful in inducing ovulation, it is often administered in combination with other agents. Human menopausal gonadotropin (hMG) in conjunction with hCG is used to stimulate ovulation in women who do not ovulate but have potentially functional ovaries. In males, hMG and hCG treatment can stimulate spermatogenesis in male patients with gonadotropin deficiency. Both endocrine and gametogenic function can be restored by this treatment.

Gonadotropins isolated from human postmenopausal urine (hMG-menotropin-Pergonal) are supplied as lyophilized powder in vials containing 75 IU of FSH and 75 IU of LH. It is dissolved in normal saline before use and injected intramuscularly. The preparation, however, has predominantly FSH-like activity and stimulates ovarian follicle development in women and spermatogenesis in men. In both sexes, it must be used with hCG (which has LH activity). Human chorionic gonadotropin is used to trigger ovulation of the primed follicle, to maintain the corpus luteum in women, and to permit testosterone production from Leydig cells in men.

The dose of hMG and the duration of treatment cannot be decided in advance and must be adjusted individually. Sensitivity to gonadotropins varies widely among patients and even in the same individual from cycle to cycle. Therefore, the amount of hMG must be carefully monitored and adjusted in each cycle. Brown et al. (73) reported a ninefold range for FSH doses among 45 patients treated.

Although varying doses are reported in the literature, the following dose is recommended by the manufacturers:

1. First treatment: One ampule each day (75 IU FSH, 75 IU LH), administered intramuscularly, for 9 to 12 days, followed by hCG 10,000 U, 1 day after the last dose of hMG. The intramuscular injection of 10,000 U hCG results in an initial blood level 20 times higher than the maximal value of LH peak during spontaneous ovulation. The $t_{1/2}\beta = 23.9$ hours, enabling persistent levels for several days to induce ovulation and maintain the corpus luteum for 14 days.

   Response to hMG is usually judged by the degree of estrogen blood level response. One developing ovum will produce an estradiol serum level of approximately 200 to 400 pg/mL. Daily estradiol levels beginning on cycle day 7 of 100 pg/mL would suggest continued dosing of hMG. By contrast, if estradiol levels on day 7 = 500 pg/mL, ultrasound monitoring may be started. Regardless of estradiol serum levels, ultrasound monitoring would begin by day 9. The injections of hMG are stopped, and an injection of hCG is given when the ovum is 18 mm in size and there is no evidence of hyperstimulation. Intercourse should be encouraged daily beginning on the day prior to administration of hCG until ovulation occurs.

2. Second treatment: If there is evidence of ovulation after the first treatment but no pregnancy, the dosing regimen is repeated at least two more times before increasing the dose. If there is no evidence of ovulation after the first treatment, the dose of hMG is increased to 150 IU FSH, 150 IU LH for 9 to 12 days, followed by 10,000 U of hCG 1 day after the last dose of hMG. The most effective dose has proven to be 150 IU of FSH/LH. If evidence of ovulation is present but pregnancy does not ensue, the same dose is repeated for two more courses.

Since gonadotropin induction of ovulation is sometimes associated with serious medical complications, including overstimulation of the ovaries, it is vital that monitoring be conducted. In hMG therapy, estrogen levels are higher than in normal cycles because more than one follicle is stimulated and each follicle secretes estrogen. The character of cervical mucus changes under the influence of estrogen. In the past, before the availability of laboratory support, clinicians tended to monitor gonadotropin therapy by physical signs: observation of the appearance and volume of cervical mucus, spinnbarkeit, ferning of cervical mucus, and vaginal cytology. Cervical mucus examination has been carefully evaluated by combining various measurements into a composite "cervical score." Although effective to a point, further increases in plasma estrogen concentration do not cause a proportional increase in cervical mucus secretion. The clinician may therefore be misled and either give hCG prematurely or delay hCG and continue hMG to the point of hyperstimulation of the ovary. For these reasons, the combination of pelvic examinations with the above clinical indices, although important, is an insufficient monitor if used alone. In combination with serum or urinary estradiol levels and ultrasonography, these indices provide an ideal means for monitoring the growth and development of follicles, timing the hCG administration, and minimizing the risk of hyperstimulation.

If the serum estradiol level is above 2000 pg/mL and more than two large follicles are present, hCG should not be administered, because the hyperstimulation syndrome is more likely to occur. Although estradiol levels can be used to assess follicular maturity among estrogen-deficient patients, the same is not true for normoestrogenic patients (e.g., polycystic ovary (PCO) or oligomenorrhea). As a result of the presence of excessive numbers of mature follicles, marked ovarian hyperstimulation and/or multiple gestations are more likely. In this group, monitoring with estradiol levels may be inadequate and frequent ultrasound studies may be mandatory. Sonographic visualization can discriminate between single and multiple follicular growth. These measurements may aid in the interpretation of estrogen levels. Evidence is accumulating that follicles with diameters greater than 16 mm will be most likely to ovulate when hCG is administered. Therefore, ultrasonic visualization is important to determine these sizes. If numerous large follicles are observed on ultrasound, hCG can be withheld to reduce the risk of multiple births.

In a group of 723 patients with hypothalamic-pituitary dysfunction who failed to ovulate or conceive on clomiphene therapy, hMG treatment led to a pregnancy rate of 21.4% (74). Although the frequencies of ovulation and pregnancy are similar to those reported for clomiphene, the frequency of multiple births is 20% and the estimate of early spontaneous abortion is 25% (72).

There is no evidence of drug-induced teratogenicity with hMG/hCG. Side effects include hyperstimulation syndrome (bloating, abdominal pain, ovarian enlargement, ascites from excessive fluid escaping from multiple rupturing follicles, hypovolemia, hemoconcentration, hypercoagulopathy, and possible shock). In addition, rupturing of an ovarian cyst (hemoperitoneum), fever, and arterial thrombosis (due to elevated estradiol levels) may occur.

Dosing in men is very different than in females. Prior to hMG, men may be treated with hCG alone (5000 U three times weekly). This treatment is continued until serum testosterone levels are within the normal range; this may require 4 to 6 months of hCG. The recommended dose of hMG is 1 amp IM three times a week and hCG 2000 U twice a week. If an increase in spermatogenesis has not occurred after 4 months, the dose may be increased to 2 amps three times a week, with no change in the dose of hCG.

Urofollitropin and Polycystic Ovarian Disease

Urofollitropin (Metrodin) is a preparation of gonadotropins extracted from the urine of postmenopausal women similar to menotropins, but without the LH. This preparation contains 75 IU FSH and is indicated for induction of ovulation in patients with polycystic ovarian disease who have an elevated LH/FSH ratio and who have failed to respond to adequate clomiphene citrate therapy.

Initial doses of urofollitropin are 75 IU/day IM for 7 to 12 days followed by 5000 to 10,000 U of hCG, one day after the last urofollitropin dose. Treatment should continue until estrogenic activity is equal to or greater than that of a normal individual. If ovaries become abnormally enlarged on the last day of therapy, do not give hCG in this cycle; this reduces the chances of developing hyperstimulation syndrome. If there is evidence of ovulation but no pregnancy, repeat the regimen for at least two more cycles before increasing the dose to 150 IU of FSH per day for 7 to 12 days. Again follow this higher dose with hCG at the same dose. If evidence of ovulation is present but pregnancy does not occur, repeat the same dose for two more courses. Larger doses are not recommended.

Hyperstimulation syndrome is reported in approximately 10% of patients. Nausea, vomiting, diarrhea, and breast tenderness have also been reported. In clinical studies, 83% of the pregnancies following therapy resulted in single births and 17% in multiple births.

GnRH

A promising new avenue for treatment of primary hypothalamic amenorrhea and infertility involves GnRH analogs. Normal release of GnRH from the hypothalamus is pulsatile. When given to induce ovulation, administration of the drug must also be pulsatile; otherwise GnRH would initially stimulate release of gonadotropins but, with continued use, would become inhibitory (see endometriosis and prostate cancer treatment). Normal pituitary and ovarian function are required for the drug to act. Gonadorelin acetate (Lutrepulse) is a synthetic decapeptide identical in amino acid sequence to GnRH approved for this use. Gonadorelin is rapidly broken down to inactive peptide fragments that are excreted in the urine ($t_{1/2}\alpha = 10$ min, $t_{1/2}\beta = 10$–40 min).

Pulses of gonadorelin are injected intravenously through a catheter, usually into a forearm vein, using a reservoir and pump available from the manufacturer that can be worn under clothing. Initial dose is 5 μg every 90 minutes for 21 days or until ovulation occurs. If pregnancy occurs, the drug may be continued for up to 2 additional weeks to maintain the corpus luteum. The cannula and IV site should be changed every 48 hours. Multiple follicular stimulation should be monitored by ultrasound. If ovulation does not occur after 3 cycles of treatment, doses can be increased to a maximum of 30 μg.

Adverse effects include infection and inflammation of the infusion site. Hyperstimulation with sudden ovarian enlargement is unlikely because pulsatile administration preserves ovarian-pituitary feedback mechanism. Multiple pregnancies have occurred in 12% of women who became pregnant with gonadorelin. Cutaneous hypersensitivity and anaphylaxis have occurred.

In anovulatory women and abnormal or absent GnRH secretion, gonadorelin can induce ovulation. The manufacturer reports that among 44 women with primary hypothalamic amenorrhea treated with pulsatile IV doses of the drug, 41 ovulated and 24 (62%) of 39 patients desiring pregnancy became pregnant.

Assisted Reproductive Technologies (ARTs)

The assisted reproductive technologies (ARTs) used in treatment of infertility are now 20 years old. Early success was obtained when one oocyte was obtained at the time of ovum aspiration. However, various methods of ovarian hyperstimulation have been employed, thereby allowing more than one embryo to be transferred at a time to the uterus. A combination of ARTs and hormonal therapies is frequently used today. Some of the beneficial additive effects of these combinations include improved ovulation timing (which in turn increases the chances of sperm and egg interaction, placing higher numbers of motile sperm in the upper genital tract) and increased numbers of ovum available for fertilization.

A sequential approach to infertility treatment, beginning with the least risky treatment, is always advised. Advances in reproductive technologies have been remarkable, with a variety of techniques being advocated. A complete discussion of other reproductive technologies is beyond the scope of this chapter. Gamete intrafallopian transfer (GIFT), direct oocyte and sperm transfer (DOST), zygote intrafallopian transfer (ZIFT), cryopreservation (freezing) of embryos and sperm, donor sperm insemination, and intrauterine insemination with washed and capacitated sperm are just some the ART forms now being used. Pregnancy rates for these procedures are highly variable, in part due to selection bias, technique variability, and lack of standardization criteria for reporting outcome. While a treatment plan should be carefully evaluated to meet the couple's own needs, long, emotionally difficult and costly procedures may only modestly increase the chance of success.

The combination of clomiphene citrate and hMG (menotropins) to cause superovulation has been used by many workers in in vitro fertilization and embryo transfer (IVF), but some groups have considerable success using hMG alone (75). Subsequently, pure follicle stimulating hormone (FSH) was used (Metrodin) instead of hMG, but results have not further improved.

All these methods of hyperstimulation are complicated by premature luteinization of the follicle or the occurrence of an endogenous LH surge in up to 20% of patients treated. Patients who receive either pure FSH or hMG require luteal phase support. Patients (except those with an endogenous LH surge) also may require hCG at the time of follicle maturity.

More recently, the GnRH agonists have been used to produce pituitary suppression and thus prevent the onset of the endogenous LH surge (76). The GnRH agonist is given immediately prior to the initial injection of hMG. An increase in gonadotropin occurs, and most groups have reported more oocytes being obtained. However, significant ovarian hyperstimulation has been noted in some patients.

CONCLUSION

The therapeutic management of common gynecologic problems, contraception, infertility, endometriosis, and toxic shock syndrome requires an understanding of the female reproductive system with its delicate balance of hormonal axis regulation and feedback control. Knowledge of the pharmacologic effects of the different components of oral contraceptives and fertility agents allows us to effectively tailor specific products for selected patients as well as identify patients in whom such therapy is contraindicated.

REFERENCES

1. Dickey RP. Managing contraceptive pill patients, 8th ed. Durant, OK: Essential Medical Information Systems, 1994.
2. Hatcher RA, Trussell J, Stewart FS, Stewart GK, Kowal D, et al. Contraceptive technology, 16th ed. New York: Irvington Publishers, 1994.
3. Realini JP, Goldzieher JW. Oral contraceptives and cardiovascular disease: a critique of the epidemiologic studies. Am J Obstet Gynecol 152:729–798, 1985.
4. Crane MG, Harris JJ, Winston W III. Hypertension, oral contraceptive agents and conjugated estrogens. Ann Intern Med 74:13, 1971.
5. Goodlin RC, Waechter V. Oral contraceptives and blood pressure. Lancet 1:1262, 1969.
6. Royal College of General Practitioners' Oral Contraception Study. Oral contraceptives and health. New York: Pitman, 1974.
7. Ramcharan S, Pellegran FA, Hoag E. The occurrence and cause of hypertensive disease in users and non-users of oral contraceptive drugs. In: Fregley MJ, Fregley MS, eds. Oral contraceptives and high blood pressure. Gainesville, FL: Dolphin Press, 1974:1.
8. Fisch IR, Frank J. Oral contraceptives and blood pressure. JAMA 237:2499, 1977.
9. Kunin CM, McCormack RC, Abernathy JR. Oral contraceptives and blood pressure. Arch Intern Med 123:362, 1969.
10. Tsai CC, Williamson HO, Kirkland BH, et al. Low-dose oral contraception and blood pressure in women with a past history of elevated blood pressure. Am J Obstet Gynecol 151:28–32, 1985.
11. Wilson ESB, Cruickshank J, McMaster M, Weir RJ. A prospective controlled study of the effect on blood pressure of contraceptive preparations containing different types and dosages of progestogen. Br J Obstet Gynaecol 91:1254–1260, 1984.
12. Saruta T, Saade GA, Kaplan NM. A possible mechanism for hypertension induced by oral contraceptives. Arch Intern Med 126:621, 1970.
13. Laragh JH, Sealey JE, Ledingham JG, et al. Oral contraceptives: renin, aldosterone, and high blood pressure. JAMA 201:918, 1967.
14. Anon. Effect on hypertension and benign breast disease of progestogen component in combined oral contraceptives: Royal College of General Practitioners' Oral Contraception Study. Lancet 1:624, 1977.
15. Hazzard WR, Spiger MJ, Bagdale JD, et al. Studies on the mechanism of increased plasma triglyceride levels induced by oral contraceptives N Engl J Med 280:471–474, 1969.
16. Davidoff F, Tishler S, Rosoff C. Marked hyperlipidemia and pancreatitis associated with oral contraceptive therapy. N Engl J Med 289:552, 1973.
17. Donde UM, Virkar K. The effect of combination and low-dose progestogen oral contraceptives on serum lipids. Fertil Steril 26:62–67, 1975.
18. Wahl P, Walden C, Knopp R, et al. Effect of estrogen/progestin potency on lipid/lipoprotein cholesterol. N Engl J Med 308:862–867, 1983.
19. Bradley DB, Wingerd J, Petti DB, et al. Serum high-density lipoprotein cholesterol in women using oral contraceptive estrogens and progestins. N Engl J Med 299:17, 1978.
20. Speroff L, De Cherney A. Evaluation of a new generation of oral contraceptives. Obstet Gynecol 81:1034–1047, 1993.
21. Spellacy W. Carbohydrate metabolism during treatment with progestogen and low-dose oral contraceptives. Am J Obstet Gynecol 142:732–734, 1982.
22. Mestman JH, Schmidt-Sarosi C. Diabetes mellitus and fertility control. Contraception management issues. Am J Obstet Gynecol 168:2012–2020, 1993.
23. Baird DT, Glasier AF. Hormonal contraception. N Engl J Med 328:1543–1549, 1993.
24. Krauss RM, Burkman RT. The metabolic impact oral contraceptives. Am J Obstet Gynecol 167:1177–1184, 1992.

25. Mann JI, Doll R, Thorogood M, et al. Risk factors for myocardial infarction in young women. Br J Prev Soc Med 30:94, 1976.

26. Collaborative Group for the Study of Stroke in Young Women. Oral contraceptives and stroke in young women: associated risk factors. JAMA 231:718, 1975.

27. Grimes DA. The saftey of oral contraceptives: epidemiologic insights from the first 30 years. Am J Obstet Gynecol 166:1950–1954, 1992.

28. Mishell DR. Contraception. N Engl J Med 320:777–787, 1989.

29. Porter JB, Hunter JR, Jick H, Stergachis A. Oral contraceptives and nonfatal vascular disease. Obstet Gynecol 66:1–4, 1985.

30. Porter JB, Jick H, Walker AM. Mortality among oral contraceptive users. Obstet Gynecol 70:29–32, 1987.

31. Mant D, Villard-Mackintosh L, Vessey MP, Yeates D. Myocardial infarction and angina pectoris in young women. J Epidemiol Community Health 41:215–219, 1987.

32. Stampfer MJ, Willett WC, Colditz GA, Speizer FE, Hennekens CH. A prospective study of past use of oral contraceptive agents and risk of cardiovascular disease. N Engl J Med 319:1313–1317, 1988.

33. Coeditz GA. Oral contraceptive use and mortality during 12 year follow up: The nurses' health study. Ann Intern Med 120:821–826, 1994.

34. Anon. Oral contraceptives and venous thromboembolic disease, surgically confirmed gallbladder disease, and breast tumors: report from the Boston Collaborative Drug Surveillance Program. Lancet 1:1399, 1973.

35. Anon. Oral contraceptives, venous thrombosis, and varicose veins: Royal College of General Practitioners' Oral Contraceptive Study. J R Coll Gen Pract 28:393, 1978.

36. Vessey MP, McPherson K, Yeates D. Mortality in oral contraceptive users. Lancet 1:549, 1981.

37. Irey NS, Manion WC, Taylor HB. Vascular lesions in women taking oral contraceptives. Arch Pathol 89:1, 1970.

38. Caspery EA, Peberdy M. Oral contraception and blood platelet adhesiveness. Lancet 1:1142, 1965.

39. Howie PW, Mallinson AC, Prentice CRM, et al. Effect of combined estrogen-progestogen oral contraceptives on antiplasmin and antithrombolic activity. Lancet 2:1329, 1970.

40. Peterson C, Kelly R, Minard B, et al. Antithrombin III: comparison of functional and immunologic assay. Am J Clin Pathol 69:500, 1978.

41. Conard J, Samama M, Salomon Y. Antithrombin III and the oestrogen content of combined oestrogen-progestagen contraceptives. Lancet 2:1148, 1972.

42. Bonnar J, Sabra A. Comparative data on the effects of low-dose oral contraceptives on coagulation. In: Elstein M, ed. Update on triphasic oral contraception. Amsterdam: Excerpta Medica, 1983:9–19.

43. Romieu I, Berlin JA, Colditz G. Oral contraceptives and breast cancer: review and meta-analysis. Cancer 66:2253–2263, 1990.

44. Centers for Disease Control Cancer and Steroid Hormone Study. Long term oral contraceptive use and the risk of breast cancer. JAMA 249:1591–1595, 1983.

45. Schlesselman JJ. Cancer of the breast and reproductive tract in relation to use of oral contraceptives. Contraception 40:1–38, 1989.

46. Khoo SK. Cancer risks and the contraceptive pill. What is the evidence after nearly 25 years of use? Med J Aust 144:185–190, 1986.

47. Speroff L, Glass RH, Kase NG. Clinical gynecologic endocrinology and infertility, 4th ed. Baltimore: Williams & Wilkins, 1989:487.

48. Grodstein F, Colditz GA, Hunter DJ, Manson JE, Willett WC, Stampher MJ. A prospective study of symptomatic gallstones in women: relation with oral contraceptives and other factors. Obstet Gynecol 84:207–214, 1994.

49. Adams, PW, Wynn V, Rose DP, et al. Effect of pyridoxine hydrochloride (vitamin B-6) upon depression associated with oral contraception. Lancet 1:897, 1973.

50. WHO Special Programme of Research, Development and Research Training in Human Reproduction. Task force on oral contraceptives: effects of hormonal contraceptives on milk volume and infant growth. Contraception 30:505–522, 1984.

51. D'Arcy PF. Drug interactions with oral contraceptives. Drug Intell Clin Pharm 20:353–362, 1986.

52. Anon. Drugs, oral contraceptives and pregnancy [Editorial]. N Z Med J 92:200, 1980.

53. Smith MB. A quantitative estimate of ocular iatrogenic disease in humans. J Am Optom Assoc 45:751, 1974.

54. Wood JR. Ocular complications of oral contraceptives. Ophthalmic Semin 2:371, 1977.

55. Chapel TA, Burns RE. Oral contraceptives and exacerbation of lupus erythematosus. Am J Obstet Gynecol 110:366, 1971.

56. Magendotz HB. Oral contraceptives. Collected Letters of the International Correspondence Society of Obstetricians and Gynecologists. 22:170, 1981.

57. Smith MA, Youngkin EQ. Current perspectives on combination oral contraceptives. Clin Pharm 3:485–522, 1984.

58. Ostergard DR. DES-related vaginal lesions. Clin Obstet Gynecol 24:379, 1981.

59. Yuzpe AA, Smith RP, Rademaker AW. A multi-center clinical investigation employing ethinyl estradiol combined with D,L-norgestrol as a post-coital contraceptive agent. Fertil Steril 37:508, 1982.

60. Kaunitz AM. Long acting injectable contraception with depot MPA. Am J Obstet Gynecol 170:1543–1549, 1994.

61. Glasier A, Thong KJ, Dewar M, Makie M, Baird DT. Mefepristone (RU486) compared top high dose estrogen and progestogen for emergency post coital contraception. N Engl J Med 327:1041–1044, 1992.

62. Louik C, Mitchell AA, Werle MM, Hanson JW, Shapiro S. Maternal exposure to spermicides in relation to certain birth defects. N Engl J Med 317:474–478, 1987.

63. Strobino B, Kline J, Lai A, Stein Z, Sussec M, Warburton D. Vaginal spermicides and spontaneous abortion of known karyotype. Am J Epidemiol 123:431–443, 1986.

64. Todd J, Fishaut M, Kapral F, et al. Toxic-shock syndrome associated with phage-group I staphylococci. Lancet 2:1116, 1978.

65. Schwartz B, Gaventa S, Broome CV, Reingold AL, Hightower AW, Perlman JA, Wolf PH. Nonmenstrual toxic shock syndrome associated with barrier contraceptives: report of a case-control study. Rev Infect Dis 2(1):S43–S49, 1989.

66. Friedrich EG. Tampon effects on vaginal health. Clin Obstet Gynecol 24:395, 1981.

67. Schreiner WE. Labhart's textbook of endocrinology. Berlin: Springer-Verlag, 1974:511.

68. WHO Technical Report Series, No. 820. Recent advances in medically assisted conception: report of a WHO scientific group. Geneva, Switzerland: WHO, 1992.

69. Abrams RM, Rayston JP. Some properties of rectum and vagina as sites for basal body temperature measurements. Fertil Steril 35:313–316, 1981.

70. Rayston JP, Abrams RM, Higgins MP, et al. The adjustment of basal body temperature measurements to allow for time of waking. Br J Obstet Gynecol 87:1123–1127, 1980.

71. Adashi EY. Clomiphene citrate: mechanism(s) and site(s) of action-a hypothesis revisited. Fertil Steril 42:331–334, 1984.

72. Rahwan RG. Antiabortifacient and fertility-inducing drugs. Am J Pharm Educ 49:86–94, 1985.

73. Brown JB, Evans JH, Adey FD, et al. Factors involved in the induction of fertile ovulations with human gonadotropins. J Obstet Gynaecol Br Commonw 76:289, 1969.

74. Lunenfeld B, Romen Y, Blankenship J. Current problems in obstetrics and gynecology: ovulation induction, vol. 5. Chicago: Year Book, 1982:55.

75. Johnston WIH, Lopata A, Pepperell RJ. The use of in vitro fertilization in the infertile couple. In: Pepperell RJ, Hudson B, Wood C, eds. The infertile couple, 2nd ed. Edinburgh: Churchill Livingstone, 263–312, 1987.

76. MacLachlan V, Besanko M, O'Shea F. A controlled study of luteinizing hormone-releasing hormone agonist (Buserelin®) for the induction of folliculogenesis before in vitro fertilization. N Engl J Med 320:1233–1237, 1989.

CHAPTER 92

DRUGS IN PREGNANCY AND LACTATION

KELLIE D. McQUEEN

A pregnant woman takes an average of 3 medications and may take up to 15 medications during her pregnancy (1, 2, 3, 4). Symptoms commonly treated include pain, nausea and vomiting, gastrointestinal upset, edema, and the common cold. Concurrent diseases such as diabetes mellitus, infections, or hypertension may also require treatment. Antimicrobial agents, cold medications, and nonnarcotic analgesics are commonly taken (5). Approximately 35 to 100% of pregnant women have taken some type of drug during pregnancy, and 40% of pregnant women have taken medications in the first trimester (6, 7, 8). These figures are impressive when considering many of these drugs are taken without medical supervision and without clear indication, and may be taken immediately after conception before the woman knows she is pregnant. Some studies suggest the majority of women take medications for nonserious conditions, perhaps without first trying nonpharmacologic measures (3).

Although many pregnant women may be unnecessarily exposed to drugs, heightened public awareness of medication use and concern for the fetus has probably improved the patterns of drug use in pregnancy. Compared to women in the mid-1960s, women in the early 1980s took less medication throughout pregnancy and less during the first trimester (9).

Little is known about the characteristics of the women who take medication, but one study identified nonwhite, unmarried, less educated women as more likely to use less medication than other groups. This may be surprising, yet the population of women taking less medication may seek prenatal care less often than their counterparts. The act of seeking medical care may itself increase the use of medications. These data could be easily biased by the study design and need confirmation by other reports, but they may serve to raise the awareness of prescribers for ensuring drugs are necessary therapy in pregnant women (3).

The number of drugs available for human use is escalating each year. Prescription drugs and over-the-counter products may be readily obtained. Attention should be paid to those drugs that may cause harm to the developing fetus. Out of nearly 1000 drugs that have been evaluated for teratogenic potential, only about 30 are proven teratogens. Examples of these are listed in Table 92.1. A teratogen is an agent that is present during critical periods of development and is able to produce a congenital defect. The term *congenital defect* refers to major and minor malformations either in structure or in function that deviate from the norm. Examples are cleft palate, behavioral variations, and latent defects such as vaginal carcinoma in offspring of women treated with diethylstilbestrol while pregnant. Minor malformations may impede or impair function but do not result in serious illness or death if not medically treated or surgically modified.

It is the responsibility of the clinician to counsel all patients with complete, accurate, and current information on the risks and benefits of using medications while pregnant. Significant harm may come to the fetus if exposed to an agent. The mother may suffer deleterious effects if not treated for certain conditions, which may also cause harm to the fetus. Thus, each patient should receive careful evaluation and counsel on her medical condition and the risks and benefits of the appropriate therapy. In reviewing the literature, the clinician should keep in mind that data on drugs in pregnancy are being updated with the publication of each new anecdotal report or review. Many times information will appear to be, and in fact may be, somewhat conflicting. Much of the data needs additional study and validation, especially that arising from case reports; it may not be generalized to all women. Sound professional medical judgment based on clinical assessment of the patient and an understanding of the literature must be combined with direct and honest patient counseling before any medication is taken during pregnancy. Patient involvement in the decision-making process is important.

This chapter will provide a general review of common issues relating to drug use in pregnancy and lactation. Other references should be consulted since this review is not meant to be all inclusive of the issues necessary in making patient-specific therapeutic decisions. Drugs and dosages are not recommendations but rather reflect what has been used. A background discussion of limitations of the literature of drug use in pregnancy will be presented. Some drug-induced syndromes will be reviewed, and common illnesses seen in pregnancy and some of the issues associated with the pharmacologic management of the diseases will also be discussed.

PREVALENCE

Approximately 3% of infants are born with major congenital malformation. This baseline measurement does not include minor malformations or defects that are mani-

Table 92.1.
Drugs Known or Suspected to Be Teratogenic in Humans

Androgenic hormones
Busulfan
Coumarin derivatives
Cyclophosphamide
Diethylstilbestrol
Etretinate
Isotretinoin
Lithium
Methimazole
Penicillamine
Phenytoin
Trimethadione
Tetracyclines (particularly during week 24-26)
Thalidomide
Valproic acid

Adapted from reference 6.

fested in later life, such as anomalies of internal organs, or behavioral or growth deficiencies. These abnormalities have been thought to double the prevalence of birth defects to around 6%. Etiologies of malformations may be classified into three main categories: (1) unknown factors, (2) genetic origin, and (3) environmental influences (10, 11). The largest cause of defects, 65%, is due to unknown factors. This includes polygenic or multifactorial causes or spontaneous errors of development. Genetic influences include chromosomal abnormalities, mutant genes, or autosomal genetic diseases. These account for up to 20% of all congenital malformations. Environmental factors can include maternal diseases such as diabetes mellitus or a poor nutritional status, as well as maternal infections with rubella, cytomegalovirus, toxoplasmosis, syphilis, or other infectious agents (10, 11, 12). Chemicals, drugs, and drug metabolites are estimated to account for roughly 3% of all defects. This 3% figure may underestimate the true percentage because many cases are presumably not reported. Furthermore, ranges of rates are reported in the literature and depend on the methods used to collect and interpret data.

LIMITATIONS IN THE LITERATURE

Since the early 1960s and the tragedy of the defects caused by thalidomide, the U.S. Food and Drug Administration (FDA) has required that before becoming commercially available, all medications must be shown to be safe and effective for the population intended to be treated. Limited knowledge of the teratogenic risk of the drug to humans can be provided through these trials. If defects have been demonstrated in several animal species, then a casual association might at least be made to the same defect being demonstrated in humans. However, there are several limitations to animal studies, and a direct extrapolation

from animal data to humans is not possible. First, differences exist in the teratogenicity of a drug between species. For example, thalidomide causes malformations in rabbits and humans, but not in rodents. The drug was not known to be teratogenic in humans until a number of infants were born with significant defects and the cause was traced to in utero thalidomide exposure. Other drugs, such as steroids and sulfonamides, have been shown to be teratogenic in animals, but at therapeutic doses have not been shown to be teratogenic in humans. Second, the pharmacokinetic properties of a drug vary between species and among the same species. Rates of absorption, biotransformation, maternal elimination, and the extent of placental transfer vary and may produce inconsistent results. Moreover, animals may react differently to environmental factors than humans, and this may also affect the susceptibility to a teratogen. In many animal studies, the agent tested is given at dosages well above the therapeutic dose used in humans, making the results almost uninterpretable.

HUMAN DATA

Most human data regarding drugs in pregnancy is anecdotal. Although this type of information is not optimal, the importance of it should not be underestimated. In fact, every known teratogen has been identified by astute clinicians who recognized possible associations between drugs used by pregnant women and resulting malformations. Thalidomide, warfarin, and isotretinoin were all first reported as teratogenic in case reports. Anecdotal reports should be evaluated carefully since they primarily report a suspected association. The majority of case reports await further study before associations can be confirmed. Unfortunately, few epidemiologic studies have been done. The Collaborative Perinatal Project is well known and was performed from 1959 to 1965. Data were collected on a cohort of 50,282 mother–child pairs to investigate the teratogenic role of drugs. Twelve centers in the United States participated. The rates of various birth defects in infants of drug-exposed women were compared to those of infants in nondrug-exposed women. The published results may serve as a useful reference for individual cases for drugs frequently used in pregnancy (13).

Yet, even among well-controlled studies, collecting teratologic information is complicated, and the data must be carefully evaluated. For many studies and reports, there is a lack of uniform definitions of malformations and diagnostic criteria. Many studies exclude the reporting of certain types of malformations, for example, stillbirths or spontaneous abortions. The majority of reporting concentrates on major anatomical abnormalities detected at birth. Minor abnormalities are often omitted, and follow-up studies to detect abnormalities in later life are rare. Similarly, surveys of pregnant women can be limiting because the maternal reporting of drugs taken during pregnancy is generally not accurate. Drugs actually taken, including over-the-counter agents, may not be accounted for by the mother, nor may the correct dose or timing of ingestion (7). Mothers of infants with birth defects tend to have more accurate reporting than those of normal infants (14). Interviews with indication-oriented and drug-oriented questions may produce better recall (15). Lastly, medical records do not generally provide accurate patient history to allow for good retrospective evaluations.

Investigator objectivity is also difficult to ensure in studies. Similar to other medical illnesses, the number of occurrences for many drug-induced birth defects may vary depending on the demographics of the patients studied. Results can be biased if a study population is significantly unbalanced in regard to its race, geographic location, genetic makeup, or diet. Facial feature changes from alcohol exposure in utero may be more difficult to diagnose in certain races. Lastly, bias may arise if the observer is aware of confounding elements. Diseases, viruses, educational status, or smoking, for example, may directly or indirectly be responsible for defects. If these influences are diagnosed by the investigator, false inferences could be made.

In summary, understanding that data regarding drug use in pregnancy is influenced by multiple confounding factors is key in assessing the relative risk of exposure for a given population.

TERATOGENIC FACTORS

The consequence of these limitations is that information specific to the case at hand is not always available. The certainty of which one can predict the precise teratogenic potential of a drug in any one patient is limited, at best. Principles of teratology have been identified and previously described by Wilson. These are outlined in Table 92.2 (16). Most important is the time during fetal development that the conceptus was exposed to the agent. Knowing the developmental stage when insult was applied can aid in predicting the possible defect. From fertilization to implantation of the ovum, days 0 through 14, most

Table 92.2.
Key Principles of Teratogens

1. The susceptibility of an embryo to a teratogen depends upon the developmental stage at which the agent is applied.
2. Each teratogen acts on a particular aspect of cellular metabolism. Different teratogenic agents, therefore, tend to produce different effects, although acting at the same period of embryonic development and on the same system.
3. The genotype influences to a degree the reaction to a teratogen.
4. An agent capable of causing malformations also usually causes an increase in embryonic mortality.
5. A teratogen need not be deleterious to the maternal organism.

Adapted from reference 16.

dangerous agents either prevent implantation of the conceptus or have no harmful effect at all. The most sensitive period is from implantation to the end of organogenesis. Exposure to agents in this period, days 18 through 60, may damage the developing organs. A classic example is thalidomide, which produces distinct deficits in limbs with exposure at 21 through 40 days after conception. During the fetal period, the time after 8 weeks to birth, morphologic changes may occur as the developmental and growth phases continue. This includes maturation of the brain. Drugs administered during labor and delivery, such as magnesium sulfate, may also enter the baby's bloodstream and produce physiologic effects and fetal compromise after delivery. Magnesium sulfate can cause neurologic depression, hyporeflexia, and shallow respirations. When a type of defect can occur anytime during pregnancy, concern regarding drug exposure throughout gestation is warranted. An example is the behavioral abnormalities that can result from alcohol exposure if it is ingested while pregnant.

Other factors that influence the outcome and association of possible insult from drugs in utero include the nature of the agent and the mechanism by which it causes the defect, exposure to a combination of agents, the maternal and fetal metabolism of the drug, the dose, duration of exposure, species, and maternal and fetal genetic makeup. The extent to which the drug crosses the placenta is also important. Most drugs will cross the placenta, primarily by simple diffusion, though other processes such as active transport play a role. Drugs with molecular weights less than 600, high lipid solubility, low protein binding, and those that are nonionized readily cross the placenta (6, 10, 17–19).

RESOURCES OF INFORMATION

When determining the risk of exposure to the fetus, in addition to considering the factors listed previously, the clinician should refer to various resources of information. Texts, journal articles, and rating systems are available. TERIS is a computer database resource that evaluates the chance of harm that could occur to the fetus if the mother takes a medication. The database is also summarized in a text, *Teratogenic Effects of Drugs: A Resource for Clinicians* (Friedman, 1994). TERIS is based on published studies, standard teratology references, and clinical experience. Ratings for agents under conventional therapeutic settings are described by teratologists as "none," "minimal," "small," "moderate," "high," and "undetermined." The quality of data used to determine the rating is described as "none," "poor," "fair," "good," or "excellent." The system relies primarily on human data and is designed to assess risk; it does not provide total therapeutic guidance because it does not address benefits of treatment or the availability of alternative therapies (20).

Table 92.3.
FDA Ratings

A: Controlled studies show no risk. Adequate, well-controlled studies in pregnant women have failed to demonstrate risk to the fetus.

B: No evidence of risk in humans. Either animal findings show risk, but human findings do not; or, if no adequate human studies have been done, animal findings are negative.

C: Risk cannot be ruled out. Human studies are lacking, and animal studies are either positive for fetal risk, or lacking as well. However, potential benefits may justify the potential risk.

D: Positive evidence of risk. Investigational or post-marketing data show risk to the fetus. Nevertheless, potential benefitis may outweigh the potential risk.

X: Contraindicated in pregnancy. Studies in animals or human or investigational or postmarketing reports have shown fetal risk that clearly outweighs any possible benefit to the patient.

In 1979, the FDA devised a system that determines the teratogenic risk of drugs by considering the quality of data from animal and human studies (21). It includes the benefits of therapy to the patient and any perinatal risks. Thus, the FDA rating system may provide some therapeutic guidance for the clinician. It does not denote a rating for all drugs, however. A description of the FDA risk factors is presented in Table 92.3. Categories denoting if the risk of therapy exceeds the benefit are described as A, B, C, D, or X. Although the A category is considered the safest category, some drugs with a B, C, or even D rating are commonly used in pregnancy. Only category X denotes that the drug is contraindicated and that there is no reason to risk using the drug in pregnancy. Isotretinoin or conjugated estrogens provide examples of this group.

A standard text, *Drugs in Pregnancy and Lactation: A Reference Guide to Fetal and Neonatal Risk,* and the quarterly updates (Briggs, 1994), is an exhaustive reference that provides an up-to-date summary of available data for specific drugs. The *Catalog of Teratogenic Agents* (Shepard, 1992) is also a standard text. Finally, reports in obstetric, teratology, genetic, pediatric, and general medicine journals may be helpful. Drug manufacturers may be a source of information also. Any rating system or reference should be used in conjunction with a complete history and physical of the patient. Specific patient risks should be fully evaluated, not just the risks associated with the therapeutic agent.

In synopsis, data describing drug use in pregnancy must be carefully evaluated before inferring results to an individual patient. With the publication of each new document, the risk to benefit ratio of a particular therapy for any one patient may change somewhat. Taking any medication while pregnant encounters some degree of risk. In general, an estimation should be made if the risk of teratogenesis from drug exposure exceeds the 3 to 6% baseline malformation rate. If it does not, then although birth defects may still occur, there is no known increased

risk with drug therapy. This concept is useful in patient counseling. Because of the lack of research on the teratogenic potential of many drugs and the lack of a good system to assess risk, conservative use of all drugs in pregnant women is warranted. The indications for any drug and the benefit of therapy should be clear, and every safeguard should be taken to decrease the risk of fetal harm.

SYNDROMES

The pathogenesis of birth defects may be divided into four different categories: deformation, disruption, dysplasia, and malformation. Abnormalities may be further classified into five subcategories, depending on their relationship to each other: single-system defects, complexes, syndromes, associations, or sequences. The discussion of these mechanisms is beyond the scope of this chapter; the reader is referred to a review by Aase (22). A group of abnormalities that develops in a consistent pattern is designated as a syndrome. Three common syndromes due to alcohol, warfarin, and phenytoin exposure are discussed.

The worldwide incidence of fetal alcohol syndrome (FAS) is estimated to be 1.9 per 1000 livebirths. Some expression of FAS is believed to occur in as many as 1 in 300 livebirths (23, 24). The syndrome is characterized with defects of the central nervous system, craniofacial abnormalities, and growth and mental deficiencies. Affected infants can display a wide range of other abnormalities. Mental retardation is the most significant consequence. The majority of affected infants are born with hypotonia, poor coordination, decreased adipose tissue, and decreased pre- and postnatal growth. A myoplastic maxilla, as well as shortened and upturned nose, may also be present. Many will demonstrate hyperactivity in childhood, retrognathia in infancy, and micrognathia in adolescence. Microcephaly, short palpebral fissures, and thin vermillion of the upper lip may also be features commonly seen. Infants can experience alcohol withdrawal symptoms such as irritability, tremors, abdominal distention, or opisthotonos. Withdrawal may occur with or without the physical disfigurements of FAS (2, 25). These defects are variable in the extent and severity of appearance. Nearly 30 to 40% of alcoholic women have infants with complete FAS, and 50 to 70% have infants with partial expression of the syndrome, referred to as fetal alcohol effects (FAE) (12). The effects may last throughout childhood and into adult life. Defects can include cardiac and renogenital abnormalities. Investigators have documented the biopsychosocial effects of FAS in adults (27, 28).

FAS and FAE are thought to be caused by ethanol or its metabolites. Investigation into the effects of acetaldehyde has been conducted, but the exact relationship between this byproduct and FAS is unclear. Additional maternal factors that may contribute to expression of the syndrome include poor nutrition, smoking, drug abuse, inadequate prenatal care, genetic predisposition, and low socioeconomic status.

The effects are dose related, but the amount of ethanol that may be ingested without causing abnormalities is unknown. Growth-retarded babies can be born to women who have one to two drinks daily, and infants exposed to the same amount of alcohol in utero can display different degrees of symptoms (29). Two drinks per day (30 ml of absolute alcohol) has been related to lower birth weights. Binge drinking (five or more drinks on one occasion per month) has been associated with adverse physical and intellectual outcomes (30, 31). Moderate consumption (more than 30 ml/week of absolute alcohol) has been associated with decreased birth weight, spontaneous abortion, and impaired motor and mental development. As many as six hard drinks (around 75 to 90 ml of absolute alcohol) per day carries a major risk for severe complications, craniofacial structural defects, and possibly stillbirth. The complete FAS is associated with alcoholic women who consume more than four drinks (60 ml of absolute alcohol) per day (11, 32). More research is needed to clearly understand the effects of moderate or low-level alcohol consumption.

Pregnant women should be informed of the dangers of alcohol and that a safe level of consumption is not known. Neither is it clear which phase of development is most susceptible to damage. Drinking in the latter stages of pregnancy increases the risk of giving birth prematurely and of having a small for gestational age baby (33). The risk of serious fetal harm is also high in the first 2 months after conception. Women should thus avoid alcohol throughout pregnancy and even when trying to conceive. Women should also not use antitussive medications with alcohol. Over-the-counter products can contain as much as 25% alcohol. Cough medications with no alcohol are available and are preferred. Any child diagnosed with FAS or FAE should receive appropriate follow-up care for the social and developmental problems displayed. All health-care workers should support education aimed at adolescents, adults, and other health-care workers on the deleterious effects on the fetus of the maternal consumption of alcohol.

The fetal warfarin syndrome is another recognizable syndrome. It is estimated to occur in 10 to 30% of infants exposed to coumarin derivatives, particularly around the 6th to 9th gestational week. Fetal warfarin syndrome is characterized primarily by nasal hypoplasia and stippling of uncalcified epiphyses. Hypoplasia of limb nails, shortened fingers, low birth weight (LBW), and severe upper airway obstruction at birth may also occur. In addition, in the second or third trimester, exposure to coumadin has been associated with other defects such as fetal central nervous system defects, spontaneous abortion, and stillbirth (10, 11, 34–36).

The fetal hydantoin syndrome is associated with anticonvulsant therapy. Although generally related to phenytoin, the FHS is not specific for any one anticonvulsant and may be seen with phenytoin, phenobarbital, carbamazepine, or a combination of these agents (37). Defects may include mental retardation; limb and craniofacial abnormalities such as cleft lip or palate, small or absent nails, or dislocated hip; cardiac abnormalities; and physical growth defects. Short neck, umbilical or inguinal hernia, strabismus, or hirsutism rarely occur (38, 39). Reports have stated there is a 5 to 10% risk for a fetus exposed to phenytoin to develop the majority of these abnormalities; whereas a one in three risk exists for only partial expression of the syndrome (38, 40). Some investigators have cited up to a 15% incidence of similar abnormalities to the FHS in untreated epileptic women (41). Hence, the exact etiology of FHS is unknown. Although the epilepsy itself may be the cause, toxicity from the antiepileptic drug, fetal genotype, or fetal exposure to the drug or its metabolites are other possible mechanisms. Maternal folic acid deficiency has been suggested to cause teratogenic effects seen with phenytoin. A combination of these factors may also play a role in FHS. Phenytoin and carbamazepine are oxidized in the liver by the enzyme epoxide hydrolase, resulting in epoxide metabolites. These metabolites have a high affinity for binding to fetal proteins, which may result in developmental defects (40, 42–44). The epoxide hydrolase activity of amniocytes may help predict which infants might be at risk for FHS. Investigators have found that phenotypes with a low epoxide hydrolase activity still expressed signs of the FHS (40).

Caffeine and Smoking

Clinicians often have the opportunity to counsel patients with regard to the use of various prescription and nonprescription medications during pregnancy. Other substances that should not be overlooked and that are commonly consumed include caffeine and cigarette smoking. If used in pregnancy, they may produce adverse fetal effects. Pregnant women should be informed of possible complications that may result from smoking or ingesting caffeine.

CAFFEINE

Caffeine is found in coffee, cola drinks, tea, cocoa, analgesics, and some other nonprescription products such as cold remedies, diet aids, and stimulants. The content of caffeine varies greatly in these products. On average, 5 ounces of coffee can have 30 to 180 mg of caffeine; 6 ounces of decaffeinated coffee, 3 to 5 mg; 12 ounces of cola drinks, 36 to 90 mg; one ounce of baking chocolate, 26 mg; and 1 ounce of milk chocolate, 6 mg. Stimulant products can have 100 to 200 mg of caffeine, whereas over-the-counter appetite suppressants contain up to 120 mg.

Caffeine is the most common drug ingested by pregnant women. An estimated 80% of women are exposed to caffeine during the first trimester. This potent CNS stimulant crosses the placenta. Caffeine is thought to damage the ovum and fetus throughout gestation because of its ability to damage chromosomes and increase cyclic adenosine monophosphate in cells. The teratogenicity associated with caffeine in animals is dose related and occurs at high doses. Caffeine has not been shown to be a major teratogen in humans, however (17). Numerous studies have been done to assess the effect of caffeine on the fetus. Some investigators have shown no association between caffeine consumption and the occurrence of congenital malformations (13, 45, 46); others have demonstrated complications in pregnancy (47, 48, 49). The consequences of perinatal exposure to caffeine through age 7 years have been considered minimal by some researchers. They detected no effects of caffeine on intelligence, attention, or physical growth (50). Additional studies evaluating similar outcomes are needed.

Studies evaluating the effects of caffeine on the fetus are difficult to interpret because of confounding variables. A positive association exists between heavy caffeine use and cigarette smoking. Other factors need to be controlled that may influence the chance of adverse fetal outcomes such as alcohol use, socioeconomic status, and other demographics (51). Findings may also be limited in that it is difficult to account for the exact dose of caffeine ingested by the gravida.

The relationship of low to moderate amounts of caffeine with a variety of effects on the fetus and infant remains in question. Fetal breathing movements and behavior, and cardiac arrhythmias in newborns have been documented with high doses of caffeine (52, 53). Focus has been given to the relationship between caffeine and the possibility of spontaneous abortion, increased risk of delivering an LBW infant, and infertility.

Some investigators have cited no association between moderate intake and low birth weight, spontaneous abortion, or abnormal fetal behavior (54–57). Yet others document positive (58, 59) associations relating high doses (6 to 8 cups a day) of caffeine use to spontaneous abortion. Others have cited that moderate to heavy consumption (151 mg/day or greater) increased the risk of late first and second trimester spontaneous abortion (60). Confounding variables may cloud the results of these studies since spontaneous abortion is susceptible to many factors. Further research is needed to define the relationship with clarity.

High doses (more than 300 mg to 450 mg/day) of caffeine may be associated with an increased risk of having an LBW infant (less than 2500 g) (61–64). LBW is associated with an increased risk of perinatal morbidity and mortality, and mothers must understand that relationship.

Other studies find no statistically significant relationship between caffeine use and LBW (65–66). Birth weight was significantly reduced in women smokers who also consume caffeine.(67)

Links to caffeine and difficulty in becoming pregnant are yet to be proved. Some studies confirm the association with heavy, recent intake (68, 69, 70). Investigators unable to confirm the association have also published their views (71). Although more research is needed, if a woman is having difficulty in conceiving, advising her to decrease or eliminate her caffeine intake would be reasonable.

In summary, current studies document conflicting results, and the limitations in the present studies make positive associations difficult. The association with low to moderate caffeine intake and congenital defects or complications in pregnancy is yet to be proved. Reduced birth weight, spontaneous abortions, and difficulty in becoming pregnant may be associated with caffeine intake. Nevertheless, women may be advised that although moderate intake is probably safe, heavy intake (greater than 300 mg/day) is not recommended. Further research is needed to establish the association between defects and caffeine intake. It is especially important for women who have other risk factors for having an LBW baby or spontaneous abortion to realize that caffeine intake may increase the chance of these outcomes.

In 1980, the FDA advised all women, based on animal data, to avoid caffeine use while pregnant. This includes all sources of caffeine such as coffee, tea, and chocolate. Until more studies are conducted to provide clear direction, this recommendation is not without merit.

SMOKING

Maternal smoking is one of the few known preventable causes of perinatal morbidity and mortality. In 1992, an estimated 14.3 million women of childbearing age (18 to 44 years) smoked cigarettes (72). Young women continue to be the target of tobacco advertisements and sociological pressures that encourage smoking even though the adverse effects of smoking on the fetus—and mother—have been well documented. Fetal, neonatal, and infant mortality is increased, birth weight and length decreased, gestation shortened, and frequency of fetal breathing movements reduced. Complications of pregnancy also may occur such as abruptio placentae, premature rupture of membranes, amnionitis, and placenta previa. Changes in uterine and placental oxygenation or blood flow may be the cause of infant death, prematurity, or spontaneous abortions. Complications in infancy and childhood may present as deficits in long-term physical growth or intellectual and behavioral performance (25, 73, 74, 75).

The effect on the placenta, uterus, fetus, and infant are dose related. Light smoking (less than one pack a day) was found to increase fetal death rate by 20% and heavy smoking (one or more packs a day) to increase the risk by 35% (25). Similarly, the more cigarettes smoked per day, the lower the birth weight. Almost half of LBW infants are born to pregnant women who smoke (75). According to the Surgeon General's 1990 report on smoking cessation, women who quit smoking within the first 3 to 4 months of pregnancy or before pregnancy reduce their risk of having a low birth weight baby to that of women who never smoked. Smoking cessation during pregnancy may also decrease the incidence of perinatal deaths and preterm deliveries. Birth weight may not be improved if a woman simply cuts down on the number of cigarettes smoked while pregnant (76).

Pregnant women who smoke should be informed of the adverse health effects not only to themselves but to their fetus. A primary target population for this education is women who have not completed high school and women who live below the poverty level (72). They are most likely to continue smoking while pregnant. All women should be encouraged to quit smoking while pregnant, and cessation programs designed for pregnant women may be beneficial.

SPECIFIC CONDITIONS

Treating a pregnant woman requires consideration of the potential risks and benefits. One of the first considerations is whether the mother's condition demands drug therapy. Many times, nonpharmacologic approaches can be effective. Drug therapy should be chosen with an understanding of the consequences of not providing treatment compared to those associated with drug therapy. Therapy is usually appropriate if the untreated maternal condition will increase fetal morbidity or mortality. However, the risk of adverse effects occurring from drug exposure in utero needs to be evaluated. Many times these risks are unknown. Some conditions commonly experienced in the pregnant woman are discussed.

Nausea and Vomiting

Nausea is the most common gastrointestinal symptom occurring during pregnancy. Nausea alone occurs in up to 80 to 90% of pregnant women. Nausea and vomiting can occur in 55 to 80% of pregnant women and may be mild to severe (77, 78). Nausea and vomiting in pregnancy (NVP) is distinguished from hyperemesis gravidarum, which is intractable vomiting leading to electrolyte imbalance, maternal weight loss, altered nutritional status, and at times, end-organ or neurologic damage. Hyperemesis gravidarum occurs in about 1 case per 1000 births and requires hospitalization (77).

Symptoms of NVP are usually first experienced during the 3rd to 7th week of pregnancy. Around 8% of women in one study reported suffering before the first missed menstrual period (79). Nausea and vomiting may last throughout the second or even third trimester, but generally it ceases within the first 4 months. "Morning sickness" is experienced in nearly 80% of women, yet many women report nausea and vomiting throughout the day (79, 80, 81). Although the symptoms are self-limiting, nearly 83% of women experiencing them take some form of medication for relief (79).

Nausea and vomiting during pregnancy do not increase the risk of harm or congenital defects to the fetus, nor do they harm the mother (78). Yet the impact of these symptoms can be great on the mother's quality of life. She may find doing household chores, taking care of other children, cooking, and other family activities difficult to perform. Social functions and work habits may also be altered or curtailed (82).

The etiology of NVP is unknown, but several possibilities are proposed, including increased concentrations of human chorionic gonadotropin hormone, progesterone, or estradiol. Neurologic, toxic, and metabolic mechanisms may also play a role. Psychosomatic reasons and unpleasant odors or sights may also contribute to NVP (77, 83). The etiology has not been clearly associated with any one of these factors, so medication therapy is chosen with consideration of the teratogenic risk of the antiemetic agent and severity of the symptoms. The goal of therapy is to eliminate the symptoms, improve the patient's quality of life, do no harm to the fetus, and prevent hyperemesis gravidarum from occurring.

Conservative nonpharmacologic measures should be tried first. Mild to moderate nausea and vomiting may be managed by such efforts as instructing the patient to eat small, frequent meals. High carbohydrate meals, crackers, or high protein snacks during the day and before bedtime may also be helpful. Spicy foods, certain beverages, and noxious odors should be avoided, and many patients find relief by lying down. Even acupressure wristbands (Sea Bands) have been tried (84).

When nondrug measures fail, or if the nutritional and metabolic health of the mother is at risk, drug therapy may be required (85). Meclizine is commonly used as the drug of choice; use in the first trimester has been shown in several reviews to be associated with low teratogenic risk (13, 86). Daily doses of 25 to 50 mg by mouth are usually effective. Dimenhydrinate 50 to 100 mg orally every 4 hours or 50 mg intramuscularly or intravenously every 3 to 4 hours has been used as an alternative with apparently low risk of adverse outcomes (87). When symptoms are not controlled, and the health of the mother and fetus remains in need of drug therapy, phenothiazines have been used in pregnancy. Conflicting results have been reported regarding the safety of individual phenothiazines. Their routine use in pregnancy is not recommended (78). No effects (83, 86, 88, 89, 90, 92) and positive associations (83, 90, 91, 92) between phenothiazine use and adverse outcomes have been documented. Promethazine 50 mg per day given orally or intramuscularly in two to four divided doses may be effective. Alternative phenothiazines such as prochlorperazine 5 to 10 mg orally or intramuscularly three to four times daily have been used, but some practitioners recommend reserving them for more severe cases or avoiding them altogether (78). Alternatively, metoclopramide 5 to 10 mg orally three times daily or 5 to 20 mg intramuscularly or intravenously three times daily is effective and appears to be safe in pregnancy. No congenital defects or other fetal or newborn complications due to metoclopramide therapy have been reported, but use has been limited. Additional data are needed to confirm the safety of metoclopramide in pregnant women. The drug has been used as early as 7 to 10 weeks of gestation and in doses of up to 60 mg per day. Droperidol is not commonly used as an antiemetic in pregnant patients, but some have used it during labor as a sedative or throughout gestation for hyperemesis gravidarum without documenting adverse effects (93). Ondansetron is a newer agent, and only two reports of it being used in pregnant women for severe nausea and vomiting were found. No adverse fetal effects were reported (94, 95).

Pyridoxine deficiency has been hypothesized to cause NVP. The demand for pyridoxine is increased during pregnancy, and women may develop a deficiency of this vitamin. In fact, dietary supplementation of pyridoxine is recommended during pregnancy to prevent deficiencies. However, the deficiency generally doesn't occur until the second or third trimester. Thus, this may not explain symptoms of nausea and vomiting that occur with normal pyridoxine levels or those experienced in the first trimester. For many years, studies have been conducted with pyridoxine, but they have not been well designed or controlled, and the efficacy of pyridoxine in eliminating symptoms has not been proved (87, 96). Other investigators have shown a beneficial effect of pyridoxine for severe NVP when 25 mg is given orally every 8 hours for 3 days (97). Lower doses of 10 to 30 mg per day have been safely administered to pregnant women for NVP.

Pyridoxine 10 mg was one ingredient in Bendectin®, the only product ever approved by the FDA for NVP in the first trimester. This product also contained doxylamine succinate 10 mg, and up until 1976, 10 mg of dicyclomine. The latter ingredient was discontinued in the product marketed in the United States because of suspected ineffectiveness. Doxylamine is currently available in over-the-counter sleep aids. Bendectin® came under considerable scrutiny because of case reports describing malformations in infants exposed to the drug in utero. For instance, congenital heart defects, limb abnormalities, and neural-tube defects were among the described abnormalities. Despite these case reports, in epidemiologic studies conducted totaling slightly over 6000 patients, no evidence of an increased risk of teratogenicity was documented. However, in 1984, the manufacturer encountered high costs in litigation and requested physicians to stop prescribing the drug. Even though there was confidence in the safety profile of Bendectin®, the product was removed from the market strictly because of the expense of legal cases (83).

Asthma

Asthma complicates about 0.4 to 4% of pregnancies (98, 99, 100). The effect pregnancy has on asthma is variable. The condition may improve, decline, or go unaltered. Women with severe asthma prior to pregnancy are more likely to have difficulty with the disease during pregnancy. Although asthma may worsen near the end of the second trimester, generally within 3 months postpartum, the gravida has returned to her baseline, prepregnancy level of severity (101).

Maternal and fetal morbidity and mortality is increased when asthma is not adequately treated. Neonatal or perinatal mortality, low birth weight, and increased risk of prematurity may be more frequent in pregnant asthmatics than normal controls. Hyperemesis gravidarum, chronic hypertension, and preeclampsia may be other maternal complications in asthmatic pregnancies (100–103). If asthma is controlled, infants are born with no greater risk for congenital abnormalities than the general population (100, 102, 104). Complications that might arise could be due to the disease or the drug therapy. Exacerbations of asthma, for example, could lead to decreased fetal oxygenation. The improved outcome of mother and child associated with treating the pregnant asthmatic supports the administration of drugs to these patients (102, 105). The goal of therapy and the drugs used are similar to those for the nonpregnant patient.

Inhaled beta-2-agonists have been used successfully in treating mild and infrequent asthmatic episodes. Systemic adverse effects are lessened by using aerosolized therapy, the preferred route of administration for pregnant women. The use of selective beta-2-agonists will also lessen adverse effects, such as cardiac abnormalities or tremor. All beta-sympathomimetics may cause fetal and maternal tachycardia, maternal hyperglycemia or hypotension, or neonatal hypoglycemia. Minor malformations, inguinal hernia, and clubfoot were associated with the sympathomimetic class of drugs when used in the first trimester (13). Of this class, metaproterenol has been commonly used in pregnant women. Albuterol, isoetharine, terbutaline, and isoproterenol are possible alternatives (99, 101, 106–109). Data using albuterol in the first trimester is limited, but use in the second and third trimester has not been linked with congenital defects (110). Terbutaline is commonly used as a tocolytic. The inhibition of labor at term when the drug is used for asthma may require that terbutaline be discontinued. All patients treated with a sympathomimetic should be monitored for adverse effects. Patients should not overuse an inhaler; a dose of two puffs every 4 to 6 hours is usually adequate. Frequent use may indicate a need for alternative therapy.

Methylxanthines are typically the drugs of choice for patients requiring continuous bronchodilator therapy. Theophylline has been used in conjunction with inhalation therapy for long-term control. Theophylline or aminophylline should be carefully administered to maintain nontoxic maternal serum concentrations. These agents cross the placenta, and fetal concentrations are about equal to maternal serum concentrations. Adverse fetal/neonatal effects reported include jitteriness, cardiac arrhythmias, hypoglycemia, vomiting, tachycardia, and feeding difficulties. Theophylline does not appear to be associated with congenital defects (13). Neonatal toxicity has been reported in women with normal to upper-end serum concentrations (111, 112). Maternal serum concentrations should be monitored throughout pregnancy, and particularly in the third trimester when a possible decrease in theophylline clearance and/or increase in volume of distribution takes place (113, 114).

If steroids are indicated, they should not be withheld (99,101,104). Oral prednisolone or prednisone have been used in severe and acute exacerbations uncontrolled by alternative medications. Doses needed to control attacks can be administered and then tapered slowly over several days to the lowest effective dose. Every-other-day dosing is optimal if continued steroid treatment is indicated. Two case reports exist describing infants exposed to prednisone through gestation. One infant was born with congenital cataracts (115) and the other with immunosuppression (116). Any association between these abnormalities and steroid therapy has not been supported by other studies, however. No evidence has confirmed that prednisone increases fetal mortality or morbidity, and the risk of prednisone to the fetus and newborn is considered to be low (99, 101). Methylprednisolone or hydrocortisone are acceptable if intravenous steroid administration is needed (101). Inhaled beclomethasone has been used in pregnant patients and will provide the advantages of topical therapy (109). Beclomethasone has been the sympathomimetic most commonly used for inhalation therapy. Defects such as spontaneous abortion, prematurity, and cardiac malformations have been documented from experience in 40 women treated with beclomethasone (117). Because of various confounding elements, including concurrent diseases and medications, the degree of association was unclear. Flunisolide or triamcinolone have also been suggested as alternative antiinflammatory agents for inhalation, but documentation on their use is sparse (101). Compared to beclomethasone, little information is published regarding the safety of triamcinolone in pregnant women.

Cromolyn sodium is indicated for the prevention of asthmatic attacks. It is administered via inhalation; therefore, significant concentrations of the drug are not achieved in the plasma. It is unknown if cromolyn crosses the placenta. There has been no evidence proving an association between this drug and congenital defects. Cromolyn has been used without adverse maternal or fetal outcomes (102–104, 108, 109, 118).

Ipratropium is an anticholinergic marketed for relief of asthma attacks. No data exists about the safety of the drug in pregnant women. Since the systemic absorption of the drug is small, adverse effects would be expected to be minimal (101).

Status asthmaticus is experienced in nearly 0.2% of pregnant women (102). This is a life-threatening condition, and treatment is the same for pregnant and nonpregnant patients.

Hypertension

Hypertension, when defined as a blood pressure measurement of over 140/80 mm Hg, complicates about 8 to 10% of all pregnancies (119, 120). Up to 20% of young women experiencing their first pregnancy and about 40 to 50% of women with twins may have complications of hypertension (120–123). Hypertension contributes significantly to maternal and perinatal morbidity and mortality (122, 124). Complications may include intrauterine growth retardation, placental insufficiency or abruptio, and preterm labor and delivery. The fetus can be deprived of oxygen and nutrients if the hypertension is severe enough to diminish the uteroplacental blood flow. The incidence of these complications increases in direct proportion to increased maternal blood pressure.

The normal gravida will have slightly lower blood pressure readings than the nongravid female. The mean diastolic values are slightly lower in early pregnancy than before conception, and approximate prepregnancy values near the time of delivery. Blood pressure readings for the gravid are carefully assessed. What are considered normal values in nonpregnant women may be abnormally high values for the gravid and indicate a need for further therapy (119, 120). Measurements taken at two different occasions that are over 130/80 mm Hg at anytime in pregnancy, or readings greater than 140/90 after 20 weeks gestation, are considered hypertensive. Increments of 30 mm Hg systolic and/or 15 mm Hg diastolic over the average value before 20 weeks gestation are also defined as hypertensive (119, 120, 125, 126). Patients with second trimester diastolic readings of 75 mm Hg and third trimester diastolic measurements of 85 mm Hg should be regarded as reaching the upper limits for uncomplicated pregnancies. Patients with readings greater than these values should be thoroughly evaluated (119, 120, 126, 127).

A committee of obstetricians and internists referred to as the Working Group on High Blood Pressure in Pregnancy, produced a consensus document that defined terminology regarding various types of hypertension in pregnancy. Four classifications were defined: (1) preeclampsia and eclampsia, (2) chronic hypertension, (3) preeclampsia superimposed on chronic hypertension, and (4) transient hypertension. The Working Group also provided recommendations for treatment of the classifications (128).

Chronic hypertension of pregnancy may be due to various causes similar to those of the nonpregnant hypertensive patient. The effect of chronic hypertension on the fetus may be serious and even fatal, depending on the underlying disease(s) of the patient and severity of hypertension. Chronic hypertensive patients are likely to develop preeclampsia, especially women older than 30 years (127). Drug therapy may prevent preeclampsia from developing although this needs further study (129).

Transient hypertension usually develops near term and can be mild to moderate with little effect on the fetus or mother (127, 129). Preeclampsia and eclampsia are a major cause of fetal and maternal morbidity and mortality. Maternal cerebral hemorrhage, pulmonary edema, liver or cardiac failure may occur. The fetus may show growth retardation due to decreased placental perfusion. Risk factors for preeclampsia include young primigravidas, multiparity, maternal age, family history, diabetes mellitus, preexisting hypertension, primary renal disease, twinning, fetal hydrops, and hydatidiform mole (124, 130). Low socioeconomic status or minority race may possibly be other risks (119, 126). Interestingly, living at high elevation (above 3100 meters) has been postulated to increase the chance of preeclampsia (119). Patients with preeclampsia can exhibit complications, other than high blood pressure, including proteinuria, edema, and coagulation abnormalities. Changes in the retinal vascular occur, and some patients experience seizure, the onset of eclampsia. This classification of hypertension requires immediate attention of a physician and hospitalization.

The etiology of preeclampsia is unknown. Theories are uteroplacental ischemia, lack of protective immunity in the mother, inadequate activity of the renin-angiotensin-aldosterone system, imbalance between prostacyclin and thromboxane A2, or other hormonal or metabolic abnormalities (119). Preventing preeclampsia with low-dose aspirin (60 to 100 mg daily) after 12 weeks gestation has been studied (120). Preliminary results are encouraging but need confirmation. Groups at risk for aspirin therapy have not been clearly identified (131). Aspirin is tried because it interferes with clotting and vasoconstriction by inhibiting thromboxane A2 production without altering prostacyclin production (119, 127).

Treatment of the hypertensive gravid is determined by considering the clinical situation of the patient and presence of complicating factors, maximum blood pressure recorded, and stage of gestation. Although the benefit of treating mild hypertensive pregnant patients with drug therapy is controversial (120, 127–129), severe hyperten-

sion requires drug treatment to reduce fetal and maternal morbidity and mortality. The goals of therapy are to decrease maternal cerebrovascular accidents and cardiac failure, yet maintain placental perfusion; target blood pressures usually being 90 to 100 mm Hg diastolic (120, 128). In general, treatment is initiated when diastolic readings are greater than 105 mm HG (120, 128).

Many patients with mild hypertension respond to nondrug therapy. Bed rest, relaxation techniques, limited physical activity, abstinence from smoking or drinking alcohol, isotonic exercises, and proper nutrition may be effective. If drug therapy is indicated, agents with the most available information regarding their use in pregnancy are preferred. The drug of choice should be carefully chosen and administered to avoid a precipitous drop in maternal blood pressure that may compromise placental perfusion.

DRUG THERAPY FOR PREECLAMPSIA-ECLAMPSIA

Hydralazine has been most commonly used to control hypertension in preeclampsia. Information on the use of the drug in all three trimesters is available. Fetal and maternal serum concentrations are similar since hydralazine readily crosses the placenta. Its use has not been clearly associated with congenital defects. Hydralazine has been used safely with other antihypertensive agents such as beta-antagonists and methyldopa. Three cases of neonatal thrombocytopenia and bleeding have been documented. It is unclear if the effect was caused by the hydralazine or the underlying hypertension (132). Patients may experience headache, tachycardia, flushing, tremors, and palpitations. A hydralazine bolus of 2 to 5 mg intravenously given slowly, then repeated carefully as needed every 20 to 30 minutes with a bolus of 2 to 10 mg has been used (126, 127). Failure to achieve normal blood pressure after maximum doses have been used may indicate the need for alternative agents.

Diazoxide has been used and reserved for patients failing to respond to other agents such as hydralazine. A 30-mg bolus has been recommended by the Working Group to avoid sudden drops in blood pressure with larger doses. Patients may experience nausea, vomiting, tachycardia, or hyperglycemia. Diazoxide may inhibit labor or cause neonatal hyperglycemia. If diazoxide is indicated, it should be used with caution to prevent sudden and significant falls in maternal blood pressure that could result in cerebral ischemia. Fatal maternal hypotension has been reported (133).

Alternatively, labetalol has been suggested (126, 128) with 10 to 20 mg intravenously as an initial dose (119, 120, 126) then 20 to 80 mg every 20 to 30 minutes until the desired response or maximum dose allowed is reached. Continuous infusion at 1 to 2 mg/min has also been employed (119, 120). Neonatal bradycardia and mild transient hypotension have been reported rarely with labetalol.

The drug apparently has no effect on uteroplacental blood flow, and it has been shown to increase production of pulmonary surfactant (134).

Nitroprusside has been used for life-threatening hypertensive emergencies. The Working Group recommends avoiding this drug unless maternal well-being dictates since the fetus is sensitive to cyanide toxicity, which can result with extensive nitroprusside therapy. Nitroprusside crosses the placenta, and the dose should be monitored closely if used in pregnant women.

Magnesium sulfate remains the recommended choice for preventing and treating seizures in the preeclamptic and eclamptic gravida, respectively (127, 128). Maternal sedation or fetal depression, which may be an effect of phenobarbital or benzodiazepines, are not a side effect of magnesium sulfate. Safety and efficacy of the drug should be monitored with serum concentrations (4 to 7 mEq/L). Patient patellar reflex, respiratory rate, and urine output should also be monitored for signs of toxicity. Neonates should be monitored for respiratory depression and hyporeflexia if exposed to magnesium sulfate over a long time.

THERAPY IN CHRONIC HYPERTENSION

If therapy is initiated during gestation for patients without preeclampsia, methyldopa has been used most frequently and remains the drug of choice of the Working Group (128). Methyldopa readily crosses the placenta, and only rare adverse effects have been documented in the newborn. Data regarding long-term effects (7.5 years) in children exposed to the drug in utero fail to document abnormalities due to the drug. Normal mental and physical development has been reported (121). Methyldopa may be given at a dose of 250 mg two or three times daily. An alternative alpha agonist is clonidine. Although not used as extensively in pregnancy as methyldopa, clonidine has been shown to be effective in severe hypertension in late pregnancy, and no reports of congenital defects have been associated with clonidine use in late gestation (135). However, it offers little to no therapeutic advantage over methyldopa. Since there is more experience with methyldopa, it is generally preferred. Hydralazine, 10 to 25 mg orally two or three times daily, has been used in conjunction with methyldopa as an alternative in chronic hypertension when needed (127).

In cases where neither methyldopa nor hydralazine is appropriate, the beta-adrenergic receptor antagonists have been used. Propranolol, atenolol, metoprolol, and labetalol have been used in pregnancy for various indications. Effects on the fetus and mother vary among these agents because of their differences in pharmacodynamic and pharmacokinetic profiles. These drugs cross the placenta, producing fetal serum levels at a steady state that approximates those of the maternal serum. Propranolol cord levels may exceed maternal serum concentrations. Antagonism of the beta receptors in the fetus can cause a decrease in fetal heart rate reactivity. Thus, the fetus exposed to these agents near delivery should be monitored for 24 to 72 hours after birth for signs of beta-adrenoreceptor blocking activity. Experience with atenolol, labetalol, and metoprolol in the first trimester is limited. Further study is needed to assess the effects with early exposure. These agents have not been found to induce premature labor or, when used in second and third trimesters, produce congenital malformations. Unlike methyldopa, no long-term follow-up studies past one year have been conducted for metoprolol, propranolol, or labetolol. The extent to which these agents may produce effects lasting throughout childhood needs to be evaluated.

Propranolol has been effective in doses of 80 to 140 mg/day; the lower doses being associated with fewer adverse effects. Intrauterine growth retardation may be associated with propranolol therapy (136). Hypoglycemia, bradycardia, and respiratory depression are some of the adverse effects that have been reported in newborns.

Metoprolol has been found to be safe at doses of 100 mg/day (120), and it has been shown to reduce perinatal mortality when compared to hydralazine therapy (137). Atenolol has been given in daily doses of 50 to 100 mg (127). Reduced birth weight has been reported; however, one-year follow-up studies have noted normal growth and development in children exposed in utero during the third trimester (138–140). Atenolol has been used primarily in late pregnancy.

Growth-retarded infants exposed to labetalol in the third trimester were documented by Sibai et al. (141). There is little documentation of using labetalol in the first trimester. The drug may be less likely to decrease cardiac output and uteroplacental blood flow because of the alpha- and beta-adrenergic receptor antagonist activities it possesses. Newborns may have transient hypotension or, rarely, bradycardia, but the majority of infants do not appear to be adversely affected (142, 143).

Limited information is available on using calcium channel blockers in pregnancy. They have been effective in treating acute hypertension near term (127), yet, in animal studies, nifedipine has been associated with fetal hypoxemia, acidosis, and decreased uterine blood flow. Nifedipine has been used only in a small number of patients in the second or third trimesters for severe hypertension (144–146). Nifedipine may increase the neuromuscular blockade properties of magnesium sulfate, and the combination of these drugs should be avoided (147, 148). Until further studies are completed to evaluate the safety of nifedipine and other calcium channel blockers, they are not recommended for general use in pregnancy (119, 120, 126, 149).

Angiotensin I converting enzyme (ACE) inhibitors are not recommended as an antihypertensive agent in pregnant patients. Use of captopril in the second and third trimester has been linked to severe and sometimes fatal fetal and neonatal anuria. Captopril may result in fetal renal compromise by inhibiting the production of angiotensin II. Decreased glomerular filtration rate resulting in fetal hypotension may, in addition, produce adverse effects such as oligohydramnios or occipital encephalocele (150). Fetal contractures and hypoplastic lung development have occurred. Other outcomes that have been observed include intrauterine growth retardation, patent ductus arteriosus, and prematurity (151, 152). The Working Group and the drug manufacturers of these products recommend ACE inhibitors not be used in pregnancy. Alternative agents with safer profiles exist such as methyldopa, labetalol, atenolol, or hydralazine. In preconception planning, use of an alternative antihypertensive agent should be employed if possible, especially in the second and third trimesters. Mothers with exposure to ACE inhibitors should receive counseling regarding the risks of oligohydramnios and other possible adverse outcomes. Infants born after in utero exposure should be closely monitored for signs and symptoms of prolonged renal failure and hypotension.

The use of diuretics in pregnant hypertensives is controversial (121). The Working Group has made recommendations on the use of diuretics. The main concern regarding diuretic use is their effect on the volume status of the patient. Diuretics cause a decrease in plasma and extracellular fluid volume, decrease in cardiac output, and decreased perfusion of the placenta and uterus. This may accentuate problems in women with previously contracted fluid volumes and preeclampsia (126). The necessary expansion of fluids during pregnancy may be counteracted by diuretic therapy, but this remains to be proved. Thiazide and loop diuretics have been rarely used in the first trimester but have been used later in gestation for refractory hypertension. Adverse fetal and neonatal effects with thiazide use in later pregnancy have included hypoglycemia, electrolyte imbalances, thrombocytopenia, decreased birth weight, and increased perinatal mortality (153). Decreased maternal weight gain may also result. Though diuretic therapy may be indicated in some clinical situations, such as pulmonary edema, normal blood pressure can usually be achieved with other agents. Thiazide and loop diuretics are not, therefore, first-line drugs of choice for initiating antihypertensive therapy during pregnancy. Some clinicians will recommend that women continue diuretic therapy throughout pregnancy if blood pressure control was achieved with a diuretic before conception (154). The Working Group endorsed that opinion (128).

Epilepsy

Less than 1% of pregnancies are complicated by seizure disorders (155). Pregnant epileptics treated with antiepileptic medications have over a 90% chance of having a normal child, but there is a two- to threefold greater risk for major congenital malformations and minor anomalies in the offspring of treated epileptics than in the nonepileptic population (156, 157). Mental retardation, stillbirth, and microcephaly have been reported to occur at increased risk in women experiencing seizures during pregnancy (158). Fetal harm is a possibility in pregnant epileptics because of several reasons. First, there is the effect of the disease on the fetus and, second, the influence of exposure to antiepileptic agents. Seizures can produce hypoxia and acidosis, which can be damaging, and adverse effects from the antiepileptic drugs may indirectly cause harm. The genetic or biochemical makeup of the epileptic mother is another component. The importance of any one of these influences is unclear because most patients present with confounding factors. However, reviews of the literature and other reports indicate that drug therapy has been associated with an increase in congenital defects (15, 160). It is also important to understand the effect of pregnancy on the patient's epilepsy. Pregnancy will improve the seizure control of nearly one-fourth of all pregnant epileptics. Similarly, one-fourth of patients will have a worsening of their disorder, whereas half of the patients will experience no change in control. Lack of control may be related to poor compliance with antiseizure medications although other factors may play a role, including the patient's history of epilepsy, patient age, and pregnancy-related changes in estrogen concentration (161, 162).

Uncontrolled seizures can be dangerous to the mother and to the fetus. Increased rates of stillbirths may occur with status epilepticus. Most offspring of epileptic mothers are exposed to antiepileptic drug (AED) because the benefit of treatment generally outweighs the risk of exposure to the AED (157, 163–165).

Further research is needed to determine which, if any, AED is clearly safest for the mother and child (165, 166). Serious risks are inherent with each agent. When drug therapy is required for control of seizures, since all AEDs have potential to cause malformations, all precautions to reduce the risk of harm should be taken. The lowest effective dose should always be used. Single agent therapy is also best if possible. In addition, the clinician should be aware that the pharmacokinetic profile of anticonvulsant medications is altered in the pregnant state. Volume of distribution increases throughout pregnancy. Renal and hepatic clearance are increased, and gastrointestinal absorption may decrease. Protein binding is decreased (156). During the postpartum period, the pharmacokinetic parameters return to normal. Thus, serum concentrations should be monitored throughout pregnancy and at least up to the 6th week postpartum.

Phenytoin is teratogenic in animals and may produce adverse effects in the fetus and newborn. Effects of the drug may be evident in childhood. The fetal hydantoin syndrome, discussed earlier, may be expressed. Serious and sometimes fatal hemorrhagic disease of the newborn can occur and may present within 1 to 2 days after delivery. It may be caused by a phenytoin-induced deficiency in fetal vitamin K-dependent clotting factors. Phenytoin may also induce thrombocytopenia. Although further research is needed to determine the best means of prevention and treatment, some clinicians recommend administering 10 to 20 mg oral vitamin K to the mother in the last 2 to 4 weeks of pregnancy, or giving vitamin K during labor. The infant could also be given vitamin K after delivery (157, 167). Phenytoin has been linked with various tumors in children whose mothers took the drug while pregnant (168). Babies should be monitored throughout childhood for any carcinogenic effects of the drug.

In summary, although the adverse effects can be serious, the lack of seizure control may do even greater harm to the fetus and mother. For instance, where phenytoin use is clearly indicated, maternal supplementation with vitamin K prior to delivery should be considered, and phenytoin serum concentrations should be carefully monitored throughout pregnancy. Both free and total phenytoin concentrations should be monitored if possible. Total concentrations may decrease in pregnancy since free concentration remains unchanged due to altered binding. The best total phenytoin concentration for maintenance of seizure control in pregnant women has not been established. Because phenytoin can induce folic acid deficiency, administration of folic acid throughout gestation is usually recommended (163, 165).

Phenobarbital has been frequently used in pregnant epileptics. Minor abnormalities have been associated with its use in the gravida. Similar to phenytoin, neonatal hemorrhage shortly after delivery, partial expression of the fetal hydantoin syndrome, and maternal folic acid deficiency may occur. Unlike phenytoin, phenobarbital may cause neonatal addiction and withdrawal symptoms such as hyperactivity and feeding problems. Withdrawal symptoms generally occur within 1 week of delivery. In this case, parents should be advised to monitor for these symptoms and to not blame themselves for the behavior of the baby or for poor parenting skills. The newborn may need to receive treatment for withdrawal symptoms.

Other anticonvulsant medications have been used in pregnant women. Ethosuximide has been used for petit mal epilepsy in pregnancy (154) although documentation on the use of this agent in pregnant women is limited. Carbamazepine has been used in the pregnant epileptic as monotherapy and in combination therapy with phenobarbital or phenytoin. Carbamazepine readily crosses the placenta and has been associated with abnormalities, including craniofacial defects, fingernail hypoplasia, and developmental delay (169, 170). A similar pattern of abnormalities to the fetal hydantoin syndrome has also

been noted with carbamazepine therapy with the appearance of minor craniofacial defects, digital hypoplasia, and delayed development. There is an estimated 1% risk of neural-tube defects with carbamazepine (171). Clinicians have recommended some patients, especially those with a family history of neural-tube defects, avoid carbamazepine and receive evaluation for using alternative AEDs (165).

Valproic acid is considered a human teratogen and should be avoided in pregnancy. It has been linked with neural-tube defects in 1 to 2% of exposures. Minor and major cardiovascular and craniofacial malformations have occurred, as have deficiencies in mental and physical development and meningomyelocele (154). Women exposed to valproic acid during pregnancy should consider prenatal testing and receive counseling (165).

To decrease the risk of adverse fetal outcome, epileptic patients should be counseled prior to pregnancy if at all possible. Patients should receive advice on adequate nutrition, including adequate folic acid intake before and during pregnancy, the importance of seizure control with the best AED regimen (an effective agent, low dose, monotherapy), and overall good prenatal health care.

Diabetes Mellitus

The risk of congenital abnormalities is three times greater in pregnant overt diabetics than in the nondiabetic pregnant population (172). Similarly, major abnormalities are more likely to occur in the diabetic population lacking control of the disease or with underlying diseases. The anomalies are significant in that 20 to 50% of perinatal deaths of offspring from diabetic women are due to birth defects. Evidence suggests that these birth defects are due to inadequate metabolic control and poor control of the blood glucose levels (173). In fact, euglycemic control of the maternal blood sugar is elemental in decreasing the incidence of perinatal mortality and morbidity (174–176). Anomalies commonly reported with maternal diabetics include macrosomia; respiratory distress syndrome; and cardiac abnormalities such as cardiomyopathy, prematurity, renal, CNS, and skeletal defects. Fetal behavioral and intellectual development may be impaired with poor management of the diabetes (177). Maternal hyperglycemia during the period of organogenesis is thought to be associated with increased incidence of congenital abnormalities. This may explain why gestational diabetics have a lessened risk of congenital abnormalities than overt diabetics. The onset of gestational diabetes does not generally occur until around the 24th week. Therefore, in the gestational diabetic, early in pregnancy the maternal blood sugar and glycosolated hemoglobin are normal, and the fetus has an increased chance of normal development.

The incidence of perinatal mortality has decreased dramatically over the last several years to around 1.6 to 4.5% (173). The decrease in mortality is largely due to tighter control of maternal blood glucose (176). Maternal mortality risk factors include clinical pyelonephritis, diabetic ketoacidosis, hypertension, preeclampsia, and lack of antenatal care (178). Diabetic ketoacidosis can occur at lower glucose concentrations than in the nonpregnant diabetic. Ketoacidosis is associated with a 50% perinatal mortality rate, and patients should be carefully monitored to prevent this from developing.

Diabetes mellitus during pregnancy is commonly categorized according to the White classification (179). This system has been used for many years and classifies patients based on the presence of vascular disease, the age of onset, and duration of diabetes mellitus in the patient. The goal of therapy in the pregnant diabetic is to achieve normalization of the blood sugar and avoid extreme fluctuations in insulin and glucose plasma concentrations. Throughout gestation, the amount of insulin required varies for insulin-dependant diabetics. During the first 24 weeks of gestation, the fetus receives its required nutrients from the mother, the transport of which can lead to maternal hypoglycemia. The mother generally requires less insulin during this part of the pregnancy. However, in the late second and third trimesters, the demand for insulin increases. This is due, in part, to an increase in placental hormones that are diabetogenic. The clinician should be aware that after delivery, the amount of insulin needed by the mother is similar to that required before conception.

If at all possible, a diabetic woman who wishes to become pregnant should carefully plan conception. Proper obstetric management would include an evaluation of the woman for the presence of complicating risk factors, including retinopathy, renal impairment, and ischemic heart disease, or a significant history of problems with previous pregnancies. Tight control of the blood sugar before conception is key in the planning process. Some patients will be recommended to achieve a glycosolated hemoglobin A (hemoglobin A_{1c}) less than 8.5% before attempting to conceive. A pregnancy test should be performed soon after the patient misses her first menstrual period. Because of the risk to the fetus of hyperglycemia, a pregnant woman should be tested for gestational diabetes around the 22nd to 26th week. If the diagnosis is not made at this time, glucose concentrations should be remeasured in the 32nd week. Ensuing a diagnosis of diabetes, patient education is important. Although there are increased nutritional needs in the pregnant patient, appropriate diet and exercise regimens that are similar for the nonpregnant diabetic should be taught to the patient. If diet fails to control blood sugar, insulin is indicated. Oral hypoglycemic agents are not recommended in pregnancy. They may induce insulin secretion from the fetal pancreas and lead to fetal hypoglycemia. As mentioned previously, the amount of insulin during gestation will vary. A mix of intermediate-acting and short-acting insulin is generally most effective.

NPH and regular can be given in a regimen specific to the patient's needs. Multiple daily injections are usually required to achieve euglycemia. Human insulin is preferred for patients not previously using insulin since it lowers the risk of developing insulin antibodies.

Patients must monitor their glucose concentration at home. The best control dictates that the blood sugar should be checked four to eight times daily. Measurements may be taken before meals, 2 hours after each meal, and at bedtime (180, 181). In some patients, once effective control is adequately demonstrated, the level could be checked twice daily. Patients should be instructed to check their glucose concentration anytime they feel it is high or low. Fasting plasma glucose concentrations near 100 mg/100 ml and postprandial concentrations of less than 120 mg/100 ml have been recommended (182). Maternal glucose concentrations will need to be carefully controlled during labor and delivery. The newborn will also need monitoring after delivery to ensure normal glucose concentrations.

Anticoagulation

Pregnancy is a "hypercoaguable state," and coagulation disorders affect around 0.2% to 0.4% of pregnant women (183, 184). Anticoagulants may be taken for a variety of indications, including thrombophlebitis, thromboembolic disease, and valvular heart prostheses (185). The high reduction of antepartum mortality rates from 13 to 1% in women with thromboembolic disease supports treatment of the pregnant patient with anticoagulant therapy (183).

The anticoagulant most commonly used as the drug of choice for the pregnant patient is heparin. It does not cross the placenta and has not been associated with congenital defects. Heparin has been used for short-term anticoagulation at doses of 5000 units subcutaneously every 12 hours, with little risk to the mother and fetus. Any risks to the fetus may be more likely related to indirect effects of the maternal disease state (186–188). Perinatal mortality rates are comparatively better for heparin therapy recipients (3.6%) than coumarin-treated patients (26.1%) (189). Although advantageous in many respects over other anticoagulants, the use of heparin is not without risks to the mother. Bleeding, particularly during delivery, may occur, and thrombocytopenia has been reported. Long-term therapy (over 3 to 6 months) proposes an increased risk of maternal osteoporosis. The effect is more likely with high-dose therapy (more than 20,000 units/day) but has been reported with lower doses and short duration (184). Safety and efficacy of heparin therapy may be assessed by monitoring platelet count periodically, prothrombin time, activated partial thromboplastin time, and hematocrit. Heparin doses may need to be decreased with significantly abnormal values and/or serious bleeding (190). Any bleeding that occurs can be readily reversed by protamine sulfate.

Coumarin derivatives are well known as teratogens, cross the placenta, and may produce significant abnormalities. Exposure during the first trimester, particularly the 6th to 9th week of gestation, can result in the characteristic fetal warfarin syndrome, described previously in this text. Central nervous system defects may be seen with exposure throughout pregnancy. Exposure to warfarin throughout pregnancy has been associated with abnormalities of the facies, skeletal system, and limbs. Stillbirths, spontaneous abortion, mental retardation, and impairment of physical growth are also possible effects. Coumarin derivatives carry serious risk to the fetus and should be avoided during pregnancy, particularly in the first and third trimesters.

Heartburn

Nearly 30 to 50% of pregnant patients complain of heartburn (191). This is generally described as a burning sensation in the substernal or epigastric region that may radiate to the back or neck. The etiology in pregnancy is not clearly understood. During pregnancy, there is increased pressure from the uterus onto the stomach, particularly during the third trimester; progesterone is thought to relax the lower esophageal sphincter tone. A decrease in gastrointestinal motility may also play a role. Patients generally do not experience any serious sequelae from heartburn, and the symptoms can usually be managed conservatively.

Nonpharmacologic therapy should be tried initially. A diet low in fat is recommended. Patients should also be instructed to avoid irritating substances such as coffee, spicy foods, orange juice, tomato juice, or peppermint. Relief is generally obtained by eating small, frequent meals and avoiding any food intake immediately before bedtime. Patients should avoid lying down immediately after eating during the day. Elevating the head of the bed is sometimes effective. Antacids provide relief for the majority of patients. Sodium bicarbonate should be replaced by oral antacid products containing aluminum hydroxide, magnesium hydroxide, or magnesium trisilicate. Tablet or liquid form has been used. Products with a combination of these ingredients appear to be safe and effective for most patients. If doses of 15 to 30 ml as needed do not relieve symptoms, dosing every 1 to 3 hours after meals and before bedtime may be effective. Patients with problems related to sodium retention should use low sodium containing antacids. Sucralfate has been used and appears to be safe in pregnancy since it is not absorbed orally. The question has been asked whether absorption of any aluminum from sucralfate would be absorbed and lead to toxicity in patients with abnormal renal function. Documentation regarding sucralfate use in pregnancy is rare (191).

Drugs used in the nonpregnant patient to manipulate the lower esophageal sphincter tone are not currently recommended for pregnant patients. Histamine 2-antagonists, bethanechol, and metoclopramide are better replaced with antacids (192). Few reports are available of women taking H$_2$-antagonists during pregnancy. Cimetidine has been used throughout pregnancy, and no reports linking it to congenital defects in humans have been cited. Concern exists over the antiandrogenic activity of cimetidine and its resultant effect on feminization of male rats. Few reports of ranitidine use are published, and none indicate an association to defects when used throughout pregnancy or near delivery (191). Neither ranitidine nor cimetidine is approved by the FDA for use in pregnancy.

Constipation

Pregnant patients commonly complain of straining, decreased frequency of bowel movements, pain during defecation, and rectal bleeding. Etiologies of constipation in pregnancy are similar to the nonpregnant state, but other possible causative factors include increased pressure on the colon, rectum, abdomen, or back muscles; increased intestinal transit time; increased progesterone; decreased motilin (a stimulating hormone); or increased colonic absorption of sodium, potassium, and water (193, 194). A good drug history should be taken to rule out any over-the-counter products that may cause constipation such as aluminum antacids. Once treatment is indicated, patients should first be counseled on increasing the amount of fiber in their diet. Daily water intake should be sufficient. Exercise and stress relaxation techniques also help in attaining regularity. Kegal exercises have been described to strengthen pelvic floor muscles (194).

Bulk-forming laxatives with psyllium appear to be safe in pregnancy. Caution should be taken not to use an over-the-counter product with unnecessary and potentially harmful inactive ingredients or combination products such as a bulk-forming laxative with mineral oil. Psyllium is readily available for patients and is safe and effective at doses of one to two tablespoons, once or twice daily. Emollients such as stool softeners may also be effective although limited information is available regarding their use in pregnancy. Docusate sodium or dioctyl sulfosuccinate 100 to 200 mg daily generally provides relief. Mineral oil should be avoided in pregnant women because of possible interference with lipid soluble vitamins. Strong laxatives, stimulants, and enemas are not recommended during pregnancy.

Common Cold

The common cold frequently affects pregnant women whose resistance is weakened. The viruses causing the common cold have not been shown to be teratogenic. However, determining the risk associated for most cold medications is difficult because of confounding variables such as the underlying illness and polypharmacy. In many patients, it is difficult to determine whether the drug, the disease, the virus, or other drugs caused the defect. Most problems associated with the common cold are the symptoms; they can be intolerable. Patients may complain of watery eyes and nose, cough, sneezing, and congestion. Although many products are available, the patient should be informed that treatment is not curative. If at all possible, medication therapy should be avoided. To limit drug exposure further, combination products should not be used when the patient can be treated with only one active component of the product.

If the patient's most bothersome symptom requires an antihistamine, both chlorpheniramine and triprolidine have commonly been used in pregnancy. A significant increased relative risk of birth defects has been documented with brompheniramine use in the first trimester, and this drug is not generally recommended. As a class of agents, use of antihistamines in the last 2 weeks of pregnancy was noted to have an increased risk of retrolental fibroplasia in exposed premature infants (195).

Sympathomimetic amines are useful in patients needing a decongestant. Minor malformations have been documented with first trimester use of this class of drugs, including club foot and inguinal hernia. Although sympathomimetic amines are not identified as human teratogens, use of this class of drugs is not without risk. Alpha-adrenergic stimulants may decrease uterine blood flow and cause fetal damage. Of the data that are available on some of the sympathomimetic amines that have been used in pregnancy, pseudoephedrine has not been associated with adverse outcomes. Phenylpropanolamine in the first trimester should be avoided if possible since significant physical deformations (eye, ear, pectus escavatum) have been positively associated with its early use (13). Further research is needed to understand the relationship between these defects and sympathomimetic amines. Epinephrine has been associated with increased incidence of major and minor birth defects with first trimester exposure and minor malformations throughout pregnancy. Epinephrine may cause constriction of blood vessels and decrease uterine blood flow. Phenylephrine may be used as a topical nasal decongestant. Although topical application is advantageous in limiting systemic exposure and toxicity, phenylephrine carries the similar risks as phenylpropanolamine. Oxymetazoline is a longer-acting topical product and has also been used in pregnancy although little documentation exists. Ephedrine has not been associated with birth defects.

Antitussives or expectorants that have been used in pregnant women include dextromethorphan and guaifenesin. There is currently little documentation about using these agents in pregnancy (13). Iodides, including saturated solution of potassium iodine, are contraindicated in pregnancy since they may induce goiter in the fetus. Available cough syrups and elixirs customarily contain some kind of sedative, sugar, and alcohol. Pregnant women

should avoid the use of products with these extra ingredients. The fetal alcohol syndrome was reported in one woman who abused cough medicine (196).

Drugs in Lactation

Since the 1970s, the incidence of women who breast-feed has increased. The subgroup of women where this increase has been most evident and easily documented is among well-educated, white, married, older women of above average income (197). Rates of women who breast-feed vary from 25 to 75% depending on geographic location, employment, socioeconomic status, education, and time from delivery. By the year 2000, the national health objective is to have 75% of women breast-feeding at hospital discharge and 50% at 6 months postpartum. Achieving a high rate of breast-fed infants is especially important in areas where medical care is insufficient, and nutrition and sanitation are poor. Breast-feeding was once commonly replaced with manufactured formulas for various reasons. Although there are specific conditions where formulas are indicated, there is no duplication for human milk. It is specific for humans and provides the total nutritional needs of the growing infant.

Knowing the importance of breast-feeding is basic in the overall management of the patient. Human milk provides several benefits to the infant that cannot be duplicated by other means. Nutrients are balanced and sufficient to the growing infant and are delivered consistently throughout each day as the baby nurses. Healthy infants are ready to suckle at birth. Nurslings are provided with unsurpassed protection against immunologic disorders and infections and protection against diseases, such as those of the gastrointestinal and respiratory system. Comparisons between bottle-fed and breast-fed babies show that the latter have a lower incidence of metabolic disorders, heart disease, obesity, and allergies and that a unique psychological bond between the infant and mother is developed. In addition, nursing enhances the maternal physiologic recovery from childbirth as body weight and hormones return to prepregnant levels (198, 199).

If a nursing woman requires drug therapy, there are numerous interrelated factors to consider so as to ensure that the therapy is rational and safe to both mother and child. Specifically, consideration must be made to the amount of drug excreted into the milk and to the amount of drug ingested by the infant. The pharmacologic handling of the drug by the mother is a primary factor. This is similar to the pregnant woman and involves evaluation of the complete dosage regimen, including drug, dose and route of administration, as well as the mother's ability to absorb, metabolize, and eliminate the drug. A second factor is in regard to the milk produced. Depending on the quantity of milk produced, the amount of drug available for the infant to ingest will also vary. Human milk is primarily made of water but also contains fat, lactose, and protein. The composition of the milk will influence the extent a drug will cross into the milk. The contents of milk varies between individuals and even among the same individual; however, the pH of human milk is generally near 7.0. Thus, a drug will distribute into the milk not only in relation to the water and fat content, but also in relation to the pH. The physicochemical properties of the drug make up a third factor to consider. Distribution of a drug into breast milk primarily occurs by passive diffusion. Other mechanisms such as carrier mediated and active transport, and possibly reabsorption, also play a role. The nature of the drug that is most important for determining transport into the milk is the pKa of the drug. The lipid and water solubility, molecular weight, and extent of protein binding will affect transport across membranes. Large molecules, such as heparin, will not pass into the milk. Ionized drugs and those that are highly bound to plasma proteins, such as warfarin, will not pass either. Acidic drugs do not enter the milk to a significant extent. Finally, the infant is another valuable part of the evaluation process. It is important to determine how much drug the infant consumes. This is influenced not only by the factors already described, but also by the amount of milk ingested by the infant. Nursing times are vital to note. If the baby nurses when the drug has reached peak concentrations in the milk, the amount ingested will be much more than if nursing occurred just before the mother took a dose. The ability of the infant to absorb, metabolize, and eliminate any consumed drug, and the resulting concentration of drug in the infant, should also be considered.

Similar to the literature addressing drugs in pregnancy, the information on drugs in lactation has several limitations. The literature consists primarily of case reports citing individual accounts of drug concentrations measured in breast milk. Many clinicians have documented adverse effects experienced in infants due to drug exposure via breast milk. Animal studies have been conducted, however, so this information is not always applicable to humans. The composition of milk varies between species, as does the pharmacokinetic handling and dosing of drugs. In many human studies, the pharmacokinetic properties of the drug are rarely taken into consideration when milk concentrations are determined. The peak concentration of the drug in breast milk may occur much later in time than that in the plasma. Further, most concentrations are taken after a single dose, and the timing of the levels in relation to the dose or stage of breast-feeding is not stated. Thus, it is difficult to estimate the actual amount of drug accumulated in the milk and ingested by the infant. In addition, studies conducted include very few patients. Drug companies have published little to no data on the distribution of their drug into breast milk and are not required by law to research this topic. Excellent reviews on the use of drugs during lactation have been published (200, 201).

The goals of therapy in a lactating woman are to treat the underlying disorder, avoid drug exposure and adverse effects in the nursing infant, and continue breast-feeding activities. Drug therapy should rarely interrupt breast-feeding. All attempts to avoid drug use in nursing women should be tried. If drug therapy is needed, steps can usually be recommended so that the goals of therapy can be achieved.

First, choose a drug that does not readily cross into breast milk, if possible. A drug rapidly eliminated will also lessen the chance of exposure to the infant. Consider also the safety profile of the agent in the infant. There may be an alternative drug that is safer for newborns. For example, acetaminophen is preferred over aspirin for analgesia because of the possibility of salicylism in the infant. Similarly, alternative drugs may exist for which there is experience using the drug in newborns. The American Academy of Pediatrics Committee on Drugs has identified some, but not all, drugs that they consider to be contraindicated during breast-feeding because of symptoms produced in the infant (202). These drugs are listed in Table 92.4. Drugs that inhibit lactation are also included in this category.

Altering the patient's drug regimen may be another option. Nursing should be avoided when the drug reaches peak concentrations in the milk and plasma. The mother should be instructed to nurse immediately before taking the medication, if at all possible. If the mother takes the medication and feeds frequently, these two activities should be spaced as far as possible from each other. Taking the medication just before the infant takes a long nap or is put to bed at night may be helpful. In certain cases, the mother may need to discontinue breast-feeding for a limited time. She can pump her breasts before beginning drug therapy, and the milk can be stored and administered to the infant during the time the medication is being

Table 92.4.
Drug Effects on Lactation

Drugs That May Suppress Lactation	
Androgens	Bromocriptine
Cloniphene citrate	Thiazide diuretics
Monoamine oxidase inhibitors	Levodopa
Ergot derivatives	High dose pyridoxine

Drugs Contraindicated During Breastfeeding	
Amphetamine	
Bromocriptine	Cocaine
Cyclophosphamide	Cyclosporine
Heroin	Ergotamine
Lithium	Marijuana
Phencyclidine	Methotrexate
Phenindione	Doxorubicin

Adapted from reference 202.

Table 92.5.
Effects of Drugs on Nursing Infants

Drugs Whose Effect on Nursing Infants Is Unknown but May Be of Concern	
Diazepam	Desipramine
Lorazepam	Doxepin
Amitriptyline	Imipramine
Amoxapine	Trazodone
Haloperidol	Chlorpromazine
Chloramphenicol	Chlorprothixene
Metronidazole	Midazolam

Drugs That Have Caused Significant Effects on Some Nursing Infants and Should Be Given to Nursing Mothers with Caution	
Aspirin	Phenobarbital
Sulfasalazine	Clemastine
Primidone	

Adapted from Reference 202.

metabolized and eliminated from the mother's body. Breast-feeding can resume once the drug is cleared. This type of intervention is recommended with metronidazole.

Regardless of interventions taken, nursing infants will need to be closely monitored. The parent(s) should be instructed to monitor for possible adverse effects, such as abnormal growth or sleeping patterns, or restlessness. Sleepiness may commonly be seen when anticonvulsant medications are given to a mother. It may be necessary to monitor milk and serum concentrations.

In summary, breast-feeding provides unsurpassed benefits to both mother and child. If drug therapy is indicated, many interrelated factors influence the extent to which the drug will pass into the milk and be ingested by the infant. These factors include the mother, the milk, the drug, and the infant. Although most drugs will enter the milk to some extent, several interventions can be made to decrease the adverse effects of the drug in the infant and yet not interrupt breast-feeding activities. Several references are available describing the use of medications during lactation. The Academy of Pediatrics has identified some drugs whose effects on nursing infants are unknown but may be of concern and others that should be given to nursing mothers with caution (202). These are presented in Table 92.5.

SUMMARY

Pregnancy is a symptom-producing condition. Pain, heartburn, nausea and vomiting, and constipation are among the possible symptoms that may require treatment. Some women will need drug therapy for chronic diseases that existed before the pregnancy, such as diabetes mellitus or hypertension. What is unique in the pregnant patient is the need to consider the effect of the ingested drug on the developing fetus. Most drugs taken by the mother will reach the fetus to some extent. It is important to assess whether the risk of a congenital defect from drug exposure exceeds the risk of a defect occurring without drug exposure. The estimated baseline rate of infants born with congenital malformations is 3%; the rate may rise to 6% if minor malformations are included. It is difficult to assess with total confidence the exact probability of which a drug may cause damage to the fetus. Information available from the literature is limited due in part to the logistical problems of data capture and analysis associated with this type of research. Anecdotal information composes the majority of the literature. One of the most important key factors to consider while assessing risk to the fetus, is the time during pregnancy of fetal drug exposure. In addition, if a maternal disease is left untreated, it may adversely affect perinatal or even maternal morbidity or mortality. No drug taken during any stage of pregnancy is without risk. The mother must be well informed of the issues surrounding drug therapy in pregnancy so that an educated decision can be made between herself and her physician. This type of communication is also important after a baby is born. Breastfeeding provides unsurpassed nutrition for the infant. Yet, many drugs will distribute into breast milk and be ingested by the nursling. Similar to the pregnant woman, it must be assessed whether or not the mother needs medication. If drug therapy is indicated, then a drug with a low milk to plasma ratio should be chosen. Drugs with a short half-life are also more desirable over long-acting medications. If necessary, the mother may need to schedule taking the drug around the breastfeeding activities. The child should be monitored for any possible adverse effects of ingested medication. Educating and communicating with the mother is vital in ensuring proper care of the mother as well as the baby.

REFERENCES

1. Doering PL, Stewart RB. The extent and character of drug consumption during pregnancy. JAMA 239:843–846, 1978.
2. Rudd CC, Brazy GE. Drugs in the perinatal period: implications for the preterm infant. Pediatr 14(20):30–37, 1988.
3. Buitendijk S, Bracken MB. Medication in early pregnancy: Prevalence of use and relationship to maternal characteristics. Am J Obstet Gynecol 165:33–40, 1991.
4. Collaborative group on drug use in pregnancy. An internatinal survey on drug utilization during pregnancy. International Risk and Safety in Medicine. 1:1, 1991.
5. Bologna-Campeanu M, et al. Prenatal adverse effects of various drugs and chemicals. Med Tox 3:307–323, 1988.
6. Anonymous. Congenital malformations and inherited disorders. In: Cunningham FG, MacDonald PC, Levenok J, Gant NF, Gilstrap LC, eds. Williams Obstetrics. Norwalk: Appleton & Lange, 1993.
7. Bodendorfer TW, Briggs GG, Gunning JE. Obtaining drug exposure histories during pregnancy. Am J Obstet Gynecol 135:490–494, 1979.
8. Bonati M, Bortolus R, Marchetti F, Romero M, Tognoni G. Drug use in pregnancy: an overview of epidemiological (drug utilization) studies. Eur J Clin Pharmacol 38:325–328, 1990.
9. Rubin CP, Craig GF, Gavin K, et al. Prospective survey of use of

therapeutic drugs, alcohol, and cigarettes during pregnancy. Br Med J 292:81–83, 1986.

10. Dicke JM. Teratology: principles and practice. Med Clin North Am 73(3):567–582, 1989.

11. Beckman DA, Brent RL. Mechanisms of teratogenesis. Ann Rev Pharmacol Toxicol 24:483–500, 1984.

12. Kalter H, Warkany J. Congenital malformations, etiological factors and their role in prevention. N Engl J Med 308(8):424–431, 1983.

13. Heinonen OP, Slone D, Shapiro S, eds. Birth defects and drugs in pregnancy. Littleton, Mass.:PSG Publishing Co,Inc., 1977.

14. Werler MM, Pober BR, Nelson K, Holmes LB. Reporting accuracy among mothers of malformed and nonmalformed infants. Am J Epidemiol 129:415–421, 1989.

15. de Jong-Van den Berg ITW, Waardenburg CM, H Aaijer-Ruskamp FM, Dukes MNG, Wesseling H. Drug use in pregnancy: a comparative appraisal of data collecting methods. Eur J Clin Pharmacol 45:9–14, 1993.

16. Wilson JG. Experimental studies on congenital malformations. J Chron Dis 10:111–114, 1959.

17. Hill LM, Kleinberg F. Effects of drugs and chemicals on the fetus and newborn, Part I. Mayo Clin Proc 59:707–716, 1984.

18. Shephard TH. Teratogenicity of therapeutic agents. Curr Probl Pediatr 10(2):3–43, 1979.

19. Scialli AR. Safe medications during pregnancy. Contemp Obstet Gynecol 22:39–65, 1983.

20. Friedman JM, Little BB, Brent RL, Cordero JF, Hanson JW, Shephard TH. Potential human teratogenicity of frequently prescribed drugs. Obstet Gynecol 75:594–599, 1990.

21. Anonymous. Fed Regist 44:37434–37467, 1980.

22. Aase JM. Principles of normal and abnormal embryogenesis. In: Aase JM, ed. Diagnostic dysmorphology. New York: Plenum Medical Book Co., 1990:5.

23. Clarren SK, Smith DW. The fetal alcohol syndrome. N Engl J Med 298(19):1063–1067, 1978.

24. Anonymous. Committee on substance abuse and committee on children with disabilities. Fetal alcohol syndrome and fetal alcohol effects. Pediatr 91(5):1004–1006, 1993.

25. Hill LM, Stern L. Drugs in pregnancy: effects on the fetus and newborn. Drugs 17:182–197, 1979.

26. Coles CA, Smith IE, Fernhoff, PM, Falek A. Neonatal ethanol withdrawal: characteristics in clinically normal, nondysmorphic neonates. J Pediatr 105:445–451, 1984.

27. Streissguth AP, Aase JM, Clarren SK, et al. Fetal alcohol syndrome in adolescents and young adults. JAMA 265:1961–1967, 1991.

28. Steinhaussen HC, Willms J, Spohr H-L. Long-term psychopathological and cognitive outcome of children with fetal alcohol syndrome. J Am Acad Child Adolesc Psychiatry 32(5):990–994, 1993.

29. Mills JL, Graubard BI, Harley EE, Rhoads GG, Berends HW. Maternal alcohol consumption and birth weight: how much drinking in pregnancy is safe? JAMA 252:1875–1879, 1984.

30. Centers for Disease Control. Frequent alcohol consumption among women of childbearing age—behavioral risk factor surveillance system, 1991. MMWR 43(18):328–335, 1994.

31. Streissguth AP, Barr HM, Sampson PD. Moderate prenatal alcohol exposure: effects on child IQ and learning problems at age 7 1/2 years. Alcohol Clin Exp Res 14:662–669, 1990.

32. Barrison IG, Waterson EF, Murray-Lyon IM. Adverse effects of alcohol in pregnancy. Br J Addiction 80:11–25, 1985.

33. Jones KL, Smith DW, Streissguth AP, Myrianthopoulos NC. Outcome in offspring of chronic alcoholic women. Lancet 1:1076–1078, 1974.

34. Jones KL. Smith's Recognizable Patterns of Human Malformations. Philadelphia: WB Saunders, 1988:504.

35. Shaul WL, Hall JG. Multiple congenital anomalies associated with oral anticoagulants. Am J Obstet Gynecol 127:191–198, 1977.

36. Briggs GG, Freeman RK, Yaffe SJ. Drugs in pregnancy and lactation. Baltimore: Williams & Wilkins, 1994:223.

37. Donaldson JO. Neurological complications. In: Burrows GN, Ferris TF, eds. Medical complications during pregnancy. Philadelphia: WB Saunders, 1988:485.

38. Jones KL, op cit, p. 495.

39. Hanson JW. Teratogen update: fetal hydantoin effects. Teratology 33:349–353, 1986.

40. Buehler BA, Delimont D, Van Waes M, Finnel RH. Prenatal prediction of risk of the fetal hydantoin syndrome. N Engl J Med 322(22):1567–1572, 1990.

41. Hanson JW, Buehler BA. Fetal hydantoin syndrome: current status. J Pediatr 101(5):816–818, 1982.

42. Kaneko S, Otani K, Fukushima Y, Ogawa Y, Nomura Y, Ono T, et al. Teratogenicity of antiepileptic drugs: analysis of possible risk factors. Epilepsia 29(4):459–467, 1988.

43. Lindhout D, Hoppener RJ, Meinardi H. Teratogenicity of antiepileptic drug combinations with special emphasis on epoxication. Epilepsia 25(1):77–83, 1984.

44. Van Dyke DC, Berg M, Olson CH. Differences in phenytoin biotransformation and susceptibility to congenital malformations: a review. DICP Annals Pharmacotherapy 25:987–992, 1991.

45. Rosenberg L, Mitchell AA, Shapiro S, Slone D. Selected birth defects in relation to caffeine-containing beverages. JAMA 247:1429–1432, 1982.

46. Linn S, Schoenbaum SC, Monson RR, Rosner B, Stubblefield PG, Ryan KJ. No association between coffee consumption and adverse outcomes of pregnancy. N Engl J Med 306:141–145, 1982.

47. Kuzma JW, Sokol RJ. Maternal drinking behaviour and decreased intrauterine growth. Alcohol Clin Exp Res 6:396–402, 1982.

48. Martin TR, Bracken MB. The association between low birth weight and caffeine consumption during pregnancy. Am J Epidemiol 126:813–821, 1987.

49. Munoz L, Lonnerdal B, Keen CL, Dewey KG. Coffee consumption as a factor in iron deficiency anemia among pregnant women and their infants in Costa Rica. Am J Clin Nutr 48:645–651, 1988.

50. Barr HM, Streissguth AP. Caffeine use during pregnancy and child outcome: a 7-year prospective study. Neurotoxicol Teratol 13(4):441–448, 1991.

51. Olsen J. Cigarette smoking, tea and coffee drinking, and subfecundity. Am J Epidemiol 133:734–739, 1991.

52. Hadeed A, Siegel S. Newborn cardiac arrhythmias associated with maternal caffeine use during pregnancy. Clin Pediatr 32:45–47, 1993.

53. Devoe LD, Murray C, Youssif A, Arnaud M. Maternal caffeine consumption and fetal behaviour in normal third-trimester pregnancy. Am J Obstet Gynecol 168:1105–1112, 1993.

54. Watkinson B, Fried PA. Maternal caffeine use before, during, and after pregnancy and effects upon offspring. Neurobehav Toxicol Teratol 7:9–17, 1985.

55. Leviton A. Caffeine consumption and the risk of reproductive hazards. J Reprod Med 33:175–178, 1988.

56. Berger A. Effects of caffeine consumption on pregnancy outcome: a review. J Reprod Med 33:945–956, 1988.

57. Mills JL, Holmes LB, Asrons JH, et al. Moderate caffeine use and the risk of spontaneous abortion and intrauterine growth retardation. JAMA 269:593–597, 1993.

58. Soyka LF. Caffeine ingestion during pregnancy: in utero exposure and possible effects. Semin Perinatol 5:305–309, 1981.

59. Hogue CJ. Coffee in pregnancy. Lancet 2:554, 1981.

60. Srisuphan W, Bracken MB. Caffeine consumption during pregnancy and association with late spontaneous abortion. Am J Obstet Gynecol 154:14–20, 1986.

61. Kuzma JW, Sokol RJ. Maternal drinking behaviour and decreased intrauterine growth. Alcohol Clin Exp Res 6:396–402, 1982.

62. Martin TR, Bracken MB. The association between low birth weight and caffeine consumption during pregnancy. Am J Epidemiol 126:813–821, 1987.

63. Munoz L, Lonnerdal B, Keen CL, Dewey KG. Coffee consumption as a factor in iron deficiency anemia among pregnant women and their infants in Costa Rica. Am J Clin Nutr 48:645–651, 1988.

64. Fenster L, Eskenazi B, Windham GC, Swan SH. Caffeine consumption during pregnancy and fetal growth. Am J Public Health 81:458–461, 1991.

65. Caan BJ, Goldhaber MK. Caffeinated beverages and low birth-weight: a case control study. Am J Public Health. 79:1299–1300, 1989.

66. Brooke OG, Anderson HR, Bland JM, Peacock JL, Stewart CM. Effects on birthweight on smoking, alcohol, caffeine, socioeconomic factors and psychosocial stress. Br Med J 298:795–801, 1989.

67. Beaulac-Baillargeon L, Desrosiers C. Caffeine-cigarette interaction on fetal growth. Am J Obstet Gynecol 157:1236–1240, 1987.

68. Wilcox A, Weinberg C, Baird D. Caffeinated beverages and decreased fertility. Lancet 2:1453–1456, 1988.

69. Christianson RE, Oechsli FW, van den Berg BJ. Caffeinated beverages and decreased fertility. Lancet 1:378, 1989.

70. Williams MA, Monson RR, Goldman MB, Mettendorg R, Ryan KJ. Coffee and delayed conception. Lancet 1:1603, 1990.

71. Joesoef MR, Beral V, Rolfs RT, Aral SO, Cramer DW. Are caffeinated beverages risk factors for delayed conception? Lancet 1:136–137, 1990.

72. Centers for Disease Control. Cigarette smoking among women of reproductive age—United States, 1987–1992. MMWR 43(43):789–797, 1994.

73. Hill LM, Kleinberg F. Effects of drugs and chemicals in the fetus and newborn, Part II. Mayo Clin Proc 59:755–765, 1984.

74. Olsen J, Pereira A, Olsen SF. Does material tobacco smoking modify the effect of alcohol on fetal growth? Am J Public Health 181:69–73, 1991.

75. Berkowitz GS. Smoking and pregnancy. In: Niebyl JR, ed. Drug use in pregnancy. Philadelphia: Lea & Febiger, 1988:173–191.

76. Centers for Disease Control. The Surgeon General's 1990 Report on The Health Benefits of Smoking Cessation (Executive Summary). MMWR 39:RR12, 1990.

77. Walters WAW. The management of nausea and vomiting during pregnancy. Med J Aust 147:290–291, 1987.

78. Baron TH, Ramirez B, Richter JE. Gastrointestinal motility disorders during pregnancy. Ann Int Med 118:366–375, 1993.

79. Vellacott ID, Cooke EJA, James CE. Nausea and vomiting in early pregnancy. Int J Gynecol Obstet 27:57–62, 1988.

80. DiIorio C. The management of nausea and vomiting in pregnancy. Nurs Pract 13(5):23–28, 1988.

81. Gadsby R, Barnie-Adshead AM, Jagger C. A prospective study of nausea and vomiting during pregnancy. Bt J Gen Prac 43:245–248, 1993.

82. O'Brian B, Naber S. Nausea and vomiting during pregnancy: effects on the quality of women's lives. Birth 19(3):138–143, 1992.

83. Niebyl JR, Maxwell KD. Treatment of nausea and vomiting of pregnancy. In: Niebyl JR, ed. Drug use in pregnancy. Philadelphia: Lea & Febiger, 1988:11–19.

84. Dundee JW, Sourial FBR, Ghaly RG, Bell PF. P6 acupressure reduces morning sickness. J R Soc Med 81:456–457, 1988.

85. Kousen M. Treatment of nausea and vomiting in pregnancy. Am Fam Physc 48(7):1279–1283, 1993.

86. Milkovich L, Van den Berg BJ. An evaluation of the teratogenicity of certain antinauseant drugs. Am J Obstet Gynecol 125:244–248, 1976.

87. Leathem AM. Safety and efficacy of antiemetics used to treat nausea and vomiting in pregnancy. Clin Pharm 5:660–668, 1986.

88. Greenberg G, Inman WH, Weatherall JA, et al. Maternal drug histories and congenital abnormalities. Br Med J 2:853–856, 1977.

89. Slone D, Siskind V, Heinonen OP, Monson RR, Kaufman DW, Shapiro S. Antenatal exposure to the phenothiazines in relation to congenital malformations, perinatal mortality rate, birth weight, and intelligence quotient score. Am J Obstet Gynecol 128(5):486–488, 1977.

90. Nelson MM, Forfar JO. Associations between drugs administered during pregnancy and congenital abnormalities of the fetus. Br Med J 1:523–527, 1971.

91. Rumeau-Rouquette C, Goujard J, Huel G. Possible teratogenic effect of phenothiazines in human beings. Teratology 15:57–64, 1977.

92. Beeley L. Adverse effects of drugs in the first trimester of pregnancy. Clin Obstet Gynaecol 8:261–274, 1981.

93. Briggs GG, et al., op cit, p. 309.

94. World MJ. Ondansetron and hyperemesis gravidarum. Lancet 341:185, 1993.

95. Guikontes E, Spantideas A, Diakakis J. Ondansetron and hyperemesis gravidarum. Lancet 340:1223, 1992.

96. Weinstein BB, Wohl Z, Mitchell GJ, Sustendal GF. Oral administration of pyridoxine hydrochloride in the treatment of nausea and vomiting of pregnancy. Am J Obstet Gynecol 47:389–394, 1944.

97. Sahakian V, Rouse D, Sipes S, Rose N, Niebyl J. Vitamin B6 is effective therapy for nausea and vomiting of pregnancy: a randomized, double-blind placebo-controlled study. Obstet Gynecol 78:33–36, 1991.

98. Perlow JH, Montgomery D, Morgan MA, Towers CV, Porto M. Severity of asthma and perinatal outcome. Am J Obstet Gynecol 167:963–967, 1992.

99. Clark SL. Asthma in pregnancy. Obstet Gynecol 82:1036–1040, 1993.

100. Weinberger SE, Weiss ST. Pulmonary disease. In: Burrow GN, Ferris TF. Medical complications during pregnancy. Philadelphia: WB Saunders, 1988:448.

101. D'Alonzo GE. The pregnant asthmatic patient. Semin Perinatol 14(2):119–129, 1990.

102. Schwartz DB. Medical disorders in pregnancy. Emerg Med Clin North Am 5(3):509–528, 1987.

103. DiMarco AF. Asthma in the pregnancy patient: a review. Ann Allergy 62(6):527–533, 1989.

104. Noble PW, Lavee AE, Jacobs MM. Respiratory disease in pregnancy. Obstet Gynecol Clin North Am 15(2):391–423, 1988.

105. Steinius-Aarniala B, Piirila P, Teramo K. Asthma and pregnancy: perspective study of 198 pregnancies. Thorax 43:12–18, 1988.

106. Schatz M, Zeiger RS, Harden KM, Hoffman CP, Forsythe AB, Chilinger LM, et al. The safety of inhaled B-agonist bronchodilators during pregnancy. J Allergy Clin Immunol 82:686–695, 1988.

107. Romero R, Lockwood C. The use of anti-asthmatic drugs in pregnancy. In: Niebyl JR, ed. Drug use in pregnancy. Philadelphia: Lea & Febiger, 1988:67–82.

108. Huff RW. Asthma in pregnancy. Med Clin North Am 73(3):653–659, 1989.

109. Greenberger PA, Patterson R. Management of asthma during pregnancy. N Engl J Med 312(14):897–902, 1985.

110. Briggs GG, et al. op cit, p 18.

111. Arwood LL, Dasta JF, Freidman C. Placental transfer of theophylline: two case reports. Pediatrics 63:844–846, 1979.

112. Yeh TF, Pildes RS. Transplancental aminophylline toxicity in a neonate. Lancet 1:910, 1977.

113. Gardner MJ, Schatz M, Cousins L, et al: Longitudinal effects of pregnancy on the pharmacokinetics of theophylline Eur J Clin Pharmacol 31:289–295, 1987.

114. Carter BL, Discoll EC, Smith GD. Theophylline clearance during pregnancy. Obstet Gynecol 68:555–559, 1986.

115. Kraus AM. Congenital cataract and maternal steroid injection. J Pediatr Opthalmol 12:107–108, 1975.

116. Cote CJ, Meuwissen HJ, Pickering RJ. Effects of the neonate of prednisone and azathioprine administered to the mother during pregnancy. J Pediatr 85:324–328, 1974.

117. Greenberger PA, Patterson R. Beclomethasone dipropionate for severe asthma during pregnancy. Ann Intern Med 98:478–480, 1983.

118. Wilson J. Use of sodium cromoglycate during pregnancy: results on 296 asthmatic women. Acta Therap 8(Suppl):45–51, 1982.

119. Goldberg CA, Schrier RW. Hypertension and pregnancy. Seminars in Nephrology 11(5):576–593, 1991.

120. Remuzzi G, Ruggenenti P. Prevention and treatment of pregnancy-associated hypertension: What have we learned in the last 10 years? Am J Kidney Diseases 18(3):285–305, 1991.

121. Drayer JI, Zegarelli EC: Hypertension and pregnancy. Cardiovascular Clinics 19(3):97–111, 1989.

122. Schoenfeld A, Segal J, Freidman S, Hirsch M, Oradia J. Adverse reactions to antihypertensive drugs in pregnancy. Obstet Gynecol Surv 41(2):67–73, 1986.

123. Doany W, Brinkman CR III. Antihypertension drugs in pregnancy. Clin Perinatol 14(4):783–805, 1987.

124. Liauw PCY. The management of hypertension in pregnancy. Sing Med J 30:590–596, 1989.

125. Ferris TF. Pregnancy complicated by hypertension and renal disease. Adv Intern Ed 35:269–288, 1990.

126. Probst BD. Hypertensive disorders of pregnancy. Emerg Med Clin North Am 12(1):73–89, 1994.

127. Lindheimer MD, Cunningham G. Hypertension and pregnancy: Impact of the working group report. Am J Kidney Diseases 21(5) Supp 2:29–36, 1993.

128. National High Blood Pressure Education Working Group: Report on High Blood Pressure in Pregnancy. Am J Obstet Gynecol 163:1689–1712, 1990.

129. Naden RP, Redman CW. Antihypertensive drugs in pregnancy. Clin Perinatol 12(3):521–538, 1985.

130. Repke JT. Pharmacologic management of hypertension in pregnancy. In: Niebyl JR, ed. Drug use in pregnancy. Philadelphia: Lea & Febiger, 1988:55–65.

131. Cunningham FG, Gant NF. Prevention of preeclampsia—a reality? N Engl J Med 321:606–607, 1989.

132. Widerlov E, Karlman I, Storsater J. Hydralazine-induced neonatal thrombocytopenia. N Engl J Med 303:1235, 1980.

133. Henrich WL, Cronin R, Miller PD, Anderson RJ. Hypotensive sequelae of diazoxide and hydralazine therapy. JAMA 237: 264–265, 1977.

134. Riley AJ. Clinical pharmacology of labetolol in pregnancy. J Cardiovasc Pharmacol 3(suppl 1):S3–S9, 1981.

135. Horvath JS, Phippard A, Korda A. Clonidine hydrochloride—a safe and effective antihypertensive agent in pregnancy. Obstet Gynecol 66:634–638, 1985.

136. Redmond GP. Propranolol and fetal growth retardation. Semin Perinatol 6:142–147, 1982.

137. Sandstrom B. Antihypertensive treatment with the adrenergic B-receptor blocker metoprolol during pregnancy. Gynecol Invest 9:195–204, 1978.

138. Dubois D, Peticolas J, Temperville B, Klepper A. Treatment with atenolol of hypertension in pregnancy. Drugs 25(Suppl 2): 215–218, 1983.

139. Rubin PC, Butters L, Clark DM, Reynolds B, Sumner DJ, Steedman D, et al. Placebo-controlled trial of atenolol in treatment of pregnancy-associated hypertension. Lancet 1:431–434, 1983.

140. Reynolds B, Butters L, Evans J, Adams T, Rubin PC. First year of life after the use of atenolol in pregnancy associated hypertension. Arch Dis Child 59:1061–1063, 1984.

141. Sibai BM, Gonzalez AR, Mabie WC, Moretti M. A comparison of labetalol plus hospitalization versus hospitalization alone in the management of preeclampsia remote from term. Obstet Gynecol 70:323–327, 1987.

142. Frishman WH, Chesner M. Beta-adrenergic blockers in pregnancy. Am Heart J 115:147–152, 1988.

143. Pickles CJ, Symonds Em, Broughton Pipkin F. The fetal outcome in a randomized trial of labetalol versus placebo in pregnancy-induced hypertension. Br J Obstet Gynecol 96:38–43, 1989.

144. Lindow SW, Davies N, Davey DA, Smith JA. The effect of sublingual nifedipine on uteroplacental blood flow in hypertensive pregnancy. Br J Obstet Gynaecol 95:1276–1281, 1988.

145. Walters BNJ, Redman CWG. Treatment of severe pregnancy-associated hypertension with the calcium antagonist nifedipine. Br J Obstet Gynaecol 91:330–336, 1984.

146. Constantine G, Beevers DG, Reynolds AL, Luesley DM. Nifedipine as a second line antihypertensive drug in pregnancy. Br J Obstet Gynaecol 94;1136–1142, 1987.

147. Snyder SW, Cardwell MS. Neuromuscular blockade with magnesium sulfate and nifedipine. Am J Obstet Gynecol 161:35–36, 1989.

148. Waisman GD, Mayorga LM, Camera MI, Vignolo CA, Martinotti A. Magnesium plus nifedipine potentiation of hypotensive effect in preeclampsia? Am J Obstet Gynecol 159:308–309, 1988.

149. Rubin PC. Treatment of hypertension in pregnancy. Clinics in Obstetrics and Gynaecology 13:307–317, 1986.

150. Piper JM, Ray WA, Rosa FW. Pregnancy outcome following exposure to angiotensin-converting enzyme inhibitors. Obstet Gynecol 80:429–432, 1992.

151. Brent RL, Beckman DA. Angiotensin-converting enzyme inhibitors, an embryopathic class of drugs with unique properties: information for clinical teratology counselors. Teratology 43:543–546, 1991.

152. Barr M, Cohen MM. ACE inhibitor fetopathy and hypocalvaria: the kidney-skull connection. Teratology 44:485–495, 1991.

153. Christianson R, Page EW. Diuretic drugs and pregnancy. Obstet Gynecol 48:647–652, 1976.

154. Feinberg LE. Hypertension and preeclampsia. In: Abrams RS, Wexler P, eds. Medical care of the pregnant patient. Boston: Little, Brown, 1983:161–182.

155. Scialli AR. Anticonvulsants in pregnancy. In: Niebyl JR, ed. Drug use in pregnancy. Phildelphia: Lea & Febiger, 1988:45–54.

156. Anonymous. Anticonvulsant and pregnancy. American Academy of Pediatrics Committee on Drugs. Pediatrics 63:331–333, 1979.

157. Patterson RM. Seizure disorders in pregnancy. Med Clin North Am 73(3):661–665, 1989.

158. Nelson KB, Ellenberg JH. Maternal seizure disorder, outcome of pregnancy, and neurologic abnormalities in the children. Neurology 32(11):1247–1254, 1982.

159. Hanson JW, Buehler BA. Fetal hydantoin syndrome: current status. J Pediatr 101:816–818, 1982.

160. Janz D. On major malformations and minor anomalies in the offspring of parents with epilepsy: review of the literature. In: Janz D, Dam M, Richens A, Bossi L, Helge H, Schmidt D, eds. Epilepsy, pregnancy and the child. New York: Raven Press, 211–222, 1982.

161. Philbert A, Dam M. The epileptic mother and her child. Epilepsia 23(1):85–99, 1982.

162. Schmidt D, Canger R, Avanzini G, Battino D, Cusi C, Beck-Mannagetta G, Koch S, Rating D, Janz D. Change of seizure frequency in pregnancy epileptic women. J Neurol Neurosurg Psychiatry 46:751–755, 1983.

163. Treiman DM. Current treatment strategies in selected situations in epilepsy. Epilepsia 34(S5):S17–S23, 1993.

164. Lindhout D, Omtzigt JGC. Pregnancy and the risk of teratogenicity. Epilepsia 33(S4):S41–S48, 1992.

165. Delgado-Escueta AV, Janz D. Consensus guidelines: preconception counseling, management, and care of the pregnant woman with epilepsy. Neurology 42(S5):149–160, 1992.

166. Waters CH, Belai Y, Gott PS, Shen P, DeGiorgio CM. Outcomes of pregnancy associated with antiepileptic drugs. Arch Neurol 51:250–253, 1994.

167. Lane PA, Hathaway WE. Vitamin K in infancy. J Pediatr 106:351–359, 1985.

168. Hanson JW. Teratogen update: fetal hydantoin effects. Teratology 33(3):349–353, 1986.

169. Janz D. Antiepileptic drugs and pregnancy: altered utilization patterns and teratogenesis. Epilepsia 23:S53–S63, 1982.

170. Jones KL, Lacro RV, Johnson KA, Adams J. Pattern of malformations in the children of women treated with carbamazepine during pregnancy. N Engl J Med 320:1661–1666, 1989.

171. Roza FW. Spina bifida in infants of women treated with carbamazepine during pregnancy. NEJM 324(10):674–675, 1991.

172. Reece EA, Hobbins JC. Diabetic embryopathy: Pathogenesis, prenatal diagnosis, and prevention. Obstet Gynecol Surv 41(6):325–335, 1986.

173. Anonymous. Endocrine disorder. In: Williams Obstetrics. Cunningham FG, MacDonald PC, Leveno KJ, Gant NF, Gilstrap LC eds. Norwalk, Connecticut: Appleton & Lange, 1993:1207.

174. Greene MF, Hare JW, Cloherty JP, Benacerraf Br, Soeldner JS. First-trimester hemoglobin A1 and risk for major malformation and spontaneous abortion in diabetic pregnancy. Teratology 39:225–331, 1989.

175. Mills JL, Knopp RH, Simpson JL, et al. Lack of relation of increased malformation rates in infants of diabetic mothers to glycemic control during organogenesis. N Engl J Med 318(11):671–676, 1988.

176. Gabbe SG. A story of two miracles: The impact of the discovery of insulin on pregnancy in women with diabetes mellitus. Obstet Gynecol 79(2):295–299, 1992.

177. Rizzo T, Metzger BE, Burns WJ, Burns K. Correlations between antepartum maternal metabolism and child intelligence. N Engl J Med 325(13):911–916, 1991.

178. Cousins L. Pregnancy complications among diabetic women:Review 1965–1985. Obstet Gynecol Surv 42(3):140–149, 1987.

179. Hare JW, White P. Gestational diabetes and the White classification. Diabetes Care 3:394–398, 1980.

180. Schneider JM, Curet LB, Olson RW, Shay G. Ambulatory care of the pregnant diabetic. Obstet Gynecol 56:144–149, 1980.

181. Bourgeois FJ, Duffer J. Outpatient obstetric management of women with type I diabetes. Am J Obstet Gynecol 163:1065–1072, 1990.

182. Coustan DR, Felig P. Diabetes mellitus. In: Burrow GN, Ferris TF, eds. Medical complications during pregnancy. Philadelphia: W.B. Saunders, 1988:34–64.

183. Goldberg E. Anticoagulants in pregnancy. In: Niebyl, JR, ed. Drug use in pregnancy. Philadelphia: Lea & Febiger, 1988:83–88.

184. Rutherford SE, Phelan JP. Clinical Management of thromboembolic disorders in pregnancy. Critical Care Clinics 7(4):809–828, 1991.

185. Hall JG, Pauli RM, Wilson KM. Maternal and fetal sequelae of anticoagulation during pregnancy. Am J Med 68:122–140, 1980.

186. Nageotte MP, Freeman RK, Garite TJ, Block RA. Anticoagulation in pregnancy. Am J Obstet Gynecol 141:472–473, 1981.

187. Flessa HC, Kapstrom AB, Glueck HI, Will JJ, Miller MA, Brinker B. Placental transport of heparin. Am J Obstet Gyenecol 93:570–573, 1965.

188. Ginsberg JS, Kowalchuk G, Hirsh J, Brill-Edwards P, Burrows R. Heparin therapy during pregnancy: risks to the fetus and mother. Arch Intern Med 149:2233–2236, 1989.

189. Ginsberg JS, Hirsh J, Turner C, et al. Risks to the fetus of anticoagulant therapy during pregnancy. Thromb Haemost 61:197:1989.

190. Greaves M. Anticoagulation in pregnancy. PharmaTher 59:311–327, 1993.

191. Baron TH, Ramirez B, Richter JE. Gastrointestinal motility disorders during pregnancy. Ann Int Med 118:366–375, 1993.

192. Key TC. Gastrointestinal diseases. In: Creasy RK, Resnik R, eds. Maternal-fetal medicine: principles and practice. Philadelphia: WB Saunders 1989:1032–1046.

193. Parry E, Shields R, Turnbull AC. The effect of pregnancy on colonic absorption of sodium, potassium and water. Br J Obstet Gynecol 77:616–620, 1970.

194. West L, Warren J, Cutis T. Diagnosis and management of irritable bowel syndrome, constipation, and diarrhea in pregnancy. Gastrointestinal Clin N Am 21(4):793–802, 1992.

195. Zierler S, Purohit D. Prenatal antihistamine exposure and tretrolental fibroplasia. Am J Epidemiol 123:192–196, 1986.

196. Chasnoff IJ, Diggs G, Schnoll SH. Fetal alcohol effects and maternal cough syrup abuse. Am J Dis Child 135:968–974, 1981.

197. MacGowan RJ, MacGowan CA, Serdula MK, Lane M, Joesoef RM, Cook FH. Breast-feeding among women attending women, infants, and children clinics in Georgia, 1987. Pediatr 87(3):361–366, 1991.

198. Lawrence RA. Breastfeeding and medical disease. Med Clin North Am 73(3):583–603, 1989.

199. Berlin CM, Jr. Drugs and chemicals: exposure of the nursing mother. Pediatr Clin North Am 36(5):1089–1097, 1989.

200. Anderson PO. Drug use during breast-feeding. Clin Pharm 10:594–624, 1991.

201. Atkinson HC, Begg EJ, Darlow BA. Drugs in human milk: clinical pharmacokinetic considerations. Clin Pharmacokinet 14:217–240, 1988.

202. Anonymous. Transfer of drugs and other chemicals into human milk. American Academy of Pediatrics. Pediatrics 93(1):137–158, 1994.

CHAPTER 93

ALZHEIMER'S DISEASE

DARLENE FUJIMOTO and SAM K. SHIMOMURA

The most common cause of dementia is a primary cerebral disorder called Alzheimer's disease or primary degenerative dementia of the Alzheimer's type, which was first described in 1907 by a neuropsychiatrist, Alois Alzheimer. Alzheimer's disease is recognized as a syndrome of clinical features characterized by a decline of memory and other cognitive functions in comparison with the patient's previous level of function (1). Alzheimer's disease has an insidious onset, is progressive, and is differentiated by the exclusion of other diseases that would account for the cognitive deterioration and personality changes. Disturbances in memory are the hallmark of this disease, but other cognitive areas such as language use, visual-spatial perception, and the ability to learn, solve problems, perform mathematical calculations, think abstractly, and make judgments are also affected (2).

EPIDEMIOLOGY

Alzheimer's disease is responsible for about 55% of the total cases of dementia and afflicts approximately 4 million people in the United States. The prevalence of dementia doubles every 5 years from age 60 to age 90. A community-based study of elderly people found that 10.3% of the population over age 65 has Alzheimer's disease. This study showed a high prevalence of Alzheimer's disease which increases with age: For those 65 to 74 years of age, the rate is 3.0%; for those 75 to 84 years of age it is 18.7%; and among those over 85 years of age it is 47.2% (3). It is estimated that over 50% of nursing home patients have dementia. More than 100,000 people die of Alzheimer's disease each year, making it the fourth most prevalent cause of death in adults, after heart disease, cancer, and stroke (4).

ETIOLOGY

Although the dementia syndrome may be caused by over 60 disorders, most cases are due to Alzheimer's disease, followed by multiinfarct dementia or a combination of the two. Other important causes of dementia include infections, other neurodegenerative disorders, toxins, and metabolic disorders (Table 93.1). The cause of up to 5% of cases of dementia remains unknown. The putative risk factors for Alzheimer's dementia include advancing age, a history of (a) serious head trauma, (b) hypothyroidism, (c) dementia in a first-degree relative, and (d) Down syndrome in a first-degree relative. Approximately one-third of Alzheimer's patients appear to have a genetic link (5).

Alzheimer's disease is correlated with diminished neuron function and a decrease in neurotransmitters. The major biochemical abnormality that is observed in Alzheimer's disease is a 40 to 90% decrease in the enzyme choline acetyltransferase in the cerebral cortex and hippocampus. The deficiency of this enzyme causes decreased synthesis of acetylcholine in the brain. The loss of acetyltransferase in the brain appears to begin within the first year of onset of the symptoms of dementia, and there seems to be a strong correlation between the degree of enzyme reduction and the decline of mental status scores.

Although acetylcholine is the primary neurotransmitter deficit associated with Alzheimer's disease, other neurotransmitters have been implicated. For example, somatostatin is often deficient in patients with Alzheimer's disease, as is the number of somatostatin receptors. There is also a study that reports a decrease in corticotropin-releasing factors (6). Variable losses in the amount of norepinephrine and the biosynthetic enzyme dopamine β-hydroxylase and decreased numbers of serotonin cells have occurred and may account for noncognitive symptoms of depression and aggression, but no consistent correlations have been shown with Alzheimer's disease.

PATHOGENESIS

From brain autopsy studies, Alzheimer's disease patients have been found to have cortical atrophy, a significant loss of neurons, an increase in neuritic plaques, and a high density of neurofibrillary tangles (Figure 93.1). Neurofibrillary tangles are abnormal neurons containing bundles of filamentous structures in the cytoplasm. These filaments are wound around each other in a helical fashion. Neuritic plaques are small spheres with an amyloid protein core surrounded by degenerating nerve terminals. Two amyloid proteins, β-amyloid protein and paired helical filament protein, are present in those hallmark lesions and may be linked to the cause of Alzheimer's disease (7). The neurofibrillary tangle consists of a ropelike filament and has a pleated-sheet formation. Certain abnormally phosphor-

Table 93.1.
Causes of Dementia Syndrome[a]

Psychiatric disorders	Metabolic diseases	Intracranial conditions
Depression	Renal failure	Hydrocephalus
Delirium	Fluid and electrolyte imbalances	Brain tumor
Paranoid states	Hypoglycemia	Multiinfarct dementia (stroke)
Schizophrenia	Hyperglycemia	Degenerative neurological disorders
Trauma	Hypothyroidism	Alzheimer's disease
Subdural hematoma	Hyperthyroidism	Pick's disease
Dementia pugilistica	Hepatic failure	Huntington's chorea
Drugs and toxins	Addison's disease	Parkinson's disease
Antidepressants	Cushing's syndrome	Cardiovascular
Lithium carbonate	Hypopituitarism	Congestive heart failure
Anticholinergics	Severe anemia	Arrhythmia
Alcohol	Hypoxia and anoxia	Vascular occlusion
Benzodiazepines	Infections	Nutritional disorders
Barbiturates	AIDS	Vitamin B_{12} deficiency
Propranolol	Neurosyphilis	Folate deficiency
Methyldopa	Meningitis	Collagen vascular disorders
Reserpine	Tuberculosis	Systemic lupus erythematosus
Heavy metal poisoning	Pneumonia	Temporal arteritis
Organophosphates	Creutzfeldt-Jakob (slow-virus) dementia	

[a]Table represents a partial list.

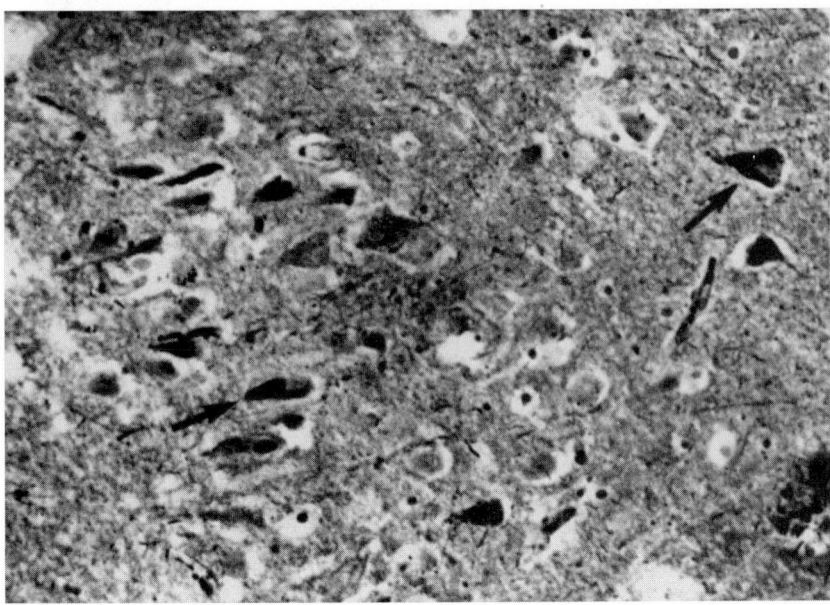

Figure 93.1. Neurofibrillary degeneration (arrows) within Sommer's sector of the hippocampus. Bielschowsky silver impregnation, ×360.

ylated proteins are components of the paired helical filaments, especially tau proteins. These abnormal proteins may interfere with nerve cell functioning. In autopsy studies, the degree of plaque formation has been highly correlated with the degree of clinical impairment observed when the patient was alive.

β-amyloid protein, an insoluble protein deposit, is an abnormal fragment from amyloid precursor protein (APP). APP overproduction may contribute to the buildup of β-amyloid. Mutations of the APP gene on chromosomes 21 and 14 have been linked to familial Alzheimer's disease (8).

Current research has shown a possible role for apolipoprotein E (ApoE) in the pathogenesis of Alzheimer's disease. It is a protein that binds to the β-amyloid that is present in neuritic plaques and tangles. The gene for ApoE is on chromosome 19, and the presence of ApoE4 allele has been identified. Because it makes amyloid deposition in plaques more likely, it is considered a risk factor for developing late onset Alzheimer's disease (9). The identification of ApoE4 allele may eventually be used as a diagnostic aid or may be used for presymptomatic testing for Alzheimer's disease.

SIGNS AND SYMPTOMS

To clarify discussions of the disease, the progression of Alzheimer's disease is divided into three stages. These stages are not clear-cut; symptoms may overlap, and there is an individual progression of symptoms. The first stage, or mild Alzheimer's disease, is characterized by signs of minimal memory impairment, especially in recall of recent events. The onset of symptoms is often overlooked or dismissed as a natural progression of aging. The loss of choline acetyltransferase begins within the first year of the onset of symptoms in these patients (10). Patients may express concern about forgetfulness but do not display a clear memory deficit during clinical interview. There may be some disorientation, impaired concentration, anxiety, and depression, all of which are fairly nonspecific symptoms. Judgment is relatively intact, and the person maintains the capacity for independent living.

In the second stage, or moderate Alzheimer's disease, memory impairment progresses, and deficits of the early stage become more pronounced. There is decreased performance in demanding employment or social situations; co-workers notice decreased performance at work. Friends, family, and co-workers may become aware of deficits before the patient does. Blunting of emotions and apathy are common. Judgment and the capacity for abstract thinking and calculation begin to wane or are lost. Patients have difficulty finding words and names. The prevalence of agitation, which can be aggressive/nonaggressive, physical or verbal, can increase with disease progression. Psychotic symptoms such as hallucinations, delusions, and paranoia may become more prevalent toward the end of this stage. Patients often become disoriented, lost, or wander, and independent living becomes hazardous.

In the final stage, or severe Alzheimer's disease, there is a disturbance of practically all intellectual function. Patients are disoriented and incapacitated. Activities of daily living are so impaired that independent living is hazardous or impossible. There are marked neurologic deficits and often increased muscle tone and akinesia, resulting in a slow, unsteady gait. There is emotional disinhibition, which may magnify problems of anxiety and agitation, with a loss of former personality traits. Patients often cannot recognize relatives or remember their own names. They eventually become bedfast, become incontinent of bowel and bladder, and suffer progressive wasting of functions. Death is usually the result of pneumonia or other infections.

DIAGNOSIS AND CLINICAL FINDINGS

The National Institute of Neurological and Communicative Disorders and Stroke and the Alzheimer's Disease and Related Disorders Association (now known as the Alzheimer's Association) established a group to refine the

Table 93.2.
DSM-IV Diagnostic Criteria for Dementia of the Alzheimer's Type

Dementia
A. The development of multiple cognitive deficits manifested by both
   1. memory impairment (impaired in the abiity to learn new information or forget previously learned information) and
   2. at least one of the follow cognitive disturbances:
      a. aphasia (language disturbance),
      b. apraxia (impaired ability to carry out motor activities),
      c. agnosia (failure to recognize or identify objects),
      d. disturbance in executive functioning (i.e., planning, organizing, sequencing).
B. The cognitive deficits cause significant impairment in social or occupational functioning and represent a significant decline from a previous level of functioning.
C. The course is characterized by gradual onset and involves continuing cognitive decline.
D. The cognitive deficits are not due to any of the following:
   1. other central nervous system conditions that cause progressive deficits in memory and cognition (cerebrovascular disease, Parkinson's disease, Huntington's disease, subdural hematoma, normal-pressure hydrocephalus, brain tumor),
   2. systemic/medical conditions that are known to cause dementia (e.g., HIV infection, hypothyroidism, vitamin B_{12} deficiency, neurosyphilis [see Table 93.2]),
   3. substance-induced conditions.
E. The deficits do not occur exclusively during the course of a delirium.
F. The disturbance is not better accounted for by another Axis I disorder (e.g., major depressive disorder).

Source: Adapted from the Diagnostic and Statistical Manual of Mental Disorders IV. Washington, DC: American Psychiatric Association, 1994.

diagnosis of Alzheimer's disease in 1984. (11). The work group's criteria are compatible with the American Psychiatric Association's *Diagnostic and Statistical Manual of Mental Disorders IV* (Table 93.2). The NINCDS/ADRDA Criteria for Clinical Diagnosis of Alzheimer's disease (Table 93.3) are used as a standard for clinical and research diagnosis. With these criteria the accuracy rate for diagnosis has increased from less than 50% to at least 90%.

There is a definite need to accurately identify any treatable or reversible causes of dementia. A thorough history and an extensive battery of tests should be performed, not to diagnose Alzheimer's disease but to identify or eliminate other causes (Table 93.4). Diagnostic errors are often made because of the failure to recognize depression or pseudodementia as a cause of memory loss and other symptoms associated with Alzheimer's disease. Depression is a potentially treatable illness that must be distinguished from Alzheimer's disease. Mental status examinations and neuropsychological testing are important in the clinical identification of depression versus dementia.

From onset of symptoms the life span of a patient with Alzheimer's disease ranges from 2 to over 20 years. The average life span after onset is about 8 to 10 years.

Table 93.3.
NINCDS/ADRDA Criteria for Clinical Diagnosis of Alzheimer's Disease[a]

Criteria for the clinical diagnosis of *probable* Alzheimer's disease include:

Dementia established by clinical examination and documented by the Mini-Mental State Examination, Blessed Dementia Scale, or some similar examination and confirmed by neuropsychologic tests

Deficits in two or more areas of cognition

Progressive worsening of memory and other cognitive functions

No disturbance of consciousness

Onset between ages 40 and 90, most often after age 65

Absence of systemic disorders or other brain diseases that could account for the progressive deficits in memory and cognition

The diagnosis of *probable* Alzheimer's disease is supported by

Progressive deterioration of specific cognitive functions such as language (aphasia), motor skills (apraxia), and perception (agnosia)

Impaired activities of daily living and altered patterns of behavior

Family history of similar disorders, particularly if confirmed neuropathologically

Laboratory results as follows: normal lumbar puncture as evaluated by standard techniques, normal pattern or nonspecific changes in EEG, such as increased slow-wave activity, and evidence of cerebral atrophy on CT with progression documented by serial observation

Other clinical features consistent with the diagnosis of *probable* Alzheimer's disese, after exclusion of causes of dementia other than Alzheimer's disease, include

Plateaus in the course of progression of the illness

Associated symptoms of depression, insomnia, incontinence, delusions, illusions, hallucinations, sexual disorders, weight loss, and catastrophic verbal, emotional, or physical outbursts

Other neurologic abnormalities in some patients especially with more advanced disease and including motor signs such as increased muscle tone, myoclonus, or gait disorder

Seizures in advanced disease

CT normal for age

Features that make the diagnosis of *probable* Alzheimer's disease uncertain or unlikely include:

Sudden, apoplectic onset

Focal neurologic findings such as hemiparesis, sensory loss, visual field deficits, and incoordination early in the course of the illness

Seizures or gait disturbances at the onset or very early in the course of the illness

Clinical diagnosis of *possible* Alzheimer's disease

May be made on the basis of the dementia syndrome, in the absence of other neurologic, psychiatric, or systemic disorders sufficient to cause dementia and in the presence of variations in the onset, presentation, or clinical course

May be made in the presence of a second systemic or brain disorder sufficient to produce dementia, which is not considered to be *the* cause of dementia

Should be used in research studies when a single, gradually progressive, severe cognitive deficit is identified in the absence of another identifiable cause

Criteria for diagnosis of *definite* Alzheimer's disease are

The clinical criteria for probable Alzheimer's disease

Histopathologic evidence obtained from a biopsy or autopsy

Classification of Alzheimer's disease for research purposes should specify features that may differentiate subtypes of the disorder, such as

Familial occurrence

Onset before age 65

Presence of trisomy 21

Coexistence of other relevant conditions, such as Parkinson's disease

[a]NINCDS = National Institute of Neurological and Communicative Disorders and Stroke; ADRDA = Alzheimer's Disease and Related Disorders Association.

Drugs often cause delirium or exacerbate an existing organic dementia. Patients with dementia are more sensitive to the central nervous system adverse effects of all medications. Although delirium tends to have a more abrupt onset and fluctuating course, its presentation may mimic dementia syndrome. Any medication the patient is taking should be evaluated for its ability to cause memory problems and confusion. The elderly use many medicines that are high in anticholinergic side effects, and they are very susceptible to the delirium these medicines might cause. Stopping the use of any unnecessary medications or changing the selection of medication to decrease side effects may be a vital therapeutic intervention.

TREATMENT

Although there are no truly successful drug therapies to be discussed in the treatment of Alzheimer's disease, it is important to be acquainted with the wide variety of drug therapies that have been tried over the years and their purported rationales. The families of Alzheimer's disease patients are often desperate to find a cure and will turn to unproven and often expensive treatment modalities. General guidelines for treating Alzheimer's patients are outlined in Table 93.5. Patients and caregivers must be guided by well-informed professionals.

There are two basic divisions of Alzheimer's drug treatment. The first, and most often used, is *symptomatic* drugs that are palliative and help to control unwanted behaviors and maintain patient functioning. These drugs consist primarily of psychotropic agents. The other division is *therapeutic*. These agents are used to stop or reverse the disease process and are largely experimental.

Symptomatic Treatment

During the course of Alzheimer's disease, patients experience memory dysfunction, progressive loss of cognitive ability, difficulties in the use of language, disorientation, confusion, disruption of the sleep-wake cycle, personality changes, and lack of emotional control that often results in anxiety and agitation. Psychotropic medicines are very often needed to alleviate some of these symptoms as the disease progresses. All psychotropics should be used with caution; those that are low in anticholinergic side effects are usually preferred. They should be started at low doses

Table 93.4.
Diagnosis of Dementia

History—from patient, relative, close associates
Mental status examination (especially mild and moderate stages)
Physical examination including vital signs
Neurologic examination
CT scan/magnetic resonance imaging
Laboratory tests
    Thyroid function tests (T_4, T_3RU, TSH)
    Serum B_{12}
    Folic acid
    CBC with RBC indices
    Syphilis serology (VDRL, FTA/MHATP)
    Glucose
    BUN/creatinine
    Calcium/phosphorus
    Albumin
    Electrolytes
    Alkaline phosphatase
    Sedimentation rate
Optional/suggested procedures and tests as indicated
    Chest radiograph
    Electrocardiogram
    Electroencephalogram
    Lumbar puncture
    Urinalysis
    Drug screens/levels

Table 93.5.
Guidelines for Treatment of Patients with Alzheimer's Disease

1. The differential diagnosis of cognitive impairment is imperative prior to treatment. Rigorously pursue the diagnosis of any treatable states that may cause dementia; especially consider depression.
2. Avoid any unnecessary use of medications. Alzheimer's disease patients have little reserve capacity against toxicities and are therefore more prone to adverse effects.
3. Individualize therapy. Each patient exhibits different behavioral and cognitive manifestations of the disease. Optimum dosages of medications used in Alzheimer's disease have not been established. Dosages must be individually titrated and monitored. Also consider that, because of the progressive nature of the disease, therapy should not be static and must be reevaluated and changed accordingly.
4. Carefully monitor patients on medications. The effects seen are usually moderate or may manifest only as a slowing of decline rather than improvement in function. Adverse effects are frequent; also note other medications (e.g., cardiac, nonsteroidal antiinflammatory, antihypertensive) may exacerbate mental decline.
5. Always be aware that medications all have toxicities that may cause or unmask the very problems they are trying to treat.
6. Discontinue ineffective or unnecessary medications.

Table 93.6.
Representative Starting Doses of Psychotropic Medications Used to Treat Symptoms of Alzheimer's Disease Patients

Antidepressants	
Fluoxetine (Prozac)	10 mg q.o.d or q.d. (A.M.)
Nortriptyline (Pamelor)	10 mg b.i.d.–t.i.d.
Paroxetine (Paxil)	10 mg q.d.
Phenelzine (Nardil)	15 mg b.i.d.
Sertraline (Zoloft)	25 mg q.d.
Trazodone (Desyrel)	25 mg q.d.–b.i.d.
Anxiolytics	
Alprazolam (Xanax)	0.25 mg q.d.–b.i.d.
Buspirone (Buspar)	5 mg b.i.d.–t.i.d.
Lorazepam (Ativan)	0.5 mg q.d.–b.i.d.
Oxazepam (Serax)	10 mg b.i.d.
Antipsychotics	
Clozapine (Clozaril)	25 mg q.d.–b.i.d.
Haloperidol (Haldol)	0.5 mg q.d.–b.i.d.
Risperidone (Risperdal)	1.0 mg q.d.
Thioridazine (Mellaril)	10 mg q.d.–bi.d.
Thiothixene (Navane)	1.0 mg q.d.–b.i.d.
Hypnotics	
Chloral hydrate (Noctec)	250–500 mg q HS
Temazepam (Restoril)	7.5 mg q HS
Triazolam (Halcion)	0.125 mg q HS
Zolpidem (Ambien)	5 mg q HS

and titrated according to therapeutic response and side effects (Table 93.6).

ANTIDEPRESSANTS

Early states of Alzheimer's disease are often accompanied by depressive symptoms, which may respond to drug therapy. Resolution of depression results in improvement of mood, functional abilities, and possibly cognitive faculties (12). All patients with dementia should be carefully evaluated for depression. Depressive symptoms such as agitation, memory loss, and insomnia can easily be confused with dementia. A therapeutic trial of antidepressants can be effective in treating a masked depression whose symptoms often mimic Alzheimer's disease. In general, antidepressants should be chosen for Alzheimer's disease patients as for any other depressed patient: by side effect profiles and trial for response. Low doses of nortriptyline or trazodone given once or twice a day are often beneficial. Sedating antidepressants such as trazodone can also be used for their calming effects to help decrease excessive excitation and agitation. A bedtime dose may alleviate insomnia. The newer serotonin-specific (SSRI) antidepressants are effective for depression and offer a preferable side effect profile, although they do have the potential of increased anxiety symptoms, agitation, and insomnia.

The clinical symptoms of Alzheimer's disease have been correlated in neurochemical studies with deficits of acetylcholine in the brain. Some clinicians are therefore wary of using drugs that have anticholinergic properties to treat these patients because of the possibility of exacerbating memory impairment and cognitive decline. In most cases, antidepressants are beneficial, and with proper titration to a therapeutic level and appropriate monitoring they can be safely recommended. (Note that most Alzheimer's patients are elderly and usually require lower doses to achieve therapeutic blood levels.)

For depressed Alzheimer's disease patients who do not respond to tricyclics, SSRIs, and other standard antidepressants or those who suffer troublesome side effects, the use of monoamine oxidase inhibitors (MAOIs) should be considered. The enzyme monoamine oxidase (MAO) has been shown to increase with age, and demented patients may have even higher levels of MAO than do age-matched controls (13). MAOIs do not adversely affect memory and cognitive function as tricyclics do. Unfortunately, postural hypotension, dietary restrictions, and the possibility of hypertensive crisis can limit their usefulness for these patients.

HYPNOTICS

Insomnia is a common complaint in the elderly, and sleep disturbances are more frequent in patients with dementia. Sleep difficulties often distress patients and caregivers and can lead to exhaustion of caregivers. Sleep disturbance can be manifested by patients being awake at night, pacing, trying to go outside, or searching for lost items. Hypnotics should be avoided if at all possible because of their widespread central nervous system depressant effects. Regulating patients' schedules, keeping them active during the day, and preventing daytime napping all help to decrease nighttime insomnia.

Sedating antidepressants such as trazodone 25 to 50 mg at bedtime may be beneficial. When a hypnotic is absolutely necessary, the lowest dose for the shortest duration should be used. The short-acting benzodiazepines (triazolam 0.125 mg, temazepam 7.5 mg) and zolpidem (5 to 10 mg) are often helpful, but they should be used judiciously because they can increase confusion and memory impairment, worsen depressive symptoms, and aggravate most other cognitive symptoms occurring in Alzheimer's disease. Longer-half-life benzodiazepines should be avoided because of their tendency to accumulate and cause oversedation and falls. Chloral hydrate in low doses (250 mg to 1 g) has been used with benefit. Chloral hydrate has many adverse side effects and more drug interactions than benzodiazepines, and as with benzodiazepines, caution should be taken because this drug can also exacerbate symptoms of Alzheimer's disease. Diphenhydramine, an antihistamine, has been used for its moderate sedating properties but has anticholinergic effects that may increase confusion and psychotic symptoms. Because of its limited efficacy and potential side effects, it is not recommended. Alcohol intake should also be discontinued or kept to a minimum because of its effects on cognition, disruption of sleep pattern, and other side effects; furthermore, drug interactions and excessive intake can cause delirium or dementia.

It is important to minimize the constant use of hypnotics. The efficacy of long-term, routine use of hypnotics has not been proven. Maintaining daytime activity and giving other sedating medications at bedtime and "as needed" hypnotics can sufficiently control insomnia.

ANXIOLYTICS

Anxiety frequently affects patients who are experiencing memory loss. The elderly often manifest their anxiety in somatic form such as agitation, motor restlessness, and insomnia. The judicious use of benzodiazepines or buspirone in treating these symptoms has been successful. Buspirone is sometimes effective for the anxiety and mild agitation of Alzheimer's disease and has minimal side effects. Doses such as 5 mg three times a day or 10 mg twice a day are often beneficial; some studies show benefit with doses up to 60 mg/day. Short-half-life benzodiazepines in low doses given once or twice a day are also useful. The use of benzodiazepines for anxiety is limited by side effects. They act on the central nervous system to produce confusion, drowsiness, and amnesia, features that mimic and confound Alzheimer's disease. They can also cause gait instability and have been correlated with an increased frequency of falls.

ANTIPSYCHOTICS

Antipsychotics are indicated for the treatment of specific psychotic symptoms such as auditory and visual hallucinations, paranoia, and delusions with suspiciousness and severe agitation, which are stressful to the patient and may interfere with the caregiver's ability to provide care for the patients. Antipsychotics do not affect higher cortical functions such as memory, judgment, and problem solving.

No single drug emerges as a superior agent. The high-potency antipsychotics (haloperidol, fluphenazine) leave the patient prone to extrapyramidal side effects such as pseudoparkinsonism and tardive dyskinesia. Low-potency (chlorpromazine, thioridazine) agents are anticholinergic and have cardiovascular side effects. The adverse effects may further impair the remaining physical and cognitive functions of Alzheimer's disease patients. Movement may be decreased, hypotension may cause falling, and sedation may exacerbate confusion. Low doses (e.g., haloperidol 0.5 to 1 mg) given once or twice a day are usually sufficient. The newer atypical antipsychotic agents (risperidone and clozaril) with effects on dopamine and serotonin have also been beneficial and may have a more desirable extrapyramidal side effect profile. (However, clozaril requires constant monitoring for blood dyscrasias.) A late afternoon or early evening dose may lessen daytime sedation and decrease "sundowning" (a phenomenon of agitation and confusion worsening in the late afternoon and evening).

Benefits of psychotropic medications are variable, and responses to agents are highly individual and limited by adverse effects. Psychotropics are useful and can improve behavior and functioning, easing patients' distress and the burden of care. The efficacy of neuroleptics in controlling agitation is modest at best. Antipsychotic use should be minimized and is indicated only for symptoms that are harmful and distressing to the patient that cannot be controlled through all other means. Antipsychotics have potentially severe and permanent side effects, and their use should be minimized. Strict monitoring is imperative to prevent more harm than benefit from the use of these medications. Developing literature has suggested alternative drugs such as carbamazepine, trazodone, and propranolol for controlling agitation and significant behavior symptoms. Benefits have been shown, but studies are preliminary and include small sample populations of patients (14).

Because the disease is progressive, therapy should be evaluated at least every 6 months to ensure that the fewest drugs are being used in the lowest effective doses. Tapering psychotropic medications in stabilized patients at regular intervals is effective in assessing the need for continued drug therapy. Families and caregivers should be counseled. They must understand that psychotropic medications may improve some symptoms but will not improve dementia or prevent further deterioration of function or progression of the disease. The caregivers' understanding of the disease process and the effects of drug therapy often lessens the need to use medication.

Therapeutic Treatments

Therapeutic drugs are being developed to slow progression of brain failure or reverse or alleviate disease symptoms in Alzheimer's disease patients. Most therapeutic treatments are investigational. When Alzheimer's disease is further characterized, treatment will probably consist of a combination of therapies. Drug therapy will probably affect the balance of cholinergic and other neurotransmitter systems because of the multiple neurochemical abnormalities and brain functions affected. Eventually, when the cause is known, therapies can be directed at reversing pathologic damage and preventing the disease progression.

METABOLIC ENHANCERS

Hydergine (ergoloid mesylates) has a Food and Drug Administration (FDA) approved indication for use in the cognitive decline of the elderly. Originally thought to act as a cerebral vasodilator, ergoloid mesylates are now classified as metabolic enhancers. Their proposed mechanisms in dementia treatment are to increase certain enzymes, alter glucose and oxygen utilization, and act as α-adrenoreceptor blockers and as serotonin and dopamine agonists. How the pharmacologic effects are related to clinical efficacy is uncertain (15).

Studies show some improvement in behavioral variables, including mood, attention, and performance of specific tasks, when ergoloid mesylates are given early in the course of dementia. This improvement may be related to a mild improvement in mood (15, 16). Once the disease has progressed and there is serious cognitive impairment, little effect is expected.

Optimal doses for Alzheimer's disease patients have not been established. However, some studies have used 6 to 12 mg/day, which is above the FDA-recommended dosage of 3 mg/day. Ergoloid mesylates can usually be safely administered with mild and occasional adverse effects of gastrointestinal upset and bradycardia. A drug trial should last at least 6 months. If no benefit is seen or if symptoms of the disease progress, the drug should be discontinued.

The efficacy and dosage of ergoloid mesylates are questionable. Despite a preponderance of studies showing positive effects, the favorable results are variable from one study to another and tend to be more statistically significant than medically important (17).

CHOLINERGIC AGENTS

At present the cholinergic deficit hypothesis provides the most viable and consistent explanation of the memory impairment that occurs in Alzheimer's disease, but it does not account for all the clinical deficits that occur. Neurochemical studies of Alzheimer's disease patients have shown a deficiency of the neurotransmitter acetylcholine and choline acetyltransferase, the enzyme that is responsible for its synthesis. A positive correlation has been reported between the degree of cognitive impairment of Alzheimer's disease patients and decreases in choline acetyltransferase and acetylcholine (18). Comparisons between Alzheimer's disease patients and age-matched controls have demonstrated neuron losses in the nucleus basalis of Meynert, an area that is thought to provide cholinergic input to the cortex and a major cholinergic pathway leading from the septum to the hippocampus, a structure that is critical to normal memory function (19).

Several pharmacologic efforts to augment cholinergic activity have focused on (a) increasing acetylcholine synthesis and release, (b) limiting acetylcholine breakdown by inhibiting acetylcholinesterase, and (c) directly stimulating acetylcholine receptors (20, 21).

Agents such as choline and lecithin (phosphatidylcholine) serve as precursors to acetylcholine, and large amounts have been shown to increase acetylcholine concentrations in the brain. Lecithin raises plasma choline levels and does not produce the foul odor that occurs with choline administration. Clinical trials of choline and lecithin have not shown convincing evidence that these substances improve cognition in Alzheimer's disease patients. This is probably because the enzyme choline acetyltransferase, which is required for these precursors to be synthesized to acetylcholine, is depleted in Alzheimer's disease.

Cholinesterase inhibitors (physostigmine, tacrine) block acetylcholinesterase (AChE) and increase the amount of available acetylcholine in the synaptic cleft by limiting its breakdown. AChE inhibitors, which have had limited success, are currently the most extensively used and studied class of drugs in the treatment of Alzheimer's disease. Physostigmine is a centrally active acetylcholinesterase inhibitor that prevents the enzymatic hydrolysis of acetylcholine released in the synapse. It has been administered both intravenously and orally with some success. Intravenous doses have shown statistically significant, moderate, and transient improvement in visual recognition memory tests (22). Although several studies corroborate improvements (23), clinical applicability is more difficult to prove, and physostigmine use is limited by the short duration of action and adverse side effects such as nausea, vomiting, diarrhea, dizziness, and headache. Oral physostigmine has resulted in modest improvements in cognitive areas, some selective memory tests, and overall functioning in certain patients. Variability of the response to oral physostigmine is due to differences in drug absorption and penetration into the central nervous systems of individual patients (24).

Tacrine (tetrahydroaminoacridine, or THA) is a centrally active, reversible cholinesterase inhibitor with a longer duration of action than physostigmine. Tacrine elevates ACh levels in the cerebral cortex and has shown encouraging results as a palliative treatment in Alzheimer's disease (25). Tacrine (Cognex), which was approved in 1993 by the FDA, is the first drug indicated to treat mild to moderate Alzheimer's disease. Tacrine has shown dose-related benefits in cognitive function such as performance of recognition and attentional tasks and improved measures of quality of life (26, 27). Improvement has not been shown in short-term memory function, and efficacy results may depend on which parameters are measured. Tacrine does not alter the course or the progress of dementia, and a slow decline in function will continue.

Adverse effects such as nausea, vomiting, diarrhea, and anorexia are common dose-related side effects and often limit tacrine use. There has been a high prevalence (30%) of abnormal liver function tests (elevated transaminase), which usually return to normal with decreases in dose or discontinuance of drug therapy. A few occurrences of liver necrosis and jaundice have been reported (28). Tacrine should be used with caution by patients with gastrointestinal disease, as it may increase gastric acid secretion and cardiovascular conditions. It has a vagotonic effect on pulse rate and can worsen bradycardia with sick sinus syndrome.

Tacrine is metabolized by the cytochrome P450 system, and most drug interactions are generally related to this. It should be used with caution for patients on phenytoin, theophylline, and cimetidine. Baseline liver function tests including bilirubin, asparate transaminase (AST), and alanine aminotransferase (ALT) are recommended. Because of its short half-life (15 to 3.5 hr), tacrine is given four times a day and should be taken on an empty stomach, since food decreases absorption. Therapy is initiated at 10 mg four times a day for 6 weeks, with transaminase levels measured every other week. If the patient tolerates the

medication, it should be increased by 40 mg/day at 6-week intervals until a dosage of 120 to 160 mg/day is reached. After each dosage increase, transaminase levels should be measured every week for 6 weeks or for the first 16 weeks of therapy; then transaminase levels should be measured monthly for 2 months and then quarterly. If alanine aminotransferase (ALT) is three to five times the upper limits of normal, it is recommended that the dose be decreased by 40 mg/day and retitrated when transaminase levels return to normal. If ALT is over five times normal, the drug should be discontinued, and a rechallenge may be considered.

Patient and family education is important so that they understand the cost of medication and monitoring (estimated to be >$2000 per year in 1994). They should be aware of the limitations of treatment and the need for continuous observation and laboratory monitoring.

There appears to be no further loss of muscarinic receptors in Alzheimer's disease patients beyond that found with normal aging (18). Bethanecol, an acetylcholine-like agonist that is given by intracranial infusion, resulted in clinical improvement in some patients (29). When improvements occurred, they were in no way dramatic, and the memory of demented patients remained impaired. The use of cholinergic agents is limited by their toxicities, including liver impairment and seizures, their short half-lives, and the fact that they do not cross the blood-brain-barrier efficiently, so administration is difficult. It is also hypothesized that acetylcholine is released in a pulsatile fashion and that replacement by infusion may not be physiologically equivalent, limiting therapeutic benefits.

The minimal benefits, systemic side effects, and difficulty of administration currently limit the applicability of most cholinergic treatments. It is still to be determined whether any or all of these cholinergic mechanisms are involved in the cognitive impairment of Alzheimer's disease patients. Ultimately, treatments using these pharmacologic strategies may have to be used in combination, with regimens individualized for each patient.

Although evidence supports the cholinergic hypothesis of memory and cognitive function, it is highly unlikely that this impairment is the sole disorder occurring in Alzheimer's disease. Alzheimer's disease represents multiple disorders or subtypes that share certain features and probably results from a combination of neuronal changes (such as decreases in protein synthesis, production of abnormal proteins, and impaired energy production) and neurotransmitter deficits in the brain. With advancing knowledge of the causes of Alzheimer's disease, new therapies can be developed. The pharmacologic efforts to treat Alzheimer's disease have been based on various theories, and the list of therapies continues to grow (30). Table 93.7 lists several of these agents. Most outcomes of these trials are moderately positive at best. Ultimately, therapy will probably consist of a combination of medica-

Table 93.7.
Drug Trials in the Treatment of Alzheimer's Disease

Drug	Mode of Action	Evaluation of Efficacy
CHOLINERGIC TREATMENTS		
Precursors to acetylcholine (ACh)		
Choline	Increase amount of ACh	Most clinical trials conclude not effective alone
Lecithin		
Acetylcholinesterase inhibitors		
Tacrine (THA)	Prevent breakdown of ACh	Clinically modest effects on selected cognitive measures
Physostigmine		Clinical trials
Velnacrine		Investigational use in rats/tissue longer half-life and increase bioavailability
Galanthamine		
Heptyl-physostigmine		Investigational, longer half-life
Cholinergic agonists		
Bethanecol	Muscarinic agonists	Some subjective improvement
OTHER THERAPEUTIC AGENTS		
Acetyl-l-carnitine	Neuroprotective/promotes acetylcholine synthesis	Less deterioration on some performance tasks
Anesthetics		
Procaine HCl	Mild CNS stimulant with local anesthetic action; weak MAO inhibitor	May have mild mood-elevating effects
(Gerovital H3)		
Cheolators	Proposed removal of toxins, calcium, and aluminum	Unproven, costly to use, dangerous
EDTA desferoxamine		
Ergofoid mesylates	Metabolic enhancer	Modest effect on clinical symptoms, possibly due to mood elevation
Nonsteroidals	Immune/inflammatory effects may cause plaque and tangle formation could prevent degeneration	Potential role supported by indomethacin study. Reduced incidence of Alzehimer's disease in rheumatoid groups versus controls
Nerve growth factor	May attenuate rate of degeneration of remaining cholinergic neurons	On the basis of animal studies, N.I.A. workgroup concluded strong rationale for clinical trials
Neuropeptides		
ACTH	Neurotransmitters may enhance activity of endogenous neurotransmitters	Little benefit, principal effects on mood and attention, not learning
Somatostatin		
Vasopressin		
Nimodipine	Inhibits calcium influx that occurs with cellular damage, may slow progression of disease	Less deterioration on several memory tests, improved cognitive effects
Nootropic agents		
Piracetam	Enhances brain metabolism/possibly neuroprotective	Equivocal results, limited clinical utility; response may improve when given with precursors
Psychostimulants		
Methylphenidate	Central nervous system stimulants	No sound evidence of therapeutic benefit; may treat symptoms of fatigue, motor retardation
Pemoline		
Pentylenetetrazol		
Selegiline (Deprenyl)	Irreversible MAO-B inhibitor	Improvements in testing. Case reports beneficial for behaviors such as anxiety, agitation, depression
Vasodilators		
Cyclandelate	Enhance blood flow to the brain	Limited clinical efficacy; may actually be detrimental by shunting blood away from brain
Isoxsuprine		
Papaverine		

tions based on cause and symptoms. The optimal therapy will prevent or reverse the disease process itself.

Environment

Besides pharmacotherapy, a comprehensive plan should include adequate nutrition, correction of sensory deficits (e.g., glasses, hearing aid), and attention to the social environment. A safe, stable, comfortable environment will minimize the strain of decreasing mental capacities and lessen confusion. Patients should be stimulated and helped to function, but choices, which may overwhelm and confuse them, should be limited. Labeling items with names and laying out one change of clothes will help maintain the patient's ability to perform the activities of daily living. Alterations in surroundings such as room changes should be minimized, as they may cause an increase in confusion and disorientation. Physical and psychosocial stressors such as minor surgery, bereavement, or institutionalization can and often will aggravate intellectual deficits in a demented patient. Within reason, familiar furnishings, diet, and routines should be maintained.

Caregiver training is important. Caregivers must understand the limitations of the patient's cognition and how that affects their behaviors and functioning. Patients are often confused and cannot process what is going on around them. A lot of the interactions between patients and caregivers can be modified to best suit the patient and prevent or minimize incidents that might lead to agitation and difficulty in caring for the patient.

Family Support

The treatment plan should provide adequate emotional support for family members and those who provide the most patient care. Referring the family to the local branch of the Alzheimer's Association and to books such as the *36 Hour Day* (31) is often as valuable as any current drug therapy. Relatives of Alzheimer's disease patients who are experiencing changes in the patient's cognitive abilities and personality and their relationship with the Alzheimer's disease patient grieve for their own loss (32). Families must be educated about the disease and expectations of therapy. There are no medical cures, and the disease waxes and wanes but is progressive. Often a rational presentation of the disease will allay fears, allow sensible expectations, and enhance the family's ability to provide support to the patient without the use of medications. It must always be remembered that all drugs have toxicities, and many may exacerbate the symptoms they are supposed to treat. Medications are often used to maintain patients in the home. Caregivers must understand the dangers of overmedication and the need to administer medications only as directed. Families and the caregivers who are closest to the patients should be included in therapeutic decisions and often provide the best monitoring information.

Because of the lack of nursing home beds and their high costs, alternative care will become even more important in the future. Patients who are in early stages of Alzheimer's disease need education and counseling. They are often responsible for their own drug therapy. When family members become involved in care, their understanding of drug therapy and the ability to comply with regimens should be evaluated. Care for the caregivers is often as important as care of the patient. Remember that an aging spouse may be on the borderline of competency and function, and the added burden of caring for a demented mate may be too much for that person to handle properly. When the caregiver gives out, the care system suffers. Social services provide some aid with home care. Day-care services are offered by various local agencies and provide different levels of supervision and activities for Alzheimer patients. Day care is especially important in providing much needed respite for the caregivers at home. Eventually, most patients will become incapacitated, many suffering from aggression, wandering, and incontinence, and will often require long-term care placement.

CONCLUSION

Alzheimer's disease is a complex, progressive, degenerative disorder with no known cure. All potentially reversible causes of dementia should be excluded or treated before a diagnosis of Alzheimer's disease is made. Management includes supportive care and control of detrimental symptoms. The goals of therapy are to maintain the most appropriate level of care and to keep the patient as functional as possible for as long as possible.

REFERENCES

1. Huppert FA, Tym E. Clinical and neuropsychological assessment of dementia. Br Med Bull 42:11–8, 1986.
2. Katzman R. Alzheimer's disease. N Engl J Med 314:964–73, 1986.
3. Evans DA, Funkenstein HH, Albert MS, et al. Prevalence of Alzheimer's disease in a community population of older persons: higher than previously reported. JAMA 262:2551–56, 1989.
4. Statistical data on Alzheimer's disease. Chicago, Illinois: Alzheimer's Association, 1992.
5. Fox JH, Heston, LL, Terry RD. Zeroing in on Alzheimer's disease. Patient Care 20:68–91, 1986.
6. Bissette G, Reynolds GP, Kilts CD, et al. Corticotropin-releasing factor-like immunoreactivity in the senile dementia of the Alzheimer type: reduced cortical and striatal concentrations. JAMA 254:3067–69, 1985.
7. Caputo CB, Salama AI. The amyloid proteins of Alzheimer's disease as potential targets for drug therapy. Neurobiol Aging 10(5):451–61, 1989.
8. Liddell M, Williams J, Bayer A, et al. Confirmation of association between the e4 allele of apolipoprotein E and Alzheimer's disease. J Med Genet 31:197–200, 1994.
9. Mayeux R, Stern Y, Ottman R, et al. The apolipoprotein e4 allele in patients with Alzheimer's disease. Ann Neurol 34:752–54, 1993.
10. Francis PT, Palmer, AM, Sims, NR, et al. Neurochemical studies of early-onset Alzheimer's disease. N Engl J Med 313:7–11, 1985.
11. McKhann G, Drachman D, Folstein, M, et al. Clinical diagnosis of Alzheimer's disease. Neurology 34:939–44, 1984.
12. Reifler BS, Larson E, Teri, L, et al. Dementia of the Alzheimer's type and depression. J Am Geriatr Soc 34:855–59, 1986.
13. Gottfried CG, Adolfsson R, Aquilonius, SM, et al. Biochemical changes in dementia disorders of Alzheimer type (AD/SDAT). Neurobiol Aging 4:261–71, 1983.
14. Schneider LS, Sobin PB. Non-neuroleptic treatment of behavioral symptoms and agitation in Alzheimer's disease and other dementias. Psychopharmacol Bull 28:71–9, 1992.
15. Hollister LE, Yesavage J. Ergoloid mesylates for senile dementias: unanswered questions. Ann Intern Med 100:894–98, 1984.
16. Thompson TL, Filley CM, Mitchell WD, et al. Lack of efficacy of hydergine in patients with Alzheimer's disease. N Engl J Med 323:445–48, 1990.
17. Schneider LS, Olin JT. Overview of clinical trials of hydergine in dementia. Arc Neurol 51:787–98, 1994.
18. Bartus RT, Dean RL, Beer B, et al. The cholinergic hypothesis of geriatric memory dysfunction. Science 217:408–14, 1982.
19. Davis, BM, Mohs, RC, Greenwald BS, et al. Clinical studies of the

cholinergic deficit in Alzheimer's disease. 1: neurochemical and neuroendocrine studies. J Am Geriatr Soc 33:741–48, 1985.

20. Hollander E, Mohs, RC, Davis, KL. Cholinergic approaches to the treatment of Alzheimer's disease. Br Med Bull 42:97–100, 1986.

21. Kumar V, Calache, M. Treatment of Alzheimer's disease with cholinergic drugs. Int J Clin Pharmacol Ther Toxicol 29:23–37, 1993.

22. Davis KL, Mohs, RC. Enhancement of memory processes in Alzheimer's disease with multiple dose intravenous physostigmine. Am J Psychol 139:1421–24, 1982.

23. Christie JE, Shering A, Ferguson J, et al. Physostigmine and arecoline effects of intravenous infusions in Alzheimer presenile dementia. Br J Psychol 138:46–50, 1982.

24. Thal LJ, Masur DM, Blau AD, et al. Chronic oral physostigmine without lecithin improves memory in Alzheimer's disease. J Am Geriatr Soc 37:42–8, 1989.

25. Summer WK, Majovski LV, Marsh GM, et al. Oral tetrahydroaminoacridine in long-term treatment of senile dementia, Alzheimer type. N Engl J Med 315:1241–45, 1986.

26. Knapp MJ, Knopman DS, Soloman PR, et al. A 30-week randomized controlled trial of high-dose tacrine in patients with Alzheimer's disease. JAMA, 271:985–91, 1994.

27. Davis KL, Thal LJ, Gamzu ER et al. A double-blind, placebo controlled multicenter study of tacrine for Alzheimer's disease. N Engl J Med 327:1253–59, 1992.

28. Gamzu ER, Hal LJ, Davis KL. Therapeutic trials using tacrine and other cholinesterase inhibitors. Adv Neurol 51:241–45, 1990.

29. Harbaugh RE, Roberts DW, Coombs DW, et al. Preliminary report: intracranial cholinergic drug infusion in patients with Alzheimer's disease. Neurosurgery 15:514–18, 1984.

30. Schneider LS, Tarlot PN. Emerging drugs for Alzheimer's disease: Mechanisms of action and prospects for cognitive enhancing medications. Med Clin North Am 78:911–34, 1994.

31. Mace NL, Rabis, PV. The 36 hour day. Baltimore: Johns Hopkins University Press, 1981.

32. Howell M. Caretakers' views on responsibilities for the care of the demented elderly. J Am Geriatr Soc 32:657–60, 1984.

CHAPTER 94

GERIATRIC DRUG THERAPY

SUSAN W. MILLER and ROBERT J. ANDERSON

Over 27 million people in the United States are more than 65 years of age. By the year 2000, it is projected that 17% of the U.S. population will be over the age of 65 years; the 75 to 84 year age group will increase by 60%, and the very old, those over the age of 85, will increase by 100%. Factors contributing to the growing numbers of elderly include the increased birth rate prior to 1920 and after World War II (1), the decrease in mortality associated with the development of antibiotics and vaccines, and improvements in sanitation and technology (2).

Because the elderly experience a higher rate of chronic conditions than the population at large, they are more likely to use health care services (3). They account for 31% of all hospital discharges and 42% of all acute care hospital days. Older patients are admitted to hospitals more than three times as often as younger patients, are hospitalized 50% longer, and use twice as many prescription medications as the general population. Although only 5% of the total elderly population resides in a nursing home, about 20% spend some time in a nursing home during their lifetime. These demographic changes will continue to have a major impact on both manpower and health care expenditures.

The use of multiple prescription medications for management of chronic diseases in the aging population increases the chances for noncompliance, drug interactions, and adverse drug reactions (ADRs) (Table 94.1). ADRs may present atypically in geriatric patients, often being confused with aging or disease progression. Cognitive impairment and behavioral changes are often the result of drug therapy; therefore, evaluation of the older patient should include a thorough review of drug therapy (4) (see Table 94.2). Classic digoxin toxicity commonly presents as anorexia and weight loss instead of nausea and vomiting; further, instead of haloes and color vision changes, the patient may complain of hazy or muddy vision. Suspected toxicity should be confirmed by electrocardiograms and appropriately drawn digoxin serum blood levels.

The inability of older patients to manage their medications at home has been attributed to one-fourth of nursing home admissions (5), and up to 9% of hospital admissions of patients above the age of 65 are attributable to ADRs (6, 7). Previously, ADRs in the elderly have been documented primarily in the nursing home setting (8, 9), but recently, the incidence of potentially inappropriate prescribing in U.S. community-dwelling elderly persons has been estimated to be 23.5% (10). For this study,

inadequate prescribing was defined as prescribing from a comprehensive set of explicit criteria based on the concepts of prescription medicines that should be entirely avoided in the elderly, excessive dosage, and excessive duration of treatment (11) (see Table 94.3). The majority of drugs on this list should be entirely avoided in the geriatric patient because they are either ineffective or more toxic than equally effective alternatives. Many of these drugs place the older patient at risk for subtle CNS dysfunction that may go unrecognized as a cause of functional impairment. Careful prescribing by the physician and drug therapy monitoring of the elderly patient by the pharmacist can have a major favorable impact on reducing both the incidence of ADRs and the costs of health care (12).

COMPLIANCE IN THE ELDERLY

Compliance is defined as the extent to which a patient's behavior coincides with a prescriber's planned medical regimen. Noncompliance with drug therapy occurs in one-half to one-third of elderly patients (13); a majority of the time they are taking too little medication (14). Although the elderly population is at risk for noncompliance because of the number of drugs that they are prescribed, studies have failed to prove that older patients, as a group, are any less compliant than the general population (15). Poor communication with health professionals, coupled with declining cognitive function, is a major reason for noncompliance in older patients. Pharmacists need to make a special effort to counsel these high-risk patients by providing both verbal reinforcement and written instructions to assure an understanding of why the drug was prescribed, its use, the proper administration time consistent with their lifestyle, and common side effects. On refill visits to the pharmacy, subtle questions related to side effects and serious adverse reactions should be asked by the pharmacist. Eliminating unnecessary or duplicative therapy in addition to simplifying the regimen will help minimize adverse drug reactions and maximize compliance. Health care professionals should be aware of the major risk factors for noncompliance and assess each patient for the presence of possible risk factors (Table 94.4).

AGE-RELATED PHYSIOLOGIC AND PHARMACOLOGIC CHANGES

It has been estimated that a majority of ADRs in the elderly are the result of dose-related pharmacokinetic

Table 94.1.
Reasons for High Frequencies of ADRs in Elderly

- Multiple chronic diseases requiring treatment with potent medications
- Several physicians prescribing therapy independently
- Inappropriate identification of ADR's
- Patient noncompliance with prescribed medications, or self-medicating inappropriately
- Inadequate patient education on prescribed and over-the-counter (OTC) drugs
- Age-related physiological changes that alter drug kinetics and pharmacological response to the prescribed medication

Table 94.2.
Medications Which Can Cause Changes in Mental Status

Cognitive Impairment	Behavioral Changes (agitation, delirium, psychosis)
Cephalosporins	Anticholinergics
Buspirone	Tricyclic antidepressants
Hydrochlorothiazide	Ranitidine
Reserpine	Barbiturates
Antipsychotics	Beta-agonists
Opiate narcotics	Digoxin
Methyldopa	Bromocriptine
Amantadine	Amantadine
Benzodiazepines	Selegiline
Anticonvulsants	Levodopa
Depression	Baclofen
Reserpine	Opiate narcotics
Methyldopa	Sympathomimetics
Beta-Blockers	Corticosteroids
Corticosteroids	Antihistamines
	Fluoxetine
	Nonsteroidal antiinflammatories
	Thyroid supplements

changes and thus may be prevented. The aging process alone can influence drug response by interfering with the fraction of drug absorbed (f), the plasma drug half-life (T 1/2), the volume of drug distribution in the body (Vd), and the metabolic and renal clearance from the body (Cl). By predicting which drugs are potentially affected by age-related pharmacokinetic changes, the proper dose and dosing interval can be better estimated. In addition to alterations in drug kinetics, age can influence the pharmacologic response of drugs.

Physiologic Changes Influencing Drug Absorption

Product formulation, inherent drug properties, and patient variables can influence the rate, and in some cases the extent, of drug absorbed in the elderly. In terms of product formulation, it is common for a geriatric patient to have difficulty in swallowing a tablet or capsule. It is frequently necessary to use a liquid dosage form or crush the tablet for administration with food or via a nasogastric tube. In general, extended-release, enteric-coated, and sublingual products should not be crushed because of adverse effects on absorption, half-life, and toxicity.

Age-related physiologic changes in the gastrointestinal tract include elevated gastric pH, delayed gastric emptying time, and decreases in both gastrointestinal motility and intestinal blood flow. These age-related physiologic

Table 94.3.
Drugs Considered Inappropriate in the Elderly[a]

Drugs	Reason	Alternative
Sedatives		
Diazepam	Impaired metabolism	Lorazepam
Chlordiazepoxide	Impaired metabolism	Lorazepam
Meprobamate	Increased side effects	Lorazepam
Hypnotics		
Flurazepam	Impaired metabolism	Oxazepam
Pentobarbital	Increased distribution Increased side effects	Temazepam
Secobarbital	Increased distribution Increased side effects	Temazepam
Antidepressants		
Amitriptyline	Increased distribution Increased side effects	Nortriptyline
NSAIDS		
Indomethacin	Increased side effects	Namebutone
Phenylbutazone	Increased side effects	Sulindac
Oral Hypoglycemics		
Chlorpropamide	Impaired elimination	Glyburide, Glipizide, Tolbutamide, Tolazamide
Analgesics		
Propoxyphene	Impaired elimination	
Pentazocine	Increased side effects	
Dementia Treatments		
Isoxsuprine	Ineffective	Tacrine
Cyclandelate	Ineffective	Tacrine
Platelet Inhibitors		
Dipyridamole	Ineffective	Aspirin, Ticlopidine
Muscle Relaxants		
Cyclobenzaprine	Increased side effects	
Methocarbamol	Increased side effects	
Carisoprodol	Increased side effects	
Orphenadrine	Increased side effects	
Antiemetics		
Trimethobenzamide	Ineffective	
Cariodvascular		
Propranolol	Increased bioavailability Increased side effects	Atenolol
Methyldopa	Increased side effects	ACEIs, CCBs
Reserpine	Increased side effects	ACEIs, CCBs

[a]Adapted from reference 10.

Table 94.4.
Major Risk Factors for Noncompliance

Chronic disease or long term therapy
Use of multiple pharmacies
Psychiatric illness
Cognitive impairment
Multiple physicians
Multiple medications
Multiple or complicated dosing schemes
Ineffective communication with health care professionals

changes alone do not seem to influence the passive transport mechanisms by which most drugs are absorbed. Drugs may, however, have reduced or enhanced bioavailability because of incomplete absorption or first-pass metabolism. Bioavailability problems have been reported with many drugs, and the issue of generic substitution is especially important to the geriatric patient because drug costs are so vital to this population (16). Studies have demonstrated wide bioavailability differences when comparing various brands of generic tolbutamide, phenytoin, prednisone, furosemide, and digoxin (17). Indiscriminate switching among generic products should be avoided, especially for drugs in critical therapeutic categories and for drugs prescribed for debilitated patients. Therapeutic interchange among sustained release preparations should also be monitored carefully.

Physiologic changes and diseases, such as acute congestive heart failure (CHF), often necessitate the use of the intravenous route of administration because of incomplete absorption via the oral and intramuscular routes. There is also a decrease in absorption of intramuscularly administered drugs in bedridden elderly patients probably due to changes in regional blood flow.

Drugs with a high intrinsic clearance in the liver are metabolized during their passage from the portal vein through the liver to the systemic circulation, thus reducing their bioavailability (see Table 94.5). The bioavailability of several beta-blockers, including labetalol (18), tricyclic antidepressants (TCAs), and verapamil (19) may be increased, presumably due to a decrease in first-pass metabolism. This would require both smaller initial and maintenance doses of these medications used to manage chronic diseases.

The age-related delay in gastric emptying allows more contact time in the stomach for potentially ulcerogenic drugs such as the nonsteroidal antiinflammatory drugs (NSAIDs), a higher frequency of antacid drug interactions providing more chance for binding, increased absorption of poorly soluble drugs, and a delay in onset action of the weakly basic drugs. The presence of achlorhydria in many elderly does not afford any protective action from NSAID-induced gastric ulcers (20).

Age does influence the active transport mechanisms involved in the absorption of sugars (galactose), vitamins (thiamine, folic acid), and minerals (calcium, iron). Because of these changes in absorption, as well as the fact that the elderly often do not consume a balanced diet for economic reasons, the use of a multivitamin and mineral supplement should be considered. To prevent osteoporosis, women should receive a daily intake of 1200 to 1500 mg of elemental calcium from the diet and supplements unless there is a history of renal stones or hypercalciuria.

Physiologic Changes Influencing Drug Distribution

Age can also change the distribution of the drug to the target organ. Although total protein is unaffected, the plasma albumin portion can often decrease in elderly debilitated patients. Albumin acts as a drug carrier, binding the drug until it is needed. If albumin is decreased, there will be a resultant increase in active, or unbound drug. In addition to age and diet, disease states such as cirrhosis, renal failure, and malnutrition can reduce albumin levels.

Decreased protein binding is also seen with phenytoin, but the drug is cleared from the plasma more rapidly as a result of an increase in the fraction of free phenytoin in the blood (21). Seizure control is expected to be seen at lower measured drug levels. In the case of meperidine, there is a decrease in binding to red blood cells with increasing age (22), thus increasing the amount of free drug available in the patient; this may result in a higher incidence of respiratory depression or, in the case of the active metabolite of meperidine, CNS stimulation. Although higher therapeutic effects of some drugs may be beneficial, the accompanying risks of toxicity are unacceptable in the geriatric patient. Initial doses of most highly protein-bound drugs (greater than 90% protein bound) should be reduced and increased slowly if there is evidence of decreased albumin. If several highly protein-bound drugs are used together, the chance of the patient suffering a drug interaction increases.

Table 94.5.
Representative Drugs Showing Low Oral Availability Due to Extensive First-Pass Hepatic Elimination

Alprenolol	Methylphenidate
Amitriptyline	Metoprolol
Despiramine	Morphine
Dextropropoxyphene	Nifedipine
Dihydroergotamine	Nitroglycerin
Diltiazem	Pentazocine
5-Fluorouracil	Propranolol
Hydralazine	Salicylamide
Labetolol	Verapamil
6-Mercaptopurine	

Adapted from Pond SM, Tozer TN. First-pass elimination: Basic concepts and clinical consequences. Clin Pharmacokin 9:1–25, 1984.

Estimation of Lean Body Weight

Males = 50 kg + 2.3 (inches in height > 5')
Females = 45 kg + 2.3 (inches in height > 5')

Figure 94.1. Estimation of lean body weight. Adapted from Devine B. Gentamicin therapy. Drug Intel Clin Pharm 8:650-655, 1974.

Table 94.6.
Examples of Fat Soluble Drugs

Most antidepressants
Barbiturates
Benzodiazepines
Calcium channel blockers
Phenothiazines

Changes in the ratio of lean body weight to fat can also alter drug distribution and thus pharmacologic response. With aging, total body water is decreased, and total body fat is increased. These changes influence the onset and duration of action of highly tissue-bound drugs such as digoxin and water-soluble drugs such as alcohol, lithium, or morphine. The dosages of most water-soluble drugs are based on an estimation of lean body weight (see Figure 94.1). If actual weight is less than estimated lean body weight, the actual weight should be utilized in dosage calculations.

Between the ages of 18 and 85 years, there is an increase in total body fat in both females and males; lean body mass will eventually decrease in both groups as well. With age, the volume of distribution of lipophilic drugs increases as a result of a decrease in total body weight, diminished protein binding, and an increase in the fat to lean muscle ratio. Fat-soluble drugs (Table 94.6), including many CNS active drugs, may have a delayed onset of action and accumulate in adipose tissue, prolonging their duration action, sometimes to the level of toxicity.

PHYSIOLOGIC CHANGES INFLUENCING DRUG ELIMINATION

Drugs are primarily cleared from the body by metabolism in the liver, excretion by the kidneys, or some combination of the two processes. A decrease in total body clearance results in higher average plasma drug concentrations and an enhanced pharmacologic response, which could lead to toxicity. Age-related physiologic changes in the kidney influence drug elimination and response in the geriatric patient to a greater extent than age-related physiologic changes that occur in the liver.

Physiologic Changes Influencing Hepatic Metabolism

Age-related physiologic changes, such as reductions in liver mass, hepatic metabolizing enzyme activity, and liver blood flow may account for the decreased elimination of some hepatically metabolized drugs in the elderly. Drugs that are biotransformed in the liver, such as NSAIDs, phenytoin, TCAs, trazodone, fluoxetine, and ACEIs, may be affected by these changes. Drug metabolism can also be affected at all ages by gender, genetics, smoking, diet, concomitant drugs, and diseases.

Hepatic metabolism is highly dependent on blood flow. From 25 to 65 years of age, there is a decrease in hepatic blood flow, and in the presence of CHF, hepatic blood flow is further compromised. With drugs that depend highly on hepatic metabolism, such as most beta-blockers, lidocaine, theophylline, and the narcotic analgesics, the decrease in liver clearance could increase the plasma concentration of the drug to toxic levels.

In addition to alterations of hepatic blood flow, age influences the hepatic clearance rate of drugs by causing changes in the intrinsic activity of selected liver enzymes. This has been shown in the oxidative or Phase I metabolism enzyme pathway. Common drugs using this pathway influenced by age include selected benzodiazepines such as diazepam, chlordiazepoxide, clorazepate, halazepam, and prazepam. The enzymatic demethylation of amitriptyline (23), imipramine (24), thioridazine (25), and theophylline (26) has also been shown to be decreased in the elderly. Drugs that undergo Phase II enzymatic biotransformation, such as oxazepam, lorazepam, and temazepam, do not appear to be adversely affected by age and are the preferred agents for use in the elderly. Unlike renal function, there are no accurate laboratory tests to directly measure liver function and thereby adjust drug doses. Nonspecific tests to monitor liver function include alanine aminotransferase (ALT), plasma albumin, and prothrombin time. Studies seem to suggest that, in elderly patients, initial doses of hepatically metabolized drugs should be reduced by one-third to one-half the usual recommended starting dose and then adjusted based on the clinical response.

Physiologic Changes Influencing Renal Elimination

The glomerular filtration rate may decrease as much as 50% with increasing age; this would directly affect the elimination of drugs, or their active metabolites, which are eliminated principally by the kidney. Serum creatinine is frequently used to monitor kidney function, but this test is of limited usefulness in monitoring the glomerular filtration rate of the geriatric patient. Significant elevations do not occur unless a majority of the kidney function has deteriorated. The production of creatinine, which depends on muscle mass, is decreased in the elderly; therefore, an apparently normal serum creatinine in a geriatric patient may not be a valid predictor of drug elimination. Blood urea nitrogen (BUN) is also not useful because it can be affected by hydration status, diet, and blood loss.

A commonly used estimation of glomerular filtration rate in the elderly population is the creatinine clearance

Estimation of Creatine Clearance

$$Cl_{cr}{}^a \ (\text{Male}) =$$

$$\frac{\text{LEAN BODY WEIGHT (KG)} \times (140 - \text{AGE IN YEARS})}{\text{SERUM CREATININE} \times 72}$$

$$Cl_{cr}{}^a \ (\text{Female}) = 0.85 \times Cl_{cr} \ (\text{Male})$$

Figure 94.2. Estimation of creatinine clearance. From Cockroft DW, Gault MH. Prediction of creatinine clearance from serum creatinine. Nephron 16:31-41, 1976.

(Cl^{cr}), which correlates well with both glomerular filtration rate and tubular secretion. Creatinine clearance can be estimated by a standard equation (see Figure 94.2), developed by Cockroft and Gault (27), that takes into consideration age, body weight, and serum creatinine in patients with stabilized renal function.

This as well as other creatinine-clearance-estimating equations in common clinical use have been reported to provide unacceptable predictions of creatinine clearance in a representative sample of healthy elderly (28). An evaluation of several methods of calculations and nomograms used to estimate clearance in older patients determined that the use of published equations and rounding low serum creatinine values up to 1.0 mg/dL caused a significant underestimation of actual creatinine clearance in older patients. This study suggested that the practice of rounding-up serum creatinine concentrations could potentially lead to underdosing of certain medications such as aminoglycosides (29). It is important to remember that mathematical equations and nomograms are simply estimates of an individual's actual renal function. Although estimates appear to be less accurate in the geriatric population, the difficulty in collecting 24-hour urine samples may preclude more accurate creatinine clearance determinations.

To avoid drug toxicity, dosages of renally excreted drugs (or their active metabolites) must be adjusted if the creatinine clearance is less than 30 ml/min. In elderly patients, the renal clearance of digoxin is reduced approximately 50% as a result of age-related changes in renal function, resulting in a longer plasma drug half-life. Other drugs that are excreted primarily unchanged by the kidneys may be found in Table 94.7.

AGE-RELATED PHARMACODYNAMIC CHANGES INFLUENCING DRUG RESPONSE

With increasing age, there is an increased intolerance to drugs as a result of altered pharmacodynamic response at the target organs. Altered response may be due to reduction in receptor number and sensitivity, depletion of neurotransmitters, the presence of disease, or physiologic changes. With aging, there is evidence of a depletion in

acetylcholine, dopamine, and serotonin; a decrease in the enzymatic degradation of monoamine oxidase; an impaired baroreceptor response to blood pressure changes; a decreased responsiveness to beta-adrenergic receptors; and increased pain tolerance (30).

Many drugs routinely prescribed for geriatric patients have adverse effects on the CNS such as cognitive impairment and memory loss. Careful monitoring of these agents is necessary in an effort to differentiate among drug effectiveness, adverse effects, or progression of the disease. Altered end-organ sensitivity may result in exaggerated pharmacologic response, as seen with the barbiturates and benzodiazepines, or diminished pharmacologic response, as seen with the beta-blockers, beta-agonists, and calcium channel blockers (CCBs). Other drug classes affected include the narcotic analgesics, antihypertensive agents, antiparkinson drugs, phenothiazines, and antidepressants. Both the incidence and irreversibility of tardive dyskinesia are increased in the elderly and may be due to age-related imbalances in neurotransmitters (31). The elderly are also more sensitive to the cardiovascular and neurologic side effects of the antipsychotics, including both clozapine and risperidone; therefore, lower initial and maintenance doses are recommended.

Increased sensitivity to warfarin in the elderly has been demonstrated (32). Recommendations for warfarin use are to reduce the average daily dosage by 30 to 40% and monitor carefully. Elderly females have been reported to be more susceptible to the bleeding complications of heparin (33). There is, however, no age-related relationship between plasma heparin concentration and its anticoagulant effect (34); thus, increased bleeding complications, if they occur, would be due to altered pharmacologic response at the receptor site level. Hematuria is a sensitive clinical parameter to monitor for potential heparin or warfarin toxicity.

Table 94.7.
Examples of Drugs Primarily Excreted by the Kidney

Acetazolamide
ACE inhibitors
Amantadine
Aminoglycosides
Cephalosporins
Chlorpropamide
Cimetidine
Digoxin
Disopyramide
Ethambutol
H_2-Antagonists
Lithium
Methotrexate
Penicillins
Procainamide
Quinidine

Dosing adjustments are often necessary since many of these same drugs are also influenced by age-related physiologic changes, especially drug distribution and elimination. The net effect in an individual patient is often difficult to predict. For example, in elderly patients, there is an increased bioavailability of beta-blockers but decreased responsiveness at the receptor site level. Another example is that the inotropic effect of theophylline is increased with age, but the bronchodilator effect is decreased (35). Numerous drug therapies require special attention when prescribed to geriatric patients.

Oral Hypoglycemics

Aging changes related to glucose metabolism include impaired pancreatic secretion of insulin, changes in the renal threshold, and impaired glucose tolerance. Because of increasing hyperglycemia with advancing age, the diagnostic criteria for diabetes mellitus in a geriatric patient requires a random blood glucose level of more than 200 mg/dl or two fasting blood glucose levels of more than 140 mg/dl (36). Most clinicians try to maintain fasting serum glucose levels less than 140 mg/dl and postprandial levels less than 200 mg/dl. Blood glucose monitoring provides the best index of control because urine glucose monitoring has been shown to be unreliable because of age-related increases in the renal threshold.

When selecting an oral hypoglycemic agent for use in elderly patients who may have impaired renal function and/or limited finances, a first-generation sulfonylurea agent such as tolbutamide or tolazamide, which are totally or partially inactivated in the liver, is safer than a longer-acting agent such as chlorpropamide, which can accumulate as a result of decreased renal elimination. In general, oral hypoglycemic doses are reduced or dosing

intervals are increased based on the pharmacokinetic profile of the drug. The second-generation agents such as glyburide and glipizide are increasingly being used because of their single daily dosing, favorable hepatic metabolism, and favorable side effect profile. The pharmacokinetics of glipizide were shown to be similar in both healthy and diabetic elderly patients compared to a younger population, so dosage alteration would not be necessary (37). Patients maintained on oral hypoglycemics should be rechallenged annually with drug withdrawal to determine if continued use, or a lower dose, is necessary.

Cardiovascular Agents

Aging produces several hemodynamic changes that may influence the choice of cardiovascular agents, such as an increase in peripheral vascular resistance, and decreases in renal blood flow, plasma volume, plasma renin, aldosterone, and cardiac output. With an increase in peripheral vascular resistance, elderly patients may exhibit an enhanced response to vasodilators, especially diuretics, CCBs, and ACEIs. Antihypertensive drug therapy should be implemented cautiously in older patients because they may be more sensitive to volume depletion and sympathetic inhibition than younger patients.

Several studies have established the value of treating Stage 2 and 3 hypertension in older patients (see Table 94.8), especially males and those with preexisting cardiovascular disease. In treating the elderly hypertensive patient, new guidelines suggest that the initial goal of therapy is to reduce the systolic blood pressure (SBP) to less than 160 mm Hg for those with SBP greater than 180 mm Hg and to lower blood pressure by 20 mm Hg for those with SBP between 160 and 179 mm Hg. If this is well tolerated, it may be appropriate to reduce the blood

Table 94.8.
Summary of Selected Research Studies on Efficacy of Treating Hypertension in the Elderly

Study	Year	Results
VA CoOp[a]	1972	decrease in cardiovascular complication from 63% to 29%
ANHS[b]	1981	31% decrease in morbidity and mortality with Stage 2 hypertension
EWPSH[c]	1985	efficacy of drugs to reduce blood pressure and fatal myocardial infarction, stroke, severe heart failure
HDFP[d]	1982	16% decrease in cardiovascular mortality with Stage 2 hypertension
STOP[e]	1991	40% decrease in all cardiovascular mortality with Stage 2 hypertension in patients age 70-84 years
SHEP[f]	1991	treatment of isolated systolic hypertension with low dose drugs decreased strokes 33%, MIs by 27%, CHF by 55%

[a]Veterans Administration Cooperative Study on Antihypertensive Agents: Effects of treatment on morbidity in hypertension. III. Influence of age on diastolic pressure and prior cardiovascular disease; further analysis of side effects. Circulation 45:991–1004, 1972.
[b]Management Committee. Treatment of Mild Hypertension in the elderly. Med J Aust 2:398–402, 1981.
[c]O'Malley K, McCormack P, O'Brien ET. Isolated systolic hypertension: data from the European Working Party on High Blood Pressure in the Elderly. J Hypertension 6(Suppl): S105–S108, 1988.
[d]Hypertension Detection and Follow-up Program Cooperative Group. The effect of treatment on mortality in "mild" hypertension: results of the Hypertension Detection and Follow-up Program. N Engl J Med 307:976–980, 1982.
[e]Dahlof B, Lindholm LH, Hansson L, et al. Morbidity and mortality in the Swedish trial in old patients with hypertension (STOP-hypertension). Lancet 338:1281–1285, 1991.
[f]SHEP Cooperative Research Group. Prevention of stroke by antihypertensive drug treatment in older persons with isolated systolic hypertension. Final results of the Systolic Hypertension in the Elderly Program (SHEP). JAMA 265:3255–3264, 1991.

pressure even further (38). All classes of antihypertensive medications have been shown to be effective in lowering blood pressure in older patients; however, only the diuretics and beta-blockers have been used in controlled trials that have shown a reduction in cardiovascular morbidity and mortality (43). Other initial therapy choices include the CCBs, ACEIs, and the alpha blockers. The impact of these agents on cardiovascular morbidity and mortality is currently under study, and the results will not be known until after the year 2000. Interimly, agents should be selected on the basis of cost, adverse effect profiles, compliance factors, and co-existing medical conditions.

The blood pressure lowering effect of different drugs appears to be affected by age and ethnicity (39). Among six different classes of antihypertensive drugs, older black males responded best to CCBs and diuretics. Elderly white males responded almost comparably to all antihypertensives, but more side effects were reported with clonidine and the alpha blocker.

With the age-related decline in renal function, the choice and dosage of a diuretic is important. Since older patients have a decreased plasma volume and lower levels of aldosterone, aggressive diuretic therapy to reduce the blood pressure is generally not indicated. Elderly, especially blacks, who are salt sensitive, exhibit an enhanced response to diuretic therapy compared to younger patients. Diuretics have been shown to be particularly effective in the treatment of isolated systolic hypertension (40).

The current recommendation is to initiate therapy with a small dose of hydrochlorothiazide (12.5 mg) or its equivalent, increasing to a maximum dose of 25 mg twice daily. Similar doses of the longer-acting diuretic, chlorthalidone, have been used successfully. If diuretic therapy is overzealous or water intake is reduced, the elderly patient is at risk of dehydration because of a diminished renal concentrating ability. With hypokalemia, the elderly may be more susceptible to sudden death from ventricular arrhythmias, especially in the presence of left ventricular hypertrophy. With a creatinine clearance of less than 30 ml/min, indapamide, furosemide, torasemide, bumetanide, or metolazone are recommended since thiazide drugs will be ineffective. Diuretic combinations with a potassium-sparing agent can be useful, but hyperkalemia may develop from reduced potassium excretion, the concurrent use of potassium supplements, or concurrent use of ACEIs.

Beta-blockers are primarily indicated in the elderly patient with a history of myocardial infarction or chronic stable angina pectoris. As a result of changes in first-pass metabolism, there is an increase in average peak plasma levels of beta-blockers in older patients (41). When selecting a beta-blocker for use in the geriatric patient, the choice of a long-acting water-soluble agent such as atenolol or nadolol may minimize the occurrence of CNS side effects and maximize patient compliance. Labetalol,

though not cardioselective, may be an alternative choice. Labetalol, with its alpha-blocking activity, is an effective antihypertensive in reducing peripheral vascular resistance and is well tolerated in the elderly without adversely compromising cardiac output. A reduction in clearance in the elderly is the justification for starting with a lower dose (42).

Calcium channel blockers have been shown to decrease blood pressure as effectively as hydrochlorothiazide, beta-blockers, or sympathetic inhibitors in elderly hypertensives but with fewer adverse reactions. With increasing age, there is evidence of a decrease in total body clearance of both verapamil and its active metabolites because of impaired renal elimination (43). The metabolism of verapamil can also be altered by CHF, liver disease, and concomitant use of cimetidine. Verapamil interferes with the tubular secretion of digoxin, sometimes leading to toxic levels (44).

In both young and elderly patients, there is a decrease in metabolism and an increase in plasma half-life of diltiazem when administered on a chronic basis. There is an increase in the incidence of edema, but the more serious effects on myocardial function do not occur (45). Increases in both bioavailability (46) and plasma half-life (47) have also been demonstrated for nifedipine. Headache, peripheral edema, and orthostatic blood pressure change are the rate-limiting side effects. Because of these age-related pharmacokinetic changes, verapamil, diltiazem, and nifedipine should be administered at lower initial and maintenance doses to minimize the incidence of side effects. Nicardipine has been shown to be safe and effective in elderly hypertensives even though both absorption and plasma levels are increased (48). Amlodipine (49) and nitrendipine (50) have been shown to have similar pharmacokinetic profiles and blood pressure lowering responses in both young and elderly hypertensives.

Captopril, and other ACEIs have been shown to reduce blood pressure in elderly hypertensive patients by reducing peripheral vascular resistance through both renin- and nonrenin-related mechanisms (51). All ACEIs appear to be equally effective in the treatment of CHF. The ACEIs are also well tolerated in the elderly without severe adverse metabolic effects though renal function must be carefully monitored. The presence of a drug-induced persistent nonproductive dry cough should be assessed by the pharmacist. Captopril has been shown to protect against deterioration in renal function in insulin-dependent diabetic nephropathy and was significantly more effective than blood pressure control alone (52). ACEIs are the preferred agents in elderly patients with CHF and/or diabetes mellitus. Enalapril, lisinopril, and some of the newer agents offer the advantage of single daily dosing.

Initial doses of ACEIs are generally less in patients with CHF in comparison to hypertension due to a high incidence of orthostatic hypotension, especially with volume depletion from diuretic therapy. To minimize side effects, dosage reductions approximating 50% are recommended for all ACEIs used in patients with moderate to severe renal impairment (creatinine clearance less than 30 ml/min), the elderly, and those with moderate to severe CHF. Fosinopril, benazapril, or quinapril may be better choices since they both have a compensatory nonrenal elimination pathway.

Older patients have an impaired baroreceptor reflex response that makes them more susceptible to hypotension. Aggressive treatment will often result in severe orthostasis leading to falls and subsequent injuries. There is evidence of a 20 mm Hg or greater drop in blood pressure in one-fourth of normal elderly patients undergoing positional changes. Drugs that interfere with the baroreceptor reflex, such as adrenergic-blocking agents, should be used cautiously because of the increased risk of falls and fractures.

Blood pressure should be measured in the standing as well as the sitting position, and antihypertensive treatments should be initiated with smaller dosages and in larger intervals than usual. Additional complications of aggressive therapy are cognitive dysfunction resulting from hypoperfusion to the brain or side effects of antihypertensive agents. In general, starting doses of antihypertensives are reduced by one-third to one-half with slow titration until desired patient response is reached.

The new clinical practice guidelines (53) regarding the management of CHF reflect the increased use of ACEIs because they have been shown to not only provide symptomatic relief with fewer side effects, but they prolong survival in patients with mild, moderate, or severe CHF. The guidelines suggest that diuretics are indicated in patients with evidence of fluid overload, and the use of cardiac glycosides is restricted to those patients with severe systolic dysfunction or who are intolerant to or unresponsive to diuretic and/or ACEI therapy. Long-term maintenance digoxin therapy may no longer be necessary. Studies (54, 55) have shown that a majority of elderly patients can be safely withdrawn from digoxin if there was no evidence of heart failure and if the heart was in normal sinus rhythm, especially with subtherapeutic plasma levels of digoxin (<0.8 ηg/ml). Signs and symptoms of atrial fibrillation and CHF should be monitored if withdrawal from digoxin is attempted.

The benefits of treatment of atrial and ventricular arrhythmias must outweigh the risks of drug toxicity—especially the development of proarrhythmias. Because of changes in hepatic and renal clearance, the geriatric patient is at higher risk of drug toxicity from the antiarrythmic agents.

For quinidine, age-related changes can decrease both hepatic and renal clearance and cause a 33% increase in plasma half-life and antiarrhythmic response (56). Active metabolites can also accumulate, contributing to both pharmacologic and toxic effects. To account for these changes, a reduction in dose or an increase in dosing interval is indicated. Instead of the standard dose of 300 mg every 6 hours, a conservative dosing regimen of 300 mg every 8 hours, or 200 mg every 6 hours may be effective. Plasma concentrations of quinidine can be increased if concurrent CHF is present.

Procainamide has an active metabolite (η-acetyl procainamide or NAPA) that is 100% excreted unchanged by the kidney. Drug accumulation may result in hypotension and heart block. Dosage recommendations for the geriatric patient are 250 mg to 375 mg of procainamide every 4 to 6 hours. Blood levels should be maintained in the 4 to 8 μg/ml range, remembering that the NAPA metabolite also possess significant antiarrythmic activity. In the presence of CHF, drug clearance is further compromised.

Lidocaine is very dependent on the liver for its metabolism, and a decrease in hepatic perfusion will alter drug kinetics. Decreases in plasma clearance occur with age as a result of a decrease in cardiac output such as a myocardial infarction, or in the presence of CHF or liver disease. If any of these risk factors are present, the patient may experience toxicity exhibited as CNS depression, hypotension, or convulsions. The rate of ADRs associated with lidocaine doubles in patients over the age of 70 compared with those under 50 years of age (57). Most of these reactions occur during the initial 2 days of therapy.

Disopyramide is primarily excreted by the kidney, with 50% excreted unchanged and 30% as metabolites, some of which have antiarrhythmic activity. Disopyramide may induce mild heart failure as a result of profound negative inotropic effect (58). This drug should be used with caution in patients with a history of heart failure and in those being maintained on beta-blockers. Urinary retention may also be aggravated by the use of this agent.

Anxiolytics, Sedatives, and Hypnotics

As many as half of the patients over the age of 50 report experiencing insomnia, and it has also been shown that hypnotic drug use increases with age. In a survey of nursing home patients, up to half of the patients received a sedative-hypnotic or anxiolytic prescription on a regular basis (59). A general guideline for dosing the sedative-hypnotics in geriatrics is to start with one-third to one-half the usual recommended starting dose or, for sedatives, increase the time interval between doses.

Geriatric patients are more sensitive to the cortical depressant effect of the benzodiazepines and can appear to be demented, depressed, or both as a result of chronic intoxication. In the older patient, benzodiazepines are effective in reducing sleep latency, but chronic or repeated use can lead to overmedication, additive side effects, or hypersomnolence. When used regularly in the elderly, benzodiazepines can cause significant toxicity, including dependence, hangover effect, dysphoria, and withdrawal on discontinuation.

An increased risk of hip fracture has been correlated directly with the use of long-acting benzodiazepines; users of short half-life benzodiazepines had no significantly increased risk compared to controls (60). The benzodiazepines are also associated with residual cognitive deficits in geriatric patients.

In selecting a benzodiazepine for use in elderly patients, considerations should include specific symptoms and needs of the patient (i.e., sleep latency, sleep maintenance, and/or early morning wakening anxiety) and the metabolic pathway of the drug. In elderly patients, the benzodiazepines that may be preferable include oxazepam, lorazepam, and temazepam. Triazolam may be used short term if the dosage is reduced by 50% from the usual dosage prescribed. Tirazolam use has been associated with anterograde amnesia. (For dosing information regarding anxiolytics, sedatives, and hypnotics, see Table 94.9.)

Buspirone, a nonbenzodiazepine anxiolytic, and zolpidem, a nonbenzodiazepine hypnotic, may be useful alternatives to the benzodiazepines in geriatric therapeutics. Buspirone does not require dosage alteration in the healthy elderly (61). Buspirone is most beneficial when

provided as a scheduled medication for 2 weeks or longer. Zolpidem has a rapid onset of action and short elimination half-life, reduces sleep latency, and prolongs the duration of sleep in patients with insomnia, yet it has no major effects on sleep stages with no evidence of withdrawal. The bioavailability, half-life, and peak concentrations are increased in the elderly; therefore, lower initial and maintenance doses are recommended.

Chloral hydrate is a cost-effective hypnotic agent for use in the geriatric patient; however, tolerance quickly develops in as little time as 1 week if the drug is used daily. Diphenhydramine is good for occasional use as a sedative in the geriatric patient, but the risk of anticholinergic delirium or worsening of the patient's cognitive state can occur if the drug is used too frequently, in excessive doses, or with other drugs that have anticholinergic activity.

Antipsychotic Agents

In the geriatric population, the antipsychotic agents are useful for treatment of psychoses and severe behavioral manifestations associated with dementia. Behavioral symptoms occurring with dementia include anxiety, agitation, aggression, paranoia, hallucinations, and combativeness. When these symptoms occur, they are disturbing to both the patient and the caregiver. Guidelines that are a part of the Omnibus Reconciliation Act (OBRA) require that prior to prescribing an antipsychotic agent for management of a dementia patient within a long-term care facility, the clinical record must contain (in addition to the diagnosis of dementia) both quantitative and qualitative documentation of associated psychotic and/or agitated behaviors that present a danger to the patient or to others. Inappropriate use of the antipsychotic agents in dementia patients includes use limited to the treatment of wandering, poor self-care, restlessness, impaired memory, anxiety, depression, insomnia, unsociability, indifference to surroundings, fidgeting, nervousness, uncooperativeness, or agitated behaviors that do not represent a danger to the resident or others. OBRA guidelines also require periodic (every 6 months) trial dosage reductions to determine the lowest effective dose for a particular patient (62).

The phenothiazines have prominent sedative, cardiovascular, anticholinergic, and neurologic side effects that are often manifested in the elderly patient; probably as a result of a decreased ability of the hepatic enzymes to metabolize the drugs to inactive metabolites and to altered receptor sensitivity. Nonphenothiazine antipsychotics are less sedating and cause less anticholinergic toxicity but can cause more neurologic adverse effects. Usual starting doses of antipsychotic agents are recommended at one-quarter to one-third those commonly prescribed for younger adults (see Table 94.10). The dosage should be gradually increased, according to the clinical response of the patient. Initially, drugs may be given in divided doses or a single

Table 94.9.
Anxiolytics, Sedatives, and Hypnotics (Oral Dosage Ranges)

	Adult	Geriatric
Benzodiazepine Anxiolytics		
Alprazolam	0.75–4 mg/d	0.25–0.75 mg/d
Chlordiazepoxide	15–100 mg/d	10–20 mg/d[a]
Chlorzaepate	15–60 mg/d	7.5–15 mg/d[a]
Diazepam	6–40 mg	1–5 mg[a]
Halazepam	60–160 mg/d	20–40 mg/d
Lorazepam	2–6 mg/d	0.5–2 mg/d
Oxazepam	30–120 mg/d	10–30 mg/d
Prazepam	20–60 mg/d	10–15 mg/d[a]
Benzodiazepine Sedative/Hypnotics		
Estalozam	1–2 mg	0.5–1 mg
Flurazepam	15–30 mg	15 mg[a]
Quazepam	7.5–15 mg	7.5 mg[a]
Temazepam	15–30 mg	15 mg
Triazolam	0.125–0.5 mg	0.0625–0.125 mg
Clonazepam	1.5–20 mg	0.5–1.5 mg
Other Anxiolytics and Sedatives		
Buspirone	15–60 mg/d	10–60 mg/d
Chloral hydrate	250–1000 mg/d	250 mg–500 mg/d
Diphenhydramine	25–200 mg/d	25–50 mg/d
Hydroxyzine	25–600 mg/d	10–50 mg/d
Zolpidem	5–20 mg/d	5–10 mg/d

[a]Not recommended for use in geriatric patients.

small dose with "as-needed orders" for repeating the dose to determine the lowest effective dose and to minimize side effects. Maximum doses should be approximately one-fourth those recommended in younger patients (Table 94.10).

Extrapyramidal symptoms have been shown to occur in up to 50% of all patients on antipsychotics between the ages of 60 and 80 years (63), and 90% of these reactions will occur within the first 10 weeks of therapy. These acute side effects can be minimized by using the lowest effective dose, or they may be treated with antiparkinson agents, such as benztropine or diphenhydramine. After 3 months of continuous therapy, most patients can be withdrawn from the antiparkinson agents without a recurrence of extrapyramidal symptoms. Antiparkinson agents should not be used prophylactically because the use of these agents may expose the patient to an increased risk of tardive dyskinesia and additional anticholinergic effects such as confusion and hallucinations. The incidence of tardive dyskinesia can be minimized by proper utilization of antiparkinson drugs by limiting the use of antipsychotic medications and by adjusting maintenance doses to the lowest effective levels.

Antidepressants

Depression is common among geriatric patients with the prevalence estimated between 5 and 43% (64). The diagnosis of depression should be made only after a thorough history and physical examination. The presentation of depression in an older patient may be atypical, presenting as cognitive impairment. The presence of iatrogenic depression should also be considered.

The heterocyclic antidepressants (amitriptyline, nortriptyline, imipramine, desipramine, doxepin, protriptyline, trimipramine, amoxapine, and maprotiline) are rarely considered drugs of first choice for treatment of depression in those geriatric patients who are not truly clinically depressed, those whose depression is long-standing and resistant to previous antidepressant therapy, and those with concomitant psychotic or delusional symptoms.

The selective serotonin reuptake inhibitors (SSRIs), which include fluoxetine, paroxetine, and sertraline, lack anticholinergic side effects and cardiotoxicity at therapeutic doses, and some clinicians favor their use in the elderly. However, these agents are more costly than the secondary amines (nortriptyline and desipramine) and can cause restlessness, anorexia, and sexual dysfunction. The SSRIs as a group are equally effective in treating depression in the elderly although their pharmacokinetic profiles differ. Sertraline may be the preferred choice because of good bioavailability, dual elimination pathways (hepatic and renal), 24-hour half-life allowing once-a-day dosing, no pharmacologically active metabolites, and low affinity for

Table 94.10.
Oral Antipsychotics Dosage Guidelines (mg/day)

	Adult (max)	Geriatric	Geriatric/Dementia (max)
Chlorpromazine	200–1600	800	400
Clozapine	50–600	450	a
Fluphenazine	5–40	20	10
Haloperidol	5–100	50	15
Loxapine	25–250	125	60
Mesoridazine	30–500	250	125
Molindone	25–225	115	55
Perphenazine	16–64	32	16
Promazine	40–1200	500	250
Risperidone	4–16	1–6	a
Thioridazine	200–800	400	200
Thiothixene	5–60	30	15
Trifluoperazine	10–80	40	20

aLimited clinical experience in this population.

the cytochrome P-450 enzyme system involved in many drug interactions. Weight loss and sleep patterns should be carefully monitored with the SSRIs.

In the treatment of depression, despiramine and nortriptyline are as efficacious as imipramine and amitriptyline, and they offer an important advantage of lessened anticholinergic, cardiovascular, and sedating side effects that is desirable in apathetic, withdrawn, or depressed elderly patients. For agitated, depressed patients, more sedating antidepressants, such as doxepin, or maprotiline may offer some advantage. Trazodone lacks anticholinergic side effects but is extremely sedating and can cause hypotension. It is recommended as an alternative antidepressant for elderly patients who have not responded to the SSRIs, desipramine, or nortriptyline (65).

Geriatric patients require lower initial doses and gradual titration of maintenance doses of the heterocyclic antidepressants because they metabolize and excrete these drugs more slowly. With nortriptyline, there are no changes in drug kinetics with age (66), but there is wide interpatient variability in drug dose, requiring careful titration and perhaps monitoring of plasma levels. Therapeutic plasma levels of imipramine, desipramine, and nortriptyline correlate with therapeutic effect. For nortriptyline, the therapeutic level in geriatric patients is between 50 and 150 ηg/ml, and for imipramine and desipramine, the therapeutic level should be at least 200 ηg/ml. Plasma levels can be used in selected patients as guidelines for dosing, and patient response should be closely monitored. The final dose depends on the clinical response and on the appearance and/or severity of side effects. The selection of an antidepressant agent for use in a geriatric patient should be based on the degree and frequency of side effects for a particular agent. (For recommended dosages of antidepressant agents, see Table 94.11.)

Table 94.11.
Antidepressants Oral Dosage Ranges (mg/day)

	Adult	Geriatric
Amitriptyline[a]	75–300	25–150
Amoxapine[a]	150–600	25–300
Bupropion	225–450	50–100
Desipramine[b]	75–300	10–100
Doxepin	75–300	10–75
Fluoxetine	20–80	10–40
Imipramine	75–300	10–150
Maprotiline	75–300	25–75
Nortriptyline[b]	75–300	10–75
Paroxetine[b]	20–50	10–30
Sertraline[b]	75–200	10–30
Trazodone	150–600	25–200
Trimipramine	75–300	25–100

[a]Not recommended for use in geriatric patients.
[b]Preferred agents in geriatric patients.

Analgesics

Geriatric patients are significantly more sensitive to the pain-relieving effect of narcotics because of alteration of receptors, changes in plasma protein binding, and prolonged clearance of these agents (67). These changes allow narcotics to be more effective in smaller doses when used in geriatric patients compared to younger patients. In the case of meperidine, there is a decrease in binding to red blood cells with increasing age, thereby increasing the amount of free drug available. This may result in a higher incidence of respiratory depression or, in the case of the active metabolite of meperidine, CNS stimulation (68). For these reasons, some clinicians do not recommend meperidine for geriatric patients. One study (69) demonstrated that in patients 70 years of age, the duration of pain relief at 4 hours was identical at doses of 8 mg and 16 mg of morphine although the incidence of side effects was higher in the high-dose group. The elderly, as a group, are more likely to develop narcotic side effects of constipation, respiratory depression, cough suppression, and clouding of mental functions. These side effects may occur at lower doses than in younger patients. Pentazocine is not a good analgesic choice in older patients due to a higher incidence of CNS side effects such as visual hallucinations, confusion, disorientation, and seizures. The adverse side effect of constipation can be serious in the elderly patient, and it can be prevented or treated by minimizing the narcotic dose or frequency of administration, using a high-bulk diet, or increasing the amount of fluid intake, and increasing activity level. Laxatives may be necessary for those patients receiving scheduled narcotics.

No evidence yet allows the choice use of one narcotic over another on the basis of age alone. The dosing of narcotic analgesics in the geriatric patient should be done by cautiously increasing the dose until the patient obtains pain relief for at least 4 hours. The dose should be administered prior to the pain occurring to avoid anticipatory anxiety and behavioral reinforcement of drug use, especially in terminally ill patients with chronic pain. Adjuvant analgesic relief may be provided by the use of tricyclic antidepressants or NSAIDs.

Nonsteroidal Antiinflammatory Drugs (NSAIDs)

Increased blood levels of naproxen, diflunisal, and salicylate have been found in the elderly, presumably as a result of this decrease in albumin protein binding (70). Increased blood levels of NSAIDs may be partially responsible for the reported higher incidence of gastric bleeding from gastric ulceration in this population (71). The risk of upper GI bleeding and perforation may differ among the NSAIDs and appears to be dose related; the incidence was six times greater with the longer-acting piroxicam than with ibuprofen in a retrospective case-control study by the Boston Collaborative Drug Surveillance Program (72). Omeprazole has been shown to be more effective than ranitidine in healing NSAID-induced gastric ulcers (73).

In addition to age, other risk factors for NSAID-induced gastric bleeding and ulcerations include smoking, history of peptic ulcer, and concurrent use of corticosteroids or anticoagulants. If NSAID use must be continued in high-risk patients, misoprostol should be considered. Dosage reductions are indicated in patients over the age of 65 for naproxen, ketoprofen, and ketorolac, especially in the presence of liver or renal disease. Newer NSAIDs, like nabumetone and etodolac, are reportedly safer to use because they do not inhibit cytoprotective prostaglandin synthesis in the stomach tissue. The efficacy and safety of the newer agent nabumetone has been shown to be similar in elderly patients when compared with younger patients (74); however, two cases of nabumetone-induced GI bleeding in elderly patients with risk factors have been recently reported (75); thus, the risk is still present.

Caution must be exercised with long-term use of the NSAIDs in elderly patients with compromised renal function. The metabolites of most NSAIDs are eliminated via the kidney. A prerenal azotemia may result from an inhibition of prostaglandin synthesis causing a reduction in renal perfusion and blood volume, especially in the presence of diuretic therapy and CHF. Sulindac has been purported to be renal sparing and may be the drug of choice in patients with mild renal failure. Fenoprofen and mefenamic acid are contraindicated in patients with preexisting renal disease. Lower doses should be used, and renal function and electrolyte levels should be monitored.

H₂ Receptor Antagonists

The bioavailability of cimetidine increases with age (76), most likely because of decreased hepatic clearance. Cimetidine is a potent inhibitor of the hepatic microsomal

1820

oxidase enzyme system, which is the mechanism responsible for the high frequency of drug interactions occurring with this agent. The decreased enzyme efficiency results in higher plasma levels of cimetidine, which may be a contributing factor to a higher rate of mental confusion in the elderly patient. The symptoms of mental confusion may range from agitation to paranoia or delusions and are usually reversible on discontinuation of the offending agent. The recommended oral dose of cimetidine should be reduced by 33 to 50%, especially in the presence of liver and/or renal impairment.

Ranitidine undergoes variable metabolism as well renal excretion of the unchanged parent drug. One study (77) reported an increase in the plasma concentration of ranitidine in the elderly that could lead to similar side effects, such as confusion, as seen with cimetidine. With renal dysfunction, a 150 mg daily dose may be sufficient for both active treatment and prophylaxis of ulceration. Because of its different chemical structure, fewer drug interactions are reported with ranitidine than with cimetidine. The efficacy as measured by ulcer healing and relapse rates, as well as incidence of side effects, is the same in elderly as in younger patients (78). Famotidine requires dose or interval adjustment only in severe renal impairment (79), and nizatidine appears to be handled much like ranitidine.

PREVENTIVE CARE

Mortality from pneumococcal pneumonia and influenza epidemics is very high in the elderly. Elderly patients show a comparable response to antibody formation to the polyvalent pneumococcal vaccine as that of a younger population (80). Revaccination of high-risk geriatric patients should be considered, primarily in the presence of low pneumococcal antibody levels. Routine revaccination is not recommended because of a higher incidence of local and systemic reactions. A favorable antibody response is likewise elicited from an annual influenza vaccine, with an efficacy of 70 to 80% against the influenza strains of the season. It usually takes 4 to 8 weeks to elicit a full antibody response, so vaccinations must be made in advance of the anticipated flu season. The majority of elderly patients with chronic disease should be immunized with a documented dose of polyvalent pneumococcal vaccine and an annual influenza vaccine.

During the first 48 hours of symptoms in a flu epidemic, high-risk, nonimmunized elderly patients may be given chemoprophylaxis with amantadine or ramantadine, and even symptomatic immunized elderly patients may benefit from treatment. Chemoprophylaxis will protect only against influenza A, which is responsible for 80% of all cases. CNS side effects such as hallucinations are common with amantadine, especially in patients with reduced renal function.

DRUG REGIMEN REVIEWS IN LONG-TERM CARE FACILITIES

Federal regulations that were implemented in 1974 and expanded under the Omnibus Reconciliation Act (OBRA) in 1987 require (1) pharmacists to provide monthly drug regimen reviews for all residents of long-term care facilities; (2) the physician and nursing staff to be made aware of any medication-related problems that are identified by the pharmacist; and (3) the nurse and/or physician to respond to the pharmacist-initiated comments. These monthly drug regimen reviews serve to identify potential medication-related problems for residents of long-term care facilities. These reviews have been shown to decrease polypharmacy, minimize duplicate drug therapy, prevent drug interactions, reduce inappropriate drug use, ensure appropriate monitoring of drug therapy, and reduce drug costs (81, 82).

Above all, communication should be encouraged among those involved in patient care—the patient, the physician, and the pharmacist. Indications and realistic goals of drug therapy must be clearly identified in the patient medical record for the purpose of achieving definite outcomes that improve a patient's quality of life. The professional responsibilities of the pharmacist must be expanded to include assuring the appropriate use of each drug prescribed and monitoring for its efficacy and toxicity. Drugs of choice and dosage adjustments must be individualized for each geriatric patient.

To minimize drug interactions and serious adverse reactions causing costly and unnecessary hospitalizations, the number of drugs on the patient profile should be minimized. The frequency of administration of PRN or as-needed drugs should be reviewed monthly and may provide clues to signs of drug toxicity; the necessity of these PRN drugs should be reassessed on a regular basis, such as quarterly.

CONCLUSION

Proper medication utilization by geriatric patients should include optimization of drug therapy to meet the patient's medical needs yet avoid drug-induced adverse effects, patient education to maximize patient adherence to drug therapy regimens, and regular review of the patient's drug therapy to screen for unnecessary or duplicate drug therapy. Above all, communication among the pharmacist, the physician, the nurse, the patient, and the patient's caregiver is of utmost importance to meeting the goal of therapy.

REFERENCES

1. Soldo BJ, Agree EM. Population Bulletin America's Elderly 1988. 43(3), Population Reference Bureau, Inc. Washington, District of Columbia, 1988.

2. Aging America Trends and Projections. Serial No. 101-E U.S. Government Printing Office, Washington, District of Columbia, 1989.

3. The Merck Manual of Geriatrics. MSD Research Laboratories, Rahway, New Jersey 193–203, 1993.

4. Anon. Drugs that cause psychiatric symptoms. Med Lett Drugs Ther 31(808):113–118, 1989.

5. Green LW, Mullen PD, Stainbrook GL. Programs to reduce drug errors in the elderly: direct and indirect evidence from patient education. J Ger Drug Ther 1:3–18, 1986.

6. Nolan L, O'Malley K. Prescribing for the elderly Part 1: sensitivity of the elderly to adverse drug reactions. J Am Ger Soc 36:142–149, 1988.

7. Gurwitz JH, Avorn J. The ambiguous relation between aging and adverse drug reactions. Ann Intern Med 114:956–966, 1991.

8. Gurwitz JH, Soumerai SB, Avorn J. Improving medication prescribing and utilization in the nursing home. J Am Ger Soc 38:542–552, 1990.

9. Ray WA, Federspiel CF, Schaffner W. A study of antipsychotic drug use in nursing homes: epidemiologic evidence suggesting misuse. Am J Pub Health 70:485–491, 1980.

10. Willcox SM, Himmelstein DU, Woolhandler S. Inappropriate drug prescribing for the community-dwelling elderly. JAMA 272:229–296, 1994.

11. Beers MH, Ouslander JG, Rollingher I, et al. Explicit criteria for determining inappropriate medication use in nursing homes. Arch Intern Med 151:1825–1832, 1991.

12. Schneider JK, Mion LC, Frengley JD. Adverse drug reactions in an elderly outpatient population. Am J Hosp Pharm 49(1):90–96, 1992.

13. Morrow D, Leirer V, Sheikh J. Adherence and medication instructions: review and recommendations. J Am Geriatr Soc 36:1147–1160, 1988.

14. Cooper JK, Love DW, Raffoul PR. Intentional prescription nonadherence (noncompliance) by the elderly. J Am Geriatr Soc 30:329–333, 1982.

15. Montamat SC, Cusack BJ, Vestal RE. Management of drug therapy in the elderly. N Engl J Med 321:303–309, 1989.

16. Miller SW, Strom JG. Drug-product selection: implications for the geriatric patient. The Consul Pharm 5:30–37, 1990.

17. Tuttle CB, Mayersohn M, Walker GC. Biological availability and urinary excretion of oral tolbutamide formulations in man. Can J Pharm Sci 8:31, 1974.

18. Kelly JG, McGarry K, O'Malley K, et al. Bioavailability of labetalol increases with age. Br J Clin Pharmacol 14:304–305, 1982.

19. Storstein L, Larsen A and Saevareid L. Pharmacokinetics of calcium channel blockers in patients with renal insufficiency and in geriatric patients. Acta Med Scandinavica 681(Suppl.1):25–30, 1984.

20. Janssen M, Dijkmans BA, Vandenbrouche JP, et al. Achlorhydria does not protect against benign upper gastrointestinal ulcers during NSAID use. Dig Dis Sci 39(2):362–365, 1994.

21. Hayes MJ, Langman MJS, Short AH. Changes in drug metabolism with increasing age. Br J Clin Pharmacol 2:73–79, 1975.

22. Mather LE, Tucker GT, Pflug AE, et al. Meperidine kinetics in man. Clin Pharmacol Ther 17:21–30, 1975.

23. Dawling S, Lynn K, Rosser R, Braithwaite R. Nortriptyline metabolism in chronic renal failure: metabolic elimination. Clin Pharm and Ther 32:322–329, 1982.

24. Abernathy DR, Greenblatt DJ, Shader RI. Imipramine and desipramine disposition in the elderly. J Pharm & Exp Ther 232:183–188, 1985.

25. Cohen BM, Sommer BR. Metabolism in thioridazine in the elderly. Journal Pharm Clinical Psychopharmacology 8:336–339, 1988.

26. Antal EJ, Kramer PA, Mercik SA, Chapron DJ, Lawson IR. Theophylline pharmacokinetics in advanced age. Brit J Clin Pharmacol 12:637–645, 1982.

27. Cockroft DW, Gault MH. Prediction of creatinine clearance from serum creatinine. Nephron 16:31–41, 1976.

28. Malmrose LC, Gray SL, Peiper CF, et al. Measured versus estimated creatinine clearance in a high-functioning elderly sample: MacArthur foundation study of successful aging. J Am Ger Soc 41:(7):715–721, 1993.

29. Smythe M, Hoffman J, Kizy K, et al. Estimating creatinine clearance in elderly patients with low serum creatinine concentrations. Am J Hosp Pharm 51:198–204, 1994.

30. Bressler R. Adverse drug reactions. In: Bressler R, Katz MD, eds. Geriatric Pharmacology. New York: McGraw Hill, 41–61, 1993.

31. Smith JM, Baldessarini RJ. Changes in prevalence, severity, and recovery in tardive dyskinesia with age. Arch Gen Psychiatry 37:1368–1373, 1980.

32. Gurwitz JH, Avorn J, Ross-Degnan D, et al. Aging and the anticoagulant response to warfarin therapy. Ann Int Med 116:901–904, 1992.

33. Jick H, Slone D, Borda IT, et al. Efficacy and toxicity of heparin in relation to age and sex. N Engl J Med 279:284–286, 1968.

34. Whitfield LR, Schentag JJ, Levy G. Relationship between concentration and anticoagulant effect of heparin in plasma of hospitalized patients: magnitude of predictability of interindividual differences. Clin Pharmacol Ther 32:503–516, 1982.

35. Feely J, Cloakley D. Altered pharmacodynamics in the elderly. Clin Geriatr Med 6(2)269–283, 1990.

36. Morley JE, Mooradian AD, Rosenthal MJ, et al. Diabetes mellitus in elderly patients, is it different? Am J Med 83:533–544, 1987.

37. Kradjan WA, Kobayashi KA, Bauer LA, et al. Glipizide pharmacokinetics: effects of age, diabetes and multiple dosing. J Clin Pharmacol 29:1121–1127, 1989.

38. Joint National Committee on Detection, Evaluation, and Treatment of High Blood Pressure. The Fifth Report of the Joint National Committee on Detection, Evaluation, and Treatment of High Blood Pressure (JNC V). Arch Intern Med 153:154–183, 1993.

39. Materson BJ, Reda DJ, Cushman WC, et al. Single-Drug Therapy for Hypertension in Men. New Engl J Med 328:914–921, 1993.

40. SHEP Cooperative Research Group. Prevention of stroke by antihypertensive drug treatment in older persons with isolated systolic hypertension. JAMA 265:3255–3264, 1991.

41. Castleden CM, George CF. The effect of aging on the hepatic clearance of propranolol. Br J Clin Pharmacol 7:49–54, 1979.

42. Abernethy DR, Schwartz JB, Plachetka JR, et al. Comparison in young and elderly patients of pharmacodynamics and disposition of labetalol in systemic hypertension. Am J Card 60(8):697–702, 1987.

43. Storstein L, Larsen A, Midtb K, et al. Pharmacokinetics of calcium blockers inpatients with renal insufficiency and in geriatric patients. Acta Med Scand 681(Suppl):25-30, 1984.

44. Pederson KE, Dorph-Pederson A, Hvidt S, et al. Digoxin-verapamil interaction. Clin Pharmacol Ther 30:311–316, 1981.

45. Abernethy DR, and Montamat SC. Acute and chronic studies of diltiazem in elderly versus young hypertensive patients. Am J Card 60(17):1161–1201, 1987.

46. Robertson DR, Waller DG, Renwick AG, et al. Age-related changes in the pharmacokinetics and pharmacodynamics of nifedipine. Br J Clin Pharmacol 25(3):297–305, 1988.

47. Scott M, Castleden CM, Adam HR, et al. The effect of aging on the disposition of nifedipine and atenolol. Br J Clin Pharmacol 25(3):289–296, 1988.

48. Forette F, McClaran J, Hervey, et al. Nicardipine in elderly patients with hypertension: a review of experience in France. Am Heart J 117(1):256–261, 1989.

49. Abernethy DR. An overview of the pharmacokinetics and pharmacodynamics of amlodipine in elderly persons with systemic hypertension. Am J Cardiol 73(3):10A–17A, 1994.

50. Baksi A, Edwards JS. Pharmacokinetics of nitrendipine in the elderly. J Cardiovasc Pharmacol 14S(10):S33–S35,S59–S62, 1989.

51. Zuzman RM. Renin and non-renin mediated antihypertensive actions of converting enzyme inhibitors. Kidney Int 25:969, 1984.

52. Lewis EJ, Hunsicker LG, Bain RP, et al. The effect of angiotensin-converting-enzyme inhibition on diabetic nephropathy. New Engl J Med. 329(20):1456–1462, 1993.

53. Heart failure: evaluation and care of patients with left ventricular dysfunction. Clinical practice guideline no. 11. Rockville, Maryland: Agency for Health Care Policy and Research, Public Health Service, U.S. Department of Health and Human Services, Jun 1994; AHCPR publication no. 94-0612.

54. Fleg JL, et al. Is digoxin really important in treatment of compensated heart failure? Am J Med 73:244, 1982.

55. Gheorghiade M, Beller GA. Effects of discontinuing maintenance digoxin therapy in patients with ischemic heart disease and congestive heart failure in sinus rhythm. Am J Cardiol 51:1243, 1983.

56. Ochs HR, Greenblatt DJ, Woo E, et al. Reduced quinidine clearance in elderly persons. Am J Cardiol 42:481–485, 1978.

57. Pfeifer HJ, Greenblatt DJ, Koch-Weser J. Clinical use and toxicity of intravenous lidocaine. Am Heart J 92:168–173, 1976.

58. Podrid P, Schoeneberger A, Lawn B. Congestive heart failure caused by oral disopyramide. N Engl J Med 302:614–617, 1980.

59. Stewart RB, May FE, Moore MT, Hale WE. Changing patterns of psychotropic drug use in the elderly: A five-year update. Drug Intell Clin Pharm 23:610–613, 1989.

60. Ray WA, Griffin MR and Dwney W. Benzodiazepines of long and short elimination half-life and the risk of hip fracture. JAMA 262:3303–3307, 1989.

61. Gammans RE, Westrick ML, Shea JP, et al. Pharmacokinetics of buspirone in elderly subjects. J Clin Pharmacol 29(1)72–78, 1989.

62. Federal Register 56(187):483, 1991.

63. Inoue F. Adverse reactions to antipsychotic drugs. Drug Intel Clin Pharm 13:198–207, 1979.

64. Abrams RC, Teresi JA, Butin DN. Depression in nursing home residents. Clin Ger Med 8:309–320, 1992.

65. Plotkin DA, Gerson SC, Jairrh LF. Antidepressant drug therapy in the elderly. In Meltzer HY (ed): Psychopharmacology: The third generation of progress. New York, Raven Press; 1149–1158, 1987.

66. Katz IR, Simpson GM, Jethanandani V. Steady state pharmacokinetics of nortriptyline in the frail elderly. Neuropharmacology 2(3):229–236, 1989.

67. Foley KM, Inturisi CE. Analgesic drug therapy in cancer pain: Principles and practice. Med Clin North Am 71:207, 1987.

68. Mather LE, Tucker GT, Pflug AE, et al. Meperidine kinetics in man. Clin Pharmacol Ther 17:21–30, 1975.

69. Kaiko RF, Wallenstein SL, Rogers AG, et al. Narcotics in the elderly. In: Reidenberg MM, ed. Med Clin North Am 66:1079–89, 1982.

70. Wallace SM, Verbeek RO. Plasma protein binding of drugs in the elderly. Clin Pharmacokinet 12:41–72, 1987.

71. Somerville K, Faulkner G, Langman M. Non-steroidal anti-inflammatory drugs and bleeding peptic ulcer. Lancet 1:462–464, 1986.

72. Rodriguez LAG, Jick H. Risk of upper gastrointestinal bleeding and perforation associated with individual non-steroidal anti-inflammatory drugs. Lancet 1994;343:769, 1989.

73. Walan A, Bader JP, Classen M, et al. Effect of omeprazole and ranitidine on ulcer healing and relapse rates in patients with benign gastric ulcer. New Engl J Med 320:69–75, 1989.

74. Morgan GJ, Poland M, DeLapp RE. Efficacy and safety of nabumetone versus diclofenac, naproxen, ibuprofen, and piroxicam in the elderly. Am J Med 95:P19S-27S, 1993.

75. Voss GS, Schweitzer P. GI bleeding associated with nabumetone. Am J Hosp Pharm 1994;51:2506-2507.

76. Redolfi A, Borgogelli E, Lodola E. Blood level of cimetidine in relation to age. Eur J Clin Pharmacol 15:257–261, 1979.

77. Greene DS, Szego PL, Anslow JA, et al. The effect of age on ranitidine pharmacokinetics. Clin Pharmacol Ther 39:300–305, 1986.

78. Mills R, Begun JM, Holland CE, et al. Ranitidine for duodenal ulcer disease in the elderly: a retrospective review of four multicenter trials. J Geriatr Soc 3(2):43–56, 1989.

79. Lin JH, Chremos AN, Yeh KL, et al. Effects of age and chronic renal failure on the urinary excretion kinetics of famotidine in man. Eur J Clin Pharmacol 34(1)41–46, 1988.

80. Ammann AJ, Schiffman G, Austrian R. The antibody responses to pneumococcal capsular polysaccharides in aged individuals. Proc Soc Exp Biol Med 164:321, 1980.

81. Kidder SW. Cost-benefit of pharmacist-conducted drug regimen reviews. Consult Pharm 1987;2:394–398.

82. Neel AB Jr, Pittman JC, Marasco RA, et al. Psychoactive drug use in Georgia nursing homes: effects of aggressive intervention. Consult Pharm 8:245–248, 1993.

83. Veterans Administration Cooperative Study on Antihypertensive Agents: Effects of treatment on morbidity in hypertension. III. Influence of age on diastolic pressure and prior cardiovascular disease; further analysis of side effects. Circulation 45:991–1004, 1972.

84. Management Committee. Treatment of Mild Hypertension in the elderly. Med J Aust 2:398–402, 1981.

85. O'Malley K, McCormack P, O'Brien ET. Isolated systolic hypertension: data from the European Working Party on High Blood Pressure in the Elderly. J Hypertension 6(Suppl):S105–S108, 1988.

86. Hypertension Detection and Follow-up Program Cooperative Group. The effect of treatment on mortality in "mild" hypertension: results of the Hypertension Detection and Follow-up Program. N Engl J Med 307:976–980, 1982.

87. Dahlof B, Lindholm LH, Hansson L, et al. Morbidity and Mortality in the Swedish Trial in Old Patients with Hypertension (STOP-Hypertension). Lancet 338:1281–1285, 1991.

88. SHEP Cooperative Research Group. Prevention of stroke by antihypertensive drug treatment in older persons with isolated systolic hypertension. Final results of the Systolic Hypertension in the Elderly Program (SHEP). JAMA 265:3255–3264, 1991.

CHAPTER 95

CRITICAL CARE THERAPY

BRADLEY A. BOUCHER and G. DENNIS CLIFTON

Critical care medicine is a multidisciplinary subspecialty that has realized remarkable growth over the last three decades, paralleling advances in life-support technologies. Individuals requiring intensive care unit (ICU) management include postoperative general surgical, cardiothoracic, and neurosurgical patients; victims of major trauma and burns; medical patients with acute respiratory failure and exacerbations of chronic diseases; and obstetrical and neonatal patients. A common feature among many of these patients is their complex pathophysiologic states and the use of a large number of pharmacologic agents in their management, many having a narrow therapeutic index. On average, these patients receive from seven to nine medications while being cared for in the ICU (1, 2). Table 95.1 lists categories of agents commonly administered to medical and surgical ICU patients. The thrust of this chapter will be to introduce the reader to the practice of critical care by outlining several general principles relevant to the care of ICU patients and highlighting the management of medical problems frequently encountered in the critically ill patient population.

USE OF THE PROBLEM-ORIENTED METHOD

Developing a problem list is an essential initial step in the process of formulating a treatment and monitoring plan for patients in general. Use of the problem-oriented approach is particularly important in the care of critically ill patients considering the relative complexities of their medical problems. Since these patients will frequently have multiorgan system involvement, it is strongly recommended that the critical care practitioner reflect on each respective organ system (e.g., central nervous system, pulmonary system, cardiovascular system) to determine whether or not a problem or potential problem amenable to pharmacologic therapy exists. In so doing, the formidable challenge of evaluating the critically ill patient as a whole will have been significantly simplified by breaking down their medical problems into more manageable pieces. Furthermore, the task of identifying appropriate monitoring parameters for treatment success or failure, including drug toxicity, will be much more easily accomplished. This latter task is aided substantially by the relative wealth of clinical and laboratory data available in critically ill patients for this purpose compared to other hospitalized patients and the ambulatory patient care environment. A more thorough discussion and examples of the problem-oriented method can be found in the companion workbook for this text.

PHARMACOKINETIC AND PHARMACODYNAMIC CONSIDERATIONS

Critically ill patients undergo a number of physiologic changes during periods of acute stress that have the potential to dramatically affect drug disposition and/or response in these patients relative to more stable patients or volunteers. Among these changes is a surge in catecholamines commonly observed in critically ill patients that can have significant effects on cardiac output (CO) and systemic vascular resistance (SVR). These effects in turn may result in increases or decreases in drug delivery to the kidneys and liver by altering renal and hepatic blood flow, respectively. Mechanical ventilation (MV) settings, especially very high positive end expiratory pressure (PEEP) may also reduce hepatic blood flow. Another important hemodynamic alteration often observed in critically ill patients is hypotension accompanying various shock states (e.g., cardiogenic, hemorrhagic, septic, neurogenic, etc.). Prolonged hypotension may not only result in acute pharmacokinetic alterations but in end organ damage as well (e.g., acute renal failure, hepatic dysfunction, bowel ischemia, etc.). In severe cases of acute renal failure, patients may require dialysis in order to sustain homeostasis which is yet another important factor to consider relative to drug disposition.

A number of other factors besides hemodynamic alterations may affect drug disposition in critically ill patients. One of these factors is the release of cytokines during the acute phase response. Several recent in vitro and animal studies have provided evidence that many of the pro-inflammatory cytokines [e.g., interleukin-1 (IL-1), interleukin-6 (IL-6), and tumor necrosis factor (TNF)] decrease cytochrome P-450 enzyme concentrations and/or activity which could affect many drugs used in the critical care setting that undergo hepatic oxidative metabolism.(4) The potential for reversal of these changes by drugs that antagonize one or more of these mediators may need to be considered in the future. Critically ill patients are also

1824

Table 95.1.
Medications Commonly Administered in Medical and Surgical Intensive Care Units

Analgesics
Antiarrhythmics
Antibiotics
Anticoagulants
Antihypertensives/vasodilators
Antipyretics (acetaminophen/aspirin)
Anxiolytics/antipsychotics
Bronchodilators
Corticosteroids
Diuretics
Inotropes/vasopressors
Insulin
Stress ulcer prophylaxis (H_2 blockers/antacids/sucralfate)

susceptible to protein binding changes as an indirect consequence of acute stress. For example, during the acute phase response, patients typically become very catabolic which can result in profound hypoalbuminemia. This may cause significant reductions in the protein binding of acidic drugs. Other patients receiving highly protein bound, basic drugs (e.g., lidocaine) may have significant increases in protein binding accompanying dramatic rises in α_1-acid glycoprotein (AAG). The pharmacokinetic implications of these protein binding changes on the total and unbound drug concentrations will be largely determined by the clearance properties of the drug in question (i.e., high extraction vs. low extraction). Finally, considering the large number of medications administered to critically ill patients, the potential for pharmacokinetic and pharmacodynamic drug interactions increases substantially. While these interactions may be well tolerated in other patient populations, the critically ill patient may be particularly susceptible to any associated adverse effects due to their unstable physiologic state.

Figure 95.1 summarizes the wide array of variables that may potentially affect drug disposition and response in critically ill patients. Superimposed on these many variables is the dynamic nature of the critically ill patient. For example, pharmacokinetic parameter estimates at one point in time may be dramatically different from those obtained only a short time later in the patient's hospital course. Thus, critical care pharmacy practitioners facing the daunting task of designing treatment regimens and monitoring therapy in these individuals need to have a keen appreciation of these many factors. In addition, surveillance of the primary literature for pharmacokinetic and pharmacodynamic investigations of specific drugs in various critically ill patient subsets is of utmost importance. Despite the difficulty in conducting these investigations because of numerous confounding variables, an ever-increasing number of studies are being published each

year. Readers are directed to the textbook entitled *The Pharmacologic Approach to the Critically Ill Patient*, 3rd ed, which focuses on drug use in the critically ill, for a more comprehensive treatment of this topic (5).

DRUG ADMINISTRATION IN THE ICU

Individual patient care plans in critically ill patients should always include assessment of the most appropriate and cost-effective route of drug administration. All routes of drug administration, including intravenous (IV), intramuscular (IM), intraarterial, epidural, subcutaneous (SC), oral, sublingual, rectal, inhalation, and topical routes, are used in the ICU setting. The route of drug administration depends on available dosage forms, intended use of the agent, functionality and availability of the gut, duration of action, urgency of treatment, and the hemodynamic stability of the patient. The duration of action of cardiovascular-acting agents is especially important when dealing with hemodynamically unstable patients. In these patients, intravenous administration of short-acting cardiovascular agents is generally preferred. The rapidity by which the desired effect takes place is also an important variable in deciding the type and route of drug administration. For example, the pharmacologic management of hyperkalemia may be performed over a period of hours by oral administration of sodium polystyrene sulfonate or more rapidly with the intravenous administration of insulin or sodium bicarbonate.

Intravascular Drug Administration

Antimicrobials, inotropes, vasopressors, vasodilators, and analgesics administered to critically ill patients are most commonly administered intravenously. Additionally, the intravenous route is often used to administer nutrition, blood products, and fluid and electrolytes. Unfortunately, intravenous drug therapy in the ICU is often complicated by large numbers of concurrent drugs, limited sites of access, fluid restriction, and drug incompatibilities. These factors require critical care practitioners to be knowledgeable about many facets of intravenous therapy.

The number of intravenous medications that must be administered simultaneously often exceeds the available number of intravenous access sites. Consequently, it is essential that the chemical compatibility of agents mixed or infused together be known. Additionally, patient's fluid restriction often requires that drugs be mixed in the minimum amount of fluid possible. The manufacturers' package inserts, along with a variety of published references (6) and charts, are available to assist clinicians in determining the compatibility and stability of various agents. These publications provide useful guidelines but do not cover all possible combinations of specific drugs, their concentrations, routes, or conditions of administration. Clinicians must be cautious and generally should avoid mixing drugs together when no compatibility or stability data exist. The absence of visual changes when two drugs are admixed or when a single drug is highly concentrated does not ensure compatibility or stability. An additional consideration is whether the infusion device to be used is able to accurately deliver a highly concentrated solution.

Most intravenous solutions administered to critically ill patients are done through peripheral veins. Central venous administration of agents is used when pharmacologic agents or electrolytes may be damaging to peripheral veins or when peripheral venous access is limited or nonexistent. Vasopressor agents (e.g., norepinephrine, dopamine) should always be administered via a central vein. Peripheral venous administration of these agents is associated with the risk of ischemic necrosis and sloughing of superficial tissues if extravasation occurs (i.e., infiltration of the catheter and solution out of the vein and into the surrounding tissues). If extravasation occurs, the medication should be discontinued and the tubing disconnected from the catheter. Phentolamine 5 to 10 mg in 10 to 15 ml of saline solution should be infiltrated through the catheter and around the site using a tuberculin needle as soon as possible (6). Highly concentrated solutions of certain agents (e.g., potassium chloride) may also be very irritating and damaging to the peripheral vein.

A major concern for central venous catheters used for drug administration is the development of infection at the puncture site. This may lead to thrombophlebitis, venous thrombosis, embolism, or septicemia. Meticulous aseptic technique is essential for inserting and caring for the catheter. A sterile dressing should be applied to the puncture site and changed every 2 to 4 days. Ointments containing povidone iodine are widely recommended with the sterile dressing; however, there is no conclusive evidence documenting their efficacy. Conflicting recommendations exist regarding the frequency with which central venous catheters should be changed. Recent recommendations suggest that catheters be changed only when there is obvious infection at the puncture site or when there is severe sepsis or fever of unknown origin. Because of the potential consequences of losing a central venous access site, it is crucial that drug preparation and administration occur under strict aseptic technique. When possible, the infusion system should be completely closed; this is essential if it is used for intravenous nutrition. Blood sampling from the line, intravenous injections into the line, and the use of stopcocks with injection ports should be avoided. Intravenous fluids and any additives should be prepared in the pharmacy under aseptic conditions whenever possible.

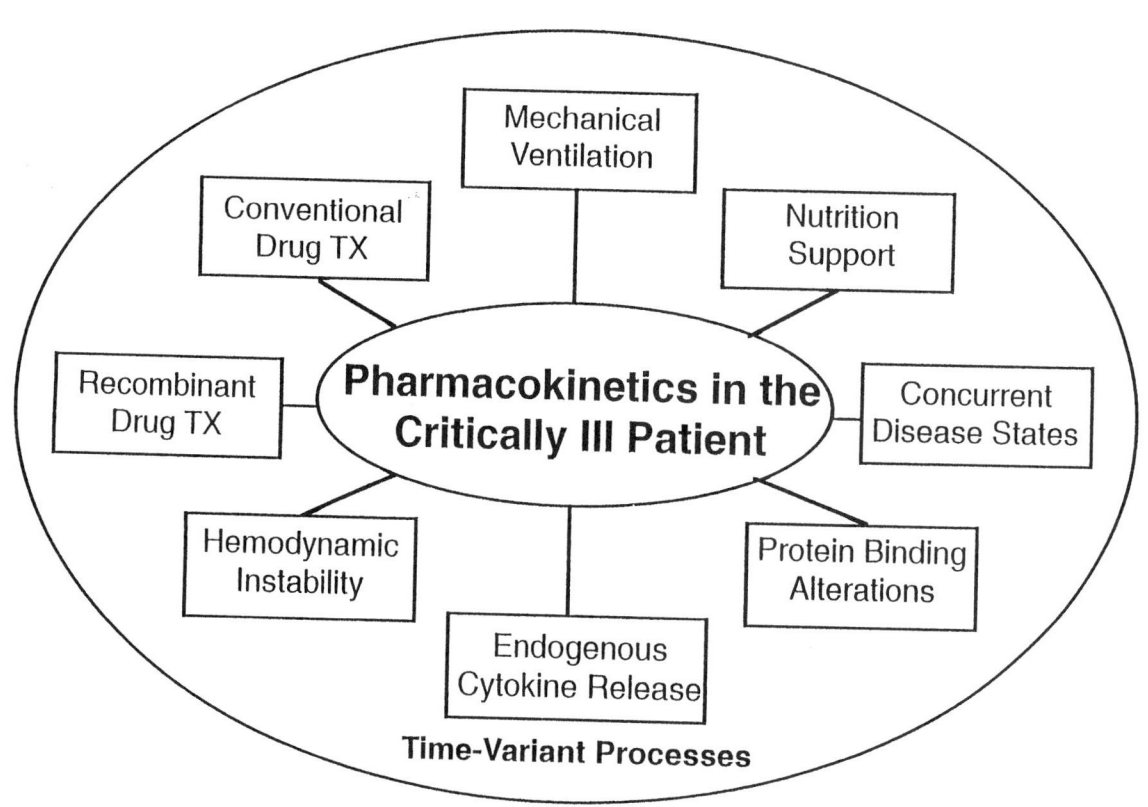

Figure 95.1. Potential factors affecting drug disposition in the critically ill patients. The possibility of temporal changes in these factors must also be considered secondary to the dynamic nature of this patient subset.

Central venous catheters may have one or more lumens. Multilumen catheters are advantageous in patients with limited insertion sites who require multiple infusions. Catheters vary in their likelihood to become thrombosed. Heparin-bonded or impregnated catheters are commercially available and decrease the incidence of thrombus formation. When a lumen is not being used, it may be filled or flushed with a heparin-containing solution and capped. Normal saline-containing heparin 0.5 to 2.0 units/ml is usually infused at a low rate (5 to 10 ml/hr) through each port to maintain catheter patency.

Occasionally, drugs may be administered directly into an artery. The most common indication for this route is for local administration of a drug. For example, thrombolytic agents may be infused through a catheter whose tip is placed near an arterial thrombus. The high pressures encountered in the arterial circulation necessitate administration of such agents via an infusion pump capable of operating under these conditions. A catheter for monitoring arterial blood pressure and obtaining arterial blood gasses is often placed in the radial or ulnar artery of critically ill patients. The patency of this catheter, or so-called "art line," is generally maintained with a slow-flowing heparinized solution (7). These lines should not be used for drug administration.

Epidural Drug Administration

Epidural administration of narcotics, particularly morphine, fentanyl, and hydromorphone, alone or in combination with local anesthetics such as bupivacaine, are very effective for the relief of acute pain. The analgesic agent(s) may be administered by continuous infusion with or without intermittent bolus doses. The incidence of pruritus, urinary retention, hypotension, vomiting, and sedation may be higher with this route of narcotic administration. Epidural analgesia is generally contraindicated in patients who have systemic infections, anticoagulant therapy, or a coagulopathy. Only preservative-free medications should be administered directly into the epidural space. Epidural doses range from 1 to 10 mg for morphine, 50 to 100 mcg for fentanyl, and 0.5 to 3 mg for hydromorphone.

Inhalational Drug Administration

The pulmonary route for local and systemic drug administration is frequently used in critically ill patients. Inhalation of beta-adrenergic and muscarinic bronchodilators, corticosteroids, mucolytics, and antibiotics are administered for their local effects in the lung. These agents, if commercially available, may be administered via metered dose inhalers (MDIs) or, alternatively, by ultrasonic or jet nebulization. The choice of technique also depends on the ability of the patient to cooperate or assist with treatment. Nebulization treatments are generally more time consuming, require the use of specialized equipment and personnel, and are more expensive (8). Nebulization treatments

and meter dose inhalers can also be used in patients that are intubated and mechanically ventilated. When meter dose inhalers are used to administer agents through the ventilator circuit, the deposition of drug in the lung may be decreased by as much as 50% compared to spontaneously breathing patients. When utilizing MDIs to administer drugs in mechanically ventilated patients, the normal dose should be doubled. Actuation of the MDI should occur at the beginning of the inspiratory phase. Holding chambers that attach to the ventilatory circuit may increase the amount of aerosol delivered to the lungs. If an in-line holding chamber is used, the inhaler should be actuated 1 to 2 seconds prior to the mechanical breath.

The administration of antimicrobials via inhalation to treat pneumonia is controversial. Agents most commonly administered in this manner include the aminoglycosides, polypeptides such as polymyxin B and colistin, amphotericin B, and pentamidine. Controlled trials of these agents for the treatment of pneumonia via this route conflict with regard to their clinical efficacy. Concerns over the selection of resistant organisms, and the ability of the agents to reach and/or penetrate the infected area of the lung, have limited the use of aerosolized antibiotics in critically ill patients. Nevertheless, select patient subsets may benefit from local antibiotic administration. Few guidelines exist with regard to the proper dose to use when administering antibiotics via inhalation, particularly through the ventilator circuit. Dosage regimens intended for inhalation should take into account that only 2 to 5% of aerosolized drug should be expected to be deposited in the lung of an intubated patient (9). Recently, various agents for the treatment of acute respiratory distress syndrome (ARDS) have also been administered via inhalation in mechanically ventilated patients. Specific examples include pulmonary surfactant and nitrous oxide.

Systemic administration of selective cardiovascular-acting agents via the endotracheal tube may be performed in emergency situations in which venous access has not yet been established. Agents in which endotracheal administration has proved to be effective include epinephrine, atropine, and lidocaine. When administered by this route, a catheter for drug administration should be advanced beyond the tip of the endotracheal tube. Two to two and a half times the normal dose should be administered followed by delivery of several quick breaths (10).

SPECIAL PROBLEMS IN THE CRITICALLY ILL PATIENT

Central Nervous System

PAIN AND ANXIETY

Two of the most common central nervous system (CNS) problems encountered in critically ill patients are acute pain and anxiety. Pain may be a consequence of direct trauma or medical and surgical procedures, or it may

Table 95.2.

Clinical Use of Selected Analgesics, Anxiolytics/Neuroleptics/Sedatives, and Skeletal Muscle Relaxants Commonly Used in Critically Ill Patients

Agent	Dose	Onset of Action	Duration of Activity
Analgesics			
Morphine	2–15 mg q 1–4 hr IV	5 min	4–5 hr
	5–30 mg/hr IV infusion	—	—
	5–10 mg q 4 hr IM/SC	10–30 min	4–7 hr
Meperidine	25–100 mg q 1–2 hr IV	5 min	2 hr
	25–100 mg q 2–4 hr IM	10–45 min	2–4 hr
Fentanyl	30–100 mcg/hr IV infusion	7–8 min	30–60 min
Anxiolytics/Neuroleptics			
Diazepam	2–20 mg q 1–4 hr IV	1–5 min	15–60 min
Lorazepam	1–4 mg q 1–6 hr IV	1–5 min	4 hr
Midazolam	1–25 mg/hr IV infusion	1–5 min	15 min–6 hr
Haloperidol	0.5–20 mg q 1–4 hr IV[a]	1 min	>24 hr
Propofol	5–50 mcg/kg/min IV infusion	<1 min	8–10 min
Skeletal Muscle Relaxants			
Pancuronium	0.06–0.1 mg/kg/hr IV	3–6 min	90–100 min
Vecuronium	0.1–0.2 mg/kg/hr IV	3–5 min	35–45 min
Atracurium	0.4–1.0 mg/kg/hr IV	2–4 min	25–35 min

[a]Not FDA approved

accompany underlying medical problems. Anxiety is often a result of fear, dependency, sleep deprivation, and unfamiliarity with the ICU environment in addition to pain. In extreme cases, these untoward feelings can progress to a state of depression, hallucinations, and paranoia sometimes referred to as ICU psychosis (11). In order to minimize suffering and emotional stress in ICU patients, it is imperative that adequate attention be given to pain relief, sedation, and management of anxiety. In general, the goal of analgesic therapy in these patients is to provide short-term symptomatic pain relief during the period of tissue healing. The tendency to undertreat acute pain has been highlighted in recent years (12). The most commonly used analgesics for acute pain within the ICU setting are parenteral opiate analgesics, most notably, morphine, meperidine, and fentanyl. Effective analgesic dosage requirements of these agents can vary tremendously, emphasizing the need for individualization of therapy while monitoring closely for adverse effects (13). The term *adverse effect* is a relative term, however, since sedation associated with the use of opiates is often an added benefit in the ICU setting. The benzodiazepines—diazepam, lorazepam, and midazolam—are the most commonly used anxiolytics or sedatives in ICU patients. Antihistamines such as diphenhydramine are also used occasionally as a sedative in the ICU. Parenteral haloperidol is another effective agent used to manage agitation, delirium, and psychosis in critically ill patients. Neuromuscular-blocking agents such as pancuronium, vecuronium, and atracurium are very important adjunctive agents in agitated patients requiring mechanical ventilation. These agents should be administered with sedative or anxiolytic therapy to prevent further emotional

distress during the paralysis period. Use of peripheral nerve stimulators for monitoring neuromuscular blockers is becoming increasingly more common in ICUs. Persistent paralysis on discontinuation is a growing concern with the use of neuromuscular-blocking agents in ICU patients (14). A relatively new drug used for short-term sedation in ICU patients is propofol. The overall role of this agent in the ICU setting is unclear at this time, especially considering its high cost (15). Table 95.2 summarizes dosing regimens, typical onset of action, and duration of activity for these selected agents.

HEAD INJURY, SPINAL CORD INJURY, AND STROKE

In contrast to the symptomatic problems of pain and anxiety frequently encountered in critically ill patients, CNS disorders that may result in ICU admission include traumatic brain injury, spinal cord injury, and stroke. Although all patients with acute neurotrauma or stroke will not require admission to an ICU, those with the most severe insults typically will require supportive care and intensive monitoring. Patients suspected of having a stroke, head injury, or SCI should undergo a thorough physical and neurologic examination along with a computerized tomography scan. The Glasgow Coma Scale (GCS) is the most widely used system to grade the arousal and functional capacity of the cerebral cortex in these patients. A GCS of 3–8, 9–12, and 13–14 is consistent with severe, moderate, and minor head injury, respectively (see Table 95.3). The possibility that ethanol, or drug intoxication, hypoglycemia, severe electrolyte disturbances, infection, hypoxia, hypotension, or spinal cord injury may alter the initial neurologic examination should always be considered. Thus,

Table 95.3.
Glasgow Coma Scale

	Response	Score
Eyes	Open spontaneously	4
	To verbal command	3
	To pain	2
	No response	1
Best Motor Response		
To verbal command	Obeys	6
To painful stimulus (pressure to nailbeds)	Localizes pain	5
	Flexion-withdrawal	4
	Flexion-abnormal (decorticate rigidity)	3
	Extension (decerebrate rigidity)	2
	No response	1
Best Verbal Response	Oriented and converses	5
(Arouse patient with painful stimulus if necessary)	Disoriented and converses	4
	Inappropriate words	3
	Incomprehensible sounds	2
	No response	1
	Total	3–15

initial laboratory tests for all patients with suspected neurologic injury should include a urine drug screen, blood ethanol concentration, complete blood count, electrolytes, glucose, BUN, and serum creatinine.

The initial management goal in these patients is to establish an adequate airway and maintain breathing and circulation during the initial period of evaluation (ABCs of resuscitation). Control of increased intracranial pressure (ICP) is also a priority in head injury patients considering its potential to decrease cerebral blood flow (CBF) and thus, cerebral oxygen delivery (CDO_2). Nonpharmacologic and pharmacologic approaches in managing increased ICP (i.e., more than 20 mm Hg) include hyperventilation; elevating the patient's head to 30°; moderate, controlled hypothermia (32° to 34° C); osmotic and loop diuretics; and barbiturate coma in refractory patients. (For a more extensive discussion of this topic, see (16).) Neurotrauma patients should generally be kept euvolemic with systemic blood pressure maintained in a normotensive range in an attempt to sustain CBF without exacerbating elevations in ICP. Patients with systemic hypertension should receive α-blockers, β-blockers, or angiotensin-converting enzyme inhibitors since they do not typically affect ICP. Use of sedatives (e.g., benzodiazepines, barbiturates) and opiate analgesics may also be effective in lowering transiently increased blood pressure. Use of the venodilators, nitroprusside and nitroglycerin, and selected calcium channel blockers (e.g., nicardipine, diltiazem) should be avoided since they may have the undesirable effect of increasing cerebral blood volume, thereby increasing ICP. In stroke patients, excepting hemorrhagic stroke, aggressive man-

agement of hypertension is generally not indicated unless the systolic or diastolic pressures exceed 220 mm Hg or 120 mm Hg, respectively.

By maintaining ventilation and CDO_2, further cerebral ischemia may be prevented or attenuated. This is of utmost importance since ischemia is thought to be the key pathophysiologic event in stroke, head injury, and SCI, triggering extension of the primary insult into uninjured tissue. Figure 95.2 outlines the postulated cascade of secondary biochemical and cellular events occurring following stroke and severe neurotrauma. In essence, cerebral ischemia results in cellular hypoxia and loss of cell membrane integrity. This in turn can lead to major intracellular and extracellular ionic shifts resulting in cytotoxic edema (with or without concurrent increased intracranial pressure), intracellular acidosis, electrical failure, and eventual generation of reactive oxygen species (e.g., oxygen free radicals). The importance of understanding the pathophysiology of secondary neuronal injury is readily apparent in light of the many promising pharmacologic strategies available or under investigation that attempt to modulate this destructive cascade of events. Early systemic and intraarterial thrombolytic therapy (e.g., alteplase) and heparinoids may be beneficial in directly reversing ischemia in selected stroke patients (17). Other strategies include high-dose corticosteroids, reactive oxygen metabolite scavengers, exogenous magnesium, NMDA receptor antagonists, calcium channel blockers, opiate antagonists, and nonsteroidal antiinflammatory drugs. Table 95.4 summarizes many of these strategies and their current status.

Unquestionably, the most significant breakthrough in the pharmacologic attenuation of secondary neuronal injury was the findings of the second National Acute Spinal Cord Injury Study (NASCIS 2) (18). In this multicenter study, SCI patients randomized to receive methylprednisolone 30 mg/kg intravenously over 15 minutes followed by a 5.4 mg/kg/hr infusion for 23 hours had a significant increase in motor and sensory function at 6 weeks and 6 months compared to placebo patients in those patients receiving therapy within *8 hours* post injury. Thus, *all* future SCI patients should receive methylprednisolone within this 8-hour treatment window since there is no alternative therapy of proven benefit at present to offer these patients.

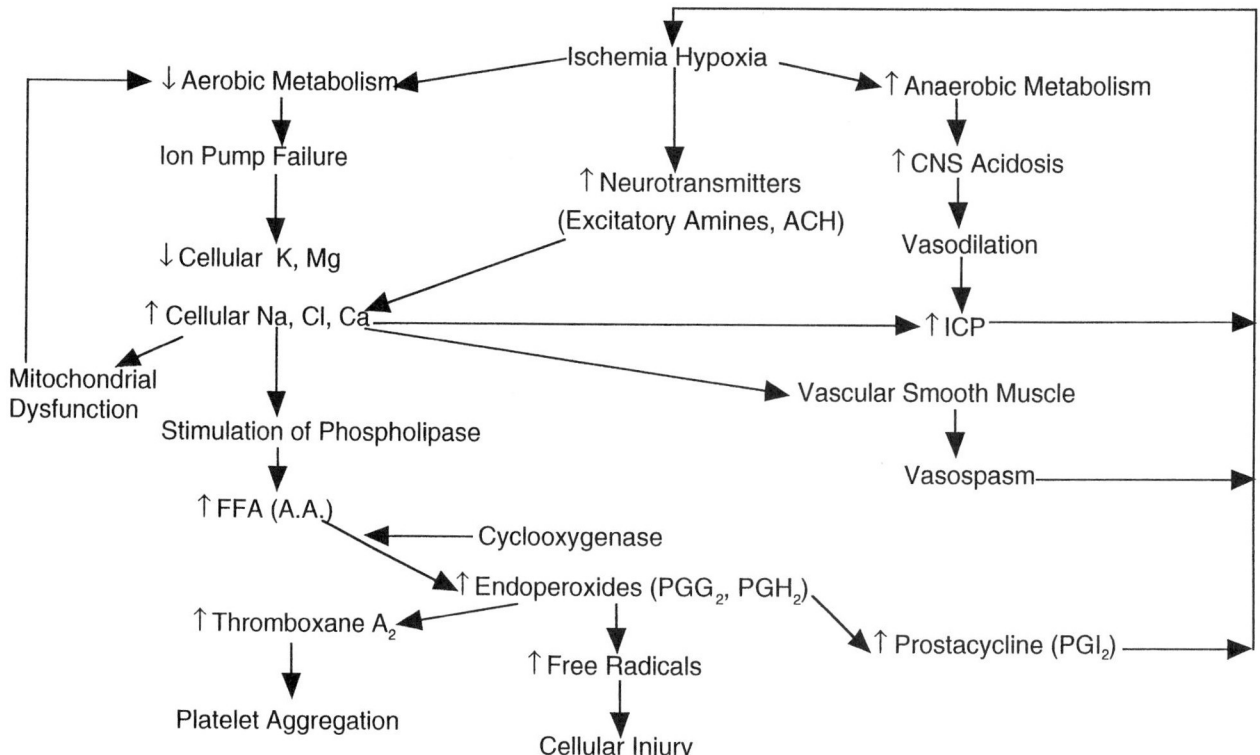

Figure 95.2. Schematic illustration of the complex cascade of biochemical events proposed to occur following severe neurotrauma. Selected abbreviations: ACH=acetylcholine, NMDA=N-methyl-D-aspartate, CCB=calcium channel blocker, FFA=free fatty acid, A.A.=arachidonic acid. (Adapted with permission from: Kirsch et al. Current concepts in brain resuscitation. Arch Intern Med 1986;146:1413–19).

Table 95.4.
Pharmacologic Attenuation of Secondary Neuronal Injury

Agent	Proposed Mechanism of Action	Injury Type°	Status†
Methylprednisolone (high dose)	Reactive oxygen metabolite scavenger	SCI	A
Tirilazad	Reactive oxygen metabolite scavenger	TBI, SCI, S	I
PEG-superoxide dismutase	Reactive oxygen metabolite scavenger	TBI	I
Vitamin E (α-tocopherol)	Reactive oxygen metabolite scavenger	TBI, SCI	I
Magnesium	Decrease intracellular calcium	TBI	A
NMDA receptor antagonists	Decrease intracellular calcium	TBI, SCI, S	I
Calcium channel blockers	Decrease intracellular calcium	TBI, SCI, S	A, I
Opiate antagonists	Endogenous opiate antagonism	SCI, S	A, I
Indomethacin	Antagonism of eicosanoid formation	SCI, TBI	A
Gangliosides	Repair of damaged neuronal tissue	SCI, S	I

°TBI = traumatic brain injury, SCI = spinal cord injury, S = stroke
†A = available for clinical use (may be off-label indication), I = investigational

SEIZURE TREATMENT AND PROPHYLAXIS

Seizures are caused by variety of conditions in ICU patients, including mechanical brain injury, cerebral hypoxia/ischemia, CNS infections, metabolic disorders, and chronic alcohol abuse (19). Of these conditions, seizures in patients with moderate to severe head injury are of particular concern since the seizure activity can greatly increase cerebral metabolism. Thus, head injury patients experiencing one or more seizures should receive initial therapy consisting of incremental intravenous doses of diazepam (5 to 40 mg) or lorazepam (2 to 8 mg) to terminate any active seizure activity followed by intravenous phenytoin to prevent seizure recurrence. In addition, prophylactic phenytoin should be considered in patients with mild to moderate injury based on a landmark study by Temkin in 1990 (20). Data from this study do not support the use of phenytoin beyond 7 days unless seizures are observed. Aggressive phenytoin therapy is recommended during the treatment period to maintain total concentrations in the range of 40 to 80 mmol/l (10 to 20 mg/l). This can generally be achieved using an adult intravenous-loading dose of 18 to 20 mg/kg followed by an initial adult daily maintenance dose of 2.5 to 3.0 mg/kg/day q12h. The potential for phenytoin's metabolism to increase as a function of time should also be considered in these patients. For a thorough discussion of managing nontrauma-related seizures, including status epilepticus, see Chapter 50.

Pulmonary System

MECHANICAL VENTILATION (MV)

A high percentage of critically ill patients are mechanically ventilated for a portion or all of their intensive care unit stay. The objectives of MV include improvement of pulmonary gas exchange, relief of respiratory distress, alteration of pressure-volume relationships (e.g., atelectasis, decreased compliance), and allowance of lung and airway healing. Basic MV settings include the fraction of inspired oxygen (FiO_2) (i.e., the percent of oxygen contained in the inhaled gas), tidal volume (usually 5 to 15 ml/kg), and ventilation rate. Because of the toxic effects of oxygen to the lung, the lowest FiO_2 that will achieve satisfactory arterial oxygenation (arterial oxygen pressure [PaO_2] of more than 60 mm Hg or arterial hemoglobin saturation [SaO_2] greater than 90%) is used. Another ventilator setting commonly adjusted is PEEP in order to maintain positive airway pressure throughout the respiratory cycle. The principal therapeutic effect of PEEP is to improve or maintain PaO_2 or SaO_2 while allowing a decline in FiO_2. Mechanical ventilation, particularly when high levels of PEEP are used, may lower cardiac output (CO), primarily as a result of decreased venous return. (For a more thorough discussion of MV therapy, see [21].)

Several important factors and variables should be considered and monitored by clinicians caring for patients who receive MV. Nosocomial pneumonia is a common complication of MV occurring in approximately 30% of patients. Nosocomial pneumonia in these patients is associated with a greater than twofold risk of mortality (22). If signs and symptoms of pneumonia appear, empiric antibiotic treatment aimed at the most likely pathogens (e.g., *Pseudomonas aeruginosa*, *Enterobacteriaceae*) should be promptly initiated. Other studies have suggested that MV may be an independent risk factor for the development of stress ulcers in critically ill patients. Mechanical ventilation can also be an uncomfortable and frightening experience. Although use of proper ventilatory settings and reassurance of the patient are the primary treatments for distress and agitation, medications are also frequently used, including analgesics, sedatives, and neuromuscular-blocking agents.

When weaning the patient from MV, a number of other factors should be considered to improve the patient's likelihood for successful extubation. These include adequate and proper nutrition (e.g., relatively high ratio of fat to carbohydrate calories) and correction of electrolyte disturbances, especially hypophosphatemia that could impair oxygen delivery and respiratory muscle function (23). Sedatives and narcotic analgesics should be used sparingly if at all when trying to wean patients from the ventilator. Optimization of bronchodilator therapy in patients with underlying obstructive or bronchospastic pulmonary disease may also aid in successful extubation of patients.

ACUTE RESPIRATORY DISTRESS SYNDROME

The acute (formerly adult) respiratory distress syndrome (ARDS) is a condition involving impaired oxygenation associated with bilateral pulmonary infiltrates on frontal chest radiograph and a pulmonary artery capillary wedge pressure (PCWP) of ≤18 mm Hg. Injury is characterized by diffuse alveolar damage, increased vascular permeability, and the development of noncardiogenic pulmonary edema. When damage is severe, the air spaces fill with fluid resulting in deterioration in gas exchange and mechanical properties of the lung (24). ARDS may result from direct lung injury such as gastric aspiration or inhalation of toxins, or indirectly from conditions such as bacterial sepsis or pancreatitis. The mortality rate associated with ARDS approaches 50%, with most patients dying from the underlying predisposing illness, severe sepsis, or multiorgan dysfunction. The current clinical management of ARDS involves primarily supportive measures aimed at maintaining gas exchange and oxygen delivery. No specific measures currently exist to correct the abnormalities associated with ARDS. Mechanical ventilation with PEEP is typically required for at least 10 to 14 days in most patients. Extracorporeal membrane oxygenation (ECMO) may be used when ventilation is ineffective in providing adequate blood oxygenation. Fluid management is also important since intravascular hydrostatic pressures may contribute to pulmonary edema. Therapy should be aimed at achieving the lowest PCWP while maintaining an adequate CO. If sepsis is presumed to be the cause of ARDS, empirical antibiotic therapy should be instituted early. The use of corticosteroids is controversial and probably should not be used early in treatment unless a significant number of eosinophils are found in the blood or bronchoalveolar lavage fluid. Some experts recommend a trial of corticosteroids beginning 1 to 2 weeks following the onset of ARDS in patients with severe disease and no sign of improvement. A variety of other antiinflammatory and vasodilatory agents have been investigated. Trials of agents such as nitric oxide, ketoconazole, and pulmonary surfactant in the treatment of ARDS are ongoing.

Cardiovascular System

PRINCIPLES OF OXYGEN DELIVERY AND CONSUMPTION

The primary goal of life-support techniques used in modern critical care units is to achieve and maintain optimal tissue oxygenation. Although traditional hemodynamic monitoring of pressures and flow are important for providing measures of tissue perfusion, they do not allow assessment of oxygenation. Several studies have shown that oxygen transport monitoring is superior to hemodynamic monitoring alone, particularly in high-risk critically ill patients (25, 26).

Oxygen demand depends on the overall rate of tissue metabolism and the intrinsic ability of tissues to extract oxygen. Generally, little can be done to alter oxygen demand. However, interventions aimed at reducing metabolic rate such as lowering body temperature, muscle paralysis, or sedation may modestly lower overall oxygen demand. Hence, most interventions are directed at improving the transportation of oxygen to tissues. The delivery of oxygen ($\dot{D}O_2$) to tissues is the product of cardiac index (CI) and arterial oxygen content (CaO_2). The actual amount of oxygen consumed at the tissue level (VO_2) may be calculated as the product of CI and the difference between CaO_2 and mixed venous oxygen content ($C\bar{v}O_2$). Arterial and venous oxygen content depend on the hemoglobin concentration, the percent oxygen saturation of arterial or mixed venous hemoglobin (SaO_2 or $S\bar{v}O_2$), and, to a minor extent, the amount of oxygen dissolved in plasma. The percentage of oxygen extracted by the tissues (O_2 ER) is calculated as ($CaO_2 - C\bar{v}O_2$) ÷ CaO_2. Oxygen transport variables, their calculation, and normal values are listed in Table 95.5. In addition to SaO_2, $S\bar{v}O_2$, CaO_2, $C\bar{v}O_2$, $\dot{D}O_2$, and VO_2, other clinical and laboratory parameters commonly used to monitor the adequacy of tissue oxygenation include arterial pH, total CO_2 content, lactic acid levels, blood pressure, heart rate, temperature, respiratory rate, urine output, and mental status.

In order to improve tissue oxygenation, oxygen delivery may be increased by altering CI and/or CaO_2. One approach to improving tissue oxygenation is outlined in Figure 95.3. Patients who are anemic, and subsequently have a low hemoglobin concentration, may benefit from transfusion of red blood cells. Commonly used methods to improve SaO_2 include increases in FiO_2 and PEEP. Improvements in CO can be achieved by assuring appropriate heart rate and stroke volume. Stroke volume depends on preload, afterload, and contractility. Pharmacologic therapies aimed at correcting these hemodynamic variables are addressed in other textbook chapters and include the use of fluids, vasodilators (e.g., nitroprusside), inotropes (e.g., dobutamine), and antiarrhythmics (including atropine, beta-blockers, and digoxin). The maneuver that will yield the greatest improvement in $\dot{D}O_2$ as determined by calculating their effect on oxygen transport variables is generally the one that should be used.

Table 95.5.
Oxygen Transport Variables, Normal and Goal Values

Parameter	Abbreviation	Calculation	Normal Value	Goal Value
Arterial Hgb saturation	SaO_2	Measured	95–99	>95
Mixed venous oxygen saturation	$S\bar{v}O_2$	Measured°	65–75%	>60
Arterial oxygen content	CaO_2	$(Hgb \times SaO_2 \times 1.34\dagger) + (PaO_2 \times 0.0031\ddagger)$	17–20 ml O_2/dl	
Venous oxygen content	$C\bar{v}O_2$	$(Hgb \times S\bar{v}O_2 \times 1.34) + (PvO_2 \times 0.00301)$	17–20 ml O_2/dl	
Oxygen delivery	$\dot{D}O_2$	$CI \times CaO_2 \times 10$	529–720 ml/min/m²	>550
Oxygen consumption	$\dot{V}O_2$	$(CaO_2 - C\bar{v}O_2) \times CI \times 10$	100–150 ml/min/m²	>167
Oxygen extraction ratio	O_2ER	$(CaO_2 - C\bar{v}O_2) \div CaO_2$	22–30%	<31%

Abbreviations: Hgb = hemoglobin (gm/dl), CI = cardiac index (l/min/m²), PaO_2 = arterial pressure of oxygen in blood (mm Hg), PvO_2 = venous pressure of oxygen in blood (mm Hg).
°Obtained from pulmonary artery blood.
†ml of O_2/l g Hgb.
‡Solubility coefficient of O_2 in plasma.

DETERMINANTS OF OXYGEN DELIVERY TO TISSUES
MEANS OF IMPROVING DELIVERY

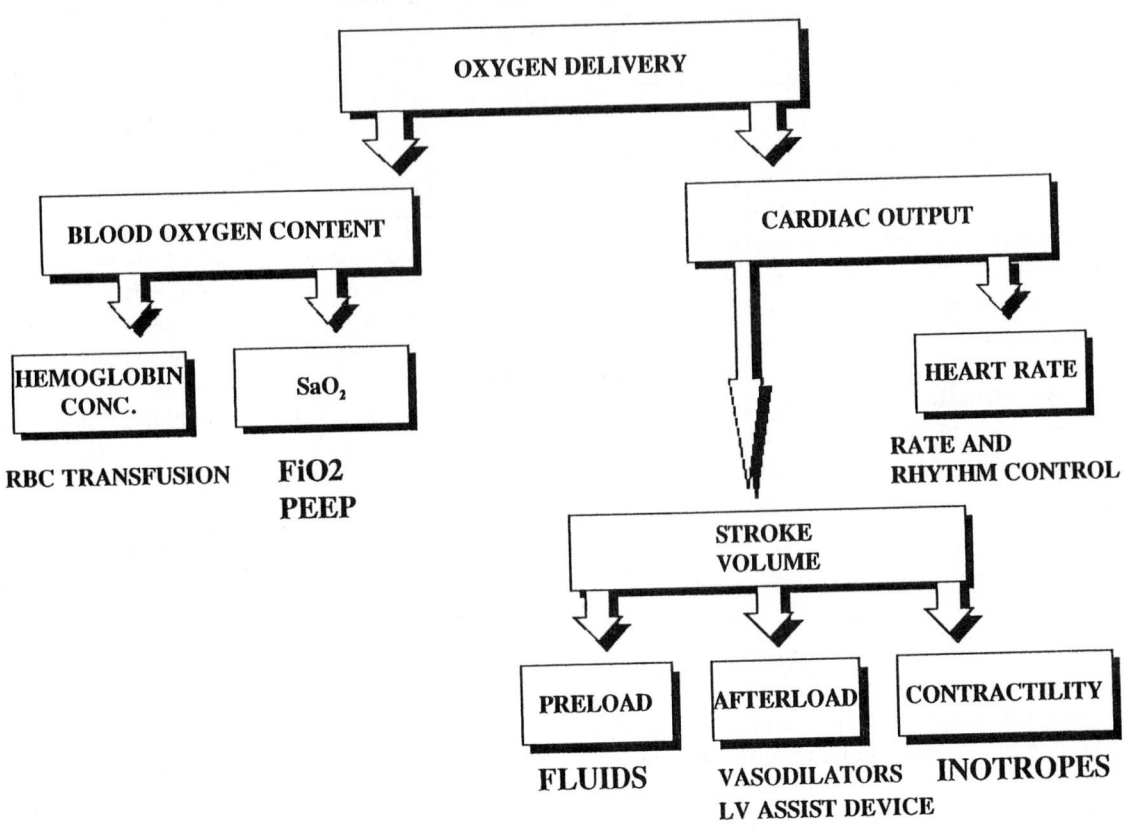

Figure 95.3.   Factors influencing oxygen delivery to tissues. Means of altering each factor for improved oxygen delivery are provided.

The drawbacks of oxygen transport monitoring, as described, are that it provides only an indication of global tissue oxygenation and may not detect regional or organ-specific mismatching of oxygen delivery and utilization. Tissue-specific markers of oxygen utilization, such as gastric intramucosal pH, have recently been developed and increasingly used to obtain evidence of regional adequacy of tissue oxygenation (27).

ACUTE MYOCARDIAL INFARCTION

The medical management of uncomplicated acute myocardial infarction (AMI) is well established and discussed in detail in Chapter 41. In the absence of contraindications, treatment with thrombolytics and aspirin should be initiated within 30 minutes of patient presentation to the hospital. Intravenous beta-adrenergic blocking agents should be administered as early as possible in the course of therapy, as should nitroglycerin. Intravenous or SC heparin should be initiated during alteplase therapy and immediately following streptokinase therapy. Oral beta-adrenergic blocking agents are ideally begun within hours of the intravenous drug and continued for at least 3 to 7 days. Oral angiotensin-converting enzyme inhibitors are indicated in patients with anterior myocardial infarctions, particularly those with ejection fractions less than 40%. Therapy is generally begun 1 to 3 days following the infarction and continued indefinitely to reduce left ventricular remodeling and development of congestive heart failure. Chronic therapy with beta-adrenergic blocking agents may also be indicated in those patients at high risk for recurrent infarction or sudden cardiac death.

CARDIOGENIC SHOCK

Cardiogenic shock can occur as a complication of AMI in 6 to 20% of survivors. A variety of other conditions such as acute myocarditis, sustained arrhythmia, and decompensation in patients with end-stage heart failure may also result in cardiogenic shock. Clinically, cardiogenic shock is defined as reduced CI (less than 2.2 $L/min/m^2$) and evidence of tissue hypoxia (i.e., O_2 ER more than 31%, oliguria, cyanosis, cool extremities, altered mentation) in the presence of adequate intravascular volume.

Specific treatment of cardiogenic shock is preceded by correcting problems of hypoxia, electrolyte abnormalities, acidosis, and restoring sinus rhythm (28). Restoration of adequate $\dot{D}O_2$ to tissues occurs primarily through improving myocardial systolic function (see Figure 95.3). Inotropic agents such as dobutamine and vasodilators such as sodium nitroprusside work to improve forward blood flow and reduce pulmonary edema. Dobutamine is preferred to dopamine and norepinephrine in cardiogenic shock; however, the latter two agents are useful in patients who are profoundly hypotensive. Sodium nitroprusside is particularly useful in reducing systemic vascular resistance (afterload), improving CI, and reducing myocardial $\dot{V}O_2$. Sodium nitroprusside and nitroglycerin also lower left ventricular filling pressures (preload), which helps reduce oxygen consumption. These agents may also improve $\dot{D}O_2$ by reducing pulmonary edema, improving gas exchange, and subsequently increasing blood oxygen content. Intraaortic balloon counterpulsation, which increases diastolic coronary filling and decreases afterload, is used in cardiogenic shock, especially in patients with high systemic vascular resistance but low blood pressures (i.e., systolic less than 90 mm Hg).

Cardiogenic shock secondary to right ventricular failure occurs less frequently and is a challenge to manage. Adequate filling pressures must be maintained since these patients are particularly sensitive to volume depletion. Dobutamine is used to increase right ventricular contractility and reduce pulmonary vascular resistance.

ACUTE CARDIAC ARRHYTHMIAS

Ventricular and supraventricular cardiac arrhythmias are frequently encountered in critically ill patients. The specific management of acute cardiac arrhythmias is covered in Chapter 39. When cardiac arrhythmias occur in critically ill patients, they are often precipitated by some other event or abnormality. Correctable causes of cardiac arrhythmias such as electrolyte abnormalities, hypoxia, acid–base disturbances, and drug toxicity should always be assessed and managed if present. Pharmacologic management of cardiac arrhythmias can generally be discontinued once the underlying abnormality is corrected or the precipitating factor removed.

HYPERTENSIVE EMERGENCIES AND URGENCIES

Immediate blood pressure reduction is necessary when hypertension is associated with symptoms or end-organ damage (hypertensive emergencies). Patients with hypertension associated with complications such as acute congestive heart failure, AMI, unstable angina, hypertensive encephalopathy, intracranial hemorrhage, dissecting aortic aneurysm, or eclampsia should be hospitalized and their blood pressure immediately lowered. Accelerated or malignant hypertension without severe symptoms or end-

organ involvement (hypertensive urgencies) should be controlled within 24 hours.

A variety of intravenous medications are available to treat hypertensive emergencies. Sodium nitroprusside and labetolol have proved to be especially effective and safe for lowering blood pressure in these situations. When hypertension is complicated by dissecting aortic aneurysm, sodium nitroprusside should be avoided and intravenous beta-adrenergic blockers, calcium channel blockers (verapamil or diltiazem), or trimethaphan camsylate used. Oral medications agents used to treat hypertensive urgencies include nifedipine, captopril, clonidine, and labetolol (29).

Renal System

Acute renal failure (ARF), defined as an abrupt decrease in the glomerular filtration rate (GFR), is a relatively common problem observed in critically ill patients. This is not surprising considering that shock, sepsis, and trauma are among the leading causes of ARF. A smaller number of patients will have exacerbation of their chronic renal failure (CRF) as the problem precipitating ICU admission or as a concurrent disease state accompanying an independent acute problem. Regardless of the circumstances, it is essential that the critical care practitioner be highly sensitized to the potential for renal insufficiency to be present or develop in ICU patients and adept at evaluating their level of renal impairment. In essence, not only may specific treatment be warranted for reversing the ARF or managing the complications of CRF, but major adjustments in drug dosing regimens, as well as fluid and electrolyte supplementation, may be needed. In addition, since critically ill patients are particularly susceptible to developing ARF, drugs that may induce renal failure should be identified and used cautiously. The most noteworthy of these agents are the aminoglycosides, amphotericin B, radiocontrast dye, cyclosporine, and nonsteroidal antiinflammatory drugs.

Key laboratory tests and monitoring parameters in patients diagnosed or suspected of having acute renal insufficiency include serum creatinine, blood urea nitrogen, urine sodium, urine osmolality, urinalysis, serum electrolytes, and urine output. Upon ruling out prerenal causes of ARF (e.g., dehydration, hemorrhage) and urinary obstruction, the primary goal of therapy should be to increase urinary output in oliguric patients since nonoliguric patients have fewer complications and improved survival. Drugs used for this purpose include mannitol 25 g intravenously repeated in 1 hour if no response, furosemide 100 mg intravenously followed by 250 mg intravenously in 1 hour if no response, and low-dose dopamine 1 to 5 mcg/kg/min (30). Restriction of fluid, dietary protein, and electrolytes, especially potassium, magnesium, and phosphorus, are also important in oliguric patients to maintain homeostasis. Treating the underlying cause of ARF such as antibiotics for infected patients and discontinuation of nephrotoxic drugs when feasible are additional considerations. General guidelines for dosage adjustments for renally eliminated drugs and/or active drug metabolites, including reference tables, can be found in Chapter 21. Nonetheless, a caveat to consider in applying these guidelines is that most equations used to estimate creatinine clearance (e.g., Cockroft and Gault) assume that the serum creatinine is at steady state. However, in ARF patients, serum creatinine may be rising rapidly. Thus, either special formulas that take this problem into account must be used (31) or an acknowledgment given that the estimates made using the conventional formulas may be significantly overestimating the creatinine clearance.

In contrast to the diagnosis of ARF, the presence of CRF will usually be identified during the patient history. When possible and appropriate, medications that the patient was receiving prior to admission should be continued as previously prescribed. Dosage adjustments for newly instituted medications should be made in a manner similar to adjustments in ARF patients although in this instance, the problem of rapidly changing serum creatinine values is usually irrelevant. In both ARF and CRF patients, dialysis therapy (i.e., hemodialysis, peritoneal dialysis, continuous arteriovenous hemodialysis) may be needed to maintain a homeostatic state. The effect of dialysis therapy on drug-dosing regimens and fluid and electrolyte supplementation is yet another important area for the critical care practitioner to understand in order to optimize care in these patients. A thorough discussion of this topic can be found in Chapter 22.

Gastrointestinal System

COLONIZATION OF THE GI TRACT AND NOSOCOMIAL INFECTIONS

It has been recognized since the early 1970s that critically ill patients are at risk to develop superficial gastroduodenal lesions that can result in major gastric bleeding if untreated. A thorough discussion of the pathophysiology and treatment alternatives can be found in Section 7. Appreciating the significant morbidity and mortality associated with major gastric hemorrhage, critically ill patients typically receive stress ulcer prophylaxis consisting of one of the following agents: antacids, H_2-antagonists, or sucralfate. In the late 1980s, however, the practice of arbitrarily choosing between these equally efficacious alternatives was called into question following a study by Driks et al., concluding that drugs raising the gastric pH (i.e., antacids and H_2-antagonists) were associated with a higher incidence of nosocomial pneumonia than sucralfate, a drug that has proved to be effective for this indication

without affecting gastric pH (32). The explanation offered for this phenomenon is that by raising the gastric pH, colonization of the stomach with Gram-negative bacteria will occur with subsequent retrograde migration of the bacteria to the lungs. Since that time, numerous other studies have been conducted to settle the ensuing controversy. A meta-analysis of these studies has suggested that though the results are equivocal, there does appear to be a higher incidence of associated nosocomial pneumonia with antacids and H_2-antagonists than with sucralfate (33). Nonetheless, both H_2-antagonists and sucralfate continue to be used extensively in critically ill patients for the prophylaxis of stress ulcers. More recently, this practice has also been questioned by some investigators arguing that many if not the majority of patients receive no benefit from these drugs (34). More studies are needed in specific ICU patient subsets to discern which critically ill patients are at greatest risk for major gastrointestinal bleeding before this practice can be advocated.

In addition to concern over bacterial colonization of the stomach secondary to stress ulcer prophylaxis therapy, the role of colonization of the oropharynx and gut relative to the development of nosocomial infections in critically ill patients, in general, continues to be a subject of investigation. In particular, the cost–benefit ratio of attempting to modulate the bacterial colonization process with local and systemic antimicrobials is a source of significant controversy. This strategy, known as selective digestive decontamination (SDD), typically involves placement of a polymyxin, tobramycin, and amphotericin B mixture into the mouth of critically ill patients as a paste and into the stomach as a solution via a nasogastric tube early in their hospital course. Intravenous antibiotics, most notably cefotaxime, are also occasionally administered. The overall goal of this empiric therapy is to block colonization of the GI tract with enteric, Gram-negative bacteria and fungi while sparing endogenous bacteria, thereby decreasing the incidence of nosocomial infections, especially nosocomial pneumonia. (For a summary of the numerous clinical investigations evaluating the effectiveness of SDDs, see references 35 and 36.) In general, the preponderance of evidence points to a benefit of SDD in preventing colonization and secondary nosocomial infection in critically ill patients. More equivocal is the effect of SDD in reducing mortality. Other remaining questions pertaining to this therapy are (1) the ideal SDD regimen (e.g., antimicrobial selection, inclusion of a parenteral antibiotic), (2) the identification of critically ill patients most likely to benefit from SDD, and (3) the pharmacoeconomic implications of SDD (25). Considering the many pharmaceutical issues related to SDD, including preparation of these extemporaneous mixtures, it behooves the critical care practitioner to be familiar with this therapy since it is the standard of care in many ICU settings throughout the world.

LIVER DYSFUNCTION

Liver dysfunction is a relatively common finding in critically ill patients. Some patients may have a history of severe chronic liver disease (e.g., alcoholic cirrhosis), whereas others may develop acute hepatic dysfunction secondary to direct trauma, infectious hepatitis, or following an ischemic insult (e.g., hemorrhagic shock). From a therapeutic standpoint, one of the most important considerations in evaluating these patients is the potential for alterations in drug metabolism. Alterations in the synthetic functions of the liver can also affect drug dosing and monitoring in these patients. For example, protein binding can be dramatically decreased for acidic, highly protein bound drugs secondary to hypoalbuminemia. Hyperbilirubinemia can result in protein binding displacement as well. The pharmacodynamic profile of certain drugs may also be altered such as anticoagulant drugs secondary to diminished clotting factor production and an increased sensitivity to CNS active drugs.

Acknowledging the potential for pharmacokinetic and pharmacodynamic alterations in critically ill patients with suspected liver disease, several challenges face critical care practitioners in designing therapeutic drug regimens for an individual patient. One issue is that few, if any, hepatic processes are performed at 100% capacity. Therefore, even though liver dysfunction may be present, the effects of this impairment on drug metabolism may be insignificant. The liver also has reparative properties allowing function to return after an acute insult. Finally, unlike creatinine clearance, which is a good estimate of the glomerular filtration rate in patients with renal dysfunction, no analogous predictor of hepatic function is available for clinical use in patients with liver disease. Laboratory tests that are useful in identifying liver disease but not necessarily the extent of damage are serum albumin, prothrombin time, bilirubin, and the "liver enzymes," aspartate aminotransferase (AST), alanine aminotransferase (ALT), and alkaline phosphatase (37). Thus, careful attention to signs and symptoms of severe liver impairment (e.g., CNS changes, hepatomegaly) in conjunction with these laboratory tests remains the most viable approach for assessing the level of residual hepatic function in a given patient. After making this assessment, tables summarizing the pharmacokinetic literature relative to the normal disposition pathway for a particular drug or citing specific clinical drug trial findings from patients with liver disease can be used as general guides for drug usage in those individuals deemed to have significant impairment (37). The possibility that induction and inhibition of hepatic enzymes may be modified is yet another consideration in these patients. The potential for drug-induced liver disease should also be evaluated in those critically ill patients with evidence of hepatic dysfunction to avoid exacerbation of the condition.

Hematologic System

Coagulation and hematologic disorders are common in the ICU population. Routine laboratory monitoring should include a daily complete blood count with platelets, activated partial thromboplastin time (APTT), and prothrombin time (PT). Commonly encountered hematologic problems include anemia, thrombocytopenia, and neutropenia. The recognition of anemia and its treatment is covered in Chapters 13 and 14. In the critical care setting, it is imperative that an adequate hematocrit and hemoglobin be maintained to ensure adequate tissue oxygenation. Transfusion of red blood cells in the form of whole blood or packed red blood cells may be necessary to provide sufficient oxygen-carrying capacity in the critically ill.

PLATELET DISORDERS

Thrombocytopenia is perhaps one of the most commonly encountered hematologic abnormalities in critically ill patients. As discussed in Chapter 15, a variety of factors exist that may be responsible for the reduction in platelets seen in this population. Heparin-induced thrombocytopenia should be considered, particularly if platelet counts begin to precipitously fall following several days of therapy (38). If suspected, heparin administration should be discontinued and removed from all flush solutions (e.g., arterial and pulmonary artery catheters). Low molecular weight heparins may be alternatives in patients suffering from thrombocytopenia due to unfractionated heparin products. Thrombocytopenia, secondary to sequestration, may also occur during extracorporeal circulation with procedures such as cardiopulmonary bypass or charcoal hemoperfusion.

Platelet dysfunction secondary to drugs and organ abnormalities such as renal failure and hepatic cirrhosis are also encountered in the critically ill. Prolonged bleeding times caused by renal failure have empirically been treated with conjugated estrogens and intravenous desmopressin at a dose of 0.3 mcg/kg. Cirrhosis-induced platelet dysfunction has also been treated with desmopressin.

DISSEMINATED INTRAVASCULAR COAGULOPATHY

Disseminated intravascular coagulopathy (DIC), as discussed in Chapter 15, is a common occurrence in critically ill patients, especially those with viral, fungal, or bacterial sepsis, severe tissue injury or ischemia, and ARDS. Microvascular thrombosis associated with DIC may lead to further end-organ damage, including focal skin necrosis, ARF, seizures, and stroke. The management of DIC includes the treatment of the underlying disease while providing supportive measures to maintain circulation and oxygenation. Transfusion of blood products and coagulation factors are frequently administered in patients who demonstrate clinical manifestations of DIC.

DEEP VENOUS THROMBOSIS

Critically ill patients, particularly those suffering major trauma, are at significant risk for the development of deep venous thrombosis (DVT) and the catastrophic occurrence of pulmonary embolism (39). Risk factors for the development of DVT include tissue injury secondary to trauma and surgery, immobilization, venous stasis, and cardiac dysfunction. Unless specific contraindications exist, all critically ill patients should receive DVT prophylaxis. Prophylaxis generally consists of SC heparin 5000 to 10,000 units every 8 to 12 hours. Compression stockings and intermittent compression boots are alternatives for DVT prophylaxis in patients with contraindications to heparin treatment.

Fluid and Electrolyte Disturbances

The homeostatic mechanisms that maintain normal electrolyte concentrations are often impaired in critically ill patients. In many instances, these abnormalities are a direct result of the patient's primary illness (e.g., hypokalemia with diabetic ketoacidosis), whereas in others the disturbance may be the result of secondary disorders or a consequence of therapy (e.g., diuretics). Proper correction of the electrolyte disorder depends on identification of its cause, estimation of the degree of abnormality, and selection of the appropriate replacement source. Electrolyte abnormalities most commonly observed in critically ill patients include decreased potassium, phosphate, magnesium and calcium, and increased potassium. The etiology of these electrolyte disorders and their manifestations in the stable patients are discussed in Chapter 9.

Hypokalemia (potassium less than 3.5 mmol/l) is one of the most common electrolyte abnormalities in the critically ill. Reductions in serum potassium may cause cardiac arrhythmias, skeletal muscle weakness, and respiratory paralysis if severe. Other relevant clinical features of hypokalemia in the critically ill include diminished pressor response to catecholamines, enhanced sensitivity to digitalis, diminished insulin activity, and impaired protein synthesis.

Treatment of hypokalemia involves correction of the underlying causes and potassium supplementation. Hypokalemia is often accompanied by other electrolyte abnormalities. Thus, serum sodium, phosphorus, magnesium, and calcium should be measured concurrently. Care should be taken not to restore potassium deficits too fast in order to prevent cardiac arrhythmias or hyperkalemia. When administered intravenously to critically ill patients, potassium should not be given faster than 40 meq/hr to avoid potentially life-threatening hyperkalemia. Guidelines for potassium administration and for other electrolytes are outlined in Table 95.6. Intravenous potassium should be administered into either a large peripheral vein or a central catheter in order to reduce the risk of sclerosis. If administering potassium through a central catheter, the tip of the catheter should not be in the atrium or ventricle to avoid localized hyperkalemia.

Hypophosphatemia (phosphorus less than 0.8 mmol/l [2.4 mg/dl]) can result from a variety of clinical disorders in the critically ill patient. Carbohydrate loading is the most common cause of hypophosphatemia in hospitalized patients and accounts for about half of all cases. Other causes of transcellular shifts in phosphorus are recovery from burns, acute alkalosis, alcoholism, diabetic ketoacidosis, severe sepsis, and recovery from malnutrition. Hypophosphatemia occurs in approximately 29% of all surgical patients and usually develops within 24 hours of surgery (40).

Severe hypophosphatemia may result in a variety of clinical conditions that affect almost every organ system in the body. Patients with serum phosphorus level near or below 0.32 mmol/l (1 mg/dl) may develop significant clinical manifestations such as respiratory insufficiency. This may prolong or prevent MV weaning especially in patients with underlying lung disease (23). Decreased phosphorus concentrations also cause a shift in the oxyhemoglobin dissociation curve to the left, which results in a greater affinity between oxygen and hemoglobin, thereby effectively reducing tissue DO_2. On rare occasions, patients can also develop cardiac insufficiency. Hematologic effects resulting from severe hypophosphatemia include hemolysis, platelet dysfunction, and leukocyte dysfunction as well as hemolytic anemia where serum phosphorus concentrations are extremely low (less than 0.16 mmol/l [0.5 mg/dl]). Muscle cell integrity is compromised at serum phosphorus concentrations of less than 0.32 mmol/l (1 mg/dl) and can result in rhabdomyolysis.

The exact amount of phosphorus necessary for adequate replacement therapy is unclear. Rapid phosphorus replacement with intravenous phosphorus products is probably required only in patients with serum phosphorus concentrations of less than 0.32 mmol/l (1 mg/dl); others should receive less aggressive replacement therapy. An exception might be the patient who has a serum phosphorus concentration of more than 0.32 mmol/l (1 mg/dl) but is symptomatic (41). Recommendations for administering intravenous phosphorus are outlined in Table 95.6.

Free, ionized calcium is the only physiologically active form of calcium. It is also the calcium fraction that is homeostatically regulated. Because serum calcium is highly protein bound, total serum calcium may not reflect ionic calcium concentrations. Equations to mathematically correct the total serum calcium concentration for alterations in circulating albumin have not proved to be satisfactory in the critically ill (42). Because of the multitude of factors that may alter the relationship between total and ionized serum calcium in this population, serum-ionized calcium concentrations should be measured.

Table 95.6.
Adult Electrolyte Infusion Guidelines for the ICU

Electrolyte	Recommended Infusion Rates	Maximum Concentration
Potassium chloride Injection: 2 meq/mL	Mild/asymptomatic hypokalemia (2–3.5 mmol/l) 10 meq/hr Moderate to severe hypokalemia (<2 mmol/l), symptomatic or ECG changes up to 40 meq/hr	PC = 60 meq/l CC = 80 meq/l (large volume parenterals)

Rates > 10 meq/hr require ECG monitoring, PC = peripheral venous catheter, CC = central venous catheter.

Electrolyte	Recommended Infusion Rates	Maximum Concentration
Potassium phosphate Injection: 3 mmol phosphate/ml and 4.4 meq potassium/ml	Mild hypophosphatemia (<0.64 mmol/l [2.4 mg/dl]): Recent/uncomplicated hypophosphatemia: 0.02 mmol/kg/hr, continue until serum phosphorus > 0.66 mmol/l (2.0 mg/dl)	6 mmol/100 ml (concentrations of 15 mmol/250 ml have been reported without apparent side effects)
Sodium phosphate Injection: 3 mmol phosphate/ml and 4.0 meq sodium/ml	Prolonged and multifactorial hypophosphatemia: 0.03 mmol/kg/hr, continue until serum phosphorus > 0.66 mmol/l (2.0 mg/dl) Moderate hypophosphatemia (0.17–0.32 mmol/l [0.5–1.0 mg/dl]): 0.06 mmol/kg/hr × 4 hrs Severe hypophosphatemia (<0.17 mmol/l [0.5 mg/dl]): 0.125 mmol/kg/hr × 4 hrs	

Dose based on ideal body weight, phosphorus serum concentrations should be checked every 6 hr during infusion and at the end of infusion.

Electrolyte	Recommended Infusion Rates	Maximum Concentration
Calcium chloride 10% Injection: 27 mg Ca^{++}/ml Calcium gluconate 10% Injection: 9 mg Ca^{++}/ml Calcium gluceptate 22% Injection: 18 mg Ca^{++}/ml	Asymptomatic hypocalcemia (ionized Ca^{++} < 1.12 mmol/l [2.24 meq/l]) 90–180 mg elemental Ca^{++} over 10 min Acute, symptomatic hypocalcemia: 90–180 mg elemental Ca^{++} over 10 min. Follow with 1.0–2.0 mg/kg hr for 6–12 hr	Calcium chloride 2% (1 gm in 50 ml D5W)

Gluconate and gluceptate salts less likely to cause thrombophlebitis.

Electrolyte	Recommended Infusion Rates	Maximum Concentration
Magnesium sulfate (50%) Injection: 49 mg Mg^{++}/ml Magnesium chloride (20%) Injection: 25.8 mg Mg^{++}/ml	Hypomagnesemia (<0.8 mmol/l [1.6 meq/ml]): 100–120 mg elemental Mg^{++} over 30 min Severe hypomagnesemia (< 0.5 mmol/l [1.0 meq/ml]): Loading: 600 mg elemental Mg^{++} over 3 hr Maintenance: 600–900 mg elemental Mg^{++}/24 hr	Dilute in > 10 ml D5W or 0.9% NaCl

If hypocalcemic, use chloride salt since sulfate may chelate Ca^{++} and further lower levels.

The more frequently encountered causes of low serum ionized calcium in the critically ill include renal failure, hypoparathyroidism, severe hypomagnesemia, hypermagnesemia, acute pancreatitis, rhabdomyolysis, tumor lysis syndrome, severe sepsis, fat embolism syndrome, burns, and toxic shock syndrome (43). Chelation of calcium may occur with rapid infusion of citrate-buffered blood. Ethylene glycol intoxication can produce hypocalcemia with widespread tissue deposition of calcium oxalate. The

clinical manifestations of hypocalcemia vary with the degree and rate of onset. An alkaline pH will increase binding of ionized calcium to albumin and increases the severity of symptoms. Cardiovascular manifestations are the most commonly encountered features of hypocalcemia seen in critically ill patients. Patients may develop hypotension, reversible heart failure, bradycardia, ventricular arrhythmias, and failure to respond to drugs that act through calcium-mediated mechanisms (e.g., catecholamines, digoxin, glucagon). The electrocardiogram (ECG) may show prolonged QT and ST interval, and T wave inversion.

Critically ill patients with suspected hypocalcemia should have a serum-ionized calcium measured along with serum phosphorus and magnesium. Symptomatic hypocalcemia should be treated as an emergency. Hypomagnesemia, if present, must be treated to correct hypocalcemia. Administration of calcium to hyperphosphatemic patients may cause calcium precipitation. Guidelines for the administration of calcium products depending on the severity of the disorder are shown in Table 95.6. Treatment is monitored by following disappearance of tetany or latent tetany, normalization of the ECG, and the patient's hemodynamic profile. Serum-ionized calcium, magnesium, phosphorus, potassium, and creatinine should be measured every 4 to 6 hours.

Magnesium depletion is a common clinical disorder but is frequently overlooked because of the multisystem problems and associated electrolyte disorders commonly seen in critically ill magnesium-deficient patients. Diffuse tubular abnormalities associated with postobstructive diuresis, the diuretic phase of ARF, and the period immediately after renal transplantation have also led to marked renal magnesium wasting and hypomagnesemia. Acute and chronic alcoholism, primarily secondary to poor intake and gastrointestinal losses, are also frequent causes of hypomagnesemia. Acute ethanol withdrawal, intravenous glucose therapy, and respiratory alkalosis may all lead to further reductions in serum magnesium levels (43). These reductions in serum magnesium, combined with hypokalemia, hypocalcemia, and metabolic alkalosis, may result in profound neurologic disturbances and contribute to the development of delirium tremens. Symptoms of magnesium depletion are generally not seen unless serum values are 0.25 to 0.38 mmol/l (0.5 to 0.75 meq/l) below the normal value 0.8 to 1.1 mmol/l (1.6 to 2.2 meq/l). Hypomagnesemia manifests clinically as alterations in neuromuscular, cardiovascular, and gastrointestinal function, and associated hypophosphatemia, hypocalcemia, and hypokalemia. Overt or severe hypomagnesemia should be treated with intravenous magnesium. Recommendations for dosing based on the degree of deficiency are given in Table 95.6. During therapy, patients require monitoring of serum magnesium level, neurologic status, respiration status, renal function, ECG, and blood pressure. Renal function should be checked prior to therapy since renal failure warrants markedly reduced therapeutic doses of magnesium.

Nutritional Support

Appropriate nutritional support enhances immune function, potentially reduces ICU days, and increases survival. Nutritional support of hospitalized patients is covered in Chapter 12. Enteral nutrition, particularly when administered postpylorically, can be given early in most critically ill patients and should be considered first-line therapy for those requiring nutritional support. Advantages of enteral nutrition in this population include a decreased rate of complications and mortality, lower cost, improved GI protection, and a lower infectious risk profile.

The selection of the specific route and formulation of the nutritional product will depend on the goals of nutritional support, caloric requirements, and the specific nutrients to be delivered. The determination and administration of caloric needs is paramount in critically ill patients. Underfeeding may result in impaired host defenses, delayed wound healing, muscle wasting, and prolonged weaning from MV. Overfeeding is associated with hepatic dysfunction, elevated blood urea nitrogen, fluid overload, and excessive carbon dioxide production. The commonly used Harris–Benedict equation is often inaccurate in critically ill patients, resulting in both under- and overprediction of caloric needs. The measurement of resting-energy expenditure by indirect calorimetry can be performed accurately in many critically ill patients and allow individualization of nutritional support.

Multiorgan Dysfunction Syndrome

During periods of acute stress, critically ill patients undergo a number of metabolic changes secondary to activation of the sympathetic nervous system and the hypothalamic-pituitary-adrenal axis. Specific mediators involved in the "acute phase response" include epinephrine, norepinephrine, cortisol, glucagon, proinflammatory cytokines such as IL-1, interleukin-2, interleukin-6 , and TNF (44). The net effect of this response is generally an acceleration of whole body metabolism proportional to the intensity of the initiating event or injury (45). If unchecked, the stress response can have pathologic consequences. Specifically, depletion of body stores of protein, fat, and carbohydrates, and/or defects in intracellular energy metabolism may contribute significantly to major organ dysfunction, including the lungs, heart, kidneys, gut, CNS, and immune system. Shock states, severe sepsis (see Chapter 76) and major trauma are other conditions that can set in motion an intense inflammatory response, known as the systemic inflammatory response syndrome (SIRS), by activating the aforementioned mediators, polymorphonuclear neutrophils (PMNs), macrophages, and the complement, kinin, and coagulation pathways that can result in organ dysfunction or failure (46). Relative tissue hypoxia and generation of reactive oxygen species may be key events in the pathogenesis of organ failure in these patients. When these pathophysiologic processes affect two or more major organs, it is referred to as the multiorgan dysfunction syndrome (MODS) (46). Regardless of the cause, MODS is a condition associated with significant morbidity and mortality in critically ill patients. Hence, intensive efforts are underway to identify strategies to prevent and/or attenuate its devastating effects.

Among the various approaches to modulate the systemic inflammatory response in critically ill patients is early and aggressive nutritional support. The goal of nutritional supplementation in this setting is to meet the increased energy and protein requirements typically present in these patients, and thus diminish NET catabolism of body tissue. Enhancement of anabolic processes is also possible. One example is administration of recombinant human growth hormone. Another exciting approach for modifying this cascade of events is through the use of monoclonal antibodies. These antibodies are typically directed at the mediators themselves (e.g., anti-TNF antibody) or at the receptor sites for the mediators (e.g., IL-1 receptor antagonist) (47). Antibodies to molecules responsible for endothelial cell adherence of PMNs during their migration following an inflammatory stimulus are also being developed to blunt their damaging effects. Despite the theoretical benefits of many of these biotechnologic products, a number of disappointing clinical investigations (e.g., antiendotoxin antibody) have dampened the initial enthusiasm generated relative to the overall impact they will have in altering the course of MODS. In essence, there still remains a tremendous amount to be learned about the complexities of the metabolic response to critical illness and injury. Thus, many promising drugs of today may be abandoned giving way to other agents as our understanding of these processes grows. Hence, the likelihood is still reasonably strong that eventually a drug or combination of drugs, effective in reversing or attenuating MODS in critically ill patients, will be identified.

PHARMACOECONOMIC CONSIDERATIONS IN CRITICAL CARE

Technological advances in medical science coupled with economic incentives over the past three decades have led to a tremendous increase in the quantity and quality of critical care therapy provided to severely ill patients. This type of care is very expensive. An estimated $62 billion of the approximate $809 billion the United States spent on health care during 1992 was allocated to reimburse charges incurred in the ICU. Intensive therapy has been reported to be 3.8 times more expensive than general ward care and to account for 20% of total hospital charges. Because of the high cost of ICU treatment, national debates over rising health care costs, and mechanisms for reimbursement, the cost-effectiveness of health care provided in this setting is under increasing scrutiny (48).

The introduction of new pharmacologic agents and an increased understanding of the properties and benefits of older agents have contributed significantly to the decrease in morbidity and mortality associated with critical illness. Considerable study has been devoted toward determining the clinical benefit of various and competing pharmacologic therapies. Unfortunately, efficacy can no longer be the sole criterion that determines whether or not a particular pharmacologic agent should be used in caring for patients. This is particularly true in the critical care setting where a patient's medication costs per day may reach into the thousands of dollars. A major question regarding the use of new and expensive agents, therefore, aside from their clinical efficacy, concerns their economic impact and added costs. If agents reduce morbidity and improve survival, any additional costs may be partially or completely obviated by reductions in other expenditures and/or improved quality of life. Rational use of new and expensive drugs will involve proper patient selection, treatment guidelines, drug use evaluation techniques, and outcome indicators. The performance of pharmacoeconomic and outcomes research by critical care practitioners is of paramount importance in the development of treatment guidelines and cost-effective use of drugs.

CONCLUSION

Medical management of the critically ill can be an intimidating and daunting task for those individuals unfamiliar with the special needs of this patient population. Nonetheless, by carefully delineating individual problems, identifying appropriate treatment regimens, and formulating a thoughtful monitoring plan, the complexity of caring for these patients can be vastly simplified. This chapter has attempted to highlight many of the problems frequently encountered in the ICU environment as a starting point in this effort. Although demanding and requiring a high level of commitment, for those individuals accepting the challenge of providing care for the critically ill, the rewards can be extremely gratifying both personally and professionally.

REFERENCES

1. Boucher BA, Kuhl DA, Coffey BC, Fabian TC. Drug use in a trauma intensive-care unit. Am J Hosp Pharm 47:805–810, 1990.
2. Smythe MA, Melendy S, Jahns B, Dmuchowski C. An exploratory analysis of medication utilization in a medical intensive care unit. Crit Care Med 21:1319–1323, 1993.
3. Majerus TC, Dasta JF. Practice of Critical Care Pharmacy. Rockville, MD: Aspen Systems, 1985.
4. Andus T, Bauer J, Gerok W. Effects of cytokines on the liver. Hepatology 13:364–375, 1991.
5. Chernow B. The Pharmacologic Approach to the Critically Ill Patient, ed. 3. Baltimore, Williams & Wilkins, 1994.
6. Trissel LA. Handbook on Injectable Drugs. Bethesda, MD. American Society of Hospital Pharmacists, 1992.
7. Clifton GD, Branson P, Kelly HJ, Dotson LR, Record KE, Phillips BA, Thompson JR. Comparison of normal saline and heparin solutions for maintenance of arterial catheter patency. Heart and Lung 20:115–118, 1991.

8. Summer W, Elston R, Tharpe L, et al. Aerosol bronchodilator delivery methods: Relative impact on pulmonary function and cost of respiratory care. Arch Intern Med 149:618–623, 1989.

9. MacIntyre NR, Silver RM, Miller CW, Schuler F, Coleman E. Aerosol delivery in intubated, mechanically ventilated patients. Crit Care Med 13:81–84, 1985.

10. Adult Advanced Cardiac Life Support. JAMA 268;2199–2241, 1992.

11. Cassem NH. Psychiatric problems of the critically ill patient. In: Shoemaker WS, Ayres S, Grenvik A, Holbrook PR, Thompson WL. Textbook of Critical Care Med, ed. 2. Philadelphia, W.B. Saunders Co., 1989:1404.

12. Agency for Health Care Policy and Research. Acute pain management: operative or medical procedures and trauma, part 1. Clin Pharm 11:309–331, 1992.

13. Stanley TH, Allen SJ, Bryan-Brown CW. Sleep, pain, and sedation. In: Shoemaker WS, Ayres S, Grenvik A, Holbrook PR, Thompson WL. Textbook of Critical Care Med, ed. 2. Philadelphia, W.B. Saunders Co., 1989:1155.

14. Hoyt JW. Persistent paralysis in critically ill patients after the use of neuromuscular blocking agents. New Horizons 2:48–55, 1994.

15. Smith I, White PF, Nathanson M, Gouldson R. Propofol. An update on its clinical use. Anesthesiology 81:1005–1043, 1994.

16. Boucher BA, Phelps SJ. Acute management of the head injury patient. In DiPiro JT, Talbert RL, Hayes PE, Yee GC, Matzke GR, Posey LM: Pharmacotherapy: A Pathophysiologic Approach, ed. 2. New York, Elsevier, 1992:904.

17. Camarata PJ, Heos RC, Latchaw RE. "Brain attack": the rationale for treating stroke as a medical emergency. Neurosurgery 34:144–158, 1994.

18. Bracken MB, Shepard MJ, Collins WF Jr, et al. A randomized, controlled trial of methylprednisolone or naloxone in the treatment of acute spinal cord injury. Results of the second National Acute Spinal Cord Injury Study. N Engl J Med 322:1405–1411, 1990.

19. Litt B, Krauss. Pharmacologic approach to acute seizures and antiepileptic drugs. In Chernow B: The Pharmacologic Approach to the Critically Ill Patient, ed. 3. Baltimore, Williams & Wilkins, 1994:484.

20. Temkin NR, Dikmen SS, Wilensky AJ, et al. A randomized, double-blind study of phenytoin for the prevention of post-traumatic seizures. N Engl J Med 323:497–502, 1990.

21. Tobin MJ. Mechanical ventilation. N Engl J Med 330:1056–1061, 1994.

22. Fagon JY, Chastre J, Domart Y, et al. Nosocomial pneumonia in patients receiving continuous mechanical ventilation: prospective analysis of 52 episodes with use of a protected specimen brush and quantitative culture techniques. Am Rev Respir Dis 139:877–884, 1989.

23. Agusti AG, Torres A, Estopa R, Agustividal A. Hypophosphatemia as a cause of failed weaning; the importance of metabolic factors. Crit Care Med 12:142–143, 1984.

24. Kollef MH, Schuster DP. The acute respiratory distress syndrome. N Engl J Med 332:27–36, 1995.

25. Shoemaker WC, Appel PL, Kram HB. Oxygen transport measurements to evaluate tissue perfusion and titrate therapy: dobutamine and dopamine effects. Crit Care Med 19:672–688, 1991.

26. Teboul JL, Graini L, Boujdaria R, Berton C, Richard C. Cardia index vs oxygen-derived parameters for rational use of dobutamine in patients with congestive heart failure. Chest 103:81–85, 1993.

27. Maynard N, Bihari D, Beale R, et al. Assessment of splanchnic oxygenation by gastric tonometry in patients with acute circulatory failure. JAMA 270:1203–1210, 1993.

28. Califf RM, Bengtson JR. Cardiogenic shock. N Engl J Med 330:1724–1730, 1994.

29. Joint National Committee on Detection Evaluation, and Treatment of High Blood Pressure. The Fifth Report of the Joint National Committee on Detection, Evaluation, and Treatment of High Blood Pressure (JNC V). Arch Intern Med 153:154–183, 1993.

30. Heim-Duthoy KL, Kalil RS, Kasiske BL. Acute renal failure. In: DiPiro JT, Talbert RL, Hayes PE, Yee GC, Matzke GR, Posey LM. Pharmacotherapy: A Pathophysiologic Approach, ed. 2. New York, Elsevier, 1992:660.

31. Lott RS, Hayton WL. Estimation of creatinine clearance from serum creatinine concentration—a review. Drug Intell Clin Pharm 12:140–150, 1978.

32. Driks MR, Craven DE, Celli BR, et al. Nosocomial pneumonia in intubated patients given sucralfate as compared with antacids or histamine type 2 blockers. New Engl J Med 317:1376–1382, 1987.

33. Cook DJ, Laine LA, Guyatt GH, Raffin TA. Nosocomial pneumonia and the role of gastric pH. A meta-analysis. Chest 100:7–13, 1991.

34. Cook DJ, Fuller HD, Guyatt GH, et al. Risk factors for gastrointestinal bleeding in critically ill patients. New Engl J Med 330:377–381, 1994.

35. Lockrem JD, Stoller JK. Selective digestive decontamination in the intensive care unit. In Chernow B: The Pharmacologic Approach to the Critically Ill Patient, ed. 3. Baltimore: Williams & Wilkins, 1994:1122.

36. van Saene HKF, Stoutenbeek CP, Stoller JK. Selective decontamination of the digestive tract (SDD) in the ICU: current status and future prospects. Crit Care Med 20:691–703, 1992.

37. Kubisty CA, Arns PA, Wedlund PJ, Branch RA. Adjustment of medications in liver failure. In: Chernow B. The Pharmacologic Approach to the Critically Ill Patient, ed. 3. Baltimore: Williams & Wilkins, 1994:95.

38. Clines DB, Kaywin P, Bina M, Tomaski A, Schreiber AD. Heparin-associated thrombocytopenia. N Engl J Med 303:788–795, 1980.

39. Geerts WH, Code KI, Jay RM, Chen E, Szalai JP. A prospective study of venous thromboembolism after major trauma. N Engl J Med 331:1601–1606, 1994.

40. Swaminathan R, Bradley P, Morgan DB, Hill GI. Hypophosphatemia in surgical patients. Surg Gynecol Obstet 148:448–454, 1979.

41. Kingston M, Al-Siba'I MB. Treatment of severe hypophosphatemia. Crit Care Med 13:16–18, 1985.

42. Zaloga GP, Chernow B, Cook D, et al. Assessment of calcium homeostasis in the critically ill patient. The diagnostic pitfalls of the McLean Hastings Nomogram. Ann Surg 202:587–594, 1985.

43. Zaloga GP, Chernow B. Divalent ions: calcium, magnesium, and phosphorus. In: Chernow B. The Pharmacologic Approach to the Critically Ill Patient, 3rd ed. Baltimore: Maryland, Williams & Wilkins, 1994:777.

44. Michelson D, Gold PW, Sternberg EM. The stress response to critical illness. New Horizons 2:426–431, 1994.

45. Bessey PQ, Downey RS, Monafo WW. Metabolic response to injury and critical illness. In: Civetta JM, Taylor RW, Kirby RR. Critical Care, ed. 2. Philadelphia: J.B. Lippincott Co, 1992:527.

46. ACCP/SCCM Consensus Conference Committee. Definitions for sepsis and organ failure and guidelines for the use of innovative therapies in sepsis. Chest 101:1644–1655, 1992.

47. Shapiro L, Gelfand JA. Cytokines and sepsis: pathophysiology and therapy. New Horizons 1:13–22, 1993.

48. Clifton GD, Blumenschein K. Improving economic efficiency in use of pharmaceuticals in critical care: The importance of outcome prediction models in economic analysis. PharmacoEconomics. In Press, 1995.

CHAPTER 96

SOLID ORGAN TRANSPLANTATION

SHIRLEY M. TSUNODA and FRANCESCA T. AWEEKA

Solid organ transplantation has become a curative option for many previously fatal diseases. The success of transplantation has only recently come to fruition owing to advances in immunology and immunopharmacology. The origin of transplantation dates as far back as the second century BC when Chinese surgeons desired to prolong life (1). Over the centuries, the many attempts at transplanting various organs failed because of the lack of surgical expertise and knowledge on ameliorating rejection. Although surgical techniques for organ transplantation became available in the early 1900s, successes in this discipline have been recent, beginning in the 1960s with the implementation of tissue typing and the development of immunosuppressive therapy (Table 96.1) (1–4). Tissue typing allowed for close matching of the donor and recipient to theoretically lessen the chances of rejection. Azathioprine was the first immunosuppressant utilized as a single agent to prevent allograft rejection. This was closely followed by the addition of steroids, which was found to have a synergistic effect (5). However, it was the discovery and clinical use of the immunosuppressive agent cyclosporine that revolutionized the field of transplantation. Survival rates have increased dramatically with 1-year cadaver kidney survival rates of 75–80% with cyclosporine compared to 50–60% without cyclosporine (6–8). Most transplant protocols today continue to use cyclosporine in combination with one or two other immunosuppressive agents for the prophylaxis of allograft rejection (see Table 96.2 for transplant nomenclature).

An increasing number of organs continue to be transplanted. The field began with kidney transplantation for the treatment of end-stage renal failure, which is now routine in many centers around the globe. Liver transplantation is the second most frequently performed transplant (9) and has become a viable treatment option for patients with end-stage liver disease. Orthotopic heart transplantation also has demonstrated improved survival rates since the first successful transplant in 1967. As surgical techniques and immunosuppressive regimens have improved, more end-stage heart failure patients are being considered as candidates for transplantation. Pancreas transplantation, which had 1-year survival rates of 21% between 1966 and 1980, now has improved 1-year survival rates of 89% (10). Transplantation of the lung has evolved over the last decade with improvements in operative techniques and rejection

surveillance. One-year survival rates of greater than 90% have been demonstrated for single-lung transplants, and greater than 85% for bilateral lung transplants (11). Small bowel transplantation has taken longer to evolve into a clinically successful treatment for intestinal failure. The availability of cyclosporine has not altered the survival rates. However, recently, with the introduction of tacrolimus, some success has been demonstrated in small bowel transplantation (12). In addition to single organ transplants, various combinations of organ transplantations have been performed, including kidney-pancreas, kidney-liver, heart-lung, and liver-small bowel.

As surgical techniques and medical management have improved, a shortage of donor organs has become an increasing problem. In 1990, the number of patients on the waiting list for renal transplantation in the United States was approximately 18,000. This number has grown to 25,000 patients as of December 1993, with the number of cadaveric organ donors remaining constant at approximately 4150 (13). Living-related transplantation has been an attempt to alleviate this shortage. For example, living-related renal transplantation accounts for approximately 20% of all renal transplants (14). Living-related liver transplantation also has shown good results, especially in the pediatric population (14). With improvements in surgical procedures and immunosuppression, continued success in this area with other organ transplants can be expected. In addition, xenotransplantation, which was an active area of research in the 1960s, is again becoming an area of renewed interest. Xenotransplantation could solve the worldwide shortage of organs; however, technological difficulties as well as ethical issues preclude its use currently (15).

TRANSPLANT IMMUNOLOGY

Advances in immunology have enabled the field of transplantation to prosper. Enhanced understanding of specific components of immune function, such as the molecular events of rejection and the major histocompatibility complex, have benefited transplant patients; however, other important factors such as the mechanisms to induce tolerance and chimerism (see Table 96.2) must be further explored. The following section summarizes the series of events that lead to allograft rejection, including a discussion of the major histocompatibility complex, the types of rejection and how they differ in various organs, and the treatment of rejection.

Table 96.1.
Historical Overview of Transplantation[a]

1905	Development of vascular suture technique
1933	First human kidney transplant attempted
1954	First successful human kidney transplant in monozygotic twins
1960	Development of tissue typing begins
1962	Azathioprine used as a single immunosuppressive agent
1963	First human liver transplant attempted
1963	Steroids and azathioprine shown to have synergistic immunosuppressive effects
1966	First human segmental pancreas transplant attempted
1966	Antilymphocyte globulin used clinically as adjunctive immunosuppressive therapy
1967	First successful human liver transplant
1967	First successful human orthotopic heart transplant
1968	First human heart–lung transplant attempted
1970	Cyclophosphamide tried as a substitute for azathioprine
1974	First clinical heterotopic heart transplant
1978	Clinical trials of cyclosporine initiated
1982	First successful human heart–lung transplant
1983	Cyclosporine approved by the FDA
1983	Clinical trials of muromonab CD3 (Orthoclone OKT3) initiated
1986	First successful double-lung transplant
1987	Orthoclone OKT3 aproved by the FDA
1987	First successful small bowel transplant performed
1988	First successful small bowel–liver transplant
1989	Clinical trials of FK506 (tacrolimus) and animal trials of rapamycin initiated
1989	First living-related liver transplant
1990	Clinical trials of RS-61443 (mycophenolate mofetil) initiated
1992	FDA places "clinical hold" on production of Minnesota Antilymphocyte Globulin (MALG)
1994	Tacrolimus approved by the FDA
1995	Mycophenolate mofetil approved by the FDA
1995	Cyclosporine (Neoral®) approved by the FDA
1995	Clinical trials of deoxyspergualin initiated

[a]Adapted from Pifarre R, Sullivan H, Montoya A, et al. Cardiac transplantation. Cardiol Clin 7:183–194, 1989; Flye MW. History of transplantation. In: Flye MW. Principles of Organ Transplantation. Philadelphia: WB Saunders, 1989:1–17; Raia S, Nery JR, Mies S. Liver transplantation from live donors. Lancet 2:497, 1989; Grant D, Wall W, Mimeaullt R, et al. Successful small-bowel/liver transplantation. Lancet 335:181–184, 1990.

Major Histocompatibility Complex

The major histocompatibility complex (MHC) consists of the genes encoding the cell surface glycoproteins that aid the immune system in recognizing self versus nonself antigens. All mammalians possess a single chromosome region that encodes for the major tissue surface antigens (16). In humans, the MHC is known as the human leukocyte antigen (HLA) complex and is located on the short arm of chromosome 6 (Fig. 96.1). The specific product that is produced by the particular gene encoded on the chromosome is called the antigen. It is the particular antigen that evokes an immune response. Many alternative forms of the gene, called alleles, produce distinct antigens for a given individual.

There are three classes of antigens within the MHC: HLA classes I, II, and III. Genes for HLA class III encode

Table 96.2.
Transplant Nomenclature

Term	Definition
Autograft	A transplant of tissue or organ taken from the recipient
Syngraft	A transplant of tissue or organ taken from a genetically identical donor (i.e., monozygotic twins)
Allograft	A transplant of tissue or organ taken from a genetically different donor of the same species
Xenograft	A transplant of tissue or organ taken from a donor belonging to a different species
Heterotopic transplant	The recipient's native organ is left in place, and the donor organ is grafted into an ectopic position or site
Orthotopic transplant	The recipient's native organ is removed, and the donor organ is placed with normal or near-normal anatomic reconstruction
Tolerance	Indefinite host unresponsiveness to an allograft without the need for long-term immunosuppression
Chimerism	The coexistence of genetic material from different individuals in one host

complement components. The HLA classes I and II are utilized in determining histocompatibility in clinical transplantation. There are three well-characterized loci on the HLA class I: HLA-A, -B, and -C. The HLA-A, -B, and -C are highly polymorphic (i.e., there is a high frequency of multiple alleles encoding different antigens), with 26, 40, and 14 defined specificities, respectively (17). The class I antigens are present on the plasma membranes of virtually all nucleated cells in the body. The class II molecules consist of HLA-DR, -DP, and -DQ. They have a more restricted distribution and are expressed primarily on B lymphocytes, antigen-presenting cells, and vascular endothelium (18). The HLA-A, -B, and -DR antigens are considered the most important in clinical transplantation (19).

Histocompatibility testing of the donor and recipient is used to minimize donor-specific immune responses to a transplanted organ. Theoretically, the more antigens that match, the less likely rejection is to occur. A donor and recipient are considered HLA identical when all detectable antigens are the same. In practice, histocompatibility matching is significant only in renal and pancreas transplantation. It is not utilized in liver, heart, or lung transplantation because of limitations on organ viability and shortage of organs. In addition, since the introduction of potent immunosuppressants such as cyclosporine, it is unclear if HLA matching has had a significant effect on survival of cadaver, living-related, and/or living-unrelated renal transplants (18). The benefit of HLA matching may be evident only in long-term graft survival rates (20). However, in the case of HLA-identical siblings, these procedures have resulted in the highest long-term survival rates, fewer complications, and less immunosuppression.

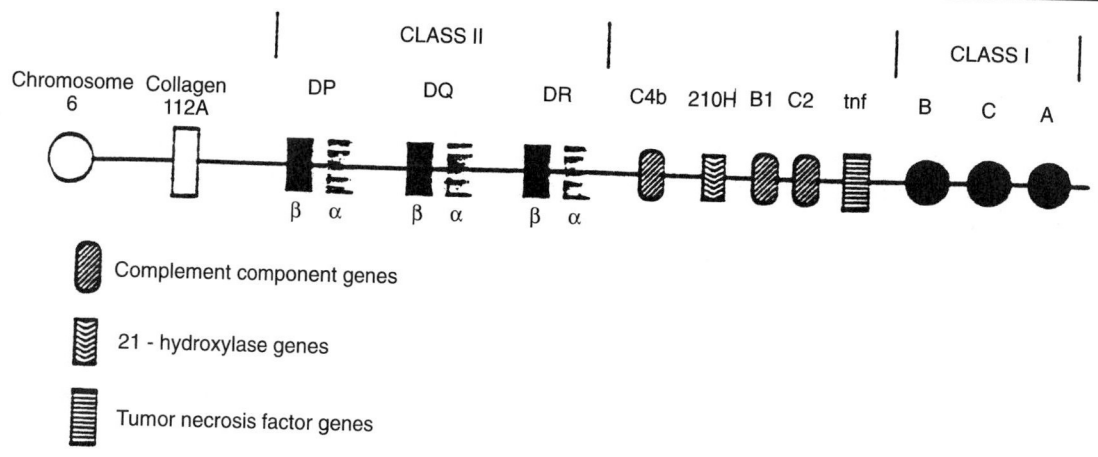

Figure 96.1 The human major histocompatibility complex (MHC). Genetic loci designated A, B, and C encode Class I MHC (HLA) antigens. Genetic region designated DP, DQ, and DR encode Class II MHC (HLA) antigens. (Reprinted with permission, WB Saunders.)

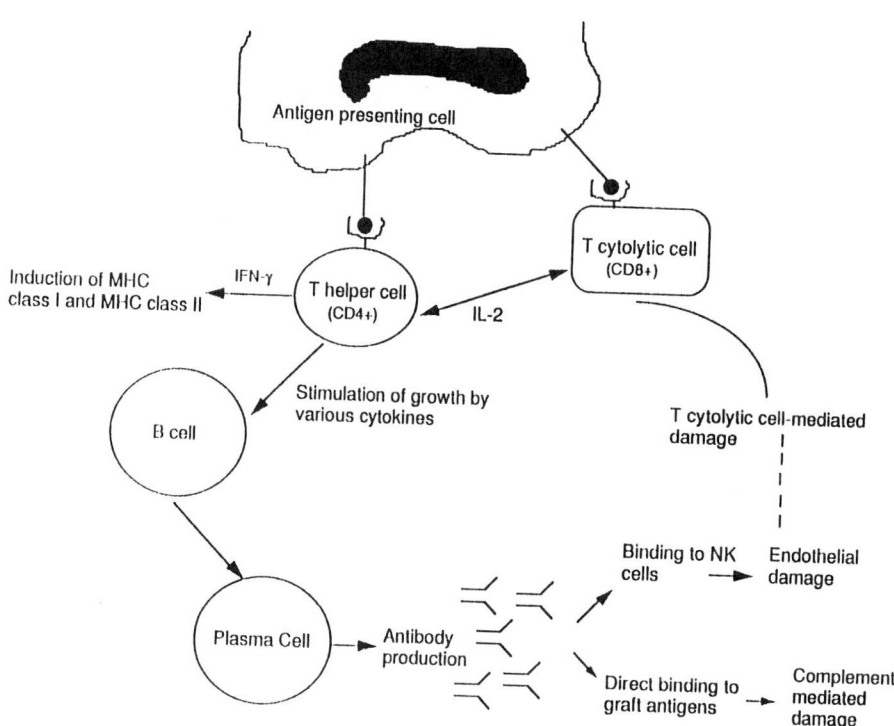

Figure 96.2 Schematic representation of an allograft undergoing rejection. (Modified from Hammond EH, ed. Mechanisms of Allograft Rejection. Philadelphia: WB Saunders, 1994. Reprinted with permission).

REJECTION

Immunology of the Rejection Response

The function of the immune system is to protect the host environment from foreign substances. When a foreign allograft is placed in a transplant recipient, antigens are released into the host environment that initiate an immune response. The immune response is the result of a complex cascade that results in the formation of antibodies (immunoglobulins) and sensitized cells (lymphocytes) that participate in specific humoral or cell-mediated responses to antigenic stimuli (Fig. 96.2). Two lines of defense exist: the humoral arm and the cellular arm. Humoral immunity is mediated by B lymphocytes that develop into antibodies in the serum, whereas cellular immunity is mediated by T lymphocytes. T lymphocytes can be further divided into subsets based on function. Helper T lymphocytes secrete cytokines, which are a diverse group of proteins that among other functions promote the proliferation and differentiation of T cells. One important cytokine secreted by T helper cells is interleukin-2 (IL-2). IL-2 stimulates the proliferation of other T helper cells as well as the differentiation of mature cytolytic T cells. Cytolytic T lymphocytes actually lyse virus-infected cells, tumor cells, and allografts. Lymphocytes are the only cells in the body that can recognize specific antigens; therefore, they are central to the response to a foreign allograft. They recognize only peptide antigens attached to the MHC (21).

When antigens from the donor graft elicit a response from the recipient's immune system, the sequence of events that ensues can be subdivided into afferent and efferent responses. The afferent limb involves the recognition of the host immune system to the graft. When the graft histocompatibility antigens elicit recognition by the host, T and B lymphocytes are activated. This initiates a complex series of intracellular events involving the proliferation and differentiation of antigen-specific T and B lymphocytes. A multitude of cytokines are released and secreted that aid in the overall rejection response (18).

The sensitized cells and antibodies initiate the efferent limb of allograft rejection. The primary effector cells are the antigen-specific T lymphocytes although other cells, such as macrophages and natural killer cells, may also be involved. These cells migrate to the graft where they interrupt vascular connections. The infiltration of lymphoid and phagocytic cells causes the graft to become necrotic. Without appropriate therapy, the result is vascular stasis, thrombosis, and necrosis of the transplanted organ (18, 22).

Classification of Rejection

Although HLA typing and improvements in immunosuppressive agents have increased survival rates, rejection remains a problem. Approximately 30–75% of renal, hepatic, cardiac, pancreatic, and pulmonary transplant recipients will experience rejection. Allograft rejection can be classified into four types: hyperacute, accelerated acute, acute, and chronic (Table 96.3) (18). Classification is based not only on the time course after transplantation but also on the histologic picture and the nature of the inflammatory reaction (21). Many cases of acute rejection will be treated effectively; however, none of the currently available immunosuppressants have to date proved to decrease the rate of chronic rejection.

Table 96.3.
Types of Rejection Reactions

Type	Time After Transplantation	Probable Mediators
Hyperacute	Minutes to 1 to 5 days	Preformed donor-specific lymphocytotoxic antibodies
Accelerated acute	7 to 10 days	Low levels of anti-class I antibodies or T-cell-mediated rejection in presensitized individuals
Acute	Weeks to 6 months	Newly developed antibodies, delayed-type hypersensitivity of helper and cytolytic T lymphocytes
Chronic	Months to years	T lymphocytes and donor-specific antibody response directed at allograft vasculature

Hyperacute rejection occurs very soon after perfusion of the transplanted organ. It is mediated by anti-HLA (donor-specific lymphocytotoxic) antibodies. Severe vascular damage occurs, including thrombosis, congestion, inflammation, and necrosis. It is presumed that this type of rejection is caused by humoral presensitization to donor ABO blood or HLA antigens (23). It occurs more frequently in kidney and heart transplant recipients. Therefore, a negative T-cell cross match (absence of donor-specific class I HLA antibodies) is required prior to these types of transplants with some exceptions. Some cases of transplantation have been successful in highly sensitized individuals after removal of anti-HLA antibodies by plasmapheresis with immunoadsorbent columns (24). Hyperacute rejection in liver transplantation occurs less frequently and occurs later, approximately 3 to 7 days after transplant. The reasons for this are unclear but may be related to the liver's capacity to absorb antibodies (18). In pancreas and lung transplantation, the propensity for hyperacute rejection is unknown at this time. The overall incidence of hyperacute rejection for all solid organ allografts has been reduced to less than 1% due to the use of pretransplantation antidonor lymphocyte-toxic antibody assays (25, 26). The only treatment option for hyperacute rejection is to immediately remove the transplanted organ.

Accelerated acute rejection occurs within 3 to 10 days of renal transplantation (18, 27). It is a reflection of host antidonor presensitization and occurs more frequently in recipients who have received blood products from the donor (donor-specific transfusions, DST), had multiple pregnancies, or had previously rejected allografts. It may be caused by low levels of anticlass I antibodies or by T-cell-mediated rejection in presensitized patients. Antirejection therapy can be successful in the short term; however, there may be an increased risk of graft failure in the long term. Allograft failure occurs in approximately 60% of cases of accelerated acute rejection (18).

Acute rejection usually occurs within the first few weeks to months after transplantation, but may occur years later (21). Although its onset is generally rapid, the clinical presentation of acute rejection differs for the various organs transplanted (see Table 96.4) (2, 12, 27–38). In general, acute rejection can be both cell and antibody mediated, involving both helper and cytolytic T lymphocytes. Infiltrating lymphocytes and macrophages cause lysis of the graft parenchymal cells. This leads to injury or destruction of certain epithelial structures of the transplanted allograft (e.g., renal tubules in the kidney, the bile duct epithelium of the liver, and monocytes in the heart). Acute rejection is usually reversible, especially if treated early.

Chronic allograft rejection is one of the main causes of graft failure later in the transplant course. It usually presents months to years after transplantation but can

Table 96.4.
Signs and Symptoms of Rejection in Specific Transplanted Organs

Organ	Clinical Signs	Laboratory Signs	Reference
Kidney	Fever, malaise, weight gain, oliguria, graft tenderness, edema, diastolic hypertension	Scr increase > 20% above baseline, increased BUN	(27, 28)
Liver	Fever, lethargy, change in color or quantity of bile in patient with biliary T-tube, graft tenderness and swelling, back pain, anorexia, ileus, tachycardia; in severe rejection: jaundice, ascites, overt encephalopathy	Abnormal LFTs: rapid rise in GGTP, increased serum bilirubin, increased alkaline phosphatase, increased serum transaminases	(29, 30)
Heart	Low-grade fever, lethargy, weakness, SOB, DOE, hypotension, tachycardia, atrial flutter, ventricular arrhythmias, pericardial friction rub	Leukocytosis	(2, 31, 32)
Pancreas	Fever, malaise, graft tenderness and swelling, abdominal pain, ileus	FBS > 11 mmol/L, leukocytosis, human C peptide < 0.7 ng/ml, urinary amylase < 167 μkat/L (bladder anastomosis)	(33–35)
Lung	Fever, impaired gas exchange, decreased FEV_1, infiltrate on chest radiograph, breathlessness, malaise, feeling of anxiety		(36, 37)
Small bowel	Fever, abdominal pain, nausea, vomiting, diarrhea, ileus, distension, acidosis, positive blood cultures for enteric organisms		(12, 38)

rarely occur within weeks of transplant surgery. Although the clinical presentation and incidence of chronic rejection varies with the organ transplanted, a common denominator in kidney, liver, and heart transplants is persistent perivascular and interstitial inflammation. There is little lymphocyte activation and a concentric distribution of graft arteriosclerosis (39, 40). The cause of chronic rejection is not fully known although it is thought to be immunologically based. Several risk factors may be associated with its development. They include histocompatibility mismatching, an increased frequency and intensity of acute rejection episodes, increased cold ischemia time (the amount of time the donor organ is without blood flow), and the presence of cytomegalovirus infection (41).

Unfortunately, cyclosporine has failed to alter the rates of chronic rejection. In kidney transplant recipients, approximately 8–10% of grafts are lost to chronic rejection (42). In liver transplantation, chronic rejection is characterized by the loss of bile ducts, called vanishing bile duct syndrome. Approximately 10–15% of patients must be retransplanted owing to this irreversible syndrome (43). Chronic rejection in heart transplant recipients is manifested by arteriosclerosis. Long-term graft survival is greatly affected by the incidence of coronary arteriosclerosis: 6–18% at 1 year, 23% at 2 years, and as high as 50% at 5 years (44, 45). Chronic lung rejection, called bronchiolitis obliterans, occurs in 20–50% of pulmonary transplant recipients and is the leading cause of morbidity and mortality after the first year of transplant (11). Chronic rejection in all organ types is in most cases irreversible with current antirejection therapy, and requires retransplantation.

Diagnosis of Rejection

Diagnosing rejection in transplant patients receiving multiple immunosuppressive agents can be difficult. Often the expected signs and symptoms are "masked" due to the patient's blunted immune system from immunosuppression. In addition, particularly with kidney transplantation, the symptoms of rejection are very similar to the signs of nephrotoxicity from cyclosporine. Therefore, the clinician must rely on multiple tools (i.e., clinical symptoms, laboratory values, imaging studies, biopsy pathology) in order to make the diagnosis of rejection. In many centers, routine biopsies (tissue samples of the transplanted organ) are taken at regular intervals as a surveillance mechanism to monitor the graft.

KIDNEY

Approximately 50% of renal transplant recipients will experience one or more rejection episodes (46). Acute renal allograft rejection usually occurs within the first 3 months after transplantation. It is characterized by a rising creatinine greater than 20% above baseline values, decreased urine output, and enlargement and tenderness of the allograft. Other symptoms include malaise, fever, peripheral and/or pulmonary edema, and diastolic hypertension (27). Since the diagnosis of rejection usually cannot be made based on clinical symptoms alone, other methods such as ultrasound, urine cultures, and cyclosporine levels may be used to rule out other causes of renal dysfunction, such as renal artery or vein stenosis, cytomegalovirus infection, or cyclosporine-induced renal toxicity (27, 28, 46). Renal biopsy is one of the best tools at confirming rejection. The predominant findings include lymphocytic infiltration and tissue damage within the interstitium (28, 47).

LIVER

Approximately 70% of liver transplant patients experience an episode of acute rejection, usually between 4 and 14 days. Approximately 75% of these patients have resolution of their rejection with antirejection therapy while the remainder will progress to chronic rejection (43). Clinical signs and symptoms include abnormal liver function tests, fever, ileus, ascites, abdominal pain, and jaundice. An increase in serum γ-glutamyl transpeptidase (GGTP) activity is an early but nonspecific indicator of acute rejection. Increases in bilirubin, alkaline phosphatase, and amyloid A protein levels may also occur, along with a change in the color and quantity of bile. The diagnosis of rejection is confirmed by core needle biopsy, which reveals a mixed inflammatory cell infiltrate of portal tracts, bile duct damage, infiltration with lymphocytes, and hepatic and portal venous endothelial inflammation. Intraoperative liver biopsies are obtained at the time of transplantation for later comparison with routine serial biopsies (29, 43, 48).

HEART

Rejection is one of the most common posttransplant complications in heart transplant recipients. In the first year after transplant, 0.5–2.5 rejection episodes occur per patient, most in the first three months (49). Most of the clinical signs and symptoms of rejection are nonspecific. They include fever, lethargy, weakness, elevated jugular venous pressure, a new S3 gallop, new dysrhythmias, shortness of breath, and hypotension. However, clinical signs are usually absent unless rejection is prolonged or severe. The transplanted heart is denervated, so angina and chest pain are not present. Therefore, routine surveillance endomyocardial biopsies are performed weekly during the early postoperative period, then less frequently at regular intervals (2, 31, 4). Histologic changes detected on biopsy that are consistent with rejection include diffuse mononuclear infiltrates.

LUNG

Acute rejection in lung transplant recipients usually occurs within the first 3 months. Most recipients experience an episode of rejection within the first few weeks, with biopsy-proven rejection occurring in 60–70% of patients in the first month (36, 50, 51). The diagnosis is usually made based on clinical symptoms that include temperature elevation with an increase of 0.5° C being significant, gas exchange impairment, decreased forced expiratory volume (FEV_1), and the development of infiltrates on chest films (11). Serial radionuclide perfusion scans that measure the proportion of blood flow to the transplanted lung may also be helpful in aiding the diagnosis of rejection (11). In addition, transbronchial biopsy is very useful when coupled with clinical signs and symptoms in diagnosing rejection (37).

PANCREAS

Many pancreas grafts are lost to rejection because there are no reliable markers of pancreatic rejection. In addition, biopsies, which are diagnostic in other types of transplants, are difficult to perform, cause morbidity, and are not easy to interpret (52). Rejection is the most common cause of pancreatic loss (53). In patients who have simultaneous kidney-pancreas transplants, kidney transplant rejection usually precedes that of the pancreas. It is uncommon to have rejection in the pancreas without concomitant rejection in the kidney. Therefore, pancreas loss in these patients has been decreased because of earlier detection of kidney allograft rejection (18). Allograft function is monitored by measuring changes in urinary amylase and percutaneous needle biopsies of the pancreas. Monitoring serum glucose has been utilized, but hyperglycemia usually occurs late in rejection, so this has not been useful (18).

SMALL BOWEL

Small bowel transplantation confers a unique immunologic problem unknown to other organ transplants. When the intestine is transplanted, within it is a large amount of lymphoid tissue rendering it very immunogenic as well as immunocompetent. Therefore, two types of immune reactions are possible after transplant: (1) recipient cells attacking the graft (rejection) and (2) graft cells attacking the recipient (graft-versus-host disease, or GVHD). Fortunately, so far, GVHD has occurred only rarely (54, 55). Rejection, however, is common after transplant and if detected early responds well to antirejection therapy (56). It is characterized by fever, abdominal pain, vomiting, and ileus. Severe rejection presents with fever, massive diarrhea, abdominal pain, distension, and positive blood cultures (due to translocation of bacteria from the gut lumen) (12, 38). Biopsy of the mucosa is the best measurement of rejection (12). Endoscopy and measuring serum levels of procoagulant factor also may aid in the diagnosis in addition to signs and symptoms and positive blood cultures (12, 38).

Strategies to Modify the Immune Response

Two strategies have been used in an effort to induce immunologic hyporesponsiveness in the recipient and thus prevent rejection. One method involves giving the recipient donor-specific-transfusion (DST) of blood prior to either cadaver or living-related or -unrelated renal transplantation. Increased survival rates have been documented in cadaver transplants (57) and living-unrelated renal transplants (58, 59) when DST was given prior to transplant in addition to cyclosporine-based immunosuppression.

Some of the disadvantages to DST administration are the potential for acquiring transfusion-related diseases such as cytomegalovirus and hepatitis, and an increased rate of recipient sensitization to the donor (57).

Another strategy involves infusing donor-specific bone marrow into the recipient prior to cadaveric renal transplantation. The basis behind this method is to induce tolerance in the recipient. Some have proposed that by using this approach, organ transplant recipients may achieve a donor-specific hyporeactivity, thereby requiring less or no immunosuppression while maintaining graft function (60, 61). Although preliminary data suggest that administering donor-specific bone marrow augments chimerism, further study is required before routine clinical use of this technology.

Treatment of Rejection

The overall goal in treating acute rejection is to minimize the intensity of the immune response toward the transplanted organ. The majority of acute rejection episodes occurring early in posttransplant are amenable to antirejection therapy. The treatment usually involves steroid pulses (bursts of high doses) followed by a recycling of steroids (resumption of induction doses). Although the exact protocols vary between transplant centers, the general practice is to increase the dose for 3 to 7 days and then taper to the maintenance or prerejection dose. The usual treatment is methylprednisolone 1 to 2 g per day for 3 days or until there is evidence of improved allograft function. Lower doses of 2 to 4 mg/kg/day have also been effective.

If the rejection cannot be controlled with high-dose steroids, more powerful immunosuppressants are used, such as polyclonal antibodies, orthoclone CD3 (OKT3), or tacrolimus. Antithymocyte globulin (ATG), a polyclonal antibody has been given for the treatment of rejection at doses of 10–20 mg/kg for 7 to 14 days. OKT3 is dosed at 5 mg per day for 7 to 14 days. Tacrolimus has also shown effectiveness in treating ongoing rejection. To date, its use has been primarily in patients who have steroid and/or OKT3-resistant rejection. Doses of 0.05–0.1 mg/kg/day intravenously have been used (see "Specific Immunosuppressive Agents").

SURGICAL CONSIDERATIONS

Criteria for Selection

The criteria used for selecting an appropriate transplant recipient can vary widely between transplant centers and often depend on the experience of the center and organ donor availability. In general, there are certain criteria in which transplantation is absolutely contraindicated. Most centers will not accept recipients who have metastatic malignancy, HIV disease or seropositivity, or anatomic anomalies precluding transplantation. In addition, patients who are active substance abusers or who are not compliant

with medications would generally not be considered transplant candidates. Beyond these conditions, the indications for transplantation are continually evolving, with each recipient's case determined individually. For instance, kidney transplantation has become so common that the guidelines used now for selecting a recipient are far less limiting than those used 10 to 20 years ago. Table 96.5 lists diseases for which transplantation has been performed (11, 12, 32, 46, 52, 62–67).

In order to maximize the utilization of potential organs for transplant, an organization called the United Network

Table 96.5.
Indications for Transplantation

Organ	Disease State
Kidney	Diabetic nephropathy
	Polycystic kidney disease
	Amyloidosis
	Renal cell carcinoma
	Lupus nephritis
	Chronic pyelonephritis
Liver	Primary biliary cirrhosis
	Primary sclerosing cholangitis
	Biliary atresia
	Fulminant and subfulminant hepatitis
	Cirrhosis due to Hepatitis B virus (HBV)[a]
	Cirrhosis due to Hepatitis C virus (HCV)[b]
	Alcoholic cirrhosis[c]
	Primary hepatocellular carcinoma[d]
	Hepato-renal syndrome
	Budd-Chiari syndrome
	Inherited metabolic disorders
Heart	Ischemic myocardial disease
	Idiopathic cardiomyopathy
	Valvular disease
	Congenital cardiac disease
	Myocardial disease (sarcoidosis, amyloidosis)
	Infection (Chagas disease)
	Drug-induced myocardial destruction
Pancreas	Type I diabetes
Lung	Emphysema (incl. α_1-antitrypsin deficiency)
	Cystic fibrosis
	Primary and secondary pulmonary hypertension
	Idiopathic pulmonary fibrosis/interstitial lung diseases
	Obliterative bronchiolitis
	Eosinophilic granuloma
	Lymphangioleiomyomatosis
	Sarcoidosis
	Bronchiectasis
Small bowel	Crohn's disease
	Radiation injury
	Neoplasm
	Strangulated hernia
	Trauma

[a]With absence of HBV replication and long-term passive Hepatitis B surface antibody (HBsAb) prophylaxis.
[b]With absence of serious complications.
[c]With documented abstinence of alcohol for a defined period.
[d]Only in certain centers in patients meeting certain criteria, often with adjunctive chemotherapy or chemoembolization.

for Organ Sharing (UNOS) was established in 1977. UNOS maintains a computerized registry of patients awaiting transplantation and coordinates the appropriate selection of donor and recipient. A scoring system based on a multitude of factors such as blood type, HLA typing, length of time on the waiting list, and degree of medical urgency is used to determine which donor organ will go to which recipient (68, 69).

Operative Procedures

The surgical techniques used for transplantation may influence the therapeutic management of patients following transplantation. Therefore, a brief overview of the procedures used for kidney, liver, heart, lung, and pancreas transplantation will be presented, including the site of organ implantation and the major arterial and venous anastomoses.

KIDNEY

In kidney transplantation, the transplanted allograft can be from either a cadaver, a living-related, or a living-unrelated (e.g., spouse) donor. In most cases, the native kidneys of the recipient remain in place. The donor kidney may be implanted retroperitoneally in either iliac fossa; however, the right is the site of choice. The external iliac or (rarely) internal iliac artery is used for the arterial anastomotic site to the renal artery, and the external iliac vein is anastomosed to the renal vein (62). The ureter is anastomosed to the bladder directly (Fig. 96.3). Revascularization of the new kidney takes about 30 minutes, with the production of urine often beginning immediately.

LIVER

Transplantation of the liver is one of the most difficult surgical procedures to perform. Contrary to the procedure in kidney transplantation, the recipient's liver is removed and replaced with the donor liver (orthotopic transplantation). The donor and recipient are generally matched for liver size (± 20%) since insertion of an excessively large liver would lead to splinting of the diaphragm and

pulmonary complications (70–72). Prior to the late 1980s, liver preservation time was limited to 6 to 8 hours. With a new preservation solution, the donor liver can be safely preserved for 15 to 24 hours (66), which eases the time limitations for transplant.

After appropriate dissection has been performed to ease excision of the recipient liver, preparations for venovenous bypass are made. During the period when the recipient is without a liver, the anhepatic phase, venovenous bypass is recommended in order to maintain venous return from the kidneys and lower extremities, and allow better hemodynamics. After removal of the recipient liver, implantation of the donor liver begins. The gallbladder is removed, and vascular anastomoses are made with the suprahepatic vena cava, the infrahepatic vena cava, the hepatic artery, and the portal vein (Fig. 96.4). When liver function has resumed, anastomosis of the biliary tract is carried out by connecting the donor's and recipient's common ducts over a drainage tube (T-tube) (73).

In response to the shortage of donor organs, different techniques of liver transplantation have been developed. These include reduced-size, split-liver (splitting one donor liver and transplanting it into two recipients), and liver-related liver transplantation. Most of these operations are performed in pediatric patients because of size constraints. Although reduced-size and split-liver transplants are performed in certain cases, difficulties with high morbidity and surgical techniques have limited their use (14). Living-related liver transplantation, however, has been successful in pediatric patients with experienced surgeons. Since its inception in 1989, more than 150 patients worldwide have been given living-related transplants (74). The benefits include the elimination of waiting time, the high quality of the donor organ, and the ability to anticipate immunologic benefits (i.e., HLA-identical siblings) (14).

HEART

Orthotopic heart transplantation is the most common heart transplant procedure performed. At the time of surgery, the patient is placed on cardiopulmonary bypass to

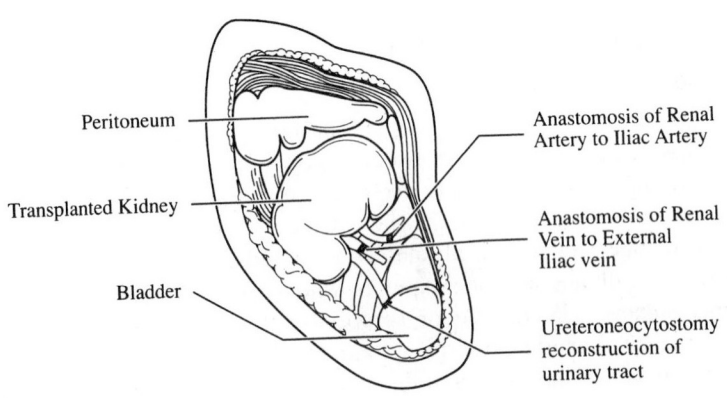

Figure 96.3 Completed kidney transplant into right iliac fossa with sites of major surgical anastomoses. (Adapted with permission, Mosby Year Book.)

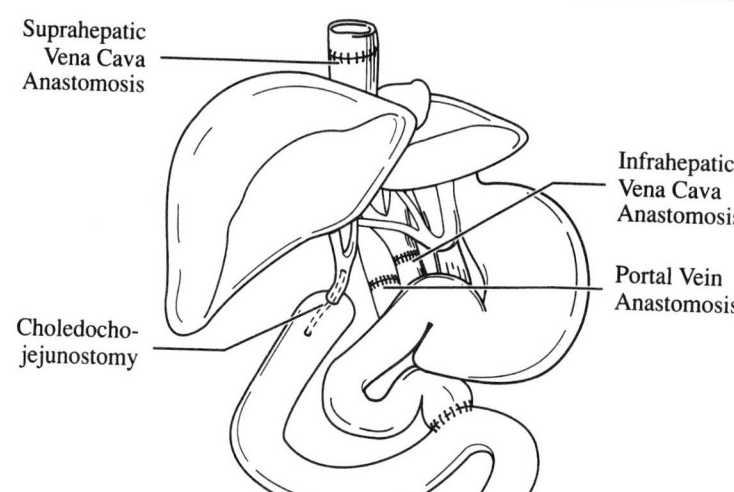

Figure 96.4 Completed liver transplant with sites of major surgical anastomoses. (Adapted with permission, Mosby Year Book.)

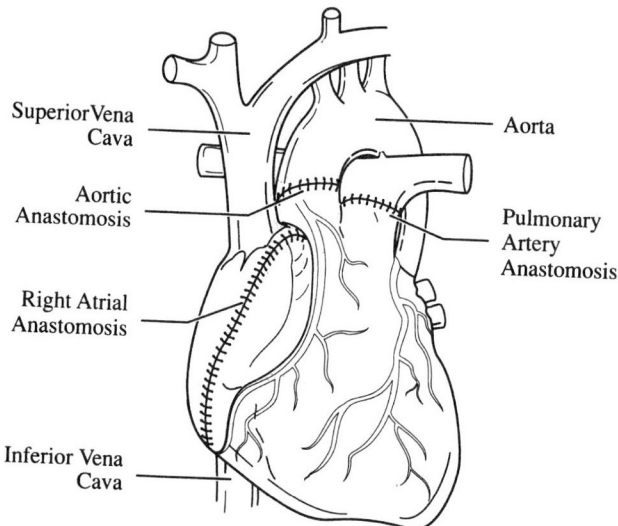

Figure 96.5 Completed heart transplant with sites of major surgical anastomoses. (Modified from Wallwork J, ed. Heart and Heart-Lung Transplantation. Philadelphia: WB Saunders, 1989. Reprinted with permission.)

maintain adequate circulation throughout the surgical procedure. Once the patient is stable, the native heart is removed (cardiectomy), leaving most of both atria and septum in place. Implantation of the donor heart is performed by anastomosis of the left atrium of the heart to the residual left atrial wall of the recipient, followed by joining of the right atrial wall and atrial septum. The main pulmonary artery is then connected to the ascending aorta (Fig. 96.5) (75).

One of the unique aspects of the transplanted heart is that it is denervated and relies on circulating catecholamines for normal function. The transplanted heart contains a right atria with two sinus nodes. Since the native atrial activity cannot cross the suture line, it is the donor

sinus node activity that is conducted through the ventricles. Therefore, cardiac transplant patients will not experience symptoms of ischemia, such as angina, and can present with myocardial infarctions or sudden death. In addition, many drugs that act predominantly via the autonomic nervous system will have no effect on the transplanted heart (2, 49).

LUNG

Lung transplantation involves either single-lung or double-lung transplant. The decision of which operation is performed depends on several factors of the recipient, including the cause of the lung failure as well as donor lung availability. For instance, a patient with cystic fibrosis or bronchiectasis would generally not be considered for a single-lung transplant since there would be a risk of infection to the nontransplanted lung (67).

After the recipient's pulmonary anatomy is dissected, a pneumonectomy is performed and the donor lung is implanted. The donor and recipient bronchus is anastomosed followed by the pulmonary artery. A left atrial cuff is made with the recipient superior and inferior pulmonary veins and anastomosed to the remnant of the donor left atrium (Fig. 96.6) (11, 76). In double-lung transplantation, the preferred technique is a bilateral, sequential lung replacement, which is basically performing two single lung transplants one after the other. It is technically simpler than an en-bloc double-lung transplant, requires less frequent use of cardiopulmonary bypass, and allows for shorter recovery periods (67, 76). Double-lung transplantation has been successfully performed in patients with cystic fibrosis, bronchiectasis, and primary and secondary pulmonary hypertension (67).

Living-related lung transplantation has also been performed in a limited number of cases, mostly for the treatment of cystic fibrosis. Although some short-term success has been achieved, with results similar to cadaver

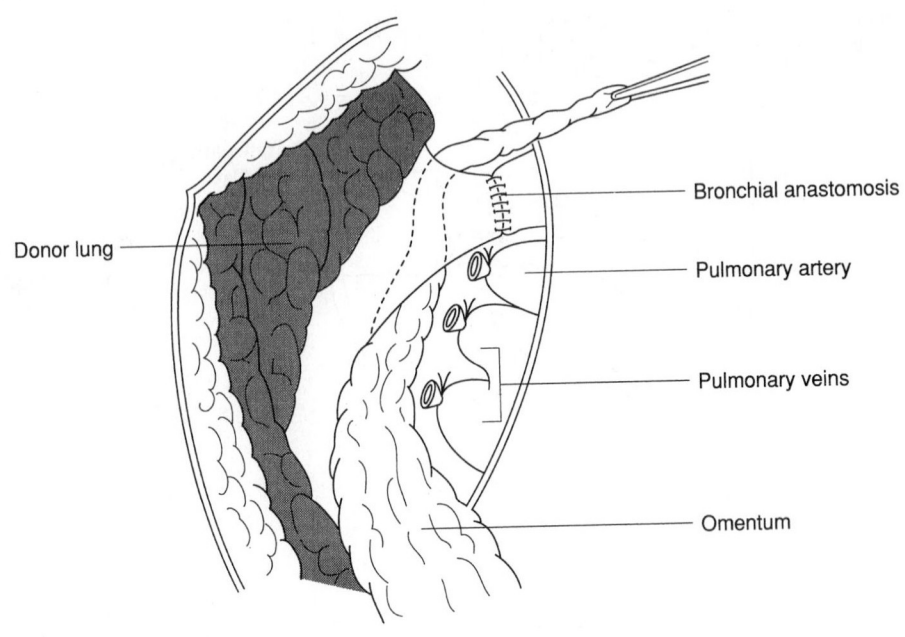

Figure 96.6 Lung transplantation after completion of the bronchial anastomosis; pulmonary artery and veins are shown ligated. (Reprinted with permission, JB Lippincott.)

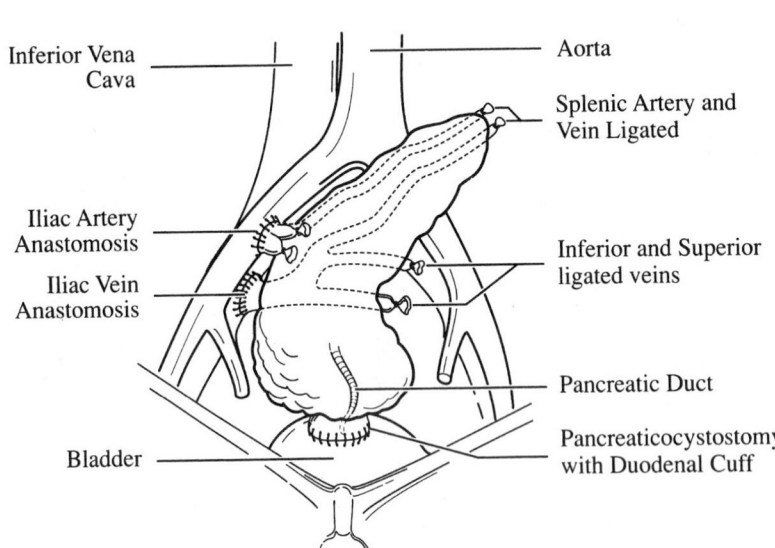

Figure 96.7 Completed whole pancreas transplant with sites of major surgical anastomoses. (Adapted with permission, Mosby Year Book.)

transplants, this procedure remains experimental at this time (11, 77).

PANCREAS

The goal of pancreas transplantation is not only to provide an endogenous source of insulin to an insulin-dependent diabetic patient, but mainly to prevent, stabilize, or reverse the long-term complications of diabetes such as neuropathy and retinopathy. Since many long-term diabetic patients eventually have compromised kidney function requiring transplantation, pancreas transplantation can be performed either alone, after successful kidney transplantation, or simultaneously with kidney transplant. Simultaneous pancreas–kidney transplantation has demonstrated the highest survival rates (78).

In pancreas transplantation, the native pancreas is left in place (heterotopic procedure). Pancreas transplants may be either segmental (tail and body) or whole organ. Segmental grafts are commonly placed extra- or intraperitoneally in the pelvis, with vascular anastomosis to the iliac vessels. The whole organ graft is obtained as a bloc dissection and includes the pancreas, spleen, and long duodenal segment. It is placed intraperitoneally where the exudates of the pancreas can be absorbed by the highly vascular peritoneum. Placed into the right iliac fossa, the arterial supply of the graft is anastomosed to the common iliac artery, and its venous drainage is anastomosed to the common iliac vein (Fig. 96.7). The exocrine duct is usually drained into the bladder for urinary excretion of pancreatic enzymes. This has been shown to be a superior technique in terms of graft survival since it allows for monitoring of urinary amylase, which can be a marker for pancreatic rejection (35, 78, 79).

PRINCIPLES OF IMMUNOSUPPRESSION

Immunosuppressive therapy is tantamount to the survival of a transplant recipient. Until the immune mechanisms of tolerance and chimerism are better understood such that the graft survives without immunosuppression, transplant recipients will require these agents to sustain life. Immunosuppression is utilized to blunt the recipient's immune response to foreign antigens on the transplanted allograft. Ideally, an immunosuppressant should specifically inhibit the cells responsible for the allograft rejection process, affecting only the lymphocyte subsets directed against donor-specific alloantigens. Unfortunately, none of the

agents currently available are capable of this (see Fig. 96.8). Various side effects associated with these drugs limit maximizing the dose. Therefore, several immunosuppressive agents with different side effect profiles and different mechanisms of action are given together in order to maximize the therapeutic benefit while minimizing side effects.

The two tenets of current immunosuppressive therapy are to prevent rejection and avoid infection, and these two objectives are in constant conflict. The clinical challenge is to balance the doses of immunosuppressive agents so that optimal immunosuppression is achieved and the risk of infection is minimized. This is not a static process, but rather an ongoing process that requires constant monitoring and adjustment in accord with the clinical course of each patient. Although the dose of immunosuppressive

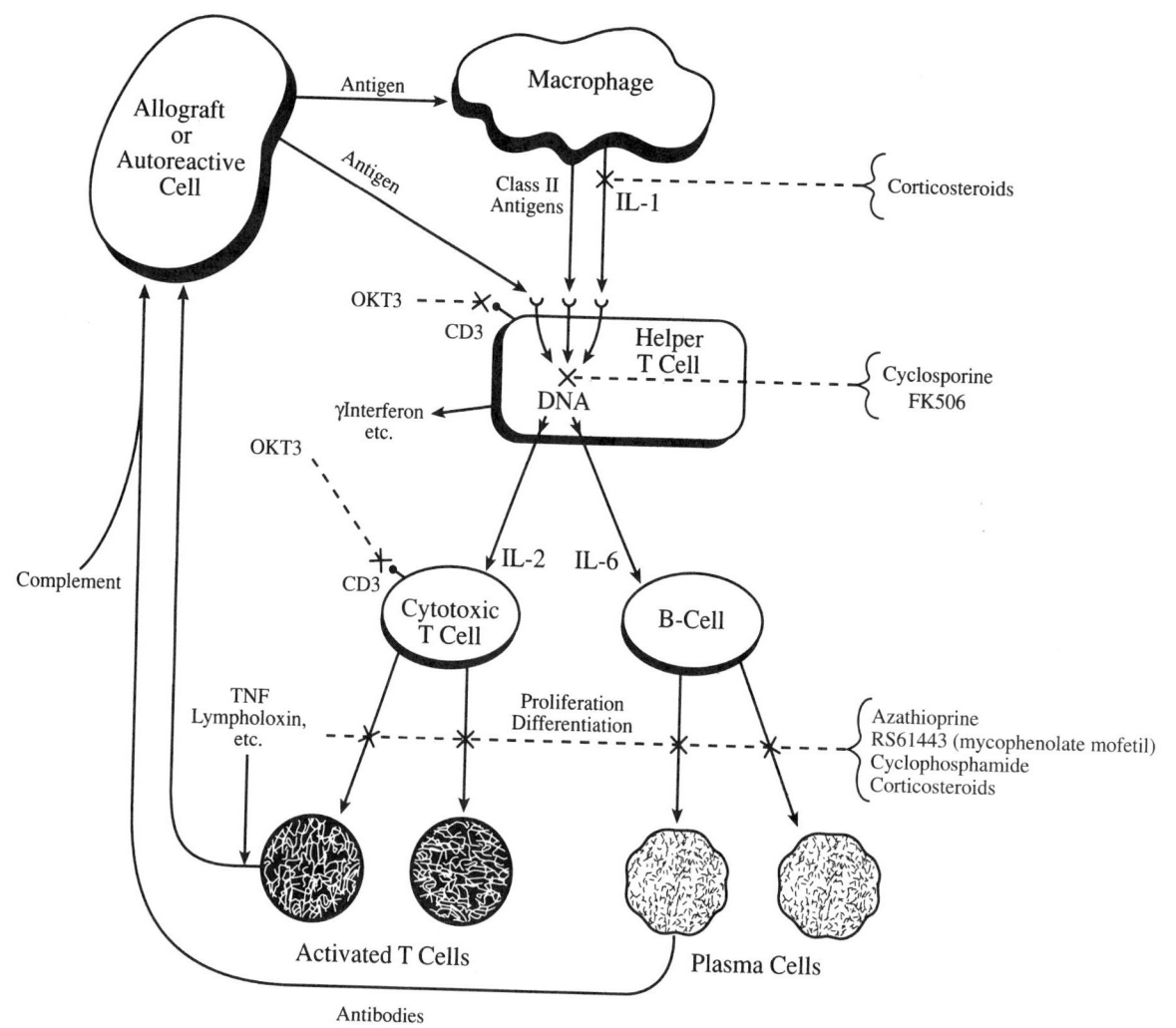

Figure 96.8 Schematic representation summarizing the mechanism of action of immunosuppressive agents. (Modified from Hundschumacher RE. Immunosuppressive agents. In: Gillman AG, Rall TW, Nies AS, Taylor P. Goodman and Gillman's The Pharmacological basis of Therapeutics, 8th ed. New York: Pergamon Press, Inc., 1990. Copyright 1990, Pergamon Press, Inc. Reprinted with permission, Macmillan Publishing Company.)

Table 96.6.
Examples of Immunosuppression Protocols for Rejection Prophylaxis[a], [b]

Kidney Transplant Protocols

Regimen A (Quadruple Therapy)		Regimen B (Triple Therapy)		Regimen C	
DAY 0–7	ATG 15 mg/kg IV qd continue until therapeutic CyA levels	DAY 0	MPred 500 mg IV × 1	INTRA-OP	MPred 500 mg IV
				DAY 1	MPred 250 mg IV
		DAY 1–5	Pred 1 mg/kg po	DAY 2–7	Pred 30 mg po bid
		DAY 6–8	Pred 0.75 mg/kg po	DAY 8–14	Pred 20 mg po bid
DAY 0	MPred 500 mg IV × 1	DAY 9–12	Pred 0.5 mg/kg po, then taper to 0.15 mg/kg at 6 months	DAY 15–21	Pred 15 mg po bid
				DAY 21–Mo 3	Pred 10 mg po bid
DAY 1–5	Pred 1 mg/kg po			Mo 3–Mo 6	Pred 15 mg po qd
DAY 6–9	Pred 0.75 mg/kg po	DAY 0–	AZA 5 mg/kg po adjust to keep WBC > 4000	> Mo 6–	Pred 10 mg po qd
DAY 10–12	Pred 0.5 mg/kg po, then taper to 0.15 mg/kg at 6 months				
				DAY 0–	CyA (Neoral) 5 mg/kg po bid
		DAY 6–	CyA 10 mg/kg/day (bid) adjust to maintain thera-peutic trough levels		
DAY 0–	AZA 2.5 mg/kg po adjust to keep WBC > 400. continue indefinitely			DAY 0–	MM 1 gm po bid; hold if WBC < 5.0
DAY 6–	CyA 10 mg/kg/day (bid) adjust to maintain thera-peutic trough levels				

Liver Transplant Protocols

Regimen D		Regimen E		Regimen F (Living Related)	
INTRA-OP	HC 1 gm × 1	DAY 0–7	MPred 5 mg/kg bid	INTRA-OP	MPred 10 mg/kg IV × 2
DAY 0	MPred 1 gm × 1	DAY 8	MPred 0.5 mg/kg/d		
DAY 1	Pred 200 mg/d (qid)			DAY 1–3	MPred 1 mg/kg IV
DAY 2	Pred 160 mg/d (qid)	DAY 0	AZA 2 mg/kg	DAY 4–6	MPred 0.5 mg/kg IV bid
DAY 3	Pred 120 mg/d (qid				
DAY 4	Pred 80 mg/d (qid)	DAY 0–2	CyA 1 mg/kg/d	DAY 7–20	Pred 0.5 mg/kg po
DAY 5	Pred 40 mg/d (qid)	DAY 3	CyA 6 mg/kg/d adjust to maintain thera-peutic blood levels	DAY 21–°°°	Pred 0.3 mg/kg po
DAY 6–13	Pred 20 mg/d			DAY 0–?	TACRO 0.03 mg/kg IV q12h until able to take po
DAY 14–20	Pred 15 mg/d				
DAY 21–27	Pred 12.5 mg/d			Day?–	TACRO 0.15 mg/kg po bid; adjust to maintain adequate drug levels
DAY 28–34	Pred 10 mg/d				
DAY 35–41	Pred 7.5 mg/d				
DAY 42	Pred 5 mg/d				
DAY 0–5	ATG 15 mg/kg IV given until adequate CyA levels obtained				
				If pt transplanted across ABO blood group:	
				DAY 0–14	OTK3 2.5 mg/kg IV
DAY 0–5	AZA 1 mg/kg/d IV				
DAY 6 or when tolerating po	AZA 2 mg/kg/d po				
DAY ? when tolerating po	CyA 10–15 mg/kg bid adjust to maintaining therapeutic blood levels				

[a]Data taken from Browne BJ, Kahan BD. Renal transplantation. Surg Clin North Am 74:1097–1116, 1994; Farges O, Samel D, Bismuth H. Optimal immunosuppressive clinical regimen in liver transplantation. Transplant Proc 26:2676–2678, 1994; Todo S, Fung JJ, Starl TE, et al. Single-center experience with primary orthotopic liver transplantation with FK506 immunosuppression; Ann Surg 220:297–309, 1994. Ueda M, Uemoto S, Inomata Y, et al. A proposal of FK506 optimal dosing in living related liver transplantations. Transplantation 60:258–264, 1995; Frazier OH, Macris MP. Progress in cardiac transplantation. Surg Clin North Am 74:1169–1182, 1994; Shumwa SJ, Bolman RM. Cardiac transplantation. In: Greenfield LJ. Surgery Scientific Principles and Practice. Philadelphia: JB Lippincott, 1993; Trulock EP. Management of lung transplant rejection. Chest 103:1566–1576, 1993; Sollinger HW, Geffner SR. Pancreas transplantation. Surg Clin North Am 74:1183–1195, 1994; Wadstrom J, Brekke B, Wramner L. et al. Triple versus quadruple induction immunosuppression in pancreas transplantation. Transplant Proc 27:1317–1318; Asfar S, Zhong R, Grant D. Small bowel transplantation. Surg Clin North Am 74:1197–1210, 1994; Todo S, Tzakis A, Abu-Elmagd K, et al. Clinical intestinal transplantation. Transplant Proc 25:2195–2197, 1993.

[b]Abbreviations: ATG, Antithymocyte globulin; CyA, cyclosporine; MPred, methylprednisolone; Pred, predisone; AZA, azathioprine; MM, mycophenolate mofetil; HC, hydrocortisone; TACRO, tacrolimus; Predlon, prednisolone.

°°° Withdrawn step-by-step within 1–9 months postop

(continued)

Table 96.6. *(Continued)*

Heart Transplant Protocols			

Regimen G		Regimen H		Regimen I	
PRE-OP	AZA 2 mg/kg po	DAY 0–10	OKT 3 5 mg IV	PRE-OP	CyA 6–10 mg po
	CyA 2–6 mg/kg po	DAY 0–10 DAY 11–	Pred 20 mg/d Increase to 2 mg/kg/d then taper to 0.5 mg/kg/d	DAY 0–2	CyA 1–2 mg/hr cont. IV infusion, if needed to maintain therapeutic CyA levels
DAY 0–11	MPred 500 mg IV taper to 30 mg/day by DAY 11	DAY 6–	AZA 2 mg/kg/day po	DAY 0–Mo 6	CyA dose to maintain a CyA trough level of 200 ± 25 ng/ml by HPLC
DAY 0–	AZA 2 mg/kg/day po adjust to WBC 5000–7000	DAY 6–10 DAY 11	CyA 5 mg/kg/day po increase dose to maintain CyA levels of 300–500 (¹²⁵I-RIA)	Mo 6–	CyA dose to maintain a trough level of 100 ng/ml by HPLC
DAY 0–	CyA 6 mg/kg/day po adjust to CyA levels of 300–500 ng/ml (¹²⁵I-RIA)			PRE-OP DAY 0–	AZA 2 mg/kg po AZA 2–2.5 mg/kg/d titrate to WBC ≥ 4000
				DAY 0 DAY 1	MPred 500 mg IV × 1 then MPred 125 mg IV q8h × 3
				DAY 2–Mo 3	Pred 1 mg/kg/d taper to 0.3 mg/kg/d
				Mo 3–Year 1	Pred 0.10–0.15 mg/kg/d

Lung Transplant Protocols			

Regimen J		Regimen K	
INTRA-OP	MPred 1 g IV	INTRA-OP	MPred 1 g IV
DAY 1–3	MPred 1 mg/kg/d IV	DAY 1–3	MPred 1 mg/kg/d IV
DAY 4–	MPred 0.5 mg/kg/d IV or Pred 0.5 mg/kg/d po	DAY 4–	MPred 0.5 mg/kg/d IV or Pred 0.5 mg/kg/d po
DAY 0–	AZA 2 mg/kg/d IV switch to oral therapy when tolerated	DAY 0–7	ATG 10–15 mg/kg/d IV
DAY 0–	CyA 2–4 mg/h IV adjusts based on levels switch to oral when tolerated	DAY 0–	AZA 2 mg/kg/d IV switch to oral therapy when tolerated
		DAY 0–	CyA 2–4 mg/kg/hr IV adjust based on levels switch to oral when tolerated

Pancreas Transplant Protocols			

Regimen L (Quadruple Therapy)		Regimen M (Quadruple Therapy)		Regimen N (Triple Therapy)	
DAY 0–14	OKT3 5 mg IV	DAY 0–8	ATG 3–5 mg/kg/d IV	INTRA-OP	MPred 500 mg IV
DAY 0	MPred 500 mg IV	INTRA-OP	MPred 500 mg IV	DAY 1–14	Predlon 100 mg/d taper to 20 mg/d
DAY 1–14	Pred taper to 30 mg/d	DAY 1–14	Predlon 100 mg/d taper to 20 mg/d	DAY 14–WK6	taper to 10 mg/d
DAY 15–Mo 6	Pred taper to 10 mg/d	DAY 14–WK 6	taper to 10 mg/d	DAY 1–	AZA 1.5–2 mg/kg/d
DAY 1–	AZA 1–2 mg/kg/d	DAY 1–	AZA 1.5–2 mg/kg/d	DAY 1–	CyA IV infusion dosed to maintain trough levels of 350–400 ng/ml switch to oral when tolerated
DAY ?	CyA begun when Scr < 3 target RIA level of 350–500 ng/ml	DAY 1–	CyA IV infusion dosed to maintain trough levels of 350–400 ng/ml switch to oral when tolerated	DAY ?–	CyA PO dosed to maintain therapeutic trough levels
		DAY ?–	CyA po dosed to maintain therapeutic trough levels		

(continued)

Table 96.6. (*Continued*)

Small Bowel Transplant Protocols			
Regimen O		**Regimen P**	
INTRA-OP	Donor blood 500 ml	INTRA-OP	MPred 1 g IV
		DAY 1	MPred 200 mg IV
INTRA-OP–	OKT3 5 mg IV	DAY 2	MPred 160 mg IV
DAY 2		DAY 3	MPred 120 mg IV
		DAY 4	MPred 80 mg IV
INTRA-OP	MPred 500 mg IV	DAY 5	MPred 60 mg IV
DAY 1–	MPred 0.5 mg/kg IV	DAY 6	MPred 20 mg IV
DAY ?	Pred 0.3 mg/kg/d started	DAY 7	steroid taper with Pred
	when enteral feeding re-		
	sumed and tapered to 0.3		
	mg/kg/d	INTRA-OP	TACRO 0.1 mg/kg/d IV cont.
			until tolerating po
INTRA-OP–	Prostaglandin E$_1$ 0.6–0.8	DAY ?	TACRO 0.3 mg/kg/d po
WEEK 2	µg/kg/h cont. IV infusion		
WEEK 3–8	Misoprostil 800 µg/d	DAY 0–(D5–25)	Prostaglandin E$_1$ 0.6–0.8
	(bid or qid)		µg/kg/h cont. IV infusion
DAY 0–	TACRO 0.3 mg/kg/d (bid)	°°	AZA given if unable to achieve
	adjust to maintain levels		adequate dosing of Tacrolimus
	of 20–40 ng/ml for 1st		
	month; then 10–20 ng/ml		
	(plasma ELISA)		

agents may be tapered with time, currently, patients must continue to use them indefinitely.

Immunosuppressive protocols exist both for rejection prophylaxis and for the treatment of established rejection. The specifics of the protocols vary, depending on the organ transplanted, the transplant center, and the collective clinical data at the time. Prophylactic regimens usually include an induction phase, where relatively high doses of immunosuppressive agents are administered early posttransplant, and a maintenance phase, where lower doses of immunosuppressants are adequate because the risk of rejection decreases with time. Most maintenance regimens include at least two or three agents used at lower doses. Table 96.6 lists some immunosuppression protocols for rejection prophylaxis. Table 96.7 summarizes the immunosuppressive agents utilized most frequently in transplantation.

SPECIFIC IMMUNOSUPPRESSIVE AGENTS

Corticosteroids

Corticosteroids such as prednisone or methylprednisolone were one of the first agents used for the prevention of rejection and continue to be part of most immunosuppressive protocols. For the treatment of rejection, high-dose intravenous methylprednisolone or prednisolone is used as first-line therapy. Oral prednisone is employed in most immunosuppressive protocols for the prophylaxis of rejection.

Corticosteroids inhibit the inductive phase of cytotoxic T cells by decreasing the production of important immunomodulating proteins such as IL-1 and IL-2, which results in diminished T lymphocyte proliferative response to alloantigens. The production of γ-interferon by T cells is also decreased (80–82). In addition, high-dose rejection therapy can decrease the expression of HLA antigens and β-2 microglobulins on peripheral blood lymphocytes. The immunogenicity of transplanted organs is thereby decreased (82, 83).

The dose of corticosteroids used in organ transplantation is empirical, and dosage adjustments are based on both therapeutic and toxic clinical responses. Although therapy is not routinely monitored by plasma levels, the pharmacokinetics of corticosteroids are complex, with changes occurring in various disease states (e.g., renal dysfunction) (Table 96.8) (84–87). Because of the widespread use of cyclosporine, steroid doses are currently lower than those used previously. Transplant protocols employ prednisone doses ranging from 20 to 140 mg/day initially. These doses are usually tapered to maintenance doses of 5 to 30 mg/day approximately 3 months posttransplantation. Maintenance doses at 12 to 18 months posttransplant range from 5 to 10 mg/day. A typical protocol includes high-dose prednisone (200 mg/day orally) at the time of transplant followed by rapid taper over 5 days to 20 mg/day. Others start with a prednisone dose of 30 mg/day orally that is slowly tapered to 7.5 to 15 mg/day at 12 to 18 months.

Adverse effects associated with corticosteroid use include fluid retention, electrolyte abnormalities, hyperglycemia, hypertension, peptic ulcers, delayed wound healing, and mental status changes. Long-term steroid use

Table 96.7.
Summary of Immunosuppressive Agents

Agent	Primary Mechanism of Action	Usual Dose	Adverse Effects	Comments
Corticosteroids	Blocks synthesis or response to IL-2, IL-1, prostaglandins and γ-interferon; reduces T-cell proliferative response to specific antigens	Initial prednisone: 0.5–2 mg/kg/day po Maintenance prednisone: 0.1–0.2 mg/kg/day po	Suppression of adrenal function, hypertension, fluid retention, hyperglycemia, psychosis, delayed wound healing, osteoporosis, cataracts	Administer with food or milk to minimize GI side effects
Azathioprine	Inhibits purine synthesis and metabolism, blocking DNA and RNA synthesis in response to antigenic stimulation	Initial: 1–4 mg/kg/day po or IV at the time of surgery Maintenance: 1–3 mg/kg/day	Bone marrow suppression megaloblastic anemia, nausea, vomiting, anorexia, diarrhea, drug fever, rash, alopecia, hepatotoxicity	Tablets may be administered with or after meals to minimize GI side effects
Cyclosporine	Inhibits T helper cell activity by decreasing IL-2 production and inhibiting T cell activitation; Also inhibits IL-1, IL-3, IL-5, and TNF-α	Initial: 0.5–5 mg/kg/day IV or 10–20 mg/kg/day po Maintenance: 2–5 mg/kg/day po; adjust dose based on measured trough levels and adverse reactions	Nephrotoxicity, hypertension, nausea, vomiting, diarrhea, hyperkalemia, hypomagnesemia, headache, tremors, paresthesias, hirsutism, gingival hyperplasia, seizures, hepatotoxocity	IV dose is ~ 1/3 the oral dose; IV administered as slow infusion (2–24 hr); Glass bottles only for administration of IV and oral solution; Oral IV solution has 12.5–32.9% alcohol, do not refrigerate
Tacrolimus	Inhibits T helper cell activity by decreasing IL-2 productoin; inhibits IL-3, IL-4, TNF-α, and IFN-γ	Initial: 0.05–0.1 mg/kg/day IV or 0.3 mg/kg/day po Maintenance: adjust based on measured trough levels and adverse reactions	Nephrotoxicity, insomnia, tremor, headache, tingling sensations, muscle aches, itching, fatigue, light sensitivity, nausea, vomiting, hypertension, hyperglycemia	IV dose is ~ 1/3 the oral dose; decrease dose in hepatic dysfunction
Mycophenolate mofetil	Inhibits de novo guanine synthesis; inhibits DNA proliferation of lymphocytes	Initial: 1 gm po bid	Gastrointestinal: diarrhea, nausea vomiting, loss of appetite, GI hemorrhage; anemia, leukopenia	Avoid co-administration of antacids, cholestyramine
Muromonab CD3 (OKT3)	Immediately decreases circulating T cells; interferes with antigen recognition by binding to CD3 cell surface	5 mg/day IV for 5–14 days	Fever, chills, tremor, headache, diarrhea, cramping, nausea, vomiting, hypotension, aseptic meningitis, pulmonary edema	Administer undiluted over 1 min; filter through a 0.22-micron filter
Antithymocyte globulin (ATG)	Complement-mediated lysis of lymphocytes, clearing of lymphocytes, alteration of T cell function	10–30 mg/kg/day for 7–14 days	Fever, chills, malaise, arthralgia, nausea, vomiting, leukopenia, thrombocytopenia, rash	Dilute in 0.45 or 0.9% normal saline; must be filtered and administered through central line

can lead to abnormalities such as osteoporosis, adrenal insufficiency, acne, and hirsutism (81). In addition, transplant patients requiring long-term steroid therapy are at increased risk for infection. To minimize steroid toxicity, alternate-day regimens are sometimes used for stable transplant recipients. The full spectrum of steroid side effects is discussed in Chapter 16, "Adrenocortical Dysfunction and Clinical Use of Steroids."

Azathioprine

First utilized in organ transplantation in 1962 (88), azathioprine remains part of many immunosuppressive protocols currently in use. It is a cytotoxic derivative of 6-mercaptopurine (6-MP). It was first synthesized in the early 1950s and was intended to be a slow-release prodrug of 6-MP (89), but was found to have a superior therapeutic index for immunosuppression. Azathioprine becomes ac-

Table 96.8.
Pharmacokinetic Parameters for Immunosuppressive Agents

Drug	CL (ml/min/kg)	Vd (L/kg)	T 1/2 (hr)	F (%)	Protein Binding (%)	Elimination	Reference
Prednisolone/ prednisone	1.6–2.8[a]	0.3–0.7	2.2	85–99	70–95[a]	Hepatic metabolism; concentration-dependent kinetics; renal excretion of metabolites; 7–15% excreted unchanged in urine	(84–87)
Azathioprine	0.81[b]	0.8	0.2	60	Unknown	Primarily metabolized to active 6-mercaptopurine (6-MP)	(96–99)
Cyclosporine	2.0–11.8	3.5	6–20	2–89 (ave. 30)	>96	Extensively metabolized liver and intestine by CYP3A4 to active and inactive metabolites	(119–126, 133, 141, 142)
Tacrolimus	5.8–103	5–65	3.5–40.5 (ave. 11)	5–67 (ave. 27)	88	Extensively metabolized in liver and intestine by CYP3A4 to active and inactive metabolites	(217, 221)

[a]Concentration dependent.
[b]Based on weight of 70 kg.

tive after it is metabolized to 6-MP and further converted to active 6-thioguanine nucleotides (90). These metabolites act by inhibiting early immune response during the proliferative cycle of effector T or B lymphocytes (91, 92). Intracellularly, they are incorporated into DNA, where they inhibit purine nucleotide synthesis and metabolism (92–95). Although useful in preventing the onset of acute rejection, azathioprine has little or no value in the treatment of ongoing rejection.

Azathioprine exhibits large interindividual variability in pharmacokinetics (96–98). It is readily absorbed from the gastrointestinal tract after oral administration, undergoes extensive first-pass hepatic metabolism, and is rapidly cleared from the blood. The pharmacokinetic parameters for azathioprine are summarized in Table 96.8 (96, 99). Azathioprine and 6-MP are rapidly metabolized in vivo to intracellular thioguanine nucleotides and to 6-thiouric acid via xanthine oxidase (100). Renal dysfunction does not impair the overall elimination of azathioprine or 6-MP (91).

The principal toxic effects of azathioprine are related to bone marrow suppression. Leukopenia is the most common manifestation although other hematologic disorders such as thrombocytopenia and megaloblastic anemia may occur. These hematologic effects appear to be dose related. Careful monitoring of the complete blood count is necessary. Other adverse effects include pruritis, dermatitis, fever, myopathy, alopecia, and pancreatitis. Gastrointestinal disturbances such as nausea, vomiting, and diarrhea may also occur, but they are most frequent in patients receiving large doses of azathioprine and may be avoided by giving the drug in divided doses or with meals. Drug-induced hepatitis has been reported as a late complication (after 6 months) of azathioprine therapy. It is manifested by low-grade jaundice with an increase in serum transaminases and bilirubin levels and is usually reversible on discontinuation of the drug (101–103).

An important drug interaction between allopurinol and azathioprine exists. By inhibiting xanthine oxidase, allopurinol prevents the metabolic formation of 6-thiouracil (6-TU) and therefore markedly prolongs the duration of action of azathioprine and 6-MP. Concomitant use of allopurinol with azathioprine can cause a marked increase in azathioprine exposure (104) and exacerbate adverse effects. Doses of azathioprine should be reduced by 25 to 50% to prevent this complication.

Clinically, azathioprine is used in conjunction with other immunosuppressive agents for the prophylaxis of allograft rejection. It is usually administered continuously since withholding the drug in the early posttransplant period has led to transplant rejection (105) although it has been withdrawn later in the posttransplant course without deleterious effects. Azathioprine is commonly administered in standard doses of 1 to 4 mg/kg at the time of surgery and then orally in doses of 1 to 3 mg/kg posttransplantation. Doses are adjusted based on the complete blood count and should be monitored throughout therapy. It has been recommended that blood counts be monitored weekly during the first 8 weeks of therapy and less frequently thereafter. It must be noted that leukopenia and thrombocytopenia can persist even after azathioprine has been discontinued (100, 106).

Cyclosporine

Cyclosporine (CyA) is a lipophilic, cyclic undecapeptide produced by the fungus *Tolypocladium inflatum gams* (107). It was discovered in 1972 from a soil sample containing the fungus and was shown to have immunosuppressive properties in 1976 (108). Initial clinical studies in renal transplant recipients began in 1978 (109). Cyclosporine revolutionized the field of transplantation because it was the first agent to produce relatively specific immunosuppression, without causing bone marrow suppression.

MECHANISM OF ACTION

Although widely used in transplant protocols around the world for more than 10 years, the exact molecular mechanism of cyclosporine remains to be elucidated. Basically, cyclosporine inhibits cytotoxic T cell activation while allowing the activation and amplification of T suppressor lymphocytes. The result is a specific immunologic unresponsiveness to the stimulating alloantigen (i.e., from the foreign allograft) (110). More specifically, cyclosporine is a prodrug, becoming active when bound to an intracellular receptor called cyclophilin. This drug-receptor complex interferes with an intermediate signaling protein called calcineurin, which appears to block a nuclear factor required for transcription of the cytokine IL-2 (111). The result is a disabling of T cell function. T cells are unable to transform and release cytokines that would normally induce and mount an immune response (112–114). Cyclosporine is also thought to have effects on many other cytokines and cell types, including IL-1, IL-3, IL-5 (115, 115), B cells, and tumor necrosis factor α (TNF α) (117). Because cyclosporine spares suppressor T cells and lacks activity against mature cytotoxic T cells, it is essentially ineffective in the treatment of ongoing rejection (118).

PHARMACOKINETICS AND METABOLISM

Cyclosporine exhibits highly variable pharmacokinetics and metabolism. The pharmacokinetics are summarized in Table 96.8. After oral administration, cyclosporine absorption is slow and incomplete. Peak concentrations occur between 1 and 8 hours after dosing. Bioavailability ranges from 2 to 89% with a mean of 30% reported in various types of transplant recipients (119–126). Several factors can influence the absorption of cyclosporine. The bioavailability of cyclosporine appears to increase with time after transplantation (127, 128). A high-fat meal has been shown to increase absorption and/or clearance (129) although standardized meals had no effect on cyclosporine pharmacokinetics (130–132). Bile is required for the absorption of cyclosporine; therefore, factors affecting bile flow such as cholestasis and biliary diversion (e.g., T-tube) can decrease cyclosporine absorption (133, 134). Finally, absorption may also be reduced in patients with liver disease, postoperative ileus, gastroparesis, and diarrhea (127, 133, 135, 136).

Cyclosporine is widely distributed in the body. The volume of distribution ranges from 0.9 to 4.8 L/kg, with an average of 3.5 L/kg (133). The highest cyclosporine concentrations are found in fat and the liver. It also sequesters in the thymus, spleen, lymph nodes, bone marrow, pancreas, kidneys, lungs, and skin (137–139). Approximately 60% of cyclosporine in the blood is bound to red blood cells. In plasma, cyclosporine is also highly bound, with 85 to 90% bound to plasma lipoproteins, mostly high-density lipoprotein (HDL) (140).

Cyclosporine is extensively metabolized in the liver and intestine by cytochrome P450 3A4 (CYP3A4) (141, 142) to more than 30 metabolites (143). Recent evidence suggests that the erratic and low bioavailability of cyclosporine may not be due to poor absorption, but rather to intestinal metabolism occurring prior to the drug reaching the systemic circulation (144). The clinical significance of the metabolites remains unclear. The most active metabolite is AM1, with approximately 10 to 20% of the immunosuppressive activity of parent cyclosporine. Other less active metabolites are AM9 and AM4N (143, 145).

Less than 1% of cyclosporine is excreted unchanged in the urine. Biliary excretion is the major route of elimination of cyclosporine, with less than 1% excreted as unchanged cyclosporine and greater than 40% appearing as metabolites (122, 133, 146). Therefore, dosage adjustment in patients with renal insufficiency is not warranted; however, patients with hepatic failure exhibit decreased cyclosporine clearances (135). Other factors that may affect cyclosporine clearance include age (pediatric patients exhibit higher clearance rates) and small bowel length in pediatric liver transplant patients (127, 147, 148).

DRUG INTERACTIONS

Because cyclosporine is metabolized extensively by CYP3A4, and because CYP3A4 may be responsible for more than 50% of the metabolism of all drugs, the potential for drug interactions is immense. Many drug interactions have been substantiated both in vitro and in vivo. Some of these are of clinical significance (see Table 96.9) (149–180). Agents such as phenytoin, phenobarbital, valproic acid, carbamazepine, and rifampin induce the cytochrome P450 system and when given concomitantly with cyclosporine will increase the metabolism of cyclosporine and cause decreased drug levels. On the other hand, agents such as ketoconazole, erythromycin, verapamil, and diltiazem inhibit the cytochrome P450 system, decreasing the metabolism of cyclosporine and increasing drug levels. In addition, alterations in intestinal metabolism can occur with oral cyclosporine given concomitantly with a known CYP3A4 inhibitor or inducer (156, 174).

In addition to the pharmacokinetic drug interactions discussed here, other pharmacodynamic interactions may occur when cyclosporine is administered concomitantly with certain therapeutic agents. Some drugs such as aminoglycosides, amphotericin B, trimethoprim-sulfamethoxazole, cephalosporins, and indomethacin can potentiate the nephrotoxicity of cyclosporine (181–186). Careful monitoring of renal function is required. The nephrotoxicity is

Table 96.9.
Drug Interactions with Cyclosporine (CyA)

Drug	Proposed Mechanism	Reference
Drugs that *increase* CyA conc.		
Erythromycin	Inhibition of CyA metabolism and biliary excretion, increased CyA absorption	(149–152)
Ketoconazole	Inhibition of CyA metabolism	(153–156)
Diltiazem	Inhibition of CyA metabolism	(157–158)
Verapamil	Inhibition of CyA metabolism	(159)
Nicardipine	Inhibition of CyA metabolism	(160, 161)
Metoclopramide	Increased CyA absorption	(162)
Methyltestosterone	Inhibition of CyA metabolism	(163)
Oral contraceptives	Inhibition of CyA metabolism	(164)
Methylprednisolone (hi dose)	Inhibition of CyA metabolism	(165)
Danazol	Inhibition of CyA metabolism	(166, 167)
Drugs that *decrease* CyA conc.		
Carbamazepine		(168)
Phenobarbitone	Induction of CyA metabolism	(169)
Phenytoin	Induction of CyA metabolism	(170, 171)
Rifampin/rifampicin	Induction of CyA metabolism, decreased CyA absorption	(172–174)
Isoniazid	Induction of CyA metabolism	(175, 176)
Nafcillin	Induction of CyA metabolism	(177)
Octreotide	Alteration of CyA absorption	(178–180)

usually reversible on discontinuation of these agents (133). Other important interactions include potentiation of other toxicities of cyclosporine, such as lovastatin increasing the incidence of rhabdomyolysis (187–189), minoxidil causing additive hirsutism (30), and nifedipine causing increased gingival hyperplasia (190).

TOXICITY PROFILE

The most common adverse effect of cyclosporine is nephrotoxicity. It is dose limiting and has been shown to occur in 50 to 70% of renal transplant patients, with similar incidence in heart and liver transplant patients (191, 192). The characteristics of cyclosporine nephrotoxicity are that it is dose and concentration dependent, involves a reduction in glomerular filtration rate, and is usually reversible on discontinuation. It presents clinically as a rise in serum creatinine often with oliguria, hyperkalemia, and decreased renal blood flow. In kidney transplant patients, it is often difficult to differentiate between cyclosporine-induced nephrotoxicity and allograft rejection.

Another serious, but less common side effect of cyclosporine is hepatotoxicity. It occurs in 4 to 7% of allograft recipients and is characterized by a rise in serum transaminases (AST and ALT), alkaline phosphatase, and total bilirubin levels (193–195). These effects appear to be dose dependent and reversible with dosage reduction.

Other side effects attributable to cyclosporine are hypertension and hypomagnesemia. Further, gingival hyperplasia, hirsutism, and a variety of neurologic syndromes such as headaches, tremor, paresthesias, and seizures can occur (196).

DRUG LEVEL MONITORING

Drug level monitoring is an important part of cyclosporine therapy and is done routinely in most transplant centers. Since cyclosporine exhibits wide inter- and intraindividual variability in pharmacokinetics and metabolism, and because of its narrow therapeutic range, tailoring therapy to a specific individual is difficult. In addition, the dose of cyclosporine correlates poorly with the resultant drug level (197). Therefore, therapeutic drug monitoring is used to help guide therapy and make dosage adjustments in order to maximize therapy while trying to minimize toxicity. Drug levels may also be utilized to monitor compliance.

Cyclosporine may be measured in either whole blood or plasma. Whole blood is the preferred medium because of analytical ease. Approximately 60% of cyclosporine is bound to red blood cells (140); therefore concentrations are higher in whole blood than plasma. In addition, the partitioning of cyclosporine in whole blood and plasma depends on temperature, hematocrit, drug concentration, and incubation time (198, 199). These factors are avoided when whole blood is used.

Many different assays exist to measure cyclosporine. Each has advantages and disadvantages that will be discussed. It is important to know which assay is being utilized to measure cyclosporine so that levels may be interpreted appropriately since all have different reference ranges. High performance liquid chromatography (HPLC) measurement of cyclosporine is the most specific assay available and is used as a reference assay against which other assays are compared (200, 201). It is a specific measure of cyclosporine in that parent cyclosporine and metabolites are measured separately. However, it is difficult to perform, requires technical expertise, expensive equipment, and takes 6 to 24 hours to analyze samples. Therefore, few centers continue to use HPLC to measure cyclosporine concentrations for clinical monitoring (202).

Radioimmunoassays (RIA) are also used for cyclosporine quantitation and can be divided into two classes: one class utilizing a "specific" monoclonal antibody to cyclosporine and one class utilizing a "nonspecific" monoclonal antibody. The specific assays measure parent cyclosporine, whereas the nonspecific assays measure parent cyclosporine as well as some metabolites. Generally, no role exists for the nonspecific class of RIAs. Two RIAs are available to measure cyclosporine more specifically, one with an iodinated tracer (^{125}I-RIA) and one with a tritiated tracer (^{3}H-RIA). Both tests are less difficult to perform than HPLC and have faster turnaround times (203). Both have demonstrated good results in measuring cyclosporine levels and are used clinically.

There are also two types of fluorescein polarization immunoassays (FPIA): one utilizing a specific monoclonal antibody and one with a nonspecific monoclonal antibody. Again, no role exists for the nonspecific FPIA; it measures cyclosporine concentrations approximately 3 to 4 times that of HPLC (204). Although cyclosporine measurements with the specific FPIA appear to be higher than ^{125}I-RIA (205–207), the FPIA appears to be technically simpler than the RIAs and has rapid turnaround times. More experience is required with this assay; however, it appears promising for use in the clinical setting.

Target concentrations of cyclosporine depend on the assay utilized, the type of transplant, the time after transplant, and the individual transplant center. In general, when measuring cyclosporine in whole blood using a specific assay such as HPLC or RIA, target concentrations are in the range of 150 to 400 ng/ml.

DOSING

The dose of cyclosporine used in the prophylaxis of allograft rejection varies depending on the institution, the organ transplanted, other concomitant immunosuppressive agents, and the time after transplantation. Initial doses of 10 to 20 mg/kg/day are commonly used.

Cyclosporine is available as 25 mg and 100 mg gelatin capsules, an oral solution of 100 mg/ml in an olive oil and alcohol base, and a parenteral solution of 250 mg/5 ml vial for dilution.

Cyclosporine doses should be administered on a consistent schedule with respect to time of day and meals. Cyclosporine oral solution may be diluted in chocolate milk to make it more palatable. In patients with nasogastric (NG) tubes, cyclosporine oral solution may be administered directly followed by flushing with water. Parenteral cyclosporine solutions may be diluted in 0.9% NaCl or

D5W and given by slow intravenous infusion over 2 to 24 hours. Intravenous doses are empirically given at approximately one-third the oral dose and titrated to the desired therapeutic level.

Cyclosporine (Neoral®)

In an effort to decrease the high variability in absorption, a new microemulsion formulation of cyclosporine has been developed and approved for use in the prophylaxis of allograft rejection. It is the same molecular compound of cyclosporine A in a formulation containing a surfactant, lipophilic and hydrophilic solvents, and ethanol. Incorporation of these components apparently allows more rapid dispersion of cyclosporine in the gut lumen, thus allowing more complete and better absorption (208). Improvement in several pharmacokinetic parameters has been demonstrated. Neoral has an average 29% higher bioavailability compared to the gelatin capsules. In addition, Neoral exhibits less within patient variability in t_{max}, C_{max}, C_{min}, and area-under-the-concentration-time curve (AUC). Finally, an improved correlation between trough concentrations and AUC was demonstrated with Neoral (209–211). Theoretically, these advantages should translate into a more efficacious compound, with fewer incidences of rejection and more optimal dosing, and allow better predictions of drug exposure based on a given dose (211).

Tacrolimus

Tacrolimus, formerly known as FK506, is a macrolide antibiotic isolated from the fungus *Streptomyces tsukubaensis* (212). It is a potent immunosuppressive agent with 10 to 100 times the activity of cyclosporine in vitro. Tacrolimus has shown comparable efficacy to cyclosporine in preventing acute rejection with a generally similar side effect profile. Some centers have demonstrated superior efficacy with tacrolimus than with cyclosporine and are using tacrolimus as first-line prophylaxis therapy, replacing cyclosporine (213–215). One significant difference in its clinical applicability compared to cyclosporine is its ability to reverse ongoing rejection as well as prevent it.

MECHANISM OF ACTION

Although structurally distinct from cyclosporine, tacrolimus possesses a similar mechanism of action. Both tacrolimus and cyclosporine act at an early step in blocking T-cell activation. Tacrolimus binds to an intracellular binding protein, FKBP, and inhibits the same intermediate signaling protein, calcineurin, as cyclosporine (111). Ultimately, tacrolimus inhibits IL-2 gene transcription, as well as IL-3, IL-4, TNF-α, and interferon-γ (IFN-γ) (216).

PHARMACOKINETICS AND METABOLISM

Tacrolimus exhibits highly variable pharmacokinetics and metabolism. After oral administration, tacrolimus has poor and erratic absorption. Its bioavailability has been reported to range from 5 to 67%, with a mean of 27% in transplant patients. Peak plasma concentrations are attained in 0.5 to 4 hours (217, 218). Coadministration of food causes a reduction in the rate and extent of absorption (219). In contrast to cyclosporine, tacrolimus absorption depends less on the presence of bile (220).

Because of its high lipophilicity, tacrolimus is extensively distributed in red blood cells and tissues. In the plasma, tacrolimus is primarily bound to α-1 acid glycoprotein in contrast to cyclosporine (bound to lipoproteins). As for cyclosporine, the distribution of tacrolimus within the blood is influenced by hematocrit, concentration, temperature, and the concentration of plasma proteins. In addition, tacrolimus sequesters in the heart, lung, spleen, kidney, and pancreas (217).

Tacrolimus is predominantly metabolized in the liver and intestine by CYP3A4 (221) to at least nine metabolites, of which two possess approximately 10% the immunosuppressive activity of the parent compound (221). Less than 5% of the dose is excreted in the bile as the parent compound, whereas the majority of the metabolites are found in the bile. Less than 1% of the dose is excreted in the urine as unchanged drug (217). Hepatic dysfunction alters the clearance of tacrolimus, and dosage adjustments must be made.

DRUG INTERACTIONS

Many drug interactions with tacrolimus have been documented as clinically significant. Interactions resulting in increased tacrolimus levels have been documented for the CYP3A4 inhibitors erythromycin, fluconazole, methylprednisolone, and clotrimazole (217). Although the experience with tacrolimus is not as vast to date, it is prudent to suspect that interactions documented with cyclosporine may occur with tacrolimus, especially if it involves CYP3A4. Tacrolimus should be monitored closely in patients receiving agents known to induce or inhibit CYP3A4.

TOXICITY

The toxicity profile of tacrolimus is similar to cyclosporine. The most common adverse effects appear to be nephrotoxicity, neurotoxicity, and diabetogenic effects. The nephrotoxicity is dose limiting and appears to have a similar incidence and presentation as cyclosporine (222). Other adverse effects in order of decreasing frequency include insomnia, tremors, headache, tingling sensations, muscle achiness, itching, fatigue, sensitivity to light, and gastrointestinal symptoms. Some side effects seen with cyclosporine appear to occur with decreased frequency in patients treated with tacrolimus, including hirsutism, gingival hyperplasia, and hypertension. In addition, patients on tacrolimus may have a decreased steroid requirement compared to patients taking cyclosporine (213).

Other side effects such as hyperglycemia and tremor have been reported to occur more frequently with tacrolimus than cyclosporine (214).

DRUG LEVEL MONITORING

Because of the wide variability in pharmacokinetics and metabolism as well as its relatively narrow therapeutic range, it is recommended that drug level monitoring be used to guide tacrolimus therapy. Analogous to the issues with cyclosporine, there are advantages to measuring tacrolimus in whole blood versus plasma: whole blood levels are higher and analysis times are faster (213). Two assays have been developed to measure tacrolimus concentrations: an enzyme-linked immunosorbent assay (ELISA) (223) and a microparticle enzyme immunoassay (MEIA) (224). Both utilize the same nonspecific monoclonal antibody to tacrolimus. Although both methods are reliable and effective in guiding tacrolimus therapy, each has advantages and disadvantages. The MEIA suffers from sensitivity problems at low tacrolimus concentrations, and the ELISA has a slower turnaround time (225). Therapeutic plasma concentrations of tacrolimus using ELISA are approximately 0.5 to 2 ng/ml, whereas whole blood levels are in the range of 5 to 20 ng/ml (226).

DOSING

Tacrolimus dosing requirements should be adjusted based on drug level monitoring, individual center protocols, concomitant immunosuppression, and adverse effects. Initial intravenous doses of 0.05 to 0.1 mg/kg/day given over 4 to 24 hours have been used with conversion to 0.3 mg/kg/day as oral therapy (214–216, 227). When changing from intravenous to oral therapy, a threefold increase in dose can be used as a guideline. Dosage requirements will generally decline with time after transplantation.

Life-threatening anaphylaxis has occurred with intravenously administered tacrolimus most likely due to the polyoxyl 60 hydrogenated castor oil vehicle. Therefore, caution must be observed, and the appropriate equipment and agents for potential anaphylaxis should be available when administering intravenous tacrolimus. Tacrolimus must be diluted in 0.9% normal saline or D5W to a concentration of 4 to 20 μg/ml prior to administration. Tacrolimus is available for intravenous use in 5 mg/ml concentrate for infusion. Oral capsules are available in 1- and 5-mg strengths.

Mycophenolate Mofetil

Mycophenolate mofetil, formerly known as RS-61443, was developed with the intention to improve the current armamentarium of immunosuppressive agents. An agent specific to lymphocytes with fewer adverse effects on other cell types was needed. Mycophenolate mofetil recently received FDA approval for the prophylaxis of renal allograft rejection. Preliminary clinical studies have shown that mycophenolate mofetil may be more effective than azathioprine in preventing acute renal allograft rejection and was better tolerated (228).

MECHANISM OF ACTION

Mycophenolate mofetil is the morpholinoethyl ester of mycophenolic acid. Mycophenolic acid is a potent, noncompetitive, reversible inhibitor of inosine monophosphate dehydrogenase. The ultimate result is inhibition of de novo purine guanosine synthesis. The antiproliferative activity of mycophenolate is specific to lymphocytes because lymphocytes depend on this de novo pathway of purine synthesis, whereas most other cells can utilize a salvage pathway (229). In vitro, mycophenolate also inhibits the proliferation of B lymphocytes, antibody formation, and the generation of cytotoxic T cells (230, 231). In animal models, mycophenolate has been shown to prevent the occurrence of chronic rejection (232). If similar results can be obtained in humans, mycophenolate would have a distinct advantage over other currently available immunosuppressive agents since none to date have been able to decrease the incidence of chronic rejection.

PHARMACOKINETICS AND METABOLISM

Preliminary studies suggest that there are substantial interindividual variations in the pharmacokinetics of mycophenolate mofetil. AUCs after 20 days of therapy were significantly higher than the first day of therapy, suggesting possible accumulation. The primary route of elimination of mycophenolate mofetil is by urinary excretion as the glucuronide metabolite. Renal impairment appears to affect the elimination of mycophenolate, with increasing renal dysfunction causing higher AUCs and decreased metabolite excretion (233, 234).

DRUG INTERACTIONS

Mycophenolate mofetil should not be administered concomitantly with azathioprine because of potentiation of adverse effects. In addition, antacids and cholestyramine cause a reduction in the absorption and systemic concentrations of mycophenolate mofetil. Therefore, it is recommended that administration of antacids be given separately from mycophenolate and that concomitant administration of mycophenolate and cholestyramine or other agents that interfere with enterohepatic recycling be avoided.

TOXICITY

The main adverse effects associated with mycophenolate mofetil are gastrointestinal. Nausea, vomiting, abdominal pain, loss of appetite, gastrointestinal hemorrhage, and pancreatitis (rare) have been reported. In addition, anemia and leukopenia may occur with mycophenolate mofetil. Other adverse events that are mild or moderate in severity include sore throat, numbness of limbs, numbness of tongue, and muscle weakness.

DOSING

Currently, mycophenolate is available orally as 250-mg capsules. The recommended dose for the prevention of allograft rejection in renal transplant patients is 1 gram orally twice daily. As with all other immunosuppressive agents, dosage adjustments should be made based on concomitant immunosuppressive therapy, adverse effects, type of organ transplanted, and time after transplantation.

Monoclonal Antibodies—OKT3

OKT3 (or muromonab CD3) is a purified murine IgG2a monoclonal antibody directed against the CD3 antigen found on the surface of all mature human T cells. Although its exact mechanism has not been fully characterized, OKT3 is thought to exert its anti-T-cell proliferative effects by two mechanisms. One mechanism is T-cell depletion, and the other is modulation of the T-cell receptor. OKT3 is thought to bind to mature T cells causing opsonization and removal by the reticuloendothelial system in the liver and spleen. Within minutes after intravenous injection of OKT3, there is a rapid clearing of CD3+ cells from the circulation, which is complete in 1 hour (235, 236). It has been shown that T-cell depletion is not the only mode of action. OKT3 cross-links with the CD3 molecule on the T cell resulting in removal of all CD3 molecules on the T-cell surface, including the T-cell receptor (T-cell modulation). The result is the production of T lymphocytes that lack the ability to function properly.

OKT3 is a very potent immunosuppressive agent that is used in the treatment of rejection as well as in some induction therapy protocols. In reversing steroid-resistant rejection, it is effective in 75 to 95% of all cases (237). It appears to be more efficacious when given as first-line treatment than when given as rescue therapy. For instance, in renal transplant patients, its reversal rate when used in primary treatment was 90 versus 71% in steroid-resistant cases (238).

OKT3 is usually reserved for the treatment of steroid-resistant rejection because of some limitations that can preclude its use. The most important shortcoming is its extensive T-cell suppression, which may cause an increase in viral infections, notably cytomegalovirus (239). In addition, antibodies can develop against OKT3 (xenosensitization), preventing further use of the agent. A first-dose "cytokine release syndrome" is common, which consists of flulike symptoms, dyspnea, tremor, chest pain, and less commonly aseptic meningitis and pulmonary edema. This is thought to be due to the release of cytokines during initial T-cell depletion (240, 241).

Immunologic monitoring can be useful in determining the efficacy of therapy with OKT3. Three tactics can be used, either alone or in combination. First, CD3+ cells can be monitored. CD3+ cells disappear from the circulation after OKT3 administration, and for optimal efficacy, they should be nearly undetectable. The problem with inferring efficacy information by this method is that only circulating CD3+ cells are measured and not those infiltrating the graft (242). It is recommended that CD3+ cells be monitored three times a week (243). If levels remain elevated, the dose of OKT3 may be increased. Second, serum OKT3 levels can be monitored. The two factors influencing the level of OKT3 are the total number of available CD3 molecules on the T-cell surface and the gradual formation of anti-OKT3 antibodies due to xenosensitization. Therefore, serum OKT3 levels should provide both information on the efficacy of OKT3 and an indirect measurement of xenosensitization. However, this method is controversial since its clinical usefulness has not been definitively proved (242). Finally, anti-OKT3 antibodies can be monitored directly in order to determine if sensitization has occurred. Most centers utilize the measurement of anti-OKT3 antibodies particularly when a patient is to receive a repeated course of OKT3. If the anti-OKT3 titer is less than 1:100 as measured by ELISA, OKT3 may still be effective; however, if the anti-OKT3 titer is greater than 1:1000, then OKT3 is not given.

The recommended dose of OKT3 is 5 mg intravenously daily for 5 to 14 days. In patients weighing less than 30 kg, the dose may be decreased to 2.5 mg. Acetaminophen, diphenhydramine, and/or steroids are given prior to the first dose, and subsequent doses are given in order to ameliorate some of the first-dose "cytokine release syndrome" effects. OKT3 should not be administered to patients whose body weight has increased more than 3% during the week prior to therapy because of the risk of pulmonary edema. OKT3 is available as 5 mg/5 ml vials.

Polyclonal Antibodies—Antithymocyte Globulin (ATG)

Prior to 1992, many transplant patients were receiving an investigational polyclonal antibody produced in Minnesota, Antilymphocyte Globulin (MALG), as induction therapy. MALG was never formally approved by the Food and Drug Administration (FDA) and is not currently available for clinical use (244). The alternative therapies currently available for induction therapy consist of (1) OKT3, (2) antithymocyte globulin (ATG), or (3) no induction therapy. Some centers have opted to forgo induction therapy with a potent agent such as OKT3 or ATG because of the risks of overimmunosuppression.

ATG is an immunoglobulin (primarily IgG) prepared from the plasma or serum of horses that have been hyperimmunized with human thymus lymphocytes. It is a potent immunosuppressant that is used for the prophylaxis and treatment of rejection. When used for prophylaxis, it is part of the induction regimen given immediately postoperatively to prevent first rejection or to protect early kidney function from the nephrotoxicity of cyclosporine. ATG also is effective in treating steroid-resistant rejection (245, 246). ATG exerts its effect against rejection by complement-mediated lysis of lymphocytes, clearing of lymphocytes by the reticuloendothelial system, and/or alteration of T-cell function (247).

One of the limitations of ATG therapy is the potential for overimmunosuppression analogous to OKT3 with subsequent risk of infections and malignancy. The most common adverse effect of ATG therapy is fever accompanied by chills. In addition, many patients experience a serum sickness reaction that resembles a flulike reaction with fever, malaise, arthralgia, nausea, vomiting, and lymphadenopathy. Acetaminophen and diphenhydramine can be given as premedications in addition to steroids to ward off this complication. Other adverse effects consist of leukopenia, thrombocytopenia, anemia, rash, pruritis, and less frequently, hypotension, hypertension, and tachycardia (247).

ATG is available in 50 mg/ml concentrated solution. It must be diluted in 0.45 or 0.9% sodium chloride prior to administration. Dextrose solutions are not recommended for dilution. ATG should be filtered and administered through a central line, arteriovenous shunt, or fistula to minimize the risk of phlebitis and tissue necrosis. For the prevention or treatment of allograft rejection, the dose given is 10 to 30 mg/kg/day for 7 to 14 days.

Immunosuppressive Regimens

Table 96.6 reviews immunosuppressive regimens published in the literature for the various organs transplanted. Historically, most immunosuppressive regimens consisted of induction therapy for the first 7 to 14 days after transplantation. More recently, some transplant centers have eliminated potent induction agents from their protocols because of risks of overimmunosuppression and availability of newer agents for maintenance immunosuppression. In general, maintenance regimens have traditionally consisted of cyclosporine, azathioprine, and prednisone. With the advent of new immunosuppressants, other combinations of agents can be utilized. For example, tacrolimus can be used in place of cyclosporine, and mycophenolate mofetil can be used in place of azathioprine.

Investigational Immunosuppressive Agents

DEOXYSPERGUALIN

15-deoxyspergualin is a 15-deoxy analog of spergualin isolated from Bacillus laterosporus. It has been developed and tested clinically in Japan since 1987 and was approved for commercial use there in 1994. Deoxyspergualin reversibly suppresses the maturation of T cells, the induction of cytotoxic T cells, and the amplification of plasma cells from B cells (248, 249). Deoxyspergualin has been given to patients in Japan for the treatment of rejection. When given in combination with methylprednisolone in a multi-central open trial, acute rejection resolved in 92% of patients. The dose recommended after a dose-finding study was 5 mg/kg/day as an intravenous infusion for 7 days. Adverse effects noted in these patients were temporary facial sensory disorders, nausea, vomiting, and leukopenia (248). Deoxyspergualin is currently undergoing clinical trials in the United States.

MIZORIBINE

Another investigational agent being used in Japan is mizoribine. It is an analog of azathioprine and, like azathioprine, is a prodrug converted to its active moiety by phosphorylation. It inhibits de novo purine synthesis in lymphocytes by blocking inosine monophosphate dehydrogenase. Preliminary results in renal transplant patients indicate that it is equally efficacious to azathioprine. Comparing mizoribine with azathioprine in triple drug regimens containing cyclosporine and prednisone, 3-year patient and graft survival rates were 100 and 92% in the mizoribine group, and 100 and 91% in the azathioprine group. The incidence of bone marrow suppression was significantly less in the mizoribine group. In addition, mizoribine also appears to have less hepatotoxic effects than azathioprine (250).

SIROLIMUS

Sirolimus, also known as rapamycin, is a macrolide antibiotic produced by *Streptomyces hydroscopicus* (251). It is structurally similar to tacrolimus and has similar potency, approximately 100-fold greater than cyclosporine.

Although sirolimus binds to the same binding protein, FK-binding protein, sirolimus does not inhibit IL-2 production. Rather, it inhibits the responses of T-cells to IL-2 and other cytokines. In addition, it may be synergistic with cyclosporine (252–255).

POSTTRANSPLANT MANAGEMENT

Two of the most important considerations in patients on lifelong immunosuppression are the subsequent risks of infection and malignancy (see "Infection" and "Malignancy"). In addition, the individual immunosuppressive agents have several side effects that often require medical management. Both cyclosporine and tacrolimus have the potential to cause hypertension, which may require antihypertensive therapy with diuretics or calcium-channel blockers. Cyclosporine can also cause electrolyte imbalances, such as hyperkalemia or hypomagnesemia, which, if severe enough, may require fludrocortisone to help retain potassium or magnesium replacement, respectively.

Infection

Several factors can influence the incidence and severity of infections posttransplantation. These include possible surgical complications; the type, intensity, and duration of immunosuppressive therapy; and the organisms encountered by the patient in the hospital and the community. There is a general time course of risk for bacterial, viral, fungal, and protozoal organisms (see Fig. 96.9). Overall, approximately 55% of posttransplant infections are due to bacteria, 30% to viruses, and 15% to fungi (18). During the first month after transplant, the majority of infections are related to the surgical procedure and are bacterial in origin. For instance, renal transplant patients are at risk for urinary tract infections, heart and lung transplant patients for

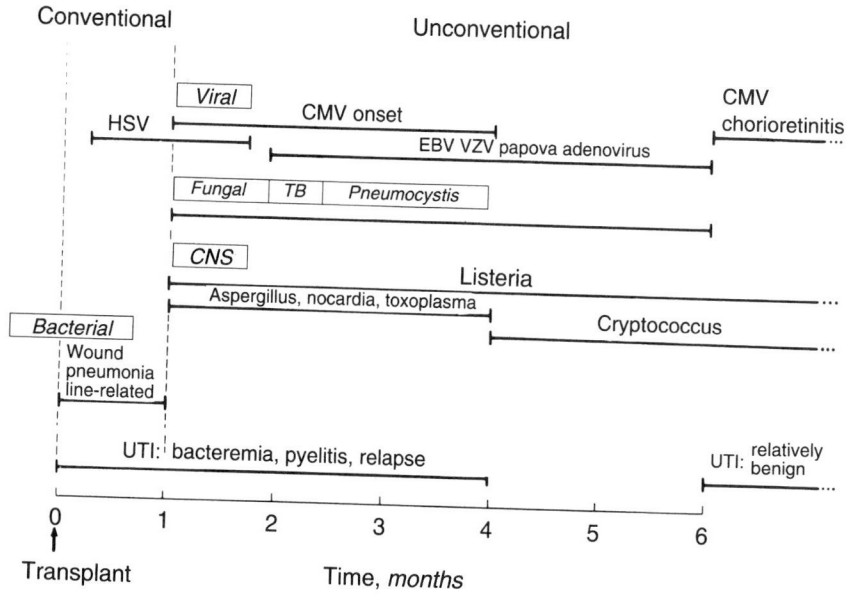

Figure 96.9 Incidence of posttransplant infections and time course in solid organ transplant patients. (Modified from Rubin RH. Kidney Int 44:221, 1993. Reprinted with permission, Blackwell Science, Inc.)

intrathoracic infections, and liver transplant patients for intraabdominal infections (256).

Viral infections pose the greatest infectious risk 1 to 6 months after transplant. The most common pathogens are from the herpes virus family, Herpes Simplex Virus (HSV), cytomegalovirus (CMV), Epstein-Barr virus (EBV), and varicella zoster virus (VZV). HSV infections usually occur during the first 6 weeks and usually present as mucocutaneous infections in and around the oral cavity. CMV infections occur in approximately 40 to 70% of transplant patients, whereas approximately 10 to 30% go on to develop significant disease (257–260). Risk factors for developing CMV disease include the use of antilymphocyte therapy (especially OKT3), retransplantation, and the donor organ being seropositive for CMV (261). Prophylaxis to prevent CMV disease is currently controversial. Prophylactic measures include high-dose oral acyclovir, ganciclovir, or CMV hyperimmune globulin. For the treatment of CMV disease, ganciclovir 5 mg/kg intravenous is given every 12 hours.

The majority of fungal infections occur in the first 2 months after transplantation. Candida and Aspergillus species account for more than 80% of these infections. The most common site for Candida infections is in the oral mucosa. Prophylaxis with clotrimazole troches or nystatin is often given to reduce the incidence of infection. If invasive disease occurs with Candida, treatment with fluconazole or amphotericin B is given. Invasive disease with Aspergillus carries a poor prognosis, with reported mortality ranging from 30 to 100%. This is due in part to the difficulty in recognizing that early infection is difficult and often ineffective therapy (256). The only therapeutic option in the face of invasive Aspergillus disease is Amphotericin B.

Pneumocystis carinii is a protozoan parasite that can cause pneumonia late in the posttransplant course. All transplant patients are placed on trimethoprim-sulfamethoxazole prophylaxis for 6 to 12 months, and this has nearly eliminated infection with this pathogen.

Malignancy

The incidence of malignancy in transplant patients is 1 to 16%, with an average of 6%, which is greater than the incidence in the general population (18, 262). The occurrence of cancer increases with time. Malignancies that are common in the general population are relatively uncommon in transplant patients. Cancer of the skin and lips is the most common type of neoplasm occurring in 39% of transplant patients, followed by lymphoma. Lymphoproliferative disease, or LPD, is a term often used to describe the type of lymphoma seen particularly in the transplant recipients. The overall incidence of this complication in renal, hepatic, cardiac, and cardiopulmonary transplant patients is 1 to 2.5%, 2.3%, 5 to 6.3%, and 33% respectively (18).

Patient Education

Patient compliance with the immunosuppressive drug regimen is one of the key factors in long-term graft survival (263). The incidence of noncompliance with medications and follow-up care in transplant patients has been reported to be 15 to 18% (263, 264). The consequences are severe, with 28% of graft losses reported at 2 years due to noncompliance, and graft loss or death in 91% of noncompliant kidney transplant patients (263, 265).

With several immunosuppressive agents, prophylactic antiinfectives, as well as medications to treat some of the adverse effects, the posttransplant medication regimen is a complicated one. It is imperative that patients be self-reliant and conscientious about their medications. They should receive adequate training on taking their medications as well as detailed information about each medication and side effects. In addition, patients should recognize the signs and symptoms of organ rejection.

CONCLUSION

Solid organ transplantation is now a common therapeutic modality for patients with end-stage organ failure. The emergence of new and better immunosuppressive agents has resulted in excellent success rates for many transplant procedures. The field of transplantation continues to grow as it benefits from the breakthroughs in the evolving field of immunology. However, transplantation still faces future challenges. The donor organ shortage remains a critical barrier to widespread salvation of all patients in need of transplantation. Finally, managing the enormous costs associated with transplantation in an era of cost-containment remains a challenge.

REFERENCES

1. Flye M. History of transplantation. In: Flye M. Principles of Organ Transplantation. Philadelphia: WB Saunders, 1989:1–17.
2. Pifarre R, Sullivan H, Montoya A, et al. Cardiac transplantation. Cardiol Clin 7:183–194, 1989.
3. Raia S, Nery JR, Mies S. Liver transplantation from live donors. Lancet 2:497, 1989.
4. Grant D, Wall W, Mimeaullt R. Successful small-bowel/liver transplantation. Lancet 335:181–184, 1990.
5. Starzl TE, Marchioro TL, Waddell WR. The reversal of rejection in human renal homografts with subsequent development of homograft tolerance. Surg Gynecol Obstet 117:385, 1963.
6. Standards Committee of American Society of Transplant Surgeons. Current results and expectations of renal transplantation. JAMA 246:1330, 1981.
7. Tilney NL, Milford EL, Araujo JL, et al. Experience with cyclosporine and steroids in clinical renal transplantation. Ann Surg 200:605–613, 1984.
8. Cecka JM, Terasaki PI. The UNOS Scientific Renal Transplant Registry. In: Terasaki PI, Cecka JM. Clinical Transplants 1992. Los Angeles, UCLA Tissue Typing Laboratory, 1993:1–16.
9. Murray JE. Human organ transplantation: background and consequences. Science 256:1411–1416, 1992.
10. Timsit J, Legendre C, Chatenoud L, et al. Pancreas and islet transplantation in man. Biomed & Pharmacother 46:71–78, 1991.

11. Davis RD, Pasque MK. Pulmonary transplantation. Ann Surg 221:14–28, 1995.

12. Asfar S, Zhong R, Grant D. Small bowel transplantation. Surg Clin North Amer 74:1197–1210, 1994.

13. Suthanthiran M, Strom TB. Renal transplantation. N Engl J Med 331:365–376, 1994.

14. Emond JC. Clinical application of living-related liver transplantation. Gastroenterol Clin North Am 22:301–315, 1993.

15. Somerville CA, D'Apice AJF. Future directions in transplantation: xenotransplantation. Kidney Int 44(suppl 42):S112–S121, 1993.

16. Monaco A. Development of clinical immunosuppression for organ transplantation. Jpn J Surg 17:119–130, 1988.

17. Committee Report. Nomenclature for factors of the HLA system. Immunol H 31:186, 1991.

18. Hanto DW, Mohanakumar T. Transplantation and immunology. In: Greenfield LJ. Surgery. Scientific Principles and Practice. Philadelphia: JB Lippincott Company, 1993:461–500.

19. Kerman RH. Relevance of histocompatibility testing in clinical transplantation. Surg Clin North Am 74:1015–1028, 1994.

20. Mickey R, Cho YW, Carnahan E. Long-term graft survival. In: Terasaki PI. Clinical Transplants 1990. Los Angeles: UCLA Tissue Typing Laboratory, 1991:45.

21. Abbas AK, Lichtman AH. Cellular and Molecular Immunology. Philadelphia: WB Saunders, 1994:Ch 1.

22. Flye MW. Transplantation immunobiology. In: Flye MW. Principles of Organ Transplantation. Philadelphia: WB Saunders, 1989:18–46.

23. Sanfilippo F, Amos DB. Mechanisms and characteristics of allograft rejection. In: Sabiston DC. Textbook of Surgery. The Biological Basis of Modern Surgical Practice. Philadelphia: WB Saunders, 1991:357–374.

24. Palmer A, Taube D, Welsh K, et al. Removal of anti-HLA antibodies by extracorporeal immunoabsorption to enable renal transplantation. Lancet 1:10–12, 1989.

25. Sibley R, Payne W. Morphologic findings in the renal allograft biopsy. Semin Nephrol 5:294–306, 1985.

26. Gordon R, Iwatsuki S, Esquive C, et al. Liver transplantation across ABO blood groups. Surgery 100:342–348, 1986.

27. Browne BJ, Kahan BD. Renal transplantation. Surg Clin North Am 74:1097–1116, 1994.

28. Barker CF, Naji A, Dafoe DC, et al. Renal transplantation. In: Sabiston DC. Textbook of Surgery. The Biological Basis of Modern Surgical Practice. Philadelphia: WB Saunders, 1991:374–393.

29. Shaw B, Stratta R, Donovan J, et al. Postoperative care after liver transplantation. Semin Liver Dis 9:202–230, 1989.

30. Starzl T, Demetris A. Liver transplantation: a 31-year perspective part II. Curr Prob Surg 27:117–178, 1990.

31. Burdine J, Fischel R, Bolman R. Cardiac transplantation. Crit Care Clin 6:927–945, 1990.

32. Frazier OH, Macris MP. Progress in cardiac transplantation. Surg Clin North Am 74:1169–1182, 1994.

33. Cook D, Sasaki T. Current status of pancreas transplantation. West J Med 150:309–313, 1989.

34. Toledo-Pereyra L, Dewan S, Mittal V, et al. Clinical pancreas transplantation. Complete review of eight years experience. Am Surg 55:576–581, 1989.

35. Sutherland D, Goetz F, Najarian J. Current status of transplantation of the pancreas. Adv Surg 20:303–311, 1987.

36. Trulock EP. Management of lung transplant rejection. Chest 103:1566–1576, 1993.

37. Bolman RM. Cardiac and cardiopulmonary homotransplants. In: Sabiston DC. Textbook of Surgery. The Biological Basis of Modern Surgical Practice. Philadelphia: WB Saunders, 1991:438–446.

38. Mayer AD. Small bowel transplantation. Baillieres Clin Gastroenterol 8:561–580, 1994.

39. Oguma S, Belle S, Starzl TE, et al. A histometric analysis of chronically rejected human liver allografts: insights into the mechanisms of bile duct loss: direct immunologic and ischemic factors. Hepatology 9:204–209, 1989.

40. Croker BP, Salomon DR. Pathology of renal allograft. In: Brenner CC, Brenner BM. Renal Pathology. Philadelphia: Lippincott, 1989:1518.

41. Hayry P, Isoniemi H, Yilmaz S, et al. Chronic allograft rejection. Immunol Rev 134:33–81, 1993.

42. Knight RJ, Kerman RH, Welsh M, et al. Chronic rejection in primary renal allograft recipients under cyclosporine-prednisone immunosuppressive therapy. Transplantation 51:355–359, 1991.

43. Adams D. Immunological aspects of clinical liver transplantation. Immunol Lett 29:69–72, 1991.

44. Gao S-Z, Alderman EL, Schroeder JS, et al. Accelerated coronary vascular disease in the heart transplant patient: coronary arteriographic findings. J Am Coll Cardiol 12:334–340, 1988.

45. Olivari MT, Homans DC, Wilson RF, et al. Coronary artery disease in cardiac transplant patients receiving triple-drug immunosuppressive therapy. Circulation 80(suppl III):111, 1989.

46. D'Alessandro AM, Sollinger HW, Kalayoglu M, et al. Indications and techniques for renal, pancreas, and liver transplantation. Compr Ther 17:32–42, 1991.

47. Rao K. Mechanism, pathophysiology, diagnosis, and management of renal transplant rejection. Med Clin North Am 74:1039–1057, 1990.

48. Demetris A. The pathology of liver transplantation. Prog Liver Dis 9:687–709, 1990.

49. DeMarco T. Cardiac transplantation. Calif J Health Sys Pharm 7:11–16, 1995.

50. Cooper JD, Patterson GA, Trulock EP, et al. Results of 131 consecutive single and bilateral lung transplant recipients. J Thorac Cardiovasc Surg 107:460–471, 1994.

51. DoHoyos A, Patterson G, Maurer J, et al. Pulmonary transplantation: early and late results. J Thorac Cardiovasc Surg 103:295–306, 1992.

52. Martin X, Dubernard JM, Lefrancois N. Pancreatic transplantation: indications and results. Baillieres Clin Gastroenterol 8:533–560, 1994.

53. Dubernard JM, Traeger J, Touraine JL, et al. Rejection of human pancreatic allografts. Transplant Proc 12:103–106, 1980.

54. Grant D, Garcia B, Wall W, et al. Graft-versus-host disease after clinical small bowel/liver transplantation. Transplant Proc 22:2464, 1990.

55. Tzakis AG, Todo S, Reyes J, et al. Clinical intestinal transplantation: focus on complications. Transplant Proc 24:1238–1240, 1992.

56. Todo S, Tzakis A, Reyes J, et al. Clinical intestinal transplantation: three-year experience [abstract 02]. Third International Symposium on Small Bowel Transplantation, Paris, 1993.

57. Alexander JW, Babcock GF, First MR, et al. The induction of immunologic hyporesponsiveness by preoperative donor-specific transfusions and cyclosporine in human cadaveric transplants. Transplantation 53:423–427, 1992.

58. Salvatierra O, McVicar J, Melzer J, et al. Improved results with combined donor-specific transfusion (DST) and sequential therapy protocol. Transplant Proc 23:1024–1026, 1991.

59. Terasaki PI, Cecka JM, Gjertson DW, et al. High survival rates of kidney transplants from spousal and living unrelated donors. N Engl J Med 333:333–336, 1995.

60. Rao AS, Fontes P, Zeevi A, et al. Augmentation of chimerism in whole organ recipients by simultaneous infusion of donor bone marrow cells. Transplant Proc 27:210–212, 1995.

61. Zeevi A, Pavlick A, Lombardozzi S, et al. Serial evaluation of immune profiles of simultaneous bone marrow and whole organ transplant recipients. Transplant Proc 27:213–215, 1995.

62. Ferguson RM, Henry ML. Renal transplantation. In: Greenfield LJ. Surgery. Scientific Principles and Practice. Philadelphia: JB Lippincott, 1993:516–524.

63. International Consensus Conference. Consensus statement on indications for liver transplantation. Hepatology 20:63S–68S, 1994.

64. Frohlich ED. Selection of patients for organ transplantation. Med Clin N Am 76:1187–1195, 1992.

65. Lake JR. Changing indications for liver transplantation. Gastroenterol Clin North Am 22:213–229, 1993.

66. Wood RP, Ozaki CF, Katz SM, et al. Liver transplantation. The last ten years. Surg Clin North Am 74:76–86, 1994.

67. Onofrio JM, Emory WB. Selection of patients for lung transplantation. Med Clin N Am 76:1207–1219, 1992.

68. Pierce GA. UNOS history. In: Phillips MG. Organ Procurement, Preservation and Distribution in Transplantation. Richmond: William Byrd Press, 1991:1–12.

69. Ferree DM. Cadaveric organ sharing: the organ center. In: Phillips MG. Organ Procurement, Preservation and Distribution in Transplantation. Richmond: William Byrd Press, 1991:129–144.

70. Starzl T, Demetris A, Van Thiel D. Liver transplantation (part I). N Engl J Med 321:1014–1022, 1989.

71. Roberts J, Forsmark C, Lake J, et al. Liver transplantation today. Annu Rev Med 40:287–303, 1989.

72. Munoz S, Friedman L. Liver transplantation. Med Clin North Am 73:1011–1039, 1989.

73. Campbell DA, Ham JM, Turcotte JG, et al. Hepatic transplantation. In: Greenfield LJ. Surgery. Scientific Principles and Practice. Philadelphia: JB Lippincott, 1993:524–541.

74. Broelsch CE, Burdelski M, Rogiers X, et al. Living donor for liver transplantation. Hepatology 20:49S–55S, 1994.

75. Shumway SJ, Bolman RM. Cardiac transplantation. In: Greenfield LJ. Surgery. Scientific Principles and Practice. Philadelphia: JB Lippincott, 1993:541–548.

76. Kaiser LR. Pulmonary transplantation. In: Greenfield LJ. Surgery. Scientific Principles and Practice. Philadelphia: JB Lippincott, 1993:548–559.

77. Barr ML, Schenkel FA, Cohen RG, et al. Living-related lobar transplantation: recipient outcome and early rejection patterns. Transplant Proc 27:1995–1996, 1995.

78. Sollinger HW, Geffner SR. Pancreas transplantation. Surg Clin North Am 74:1183–1195, 1994.

79. Rosenberg L. Pancreatic and islet transplantation. In: Greenfield LJ. Surgery. Scientific Principles and Practice. Philadelphia: JB Lippincott, 1993:559–571.

80. Goodwin J, Durgaprasadarao A, Sierakowski S, et al. Mechanism of action of glucocorticosteroids. J Clin Invest 77:1244–1250, 1986.

81. Haynes RC. Adrenocorticotropic hormone: adrenocortical steroids and their synthetic analogs; inhibitors of the synthesis and actions of adrenocortical hormones. In: Goodman Gilman A, Rall TW, Nies AS, et al. The Pharmacological Basis of Therapeutics, 8th ed. New York: Pergamon Press, 1990:1431–1462.

82. Cupps T, Fauci A. Corticosteroid-mediated immunoregulation in man. Immunol Rev 65:113–155, 1982.

83. Dupont E, Wybran J, Toussaint C. Corticosteroids and organ transplantation. Transplantation 37:331–335, 1984.

84. Gambertoglio J, Frey F, Holford N, et al. Prednisone and prednisolone bioavailability in renal transplant patients. Kidney Int 21:621–626, 1982.

85. Uribe M, Summerskill W, Go V. Comparative serum prednisone and prednisolone concentrations following administration to patients with chronic active liver disease. Clin Pharmacokinet 7:452–459, 1982.

86. Uribe M, Go V. Corticosteroid pharmacokinetics in liver disease. Clin Pharmacokinet 4:233–240, 1979.

87. Uribe M, Schalm S, Summerskill W, et al. Oral prednisone for chronic active liver disease: dose responses and bioavailability studies. Gut 19:1131–1135, 1978.

88. Murray J, Merrill J, Harrison J, et al. Prolonged survival of human kidney homografts by immunosuppressive drug therapy. N Engl J Med 268:1315–1323, 1963.

89. Chan G, Gruber S, Skjei K, et al. Principles of immunosuppression. Crit Care Clin 6:841–891, 1990.

90. Ahmed A, Mory R. Azathioprine. Int J Dermatol 20:461–467, 1981.

91. Chan G, Canafax D, Johnson C. The therapeutic use of azathioprine in renal transplantation. Pharmacotherapy 7: 165–177, 1987.

92. Tidd DM, Paterson ARP. A biochemical mechanism for the delayed cytotoxic reaction of 6-mercaptopurine. Cancer Res 34:738–746, 1974.

93. Schutz E, Gummert J, Mohr FW, et al. Azathioprine myelotoxicity related to elevated 6-thioguanine nucleotides in heart transplantation. Transplant Proc 27:1298–1300, 1995.

94. Lennard L, Maddocks JL. Assay of 6-thioguanine nucleotide a major metabolite of azathioprine, 6-mercaptopurine and 6-thioguanine, in human red cells. J Pharm Pharmac 35:15–18, 1983.

95. Bergan S, Rugstad HE, Bentdal Ø, et al. Monitoring of azathioprine treatment by determination of 6-thioguanine nucleotide concentrations in erythrocytes. Transplantation 58:803–808, 1994.

96. Lin S-N, Jessup K, Floyd M, et al. Quantitation of plasma azathioprine and 6-mercaptopurine levels in renal transplant patients. Transplantation 29:290–294, 1980.

97. Odlind B, Hartvig P, Lindstrom B, et al. Serum azathioprine and 6-mercaptopurine levels and immunosuppressive activity after azathioprine in uremic patients. Int J Immunopharmac 8:1–11, 1986.

98. Ohlman S, Lafolie P, Lindholm A, et al. Large interindividual variability in bioavailability of azathioprine in renal transplant recipients. Clin Transplant 7:65–70, 1993.

99. Ding T, Gambertoglio J, Amend W, et al. Azathioprine bioavailability and pharmacokinetics in kidney transplant patients. Clin Pharmacol Ther 27:250, 1980.

100. Lennard L. The clinical pharmacology of 6-mercaptopurine. Eur J Clin Pharmacol 43:329–339, 1992.

101. Soko J, Arunas S. Liver disease in renal transplant patients. Am J Med 64:139–146, 1978.

102. Delphin E. Principles of immunosuppression. Surg Clin North Am 12:283–298, 1979.

103. Berne T, Chaterjee S, Craig J, et al. Hepatic dysfunction in recipients of renal allografts. Surg Gynecol Obstet 141:171–175, 1975.

104. Zimm S, Collins JM, Riccardi R, et al. Inhibition of first-pass metabolism in cancer chemotherapy. Clin Pharmacol Ther 34:810–817, 1983.

105. Oncevski A, Rostoker G, Buisson C. Is long-term triple-drug therapy required for maintaining kidney allograft tolerance? Effect of azathioprine withdrawal at 3 months post-transplantation. Transplant Proc 21:1625–1626, 1989.

106. Winkelstein A. The effects of azathioprine and 6MP on immunity. J Immunopharmacol 1:429–454, 1979.

107. Borel JF, Feurer C, Gubler HU, et al. Biological effects of cyclosporine A: a new antilymphocyte agent. Agents Actions 6:468–475, 1976.

108. Borel J. Comparative study of in vitro and in vivo drug effects on cell mediated cytotoxicity. Immunology 31:631–641, 1976.

109. Calne RY, White DJG, Thiru S, et al. Cyclosporine A in patients receiving renal allografts from cadaver donors. Lancet 2:1323–1327, 1978.

110. Hess AD, Esa AH, Colombani PM. Mechanisms of action of cyclosporine: effect on cells of the immune system and on subcellular events in T cell activation. Transplant Proc 20(2 suppl 2):29–40, 1988.

111. Schreiber SL, Crabtree GR. The mechanism of action of cyclosporine and FK506. Immunol Today 13:136–142, 1992.

112. Borel J. Pharmacology of cyclosporine (Sandimmune). Pharmacol Rev 41:259–371, 1989.

113. Hess A, Turschka P, Santos G. Effect of cyclosporine A on human lymphocyte response in vitro. J Immunol 128:355–359, 1982.

114. Larsson E. Cyclosporin A and dexamethasone suppress T cell response by selectively acting at distinct sites of the triggering process. J Immunol 124:2828–2833, 1980.

115. Kahan BD. Cyclosporine: the agent and its actions. Transplant Proc 27(4 suppl 1):5–18, 1985.

116. Cirillo R, Triggiani M, Siri L. Cyclosporin A rapidly inhibits mediator release from human basophils presumably by interacting with cyclophilin. J Immunol 144:3891–3897, 1990.

117. Sung SS, Jung LK, Walters JA, et al. Production of tumor necrosis factor/cachectin by human B cell lines and tonsillar B cells. J Exp Med 168:1539–1551, 1988.

118. Lillehoj H, Malek T, Shevach E. Differential effect of cyclosporin A on the expression of T and B lymphocyte activation antigens. J Immunol 133:244–250, 1984.

119. Ptachcinski RJ, Venkataramanan R, Rosenthal JT, et al. Cyclosporine kinetics in renal transplantation. Clin Pharmacol Ther 38:296–300, 1985.

120. Ptachcinski RJ, Burckart GJ, Rosenthal JT, et al. Cyclosporine pharmacokinetics in children following cadaveric renal transplantation. Transplant Proc 18:766–767, 1986.

121. Reynolds KL, Grevel J, Gibbons SY, et al. Cyclosporine pharmacokinetics in uremic patients: influence of different assay methods. Transplant Proc 20(suppl 2):462–465, 1988.

122. Venkataramanan R, Burckart GJ, Ptachcinski RJ, et al. Cyclosporine pharmacokinetics in heart transplant patients. Transplant Proc 18:768–770, 1986.

123. Burckart GJ, Venkataramanan R, Ptachcinski RJ, et al. Cyclosporine absorption following orthotopic liver transplantation. J Clin Pharmacol 26:647–651, 1986.

124. Frey FJ, Horber FF, Frey BM. Trough levels and concentration time curves of cyclosporine in patients undergoing renal transplantation. Clin Pharmacol Ther 43:55–62, 1988.

125. Lindberg A, Odlind B, Tufveson G, et al. The pharmacokinetics of cyclosporine A in uremic patients. Transplant Proc 18 (suppl 5):144–152, 1986.

126. Morse GD, Holdsworth MT, Venuto RC, et al. Pharmacokinetics and clinical tolerance of intravenous and oral cyclosporine in the immediate postoperative period. Clin Pharmacol Ther 44:654–664, 1988.

127. Kahan BD, Kramer WG, Wideman C, et al. Demographic factors affecting the pharmacokinetics of cyclosporine estimated by radioimmunoassay. Transplantation 41:459–464, 1986.

128. Awni WM, Kasiske BL, Heim-Duthoy K, et al. Long-term cyclosporine pharmacokinetic changes in renal transplant recipients: effects of binding and metabolism. Clin Pharmacol Ther 45:41–48, 1989.

129. Gupta SK, Manfro RC, Tomlanovich SJ, et al. Effect of food on the pharmacokinetics of cyclosporine in healthy subjects following oral and intravenous administration. J Clin Pharmacol 30:643–653, 1990.

130. Lindholm A, Henricsson S, Dahlqvist R. The effect of food and bile acid administration on the relative bioavailability of cyclosporine. Br J Clin Pharmacol 25:541–548, 1990.

131. Keown PA, Stiller CR, Sinclair NR, et al. The clinical relevance of cyclosporine blood levels as measured by radioimmunoassay. Transplant Proc 15:2438–2441, 1983.

132. Keogh A, Day R, Critchley L, et al. The effect of food and cholestyramine on the absorption of cyclosporine in cardiac transplant recipients. Transplant Proc 20:27–30, 1988.

133. Ptachcinski RJ, Venkataramanan R, Burckart GJ. Clinical pharmacokinetics of cyclosporine. Clin Pharmacokinet 11:107–132, 1986.

134. Naoumov NV, Tredger JM, Steward CM, et al. Cyclosporin A pharmacokinetics in liver transplant recipients in relation to biliary T-tube clamping and liver dysfunction. Gut 30:391–396, 1989.

135. Venkataramanan R, Starzl T, Ptachcinski R, et al. Cyclosporine kinetics in liver disease. Clin Pharmacol Ther 37:234–239, 1985.

136. Atkinson K, Britton K, Palul P, et al. Detrimental effect of intestinal disease on absorption of orally administered cyclosporine. Transplant Proc 15(suppl 1):2446–2449, 1983.

137. Atkinson K, Boland J, Britton K, et al. Blood and tissue distribution of cyclosporine in humans and mice. Transplant Proc 15(suppl 1):2430–2433, 1983.

138. Kahan BD, Van Buren CT, Boileau M, et al. Levels in cadaveric renal allograft recipient. Transplantation 35:96–99, 1983.

139. Niederberger W, LeMarie M, Maurer G, et al. Distribution and binding of cyclosporine in blood and tissues. Transplant Proc 15:2419–2421, 1983.

140. Lemaire M, Tillement J. Role of lipoproteins and erythrocytes in the in vitro binding and distribution of cyclosporine A in the blood. J Pharm Pharmacol 34:715–718, 1982.

141. Kronbach T, Fischer V, Meyers UA. Cyclosporine metabolism in human liver: identification of cytochrome p-450 III gene family as the major cyclosporine-metabolizing enzyme explains interactions of cyclosporine with other drugs. Clin Pharmacol Ther 43:630–635, 1988.

142. Kolars JC, Stetson PL, Rush BD, et al. Cyclosporine metabolism by P450IIIA in rat enterocytes—another determinant of oral bioavailability? Transplantation 53:596–602, 1992.

143. Christians U, Sewing K-F. Cyclosporin metabolism in transplant patients. Pharmacol Ther 57:291–345, 1993.

144. Wu C-Y, Benet LZ, Hebert MF, et al. Differentiation of absorption, first pass gut and hepatic metabolism in man: studies with cyclosporine. Clin Pharmacol Ther 58:1995.

145. Yatscoff RW, Rosano TG, Bowers LD. The clinical significance of cyclosporine metabolites. Clin Biochem 24:23–35, 1991.

146. Venkataramanan R, Starzl TE, Yang S, et al. Biliary excretion of cyclosporine in liver transplant patients. Transplant Proc 17:286–289, 1985.

147. Yee G, Lennon T, Gmar D, et al. Effect of age on cyclosporine kinetics in marrow transplant recipients. Transplant Proc 19:1704–1705, 1987.

148. Whitington PF, Emond JC, Whitington SH, et al. Small-bowel length and the dose of cyclosporine in children after liver transplantation. N Engl J Med 322:733–738, 1990.

149. Ptachcinski RJ, Carpenter BJ, Burckart GJ, et al. Effect of erythromycin on cyclosporine levels. N Engl J Med 313:1416–1417, 1985.

150. Gonwa T, Nghiem D, Schulak J, et al. Erythromycin and cyclosporine. Transplantation 41:797–799, 1986.

151. Martell R, Heinrichs D, Stiller C, et al. The effect of erythromycin in patients treated with cyclosporine. Ann Intern Med 104:660–661, 1986.

152. Gupta S, Bakran A, Johnson W, et al. Erythromycin enhances the absorption of cyclosporine. Br J Clin Pharm 25:401–402, 1988.

153. Ferguson RM, Sutherland DER, Simmons RL, et al. Ketoconazole, cyclosporine, metabolism and renal transplantation. Lancet 2:882–883, 1982.

154. Dieperink H, Moller J. Ketoconazole and cyclosporine. Lancet 2:1217, 1982.

155. White D, Blatchford N, Canwenbergh G. Cyclosporine and ketoconazole. Transplantation 37:214–215, 1984.

156. Gomez DY, Wacher VJ, Tomlanovich SJ, et al. The effects of ketoconazole on the intestinal metabolism and bioavailability of cyclosporine. Clin Pharmacol Ther 58:15–19, 1995.

157. Pochet JM, Pirson Y. Cyclosporine-diltiazem interaction. Lancet 1:979, 1986.

158. Grino JM, Sebate I, Castelao AM, et al. Influence of diltiazem on cyclosporine clearance. Lancet 1:1387, 1986.

159. Lindholm A, Henriscsson S. Verapamil inhibits cyclosporine metabolism. Lancet 1:1262–1263, 1987.

160. Cantarovich M, Hiesse C, Lockiec F, et al. Confirmation of the interaction between cyclosporine and the calcium channel blocker nicardipine in renal transplant patients. Clin Nephrol 28:190–193, 1987.

161. Kessler M, Netter P, Renoult E, et al. Influence of nicardipine on renal function and plasma cyclosporine in renal transplant patients. Eur J Clin Pharmacol 36:637–638, 1989.

162. Wadhwa N, Schroeder T, O'Flaherty E, et al. The effect of oral metoclopramide on the absorption of cyclosporine. Transplantation 43:211, 1987.

163. Moller B, Ekelund B. Toxicity of cyclosporine during treatment with androgens. N Engl J Med 313:1416, 1985.

164. Deray G, LeHoang P, Cacoub P, et al. Oral contraceptive interaction with cyclosporine. Lancet 1:158–159, 1987.

165. Klintmalm G, Sawe J. High dose methylprednisolone increases plasma cyclosporin levels in renal transplant recipients. Lancet 1:731, 1984.

166. Koneru B, Hartner C, Iwatsuki S, et al. Effect of danazol on cyclosporine pharmacokinetics. Transplantation 45:1001, 1988.

167. Ross W, Roberts D, Griffin P, et al. Cyclosporine interaction with danazol and norethisterone. Lancet 2:330, 1986.

168. Lele P, Peterson P, Yang S, et al. Cyclosporine and Tegretol— another drug interaction. Kidney Int 27:344, 1985.

169. Carstensen H, Jacobsen N, Dieperink H. Interaction between cyclosporin A and phenobarbitone. Br J Clin Pharmacol 21:550–551, 1986.

170. Freeman DJ, Laupacis A, Keown PA, et al. Evaluation of cyclosporine-phenytoin interaction with observation on cyclosporine metabolites. Br J Clin Pharm 18:887, 1984.

171. Rowland M, Gupta SK. Cyclosporine-phenytoin interaction: re-evaluation using metabolite data. Br J Clin Pharm 24:329–334, 1987.

172. Allen R, Hunnisett A, Morris P. Cyclosporine and rifampicin in renal transplantation. Lancet 1:980, 1985.

173. Cassidy M, Van Zyl-Smit R, Pascoe M, et al. Effect of rifampicin on cyclosporine A. Blood levels in a renal transplant recipient. Nephron 41:207–208, 1985.

174. Hebert MF, Roberts JP, Prueksaritanont T, et al. Bioavailability of cyclosporine with concomitant rifampin administration is markedly less than predicted by hepatic enzyme induction. Clin Pharmacol Ther 52:453–457, 1992.

175. Langhoff E, Madsen S. Rapid metabolism of cyclosporine and prednisone in kidney transplant patients on tuberculostatic treatment. Lancet 2:1031, 1983.

176. Coward R, Raftery A, Brown C. Cyclosporine and antituberculous therapy. Lancet 1:1342–1343, 1985.

177. Veremis SA, Maddux MS, Pollack R, et al. Subtherapeutic cyclosporin concentrations during nafcillin therapy. Transplantation 43:913–915, 1987.

178. Rosenberg L, Dafoe D, Schwartz R, et al. Administration of somatostatin analog (SMS 201-995) in the treatment of a fistula occurring after pancreas transplant: interference with cyclosporine immunosuppression. Transplantation 43:764–766, 1987.

179. Landgraf R, Landgraf-Leurs M, Nusser J, et al. Effect of somato-statin analog (SMS 201-995) on cyclosporine levels. Transplantation 44:724–725, 1987.

180. Stratta RJ, Taylor RJ, Lowell JA, et al. Selective use of Sandostatin in vascularized pancreas transplantation. Am J Surg 166:598–604, 1993.

181. Termeer A, Hoitsma A, Koene R. Severe nephrotoxicity caused by the combined use of gentamicin and cyclosporine in renal allograft recipients. Transplantation 42:220–221, 1986.

182. Gluckman E, Devergie A, Lokiec F, et al. Role of immunosuppres-sive drugs for prevention of graft-v-host-disease after HLA matched bone marrow transplantation. Transplant Proc 19(suppl 7): 61–65, 1987.

183. Hows J, Palmer S, Want S, et al. Serum levels of cyclosporine A and nephrotoxicity in bone marrow transplant patients. Lancet ii:145–146, 1981.

184. Tutschka PJ, Beschorner W, Hess A, et al. Cyclosporine-A to prevent graft-versus-host disease. A pilot in 22 patients receiving allogenic marrow transplants. Blood 61:318–325, 1983.

185. Kennedy M, Deeg H, Siegal M, et al. Acute renal toxicity with combined use of amphotericin B and cyclosporine after marrow transplantation. Transplantation 35:211–215, 1983.

186. Gluckman E, Devergie A, Poirier O, et al. Use of cyclosporine as prophylaxis of graft-vs-host disease after human allogenic bone marrow transplantation: report of 38 patients. Transplant Proc 15 (suppl 1):2628–2633, 1983.

187. East C, Alizvizatos P, Grundy S, et al. Rhabdomyolysis in patients receiving lovastatin after cardiac transplantation. N Engl J Med 318:47–48, 1988.

188. Norman D, Illingworth D, Munson J, et al. Myolysis and acute renal failure in a heart transplant recipient receiving lovastatin. N Engl J Med 318:46–47, 1988.

189. Tobert J. Rhabdomyolysis in patients receiving lovastatin after cardiac transplantation (Letter). N Engl J Med 318:47–48, 1988.

190. Slavin J, Taylor J. Cyclosporine, nifedipine, and gingival hyperplasia. Lancet ii: 739, 1987.

191. Klintmalm G, Iwatsuki S, Starzl T. Nephrotoxicity of cyclosporine A in liver and kidney transplant patients. Lancet 1:470–471, 1981.

192. Hamilton D, Calne R, Evans R, et al. Effects of long-term cyclosporine A on renal function. Lancet 1:1218–1219, 1981.

193. Klintmalm G, Iwatsuki S, Starzl T. Cyclosporine A hepatotoxicity in 66 renal allograft recipients. Transplantation 32:488–499, 1981.

194. Rodger R, Turney J, Haines I, et al. Cyclosporine and liver function in renal allograft patients. Transplant Proc 15(suppl 1):2754–2756, 1983.

195. Schade R, Gugliemi D, Van Thiel D, et al. Cholestasis in heart transplant recipients treated with cyclosporine. Transplant Proc 1 (suppl 1):2757–2760, 1983.

196. Kahan BD. Cyclosporine. N Engl J Med 321:1725–1738, 1989.

197. Kahn D, Cervio G, Mazzaferro V, et al. Relationship between the dose and whole blood level of cyclosporine after liver and kidney transplantation. J Clin Lab Immunol 37:163–171, 1992.

198. Legg B, Gupta SK, Rowland M, et al. Cyclosporin: pharmacokinetics and detailed studies of plasma and erythrocyte binding during intravenous and oral administration. Eur J Clin Pharmacol 34:451–460, 1988.

199. Lensmeyer GL, Wiebe DA, Carlson IH. Distribution of cyclosporin A metabolites among plasma and cells in whole blood: effect of temperature, hematocrit, and metabolite concentration. Clin Chem 35:56–63, 1989.

200. Kahan BD, Shaw LM, Holt D, et al. Consensus document: Hawk's Cay meeting on therapeutic drug monitoring of cyclosporine. Clin Chem 36:1510–1516, 1990.

201. Shaw LM, Bowers L, Demers L, et al. Critical issues in cyclosporine monitoring: report of the task force on cyclosporine monitoring. Clin Chem 33:1269–1288, 1987.

202. Holt DW, Marsden JT, Johnston A. Quality assessment of cyclo-sporine measurements: comparison of current methods. Transplant Proc 22:1234–1239, 1990.

203. Napoli KL, Kahan BD. Considerations for monitoring cyclosporine in transplant recipients. Clin Lab Med 11:671–691, 1991.

204. Lee SF, Yang WC, Shann TY, et al. Comparison of non-specific radioimmunoassay, high-performance liquid chromatog-raphy, and fluorescence polarization immunoassay for cyclosporine monitoring in renal transplantation. Ther Drug Monit 13: 152–156, 1991.

205. Wacke R, Drewelow B, Hehl E-M, et al. Measurement of cyclosporin A in whole blood by RIA, EMIT and FPIA: a comparative study. Int J Clin Pharmac Ther Tox 30:502–503, 1992.

206. Winkler M, Schumann G, Petersen D, et al. Monoclonal fluorescence polarization immunoassay evaluated for monitoring cyclosporine in whole blood after kidney, heart, and liver transplantation. Clin Chem 38:123–126, 1992.

207. Sabate I, Gracia S, Diez O, et al. Comparison of cyclosporine blood concentrations measured by radioimmunoassay and two nonisotopicimmunoassays using monoclonal antibodies. Clin Chem 38:1187–1188, 1992.

208. Holt DW, Mueller EA, Kovarik JM, et al. Sandimmune Neoral pharmacokinetics: impact of the new oral formulation. Transplant Proc 27:1434–1436, 1995.

209. Kovarik JM, Mueller EA, van Bree JB, et al. Cyclosporine pharmacokinetics and variability from a microemulsion formulation—a multicenter investigation in kidney transplant patients. Transplantation 58:658–663, 1994.

210. Mueller EA, Kovarik JM, van Bree JB, et al. Pharmacokinetics and tolerability of a microemulsion formulation of cyclosporine in renal allograft recipients—a concentration-controlled comparison with the commercial formulation. Transplantation 57:1178–1182, 1994.

211. Kahan BD, Dunn J, Fitts C, et al. The Neoral formulation: improved correlation between cyclosporine trough levels and exposure in stable renal transplant recipients. Transplant Proc 26:2940–2943, 1994.

212. Kino T, Hatanaka H, Miyata S, et al. FK 506, a novel immunosuppressant isolated from a Streptomyces. Immunosuppressive effect of FK506 in vitro. J Antibiot 40: 1256–1265, 1987.

213. Fung JJ, Starzl TE. FK 506 in solid organ transplantation. Transplant Proc 26:3017–3020, 1994.

214. European FK 506 Multicentre Liver Study Group. Randomised trial comparing tacrolimus (FK 506) and cyclosporin in prevention of liver allograft rejection. Lancet 344:423–428, 1994.

215. Todo S, Fung JJ, Starzl TE, et al. Single-center experience with primary orthotopic liver transplantation with FK 506 immunosuppression. Ann Surg 220:297–309, 1994.

216. Peters DH, Fitton A, Plosker GL, et al. Tacrolimus. A review of its pharmacology, and therapeutic potential in hepatic and renal transplantation. Drugs 46:746–794, 1993.

217. Venkataramanan R, Jain A, Warty VS, et al. Pharmacokinetics of FK 506 in transplant patients. Transplant Proc 23:2736–2740, 1991.

218. Venkataramanan R, Jain A, Warty VS, et al. Pharmacokinetics of FK 506 following oral administration : a comparison of FK 506 and cyclosporine. Transplant Proc 23:931–933, 1991.

219. Sewing K-F. Pharmacokinetics, dosing principles, and blood level monitoring of FK 506. Transplant Proc 26:3267–3269, 1994.

220. Jain AB, Venkataramanan R, Cadoff E, et al. Effect of hepatic dysfunction and T tube clamping on FK 506 pharmacokinetics and trough concentrations. Transplant Proc 22(suppl 1):57–59, 1990.

221. Sattler M, Guengerich FP, Yun C-H, et al. Cytochrome P-450 3A enzymes are responsible for biotransformation of FK 506 and rapamycin in man and rat. Drug Metab Dispos 20:753–761, 1992.

222. McCauley J. The nephrotoxicity of FK 506 and compared with cyclosporine. Curr Opin Nephrol Hyperten 2:662–669, 1993.

223. Tamura K, Kobayashi M, Hashimoto K, et al. A highly sensitive method to assay FK 506 levels in plasma. Transplant Proc 19:23–29, 1987.

224. Grenier FC, Luczkiw J, Bergmann M, et al. A whole blood FK 506 assay for the IMx® analyzer. Transplant Proc 23:2748–2749, 1991.

225. Jusko WJ, Thomson AW, Fung J, et al. Consensus document: therapeutic monitoring of tacrolimus (FK 506). Ther Drug Monit 1995. In press.

226. D'Ambrosio R, Girzaitis N, Jusko WJ. Validation and quality assurance program for monitoring tacrolimus (FK 506) concentrations in plasma and whole blood. Ther Drug Monit 15:414–426, 1993.

227. McDiarmid SV, Busuttil RW, Ascher NL, et al. FK 506 (tacrolimus) compared with cyclosporine for primary immunosuppression after pediatric liver transplantation. Transplantation 59:530–536, 1995.

228. HW Sollinger for the US Renal Transplant Mycophenolate Mofetil Study Group. Mycophenolate mofetil for the prevention of acute rejection in primary cadaveric renal allograft recipients. Transplantation 60:225–232, 1995.

229. Allison AC, Eugui EM. Immunosuppressive and other effects of mycophenolic acid and an ester prodrug, mycophenolate mofetil. Immunol Rev 136:5–28, 1993.

230. Eugui EM, Almquist SJ, Muller CD, et al. Lymphocyte-selective cytostatic and immunosuppressive effects of mycophenolic acid in vitro: role of deoxyguanosine nucleotide depletion. Scand J Immunol 33:161–173, 1991.

231. Eugui EM, Mirkovich A, Allison AC. Lymphocyte-selective antiproliferative and immunosuppressive effects of mycophenolic acid in mice. Scand J Immunol 33:175–183, 1991.

232. Morris RE, Hoyt EG, Murphy MP, et al. Mycophenolic acid morpholinoethylester (RS-61443) is a new immunosuppressant that prevents and halts heart allograft rejection by selective inhibition of T and B cell purine synthesis. Transplant Proc 22:1659–1662, 1990.

233. Sollinger HW, Deierhoi MH, Belzer FO, et al. RS-61443—a phase I clinical trial and pilot rescue study. Transplantation 53:428–432, 1992.

234. Shah J, Bullingham R, Rice P, et al. Pharmacokinetics of oral mycophenolate mofetil (MMF) and metabolites in renally impaired patients [abstract]. Clin Pharmacol Ther 57:149, 1995.

235. Chatenoud L, Baudrihaye MF, Kreis H, et al. Human in vivo antigenic modulation induced by the anti-T cell OKT3 monoclonal antibody. Eur J Immunol 12:979–982, 1982.

236. Cosimi AB. Clinical development of Orthoclone OKT3. Transplant Proc 14(suppl 1):7–16, 1987.

237. Todd PA, Brogden RN. Muromonab CD3. A review of its pharmacology and therapeutic potential. Drugs 37:871–899, 1989.

238. Hooks MA, Wade CS, Millikan WJ. Muromonab CD3: a review of its pharmacology, pharmacokinetics, and clinical use in transplantation. Pharmacotherapy 11:26–37, 1991.

239. Cosimi AB. Future of monoclonal antibodies in solid organ transplantation. Dig Dis Sci 40:65–72, 1995.

240. Ortho Multicenter Transplant Study Group. A randomized clinical trial of OKT3 monoclonal antibody for acute rejection of cadaveric renal transplants. N Engl J Med 313:337–342, 1985.

241. Roitt IM. OKT3: immunology, production, purification, and pharmacokinetics. Clin Transplantation 7:367–373, 1993.

242. Chatenoud L. Immunologic monitoring during OKT3 therapy. Clin Transplant 7:422–430, 1993.

243. Kreis H, Legendre C, Chatenoud L. OKT3 in organ transplantation. Transplant Rev 5:181–199, 1991.

244. Anderson C. Scandal scars Minnesota medical school. Science 262:1812–1813, 1993.

245. Widmer U, Frei D, Keusch G, et al. OKT3 treatment of steroid- and/or anti-thymocyte globulin-resistant renal allograft rejection occurring on triple baseline immunosuppression including cyclosporine A. Transplant Proc 20:90–95, 1988.

246. Hoitsma AJ, Wetzels JFM, et al. Antirejection treatment with anti-thymocyte globulin in renal transplant recipients treated with cyclosporine as basic immunosuppression. Transplant Proc 20 (suppl 6):12–13, 1988.

247. Barry JM. Immunosuppressive drugs in renal transplantation. Drugs 44:554–566, 1992.

248. Amemiya H, Japanese Collaborative Transplant Study Group of NKT-01. Immunosuppressive mechanisms and action of deoxyspergualin in experimental and clinical studies. Transplant Proc 27:31–32, 1995.

249. Takahashi K, Tanabe K, Ooba S, et al. Prophylactic use of a new immunosuppressive agent, deoxyspergualin, in patients with kidney transplantation from ABO-incompatible or performed antibody-positive donors. Transplant Proc 27:1078–1082, 1995.

250. Uchida H, Mita K, Bekku Y, et al. Advantages of triple therapy with mizoribine, cyclosporine and prednisolone over other types of triple and/or double therapy including cyclosporine for renal transplantation. J Tox Sci 16:181–190, 1991.

251. Sehgal SN, Baker H, Vezina C. Rapamycin (AY-22,989) a new antifungal antibiotic II. Fermentation, isolation and characterization. J Antibiot 28:727, 1975.

252. Thomson AW. The immunosuppressive macrolides FK 506 and rapamycin. Immunol Lett 29:105–112, 1991.

253. Kimball PM, Kerman RH, Kahan BD. Production of synergistic, but non-identical mechanisms of immunosuppression by rapamycin and cyclosporine. Transplantation 51:486–490, 1991.

254. Metcalfe SM, Richards FM. Cyclosporine, FK 506 and rapamycin: some effects on early activation events in serum-free, mitogen-stimulated mouse spleen cells. Transplantation 49:798–802, 1990.

255. Dumont FJ, Staruch MJ, Koprak SL, et al. Distinct mechanisms of suppression of murine T-cell activation by the related macrolides FK 506 and rapamycin. J Immunol 144:251–258, 1990.

256. Nicholson V, Johnson PC. Infectious complications in solid organ transplant recipients. Surg Clin North Am 74:1223–1245, 1994.

257. Dummer SJ. Cytomegalovirus infection after liver transplantation. Rev Infect Dis 12:767–775, 1990.

258. Dunn DL, Najarian JS. New approaches to the diagnosis, prevention, and treatment of cytomegalovirus infection after transplantation. Am J Surg 161:250–255, 1991.

259. Lewis RM, Johnson PC, Golden D, et al. The adverse impact of cytomegalovirus infection on clinical outcome in cyclosporine-prednisone treated renal allograft patients. Transplantation 45:353–359, 1988.

260. Stratta RJ, Schaefer MS, Markin RS, et al. Clinical patterns of cytomegalovirus disease after liver transplantation. Arch Surg 124:1443–1450, 1989.

261. Stratta RJ, Shaeffer MS, Markin RS, et al. Cytomegalovirus infection and disease after liver transplantation. Dig Dis Sci 37:673–688, 1992.

262. Penn I. Malignancy. Surg Clin North Am 74:1247–1257, 1994.

263. Schweizer R, Rovelli M, Palmieri D, et al. Noncompliance in organ transplant recipients. Transplantation 49:374–377, 1990.

264. Christopherson L. Cardiac transplantation: a psychological perspective. Circulation 75:57–62, 1987.

265. Dunn J, Golden D, Van Buren C, et al. Causes of graft loss beyond two years in the cyclosporine era. Transplantation 49:349–353, 1990.

INDEX

Page numbers in italics denote figures; those followed by "t" denote tables.